Critical Care Nephrology

Claudio Ronco, MD
Director, Department of Nephrology, Dialysis, and Transplantation
St. Bortolo Hospital
Vicenza, Italy

Rinaldo Bellomo, MD, MB BS(Hons), FRACP, FCCP
Professor
University of Melbourne
Director of Intensive Care Research
Austin Hospital
Melbourne, Victoria, Australia

John A. Kellum, MD, FCCM, FACP
Professor and Vice Chair
Department of Critical Care Medicine
University of Pittsburgh School of Medicine
Pittsburgh, Pennsylvania

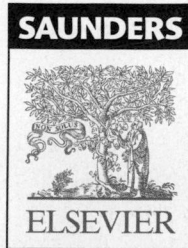

SAUNDERS

ELSEVIER

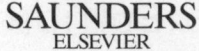

SAUNDERS
ELSEVIER

1600 John F. Kennedy Boulevard
Suite 1800
Philadelphia, PA 19103-2899

CRITICAL CARE NEPHROLOGY   ISBN: 978-1-4160-4252-5

Notice

Knowledge and best practice in this field are constantly changing. As new research and
experience broaden our knowledge, changes in practice, treatment, and drug therapy may
become necessary or appropriate. Readers are advised to check the most current information
provided (i) on procedures featured or (ii) by the manufacturer of each product to be
administered, to verify the recommended dose or formula, the method and duration of
administration, and contraindications. It is the responsibility of practitioners, relying on
their own experience and knowledge of their patients, to make diagnoses, to determine
dosages and the best treatment for each individual patient, and to take all appropriate safety
precautions. To the fullest extent of the law, neither the Publisher nor the Editors assume
any liability for any injury and/or damage to persons or property arising out of or related to
any use of the material contained in this book.

The Publisher

Library of Congress Cataloging-in-Publication Data

Critical care nephrology / [edited by] Claudio Ronco, Rinaldo Bellomo, John A. Kellum.
—2nd ed.
     p. ; cm.
   Includes bibliographical references and index.
   ISBN 978-1-4160-4252-5
 1. Renal intensive care.   I. Ronco, C. (Claudio)   II. Bellomo, R. (Rinaldo)
III. Kellum, John A.
   [DNLM: 1. Kidney Diseases—therapy.   2. Critical Care.   3. Kidney Diseases—
complications. WJ 300 C934 2009]
RC903.C75 2009
616.6′1028—dc22   2008001015

Acquisitions Editor: Adrianne Brigido
Developmental Editor: Arlene Chappelle
Publishing Services Manager: Frank Polizzano
Project Manager: Lee Ann Draud
Design Direction: Steve Stave

Printed in Canada

Last digit is the print number: 9 8 7 6 5 4 3 2 1

CONTRIBUTORS

Cataldo Abaterusso, MD
Assistant Professor of Nephrology, School of Medicine, University of Verona; Assistant Professor, Division of Nephrology, Ospedale Civile Maggiore, Verona, Italy
Endothelial Progenitor Cells in Acute Renal Injury

Stéphane P. Ahern, MD, PhD, FRCPC
University of Montreal Faculty of Medicine; Critical Care Division, Maisonneuve-Rosemont Hospital, Montreal, Quebec, Canada
Urinary Tract Infections in the Intensive Care Unit

Maria Cristina Aisa, PhD
Department of Internal Medicine, University of Perugia Faculty of Medicine, Perugia, Italy
Oxidative Stress in Acute Kidney Injury and Sepsis

Robert C. Albright, Jr., DO
Assistant Professor, Mayo Graduate School of Medicine; Director of Dialysis, Mayo Clinic, Rochester, Minnesota
Cardiovascular Problems in Acute Renal Failure

Vicente Alfaro, PhD, MSc
Associate Professor of Physiology, School of Biology, University of Barcelona, Barcelona, Spain
Acid-Base Disorders in Chronic Lung Diseases

Ali Al-Khafaji, MD, MPH
Assistant Professor of Critical Care Medicine, University of Pittsburgh School of Medicine, Pittsburgh, Pennsylvania
Infectious Complications of Renal Transplantation

Jean-Christophe Allo, MD
Assistant Professor, Department of Emergency Medicine, Medical School, Université Paris Descartes; Department of Emergency and Critical Care Medicine, Hôpital Cochin, Paris, France
The Coagulation System in Inflammation

Richard Amerling, MD
Associate Professor of Clinical Medicine, Albert Einstein College of Medicine of Yeshiva University, Bronx; Director of Outpatient Dialysis and Continuous Renal Replacement Therapy, Beth Israel Medical Center, New York, New York
Continuous-Flow Peritoneal Dialysis as Acute Therapy; Anticancer Drugs and the Kidney

Alessandro Amore, MD, PhD
Professor of Nephrology, University of Turin Faculty of Medicine and Surgery; Director of Dialysis, Regina Margherita University Hospital, Turin, Italy
Antibiotics and Antiviral Drugs in the Intensive Care Unit

Robert J. Anderson, MD
Professor and Chair, Department of Medicine, University of Colorado Denver School of Medicine; Attending Physician, University Hospital, Denver, Colorado
Assessment of Fluid and Electrolyte Problems: Urine Biochemistry

Michele Andreucci, MD, PhD
Associate Professor of Nephrology and Chair, Department of Nephrology, Faculty of Medicine and Surgery, Università "Magna Graecia," Catanzaro, Italy
Acute Interstitial Nephritis

Vittorio E. Andreucci, MD
Professor of Nephrology and Chair, Department of Nephrology, Faculty of Medicine and Surgery, Università "Federico II," Naples, Italy
Acute Interstitial Nephritis

Emilios Andrikos, MD
Consultant in Nephrology, Department of Nephrology, G. Hatzikosta General Hospital, Ioannina, Greece
Pharmacological Treatment for Hepatorenal Syndrome

Vicente Arroyo, MD
Professor of Medicine, University of Barcelona Faculty of Medicine, Barcelona, Spain
Spontaneous Bacterial Peritonitis and Hepatorenal Syndrome

John M. Arthur, MD, PhD
Attending Physician, Medical University of South Carolina, Charleston, South Carolina
Proteomics and Acute Renal Failure

Stephen R. Ash, MD
Clarian Arnett Health; Ash Access Technology, Inc.; and Hemo Cleanse, Inc., Lafayette, Indiana
Indications, Contraindications, and Complications of Peritoneal Dialysis in Acute Renal Failure

Emilio Assanelli, MD
Deputy Director, Intensive Cardiac Care Unit, Centro Cardiologico Monzino, Institute of Cardiology, University of Milan, Milan, Italy
Intermittent Hemofiltration for Management of Fluid Overload and Administration of Contrast Media

Filippo Aucella, MD
Head, Dialysis Unit, Lastaria Hospital, Foggia, Italy
Environment, Smoking, Obesity, and the Kidney

Sean M. Bagshaw, MD, MSC, FRCPC
Assistant Professor, Division of Critical Care Medicine, University of Alberta Faculty of Medicine and Dentistry, Edmonton, Alberta, Canada
Septic Acute Renal Failure; Kidney Function Tests and Urinalysis in Acute Renal Failure; Disorders of Sodium and Water Balance; Renal Replacement Therapy in Acute Renal Failure Secondary to Sepsis; Dialysis Disequilibrium Syndrome

Olga Balafa, MD
Registrar in Nephrology, Department of Nephrology, G. Hatzikosta General Hospital, Ioannina, Greece
Pharmacological Treatment for Hepatorenal Syndrome

André Luís Balbi, MD
Assistant Professor of Nephrology, Botucatu Medical School, São Paulo State University, Botucatu, São Paulo, Brazil
Nursing Issues and Procedures in Acute Peritoneal Dialysis

Ian Baldwin, PhD, RN
Adjunct Professor, Division of Nursing, RMIT University; Postgraduate Educator, Department of Intensive Care, Austin Hospital, Melbourne, Victoria, Australia
Daily Dialysis in the Intensive Care Unit: Nursing Perspectives; Strategies to Prevent Coagulation of the Extracorporeal Circuit

Marco Ballestri, MD
Division of Nephrology, Dialysis, and Renal Transplantation, Policlinico di Modena, Modena, Italy
Nanoparticles: Potential Toxins for the Organism and the Kidney?

Joanne M. Bargman, MD, FRCPC
Professor of Medicine, University of Toronto; Staff Nephrologist and Director, Home Peritoneal Dialysis, University Health Network, Toronto, Ontario, Canada
Efficiency and Adequacy of Peritoneal Dialysis in Acute Renal Failure

Gina-Marie Barletta, MD
Assistant Professor, Michigan State University College of Human Medicine, Lansing; Pediatric Nephrologist, Helen DeVos Children's Hospital, Grand Rapids, Michigan
Drug Dosing in Pediatric Acute Kidney Insufficiency and Renal Replacement Therapy

Jeffrey F. Barletta, PharmD
Adjunct Assistant Professor, Ferris State University College of Pharmacy; Clinical Specialist, Critical Care, Spectrum Health, Grand Rapids, Michigan
Drug Dosing in Pediatric Acute Kidney Insufficiency and Renal Replacement Therapy

Libero Barozzi, MD
Director of Radiology and Attending Physician, San Orsola University Hospital, Bologna, Italy
Computed Tomography and Magnetic Resonance Imaging in Acute Renal Failure

Rashad S. Barsoum, MD, FRCP, FRCPE
Professor, Department of Internal Mecicine, Cairo University School of Medicine; Chairman; The Cairo Kidney Center, Cairo, Egypt
Tropical Infections Causing Acute Kidney Injury

Monica Beaulieu, MD, FRCPC
Clinical Assistant Professor of medicine, University of British Columbia Faculty of Medicine; Staff Physicsian, Providence Health Care, Vancouver, British Columbia, Canada
Management of Patients with Diabetes in the Intensive Care Unit

Donna Beer-Stolz, PhD
Department of Cell Biology and Physiology, University of Pittsburgh School of Medicine, Pittsburgh, Pennsylvania
Epithelial Barrier Dysfunction as a Mechanism Underlying the Pathogenesis of Multiple-Organ Dysfunction

Rinaldo Bellomo, MD, MB BS(Hons), FRACP, FCCP
Professor, University of Melbourne; Director of Intensive Care Research, Austin Hospital, Melbourne, Victoria, Australia
What Is Acute Kidney Injury?; Basic Principles of Renal Support; Glomerular Filtration Rate and Renal Functional Reserve; Septic Acute Renal Failure; Renal Blood Flow and Perfusion Pressure; Animal Models of Septic Acute Renal Failure; Kidney Function Tests and Urinalysis in Acute Renal Failure; Vasoactive Drugs and Acute Renal Failure; Dopamine Receptor Agonists; Disorders of Sodium and Water Balance; Acid-Base Disorders Secondary to Renal Failure; Blood Glucose Control in Critical Care; Renal Replacement Therapy in Acute Renal Failure Secondary to Sepsis; Blood Purification for Sepsis; Dialysis Disequilibrium Syndrome; Renal Replacement Techniques: Descriptions, Mechanisms, Choices, and Controversies; The Concept of Renal Replacement Therapy Dose and Efficiency; Current Nomenclature; Continuous Renal Replacement Therapy: Hemofiltration, Hemodiafiltration, or Hemodialysis?; Multiple-Organ Support Therapy for the Critically Ill Patient

Jose Bernardo, MD
Assistant Professor of Medicine, University of Pittsburgh School of Medicine; Attending Physician, University of Pittsburgh Medical Center, Pittsburgh, Pennsylvania
Short- and Long-Term Management after Kidney Transplantation

Michele Bertolotto, MD
Assistant Professor, Department of Radiology, University of Trieste; Attending Physician, Ospedale di Cattinara, Trieste, Italy
Ultrasonography and Doppler Techniques in Acute Kidney Injury; Contrast-Enhanced Renal Ultrasonography

John T. Bestoso, MD
Nephrologist, San Diego,
California
*Starting and Stopping Renal
Replacement Therapy in the
Critically Ill*

Gerard A. Betro, MD
Clinical Instructor of Surgery,
Yale University School of
Medicine; Attending Surgeon
(Clinical Instructor), Yale–New
Haven Hospital, New Haven,
Connecticut
Abdominal Compartment Syndrome

Mallar Bhattacharya, MD, MSc
Clinical Fellow, Pulmonary and
Critical Care Medicine,
University of California, San
Francisco, School of Medicine,
San Francisco, California
*Acute Respiratory Distress Syndrome
and the Kidney: Lung and Kidney
Crosstalk*

Geoffrey R. Bihl, MB, BCh
Consultant Nephrologist and
Clinical Director, Winelands
Kidney and Dialysis Center,
Somerset West, South Africa
Acute Lupus Nephritis

Stijn I. Blot, PhD
Attending Physician; Infectious
Diseases Department, Ghent
University Hospital, Ghent,
Belgium
*Immunological and Infectious
Complications of Acute Kidney Injury*

Willem Boer, MD
Nephrologist and Consultant,
Intensive Care Unit, Atrium
Medical Center Heerlen, Heerlen,
The Netherlands
*Removal of Mediators of
Inflammation by Continuous Renal
Replacement Therapy: An Open
Debate of Pros and Cons*

Mirian A. Boim, PhD
Affiliated Professor, Renal
Division, Department of
Medicine, Federal University of
São Paulo, São Paulo, Brazil
*The Physiology of the Glomerular
Tuft*

Monica Bonello, MD
Specialist in Nephrology,
Ospedale Civile di Amaghi,
Frosinone, Italy
*Acute Renal Failure in Oncological
Disorders and Tumor Lysis
Syndrome; Acute Renal Failure in
the Elderly Critically Ill Patient*

Joseph V. Bonventre, MD, PhD
Robert H. Ebert Professor of
Medicine and Health Sciences
and Technology, Harvard Medical
School and Massachusetts
Institute of Technology; Chief,
Renal Division, Brigham and
Women's Hospital, Boston,
Massachusetts
*Models of Ischemic Renal Injury;
Biomarkers in Acute Kidney Injury*

A. D. Booth, MB, FRCP
Clinical Scholar, University of
British Columbia Faculty of
Medicine, Vancouver, British
Columbia, Canada
Statins and the Kidney

Edmund Bourke, MD
Professor and Chair, Department
of Medicine, State University of
New York Downstate Medical
Center, Brooklyn, New York
Pulmonary Renal Syndromes

**George Braitberg, MB, BS,
FACEM**
Professor of Emergency Medicine,
Monash University Faculty of
Medicine, Nursing, and Health
Sciences; Director, Emergency
Medicine, Southern Health,
Melbourne, Victoria, Australia
*Drugs and Antidotes in Acute
Intoxication*

Diego Brancaccio, MD
Professor of Nephrology,
University of Milan Faculty of
Medicine; Attending Physician,
San Paolo Hospital, Milan, Italy
Calcium and Phosphate Physiology

Alessandra Brendolan, MD
Chief of Hemodialysis Section,
Department of Nephrology,
Dialysis, and Transplant, St.
Bortolo Hospital, Vicenza, Italy
*Pulse High-Volume Hemofiltration in
Management of Critically Ill Patients
with Severe Sepsis or Septic Shock;
Multiple-Organ Support Therapy for
the Critically Ill Patient*

Brigida Brezzi, MD
Consultant Nephrologist, IRCCS
Fondazione Ospedale Maggiore
Policlinico Mangiagalli e Regina
Elena, Milan, Italy
*Alterations in Calcium and
Phosphorus Metabolism in Critically
Ill Patients*

James C. Brodie, PhD
University of Edinburgh,
Edinburgh, United Kingdom
Stem Cells and Renal Repair

Patrick D. Brophy, MD, BSc
Associate Professor of Pediatrics,
University of Iowa Carver College
of Medicine; Division Director,
Pediatric Nephrology, Dialysis,
and Transplantation, University
of Iowa Children's Hospital, Iowa
City, Iowa
*Technical Aspects of Pediatric
Continuous Renal Replacement
Therapy; Inborn Errors of Metabolism
and Continuous Renal Replacement
Therapy*

Ryan Brown, MD
Nephrologist, Muhlenberg
Regional Medical Center,
Plainfield; Nephrologist, Overlook
Hospital, Summit, New Jersey
*Correction of Water, Electrolyte, and
Acid-Base Derangements by
Hemodialysis and Derived
Techniques*

Richard Bucala, MD, PhD
Department of Medicine, Yale
University School of Medicine;
Attending Physician, Yale–New
Haven Hospital, New Haven,
Connecticut
*The Macrophage in Innate and
Adaptive Immunity*

**Jonathan Buckmaster, MB,
BS (Melb)**
Honorary Senior Fellow, Faculty
of Medicine, Austin Hospital
Clinical School, University of
Melbourne; Staff Specialist in
Intensive Care, Austin Health,
Melbourne, Victoria, Australia
Intravascular Volume Depletion

Milos N. Budisavljevic, MD
Nephrologist, Medical University
of South Carolina, Charleston,
South Carolina
Proteomics and Acute Renal Failure

Timothy E. Bunchman, MD
Professor of Pediatric
Nephrology, Helen DeVos
Children's Hospital, Grand
Rapids, Michigan
*Epidemiology of Pediatric Acute
Kidney Injury*

**Emmanuel A. Burdmann, MD,
PhD**
Associate Professor of
Nephrology, São José do Rio
Preto Medical School, São José
do Rio Preto, Brazil
Drug-Induced Acute Renal Failure

Benedetta Bussolati, MD, PhD
Associate Professor of
Nephrology, University of Turin
Faculty of Medicine and Surgery,
Turin, Italy
Stem Cells and the Kidney

Matthew A. Butkus, PhD
University of Pittsburgh Medical
Center, Pittsburgh, Pennsylvania
*Genetic Variation and Critical Illness;
Acid-Base Disorders Secondary to
Renal Failure; Disorders of Chronic
Metabolic Alkalosis*

Daniela Buzzelli
Department of Internal Medicine,
University of Perugia Faculty of
Medicine, Perugia, Italy
*Oxidative Stress in Acute Kidney
Injury and Sepsis*

Paolo Calzavacca, MD
Research Fellow, Department of
Intensive Care, Austin Hospital
Clinical School, Melbourne,
Victoria, Australia
*Renal Blood Flow and Perfusion
Pressure; Dopamine Receptor
Agonists; Acid-Base Disorders
Secondary to Renal Failure*

Giovanni Camussi, MD
Professor of Nephrology,
University of Turin Faculty of
Medicine and Surgery, Turin,
Italy
Stem Cells and the Kidney

Bernard Canaud, MD, PhD
Professor of Nephrology,
Montpelier University School of
Medicine; Head of Nephrology,
Dialysis, and Intensive Care Unit,
Lapeyronie University Hospital,
Montpelier, France
*Vascular Access for Intermittent
Renal Replacement Therapy;
Vascular Access for Continuous
Renal Replacement Therapy*

Noël J. M. Cano, MD, PhD
Director, Centre de Recherche en
Nutrition Humaine d'Auvergne,
University Hospital of Clermont-
Ferrand, Clermont-Ferrand,
France
*Nitrogen Balance and Nutritional
Assessment*

Vincenzo Cantaluppi, MD
Research Associate, School of
Nephrology, University of Turin
Faculty of Medicine and Surgery,
Turin, Italy
Humoral Mediators in Sepsis

Giovambattista Capasso, MD
Professor of Nephrology, School
of Medicine, Second University
of Naples, Naples, Italy
The Physiology of the Loop of Henle

Gianni Cappelli, MD
Nephrology, Dialysis, and Renal
Transplantation Unit, University
Hospital of Modena, Modena,
Italy
*Nanoparticles: Potential Toxins for
the Organism and the Kidney?*

Eleonora Carlesso, MSc
Istituto di Anestesiologia e
Rianimazione, Università Degli
Studi di Milano, Milan, Italy
Arterial and Venous Blood Gases

Francesco G. Casino, MD
Nephrologist, Division of
Nephrology and Dialysis,
Ospedale Madonna delle Grazie,
Matera, Italy
*Quantification of Acute Renal
Replacement Therapy*

Leticia Castillo, MD
Associate Professor of Pediatrics,
Baylor College of Medicine,
Houston, Texas
*Nutrition of Critically Ill Children
with Acute Renal Failure*

Roberta Cerutti, MD
Consultant Nephrologist, IRCCS
Fondazione Ospedale Maggiore
Policlinico Mangiagalli e Regina
Elena, Milan, Italy
*Alterations in Calcium and
Phosphorus Metabolism in Critically
Ill Patients*

Lakhmir S. Chawla, MD
Assistant Professor of Medicine,
George Washington University
School of Medicine and Health
Sciences; Attending Physician,
George Washington University
Hospital, Washington, DC
*Human Immunodeficiency Virus
Infection and Acute Renal Failure*

**Chang Yin Chionh, MB, BS,
MRCP(UK)**
Fellow, Department of
Nephrology, St. Bortolo Hospital,
Vicenza, Italy; Associate
Consultant, Renal Unit,
Department of General Medicine,
Tan Tock Seng Hospital,
Singapore
*Adjustment of Antimicrobial
Regimen in Septic Patients
Undergoing Continuous Renal
Replacement Therapy in the
Intensive Care Unit; Sorbents: From
Basic Structure to Clinical
Application*

**Alexander Chiu, MBChB,
MRCP(UK), FHKCP**
Honorary Assistant Professor,
Department of Anesthesiology;
Associate Consultant, Adult
Intensive Care Unit, Queen Mary
Hospital, Hong Kong, China
*Clinical Outcomes with the
Molecular Adsorbent Recirculating
System*

May T. Chow, MD, FACP, FASN
Attending Physician
(Nephrologist), La Grange
Memorial Hospital, La Grange,
Illinois
*Gastrointestinal Problems in Acute
Renal Failure*

Kirpal S. Chugh, MD, FRCP
Emeritus Professor of
Nephrology, Postgraduate
Institute of Medical Education
and Research, Chandigarh, India
Acute Kidney Injury in Malaria

Bruno Cianciaruso, MD
Associate Professor and Chair of Nephrology, University "Federico II" of Naples School of Medicine; Director, Outpatient Clinic for Chronic Kidney Disease, Azienda Ospedaliera Universitaria "Federico II" of Naples, Naples, Italy
Carbohydrates and Lipids

Mauro Cignarelli, MD
Professor of Endocrinology and Metabolic Diseases, University of Foggia School of Medicine; Head, Unit of Endocrinology and Metabolic Diseases, OORR Hospital, Foggia, Italy
Environment, Smoking, Obesity, and the Kidney

Yann-Erick Claessens, MD, PhD
Assistant Professor, Emergency Medicine, Medical School, Université Paris Descartes; Department of Emergency and Critical Care Medicine, Hôpital Cochin, Paris, France
The Coagulation System in Inflammation

John A. Clark, MD
Nephrology Consultants, Hampton Cove, Alabama
Practical Aspects of Hybrid Dialysis Techniques

William R. Clark, MD
Gambro Renal Products, Indianapolis, Indiana
Solute and Water Transport across Artificial Membranes in Conventional Hemodialysis; Predilution and Postdilution Reinfusion Techniques; Solute and Water Kinetics in Continuous Therapies; Nonrenal Applications of Extracorporeal Treatments: Heart Failure and Liver Failure

David J. Cohen, MD
Professor of Medicine, Columbia University College of Physicians and Surgeons, New York, New York
Renal Function and Acute Renal Failure in the Setting of Heart and Heart-Lung Transplantation

Scott D. Cohen, MD, MPH
Nephrology Fellow, George Washington University School of Medicine and Health Sciences, Washington, DC
Human Immunodeficiency Virus Infection and Acute Renal Failure

Peter Constable, PhD, MS, BVSc
Professor and Head, Department of Veterinary Clinical Sciences, Purdue University, West Lafayette, Indiana
Clinical Acid-Base Chemistry

Rosanna Coppo, MD
Professor of Nephrology, University of Turin Faculty of Medicine and Surgery; Director, Nephrology Dialysis Transplantation Department, Regina Margherita University Hospital, Turin, Italy
Antibiotics and Antiviral Drugs in the Intensive Care Unit

Howard E. Corey, MD
Director, Children's Kidney Center of New Jersey, Goryeb Children's Hospital of Morristown Memorial Hospital, Morristown, New Jersey
Renal Acid-Base Physiology; Metabolic Acidosis

Mario Cozzolino, MD, PhD
Professor of Nephrology, University of Ferrara Faculty of Medicine; Attending Physician, San Paolo Hospital, Milan, Italy
Calcium and Phosphate Physiology

Maureen Craig, RN, MSN, CNN, CCNS
Clinical Nurse Specialist, Nephrology, University of California Davis Medical Center, Sacramento, California
Practical Aspects of Hybrid Dialysis Techniques

Carl H. Cramer II, MD
Department of Pediatrics, Mayo Clinic, Rochester, Minnesota
Technical Aspects of Pediatric Continuous Renal Replacement Therapy

Mark Crandall, MD
Third-Year Resident, Mayo Clinic Graduate School of Medical Education; Resident Physician, Internal Medicine, Mayo Clinic, Rochester, Minnesota
Renal Function in Congestive Heart Failure

Paolo Cravedi, MD
Division of Nephrology and Dialysis, Azienda Ospedaliera Ospedali Riuniti di Bergamo and Mario Negri Institute for Pharmacological Research, Bergamo, Italy
Acute Renal Failure in Kidney Transplant Recipients

Carlo Crepaldi, MD
Associate of Clinical Nephrology, Department of Nephrology, St. Bortolo Hospital, Vicenza, Italy
Myoglobin as a Toxin

R. John Crew, MD
Assistant Professor of Medicine, Columbia University College of Physicians and Surgeons, New York, New York
Renal Function and Acute Renal Failure in the Setting of Heart and Heart-Lung Transplantation

Donald F. Cronin, MD
Associate Clinical Professor of Medicine, Division of Nephrology, University of California, San Diego, Medical Center, San Diego, California
Principles of Anticoagulation in Extracorporeal Circuits

Dinna N. Cruz, MD, MPH
Nephrologist, St. Bortolo Hospital, Vicenza, Italy
The Role of Extracorporeal Blood Purification Therapies in the Prevention of Radiocontrast-Induced Nephropathy Effect of Renal Replacement Therapy on the Brain; Sorbents: From Basic Structure to Clinical Application; The Toraymyxin and Other Endotoxin Adsorption Systems

Antonio Dal Canton, MD
Professor of Nephrology, University of Pavia School of Medicine; Director, Department of Nephrology Dialysis Transplantation, Pavia, Italy
Growth Factors

Maurizio Dan, MD
Department of Anesthesia and
Intensive Care, Ospedale Civile,
Verona, Italy
*Ethical Considerations in Acute
Renal Replacement Therapy*

Angela D'Angelo, MD
Professor and Director,
Nephrology Unit, University of
Padua School of Medicine,
Padua, Italy
Acute Obstructive Nephropathy

Andrew Davenport, MD, FRCP
Honorary Senior Lecturer, Royal
Free and University College
Medical School; Consultant
Nephrologist, Royal Free
Hospital, London,
United Kingdom
*Neurological Problems in Acute
Renal Failure; Treatment of
Combined Acute Renal Failure and
Cerebral Edema; Dialysis
Disequilibrium Syndrome; Effect of
Renal Replacement Therapy on the
Brain*

**Andrew R. Davies, MB, BS,
FRACP**
Deputy Director, Intensive Care,
Alfred Hospital, Melbourne,
Victoria, Australia
*Disorders of Trace Elements and
Vitamins; Enteral Nutrition*

James W. Dear, PhD, MRCP
Clinical Lecturer, Centre for
Cardiovascular Science,
Edinburgh University, Edinburgh,
United Kingdom
*New Imaging Techniques for Acute
Kidney Injury*

Andrea De Gasperi, MD
Director of Transplantation
Department, Niguarda Ca'Granda
Hospital, Milan, Italy
*Hematological Malignancies and
Critical Illness*

Roberto Dell'Aquila, MD
Section Chief, Peritoneal Dialysis,
Department of Nephrology,
Dialysis, and Transplantation, St.
Bortolo Hospital, Vicenza, Italy
*Peritoneal Access for Acute
Peritoneal Dialysis*

Giorgio Della Rocca, MD
Professor of Anaesthesia and
Intensive Care, University of
Udine School of Medicine; Chief,
Department of Anaesthesia and
Intensive Care Unit, Azienda
Ospedaliero Universitaria,
University of Udine, Udine, Italy
Vasoactive Drugs and Renal Function

Dorella Del Prete, MD, PhD
Researcher, Department of
Medical and Surgical Sciences,
Nephrology Unit, University of
Padua School of Medicine,
Padua, Italy
Acute Obstructive Nephropathy

Russell L. Delude, PhD
Associate Professor of Critical
Care Medicine and Pathology,
University of Pittsburgh School
of Medicine; CRISMA Laboratory,
University of Pittsburgh Medical
Center, Pittsburgh, Pennsylvania
*Innate Mechanisms of Host Defense;
High Mobility Group Box 1 Protein;
Epithelial Barrier Dysfunction as a
Mechanism Underlying the
Pathogenesis of Multiple-Organ
Dysfunction*

Thomas Depner, MD
Professor of Medicine and
Director of Dialysis Services,
Division of Nephrology,
University of California Davis
Medical Center, Sacramento,
California
*Urea Kinetics, Efficiency, and
Adequacy of Hemodialysis and Other
Intermittent Treatments*

Lorenzo E. Derchi, MD
Professor and Chairman,
Department of Radiology, DICMI
University of Genova; Attending
Physician, Ospedale San Martino,
Genova, Italy
*Ultrasonography and Doppler
Techniques in Acute Kidney Injury*

Prasad Devarajan, MD
Louise M. Williams Endowed
Chair, Professor of Pediatrics and
Developmental Biology,
University of Cincinnati College
of Medicine; Director of
Nephrology and Hypertension,
Director of Clinical Nephrology
Laboratories, and CEO of Dialysis
Unit, Cincinnati Children's
Hospital Medical Center,
Cincinnati, Ohio
*Apoptosis and Necrosis;
Pathophysiology of Pediatric Acute
Kidney Injury*

Jan J. De Waele, MD
Surgical Intensive Care,
University Hospital Ghent, Ghent,
Belgium
*Immunological and Infectious
Complications of Acute Kidney Injury*

**Jean-François Dhainaut, MD,
PhD**
Professor, Intensive Care, Medical
School, Université Paris
Descartes; Department of
Emergency and Critical Care
Medicine, Hôpital Cochin, Paris,
France
*The Coagulation System in
Inflammation; Indications for and
Contraindications to Intermittent
Hemodialysis in Critically Ill Patients*

José A. Diaz-Buxo, MD
Home Therapies Development,
Fresenius Medical Care,
Charlotte, North Carolina
*Technology of Peritoneal Dialysis in
the Intensive Care Unit*

Lucia Di Micco, MD
Nephrology Fellow, Azienda
Ospedaliera Universitaria
"Federico II" of Naples, Naples,
Italy
Carbohydrates and Lipids

**José Carolina Divino-Filho, MD,
PhD**
Divisions of Baxter Novum and
Renal Medicine, Karolinska
Institutet, Stockholm, Sweden;
Vice President of Medical Affairs,
Baxter Health Care Latin
America, Mexico City, Mexico
*Nursing Issues and Procedures in
Acute Peritoneal Dialysis*

Sarah Doernberg, MD
Yale University School of
Medicine, New Haven,
Connecticut
*The Macrophage in Innate and
Adaptive Immunity*

Gordon S. Doig, DVM, PhD, MSc
Senior Lecturer in Intensive Care,
Northern Clinical School,
University of Sydney; Clinical
Epidemiologist, Royal North
Shore Hospital, Sydney,
New South Wales, Australia
Parenteral Nutrition

David J. Dries, MD, MSE
John F. Perry, Jr., Professor of
Surgery, University of Minnesota
Medical School; Assistant
Medical Director, Surgical Care,
HealthPartners Medical Group,
Minneapolis, Minnesota
Mechanical Ventilation

Francesco Maria Drudi, MD
Senior Assistant, University
Hospital "La Sapienza" Roma,
Rome, Italy
*Computed Tomography and
Magnetic Resonance Imaging in
Acute Renal Failure*

Wilfred Druml, MD
Professor of Medicine, Medical
University of Vienna; Director,
Acute Dialysis Unit, Vienna
General Hospital, Vienna, Austria
*Amino Acid and Protein Turnover
and Metabolism in Acute Renal
Failure; Nutritional Support in the
Critically Ill with Acute Renal Failure*

**Graeme Duke, MD, FJICM,
FANZCA**
University of Melbourne Faculty
of Medicine, Dentistry, and
Health Sciences; Director, Critical
Care Department, Northern
Hospital, Victoria, Australia
Glomerulonephritis

**Andrew Durward, MBChB (Cape
Town), FCP**
Consultant in Paediatric Intensive
Care, Evelina Children's Hospital,
London, United Kingdom
Diabetic Ketoacidosis

Morltoki Egi, MD
Clinical Research Fellow,
Okayama University; Clinical
Fellow, Department of Intensive
Care, Okayama University
Hospital, Okayama, Japan
*Blood Glucose Control in Critical
Care*

Ciro Esposito, MD, PhD
Associate Professor of
Nephrology, University of Pavia
School of Medicine; Senior
Assistant, Department of
Nephrology, Dialysis, and
Transplantation, IRCCS
Policlinico San Matteo, Pavia,
Italy
Growth Factors

Pieter Evenepoel, MD, PhD
Associate Professor, Department
of Pathophysiology, Catholic
University; Department of
Medicine, Division of
Nephrology, University Hospital
Leuven, Leuven, Belgium
Toxic Acute Renal Failure

Teresa Faga, MD
Attending Physician in
Nephrology, Renal Unit, Hospital
of Soverato, Soverato, Italy
Acute Interstitial Nephritis

**Sheung Tat Fan, MD, PhD, DSc,
FRCS, FACS**
Professor and Chair, Department
of Surgery, University of Hong
Kong; Chief of Service,
Department of Surgery, Queen
Mary Hospital, Hong Kong, China
*Clinical Outcomes with the
Molecular Adsorbent Recirculating
System*

Donald A. Feinfeld, MD
Professor of Clinical Medicine,
Albert Einstein College of
Medicine of Yeshiva University,
Bronx; Director of Nephrology
Training, Beth Israel Medical
Center, New York, New York
*Hemodialysis, Hemofiltration, and
Hemoperfusion in Acute Intoxication
and Poisoning*

Eric Féraille, MD, PhD
Maître d'Enseignement et de
Recherche, University of Geneva,
Geneva, Switzerland
*The Physiology of the Collecting
Ducts*

Javier Fernández, MD
Liver Unit, Hospital Clinic of
Barcelona, Barcelona, Spain
*Spontaneous Bacterial Peritonitis
and Hepatorenal Syndrome*

**Simon Finfer, MB, BS, FRCP,
FRCA**
Professor, The George Institute
for International Health,
University of Sydney Faculty of
Medicine; Senior Staff Specialist
in Intensive Care, Royal North
Shore Hospital, Sydney, New
South Wales, Australia
Crystalloids and Colloids

Mitchell P. Fink, MD
Professor, Departments of Critical
Care Medicine, Surgery, and
Pharmacology, University of
Pittsburgh School of Medicine,
Pittsburgh, Pennsylvania;
President and CEO, Logical
Therapeutics, Inc., Waltham,
Massachusetts
*Epithelial Barrier Dysfunction as a
Mechanism Underlying the
Pathogenesis of Multiple-Organ
Dysfunction*

Kevin W. Finkel, MD
Professor and Vice-Chairman of
Medicine and Director, Division
of Renal Diseases and
Hypertension, University of
Texas Medical School at
Houston, Houston, Texas
Acute Tubular Necrosis

Michael F. Flessner, MD, PhD
University of Mississippi Medical
Center, Jackson, Mississippi
*Solute and Water Transport across
the Peritoneal Membrane*

Marco Formica, MD
Director, Nephrology and Dialysis
Unit, Santa Croce and Carle
Hospital, Cuneo, Italy
*Extracorporeal Blood Purification
Techniques beyond Dialysis: Coupled
Plasmafiltration-Adsorption*

Lui G. Forni, PhD, MRCPI
Honorary Senior Lecturer,
Brighton and Sussex Medical
School, Sussex; Consultant
Intensivist/Physician, Department
of Critical Care, Worthing and
Southlands Hospital Trust,
West Sussex, United Kingdom
*Unmeasured Anions in Metabolic
Acidosis*

James D. Fortenberry, MD
Associate Professor of Pediatrics and Chief of Division of Critical Care, Emory University School of Medicine; Medical Director, Pediatric Extracorporeal Membrane Oxygenation and Advanced Technologies, and Medical Director, Clinical Research, Children's Healthcare of Atlanta, Atlanta, Georgia
Continuous Renal Replacement Therapies in Combination with Other Extracorporeal Therapies

Craig French, MD
Department of Intensive Care, Western Hospital, Melbourne, Victoria, Australia
Blood and Blood Products; Anemia of Critical Illness

Roberto Fumagalli, MD
Associate Professor, Department of Experimental Medicine, University of Milan; Director, Department of Perioperative and Critical Care Medicine, San Gerardo Hospital, Milan, Italy
Extracorporeal Support and Renal Function; Indications for Renal Replacement Therapy in the Critically Ill Patient

Mario Furlanut, MD
Institute of Clinical Pharmacology and Toxicology, Department of Experimental and Clinical Pathology and Medicine, University of Udine, Udine, Italy
Principles of Pharmacodynamics and Pharmacokinetics of Drugs Used in Extracorporeal Therapies

Micheline Djouguela Fute, MD
Resident, Department of Radiology, University of Trieste; Attending Physician, Ospedale di Cattinara, Trieste, Italy
Contrast-Enhanced Renal Ultrasonography

Daniela Ponce Gabriel, MD
Assistant Professor of Nephrology, Botucatu Medical School, São Paulo State University, Botucatu, SP, Brazil
Nursing Issues and Procedures in Acute Peritoneal Dialysis

Andrea Galassi, MD
Attending Physician, San Paolo Hospital, Milan, Italy
Calcium and Phosphate Physiology

Miriam Galbusera, BiolSciD
Head, Unit of Platelet-Endothelial Cell Interaction, Negri Bergamo Laboratories, Mario Negro Institute for Pharmacological Research, Bergamo, Italy
Bleeding and Hemostasis in Acute Renal Failure

Francesco Galli, PhD
Research Scientist, Department of Internal Medicine, University of Perugia Faculty of Medicine, Perugia, Italy
Oxidative Stress in Acute Kidney Injury and Sepsis

Giovanni Galli, MD
Department of Nephrology, University of Trieste; Attending Physician, Ospedale di Cattinara, Trieste, Italy
Contrast-Enhanced Renal Ultrasonography

Maurizio Gallieni, MD
Professor of Nephrology, University of Milan Faculty of Medicine; Attending Physician, San Paolo Hospital, Milan, Italy
Calcium and Phosphate Physiology

Giampiero Gallo, MD
Attending Physician, Department of Anaesthesiology and Intensive Care, St. Bortolo Hospital, Vicenza, Italy
Diagnosis and Management of the HELLP Syndrome

Giovanni Gambaro, MD, PhD
Associate Professor of Nephrology, School of Medicine, University of Verona; Associate Professor, Division of Nephrology, Ospedale Civile Maggiore, Verona, Italy
Endothelial Progenitor Cells in Acute Renal Injury

Hilary S. Gammill, MD
Acting Assistant Professor, University of Washington School of Medicine; Research Associate, Fred Hutchinson Cancer Research Center, Seattle, Washington
Acute Renal Failure in Pregnancy

Ezio Nicola Gangemi, MD
Fellowship, Department of Plastic Surgery, Burn Unit, CTO Hospital, Turin, Italy
Burns and Acute Renal Failure

Dayong Gao, PhD
Professor of Engineering, University of Washington, Seattle, Washington
Solute and Water Transport across Artificial Membranes in Conventional Hemodialysis; Predilution and Postdilution Reinfusion Techniques; Solute and Water Kinetics in Continuous Therapies

Susan Garwood, MBChB
Associate Professor, Yale University School of Medicine; Attending Anesthesiologist, Yale–New Haven Hospital, New Haven, Connecticut
Ischemic Acute Renal Failure; Osmotic Diuretics

Francesco Garzotto, BD
Technician, Department of Nephrology, Dialysis, and Transplantation, St. Bortolo Hospital, Vicenza, Italy
Information Technology and Therapy Delivery in Continuous Renal Replacement Therapies

Antonietta M. Gatti, MD
Department of Neurosciences, University of Modena and Reggio Emilia, Modena, Italy
Nanoparticles: Potential Toxins for the Organism and the Kidney?

Luciano Gattinoni, MD, FRCP
Professor of Anesthesiology and Intensive Care Medicine, Istituto di Anestesiologia e Rianimazione, Università Degli Studi di Milano; Chief, Dipartimento di Anestesia, Rianimazione, e Terapia del Dolore, IRCCS Fondazione Ospedale Maggiore Policlinico Mangiagalli e Regina Elena, Milan, Italy
Arterial and Venous Blood Gases

John P. Geibel, MD, DSc
Vice Chairman and Professor, Department of Surgery; Director of Surgical Research; and Professor of Cellular and Molecular Physiology, Yale University School of Medicine, New Haven, Connecticut
Distal Tubular Physiology

Stephen George, PhD, MRCPath
Honorary Lecturer, School of Biosciences, University of Birmingham; Consultant Clinical Scientist, West Midlands Toxicology Laboratory, City Hospital, Birmingham, United Kingdom
Laboratory Testing in Toxicology

Loreto Gesualdo, MD
Professor of Nephrology, University of Foggia School of Medicine; Chief, Division of Nephrology, Dialysis, and Transplantation, Teaching Hospital, Foggia, Italy
Environment, Smoking, Obesity, and the Kidney

R. T. Noel Gibney, MB, FRCP(C), FRCPI
Professor and Director, Division of Critical Care Medicine, University of Alberta Faculty of Medicine and Dentistry; Regional Program Medical Director, Critical Care Program, Capital Health, Edmonton, Alberta, Canada
Continuous Venovenous Hemodialysis and Continuous High-Flux Hemodialysis

Debbie S. Gipson, MD, MS
Associate Professor, Departments of Medicine and Pediatrics, Division of Nephrology and Hypertension, University of North Carolina at Chapel Hill School of Medicine, Chapel Hill, North Carolina
Pathophysiology of Vasculitis

Ilya G. Glezerman, MD
Assistant Professor of Clinical Medicine, Weill Cornell Medical College; Assistant Clinical Member, Memorial Sloan-Kettering Cancer Center, New York, New York
Anticancer Drugs and the Kidney

Griet Glorieux, PhD, MSc
Attending Physician, University Hospital Ghent, Ghent, Belgium
Metabolic Waste Products in Acute Uremia; Granulocyte-Inhibitory Proteins and Other Proteinaceous Molecules in Acute Kidney Injury

Stuart L. Goldstein, MD
Associate Professor of Pediatrics, Baylor College of Medicine; Medical Director, Renal Dialysis Unit and Pheresis Service, Texas Children's Hospital, Houston, Texas
Epidemiology of Pediatric Acute Kidney Injury; Outcome of Pediatric Acute Kidney Injury

Thomas A. Golper, MD
Professor of Medicine (Nephrology), Vanderbilt University School of Medicine, Nashville, Tennessee
Hybrid Dialysis Techniques in the Intensive Care Unit; Practical Aspects of Hybrid Dialysis Techniques

Manjula Gowrishankar, MD, FRCP(C)
Professor, University of Alberta Faculty of Medicine; Pediatric Nephrologist, Stollery Children's Hospital, Edmonton, Alberta, Canada
Regulatory Mechanisms of Water and Sodium Balance

Fabio Grandi, PhD.
Gambro Dasco S.P.A., Medolla, Italy
Information Technology and Therapy Delivery in Continuous Renal Replacement Therapies

Cesare Gregoretti, MD
Head, Emergency Department, Intensive Care Unit, CTO Hospital, Turin, Italy
Burns and Acute Renal Failure

Brian W. Grinnell, PhD
Distinguished Research Fellow, Eli Lilly and Company, Indianapolis, Indiana
Activated Protein C Therapy and Sepsis-Associated Acute Kidney Injury

A. B. Johan Groeneveld, MD, PhD
Intensivist and Professor of Intensive Care, VU University Medical Center, Amsterdam, The Netherlands
The Kidney during Mechanical Ventilation

Steven J. Gruber, MD
Assistant Professor of Clinical Medicine, Albert Einstein College of Medicine of Yeshiva University, Bronx; Director, Nephrology Development, Beth Israel Medical Center, New York, New York
Hemodialysis, Hemofiltration, and Hemoperfusion in Acute Intoxication and Poisoning

Gualtiero Guadagni, PhD
Department of Bioengineering, Politecnico di Milano, Milan, Italy
The Toraymyxin and Other Endotoxin Adsorption Systems

Kyle J. Gunnerson, MD
Associate Professor of Anesthesiology and Emergency Medicine, Virginia Commonwealth University School of Medicine; Director of Critical Care Anesthesiology; Medical Director of Cardiac Surgery, Intensive Care Unit; and Senior Investigator, VCURES Laboratory, Virginia Commonwealth University Medical Center, Richmond, Virginia
Impact of Acid-Base Disorders on Different Organ Systems; Acid-Base Disorders Secondary to Poisoning

Akanksha Gupta
Research Scientist, Eli Lilly and Company, Indianapolis, Indiana
Activated Protein C Therapy and Sepsis-Associated Acute Kidney Injury

Victor Gura, MD
Chief Scientist and Director, Xcorporeal, Inc., Irvine, California
Continuous Ultrafiltration and Dialysis with a Wearable Artificial Kidney

Isabella Guzzo, MD
Dialysis Unit, Department of Nephrology and Urology, Ospedale Pediatrico Bambino Gesu, Instituto di Ricerca Scientifica, Rome, Italy
Multiple Organ Dysfunction in the Pediatric Intensive Care Unit

Richard Hackbarth, MD
Division of Pediatric Critical
Care, DeVos Children's Hospital,
Grand Rapids, Michigan
*Technical Aspects of Pediatric
Continuous Renal Replacement
Therapy*

**Mitchell L. Halperin, MD, FRCPC,
FRS**
Emeritus Professor of Medicine,
University of Toronto Faculty of
Medicine; Attending Staff,
Department of Nephrology,
St. Michael's Hospital, Toronto,
Ontario, Canada
*Regulatory Mechanisms of Water and
Sodium Balance*

Nikolas Harbord, MD
Attending Nephrologist, Beth
Israel Medical Center, New York,
New York
*Hemodialysis, Hemofiltration, and
Hemoperfusion in Acute Intoxication
and Poisoning*

Jean-Philippe Haymann, MD
Assistant Professor, Pierre and
Marie Curie Faculty of Medicine;
Attending Physician, Tenon
Hospital, Paris, France
*Other Experimental Interventions
for the Management of Acute
Renal Failure*

Alan C. Heffner, MD
Division of Critical Care,
Department of Emergency
Medicine, Carolinas Medical
Center, Charlotte, North Carolina
*Diagnosis and Therapy of Metabolic
Alkalosis*

**Anthony J. Hennessy, MB BCh,
MRCPI**
Senior Registrar, Anaesthesia and
Intensive Care, Cork University
Hospital, Cork, Ireland
*Disorders of Trace Elements and
Vitamins; Enteral Nutrition*

Samuel N. Heyman, MD
Professor of Medicine, Hadassah
Hebrew University Medical
School; Senior Physician,
Department of Medicine,
Hadassah University Hospital,
Jerusalem, Israel
*Critical Assessment of Animal
Models of Acute Renal Failure*

**Graham L. Hill, MD, FRCS,
FRACS, FACS**
Emeritus Professor of Surgery,
University of Auckland Faculty
of Medical and Health Sciences,
Auckland, New Zealand
*Energy Requirement and
Consumption in the Critically Ill
Patient*

Philip J. Hilton, MD, FRCP
Consultant Physician and
Research Director, Renal
Laboratory, St. Thomas' Hospital,
London, United Kingdom
*Unmeasured Anions in Metabolic
Acidosis*

Jonathan Himmelfarb, MD
Director, Division of Nephrology,
Maine Medical Center, Portland,
Maine
*Oxidative Stress in Acute Kidney
Injury; The Kidney in Sepsis*

Hiroyuki Hirasawa, MD, PhD
Professor Emeritus, Chiba
University Graduate School of
Medicine, Chiba City, Japan
*Slow Plasma Exchange plus CHDF
for Liver Failure and CHDF Alone for
Severe Acute Pancreatitis*

Nicholas A. Hoenich, PhD
Honorary Lecturer, School of
Clinical Medical Sciences,
Faculty of Medical Sciences,
Newcastle University, Newcastle-
upon-Tyne, United Kingdom
*Poisoning: Kinetics to Therapeutics;
Membranes and Filters for Use in
Acute Renal Failure; Biocompatibility
of the Dialysis System*

**Stephen R. Holdsworth, MB BS,
MD, PhD**
Head, Southern Clinical School,
and Head, Department of
Medicine, Monash University
Faculty of Medicine, Nursing,
and Health Sciences; Director of
Clinical Immunology and
Consultant Physician in Clinical
Immunology, General Medicine,
and Nephrology, Southern
Health, Monash Medical Centre,
Clayton, Victoria, Australia
Pulmonary Renal Syndromes

**Anthony Holley, MB BCh,
FACEM**
Senior Lecturer, The School of
Medicine, University of
Queensland; Staff Specialist,
Department of Intensive Care
Medicine, Royal Brisbane and
Women's Hospital, Brisbane,
Queensland, Australia
*Principles of Pharmacology in the
Critically Ill*

Patrick M. Honoré, MD
Consultant and Director,
Intensive Care Unit, St. Pierre
Para-University Hospital,
Ottignies-Louvain-La Neuve,
Belgium
*High-Volume Hemofiltration in the
Intensive Care Unit; Removal of
Mediators of Inflammation by
Continuous Renal Replacement
Therapy: An Open Debate of Pros
and Cons*

Eric A. J. Hoste, MD, PhD
Department of Internal Medicine,
Ghent University; Head of Clinic,
Ghent University Hospital, Ghent,
Belgium
*What Is Acute Kidney Injury?;
Epidemiology of Nosocomial Acute
Kidney Injury; Epidemiology of End-
Stage Renal Disease in Patients with
Critical Illness Admitted to Intensive
Care Units; Immunological and
Infectious Complications of Acute
Kidney Injury; Outcome of
Intermittent Dialysis in Critically Ill
Patients with Acute Renal Failure*

Andrew A. House, MD
Division of Nephrology,
Department of Medicine,
London Health Sciences Center–
University Hospital, London,
Ontario, Canada
*Anti-inflammatory Drugs and the
Kidney*

David T. Huang, MD, MPH
Assistant Professor, CRISMA
Laboratory, Critical Care
Medicine, University of
Pittsburgh Medical Center,
Pittsburgh, Pennsylvania
Septic Shock

Zhongping Huang, PhD
Department of Mechanical Engineering, Widener University, Chester, Pennsylvania
Solute and Water Transport across Artificial Membranes in Conventional Hemodialysis; Predilution and Postdilution Reinfusion Techniques; Solute and Water Kinetics in Continuous Therapies

Rolf D. Hubmayr, MD
Walter and Leonore Annenberg Professor in Cardiology and Critical Care and Professor of Medicine and Physiology, Mayo Clinic College of Medicine, Rochester, Minnesota
Respiratory Monitoring

Alun D. Hughes, MB BS, PhD
Professor of Clinical Pharmacology, National Heart and Lung Institute, Faculty of Medicine, Imperial College, London, London, United Kingdom
Thiazide Diuretics

H. David Humes, MD
Professor, Department of Internal Medicine, Division of Nephrology, University of Michigan Medical School, Ann Arbor, Michigan
The Bioartificial Kidney

T. Alp Ikizler, MD
Catherine McLaughlin Hakim Professor of Medicine, Director of Clinical Research in Nephrology, and Medical Director of Vanderbilt Outpatient Dialysis Unit, Division of Nephrology, Vanderbilt University Medical Center, Nashville, Tennessee
Oxidative Stress in Acute Kidney Injury

Barbara Imberti, PhD
Laboratory of Cell Biology and Xenotransplantation, Negri Bergamo Laboratories, Mario Negri Institute for Pharmacological Research, Bergamo, Italy
Mesenchymal Stem Cells and Their Use in Acute Renal Injury

Todd S. Ing, MD
Professor Emeritus of Medicine, Loyola University Chicago Stritch School of Medicine; Attending Physician, Loyola University Medical Center, Maywood, Illinois
Gastrointestinal Problems in Acute Renal Failure; History and Development of Acute Dialysis Therapy

Bertrand L. Jaber, MD, MS
Associate Professor of Medicine, Tufts University School of Medicine; Vice Chair, Clinical Affairs, Department of Medicine, Caritas St. Elizabeth's Medical Center, Boston, Massachusetts
Genetic Factors Influencing Acute Kidney Injury

Gérard Janvier, MD, PhD
Professor Department of Anesthesia, University Hospital of Bordeaux, Pessoc, France
High-Volume Hemofiltration in the Intensive Care Unit

Arundhathi Jeyabalan, MD, MSCR
Assistant Professor, University of Pittsburgh School of Medicine, Pittsburgh, Pennsylvania
Acute Renal Failure in Pregnancy

Vivekanand Jha, MD, DM
Professor of Nephrology, Postgraduate Institute of Medical Education and Research, Chandigarh, India
Acute Kidney Injury in Malaria

Olivier Joannes-Boyau, MD
Consultant, Department of Anesthesia, University Hospital of Bordeaux, Pessoc, France
High-Volume Hemofiltration in the Intensive Care Unit; Removal of Mediators of Inflammation by Continuous Renal Replacement Therapy: An Open Debate of Pros and Cons

Michael Joannidis, MD
Professor of Internal Medicine, Medical University Innsbruck; Director, Intensive Care Unit, Department of Internal Medicine, University Hospital, Innsbruck, Austria
Long-Term Outcomes of Acute Kidney Injury; Indications for Renal Replacement Therapy in the Critically Ill

Daryl A. Jones, BSc(Hons), MB BS
Honorary Senior Research Fellow, Department of Epidemiology and Preventive Medicine, Monash University Faculty of Medicine, Nursing, and Health Sciences; Senior Intensive Care Registrar, Department of Intensive Care, Alfred Hospital, Melbourne, Victoria, Australia
Crystalloids and Colloids; Dysfunction in the Critically Ill: Doubts and Controversies

Achim Jörres, MD
Immunomodulation and Biological Effects of Continuous Renal Replacement Therapy

Kamel S. Kamel, MD, FRCPC
Professor of Medicine, University of Toronto Faculty of Medicine; Division Head, Nephrology, St. Michael's Hospital, Toronto, Ontario, Canada
Regulatory Mechanisms of Water and Sodium Balance

Ryan C. Kamp, MD
Fellow, Pulmonary and Critical Care, University of Chicago Medical Center, Chicago, Illinois
Characteristics, Pathophysiology, and Effects of Common Toxic Substances

Neeta Kannan
University of Pittsburgh Medical Center, Pittsburgh, Pennsylvania
Genetic Variation and Critical Illness

Lewis J. Kaplan, MD, FACS, FCCM, FCCP
Associate Professor, Department of Surgery, Section of Trauma, Yale University School of Medicine; Director, Surgical Intensive Care Unit and Surgical Critical Care Fellowship Program, Yale–New Haven Hospital, New Haven, Connecticut
Abdominal Compartment Syndrome

Özgür Karacan, MD
Associate Professor, Department of Pulmonary Diseases, Baskent University Hospital, Ankara, Turkey
Lung Function in Uremia

Vijay Karajala-Subramanyam, MD
Assistant Program Director, McKeesport Internal Medicine Residency Program, University of Pittsburgh Medical Center, Pittsburgh, Pennsylvania
Nonpharmacological Management of Acute Renal Failure; Use of Diuretics in Acute Renal Failure; The Kidney in Acute Heart Failure Syndromes and Cardiogenic Shock

Gur P. Kaushal, PhD
Professor of Internal Medicine, Division of Nephrology, and Professor of Biochemistry and Molecular Biology, University of Arkansas for Medical Sciences College of Medicine; Research Health Scientist, John L. McClellan Memorial Veterans Hospital, Little Rock, Arkansas
Antiapoptotic Agents

John A. Kellum, MD, FCCM, FACP
Professor and Vice Chair, Department of Critical Care Medicine, University of Pittsburgh School of Medicine, Pittsburgh, Pennsylvania
Genetic Variation and Critical Illness; What Is Acute Kidney Injury?; Basic Principles of Renal Support; Glomerular Filtration Rate and Renal Functional Reserve; Oliguria; Nonpharmacological Management of Acute Renal Failure; Use of Diuretics in Acute Renal Failure; Adenosine Antagonists; Principles of Fluid Therapy; Anion Gap and Strong Ion Gap; Diagnosis and Therapy of Metabolic Alkalosis; Complex (Mixed) Acid-Base Disorders; Acid-Base Disorders Secondary to Renal Failure; Disorders of Chronic Metabolic Alkalosis; Renal Replacement Therapy in Acute Renal Failure Secondary to Sepsis; Blood Purification for Sepsis; The Kidney in Acute Heart Failure Syndromes and Cardiogenic Shock; The Liver in Kidney Disease; The Concept of Renal Replacement Therapy Dose and Efficiency; Current Nomenclature

Markus J. Kemper, MD
Professor of Pediatrics, University Medical Center Hamburg-Eppendorf, Hamburg, Germany
Potassium and Magnesium Physiology

Asjad Khan, MD
Pediatric Endocrinology, Brooklyn, New York
Septic Shock

Ramesh Khanna, MD
Professor, University of Missouri School of Medicine, Columbia, Missouri
Comparison of Peritoneal Dialysis with Other Treatments for Acute Renal Failure

Vijay Kher, MD, DM, FRCPE
Director, Department of Nephrology and Transplant Medicine, Fortis Hospital, New Delhi, India
Clinical Results and Complications of Peritoneal Dialysis in Acute Renal Failure

Paul L. Kimmel, MD
Professor of Medicine, George Washington University School of Medicine and Health Sciences; Attending Physician, George Washington University Hospital, Washington, DC
Human Immunodeficiency Virus Infection and Acute Renal Failure

Detlef Kindgen-Milles, MD
Department of Anaesthesiology, University Hospital Düsseldorf, Dusseldorf, Germany
Acute Dialysis with the GENIUS System

A. Richard Kitching, MBChB, PhD
Associate Professor, Department of Medicine, Southern Clinical School, Monash University Faculty of Medicine, Nursing, and Health Sciences; Consultant Physician in Nephrology and Paediatric Nephrology, Southern Health, Monash Medical Centre, Clayton, Victoria, Australia
Pulmonary Renal Syndromes

Carl M. Kjellstrand, MD, PhD
Clinical Professor of Medicine, Loyola University Chicago Stritch School of Medicine, Maywood, Illinois
History and Development of Acute Dialysis Therapy

Orly F. Kohn, MD
Associate Professor of Medicine, University of Chicago Pritzker School of Medicine; Medical Director, Home Dialysis Program, University of Chicago Medical Center, Chicago, Illinois
Gastrointestinal Problems in Acute Renal Failure; History and Development of Acute Dialysis Therapy

Laura A. Kooienga, MD
Denver Nephrology, PC, Denver, Colorado
Correction of Fluid, Electrolyte, and Acid-Base Derangements by Peritoneal Dialysis in Acute Renal Failure

Jeroen P. Kooman, MD, PhD
Associate Professor of Internal Medicine and Nephrology, Maastricht University Medical Center, Maastricht, The Netherlands
Hypertensive Emergencies

Peter Kotanko, MD
Senior Lecturer, Medical University Innsbruck, Innsbruck, Austria; Renal Research Institute, New York, New York
Assessment of Fluid Status and Body Composition, and Control of Fluid Balance with Intermittent Hemodialysis in the Critically Ill Patient

Raymond T. Krediet, MD, PhD
Professor of Nephrology, University of Amsterdam; Head, Division of Nephrology, Department of Medicine, Academic Medical Center, University of Amsterdam, Amsterdam, The Netherlands
Choice of Peritoneal Dialysis Technique: Intermittent or Continuous

A. A. Kroon, MD, PhD
Associate Professor of Internal Medicine, Cardiovascular Research Institute, Maastricht University Medical Center, Maastricht, The Netherlands
Hypertensive Emergencies

Dingwei Kuang, MD
Department of Nephrology, St. Bortolo Hospital, Vicenza, Italy; Department of Nephrology, Huashan Hospital, Fudan University, Shanghai, China
Poisoning: Kinetics to Therapeutics; Adjustment of Antimicrobial Regimen in Septic Patients Undergoing Continuous Renal Replacement Therapy in the Intensive Care Unit; Sorbents: From Basic Structure to Clinical Application

Martin K. Kuhlmann, MD
Department of Medicine, Division of Nephrology, Vivantes Klinikum im Friedrichshain, Berlin, Germany
Cardiovascular Problems in Acute Renal Failure

Jan Willem Kuiper, MD, MSc
Resident in Pediatrics, Department of Pediatric Intensive Care, VU University Medical Center, Amsterdam, The Netherlands
The Kidney during Mechanical Ventilation

Man-Fai Lam, MB BS, MRCP(UK), FHKCP, FHKAM
Honorary Assistant Professor, Department of Medicine, University of Hong Kong; Associate Consultant, Queen Mary Hospital, Hong Kong, China
Treatment of Peritonitis and Other Clinical Complications of Peritoneal Dialysis in the Critically Ill Patient

Olga Lamacchia, MD
Attending Physician, Unit of Endocrinology and Metabolic Diseases, OORR Hospital, Foggia, Italy
Environment, Smoking, Obesity, and the Kidney

Norbert Lameire, MD, PhD
Emeritus Professor of Medicine; Emeritus Professor of Nephrology, University Hospital Ghent, Ghent Belgium
Epidemiology of End-Stage Renal Disease in Patients with Critical Illness Admitted to Intensive Care Units; Metabolic Waste Products in Acute Uremia; Granulocyte-Inhibitory Proteins and Other Proteinaceous Molecules in Acute Kidney Injury; Outcome of Intermittent Dialysis in Critically Ill Patients with Acute Renal Failure

Christoph Langenberg, MD, PhD
Research Fellow, Howard Florey Institute, University of Melbourne, Melbourne, Victoria, Australia
The Physiology of the Afferent and Efferent Arterioles; Septic Acute Renal Failure; Animal Models of Septic Acute Renal Failure

Gianfranco Lauri, MD
Deputy Director, Intensive Cardiac Care Unit, Centro Cardiologico Monzino, Institute of Cardiology, University of Milan, Milan, Italy
Intermittent Hemofiltration for Management of Fluid Overload and Administration of Contrast Media

Martine Leblanc, MD, FRCPC
Associate Professor, University of Montreal Faculty of Medicine; Chief of Medicine, Maisonneuve-Rosemont Hospital, Montreal, Quebec Canada.
Disorders of Potassium Balance; Disorders of Magnesium Balance; Urinary Tract Infections in the Intensive Care Unit

Ingrid Ledebo, PhD
Director, Scientific Affairs, Gambro AB, Lund, Sweden
Principles of Fluid Manufacturing and Sterilization for Renal Replacement Therapy in the Intensive Care Unit

Paolo Lentini, MD
Department of Nephrology, St. Bortolo Hospital, Vicenza, Italy
Lead and Heavy Metals and the Kidney

Edward F. Leonard, PhD
Professor, Departments of Chemical and Biomedical Engineering, Columbia University, New York, New York
The Bases of Mass Separation Processes

Jeffrey J. Letteri
Gambro Renal Products, Lakewood, Colorado
Solute and Water Transport across Artificial Membranes in Conventional Hemodialysis; Predilution and Postdilution Reinfusion Techniques; Solute and Water Kinetics in Continuous Therapies

Karel M. Leunissen, MD, PhD
Professor of Internal Medicine and Nephrology, Maastricht University Medical Center, Maastricht, The Netherlands
Hypertensive Emergencies

Xavier M. Leverve, MD, PhD
Professor of Nutrition, Joseph Fourier University School of Medicine; University Hospital of Grenoble, Grenoble, France
Nitrogen Balance and Nutritional Assessment

Adeera Levin, MD, BSc, FRCPC
Professor of Medicine, University of British Columbia Faculty of Medicine; Director of Clinical Research and Attending Physician, Providence Health Care, Vancouver, British Columbia, Canada
Management of Patients with Diabetes in the Intensive Care Unit; Statins and the Kidney

John K. Leypoldt, PhD
Renal Division, Baxter Healthcare Corporation, McGaw Park, Illinois
Intermittent Techniques for Acute Dialysis

Orfeas Liangos, MD, FASN
Assistant Professor of Medicine, Department of Nephrology, Tufts University School of Medicine; Director, Acute Renal Failure Research Programs, Kidney and Dialysis Research Laboratory, Caritas St. Elizabeth's Medical Center, Boston, Massachusetts
Genetic Factors Influencing Acute Kidney Injury

Elisa Licari, MD
Research Fellow, Department of
Intensive Care, Austin Hospital
Clinical School, Melbourne,
Victoria, Australia
*Renal Blood Flow and Perfusion
Pressure; Dopamine Receptor
Agonists; Acid-Base Disorders
Secondary to Renal Failure*

Wilfred Lieberthal, MD
Professor of Medicine, Stony
Brook Medical Center, Stony
Brook, New York
Models of Toxic Acute Renal Failure

Peter K. Linden, MD
Professor of Critical Care
Medicine, University of
Pittsburgh School of Medicine;
Director, Transplant Intensive
Care Unit, University of
Pittsburgh Medical Center,
Pittsburgh, Pennsylvania
*Microbiological Considerations in the
Intensive Care Patient; Laboratory
Testing in Infectious Diseases;
Infectious Complications of Renal
Transplantation*

Jeffrey Lipman, MB BCh, MD
Professor and Head, Discipline of
Anaesthesiology and Critical
Care, The School of Medicine,
University of Queensland;
Director, Department of Intensive
Care Medicine, Royal Brisbane
and Women's Hospital, Brisbane,
Australia
*Principles of Pharmacology in the
Critically Ill*

Kathleen D. Liu, MD, PhD, MCR
Assistant Professor, Departments
of Medicine and Anesthesia,
Division of Nephrology and
Critical Care, University of
California, San Francisco, School
of Medicine, San Francisco,
California
Renal Repair and Recovery

Shiguang Liu, MD, PhD
University of Kansas Medical
Center, Kansas City, Kansas
*Epithelial Barrier Dysfunction as a
Mechanism Underlying the
Pathogenesis of Multiple-Organ
Dysfunction*

Sergio Livigni, MD
Director, Intensive Care Unit, San
Giovanni Bosco Hospital, Turin,
Italy
*Extracorporeal Blood Purification
Techniques beyond Dialysis: Coupled
Plasmafiltration-Adsorption*

**Wai-Kei Lo, MB BS, FHKCP,
FHKAM, FRCP**
Honorary Associate Clinical
Professor, Department of
Medicine, University of Hong
Kong; Consultant Physician,
Department of Medicine, Tung
Wah Hospital, Hong Kong, China
*Treatment of Peritonitis and Other
Clinical Complications of Peritoneal
Dialysis in the Critically Ill Patient*

Manuela Lugano, MD
Attending Physician, Department
of Anaesthesia and Intensive Care
Unit, Azienda Ospedaliero
Universitaria, University of
Udine, Udine, Italy
Vasoactive Drugs and Renal Function

**Sing-Leung Lui, MB BS, MD,
FRCPE**
Honorary Clinical Associate
Professor, Department of
Medicine, University of Hong
Kong; Senior Medical Officer,
Tung Wah Hospital, Hong Kong,
China
*Treatment of Peritonitis and Other
Clinical Complications of Peritoneal
Dialysis in the Critically Ill Patient*

Antonio Lupo
Professor of Nephrology, School
of Medicine, University of
Verona; Director, Division of
Nephrology and Professor of
Nephrology, Ospedale Civile
Maggiore, Verona, Italy
*Endothelial Progenitor Cells in Acute
Renal Injury*

Valerie A. Luyckx, MB BCh
Assistant Professor, University of
Alberta Faculty of Medicine and
Dentistry; Assistant Professor,
University of Alberta Hospital,
Edmonton, Alberta, Canada
*Models of Ischemic Renal Injury;
Biomarkers in Acute Kidney Injury*

William L. Macias
Senior Medical Fellow II, Eli
Lilly and Company, Indianapolis,
Indiana
*Activated Protein C Therapy and
Sepsis-Associated Acute Kidney
Injury*

Nicholas Madden, MD
CRISMA Laboratory, Department
of Critical Care Medicine,
University of Pittsburgh Medical
Center, Pittsburgh, Pennsylvania
*Diagnosis and Therapy of Metabolic
Alkalosis; Acid-Base Disorders
Secondary to Renal Failure;
Disorders of Chronic Metabolic
Alkalosis*

François Madore, MD, MSc
Associate Professor, University of
Montreal Faculty of Medicine;
Nephrologist, Hôpital du Sacré-
Couer de Montréal, Montreal,
Quebec, Canada
*Plasmapheresis in Acute Intoxication
and Poisoning*

Daniel S. Majors, RN
Senior Nurse, Acute
Hemodialysis/Apheresis Unit,
Vanderbilt University Medical
Center, Nashville, Tennessee
*Practical Aspects of Hybrid Dialysis
Techniques*

Elena Mancini, MD
Attending Physician, Nephrology,
Dialysis, and Hypertension Unit,
Policlinico San Orsola-Malpighi,
Bologna, Italy
*Pathophysiology of the Hepatorenal
Syndrome*

Filippo Mangione, MD
Fellow in Nephrology, University
of Pavia School of Medicine;
Junior Assistant, Department of
Nephrology, Dialysis, and
Transplantation, IRCS Policlinico
San Matteo, Pavia, Italy
Growth Factors

Sunil Mankad, MD
Associate Professor of Medicine,
Mayo Clinic College of Medicine;
Associate Professor of Medicine,
Department of Cardiovascular
Diseases, Mayo Clinic, Rochester,
Minnesota
*Renal Function in Congestive Heart
Failure*

Pier Paolo Manzini
Gambro Dasco S.P.A., Medolla, Italy
Information Technology and Therapy Delivery in Continuous Renal Replacement Therapies

Martino Marangella, MD
Nephrology Division and Renal Stone Center, Mauriziano Hospital, Torino, Italy
Granulocyte Inhibitory Proteins and Other Proteinaceous Molecules in Acute Kidney Injury; Uric Acid as a Toxin

Giancarlo Marenzi, MD
Director, Intensive Care Unit, Centro Cardiologico Monzino, Institute of Cardiology, University of Milan, Milan, Italy
Intermittent Hemofiltration for Management of Fluid Overload and Administration of Contrast Media

Filippo Mariano, MD
Vice-Head, Department of Medicine Area, Nephrology, and Dialysis Unit, CTO Hospital, Turin, Italy
Humoral Mediators in Sepsis; Burns and Acute Renal Failure

Paul E. Marik, MB BCh, FCP(SA), FRCP(C), FCCP, FACP
Professor of Medicine, Jefferson Medical College of Thomas Jefferson University; Director of Pulmonary and Critical Care Medicine, Thomas Jefferson University Hospital, Philadelphia, Pennsylvania
Endocrinology of the Stress Response during Critical Illness; Diagnosis and Management of Critical Illness–Related Corticosteroid Insufficiency

John J. Marini, MD
Professor of Medicine, University of Minnesota Medical School; Director of Translational Research, HealthPartners Research Foundation, Minneapolis, Minnesota
Mechanical Ventilation

François Marquis
Montreal, Quebec, Canada
Urinary Tract Infections in the Intensive Care Unit

John C. Marshall, MD, FRCSC
Professor of Surgery, University of Toronto Faculty of Medicine; Acute Care Surgeon and Intensivist, St. Michael's Hospital, Toronto, Ontario, Canada
The Neutrophil and Inflammation

Mark R. Marshall, MD
Honorary Senior Lecturer, University of Auckland Faculty of Medical and Health Sciences; Clinical Head, Department of Renal Medicine, Middlemore Hospital, Auckland, New Zealand
Quantification of Acute Renal Replacement Therapy; Hybrid Dialysis Techniques in the Intensive Care Unit; Practical Aspects of Hybrid Dialysis Techniques

Roy Mathew, MD
Division of Nephrology, Department of Medicine, University of California, San Diego, School of Medicine, San Diego, California
Starting and Stopping Renal Replacement Therapy in the Critically Ill; Anticoagulation Strategies for Continuous Renal Replacement Therapies

Kenichi Matsuda, MD, PhD
Professor, Department of Emergency and Critical Care Medicine, University of Yamanashi School of Medicine; Chairman, Department of Emergency and Critical Care Medicine, Yamanashi University Hospital, Chuo City, Yamanashi, Japan
Slow Plasma Exchange plus CHDF for Liver Failure and CHDF Alone for Severe Acute Pancreatitis

Michael A. Matthay, MD
Professor of Medicine and Anesthesia and Director of Critical Care Medicine Training, University of California, San Francisco, School of Medicine, San Francisco, California
Acute Respiratory Distress Syndrome and the Kidney: Lung and Kidney Crosstalk

Norma J. Maxvold, MD, FCCH, FCCP
Associate Professor of Pediatrics, Michigan State University College of Human Medicine, Lansing; Attending Physician, Pediatric Critical Care Medicine, Helen DeVos Children's Hospital, Grand Rapids, Michigan
Nutrition of Critically Ill Children with Acute Renal Failure

Clive N. May, PhD
Senior Research Fellow, National Health and Medical Research Council, Howard Florey Institute, University of Melbourne, Melbourne, Victoria, Australia
The Physiology of the Afferent and Efferent Arterioles; Septic Acute Renal Failure; Animal Models of Septic Acute Renal Failure; Vasoactive Drugs and Acute Renal Failure

Jerry McCauley, MD, MPH
Professor of Medicine and Surgery, University of Pittsburgh School of Medicine; Medical Director, Kidney and Islet Cell Transplantation, University of Pittsburgh Medical Center, Pittsburgh, Pennsylvania
Patient Selection and Pretransplantation Care for Kidney Transplant Recipients; Kidney Support and Perioperative Care in Kidney Transplantation; Short- and Long-Term Management after Kidney Transplantation

Maureen McCunn, MD, MIPP
Associate Professor, Department of Anesthesiology, University of Pennsylvania School of Medicine, Philadelphia, Pennsylvania
Continuous Renal Replacement Therapy in Trauma

Joseph McKenna, MD
Maine Medical Center, Portland, Maine
The Kidney in Sepsis

Ravindra L. Mehta, MB BS, MD, DM, FACP, FASN
Professor of Clinical Medicine and Associate Chair, Clinical Affairs, Department of Medicine, University of California, San Diego, San Diego, California
Epidemiology of Community-Acquired Acute Kidney Injury; Principles of Anticoagulation in Extracorporeal Circuits; Starting and Stopping Renal Replacement Therapy in the Critically Ill; Anticoagulation Strategies for Continuous Renal Replacement Therapies

Caterina Mele, MD
Department of Immunology and Genetics of Organ Transplantation and Rare Diseases, Negri Bergamo Laboratories, Mario Negri Institute for Pharmacological Research, Bergamo, Italy
Hemolytic Uremic Syndrome

Aicha Merouani, MD
Assistant Clinical Professor of Pediatrics, University of Montreal Faculty of Medicine; Director of Peritoneal Dialysis, Division of Nephrology, Hôpital Ste-Justine, Montreal, Quebec, Canada
Continuous-Flow Peritoneal Dialysis as Acute Therapy

Laurent Mesnard, MD
Assistant Professor, Pierre and Marie Curie Faculty of Medicine; Attending Physician, Tenon Hospital, Paris, France
Other Experimental Interventions for the Management of Acute Renal Failure

Piergiorgio Messa, MD
Teaching Professor, University of Milan Faculty of Medicine; Director of Nephrology, Dialysis, and Renal Transplant Unit, IRCCS Fondazione Ospedale Maggiore Policlinico Mangiagalli e Regina Elena, Milan, Italy
Alterations in Calcium and Phosphorus Metabolism in Critically Ill Patients

Philipp G. H. Metnitz, DEAA, EDIC
Professor of Anesthesia and Intensive Care Medicine, Medical University of Vienna, Vienna, Austria
Long-Term Outcomes of Acute Kidney Injury

Madhukar Misra, MD, FRCP(UK), FACP, FASN
Associate Professor of Clinical Medicine, University of Missouri School of Medicine, Columbia, Missouri
Technical and Clinical Complications of Intermittent Hemodialysis in the Intensive Care Unit

Steffen R. Mitzner, MD
Professor of Medicine, Division of Nephrology, University of Rostock, Rostock, Germany
Albumin Dialysis with Molecular Adsorbent Recirculating System in the Treatment of Liver Failure

Barry A. Mizock, MD
Associate Professor of Medicine, University of Illinois at Chicago Medical School; Senior Attending Physician, Department of Medicine, University of Illinois Medical Center, Chicago, Illinois
Pathophysiology of Hyperlactatemia; Lactic Acidosis—Clinical Syndrome

Babak Mokhlesi, MD
Assistant Professor of Medicine, Section of Pulmonary and Critical Care, University of Chicago Pritzker School of Medicine, Chicago, Illinois
Characteristics, Pathophysiology, and Effects of Common Toxic Substances

Bruce A. Molitoris, MD
Professor of Medicine, Director of Nephrology, and Director of Indiana Center for Biological Microscopy, Indiana University School of Medicine, Indianapolis, Indiana
New Imaging Techniques in Acute Kidney Injury

Andrea Morelli, MD
Assistant Professor, Department of Anesthesiology and Intensive Care, La Sapienza University of Rome School of Medicine, Rome, Italy
Monitoring Kidney Function in the Intensive Care Unit

Thomas John Morgan, FJFICM
Senior Intensive Care Specialist, Mater Health Services, Brisbane, Queensland, Australia
Iatrogenic Hyperchloremic Metabolic Acidosis

Marina Morigi, PhD
Head, Laboratory of Cell Biology and Xenotransplantation, Negri Bergamo Laboratories, Mario Negri Institute for Pharmacological Research, Bergamo, Italy
Mesenchymal Stem Cells and Their Use in Acute Renal Injury,

Peter Mount, PhD, FRACP
University of Melbourne Faculty of Medicine, Dentistry, and Health Sciences; Department of Medicine, The Northern Hospital, Epping, Victoria, Australia
Poststreptococcal Glomerulonephritis

Roberto Pozzi Mucelli, MD
Professor of Radiology, School of Medicine, University of Verona; Chairman, Department of Radiology, Policlinico G. B. Rossi, Verona, Italy
Nephrotoxicity of Contrast Media

Bruce A. Mueller, PharmD
Professor and Chair, Clinical, Social, and Administrative Sciences, University of Michigan College of Pharmacy, Ann Arbor, Michigan
Drug Dosing in Patients with Acute Kidney Injury and in Patients Undergoing Renal Replacement Therapy

Patrick Murray, MD
Professor of Medicine, University of Chicago Pritzker School of Medicine, Chicago, Illinois
Correction of Water, Electrolyte, and Acid-Base Derangements by Hemodialysis and Derived Techniques

Raghavan Murugan, MD, MS, MRCP(UK)
Assistant Professor, Department of Critical Care Medicine, University of Pittsburgh School of Medicine; Intensivist, University of Pittsburgh Medical Center, Pittsburgh, Pennsylvania
Anion Gap and Strong Ion Gap; Diagnosis and Therapy of Metabolic Alkalosis; Complex (Mixed) Acid-Base Disorders; Acid-Base Disorders Secondary to Renal Failure; Disorders of Chronic Metabolic Alkalosis; Alarm Phase Cytokines

Masataka Nakamura, MD
Assistant Professor, Department of Emergency and Critical Care Medicine, Chiba University Graduate School of Medicine, Chiba City, Japan
Slow Plasma Exchange plus CHDF for Liver Failure and CHDF Alone for Severe Acute Pancreatitis

Federico Nalesso, MD, PhD
Staff Nephrologist, St. Bortolo Hospital, Vicenza, Italy
The Plasmafiltration-Adsorption-Dialysis System

Carla M. Nester, MD, MSA
Assistant Professor, Departments of Medicine and Pediatrics, Division of Nephrology, University of Iowa Carver College of Medicine, Iowa City, Iowa
Pathophysiology of Vasculitis

Allen Nissenson, MD, FACP
Professor of Medicine and Associate Dean, Division of Nephrology, David Geffen School of Medicine at UCLA; Director, Dialysis Program, UCLA Dialysis Unit, Los Angeles, California
Renal Replacement Therapy in the Intensive Care Unit

Karl Nolph, MD
Professor Emeritus, University of Missouri School of Medicine, Columbia, Missouri
Comparison of Peritoneal Dialysis with Other Treatments for Acute Renal Failure

Catalina Ocampo, MD
Temporary Fellow, Department of Nephrology, St. Bortolo Hospital, Vicenza, Italy
Dialysis Disequilibrium Syndrome; Effect of Renal Replacement Therapy on the Brain; Myoglobin as a Toxin

Shigeto Oda, MD, PhD
Professor, Department of Emergency and Critical Care Medicine, Chiba University Graduate School of Medicine; Chairman, Department of Emergency and Critical Care Medicine, Chiba University Hospital, Chiba City, Japan
Slow Plasma Exchange plus CHDF for Liver Failure and CHDF Alone for Severe Acute Pancreatitis

Mark D. Okusa, MD
John C. Buchanan Distinguished Professor of Medicine, University of Virginia School of Medicine; Attending Physician, University of Virginia Health System, Charlottesville, Virginia
Adenosine 2A Receptor Agonists in Acute Kidney Injury

Steven M. Opal, MD
Professor of Medicine, Warren Alpert Medical School of Brown University, Providence; Chief, Infectious Diseases Division, Memorial Hospital of Rhode Island, Pawtucket, Rhode Island
Endotoxin Recognition

Helen Opdam, MB BS, FRACP, FJFICM
Intensive Care Specialist, Austin Hospital, Melbourne, Victoria, Australia
Renal Protection in the Organ Donor

Hartmut Osswald, MD
Professor of Pharmacology, Chairman, Department of Pharmacology and Toxicology, Medical Faculty, University of Tübingen, Tübingen, Germany
Adenosine and Tubuloglomerular Feedback in the Pathophysiology of Acute Renal Failure

Heleen M. Oudemans–van Straaten, MD, PhD
Intensivist and Deputy Head of Medical Education in Intensive Care, Onze Lieve Vrouwe Gasthuis, Amsterdam, The Netherlands
Continuous Venovenous Hemofiltration

Massimo A. Padalino, MD, PhD
Assistant Professor of Cardiovascular Surgery, University of Padua Medical School; Consultant in Pediatric Cardiac Surgery, Azienda Ospedaliera Padova, University Hospital, Padua, Italy
Modified Ultrafiltration in Pediatric Heart Surgery

Matthew L. Paden, MD
Assistant Professor of Pediatrics, Division of Critical Care, Emory University School of Medicine; Associate Director, Pediatric Extracorporeal Membrane Oxygenation and Advanced Technologies, Children's Healthcare of Atlanta, Atlanta, Georgia
Continuous Renal Replacement Therapies in Combination with Other Extracorporeal Therapies

Emil P. Paganini, MD, FACP
Head, Section of Dialysis and Extracorporeal Therapy, Cleveland Clinic, Cleveland, Ohio
Acute Renal Failure after Cardiac Surgery

Paul M. Palevsky, MD
Professor of Medicine, Renal-Electrolyte Division, University of Pittsburgh School of Medicine; Chief, Renal Section, Veterans Affairs Pittsburgh Healthcare System, Pittsburgh, Pennsylvania
Risk Factors for Nosocomial Renal Failure

Mani John Panat, MB BS, MD, DM
Adjunct Senior Lecturer, University of New England, Armidale; Senior Lecturer, University of Newcastle, Newcastle; Staff Specialist Physician, Tamworth Rural Referral Hospital, Tamworth, New South Wales, Australia
Dialysis for Acute Renal Failure in Developing Countries

Francesco Paolini, PhD
Gambro Dasco S.P.A., Medolla, Italy
Information Technology and Therapy Delivery in Continuous Renal Replacement Therapies

Dipen Parikh, MD
Renal Fellow, Duke University
Medical Center, Durham, North
Carolina
Cardiac Surgery and the Kidney

Nicolò Patroniti, MD
Researcher, Department of
Experimental Medicine,
University of Milan; Department
of Perioperative and Critical Care
Medicine, San Gerardo Hospital,
Milan, Italy
*Extracorporeal Support and Renal
Function*

Pietro Pavlica, MD
Attending Physician, San Orsola
University Hospital, Bologna,
Italy
*Computed Tomography and
Magnetic Resonance Imaging in
Acute Renal Failure*

Didier Payen de La Garanderie
Department of Anesthesiology
and Critical Care and SAMU,
Lariboisiere University Hospital,
Paris, France
*Hemodynamic and Biological
Response to Continuous Renal
Replacement Therapies*

Federico Pea, MD
Institute of Clinical Pharmacology
and Toxicology, University of
Udine, Udine, Italy
*Principles of Pharmacodynamics and
Pharmacokinetics of Drugs Used in
Extracorporeal Therapies*

Zhiyong Peng, MD, PhD
Visiting Researcher, Department
of Critical Care Medicine,
University of Pittsburgh Medical
Center, Pittsburgh, Pennsylvania
*Genetic Variation and Critical Illness;
Blood Purification for Sepsis*

Mark A. Perazella, MD
Associate Professor of Medicine
and Director, Nephrology
Fellowship Program, Yale
University School of Medicine;
Director of Acute Dialysis
Program, Yale–New Haven
Hospital, New Haven,
Connecticut
*Vulnerability of the Kidney to
Nephrotoxins; The Role of
Extracorporeal Blood Purification
Therapies in the Prevention of
Radiocontrast-Induced Nephropathy*

Angelo F. Perego, MD
Chief, Renal Unit, Department of
Medicine, Ospedale Civile,
Monselice, Italy
*Hematological Malignancies and
Critical Illness*

Estela Regina Pereira, RN
Nurse, Dialysis Unit, Botucatu
Medical School, São Paulo State
University, Botucatu, Brazil
*Nursing Issues and Procedures in
Acute Peritoneal Dialysis*

**Evans R. Fernández Pérez, MD,
MSc**
Assistant Professor of Medicine,
National Jewish Medical and
Research Center, Denver,
Colorado
Respiratory Monitoring

Norberto Perico, MD
Director, Laboratory of Drug
Development, Mario Negri
Institute for Pharmacological
Research, Bergamo, Italy
*Acute Renal Failure in Kidney
Transplant Recipients*

Nicoletta Pertica, MD
PhD student, School of Medicine,
University of Verona, and
Ospedale Civile Maggiore,
Verona, Italy
*Endothelial Progenitor Cells in Acute
Renal Injury*

Giovanni Pertosa, MD
Professor of Nephrology,
University of Bari School of
Medicine; Head of Dialysis Unit,
Azienda Ospedaliera
Universitaria Consorziale
"Policlinico di Bari," Bari, Italy
*Calcineurin Inhibitors and Other
Immunosuppressive Drugs and the
Kidney*

Licia Peruzzi, MD, PhD
Nephrologist, Regina Margherita
University Hospital, Turin, Italy
*Antibiotics and Antiviral Drugs in
the Intensive Care Unit*

Dimitris Petras, MD
Department of Nephrology, St.
Bortolo Hospital, Vicenza, Italy
*Acute Renal Failure in the Elderly
Critically Ill Patient*

Phuong-Chi Pham, MD
Associate Clinical Professor of
Medicine, David Geffen School of
Medicine at UCLA, Los Angeles,
California
*Kidney Dysfunction after Liver
Transplantation*

Phuong-Thu Pham, MD
Division of Nephrology, Kidney,
and Pancreas Transplantation,
David Geffen School of Medicine
at UCLA, Los Angeles, California
*Kidney Dysfunction after Liver
Transplantation*

Richard K. S. Phoon
Centre for Inflammatory Diseases,
Monash University Faculty of
Medicine, Nursing, and Health
Sciences, Monash Medical
Centre, Clayton, Victoria,
Australia
Pulmonary Renal Syndromes

Stefano Picca, MD
Department of Nephrology and
Urology, Dialysis Unit, Ospedale
Pediatrico Bambino Gesu,
Instituto di Ricerca Scientifica,
Rome, Italy
*Multiple Organ Dysfunction in the
Pediatric Intensive Care Unit*

Pasquale Piccinni, MD
Head, Department of
Anaesthesiology and Intensive
Care, St. Bortolo Hospital,
Vicenza, Italy
*Multiple Organ Dysfunction
Syndrome; Diagnosis and
Management of the HELLP
Syndrome; Early High-Volume
Hemofiltration to Prevent Invasive
Ventilation in Critically Ill Patients;
Ethical Considerations in Acute
Renal Replacement Therapy*

Maury N. Pinsk, MD, BSc, FRCP
Assistant Professor of Pediatrics,
University of Alberta Faculty of
Medicine and Dentistry; Pediatric
Nephrologist, Stollery Children's
Hospital, Edmonton, Alberta,
Canada
*Medical Informatics in Disaster
Response*

Michael R. Pinsky, MD, FCCP, FCCM
Professor of Critical Care Medicine, Bioengineering, Cardiovascular Diseases, and Anesthesiology, University of Pittsburgh School of Medicine, Pittsburgh, Pennsylvania
The Critically Ill Patient; Hemodynamic Monitoring in the Intensive Care Unit; Alarm Phase Cytokines

Marta Piroddi, PhD
Department of Internal Medicine, University of Perugia Faculty of Medicine, Perugia, Italy
Oxidative Stress in Acute Kidney Injury and Sepsis

Isabelle Plamondon, MD
Fellow in Intensive Care, University of Montreal Faculty of Medicine, Montreal, Quebec, Canada
Disorders of Potassium Balance; Disorders of Magnesium Balance

Lindsay D. Plank, DPhil, MSc
Associate Professor, Department of Surgery, University of Auckland Faculty of Medical and Health Sciences, Auckland, New Zealand
Energy Requirement and Consumption in the Critically Ill Patient

Frans B. Plötz, MD, PhD
Department of Pediatric Intensive Care, VU Medical Center, Amsterdam, The Netherlands
The Kidney during Mechanical Ventilation

Lusine Poghosyan, PhD, MPH, RN
Assistant Professor of Nursing and Public Health, Northeastern University Bouvé College of Health Sciences, School of Nursing and School of Health Professions, Boston, Massachusetts
Lead and Heavy Metals and the Kidney

Natalia Polanco
Department of Nephrology, St. Bortolo Hospital, Vicenza, Italy
Dialysis Disequilibrium Syndrome; Effect of Renal Replacement Therapy on the Brain

Patricio M. Polanco, MD
Surgery Resident (Trauma), University of Pittsburgh Medical Center, Pittsburgh, Pennsylvania
Hemodynamic Monitoring in the Intensive Care Unit

Hans Dietrich Polaschegg, Dipl.Ing.
Medical Devices Consultant, Koestenberg, Austria
Evolution of Machines for Acute Renal Replacement Therapy; History and Development of Continuous Renal Replacement Therapy

Rafael Ponikvar, MD, PhD
Professor of Internal Medicine, University of Ljubljana Medical School; Head of Dialysis Center, Department of Nephrology, Univesity Medical Center, Ljubljana, Slovenia
Hemoperfusion

Silvia Porecca, MD
Fellow in Nephrology, Azienda Ospedaliera Universitaria Consorziale "Policlinico di Bari," Bari, Italy
Calcineurin Inhibitors and Other Immunosuppressive Drugs and the Kidney

Didier Portilla, MD
Professor of Internal Medicine, Division of Nephrology, University of Arkansas for Medical Sciences College of Medicine; Staff Physician, University of Arkansas for Medical Sciences Medical Center and John L. McClellan Memorial Veterans Hospital, Little Rock, Arkansas
Antiapoptotic Agents

T. Brian Powell
Department of Medicine, Medical University of South Carolina; Department of Medicine, Ralph H. Johnson Veterans Affairs Medical Center, Charleston, South Carolina
Proteomics and Acute Renal Failure

Raymond Quigley, MD
Professor of Pediatrics, University of Texas Southwestern Medical Center; Medical Director, End-Stage Renal Disease, Children's Medical Center, Dallas, Texas
The Physiology of the Proximal Tubule

Hamid Rabb, MD
Professor of Medicine, Johns Hopkins University School of Medicine; Director, Transplant Nephrology, Johns Hopkins Health System, Baltimore, Maryland
Acute Respiratory Distress Syndrome and the Kidney: Lung and Kidney Crosstalk

Maximilian Ragaller, MD
Professor of Anaesthesiology and Critical Care Medicine, Medical Faculty Carl Gustav Carus, Technical University of Dresden; Vice Chairman and Head of Intensive Care Unit, University Hospital, Technical University of Dresden, Dresden, Germany
Colloid Osmotic Pressure

Teresa Rampino, MD
Deputy Director, Department of Nephrology, Dialysis, and Transplantation, IRCCS Policlinico San Matteo, Pavia, Italy
Growth Factors

Reena Ranpuria, MD
Renal Fellow, Renal-Electrolyte Division, University of Pittsburgh School of Medicine, Pittsburgh, Pennsylvania
Risk Factors for Nosocomial Renal Failure

Anjay Rastogi, MD, PhD
Assistant Professor, Division of Nephrology, David Geffen School of Medicine at UCLA, Los Angeles, California
Renal Replacement Therapy in the Intensive Care Unit

Ranistha Ratanarat
Division of Critical Care, Department of Medicine, Siriraj Hospital, Mahidol University, Bangkok, Thailand
Pulse High-Volume Hemofiltration in Management of Critically Ill Patients with Severe Sepsis or Septic Shock

Naem Raza, MD
Department of Critical Care Medicine, University of Pittsburgh School of Medicine, Pittsburgh, Pennsylvania
The Liver in Kidney Disease

Michael C. Reade, MB BS, MPH, DPhil, FANZCA
Associate Professor, University of Melbourne Faculty of Medicine; Consultant Intensivist, Austin Hospital, Melbourne, Victoria, Australia
Respiratory Acid-Base Physiology; Respiratory Acid-Base Disorders

John H. Reeves, MB BS, MD, FANZCA, FJFICM
Honorary Senior Lecturer, Academic Board of Anaesthesia and Perioperative Medicine, Monash University Faculty of Medicine, Nursing, and Health Sciences, Melbourne; Director of Intensive Care, Cabrini Hospital, Malvern, Victoria, Australia
Plasmapheresis in Critical Illness

Karl Reiter, MD
Consultant Pediatric Intensivist, Pediatric Intensive Care Unit, University Children's Hospital, Munich, Germany
The Role of Renal Replacement Therapy in the Management of Acid-Base Disorders

Giuseppe Remuzzi, MD, FRCP
Professor of Nephrology and Director, Negri Bergamo Laboratories, Mario Negri Institute for Pharmacological Research; Director, Department of Medicine and Transplantation, Ospedali Riuniti of Bergamo, Bergamo, Italy
Mesenchymal Stem Cells and Their Use in Acute Renal Injury; Hemolytic Uremic Syndrome; Bleeding and Hemostasis in Acute Renal Failure; Acute Renal Failure in Kidney Transplant Recipients

Zaccaria Ricci, MD
Consultant, Department of Pediatric Cardiac Surgery, Bambino Gesù Hospital, Rome, Italy
Multiple Organ Dysfunction Syndrome; Renal Replacement Techniques: Descriptions, Mechanisms, Choices, and Controversies; The Concept of Renal Replacement Therapy Dose and Efficiency; Current Nomenclature; Clinical Effects of Continuous Renal Replacement Therapies; Acute Renal Failure in the Elderly Critically Ill Patient

Sven-Erik Ricksten, MD, PhD
Professor, The Sahlgrenska Academy, University of Gothenburg; Consultant, Department of Cardiothoracic Anesthesia and Intensive Care, Sahlgrenska University Hospital, Gothenburg, Sweden
Atrial Natriuretic Peptide in Acute Renal Failure

Christophe Ridel
Service de Réanimation Médicale, Centre Hospitalo-Universitaire de Bicêtre, Assistance Publique-Hôpitaux de Paris, Université Paris XI, Paris, France
Indications for and Contraindications to Intermittent Hemodialysis in Critically Ill Patients

Kinan Rifai, MD
Department of Gastroenterology, Hepatology, and Endocrinology, Hannover Medical School, Hannover, Germany
The Prometheus System

Troels Ring, MD
Consultant, Department of Nephrology, Aalborg Hospital, Aalborg, Denmark
Renal Tubular Acidosis

Julie Riopel, MD, FRCPC
Department of Pathology, Laval University Faculty of Medicine, Quebec City; University of Alberta Hospital, Edmonton, Alberta, Canada
Histopathological and Electronic Microscopy Findings in Acute Renal Failure

Eduardo Rocha
Nephrology Department, Universidade Federal do Rio de Janeiro, Rio de Janeiro, Brazil
Nonrenal Applications of Extracorporeal Treatments: Heart Failure and Liver Failure

Eric Roessler, MD
Adjunct Instructor, Department of Nephrology, Pontificia Universidad Católica de Chile Faculty of Medicine; Staff Member, Nephrology Laboratory, Hospital Clinic, Pontificia Universidad Católica de Chile, Santiago, Chile
Pulse High-Volume Hemofiltration in Management of Critically Ill Patients with Severe Sepsis or Septic Shock

Roberto Rona, MD
Department of Perioperative and Critical Care Medicine, San Gerardo Hospital, Milan, Italy
Indications for Renal Replacement Therapy in the Critically Ill Patient

Claudio Ronco, MD
Director, Department of Nephrology, Dialysis, and Transplantation, St. Bortolo Hospital, Vicenza, Italy
What Is Acute Kidney Injury?; Basic Principles of Renal Support; Glomerular Filtration Rate and Renal Functional Reserve; Multiple Organ Dysfunction Syndrome; Oliguria; Acute Renal Failure in Oncological Disorders and Tumor Lysis Syndrome; Renal Replacement Therapy in Acute Renal Failure Secondary to Sepsis; Blood Purification for Sepsis; Poisoning: Kinetics to Therapeutics; The Role of Extracorporeal Blood Purification Therapies in the Prevention of Radiocontrast-Induced Nephropathy; Effect of Renal Replacement Therapy on the Brain; Uric Acid as a Toxin; Myoglobin as a Toxin; Renal Replacement Techniques: Descriptions, Mechanisms, Choices, and Controversies; Membranes and Filters for Use in Acute Renal Failure; Evolution of Machines for Acute Renal Replacement Therapy; The Concept of Renal Replacement Therapy Dose and Efficiency; Solute and Water Transport across Artificial Membranes in Conventional Hemodialysis; Flow Distribution and Cross Filtration in Hollow-Fiber Hemodialyzers; Composition of Hemodialysis Fluid; Current Nomenclature; History and Development of Continuous Renal Replacement Therapy; Continuous Renal Replacement Therapy: Hemofiltration, Hemodiafiltration, or Hemodialysis?; Predilution and Postdilution Reinfusion Techniques; Solute and Water Kinetics in Continuous Therapies; Pulse High-Volume Hemofiltration in Management of Critically Ill Patients with Severe Sepsis or Septic Shock; Nonrenal Applications of Extracorporeal Treatments: Heart Failure and Liver Failure; Clinical Effects of Continuous Renal Replacement Therapies; Immunomodulation and Biological

Effects of Continuous Renal Replacement Therapy; Continuous Ultrafiltration and Dialysis with a Wearable Artificial Kidney; Information Technology and Therapy Delivery in Continuous Renal Replacement Therapies; Adjustment of Antimicrobial Regimen in Septic Patients Undergoing Continuous Renal Replacement Therapy in the Intensive Care Unit; The Peritoneal Dialysis System; Peritoneal Access for Acute Peritoneal Dialysis; Sorbents: From Basic Structure to Clinical Application; Extracorporeal Blood Purification Techniques beyond Dialysis: Coupled Plasmafiltration-Adsorption; The Toraymyxin and Other Endotoxin Adsorption Systems; The Plasmafiltration-Adsorption-Dialysis System; Multiple-Organ Support Therapy for the Critically Ill Patient; Acute Renal Failure in the Elderly Critically Ill Patient; Anti-inflammatory Drugs and the Kidney; Lead and Heavy Metals and the Kidney; Erythropoietin Therapy in Critically Ill Patients

Eric Rondeau, MD
Professor, Pierre and Marie Curie Faculty of Medicine; Attending Physician, Tenon Hospital, Paris, France
Other Experimental Interventions for the Management of Acute Renal Failure

Seymour Rosen, MD
Professor of Pathology, Harvard Medical School; Director, Surgical Pathology, Beth Israel Deaconess Medical Center, Boston, Massachusetts
Critical Assessment of Animal Models of Acute Renal Failure

Christian Rosenberger, MD
Consultant in Internal Medicine, Nephrology and Medical Intensive Care, Charité University Clinic, Berlin, Germany
Critical Assessment of Animal Models of Acute Renal Failure

Shane Rowan, MD
Fellow, Cardiology, Vanderbilt University School of Medicine; Fellow, Cardiology, Vanderbilt University Hospital, Nashville, Tennessee
Assessment of Fluid and Electrolyte Problems: Urine Biochemistry

Thomas Roy
Research and Development, Fresenius Medical Care Deutschland GmbH, Bad Homburg, Germany
Acute Dialysis with the GENIUS System

Georges Saab, MD
Assistant Professor of Medicine, University of Missouri School of Medicine; Attending Physician, Harry S. Truman Veterans Affairs Hospital, Columbia, Missouri
Comparison of Peritoneal Dialysis with Other Treatments for Acute Renal Failure

Tomohito Sadahiro, MD, PhD
Associate Professor, Department of Emergency and Critical Care Medicine, Chiba University Graduate School of Medicine, Chiba City, Japan
Slow Plasma Exchange plus CHDF for Liver Failure and CHDF Alone for Severe Acute Pancreatitis

Carla Sala, MD
Assistant Professor, Istituto di Medicina Cardiovascolare, University of Milan; Assistant Professor, Unità Operativa di Medicina Cardiovascolare, Fondazione IRCCS Ospedale Policlinico Mangiagalli e Regina Elena, Milan, Italy
Nephrotic Syndrome

Chiara Sala, MD
Resident, School of Anesthesia and Intensive Care, San Gerardo Hospital, Milan, Italy
Extracorporeal Support and Renal Function

Alan D. Salama, MB BS, PhD, FRCP
Senior Lecturer, Imperial College London; Consultant Nephrologist, Hammersmith Hospital, London, United Kingdom
Indications for Renal Biopsy in Acute Renal Failure

Adrian Salmon, MD
Department of Critical Care Medicine, University of Pittsburgh School of Medicine, Pittsburgh, Pennsylvania
The Kidney in Acute Heart Failure Syndromes and Cardiogenic Shock

Gabriela Salvatori, MD
Anesthesiologist and Intensive Care Physician, San Pietro Fatebenefratelli Hospital, Rome, Italy
Slow Continuous Ultrafiltration

Ramin Sam, MD
Associate Clinical Professor, University of California, San Francisco, School of Medicine; Attending Physician, San Francisco General Hospital, San Francisco, California
Gastrointestinal Problems in Acute Renal Failure

Ruben M. Sandoval, MS
Research Associate, Indiana University School of Medicine, Indianapolis, Indiana
New Imaging Techniques in Acute Kidney Injury

Antonio Santoro, MD
Chief, Nephrology, Dialysis, and Hypertension Unit, Policlinico San Orsola-Malpighi, Bologna, Italy
Pathophysiology of the Hepatorenal Syndrome

Takao Saotome, MD
Howard Florey Institute, University of Melbourne Faculty of Medicine, Dentistry, and Health Sciences, Melbourne, Australia
Septic Acute Renal Failure

Penny L. Sappington, MD
Assistant Professor, University of Pittsburgh Medical Center, Pittsburgh, Pennsylvania
Epithelial Barrier Dysfunction as a Mechanism Underlying the Pathogenesis of Multiple-Organ Dysfunction; Principles of Antibiotic Prescription in Intensive Care Unit Patients and Patients with Acute Renal Failure

J. Vidya Sarma, PhD
Research Assistant Professor, Department of Pathology, University of Michigan Medical School, Ann Arbor, Michigan
The Role of Complement in Sepsis

Judy Savige, PhD, MSc, FRCP, FRACP, FRCPA
University of Melbourne Faculty of Medicine, Dentistry, and Health Sciences; Chair, Division of Medicine, Northern Hospital, Victoria, Australia
Glomerulonephritis; Poststreptococcal Glomerulonephritis

Francesco Paolo Schena, MD
Professor of Nephrology, University of Bari School of Medicine; Head of Renal, Dialysis, and Transpslant Unit, Azienda Ospedaliera Universitaria Consorziale "Policlinico di Bari," Bari, Italy
Calcineurin Inhibitors and Other Immunosuppressive Drugs and the Kidney

Eva Schepers, MBScE
University Hospital Ghent, Ghent, Belgium
Metabolic Waste Products in Acute Uremia; Granulocyte-Inhibitory Proteins and Other Proteinaceous Molecules in Acute Kidney Injury

Miet Schetz, MD, PhD
Associate Professor of Medicine, Catholic University Leuven; Attending Physician, Department of Intensive Care Medicine, University Hospitals Leuven, Leuven, Belgium
Use of Diuretics in Acute Renal Failure; Assessment of Volume Status; Loop Diuretics

Gregory A. Schmidt, MD
Professor of Medicine, University of Iowa Carver College of Medicine; Director, Critical Care Medicine, University of Iowa Hospitals, Iowa City, Iowa
Alkalinizing Therapy in the Management of Acid-Base Disorders

Nestor Schor, MD, PhD
Professor, Renal Division, Department of Medicine, Federal University of São Paulo, São Paulo, Brazil
The Physiology of the Glomerular Tuft

Nicola Schusterschitz, MD
Medical University Innsbruck; Resident, Intensive Care Unit, Department of Internal Medicine, University Hospital, Innsbruck, Austria
Long-Term Outcomes of Acute Kidney Injury

Giuseppe Segoloni, MD
Professor of Nephrology, University of Turin Faculty of Medicine and Surgery; Department of Nephrology, Dialysis, and Transplantation, Molinette Hospital, Turin, Italy
Humoral Mediators in Sepsis

Nirva Shah, MD
Assistant Professor of Medicine, University of Pittsburgh Medical Center, Pittsburgh, Pennsylvania
Patient Selection and Pretransplantation Care for Kidney Transplant Recipients; Kidney Support and Perioperative Care in Kidney Transplantation; Short- and Long-Term Management after Kidney Transplantation

Shamik H. Shah, MB BS, MD
Postdoctoral Scholar, University of California, San Diego, School of Medicine, San Diego, California
Epidemiology of Community-Acquired Acute Kidney Injury

Sudhir V. Shah, MD
Professor of Internal Medicine, Division of Nephrology, University of Arkansas for Medical Sciences College of Medicine; Director, Division of Nephrology, University of Arkansas for Medical Sciences Medical Center; Chief, Renal Section, John L. McClellan Memorial Veterans Hospital, Little Rock, Arkansas
Antiapoptotic Agents

Asif A. Sharfuddin, MD
Assistant Professor of Clinical Medicine, Indiana University School of Medicine; Staff Physician (Nephrologist), Veterans Affairs RLR Medical Center, Indianapolis, Indiana
New Imaging Techniques in Acute Kidney Injury

Andrew Shaw, MD, FRCA, FCCM
Associate Professor, Department of Anesthesiology, Duke University Medical Center, Durham, North Carolina
Cardiac Surgery and the Kidney

Hidetoshi Shiga, MD, PhD
Professor, Emergency and Intensive Care Center, Teikyo University Chiba Medical Center, Ichihara City, Chiba, Japan
Slow Plasma Exchange plus CHDF for Liver Failure and CHDF Alone for Severe Acute Pancreatitis

Hisataka Shoji
Division of Planning and Science, Department of Blood Purification Medical Devices, Toray Medical Company, Tokyo, Japan
The Toraymyxin and Other Endotoxin Adsorption Systems

Ashutosh Shukla, MD, MB BS, DM, DNB
Clinical Fellow in Nephrology, University of Toronto Faculty of Medicine, Toronto, Ontario, Canada
Efficiency and Adequacy of Peritoneal Dialysis in Acute Renal Failure

Fiona Simpson, MND, BSc
Clinical Associate Lecturer, Human Nutrition Unit, School of Molecular and Microbial Biosciences, University of Sydney; Senior Research Fellow, Intensive Care Unit, Royal North Shore Hospital, Sydney, New South Wales, Australia
Parenteral Nutrition

Kai Singbartl, MD
Assistant Professor of Critical Care Medicine and Anesthesiology, Department of Critical Care Medicine, University of Pittsburgh School of Medicine; Attending Physician, Department of Critical Care Medicine, University of Pittsburgh Medical Center, Pittsburgh, Pennsylvania
Antioxidants

Mervyn Singer, MB BS, MD, FRCP(Lon), FRCP(Edin)
Professor of Intensive Care Medicine, University College London, London, United Kingdom
Fundamentals of Oxygen Delivery

Kim Solez, MD, FRCPC
Professor of Pathology, Department of Laboratory Medicine, University of Alberta Faculty of Medicine and Dentistry; Pathologist, University of Alberta Hospital, Edmonton, Alberta, Canada
Histopathological and Electronic Microscopy Findings in Acute Renal Failure; Medical Informatics in Disaster Response

Kevin M. Sowinski, PharmD, FCCP
Associate Professor of Pharmacy Practice, Purdue University School of Pharmacy and Pharmaceutical Sciences; Adjunct Associate Professor of Medicine, Indiana University School of Medicine, Indianapolis, Indiana
Drug Dosing in Patients with Acute Kidney Injury and in Patients Undergoing Renal Replacement Therapy

Mark Stafford-Smith, MD, FRCP(C), FASE
Professor of Anesthesiology, Duke University Medical Center, Durham, North Carolina
Cardiac Surgery and the Kidney

Jan Stange, MD
Professor of Medicine, Division of Nephrology, University of Rostock, Rostock, Germany
Albumin Dialysis with Molecular Adsorbent Recirculating System in the Treatment of Liver Failure

Luca Stefanelli
Department of Internal Medicine, University of Perugia Faculty of Medicine, Perugia, Italy.
Oxidative Stress in Acute Kidney Injury and Sepsis

Deborah M. Stein, MD, MPH, FACS
Assistant Professor of Surgery, University of Maryland School of Medicine; Attending Surgeon, Program in Trauma/Division of Critical Care, and Medical Director, Neurotrauma Critical Care Unit, R. Adams Cowley Shock Trauma Center, University of Maryland Medical Center, Baltimore, Maryland
Continuous Renal Replacement Therapy in Trauma

Maurizio Stella, MD
Head, Department of Plastic Surgery, Burn Unit, CTO Hospital, Turin, Italy
Burns and Acute Renal Failure

Giovanni Stellin, MD
Professor of Cardiovascular Surgery, University of Padua Medical School; Chief of Pediatric and Congenital Cardiac Surgery Unit, Azienda Ospedaliera Padova, University Hospital, Padua, Italy
Modified Ultrafiltration in Pediatric Heart Surgery

David A. Story, MB BS (Hons), BMedSci(Hons), MD, FANZCA
Associate Professor, Department of Surgery, Austin Hospital Clinical School, University of Melbourne; Head of Research, Department of Anaesthesia, Austin Health, Melbourne, Victoria, Australia
Blood Biochemistry: Measuring Major Plasma Electrolytes; Respiratory Acid-Base Physiology; Respiratory Acid-Base Disorders

Sanjay Subramanian, MD
Staff Intensivist, Everett Clinic, Everett, Washington
Oliguria

Kristina Swärd, MD, PhD
Associate Professor, The Sahlgrenska Academy, University of Gothenburg; Consultant, Department of Cardiothoracic Anesthesia and Intensive Care, Sahlgrenska University Hospital, Gothenburg, Sweden
Atrial Natriuretic Peptide in Acute Renal Failure

Jordan M. Symons, MD
Associate Professor of Pediatrics, University of Washington School of Medicine; Attending Nephrologist, Seattle Children's, Seattle, Washington
Renal Replacement Therapy for the Critically Ill Infant

Kian Bun Tai, MBChB, MRCP, FHKAM
Honorary Clinical Assistant Professor, Department of Medicine and Therapeutics, Chinese University of Hong Kong; Associate Consultant, Department of Medicine, Alice Ho Miu Ling Nethersole Hospital, Hong Kong, China
Alternative Medicine and Chinese Herbs and the Kidney

James Tattersall
Information Technology Manager and Nephrologist, Department of Renal Medicine, St. James's University Hospital, Leeds, United Kingdom
Information Technology in Renal Replacement Therapy

Luisa Tedeschi, MD
Vice-Head, Emergency Department, Intensive Care Unit, CTO Hospital, Turin, Italy
Burns and Acute Renal Failure

Isaac Teitelbaum, MD
Professor of Medicine, University of Colorado Denver School of Medicine; Medical Director, Acute and Home Dialysis Programs, University of Colorado Hospital, Aurora, Colorado
Correction of Fluid, Electrolyte, and Acid-Base Derangements by Peritoneal Dialysis in Acute Renal Failure

Vicente P. Castro Teixeira, MD, PhD
Affiliated Professor, Renal Division, Department of Medicine, Federal University of São Paulo, São Paulo, Brazil
The Physiology of the Glomerular Tuft

Ciro Tetta, MD
Contract Professor of Nephrology, University of Bologna Faculty of Medicine, Bologna, Italy; Director, Extracorporeal Therapies Research, International Research and Development, Fresenius Medical Care, Bad Homburg, Germany
Humoral Mediators in Sepsis; Acute Dialysis with the GENIUS System; Hemodynamic and Biological Response to Continuous Renal Replacement Therapies

Charuhas V. Thakar, MD, FASN
Assistant Profesor of Medicine, Division of Nephrology, University of Cincinnati College of Medicine; Chief, Section of Nephrology, Cincinnati Veterans Affairs Medical Center, Cincinnati, Ohio
Acute Renal Failure after Cardiac Surgery; Renal Function during Cardiac Mechanical Support and the Artificial Heart

Hermann Theilen, MD
Assistant Professor of Anaesthesiology and Critical Care Medicine, Medical Faculty Carl Gustav Carus, Technical University of Dresden; Head of Neuroanesthesia, University Hospital, Technical University of Dresden, Dresden, Germany
Colloid Osmotic Pressure

Karl W. Thomas, MD
Associate Clinical Professor, University of Iowa Carver College of Medicine; Director, Primary and Specialty Medicine, Veterans Affairs Medical Center, Iowa City, Iowa
Alkalinizing Therapy in the Management of Acid-Base Disorders

Ashita Tolwani, MD, MS
Associate Professor of Medicine, University of Alabama at Birmingham School of Medicine, Birmingham, Alabama
Extracorporeal Liver Support and the Kidney

Francesco Trepiccione
Postgraduate Fellow in Nephrology, Second University of Naples, Naples, Italy
The Physiology of the Loop of Henle

Giorgio Triolo, MD
Head, Department of Medicine, Nephrology and Dialysis Unit, CTO Hospital, Turin, Italy
Burns and Acute Renal Failure

Jennifer L. Y. Tsang, MD, FRCPC
Fellow, Critical Care Medicine, University of Toronto Faculty of Medicine and St. Michael's Hospital, Toronto, Ontario, Canada
The Neutrophil and Inflammation

Emre Tutal, MD
Specialist of Internal Medicine and Nephrology, Baskent University Hospital, Ankara, Turkey
Lung Function in Uremia

Shigehiko Uchino, MD
Staff Specialist in Intensive Care, Department of Anesthesiology, Jikei University School of Medicine, Tokyo, Japan
Kidney-Specific Severity Scores; Beginning and Ending Continuous Therapies in the Intensive Care Unit

Mark Unruh, MD, MSc
Assistant Professor of Medicine, University of Pittsburgh School of Medicine, Pittsburgh, Pennsylvania
Patient Selection and Pretransplantation Care for Kidney Transplant Recipients; Kidney Support and Perioperative Care in Kidney Transplantation; Short- and Long-Term Management after Kidney Transplantation

G. Matthew Vail
Medical Adviser, Eli Lilly and Company, Indianapolis, Indiana
Activated Protein C Therapy and Sepsis-Associated Acute Kidney Injury

Massimo Valentino, MD
Attending Physician, San Orsola University Hospital, Bologna, Italy
Computed Tomography and Magnetic Resonance Imaging in Acute Renal Failure

Volker Vallon, MD
Associate Professor, Department of Medicine, University of California, San Diego, School of Medicine, San Diego, California
Adenosine and Tubuloglomerular Feedback in the Pathophysiology of Acute Renal Failure

Wim Van Biesen, MD, PhD
Professor, Faculty of Medicine and Health Sciences, Ghent University; Chief Clinician, Renal Division, University Hospital Ghent, Ghent, Belgium
Epidemiology of End-Stage Renal Disease in Patients with Critical Illness Admitted to Intensive Care Units; Metabolic Waste Products in Acute Uremia; Granulocyte-Inhibitory Proteins and Other Proteinaceous Molecules in Acute Kidney Injury; Outcome of Intermittent Dialysis in Critically Ill Patients with Acute Renal Failure

Frank M. van der Sande, MD, PhD
Associate Professor of Internal Medicine and Nephrology, Maastricht University Medical Center, Maastricht, The Netherlands
Hypertensive Emergencies

Dominique M. Vandijck, MSc, MA, RN
Department of Intensive Care Medicine, University Hospital Ghent, Ghent, Belgium
Immunological and Infectious Complications of Acute Kidney Injury

Raymond Vanholder, MD, PhD
Professor, Faculty of Medicine and Health Sciences, Ghent University; Head, Renal Division, University Hospital Ghent, Ghent, Belgium
Epidemiology of End-Stage Renal Disease in Patients with Critical Illness Admitted to Intensive Care Units; Metabolic Waste Products in Acute Uremia; Granulocyte-Inhibitory Proteins and Other Proteinaceous Molecules in Acute Kidney Injury; Outcome of Intermittent Dialysis in Critically Ill Patients with Acute Renal Failure

Sanju A. Varghese, MD
Department of Medicine, Medical University of South Carolina; Department of Medicine, Ralph H. Johnson Veterans Affairs Medical Center, Charleston, South Carolina
Proteomics and Acute Renal Failure

Ramesh Venkataraman, MD, FACP, FCCP
Consultant, Critical Care Medicine, Chennai Critical Care Consultants Group, Apollo Hospitals, Chennai, India
Nonpharmacological Management of Acute Renal Failure; Use of Diuretics in Acute Renal Failure; Adenosine Antagonists; Principles of Fluid Therapy

Bala Venkatesh, MB BS, MD, FRCA, FFARCSI(Dubl)
Professor in Intensive Care, Division of Anesthesiology and Critical Care, University of Queensland School of Medicine; Staff Specialist, Department of Intensive Care, Princess Alexandra and Wesley Hospitals, Brisbane, Queensland, Australia
Dysfunction in the Critically Ill: Doubts and Controversies

Anton Verbine
Department of Nephrology, St. Bortolo Hospital, Vicenza, Italy
Composition of Hemodialysis Fluid; Erythropoietin Therapy in Critically Ill Patients

Jean-Louis Vincent, MD, PhD
Professor of Intensive Care, Free University of Brussels; Head, Department of Intensive Care, Erasme University Hospital, Brussels, Belgium
General Illness Severity Scores; The Sepsis Syndrome

Christophe Vinsonneau, MD
Assistant Professor, Intensive Care, Medical School, Université Paris Descartes; Department of Emergency and Critical Care Medicine, Hôpital Cochin, Paris, France
The Coagulation System in Inflammation; Indications for and Contraindications to Intermittent Hemodialysis in Critically Ill Patients

Ravindran Visvanathan, MB BS, FRCP(Edin)
Consultant Nephrologist, Hospital Kuala Lumpur, Kuala Lumpur, Malaysia
Clinical Results and Complications of Peritoneal Dialysis in Acute Renal Failure

Alexandra Voinescu, MD
Assistant Professor of Medicine, St. Louis University Hospital, St. Louis, Missouri
Technical and Clinical Complications of Intermittent Hemodialysis in the Intensive Care Unit

Scott Walters, MD
Clinical Assistant Professor of Pediatrics, University of Michigan Medical School; Staff Physician, C. S. Mott Children's Hospital and University of Michigan Medical Center, Ann Arbor, Michigan
Inborn Errors of Metabolism and Continuous Renal Replacement Therapy

Li Wan, MD
Research Fellow, Department of Intensive Care, Austin Hospital, Melbourne, Victoria, Australia
Septic Acute Renal Failure; Animal Models of Septic Acute Renal Failure; Vasoactive Drugs and Acute Renal Failure

Peter A. Ward, MD
Godfrey D. Stobbe Professor, Department of Pathology, University of Michigan Medical School, Ann Arbor, Michigan
The Role of Complement in Sepsis

Richard A. Ward, PhD
Professor of Medicine, University of Louisville School of Medicine, Louisville, Kentucky
Principles of Extracorporeal Circulation

Stephen Warrillow, MB BS, FRACP
Clinical Tutor, University of Melbourne; Intensive Care Physician, Austin Hospital, Melbourne, Victoria, Australia
Aldosterone Antagonists, Amiloride, and Triamterene; Carbonic Anhydrase Inhibitors

Steve Webb, MB BS, PhD, MPH, FRACP, FJFICM
Clinical Associate Professor, School of Medicine and Pharmacology and School of Population Health, University of Western Australia; Senior Staff Specialist, Department of Intensive Care, Royal Perth Hospital, Perth, Western Australia, Australia
Dysfunction in the Critically Ill: Doubts and Controversies

Kenneth Scott Whitlow, DO, FAAEM
Assistant Professor of Emergency Medicine, Virginia Commonwealth University School of Medicine; Associate Medical Director, Virginia Poison Center, Richmond, Virginia
Acid-Base Disorders Secondary to Poisoning

Anders Wieslander, PhD
Director of Research, Gambro AB, Lund, Sweden
Principles of Fluid Manufacturing and Sterilization for Renal Replacement Therapy in the Intensive Care Unit

Alan H. Wilkinson, MD, FRCP
Professor of Medicine, David Geffen School of Medicine at UCLA; Director, Kidney and Pancreas Transplantation, UCLA Medical Center, Los Angeles, California
Kidney Dysfunction after Liver Transplantation

Keith Wille, MD
Assistant Professor of Medicine, University of Alabama at Birmingham School of Medicine, Birmingham, Alabama
Extracorporeal Liver Support and the Kidney

James Frank Winchester, MD, FRCP(Glas), FACP
Professor of Clinical Medicine, Albert Einstein College of Medicine of Yeshiva University, Bronx; Chief, Division of Nephrology and Hypertension, and Vice-Chair, Department of Medicine, Beth Israel Medical Center, New York, New York
Hemodialysis, Hemofiltration, and Hemoperfusion in Acute Intoxication and Poisoning

Christine Wu, MD
Assistant Professor of Medicine, University of Pittsburgh School of Medicine, Pittsburgh, Pennsylvania
Patient Selection and Pretransplantation Care for Kidney Transplant Recipients; Kidney Support and Perioperative Care in Kidney Transplantation; Short- and Long-Term Management after Kidney Transplantation

James Yassin, MB BS, FRCA
Consultant in Anaesthesia and Intensive Care Medicine, Royal Sussex County Hospital, Brighton, United Kingdom
Fundamentals of Oxygen Delivery

Jane Y. Yeun, MD
Professor of Medicine, Division of Nephrology, University of California Davis Medical Center; Professor of Medicine, Veterans Affairs Sacramento Medical Center, Sacramento, California
Urea Kinetics, Efficiency, and Adequacy of Hemodialysis and Other Intermittent Treatments

Terence Pok-Siu Yip, MB BS, MRCP(UK), FHKCP, FHKAM
Specialist in Nephrology, Queen Mary Hospital, Hong Kong, China
Treatment of Peritonitis and Other Clinical Complications of Peritoneal Dialysis in the Critically Ill Patient

Alex W. Yu, MD, FRCP
Honorary Clinical Professor, Department of Medicine and Therapeutics, Chinese University of Hong Kong; Chief-of-Service and Consultant Physician, Department of Medicine, Alice Ho Miu Ling Nethersole Hospital, Hong Kong, China
Alternative Medicine and Chinese Herbs and the Kidney

Miriam Zacchia, PhD
Postgraduate Fellow in Nephrology, Second University of Naples, Naples, Italy
The Physiology of the Loop of Henle

Najam Zaida, MD
Clinical Assistant Professor, Warren Albert Medical School of Brown University, Providence; Attending Physician, Kent County Memorial Hospital, West Warwick, Rhode Island
Endotoxin Recognition

Nereo Zamperetti, MD
Department of Anesthesia and Intensive Care, St. Bortolo Hospital, Vicenzo, Italy
Early High-Volume Hemofiltration to Prevent Invasive Ventilation in Critically Ill Patients; Ethical Considerations in Acute Renal Replacement Therapy; Acute Renal Failure in the Elderly Critically Ill Patient

Michael Zappitelli, MD, MSc
Assistant Professor of Pediatrics, Division of Nephrology, McGill University Faculty of Medicine; Pediatric Nephrologist, Montreal Children's Hospital, Montreal, Quebec, Canada
Nutrition of Critically Ill Children with Acute Renal Failure

Alexander Zarbock, MD
Resident in Anesthesiology and Critical Care Medicine, Department of Anesthesiology and Critical Care Medicine, University of Muenster, Muenster, Germany
Antioxidants

PREFACE

Critical care nephrology is a new discipline formally born in 1998 from a group of scientists and physicians who established its definition as a multidisciplinary branch of medicine dealing with issues at the crossroad of intensive care medicine and nephrology. The discipline became established thanks to a growing appreciation of the importance of this field, an expanding body of laboratory and clinical research in this area, editorials (C Ronco, R Bellomo: Critical Care Nephrology: the time has come. Nephrol Dial Transplant, 13, 264-267, 1998), International Congresses (First- Second and Third International Courses on Critical Care Nephrology, Vicenza Italy, 1998-2001-2004 and 2007), and the first dedicated textbook (*Critical Care Nephrology*, Kluwer Academic Publishers, 1998). This book, unique in its nature, reach, and content was well received by the scientific and clinical community. Now, 10 years after the first edition, we are pleased to present the second edition, enriched, updated, and expanded to take into account the very large body of work carried out in the last 10 years.

The unrelenting advance of medical progress opens new areas of interest and opportunity. Such areas must be explored and explained by experts with appropriate reference tools and information sources to help clinicians practice at the very best level. Thus, after much clinical and experimental research experience in the field of *critical care medicine and nephrology*, we have decided to undertake the effort of producing a second and revised edition of a book dealing with this subject. Common guidelines, standardized approaches, and appropriate literature dealing with a multidisciplinary approach to kidney diseases in critically ill patients are emerging and growing significantly. Internists, surgeons, critical care physicians, and nephrologists all treat critically ill patients with acute renal failure and the multiple system organ dysfunction syndromes. The approach varies from hospital to hospital and often within hospitals. It depends on the structure of the institution, the tradition of the medical school, the financial status of the facility, and the heterogeneity of training and experience of clinicians. Doctors from different fields write notes without searching for a common multidisciplinary approach to the patient. Often, they hardly meet at the bedside and various prescriptions are made in absence of a common decision-making process.

A comprehensive review of the state of the art on this matter is definitely needed both in academic and clinical medicine. *Critical Care Nephrology* should provide such a comprehensive review. It will inevitably become a useful reference tool both for nephrologists and intensivists. The title *Critical Care Nephrology* has been chosen to stress the aim of the book: to provide a comprehensive and state-of-the art description and understanding of the problems related to kidney diseases and blood purification in critically ill patients. This review includes the pathophysiological foundations of major syndromes, the basis of laboratory investigations pertinent to this field, clinical approaches to complex patient management, interactions between renal and other organ system failure, monitoring techniques, therapeutical interventions, supportive treatments, new and advanced blood purification technologies, and the principles of management for various relevant derangements. The title is also intended to draw the reader's attention to the multidisciplinary nature of this complex subject matter and to the need for maximal cooperation between experts in intensive care and nephrology.

The book has three major parts: the first deals with basic sciences—biology, chemistry, physics, molecular biology, genomics, proteomics, and immunology—as they pertain to this field. All these are dealt with in chapters with a strong attention to the clinical setting and the application of such principles to daily clinical practice. Experimental research and evidence-based concepts are also discussed. The second part describes all relevant clinical syndromes with particular attention to pathophysiology, diagnosis, and clinical care, and the third part deals with diagnostic tools and the application of technology to therapeutical strategies and future trends.

Critical Care Nephrology deals with general information, definitions of critical illness, epidemiology, monitoring and diagnostic procedures, pathophysiology of organ systems in relation to kidney function, concepts of renal physiological and pathological responses to various derangements, oxygen transport and cardiovascular adaptations, hemodynamic parameters, respiratory parameters, mechanical ventilation and cardiac support, and severity score parameters as they relate to the complex care of patients with kidney injury or the requirement of advanced blood purification technology. This book is also devoted to all forms of acute renal failure, with specific reference to intensive care patients. Prerenal, renal, and postrenal acute renal failure are discussed in terms of etiology, frequency, mechanisms, pathophysiology, tissue lesions, biopsy patterns, diagnostic procedures, and management. The nature of the multiple organ dysfunction syndrome is discussed, with special emphasis on the impact of different organs dysfunction and kidney failure. Poisoning, infections (in general and of the urinary tract), drug-induced renal failure, and sepsis are all discussed in this part, with focus on the pathophysiological foundations of these syndromes. Kidney function and acute renal failure in patients with kidney, liver, and heart transplants are also discussed in detail, as is acute illness occurring in long-term hemodialysis patients. Finally, issues related to special patients such as children, diabetics, and elderly subjects are carefully analyzed in a specific session offering an important reference to pediatric critical care nephrology specialists.

Special emphasis has been placed on therapeutical interventions and treatment procedures. Different forms of extracorporeal organ support are discussed in detail, including liver, lung, and cardiac support. Artificial renal support is conceived and discussed first in terms of preventive measures to avoid renal failure and then as supportive treatment to replace renal function in different conditions. Thus, the use and pharmacokinetics of drugs in the critically ill patient is thoroughly explored. Various forms of extracorporeal therapies are discussed in detail, including hemodialysis, hemofiltration, hemoperfusion, and extracorporeal membrane oxygenation. Mechanical ventilation, mechanical cardiac support, and the total artificial heart are discussed in relation to kidney function.

Recent advances in the therapy of the sepsis syndrome are presented, and new insights on future trends in terms of extracorporeal treatments are provided.

Replacement of renal function by dialysis has been carried out for many years either in acute or chronic renal failure patients. The use of continuous renal replacement techniques has permitted new achievements in the correction of the metabolic and clinical derangements observed in critically ill patients. Today, extracorporeal techniques seem to display important beneficial effects that may overcome the classic indications of urea removal and fluid regulation. For this reason, a series of new techniques are appearing on the scene, with the specific aim of designing a treatment suitable for patients with multiple organ failure. Selective removal of cytokines and pro-inflammatory mediators, plasma adsorption, and other techniques have been used in vitro, in animal models, and sometimes in patients. There is a need to summarize all the current experience in the field and to deliver a comprehensive review of most of the experimental and clinical work carried out so far. We believe this book achieves such a goal.

The multidisciplinary nature of the subject and the rapid evolution of the knowledge in the field make this second revised edition necessary. Because of its uniqueness, we believe this book will become a "classic" in the field as did its predecessor and will be an important reference tool for nephrologists and intensive care specialists. It is no coincidence that the editors of the book are themselves specialists in these particular fields and are stragegically located throughout the world.

In conclusion, the aim of this book is to provide a comprehensive and educational review of the field of critical care nephrology. *Critical Care Nephrology* aims to create a complete reference book for colleagues who are dealing every day with critically ill patients suffering from kidney diseases, electrolyte and metabolic imbalances, poisoning, severe sepsis, major organ dysfunction, and other pathological events that require a multidisciplinary approach, a deep knowledge of extracorporeal organ support techniques, and a deep understanding of human knowledge in this field.

The book seeks to facilitate the process of developing common definitions and approaches to patient management in nephrology and critical care medicine, so that physicians think the same way and speak the same language. As such, it aims to present a comprehensive review of the recent evolution of the indications, applications, and mechanisms of function of the most recent extracorporeal techniques both for the treatment of acute renal failure and for the management of related disorders in the critically ill patient. Given these premises, the book may also be helpful for residents, fellows, and advanced trainees in nephrology and critical care medicine, as well as for staff physicians and members of the academic and scientific community involved in practice and research in the field of critical care nephrology.

We are grateful to all contributors who made this book possible, and we especially thank the editorial team at Elsevier who managed the production of the book with great professionalism and enthusiasm. We hope our readers will find that this effort has been worth it and sincerely hope that it will contribute to improving the care of acutely ill patients worldwide.

Claudio Ronco
Rinaldo Bellomo
John A. Kellum

CONTENTS

Color plates appear immediately after the front matter.

Color Plates

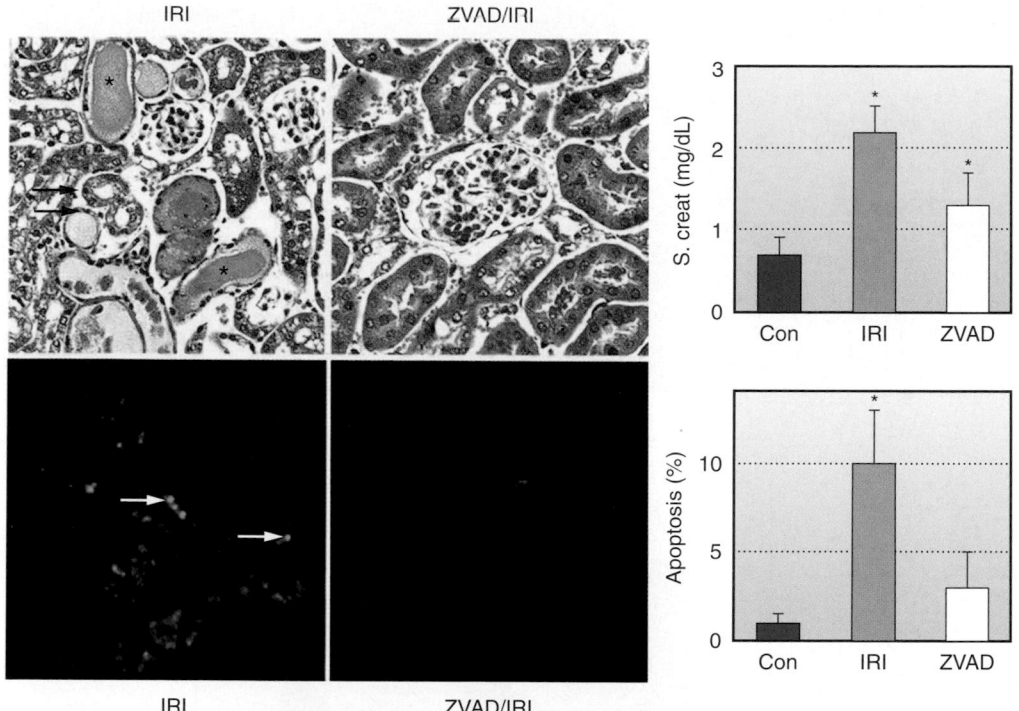

FIGURE 34-1. Morphology of apoptosis in acute kidney injury. Sections from mouse kidneys following ischemia-reperfusion injury (IRI) stained with hematoxylin-eosin (*top panel*) to reveal general morphology, and with TUNEL (terminal deoxynucleotidyl transferase biotin–d-uridine triphosphate nick end-labeling) (*bottom panel*) to identify apoptotic nuclei. *Arrows* show apoptotic nuclei, and *asterisks* (*) represent dilated tubules with flattened epithelium and intratubular cast formation. Pretreatment with the pan-caspase inhibitor ZVAD completely abrogated the apoptosis and resulted in partial functional protection. Con, control.

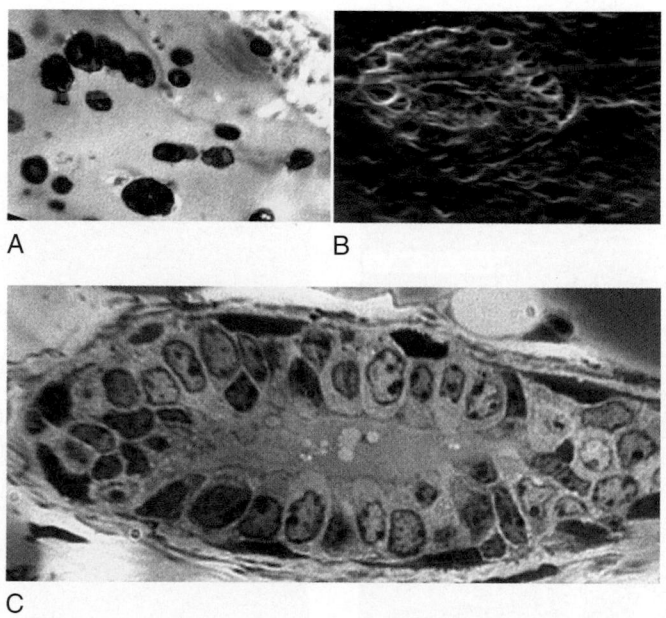

FIGURE 39-1. In vivo differentiation of human renal CD133⁺ progenitor cells in tubular structures. Undifferentiated CD133⁺ cells were injected subcutaneously in the solubilized basement membrane preparation Matrigel in nonimmunocompetent SCID mice (mice with severe combined immune deficiency). **A,** Immunohistochemistry showed that the tubular structures were positive for cytokeratin, indicating their epithelial differentiation. **B** and **C,** The morphological aspect of tubular structures on scanning electron microscopy (**B**) and toluidine blue staining of semithin sections (**C**). (Original magnifications: **A,** ×150; **B,** ×450; **C,** ×600.)

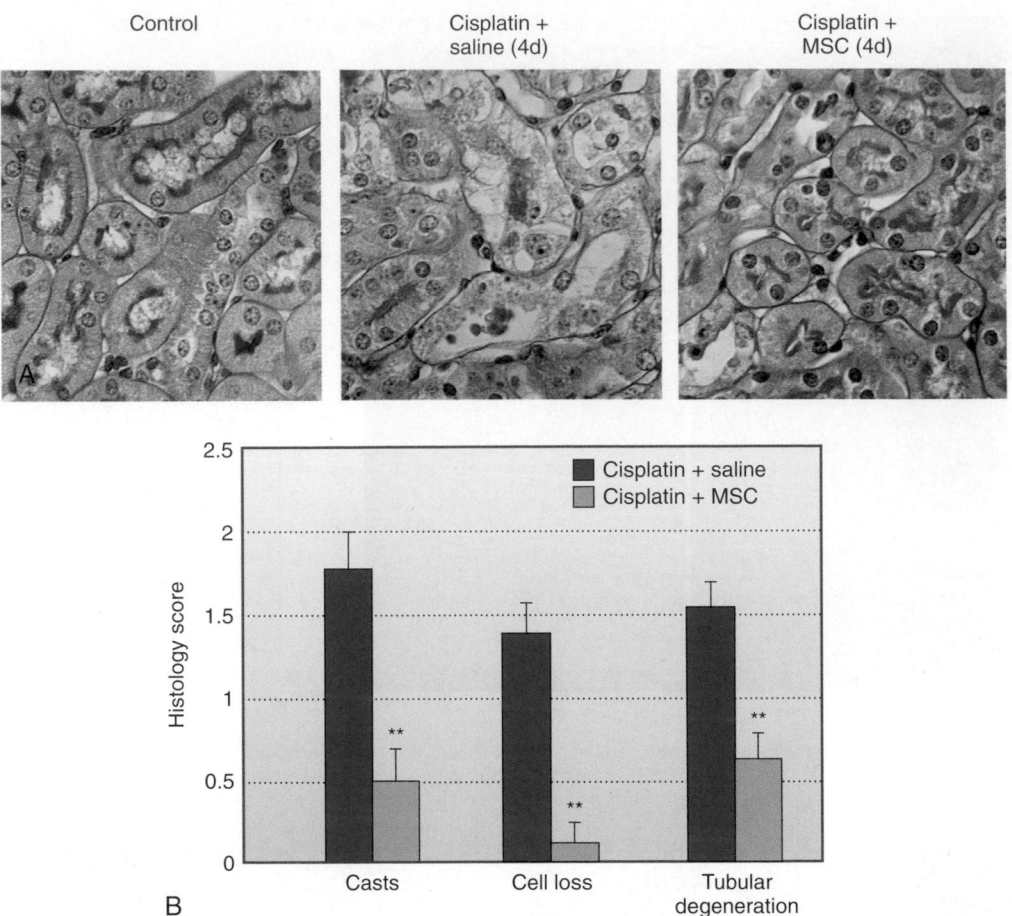

Control   Cisplatin + saline (4d)   Cisplatin + MSC (4d)

FIGURE 40-1. A, Renal histology of C57BL6/J control or cisplatin-treated mice that received saline or mesenchymal stem cells (MSCs). *Left,* Normal mouse kidney (control). *Center,* Cisplatin-treated mice at 4 days (d): Severe tubular changes (epithelial cell flattening and loss) are visibile in addition to loss of brush border and cell debris. *Right,* Cisplatin-mouse injected with MSCs shows, at 4 days, less severe tubular damage. (Original magnification ×400.) **B,** Effect of MSCs on renal histology. Semiquantitative analysis of tubular injury (at day 4 after administration of cisplatin) was performed by light-microscopic examination of renal tissues in cisplatin-treated mice given saline or injected with MSCs. Histology data are mean scores ± SE. *$P < .05$ vs cisplatin + saline; **$P < .01$.

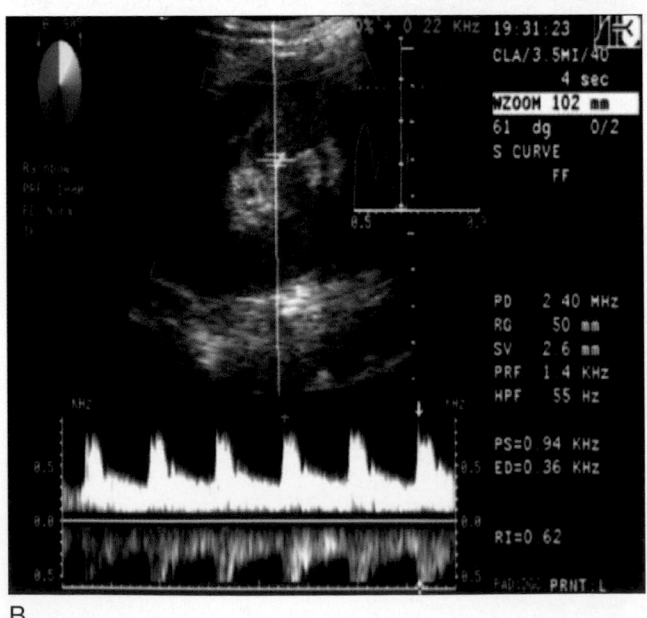

FIGURE 48-3. B, Follow-up examination demonstrates return to a normal RI of 0.62.

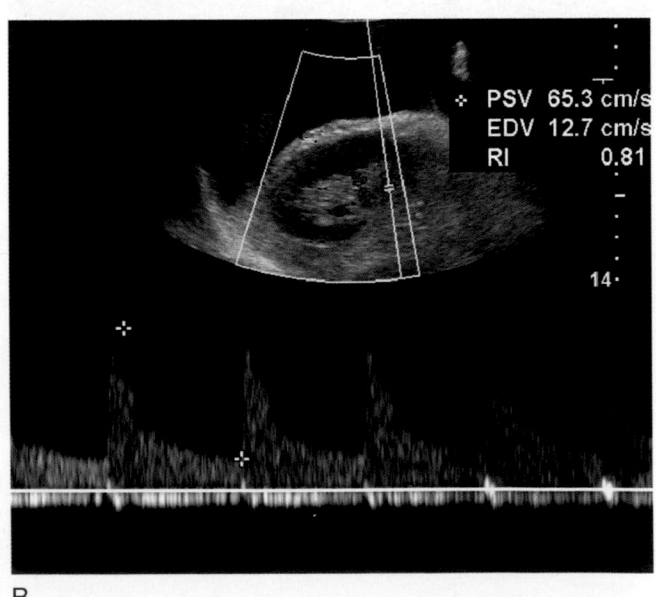

FIGURE 48-4. B, Duplex Doppler ultrasound image shows an increased resistive index (RI). Hepatorenal syndrome developed subsequently. EDV, end diastolic velocity; PSV, peak systolic velocity.

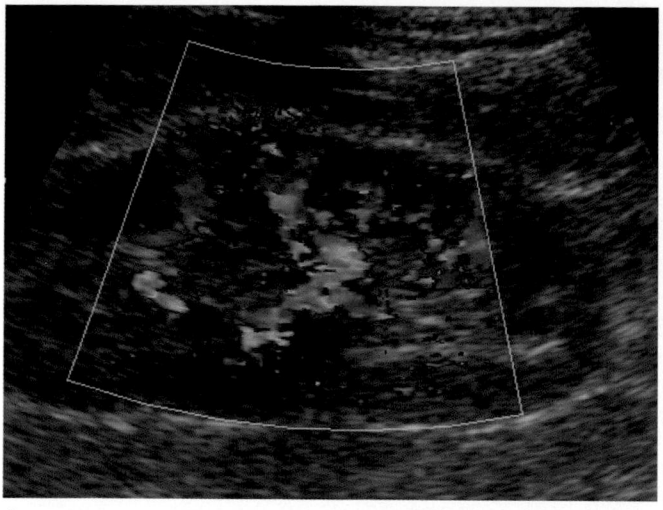

A

FIGURE 49-5. Atheroembolic renal disease, right kidney. **A,** Color Doppler ultrasound examination shows reduced renal vascularity *(outlined area).*

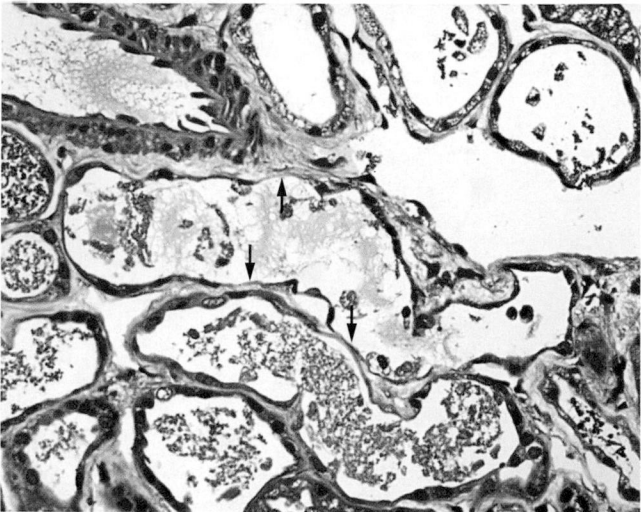

FIGURE 54-3. Portion of same photomicrograph as in Figure 54-2, at higher magnification. (Hematoxylin-eosin stain, 400×.) Tubular lumina are dilated and bordered by a flattened epithelium. Focal tubular cell loss is seen as a portion of denuded basement membrane *(arrows).* Granular debris and desquamated epithelial cells are present in tubular lumina.

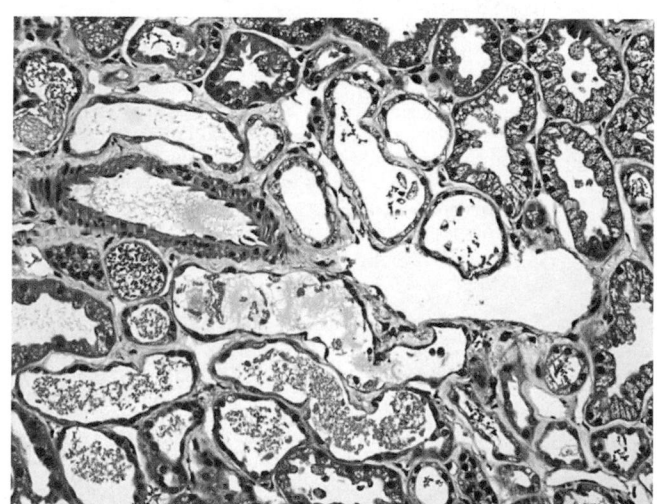

FIGURE 54-2. Histological evidence of acute tubular injury in a native kidney. (Hematoxylin-eosin stain, 200×.) Note the presence of dilated tubules with an attenuated epithelium and granular debris in tubular lumina.

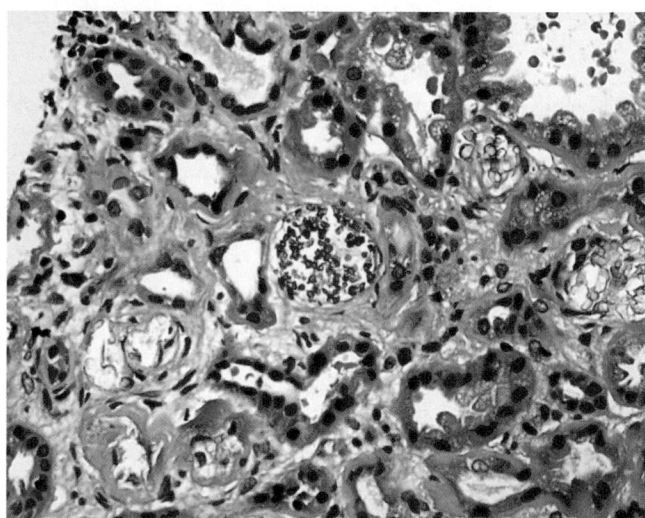

FIGURE 54-4. Histological evidence of acute tubular injury in a native kidney. (Hematoxylin-eosin stain, 400×.) Bluish calcifications are seen replacing tubules.

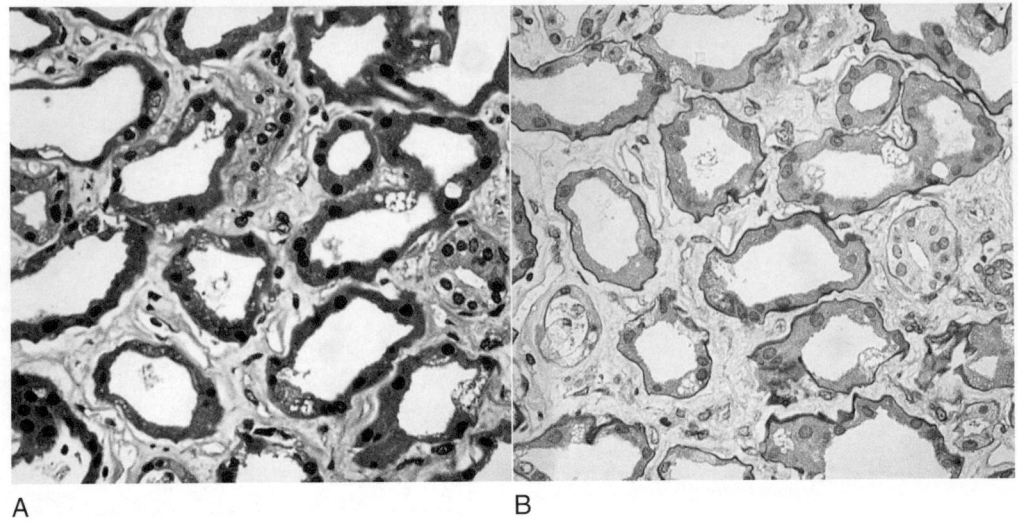

FIGURE 54-5. Acute tubular injury in a native kidney seen with staining by hematoxylin-eosin (**A**) and periodic acid–Schiff (PAS) (**B**). (400×.) Tubular lumina are dilated. The tubular epithelium is attenuated and shows focal vacuolization. The PAS-positive brush border is lost. Note the presence of interstitial edema.

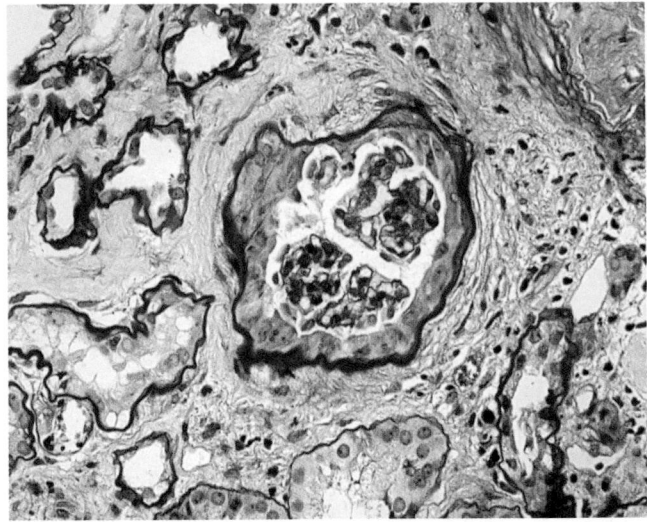

FIGURE 54-6. Tubularization of Bowman's capsular epithelium in a case of acute tubular injury in a native kidney. (Periodic acid–Schiff stain, 400×.)

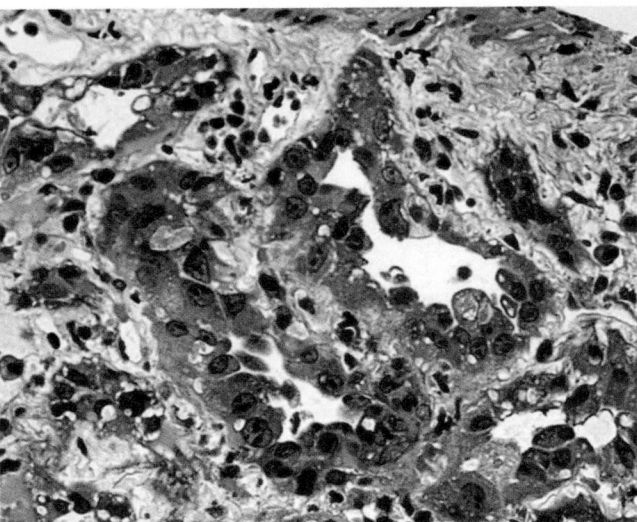

FIGURE 54-8. Nephrotoxic acute tubular injury in a native kidney showing prominent tubular damage with evidence of regeneration (basophilic cytoplasm, nucleoli, variations in cell size and shape). (Hematoxylin-eosin stain, 400×.)

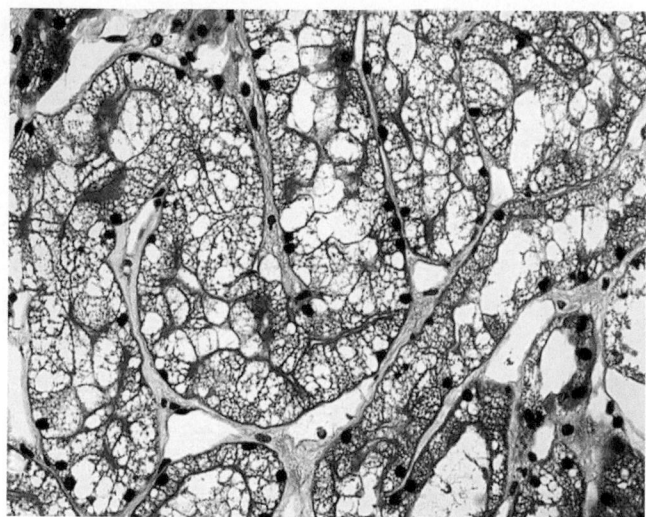

FIGURE 54-9. Nephrotoxic acute tubular injury in a native kidney, showing prominent tubular vacuolization. (Hematoxylin-eosin stain, 400×.) Of note, the vacuoles vary widely in size, unlike the isometric vacuolization caused by cyclosporine toxicity.

FIGURE 55-1. Texas Red–labeled gentamicin uptake in proximal tubule cells. A Munich-Wistar rat was given an intravenous injection of Texas Red gentamicin (TRG) and a 10-kD fluorescent dextran 24 hours before imaging. In **A,** a 10-μm-thick projection of the two probes (TRG in *red* and the 10-kD dextran in *blue*) shows the accumulation patterns in two different proximal tubule segments. In **B,** the single channel for TRG accumulation is shown in pseudo-color (see scale index correlating signal intensity and color in **D**). The two tubules are divided into two regions for analysis; note that the overall intensity for TRG is approximately the same in the two regions. In **C,** the single channel for the 10-kD fluorescent dextran is shown in pseudo-color; note the decreased accumulation of this probe in region 2.

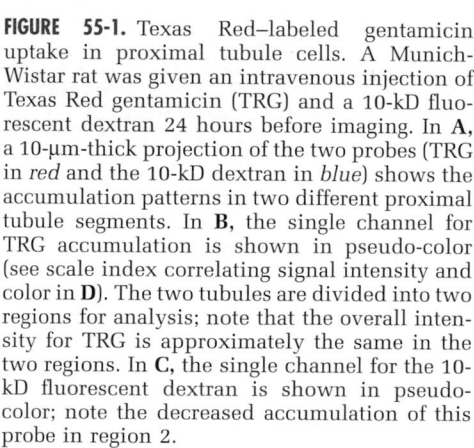
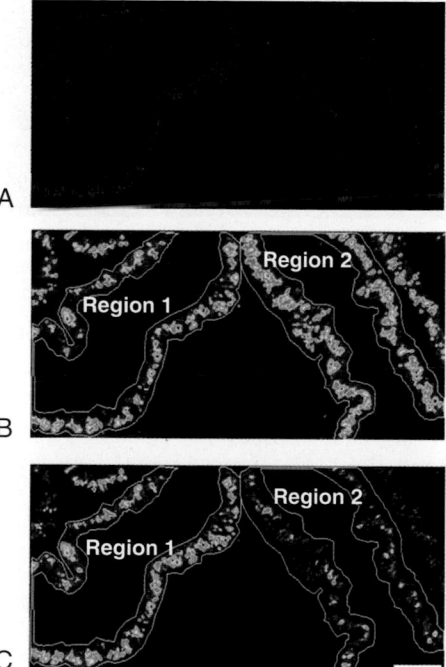
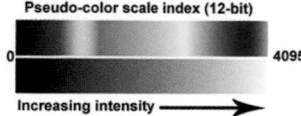

Pseudo-color scale index (12-bit)

0   4095

Increasing intensity ⟶

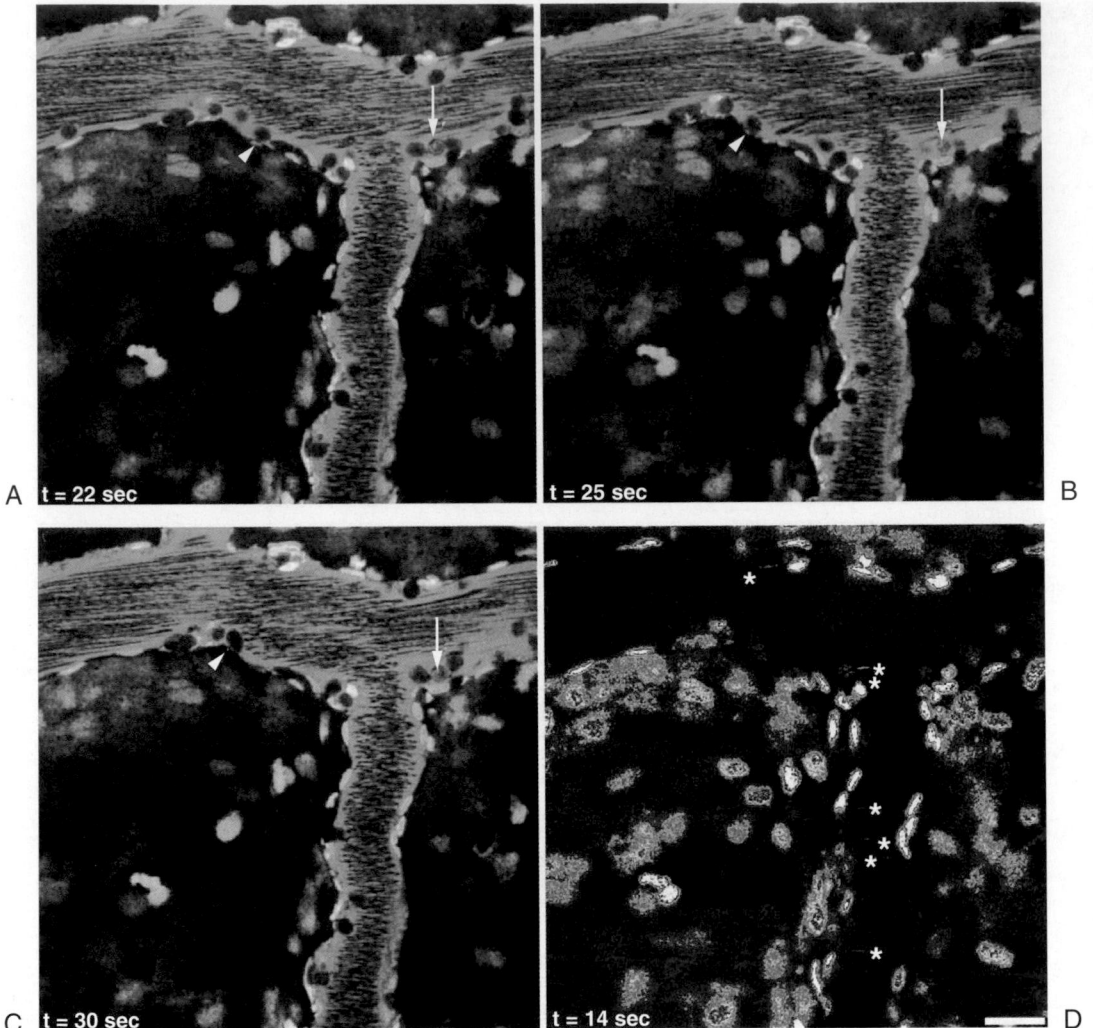

FIGURE 55-3. White blood cell (WBC) movement in the superficial microvasculature of a rat kidney. A Sprague-Dawley rat was injected with a fluorescein dextran with a molecular weight of 500,000 (*green*) along with a nuclear dye (Hoechst 33342, *cyan*), and images were acquired at a rate of 1 frame per second. The dextran fills the plasma in the blood but not the red blood cells (RBCs) or WBCs; hence, RBCs appear as *dark oblong shadows* within the vessel, whereas adherent or rolling WBCs appear as *dark circles* with some nuclear *(cyan)* staining. In **A** to **C**, numerous WBCs can be seen localized to the edge of a large vessel in frames acquired at 22, 25, and 30 seconds, respectively. A rolling WBC *(arrowhead)* moves approximately 15 μm during the elapsed 8-second period for the images in **A** through **C**. An adherent WBC *(arrow)* can be seen localized to the same area for the duration of the imaged sequence. In **D**, a pseudo-color image of the nuclear staining shows rapidly moving WBCs flowing within the vessel. Because the speed at which the WBCs are traveling far exceeds the acquisition rate of the microscope, the well-defined nucleus seen in static or rolling WBCs appears as a *small dash* within the vessel *(yellow asterisks)*. In this frame (14 seconds into the sequence), seven WBCs not seen in the previous or following frame appear with the vessel as *faint streaks*. Speeds of RBC/WBC flow within these larger vessels have been documented at well over 1.5 mm/second. See Figure 55-1 for pseudo-color scale index. (Bar = 20 μm.)

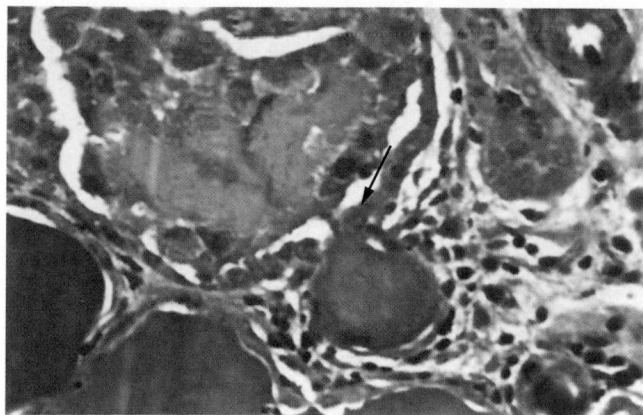

FIGURE 65-1. Ruptured tubular basement membrane. Periodic acid–Schiff (PAS)–positive cast-like material flows from the tubular lumen into the adjacent interstitium (*arrow*). This extravasation of tubular cast material often is noted in patients with renal obstruction (intrarenal or extrarenal). (From D'Agati VD, Jennette JC, Silva FG [eds]: Atlas of Nontumor Pathology: Non-Neoplastic Kidney Diseases, Vol 4. Washington, DC, ARP Press, 2005.)

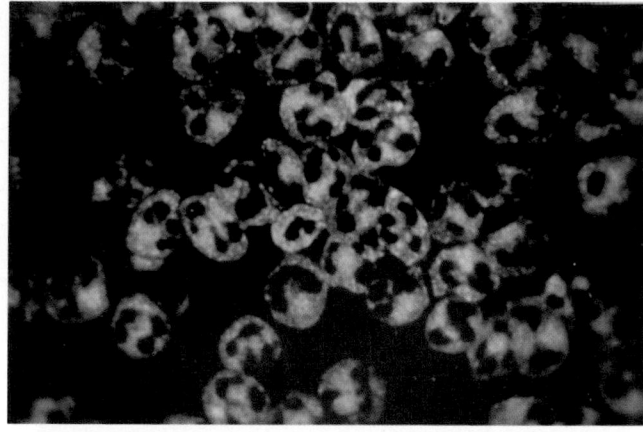

A

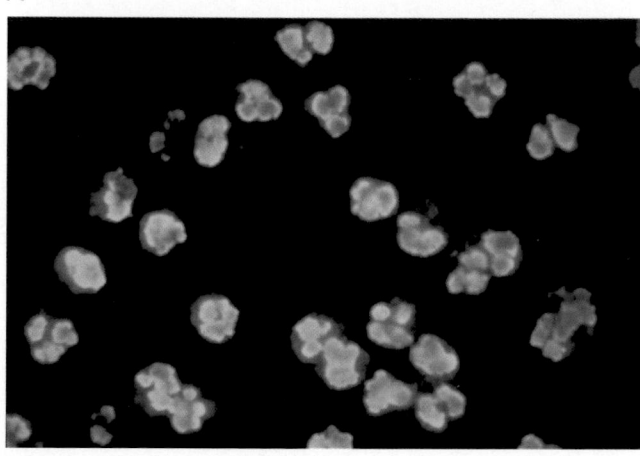

B

FIGURE 66-2. A, Cytoplasmic ANCA (C-ANCA) with coarse granular fluorescence of the neutrophil cytoplasm and interlobular accentuation. **B,** Perinuclear ANCA (P-ANCA) with perinuclear staining with nuclear extension. ANCA, antineutrophil cytoplasmic antibodies.

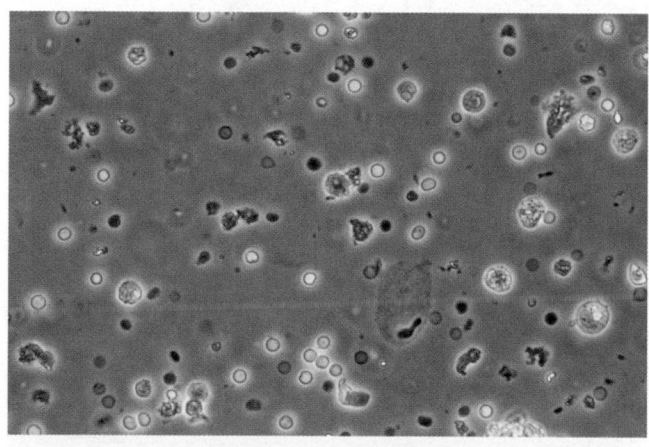

A

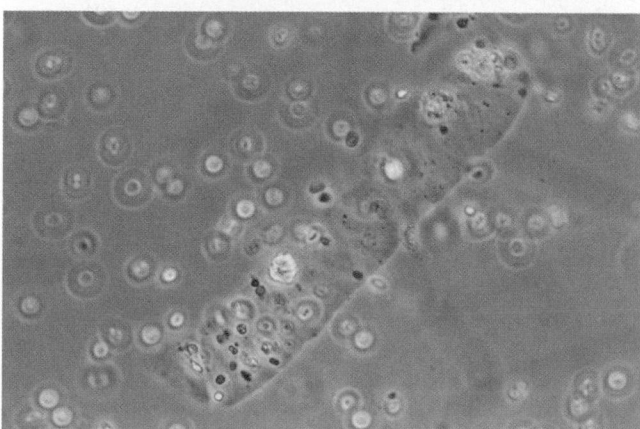

B

FIGURE 66-1. Phase contrast microscopy of the urinary sediment showing a mixed population of dysmorphic or "glomerular" red blood cells with fragments of varying size, shape, and hemoglobin content (**A**) and a cast containing red blood cells and red cell debris (**B**).

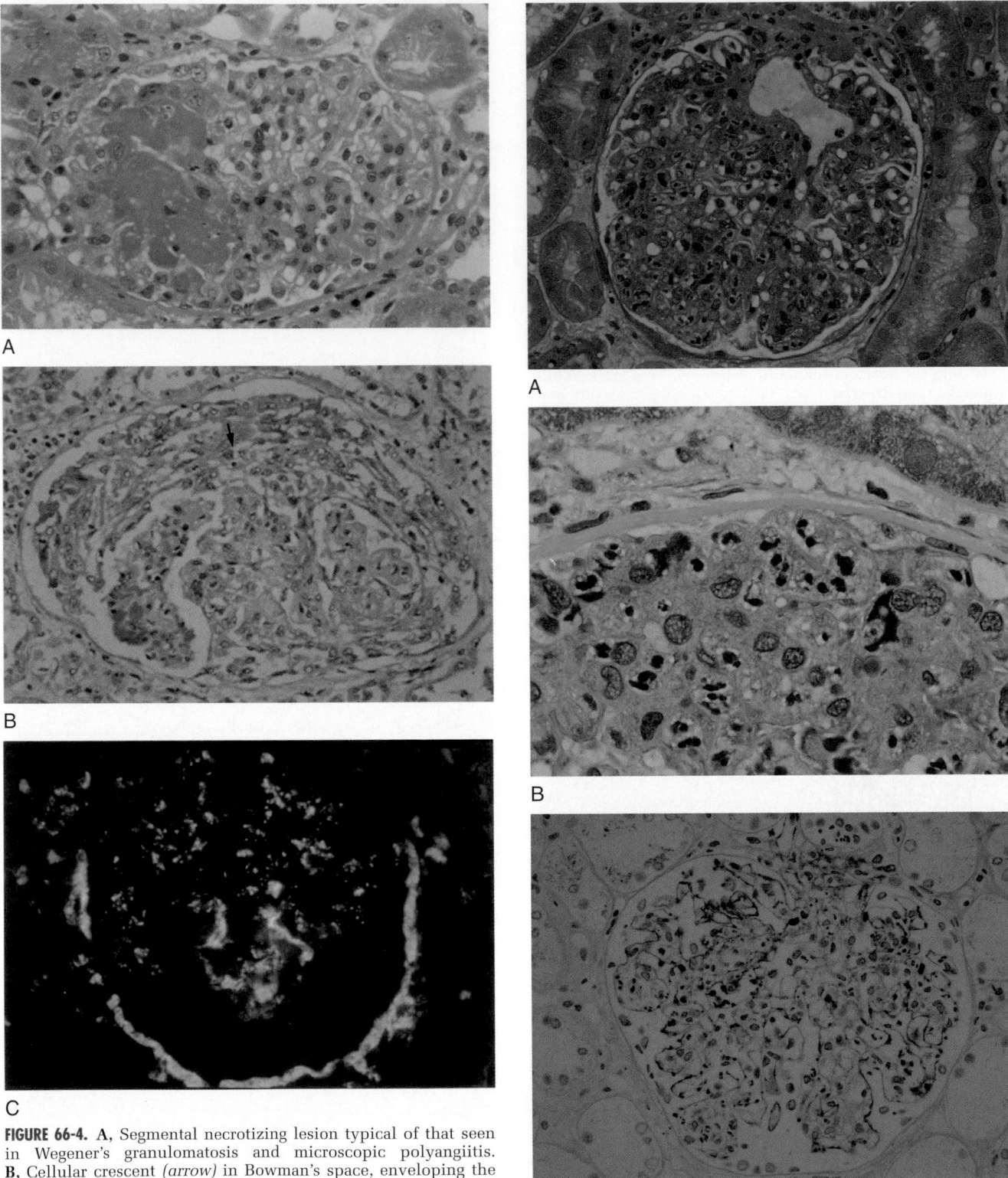

FIGURE 66-4. A, Segmental necrotizing lesion typical of that seen in Wegener's granulomatosis and microscopic polyangiitis. **B,** Cellular crescent *(arrow)* in Bowman's space, enveloping the glomerular tuft. **C,** "Pauci-immune" pattern, with only a few scattered C3 deposits in the glomerulus.

FIGURE 165-1. A, Diffuse endocapillary glomerulonephritis with glomerular hypercellularity due to increased numbers of endothelial and mesangial cells and a neutrophil infiltrate (hematoxylin and eosin, ×400). **B,** Occasional small subepithelial humps (*stained red*) outline the slightly irregular glomerular basement membrane and protrude into Bowman's space (Masson, ×1000). **C,** Granular staining of the capillaries for C3 (×400). (**A-C** courtesy of Dr. Moira Finlay, Department of Anatomical Pathology, Melbourne Health, Parkville, Victoria, Australia.)

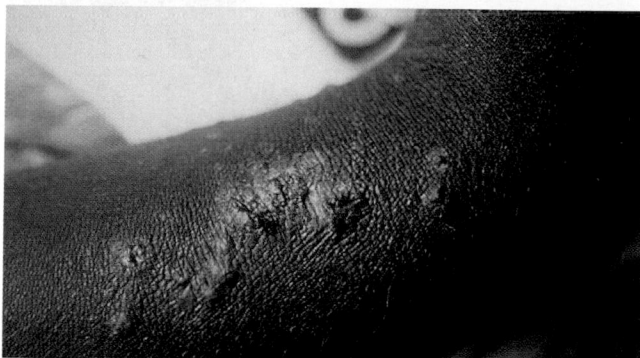

FIGURE 165-2. Streptococcal impetigo in an Australian Aboriginal child. (Courtesy of Dr. Bart Currie, Menzies School of Health Research, Darwin, Northern Territory, Australia.)

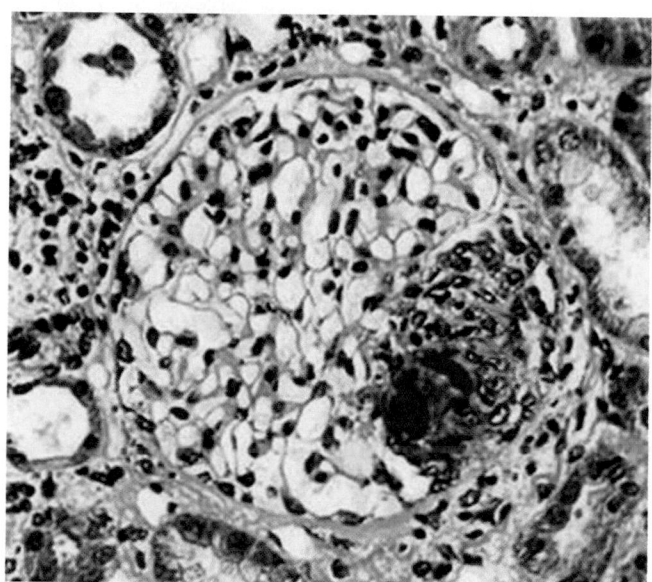

FIGURE 167-1. Leptospirosis. Note the interstitial infiltration, tubular necrosis, and blood casts.

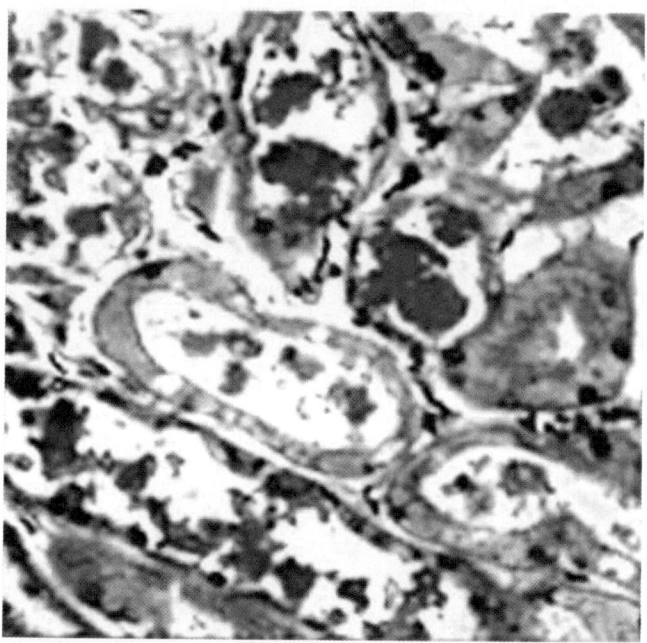

FIGURE 167-2. Hepatitis B; ANCA-negative vasculitis. Note the small cellular crescent adjacent to the focus of fibrinoid necrosis. ANCA, antineutrophil cytoplasmic antibody.

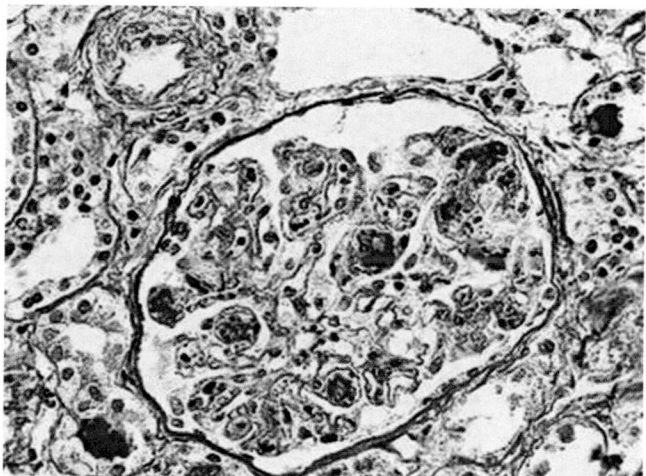

FIGURE 167-3. Shigella dysentery; glomerular capillary thrombi associated with the hemolytic uremic syndrome.

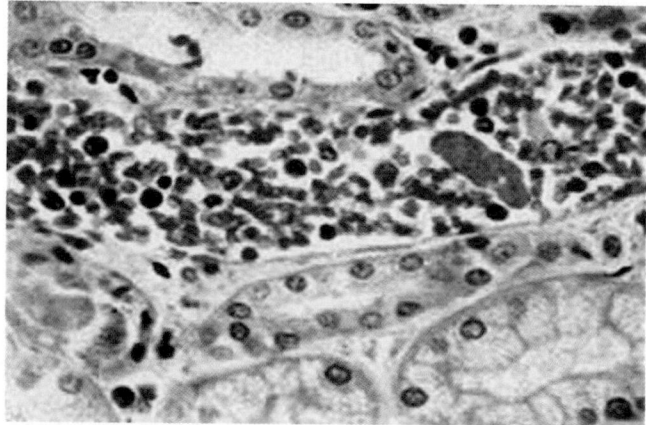

FIGURE 167-4. Malaria; sludging of red cells and platelets in a renal venule.

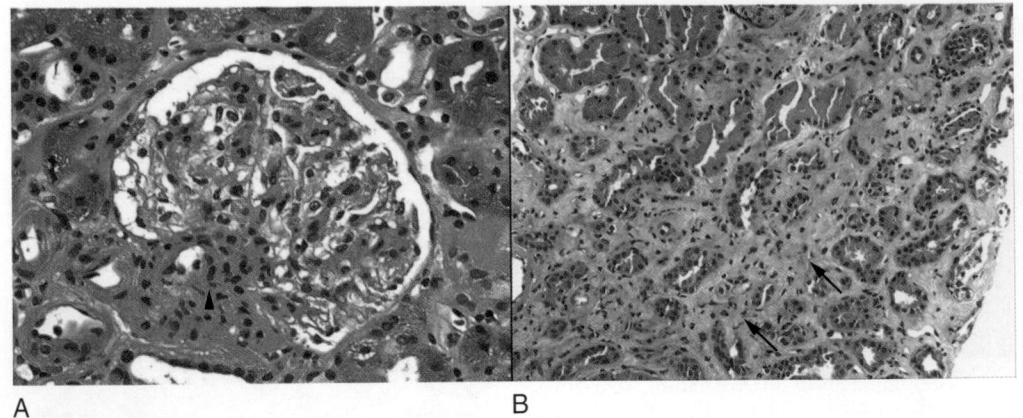

FIGURE 181-1. Pathological features of ischemic nephropathy in heart failure. **A,** The *arrowhead* marks the hypertrophied juxtaglomerular apparatus. **B,** *Arrows* identify the severe tubular atrophy and interstitial fibrosis present in a different high-power field.

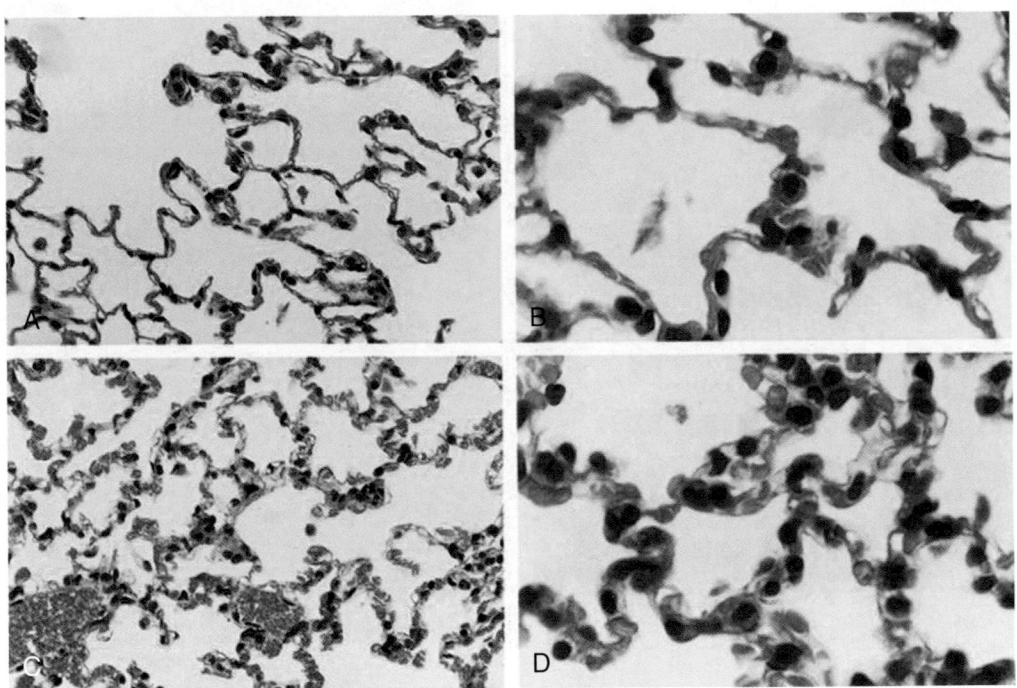

FIGURE 188-3. Increased interstitial edema in lung in response to renal ischemia-reperfusion. Preparations from sham-operated rats display clear alveolar spaces and minimal fluid or blood cells in the interstitial spaces at low (20×) and at high (40×) power (**A** and **B**). By contrast, preparations from rats with ischemic acute kidney injury exhibit lung interstitial edema, leukocyte sludging, and erythrocyte rouleaux formation, with occasional areas of alveolar hemorrhage (**C** and **D**). (From Kramer AA, Postler G, Salhab KF, et al: Renal ischemia/reperfusion leads to macrophage-mediated increase in pulmonary vascular permeability. Kidney Int 1999;55:2362.)

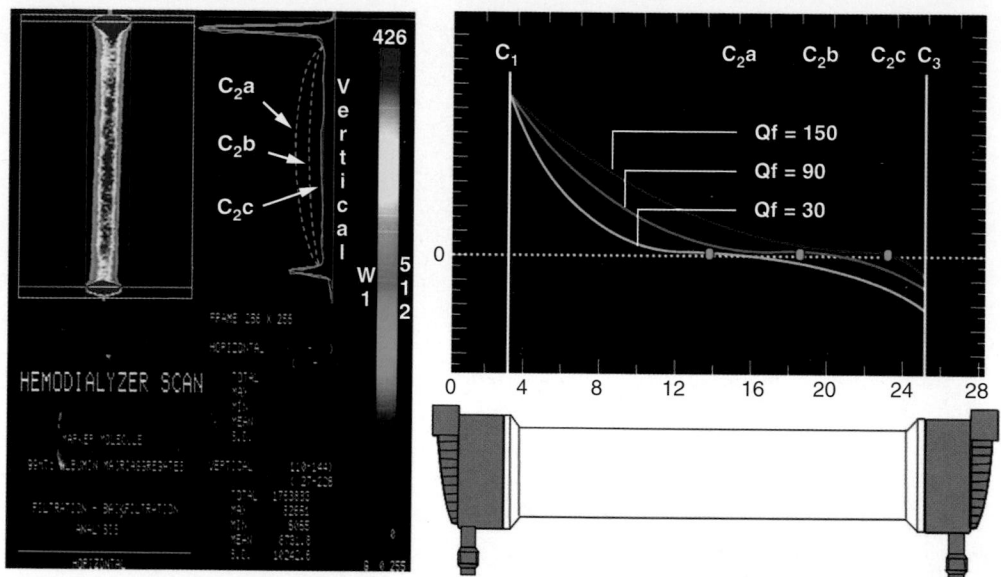

FIGURE 224-7. *Left,* Images of a dialyzer filter analyzed with the gamma camera after injection of a specific marker molecule in blood. The increased concentration of the labeled nondiffusible marker molecule in the central portion of the hemodialyzer can be visually captured from the change in color. The curve of the radioactive count is displayed on the right side of the filter image. The peak changes in concentration C_2a, C_2b, C_2c differ according to the net filtration rates. The lower the filtration rate is, the higher the peak concentration change and the higher the internal filtration-backfiltration (*right*). The different lines describe the local cross-filtration along the length of the fiber bundle. In the proximal portion (*left*), the cross-filtration is positive, and in the distal portion (*right*) the cross-filtration is negative (backfiltration).

Part I

Basic Clinical Problems

The Critically Ill Patient

Basic Principles of Care

The Critically Ill Patient

Michael R. Pinsky

OBJECTIVES

This chapter will:
1. Place acute severe illness on the continuum of health and chronic disease.
2. Describe the phenotype of critical illness.
3. Identify the initiating and sustaining immune effector cellular response to acute illness.
4. Identify the major humoral mediators that modulate the inflammatory response.
5. Describe how organ injury and immune effort cell activation and adhesion to the vascular endothelium are linked.
6. Elucidate the pro-inflammatory versus anti-inflammatory balance that is acute illness and how it affects response to treatment and outcome.
7. Explain the concept of immune reprogramming as a central aspect of acute illness.
8. Describe the interaction between the pro-inflammatory and anti-inflammatory intracellular promoters of gene induction and the cellular response to sepsis.
9. Demonstrate the linkage between cellular health and mitochondrial function in critical illness and how it is linked to the pro-inflammatory versus anti-inflammatory intracellular processes.

ACUTE CARE MEDICINE— A PERSPECTIVE

Acute care medicine has evolved greatly over the past 50 years from the former mix of specialized cardiovascular monitoring beds for postoperative patients and ventilatory support for patients with acute and chronic respiratory failure. Now it comprises an integrated acute care service whose direct influence spans the entire breadth of the hospital through intensive care units, intermediate care, and general patient support via medical emergency response teams as well as beyond the hospital walls via protocolized care in the field by paramedics. These changes have paralleled the advances in medical science that have enabled more effective and aggressive therapies for cancers,

continuous hemofiltration, minimally invasive surgery and angioplasty, organ transplantation, and gamma knife neurosurgery. Monitoring techniques have similarly advanced, with bedside ultrasound scanning becoming routine for procedures such as intravascular catheter insertion, cardiac functional analysis and tissue blood flow, and visceral organ analysis, to name a few. Hemodynamic monitoring has progressed from merely defining static variables of questionable diagnostic and therapeutic significance to functional hemodynamic monitoring that drives treatment protocols with documented improved outcome.

Yet with all these marvelous advances, disease has kept pace. The changes in diagnosis and treatment options have created a growing population of patients whose lives would otherwise have ended earlier. The result of this health dividend is an aging population. Thus, older patients, who have benefited from the miracles of modern science that have controlled hypertension, diabetes, blood cholesterol levels, severe infections, and a vast variety of chronic disease processes, are now becoming its victims. Because of the development of better emergency transport systems and trauma services, younger patients with more severe injury after trauma now survive long enough to be treated. Furthermore, patients with profound immunological compromise due to chronic disease, organ failure, or immunosuppression present to hospitals either with complications of a primary disease or with new disease processes that may be lethal in weakened hosts. Finally, bacteria have been winning the battle of drug resistance because of the combination of the use of massive amounts of antibiotics in agriculture and the indiscriminate use of newer antibiotics in hospitals.

This tension between advances in medical science and greater patient challenges is occurring within the context of increased rationing of health care resources in the civilized world. Health care providers are being required by health care payers to shorten length of hospital stay, minimize diagnostic investigations, and reduce overall hospital costs while maintaining a constant risk-adjusted mortality rate. This seemingly paradoxical situation is complicated by the fact that most of the therapeutic options available to the acute care physician are supportive rather than curative in nature. Artificial ventilation supports gas exchange but cannot treat acute lung injury, and hemodialysis supports the internal milieu without restoring renal function. This non–steady state health delivery equation is being addressed with different results in different countries and across regions of the same country. Thus, what appears to be the health care economic approach today will probably change in the near future as economies, demographics, and science evolve.

The challenge to the health care profession is to embrace these changes, understand their economic underpinnings, and revise practice while maintaining a firm commitment to patient welfare. This balance is imperfect and is made even more difficult by the alterations that occur in patients when they become critically ill. This chapter discusses (1) how the patient changes during the process of critical illness and recovery and (2) the effects of these changes on diagnosis and management.

CRITICAL ILLNESS

Patient care is always individualized, being adjusted to meet the needs of the patient and his or her response to treatment. In reality, however, the critically ill patient is not just a healthy person with a single important physiological impairment but, rather, is a new type of species whose response to the treatments and physiological challenges are different from the responses the patient would have if healthier. Thus, the critically ill patient is unique in the health care system. Surprisingly, from a wide variety of sources a certain amount of reductionist thinking seems reasonable in assessing critically ill patients.[1] First, subjects with acute disease processes that involve single organ systems have a better prognosis than those with a chronic process in which similar levels of organ failure occur or in whom less severe organ dysfunction occurs but in more than one organ at a time. Furthermore, if organ failure is sustained or progresses over time in spite of high-quality supportive therapy, the prognosis is worse still. Importantly, once a patient has been critically ill for more than 24 hours, complex but common cellular changes occur in the host inflammatory response and in the rest of the body that make these cases more common than the primary diagnoses would lead one to believe.[2] Most of the critically ill patients in whom initial resuscitative efforts are successful but who nevertheless die during their hospitalization do so because of progressive multiple-organ failure and, ultimately, cardiovascular collapse.[3] This inflammatory process masks the individual personalities of the various disease states in patients who remain critically ill despite appropriate and aggressive therapy. Accordingly, an understanding of the processes that induce this generalized inflammatory response, its effect on the body, and the potential biological markers of this process are important for the bedside clinician.

The body has evolved certain preprogrammed responses to specific insults and stresses. Profound injury, infection, and single organ failure induce inactivity, cause remote organ system shutdown (e.g., coma, ileus), and alter the basic metabolic machinery of the body to produce acute phase reactants to minimize inflammation and cellular injury at the expense of anabolic activities, such as albumin synthesis. The usual presentation of this process involves nonspecific aspects of acute inflammation common to trauma, myocardial infarction, and influenza virus infections. They are fever, leukocytosis, tachycardia, and increased metabolic activity. In the extreme, exactly opposite physiological changes can occur, such as hypothermia, leukopenia, bradycardia, and depressed metabolic activity. This clinical syndrome has been called *sepsis* or *sepsis syndrome* when it occurs with or without a clear source of infection, respectively. If cardiovascular insufficiency also develops, the condition is referred to as *septic shock*.

Systemic inflammatory response syndrome (SIRS) has been suggested to underscore the presumed common inflammatory etiology that multiple initiating processes create.[4] Furthermore, the deterioration of multiple organ systems associated with SIRS is referred to as *multiple-organ dysfunction syndrome* (MODS) so as to underscore the concept that organ dysfunction is a continual process rather than a threshold phenomenon. This syndrome is analogous to a total "tumor burden" used in oncology. Viewed from this perspective, SIRS can be regarded as a system-wide inflammatory response that results in systemic endothelial and parenchymal cellular injuries. Evidence now suggests that primary energy failure at the mitochondrial level is a central aspect of the terminal events of MODS. In support of this view, Knaus and associates[5] continue to document that in critically ill patients, the overall level of organ dysfunction is a more important variable defining survivorship than the functional status of a single organ.

INSULT AND MALIGNANT INTRAVASCULAR INFLAMMATION

Is there an underlying "theme" for all critically ill patients? Probably, although the initiating events that ultimately lead to this process are quite varied and define unique time courses and levels of organ system dysfunction. Pinsky and Matuschak[6,7] proposed a different term to describe the primary process that creates the observed end-organ dysfunction. Our concept was that SIRS and MODS reflect varying stages of a *malignant intravascular inflammatory process*. We reasoned that it was *malignant* because it is uncontrolled, rather than overwhelming, in its unregulated and self-sustaining nature; *intravascular* because it represents the blood-borne spread of what is usually a cell-cell interaction in the interstitial space; and *inflammation* because all the primary processes that characterize the response are part of the host's normal inflammatory response. The "normal process" of inflammation is a controlled or balanced activation of the host's cellular immune response (Table 1-1). The activation of this response in uncontrolled fashion and in the bloodstream makes this process virulent. Cytokine upregulation,[8,9] leading to activation of both immune effector cells[10] and vascular endothelium, characterizes the initiating inflammatory processes. Activated polymorphonuclear leukocytes (PMNs) and platelets stick to vascular endothelium, with subsequent capillary occlusion and/or endothelial disruption, transcapillary migration of immune effector cells, and damage to the parenchymal cells by both ischemic and cytotoxic processes. Interestingly, since my colleague and I proposed this term more than 15 years ago, no new information has surfaced to suggest that it is not completely correct.

Inflammation requires activation of cells capable of inducing further pro-inflammatory mediators and inducing injury themselves. Trauma, gram-negative, gram-positive, fungal, and anaphylactic initiating stimuli all

TABLE 1-1

Hierarchy of Immune Response: The Pro-inflammatory Initiation Cascade

SKIN	LYMPHATICS AND REGIONAL LYMPH NODES
Gut mucosa	Gut-associated lymphatic tissue (GALT)
Tissue	Tissue macrophages
Bloodstream	Innate immunity:
	Polymorphonuclear leukocytes (PMNs)
	Complement, endotoxin-binding protein
	(LBP)
Cell surface	CD14, Toll-like receptors 2 and 4, CD11b/
	CD18, HLA-DR2
Intracellular	Nuclear factor-κB

create different patterns of initiating pro-inflammatory mediators and reactive anti-inflammatory processes. Loss of skin or gut barrier function, atrophy of the gut-associated lymphatic tissue (GALT), and iatrogenic immune suppression all accelerate this process by different mechanisms that allow common activation of inflammation. However, the general principles characterized by lipopolysaccharide (LPS) challenge tend to reflect both a well-described model and many of the elements commonly seen in clinical studies. On the basis of those studies, the following construct can be developed. LPS, or endotoxin, is the complex surface molecule of gram-negative bacilli. Activation of immunocompetent tissue macrophages by LPS induces an upregulation of tumor necrosis factor (TNF) gene transcription, TNF synthesis, and subsequent release of TNF-α into the microenvironment around the cell.[11] This initial process is central to innate immunity and requires approximately 20 minutes to occur. Thus, any immediate systemic effects of LPS infusion must represent the systemic release of preformed mediators rather than an immunological response. Histamine release is a major component of the immediate response to LPS or other noxious stimuli. TNF is the initiator pro-inflammatory cytokine of the inflammatory process.

Released TNF can auto-stimulate the cell that secreted it through binding to that cell's surface TNF receptors. Self-stimulation by release of mediators is referred to as an *autocrine process*. Autocrine stimulation is an important process by which an immunocompetent cell's level of activation is sustained. The effect of autocrine stimulation is to amplify the initiator inflammatory signal of the sentinel immunocompetent cell. In doing so, it induces synthesis and release of more TNF as well as of a novel cytokine, interleukin-1β (IL-1β). The combined stimulatory effect of TNF and IL-1β on immunocompetent cells is approximately 20 to 50 times more powerful than that of TNF alone, in terms of eliciting further mediator synthesis and release.[12] TNF has direct effects on cellular function and indirect effects mediated by other cytokine and lipid inflammatory molecules.[13,14] It induces the production of numerous additional mediators of inflammation, such as IL-1β,[14] platelet-activating factor, IL-2, IL-6, IL-8, IL-10, interferon-γ, and eicosanoids, in addition to activation of PMNs, tissue macrophages, and lymphocytes.[15,16] In fact, just as the initial activation of intracellular pathways is occurring, the immunocyte is releasing large amounts of the cell surface receptor of TNF into the circulation. This shedding has three primary effects. First, it induces binding of free TNF to its receptor, making it less capable of inducing cell activation. Second, it decreases the possible

response of the stimulated cell to subsequent restimulation, either in an autocrine fashion or from remote cell sources. Finally, these soluble TNF receptors may potentially adsorb onto naive cells, making them responsive to TNF, in a fashion analogous to CD14 sensitization of naive cells.

The increased levels of mediator release aid in recruitment of adjacent cells, such as other fixed tissue macrophages and circulating immune effector cells, as well as parenchymal cells. This sort of mediator interaction is referred to as a *paracrine process*.[14] Paracrine processes represent powerful means by which complex signaling occurs among adjacent cells and are central to the natural processes of life. For example, stimulated Kupffer cells interact with hepatocytes to change hepatocytic synthetic activity through cytokine release, vascular endothelium interacts with vascular smooth muscle cells to alter vascular tone through nitric oxide release, and neurons interact with other neurons to consolidate memory through a variety of mechanisms, including nitric oxide and related neurotransmitter substances.

If mediator release exceeds the boundaries of the local environment, seeping into the lymphatics or bloodstream, a more generalized activation occurs via cellular processes similar to those described for both autocrine and paracrine functions. When inflammatory mediators spread beyond paracrine into *endocrine* interactions, inflammation becomes a generalized process.[17] Accordingly, one can regard SIRS as an inflammatory process exceeding the level of paracrine activation. Because SIRS commonly occurs in many nonfatal processes, such as minor viral prodromes and allergic reactions, and during uneventful recovery from trauma and surgery, its presence may not represent a maladaptive process. SIRS is part of the overall systemic response to biological stress necessary for the speedy clearance of noxious stimulants and repair of tissue. Fever tends to retard bacterial growth, and leukocytosis aids in recruitment of PMNs to sites of inflammation. Unfortunately, it is not clear at what point SIRS stops being beneficial to the host and starts being detrimental.

If some level of SIRS is necessary as part of the overall effective response to severe biological stress, preventing the expression of SIRS may not be desirable. If SIRS-induced MODS is reversible but end-stage organ failure is not, stratifying patients according to level of MODS may not identify those patients in whom suppression of excessive SIRS is inducing MODS from those in whom suppression of SIRS will have minimal effect on MODS. Similarly, if SIRS is a natural process that confers a survival advantage to the host, as most data suggest, suppression of SIRS in critically ill patients may not have an overall benefit in terms of morbidity or mortality. This is because both good and bad effects of suppression of the systemic inflammatory response will be combined into a single group analysis. These complexities illustrate the quandary faced by researchers striving to study the effects of immunomodulating agents in the treatment of critically ill patients with SIRS and MODS.

MEDIATORS OF THE INFLAMMATORY RESPONSE: THE CYTOKINE HYPOTHESIS

Both SIRS and MODS appear to be due to host-initiated damage to vascular endothelial cells and parenchymal cells through activation of the normal immune effector limb of the inflammatory cascade. The process matures through microvascular sequestration of activated-formed cellular elements (PMNs, monocytes, and lymphocytes), microvascular thrombosis, and immune effector cell–mediated cytotoxic and complement-mediated endothelial and parenchymal cell injuries. Blood levels of both TNF and IL-6 rise in subjects challenged with endotoxin.[18,19] TNF elevations occur prior to the systemic febrile response and leukocytosis that are seen after endotoxin infusion. Furthermore, distal suppression of fever by ibuprofen, a cyclooxygenase inhibitor, does not abolish either TNF release or leukocytosis in response to endotoxin infusion,[18,20,21] although pretreatment minimizes the systemic effects of endotoxemia. Furthermore, blood levels of TNF and IL-6 are high in septic patients,[22,23] although the metabolic abnormalities seen during experimental endotoxic shock are prevented by anti-TNF antibodies.[11] Maximal levels of TNF and IL-6 are crudely predictive of mortality in children with meningococcal sepsis.[24,25] Finally, persistence of TNF and IL-6 in the blood, rather than absolute blood levels of TNF and IL-6, predicts which patients with similar initial levels of cardiovascular insufficiency will experience MODS and/or die.[8]

Rather than being the cause of tissue injury, elevations of cytokines in the blood may reflect disease severity in a more readily measurable form. Intravascular cytokine levels could be a marker of, not the cause of, critical illness, just as smoke is a marker of fire but not the cause of burn injury. This concept has been referred to as the "smoking gun hypothesis," in that it suggests an association but does not prove it. Additional data are needed to solidify the argument that malignant intravascular inflammation induces MODS. These data will come from related studies of upregulation of circulating immune effector cells. Activated immunocompetent PMNs or monocytes can induce cell injury directly; they are the "bullets" from which the "smoking gun" theory of sepsis must be developed if it is to be proven. Thus, studies correlating cytokine levels with activation of circulating immune effector cells and subsequent organ system dysfunction or recovery are required to validate the cytokine hypothesis of SIRS.

CELL ADHESION AND ORGAN FAILURE

A complex and highly variable surface, or glycocalyx, covers the free cell surface of most cells. This covering is composed of numerous lipid-carbohydrate-protein moieties that extend out from the cell, attach to the cell surface, and may cross the cell membrane once or several times. This surface is not a passive barrier to diffusion, although it can function in that way as well. It is primarily a major recognition and attachment site for cell interactions that, for inflammation, translates into a ligand binding site with functional inflammatory transduction characteristics. Such binding must activate an intracellular process that results in upregulation of gene expression, synthesis of new protein, and phenotypic changes characteristic of inflammation that can be measured outside the cell.

As an initiating receptor, the cell surface receptor CD14 plays a pivotal role in the recognition of many microbiological toxins, host-derived mediators, and, probably, more molecular species with immune-modulating characteristics. To activate the CD14 receptor, LPS in the bloodstream binds to an LPS binding protein (LBP), the complex of which can then bind to CD14.[26] CD14 exists as a superficial receptor that has no cross-membrane component.[27] Presumably, CD14 functions to present the LPS-LBP complex to Toll-like receptor-4 (TLR-4), which internalizes the LPS moiety. Cells without CD14 do not react to LPS exposure.[28] Interestingly, CD14 can be shed into the circulation and bind LPS-LBP complexes. This trimer can bind to otherwise non-CD14 cells, conferring LPS sensitivity. The significance of this finding is currently unknown but is probably a cause of increased apoptosis of otherwise non–immunologically competent tissues, such as cardiac myocytes. The cell surface complex of LPS, LBP, and CD14 interacts with the transmembrane protein TLR-4 to induce intracellular signal transduction for the synthesis of new TNF and, probably, other pro-inflammatory cytokines (Table 1-2).[27] The initial central point in the first steps of intracellular activation is activation of serine kinases. Activated serine kinases eventually activate nuclear factor-κB (NF-κB), which cleaves its inhibitory component,

TABLE 1-2

Partial List of Inflammatory Mediator Balance

PRO-INFLAMMATORY MEDIATORS	ANTI-INFLAMMATORY MEDIATORS	VARIABLE MEDIATORS	PROMOTER	PRODUCT
Extracellular				
TNF	Transforming growth	IL-6	NF-κB	IL-1β, TNF
IL-1, IL-2, IL-8	factor-α		AP1	IL-8
	IL-4, IL-10		Sp1	IL-10
			HSFs	Heat shock protein (HSP) 70
Intracellular				
NF-κB, AP1	Sp1, HSFs			

AP, activating protein; HSFs, heat shock factors; IL, interleukin; NF, nuclear factor; Sp, specificity protein; TNF, tumor necrosis factor.

migrates into the nucleus, and binds to promoter sites on the genome coding for the synthesis of messenger RNA of various inflammatory protein species, including TNF.

Release of pro-inflammatory cytokine stimulates endothelial cells and circulating immune effector cells to change the expression of their cell surface adhesion molecules. The initial proadhesion cell surface receptors expressed are from the family of molecules called *selectins*. They allow for loose binding of circulating PMNs to the endothelium. The initial site of binding is in the postcapillary venule, where radial dispersive forces and low flow rate–shear forces promote cell-cell contact. This initial binding is weak, and if local endothelial activation induces expression of L-selectin–specific ligands along the endothelial surface, normal vessel flow induces the PMNs to roll along the vascular endothelium. If there is minimal endothelial activation, the PMNs dislodge and reenter the circulation. This transient binding of PMNs to the endothelium is the cause of initial leukopenia in response to dialysis-induced PMN activation and other related phenomena. If the endothelium has been strongly stimulated either by systemic pro-inflammatory mediators or local injury/inflammation, it will express a second family of cell adhesion molecules called *integrins*, of which intercellular adhesion molecules (ICAMs) are a subclass. ICAM expression on vascular endothelial cells occurs at the expense of selectin expression. Other integrins, such as CD11b and CD18, are upregulated on PMNs during sepsis. The strongly negatively charged selectins are cleaved into the circulation early in a septic challenge and may represent a major component in the initial acidosis seen in sepsis.[28]

Endothelial cell activation induces expression of L-selectin and, if sustained, of ICAM. Both adhesion molecules promote platelet binding rather than repulsion, which is the reason for the development of the procoagulant activity of the endothelium during inflammation. Activated endothelium expresses IL-8, a potent PMN chemoattractant, into its microenvironment. IL-8 suppresses the subsequent activation of immune effector cells in response to subsequent exposure to TNF. ICAM expression promotes firm binding of those PMNs that are also activated. Tight adhesion mediated through ICAM binding allows for prolonged PMN-endothelial contact. Activated PMNs bound to activating endothelium is a deadly combination for the endothelial cell. Release of toxic oxygen species and proteases by the PMNs into the microenvironment between these two cell types promotes lipid peroxidation and damage to the endothelial barrier of the vessel. In a less well-defined process, chemoattractants within the site of inflammation induce the migration of other PMNs into the parenchyma once endothelial damage has occurred.

Using the Goris Organ Failure Score in septic patients with end-stage liver failure, Rosenbloom and associates[10] correlated change in adhesion molecule activity with subsequent development of organ failure.[8] They found that mild sepsis was associated with slight elevations in L-selectin on PMNs, whereas severe sepsis was associated with a decreased L-selectin expression, a markedly increased CD11b expression, and a slightly increased CD35 expression (complement-binding receptor). Furthermore, although both IL-6 serum levels and CD11b PMN levels were highly variable among patients and even variable over time, most of the variability in CD11b expression could be explained by paired variations in IL-6. Finally, levels of CD11b and CD35 on circulating PMNs predicted subsequent organ failure. Accordingly, variations in CD11b over time related to variations in IL-6 serum level and to the severity of intravascular inflammation, as assayed by CD11b upregulation predicted subsequent MODS.

YIN AND YANG OF INJURY AND INFLAMMATION: THE ANTI-INFLAMMATORY RESPONSE

Importantly, both pro-inflammatory cytokines, such as TNF, IL-1β, IL-6, and IL-8, and anti-inflammatory species, such as IL-1 receptor antagonist (IL-1ra), IL-10, and the soluble TNF receptors I and II (sTNFrI and sTNFrII, respectively) coexist in the circulation in patients with established sepsis and presumably within the tissues (see Table 1-2).[29-31] Thus, sepsis may be more accurately described as a dysregulation of the innate immunity rather than as merely the overexpression of pro-inflammatory substances. This interaction of pro- and anti-inflammatory mediators may explain the observed failures of all the major anti-inflammatory drug trials in the treatment of septic shock.[32] Accordingly, Pinsky[33] proposed *malignant intravascular inflammation* to describe the systemic process of severe sepsis. This paradoxical expression in the blood of pro-inflammatory mediators and anti-inflammatory species creates an internal milieu that, in sustained sepsis, induces impairment of host immunity. Experimentally, this altered immune response state resembles *endotoxin tolerance*. Cavaillon[34] termed this blunted immune response *inflammatory stimuli–induced anergy*, because it is universally seen in severe stress states and can be induced by prior exposure to low levels of one of many pro-inflammatory stimuli, not only endotoxin. Hence, its original name, *endotoxin tolerance*, is misleading, although it is used here to describe this nonspecific response. Inflammatory stimuli–induced anergy can be induced by anti-inflammatory cytokines, such as tumor growth factor-β (TGF-β), IL-10, and IL-4, and somewhat by IL-1β, but not by TNF, IL-6, or IL-8. Furthermore, it is associated with altered intracellular metabolism of the important regulatory protein NF-κB. Leukocyte dysfunction also occurs in sepsis and in endotoxin-tolerant states and may be a central determinant of outcome.[35-38]

Presumably, inflammatory stimuli–induced anergy minimizes the inflammatory response, preventing a chain-reaction, system-wide activation of the inflammatory processes. However, it also limits subsequent ability to mount an appropriate inflammatory defense to infection. Because endotoxin tolerance usually requires a few hours to develop in isolated cells and 4 to 10 hours in intact animals, its expression parallels that of clinical sepsis. Thus, my colleagues and I have previously hypothesized that endotoxin tolerance carries most if not all of the intracellular qualities of fully developed severe sepsis.[33] However, the intracellular mechanisms of inflammatory stimuli–induced anergy are poorly understood, although they reflect, in large part, intracellular change in the activation of the inflammatory pathways. Thus, the severely ill patient represents a dysequilibrium between pro-inflammatory stimuli and anti-inflammatory counterregulation that leaves him or her with ongoing inflammatory tissue damage and decreased immune responsiveness. The hallmarks of critical illness are nonspecific inflammation and reduced host defense.

The exact nature of the blunted inflammatory response seen in severe illness and characterized by sepsis is not known. Some innate responses, such as IL-10 activation, are not impaired. Thus, the entire process may be more appropriately called *immunological reprogramming* rather than immune suppression. However, several humoral and cell surface anti-inflammatory processes are present in both endotoxin tolerance and severe illness. First, increased serum levels of soluble CD14, LBP, and phospholipids are seen as part of the acute phase response to severe illness. All of these processes tend to reduce the presence of biologically active LPS in the circulation. Second, LPS binds to a specific transmembrane receptor, TLR-4, which initiates the intracellular signaling that induces synthesis and release of pro-inflammatory mediators. Pro-inflammatory stimuli decrease TLR-4 activity, reducing the stimulatory effects of circulating LPS.[39] Cross-tolerance among TLR species (e.g., TLR-1, -2, -3, -4, and -5) has also been reported.

THE BATTLE INSIDE THE CELL: PRO-INFLAMMATORY AND ANTI-INFLAMMATORY RESPONSES

NF-κB is an oxidant-inducible promoter protein of the pro-inflammatory response of immune effector cells.[40] Although other intracellular pro-inflammatory promoters are also present, none has the breadth of gene activation or complex feedback control mechanisms described for NF-κB. NF-κB–inducible proteins include TNF, IL-1β, and IL-8 plus the pro-inflammatory enzymes inducible nitric oxide synthase (iNOS) and cyclooxygenase 2 (COX-2).[34] When viewed from a purely regulatory perspective, NF-κB is an excellent target for modulating the cellular inflammatory response. It is not surprising, therefore, that several intracellular mechanisms modulate NF-κB activity.

What is endotoxin tolerance and why can it be used to study the molecular mechanisms of sepsis? As previously described, exposure to small amounts of endotoxin induces an endotoxin-tolerant state in both cell culture in 4 hours and animal models in about 8 hours.[41] In this state, subsequent exposure to a previously lethal dose of endotoxin does not induce the fatal pro-inflammatory state. The endotoxin-tolerant state lasts in decreasing strength for between 24 and 36 hours, depending on the species and the initial dose of endotoxin. Interestingly, after the induction of an endotoxin-tolerant state, the initial steps of pro-inflammatory signal transduction up to cleavage of the cytoplasmic inhibitor protein IκB, which thereby releases NF-κB, can still occur. However, the liberated NF-κB appears to be dysfunctional.[40] The reasons for this dysfunction are multiple and not fully defined. However, some specific interactions have been identified that speak to the significance of the pro- and anti-inflammatory interactions. Importantly, there is much similarity between endotoxin tolerance and human sepsis. First, sepsis rarely starts with a massive exposure to an overwhelming noxious stimulus. Usually, infection and its associated inflammation build over hours. Thus, the host is exposed to low levels of pro-inflammatory species with a time course similar to that in classic endotoxin tolerance. Second, just as endotoxin tolerance minimizes the subsequent pro-inflammatory response to an additional pro-inflammatory stimulation, sepsis is characterized by a blunted immune effector cell response. By what mechanisms do pro-inflammatory stimuli induce an apparently anti-inflammatory response? The answer appears to relate to the complex mechanisms by which NF-κB is activated and binds to the pro-inflammatory promoter regions.

The activation of NF-κB is central to the activation of immune effector cells. Endotoxin can induce the initial steps of signal transduction up to NF-κB, but NF-κB activation is required for much of the subsequent intracellular signaling. The phosphorylation of the IκB-α subunit of the NF-κB complex after intracellular oxidative stress frees the dimer to translocate into the nucleus[42] through activation of the Iκ kinase (IKK).[43] The phosphorylated IκB-α is rapidly degraded by proteasomes. The p65 moiety has a DNA-binding domain that allows it to bind to numerous specific DNA sites throughout the genome, regulating gene transcription for most, if not all, of the pro-inflammatory species, including TNF,[44] IL-1β, inducible nitric oxide synthase,[45] lipoxygenase, and cyclooxygenase.

IκB-α is a heat shock protein (HSP). An increase in synthesis of IκB-α also downregulates NF-κB activation by dissociating the p65-p50 heterodimer from its responsive elements on the genome and keeping it in an inactive form in the cytoplasm.[46] NF-κB's DNA binding activity can also be downregulated by excess p50 synthesis. The NF-κB dimer can exist in one of two forms, the p65-p50 dimer and a p50-p50 homodimer. The p65 subunit has DNA binding activity, whereas the p50 subunit does not. Activation of p65-p50 dimers results in markedly increased transcription of messenger RNA after binding, whereas p50-p50 activation only minimally increases transcription rates. NF-κB dysfunction reflects both an excess p50 homodimer production, which has impaired transcription activity,[40] and excess synthesis of IκB-α.[46] The balance of NF-κB species is very sensitive to transcription rates; a ratio of NF-κB p50-p65 heterodimer to p50 homodimer of 1.8 ± 0.6 confers activation of the inflammatory pathways, whereas a ratio of 0.8 ± 0.1 confers lack of stimulation in response to LPS (i.e., endotoxin tolerance). The p50 subunit may inhibit synthesis of TNF messenger RNA. However, these p65-p50/p50-p50–related processes can explain only the downregulation of the overall inflammatory process. They cannot explain why activation of both pro- and anti-inflammatory processes is sustained in severe sepsis or why immune suppression, a common characteristic of sepsis, coexists with a heightened inflammatory state.

Downregulation of NF-κB–related intercellular processes is an important aspect of the overall intracellular inflammatory response. Potentially, if anti-inflammatory pathways were activated by the same stimuli that activate pro-inflammatory pathways, an intrinsic mechanism would exist to autoregulate the inflammatory response on a cellular level. This system might be induced by much of the same stimuli and act through parallel intracellular processes. The cell does have several intrinsic anti-inflammatory processes, including antiproteases, melanoproteins, and free radical scavengers. However, the HSP system is by far the most prevalent in terms of mass of protein and scope of oversight.

THE STRESS RESPONSE AND SURVIVAL

The HSP system is the oldest-identified phylogenetic cellular defense mechanism. It has widespread and overarching basic roles in cellular defense against numerous stresses, such as fever, trauma, and inflammation.[47] Intracellular chaperone proteins of the HSP family appear to be pivotal in the regulation of the cellular response to inflammatory signals and external injury. An initial step in the intracellular activation of the inflammatory pathway is the production of reactive oxygen species (ROS). Mitochondria not only are very sensitive to oxidative stress from ROS but also are a primary intracellular site of free radical production. Thus, measuring mitochondrial membrane potential ($\Psi\Delta$) allows one to monitor the degree of intracellular oxidative stress over time.[48] Detection of the mitochondrial permeability transition event also provides an early indication of the initiation of cellular apoptosis. This process is typically defined as a collapse in the mitochondrial membrane electrochemical gradient, as measured by the change in the $\Psi\Delta$. The literature clearly documents that HSPs are a basic cellular defense mechanism against numerous stresses, such as fever, trauma, and inflammation.[47,49] They also minimize nitric oxide, ROS, and streptozotocin cytotoxicity.[50,51] HSP70 is also an inducible protective agent in myocardium against ischemia, reperfusion injury, and nitric oxide toxicity,[52] although it requires some initial trigger for activation. Thus, the intracellular pathway mobilized upon heat shock may be important in modulating the intracellular inflammatory signal acting at the level of NF-κB and appears to have many of the immune-modulating characteristics of endotoxin tolerance. Because heat shock is a primordial cellular defense mechanism, is upregulated in a matter of minutes, and rapidly confers an immune-depressed state, its actions reflect a relatively pure antioxidant, anti-inflammatory response. Although the time courses for production of endotoxin tolerance and heat shock are different, similar gene activation and inhibition occur with the two processes.

The heat shock factors (HSFs), particularly HSF1, are primarily responsible for inducing the transcription of HSP genes and can be considered the NF-κB equivalent for HSP synthesis. HSFs exist preformed in the cytosol, bound to HSP70. The presence of denatured protein—resulting, for example, from heat or ROS-induced protein damage—strips the HSP70 proteins from HSF as HSP70 binds to the damaged proteins. Trimerized HSF migrates into the nucleus to bind to numerous regions within the genome. Although HSF1 and NF-κB are not structurally related, the DNA recognition elements for the two factors can be somewhat similar.[53] Thus, the possibility exists that some NF-κB sites may be recognized by HSF1.

Putative recognition of specific NF-κB response elements by HSF1 does not necessarily imply that transcription would ensue. Transcriptional activation by DNA-bound HSF1 requires site-specific phosphorylation, which apparently is brought about by the precise coordination of multiple stress-activated kinases. Indeed, HSF1 has been implicated in transcriptional repression of the IL-1β gene promoter.[48] The mechanism for this repression appears to require the binding of HSF1 to a heat shock element (HSE)–like sequence within the IL-1β promoter. One of the phenotypes observed in HSF1 knockout mice also supports a role for HSF1 in transcriptional repression of pro-inflammatory genes. Following an endotoxic challenge (i.e., *E. coli* LPS) in one study, HSF1 knockout mice exhibited a potentiation of pro-inflammatory TNF-α production.[54] Because HSP induction is severely limited in the HSF1 knockout mice, the effect of HSF1 on TNF-α induction does not appear to require an HSF1–induced HSP such as HSP70. Thus, although HSP70 stabilization of IκB-α has been postulated to participate in downregulation of NF-κB,[55] other levels of control may operate under conditions of endotoxic shock. The IκB-α promoter region has a NF-κB recognition site, and NF-κB activation increases IκB-α synthesis in a negative-feedback-loop fashion.[56,57] Potentially, HSF1 may inhibit NF-κB–induced transcription promotion via tethering of NF-κB to its responsive element, much like glucocorticoids do.[58]

HSP activation confers a survival advantage to the host. Thermal pretreatment was found to be associated with attenuated lung damage in a rat model of acute lung injury induced by intratracheal instillation of phospholipase A₂.[59] Thermal pretreatment reduces mortality rate and the extent of sepsis-induced acute lung injury produced by cecal ligation and perforation.[60] The subsequent higher expression of a broad variety of HSPs not only confers a nonspecific protection against subsequent oxidative stress but also minimizes the cellular response to pro-inflammatory stimuli. Survival in cold-blooded animals given an infectious inoculum is linearly related to body temperature. Finally, if specific HSPs are depleted, multiple intracellular signaling processes can be affected.

MITOCHONDRIA AS MARKERS AND TARGETS OF INJURY

An initial step in the intracellular activation of the inflammatory pathway between mediator binding to the cell surface and inflammatory gene activation is the production of ROS and an associated oxidative stress on the mitochondria.[61] Mitochondria operate by generating a chemi-osmotic gradient via the Krebs cycle inside their inner membrane that is necessary to drive adenosine triphosphate formation across this membrane. Essentially, they are intracellular batteries whose charge or polarization level defines their ability to create adenosine triphosphate. Loss of internal membrane polarization induces release of cytochrome c from the mitochondria into the cytosol. Importantly, cytochrome c activates the intrinsic caspase system to initiate apoptosis, or programmed cell death. Thus, preventing mitochondrial depolarization would be an important function for HSPs if their role were to aid in cell survival. HSP70 prevents this mitochondrial oxidative stress and blunts the inflammatory response.[50] Consistent with the pluripotential effects of the heat shock response as described previously, HSP70 is also an inducible protective agent in myocardium against ischemia, reperfusion injury, and nitric oxide toxicity.[52] Evidence that HSP70 may be active in human sepsis comes from the observation that higher HSP70 expression is seen in peripheral mononuclear cells in septic patients. Although not conclusive, these data strongly suggest that HSPs, and HSP70 in particular, may be important in modulating the intracellular inflammatory signal acting at the level of NK-κB. Importantly, Wong and colleagues[62] identified a potential heat shock–responsive element in the IκB-α promoter that can be activated by HSFs after heat shock. Moreover, the heat shock response can also modulate NF-κB inactivation via this increase in IκB-α expression. Thus, the primary inhibitor of NF-κB activation, IκB-α, is itself an HSP.

SEPSIS: THE GREAT DISEQUILIBRIUM

Given that both pro- and anti-inflammatory processes are ongoing in the cell and that both pro- and anti-inflamma-

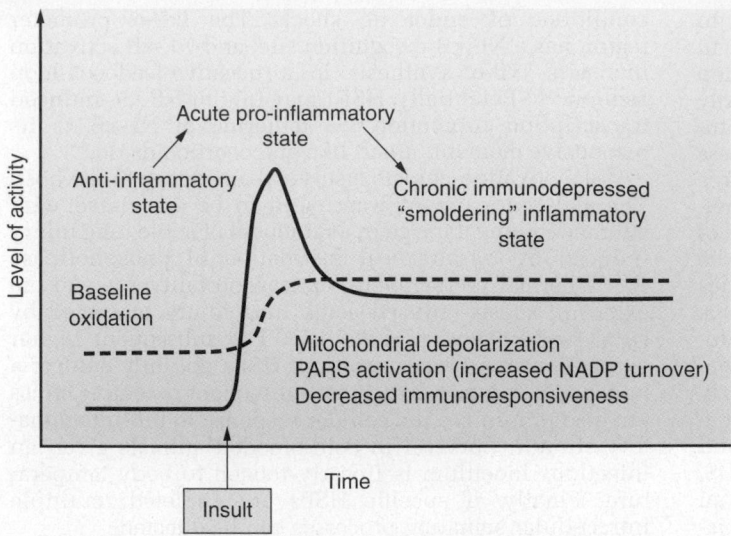

FIGURE 1-1. Schematic representation of the pro-inflammatory (*solid line*) and anti-inflammatory (*dashed line*) intracellular activity before and during the response to a foreign insult, such as sepsis or trauma. NADP, nicotinamide adenine dinucleotide phosphate; PARS, poly (ADP-ribose) synthase.

tory mediators are present in the bloodstream, it is reasonable to assume that the immune effector cells are also receiving mixed messages and undergo immunological reprogramming. This concept is illustrated schematically in Figure 1-1. However, the phenotypic response that they make is more difficult to predict. The normal cellular inflammatory response is essential to survival. It localizes and eliminates foreign material, including microorganisms. Similarly, some degree of systemic inflammatory response is useful. Fever reduces microorganism growth, malaise causes the host to rest, and secretion of acute phase proteins minimizes oxidative injury. Inflammation is also destructive, however; local abscess formation and multiple-system organ failure are its very real byproducts. Sepsis also carries a strong anti-inflammatory response. The exact balance or interaction among these two processes with their multiple layers of feedback, activation, and control, is difficult, if not impossible, to assess clinically.

Prior studies have documented that sepsis and all acute severe processes result in the expression of cytokines in the systemic circulation. However, it is difficult to assess the extent of inflammatory stimulation by measuring serum cytokine levels, because they can change within minutes and may be very different in adjacent tissue compartments.[63] Although serum levels of TNF and IL-6 are excellent markers of disease severity and good positive predictors of the subsequent development of remote organ system dysfunction, measuring blood levels of cytokines does not aid in defining the balance between pro- and anti-inflammatory processes in predicting response to therapy.

Attention has subsequently shifted to examination of the functional status of circulating immune effector cells. Because activation and localization of PMNs represent the initial cellular host defense against infection, their tight control is essential to prevent widespread nonspecific injury. Subsequently, monocytes localize at the site of inflammation. Their activity appears to become the predominant process in both host defense and repair, especially from the second or third day onward in the course of acute illness. Thus, inhibition of monocyte immune responsiveness is a powerful mechanism to downregulate the inflammatory response. Anergy, a cardinal characteristic of severe illness, reflects macrophage inhibition of

antigen processing. Importantly, antigen processing reflects a primary aspect of this cellular response. In this regard, the cell surface receptor family HLA-DR is responsible for antigen presentation to antigen-processing cells. Immature monocytes cannot process antigen and have lower cell surface levels of HLA-DR. Docke and associates demonstrated that monocytes require HLA-DR levels higher than 20% for normal cell-mediated immunity. Lower levels of HLA-DR expression confirm immune suppression.[64] Consistent with the overall theme of increased anti-inflammatory responses in severe sepsis, these researchers and others have found a profound decrease in HLA-DR expression on circulating monocytes obtained from patients with sepsis.

A primary determinant of innate immunity and clearance of bacteria as well as the subsequent development of endothelial injury and organ dysfunction is the activation of circulating immune effector cells (e.g., PMNs, monocytes). Clearly, PMNs can be both overactive[65] and dysfunctional,[35] and their CD11b display, as a marker of activation, can be either decreased[66] or increased[67] in critically ill patients. Furthermore, the de novo display of CD11b on circulating PMNs and its subsequent change in expression of both total CD11b and its avid form, CBRM1/5 epitope, in response to in vitro stimulation by TNF can be used to characterize the in vivo state of PMN activation and responsiveness. Circulating PMNs of septic humans have a similar phenotype, characterized by high CD11b and low L-selectin expression.[68] Thus, severe sepsis is associated with increased de novo activation of circulating immune effector cells. Paradoxically, however, in a sustained inflammatory state, those same PMNs are impaired in the ability to upregulate CD11b further or to change surface CD11b to the avid state[69] in response to an *ex vivo* challenge through exposure to biologically significant levels of TNF. Furthermore, circulating PMNs in subjects with severe sepsis have impaired phagocytosis, reduced oxygen burst capacity, and diminished in vitro adhesiveness.[70] This desensitization to exogenous TNF is due not to a loss of TNF receptors but to downregulation of cell surface TLR-4 levels.

Finally, in analyzing peripheral blood monocytes from septic subjects for NF-κB activity and in vitro responsiveness to LPS, Adib-Conquy and colleagues[41] observed an NF-κB pattern of response similar to that seen with endotoxin tolerance. The cause of the reduced nuclear translocation of NF-κB was not an excess of IκB but, rather, an increase in the proportion of the inactive p50-p50 heterodimers relative to the active p65-p50 homodimers. Interestingly, survivors had higher levels of NF-κB than nonsurvivors, suggesting that although downregulation of inflammation is a normal aspect of sepsis, excessive inhibition of the process is associated with a poor prognosis. Clearly, this is an area of active investigation, and the complex interactions among pro- and anti-inflammatory processes are just now being teased out.

CRITICAL ILLNESS, ORGAN FAILURE, AND SURVIVAL

One may reasonably ask, "Why would the body create a system of mutual immune suppression and self-destruction in response to severe illness? Is this just a misplaced adaptive response, like the fluid retention and vasoconstriction seen in congestive heart failure, wherein reversal of this natural response improves survival?" Potentially, the answer to the second question is "Yes," because one could imagine that keeping severely injured members of a group alive when resources were limited would limit the overall fitness of the group. Having those poor individuals die quickly if it were clear that their survival was doubtful would be an extremely efficient means to sustain group health. And Nature is not known for her sentimentality. The argument can be made that no organism was expected to survive severe illness, and death was the appropriate outcome. In essence, Nature did not consider medical care when developing its own internal mechanisms to sustain life. In this context, multiple-system organ failure may be regarded as a manufactured disease, one created by our ability to sustain and support the severely injured individual without eradicating the primary cause of the illness or its protean sequelae. This argument is supported by the studies showing that preventing further injury, rather than reversing acute processes, improves survival rates. Examples are the use of low tidal-volume ventilation in acute respiratory distress syndrome to minimize barotrauma and continuous venovenous hemofiltration in acute renal failure to limit hypotension-induced acute tubular necrosis during recovery.

However, one may look at this process with the opposite perspective as well. Ill subjects tend to markedly restrict their physical activity and to rest or sleep a lot. Acute renal failure shuts down the kidney but is often associated with complete renal recovery if the subject can tolerate the uremia that follows for a defined interval. Similarly, myocardium starved of oxygen goes into hibernation and fails to contract rather than becoming necrotic, and then is completely normal on revascularization. Singer and coworkers[71] have suggested that mitochondrial shutdown in sepsis may be this same process on a cellular level. The logic develops along the following lines: Sepsis and other critical illnesses produce a biphasic inflammatory, immune, hormonal, and metabolic response. The acute phase is marked by an abrupt rise in the secretion of stress hormones with an associated increase in mitochondrial and metabolic activity. The combination of severe inflammation and secondary changes in endocrine profile diminish energy production, metabolic rate, and normal cellular processes, leading to multiple-organ dysfunction. Potentially, the presumed organ failure might be a potentially

protective mechanism, because reduced cellular metabolism could improve the chance of survival of cells and, thus of organs in the presence of an overwhelming insult. According to this hypothesis, the decline in organ function is triggered by a decrease in mitochondrial activity and oxidative phosphorylation, leading to reduced cellular metabolism.

If this hypothesis proves correct, forcing organs to work during repair from injury, with its associated mitochondrial dysfunction, may worsen outcome. Clearly, protecting viable tissue is a cornerstone of acute care management. It is not clear, however, how sustaining blood flow to organs with mitochondrial dysfunction alters their outcome. Potentially greater oxygen supply might increase free radical production and cellular injury, whereas worsening ischemia may hasten necrotic cell death. At present, the most prudent therapeutic philosophy is to aggressively resuscitate critically ill patients at initial presentation prior to organ injury but, once organ injury has developed, to sustain only minimal oxygenation, blood flow, and perfusion pressure with the least artificial support needed to achieve these goals. The big problem for the practicing clinician is to know when to switch from acute rescue resuscitation to maintaining recovery mode. The literature has yet to address this question, let alone suggest a solution.

Key Points

1. The inflammatory response is part of innate immunity.
2. The inflammatory response is complex and involves soluble mediators, adhesion molecules, hormones, paracrine events, intracellular gene promoters, and multiple interactions.
3. The primacy of one response system over another is not known.
4. Inflammation and counterinflammation can occur sequentially or simultaneously.
5. Counterinflammation can lead to immune suppression and opportunistic infection.
6. The mammalian response to sepsis may be directed toward individual death for the benefit of the herd.
7. Multiple-organ dysfunction may reflect a kind of hibernation that organs undergo to protect themselves. The task of the physician may be to wait and to avoid additional organ injury.
8. The big problem for the practicing clinician is to know when to switch from acute rescue resuscitation to maintaining recovery mode. No data exist in the literature to guide doctors in making this choice.

Key References

8. Pinsky MR, Vincent JL, Deviere J, et al: Serum cytokine levels in human septic shock: Relation to multiple systems organ failure and mortality. Chest 1993;103:565-575.
10. Rosenbloom A, Pinsky MR, Bryant JL, et al: Leukocyte activation in the peripheral blood of patients with cirrhosis of the liver and SIRS: Correlation with serum interleukin-6 levels and organ dysfunction. JAMA 1995;274:58-65.

29. Goldie AS, Fearon KC, Ross JA, et al: Natural cytokine antagonists and endogenous anti-endotoxin core antibodies in sepsis syndrome. The Sepsis Intervention Group. JAMA 1995;74: 172-217.

49. Polla BS, Kantegwa D, François S, et al: Mitochondria are selective targets for the protective effects of heat shock against oxidative injury. Proc Natl Acad Sci U S A 1996;93:6458-6463.

71. Singer M, De Santis V, Vitale D, Jeffcoate W: Multiorgan failure is an adaptive, endocrine-mediated, metabolic response to overwhelming systemic inflammation. Lancet 2004;364: 545-548.

See the companion Expert Consult website for the complete reference list.

CHAPTER 2

Genetic Variation and Critical Illness

Zhiyong Peng, Matthew A. Butkus, Neeta Kannan, and John A. Kellum

OBJECTIVES

This chapter will:
1. Define gene polymorphisms.
2. Illustrate potential markers related to critical illness.
3. Describe gene polymorphisms and their potential impact on conditions commonly encountered in critically ill patients.
4. Discuss the limitations and future directions of the study of gene polymorphisms.

With the development of molecular techniques that allow screening for a wide variety of genetic factors, attention is shifting toward the influence of genes on susceptibility to and severity of illness. The diathesis-stress model of illness has long been advocated in internal medicine and behavioral health, but the complexity of the interaction has remained elusive. Historically, genetics has been a useful tool for exploring the etiology and pathogenesis of illness and disease. The advent of gene-based therapies and diagnostics, however, has provided a significant amount of information on correlative and causative disease mechanisms, and it is anticipated that genetic interventions may offer powerful preventive, diagnostic, and therapeutic tools. In addition to genetic roles in disease processes, current research is exploring genetic responsiveness to pharmacological therapies, host responses to illness, and drug metabolism.

Only a small fraction of the human genome codes for proteins; instead, most cellular DNA has been labeled "junk DNA," an increasingly inaccurate term. This noncoding DNA appears to offer information useful for population genetics as well as to provide mechanisms for changes in coding regions of DNA and, hence, to implicate them in the etiology of illness.[1] Additionally, coding gene sequences are not evenly distributed; for instance, coding sequence clusters have been found to be especially prevalent on chromosomes 17, 19, and 22, and relatively less dense on 4, 8, 13, 18, and Y.

In humans, two unrelated people share more than 99.9% of their DNA sequences. The remaining 0.1% of variants, known as *gene polymorphisms*, are markers of biological diversity, and some genotypic variations correlate with specific phenotypes relevant to human disease. Polymorphism of human genes may be observed at one or more of the following sites: (1) the promoter or 5′-flanking region, (2) the exon or gene-coding sequences, (3) the intron or gene-intervening sequences, and (4) the 3′-untranslated region.

Genetic susceptibility to disease occurs through multiple means. In addition to dominant and recessive inheritance patterns producing illness (e.g., inheritance of two recessive and deleterious alleles), disease can arise through changes in DNA sequencing (*mutation*). These mutations can have a variety of morphological effects (both visible and invisible) and can accrue slowly over time despite cellular defense mechanisms.[2] Recognized pathways for mutation include single-nucleotide polymorphism (SNP), variable number of tandem repeats (VNTRs), and microsatellites. Additionally, genetic etiologies of disease involve *trisomies* (incomplete chromosomal separation during cellular division), *imprinting* (both chromosomes are inherited from one parent), *mosaicism* (tissues are composed of cells with different genetic sequences), and *mitochondrial disorders* (in which the genetic illness is located in the mitochondrial DNA rather than the host DNA); about 1000 gene mutations have been causally linked to disease etiologies.

Many mutations produce no overt phenotypic consequences. Those that do produce phenotypic change are generally categorized as *loss-of-function* or *gain-of-function* mutations, which may or may not be deleterious or advantageous to the organism. Functional changes can be produced by an alteration in the protein produced (e.g., a gene sequence that coded for arginine may code instead for serine owing to a point mutation) or by disruption of the chain of proteins coded by conversion of a protein codon to a stop codon. These functional shifts (and subsequent protein alterations) can affect sensitivity to other physicochemical stimuli, producing drug sensitivities, reactions, or ineffectual therapies (e.g., a plausible explanatory mechanism for the relative lack of a panacea in pharmacotherapy).[3] These shifts can also produce significant changes in physiology and immune response to trauma and insult. This is not to suggest that there is a strict causal pathway between gene sequence and phenotype; gene expression requires multiple intermediate steps, including messenger RNA processing, translation, and

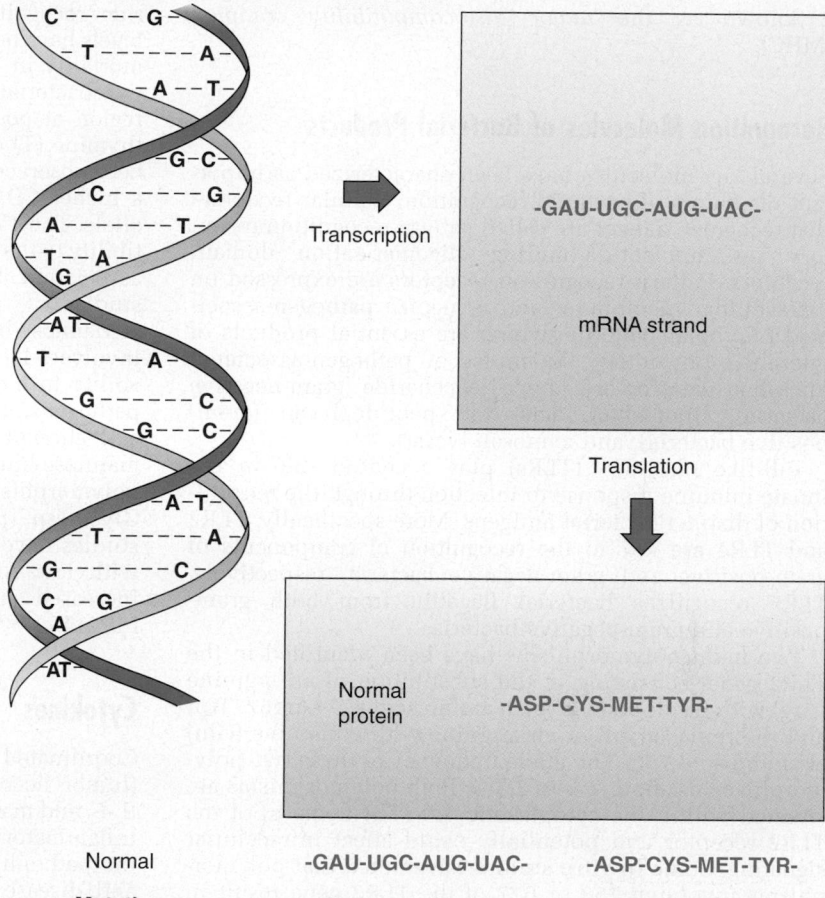

FIGURE 2-1. Normal gene sequences and polymorphisms. The normal messenger RNA (mRNA) strand and its subsequent protein are coded in *dark blue*. Mutations have been introduced (SNPs, VNTRs, and sequence inversion), with the mutations and corresponding protein changes coded in *light blue*.

Normal	-GAU-UGC-AUG-UAC-	-ASP-CYS-MET-TYR-
Mutation	**Sequence Change**	**Resultant Protein**
Single-nucleotide polymorphism (SNP)	-GAU-UGA-AUG-UAC-	-ASP-TER (stop)
Variable number of tandem repeats (VNTRs)	-GAU-UGU-GUG-CAU-	-ASP-CYS-VAL-HIS-
Microsatellite sequence inversion	-GAU-CAU-GUA-CGA-	-ASP-HIS-ASP-ARG-

additional post-translational influences like methylation and histone modification. In addition, multiple genotypes can code for the same phenotype (i.e., minor differences in messenger RNA sequences can produce the same end proteins). Examples of potential mutations are shown in Figure 2-1.

The current chapter explores the impact of genetic variation on critical illness. Contemporary research is focusing on mutation in disease susceptibility and outcomes. For instance, significant research is being conducted on SNPs in cytokine and cytokine receptors as markers of critical illness and prognosticators of clinical outcome. Although some researchers have suggested that there are systemic problems with these causative/correlational studies,[4] and others have proposed that SNPs may actually be biomarkers for regions in which the deleterious mutations are occurring (instead of causative agents),[5] research suggests that specific sequences, alone and in tandem, offer compelling correlational models of illness and mortality[6-8] and provide possible therapeutic interventions.[9-11]

CANDIDATE GENETIC MARKERS RELATED TO CRITICAL ILLNESS

There is mounting evidence to support the important role of systemic inflammatory response in the pathogenesis of critical illness. The systemic inflammatory disorder is the result of an interaction between environmental factors and the host immune response. Genetic factors in the host immune response may determine the susceptibility to, severity of, and clinical outcomes of the systemic inflammatory response. The study of polymorphisms among immune response genes has become the subject of intense interest, as these genetic markers may be potential determinants of susceptibility to or severity of acute illness. Because the systemic inflammatory response involves the recognition molecules, inflammatory cytokines, and coagulation cascade, a review of these gene variations is first necessary. Most of the candidate genes hypothesized to influence the intensity of the inflammatory response are located on the highly polymorphic region of chromosome

6 known as the *major histocompatibility complex* (MHC).[12,13]

Recognition Molecules of Bacterial Products

Several key molecules have been characterized as important mediators of bacterial recognition. Cellular receptors that recognize danger are called pattern recognition receptors and nucleotide-binding oligomerization domain receptors. Pattern recognition receptors are expressed on extracellular membranes and recognize pathogen-associated microbial patterns, which are essential products of microbial physiology. Examples of pathogen-associated microbial patterns are lipopolysaccharide (gram-negative bacteria), lipotechoic acid and peptidoglycan (gram-positive bacteria), and zymosan (yeast).[14,15]

Toll-like receptors (TLRs) play a central role in the innate immune response to infection through the recognition of distinct bacterial antigens. More specifically, TLR2 and TLR4 are key to the recognition of components of gram-positive and gram-negative bacteria, respectively. TLR5 recognizes bacterial flagellin from both gram-positive and gram-negative bacteria.

Two main polymorphisms have been identified in the TLR2 gene, consisting of the substitution of an arginine (Arg) with tryptophan (Trp) at amino acid 677 (Arg677Trp) and the replacement of an arginine with glutamine (Gln) at amino acid 753. The allele frequency of these two polymorphisms is about 2% to 2.5%. Both polymorphisms are situated within the cytoplasmic tail (TIR domain) of the TLR2 receptor and potentially could affect intracellular signaling. Some in vitro studies have noted that polymorphisms involving 753 or 677 of the TLR2 gene result in reduced nuclear factor-κB–dependent transcriptional activity in response to a variety of gram-positive bacteria–derived products. Clinical studies from small sample populations illustrated that a defective TLR2 gene may predispose susceptible individuals to certain gram-positive infections leading to shock syndrome.[7,8,14,15]

TLR4 is one of the promising candidate genes. Studies have focused on several candidate polymorphisms at the TLR4 locus, including two missense SNPs, which confer alterations in the extracellular domain of the receptors. These consist of a substitution of the conserved aspartic acid (Asp) to glycine (Gly) at amino acid 299 (Asp299Gly; frequency 5%) and the replacement of threonine (Thr) by isoleucine (Ile) at amino acid 399 (Thr399Ile). These mutations in TLR4 attenuate response to gram-negative bacteria or endotoxin exposure in vivo and in vitro. In some studies, however, no association was shown between the TLR4 299/399 alleles and sepsis. These findings suggest that individuals with TLR4 299/399 polymorphisms may have an aberrant response to certain, but not all, gram-negative bacterial infections, resulting in an increased susceptibility to infection and severity of disease.[7,8,14,15]

A stop codon polymorphism at amino acid 392 from Arg to TER (termination) has been identified in the TLR5 gene and is associated with a greater susceptibility to Legionnaires' disease. A TLR5 392 from Arg to TER polymorphism may also increase the susceptibility to pneumonia associated with flagellated organisms.[14]

CD14 is a membrane glycoprotein with high-affinity receptors for lipopolysaccharide that is mainly expressed on the surface of macrophages, monocytes, neutrophils, and other nonmyeloid cells or is found in soluble form (sCD14). CD14 and TLR4 are part of the lipopolysaccha-ride recognition/response unit. Increased serum CD14 levels have been shown to correlate with shock and greater mortality in patients with gram-positive and gram-negative bacterial infections. The SNPs within the promoter region at positions −159 and −260 from cytosine (C) to thymine (T) of the CD14 gene have been detected. It has been observed that the TT homozygous individuals present a higher CD14 serum level than individuals with the C allele. The TT genotype can result in a differential susceptibility to the development of severe diseases, although the association has not been verified in all populations studied.[7,14]

Mannose-binding lectin is an acute-phase protein involved in the innate immune responses. It has the ability to bind carbohydrate structures on the microbial pathogens, enhancing phagocytosis, and promotes the activation of the complement system. Within exon 1 of the mannose-binding lectin gene, the following three different polymorphisms have been described: Arg52Cys (D allele), Gly54Asp (B allele), and Gly57Glu (C allele). Several studies have shown that all the variations are associated with low serum levels of mannose-binding lectin and increased susceptibility to a wide range of bacterial infections.[7,14]

Cytokines

Coordinated production of pro-inflammatory cytokines (tumor necrosis factor-α [TNF-α], interleukins IL-1 and IL-6, and macrophage migration inhibitory factor and anti-inflammatory cytokines [IL-10, etc.]) plays a major role in the pathophysiology of systemic inflammatory responses and diseases. Genetic polymorphisms in some of these cytokines have been identified.

There have been three TNF-α polymorphisms, at positions −308, −376, and −238 in the promoter region of the TNF-α gene, each of which consists of a nucleotide guanine (G) in the common allele and an adenosine (A) in the uncommon allele, modifying gene expression. The TNF-α −308A allele has a prevalence of approximately 30% in the general white population. In vitro studies show that a TNF-α −308A variant displays increased gene transcription than in the wild-type allele and is associated with adverse outcome in a variety of infectious and inflammatory diseases, including cerebral malaria, meningococcal disease, and celiac disease. There are few function studies on the TNF-α polymorphisms at positions −376 and −238, but a higher frequency of the mutation at −376 was shown to be present in nonsurvivors of septic shock. The polymorphism at −238 was also reported to be associated with community-acquired pneumonia. The TNF-α promoter gene is in linkage dysequilibrium with several HLA alleles that either may be involved with the control of TNF-α secretion or may be independent risk factors for the development of meningococcal disease or other forms of sepsis.[7,8,12,14,15]

SNPs at positions 1069 and 252 (G to A) in the first intron of the TNF-β gene have been characterized. These variations have been associated with increased secretion of TNF-α in response to sepsis as well as greater susceptibility to severe sepsis and post-traumatic sepsis.[7,8,15-17]

The IL-1 gene complex codes for three different proteins: IL-1α, IL-1β, and IL-1 receptor antagonist (IL-1ra). IL-1 exists in two forms, IL-1α and IL-1β, and is one of the most potent inflammatory agents. IL-1ra, an acute-phase protein produced in response to infection and trauma, appears to protect against these deleterious effects.

There are two biallelic base-exchange polymorphisms within the IL-1β gene. The first, at position −511 in the promoter region (*Ava*I polymorphism), has been associated with febrile seizures in children, variation in serum C-reactive protein CRP level, and severity of meningococcal disease. The second is at 3953 in the fifth axon (*Taq*I polymorphism); the presence of this rare polymorphism has been demonstrated to be associated with higher endotoxin-induced IL-1β production in vitro. In addition, a polymorphic region in the IL-1α gene (intron 6: VNTR, 46 base pairs) has been identified, but functional studies involving this polymorphism have not been described. No association between IL-1α and IL-1β polymorphisms and susceptibility to sepsis has been shown. The IL-1ra gene contains a VNTR of 86 base pairs within intron 2, giving rise to a penta-allelic minisatellite polymorphism. The uncommon allele 2, which consists of two 86–base pair repeats, has been associated with increased IL-1β production. Several studies have demonstrated that a higher frequency of the A2 allele correlates with diverse inflammatory diseases.[7,8,12,14,15]

IL-6 plays an important role in bacterial clearance and initiation of the adaptive immune responses. IL-6 has also been demonstrated to be a marker of severity in sepsis. The G to C polymorphisms at positions −174 and −572 within the promoter region of the IL-6 gene have been identified. The frequency of the IL-6 −174 C allele has been estimated at 40% in a white population. The presence of the C allele in healthy subjects has been associated with lower serum levels of IL-6. In in vitro study, the C allele resulted in suppression of IL-6 transcription in response to endotoxin or IL-1β. Studies also suggested that IL-6 polymorphism is not associated with susceptibility to sepsis, although some studies showed that patients with the −174 GG genotype had a better survival rate than those with the CC genotype.[7,8,14,15]

IL-10 is an anti-inflammatory cytokine that inhibits the innate and adaptive immune response and decreases the production of IL-1, IL-6, and TNF-α by human monocytes. There are three polymorphisms in the promoter region of the IL-10 gene, occurring at −1082 (G to A), −819 (C to T), and −592 (C to A). IL-10 −1082 polymorphic alleles have been associated with susceptibility to meningococcal disease and with adverse clinical outcomes and greater severity of illness in community-acquired pneumonia. Polymorphisms at the other two sites have variably been linked to regulation of gene transcription and are in linkage dysequilibrium.[8,14,15]

Migration inhibitory factor (MIF) is a pro-inflammatory cytokine that plays an important role in the activation of innate and adaptive immune responses by inducing the release of TNF-α, IL-β, and nitric oxide as well as suppressing the glucocorticoid release of anti-inflammatory mediators. Elevated circulating MIF concentrations are seen in humans with severe sepsis and correlate with reduced survival. Polymorphisms in the promoter region of the MIF gene have been identified and include −173 G to C and −794 VNTR of five to eight repeats. The polymorphism at the −173 promoter site (−173 G to C) within the MIF gene is associated with increased MIF expression in healthy subjects and in people with inflammatory arthritis. A higher frequency of the C allele has also been shown in patients with sepsis or sepsis-induced acute lung injury than in controls.[14]

Chemokines

IL-8 and monocyte chemotactic protein-1 (MCP-1) are two potent neutrophil and monocyte chemokines. The IL-8 genetic polymorphism (T to A) in the promoter region at position −251 has been identified. This polymorphism was shown to be associated with increased IL-8 production in whole blood stimulated with lipopolysaccharide. Furthermore, it was associated with some diseases, such as enteroaggregative *Escherichia coli* diarrhea, respiratory syncytial virus infection, and multiple-system atrophy.[8,14]

A genetic polymorphism (G to A) in the 5-flanking region of the MCP-1 gene at position −2518 has been shown to affect MCP-1 expression. The MCP-1 −2518 G allele is associated with higher levels of MCP-1 production by human monocytes. Moreover, the MCP-1 −2518 GG genotype has been found to be associated with higher plasma and urinary MCP-1 levels in patients with lupus nephritis and has been linked to a higher risk for premature failure of kidney grafts.[8]

Coagulation Factors

Cross-talk exists between the inflammatory cascade and the coagulation cascade. Several genetic polymorphisms related to critical illness have been described in genes of hemostatic factors, including factor V and plasminogen activator inhibitor-1 (PAI-1).

Three independent SNPs of factor V in different populations have been described: factor V Cambridge (Arg306Thr), factor V Hong Kong (Arg306Gly), and factor V Leiden (Arg-506Gln). All of the SNPs make factor Va partially resistant to inactivation by activated protein C, thereby yielding a prothrombotic state. The frequency of polymorphism of factor V Leiden is about 5% in white populations. Factor V Leiden heterozygosity was associated with increased incidence of purpura fulminans in children with meningococcal disease. In septic patients, factor V Leiden carrier was associated with lower 28-day mortality and less vasopressor use.[7]

PAI-1 is an important mediator to regulate the fibrinolytic system. It has been reported that PAI-1 plasma concentrations are very high in children with meningococcal sepsis, and the highest concentration was found in severe and fatal disease states. A common functional polymorphism exists in the promoter region of the PAI-1 gene: a single–base pair insertion (5G) or deletion (4G). This polymorphism is important in regulating the expression of the PAI-1 gene and, in response to interleukin 1, laboratory constructs containing the 4G allele have a sixfold increase in the rate of transcription compared to constructs containing the 5G allele. Clinical studies strongly support an association between PAI-1 4G/4G genotype and poor outcome in meningococcal or trauma-induced sepsis.[7,12,18,19]

Other Candidates

Angiotensin-converting enzyme (ACE) is involved in cardiovascular homeostasis, inflammation, and wound healing. An insertion (I)/deletion (D) of a 287–base pair, repeat sequence, restriction fragment length polymorphism was found in the noncoding region of human ACE gene.[7] High plasma and tissue ACE concentrations have been shown to be associated with DD genotype. ACE DD genotype was associated with significantly higher predicted mortality and worse disease severity in patients with meningococcal disease. Patients with acute respiratory distress syndrome (ARDS) had significantly higher frequency of DD genotype and higher mortality compared with ARDS patients with ACE wild type.[20]

Conclusion

In the preceding summaries of the potential candidate genes (listed in Table 2-1), positive or negative associations between a polymorphism and outcome have been identified in studies involving patients with critical illness, but the confidence in such conclusions is often tenuous because of small sizes. Thus, it is unlikely that one polymorphism will result in a particular phenotype, but when several or many polymorphisms act together in the presence of an infection, the disease phenotype associated with a defined outcome, such as increased risk for death, may be apparent.

GENE POLYMORPHISM AND COMMON CRITICAL ILLNESS SYNDROMES

Sepsis/Septic Shock

Sepsis is a systemic response to severe infection. In severe cases, sepsis is complicated with refractory shock and multiple-organ failure and is a leading cause of death in noncoronary patients in intensive care units. The systemic inflammatory response induced by the host innate immune response and the invader is the main pathophysiology of sepsis.

Most patients with infection do not experience severe sepsis and septic shock, but some do have a significantly higher risk of death. In at least one seminal study about adoption and twins, there was a fivefold higher risk of death from infection for a patient whose biological parent died of the same infection.[21] More and more genetic epidemiological studies suggest a strong genetic influence on the outcome of sepsis.

With advances in molecular genetic research leading to an ever-expanding appreciation of the potential role of genetic variation in predisposition to disease, new discoveries have provided insight into susceptibility to a wide range of conditions, including many cancers and autoimmune inflammatory conditions. The discovery of various common genetic polymorphisms in genes that control the inflammatory response has lent credence to this hypothesis. The identified genetic polymorphisms include TNF-α, TNF-β, the IL-1 family, IL-10, CD-14, ACE, mannose-binding lectin, TLR-4, TLR-2, PAI-1, and the factor V mutation (discussed previously). These polymorphisms are reported to be associated to different extents with the outcome of sepsis.

Acute Lung Injury–Acute Respiratory Distress Syndrome

Acute lung injury–acute respiratory distress syndrome (ALI/ARDS) is also common in the intensive care unit. It is characterized by severe hypoxemia and an unacceptably high mortality. ALI is different from ARDS in severity of injury. ARDS is the severe stage of ALI. Survival of ALI appears to be influenced by the stress generated by trauma and by sepsis-associated factors, which initiate and amplify the inflammatory response in the disease. Emerging evidence also suggests that genetic factors are associated with susceptibility to ALI. Both a nonsynonymous SNP in the surfactant protein B gene and an intronic SNP in the ACE gene have been reported to contribute to the susceptibility and outcome of patients with ALI.[22] However, the sporadic nature of ALI and the lack of family-based cohort studies preclude conventional genomic approaches such as linkage mapping. A newer strategy, the candidate gene approach discussed previously, is a robust method to identify novel biochemical and genetic markers and may provide unique insights into the pathogenic mechanisms and the genetic basis of ALI. This approach uses extensive gene expression profiling studies in animal and human models of ALI to identify potential ALI candidate genes associated with sepsis and ventilator-associated lung injury. These studies suggest that both novel (pre–B cell colony-enhancing factor, myosin light chain kinase) and previously identified (IL-6, MIF) gene candidates contribute to susceptibility to and outcome of ALI.[22-25]

CURRENT RESEARCH LIMITATIONS AND FUTURE DIRECTIONS

Until now, case-control studies were the primary methods by which genetic polymorphism research was conducted. Case-control studies involve comparing the prevalence of a genetic marker in a group of unrelated people to the prevalence of the same marker in a healthy control population. The major limitations of such studies are the small sample sizes, because the results are accounted for by chance. Results of such studies are often applied to the general population, even though they may be biased owing to variance in the frequency of genetic polymorphisms in some ethnic or geographic groups but not others. The solution to this problem would be to carefully select cases and controls for the studies. In particular, information about age, gender, environmental factors, and infections should all be accessible for better understanding of the case study. Another way of ensuring the accuracy of a case study of a population is to make sure that the control group is in Hardy-Weinberg equilibrium. If it is not, unusual genetic instances, such as new mutations, inbreeding, and genetic drift, occur.[4,8]

Survival bias is also a concern in genetic polymorphism research. It occurs when genetic markers are the basis by which mortality is evaluated. In order to avoid this bias, case-control studies that have considered and matched variables such as age should be conducted. Another bias common in genetic association studies is observer bias, which can stem from genotyping error. This issue can be easily resolved through the use of two independent genotypers. It is also necessary to repeatedly carry out the genotyping in different, randomly chosen subgroups in order to ensure accuracy.

Currently, two types of complementary screening strategies are available. These techniques allow for the understanding of the genetic basis in complicated diseases such as sepsis. One method is to screen a high number of alleles in a few patients with techniques such as oligonucleotide microarrays. Although expensive, this method allows for the confirmation of the interactive role of genes.

TABLE 2-1

Potential Gene Polymorphisms Related to Critical Illness

GENES	SITE	POSITION(S)	VARIATIONS	FREQUENCY (%)	FUNCTION	ASSOCIATION
Recognize Molecules						
TLR2	Exon	+677	Arg → Trp	2	Decreased production of IL-12 Inhibition of NF-κB activation	Susceptibility to leprosy Risk factor for *Mycobacterium tuberculosis*
TLR4	Exon	+753	Arg → Gln	2.5	Decreased NF-κB activation	Risk for deadly infection
	Exon	+299	Asp → Gly	5	Inhibition of NF-κB translocation	Susceptibility to gram-negative infection
		+399	Thr → Ile		Reduced IL-1α	Severe infections
TLR5	Exon	+392	Arg → TER	7.5	Decreased NF-κB activation	Association with legionnaire's disease
CD14	Promoter	+159	C to T	43	Increased levels of soluble CD14	Association with susceptibility and mortality in septic shock
MBL	Exon	+52	Arg → Cys (variant D)	5	Low MBL serum levels	Deficiency associated with susceptibility to infections
	Exon	+54	Gly → Asp (variant B)	14		
	Exon	+57	Gly → Glu (variant C)	5		
Cytokines						
TNF-α	Promoter	−308	G to A	30	Increased circulating TNF-α	Increased susceptibility and mortality to septic shock Associated with death from meningococcal disease
TNF-β	Intron	+1069	G to A	Unknown	Increased circulating TNF-α	Susceptibility to severe sepsis and posttraumatic sepsis
IL-1 receptor agonist	Intron	Intron 2	86–base pair VNTRs	23	Increased IL-1β production	Susceptibility to sepsis Endothelial activation markers in acute coronary syndrome
IL-6	Promoter	−174	G to C	40	Lowered IL-6 serum level	Possible association of GG genotype with improved survival
IL-10	Promoter	−592	C to A	33	Reduced IL-10 levels	Increased mortality with sepsis
		−1082	G to A	49		Severity of illness in community-acquired pneumonia
		−819	C to T	21		Greater risk with sepsis
Migration inhibitory factor (MIF)	Promoter	−173	G to C	19	Reduced MIF levels	Increased frequency in the C allele in sepsis
Chemokines						
IL-8	Promoter	−251	A to T	36	Increased IL-8 production	Related to respiratory syncytial virus bronchiolitis
		−845	C to T			Severity of lupus nephritis
MCP-1	Promoter	−2518	G to A	4.3	Increased MCP-1 production	Association of GG genotype with higher risk for premature kidney graft failure
Coagulation Factors						
Factor V	Exon	+506	Arg → Gln	5	Lower mortality in factor V Leiden mice than in wild-type controls	Lower mortality, lesser vasopressor use in heterozygotes
PAI-1	Promoter		4G/5G	13	Increased PAI-1 transcription	Strong association of 4G allele with poor outcome of sepsis
Other						
ACE	Promoter		I/D	II: 52 ID: 40 DD: 8	Higher ACE level with DD genotype	DD genotype associated with higher mortality in sepsis and acute respiratory distress syndrome

A, adenine; ACE, angiotensin-converting enzyme; Arg, arginine; Asp, aspartic acid; C, cytosine; D, deletion; G, guanine; Gln, glutamine; Gly, glycine; I, insertion; IL, interleukin; Ile, isoleucine; MCP-1, monocyte chemotactic protein-1; MLB, mannose-binding lectin; NF-κB, nuclear factor-κB; PAI-1, plasminogen activator inhibitor-1; T, thymine; TER, termination; TLR, Toll-like receptor; TNF, Tumor necrosis factor; Trp, tryptophan; VNTRs, variable number of tandem repeats.

Eventually, this method of screening will also be used to identify new genetic markers. The second method of screening involves using techniques such as template-directed insertion and fluorescence detection, which search for a few markers in a large group of people. This method studies and either confirms or excludes the specific roles of certain alleles as they pertain to the pathogenesis of diseases such as sepsis. This method is beneficial owing to its inexpensive nature and its application in large-scale analysis. Unfortunately, a drawback is that it cannot detect new genetic markers.

The use of haplotypes, which are inherited sets of linked SNPs, as the units of genetic variation in association studies and the marking of these haplotypes with unique "tag SNPs" may help narrow the search for causal SNPs. The associations and the identification of a few alleles of a haplotype bloc can unambiguously identify all other polymorphic sites in its region. With simultaneous examination of multiple markers in a haplotype, the overall linkage dysequilibrium is less variable and exists in simpler patterns.

In brief, genetic epidemiology studies may help unravel the relative importance of genetic markers in predicting the development of critical illness. Future studies on genetic variation and critical illness would be large prospective cohort studies with strong correlation between these genetic markers and the progression of critical illness. Function studies and careful characterization of intermediate phenotypes must be done to lend biological plausibility to genotype-phenotype associations. Examination of associations between genetic polymorphisms and critical illness promises to provide clinicians with new tools to evaluate prognosis, to intervene early and aggressively in treating high-risk patients, and to avoid the use of therapies with adverse effects in treating low-risk patients.[12,26,27]

Key Points

1. Genetic polymorphisms can affect the systemic inflammation response.
2. Some potential gene polymorphisms, such as tumor necrosis factor-α, Toll-like receptor-4, CD14, and interleukin-6, have been shown to alter the susceptibility to and outcome of critical illness in small studies.
3. Inconsistencies exist in the literature regarding the association between genetic variants and disease susceptibility and prognosis. The reasons for these are multifactorial and include study design and the complexities introduced by background genetic heterogeneity.
4. Future study of genetic variation would be improved by large prospective cohort studies with strong correlation between the genetic markers and progression of critical illness.
5. Future treatment regimens for critically ill patients are likely to be designed to target specific genotypes and associated cellular responses, maximizing clinical response and patient safety.

Key References

3. Villar J, Maca-Meyer N, Pérez-Méndez L, Flores C: Bench-to-bedside review: Understanding genetic predisposition to sepsis. Crit Care 2004;86:180-189.
8. Jaber BL, Pereira BJ, Bonventre JV, Balakrishnan VS: Polymorphism of host response genes: Implications in the pathogenesis and treatment of acute renal failure. Kidney Int 2005;67:14-33.
9. Vitali SH, Randolph AG: Assessing the quality of case-control association studies on the genetic basis of sepsis. Pediatr Crit Care Med 2005;6:S74-S77.
12. Tabrizi AR, Zehnbauer BA, Freeman BD, Buchman TG: Genetic markers in sepsis. J Am Coll Surg 2001;192:106-117.

See the companion Expert Consult website for the complete reference list.

CHAPTER 3

Fundamentals of Oxygen Delivery

James Yassin and Mervyn Singer

OBJECTIVES

This chapter will:
1. Explain the need for oxygen.
2. Discuss factors influencing arterial oxygen tension.
3. Describe the calculation of global oxygen delivery.
4. Discuss the causes of hypoxia.

A proportion of oxygen consumed by the body is required for generation of reactive oxygen species by leukocytes and for intracellular and intercellular signaling; some is utilized for enzymatic reactions, for example oxidases; however, more than 90% of oxygen is used for oxidative phosphorylation by the mitochondrion for generation of energy in the form of adenosine triphosphate (ATP) and heat.

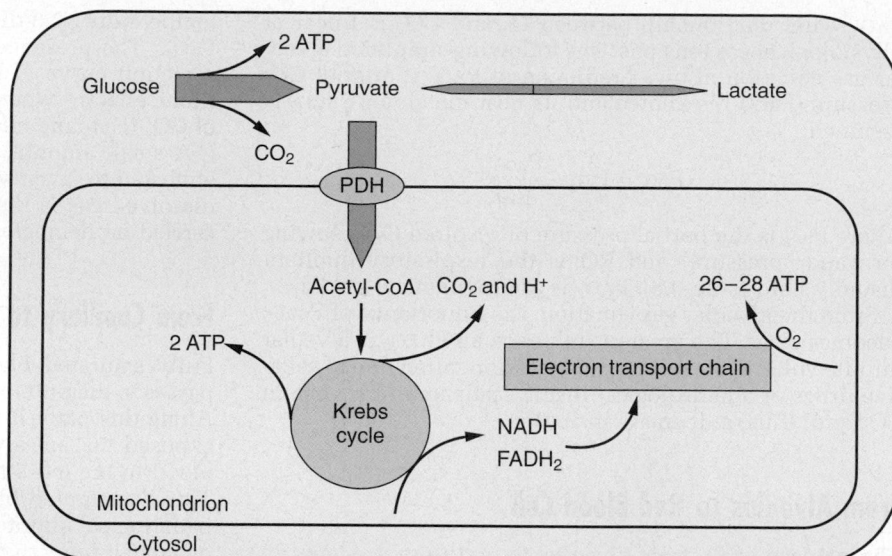

FIGURE 3-1. Aerobic and anaerobic generation of adenosine triphosphate (ATP) from glucose. CoA, coenzyme A; $FADH_2$, flavin adenine dinucleotide hydroxide [reduced form]; NADH, nicotinamide adenine dinucleotide, reduced; PDH, phosphate dehydrogenase.

Aerobic metabolism maximizes energy generation from available substrate. For every mole of glucose, 2 molecules of ATP are generated by glycolysis, 2 by the Krebs cycle, and 26 to 28 by the electron transport chain (Fig. 3-1). Apart from certain cells, such as erythrocytes, which rely totally on glycolytic ATP, and neutrophils, which are predominantly glycolytic, most cell types rely on aerobic ATP production for most of their functions.

Failure of aerobic metabolism, because of either insufficient delivery of O_2 or reduced cellular utilization, results in a greater dependence on anaerobic metabolism. Although glycolytic activity can upregulate to a certain degree, this process has the disadvantage of a greatly reduced energy generation per unit of substrate and a potential inability to meet any shortfall in cellular energy requirements. Enhanced glycolysis also increases production of byproducts such as hydrogen ions (H^+), carbon dioxide (CO_2), and lactate through increased activity of lactate dehydrogenase and decreased activity of pyruvate dehydrogenase.[1] Although traditionally perceived as negative, these byproducts serve adaptive roles that may assist cell function and integrity in critical illness—for example, a right shift of the oxyhemoglobin dissociation curve, alternative substrate provision through lactate, and vasodilatation through activation of targeted ion channels.

OXYGEN DELIVERY

Oxygen delivery to the cells occurs in the following stages:
1. Passage of O_2 to the alveolus.
2. Transfer of O_2 from the alveolus to the red blood cell.
3. Movement of O_2 from the alveolar capillary to the pulmonary vein.
4. Transport of O_2 to the tissues.
5. Cellular uptake of O_2.

Figure 3-2 shows the "oxygen cascade." O_2 tension falls progressively from inspired air (approximately 21 kPa) to the level of the mitochondrion (estimated to be 0.1-1 kPa), with shunt and diffusion being represented within the lungs.

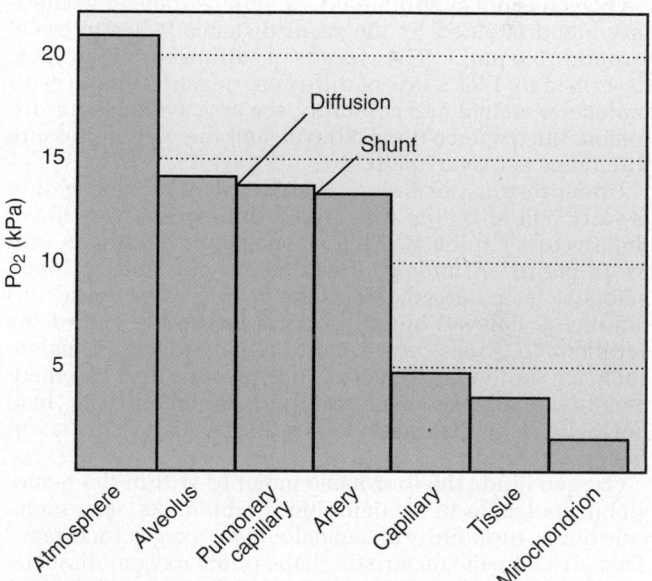

FIGURE 3-2. "Oxygen cascade" from air to mitochondrion.

Alveolar Oxygen

The partial pressure of O_2 in the alveolus (PA_{O_2}) is influenced by a number of factors. At sea level, PO_2 is 21 kPa, (21% of atmospheric pressure [P_{atm}]). Under physiological conditions, a tidal breath passes to the carina, and the air is warmed and humidified. As a result of the addition of saturated vapor pressure (6 kPa), the PO_2 drops to 19.7 kPa (= 21 × [100 − 6]). This drop is not significant at sea level but becomes very important to a person breathing rarefied air, for example, at the summit of Mount Everest.

Under conditions of constant O_2 utilization and CO_2 production, PA_{O_2} is influenced primarily by PA_{CO_2}, because the partial pressures of the other constituents of air (mostly nitrogen) are relatively stable. An increase in PA_{CO_2} as a result of reduced alveolar ventilation (V_A), increased physiological dead space, or increased CO_2 production decreases

PaO_2. This relationship between O_2 and CO_2 is linear at physiological gas tensions. The following simplified alveolar gas equation allows prediction of PaO_2 if arterial CO_2 pressure ($PacO_2$) is known and its near match for $PacO_2$ is assumed:

$$PaO_2 = PIO_2 - \frac{PacO_2}{RQ}$$

where PIO_2 is the partial pressure of inspired O_2 (allowing for vapor pressure) and RQ is the respiratory quotient (usually held to be 0.8). PaO_2 is approximately 13 kPa.

From the alveolar gas equation, the importance of $PacO_2$ becomes clear. The greatest influence on $PacO_2$ is alveolar minute volume. Respiratory depression, often due to sedative drugs or a neurological insult, leads to an increase in CO_2 and, thus, a decrease in PaO_2.

From Alveolus to Red Blood Cell

The passage of O_2 from alveolus to erythrocyte occurs in two stages. First, the gas diffuses across the basement membrane into the capillary and, second, the O_2 binds to hemoglobin.

Oxygen is not as soluble as CO_2, and its transfer to capillary blood is aided by the small distance it has to travel (around 0.6 μm).[2] The speed of diffusion of oxygen, described by Fick's law of diffusion, depends on oxygen's molecular weight and solubility, the area available for diffusion, the distance it must travel, and the partial pressure difference across its path.

Under resting physiological circumstances, hemoglobin is fully bound by the time it is a third of the way down the alveolar capillary.[3] Thus, hemoglobin binding is said to be *perfusion limited*. If cardiac output, and so blood velocity, is increased, for example during exercise, full binding is delayed but still occurs before the end of the capillary. In disease, any condition that reduces diffusion, such as pulmonary edema, lung fibrosis, or basement membrane disease, may result in an inability to load hemoglobin by the time it leaves the capillary. This is *diffusion limitation*.

Oxygen binds the four heme moieties within the hemoglobin molecule in a homotropic fashion. As each molecule binds, the affinity of hemoglobin for oxygen increases.[4] This gives the characteristic shape of the oxygen dissociation curve (Fig. 3-3). Hemoglobin's affinity for O_2 is also heterotropic and is influenced by the H^+ concentration,

temperature, 2,3-diphosphoglycerate concentration, and PcO_2.[5] The presence of H^+ and CO_2 shifts the oxygen dissociation curve to the right and so facilitates O_2 release (Bohr effect),[6] whereas binding of O_2 leads to the release of CO_2 (Haldane effect).[7]

A small amount of O_2 also dissolves in blood. At one atmosphere, even when supplementary O_2 is given, this dissolved gas is insignificant compared with the amount carried on hemoglobin.

From Capillary to Pulmonary Vein

Fully saturated blood leaves the alveolar capillary and passes to the pulmonary vein and thence to the left atrium. Along this path, it is mixed with blood that has not been exposed to an alveolus, so the overall saturation of blood in the left atrium is lower than would be expected. This desaturated blood is the result of physiological and pathological shunt (*true* shunt) and ventilation-perfusion mismatch (*effective* shunt). The desaturated blood, called *venous admixture*, is the theoretical volume of blood that would need to be added to fully saturated arterial blood to produce the observed arterial oxygen saturation (SaO_2).

Physiological shunt allows desaturated venous blood into the systemic circulation via normal vascular anatomy, for example, thebesian veins and venous drainage of the bronchial tree. This is usually a small fraction of cardiac output.

Pathological shunt may be caused by pulmonary arteriovenous malformations or right-to-left cardiac septal defects. This shunt also depresses the arterial PO_2 but, importantly for both physiological and pathological shunts, neither can be improved by the administration of 100% O_2, because nowhere in its path would the blood be exposed to the oxygen, and the increased PIO_2 would have little effect on the already fully saturated blood passing through the alveoli.

Under physiological conditions in the standing subject, ventilation and perfusion of the lung are approximately matched. Thus, alveoli with a good blood supply are well ventilated, and vice versa. Both ventilation and perfusion are greater in the dependent parts of the lung. This effect is due, in part, to the action of gravity on the weight of the lung tissue itself and the column of blood.[8] Any condition that alters the ratio of ventilation and perfusion may allow desaturated blood to reach the systemic circulation.

Transfer to the Tissues

The amount of oxygen delivered to the tissues is a product of the oxygen content per unit volume of blood and the cardiac output. The arterial O_2 content (CaO_2) depends on the amount of hemoglobin and its saturation. There is also a small addition for the O_2 dissolved in plasma, as discussed earlier. Arterial oxygen content is calculated as follows:

$$CaO_2 = (Hb \times SaO_2 \times 1.39) + (PaO_2 \times 0.02)$$

where CaO_2 is the arterial O_2 content in mL per 100 mL of blood; Hb is the hemoglobin concentration in g/dL; PaO_2 is the arterial PO_2 in kPa; and 1.39 is Huffner's constant, which refers to the amount of O_2 (mL) that a gram of hemoglobin can hold.

Every liter of blood in a healthy subject breathing room air at one atmosphere carries approximately 200 mL of O_2. If this amount is then multiplied by cardiac output (CO),

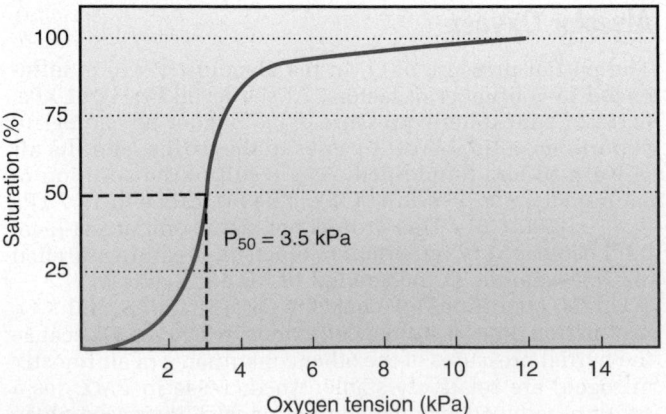

FIGURE 3-3. Oxyhemoglobin dissociation curve.

the global O_2 delivery (DO_2) in a resting adult is approximately 1000 mL/min, calculated as follows:

$$DO_2 = Cao_2 \times CO$$

A thousand milliliters of O_2 is ejected from the left ventricle every minute. This represents the global O_2 delivery but does not indicate delivery to individual vascular beds—splanchnic, renal, cerebral, and so on. Each of these beds can regulate its own blood flow[9-11] and, with the exception of the coronary system, can alter the amount of O_2 removed from its regional circulation.[12]

Cellular Uptake

The PO_2 within mitochondria is extremely low, being estimated on the order of 0.1 to 1 kPa.[13] This varies between cell types and is intimately related to cytosolic PO_2. In order to enter the cell, the O_2 molecules must first dissociate from the erythrocyte hemoglobin. This process is aided by the presence of CO_2 and H^+ ions in the capillary, as previously described.[14] Once released, O_2 can then diffuse down its "tension gradient" into the cell, and thus becomes available to the mitochondrion.

The site of O_2 transfer into the tissue is the subject of current research. Investigators have measured a large drop in PO_2 across the terminal arteriole—less change in the capillary than might be expected—and an increase in PO_2 in the postcapillary venule.[15] The reasons for this finding are unclear, but suggestions include protection of the capillary bed from hyperoxia (and thus increased free radical production) by a "countercurrent" transfer of O_2 from arteriole to venule.[16] The countercurrent transport of CO_2 also allows the capillary pH to remain low and so increases the efficiency of O_2 offloading from hemoglobin for a given PO_2.[17] This process may be affected by anything that prevents unloading of O_2 from the red cell, by increased distance from the capillary to the mitochondrion, or by any inability of the mitochondrion to use the O_2 for aerobic respiration.

HYPOXIA

Hypoxia is defined as the point at which aerobic respiration ceases, further metabolism continuing anaerobically. Hypoxia may occur with a "normal" PaO_2. *Hypoxemia* is defined as a low arterial oxygen tension, using an arbitrary cutoff of 8 kPa in room air. The two terms are not interchangeable, and this chapter discusses only hypoxia and its causes.

According to the staging system of oxygen delivery already described, the causes of hypoxia can be categorized as hypoxic, anemic, or circulatory hypoxia and cytopathic dysoxia (Table 3-1).

Hypoxic hypoxia is the result of a failure of gas exchange and/or an increase in venous admixture. Its causes are many, including chronic obstructive pulmonary disease (COPD), collapse/consolidation, lung fibrosis, and intracardiac shunts. This condition may respond to administration of oxygen, provided that shunt is not a predominant feature.

Anemic hypoxia may be treated by infusion of red blood cells. The hemoglobin concentration at which oxygen delivery is insufficient depends on oxygen requirements. In healthy volunteers a concentration of 3 g/dL may be tolerated.[18] In the critically ill population, a target of

TABLE 3-1

Causes of Hypoxia

MECHANISM	EXAMPLES OF CAUSES
↓ O_2 content:	
↓ PAO_2	↓ inspired O_2
	↓ minute ventilation
↓ diffusion	Pulmonary edema
	Pneumonia
	Fibrosis
↓ binding to hemoglobin	Abnormal hemoglobin
	Carbon monoxide poisoning
	Acidosis
↑ admixture anemia	↑ venous admixture
↓ cardiac output	Hypovolemia
	Heart failure
↓ peripheral O_2 offloading	Alkalosis
↓ cellular utilization	Sepsis
	Cyanide poisoning
	Carbon monoxide poisoning
	Drugs with mitochondrial toxicity, e.g., non-nucleoside reverse transcriptase inhibitors used in therapy for human immunodeficiency virus

7 g/dL has been shown to be sufficient for most patients,[19] but uncertainty remains about the optimal value in patients with cardiorespiratory failure. An outcome study investigating early, goal-directed resuscitation of patients with early sepsis targeted a hematocrit value of 30%.[20]

Circulatory hypoxia refers to hypoxia in the patient with an inadequate cardiac index, although it can perhaps be extended to microcirculatory dysfunction, in the light of new information about regional microcirculatory disturbances despite an apparently adequate macrocirculation.[21] If the problem is due to inadequate ventricular filling, blood or another intravenous fluid should be administered. Low cardiac output due to poor ventricular function (left or right) may respond to vasoactive drugs; the cause should be identified and, if possible, specifically treated, for example with revascularization.

Cytopathic dysoxia, the final cause to consider, results from an inability of the mitochondrial electron transport chain to utilize available O_2. It may be caused by damage to or inhibition of the respiratory enzymes involved in oxidative phosphorylation. In sepsis, the electron transport chain is inhibited (or damaged) by nitric oxide and other reactive species.[22,23] Other causes are cyanide or carbon monoxide poisoning, owing to the binding of these substances to the ferric ion of cytochrome oxidase (complex IV of the electron transport chain) which thereby inhibits its ability to function normally.[24]

CONCLUSION

A series of steps is needed to transport oxygen from the atmosphere to the mitochondrion, where the bulk of it is used for generation of energy. Understanding of this pathway greatly aids the diagnosis and management of the hypoxic patient. Cellular uptake of O_2 is still incompletely characterized, and further research will better elucidate physiological control mechanisms and processes that occur during pathological states.

Key Points

1. Oxygen is vital for effective respiration.
2. An understanding of the stages of oxygen delivery allows diagnosis of the cause of hypoxia.
3. Appreciation of the cause of hypoxia leads to effective treatment.

Key References

7. Christiansen J, Douglas CG, Haldane JS: The absorption and dissociation of carbon dioxide by human blood. J Physiol (Lond) 1914;48:244-271.

10. Navar LG: Renal autoregulation: Perspectives from whole kidney and single nephron studies. Am J Physiol Renal Physiol 1978;234:F357-F370.
21. Elbers PW, Ince C: Mechanisms of critical illness—classifying microcirculatory flow abnormalities in distributive shock. Crit Care 2006;10:221.
22. Boekstegers P, Weidenhofer S, Kapsner T, Werden K: Skeletal muscle partial pressure of oxygen in patients with sepsis. Crit Care Med 1994;22:640-650.
23. Brealey D, Brand M, Hargreaves I, et al: Association between mitochondrial dysfunction and severity and outcome of septic shock. Lancet 2002;360:219-222.

See the companion Expert Consult website for the complete reference list.

CHAPTER 4

Mechanical Ventilation

David J. Dries and John J. Marini

OBJECTIVES

This chapter will:
1. Describe the physiological basis of mechanical ventilatory support.
2. Discuss pressure- and volume-targeted ventilation.
3. Review common modes of mechanical ventilation.
4. Present principles of ventilator care for common forms of pulmonary dysfunction.
5. Introduce applications of noninvasive ventilation.

PHYSIOLOGY

Positive-pressure ventilation as currently known came into its own during the poliomyelitis epidemics of the 1950s.[1] Since that time, mechanical ventilatory support has become emblematic of critical care medicine. Early ventilation used neuromuscular blocking agents to control patient respiratory efforts. Today, maintaining patient control of ventilation is encouraged, and awareness of the complications associated with neuromuscular blockade is growing.[2] Importantly, the increasing recognition that ventilators can induce various forms of lung injury has led to reappraisal of the goals of ventilatory support.[3] Although it seems that intricate new modes of mechanical ventilation have been introduced to clinical practice, the fundamental principles of ventilatory management of critically ill patients remain unchanged.

Positive-pressure ventilation can be lifesaving in patients with hypoxemia or respiratory acidosis that is refractory to simpler measures (Fig. 4-1). In patients with severe cardiopulmonary distress and excessive work of breathing, mechanical ventilation effectively augments the force of the respiratory muscles.[4] In the setting of respiratory distress, ventilatory muscles may account for as much as 40% of total oxygen consumption.[5] Under these circumstances, relief of the breathing workload by mechanical ventilation allows diversion of oxygenated blood to other tissue beds that may be vulnerable to ischemia. Reversal of fatigue, which may contribute to respiratory failure, depends on the respiratory muscle rest that mechanical ventilation affords. Positive-pressure ventilation can reverse or prevent atelectasis through recruitment and prevention of collapse. Although mechanical ventilation is not therapeutic in and of itself, improved gas exchange and relief from excessive respiratory muscle work give the lungs and airways a chance to heal. Conversely, high ventilatory pressures may aggravate or initiate alveolar damage. These dangers of ventilator-induced lung injury have led to reappraisal of the objectives of mechanical ventilation. Rather than seeking normal arterial blood gas values, it is often better to accept a degree of respiratory acidosis and, possibly, relative hypoxemia so as to avoid large tidal volumes and high inflation pressures.

Mechanical ventilation strategies should be tailored to the underlying pulmonary disease. For example, in patients with acute respiratory failure, chronic obstructive pulmonary disease, asthma, or other conditions associated with a high minute ventilation, gas trapping develops in alveoli because patients have inadequate expiratory time available before the next breath begins. Patients experiencing this "breath stacking" have residual positive end-expiratory pressure (PEEP) that was not set by the clinician, termed *auto-PEEP*. Retained peripheral gas makes triggering the ventilator difficult, because the patient must generate a negative pressure equal in magnitude to the level of auto-PEEP in addition to the trigger threshold of

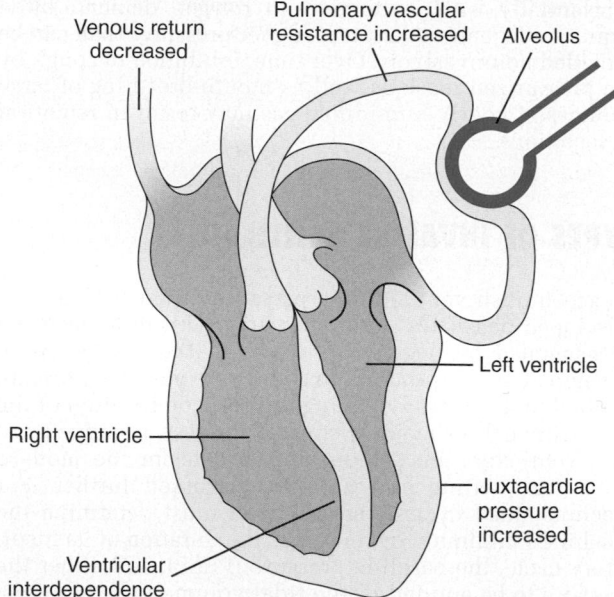

FIGURE 4-1. Factors responsible for the hemodynamic effects seen with positive-pressure ventilation. A drop in intrathoracic pressure compresses the vena cava and thus decreases venous return. Alveolar distention compresses the alveolar vessels, and the resulting increases in pulmonary vascular resistance and right ventricular afterload produce a leftward shift in the interventricular septum. Left ventricular compliance is reduced by both the bulging septum and the higher juxtacardiac pressure resulting from distended lungs. (Adapted from Tobin MJ: Mechanical ventilation. N Engl J Med 1994;330:1056-1061.)

the machine. This is one factor that may contribute to a patient's inability to trigger the ventilator despite obvious respiratory effort. Auto-PEEP may remain undetected (on the pressure tracing) because it is not routinely registered during tidal cycles. Persistent end-expiratory flow driven by the excess pressure provides the clue. Newer machines have software to detect auto-PEEP under controlled conditions. In older machines, occluding the expiratory port of the circuit at the end of expiration in a fully relaxed patient causes pressure in the lungs and ventilator circuit to equilibrate and the level of auto-PEEP to be displayed on the manometer.[6] If auto-PEEP or breath stacking is detected, improving airflow resistance, extending the expiratory time, and reducing the minute ventilation help reverse the process.

INDICATIONS FOR MECHANICAL VENTILATION

Although often made concurrently, the decisions to institute or withdraw mechanical support should be made independently of those to perform tracheal intubation or use positive end-expiratory pressure. This statement is especially true in light of improved noninvasive (nasal and mask) options for supporting ventilation with continuous positive airway pressure (CPAP).[7] As the ventilator assumes the work of breathing, important changes occur in pleural pressure, ventilation distribution, and cardiac output. Mechanical assistance may be needed because

oxygenation cannot be achieved with an acceptable F_{IO_2} without manipulation of PEEP, mean airway pressure, and the pattern of ventilation or because spontaneous ventilation places excessive demands on ventilatory muscles or on a compromised cardiovascular system.[8] Relief of the work of breathing simultaneously reduces the associated need for cardiac output, diminishes oxygen extraction, and improves oxygenation efficiency.

Inadequate Alveolar Ventilation

When other therapeutic measures are insufficient to avert apnea and ventilatory deterioration, mechanical breathing assistance is clearly indicated. In such cases, there are usually signs of respiratory distress or advancing obtundation, and serial blood gas measurements show a falling blood pH and a stable or rising $PaCO_2$. Although few clinicians would withhold mechanical assistance in the patient in whom blood pH trends steadily downward and there are signs of physiological intolerance, there is less agreement about the absolute values of $PaCO_2$ and blood pH that warrant such intervention; these values clearly vary with the specific clinical setting and the duration of the abnormality. In fact, after intubation has been accomplished, pH and $PaCO_2$ values may be deliberately allowed to drift far outside the normal range to avoid the high ventilating pressures and tidal volumes that tend to induce lung damage. This strategy—*permissive hypercapnia*—is now considered integral to a lung-protective ventilatory approach to the acute management of severe asthma and adult respiratory distress syndrome.[9] Acute hypercapnia has well-known and potentially adverse physiological consequences. Nonetheless, experimental work in varied models of clinical problems—notably, ischemia-reperfusion and ventilator-induced lung injury—clearly indicates that certain forms of cellular injury are actually attenuated by hypercapnia. Whether it is hypercapnia itself or the associated change in hydrogen ion concentration that exerts the attenuating effect is still a subject of investigation.

Blood pH is generally a better indicator than $PaCO_2$ of the need for ventilatory support. Hypercapnia per se should not prompt aggressive intervention if pH remains acceptable and the patient remains alert, especially if CO_2 retention occurs slowly. Many patients require ventilatory assistance despite levels of alveolar ventilation that would be appropriate to normal resting metabolism. For example, in patients with metabolic acidosis and neuromuscular weakness or airflow obstruction, $PaCO_2$ may drop to 40 mm Hg or less but not sufficiently to prevent acidemia. The physiological consequences of altered pH are still debated and clearly depend on the underlying pathophysiology and comorbidities. However, if not quickly reversible by simpler measures, a sustained pH greater than 7.65 but less than 7.10 is often considered sufficiently dangerous in itself to require correction by mechanical ventilation. Inside these extremes, the threshold for initiating support varies with the clinical setting.[8] For example, a lethargic patient with asthma who is struggling to breathe can maintain a normal pH until shortly before suffering a respiratory arrest, whereas in an alert cooperative patient with chronically blunted respiratory drive, pH may fall to 7.25 or lower before the patient recovers uneventfully in response to aggressive bronchodilation, corticosteroids, and oxygen. In less obvious situations, the decision to ventilate should be guided by trends in pH, arterial blood gas values, mental status, dyspnea, hemodynamic stability, and response to therapy. The ongoing need for ventilatory assistance must be repeatedly assessed.

Inadequate Oxygenation

Arterial oxygenation results from complex interactions between systemic oxygen demand, cardiovascular adequacy, and the efficiency of pulmonary oxygen exchange. Improving cardiovascular performance and minimizing O_2 consumption (by reducing fever, agitation, pain, etc.) may dramatically improve the balance between delivery and consumption of oxygen. Transpulmonary oxygen exchange can be aided by supplementing FIO_2 by using PEEP, by changing the pattern of ventilation to increase mean airway pressure (and consequently, mean alveolar pressure and average lung size), or by prone positioning. In patients with edematous or injured lungs, relief of an excessive breathing workload may improve oxygenation by relaxing the expiratory muscles and allowing mixed venous O_2 saturation to improve, thereby reducing the venous admixture.[10]

Modest fractions of inspired oxygen are administered to nonintubated patients by means of masks or nasal cannulas. Controlled O_2 therapy is best delivered to the nonintubated patient with a well-fitting Venturi mask, which keeps FIO_2 nearly constant despite changes in inspiratory flow requirements. Without tracheal intubation or a sealed noninvasive ventilation interface, delivery of high FIO_2 can be achieved only with a tight-fitting, nonrebreathing mask that is flushed with high flows of pure O_2. Unfortunately, apart from the risk of O_2 toxicity, such a mask often becomes displaced or must be removed intentionally for eating or expectoration. Intubation facilitates the application of PEEP and CPAP needed to avert oxygen toxicity and enables extraction of airway secretions.

Excessive Respiratory Workload

A common reason for mechanical assistance is to amplify ventilatory power. The respiratory muscles cannot sustain tidal pressures greater than 40% to 50% of their maximal isometric pressure. Respiratory pressure requirements rise with minute ventilation and the impedance to breathing. Patients with hypermetabolism or metabolic acidosis often need ventilatory support to avoid decompensation. Impairment of ventilatory drive or muscle strength diminishes ventilatory capacity and reserve.

Although little effort is expended by normal subjects who breathe quietly, the O_2 demands of the respiratory system account for a very high percentage of total body oxygen consumption ($\dot{V}O_2$) during periods of physiological stress.[5,10] Experimental animals in circulatory shock that receive mechanical ventilation survive longer than their unassisted counterparts. Moreover, in patients with combined cardiorespiratory disease, attempts to withdraw ventilatory support for cardiac rather than respiratory reasons often fail. Such observations demonstrate the importance of minimizing the ventilatory O_2 requirement during cardiac insufficiency or ischemia to rebalance myocardial O_2 supply with requirements and/or allow diaphragmatic blood flow to be redirected to other oxygen-deprived vital organs. Moreover, reducing ventilatory effort may improve afterload to the left ventricle. Although it is possible to use noninvasive ventilation or CPAP alone in patients affected by cardiac insufficiency, fatigue often sets in unless underlying oxygen requirements are reduced

substantially; such reduction in oxygen demand often requires adequate sedation or higher pressures than can be provided noninvasively. Over time, inhibition of cough by the pressurized mask as well as mouth-breathing of large volumes of poorly humidified gas may result in retention of secretions.

TYPES OF INVASIVE VENTILATION

To accomplish ventilation, a pressure difference must be developed phasically across the lung. This difference can be generated by negative pressure in the pleural space developed by respiratory muscles, by positive pressure applied to the airway opening, or by a combination of the two. Although of major historical interest, negative-pressure ventilators are seldom appropriate for the modern acute care setting and are not discussed further. For machine-aided cycles, the clinician must determine the machine's minimum cycling rate, the duration of its inspiratory cycle, the baseline pressure (PEEP), and either the pressure to be applied or the tidal volume to be administered, depending on the mode selected.[4]

Positive-pressure inflation can be achieved with machines that control *either* of the two determinants of ventilating power—pressure or flow—and that terminate inspiration according to pressure, flow, volume, or time limits.[4,11-13] The waveforms of both flow and pressure cannot be controlled *simultaneously*, however, because pressure is developed as a function of flow and the impedance to breathing, which is unalterably determined by the uncontrolled parameters of resistance and compliance. Thus, the clinician has the choice of controlling pressure, with tidal volume as a resulting (dependent) variable, or of controlling flow, with pressure as the dependent variable. Although older ventilators offered only a single control variable and single cycling criterion, positive-pressure ventilators of the latest generation enable the clinician to select freely among multiple options.

Pressure-Preset (Pressure-Targeted) Ventilation

Modern ventilators provide pressure-preset or pressure-targeted (e.g., pressure-control or pressure-support) ventilatory modes as options for full or partial ventilatory assistance. After the breath is initiated, these modes quickly attain a targeted amount of pressure at the airway opening until a specified time (pressure-control) or flow (pressure-support) cycling criterion is met. Maximal pressure is controlled, but tidal volume is a complex function of applied pressure and its rate of approach to target pressure, available inspiratory time, and the impedance to breathing (compliance, inspiratory and expiratory resistance, and auto-PEEP). High–flow capacity, pressure-targeted ventilation compensates well for small air leaks and is therefore quite appropriate for use with leaking or uncuffed endotracheal tubes, as in neonatal or pediatric applications.

Because of its virtually "unlimited" ability to deliver flow and its decelerating flow profile, pressure-targeted ventilation also is an appropriate choice for spontaneously breathing patients with high or varying inspiratory flow demands, which usually peak early in the ventilatory cycle. The decelerating flow profiles of pressure-targeted

TABLE 4-1

Comparison of Pressure-Control and Volume-Control Breaths: Fundamental Dichotomy between Pressure and Volume Strategies in Mechanical Ventilatory Support, Showing Dependent and Independent Variables with Points for Clinician Input

VARIABLE	VOLUME CONTROL BREATH	PRESSURE CONTROL BREATH
Tidal volume	Set by clinician Remains constant	Variable with changes in patient effort and respiratory system impedance
Peak inspiratory pressure	Variable with changes in patient effort and respiratory system impedance	Set by clinician Remains constant
Inspiratory time	Set directly or as a function of respiratory frequency and inspiratory flow settings	Set by clinician Remains constant
Inspiratory flow	Set directly or as a function of respiratory frequency and inspiratory flow settings	Variable with changes in patient effort and respiratory system impedance
Inspiratory flow waveform	Set by clinician Remains constant Can use constant, sine, or decelerating flow waveform	Variable with changes in patient effort and respiratory system impedance Flow waveform always is decelerating

Adapted from Branson RD, Campbell RS: Modes of ventilator operation. In MacIntyre NR, Branson RD (eds): Mechanical Ventilation. Philadelphia, WB Saunders, 2001, p 55.

modes also improve the distribution of ventilation in lungs with heterogeneous mechanical properties (widely varying time constants). Apart from limiting the lung's potential exposure to high airway pressure and the risk of barotrauma, pressure-targeted modes of ventilation often prove helpful for the adult patient whose airway cannot be completely sealed (e.g., in bronchopleural fistula).

Flow-Controlled, Volume-Cycled Ventilation

For many years, flow-controlled, volume-cycled (assist-control) ventilation has been the technique of choice for support of seriously ill adult patients. Flow can be controlled by selecting a waveform (e.g., constant or decelerating) and setting a peak flow value or by selecting a flow waveform and setting the combination of tidal volume and inspiratory time. Every breath triggered by patient effort is met with a cycle that has an identical flow trajectory for a fixed inspiratory period. Through control of the tidal volume and backup frequency, a certain lower limit for minute ventilation can be guaranteed, but the pressure required to ventilate varies widely with the impedance to breathing. Moreover, once this mode is chosen, the preset flow profile remains inflexible to increased (or decreased) inspiratory flow demands. The high-pressure alarm is often triggered by expiratory efforts that begin during the ventilator's time-determined inflation phase.

Differences between Pressure-Targeted and Volume-Targeted Ventilation

After the decision has been made to initiate mechanical ventilation, the clinician must decide to use either pressure-controlled or volume-cycled ventilation. For a well-monitored, passively ventilated patient, pressure-targeted and volume-targeted modes can be used with virtually identical effects. With either method, FIO_2, PEEP, and backup frequency must be selected. If pressure control (sometimes referred to as pressure assist-control) is used, the targeted inspiratory pressure (above PEEP) and the inspiratory time (T_I) must be selected (usually with consideration of the desired tidal volume). Although the exha-

lation valve remains closed, flow may cease when thoracic recoil pressure equals the pressure target. An "inspiratory hold" will then occur for the remainder of the set T_I. Pressure support differs from pressure control, in that each pressure-supported breath must be initiated ("triggered") by the patient. Furthermore, the off-cycling criterion for pressure support is flow rather than time, so that cycle length is free to vary with patient effort. If volume-cycled ventilation is used, the clinician may select (depending on ventilator) either tidal volume and flow delivery pattern (waveform and peak flow) or flow delivery pattern and minimum minute ventilation (with tidal volume the resulting quotient of expiratory volume [V_E] and backup frequency) (Table 4-1).

The fundamental difference between pressure-targeted and volume-targeted ventilation is implicit in their names; pressure-targeted modes guarantee pressure at the expense of letting tidal volume vary, and volume-targeted modes guarantee flow—and, consequently, the volume provided to the closed circuit in the allowed inspiratory time (tidal volume)—at the expense of letting airway pressure vary. This distinction governs how the two modes are used in clinical practice.

MODES AND SETTINGS

Technological developments have provided a wide variety of modes by which a patient may be mechanically ventilated.[14] Various modes have been developed with the hope of improving gas exchange, patient comfort, or rapid return to spontaneous ventilation. Almost any of these newer modes, however, can be adjusted to allow full rest of the patient on the one hand and periods of exercise on the other. Thus, in the great majority of patients, choice of mode is merely a matter of clinician or patient preference. Because controlled ventilation with abolition of spontaneous breathing rapidly leads to deconditioning or gradual atrophy of respiratory muscles, various assisted modes that are triggered by inspiratory efforts are preferred.[2] The most common triggered modes are assist-control ventilation, intermittent mandatory ventilation, and pressure-support ventilation. Because of their importance and ubiquity, these modes are detailed here.

Assist-Control Ventilation

In assist-control ventilation (or assisted mechanical ventilation [AMV]), each inspiration triggered by the patient is powered by the ventilator by means of either volume-cycled or pressure-targeted breaths.[4] When pressure is the targeted variable and inspiratory time is preset, the mode is known as pressure-control or, less commonly, pressure assist-control ventilation. Sensitivity to inspiratory effort can be adjusted to require a small or large negative pressure deflection below the set level of end-expiratory pressure to initiate mechanical inspiration. Most of the newest machines can be flow-triggered, initiating a cycle when a flow deficit is sensed in the expiratory limb of the circuit relative to the inspiratory limb during exhalation. As a safety mechanism, a backup rate is set so that if the patient does not initiate a breath within the number of seconds dictated by that backup frequency target, the machine cycle begins automatically. A backup rate set high enough to cause alkalosis blunts respiratory drive and terminates the patient's efforts to breathe at the apneic threshold for PCO_2. In awake, normal subjects, this threshold is usually achieved when the $PaCO_2$ is abruptly lowered to 28 to 32 mm Hg; it may be considerably higher during sleep. Changes in machine frequency have no effect on minute ventilation unless the backup frequency is set sufficiently high to terminate patient respiratory efforts. Thus, assist-control ventilation is not appropriate for use in weaning.

Synchronized Intermittent Mandatory Ventilation

In a passive patient, synchronized intermittent mandatory ventilation (SIMV) cannot be distinguished from assist-control ventilation; ventilation is then determined by the mandatory frequency and tidal volume.[15] If the patient initiates effort within the mandated interval, a different type of breath, usually pressure-supported, is allowed. Thus, when a breath is initiated outside the mandated synchronization "window," tidal volume, flow, and inspiratory-to-expiratory time ratio are determined by patient effort, any pressure support, and respiratory system mechanics, not by ventilator settings.[16] These spontaneous breaths tend to be of small volume and are highly variable from breath to breath. Respiratory work associated with these breaths may be significant, particularly for the patient with underlying cardiopulmonary disease. The SIMV mode is often used in weaning to gradually augment the patient's work of breathing by lowering the mandatory breath frequency. The mandated breaths may be pressure- or flow-targeted and are often selected to be somewhat larger than the patient's own pressure-supported breaths.

Pressure-Support Ventilation

Pressure-support ventilation (PSV) is a method in which each breath taken by a spontaneously breathing patient receives a pressure boost. The patient must trigger the ventilator to activate this mode; thus, PSV is not applied in passive, paralyzed, or sedated patients. Ventilation is determined by preset inspiratory pressure, patient-determined rate, and patient effort. Once a breath is triggered, the ventilator attempts to maintain inspiratory pressure at the clinician-determined level using whatever flow is necessary to accomplish this goal.[17,18] As tidal volume rises, eventually, flow begins to fall as a result of either cessation of patient inspiratory effort or increasing elastic recoil of the respiratory system. The ventilator maintains inspiratory pressure until inspiratory flow falls by an arbitrary amount (for example, to 25% of initial flow) or below an absolute flow rate. Apart from the selected level of pressure support, the clinician can vary the rate of rise to the targeted pressure and, perhaps more importantly, the flow off-switch. The patient's work of breathing can be increased by lowering the inspiratory pressure or making the trigger less sensitive. The work of breathing can inadvertently increase if respiratory system mechanics change with no change in ventilator settings. A potential advantage of PSV is greater patient comfort and, for some patients with very high respiratory drive, reduced work of breathing compared with volume-preset modes.

PSV hybridizes the power of the machine and the patient, providing assistance that ranges from no support at all to fully powered ventilation depending on the machine's developed pressure relative to patient effort.[19] Because the depth, length, and flow profile of the breath are influenced by the patient, well-adjusted PSV tends to be relatively comfortable in comparison with time-cycled modes. Adaptability to the vagaries of patient cycle length and effort can prove especially helpful for patients with erratic breathing patterns that otherwise would be difficult to adapt to a fixed flow profile or set inspiratory time (e.g., because of chronic obstructive pulmonary disease, anxiety, or Cheyne-Stokes breathing). Because the cycle length is flow-adjustable by the patient, it is not uncommon for high-level PSV to be the only commonly available mode that can be tolerated during severe dyspnea. The transition to spontaneous breathing is eased by the gradual removal of machine support. Although PSV has widespread application as a weaning mode, it also is valuable in offsetting the resistive work required to breathe spontaneously through an endotracheal tube, such as during CPAP or SIMV. When used to support ventilation, the pressure support level should be adjusted to maintain adequate tidal volume at an acceptable frequency (<30 breaths/min). In theory, PSV would provide sufficient power for the entire work of breathing if it were set to meet or exceed the average inspiratory pressure required per breath (P_{req}). For a normal subject breathing at a moderate rate, P_{req} is amazingly small, seldom exceeding 7 cm H_2O. For patients who are candidates for weaning from ventilation, V_E usually approximates 10 L/min or less, and P_{req} commonly does not exceed 10 to 15 cm H_2O. This explains why patients seem to be "weaning smoothly" until some rather low threshold value of PSV is reached, at which point further reductions precipitate sudden decompensation.[8]

Routine Settings

Ventilator settings are based on the patient's size and condition. The risk of toxic oxygen effects is minimized by using the lowest fraction of inspired oxygen that can satisfactorily oxygenate arterial blood. The usual goal is an arterial oxygen tension (PaO_2) of 60 mm Hg or an oxygen saturation of 90%, because higher values do not substantially enhance tissue oxygenation and because slight reductions in PaO_2 cause oxygen saturation and content to fall precipitously below that value.[4]

Historical practice has involved setting tidal volumes at 10 to 15 mL per kg body weight, which is two to three times normal.[4] This approach is now considered inappropriate in light of convincing data from experiments indicating that alveolar overdistention can produce endothelial, epithelial, and basement membrane injuries associated with increased microvascular permeability and lung injury (ventilator-induced lung injury).[3] To reduce this risk, one would ideally like to monitor alveolar volume, which is not feasible. A reasonable substitute is to monitor peak alveolar pressure, as obtained from the plateau pressure measured in a relaxed patient by briefly occluding the ventilatory circuit at end-inspiration. The incidence of ventilator-induced lung injury rises markedly when plateau pressure is high. In patients with severe underlying pulmonary dysfunction, there is a growing tendency to limit the tidal volume delivered to less than 7 mL/kg to achieve a plateau (alveolar) pressure no higher than 30 cm H_2O. In patients with very noncompliant chest walls, this upper limit value in plateau pressure may be relaxed somewhat. Such an approach may lead to an increase in $PaCO_2$. Acceptance of elevated carbon dioxide tension in exchange for controlled alveolar pressure, as previously discussed, is termed permissive hypercapnia. It is important to focus on pH rather than arterial PCO_2 if this approach is employed. In a patient in whom the pH falls below 7.20, some clinicians would increase minute ventilation or administer bicarbonate.

Flow-Targeted, Volume-Controlled Ventilation

The rate of ventilation that is set depends both on the mode and on patient requirements. With assist-control ventilation, a backup rate should be about 4 breaths/min less than the patient's spontaneous rate; this setting ensures that the ventilator will continue to supply adequate minute ventilation if there is a sudden decrease in output from the patient's respiratory centers. With SIMV, the rate is typically high at first and then gradually decreased in accordance with patient tolerance.

A peak flow rate of about three times the minute ventilation is commonly selected for the constant inspiratory flow profile, or about four to six times minute ventilation if the profile is decelerating. Peak inspiratory flow rate should be fast enough to satisfy peak flow demand but not so high as to produce discomfort or excessive shearing stress. An inspiratory flow rate of 40 to 60 L/min is appropriate if the minute ventilation is 12 L/min and the profile is square (50-70 L/min if the profile is decelerating).[20] In certain patients with obstructive pulmonary disease, better gas exchange may be achieved by higher flow rates, probably because the resulting increase in expiratory time allows for more complete emptying of regions of gas trapping. Patients with severe airflow obstruction may prefer a constant flow profile. If the flow rate is insufficient to meet the patient's ventilatory requirements, the patient will strain against his/her own pulmonary impedance and that of the ventilator, with a consequent increase in the work of breathing.[21] Examination of the monitoring waveform for airway pressure may be helpful when flow rate and ventilator trigger sensitivity are adjusted.

Few aspects of ventilator management are more controversial than the use of PEEP. In patients with acute respiratory distress syndrome (ARDS), a higher PEEP substantially improves oxygenation. The reason is probably a reduction in intrapulmonary shunting as a result of recruitment (prevention of collapse) and redistribution of lung water from alveoli to the perivascular interstitial space.[22] PEEP does not decrease total extravascular lung water. Provided that the improvement in PaO_2 is not offset by decline in cardiac output, FIO_2 can be decreased. The addition of PEEP influences lung mechanics. Patients with acute lung injury commonly have reduced end-expiratory lung volume, so their tidal breathing occurs on the low flat portion of the pressure-volume curve. By shifting tidal breathing to a more compliant portion of the curve, PEEP can reduce the work of breathing.[23] In patients with airflow limitation, auto-PEEP, and difficulty triggering the ventilator, the addition of external PEEP (to a level not exceeding the level of auto-PEEP) can help counteract dynamic hyperinflation, because under these specific circumstances, the patient needs only to decrease alveolar pressure to 1 to 2 cm H_2O below the level of external PEEP, rather than below zero.[24] An appropriate PEEP setting applied to bedridden adults without significant coexisting pulmonary problems is 3 to 7 cm H_2O, but this value can range to 15 to 20 cm H_2O or higher in the setting of ARDS or acute lung injury.

Other Settings

Flow-controlled, volume-cycled ventilators allow the clinician to choose the inspiratory flow rate and define its contour (constant "square" or decelerating).[25] Inappropriately rapid inspiratory flow rates may worsen the distribution of ventilation in some patients; however, a decelerating flow waveform helps satisfy rapid early inspiratory flow demand. Although peak pressure rises as flow rate increases, the mean airway pressure averaged over the entire ventilatory cycle may remain unchanged or may even fall as flow rate increases. Longer exhalation time is a marked advantage for some patients with airflow obstructions. The extent to which the ventilator takes up the inspiratory work of breathing is a function of the margin by which flow delivery exceeds flow demand. It is mandatory that the flow metered by the ventilator meets or exceeds the patient's flow demand throughout inspiration. Otherwise, the ventilator not only fails to reduce the work of breathing but also may force the patient to pull against the resistance of the ventilator circuitry as well as against his/her own internal impedance to airflow and chest expansion.[26]

Comfortably rapid inspiratory flow rates also are desirable to ensure that the machine completes inflation before the patient's own ventilatory rhythm cycles into its exhalation phase. Delayed opening of the exhalation valve causes the patient to "fight the ventilator." As a very general rule of thumb, the ventilator's *average* inspiratory flow should approximate four times the minute ventilation, as already noted. Peak flow should be set 20% to 30% higher than this average value when the decelerating waveform is used. Peak airway pressure is influenced by inspiratory flow rate, airway resistance, tidal volume, and total thoracic compliance. During an end-inspiratory pause, the plateau airway pressure reflects the maximum stretching force applied to a typical alveolus and its surrounding chest wall. To avoid barotrauma, maximum pressure (alarm pressure) should be set at no more than 15 to 20 cm H_2O above the peak pressure observed during a typical breath during constant flow. The pop-off alarm should be set closer than this (within 10 cm H_2O) if a decelerating flow waveform or pressure control is used, because under those conditions, end-inspiratory dynamic and static (plateau) pressures are not as widely separated (Table 4-2).

TABLE 4-2

Outline of Ventilator Classification Systems

Input	Electrical
	Pneumatic
Control scheme	Control variables:
	Pressure
	Volume
	Flow
	Phase variables:
	Trigger
	Limit
	Cycle
	Baseline
	Conditional variables
	Control subsystems:
	Control circuit
	Drive mechanism
	Output control valve
	Modes of ventilation
Output	Waveforms:
	Pressure
	Volume
	Flow
	Displays
Alarm systems	Input power alarms
	Control circuit alarms
	Output alarms

Adapted from Chatburn RL, Branson RD: Classification of mechanical ventilators. In MacIntyre NR, Branson RD (eds): Mechanical Ventilation. Philadelphia, WB Saunders, 2001, p 3.

PATIENT MANAGEMENT

Initial ventilator settings depend on the goals of ventilation (full respiratory muscle rest vs. partial exercise) as well as the patient's respiratory system mechanics and minute ventilation needs. In all patients, the initial FIO_2 should usually be 0.5 to 1.0 to ensure adequate oxygenation, although it can usually be lowered within minutes when guided by pulse oximetry and, in the appropriate setting, with application of PEEP.[27] In the first minutes after institution of mechanical ventilation, the clinician should be alert for several common problems, most notably airway malposition, aspiration, and hypotension. Positive-pressure ventilation may reduce venous return. Cardiac output reduction is especially likely in patients with low mean systemic pressure (hypovolemia, vasodilating drugs, decreased sympathetic tone) or a very high ventilation-related pleural pressure (chest wall restriction, high PEEP, high auto-PEEP). If hypotension occurs, care should be taken to rule out mainstem intubation. Intravascular volume should then be expanded and pleural pressure reduced through a decrease in tidal volume and/or minute ventilation. Although uncommon, tension pneumothorax may be catastrophic in this setting.

For patients with relatively normal respiratory mechanics and gas exchange, initial ventilator orders should be as follows: FIO_2 0.5 to 1.0, tidal volume 7 to 10 mL/kg, backup rate 8 to 12, and inspiratory flow rate 40 to 60 L/min. Alternatively, if the patient has sufficient drive and is not profoundly weak, PSV may be used. This is a particularly good strategy when the patient's respiration is otherwise overtly dyssynchronous with flow-controlled modes. The level of pressure support is adjusted (frequently in the range 10 to 20 cm H_2O above PEEP) to bring respiratory rate down to 20 to 25 breaths/min, corresponding to

a tidal volume of approximately 400 mL in the adult. If gas exchange is normal, FIO_2 may be further reduced on the basis of pulse oximetry or arterial blood gas determinations.

Severe airflow obstruction is often seen in patients with asthma or exacerbated chronic obstructive disease but may also be encountered in individuals sustaining inhalation injury, voluminous aspiration or pulmonary edema, or central airway lesions (e.g., tumor or foreign body) that are not bypassed by the endotracheal tube. These patients are frequently anxious and distressed. Deep sedation should be provided in such instances, supplemented in the occasional individual by therapeutic administration of muscle relaxants. Notably, the use of such agents may cause long-lasting weakness, especially when profound paralysis is extended for more than 4 hours.[2] These interventions help reduce oxygen consumption and carbon dioxide production, lower airway pressures, and decrease the risk of self-extubation. Because gas exchange abnormalities in patients with severe airflow obstruction often result primarily from ventilation-perfusion mismatching, an FIO_2 setting of 0.5 will be adequate in the majority of cases.[28] Ventilation is most commonly initiated using the assist-control mode (or SIMV), the tidal volume should be small (5-7 mL/kg), and the backup respiratory rate set at 12 to 15 breaths/min. If constant flow is the waveform, a peak flow setting of 60 L/min is recommended because higher flow rates do little to increase expiratory time. These patients are at significant risk for development of auto-PEEP, and the minimum acceptable minute ventilation is frequently employed when breathing is controlled. If the patient is triggering the ventilator, PEEP may be added to reduce the work of triggered inspiration. In general, auto-PEEP does not increase as long as PEEP is not set higher than about 85% of the initial auto-PEEP level. Goals in this situation are to minimize alveolar overdistention (plateau pressure <30 cm H_2O) and minimize dynamic hyperinflation (auto-PEEP < 15 cm H_2O). Reducing minute ventilation to achieve these goals may cause arterial PCO_2 to rise above 40 mm Hg, often to 50 to 70 mm Hg or even higher. Although this situation requires sedation, such permissive hypercapnia is tolerated well except in patients with increased intracranial pressure and, perhaps, those with critical pulmonary hypertension or significant ventricular dysfunction.

A third group of patients of particular importance are those experiencing acute hypoxemic respiratory failure. This situation is created by alveolar filling with blood, pus, or edema and by atelectasis, which results from the altered mechanics and body positioning. The end result is impairment of lung mechanics and gas exchange. Gas exchange impairment results from intrapulmonary shunt that is largely refractory to oxygen therapy. In ARDS, the reduced functional residual capacity arising from alveolar flooding and collapse leaves many fewer alveoli to accept the tidal volume, making the lung appear stiff and dramatically increasing the work of breathing.[29] The ARDS lung should be viewed as a small lung, however, rather than a stiff lung. In line with this current concept of ARDS, it is clearly established that extensive distention of functioning alveoli in the ARDS lung compounds lung injury and may induce systemic inflammation.[30] The goals of ventilation are to reduce work of breathing, avoid toxic concentrations of oxygen, and choose ventilator settings that do not amplify lung damage. Initial FIO_2 should be high in view of hypoxemia. PEEP is indicated in patients with diffuse lung lesions but may be less helpful in patients with focal infiltrates such as lobar pneumonia. In patients with

ARDS, PEEP should be instituted immediately and its level adjusted to the lowest level necessary to produce a net arterial saturation of 90%. Tidal volume should be adjusted to keep plateau pressure within acceptable limits (generally <30 cm H_2O). Pressure-control ventilation can be used as well, but parameters for this mode that ensure lung-protective ventilation have not been rigorously examined. The inspiratory pressure target proposed is 30 to 35 cm H_2O (PEEP plus inspiratory driving pressure). In either mode, respiratory rate should be set as high as 24 to 28 breaths/min in the absence of auto-PEEP. An occasional consequence of lung-protective ventilation of this kind is hypercapnia. As previously discussed, this approach, of preferring hypercapnia to alveolar overdistention, is well tolerated.

A final important group of patients requiring mechanical ventilation, consists of those with restriction of pulmonary excursion, frequently associated with chest wall edema (massive fluid resuscitation), recent abdominothoracic surgery, extensive burns, or morbid obesity. A small tidal volume (5-7 mL/kg) and relatively rapid respiratory rate (18-24 breaths/min) are valuable in this patient group in order to minimize the hemodynamic consequences of positive-pressure ventilation and reduce the likelihood of injury to the lung.[27] The F_{IO_2} setting needed to maintain appropriate oxygenation is determined by the extent of alveolar filling or collapse. When the restrictive abnormality involves the chest wall (may include the abdomen), a large ventilation-induced rise in pleural pressure has the potential to compromise cardiac output. This compromise would in turn reduce mixed venous P_{O_2} and, in the setting of ventilation-perfusion mismatch or shunt, PaO_2 as well.

WEANING

Discontinuation of mechanical ventilation can be easy in patients needing short-term support. However, it can be quite difficult in patients recovering from a major episode of acute respiratory failure, a complicated operative procedure, or major torso trauma. Weaning such patients from ventilation is a major clinical challenge and constitutes a significant workload in the intensive care unit.[4,31]

Timing is important in the separation of a patient from mechanical ventilation. If weaning is delayed unnecessarily, the patient remains at risk for ventilator-associated complications. If weaning is performed prematurely, cardiopulmonary decompensation may delay further extubation.[32,33] In general, discontinuation of mechanical ventilation is not attempted in a patient who has not regained consciousness or who has cardiopulmonary instability or an arterial P_{O_2} value lower than 60 mm Hg with a F_{IO_2} value of 0.40 or higher. Satisfactory oxygenation, however, does not reliably predict successful weaning. A more important determinant of weaning outcome is the ability of respiratory muscles to address the respiratory work requirements. Similarly, parameters traditionally gathered by respiratory care practitioners, including maximal inspiratory pressure, vital capacity, and minute ventilation, have been used to evaluate a patient's readiness for weaning, but these parameters have limited predictive accuracy. The ratio of respiratory frequency to tidal volume during 1 minute of spontaneous breathing (Rapid Shallow Breathing Index) is a useful but not infallible predictor. A value less than 100 indicates that a weaning attempt is more likely to be successful.[34] Two widely quoted clinical studies compared ventilator

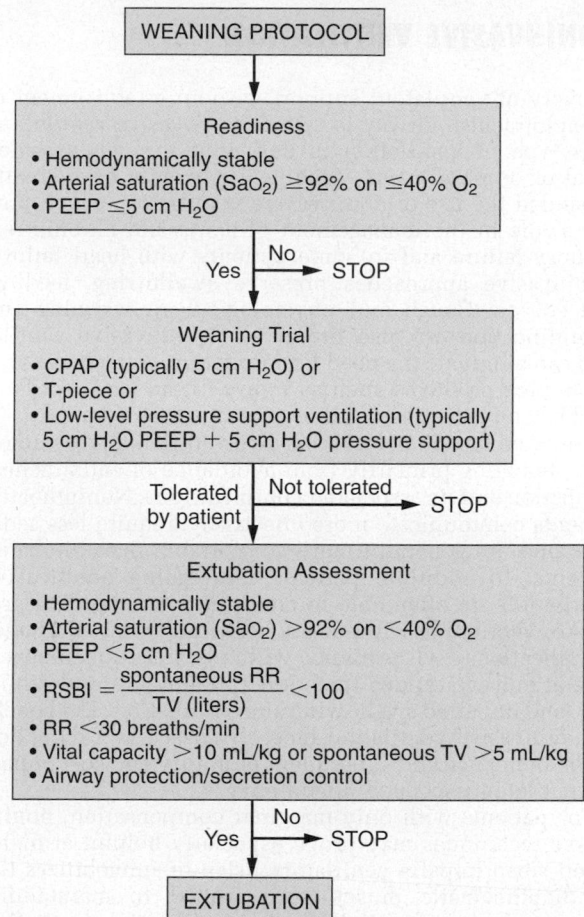

FIGURE 4-2. Algorithm for mechanical ventilation weaning protocol. CPAP, continuous positive airway pressure; PEEP, positive end-expiratory pressure; RSBI, Rapid Shallow Breathing Index; RR, respiratory rate; TV, tidal volume.

modes used in weaning the patient who does not immediately separate from mechanical ventilation. T-piece trials, SIMV, and PSV were compared. These studies demonstrated that choice of weaning mode does affect outcome in the patient with complex respiratory problems. Modes providing equal treatment of each breath (T-piece trials and PSV) gave better results than SIMV.[35,36] Whatever method is chosen, the daily trial of unassisted breathing is integral to the evaluation.[37]

The process of weaning begins by determining patient readiness (Fig. 4-2). In addition to applying the recommendations from the Task Force for Evidence-Based Guidelines for Weaning and Discontinuing Ventilatory Support, patients should be carefully screened for mental status, respiratory muscle strength, consistent and adequate wakefulness, ability to manage secretions, state of nutritional repletion, and acid-base and electrolyte status. Particular attention should be given to acceptance of hypercapnia if chronically present. Finally, normality of levels of electrolytes affecting muscle function and cardiac status (calcium, phosphate, and potassium) should be assured. If the aforementioned conditions are addressed, weaning may be attempted. A protocol utilizing the Rapid Shallow Breathing Index in the separation of patients from mechanical ventilation has been evaluated.[38]

NONINVASIVE VENTILATION

Delivery of ventilatory support without establishment of an endotracheal airway is called *noninvasive ventilation.* This type of ventilation is delivered through a sealed nasal or oronasal mask. Technical advances have greatly expanded the use of noninvasive ventilation, which now has a role in the management of acute and chronic respiratory failure and in some patients with heart failure. Noninvasive approaches preserve swallowing, feeding, and speech. Cough and physiological air warming and humidification are also preserved. Noninvasive ventilation can eliminate the need for intubation or tracheostomy, preventing problems such as injury to the vocal cords or trachea and infections of the lower respiratory tract.

Reported benefits of noninvasive ventilation are numerous, stemming primarily from avoidance of endotracheal intubation and its associated complications. Nonintubated patients communicate more effectively, require less sedation, and are generally more comfortable than intubated patients. In addition, patients undergoing noninvasive ventilation are often able to continue with standard oral intake. Ventilation without tracheal intubation eliminates complications such as trauma with tube insertion, mucosal ulceration, aspiration, infection (pneumonia and sinusitis), and impaired swallowing after extubation. The benefit of noninvasive ventilation most discussed is a reduction in the incidence and subsequent mortality and cost impact of ventilator-associated pneumonia.[39]

For patients with only marginal compensation, noninvasive techniques may prove especially helpful at night, when sleep impairs ventilatory drive or immobilizes the nondiaphragmatic musculature crucial to maintaining adequate ventilation. Indeed, nocturnal nasal ventilation (by nasal mask or other occlusive fitting) seems to be useful over extended periods for selected patients with irreversible neuromuscular disease, sleep apnea, and airflow obstruction. Intermittent rest of fatigued respiratory muscles and, in a minority of cases, improved lung compliance may result. The precise reason for nocturnal noninvasive ventilation's benefit during waking hours remains undetermined. It has been suggested that nocturnal support may allow the sleep quality needed to preserve adequate ventilatory drive and muscle strength.

In published studies, alert, cooperative, spontaneously breathing patients fare much better with noninvasive ventilation than patients without those characteristics. The patient must be able to protect the airway. Hemodynamic or electrocardiographic instability or an unstable airway argues against the use of noninvasive ventilation; thus, the unconscious trauma patient with multiple injuries including maxillofacial fractures is not a candidate for noninvasive ventilation. A further contraindication is compromise of cough and secretion clearance. A common reason for failure of noninvasive ventilation has been abundant secretions secondary to pneumonia. Relative contraindications include the inability to adequately fit and seal the mask or to cough with prompting and difficulty with removal of the mask in the event of emesis. Most investigators now believe that patients with cardiogenic pulmonary edema may improve with the aid of noninvasive ventilation to help unload respiratory muscles and decrease work and oxygen cost of breathing as well as to recruit lung units and reduce alveolar edema.[40]

The primary complication of noninvasive ventilation is focal skin necrosis secondary to prolonged pressure from the mask on the underlying skin.[7] The necrosis typically occurs over the bridge of the nose but may also occur over the zygoma; it is prevented by avoidance of excessive pressure when the straps are tightened to the mask. The straps should be just tight enough to seal any large air leaks. Skin necrosis can be further prevented by the prophylactic placement of hydrocolloid dressing (DuoDerm) or a similar product on the bony contact points. Facial soft tissue sores occur in 7% to 10% of patients receiving full–face mask noninvasive ventilation. The other complications, which all seem to occur at approximately a 1% to 2% incidence, are gastric distention (avoided by ventilating with pressures below 30 cm H_2O), aspiration, and pneumothorax. Conceptual concerns with gastric distention are subsequent vomiting, aspiration, and pneumonia. However, in studies addressing gastric distention, there did not appear to be a direct correlation between gastric distention and the development of pneumonia. Patients in whom gastric distention developed did not suffer subsequent aspiration and pneumonia. Prophylactic placement of a nasogastric tube did not prevent gastric distention. Furthermore, it has been hypothesized that the use of noninvasive ventilation in patients after recent upper gastrointestinal surgery could lead to air swallowing and disruption of anastomotic suture lines; to date, however, this occurrence has not been reported.

Less common complications of noninvasive ventilation are pneumothorax requiring a chest tube and conjunctivitis, which may develop secondary to air leaks near the eyes in about 2% of patients.[41] Treatment of the latter problem consists of correction of the air leak and administration of synthetic eye lubricants. The most serious complication is failure to recognize when noninvasive ventilation is not giving a patient adequate ventilation, oxygenation, or airway support. Delayed intubation may encourage continued deterioration of the patient. Whether noninvasive ventilation is working is generally evident within the first minutes to hours of its application.

CONCLUSION

Positive-pressure ventilation is a lifesaving intervention in patients with excessive respiratory work, ventilation failure, or oxygenation deficits. Mechanical ventilation is not therapeutic in and of itself, but lung healing is enhanced with optimal settings. Research now suggests that ventilatory settings that use excessive tidal volumes and airway pressures may, in fact, be deleterious to the critically ill patient. Thus, acceptance of hypercapnia and lower tidal volumes than traditionally employed is now common. Although a variety of modes have been introduced on newer ventilators, traditional modes such as assist-control ventilation, SIMV, and PSV are most commonly employed. Separation of the patient from mechanical ventilation can usually be achieved rapidly if the presenting problems that required critical care are resolved or stable. Simple evaluation of patient's respiratory rate and tidal volume gives significant insight into readiness for separation from the ventilator. Finally, complications of invasive mechanical ventilation are avoided in a growing number of patients through the use of noninvasive ventilation through nasal or oronasal masks. Effectiveness of noninvasive ventilation is generally determined within minutes from the clinical response to the application of this therapy.

1. Mechanical ventilation can be lifesaving in patients with hypoxemic or hypercarbic respiratory failure. This therapy allows relief of cardiopulmonary distress and diversion of oxygen delivery to other vital organs.
2. Patients may be ventilated with pressure-targeted or volume-targeted ventilation. Pressure-targeted modes of ventilation guarantee airway pressure at the expense of tidal volume fluctuation, and volume-targeted modes fix tidal volume but allow airway pressure to vary.
3. The most commonly used modes of ventilation in the acute phase of critical illness are assist-control ventilation and synchronized intermittent mandatory ventilation (frequently in combination with pressure-support ventilation).
4. Weaning of mechanical ventilatory support begins after acute problems faced by the patient are resolved or stable. Although many parameters predictive of successful weaning have been proposed, none used alone is perfect. The most widely applied is the Rapid Shallow Breathing Index, which is obtained by dividing the respiratory rate in breaths per minute by the tidal volume in liters; a value lower than 100 suggests that weaning is likely to be successful.
5. Ventilatory support delivered without an endotracheal airway is noninvasive ventilation. Benefits of this therapy are numerous and include more effective communication, lower sedation requirements, continuation of oral intake, and reduction of complications such as pneumonia.

Key References

 3. Dreyfuss D, Saumon G: Ventilator-induced lung injury: Lessons from experimental studies. Am J Respir Crit Care Med 1998;157:294-323.
31. Tobin MJ: Advances in mechanical ventilation. N Engl J Med 2001;344:1986-1996.
36. Esteban A, Frutos F, Tobin MJ, et al: A comparison of four methods of weaning patients from mechanical ventilation. N Engl J Med 1995;332:345-350.
37. Kress JP, Pohlman AS, O'Connor MF, et al: Daily interruption of sedative infusions in critically ill patients undergoing mechanical ventilation. N Engl J Med 2000;342:1471-1477.
39. Meduri GU: Noninvasive positive-pressure ventilation in patients with acute respiratory failure. Clin Chest Med 1996;17:513-553.

See the companion Expert Consult website for the complete reference list.

CHAPTER 5

Principles of Pharmacology in the Critically Ill

Anthony Holley and Jeffrey Lipman

OBJECTIVES

This chapter will:
 1. Define the major pharmacologic concepts.
 2. Review the main principles of pharmacokinetics related to the critically ill patient.
 3. Review the main principles of pharmacodynamics related to the critically ill patient.
 4. Relate the physiological changes in critical illness to their potential impact on pharmacotherapy.
 5. Consider strategies for safe and effective pharmacotherapy in critical illness.

Patients in the intensive care unit (ICU) are often being given multiple drugs. Intensivists prescribing these drugs need to consider the pharmacologic implications of deranged physiology, underlying disease, and drug-drug interactions. Physiological changes resulting from critical illness may alter several aspects of both pharmacokinetics and pharmacodynamics in a manner that is often difficult to predict on the basis of available information. Furthermore, these patients routinely receive multiple medications, and the potential for adverse drug reactions, particularly drug-drug interactions, increases in proportion to the number of agents received. Rational therapeutics is a major component of providing cost-effective critical care, as a substantial fraction of such patient's costs are directly attributable to drugs.[1] New drugs and the use of old drugs for new indications are becoming more commonplace. After a rational drug regimen is implemented, therapeutic drug monitoring may be necessary to ensure maintenance of the desired outcome as well as for potential toxicity and adverse events. Application of pharmacologic principles can guide the design of a rational drug regimen to achieve rapid and beneficial effects, thereby minimizing adverse events. This chapter reviews the basic principles of pharmacology, including pharmacokinetics and pharmacodynamics (Fig. 5-1), with particular reference to the critically ill patient and the more complex application of these principles to optimize both patient care and patient safety.

CRITICAL ILLNESS AND PHARMACOKINETICS

Pharmacokinetics describes the absorption, distribution, metabolism, and elimination of drugs[2]—essentially, what the body does to the drug. Critical illness results in a number of physiological alterations that may subsequently influence absorption and bioavailability of drugs.

Absorption and Bioavailability

The method of administration of drugs to critically ill patients is determined by factors such as the onset of action, reliability of delivery, and titratability of available preparations. Gastrointestinal dysfunction and reliability of the parenteral route commonly result in intravenous administration of drugs in ICU, but with renewed emphasis on enteral feeding, oral administration is increasingly an option. Medications are often administered with intended immediate effect. The intravenous route is rapid and reliable. Slow or sustained-release medications are convenient in ambulatory patients but lack the titratability that is often required in patients receiving intensive care. When a route other than intravenous is employed, the clinician must consider alterations that may impair or exaggerate drug absorption and/or drug bioavailability.

The extent of absorption, or *bioavailability* (F), describes the fraction of administered drug that reaches the central circulation unchanged. Drugs administered by the intravenous route have complete bioavailability (F = 1.0).[3] For all other routes of administration, F is less than or equal to 1.0 because of incomplete absorption or, for some enterally administered drugs, because of presystemic metabolism. Bioavailability after administration by enteral, topical, subcutaneous, or intramuscular routes may be affected by a variety of factors, such as edema and inflamed tissue (Table 5-1).

Drugs that are administered via an enteral route depend on the gut's absorptive function and motility for adequate absorption. Before they enter the systemic circulation, enterally administered drugs may be subject to first-pass metabolism. Gastrointestinal flora, intestinal enzymes, and hepatic enzymes can alter parent drugs and render them inactive (e.g., propranolol) or indeed can activate prodrugs (e.g., enalapril to enalaprilat).[4] The small intestine has the fastest and most extensive absorption owing to its small lumen and the presence of microvilli. Normal peristaltic movements are important in dividing and dispersing the drug mass. Delayed gastric emptying, often a feature of the critically ill patient, as well as alterations in intestinal transit, permeability, integrity, and surface may lead to unpredictable and erratic drug absorption.

Distribution

Following entry into the systemic circulation, the administered drug is distributed to the body's tissues. Distribution is not uniform, however, reflecting the differences in tissue binding, solubility, tissue perfusion, permeability of cell membranes, and local pH.[5]

The *volume of distribution* (V_d; measured in liters) may be regarded as the theoretical volume of fluid into which the total drug administered would have to be diluted to produce the concentration in plasma. This reflects a theoretical space that allows estimation of the initial drug dose required to reach a therapeutic plasma concentration,[4] as follows:

$$\text{Volume of distribution } (V_d) = \text{Amount of drug in body} \div \text{Plasma drug concentration}$$

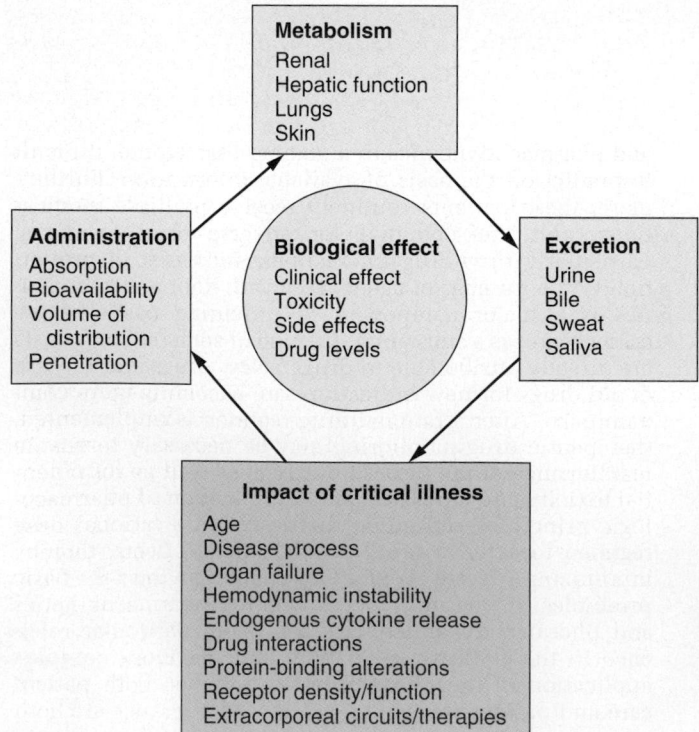

FIGURE 5-1. Pharmacologic considerations in critical illness.

TABLE 5-1

Drugs and Critical Illness

Factors determining bioavailability	Drug molecule size
	Solubility
	Extent of lipophilicity
	pKa
	Drug stability
	pH
	Blood flow
	Surface area
	Gastrointestinal motility
	Gastrointestinal absorption
	Pathological conditions— inflammation/edema
Factors determining volume of distribution	Fluid shifts
	Protein binding
	Local pH
	Drug ionization
	Cell membrane permeability
Factors determining drug metabolism in critical illness	Intrinsic clearance
	Hepatic blood flow
	Protein binding

Knowledge of the V_d for a drug allows estimation of an appropriate loading dose (LD) to achieve a desired serum concentration ([C], in mg/L), as follows:

$$LD = [C] \times Vd$$

Drug distribution during critical illness is influenced primarily by alterations in protein binding and extracellular fluid volume (see Table 5-1).[5] Increased capillary permeability and decreased oncotic pressure together with large volumes of resuscitation fluids typically seen in septic shock result in massive fluid shifts. The end result is leakage of large volumes into the interstitium, generating a new compartment where hydrophilic drugs may accumulate with an increased V_d. Drugs that have a small V_d, for example, the aminoglycosides, are most affected by these volume shifts.[6,7] Changes in V_d have been well documented in the administration of antibiotics to the critically ill.[7-9] The entry rate of a drug into a tissue depends on the rate of blood flow to the tissue, the tissue mass, and partition characteristics between blood and tissue. Distribution for poorly perfused tissues (e.g., fat), is very slow, particularly if there is high tissue affinity for the drug. Only after *distribution equilibrium* (state in which entry and exit rates are the same) is reached are drug concentrations in tissues and in extracellular fluids reflected by the plasma concentrations.[5]

Changes in distribution of highly protein-bound drugs are to be expected in the critically ill patient. Decreased albumin concentrations result in a higher free fraction of drugs such as phenytoin,[8] ceftriaxone,[10] and diazepam,[11] which normally are extensively bound by albumin. Increased α_1-acid glycoprotein concentrations result in a decreased free fraction of α_1-acid glycoprotein–bound drugs, such as propranolol, meperidine, and lidocaine. It has been repeatedly demonstrated that albumin decreases and α_1-acid glycoprotein synthesis increases during physiological stress.[12,13] This fact suggests the need to monitor the free or unbound concentrations of highly bound drugs in the critically ill patient and to be cognizant of their implications. Although the overall number of agents for which alterations in protein binding significantly affect drug exposure has been found to be limited,[14] several com-

monly prescribed agents are affected, including fentanyl, nicardipine, verapamil, milrinone, haloperidol, itraconazole, erythromycin, ceftriaxone, cloxacillin, and propofol.

pH is frequently altered in the critically ill. Most drugs are weak organic acids or bases existing in un-ionized and ionized forms in an aqueous environment. The un-ionized form is usually lipid soluble (lipophilic) and diffuses readily across cell membranes. The ionized form has low lipid solubility, but high water solubility (hydrophilic) and high electrical resistance, and thus cannot penetrate cell membranes easily. The *pKa* is the pH at which concentrations of ionized and un-ionized forms are equal. When the pH is lower than the pKa, the un-ionized form of a weak acid predominates, but the ionized form of a weak base predominates. Therefore, pH-generated alterations in the ionized state can increase or decrease the extent of distribution or penetration of a drug.[15]

Metabolism

The liver is the principal site of drug metabolism, and critical illness can profoundly affect liver function and, hence, metabolism. Although metabolism typically inactivates drugs, some drug metabolites are pharmacologically active. Drugs are metabolized by oxidation, reduction, hydrolysis, hydration, conjugation, condensation, or isomerization. Regardless of the metabolic mechanism, the process makes drug excretion more effective. Metabolism of a drug often occurs in two phases.[2] *Phase I reactions* involve formation of a modified functional group by oxidation, reduction, or hydrolysis, and these reactions are nonsynthetic. The most important enzyme system of phase I metabolism is the cytochrome P-450 system, a microsomal superfamily of isoenzymes that catalyze the oxidation of many drugs. *Phase II reactions* are synthetic and utilize conjugation with an endogenous substance (e.g., glucuronic acid, sulfate, glycine). Metabolites formed in these synthetic reactions are more polar and thus readily excreted by the kidneys. Glucuronidation, the most common phase II reaction, is the only one that occurs in the liver's microsomal enzyme system.

The rate of elimination may be described by *first-order kinetics*, whereby the metabolic rate is a constant fraction of the drug remaining in the body (rather than a constant amount of drug per hour). *Zero-order kinetics* describes metabolism that occurs at its maximal rate and does not change in proportion to drug concentration; thus, a fixed amount of drug is metabolized per unit time.[2,16] Phenytoin and alcohol are examples of drugs whose metabolism may move from first-order to zero-order kinetics as their concentration increases.

A drug's half-life ($t_{1/2}$) is the time required for its serum concentrations to decline by 50% after absorption and distribution are complete. Half-life determines the dosage interval as well as the time it takes to reach steady-state concentrations. Approximately 90% of steady-state concentration is attained after three half-lives, so therapeutic drug monitoring is often performed in connection with the third dose.[2,16] Changes in half-life can result from a change in either V_d or clearance, as reflected in the following equation:

$$t_{1/2}(\text{hours}) = 0.693 \times V_d \ (L)/Cl \ (L/hour)$$

where *Cl* is clearance (see later). V_d and clearance are both affected in the critically ill. This situation needs to be identified, and the appropriate dosage adjustments instituted.

Clearance (Cl) is the theoretical volume of blood that is emptied of drug in a given period and is expressed in volume per unit of time.[2,5,16] It determines the steady-state concentration for a given dose. Clearance is determined by blood flow to the organ that metabolizes or eliminates drug and the efficiency of the organ at extracting drug from the bloodstream (see Table 5-1).

Clearance is a measure of the efficiency of drug removal that encompasses both drug metabolism and drug excretion. Extraction ratios are determined by the drug-metabolizing capacity of hepatic enzymes and protein binding.[17] Clearance is affected when blood flow is altered or when the extraction ratio changes. Disease states and interventions that increase hepatic blood flow result in enhanced clearance of high-extraction drugs; those that decrease hepatic blood flow result in decreased elimination. The extraction ratio rises when enzyme inducers increase the amount of drug-metabolizing enzyme[5,17] and drops when enzyme inhibitors inhibit drug-metabolizing enzymes or there is parenchymal loss. In the case of low-extraction drugs, hepatic clearance is primarily a function of intrinsic hepatocyte metabolic activity and, to a lesser degree, protein binding.[15]

Critical illness can lead to profound changes in hepatic blood flow,[15] which may then affect drug metabolism by increasing or decreasing drug delivery to the hepatocyte. In the hyperdynamic stage of sepsis, cardiac output often increases and blood flow distribution changes to shunt blood flow to vital organs. Hepatic blood flow reductions may also occur, although late in sepsis, thus decreasing the clearance of drugs. Hypovolemic shock, myocardial infarction, and acute heart failure are other problems frequently encountered in the patient receiving intensive care for which one can anticipate a decrease in drug clearance for high-extraction drugs.

Hepatic blood flow and, consequently, drug clearance are modified by the action of certain drugs.[18] Vasoconstrictors, including adrenaline, noradrenaline, phenylephrine, vasopressin, and dopamine, can produce hepatic arterial and portal vein vasoconstriction with a subsequent decrease in hepatic blood flow. Conversely, nitroglycerin may increase hepatic blood flow by decreasing portal and hepatic vein resistance. Inotropes such as dopamine and dobutamine have also been shown to increase hepatic blood flow by raising cardiac output. Physical factors such as the application of positive end-expiratory pressure also affect hepatic blood flow, possibly producing significant alterations in the clearance of drugs whose elimination has blood flow–dependent characteristics.[19]

Critically ill patients often have significant elevations of stress hormones, such as noradrenaline, adrenaline, and cortisol, as well as acute-phase proteins, including α_1-acid glycoprotein and C-reactive protein. Cytokines have variable effects on the cytochrome P-450 enzymes, depending on the specific cytokine and enzyme subgroup combination evaluated. Most studies conclude that enzyme inhibition does occur and may result in decreased clearance of low-extraction drugs.[20] Endotoxin release during sepsis is also a potent inhibitor of hepatic enzyme activity, and traumatic injury enhances phase I oxidative metabolism, resulting in increased drug clearance.[21] Phase II reactions may also be altered, but to a lesser extent. Human experimental data show that the inflammatory response to even a very low dose of lipopolysaccharide significantly reduces hepatic cytochrome P-450–mediated drug metabolism, and this effect evolves over 24 hours.[21] It is likely that patients with sepsis and much higher exposures to endotoxin have more profound inhibition of drug metabolism. Nitric oxide, an important mediator during septic conditions, inhibits the activity of the iron-containing cytochrome P-450. Metabolism of drugs that depend on cytochrome P-450 is therefore affected by septic conditions.[22]

Ideally, drug doses should be reduced initially and then raised slowly in the presence of liver disease; however, this approach might not be practical in the ICU setting. If available, therapeutic drug monitoring of plasma levels may provide a guide to dosage adjustments for drugs with low therapeutic indices in patients with liver dysfunction.

Pharmacodynamic monitoring methods, such as daily assessment of time-to-awakening after sedation withdrawal, may permit safe and effective use of hepatically metabolized drugs in the patient with liver disease.[20]

Excretion

Excretion and elimination of drugs occur primarily via the kidneys. Biliary secretion, plasma esterases, and minor pathways are other, less common routes of elimination.

Renal excretion of drugs occurs through glomerular filtration, tubular secretion, and reabsorption; it is influenced by renal blood flow, glomerular filtration rate (GFR), and urinary flow rate. Glomerular elimination is influenced by both the level of protein binding and the molecular size of drug, whereas tubular secretion of drugs is higher for those that are protein bound and increases with uremia.

The use of pharmacokinetic principles is important to the understanding of dosage modification for drugs in patients with renal failure. GFR is a useful measure of renal function, so measurement (or accurate estimation) of GFR is crucial to appropriate drug dosing.[4] Estimation of GFR through 24-hour or 8-hour urine creatinine collection and serum creatinine concentration is simple and reliable except when the GFR is very low.

Renal elimination of drugs has particular significance in the critically ill, in whom acute renal failure is common, with approximately 5% to 10% of ICU patients requiring renal replacement therapy.[23] Renal clearance of drugs with extensive renal elimination is decreased, with associated toxicity or exaggerated clinical effect.[24,25] Conversely, pathologically elevated cardiac output may be a feature of certain critical illness, for example, head injury, sepsis, and burns; in these pathological situations, creatinine clearance and therefore drug clearance may be markedly elevated.[26]

Modification of dosage is required in renal dysfunction, especially for a drug with a low therapeutic index or for which renal mechanisms play a major role in elimination.[27] If the renal clearance of a drug is normally less than 25% to 30% of total body clearance, impaired renal function is unlikely to have clinically significant influence on drug removal.[4] Identifying and developing a strategy for effective prescribing in renal failure require a rational approach (Table 5-2).

The intensive care patient requiring continuous renal replacement therapy (CRRT) is at risk for both drug overdose as a result of acute renal failure, and for underdosing, for example, with antibiotics, with potentially severe consequences.[23] Protein binding of the substance, together with dialysate and filtrate flow rates, determine drug clearance (Table 5-3). The relevance of this extracorporeal

TABLE 5-2

An Approach to Pharmacotherapy in Critical Illness Complicated by Renal Failure

1. Quantify renal function.
2. Establish hepatic functional integrity.
3. Determine therapeutic index.
4. Consider implications of underdosing.
5. Consider implications of overdosing.
6. Establish loading dose.
7. Determine maintenance dose (dosing interval or dose adjustment).
8. Monitor clinical effect.
9. Measure drug levels (if available).
10. Regularly modify therapy on basis of preceding factors.

TABLE 5-3

Factors Enhancing Drug Removal during Continuous Renal Replacement Therapy

Small volume of distribution (V_d <250 L or <4 L/kg)
Lower protein-binding value (<90%)
Molecular size (<500 d for traditional membranes; <5000 d for high-flux membranes)
Intrinsic clearance of the drug (<500 mL/70 kg/min)
High blood flow
High dialysate flow
Prolonged duration of continuous renal replacement therapy
High water solubility

Adapted from Perazella MA, Parikh C: Pharmacology. Am J Kidney Dis 2005;46:1129-1139.

clearance for overall drug removal, however, also depends on concurrent drug clearance by residual renal function, the liver, or other nonrenal mechanisms.[23] For the majority of drugs, there are still no studies available that investigated pharmacokinetics in patients receiving CRRT. Because of the numerous variations in CRRT modality, it is difficult to find dosing guidelines that fit both the individual patient and the specific method of treatment.

PHARMACODYNAMICS IN CRITICAL ILLNESS

Pharmacodynamics refers to the interaction of a drug with its target site (receptor), which results in a pharmacologic response[2] and may be considered "what the drug does to the body." It reflects the relationship between drug concentrations at the receptor or target site and subsequent pharmacologic response. *Receptors* are macromolecules involved in chemical signaling between and within cells. They may be located on the cell surface membrane or within the cytoplasm. The activated receptors directly or indirectly regulate cellular biochemical processes, such as protein phosphorylation, ion conductance alterations, and nucleic acid transcription. Drugs, hormones, and neurotransmitters that bind to a receptor are referred to as *ligands*. A ligand may activate or inactivate a receptor, and the activation may either increase or decrease a particular cell function. Few if any drugs are absolutely specific for one receptor or subtype, but most have relative selectivity.

TABLE 5-4

Pharmacodynamic Changes Associated with Critical Illness

Decreased receptor numbers
Decreased receptor binding
Altered signal transduction
Drug-drug interactions

The pharmacodynamic effect of a drug (as measured by onset, intensity, and duration) depends not only on pharmacokinetic factors but also on the ability of the target organ to respond to receptor activation, the number of receptors at the target organ, and counter-regulatory influences at those receptors (Table 5-4).

Drug Monitoring

The use of pharmacokinetic principles may aid in the development of a safe and effective dosing regimen for a drug; nevertheless, therapy requires frequent monitoring and titration to optimize the desired effect. Assessment of drug effect can consist of clinical measurements, such as level of sedation, analgesia, blood pressure change, or heart rate, or direct monitoring, such as measurement of plasma levels of drug or metabolites. Although direct plasma drug level monitoring is possible for some drugs, it is not available for most. Furthermore, many considerations are involved in the decision to assay a drug level—for example, the difference between free and bound drug may be significant, but the timing of the plasma drug level in relation to the time of the last dose is important and varies for individual agents. In some situations, measurement of the peak plasma concentration is required (carbamazepine or lithium toxicity), whereas for therapeutic monitoring of cyclosporine or tacrolimus, the plateau drug concentration may be utilized to assess effective dosing.[15] Other drugs may require measurement of both peak and trough levels for adequate monitoring of efficacy and potential toxicity; one example is the aminoglycosides.[7]

CONCLUSION

The ICU is an environment of extreme monitoring of physiological variables and therefore should be an environment for intensive monitoring and individualization of drug therapy through the knowledge and application of pharmacodynamic/pharmacokinetic principles. The intensivist must be aware of individual patient characteristics and illness severity as well as particular drug kinetics, dynamics, and interactions in order to prescribe rationally. Despite diligent practice, errors occur, and practical strategies to minimize these errors must be employed. These strategies largely use pharmacologic principles but may also include other aspects of care. Computerized physician order entry has been shown to reduce the rate of serious medication errors by more than half.[28] Furthermore, including a clinical pharmacist on intensive care ward rounds, as is the practice in our institution, further enhances the quality and safety of prescribing.[29] This chapter has considered both pharmacokinetics and pharmacodynamics in the context of critical illness, providing a broad overview. For every agent prescribed, the intensivist must ask the following questions: How is this drug best administered? What is its expected bioavailability? Will metabolism or excretion be compromised by the patient's illness? and How will this drug work in the altered milieu of critical illness?

Key Points

1. Absorption, bioavailability, and volume of distribution are often altered by critical illness.
2. Metabolism of drugs may be impaired by diminished hepatocyte function or decreased hepatic blood flow.
3. Excretion of drug metabolites may be altered in critical illness, raising a potential for toxicity.
4. Pharmacodynamics is affected in critical illness by changes in receptor number, binding, and signal transduction.
5. Rational prescribing in the intensive care unit requires an understanding of potential drug interactions.

Key References

3. Murray P, Corbridge T: Critical care pharmacology. In Hall JB, Schmidt GA (eds): Principles of Critical Care, 2nd ed. New York, McGraw-Hill, 1998, p 1529.
4. Perazella MA, Parikh C: Pharmacology. Am J Kidney Dis 2005;46:1129-1139.
5. Boucher BA, Wood GC, Swanson JM: Pharmacokinetic changes in critical illness. Crit Care Clin 2006;22:255-271, vi.
15. Krishnan V, Murray P: Pharmacologic issues in the critically ill. Clin Chest Med 2003;24:671-688.
17. McKindley DS, Hanes S, Boucher BA: Hepatic drug metabolism in critical illness. Pharmacotherapy 1998;18:759-778.

See the companion Expert Consult website for the complete reference list.

CHAPTER 6

Hemodynamic Monitoring in the Intensive Care Unit

*Patricio M. Polanco and Michael R. Pinsky**

OBJECTIVES

This chapter will:
1. Explain the rationale for and physiological basis of hemodynamic monitoring.
2. Describe the principal hemodynamic variables, parameters, and monitoring techniques.
3. Review the interpretation and clinical application of hemodynamic monitoring.

Hemodynamic monitoring is a central component of the overall management approach to the critically ill patient. The utilization of different monitoring techniques, procedures, and devices is essential for the effective assessment and management of the patient receiving critical care. The level of complexity of this hemodynamic monitoring varies among patients according to the pathophysiology of the disorder to be treated, the stability of the patient, the competence of the staff, and the resources of each unit. The utilization of hemodynamic monitoring is vital not only in assessing the patient's condition but also in close titration of therapies guided by these data. Implicit in this approach are the assumptions that (1) physiological assessment of the subject's cardiopulmonary status can be made and (2) its trends over time reflect both known pathophysiological processes and the effect of treatment on them.

The level of invasiveness required to measure specific physiological variables and the frequency of those measurements are functions of the accuracy required and the expected rate of change of these variables over time. For example, arterial pressure can be monitored with a sphygmomanometer to derive mean, systolic, and diastolic arterial pressure values up to a frequency of every 5 minutes. However, if information about arterial pulse pressure variation is required or the blood pressure may vary widely over 5 minutes, continuous arterial pressure monitoring, which involves arterial catheterization or more sophisticated noninvasive monitoring, is needed.

Although several novel approaches of hemodynamic monitoring have appeared over the last few decades, only a few monitoring techniques and associated therapeutic interventions have demonstrated a truly beneficial effect on patients' conditions. Therefore, their use in the management of the critically ill patient can not be recommended except under specific conditions.

RATIONALE FOR HEMODYNAMIC MONITORING

In generic and pragmatic terms, hemodynamic monitoring is used to assess cardiovascular insufficiency and sufficiency and to direct therapies to maintain adequate tissue perfusion and organ system function. A fundamental means of attaining tissue wellness is to sustain adequate amounts of oxygen delivery (DO_2) to the tissues. Because there is no clear evidence that maintaining target levels of DO_2 will ensure adequate oxygen delivery to all tissues in critically ill patients, justification for the use of specific types of monitoring has been divided into three *levels of defense*, as described by Bellomo and Pinsky,[1] on the basis of the strength of validation. The basic level of defense argues on the basis of historical controls, in whom prior experience using similar monitoring was traditionally used and presumed to be beneficial; the mechanism by which the benefit is achieved need not be understood or even postulated. The second level of defense uses arguments based on an understanding of the pathophysiology of the process being treated. This physiological argument is stated as "knowledge of how a disease process creates its effect and thus preventing the process from altering measured bodily functions should prevent the disease process from progressing or injuring remote physiological functions." Most of the rationale for hemodynamic monitoring resides at this level. The third level of defense is

---

*This work was supported by NIH funding HL67181 and HL0761570.

based on documentation that the monitoring device, by altering therapy in otherwise unexpected ways, improves outcome in terms of survival and quality of life. In reality, few therapies performed in medicine can claim benefit at this level. Thus, we are left with the physiological rationale as the primary defense for the monitoring of critically ill patients.

PHYSIOLOGICAL BASIS AND APPLICATION OF HEMODYNAMIC MONITORING

Hemodynamic monitoring of critically ill patients has a dual function. First, it can be used to document hemodynamic stability and the lack of need for acute therapeutic interventions. Second, through monitoring, we can measure variables and define the extent to which they vary from their baseline values. Thus hemodynamic monitoring must be able to define both stability and change.

Hemodynamic monitoring can be either invasive or noninvasive and either continuous or intermittent, and can report either directly measured events or processed signals. Monitoring devices can measure physiological variables directly or can derive these variables through signal processing. Signal processing does not minimize the usefulness of physiological variable analysis; it merely separates the output data from the patient through the use of the data processor. The signal processing physiological variable measurement most commonly used clinically is electrocardiography; although the electrocardiogram reflects a highly processed signal, it is both well described and clinically useful.

The variables that can be measured noninvasively are body temperature, heart rate, systolic and diastolic arterial blood pressures, and respiratory frequency. Noninvasive variable measurements that use signal processing are electrocardiography, transcutaneous pulse oximetry (SpO_2), expired carbon dioxide, transthoracic echocardiography, and noninvasive respiratory plethysmography. Invasive monitoring involves intravascular catheter insertion, transesophageal echocardiographic probe insertion, and blood component analysis. Invasive hemodynamic monitoring of vascular pressures is usually performed via the percutaneous insertion of catheters into a vascular space and transduction of the pressures sensed at the distal ends. This approach allows for the continuous display and monitoring of the complex waveforms. Similar, intrapulmonary vascular catheters may derive thermal signals and mixed venous oxygen saturation (SvO_2), which are needed to assess cardiac output (CO) and the adequacy of oxygen delivery, respectively. Summaries of all the possible unitary and calculated measures derived from invasive hemodynamic monitoring are shown in Tables 6-1 and 6-2, respectively.

In order to appreciate the potential benefits, limitations, and common misinterpretations of the different hemodynamic measurements, one must understand some physiological concepts. Therefore, for each of the primary hemodynamic variables, we describe the physiological determinants, the monitoring techniques, and their application in the care of the critically ill patient.

Arterial Pressure

After pulse rate, arterial pressure is the most commonly monitored and recorded hemodynamic variable. Arterial

TABLE 6-1

Unitary Measures of Physiological Variables Derived from Invasive Monitoring and Their Physiological Relevance

MEASURE	SIGNIFICANCE
Arterial Pressure	
Mean arterial pressure (MAP)	Organ perfusion inflow pressure
Arterial pulse pressure and its variation during ventilation	Left ventricular (LV) stroke volume changes and pulsus paradoxus
	Preload responsiveness (if assessed during intermittent positive-pressure ventilation)
Arterial pressure waveform	Aortic valvulopathy, input impedance, and arterial resistance
	Used to calculate stroke volume by pulse contour technique
Central Venous Pressure (CVP)	
Mean CVP	If elevated, that effective circulating blood volume is not reduced
CVP variations during ventilation	Tricuspid insufficiency, tamponade physiology
	Preload responsiveness (if assessed during spontaneous breathing)
Pulmonary Arterial Pressure (Ppa)	
Mean Ppa	Pulmonary inflow pressure
Systolic pulmonary artery pressure	Right ventricular (RV) pressure load
Diastolic pulmonary artery pressure, pulse pressure, and their variations during ventilation	RV stroke volume, pulmonary vascular resistance
	Diastolic pressure tract changes in intrathoracic pressure during ventilation
Pulmonary Artery Occlusion Pressure (Ppao)	
Mean Ppao	Left atrial and left ventricular intraluminal pressure and by inference, LV preload
	Backpressure to pulmonary blood flow
Ppao waveform and its variation during occlusion and ventilation	Mitral valvulopathy, atrial or ventricular etiology of arrhythmia, accuracy of mean Ppao to measure intraluminal LV pressure, and pulmonary capillary pressure (Ppc)

TABLE 6-2

Calculated Measures of Physiological Variables Derived from Invasive Monitoring and Their Physiological Relevance*

Vascular resistances	Total peripheral resistance = MAP/COtd
	Systemic vascular resistance = (MAP − CVP)/COtd
	Pulmonary arterial resistance = (mean Ppa − Ppc)/COtd
	Pulmonary venous resistance = (Ppc − Ppao)/COtd
	Pulmonary vascular resistance (PVR) = (mean Ppa − Ppao)/COtd
Vascular pump function	Left ventricular stroke volume (SVlv) = COtd/HR
	Left ventricular stroke work (SWlv) = (MAP − Ppao)/SVlv
	Preload-recruitable stroke work = SWlv/Ppao
Oxygen transport and metabolism	Global oxygen transport or delivery (Do_2) = CaO_2/COtd
	Global oxygen uptake (VO_2) = (CaO_2 − CvO_2)/COtd
	Venous admixture
	Ratio of dead space to total tidal volume (V_D/V_T) = $PaCO_2$/($PaCO_2$ − $PetCO_2$)
Right ventricular function using RV ejection fraction (EFrv) catheter-derived data	Right ventricular end-diastolic volume (EDVrv) = SV/EFrv
	Right ventricular end-systolic volume (ESVrv) = EDVrv − SV

CaO_2, arterial oxygen concentration; COtd, cardiac output as determined by thermodilution; CvO_2, venous oxygen concentration; CVP, central venous pressure; HR, heart rate; MAP, mean arterial pressure; $PaCO_2$, arterial partial pressure of carbon dioxide; $PetCO_2$, end-tidal CO_2 pressure; Ppa, pulmonary arterial pressure; Ppao, pulmonary artery occlusion pressure; Ppc, pulmonary capillary pressure; SV, stroke volume.
*Calculated measures using multiple measured variables, including COtd, arterial blood gases (ABGs), and mixed venous blood gases (VBGs).
Adapted from Bellomo R, Pinsky MR: Invasive monitoring. In Tinker J, Browne D, Sibbald W (eds): Critical Care: Standards, Audit and Ethics. London, Hodder Arnold, 1996, pp 82-104.

pressure is a function of both vasomotor tone and CO. The local vasomotor tone also determines blood flow distribution, which itself is usually determined by local metabolic demands. For a constant vasomotor tone, vascular resistance can be described from the relationship between changes in both arterial pressure and CO. The body defends organ perfusion pressure above all else in its autonomic hierarchy through alterations in α-adrenergic tone, which are mediated through baroreceptors located in the carotid sinus and aortic arch. This supremacy of arterial pressure in the adaptive response to circulatory shock exists because both coronary and cerebral blood flows depend on perfusion pressure alone. The cerebral vasculature has no α-adrenergic receptors, and the coronary circulation only a few. Accordingly, hypotension always reflects cardiovascular embarrassment, but normotension does not exclude it. Hypotension decreases organ blood flow and stimulates a strong sympathetic response that induces a combined α-adrenergic (increased vasomotor tone) and β-adrenergic (increased heart rate and cardiac contractility) effect and causes a massive adrenocorticotropic hormone (ACTH)–induced release of cortisol from the adrenal glands. Thus, to understand the determinants of arterial pressure, one must know both blood flow and the level of vasomotor tone.

The difference between systolic and diastolic arterial pressures is the *pulse pressure*. On a beat-to-beat basis, the changes in arterial pulse pressure reflect only changes in left ventricular (LV) stroke volume, because arterial input impedance and output resistance do not vary over this short interval. *Hypotension* is usually defined as systolic pressure less than 90 mm Hg or a mean arterial pressure (MAP) less than 65 mm Hg. No firm data supporting any one limit of arterial pressure or CO or use of therapeutic approaches based on these values has proved more beneficial than any other. Accordingly, empiricism is the rule regarding target values of both MAP and CO during resuscitation. At present, the literature suggests that keeping MAP above 65 mm Hg through the use of fluid resuscitation and subsequent vasopressor therapy is an acceptable target in a patient who was not previously hypertensive. Previously hypertensive subjects need a higher MAP to ensure the same degree of blood flow.[2] There is no proven value in forcing either arterial tone or CO to higher levels to achieve an MAP value greater than this threshold. In fact, data suggest that further resuscitative efforts using vasoactive agents markedly increases mortality.[3] The relatively new concept of "delayed resuscitation" or "hypotensive resuscitation" for traumatic hemorrhagic shock has been shown to improve outcome in some clinical and experimental studies, presumably because the risks of hypoperfusion are less than the risks of excessive bleeding after trauma.[4-6] However, these studies were performed in trauma patients with penetrating wounds and no immediate access to surgical repair. Once a patient is in the hospital and the sites of active bleeding have been addressed, aggressive fluid and vasopressor resuscitation is indicated.

Another very important application of the continuous display of the arterial waveform (using arterial catheterization) is the interpretation of the heart-lung interactions during ventilation. The commonly observed variations in arterial pressure and aortic flow seen during positive-pressure ventilation have been analyzed as a measure of preload responsiveness.[7] The rationale for this approach is that positive-pressure ventilation–induced changes in either systolic arterial pressure (used to describe pulsus paradoxus), arterial pulse pressure, or stroke volume can predict which subjects will display an increase in CO in response to fluid resuscitation. Ventilation-induced changes in systolic arterial pressure (pulsus paradoxus) and arterial pulse pressure are easy to measure from arterial pressure recordings. The greater the variation in systolic arterial pressure or pulse pressure over the respiratory cycle, the greater the rise in CO in response to a defined fluid challenge. Also, Monnet and colleagues[8] have shown that measuring the mean change in aortic blood flow during passive leg raising in spontaneously breathing patients has proved accurate in predicting preload responsiveness.[8] Although arterial pressure variations are a measure of preload responsiveness,[9] the "traditional" preload measures, such as right atrial pressure (Pra), pulmonary artery occlusion pressure (Ppao), right ventricular (RV) end-diastolic volume, and intrathoracic blood volume, reflect preload responsiveness poorly.[10] In essence, preload is not preload responsiveness.

Blood pressure is usually measured noninvasively with a sphygmomanometer and the auscultation technique. It is important to remember that in very large and obese subjects in whom the upper arm circumference exceeds the width limitations of a normal blood pressure cuff, a normal cuff will record erroneously high pressures. In such patients, using the large thigh blood pressure cuff on the upper arm commonly resolves this problem. Blood pressure can be measured automatically with computer-driven devices (e.g., Dinamap [Wipro GE Healthcare]), which greatly reduce nursing time. Blood pressure values measured with the sphygmomanometer are slightly higher for systolic and lower for diastolic pressures than values derived simultaneously via indwelling arterial catheters. The MAPs are usually similar with the two methods, and the actual systolic and diastolic pressure differences are often small except in the setting of increased peripheral vasomotor tone. If perfusion pressure of the finger is similar to arterial pressure, both blood pressure and pressure profile may be recorded noninvasively and continuously with an optical finger probe (Finapres; see later). However, finger perfusion is often compromised during hypovolemic shock and hypothermia, limiting this monitoring technique to use in relatively well-perfused patients.

Accurate and continuous measurements of arterial pressure can be made through arterial catheterization of easily accessible arterial sites in the arm (axillary, brachial, or radial artery) or groin (femoral artery). Usually, neither axillary nor brachial arterial sites are used because of fear of causing downstream ischemia, although data supporting such fear are nonexistent. Arterial catheterization with continuous display of arterial pressure waveforms enables arterial waveform analysis, which is essential in calculating pulse pressure, pulse pressure variations, and CO.

There is no evidence to support the routine use of pulmonary arterial catheterization (PAC) upon admission to the intensive care unit for continuous monitoring of blood pressure and repetitive measurements of blood gases. Probably the only proven indication for PAC is to synchronize the intra-aortic balloon for counterpulsation, although the information obtained from this technique is also valuable in the assessment and treatment of the patient with cardiovascular instability or for the use of vasopressors or vasodilators during resuscitation. PAC is an invasive procedure that is not free of complications. A systematic review of a large number of cases showed, however, that most of the complications were minor, including temporary vascular occlusion (19.7%) and hematoma (14.4%); permanent ischemic damage, sepsis, and pseudoaneurysm formation occurred in less than 1% of cases.[11]

Central Venous Pressure or Right Atrial Pressure

In this chapter we use the terms central venous pressure (CVP) and right atrial pressure interchangeably. Starling demonstrated the relationship between CO, venous return, and CVP, showing that increasing the venous return (and preload) raises the stroke volume (and CO) until a plateau is reached (Fig. 6-1). CVP is clearly influenced by the volume of blood in the central compartment and its venous compliance. Several physiological and anatomical factors, however, can influence its measurement and waveform, such as the vascular tone, RV function, intrathoracic pressure changes, tricuspid valve disease, arrhythmias, and either myocardial or pericardial disease.

Central venous pressure is the pressure in the large central veins proximal to the right atrium relative to atmosphere. In the intensive care unit, CVP is usually measured with a fluid-filled catheter (central venous line or pulmonary artery catheter), with the distal tip located in the

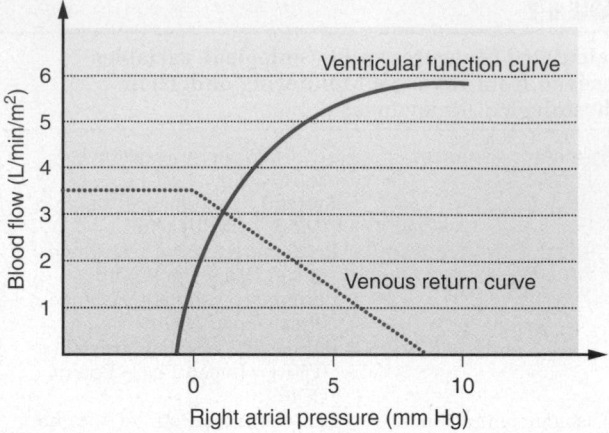

FIGURE 6-1. Interaction of venous return and ventricular function.

superior vena cava and the proximal end connected to a manometer or, more often, to the pressure transducer of a monitor, which displays the waveform in a continuous fashion. CVP can also be measured noninvasively as jugular venous pressure, which is indicated by the height of the column of blood distending the internal and external jugular veins when the subject is sitting in a semi-reclined position, such that small elevations in CVP are reflected in a persistent jugular venous distention.

CVP has been used as a monitor of central venous blood volume and an estimate of right atrial pressure for many years, being wrongly regarded as a parameter for and sometimes a goal in replacement of intravascular volume in shock. Numerous studies have negated the validity of this measure as an index of RV preload. It has been shown that CVP has a poor correlation with cardiac index, stroke volume, and LV or RV end-diastolic volume.[12-14]

Although a very high CVP demands a certain level of total circulating blood volume, one may have a CVP of 20 mm Hg and still have an underfilled left ventricle that is responsive to fluid replacement. For example, in the setting of acute RV infarction, CVP can be markedly elevated, whereas CO often increases further with volume loading. In reported series, some patients with low CVP showed no response to fluids, and some patients with high CVP showed a response to challenge with fluids.[15] On the basis of these findings and the poor correlations described previously, it is impossible to define ideal values for CVP. However, there is some evidence that volume loading in patients with CVP higher than 12 mm Hg is very unlikely to improve CO.[16] Thus, the only usefulness of CVP is to define relative hypervolemia, because elevated CVP occurs only in disease. Two clinical studies showed a potential benefit in specific groups of surgical patients (those undergoing hip replacement or renal transplantation),[17,18] in whom CVP was used to guide therapy; however, there is no clinical evidence that CVP monitoring improves outcome in critically ill patients, and attempts to normalize CVP in early goal-directed therapy during resuscitation do not have any benefit.[19]

Pulmonary Artery Catheterization and Its Associated Monitored Variables

PAC allows the measurement of many clinically relevant hemodynamic variables (see Tables 6-1 and 6-2). One can

TABLE 6-3

Complications of the Pulmonary Artery Catheter

Arrhythmia
Complete heart block
Catheter malpositioning:
  Extracardiac
  Catheter knotting
  Catheter fragmentation and meteorism
Pulmonary infarction
Pulmonary artery rupture
Thrombosis
Vascular infection

measure the intrapulmonary vascular pressures, including CVP, pulmonary arterial pressure (Ppa), and, by intermittent balloon occlusion of the pulmonary artery, Ppao, and pulmonary capillary pressure (Ppc). Furthermore, with use of the thermodilution technique and the Stewart-Hamilton equation, one can estimate CO and RV ejection fraction (RVef), global cardiac volume, and intrathoracic blood volume. Finally, one can measure SvO_2 either intermittently, by direct sampling of blood from the distal pulmonary arterial port, or continuously, via fiberoptic reflectometry. Assuming that the hemoglobin concentration is known and that arterial oxygen saturation (SaO_2), easily estimated noninvasively by pulse oximetry as transcutaneous pulse oximetry (SpO_2), can be tracked, one can calculate numerous derived variables that accurately describe the global cardiovascular state of the patient. These derived variables include total oxygen delivery (DO_2), whole-body oxygen consumption (VO_2), venous admixture (as an estimate of intrapulmonary shunt), pulmonary and systemic vascular resistances, RV end-diastolic and end-systolic volumes, and both RV and LV stroke work indices.

Although PAC is still commonly used in assessing cardiac function, global DO_2, intravascular volume status, and pulmonary pressures, there are currently no proven indications for its use. Despite some exciting initial reports, in uncontrolled studies, of markedly improved outcome in high-risk surgical patients,[20,21] further well-controlled studies in both high-risk surgical patients[22] and trauma patients[23,24] failed to document any improvement in survivability when patients were treated on the basis of PAC-derived data. Like other invasive monitoring techniques, PAC has potentially serious complications. Two large prospective multicenter studies showed a complication incidence of 5% to 10%.[25,26] The most common complications described in these series were hematomas, arterial puncture, arrhythmias, and PAC-related infections, although many others have been described (Table 6-3). No deaths attributable to PAC were found in these series, but other researchers have previously reported deaths, generally due to right heart and pulmonary artery perforation.[27,28]

Pulmonary Arterial Pressure

The determinants of Ppa are the volume of blood ejected to the pulmonary artery during systole, the resistance of the pulmonary vascular bed, and the downstream left atrial pressure. The pulmonary vascular bed is a low-resistance circuit with a large reserve that allows increases in CO with minor changes in the Ppa. On the other hand,

rises in the downstream venous pressure (e.g., LV failure) or in the flow resistance (e.g., lung diseases) raise Ppa. Increases in CO alone do not cause pulmonary hypertension, but in patients with greater vascular resistance, the Ppa can be increased because of changes in CO. Given these considerations, Ppa should not be regarded as a reliable parameter of ventricular filling in several lung diseases that cause changes in the vascular tone and CO. The normal range of values for Ppa are systolic, 15 to 30 mm Hg; diastolic, 4 to 12 mm Hg; and mean, 9 to 18 mm Hg.[29]

Pulmonary Artery Occlusion Pressure

When the pulmonary artery catheter is adequately positioned and the balloon tip is inflated, completely occluding the pulmonary artery, the pressure of the left atrium becomes the main determinant of pressure distal to the inflated balloon, because of a static column of blood between the distal tip of the balloon-occluded catheter and the left atrium. Thus, Ppao reflects the LV filling pressure or preload. In order for one to obtain an accurate measurement, two primary aspects of Ppao must be considered: a decrease in diastolic pressure values to less than diastolic Ppa and the damping of the pressure signal (Fig. 6-2). Ppao has been described in multiple clinical scenarios, being used most often in the bedside assessment of pulmonary edema, pulmonary vasomotor tone, intravascular volume status, LV preload, and LV performance.

Pulmonary edema can be caused by either elevations of pulmonary capillary pressure, referred to as *hydrostatic* or *secondary pulmonary edema*, or increased alveolar capillary or epithelial permeability, referred to as *primary pulmonary edema*. Although there are exceptions not addressed in this chapter, it is generally correct that Ppao values less than 18 mm Hg suggest a nonhydrostatic cause, and values greater than 20 mm Hg a hydrostatic cause, of pulmonary edema.[30]

Pulmonary vascular resistance (PVR) can be estimated, with the use of Ohm's law, as the ratio of the pulmonary vascular pressure gradient (mean Ppa – Ppao) and CO; that is, PVR = (mean Ppa – Ppao)/CO. Normal PVR is between 2 and 4 mm Hg/L/min/m^2. Usually these values are multiplied by 80 to give a normal PVR range of 150 to 250 dynes · sec/cm^5. Either an increased PVR or a passive pressure buildup from the pulmonary veins can induce pulmonary hypertension. If pulmonary hypertension is associated with an increased PVR, the causes are primarily within the lung; diagnoses such as pulmonary embolism, pulmonary fibrosis, essential pulmonary hypertension, and pulmonary veno-occlusive disease must be excluded. If PVR is normal, however, LV dysfunction is a more likely cause of pulmonary hypertension.[31]

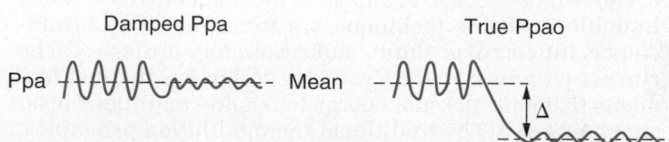

FIGURE 6-2. Differential characteristics of a damped pulmonary artery pressure (Ppa) and a true wedge or pulmonary artery occlusion pressure (Ppao) during balloon inflation. Notice the flattening of the waveform on the damped Ppa tracing (*left*) without a decrease in mean pressure; in the true Ppao tracing (*right*), there is a substantial decrease in mean pressure (Δ).

Ppao is often taken to reflect LV filling pressure and, by inference, LV end-diastolic volume. The patient with cardiovascular insufficiency and a low Ppao is presumed to be hypovolemic and is initially treated with fluid resuscitation, whereas the patient with a similar presentation but elevated Ppao is presumed to have impaired contractile function. Although there are no accepted high and low Ppao values for presence and absence, respectively, of LV underfilling, a Ppao value less than 10 mm Hg is commonly regarded as presumed evidence of a low LV end-diastolic volume, whereas a value greater than 18 mm Hg suggests a distended LV.[32] There are multiple documented reasons for this observed inaccuracy, which relate to individual differences in LV diastolic compliance and contractile function[33] and to undefined relations among absolute values of Ppao and LV end-diastolic volume and their changes.[34] Because Ppao is a poor predictor of preload responsiveness, its use to predict response to fluid resuscitation in critically ill patients is not recommended.

The four primary determinants of LV performance are preload (LV end-diastolic volume), afterload (maximal LV wall stress), heart rate, and contractility. Ppao is often used as a substitute for LV end-diastolic volume in the construction of Starling curves (i.e., relationship between changing LV preload and ejection phase indices). Usually, one plots Ppao versus LV stroke work (LV stroke volume × developed pressure). With this construct, patients with heart failure can be divided into four groups according to Ppao value (greater or less than 18 mm Hg) and cardiac index value (greater or less than 2.2 L/min/m^2).[32] Patients with low cardiac indices and high Ppao are presumed to have primary heart failure, and those with low CO and low Ppao are presumed to have hypovolemia. Those with high cardiac indices and high Ppao are presumed to be volume overloaded, whereas those with high CO and low Ppao to have increased sympathetic tone. Although this construct may be useful in determining diagnosis, treatment, and prognosis for patients with acute coronary syndrome, it predicts cardiovascular status in other patient groups poorly. As described previously, if LV end-diastolic volume and Ppao do not trend together in response to fluid loading or inotropic drug infusion, inferences about LV contractility based on this Ppao–LV stroke work relation may be incorrect. The same limitations on the use of Ppao in assessing LV preload must apply to its use in assessing LV performance.

Cardiac Output

CO can be estimated with many techniques, including PAC. Both pulmonary blood flow using a balloon flotation pulmonary artery catheter equipped with a distal thermistor and transpulmonary blood flow using an arterial thermistor, both using a central venous cold volume injection, can be employed. Using an average of multiple determinations minimizes confounding factors of the ventilatory cycle, is more accurate, and so is recommended.[35,36] Some limitations of this technique are tricuspid valve insufficiency, intracardiac shunt, and respiratory artifacts.[36] The current pulmonary artery catheter design has thermal filaments that emit thermal energy to obtain continuous measurements of CO by traditional thermodilution principles. The advantage of both the continuous CO technique and the transpulmonary technique is that neither is influenced greatly by ventilation-induced swings in pulmonary blood flow. The other techniques available to measure CO are described later.

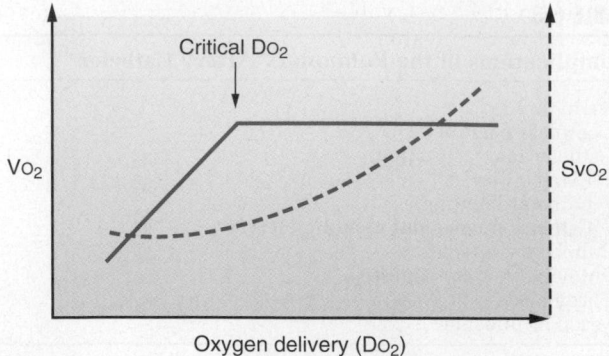

FIGURE 6-3. Interrelationship of the determinants of mixed venous oxygen saturation (SvO$_2$). The decrease in oxygen delivery under invariable oxygen consumption (VO$_2$) by the tissues will cause a decrease in SvO$_2$ to a critical point, at which the consumption becomes dependent on the delivery in an almost linear fashion; in this way, the SvO$_2$ remains stable.

Mixed Venous Oxygen Saturation

SvO$_2$ obtained from PAC reflects the pooled venous oxygen saturation—in other words, saturation of the entire body, being an important parameter in the assessment of the adequacy of oxygen delivery (DO$_2$) and its relation to oxygen consumption (VO$_2$). Decrease in SvO$_2$ could be due to a decrease on DO$_2$ or any of the parameters that determine it, such as CO, hemoglobin, and saturation (SaO$_2$), and also to an increase in VO$_2$. A decrease in DO$_2$ is followed by stable VO$_2$ with a consequent decrease in the SvO$_2$ until a critical value of DO$_2$ is reached; at that value, the tissues are no longer able to compensate, having a constant VO$_2$, and VO$_2$ becomes dependent on DO$_2$ in an almost linear fashion. At this level, although SvO$_2$ continues to decrease, it becomes less sensitive to changes in tissue perfusion (Fig. 6-3).

SvO$_2$ measured in blood drawn from the distal tip of a pulmonary artery catheter represents the true mixed venous value of the blood blended in the right ventricle. Care must be taken to withdraw blood slowly so that it is not aspirated from the downstream pulmonary capillaries. Currently, fiberoptic reflectance spectroscopy enables continuous measurements of SvO$_2$.

Central Venous Oxygen Saturation

Over the last few years, interest in superior vena cava oxygen saturation (ScvO$_2$) has been renewed because of results of a study by Rivers and associates.[37] This study demonstrated that in patients with septic shock or severe sepsis who were admitted to the emergency department, early and aggressive resuscitation guided by ScvO$_2$, CVP, and MAP values reduced 28-day mortality from 46.5% to 30.5%. Although both SvO$_2$ and SvcO$_2$ are used, the first one remains the gold standard for measurement of minimal oxygen delivery. This is because although they seem to follow a parallel tracking, ScvO$_2$ may be 5% or more higher or lower than SvO$_2$ during dynamic changes in CO as occur in shock states.[38] This fact limits the use of ScvO$_2$ to determine when to start or stop resuscitation in a critically ill patient. Still, this measurement does not require major invasive techniques; it could be clinically useful at lower threshold values in the early detection of tissue hypoxia, because a low $ScvO_2$ value (<65%) is invariably associated with a low SvO_2 value (<72%).

ALTERNATIVE TECHNIQUES TO MEASURE CARDIAC OUTPUT

Esophageal Doppler Monitoring

Since the first description by Christian Doppler in 1842, multiple uses have been described for the Doppler effect in several areas of science. Although suprasternal and transtracheal techniques are available, esophageal Doppler monitoring stands as the most relevant and most accurate measurement of CO. This minimally invasive approach estimates CO by measuring (1) blood flow velocity at the aortic valve and (2) descending aortic flow. Numerous studies comparing this technique with thermodilution, echocardiography, and dye dilution have validated it.[39-41] Although esophageal Doppler monitoring is a simple technique that requires a brief training, operator efficiency has been cited as affecting accuracy.[42] Besides the measurement of flow and calculation of CO, further information regarding the hemodynamic status can be obtained from interpretation of the size and shape of the waveform (Fig. 6-4).

Arterial Pulse Contour Analysis

Pulse contour analysis estimates LV stroke volume, and therefore CO, from the arterial pressure waveform. Arterial pressure and arterial pulse pressure are functions of the rate of LV ejection, LV stroke volume, and the resistance, compliance, and inertance characteristics of the arterial tree and the blood. If tone remains constant, changes in pulse pressure most proportionally reflect changes in LV stroke volume. Thus, caution must be applied when pulse contour analysis is used to monitor patients with hemodynamic instability and rapid changes in arterial tone. Pulse contour–derived estimates of stroke volume variation can also be used to determine preload responsiveness.[43,44]

Three different monitoring devices using pulse contour analysis of an arterial line waveform to obtain continuous CO are currently available and approved for clinical use—PiCCO (Pulsion Medical Systems AG, Munich), LIDCO-plus (LIDCO Ltd, Cambridge, UK), and Flo Trac–Vigileo (Edwards Life Sciences LLC, Irvine, CA). The technique's minimal invasiveness and the correlation with "standard" methods of measuring CO in clinical and experimental studies makes it a promising tool for hemodynamic monitoring.[45-47] Both the PiCCO and LiDCO-plus monitoring systems have been shown to help drive resuscitation protocols and improve outcome of critical illness.

FUTURE DIRECTIONS OF HEMODYNAMIC MONITORING

In order to succeed as diagnostic and therapeutic tools, future monitoring techniques for the critically ill patient must be continuous and noninvasive and must yield metabolic assessment to some extent. Several technologies that have been available during the last 20 years partially meet these criteria and may represent the future direction of intensive care monitoring, so they are briefly described here. Although they are not new concepts, their translation from basic scientific understanding and laboratory experimentation to the clinical setting has been challenging and requires further improvement and validation.

Finger Pulsometry

Finapres (from finger arterial pressure; Finapres Medical Systems, Amsterdam) is the proprietary name for a device that measures beat-to-beat arterial blood pressure continuously and noninvasively through photoplethysmography in the finger. This technique is based on detection of the pulsatile unloading of the finger arterial walls using an inflatable finger-cuff with a built-in photoelectric plethysmograph. Pulse rate and systolic, diastolic, and mean pressures are obtained from the finger-pressure waveform in a beat-to-beat fashion.

Many studies described the accuracy of the device in comparison with invasive or noninvasive blood pressure measurements. Although the Finapres has some limitations that affect mostly the systolic and mean pressures (because finger arteries are affected by contraction and dilatation in relation to psychological and physical heat,

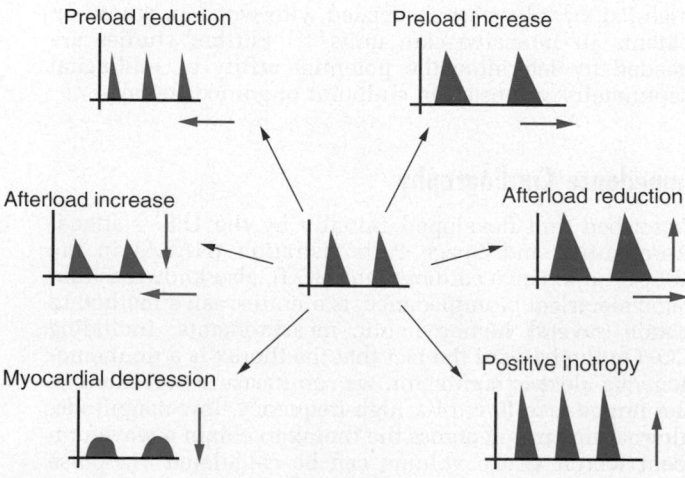

FIGURE 6-4. Interpretation of aortic Doppler waveform changes. (Adapted from Singer M: Esophageal Doppler monitoring. In Pinsky MR, Payen D [eds]: Functional Hemodynamic Monitoring. Berlin, Springer-Verlag, 2006, p 101.)

cold, blood loss, orthostasis, and stress), its precision and accuracy allow for reliable tracking of changes in blood pressure.[48]

Near-Infrared Spectroscopy with Tissue Oxygen Saturation

Near-infrared spectroscopy with tissue oxygen saturation (StO_2) quantifies the oxyhemoglobin fraction of the capillaries of the observed muscle, making use of the oxygenation-dependent characteristics of hemoglobin. Studies have shown that this measurement correlates well with SvO_2 and the severity of hemorrhagic shock and that it can track changes in systemic oxygen delivery in trauma patients.[49-51] One report indicates that measuring tissue oxygen saturation in the thenar muscle and estimating StO_2 debt may allow prediction of developing multiple-organ dysfunction in trauma patients with hemorrhagic shock.[52]

Gastric and Sublingual Capnometry

Because increases in partial pressure of tissue carbon dioxide (PCO_2) represent insufficient oxygen supply to the cells, it makes perfect sense to monitor tissue PCO_2 to identify perfusion abnormalities and guide therapy to correct them. Gastric tonometry and sublingual capnometry are techniques developed to achieve this goal. Gastric tonometry measures PCO_2 in the stomach, which, like the gut, has been described as an early alarm ("canary of the body") in situations of circulatory insufficiency. Gastric PCO_2, like derived gastric intramucosal pH (pHi) and the gradient or gap between gastric PCO_2 and arterial PCO_2, or $P(g-a)CO_2$, has been shown to be a reliable index of hypoperfusion with prognostic value in critically ill patients.[53-55] Although the results are promising, the technique has never been implemented because of technical limitations and artifacts during measurements.

Sublingual capnometry is a noninvasive technique to measure sublingual mucosal PCO_2 ($PslCO_2$) using carbon dioxide–sensing optodes or microelectrodes. Experimental studies showed that $PslCO_2$ correlates with organ blood flows and systemic markers of hypoperfusion such as MAP, cardiac index, and arterial lactate value.[56-58] Weil and associates[59] suggested a range of 43 to 47 mm Hg for $PslCO_2$ in normal subjects and a threshold of 70 mm Hg as a predictor of hospital survival in a study of 46 critically ill patients. Other clinical studies have demonstrated that high $PslCO_2$ values are associated with worse prognosis in patents in intensive care units.[60,61] Further studies are needed to determine the potential utility of sublingual capnometry values as an endpoint of guided therapy.

Impedance Cardiography

Described and developed initially by the U.S. National Aeronautics and Space Administration (NASA) in the 1960s, impedance cardiography (ICG), also known as thoracic electrical bioimpedance, is a noninvasive method to obtain several hemodynamic measurements, including CO. On the basis of the fact that the thorax is a nonhomogeneous electric conductor, we can measure variations in the impedance flow of a high-frequency, low-magnitude, alternating current across the thorax to obtain a waveform from which stroke volume can be calculated via pulse contour analysis.[62] More than 200 studies correlate ICG with other measurements of CO. Although several do not show good correlation, some meta-analyses of the literature on ICG found correlations (r) of 0.82 to 0.93.[63,64] However, owing to several limitations described for this technique, such as electrocardiographic signal abnormalities, movement artifacts, excessive thoracic fluid states (congestive heart failure, hemothorax, pulmonary edema, etc.) and arrhythmias, the reliability of ICG and its application in critically ill patients are still limited.[65]

CONCLUSIONS

The principal objective of hemodynamic monitoring as a therapeutic tool is to maintain an adequate tissue perfusion through oxygen delivery, with the ultimate goal to decrease morbidity and mortality in the critically ill patient. The physiological rationale is still the primary level of defense for using hemodynamic monitoring in critically ill patients.

PAC to monitor arterial pressure is a safe procedure with a low complication rate. However, it should be used only when clear indications exist. There is no evidence that achieving pressures higher than 65 mm Hg improves organ perfusion or favors outcome. The analysis of pulse pressure variation is a useful method to assess preload responsiveness and a potential tool for resuscitation. CVP values have been wrongly used as goals for replacement of intravascular volume in patients with shock. Volume loading in patients with CVP values higher than 12 mm Hg is unlikely to increase CO, and attempts to normalize CVP in early goal-directed therapy during resuscitation have no proven benefit.

The use of PAC provides direct assessment of several physiological parameters, as both raw data and derived measurements (CO, SvO_2, DO_2). Ppao is often used as bedside assessment of pulmonary edema, pulmonary vasomotor tone, intravascular volume status, LV preload, and LV performance. Although PAC is used extensively, there are no clear indications or benefits for its use.

SvO_2 and $ScvO_2$ are important parameters in the assessment of the adequacy of oxygen delivery (DO_2) and its relation to oxygen consumption (VO_2). $ScvO_2$ is a less invasive technique that could be clinically useful in the early detection of tissue hypoxia and as a parameter for therapeutic interventions. The trend of future hemodynamic monitoring devices is moving toward continuous, less invasive, and metabolic assessment techniques, many of which currently require further improvement before they can be used clinically.

Key Points

1. The physiological rationale is the primary level of defense for the use of hemodynamic monitoring in critically ill patients.
2. Arterial catheterization should be used only when clear indications exist. There is no evidence that achieving mean arterial pressures higher than 65 mm Hg improves organ perfusion or favors outcome.
3. Central venous pressure values have been wrongly used as goals for replacement of intravascular volume in patients with shock.

4. There are no clear indications for or proven benefits of the use of the pulmonary artery catheter in hemodynamic monitoring.
5. Mixed venous oxygen saturation and superior vena cava oxygen saturation are important parameters in the assessment of the adequacy of oxygen delivery and its relation to oxygen consumption.

Key References

8. Monnet X, Rienzo M, Osman D, et al: Passive leg raising predicts fluid responsiveness in the critically ill. Crit Care Med 2006;34:1402-1407.

10. Michard F, Teboul JL: Predicting fluid responsiveness in ICU patients: A critical analysis of the evidence. Chest 2002;121:2000-2008.
34. Kumar A, Anel R, Bunnell E, et al: Pulmonary artery occlusion pressure and central venous pressure fail to predict ventricular filling volume, cardiac performance, or the response to volume infusion in normal subjects. Crit Care Med 2004;32:691-699.
47. Pinsky MR, Payen D: Functional hemodynamic monitoring. Crit Care 2005;9:566-572.
52. Cohn SM, Nathens AB, Moore FA, et al: Tissue oxygen saturation predicts the development of organ dysfunction during traumatic shock resuscitation. J Trauma 2007;62:44-55.

See the companion Expert Consult website for the complete reference list.

CHAPTER 7

Respiratory Monitoring

Evans R. Fernández Pérez and Rolf D. Hubmayr

OBJECTIVES

This chapter will:
1. Describe the difference between diagnostic testing and monitoring.
2. Discuss the goals and benefits of as well as indications for respiratory monitoring.
3. Describe the limitations of commonly used respiratory monitoring systems and monitored data.

This chapter discusses the indications, limitations, and benefits of traditional and some investigational methods of respiratory monitoring. We will be careful to distinguish between monitoring and diagnostic testing even though the instrumentation and measured variables for the two activities are often identical. Monitoring is continuous and is usually linked to alarm functions, whereas diagnostic testing is intermittent and generally does not alert the provider of a change in system performance. This latter issue is important because some devices are extremely useful diagnostic adjuncts for the management of critically ill patients yet fail to maintain adequate calibration or lack sensitive and specific alarm trigger algorithms enabling them to serve as monitors of respiratory performance.

RESPIRATORY SERIAL DIAGNOSTIC TESTING AND MONITORING

To monitor or *monitoring* generally means to be aware of the state of a system. For the purpose of this chapter, we have narrowed this definition to the continuous measurement of patient variables coupled to some kind of alarm function. Monitoring commonly overlaps with serial intermittent diagnostic testing. Although the frequency of testing is generally determined by the stability of the patient and hence the likely rate of change in the function being assessed, there is rarely unanimity of opinion about the optimal interval between measurements. In fact, the distinction between diagnostic testing and monitoring is sometimes blurred and commonly depends on the clinical context. For example, a pulse oximeter left in place to monitor changes in oxygen-hemoglobin saturation in response to therapy (e.g., recruitment maneuver) constitutes a different type of surveillance from serial arterial blood gas determinations in a patient with chronic respiratory failure.

Respiratory monitoring in the intensive care unit (ICU) revolves around the information recorded by electronic devices. Although integrated monitoring systems, such as knowledge-based systems for automatic ventilatory management, can increase the rate of accurate signal processing and of clinically significant alarms,[1] current monitoring devices typically incorporate alarm functions that are triggered when a value exceeds a predefined limit. These boundary-based devices (e.g., pulse oximeter) have a good sensitivity but high false-positive rate or low positive predictive value,[2] and for the most part, their diagnostic capacity depends on the type of device.[3] In contrast, the predictive power of diagnostic procedures is high but largely depends on the clinical context (e.g., postintubation chest radiographs).[4]

The clinical utility of a monitoring device is often promoted in terms of the precision and accuracy of its output. Needless to say, these attributes are meaningless unless the management decisions that are made from the results of monitoring or serial testing improve patient outcomes. Unfortunately, conclusive outcomes data are often hard to come by, as the 2001 reassessment of the hemodynamic monitoring practice vividly demonstrated.[5]

CLINICAL DECISION FOR RESPIRATORY MONITORING

The decision to monitor respiration rests on the following assumptions: (1) a decline in respiratory system function warrants a rapid intervention, (2) the intervention is efficacious, and (3) intermittent clinical observation, patient-initiated alerts such as pressing a call button, and alerts from commonly monitored measures of cardiovascular performance such as heart rate are neither sensitive nor specific enough to trigger the warranted intervention. Although it is easy to make the case for the first two assumptions, data in support of the third assumption are few and far between. For example, in a prospective, randomized, observational study of mechanically ventilated patients, a strategy calling for daily routine chest films was associated with neither reductions in ICU and hospital mortality or shorter ICU and hospital length of stay.[6] Arguments in favor of pulse oximetry often focus on the difficulty of detecting hypoxia or hypoventilation by clinical means alone.[7,8] Yet a prospective, randomized evaluation of pulse oximetry in 20,802 surgical patients, although revealing a 19-fold increase in the detection of hypoxemia, failed to demonstrate reductions in the number of postoperative complications, including death.[9]

Features of an ideal monitoring system are reliability, high technical reproducibility, and accuracy, specificity, and sensitivity for detection of clinically relevant changes in system function that lead to improved patient safety and cost-effectiveness of care.[10] In the absence of respiratory monitoring devices that unequivocally fulfill all these specifications, the medical community has come to accept somewhat lesser goals. For example, respiratory monitoring is employed when a therapy cannot be delivered safely without a monitor (e.g., titration of positive end-expiratory pressure [PEEP] in a patient with hypoxic respiratory failure) or when it can help detect relevant physiological alterations (e.g., increased airway pressure in patients at risk for barotrauma) or direct management (e.g., noninvasive ventilation in a hypercapnic patient). Because of the expectation of improvement in patient outcome, monitoring is subject to closer scrutiny than most other diagnostic procedures. However, there is a general lack of randomized and controlled trials documenting that any specific respiratory monitoring or diagnostic technique improves patient outcome.

Pulse Oximetry

The pulse oximeter is probably the most frequently used monitor of respiration in critically ill patients. Despite its widespread use, a UK survey revealed that 97% of critical care providers did not understand how a pulse oximeter worked or what factors influenced its output.[11] Oximeters are diode probes that emit light at two wavelengths, 660 nm (red band) and 940 nm (infrared band).[12] Light penetrates the tissue and is sampled with a photodetector. The oxygen saturation of hemoglobin is derived from the relative rates of absorption of red light (by oxygen-bound hemoglobin) and infrared light (by hemoglobin without oxygen) during the capillary pulse wave under the sensor probe.[13]

The safety and simplicity of pulse oximetry compared with intermittent sampling of arterial blood for gas analysis have led some to promote use of the former as a "fifth vital sign." Pulse oximeters are probably most valuable in patients at risk for hypoxemia in operating and recovery rooms, in emergency units, and in the ICU.[14-16] Pulse oximetry provides near–real-time feedback about the effects of ventilator manipulations on pulmonary gas exchange and acts as a safeguard against serious unrecognized hypoxemia during endoscopic procedures, patient transport, and narcotic- and sedative-induced exacerbations of sleep-related breathing disorders in the critically ill.[17,18]

Most manufacturers report a ±4% accuracy at an oxygen saturation value (SpO_2) of 90% or more. Oximetry is much less reliable at saturation values below 80%, because the device must rely on extrapolated values for which there are no primary source data.[19,20] On the other hand, there is hardly a clinical scenario in which medical decision-making requires a high level of precision when hypoxemia is that severe. Given the sigmoid shape of the oxyhemoglobin dissociation curve, the oximeter has limited use for detection of hyperoxemia.[21] In contrast to co-oximeters, which emit and sample four wavelengths of light to distinguish among adult hemoglobin species (oxygenated, deoxygenated, carboxyhemoglobin, and methemoglobin), the pulse oximeter cannot detect reductions in oxygenation in the presence of dyshemoglobinemias such as carboxyhemoglobinemia and methemoglobinemia. Hyperbilirubinemia generally does not affect the accuracy of the pulse oximeter. However, carbon monoxide is a byproduct of heme metabolism, and icteric patients tend to have higher levels of carboxyhemoglobin. Carbon monoxide competes with hemoglobin for oxygen-binding sites and has optical absorbance characteristics similar to those of oxyhemoglobin. Therefore, the oximeter may overestimate the oxygen saturation in such patients.[22,23]

When using pulse oximetry, one must validate the signal quality by ensuring an acceptable pulse waveform on the photoplethysmographic tracing. Motion artifacts (e.g., from shivering, patient transport) and low perfusion states are the most common sources of artifact and erroneous readings.[24,25] Also, dark skin pigmentation, nail polish, venous pulsation associated with arteriovenous anastomoses or severe right heart failure, administration of methylene blue or indocyanine, fluorescent lighting, and xenon surgical lamps can result in erroneous SpO_2 signals.[26,27] Data acquisition can also affect the timing and depth of recorded desaturation.[28] Real-time oximeters report the average SpO_2 value from a moving window of data points. The output is updated every 0.5 to 2 seconds. Processing data in this way does not display the magnitude of changes in SpO_2. In a trend mode, SpO_2 values are stored every 3 to 12 seconds, depending on the device's manufacturer. Hence, systematic error is introduced with the signal being regressed to the mean. Furthermore, major variations in tracing can be appreciated (Fig. 7-1).[28,29]

The widespread use of pulse oximetry has probably led to a more liberal use of supplemental oxygen, mask ventilation, continuous PEEP, and, on occasion, even mechanical ventilation with the resulting large, potentially injurious tidal volumes. Episodes of hypoxemia in the critically ill are often short lived and related to activity and nursing interventions, so may not require sustained increases in fraction of inspired oxygen (FIO_2) or ventilator settings. Although there is a general consensus that a sustained decrease in oxygen saturation below 88% is to be avoided, this consensus reflects empiricism as much as evidence. It is simply hard to ignore an abnormal reading even though corrective interventions may not be efficacious, and in some instances, as with high tidal volume ventilation, could even prove harmful.

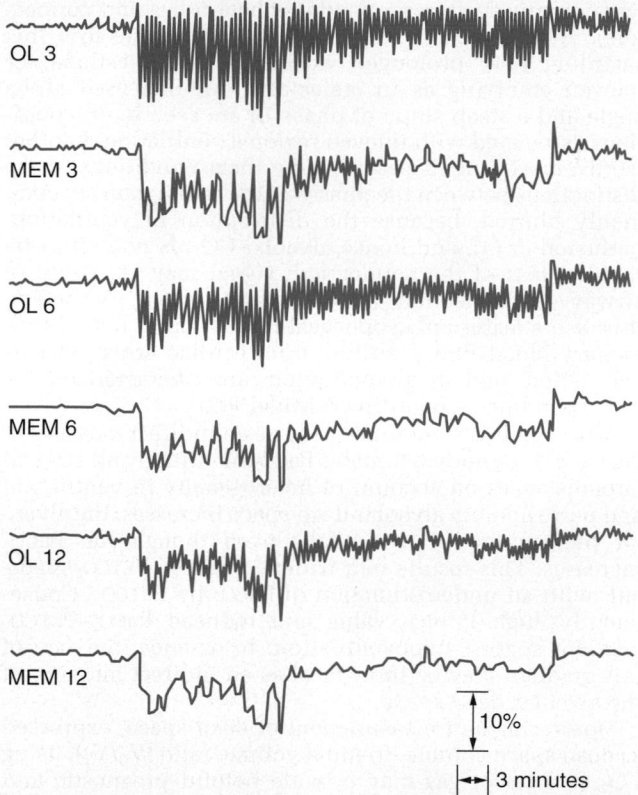

FIGURE 7-1. A segment of a pulse oximeter oxygen saturation (SpO_2) tracing from a single patient, acquired simultaneously in "online" real-time fashion at three different recording settings. Although the overall morphology of the three online traces is quite similar, there is an apparent loss of resolution from the 3-second to 6-second to 12-second recording settings. OL 3, OL 6, and OL 12 correspond to online recording with the oximeter averaging time set at 3, 6 and 12 seconds, respectively. This figure also allows direct comparison of the SpO_2 tracings acquired online with those obtained from the memory of the oximeter; MEM 3, MEM 6, and MEM 12 show the corresponding values from the output stored in the memory. The memory tracings appear similar to the online versions but show a consistent loss of detail in the signal at each recording setting. (From Davila DG, Richards KC, Marshall BL et al: Oximeter performance: The influence of acquisition parameters. Chest 2002;122:1654-1660.)

Transcutaneous and Transconjunctival Oxygen Monitoring

Transcutaneous PO_2 (TcPO$_2$) and transconjunctival PO_2 measurement devices employ polarographic electrodes, which measure the current resulting from a chemical reaction at the sensor surface.[30,31] A platinum cathode and a silver anode maintain a polarizing potential while immersed in an electrolyte solution. Oxygen, which diffuses from the epithelial surface across a semipermeable membrane, generates hydroxyl ions at the cathode, producing a proportional current. These methods provide information about gas tension rather than hemoglobin oxygen saturation and may therefore be used to guard against hyperoxia. Moreover, TcPO$_2$ measurements are not biased by the presence of abnormal hemoglobins.

The transcutaneous device contains a heating element to induce local vasodilatation, because in unstimulated

skin, epidermal PO_2 is nearly zero.[21] In contrast, measurement of transconjunctival PO_2 does not require warming. TcPO$_2$ monitoring has been used to determine the optimal level of amputation in diabetic patients with foot ulcers[32] and to evaluate the outcome of vascular reconstruction.[33] Moreover, this method has gained popularity as a noninvasive tool for selecting candidates with critical limb ischemia for hyperbaric oxygen therapy.[34] In premature infants, the device is often used to monitor hemodynamic performance and to help prevent retinopathy from inadvertent hyperoxemia.[35]

Technical limitations of these methods are prolonged stabilization time after electrode placement and improper calibration due to trapped air bubbles and damaged membranes, which may be difficult to detect. Discrepancies between arterial and transcutaneous PO_2 values are common in states associated with local hypoperfusion.[36]

Transcutaneous Carbon Dioxide Monitoring

In heated skin, CO_2 diffuses readily from capillaries through the avascular stratum corneum, providing a means to estimate and/or identify a trend in changes in arterial CO_2 tension (PaCO$_2$).[37] Transcutaneous carbon dioxide (TcPCO$_2$) is the CO_2 tension of heated skin. TcPCO$_2$ monitoring is the most commonly used noninvasive means of monitoring CO_2 in neonatal intensive care and has been shown to accurately predict PaCO$_2$ and track CO_2 trends.[38,39] TcPCO$_2$ monitoring has many of the same limitations as TcPO$_2$ monitoring.[36] Device calibration is cumbersome, and local skin warming is required. The latter precludes rapid TcPCO$_2$ assessment and may predispose to first-degree burns. The device is costly and sensitive to changes in skin perfusion, which may limit its usefulness in hemodynamically unstable patients. Nevertheless, some studies have reported acceptable correlations between TcPCO$_2$ and PaCO$_2$ values in patients presenting to an emergency department,[40] in stable patients during weaning from mechanical ventilation, in neurosurgical patients, in pediatric patients receiving high-frequency oscillatory ventilation,[41,42] and in older adults in intermediate care units in whom frequent PaCO$_2$ monitoring is desired.[43] TcPCO$_2$ monitoring has also been used during apnea tests for determining brain death.[44]

Capnograph

A *capnograph* is a device for measuring the CO_2 content of inspired and expired gas. The PCO$_2$ can be displayed as a numeric reading (capnometry) and/or as a graphic waveform called a *capnogram*.[45] Time-based capnography expresses the CO_2 signal as a function of time, and from this plot, mean expiratory or end-expiratory (end-tidal) CO_2 values can be obtained. The integration of the volume signal using a flow sensor (pneumotachograph) and CO_2 signal is known as *volumetric capnography*.

Several methods of monitoring and measuring CO_2 are mass spectroscopy, Raman spectroscopy, and infrared light absorption spectroscopy. The most common method of measuring CO_2 is by infrared spectroscopy. Infrared capnographs are configured as either mainstream or sidestream analyzers.[45] Mainstream analyzers attach directly to the oral end of the tracheal tube, thereby minimizing delays between gas sampling and analysis. Their dead space tends to be small, the sample lumen large, and

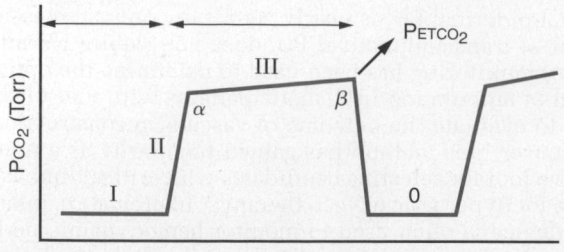

FIGURE 7-2. The phases of a capnogram. Phase I is the inspiratory baseline, which is normally devoid of carbon dioxide and represents the anatomical dead space. A rising baseline suggests that the patient is rebreathing CO_2. Phase II is the expiratory upstroke occurring as existing alveolar gas mixes with dead-space gas; the slope in this phase is more upward and rounded ascending in patients with airflow obstruction (shark-fin morphology). Phase III is the alveolar plateau. The terminal and highest portion of the plateau is called the $PETCO_2$ (concentration of carbon dioxide reached at the end of exhalation). The slope of phase III is slightly positive and is due mainly to differences in time constants and the ventilation-perfusion ($\dot{V}/\dot{Q}$) ratio in various lung segments. Phase IV is the inspiratory waveform decay as inspiration begins. The alpha angle (α) is the angle between phases II and III. This angle is an indirect indication of the $\dot{V}/\dot{Q}$ status of the lung. It tends to be blunted and larger in the setting of airflow obstruction. The beta angle (β) is the angle between phases III and IV. It can be used to assess the extent of rebreathing. During rebreathing, there is an increase in beta angle from the normal 90°.

effects on the work of breathing minimal. Unfortunately, some analyzers are heavy and must be supported to prevent tracheal tube kinking or dislodgment. The analyzer is warmed to prevent condensation, and caution must be taken to prevent burns. Sidestream analyzers connect via small-bore tubing to a bedside monitor and withdraw gas at a constant rate from the ventilator circuit. Because the sampling tubing diameter is small, secretions often block it. Because of the added dead space and continuous sampling, sidestream analyzers exhibit a slower response time and spuriously decrease exhaled tidal volume measurements.

As with other monitoring techniques, several technical limitations can cause errors and inaccuracies in infrared capnograph readings. High concentrations of oxygen, nitrous oxide, and water vapor can change CO_2 concentration because of spectral overlap.[46,47] In addition, high airway pressures can cause a false increase in PCO_2 readings because of transmission of pressure to the cuvette of the capnometer.[46,47]

Monitoring the characteristic abnormalities in the capnographic waveform and measurement of the arterial–to–end-tidal PCO_2 concentration difference and dead space ventilation are useful clinical applications of the capnograph. The capnogram of expired gas has a typical pattern (Fig. 7-2). Phase I represents the anatomical dead space—that is, gas exhaled from the large conducting airway, which normally is devoid of CO_2. Phase II is the expiratory upstroke in which alveolar gas mixes with gas from the conducting airways. The angle between phase II and phase III is the alpha angle. During phase III, the CO_2 concentration curve increases only gradually (alveolar plateau) with a slope that is largely determined by the heterogeneity in alveolar CO_2 tension. The terminal and highest portion of the plateau is called the end-tidal CO_2 ($PETCO_2$). Phase IV is the waveform decay as inspiration begins.

A high baseline CO_2 concentration (phase I) suggests rebreathing of previously expired CO_2 on account of a

large circuit dead space (endotracheal tubes and connectors). A slow upstroke of phase II can be due to a low sampling rate, prolonged expiration as in asthma, or uneven emptying as in atelectasis. An increased alpha angle and a steep slope of phase III are seen in all conditions associated with uneven regional ventilation, in other words, most lung diseases. Under those conditions, sharp distinctions between the phases of the capnogram are commonly blurred, because the distribution of ventilation-perfusion ($\dot{V}/\dot{Q}$), and hence alveolar CO_2, is non-uniform. Sudden loss of the capnograph signal may be a sign of airway disconnection or of sample tubing occlusion. It is also a feature of esophageal intubation or loss of pulmonary blood flow resulting from cardiac arrest. Hyperventilation and hypoventilation are characterized by corresponding changes in end-tidal PCO_2.

Although it is sometimes used as an indirect measure of $PaCO_2$, $PETCO_2$ underestimates $PaCO_2$ in virtually all clinical circumstances on account of heterogeneity in ventilation and perfusion. As alveolar dead space increases, the alveolar plateau (and $PETCO_2$) falls even though the $PaCO_2$ increases. This results in a widened $PaCO_2$–$PETCO_2$ gradient, with an underestimation of $PaCO_2$ by $PETCO_2$. Consequently, high $PETCO_2$ value and reduced $PaCO_2$–$PETCO_2$ gradient suggest hypoventilation. In essence, the size of this gradient may be thought of as an indirect measure of the alveolar dead space.

Monitoring and measurement of dead space, expressed as dead space volume–to–tidal volume ratio (V_D/V_T), using CO_2 as a tracer gas may provide helpful prognostic and diagnostic information in mechanically ventilated patients with lung disease. Mixed expired CO_2 tension ($PECO_2$) has been measured to derive *physiologic dead space* (sum of the anatomic and alveolar dead space). Physiologic dead space calculated from the Enghoff modification of the Bohr equation uses $PaCO_2$ with the assumption that $PaCO_2$ is similar to alveolar PCO_2 ($PACO_2$), such that:

$$V_D/V_T = (PaCO_2 - PECO_2)/PaCO_2$$

In healthy patients, the normal V_D/V_T varies from 0.25 to 0.3. The lower the $PECO_2$, the greater the ratio of dead space to alveolar ventilation for any given level of alveolar CO_2 tension. For example, in patients requiring mechanical ventilation for acute respiratory distress syndrome (ARDS), V_D/V_T has been shown to decrease as the lung is recruited but to increase with lung overdistention during PEEP titration.[48] Furthermore, at least one study demonstrated that V_D/V_T predicts the risk of death independently when measured early in the course of ARDS (for every 0.05 increase in V_D/V_T, the odds of death rose by 45%).[49] In pediatric patients, a V_D/V_T value of 0.50 or less is thought to predict successful extubation, whereas a V_D/V_T value higher than 0.65 tends to be associated with weaning failure.[50] Although capnography is an attractive monitoring modality in critically ill patients, its efficacy remains to be established.

Monitoring Respiratory Rate and Use of Apnea Monitors in Non-Intubated Patients

Acute respiratory failure is a life-threatening condition that is usually preceded by air hunger and changes in respiratory rate and effort. Thus, monitoring of respiratory activity is common practice in patients at risk for respiratory decompensation. Indeed, dyspnea, tachypnea, and apnea are universally accepted triggers of "rapid response team" consultations, which are intended to reduce mortality associated with unwitnessed cardiopulmonary arrest in the hospital.[51,52] Historically, respiratory rate has been used as a component of clinical scoring systems and has proved to be a sensitive marker of acute respiratory dysfunction.[53-55] In one study, for example, a respiratory rate of less than 6 breaths/minute was associated with a 6.8-fold increase in the risk of unexpected in-hospital cardiac arrest and death.[56]

Because a substantial proportion of ICU patients are admitted for monitoring only, there has been interest in identifying which patients can be safely and effectively admitted to intermediate care or "step-down" units, in which monitoring is performed noninvasively. Although pulse oximetry and capnography have received wide acceptance, monitoring devices that detect airflow (e.g., temperature, humidity, and CO_2 sensors) or respiratory effort (e.g., transthoracic impedance, inductance plethysmography) are also available and have been evaluated in small observational studies.[57-59] Airflow can be measured with a pneumotachograph, but this approach requires a tight-fitting face mask and is not practical in critically ill patients. Thermal sensors or nasal pressure monitors are viable alternatives. Thermistors and piezoelectric polymer transducers attached to a nasal cannula or oxygen mask record temperature changes between inspired and expired air. A CO_2 analyzer may be used in a similar fashion. In general, these devices are inexpensive, noninvasive, disposable, and safe but have the drawbacks of inaccuracy and instability. These techniques do not measure airflow quantitatively; instead, changes in the amplitude of the signals reflect relative alterations in flow. These devices are particularly suited to monitor apnea because their signal is not deceived by the confounding influences of patient thoracoabdominal movement.

Respiratory effort may be inferred from recordings of thoracoabdominal motion. Thorax and abdominal wall displacement can be measured with strain gauges or derived from changes in the electrical impedance of wires attached to elastic bands and placed around the rib cage and abdomen. Normally, the thorax and abdomen expand during inspiration. In the presence of upper airway obstruction or respiratory distress and in patients with diaphragm paralysis or cervical spinal cord transection, these structures may move in opposite directions (i.e., paradoxical movement). Chest wall motion monitors help identify apnea (absence of airflow for at least 10 seconds) as central as opposed to obstructive,[60,61] with the caveat that cardiac oscillations may be misinterpreted as ventilatory efforts. Volumetric calibration of respiratory inductive plethysmographs requires patients to perform isovolume maneuvers (moving the chest with closed glottis) a maneuver that requires cooperation and is often impossible for critically ill patients. Monitoring of respiratory rate using single-point impedance devices is common practice, but at present, inductive plethysmography for monitoring respiratory effort must be considered investigational.

Monitoring Respiratory Mechanics during Mechanical Ventilation

The assessment of patient-ventilator interactions is the most informative component of the physical examination of the patient with respiratory failure. A careful inspection of volume, pressure, and flow waveforms, which are displayed by virtually all modern mechanical ventilators, can alert the provider to important changes in lung and respiratory system functions that often require targeted interventions. These include identifying patient-ventilator dyssynchrony, inappropriate and injurious ventilator settings, dynamic hyperinflation, airflow obstruction and decreases in respiratory system compliance, which in turn ought to raise suspicion for barotrauma, mainstem intubation, alveolar collapse, and/or widespread alveolar flooding.

Accurate clinical decision-making based on the information provided by monitoring respiratory mechanics during mechanical ventilation requires an appreciation of pressure, volume, and flow waveforms and the factors that influence them. Assessment of the inspiratory phase can help identify patients at risk for ventilator-induced lung injury. Alternatively, the expiratory phase may provide diagnostic information about the presence of dynamic hyperinflation and gas trapping. Careful inspection of so-called ventilator waveforms may reveal that a patient generates inspiratory efforts far in excess of machine rate or that there is no appreciable temporal relationship between efforts and machine breaths (i.e., patient-ventilator dyssynchrony).

Inspection of the Airway Pressure Tracing

The rules that govern the interactions among pressure, volume, and flow are derived from newtonian physics, and as such, they apply to any mode of mechanical ventilation. Nevertheless, the information contained in the airway-pressure time tracing is easiest to interpret in patients who are relaxed and mechanically ventilated in a volume-preset mode with constant (square wave) inspiratory flow. If one regards the intubated respiratory system as a single unit (and ignores small-scale heterogeneity and nonlinear behavior), the inflation pressure generated by the mechanical ventilator may be decomposed into its resistive (Pres) and elastic (Pel) components. According to Ohm's law, Pres is determined by flow and the resistance of the intubated airways, whereas Pel reflects lung volume and the stiffness of lungs and chest wall. During volume-preset ventilation with constant inspiratory flow and a short postinflation pause, the resulting airway pressure (Paw) tracing has three distinct phases: (1) an initial step change proportional to Pres, (2) a ramp that reflects the increase in Pel as the lungs fill to their end-inflation volume, and (3) a sudden decay from a pressure maximum (Ppeak) to a plateau (Pplat) that reflects the elastic recoil (Pel) of the relaxed respiratory system at the volume at end-inflation.[62] If flow is held constant throughout inflation, Pres must remain constant unless flow resistance changes with volume and time. Consequently, the initial step-change in Paw and its decay from Ppeak to Pplat are of similar magnitude.[62] Figure 7-3 demonstrates these features.

All mechanical ventilators monitor Ppeak on a breath-by-breath basis and trigger alarms at deviations from accepted norms. The long-standing rationale for this safety/alarm function is concern for barotrauma. Although the literature on ventilator-associated lung injury has appropriately focused on the avoidance of large tidal volumes and the maintenance of a safe Pplat, there are no ventilators with distinct—that is, Ppeak-independent—Pplat alarm functions. To the extent to which the variance in Pres is small, monitoring of Ppeak may be considered an adequate surrogate of Pplat monitoring. Nevertheless, no comprehensive studies have addressed this issue. Even

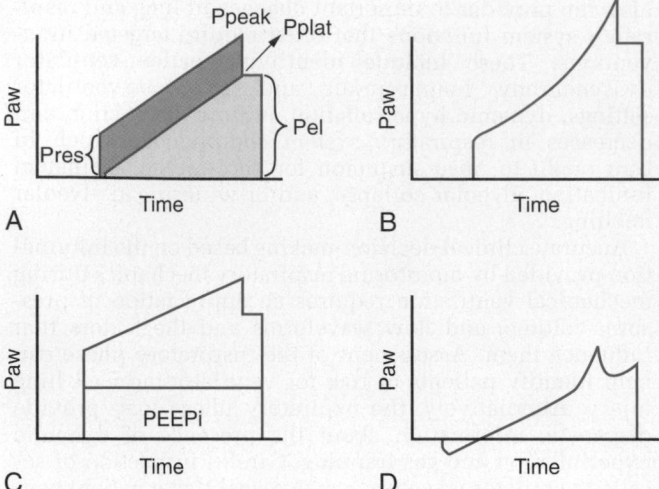

FIGURE 7-3. Schematic illustration of the Paw (airway pressure) profile with time during constant-flow, volume-cycle ventilation. **A,** Passive respiratory system with normal elastance and resistance. Work to overcome the resistive forces is represented by the *dark-shaded area*, and the work to overcome the elastic forces by the *light-shaded area*. Pel, elastic pressure; Ppeak, pressure maximum; Pplat, pressure plateau. **B,** Upsloping of the Paw tracing representing increased respiratory system elastance. **C,** Paw tracing in the presence of inadvertent positive end-expiratory pressure (PEEPi). **D,** Scalloping of the Paw tracing generated by a large patient effort. (From Fernandez Perez ER, Hubmayr RD: Interpretation of airway pressure waveforms. Intensive Care Med 2006;32:658-659.)

less tested is the analysis of the pressure ramp (ΔPel/Δt, where *t* is time) for detecting alveolar recruitment and overdistention. An increase in respiratory compliance during inflation, as reflected by a concavity of the pressure tracing with the time axis, is consistent with progressive alveolar recruitment and may warrant an increase in PEEP therapy. Alternatively, a progressive upward deflection of the pressure-time ramp consistent with stiffening should alert the provider to the dangers of overinflation (see Fig. 7-3).

In an otherwise relaxed patient, monitoring of the pressure-time tracing can also alert the clinician to the presence of dynamic hyperinflation and provide an estimate of the extrinsic PEEP necessary to minimize the effort required to initiate a machine breath.[62] When inadvertent PEEP (PEEPi) is present, the initial step-change in Paw exceeds the peak-to-plateau pressure difference. Pres appears to have decreased as a function of lung volume, but that is not the case. PEEPi would drive expiratory flow were it not for the opposing inflation pressure generated by the mechanical ventilator. Therefore, PEEPi must contribute in addition to Pres to the step-change in Paw at the beginning of a ventilator-initiated lung inflation.[62,63] This method of estimating PEEPi is valid only during volume-preset mechanical ventilation with constant flow, which is the only form of mechanical ventilation during which Pres may be assumed to remain constant with volume and time. Relaxation is not strictly required (the patient may trigger the ventilator) as long as the initial step-change can be extrapolated with reasonable confidence from the slope of the airway pressure ramp.

Inspection of the Flow-Time Tracing and Flow-Volume Curves

During pressure-preset mechanical ventilation, one may deduce the following from the inspiratory flow tracing: (1) A low peak flow may be caused by inadvertent PEEP or a high inspiratory resistance and (2) a decreased slope of the flow time tracing associated with persistence of inspiratory flow throughout the inflation cycle indicates a long time constant. The *time constant* is the time required for the lungs to fill or empty to 63% of their final volume. In linear systems the time constant is determined by the product of resistance and compliance. The longer the time constant, because of either increased resistance (bronchial obstruction, endotracheal tube obstruction) or high compliance (emphysema), the longer it will take for airway and alveolar pressures to equilibrate and hence for the lungs to either fill or empty.[64]

The following may be inferred from the expiratory flow tracing:

1. Unless ventilator tubing and other apparatus dampen the signal, dynamic airway collapse is associated with a large flow transient (flow spike) at the beginning of expiration. This is because gas residing in the collapsing airways is being expelled at a high rate before flow limitation sets in.
2. Persistent flow at end-expiration is seen in the presence of tachypnea, active expiration, or dynamic hyperinflation.[63]

Pressure–Volume Curves

The pressure-volume (P-V) curve has been studied most extensively in patients with ARDS, in hopes that it might allow clinicians to follow the course of disease, individualize ventilator settings, and thereby protect the patient from ventilator-induced lung injury.[65] P-V curves of patients with injured lungs have the following distinguishing features: (1) reduced volume range (i.e., inspiratory capacity), (2) increased recoil pressure at any given volume, (3) reduced cord compliance (i.e., a decrease in the rate of volume change per unit of pressure change, and (4) increased hysteresis (i.e., difference between inflation and deflation characteristics). Although the last feature is generally interpreted as evidence of alveolar recruitment and derecruitment, volume-dependent changes in interfacial tensions would produce the same pattern.

The many descriptors of P-V curve shape, such as resistance, compliance, hysteresis, and inflection point, can vary considerably with measurement method. The P-V curve of a ventilated patient can be constructed with use of the supersyringe method (gold standard),[65] the low-flow inflation technique,[66] and the multiple-occlusion technique.[67] Because static measurements are cumbersome to perform, introduce errors on account of net gas uptake by the lungs during airway occlusion, and require stopping of therapeutic ventilation, some investigators advocate the use of dynamic methods such as the slice method[68] and the dynastic algorithm.[69]

During volume-controlled ventilation with constant inspiratory flow, the total resistance of the respiratory system is related to respiratory circuits, endotracheal tube, conducting airways, and lung parenchyma. The resistive component related to the endotracheal tube can be easily bypassed by direct measurement of the intratracheal pressure.[70] Because airway resistance, the inhomogeneity of regional time constants, and the viscoelastic behavior of the lung tissue are permanent sources of resistive pressure loss, however, all dynamic methods tend to overestimate recoil pressure and, along with it, shape characteristics such as inflection points to some extent.[66,70] The physiological basis of P-V changes with volume and time and the benefit of aggressive lung recruitment remain controversial, so currently, the value of monitoring the P-V relationships in ARDS is unclear.

Electrical Impedance Tomography

Electrical impedance tomography (EIT) is a noninvasive, radiation-free method used to assess regional lung aeration at the bedside. EIT is particularly popular among investigators who endorse aggressive lung recruitment as the surrogate endpoint of optimal ventilator management. Although other modalities, such as computed tomography and magnetic resonance imaging, provide superior spatial resolution, they require patient transport to an imaging suite and are therefore not suitable for frequent monitoring of regional lung function.

EIT consists of two-dimensional maps of potential differences between multiple pairs of circumferentially applied thoracic surface electrodes. The impedance maps correspond to the topographical distributions of regional lung gas. In patients with acute lung injury, EIT images have been found to correlate well ($r^2 = 0.92$) with changes in lung density detected by computed tomography.[71] Anecdotal proof of concept data supporting EIT-guided ventilator management are available in adults and pediatric patients.[72] However, the signal-to-noise ratio tends to be low,[21] and definitive outcome data are lacking.

CONCLUSION

In this chapter, we have provided an overview of traditional as well as some investigative respiratory monitoring devices. Strictly speaking, not even use of the most widely employed device, the pulse oximeter, is supported by level I clinical evidence. Given the catastrophic consequences of failure to recognize severe or sustained hypoxia, it is unlikely that respiratory monitoring modalities will be subjected to the kind of scrutiny hemodynamic monitoring has undergone. In the absence of validated indications—risk-to-benefit statistics pertaining to specific target populations—the provider must nevertheless understand the principles of device operations, must appreciate the physiological determinants of the monitored variables, and must avoid knee-jerk responses that focus on the monitored variable rather than patient benefit.

Key Points

1. Monitoring of oxygenation with pulse oximetry has become the standard of care in critically ill patients.
2. Pulse oximetry is safe, noninvasive, and particularly helpful for detecting hypoxemia during patient transport and invasive procedures.
3. Pulse oximetry is unreliable in the presence of abnormal hemoglobins (e.g., carboxyhemoglobinemia and methemoglobinemia), and its accuracy decreases substantially when the oxygen saturation falls below 85%.
4. Pulse oximetry is often unreliable in shock states associated with peripheral hypoperfusion and is subject to motion artifacts.
5. Measurements of transcutaneous oxygen tension ($TcPO_2$) have been used for monitoring of limb blood flow and hyperoxemia in premature infants.
6. In neonates, transcutaneous CO_2 is the most commonly used noninvasive method to monitor alveolar ventilation and, in this population, predicts arterial CO_2 tension ($PaCO_2$) with reasonable accuracy.
7. Measurements of end tidal CO_2 tension ($PETCO_2$) are often used to differentiate esophageal from tracheal intubation, to assess the adequacy of pulmonary blood flow during cardiopulmonary resuscitation, and, occasionally, to monitor alveolar ventilation during weaning of a patient from mechanical ventilation.
8. In intubated and mechanically ventilated patients, monitoring of airway pressure (Paw), volume (V), and flow (F) is not only integral to machine operation but also essential for assuring lung protection.
9. A formal diagnostic evaluation of respiratory system mechanics and patient-ventilator interactions is useful for estimating the severity of lung impairment and can be a helpful guide in ventilator management.
10. Electrical impedance tomography (EIT) is a new and promising imaging modality for bedside monitoring of regional lung aeration and has been used to adjust positive end-expiratory pressure settings.

Key References

18. AARC (American Association for Respiratory Care) clinical practice guideline: Pulse oximetry. Respir Care 1991;36:1406-1409.
19. Jubran A: Advances in respiratory monitoring during mechanical ventilation. Chest 1999;116:1416-1425.
45. AARC (American Association for Respiratory Care) clinical practice guidelines: Capnography/capnometry during mechanical ventilation. Respir Care 1995;40:1321-1324.
63. Grasso S, Terragni P, Mascia L, et al: Airway pressure-time curve profile (stress index) detects tidal recruitment/hyperinflation in experimental acute lung injury. Crit Care Med 2004;32:1018-1027.
64. de Chazal I, Hubmayr RD: Novel aspects of pulmonary mechanics in intensive care. Br J Anaesth 2003;91:81-91.

See the companion Expert Consult website for the complete reference list.

CHAPTER 8

Monitoring Kidney Function in the Intensive Care Unit

Andrea Morelli

OBJECTIVES

This chapter will:
1. Discuss the best parameters for monitoring kidney function in clinical practice.
2. Describe the role of traditional biomarkers.
3. Detail the role of new biomarkers.

Monitoring of kidney function in the intensive care unit (ICU) is of paramount importance because it facilitates early intervention, evaluates the effectiveness of the therapeutic intervention, and thus might reduce both the need for renal replacement therapy and the rates of morbidity and mortality. Research into new techniques, such as magnetic resonance imaging and new biomarkers for monitoring kidney function, is evolving rapidly as modern technologies make headway. New biomarkers such as neutrophil gelatinase–associated lipocalin, and urinary interleukin-18 might detect injury early on, identify subclinical injury, pinpoint the most affected nephron segments, and thus detect kidney dysfunction at an early stage. Most new biomarkers must still undergo prospective evaluation in a large population and so cannot be used routinely at this time in the ICU. Despite their promising results, however, new sophisticated imaging techniques such as magnetic resonance imaging cannot be regarded as part of the routine bedside evaluation of kidney function. Currently in clinical practice, the monitoring of kidney function in the ICU routinely consists of measurements of the traditional blood (serum creatinine, urea nitrogen) and urine (casts, fractional excretion of filtered sodium) markers of kidney injury. Acute renal failure (ARF) and its severity can be inferred from a decrease in urinary output and an elevation in serum creatinine and/or blood urea nitrogen values, which are correlated with a decline in glomerular filtration rate (GFR) (Table 8-1).[1,2]

MONITORING KIDNEY FUNCTION WITH CURRENTLY AVAILABLE URINE MARKERS

Urinary indices, such as the fractional excretion of filtered sodium, may help distinguish between the two main causes of ARF, prerenal failure and acute tubular necrosis (ATN).[1,2] The passing from prerenal failure to renal failure is usually associated with a rise of (low) fractional sodium and urea excretion rates.[3] However, because of their poor sensitivity and specificity, the use of these indices is quite limited, although a high fractional excretion of urea during ARF (versus prerenal failure) is less influenced by diuretic therapy and thus might be a more sensitive and specific index of kidney function than the fractional excretion of filtered sodium.[3] Characteristics of the urine sediment may also help distinguish between prerenal state and ARF. In prerenal failure, the sediment might appear normal with occasional hyaline or finely granular casts, and the presence of microproteinuria might be detected.[1] In ARF, renal tubular and collecting duct epithelial cells might be detected in addition to granular, leukocytic, waxy, and muddy brown, pigmented casts.[1,2] Nevertheless, the presence of tubular epithelial cells in the urine can reveal only an advanced damage to the renal tubuli, whereas the lack of these findings does not enable renal tubular injury to be excluded. Thus, the urinary sediment lacks specificity and sensitivity for the detection of tubular injury or kidney dysfunction, especially at a very early stage.[1]

MONITORING KIDNEY FUNCTION WITH RENAL PLASMA FLOW

Hemodynamic alterations are a common feature in ICU patients and are important in the pathogenesis of ARF. Thus the estimation of renal plasma flow should be of great importance in monitoring kidney function. However, the renal plasma flow is not a reliable index of kidney function. First, because urinary *p*-aminohippurate clearance, which has traditionally been used as a test of renal plasma flow, may underestimate renal plasma flow in patients with ARF.[4] Second, total renal plasma flow is relatively normal or only modestly decreased during the extension, maintenance, and recovery stages of ischemic renal injury despite a disproportionately profound depression of GFR.[4]

MONITORING KIDNEY FUNCTION WITH GLOMERULAR FILTRATION RATE

Given the preceding observations, the best global index for the monitoring of renal function is GFR. GFR is commonly measured using plasma or renal clearance of marker solutes administered as a bolus or continuous infusion.[5] Inulin clearance has been indicated as the reference standard for GFR measurement because inulin fulfills the criteria for an ideal GFR marker (i.e., its production rate is stable, its circulating levels are not affected by other patho-

TABLE 8-1

Proposed Classification Scheme for Acute Renal Failure*

CLASSIFICATION	GLOMERULAR FILTRATION RATE	SERUM CREATININE CONCENTRATION	URINE OUTPUT
Risk	>25% decrease	Increased 1.5 times	<0.5 mL/kg/hr for 6 hr
Injury	>50% decrease	Increased 2.0 times	<0.5 mL/kg/hr for 12 hr
Failure	>75% decrease	Increased 3.0 times	<0.3 mL/kg/hr for 24 hr
		or	*or*
		>355 µmol/L with acute rise >44 µmol/L^{-1}	Anuria for 12 hr
Loss	Persistent acute renal failure = complete loss of kidney function for >4 wk		
End-stage renal disease	Persistent acute renal failure = complete loss of kidney function for >3 months		

*The classification system includes separate criteria for creatinine and urinary output.
Modified from Trof RJ, Di Maggio F, Leemreis J, Groeneveld AB: Biomarkers of acute renal injury and renal failure. Shock 2006;26:245-253.

logical changes, and it is freely filtered at the glomerulus without tubular reabsorption or secretion). The clearances of radioisotope-labeled substances, such as chromium Cr 51–labeled ethylenediaminetetraacetic acid (EDTA) (^{51}Cr-EDTA) and technetium Tc 99m–labeled diethylene-triamine pentaacetic acid (^{99m}Tc-DTPA), or of nonlabeled trace quantities of iothalamate or iohexol, have been accepted as accurate substitutes for inulin clearance.

GFR can be measured by continuous infusion method, standard clearance method, or plasma clearance method. When GFR is estimated with the infusion method without urine collection, a known concentration of GFR marker is infused at a constant rate, generally after a bolus loading dose, in order to achieve a steady state. However, if GFR is highly unstable, a steady state may not be achieved. In estimation of GFR with the standard clearance method, bolus administration and infusion of a GFR marker are performed exactly as described previously. In addition, urine is collected at fixed intervals. Urine flow rate (V) and urinary marker concentration (U) are recorded. Peripheral venous blood is drawn immediately before and after the urine collection period for measurement of plasma marker concentrations. Renal clearance can be calculated with application of the following formula:

$$\text{GFR} = \frac{U \times V}{P}$$

where P is the logarithmic average of the plasma marker concentration before and after the collection period. Collection of urine and plasma at fixed-time intervals enables rapid changes in GFR to be detected. With estimation of GFR using the plasma clearance method, a bolus dose of a marker is administered, and then multiple plasma samples are collected to enable calculation of the disappearance rate of the marker.

Although the exact estimation of GFR would be desirable for determination of drug dosages, timing of dialysis, and prediction of prognosis, the previously mentioned GFR markers are not easily assayed in laboratories, and the methods are difficult to perform at the bedside in a critical care setting.[5] GFR can also be assessed through measurement of the clearance of endogenous markers, such as creatinine and urea, or through determination of their plasma concentrations or their reciprocals, mainly of serum creatinine and serum cystatin C.[5-7] Although serum creatinine is widely used as such a marker, its limitations are well known. The serum creatinine concentration depends on dietary intake, and its value is not a very accurate predictor of GFR in very elderly patients because creatinine production decreases as muscle mass decreases

with age. Moreover, serum creatinine concentration alone provides for inaccurate information of estimated GFR when GFR is rapidly changing or before it reaches an equilibrium value. Indeed, changes in serum creatinine concentration lag several days behind actual changes in GFR. Moreover, the alterations in serum creatinine concentration are not particularly sensitive or specific for small changes in GFR. In addition, creatinine clearance overestimates GFR because of tubular secretion of creatinine. Oral administration of cimetidine, a blocker of tubular creatinine secretion, may improve the accuracy of measurement of creatinine clearance but requires a pretreatment period that is not useful in routine monitoring of kidney function in ICU patients. Moreover, this technique has not been validated in patients with ARF. Equations such as the Cockcroft-Gault equation and the more recent Modification of Diet in Renal Disease (MDRD) Study equation are available to estimate creatinine clearance from a patient's age, body weight, and serum creatinine concentration.[8] The Cockcroft-Gault equation might underestimate renal function in older people because of a too strong effect of age. However, these equations should not be used in the patient with rapid modifications of GFR—which are quite common in ARF or in unstable critically ill patients—because they start from the value of serum creatinine.

Many low-molecular-weight serum proteins have been investigated as suitable endogenous markers of GFR. Among these, attention has been particularly focused on serum cystatin C, a nonglycosylated, low-molecular-weight protein containing 120 amino acids. Serum cystatin C is steadily produced by all human nucleated cells, and importantly, it does not depend on muscle mass, body mass index, hydration status, or gender. Cystatin C is freely filtered by the glomerulus and is catabolized in the proximal tubules.[9] A decline in renal function is associated with an increase in serum cystatin C concentrations. In contrast to the past, cystatin C can now be easily measured by immunometric/nephelometric methods, and thus, its concentration can be routinely used in clinical practice. There are still conflicting findings as to the predictive value of serum cystatin C values in critically ill patients. A change in serum cystatin C has been reported to be more sensitive than a change in serum creatinine concentration as a marker of changes in glomerular filtration. A meta-analysis confirmed the superiority of serum cystatin C concentration over serum creatinine concentration as a measure of GFR.[10] Cystatin C was also evaluated as an early marker of decreased glomerular filtration and ARF in critically ill patients. Serum cystatin C levels were able to predict the development of ARF 1 or 2 days earlier than serum creatinine concentrations.[11] Nevertheless, these results were not confirmed in other studies. Cystatin C can also be detected in the urine. Normally, cystatin C is present in the urine at concentrations 10-fold lower than in plasma; it has been reported, however, that in the presence of renal tubular injury, urinary cystatin C concentrations increase approximately 200 times.[12] Herget-Rosenthal and associates[13] found that increased urinary excretion of cystatin C had a higher sensitivity and specificity for renal injury than did the α_1-microglobulin N-acetyl-glucosaminidase level in predicting the need for renal replacement therapy. Because cystatin C levels do not demonstrate a circadian rhythm, there is no need for a 24-hour urine collection. This substance can be measured in a single urine sample.

MONITORING KIDNEY FUNCTION WITH NEW SERUM AND URINE BIOMARKERS

N-Terminal prohormone of the atrial natriuretic peptide, proANP(1-98), has been extensively analyzed in patients with chronic renal failure. Its level has been found to be closely related to renal function. In septic patients on their first day in the ICU, proANP(1-98) measurements were found to have better predictive value for the occurrence of renal failure than diuresis, calculated creatinine clearance, or serum cystatin C levels. Interestingly, proANP(1-98) was also higher in nonsurvivors in this study.[14]

Several tubular enzymes have been investigated mainly as markers of tubular damage and, indirectly, of early kidney dysfunction, because enzymuria seems to be directly related to a rise in serum creatinine concentration, a reduction in creatinine clearance, and thus, a decrease in GFR.[15] The best-characterized tubular enzymes for detection of tubular injury are glutathione S-transferases (GSTs), γ-glutamyl transferase (γ-GT), alkaline phosphatase, lactate dehydrogenase, N-acetyl-D-glucosaminidase (NAG), fructose-1,6-bisphosphatase, and Ala-(Leu-Gly)-aminopeptidase. The α- and π-glutathione S-transferase (α-GST and π-GST) isomers are cytoplasmic enzymes found in the proximal and distal tubular epithelial cells, respectively. One of the major limiting factors to the use of enzymuria in clinical practice is the low threshold for the release of tubular enzymes, even in response to injury that may not proceed to ARF. Moreover, enzymes are also released during chronic glomerular diseases, a characteristic that might limit their use as specific markers of tubular injury or in monitoring renal function. In this regard, the use of NAG is limited by the fact that urinary excretion of the enzyme is also elevated in glomerular diseases such as diabetic nephropathy.[16] As Herget-Rosenthal and associates[17] reported, tubular enzymuria can detect tubular damage 12 to 14 days earlier than the currently available parameters of renal function.

CONCLUSION

In the future, new biomarkers in urine and serum will enable routine monitoring of kidney function in the ICU and detection of kidney dysfunction at an early stage, before a decline in GFR is reflected by an increase in serum creatinine concentration. Nevertheless, at present, the serum cystatin C level is becoming easier to assay and seems to be superior to serum creatinine concentration in monitoring kidney function in the ICU.

Key Points

1. Glomerular filtration rate is the best index for monitoring renal function.
2. Changes in serum creatinine concentration lag several days behind actual changes in the glomerular filtration rate, and the alterations in serum creatinine concentration are not particularly sensitive or specific for small changes in this rate.
3. An increase in serum creatinine concentration is not directly related to tubular injury but it is the effect of a loss of the filtration function that occurs with acute renal injury.
4. Serum cystatin C levels reflect glomerular filtration rate with great sensitivity and specificity.
5. Serum cystatin C concentration is becoming easier to assay and seems to be superior to serum creatinine concentration for monitoring kidney function in the intensive care unit.

Key References

1. Thadhani R, Pascual M, Bonventre JV: Acute renal failure. N Engl J Med 1996;334:1448-1458.
4. Corrigan G, Ramaswamy D, Kwon O, et al: PAH extraction and estimation of plasma flow in human postischemic acute renal failure. Am J Physiol 1999;277:F312-F318.
5. Price CP, Finney H: Developments in the assessment of glomerular filtration rate. Clin Chim Acta 2000;297:55-56.
10. Herget-Rosenthal S, Markggraf G, Hüsing J, et al: Early detection of acute renal failure by serum cystatin C. Kidney Int 2004;66:1115-1122.
14. Westhuyzen J, Endre ZH, Reece G, et al: Measurement of tubular enzymuria facilitates early detection of acute renal impairment in the intensive care unit. Nephrol Dial Transplant 2003;18:543-551.

See the companion Expert Consult website for the complete reference list.

The Critically Ill Patient: Severity Scores

CHAPTER 9

General Illness Severity Scores

Jean-Louis Vincent

OBJECTIVES

This chapter will:
1. Define the general illness severity scores currently used in critically ill patients.
2. Discuss studies comparing these various severity scores.
3. Propose future developments in general illness severity scoring.

Characterizing patients being treated in the intensive care unit (ICU) according to the severity of their illness is clearly important in terms of prognostication, ICU organization, and resource allocation as well as for developing inclusion criteria for and interpreting data from clinical trials. However, the ideal tool for determining disease severity has been a matter of some debate.

Characterizing severity of illness in ICU patients has taken the following approaches:
- Admission outcome prediction scores (APACHE, SAPS, MPM)
- Admission organ failure score (LODS)
- Organ dysfunction scores (MODS, SOFA)
- Scores that define severity according to resource use (TISS, NEMS)

ADMISSION OUTCOME PREDICTION SCORES

Acute Physiology and Chronic Health Evaluation

The Acute Physiology and Chronic Health Evaluation (APACHE) score was first developed in 1981 by Knaus and colleagues[1] using a nominal group process. This score and its offspring, APACHE II through IV, have become the most commonly used ICU survival prediction model. The purpose of the APACHE system as it was developed was not to prognosticate for individual patients but to classify groups of patients according to severity of illness.[1] The original APACHE score was divided into two sections, a

physiology score designed to measure the level of acute illness and a preadmission health status evaluation designed to determine the chronic health status of the patient. The physiology portion assessed abnormalities in 34 physiological variables over the first 32 hours of admission and awarded each a weighted score such that the higher the score, the sicker the patient. The preadmission health status portion reviewed functional status, medical attention, and presence of chronic diseases over the 6 months prior to admission and allocated patients to one of four chronic health categories from A (prior good health) to D (severe restriction of activity due to disease). A patient's APACHE classification would, therefore, consist of a number (the physiology score) and a letter (the chronic health status), for example, 33-D. In 1985, Knaus and colleagues[2] revised and simplified the original APACHE model to create APACHE II. APACHE II reduced the number of physiological measurements from 34 to just 12 using a multivariate comparison of the original APACHE, with each proposed revision to ensure that the model remained valid. Weightings and thresholds were also altered in some cases. Another major change was that the effects of age and chronic health status were incorporated directly into the model, with weighting according to their relative impacts. The recorded value is based on the worst value recorded during the first 24 hours of a patient's admission to the ICU. The maximum possible APACHE II score is 71, and rising scores correlate with increasing mortality rates.[2]

APACHE III was developed in 1991[3] and was validated and further updated in 1998.[4] APACHE III was a more complex score, and partly owing to its lack of free availability, it never became as popular as APACHE II. Most recently, APACHE IV was developed in an attempt to improve the prognostic accuracy of the system. ICU patient populations have changed over the last 10 to 15 years, since the last update was created, and the accuracy of the APACHE system and, indeed other predictive systems, has deteriorated in that time.[5] APACHE IV has been developed through remodeling of APACHE III using the same physiological variables and weights but different predictor variables and refined statistical methods.[5] Importantly, APACHE IV is available in the public domain, but it is a complex system, and because it has been developed and validated in ICUs in the United States, it may not be as accurate in mortality prediction in other countries with different ICU organization or different patient populations.

Simplified Acute Physiology Score

The Simplified Acute Physiology Score (SAPS), first developed and validated in 1984 in France, used 13 weighted physiological variables and age to indicate the risk of death for ICU patients.[6] Like the APACHE score, SAPS was calculated from the worst values obtained during the first 24 hours after ICU admission and was not designed for individual prognostication. In 1993, SAPS II was developed through the use of logistic regression analysis to select and weight the variables.[7] SAPS II consists of 17 variables: 12 physiological variables, age, type of admission (scheduled surgical, unscheduled surgical, or medical), and 3 variables related to underlying disease (acquired immunodeficiency syndrome, metastatic cancer, and hematologic malignancy). For the physiological variables, the worst value during the first 24 hours of ICU admission is used for the calculation. The SAPS II score was validated with data from consecutive admissions to 137 ICUs in 12 countries.[7]

As with the APACHE, the realization that the SAPS II had lost some of its accuracy over time led to attempts to improve its accuracy. An extended version was created and published in 2005,[8] with the addition of 6 admission variables: age, sex, length of pre-ICU hospital stay, patient location before ICU, clinical category, and presence of drug overdose. This model had better calibration, discrimination, and uniformity of fit than the original SAPS II. Also in 2005, a completely new SAPS model, SAPS III, was created from a database of 16,784 patients from 303 ICUs in 35 countries that had been established in 2002.[9] Complex statistical techniques were used to select and weight variables. The SAPS III score consists of 20 variables and is divided into two parts: the SAPS III admission score, and the SAPS III probability of death at hospital discharge. The SAPS III admission score (range 0-217) is the total of three subscores related to patient characteristics before admission, the circumstance of the admission, and the extent of physiological derangement within 1 hour before or after ICU admission. Interestingly, unlike any of the other scores, SAPS III has customized equations for prediction of hospital mortality in the following seven geographical regions: Australasia; Central and South America; Central and Western Europe; Eastern Europe; North Europe; Southern Europe and the Mediterranean; and North America. Use of a regional score potentially enables better comparison with other ICUs in the same geographic region, although it also reduces the accuracy of comparison with ICUs in different geographical zones. The SAPS III score has been shown to exhibit satisfactory discrimination, calibration, and goodness of fit.[9]

Mortality Probability Model

The first Mortality Probability Model (MPM) was published in 1985 with the use of data from patients in one ICU. It consisted of an admission model comprising 7 admission variables, none of which was treatment related, and a 24-hour model using seven 24-hour variables reflecting treatments and patients' conditions in the ICU.[10] Predicted outcomes using these two models were closely correlated with actual outcomes. MPM II, published in 1993 as a revision of the earlier MPM, used logistic regression techniques on a large database of 12,610 ICU patients from 12 countries.[11] MPM II also consists of two scores: MPM_0, the admission model, which contains 15 variables; and MPM_{24}, the 24-hour model, which contains 5 of the admission variables and 8 additional variables and is designed for patients who are in the ICU for more than 24 hours. Unlike with the APACHE and SAPS systems, each variable in MPM II, apart from age, which is entered as the patient's age in years, is designated as present or absent and given a score of 1 or 0 accordingly. A logistic regression equation is used to provide the user with a probability of hospital mortality. Models were also created using the same 13 variables as MPM_{24} but with different constants in the equation to reflect increasing mortality with lengthening ICU stay, to estimate the probability of hospital mortality at 48 hours (MPM_{48}) and 72 hours (MPM_{72}).[12] MPM_0 has been updated with use of data from 124,855 patients collected in 2001 through 2004.[13]

Summary

Differences in the baseline characteristics of admitted patients, in the circumstances of the ICU admission, in the availability and use of general and specific therapeutic measures, and in the use of withdrawing and withholding decisions have been recognized as introducing a growing gap between actual and predicted mortality in recent years.[14] This observation has led to updates of all three of the major prediction systems in this category with more recent patient data. Interestingly, determinants of hospital mortality have changed since the 1990s, with chronic health status and circumstances of ICU admission becoming relatively more important in prognostication.[9] All three scoring systems currently have good calibration, but as further advances are made in critical care medicine and patient populations change, the systems must undergo periodic review to ensure continued accuracy.

Although prediction scores, by providing an estimation of risk of mortality, can offer some information about disease severity, they have not been validated for this purpose. In addition, they cannot be used to predict prognosis in individual patients. Nevertheless, mortality prediction scores are widely used as a means of characterizing and comparing patients in clinical trials.[15-18]

ADMISSION ORGAN FAILURE SCORES

Logistic Organ Dysfunction Score

The Logistic Organ Dysfunction Score (LODS) was developed in 1996 from a large database of 13,152 admissions to 137 ICUs in 12 countries.[19] With use of a multiple logistic regression technique, a combination of 12 variables was selected and weighted for six organ systems (neurologic, cardiovascular, renal, pulmonary, hematologic, and hepatic). To determine the score, the worst value for each variable in the first 24 hours of admission is recorded. For each system, a score of 0 indicates no dysfunction and a score of 5 represents maximum dysfunction; however, the LODS is a weighted system, so for the respiratory and coagulation systems, the maximum score allowed is 3, and for the liver, the maximum score is 1. The range of LODS values is, therefore, from 0 to 22. As a scoring system, the LODS falls somewhere between the mortality prediction scores and the organ dysfunction scores because it combines a global score that summarizes the combined dysfunction of the organ systems, and a logistic regression equation that can be used to translate the score into a probability of death. The LODS score indeed showed good correlation with mortality, an LODS score of 22 being associated with a mortality rate of 99.7%.[19] Within organ systems, higher levels of the severity of organ dysfunction were consistently associated with higher mortality.[20] Although not initially validated for repeated use during a patient's ICU stay, the LODS has been used to characterize the progression of multiple-organ dysfunction during the first week of ICU stay.[21]

ORGAN DYSFUNCTION SCORES

Organ failure scores are designed to describe organ dysfunction and, hence, disease severity more than to predict survival. The first scoring system to classify organ dysfunction was developed more than 30 years ago,[22] but interest seemed to dwindle with the development of the outcome prediction scores. However, with the realization of the importance of (multiple) organ failure on mortality and increasing dissatisfaction with death as a sole endpoint for clinical trials, interest in organ dysfunction scores has been rekindled.

The aim of all these systems is to describe organ failure as a continuous variable rather than a present/absent phenomenon. Organ (dys)function can vary hugely among individuals and within an individual over time; for example, a patient with a slightly raised urea level may not have normal renal function, but the extent of this patient's organ dysfunction is very different from that of a patient who has no remaining renal function and requires continuous dialysis or renal transplantation. Individuals can have abnormal function of one or several organs, and scoring systems thus must be able to separate out the different organ systems. In addition, organ function varies over time, and organ dysfunction scores must be able to be reevaluated at regular intervals to reflect this dynamic process.

Although the rationale for measuring organ dysfunction is not to predict outcome but to describe morbidity as it evolves over time, the ability of organ dysfunction scores to predict mortality has been used as a measure of their accuracy because there is no gold standard organ dysfunction scoring system to compare them to.

Many organ dysfunction scores have been developed,[19,23-30] but most are less commonly used today because they do not allow the study of the time course of organ dysfunction. The two modern scores designed for repeated use are the multiple organ dysfunction score (MODS) and the sequential organ failure assessment (SOFA).

Multiple Organ Dysfunction Score

Marshall and associates[29] developed the MODS by performing a literature review of all the studies of multiple organ failure published between 1969 and 1993. These researchers determined characteristics that had been used to define organ failure in other studies, and then selected seven organ systems for further analysis (respiratory, cardiovascular, renal, hepatic, hematological, central nervous, and gastrointestinal); they later eliminated the gastrointestinal system because they could find no reliable, continuous descriptor. Variables used to define the function of each organ system were selected according to a set of "ideal descriptor" criteria established by the researchers. For the cardiovascular system, Marshall and associates[29] created an artificial variable, the pressure-adjusted heart rate (heart rate × central venous pressure/mean blood pres-

sure), which can limit the use of the score in patients who do not have a central line. For each of the six organs, the first parameters of the day are recorded to calculate the score, and a score of 0 (normal) to 4 (most dysfunction) is awarded, for a total maximum score of 24. A high initial MODS has been shown to correlate well with death in the ICU, but the delta MODS—defined as the difference between the MODS score at admission and the maximum score—was even more predictive of outcome.[29]

Sequential Organ Failure Assessment

The SOFA was derived from the MODS score. It was developed in 1994 during a consensus conference involving 51 leaders in intensive care medicine (Table 9-1).[30] Originally called the sepsis-related organ failure assessment score, the name was soon changed to sequential organ failure assessment as it became apparent that this evaluation of organ function was not specific to sepsis but could be used in all critically ill patients. The same six organ systems (respiratory, cardiovascular, renal, hepatic, central nervous, and coagulation systems) were selected, and each is scored from 0 (normal function) to 4 (most abnormal). The worst values obtained on each day are recorded. The major difference from the MODS score is in the cardiovascular component, for which the SOFA score uses a treatment-related variable (dose of vasopressor agents) instead of the artificial pressure-adjusted heart rate used in MODS. The use of a treatment-related variable is not ideal, because treatment protocols may vary among institutions and even among patients, but is difficult to avoid, especially for the cardiovascular system, in which treatment-independent variables are difficult to define. Moreover, the severity of shock states is assessed not by vital signs like arterial pressure or heart rate, but by the vasopressor requirements of the patient.

The SOFA score was validated in the general ICU population[31] and has since been validated and applied in various specific patient groups, including medical and surgical cardiovascular ICU patients[32,33] and trauma patients.[34] Although individual organ scores are important in describing the changing pattern of organ dysfunction in individual patients, the total maximum score can be used for outcome assessment because it evaluates the cumulative amount of organ dysfunction sustained by a patient during the ICU stay. In a prospective analysis of 1449 patients, a maximum total SOFA score higher than 15 correlated with a mortality rate of 90%.[35] In a study of 873 patients from 10 ICUs in Scotland, Nfor and colleagues[36] reported that the odds of ICU death within 7 days doubled for each 5-unit increase in total SOFA score on the day of admission. Changes in SOFA score over time are also useful in predicting outcome. In a prospective study of 352 ICU patients, a rise in SOFA score during the first 48 hours in the ICU, independent of the initial score, predicted a mortality rate of at least 50%, whereas a decrease was associated with an ICU mortality rate of just 27%.[37] In a prospective observational study of 1340 patients with multiple organ dysfunction syndrome, Cabré and coworkers reported 100% mortality for patients who were older than 60 years, with a total maximum SOFA score greater than 13 on any of the first 5 days of ICU admission, a minimum SOFA score lower than 10 at all times, and a SOFA score that demonstrated a positive trend or was unchanged over the first 5 days of ICU admission.[38]

One key advantage that the organ dysfunction scores have over the outcome prediction models is that they can

TABLE 9-1

The Sequential Organ Failure (SOFA) Score

FEATURE ASSESSED	ASSESSMENT USED	SOFA SCORE				
		0	1	2	3	4
Respiration	PaO_2/FiO_2, mm Hg	>400	≤400	≤300	≤200	≤100
					With respiratory support	
Coagulation	Platelets, × $10^3/mm^3$	>150	≤150	≤100	≤50	≤20
Liver function	Bilirubin, mg/dL (µmol/L)	<1.2 (<20)	1.2-1.9 (20-32)	2.0-5.9 (33-101)	6.0-11.9 (102-204)	>12.0 (>204)
Cardiovascular function	Presence of hypotension	No hypotension	Mean arterial pressure <70 mm Hg	Dopamine ≤5 *or* Dobutamine (any dose)*	Dopamine >5 *or* Epinephrine ≤0.1 *or* Norepinephrine ≤0.1*	Dopamine >15 *or* Epinephrine >0.1 *or* Norepinephrine >0.1*
Central nervous system function	Glasgow Coma Scale score	15	13-14	10-12	6-9	<6
Renal function	Serum creatinine, mg/dL (µmol/L), *or*	<1.2 (<110)	1.2-1.9 (110-170)	2.0-3.4 (171-299)	3.5-4.9 (300-440)	>5.0 (>440)
	Urine output				<500 mL/d	<200 mL/d

*Adrenergic agents administered for at least 1 hour (doses given are in µg/kg/min).
Adapted from Vincent JL, Moreno R, Takala J, et al: The SOFA (Sepsis-related Organ Failure Assessment) score to describe organ dysfunction/failure. On behalf of the Working Group on Sepsis-Related Problems of the European Society of Intensive Care Medicine. Intensive Care Med 1996;22:707-710.

separate out and follow the patterns of individual organ dysfunction over time. Multiple organ failure is by definition a combination of failure of more than two organ systems. The cardiovascular and respiratory systems are most commonly involved,[36] and in a study using data from 1449 patients from 40 ICUs, the cardiovascular SOFA component was associated with the highest relative contribution to outcome (odds ratio 1.68), followed by the renal component (odds ratio 1.46).[31]

The SOFA Score in Patients with Acute Renal Failure

The SOFA score has also been used to define profiles of and trends in patients with acute renal failure (ARF). Analysis of a database of 1411 ICU patients from 40 ICUs reported that ARF, defined as a renal SOFA score of 3 or 4, developed in 348 patients during their ICU stays.[39] Mortality was three times higher in these patients than in those in whom ARF did not develop. Of the 348 patients, 241 had failure of at least one other organ. Association of cardiovascular dysfunction with ARF was associated with the highest mortality (Fig. 9-1), and the maximum cardiovascular score in patients with ARF was an independent risk factor for mortality.[39] In patients with ARF undergoing renal replacement therapy, a greater increase in SOFA score over the first 24 hours was independently associated with a greater risk of death (odds ratio 1.7; 95% confidence interval 1.2-2.6; $P = .013$).[40] SOFA was developed to be used in heterogeneous groups of ICU patients, and although SOFA scores have been applied to the subgroup of patients with renal disease, their accuracy in this situation may be questioned, and disease-specific scoring systems are now being developed. In a 2005 study in patients with ARF, admission SOFA and APACHE II scores performed better

than renal-specific severity scores, and the admission SOFA score was an independent predictor of mortality.[41] However, in a study published by the BEST Kidney (Beginning and Ending Supportive Therapy for the Kidney) investigators,[42] none of six scores—SOFA, SAPS II, and four renal-specific severity scores—had a high level of discrimination or calibration to predict mortality in patients with ARF.

Comparison of Organ Dysfunction Scores

Relatively few studies have directly compared the various scoring systems. Jacobs and associates[43] reported that the maximum MODS and delta MODS were able to mirror organ dysfunction and describe outcome groups better than APACHE II and the organ failure score. Pettila and colleagues[44] reported that the area under receiver operating curve (AUC) values for prediction of hospital mortality for day 1 scores were 0.825 for APACHE III, 0.805 for LODS, 0.776 for SOFA, and 0.695 for MODS with no statistical differences between the total maximum scores. Peres Bota and coworkers[45] reported no significant differences between MODS and SOFA for mortality prediction, although when using the cardiovascular component, outcome prediction was better for the SOFA score at all time intervals compared to the MODS. However, Zygun and associates,[46] in their study of 1436 ICU patients in Canada, noted that the SOFA scores and MODS values had only a modest ability to discriminate between survivors and nonsurvivors. In a later study, these same researchers reported that in patients with brain injury, the SOFA system was superior to the MODS system in discriminative ability for hospital mortality and unfavorable neurologic outcome.[47]

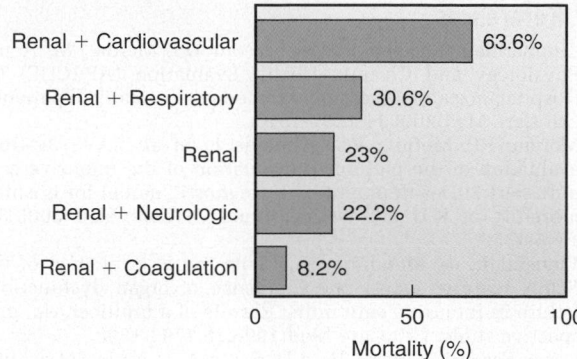

FIGURE 9-1. Association between intensive care unit mortality rate (*bars*) and presence of organ failures in patients with acute renal failure. The association of acute renal failure with acute cardiovascular failure carries the highest mortality rate. (From de Mendonça A, Vincent JL, Suter PM, et al: Acute renal failure in the ICU: Risk factors and outcome evaluated by the SOFA score. Intensive Care Med 2000;26:915-921.)

Summary

Organ dysfunction scoring systems can have several applications in critically ill patients in addition to providing a quantitative means of assessing ongoing organ dysfunction and disease evolution in individual patients, including use in clinical trials to evaluate the effects of new (or old) treatments on morbidity[48-51] and use in epidemiological studies to describe characteristics of patient populations.[52,53] Evaluation of the evolution of organ dysfunction scores during critical illness can also help improve understanding of both the pathogenesis and natural history of multiple organ failure and the interaction between various organ failures.

SCORING OF SEVERITY ACCORDING TO RESOURCE USE

One of the aims of the original therapeutic intervention scoring system (TISS) was, indeed, to stratify severity of illness. Since the development of more specific tools for this purpose, however, resource use scores have become more a management aid to assess nursing workload and associated ICU costs.

Therapeutic Intervention Scoring System

The TISS, which was developed in 1974,[54] essentially evaluates needs in staffing and assesses utilization of ICU facilities. Because sicker patients are more likely to need more interventions, a higher TISS score usually implies a more severely ill ICU patient. The original score and its update in 1983[55] involved 76 selected therapeutic activities, which made its use somewhat time-consuming. A simplified version, containing just 28 items, was developed in 1996.[56] These 28 items are weighted, giving a total possible score of 88. TISS scores correlate well with ICU costs[57,58] and may be a useful tool in the management of nursing manpower in the ICU.[56]

TABLE 9-2

The Nine Equivalents of Nursing Manpower Use Score

ITEM	POINTS
1. Basic monitoring: hourly vital signs, regular record and calculation of fluid balance.	9
2. Intravenous medication: bolus or continuous, not including vasoactive drugs.	6
3. Mechanical ventilatory support: any form of mechanical/assisted ventilation, with or without positive end-expiratory pressure (e.g., continuous positive airway pressure), with or without muscle relaxants.	12
4. Supplementary ventilatory care: patient is breathing spontaneously through endotracheal tube; supplementary oxygen via any method, except if #3 applies.	3
5. Single vasoactive medication: any vasoactive drug.	7
6. Multiple vasoactive medications: more than one vasoactive drug, regardless of type and dose.	12
7. Dialysis techniques: all	6
8. Specific interventions in the intensive care unit (ICU): e.g., endotracheal intubation, introduction of pacemaker, cardioversion, endoscopy, emergency operation in the past 24 hours, gastric lavage. Routine interventions, such as radiography, echocardiography, electrocardiography, dressings, and introduction of venous or arterial lines, are not included.	5
9. Specific interventions outside the ICU: e.g., surgical intervention or diagnostic procedure; the intervention/procedure is related to the patient's severity of illness and makes an extra demand upon manpower efforts in the ICU.	6

Modified from Reis MD, Moreno R, Iapichino G: Nine Equivalents of Nursing Manpower Use Score (NEMS). Intensive Care Med 1997;23:760-765.

Nine Equivalents of Nursing Manpower Use Score

The Nine Equivalents of Nursing Manpower Use Score (NEMS) was derived from the TISS-28 as a simpler version that would therefore be more widely used.[59] Nursing activities are separated into just nine categories (Table 9-2) and each is awarded weighted points, giving a maximum score of 66. NEMS has been validated in large cohorts of ICU patients and is easy to use with almost no interrater variability.[60] It does, however, have less discriminative power for individual patients than the TISS-28 and is indicated for measuring and comparing nursing workload in large groups of patients.

CONCLUSION

General illness severity scores can be divided into three complementary groups: those that assess resource use, those that predict outcome, and those that characterize organ dysfunction. These last scores are most useful in the ongoing clinical evaluation of individual patients and their evolution during their ICU stays. All of these scores were developed to be used in heterogeneous groups of ICU patients, but there is no reason not to apply them to specific subgroups of ICU patients, including those with renal disease. Nevertheless, disease-specific scoring systems may also be helpful. Importantly, these systems should be seen as complementary rather than competitive, and used together they will provide the most accurate assessment of the severity of the disease and the prognosis. As populations change and new therapies and prognostic techniques become available, severity of illness scores may have to be updated and revalidated.

Key Points

1. Severity of illness has been assessed by means of resource use scores, prediction of outcome scores, and organ dysfunction scores.
2. Organ dysfunction is a dynamic process and should be assessed repeatedly.
3. The variables used to assess organ dysfunction should be objective, simple, widely available, specific to the organ in question, and, ideally, patient- and treatment-independent.
4. Despite the differences among the various organ dysfunction scoring systems, their prognostic values seem to be similar in terms of mortality prediction.

Key References

5. Zimmerman JE, Kramer AA, McNair DS, Malila FM: Acute Physiology and Chronic Health Evaluation (APACHE) IV: Hospital mortality assessment for today's critically ill patients. Crit Care Med 200634:1297-1310.
9. Moreno RP, Metnitz PG, Almeida E, et al: SAPS 3—from evaluation of the patient to evaluation of the intensive care unit. Part 2: Development of a prognostic model for hospital mortality at ICU admission. Intensive Care Med 2005;31: 1345-1355.
35. Vincent JL, de Mendonça A, Cantraine F, et al: Use of the SOFA score to assess the incidence of organ dysfunction/ failure in intensive care units: Results of a multicentric, prospective study. Crit Care Med 1998;26:1793-1800.
37. Lopes Ferreira F, Peres Bota D, Bross A, et al: Serial evaluation of the SOFA score to predict outcome. JAMA 2001;286: 1754-1758.
53. Vincent JL, Sakr Y, Sprung CL, et al: Sepsis in European intensive care units: Results of the SOAP study. Crit Care Med 2006;34:344-353.

See the companion Expert Consult website for the complete reference list.

CHAPTER 10

Kidney-Specific Severity Scores

Shigehiko Uchino

OBJECTIVES

This chapter will:
1. Review published kidney-specific severity scores.
2. Evaluate accuracy of severity scores for acute renal failure.
3. Summarize risk factors for hospital death in patients with acute renal failure.

Despite continuing progress in medical treatment, acute renal failure (ARF) in critical illness carries a hospital mortality of more than 60%.[1] Several randomized controlled trials have been unsuccessful in decreasing such mortality.[2,3] One of the difficulties with the conduct of clinical trials in ARF is that there is no reliable scoring system to stratify patient selection and confirm balanced randomization. General severity scores do not reliably predict outcome of patients with ARF,[4] partly because data from only a few patients with ARF were collected to generate these scores. Multiple epidemiological studies have looked at risk factors for hospital mortality in patients with ARF,[1,5-14] and in some of these studies, kidney-specific severity scores have been published.[15-26] However, these scores also have problems and limitations, mainly because they are based on small populations.

In this chapter, published kidney-specific severity scores and their problems are reviewed. Then, major risk factors for hospital mortality in patients with ARF are discussed in order to provide information for the future development of more accurate kidney-specific severity scores.

KIDNEY-SPECIFIC SEVERITY SCORES AND THEIR EXTERNAL VALIDATION

Multiple kidney-specific severity scores have been published in the literature; they are listed in Table 10-1. Most of these scores were developed in single centers or, if multicenter, in single countries. Although one study was conducted in a multicenter setting,[23] it was originally a randomized controlled study of atrial natriuretic peptide for ARF,[27] and the sample size was smaller than that of other, later studies.[24-26]

The following ARF scores are based on larger samples than others, have been often validated externally, or have been recently published.

TABLE 10-1

Studies Reporting Kidney-Specific Severity Scores

STUDY (YEAR)	COUNTRY(IES)	NUMBER OF CENTERS	NUMBER OF PATIENTS	POPULATION	REQUIREMENT FOR RENAL REPLACEMENT THERAPY (%)	HOSPITAL MORTALITY (%)	NUMBER OF VARIABLES	EXTERNAL VALIDATION STUDIES*
Cioffi et al (1984)[15]	US	1	65	Surgical	100	81	8	29
Bullock et al (1985)[16]	US	1	462	Hospital	62	68	6	29
Rasmussen et al (1985)[17]	Australia	1	148	Hospital	—	53	10	30
Lohr et al (1988)[18]	US	1	126	Hospital	100	75	5	29, 30
Schaefer et al (1991)[19]	Germany	1	134	Intensive care unit (ICU)	100	57	6	24, 30
Liaño et al (1993)[20]	Spain	1	328	Hospital	51	53	9	20, 24-26, 30, 33
Barton et al (1993)[21]	UK	1	250	ICU	100	51	5	—
Paganini et al (1996)[22]	US	1	512	ICU	100	67	8	23, 24, 26, 33
Chertow et al (1998)[23]	US, Canada	48	256	Hospital	42	36	9	24, 33
Mehta et al (2002)[24]	US	4	605	ICU	50	52	9	33
Lins et al (2004)[25]	Belgium	8	293	ICU	37	51	8	24
Chertow et al (2006)[26]	US	5	618	ICU	64	—	5-8	—

*Superscript numbers are chapter references.

Bullock's Score

Bullock and associates[16] generated their score with data from a population of 462 patients with ARF who were admitted to a single center in the United States from January 1971 to January 1978. ARF was diagnosed when a serum creatinine (SCr) value of 2.5 mg/dL or greater and/or a blood urea nitrogen (BUN) concentration of 100 mg/dL or greater was found during the clinical course. Patients with chronic renal insufficiency were included if their SCr values rose by at least 2.5 mg/dL over baseline levels. Bullock's score was calculated as follows:

$$\text{Log odds of death} = -1.765 - 0.687 \times (CP1 + 0.037) + 0.822 \times (CP2 + 0.100) + 1.053 \times ([\text{pulmonary complications}] - 0.087) + 0.050 \times (\text{age} - 61.1) + 0.7 \times ([\text{jaundice}] + 0.143) + 0.608 \times ([\text{cardiovascular complications}] - 0.247) + 0.365 \times ([\text{hypercatabolism}] + 0.0303)$$

where *CP1* and *CP2* are categorical variables for nonoliguria and anuria, respectively (e.g., a patient with anuria would have CP1 = 0 and CP2 = 1).

Although this score was published two decades ago, data from more than 400 patients were used to generate it. However, only one external validation has been conducted so far, making it difficult to evaluate the score's accuracy. Halstenberg and colleagues[28] validated three kidney-specific severity scores (Lohr's,[18] Bullock's, and Cioffi's[15]) and the second Acute Physiology and Chronic Health Evaluation (APACHE-II) score[29] through the use of a registry of 512 patients who received acute dialysis at their institution between 1988 and 1992. Using the same population, this group generated another kidney-specific sever-

ity score.[22] When they tested the Bullock's score in their population, the Q statistic was only 20%, compared with 77% in the original population. (Q values greater than 50% are associated with good discriminatory power.)

Liaño's Score

The population that Liaño and coworkers[20] used to generate their score consisted of 328 patients with ARF who were admitted to a single hospital in Madrid from November 1977 to June 1988. ARF was diagnosed when a sudden rise in SCr to more than 2 mg/dL was found in subjects with prior normal renal function as documented by an SCr value less than 1.5 mg/dL. No patients with previous reduction in renal function were included. The researchers used two models of multiple regression analysis, linear and logistic, comparing the models' ability to predict hospital mortality. They found that the linear regression model's receiver operating characteristic (ROC) curve was better than that for the logistic regression model, so they adopted the equation from linear regression as their final model of the score, as follows:

$$\text{Probability of death} = (0.032 \times \text{age in decades}) - (0.086 \times [\text{male}]) - (0.109 \times [\text{nephrotoxic}]) + (0.109 \times [\text{oliguria}]) + (0.116 \times [\text{hypotension}]) + (0.122 \times [\text{jaundice}]) + (0.150 \times [\text{coma}]) - (0.154 \times [\text{consciousness}]) + (0.182 \times [\text{assisted respiration}]) + 0.210$$

Liaño and coworkers[20] found that there were no survivors above a discriminant score of 0.9, and at this level, the sensitivity of the score was 28%, the specificity 100%, and the positive predictive value 100%. Finally, they applied the score to 25 patients in another hospital in Spain for external validation; in this population as well, there were no survivors above a discriminant score of 0.9.

Of all the kidney-specific severity scores published, Liaño's score has been externally validated in other populations most frequently. For example, Douma and associates[30] retrospectively examined 238 patients who were treated with renal replacement therapy (RRT) for ARF in their unit. They evaluated several general severity scores and four kidney-specific severity scores (Rasmussen's,[17] Lohr's,[18] Schaefer's,[19] and Liaño's), reporting that Liaño's score had the highest area under the receiver operating curve (AUROC) (Rasmussen's,[17] 0.63; Lohr's,[18] 0.65; Schaefer's,[19] 0.69; Liaño's, 0.78).[31] (AUROC values greater than 0.7 are associated with good discriminatory power.) They also found that patients in the highest quintile of Liaño's score had a near-100% mortality (98%). However, Mehta and colleagues[24] and Chertow and associates[26] reported much lower AUROC values for Liaño's score, 0.630 and 0.53 to 0.56, respectively.

Mehta's Score

Mehta and colleagues[24] generated their kidney-specific severity score from a population of 605 patients who had undergone nephrology consultation for ARF in intensive care units (ICUs) at four hospitals in Southern California between October 1989 and September 1995. ARF was defined either as a BUN value greater than 40 mg/dL or as an SCr value greater than 2 mg/dL for patients with no prior history of kidney disease. For patients with preexisting renal insufficiency, ARF was defined as a sustained rise in SCr value of more than 1 mg/dL over baseline level. Multiple logistic regression analysis was used to generate the score as follows:

$$\text{Log odds of death} = (0.0170 \times \text{age}) + (0.8605 \times [\text{male}]) + (0.0144 \times \text{BUN}) - (0.3398 \times \text{SCr}) + (1.2242 \times [\text{hematologic failure}]) + (1.1183 \times [\text{liver failure}]) + (0.9637 \times [\text{respiratory failure}]) + (0.0119 \times \text{heart rate}) - (0.4432 \times \log(\text{urine output})) - 0.7207$$

Using the same population, these researchers compared the AUROC and Hosmer-Lemeshow goodness-of-fit[32] of their score with those of several general severity scores and kidney-specific severity scores (Schaefer's,[19] Liaño's, Paganini's,[22] Chertow's,[26] and SHARF-I/SHARF-II [see later]). Mehta's score had the best discrimination (AUROC 0.832) and calibration ability of all scores tested. However, the Beginning and Ending Supportive Therapy for the Kidney (BEST Kidney) study[33]—a multinational epidemiological study of ARF conducted at 54 centers in 23 countries and involving more than 1700 patients—found that none of the scores tested, including Mehta's score, had good discrimination or calibration ability (AUROC for Mehta's score, 0.670).

SHARF-II Score

The SHARF-II score is a modified version of a previously published kidney-specific severity score, Stuivenberg Hospital Acute Renal Failure (SHARF-I). Originally, Lins and coworkers[34] generated a score on the basis of data from 197 patients treated in a single center in Belgium from March 1996 to April 1997. ARF was defined as an SCr value more than 2 mg/dL or an increase in SCr value of more than 50% observed in patients with previous mild-to-moderate

chronic renal failure. Data were collected at study inclusion (T_0) and 48 hours later (T_{48}) and two scores were generated for each data collection point (SHARF-I_0 and SHARF-I_{48}). Both of these scores involved the same five variables—age, albumin level, prothrombin time, mechanical ventilation, and heart failure. Both scores showed good discrimination ability (AUROC 0.87 and 0.89, respectively) and good calibration ability (goodness-of-fit C P values 0.83 and 0.28, respectively) in the study population.

When Lins and coworkers[34] reevaluated validation of these scores in eight ICUs using the same inclusion criteria (from September 1997 to March 1998, 293 patients), however, they found that the discrimination ability of the original SHARF scores was not as strong as in the original population (AUROC 0.67 and 0.78, respectively). They also found three additional variables, bilirubin, sepsis, and hypotension, related to hospital mortality. Therefore, they generated new scores (SHARF-II) at T_0 and T_{48}. For example, SHARF-II at T_0 (SHARF-T_0) is as follows:

$$\text{SHARF-II}_0 = (3.0 \times \text{age in decades}) + (2.6 \times [\text{albumin category}]) + (1.3 \times [\text{prothrombin category}]) + (16.8 \times [\text{mechanical ventilation}]) + (3.9 \times [\text{heart failure}]) + (2.8 \times [\text{bilirubin}]) + (27 \times [\text{sepsis}]) + (21 \times [\text{hypotension}]) - 17$$

AUROC values for these new scores (AUROC 0.82 and 0.83, respectively) were significantly better than those of the original scores. SHARF II_0 was externally validated by Mehta and colleagues,[24] who found that it showed fairly good discrimination ability (AUROC 0.733) but bad calibration ability (goodness-of-fit C P value 0.03).

PICARD Score

The newest kidney-specific severity score, the Program to Improve Care in Acute Renal Disease (PICARD) score, was also generated from the largest population in the literature. This score was published as a substudy of the PICARD study, which was conducted in five centers in the United States from February 1999 to August 2001 and involved 618 patients. ARF was defined as an increase in SCr value of more than 0.5 mg/dL in patients with baseline values lower than 1.5 mg/dL or an increase in SCr of more than 1.0 mg/dL in patients with baseline SCr values greater than 1.5 mg/dL but less than 5.0 mg/dL. Patients with baseline SCr values greater than 5.0 mg/dL were not included. Using multiple logistic regression analysis, Chertow and associates[26] created three scores: on day of ARF diagnosis, on day of consultation, and on day of first RRT. For example, the score on day of consultation had eight variables, including adult respiratory distress syndrome (ARDS), as follows:

$$\text{Log odds of death} = (0.1241 \times \text{age in decades}) - (0.2063 \times \log \text{urine output}) + (0.6900 \times [\text{SCr} < 2 \text{ mg/dL}]) + (0.0828 \times \text{BUN per 10 mg/dL}) + (0.4811 \times [\text{liver failure}]) + (0.5800 \times [\text{ARDS}]) + (0.5074 \times [\text{platelet count} < 150 \times 10^6/\text{L}]) + (0.4083 \times [\text{sepsis}]) - 1.2563$$

Using the study population, these researchers compared the AUROC value of their score with that of several general severity scores and kidney-specific severity scores (Liaño's, Paganini's,[22] and SHARF-I). Surprisingly, the AUROC of their score was only 0.68 at day of consultation, which was lower than that of APACHE-III,[35] the second Simpli-

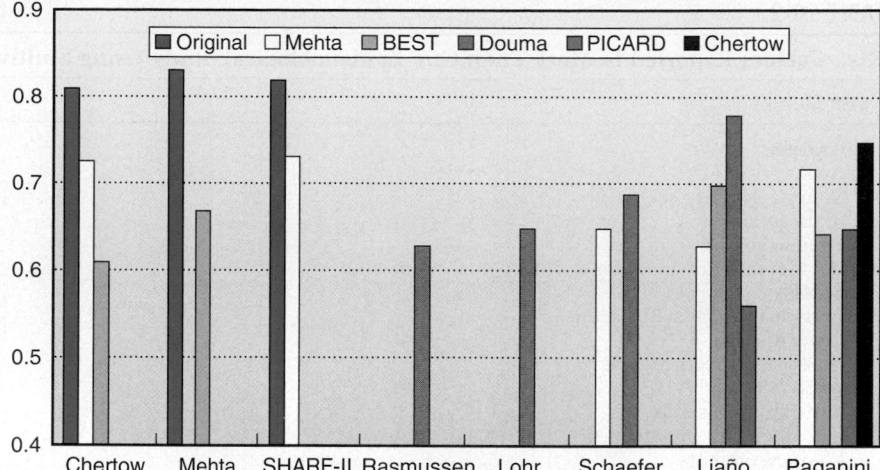

FIGURE 10-1. Area under the receiver operating curve (AUROC) values for hospital mortality reported in the original studies and external validation studies. *Black column* indicates AUROC values in original articles, and others are from external validation studies. BEST, Beginning and Ending Supportive Therapy for the Kidney (BEST Kidney) study; PICARD, Program to Improve Care in Acute Renal Disease (PICARD) study.

fied Acute Physiology Score (SAPS-II),[36] and the Sepsis-Related Organ Failure Assessment (SOFA) score[37] (AUROC values for all, 0.70). Because this score is fairly new, no external validation study has been conducted to date.

PROBLEMS OF CURRENTLY AVAILABLE KIDNEY-SPECIFIC SEVERITY SCORES

For general severity scores—SAPS-II, APACHE-II, and APACHE-III—several external validation studies have been conducted.[38,39] These studies have usually found that general severity scores have good discrimination ability in different settings, with an AUROC value greater than 0.8. However, their calibration abilities were not as good as their discrimination abilities, and recalibration to fit these scores to each center or country has been recommended.[39]

Kidney-specific severity scores have not reached this level of assessment. External validation studies have shown that no kidney-specific severity score has good calibration or discrimination ability.[29,32] Figure 10-1 shows reported AUROC values for ARF scores in the literature. For three scores (Chertow's,[26] Mehta's, and SHARF-II), the reported AUROC values from the study populations exceeded 0.8, indicating good discrimination. However, AUROC values reported in external validation studies for these scores were lower. AUROC values for other scores in external validation studies were also low. No score had an AUROC value greater than 0.8, and the values were often lower than 0.7, suggesting poor discrimination ability (see Fig. 10-1).

One of the major reasons for such a difference between general and kidney-specific severity scores is size of population. General severity scores were based on multicenter, multinational databases involving more than 5000 patients. Most of the kidney-specific scores were generated from populations in one center, and none of them involved more than 700 patients. Therefore, a large database collected from multiple centers in many nations would be required to generate more accurate severity scores for ARF.

Risk Factors for Hospital Death in Patients with Acute Renal Failure

Because of differences in case mix, collected variables, sample size, and statistical power in the studies, reported risk factors for hospital death in patients with ARF are quite variable. To determine common and relevant risk factors, Table 10-2 lists such factors that have been reported in more than one epidemiological study that used multivariate regression analysis. The most frequently reported risk factor is age, followed by mechanical ventilation, oliguria, sepsis/septic shock, and high serum bilirubin value. When hypotension and vasoactive medication are combined as a single risk factor, this factor also becomes common. Most of these risk factors are included in general severity scores as well, except for sepsis/septic shock.

Sepsis has been reported to be a leading precipitant of ARF, with 50% to 70% of cases of ARF being related to sepsis.[1,13] However, only a few studies have looked at this relationship specifically. Neveu and coworkers[40] reported that ARF was of septic origin in 50% of the cases they studied and was associated with a significantly higher hospital mortality than nonseptic ARF. Hoste and colleagues,[11] observing 185 septic patients in a surgical ICU, found that 16.2% of the patients had ARF and 70% of those patients required RRT. Therefore, sepsis is an important condition for both development of ARF and hospital mortality. Any researchers planning to develop new kidney-specific severity scores should probably include sepsis as a variable.

Several risk factors are related to renal function: oliguria, low SCr value, high BUN value, and RRT requirement. Among them, low SCr value seems to be unique because general severity scores usually classify higher SCr value as a risk factor.[28,35,37] Low SCr value could be related to diminished muscle mass or hemodilution due to volume overload. Therefore, low SCr value with high BUN value (marker of renal dysfunction) can be found as an independent variable when both values are entered in multiple regression analysis. This is the case in the three out of four studies that identified low SCr value as a risk factor.[22,24,26] In the fourth study, reported by Barton and colleagues,[21] the association between low SCr value and poor prognosis was attributed to the clinical decision by ICU care providers to request early RRT for sicker patients. For this reason,

TABLE 10-2

Risk Factors Reported in More Than One Epidemiological Study Using Multivariate Regression Analysis

RISK FACTORS	CHAPTER REFERENCES
Demographics	
Age	1, 7, 9, 11, 12, 14-16, 20, 21, 24-26
General severity scores	1, 7, 9, 10, 12-14
Male gender	15, 22-24
Female gender	12, 20
Development of acute renal failure after admission	1, 7, 12
Comorbidity	
Previous health status scores	7, 9, 13
Liver disease	13, 19
Preexisting heart disease	17, 18
Diagnosis	
Sepsis/septic shock	1, 5, 7, 8, 13, 18, 25, 26
(Hematologic) malignancy	1, 6, 17
Medical patients	12, 22
Surgical patients	12, 15, 17
Acute cardiac illness	17, 23
Organ Failure	
Oliguria	7-9, 12, 16, 17, 20, 21, 23, 24, 26
Hypotension	18-20, 25
Consciousness disturbance	17, 20
Respiratory failure	16, 17, 24, 26
Heart failure	1, 16, 25
Liver failure	24, 26
Number of organ failure	12, 22
Laboratory Data	
High bilirubin	16, 20, 21-23, 25
Low creatinine	21, 22, 24, 26
High urea	22, 24, 26
Low albumin	8, 23, 25
Metabolic acidosis	10, 21, 23
Low platelet count	22, 26
Treatment	
Mechanical ventilation	1, 6, 10-12, 18-23, 25
Vasoactive medication	1, 10, 11, 21
Renal replacement therapy requirement	9, 11, 13

Barton and colleagues[21] eliminated serum SCr value from their final model of the severity score. When two variables with strong colinearity are entered in multiple regression analysis, they weaken each other's explanatory powers, and estimating their separate effects can be difficult. Therefore, it does not seem to be correct to enter both low SCr value and high BUN value in multiple regression analysis, because these two variables have obviously strong colinearity. If one wants to evaluate SCr or BUN as a possible variable for a severity score, SCr value adjusted for body weight and/or gender might be useful.

Three studies reported that development of ARF after ICU or hospital admission was related to mortality. For example, the BEST Kidney researchers found that the odds ratio of duration between hospital admission and study inclusion, in 1-day increments, was as high as 1.02 ($P < .001$).[1] A possible explanation for the relationship between development of ARF and poor prognosis is that patients in whom ARF developed after hospital or ICU admission had a worsened clinical condition despite supportive therapy.

It might be intuitive that RRT requirement is a marker of severe renal dysfunction, which should relate to higher hospital mortality. However, of the six studies generating ARF severity scores that included patients who were not treated with RRT, none included RRT requirement in the score. Possible explanations are that some patients were too sick to receive RRT or that RRT was not given because

of expected poor prognosis. For example, in the BEST Kidney study, hospital mortality rates for patients with and without RRT were 62.1% and 55.7%, respectively ($P = .021$).[1] This slight difference was eliminated by multiple regression analysis, thus removing RRT requirement as a risk factor.

Key Points

1. Currently available kidney-specific severity scores have good discrimination and calibration ability in their study populations.
2. This accuracy is not demonstrated when the scores are validated externally.
3. The discrepancy might be due to the small sample size.
4. A large multinational database will be required to generate a more precise kidney-specific severity score.
5. Several major risk factors—age, mechanical ventilation, oliguria, sepsis/septic shock, high serum bilirubin level, and ARF that developed while the patient was in the ICU—should be included in such a score.

Key References

20. Liaño F, Gallego A, Pascual J, et al: Prognosis of acute tubular necrosis: an extended prospectively contrasted study. Nephron 1993;63:21-31.

24. Mehta RL, Pascual MT, Gruta CG, et al: Refining predictive models in critically ill patients with acute renal failure. J Am Soc Nephrol 2002;13:1350-1357.

26. Chertow GM, Soroko SH, Paganini EP, et al: Mortality after acute renal failure: Models for prognostic stratification and risk adjustment. Kidney Int 2006;70:1120-1126.

30. Douma CE, Redekop WK, van der Meulen JH, et al: Predicting mortality in intensive care patients with acute renal failure treated with dialysis. J Am Soc Nephrol 1997;8:111-117.

33. Uchino S, Bellomo R, Morimatsu H, et al; Beginning and Ending Supportive Therapy for the Kidney (BEST Kidney) investigators: External validation of severity scoring systems for acute renal failure using a multinational database. Crit Care Med 2005;33:1961-1967.

See the companion Expert Consult website for the complete reference list.

Epidemiology of Kidney Disease in the Intensive Care Unit

Basic Principles

CHAPTER 11

What Is Acute Kidney Injury?

Eric A. J. Hoste, John A. Kellum, Rinaldo Bellomo, and Claudio Ronco

---

OBJECTIVES

This chapter will:
1. Explain the rationale for having a uniform definition for acute kidney injury.
2. Elucidate the RIFLE consensus classification for acute kidney injury and the proposed modifications.
3. Emphasize that increasing severity of acute kidney injury is associated with worse outcome.
4. Discuss the limitations of the RIFLE classification.
5. Describe the opportunities for and future directions in acute kidney injury research.

The clinical picture of acute renal failure (ARF) has undergone considerable change over the last 30 years. The spectrum has changed from a single-organ disease that was managed predominantly by nephrologists on the ward to a disease that occurs predominantly in patients in intensive care units (ICUs) and is managed by both intensivists and nephrologists.[1] This difference can be explained by the gradual change in practice patterns and patient comorbidity. For example, in much of the world there has been a dramatic rise in the incidence of severe sepsis.[2,3] Kidney dysfunction occurs in roughly half of patients with severe sepsis, and 11% to 20% of patients with sepsis are treated with renal replacement therapy (RRT).[4,5] ARF treated by RRT has undergone the same trend: The proportion of patients with ARF who are treated with RRT is also rising.[6-8] Data show that approximately 5% of general ICU patients are now treated with RRT for ARF.[9,10] Another important finding is that the growing evidence that small changes of kidney function can affect outcome, even in severely ill patients with multiple-organ dysfunction.[11-14] Hence, the term *acute kidney injury* (AKI) was introduced

by the Acute Kidney Injury Network (AKIN) during their first consensus meeting in 2005.[15]

THE "BIRTH" OF THE RIFLE CLASSIFICATION AND STAGES OF ACUTE KIDNEY INJURY

A significant limitation to advances in research in AKI has been the absence of a uniform definition. In 2002, more than 35 different definitions for AKI and ARF were used in the literature describing populations with wide differences in severity and outcome.[16] After initial calls for a uniform definition of AKI,[17] the Acute Dialysis Quality Initiative (ADQI), a consortium comprising nephrologists and intensivists specialized in AKI from around the world, formulated a consensus definition, the risk, injury, failure, loss, end-stage renal disease (RIFLE) classification for AKI (Fig. 11-1). This classification defines three increasing severity grades of AKI (risk, injury, and failure), and two outcome classes (loss and end-stage renal disease). The RIFLE criteria were published first as an electronic conference report on the ADQI website on June 8, 2003,[18] and 1 year later as a peer-reviewed publication.[19] Later, the AKIN, an organization dedicated to improving outcomes for patients with AKI, sought and found worldwide endorsement from the major nephrology and critical care societies. During the first AKIN consensus meeting (Amsterdam, September 2005), small modifications were proposed to the RIFLE system on the basis of new data from the literature (Table 11-1).[15] The primary change was to include a 0.3-mg/dL rise in serum creatinine even if it was less than a 50% increase from baseline. Another proposal was to change the terminology of RIFLE (risk,

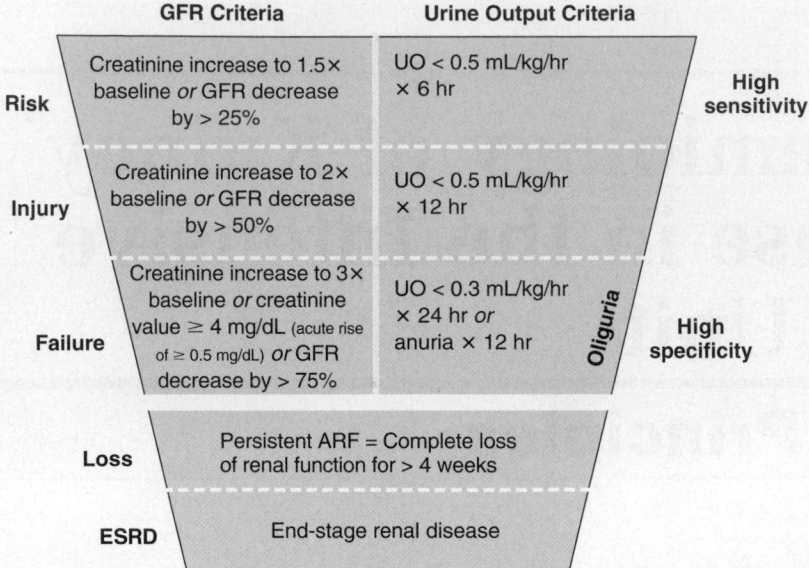

FIGURE 11-1. The RIFLE classification scheme for acute kidney injury. The classification system consists of separate criteria for serum creatinine and urine output. The criterion that leads to the worst possible classification should be used. Note that the RIFLE failure classification is used even if the increase in serum creatinine value is less than three times the baseline value, as long as the new creatinine value is ≥4.0 mg/dL (350 μmol/L) in the setting of an acute increase of at least 0.5 mg/dL (44 μmol/L). The shape of the figure denotes the fact that more patients (high sensitivity) are assigned to the "mild" category, including some who do not actually have renal failure (less specificity). In contrast, at the bottom, the criteria are strict and therefore specific, but some patients are missed. ARF, acute renal failure; GFR, glomerular filtration rate. (Modified from Bellomo R, Ronco C, Kellum JA, et al; Acute Dialysis Quality Initiative workgroup: Acute renal failure—definition, outcome measures, animal models, fluid therapy and information technology needs: The Second International Consensus Conference of the Acute Dialysis Quality Initiative [ADQI] Group. Crit Care 2004;8:R204-R212.)

injury, and failure to AKI stages 1, 2, and 3, in analogy to the staging system for chronic kidney disease (CKD). Finally, a 48-hour window was proposed in order for the first AKI criterion to be achieved (staging according to Table 11-1 would then be based on the worst values during the hospital stay).[15] Although these proposals incorporate wider consensus than the original RIFLE criteria, they have not yet been validated and may not offer any advantage over the existing system.

USE OF THE RIFLE CLASSIFICATION

A consensus definition can be successful only when it is indeed accepted by the medical community. In this respect, the RIFLE classification has already reached its goal. Since its introduction, the RIFLE criteria have been increasingly used in studies on AKI.[20] Not all studies use the classifications as they were designed, however.[14] Because urine output data are lacking in most retrospective studies, or in studies on hospitalized, non-ICU patients, many studies use a customized form of the classification in which patients are classified only according to increased creatinine levels. Two studies used the RIFLE classification to classify severity of AKI in patients who were started on renal replacement therapy.[21,22]

ACUTE KIDNEY INJURY ACCORDING TO THE RIFLE CLASSIFICATION

High Incidence of AKI

As a consequence of the high sensitivity of the RIFLE classification for detection of AKI, all studies invariably report

TABLE 11-1

Classification/Staging System for Acute Kidney Injury (AKI)*

AKI STAGE	SERUM CREATININE CRITERIA	URINE OUTPUT CRITERIA
1	Absolute increase ≥0.3 mg/dL *or* Value is 1.5-2× baseline value	<0.5 mL/kg/hr for >6 hr
2	Value is 2-3× baseline value	<0.5 mL/kg/hr for >12 hr
3	Value ≥3× baseline value *or* Value ≥4.0 mg/dL with absolute increase ≥0.5 mg/dL *or* Patient is receiving renal replacement therapy	<0.3 mL/kg/hr × 24 hr *or* Anuria ×12 hr

*According to the 2005 AKIN (Acute Kidney Injury Network) Consensus Meeting modification of the RIFLE (Risk, Injury, Failure, Loss, End-stage renal disease) classification.[15] Only one criterion (serum creatinine or urine output) has to be fulfilled for the case to qualify for a stage.

a high occurrence rate for AKI. In 2007, Ali and coworkers[23] found the annual incidence of AKI to be 2147 per million population (pmp) in the Grampian region in Scotland. Not surprisingly, this figure is considerably higher than the incidence of ARF reported in the same region in the mid-1990s.[24] Similarly, Uchino and colleagues[25] found that AKI as defined by RIFLE criteria occurred in 18% of hospitalized patients; this figure compares to 7.2% as reported in the landmark study of

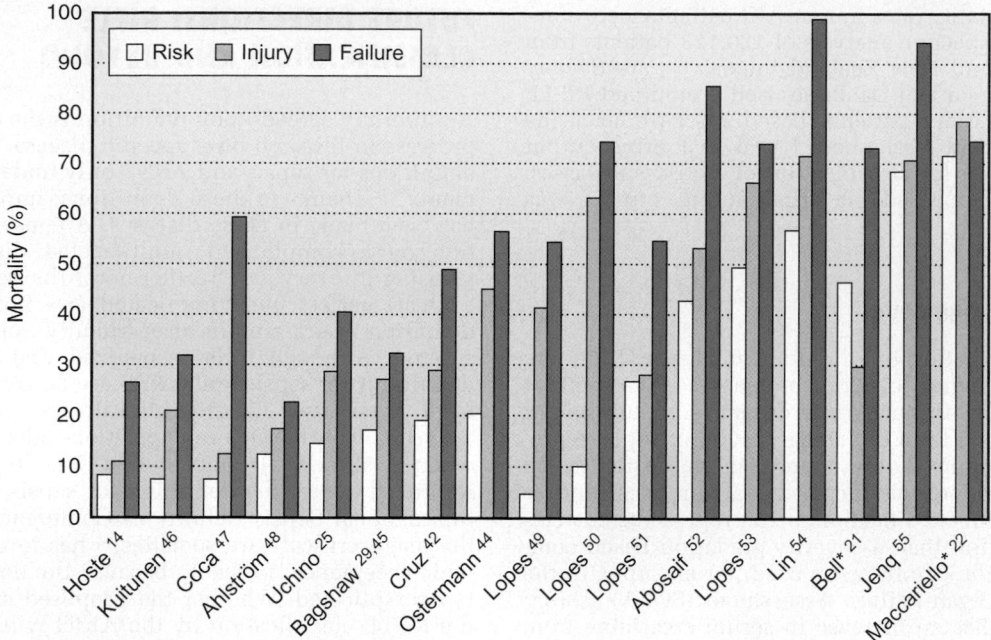

FIGURE 11-2. Increasing mortality associated with higher RIFLE class in different studies. *Study that classified patients who had been started on renal replacement therapy.

ARF performed by Nash and associates.[26] Hoste and coworkers[14] found that as many as two thirds of general ICU patients in a large U.S. tertiary care hospital demonstrated AKI during an ICU stay. The RIFLE classification has proved to be a very sensitive classification for AKI, rendering a high incidence.

Worse Outcomes of AKI

Despite the increased incidence of AKI according to RIFLE classification, the clinical relevance remains high. Hoste and coworkers[14] found that higher RIFLE class was associated with longer length of stay in the ICU and the hospital and, therefore, a greater use of hospital resources.[14]

All studies on the RIFLE classification published to date found that patients with AKI had a lower survival than patients without AKI, and with the exception of two reports, there was a stepwise increase in in-hospital mortality in relation to higher RIFLE class (Fig. 11-2). The two exceptions studied patients who were started on renal replacement therapy rather than all patients with AKI,[21,22] and, thus, focused on a specific subgroup of patients for whom AKI staging was nondiscriminative.

LIMITATIONS OF THE RIFLE CLASSIFICATION

Urine Output Criteria

Although at first glance urine output may seem the most obvious, most available, cheapest, and most specific and sensitive biomarker for detection of decreased kidney function, the use of urine output criteria is less widespread that that of serum creatinine criteria. Practical consider-

ations may play an important role in this situation. Precise measurement of urine output over 6, 12 or 24 hours requires the use of a urinary bladder catheter; this is a routine practice in ICU patients that is used less often in hospitalized non-ICU patients and obviously never in outpatients. Also, there may be many reasons that prevent exact timing and measurement of urine output—for example, obstruction of the urine bladder catheter by debris or blood clots and kinking of the catheter. Another practical issue that may hamper the use of urine output criteria is the use of diuretics. Diuretics are commonly used in patients with decreasing urine output or AKI (reported incidences from 59% to 70%),[27,28] but the sensitivity and specificity of the RIFLE classification may be lost when diuretics are used. However, the use of diuretics is not explicitly addressed in the RIFLE criteria, nor in the recent AKIN modifications, and studies including urine output continue to show very good calibration despite a high likelihood that they included many patients receiving diuretics.[14]

Finally, it is uncertain whether urine output and creatinine criteria are well balanced for the RIFLE classes of risk, injury, and failure. In other words, "risk" patients identified according to creatinine criteria may be more or less severely ill than "risk" patients identified according to urine output criteria. If we consider the two large studies on the epidemiology of AKI as defined by RIFLE classification, those performed by Hoste and coworkers[14] (creatinine and urine output criteria) and Uchino and colleagues[25] (creatinine criteria only), there are some indications that urine output criteria may be more sensitive than creatinine criteria. Increasing RIFLE class had a less pronounced impact in the Hoste study; mortality in the risk, injury, and failure groups was much higher in the cohort studied by Uchino and colleagues,[25] despite (1) the fact that the latter was a hospital-wide population and the former studied a general ICU population and

(2) baseline mortality rates in non-AKI patients were comparable. A retrospective analysis of 120,123 patients from the Australian and New Zealand Intensive Care Society (ANZICS) Adult Patient Database used a modified RIFLE algorithm to classify patients based on 24-hour urine output values. The researchers found that urine output was less sensitive for classification of RIFLE subclasses, but that outcome based on urine output criteria was worse.[29]

Baseline Creatinine Level

An inherent limitation to all definitions for AKI that are based on the changing level of a biomarker is the need for a baseline value for this marker. In order to sort out whether a serum creatinine level of 3.0 mg/dL, for example, represents AKI, one must know a previous value for serum creatinine. A proportional increase in serum creatinine, as used in the RIFLE classification, better represents changes in kidney function than a severity gradation based completely on specific cutoffs, as is used, for example, in the Sepsis-related Organ Failure Assessment (SOFA) score.[30] A patient who has an increase in serum creatinine from 0.5 mg/dL to 1.1 mg/dL has a 60% decrease in GFR, and would be classified as RIFLE class injury; the same patient would have a renal SOFA score of 0. Baseline serum creatinine levels are very difficult to establish, however. Serum creatinine may be falsely elevated on admission owing to early kidney dysfunction, previous levels such as those available in the hospital information system may be falsely low because of loss of muscle mass after a period of immobilization during hospitalization,[31] and finally, serum creatinine levels may vary considerably, depending on the calibration of the particular assay used.[32] In patients without a history of chronic kidney disease, a standard baseline creatinine level can be estimated from the Modification of Diet in Renal Disease (MDRD) Study equation, as suggested by the ADQI workgroup.[19] However, besides the fact that this approach can provide only an approximation, there may also be a question of its validity. The MDRD study equation was validated in a large dataset of U.S. patients with moderate chronic kidney insufficiency, and its applicability to patients without chronic kidney insufficiency or patients with ethnicities not well represented in the original dataset remains uncertain. Later reports from different parts of the world confirm the validity of the MDRD study equation in other groups of patients and ethnicities.[33-35] With this approach also, however, calibration of the specific serum creatinine assay may influence the results.[36]

Other Biomarkers for Kidney Function

Another issue was raised by Herget-Rosenthal and associates,[37] who demonstrated that serum cystatin C levels allow for earlier determination of AKI than serum creatinine levels. Although serum creatinine has its limitations, it has been the biomarker of choice for evaluation of kidney function for many years. The AKIN has also extended this concept in its second conference (September 2006, Vancouver, Canada) and recognizes different phases in the development of AKI, including an early phase with "damage," without injury or decreased kidney function, which may be measured by future biomarkers.[38] Other biomarkers for detection of AKI have also emerged.

FUTURE DIRECTIONS: RIFLE CLASSIFICATION AND BEYOND

A uniformly agreed-upon definition is the cornerstone for progress in research on a specific disease. The consensus definitions for sepsis and ARDS only underline this statement.[39,40] Thanks to these definitions, important progress has been made in these diseases. A consensus classification on a complicated, multifaceted disease is never pleasing to everyone. Furthermore, the balance between a (near) perfect but complicated and non–user-friendly definition and a simple, user-friendly one must be considered. Although it is recognized that the consensus definitions for sepsis and ARDS are far from perfect, they have been used worldwide already for more than 10 years. The PIRO (predisposition–infection–response–organ dysfunction) concept that was introduced as an improved consensus definition for sepsis in 2001 by the International Sepsis Definitions Conference (endorsed by the major critical care societies)[41] has to date not gained wide acceptance, probably because the definition proved too complicated. Whether the proposed modifications of the RIFLE classification by the AKIN will also prove too cumbersome or whether they will indeed be helpful remains to be seen.

The growing use of the RIFLE classification is therefore an important step. The epidemiology of AKI defined by the RIFLE classification has been assessed in many single-center studies, each with its specific cohort characteristics. The next step is to perform multicenter studies of AKI in the ICU setting, the hospital-wide setting, and the outpatient setting. These studies may also allow for the evaluation and calibration of the creatinine and the urine output criteria as well as of the AKIN modifications concerning the inclusion of an absolute 0.3-mg/dL serum creatinine increase and a 48-hour window. Already, several multicenter studies and one population-based study have been published.[21,23,26,42-45] However, all studies except those by Cruz and coworkers and Bell and coworkers used modified criteria to correct for the absence of detailed urine output data.

The RIFLE classification allows not only for comparisons between cohorts in different settings (e.g., ICU patients vs. hospitalized patients vs. outpatients vs. pediatric patients), but also for evaluation of whether different causes of AKI (e.g., cardiogenic shock, sepsis, acute interstitial nephritis) have different outcomes. Many other important improvements can be realized when a uniform classification system is used. Insight into the pathophysiology of the disease can grow when the cohort is well defined. This classification also allows for intervention studies, for example, on timing of the initiation of renal replacement therapy or on pharmacological interventions in patients with comparable severity of AKI. Obviously, new biomarkers for the assessment of kidney function must be considered for replacement of the current markers, on the condition that they are cheap, easily assessable, and widely available—comparable to serum creatinine and urine output. Finally, only one study to date has evaluated outcome criteria for RIFLE classes loss and end-stage renal disease. Because we now know that so many patients are affected by AKI, which has significant impact on short-term outcome, it is of utmost importance to also evaluate long-term outcomes in patients with different grades of AKI.

Key References

6. Xue JL, Daniels F, Star RA, et al: Incidence and mortality of acute renal failure in Medicare beneficiaries, 1992 to 2001. J Am Soc Nephrol 2006;17:1135-1142.
7. Waikar SS, Curhan GC, Wald R, et al: Declining mortality in patients with acute renal failure, 1988 to 2002. J Am Soc Nephrol 2006;17:1143-1150.
9. Metnitz PG, Krenn CG, Steltzer H, et al: Effect of acute renal failure requiring renal replacement therapy on outcome in critically ill patients. Crit Care Med 2002;30:2051-2058.
10. Uchino S, Kellum JA, Bellomo R, et al: Acute renal failure in critically ill patients: A multinational, multicenter study. JAMA 2005;294:813-818.
14. Hoste EA, Clermont G, Kersten A, et al: RIFLE criteria for acute kidney injury are associated with hospital mortality in critically ill patients: A cohort analysis. Crit Care 2006;10: R73.
19. Bellomo R, Ronco C, Kellum JA, et al; Acute Dialysis Quality Initiative workgroup: Acute renal failure—definition, outcome measures, animal models, fluid therapy and information technology needs: The Second International Consensus Conference of the Acute Dialysis Quality Initiative (ADQI) Group. Crit Care 2004;8:R204-R212.

See the companion Expert Consult website for the complete reference list.

CHAPTER 12

Basic Principles of Renal Support

Rinaldo Bellomo, John A. Kellum, and Claudio Ronco

OBJECTIVES

This chapter will:
1. Present the principles of clinical assessment in acute kidney injury.
2. Review the classification of acute kidney injury and the diagnostic tools that are appropriate in different clinical situations.
3. Describe the principles of kidney resuscitation.
4. Discuss the principles of management of established acute kidney failure.

Acute renal failure (ARF) remains one of the major therapeutic challenges for the critical care physician. The term describes a syndrome characterized by a rapid (hours to days) decrease in the kidney's ability to eliminate waste products. Such loss of excretory function is clinically manifested by the accumulation of end products of nitrogen metabolism (urea and creatinine), which are routinely measured in patients in the intensive care unit (ICU). Other typical clinical manifestations are decreased urine output (not always present), accumulation of nonvolatile acids, and an increased potassium concentration.

According to the recent RIFLE (risk, injury, failure, loss, end-stage renal disease) consensus criteria for the definition of acute kidney injury and fully developed advanced ARF,[1] these conditions have been reported to occur in 27% and 28% of ICU patients, respectively.[2] In hospitalized patients, their incidence has been reported at 5% and

3.7% respectively.[3] Acute kidney injury (albuminuria, loss of small tubular proteins, inability to excrete a water load or a sodium load or amino acid load) is almost ubiquitous in critically ill patients. There is some evidence, however, that, when dialysis becomes necessary, mortality is increased.

There is limited evidence that another frequently used term, acute tubular necrosis (ATN), has any clinical implications or that it describes the histopathology of what we now see in a modern ICU. The term acute tubular necrosis comes from animal models that poorly reflect clinical situations and from old biopsy data. Even in such cases, tubular "necrosis" is patchy and mostly isolated to the thick ascending loop of Henle. Furthermore, cells found in the urinary "tubular casts" of patients diagnosed with ATN are viable on staining studies, thus partly invalidating the term "necrosis."

ASSESSMENT OF RENAL FUNCTION

Irrespective of the definition and histopathology of the syndrome called ARF, the first aspect of the basic principles of renal support relates to the assessment of kidney function. Renal function is complex (control of calcium and phosphate, acid-base balance, water balance, erythropoiesis, etc.). In the clinical context, monitoring of renal function is reduced to assessment of glomerular filtration rate (GFR) by the measurement of urea and creatinine in blood. These waste products are insensitive markers of GFR and are heavily modified by nutrition, the use of corticosteroids, and the presence of gastrointestinal blood or muscle injury. Furthermore, their levels become abnormal only when there is a decrease of more than 50% of GFR, do not reflect dynamic changes in GFR, and are grossly modified by aggressive fluid resuscitation. The use of creatinine clearance (2- or 4-hour collections) or calculation of creatinine clearance by means of formulas increases the accuracy of the evaluation of GFR but rarely, if ever, changes clinical management. The use of more sophisticated radionuclide-based tests is cumbersome in the ICU and useful only for research purposes. Serum cystatin C measurement has emerged as a potentially useful measure of GFR[4]; however, its accuracy in critically ill patients is not yet clear, and its potential practical advantages over serum creatinine measurement are untested.

DIAGNOSIS AND CLINICAL CLASSIFICATION

The second important principle of renal support is to correctly diagnose the cause or causes of renal injury and to correctly classify the "source" of renal injury. The most practically useful approach to the etiological diagnosis of ARF is to divide its causes according to the probable "source" of renal injury: prerenal, renal (parenchymal) and postrenal.

So-called prerenal ARF is by far the most common entity in ICU. The term indicates that the kidney malfunctions predominantly because of systemic factors that diminish renal blood flow and decrease GFR or alter intraglomerular hemodynamics and thereby also decrease GFR. This is not to be confused with another concept, that of prerenal azotemia, in which the term prerenal is used to indicate that no structural injury has occurred to the kidney and that the loss of GFR is entirely functional and can be rapidly reversed by the administration of adequate resuscitation. The usefulness of this concept, at least in septic patients, has been recently called into question.[5]

Renal blood flow or effective glomerular filtration pressure can be diminished because of decreased cardiac output, hypotension, or raised intra-abdominal pressure. The last condition can be suspected on clinical grounds and confirmed by measurement of bladder pressure with a urinary catheter. A pressure of more than 25 to 30 mm Hg above the pubis should prompt consideration of decompression.

If the systemic cause of renal failure is rapidly removed or corrected, renal function improves and GFR returns to near normal levels relatively rapidly. However, if intervention is delayed or unsuccessful, renal injury becomes established, and several days or weeks are then necessary for recovery. Several tests have been used to help clinicians identify the development of such "established" ARF. The clinical utility and accuracy of these tests in ICU patients or patients with sepsis who receive vasopressors, massive fluid resuscitation and, increasingly, loop diuretic infusions are questionable; systematic reviews have found them to be poor.[5,6] Furthermore, it is important to observe that prerenal ARF and established ARF are part of a continuum, and their separation has limited clinical implications.[7] The therapy is the same: treatment of the cause along with prompt resuscitation of the patient and use of invasive hemodynamic monitoring to guide therapy.[8]

TABLE 12-1

Causes of Parenchymal Acute Renal Failure

Glomerulonephritis
Vasculitis
Interstitial nephropathy
Malignant hypertension
Pelvicaliceal infection
Bilateral cortical necrosis
Amyloidosis

TABLE 12-2

Drugs Commonly Used in the Intensive Care Unit or Operating Room That May Cause Acute Renal Failure

Radiocontrast agents
Aminoglycosides
Amphotericin
Nonsteroidal anti-inflammatory drugs
β-lactam antibiotics (interstitial nephropathy)
Methotrexate
Cisplatin
Cyclosporin A
FK-506 (tacrolimus)

Parenchymal renal failure is used to define a syndrome whereby the principal source of damage is within the kidney and typical structural changes can be seen on microscopy. Disorders of the glomerulus or the tubule can be responsible (Table 12-1). Among these, nephrotoxins are particularly important, especially in hospitalized patients. The most common nephrotoxic drugs affecting ICU patients are listed in Table 12-2. Many cases of drug-induced ARF rapidly improve upon removal of the offending agent. Accordingly, a careful history of drug administration is *mandatory* in all patients with ARF. In some cases of parenchymal ARF, a correct working diagnosis can be obtained from history, physical examination, and radiological and laboratory investigations. In such cases, the clinician can proceed to a therapeutic trial without resorting to renal biopsy. However, prior to aggressive immunosuppressive therapy, renal biopsy is recommended to allow histological confirmation of the etiology of ARF. Renal biopsy performed under ultrasound guidance in ventilated patients does not carry additional risks compared with biopsy performed under standard conditions.

More than a third of patients in whom ARF develops have chronic renal dysfunction owing to factors such as age-related changes, long-standing hypertension, diabetes, and atheromatous disease of the renal vessels. They may have a raised serum creatinine value. However, this is not always the case. Often, what may seem to the clinician to be a relatively trivial insult that does not fully explain the onset of ARF in a normal patient is sufficient to unmask lack of renal functional reserve in another patient.

Obstruction to urine outflow causes so-called postrenal renal failure, the most common cause of functional renal impairment in the community. Typical causes of obstructive ARF are bladder neck obstruction from an enlarged prostate, ureteric obstruction from pelvic tumors or retroperitoneal fibrosis, papillary necrosis, and large calculi. The clinical presentation of obstruction may be acute or acute-on-chronic in patients with long-standing renal calculi. It may not always be associated with oliguria. If obstruction is suspected, ultrasonography can be easily performed at the bedside. However, not all cases of acute obstruction have abnormal ultrasonography findings, and in many cases, obstruction occurs in conjunction with other renal insults (e.g., staghorn calculi and severe sepsis of renal origin).

PRINCIPLES OF RENAL SUPPORT

The fundamental principle of renal support is to treat the cause of renal injury. If prerenal factors contribute, these must be identified, and hemodynamic resuscitation quickly instituted. Intravascular volume must be maintained or rapidly restored; in critically ill patients, this step is often best initiated immediately and then completed by means of invasive hemodynamic monitoring (central venous catheter, arterial cannula, and, in some cases, pulmonary artery catheter or pulse contour cardiac output catheter). Oxygenation must be maintained. An adequate hemoglobin concentration (at least 80 g/L) must be maintained or immediately restored. Once intravascular volume has been restored, some patients remain hypotensive (mean arterial pressure [MAP] < 75 mm Hg); in these patients, autoregulation of renal blood flow may be lost. Restoration of MAP to near normal levels is likely to maintain GFR and prevent ischemic renal injury.[9] Such elevations in MAP require the addition of vasopressor drugs. In patients with hypertension or renovascular disease, an MAP of 70 mm Hg may still be inadequate. The nephroprotective role of additional fluid therapy in a patient with normal or increased cardiac output and blood pressure values is questionable. Despite these measures, renal failure may still develop if cardiac output is inadequate. This development may require a variety of interventions, from the use of inotropic drugs to the application of ventricular assist devices.

Following hemodynamic resuscitation and removal of nephrotoxins, it is unclear whether the use of additional pharmacological measures is of further benefit to the kidneys. A large phase III trial in critically ill patients showed low-dose dopamine to be ineffective in the prevention of renal dysfunction.[10] In a patient with a low cardiac output, however, the administration of β-dose dopamine (such as dobutamine or milrinone) may increase cardiac output, renal blood flow, and GFR. A biological rationale exists for the use of mannitol, as is the case for dopamine. However, no controlled human data support its clinical use. Loop diuretics are widely used, but their role remains controversial because no adequately powered and designed study has yet been conducted for its use in ICU patients with early evidence of renal injury.

In patients receiving arterial radiocontrast agents, there is a consensus view that isotonic saline infusion is likely to attenuate renal injury and that low-osmolality agents should be used. There are insufficient data to recommend other interventions at this time.[11]

An etiological diagnosis of ARF must always be established. Such a diagnosis may be obvious on clinical grounds. In many patients, however, it is best to consider all possibilities and exclude common treatable causes by simple investigations. Such investigations include the examination of urinary sediment and exclusion of a urinary tract infection (most if not all patients), the exclusion of obstruction when appropriate (some patients), and the careful exclusion of nephrotoxins (all patients).

In specific situations, other investigations are necessary to establish the diagnosis, such as measurement of creatine kinase and free myoglobin for possible rhabdomyolysis. A chest radiograph, a blood film analysis, the measurement of nonspecific inflammatory markers, and the measurement of specific antibodies (e.g., anti-glomerular basement membrane, anti-neutrophil cytoplasm, anti-DNA, anti-smooth muscle) are extremely useful screening tests to help support the diagnosis of vasculitis or of certain types of collagen disease or glomerulonephritis. If thrombotic thrombocytopenic purpura is suspected, the additional measurement of serum levels of lactic dehydrogenase, haptoglobin, unconjugated bilirubin, and free hemoglobin is needed. In some patients, specific findings (cryoglobulins, Bence-Jones proteins) are almost diagnostic. In a few rare patients, a renal biopsy becomes necessary.

MANAGING ESTABLISHED ACUTE RENAL FAILURE

The principles of management of established ARF are the treatment or removal of its cause and the maintenance of physiological homeostasis while recovery takes place. Complications such as severe encephalopathy, pericarditis, myopathy, neuropathy, electrolyte disturbances, and other major electrolyte, fluid, or metabolic derangement should never occur in a modern ICU. Their prevention may consist of several measures varying in complexity from fluid restriction to the initiation of extracorporeal renal replacement therapy (RRT).

Nutritional support should be started early and must contain adequate calories (30-35 kcal/kg/day) as a mixture of carbohydrates and lipids. Adequate protein (≈1-2 g/kg/day)[12] should be administered. There is no evidence that specific renal nutritional solutions are useful. Vitamins and trace elements should be administered at least according to their recommended daily allowances. The enteral route is preferred to the use of parenteral nutrition.

Hyperkalemia (serum potassium > 6 mmol/L) must be promptly treated with either administration of insulin and dextrose (after exclusion of spurious hyperkalemia secondary to hemolysis, thrombocytosis, and a very high white cell count), the infusion of bicarbonate if acidosis is present, and/or the administration of nebulized salbutamol. If the "true" serum potassium level is greater than 7 mmol/L or electrocardiographic signs of hyperkalemia appear, calcium gluconate (10 mL of 10% solution given intravenously) should also be administered. These measures are temporizing actions taken while RRT is being initiated. The presence of hyperkalemia is a major indication for the immediate institution of RRT.

Metabolic acidosis is almost always present but rarely requires treatment per se. Anemia must be corrected to maintain a hemoglobin level greater than 70 g/L. More aggressive transfusion requires individual patient assessment. Drug therapy must be adjusted to take into account the effect of the decreased clearances associated with loss of renal function. Stress ulcer prophylaxis is advisable and should utilize histamine H_2 receptor antagonists or proton pump inhibitors in selected cases. Assiduous attention should be paid to the prevention of infection.

Fluid overload can be prevented by the use of loop diuretics in patients with polyuria. However, if the patient is oliguric, the only way to avoid fluid overload is to institute RRT at an early stage (see Chapter 208). Marked azotemia (serum urea > 40 mmol/L or serum creatinine > 400 µmol/L) is undesirable and should probably be treated with RRT unless recovery is imminent or already under way and a return toward normal values is expected within 24 hours.[12] This recommendation is made, however, with the recognition that no controlled studies exist to define the ideal time for intervention with artificial renal support.

RENAL REPLACEMENT THERAPY

When ARF is severe, its resolution can take several days or weeks. In such cases, extracorporeal techniques of blood purification must be applied to prevent complications. The criteria for the initiation of RRT in patients with chronic renal failure may be inappropriate in the critically ill. A set of modern criteria for the initiation of RRT in the ICU is presented in Table 12-3.

There is controversy about the "adequate" intensity of dialysis and the best modality of treatment.[13,14] However, any form of artificial support should achieve maintenance of homeostasis in all of the following areas:

- Hemodynamics
- Fluid status
- Biocompatibility
- Risk of infection
- Uremia
- Cerebral water content
- Electrolytes
- Nutritional support
- Acid-base balance

Finally, ARF and RRT profoundly affect drug clearance. A comprehensive description of changes in drug dosage according to the technique of RRT, residual creatinine clearance, and other determinants of pharmacodynamics

is beyond the scope of this chapter and can be found in Chapter 219. The important principle, however, remains that prescription must take into account the effect of renal failure and renal support on pharmacokinetics.

TABLE 12-3

Modern Criteria for the Initiation of Renal Replacement Therapy (RRT) in the Intensive Care Unit*

- Oliguria (urine output < 200 mL/12 hours)
- Blood urea nitrogen > 80 mg/dL
- Serum creatinine > 3 mg/L
- Serum potassium > 6.5 mmol/L or rapidly rising
- Pulmonary edema unresponsive to diuretics
- Uncompensated metabolic acidosis (pH < 7.1)
- Temperature > 40° C
- Uremic complications (encephalopathy/myopathy/neuropathy/pericarditis)
- Overdose with a dialyzable toxin (e.g., lithium)

*If one criterion is present, RRT should be considered. If two criteria are simultaneously present, RRT is strongly recommended.

Key Points

1. Early detection of acute kidney injury is vital to prompt supportive therapy.
2. Immediate fluid resuscitation to restore circulating volume is vital to renal protection.
3. In critically ill patients, optimal resuscitation typically requires invasive monitoring.
4. Vasopressor drugs are often needed to optimize perfusion pressure.
5. Nephrotoxins must be avoided or rapidly removed.
6. The cause of renal injury must be rapidly identified and removed or treated.
7. If artificial renal support appears likely, it should be started early to avoid the complications of uremia, fluid overload, and electrolyte and acid-base disorders.

Key References

1. Bellomo R, Ronco C, Kellum JA, et al; Acute Dialysis Quality Initiative workgroup: Acute renal failure: Definition, outcome measures, animal models, fluid therapy and information technology needs. The Second International Consensus Conference of the Acute Dialysis Quality Initiative (ADQI) Group. Crit Care 2004;8:R204-R212.
3. Uchino S, Bellomo R, Goldsmith D, et al: An assessment of the RIFLE criteria for acute failure in hospitalized patients. Crit Care Med 2006;34:1913-1917.
10. Bellomo R, Chapman M, Finfer S, et al: Low-dose dopamine in patients with early renal dysfunction: A placebo-controlled randomised trial. Australian and New Zealand Intensive Care Society (ANZICS) Clinical Trials Group Lancet 2000;356:2139-2143.
12. Bellomo R, Ronco C: Adequacy of dialysis in the acute renal failure of the critically ill: The case for continuous therapies. Int J Artif Organs 1996;19:129-142.
13. Ronco C, Bellomo R, Homel P, et al: Effects of different doses in continuous veno-venous haemofiltration on outcomes of acute renal failure: A prospective randomised trial. Lancet 2000;355:26-30.

See the companion Expert Consult website for the complete reference list.

CHAPTER 13

Genetic Factors Influencing Acute Kidney Injury

Orfeas Liangos and Bertrand L. Jaber

OBJECTIVES

This chapter will:
1. Outline current knowledge on the role of genetic polymorphisms in acute kidney disease.
2. Describe selected candidate gene polymorphisms and their possible role in the development and severity of acute kidney disease.
3. Discuss the strengths and limitations of a genetic approach to acute kidney disease.
4. Consider potential implications for future clinical practice.

The role of host immune and inflammatory responses in the development and manifestation of acute kidney injury (AKI) is increasingly recognized. Local and systemic inflammatory mechanisms are likely the result of the interplay between environmental influence and genetic factors, which might play an important role in the pathophysiology of AKI. Therefore, if identified, predisposing genetic factors might serve as risk markers for the susceptibility to and/or the severity of AKI in specific individuals and, as such, might have important future implications for clinical practice.

GENETIC POLYMORPHISM IN HEALTH AND DISEASE

Among humans, 99.9% of the DNA sequences are identical.[1] The remaining 0.1% of the human genome, which accounts for interindividual variability, has become the subject of intense investigation in the past decade in both the academic and commercial sectors.[2] This interindividual variability, known as *gene polymorphism*, is responsible for the biological diversity within one species and might therefore be relevant to the study of susceptibility risk factors of or markers for complex diseases.[3,4]

Genetic polymorphism can be observed along a human gene at one of the following locations: (1) the promoter or 5′-flanking region, (2) the *exon* or gene-coding sequences, (3) the *intron* or gene-intervening sequences, and (4) the 3′-untranslated region. Polymorphism of the promoter region of a gene can affect its function by influencing transcriptional activity.[1] Polymorphism of the coding region, however, does not always affect gene expression; it may be silent or may affect the structure, binding, or

trafficking of the gene product. Introns are initially transcribed, but subsequently removed from the messenger RNA (mRNA) before translation. Consequently, polymorphism involving the intron may impair mRNA processing. Finally, polymorphism in the 3′-untranslated region may affect gene expression by affecting the RNA half-life or influencing mRNA's translation into protein.[5]

Three forms of human gene polymorphisms have been described.[1] *Single-nucleotide polymorphism* (SNP), the most common form, typically consists of a single nucleotide substitution. SNPs in the promoter region of a gene may affect gene expression through changes in its affinity for transcription factors. *Variable number of tandem repeats* (VNTR), also known as minisatellite polymorphism, is caused by in-tandem insertion of multiple repeats of a nucleotide sequence of less than 100 base pairs. Because the number of minisatellite tandem repeats represents one allele, this form of polymorphism is characterized by many alleles.[1] Finally, *microsatellite polymorphism* is formed by several repeats of a short motif of one to five nucleotides. In this instance, the dinucleotide repeat of cytosine and adenine (CA) is the most commonly observed form of microsatellite polymorphism.

THE CANDIDATE GENE APPROACH

A traditional approach for the identification of the genetic etiology of a disease is *linkage analysis*, whereby the co-inheritance of a disease phenotype along with a specific region of the genome is identified in families afflicted by the disease. These analyses have proved successful for the identification and description of *monogenic* conditions, such as polycystic kidney disease, in which environmental factors play only a minimal role.

The *candidate gene approach* is more relevant for the study of AKI, whereby susceptibility genes for common *polygenic* diseases are identified. This approach, however, requires the biological plausibility for a potential role of likely candidate genes for a specific disease. In this approach, gene-environment interactions play a critical role in disease expression, and candidate genes are selected if they are likely to modify individual host responses to environmental stimuli—for example, the study of cytokine genes for their role in sepsis and AKI. It is important to note, however, that such an approach does not clearly identify a cause-and-effect relationship. Indeed, specific genetic polymorphisms that are associated with a disease might be merely located in proximity to other, pathogenic genetic factors, a phenomenon known as *linkage dysequilibrium*.

GENETIC POLYMORPHISM IN CLINICAL AND EXPERIMENTAL ACUTE KIDNEY DISEASE

Inflammatory Cytokine Genes

The important role of inflammation in the pathophysiology of AKI is now well recognized and accepted within the scientific and clinical communities.[6] It is useful to conceptualize and structure the host inflammatory processes into two complex, antagonizing axes of pro- and anti-inflammatory responses (Fig. 13-1).

The Pro-inflammatory Axis

The systemic inflammatory response syndrome is a maladaptive response pattern that consists of exaggerated acute host defense reactions to various infectious and non-infectious triggers.[7] This response results in the release of biologically active mediators, which in turn lead to organ dysfunction, including AKI.[8]

Pro-inflammatory cytokines, such as tumor necrosis factor-α (TNF-α), interleukin-10 (IL-10), and IL-6, are released by monocytes. TNF-α and IL-1β exert systemic effects via vascular endothelium–derived stimulation of platelet-activating factor, prostanoid, and nitric oxide synthesis, which result in vasodilatation and capillary leak, intravascular coagulation, systemic hypotension, and organ dysfunction. Chemokines such as IL-8 facilitate recruitment of neutrophils to inflammatory sites, where they exert toxic effects through the release of reactive oxygen species and proteolytic enzymes. IL-6 induces hepatically derived positive acute-phase proteins, such as C-reactive protein, and suppresses negative acute-phase proteins, such as albumin.[9] TNF-α and IL-6 also induce a metabolic state of protein catabolism.[10] As

observed in patients with acute inflammatory states, pro-inflammatory cytokines are associated with adverse clinical outcomes.[11,12]

The Anti-Inflammatory Axis

A compensatory anti-inflammatory response that can be observed in response to the systemic inflammatory response syndrome might play an important role in limiting pro-inflammatory responses. Immunomodulatory mediators, including monocyte-derived IL-10, IL-1 receptor antagonist (IL-1ra), and soluble TNF receptors (sTNF-R), play a critical role in the development of the compensatory anti-inflammatory response.[13] IL-10, one of the most potent anti-inflammatory molecules,[14] inhibits the production of TNF-α, IL-1β, and IL-6.[15,16] IL-1ra, a competitive inhibitor of IL-1β,[17] is released primarily by monocytes, and 1000-fold excess of this molecule is required to inhibit the hemodynamic effects of IL-1β.[18]

The balance of the aforementioned pro- and anti-inflammatory cascades might determine the extent of host inflammatory responses, and their modulation might allow for the development of therapeutic strategies.[19,20]

Candidate Genes Altering the Intensity of the Inflammatory Response

This section reviews polymorphisms of genes that code for key immune-regulatory molecules and may have an influence on the susceptibility to or severity of host inflammatory responses. Summaries of known genetic polymorphisms and their associations with acute inflammatory and infectious disorders are shown in Tables 13-1 and 13-2.[21]

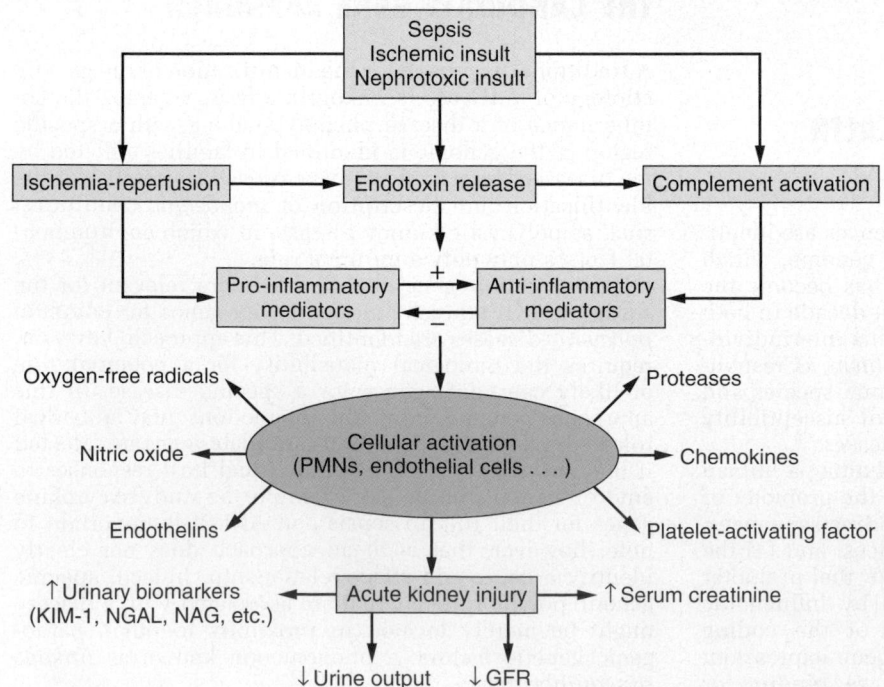

FIGURE 13-1. Schematic representation of the inflammatory response to sepsis, ischemia reperfusion injury, or toxic insult and resulting kidney injury. GFR, glomerular filtration rate; KIM-1, kidney injury molecule-1; NAG, N-acetyl-β-(D)-glucosaminidase; NGAL, neutrophil gelatinase-associated lipocalin; PMN, polymorphonuclear leukocyte. (From Jaber BL, Liangos O, Pereira BJ, Balakrishnan VS: Polymorphism of immunomodulatory cytokine genes: Implications in acute renal failure. Blood Purif 2004;22:101-111.)

TABLE 13-1

Selected List of Polymorphisms of Immune Response Genes in Humans

GENE	Polymorphism SITE	CLASS	POSITION	GENE EXPRESSION OR FUNCTION	CHAPTER REFERENCE(S)
Cytokines					
TNF-α	Promoter	SNS (G to A)	−238	Affected	22
TNF-α	Promoter	SNS (G to A)	−308	Affected	24, 27, 106
TNF-β (LT-α)	Intron	SNS (G to A)	+250 (intron 1)	Affected*	30
TNF-β (LT-α)	Intron	SNS (G to A)	+1069 (intron 1)	Affected*	29
IL-1α	Promoter	SNS (C to T)	−889	Affected	46
IL-1α	Intron	46-bpVNTR	Intron 6	Unknown	107
IL-1β	Exon	SNS (C to T)	+3953 (exon 5)	Affected	108
IL-1β	Promoter	SNS (C to T)	−511	Affected	47
IL-1ra	Intron	86-bp VNTR	Intron 2	Affected	53
IL-6	Promoter	SNS (G to C)	−174	Affected	59-61
IL-6	Promoter	SNS (G to C)	−572	Affected	109
IL-10	Promoter	SNS (G to A)	−1082	Affected	66, 67
IL-10	Promoter	SNS (C to T)	−819	Affected	23, 67
IL-10	Promoter	SNS (C to A)	−592	Affected	23
Chemokines					
IL-8	Promoter	SNS (A to T)	−251	Affected	76, 77
IL-8	3′ UTR	SNS (G to A)	+2767	Affected	79, 110
IL-8	Promoter	SNS (C to T)	−845	Affected	111
Monocyte chemotactic protein-1	Promoter	SNS (G to A)	−2518	Affected	112, 113
Toll-like Receptors					
TLR2	Exon	SNS (C to T)	+2029	Affected	114
TLR2	Exon	SNS (G to A)	+2251	Affected	115
TLR4	Exon	SNS (A to G)	+896	Affected	116
Heat Shock Proteins					
HSP70-2	Exon	SNS (G to A)	+1267	Affected	117
HSP70-2	Exon	SNS (G to A)	+1538	Unknown	118
HSP70-Hom	Exon	SNS (C to T)	+2437	Unknown	118
Oxidant Stress–Related Enzymes					
HO-1	Promoter	MSR (GT)n	−263, −185	Affected	119, 120
NADPH oxidase p22phox	Exon	SNS (C to T)	+242 (exon 4)	Affected	93
NADPH oxidase p22phox	3′ UTR	SNS (A to G)	+640	Unknown	93
Myeloperoxidase	Promoter	SNS (G to A)	−463	Affected	121, 122
Superoxide dismutase-3	Exon	SNS (C to G)	+637	Affected	123
Catalase	Promoter	SNS (C to T)	−262	Affected	96
GPX1	Exon	MSR (GCG)n	Exon 1	Unaffected	124
GPX1	Exon	SNS (C to T)	+593	Unaffected	125
Glutathione S-transferase M1	Exon†	—	—	Affected	126, 127
Inducible nitric oxide synthase	Promoter	SNS (C to T)	−1173	Affected	128

*TNF-α production is affected.
†Gene deletion prevalent in up to 50% of humans.
A, adenine; bp, base pair; C, cytosine; G, guanine; GPX, glutathione peroxidase; HO, hemeoxygenase; HSP, heat shock protein; IL, interleukin; LT, lymphotoxin; MSR, microsatellite repeats; NADPH, nicotinamide adenine dinucleotide phosphate; ra, receptor antagonist; SNS, single-nucleotide substitution; T, thymine; TNF, tumor necrosis factor; TLR, Toll-like receptor; UTR, untranslated region; VNTR, variable number of tandem repeats.
Modified from Jaber BL, Pereira BJ, Bonventre JV, Balakrishnan VS: Polymorphism of host response genes: Implications in the pathogenesis and treatment of acute renal failure. Kidney Int 2005;67:14-33.

The Tumor Necrosis Factor Locus

The TNF-α and TNF-β (also known as lymphotoxin-α [LT-α]) genes are located on the short arm of chromosome 6. Polymorphism within the 5′-flanking region of the TNF-α gene at positions −238 (G [glycine] to A) and −308 (G to A) has been reported, and the −308 A-allele, also referred to as the TNF-α2 allele, is associated with high promoter activity.[22-24] Moreover, the TNF-α2 allele has been found to correlate with increased TNF-α production.[25-28]

The gene coding for TNF-β is in proximity to the TNF-α gene. SNS at position +1069 (G to A) in the first intron of the gene has been characterized.[29] The A or TNF-β2 allele is more common than the G or TNF-β1 allele. The TNF-β2 allele is associated with higher IL-1β and TNF-α production in monocytes[30] and with adverse clinical outcomes in patients with sepsis.[31,32] However, strong linkage dysequi-librium between TNF-α −308 (G to A) and TNF-β polymorphism might exist.[33]

Polymorphism in the TNF-α gene is associated with adverse clinical outcomes in various acutely ill patient populations, such as those with sepsis[34-36] and with several acute infections.[37-40]

In addition, polymorphism in the TNF-α[41,42] and TNF-β[43] genes affects expression of TNF-α in patients exposed to cardiopulmonary bypass during coronary artery bypass graft surgery. The TNF-β +250 G-allele was found to be associated with prolonged mechanical ventilation,[41,42] and the TNF-α −308 G-allele with a slower rate of body temperature normalization after cardiopulmonary bypass.[44] In another study, carriers of the TNF-α −308 A-allele who required dialysis for AKI had higher levels of monocyte-derived TNF-α production, higher disease severity scores, and greater mortality.[45]

TABLE 13-2

Positive Associations between Polymorphisms of Immune Response Genes and Acute Infectious and Inflammatory Disorders

GENE	POLYMORPHIC ALLELE	ACUTE ILLNESS	CHAPTER REFERENCE(S)
Cytokines			
TNF-α	−308 A-allele (TNFα2)	Sepsis/septic shock	31, 33, 34-36
TNF-α	−308 A-allele (TNFα2)	Meningococcal disease	38
TNF-α	−308 A-allele (TNFα2)	Cerebral malaria	39
TNF-α	−308 A-allele (TNFα2)	Mucocutaneous leishmaniasis	40
TNF-α	−308 A-allele (TNFα2)	Rate of body temperature normalization after CPB	44
TNF-α	−308 A-allele (TNFα2)	Neonatal acute renal failure	65
TNF-α	−308 A-allele (TNFα2)	Severe acute kidney-pancreas transplant rejection episodes	69
TNF-α	−308 A-allele (TNFα2)	Increased risk of death in dialysis-requiring AKI	45
TNF-α	−238 A-allele	Malarial anemia	114
TNF-β*	+250 AA genotype	Septic shock in community-acquired pneumonia	37, 129
TNF-β	+250 G-allele	Prolonged mechanical ventilation after CPB	41
TNF-β	+1069 (NcO1) allele-2/2	Septic shock after acute biliary pancreatitis	130
TNF-β	+1069 (NcO1) allele-2/2	Higher circulating TNF-α levels after CPB	43
TNF-β	+1069 (NcO1) allele-2/2	Increased mortality in severe sepsis	31
TNF-β	+1069 (NcO1) allele-2/2	Susceptibility to severe post-traumatic sepsis	32
IL-1α	−889 TT genotype	Osteomyelitis	131
IL-β	+3953 TT genotype	Osteomyelitis	131
IL-1β	−511 allele-2/2	Febrile seizure in children	48
IL-1β	+3953 allele-2	Increased risk of ESRD in PR3-ANCA vasculitis	57
IL-1β	−511 allele-1/2	Survival in meningococcal disease	132
IL-1ra	86-bp VNTR (allele 2)	Susceptibility to sepsis	54, 55
IL-1ra	86-bp VNTR (allele 2)	Reduced Mantoux response to purified protein derivative of *Mycobacterium tuberculosis*	133
IL-1ra	86-bp VNTR (allele 2)	Increased risk of ESRD in PR3-ANCA vasculitis	57
IL-1ra	86-bp VNTR (allele 2)	Severity of Henoch-Schönlein purpura–associated nephritis	79
IL-1ra	86-bp VNTR (allele 2)	High levels of soluble endothelial activation (von Willebrand factor and E-selectin) markers in acute coronary syndromes	134
IL-6	−174 GG genotype	Improved survival in sepsis	62
IL-6	−174 C-allele	Neonatal acute renal failure	65
IL-6	−572 C-allele	Higher serum C-reactive protein level	109
IL-10	−1082 GA genotype	Meningococcal disease	68
IL-10	−1082 G-allele	Severity of illness in community-acquired pneumonia	63
IL-10	−1082 G-allele	Severe acute kidney-pancreas transplant rejection episodes	69
IL-10	−1082 GA genotype	Susceptibility to pulmonary tuberculosis	135
IL-10	−1082 G-allele	Decreased risk of death in dialysis-requiring acute renal failure	45
IL-10	−592 A-allele	Increased mortality in sepsis	71
IL-10	−592 AA genotype	Decreased risk of acute graft-versus-host disease and death	136
Chemokines			
IL-8	+2767 A-allele	Henoch-Schönlein purpura–associated nephritis	79
IL-8	−251 A-allele	Enteroaggregative *Escherichia coli* diarrhea	76
IL-8	−251 A-allele	Respiratory syncytial virus bronchiolitis	77
IL-8	−845 C-allele	Severity of lupus nephritis	111
Monocyte chemotactic protein-1	−2518 G allele	Premature kidney graft failure	78
Toll-like Receptors			
TLR2	Arg753Gln	Gram-positive bacterial sepsis	115
TLR2	Arg677Trp	Susceptibility to lepromatous leprosy	137
TLR4	Asp299Gly Thr399Ile	Gram-negative bacterial sepsis	138
TLR4	Asp299Gly	Sepsis and septic shock	139, 140

TABLE 13-2

Positive Associations between Polymorphisms of Immune Response Genes and Acute Infectious and Inflammatory Disorders—cont'd

GENE	POLYMORPHIC ALLELE	ACUTE ILLNESS	CHAPTER REFERENCE(S)
Heat Shock Proteins			
HSP70-2	+1267 GG genotype	Neonatal acute renal failure	117
HSP70-2	+1267 AA genotype	Increased risk of septic shock	129
HSP70-Hom	+1538 CT genotype	Multiple-organ failure after trauma	118
Oxidant Stress–Related Enzymes			
HO-1	Long $(GT)_n$ repeats	Increased susceptibility to coronary artery disease in diabetic patients	120
HO-1	Long $(GT)_n$ repeats	Increased risk of restenosis after percutaneous transluminal coronary angioplasty	141
HO-1	Long $(GT)_n$ repeats	Increased risk for development of abdominal aortic aneurysm	142
HO-1	Long $(GT)_n$ repeats	Greater susceptibility to pulmonary emphysema in cigarette smokers	143
NADPH oxidase p22phox	+242 CC genotype	Higher oxidized high-density lipoprotein cholesterol in type 2 diabetes mellitus	144
NADPH oxidase p22phox	+242 CC genotype	Increased plasma nitrotyrosine concentration and prolonged hospital stay in AKI	98
Catalase	−262 T allele	Reduced whole-blood catalase activity in AKI	98
Myeloperoxidase	−463 GG genotype	Higher prevalence of cardiovascular disease and higher circulating levels of pentosidine in ESRD	122
GST	GSTM1-0 genotype	Increased risk for lung cancer in heavy smokers	145
GST	GSTM1-B allele carrier	Decreased risk of delayed graft function	146
Inducible nitric oxide synthase	−1173 T allele carrier	Decreased risk of malarial complications	128

*TNF-β = Lymphotoxin-α (LT-α).

A, alanine; AKI, acute kidney disease; Arg, arginine; Asp, aspartic acid; bp, base pair; C, cytosine; CPB, cardiopulmonary bypass; ESRD, end-stage renal disease; G, guanine; Gln, glutamine; Gly, glycine; GST, glutathione-S-transferase; HO, hemeoxygenase; HSP, heat shock protein; IL, interleukin; Ile, isoleucine; NADPH, nicotinamide adenine dinucleotide phosphate; PR3-ANCA, proteinase 3 anti-neutrophilic cytoplasmic antibody; T, thymine; Thr, threonine; TNF, tumor necrosis factor; Trp, tryptophan.

Modified from Jaber BL, Pereira BJ, Bonventre JV, Balakrishnan VS: Polymorphism of host response genes: Implications in the pathogenesis and treatment of acute renal failure. Kidney Int 2005;67:14-33.

The Interleukin-1 Family

An entire family of genes related to the important inflammatory mediator IL-1 consists of IL-1α, IL-1β, IL-1 receptors (I and II), and IL-1ra. The genes coding for the IL-1α, IL-1β, and IL-1ra proteins are located on the short arm of chromosome 2, and the IL-1 receptor gene is located on the long arm of chromosome 2.

Functionally relevant polymorphisms of the IL-1α gene[45] and the IL-1β gene at position +3953 (C to T [thymine])[23] have been described. Another polymorphism of the gene at position −511 (C to T)[47] has been associated with clinical manifestations of infectious and inflammatory diseases.[47-49]

The IL-1ra gene contains both a penta-allelic minisatellite and a SNP, which are in linkage dysequilibrium with each other.[50] The less common allele-2 has been associated with increased IL-1β production.[51-53] Clinical manifestations associated with this polymorphism included an increased susceptibility to sepsis[54,55] and greater disease severity of acute glomerulonephritis.[56]

Interactions between the products of the IL-1 gene cluster suggest that a combined evaluation of IL-1β and IL-1ra polymorphism including using a ratio of these two gene products could be used to estimate the effect on inflammatory host response.[57]

Interleukin-6

Interleukin-6 possesses both pro- and anti-inflammatory properties and is therefore considered pleiotropic.[58] The SNP at position −174 (G to C)[59] is associated with altered IL-6 expression.[59] Presence of the C-allele has also been associated with lower serum levels of IL-6 in healthy subjects,[60] which is consistent with in vitro observations of reduced gene promoter activity.[59]

Although several studies failed to link this IL-6 gene polymorphism with relevant clinical outcomes in patients with trauma,[61] sepsis,[62] or pneumonia,[63] other reports did demonstrate an association with sepsis,[62] the inflammatory response to coronary artery bypass grafting,[64] and AKI in low-birth-weight infants.[65] The pleiotropic nature of IL-6 as a promoter or inhibitor of inflammation might explain the conflicting clinical results of the aforementioned association studies.

Interleukin-10

Most of the variability in IL-10 gene expression appears to be genetically determined and controlled at the transcriptional level.[66] A single–base pair substitution polymorphism (G to A) at position −1082 in the IL-10 5′-flanking region affects gene transcription.[67] Three levels of IL-10 expression based on the two alleles G and A at position −1082 have been described: high- (GG), intermediate- (GA), and low-producer (AA) genotypes.[23,67] Although additional polymorphisms at positions −819 (C to T) and −592 (C to A), which are also in linkage dysequilibrium, have been described, they have not consistently been linked to gene expression.[23,67]

Clinically, IL-10 gene polymorphism at position −1082 has been associated with susceptibility to and clinical manifestation of meningococcal disease,[68] severity of illness in community-acquired pneumonia,[62] kidney-pancreas transplant rejection,[69] and disease severity and mortality in dialysis-requiring AKI.[70] Presence of the IL-10 −592 A-allele has also been associated with higher mortality in sepsis.[71]

Chemokine Genes

Chemokines are small chemotactic cytokines that are secreted for the recruitment of subsets of leukocytes to areas of inflammation. An ever-increasing number of chemokines has been identified, and chemokines have now been found to be expressed in renal tissue and may thus play a pivotal role in the mediation of tissue injury in response to systemic and local inflammatory conditions. The role of chemokines and chemokine receptors in renal disease has been extensively reviewed.[72,73] Upregulation of several chemokines in animal models of renal ischemia and reperfusion appear to induce early neutrophil influx into the renal tissue and to increase disease severity and mortality.[74] The strong expression of chemokine genes, specifically IP-10 (interferon-gamma inducible protein-10), MIP-2 (macrophage inflammatory protein-2), MIP-1α, MIP-1β, MCP-1 (monocyte chemoattractant protein-1), and RANTES (regulated on activation, normal T cell expressed and secreted), observed in kidney tissue of a murine model of AKI due to polymicrobial sepsis[75] underscores the importance of the activity and regulation of these genes in the pathogenesis of experimental AKI. Genetic polymorphism has been described for several chemokine genes and found to be associated with acute infectious diarrhea and respiratory tract infection,[76,77] renal allograft rejection,[78] and acute glomerulonephritis.[72,79]

Oxidative Stress–Related Genes

In a healthy state, pro-oxidant and antioxidant mechanisms are typically in balance. Endogenous antioxidant compounds present in three main locations—intracellular compartment, cell membrane, and extracellular compartment—prevent the accumulation of noxious reactive oxygen species.[80]

The cell membrane-bound nicotinamide adenine dinucleotide phosphate (NADPH) oxidases, which are present in neutrophils and endothelial cells,[81] facilitate the production of superoxide and might play a role in sepsis and AKI.[82] The release of myeloperoxidase from neutrophils and monocytes is required for the synthesis of hypochlorous acid and is associated with tissue injury in ischemia-reperfusion injury.[83] The lipophilic α-tocopherol is another important membrane-bound antioxidant.[82] Glutathione peroxidases are intracellular antioxidant enzymes[84] that require glutathione as a cofactor to reduce hydrogen peroxide, lipid peroxides,[85] and peroxynitrite.[86] There are also

several different forms of superoxide dismutases, which scavenge superoxide anion.[87,88] Excessive reactive oxygen species production, inadequate reactive oxygen species degradation, or both can alter this balance and allow for oxidative stress to occur. Suboptimal levels or function of oxidant stress–related enzymes superoxide dismutases, catalase, and glutathione peroxidases are influenced by genetic factors.

Evidence is mounting that assigns oxidative stress an important role in the pathophysiology of AKI,[89] whereby antioxidant defenses might modulate ischemic or toxic acute renal injury.[82,90-92]

Genetic variation in the expression of two key pro-oxidant and antioxidant enzymes, the NADPH oxidase p22phox subunit at position +242 (C to T),[93-95] and human catalase, consisting of a promoter polymorphism at position −262 (C to T), has been well described and found to be of functional relevance for protein expression and enzyme activity[96,97] and might partly account for the inter-individual variability observed in the manifestation of acute organ injury.[87] The importance of these two genetic polymorphisms for the development of clinical manifestations of AKI has been demonstrated: A genotype-phenotype association was demonstrable between the NADPH oxidase p22phox genotypes (+242 C to T) and plasma nitrotyrosine level, as well as between the catalase genotypes (−262 C to T) and whole blood catalase activity.[98] In this study, polymorphism in the gene encoding the NADPH oxidase p22phox subunit at position +242 was also associated with dialysis requirement or hospital death among patients with AKI.[98]

LIMITATIONS OF THE SINGLE CANDIDATE GENE APPROACH

Commonly, clinical genetic association studies are designed as case-control studies and compare the prevalence rates of a genetic marker in subjects with a relevant clinical manifestation and in a control group. Small sample size, patient selection, and the lack of physiological plausibility may favor the detection of false-positive results in many such studies. In addition, the statistical association of a disease manifestation with a specific genetic variant may be due to linkage with another, yet unidentified polymorphism.[99] Detection of such an association may require the use of linkage analyses and comprehensive knowledge of other candidate genes located in proximity to the marker. In addition, clinical studies of cytokine gene polymorphisms are frequently restricted to one center or one geographic region, not taking into account ethnic or geographic differences in allelic distribution.[100] Indeed, certain genetic variants are uncommon in some but not other ethnic groups.

Survival bias may alter the frequency of some genetic risk markers if they are evaluated as predictors of mortality, making the use of a case-control design all the more problematic. Therefore, prospective cohort studies that link genetic polymorphism to clinical outcomes over time should be the preferred approach.[101]

Specific quality criteria should therefore govern clinical research into genetic polymorphism. In addition to a plausible hypothesis of the research, the gene polymorphism in question should alter the expression of the gene product, the study sample must be large enough, and the beneficial or harmful phenotypes under study must be clearly defined.[102]

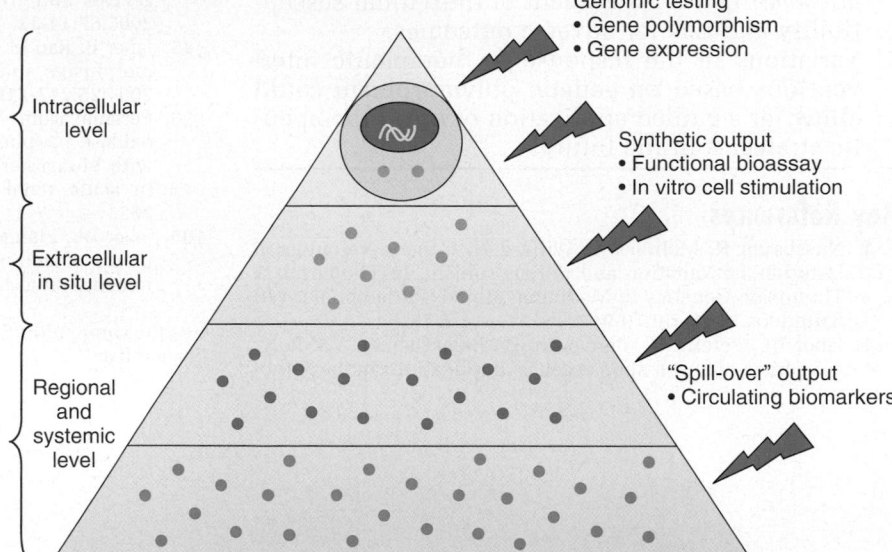

FIGURE 13-2. Schematic representation of genotype-phenotype interactions for the expression of gene products in response to noxious stimuli. (From Jaber B: The cytokine network in acute renal failure. Nephrology Rounds [Brigham and Women's Hospital] 2005;31-36.)

Other criteria that indicate good quality results are as follows:

- Reproducibility in several, diverse populations
- Choice of an appropriate control group if applicable
- Prospective design, adequate size, and generalizability of the study sample
- Precise phenotype definition
- Correction for confounders
- High strength of the genotype-phenotype association
- Specificity of the clinical effect
- Presence of a biological gradient
- A gene-dose effect
- Appropriate temporal association

FUTURE OUTLOOK

The successful translation of current and future discoveries of susceptibility genes in AKI into the clinical context could include a diverse array of novel clinical applications for the management of AKI as previously reviewed.[103,104] The early and more accurate diagnosis of certain clinically important manifestations of AKI, such as acute tubular necrosis, could be aided by detecting gene expression patterns specific for this condition. One example would be an early, noninvasive diagnostic test for primary nonfunction of a kidney transplant that would discriminate between acute rejection and tubular necrosis.

However, genetic susceptibility profiles may lend themselves better to performing accurate outcome predictions compared with physiologic assessments and protein biomarkers because of the profiles' stability over the course of time and their independence from gene product expression, which could occur at the local tissue level and might not be amenable to clinical evaluation, such as serum or urinary measurement (Fig. 13-2). The genetic predisposition of individuals to AKI may assist clinicians with the planning of procedures that carry a moderate to high risk of AKI as a complication, such as radiocontrast administration and surgical procedures. Although less concrete and more speculative at this juncture, the molecular design of therapeutic drugs could be based on the genetic susceptibility profile of an individual patient.[105] The use of gene therapy techniques to block specific maladaptive responses in the kidney parenchyma, for example with antisense oligonucleotide therapy, should be mentioned in this context. The pharmacogenomic design of so-called custom drugs could also be based on individual genetic profiles that would contain a vast array of susceptibility genes and their polymorphisms and, thus, would allow for tailoring an individualized approach directed at patients most likely to benefit.

CONCLUSION

The study of polymorphism of immune response genes in AKI may improve the understanding of variations in susceptibility and manifestations of this complex disorder. The identification of potential markers of susceptibility, improved prediction of severity of disease and clinical outcomes, and the identification of potential markers predicting a response to therapy are potential goals of this approach.

Key Points

1. The pathogenesis and manifestation of acute kidney injury are largely governed by host immunological responses to systemic or local noxious stimuli.
2. The expression of mediators of host immune responses is to a considerable degree determined by genetic factors.
3. Genetic polymorphism of immune response genes may affect disease severity, pathophysiological manifestations, and outcomes in acute kidney injury.
4. The discovery and description of genetic polymorphism relevant to acute kidney injury may

allow for better assessment of individual susceptibility and risk for adverse outcomes.

5. Variations in the response to therapeutic interventions based on genetic polymorphism could allow for a guided application of novel therapeutic strategies in the future.

Key References

1. Nussbaum R, McInnes R, Willard H: Genetic variation in individuals: Mutation and polymorphism. In Thompson & Thompson Genetics in Medicine, 6th ed. Philadelphia, WB Saunders, 2001, pp 79-94.
21. Jaber BL, Pereira BJ, Bonventre JV, Balakrishnan VS: Polymorphism of host response genes: Implications in the pathogenesis and treatment of acute renal failure. Kidney Int 2005;67:14-33.
45. Jaber B, Rao M, Guo D, et al: Cytokine promoter gene polymorphisms and mortality in acute renal failure. Cytokine 2004;25:212-219.
98. Perianayagam M, Liangos O, Kolyada A, et al: NADPH oxidase p22phox and catalase gene variants are associated with biomarkers of oxidative stress and adverse outcomes in acute renal failure. J Am Soc Nephrol 2007;18:255-263.
105. Jaber BL, Liangos O, Pereira BJ, Balakrishnan VS: Polymorphism of immunomodulatory cytokine genes: Implications in acute renal failure. Blood Purif 2004;22:101-111.

See the companion Expert Consult website for the complete reference list.

Clinical Syndromes

CHAPTER 14

Epidemiology of Community-Acquired Acute Kidney Injury

Shamik H. Shah and Ravindra L. Mehta

OBJECTIVES

This chapter will:
1. Describe the epidemiology of community-acquired acute kidney injury.
2. Discuss factors affecting changes in the epidemiology of acute kidney injury.

Acute kidney injury (AKI) is a common and devastating problem in clinical medicine that is associated with high mortality and has a separate, independent effect on the risk of death.[1] Traditionally, *acute kidney injury* has been defined as a rapid (i.e., over hours to weeks) and usually reversible decline in glomerular filtration rate.[2,3] Although AKI has been the focus of extensive clinical and basic research efforts over the last decades, there is no consensus on the definition. More than 30 definitions had been published as of 2002.[4]

The epidemiology of chronic kidney disease is well characterized, and the disease has been defined by the Kidney Disease Outcomes Quality Initiative (K/DOQI) guidelines with stages based on estimates of glomerular filtration rate.[5] The United States Renal Data System (USRDS) provides ongoing analysis of the incidence, prevalence, treatment, morbidity, and mortality of end-stage renal disease based on systematic data collection. Similar national data on the epidemiology of AKI are limited.

In 2005, the International Acute Dialysis Quality Initiative (ADQI) group proposed new criteria for classifying acute kidney injury on the basis of serum creatinine and/or urine output values.[6] This classification system defines three increasingly severe levels of renal dysfunction. Patients are classified according to their *risk* of renal dysfunction, type of kidney *injury*, and extent of renal *failure* associated with two clinical outcomes: *loss* and *end-stage* renal disease (RIFLE).[7] Although serum creatinine and urine output values may not clearly delineate the timing, nature, and pathophysiological basis of AKI, the data obtained from the RIFLE classification suggest a strong relationship of the magnitude of renal dysfunction with adverse outcomes.[8]

A collaboration of more than 25 international societies in nephrology and critical care has led to the creation of an Acute Kidney Injury Network (AKIN). This group proposed a new definition and staging system for AKI based on the RIFLE criteria[9] (see Chapter 11).

COMMUNITY-ACQUIRED ACUTE KIDNEY INJURY IN DEVELOPED COUNTRIES

The majority of the epidemiological studies on AKI have been published with data from developed countries (Table 14-1). A 1991 study from the United States by Kaufman and colleagues[10] found that community-acquired AKI was responsible for 1% of all hospital admissions and that prerenal azotemia and exacerbation of chronic kidney disease were the major causes.

Feest and coworkers[11] published a prospective study in 1993 that looked at community-acquired AKI in England. They found that the incidence of severe acute kidney injury in the community was at least twice as high as that reported from renal unit–based studies. Another interesting observation was that 72% of the patients were older than 70 years. The survival rate at the end of 2 years was 34%.

The Madrid Acute Renal Failure Study Group defined *renal failure* as a sudden rise in serum creatinine to more than 177 µmol/L or sudden increase in serum creatinine by more than 50% in patients in whom prior renal function was normal. This 1996 study found the incidence of acute kidney injury to be 209 per million population (pmp).[12] Using a serum creatinine level greater than 300 µmol/L as a definition for AKI, Khan and associates[13] reported an incidence of 602 pmp in Scotland in 1997. These figures appear to show that the incidence of community-acquired AKI has been rising over the years.

Table 14-2 lists the most common causes of community-acquired AKI in developed and developing countries.

RADIOCONTRAST MEDIA–INDUCED ACUTE KIDNEY INJURY

In developed countries, it is estimated that 6000 diagnostic and 2000 therapeutic coronary catheterizations are performed per million population every year. The proportion of procedures that require the use of radiocontrast media has increased over time, and the population submitted to it is growing older, presenting more comorbidities.[14,15]

TABLE 14-1

Epidemiology of Community-Acquired Acute Kidney Injury

COUNTRY	STUDY*	TYPE OF STUDY	STUDY PERIOD	DEFINITION OF ACUTE RENAL FAILURE	STUDY POPULATION (MILLIONS)	INCIDENCE (PER MILLION POPULATION PER YEAR)
Israel	Eliahou et al, 1973[55]	Prospective	1965-1966 (2 yr)	Unknown	2.2	52
Kuwait	Abraham et al, 1989[56]	Prospective	1984-1986	Unknown	0.4	95
United States	Kaufman et al, 1991[10]	Prospective	17 mo	Serum creatinine >2 mg/dL		1% of all hospital admissions
United Kingdom	McGregor et al, 1992[57]	Prospective	1986-1988		0.94	185
	Feest et al, 1993[11]	Prospective		Serum creatinine >500 µmol/L	0.44	175
France	Chanard et al, 1994[58]	Prospective	1991	Requirement for dialysis		104
Spain	Liaño & Pascual, 1996[12]	Prospective	9 mo	Sudden increase in serum creatinine by >177 µmol/L or sudden increase in serum creatinine by >50% when prior renal function was normal	4.2	209
Scotland	Khan et al, 1997[13]			Serum creatinine >300 µmol/L		620
England	Stevens et al, 2001[59]	Prospective	1 year	Serum creatinine >300 µmol/L	0.59	486
Canada	Bagshaw et al, 2005[60]	Prospective	3 years	New requirement for renal replacement therapy with evidence of renal dysfunction (serum creatinine ≥150 µmol/L)	1	11 per 100,000 per year
Scotland	Ali, 2007[61]	Retrospective	6 months	Rise of serum creatinine to >1.5× baseline times or drop in glomerular filtration rate of 25%	0.52	1811

*Superscript numbers indicate chapter references.

TABLE 14-2

Causes of Community-Acquired Acute Kidney Injury in Developed and Developing Countries

Common causes	Crush syndromes Earthquakes Accidents
In developed countries	Infections Community-acquired pneumonia Urosepsis Drugs Nonsteroidal anti-inflammatory drugs Antibiotics Antiretroviral agents
In developing countries	Infections Diarrheal diseases: cholera Parasitic: malaria, dengue Drugs Herbs and indigenous medicines Industrial exposure to chemicals Hemolytic: snake bite Obstetrical: septic abortion

Depending on the definition used, the incidence of AKI due to use of radiocontrast media has been reported to be as high as 40% to 90% in high-risk groups.[16,17]

Radiocontrast media–induced AKI typically is asymptomatic and nonoliguric.[18] Serum creatinine concentration usually rises 24 to 72 hours after exposure, peaks at 3 to 5 days and returns to baseline in 7 to 14 days.[19,20]

Studies have shown that outpatient coronary catheterization is safe and feasible in selected groups.[21,22] Most patients undergoing the procedure have been discharged home just when their serum creatinine level would have begun to rise if they were to experience radiocontrast media–induced AKI. Hence, it is important to ensure that the serum creatinine level is measured within 24 to 48 hours after this procedure and then followed up to check for possible AKI.

COMMUNITY-ACQUIRED PNEUMONIA AND ACUTE KIDNEY INJURY

Community-acquired pneumonia is the seventh leading cause of death overall and the most common cause of death from infectious diseases in the United States. About 1.2 million U.S. patients are hospitalized for treatment of community-acquired pneumonia every year.[23] AKI is observed in 11% to 24% patients with this type of pneumonia.[24,25] One multicenter, international study found that AKI was one of the three independent variables significantly associated with death in patients who had community-acquired pneumonia requiring mechanical ventilation.[25]

MALARIA AND ACUTE KIDNEY INJURY

Malaria is widespread throughout the world. It affects close to 400 million people every year, most of whom live in Africa, India, Southeast Asia, and Latin America.[26] Of these, 2 to 3 million die from complications of the disease.[27] The case-fatality rate due to severe malaria has been known to rise in the presence of renal failure and pulmonary complications.[28]

The incidence of AKI due to malaria has been reported to be between 2% and 39%.[29-31] This wide variation may be due to the local prevalence of the disease, the relative preponderance of other causes, patient referral policy, and other factors. Of patients with malarial AKI, between 60% and 80% need immediate dialysis at presentation.[30-32]

Late referral, high parasitemia, and presentation with multisystem involvement, hepatitis, or acute respiratory distress are all risk factors for death from malarial AKI, the rate of which has been reported as between 15% and 45%.[26]

The prevention of malarial infection and early diagnosis are the only measures likely to decrease malarial AKI in developing countries. Early referral to centers equipped to provide renal replacement therapy, along with antimalarial therapy and support, could further reduce mortality and enhance recovery of renal function.

DRUGS AND ACUTE KIDNEY INJURY

Nonsteroidal anti-inflammatory drugs (NSAIDs) are prescribed commonly as analgesics and anti-inflammatory drugs in the general population. Various adverse effects of NSAIDs, such as gastrointestinal bleeding, have been studied widely and quantified, but much less is known about the renal effects of these agents as used in the general population. The incidence of NSAID-induced AKI in the community has been reported as 1.1 per 10,000 patient-years[33] to 2 per 100,000 patient-years.[34]

A 2005 nested case-control study from the United Kingdom showed that NSAID users had a threefold greater risk for development of AKI than nonusers in the general population. The use of diuretics and angiotensin-converting enzyme inhibitors was independently associated with an increased risk for AKI and the risk was even greater with the concomitant use of NSAIDs and diuretics or calcium channel blockers.[33]

A few other epidemiological studies have looked at the association of NSAID use and AKI in the general population.[35,36] A history of hypertension, diabetes, or heart failure, and use of cardiovascular drugs are risk factors for renal failure.[33,35,36]

In another study, Schneider and associates[37] looked at the association between exposure to conventional NSAIDs and cyclooxygenase-2 inhibitors and hospitalization for AKI. They found the risk of AKI with low-dose rofecoxib comparable to that with conventional NSAIDs. For celecoxib also, the risk appears to be dose dependent.[37]

SEPSIS AND ACUTE KIDNEY INJURY

Martin and colleagues[38] studied the epidemiology of sepsis in the United States over a 22-year period. They found that the incidence of sepsis rose during that time from 82.7 to 240.4 cases per 100,000 population, for an annualized increase of 8.7%. Kidney failure was observed in 15% of cases.

Angus and coworkers,[39] analyzing more than 6 million hospital discharge records from seven states in the United States, estimated that 751,000 cases of severe sepsis occur annually, with a mortality rate of 28.6%. Renal involvement was observed in 22% of cases. To the best of our knowledge, these two studies are the only ones that describe the population incidence of sepsis.

HUMAN IMMUNODEFICIENCY VIRUS INFECTION AND ACUTE KIDNEY INJURY

Acute kidney injury is a common finding in people infected by human immunodeficiency virus (HIV) and is associated with advanced stages of HIV infection (i.e., CD4 cell count less than 200 per mm^3 and HIV RNA level greater than 10,000 copies/mL), hepatitis C virus coinfection, and a history of antiretroviral treatment.[40] A 2005 prospective analysis of 754 ambulatory HIV-infected patients reported an incidence of 5.9 cases of AKI per 100 patient-years.[40] Aminoglycosides, amphotericin, foscarnet, trimethoprim-sulfamethoxazole, tenofovir, indinavir, and acyclovir—all drugs used in treatment of patients with HIV infection—can potentially cause AKI.[41] Furthermore, AKI may be related to thrombotic thrombocytopenic purpura–hemolytic uremic syndrome due to the HIV disease process.[42]

COMMUNITY-ACQUIRED ACUTE KIDNEY INJURY IN DEVELOPING COUNTRIES

There are no reliable statistics about the true incidence of community-acquired AKI in developing countries. It is believed that the incidence is 150 per million population.[43] This incidence is based on sporadic regional reports, however, and is probably biased because it represents only the cases encountered in large hospitals by enthusiastic physicians who want to report them. Moreover, the majority of the causes of AKI are medical, as opposed to the surgical or trauma causes observed in the developed world.

Chugh and colleagues[44] have shown that obstetrical and hemolytic causes of AKI tend to decrease in an area or country as economic power and availability of hospitalization improve with time. Jayakumar and colleagues published 10-year data on AKI at a tertiary care hospital in South India.[45] The interesting findings in this paper were the younger age of patients (37.8 years) and an overwhelming majority of medical causes (87%). Obstetrical causes were not significantly different from those observed in 1987, accounting for 8.9% of cases of AKI.

Similar findings are seen in publications from Africa. The patients in whom AKI develops are young, and the predominant causes of AKI are infections, toxins, and herbal medications.[46-48]

In conclusion, the economic level of a country determines the spectrum of AKI causes observed. When a developing country improves its economic situation, the spectrum moves toward that observed in developed countries, and great differences in AKI causes can be observed in developing countries.[44,48,49]

ACUTE KIDNEY INJURY IN THE ELDERLY POPULATION

Several groups have reported a gradual increase in the mean or median age of population with AKI.[11,50-52] In the next few decades, demographic projections in developed countries have predicted a large increase in the proportion of patients older than 65 years. This population also has a dropping glomerular filtration rate owing to the structural and functional changes that occur in the kidneys with age. Also, elderly persons are more likely both to consume medications and to have comorbidities, such as dehydration.

CONCLUSIONS

Thus, in population studies, the incidence of AKI has risen in the last two decades. This rise appears to be multifactorial, being due to improved survival of patients with diabetes mellitus and ischemic heart disease, a growing elderly population, and better care of high-risk surgical and intensive care patients. The incidence of isolated AKI is reported to be decreasing, while AKI is more commonly encountered in patients with multiple organ failure. The rising incidence of opportunistic infections and nonrenal solid-organ transplantations has changed the spectrum of AKI.[53]

Acceptance of consensus criteria will be an important factor determining new multiple-center prospective studies. The AKIN criteria seem to be the first important step in this direction.[9] As in studies looking at sepsis and ARDS,[54] we anticipate that the publication of the AKIN criteria will prompt additional studies.

Key Points

1. The incidence of acute kidney injury is rising worldwide and is more likely to be associated with other organ failure.
2. The spectrum of acute kidney injury has evolved over the years and is different in developing and developed countries.
3. Various factors in the management of acute kidney injury influence its course and duration and contribute to the differences seen in the developed world.
4. Acceptance of consensus criteria for diagnosis and staging of acute kidney injury will be an important factor determining new multiple-center prospective studies.

Key References

7. Bellomo R, Ronco C, Kellum JA, et al: Acute renal failure—definition, outcome measures, animal models, fluid therapy and information technology needs: The Second International Consensus Conference of the Acute Dialysis Quality Initiative (ADQI) Group. Crit Care 2004;8:R204-R212.
9. Mehta RL, Kellum JA, Shah SV, et al: Acute Kidney Injury Network: Report of an initiative to improve outcomes in acute kidney injury. Crit Care 2007;11:R31.
51. Akposso K, Hertig A, Couprie R, et al: Acute renal failure in patients over 80 years old: 25-years' experience. Intensive Care Med 2000;26:400-406.
53. Lameire N, Van Biesen W, Vanholder R: The changing epidemiology of acute renal failure. Nature Clin Pract 2006;2:364-377.

See the companion Expert Consult website for the complete reference list.

CHAPTER 15

Epidemiology of Nosocomial Acute Kidney Injury

Eric A. J. Hoste

OBJECTIVES

This chapter will:
1. Discuss the multiple definitions of acute renal failure and consensus criteria for acute kidney injury.
2. Consider the association between small changes in kidney function and increased mortality.
3. Explain that incidence and outcome depend on the definition and the cohort studied.
4. Discuss the incidences of acute renal failure and acute kidney injury in a general intensive care unit setting.
5. Emphasize that mortality remains high even though it appears to be decreasing.

The clinical picture of acute renal failure (ARF) has undergone considerable change over the last 30 years. The spectrum has changed from that of a single-organ disease managed principally by nephrologists on the hospital ward to a disease that occurs predominantly in critically ill patients and is managed by both intensivists and nephrologists.[1] Another important finding is the growing evidence that small changes in kidney function can affect outcome, even in severely ill patients with multiple-organ dysfunction.[2-5] Hence, the term acute kidney injury (AKI) was introduced by the Acute Kidney Injury Network during the first consensus meeting in 2005.[6] This new term allows the differentiation of patients with moderate kidney injury (AKI) from those with severe kidney failure (ARF).

Even a cursory review of the literature reveals a wide array of quoted incidences of AKI, from as low as less than 1% to more than 80%. The incidence may vary according to the definition of ARF or AKI and the cohort studied. Kellum and associates[7] found that at least 35 different definitions for impairment of kidney function have been used in the medical literature. These definitions cover the entire scope of impairment of kidney function, from moderately decreased kidney function (e.g., 25% increase in serum creatinine value, or increase in serum creatinine with 0.3 mg/dL) to severe impairment (e.g., ARF treated with renal replacement therapy [RRT]). These investigators could even demonstrate a correlation between the definition used in different studies and the outcome: The more severely kidney function is impaired, the worse the prognosis. That different definitions can lead to major differences in epidemiology was also demonstrated by Chertow and colleagues,[4] who evaluated the epidemiology of AKI in a general hospital population. In this study, nine different definitions for AKI, defined as an absolute or relative increase in serum creatinine value, were evaluated in a cohort of 9205 patients who were admitted to a general hospital and in whom two or more measurements of serum creatinine were performed during their hospitalization.[4] All definitions were clinically relevant, because they were all associated with greater mortality and higher cost. Depending on the definition, the incidence of AKI in this cohort ranged from 1% to 44%.

Correct interpretation of the epidemiology of AKI is hindered not only by the multitude of definitions but also by differences in case mix. Patients who are hospitalized but not treated in ICUs are different from patients treated in ICUs. A general ICU population in a tertiary care center differs from that in a rural hospital setting; patients who have undergone cardiac surgery are different from patients with decompensated liver cirrhosis, and so on. Also, community-acquired AKI, predominantly a single-organ disease, probably has a different impact on outcome from that of nosocomial AKI acquired in the course of multiple-organ dysfunction during hospital admission.

Nosocomial comes from the Greek words *nosos* (disease) and *komeion* (to take care of). The term is most often used in discussions of infectious disease. Nosocomial infections are infections that occur during hospital stay or result from treatment during hospital stay.[8] Application of nosocomial to ARF or AKI implies knowledge of the precise start of the deterioration of kidney function. This date may sometimes be known, for example, in contrast nephropathy after elective coronary angiography; however, in many cases, the start of deterioration is not so clear-cut. An important limitation for detection of decreases in kidney function is the important lag time in serum creatinine value, the biomarker currently most often used for detection of AKI.[9] AKI diagnosed 24 hours after hospital admission may very well have already started outside the hospital. The same problem exists for the diagnosis of infections. In order to improve the specificity of the diagnosis of nosocomial infection, appearance of the infection 48 hours or longer after hospital admission or longer is advised.[10] With application of the same line of reasoning to AKI, this disorder can be classified as nosocomial if it occurs 48 hours or more after hospital admission. The 48-hour time frame is concordant with that used for the diagnostic criteria for AKI.

INCIDENCE OF ACUTE KIDNEY INJURY AND ACUTE RENAL FAILURE

Very few studies report what proportion of patients has community-acquired AKI and what proportion nosocomial AKI. The true incidence of community-acquired AKI is most probably grossly underestimated. Outpatients may die or may be cured of AKI in whom blood sampling on which the diagnosis could have been made has not occurred. Also, retrieval of all blood samples in a certain region can be difficult because samples can be analyzed in different laboratories. Only a limited number of studies report in detail on the proportion of hospitalized patients with community-acquired AKI.[11-13] Because the median length of stay in the hospital before occurrence of AKI is in most studies at least 1 or 2 days, however, the proportion of community-acquired AKI will be low, and the majority of patients described actually have nosocomial AKI.

Incidence of Acute Renal Failure Treated with Renal Replacement Therapy

Data from two large multicenter studies have shown that approximately 4% to 6% of general ICU patients are treated with RRT for ARF.[14,15] However, there may be large variation between centers; in the Beginning and Ending Supportive Therapy for the Kidney (BEST Kidney) trial, the center-specific incidence ranged between 1.4% and 25.9%.[15] The most plausible explanation for this variation is a difference in baseline characteristics of the ICU population.

Over a period of almost 20 years, the incidence of ARF treated with RRT has more than doubled. Two studies found, in a cohort from the late 1980s, that the incidence of patients with ARF treated with RRT was less than 50 patients per million population (pmp).[16,17] Studies from the beginning of this century report incidence rates of 110 to even 283 pmp.[16-27] Why is it that the incidence for ARF treated with RRT has increased so much? Ostermann and coworkers[28] noted, in a cohort of patients undergoing cardiac surgery in the period 1997-1998, older age as well as higher incidences of diabetes, hypertension, preoperative renal dysfunction, repeat surgery, and emergency surgery than in a cohort of patients undergoing similar procedures in the period 1989-1990. Many studies confirm that patients treated in recent years are older, have more comorbid disease, and are more severely ill at the start of RRT.[29-33]

Selection bias may also explain differences in incidence. In the period between 2000 and 2003, three groups from Scotland studied the incidence of AKI in different regions. Metcalfe and colleagues[18] found in 2000, in the Grampian, Highland, and Tayside regions (1,112,200 inhabitants), an incidence for AKI treated with RRT of 203 pmp. Prescott and associates[27] found in 2002, in the whole of Scotland (5,054,800 inhabitants), an incidence of 286 pmp, the same incidence found by Ali and coworkers[34] in 2003 in the Grampian region alone (523,390 inhabitants).

Incidence of Acute Kidney Injury

The scarce data available indicate that the majority of AKI episodes are community-acquired. In a study of patients treated in all hospitals in Madrid, in the mid-1980s, 40.5% of all patients with AKI had normal renal function on admission (nosocomial AKI).[20] Therefore, 59.5% of all ARF episodes in Madrid during the study period were potentially community-acquired AKI. Severe community-acquired ARF (serum creatinine value >3.0 mg/dL) was present in 25% of all ARF patients. The mortality of patients with nosocomial AKI was higher than that for patients with severe community-acquired AKI (50.8% vs. 29.8%, respectively; $P < .001$). Obialo and colleagues[13] found, in a cohort of African-American patients admitted to one hospital in the United States, that the incidence of community-acquired AKI was 3.5 times higher than the incidence of nosocomial AKI (0.55% vs. 0.15% of all admissions, respectively).[13] In Peking, a single-center study also confirmed that community-acquired AKI accounted for the majority of cases of AKI (59.4%) admitted to the hospital.[11,12] Patients with community-acquired AKI are also less severely ill: There is less oliguria, fewer patients have sepsis and multiple-organ dysfunction (24%, vs. 59% for patients with nosocomial AKI; $P = .002$), and fewer are hospitalized in an ICU (6% vs. 55%, respectively; $P < .001$).[13]

As discussed previously, the incidence of ARF treated with RRT has risen over time. This change can probably be explained by a change in indications for initiation of RRT. Increasing age and comorbidity of hospitalized patients and changes in medical practice may also have led to an increase in the incidence of nosocomial AKI. The incidence of AKI is indeed rising, as demonstrated by two large multicenter, longitudinal databases in the United States. Both studies used administrative databases and scored the occurrence of AKI on the basis of reporting of codes from International Statistical Classification of Diseases and Related Health Problems, 9th revision (ICD-9), for acute renal failure.[17,35] Waikar and colleagues[17] reported that the incidence quadrupled from 61 to 288 patients per 100,000 population during their 15-year study period.[17] Xue and coworkers[35] found that during the period 1992 to 2001, there was an 11% yearly increase in the diagnosis of AKI as well as an overall incidence rate of 23.8 patients per 1000 hospital discharges.[35] A limitation of these studies may be that ICD-9 coding does not define strict cutoffs for AKI. Consequently, sensitivity to detect AKI is low or, in other words, many patients with AKI are missed when epidemiology is based on administrative databases.[36] Also, reporting of AKI may vary among hospitals and during different periods.

An important part of the rise in incidence of AKI is probably explained by an increase in nosocomial AKI. It has been demonstrated in different settings that the incidence of nosocomial AKI is indeed growing. Two study groups, applying the same definition for AKI in one hospital in the United States in 1979 and 1996, reported that the incidence increased from 4.9% to 7.2% of all hospital admissions.[37,38] Also, Wang and colleagues[11] found that the incidence of nosocomial AKI increased from 26% in the period 1994-1998, to 49.8% in the period 1999-2003 in Beijing.[11]

Recently, as described in Chapter 11, the RIFLE (risk, injury, failure, loss, end-stage renal disease) classification has been used to classify AKI according to changes in serum creatinine or urine output values. A single-center study in Melbourne, Australia, examining a cohort of more than 20,000 patients, reported that 18% had AKI according to RIFLE criteria.[39] The maximum severity of AKI was I (R) in 9.1% of patients, II (I) in 5.2%, and III (F) in 3.7%. Hoste and associates[5] evaluated the incidence of AKI in a cohort of ICU patients admitted during a 1-year period to a tertiary-care hospital. In this cohort of 5383 patients, 67% had AKI according to the RIFLE classification, 12.4% had maximum RIFLE class risk, 26.7% had maximum RIFLE class injury, and 28.1% had maximum RIFLE class failure.[5] Several other groups have used the RIFLE classification to evaluate the epidemiology in specific cohorts.[40-47] The incidence of AKI defined by RIFLE criteria ranged from 10.8% in a general ICU setting, to 15.4% in a cohort of cardiac surgery patients,[43] to 78% in a small cohort of patients treated with extracorporeal membrane oxygenation.[42]

Acute Kidney Injury and Acute Renal Failure in Specific Settings

Because the data on nosocomial AKI are so scarce, this chapter discusses the two settings in which AKI is with near certainty of nosocomial etiology: after cardiac surgery and with contrast-induced nephropathy.

After Cardiac Surgery

The incidence of ARF with the need for RRT in a post-cardiac surgery setting is less than 2%.[48-52] A detailed discussion on AKI after cardiac surgery can be found in Chapter 180. Data on less severe forms of AKI after cardiac surgery are relatively scarce. Only recently has there been more interest in the impact of AKI in this patient group. Lassnigg and coworkers[3] reported that in total, 41% of patients in their study group had an increase in serum creatinine value—36% of patients had an increase of only 0 to 0.5 mg/dL, and 5% an increase greater than 0.5 mg/dL. Both groups had worse outcomes than patients with a moderate decrease in serum creatinine.[3] This difference remained even after correction for covariates. A later study reported the use of RIFLE criteria to evaluate the incidence of AKI.[40] In the study's single-center cohort of 813 patients, 19.3% of patients had AKI. The RIFLE criteria defined a clinically relevant population, because RIFLE classification was an independent risk factor for in-hospital mortality.

Contrast-Induced Nephropathy

Nephrotoxic radiocontrast media are used daily worldwide in an enormous number of procedures, for example, in coronary angiography. Small changes in kidney function after contrast exposure are associated with increased mortality.[2] Depending on the cohort studied, the procedure performed, and the definition of AKI used, the incidence of AKI after radiocontrast exposure varies from 5.7% to 45%.[53]

ETIOLOGY OF NOSOCOMIAL ACUTE KIDNEY INJURY

In the majority of patients, nosocomial AKI develops as a consequence of severity of underlying disease (in combination with underlying comorbidity), with sepsis-decreased renal perfusion and major surgery as the primary etiolo-

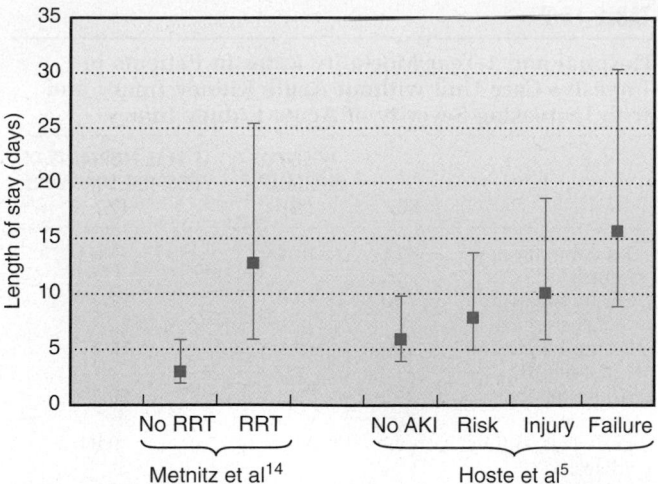

FIGURE 15-1. Length of stay in the hospital for ICU patients treated in intensive care units, stratified according to severity of acute kidney injury.

gies.[13,15,38] Radiocontrast media and medications, predominantly anti-infective agents, constitute the second most important etiology for nosocomial AKI.

OUTCOME OF ACUTE RENAL FAILURE AND ACUTE KIDNEY INJURY

Length of Stay

Patients with AKI or ARF are among the most severely ill in the ICU.[5,14] Therefore, it is not surprising that ICU patients with AKI or ARF have a longer length of stay in the ICU and in the hospital compared with ICU patients who do not have either renal condition. In one study, patients with ARF who were treated with RRT had a median ICU stay of 13 days, compared with 3 days for patients without ARF treated with RRT.[14] In addition, patients with less severe forms of AKI have greater length of in-hospital stay than patients without AKI, and a stepwise increase in length of stay according to severity of AKI determined by RIFLE criteria can be demonstrated (Fig. 15-1).[5]

Patients with nosocomial AKI also stay longer in the hospital than patients with community-acquired AKI. In a U.S. study, the mean length of stay was 2 weeks longer for patients with nosocomial AKI (26 days, standard deviation [SD] 28, vs. 12 days/SD 11, respectively; $P < .001$).[13]

Need for Renal Replacement Therapy after Hospital Discharge, Loss, and End-Stage Kidney Disease

Although the majority of survivors of AKI regain kidney function, some patients do not recover by hospital discharge and some go on to have end-stage kidney disease (ESKD) with permanent need for RRT. In 13.8% (95% confidence interval [CI], 11.2% to 16.3%) of survivors in the large multicenter BEST Kidney study, renal function

had not returned by hospital discharge[15]; unfortunately, the number in whom function recovered after discharge is unknown. Several other smaller studies found comparable proportions. Ten percent of survivors in a cohort of patients with ARF treated with continuous RRT had persistent AKI (L or E class of the RIFLE criteria) in a study by Morgera and colleagues.[54] In the Belgian SHARF (Stuivenburg Hospital Acute Renal Failure) study, 14 of 105 survivors (13.3%) had not recovered AKI by hospital discharge.[55] On follow-up of these patients, 4 became RRT-independent within 1 year, whereas 3 patients (2.9%) had ESKD. In contrast to these numbers are the findings by the Scottish Society of Intensive Care Audit Group in their study on ICU patients treated with RRT and mechanical ventilation. Of 199 hospital survivors, only 7 patients (3.5%) did not recover renal function by hospital discharge.[56] On the other end of the spectrum are the findings reported by Leacche and coworkers[57] in a small study (n = 40) on development of ARF after cardiac surgery. In this cohort, 7 of 11 survivors (63%) did not recover renal function by hospital discharge. Again, the most obvious explanation for this variation is differences in baseline characteristics. More specifically, preexisting chronic kidney disease may play an important role in development of AKI and persistence in need for RRT after AKI. Metcalfe and associates[18] reported that 16.7% of patients with acute-on-chronic disease were dialysis dependent at 90 days (RIFLE-E), compared with 2.9% of patients who had not had preexisting kidney insufficiency.[18]

Mortality

Wang and colleagues[11,12] found that mortality for community-acquired AKI was lower than that for hospital-acquired AKI (21.6 vs. 63.1%, respectively; $P < .001$). The in-hospital mortality rate for general ICU patients with AKI who are treated with RRT approaches 60%.[14,15,19] The mortality rate for ICU patients with AKI depends on severity of AKI and case mix.[15] Despite advances in treatment, the published mortality rates for patients with AKI in individual studies have remained more or less constant from 1956 on.[58] However, several longitudinal studies performed within single institutions found an improvement in prognosis over the years (Table 15-1). In addition, the aforementioned two large databases in which AKI was classified by means of administrative data also showed an improvement in outcome.[17,35]

Nosocomial AKI carries a greater mortality than community-acquired AKI, although the difference between them may vary according to case mix. In the study in African-American patients, 120-day mortality rates were 57% for nosocomial AKI and 34% for community-acquired AKI ($P = .05$),[13] whereas in the Chinese study, the difference was much greater (21.6% vs. 63.1%, respectively; $P < .001$).[11]

Long-Term Outcome

Increasing severity of AKI is associated with a rising 1-year mortality rate, and patients with AKI have a worse 1-year survival than those without AKI.[59] However, hospital survivors with different severities of AKI appear to have comparable 1-year mortality rates (Table 15-2 and Fig. 15-2).[55,59] However, few studies have examined this question in detail.

TABLE 15-1

Temporal Trend of Outcome in Patients with Acute Renal Failure within Single Institutions

STUDY*	OBSERVATION PERIOD(S)	NO.	MORTALITY (%)
Abreo et al[29]	1962-1969	55	54.5
	1979-1981	46	71.7
Turney et al[30]	1956-1959	101	51.2
	1985-1989	227	42.1
McCarthy[32]	1977-1979	71	68
	1991-1992	71	48
Biesenbach et al[31]	1975-1979	227	69
	1980-1984	240	24
	1985-1989	243	48
Druml et al†	1975-1990	243	>70 to <50
Wang et al[11]	1994-1998	173	39.7
	1999-2003	136	37.5
Desegher et al‡	1995	122	72.1
	2004	156	52.6

*Superscript numbers indicate chapter references.
†Druml W, Lax F, Grimm G, et al: Acute renal failure in the elderly 1975-1990. Clin Nephrol 1994;41:342-349.
‡Desegher A, Reynvoet E, Blot S, et al: Outcome of patients treated with renal replacement therapy for acute kidney injury. Critical Care 2006;10: P296.

TABLE 15-2

Hospital and 1-Year Mortality Rates in Patients in Intensive Care Unit without Acute Kidney Injury and with Increasing Severity of Acute Kidney Injury

	NO.	HOSPITAL MORTALITY (%)	1-YEAR MORTALITY OF HOSPITAL SURVIVORS (%)
No acute kidney injury	4411	13.4	4.5
Serum creatinine 1.7-3.4 mg/dL	790	40.0	11.4
Serum creatinine ≥3.4 mg/dL	160	40.6	12.6
Acute renal failure	240	59.6	10.3
End-stage kidney disease	92	33.7	9.8

Modified from Bagshaw SM, Mortis G, Doig CJ, et al: One-year mortality in critically ill patients by severity of kidney dysfunction: A population-based assessment. Am J Kidney Dis 2006;48:1038-1048.

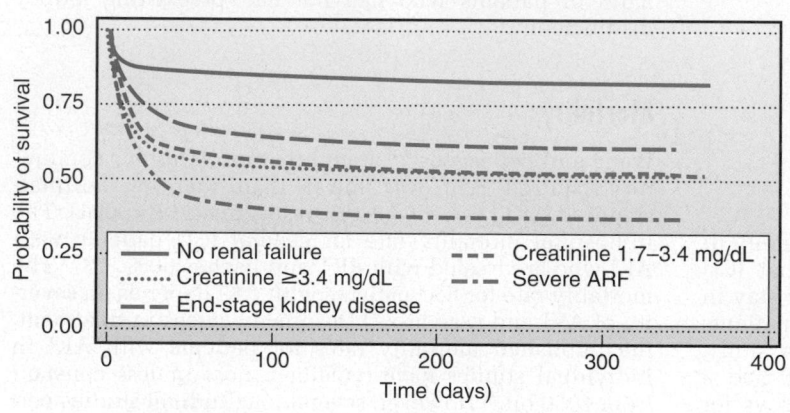

KAPLAN-MEIER ESTIMATES BY KIDNEY DYSFUNCTION

Legend:
— No renal failure
⋯ Creatinine ≥3.4 mg/dL
– – End-stage kidney disease
--- Creatinine 1.7–3.4 mg/dL
-·- Severe ARF

FIGURE 15-2. Long-term survival in patients receiving intensive care, stratified according to severity of acute kidney injury. ARF, acute renal failure. (Modified from Bagshaw SM, Mortis G, Doig CJ, et al: One-year mortality in critically ill patients by severity of kidney dysfunction: A population-based assessment. Am J Kidney Dis 2006;48:402-409.)

Patients Die of Acute Kidney Injury

Optimism from the past, dictating that renal function could be substituted by RRT and, therefore, patients died *with* ARF but not *because of* ARF, has been replaced by realism. Observed mortality in patients with ARF or AKI is higher than expected. This statement applies to the whole spectrum of AKI and to both patients treated in ICUs and patients treated in hospital. Levy and associates[2] reported that patients with a 25% increase in serum creatinine value after undergoing radiocontrast procedures have an in-hospital mortality of 34%, compared with 7% for carefully matched patients without an increase in serum creatinine value (odds ratio [OR] 5.5).[2] Several other groups have also confirmed the association of small absolute or relative increases in serum creatinine value in hospitalized (non-ICU) patients and in-hospital mortality.[4] In ICU patients, minor severity of AKI is also associated with worse outcome, even after correction for covariates; this association has been demonstrated in several studies using the RIFLE classification for AKI as well as studies evaluat-

ing small absolute increases in serum creatinine value.[3,5,60] The observed mortality of patients with ARF treated with RRT is higher than the expected mortality based on general ICU severity scoring systems. In the multicenter cohort of the BEST Kidney investigators, expected mortality based on SAPS II (Simplified Acute Physiology Score, revised) value was 45.6%, whereas observed mortality was as high as 60.3% (*P* < .001).[15] Metnitz and colleagues[14] performed a case-control study in which they matched each patient with ARF, on the basis of age and SAPS II value, with a patient without ARF who was treated in the ICU. Mortality rates in cases and controls (ARF vs. non-ARF patients) were, respectively, 62.8% and 38.5%, rendering an attributable mortality rate of 24.3% (*P* < .001).[14]

Key Points

1. Small changes in kidney function are associated with worse outcome, even after correction for case mix.

2. In the past, the epidemiology of acute kidney injury has been difficult to describe, given differences in definitions and characteristics of the cohorts studied.
3. The incidence of acute kidney injury appears to be increasing.
4. Despite improvement in care, mortality rates for acute kidney injury and acute renal failure remain high, but may be decreasing.

Key References

2. Levy EM, Viscoli CM, Horwitz RI: The effect of acute renal failure on mortality: A cohort analysis. JAMA 1996;275:1489-1494.
5. Hoste EA, Clermont G, Kersten A, et al: RIFLE criteria for acute kidney injury are associated with hospital mortality in critically ill patients: A cohort analysis. Crit Care 2006;10:R73.
7. Kellum JA, Levin N, Bouman C, Lameire N: Developing a consensus classification system for acute renal failure. Curr Opin Crit Care 2002;8:509-514.
15. Uchino S, Kellum JA, Bellomo R, et al: Acute renal failure in critically ill patients: A multinational, multicenter study. JAMA 2005;294:813-818.
20. Liaño F, Pascual J; the Madrid Acute Renal Failure Study Group: Epidemiology of acute renal failure: A prospective, multicenter, community-based study. Kidney Int 1996;50:811-818.

See the companion Expert Consult website for the complete reference list.

Risk Factors for Nosocomial Renal Failure

Reena Ranpuria and Paul M. Palevsky

OBJECTIVES

This chapter will:
1. Identify the common causes of acute kidney injury in critically ill patients.
2. Recognize the factors that generally predispose to the development of nosocomial acute kidney injury in critically ill patients.
3. Recognize risk factors associated with specific etiologies of nosocomial acute kidney injury.
4. Understand the use and limitations of risk stratification indices in the prediction of nosocomial acute kidney injury.

Acute kidney injury (AKI) is a serious complication in hospitalized patients, particularly in critically ill patients with multiple other organ dysfunctions. AKI is associated with increased mortality, prolongation of hospital length of stay, and higher costs of care. There is a graded relationship between changes in kidney function and mortality risk. Increases in serum creatinine level of 0.3 mg/dL or more are associated with a more than fourfold increase in risk mortality, increases of 1 mg/dL or more with a nearly 10-fold increase in mortality risk, and increases of 2 mg/dL or more with a greater than 16-fold increase in mortality risk, after adjusting for demographic and comorbid conditions.[1]

Epidemiological studies have suggested that there has been a progressive increase in the incidence of AKI over the past two decades.[2,3] Using administrative data from the Medicare database in the United States, Xue and colleagues[2] observed a rise in the incidence rate of AKI from 14.6 cases per 1000 discharges in 1992 to 36.4 cases per 1000 discharges in 2001, a change of approximately 11%

per year. Similarly, from an administrative database that included both Medicare and non-Medicare patients, Waikar and associates[3] reported an increase in AKI from 61 to 288 cases per 100,000 population over the period from 1988 to 2002. These rates are somewhat higher than the 209 cases per million population observed by Liaño and Pascual[4] in a prospective observational study conducted in Madrid in 1991 and 1992. The epidemiological studies of AKI in critically ill patients are more limited. In the largest study, Uchino and colleagues[5] observed a 5.7% period prevalence of AKI in a cohort of more than 29,000 critically ill patients at 54 hospitals in 23 countries in the period spanning September 2000 through December 2001. Hospital mortality in this cohort with AKI was 60.3%.

Given both the rising incidence of and high mortality rate associated with AKI, it is important to understand the risk factors predisposing to its development. These risk factors can be divided into specific etiological factors that represent the proximate cause of AKI, such as sepsis, trauma, major surgery, and nephrotoxic medications and diagnostic agents, and more general risk factors predisposing to the development of AKI, such as preexisting chronic kidney disease and increasing age.

HOSPITAL-ACQUIRED VERSUS COMMUNITY-ACQUIRED ACUTE KIDNEY INJURY

There are significant differences between the etiologies of nosocomial, or hospital-acquired, AKI and those of community-acquired AKI.[6-8] In a single-center study from the 1970s, Hou and associates[6] identified decreased renal perfusion as the most common cause of hospital-acquired AKI (41.9%), followed by postoperative AKI (17.8%), radiocontrast agent–induced nephrotoxicity (RCN) (12.4%), and aminoglycoside administration (7%). In a similar study nearly two decades later, Nash and colleagues[8] again found decreased renal perfusion (38.7%) to be the most common form of hospital-acquired AKI, followed by medication-associated toxicity (16%), RCN (11.3%), postoperative AKI (9.2%), and sepsis (7.4%). A weakness of both of these studies was the failure to differentiate between decreased renal perfusion resulting in reversible, hemodynamically mediated renal dysfunction (i.e., prerenal disease) and alterations in renal perfusion that caused ischemic renal injury (acute tubular necrosis). A markedly different pattern in etiologies of AKI was observed by Kaufman and associates[7] in a study of patients with community-acquired disease. In this study's cohort of 100 consecutive patients admitted with AKI, prerenal azotemia accounted for 70% of cases, obstructive renal disease for 17%, and intrinsic renal disease for only 11%.

CAUSES OF ACUTE KIDNEY INJURY IN THE INTENSIVE CARE UNIT

The causes of AKI in critically ill patients differ from those of AKI in the general hospitalized population. Of 748 patients with AKI identified by Liaño and coworkers[4,9] in their observational study of AKI in Madrid, 253 cases occurred in critically ill patients. Acute tubular necrosis accounted for 75.9% of intensive care unit (ICU) cases, compared with only 37.6% in non–critically ill patients. In contrast, prerenal azotemia accounted for 17.8% and obstructive disease for less than 1% of cases of AKI in the ICU, compared with 28.1% and 14.7% of cases, respectively, in non–critically ill patients. The etiologies of acute tubular necrosis in the ICU also differed from those observed in non–critically ill patients. Sepsis (35.4%) and medical causes (35.4%) of acute tubular necrosis predominated in the ICU, whereas nephrotoxic etiologies (51.6%) accounted for a majority of the non-ICU cases.[9] A similar pattern of causes of AKI were reported by Uchino and colleagues[5] in the Beginning and Ending Supportive Therapy for the Kidney (BEST Kidney) study. These researchers identified septic shock (47.5%), major surgery (34.3%), cardiogenic shock (26.9%), and hypovolemia (25.6%) as the four most common contributing factors for the development of AKI in a cohort of more than 29,000 ICU patients.

GENERAL RISK FACTORS FOR THE DEVELOPMENT OF NOSOCOMIAL ACUTE KIDNEY INJURY

A variety of demographic and clinical risk factors are associated with an increased risk for development of AKI (Table 16-1). In large epidemiological studies, increasing age, male gender, and black race are strongly associated with higher rates of AKI.[2,10] In an analysis of the 2001 National Hospital Discharge Survey (NHDS), containing data from more than 330,000 hospital discharges, Liangos and associates[10] found the median age of patients with a discharge diagnosis of AKI to be 73 years, whereas that in

TABLE 16-1

General Risk Factors Predisposing to the Development of Acute Kidney Injury

Underlying chronic kidney disease
Increasing age
Male gender
Black race
Chronic comorbidities
  Diabetes mellitus
  Congestive heart failure
  Chronic lung disease
  Human immunodeficiency virus infection
Volume depletion
Use of nonsteroidal anti-inflammatory medications

the overall cohort was only 58 years; 51.8% of patients with AKI were male, compared with 37.9% in the overall cohort. Similarly, 62.3% were white and 14.4% were black in the group with AKI, whereas 62.7% were white and 11.2% were black in the overall cohort.

Similar results were reported by Xue and colleagues[2] in their analysis of the US Medicare database. They observed a progressive increase in rates of AKI with rising age, with rates of 18.5, 20.8, 25.8, and 28.6 cases per 1000 discharges for patients aged 64 years or less, 65 to 74, 75 to 84, and 85 years or older, respectively. These researchers also observed a higher rate of AKI in men than in women (28.3 vs. 20 cases per 1000 discharges, respectively) and in black patients than in white patients and in patients of other racial background (34.4, 22.3, and 24.3 cases per 1000 discharges, respectively).

The clinical factor most strongly associated with the development of AKI is preexisting chronic kidney disease (CKD). In the analysis of the 2001 National Hospital Discharge Survey data, Liangos and associates[10] found CKD to be an underlying diagnosis in 30.6% of patients with AKI but in only 4.6% of the overall cohort. Other chronic comorbidities associated with the development of AKI were congestive heart failure, chronic lung disease, and human immunodeficiency virus infection.[10] Acute hospital-related factors included sepsis, cardiac surgery, and any acute nonrenal organ system dysfunction.

In addition to being a direct cause of AKI, particularly in elderly patients and in patients with impaired kidney function, nonsteroidal anti-inflammatory drugs (NSAIDs) are known to potentiate the risk for other causes of AKI.[11-13] NSAID use is associated with an incidence of AKI of approximately 2 cases per 100,000 person-years and is associated with a greater than fourfold increase in the odds ratio for development of AKI, a risk that is more than doubled in the first month of NSAID use.[11,13] The risks associated with NSAIDs are also increased in patients with reductions in effective circulating blood volume, including those with volume depletion, liver failure, congestive heart failure, hypertension, and diabetes mellitus.

Risk Factors for Acute Kidney Injury in Critically Ill Patients

De Mendonça and coworkers[14] evaluated risk factors for the development of AKI in a cohort of 1449 critically ill patients at 40 centers in 16 countries over a 1-month period, excluding patients with preexisting end-stage renal disease. AKI developed in 348 patients in this cohort

(24.7%). Using logistic regression, these researchers found that risk factors for the development of AKI were age 65 years or more, the presence of infection on admission, cardiovascular failure, cirrhosis, respiratory failure, chronic heart failure, and lymphoma or leukemia. Although de Mendonça and coworkers[14] did not identify CKD as a risk factor for AKI, 29.5% of the patients with AKI in the BEST Kidney study had underlying chronic renal impairment.[5] The rate of CKD in the overall cohort of critically ill patients was not reported in the BEST Kidney study, but given the epidemiology of CKD, it is unlikely to have been present in such a large proportion of the cohort.

Chawla and associates[15] identified cohorts of critically ill patients who were at either high or low risk for the development of AKI through the use of a combination of chronic major risk factors (advanced age, diabetes mellitus, atherosclerotic cardiovascular disease, and CKD), chronic minor risk factors (hypertension, morbid obesity, elevated bilirubin, history of a cerebrovascular accident, human immunodeficiency virus infection, and cancer) and acute risk factors (hypovolemia, hypotension, high-risk surgery, nephrotoxin exposure, systemic inflammatory response syndrome, and sepsis). The high-risk group was defined as having at least one acute and one chronic major risk factor, one acute and two chronic minor risk factors, or two acute risk factors; the low-risk group was defined as either having no acute risk factors independent of the number of chronic risk factors or having a single acute risk factor with no associated chronic risk factors. The incidence of AKI was 27.1% in the high-risk group and 3.9% in the low-risk group. Using multiple logistic regression analysis, these researchers found that an increased alveolar-to-arterial (A–a) oxygen gradient, a decreased serum albumin value, and the presence of cancer were independent predictors of the development of AKI.[15]

Risk Factors for Acute Kidney Injury in Specific Settings
Sepsis

Sepsis is a common predisposing factor for the development of AKI—having been reported as contributing to the development of 35% to 50% of cases of AKI in ICUs.[5,9,16,17] Clinical and biochemical risk factors for the development of AKI in patients with sepsis are poorly defined. In a cohort of 185 septic patients at a single center, Hoste and colleagues[18] identified only 30 (16.2%) in whom AKI developed. Numerous factors present on the first day of sepsis, including mean arterial pressure, need for vasoactive therapy, ratio of arterial oxygen pressure to fraction of inspired oxygen (PaO_2/FiO_2 ratio), serum creatinine concentration, blood pH, urinary volume, and positive fluid balance all correlated with the development of AKI on univariate analysis; only arterial blood pH less than 7.35 and serum creatinine concentration higher than 1 mg/dL, however, were statistically significant in a multivariate logistic regression model. Similarly, Chawla and associates,[19] analyzing data from the control arm of the Prospective Recombinant Human Activated Protein C Worldwide Evaluation in Severe Sepsis (PROWESS) study, identified increasing age, lower serum albumin, dependency as indicated by activities of daily living (ADL) score, higher baseline Sepsis-Related Organ Failure Assessment (SOFA) scores (except cardiovascular and hepatic subscores), higher baseline second Acute Physiology and Chronic Health Evaluation (APACHE-II) score, and higher interleukin-6 levels as predictors of the development of AKI on univariate analysis. On multivariate analysis, however, only APACHE-II score and interleukin-6 level remained statistically significant in this study.[19]

Trauma

Although the incidence of AKI after major trauma is relatively low, ranging from less than 1% to 8.4%,[20,21] the development of AKI in patients with major trauma is associated with mortality rates in excess of 50%.[20] In a series of 153 patients with multiple trauma, Vivino and coworkers[22] identified increased age, Glasgow Coma Scale score lower than 5, Injury Severity Score (ISS) higher than 17, respiratory failure requiring mechanical ventilation with positive end-expiratory pressure (PEEP) greater than 6 cm H_2O, rhabdomyolysis with serum creatine phosphokinase (CPK) value higher than 10,000 U/L, hemoperitoneum, and long-bone fracture as risk factors for AKI.

Cardiac Surgery

The incidence of AKI after cardiac surgery, defined as the need for postoperative renal replacement therapy, ranges between 0.5% and 15%.[23-27] The development of AKI is associated with a marked increase in mortality. In an analysis of more than 42,000 cardiac surgery procedures, Chertow and colleagues[28] reported a mortality rate of 63.7% in the 460 patients (1.1%) in whom dialysis-dependent renal failure developed, compared with only 4.3% in patients without AKI. After adjustment for demographic factors, comorbidities, and other postoperative complications, the adjusted odds ratio for death was 7.9.

Identified risk factors for post–cardiac surgery AKI include high baseline serum creatinine concentration, presence of diabetes mellitus, chronic obstructive pulmonary disease (COPD), previous cardiac surgery, markers of severe cardiovascular disease, female gender, and prolonged cardiopulmonary bypass time.[23-25,27] Risk stratification algorithms to estimate the risk for postoperative AKI have been developed through the use of multivariate models (Table 16-2).[23,24,27] Unfortunately, although these models are able to identify high-risk subsets, they have relatively low sensitivity. For example, according to the risk stratification score developed by Thakar and associates,[27] a score of 9 or higher is associated with a greater than 20% risk of postoperative AKI. Although a score of 3 to 5 is associated with only a 1.8% risk of AKI, three times as many patients in whom AKI develops have a score of 3 to 5 as have a score of 9 or higher. Thus, these risk prediction algorithms are insufficiently sensitive to be useful for clinical decision-making.

Radiocontrast Agent–Induced Nephropathy

RCN represents one of the most common etiologies of nosocomial AKI. The development of RCN is of greatest consequence in the critical care setting in patients undergoing diagnostic coronary angiography and percutaneous coronary interventions. The most important risk factor for the development of RCN is preexisting renal disease, particularly diabetic nephropathy.[29-31] McCullough and associates[29] reported a progressive increase in the risk for RCN from 0.04% at a creatinine clearance rate (CCR) of 50 mL/min to 12% at a CCR of 20 mL/min to 48% at a CCR of

TABLE 16-2

Risk Stratification for Acute Kidney Injury after Cardiac Surgery

RISK FACTORS	Score* SYSTEM OF CHERTOW ET AL[23]	SYSTEM OF THAKAR ET AL[27]
Female gender	—	1
Cardiac function:		
Congestive heart failure	—	1
Pulmonary rales	2	—
Left ventricular ejection fraction <35%	2	1
New York Heart Association functional class 4	2	—
Preoperative use of intra-aortic balloon pump	5	2
Comorbid conditions:		
Chronic obstructive pulmonary disease	2	1
Insulin-requiring diabetes	—	1
Peripheral vascular disease	2	—
Surgical characteristics:		
Previous cardiac surgery	3	1
Emergency surgery	—	2
Valve surgery	3	1
Combined coronary artery bypass grafting (CABG) + valve surgery	3	2
Other cardiac procedures	—	2
Preoperative renal function:		
Serum creatinine (mg/dL):		
1.2 to 2.1	—	2
≥2.1	—	5
Creatinine clearance (mL/min):		
80-99	2	—
60-79	3	—
40-59	5	—
<40	9	—
Systolic blood pressure (mm Hg):		
<120 + valve surgery	2	—
≥160 + CABG	3	—

*Superscript numbers refer to chapter references.

10 mL/min in nondiabetic patients. In contrast, the comparable risks in diabetic patients were significantly greater, increasing from 0.2% at a CCR of 50 mL/min to 43% at a CCR of 20 mL/min to 84% at a CCR of 10 mL/min. Other risk factors for the development of RCN are intra-arterial rather than intravenous administration, the use of high-osmolar rather than low-osmolar and iso-osmolar contrast agents, increasing age, and greater volume of radiocontrast media used.[30,31] In addition, intravascular volume depletion, cardiac dysfunction, need for urgent procedure, and use of an intra-aortic balloon pump are associated with a higher risk for RCN.[30,31] Several scoring systems have been developed to predict the risk of RCN after coronary angiography (Tables 16-3 and 16-4).[30,31] Although the precise details of these scoring systems differ, there is significant overlap in their major predictive components.

CONCLUSION

Hospital-acquired AKI is a serious complication that is associated with increases in morbidity, mortality, and length of hospitalization. Risk factors for the development of AKI can be categorized into specific etiologic processes, which are associated with the development of renal dysfunction, such as sepsis, cardiac surgery and the use of potentially nephrotoxic medications and general risk factors, which contribute to the development of AKI independent of the proximate cause. These latter risk factors include the presence of chronic kidney disease, increasing

age, and demographic factors such as gender and race. Comorbid conditions, particularly when associated with decreased effective circulatory volume, and concomitant administration of medications that alter renal hemodynamics, such as NSAIDs, also contribute to the development of nosocomial AKI.

Key Points

1. The etiologies of AKI vary according to clinical setting, with rates of intrinsic AKI rising from community-acquired, to hospital-acquired, to ICU-associated AKI.
2. Risk factors for the development of nosocomial AKI can be categorized into specific proximate etiologies and more general predisposing risk factors.
3. The major predisposing factors for the development of nosocomial AKI include increasing age and preexistent chronic kidney disease.
4. Comorbid conditions that are associated with compromised renal perfusion raise the risk of nosocomial AKI.
5. Risk stratification scores can identify patients at increased risk for development of specific etiologies of AKI; current risk stratification scores have low sensitivity.

TABLE 16-3

Risk Stratification for Development of Radiocontrast Agent–Induced Nephropathy*

| | Score | | |
| | SYSTEM OF MEHRAN ET AL,[31] MODEL A | SYSTEM OF MEHRAN ET AL,[31] MODEL B | SYSTEM OF BARTHOLOMEW ET AL[30] |
RISK FACTORS			
Renal function:			
Serum creatinine > 1.5 mg/dL	4	—	—
Estimated glomerular filtration rate (mL/min/1.73 m²):			
40 to 60	—	2	—
20 to 40	—	4	—
<20	—	6	—
Creatinine clearance < 60 mL/min	—	—	2
Hypotension	5	5	—
Intra-aortic balloon pump use	5	5	2
Congestive heart failure	5	5	1
Urgent/emergency procedure	—	—	2
Age > 75 years	4	4	1
Diabetes mellitus	3	3	—
Anemia	3	3	—
Peripheral vascular disease	—	—	1
Volume of contrast agent:			
For every 100 mL used	1	1	—
>260 mL used	—	—	1

*See Table 16-4 for significance of total scores.

TABLE 16-4

Significance of Total Score in Risk of Radiocontrast Agent–Induced Nephropathy (RCN)*

TOTAL SCORE	RISK OF RCN (%)
System of Mehran et al (Models A and B)[31]	
≤5	7.5
6-10	14.0
11-16	26.1
≤16	57.3
System of Bartholomew et al[30]	
0-4	0.5
5-6	5.5
7-8	18
9-11	43

*See Table 16-3 for details of scoring systems.

Key References

5. Uchino S, Kellum JA, Bellomo R, et al: Acute renal failure in critically ill patients: A multinational, multicenter study. JAMA 2005;294:813-818.
8. Nash K, Hafeez A, Hou S: Hospital-acquired renal insufficiency. Am J Kidney Dis 2002;39:930-936.
9. Liaño F, Junco E, Pascual J, et al: The spectrum of acute renal failure in the intensive care unit compared with that seen in other settings. The Madrid Acute Renal Failure Study Group. Kidney Int Suppl 1998;66:S16-S24.
10. Liangos O, Wald R, O'Bell JW, et al: Epidemiology and outcomes of acute renal failure in hospitalized patients: A national survey. Clin J Am Soc Nephrol 2006;1:43-51.
15. Chawla LS, Abell L, Mazhari R, et al: Identifying critically ill patients at high risk for developing acute renal failure: A pilot study. Kidney Int 2005;68:2274-2280.

See the companion Expert Consult website for the complete reference list.

CHAPTER 17

Etiology of Acute Renal Failure in the Intensive Care Unit

François Marquis, Stéphane P. Ahern, and Martine Leblanc

OBJECTIVES

This chapter will:
1. Describe the various etiologies of acute renal failure occurring in critical illness.
2. Discuss risk factors (intrinsic or modifiable) for the development of acute kidney injury or failure.
3. Provide an overview of the different mechanisms leading to acute renal failure.

Acute renal failure (ARF) affects as many as 25% of patients admitted to intensive care units (ICUs); however, its incidence may vary from 1% to 25%, depending on the criteria used for the definition of ARF and the population surveyed.[1-4] Until recently, there was a major lack of uniformity in the definition of ARF; the RIFLE (risk, injury, failure, loss, end-stage renal disease) criteria that have been proposed (see Chapter 11) are very useful and present many advantages over other classification systems used for acute kidney injury (AKI).

Sepsis accounts for most cases of ARF in critically ill patients. A prospective, single-center, observational study of 257 patients with systemic inflammatory response syndrome (SIRS) or overt sepsis who were admitted to medical and surgical ICUs during a 1-year period found an incidence of 11% for AKI.[5] Others have reported that ARF develops in approximately 50% of patients with septic shock and positive blood culture results.[6]

A prospective observational study of 29,269 patients admitted to the ICUs of 54 hospitals in 23 countries between September 2000 and December 2001 reported that 1738 patients had ARF during their ICU stays (ARF occurrence of 5.7%; 95% confidence interval ([CI] 5.5%-6.0%), and that the majority (1260 patients) were treated with renal replacement therapy.[7] Septic shock was the most common contributing factor to ARF (47.5%; 95% CI 45.2%-49.5%); other contributing factors were major surgery (34.3%), cardiogenic shock (26.9%), hypovolemia (25.6%) and medications (19%). Preadmission renal dysfunction was found in nearly 30% of patients.[7]

RISK FACTORS FOR DEVELOPMENT OF IN-HOSPITAL ACUTE RENAL FAILURE

Preadmission risk factors, clinical conditions, and nephrotoxic agents have been associated with the development of AKI in hospitalized patients in several epidemiological studies.[8] Although older age, underlying renal insufficiency, diabetes, and heart failure all predispose to ARF,

"diabetic nephropathy" or "diabetes with renal failure" represents probably the highest risk at baseline.

Sepsis and ARF are clearly related.[6] Hypotension and hypovolemia both contribute to ARF. Open heart surgery (especially valve replacement), acute or acute-on-chronic liver failure, and rhabdomyolysis predispose to ARF. The risk for development of AKI appears higher in mechanically ventilated patients,[9,10] although several confounding factors may play a role in complex clinical situations associated with critical illness. Intra-abdominal hypertension in the so-called abdominal compartment syndrome may lead to ARF by decreasing venous return and renal perfusion pressure and obstructing renal outflow.[11,12]

AKI in hospitalized patients is usually caused by hypoperfusion (prerenal azotemia) or acute tubular necrosis (ATN). Prerenal azotemia can result in ischemic ATN if renal hypoperfusion is severe and prolonged. Therefore, these two conditions may be seen as a continuum. Simple clinical indices may help distinguish prerenal azotemia from ATN (Table 17-1).

PRERENAL AZOTEMIA

Prerenal azotemia corresponds to a large proportion of cases of ARF occurring in hospitalized patients. Any reduction in renal perfusion can induce prerenal ARF; it is usually caused by either a reduction in effective circulating volume or a relative hypotension. The renal response to hypoperfusion is characterized by rapid and reversible increases in serum urea and creatinine levels. If renal perfusion is restored after only a short delay, renal parenchyma remains intact and renal function returns to normal. Renal perfusion and glomerular filtration are maintained during moderate hypovolemia and hypotension by different autoregulation mechanisms that are effective until the mean arterial pressure falls below 60 to 70 mm Hg.[13] Autoregulation of renal blood flow is achieved by afferent arteriolar vasodilatation (triggered by a decrease in myogenic tone within the vessel wall), by synthesis of intrarenal vasodilators (prostaglandins and nitric oxide), and by efferent arteriolar vasoconstriction (angiotensin II), with the purpose of keeping the glomerular filtration rate (GFR) constant.[14] In addition, proximal sodium reabsorption is enhanced, reducing the load to the distal tubule and generating a "reflex" dilatation of the glomerular afferent arteriole to sustain GFR; thus, there is a complex communication between the macula densa and the glomerular circulation.

Nephrotoxicity of nonsteroidal anti-inflammatory drugs (NSAIDs) and cyclooxygenase-2 (COX-2) inhibitors is enhanced in situations of renal hypoperfusion (i.e., dehydration, diuretics, cyclosporin, and heart and liver failure). As well, angiotensin-converting enzyme (ACE) inhibitors

Biochemical Parameters That Might Help Differentiate Prerenal Azotemia and Acute Tubular Necrosis (ATN)

PARAMETER	PRERENAL AZOTEMIA	ATN
Urinary osmolality (mOsm/kg)	>500	<400
Urinary sodium content (mmol/L)	<20	>40
Serum urea-to-creatinine ratio	>0.1	<0.05
Urinary-to-serum creatinine ratio	>40	<20
Urinary-to-serum osmolality ratio	>1.5	>1
Fractional excretion (%):		
Sodium	<1	>2
Urea	<35	>35

may induce renal failure in cases of renal hypoperfusion (i.e., volume depletion, bilateral renal artery stenosis).[15] The combined use of NSAIDs or cyclooxygenase-2 inhibitors plus ACE inhibitors should be avoided in the elderly.[16]

ACUTE TUBULAR NECROSIS

The most common cause of intrinsic ARF is ischemic ATN. Interruption of renal blood flow by cross-clamping for 60 minutes induces clinical and histopathologic features of ischemic ATN in animals.[17] Most susceptible tubular segments are situated in the outer medulla, a zone more prone to ischemia because of its relatively low partial oxygen tension (around 20 mm Hg) and its high energy requirements (due to important tubular epithelial transport) (Fig. 17-1). Epithelial tubular cells respond in multi-

ple ways to an insult, either ischemic or toxic; in ATN, injured cells predominantly evolve to necrosis. Sublethally injured cells contribute to the tubular dysfunction but, on the other hand, begin reparation. The distribution of tubular lesions has been described as patchy during ischemic insult, whereas a toxic insult affects tubular segments in a more evenly distributed pattern.

With a sustained ischemic insult, intrarenal hemodynamic alterations also contribute to the drop in GFR, because persistent hypoperfusion leads to afferent arteriole vasoconstriction and reduction of glomerular filtration coefficient owing to mesangial contraction.

ATN secondary to the administration of aminoglycosides was reported to occur in 10% to 20% of treated patients two decades ago.[18] Its incidence appears to have declined since then, owing to the introduction of several newer antibiotics used for coverage against gram-negative organisms. Aminoglycosides are polycationic molecules that can be transported into the lysosomes of proximal tubular cells by pinocytosis. Nephrotoxicity operates at the level of proximal tubular cells, creating a tubular dysfunction similar to that in Fanconi's syndrome. Tissue half-life exceeds plasma half-life, thus contributing to cortical accumulation. Risk factors for renal toxicity include treatment duration exceeding 7 days, underlying renal hypoperfusion resulting from hypovolemia or hypotension, concomitant diuretic use, other nephrotoxins such as NSAIDs, predose serum levels more than 2 to 3 μg/mL, and liver insufficiency. To avoid toxicity, it is of primary importance to adjust the dosage appropriately, especially in patients with renal impairment. Although formulation of toxicity profiles for aminoglycosides according to their cationic charges remains controversial, once-daily dosage appears safer from a renal perspective than multiple daily doses.

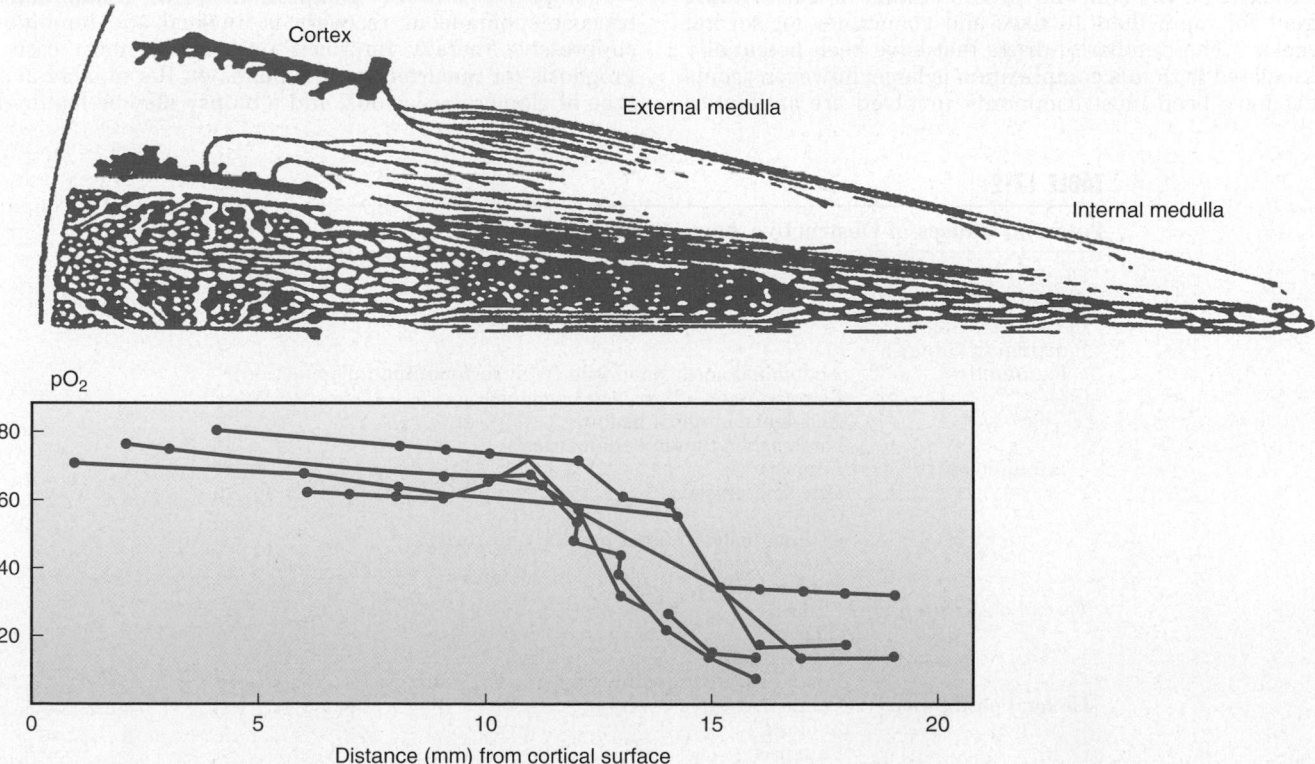

FIGURE 17-1. Schema of intrarenal oxygenation. The medulla is at risk for ischemia because of a lower oxygenation than the cortex.

CORTICAL NECROSIS

Cortical necrosis corresponds to ischemia of the cortex, where glomeruli are located. It indicates a prolonged ischemic insult (i.e., profound shock, circulation arrest, grave hypoxemia). Usually irreversible, cortical necrosis is associated with total anuria.

OBSTRUCTIVE ACUTE RENAL FAILURE

Obstructive uropathy is responsible for less than 10% of all cases of ARF in hospitalized patients. It is even less common in the ICU because the majority of patients have urinary catheters in place. However, extraureteral or intraureteral obstruction may occur on rare occasions; potential causes of obstructive ARF that may be encountered are listed in Table 17-2. Acyclovir and indinavir can precipitate acute crystal nephropathy, particularly if high doses are administrated rapidly to a volume-depleted patient. Nephrocalcinosis (intratubular calcium phosphate deposits) has been described after the ingestion of sodium phosphate solution as bowel preparation or purgative. Such phosphate nephropathy is potentially irreversible.[19]

OTHER CAUSES OF ACUTE RENAL FAILURE

Acute Interstitial Nephritis

Acute interstitial nephritis is a relatively rare form of ARF. It usually occurs after the administration of an offending agent for more than 10 days and sometimes for several weeks.[20] The number of drugs that have been potentially associated with this complication is large; however, agents that have been most commonly involved are antibiotics (penicillin-like compounds, cephalosporins, rifampicin, ciprofloxacin, sulfonamides, interferon), NSAIDs, and phenytoin. In the ICU, this disorder is usually seen after a long course of antibiotics given for a significant infectious process.

The clinical presentation may involve fever, cutaneous rash, and arthralgias (Table 17-3). Eosinophilia and eosinophiluria are present in many but not all cases, and serum immunoglobulin (Ig) E values may occasionally be elevated. Kidneys may be enlarged on imaging studies because of diffuse renal swelling; results of a radioactive gallium scan are usually positive because of the inflammatory cell infiltrate of renal tissues. Renal function should improve shortly after discontinuation of the offending agent, but a trial of corticosteroids for 2 or 3 weeks may be required for return of renal function. Kidney biopsy, which will confirm the suspected etiology, can be performed in doubtful situations or when there is no recovery despite cessation of suspected drug ingestion, in order to avoid irreversible damage.

Acute Glomerulonephritis

A few decades ago, acute glomerulonephritis was held responsible for 10% of cases of ARF.[21] This estimation may not be accurate anymore with the relative changes in ARF epidemiology.

Nonetheless, the most common types of glomerulonephritis manifesting as ARF are microscopic polyarteritis and Wegener's granulomatosis, in both of which circulating anti–neutrophil cytoplasm antibodies (ANCAs) are found. Systemic lupus erythematosus, anti–glomerular basement membrane disease, and mesangioproliferative glomerulonephritis can also manifest in an "ARF mode." Berger's disease and postinfectious glomerulonephritis relatively rarely manifest as ARF.

Prompt recognition of glomerulonephritis is important, because spontaneous recovery is unusual and immunosuppressive therapy improves outcome in most cases. Prognosis for renal recovery depends on the number and type of glomerular lesions, and a biopsy may be required

TABLE 17-2

Potential Causes of Obstructive Acute Renal Failure

Ureteral obstruction (bilateral or unilateral in case of a single functioning kidney):	
Extraureteral	Abdominal aortic aneurysm (with surrounding inflammation)
	Retroperitoneal fibrosis or hematoma
	Accidental surgical ligature
	Large pelvic tumor, endometriosis
Intraureteral	Lithiasis
	Uric acid crystals
	Clots
	Cellular material (after papillary necrosis)
	Massive edema
	Fungus ball
Vesical obstruction	Lithiasis
	Clots
	Pelvic tumor
	Functional (neuropathy, drugs)
Ureteral obstruction	Congenital valve
	Stenosis
	Phimosis
	Iatrogenic cause

TABLE 17-3

Clinical Presentation of Acute Interstitial Nephritis

Acute or subacute elevation of serum creatinine concentration
Suspected drug administered for more than 10 days (or 3-5 days if for a second course)
Fever (75% of cases, not with nonsteroidal anti-inflammatory drugs)
Cutaneous rash (50% of cases)
Eosinophilia (30% of cases)
Urinalysis:
  Eosinophiluria (85% of cases)
    White cell casts
    Unspecific findings:
      Mild proteinuria (<1 g/day)
      Red and white blood cells
Positive radioactive gallium scan result

TABLE 17-4

Risk Factors for Radiocontrast Agent–Induced Nephropathy

Nonmodifiable factors	Preexisting renal dysfunction
	Diabetes
	Older age
	Congestive heart failure
	Cardiogenic shock
	Acute myocardial infarction
	Renal transplant
	Low left ventricular ejection fraction
Modifiable factors	Dehydration
	Volume of contrast agent used
	Type of contrast agent used
	Nonsteroidal anti-inflammatory drugs
	Angiotensin-converting enzyme inhibitors, angiotensin II receptor blocker
	Nephrotoxic antibiotics
	Diuretics
	Anemia
	Low serum albumin level (<35 g/L)
	Intra-aortic balloon pump

Adapted from Mehran R, Nikolsky E: Contrast-induced nephropathy: Definition, epidemiology, and patients at risk. Kidney Int 2006;69: S11-S15.

to assess precisely not only the type of disease but also the extent of tissue damage.

Clinical presentation includes microscopic or macroscopic hematuria, proteinuria, and active urine sediment (red cells that may be dysmorphic, red cell casts, and/or white cell casts). Other manifestations are hypertension, fever, anemia, unspecific inflammatory indices, systemic symptoms, and hemoptysis (depending on the type of glomerulonephritis). Rapidly progressive glomerulonephritis appears with renal deterioration over a few days and requires prompt management. Characteristic glomerular findings are crescentic changes and necrotizing lesions.

Clinical Conditions Associated with Acute Kidney Injury

Use of Radiocontrast Agents

The incidence of radiocontrast agent–induced nephropathy (RCN) does not appear to have changed significantly over the last 30 years; it remains the third leading cause of hospital-acquired ARF, corresponding to 11% of cases in a 2006 survey.[22] The incidence of RCN is estimated between 1% and 2% in the general population, but it may exceed 50% in high-risk groups.[23] The most important risk for the development of RCN is preexisting renal impairment with a GFR less than 60 mL/min/1.73 m². Diabetes clearly amplifies that risk. Cardiovascular disease, hemodynamic instability, use of nephrotoxic drugs, and anemia have also been found to enhance the risk of RCN.[24] Multiple risk factors are additive, leading to a high probability of ARF; they are contrast volume, type of contrast medium used, and intra-arterial administration (Table 17-4). The tolerable dose of contrast depends on preexisting kidney function; amounts greater than 100 mL enhance the risk.[25] The risk of RCN can be minimized by using less than 30 mL of contrast medium in an azotemic diabetic patient.[26] Non-ionic iso-osmolar contrast agents may cause less damage than hyperosmolar media and should be preferred in high-risk patients.[27]

Radiocontrast agent–induced kidney damage occurs from a combination of toxic injury to the renal tubules and ischemic injury mediated in part by reactive oxygen species; low blood medullary flow might result from greater perivascular hydrostatic pressure, high blood viscosity, and impaired vasodilatation.

Pigments

Most cases of myoglobinuric ARF encountered in our ICUs are related to nontraumatic muscle injury rather than crush injury and severe trauma. Common causes are rather prolonged immobilization and compression during drug overdose, seizures, peripheral arterial disease with compartment syndrome, strenuous exercise, and alcohol or drug toxicity. Pharmacologic agents involved in rhabdomyolysis include statins, fibrates, foscarnet, and stimulants such as cocaine.

Although the suggestion is controversial, the serum level of creatinine phosphokinase at admission may be predictive of AKI. In a series of 72 patients with rhabdomyolysis, initial serum creatinine phosphokinase level greater than 25,000 U/L was associated with a higher risk of AKI.[28] Another study reported that abnormal initial serum creatinine concentration was most predictive of AKI or need for renal replacement therapy.[29] Propofol myotoxicity may occur with prolonged (>48 hours) and high-dose (>5 mg/kg/hr) administration of this agent in sepsis or neurologic injury.[30]

Hemoglobinuric ARF is rare; it may be found with valve leaks and may contribute to AKI in hemolytic-uremic syndrome/thrombotic thrombocytopenic purpura.

Open Heart Surgery

Open heart surgery for myocardial revascularization substantially raises the risk of ARF,[31,32] and valve replacement appears to raise it further. Because both the duration of aortic cross-clamping and use of cardiopulmonary bypass are independent determinants for the risk of ARF,[17] "off-pump" techniques have been recommended, especially for patients with underlying renal dysfunction. However, these approaches may not reduce the risk significantly.[33]

Bone Marrow Transplantation

The reported incidence of ARF after bone marrow transplantation ranges from 30% to 80%.[34,35] Causes of ARF differ with the time since transplantation; early ARF is usually due to ATN, veno-occlusive disease, tumor lysis, or nephrotoxic drugs, whereas late-onset ARF is due to graft-versus-host disease, hemolytic-uremic syndrome, or cyclosporin toxicity.[36] Among 57 patients who had received bone marrow transplants and were admitted to our ICUs for respiratory distress and hypotension, the incidence of ARF was 74%, and ARF was more common with allogeneic than autologous bone marrow. The rates of sepsis (83%) and liver failure (69%) were significantly higher in patients in whom ARF developed than in those without ARF.[37]

Tumor Lysis Syndrome

Tumor lysis syndrome results from massive cell death leading to metabolic disturbances (hyperuricemia, hyperphosphatemia, hyperkalemia, hypocalcemia) and ARF. Patients with tumors that have high cell turnover, such as high-grade lymphomas, high–leukocyte count leukemias, and, rarely, solid tumors are particularly at risk, usually during cell destruction by chemotherapy. Extracellular volume depletion and overload of uric acid and phosphate both contribute to ARF, which is frequently oliguric. Hyperphosphatemia promotes the precipitation of calcium-phosphate complexes within the tubular/interstitial parenchyma, producing acute nephrocalcinosis. Hyperuricemia, due to purine release from nucleic acid breakdown and catabolism of hypoxanthine and xanthine, increases renal elimination burden of uric acid, which is less ionized and less soluble in renal tubules, especially at an acid pH. Indeed, urate crystals may form in the distal collecting system, leading to luminal obstruction and consequently reduced GFR. Adenosine released from neoplastic cells seems also to contribute to ARF, by facilitating arterial vasoconstriction.

Liver Disease

Prerenal azotemia, ATN, and hepatorenal syndrome (HRS) represent three common causes of ARF in patients with liver failure. Among 355 patients with cirrhosis and ARF, prerenal azotemia was found in 38%, ATN in 42%, and HRS in 20%.[38] Decreased splanchnic/systemic vascular resistance, hyperdynamic circulation, and neurohumoral vasoconstrictors are involved in renal injury in HRS.[39] Type I HRS is characterized by an abrupt decrease in renal function after a precipitating event (i.e., peritonitis, bleeding, paracentesis) during hospitalization and carries a poor prognosis, whereas type II HRS develops more slowly in the context of refractory ascites and diuretic resistance.

Atheroembolic Acute Renal Failure

Atheroembolic renal disease results from occlusion of small renal arteries by showers of cholesterol crystals from an atherosclerotic aorta. It is increasingly recognized as an iatrogenic complication after an invasive vascular procedure or surgery. However, atheroembolic ARF may also be precipitated by anticoagulation or fibrinolytic therapy or, rarely, may be spontaneous. Older patients and smokers are more at risk, as are hypertensive patients with vascular disease. Atheroembolic disease may lead to various degrees of renal impairment, because ARF may be mild or severe enough to require dialysis. An abrupt renal deterioration may occur, although subacute renal failure usually appears progressively over weeks and evolves in steps.[40] Extrarenal manifestations (especially at the skin level, with livedo reticularis and blue toes) and clinical circumstances are of help in making the diagnosis. In addition, eosinophilia and hypocomplementemia are relatively common. Biopsy of the target organs may be necessary to confirm the diagnosis. Renal recovery is not infrequent, but the overall outcome is difficult to predict.

In 2003, Thériault and colleagues[41] identified 43 patients with atheroembolic ARF severe enough to require dialysis. Most patients had at least one precipitating event (58% coronary angiography, 26% peripheral angiography, 16% vascular surgery, 2% anticoagulation). More than 90% had underlying hypertension and chronic renal dysfunction, with a mean baseline serum creatinine level of 195 ± 81 µmol/L. Acute-on-chronic renal failure was nonoliguric in 80% of cases, and 12 patients (28%) were able to discontinue dialytic support after variable periods.[41]

Key Points

1. Acute renal failure or injury is a common issue in the intensive care unit and carries a high morbidity and mortality.
2. Recognized risk factors for acute renal failure are older age, baseline renal impairment, diabetic nephropathy, open heart surgery, and acute liver failure.
3. Sepsis is an important risk factor for acute kidney injury and may be preventable with early aggressive therapy.
4. Radiocontrast agent–induced nephropathy is an important cause of acute renal failure in high-risk groups.

Key References

5. Yegenaga I, Hoste E, Van Biesen W, et al: Clinical characteristics of patients developing ARF due to sepsis/systemic inflammatory response syndrome: Results of a prospective study. Am J Kidney Dis 2004;43:817-824.
7. Uchino S, Kellum JA, Bellomo R, et al; Beginning and Ending Supportive Therapy for the Kidney (BEST Kidney) Investigators: Acute renal failure in critically ill patients: A multinational, multicenter study. JAMA 2005;294:813-818.
22. McCullough PA, Adam A, Becker CR, et al; CIN Consensus Working Panel: Epidemiology and prognostic implications of contrast-induced nephropathy. Am J Cardiol 2006;98(Suppl 1):5-13.
31. Thakar CV, Liangos O, Yared JP, et al: ARF after open-heart surgery: Influence of gender and race. Am J Kidney Dis 2003;41:742-751.
42. Mehran R, Nikolsky E: Contrast-induced nephropathy: Definition, epidemiology, and patients at risk. Kidney Int 2006;69: S11-S15.

See the companion Expert Consult website for the complete reference list.

CHAPTER 18

Epidemiology of End-Stage Renal Disease in Patients with Critical Illness Admitted to Intensive Care Units

Norbert Lameire, Wim Van Biesen, Eric A. J. Hoste, and Raymond Vanholder

---

OBJECTIVES

This chapter will:
1. Review the few studies describing the epidemiology of critical illness in patients undergoing long-term hemodialysis, of whom between 8% and 12% require intensive care.
2. Discuss the most common causes of critical illness in patient undergoing long-term dialysis—acute postoperative complications, cardiac resuscitation, neurological syndromes, sepsis, and major gastrointestinal bleeding.

The precise number of patients with stage 5 kidney disease (end-stage renal disease [ESRD]) worldwide is unknown, but the number of patients being treated for ESRD reached about 1.9 million at the end of 2005. With a 6% yearly growth rate, this number continues to rise at a significantly higher rate than the world population.[1]

Of the 1.9 million patients being treated with ESRD in 2005, more than 1.45 million were undergoing renal replacement therapy (RRT), either hemodialysis or peritoneal dialysis, and about 445,000 people were living with a functioning kidney transplant.

The prevalence of treated patients with ESRD in the general population shows a high global variation, ranging from less than 100 to more than 1600 patients per million population (pmp). ESRD prevalence exceeds 2100 pmp in Japan and 1600 pmp in the United States but averages 900 pmp in the European Union.[1] The much lower global average, 290 pmp, strongly suggests that access to treatment is still limited in many countries and that a significant number of patients with terminal renal failure do not receive treatment. The rise in global prevalence rates over the last years, however, indicates a gradual improvement in the situation.

The epidemiology of long-term dialysis shows that growing numbers of patients are becoming older and sicker and, at least in the developed world, have nonrenal comorbid conditions. These patients frequently have cardiovascular complications,[2-4] hematological abnormalities with bleeding tendencies such as gastrointestinal (GI) bleeding, bacterial infections, and malnutrition, all of which contribute to their morbidity and mortality.

Besides the often important comorbidity at the moment of initiation of chronic dialysis, many complications of the dialysis procedure per se present unique challenges, so many patients require hospitalization, including admission to the intensive care unit (ICU).[5] Few data exist on the actual admission rate of patients with ESRD in ICUs, however, because most studies on renal failure in the critically ill patient exclude subjects with ESRD from analysis.[6] Of the 19,124 patients enrolled to develop and validate the Mortality Probability Model II (MPM II), only 888 (4.6%) had chronic renal insufficiency on admission.[7]

As summarized by Hoste and colleagues,[8] relatively few studies have evaluated the incidence of supplementary renal insults leading to ARF superimposed on chronic renal failure (CRF). Interestingly, few reports suggest a negative impact of preexisting CRF on patient survival related to ARF, and most studies could not find a specific additional impact. In some studies, a more favorable immediate outcome has been reported for ARF in patients with preexisting CRF.[9] On the other hand, in many series on ARF, even relatively mild chronic kidney disease is found to be a strong risk factor for the development of acute kidney injury (AKI). This underlying chronic kidney disease, often unknown, contributes substantially to the changing epidemiology of acute kidney injury over the last decade.[10]

This chapter summarizes the epidemiology and outcomes of patients undergoing long-term dialysis in whom critical illness develops and requires their admission to an ICU. The intensive care management of the renal transplant recipient has been discussed elsewhere[11] and is covered in other chapters of this book.

EPIDEMIOLOGY OF ACUTE CRITICAL ILLNESS IN PATIENTS WITH END-STAGE RENAL DISEASE

We performed a preliminary analysis of the epidemiology of 389 patients with ESRD and undergoing hemodialysis at the University Hospital in Gent. The analysis shows that from January 2004 until the end of September 2006, 76 patients (19.5%) needed general hospitalization and 42 (10.8%) required admission to the ICU. Table 18-1 indicates that 36% of the patients were admitted to the ICU for acute cardiovascular problems, 21% for acute respiratory problems, and 18% for sepsis or septic shock. A minority of the patients suffered from hypovolemia, bleeding (1 GI, 1 cerebral hemorrhage), cholecystectomy, or abdominal pain or were admitted for miscellaneous or unknown reasons.

Clermont and associates[12] were the first researchers to include patients with ESRD in their epidemiology study

TABLE 18-1

Major Causes of Admission to the Intensive Care Unit in 42 Patients Undergoing Long-Term Hemodialysis at The University Hospital, Gent, Belgium (January 2004 to October 2006)

CAUSE	Patients Affected	
	NO.	PERCENTAGE
Cardiovascular problems:	15:	36
Arrhythmias	6	
Angina	5	
Peripheral thrombosis	3	
Pericarditis	1	
Respiratory problems:	9:	21
Acute respiratory insufficiency	7	
Acute pulmonary edema	2	
Sepsis, septic shock	7	18
Hypovolemia after dialysis	3	7
Bleeding	2	4
Cholecystectomy	1	2
Abdominal pain	1	2
Miscellaneous/unknown	4	10

of ARF in the ICU. In a total of 1530 patients admitted to eight ICUs over a 10-month period, 254 (16.6%) were diagnosed as having ARF on the basis of the definitions used by Hou and coworkers[13] and 57 (3.7% of total, but 22.4% of those with ARF) had preexisting ESRD. Unfortunately, reasons for admission and/or diagnosis of critical illness are not given in this study. In roughly half the patients with ARF, the disease already existed at admission to the ICU; in the other half, ARF developed during the ICU stay. As expected, patients with ARF had significantly higher acute illness severity scores than those without renal failure, whereas patients with preexisting ESRD had intermediate severity scores. Interestingly, ICU mortality was 23% for patients with de novo ARF, 11% for those with preexisting ESRD, and only 5% for those without renal failure. There was no difference in outcome between patients who had ARF at ICU admission and those in whom ARF developed in the ICU. However, the Acute Physiology and Chronic Health Evaluation (APACHE) III scoring system predicted outcome very well in patients without renal failure and patients with ARF at the time of scoring, but underpredicted mortality in those in whom ARF developed after ICU admission and overestimated mortality in those patients with ESRD. This pattern could explain why the moment of scoring in these patients influenced outcome in the ICU.

A second, more comprehensive study on epidemiology of critical illness in patients with ESRD used a prospectively collected national database of all patients treated with RRT in Australian ICUs over 3 months.[14] Thirty-eight patients with ESRD received RRT in an ICU over the study period, representing 11.2% of all ICU patients treated with RRT in Australian ICUs. Given an adult population of 15.85 million at the time of the investigation in Australia, the incidence of patients with ESRD requiring ICU admission and acute RRT was calculated as approximately 10.4 per million adults per year. Furthermore, given a prevalence of 530 patients with ESRD per million population, these calculations indicate that 2.0% of such patients are admitted to an ICU requiring RRT every year. The investigators of this study pointed out that this value is likely to represent an underestimate of the percentage of all patients with ESRD who require ICU admission every year, because some of these patients may require only a short ICU stay and do not receive RRT during that time. Data from units participating in an Australian national database project suggest that approximately 70,000 to 80,000 patients are admitted to ICUs in Australia every year. From this information, it appears that the diagnosis of ESRD confers more than a fourfold increase of the yearly risk of combined ICU admission and need for RRT.

This study also gives information on the most important diagnostic categories for these 38 patients. Eight of the 38 (21%) were admitted for septic shock, 10 (26%) for cardiovascular problems (the majority being coronary surgery), 4 for respiratory diseases (pulmonary edema and pneumonia), and 6 (16%) for GI problems, among them bleeding, perforation, and neoplasm.

To analyze the prognosis, the investigators compared these acutely ill patients with ESRD, all of whom underwent dialysis and continuous RRT, with matched controls with ARF but without preexisting ESRD who were also treated with continuous RRT. The mean APACHE II score in the patients with ESRD was 21.8 (predicted mortality, 37%), the Simplified Acute Physiology Score (SAPS) II value was 44.7 (predicted mortality, 37%), and the hospital mortality rate was 34%. Receiver operating characteristic (ROC) curves showed good discriminating ability for hospital mortality for these two scores (area under the curve [AUC], 0.81 for APACHE II and 0.84 for SAPS II). Using admission diagnosis and SAPS II scores, 32 patients with ESRD and treated with CRRT were matched with 32 ARF patients also treated with CRRT. ICU mortality (22% vs. 38%) and hospital mortality (38% vs. 38%) were comparable between the two groups. On the other hand, the presence of systemic inflammatory response syndrome and the need for vasopressor medication were less common, and the duration of stay in the ICU and hospital was significantly shorter, in patients with ESRD.

To describe the clinical course of patients with ESRD admitted to the ICU and to compare the performance of APACHE III and Sequential Organ Failure Assessment (SOFA) in predicting their outcome, Dara and colleagues[15] analyzed a retrospective cohort consisting of patients with ESRD who were admitted to three ICUs between January 1, 1997, and November 30, 2002. Data on demographics, APACHE III score, SOFA score, development of sepsis and organ failure, use of mechanical ventilation, and mortality were collected. Of the 476 patients with ESRD, 93 (20%) required admission to the ICU during the study period. The most common ICU admission diagnosis was GI bleeding. The observed ICU, hospital, and 30-day mortality rates were 9%, 16%, and 22%, respectively. Nonrenal organ failure developed in 48 (52%) and sepsis in 15 (16%) of these patients. Mechanical ventilation was required in 26 patients (28%). The area under the receiver operating characteristic curve for the first-day APACHE III probability of hospital death in predicting 30-day mortality was 0.78 (95% confidence interval [CI], 0.68-0.86), compared with 0.66 (95% CI, 0.55-0.76) for the SOFA score.

In 38 patients with "established" CRF who were admitted to the ICU of the Hinduja hospital in Mumbai, India, in 2001, the major precipitating diseases were sepsis in 6 patients, left ventricular failure in 10 patients, and noncardiac pulmonary edema in 14; 8 were described as being admitted for "other causes."[16] The observed hospital mortality for these patients was rather low (11/38).

Manhes and associates[17] reported on their study seeking to determine the epidemiology and outcome of patients undergoing long-term dialysis in an ICU setting and to test the performance of SAPS II in predicting hospital mortality in this population. All patients undergoing long-term dialysis who were consecutively admitted to an adult, 10-bed medical-surgical ICU at a university hospital between January 1996 and December 1999 were included in this prospective observational study. During this period, 1257 ICU admissions were recorded, consisting of 1149 admissions of patients without ESRD and 108 admissions (8.6%) in a total of 92 patients undergoing dialysis, 16 on peritoneal dialysis and 76 on hemodialysis. The reasons for ICU admission were requirement for life-sustaining support in most patients—severe sepsis (n = 28), heart failure or fluid overload (n = 17), hemorrhage (n = 12), surgery (n = 8), cardiac arrest (n = 6), arterial thrombosis (n = 5), stroke (n = 5), hyperkalemia (n = 4), abdominal crisis (n = 2), drug overdose (n = 2), pancreatitis (n = 1), malaise (n = 1) and anaphylactic shock (n = 1). Organ system failure in addition to renal failure in the patients at ICU admission were cardiovascular failure (n = 27), respiratory failure (n = 56), hematological failure (n = 8), and neurological failure (n = 15); in 30 patients, only renal failure was observed. The main reason for ICU admission was sepsis, and the mean ICU length of stay 6.2 ± 9.9 days. In 35 patients (38.0%), mechanical ventilation was required for a mean duration of 5.1 ± 5.4 days. Twenty-six of the 92 patients died (28.3%), and the mortality rate was associated in multivariate analysis with SAPS II, duration of mechanical ventilation, and either high or low serum phosphorus values. Nine additional deaths were recorded before hospital discharge, giving an overall hospital mortality of 38.0%. Five of the 57 hospital survivors (8.8%) were lost to follow-up after hospital discharge. Of the remaining 52 patients, 4 died during the 6-month follow-up period, all of whom had diabetes and/or vascular disease. Thus, the 6-month ICU survival rate was 52.2%.

In this study, the patients undergoing long-term dialysis formed a subgroup with a greater illness severity and a higher mortality than observed in the patients in ICU who did not need dialysis. This higher severity may be related to the frequency of associated comorbidity, especially cardiovascular disease, that occurs in almost all of this population. However, half of the patients undergoing long-term dialysis were 6-month survivors, showing that intensive care can be successful and should not be dismissed as useless for patients in this clinical situation. No previous study has reported long-term survival after ICU discharge of patients undergoing long-term dialysis.

Bagshaw and colleagues[18] published the results of a population-based surveillance of adult residents of the Calgary Health Region (population, 1 million) admitted to any multidisciplinary ICU or cardiovascular surgery ICU from May 1, 1999, to April 30, 2002. Of a total of 5693 adult admissions, 92 (1.62%) occurred in patients who had ESRD treated with RRT. The distribution of the admission type was 48% medical, 28% noncardiac surgery, and 24% postcardiac surgery. It was remarkable that the immediate ICU prognosis in the patients with ESRD was much better that in those with moderate and severe ARF; the same study found that critically ill patients with ESRD had a mortality rate at 1 year similar to those with no kidney dysfunction after adjustment for age, severity of illness, and admission type.

Two of the studies discussed previously proposed that the severity of illness and organ dysfunction scoring systems APACHE II and SAPS II reliably predict hospital mortality[14,17]; however, in the study performed by Bagshaw and colleagues,[18] APACHE II scores of patients with ESRD were considerably higher despite similar hospital mortality. This finding is not surprising because renal function is included in the calculation of the APACHE II score. Therefore, APACHE II scores and SAPS II values likely underestimate hospital mortality, as also suggested in the Beginning and Ending Supportive Therapy for the Kidney (BEST Kidney) study.[19] The apparent better outcome of patients with ESRD in the Bagshaw study may be accounted for by a larger sample size of such patients and adjustment for severity of illness and admission type. Also, a greater proportion of the patients with ESRD underwent cardiac surgery. It is known that the case-fatality rate in post–cardiac surgery patients admitted to the ICU is lower than in those with medical admissions, likely because of the routine and elective postoperative admission of such patients. In light of these findings, further investigations into the outcome of critically ill patients with ESRD are warranted.

SELECTED CRITICAL ILLNESSES OR CONDITIONS IN PATIENTS WITH END-STAGE RENAL DISEASE

The most common causes for ICU admission of patients undergoing dialysis are cardiac surgery, cardiac resuscitation, sepsis, and GI bleeding.

Cardiovascular Surgery

Because of the growing numbers of elderly patients who are entering dialysis programs today, the number of patients receiving dialysis who will require myocardial revascularization is expected to increase. There are many complications in the surgical treatment of ischemic heart disease in patients undergoing dialysis, such as poor general condition before surgery, poor water and electrolyte control, calcification of the aorta and peripheral arterial trees, and the necessity for simultaneous operations. It can be estimated that 0.5% to 1.5% of patients undergoing coronary operations are uremic, and their perioperative mortality is between 8% and 30%.[20]

Coronary artery bypass grafting (CABG) has become the standard treatment for coronary artery disease in patients with ESRD because it yields better overall and angina-free survival than percutaneous coronary intervention (PCI).[21,22] In particular, the rate of restenosis after percutaneous coronary intervention is higher in uremic than in nonuremic patients. Despite suboptimal results in comparison with results of bypass surgery, PCI remains a viable option, especially for patients who are not candidates for surgery and those with disabling angina despite antianginal therapy. Regardless of the revascularization strategy used, outcomes of CABG or PCI in these patients are significantly worse than outcomes in the population without renal disease.[23]

Whether or not CABG is safe for patients undergoing long-term dialysis remains a great concern. Kan and Yang,[24] retrospectively reviewing all cases of elective or urgent isolated CABG performed from January 1, 1998, through March 31, 2003, at the National Cheng Kung University Hospital in Taiwan, identified 23 consecutive patients with dialysis-dependent renal disease, 22 undergoing hemodialysis, and 1 peritoneal dialysis. The mean duration of dialysis was 19.2 ± 22.5 months. These researchers chose 69 matched patients not receiving dialysis who underwent CABG in 2001 to serve as control group. Preoperative, operative, and postoperative data on these patients were compared. There were no significant differences between the two groups in preoperative factors, intubation time, intensive care unit stay, major complications, or 30-day mortality. However, uremic patients had a greater tendency to bleed, longer postoperative hospital stays, and more late deaths. Kan and Yang[24] concluded that with a well-prepared dialysis program and meticulous perioperative management, CABG can be performed in dialysis-dependent patients, with increased but acceptable perioperative morbidity and mortality risks. Nevertheless, management of the water-electrolyte balance in these patients remains an important issue. Through close cooperation between cardiac surgeons and nephrologists and the use of ultrafiltration, routine dialysis protocols were observed and surgery was integrated into the patient's routine schedule.

Witczak and coworkers[25] evaluated results of cardiovascular surgery in patients with CRF (serum creatinine >200 µmol/L or established dialysis) from 1990 to 2000 at Rikshospitalet University Hospital in Norway. One hundred and six patients with CRF underwent various cardiovascular procedures—56 coronary artery bypass operations, 25 valve replacements with or without coronary bypass, and 25 other major cardiovascular operations (8 thoracic aorta, 10 abdominal aorta, 7 other). Matched controls were selected (n = 106) on the basis of age, sex, year and type of operation, and occurrence of diabetes. The study group consisted of 88 men and 18 women with a mean age of 64 ± 10 years (standard deviation). Demographic features did not differ between CRF and control patients, except for hypertension, which was more prevalent in those with CRF. Rate of intraoperative hemorrhage, perfusion and ischemia time, and rate of reoperation did not differ between the groups. Patients with CRF received more transfusions of red blood cells, plasma, and platelets ($P < .02$). Ventilation support time, ICU stay, and hospital stay were significantly longer in patients with CRF. Early mortality rates were 16% for patients with CRF and 6.6% for the control group, and 5-year mortality rates were 79% and 39%, respectively. Independent preoperative risk factors of mortality were age greater than 70 years (relative risk [RR] = 2.32), chronic obstructive pulmonary disease (RR = 2.59), diabetes (RR = 1.80), and dialysis (RR = 2.03). Patients with CRF suffered more postoperative complications and had substantially higher short-term and long-term mortality rates.

Abdominal Surgery in Patients Undergoing Hemodialysis

Wind and associates[26] performed a 7-year retrospective study involving 43 patients undergoing long-term hemodialysis who had abdominal surgery in the Necker Hospital in Paris. The patients were separated into elective surgery and emergency surgery groups. In the elective surgery group (18 patients), the most common reasons for operation were colorectal cancer, symptomatic gallbladder stones, and hernia. There was no death related to surgery in this group, and only 1 patient had a complication (5%). In the emergency surgery group (25 patients), the most common reasons for operation were mesenteric ischemia and GI bleeding from angiodysplasia. Complications occurred in 10 patients (total morbidity rate, 40%), 6 of whom died (mortality rate, 24%). Elective GI surgery in patients undergoing long-term hemodialysis can therefore be performed with low morbidity and low mortality. The emergency surgery group was differentiated by the high prevalence of bleeding from angiodysplasia and mesenteric infarction as well as by the high surgical mortality rate.

Neurological Syndromes

A variety of disorders may cause acute neurological problems, such as headache, confusion, delirium, seizures, altered level of consciousness, and focal neurological deficits (e.g., hemiplegia).[27] Dialysis dysequilibrium is rare nowadays but may generally be encountered during or immediately after the initial few hemodialysis sessions. Stroke (ischemic or hemorrhagic) is common in patients undergoing dialysis, mainly owing to greater prevalence and severity of hypertension and cerebral atherosclerosis, heparinization during the procedure, and uremic platelet dysfunction in these patients.

For example, in the trial of atorvastatin in patients who had type 2 diabetes and were undergoing hemodialysis, 70 cerebrovascular events were noted in a total of 636 patients (11%) in the placebo group.[28] These events included fatal and nonfatal strokes, transient ischemic attacks, and prolonged reversible ischemic neurological deficits.

Subdural hematomas occur with greater frequency in patients with ESRD, probably owing to the hemostatic abnormalities previously mentioned. In addition to acute neurological symptoms, chronic dementia may result from subdural hematoma. A low threshold for neuroimaging is recommended in patients undergoing dialysis, because subdural hematoma can be effectively treated.[27]

Other etiologies of acute neurological syndromes in patients undergoing dialysis are hypertensive encephalopathy, uremia due to inadequate dialysis, hypercalcemia, various meningoencephalitides, hypoglycemia, hyponatremia or hypernatremia, hepatic or respiratory failure, and adverse effects of a variety of drugs (penicillins, cephalosporins, acyclovir, amantadine, and quinolones) with altered pharmacokinetics in ESRD (if the dose is not reduced appropriately).[27]

Cardiopulmonary Resuscitation in Patients with End-Stage Renal Disease

Acute myocardial infarction (AMI) is associated with poor long-term survival in patients undergoing dialysis, the 2-year survival rate of 25% remaining unchanged over the past two decades. Although underuse of appropriate therapies likely contributes to adverse outcomes, data also suggest that patients undergoing dialysis who have AMI are more likely to have clinical presentations atypical for acute coronary syndrome. The risks for cardiac arrest and in-hospital death after AMI are increased in patients undergoing dialysis compared with a cohort not requiring dialysis. The phenomenon of higher MI mortality in patients with CKD is not restricted to ESRD because there is a gradient of mortality risk related to decreased renal function. Sudden cardiac death is the single largest cause of mortality in patients undergoing dialysis. Such patients are vulnerable to sudden cardiac death, and myocardial ischemia likely plays a major role. Nevertheless, even after apparently successful percutaneous and surgical coronary revascularization, patients undergoing dialysis remain at high risk for sudden cardiac death after MI, implying that other factors in addition to myocardial ischemia are important.[29]

The information in the medical literature about outcomes of cardiopulmonary resuscitation in patients with renal failure is rather limited. Moss and coworkers[30] described their 8-year experience with CPR in patients undergoing dialysis at a university dialysis program. These investigators used a control group of patients without dialysis who were undergoing CPR during the same period in the same hospital. Of 221 patients undergoing dialysis, 74 (34%) had CPR compared with 247 (21%) of 1201 control patients (P = .0002). Six of 74 patients undergoing dialysis (8%; 95% CI, 2% to 14%) survived to hospital discharge, compared with 30 of 247 control patients (12%; 95% CI, 8% to 16%; difference not significant). At 6 months after CPR, 2 (3%) of the dialysis group were still alive, compared with 23 (9%) of the controls; this significant difference was not explained by age or comorbid conditions. Twenty-one (78%) of the 27 successfully resuscitated patients undergoing dialysis died a mean of 4.4 days after CPR; 95% were receiving mechanical ventilation in an ICU at the time of death. This study suggests that only 10% or even fewer of patients with renal failure, particularly those undergoing dialysis, needing CPR survive to hospital discharge. The quite pessimistic conclusion of this study was that CPR rarely results in extended survival for patients undergoing dialysis.

Karnik and associates[31] reported on 400 cardiac arrests on dialysis units. They compared the patients experiencing cardiac arrest with the nationally representative Fresenius Medical Care North America (FMCNA) cohort of patients undergoing dialysis. Older age, diabetes, and catheter use for vascular access were all risk factors for cardiac arrest in dialysis units. Age was not found to be a predictor of cardiac arrest in this series; indeed, it is not always reported as a factor for sudden death in patients undergoing dialysis.[32] In a study on CPR in dialysis units, Bleyer and colleagues[32] found a higher incidence of cardiac and sudden deaths on Mondays and Tuesdays in the United States Renal Data System (USRDS) cohort. They hypothesized that greater fluid overload as well as greater electrolyte and toxin fluctuations on the 3-day dialysis-free intervals contribute to an enhanced risk.

In a later study, Lafrance and associates[33] retrospectively reviewed all calls for CPR occurring in their dialysis unit between August 1997 and December 2004 and compared data with those in a control cohort of patients undergoing long-term hemodialysis. A total of 38 calls occurred over 307,553 sessions, corresponding to an incidence of 0.012%. Statistically significant predictors of a call for CPR were ischemic heart disease, heart failure, and female gender. Patients for whom a call for CPR was made had a lower dialysis vintage than control patients. Twenty of the 38 events presented on Mondays or Tuesdays; 78% occurred during hemodialysis, compared with 14% immediately after dialysis and 8% immediately before dialysis while patients were at the unit, respectively. Of the 38 events, 24 were true cardiopulmonary arrests. Cardiac causes were the most common (34%), and only 4 events were attributed to potassium disorders. One quarter of patients were dialyzed against a dialysate potassium concentration of 1 mmol/L or less. An arrhythmia was identified in 19 patients; a malignant ventricular fibrillation or ventricular

tachycardia was most commonly found (32%), followed by severe bradycardia (26%). For the whole group, there were 6 deaths (16%) within 48 hours; 30 patients (79%) were alive at 30 days and had been discharged from the hospital. Among the 24 patients with cardiopulmonary arrests, there were 4 deaths (17%) within 48 hours; 18 patients (75%) were alive at 30 days and had been discharged from the hospital. There was a trend for worse prognosis at 60 days for patients in whom true cardiopulmonary arrest had occurred.

This study confirms thus that alerts for cardiopulmonary arrest occur more frequently on Mondays and Tuesdays in a hemodialysis unit. Survival after such an alert appears to be better than in certain other circumstances, probably in part because of the presence of witnesses, physicians, and equipment, and the ready availability of vascular access. Thus it seems that over the last few years the prognosis of patients with ESRD who need CPR has improved considerably.

Sepsis

Patients undergoing dialysis are particularly susceptible to infection because the uremic internal milieu leads to impaired chemotaxis, reactive oxygen species production, and phagocytosis as well as to accelerated apoptosis of granulocytes.[34]

In a historical cohort study of 393,451 U.S. dialysis patients, Foley and colleagues[35] used discharge diagnosis codes from the International Classification of Disease, Ninth Revision, Clinical Modification (ICD 9 CM) to compare first-year septicemia admission rates in annual incident cohorts from 1991 to 1999 and to calculate subsequent cardiovascular event and mortality rates. Hemodialysis (compared with peritoneal dialysis) as initial therapy and starting dialysis in more recent years were the principal antecedents of septicemia. In hemodialysis patients, adjusted first admission rates (expressed as first episodes per 100 patient-years) rose by 51%, from 11.6 in 1991 to 17.5 in 1999. In patients undergoing peritoneal dialysis, rates were 5.7 in 1991, peaked at 9.2 in 1997, and declined to 8.0 in 1999. Mortality rates after septicemia were similar to those after major cardiovascular events. Septicemia was associated with developing myocardial infarction, congestive heart failure, stroke, and peripheral vascular disease, with adjusted risk ratios of 4.1, 5.5, 4.1, and 3.8, respectively in the first 6 months after admission for septicemia and 1.7, 2.0, 2.0, and 1.6, respectively, after 5 years.

Gastrointestinal Bleeding

It has been estimated that GI bleeding accounts for 3% to 7% of all deaths in patients with ESRD.[36] The reasons for this high incidence are not known. In particular, the role in the dialysis population of factors that raise the risk for GI bleeding in the general population—such as age, gender, alcohol use, smoking, ulcer disease, cardiovascular disease, immobilization, and intake of anti-inflammatory drugs—is unknown.[37] In addition, several dialysis-specific factors have been postulated to increase the risk of gastrointestinal bleeding, including heparin exposure, poor platelet function due to uremia,[38] mucosal abnormalities of the GI tract, and hypergastrinemia.[36,39,40]

Wasse and colleagues[37] analyzed data from the United States Renal Data System Dialysis Morbidity and Mortality Studies, Waves 2 through 4, to identify risk factors for incidence of upper GI bleeding among patients with ESRD. Over a total of 30,648 patient-years of follow-up, 698 cases of upper GI bleeding were observed. After adjustment for confounding factors, African-American race was associated with a lower risk of upper GI bleeding (RR = 0.90; CI 0.82, 0.98), and current smoking (RR = 1.11; CI 1.03, 1.19), history of CVD (RR = 1.32; CI 1.10, 1.59), and inability to ambulate independently (RR = 1.32; CI 1.07, 1.63) were associated with a higher risk. Age, gender, diabetes, lower serum albumin value, nutritional status, dialysis modality, and use of aspirin, nonsteroidal anti-inflammatory drugs, and antiplatelet or anticoagulant medications were not found to be significantly related to the risk for upper GI bleeding. Gastric ulcers were found to be the most common source of bleeding (7.0 per 1000 persons per year), and bleeding due to a gastrojejunal ulcer to be least common (0.1 per 1000 persons per year). Duration of hospital stays for patients diagnosed with upper GI bleeding ranged between 1 and 87 days, with a median of 5 days.

It should be noted that of the 93 patients with ESRD admitted to the ICU in an analysis from the Mayo Clinic, the main reasons for admission were GI bleeding (10 from the upper GI tract and 7 from the lower GI tract).[15] The researchers of this study did not investigate the underlying source of bleeding in these patients. Although the differential diagnosis of GI bleeding is diverse, erosive gastritis is more common, and the mortality rate is significantly higher in patients with ESRD than in the general population.[41] Whether the greater use of newer antiplatelet agents or changes in intradialytic anticoagulation regimens have had a bearing on these data remains speculative but intriguing. Whether preventive strategies can reduce the incidence of GI bleeding in patients with ESRD must be studied prospectively.

Key Points

1. Between 8% and 12% of a long-term hemodialysis population per year are estimated to need admission to an intensive care unit for treatment for intercurrent critical illness.

2. The most common causes of critical illness in patients undergoing long-term dialysis are acute complications of cardiovascular surgery, cardiac resuscitation, neurological syndromes, sepsis, and major gastrointestinal bleeding.

3. In particular, elective cardiovascular and abdominal surgery in patients undergoing dialysis is associated with low morbidity and mortality rates, but emergency surgery is associated with a high mortality rate.

4. Patients undergoing either long-term hemodialysis or peritoneal dialysis are prone to septicemia, which is often associated with major cardiovascular events such as myocardial infarction, congestive heart failure, stroke, and peripheral vascular disease.

5. It is very difficult to predict the outcome in the individual patient with ESRD undergoing long-term dialysis who has a critical illness, so such a patient should be offered the chance for intensive care treatment.

Key References

10. Lameire N, Van Biesen W, Vanholder R: The changing epidemiology of acute renal failure. Nature Clin Pract Nephrol 2006;2:364-377.
12. Clermont G, Acker CG, Angus DC, et al: Renal failure in the ICU: Comparison of the impact of acute renal failure and end-stage renal disease on ICU outcomes. Kidney Int 2002; 62:986-996.
14. Uchino S, Morimatsu H, Bellomo R, et al: End-stage renal failure patients requiring renal replacement therapy in the intensive care unit: incidence, clinical features, and outcome. Blood Purif 2003;21:170-175.
17. Manhes G, Heng AE, Aublet-Cuvelier B, et al: Clinical features and outcome of chronic dialysis patients admitted to an intensive care unit. Nephrol Dial Transplant 2005;20:1127-1133.
33. Lafrance JP, Nolin L, Senecal L, Leblanc M: Predictors and outcome of cardiopulmonary resuscitation (CPR) calls in a large haemodialysis unit over a seven-year period. Nephrol Dial Transplant 2006;21:1006-1012.

See the companion Expert Consult website for the complete reference list.

CHAPTER 19

Long-Term Outcomes of Acute Kidney Injury

Michael Joannidis, Nicola Schusterschitz, and Philipp G. H. Metnitz

---

OBJECTIVES

This chapter will:
1. Review the hospital mortality of acute kidney injury.
2. Describe the long-term outcome of patients discharged from hospital after acute kidney injury.
3. Discuss the factors influencing long-term outcome of acute kidney injury.
4. Consider the dependency on renal replacement therapy after acute kidney injury.
5. Review patient's quality of life after acute kidney injury.

Acute kidney injury (AKI) is an entity associated with significant morbidity and mortality. Consequently, the diagnosis of AKI has a significant effect on the patient's prognosis in the intensive care unit (ICU). However, for those patients who survive AKI, issues of major importance are questions such as whether they will be dependent on dialysis and whether they must face a higher risk of dying during the following years. This chapter focuses on these issues.

INTENSIVE CARE UNIT AND HOSPITAL MORTALITY RATES

On the basis of currently available data, the occurrence of acute renal failure is associated with an excess mortality rate compared with the rate predicted through the use of conventional ICU scores like the second Simplified Acute Physiology Score (SAPS-II) and the second or third Acute Physiology and Chronic Health Evaluation (APACHE-II or APACHE-III) score.[1-7] ICU mortality is reported as between 20% and 70%, and hospital mortality as slightly higher, between 25% and 80%.

There is an ongoing debate on whether excess mortality is already occurring in mild cases of AKI. Nash and coworkers[8] could establish a positive correlation between an increase in serum creatinine concentration (SCr) and mortality in their prospective study involving 4622 patients admitted consecutively to the medical and surgical services of an urban tertiary care hospital.[8] These findings are supported by a later study of patients undergoing cardiovascular surgery in whom a moderate rise in SCr (>0.5 mg/dL) was already associated with a more than 18-fold increase in 28-day mortality (i.e., 36%).[9] Further support of this hypothesis results from a recent U.S. study on 19,982 patients, in which a relative modest increase in SCr, between 0.3 and 0.4 mg/dL, was associated with a 70% higher risk of death.[10]

Nevertheless, the need for renal replacement therapy (RRT) appears to be a crucial factor with regard to prognosis. A study from the Program to Improve Care in Acute Renal Disease (PICARD) program in ICU patients demonstrated significantly lower mortality in patients with AKI who did not require dialysis than in patients who underwent RRT (24% vs. 45%, respectively).[11] Furthermore, patients who had acute renal failure classified as an increase in SCr[12] but did not require RRT had a hospital mortality of 31%, compared with 57% for those requiring dialysis. One of the largest trials, involving 17,126 patients admitted to 30 ICUs in Austria, showed a roughly fourfold higher mortality in patients with AKI requiring RRT than in patients with the same level of severity of illness as assessed by SAPS-II value (62.8% vs. 15.8%; $P < .01$) who did not require RRT.[13] Even after adjustments were made for age, severity of illness, and treatment center, AKI still conferred an about 1.7-fold higher mortality in comparison with matched controls without renal failure. Similar results were found in a study performed in the United States, in which ICU patients with AKI had an about 50% higher mortality than patients with preexistent end-stage renal disease despite comparable APACHE-III scores. Interestingly, ICU mortality rates for patients with end-stage renal disease were similar to those for patients without renal failure.[14] This finding demonstrates that death in acute renal failure is not just a matter of organ loss. This assumption is further undermined by the findings that AKI in the ICU is highly associated with the development of multiple-organ failure. A multicenter trial performed in 40 ICUs in 16 countries involving 1411 patients and using Sepsis-Related Organ Failure Assessment (SOFA) scores revealed that multiple-organ failure developed in about 70% of the patients with AKI but in only 10% of the patients without AKI.[15]

In some instances, the occurrence of AKI requiring RRT is associated with an extremely bad prognosis, as described for ICU patients with underlying liver cirrhosis[16] or hematological malignancy[17] and reported mortalities of 89% and 88%, respectively. Similarly, in a cross-sectional study of 420 patients admitted with cardiac arrest, renal failure after cardiopulmonary resuscitation was associated with a mortality of 93.7%.[18]

FACTORS PREDICTING SURVIVAL TO DISCHARGE FROM HOSPITAL

Very few studies have investigated the factors influencing outcome of AKI in a systematic and prospective manner. In a Canadian study,[19] 38% of the 87 patients with AKI requiring RRT survived to discharge. Absence of oliguria, a better premorbid renal function, and a shorter period of dependence on RRT were factors associated with better prognosis. In patients who survived to hospital discharge, independence from RRT could be achieved in more than 90%. An Australian study involving 299 patients with AKI in an ICU setting showed a mortality rate of roughly 47%. Survival was associated with lower age, absence of mechanical ventilation, and less need for vasoactive drugs. Only about 16% of patients discharged from the hospital needed further dialysis treatment.[20] Similar mortality rates (49%) were obtained from another Australian multicenter trial performed in 116 IUC patients with AKI requiring RRT. Only 19% of the surviving patients needed dialysis after discharge from the hospital.[21]

The choice of initial technique of RRT and its possible impact on survival remain a constant matter of debate. A prospective multinational study analyzed data of 1218 patients and compared outcome of AKI in patients treated with continuous RRT (CRRT) and patients treated with intermittent RRT.[22] In 80% of the patients, CRRT was the initial treatment form chosen; these patients presented with higher SAPS-II values and lower mean blood pressures, required higher doses of vasoactive drugs, and had higher rates of mechanical ventilation than those patients treated with intermittent RRT. Not surprisingly, mortality in patients receiving CRRT was higher, but after data were adjusted for illness severity, no difference in survival was found. This finding corresponds to those from several larger prospective randomized trials, which were unable to prove a significant survival benefit for CCRT over intermittent RRT.[23-25]

LONG-TERM PROGNOSIS

Although in-hospital survival of critically ill patients with AKI is poor, long-term prognosis for those patients who survive is not bad (Table 19-1). Mortality rate after hospital discharge increases only slightly, and renal function recovers in the majority of the cases. The number of studies investigating long-term outcome after AKI, however, is relatively low. A German study involving 979 ICU patients treated with CRRT found that although only 31% of the patients survived to hospital discharge; the probability to survive the first 6 months after discharge was 77%.[26] In patients who survived this period, the probability to survive the next 6 months was 89%. Five year survival probability, however, did not surpass 50%. Etiology of AKI had no impact on long-term survival probability, whereas age and comorbidity before hospitalization were associated with worse outcome. Patients with sepsis had the greatest in-hospital mortality (75%) and required RRT significantly longer than patients without sepsis; interestingly, patients with sepsis showed a tendency toward better long-term outcome. Fifty-nine percent of the surviving patients regained normal renal function. Of the remaining 41% with residual renal impairment, only 10% required long-term dialysis. Seventy-seven percent of the surviving patients reported good-to-excellent health status.

Bagshaw and associates[27] investigated the epidemiology and long-term outcomes of 240 patients with AKI requiring RRT. ICU and hospital mortality rates in these patients were 50% and 60%, respectively. Of the surviving patients, 38% were independent of RRT at discharge from the ICU, and 68% at the time of hospital discharge. There was only a minor increase in mortality after 1 year, from 60% to 64%, whereas 28% of the patients were alive and inde-

pendent of RRT. Factors independently associated with 1-year mortality were preexisting comorbidities, liver disease, need for continuous RRT, septic shock, older age, and a higher APACHE-II score at ICU admission. Schiffl[28] reported a similar 1-year survival rate, roughly 35%, in patients who had AKI treated with RRT.

A Finnish study investigating 703 patients with acute renal failure receiving RRT reported a mortality rate of 41% at 28 days, 57% at 1 year, and 70% at 5 years.[29] There was a significant difference in 1-year mortality between patients treated in the ICU (57%) and patients treated on hospital wards (47%). Independent predictors for the 1-year mortality were SOFA score, age, and need for continuous RRT. Korkeila and associates[30] found mortality rates in 62 patients with AKI that was treated with RRT to be 45% at hospital discharge, 55% at 6 months, and 65% at 5 years. Renal function was restored in 82% of the survivors. Three days after start of RRT, oliguria had been present in 82% of the nonsurvivors but in only 43% of the surviving patients, implying that oliguria is a risk factor for bad outcome. Eighty percent of the patients who died within 6 months had multiple-organ dysfunctions at the time RRT was initiated.

Three studies also investigated the effect of moderate renal functional impairment on long-term prognosis. In the setting of cardiac surgery, perioperative or postoperative deterioration in renal function, characterized by an increase in SCr of at least 25%, carried a significant risk of higher mortality over an observation period of 8 years—that is, a hazard risk of 1.83 in comparison with the patient group who did not show perioperative deterioration in renal function.[31] A study by Bagshaw and associates[32] analyzed 1-year mortality in critically ill patients according to severity of kidney dysfunction at ICU admission in a cohort of 5693 patients. Kidney function was stratified as no renal failure (SCr < 1.7 mg/dL), mild renal dysfunction (SCr 1.7-3.4 mg/dL), moderate renal dysfunction (SCr ≥ 3.4 mg/dL), severe renal failure (requirement for RRT), and end-stage renal disease requiring long-term RRT before ICU admission. Hospital mortality rates were 13%, 40%, 41%, 60%, and 34%, respectively, for the kidney function groups. Although AKI requiring RRT was associated with a significantly higher hospital mortality, 1-year survival rates for patients discharged from hospital were comparable for all groups: 89% in patients with mild renal dysfunction, 87% in those with moderate renal dysfunction, and 90% in those with either severe AKI requiring RRT or end-stage renal disease. Similar findings were reported by Lins and coworkers,[33] who showed that there was no difference in 1-year survival after hospital discharge between patients who had AKI treated with RRT and those who did not.

RECOVERY OF RENAL FUNCTION

All of the preceding studies show that the majority of the patients who survive AKI can be discharged from hospital and remain independent from further RRT (see Table 19-1). In the two Australian studies, less than 20% of the patients required further renal support after hospital discharge, most of whom (80%) had a history of chronic renal impairment.[20,21] Bagshaw and associates[27,32] reported independence from RRT 1 year after diagnosis of AKI in 78% of the surviving patients in their series. Renal recovery appeared to peak by 90 days, with the number of patients requiring RRT being more or less the same at 1 year. The

TABLE 19-1

Studies of Long-Term Outcome of Acute Kidney Injury Treated with Renal Replacement Therapy (RRT)

STUDY	PATIENTS (N)	HOSPITAL SURVIVAL (%)	28-DAY SURVIVAL (%)	90-DAY SURVIVAL (%)	INDEPENDENCE FROM RRT AT HOSPITAL DISCHARGE (% OF SURVIVORS)	6-MONTH SURVIVAL (%)	1-YEAR SURVIVAL (%)	5-YEAR SURVIVAL (%)
Wald et al (2006)[19]	87	38	—	—	90	—	—	—
Silvester et al (2001)[20]	299	53	—	—	84	—	—	—
Cole et al (2000)[21]	116	51	—	—	81	—	—	—
Morgera et al (2002)[26]	979	31	—	—	90	24	21	15
Bagshaw et al (2005)[27]	240	40	49	40	68	—	36	—
Ahlstrom et al (2005)[29]	703	—	59	—	95	—	43	30
Lins et al (2006)[33]	293	—	49	—	—	—	90	—
Schiffl (2006)[28]	443	53	—	—	90	—	35	—
Korkeila et al (2000)[30]	62	55	—	—	82	45	—	35

majority of patients remaining dependent on RRT were found to have suffered from preexisting chronic renal dysfunction. Analysis of the data on renal function at 90 days showed that a diagnosis of sepsis and septic shock, lower SCr and blood urea level prior to RRT, male sex, and fewer comorbidities were independently associated with renal recovery. Patients with cardiac disease, diabetes mellitus, peripheral vascular disease, and chronic kidney disease were less likely to regain renal function. No impact on renal recovery was found for type of admission, severity of illness, need for mechanical ventilation and vasopressor therapy, oliguria, or exposure to nephrotoxins. One study investigated patients who did not regain renal function after AKI, which was the case for 16% of the surviving patients.[34] When data were analyzed according to cause of AKI, these researchers found a 3% to 41% rate of dialysis dependency, with the highest rates occurring in AKI due to parenchymal disease. Only one study reports a recurrence of need for RRT, in a single patient (<1%), who had had incomplete recovery of renal function at hospital discharge.[28]

Because the choice of technique of RRT remains controversial, several studies investigated the effect of RRT modality on renal recovery. Although mortality in patients treated with CRRT tends to be higher owing to the feasibility of performing this modality also in unstable and more severely ill patients, initial CRRT was found to be associated with significantly higher rates of renal recovery in surviving patients than in patients treated with intermittent hemodialysis (92% in CRRT vs. 59% in intermittent hemodialysis).[23] This finding is supported by results obtained from the study reported by Uchino and colleagues,[35] who demonstrated that CRRT as initial treatment predicted renal recovery in surviving patients. This finding suggests that hypotension, which was more frequently observed during intermittent hemodialysis in this study, might contribute to the persistence of renal dysfunction and subsequent higher rate of dependence on RRT in patients treated with intermittent hemodialysis.

QUALITY OF LIFE

In addition to survival and dialysis dependency, quality of life (QOL) is of major importance to patients with AKI.

Korkeila and associates[30] tried to evaluate QOL by sending questionnaires to patients who had survived AKI at 6 months after their ICU admission. The majority reported an acceptable QOL as assessed by the Nottingham Health Profile (NHP). The most common complaints were loss of energy and a limited physical mobility. Most of the patients were able to manage everyday life on their own, with 36% being dependent on external help. Another Finnish study[29] evaluated QOL with the Euro QOL (EQ-5d) instrument, which included a visual analogue scale (VAS) score to assess the patient's perceived health. Although survivors had a lower health-related QOL than an age- and gender-matched general population, patients themselves were as satisfied with their health as the general population.

Gopal and coworkers[36] reported that survivors of combined multiple-organ failure and AKI treated with RRT have a relatively good state of health and an acceptable QOL. The majority of the patients in their study responded that they would undergo the same treatment again, if necessary. Maynard and colleagues[37] used the Medical Outcomes Study Short Form-36 Health Survey (SF-36) to evaluate health-related QOL at 6 months after hospital discharge in 12 patients treated with RRT. Although health status was not perceived to be very good, health-related QOL was reported as fairly satisfying. No correlation was found between SF-36 score and APACHE-III score at ICU admission, indicating that severity of illness does not predict QOL in survivors; this finding corresponds to those of other studies.[38,39]

CONCLUSIONS

Although patients with AKI have very high ICU and hospital mortality rates, those who survive to hospital discharge have a good long-term prognosis. Most of the patients regain renal function along with an acceptable health status. The patients who continue to receive dialysis frequently had a history of chronic renal disease before the ICU admission for AKI. The majority of patients who have survived AKI are capable of managing everyday life without external help, and their perception of quality of life is comparable to that of the age- and gender-matched general population.

Key Points

1. In patients with acute kidney injury severe enough to warrant renal replacement therapy, the rate of hospital survival is 38% to 55%, the 1-year survival is 21% to 48%, and the 5-year survival is 15% to 35%.
2. Eighty percent to 90% of surviving patients do not require further renal replacement therapy.
3. Most patients who survive acute kidney injury report a satisfying quality of life.

Key References

26. Morgera S, Kraft AK, Siebert G, et al: Long-term outcomes in acute renal failure patients treated with continuous renal replacement therapies. Am J Kidney Dis 2002;40:275-279.
29. Ahlstrom A, Tallgren M, Peltonen S, et al: Survival and quality of life of patients requiring acute renal replacement therapy. Intensive Care Med 2005;31:1222-1228.
30. Korkeila M, Ruokonen E, Takala J: Costs of care, long-term prognosis and quality of life in patients requiring renal replacement therapy during intensive care. Intensive Care Med 2000;26:1824-1831.
33. Lins RL, Elseviers MM, Daelemans R: Severity scoring and mortality 1 year after acute renal failure. Nephrol Dial Transplant 2006;21:1066-1068.
37. Maynard SE, Whittle J, Chelluri L, Arnold R: Quality of life and dialysis decisions in critically ill patients with acute renal failure. Intensive Care Med 2003;29:1589-1593.

See the companion Expert Consult website for the complete reference list.

SECTION 3

Principles of Applied Renal Physiology

CHAPTER 20

Glomerular Filtration Rate and Renal Functional Reserve

Claudio Ronco, John A. Kellum, and Rinaldo Bellomo

OBJECTIVES

This chapter will:
1. Describe the process of glomerular filtration.
2. Characterize the mechanisms involved in glomerular filtration.
3. Discuss the methods of measurement for baseline and estimated glomerular filtration rate and for renal functional reserve.
4. Summarize the pathophysiological changes of glomerular filtration rate that occur in acute kidney injury.

Glomerular filtration rate (GFR) is usually accepted as the best overall index of kidney function in health and disease. Normal GFR varies with age, sex, and body size. It is approximately 120 to 130 mL/min/1.73 m^2 in young adults and declines with age.[1] A decrease in GFR precedes the onset of clinical kidney failure; therefore, a persistently reduced GFR is a specific indication of chronic kidney disease (CKD), whereas an abrupt reduction of GFR that is possibly transient in nature may be used to describe acute kidney injury (AKI). With a GFR less than 60 mL/min/1.73 m^2, the prevalence of complications and the risk of cardiovascular disease seem to be higher in both CKD and AKI.[2-4]

The physiological mechanism of glomerular filtration is generally clearly understood. A more complex issue, however, is the measurement of GFR in clinical practice and especially the definition of "normal" renal function. In fact, one cannot define *renal function* solely from GFR, because the convective transport of solutes in Bowman's space is just one of the many functions of the kidney. Furthermore, the measurement of GFR or its calculation from derived equations can be complex and faulty. Finally, GFR may not be a fixed function but, rather, may display significant variations among individuals or even at different times within one individual. All of these aspects have an important impact on the diagnosis and staging of CKD,

but they are similarly important in the evaluation of kidney function in patients in intensive care units (ICUs) with or without AKI. In this chapter, we try to elucidate some of the aspects related to GFR in the clinical setting.

THE MECHANISM OF GLOMERULAR FILTRATION

The process of glomerular filtration[1] is a typical model for transcapillary ultrafiltration. *Ultrafiltration* is a process whereby plasma water, which contains solutes and crystalloids but not cells or colloids, is separated from whole blood by means of a pressure gradient through a semipermeable membrane. The pressures involved in the process are typical Starling forces—that is, hydrostatic and colloid osmotic (oncotic) pressures.

The filtration gradient results from the net balance between the transcapillary hydraulic pressure gradient (ΔP) and the transcapillary colloid osmotic pressure gradient ($\Delta \pi$). Such pressure, multiplied by the hydraulic permeability of the filtration barrier (K), determines the rate of fluid movement (ultrafiltration = J_w) across the capillary wall, as follows:

$$J_w = K(\Delta P - \Delta \pi)$$

Obviously, J_w results from the sum of different local fluid movements along the length of the capillary, and thus, the equation describes an average phenomenon.

The product of the surface area for filtration (S) and average values along the length of the glomerular capillary determines the single-nephron glomerular filtration rate (SNGFR), as follows:

$$\text{SNGFR} = KS\ (\Delta P - \Delta \pi) = K_f P_{uf}$$

where K_f is the glomerular ultrafiltration coefficient and P_{uf} is the mean net ultrafiltration pressure.

The barrier for ultrafiltration is complex, consisting of the glomerular capillary endothelium with its fenestra-

111

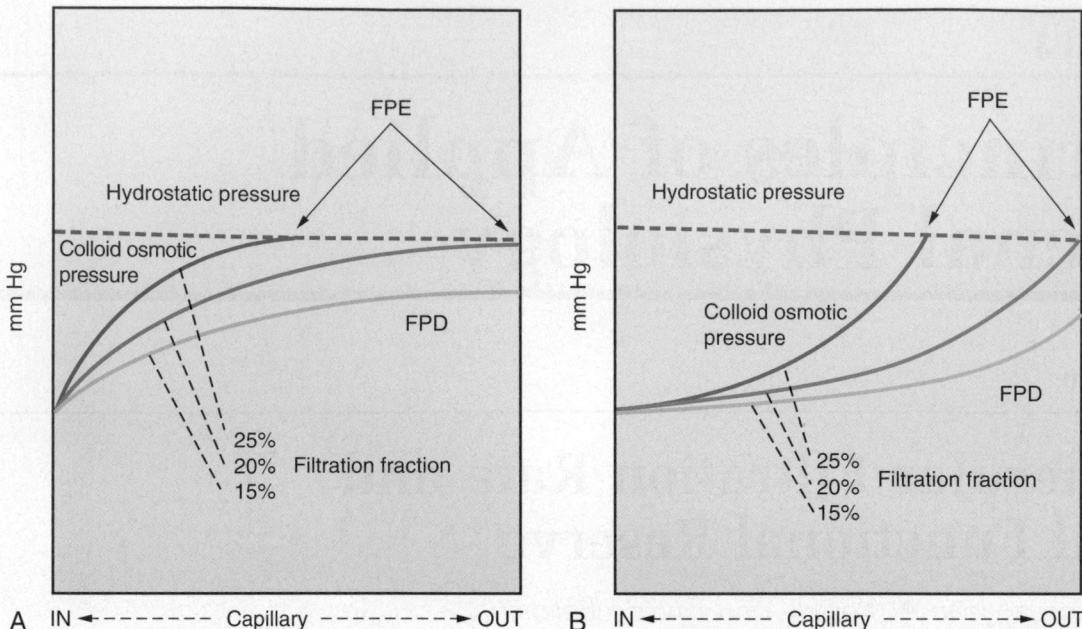

FIGURE 20-1. The concept of filtration pressure equilibrium (FPE) in the glomerular capillary. As blood moves through the capillary, water is removed from blood by ultrafiltration. The resulting progressive increase in protein concentration is paralleled by a rise in colloid osmotic pressure. Two possible profiles of colloid osmotic pressure have been hypothesized, one in which the increase is steep in the proximal part of the capillary, reaching a plateau in the distal part **(A)**, and another in which the increase is slow in the proximal part, becoming exponential in the distal part **(B)**. There is no agreement as to which profile more accurately reflects the real phenomenon. Independent of the profile, colloid osmotic pressure rises until it equals the hydraulic pressure inside the capillary, and filtration ceases. The point of FPE moves along the length of the capillary in response to different blood flows. While FPE is maintained, filtration fraction is fairly constant. When FPE is lost (FP dysequilibrium [FPD]), the filtration fraction changes. These findings relate mostly to the patient's hydration status and to the flow autoregulation mechanism.

tions, the glomerular basement membrane, and the filtration slits between the glomerular epithelial cell foot processes. Anatomic alterations in various components of the glomerular filtration barrier play a crucial role in determining glomerular hydraulic conductivity and, hence, glomerular filtration in disease states.

The surface of a single glomerular loop is difficult to assess because of the variable number of capillaries, the varying proportion of capillaries that are perfused, and the extent of stretching of the capillaries.

For the same reason, the permeability coefficient is difficult to determine, but calculations can be made with specific techniques in selected experimental animals for single nephrons. The glomerular ultrafiltration coefficient is reduced in a variety of kidney diseases. Experimental glomerulonephritis, acute renal failure (ARF), chronic ureteral obstruction, puromycin aminonucleoside–induced nephrosis, and chronic protein malnutrition can all affect K_f. In addition, the hydraulic permeability of the glomerular basement membrane is inversely related to ΔP, suggesting that K_f may be directly affected by ΔP. The hydraulic conductivity of the glomerular basement membrane and K_f are also affected by the plasma protein concentration.

The behavior of the pressure in the glomerular capillary is interesting, and it has been considered similar to the behavior that can be experimentally determined in artificial hollow fibers of hemofilters. As blood moves through the capillary, water is removed by ultrafiltration. This results in a progressive decrease of hydraulic pressure in the blood compartment with a parallel increase in the counterpressure generated by the progressive increase in plasma proteins. Different profiles can be postulated for

the colloid osmotic pressure (Fig. 20-1), but it has been demonstrated that in fluid-depleted animals, filtration pressure equilibrium (FPE) occurs along the length of the capillary.[1] This means that hydrostatic and colloido-osmotic pressures equalize at a given point and filtration stops before the end of the capillary. Progressive expansion of the extracellular fluid volume (or progressive increase in extracorporeal blood flow in artificial fibers) results in a progressive shift of the FPE points toward the end of the capillary until such equilibrium does not occur any more.

Changes in GFR and *filtration fraction* (the ratio between the GFR and the plasma flow rate) as a function of selective alterations in plasma flow, hydrostatic pressure, or oncotic pressure at the inlet of the capillary can be predicted by a mathematical model consisting of a system of identical capillaries in parallel (homogeneous model). Such an approach obtained relatively good correlation with experimental data in animals.[1] The anatomy of the glomerular capillary network is far more complex, however, with capillary loops varying in length. Even when the data suggest that the overall network is at filtration pressure dysequilibrium, FPE may be achieved in some parts of the capillary network. Using a mathematical model based on a capillary network reconstructed from serial sections of the glomerulus (network model), it was found that calculated values of K_f from the homogeneous model were somewhat lower than those obtained from the network model.[1] This discrepancy became greater as FPE was approached. Therefore, it is evident that the permeability coefficient of the glomerular membrane can be studied only in conditions in which FPE does not occur. In these conditions, in fact, the entire surface of the capillary is not used for filtration, and the real effective surface used for filtration cannot be determined.

Different points of FPE along the length of the capillary correspond to different levels of filtration fraction and have significant effects on the proximal and distal tubular physiological response. At the same time, it becomes clear that all conditions altering blood flow to the capillary (ischemia, sepsis, cardiac dysfunction) can be tolerated only while renal blood flow autoregulation is intact. When autoregulation is lost or the delicate equilibrium between afferent and efferent arteriolar tone is altered, both blood flow and filtration fraction are altered, as are the intraglomerular hemodynamics and the process of ultrafiltration. This issue is especially important if we consider that most of the preglomerular pressure drop between the arcuate artery and the glomerulus occurs along the afferent arteriole, whereas approximately 70% of the hydraulic pressure drop between the glomerular capillaries and the renal vein takes place along the efferent arterioles. Thus, these two anatomic sites are important determinants of the intraglomerular hemodynamics.

Another important concept to underline is tubular-glomerular feedback. The macula densa region of the nephron is a specialized segment of the nephron lying between the end of the thick ascending limb of the loop of Henle and the early distal convoluted tubule. It runs between the angle formed by the afferent arteriole and the efferent arteriole, adjacent to the glomerulus of the same nephron. This anatomic arrangement, the juxtaglomerular apparatus, is ideally suited for a feedback system whereby a stimulus received at the macula densa might be transmitted to the arterioles of the same nephron to alter GFR. Changes in the delivery and composition of the fluid flowing past the macula densa have now been shown to elicit rapid changes in glomerular filtration of the same nephron, with increases in the delivery of fluid out of the proximal tubule resulting in reductions in filtration rate of the same nephron. This process is called *tubular-glomerular feedback*. Agents that interfere with sodium chloride transport in the macula densa cells inhibit the feedback response and consequently alter the physiological regulation of GFR.

Another important mechanism is the neural regulation of GFR. The renal vasculature—the afferent and efferent arterioles, the macula densa cells of the distal tubule, and the glomerular mesangium—are richly innervated. Innervation is supplied by renal efferent sympathetic adrenergic nerves and renal afferent sensory fibers. Neurological stimuli may contribute to the alteration of vascular tone and tubular-glomerular feedback as well as vasoconstriction mediated by renin secretion.

A variety of hormonal and vasoactive substances influence glomerular ultrafiltration, modifying the tone in the arcuate arteries, interlobular arteries, and afferent and efferent arterioles. Vasoconstricting or vasodilating substances thereby regulate the tone of preglomerular and postglomerular resistance vessels to control renal blood flow (RBF) as well as glomerular capillary hydraulic pressure and the glomerular transcapillary hydraulic pressure gradient. Glomerular filtration can also be regulated by mesangial cell activity (production of a substance or proliferation and contraction) and by glomerular epithelial cells (podocytes). The renal vasculature and glomerular mesangium respond to a number of endogenous hormones and vasoactive peptides through vasoconstriction and reductions in the glomerular ultrafiltration coefficient. Among these compounds are angiotensin II, norepineph-

rine, leukotrienes C_4 and D_4, platelet-activating factor (PAF), adenosine triphosphate (ATP), endothelin, vasopressin, serotonin, and epidermal growth factor.

A special mention should be made of norepinephrine, because its use in the critically ill patient with septic shock and AKI is often questioned but is necessary. Norepinephrine is a potent vasoconstrictor that promptly increases arterial blood pressure when administered systemically. In the kidney, norepinephrine induces vasoconstriction of the preglomerular vessels and efferent arteriole, theoretically decreasing blood flow. A rise in intraglomerular pressure, however, prevents a flow-induced decrease in GFR and frequently preserves diuresis in septic patients.

Among vasodilator substances, nitric oxide influences glomerular filtration. Endothelial cells of both arteries and veins release an endothelium-derived relaxing factor (EDRF) that is either nitric oxide or an unstable nitroso-compound that yields nitric oxide. EDRF formation in the vascular endothelium is stimulated by an excess of vasoconstricting agents. EDRF plays a major role in modulating renal hemodynamics and systemic blood pressure, and it is also involved in the mechanism of hyperfiltration in some conditions, such as diabetes. Other vasodilators are prostaglandins: The vasodilator prostaglandins PGE_1 and PGE_2 and prostacyclin generally increase RPF, but not necessarily GFR because they may not affect intraglomerular pressure.

Histamine, a potent vasodilator of the renal circulation, promotes large increases in RPF and RBF mediated by histamine H_2 receptors. This substance activates adenylate cyclase, increasing cellular concentrations of the vasodilator cyclic adenosine monophosphate (cAMP). Despite this, histamine does not substantially alter GFR. Bradykinin, another potent renal vasodilator, produces large increases in renal and glomerular blood flow mediated through the bradykinin B_2 receptor. Much like PGE_2 and prostacyclin, however, bradykinin does not substantially increase GFR. Acetylcholine raises urinary excretion of cyclic guanosine monophosphate (cGMP), and the renal and systemic vasodilation induced by acetylcholine is now thought to be mediated to a large extent through the stimulation of EDRF production. Acetylcholine also does not significantly alter GFR. Insulin and glucocorticoids also increase renal blood flow and possibly GFR. The effect seems to be EDRF mediated. Other vasodilating factors are insulin-like growth factor, calcitonin-gene related peptide, and cyclic adenosine monophosphate. Finally, another series of hormones seen to affect GFR are parathyroid hormone (PTH), PTH-related protein, natriuretic peptides, adenosine, and adrenomedullin.

MEASUREMENT OF GLOMERULAR FILTRATION RATE

It is well known that we use "clearance" as a tool to estimate GFR. Why? Human beings were not created equal. Teleologically speaking, however, human organ function is designed to maintain life parameters as close as possible to normal. Kidneys are not an exception to this rule. They might be bigger or smaller but they are designed to maintain the internal milieu, as Claude Bernard suggested. A simple measure of solute concentration in blood or of solute excretion or urine output cannot describe the real "function" of the organ. It takes an integration of all these parameters, appropriately combined, to enable a simple computation of "clearance."[5,6] Thus, clearance is a tool for comparing renal function among different individuals independently (at least in great part) of urine flow, body size, and solute concentration in blood. Of course, along the nephron, the fluid filtrated by the glomerulus is manipulated, varying its final composition. Therefore, for the computation of clearance as a surrogate of GFR, we need a molecule with ideal features: full filtration by the glomerular membrane (sieving = 1), absence of reabsorption or secretion in the tubular part of the nephron, and ease of measurement; and if we use an exogenous substance, it must be nontoxic for the organism.[7]

In 2006, Stevens and colleagues[8] reported that measuring GFR with the ideal exogenous marker molecules is expensive and complex and that it leads to a 5% to 20% error in various daily measurements. On the other end, the measurement of clearance with endogenous filtration markers such as creatinine is cheaper but also subject to errors, especially when timed or 24-hour urine collection is involved. In a steady state condition, the serum level of an endogenous marker is correlated with the reciprocal of the level of GFR, making it possible to estimate GFR without urine collection.[9,10] For creatinine, however, variations in the amounts of tubular secretion, altered extrarenal elimination, and variable generation rates make the use of a single reference range for serum creatinine value inadequate to distinguish between normal and abnormal GFR.[11] Other researchers have proposed cystatin C as a better filtration marker than creatinine, but this suggestion is still controversial, and no definitive statements can be made.[12,13] Certainly it would be useful to have a direct measure of the concentration of the marker molecule in the filtrate. Indeed, this is exactly what can be done in some forms of renal replacement therapy, such as hemofiltration, in which clearance can be quantitated precisely. This measurement, unfortunately, can be used only to compare efficiency of different treatments in a given moment, not as a tool to establish the effect of treatment on the patient. The reason is that extracorporeal clearance cannot be compared with a GFR unless the treatment is continuous, as in continuous venovenous hemofiltration (CVVH) or continuous ambulatory peritoneal dialysis (CAPD). In all other techniques, serum levels are far from being in steady state conditions, and similar clearances lead to different mass removal rates.

The National Kidney Disease Education Program (NKDEP) of the National Institute of Diabetes and Diseases of the Kidney (NIDDK), the National Kidney Foundation (NKF), and the American Society of Nephrology (ASN) recommend estimation of GFR (eGFR) from serum creatinine using the Modification of Diet in Renal Disease (MDRD) Study equation.[2,14-16] This equation uses the serum creatinine value in combination with age, sex, and race to estimate GFR, and thereby avoids several of the limitations to the use of the serum creatinine value alone.[16] The MDRD Study equation, which has been rigorously developed and validated, is more accurate than measured creatinine clearance from 24-hour urine collections.[15,16]

The equation is as follows:

$$GFR = 186 \times (P_{Cr})^{-1.154} \times (age)^{-0.203} \times (0.742 \text{ if female}) \times (1.210 \text{ if black})$$

where GFR is expressed in mL/min/1.73 m², P_{cr} is serum creatinine expressed in mg/dL, and age is expressed in years. The four-variable equation has an R^2 value of 89.2%; 91% and 98% of the estimated values in the MDRD Study fell within 30% and 50% of measured values, respectively.

Thus, GFR can be estimated using different equations that take account of race, gender, age, and body size.

The MDRD Study equation, derived from the study carried out in 1999,[15] was reasonably accurate and probably more precise than the previous Cockcroft-Gault equation developed in 1973[10] for patients with CKD. Both equations, however, have been reported to be less accurate in patients without CKD.[8,17] In several conditions, eGFR from the MDRD Study equation can be significantly lower than direct measurements of renal clearance, potentially leading to a false-positive diagnosis of chronic renal disease (eGFR < 60 mL/min/1.73 m²) with important consequences.[17] This phenomenon has been more evident in Europe than in the United States, and a possible explanation is different calibrations of serum creatinine assays among laboratories.[18]

The MDRD Study equation was validated in a group of patients with CKD (mean GFR 40 mL/min/1.73 m²) who were predominantly white and did not have diabetic kidney disease or kidney transplants.[15] This equation has now been validated in diabetic kidney disease, kidney transplant recipients, and African Americans with nondiabetic kidney disease.[19,20] It has not been validated, however, in children (age < 18 years), pregnant women, elderly patients (age > 70 years), racial or ethnic subgroups other than white and African American, individuals with normal kidney function who are at increased risk for CKD, or normal individuals. Furthermore, any of the limitations of the use of serum creatinine, as related to nutritional status or medication use, are not accounted for in the MDRD Study equation.[8,15,16] Despite these limitations, GFR estimates using this equation are more accurate than serum creatinine alone. Understanding these limitations should help clinicians interpret GFR estimates. If more accurate estimation of GFR is needed, one should obtain a clearance measurement (e.g., creatinine, iothalamate, iohexol, inulin).

At this time, two important points must be clarified. First, we know from different studies that even minimal reductions in GFR may result in an increased risk of death, cardiovascular disease, and hospitalization.[21,22] The evaluation and management of such complications definitely pertains to the nephrologist, who is well aware of the full spectrum of problems in these circumstances. An early referral to a nephrologist may result in better management of CKD and its complications but also may have a significant impact on the administration of appropriate medications and, ultimately, on the progression of the nephropathy. For these reasons, monitoring GFR and identifying an early reduction in GFR may become quintessential in the prevention of kidney and cardiovascular disease. The effect on health care systems and providers, together with the benefits for the entire population, is clearly evident. Second, on the basis of potential GFR underestimation from inaccurate serum creatinine measurements (or, better, calibrations), we might be facing a "false epidemic" of mild CKD with a tremendous overload of nephrological centers through a series of referrals made by general practitioners according to nephrologists' suggestions and guidelines. What should we then do? We know that GFR estimates can be inaccurate under some circumstances, such as dietary disorders, altered muscle mass, exercise, and laboratory calibration changes. Such inaccuracies may have a little impact on a subject with overt renal dysfunction but might be crucial in subjects with GFR estimates between 60 and 90 mL/min/1.73 m². In these latter cases, exogenous marker clearance may be the solution or at least may represent an important auxiliary tool.[7]

GFR declines with aging. Although the age-related decline in GFR has been considered part of normal aging, decreased GFR in the elderly is an independent predictor of adverse outcomes such as death and cardiovascular disease.[22] In addition, decreased GFR in the elderly requires adjustment in drug dosages, as in other patients with CKD. Generally, drug dosing is based on GFR levels that are not adjusted for body surface area (BSA). In practice, adjusted GFR estimates are adequate except in patients whose body size differs considerably from average. In these patients, unadjusted estimated GFR can be computed by the following formulas:

$$\text{GFR [estimate (mL/min)]} = \text{GFR estimate} \\ (\text{mL/min/1.73 m}^2) \times \text{BSA}$$

$$\text{BSA} = W^{0.425} \times H^{0.725} \times 0.007184/1.73 \text{ m}^2$$

where W is weight and H is height. All of these issues must be considered once GFR is evaluated in the critically ill patient in whom a preexisting GFR decline could have been present, in whom hormonal and nutritional disorders are present, or who is receiving significant pharmacological support, with the enormous potential of physiological interactions.

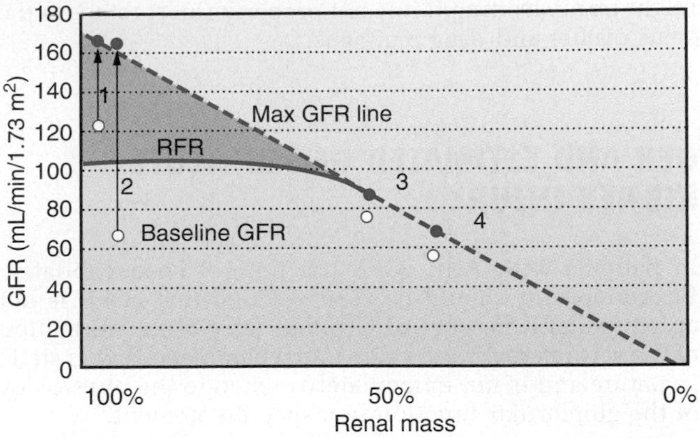

RENAL FUNCTIONAL RESERVE

In all this discussion, we have taken for granted a series of aspects that deserve a more detailed analysis. Is clearance of an appropriate molecule a good measure of GFR and therefore of kidney function? If so, can we define a "normal" kidney function from GFR under normal circumstances? Or, even better, is a normal GFR a sign of normal kidney function?

We know that so-called normal values are related to age, sex, and body size and that they are identified as 130 mL/min/1.73 m² in men and 120 mL/min/1.73 m² in women. But can we really give a number for normal GFR in a single measurement? Above all, can we extrapolate the presence of normal kidney condition from a normal GFR?

GFR is not a fixed parameter in subjects with normal renal function. Because several factors may affect the regulation of the afferent and efferent arteries and, thus, filtration fraction, GFR may vary even in the presence of a normal glomerulus and a normal kidney.

Experiments performed on normal subjects in 1983[23] demonstrated that there is a baseline GFR, the value of which (in the absence of disease) depends on several factors, including circulating prostaglandins and other vasoactive substances and, ultimately, at steady state, the level of protein intake. Subjects consuming vegetarian diets have GFR values as low as 45 to 50 mL/min, whereas subjects with high intake of animal protein may have GFR values as high as 140 to 150 mL/min/1.73 m².[24]

In all subjects, baseline GFR can be increased by an exogenous stimulus that causes a constriction in the efferent artery or a vasodilation in the afferent artery. This effect is exactly the opposite of the one observed when angiotensin-converting enzyme (ACE) inhibitors are administered to a subject who is in a condition of hyperfiltration. In this latter circumstance, the already vasoconstricted efferent artery is dilated by the ACE inhibitor, filtration fraction ceases, and the GFR falls.[25]

The maximal value of GFR is not clear, but it can certainly be approached in a subject receiving an acute load of at least 1.2 g of animal protein or an intravenous infu-

FIGURE 20-2. The concept of renal functional reserve (RFR). Four examples (patients *1* through *4*; see text for explanation) are shown. The baseline glomerular filtration rate (GFR) depends on many factors, including diet and fluid intake. Nevertheless, each person has the capability to increase GFR in response to different stimuli. The difference between maximum GFR (Max GFR) and baseline GFR describes the renal functional reserve. When renal mass is lost, Max GFR declines in an almost linear function. RFR is still present any time the baseline GFR is lower than the Max GFR at a given value for functioning renal mass.

sion of a mixture of essential amino acids with the addition of histidine. The concept of a baseline and maximal GFR in humans has been defined by the so-called renal functional reserve (RFR).

In order to better explain this concept, let us consider GFR in four different patients in a GFR/functioning renal mass domain graph, as in Figure 20-2. GFR can be considered a continuous function that is maximal in subjects with 100% renal mass and absent in anephric patients. In a patient with a monolateral nephrectomy, renal mass is by definition 50%. Once the curve of maximal GFR has been drawn, various conditions of baseline GFR can be imagined.

Patient 1 has a baseline GFR of 120 mL/min. The renal mass is intact, and if stimulated, this patient can increase GFR to values as high as 170 mL/min.[23-26] Patient 2 is a vegetarian whose baseline GFR is 65 mL/min. When stimulated, this patient can also increase GFR to values close to 170 mL/min. In other words, the RFR in these two patients is different because they are using their GFR capacities at different levels, as indicated by their baseline GFR values. Nevertheless, baseline GFR cannot tell us whether either patient's renal function is fully preserved.

Patient 3 has undergone monolateral nephrectomy because of a renal cancer. The baseline GFR corresponds to this patient's maximal GFR under unrestricted dietary conditions. If moderate protein restriction is applied to the diet, the baseline GFR may decrease, and some RFR becomes evident. The same concept is true for patient 4, although for this patient, the only way to restore some functional reserve is to apply a severe protein restriction. In some cases, even a regimen of ultra-low protein intake cannot restore RFR.

One can conclude that baseline GFR does not necessarily correspond to the extent of functioning renal mass. A test of stimulation to reach maximal GFR might be helpful to define the real situation of the patient in terms of renal function. Only this maximal "test" GF value fully describes the level of renal function, and the baseline GFR value might be misleading if it is not properly interpreted on the basis of diet and drug regimens.

GFR AND ESTIMATED GFR IN ACUTE KIDNEY INJURY

In patients with AKI, eGFR has not yet been validated; furthermore, it should be clearly stated that eGFR is not an equivalent measure of GFR but only a transformation of the serum creatinine value into a parameter that is static in nature and is not immediately related to the physiology of the glomerular function in a specific moment.[27]

Accurate estimation of GFR from serum creatinine values requires a steady state of creatinine balance; that is, serum creatinine concentration is stable from day to day. This is true whether the serum creatinine value is used alone, in the MDRD Study equation, or in other estimating equations such as the Cockcroft-Gault formula. However, the serum creatinine value can provide important information about the level of kidney function even when it is not in a steady state. Estimated GFR overestimates true GFR when serum creatinine levels are rising, and underestimates GFR when serum creatinine levels are falling. In general, if the serum creatinine value doubles within one day, the GFR is near zero.

On the basis of these concepts, the definition of ARF should include the physiological concepts of "normality," the presence of residual RFR, and, finally, the dynamic modifications of GFR within hours during the clinical course. Therefore, estimated GFR is not a parameter that can be used to define or classify ARF.

Regulation and Measurement of Glomerular Filtration Rate in Acute Kidney Injury

In different clinical conditions, renal blood flow is maintained at steady levels through autoregulation (Fig. 20-3). Significant variations in blood pressure are counterbal-

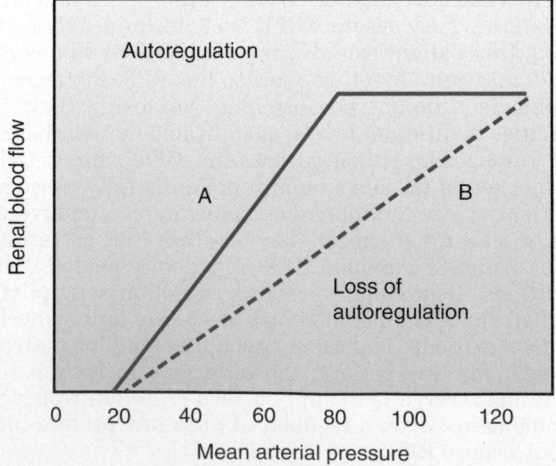

FIGURE 20-3. The concept of renal blood flow autoregulation. Renal blood flow is kept fairly constant in the presence of significant variations of renal perfusion pressure (*line A*). When a pathological event occurs, the mechanism is lost, and even small variations in perfusion pressure result in significant variations of renal blood flow (*line B*).

anced by changes in the renal vascular tone, and the final result is the maintenance of blood flow within normal ranges.[1] The same is true for GFR, which is also kept constant by tubular-glomerular feedback, as already described.[1] In detail, GFR depends on the transcapillary pressure gradient, which is regulated by a fine tuning of the tone of afferent and efferent arteries. This mechanism enables compensation for changes in plasma flow through a variation in filtration fraction. Although this parameter is regulated to keep it around 20%, significant variations in filtration fraction may allow GFR to remain stable in the presence of plasma flow variations. The combined effect of autoregulation and filtration fraction determines the quantity and composition of the urine. In the so-called syndrome of prerenal dysfunction, the loss in renal perfusion due to arterial underfilling produces a temporary decrease in glomerular filtration and lower sodium content in the tubular lumen, which is rapidly counterbalanced by an increase in reabsorption of sodium and water (leading to a reduced fractional secretion of sodium, high urine osmolality, and oliguria), whereas glomerular hemodynamics are adjusted to increase filtration fraction even though GFR may decrease and the serum creatinine level may rise.

If the patient receives a fluid infusion and extracellular volume expansion therapy, these conditions may be reversible, and the original equilibrium can be restored. In some pathological conditions, however, or when arterial underfilling remains untreated for longer times, the original alteration, which is functional in nature, may become structural, and parenchymal damage may occur. In such conditions, autoregulation is lost, glomerular hemodynamics and the tubular glomerular feedback are altered, and so is the modulation of filtration fraction. The GFR decreases with a progressive increase in the fractional excretion of sodium and a progressive reduction in urine osmolality.

It should be speculated that subjects with partial or total loss of RFR due to previous damage or loss of nephron mass are more likely than others to demonstrate a rapid passage from the prerenal to the renal phase of AKI. In the absence of previous baseline and test GFR determinations, this possibility might explain the variability of responses observed to ischemic insults, to hypovolemia, and to fluid infusion.

Urea and blood urea nitrogen (BUN) values are nonspecific indicators of renal function; they are very poor markers of GFR relative to creatinine and thus are not discussed further. However, a serum creatinine value of 1.5 mg/dL (133 µmol/L), in a steady state, corresponds to a GFR of about 36 mL/min in an 80-year-old white woman but to a GFR of about 77 mL/min in a 20-year-old black man. Similarly, a serum creatinine value of 3.0 mg/dL (265 µmol/L) in a patient in whom renal impairment is suspected would reflect a GFR of 16 mL/min in the elderly woman but 35 mL/min in the young man. In both cases, a doubling of the serum creatinine value corresponds to a decrease in GFR of approximately 50% (exactly a 55% decrease in the preceding example), because there is an inverse relationship between GFR and serum creatinine value. Thus, although every classification of ARF in the literature relies on some threshold value for serum creatinine value, *no single creatinine value corresponds to a given GFR in all patients.*[27] Therefore, it is *the change* in creatinine that is useful in determining the presence of ARF.

Unfortunately, like creatinine clearance, the serum creatinine value is not an accurate reflection of GFR in the non–steady state condition of ARF. During the evolution of dysfunction, the serum creatinine will *underestimate* the level of dysfunction. Nonetheless, the extent to which the serum creatinine value changes from baseline (and perhaps the rate of change as well) to some degree reflects the change in GFR. Serum creatinine is readily and easily measured as well as reasonably specific for renal function. Thus, serum creatinine (or creatinine clearance) is a reasonable approximation of GFR in most patients with normal renal function.[8] Creatinine is formed from nonenzymatic dehydration of creatine in the liver, and 98% of the creatine pool is in muscle. Critically ill patients may have abnormalities in liver function and markedly decreased muscle mass.[4] Additional factors influencing creatinine production are conditions of increased production, such as trauma, fever, and immobilization, and conditions of decreased production, including liver disease, reduced muscle mass, and aging. In addition, tubular reabsorption ("backleak") may occur in conditions associated with low urine flow rate. Finally, the volume of distribution (V_D) for creatinine (total body water) influences the serum creatinine value and may be dramatically increased in critically ill patients. There is currently no information on extrarenal creatinine clearance in ARF, and a non–steady state condition often exists.[27]

Once glomerular filtration has reached a steady state, it can be quantified by measurement of 24-hour creatinine clearance. Unfortunately, the accuracy of a creatinine clearance (even when collection is complete) is limited because, as GFR falls, creatinine secretion is increased and thus the rise in serum creatinine value is less.[6,10,11] Accordingly, creatinine excretion is much greater than the filtered load, resulting in a potentially large overestimation of the GFR (as much as a two-fold difference). Therefore creatinine clearance represents the upper limit of what the true GFR is under steady state conditions. A more accurate determination of GFR would require measurement of the clearance of inulin or a radiolabeled compound.[7] Unfortunately, these tests are not routinely available. However, for clinical purposes, *determining the exact GFR is rarely necessary.* Instead, it is important to determine whether renal function is stable or getting worse or better—which can usually be accomplished by monitoring serum creatinine value alone.[8] Furthermore, because patients with ARF are not in a steady state, creatinine clearance does not accurately reflect GFR.

When the patient has preexisting renal disease, the baseline GFR and serum creatinine value are different from those predicted by the MDRD Study equation. Also, the relative decrease in renal function required to reach a level consistent with the diagnosis of ARF is less than that in a patient without preexisting disease. For example, a patient with a baseline serum creatinine value of 1 mg/dL (88 µmol/L) has a steady state serum creatinine value of 3 mg/dL (229 µmol/L) once 75% of GFR is lost. By contrast, in a patient perfectly matched with the preceding one for age, race, and sex who has a baseline creatinine of 2.5 mg/dL (221 µmol/L), a mere 50% decrease in GFR corresponds to a serum creatinine value of 5 mg/dL (442 µmol/L). The problem with these criteria is that the first patient may have had a baseline GFR of 120 mL/min decreasing to 30 mL/min, and the second patient a baseline GFR of 40 mL/min decreasing to 20 mL/min. It would be confus-

ing to regard the first patient, with a GFR of 30 mL/min, as having ARF, and the patient with a GFR of 20 mL/min as not having ARF. Thus, it seems that either a different set of criteria is needed in patients with preexisting disease or some absolute creatinine criteria must be integrated into the classification system. One possible approach would be to use a relative change in creatinine (e.g., threefold) as the primary criterion, with an absolute cutoff (e.g., 4 mg/dL or about 350 µmol/L) as a secondary criterion when the baseline serum creatinine value is abnormal. Separate criteria should be used for the diagnosis of ARF superimposed on chronic renal disease. An acute rise in serum creatinine (of at least 0.5 mg/dL or 44 µmol/L) to more than 4 mg/dL (350 µmol/L) serves to identify most patients with ARF whose baseline serum creatinine values are abnormal.

All of these considerations have been used to come up with a definition of ARF or AKI that could serve for prospective studies as well as for stratification of patients according to severity of the syndrome and of the organ damage.[27] The issue of AKI definition is treated in Chapter 11.

Key Points

1. Glomerular filtration rate is the main parameter to describe kidney function.
2. The mechanisms that regulate glomerular ultrafiltration are numerous and complex. The final regulation is achieved through a fine regulation of the transcapillary pressure gradient and the membrane permeability coefficient.
3. The measurement of glomerular filtration rate is complicated, and in clinical settings, simplified methods or even estimations from serum creatinine using special formulas can be used.
4. Baseline and maximal glomerular filtration capacities may be different. The difference between the two values describes a third parameter called renal functional reserve.
5. Measurement of glomerular filtration rate and its modification over time is an important method in determining the level of acute kidney injury.

Key References

1. Maddox DA, Brenner BM: Glomerular ultrafiltration. In Brenner BM (ed): Brenner and Rector's The Kidney, 7th ed. Philadelphia, WB Saunders, 2004, pp 353-412.
5. Levey AS: Measurement of renal function in chronic renal disease. Kidney Int 1990;38:167-173.
10. Cockroft D, Gault M: Prediction of creatinine clearance from serum creatinine. Nephron 1976;16:31-41.
15. Levey A, Bosch J, Lewis JB, et al: A more accurate method to estimate glomerular filtration rate from serum creatinine: A new prediction equation. Ann Intern Med 1999;130: 461-470.
25. Bosch JP, Saccaggi A, Lauer A, et al: Renal functional reserve in humans: Effect of protein intake on glomerular filtration rate. Am J Med 1983;75:943-950.

See the companion Expert Consult website for the complete reference list.

CHAPTER 21

The Physiology of the Afferent and Efferent Arterioles

Clive N. May and Christoph Langenberg

OBJECTIVES

The chapter will:
1. Explain why preglomerular and postglomerular resistances are controlled differentially.
2. Describe the effect of this differential control on renal blood flow and glomerular filtration rate.
3. Discuss the preferential actions of circulating vasoactive peptides on the afferent and efferent arteriole.
4. Explain how paracrine agents alter afferent and efferent arteriole tone.
5. Describe how the sympathetic nervous system can selectively alter preglomerular and postglomerular resistances.
6. Discuss the effect of several drugs on preglomerular and postglomerular resistances.

Major functions of the kidney are to maintain fluid and electrolyte homeostasis and to excrete metabolites. To accomplish this, plasma is filtered in the glomerular tuft of the nephron into the proximal tubules. One of the driving forces for glomerular filtration pressure is the hydrostatic pressures in the glomerulus, which are regulated mainly by the balance in vascular tone of the two glomerular resistance vessels, the afferent and efferent arterioles.

ROLE OF AFFERENT AND EFFERENT ARTERIOLES

The kidneys have a sophisticated autoregulatory system to keep their blood flow and perfusion constant over a wide range of systemic blood pressures. Unlike perfusion of all other organs, perfusion of the kidney is not necessarily regulated to maintain organ nutrition but to retain its functions in terms of filtration. The filtration pressure is determined by the hydrostatic pressure within the glomerulus, the glomerular oncotic pressure, and the tubular oncotic pressure. The glomerular hydrostatic pressure, which is the predominant factor, is regulated mainly by the balance of vascular tone in the afferent and efferent arterioles. These vessels form two capillary resistance beds in series that almost entirely control renal resistance.[1,2] Owing to this exceptional arrangement of resistance vessels in series, before and after the glomerulus, renal blood flow (RBF) and glomerular filtration rate (GFR) can be regulated independently. A selective increase in afferent resistance decreases RBF, the blood flow into the glomerulus, and

the glomerular filtration pressure, a primary force for plasma ultrafiltration. On the other hand, constriction of the efferent arteriole raises glomerular filtration pressure, thereby maintaining or even increasing GFR despite a drop in RBF and thus causing an increase in filtration fraction (GFR/RBF) (Fig. 21-1).

The vascular tone of these preglomerular and postglomerular vessels is regulated by several systems, including circulating hormones, paracrine factors, and the renal sympathetic nerves. It is not possible to measure the tone of these vessels in vivo, but a number of studies have used the relation of RBF and GFR to provide indirect evidence of preferential actions of different agents on the afferent and efferent arterioles. It should be noted that results of in vivo studies may be confounded by changes in renal perfusion pressure and the influences of other neurohumoral factors in response to the treatments being studied. Experimental studies have used many different techniques, including isolated arterioles, micropuncture, and morphometric studies. It is important, however, to recognize the limitations of in vitro studies and note that the physiological relevance of the different models is not certain. Also, how the levels of the different hormones used in the in vitro studies relate to the physiological and pathological levels found in the kidney is unclear.

Studies that have investigated the endocrine, paracrine, and neural mechanisms controlling afferent and efferent vascular tone, as well as the actions of some drugs, are discussed in the following sections.

HUMORAL MECHANISMS CONTROLLING AFFERENT AND EFFERENT ARTERIOLAR RESISTANCE

A number of circulating hormones have been shown to have differential actions on the afferent and efferent arterioles. These hormones play important roles in the normal physiological control of RBF and GFR and may also exert significant beneficial or detrimental actions in disease.

Angiotensin II

Angiotensin II, a potent vasoconstrictor, has a more powerful action on the vasculature in the kidney than that in other organs.[3] It is a critical mediator of the regulation of glomerular filtration through its combined control of the vascular tone in the afferent and efferent arterioles. In both human and animal studies, angiotensin II has been consistently demonstrated to cause a rise in filtration fraction,[4-6] suggesting that functionally, this vasoconstrictor has a

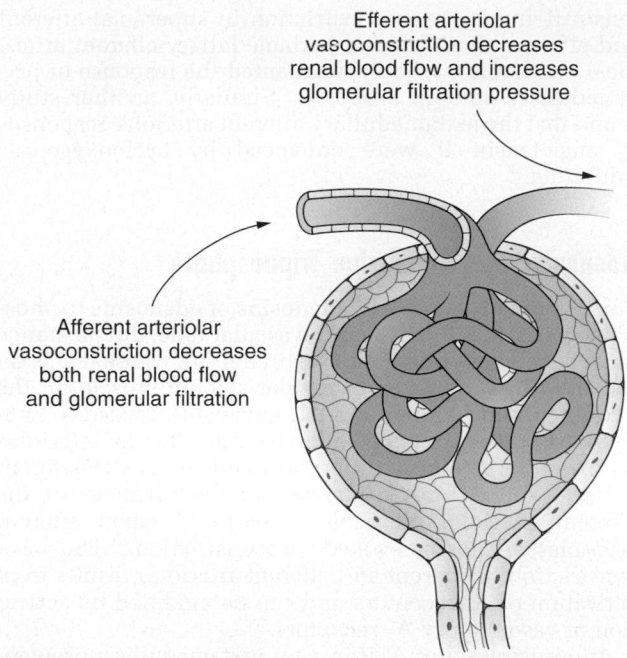

Efferent arteriolar
vasoconstriction decreases
renal blood flow and increases
glomerular filtration pressure

Afferent arteriolar
vasoconstriction decreases
both renal blood flow
and glomerular filtration

FIGURE 21-1. Diagram showing the functional consequences of selective afferent or efferent arteriolar vasoconstriction.

predominant action on the efferent arteriole. The effects of angiotensin II are mediated by two receptors, AT-1 and AT-2. The renal AT-1 receptors mediate vasoconstriction, whereas the AT-2 receptors mediate vasodilation.[7]

Although it is agreed that angiotensin II has potent actions on the renal vasculature, there is still debate about the proposal that it has a preferential vasoconstrictor action on efferent over afferent arterioles. The controversy probably relates to the wide variety of techniques that have been used in functional studies, including the different protocols, species, and doses of angiotensin II employed.

Using an in vitro model to study isolated rabbit arterioles, and so avoiding the influence of neurohumoral variables, Edwards[8] found that efferent arterioles were extremely sensitive to angiotensin II, whereas the afferent arterioles were completely unresponsive. A unique sensitivity of the efferent arterioles to angiotensin II was also found in two studies using isolated perfused rat kidneys.[9,10] A greater sensitivity of the efferent arteriole to angiotensin II was found in studies using microperfused rabbit arterioles[11] and in isolated rat glomerular arterioles.[12] A similar effect of angiotensin II on both arterioles has been reported in two micropuncture studies in rats.[13,14] If renal perfusion pressure was kept constant during angiotensin II, one study found, the afferent arteriolar vasoconstriction was largely prevented, suggesting that this response was autoregulatory in response to the increase in pressure, and not an effect of angiotensin II.[14]

Data from morphometric studies provide evidence that angiotensin II causes a preferential increase in efferent resistance. Denton and colleagues[15] measured the diameters of the afferent and efferent arterioles in perfusion-fixed kidneys from rabbits by morphometric analysis using transmission electron microscopy.[15] In the outer cortex, angiotensin II caused a greater reduction in the diameters of the afferent than the efferent arterioles. But because of the smaller resting diameter of the efferent arterioles, and because resistance is inversely proportional to the fourth power of the radius (Poiseuille's relationship), this

translated into a greater increase in vascular resistance in the efferent arterioles. A later study by the same group reported similar findings when they infused angiotensin II intrarenally to avoid changes in systemic pressure.[4] They also extended their original findings to show that angiotensin II preferentially increased the resistance of efferent arterioles in the mid-cortex as well as in the outer cortex.

Endothelin

The endothelins are a family of potent vasoconstrictor peptides whose vasoconstrictor actions are mediated usually through ET_A receptors but in some tissues, including the kidney, through ET_B receptors. At the whole kidney level, endothelin-1 (ET-1) causes renal vasoconstriction and a decrease in RBF.[16]

At the level of the arterioles, both ET-1 and ET-3 have been found to cause vasoconstriction of isolated rabbit afferent and efferent arterioles.[17] In a study by Inscho and associates,[18] arteriolar responses to ET-1 in a rat kidney blood-perfused juxtamedullary nephron preparation demonstrated that the afferent arteriole is more sensitive to the vasoconstrictor action of ET-1 than the efferent arteriole. The vasoconstriction in both afferent and efferent arterioles was mediated largely by ET_A receptors. These investigators found evidence for ET_B receptor–mediated vasoconstriction in the afferent arteriole and for ET_B receptor–mediated vasodilation in the efferent arteriole. Other studies using perfusion fixed kidneys and hydronephrotic kidneys also demonstrated a much greater vasoconstriction in response to ET-1 in afferent arterioles than in efferent arterioles.[19,20] In yet other reports, however, afferent arterioles were less or similarly responsive to ET compared with efferent arterioles.[21,22]

In patients with renal failure, ET values are often elevated, possibly endangering renal function, and treatment with ET-1 antagonists may be beneficial.[23]

Atrial Natriuretic Peptide

The reported effects of atrial natriuretic peptide (ANP) on renal arterioles are more consistent, with a consensus that it causes afferent arteriolar vasodilation and efferent arteriolar vasoconstriction.[24] In anesthetized rats, intravenous infusion of rat ANP (126-149) reduced renal vascular resistance but increased GFR and filtration fraction. The greater GFR resulted from a rise in glomerular pressure, which was due to afferent dilation and efferent arteriolar vasoconstriction.[25] Similar findings have been reported from the use of morphometric analysis of renal vascular casts.[26] ANP has also been shown to reverse noradrenaline-induced afferent vasoconstriction and to potentiate its efferent arteriolar vasoconstriction.[27]

This action of ANP has been suggested to help maintain GFR in heart failure,[28] in which ANP values are elevated and renal perfusion pressure is reduced. Long-term infusion of ANP has been demonstrated to improve both RBF and GFR in patients with acute renal impairment after cardiac surgery.[29]

Arginine Vasopressin

Arginine vasopressin (AVP) is a potent vasoconstrictor, particularly in the mesenteric circulation, with less effect on the kidney. In isolated rabbit arterioles, AVP caused a reduction in the lumen diameter of efferent arterioles, an effect blocked by a specific V_1 receptor antagonist, but AVP had no effect on afferent arterioles.[30] In contrast, in rat blood-perfused medullary nephrons, the afferent arterioles were more sensitive to the vasoconstrictor actions of AVP than the efferent arterioles,[31] whereas in rat hydronephrotic kidneys, AVP constricted only the interlobular and arcuate arteries, not the afferent nor efferent arterioles.[32]

Conclusion

With all these hormones, the contrasting findings of different groups may be due to the differences in species or nephron populations studied and to the different levels of hormones in the preparations used. Also, interactions among the humoral, paracrine, and neural systems controlling glomerular function are disrupted to different degrees in different preparations. For example, in isolated microvessel preparations, there is little flow through the lumen, but flow-induced shear stress is a stimulus for endothelial production of nitric oxide and prostaglandins, both of which have modulatory actions on the responses to these hormones.

PARACRINE AGENTS

Nitric Oxide

It is well established that nitric oxide (NO), synthesized from L-arginine by a number of isoforms of nitric oxide synthase (NOS), is a potent renal vasodilator. Microperfusion studies indicate that the afferent arteriole is more sensitive than the efferent arteriole to the vasodilator effects of NO.[11] In microperfused rabbit arterioles, inhibition of NOS with the nonselective inhibitor L-NAME (nitro-L-arginine methyl ester) caused a greater decrease in diameter in the afferent than in the efferent arteriole.[11] In addition, the effects of NOS inhibition have been studied extensively in vivo. Short-term and long-term nonspecific inhibition of all NOS isoforms significantly increases renal vascular resistance,[33,34] and a preferential vasodilator action of NO on the afferent arteriole was proposed on the basis of the changes in RBF and GFR.[33]

The main action of NO may well be to modulate the action of angiotensin II and other vasoconstrictors. In microperfused rabbit arterioles, L-NAME significantly augmented the vasoconstrictor action of angiotensin II in afferent but not efferent arterioles,[11] indicating that NO modulates the action of angiotensin II in afferent but not efferent arterioles. Studies in mice suggest, however, that L-NAME increases the sensitivity to angiotensin II in both efferent and afferent arterioles.[35]

Prostaglandins

Matsuda and colleagues[36] found that indomethacin had no effect on baseline renal function (GRF, filtration fraction) or renal hemodynamics (RBF and afferent and efferent arteriolar diameters) in canine arterioles.[36] As with NO, it seems likely that the major action of prostaglandins is to modulate the actions of vasoconstrictors. These researchers also found that indomethacin had no effect on angio-

tensin II–induced vasoconstriction in superficial afferent and efferent arterioles and juxtamedullary efferent arterioles, but that it markedly augmented the response of juxtamedullary afferent arterioles. Similarly, another study found that the juxtamedullary afferent arteriolar responses to angiotensin II were enhanced by cyclooxygenase inhibition.[37]

Adenosine and Adenosine Triphosphate

For intrarenally generated adenosine or adenosine triphosphate (ATP) to influence microvascular tone, the substance must be released into the interstitial fluid, where it acts on the adventitial surface of vascular smooth muscle. In the hydronephrotic kidney model, adenosine caused a transient vasoconstriction of afferent and efferent arterioles followed by a return to normal diameter in the afferent arteriole but a further increase in the diameter of the efferent arteriole.[38] In isolated perfused rabbit afferent arterioles, adenosine evoked vasoconstriction.[39] The vasoconstriction of afferent and efferent arterioles results from activation of A_1 receptors and can be modified by activation of vasodilatory A_2 receptors.[40]

Administration of ATP in a rat juxtamedullary preparation causes afferent vasoconstriction but has no effect on efferent arterioles.[41] Afferent vasoconstriction in response to ATP has also been observed in rabbit afferent arterioles.[40] This selective action of ATP on afferent arterioles fits well with the finding that $P2X_1$ purinoreceptors appear only on preglomerular microvessels.[42]

CONTROL BY THE SYMPATHETIC NERVOUS SYSTEM

The kidney receives sympathetic innervation that extends to the vascular smooth muscle cells, juxtaglomerular renin-secreting cells, and mesangium as well as the proximal and distal tubules and the loop of Henle.[43,44] In spite of this extensive innervation, the important role that the sympathetic nervous system plays in the control of renal function and renin release has been accepted only relatively recently.[45]

Studies now indicate that the afferent arterioles are threefold more densely innervated than the efferent arterioles. Two distinct types of sympathetic axons have been found to innervate the renal arterioles; type I axons almost exclusively innervate the afferent arteriole, whereas type II axons are equally distributed on the two arterioles.[46] Being sympathetic fibers, both axon types contain noradrenaline, but these authors demonstrated that only type II axons contained the cotransmitter neuropeptide Y. The finding of differential innervation of the afferent and efferent arterioles indicates that the sympathetic nervous system may evoke selective changes in preglomerular and postglomerular resistance to regulate GFR and renal function. Differential control of sympathetic outflow to different organs is well established, but there is no definitive evidence that type I or type II axons can be independently regulated.

The finding that noradrenaline has similar vasoconstrictor actions on isolated rat efferent and afferent arterioles[12] suggests that any differential action of the sympathetic nervous system on the preglomerular and postglomerular vessels must result from the different levels of innervation of the two types of vessel.

EFFECTS OF DRUGS

Calcium Antagonists

Several lines of evidence indicate that calcium antagonists cause preferential vasodilation of the afferent arteriole, with only a minor action on the efferent arteriole.[47,48] Dietz and colleagues[49] found that nifedipine caused a greater increase in GRF than in renal plasma flow, leading to an increase in filtration fraction in anesthetized dogs, supporting the notion of a greater vasodilator action on the afferent arteriole. The finding that voltage-dependent L-type and T-type calcium channels are expressed in cortical afferent arterioles but not cortical efferent arterioles indicates that calcium influx via voltage-gated calcium channels regulates afferent arteriole resistance. In contrast, efferent resistance is mediated primarily by calcium ion (Ca^{2+}) entry pathways as well as intracellular Ca^{2+} mobilization. Organic calcium antagonists are therefore potent afferent arteriolar vasodilators, with little effect on efferent resistance. These findings suggest that this action of a calcium antagonist may cause glomerular hypertension that could lead to the progression of renal diseases. The extent of preferential afferent vasodilation can vary according to the particular Ca^{2+} antagonist used, with some novel antagonists having a dilator action on both efferent and afferent arterioles.[50]

Interestingly, Ca^{2+} channel blockers prevent the vasoconstrictor action of angiotensin II on afferent, but not efferent, arterioles,[47] suggesting different mechanisms for vascular contraction by angiotensin II of the preglomerular and postglomerular arterioles. This suggestion is supported by the finding that nifedipine prevented the calcium influx caused by angiotensin II only in the afferent arteriole.[51] These findings suggest that in the afferent arteriole, angiotensin II activates dihydropyridine-sensitive L-type calcium channels, presumably by membrane depolarization, whereas in the efferent arteriole, angiotensin II appears to stimulate calcium entry via store-operated calcium influx,[57] a process by which the emptying of intracellular Ca^{2+} stores activates Ca^{2+} influx into the cell.

Angiotensin-Converting Enzyme Inhibitors/ Angiotensin AT-1 Antagonists

Studies that have examined the effects of angiotensin-converting enzyme (ACE) inhibitors and AT-1 receptor antagonists on renal function support the proposition that angiotensin II has a preferential vasoconstrictor action on the efferent arteriole. Heller and colleagues[52] found, in anesthetized dogs, that an active metabolite (EXP 3174) of the AT-1 receptor antagonist losartan increased RBF and GFR and decreased filtration fraction, through a reduction in total renal resistance that was mainly due to a decrease in efferent resistance. Addition of captopril, an ACE inhibitor, caused a further increase in renal blood flow, which was probably mediated by kinins because the effect was prevented by a bradykinin B_2 antagonist. Treatment of mild hypertensive patients with valsartan, an AT-1 antagonist, was also shown to increase resistance more in efferent than in afferent arterioles.[53]

Dopamine

Low-dose dopamine causes renal vasodilation and has been used to prevent or alter the course of acute renal failure, although there is much evidence that argues against its effectiveness.[54,55] At the level of the glomerular arterioles, dopamine has been shown to cause a dose-dependent relaxation of noradrenaline-induced tone in both afferent and efferent arterioles from rabbit kidney.[56] Studies in the split hydronephrotic rat kidney found that dopamine produced dilation of the afferent arterioles and a smaller degree of dilation of the efferent arterioles near the glomeruli. Higher doses of dopamine caused vasodilation of both afferent and efferent arterioles away from the glomeruli.[57]

CONCLUSION

At present there remains considerable controversy regarding the mechanisms leading to this differential control, some of the reasons for which have been discussed. Unfortunately, because it is not possible to conduct the required experiments in vivo, there is only indirect supporting data from human studies. A number of conclusions can be drawn from the available data, which in some cases are limited to a single species or technique (Table 21-1).

Many of these differential actions probably depend on the different distribution of receptors on the afferent and efferent arterioles as well as the different calcium activation mechanisms in the two vessels.

TABLE 21-1

Relative Actions of Vasoactive Agents and Drugs on the Afferent and Efferent Arterioles*

COMPOUND	VASCULAR ACTIONS
Angiotensin II	Afferent constriction < efferent constriction
Noradrenaline	Afferent constriction = efferent constriction
Endothelin-1	Afferent constriction > efferent constriction
Atrial natriuretic peptide	Afferent dilation; efferent constriction
Nitric oxide	Afferent dilation > efferent dilation
Adenosine triphosphate	Afferent constriction; no efferent effect
Ca^{2+} antagonists	Afferent dilation > efferent dilation
Angiotensin blockers	Afferent constriction < efferent constriction
Dopamine	Afferent dilation = efferent dilation

*Data are a consensus view from published work, although in some cases there remains controversy about the relative actions on the preglomerular and postglomerular arterioles.

Key References

2. Thurau KW: Autoregulation of renal blood flow and glomerular filtration rate, including data on tubular and peritubular capillary pressures and vessel wall tension. Circ Res 1964; 15:(Suppl):132-141.
11. Ito S, Arima S, Ren YL, et al: Endothelium-derived relaxing factor/nitric oxide modulates angiotensin II action in the isolated microperfused rabbit afferent but not efferent arteriole. J Clin Invest 1993;91:2012-2019.
15. Denton KM, Fennessy PA, Alcorn D, Anderson WP: Morphometric analysis of the actions of angiotensin II on renal arterioles and glomeruli. Am J Physiol 1992;262:F367-F372.
17. Edwards RM, Trizna W, Ohlstein EH: Renal microvascular effects of endothelin. Am J Physiol 1990;259:F217-F221.
48. Carmines PK, Navar LG: Disparate effects of Ca channel blockade on afferent and efferent arteriolar responses to angiotensin II. Am J Physiol 1989;256:F1015-F1020.

See the companion Expert Consult website for the complete reference list.

CHAPTER 22

The Physiology of the Glomerular Tuft

Mirian A. Boim, Vicente P. Castro Teixeira, and Nestor Schor

OBJECTIVES

This chapter will:
1. Review the structure and function of the glomerular tuft.
2. Discuss regulation of the hemodynamics of glomerular ultrafiltration.
3. Describe the selectivity of the glomerular capillary wall.
4. Discuss the functions of endothelial, mesangial, and epithelial cells.

The glomerulus is a sophisticated renal structure responsible for plasma ultrafiltration, the initial process in formation of urine, the stability of which depends on the cooperative function of its components. It is a network of capillaries held together by connective tissue and essentially composed of three distinct cell types: endothelial cells, mesangial cells, and glomerular visceral epithelial cells (podocytes). In addition, three extracellular matrices make up part of the glomerulus's organization; the major constituents of all three are components of the basement membrane.

Kidney impairment can have diverse causes, but the glomerular filtration barrier is usually the main location of damage. This barrier is a trilaminar structure composed of a fenestrated endothelium, the hydrated meshwork of the glomerular basement membrane (GBM), and the filtration slit formed by pedicel interdigitation (see later). In the last 25 years, the understanding of the physiology and pathophysiology of the glomerulus has increased enormously. Most of this knowledge has been acquired from exploration of the structure and function of the glomerular cells with new techniques of cell and molecular biology. This chapter reviews the structure and function of the glomerular tuft, focusing on regulation of ultrafiltration by hemodynamic factors and glomerular structures such as endothelial, mesangial, and epithelial cells.

Each human kidney contains approximately 1 million glomeruli. The glomerulus consists of a capillary tuft that is surrounded by Bowman's capsule, which passes the filtered primary urine to the tubular system. Basically, the characteristics of glomerular microcirculation determine how much fluid will be filtered and the highly specialized glomerular capillary wall (as discussed later) determines what will be filtered, conferring selectivity to the glomerular ultrafiltration process.

The main determinants of single-nephron glomerular filtration rate (SNGFR) are the hydraulic permeability of the glomerular capillary wall and the effective filtration pressure gradient across the glomerular capillary, which is determined mainly by glomerular capillary hydraulic pressure (P_{GC}) and intracapillary oncotic pressure (π_{GC}). Thus, the primary force driving SNGFR is P_{GC}, the precise control of which is important because significant drops in P_{GC} can lead to acute renal failure, and a long-term increase in P_{GC} causes irreversible glomerular damage resulting in sclerosis and chronic renal disease.

The P_{GC} is kept relatively constant through the glomerular capillary in spite of the glomerular filtration. This phenomenon is explained by the existence of differences in diameter of the efferent and afferent arterioles for the majority of glomeruli. The resistance of the efferent arterioles is higher than that of the afferent arterioles. Variations in the diameter of the preglomerular and postglomerular arterioles directly affect P_{GC} and glomerular plasma flow. These variations also indirectly affect SNGFR, which increases if the ratio of afferent arteriolar resistance to efferent arteriolar resistance drops and decreases if this resistance ratio rises. In contrast, the ultrafiltration process is limited by the intraglomerular oncotic pressure (π_{GC}), because this pressure rises as protein-free ultrafiltrate is formed.[1,2]

Under normal conditions, afferent arteriolar resistance is regulated so it increases with systemic pressure elevation,[3] and thus, P_{GC} remains constant. This is the major mechanism by which SNGFR is autoregulated, and it involves an afferent arteriolar myogenic response to variations in perfusion pressure. The loss of autoregulation ability results in glomerular hypertension and hyperfiltration, and as proposed by several researchers, this abnormality of glomerular hemodynamics, especially elevated glomerular capillary pressure, plays an important role in the progression of renal failure.[4,5] Afferent arteriole autoregulation is impaired in many clinical and experimental conditions.[6] In rats subjected to subtotal nephrectomy, compensatory hyperfiltration of the remnant nephrons helps maintain overall GFR; however, this adaptation also leads to glomerular hypertension, proteinuria, and progressive chronic renal failure.[7] Clinical and experimental data show that early diabetes is associated with elevated GFR, owing to increases in glomerular capillary hydraulic pressure and hyperfiltration. These increases occur despite normal systemic pressure,[8,9] which is in turn a result of a proportionally greater reduction in the ratio of afferent to efferent arteriolar resistances.[10] Glomerular hypertension is also present in human patients with diabetes; a correlation has been demonstrated between urine albumin excretion and the glomerular pressure but not systemic pressure.[11] Thus, as in the remnant kidney model, glomerular hypertension in diabetic nephropathy itself plays a key role in the chronic decline in GFR.

The balance of vascular tone in preglomerular and postglomerular arterioles is a crucial determinant of glomerular hemodynamics, because both glomerular pressure and plasma flow are controlled by adjustments of these arterioles. The tone of both vessels results from the influence of nerves and humoral and paracrine factors, through a balance of constrictor and dilator systems. Angiotensin II, nitric oxide, and prostaglandins are important factors determining vascular tone. Angiotensin II constricts both afferent and efferent arterioles, although most of the data point to a higher sensitivity of efferent arterioles to angiotensin II.[2,12-14] Moreover, tone in afferent and efferent arterioles is modulated by different mechanisms. As discussed previously, the control of afferent arteriolar tone by the myogenic response, together with tubuloglomerular feedback, plays a dominant role in keeping GFR at a constant level over a wide range of renal perfusion pressures. In addition, an interaction between tubuloglomerular feedback and angiotensin II seems to be essential to maintaining GFR despite large variations in daily intake of salt and water. Experimental evidence has shown that these two mechanisms are modulated mainly by nitric oxide[14,15] derived from glomerular endothelial cells.[16] In contrast, in the efferent arteriole, neither myogenic response nor tubuloglomerular feedback seems to be important. Angiotensin II, however, is one major factor involved in the control of efferent vascular resistance, which appears to be modulated primarily by prostaglandin largely produced by the upstream glomerulus.[17] Thus, the differential response of preglomerular and postglomerular arterioles to vasoactive substances locally produced by the glomerular cells may constitute the mechanism whereby the glomerulus controls its own capillary pressure by releasing and thereby adjusting the resistance of afferent and efferent arterioles.

It is well known that the vasoconstrictor action of angiotensin II is mediated by its interaction with the angiotensin type 1 (AT_1) receptor. However, angiotensin II can also induce vasodilation via the angiotensin II type 2 receptor (AT_2).[18] Data have shown that arteriolar activation of the AT_2 receptor causes endothelium-dependent vasodilation, which modulates the vasoconstrictor action mediated by AT_1 receptors.[14] Such modulator mechanisms that regulate tone in both afferent and efferent arterioles may play an important role in the precise control of glomerular hemodynamics, and their alterations may contribute to the pathophysiology of renal diseases, including hypertension and diabetic nephropathy.

In addition to these intraglomerular hemodynamic factors, SNGFR is also influenced by the glomerular capillary ultrafiltration coefficient (K_f), which represents the product of the glomerular filtration surface area (S) available for filtration and the hydraulic permeability of the glomerular wall (k), which is very high compared with the permeability of other capillaries. K_f has been shown to decrease in response to a number of vasoactive stimuli, although the mechanisms are not well understood. Like other capillaries, the glomerular capillary wall has no vascular smooth muscle cells, and thus, glomeruli do not constrict or relax. However, the glomerular capillary lumen may be affected by the mesangial cell contraction or relaxation. Moreover, mesangial cell function is involved in the control of glomerular filtration surface and therefore of K_f.

MESANGIAL CELLS

In reality, there are two distinct populations of mesangial cells. The first population makes up about 85% to 95% of resident mesangial cells and has as the main characteristic the presence of a network of contractile elements, such as actin, myosin, and tropomyosin, comparable to those in smooth muscle cells. The second population, representing 5% to 15% of resident mesangial cells, exhibit features of monocytes/macrophages and are derived from bone marrow.[19]

The covering of the capillaries by the GBM is partial. Because they are located inside the glomerulus, surrounding glomerular capillaries and contiguous to the fenestrated endothelium, mesangial cells account for the completion of the capillary covering. Actually, in addition to completing the mechanical enclosure of the capillary, mesangial cells form loops that completely encircle the capillaries.[20] Furthermore, there are multiple contact points between mesangial cell contractile apparatus, the mesangial extracellular matrix, and the basement membrane via an extensive intertwined three-dimensional meshwork formed by bundles of extracellular fibrils. Those contacts establish a sort of biomechanical unit, with the basement membrane serving as the effector site and mesangial cells as the contractile motor.[21] In this regard, these contacts permit the mesangial cells to support the mesangium and regulate the capillary surface area and glomerular volume, influencing glomerular hemodynamics. Therefore, mesangial cells can modulate GFR partly by changing the capillary surface area and partly by redistributing blood volume in glomerular capillaries through the actions of mesangial loops. These mechanisms may enable mesangial cells to exert static and dynamic regulation of GFR.

Furthermore, mesangial cells present numerous receptors for many distinct biomolecules that modulates several of their actions. Generally, contraction of a mesangial cell occurs in response to hormones, vasoactive compounds, and growth factors through G protein–associated receptors that activate phospholipase C, resulting in an increase in intracellular calcium concentration. On the other hand, hormones using the cyclic adenosine monophosphate and cyclic guanosine monophosphate cascades as second messengers normally relax mesangial cells through direct effects or through antagonism of the previously mentioned contracting substances (Table 22-1).[22]

Mesangial cell dysfunction has been implicated in the pathogenesis of many forms of progressive renal disease, including diabetic nephropathy. The increase in the mesangial matrix and protein deposition (collagen types I, IV, V, and VI, fibronectin, and laminin) at the glomerular level leads to mesangial expansion, basement membrane thickening, and glomerular sclerosis.[23] Moreover, low enzymatic degradation of extracellular matrix contributes to an excessive accumulation.[24] Particular attention has been paid to the role of transforming growth factor β_1 (TGFβ_1) in the mesangial expansion and glomerular sclerosis. This cytokine, synthesized by different cell types, including mesangial cells, is one of the most important regulators of extracellular matrix synthesis and degradation.[25] In addition, local synthesis of angiotensin II by mesangial cells has also been implicated in the mesangial dysfunction observed in the progression of renal disease, particularly diabetic nephropathy.[26]

GLOMERULAR FILTER

Glomerular capillary conductance differs from conductance in other fenestrated and nonfenestrated capillary beds in several ways, including control of intraglomerular

TABLE 22-1

Substances Affecting Mesangial Cells' Tone

Contraction	Hormones:
	Angiotensin II
	Arginine vasopressin
	Endothelin-1
	Norepinephrine
	Growth factors:
	Platelet-derived growth factor
	Platelet-activated factor
	Autacoids:
	Thromboxane A_2
	Prostaglandin $F_{2\alpha}$
	Leukotriene C_4
	Leukotriene D_4
	Cytokines:
	Interleukin-1
	Interleukin-6
Relaxation	Hormones:
	Atrial natriuretic peptide
	Nitric oxide
	Autacoids:
	Prostaglandin I_2
	Prostaglandin E_2

hydraulic pressure and flow and the unique anatomical characteristics of the capillary wall, which is crucial to limiting the passage of fluid and solute. Understanding of the glomerular filters as a highly size- and charge-selective barrier has substantially improved, and data now point to the crucial role of the podocytes in restricting the passage of albumin. Moreover, there is growing evidence that the highly fenestrated endothelial cells are important elements contributing to glomerular permselectivity.

Endothelial Cell

As previously discussed, the glomerular filter is a size- and charge-selective barrier.[27] The fenestrae of glomerular endothelia do not have visible diaphragms, although findings now suggest that the glomerular endothelial fenestrae may be covered by a diaphragm formed by a thick cell coat (glycocalyx).[28,29] This layer is a matrix-like gel composed of proteoglycans, with negatively charged as well as neutral glycosaminoglycans, glycoproteins, and plasma proteins carrying a negative charge. It has been suggested that the endothelial glycocalyx could potentially contribute to a primary glomerular anionic barrier, reducing the load of macromolecules on the GBM. Thus, the glycocalyx may represent an initial charge barrier in the glomerular filter and may also, to some extent, function as a size-selective barrier.[29]

GLOMERULAR BASEMENT MEMBRANE

The GBM is an especially thick membrane that lies between the endothelial cells and the visceral epithelium (podocytes). The main components of the GBM are triple-helical type IV collagen, proteoglycans, laminin, and entactin.[30,31] According to the current understanding of basement membrane structure, two main independent networks formed by collagen type IV and laminin are connected through entactin and other GBM components to form a tight, cross-linked mesh that is porous but does not have pores of defined size.[32] The GBM was previously considered to represent the size- and charge-selective macromolecular barrier.[27] This notion is supported by the fact that mutations in type IV collagen lead to Alport's syndrome, characterized by altered GBM; however, most patients with Alport's have hematuria but only a mild proteinuria.[33] Moreover, GBM contains negatively charged perlecan, a proteoglycan rich in heparan sulfate, which was thought to contribute to the charge selectivity of the GBM[34]; later studies, however, have shown that mice containing heparan sulfate–deficient perlecan had no visible defects in GBM and no signs of proteinuria.[35] Finally, in vitro studies have suggested that the GBM has some size selectivity but lacks charge selectivity.[36] Thus, current understanding points to a limited role for the GBM in the glomerular barrier.

Glomerular Visceral Epithelial Cells (Podocytes)

Podocytes are terminally differentiated cells with complex organization that have both epithelial and mesenchymal features. Structurally, podocytes can be divided into three distinct functional segments: cell body, primary processes, and secondary processes, also known as foot processes or pedicels. These cells are located at the external surfaces of glomerular capillaries, which they cover with pedicels. The covering of capillaries is achieved by interdigitation of pedicels derived from adjacent podocytes, forming between them filtration slits that are bridged by a specialized cell junction, called slit diaphragms, which represent the last filtration barrier to proteins. Three membrane domains can be defined in pedicels: apical, facing the urinary space; basal, adhered to the GBM, and lateral, composed by slit diaphragm protein complex. The subplasmalemmal region of all three domains is connected to the pedicel's actin cytoskeleton.

Podocytes have a well-developed cytoskeleton with several levels of structural organization that are responsible for their shape and the maintenance of primary and secondary processes. The cell body and primary processes are mainly constituted by microtubules and intermediate filaments, whereas pedicels contain a dense network of actin microfilament bundles associated with myosin II, α-actin, talin, and vinculin, forming a complex contractile apparatus. Consequently, podocytes have all the necessary elements to generate tensile strength and stabilize glomerular architecture by counteracting the hydrostatic forces causing distentions of glomerular capillaries. Moreover, these cells are responsible for approximately 40% of the hydraulic resistance of the filtration barrier.[37] These microfilament bundles are linked at one side with the microtubules and intermediate filament system in primary processes and connected at the other side by linker proteins with the slit membrane complex and GBM proteins. In addition to providing mechanical stability, the actin cytoskeleton and cytoskeleton reorganization serve a variety of other functions, including transduction of mechanical forces into changes of membrane potential, protein kinase activation, and gene expression.[38] In podocytes, reorganization of the actin cytoskeleton has been implicated in the action of vasoactive

hormones on the permeability of the glomerular filtration barrier.[39]

Podocytes also present receptors for several contracting and relaxing factors, suggesting that some podocyte functions may be modulated by vasoactive agents. Indeed, it was already demonstrated that they are a target for a variety of vasoactive substances, such as angiotensin II, arginine vasopressin, norepinephrine, adenosine triphosphate, bradykinin, atrial natriuretic peptide, nitric oxide, endothelin, prostaglandins, and parathormone (Table 22-2). Those substances using intracellular calcium, cyclic adenosine monophosphate, and cyclic guanosine signaling pathways might have several effects on podocyte physiology.[40] For example, the renin-angiotensin system (RAS) plays an important role in regulation of glomerular hemodynamics through modulation of the tone of the glomerular arterioles with a decrease in ultrafiltration coefficient. Human podocytes present a functionally active local RAS, expressing messenger RNA for angiotensinogen, renin, angiotensin-converting enzyme type 1, and the AT_1 and AT_2 angiotensin receptor types. They not only respond to angiotensin II but also are able to directly produce angiotensin II, implicating this local RAS in physiological and pathophysiological processes.[41,42] As a matter of fact, it has been long proposed that hormone-induced cellular signaling might alter the contractile structures of pedicels, resulting in change of ultrafiltration coefficient.[39,43] Infusion of norepinephrine into the renal artery has been found to cause acute renal failure and lesions of the filtration barrier, with changes in podocyte morphology.[44]

Progress in molecular cell biology and genomic analyses has expanded the comprehension of podocyte morphology and function, mainly in relation to the slit diaphragm structure (Fig. 22-1). The slit diaphragm shares many structural similarities with epithelial apical adhesion junctions and is considered a modified adherens junction,[45] and knowledge about its constitution has grown in the last few years. The slit diaphragm, the only contact between contiguous podocytes, is formed by several proteins arranged in a zipper-like pattern 30 to 40 nm in width and is regarded as the ultimate filter for proteins. Proteins of the immunoglobulin family, such as nephrin and NEPH1, the cadherin family, such as P-cadherin and FAT, and the stomatin family, such as podocin, make up part of the slit diaphragm's organization. At the cytoplasm side, CD2-associated protein (CD2AP) and zonula occludens-1 (ZO-1) are also associated with slit diaphragms.

Another relatively new discovery is that the slit diaphragm not only provides a structural element, serving as a static molecular sieve, but also is a dynamic multifunctional protein complex that functions as a signaling platform for the podocyte. Studies have shown that the slit diaphragm is located in lipid rafts, a microdomain of plasma membrane enriched in cholesterol and glycosphingolipids that recruits and clusters membrane proteins in a selective and dynamic way, providing molecular frameworks for several cell biological processes, including signal transduction. Nephrin, podocin, and CD2AP are known to be associated, together with actin cytoskeleton, in a lipid raft complex at the slit diaphragm. In this respect, it has already been shown that nephrin undergoes tyrosine phosphorylation by the src kinase Fyn, resulting in increased podocin binding and nephrin signaling. Deletion of Fyn results in reduced nephrin phosphorylation and coarsening of pedicel morphology, suggesting complex regulation of nephrin signaling.[46] The very survival of podocytes seems to depend partially on signaling originated in slit diaphragms. For example, nephrin can activate the AKT

TABLE 22-2

Signaling Pathways Stimulated by Several Hormones in Podocytes

HORMONE	TYPE OF RECEPTOR	CELLULAR EVENT
Angiotensin II	AT_1/AT_2	$cAMP\uparrow$
		$[Ca^{2+}]_i\uparrow$
		Cl^- channel$\uparrow$
Acetylcholine	M5	$[Ca^{2+}]_i\uparrow$
		Cl^- channel$\uparrow$
Arginine-vasopressin, oxytocin	V_{1a}, unknown	$cAMP\uparrow$
		$[Ca^{2+}]_i\uparrow$
Bradykinin	BK_2	$[Ca^{2+}]_i\uparrow$
		$IP3\uparrow$
Adenine triphosphate	P2Y2	$[Ca^{2+}]_i\uparrow$
		$IP3\uparrow$
Endothelin	ET_A	$[Ca^{2+}]_i\uparrow$
		$IP3\uparrow$
Histamine	H_1	$[Ca^{2+}]_i\uparrow$
		$IP3\uparrow$
Norepinephrine	α_1	$[Ca^{2+}]_i\uparrow$
Prostaglandin E_2	EP1	$[Ca^{2+}]_i\uparrow$
Prostaglandin $F_{2\alpha}$	FP	$[Ca^{2+}]_i\uparrow$
		Cl^- channel$\uparrow$
Thromboxane	A_2 agonist	$[Ca^{2+}]_i\uparrow$
Thrombin	Unknown	$[Ca^{2+}]_i\uparrow$
		$IP3\uparrow$
Prostaglandin E_2	EP_4	$cAMP\uparrow$
Dopamine	D_1-like	$cAMP\uparrow$
Epinephrine	β_2	$cAMP\uparrow$
Atrial natriuretic peptide	Unknown	$cGMP\uparrow$
Parathormone	PTH/PTHrP	$cAMP\uparrow$

$[Ca^{2+}]_i$, cytosolic Ca^{2+} concentration; cAMP, cyclic adenine monophosphate; cGMP, cyclic guanosine monophosphate; IP3, inositol 1,4,5-trisphosphate; $\uparrow$, increase; $\downarrow$, decrease.
Adapted from Pavenstadt H, Kriz W, Kretzler M: Cell biology of the glomerular podocyte. Physiol Rev 2003;83:253-307.

pathway in a phosphoinositide 3-OH kinase (PI3K)–dependent manner, giving protection against apoptosis.[47] In addition, stimulation of nephrin by vascular endothelial growth factor (VEGF) can also protect podocytes against apoptosis via AKT-independent mechanisms.[48]

The interaction of podocytes and GBM is another aspect to be considered in the integrity of pedicel architecture and, hence, proper functioning of slit diaphragms. Transmembrane matrix receptors, such as integrins, in addition to fastening pedicels to GBM, are involved in transduction of signals originated upon ligation of integrins by the GBM and also function as downstream effectors in cell responses. The relevance of these receptors can be underscored by the fact that knockout mice lacking the α3β1 integrin showed effacement of foot processes and immature GBM. Integrins are coupled to the podocyte cytoskeleton through adapter and scaffolding proteins necessary to transmission and amplification of the signaling. Integrin-linked kinase (ILK) is involved in a variety of biological processes, such as differentiation and cell cycle and survival, and its stimulation was found to be a common characteristic in podocyte damage.[49,50]

Finally, podocytes seem to play a crucial role in the development of the entire glomerular tuft, mainly through production of angiogenic factors. During glomerular development, they express vascular endothelial growth factor-A (VEGF-A), whereas the endothelial and mesangial cells express the VEGF receptors. In mice, podocyte-specific homozygous deletion of VEGF-A has been shown to result in perinatal lethality, and the kidneys showed a marked reduction in endothelial cell migration, differentiation, and survival.[51] Another study demonstrated that VEGF-A production in the podocyte is also essential for mesangial cell survival and differentiation.[52]

Key Points

1. The glomerular filtration barrier is the main location of kidney damage.
2. The main determinants of glomerular ultrafiltration are glomerular capillary hydraulic pressure (P_{GC}), intracapillary oncotic pressure (π_{GC}), and the ultrafiltration coefficient (K_f).
3. Control of the single-nephron glomerular filtration rate depends on the balance between preglomerular and postglomerular arteriolar resistances.
4. Mesangial cell dysfunction is implicated in glomerular sclerosis.
5. The selectivity of the glomerular filter depends on the interaction among its capillary wall layers.
6. Endothelial glycocalyx contributes to the charge selectivity of the glomerular barrier.
7. Podocytes stabilize the glomerular architecture and may constitute the major size selectivity of the glomerular barrier.

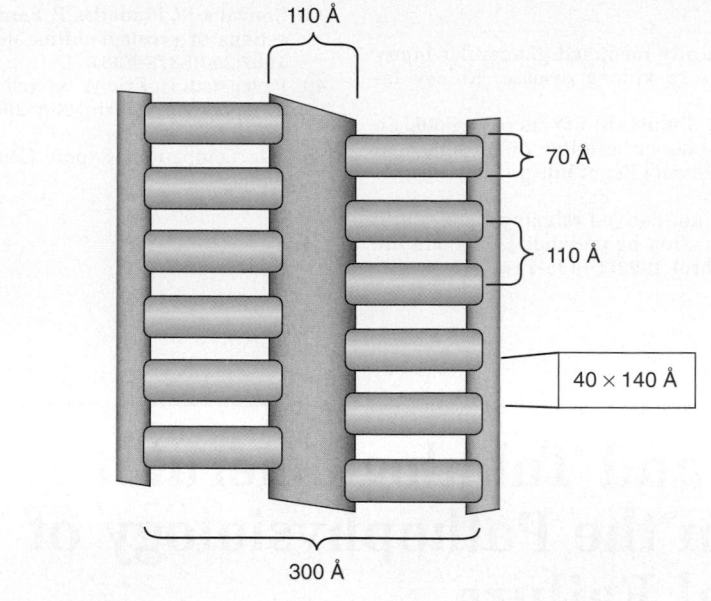

A

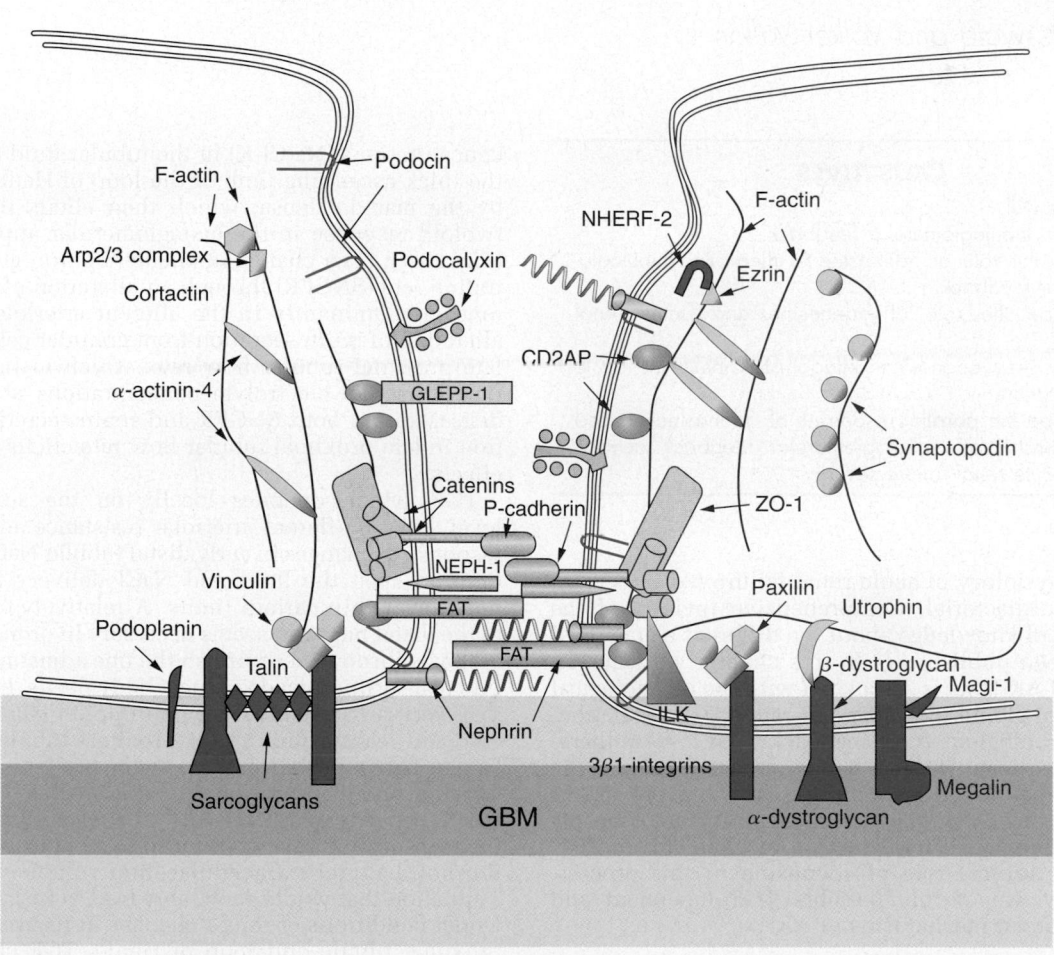

B

FIGURE 22-1. Changes in understanding of the podocyte slit diaphragm over 30 years. **A,** Model proposed by Rodewald and Karnovsky in 1974. **B,** Regulation of the key molecules of glomerular ultrafiltration in proteinuric models as determined by 2002. Arp2/3, actin-related protein-2/3; CD2AP, CD2-associated protein; FAT, fatty acid transporter tumor suppressor homolog; GBM, glomerular basement membrane; GLEPP-1, glomerular epithelial protein-1; Magi-1, membrane-associated guanylate-kinase with an inverted arrangement of protein-protein interaction domain 1; NEPH-1, nephrin-like Ig cell adhesion molecule; NHERF-2, Na$^+$/H$^+$-exchanger regulatory factor 2; ZO-1, zonula occludens-1. (Modified from Luimula P, Sandstrom N, Novikov D, Holthofer H: Podocyte-associated molecules in puromycin aminonucleoside nephrosis of the rat. Lab Invest 2002;82:713-718.)

Key References

4. Brenner BM: Hemodynamically mediated glomerular injury and the progressive nature of kidney disease. Kidney Int 1983;23:647-655.
12. Denton KM, Anderson WP, Sinniah R: Effects of angiotensin II on regional afferent and efferent arteriole dimensions and the glomerular pole. Am J Physiol Regul Integr Comp Physiol 2000;279:R629-R638.
16. Raij L, Shultz PJ: Endothelium-derived relaxing factor, nitric oxide: Effects on and production by mesangial cells and the glomerulus. J Am Soc Nephrol 1993;3:1435-1441.
17. Bonvalet JP, Pradelles P, Farman N: Segmental synthesis and actions of prostaglandins along the nephron. Am J Physiol 1987;253:F377-F387.
40. Pavenstadt H, Kriz W, Kretzler M: Cell biology of the glomerular podocyte. Physiol Rev 2003;83:253-307.

See the companion Expert Consult website for the complete reference list.

CHAPTER 23

Adenosine and Tubuloglomerular Feedback in the Pathophysiology of Acute Renal Failure

Hartmut Osswald and Volker Vallon

OBJECTIVES

This chapter will:
1. Explain tubuloglomerular feedback.
2. Define the role of adenosine in mediating tubuloglomerular feedback.
3. Describe the role of adenosine and acute renal failure.
4. Clarify how adenosine antagonists ameliorate acute renal failure.
5. Describe the parallel responses of adenosine-induced vasoconstriction, tubuloglomerular feedback activity, and acute renal failure severity.

The pathophysiology of acute renal failure (ARF) is complex and multifactorial. Comprehensive reviews of the current state of knowledge about the different elements of ARF have been published.[1-3] In this chapter we focus on one aspect of ARF that is associated with the physiological mechanism of glomerular filtration rate (GFR) regulation, known as tubuloglomerular feedback (TGF). New therapeutic options result from a better understanding of the pathophysiology of ARF, including possible preventive measures. In this chapter, we discuss the current concepts involved in the signal transduction mechanisms of TGF, stressing the critical role of adenosine in this process. Subsequently, we outline possible TGF-dependent and TGF-independent mechanisms of ARF.

ADENOSINE AND TUBULOGLOMERULAR FEEDBACK

TGF consists of a series of events whereby changes in the sodium (Na^+), chloride (Cl^-), and potassium (K^+) ion concentrations (Na-Cl-K) in the tubular fluid at the end of the thick ascending limb of the loop of Henle are sensed by the macula densa, which then elicits the following twofold response in the juxtaglomerular apparatus (JGA) (Fig. 23-1): (1) a change in single-nephron glomerular filtration rate (SNGFR) through an alteration of the vascular tone, predominantly in the afferent arteriole and (2) an alteration of renin secretion from granular cells.[4] A rise in late proximal tubular flow rate, which in turn increases the respective electrolyte concentrations at the macula densa, lowers both SNGFR and renin secretion; a reduction in late proximal tubular flow rate elicits the opposite effects.

TGF, which operates locally on the single-nephron level, adjusts afferent arteriolar resistance and SNGFR in response to changes in early distal tubular NaCl concentrations to keep the fluid and NaCl delivery to the distal nephron within certain limits. A relatively constant load to the distal nephron seems necessary in order for this part of the nephron to accomplish the fine adjustments in absolute reabsorption made to meet body needs. In this regard, TGF serves to establish an appropriate balance between GFR and reabsorption in the proximal tubule and loop of Henle. The importance of the symmetry between nephron filtration and reabsorption can be appreciated from the fact that a disparity of as little as 5% between filtered load and the reabsorption rate would lead to a net loss of about one third of the total extracellular fluid volume within 1 day, a situation that would inevitably lead to vascular collapse. Under conditions of minor changes in reabsorption in the proximal tubule and loop of Henle, TGF contributes to autoregulation of GFR by adjusting afferent arteriolar resistance and SNGFR in order to keep early distal tubular fluid and NaCl delivery constant. Because the amount of fluid and NaCl filtered in the glomeruli determines reabsorption and, thus, energy demand in the tubular and collecting duct system, TGF, by affecting GFR, contributes to the *metabolic control* of kidney function (for a review, see also Vallon et al[5]).

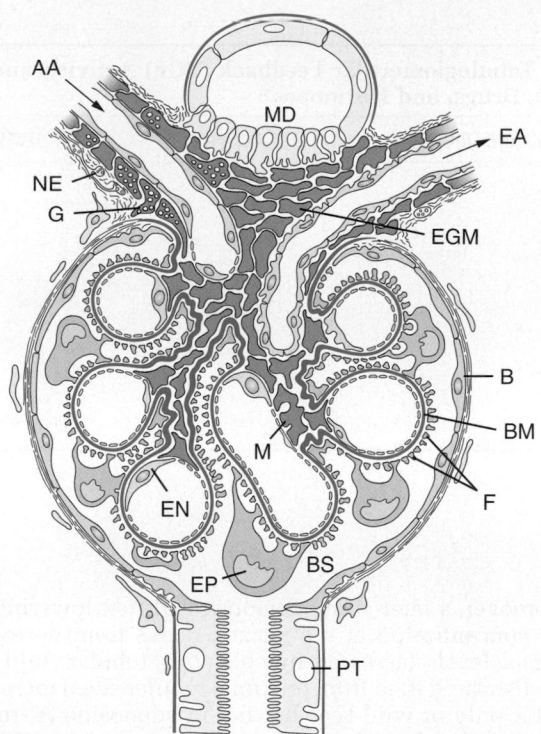

FIGURE 23-1. Schematic drawing of a cross-section through a glomerulus. The macula densa (MD) segment of the tubular epithelium at the end of the thick ascending limb of the loop of Henle is located at the vascular pole, with the afferent arteriole (AA) entering and the efferent arteriole (EA) leaving the glomerulus. The renin-secreting granular cells (G) in the wall of the afferent arteriole are in close proximity to sympathetic nerve endings (NE) and to the extraglomerular mesangium (EGM), which is connected to the intraglomerular mesangium (M). B, Bowman's capsule; BM, glomerular basement membrane; BS, Bowman's space; EN, fenestrated endothelial cells; EP, epithelial podocytes with foot processes (F); PT, cell from the proximal tubule at its beginning. (Courtesy of Dr. Wilhelm Kriz, Rolf Nonnenmacher, and Dr. Brigitte Kaissling.)

TGF can be divided into the following steps:
1. The luminal signal in the tubular fluid, which is sensed by the macula densa.
2. Signal transduction by the macula densa/extraglomerular mesangium to generate factors that act in step 3.
3. These factors ultimately exert effects at the afferent arterioles, including vascular smooth muscle cells and renin-containing cells (see Fig. 23-1).

There is agreement that the luminal signal is *primarily* recognized by the Na^+-$2Cl^-$-K^+ cotransporter, which is located in the luminal membrane of macula densa cells. By which mechanism the macula densa cells transform this signal to generate the mediators, however, is not fully understood.

Various factors have been suggested to be involved in signal transmission of the TGF response. What would be the functional requirements for a factor that could mediate these minute-to-minute responses? First, the factor must have a rapid (within seconds) onset of action, because the change in vascular tone after an increase in luminal electrolyte concentration in the tubular fluid at the macula densa occurs with a delay of only a few seconds.[6,7] Second, the duration of the vascular response

has to be short and must be fully reversible within seconds.[7] Third, the factor must be generated locally in the JGA, because other nephrons in close proximity to the perfused nephron do not respond to the stimulus if the blood supply originates from a different cortical radial artery.[5,8-10] Fourth, the factor must be generated or released independent of the Na^+-$2Cl^-$-K^+ cotransporter at the macula densa. Furthermore, substances acting synergistically with the factor should enhance the TGF response, whereas substances acting antagonistically to the factor should be inhibitory. Because the TGF response includes an inhibition of renin secretion after an elevation in NaCl concentration at the macula densa, the factor may also have an inhibitory action on renin release. As outlined in the next section, experimental evidence has been reported that adenosine fulfills the preceding criteria. The review by Vallon and associates[5] describes the renal actions of adenosine in more detail.

Altering Tubuloglomerular Feedback Responses by Manipulating Adenosine Receptor Activation or Adenosine Formation

Adenosine may contribute to signal transduction in TGF because (1) it reduces glomerular capillary pressure and SNGFR by predominant afferent arteriolar vasoconstriction and (2) this response is rapid in onset and short in duration when the adenosine delivery is discontinued.[7,11-19] Table 23-1 summarizes the interactions between different conditions and factors and the renal vasoconstriction mediated by adenosine as well as TGF activity. Furthermore, adenosine inhibits renin release even at concentrations that are well below those inducing vasoconstriction.[19-25] Most importantly, with the use of *unselective* adenosine receptor antagonists, such as theophylline or PSPX, it is possible to inhibit the TGF response of the nephron.[19,26,27] Subsequent studies, using selective adenosine A_1 receptor antagonists like DPCPX, KW-3902, CVT-124, and FK838, revealed a predominant role for adenosine A_1 receptors in the TGF mechanism.[13,28-31]

Manipulating local adenosine formation, Osswald and associates[18] observed that infusion of the adenosine deaminase inhibitor erythro-9-(2-hydroxy-3-nonyl)adenine, which is supposed to reduce adenosine degradation, potentiated the TGF response. Similarly, dipyridamole, which inhibits cellular adenosine uptake and thus elevates extracellular adenosine levels, potentiated the maximum TGF response.[19] With regard to aspects of pathophysiology, it has been shown that the activity of TGF is reduced in early experimental diabetes mellitus.[32,33] In this condition, long-term dipyridamole treatment not only normalized maximum TGF responses but also prevented glomerular hyperfiltration and lowered proteinuria.[33] In contrast to the previously described experiments with dipyridamole, infusion of adenosine deaminase, which is supposed to degrade adenosine and thus lower extracellular adenosine concentrations, attenuated the TGF-mediated drop in SFP.[18] Similarly, local application of the ecto-5'-nucleotidase inhibitor α,β-methyleneadenosine-5'-diphosphate (AMPCP), which inhibits the conversion of AMP to adenosine, was found to attenuate the TGF response.[31,34] Thus, maneuvers that lower local adenosine concentrations also reduce TGF responses, and maneuvers that raise local adenosine concentrations enhance TGF responses.

TABLE 23-1

Parallel Response of Adenosine (ADO)–Induced Vasoconstriction, Tubuloglomerular Feedback (TGF) Activity, and Severity of Acute Renal Failure (ARF) to Experimental Conditions, Drugs, and Hormones*

	ADO-INDUCED VASOCONSTRICTION	TGF ACTIVITY	ARF SEVERITY
Conditions			
Low-salt diet, volume depletion, or hemorrhage	↑[114]	↑[75-78]	↑[1,2]
High-salt diet or volume expansion	↓[25,114]	↓[128]	↓[1,2]
Drugs/hormones			
ADO A1 receptor antagonists	↓[125,129]	↓[13,18,19]	↓[84-92,94-104]
Angiotensin II	↑[114,130-132]	↑[69-74]	↑[1,2,148]
Angiotensin II blockade	↓[18,132,133]	↓[140-142]	↓[149]
Nitric oxide synthase inhibition	↑[134]	↑[79-83]	↓↔↑[150-152]
Cyclooxygenase inhibition	↑[135-137]	↑[143-145]	↑[153-160]
Reduction in ADO reuptake	↑[7,129,138]	↑[18,19,32]	↑[129]
Calcium antagonists	↓[139]	↓[146,147]	↓[161-166]

*Superscript numbers indicate chapter references.
↑, increased; ↓, decreased; ↔, no change.

Absence of Tubuloglomerular Feedback Response in Adenosine A₁ Receptor–Deficient Mice

In 2001, two groups investigated the role of adenosine A₁ receptors in TGF response by generating independently knockout mice for the adenosine A₁ receptor (Fig. 23-2B and C). Sun and colleagues[35] observed that the TGF response, assessed as the fall in SFP or early proximal flow rate during an increase in loop of Henle perfusion from 0 to 30 nL/min, was completely absent in adenosine A₁ receptor–deficient mice. Similarly, Brown and coworkers[36] showed that the TGF response, assessed as the fall in SFP during perfusion of Henle's loop at 0 and 35 nL/min, was abolished in adenosine A₁ receptor–deficient mice.[36]

Moreover, a later study demonstrated that lowering the NaCl concentration at the macula densa from normal to minimal levels (assessed by collecting tubular fluid first from distal and then from proximal tubular sites) increased SNGFR only in wild-type but not in adenosine A₁ receptor–deficient mice. These results indicate a tonic, SNGFR-depressing effect of the NaCl concentration at the macula densa that depends on intact adenosine A₁ receptors.[37] Further experiments in these knockout mice demonstrated the role of adenosine A₁ receptor– and TGF-mediated control of GFR in stabilizing the Na⁺ delivery to the distal tubule and showed a lack of *spontaneous* oscillations in proximal tubular hydrostatic pressure in knockout mice[38,39]—which, as suggested originally by Leyssac and coworkers,[38] are caused by the operation of TGF. Presumably in relation to the absence of TGF regulation, autoregulation of renal vascular resistance is reduced in adenosine A₁ receptor–knockout mice.[40]

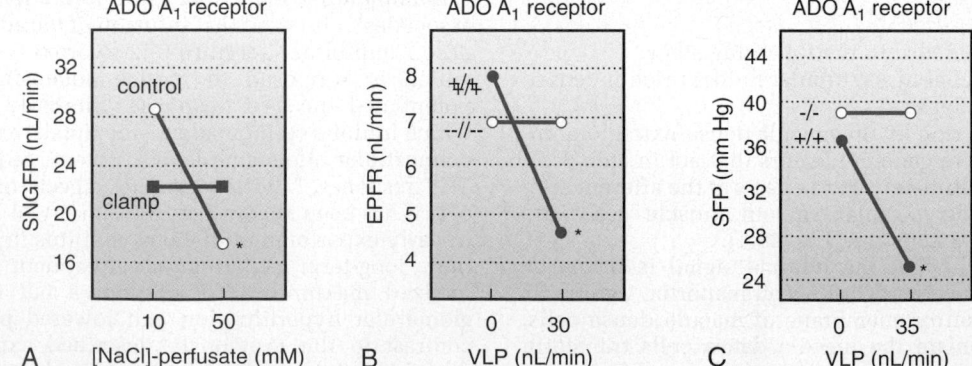

FIGURE 23-2. Tubuloglomerular feedback responses in rats with inhibition of ADO A₁ receptor activation (**A**), and in wild-type mice (+/+) and mice deficient (–/–) in adenosine (ADO) A₁ receptor (**B** and **C**). **A**, Clamping of ADO A₁ receptor activation (see text for procedure) blunted TGF response, which was assessed as the change in single-nephron GFR (SNGFR; measured by paired proximal collections) during retrograde perfusion of the macula densa segment from the early distal tubule with artificial tubular perfusate containing either 10 or 50 mM NaCl to induce minimum and maximum stimulation of TGF. *P < .05 vs. 10 mM. (Adapted from Thomson S, Bao D, Deng A, Vallon V: Adenosine formed by 5′-nucleotidase mediates tubuloglomerular feedback. J Clin Invest 2000;106:289-298.) **B** and **C**, The response in early proximal flow rate (EPFR) or proximal stop-flow pressure (SFP) to an increase in loop of Henle perfusion rate (VLP) is blunted in –/– mice. *P < .05 vs. 0 nL/min loop perfusion. (Adapted from Sun D, Samuelson LC, Yang T, et al: Mediation of tubuloglomerular feedback by adenosine: Evidence from mice lacking adenosine 1 receptors. Proc Natl Acad Sci U S A 2001;98:9983-9988; and Brown R, Ollerstam A, Johansson B, et al: Abolished tubuloglomerular feedback and increased plasma renin in adenosine A₁ receptor-deficient mice. Am J Physiol Regul Integr Comp Physiol 2001;281:R1362-R1367.)

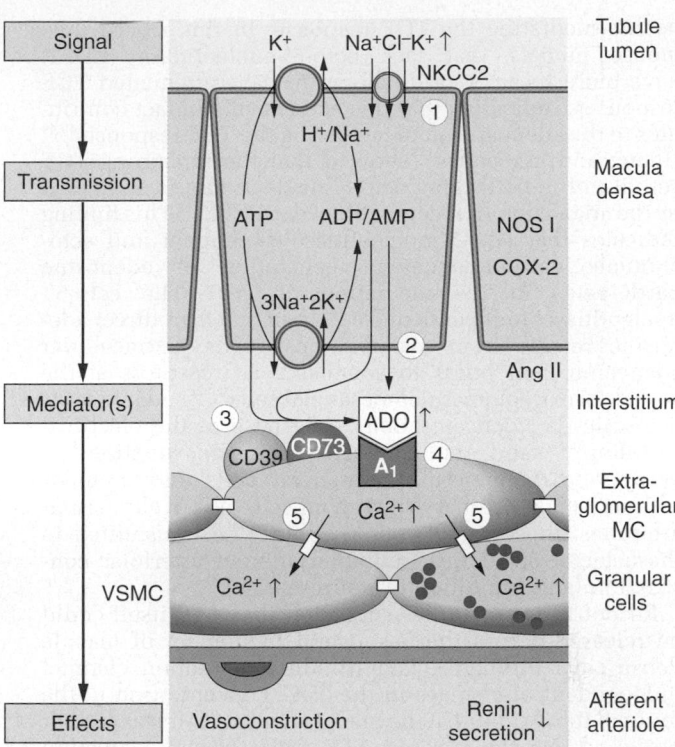

FIGURE 23-3. Proposed mechanism of adenosine acting as a *mediator* of tubuloglomerular feedback. Numbers in *circles* refer to the following sequence of events: *1*, Increase in concentration-dependent uptake of Na^+, K^+, and Cl^- via the furosemide-sensitive Na^+-K^+-$2Cl^-$ cotransporter (NKCC2); *2* and *3*, transport-dependent, intracellular and/or extracellular generation of adenosine (ADO); the extracellular generation involves ecto-NTPDase$_1$ (CD39) and ecto-5'-nucleotidase (CD73); *4*, extracellular ADO activates adenosine A_1 receptors, triggering an increase in cytosolic Ca^{2+} in extraglomerular mesangium cells (MC); *5*, the intensive coupling between extraglomerular MC, granular cells containing renin, and smooth muscle cells of the afferent arteriole (VSMC) by gap junctions allows propagation of the increased Ca^{2+} signal, resulting in afferent arteriolar vasoconstriction and inhibition of renin release. Factors such as nitric oxide, arachidonic acid breakdown products, and angiotensin (Ang) II *modulate* the described cascade. ADP, adenosine diphosphate; AMP, adenosine monophosphate; ATP, adenosine triphosphate; COX-2, cyclooxygenase-2; NOS I, neuronal nitric oxide synthase. See text for further explanation. (Adapted from Vallon V, Muhlbauer B, Osswald H: Adenosine and kidney function. Physiol Rev 2006;86:901-940.)

Adenosine Is a Mediator of Tubuloglomerular Feedback

The preceding findings demonstrate that adenosine and adenosine A_1 receptors are involved in macula densa control of GFR. The exact role of adenosine, however, was not addressed in the experiments described. Adenosine in the interstitium of the JGA could establish a relatively constant vasoconstrictor tone that provides a necessary background for another mediator to elicit the TGF response; thus, adenosine may act as a *modulator* of TGF. Alternatively, intact TGF may require local adenosine concentrations in the JGA to fluctuate directly independent of the luminal NaCl concentrations at macula densa, implying that adenosine is a *mediator* of TGF. To address this issue, Thomson and colleagues performed micropuncture experiments in which local adenosine A_1 receptor activation at the JGA was clamped through a combination of pharmacological inhibition of ecto-5'-nucleotidase (and thus adenosine generation) by AMPCP and adding back constant amounts of the adenosine A_1 receptor agonist CHA.[31] If local adenosine merely induces a relatively constant adenosine A_1 receptor–mediated vasoconstrictor tone to establish a necessary background for another mediator to elicit the TGF response, the preceding maneuver should not inhibit the TGF response. It was observed, however, that this maneuver significantly reduced the slope of the TGF curve (i.e., SNGFR responses to small changes in late proximal flow rate) in free-flow experiments. Moreover, inhibition of adenosine A_1 receptor activation as described completely inhibited the fall in SNGFR in response to retrograde perfusion of the macula densa segment from early distal tubular site with low and then high NaCl concentrations in the perfusate (see Fig. 23-2A).[31] Thus, TGF is attenuated by adenosine A_1 receptor blockade or inhibition of ecto-5'-nucleotidase–mediated generation of ade-

nosine and cannot be restored by establishing a constant adenosine A_1 receptor activation. These findings suggest that local adenosine concentration must fluctuate for normal TGF to occur, indicating that adenosine is a *mediator* of TGF.[31]

The concept proposed by Osswald and colleagues in 1980,[19] that adenosine couples energy metabolism with the control of GFR (and renin secretion)—that is, adenosine acts as a *mediator* of TGF—could be realized in the following manner (Fig. 23-3): Transport-dependent hydrolysis of ATP in macula densa cells (or in the cells of the thick ascending limb in close proximity to the JGA) would lead to enhanced generation of AMP. Involved ATPases include basolateral Na^+-K^+-ATPase, which extrudes the Na^+ taken up across the apical membrane. A 2006 study provided evidence for the role of basolateral Na^+-K^+-ATPase in the TGF response.[41] In addition, Na^+ may leave the macula densa cells via an $(Na^+)H^+/K^+$-ATPase that is expressed in the apical membrane (see Fig. 23-3).[42,43] The AMP generated by these ATPases is dephosphorylated in the cell to adenosine by cytosolic 5'-nucleotidase and the generated adenosine could be released through a nucleoside transporter into the interstitium of the extraglomerular mesangium. NaCl transport–dependent release of endogenous adenosine has been demonstrated in the perfused shark rectal gland, a model epithelium for hormone-stimulated electrolyte transport[44] as well as medullary thick ascending limb.[45,46] Alternatively or in addition, AMP may leave the macula densa cells, and then plasma membrane-bound ecto-5'-nucleotidase may convert it to adenosine in the interstitium.

The 5'-nucleotidase inhibitor AMPCP, which was shown by previously described micropuncture studies[31] to inhibit TGF, is supposed to inhibit plasma membrane–bound ecto-5'-nucleotidase but not AMP-specific cytosolic 5'-nucleotidase.[47] Thus, plasma membrane–bound ecto- or cytosolic 5'-nucleotidase may serve to generate the adenosine mediating the TGF response. In this regard, two mouse models that lack ecto-5'-nucleotidase (CD73) have more recently been shown to have attenuated TGF responses, indicating that this ectoenzyme in fact contributes to the adenosine pool mediating the TGF response.[48,49] Huang and associates[49] showed that the remaining TGF activity of mice lacking ecto-5'-nucleotidase is abolished by the adenosine A_1 receptor blocker DPCPX.[49] This finding indicates that ecto-5'-nucleotidase–dependent and ecto-5'-nucleotidase–independent generation of adenosine participates in the mediation of TGF. The ecto-5'-nucleotidase–independent fraction may reflect direct adenosine release from macula densa cells. Extracellular adenosine then binds to adenosine A_1 receptors at the surface of extraglomerular mesangial cells[50-53] and increases cytosolic Ca^{2+} concentrations.[54] Because of the electrical coupling[55,56] and the connection by gap junctions[57,58] between extraglomerular mesangial cells and granular cells as well as ordinary smooth muscle cells of glomerular arterioles, these signals could rapidly be transmitted to these target structures, inducing afferent arteriolar constriction (and inhibition of renin release).

Recent in vitro studies suggested that ATP itself could be released across the basolateral membrane of macula densa cells through a large-conductance anion channel independent of changes in the NaCl concentration in the luminal tubular fluid at the macula densa.[59,60] It was further proposed that the released ATP itself, through activation of purinergic P_2 receptors, triggers an increase in cytosolic Ca^{2+} in the extraglomerular mesangium cells and/or the smooth muscle cells of the afferent arteriole, and thus, ATP acts as the principal *mediator* of TGF.[60,61] Even though substantial evidence points to a role for ATP and P_2X_1 receptors in renal autoregulation,[34,62] the role of P_2 receptors in the TGF response remains unclear. Ren and colleagues,[34] microperfusing rabbit afferent arterioles and attached macula densa cells simultaneously in vitro, found that adding the P_2 purinergic receptor inhibitor suramin to both arteriole lumen and bath did not significantly inhibit the TGF response.[34] If, however, one considers the previously described existing evidence for adenosine, ecto-5'-nucleotidase, and adenosine A_1 receptors in *mediating* TGF, it seems possible that ATP being released from the macula densa is converted in the interstitium by ecto-ATPase and ecto-5'-nucleotidase to adenosine. In fact, mice lacking ecto-NTPDase1/CD39, an enzyme that converts ATP and ADP to AMP,[63] also have an attenuated TGF response.[64] Thus, a model could be envisioned in which both ATP and adenosine would be considered *mediators* of TGF because both are released and generated, respectively, independent of the NaCl concentration at the macula densa and both are part of a signaling cascade in which adenosine via adenosine A_1 receptor activation triggers the final effects of the TGF response, that is, preglomerular vasoconstriction. This concept does not exclude the possibility that other factors, such as prostaglandins and nitric oxide, may be involved in the process of TGF signaling.

ACUTE RENAL FAILURE

Intrarenal Tubuloglomerular Feedback– Dependent Mechanisms

Acute renal failure is a syndrome in which GFR is greatly reduced with the consequence that the kidney cannot

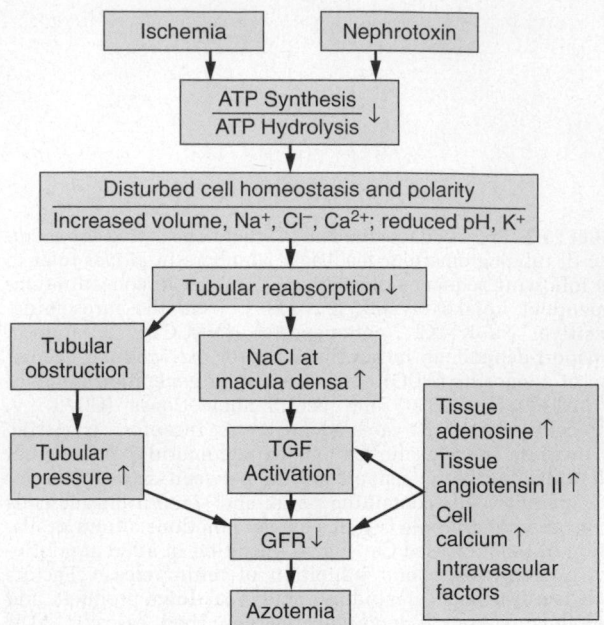

FIGURE 23-4. Schematic illustration of intrarenal mechanisms in acute renal failure. ATP, adenosine triphosphate; GFR, glomerular filtration rate; TGF, tubuloglomerular feedback. ↑, increased; ↓, decreased. See text for further explanation.

excrete metabolic waste products even though renal blood flow and urine flow can be maintained. Here we discuss mainly those forms of ARF that are caused by intrarenal mechanisms. Renal ischemia or administration of nephrotoxic substances can lead to ARF. As depicted schematically in Figure 23-4, both ischemia and nephrotoxic substances damage kidney cells and impair cellular phosphorylation potential through a decrease in ATP synthesis and/or an increase in ATP hydrolysis. The immediate result of a reduced phosphorylation potential is impaired tubular reabsorption of electrolytes, which in turn leads to an increase in the NaCl concentration in the tubular fluid at the macula densa, followed by a TGF-mediated drop in GFR.[65-68]

Under normal conditions, maximal TGF activation lowers ambient GFR by approximately 20%. Such a reduction of GFR could not account for severe forms of ARF. In addition, a sustained increase in late proximal tubular flow rate (causing a parallel change in the NaCl concentration in the tubular fluid at the macula densa) has been shown to attenuate TGF activity within 30 minutes by resetting the mechanisms of TGF.[69] Thus, in order for TGF to play a substantial role in the reduction of GFR in ARF, additional mechanisms that may increase maximal TGF activity or affect TGF resetting must be involved. Factors that can increase the activity of TGF are activation of the renin-angiotensin system,[70-75] contraction of the extracellular volume as seen also in hemorrhage,[76-78] nitric oxide synthase inhibition,[79-83] and maneuvers that increase interstitial adenosine concentration.[18,19,32]

As shown in Table 23-1, these factors also aggravate ARF. Most of the factors that attenuate TGF activity, such as extracellular volume expansion, calcium antagonists, and adenosine antagonists, ameliorate renal function in different models of ARF (see Table 23-1 for references). Theophylline or other adenosine receptor antagonists, for instance, have been used to treat ARF in laboratory animals and humans (for review, see also Vallon and colleagues[5]). Adenosine antagonists have been found to improve renal function in the following models of ARF: 1-hour renal artery clamping,[84-87] administration of glycerol,[88-92] uranyl nitrate,[85] radiological contrast media,[83,93-97] amphotericin B administration,[98] cisplatin application,[99-102] myoglobinuric ARF,[103] and endotoxin-induced ARF.[104]

Intrarenal "Tubuloglomerular Feedback–Independent" Mechanisms

TGF is a mechanism that operates in a highly specialized local structure. In ARF, however, some of the known elements in the cascade of TGF signal transmission, such as angiotensin II and adenosine, can be generated and act independently of TGF. Tubular cells in close proximity to the afferent arteriole could release vasoactive autacoids (adenosine, angiotensin II, prostaglandins, nitric oxide) at an enhanced rate *independent* of macula densa signal. Those autacoids can reduce GFR not only through vasoconstriction of the afferent arteriole or by decreasing glomerular ultrafiltration coefficient (K_f) but also through postglomerular vasodilation resulting in a drop in hydrostatic pressure of the glomerular capillaries. Thus, adenosine, which can induce postglomerular vasodilatation at micromolar concentrations,[105-108] could contribute to a more pronounced fall in GFR. This sequence of events, preglomerular vasoconstriction and postglomerular vasodilatation, was considered most important in the pathophysiology of ARF in humans.[109] Thus, translation of results obtained in experimental animals into the situation in humans appears to be justified because the vascular response of human kidneys to adenosine is very similar to that of dog or rat kidneys.[110-114]

The time course of ARF allows differentiation of initiating and sustaining factors. If, for instance, the actual sensitivity of the renal vasculature to constricting factors such as adenosine is markedly enhanced, resulting in local ischemia, a vicious circle might be initiated, consisting of ischemia, fall in ATP, enhanced adenosine generation,[45,115-117] and further vasoconstriction (see Fig. 23-4). Nephrotoxic substances and ischemia can lead, through cell damage, to disintegration and formation of cellular debris such as detached brush-border membranes. This material may lead to tubular obstruction, especially when tubular flow rate is low as in oliguric-anuric forms of ARF. The acute tubular obstruction can eventually stop glomerular filtration. Constant tubular obstruction for 24 hours at the nephron and whole kidney level leads to sustained preglomerular vasoconstriction.[118,119] This condition is accompanied by a 100-fold increase in potency of the vasoconstriction of adenosine.[119] Additional factors, such as the renin-angiotensin system and thromboxane, could contribute to changes in renal function in chronic ureteral obstruction.[120-123] Also, physical factors like cell swelling of tubule epithelial cells and vascular endothelium can interfere with the normal flow through renal tubules and blood vessels[124-126] independent of TGF. Taken together, the factors being generated by damaged tissue disturb the balance between vasoconstrictors and vasodilators that control the homeostasis of GFR. During the maintenance phase of ARF, the balance of these factors can be even more deranged owing to an inflammation-like reaction to the damaged tissue.

Because the TGF mechanism serves to establish a relatively constant delivery to the early distal tubule, a reduction in filtration rate would be an appropriate response to a signal indicating failure of volume reabsorption. This glomerular shutdown can, therefore, be considered an intrarenal reflex to conserve volume. Without this reflex, an unchanged high GFR in the presence of a reduced capability of the tubular epithelium to reabsorb would lead to massive urinary volume loss.[127] This advantage of the initial shutdown of GFR, however, if not reversible, would turn into the disadvantage of end-stage renal failure. Therefore, the therapeutic aim should be directed at reversing the initial phase of ARF.

CONCLUSION

In summary, activation of TGF can contribute to but may not fully account for the observed marked reduction of GFR in ARF. Sustaining factors can differ from initiating factors of ARF. In the early phase of ARF, therapeutic strategies directed to attenuation of TGF activity may be successful. To what extent TGF activity contributes to impairment of renal function during the maintenance phase of ARF is unclear at present.

Key Points

1. Tubuloglomerular feedback is an intrarenal mechanism to keep glomerular filtration rate constant.
2. The anatomical basis for tubuloglomerular feedback is the juxtaglomerular apparatus: the macula densa, cells of the extraglomerular mesangium, and the distal part of the afferent arteriole.
3. Tubuloglomerular feedback responds to the composition of the tubular fluid near the macula densa.
4. The macula densa cells release mediators that elicit vasoconstriction of the afferent arteriole and reduce renin release when sodium, chloride, and potassium concentrations rise in the tubular fluid.
5. Adenosine, the final mediator of the tubuloglomerular feedback response, is generated from enzymatic adenosine triphosphate hydrolysis by intracellular and extracellular pathways.
6. Blockade of adenosine A_1 receptors and inhibition of adenosine triphosphate–hydrolyzing enzymes abolish or attenuate tubuloglomerular feedback.
7. When nephrotoxic substances or ischemia reduces electrolyte reabsorption, tubuloglomerular feedback prevents loss of electrolytes and fluid.
8. Independent of tubuloglomerular feedback, a global increase of adenosine concentration in the kidney can elicit preglomerular vasoconstriction.
9. Enhanced tubuloglomerular feedback activity is associated with severity of acute renal failure in a large variety of experimental conditions, and adenosine may be an important pathophysiological factor in acute renal failure.

Acknowledgments

Work of the authors was supported by grants from the Deutsche Forschungsgemeinschaft (DFG OS 42/1- 42/7, DFG VA 118/2-1), the U.S. Department of Veterans Affairs (VV), and the National Institutes of Health (VV; DK56248 & DK28602).

Key References

5. Vallon V, Muhlbauer B, Osswald H: Adenosine and kidney function. Physiol Rev 2006;86:901-940.
31. Thomson S, Bao D, Deng A, Vallon V: Adenosine formed by 5'-nucleotidase mediates tubuloglomerular feedback. J Clin Invest 2000;106:289-298.

94. Erley CM, Duda SH, Schlepckow S, et al: Adenosine antagonist theophylline prevents the reduction of glomerular filtration rate after contrast media application. Kidney Int 1994;45:1425-1431.
100. Benoehr P, Krueth P, Bokemeyer C, et al: Nephroprotection by theophylline in patients with cisplatin chemotherapy: A randomized, single-blinded, placebo-controlled trial. J Am Soc Nephrol 2005;16:452-458.
131. Weihprecht H, Lorenz JN, Briggs JP, Schnermann J: Synergistic effects of angiotensin and adenosine in the renal microvasculature. Am J Physiol Renal Physiol 1994;266: F227-F239.

See the companion Expert Consult website for the complete reference list.

CHAPTER 24

The Physiology of the Proximal Tubule

Raymond Quigley

> ### OBJECTIVES
>
> This chapter will:
> 1. Explore the normal transport functions of the proximal tubule.
> 2. Describe the metabolic functions of the proximal tubule.
> 3. Explain the regulation of transport in the proximal tubule.
> 4. Review the pathophysiological disturbances of transport in the proximal tubule.

The kidney excretes nitrogenous wastes by filtering the blood. Clearance of the necessary amounts of waste products in an adult human requires that the kidneys filter about 150 liters per day. This places a large demand on the renal tubules to reclaim most of the filtered solutes and water so that the final urine volume is about 1% to 2% of the filtered load. The proximal tubule reabsorbs approximately two thirds to three fourths of the filtered load of fluid and sodium and more than 80% of some of the solutes, such as bicarbonate and glucose. In addition, the proximal tubule actively secretes several solutes and is involved in a number of metabolic functions. This chapter reviews the processes by which the proximal tubule achieves these functions as well as regulation of transport in the proximal tubule and the pathophysiological conditions that affect the proximal tubule.

STRUCTURE OF THE PROXIMAL TUBULE

The proximal tubule receives the ultrafiltrate from the glomerulus. This fluid is normally free of protein, and its electrolyte and solute composition is essentially the same as that of serum. The proximal tubule is an epithelium consisting of a single layer of cells that are oriented so that they separate the luminal fluid that eventually becomes urine and the interstitial fluid. The membrane surface in contact with the luminal compartment (*apical membrane*) has microvilli (*brush border*), and the surface in contact with the interstitium (*basolateral membrane*) has multiple infoldings to maximize the total surface area available for transport. The basolateral portion of the proximal tubule cells is rich in mitochondria, which provide the energy for its transport functions. The intercellular junctions have specialized proteins for maintaining the passive permeabilities across the epithelium. Thus, transport can be divided into active, transcellular transport and passive, paracellular transport. The advantage of active transport is that it can be highly regulated and the energy expenditure can be used to transport solutes against an electrochemical gradient. The advantage of passive transport is that it requires no additional energy.

The early part of the proximal tubule (proximal convoluted tubule) is located in the cortex of the kidney, a feature that is critical because the proximal convoluted tubule has a higher transport rate than the proximal straight tubule—the late portion of the proximal tubule—and thus has a higher energy demand. The cortex of the kidney receives the bulk of the renal blood flow and so can provide more energy to sustain the metabolic demand of the proximal convoluted tubule cells as well as carry the reabsorbed fluid and solutes into the bloodstream. The proximal straight tubule is located in the outer medulla, which receives less blood supply and has a lower oxygen tension than the cortex. This difference can present a problem during ischemia because the blood flow and oxygenation reaching the outer medulla can be more easily compromised. Therefore, the proximal straight tubule is more susceptible to ischemic damage, resulting in acute tubular necrosis.

TRANSPORT IN THE PROXIMAL TUBULE

Transport in the proximal tubule is driven primarily by sodium-potassium adenosine triphosphatase (ATPase), which is located in the basolateral membrane of the cell.[1,2] This enzyme maintains a low intracellular sodium concentration, which can then be used by transporters located in the apical membrane for secondary active transport (see Figs. 24-1 and 24-3). Most of the active transport processes in the proximal tubule are driven by this low intracellular sodium concentration by way of sodium-coupled transporters. I will discuss first the mechanisms involved in the reabsorption of bicarbonate and then the transport of the other principal solutes, namely chloride, glucose, phosphate, and amino acids.

Bicarbonate Transport

Most of the sodium crosses the proximal tubule cell's apical membrane by way of the sodium-hydrogen exchanger (NHE3).[3-5] This process exchanges one hydrogen ion (proton; H^+) for each sodium ion that enters the cell and is the first step in the reabsorption of bicarbonate (Fig. 24-1). Once the hydrogen ion enters the lumen of the tubule, it combines with a bicarbonate ion to form carbonic acid, as indicated in the following equation:

$$H^+ + HCO_3^- \leftrightarrow H_2CO_3 \xleftarrow[\text{anhydrase}]{\text{carbonic}} H_2O + CO_2$$

In the presence of carbonic anhydrase, located in the brush-border membrane, the carbonic acid is converted to

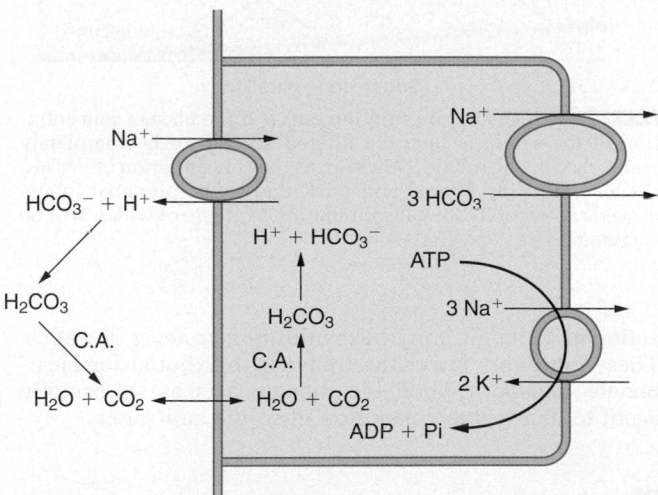

FIGURE 24-1. Bicarbonate reabsorption in the proximal tubule begins with proton (H^+) secretion via the sodium-hydrogen exchanger (NHE3). The proton then combines with bicarbonate (HCO_3^-) in the lumen to form carbonic acid (H_2CO_3), which is converted to carbon dioxide (CO_2) and water (H_2O) in the presence of carbonic anhydrase (C.A.). The CO_2 and H_2O enter the cell and recombine to form carbonic acid (also in the presence of intracellular C.A.), which then ionizes to bicarbonate and a hydrogen ion. The bicarbonate exits the cell via the basolaterally located sodium-bicarbonate cotransporter, NBC1. ADP, adenosine diphosphate; ATP, adenosine triphosphate; K^+, potassium ion; Na^+, sodium ion; Pi, phosphate.

carbon dioxide (CO_2) and water, which then enter the cell.[6,7] Intracellular carbonic anhydrase then catalyzes the recombining of the CO_2 and water into carbonic acid, which ionizes into bicarbonate and a hydrogen ion. The bicarbonate then exits the cell via the basolaterally located sodium-bicarbonate cotransporter (NBC1).[8-10] The proton can then be transported again through the apical membrane. By the end of the proximal tubule, about 80% of the filtered bicarbonate has been reabsorbed. In addition to the sodium-hydrogen exchanger, there is a proton pump (H^+-ATPase) located in the apical membrane that also secretes hydrogen ions through direct hydrolysis of ATP. It has been estimated that up to one third of the hydrogen ion secretion in the proximal tubule occurs via the H^+-ATPase.[11]

Sodium Chloride Transport

The sodium-hydrogen exchanger can also be used to transport sodium chloride actively through the tubule cell. This occurs because the intracellular pH rises after the hydrogen ion is transported into the lumen, providing a pH gradient for the chloride-base exchanger to allow the entry of a chloride ion into the cell through the apical membrane. The overall process of these parallel exchangers is to actively reabsorb sodium chloride in an electroneutral fashion.[12] There is evidence for a chloride-formate exchanger that secretes formate into the lumen of the tubule. The formate then becomes protonated and can diffuse back into the cell, where it ionizes back into formate and a hydrogen ion. The preceding process is the probable mechanism by which formate stimulates sodium chloride reabsorption in the proximal tubule.[13,14]

Passive Sodium Chloride Reabsorption

Another mechanism for reabsorption of sodium chloride in the proximal tubule is passive, paracellular transport. It occurs as a result of the preferential reabsorption of bicarbonate. In the early proximal tubule, there is more bicarbonate than chloride is reabsorbed. Thus, as the fluid travels along the length of the proximal tubule, the bicarbonate concentration decreases and the chloride concentration increases (Fig. 24-2). This provides a favorable gradient for the reabsorption of chloride through the intercellular junctions.[2] The junctions contain the appropriate tight junction proteins that allow for passive chloride reabsorption. The advantage to having passive reabsorption of sodium chloride is the conservation of energy.

Glucose Transport

The energy of the sodium gradient is used for reabsorption of most of the solutes that the proximal tubule reabsorbs. Glucose is a classic example. Early in the proximal tubule, there is a sodium-glucose cotransporter (SGLT2) that transports one sodium ion and one glucose molecule.[15,16] SGLT2 is a high-capacity, low-affinity transporter that is responsible for the bulk of glucose reabsorption. As the proximal tubule intracellular glucose concentration rises, glucose diffuses out through the basolateral membrane by means of a facilitative transporter (GLUT2).[17] As the luminal glucose concentration diminishes along the length of the tubule, the energy required for active transport across the apical membrane increases owing to the higher

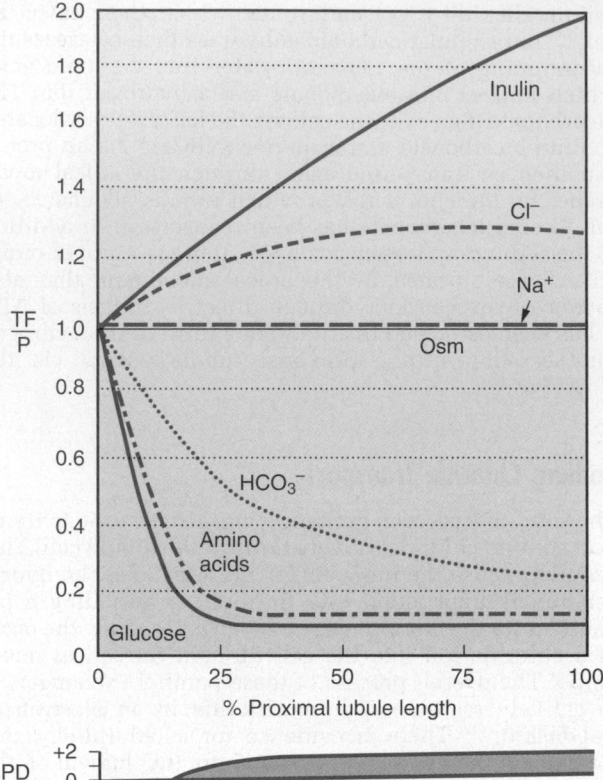

FIGURE 24-2. Concentrations of solutes found in the tubular fluid compared with plasma (TF/P) along the length of the proximal tubule. As can be seen, early in the proximal tubule, the TF/P value of these solutes is 1. Preferential reabsorption of bicarbonate (HCO_3^-) decreases the bicarbonate concentration along the tubule, whereas the concentration of chloride (Cl^-) rises as a consequence of fluid reabsorption. This process then provides a favorable gradient for passive reabsorption of chloride in the late proximal tubule. PD, potential difference. (From Rector FC: Sodium, bicarbonate, and chloride absorption by the proximal tubule. Am J Physiol Renal Physiol 1983;244:F461-F471.)

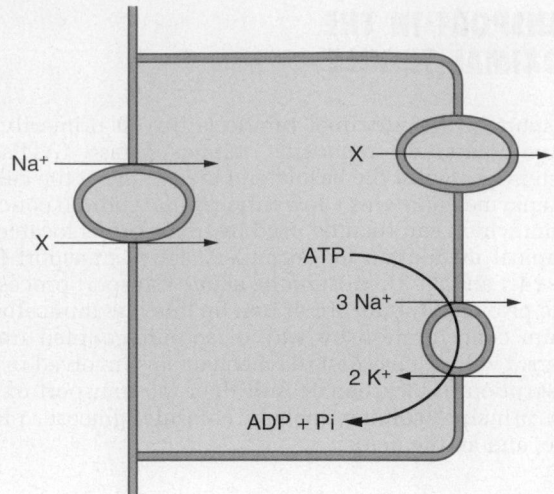

FIGURE 24-3. Sodium coupled reabsorption of solute X (e.g., glucose). The solute is taken up into the cell across the apical membrane because of the driving force of the sodium concentration gradient. The high intracellular concentration of the solute then allows for passive diffusion across the basolateral membrane via a facilitative transporter. ADP, adenosine diphosphate; ATP, adenosine triphosphate; K^+, potassium ion; Na^+, sodium ion; Pi, phosphate.

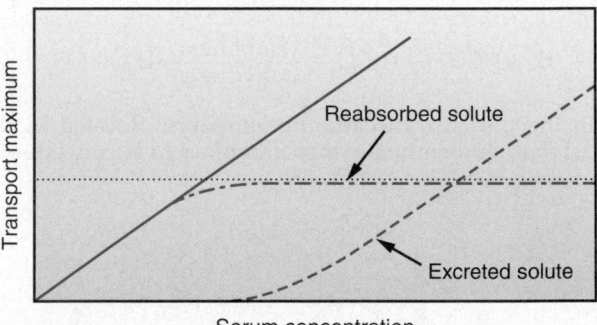

FIGURE 24-4. Reabsorption titration curve. If the plasma concentration of the solute is low, the filtered solute can be completely reabsorbed by the tubule. However, as the concentration increases, the amount being filtered and presented to the proximal tubule exceeds its capacity to reabsorb the solute, some of which will be excreted.

gradient for glucose transport. To provide this additional energy, the transporter in the final portion of the proximal tubule has a stoichiometry of two sodium ions to one glucose molecule (SGLT1). With this transporter, the proximal tubule can reabsorb virtually all of the filtered glucose. This process is illustrated in Figure 24-3. The mechanism is the model for reabsorption of most of the solutes that are reabsorbed in the proximal tubule and hence are represented as Na and *X* on the cotransporters. The stoichiometry varies according to the transporter involved.

One feature of this mechanism that is true for most of these solutes, including bicarbonate, is that the process is saturable. The rates at which the transporters can carry the solutes from the lumen of the tubule across to the interstitial fluid are finite. If the tubule is presented with more solute than it is capable of transporting, reabsorption is incomplete and the solute appears in the final urine (Fig. 24-4). As long as the filtered load of solute remains below the transport maximum, all of the filtered solute is reabsorbed. Once the transport maximum is exceeded, the excess solute is excreted. This is the basis for the osmotic diuresis found in the diabetic patient when the serum glucose concentration is elevated and exceeds the transport maximum for glucose. It is also the mechanism of

action for carbonic anhydrase inhibitors to act as diuretics. These inhibitors lower the transport maximum for bicarbonate transport. Then bicarbonate acts as an osmotic agent to increase the excretion of solute and water.

Phosphate Transport

Phosphate homeostasis in the body is regulated primarily by alterations in proximal tubule transport of phosphate. Under normal conditions, about 85% of the filtered phosphate is reabsorbed by the proximal tubule by means of the sodium-phosphate cotransporter (NaPi2).[18] The reabsorption can be significantly increased under conditions of low phosphate intake so that the body conserves phosphate. In the setting of a high phosphate intake, the tubule reabsorbs less of the filtered phosphate and a larger fraction is excreted. A number of hormones play a role in this regulation. Parathyroid hormone (PTH), one of the most potent hormonal regulators of phosphate transport, promotes renal excretion of phosphate. It has now become clear that the mechanism of action of PTH is to stimulate endocytosis of the NaPi2 cotransporters from the apical membrane of the proximal tubule cells.[18,19] The PTH receptor is a G protein–coupled receptor that stimulates the production of cyclic adenosine monophosphate (cAMP). Activation of protein kinase A (PKA) by cAMP then causes internalization of NaPi2. The mechanism by which this occurs serves as a paradigm for regulation of transport in the proximal tubule and has revealed the coordinated interaction of scaffolding proteins in the apical membrane of the tubule.[20-23]

Phosphotonins are another newly discovered class of regulators for phosphate transport.[24] Briefly, these factors inhibit phosphate transport and therefore promote phosphate excretion independently from PTH. They play a role in tumor-induced osteomalacia and in X-linked and autosomal dominant forms of hypophosphatemic rickets.[24]

Amino Acid Transport

Reabsorption of amino acids by the proximal tubule is much more complicated than that of glucose or phosphate. First, there are a number of different transporters for the various classes of amino acids (i.e., neutral, acidic, basic, dibasic).[25-28] Second, some of the transport proteins involved in amino acid transport exchange amino acids. Thus, although some amino acids are initially taken up by the cell, they are then secreted in exchange for another amino acid. In addition, some of the proteins that have been identified to participate in amino acid transport probably serve as accessory proteins and might not be directly involved in the uptake of the amino acid (e.g., rBAT [rat hepatic bile acid coenzyme A–amino acid N-acyltransferase] and cystine). Defects in amino acid transporters can lead to renal wasting of the involved amino acids. Hartnup's disease is an example of a defect in the neutral amino acid transporter.[27] Cystinuria is caused by a defect in the transporter for cystine.[29]

SECRETION IN THE PROXIMAL TUBULE

A number of organic molecules are actively secreted in the proximal tubule. The mechanism of secretion is similar to that of reabsorption, except that the transporters for uptake are located in the basolateral membrane.[30-33] The principal molecules that are secreted include creatinine and many drugs (e.g., penicillins). Probenecid has been used as an inhibitor for these transport processes. Other drugs, such as trimethoprim and cimetidine, also inhibit the transporters.

TRANSPORT OF WATER

Active transport of solutes in the proximal tubule leads to an intraluminal fluid that is hypo-osmotic compared with the blood. This state establishes a small but measurable osmotic gradient.[34] The proximal tubule has a very high osmotic water permeability, which is due, in part, to the presence of aquaporin 1 (water channels) in its apical and basolateral membranes.[35] Thus, the high permeability allows for the rapid movement of water and the nearly iso-osmotic reabsorption of the glomerular filtrate. In mice that lack the aquaporin 1 water channels, the water permeability of the proximal tubule is much lower than in the control mice, and these deficient mice have trouble conserving water.[36,37] However, the significance of the aquaporin 1 water channels in humans is not entirely clear. There are humans with mutations of the water channel who lead fairly normal lives.[38] The physiology and molecular biology of water channels have been the focus of a number of reviews.[39-41]

METABOLIC FUNCTIONS

In addition to the transport of solute and water, the proximal tubule has a number of metabolic functions. One of the more important is ammoniagenesis. Although the proximal tubule can reabsorb the bulk of the filtered load of bicarbonate, the reabsorption does not result in overall acid secretion but can only conserve the bicarbonate that is already in the body. In addition, if the body has accumulated acid (or has lost base equivalents in diarrhea), it must generate new bicarbonate. It does so by generating ammonia, which is then secreted into the lumen of the tubule for eventual excretion in the form of ammonium chloride. The enzymes for ammoniagenesis are located in the proximal tubule and are under the control of the acid-base balance.[42-44] Under conditions of acidosis, the kidney can more than double its production of ammonia so that the body can repair the base deficit that has accumulated.

Gluconeogenesis

The proximal tubule has all the enzymes for gluconeogenesis. The rate of glucose production by the kidney is second only to that by the liver. Thus, the kidney can play a crucial role in energy balance during states of hypoglycemia.

Vitamin D Synthesis

The proximal tubule is the site in the kidney for the 1α-hydroxylase enzyme in the synthetic pathway for vitamin D activation. This enzyme is primarily under the control of PTH.

REGULATION OF TRANSPORT

Transport in the proximal tubule is controlled by several factors. The ultimate goal is to preserve the body's volume status during times when the body is losing salt and water and is at risk for development of significant volume depletion such as diarrhea. The overall role of the proximal tubule in this setting is to reclaim a larger fraction of the filtered sodium and chloride to help preserve the extracellular fluid volume.

When the body becomes volume depleted, a number of events occur that prevent the ongoing loss of fluid through the kidney. First, the kidney secretes renin, ultimately leading to the production of angiotensin II, which has a number of effects. Angiotensin II affects the glomerular circulation by causing vasoconstriction of the efferent arteriole and increasing the filtration fraction (glomerular filtration rate/renal blood flow). As a result, the blood in the efferent arteriole has a higher than normal protein concentration. Thus, the peritubular capillaries have a higher oncotic pressure, which enhances the movement of fluid from the interstitium to the circulation, improving reabsorption of the glomerular filtrate by the proximal tubule.

Angiotensin II has also been shown to have direct effects on transport in the proximal tubule.[45] Receptors for this hormone are located in the proximal tubule. Direct effects of angiotensin II on proximal tubule transport were first demonstrated in isolated microperfused rabbit proximal tubules as well as in vivo microperfusion of rat tubules.[46-48] The effect was found to be biphasic, with a stimulation occurring at low concentrations and inhibition occurring at higher concentrations. The role of locally produced angiotensin II has also been investigated.[49] The proximal tubule contains all of the components needed to produce angiotensin II.[50] It then can directly affect transport in the proximal tubule. Under conditions of volume depletion, the angiotensin II stimulates a larger fraction of the transport, whereas volume expansion will blunt this response.

The second system that plays a role in increasing proximal tubule transport is the renal nerves.[51-53] The renal nerves are activated during volume depletion, and the norepinephrine causes the tubule to increase its transport rate. Norepinephrine has been shown to directly stimulate transport in the proximal tubule. The renal nerves might also regulate the local renin-angiotensin system.[51]

One factor that serves as a counterregulatory factor is dopamine. Dopamine has almost no effect on proximal tubule transport in the control state.[54] However, if the tubule is stimulated with norepinephrine, dopamine inhibits transport. The clinical significance of these findings is unclear at this time.

Another factor that controls transport in the proximal tubule is acid-base status. If the body becomes acidotic (e.g., as a result of diarrhea), the proximal tubule increases reabsorption of bicarbonate and bicarbonate equivalents such as citrate. When respiratory acidosis develops, the kidney attempts to correct the condition by reabsorbing more bicarbonate. During alkalosis, the transport of bicarbonate decreases to help correct the alkalosis. However, a number of factors limit the ability to excrete bicarbonate. The GFR is generally low because of volume depletion. Transport is also generally increased during volume depletion because of the previously mentioned factors. Thus, maintenance of metabolic alkalosis generally occurs because of continued volume depletion.

PATHOPHYSIOLOGICAL DISTURBANCES OF TRANSPORT IN THE PROXIMAL TUBULE

Because the proximal tubule reabsorbs the bulk of the glomerular filtrate, any dysfunction of the proximal tubule can lead to wasting of large amounts of fluid and solute. Global dysfunction of the proximal tubule, termed Fanconi's syndrome, results in bicarbonaturia (proximal renal tubular acidosis), glucosuria, phosphatu-

TABLE 24-1

Common Causes of Fanconi's Syndrome

Inherited causes	Cystinosis
	Tyrosinemia
	Inherited fructose intolerance
	Defects in glucose transporter GLUT2
	Defects in hepatocyte nuclear factor HNF1-α
Acquired causes	Gentamicin
	Valproic acid
	Ifosfamide
	Heavy metals (particularly, cadmium)
	Multiple myeloma

ria, and amino aciduria. Fanconi's syndrome can be caused by inherited disorders, drugs, or disease states (Table 24-1). The most common inherited cause of Fanconi's syndrome is cystinosis.[55,56] Common drugs that are associated with Fanconi's syndrome are gentamicin and valproic acid.

Another disease that affects the proximal tubule is Dent's disease. It is caused by defects in the CLC5 chloride channel. The exact mechanism by which the defect causes disease is not entirely clear, but it leads to low-molecular-weight proteinuria and, eventually, to Fanconi's syndrome and renal failure.[57]

As discussed previously, the proximal tubule has very high transport rates and consumes a large amount of energy. During shock, the proximal tubule (the proximal straight tubule in particular) is susceptible to the development of ATN. The proximal tubule is also sensitive to damage from a number of heavy metals, particularly cadmium.[58,59] Other drugs that cause proximal tubular dysfunction are cisplatinum and methotrexate.[60]

Key Points

1. The proximal tubule reabsorbs the bulk of the filtered load of solutes and water—for instance, 80% of filtered bicarbonate.
2. The proximal tubule is the primary regulator of the serum phosphate concentration.
3. The proximal tubule is responsible for ammoniagenesis and is a key player in acid-base regulation.
4. The proximal tubule activates vitamin D through the activity of the 1α-hydroxylase enzyme.
5. The proximal tubule participates in gluconeogenesis.
6. The proximal straight tubule is susceptible to ischemic injury and is a major site of acute tubular necrosis.
7. Injury to the proximal tubule can lead to Fanconi's syndrome, which can be difficult to treat because of the high rate of solute loss.

Key References

18. Forster IC, Hernando N, Biber J, Murer H: Proximal tubular handling of phosphate: A molecular perspective. Kidney Int 2006;70:1548-1559.

24. Schiavi SC, Moe OW: Phosphatonins: A new class of phosphate-regulating proteins. Curr Opin Nephrol Hypertens 2002;11:423-430.

29. Goodyer P: The molecular basis of cystinuria. Nephron Exp Nephrol 2004;98:e45-e49.

41. Nielsen S, Agre P: The aquaporin family of water channels in kidney. Kidney Int 1995;48:1057-1068.

56. Kalatzis V, Nevo N, Cherqui S, et al: Molecular pathogenesis of cystinosis: Effect of CTNS mutations on the transport activity and subcellular localization of cystinosin. Hum Mol Genet 2004;13:1361-1371.

See the companion Expert Consult website for the complete reference list.

CHAPTER 25

The Physiology of the Loop of Henle

Giovambattista Capasso, Francesco Trepiccione, and Miriam Zacchia

OBJECTIVES

This chapter will:

1. Define the structural-function correlation of the loop of Henle.
2. Discuss sodium transport and the countercurrent system.
3. Analyze, at the molecular level, the mechanisms and factors regulating bicarbonate reabsorption.
4. Examine the role of the loop of Henle in the renal handling of ammonia/ammonium ion.
5. Discuss the reabsorption of divalent cations.

The loop of Henle is a very complex segment characterized by at least two peculiar properties, its extreme heterogeneity and its particular anatomical configuration. This structure is defined anatomically as composing the pars recta of the proximal tubule (thick descending limb), the thin descending and ascending limbs, the thick ascending limb (TAL), and the macula densa. The loop of Henle is surrounded by tissue with increasing interstitial osmolality,[1] resulting from the noticeable addition of sodium, chloride, and urea contents,[2] which is accomplished through the countercurrent system. As shown by several investigators, medullary cells utilize cellular osmolytes to survive in this hypertonic environment.[2a] In addition to its role in continuing the reabsorption of solutes, this part of the nephron is responsible for the kidney's ability to generate a concentrated or dilute urine.[1,3]

SODIUM TRANSPORT AND THE COUNTERCURRENT SYSTEM

A major function of the loop of Henle is the creation and maintenance of the interstitial osmotic gradient that increases from the renal cortex ($\approx$290 mOsm/kg) to the tip of the medulla ($\approx$1200 mOsm/kg). The anatomical loop of Henle reabsorbs approximately 40% of filtered sodium, mostly in the TAL, and approximately 25% of filtered water in the pars recta and thin descending limb. The thin descending limb is permeable to water but relatively impermeable to sodium, whereas both the thin ascending limb and TAL are essentially impermeable to water.[4] Sodium is reabsorbed passively in the thin ascending limb but actively in the TAL. Active sodium reabsorption in the TAL is driven by the basolateral sodium pump (Na$^+$,K$^+$–adenosine triphosphatase [ATPase]), which maintains a low intracellular sodium concentration, allowing sodium entry from the lumen, mainly via the Na$^+$,K$^+$,2Cl$^-$ cotransporter.[5] This transporter, which is exclusively expressed along the loop of Henle, is the site of action of loop diuretics like furosemide. Sodium exits the cell via the sodium pump, and chloride and potassium exit via basolateral ion channels and a K$^+$,Cl$^-$ cotransporter. Potassium also recycles through apical membrane ROMK (renal outer medullary potassium) channels. Reentry of potassium into the tubular lumen is necessary for normal operation of the Na$^+$,K$^+$,2Cl$^-$ cotransporter, presumably because the availability of potassium is a limiting factor for the cotransporter.[6] Potassium recycling is also partly responsible for generating the lumen-positive potential difference (transepithelial voltage [V_{te}]) found in this segment. This V_{te} drives additional sodium reabsorption through the paracellular pathway: For each sodium ion reabsorbed transcellularly, another one is reabsorbed paracellularly. Other cations (potassium, calcium, magnesium) are also reabsorbed by this route. The reabsorption of sodium chloride along the TAL, in the absence of significant water reabsorption, is responsible for the hypertonicity of the tubular fluid leaving this segment—hence its other name: the diluting segment (Fig. 25-1).

The U-shaped, countercurrent arrangement of the loop of Henle, the differences in permeability of the descending and ascending limbs to sodium and water, and the active sodium reabsorption in the TAL are the basis of countercurrent multiplication and generation of the medullary osmotic gradient. Fluid entering the descending limb from the proximal tubule is isotonic ($\approx$290 mOsm/kg). However, the raised medullary osmolarity, resulting from sodium chloride reabsorption in the water-impermeable ascending limb, induces water reabsorption from the thin descending limb, thereby raising both the osmolarity and sodium chloride concentration of the fluid delivered to the ascending limb. These events, combined with continuing sodium chloride reabsorption in the ascending limb, result in a progressive increase in medullary osmolarity from corti-

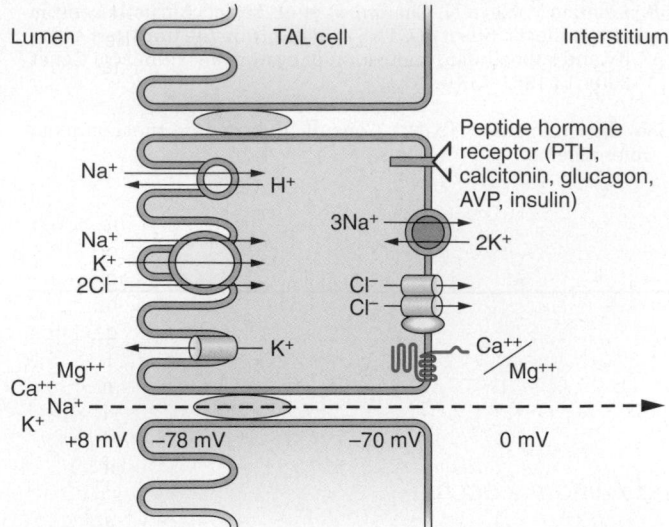

FIGURE 25-1. Schema of the thick ascending limb (TAL) cells with the main ion transport proteins localized on the luminal and basolateral membranes. Note the lumen's positive transepithelial potential difference. AVP, arginine vasopressin; Ca²⁺, calcium ion; Cl⁻, chloride ion; H⁺, hydrogen ion; K⁺, potassium ion; Mg⁺⁺, magnesium ion; mV, millivolt(s); Na⁺, sodium ion; PTH, parathyroid hormone.

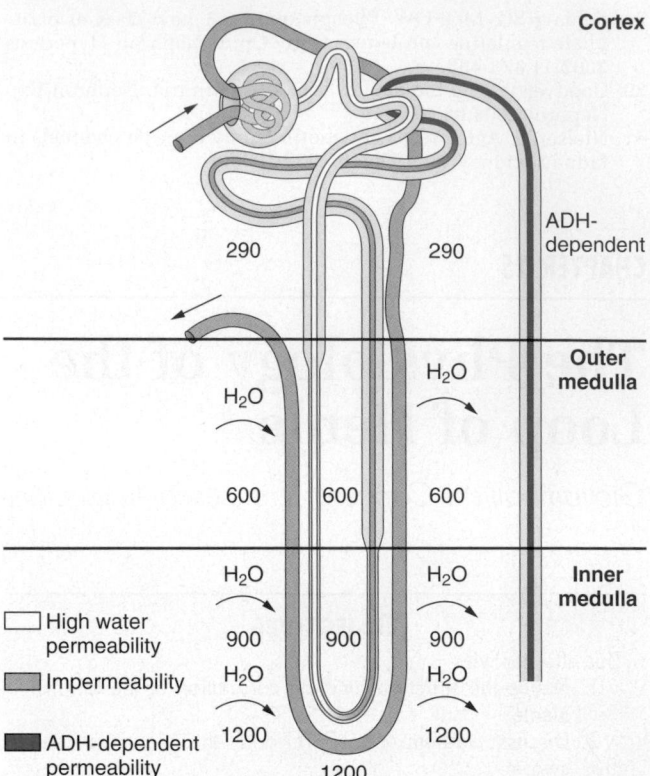

FIGURE 25-2. The U-shaped arrangements of the loop of Henle and vasa recta. The interstitial osmolality increases from the cortex (290 mOsm/kg H_2O) to the medulla (up to 1200 mOsm/kg H_2O). ADH, antidiuretic hormone; H_2O, water molecule.

comedullary junction to papillary tip. Thus, hypotonic (≈100 mOsm/kg) fluid is delivered to the distal tubule. It must be pointed out that the principal cause of countercurrent multiplication is active sodium reabsorption in the TAL (Fig. 25-2).

As already indicated, sodium reabsorption in the thin ascending limb is passive; this is likely due to a mechanism involving urea.[2] The thin limbs of the loop of Henle are relatively permeable to urea, but more distal nephron segments—TAL and beyond, up to the final part of the inner medullary collecting duct—are urea impermeable. By this stage, vasopressin-dependent water reabsorption in the collecting ducts has led to a high urea concentration within the lumen, which in turn leads to reabsorption of urea into the interstitium by vasopressin-sensitive urea transporters along the terminal portion of the inner medullary collecting duct. The interstitial urea exchanges with vasa recta capillaries, in which uptake is facilitated by a specific urea carrier, and some urea enters the S3 segment of the pars recta and the descending and ascending thin limbs of the loop of Henle; it returns to the inner medullary collecting ducts to be reabsorbed. The net result of this recycling process is to add urea to the inner medullary interstitium, thereby raising interstitial osmolality, in turn increasing water abstraction from the thin descending limb of the loop of Henle. This process raises the intraluminal sodium concentration in the thin descending limb and explains the passive sodium diffusion from the thin ascending limb into the surrounding inner medullary interstitium.

The capillaries that supply the medulla also have a special anatomical arrangement. If they passed through the medulla as a more usual capillary network, they would soon dissipate the medullary osmotic gradient owing to equilibration of the latter with the isotonic capillary blood. This does not happen to any appreciable extent because the U-shaped arrangement of the vasa recta ensures that solute entry and water loss in the descending vasa recta

are offset by solute loss and water entry in the ascending vasa recta. This is the process of countercurrent exchange, which is entirely passive.

ACID-BASE TRANSPORT

The maintenance of a correct acid-base balance is essential for normal cell function. The kidney plays a central role in this process through several mechanisms, including the almost complete tubular reabsorption of filtered bicarbonate. Various nephron segments participate in this task; there is general agreement about the importance of the proximal tubule in bicarbonate reabsorption. However, other downstream segments participate in this process as well.[7] Thus, the loop of Henle is potentially an important site of acid-base regulation because it reabsorbs, under physiological conditions, a significant fraction (about 15%) of the filtered bicarbonate.

Studies on bicarbonate transport along the loop of Henle in the rat in vivo indicate that the descending limb of Henle's loop has low bicarbonate permeability.[8] Accordingly, it is unlikely to play a major role in the overall process of bicarbonate reabsorption. In contrast, perfusion studies of the S3 segment of the proximal tubule have demonstrated its ability to reabsorb bicarbonate. On the basis of these observations, two portions of the loop of Henle, the S3 segment of the proximal tubule and the TAL, participate significantly in the overall reabsorption of bicarbonate. However, it is possible that under physiological conditions, the contribution of the S3 segment to bicarbonate reabsorption is only modest because the concentration of bicarbonate of the fluid entering this nephron segment is low (about 5 mM) as a consequence of avid bicarbonate reabsorption in the early segments (S1 and S2) of the proximal tubule.

The situation is different in the TAL. Micropuncture studies have shown that, by the time fluid has reached the tip of Henle's loop, the concentration of bicarbonate rises significantly.[9] As a consequence, bicarbonate reabsorption in the TAL is greatly facilitated. The reabsorption of water in excess of bicarbonate in the descending limb of Henle and the transfer of bicarbonate in a concentration-dependent manner in the TAL constitute a potent system of bicarbonate retrieval along the TAL. It may be concluded that under physiological conditions, bicarbonate reabsorption along the loop of Henle is largely a function of the TAL.[10]

At the molecular level, in vivo perfusion studies of the LOH have identified the Na^+,H^+ exchanger as the major proton-secreting mechanism responsible for bicarbonate reabsorption, thus confirming previous experiments performed in vitro on isolated TALs.[11,12] This antiporter is a ubiquitous membrane protein that pumps protons against an electrochemical gradient by utilizing a downhill sodium gradient. Starting from the seminal work of Sardet and associates,[13] at least eight membrane isoforms (NHEs) have been cloned. Along the TAL, NHE3 has been localized to the luminal membrane and has been identified as the major proton-secreting NHE along this segment.[14] In addition, NHE2 has also been found along the TAL.[15] The role of NHE2 is unknown, but it has been postulated to offset the loss of function of NHE3. The transport process of bicarbonate is active in nature because its concentration in the fluid emerging from the loop is much lower than that measured at the tip of Henle's loop.[8] The TAL can lower luminal bicarbonate concentration to a limiting value of about 5 mM. Moreover, as demonstrated by both loop perfusions in vivo and perfusion studies of TAL in vitro, the transport of bicarbonate is concentration-dependent and sharply decreases following administration of a carbonic anhydrase inhibitor such as acetazolamide or methazolamide.[11] Maneuvers that interfere with the activity of basolateral Na^+,K^+-ATPase, such as the removal of either sodium from the basolateral and lumen, or of potassium from the basolateral, lead to almost complete cessation of bicarbonate reabsorption in perfused TAL in vitro. It is of interest that both furosemide and bumetanide, inhibitors of $Na^+,K^+,2Cl^-$ cotransport in the apical membrane of cells lining the TAL, stimulate bicarbonate reabsorption.[11] This effect is best explained by the fall in cell sodium concentration after exposure to inhibitors of $Na^+,K^+,2Cl^-$ transport and the rise of the sodium gradient across the apical membrane, which would be responsible for increasing the rate of Na^+-H^+ exchange.[12] Results from perfusion studies of the loop of Henle in vivo are consistent with the conclusion that NHE3 is the predominant isoform of the sodium-hydrogen exchanger involved in bicarbonate reabsorption, because such studies show that bicarbonate transport is sharply reduced by a specific NHE3 inhibitor but not by HOE 694, an agent known to block NHE2 exclusively.[16,17]

The role of additional transporters participating in bicarbonate transport along the loop of Henle is uncertain. Conceivably, H^+ transport by H^+-ATPase could mediate some bicarbonate reabsorption in the S3 segment of the proximal tubule and the TAL.[11] Microperfusion studies performed on LOH with the use of bafilomycin, an inhibitor of electrogenic H^+-ATPase, have demonstrated the presence of a modest, but functionally significant active H^+-ATPase. Moreover, immunohistochemical evidence for the presence of proton ATPase along the TAL has been reported.[18]

Basolateral Membrane

Tubular cells are specialized for selective ions and water transport, resulting in the generation of concentrated urine and in maintaining hydroelectrolyte and acid-base balance. Epithelial polarity of these cells plays the main role in those processes by generating the osmotic gradient cell-to-lumen and cell-to-interstitium that modulate the trafficking of many solutes. Transcellular bicarbonate reabsorption depends also on effective mechanisms of base exit across the basolateral membranes of bicarbonate-transporting tubule cells. Experimental evidence, obtained both in perfused TAL and in fused cells of the frog's diluting segment, have demonstrated the presence of an electrogenic sodium bicarbonate cotransporter that shares many properties with a cotransporter in the basolateral membrane of proximal tubule cells.[19,20] Ultimately, this electrogenic transporter's activity depends on the cell's negative potential and, thus, on the ubiquitous Na^+,K^+-ATPase and passive potassium efflux from tubule cells. Additional transporters, such as chloride-bicarbonate exchange and a potassium-bicarbonate cotransport, have also been reported to play a role in the exit of base from the basolateral membrane.[21]

Some properties of the basolateral acid-base transporters deserve mention. First, basolateral sodium-hydrogen exchange, maintained by the NHE1 isoform of the Na^+-H^+ transporter family, has been identified in the TAL,[22] and its activity has been shown to alter apical Na^+-H^+ exchange and, thus, net bicarbonate reabsorption. Perfusion experiments in which both net transport of bicarbonate and cell pH were monitored showed that basolateral Na^+-H^+ exchange enhances transepithelial bicarbonate reabsorption. These results are unexpected because stimulation of basolateral Na^+-H^+ exchange should increase cell pH and thus lower apical Na^+-H^+ exchange. The mechanism of such "cross-talk" between basolateral and apical membrane Na^+-H^+ exchanges, and their coordination, is incompletely understood. However, the identification of basolateral Na^+-H^+ exchange as a potential site of physiological regulation of luminal acidification and of bicarbonate transport across the TAL is of great interest.

In addition to NHE1, NHE4 has been localized on the basolateral membrane of TAL. Functional experiments have led to the hypothesis that this particular isoform may be specifically involved in ammonium transport across the basolateral membrane of TAL.[23]

Cell pH and Bicarbonate Transport

The regulation of transepithelial bicarbonate reabsorption by intracellular pH (pH_i) and hyperosmolarity is also a subject of study. Compared with the behavior of Na^+-H^+ exchange in most epithelia, the NHE3-mediated Na^+-H^+ exchange in the apical membrane of TAL has a much higher apparent affinity for intracellular H^+.[24] Thus, exchange activity is relatively insensitive to changes in cell pH over the physiological range, and the turnover rate of the transporter is already near maximum at normal cell pH and does not respond to pH changes (pH_i between 6.5 and 7.2). This situation contrasts with the characteristics of Na⁺-H⁺ exchanges in other epithelia, in which transport activity drops sharply when pH is altered in the range of 6.5 to 7.1.[25] It has been suggested that the insensitivity of apical Na⁺-H⁺ exchange in the TAL reflects an adaptation to prevent fluctuations of transepithelial bicarbonate transport during changes in pH_i that may be related to ammonium (NH_4^+) transport. NH_4^+ entry into cells of the TAL has been shown to occur by carrier-mediated electroneutral $NH_4^+,2Cl^-$ transport (NH_4^+ replacing Na⁺ and K⁺ on the Na⁺,K⁺,2Cl⁻ transporter; see later) and may lead to fluctuations of pH_i. Insensitivity of the apical Na⁺-H⁺ exchanger to pH_i changes would thus uncouple bicarbonate reabsorption from NH_4^+ excretion. Changes in external osmolality also modulate apical Na⁺-H⁺ exchange and bicarbonate absorption in TAL.[26] External hyperosmolarity lowers transepithelial bicarbonate transport, whereas hypotonicity stimulates transport.[27] It appears that the mechanism by which hyperosmolarity reduces apical Na⁺-H⁺ exchange involves an acid shift in the pH_i dependence of bicarbonate transport and a decrease in the transporter's sensitivity to the stimulating effect of pH_i. The opposite effect, stimulation of Na⁺-H⁺ exchange and bicarbonate reabsorption during decrease in medullary osmolarity, may play a role in greater urinary acidification and diminished bicarbonate excretion when loop diuretics affect medullary washout of solutes.[28]

Other Regulating Factors

Systemic acid-base disturbances also modulate bicarbonate transport: Acidosis increases bicarbonate reabsorption, whereas metabolic alkalosis has the opposite effect.[29] The loop of Henle can participate in the tubular adaptation to an increase in filtered load of bicarbonate by increasing net loop of Henle bicarbonate transport. In this setting, at the molecular level, NHE3 RNA and protein abundance were also stimulated and, accordingly, NHE3 activity increased.[30] Finally NHE3 expression and abundance were

highly stimulated in the early phase of diabetes, which is characterized by increased glomerular filtration rate.[31]

AMMONIA/AMMONIUM ION TRANSPORT

Ammonium ion (NH_4^+) is generated by proximal tubular cells and is partly secreted within the tubular fluid. NH_4^+ then reaches the TAL of Henle's loop, where it is largely reabsorbed. Absorption of NH_4^+ and ammonia (NH_3) by the medullary TAL (MTAL) in absence of water transport provides the energy for total ammonia accumulation (the sum of NH_4^+ and NH_3) in the medullary interstitium, which favors ammonia secretion into the tubular fluid of adjacent medullary collecting ducts. Thus, a major part of the NH_4^+ excreted in urine derives from the NH_4^+ synthesized by proximal tubular cells and absorbed by the MTAL. The diffusion of NH_3 coupled to H⁺ transport and trapping as NH_4^+ in the acidic lumen of the collecting duct make up an important mechanism of transepithelial ammonium transport (Fig. 25-3).[32]

As stated earlier, a major fraction of the NH_4^+ delivered by the proximal tubule must be reabsorbed by the MTAL in order to accumulate in the medullary interstitium and to be directly secreted in contiguous collecting ducts. Total ammonia is absorbed by the MTAL primarily as NH_4^+ by means of secondary active transporters. Diffusion of NH_4^+ from lumen to peritubular space also takes place through the paracellular pathway as a consequence of the lumen-positive transepithelial voltage of the MTAL. NH_4^+ absorption is regulated by the acid-base status. Indeed, the ability of the MTAL that has been isolated and perfused in vitro to absorb total ammonia is increased during chronic metabolic acidosis (CMA).[33] The Na⁺,K⁺(NH_4^+),2Cl⁻ cotransporter is the main apical NH_4^+ carrier and is responsible for 50% to 65% of NH_4^+ luminal uptake. An

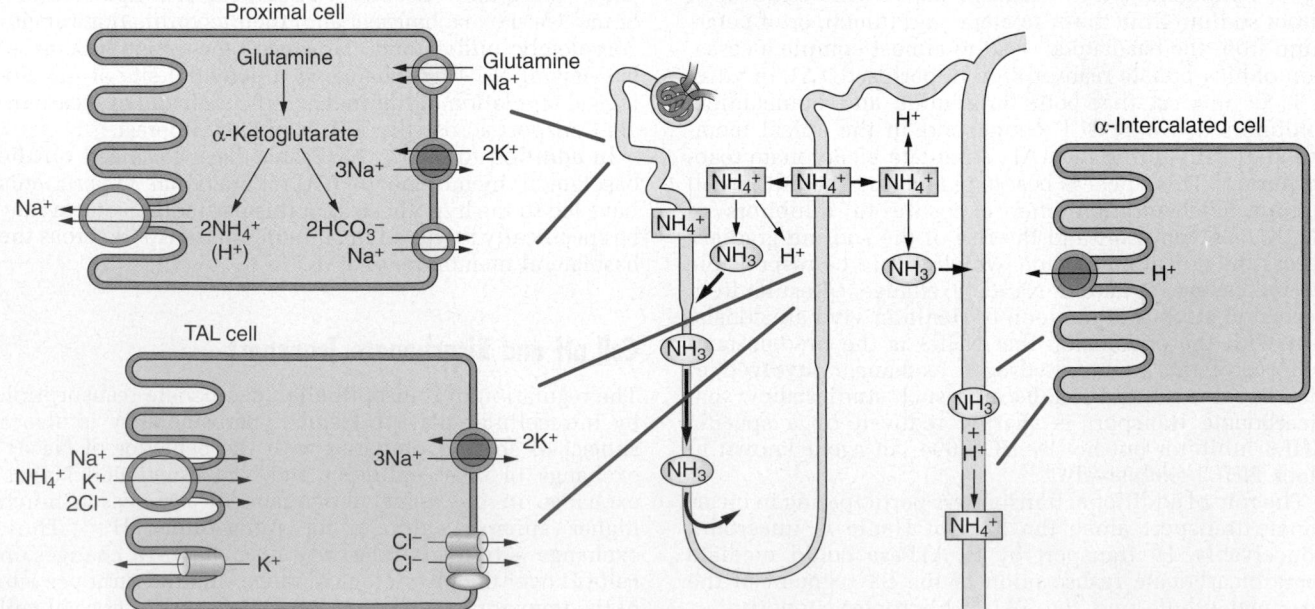

FIGURE 25-3. Renal handling of ammonia (NH_3) and ammonium ion (NH_4^+). For details see text. Cl⁻, chloride ion; H⁺, hydrogen ion; HCO_3^-, bicarbonate ion; K⁺, potassium ion; Na⁺, sodium ion.

electroneutral barium- and verapamil-sensitive $K^+, NH_4^+(H^+)$ antiport mechanism is responsible for the rest of the MTAL NH_4^+ luminal uptake. On the basolateral side of TAL cells, the Na^+-H^+ exchanger NHE1 of the MTAL significantly contributes to the cell-to-peritubular space NH_4^+ transport. As previously stated, the capacity of the MTAL to absorb NH_4^+ increases during chronic metabolic acidosis, and this adaptation favors the renal elimination of an acid load.[34] The mechanism explaining this MTAL adaptation is the increased expression and activity of $Na^+,K^+(NH_4^+),2Cl^-$ by metabolic acidosis.[35]

THE FUNCTION OF THE MACULA DENSA

The *macula densa* is a region of specialized epithelial cells of the TAL where there is close anatomical contact between the TAL and the vascular pole of its own glomerulus.[36] Macula densa cells differ from the other cells of the TAL; they have large nuclei and are closely packed, thus looking like a plaque (leading to the term macula densa). They are part of the juxtaglomerular apparatus, which consists of the extraglomerular matrix (secreted by the mesangial cells of the glomerulus) and the granular cells of the afferent arterioles, which are the site of production, storage, and release of renin (Fig. 25-4). The juxtaglomerular apparatus is a part of a complex feedback mechanism that regulates renal blood flow, glomerular filtration rate, and sodium balance. The complex mechanism matches the amount of sodium that escapes the proximal tubule, and thus is delivered to the TAL, with the capacity of more distal nephron segments to reabsorb sodium; it does so by altering the glomerular filtration rate and the filtered load of sodium, a process known as *tubuloglomerular feedback*.

Macula densa cells detect changes in luminal sodium chloride concentration through a complicated series of ion transport–related intracellular events. Sodium chloride entry via an $Na^+,K^+,2Cl^-$ cotransporter and exit of chloride ions through a basolateral channel lead to cell depolarization and elevations in cytosolic calcium.[37] Communication from macula densa cells to the glomerular vascular ele-

ments involves the release of ATP across the macula densa basolateral membrane through an axion channel with high conductance. Increased sodium and fluid delivery to the TAL and macula densa region signals the cells of the juxtaglomerular apparatus to release renin and produce angiotensin II locally as well as other vasoconstrictors, which act on the afferent arteriole to decrease filtration and thereby sodium and fluid delivery to the TAL and beyond.[38]

TRANSPORT OF DIVALENT CATIONS

Calcium Transport

Plasma calcium is approximately 50% protein bound; only the remaining 50% is filterable. The proximal tubule is the major site of calcium ion (Ca^{2+}) transport, reabsorbing around 65% of the filtered load. Along the loop of Henle, the thin limbs have a minor role, whereas the TAL transports calcium mainly paracellularly, driven by a substantial lumen-positive V_{te}. However, a significant component of calcium reabsorption along the TAL is transcellular, as indicated by the finding that the loss of V_{te} does not completely suppress calcium transport and by the presence of Ca^{2+}-ATPase in the basolateral membrane.[39] Calcium transport is affected by parathyroid hormone, which stimulates calcium transport along the TAL and distal tubule through accumulation of cyclic adenosine monophosphate. However, when parathyroid hormone is present in excess, its anticalciuretic effect is offset by the increased filtered load of calcium due to enhanced gastrointestinal absorption of calcium and its release from bone. The action and importance of calcitonin as a regulator of calcium excretion are uncertain, but it is probably also anticalciuretic, acting (like parathyroid hormone) at the TAL and distal tubule. In contrast to thiazides, which induce hypocalciuria, loop diuretics such as furosemide increase calcium excretion, presumably because of their predominant action on the TAL's V_{te}-dependent paracellular calcium reabsorption. Clinical correlates of the differing effects of thiazide and loop diuretics on calcium excretion are Gitelman's and Bartter's syndromes, characterized by hypocalciuria and hypercalciuria, respectively.[40]

Changes in acid-base balance also affect calcium excretion. Metabolic acidosis is associated with an increase in calcium excretion, whereas metabolic alkalosis has the opposite effect. Although there is evidence that the calcium channels in the distal tubule are pH sensitive, much of the effect on calcium excretion occurs through alterations in filtered load. The buffering of hydrogen ions by the skeleton leaches calcium from bone, and additionally, a fall in plasma pH reduces calcium binding by proteins and thereby increases free calcium ions; these effects both increase the filtered load of calcium.

Magnesium Reabsorption

Magnesium is the fourth most abundant cation in the body and the second most common cation in the intracellular fluid. The kidney provides the most sensitive control for magnesium balance. About 80% of the total serum magnesium is ultrafilterable through the glomerular membrane. The proximal tubule of the adult animal reabsorbs only a small fraction (10%-15%) of the filtered magne-

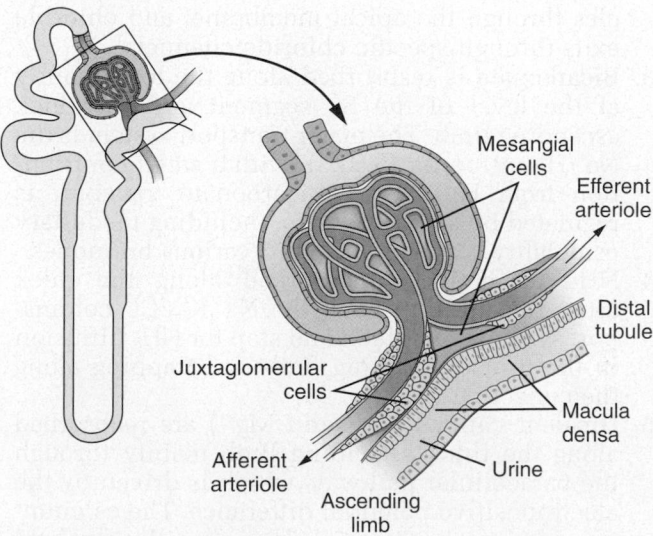

FIGURE 25-4. Schematic view of the juxtaglomerular apparatus.

sium. Micropuncture experiments indicate that approximately 60% of the filtered magnesium is reabsorbed in the loop of Henle.[41] Magnesium reabsorption in the loop occurs within the cortical thick ascending limb (CTAL) by passive means. The driving force for paracellular magnesium reabsorption is the lumen-positive voltage of the TAL.[42] Along this segment, a specific tight junction protein called claudin 16 (paracellin 1) is necessary for paracellular magnesium reabsorption.[43] Support for the importance of such protein comes from finding that mutations of the claudin 16 gene are associated with severe renal magnesium wasting.[44]

Many hormones (parathyroid hormone, calcitonin, glucagons, arginine vasopressin) and nonhormonal factors (magnesium restriction, acid-base balance, potassium depletion) influence renal reabsorption of magnesium to variable extents in the CTAL. Dietary magnesium restriction leads to renal magnesium conservation with diminished urinary magnesium excretion. Adaptation of magnesium transport with dietary magnesium restriction occurs in both the CTAL and distal tubule. Elevation of plasma magnesium and calcium concentrations inhibits magnesium and calcium reabsorption, leading to hypermagnesuria and hypercalciuria. The identification of a calcium-magnesium–sensing receptor located on the peritubular sides of TAL and distal tubule cells explains this phenomenon (see later). Loop diuretics, such as furosemide and bumetanide, diminish salt absorption in the CTAL. Finally, metabolic acidosis, potassium depletion, or phosphate restriction can diminish magnesium reabsorption within the loop and distal tubule.[45]

The Calcium-Magnesium–Sensing Receptor

Calcium and magnesium transport in the TAL are influenced by the calcium-magnesium–sensing receptor, which has been localized to the basolateral membrane. When activated by a rise in plasma calcium/magnesium concentration, it causes reductions in sodium chloride reabsorption and V_{te}, thereby inhibiting reabsorption of calcium and magnesium.[46]

The signal transduction pathway includes stimulation of arachidonic acid (AA) production through direct or indirect activation of phospholipase A_2 (PLA_2), which is metabolized via the cytochrome P450 pathway to an active metabolite that inhibits the apical potassium channel and, perhaps, the $Na^+,K^+,2Cl^-$ cotransporter (Fig. 25-5). Both actions lower overall cotransporter activity, thereby reducing the lumen-positive voltage and paracellular transport of divalent cations. The calcium-magnesium–sensing receptor probably also directly or indirectly (by raising intracellular Ca^{2+}) inhibits adenylate cyclase and causes decrease of hormone-stimulated divalent cation transport.[47]

CONCLUSION

The loop of Henle is an important segment for fluid and ion transport. It participates in the generation of concentrated urine and is involved in the reabsorption of sodium, potassium, and chloride. The major and unique transport system is the $Na^+,K^+,2Cl^-$ transporter, the site of action of the loop diuretics. Along this segment, about 15% of the filtered bicarbonate is reabsorbed mainly through Na^+-H^+ exchange; in addition, the TAL actively reabsorbs NH_4^+, an important step for the diffusion of NH_3 in the thin descend-

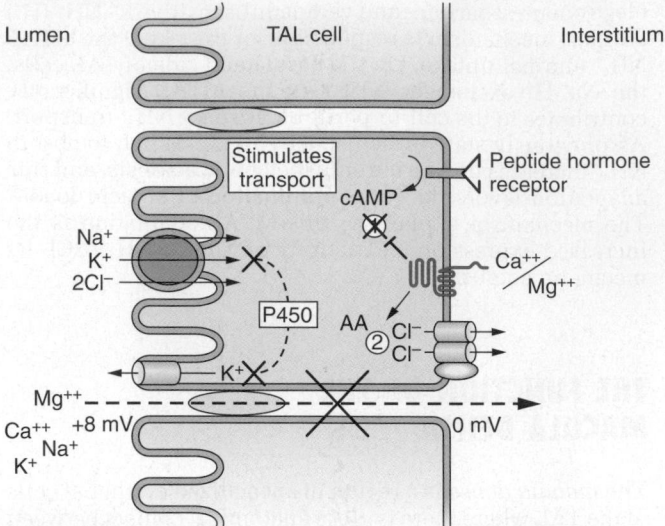

FIGURE 25-5. Cell signaling of the calcium/magnesium sensing receptor. For details see text. *1*, adenylate cyclase; *2*, phospholipase A_2; AA, arachidonic acid; cAMP, cyclic adenosine monophosphate; Ca^{2+}, calcium ion; Cl^-, chloride ion; H^+, hydrogen ion; K^+, potassium ion; Mg^{++}, magnesium ion; mV, millivolt(s); Na^+, sodium ion; P450, cytochrome P450; TAL, thick ascending limb.

ing limb and for its trapping along the collecting ducts. Finally, the TAL is responsible for a significant fraction of calcium and magnesium reabsorption.

Key Points

1. The loop of Henle is an important site for fluid and solute reabsorption. Moreover, it is the segment that actively participates in the concentration of the urine through the countercurrent system.
2. Ions transport is localized mainly along the thick ascending limb, where a complex system links basolateral Na^+,K^+-ATPase to the luminal $Na^+,K^+,2Cl^-$ transporter, whereas potassium recycles through the apical membrane, and chloride exits through specific chloride channels.
3. Bicarbonate is reabsorbed along the loop mainly at the level of the S3 segment and the thick ascending limb. The major transport system is the Na^+/H^+ antiporter (NHE3), with a small contribution from H^+-ATPase. Bicarbonate transport is regulated by several factors, including medullary osmolality, systemic pH, and various hormones.
4. $NH4^+$ is actively reabsorbed along the thick ascending limb through the $Na^+,K^+,2Cl^-$ cotransport system, a fundamental step for NH_3 diffusion in the thin descending limb and trapping along the collecting duct.
5. Divalent cations (Ca^{2+} and Mg^{2+}) are reabsorbed along the thick ascending limb mainly through the paracellular pathway, which is driven by the electropositive potential difference. The calcium-magnesium–sensing receptor is greatly involved in the regulation of the divalent ions transport.

Key References

11. Capasso G, Unwin R, Agulian S, Giebisch G: Bicarbonate transport along the loop of Henle. I: Microperfusion studies of load and inhibitor sensitivity. J Clin Invest 1991;88:430-437.
21. Blanchard A, Leviel F, Bichara M, et al: Interactions of external and internal K+ with K+HCO3- cotransporter of rat medullary thick ascending limb. Am J Physiol 1996;271:C218-C225.
29. Capasso G, Unwin R, Ciani F, et al: Bicarbonate transport along the loop of Henle. II: Effects of acid-base, dietary and neurohumoral determinants. J Clin Invest 1994;94:830-838.

30. Capasso G, Rizzo M, Pica A, et al: Bicarbonate reabsorption and NHE-3 expression: Abundance and activity are increased in Henle's loop of remnant rats. Kidney Int 2002;62:2126-2135.
33. Good D: Adaptation of bicarbonate and ammonium transport in the rat medullary thick ascending limb: Effects of chronic metabolic acidosis and sodium intake. Am J Physiol 1990;258:F1345-F1353.

See the companion Expert Consult website for the complete reference list.

CHAPTER 26

Distal Tubular Physiology

John P. Geibel

OBJECTIVES

This chapter will:
1. Review the components of the distal tubule.
2. Explain the distribution of cell types in the distal tubule.
3. Discuss the role of several proteins in the process of urine acidification.
4. Consider the hormonal regulation of tubular acidification.
5. Explain the mechanisms of proton secretion.
6. Discuss the mechanisms of bicarbonate excretion and reabsorption.

Distal tubule defines the terminal section of the renal tubule. This segment of the nephron is composed of the following four separate segments, each of which has one or more distinct cell types:
- Distal tubule
- Connecting segment (previously defined as being part of the distal tubule)
- Collecting duct
- Medullary collecting tubule

This section of the nephron has also been considered the area where the maximal concentration and acidification of the urine occurs. This potential is due to the fact that most reabsorption takes place in the proximal tubule and other nephron segments. The cortical collecting duct can secrete either net acid or net base,[1,2] depending on the physiological state of the animal, as illustrated in conditions of acidosis or alkalosis,. These functions are believed to be accomplished in the cortical collecting duct by type A and type B intercalated cells, respectively.[3,4] Type A intercalated cells are associated with net proton secretion, allowing for replenishment of body bicarbonate levels; conversely, type B intercalated cells modulate bicarbonate concentration during metabolic alkalosis by varying their level of bicarbonate secretion. The medullary collecting ducts are capable of only net acid secretion, and for that reason, only type A intercalated cells are detectable in the medulla.[5-8]

Regulation of acidification along the collecting duct requires the ability to secrete protons and reabsorb bicarbonate. Secretion of protons is carried out predominantly by the H+-ATPase, with an additional contribution from Na+-H+ exchangers and also, potentially, to a small extent, by the H+,K+-ATPase.

The remainder of this chapter, because of space limitations, consists of a brief overview of localization of these transport proteins and their roles in the complex process of distal tubule acidification. The focus of the discussion is the collecting duct, where the majority of the acidification and alkalinization of the tubular fluid occurs.

COLLECTING DUCT

The intercalated cells of the collecting duct contain the highest levels of vacuolar H+-ATPases of all acid-base transporting cells in the kidney (Fig. 26-1). However, the ability to provide a simple classification of intercalated cells is not possible until more information is acquired about their functional properties. An attempt has been made to combine the nomenclature that has been used to define the cells found along this segment and to simply call the cell that predominantly is an acid-secreting cell the A cell and the cell that predominantly secretes base the B cell. In an early study investigating the cellular distribution of the vacuolar H+-ATPase in different intercalated cells, it was determined that in addition to showing positive staining response for numerous cytoplasmic vesicles in most intercalated cells, A cells also showed positive apical staining response for the vacuolar H+-ATPase. B cells showed positive staining at the basolateral membrane for vacuolar H+-ATPase; of note was that many of these cells had a pattern of diffuse or even bipolar vacuolar H+-ATPase distribution.[9,10] The outer stripe of the outer medulla displays a predominance of A cells with only a few residual B cells. In contrast, the inner stripe of the outer medulla has only A cells, which represent about 40% of the epithelial cell population of the collecting duct. The epithelium of the inner medulla contains 5% to 10% A intercalated cells in the initial section of the

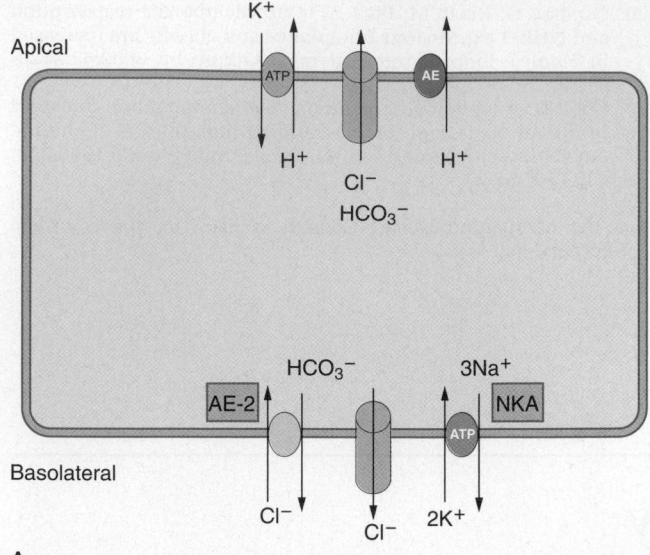

A

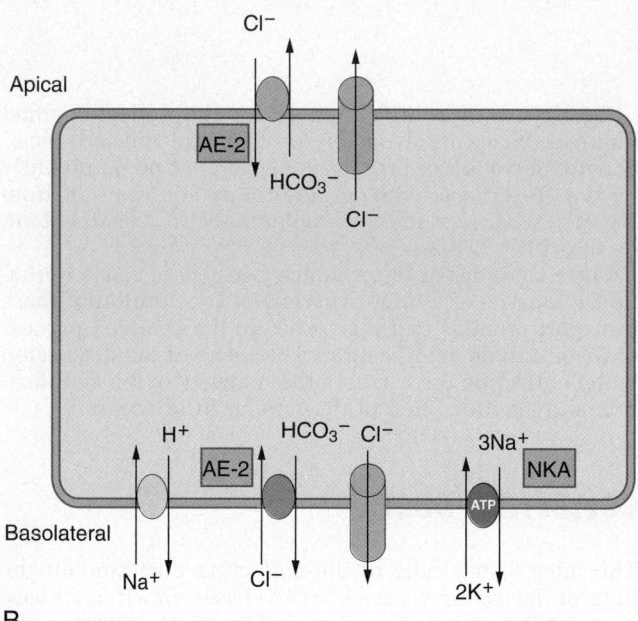

B

FIGURE 26-1. Schematic representations of cortical collecting duct A cell (intercalated cell type A) (**A**) and B cell intercalated cell type B) (**B**). AE, anion exchanger; ATP, adenosine triphosphate; NKA, sodium potassium ATPase.

segment; these cells do not appear in the middle and terminal portions of the inner medullary collecting duct.[11,12]

If one wishes to distinguish the A from B intercalated cells in this segment, it is necessary only to look for cells that stain positive for the anion exchanger AE-1 (band 3) on the basolateral plasma membrane (see Fig. 26-1). The AE-1 protein is virtually undetectable in typical B intercalated cells.[13] Thorough studies have shown that cells with discrete basolateral vacuolar H+-ATPase staining are AE-1–negative; of interest is the fact that, in addition, those cells having a more diffuse or bipolar H+-ATPase staining pattern were also AE-1–negative.[9,13]

These rather complex results could help explain the previous controversies about whether an additional cell type existed; it was possible to observe intercalated cells having unique apical and basolateral staining as well as combinations of both apical and basolateral staining.[9] The original study by Al-Awqati and colleagues was the first to suggest that some of the cells found in this segment might be interconvertible due to the unique plasticity of intercalated epithelial cell polarity.[79] The demonstration of vacuolar H+-ATPase on numerous intracellular vesicles that would allow for shuttling of the protein to and from the plasma membrane adds credence to this original plasticity theory. The complexity of this relationship of cell types and ratios of the different intercalated cell phenotypes becomes even more complicated as the relative proportions of different phenotypical intercalated cell variants on the cortical region differ among species,[7] along with the fact that the ratio and patterns being found can be further modulated by dietary factors.

Medullary Collecting Duct

The medullary collecting duct is composed of several functionally and morphologically distinct subsegments. The outer medullary collecting duct (OMCD) is composed of two main cell types, acid-secretory A type[13] intercalated cells and principal cells that are involved in water, Na+, and K+ transport. The proton secretion found in this segment is mediated by vacuolar H+-ATPases, first demonstrated through in vitro perfusion studies of isolated OMCDs. Bicarbonate absorption via the basolateral Cl−–HCO3− exchanger AE-1/band 3[15] found in this segment is Cl− dependent. Conversely, apical bicarbonate reabsorption is not Cl− dependent. The levels of both proton secretion and bicarbonate absorption in perfused tubules are modulated by the acid-base status of the animal. The rates of both proton secretion and bicarbonate absorption are stimulated in animals with metabolic acidosis and reduced in animals with metabolic alkalosis.

An additional yet equally important function of the medullary collecting duct is to buffer excreted protons using titratable acids, phosphate, citrate, and ammonia/ammonium.[16,17] The buffering of protons is critical to maintaining a favorable proton gradient across the apical membrane, which facilitates vacuolar H+-ATPase activity. If these titratable acids were absent and not available to act as a buffer, the proton gradient would exceed more than 3 to 4 pH units, which would result in reduced efficiency of urinary acidification. Citrate and phosphate are both freely filtered and, for the most part, reabsorbed in the proximal tubule, thereby restricting their availability under normal conditions. Ammonia (NH3) and ammonium (NH4+), on the other hand, are generated in the proximal tubule during the metabolism of glutamine and glutamate, resulting in the generation of bicarbonate ions.[18] The NH4+ that is produced is secreted into urine via the Na+-H+ exchanger (with NH4+ substituting for H+), but NH3 passes into the tubular lumen via simple diffusion, where it becomes protonated, resulting in the generation of NH4+. The secreted NH4+ is then reabsorbed in the thick ascending limb via the Na+-K+-2Cl− symporter NKKC2/BSC1 (NH4+ substitutes for K+) and accumulates in the medullary interstitium. The NH4+ thus reaches a chemical equilibrium with NH3, which in turn can freely diffuse across the medullary collecting duct epithelium and into the tubule lumen. The accumulated NH3 is then protonated to generate NH4+ after proton secretion by intercalated cells. The generated NH4+ is trapped in the collecting duct lumen owing to a lack of apical permeability to NH4+.

Both NH_3 and NH_4^+ are actively taken up and secreted by cells along the length of the medullary collecting duct. Several transport pathways have been postulated as potential transporters in the collecting duct, including the Na^+/K^+-ATPase,[19,20] the Na^+-K^+-$2Cl^-$ cotransporter NKCC1 (SLC12A2),[21] and members of the Rhesus surface antigen–determining Rh protein family, RhGB and RhCB.[22-28] In addition, the vacuolar H^+-ATPases, and more recently an H^+/K^+-ATPase, have been identified in OMCDs on the basis of immunohistochemistry[29-31] and inhibition of proton secretion by SCH28080, a selective inhibitor of H^+/K^+-ATPase,[32,33] both of which could also play a role in the transport of NH_3 and NH_4^+. Still controversial at this time is which isoform(s) of the H^+/K^+-ATPase are active—colonic, gastric, or both. These conflicting results are based on which of the various pharmacological tools (ouabain, SCH28080, or omeprazole) was selected, along with which molecular tool(s) (immunohistochemistry, Northern blot analysis, in situ hybridization)[30,34-41] was selected. What is agreed by all parties is that the contribution of H^+/K^+-ATPases to overall proton secretion in this segment, and thus to bicarbonate reabsorption, is minor and that H^+/K^+-ATPases may rather play an important role as potassium scavengers during systemic potassium depletion.[42-45]

Inner Medullary Collecting Duct

The inner medullary collecting duct (IMCD) can be subdivided into at least two separate segments, the initial portion and the terminal region constituting approximately the last two thirds of the IMCD.[46,47] The initial third of the IMCD contains intercalated cells, which gradually disappear in the more distal portions of this segment. In the latter and terminal portions there are only the so-called IMCD cells (the "principal cells" in the IMCD are sufficiently distinct from principal cells found in the outer medulla to warrant a different distinct name). These latter IMCD cells express aquaporin-2 (AQP 2) and play a role in establishing the final concentration of urine. Investigators using a knockout mouse model for AQP-1 determined that these animals produced surprisingly only partially acidic urine. In these same animals, expression of vacuolar H^+-ATPases in the inner medulla was increased, and again surprisingly, IMCD cells with strong apical expression of vacuolar H^+-ATPases were detected.[48]

In the collecting duct, intercalated cells express high levels of vacuolar H^+-ATPase in a pool of intracellular vesicles and/or on their plasma membrane(s); as discussed in some detail previously, the phenotype and distribution of intercalated cells varies along the collecting duct and is regionally dependent. The definition of the ratio of membrane to vesicular pools is especially complex in the cortical collecting duct and the connecting segment of the urinary tubule. Because it appears that all intercalated cells can modulate cell surface expression of vacuolar H^+-ATPase by vesicle trafficking, the levels of surface expression of the H^+-ATPases are constantly changing at any given time and with the acid-base status of the lumen of the nephron. When confronted with the physiological conditions of acidosis or alkalosis, the cortical collecting duct can secrete either protons or bicarbonate so as to modulate the net acid or net base status, respectively.[1,2] In the most straightforward scenario, these functions are achieved by type A and type B intercalated cells, respectively.[47,49] Net proton secretion conducted by type A intercalated cells acts to replenish body bicarbonate levels, whereas bicarbonate secretion is conducted by type B intercalated cells,

which can aid in restoring bicarbonate concentrations during metabolic alkalosis. In contrast, medullary collecting ducts are capable only of net acid secretion, and therefore, only A cells are detected in the medulla.[5-8]

MODULATIONS IN CELL NUMBERS DURING ACID-BASE REGULATION IN INTERCALATED CELLS

As described previously, proton secretion by intercalated cells is regulated to a great extent by alterations in the levels of cell surface vacuolar H^+-ATPase expression. H^+-ATPase proteins are shuttled to and from the apical membrane via dedicated intracellular acidic vesicles.[9,47,49-57] Previous studies on mice, rats, and rabbits demonstrated that the induction of systemic acidosis resulted in a modulation of the number of cortical intercalated cells with apical membrane vacuolar H^+-ATPase expression (increased expression) and the number of cells with basolateral vacuolar H^+-ATPase expression (decreased expression).[9,47,55,56] Induction of a systemic alkalosis results in a reversal of expression patterns, with the number of cells having basolateral vacuolar H^+-ATPase expression increasing and of those having apical vacuolar H^+-ATPase expression decreasing. This configuration would facilitate an increase in net acid secretion to compensate for acidosis or in net bicarbonate secretion to compensate for metabolic alkalosis. Different mechanisms could operate that would cause the aforementioned cellular changes, although the physiological result would be the same in all cases.

Intercalated Cell Plasticity

Al-Awqati, in his initial study on proton secretion by intercalated cells, proposed that A and B cells were functionally discrete copies generated from a single type of intercalated cell.[57] Consequently, A cells that had apical vacuolar H^+-ATPase and basolateral anion exchanger (AE-1) can repolarize, presumably by transcytosis, to generate B cells, expressing the mirror image of polarity, namely, basolateral vacuolar H^+-ATPase and apical AE-1. This interesting hypothesis has received considerable support from studies demonstrating that a novel matrix protein, hensin, could reverse the functional phenotype of cultured intercalated cells.[57] One study presented convincing data that cultured bicarbonate-secreting intercalated cells were converted to proton-secreting cells when grown on a matrix containing hensin.[58] Other studies in collecting ducts incubated in vitro show that anti-hensin antibodies applied in the basolateral bathing medium could inhibit the induction of acid secretion and bicarbonate reabsorption that would normally occur after exposure to acidic medium.[59] Hensin is postulated to induce terminal differentiation in intercalated cells, which was reflected by the typical A-cell phenotypic conversion after acid exposure, a process that was inhibited when hensin function was blocked by antibodies. Such plasticity changes in functional activity of intercalated cells are proposed to involve the concerted action of microtubules and microfilaments, and de novo protein synthesis.[59]

Although there are now several supportive observations as to the interconversion of the various cells, some issues must still be reconciled with the simple notion that A and B cells are phenotypical variants of the same cell type that can, under appropriate conditions, rapidly remodel. The complexity of this issue is shown by some examples of medullary A cells with the appearance of B cells, an observation never formally described in the adult kidney. Furthermore, intercalated cells in the medulla retain their A cell phenotype under all experimental conditions. This finding may indicate either that their A cell phenotype is irreversibly fixed or that appropriate experimental conditions in vivo have not been found that would cause them to convert to B cells. The prospective for plasticity is demonstrated by the facts that both A and B intercalated cells are present in the inner medulla of neonatal rats and that the number of B cells is greater in pups from alkalotic mothers.[3,50,67] In addition, the relative numbers of A and B cells in the cortex appear to be constantly changing in response to modulations of the acid-base status.

An apical anion exchanger in B cells was also a matter of considerable debate because it was not detectable with antibodies against AE-1[13] and because AE-1 messenger RNA was expressed only at very low levels in immunosorted B cells.[60] Cultured intercalated cells have been shown to express AE-1 as the apical anion exchanger,[61] whereas in the kidney, pendrin has been identified as at least one major participant responsible for apical anion exchange in type B intercalated cells.[62-64] Additionally, apical pendrin becomes relocated to the cytosol of B cells in the acid-loaded mouse kidney; this finding is consistent with previous reports of acid-induced apical anion exchanger internalization in rabbit collecting ducts.[65]

Principal Cell and Intercalated Cell Plasticity

An intriguing hypothesis would allow for the conversion of intercalated cells to principal cells in order to gain additional flexibility to adapt to physiological stress. Early reports present evidence that the number of cells identified as intercalated or principal cells could vary under a variety of physiological conditions, such as acid-base changes, dietary potassium intake, and the hydration state of the animal.[66] It should be pointed out that these studies were conducted with the use of light and electron microscopic examination showing cellular appearance only, and without the use of antibodies. Studies conducted in neonatal rats showed that intercalated cells are found in the tip of the papilla but gradually disappear from this region as the pups develop.[67,68] One potential explanation for this loss could be attributed to either selective shedding or apoptosis,[69] although a conversion to principal cells has not been ruled out. However, the following findings give strong support to the "conversion" process between principal and intercalated cells:

- Some cells expressing principal and intercalated cell markers (AQP-2 and vacuolar H+-ATPase) can be identified in the cortical regions of neonatal rats.[70]
- Inhibition of carbonic anhydrases with acetazolamide treatment in adult rats increases the number of intercalated cells and decreases the number of principal cells in the collecting duct.[71]
- The number of intercalated cells can be significantly increased in collecting ducts of rats exposed to lithium, which elicits a marked water diuresis and altered renal acid-base handling.[72]
- Under conditions of cell culture, it has been shown through the use of cell-specific monoclonal antibody markers that type B intercalated cells could differentiate to both type A intercalated cells and principal cells.[73]

Furthermore, other studies have concluded that intercalated and principal cells are derived from a common

precursor cell[74] and that the cellular composition of developing collecting ducts can be modified by the ionic composition of the environment in vitro.[75]

ELECTROLYTE DISTURBANCES

Modulations of electrolyte homeostasis are often linked with changes of systemic acid-base balance associated with altered renal transport processes in addition to a shift of electrolytes between intracellular and extracellular compartments in exchange for protons.

One such instance is hypokalemia, which leads to metabolic alkalosis caused in part by the shift of intracellular potassium to the extracellular space, resulting in the uptake of protons into cells. Typically, hypokalemia can be induced by either a low-potassium diet or more swiftly by application of loop diuretics.[76] Hypertrophy of intercalated cells is observed in the distal tubule and cortical collecting duct,[22,77] with a more pronounced apical location of the vacuolar H+-ATPase associated with increased activity.[71,78,79] These enhanced transport mechanisms are likely to contribute to the development of metabolic alkalosis under these conditions.

In studies involving a rat model for acute chloride depletion alkalosis, a redistribution of vacuolar H+-ATPases has been noted during the compensatory bicarbonate secretion that is consistent with activation of type B intercalated cells and inactivation of type A intercalated cells.[33,80] Vacuolar H+-ATPases appeared to be strongly associated with the basolateral membrane in type B intercalated cells and were mainly found in subapical storage vesicles in type A intercalated cells.[80]

HORMONAL REGULATION OF VACUOLAR H+-ATPASE ACTIVITY

The end product of hormonal regulation of vacuolar H+-ATPase activity in the kidney has not been extensively studied. A wide variety of conclusions have been made as to the effects of exposure to one of several hormones (including angiotensin and aldosterone). The results of these studies have been rather indirect, with the purported actions on bicarbonate reabsorption or secretion in the respective nephron segments or cells.

Angiotensin

A variety of studies by several different groups have shown either in whole animal or cell culture models that angiotensin II is a potent activator of bicarbonate-reabsorbing and proton-secreting mechanisms along the nephron, and thereby stimulates overall bicarbonate reabsorption. The target transport mechanism in the distal convoluted tubule and intercalated cells of the cortical collecting duct is the vacuolar H+-ATPase.[81-84] Studies performed in whole animals and in humans showed a stimulatory effect of angiotensin II on acid secretion and bicarbonate reabsorption,[81,85,86] with the stimulation occurring via angiotensin type 1 (AT$_1$) receptors.[85] However, conflicting views remain on how the effects of angiotensin II modify net bicarbonate transport. One study reported that a reduction in cortical collecting duct vacuolar H+-ATPase enzymatic activity occurred in response to exposure to angiotensin II[87]; in another study, however, an increase of bicarbonate secretion in isolated rabbit cortical collecting duct[17] was observed after hormone application. In an additional series of studies using perfused rat OMCD, a reduction in bicarbonate reabsorption was found after application of angiotensin II.[20] Two groups reported that the hormone-induced stimulation of vacuolar H^+-ATPase was prevented by application of colchicine, thereby disrupting the microtubular network.[83,84] These results suggest that vacuolar H^+-ATPase, or some of its subunits or other stimulatory proteins, may be trafficked to the membrane, resulting in upregulation.

Aldosterone

Mineralocorticoid receptors are expressed along the entire length of the collecting duct and connecting segment, with only a small fraction of cells having a negative staining pattern.[88,89] The effects of aldosterone has two primary modes of action on the regulation of cell and transport functions, occurring through both rapid, nongenomic effects and through transcription-dependent mechanisms that occur early (within 30 min), occur up to several hours after (early genes), or start only after several hours (late genes).[90-93] At the functional level, there are several strong links between aldosterone and proton secretion in the collecting duct, as follows:

1. Stimulation of electrogenic Na^+ reabsorption through luminal epithelial Na^+ channels is stimulated by aldosterone.[91,93] This activation results in a lumen negative potential, which is thought to raise the electrical driving force for H^+ secretion in the cortical collecting duct.[94,95]
2. Direct actions of aldosterone on H^+ secretion via transcriptional/translational pathways have been revealed in turtle bladder and in rat medullary collecting duct.[96,97]
3. Whole animal studies using an Na^+ depletion model caused increased urinary H^+ secretion that is independent of the concomitant hypokalemia.[98]
4. A number of monogenic diseases that interfere with aldosterone synthesis, signaling, or its target proteins affect H^+ secretion in the collecting duct, causing either metabolic acidosis or alkalosis.[11,13,42]

Exposure to aldosterone stimulates H^+-ATPase–dependent bicarbonate reabsorption in all collecting duct segments, although different sensitivities of vacuolar H^+-ATPase enzymatic activity have been described in distinct collecting duct segments.[50] Aldosterone's effect on H^+-ATPase enzymatic activity was independent of Na^+ in medullary collecting ducts perfused in vitro, pointing to mechanisms in addition to changes in electrical driving force.[97] Studies performed in isolated collecting duct segments demonstrated that the action of aldosterone (incubation over several hours) could be blocked by inhibitors of RNA and protein synthesis.[50] Wax and colleagues[99] demonstrated a rapid nongenomic effect of aldosterone on vacuolar H^+-ATPase–mediated proton secretion in intercalated cells in isolated mouse OMCDs. The stimulatory effect of aldosterone on proton secretion could not be prevented by either the mineralocorticoid receptor blocker spironolactone or by inhibition of RNA or protein synthesis. Application of colchicine, an agent that disrupts microtubular trafficking, did inhibit the aldosterone-induced stimulation. These results suggested the involvement of trafficking processes in aldosterone-sensitive proton secretion. In addition, application of chlerythrine, a known protein kinase C–dependent process inhibitor,

abolished the stimulatory effect of aldosterone, thus pointing to a role for protein kinase C in the signaling cascade.[99]

CONCLUSION

The distal tubule remains a complex epithelium composed of at least three cell types with defined and distinct functions, which can, through either the metabolic or the hormonal state of the animal, express a certain degree of plasticity and remodeling that will aid in maintaining the metabolic state of the organism.

Key Points

1. Secretion of protons is carried out predominantly by the H^+-ATPase, with an additional contribution from Na^+-H^+ exchangers and also potentially, to a small extent, by the H^+,K^+-ATPase.
2. The outer medullary collecting duct is composed of two main cell types, acid-secretory type A[20] intercalated cells and principal cells that are involved in water, Na^+, and K^+-transport. The proton secretion found in this segment is mediated by vacuolar H^+-ATPases.
3. Net proton secretion conducted by type A intercalated cells acts to replenish body bicarbonate levels, whereas bicarbonate secretion is conducted by type B intercalated cells that can aid in restoring bicarbonate concentrations during metabolic alkalosis.
4. Medullary collecting ducts are capable only of net acid secretion, and therefore only type A intercalated cells are detected in the medulla.
5. Angiotensin II is a potent activator of bicarbonate-reabsorbing and proton-secreting mechanisms along the nephron, thereby stimulating overall bicarbonate reabsorption.
6. Pendrin has been identified as at least one major participant responsible for apical anion exchange in type B intercalated cells.

Key References

44. Geibel J, Giebisch G, Boron WF: Angiotensin II stimulates both Na^+/H^+ exchange and Na^+. Proc Natl Acad Sci U S A 1990;87:7917-7920.
58. Stockand JD: New ideas about aldosterone signaling in epithelia. Am J Physiol Renal Physiol 2002;282:F559-F576.
77. Smith AN, Skaug J, Choate KA, et al: Mutations in ATP6N1B, encoding a new kidney vacuolar proton pump 116-kD subunit, cause recessive distal renal tubular acidosis with preserved hearing. Nat Genet 2000;26:71-75.
90. Levine DZ, Iacovitti M, Luck B, et al: Surviving rat distal tubule bicarbonate reabsorption: effects of chronic AT_1 blockade. Am J Physiol Renal Physiol 2000;278:F476-F483.
94. Bailey M, Capasso G, Agulian S, et al: The relationship between distal tubular proton secretion and dietary potassium depletion: evidence for up-regulation of H^+-ATPase. Nephrol Dial Transplant 1999;14:1435-1440.

See the companion Expert Consult website for the complete reference list.

CHAPTER 27

The Physiology of the Collecting Ducts

Eric Féraille

OBJECTIVES

This chapter will:
1. Describe the general functional properties of collecting ducts.
2. Discuss the mechanisms of sodium reabsorption and potassium secretion.
3. Explain the mechanisms of water reabsorption.
4. Describe the mechanisms of acid-base transport.
5. Illustrate how human monogenic diseases contribute to the understanding of renal physiology.

The reabsorption process occurring along renal tubules results in the daily generation of 1 to 2 liters of urine, corresponding to 5% to 10% of the glomerular ultrafiltrate containing 1% to 5% of the filtered sodium ion (Na^+) load. Collecting ducts represent the final checkpoint for water and Na^+ reabsorption as well as potassium and acid secretion, their function being tightly controlled by hormones and nonhormonal factors in order to meet homeostatic requirements.

GENERAL TRANSPORT PROPERTIES OF COLLECTING DUCTS

The collecting duct derives from the embryonic ureteral bud and can be divided in three individual portions: cortical, outer medullary, and inner medullary. Cortical and outer medullary collecting ducts are made up of two different cell types. Principal cells are responsible for water and sodium reabsorption as well as potassium secretion, and intercalated cells are involved in acid-base regulation.

Figure 27-1 summarizes the functional organization of the collecting duct principal cell. Active electrogenic Na^+ transport generates a lumen-negative transepithelial voltage (0 to −60 mV), which is higher in more cortical segments of the collecting duct (−10 to −60 mV) and which decreases in the deeper segments as a result of decreased Na^+ reabsorption by principal cells combined with increased electrogenic H^+ secretion by intercalated cells. Na^+ reabsorption in principal cells is linked to K^+ secretion through a two-step mechanism: K^+ transport in and Na^+ transport out of the cell under the control of basolateral sodium ion–potassium ion adenosine triphosphatase (Na^+,K^+-ATPase) generates the driving forces for apical Na^+ entry and K^+ exit. K^+ exit occurs through apical (ROMK [renal outer medullary potassium]) and basolateral potas-

sium channels. Through this mechanism, K^+ secretion is primarily coupled to Na^+ reabsorption at a 2 K^+–to–3 Na^+ stoichiometry via Na^+,K^+-ATPase. The lumen-negative transepithelial voltage also favors paracellular chloride ion (Cl^-) reabsorption.

Apical Na^+ influx is mediated by the amiloride-sensitive Na^+ channel (ENaC), and intracellular Na^+ is then extruded by basolateral Na^+,K^+-ATPase, which provides the driving force for Na^+ entry and for secondary active transport of other solutes. The major role played by ENaC in primary Na^+ reabsorption and secondary K^+ secretion is illustrated by hyperkalemic hypotensive (autosomal recessive pseudohypoaldosteronism type 1) or hypokalemic hypertensive (Liddle's syndrome) monogenic diseases associated with mutations that lead to loss of function or gain of function of the channel, respectively.[1] Long-term regulation of Na^+ and K^+ transporters relies mainly on altered subunit expression, whereas short-term control is mediated by changes in functional properties and/or subunit redistribution between intracellular compartments and the cell surface. The two major hormonal factors that induce Na^+ reabsorption and K^+ secretion are aldosterone and arginine vasopressin (AVP). In addition, insulin may play a significant role during the postprandial period.[2] Moreover, proteases play an important role in controlled ENaC activity. Limited intracellular proteolysis of ENaC subunits is part of the maturation process leading to ENaC activation,[3] and secreted extracellular proteases increase ENaC .activity.[4] Direct proteolysis of ENaC subunits remains to be demonstrated.

Luminal K^+ secretion through ROMK is mostly driven by negative transepithelial voltage generated by Na^+ reabsorption. However, ROMK is subjected to specific regulation by various protein kinases. It is interesting to mention that SGK1, an aldosterone-induced protein kinase, increases ROMK cell surface expression and may therefore participate in the kaliuretic effect of aldosterone.[5] Moreover, WNK4, a protein kinase mutated in Gordon's syndrome (hypertension, hyperkalemia, and metabolic acidosis), decreases ROMK cell surface expression.[6]

Water reabsorption along the collecting duct is a facilitated process that occurs through specific water channels of the aquaporin family. As depicted in Figure 27-1, water enters the luminal (apical) side via aquaporin 2 (AQP2) water channels and leaves the cell through basolateral AQP3 and AQP4 water channels. Although the driving force for water reabsorption is provided mainly by the osmotic gradient generated by countercurrent concentrating mechanism in the loop of Henle, Na^+ reabsorption along the collecting duct, especially in cortical regions, dilutes luminal fluid and contributes to the generation of an osmotic gradient favorable to water reabsorption. Water reabsorption along the collecting duct is controlled chiefly by vasopressin and secondarily by additional factors such as extracellular tonicity, aldosterone, insulin, and extracellular calcium.[7]

The collecting duct is the major site of acid secretion (40-60 mMol H^+/day) and coupled bicarbonate (HCO_3^-) reabsorption (regeneration). Intercalated cells compose about 40% of the overall cell population in cortical, outer medullary, and initial inner medullary collecting ducts,

whereas these cells are absent in deeper portions of inner medullary collecting ducts. At least two subtypes of intercalated cells are located along the collecting ducts: Type A (or α) intercalated cells are involved in acid and HCO_3^- secretion, and type B (or β) intercalated cells are involved in bicarbonate secretion and chloride reabsorption. Figure 27-2 shows that type A intercalated cells express apical V-type H^+-ATPase and basolateral AE1 (Cl^-/HCO_3^- exchanger). H^+ and HCO_3^- are generated from carbon dioxide (CO_2) and water (H_2O) by a cytoplasmic type II carbonic anhydrase. The luminal secretion of H^+ is coupled to the basolateral exit of HCO_3^-. Cl^- exchanged with HCO_3^- is recycled back to the interstitium via basolateral Cl^- channels. Type B intercalated cells (see Fig. 27-2) exhibit apical Cl^-/HCO_3^- exchangers (pendrin and AE4), and a basolateral V-type H^+-ATPase. Luminal Cl^- exchanged with intracellular HCO_3^- leaves the cell via basolateral Cl^- channels.[8]

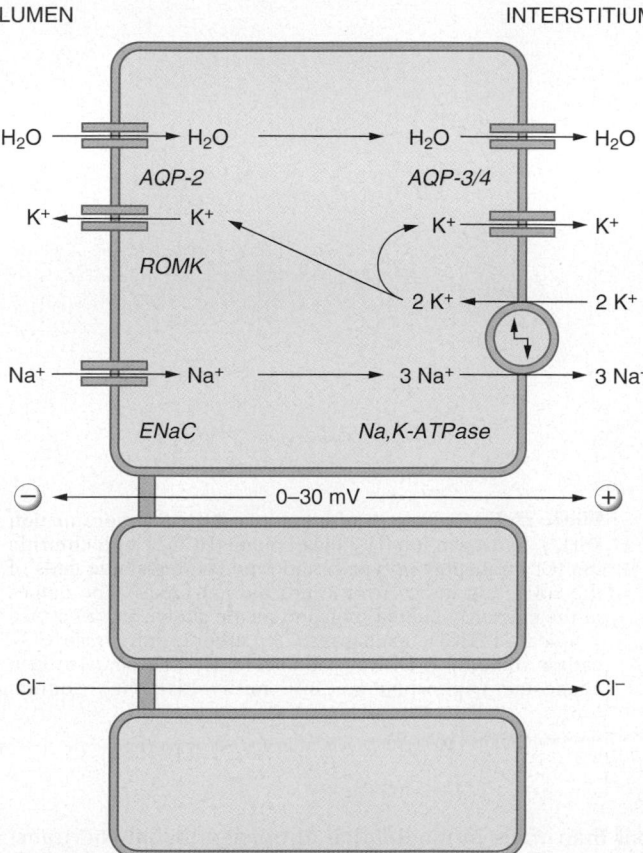

FIGURE 27-1. Mechanism of sodium ion (Na^+), potassium ion (K^+), chloride (Cl^-), and water (H_2O) transport in principal cells of the collecting duct. *Arrows* indicate net fluxes of water and ions. The names of the currently cloned transporters are shown in *italic*. AQP, aquaporin; Ca^{2+}, calcium ion; ENaC, amiloride-sensitive sodium channel; H^+, hydrogen ion; mV, millivolt(s); Na,K-ATPase, sodium-potassium-exchanging adenosine triphosphatase; ROMK, renal outer medullary potassium channel.

SODIUM ION REABSORPTION AND POTASSIUM ION SECRETION BY COLLECTING DUCT PRINCIPAL CELLS

Table 27-1 summarizes the effect of various hormones on transport of ions and water in the collecting ducts.

Aldosterone

The major physiological role of the mineralocorticoid hormone aldosterone is to increase extracellular volume in response to volume depletion signaled by the renin-angiotensin system. Aldosterone also plays an important role in K^+ homeostasis: On the one hand, high extracellular K^+ stimulates aldosterone secretion, and on the other hand, K^+ secretion into the kidney tubule is directly linked to aldosterone-regulated Na^+ reabsorption, which generates the electrical driving force for K^+ secretion.[2] The effects of aldosterone are mostly, if not exclusively, dependent on binding to the mineralocorticoid receptor (MR), which itself binds to specific sequences along the promoter of aldosterone-responsive genes. The key role of MR in mediating aldosterone effects is highlighted by loss of function and gain of function mutations leading to hyperkalemic hypotension (autosomal dominant pseudohypoaldosteronism type I) and hypokalemic hypertension (hypertension exacerbated in pregnancy), respectively.[1,6] In vivo,

TABLE 27-1

Hormonal Control of Sodium, Potassium, Hydrogen, and Water Transport in the Collecting Duct

HORMONE	Effect on			
	Na^+ REABSORPTION	K^+ SECRETION	H^+ SECRETION	H_2O REABSORPTION
Aldosterone	Increases	Increases	Increases	Increases
Vasopressin	Increases	Increases	?	Increases
Insulin	Increases	Increases	?	Increases
Endothelin	Decreases	?	Increases	Decreases
Prostaglandin E_2	Decreases	?	?	Decreases
Bradykinin	Decreases	?	?	Decreases
Dopamine	Decreases	?	?	Decreases

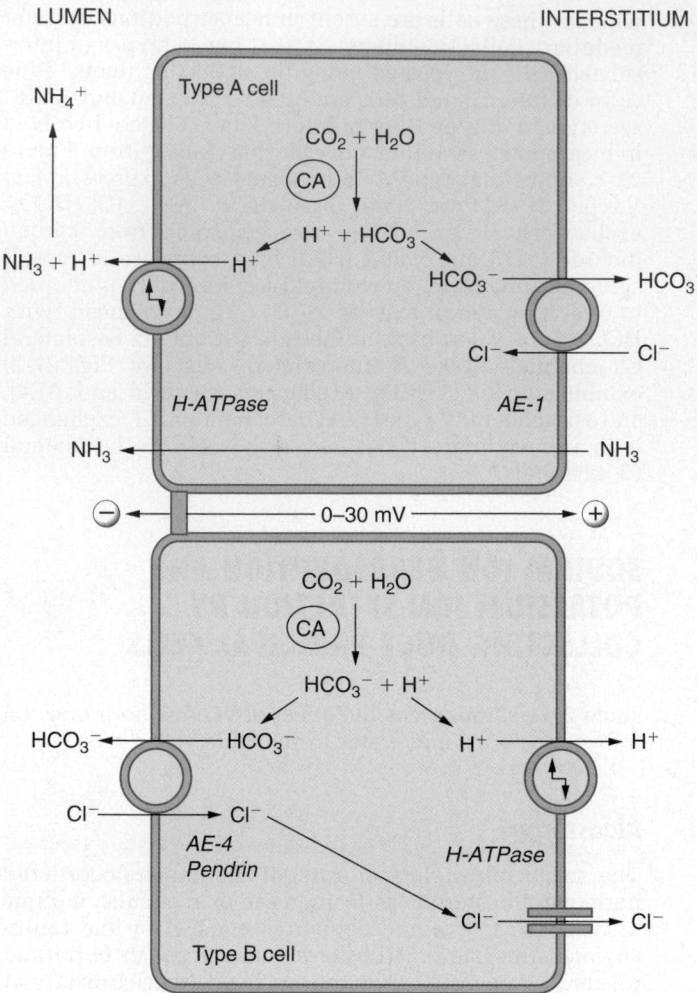

FIGURE 27-2. Mechanism of ammonia (NH_3)/ammonium ion (NH_4^+), hydrogen ion (H^+), bicarbonate (HCO_3^-), and chloride ion (Cl^-) transport in type A and type B intercalated cells of the collecting duct. *Arrows* indicate net fluxes. The names of the currently cloned transporters are shown in *italic*. AE-1, apical Cl^-/HCO_3^- exchanger; CA, carbonic anhydrase; CO_2, carbon dioxide; H_2O, water molecule; H^+-ATPase, hydrogen adenosine triphosphatase; mV, millivolt(s); Na^+, sodium ion.

glucocorticoids circulate at a concentration up to 1000-fold higher than that of mineralocorticoids, whereas in vitro, cortisol and aldosterone bind equally well to MR. In "aldosterone-sensitive" tissues, 11β-hydroxysteroid-dehydrogenase type 2 metabolizes cortisol to cortisone, which does not efficiently bind to MR.[9] The major role of this enzyme is illustrated by loss of function mutations leading to the syndrome of apparent mineralocorticoid excess associated with hypokalemic hypertension.[1]

Aldosterone controls Na^+ reabsorption in collecting duct principal cells through coordinated stimulation of apical ENaC and basolateral Na^+,K^+-ATPase necessary to maintain the stability of the intracellular Na^+ concentration ($[Na^+]_i$). The physiological response to aldosterone action can be separated into short-term and long-term effects, both effects being mediated by MR. The short-term (early) aldosterone effect on Na^+ reabsorption (and on K^+ secretion) can be observed after 30 minutes of aldosterone stimulation. This effect relies mostly on increased expression of active ENaC[10] and Na^+,K^+-ATPase[11,12] in the apical and basolateral plasma membrane, respectively. The long-term (late) effect of aldosterone induces a more sustained increase in the transport capacity of target cells via greater synthesis of ENaC and Na^+,K^+-ATPase subunits.[11,12]

Short-term stimulation of Na^+ reabsorption by aldosterone requires de novo transcription and translation.[2] Several aldosterone-induced genes have been identified,

but their roles in modulation of transepithelial Na^+ transport remain to be established. Serum- and glucocorticoid-regulated kinase 1 (SGK1) has received much attention. SGK1 messenger RNA and protein are induced 2 hours after administration of aldosterone in collecting duct principal cells of adrenalectomized rats.[10] Moreover, coexpression of SGK1 and ENaC subunits in the *Xenopus* oocyte expression system strongly stimulates ENaC activity and cell surface expression.[13] SGK1 binds and phosphorylates the ubiquitin-ligase Nedd4-2, thereby reducing its interaction with ENaC and leading to enhancement of ENaC cell surface expression.[14] Taken together, these effects strongly suggest a role for SGK1 in aldosterone-induced ENaC cell surface recruitment in collecting ducts. However, induction of SGK1 per se is not sufficient to recruit ENaC to the cell surface. Indeed, SGK1 is induced throughout the connecting tubule and collecting ducts, whereas ENaC is translocated to the cell surface in the connecting tubule and cortical collecting duct only.[10] In addition to the modulation of ENaC activity, SGK1 also increases Na^+,K^+-ATPase cell surface expression.[15,16] The physiological control of renal Na^+ handling by SGK1 has been highlighted by the generation of SGK1-knockout mice, which exhibit impaired ability to reduce urinary Na^+ excretion in response to dietary Na^+ restriction.[16] The mechanisms of action of aldosterone are summarized in Figure 27-3.

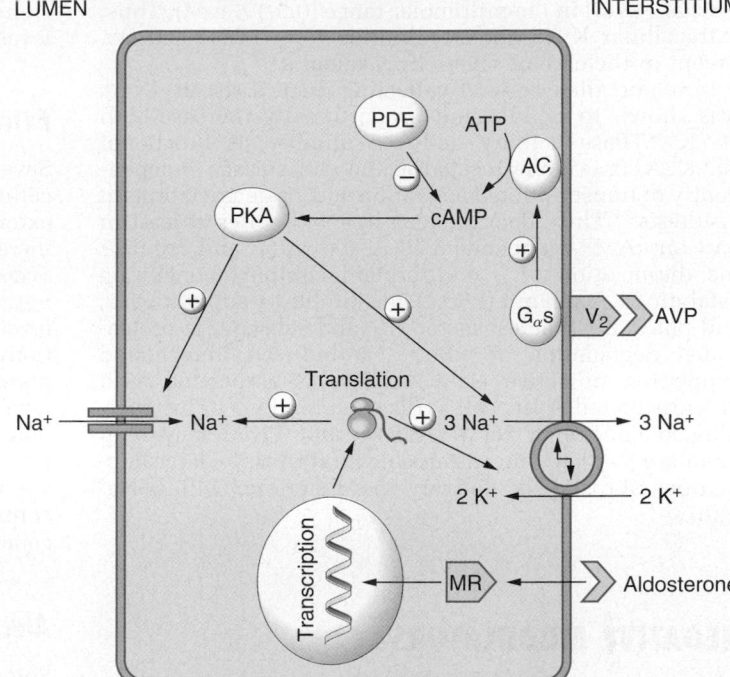

FIGURE 27-3. Schematic overview of aldosterone and vasopressin signaling pathways that control sodium ion (Na$^+$) and potassium ion (K$^+$) transport in collecting duct principal cells. *Arrows* indicate direction of the signaling cascade and the resulting stimulatory (+) or inhibitory (–) effects on their targets. AC, adenylyl cyclase; AVP, arginine vasopressin; G$_\alpha$s, G protein alpha subunits; MR, mineralocorticoid receptor; PDE, phosphodiesterase; PKA, protein kinase A; V2, vasopressin V2 receptor.

Vasopressin

Through vasopressin V2 receptor coupled to adenylyl cyclase, AVP stimulates the cyclic adenosine monophosphate–protein kinase A (cAMP/PKA) signaling pathway in collecting duct principal cells. In addition to water reabsorption (see previous discussion), AVP stimulates renal Na$^+$ reabsorption.[17] In both isolated mammalian collecting ducts and cultured collecting duct cells, AVP as well as cAMP analogues rapidly stimulate Na$^+$ reabsorption through coordinated activation of ENaC and Na$^+$,K$^+$-ATPase.[18,19] Patch-clamp experiments performed on principal cell apical membranes derived from isolated rat cortical collecting duct show that cAMP treatment increases the density of active ENaC.[18] Similarly, stimulation of Na$^+$,K$^+$-ATPase in response to cAMP was associated with a proportional increase of Na$^+$,K$^+$-ATPase cell surface expression without altering the total Na$^+$,K$^+$-ATPase cellular pool.[19] In addition to these short-term (minutes) effect on apical Na$^+$ conductance, long-term (hours) vasopressin stimulation increased expression of ENaC β- and γ-subunits in AVP-supplemented Brattleboro rats (a rat strain exhibiting a spontaneous knockout of the AVP gene).[20] These reports demonstrate that AVP controls the synthesis, plasma membrane expression, and activity of Na$^+$ transporters in mammalian collecting duct principal cells. The mechanisms of AVP control of Na$^+$ are summarized in Figure 27-3.

Cyclic AMP classically binds to the regulatory subunits of the PKA holoenzyme and releases active catalytic PKA subunits (PKAc) by alleviating autoinhibitory contacts. The PKA-dependent activation of ENaC may involve direct phosphorylation of ENaC β- and γ-subunits.[21] In cultured collecting duct principal cells, PKA inhibition by either protein kinase inhibitor H89 or myristoylated PKI (protein kinase A inhibitor) prevents the AVP-induced recruitment of Na$^+$,K$^+$-ATPase to the cell surface. However, direct phosphorylation of the Na$^+$,K$^+$-ATPase α$_1$-subunit by PKA is not involved in the stimulatory effect of AVP.[22]

Insulin

An antinatriuretic effect of insulin that is independent of glycemic status was first demonstrated in healthy humans and confirmed in an isolated perfused dog kidney preparation, indicating that insulin may directly control renal handling of Na$^+$. However, in in vitro perfused rabbit cortical collecting duct, insulin was shown to inhibit both K$^+$ secretion and Na$^+$ reabsorption, whereas it stimulates Na$^+$,K$^+$ pump–mediated cation transport in a time- and concentration-dependent manner in isolated rat cortical collecting duct. The reason for this discrepancy remains unexplained, because in every system studied so far, insulin stimulates Na$^+$,K$^+$-ATPase–coupled Na$^+$ transport.[2]

Intracellular Na$^+$ Concentration

[Na$^+$]$_i$ is the most important nonhormonal factor regulating Na$^+$,K$^+$-ATPase activity, which energizes Na$^+$ reabsorption and K$^+$ secretion processes. Na$^+$,K$^+$-ATPase is kinetically stimulated by Na$^+$, acting at the cytosolic side of the membrane, with an apparent affinity constant (K0.5) in the range of 5 to 15 mM in the presence of 5 to 10 mM of K$^+$. Under these conditions, maximal enzyme velocity (Vmax) is achieved at 60 to 100 mM Na$^+$. Because [Na$^+$]$_i$ ranges between 5 and 20 mM, Na$^+$,K$^+$-ATPase works well below its Vmax (20%-30%), and [Na$^+$]$_i$ is the major rate-limiting factor for Na$^+$,K$^+$-ATPase activity in intact cells. Thus, any increase in [Na$^+$]$_i$ stimulates Na$^+$,K$^+$-ATPase, which in turn pumps more Na$^+$ out of the cell and thereby contributes to restoration of initial [Na$^+$]$_i$. Conversely, any decrease in [Na$^+$]$_i$ reduces Na$^+$,K$^+$-ATPase activity. This autoregulatory process is highly efficient because Na$^+$ activation of Na$^+$,K$^+$-ATPase displays positive cooperativity; thus, small variations of [Na$^+$]$_i$ around K0.5 induce large variations of Na$^+$,K$^+$-ATPase activity. On the extracellular side, Na$^+$,K$^+$-ATPase is stimulated by K$^+$, with an apparent Michaelis constant (Km) in the millimolar range (0.5-1.5 mM). Thus, extracellular K^+ is not rate-limiting for ATPase activity, except in the case of severe hypokalemia.[2]

In mammalian cortical collecting duct, a rise in $[Na^+]_i$ was shown to rapidly and proportionally increase both Na^+,K^+-ATPase activity and the number of functional Na^+,K^+-ATPase units located at the cell surface independently of transcriptional activation and/or de novo protein synthesis.[23] This effect induced by $[Na^+]_i$ relies at least in part on cAMP-independent PKA activation and requires the dissociation of a multiprotein complex containing catalytic PKA subunit (PKAc), the inhibitory subunit $I\kappa B\alpha$, and p65/RelA (nuclear factor-κB), and subsequent proteasomal degradation of $I\kappa B\alpha$.[24] Na^+-induced upregulated expression of active Na^+,K^+-ATPase is associated with downregulated ENaC cell surface expression.[25] This coordinated control of Na^+,K^+-ATPase and ENaC may help maintain $[Na^+]_i$ within sustainable limits despite large fluctuations of distal Na^+ delivery and, therefore, cellular Na^+ influx.

NEGATIVE MODULATORS

The stimulatory effect of AVP Na^+,K^+-ATPase is counteracted by several negative modulators, such as prostaglandins, α_2-adrenergic agonists, endothelin, dopamine, and bradykinin. Most of these mediators modulate intracellular concentration of cAMP at the level of its production and/or degradation, thereby indirectly controlling ENaC and Na^+,K^+-ATPase activity.[2]

Water Reabsorption by Collecting Duct Principal Cells

Fine regulation of water reabsorption along the collecting duct is largely achieved through AVP-regulated expression and trafficking of AQP2 expressed in collecting duct principal cells.[7] In addition, AVP-independent factors, including extracellular tonicity, aldosterone, and extracellular calcium, modulate collecting duct water permeability and AQP2 expression.

Vasopressin

As summarized by Figure 27-3, AVP participates in both short-term (minutes) and long-term (hours or days) regulation of collecting duct water permeability by binding to basolateral V2 receptors of collecting duct principal cells, which in turn leads to activation of the $Gs\alpha$–adenylyl cyclase system, higher concentrations of intracellular cAMP, and PKA activation. Sudden increases in plasma AVP concentration cause AQP2-containing intracellular vesicles to rapidly fuse to the apical plasma membrane, consequently raising the water permeability of the collecting ducts. In addition to its rapid action, prolonged increases in circulating AVP increase AQP2 and AQP3 expression and thereby increase maximal collecting duct water permeability.[7] Prolonged infusion with AVP increases the water permeability of renal collecting duct in normal and AVP-deficient Brattleboro rats, an effect that correlates well with higher levels of whole cell AQP2.[26] Cell culture studies have shown that AVP stimulates AQP2 expression at both transcriptional and translational levels.[27]

Extracellular Osmolarity

Several pieces of experimental evidence suggest that extracellular osmolarity regulates AQP2 abundance. First, both extracellular osmolarity and AQP2 expression gradually increase along the corticopapillary osmotic gradient.[28] Second, water restriction increases AQP2 content in normal animals[28] and returns AQP2 expression to normal levels in animals treated with a V2-receptor antagonist.[29] Conversely, water loading decreases AQP2 content in normal animals[28] and reduces elevated AQP2 expression levels despite ongoing V2-receptor stimulation.[30] Furthermore, in collecting duct cell cultures, extracellular osmolarity has been shown to regulate AQP2 gene transcription via activation of the transcription factor TonEBP,[31] which controls the expression of several hypertonicity-induced genes.

Aldosterone

Some evidence suggests that aldosterone influences water reabsorption as well as Na^+ transport. Like patients with chronic adrenal insufficiency, adrenalectomized rats are unable to generate maximally concentrated urine,[32] and administration of the aldosterone antagonist spironolactone increases dilute urine production in patients with severe congestive heart failure.[33] Cell culture studies have shown that aldosterone increases AQP2 expression via increased translation of AQP2 messenger RNA.[34]

Extracellular Calcium

Hypercalcemia is associated with nephrogenic diabetes insipidus. Studies performed in rat models of vitamin D–induced hypercalcemia and hypercalciuria have shown that AQP2 expression and water permeability are decreased via activation of a luminal extracellular calcium receptor.[35] In addition, cell culture studies indicate that activation of the extracellular calcium receptor decreases AVP-induced translocation of AQP2 from intracellular stores to the plasma membrane.[36] This negative feedback may increase urine volume and thereby reduce the risk of urolithiasis in the presence of hypercalciuria.

ACID-BASE TRANSPORT BY COLLECTING DUCT INTERCALATED CELLS

General Mechanisms of Acid-Base Transport

The cortical collecting duct can secrete both H^+ and HCO_3^-, but the medullary collecting duct can secrete only H^+. This dual potential of the cortical collecting duct relies on the presence of both type A and type B intercalated cells. The relative abundance of these subtypes of intercalated cells varies as a function of diet and systemic acid-base status. Although interconversion of type B and type A cells has been observed in vitro,[37] this mechanism remains to be demonstrated in vivo.

H^+, derived from CO_2 and H_2O, is secreted by type A intercalated cells via the multimeric apical V-type H^+-ATPase, whereas HCO_3^- is exchanged for Cl^- by basolateral AE1 Cl^-/HCO_3^- exchanger. The importance of these mechanisms is illustrated by inherited forms of type I (distal hypokalemic) tubular acidosis caused by mutations of the B1 or a4 subunits of V-type H^+-ATPase, and of the AE1 gene. In addition, type II carbonic anhydrase deficiency leads to type 3 (proximal and distal) renal tubular acidosis.[38]

In the cortical collecting duct, H^+ secretion is favored by luminal negative transepithelial potential generated by Na^+ reabsorption. Disruption of luminal negative transepithelial potential due to decreased Na^+ reabsorption (aldosterone deficiency or potassium-sparing diuretic treatment) or increased Cl^- reabsorption (Gordon's syndrome) leads to type 4 (distal hyperkalemic) renal tubular acidosis.[39] This mechanism does not occur in medullary collecting duct because transepithelial potential becomes positive due to low Na^+ reabsorption, which does not compensate the flow of positive charges arising from H^+ and K^+ secretion.

After its secretion, H^+ is buffered by titratable acids (phosphate and creatinine) and by secreted ammonia (NH_3). Excretion of titratable acids is mostly constitutive, but secretion of NH_3 is tightly controlled. NH_3 is generated in the proximal tubule through deamination of glutamine, is reabsorbed by the thick ascending limb of the loop of Henle via the luminal $Na^+,K^+,2Cl^-$ cotransporter (NKCC2), is accumulated along the corticopapillary axis via the countercurrent mechanism, and, finally, is secreted by the collecting duct. The contribution of non-erythroid Rhesus protein homologues (RhBG and RhCG) expressed in collecting duct cells[40] remains to be determined.

Regulation of Acid-Base Transport

Systemic acid-base status is the major mechanism controlling acid-base secretion by the collecting duct. Metabolic as well as respiratory acidosis increases whole cell V-type H^+-ATPase expression and induces recruitment of an inactive intracellular pool to the apical membrane of type A intercalated cells. In addition, carbonic anhydrase expression and activity are increased, and HCO_3^- secretion by type B intercalated cells is inhibited. A mirror image of this situation is observed during alkalosis.[8]

Several hormonal and local factors also contribute to regulated acid-base transport along the collecting duct. Angiotensin II increases HCO_3^- reabsorption along the collecting duct via AT1 receptor–induced recruitment of V-type H^+-ATPase.[8] On the other hand, aldosterone increases H^+ secretion via (1) increased Na^+ reabsorption and thereby luminal-negative transepithelial potential[2] and (2) stimulation of V-type H^+-ATPase activity.[41] Finally, endothelin 1 stimulates HCO_3^- reabsorption and H^+ secretion along the collecting duct via A-type endothelin receptors.[42]

Key Points

1. Fine tuning of Na^+ and water reabsorption as well as K^+ and H^+ secretion occurs along the collecting ducts.
2. Principal cells are responsible for Na^+ and water reabsorption and K^+ secretion, whereas intercalated cells account for H^+ secretion as well as HCO_3^- and Cl^- reabsorption.
3. Na^+ reabsorption generates a luminal-negative transepithelial potential, which drives K^+ and H^+ secretion.
4. Aldosterone is the major stimulatory factor of Na^+ reabsorption and K^+ secretion.
5. Vasopressin and interstitial osmolarity are the major factors controlling aquaporin 2 expression levels and, thereby, water reabsorption.

Key References

1. Lifton RP, Gharavi AG, Geller DS: Molecular mechanisms of human hypertension. Cell 2001;104:545-556.
2. Féraille E, Doucet A: Sodium-potassium-adenosinetriphosphatase-dependent sodium transport in the kidney: Hormonal control. Physiol Rev 2001;81:345-418.
7. Nielsen S, Frokiaer J, Marples D, et al: Aquaporins in the kidney: From molecules to medicine. Physiol Rev 2002;82:205-244.
9. Ferrari P, Krozowski Z: Role of the 11beta-hydroxysteroid dehydrogenase type 2 in blood pressure regulation. Kidney Int 2000;57:1374-1381.
39. Rodriguez Soriano J: Renal tubular acidosis: The clinical entity. J Am Soc Nephrol 2002;13:2160-2170.

See the companion Expert Consult website for the complete reference list.

Acute Renal Failure: Pathophysiological Principles

Pathophysiology

CHAPTER 28

Ischemic Acute Renal Failure

Susan Garwood

OBJECTIVES

This chapter will:

1. Explain how prerenal azotemia progresses to ischemic acute renal failure.
2. Provide diagnostic criteria for differentiating between prerenal azotemia and ischemic renal failure.
3. Describe the pathophysiological changes in tubular epithelial cells that contribute to the profound reduction in glomerular filtration rate typical of ischemic acute renal failure.
4. Discuss the pathophysiological principles of renal vascular endothelial activation, which serve to reduce renal blood flow further and extend cellular injury.
5. Set the scene for an understanding of the dual role of nitric oxide and oxidant injury discussed in later chapters.

Ischemic acute renal failure (ARF) spans the range from prerenal azotemia to acute tubular necrosis (ATN) and accounts for most cases of ARF seen in the community and for approximately three quarters of hospital-acquired cases of acute renal failure.[1] Prerenal azotemia may be completely reversible if the underlying causes are corrected, but prolonged or untreated prerenal azotemia often progresses to ATN, which continues to have substantial morbidity and mortality rates. Although ischemic ARF is frequently associated with multiple-organ failure, the presence of ARF carries an independent risk for death.[2] The ischemic burden necessary before prerenal azotemia develops into full-blown ATN is well characterized in animal experimental models, but the equivalent is unknown in humans. An understanding of the pathophysiology and adaptive responses in the varying stages of ischemic kidney injury may enable early diagnosis and treatment of prerenal azotemia, before ATN ensues,

and may help further the search for better treatment modalities.

PRERENAL AZOTEMIA

Prerenal azotemia is caused by an absolute or relative reduction in renal perfusion, effecting a modest reduction in glomerular filtration rate (GFR) and increases in serum creatinine and blood urea nitrogen levels. It is generally, but not exclusively, accompanied by oliguria (see later). This disorder occurs as a physiological response to lowered renal perfusion, which may result from a globally or regionally reduced blood flow to the kidney (Table 28-1). Regardless of the cause, the initial compensatory mechanisms correct renal blood flow (RBF) and bring GFR toward normal. The ability of the kidney to autoregulate RBF and GFR was first demonstrated 60 years ago.[3] Since then it has become well established that the renal microvasculature exhibits a highly efficient, autoregulatory behavior such that steady-state renal blood flow, GFR, glomerular pressure, proximal tubule pressure, and peritubular capillary pressure remain relatively unchanged over a wide range of renal arterial perfusion pressures.[4] Autoregulation has been demonstrated in denervated and isolated kidneys, so autoregulation of both RBF and GFR is thought to be intrinsic to the kidney, residing predominantly in the afferent arteriole. It is believed to be partly mediated by an intrinsic myogenic response to changes in renal arterial perfusion pressure, allowing a gradual vasodilation of the preglomerular arteriole, and partly to the tubuloglomerular feedback mechanism, both of which stabilize GFR and fluid delivery to the distal nephron (see also Chapters 25, 27, and 36).[4]

In addition to engendering renal autoregulation, global hypotension or hypoperfusion stimulates the baroreceptors in the carotid sinus and aortic arch. This initiates activation of the sympathetic nervous system and the renin-angiotensin-aldosterone system (RAAS) and also stimulates release of vasopressin from the posterior pitu-

TABLE 28-1

Causes of Reduced Renal Perfusion

Global Causes

Decreased cardiac output:	
Hypovolemia	Hemorrhage
	Reduced fluid intake
	Diarrhea
	Hyperemesis
	Polyuria (diuretics, hyperglycemia, central diabetes insipidus)
	Excessive sweating
	Burns
	Third spacing (bowel obstruction or surgery, peritonitis, pancreatitis)
	Enterocutaneous fistula
	Adrenal insufficiency
Cardiac failure (left- and/or right-sided)	Cardiac arrest
	Ischemia
	Arrhythmia
	Cardiomyopathy
	Myocarditis
	Valvular disease
	Pulmonary hypertension
	Tamponade (effusion, restrictive pericarditis)
	Pulmonary embolus
Increased systemic vascular resistance	Hypovolemia
	Cardiogenic shock
	Vasoconstrictor drugs
	Atheromatous aortic disease
	Hypothermia
	Coarctation of the aorta
	Pheochromocytoma
	Vascular ring
Decreased systemic vascular resistance	Sepsis
	Toxemia
	Systemic inflammatory response
	Vasodilator drugs
	Hyperthermia
	Cirrhosis
	Arteriovenous fistula
	Anaphylaxis
Cardiopulmonary bypass	Pulsatile flow
	Nonpulsatile flow
	Deep hypothermic circulatory arrest

Regional Causes

Aorta and/or renal artery or renal vein	Atheroma
	Dissection
	Thrombus
	Embolus
	Surgical cross-clamping
	External compression (hematoma, tumor)
	Vasculitis
	Phlebitis
Intrarenal	Arteriosclerosis
	Vasculitis
	Vasoconstrictor drugs
	Increased renin-angiotensin-aldosterone system state

itary—a net effect of increased proximal and distal tubule reabsorption—so that autoregulation of RBF and GFR takes place in a milieu of generalized vasoconstriction and an upregulated RAAS, which also serve to normalize systemic blood pressure during hypotension.

If hypoperfusion continues, vasoconstriction at the postglomerular arteriole also takes place under the influence of angiotensin II, maintaining a constant glomerular capillary hydrostatic pressure. During this phase, a number of intrarenal and extrarenal vasodilators are also activated, mitigating the effects of unrestricted renal vasoconstriction and further adding to the maintenance of RBF and GFR. The vasoconstrictive effects of angiotensin II are counteracted locally by the intrarenal production of prostaglandins and nitric oxide (NO), which in the systemic circulation are direct vasodilators but, within the renal circulation, probably mediate their activity as antagonists of the vasoconstrictor effects of angiotensin II and renal adrenergic nerve activity. The effects of both angiotensin II and NO are complex within this context, and although NO generally antagonizes the effects of angiotensin II, it also stimulates the RAAS, so that chronic reductions in NO activity can result in reduced intrarenal generation of angiotensin II.[5]

In hypotension secondary to congestive heart failure, atrial stretch receptors stimulate the release of atrial natriuretic peptide (ANP) prohormone,[6] which in its active forms attenuates the production of renin, angiotensin II, angiotensin II–stimulated aldosterone release, and sympathetic nervous system activity.[7,8] ANP also inhibits Na^+,K^+-ATPase by enhancing the production of intrarenal prostaglandin E_2. The gene for the ANP prohormone is present in the kidney as well as the cardiac atria and is upregulated in early renal failure; however, intrarenal post-translational processing of the ANP prohormone results in urodilatin (rather than ANP), which exerts similar local effects.[9] Increased circulating levels of ANP stimulate intrarenal production of urodilatin, which probably accounts for much of the renal effects of circulating ANP.[10]

Throughout the period of prerenal azotemia, this balance of vasoconstrictor and vasodilator regulatory systems maintains RBF and GFR at the expense of increased water and urea resorption under the influence of vasopressin—hence the typical clinical picture of an increased blood urea nitrogen (BUN) level with a high BUN-to–serum creatinine ratio and oliguria (Table 28-2). Serum and urine osmolality values are high, with urinary sodium level typically less than 20 mEq/L. On the basis of history, physical examination, and serum and urinary testing, this clinical entity is therefore not too difficult to diagnose; however, the picture may be confused in patients in whom there are renal concentrating defects[11] or in catabolic states such as burns, trauma, and postoperative recovery, in which the obligatory excretion of urea causes polyuria.[12]

ACUTE ISCHEMIC RENAL FAILURE

As noted previously, the duration or intensity of ischemia required for the transition from prerenal azotemia to ATN is unknown in humans. Typically in animal experimental ATN, a single maneuver such as renal artery clamping or intrarenal infusion of high-dose norepinephrine for 30 to 60 minutes effects profound ischemia, predictably leading to ATN. Clinical ischemic ARF is somewhat different. It is often multifactorial, and seemingly minor deviations from baseline perfusion may result in renal failure in particular populations of patients, especially the elderly, diabetic patients, and patients with some prior renal dysfunction.[2]

TABLE 28-2

Serum and Urinary Tests Used to Differentiate Prerenal Azotemia and Ischemic Acute Renal Failure

TEST	Result	
	IN PRERENAL AZOTEMIA	**IN ISCHEMIC ACUTE RENAL FAILURE**
Blood urea nitrogen/creatinine ratio	15 : 1 to 20 : 1	≤10 : 1
Urinary sediment	Normal, occasional hyaline or fine granular casts	Renal tubular epithelial cells; granular and muddy-brown casts
Urine osmolality (mOsm/L)	>500	<350
Urine/plasma osmolality ratio	>1.4	<1
Urine specific gravity	>1.020	≈1.010
Urinary sodium (mEq/L)	<20	>40
Urine creatinine/plasma creatinine ratio	>40	<20
Fractional excretion of sodium (Fe_{Na}) (%)*	<1	>1
Fractional excretion of urea (FE_{urea}) (%)*	<35	>35
Fractional excretion of uric acid (Fe_{UA}) (%)*	<7	>15
Fractional excretion of lithium (Fe_{Li}) (%)*	<7	>20
Low-molecular-weight protein values[†]	Low	High
Brush-border enzyme values[‡]	Low	High
Renal failure index	<1	>2

*Fractional excretion calculated from standard formulas, as follows:

$$FE_{substance} = \frac{urinary\ substance}{plasma\ substance} \times \frac{plasma\ creatinine}{urinary\ creatinine} \times 100$$

Renal failure index = ([urinary sodium] × [plasma creatinine])/[urinary creatinine].
[†]For example, β_2-microglobulin, amylase, α_1-microglobulin.
[‡]For example, alkaline phosphatase, N-acetyl-β-glucosaminidase, alanine aminopeptidase.

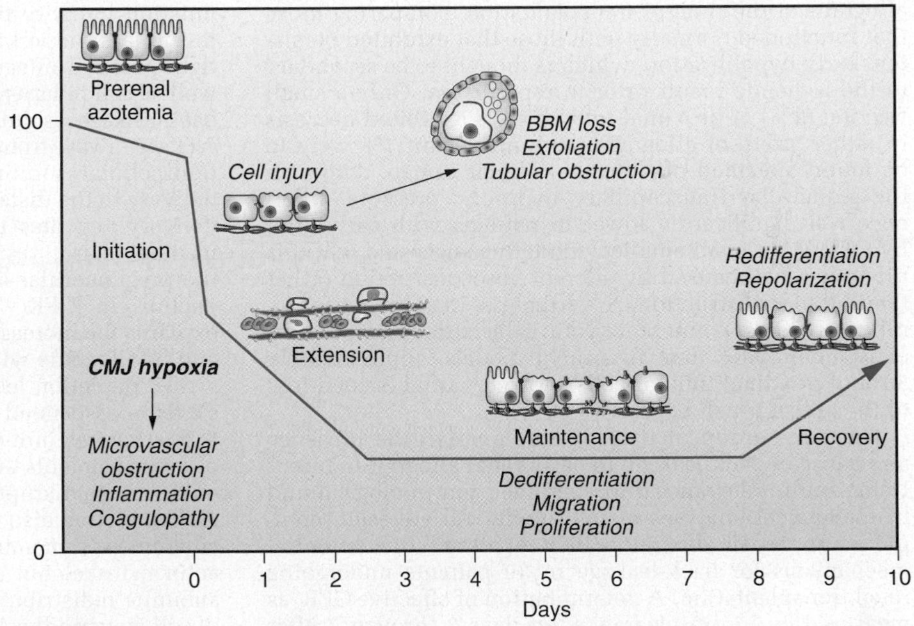

FIGURE 28-1. Stages of ischemic acute renal failure. BBM, brush-border membrane; CMJ, corticomedullary junction; GFR, glomerular filtration rate. (From Sutton TA, Fisher CJ, Molitoris BA: Microvascular endothelial injury and dysfunction during ischemic acute renal failure. Kidney Int 2002;62:1532-1539.)

The key sign of clinical ischemic ARF is a rapidly progressive and profound reduction in GFR, which has been noted to continue and even progress after the return of renal perfusion to baseline. This observation has led to the addition of an extension phase to the traditional paradigm of renal injury, which originally consisted of initiation, maintenance, and recovery (Fig. 28-1).[13] During prerenal azotemia, renal tubules and microvasculature remain intact; in ischemic ARF, marked pathophysiological changes occur in both the tubules and the renal vasculature.

In the early phase of ischemic ARF (*initiation phase*), autoregulatory mechanisms, which were effective in pre-renal azotemia, begin to fail, and RBF declines with GFR while adenosine triphosphate (ATP) stores become depleted. Inappropriate and selective renal vasoconstriction occurs in response to sympathetic nervous system stimulation and to RAAS. There is heightened sensitivity of the vascular endothelium to these two systems and a number of other vasoconstrictors, such as thromboxane, endothelin, and leukotrienes.[14-16] Furthermore, vasorelaxation in response to stimuli that normally generate endothelium-dependent vasodilators is also inhibited,[17] a development that may be attributable to the increased cytosolic and mitochondrial calcium concentrations noted at this stage.[14]

TUBULAR PATHOPHYSIOLOGY IN ISCHEMIC ACUTE RENAL FAILURE

The existence of tubular injury in ischemic ARF is evident from the disruption of normal function; tubular sodium resorption is decreased (fractional excretion of sodium [FE_{Na}] > 2), water reabsorption is impaired, and GFR falls precipitously. Structural and functional changes take place, but these may be different in animal experimental models and clinical forms of ischemic ARF in humans. In animal models, the decrease in GFR is attributed predominantly to the obstruction of tubules by necrotic cell debris with a resultant rise in the upstream hydraulic pressure in Bowman's space.[18] Afferent arteriolar vasoconstriction lowers glomerular capillary hydraulic pressure, depressing the glomerular transcapillary hydraulic pressure difference even further. Animal models of ischemic ARF are characterized by a reduction in the *effective GFR*, which is defined as the rate at which filtrate is delivered into final urine. Effective GFR is a consequence of transtubular backleakage of a fraction of the filtrate that is formed, a phenomenon that is attributable to a loss of those properties that normally render the tubule cell monolayer impermeable to certain components of filtrate.

To investigate the cause of the suspected reduced glomerular transcapillary hydraulic pressure in man, Alejandro and colleagues[19] examined living related renal allografts at the time of transplantation, comparing those that functioned normally with those that exhibited persistent early hypofiltration, which is thought to be secondary to the ischemic insult prior to reperfusion. Only a small fraction (2%) of proximal tubular cells exhibited necrosis in either group of allografts, and only about 1% were to be found sloughed off into the tubular lumen. Although the glomerular transcapillary hydraulic pressure difference was significantly lower in patients with early graft hypofiltration, mathematical modeling suggested that this difference was caused by afferent vasoconstriction rather than tubular obstruction. Nevertheless, in spite of the significantly lower count of necrotic cells in this clinical form of ischemic ARF than in animal models, approximately 50% of proximal tubular cells showed partial or total loss of the apical brush border.[19]

The same group of investigators queried the presence and cause of back-leakage in early renal allograft failure.[20] Using inulin clearance and combined morphological and histochemical analyses of the tubule cell adhesion complexes in renal allografts, they explored the potential mechanisms for back-leakage in 39 patients undergoing renal transplantation. A determination of effective GFR, as measured by inulin clearance, on days 3 through 7 after transplantation was used to divide the patients into two groups, those with sustained ARF and those with recovering ARF. Long-standing recipients of living donor kidneys that had never undergone rejection served as functional controls, and living related donors of healthy kidneys as structural controls. A transtubular back-leakage of almost 60% of filtrate was demonstrated in sustained ARF, but no back-leakage was detected in recovering ARF. Histochemical analysis of membrane-associated adhesion complexes confirmed a marked abnormality of proximal but not distal tubule cells in sustained ARF but, again, not in recovering ARF. Staining for the zonula occludens complex and adherens complex revealed diminished intensity and redistribution of cytoskeletal proteins from the apicolateral membrane boundary. The researchers concluded that impaired integrity of tight junctions and cell-cell adhesion

in the proximal tubule may provide a paracellular pathway through which filtrate leaks back in sustained allograft ARF. Consistent with the group's previous findings, electron microscopy showed disruption of both apical and basolateral membranes of proximal tubule cells in both sustained and recovering ARF, but negligible cell exfoliation and tubule basement membrane denudation.

Further investigations into delayed graft function in renal transplants also revealed that in allografts that suffered ischemic injury and persistent hypofiltration, there was a loss of polarity of proximal tubule cells with relocation of Na^+,K^+-ATPase and other cytoskeletal proteins from the basolateral membrane to the cytoplasm—abnormalities that were confined to proximal tubule cells.[21] This finding confirmed earlier reports of animal models of renal ischemia, in which Na^+,K^+-ATPase relocated to the apical membrane when cellular morphology was otherwise intact and apical sodium permeability, sodium-coupled cotransport, intracellular pH, and single-nephron filtration rates were normal.[22] Such an abnormal redistribution of Na^+,K^+-ATPase to the apical membrane domain could well explain the reduction in sodium and water reabsorption observed after ischemic injury. Furthermore, functionally normal Na^+,K^+-ATPase has been found to be necessary for the development of cellular polarity and the formation of tight junctions in renal epithelial cells.[23] During renal ischemia, renal tubular ATP is rapidly depleted, resulting in inhibition of Na^+,K^+-ATPase. It is thought that the loss of tight junction integrity that is seen during renal ischemia[20] is due at least in part to inhibition of Na^+,K^+-ATPase. Loss of tight junction integrity alters paracellular permeability as well as cell polarity, increasing permeability and therefore back-leakage as noted above. The relocation of Na^+,K^+-ATPase away from the basolateral membrane reduces transcellular sodium transport, causing greater sodium delivery to the distal tubule. This enhanced distal sodium delivery activates the tubuloglomerular feedback at the macula densa, resulting in further vasoconstriction of the preglomerular arterioles and thus contributing to the decline in GFR. The mislocated Na^+,K^+-ATPase also explains the increased FE_{Na} in patients with ischemic ARF and in allografts with delayed graft function.

ATP depletion leads to early changes in the actin cytoskeleton associated with increased intracellular calcium-activating, calcium-dependent cysteine proteases. Severing of actin filaments and digestion of actin-binding proteins ensues, with disruption of the cortical actin cytoskeleton.[24] ATP depletion also disrupts the adherens junction, which contains transmembrane cadherin proteins that link to the actin cytoskeleton and signaling proteins,[25] and integrin subunits redistribute to the apical membrane with a loss of cell matrix adhesion, facilitating cell exfoliation into the luminal space.[26] These apically displaced integrin units remain functionally active and may be responsible for trapping of exfoliated cells or pieces of disrupted brush-border membrane.[27] Although obstructing cellular debris is not reported to be a prominent feature of post-transplantation hypofiltration,[20,21] cellular casts are seen in the urinary sediment of patients with clinical ischemic ARF.

In addition to structural changes of the tubular epithelial cell cytoskeleton, ATP depletion during renal ischemia induces the elaboration of adhesion molecules and chemokines by epithelial cells.[28] A large number of chemokines that attract mononuclear and polymorphic cells have been shown to be produced by proximal tubular epithelial cells in vitro[29,30] and in animal models of renal transplantation.[31] Levels of chemokines that attract neutrophils, mac-

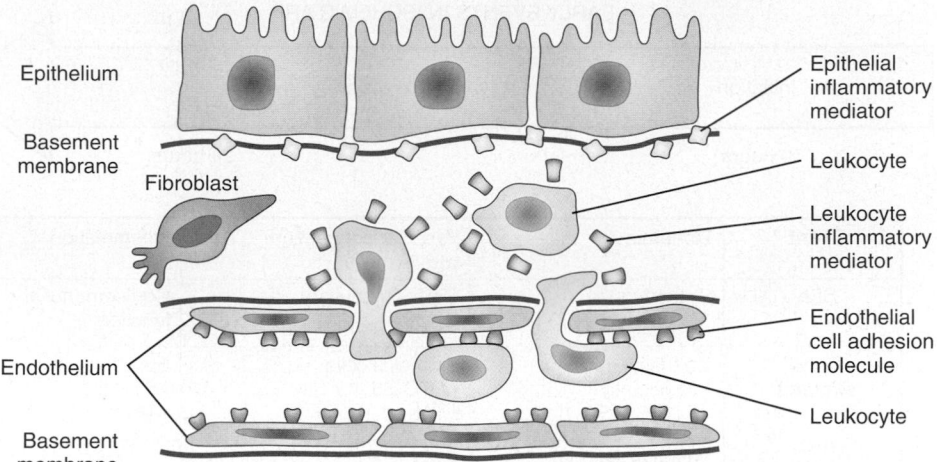

FIGURE 28-2. Inflammatory mediators elaborated by renal tubular epithelial cells attract and activate leukocytes, producing a positive feedback of inflammation and cellular injury. Adhesion molecules expressed on the surface of activated endothelial cells trap leukocytes and initiate leukocyte rolling and extravasation.

rophages, and T cells have been found to be increased in human renal allografts at the time of reperfusion, and their expression is correlated with ischemic time.[32] The activated tubular epithelial cells and leukocytes attracted into the interstitium serve to produce a positive feedback pathway of inflammation and cellular damage, not only to the epithelial cells but also to the vascular endothelial cells (Fig. 28-2 and later).

VASCULAR PATHOPHYSIOLOGY IN ISCHEMIC ACUTE RENAL FAILURE

Under normal physiological circumstances, the renal vascular endothelium regulates a number of functions; vascular permeability, vasoconstriction and vasorelaxation, the inflammatory response, and hemostasis are all modulated by endothelial cells. Injury to the endothelial cells during ischemia and reperfusion can contribute to the further impairment of renal perfusion and oxygenation, tubular epithelial cell injury, and reduced GFR that are all the hallmarks of ischemic ARF.

As noted previously, regional renal vasoconstriction occurs in response to sympathetic nerve stimulation and to RAAS as a result of heightened sensitivity of the vascular endothelium to vasoconstrictors during ischemic ARF.[14-16] Alejandro and colleagues[19] found that renal blood flow may be reduced as much as 50% within an hour after reperfusion in patients in whom delayed graft function develops after kidney transplantation, even though hemodynamics in such patients is similar to that in patients whose allografts functioned immediately. In patients with delayed graft function, this group found renal vascular resistance to be significantly increased even though plasma renin activity and endothelin levels were no different from those in patients with normal allograft function.[19] The loss of autoregulation in the ischemic kidney is thought to be related to increased cytosolic calcium observed in the afferent arterioles; the administration of intrarenal calcium channel blockers can reverse the loss of autoregulation and the abnormal sensitivity to renal nerve stimulation in norepinephrine-induced ARF in rats,[14] and a protective effect against delayed graft function has been shown in patients receiving diltiazem perioperatively for cadaveric kidney transplantation.[33]

The reduction of RBF during and after ischemic ARF demonstrates a heterogeneous pattern, with the corticomedullary region experiencing a more profound decrease in blood flow than other regions, at least in animal models.[34] A number of causes are thought to be responsible for this heterogeneity, including (1) differing regional sensitivities to endogenous vasoactive substances, (2) cell trapping in the outer medullary region resulting in stasis, and (3) localized responses to inflammatory mediators causing cellular injury to endothelial cells, swelling, and further impedance to flow. The outer medulla continues to remain hypoperfused with ongoing hypoxia even after the resumption of normal RBF, repair, and regeneration in the cortex.

The outer medullary vascular congestion, including the accumulation of intravascular leukocytes, is known to be an important component of ischemic ARF in both animal models and humans.[35,36] Activation of endothelial cells by ischemic injury, which promotes upregulation of the adhesion molecules P-selectin, E-selectin, and intercellular adhesion molecule-1 (ICAM-1) on the surfaces of endothelial cells, is thought to be responsible for the trapping of thrombocytes and leukocytes.[37-39] Inhibition of ICAM-1[37] and selectins[38-40] in animal models of ischemic ARF ameliorates renal dysfunction and improves survival. In addition to physically blocking the microcirculation, activated leukocytes engage in an inflammatory cascade that leads to further endothelial injury and alterations of the endothelial permeability barrier through the release of cytokines, proteases, and mediators of oxidant injury.[41,42] Animal depletion models show protection against ischemic ARF, and models lacking neutrophils[43] and/or T cells[44,45] have variously demonstrated protection. Natural killer cells and macrophages have also been implicated in ischemic renal injury.[46,47] However, it should be noted that lymphocyte trafficking into the kidney also occurs in sham-operated mice that have not been exposed to renal ischemia; abdominal surgery alone leads to lymphocyte migration to the kidney,[47] so some of the cellular trafficking noted in animal models of renal ischemia may be due to surgery alone.

Both endothelial and smooth muscle cells of the renal vasculature have a dynamic cytoskeleton that, like the tubular epithelial cells, is affected by ischemia. In the arterial clamp model, Sutton and associates[48] found that ischemia-reperfusion injury caused polymerization and aggregation of actin filaments in the basal and basolateral

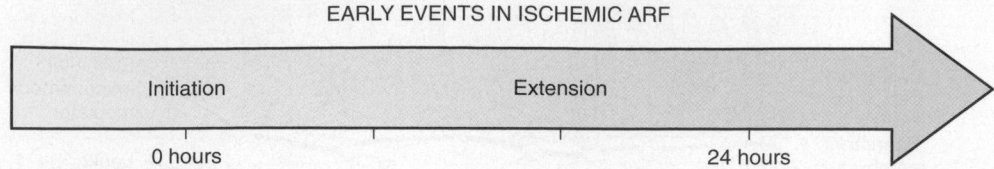

EARLY EVENTS IN ISCHEMIC ARF

	Initiation	Extension	
	0 hours		24 hours

Event	Ischemia	Vascular congestion with hypoxia	Inflammation
Site	Entire kidney	Corticomedullary junction	Corticomedullary junction
Cells affected	Epithelial cells • Especially PTC S1–S3	Epithelial cells • PTC S3 • TAL	Epithelial cells • PTC S3 • TAL
	Vascular smooth muscle cells		
	Endothelial • Large and small vessels	Endothelial cells • Small vessels	Endothelial cells • Small vessels

FIGURE 28-3. Sequence of events during the initiation and extension phases of ischemic acute renal failure (ARF). PTC, proximal tubular cell; S1, first segment of loop of Henle; S3, third segment of loop of Henle; TAL, thick ascending limb. (From Sutton TA, Fisher CJ, Molitoris BA: Microvascular endothelial injury and dysfunction during ischemic acute renal failure. Kidney Int 2002;62: 1532-1539.)

aspects of the vascular endothelial cells in the corticomedullary junction, altering barrier function, allowing leakage of plasma from the vascular space, and causing increased interstitial edema and a further reduction of already diminished medullary blood flow. Furthermore, oxidant injury as would expected during an inflammatory reaction has been shown to cause an increase in human renal endothelial cell solute permeability that is accompanied by a loss of occludin localization from endothelial cell-cell tight junctions.[49]

Endothelial cell injury is also associated with loss of the regulatory function of NO, as is demonstrated by a blunted NO response to endothelium-dependent vasodilators.[17] Uncoupling of endothelial nitric oxide synthase and a defective production of NO result in impaired vasorelaxation, diapedesis of polymorphonuclear leukocytes and monocytes, and local procoagulant and proaggregant conditions.[50] Furthermore, NO in the presence of reactive oxygen species results in the formation of peroxynitrite, which is capable of causing lipid peroxidation and DNA damage.

CONCLUSION

Ischemic ARF exists as a continuum from prerenal azotemia to ATN. Although the early stages of prerenal azotemia are completely reversible if the underlying causes are corrected, established ischemic ARF is associated with considerable morbidity and mortality. Clinical acumen is important in detecting prerenal azotemia before it progresses to ATN, and a number of serum and urinary test are available to help with diagnoses.

Autoregulatory mechanisms maintain RBF and cellular integrity at the expense of a modest decline in GFR and rising blood urea nitrogen during prerenal azotemia, but ischemic ARF is accompanied by a profound depression of GFR, greatly reduced RBF, and changes in tubular epithelium and vascular endothelium heralded by vascular congestion and hypoxia in the corticomedullary region

(Fig. 28-3). Ischemic injury and ATP depletion are associated with collapse of the actin cytoskeleton, loss of epithelial cellular polarity, disruption of tight junctions with ensuing loss of tubular fluid and plasma, expression of adhesion molecules and cytokines by both the epithelial and endothelial cells, and an influx of inflammatory mediators and leukocytes. Loss of the regulatory functions of endothelial NO and the production of peroxynitrite add to the ongoing vasoconstriction and inflammatory cascade. All of these events are more pronounced in the corticomedullary region, and this positive feedback of cellular injury is thought to continue after reperfusion and even to progress while other regions are undergoing repair and regeneration.

Key Points

1. Ischemic acute renal failure exists within the continuum of prerenal azotemia to acute tubular necrosis.
2. Autoregulation maintains renal blood flow and cellular integrity at the expense of a modest decrease in glomerular filtration rate and an increase in serum urea concentration during prerenal azotemia.
3. Prerenal azotemia is reversible if underlying causes are corrected before ischemic injury occurs to the tubular epithelium and vascular endothelium.
4. Depletion of adenosine triphosphate during ongoing ischemia causes changes in the cytoskeleton of both the tubular epithelium and vascular endothelium and disruption of tight junctions. This allows even further loss of tubular filtrate and plasma and decreases in glomerular filtration rate and renal blood flow.
5. Ischemic tubular epithelial cells express cytokines and adhesion molecules, which attract and

upregulate leukocytes. Vascular endothelial cells become activated and express adhesion molecules, trapping red cells and leukocytes particularly in the vessels of the corticomedullary junction.

6. Because of this inflammatory reaction, the process of cellular hypoxia and injury may continue and may even progress in the corticomedullary region after perfusion has been restored and repair and regeneration have begun in other regions.

Key References

13. Sutton TA, Fisher CJ, Molitoris BA: Microvascular endothelial injury and dysfunction during ischemic acute renal failure. Kidney Int 2002;62:1539-1549.

20. Kwon O, Nelson WJ, Sibley R, et al: Backleak, tight junctions, and cell-cell adhesion in postischemic injury to the renal allograft. J Clin Invest 1998;101:2054-2064.
21. Alejandro VS, Nelson WJ, Huie P, et al: Postischemic injury, delayed function and Na+/K+-ATPase distribution in the transplanted kidney. Kidney Int 1995;48:1308-1315.
28. Li H, Nord EP: CD40 ligation stimulates MCP-1 and IL-8 production, TRAF6 recruitment, and MAPK activation in proximal tubule cells. Am J Physiol 2002;282:F1020-F1033.
42. Bonventre JV, Zuk A: Ischemic acute renal failure: An inflammatory disease? Kidney Int 2004;66:480-485.

See the companion Expert Consult website for the complete reference list.

CHAPTER 29

Septic Acute Renal Failure

Li Wan, Sean M. Bagshaw, Christoph Langenberg, Takao Saotome, Clive N. May, and Rinaldo Bellomo

OBJECTIVES

This chapter will:
1. Explore the epidemiology of septic acute renal failure.
2. Discuss the prognosis of septic acute renal failure.
3. Describe current controversies about the pathogenesis and pathophysiology of septic acute renal failure.
4. Consider the possible role of the renal vasculature in the development of septic acute renal failure.
5. Present the principles of treatment of septic acute renal failure.

Acute renal failure (ARF) affects 5% to 7% of all hospitalized patients.[1-3] Sepsis and septic shock remain the most important cause of acute renal failure in critically ill patients and account for more than 50% of cases of ARF in the intensive care unit.[4,5]

Despite our growing ability to support vital organs and resuscitate patients, the incidence and mortality of septic ARF remain high.[5] A possible explanation why, despite treatment, ARF is so common in severe sepsis and septic shock and mortality has remained high might relate to our minimal understanding of septic ARF and its pathogenesis. It is therefore very important for critical care physicians to have an appreciation of what is known and not known about this condition in order to implement rational therapies. This chapter reviews current knowledge in the field and highlights new developments in our understanding of septic ARF.

DEFINITION

Until recently, there was no agreed way to define, identify, and classify septic ARF. However, the Acute Dialysis Quality Initiative has developed a consensus definition of acute renal failure that uses the acronym RIFLE.[6] This definition and classification system are described in detail elsewhere in this book. The relevance here is that the RIFLE classification and the widely established consensus definition for sepsis, severe sepsis, and septic shock that has been in use for more than 15 years together provide a standardized way to define septic ARF. Thus, septic ARF is ARF occurring in the simultaneous presence of both the RIFLE criteria for ARF and the consensus criteria for sepsis and in the absence of other clear and established, non–sepsis-related (e.g., radiocontrast, other nephrotoxins) cause of ARF.

PATHOGENESIS

The understanding of the pathogenesis of human ARF in general is markedly affected by the lack of histopathological information on what happens to the human kidney as glomerular filtration rate (GFR) decreases and oliguria develops in a variety of clinical settings. This lack of information stems from the risks associated with renal biopsy (especially with repeat renal biopsy), which make it ethically unjustifiable to obtain tissue from patients who do not have suspected parenchymal disorders and whose ARF is considered secondary to so-called prerenal factors. In the absence of such information, the clinician relies on indirect assessments of what might be happening to the

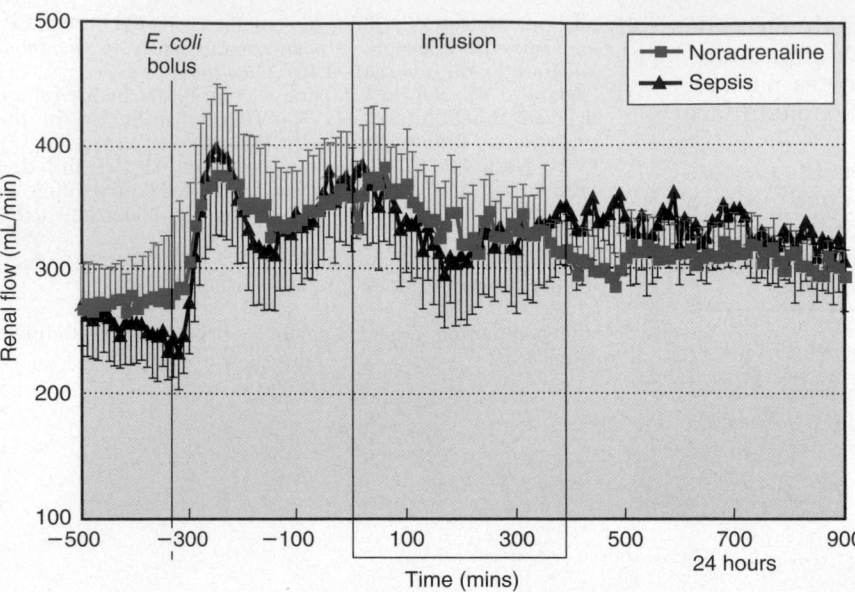

FIGURE 29-1. Changes in renal blood flow in a hyperdynamic model of sepsis with or without norepinephrine (noradrenaline) infusion. Renal blood flow is markedly increased.

kidney. Such assessments are based on results of blood tests and urine tests and force the clinician to "guess" what might be happening to kidney cells by using indirect forms of assessment, such as urine output, urinary sodium concentration, fractional excretion of sodium, and fractional excretion of urea. It is not surprising, therefore, that the understanding of septic human ARF has advanced very little in the last 50 years. To overcome such limitations, animal models of ARF have been developed that enable more sophisticated and invasive measurements to be made. Unfortunately, as highlighted in a 2002 report,[7] these animal models have been mostly based on ischemia-reperfusion injury or drug-induced injury. They are not relevant to septic ARF, and information obtained from them may be misleading when applied by the clinician to interpret what might be happening to an intensive care unit patient with sepsis in whom ARF is developing.

The Primacy of Renal Blood Flow

A major paradigm that has been derived from observations in animals and humans with hypodynamic shock (hemorrhagic, cardiogenic, or even septic) is that ARF is due to renal ischemia. This construct implies that restoration of adequate renal blood flow (RBF) should therefore be the primary means of renal protection in critically ill patients. Whether, in the presence of a normal or increased cardiac output, RBF actually decreases significantly or remains stable or even increases remains controversial.

In several experimental studies of septic ARF, global RBF was found to decline after induction of sepsis or endotoxemia.[8,9] This may result not only in a reduction in glomerular filtration but also, if hypoperfusion is severe and prolonged, in metabolic deterioration and diminished levels of high-energy phosphates, possibly causing cell death, ATN, and ARF.

Other studies show, however, that the renal circulation participates in the systemic vasodilatation seen during severe sepsis/septic shock, so that RBF and glomerular filtration do not diminish and the development of septic ARF occurs not in the setting of renal hypoperfusion but

of adequate and even increased renal perfusion. Ravikant and Lucas,[10] for example, studied a pig model of sepsis and showed that during hyperdynamic sepsis, there were increases in both global RBF and medullary blood flow. Brenner and colleagues[11] developed and studied a percutaneously placed thermodilution RBF catheter in eight critically ill patients. They demonstrated that sepsis-induced acute renal dysfunction occurred despite normal values for total RBF. Furthermore, during human sepsis, patients typically show a hyperdynamic state. Observations in hyperdynamic models of sepsis may, therefore, be much more relevant to human septic shock. Indeed, the reason that the results of experimental studies are so different in terms of renal perfusion may be related entirely to the animal models used (including animal type and type of insult), different methods of measurement, time and frequency of measurements and, most importantly, the state of the systemic circulation (hypodynamic or hyperdynamic). In fact, the consistent observation is that once a hyperdynamic state exists, global renal hypoperfusion/ischemia is *not* the norm (Fig. 29-1).

A comprehensive review of electronic reference libraries, focusing on experimental models of sepsis and ARF, was published in 2006.[12] This systematic review found that 160 experimental studies had been conducted that induced sepsis and focused on aspects of renal function or dysfunction and in which RBF was measured by one of several available techniques. Close to a third of these studies showed that RBF was either preserved or increased in experimental sepsis. To further investigate what factors might influence RBF in experimental sepsis, the investigators assessed which experimental variables were associated with preserved or increased RBF. They found that several aspects of the model (awake animal, time from surgery, use of endotoxin, cardiac output) predicted RBF during the experiment. When multivariable logistic regression analysis was used, cardiac output alone remained as the predictor of RBF. High–cardiac output sepsis was associated with preserved or increased RBF; conversely, low–cardiac output sepsis (mixed septic and cardiogenic shock) was associated with a low RBF. It is worthy of note that most patients seen in the intensive care unit with sepsis have a high–cardiac output state. In experimental studies in sheep in which both cardiac output and RBF were measured continuously and high–cardiac output septic state was induced by the infusion of *Escherichia coli*, Langenberg and associates[13] were able to simulate the typical clinical and hemodynamic state seen in severe sepsis or septic shock. Using this model, they showed that in hyperdynamic sepsis in an awake large mammal, RBF is markedly increased, renal vascular resistance is notably decreased, and GFR is significantly diminished, with a threefold increase in serum creatinine concentration and an equivalent decrease in creatinine clearance. They also found that renal recovery from this form of septic ARF was associated with decreases in cardiac output and RBF and an increase in renal vascular resistance.

These observations suggest that changes in renal vascular activity may be important in the loss of glomerular filtration pressure during the first 24 to 48 hours of sepsis. They also provide proof of the concept that glomerular filtration pressure can be lost in sepsis in the setting of markedly increased RBF. Put another away, septic ARF may represent a unique form of ARF, hyperemic ARF. Such understanding requires a further logical step—an appreciation that GFR is determined by glomerular filtration pressure, which in turn is determined by the relationship between the afferent and efferent arterioles. If the afferent arteriole constricts, glomerular filtration pressure falls, as do urine output and GFR. However, if the afferent arteriole dilates and the efferent arteriole dilates even more, RBF increases markedly, yet pressure within the glomerulus and GFR decrease. This may be the case in human sepsis.

Unfortunately, little is known about what happens to RBF in humans during severe sepsis or septic shock. The reason is that measurement of RBF requires invasive approaches. When RBF was measured in a small cohort of patients in humans, it was found to be either preserved or increased.[14] To put it bluntly, we simply do not yet know what happens to RBF in hyperdynamic human sepsis. This issue must be the focus of future investigations of the pathogenesis of septic ARF.

In conclusion, renal hypoperfusion might be important in hypodynamic states but may not play a key role in the development of ARF during hyperdynamic sepsis (the state seen in the vast majority of critically ill, septic patients with severe ARF). Further work is needed in humans to enable better understanding of the changes in RBF that occur during sepsis.

Intrarenal Hemodynamic Change

It is possible that even though global RBF is preserved or increased in hyperdynamic sepsis, internal redistribution of blood flow favoring the cortex may occur.[12] Unfortunately, no studies have looked at medullary and cortical blood flow in hyperdynamic sepsis with technology that allows continued measurement over time. An investigation by our group used laser Doppler flowmetry to continuously monitor medullary and cortical flows in hyperdynamic septic sheep (Fig. 29-2).[15] We found that both flows remain unchanged and that the administration of vasopressor (vasoconstrictor) therapy (norepinephrine) induced a significant increase in such flows. These observations challenge the view that the medulla is ischemic during hyperdynamic sepsis but simultaneously highlight that hemodynamic factors are indeed at work that can be modified by interventions affecting systemic blood pres-

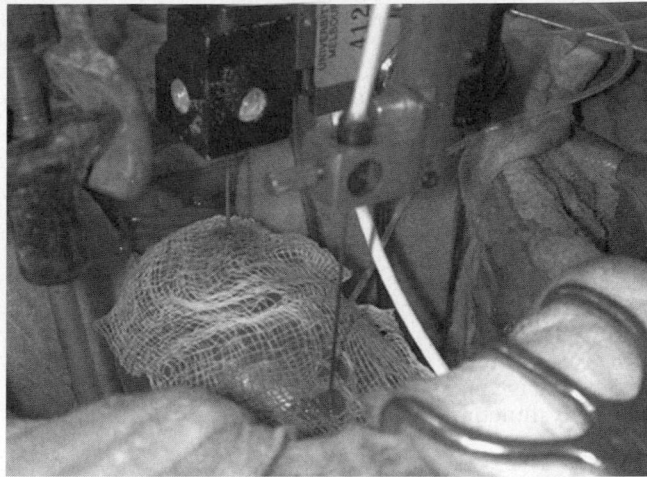

FIGURE 29-2. Photograph illustrating the technology of intrarenal Doppler flowmetry to measure relative changes in renal blood flow with sepsis in the medulla and cortex.

sure and cardiac output. In additional work using magnetic resonance spectroscopy technique with simultaneous measurement of RBF, we were also able to show that adenosine triphosphate is preserved during septic shock in the sheep, further supporting the notion that ischemia or bioenergetic failure may not be the primary cause of loss of GFR in sepsis.[16] Thus, intrarenal hemodynamic events do occur that might affect function. However, their favorable modification by vasoconstrictor therapy challenges the widely held view of what optimal renal resuscitation in sepsis is. Furthermore, even though hemodynamic changes might be important, they are likely to represent only part of the mechanisms responsible for loss of function. Other mechanisms may be at work.

URINE CHANGES IN SEPTIC ACUTE RENAL FAILURE

A variety of textbooks suggest that it is possible to use urinary tests to distinguish ATN (structural injury) from so-called prerenal ARF (functional injury). However, this aspect of septic ARF has not been adequately assessed. Our group has completed a systematic review of the urinary findings seen in experimental models of sepsis and assessed their diagnostic and prognostic value. We found that all the tests widely promoted as useful did not have sufficient data to support diagnostic accuracy, prognostic value, or clinical utility.[17] Similarly, in a systematic review of the value of such tests in humans, we found significant lack of data and a wide variety of findings in septic ARF.[18] All of these observations strongly support the concept that in the patient with septic ARF, biochemical analysis of urine using standard measurements of sodium, urea, and creatinine and calculating various indices of tubular function is not diagnostically accurate, prognostically valuable, or clinically useful. More research is needed in this field to improve understanding of the role of urinalysis in sepsis. In this regard, emerging biomarkers of kidney injury may prove more valuable.[19]

Nonhemodynamic Injury

From the preceding discussion, it is evident that neither global renal nor intrarenal hemodynamic changes can be consistently shown to be the sole contributors to sepsis-induced ARF. There must, therefore, be other mechanisms at work that are not hemodynamic in nature. Such factors that contribute to ARF in sepsis might be immunological or toxic.

Sepsis is characterized by the release of a vast array of inflammatory cytokines, arachidonate metabolites, vasoactive substances, thrombogenic agents, and other biologically active mediators. A large body of experimental data suggests that these various mediators and neuroendocrine mechanisms might be involved in the pathogenesis of organ dysfunction in sepsis.[20]

Tumor Necrosis Factor and Acute Renal Failure

Tumor necrosis factor (TNF) has been demonstrated to play a major role in the pathogenesis of gram-negative septic shock, mediating a broad spectrum of host responses to endotoxemia. In the kidney, endotoxin stimulates release of TNF from glomerular mesangial cells.[21] The direct toxic role of TNF in the kidney has also become clear. Knotek and colleagues,[22] using tumor necrosis factor p55 receptor (TNFsRp55)–based neutralization of TNF, achieved protection against renal failure induced by lipopolysaccharide (LPS) in wild-type mice. With pretreatment using TNFsRp55, GFR decreased only by 30%, compared with 75% decrease in the absence of TNF neutralization, suggesting that TNF plays an important role in septic ARF. Furthermore, van Lanschot and coworkers[23] reported that infusion of TNF in sublethal doses in dogs induced an increase in water and sodium excretion, an effect that could be prevented by prior cyclooxygenase inhibition, suggesting that vasodilatory prostaglandins mediated some of the renal response to sublethal TNF in this model. Cunningham and associates,[24] using *Escherichia coli* LPS in an intraperitoneal injection to establish a mice model of sepsis, showed that LPS-induced ARF can be attributed to the direct action of TNF on its receptor, TNFR1, in the kidney. Mice deficient in TNF receptor were resistant to LPS-induced renal failure and had less tubular apoptosis and fewer infiltrating neutrophils.[22] Although TNF receptor–positive kidneys transplanted into TNF receptor–negative mice developed LPS-induced renal failure, TNF receptor–negative kidneys implanted into TNF-positive mice did not. TNF thus seems to be an important direct mediator of endotoxin's effects during sepsis-induced ARF. These observations suggest that toxic/immunological mechanisms are important in mediating renal injury during sepsis and that hemodynamic factors do not operate in isolation and may not even be of major importance.

A New Concept in Septic Acute Renal Failure: Apoptosis

Apoptosis is a form of cell death that is mediated by a genetically determined biochemical pathway and characterized morphologically by cell shrinkage, plasma membrane blebbing, chromatin condensation, and nuclear fragmentation.[25-29] Cells can die by one of two pathways, necrosis or apoptosis. *Necrosis* results from severe depletion of adenosine triphosphate, which leads to rapid, uncoordinated collapse of cellular homeostasis. *Apoptosis* is an energy-requiring and genetically directed process.

There is now strong evidence to show that human renal tubular cells die by apoptosis as well as necrosis in experimental models of acute ischemic and toxic renal injury.[26-29] The endothelial cells can undergo apoptosis in response to a variety of stimuli, especially immune-mediated cell injury via TNF and Fas ligand.

Schumer and colleagues[29] have demonstrated that following a very brief period of ischemia (5 minutes), apoptotic bodies could be found 24 and 48 hours after reperfusion, and without any evidence of necrosis. Following more prolonged periods of ischemia, areas of necrosis became evident, but substantial numbers of apoptotic bodies were still seen after 24 to 48 hours of reflow. Whether or not apoptosis plays an important role in tubular injury in vivo remains controversial, with particular disagreement about whether renal cell apoptosis occurs during sepsis. However, Jo and associates[30] have shown that apoptosis of tubular cells by inflammatory cytokines and LPS is a possible mechanism of renal dysfunction in endotoxemia. They found that if high-dose TNF was added to cultured kidney proximal tubular cells, there was increased expression of Fas mRNA and of the Fas-associated death domain (FADD) protein as well as greater DNA fragmentation. Messmer and coworkers[31] have also shown that TNF and LPS elicit apoptotic cell death of cultured bovine glomerular endothelial cells, which is time and concentration dependent. The effect of these substances was characterized by an increase in proapoptotic proteins and a decrease in antiapoptotic proteins such as Bcl-xL. Unfortunately, TNF blockade with monoclonal antibodies fails to protect animal or kidney during endotoxemia.[32] Preliminary experimental observations by our group in septic sheep also show that after only 3 hours of sepsis induced by intravenous injection of *E. coli*, there was expression of early-phase proapoptotic proteins such as BAX as well as counterbalancing antiapoptotic proteins such as Bcl-xL in the tubular cells, indicating early activation of the apoptotic cascade in septic kidneys. Clearly, it would be helpful to have therapies that can favorably modulate the development of apoptosis.

ORGAN-PROTECTIVE THERAPY IN SEPTIC ACUTE RENAL FAILURE

The major principles of the management of septic ARF have remained unaltered for many years. They are (1) prompt resuscitation with fluid and vasopressors to maintain an adequate cardiac output and mean arterial pressure, (2) simultaneous culture of body fluids for the identification of a causative organism, and immediate administration of appropriate antibiotics thereafter, and (3) investigations targeted at identifying a focus of infection and prompt drainage if such a focus is found. Other possible avenues of treatment, summarized here, have also emerged.

Activated Protein C

Activated protein C (APC), an endogenous protein that promotes fibrinolysis and inhibits thrombosis and inflammation, is an important modulator of the coagulation and inflammation associated with severe sepsis. During sepsis, reduced levels of APC are associated with rising risk of death. Bernard and colleagues[33] demonstrated a significant drop in 28-day mortality in 1690 patients with sepsis; the rate was 30.8% in the placebo group and 24.7% in the group receiving drotrecogin alfa (activated)—also known as recombinant human APC (rhAPC). The efficacy of APC in septic patients may be due to its anticoagulation effect. However, a study by Joyce and colleagues[34] showed that rhAPC directly modulated patterns of endothelial cell gene expression clustering into anti-inflammatory and cell survival pathways and modulated several genes in the endothelial apoptosis pathway, including the Bcl-2 homologue protein, an inhibitor of apoptosis. Also, Cheng and coworkers[35] have demonstrated that APC blocks p53-mediated apoptosis of human brain endothelium in vitro; APC normalized the Bax/Bcl-2 ratio and reduced caspase-3 signaling. Their study creates a new link between coagulation, inflammation, apoptosis and cell death and provides insight into the molecular basis for the efficacy of APC in systemic inflammation and sepsis. Simultaneously, at a clinical level, there has been much controversy about the efficacy of APC.[36] Such controversy has led to calls for more randomized controlled studies in septic patients. A repeat of the initial Recombinant human protein C Worldwide Evaluation in Severe Sepsis (PROWESS) study will soon be under way and may enable better understanding of the systemic and renal effects of APC.

Caspase Inhibitors

Caspases are enzymes believed to play a key role in apoptosis. Caspase inhibitors have been developed as antiapoptotic agents. Fauvel and coworkers[36] developed an animal model showing myocardial dysfunction after endotoxin administration. These researchers demonstrated that a broad-spectrum caspase inhibitor (z-VAD.fmk) and a caspase-3 inhibitor (z-DEVD.fmk) decreased myocardial dysfunction, reduced caspase activation, and reduced nuclear apoptosis 2 hours after experimental endotoxemia. Neviere and colleagues,[38] using z-VAD.fmk 4 hours or even 14 hours after endotoxin administration in rats, showed not only that there was reduced caspase activity and nuclear apoptosis but also that endotoxin-induced myocardial dysfunction could be completely prevented. Because myocardial dysfunction can be prevented by antiapoptotic treatment, it is possible that future studies will show that the kidney is another organ that could benefit from caspase inhibitors. However, the complexity of the balance of factors involved in apoptosis and the response to sepsis is highlighted by the possibility that caspase inhibition may actually cause harm. Cauwels and associates[39] have demonstrated, in a model of TNF-induced shock in mice, that caspase inhibition is in fact associated with enhanced oxidative stress, mitochondrial damage, hyperacute hemodynamic collapse, kidney failure, and death. These investigators found a radical oxygen species (ROS)–mediated pathway to lethal TNF-induced shock. Once caspase was inhibited, a caspase-dependent protective feedback on excessive ROS formation was removed, increasing its lethality. These observations highlight how far investigators must travel to understand the significance and complex biology of apoptosis in sepsis. Nonetheless, despite limited understanding, some promising results have emerged from the use of lysophosphatidic acid, an endogenous phospholipid growth factor with antiapoptotic properties. In a mouse model of ischemia/reperfusion, lysophosphatidic acid prevented tubular cell apoptosis, loss of brush-border integrity, neutrophil influx, complement activation, and loss of renal function.[40]

Insulin and Acute Renal Failure

In a trial reported by Van den Berghe and coworkers,[41] use of aggressive insulin therapy aimed at achieving euglycemia in critically ill patients was shown to significantly reduce mortality.[41] Among the other important findings of this trial there was a dramatic reduction in the development of severe ARF requiring renal replacement therapy. A possible explanation for this finding may relate to the fact that insulin may play an important anti-inflammatory role in sepsis.[42-45] Thus, some of the beneficial effects of insulin therapy may be immune rather than endocrine. As such, they would fit in well into the paradigm that septic ARF or ARF of critical illness may represent an immunological/toxic state. It is also of interest that insulin has a powerful antiapoptotic effect[45] and that, conversely, a high glucose concentration induces oxidative stress–mediated apoptosis in tubular epithelial cells.[45] A very large multicenter, randomized, controlled study assessing the effectiveness of intensive insulin therapy in critically ill patients is currently under way[46] and will likely further elucidate whether tight glucose control does indeed benefit the kidney in critical illness and sepsis.

Low–Tidal Volume Ventilation and Acute Renal Failure

Ventilation of patients with acute respiratory distress syndrome (ARDS) by means of a low–tidal volume strategy has been shown to reduce mortality.[47] The mechanisms for such reduced mortality, however, remain unknown. It is possible that protective ventilator strategies might affect the well-being of other organs. In a fascinating series of studies, Imai and colleagues[48] demonstrated that low–tidal volume ventilation might protect the kidney from injury in the setting of experimental and clinical ARDS. Using a rabbit model of ARDS, these investigators found that animals randomly assigned to an injurious ventilator strategy had greater epithelial cell apoptosis in the kidney as well as the small intestine. Furthermore, such animals showed evidence of renal dysfunction. When renal cells were incubated in vitro with plasma from rabbits exposed to an injurious ventilator strategy, apoptosis of such cells was induced and was markedly greater than that seen with exposure to control plasma. Hypothesizing that Fas ligand might be responsible for these changes, Imai and colleagues[48] used Fas:Ig (a fusion protein that blocks soluble Fas ligand) to test the hypothesis. They found that Fas ligand blockade attenuated in vitro apoptosis of renal cells. To further confirm such an association, they obtained plasma from patients enrolled in a previous study of acute respiratory distress syndrome that compared the effects of ventilation with low and traditional levels of tidal volume; these investigators reported a significant correlation between changes in soluble Fas ligand and changes in creatinine.

CONCLUSION

Although hemodynamic factors might play a role in the pathogenesis of sepsis-induced ARF, they may not relate to ischemia. Septic ARF may represent a unique form of

ARF: hyperemic ARF. In addition, other immunological, toxic, and inflammatory mechanisms are likely to be at work. Among these mechanisms, apoptosis may turn out to be important. Indeed, organ-protective strategies reported in animal and human studies may work by inhibiting the development of the apoptotic cascade. It is possible that as evidence accumulates, the paradigms currently used to explain ARF in sepsis will shift from ischemia and vasoconstriction to hyperemia and vasodilatation and from acute tubular necrosis to acute tubular apoptosis. If this were to happen, therapeutic approaches would also be profoundly altered.

Key Points

1. Septic acute renal failure is the most common form of acute renal failure in critically ill patients.
2. Septic acute renal failure has a particularly unfavorable prognosis.
3. The pathophysiology of this disease is poorly understood. The currently dominant paradigm of ischemia and acute tubular necrosis may be incorrect.
4. Changes in renal blood flow are probably important in inducing loss of glomerular filtration rate in sepsis. These changes may be secondary to efferent

arteriolar vasodilatation with hyperemia and loss of intraglomerular filtration pressure.
5. Although new approaches to the treatment of septic acute renal failure are slowly emerging, the only accepted principles remain the same: prompt resuscitation, prompt antibiotic therapy, and prompt drainage of the septic focus when appropriate.

Key References

1. Uchino S, Kellum JA, Bellomo R, et al: Beginning and Ending Supportive Therapy for the Kidney (BEST Kidney) Investigators: Acute renal failure in critically ill patients: A multinational, multicenter study. JAMA 2005;294:813-818.
11. Brenner M, Schaer GL, Mallory DL, et al: Detection of renal blood flow abnormalities in septic and critically ill patients using a newly designed indwelling thermodilution renal vein catheter. Chest 1990;98:170-179.
12. Langenberg C, Bellomo R, May CN: Renal vascular resistance in sepsis. Nephron Physiol 2006;104:1-11.
13. Langenberg C, Wan L, Egi M, et al: Renal blood flow in experimental septic acute renal failure. Kidney Int 2006;69:1996-2002.
48. Imai Y, Parodo J, Kajikawa O, et al: Injurious mechanical ventilation and end-organ epithelial cell apoptosis and organ dysfunction in an experimental model of acute respiratory distress syndrome. JAMA 2003;289:2104-2112.

See the companion Expert Consult website for the complete reference list.

CHAPTER 30

Toxic Acute Renal Failure

Pieter Evenepoel

OBJECTIVES

This chapter will:
1. Describe the epidemiology of nephrotoxic acute kidney injury.
2. Explore the pathophysiological mechanisms underlying drug-induced nephrotoxicity.
3. Detail the roles of altered renal hemodynamics, tubular toxicity mediated by reactive oxygen species, allergic interstitial inflammation, obstructive tubulopathy, vasculopathy, and osmotic nephrosis in the development of nephrotoxicity.
4. Explain the implications of a better knowledge of the pathophysiological mechanism(s) involved in nephrotoxic acute kidney injury.

Acute renal failure (ARF), defined as a 50% increase in the serum creatinine concentration from baseline, occurs in approximately 5% of hospitalized patients. Surgical patients are particularly predisposed to ARF because of the physiological insult induced by major surgical procedures, preexisting comorbidity, and sepsis. Patients at risk

for development of perioperative ARF include those with reduced renal functional reserve, arterial hypertension, cardiac disease, peripheral vascular disease, diabetes mellitus, jaundice, and advanced age. The type of surgery is also an important determinant. Other risk factors are hypothermia, hypoxia, unstable hemodynamics, and cardiopulmonary bypass.[1,2]

Etiologically, ARF can be divided into three categories: prerenal azotemia, postrenal azotemia, and intrinsic renal failure. *Prerenal azotemia*, defined as reversible renal failure caused by decreased effective arterial blood flow to the kidney, accounts for 60% of inpatient cases of ARF. Anesthesia, blood and volume losses, volume overload and heart failure, and peripheral shunting of blood due to vasodilatation from sepsis are all common causes of prerenal azotemia in the perioperative period. Obstructive nephropathy accounts for 10% of inpatient cases of ARF. Intrinsic causes, finally, account for approximately 30% of inpatient cases of ARF.[3] Ninety percent of cases of intrinsic ARF in adults are due to acute tubular necrosis (ATN), and ischemic ATN is the most common cause of intrinsic renal failure in the surgical setting.

Finally, a wide range of toxins can provoke ARF or contribute to its onset and severity.[4] Drug-induced nephrotoxicity accounts for more than 2% of cases of ARF in patients admitted to the hospital and for 15% of cases in those in intensive care units (ICUs).[5,6] Drug-induced ARF is encountered in a growing number of hospitalized patients as a result of a more aggressive diagnostic and therapeutic approach in an aging and multimedicated patient population that is increasingly vulnerable (because of greater comorbidity). Beside the risk factors already mentioned, drug interactions should be considered an important risk factor. The mechanisms involved are an increase in blood and/or tissue half-life of the nephrotoxic drug (through interference with its metabolism and/or elimination) and/or an additive nephrotoxicity. The kidney is extremely susceptible to drug-induced toxicity because of its high blood flow (approximately 25% of the resting cardiac output), its capacity to concentrate drugs to levels considerably higher than those in blood, and its ability to degrade drugs, which often results in the formation of reactive metabolites.

The purpose of this chapter is to summarize common pathophysiological mechanisms underlying the nephrotoxicity of drugs that are relevant in the intensive care setting. As is evident from Table 30-1, many nephrotoxins may cause injury through different pathways.

PATHOPHYSIOLOGICAL MECHANISMS OF DRUG-INDUCED NEPHROTOXICITY

Altered Renal Hemodynamics

Glomerular filtration rate (GFR) is an important parameter of renal function. Glomerular filtration depends on renal blood flow, effective glomerular capillary pressure, and the hydraulic permeability of the glomerular basement membrane. Glomerular pressure (and GFR) can be modulated by changes in the resistance of the afferent and efferent glomerular arterioles: Vasoconstriction of the former and vasodilatation of the latter lowers the intraglomerular pressure, whereas the reverse situation raises it.

In normal circumstances, several mechanisms operate to keep GFR and renal blood flow at optimal, stable levels, the most important being renal autoregulation by intrinsic mechanisms. However, in situations of decreased renal perfusion pressure, hormonal mechanisms come into play, of which the renin-angiotensin and renal prostaglandin systems are the most important. Angiotensin II predominantly causes vasoconstriction of the efferent arteriole, thus preserving GFR in cases of lowered renal blood flow, whereas prostaglandins act as vasodilators of the afferent arteriole. In view of the regulatory functions of these hormone systems, it is not surprising that drugs that interfere with either system can have an important influence on renal function.[4]

Nonsteroidal anti-inflammatory drugs (NSAIDs) are widely used in the treatment of mild to moderate postoperative pain. Their opioid-sparing effect and availability for parenteral use (ketorolac) render them ideal for administration in the setting of elective day-only and short-stay surgery. These agents act by inhibiting cyclooxygenase (COX), the enzyme that converts arachidonic acid into prostaglandins. Although the selective COX-2 inhibitors have a lower incidence of gastrointestinal side effects, they appear to offer no advantage with respect to hemodynamically mediated ARF.[7-9] Angiotensin-converting enzyme inhibitors and angiotensin II receptor antagonists, which are commonly used in the treatment of hypertension and chronic heart failure, act by blocking the activity of angio-

TABLE 30-1

Common Medications Associated with Acute Renal Failure*

PATHOPHYSIOLOGY	MEDICATIONS
Hemodynamic	Amphotericin B
	Angiotensin-converting enzyme inhibitors and angiotensin receptor blockers
	Calcineurin inhibitors
	Nonsteroidal anti-inflammatory drugs (NSAIDs)
	Radiocontrast agents (?)
Tubulotoxic	Acyclovir
	Aminoglycosides
	Amphotericin B
	Calcineurin inhibitors
	Carbamazepine
	Carboplatin
	Cidofovir
	Cisplatin
	Foscarnet
	Ifosfamide
	Radiocontrast agents
	Vancomycin
Immunological	Allopurinol
	Cephalosporins
	Cimetidine
	Cytosine arabinoside
	Furosemide
	NSAIDs
	Penicillins
	Phenytoin
	Proton pump inhibitors
	Quinolones
	Rifampicin
	Sulfonamides
	Thiazide
Tubulo-obstructive	Acyclovir
	Indinavir
	Methotrexate
	Sulfonamides
	Triamterene
Vascular	Calcineurin inhibitors
	Clopidogrel
	Gemcitabine
	Mitomycin C
	Quinine/quinidine
	Rapamycin
	Ticlopidine
Nephrotic	Dextran
	Hydroxyethyl starch
	Immunoglobulins
	Mannitol
	Radiocontrast agents
	Sucrose

*Nonexhaustive list.

tensin II. Several reports have implicated these classes of drugs as the cause of ARF in patient groups in whom the hormonal mechanisms already mentioned were stimulated by a depleted "true" or "effective" circulatory volume (chronic heart failure, cirrhosis, nephrotic syndrome). Renal failure in these patients is purely functional. After discontinuation of the offending drug and restoration of the effective circulatory volume, the renal failure can usually be reversed quickly. If the reduction of renal blood flow and GFR is more profound and sustained, however, ischemic ATN may ensue.

Calcineurin inhibitors may also cause an acute, functional, and dose-dependent decrease in renal blood flow and GFR. The current hypothesis is that calcineurin inhibitors cause predominantly afferent arteriolar vasoconstriction and thereby alter renal hemodynamics. The vasoconstriction is, in part, related to an imbalance of prostaglandin E_2 (vasodilation) and thromboxane A_2 (vasoconstriction). In addition, cyclosporine may interfere with the production of nitric oxide and increase systemic vascular resistance through activation of the sympathetic nervous system. After discontinuation of calcineurin inhibitors, renal function returns to baseline without any major histologic or cytologic abnormalities. However, prolonged vasoconstriction may cause ATN and lead to tubulointerstitial lesions consistent with chronic and irreversible nephrotoxicity.[10]

Radiocontrast agents induce a biphasic hemodynamic response in the kidney, an initial increase being followed by a modest and transient decrease in blood flow. This response, however, is also noted after injection of mannitol and has been acknowledged to be nonnephrotoxic. Contrast agents may also induce disturbances in intrarenal hemodynamics that result in medullary ischemia.[11] Clinical data question the relevance of these disturbances in the pathogenesis of contrast-induced ARF, however. Indeed, fenoldopam mesylate, a unique vasodilator that selectively increases both renal cortical and outer medullary blood flow, has been shown to be ineffective in preventing deterioration of renal function in patients with chronic renal failure who receive contrast agents.[12] Overall, current evidence points to direct tubular cell injury as the major pathway leading to renal failure in patients receiving contrast agents (see later).

In addition to alterations in tubular function, amphotericin B may induce changes in renal hemodynamics. By changing vascular smooth muscle cell permeability, amphotericin B may cause cell depolarization with the resultant opening of voltage-dependent calcium channels and muscle contraction. Higher intracellular calcium concentration may activate arachidonic acid metabolism and lead to the accumulation of vasoactive substances with a net vasoconstrictive effect. Renal vasoconstriction appears to play a major role in the amphotericin B–induced reduction in GFR, and recurrent ischemia may lead to structural and tubular damage and permanent nephrotoxic effects.[13]

Allergic Interstitial Inflammation

Acute interstitial nephritis was formerly related to a variety of infections but is now increasingly associated with drug therapy.[14] Although many drugs have been implicated in clinical cases of acute interstitial nephritis (AIN), the frequency with which individual drugs are implicated varies widely. The prototype agent for drug-induced AIN is methicillin. As a result of its propensity to cause AIN (in up to 17% of patients who have been treated for more than 10 days), this agent is rarely used any more in clinical practice. The number of drugs associated with AIN exceeds 50 and is still rising. Medication groups most commonly implicated in drug-induced AIN include penicillins, cephalosporins, sulfonamides, and nonsteroidal anti-inflammatory drugs.[14]

Acute interstitial nephritis usually occurs on an allergic basis in an idiosyncratic and non–dose-dependent manner. The pathogenesis of the majority of cases involves a cell-mediated hypersensitivity reaction. This process is supported by the observation that T cells are the predominant cell type in the interstitial infiltrate. Most probably, the offending drugs behave like haptens, which may bind to serum or cellular proteins and subsequently are processed and presented by major histocompatibility complex molecules as hapten-modified peptides. Alternatively, some drugs, such as sulfamethoxazole, may be able to bind directly to major histocompatibility complex molecules. Once helper T cells have been activated, both antigen-specific and antigen-nonspecific effector mechanisms of injury are activated. Antigen-specific mechanisms include activation of both B and T cells. B cells are induced to differentiate into plasma cells and make antibody, which can react with a kidney antigen or can be deposited as antigen-antibody complexes. Helper T cells can induce effector T cells, which may be either cytotoxic to tubular epithelial cells, leading to necrosis or apoptosis, or inflammatory, leading to mononuclear cell infiltration. In addition, several cytokines are produced that amplify the immune response.[14]

A humoral response underlies rare cases of AIN in which a portion of a drug (i.e., methicillin) may act as a hapten, bind to the tubular basement membrane, and elicit anti–tubular basement membrane antibodies.[8] There is no strong evidence that the deposition of such antibodies alone results in injury to renal tubular epithelial cells. However, the deposition of antibodies can recruit nonspecific cytotoxic effector cells to the site. Activated macrophages can release a number of potentially harmful secretory products, including reactive oxygen species (see later). AIN is usually self-limiting, and spontaneous recovery occurs after withdrawal of the offending drug.

Tubular Toxicity (Mediated by Reactive Oxygen Species)

A substantial body of evidence attests to the involvement of reactive oxygen species (ROS) in the pathogenesis of nephrotoxic types of ATN, including heme protein-induced ATN as occurs in severe rhabdomyolysis and hemolysis, sepsis-associated ATN, and drug-induced ATN.[15,16] ROS commonly incriminated in the pathogenesis of renal and other forms of tissue injury include the superoxide anion (O_2^-), hydrogen peroxide (H_2O_2), hypochlorous acid (HOCl) and the hydroxyl radical (OH). The basic constituents of cells and their organelles—lipids, carbohydrates, proteins, and nucleic acids—can all be altered by ROS. Such oxidant-induced alterations can profoundly affect cellular function and vitality. Oxidative stress is the result of enhanced generation of ROS and/or deficient neutralization by antioxidant defenses, such as superoxide dismutase, catalase, and glutathione peroxidase. Possible sources of ROS include increased xanthine and nicotinamide adenine dinucleotide (reduced)/nicotinamide adenine dinucleotide phosphate (reduced) (NADH/NADPH) oxidase activity, and disabled mitochondrial respiration. Iron salts play a catalytic role in the generation of the highly reactive hydroxyl radical through the metal-catalyzed Haber-Weiss/Fenton reaction. Substantial evidence also supports the involvement of nitric oxide, which is generated in large amounts by the inducible form of nitric oxide synthase.[15]

ROS exert a variety of vasoactive effects, depending on the specific ROS, its rate of generation, and the vascular bed to which it is exposed. Superoxide anion mainly causes vasoconstriction as a result of its capacity to scavenge nitric oxide; hydrogen peroxide, however, may exert vasodilatory or vasoconstrictive effects. Additionally, ROS can influence the expression or activity of numerous vasoactive species (including endothelin, isoprostanes, and thromboxanes), can induce endothelial dysfunction, and can profoundly disturb vascular reactivity because of ROS-mediated effects on intracellular calcium handling in smooth muscle cells. Finally, ROS can promote leukocytic adherence to the endothelium.[15] Besides contributing to many of the renal hemodynamic and vascular abnormalities observed during the initiation and established phases of ATN, ROS may induce either sublethal or lethal cell injury (necrosis or apoptosis).[15] ROS-induced cell injury reflects the capacity of ROS to impair availability and/or synthesis of adenosine triphosphate, to destabilize the cytoskeleton, and to damage plasma and intracellular membranes. The destabilization of the cytoskeleton predisposes to shedding of tubular epithelial cells. This effect may ultimately compromise the patency of the tubular lumen as exfoliated cells become attached to one another as well as to the injured epithelial cells still attached to the tubular basement membrane. Thus, oxidative stress can also promote the formation of obstructing urinary casts.[15]

Oxidative stress, furthermore, can provoke inflammatory responses. Inflammatory processes are increasingly believed to be critical participants in the pathogenesis of ATN. ROS can induce other genes involved in the adhesion, and rolling of leukocytes on the endothelium ROS can also activate nuclear factor-κB, which in turn stimulates the production of tumor necrosis factor-α. Increased tumor necrosis factor-α leads to the recruitment and accumulation of inflammatory cells, including neutrophils, monocytes, natural killer cells, and T lymphocytes. These white blood cells secrete lysosomal enzymes, ROS, and proteases, which can directly injure surrounding renal tissue. In addition, the activation of these leukocytes may lead to further production of cytokines or chemokines and greater recruitment of leukocytes to the focus of inflammation, thus amplifying the renal inflammatory response.[15]

All of these mechanisms may contribute to a reduction of the GFR. Although an area largely unexplored to date, it is conceivable that ROS may also influence reparative and regenerative responses involved in the recovery from ATN. These responses are highly complex and involve the following processes: resolution of hemodynamic and vascular abnormalities, repair of injured cells, replacement of cells lost by apoptosis and necrosis, appropriate cellular differentiation dictated by the specific characteristics of the particular nephron segment, reestablishing cellular contacts with neighboring cells and the adjacent matrix, abatement and resolution of inflammatory processes, and recovery of luminal patency in obstructed nephrons. ROS thus not only may contribute to the pathogenesis of ATN, but, surprisingly, also may be involved in the reparative and regenerative events that nurse the kidney with ATN back to normality. Such considerations, as yet largely unexplored, raise the cautionary note that antioxidant strategies may not necessarily be beneficial when introduced after ATN is already established.[15]

ROS have been invoked in the pathogenesis of ATN induced by a number of drugs, including aminoglycosides,[17] carboplatin,[18] and cisplatin,[19-23] vancomycin,[24] amphotericin B,[13] calcineurin inhibitors (cyclosporine and tacrolimus),[25,26] and antiviral[27] and radiocontrast agents.[11,12,28] The origin, severity, and type of oxidative stress depends on the specific nephrotoxin.

It should be emphasized that whether the generation of ROS is the primary cause of tubular cell damage rather than a sequel of a direct tubular toxic effect is not always clear.[28] Radiocontrast agents, for example, may harm the tubular cell directly by altering plasma cell permeability or transport processes.[29]

The specificity of most of previously listed drugs for renal toxicity is related to their preferential accumulation in the renal proximal tubules. The intracellular concentration in the proximal tubules may be several times higher than the plasma concentration. Intracellular drug concentration is the major factor underlying the tubular toxicity. Low–protein-binding drugs such as aminoglycosides are freely filtered through the glomerulus. Most of the administered dose is excreted in urine, whereas a sizable portion is selectively accumulated in the renal cortex. At the brush-border membrane of the proximal tubule (cationic), aminoglycosides are bound to anionic phospholipids; they are then delivered to an anionic protein called megalin (glycoprotein 330) and undergo endocytic uptake into the cell.[30] Renal excretion of protein-bound drugs (e.g., antiviral agents, cisplatin), conversely, occurs through human organic anion/cation transporter-controlled mechanisms at the basolateral membrane and through multiple-drug resistance–associated protein (MRP)–controlled mechanisms at the luminal membrane of the proximal tubular cells.[27] It may be hypothesized that factors interfering with normal transport mechanisms modulate renal toxicity substantially (e.g., drug interactions).

In addition, the renal proximal tubules have a high dependence on oxidative phosphorylation for energy production and, thus, may be susceptible to oxidative stress. This feature also explains why ischemia sensitizes the kidney to oxidative injury.

Vasculopathy

A variety of drugs, including antineoplastics, immunotherapeutics, and antiplatelet agents, have been associated with thrombotic microangiopathy. In most series, the proportion of cases of thrombotic thrombocytopenic purpura/hemolytic uremic syndrome attributed to drugs has been small—less than 15%. In many instances it is difficult to separate the effect of the drug from the role of the underlying disorder (e.g., cancer). Although a direct causal effect has usually not been proven, the cumulative evidence linking several drugs with thrombotic microangiopathy is strong. As with idiopathic cases of thrombotic thrombocytopenic purpura/hemolytic uremic syndrome, basic science discoveries in the late 1990s suggest that the likely mechanisms by which these agents lead to a thrombotic microangiopathy include either an immune-mediated phenomenon involving the ADAMTS13 metalloprotease (quinine/quinidine, ticlopidine, and clopidogrel) or direct endothelial toxicity (mitomycin C and calcineurin inhibitor).[31-33]

Obstructive Tubulopathy

Several medications—notably acyclovir, sulfonamides, methotrexate, indinavir, and triamterene—are associated with the production of crystals that are insoluble in human urine.[19,27] Intratubular precipitation of these crystals can lead to acute renal insufficiency through obstructive tubulopathy. Many patients who require treatment with these medications have additional risk factors, such as true or effective intravascular volume depletion, underlying renal insufficiency, and metabolic perturbation (acidosis and electrolyte depletion), that increase the likelihood of drug-induced intrarenal crystal deposition.[34] Major preventive measures include adequate (pre)hydration and induction of high urinary flow rates (100-150 mL/hr), dose adjustment for renal function, and slowing down of the infusion rate.

Osmotic Nephrosis

Osmotic nephrosis is a distinct pattern of acute tubular injury observed after parenteral infusion of hyperoncotic solutions. Cellular injury begins with the uptake of nonmetabolizable molecules by pinocytosis into proximal tubule cells. The molecules create an oncotic gradient, leading to the accumulation of intracellular water, severe cytoplasmic swelling and vacuolization, and disruption of cellular integrity. Osmotic nephrosis is associated with ARF and a clinical presentation similar to that of ATN. The distinctive pattern of osmotic nephrosis may be recognized only histologically.[8,35]

Several therapeutic agents have been associated with osmotic nephrosis. They include sucrose, mannitol, intravenous immunoglobulin, radiocontrast agents, dextran, and hydroxyethyl starch (HES). HES is a volume expander that is increasingly used in the perioperative and intensive care setting. Multiple HES solutions are available and differ in their molecular weight and extent of substitution (hydroxyethylations at carbon positions C2, C3, and C6).[36] These characteristics determine the toxicity profile because they affect the time to elimination from the intravascular space and the degree of macromolecule accumulation.[36] Studies comparing the renal toxicity of gelatin and HES have provided conflicting results. In patients with severe sepsis, the use of HES 200/0.6 was associated with a significantly higher risk of ARF than with gelatin.[37] Conversely, similar (limited) alterations in renal function and structural cell injury were observed in elderly patients undergoing cardiac surgery treated with either HES 130/0.4 or gelatin.[38] The use of different HES preparations with different toxicity profiles may at least partly explain this controversy. It is probably wise to employ low-molecular-weight HES with low extent of substitution (e.g., HES 130/0.4) and to administer doses below their recommended upper limits (50 mL/kg/day) in at-risk patients.

Key Points

1. Drug-induced nephrotoxicity accounts for more than 15% of cases of acute renal failure in patients admitted to intensive care units.
2. The pathophysiological mechanisms underlying drug-induced nephrotoxicity remain, to a large extent, poorly understood.
3. Common pathophysiological mechanisms are altered renal hemodynamics, tubular toxicity (mediated by reactive oxygen species), allergic interstitial inflammation, obstructive tubulopathy, vasculopathy, and osmotic nephrosis.
4. A better knowledge of the pathophysiological mechanisms may help identify patients at risk and may provide a rationale for preventive measures.

Key References

16. Baliga R, Ueda N, Walker PD, Shah SV: Oxidant mechanisms in toxic acute renal failure. Am J Kidney Dis 1997;29:465-477.
27. Izzedine H, Launay-Vacher V, Deray G: Antiviral drug-induced nephrotoxicity. Am J Kidney Dis 2005;45:804-817.
31. Zakarija A, Bennett C: Drug-induced thrombotic microangiopathy. Semin Thromb Hemost 2005;31:681-690.
34. Perazella MA: Crystal-induced acute renal failure. Am J Med 1999;106:459-465.
35. Ebcioglu Z, Cohen DJ, Crew RJ, et al: Osmotic nephrosis in a renal transplant recipient. Kidney Int 2006;70:1873-1876.

See the companion Expert Consult website for the complete reference list.

CHAPTER 31

Renal Blood Flow and Perfusion Pressure

Elisa Licari, Paolo Calzavacca, and Rinaldo Bellomo

OBJECTIVES

This chapter will:
1. Explain the physiology of renal blood control.
2. Explore the concept of autoregulation of renal blood flow and how it changes in disease states.
3. Clarify the possible effect of changes in perfusion pressure on renal blood flow.
4. Describe the effect of increased intrarenal pressure on renal blood flow.
5. Discuss the effects of changes in intra-abdominal pressure on renal blood flow.

Renal blood flow (RBF) is a major determinant of glomerular capillary filtration pressure (P_{GC}). P_{GC} is the driving force that generates filtration and, ultimately, urine output. In normal humans, RBF approximates 1200 mL/min and represents close to 20% of cardiac output. It is needed to generate the 180 L of ultrafiltrate the kidney produces every day. However, such blood flow shows great spontaneous physiological variability, with values varying from 12% to as high as 30% of cardiac output in the resting human. Within the glomeruli, Starling's forces drive ultrafiltration across the glomerular capillaries as they do elsewhere in the body. The unique features of the glomerular capillaries are that their *permeability is much greater* than normal capillaries and that *the filtration pressure is also greater*. This situation allows the extraordinary ultrafiltration rate needed to achieve blood purification 24 hours a day. Maintaining adequate renal blood flow, therefore, is of great importance in maintaining the kidney's blood purification function. Blood flow to the kidney mostly subserves its blood purification function rather than organ perfusion.

The control of RBF is modulated by several local neurohormonal factors. Their physiological goal is to keep RBF relatively constant. All aspects of such factors and their interactions and effects are encompassed by the term *autoregulation* and are discussed in detail in Chapter 23. However, RBF is also modulated by systemic factors. One fundamental systemic factor is renal perfusion pressure (the systemic driving force for RBF). In this chapter, we focus on what is known about renal perfusion pressure (RPP) and discuss how changes in RPP, as seen in different pathophysiological conditions, can affect RBF and renal function. We also discuss how manipulation of RPP may or may not affect renal function in such settings.

STRUCTURE AND FUNCTION OF THE KIDNEY

Structure and function are strictly related in the kidney. Understanding the kidney's microscopic vascular anatomy is a prerequisite to understanding its vascular physiology, the concept of GFR, glomerular filtration pressure, and the role of perfusion pressure. The nephron is the functional part of the kidney.[1] The human kidney contains about 0.4×10^6 to 1.2×10^6 nephrons.[2] The essential vascular component of the nephron is the glomerulus. The major physiological function of the glomerulus is to filter plasma. Ultrafiltration of plasma from the glomerular capillary into Bowman's space is the first step in urine formation. *Ultrafiltration* refers to the convective movement of plasma water from the glomerular capillaries into Bowman's space. Such solvent (water) movement is associated with solute movement (solvent drag), thus enabling the first step in solute removal.

PRINCIPLES OF VASCULAR GLOMERULAR PHYSIOLOGY

The major force responsible for glomerular filtration is the hydrostatic pressure in the glomerular capillaries (P_{GC}). Because the reflection coefficient for protein across the glomerular capillary is close to 1, the glomerular ultrafiltrate is mostly protein free, and the oncotic pressure of Bowman's space (P_{BS}) is low.

As shown in Table 31-1, the net ultrafiltration pressure changes from the afferent arteriole to the efferent arteriole. Importantly, P_{GC} decreases along the length of the capillary because of the resistance to flow. Simultaneously, intraglomerular plasma oncotic pressure increases along the length of the capillary because water is filtered and protein is retained in the glomerular capillary. Thus, filtration is greater closer to the afferent arteriole and decreases as blood reaches the efferent arteriole.

GFR is proportional to the sum of Starling's forces across the capillaries multiplied by the ultrafiltration coefficient, as follows:

$$GFR = K_f([P_{gc} - P_{bs}] - \sigma(\pi_{gc} - \pi_{bs}])$$

where K_f is the product of the intrinsic permeability of the membrane and the glomerular surface area available for filtration, P_{gc} is the capillary hydrostatic pressure, P_{bs} is the interstitial hydrostatic pressure in Bowman's space, σ is the reflection coefficient for a given molecule, π_{gc} is the oncotic pressure in the glomerular capillaries, and π_{bs} is the oncotic pressure in Bowman's space.

It is vital to understand that the K_f of the glomerular capillaries is *100 times higher* than that of systemic capillaries and that the hydrostatic pressure in the glomerular capillaries is approximately *twice as great* as that of systemic capillaries.

The GFR can be altered by changing either K_f or Starling's forces. In normal individuals, the GFR is regulated by alterations in P_{GC} that are mediated mainly by changes in afferent and efferent arteriolar resistance. These changes, together with mean arterial pressure and the process of autoregulation, control overall RBF.

REGULATION OF RENAL BLOOD FLOW

Blood flow through the kidneys indirectly determines GFR, modifies the rate of solute or water reabsorption by the proximal tubule, participates in the concentration and dilution of urine, delivers oxygen, nutrients, and hormones to the cells of the nephron, returns carbon dioxide and reabsorbed fluid and solutes to the general circulation, and delivers substrates for excretion in the urine. Blood flow through any organ, including the kidney, may be represented by the following equation:

$$Q = \Delta P/R$$

where Q is blood flow; ΔP is mean arterial pressure minus venous pressure for that organ; and R is resistance to flow through that organ.

TABLE 31-1

Changes in Pressure (mm Hg) Along the Glomerulus

	AFFERENT ARTERIOLE END	EFFERENT ARTERIOLE END
Hydrostatic pressure in the glomerular capillary	60	58
Oncotic pressure in Bowman's space	0	0
Hydrostatic pressure in Bowman's space	−15	−15
Oncotic pressure in the glomerular capillary	−28	−35
Net ultrafiltration pressure	17	8

TABLE 31-2

Major Hormones That Influence Glomerular Filtration Rate and Renal Blood Flow

	STIMULUS	EFFECT ON GFR	EFFECT ON RBF
Vasoconstrictors			
Sympathetic nerves	↓ ECFV	↓	↓
AII	↓ ECFV	↓	↓
Endothelin	↑ Stretch, bradykinin, epinephrine, AII ↓ ECFV	↓	↓
Vasodilators			
Prostaglandins (PGE$_1$, PGE$_2$, PGI$_2$)	↓ ECFV ↑ Shear stress, AII	No changes/↑	↑
Nitric oxide (NO)	↑ Shear stress, acetylcholine, histamine, bradykinin, adenosine triphosphate	↑	↑
Bradykinin (BDK)	Prostaglandins (PGL) ↓ ACE	↑	↑
Natriuretic peptides (atrial [ANP], brain [BNP])	↑ ECFV	↑	No changes

ACE, angiotensin-converting enzyme; AII, angiotensin II; ECFV, extracellular fluid volume; GFR, glomerular filtration rate; RBF, renal blood flow; ↑, increase(s); ↓, decrease(s).

Accordingly, RBF is determined by the pressure difference between the renal artery and the renal vein divided by the renal vascular resistance. The major resistance vessels in the kidney are the afferent arteriole, the efferent arteriole, and the interlobular artery.

At least two mechanisms are responsible for the remarkably accurate autoregulation of RBF and renal perfusion pressure: the myogenic response of the renal vascular smooth muscle cells[3,4] and the tubuloglomerular feedback.[5,6] However, studies now suggest that a third regulatory mechanism significantly contributes to RBF autoregulation.[7] These mechanisms are described in detail in Chapter 23. Together they maintain a constant blood flow level over a wide pressure range. However, the basic assumption that RBF does not change within a large range of perfusion pressure is not fully true.[8] Oscillations of even several seconds' duration cannot be buffered by the compensatory action of the renal vasculature. The question is whether these variations in RBF have any physiological or pathophysiological significance. A number of studies have made it clear that blood pressure variability is an important risk factor in several forms of cardiovascular and renal disorders.[9]

A vasodilator system also protects against hypervolemia and hypertension; it consists of prostaglandins, atrial natriuretic peptide, and nitric oxide.[10] On the other hand, vasoconstrictor responses in the arteriolar smooth muscle and the glomerular mesangium act by way of a G protein–coupled phospholipase C receptor. This responds not only to α-adrenergic stimulation but also to many other hormones and peptides, including angiotensin II, arginine vasopressin, endothelin, platelet-activating factor, and leukotrienes.[11]

The concept of renal autoregulation, or the maintenance of RBF and GFR at a constant level over a wide range of renal arterial perfusion pressure, has been established for five decades. In 1951, Shipley and Study[12] demonstrated that the canine kidney has an autoregulatory range between 80 and 180 mm Hg. What is not generally understood, however, is that urinary flow rate is not autoregulated but is, to a degree, subject to perfusion pressure. The reason is that the hydrostatic pressure in the peritubular capillaries influences tubular water reabsorption, the primary determinant of urinary flow rate. In addition, even small increases in renal blood flow induced by greater perfusion pressure can induce a much more pronounced increase in urine output. Oliguria associated with hypotension usually is reversed to some extent when arterial blood pressure is restored toward normal. Whether such improved urine output reliably reflects better GFR is impossible to tell over the short term in the clinical situation. *Clinicians should be careful not to confuse pressure diuresis with improved GFR in such circumstances.*

Renal autoregulation seems to be mediated largely by the variable resistance of the preglomerular afferent arteriole. Renal vascular resistance diminishes with decreasing mean arterial pressure, but RBF and GFR are maintained. Several factors and hormones affect GFR and RBF (Table 31-2).

RENAL BLOOD FLOW IN PATHOPHYSIOLOGICAL STATES

The normal physiological situation of autoregulation, in which changes in perfusion pressure either up or down are compensated for by adjustments in the tone of the afferent and efferent arterioles, can be disrupted in a variety of pathophysiological states.

Severe Sepsis and/or Septic Shock

Severe sepsis is typically associated with some level of hypotension. When such hypotension becomes severe and unresponsive to fluid resuscitation, the patient is said to have septic shock. Under these circumstances of hypotension, renal function typically deteriorates with rising serum creatinine and urea concentrations, implying loss of GFR. The mechanism for the loss of GFR remains unclear; however, it is possible that loss of perfusion pressure participates in the pathogenesis. According to this paradigm, the drop in systemic blood pressure would reduce renal perfusion pressure when, because of the patient's illness, the kidney may be unable to autoregulate blood flow and thus compensate for the effects of a systemic decrease in blood pressure. Alternatively, the autoregulatory response may be intact but the decrease in mean arterial pressure (MAP) may, in some cases, be so great that autoregulation alone cannot keep RBF within normal or adequate values.

A further possible explanation for the loss of GFR in sepsis may relate to neurohumoral activation in response to systemic hypotension. This activation could, in turn, lead to afferent arteriolar vasoconstriction as part of a response dedicated to the preservation of an effective intravascular volume. Under such circumstances, hypotension would lead to a decrease in RPP, which would be combined not only with loss of autoregulation but also with actual vasoconstriction, thus exacerbating the decrease in RBF and inducing an even more marked loss of GFR. Unfortunately, because the measurement of RBF in septic shock is not routinely possible, we do not know which mechanisms may be operative in these circumstances in humans.

Given the preceding observations, increasing RPP by raising MAP appears desirable in septic shock. Such an increase may restore sufficient circulatory stability to diminish neurohormonal activation, achieve a degree of afferent arteriolar vasodilatation, and thereby restore GFR. Alternatively, by restoring RPP to near normal levels, such corrections may restore RBF to the autoregulatory range, thereby returning the kidney to near normal physiology or, if autoregulation is impaired, achieving sufficient RPP to compensate for the loss. By definition, in septic shock, the restoration of MAP and RPP can be achieved only with the administration of vasopressor drugs. However, what the renal perfusion pressure target should be for vasopressor drug infusions remains unclear.

In a small prospective, randomized, controlled study, Bourgoin and colleagues examined the effects of titrating norepinephrine to two different levels of MAP (and therefore RPP) on renal function. MAP was modified from 65 mm Hg to 85 mm Hg. Raising MAP by increasing the dose of norepinephrine infusion was accompanied by significant rises in cardiac index, systemic vascular resistance index, and left and right ventricular stroke work indices. However, renal functional variables (urine flow, serum creatinine level, creatinine clearance) were not improved by this 20 mm Hg increase in RPP.[13] These observations imply that changing RPP from 65 to 85 mm Hg with a vasopressor drug has a limited effect on RBF. In a similar study, LeDoux and associates[14] assessed the effect of raising MAP from 65 to 75 to 85 mm Hg in ten patients with septic shock. They found that, although raising MAP with norepinephrine increased the cardiac index, it had no significant effect on urine output. These studies, however, did not assess the effect on raising MAP in patients with more severe hypotension (MAP < 60 mm Hg). In 14 such patients, Albanese and coworkers[15] found that norepinephrine infusion reestablished urine output in 12 cases, with a decrease in serum creatinine and an increase in creatinine clearance. In another cohort of 16 septic patients, restoration of RPP by means of norepinephrine infusion was successful in restoring urine output in 15 cases.[16] These observations strongly suggest that, in septic patients with very low arterial RPP (MAP < 60 mm Hg), restoration of MAP values to more than 70 mm Hg is beneficial to renal function and, probably, RBF. On the other hand, raising RPP from 65 to 85 mm Hg does not appear to have a clinically important effect on renal function or, by implication, RBF.

Several explanations can be advanced for these findings. One is that renal vasoconstriction is so intense in this setting that raising RPP by 20 mm Hg is insufficient to alter intraglomerular pressure. Another is that norepinephrine itself induces renal vasoconstriction. According to this paradigm, the beneficial RBF effects of restoring RPP are offset by norepinephrine-induced afferent arteriolar vasoconstriction, resulting in no appreciable change in overall RBF and intraglomerular pressure. A third explanation is that marked afferent and efferent arteriolar vasodilation has occurred and has induced a rightward shift in the pressure-flow relationship for the kidney such that organ flow is maintained at lower perfusion pressures and autoregulation works at lower levels of RPP. A 2006 experimental study in septic dogs and sheep supports this view.[16]

Thus, the beneficial effects of modulating MAP (and RPP) to higher levels appear to depend on the baseline level of perfusion pressure. In their aggregate, the observations described suggest that MAP values of 65 to 70 mm Hg may deliver a level of RBF that cannot be appreciably improved by further increases of 15 to 25 mm Hg.

Because RPP is equal to MAP minus backup pressure (estimated to be somewhere around 13 mm Hg in normal mammals), the preceding consideration applies only to patients who do not have increased tissue/venous pressure. In patients with cardiac failure and increased right-sided pressures or tricuspid valve regurgitation or in patients with increased intra-abdominal pressure (IAP), RPP can be dramatically decreased even in the presence of a normal or near normal blood pressure.

Right-Sided Heart Failure

In situations that cause the pressures to rise in the right side of the heart, the backup venous pressure in all abdominal organs (kidney included) also rises. To ensure venous return, there must be a sufficient gradient between the mean circulatory filling pressure and the right atrial pressure.[17] The value for such differential pressure is typically in the range of 7 to 8 mm Hg. Thus, if the right atrial pressure is 20 mm Hg, the estimated backup venous pressure in organs like the kidney may be close to 30 mm Hg. Under those circumstances, in the presence of an MAP of 65 mm Hg, the RPP would be approximately 35 mm Hg. This perfusion pressure value is clearly well below the autoregulation threshold of the kidney and will result in marked hypoperfusion and rapid loss of GFR. This situation is typically aggravated by the associated decrease in cardiac output and the marked activation of a vasoconstrictive neurohormonal response. Acute renal failure develops very rapidly under these circumstances, as seen clinically in the setting of cardiac tamponade, right-sided myocardial infarction, and massive or submassive pulmonary embolism. The treatment of such low RPP–related acute renal failure is directed at treatment of its etiology (decompression of tamponade, thrombolysis or embolectomy, and inotropic or mechanical support for the failing right ventricle). However, maintenance of adequate vital organ perfusion pressure with norepinephrine is often life-saving while such therapies are implemented and may well attenuate the attendant decrease in RBF.

Cardiogenic Shock, Hemorrhagic Shock, and Anaphylactic Shock

In cardiogenic, hemorrhagic, or anaphylactic shock, maintenance of vital organ perfusion pressure while the cause of shock is addressed is important and, at times, lifesaving. Although the RBF effects of such vasopressor-dependent support of the MAP have not been studied in humans, experimental evidence supports a beneficial effect on renal oxygenation.[18]

Increased Intra-abdominal Pressure

Another clinical situation in which tissue and venous pressures are raised and thus decrease RPP is that of increased IAP. Various clinical conditions can raise pressure in a closed abdominal compartment (trauma, colonic dilation, pseudo-obstruction, mechanical obstruction, gastric dilation, retroperitoneal hemorrhage, tense ascites). Irrespective of the etiology, one of the major mechanisms responsible for acute renal failure in this context is similar—decreased RPP. Of course, many patients with increased IAP have other associated pathophysiological problems that contribute to acute renal failure (trauma, bleeding, rhabdomyolysis, sepsis, shock). Nevertheless, the effect of changes in IAP on renal function is marked, as can be shown in experimental animal studies. Experimentally increasing and decreasing IAP via the intra-abdominal administration of fluid or gas rapidly induces anuria and restoration of urine output, respectively. The treatment of decreased RBF in the context of IAP is treatment of the cause of increased IAP itself (removal of clot, decompression of inflated colon, removal of tense ascites).[19] The timing and advantages or disadvantages of specific decompressive interventions require consideration not only of kidney function but also of many other clinical aspects and are not discussed in detail here.

CONCLUSION

Renal perfusion pressure is a major determinant of RBF, glomerular filtration pressure, and GFR. Although normally the kidney is able to regulate RBF via neurohormonal mechanisms within a wide range of RPP values, such autoregulation may fail to achieve successful compensation in specific pathophysiological states. Through different mechanisms, sepsis, cardiogenic shock, increased right-sided heart pressures, and increased IAP can all decrease RPP and induce renal failure. Restoration of adequate perfusion pressure (at least 65 mm Hg in the absence of increased IAP) by means of vasopressor infusion is an important intervention that can protect all vital organs from inadequate blood flow and, in particular, is likely to keep RBF within an acceptable range.

Key Points

1. Renal perfusion pressure is an important determinant of renal blood flow.
2. In normal humans, changes in renal perfusion pressure within a certain range of values do not lead to major changes in renal blood flow.
3. When mean arterial pressure is low (<60 mm Hg), renal blood flow is likely to fall. Restoration of adequate perfusion pressure is likely to improve renal blood flow and function.
4. If intra-abdominal pressure rises, so does backup pressure within the kidneys. Under such circumstances, a normal mean arterial pressure value cannot ensure adequate renal perfusion pressure or blood flow. Decompression of the intra-abdominal compartment is needed to restore renal perfusion.
5. In septic shock, keeping mean arterial pressure above 65 mm Hg seems desirable. Further rises may not significantly increase renal blood flow.

Key References

5. Welch WJ, Tojo A, Lee JU, et al: Nitric oxide synthase in the JGA of the SHR: Expression and role in tubuloglomerular feedback. Am J Physiol Renal Physiol 1999;277:F130-F138.
7. Just A, Ehmke H, Toktomambetowa L: Dynamics characteristics and underlying mechanism of renal blood flow autoregulation in the conscious dog. Am J Physiol 2001;280: F1062-F1071.
8. Persson PB: Renal blood flow autoregulation in blood pressure control. Curr Opin Clin Nephrol Hypertens 2002;11: 67-72.
14. LeDoux D, Astiz ME, Carpati CM, Rackow EC: Effects of perfusion pressure on tissue perfusion in septic shock. Crit Care Med 2000;28:2729-2732.
15. Albanese J, Leone M, Garnier F, et al: Renal effects of norepinephrine in septic and nonseptic patients. Chest 2004;126: 534-539.

See the companion Expert Consult website for the complete reference list.

CHAPTER 32

Vulnerability of the Kidney to Nephrotoxins

Mark A. Perazella

OBJECTIVES

This chapter will:
1. Review the vulnerability of the kidney to nephrotoxins including therapeutic medications, diagnostic agents, natural products and supplements, and environmental exposures.
2. Review the patient-specific, kidney-specific, and drug-specific factors that increase the vulnerability of the kidney to nephrotoxins.
3. Describe the nephron segments and collecting duct system as all vulnerable to nephrotoxicity of drugs.
4. Describe the clinical syndromes associated with drug nephrotoxicity including acute kidney injury, nephrotic syndrome/proteinuria, tubulopathies, and chronic kidney disease.

The kidney serves many roles and performs a number of essential functions as a major end-organ in the body. It clears endogenous waste products, controls volume status through balanced excretion of sodium and water, modulates electrolyte and acid-base balance, and acts as an endocrine organ. Other major functions are the metabolism and excretion of exogenously administered therapeutic and diagnostic agents and of substances that humans are exposed to in the environment. In its role as the primary excretor of exogenous drugs and toxins, the kidney is vulnerable to various forms of injury. This chapter reviews the important nephrotoxins that the kidney is exposed to, the factors that increase vulnerability of the kidney to potential toxins, the renal compartments afflicted by toxins, and the clinical renal syndromes promoted by these nephrotoxins.

POTENTIAL NEPHROTOXINS

Humans are exposed to a variety of potential nephrotoxic substances. The first step in the development of nephrotoxicity requires adequate exposure to the potential offending agent. Clearly, humans are exposed to such substances frequently (Table 32-1). Several therapeutic agents have known nephrotoxic potential. Classic examples are antimicrobial agents, chemotherapeutic agents, analgesics, and immunosuppressive agents.[1-8] Most are prescribed by physicians, and many others are available over the counter. Numerous new drugs with unknown toxic potential are also being released for use in clinical practice. Diagnostic agents, in particular radiocontrast agents and high-dose gadolinium, are another source of nephrotoxin exposure.[9,10]

Important and unregulated sources of potentially nephrotoxic substances are alternative/complementary products, which include herbal remedies, natural products, and nutritional supplements widely available at most health food stores.[11,12] More concerning are the harmful contaminants and chemicals contained in such products (adulterants) that are not listed on the label.[11,12] Interaction of herbal products with conventional drugs is also a potential source of toxicity. Examples of nephrotoxic alternative products are aristolochic acid, *Ephedra* species, *Glycyrrhiza* species, *Akebia* species, and Cape aloes.[11,12] Adulteration of these products with dichromate, cadmium, and phenylbutazone also causes significant renal injury.[11,12]

Finally, environmental exposure to various nephrotoxins (lead, cadmium, mercury) remains a problem.[13-15] A classic and growing nephrotoxicity concern is lead exposure, even at levels that are considered safe and acceptable by governing bodies. Low-level lead exposure appears to exacerbate underlying chronic kidney disease (CKD), leading to more rapid progression to advanced stages of CKD and end-stage renal disease (ESRD).[13-15]

RISK FACTORS FOR NEPHROTOXICITY

For a simpler approach to understanding of the renal vulnerability to nephrotoxins, risk factors can be artificially separated into three major categories (Table 32-2). Each category or specific risk factor contributes to the enhanced development of kidney injury. In general, more than one type of risk factor is acting to promote renal injury. Most often, at least two or all three types conspire to cause clinical kidney disease.

Patient-Specific Characteristics

The first risk factor category comprises underlying patient-specific characteristics (see Table 32-2). The patient exposed to drugs and other substances is predisposed to development of nephrotoxicity when certain underlying risk factors are present. Many of these factors are nonmodifiable, such as older age and female gender. Risk in the elderly and females occurs through changes in total body water (reduced in the setting of decreased lean body mass), which leads to drug overdose, unrecognized lower glomerular filtration rate (despite normal serum creatinine concentration), and reduced drug binding to proteins (hypoalbuminemia), resulting in increased free drug concentrations.[16-19] The elderly also have greater propensity for vasoconstriction (angiotensin II, endothelin) and higher levels of oxidatively modified biomarkers.[16] These factors combine to expose the patient to excess drug concentration and risk of nephrotoxicity. Along these same lines,

TABLE 32-1

Commonly Encountered Nephrotoxic Agents and Exposures

Therapeutic agents	Antimicrobial:
	Aminoglycosides
	Amphotericin B
	Antiviral agents
	Colistin
	Chemotherapeutic:
	Cisplatin
	Carboplatin
	Oxaliplatin
	Ifosfamide
	Methotrexate
	Mitomycin
	Gemcitabine
	Pentostatin
	Interleukin-2
	Anti–vascular endothelial growth factor (bevacizumab and others)
	Analgesic:
	Nonsteroidal anti-inflammatory drugs/cyclooxygenase-2 inhibitors
	Analgesic combinations
	Immunosuppressive:
	Calcineurin inhibitors
	Other:
	Statins
	Angiotensin-converting enzyme inhibitors/angiotensin receptor blockers
	Methoxyflurane
	Colloids
	Pamidronate, zolendronate
Diagnostic agents	Radiocontrast:
	High-osmolar
	Low-osmolar
	Iso-osmolar
	Other:
	Gadolinium (in high dose)
	Oral sodium phosphate solution
Alternative products	Herbal remedies:
	Akebia sp
	Aristolochic acid
	Ephedra sp (ma huang)
	Cape aloes
	Taxus celebica
	Uno degatta
	Glycyrrhiza sp
	Datura sp
	Adulterants:
	Mefenamic acid
	Dichromate
	Cadmium
	Phenylbutazone
Environmental exposures	Heavy metals:
	Lead
	Mercury
	Cadmium
	Uranium
	Copper
	Bismuth
	Solvents:
	Hydrocarbons
	Other toxins:
	Silicon
	Germanium

TABLE 32-2

Specific Risk Factors That Increase Vulnerability to Nephrotoxins

Patient characteristics	Old age
	Female sex
	Acute/chronic kidney disease
	Nephrotic syndrome
	Cirrhosis/obstructive jaundice
	True or effective volume depletion:
	Decreased glomerular filtration rate
	Enhanced proximal tubular toxin reabsorption
	Sluggish distal tubular urine flow rates
	Metabolic perturbations:
	Hypokalemia
	Hypomagnesemia
	Hypercalcemia
	Alkaline or acid urine pH
	Immune response genes
	Pharmacogenetics favoring drug toxicity:
	Gene mutations in hepatic and renal P450 systems and in renal transporters and transport proteins
Kidney-specific factors	High rate of blood delivery (20% of cardiac output)
	High metabolic rate of tubular cells (loop of Henle)
	Increased toxin concentration in renal medulla and interstitium
	Biotransformation of substances to reactive oxygen species
	Proximal tubular uptake of toxins:
	Apical uptake via endocytosis/pinocytosis
	Basolateral transport via organic anion transporters and organic cation transporters
Drug/toxin– specific factors	Prolonged dosing periods and toxin exposure
	Insoluble parent compound and metabolite with intratubular crystal precipitation
	Combinations of toxins/drugs enhancing nephrotoxicity
	Competition between endogenous and exogenous toxins for transporters, increasing toxin accumulation within the tubular cell
	Potent direct nephrotoxic effects of the drug or compound

both underlying acute kidney injury (AKI) and CKD are important risk factors for increasing vulnerability to nephrotoxic injury.[17-19] Excessive drug dosing, exposure of a reduced number of functioning nephrons to toxins, and more robust renal oxidative injury response to toxins are all contributors in these settings.

Nephrotic syndrome and cirrhosis raise risk through multiple mechanisms that include altered renal perfusion (reduced effective volume), hypoalbuminemia with higher free circulating drug, and unrecognized renal impairment.[17-20] Obstructive jaundice also enhances toxicity of aminoglycosides through altered hemodynamics (decreased renal blood flow) and direct effects of bile salts on tubular epithelia.[21] Both true volume depletion (vomiting, diarrhea, diuretics) and effective volume depletion (congestive heart failure, sepsis) increase renal vulnerability to various agents. Through induction of renal hypoperfusion, these underlying processes enhance nephrotoxicity of many drugs and substances, in particular those excreted primarily by the kidney (excessive drug dosing), those reabsorbed in the proximal tubule (increased intracellular concentration), and those that tend to be insoluble in the urine (crystal precipitation within distal tubular lumens with sluggish flow).[17-20,22]

Metabolic perturbations also worsen renal vulnerability to certain drugs and potential toxins. Hypokalemia, hypomagnesemia, and hypocalcemia are electrolyte and divalent ion disturbances that heighten the renal toxicity associated with aminoglycosides.[17-19] Severe hypercalcemia induces afferent arteriolar vasoconstriction and renal sodium/water wasting, leading to prerenal physiology, which enhances nephrotoxic drug injury. Patients with metabolic disorders that alter urine pH are at risk for intratubular crystal deposition when certain drugs and substances precipitate within tubular lumens in the distal nephron.[22,23] Systemic metabolic acidosis or alkalosis may lower or raise urine pH, whereas proximal and distal renal tubular acidoses are associated with alkaline urine due to impaired renal ability to excrete hydrogen ion. Acidic urinary pH (<5.5) increases crystal deposition of certain drugs (sulfadiazine, methotrexate) that are insoluble in a low-pH environment.[22,23] Alkaline urine (pH >6.0) increases crystal precipitation within tubular lumens of drugs such as indinavir and insoluble endogenous substances such as xanthine (precursor of uric acid) and calcium phosphate.[22,23]

Finally, the underlying genetic makeup of the host can enhance renal vulnerability to potential nephrotoxins.[24-26] The drug or its metabolite forms adducts that modify the physical structure, making it more immunogenic. There is, however, significant heterogeneity in the response of patients to drugs and exogenous exposures. One obvious example is the heightened allergic response of some patients. It is likely that differences in innate host immune response genes predispose certain patients to mount an allergic response to a substance. The variability of immune responses has been demonstrated in patients with drug-induced interstitial nephritis, which appears to be a T cell–driven process.[27] This translates into enhanced vulnerability to an allergic response in the kidney and development of an acute interstitial nephritis.

Better studied and an area of intense interest is the role of pharmacogenetics in the heterogeneous response of patients to xenobiotics as it relates to efficacy and toxicity.[24-26] The hepatic cytochrome P450 enzyme system has been well studied, and several cytochrome P450 enzyme gene polymorphisms are associated with reduced metabolism and subsequent end-organ toxicity. The kidney also possesses cytochrome P450 enzymes that participate in drug metabolism.[24-26] One would expect that gene polymorphisms favoring reduced metabolism could increase nephrotoxic risk as well. Polymorphisms of genes encoding proteins involved in the metabolism and subsequent renal elimination of drugs have been described and are correlated with various levels of drug sensitivity. Specific to the discussion of nephrotoxicity, loss-of-function mutations in apical secretory transporters, and mutations in kinases that regulate drug carrier proteins can impair drug elimination and promote toxicity (elevated intracellular toxin concentrations).[25] In the future, more information about how patients differ in the function and regulation of channels, transporters, and carriers that regulate elimination of drugs and other compounds cleared by the kidney will be brought to light.

Kidney-Specific Factors

The next category of risk relates to the mechanism by which the kidney metabolizes and excretes various substances. Significant renal exposure to nephrotoxins occurs owing to the high rate of drug and toxin delivery to the kidney, a result of the high blood flow to the kidney, which is 20% to 25% of cardiac output. Many renal cells, particularly those in the loop of Henle, maintain high metabolic rates to actively transport many solutes (Na^+,K^+-ATPase–driven transport) while existing in a relatively hypoxic environment. This excess cellular workload promotes greater sensitivity to injury when exposure to potentially nephrotoxic substances occurs.[28,29] Another factor that enhances renal nephrotoxicity is the high concentration of parent compounds and their metabolites that develop in the renal medulla and interstitium from the enormous concentrating ability of the kidney.[28,29] Elevated tissue concentration of these toxins promotes injury through both direct toxicity and ischemic damage.

Biotransformation of drugs, xenobiotics, and other substances by multiple renal enzyme systems, including cytochrome P450 and flavin-containing mono-oxygenases, favors the formation of toxic metabolites and reactive oxygen species.[28-30] The presence of these byproducts of metabolism tilts the balance in favor of oxidative stress, which outstrips natural antioxidants and increases renal injury via nucleic acid alkylation or oxidation, protein damage, lipid peroxidation, and DNA strand breaks.[28-30]

Enhanced toxicity in proximal tubular cells occurs through the extensive cellular uptake of potential toxins and drugs by both apical and basolateral transport systems (Fig. 32-1A). Apical uptake of substances occurs via endocytosis and other transport pathways.[31-35] Examples are the polycationic aminoglycosides (Fig. 32-1B), heavy metals, and various complex sugars and starches (Fig. 32-1C). After endocytosis of aminoglycosides, which involves the endocytic receptor (megalin) for cationic ligands, these drugs are translocated into the lysosomal compartment, where they accumulate and subsequently form myeloid bodies.[28,29,31] These bodies are membrane fragments and damaged organelles formed as a consequence of aminoglycoside inhibition of lysosomal enzymes. This apical pathway of uptake leads to accumulation of a critical concentration of aminoglycoside within cells, which triggers an injury cascade leading to cell injury and death. Another pathway of proximal tubular cell toxin exposure occurs via basolateral delivery of endogenous and exogenous organic ions (anions and cations) by peritubular capillaries.[34,35] Toxicant delivery via peritubular capillaries is followed by uptake into proximal tubular cells via a family of transporters, including human organic anion transporters (HOATs) and human organic cation transporters (HOCTs).[34,35] As classic examples, acyclic nucleotide phosphonates are transported via HOATs,[34] whereas cisplatin is transported via HOCTs. Transport of toxicants into cells, followed by movement through the intracellular space via various regulated carrier proteins and subsequent exit from the cells via apical transport proteins (Fig. 32-1D), enhances toxicity in proximal tubular cells.[35] Loss-of-function mutations in and competition for apical secretory transporters,[36] which reduces toxin efflux from cell into urine, may promote accumulation of toxic substances within proximal tubular cells and cause cellular injury (apoptosis or necrosis). This extensive trafficking of substances increases exposure and risk for elevated concentration of toxin when other risk factors (as discussed) supervene.

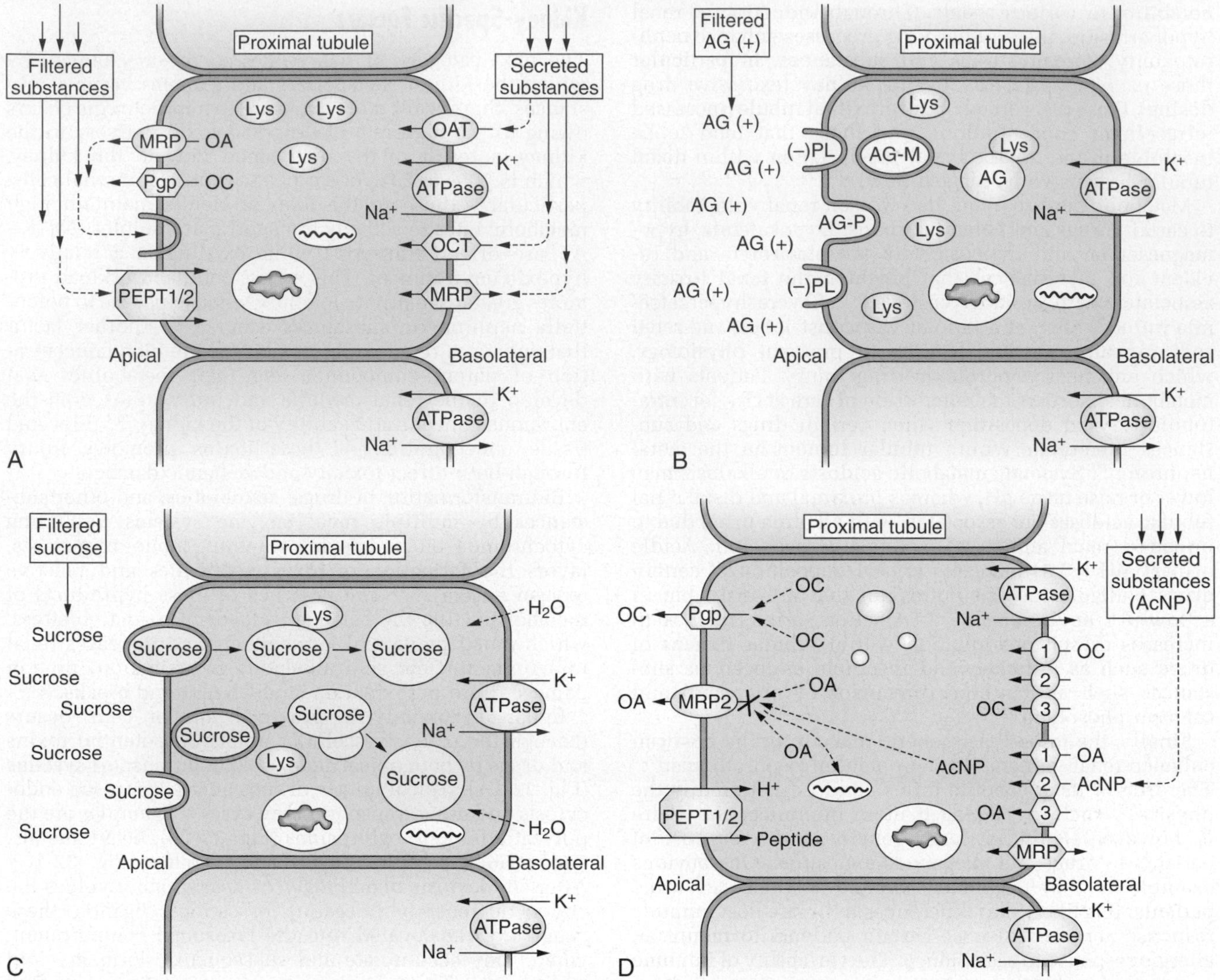

FIGURE 32-1. A, General proximal renal tubular cell handling of filtered substances and substances delivered via peritubular capillaries to the basolateral membrane. **B,** Apical membrane handling of substances, in this example aminoglycosides (AG(+)), by proximal tubular cells. Aminoglycosides interact with anionic phospholipids ((–)PL)/megalin (M) on the apical surface, where they are endocytosed and enter the cell. The drug is then translocated into lysosomes (Lys), where it is associated with various forms of cellular injury. **C,** Apical membrane handling of substances, in this example sucrose, by proximal tubular cells. Sucrose is taken up via pinocytosis into the cell, where it is translocated into the lysosomal compartment. In the absence of cellular enzymes capable of metabolizing sucrose, this substance accumulates within the cell and through its osmolar properties increases diffusion of water (H_2O) into the cell, resulting in cellular swelling and injury. **D,** Basolateral handling of substances, in this example the acyclic nucleotide phosphonates (AcNP), by proximal tubular cells. The acyclic nucleotide phosphonates are delivered to the basolateral membrane, transported into the cell via the organic anion transporter-1 (OAT-1), and excreted by various apical transporters into the urinary space. In this example, transport by the multidrug resistance protein (MRP2) transporter is inhibited, causing intracellular accumulation of drug and nephrotoxicity. K^+, potassium; Na^+, sodium; OA, organic anions; OC, organic cations; OCT, organic cation transporter; PEPT1/2, peptide transporters; Pgp, P-glycoprotein.

Drug/Toxin-Specific Factors

The underlying characteristics of the offending agent also play an important role in the development of nephrotoxicity. From a practical standpoint, prolonged therapy at high doses with toxic substances enhances renal injury on the basis of excessive renal exposure in the absence of other risks. Exogenous substances and their metabolites (drugs and toxins) that are insoluble in human urine may cause renal injury. In addition to unique characteristics of the offending agent that induce insolubility, factors such as urine pH, sluggish tubular urine flow rates, and rapid

parenteral or excessive dosing (high peak serum and urine concentrations) enhance risk for the agent's precipitation and crystal formation in distal nephron tubular lumens.[18-20] Aminoglycosides with more positive charge (neomycin > gentamicin > amikacin) are more likely to cause nephrotoxicity, perhaps due to enhanced interactions with negatively charged membrane phospholipids and megalin.[7,31] Drug combinations also raise the risk of nephrotoxicity. Combinations such as aminoglycosides and cephalothin, nonsteroidal anti-inflammatory drugs and radiocontrast agents, and cisplatin and aminoglycosides are a few examples of enhanced nephrotoxic risk with concurrent administration of drugs.[17-20] As mentioned previously, various toxins (and endogenous molecules) can compete for transport proteins in the proximal tubular cells, thereby reducing renal elimination and increasing intracellular concentration.[1,3,5,22] This situation favors development of nephrotoxicity.

Several drugs and toxins maintain extensive toxic potential that enhances renal injury, even with brief or low-level exposure. Examples are the aminoglycosides (in particular neomycin), amphotericin B, the polymyxins, zolendronate, and the antiviral agents adefovir and cidofovir.[1,3,5-7,37-39] Aminoglycosides are classic nephrotoxins. Accumulation of high concentrations within lysosomes (formation of myeloid bodies) and their release into the cell cytoplasm promote phospholipid membrane interruption, oxidative stress, and mitochondrial injury, which cause proximal tubular cell apoptosis and necrosis, leading to clinical AKI. Amphotericin B, and the lipid/liposomal formulations to a lesser degree, disrupt cellular membranes and increase permeability to cations, resulting in tubular dysfunction due to cell swelling and lysis.[37] The polymyxin antimicrobials colistin and polymyxin B are extremely nephrotoxic with a very narrow therapeutic window. Their toxicity appears to be due to the D-amino content and fatty acid component, which increase membrane permeability and influx of cations.[38] As seen with amphotericin B, cell swelling and lysis result. The acyclic nucleotide phosphonates enter the cell via basolateral human organic anion transporter-1 and promote cellular injury through multiple mechanisms.

Mitochondrial injury (as manifested by mitochondrial enlargement, clumped cristae, and convoluted contours) occurs with adefovir through inhibition of DNA polymerase gamma, the sole DNA polymerase in mitochondria.[3,5] Cidofovir, which forms cidofovir-phosphocholine (analogue of cytidine 5-diphosphocholine) within cells, interferes with synthesis and/or degradation of membrane phospholipids, resulting in proximal tubular injury.[3,5] Although currently unknown, tenofovir may impair cellular energetics through mitochondrial disruption or some other intracellular process.[3,5,22] A unique and newly recognized form of nephrotoxicity has been described with antivascular endothelial growth factor therapy.[40] Induction of proteinuria occurs from endothelial injury and a reduction in glomerular nephrin expression, which promote loss of slit diaphragm function, causing leakage of protein across the glomerular basement membrane.[41]

RENAL COMPARTMENTS AND NEPHROTOXIN INJURY

Nephrotoxic substances produce disease in all compartments of the kidney. As seen in Figure 32-2, the entire nephron and collecting duct systems are capable of being injured by various nephrotoxins. For ease of classification, they can be divided into the following renal compartments and the associated disease components: (1) hemodynamic (prerenal disease), (2) renal parenchyma (intrinsic renal disease), and (3) collecting system (postrenal disease).

Hemodynamic Disturbances

Hemodynamic disturbances induced by certain medications may produce a prerenal form of kidney injury in

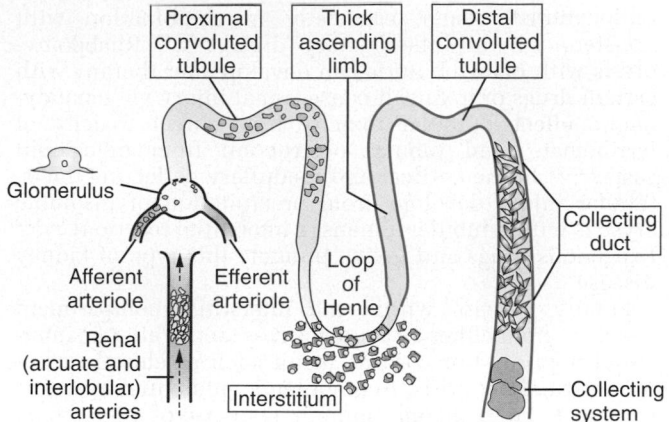

FIGURE 32-2. Nephron segments with various categories of drug or toxin-induced injury. Examples are thrombotic microangiopathy from drugs/toxins (renal arterioles), drug-induced glomerular disease (glomerulus), acute tubular necrosis from nephrotoxins (proximal tubule), acute tubulointerstitial nephritis from drugs (interstitium), drug-induced crystal nephropathy (collecting duct), and urinary obstruction from drug-induced stone formation.

patients at risk. Increased afferent arteriolar tone (vasoconstrictors) and reduced efferent arteriolar tone (angiotensin-converting enzyme inhibitors and angiotensin receptor blockers) in patients with true or effective volume depletion or underlying kidney disease alter renal hemodynamics.[1,5,6] They do so by reducing intrarenal perfusion and lowering intracapillary hydraulic pressure, thereby reducing the filtration fraction and, ultimately, the glomerular filtration rate.

Renal Parenchyma

Intrinsic kidney disease due to exogenous nephrotoxins may occur in several compartments. Medium- and small-vessel vascular disease may result from toxin- or drug-induced thrombotic microangiopathy (TMA) from endothelial injury or antibody formation against von Willebrand factor–cleaving protease or induction of a hypercoagulable state. Glomerular disease (decreased glomerular filtration rate, proteinuria) develops from a wide array of toxins and drugs.[1,5,22] Injury occurs via damage to glomerular endothelial cells, visceral epithelial cells, microthrombi within glomerular capillaries, or immune complex deposition within glomerular capillary basement membranes from formation of a drug antigen–inducing antibody.[1,5,22]

Tubular disease, particularly in the proximal tubule, is a common complication of prescribed nephrotoxins and environmental exposures. As was previously reviewed, the mechanism by which the proximal tubule handles substances contributes to enhanced nephrotoxicity in this nephron segment. Proximal cell tubular toxicity develops through direct nephrotoxic effects (mitochondrial dysfunction, lysosomal hydrolase inhibition, phospholipid damage, increased intracellular calcium concentration), formation of reactive oxygen species with injurious oxidative stress, and osmolar effects with loss of normal cell-cell contact and tubular luminal occlusion.[22,28]

In the loop of Henle, ischemic injury from reduced medullary oxygen delivery (shunting blood to the cortex) and enhanced tubular cell metabolic rate can occur with radiocontrast agents, especially in combination with nonsteroidal anti-inflammatory drugs.[1,5,22,28] Rhabdomyolysis with myoglobinuria can develop after therapy with certain drugs or toxins. It causes renal injury via hemodynamic effects, tubular toxicity from direct toxicity of ferrihemate, and tubular obstruction from myoglobin casts.[1,22,28] In the cortical and medullary collecting ducts, tubular injury develops from precipitation of insoluble crystals within tubular lumens (± interstitial reaction).[1,3,5,22] Exogenous drugs and toxins promote this type of kidney disease.

Finally, disease within the interstitial compartment develops from either an acute process (acute/allergic interstitial nephritis) or chronic insult such as chronic tubulointerstitial nephritis. Acute/allergic interstitial nephritis represents an exuberant immune response of a host to an exogenously administered substance (medications and other toxins).[1,5,22] Chronic tubulointerstitial nephritis develops from persistent, untreated inflammation associated with acute/allergic interstitial nephritis or chronic ischemia/toxicity from certain analgesic combinations, heavy metals, or nephrotoxic alternative/herbal medications.[1,2,22,42]

Collecting System

Disease of the collecting system (postrenal disease) represents the last compartment of kidney injury that occurs from certain medications or toxins. Both AKI and CKD result from obstructive disease.[1,22] Many drugs and toxins cause either intrinsic or extrinsic urinary obstruction, from structural problems (stone formation, retroperitoneal disease) or functional disturbances (bladder dysfunction with urinary retention).[1,22]

CLINICAL SYNDROMES OF NEPHROTOXICITY

The various injuries from toxic substances that occur along most nephron segments and the collecting duct system cause recognizable clinical renal syndromes that may be divided into four major categories (Table 32-3). These clinical renal syndromes—AKI, nephrotic/proteinuric disease, tubulopathies, and CKD—are reviewed in detail in other chapters of this textbook,

CONCLUSION

The kidney is vulnerable to various substances with nephrotoxic potential. Numerous known and potential nephrotoxins are prescribed to patients, available without prescription at health food and other stores, and present in the environment. Recognizing that these substances maintain nephrotoxic potential is the first step in avoiding or reducing renal injury. Awareness of the factors that enhance nephrotoxic risk is important. These factors are specific patient characteristics, renal handling of the offending agents, and the nephrotoxicity of the substance itself. Importantly, all compartments of the kidney are subject to injury by these substances. Injury by these nephrotoxins results in recognizable clinical renal syndromes, including AKI, nephrotic syndrome and proteinuric renal

TABLE 32-3

Clinical Renal Syndromes Caused by Nephrotoxins

Acute kidney injury	Hemodynamic disturbances
	Parenchymal disease
	Collecting system disease
Nephrotic syndrome/ proteinuria	Glomerular disease:
	Minimal change
	Focal segmental glomerulosclerosis
	Membranous glomerulonephritis
	Others
	Thrombotic microangiopathy:
	Hemolytic-uremic syndrome
	Thrombotic thrombocytopenic purpura
Tubulopathies	Renal tubular acidosis/Fanconi syndrome
	Sodium wasting
	Potassium wasting
	Nephrogenic diabetes insipidus
Chronic kidney disease	Analgesic nephropathy
	Chronic tubulointerstitial nephritis
	Secondary progression of toxin-induced kidney disease

disease, tubular dysfunction syndromes, and CKD. Putting these data together allows one to predict potential for nephrotoxicity and reduce development of kidney impairment.

Key Points

1. The kidney is frequently exposed to a variety of potentially nephrotoxic substances.
2. Vulnerability of the kidney to nephrotoxins is predictable from underlying patient characteristics, renal handling of substances, and factors specific to the culprit toxin or drug.
3. All nephron segments as well as the collecting duct system are at risk for development of injury from potentially nephrotoxic substances.
4. Clinical renal syndromes induced by nephrotoxins may be classified as acute kidney injury, nephrotic/proteinuric syndromes, tubulopathies, and chronic kidney disease.
5. Recognition of the vulnerability of the kidney to various nephrotoxins and the factors that enhance risk allows prevention and/or reduction of the severity of renal injury that occurs.

Key References

1. Schetz M, Dasta J, Goldstein S, Golper T: Drug-induced acute kidney injury. Curr Opin Crit Care 2005;11:555-565.
5. Perazella MA: Drug-induced nephropathy: An update. Expert Opin Drug Saf 2005;4:689-706.
13. Van Vleet TR, Schnellmann RG: Toxic nephropathy: environmental chemicals. Semin Nephrol 2003;23:500-508.
22. Markowitz GS, Perazella MA: Drug-induced renal failure: A focus on tubulointerstitial disease. Clin Chimica Acta 2005;351:31-47.
36. Lang F: Regulating renal drug elimination. J Am Soc Nephrol 2005;16:1535-1536.

See the companion Expert Consult website for the complete reference list.

CHAPTER 33

Humoral Mediators in Sepsis

Ciro Tetta, Vincenzo Cantaluppi, Filippo Mariano,
and Giuseppe Segoloni

OBJECTIVES

This chapter will:
1. Identify the complex imbalance of pro-inflammatory and anti-inflammatory mediators in sepsis.
2. Describe the biological actions of the most prominent classes of mediators associated with sepsis.
3. Review the involvement of inflammatory cells (endothelium, monocytes/macrophages, polymorphonuclear neutrophils).

Local infection may develop into a systemic inflammatory response syndrome that encompasses a complex mosaic of interconnected events, including the so-called compensatory anti-inflammatory response syndrome.[1] A 2002 hypothesis holds that a defective host innate response may render bacteria resistant to host recognition and defense mechanisms, leading to systemic infection and sepsis.[2] In higher organisms, a variety of host defense mechanisms control the resident microflora and, in most cases, effectively prevent invasive microbial disease. Many microbial pathogens avoid host recognition or dampen the subsequent immune activation through sophisticated interactions with host responses, but some pathogens even benefit from the inflammatory reaction. The defective response of the host may depend on a unique genetic makeup of a pathogen that can render it more resistant to antibiotics or on disturbances in the integrated response of both the innate arm and the adaptive arm of the immune system. Differences in reactivity of dendritic cells to microbial molecules through Toll-like receptors (TLRs) are associated with susceptibility and resistance to microbes.[3]

HUMORAL MEDIATORS IN THE PATHOGENESIS OF SEPSIS

Molecules such as bacterial lipopolysaccharides (LPSs), microbial lipopeptides, microbial DNA, peptidoglycan, and lipoteichoic acid trigger the interaction with the Toll-like receptors and related molecules (MD-2, MyD88), the principal sensors of the innate immune response.[4-6] Plasma DNA has been indicated as a predictor of mortality.[7]

Stimulus-receptor coupling activates different signal transduction pathways, leading to exacerbated generation of cytokines, and phospholipase A_2–dependent, arachidonic acid–derived platelet-activating factor (PAF), leukotrienes, and thromboxanes (Fig. 33-1). At the plasma level, activation of the complement (C3a, C5a, and their desarginated products) and coagulation pathways interacts with the process, because products generated in the fluid phase may in turn trigger and sustain cell activation.

Other agents play a role in the pathophysiology of sepsis, such as surface-expressed and soluble adhesion molecules, kinins, thrombin, myocardial depressant substances, endorphin, and heat shock proteins.

In physiological conditions, the biological activity of sepsis-associated mediators is under the control of specific inhibitors that may act at different levels. In sepsis, the homeostatic balance is altered and a profound disturbance of relative production of different mediators may be observed (as reviewed by Cavaillon and associates[8]). On one side, the spillover into the circulation of mediators intended to have autocrine or paracrine effects generates systemic effects, including endothelial damage,[9] procoagulant and fibrinolytic effects, complement activities, hemodynamic shock, and vasoparalysis.[10-16] On the other side, monocytes demonstrate a profound inability to produce cytokine when they are challenged with different stimuli *ex vivo*.[17,18]

Coagulation Cascade Activation in Sepsis: The Role of Platelet-Activating Factor

Coagulopathy can be seen in essentially all patients with severe sepsis. The earliest signs of consumptive coagulopathy in sepsis are a decrease in protein C level and an increase in D-dimer level. In patients with more severe consumptive coagulopathy, prothrombin time and partial thromboplastin time increase, with drops in fibrinogen level and platelet count. In addition, fibrinolysis is also impaired in severe sepsis.[19] LPSs cause a direct activation of coagulation through the upregulation of tissue factor on the surface of endothelial cells and monocytes. The tissue factor expression in turn activates factor VII of the extrinsic system, leading to thrombin formation and generation of fibrin clots. Thrombin is a multifunctional serine protease with the primary function of cleavage of circulating protein substrates—for example, conversion of fibrinogen to fibrin monomer or activation of protein C. However, thrombin also has important actions on cells. It is a potent activator of platelets and causes endothelial cells to deliver the leukocyte adhesion molecule P-selectin to their surfaces, to secrete von Willebrand factor, to elaborate growth factors and cytokines, and to synthesize PAF. Such cellular actions of thrombin may account for its role in controlling early cellular behavior during sepsis.[20]

On the other hand, an indirect activation of the coagulation cascade on the surface of endothelial cells can be triggered by pro-inflammatory mediators generated by sepsis, including tumor necrosis factor (TNF), interleukin-1 (IL-1), complement fragments, and PAF. In addition, activation of coagulation in sepsis can also occur indirectly throughout the activation of the contact system.

Many experimental and clinical observations suggest that PAF or PAF-like lipids are involved in the unregu-

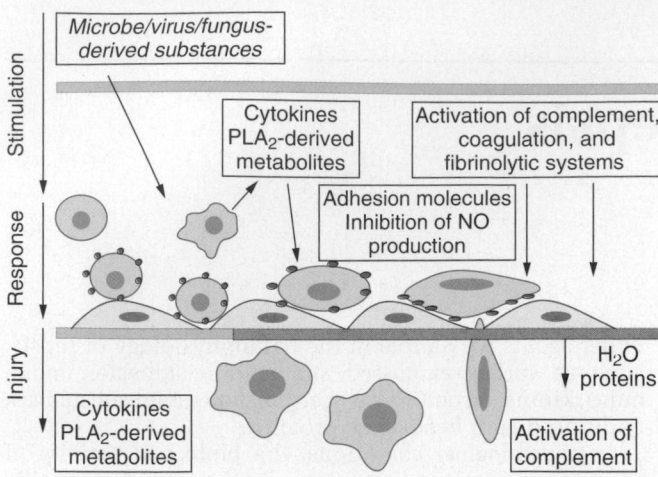

FIGURE 33-1. The drawing schematically represents the leukocyte-endothelium as a result of cytokine production and fluid phase activation. Rolling, tethering, and, finally, attachment of leukocytes to the endothelium layer is mediated by the expression of several adhesion molecules and the platelet-activating factor, release of proteolytic enzymes, and cationic proteins that enhance vascular permeability. Similar mechanisms induce cell activation (mediator production) and complement activation, leading to tissue injury by resident or recruited circulating cells. H_2O, water; NO, nitric oxide; PLA_2, phospholipase A_2.

lated inflammation and pathological thrombosis observed in septic shock.[21] PAF contributes to acute sequestration and endothelial adhesion of neutrophils and to induction of nitric oxide synthase in experimental endotoxemia.[22] In mice, the overexpression of the PAF receptor increases lethality in response to administration of LPS.[23] However, disruption of the PAF receptor gene in mice caused a marked reduction in systemic anaphylactic symptoms, but mice remained sensitive to bacterial endotoxin.[24]

In humans, several studies have shown the presence of intravascular PAF activity in septic patients.[25-27] PAF is present at high concentrations in blood and bronchoalveolar lavage fluid and occupies specific platelet receptors, and the rate of its catabolism is reduced.[26] In patients with acute renal failure (ARF) associated with septic shock, PAF was present in high concentration in plasma, in association with platelets, and in urine. Plasma concentration of PAF correlated with the severity of renal failure and with indexes of renal inflammatory injury, such as urine IL-6 and IL-8 levels. Interestingly, a negative correlation between concentration of PAF in blood and number of circulating platelets was observed, suggesting a PAF-dependent activation of platelets during septic shock.[25,27]

Pro-inflammatory and Anti-inflammatory Cytokine Network during Sepsis

The pathogenesis of sepsis was initially described as an overproduction of pro-inflammatory factors in the host. The concept was established on the basis of several studies. The injection of LPS into experimental animals and healthy human subjects reproduces the initial phase of bacterial infection.[28] In human subjects, LPS alters capillary integrity and affects the cardiovascular system,[29] causes production of cytokines,[29-31] and activates the coagulation-fibrinolytic pathways.[32] Peak concentrations of IL-1, TNF-α, IL-6, and IL-8 occur within 2 to 3 hours of LPS infusion.[19,20] Studies on knockout mice have shown that intercellular adhesion molecule-1 (ICAM-1) mutant mice are resistant to the lethal outcome of endotoxin-induced pneumonitis.[33]

What is the relevance of circulating cytokines? The presence or absence of detectable levels of cytokines within biological fluids reflects a rather complex balance between enhancing and inhibitory signals acting on producer cells, between production and catabolism, and between the

binding of cytokines to the target cells and the modulation of their receptors on the cell surface.[34] Furthermore, the presence of cytokines does not necessarily parallel their activity, and a possible interplay between a given cytokine and its relative inhibitor (if known) should be considered. Cavaillon and associates[8] called the expression of circulating cytokines "the tip of the iceberg," implying that neither the presence nor the absence of cytokines can reflect the complex interplay at the tissue level. Despite the fact that the peak concentrations of cytokines may reflect an exacerbated production, these levels do not necessarily represent enhanced bioactivity.

The concept of sepsis as a simply pro-inflammatory event has been subsequently challenged (Fig. 33-2).[35] In sepsis and systemic inflammatory response syndrome, cell-associated cytokines in peripheral blood mononuclear cells are decreased, as is the capacity of these cells to produce several cytokines, such as TNF-α and interleukins 10, 1β, 6, and 12[36-38] although not IL-1 receptor antagonist.[39] Terms such as monocyte deactivation, immunoparalysis and, more simply, cell hyporesponsiveness all indicate the inability of cells to respond *ex vivo* to LPS stimuli owing to overproduction of anti-inflammatory cytokines. Hyporesponsiveness not only is present in mononuclear cells but also occurs in whole blood[29] and is associated with increased plasma levels of IL-10 and prostaglandin E_2, which are potent inhibitors of the production of pro-inflammatory cytokines.[40] Adib-Conquy and colleagues[41] demonstrated that, upon LPS activation, peripheral mononuclear cells from patients with systemic inflammatory response syndrome show patterns of nuclear factor-κB expression that resemble those reported during LPS tolerance: global downregulation of nuclear factor-κB in survivors of sepsis and patients with trauma and the presence of large amounts of the inactive homodimer in the nonsurvivors of sepsis.

In intensive care medicine, blocking one mediator has not led to measurable outcome improvement in patients with sepsis.[42] Possibly more rigidly defined subgroups would profit from TNF-antagonizing treatments.[43] On the other hand, it has been shown that antagonizing a cytokine may lead to deleterious consequences, which in turn leads to substantially higher mortality.[44] A low-level TNF-α response seems to be necessary for the host defense to infection,[45] and high levels of TNF-α apparently must be modulated by anti-inflammatory feedback. In sepsis, however, impaired regulation may cause an excessive anti-inflammatory response, which generates monocyte "immu-

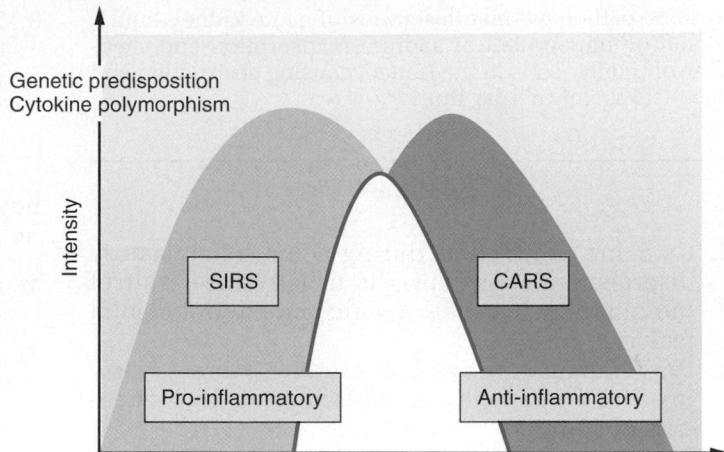

FIGURE 33-2. The first response to an inflammatory response is characterized by the prompt production of several pro-inflammatory mediators. The extent of this response is important because a reduced early inflammatory response is associated with the unconstrained invasion of the invading organism. The response, which acts at first at a local level, may extend to the systemic level, giving rise to the so-called systemic inflammatory response syndrome (SIRS). As a result of a counterbalanced effect, production of anti-inflammatory cytokines begins, which antagonizes the inflammatory response (compensatory anti-inflammatory response syndrome [CARS]).

noparalysis" and exposes the host to further infections. Both processes (inflammation and anti-inflammation) are designed to act in response to specific stimuli in a well-balanced fashion defined as immune homeostasis.

Furthermore, the time of therapeutic intervention in sepsis seems to be crucial.[46] Because the network acts like a cascade, early intervention would seem most beneficial. Sepsis shows complex and multiple rises in mediator levels that change over time. Neither single mediator–directed nor one-time interventions therefore seem appropriate. One of the major criticisms of continuous blood purification treatment in sepsis—its lack of specificity—could turn out to be a major strength. Unspecific removal of soluble mediators—be they pro-inflammatory or anti-inflammatory—without complete elimination of their effect may be the most logical and adequate approach to a complex and long-running process like sepsis.[47,40]

The contribution of inflammatory cytokines to the determination of hemodynamic alterations with consequent tissue hypoperfusion and injury acquires a particular relevance in the clinical setting of multiple-organ failure. Several causes of injury in distant organs can also induce kidney damage. Furthermore, studies show that the damaged kidney is able to release further peaks of inflammatory mediators that perpetuate organ injury. However, the importance of ARF in the induction of functional alterations in distant organs (organ cross-talk) has only lately emerged and is discussed in other chapters.

Cytokine production during acute inflammatory disorders such as sepsis is usually the result of the interplay between genetic and environmental factors. Studies on genetic polymorphism of the host immune response might help in identifying patients with a higher susceptibility to developing acute inflammatory disorders.[49] In this clinical setting, a wide range of studies over the last decades tried to identify the specific mediator responsible for organ damage, without success. On the basis of the proven absence of a "magic bullet" to interfere with these detrimental processes, extracorporeal techniques, which achieve unspecific increases in cytokine clearance, have acquired a primary importance.[50-52]

Pro-inflammatory cytokines induce a direct injury to several cell types, in particular via the activation of the apoptotic processes. It has been shown that lymphocyte apoptosis is a potential mechanism for immunosuppression during sepsis.[53] Endotoxin and inflammatory cyto-

kines induce apoptosis in the myocardium, contributing to cardiac dysfunction.[54]

Several studies demonstrated that apoptosis and necrosis are typical features of acute septic, ischemic and nephrotoxic ARF.[55] Indeed, ischemia, growth factor deficiency, loss of cell-matrix or cell-cell interactions, oxidant stress, and several pharmacological compounds (e.g., cisplatin, antibiotics, calcineurin inhibitors) are all potential causes of apoptosis in tubular cells. Some other molecules, such as TNF-α, Fas-ligand, and angiotensin, can induce tubular apoptosis via the activation of specific receptors located on tubular cells. Given the described increase in inflammatory cytokine levels in ARF, the direct involvement of such cytokines in tissue injury seems probable. Thus, inflammatory cytokines are able to activate tubular apoptosis through the upregulation of Fas and the activation of caspases. In addition, these substances cause shedding of tubular cells from the basal membrane, with consequent lumen obstruction and possible back-leakage of tubular fluid in the interstitial spaces.

The altered function induced by different causes in distant organs can result in the systemic release of inflammatory mediators that are potentially involved in kidney injury through the activation of apoptotic processes. Moreover, tubular cells regulate cytokine handling and can cause a further increase in these substances, as reported after renal ischemia-reperfusion injury.[56]

Inflammatory cytokines are also able to effect a variety of nonlethal alterations in epithelial and endothelial cells, in particular loss of cellular polarity and tight junction dysfunction.[57,58] Epithelial tight junction proteins have some major functions, working as a regulatory barrier that separates and maintains biological fluid compartments of different composition. In addition, tight junction proteins play a key role in the maintenance of polarity, cell growth, and differentiation. In different epithelial districts, inflammatory cytokines are known to increase permeability, via a nitric oxide–dependent mechanism, by altering the expression of some tight junction proteins, such as zona occludens-1 (ZO-1), ZO-2, ZO-3, and occludin.[59-61] ARF has been shown to involve alteration in tight junction proteins and disruption of actin cytoskeletal fibers. These changes lead to a misleading expression of apicobasal molecules, such as the integrins that anchor tubular cells to basal membrane or Na^+,K^+–ATPase, which regulates tubular sodium handling. Such alterations can contribute to some pathologic manifestations of acute kidney injury, including impairment of sodium readsorption and shedding of tubular cells in the lumen, causing obstruction and back-leakage of tubular fluid.[62]

Key Points

1. Cytokine production during acute inflammatory disorders such as sepsis is usually the result of the interplay between genetic and environmental factors.
2. Pro-inflammatory cytokines induce a direct injury to several cell types, in particular via the activation of apoptotic processes.

---

3. The contribution of inflammatory cytokines to the determination of hemodynamic alterations, with consequent tissue hypoperfusion and injury, acquires a particular relevance in the clinical setting of multiple-organ failure.

Key References

8. Cavaillon JM, Munoz C, Fitting C, et al: Circulating cytokines: The tip of the iceberg? Circ Shock 1992;38:145-152.
53. Hotchkiss RS, Nicholson DW: Apoptosis and caspases regulate death and inflammation in sepsis. Nat Rev Immunol 2006;6:813-822.
62. Lee DB, Huang E, Ward HJ: Tight junction biology and kidney dysfunction. Am J Physiol Renal Physiol 2006;290:20-34.

See the companion Expert Consult website for the complete reference list.

CHAPTER 34

Apoptosis and Necrosis

Prasad Devarajan

OBJECTIVES

This chapter will:
1. Present the basic differences between apoptosis and necrosis.
2. Discuss the critical molecular mechanisms underlying apoptosis and necrosis.
3. List the evidence for apoptosis in human acute kidney injury.
4. Discuss the role of apoptosis in human acute kidney injury.
5. Consider the potential therapeutic implications of pharmacologically manipulating apoptosis in human acute kidney injury.

For certain is death for the born
And certain is birth for the dead;
Therefore over the inevitable Thou shouldst not grieve.
The Bhagavad Gita

In this world nothing can be said to be certain, except death and taxes.

Benjamin Franklin, in a letter to
Jean-Baptiste Leroy, 1789

Although the inevitability of an organism's demise has been philosophically recognized for several centuries, the paradoxical but critical role of cellular death in the optimization of life has emerged only in the past two decades. Cells that have served their purpose during morphogenesis, have reached the end of their natural lifespan, or have become injured or stressed or dysregulated die in order to maintain the organism's life and homeostasis. Each living cell is equipped with a remarkable array of mechanisms

to commit suicide when the time is right, via carefully orchestrated, genetically defined pathways collectively referred to as *programmed cell death*.

Historically, although the morphological characteristics of programmed cell death have been known to developmental biologists for several decades, the recognition of this basic biological process in a wide variety of mature tissues and life forms is commonly attributed to Kerr and colleagues.[1] In 1972, they coined the term *apoptosis* (from the Greek words *apo* [from] and *ptosis* [falling]) to signify the resemblance of these dying cells to the shrinking and crumbling leaves that have fallen from trees. The subsequent identification of the genetic pathways that mediate apoptosis led to the awarding of the 2002 Nobel Prize in Physiology or Medicine to researchers Sidney Brenner, John Sulston, and Robert Horvitz.[2] The ensuing explosion in apoptosis research has markedly advanced our understanding of basic cellular processes, their physiological controls, their alterations and roles in a variety of disease states, and their therapeutic implications in clinical situations.

MECHANISMS OF CELL DEATH: APOPTOSIS VERSUS NECROSIS

Apoptosis, or programmed cell death, is the mechanism by which most cells die, both physiologically and pathologically. It is a quiet, orderly demise typified by cytoplasmic and nuclear shrinkage, DNA fragmentation, and breakdown of the cell into membrane-bound apoptotic bodies that are rapidly cleared by phagocytosis. Necrosis, on the other hand, is an explosive, chaotic process characterized by loss of membrane integrity, cytoplasmic swelling, and cellular fragmentation with an ensuing

TABLE 34-1

Morphologic Characteristics That Distinguish Apoptosis from Necrosis

FEATURE	APOPTOSIS	NECROSIS
Cell volume	Decreased	Increased
Plasma membrane integrity	Preserved	Lost
Plasma membrane structure	Characteristic blebbing	Ruptured
Cell-cell adhesion	Lost early	Typically preserved
Cell-matrix adhesion	Lost early	Lost late
Exfoliation of cells	Early, as single cells	Late, as sheets of cells
Pattern in tissues	Discrete, asynchronous	Contiguous, synchronous
Chromatin	Discrete, condensed	Preserved
Nuclear fragmentation	Characteristic	Absent
Cytosolic contents	Preserved	Released
Apoptotic bodies	Characteristic	Absent
Phagocytosis	Characteristic	Absent
Inflammatory response	Absent	Characteristic

TABLE 34-2

Biochemical Characteristics That Distinguish Apoptosis from Necrosis

FEATURE	APOPTOSIS	NECROSIS
Process	Active, energy-dependent	Passive, due to energy loss
Adenosine triphosphate dependence	Yes	No
Caspase dependence	Yes	No
DNA cleavage	180–base pair ladder pattern	Random, smear pattern
Cellular pH	Acidification	Unchanged
Mitochondrial permeability	Moderate loss	Severe loss
Mitochondrial potential	Transient loss	Permanent loss
Membrane phospholipid	Phosphatidylserine externalization	Unchanged

inflammatory response. These two forms of cell death can coexist and are considered two extremes of a spectrum. The predominant mode of cell death depends primarily on the severity of the insult, the extent of energy depletion, and the resistance of the cell type. Necrosis usually occurs after more severe injury, after profound energy depletion, and in more susceptible cell populations. Apoptosis is an energy-dependent process that predominates during physiological cell death and after less severe injuries typically encountered in clinical medicine. Apoptosis can be followed by *secondary necrosis*, especially if the apoptotic cells are not rapidly removed. The major characteristics that distinguish apoptosis from necrosis are listed in Tables 34-1 and 34-2. Commonly utilized laboratory methods for the detection and quantitation of apoptosis are summarized in Table 34-3. It should be noted that the assays commonly employed for apoptosis (TUNEL [terminal deoxynucleotidyl transferase biotin–d-uridine triphosphate nick end-labeling] assay and DNA laddering) do not adequately distinguish between apoptosis and necrosis. Strict morphological criteria are desirable for the detection and quantitation of apoptosis, including nuclear (condensation and fragmentation) and cytoplasmic (cell shrinkage, blebbing) changes.

PATHWAYS LEADING TO APOPTOSIS

Over the past decade, specific proteases belonging to the caspase family have surfaced as crucial initiators and effectors of apoptosis.[3-5] Members of this family are expressed as proenzymes and require activation by upstream stimuli in order to commit a cell to the execution phase of apoptosis. The downstream targets of activated caspases include cytoskeletal proteins such as actin, fodrin, and β-catenin (which lead to blebbing and disruption of cell-cell and cell-matrix adhesions), nuclear envelope proteins such as lamins (which result in nuclear condensation and fragmentation), and DNA repair enzymes such as poly([adenosine diphosphate]-ribose) polymerase (PARP).

The major intracellular apoptotic pathways may be classified according to the type of initiator pro-caspase that is activated. Activation of the initiator pro-caspase 8 results from signaling via cell surface death receptors such as Fas (the "extrinsic" pathway) and their ligands such as FADD (fas-associated death domain).[6] A very large number of physiological and noxious extracellular stimuli can initiate this signal transduction pathway. On the other hand, activation of the initiator pro-caspase 9 depends primarily on "intrinsic" mitochondrial signaling pathways regulated by members of the Bcl-2 family of proteins.[7] Activation of pro-apoptotic Bcl-2 family members triggers a sequence of events leading to release of mitochondrial cytochrome *c* into the cytosol, binding of cytochrome c with the adapter molecule Apaf-1 (apoptotic protease activating factor 1) to form the "apoptosome," and subsequent activation of pro-caspase 9.[4] The intrinsic pathway is typically activated after intracellular stress. The majority of mammalian cell death proceeds via the mitochondrial pathway.

TABLE 34-3

Methods Commonly Used for the Detection and Quantitation of Apoptosis

FEATURE	METHODS	COMMENTS
Cell morphology	Basic histochemistry	Rounding and shrinkage of cells; detachment of cells
	Phase-contrast microscopy	
Cell volume	Flow cytometry	Both methods provide quantitative results
	Laser scanning cytometry	
Chromatin condensation	Epifluorescence, confocal, and electron microscopy	DNA-binding dyes such as DAPI (4',6-diamidino-2-phenylindole) and Hoechst should be used
DNA fragmentation	Laddering by agarose gels	Poor sensitivity
	TUNEL (terminal deoxynucleotidyl transferase biotin–d-uridine triphosphate nick end-labeling) or ISEL (in situ end-labeling) assays	End-label fragmented DNA
	Flow cytometry	Measures hypoploid DNA
Plasma membrane integrity	Dye exclusion tests	Trypan blue, propidium iodide, etc., should be used
Externalization of phosphatidylserine	Annexin V labeling	Often combined with dye exclusion tests
Mitochondrial permeability	Release of cytochrome c or SMAC (second mitochondria-derived activator of caspase) into the cytosol	Immunocytochemistry or Western blots
Mitochondrial transmembrane potential	Voltage-sensitive dyes	Fluorescence microscopy or flow cytometry
Caspase activity	Enzyme assays	Colorimetric or fluorimetric
	Immunohistochemistry	Antibodies to activated caspases
	PARP (poly [adenosine diphosphate–ribose] polymerase) cleavage	Antibodies to cleaved product
Other	Activity and localization of proteins Bcl-2, Bax, and p53	Immunocytochemistry or Western blots

At least four potential levels of "cross-talk" exist between the extrinsic and intrinsic apoptotic pathways. First, Fas is also known to interact with Daxx (death-associated protein), with resultant activation of the ASK1/JNK signal transduction pathway that culminates in the release of cytochrome c and activation of caspase 9.[8] Second, initial activation of caspase 8 (via Fas) or of caspase 2 (by unclear mechanisms) can induce the mitochondrial translocation of BID, a pro-apoptotic member of the Bcl-2 family, with resultant release of cytochrome c and activation of caspase 9.[9] Third, the p53 gene is a potent transcription factor that regulates apoptosis most notably by activating pro-apoptotic Bcl-2 family members as well as the Fas-dependent axis.[7] Fourth, both pathways culminate in the activation of caspase 3, with subsequent entry into the "execution" phase of apoptosis, resulting in DNA fragmentation and cellular morphologic changes characteristic of apoptosis.[3-5] The anti-apoptotic Bcl-2 family members, such as Bcl-2 itself, play a pivotal protective role by preserving mitochondrial structure and inhibiting cytochrome c release.[4]

It should be noted that the general initiator and effector paradigm of caspase activation just outlined is not universal and that both cell death without caspase activation and caspase activation without cell death have been described.[5] Also, apoptosis occurs only after a complex sequence of activation and signal transduction events, all of which require cellular energy.

PATHWAYS LEADING TO NECROSIS

When a cell is severely stressed such that adenosine triphosphate (ATP) levels are profoundly depleted, it defaults into a state of biochemical collapse and necrosis.[11] In morphological terms, severe mitochondrial dysfunction leads to mitochondrial swelling and rupture, followed by osmotic swelling and lysis of the cell, invasion of inflammatory cells, and eventual removal of the debris.

From a functional viewpoint, severe ATP depletion has three major metabolic consequences.[11] First, it leads to mitochondrial injury, loss of mitochondrial membrane potential, and impaired oxidative phosphorylation, all of which further deplete cellular energy stores. Second, ATP depletion causes impaired calcium sequestration within the endoplasmic reticulum as well as diminished extrusion of cytosolic calcium into the extracellular space, leading to a rise in free intracellular calcium. Potential downstream complications include activation of proteases and phospholipases, and degradation of the cytoskeleton. Third, ATP depletion causes the generation of reactive oxygen molecules, with resultant apoptotic and necrotic cell death.

APOPTOSIS AND NECROSIS IN ACUTE KIDNEY INJURY

Both experimental and human studies indicate that tubule epithelial cells can suffer one of three distinct fates after acute kidney injury (AKI). The majority of cells remain viable, suggesting that they either entirely escape injury or are only sublethally injured and undergo recovery. A subset of tubule cells display patchy cell death resulting from apoptosis or necrosis. In AKI, the mode of cell death depends primarily on the severity of the insult and the resistance of the cell type. Necrosis usually occurs after more severe injury and in the more susceptible proximal tubule cells, whereas apoptosis predominates after less

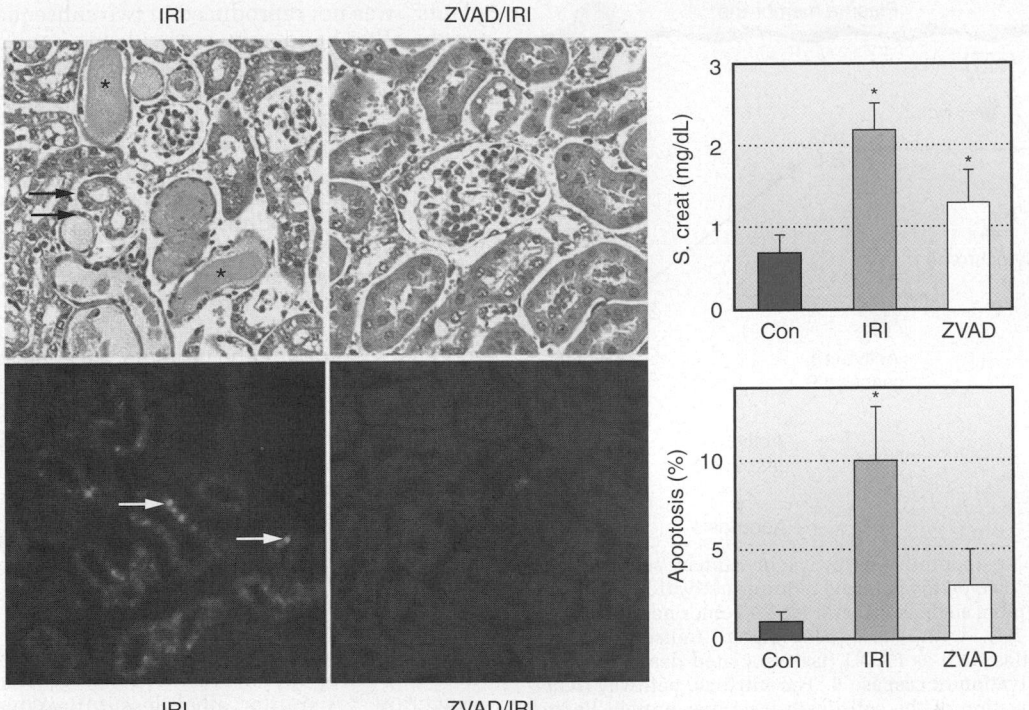

FIGURE 34-1. See also color plates. Morphology of apoptosis in acute kidney injury. Sections from mouse kidneys following ischemia-reperfusion injury (IRI) stained with hematoxylin-eosin (*top panel*) to reveal general morphology, and with TUNEL (terminal deoxynucleotidyl transferase biotin–d-uridine triphosphate nick end-labeling) (*bottom panel*) to identify apoptotic nuclei. *Arrows* show apoptotic nuclei, and *asterisks* (*) represent dilated tubules with flattened epithelium and intratubular cast formation. Pretreatment with the pan-caspase inhibitor ZVAD completely abrogated the apoptosis and resulted in partial functional protection. Con, control.

severe injury and especially in the ischemia-resistant distal nephron segments.

Mounting evidence now indicates that apoptosis is the major mechanism of early tubule cell death in contemporary clinical AKI.[12-14] Several animal models of ischemic and nephrotoxic AKI have consistently and unequivocally demonstrated the presence of apoptotic changes in tubule cells, using a variety of sensitive assays[15-20] (Fig. 34-1). Importantly, this demonstration has now been confirmed by several investigators in human models of AKI.[21-26] Several scenarios may be envisioned to explain the loss of renal function following tubule cell apoptosis.[11] First, the apoptotic cells are rapidly phagocytosed (either by neighboring cells or by macrophages), which can result in denuded areas of dysfunctional tubular epithelium. Second, the apoptotic cells undergo sloughing and desquamation, with resultant luminal obstruction. Third, although apoptosis is generally not associated with an inflammatory response, apoptotic kidney tubule cells may mount a "maladaptive response" by upregulating pro-inflammatory and chemotactic cytokines that mediate the inflammation prominently seen in ischemic AKI.

Nevertheless, controversies still exist regarding the contribution of apoptosis to the syndrome of AKI. First, most estimates place the peak incidence of apoptosis at only about 3% to 5% of tubule cells after ischemic or nephrotoxic injury, which is arguably insufficient to explain the profound renal dysfunction. A response to this skepticism is the fact that the extent of apoptosis is vastly underestimated because it is a rapidly occurring, heterogeneously distributed event that is notoriously difficult to identify and quantitate in tissues. Second, apoptosis is more commonly encountered in the distal tubule, whereas loss of

viable cells occurs predominantly in proximal segments. Reconciliation of this argument is provided by the demonstration of both necrosis and apoptosis in the proximal tubule, where these processes may represent a continuum. Third, apoptosis is generally regarded as a physiological process that removes damaged cells and may therefore be beneficial to the organ and organism. The counterpoint to this supposition is that apoptosis is a double-edged sword in that it occurs in two waves, at least in animal models of AKI. The first wave is detectable within 6 to 12 hours of the insult, peaks at about 3 days, and rapidly diminishes. This phase deletes previously healthy tubule cells, thereby contributing to the ensuing renal dysfunction. The second wave, which becomes apparent about 1 week later, removes hyperplastic and unwanted cells and may therefore play a role in the remodeling of injured tubules.

Because the evidence is overwhelmingly in favor of apoptosis as a pathogenetic mechanism in AKI, considerable attention has been directed toward dissecting out the signal transduction pathways and the molecular core machinery involved. A multitude of pathways, including the intrinsic (Bcl-2 family, cytochrome *c*, caspase 9), extrinsic (Fas, FADD, caspase 8), and regulatory (p53, nuclear factor-κB) factors appear to be activated in tubule cells after human AKI, as illustrated in Figure 34-2. The role of the Fas-FADD pathway—a leading contender for many years—in animal models has been reaffirmed by demonstration of upregulation of these proteins in apoptotic tubule cells after ischemia[17] and by the functional protection afforded by small interfering RNA duplexes targeting the *Fas* gene.[18] However, convincing human data are lacking, because the induction of the *Fas* gene demonstrated in one study of human cadaveric kidney trans-

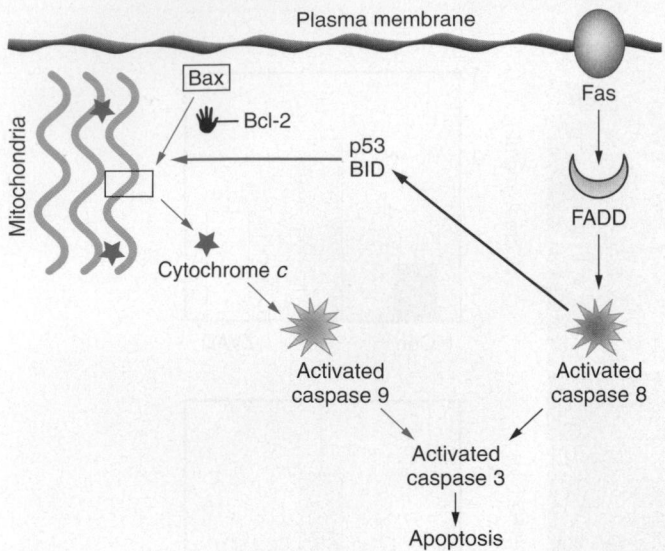

FIGURE 34-2. Major apoptotic pathways in human acute kidney injury. The extrinsic pathway (*gray*) requires activation of plasma membrane receptors such as Fas and type 1 tumor necrosis factor receptor (TNF-R1), with subsequent signal transduction via adapter molecules such as FADD (fas-associated death domain), resulting in activation of caspase 8. The intrinsic pathway (*blue*) requires translocation of the cell death promoter protein Bax to the mitochondria, thereby forming pores for the release of cytochrome *c* and activation of caspase 9. Cross-talk between these pathways is provided by two pro-apoptotic substances, Bcl-2 family protein BID and transcription factor p53. Bax translocation is normally prevented by cell survival promoter proteins Bcl-2 and Bcl-xL. Both caspases 8 and 9 activate caspase 3, which initiates the final morphologic cascades of apoptosis. The hand symbol indicates an inhibitory influence. The forward arrows indicate a positive cascade.

plants[24] was not reproduced in two subsequent studies.[25,26] On the other hand, growing evidence implicates an imbalance between the pro-apoptotic (Bax, Bid) and anti-apoptotic (Bcl-2, Bcl-xL) members of the Bcl-2 family in both animal and human models.[24-26] Of the regulatory factors, the pro-apoptotic transcription factor p53 has been shown to be induced at the mRNA[15] and protein[14] levels. Animal studies have demonstrated that inhibition of p53 by pifithrin-alpha suppresses ischemia-induced apoptosis by inhibiting transcriptional activation of Bax and mitochondrial translocation of p53.[16] However, pifithrin-alpha is an unlikely candidate for therapeutic consideration in humans because generalized inhibition of p53-dependent apoptosis would likely promote survival of damaged or mutation-bearing cells in other organ systems.

The concept of endothelial cell apoptosis in AKI has been proposed.[11] Disruptions of the actin cytoskeleton and junctional complexes, similar to those previously described in tubule epithelial cells, have been documented in endothelial cells in experimental AKI.[27] Consequent endothelial cell swelling, blebbing, death, and detachment of viable cells occur, and circulating endothelial cells have been demonstrated in humans with septic shock.[28] Systemic or intrarenal administration of fully differentiated endothelial cells into postischemic rat kidneys, to replace those lost via apoptosis, resulted in a significant functional protection.[29] A similar, albeit less impressive amelioration was achieved by the use of surrogate cells expressing endothelial nitric oxide synthase.[29] Furthermore, ischemic injury leads to a marked upregulation of angiostatin, a well-known anti-angiogenic factor that induces apoptosis of endothelial cells.[30] Collectively, these findings provide a rationale for the use of pro-angiogenic agents that can increase the pool or mobilization of endothelial progenitor cells, such as erythropoietin, bone morphogenic protein, vascular endothelial growth factor (VEGF), and statins.[11]

Inhibition of apoptosis holds significant promise in human AKI[31-36] (Table 34-4). Caspase activation is by and

TABLE 34-4

Promising Pharmacologic Inhibitors of Apoptosis

DRUG AND SOURCE	TYPE OF COMPOUND AND MECHANISM	INDICATION(S) AND CURRENT RESEARCH/ DEVELOPMENT STATUS
IDN-6556 (Pfizer Inc., New York, NY)	Small-molecule, pan-caspase inhibitor	Liver transplant (phase 2 clinical trials) Hepatitis C (phase 2)
IDN-6734 (Pfizer Inc.)	Small-molecule, pan-caspase inhibitor	Acute myocardial infarction (phase 1)
Minocycline (neuroapoptosis)	Small compound; inhibits cytochrome *c* release	Amyotrophic lateral sclerosis (phase 3) Huntington's disease (phase 2)
Amifostine (Ethyol; MedImmune, Inc., Gaithersburg, MD)	Small molecule; inhibits p53	Reduction of cisplatin nephrotoxicity (FDA approved)
Adalimumab (Humira; Abbott Laboratories, Abbott Park, IL)	Anti–TNF-α neutralizing monoclonal antibody	Rheumatoid arthritis, psoriasis, Crohn's disease (FDA approved)
Infliximab (Remicade; Centocor Inc., Horsham, PA)	Anti–TNF-α neutralizing monoclonal antibody	Rheumatoid arthritis, Crohn's disease (FDA approved)
Etanercept (Enbrel; Amgen Inc, Thousand Oaks, CA, and Wyeth Pharmaceuticals, Madison, NJ)	Type 2 TNF receptor (TNF-R2)/ immunoglobulin G fusion protein, inhibits TNF-α	Rheumatoid arthritis, Crohn's disease (FDA approved)
INO-1001 (Inotek Pharmaceuticals, Beverly, MA)	Small molecule; inhibits PARP (poly [adenosine diphosphate–ribose] polymerase)	Ischemia-reperfusion injury (phase 1)
Edavarone (Mitsubishi Pharmaceutical Corporation, Osaka, Japan)	Small molecule; free radical scavenger; antioxidant	Acute myocardial infarction (phase 3) Approved in Japan for stroke

FDA, U.S. Food and Drug Administration; TNF, tumor necrosis factor.

large the final common "execution" step in apoptosis, and cell-permeant caspase inhibitors have provided particularly attractive targets for study.[37] Currently available inhibitors have largely been investigated only in animals, provide only partial protection, and are most effective when administered before the injury (see Fig. 34-1). However, these characteristics render caspase inhibition as a potentially attractive approach to reducing apoptotic damage during cold storage of deceased donor kidneys prior to transplantation, as has been demonstrated in animal models.[38] In this regard, an orally active small molecule pan-caspase inhibitor, IDN-6556 (Pfizer Inc., New York, NY), has been developed and shown to be effective in preventing injury after lung and liver transplantation in animals.[39,40] IDN-6556 is currently undergoing evaluation in phase 2 clinical trials for prevention of ischemia-reperfusion injury in human liver transplantation (see Table 34-4). Another small-molecule pan-caspase inhibitor (IDN-6734, Pfizer) is being evaluated in phase 1 studies of acute myocardial infarction.[37]

Several other modalities ameliorate apoptosis and AKI in experimental situations. Pretreatment with erythropoietin confers structural and functional protection, inhibition of apoptosis, and upregulation of the anti-apoptotic transcription factor nuclear factor-κB.[41] However, inhibition of this factor by intrarenal transfection of decoy oligonucleotides resulted in a paradoxical attenuation of ischemic AKI, perhaps by inhibiting transcription of pro-inflammatory factors.[42] α1-acid glycoprotein (an acute-phase protein of unknown function), minocycline, tumor necrosis factor-α antagonists, adenosine A_1 receptor agonists, peroxisome proliferator–activated receptor β ligands, geranylgeranylacetone (an inducer of heat shock proteins), and PARP inhibitors have all provided encouraging functional protection from AKI with inhibition of apoptosis and inflammation.[11] Some of these agents are already widely available and safely utilized in other human conditions (see Table 34-4), and results of their use in AKI should be forthcoming. Challenges for the future clinical use of apoptosis inhibition in AKI include determining the best timing of therapy, optimizing the specificity of inhibitor, minimizing the extrarenal side effects, and tubule-specific targeting of the apoptosis-modulatory maneuvers.

Key Points

1. Apoptosis is the major mechanism of early tubule and endothelial cell death in acute kidney injury and an important contributor to the ensuing renal dysfunction.
2. Both the intrinsic (mitochondrial) and extrinsic (death receptor) apoptotic pathways are activated in human acute kidney injury.
3. Necrotic tubule cell death, which occurs primarily in the most severe cases, results from mitochondrial damage, increased intracellular calcium, and generation of reactive oxygen molecules.
4. Apoptosis and necrosis can coexist and are considered two extremes of a spectrum.
5. It is very likely that pharmacological modulation of apoptotic pathways will become an important component of medicine's armamentarium in the battle against acute kidney injury, especially in the intensive care setting.

Key References

11. Devarajan P: Update on mechanisms of ischemic acute kidney injury. J Am Soc Nephrol 2006;17:1503-1520.
13. Kaushal GP, Basnakian AG, Shah SV: Apoptotic pathways in ischemic acute renal failure. Kidney Int 2004;66:500-505.
15. Supavekin S, Zhang W, Kucherlapati R, et al: Differential gene expression following early renal ischemia/reperfusion. Kidney Int 2003;63:1714-1724.
25. Castaneda MP, Swiatecka-Urban A, Mitsnefes MM, et al: Activation of mitochondrial apoptotic pathways in human renal allografts following ischemia-reperfusion. Transplantation 2003;76:50-54.
34. Green DR, Kroemer G: Pharmacologic manipulation of cell death: Clinical applications insight? J Clin Invest 2005;115:2610-2617.

See the companion Expert Consult website for the complete reference list.

CHAPTER 35

Oxidative Stress in Acute Kidney Injury and Sepsis

Marta Piroddi, Luca Stefanelli, Daniela Buzzelli, Maria Cristina Aisa, and Francesco Galli

---

OBJECTIVES

This chapter will:
1. Describe the main concepts in oxidative stress, biomolecule damage products, and the most useful hallmarks used in clinical research.
2. Provide an overview of the literature on oxidative stress in acute kidney injury (or acute renal failure) and sepsis.
3. Critically examine possible pathogenic roles and clinical relevance of oxidative stress in sepsis, multiple-organ failure, and acute kidney injury.

Sepsis-induced multiple-organ failure (MOF) is the most relevant cause of acute kidney injury (AKI), and the association of these two conditions produces the highest mortality (up to 70%).[1] MOF is caused primarily by the release of a great quantity of bacterial endotoxins from gram-negative organisms with generalized activation and systemic expression of the host's inflammatory pathways. This response, often referred to as systemic inflammatory response syndrome (SIRS),[2] is characterized by the release of inflammatory mediators into the circulation and by oxidative stress by extensive phagocyte activation and metabolic disturbance of target tissues.

Oxidative stress is believed to play a key role in the pathogenesis of sepsis-induced AKI (Fig. 35-1),[3] but it is also well known to contribute to other causes of kidney damage, such as ischemic and toxic renal tubular injury.[4,5] In this respect, oxidative stress has to be regarded mainly as an intrarenal event. Indeed, the renal tissue is particularly susceptible to the injurious effects of reactive oxygen species (ROS)[6] because of a rich vascularization and sustained metabolic activity with high oxygen tension and a relative abundance of oxidative stress contributors, such as transition metals and heme-containing proteins.

However, during SIRS and MOF, systemic (extrarenal) oxidative stress is present and could contribute to an underlying event in AKI (see Fig. 35-1). The extensive molecular degeneration that results from oxidative stress can raise circulating levels of byproducts (e.g., through glycation and oxidation reactions, increased protein turnover, generation of activated lipids, impaired nitric oxide metabolism) that have specific biological roles of possible relevance in acute renal cell injury through metabolic overload, expression of cytokines, growth factors, adhesion molecules and chemotaxis agents, abnormal activation of detoxification, and stress response pathways.

This chapter presents an overview of the literature concerning the multiple pathogenic roles that oxidative stress can play in AKI, the molecular and biological nature of some of which remain poorly understood.

OXIDATIVE STRESS

General Concepts and Biological Implications

The chemistry of oxidative reactions has both physiological and toxicological implications that have been extensively investigated in the last decades as documented by an impressive number of publications in literature (reviewed by Galli et al[6] and Halliwell et al[7]). High fluxes of ROS are produced in the presence of a high oxygen tension and metabolic activity, and particularly during phagocyte respiratory burst, which is an essential event that accomplishes phagocytosis and cell killing with generation of superoxide ($O2^-\bullet$) as a consequence of nicotinamide adenine dinucleotide phosphate (NADPH) oxidase enzyme activity, and other relevant pro-oxidant species including peroxynitrite ($ONOO^-$), the product of a reaction between nitric oxide (NO) and superoxide, and hypochlorous acid ($HClO$), formed when hydrogen peroxide (H_2O_2) interacts with neutrophil myeloperoxidase.

Although a sustained production and the reactions of ROS with biomolecules can have toxic effects, moderate and controlled production of these species is an expression of the physiological metabolism of all the aerobic organisms and is involved in the control of several important functions, including signal transduction and gene expression regulation, cell proliferation and differentiation, and apoptosis. Therefore, the concept of oxidative stress describes a biochemical condition in which pro-oxidant species are produced in excess and overcome protection systems. This exacerbates ROS toxicity toward the entire spectrum of biomolecules (i.e., proteins, lipids, sugars and nucleic acids), hence leading to degenerative effects in the components of cells and biological fluids. ROS toxicity provides a well-accepted mechanism to explain the key pathogenic function that oxidative stress can play in several inflammation-derived and age-related conditions: cardiovascular disease, neurodegeneration, autoimmune conditions such as rheumatoid arthritis, cancer, diabetes, and kidney disease.[6]

Cells are equipped with protection systems that counterbalance the pleiotropic effects of inflammatory mediators and ROS. This protection occurs through the activation of compensation, adaptation, and repair genes that are organized in a concerted response to control metabolic (and pro-oxidant) enzymes, tissue cytokines, antioxidant and detoxification enzymes, stress proteins, and so on. However, when these cellular mechanisms are extensively

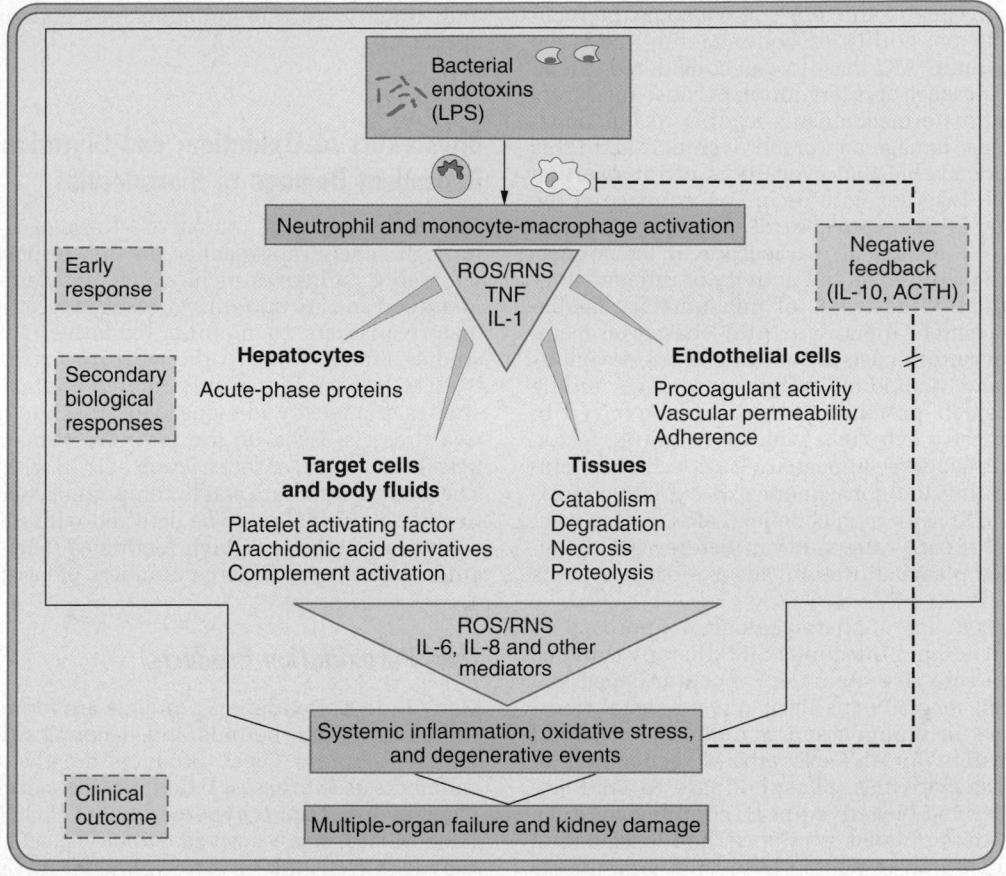

FIGURE 35-1. Biological consequences of inflammation and oxidative stress in sepsis and in acute kidney injury associated with multiple-organ failure. ACTH, adrenocorticotropic hormone; IL, interleukin; LPS, lipopolysaccharide; RNS, reactive nitrogen species; ROS, reactive oxygen species.

stimulated, effects of their protective effect could paradoxically turn to toxicity through maximized metabolic expenditure and activation of apoptotic signals.

Biological and Clinical Relevance in Acute Kidney Injury and Sepsis

Oxidative stress is an intimate consequence of uncontrolled inflammation and SIRS, hypercatabolism, and metabolic derangement of MOF (see Fig. 35-1), all of which are highly prevalent in sepsis-derived ARF. Furthermore, oxidative events can lead to metabolic disturbances of kidney tissue and decreased renal clearance of inflammation and hypercatabolism byproducts, and these specific events bring oxidative stress to attain the characteristics of a systemic self-feeding comorbidity with important pathogenic implications in ARF.

Accordingly, activation of inflammatory cells with secretion of inflammatory molecules—mainly the pro-inflammatory cytokines interleukin 1β (IL-1ß), tumor necrosis factor-α (TNF-α), and IL-6—and oxidative stress hallmarks has been observed in patients with ARF.[3,8] Nitric oxide–derived species have been also described to contribute to the inflammatory comorbidity of sepsis and ARF. The cytokine-mediated induction of NO synthesis that occurs in sepsis decreases systemic vascular resistance, thereby producing arterial vasodilatation that predisposes patients

with sepsis to ARF and to the need for mechanical ventilation and is considered to increase mortality.[1]

It remains unclear, however, whether an increase in ROS production could be an early causal event or rather a late contributor to MOF and SIRS, as well as to the chronic kidney disease of patients recovering from sepsis.

An oxidation-reduction unbalance is observed in vivo as a common underlying event of acute kidney damage induced by different types of agents, including toxic agents, immune reactions, and ischemia. Reduced renal perfusion in ARF has been proposed to be the cause of tissue damage mediated by cytokines and ROS.[9] Noninvasive in vivo studies in animal models of ischemia-reperfusion AKI performed by electron paramagnetic resonance (EPR) imaging,[10] in agreement with ex vivo analysis of lipid peroxidation hallmarks, have confirmed impairment of post–ischemia-reperfusion radical-reducing activity of the kidney tissue, and have demonstrated that this activity remains largely impaired even when parameters of renal function, such as serum creatinine and blood urea nitrogen levels, have recovered. The application of this in vivo imaging technique in Adriamycin-treated rats, a model of minimal-change nephropathy, demonstrated a transient decline of renal radical-reducing ability, which was related to mitochondria dysfunction and occurred before the appearance of continuous urinary protein.[11]

Therefore, these pieces of evidence seem to confirm the pathogenic relevance of oxidative stress in both AKI and kidney diseases in general and may suggest some intervention criteria. The possibility of counteracting oxidative stress in sepsis and AKI has to be considered as an extremely early measure of intervention because this stress is part of the intimate mechanisms leading to inflammation-derived tissue damage and organ dysfunction. In this context, it is conceivable that every type of intervention must be adopted, together with or in consequence of the main therapy that is chosen to control systemic inflammation essentially by means of extracorporeal techniques, which can lower the number and activity of inflammatory cells, and eventually, the levels of inflammatory mediators. Renal replacement therapy in ARF—based on membrane technology and the use of continuous arteriovenous hemofiltration and hemodiafiltration to remove middle molecules and small proteins and peptides involved in inflammation (mostly cytokine, platelet-activating factor, and complement factors)—appears to have a limited efficacy in ameliorating the consequence of oxidative stress in patients with ARF, although beneficial effects have been reported for use of early intervention, before ARF develops, with coupled plasma filtration–adsorption in patients with severe sepsis.

Advanced targets for a pharmacological approach to sepsis-associated and noninfectious SIRS therapy could be identified in the selective control of receptor-dependent and -independent mechanisms that activate signal transduction pathways in immune and nonimmune cells and that are responsible for the exacerbated generation of mediators such as cytokines, phospholipase A_2, and arachidonic acid–derived bioactive lipids, complement (C3a, C5a, and their desarginated products) and coagulation activation products, liver acute-phase and granulocyte proteins, and so on. The use of soluble ligands and antibodies against pro-inflammatory cytokines are examples of this strategy, although they are far from being routinely employed. On the contrary, the selective capturing of activated immune cells by sorbents or membranes seems to represent a more realistic possibility with a sure and selective effect on the oxidative stress mechanisms of ARF.

Antioxidants and targeted therapy finalized to increase renal and extrarenal protection systems may represent accessory measures that could help reduce such adverse effects. For instance, the administration of N-acetylcysteine has been suggested to be beneficial in restoring or preserving renal function in patients at risk for ARF and may also reduce inflammation during critical illness.[12] Durant and colleagues[13] suggested that vitamin E and statins can lessen the nicotinamide adenine dinucleotide phosphate (NADPH) oxidase–induced overproduction of superoxide in septic patients. However, the real effectiveness and clinical impact of antioxidant therapy in acute patients remain poorly understood, and biochemical and molecular mechanisms of renal protection are still undisclosed. These aspects could be of particular relevance in sepsis-independent AKI, in which timely and specific actions to remove the cause of damage and increase protection against tissue oxidative burden and its ultimate degenerative consequences appears much more important.

Importantly, therapies should be developed also to protect cells against chronic inflammation and degenerative events due to oxidative stress and cytokines, which may play a role in the late responses to acute inflammation.[14] For instance, inflammation-induced immune cell anergy may characterize much of the immunological imbalance seen in patients with severe SIRS.[2,15] This imbalance can lead to greater susceptibility to infections and, thus, to further inflammatory and oxidative stress events.

Biomarkers of Oxidation- and Glycation-Dependent Damage to Biomolecules

The assessment of oxidative stress can be performed through several approaches. In this respect, specific and affordable hallmarks of biomolecular damage have been identified and are currently measured together with inflammatory markers to monitor oxidative stress in clinical studies (Table 35-1). Although direct analyses of short-lived ROS have found only limited application in human studies, the most widely used approach to quantify oxidative stress is based on the indirect estimation of byproducts (biomarkers) of the reaction of ROS with biomolecules. These byproducts are stable compounds, usually produced in amounts sufficient to be detected with relatively simple analytical methods, which facilitates their application in clinical studies with large numbers of cases.

Lipid Peroxidation Products

Many lipid peroxidation products are formed during ROS attack on double bounds and decomposition of polyunsaturated lipids. These products are the most common hallmarks used to assess oxidative stress in clinical studies. They include lipid hyperperoxides (LOOH) and conjugated dienes, some derived carbonyls, such as malondialdehyde (MDA) and 4-hydroxynonenal (HNE), and the gold standard in lipid peroxidation studies, F_2-isoprostanes, which are formed from the nonenzymatic oxidation of arachidonic acid and detected with the hallmark 8-iso-PGF_2-α.[16] These products are often assessed by means of liquid and/or gas chromatography techniques coupled with mass detection, but immunodetection methods are also available and may be easier to apply in clinical studies owing to simplified sample preparation and test execution. Other methods to assess lipid peroxidation in vivo have been proposed, including gas chromatographic analysis of volatile hydrocarbon gases (e.g., ethane and pentane) in expired air.

DNA Oxidation Products

Indices of DNA damage include direct footprint of molecular derangement and fragmentation, and end products of base damage and/or products of repair and reaction with other biomolecules. The direct assays essentially detect the presence of strand breaks with formation of discrete fragments; they include single-cell micro-gel/gel electrophoresis (comet assay), and terminal uridine nick end-labeling (TUNEL) assay. All of these methods, however, are more suitable for biological and in vitro studies, providing essentially qualitative or semiquantitative results, and have relatively poor specificity.

Useful hallmarks of DNA damage and repair in blood or in urine samples have been found to be useful tools in clinical studies. They include the oxidative products of guanine and uracil, 8-hydroxydeoxyguanosine (8-OH-dG, 8OH), 7-hydroxy-8-oxo-2-deoxyguanosine (8-oxo-dG, 8OX) and 5-hydroxymethyl-2-deoxyuridine (5-OH-mdU, HMD), and the glycation product N2-carboxyethyl-2′-deoxyguanosine.[17] These molecules can be assessed by

TABLE 35-1

Some Relevant Hallmarks of Inflammation and Oxidative Stress in Acute Kidney Injury

SERUM INFLAMMATORY MARKERS	CHAPTER REFERENCE(S)
Pro-inflammatory cytokines:	3, 8
Interleukin-1β	
Tumor necrosis factor-α	
Interleukin-6	
Acute-phase proteins (e.g., C-reactive protein and fibrinogen)	
Protidemia and serum albumin	
Protein oxidation and glycoxidation:	
Protein carbonyls (as 2,4-dinitrophenylhydrazine reactants or specific epitopes by mass analysis)	20, 21, 25, 26
Advanced oxidation protein products (as di-Tyr absorbance at 340 nm in a spectrophotometric assay)	
3-Nitrotyrosine	
Advanced glycation end-products:	31, 32
Pentosidine	
Carboxymethylysine	
Carboxyethylisine	
Lipid peroxidation:	16
Malondialdehyde	
4-Hydroxynonenal	
F_2-isoprostanes (as 8-iso-PGF$_2$-α)	
DNA oxidation:	17
8-Hydroxydeoxyguanosine	
7-Hydroxy-8-oxo-2-deoxyguanosine	
5-Hydroxymethyl-2-deoxyuridine	
N_2-carboxyethyl-deoxyguanosine (DNA glycoxidation)	

specific immunometric assays, such as enzyme-linked immunosorbent assay, as well as by chromatographic methods, such as high-performance liquid or gas chromatography coupled with mass spectrometry.

GENERAL HALLMARKS OF PROTEIN DAMAGE BY REACTIVE OXYGEN SPECIES

Hydroxylation of aromatic groups and aliphatic amino acid side chains, nitration of aromatic amino acid residues, nitrosylation of sulfhydryl groups, sulfoxidation of methionine residues, chlorination of aromatic groups and primary amino groups, and cross-linking and conversion of some amino acid residues to carbonyl derivatives are some of the main reactions that occur when protein epitopes are exposed directly to ROS or reactive nitrogen species (RNS) (reviewed by Stadtman and Levine[18]). However, oxidative modifications can be induced by indirect, or secondary, events associated with ROS/RNS chemistry and oxidative stress byproduct formation.

Among the several products of protein damage by ROS/RNS, some have been extensively used as oxidative stress hallmarks. These include protein carbonyls, advanced oxidation protein products (AOPPs), and adducts formed between amino groups and free carbonyls or other molecules as lipid oxidation products, organic acids, and reducing sugars.[19]

Protein carbonyl assay is often used as an indicator of a severe oxidative stress associated with pathological conditions. This type of protein damage product can derive from a number of reaction pathways, including the direct oxidative attack on lysine, arginine, or threonine and secondary reactions of cysteine, histidine, or lysine residues with reactive carbonyl compounds. A generic but widely employed assay method for protein carbonyl measurement is the spectroscopic analysis of the stable dinitrophenyl hydrazone that these substances form after reaction with the reagent 2,4-dinitrophenylhydrazine (DNP), with maximum absorbance at 370 nm. This adduct can be also assessed with the use of anti-DNP antibodies and enzyme-linked immunosorbent assay, histochemistry, or Western blotting methods. It has been demonstrated that severe sepsis stimulates early oxidation processes, resulting in carbonylation of plasma proteins,[20,21] and there is a strong correlation between serum levels of free carbonyls, protein carbonyls, and myeloperoxidase (an index of neutrophil activation). These data confirm the key role of neutrophil oxidants in the molecular derangements observed in patients with sepsis as well as in patients with chronic renal failure.[22,23]

Oxidation and nitration of phenylalanine and tyrosine (Tyr) produce several stable products and useful oxidant stress hallmarks, such as ortho-Tyr (o-Tyr), di-Tyr, and 3-nitro-Tyr (3NT).[24-26] Di-Tyr has been described as the predominant epitope in AOPPs.[26] The compound 3NT, a marker of nitration that remains stable in protein and peptides, is universally considered an overall in vivo indicator of nitrosative stress mostly associated with overproduction of peroxynitrite. The reaction of hypochlorous acid with tyrosine can form the hallmark chlorotyrosine. Assays for these products are very sensitive and specific, and, in some cases, they can serve to identify the individual oxidation pathways and ROS species involved. Chlorotyrosyl moieties are considered specific markers of hypochlorous acid–mediated oxidation, hence reflecting neutrophil activation and myeloperoxidase catalysis. Similarly, 3NT residues indicate the production of peroxynitrite and then may indicate generation of nitric oxide and superoxide by activated monocyte-macrophages.[27] This post-translational modification has been studied with different techniques in plasma proteins of uremic patients by means of recently developed proteomics techniques, called redoxomics.[19,28]

Other hallmarks are products derived from modifications of protein thiols. Cysteine and methionine are particularly prone to oxidative attacks by almost all ROS/RNS species, and in some cases, they give origin to stable end products that can be measured in biological fluids and tissues. For instance, serum albumin plays a major role in the control of blood thiol oxidation-reduction with the formation of mixed disulfides and oxidation products that have been the subject of intensive investigation by several groups (reviewed by Piroddi and colleagues[28]).

CARBONYLATION AND PROTEIN GLYC(OXID)ATION PATHWAYS: THE ADVANCED GLYCATION END PRODUCTS

As introduced in the previous section, several oxidative pathways and products that originate from lipid peroxidation, carbohydrate oxidation, and so on, can generate protein carbonyls. In this context, two main groups of protein damage products are commonly described and identified for systematic purposes, advanced lipoxidation end products (ALEs) and advanced glyc(oxid)ation end products (AGEs). The ALE group includes epitopes generated by the covalent binding between lipid peroxidation products, such as hydroxoxynenal, malondialdehyde or acrolein, and the amino acids lysine, histidine, and cysteine. AGE compounds are a large group of epitopes that originate from one of the most notorious nonenzymatic modifications of proteins, the Maillard (or browning) reaction, which contributes not only to protein aging but may also play an important role in both physiological responses and pathological processes.[29] In this reaction, initially investigated by food chemists and identified to proceed through a complex series of steps, a large number of intermediates and AGE structures are formed by enolization, dehydration, cyclization, fragmentation, and oxidation reactions. Some AGEs, such as fluorescent vesperlysine and cross-links, retain the intact carbon structure of glucose and appear to be derived directly from glucose. In contrast, glucose-derived pentosidine requires oxidative cleavage and loss of one carbon atom. Other AGEs, such as carboxymethyllysine (CML) and carboxyethylisine (CEL), require oxidative fragmentation of the glucose carbon skeleton.

The role of free reactive carbonyls and oxidative stress in the genesis of AGEs has been unquestionably demonstrated. Reactive carbonyls can derive from polyunsaturated fatty acids, sugars and glycolytic intermediates, ascorbic acid, and some free amino acids through the contribution of oxidative stress and some cofactors, such as transition metals. Therefore, carbonyl and oxidative stress conspire to produce AGEs and ALEs. For instance, reactive aldehyde generation requires neutrophil activation and the free hydroxyl moiety of an amino acid. The generation of glycoaldehyde, 2-hydroxypropanal, and acrolein by activated phagocytes may thus play a role in AGE formation and tissue damage at sites of inflammation through the activity of the myeloperoxidase-H_2O_2-chloride system.[27,30]

Importantly, the two groups of markers identified as AGEs and ALEs contain protein products that can form cross-links and, thus, macromolecular aggregates with immunogenic and pro-inflammatory activity.[28] Moreover, they can give origin to changes in protein turnover (molecular aging) by influencing the susceptibility to protease-dependent cleavage or recognition and to elimination by scavenger cells (phagocytes).

Some AGE epitopes are fluorescent and so can be directly assessed with suitable detection equipment after purification and separation with chromatographic methods, but nonfluorescent compounds must be measured by immunoenzymatic methods or mass spectrometry coupled with liquid or gas chromatography separation.

Early evidence has confirmed high levels of circulating AGEs in animal models of and patients with ARF.[31,32] In experimental ARF in rats, circulating AGEs were found to undergo a substantial rise within a short time, a process that might derive from the lack of kidney function, accelerated synthesis of AGEs under enhanced oxidative/carbonyl stress, and liberation of AGEs from tissues through protein catabolism. Accumulation of AGEs in human ARF remains poorly documented, but it is believed to contribute to acute toxicity and/or development of late complications.[32] In general, evidence obtained in diabetes and uremia demonstrated that when protein damage occurs in vivo via the Maillard reaction, it essentially derives from inflammatory and oxidative events that combine with defective metabolism, clearance, and reactivity of free carbonyls and reducing sugars.[28] The duration and intensity of this biochemical perturbation can critically affect the tissue defense systems and repair mechanisms available to prevent irreversible damage and functional impairment. Thus, AGE formation might represent a key pathogenic mechanism in MOF and a contributor to chronic kidney damage that can accompany as late event the clinical evolution of ARF as often observed in patients recovering from septic shock.[31] In the latter case, clinical implications of AGE accumulation may include the occurrence of degenerative effects and the onset of self-feeding inflammatory loops and vascular complications as described in patients with end-stage renal disease.[28]

Key Points

1. The abnormal inflammatory response in patients with acute renal failure and sepsis is the cause of tissue damage mediated by cytokines and reactive oxygen species.
2. Oxidative stress takes place in acute renal failure mediated by other causes, such as toxic agents, immune reactions, and ischemia, and thus may represent a main pathogenic event in kidney damage.
3. As a consequence, patients with acute renal failure accumulate oxidative stress hallmarks such as lipoperoxidation markers, free and protein-associated carbonyls, and advanced glyc(oxid)ation end products.
4. Specific extracorporeal therapies and novel pharmacological approaches, including antioxidant therapy, are now available. These aim to provide a better control of the inflammatory burden in patients with acute renal failure, particularly those with septic shock, but their ability to limit kidney damage and offset the systemic effects of inflammation and oxidative stress is to be further investigated by the analysis of specific

hallmarks, such as neutrophil activation and myeloperoxidase-derived products, cytokines, and acute-phase proteins.

5. Experiments on animal models have suggested that acute renal failure is associated with acute accumulation of blood advanced glyc(oxid)ation end products, but this possibility has not been sufficiently investigated in human acute renal failure and sepsis. However, it is suspected that this AGE accumulation is caused by the lack of kidney function and the combination of oxidative stress, carbonyl accumulation, and enhanced activity of reducing sugars. Other contributing factors could be the catabolism and release of tissue advanced glyc(oxid)ation end products.

6. Accumulation of advanced glyc(oxid)ation end products in humans has been demonstrated to have major adverse effects, such as endothelial dysfunction and lowered arterial elasticity, through impairment of nitric oxide metabolism, activation by receptor-dependent mechanisms of inflammatory and vascular cells, and increased susceptibility to oxidative stress and degeneration of tissue components. Therefore, further studies are required to confirm and better characterize the biological implications of such damage to biomolecules and particularly of the formation of oxidation and advanced glyc(oxid)ation end products in the blood and tissues of patients with acute renal failure.

Key References

2. Pinsky MR: Pathophysiology of sepsis and multiple organ failure: Pro- versus anti-inflammatory aspects. Contrib Nephrol 2004;144:31-43.
3. Himmelfarb J, McMonagle E, Freedman S, et al: Oxidative stress is increased in critically ill patients with acute renal failure. J Am Soc Nephrol 2004;15:2449-2456.
6. Galli F, Piroddi M, Annetti C, et al: Oxidative stress and reactive oxygen species. Contrib Nephrol 2005;149:240-260.
9. Jaber BL, Rao M, Guo D, et al: Cytokine gene promoter polymorphisms and mortality in acute renal failure. Cytokine 2004;25:212-219.
32. Sebekova K, Blazícek P, Syrová D, et al: Circulating advanced glycation end product levels in rats rapidly increase with acute renal failure. Kidney Int Suppl 2001;78:S58-S62.

See the companion Expert Consult website for the complete reference list.

CHAPTER 36

Pathophysiology of Vasculitis

Carla M. Nester and Debbie S. Gipson

OBJECTIVES

This chapter will:
1. Identify two factors leading to susceptibility to a vasculitic environment.
2. Describe three mechanisms associated with the induction of vasculitis.
3. Identify three mediators of the maintenance of vascular inflammation.
4. Describe the potential mechanistic role of the various therapies currently used in the treatment of vasculitis.

The vasculitides comprise a collection of diseases characterized by inflammation, vessel wall necrosis, and, often, occlusion of blood vessels. Their clinical manifestations in the critical care setting depend on the localization and size of the involved blood vessels as well as on the nature of the inflammatory process.

The purpose of this chapter is to consider the proposed pathophysiological explanations of vasculitis as a whole, rather than as individual disorders, which will be covered in subsequent chapters. The discussion is framed in terms of the *susceptibility* to vasculitis, the immunopathological mechanisms of *induction*, the *maintenance* of the inflammatory state, and, finally, *resolution* or treatment considerations (Fig. 36-1).

SUSCEPTIBILITY

Susceptibility to vasculitis refers to host factors that put a particular individual at risk for vasculitis. They may include a genetic susceptibility to disease or an environmental exposure such as to a chemical or infection. These factors prepare the individual to respond to inducing mechanisms in a way that results in a vasculitic syndrome.

Patients with vasculitis have characteristics in common beyond those required to define the particular form of vasculitis. For example, the clustering of some of the vasculitic syndromes into sex- or race-predominant populations suggests the possibility of a genetic susceptibility in that population. Over the last several years, more specific associations have been made with a number of genes that appear to point to a host susceptibility to vasculitis.

One example of a specific genetic association with vasculitis is the abnormalities noted in the complement system that have been associated with Henoch-Schönlein purpura (HSP).[1-3] Two independent studies have shown that patients with HSP nephritis and the ACE D polymorphism of the angiotensin-converting enzyme (ACE) gene are more likely to have persistent or heavier proteinuria.[4,5] Additionally, studies showing an association with both cytokine polymorphisms[6] and HLA antigens and HSP[7,8] have also been reported.

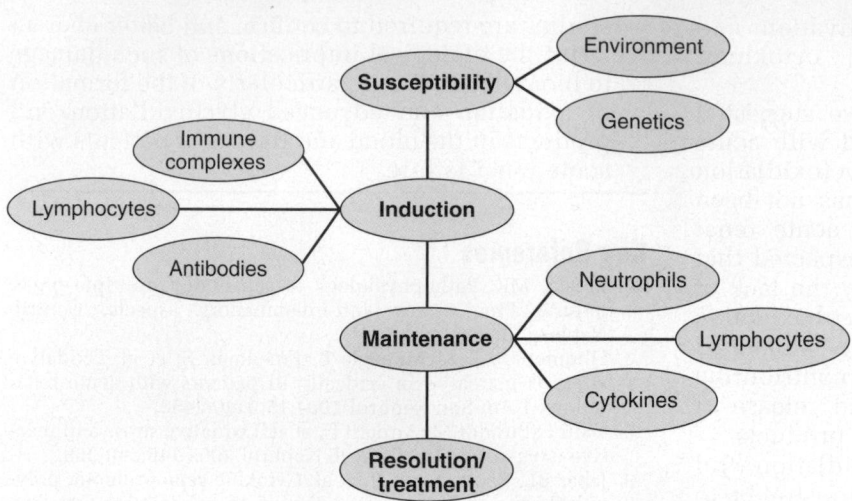

FIGURE 36-1. Key elements in the pathophysiology of vasculitis.

The link between genetics and the diseases that have antineutrophil cytoplasmic autoantibodies (ANCAs) have been somewhat more difficult to prove. It has been shown that the expression of the target antigen on the neutrophil cell surfaces of patients with ANCA vasculitis may be genetically determined,[9,10] and an increased expression of this antigen on the cell surface of the neutrophil portends an increased risk for disease. Genetic polymorphisms for α_1-antitrypsin have been variably associated with ANCA vasculitis.[11,12] One addition to defining the susceptibility to ANCA vasculitis has been the finding that a single-nucleotide polymorphism in a gene encoding a protein tyrosine phosphatase (PTPN22) has been associated with disease.[13] The full significance of this finding remains to be elucidated.

To date, there are no confirmed genetic links to polyarteritis nodosa, giant cell arteritis, or Takayasu's arteritis. However, the relative age predominance of Takayasu's arteritis in younger people and of giant cell arteritis in older populations implies the need for an age-specific event that may relate to the temporal expression of gene products.

Similarly, the female predominance of the vasculitic syndrome systemic lupus erythematosus (SLE) may indicate a sex-specific genetic susceptibility to the disease. A number of more specific susceptibility loci for SLE have been identified by genome-wide scanning,[14] and a familial disease prevalence of 12% has been reported.[14,15] Additionally, a number of HLA class I and class II major histocompatibility complex (MHC) genes have a greater frequency in patients with SLE than in the general population,[16,17] again suggesting a genetic component to the disease.

Genetic susceptibility to vasculitis appears to be important, but it is not sufficient to cause disease by itself; not all patients with abnormal polymorphisms or genes have disease. Parallel research suggests that the presentation of some of the vasculitides requires an additional event, which may be environmental. The hypothesis that there is some preceding environmental or infectious exposure has been difficult to substantiate. However, there are compelling associations to consider. A number of studies have shown that a variety of environmental factors, such as farming, solvent exposures, and earthquakes, may be linked to the development of vasculitis.[18] Silica has been reported as an environmental factor associated with ANCA vasculitis, with an odds ratio of 4.5.[19,20] Cigarette smoking has variably been shown to be associated with vasculitis.[21-23]

The fact that 90% of patients with vasculitic events report a "flu-like illness"[24] shortly before presentation suggests a potential for viral or other infectious triggers in the vasculitic patient's environment. The link between a virus and vasculitis has been demonstrated convincingly with respect to cryoglobulinemic vasculitis and hepatitis C.

It has been noted that a number of human viral infections, including those caused by Epstein-Barr virus, cytomegalovirus, human immunodeficiency virus, and hepatitis C virus (HCV), seem to elicit antibody responses to nonviral antigens, including self-antigens. This presumed polyclonal B-cell activation associated with a virus infection is of great medical interest because it may be involved in the initiation of autoimmunity and subsequent vasculitis.[25-29]

Infectious agents may also play a key role in the development of vasculitis through their ability to prime the microenvironment by triggering the production of the pro-inflammatory cytokine tumor necrosis factor-α (TNF-α).[30]

Nasal *Staphylococcus* carriage has been demonstrated to be associated with ANCA small vessel vasculitis indirectly, because prevention of carriage with antibiotics appears to limit relapse of sinus disease.[31] It has been postulated that *Staphylococcus* carriage functions as a bacterial prime—leading to a pro-inflammatory state and susceptibility to relapse. Additionally, patient exposure to propylthiouracil, minocycline, or penicillamine, which might be considered a form of environmental exposure, has also been linked to ANCA vasculitis via unclear mechanisms.

The result of the confluence of several conditions, such as genetic susceptibility and environmental exposure, is that the microenvironment becomes primed to development of vasculitis. This priming includes the exposure of antigens that are not exposed in the native state and the release of pro-inflammatory cytokines, with the resultant upregulation of the other mediators of inflammation that will play subsequent roles in perpetuating the disease process.

INDUCTION

The stimuli that induce vessel injury have been categorized as immune complexes, T lymphocytes, and antibodies.

Immune Complexes

Circulating immune complexes are typically cleared by complement-mediated mechanisms. It is only the abnormal production of these complexes and/or their abnormal deposition onto endothelial cell walls that results in vasculitis. Characteristics of the complex or the environment that cause abnormal deposition are not well defined. The sequence of events initiated by immune complex deposition includes the activation of complement and, often, the engagement of Fc receptors. Activation of complement leads to formation of the C5b-9 membrane attack complex and production of chemotactic factors, which then recruit neutrophils and monocytes into the area; it also stimulates the clotting and kinin pathways, leading to vessel thrombosis and further inflammation. Activation of Fc receptors leads to a number of intracellular events that in turn induce the release of cytokines, oxygen radicals, and proteolytic enzymes, which further advance the vascular injury.

Examples of primary immune complex–mediated diseases that may be seen in the critical care setting are hepatitis B–associated polyarteritis nodosa, HSP, and essential mixed cryoglobulinemia. In all three diseases, there is evidence of circulating immune complexes, and deposits of complement and immunoglobulin can often be found at the injured vessel wall. The hepatitis B antigen has been well described as the inciting antigen for polyarteritis nodosa[32] and has been demonstrated in circulating and tissue-bound immune complexes. Glomerular deposition of an abnormally glycosylated immunoglobulin, IgA1, accounts for the vasculitic renal disease in HSP. Circulating IgA-containing immune complexes in HSP patients tend to also contain IgG. It has been postulated that this subset of immune complexes may be more effective in eliciting an inflammatory neutrophil response.[33] The HDV antigen plays an integral role in the majority of cases of mixed cryoglobulinemia.[34,35] HCV RNA and antibodies to hepatitis C are present in serum cryoprecipitates,[35] and complexes of HCV-associated antigens and antibodies are present in vasculitic skin lesions of HCV-infected patients with mixed cryoglobulinemia.[34]

T Lymphocytes

T cells appear to be the inducers of the vasculitic process in a number of the vasculitic syndromes. For example, Cid and associates[36] reported that lymphocyte phenotyping in temporal artery biopsy specimens from patients with giant cell arteritis revealed the inflammatory infiltrate to be primarily CD4+ lymphocytes and macrophages. They concluded from this finding that the presence of these cells with activation markers suggested an autoimmune response to an antigen in the vessel wall. Similarly, the inflammatory infiltrate of Takayasu's arteritis consists primarily of various types of lymphocytes.[37] The pattern of inflammation in Kawasaki's diseases also includes CD8+ T cells and macrophages with little or no polymorphonuclear leukocytes.[38]

Finally, the presence of granulomatous inflammation in a number of vasculitic diseases (Wegener's granulomatosis, Churg-Strauss syndrome, giant cell arteritis, and Takayasu's arteritis) suggests a role for lymphocytes in the pathogenesis of disease. Granuloma formation, which is mediated by sensitized CD4+ T cells and macrophages, involves the accumulation of macrophages, epithelioid cells, lymphocytes, and multinucleated giant cells at the site of vascular injury. The presence of activated T cells and macrophages is consistent with a cell-mediated response to a foreign antigen or as a result of an innate inflammatory response. In ANCA vasculitis, autoreactive T cells have been demonstrated that are capable of proliferating in response to myeloperoxidase and proteinase 3.[39,40] This event may play a role in both induction of vasculitis and the maintenance of the inflammatory response to ANCAs.

Although SLE is a well-described immune complex disease, there is evidence that defective T-cell functions also play a role in allowing this autoimmune disease to occur.[41-43] The total number of peripheral T cells is usually reduced in patients with SLE,[44] and there is a skewing of T cells toward those that are B-cell helpers.[45] B-cell help leads to an increase in production of antibodies, some portion of which may be autoantibody in nature. Furthermore, it has been shown that patients with active SLE are often incapable of downregulating this polyclonal immunoglobulin synthesis and autoantibody production.[45]

Antibodies

Another mechanism of vessel damage is the ANCAs seen in Wegener's granulomatosis, Churg-Strauss syndrome, and microscopic polyangiitis. Experimental evidence suggests that cytokine-primed neutrophils and monocytes release granule enzymes and toxic reactive oxygen species when incubated with ANCA IgG, resulting in a cascade of inflammatory events characteristic of the maintenance phase of vasculitis.[46] Alternatively, ANCAs may interact with myeloperoxidase or proteinase 3 passively adsorbed onto endothelial cells, forming an immune complex that then damages the vessel wall.[47] Finally, endothelial cell killing by ANCA-activated neutrophils has been well documented.[48,49] Pauci-immune crescentic glomerulonephritis and small vessel vasculitis can be induced in mice by intravenous injection of ANCAs with myeloperoxidase-IgG specificity.[50]

The observation that abnormal ANCA titers are seen with disease, the correlation of ANCA titers with disease activity in some patients, and the higher risk for disease in persons with higher levels of ANCA antigens expressed on neutrophil surfaces support the hypothesis that ANCA antibodies are pathogenic. Transplacental passage of myeloperoxidase ANCA IgG has been associated with neonatal glomerulonephritis and pulmonary hemorrhage.[51]

Another group of antibodies, the anti-endothelial antibodies, have been noted in a number of vasculitic syndromes, although whether they are epiphenomena or are somehow pathogenic remains unclear. They have been detected in patients with Kawasaki's vasculitis, and binding of these antibodies to endothelial cells induces monocyte adhesion, a prerequisite to the primary monocytic inflammatory infiltrate seen in Kawasaki's disease.[52] Anti-endothelial antibodies have been described in SLE in association with active vasculitis and nephritis and appear to correlate with disease activity.[53] The exact specificities of the anti-endothelial antibodies in SLE are unknown, but it has been suggested that, as in the case of Kawasaki's disease, binding of these antibodies to the endothelium may play a role in the vascular injury of SLE.

MAINTENANCE

After the environment has been primed and injury to the blood vessel wall has occurred, the maintenance phase of inflammation begins (Fig. 36-2). The nature of the inducing event and, to some degree, the local environment determine whether the predominant infiltrating cell, and therefore the destructive force, is a lymphocyte, monocyte, neutrophil, or eosinophil. As described earlier, in each of the vasculitic syndromes, the infiltrate tends to have a predominant cell type. It appears that the receptivity of each cell type to the distinct signals in a particular inflammatory process determines the leukocyte class that responds,[54] but why certain signals predominate is not well understood. Regardless of the infiltrating cell type, the process requires an upregulation of adhesion molecules and chemoattractants as well as the expression of pro-inflammatory cytokines.

Neutrophilic Infiltrates

Central to the inflammatory process in SLE and ANCA vasculitis is the accumulation of a neutrophilic inflammatory infiltrate. Neutrophils possess enormous destructive powers, and it is their presence in the vasculitic lesion that is responsible for the ongoing inflammation. Critical to the accumulation of the neutrophil infiltrate is the binding of the neutrophil to the vascular endothelium and its subsequent transmigration into the extracellular matrix surrounding the endothelium. These events require the orchestration of a number of cellular responses and the activation of a number of chemical mediators (Table 36-1).

Selectin molecules (E-selectin and P-selectin) on the endothelium bind to carbohydrate ligands on neutrophils and are responsible for the initial tethering of a circulating leukocyte to the vessel wall.[54] Tethering brings leukocytes into proximity with chemoattractants that are displayed on or released from the endothelial lining of the vessel wall. These chemoattractants—e.g., C5a, monocyte chemotactic protein-1 (MCP-1), RANTES (regulated upon activation, normal T cell expressed and secreted), macrophage inflammatory protein (MIP-1)—bind to membrane-spanning receptors on the leukocytes and trigger G-protein activity, resulting in the activation of another set of adhesion molecules known as integrins—leukocyte function antigen-1 (LFA-1), Mac-1, and very late antigens VLA-4

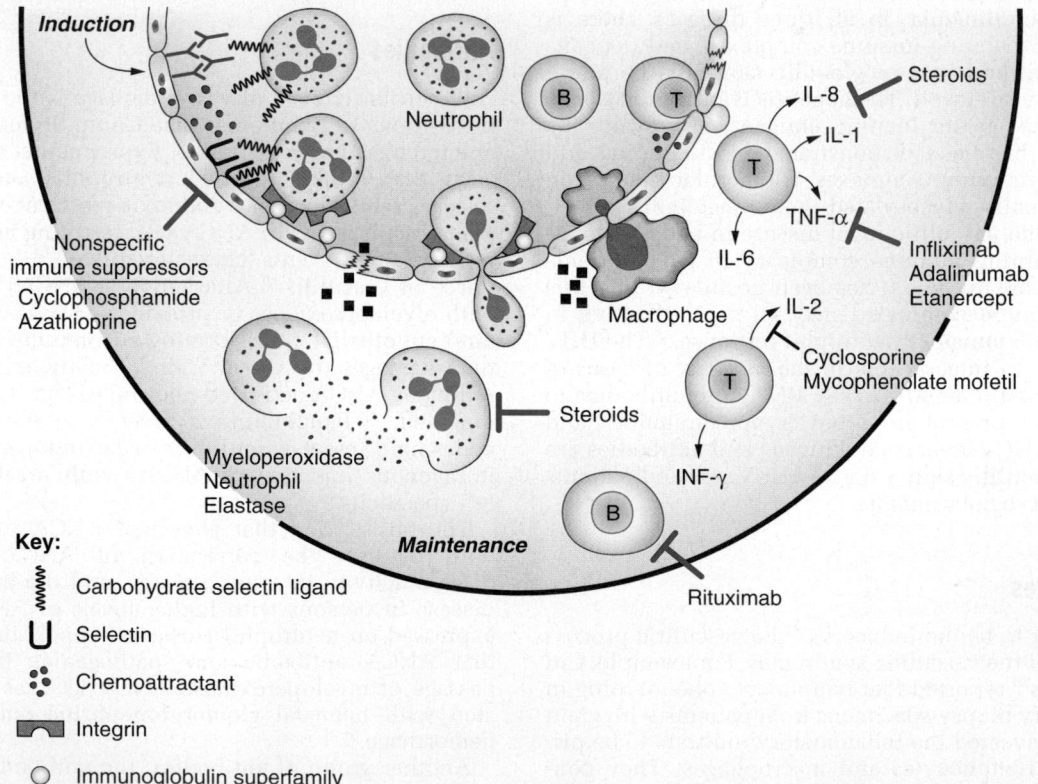

FIGURE 36-2. Cellular and chemical mediators of vasculitis. Various stimuli (immune complexes, antibodies, or lymphocytes) cause injury to the endothelium and provoke a pro-inflammatory state in and around the blood vessel wall. Inflammatory cytokines are released, and adhesion molecules are upregulated. Both lymphocytes and leukocytes migrate across the endothelial barrier, perpetuating the inflammatory process via the local release of additional cytokines and the release of granular enzymes and reactive oxygen species, respectively. Pharmacological attempts to control inflammation include blocking immune cell function (1) nonspecifically, with steroids, cyclophosphamide, or azathioprine, or (2) through more directed targeting of the components of the inflammatory process, such as the use of rituximab against B cells; of etanercept, infliximab, or adalimumab against tumor necrosis factor-α (TNF-α); and of cyclosporine and mycophenolate mofetil against interleukin-2 (IL-2). B, B lymphocyte; INF, interferon; T, T lymphocyte.

TABLE 36-1

Adhesion Molecules with Localization: Associated Ligand(s) and Reported Function

ADHESION MOLECULE	LOCALIZATION	LIGAND(S)	FUNCTION
P-selectin	Endothelial cells and platelets	Sialylated Lewis X glycoproteins	Leukocyte rolling
L-selectin	Leukocytes	Sialylated Lewis X glycoproteins	Leukocyte rolling
E-selectin (CD62E)	Endothelial cells	L-selectin	Leukocyte rolling
		CLA	
		SSEA-1	
		250-kD ESL	
CD11a/CD18 (LFA-1)	All leukocytes	ICAM-1	Adherence/emigration
CD11b/CD18 (Mac-1)	Granulocytes and monocytes	ICAM-1, iC3b	Adherence/emigration
		Fb	
CD11c/CD18 (p150,95)	Granulocytes and monocytes	iC3b	Adherence/emigration?
		Fb?	
CD49d/CD29 (VLA-4)	Lymphocytes, monocytes, eosinophils, basophils	VCAM- Extracellular matrix molecules	Adherence
ICAM-1 (CD54a)	Endothelium and monocytes	CD11a/CD18 (LFA-1)	Adherence/emigration
VCAM-1 (CD106)	Endothelium	CD49d/CD29 (VLA-4)	Adherence

CLA, cutaneous lymphocyte antigen; ESL, E selectin ligand; ICAM, intercellular adhesion molecule; VCAM, vascular cell adhesion molecule; LFA, leukocyte function antigen; VLA, very late antigen.

and VLA-5). Integrin molecules on the leukocytes in turn bind to immunoglobulin superfamily members on the endothelium (intercellular adhesion molecule-1 [ICAM-1], vascular cell adhesion molecule-1[VCAM-1], and platelet endothelial cell adhesion molecule [PECAM-1]), increasing the adhesiveness of the leukocyte-endothelial interaction. Using the integrins for traction, leukocytes can then pass the endothelial lining of the blood vessel and enter the tissue to begin the intracellular matrix damage that is noted in vasculitis.

With establishment of a neutrophilic infiltrate, the destruction of the surrounding tissues ensues. Two major functions of the neutrophil are important to this inflammatory damage, the respiratory burst and degranulation. The *respiratory burst* is the production and release of reactive oxygen species resulting from the reduction of leukocyte nicotinamide adenine dinucleotide phosphate (NADPH). These oxygen species (O_2^-, H_2O_2, and -OH), have the cumulative effect of causing cellular dysfunction and death. *Degranulation* refers to the release of leukocyte cytoplasmic granule contents into the local environment. Leukocyte granules contain a number of enzymes that can cause widespread digestion of local tissues.

Lymphocytic Infiltrates

When T cells are the predominant cell type in an inflammatory infiltrate, their presence there is guided by a sequence of events similar to that noted in neutrophil-dominant disorders. Adhesion molecules, chemoattractants, and cytokines play similar roles. However, T cells do not have a respiratory burst, nor do they degranulate. Nonetheless, they have significant destructive properties by virtue of their actions.

T-cell function at the site of inflammation can vary depending on whether the process is a primarily T cell–mediated process, such as giant cell arteritis, or whether the T cells are playing a supporting role, such as in diseases triggered by antibody interactions. Lymphocytes continually recirculate from blood, through tissue, into lymph, and back to blood. Activated T cells play a role in the vascular injury in a number of diseases. For instance, CD4+ T cells that encounter antigen differentiate into cytokine-producing effector cells, type 1 or type 2 helper T

cells. This differentiation results in a cascade of cytokine elucidation that is responsible for further recruitment of inflammatory mediators. T cells play a role in facilitating apoptosis in target cells, such as the endothelium and smooth muscle cells of the vascular bed. Alternatively, after triggering of the T-cell receptor by antigen, T cells transiently express cell surface molecules and can thereby interact with and activate resident cells and other immune cells. These functions facilitate the ongoing inflammation.

Cytokines

Cytokines are soluble proteins that play a key role in the normal immune response; however, they are equally critical in generating and maintaining the inflammatory response that is pathogenic in the vasculitides (Table 36-2). Regardless of the induction mechanism, the environment becomes further primed by cytokines, making it even more susceptible to vascular damage. Interleukin-1 (IL-1) and TNF-α are key examples of pro-inflammatory cytokines whose expression is greater after the induction of inflammation. These cytokines have a broad effect on both neutrophils and endothelial cells. TNF-α is integral to the priming process and can trigger endothelial cell activation and the induction of the expression of adhesion molecules by endothelial cells. This induction facilitates leukocyte activation, adhesion, and migration to the inflamed area. IL-1 acts as a co-stimulant for T- and B-cell proliferation. TNF-α and IL-1 are also integral to the induction of other cytokines, such as IL-6 and IL-8. IL-6 promotes the growth and differentiation of T and B cells and has endogenous pyrogen activity. IL-8 increases the adherence of leukocytes to endothelial cells, is chemotactic for both neutrophils and T cells, and plays a role in leukocyte activation. IL-2 induces the proliferation and differentiation of T and B cells and has some cytotoxicity effects.

RESOLUTION—TREATMENT

Traditional therapeutic interventions in the vasculitides are often nonspecific in their effect and in general suppress immune system function. Cyclophosphamide cross-links

TABLE 36-2

Cytokines and Growth Factors Relevant to the Pathogenesis of Vasculitis

CYTOKINE	SOURCE(S)	BIOLOGICAL EFFECTS
Interferon-γ (IFN-γ)	T cells, natural killer (NK) cells	Increases expression of major histocompatibility complex (MHC) class I and class II molecules Macrophage activation Antiviral activity
Interleukin-1 (IL-1)	Macrophage, neutrophils, endothelial cells, T and B cells, NK cells, fibroblasts, smooth muscle cells	Acts as costimulant for T- and B-cell proliferation, activates endothelial cells Induces hepatic synthesis of acute-phase proteins and endogenous pyrogen activity Increases adhesion molecule expression on endothelial cells
IL-2	T cells	Induces proliferation and differentiation of T cells and B cells Stimulates cytotoxicity of NK cells
IL-6	T cells, endothelial cells, macrophages, fibroblasts	Promotes growth and differentiation of T and B cells Induces hepatic synthesis of acute-phase proteins and endogenous pyrogen activity
IL-8	Macrophages, neutrophils, endothelial cells, T cells, fibroblasts	Chemotactic factor for neutrophils and T cells Activates neutrophils Increases adherence of leukocytes to endothelial cells
Tumor necrosis factor-α (TNF-α)	Macrophages, neutrophils, endothelial cells, T and B cells	Acts as costimulant for T- and B-cell proliferation Activates endothelial cells Induces hepatic synthesis of acute-phase proteins and endogenous pyrogen activity Increases adhesion molecule expression on endothelial cells
Platelet-derived growth factor (PDGF)	Platelets, macrophages, endothelial cells, fibroblasts, smooth muscle cells	Promotes growth of fibroblasts, smooth muscle cells, and endothelial cells Chemotactic factor for fibroblasts, smooth muscle cells, neutrophils, and monocytes Stimulates degranulation of neutrophils and monocytes
Vascular endothelial growth factor (VEGF)	Platelets, macrophages, endothelial cells, fibroblasts, smooth muscle cells	Induces endothelial cell proliferation and permeability Promotes cell migration Inhibits apoptosis

DNA strands and inhibits cell division, thereby limiting the immune cell interactions that may perpetuate the disease. Steroid therapy decreases inflammation by suppressing the migration of neutrophils and by reversing the increased capillary permeability noted in inflammation. These actions are likely to be secondary to glucocorticoid binding to and activation of the glucocorticoid receptor, which positively or negatively regulates the expression of specific genes. Other nonspecific therapeutic agents are azathioprine and mycophenolate mofetil. Through their effect on purines, these drugs appear to alter nucleic acid synthesis and therefore also disrupt immune cell function.

A number of more directed therapies attack very specific components of the inflammatory process. Rituximab, one of the newer biologicals used to treat ANCA–small vessel vasculitis, is a chimeric monoclonal antibody to CD20 on B cells that functions to deplete these B cells and decrease circulating ANCAs.[55] Cyclosporine, an older, selective immunosuppressant drug, inhibits T lymphocytes by inhibiting expression of IL-2 and its receptors.

Another approach to treatment is TNF-α blockade. TNF-α not only is responsible for activating neutrophils but also encourages a pro-inflammatory phenotype of the endothelium.[56] Infliximab, a chimeric monoclonal anti–TNF-α antibody, inhibits both cell-associated and secreted TNF-α and consequently all downstream effects, including the production of other cytokines. It also inhibits the upregulation of adhesion molecules. Etanercept, a soluble TNF-α receptor fusion protein, has a longer circulating half-life. Adalimumab is the newest anti–TNF-α drug available.

An additional therapeutic measure that has been considered in the treatment of vasculitis is plasmapheresis. This process was theorized to function to remove circulating antibodies or immune complexes that may cause endothelial injury, but in practice, plasmapheresis is not used except for life-threatening pulmonary hemorrhage syndromes and for ANCA vasculitis that manifests as complete renal failure.

CONCLUSION

Current research suggests that the clinical manifestation of vasculitis depends on a combination of environmental exposure and susceptibility to disease. Regardless of the inducing agent (antibody, lymphocyte or immune complex), the cascade of events results in the upregulation of adhesion molecules and cytokines. The effect is a series of inflammatory processes that is maintained until spontaneous resolution occurs, treatment has been effective, or, alternatively, permanent organ damage has occurred. Although the initiating event may differ in individuals or specific diseases, there are some similarities between the vasculitides in how the inflammatory process is perpetuated with respect to how both leukocytes and endothelial cells respond to the initiating injury. The same set of cytokines plays a role in both the normal immune surveillance and the pathology of vasculitis. Ultimately, more study is required not only to better define the mechanism of initiation but also to further delineate each of the key components in the inflammatory process. A more complete understanding of vasculitis would allow physicians to direct therapy more specifically at those components in the process, perhaps enabling more effective induction and maintenance of remission and avoiding the side effects of some of the currently used nonspecific immune therapies.

Key Points

1. The presentation of vasculitis may be influenced by environmental exposures and by a genetic susceptibility to disease.
2. Vasculitis results from vessel injury induced by antibodies, lymphocytes, or immune complexes.
3. The different vasculitides are distinguished by different cell types in their inflammatory infiltrates.
4. Leukocyte and endothelial cell adhesion molecules are upregulated as part of the vasculitic process.

5. Cytokines play a role in normal immune response and in the maintenance of pathological inflammation of vasculitis

Key References

16. Pisetsky DS: Systemic lupus erythematosus: epidemiology, pathology, and pathogenesis. In Klippel JH, Stone JH, Crofford LJ, White P (eds): Primer on the Rheumatic Diseases, 11th ed. Atlanta, Arthritis Foundation, 1997, pp 246-251.
38. Burns JC, Glode MP: Kawasaki syndrome. Lancet 2004;364: 533-544.
46. Falk RJ, Terrell RS, Charles LA, Jennette JC: Anti-neutrophil cytoplasmic autoantibodies induce neutrophils to degranulate and produce oxygen radicals in vitro. Proc Natl Acad Sci U S A 1990;87:4115-4119.
54. Springer TA: Traffic signals for lymphocyte recirculation and leukocyte emigration: The multistep paradigm. Cell 1994;76:301-314.
56. Bratt J, Palmblad J: Cytokine-induced neutrophil-mediated injury of human endothelial cells. J Immunol 1997;159: 912-918.

See the companion Expert Consult website for the complete reference list.

CHAPTER 37

Renal Repair and Recovery

Kathleen D. Liu

OBJECTIVES

This chapter will:
1. Describe common aspects of the pathophysiology of acute kidney injury (e.g., septic, nephrotoxic, ischemic).
2. Summarize what is known about the role of renal tubular epithelial cells, renal-specific progenitor cells, and mesenchymal stem cells in renal recovery.
3. Explain additional mechanisms that contribute to repair of renal injury: growth factors, endothelium, other tubular epithelial cells.
4. Describe how renal replacement therapy may impact renal recovery.

Acute kidney injury (AKI) has several distinct etiologies, including sepsis, ischemia, and nephrotoxins. Our understanding of the pathophysiology of these diseases is based largely on animal models. These models have important strengths and limitations, including uncertainty as to how well they replicate human disease. Our understanding of repair and recovery is significantly predicated on these models. This chapter reviews common elements of the pathophysiology of different types of AKI and then discusses what is known about mechanisms of repair and recovery. It is also increasingly clear from human studies and animal models that AKI can lead to chronic kidney disease. The chapter also briefly discusses the role of growth factors in this process. Last is a summary of the

impact of renal replacement therapy on recovery from AKI.

NORMAL RENAL ARCHITECTURE

Under normal conditions, renal tubule cells are highly polarized epithelial cells (described by Fish and Molitoris[1]). The apical side is characterized by microvilli that extend into the tubular lumen; these microvilli contain bundled F-actin filaments. The actin cytoskeleton is a dynamic structure characterized by a highly regulated, steady state equilibrium between F-actin filaments and G-actin monomers. Cells are connected one to another near their apical surfaces by a junctional complex that is made up of both tight junctions and adherens junctions. The tight junction is a multimeric protein complex (including occludin, zona occludens-1 [ZO-1], ZO-2 and cingulin) that forms the border between the apical and basolateral surfaces of the cell, segregates proteins and phospholipids to the appropriate cell surface (gate function), and blocks paracellular permeability (fence function).

The basolateral surface of the cell is also characterized by distinct proteins and phospholipids. For example, the Na^+,K^+–adenosine triphosphatase (ATPase) is localized to the basolateral side of the cell and is critical for sodium ion (Na^+) reabsorption from the tubular lumen and transport to the interstitium. Transmembrane integrins bind to extracellular matrix proteins via arginine-glycine-asparagine (R-G-D) peptide sequences. Epithelial cells also have specialized protein complexes at extracellular matrix binding sites called *focal adhesion complexes*. Together, these interactions cause the renal tubular epithelial cell to be firmly adherent to the basement membrane.

ACUTE KIDNEY INJURY: COMMON PATHOPHYSIOLOGICAL MECHANISMS OF INJURY AND REPAIR

Cellular damage in AKI involves three forms of injury: sublethal damage resulting in depolarization of cells (and therefore loss of appropriate cellular functions), as well as cell death through apoptosis and cell death through necrosis.[2-4] Although there has been controversy about which segment of the tubule is the most affected, it is clear that the proximal tubule, and in particular the S3 segment, undergoes significant morphological changes, and it therefore has been the subject of much study.[5]

Specific animal models and human disease vary with regard to the relative balance of these pathophysiological processes. In renal biopsy specimens from patients with ischemic kidney injury (e.g., after cadaveric kidney transplantation), the majority of tubules may appear fairly normal, with limited overt cellular necrosis. However, in animal models of either toxin-mediated or ischemic kidney injury, necrosis is typically widespread. These differences may be due to the fact that in animal models, severe ischemia is induced by exposure to high doses of a nephrotoxin or by cross-clamping of the renal artery. In animal models of septic AKI, cellular morphology often appears relatively normal.[6] These differences highlight an important distinction between the clinical entity of AKI and animal models[7-9] and may partially explain why many of the successful interventions for AKI in animal models have not been efficacious in clinical trials.

Despite these differences, common injury processes underlie all forms of AKI, and in order for recovery to occur, these injuries must be repaired. At one end of the spectrum, epithelial cells die through apoptosis and necrosis, resulting in loss of tubular integrity. As discussed in Chapter 34, apoptosis is a form of programmed cell death that is characterized by cell shrinkage, nuclear condensation and fragmentation, and rapid clearance by phagocytosis. Most normal cells constitutively express the machinery necessary for apoptosis but are prevented from undergoing apoptosis by the presence of survival factors. Loss of these survival, or growth, factors leads to triggering of apoptosis via a "default" pathway.[4] Depending on the nature and duration of injury, cells may also undergo necrosis. In addition, viable renal tubular epithelial cells are shed into the lumen of the tubule,[10] contributing to the loss of epithelial integrity. Thus, one of the first steps in renal recovery is the dedifferentiation of surviving epithelial cells as well as migration of appropriate epithelial cell precursors to the damaged tubules. As explored later in more detail, the precise nature of these precursor cells remains controversial. Three different types of cells have been shown to play a role in this process in various model systems: renal tubular epithelial cells, renal-specific progenitor cells, and bone marrow–derived mesenchymal stem cells.

Sublethal cellular injury has been described both in animal models and in human renal allografts. In animal models, short ischemic times lead to both loss and fusion of the apical microvilli, whereas longer ischemic times result in shedding of microvilli into the tubular lumen, loss of integrity of the actin cytoskeleton, and, ultimately, cell death.[11] Junctional complexes are disrupted after AKI, leading to increased paracellular permeability due to loss of the gate function as well as loss of cell polarity due to loss of the fence function. For example, the Na^+,K^+-ATPase that is typically localized exclusively on the basolateral surface can be found on the apical surface after ischemic injury. Mislocalization of these channels contributes to the inability of the proximal tubule to reabsorb Na^+, as is commonly seen in AKI.[12] Thus, the recovery process must result in reestablishment of polarity of sublethally injured cells and establishment of polarity in the de novo epithelial cells. Reestablishment of polarity appears to require signaling cues from adjacent cells as well as from the extracellular matrix.

In addition, AKI is frequently characterized by damage to other cellular compartments. Microvascular injury plays a critical role in both septic and ischemic AKI.[13,14] Given the enormous oxygen tension gradient within the normal kidney, small changes in oxygen delivery may greatly exacerbate tissue hypoxia. Furthermore, endothelial cell damage may lead to leukocyte activation and sludging within the capillaries and to release of inflammatory mediators. In ischemic AKI, neutrophils and T cells are recruited to the injured tissue and modulate injury.[15]

Recovery from acute tubular injury is as yet a poorly understood process, although it is known to involve recruitment of inflammatory cells, which may be important sources of paracrine growth factors, as well as proliferation and differentiation of surviving cells to form polarized epithelial tubules.[16] Growth factors may exert important antiapoptotic and proliferative effects on damaged cells. Renal-specific or bone marrow–derived mesenchymal stem cells may accelerate the repopulation of tubules through either direct proliferation or paracrine effects. Thus, the recovery process may recapitulate many aspects of renal development[17]; indeed, a number of proteins expressed in the developing kidney are reexpressed after acute renal injury.

RECOVERY FROM ACUTE KIDNEY INJURY

What Is the Progenitor Cell?

After ischemic injury, surviving renal tubular epithelial cells dedifferentiate.[17] Proliferation and migration of existing renal tubular epithelial cells clearly contribute to the recovery process. Following renal injury, proximal tubular cells express vimentin, an intermediate filament protein that is found in undifferentiated mesenchymal cells but not differentiated kidney cells; these cells also express proliferating cell nuclear antigen (PCNA), a marker of mitogenic activity.[18] In contrast, injured cells do not express either vimentin or PCNA. In the studies yielding these findings, the majority of surviving cells expressed vimentin, suggesting that many cells dedifferentiated as part of the repair/recovery process. Thus, surviving renal tubular epithelial cells play a critical role in the regeneration process.

A number of studies have examined the potential role of organ-specific stem cells as well as mesenchymal stem cells in renal repair (Fig. 37-1; reviewed by Cantley[19]). The role of stem cells in the kidney is described in more detail in Chapter 39. Renal-specific stem cells have been described by several independent groups. These cells can

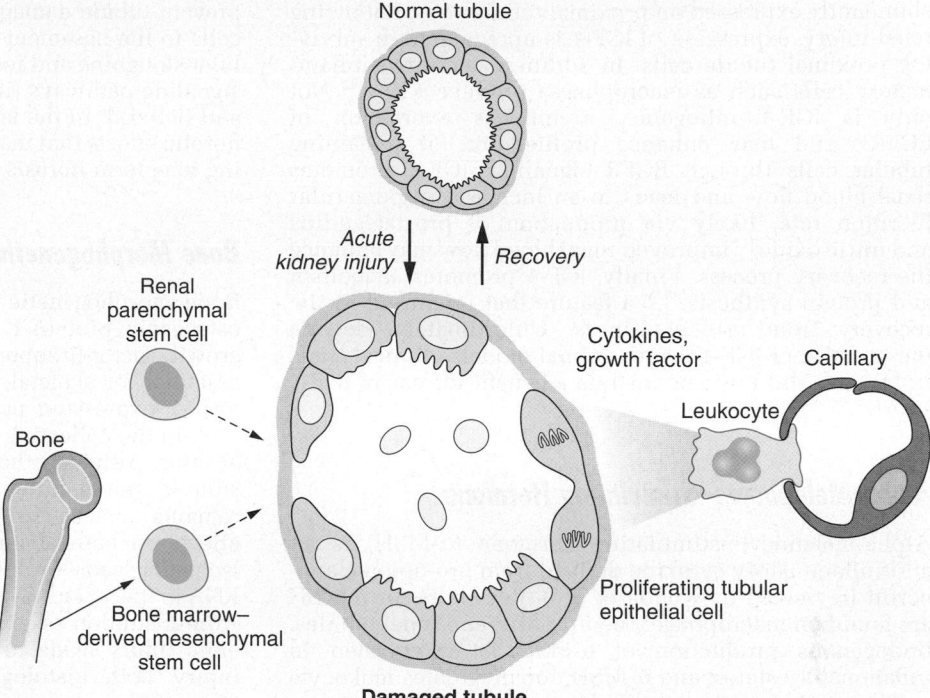

Normal tubule

Acute kidney injury   *Recovery*

Renal parenchymal stem cell

Bone

Cytokines, growth factor

Capillary

Leukocyte

Bone marrow–derived mesenchymal stem cell

Proliferating tubular epithelial cell

Damaged tubule

FIGURE 37-1. Critical mediators of renal recovery and repair. After renal injury, multiple cell types participate in the reconstitution and repolarization of the tubular epithelium.

be identified through the use of bromo-deoxyuridine (BrdU) to label cells that are slowly going through the cell cycle. Such cells have been found in the renal tubules as well as the papilla.[20,21] Moreover, these renal progenitor cells have phenotypic plasticity and are capable of expressing epithelial markers in vitro when subjected to appropriate extracellular cues.[20,21] After ischemic renal injury, renal-specific stem cells proliferate and appear to contribute to repopulation of the tubule in animal models. However, study of the role of such cells in renal repair has been limited by the lack of markers to specifically identify this cell population.

Similarly, a number of studies have focused on the role of bone marrow–derived mesenchymal stem cells in renal recovery. Clinical transplantation studies originally suggested that recipient-derived cells can be isolated from the donor kidney following engraftment, suggesting that stem cells might play a role in tissue homeostasis.[22,23] In animal models of renal ischemia, bone marrow–derived mesenchymal stem cells migrate to the kidney and are capable of repopulating the tubule. Administration of exogenous stem cells at the time of renal injury accelerates the recovery process. However, the contribution of these cells to repopulation of the tubule has varied in different experimental systems, depending on how the stem cells are identified as "foreign" (e.g., by the presence of a y chromosome in an xx animal or by β-galactosidase expression).[24,25] Thus, epithelial regeneration does not appear to be the predominant mechanism of mesenchymal stem cell benefit. Additional studies suggest that mesenchymal stem cells may exert their beneficial effects via paracrine mechanisms rather than through tubular engraftment and proliferation.[26,27]

Role of Growth Factors

A number of growth factors enhance proliferation of tubular epithelial cells in animal models as well as cell culture systems.[9,28] In animal models, administration of exogenous growth factors has been shown to accelerate renal recovery from injury. Although some of these polypeptide growth factors have been studied in clinical trials and have not been shown to have any significant benefit, the studies highlight important components of the process of renal recovery. Differences in treatment effect between animal models and clinical trials may be attributable to differences in the timing of growth factor administration in relation to injury; in animal models, growth factors are typically administered at the time of or immediately after injury. In clinical trials, however, AKI is typically advanced when therapy is initiated.[9]

Epidermal Growth Factor

Epidermal growth factor (EGF) is a ubiquitous polypeptide growth factor capable of stimulating proliferation of many types of epithelial cells. It activates cellular signaling by engaging the EGF receptor (EGFR), a receptor tyrosine kinase. EGFR is expressed in the adult kidney, and administration of EGF to animals with ischemic or toxin-mediated AKI shortens recovery time.[29] This finding is likely due to downstream activation of cell survival pathways, including phosphoinositide 3-kinase (PI3K)/Akt and extracellular signal–regulated kinase. Both renal epithelial cells and progenitor cells have been shown to proliferate in response to EGF.[21,30] Mice with a targeted mutation in the EGFR demonstrate delayed recovery from nephrotoxic AKI,[31] suggesting that this pathway may play an important role in renal repair.

Insulin-like Growth Factor-1

Although insulin-like growth factor-1 (IGF-1) is minimally expressed in the adult human kidney, its receptor is abundantly expressed on proximal tubule cells. Following renal injury, expression of IGF-1 is upregulated in surviving proximal tubule cells. In addition, recruited inflammatory cells such as macrophages produce IGF-1.[32] Not only is IGF-1 mitogenic; it induces expression of EGFR[33] and may enhance proliferation of remaining tubular cells through EGFR signaling. IGF-1 promotes renal blood flow and leads to an increase in glomerular filtration rate, likely via production of prostaglandins and nitric oxide[34]; improved renal blood flow may enhance the recovery process. Finally, IGF-1 promotes anabolism and protein synthesis,[35,36] a feature that might aid in the recovery from critical illness. Unfortunately, despite the promise of IGF-1 use in animal models, clinical trials in humans did not demonstrate a benefit for use of IGF-1 in AKI.[37]

Alpha-Melanocyte–Stimulating Hormone

Alpha-melanocyte-stimulating hormone (α-MSH) is an anti-inflammatory cytokine derived from pro-opiomelanocortin (reviewed by Kohda et al[38]). Receptors for α-MSH are found on macrophages, neutrophils, and renal tubules. Endogenous production of α-MSH is upregulated in inflammatory states, and α-MSH downregulates leukocyte activation. Interestingly, this hormone is protective even in animals deficient in intercellular adhesion molecule-1 (ICAM-1), in which neutrophil recruitment is attenuated.[39] α-MSH also appears to have direct effects on renal tubules, including downregulation of inducible nitric oxide synthase, which may attenuate the extent of injury. However, the role of endogenous α-MSH in renal repair and recovery remains unclear.

Erythropoietin

Erythropoietin has been shown to accelerate recovery from ischemic AKI (reviewed by Sharples et al[40]). It has been proposed that this finding is in part due to improved endothelial cell survival and function, which results in improved oxygen delivery to the renal tubular epithelium. Erythropoietin also promotes proliferation of tubular epithelial cells in a cisplatin model of AKI. However, data suggesting that erythropoietin therapy can attenuate human injury are limited; furthermore, the role of endogenous erythropoietin in renal repair remains unclear.

Hepatocyte Growth Factor

As the name implies, hepatocyte growth factor (HGF) was initially identified as a mitogenic factor for hepatocytes. It was subsequently shown to have additional properties, including mitogenic, morphogenic, motogenic, and differentiating effects in the kidney and in kidney-derived cell lines.[41,42] HGF binds to c-met, a receptor tyrosine kinase. Activation of c-met leads to the induction of a number of signaling pathways, such as mitogen-activated protein kinase, phosphoinositide 3-kinase (PI3K), Src, and Grb2/Sos/Ras. Renal injury leads to rapid activation of both HGF and c-met within the kidney.

In animal models of toxic and ischemic AKI, HGF therapy at the time of injury markedly accelerated functional and histological recovery.[43,44] Not only does HGF have important effects on cellular proliferation; it may prevent tubule damage by promoting adhesion of tubular cells to the basement membrane (thereby preventing cellular sloughing and loss)[45] and by activating anti-apoptotic signaling pathways (including phosphoinositide 3-kinase and Bcl-xl).[46] In the late phases of recovery, HGF has antifibrotic effects that may have an important role in preventing long-term fibrosis and scarring.[42]

Bone Morphogenetic Protein-7

Bone morphogenetic protein-7 (BMP-7), also known as osteogenic protein-1, is a member of the transforming growth factor-β superfamily that has been shown to be essential for skeletal, kidney, and ocular development.[47] BMP-7 expression persists in the adult kidney, particularly in the collecting tubule, the glomeruli, and the renal arteries. Although the role of endogenous BMP-7 expression in the maintenance of normal renal architecture remains unclear, a number of studies have examined its effects on both acute and chronic kidney injury. Renal ischemia leads to decreased levels of BMP-7 messenger RNA in the rat kidney, likely owing to local tissue damage.[48] Administration of exogenous BMP-7 at the time of ischemic injury leads to attenuation of the severity of the injury, both histologically and biochemically.[49] In the same study, administration of BMP-7 also reduced levels of ICAM-1 expression in the damaged kidney, an effect that may limit inflammatory cell–mediated injury. In cell culture models, BMP-7 appears to downregulate pro-inflammatory cytokines, including interleukin-6, interleukin-8, monocyte chemotactic protein-1, and endothelin-2, a potent vasoconstrictor.[50] Like HGF, BMP-7 appears to have important antifibrotic effects in the recovering kidney.[51]

Transforming Growth Factor-β

Transforming growth factor-β (TGF-β), a profibrotic growth factor, is a critical mediator of the epithelial to mesenchymal cell transition.[51] Although TGF-β receptor expression is upregulated after injury, this mediator does not appear to play a critical role in early renal recovery, because immediate treatment with TGF-β–neutralizing antibodies does not slow renal recovery.[52] However, treatment with such antibodies results in reduced capillary dropout and interstitial inflammation, suggesting that TGF-β may play a critical role in the long-term effects of AKI. Indeed, TGF-β appears to be an important mediator of renal fibrosis in many different contexts.

Role of Adjacent Cells and Extracellular Matrix

Cellular contact with adjacent cells and with the extracellular matrix appears to protect cells from apoptosis. Following injury, major structural components of the basement membrane, including laminin, fibronectin III, and the cell surface receptors for these basement membrane proteins (e.g., integrins), are upregulated.[53,54] Integrins are also mislocalized after renal injury; this effect has been suggested to allow epithelial cells to migrate as part of the recovery process.[17] Normal cell-cell contact via cadherins also provides an anti-apoptotic signal in proximal tubular cells.[55]

Role of Endothelium

At present, specific mechanisms of endothelial repair and recovery remain undefined. However, it is clear that endothelial injury plays a critical role in the pathogenesis of AKI.[13] Furthermore, the endothelium regulates leukocyte recruitment to areas of injury. Endothelial adhesion molecules, including E-selectin, P-selectin, and ICAM-1, become upregulated and recruit leukocytes to the site of injury.[17] As a result, leukocytes migrate from the vessel lumen to the surrounding tissue and helper T cells are stimulated. Use of multiple strategies to block ICAM-1, including anti–ICAM-1 antibodies and antisense oligonucleotides directed against ICAM-1, and studies in ICAM-1–deficient mice have shown that ICAM-1 blockade is protective in the setting of AKI. Interestingly, one study has demonstrated that statins ameliorate ischemic renal damage. In this study, inflammatory cell infiltration, upregulation of ICAM-1, and increased production of inducible nitric oxide synthase were attenuated by statin administration.[56] Modulation of the coagulation cascade by activated protein C may reduce renal injury; activated protein C also has potent anti-inflammatory effects that may limit the extent of tubular damage. Thus, renal injury clearly results in damage to the endothelial compartment, which in turn promotes tubular injury; the mechanisms of cellular repair require further study.

STRATEGIES TO ACCELERATE RENAL RECOVERY: HUMAN STUDIES

A number of clinical treatments have been proposed to enhance renal recovery from acute injury.[9] They include strategies (1) to increase urine flow and decrease tubular obstruction, such as the use of osmotic and loop diuretics, (2) to increase renal blood flow, such as the use of low-dose dopamine and atrial natriuretic peptide, and (3) to promote renal recovery using growth factors, including IGF-1. Unfortunately, none of these strategies has shown clinical benefit in human clinical trials.

Therefore, dialysis is the primary supportive therapy administered to patients with severe AKI. The impact of renal replacement therapy on renal recovery has been reviewed.[57] In brief, the effect of several aspects of the dialysis prescription, including the timing of initiation of dialysis and the dialysis dose, remain controversial or unknown. Both the timing and dose of dialysis may affect levels of inflammation and, therefore, renal recovery. A number of studies have focused on the effects of dialyzer membranes on mortality and renal recovery because the original cellulose-containing membranes activate complement and coagulation factors; these are frequently called bioincompatible membranes. Newer synthetic membranes (polyacrylonitrile, polymethyl methacrylate, polysulfone) as well as cellulose membranes containing synthetic side-groups are more "biocompatible" and therefore cause less complement activation. Although these latter membranes were initially shown to have a positive effect on renal recovery and mortality, subsequent studies did not support these results. Several meta-analyses have been published, with varying conclusions; the impact of biocompatible membranes on renal recovery appears to be limited, at best.[58]

Also, the modality of dialysis may affect renal recovery. Continuous renal replacement therapy has a number of features that may result in better renal recovery than intermittent hemodialysis[59]; they are (1) superior control of uremia, (2) prevention of intradialytic hypotension and thereby reduced risk of extending ischemic renal damage, (3) enhanced clearance of inflammatory mediators, and (4) better ability to provide nutritional support. The effect of modality on renal recovery has varied in studies to date; furthermore, modality does not appear to improve overall survival.[57] Thus, at present, these benefits for renal recovery must be considered largely theoretical.

CONCLUSION

AKI is a complex process, involving sublethal cell injury, apoptosis, and necrosis of tubular cells, with a resultant need for repair, proliferation, and repolarization of remaining tubule cells. In addition, changes in the renal microvasculature contribute to tubular injury. Renal tubular epithelial cells and renal-specific and mesenchymal stem cells appear to contribute to the recovery process, although the mesenchymal stem cells seem to have a primarily paracrine effect. A number of peptide growth factors have been studied in animal models and shown to play a role in the recovery process or to accelerate recovery, although new therapies for human disease based on this work have not yet been possible. Adjacent cells and the endothelium play critical roles in the recovery process. Additional studies are needed to clarify the effects, both positive and negative, of renal replacement therapy on recovery from AKI.

Key Points

1. The pathogenesis of AKI involves both sublethal tubular cell injury and cell death (apoptosis and necrosis).
2. Tubular epithelial cells, renal-specific progenitor cells, mesenchymal stem cells, and leukocytes all appear to play roles in the recovery process.
3. Although the mechanisms of endothelial repair are not well understood, it is clear that endothelial injury is a critical mediator of AKI.
4. Growth factors also appear to play a critical role in tubular repair/recovery.
5. The impact of renal replacement therapy on renal recovery is not well understood.

Acknowledgments

The author wishes to acknowledge the helpful comments of Paul Brakeman, Daniel Burkhardt, Naveen Gupta, and Kristina Kordesch as well as the assistance of Heather Deacon with graphics. The author's work was supported by grant K12 RR024130 from the National Center for Research Resources (NCRR), a component of the National Institutes of Health (NIH) and the NIH Roadmap for Medical Research.

Key References

3. Sheridan AM, Bonventre JV: Cell biology and molecular mechanisms of injury in ischemic acute renal failure. Curr Opin Nephrol Hypertens 2000;9:427-434.
9. Star R: Treatment of acute renal failure. Kidney Int 1998; 54:1817-1831.

13. Sutton TA, Fisher C, Molitoris BA: Microvascular endothelial injury and dysfunction during ischemic acute renal failure. Kidney Int 2002;62:1539-1549.
19. Cantley LG: Adult stem cells in the repair of the injured renal tubule. Nat Clin Pract Nephrol 2005;1:22-32.
57. Palevsky PM, Baldwin I, Davenport A, et al: Renal replacement therapy and the kidney: Minimizing the impact of renal replacement therapy on recovery of acute renal failure. Curr Opin Crit Care 2005;11:548-554.

See the companion Expert Consult website for the complete reference list.

CHAPTER 38

Stem Cells and Renal Repair

James C. Brodie

OBJECTIVES

This chapter will:
1. Give an accurate assessment of the current state of the literature on the existence of renal stem cells.
2. Consider the evidence for putative stem cell involvement in renal regeneration.
3. Indicate how the field is likely to progress on the basis of the gaps that remain in our understanding of renal stem cells.

The role of stem cells in renal repair is far from understood and remains a very active topic of research. Although a definitive adult renal stem cell has yet to be identified, analogy with other organ systems suggests that its existence is a distinct possibility,[1] and there is evidence to support this conjecture. The field is currently at an interesting stage of development, with the nature and even the very existence of adult renal stem cells still a matter of debate.

Several reports have claimed identification of adult renal stem cells (Table 38-1), and although they differ in some respects, they have certain overlaps. Before consideration of the question whether adult renal stem cells exist, it is useful to have in mind the qualities such an entity must possess in order to conform to the classic definition of a stem cell. Briefly, a *stem cell* should be capable of self-renewal as well as giving rise to multiple mature differentiated cell types (the accepted proof being their generation from a clonally isolated cell). In the context of its native tissue, a stem cell should be responsive to signals maintaining homeostasis and promoting repair.

THE SEARCH FOR THE ADULT RENAL STEM CELL

Embryonic Tissue Approach

One approach to renal stem cell identification involves starting in the embryo, where there is already good evidence for the existence of such cells.[2-5] The rationale behind this approach is that adult renal stem cells may have a molecular profile and surface markers similar to those of their embryonic counterparts. Thus, characterization of stem cells in the more experimentally accessible embryonic system may facilitate their identification and isolation from adult tissue.

Metanephric development in the mouse is initiated on the 11th day after fertilization (around embryo stage 30 [E30] in the human embryo, E13 in the rat) as the ureteric bud (UB), an offshoot of the nephric duct, invades the metanephric mesenchyme (MM). Morphogenesis proceeds by reciprocal induction events between these two tissues.[6] Prior to induction by the UB, the MM consists of several thousand morphologically similar mesenchymal cells that, together with the UB, give rise to the 26 or so cell types that make up the mature kidney.[1]

That single cells within the MM have the potential to generate all the epithelial elements of the nephron was first demonstrated in the early 1990s in a series of elegant studies in which the progeny of genetically tagged cells were subsequently detected within all segments of the nephron.[2,3] These findings are supported by later work demonstrating that single MM cells in culture can give rise to cell types of all nephron segments, as assayed by expression of molecular markers.[7] It has also been suggested that embryonic renal stem cells may have a broader differentiation potential, with the expression of markers indicative of smooth muscle cell, myofibroblast, and endothelial fates having been observed in culture.[5] It should be noted, however, that the cells used in this study were of an immortalized MM cell line and that the conclusions reached should therefore be treated with caution.

In a study by Challen and colleagues,[4] complementary DNA (cDNA) microarrays were used to identify genes specifically upregulated in the embryonic renal progenitor population.[4] A relatively modest total of 21 genes were identified in this way, including the cell surface markers CD24 and cadherin-11. As discussed previously, the hope is that characterization of the molecular profile of embryonic renal stem cells will aid in the identification/isolation of their adult counterparts. It is possible, however, that there will be significant phenotypical differences between the embryonic and any putative adult renal stem cells, as is the case with hematopoietic stem cells.[8]

Adult Tissue Approaches

Another approach to renal stem cell identification lies in a method already used successfully in other tissues that is based on the premise that resident stem cells represent a slow-cycling population within the tissue. In this method,

TABLE 38-1

Proposed Adult Renal Stem/Progenitor Cells in the Current Literature

DESIGNATION	DETECTED BY	LOCALIZED TO	CHAPTER REFERENCE(S)
Label-retaining cell in proximal or distal tubule (PT-LRC)	Retention of BrdU (bromodeoxyuridine) label	Proximal tubules	9, 11
Label-retaining cell in renal papilla (RP-LRC)	Retention of BrdU label	Renal papilla	10
Side population (SP) cell	Efflux of Hoechst dye	Proximal tubules (suspected)	12
CD133⁺	Expression of CD133	Interstitium	15
Multipotent renal progenitor cell (MRPC)	Survival in long-term culture under specialized conditions	Proximal tubules (suspected)	18

bromodeoxyuridine (BrdU), a thymidine nucleoside analogue detectable by immunohistochemistry, is administered over a "pulse" period, during which it is incorporated into replicating DNA during cell division. There follows a BrdU-free "chase" period, during which labeled cells undergoing further rounds of division dilute out the BrdU signal, whereas those remaining quiescent retain the label (and are thus often referred to as label-retaining cells [LRCs]). Using this technique, two groups have identified LRC populations in the adult kidney that they suggest represent progenitor or stem cells.[9-11]

Oliver and associates[10] administered BrdU to 3-day-old rat and mouse pups (at which stage nephrogenesis is still ongoing) twice daily for a pulse period of 3.5 days.[10] After a long chase period of 2 to 10 months, a few scattered LRCs were noted throughout the cortex and medulla, but the bulk of them were found in the renal papilla (RP-LRCs). These researchers went on to demonstrate that renal papillary cells in culture could form spherical aggregates similar to those seen with neural and embryonic stem cells and that some cells derived from clonally isolated papillary cells expressed neuronal markers, suggesting that they may have the capacity to differentiate into nonrenal lineages. They also showed that papillary cells sometimes incorporate into renal tubules after being injected beneath the kidney capsule into the cortex.

Maeshima and coworkers,[9,11] taking a slightly different approach with the same technique, administered BrdU to adult rats for a 1-week pulse period and then analyzed the kidneys after a 2-week chase period. In this case, LRCs were found only in scattered proximal and distal tubules (PT-LRCs). Taking advantage of the fact that BrdU-labeled cells resist labeling by the nuclear stain Hoechst 33342, these researchers isolated the PT-LRCs by fluorescence-activated cell sorting.[11] The following interesting differences between PT-LRCs and non-label-retaining cells (non-LRCs) were then demonstrated:

1. When treated with medium conditioned by an MM cell line, PT-LRCs proliferated significantly faster than non-LRCs.
2. PT-LRCs and non-LRCs responded differently to growth substrates.
3. PT-LRCs could be induced to form tubular structures in collagen gel after treatment with hepatocyte growth factor (HGF) or MM cell line–conditioned medium.
4. Furthermore, when PT-LRCs and non-LRCs were injected into embryonic kidneys in culture, only the PT-LRCs were found to incorporate (although rarely) into developing nephrons and collecting ducts.

The use of reduced Hoechst staining as a criterion for cell sorting (the Hoechst low population) raises the possibility of overlap between the cell populations identified by Maeshima and associates[9,11] and Challen and coworkers.[12] First in the bone marrow and subsequently in a wide variety of other tissues, it has been found that stem cells may be enriched on the basis of their ability to rapidly efflux Hoechst 33342 via membrane transport pumps (reviewed by Challen and Little[13]). Cells sorted on this basis are known as side population or SP cells. The mouse kidney SP cell has been variously estimated to represent from 0.14% to 5% of viable cells in the adult organ.[12,14] Microarray comparison of expression profiles between renal SP and main population cells (MP; the cells remaining after removal of the SP) showed that SP cells differentially express more than 700 genes. Although the SP was found to be a heterogeneous cell population, many differentially expressed genes were detected in proximal tubule cells by in situ hybridization.[12] The SP cells isolated by Challen and coworkers[12] were also found to be multipotent in vitro (could be induced to undergo adipogenic/chondrogenic differentiation) and to incorporate into MM- and UB-derived structures when injected into cultured embryonic kidneys.

By contrast, the SP cells identified by Hishikawa and associates[14] were found to reside in the interstitium and specifically to express musculin/MyoR (a basic helix-loop-helix protein previously known only as a repressor of myogenesis) and BRCP1/ABCG2 (a membrane transporter that they showed may protect SP cells from apoptosis).

Taking a different approach, Bussolati and colleagues[15] isolated a possible renal progenitor population from adult human kidneys on the basis of the expression of CD133, a marker of numerous somatic stem cell lineages and cancer cells (reviewed by Shmelkov and coworkers[16]). CD133⁺ cells in the kidney were found to be located in the interstitium, representing approximately 0.1% of the renal cortex cell population excluding glomeruli. After isolation of CD133⁺ cells by fluorescence-activated cell sorting, the Bussolati group further characterized the cells' origin by showing that they did not express CD34 or CD45 (and are therefore unlikely to belong to the hematopoietic lineage) and that they did express Pax-2—an important molecular marker in the developing kidney.[17] After clonal isolation, progeny of renal CD133⁺ cells could be differentiated in vitro and in vivo into renal epithelium-like or endothelial cells.[15]

Lastly, Gupta and coworkers[18] employed a technique similar to that used by Jiang and colleagues[19] in the isolation of a mesenchymal stem cell lineage from the bone marrow (called multipotent adult progenitor cells [MAPCs]) to derive a cell population they call multipotent renal progenitor cells (MRPCs) from adult rat kidneys.[18,19] These

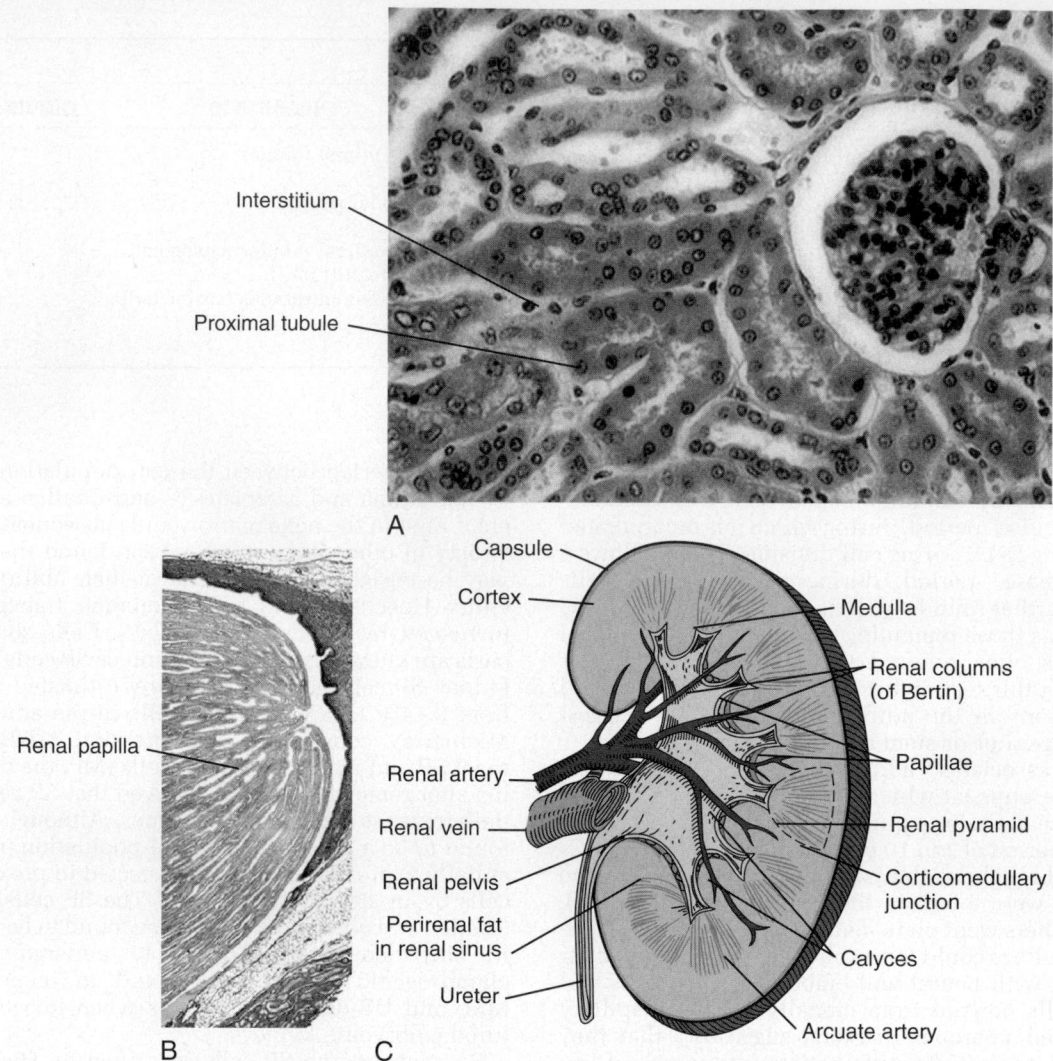

FIGURE 38-1. Proposed stem cell niches in the adult kidney: **A,** interstitium[15] and proximal tubule[9,11,18]; **B,** renal papilla.[10] **C,** An overview of kidney structures and relative locations. (Micrographs in **A** and **B** from http://lifesci.rutgers.edu/~babiarz/kid.htm/. Diagram of kidney in **C** from Brenner BM: Brenner & Rector's The Kidney, 8th ed. Philadelphia, Elsevier, 2008, p 27.)

cells appear to be able to undergo indefinite clonal expansion in vitro and express the stem cell marker Oct4 as well as Pax-2 (though not CD133).[18] Gupta's group also demonstrated that MRPCs could be induced in vitro to express endothelial, hepatocyte, and neural markers, representing the three germ layers of the embryo and suggesting that they may have pluripotentiality. Some evidence was presented to show that MRPCs form tubular structures and incorporate into renal tubules after being injected beneath the kidney capsule in adult rats.[18]

Using a transgenic rat line with a genetic marker (β-Geo) under the control of the Oct4 promoter, Gupta and associates located Oct4-expressing cells within the proximal renal tubules,[18] which they suggest may represent the MRPCs isolated by their culture technique.

It is difficult to reconcile these disparate reports of renal stem/progenitor cell identification. Use of different animal models, isolation techniques, and assay criteria likely account for some of the confusion, but it is probable that the accumulation of further data will exclude the findings of some of these early reports. Perhaps the best approach at this stage is to group the accounts according to their

similarities and consider the evidence presented in each case for a role in repair after injury.

Broadly speaking, the putative stem/progenitor cells reported so far can be divided into three groups on the basis of their locations (known or postulated) within the kidney: proximal tubular,[9,11,12,18] interstitial,[14,15] and papillary (Fig. 38-1).[10]

EVIDENCE FOR A STEM CELL ROLE IN RENAL REPAIR

Repair after Acute Injury

The kidney's capacity for regeneration after even rather severe damage caused by ischemic or nephrotoxic insult indicates the existence of an efficient mechanism for the production of new tubular epithelial cells to replace those lost through necrosis or shed in the urine. Impressive as this regenerative capacity undoubtedly is, the mortality rate associated with acute renal failure remains high, at between 50% and 80%,[20] suggesting that it could be improved.

The primary site of damage is thought to be the S3 segment of the proximal tubule.[21-25] Although the positive identification of an adult renal stem cell may change this view, the best evidence so far indicates that regeneration proceeds through dedifferentiation of remaining tubular cells, followed by proliferation and redifferentiation to reconstruct functional tubules.[25-31]

Renal Tubule–Located Stem/Progenitor Cells

Although it is unknown whether the PT-LRC, SP cell, and MRPC represent the same cell population, the possibility that they do is certainly attractive. The location of a stem/progenitor cell within the renal tubule itself would seem to be most compatible with earlier models of tubular regeneration, although it would be difficult to reconcile with the traditional view of stem cell phenotype.

In support of their hypothesis that PT-LRCs are involved in renal repair, Maeshima and colleagues[9] note that the numbers of LRCs approximately double in the 24 hours after renal ischemia, indicating that they enter the cell cycle in response to renal damage.[9] Furthermore, approximately 85% of cells that were positive for PCNA (proliferating cell nuclear antigen, a molecular marker of cells in S-phase) observed 24 hours after ischemia were also positive for BrdU, suggesting that PT-LRCs may be responsible for the bulk of proliferation after injury.[11] Interestingly, some BrdU-labeled cells were observed to express vimentin, a mesenchymal marker considered an indicator of dedifferentiation in the renal epithelia,[25] within 24 hours of ischemic injury.

Using an Adriamycin model of mouse kidney damage, Challen and associates[12] demonstrated that administration of SP cells, by direct injection into the outer cortex (2 × 10⁵ cells) and infusion into the circulation via the tail vein (1 × 10⁵ cells), resulted in decreased levels of albuminuria during progression of renal damage. Injection/infusion of MP cells had a similarly beneficial effect, however, and although the albuminuria reduction appeared to be greater with SP cells than with MP cells, the differences were not statistically significant. In examining the kidneys for the presence of donor cells, the researchers found that most remained in the interstitium in the vicinity of the injection site and that SP cells engrafted at low frequency into proximal tubules, distal tubules, and collecting ducts, and very rarely into glomeruli, whereas MP cells very rarely engrafted into distal tubules and collecting ducts only.[12]

Gupta and coworkers[18] found no difference in serum creatinine concentration or creatinine clearance rate between rats injected with MRPCs (subcapsular injection of 10⁶ cells) and controls after ischemia-reperfusion.[18]

Interstitial Stem/Progenitor Cells

Hishikawa and associates[14] injected SP cells (1 × 10⁴) into the tail veins of mice after induction of acute renal failure with cisplatin. Cell injection at 1 day after cisplatin administration resulted in significant reductions in the peak blood urea nitrogen and serum creatinine levels at 7 days after treatment. Interestingly, cisplatin treatment was found to result in reduced numbers of musculin/MyoR–positive cells in the interstitium at 7 days, but injection of SP cells reversed this trend, leading to higher numbers of musculin/MyoR–expressing cells, even compared with numbers in untreated controls. As a possible basis for a mechanism explaining the beneficial effect of interstitial musculin/MyoR–expressing cells on the progression of acute renal failure, these investigators noted that SP cells expressed significantly higher levels of hepatocyte growth factor, vascular endothelial growth factor, bone morphogenetic protein-7, and leukemia-inhibiting factor (all secreted molecules that have been implicated in renal regeneration) in cisplatin-treated animals than in untreated animals. This paracrine role would appear to exclude these cells from consideration as possible renal stem cells.

Using a model of acute tubular injury induced by intramuscular glycerol injection in SCID mice, Bussolati and colleagues[15] found that human HLA class I–positive cells were detectable in proximal and distal tubules (and rarely in glomeruli) after injection of 10⁶ CD133⁺ human renal cells into the tail veins 3 days after glycerol treatment—the time of maximal tubular injury in this model. Although they did not present quantitative data, the researchers noted that control donor cells were only very rarely found engrafted in uninjured animals. They did not attempt to assay the effect of CD133⁺ cell treatment on renal function after injury.

Papillary Stem/Progenitor Cells

Oliver and coworkers[10] used the unilateral ischemia-reperfusion model of acute renal failure to test the response of RP-LRCs to kidney damage. Their initial comparison of RP-LRC numbers between damaged and control kidneys revealed a drop from 36% of cells to 4%, which took place in the absence of apoptosis and, apparently, without migration of the LRCs elsewhere. Immunofluorescence staining for the proliferation antigen Ki-67 showed that a burst of proliferation took place in the papilla beginning in the first 36 hours after ischemia and that many of the dividing cells were also BrdU-labeled.[10] This high level of proliferative activity within the papilla is certainly interesting, given that this region appears to be largely resistant to ischemic insult. It is tempting to speculate that the proliferating cells migrate to the site of injury, but direct evidence to support this possibility has not yet been presented.

DISCUSSION

Much of the evidence supporting the existence of adult renal progenitor/stem cells in the literature at present is indirect and, although undoubtedly suggestive, is hardly conclusive. Retention of the BrdU label, for example, indicates merely that a cell divided during the pulse period and not during the subsequent chase period. Indeed small, although significant, rates of proliferation have been measured for numerous cell populations in the normal human adult kidney, including proximal tubules at a rate of approximately 23 dividing cells per thousand counted (determined by expression of proliferation antigens PCNA and Ki-67).[32] Careful observation of dividing proximal tubular cells in healthy juvenile rat kidneys has shown them to be indistinguishable from neighboring cells, both morphologically and in expression of molecular markers of fully differentiated proximal tubules.[33]

Nevertheless, the behavioral differences between PT-LRCs and other tubular cells noted by Maeshima and colleagues[9] (and those between SP and MP cells observed by Challen and associates[12]) suggest that these cells have unique and potentially clinically interesting properties. The answer may lie in an observation made by the Maeshima group that most PT-LRCs are associated with capillary endothelial cells. Capillary endothelial cells are known to produce activin A,[34] a factor that was demonstrated in earlier work to be involved in tubular regeneration after renal ischemia[29] and that inhibits proliferation of renal tubule cells.[35,36] The simplest interpretation of the data suggests the association between proximal tubular and capillary endothelial cells may protect the tubule cell from ischemic injury, ensuring its survival for participation in regeneration. It is also conceivable that this relationship confers additional properties on the tubule cell, in effect representing a sort of niche.

Clearly this model would not conform to the classic view that a stem cell represents a relatively undifferentiated precursor, giving rise to transit-amplifying cells, and so on. Rather, a broadening of the definition of a stem cell may be necessary as, for example, in the nervous system, where apparently fully differentiated neurons have been shown to possess stem cell properties.[37]

Amelioration of the effects of renal injury, as seen after the injection of (mainly proximal tubular) SP cells by Challen and associates,[12] is interesting and encouraging but unlikely to be due to the low level tubular engraftment of donor cells seen in such experiments. Similar results have been observed, and shown to be independent of donor cell contribution to regenerating tubules, after injection of multiple cell types.[38-40] The mechanism behind this beneficial effect is not yet known but may be due to paracrine actions similar to those proposed by Hishikawa and associates.[14]

The interstitial CD133+ cells described by Bussolati and colleagues[15] are promising renal stem cell candidates, but their case would be strengthened further by functional data showing that the progression of renal failure is favorably modified by the administration of such cells; quantitation of their level of contribution to regenerating tubules would also be welcome.

The data for RP-LRCs are also very suggestive.[10] Isolation, labeling, and reintroduction should be the top priority for the further characterization of these cells, along with an assessment of their functional impact on renal injury models.

CONCLUSION

The best candidate cell population for a role in renal repair is, at present, the PT-LRC identified by Maeshima and coworkers.[9,11] Although functional data regarding their impact on renal injury are still needed, the fit of this model with earlier conceptions of renal regeneration is compelling. It is possible, of course, that there are multiple progenitor or stem cell populations within the kidney, and none of the possibilities here can yet be formally excluded. The question whether any of the cells considered here may prove suitable for cell therapy applications remains very much an open one, and it seems unlikely that the development of such treatments can be expected soon. It is very much to be hoped that, although stem cell injections may not be used yet to treat renal injury, improvements in the basic understanding of renal regeneration at the cellular level will lead, in the nearer term, to treatments that stimulate the endogenous repair process.

Key Points

1. The existence of an adult renal stem/progenitor cell has not yet been proven.
2. There are several proposed candidates in the current literature.
3. Evidence of a role in renal repair for several of these candidates is strongly suggestive but not yet conclusive.
4. The balance of evidence currently available suggests that the adult kidney stem cell does not conform to classic stem cell models.
5. The field is likely to undergo clarification/rationalization in the near future.

Key References

7. Osafune K, Takasato M, Kispert A, et al: Identification of multipotent progenitors in the embryonic mouse kidney by a novel colony-forming assay. Development 2005;133:151-161.
11. Maeshima A, Sakurai H, Nigam SK Adult kidney tubular cell population showing phenotypic plasticity, tubulogenic capacity and integration capability into developing kidney. J Am Soc Nephrol 2006;17:188-198.
25. Witzgall R, Brown D, Schwarz C, Bonventre JV: Localization of proliferating cell nuclear antigen, vimentin, c-fos, and clusterin in the postischemic kidney: Evidence for a heterogeneous genetic response among nephron segments, and a large pool of mitotically active and dedifferentiated cells. J Clin Invest 1994;93:2175-2188.
31. Duffield JS, Park KM, Hsiao LL, et al: Restoration of tubular epithelial cells during repair of the postischemic kidney occurs independently of bone marrow-derived stem cells. J Clin Invest 2005;115:1743-1755.
40. Stokman G, Leemans JC, Claessen N, et al: Hematopoietic stem cell mobilization therapy accelerates recovery of renal function independent of stem cell contribution. J Am Soc Nephrol 2005;16:1684-1692.

See the companion Expert Consult website for the complete reference list.

CHAPTER 39

Stem Cells and the Kidney

Benedetta Bussolati and Giovanni Camussi

OBJECTIVES

This chapter will:
1. Discuss the search for embryonic stem cells in the kidney.
2. Describe the identification of adult resident stem cells in rodents: resident stem cells in rat papilla and rat tubules, and resident mesenchymal stem cells in rat and mouse kidneys.
3. Consider adult resident stem cells in human kidneys.
4. Describe a side cell population in human and mouse kidneys.
5. Discuss the role of bone marrow–derived cells in renal regeneration.

The presence of adult multipotent stem cells is considered critical for the turnover of many tissues. Adult stem cells have now been isolated from several tissues and organs, including the central nervous system, bone marrow, retina, skeletal muscle, and skin.

No definitive data, however, established the existence of a unique stem cell population for the kidney. The requirement for the definition of stem cells is the presence of a long-term self-renewing cell population able to undergo asymmetrical division and to present multiple differentiation capabilities, including differentiation into resident mature renal cells.

Different approaches have been used in the attempt to identify a renal stem cell. In particular, studies first addressed the presence of embryonic stem cells in the kidney and then focused on adult stem cells, exploiting functional characteristics or specific surface and nuclear markers of stem cells. Taken altogether, the results obtained suggest the presence of different progenitor/stem cell populations in the kidney with different degrees of commitment and differentiation.

The aim of this chapter is to review data relative to the characterization of embryonic and adult stem cells present in the kidney, including nonrenal adult stem cells and renal resident stem cells.

EMBRYONIC STEM CELLS

A study published in 2002 demonstrated that the embryonic rat metanephric mesenchyme possesses organ-specific progenitor cells capable of differentiating into epithelia, myofibroblasts, and smooth muscle cells, indicating the presence of embryonic renal stem cells.[1] Data are unclear about the possible origin of renal endothelial cells. Contradictory evidence suggests either a possible colonization of kidney by exogenous angioblasts or a common origin of renal endothelial cells with other renal cell types.[2,3]

In the attempt to identify markers specific for a renal progenitor population, Challen and associates[4] compared the expression profile of metanephric mesenchyme with that of the adjacent intermediate mesenchyme. This study identified the specific expression of transmembrane proteins such as CD24a and cadherin 11 in the metanephric mesenchyme of the rat embryo, which could also be used for the identification of stem cells in the adult kidney.

RESIDENT RENAL STEM CELLS IN RAT PAPILLA

In searching for stem cells in the adult kidney, Oliver and colleagues[5] tried to identify slow-cycling stem cells, on the basis of the assumption that, in tissues, stem cells are characterized by a low proliferating rate that maintains the self-renewal of the population. Cells with slow cycling time could be identified from the retention of administered bromodeoxyuridine (BrdU), which is incorporated in cell DNA during its synthesis. Using this approach, these researchers found that BrdU-retaining cells were concentrated mainly in the renal papilla in the rat. A few scattered BrdU-retaining cells were also found in the renal cortex. During recovery from transient renal ischemia, these cells proliferated, and the BrdU "signal" rapidly disappeared, suggesting a contribution of these cells to tubular regeneration. When isolated and cultured in vitro, these cells showed multilineage differentiation and the ability to organize into spheroplasts. On the basis of these observations, Oliver and colleagues[5] proposed that the renal papilla is a niche for adult kidney stem cells. In their study, the clonogenicity of the cells was not established, and the possibility that these cells represent a transiently amplifying cell population recruited in the kidney during injury was not excluded.

RESIDENT RENAL STEM CELLS IN RAT TUBULES

Using the same approach as the previous study, pulse administration of BrdU, Maeshima and coworkers[6] identified BrdU-labeled cells in the renal tubules of adult rats. These cells, termed *renal progenitor–like tubular cells*, were shown to be able to reenter mitosis in response to renal injury. In addition, these investigators showed the potential of these cells to generate proximal tubules and collecting duct cells or fibroblasts when transplanted into the metanephric kidney. These findings indicate a plasticity and tubulogenic capacity of these cells that enable them to integrate into a developing kidney.

Kitamura and associates[7] established and characterized a distinct population of renal progenitor cells from the S3 segment of the nephron in the rat adult kidney. They showed these cells to be capable of self-renewal and expression of renal embryonic markers such as Pax-2, Wtn4, and Wtn1. In addition, they demonstrated the ability of the cells to differentiate into mature epithelial cells, expressing aquaporin-1 and -2 and being responsive to parathyroid hormone and vasopressin. When engrafted into kidneys of rats with ischemia-reperfusion injury, these cells contributed to tubular regeneration and improved renal function. S3 segment–derived progenitor cells can be considered epithelial precursors rather than stem cells because they differentiate only toward the epithelial lineage.

RESIDENT MESENCHYMAL STEM CELLS IN MICE AND RATS

It has been proposed that mesenchymal stem cells reside in almost all organs and tissues. In the adult rat kidney, Gupta and colleagues[8] demonstrated the presence of a renal resident population expressing mesenchymal stem cell markers that were capable of self-renewal and multipotent differentiation. In addition, these cells expressed embryonic stem cell markers such as Octa-4 and Pax-2. When injected under the capsule of uninjured kidneys, or intra-arterially after ischemia-reperfusion injury, these cells were capable of tubular differentiation. Using a transgenic model of Octa4-X-gal, these investigators found that Octa4-positive cells were associated with the proximal tubules and were absent in the medulla. Whether these cells are an embryonic residual population or rather a bone marrow–derived population of mesenchymal stem cells conditionally modified by the renal microenvironment remains to be determined.

A mesenchymal stem cell population has been also identified in the glomeruli of mice.[9] These cells were shown to be multipotent and to express smooth muscle myosin, like mesangial cells.

RESIDENT RENAL STEM CELLS IN HUMAN CORTEX

The first demonstration of the presence of resident progenitor/stem cells in the human adult kidney was obtained by our group using CD133 as a stem cell marker.[10] CD133 is known mainly as a marker of hematopoietic stem cells/endothelial progenitors,[11] but later reports indicate its expression in tissue stem cells such as those present in the prostate and brain. We found a rare population of CD133+ cells in the interstitium in proximity of proximal tubules and glomeruli, or within tubules. Once isolated, these cells lacked the expression of hematopoietic markers (CD34 and CD45), whereas they did express some mesenchymal stem cell markers, such as CD29, CD90, CD44, and CD73. Moreover, they expressed Pax-2, an embryonic renal marker, suggesting their renal origin. These cells were shown to undergo epithelial and endothelial differentiation both in vitro and in vivo. We obtained the epithelial differentiation in vitro by culturing the cells in the presence of

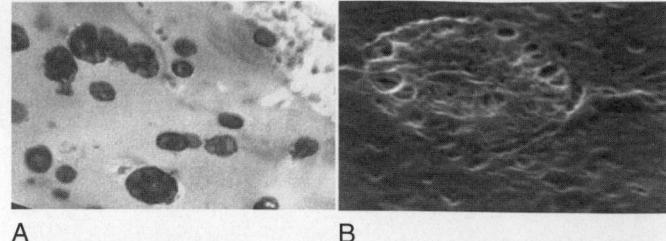

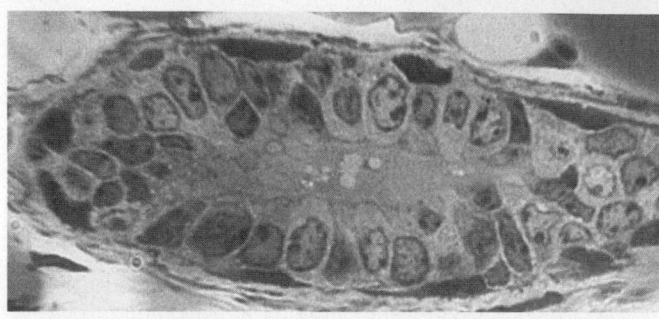

FIGURE 39-1. See also color plates. In vivo differentiation of human renal CD133+ progenitor cells in tubular structures. Undifferentiated CD133+ cells were injected subcutaneously in the solubilized basement membrane preparation Matrigel in nonimmunocompetent SCID mice (mice with severe combined immune deficiency). **A,** Immunohistochemistry showed that the tubular structures were positive for cytokeratin, indicating their epithelial differentiation. **B** and **C,** The morphological aspect of tubular structures on scanning electron microscopy (**B**) and toluidine blue staining of semithin sections (**C**). (Original magnifications: **A,** ×150; **B,** ×450; **C,** ×600.)

hepatocyte growth factor and fibroblast growth factor-4. The cells expressed proximal and distal tubular markers and, when cultured in transwell filters, formed a polarized layer showing apical microvilli and junctional complexes. When injected in vivo subcutaneously in the solubilized basement membrane preparation Matrigel (BD Biosciences, San Jose, CA), CD133+ cells spontaneously differentiated into tubular structures expressing proximal and distal tubular epithelial markers (Fig. 39-1). The endothelial differentiation was obtained in vitro by culture of the cells in the presence of vascular endothelial growth factor. In vitro, the cells expressed endothelial markers and organized into capillary-like structures (Fig. 39-2A). In vivo, when injected subcutaneously in Matrigel, endothelial differentiated CD133+ cells formed vessels connected with the mouse vasculature (Fig. 39-2B). Moreover, when injected into mice with glycerol-induced acute renal injury, CD133+ renal progenitors homed to the kidney and integrated into proximal and distal tubules during the repair.

Sagrinati and colleagues[12] isolated and characterized a population of CD133+, CD24+ cells from the Bowman's capsule of adult human kidneys. These cells exhibited a multipotent differentiation ability, enabling them to generate mature tubular epithelial cells, osteogenic cells, adipocytes, and neuronal cells. When injected into mice with glycerol-induced acute renal injury, CD133+, CD24+ stem cells contributed to tubular regeneration.

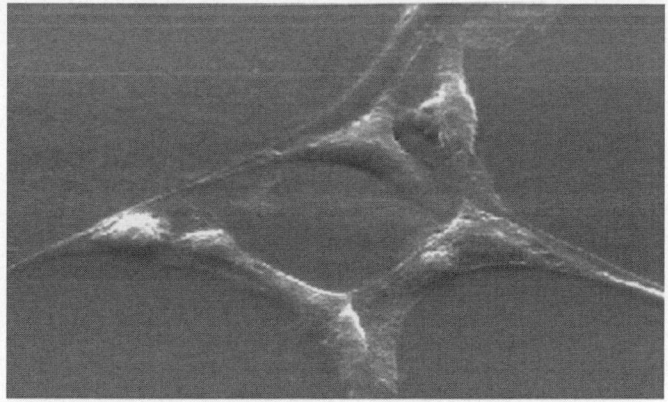

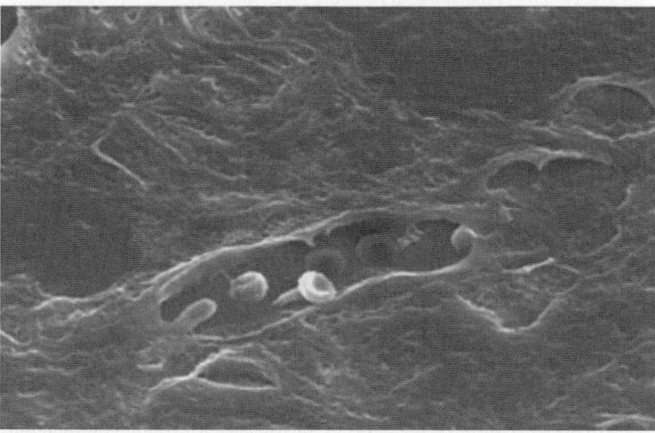

FIGURE 39-2. In vitro and in vivo differentiation of human renal CD133+ progenitor cells in endothelial cells. **A,** Endothelial differentiated cells, when cultured on surfaces coated with the solubilized basement membrane preparation Matrigel, organized into capillary-like structures. **B,** Endothelial differentiated cells injected subcutaneously in SCID mice (mice with severe combined immune deficiency) formed functional vessels as seen by scanning electron microscopy. (Original magnifications: **A,** ×750; **B,** ×1500.)

SIDE POPULATION

In hematopoietic cells, the presence of a stem cell population—so-called side population—defined by the unique ability to extrude Hoechst dye, has been reported. Side population cells express the ABCG2 transporter, a transmembrane protein, which allows them to actively extrude Hoechst dye in this specific manner.[13] When examined by fluorescence-activated cell sorting (FACS) analysis, these cells fall within a separate population to the side of the rest of the cells on a dot plot of emission data, in the blue rather than the red spectrum. Side population cells are also present in tissues.[14] Data are conflicting: Some researchers suggest that side population cells can be tissue-specific stem cells, and others hold that they are actually bone marrow–derived cells lodged within tissues.

Iwatani and coworkers[15] described the presence of a side population in the adult rat kidney, although they excluded these cells' differentiation into renal tissue, suggesting a hematopoietic origin. Hishikawa and associates,[16] on the contrary, reported the ability of cells of the side population to differentiate into renal and several other cell lineages in vitro. However, no integration into the renal structures was observed when the side population cells were injected in rats with Thy-1 glomerulonephritis. A later study by Challen and colleagues[17] detected a side population in mouse embryonic and adult kidney, in particular in the tubular compartment, that was characterized as a heterogeneous population. Some progenitor cells within this population displayed characteristics of resident renal stem cells and were different from bone marrow–derived side population cells in terms of surface marker and gene expression. In addition, side population cells from murine adult kidney showed multipotent differentiation ability and contributed to the repair of renal tissue in a doxorubicin nephropathy model, although no integration into the tissue was observed.

BONE MARROW–DERIVED CELLS IN THE KIDNEY

The possibility that bone marrow–derived stem cells might functionally contribute to the renal tubule regeneration is still a matter of debate. Three studies have demonstrated that when female kidneys are transplanted into male recipients, Y chromosome–bearing cells are found in the transplanted kidney.[18-20] However, in two of the studies, these cells represented only a small percentage of the total cells present, and in one, they were believed to represent interstitial lymphocytes rather than tubular epithelial cells. Using whole–bone marrow transplantation in the mouse, Poulsom and coworkers[18] demonstrated that bone marrow–derived cells could populate the renal tubular epithelium. Bone marrow–derived cells were also shown to ameliorate the renal disease in a mouse model of Alport's syndrome.[21,22] In particular, the recruitment of bone marrow–derived progenitor cells within the damaged glomerulus and their differentiation into podocytes and mesangial cells led to a partial restoration of expression of the type IV collagen alpha$_3$ chain.

Several studies demonstrated that stem cells expanded in vitro may protect against and reverse acute renal injury.[23-28] Experiments by Morigi and colleagues[27] demonstrated that the beneficial effect of bone marrow–derived cells is ascribed not to the hematopoietic stem cells but, rather, to the mesenchymal stem cells. In addition, the hematopoietic stem cells were reported to have a potential detrimental effect on kidney regeneration, as inferred from experiments in bone marrow mobilization.[29]

In two studies, the infusion of mesenchymal stem cells expanded in vitro protected and improved the recovery from acute tubular injury induced by cisplatin and glycerol.[27,28] In the two models, localization of mesenchymal stem cells within regenerating tubules was observed. Both models are characterized by extensive necrosis of proximal and distal tubules that may favor migration of mesenchymal stem cells within regenerating tubules. Herrera and associates[28] found that injection of transgenic green fluorescent protein (GFP) mesenchymal stem cells rapidly induced functional recovery and GFP+ cells were detectable in the interstitium and later also in tubules. The increase in proliferating cell nuclear antigen–positive tubular cells throughout the kidney suggests a trophic effect of mesenchymal stem cells on resident tubular cells that survived the injury. Also, Duffield and colleagues[30] observed a beneficial effect of mesenchymal stem cell infusion on acute renal injury induced by ischemia-reperfusion injury. However, they found that culture conditions favoring in vitro differentiation into endothelial cells was required for the in vivo protecting effect in this model. In addition, they found only interstitial localization of stem cells, without incorporation into tubules or endothelium. The discrepancy in the results of mesenchymal stem cell integration into tubules in this study may be explained by the different severity of the model used. Despite the low numbers of mesenchymal stem cells that differentiated into epithelial cells in this last study, there is a general agreement that the beneficial effect of mesenchymal stem cell infusion in acute renal injury is due to the ability of these cells to create a beneficial environment favoring proliferation of dedifferentiated epithelial cells that survive the injury or of resident stem cells.[24]

CONCLUSION

Different populations of progenitor/stem cells have been identified in the adult kidney. These cells may represent a remnant of embryonic stem cells in the adult tissue or populations of bone marrow–derived stem cells homed within the kidney and modified by the local microenvironment. This difference may implicate a partial commitment or different degrees of maturation of the different stem cell populations. Resident stem cells may account for the growth of the organ during development as well as for the physiological cell turnover. During renal injury, resident stem cells as well as stem cells derived from the circulation may contribute to tissue repair. Preliminary studies suggest the possibility of exploiting this regenerative potential of stem cells for therapeutic purposes, either through administration of stem cell populations expanded ex vivo or with strategies aimed to expand and differentiate local progenitor/stem cell populations.

Key Points

1. Different types of progenitor/stem cells are present in the kidney.
2. In the human kidney, CD133+ progenitor/stem cells with regenerative potential have been identified.
3. Mesenchymal stem cells are also present in the kidney and may originate from bone marrow or may be an embryonic residue.
4. During renal injury, resident stem cells as well as stem cells derived from the circulation may contribute to tissue repair.
5. Stem cells expanded ex vivo may be used in the future for therapeutic purposes.

Key References

8. Gupta S, Verfaillie C, Chmielewski D, et al: Isolation and characterization of kidney-derived stem cells. J Am Soc Nephrol 2006;17:3028-3040.
10. Bussolati B, Bruno S, Grange C, et al: Isolation of renal progenitor cells from adult human kidney. Am J Pathol 2005; 166:545-555.
17. Challen GA, Bertoncello I, Deane JA, et al: Kidney side population reveals multilineage potential and renal functional capacity but also cellular heterogeneity. J Am Soc Nephrol 2006;17:1896-1912.
21. Prodromidi EI, Poulsom R, Jeffery R, et al: Bone marrow derived-cells contribute to podocyte regeneration and amelioration of renal disease in a mouse model of Alport syndrome. Stem Cells 2006;24:2448-2455.
27. Morigi M, Imberti B, Zoja C, et al: Mesenchymal stem cells are renotropic, helping to repair the kidney and improve function in acute renal failure. J Am Soc Nephrol 2004;15: 1794-1804.

CHAPTER 40

Mesenchymal Stem Cells and Their Use in Acute Renal Injury

Barbara Imberti, Marina Morigi, and Giuseppe Remuzzi

OBJECTIVES

This chapter will:
1. Describe the pathogenesis of acute renal failure.
2. Discuss bone marrow–derived stem cells and the kidney.
3. Explain how mesenchymal stem cells populate the kidney.
4. Consider the functional effect of mesenchymal stem cells in experimental acute renal failure.

The quest for a pharmacological therapy to ameliorate survival after episodes of acute renal failure (ARF) has been largely unsuccessful. New therapeutic approaches for renal tissue regeneration have emerged, and one of the most promising is the use of stem cells to direct the replacement of damaged cells. In animal models and humans, there is evidence that extrarenal cells of bone marrow origin can participate in kidney repair. Ischemic or toxic injury to the kidney can be sensed by bone marrow–derived mesenchymal stem cells (MSCs), which are able to engraft the damaged organ and to promote structural and functional repair. The mechanisms underlying this protective effect are still controversial. Although the cross-lineage differentiation of MSCs takes place in the kidney, this phenomenon is limited in proportion and cannot completely account for the observed reparative capacity of MSCs. Some evidence supports the idea that MSCs could contribute to renal tissue repair after acute injury by stimulating the proliferation of resident cells via a paracrine mechanism involving the production of growth factors and/or anti-inflammatory cytokines. MSCs, by virtue of their renotropic property and tubular regenerative potential, could represent an advantageous and powerful therapeutic approach for the cure of ARF.

ACUTE RENAL FAILURE

Acute renal failure is a syndrome characterized by the rapid deterioration of renal function, with a decrease in glomerular filtration rate (GFR) accompanied by azotemia. ARF occurs in approximately 7% of hospitalized patients, especially those in medical and surgical intensive care units.[1] Although functional outcome among the surviving patients after ARF is usually good, the mortality rate is high. Over the last 30 years, despite advances in supportive care, very little clinical progress has been made in reducing the renal dysfunction of ARF as well as its mortality, which ranges from 30% to 80%. Unfortunately, at the moment no pharmacological therapy can improve the survival after ARF. Dopamine, furosemide, mannitol, calcium channel blockers, atrial natriuretic peptide, and several other hormonal or pharmacological substances have proved effective in experimental models but almost invariably failed in clinical protocols.[2,3]

ARF ensues upon ischemic or nephrotoxic insult to the kidney, and it is potentially reversible. However, the time course and extent of recovery of renal function depend on the nature of the underlying pathology. The hallmark of ischemic and toxic damage is cellular adenosine triphosphate depletion, which is associated with several intracellular events responsible for proximal tubular injury. Actin cytoskeletal dysregulation and loss of brush border are followed by alterations in junctional membrane proteins and detachment of cell-cell and cell-substrate adhesion. Sublethally, necrotic or apoptotic cells are shed and can occlude the tubular lumen, thus increasing intratubular pressure; the higher pressure, along with back-leakage of filtrate, may contribute to dysfunction.[4] In experimental models, proximal tubular epithelium has a remarkable capacity to recover. The rate of recovery depends strictly on the ability of tubular cells to replace damaged and/or dead epithelium with a new, functioning one. The contributions of growth factors such as insulin-like growth factor-1 (IGF-1), hepatocyte growth factor (HGF), and epidermal growth factor-1 (EGF-1) have been described to potentiate tubular regeneration in animal models of ARF.[5] The damaged nephrons are initially repopulated by cells with an epithelial precursor phenotype. The identity of these regenerating cells is still under investigation, but the following possibilities can be considered:

- Adult resident cells, through an initial process of dedifferentiation, migrate and then proliferate, thus redifferentiating into adult proximal tubular cells.
- Undifferentiated resident precursor/stem cells can generate terminally differentiated tubular cells.
- Some reports indicate the peritubular area and the renal papilla as a possible niche for renal progenitor cells.[6,7]

- Another possibility—that bone marrow–derived stem cells play a role in tubular repair—has been consistently documented.[8]

PLASTICITY OF BONE MARROW–DERIVED STEM CELLS AND THEIR CONTRIBUTION TO THE KIDNEY

In the last few years it has become very clear that adult bone marrow–derived stem cells have remarkable plasticity, to the extent that they can differentiate into multiple lineages other than their tissue of origin. Cells derived from bone marrow can differentiate into other cells, such as hepatocytes, cardiac muscle cells, endothelial cells, and pancreatic cells.[9] A single cell isolated from bone marrow has been reported to exhibit a multiple-organ, multiple-lineage engraftment capacity. Indeed, it was able to reconstitute all the blood elements and also to differentiate into epithelial cells in the lung, liver, intestine, and skin, even in the absence of marked injury.[10]

The contribution of adult bone marrow–derived cells to the turnover and regeneration of several cell types in the kidney has been established.[11] Several groups reported that bone marrow–derived cells can supply mesangial cells, podocytes, and endothelial cells.[12-14] Poulsom and associates[14] demonstrated that bone marrow cells can pass into the kidney and participate in normal tubular epithelial cell turnover. Kidney cells obtained from female mice recipients of male bone marrow showed colocalization of Y chromosomes and the tubular epithelial marker *Lens culinaris* lectins in up to 8% of tubular epithelial cells.[14] These researchers also reported that in men receiving kidney transplants from female donors, Y chromosome–positive tubular epithelial cells were observed in the kidneys suffering damage as a consequence of acute tubular necrosis.[14] Moreover, bone marrow–derived cells were found within the glomeruli, where they expressed vimentin, suggesting a podocyte phenotype.[14] Gupta and colleagues[15] examined the origin of tubular cells in men with resolving acute tubular necrosis who had received a kidney transplant from a female donor.[15] These investigators documented that 1% of the tubular cells were Y chromosome–positive in the kidneys after injury, because the cells were positive for cytokeratin but negative for CD45, a marker for white cells. Although the presence of male tubular cells after acute renal injury was a rare event, this finding supported the hypothesis that extrarenal cells can participate in the regeneration of tubules.[15] The origin of these cells, however, was not explained: They could come directly from the bone marrow, could represent circulating stem cells, or could derive from other organs. It is not clear whether these cells, eventually coming from the bone marrow, are already present in the kidney prior to injury, functioning as resident stem cells, or whether they are recruited to the kidney at the time of injury.

Mengel and coworkers[16] observed tubular epithelial chimerism and semiquantitatively evaluated it by means of in situ hybridization for the Y chromosome in kidney biopsy specimens from men receiving sex-mismatched kidney transplants. The group demonstrated that 72% of the patients had a stable chimerism in the kidney although the proportion of chimerical tubular cells ranged from 2.4% to 6.6%.[16]

Another study confirmed the existence of renal tubular cells that originate from transplanted bone marrow.[17] Bone marrow–derived cells recruited to the kidney have the ability to proliferate not only during the normal turnover of the renal tubular cells but also after acute tubular injury induced by folic acid treatment. In this ARF animal model, renal tubular cells and glomerular mesangial cells were found to originate from transplanted bone marrow.[17] The severity of renal damage is an important modulator of the extent of engraftment of bone marrow–derived cells into tubules after ischemia-reperfusion injury in rats. If the damage worsens, the need for repair increases and is matched by augmentation of bone marrow–derived cell engraftment.[18]

MESENCHYMAL STEM CELLS POPULATE THE KIDNEY TISSUE

Particular attention has been given to bone marrow–derived MSCs as an easy source for regenerative therapy. MSCs are multipotent cells that can give rise, in vitro and in vivo, to mesenchymal and nonmesenchymal tissues. MSCs are distributed throughout the postnatal organism and can be derived not only from the bone marrow but also from different organs and tissues, such as brain, spleen, liver, kidney, lung, muscle, thymus, and pancreas.[19]

Bone marrow stroma–derived MSCs are progenitors of skeletal tissue components, such as bone, cartilage, hematopoiesis-supporting stroma, and adipocytes.[20] After transplantation, MSCs have been shown to transdifferentiate into cardiomyocytes, neuroectodermal cells, and hepatic epithelium.[9] Devine and associates[21] demonstrated that in vitro expanded MSCs, labeled with green fluorescent protein and infused into irradiated baboons, distributed to a variety of nonhematopoietic organs, including kidney, liver, lung, thymus, and skin. Within these tissues, these cells could exhibit the capacity to proliferate, thereby participating in ongoing cellular turnover.

That MSCs can participate in kidney development and give origin to the organ tissues was demonstrated in another study.[22] Human MSCs were implanted at the nephrogenic site of developing rodent embryos that were first cultured in vitro and thereafter microdissected to isolate kidney rudiments that continued to be grown in vitro. In such an experimental setting, human MSCs were reprogrammed and developed into cells that were morphologically identical to endogenous renal cells, such as glomerular epithelial cells and tubular epithelial cells; thus, the MSCs contributed to the structure of the kidney. In some cases, entire nephrons were derived from human MSCs. The human MSCs found in the nephron were viable and, when injected into mice with Fabry's disease that did not express a gene encoding the enzyme α-galactosidase, produced nephrons that expressed significantly higher amounts of α-galactosidase than nephrons in untreated Fabry mice. This approach might have important implications for generating specific cells or tissues from autologous MSCs. The same research group has gone a step further.[23] Metanephroi, dissected from in vitro culture of whole embryos previously injected with human MSCs, have been transplanted into the omentum of a uninephrectomized rat and grown for 2 weeks. Results show that human MSCs may differentiate into functional kidney units, termed "neo-kidney," that may produce urine.

Murine MSCs that have been tagged in vitro via transduction with a lentiviral construct expressing the eGFP reporter gene were studied in order to prove their ability to generate renal cells in vivo.[24] This work proved the multipotential capacity of MSCs in vivo by demonstrating their differentiation into various cell types (hepatocytes, lung epithelial cells, myofibroblasts, myofibers) when administered systemically to sublethally irradiated mice. These eGFP cells have been identified at low frequency in the kidney, where they exhibited tubular cell morphology and tested positive for tubular markers such as *Ricinus communis* and *Lotus tetragonolobus* lectins.[24]

FUNCTIONAL ROLE OF MESENCHYMAL STEM CELLS IN RENAL RECOVERY AFTER ACUTE INJURY

The role of MSCs in ARF has been highlighted by several studies. Morigi and associates[25] documented for the first time that a cell population of male MSCs, once transplanted into female mice with cisplatin-induced ARF, restored both renal function as evaluated by measurement of blood urea nitrogen (Table 40-1) and tubular structures (Fig. 40-1).[25] Y chromosome–positive cells were detected in the context of tubular epithelial lining and displayed binding sites for *L. culinaris* lectins, thus indicating that MSCs engraft the damaged tubules and can differentiate into tubular epithelial cells. Moreover, this study showed that MSCs significantly accelerated tubular cell proliferation, assessed as numbers of Ki-67–positive cells, to a remarkable extent in response to cisplatin damage.[25] A protective effect of MSCs was also documented in another mouse model of ARF induced by glycerol.[26] In this study, intravenously injected MSCs that were positive for green fluorescent protein contributed to renal recovery and localized in tubules expressing cytokeratins. Altogether, these data prove the effectiveness of MSCs in acute kidney damage, although the mechanisms underlying this effect are not fully understood. One possibility is that tubular protection is the consequence of the capacity of MSCs to engraft the damaged kidney and integrate/differentiate within tubules (Fig. 40-2). That most kidney cells originate from mesenchymal-epithelial transdifferentiation is well known,[27] and this feature could be the basis for the theory that tubular epithelial cells derive from mesenchymal stem cells. Another mechanism suggested

TABLE 40-1

Mesenchymal Stem Cells Protect Cisplatin-Treated Mice from Renal Function Impairment*

	Blood Urea Nitrogen (mg/dL)	
DAY	CISPLATIN + SALINE	CISPLATIN + MESENCHYMAL STEM CELLS
0	17.02 ± 1.0	19.22 ± 1.25[‡]
4	82.54 ± 5.12[†]	33.43 ± 3.06[‡]
7	46.44 ± 8.89	25.87 ± 2.05
29	4.57 ± 1.61	5.03 ± 1.30

*Data are expressed as mean ± SE.
[†]$P < .01$ vs. day 0.
[‡]$P < .01$ vs. cisplatin + saline at day 4.

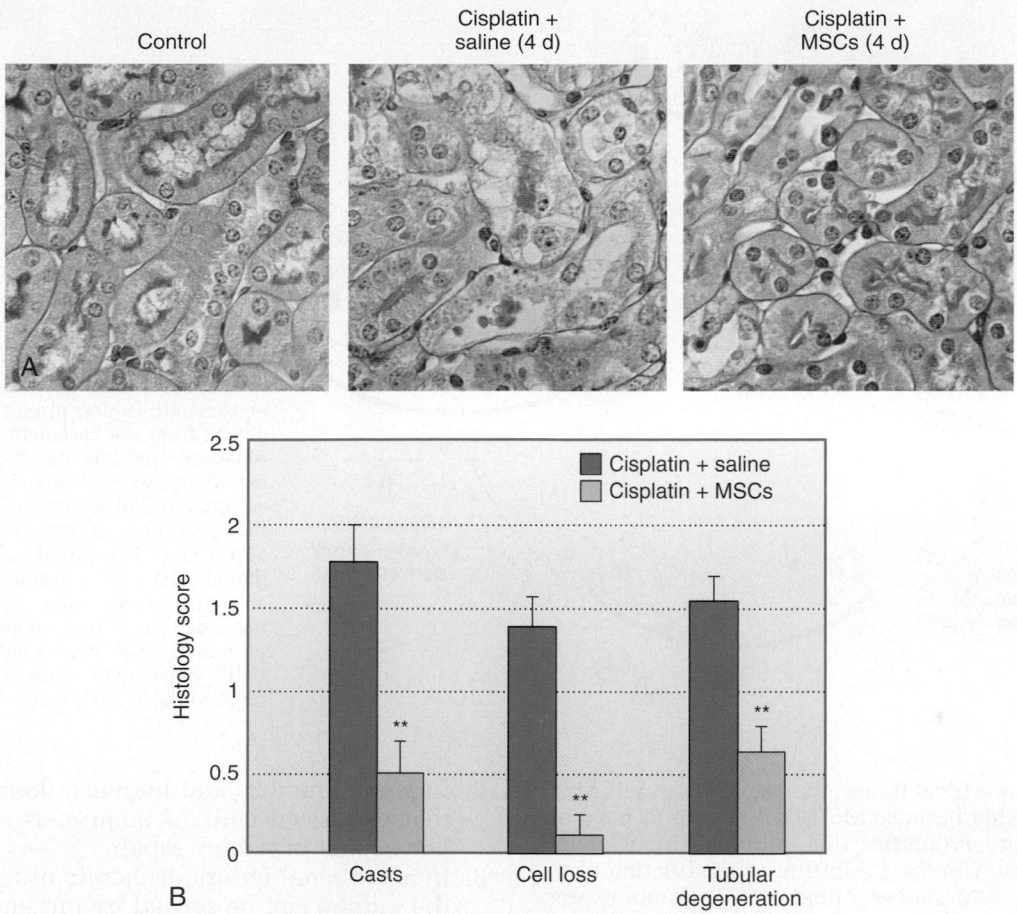

FIGURE 40-1. See also color plates. **A,** Renal histology of C57BL6/J control or cisplatin-treated mice that received saline or mesenchymal stem cells (MSCs). *Left,* Normal mouse kidney (control). *Center,* Cisplatin-treated mice at 4 days (d): Severe tubular changes (epithelial cell flattening and loss) are visibile in addition to loss of brush border and cell debris. *Right,* Cisplatin-mouse injected with MSCs shows, at 4 days, less severe tubular damage. (Original magnification ×400.) **B,** Effect of MSCs on renal histology. Semiquantitative analysis of tubular injury (at day 4 after administration of cisplatin) was performed by light-microscopic examination of renal tissues in cisplatin-treated mice given saline or injected with MSCs. Histology data are mean scores ± SE. *$P < .05$ vs cisplatin + saline; **$P < .01$.

to explain the functional benefit of MSCs can be related to their ability to produce high levels of growth, angiogenic and trophic factors.[28] That local production of stem cell factors might occur and might play a role in kidney tissue repair has been suggested by data obtained in a rat model of ischemia-reperfusion injury. Tögel and coworkers[29] showed that administration of MSCs resulted in improved renal function, increased tubular proliferation, and decreased apoptotic index. Scarce numbers of MSCs were found in the kidney, mainly in peritubular capillaries, thus excluding the possibility that these cells could physically replace lost tubular cells. This study supports the idea that MSCs could contribute to tubular repair by stimulating the proliferation of resident cells via a paracrine mechanism (see Fig. 40-2) involving mesenchymal production of hepatocyte growth factor, vascular endothelial growth factor, and insulin-like growth factor-1, as well as anti-inflammatory and organ-protective interleukin-10, basic fibroblast growth factor, and Bcl-2 protein.[29]

Bone marrow–derived MSCs as the origin of tubular cells have been challenged by Duffield and colleagues.[30] These investigators reported that bone marrow–derived MSCs ameliorated ischemic injury in mice but that MSCs were not found in renal structures. Other groups have reported that in folic acid–induced ARF, the administra-

tion of bone marrow–derived cells helped kidney regeneration; however, most (90%) of the proliferating cells were indigenous tubular cells.[17]

Besides the differentiation or paracrine mode (see Fig. 40-2) by which MSCs might provide beneficial effects in ARF, another mechanism to explain MSCs' therapeutic effect could reside in the cell fusion between mesenchymal stem cells and renal cells. This issue has been poorly investigated; however, the few data available show that in the kidney, fusion events account for a very small number.[17]

Whatever their mechanism of action, MSCs can potentially represent a valid therapeutic alternative for future application in humans. On the other hand, because ARF is a sudden phenomenon, it would not be feasible to use the patient's own MSCs because it takes too long to isolate them and then expand them in vitro. It will eventually be more feasible to use allogeneic cells previously isolated from donors and grown in vitro. This latter approach must be considered carefully, however, because in vitro expansion could lead to phenotypic and functional changes in the MSCs. Moreover, in vitro culture might modify the MSCs' migratory responses[31] and properties that affect their therapeutic efficacy. Therefore, new strategies for the in vitro expansion of MSCs are needed.

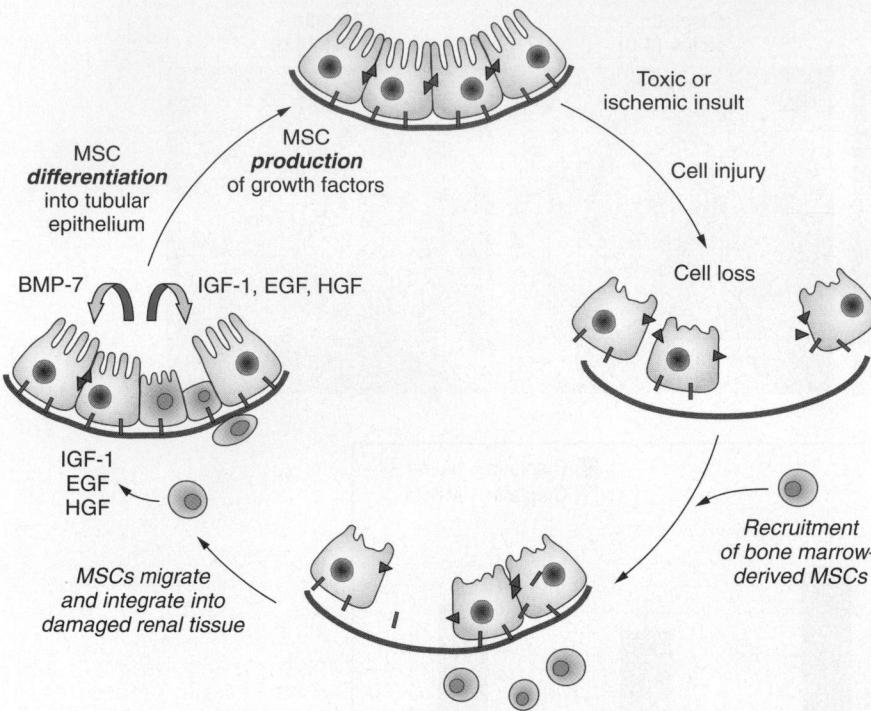

FIGURE 40-2. Proposed mechanisms of tubular repair after acute injury. After toxic or ischemic injury, proximal tubular cells detach from the basement membrane. The reparative process can be carried out by mesenchymal stem cells (MSCs), which are sensitive to kidney damage and migrate to the proximity of injured tubules. Here, MSCs may differentiate into tubular epithelial cells and/or produce growth factors able to accelerate the process of tubular regeneration. BMP-7, bone morphogenetic protein-7; EGF, epidermal growth factor; HGF, hepatocyte growth factor; IGF-1, insulin-like growth factor-1.

As for immunological issues, the use of allogeneic MSCs would be possible because MSCs are known to have immunomodulatory properties that, although incompletely understood, result in the inhibition or modulation of the T-cell response.[32] Moreover, human MSCs do not express major histocompatibility class (MHC) class II antigen (it can be induced by interferon-γ treatment),[33] do not express co-stimulatory molecules B7-1, B7-2, CD40, or CD40L, and do not activate alloreactive T cells.[33,34] This behavior might allow transplantation of allogeneic MSCs with a reduced or no need for host immunosuppression.

CONCLUSION

In the effort to enhance recovery from ARF, therapeutic strategies using stem or progenitor cells have been under development. The renotropic and regenerative potential of bone marrow–derived MSCs has been clearly demonstrated, and this finding might have huge implications in the treatment of ARF in humans. From a therapeutic point of view, future studies are needed to investigate the best route for delivering MSCs to the target tissues and the strategies for modulating their response to local pathological environment. Last but not least, the renotropism of MSCs could also be exploited to deliver anti-inflammatory molecules, drugs, and, eventually, vehicle genes to the kidney by means of genetically engineered MSCs.

Key Points

1. Acute renal failure is a syndrome characterized by the rapid deterioration of renal function with a mortality that still ranges from 30% to 80%. Pharmacological therapies have been largely unsuccessful.

2. In animal models and humans, there is evidence that extrarenal cells of bone marrow origin can participate in kidney repair.

3. In acute renal failure, ischemic or toxic injury to the kidney can be sensed by mesenchymal stem cells, which are able to engraft onto the damaged organ and promote structural and functional repair.

4. The mechanisms underlying the protective effect of these mesenchymal stem cells are still controversial. Such cells might contribute to recovery from acute renal failure through differentiation into renal cells or by supplying growth factors that stimulate the regeneration of resident cells.

Key References

11. Poulsom R, Alison MR, Cook T, et al: Bone marrow stem cells contribute to healing of the kidney. J Am Soc Nephrol 2003;14(Suppl 1):S48-S54.
24. Anjos-Afonso F, Siapati EK, Bonnet D: In vivo contribution of murine mesenchymal stem cells into multiple cell-types under minimal damage conditions. J Cell Sci 2004;117:5655-5664.
25. Morigi M, Imberti B, Zoja C, et al: Mesenchymal stem cells are renotropic, helping to repair the kidney and improve function in acute renal failure. J Am Soc Nephrol 2004;15:1794-1804.
29. Tögel F, Hu Z, Weiss K, et al: Vasculotropic, paracrine actions of infused mesenchymal stem cells are important to the recovery from acute kidney injury Am J Physiol Renal Physiol 2007;292:F1626-F1635.
30. Duffield JS, Park KM, Hsiao LL, et al: Restoration of tubular epithelial cells during repair of the postischemic kidney occurs independently of bone marrow-derived stem cells. J Clin Invest 2005;115:1743-1755.

See the companion Expert Consult website for the complete reference list.

CHAPTER 41

Endothelial Progenitor Cells in Acute Renal Injury

Nicoletta Pertica, Cataldo Abaterusso, Antonio Lupo, and Giovanni Gambaro

---

OBJECTIVES

This chapter will:
1. Define the main repair process in acute renal failure.
2. Explain different kinds of stem and mesenchymal cells that take part in renal tissue repair.
3. Provide a biological and physiological characterization of endothelial progenitor cells.
4. Discuss the role of endothelial progenitor cells in repairing acute renal damage.

Acute renal failure (ARF) is frequently due to a transient decrease in regional or total blood flow to the kidneys because of a drop in arterial blood pressure.[1,2] The secondary dysfunction and loss of tubular epithelial cells play a relevant part in the pathophysiological consequences of the syndrome. The role of the impairment to the renal microvasculature in ARF has also been recognized since the demonstration that endothelial cells swell early in ARF, causing a narrowing of the vascular lumen with prolonged hypoperfusion and delayed functional recovery.[1,3,4] The dysfunctional endothelium and tubular epithelium have a remarkable capacity to recover, however.[1,5]

With growing knowledge of stem cell biology, our understanding of these regenerative mechanisms in the kidney has also advanced. It has become evident that the cells responsible not only for tubular but also for endothelial regeneration include proliferating mature renal cells and specialized progenitor or precursor cells; the latter can be derived from either resident or circulating cells.[6,7]

RENAL TUBULAR INJURY AND STEM CELLS

The role of tubular dysfunction and tubular epithelial cell loss is central in the process leading to renal failure after ischemic or toxic damage.[3,8] The tubular epithelium has a remarkable capacity for recovery. In animal models, its rate of recovery depends on the substitution of damaged and/or dead epithelium by new functioning cells. Growth factors—insulin-like growth factor-1, hepatocyte growth factor, epidermal growth factor (EGF), and neutrophil gelatinase–associated lipocalin—have been used to potentiate tubular regeneration in experimental ARF.[1,9] Their activity may relate both to stimulatory actions on the regenerative potential of surviving cells and to cell "rescue" mechanisms. A major limitation to such healing effects lies in the need for a critical number of surviving cells for struc-

tural integrity to be restored. Other healing mechanisms most likely rely on the local supply of new cells to replace damaged cells.

Cell turnover in the adult kidney is low under physiological conditions, but after injury, increased cell proliferation is the driving event that leads to tissue recovery. This behavior supports the hypothesis that resident cells are involved in restoring structure and function by means of cell division and/or differentiation. Tubular epithelial cells that survive damage are able to proliferate, generate identical cells, and/or dedifferentiate, and subsequently to reenter the cell cycle. Tubular cell dedifferentiation is a well-known phenomenon in which the tubular cells acquire an immature mesenchymal phenotype. Stem cells (both resident and circulating) may also be involved in renal tissue healing, however.[1]

RENAL PROGENITOR/STEM CELLS IN THE ADULT KIDNEY

Tissue-based stem cells have been found to give rise to mature cells during physiological cell turnover or after tissue damage. During the healing process after ischemia, renal stem cells express mesenchymal cell markers and divide, suggesting the existence of progenitor-like cells that take part in kidney repair. Two different renal stem cells have been recognized so far. Oliver and associates[10] discovered that the renal papilla is a niche for kidney stem cells. The number of these cells declined in the papilla during recovery from ischemia, suggesting that they are involved in kidney repair. Cells with the features of renal progenitor cells have also been isolated from the tubular fraction of normal renal cortex by targeting CD133, a marker known to be expressed by hematopoietic stem and progenitor cells, and embryonic kidney[1,11]; these cells are able to differentiate in vitro into epithelial and endothelial lineages.

ADULT BONE MARROW–DERIVED STEM CELLS

Adult bone marrow–derived stem cells contribute to the turnover and regeneration of several compartments of the kidney.[1,12] Female mice recipients of male bone marrow grafts showed colocalization of Y chromosomes and the tubular epithelial marker *Lens culinaris* lectin in up to 8% of tubular epithelial cells, suggesting that bone marrow cells can traffic into the kidney and participate in normal tubular epithelial cell turnover.[12] In males receiving renal transplants from female donors, tubular epithelial cells containing Y chromosomes were observed in kidneys suffering from acute tubular necrosis.[12] Similarly, after injury in patients with sex-mismatched renal transplants, 1% of tubular cells in their kidneys were positive for Y chromosomes.[13]

Bone marrow–derived hematopoietic stem cells (HSCs) have therapeutic potential in liver, heart, and brain disorders,[1,14] and strategies have been proposed to enhance the circulation of HSCs in the kidney to treat acute tubular necrosis.[1,14]

Bone marrow stroma–derived mesenchymal stem cells (MSCs) are progenitors of skeletal tissue components, such as bone, cartilage, hematopoiesis-supporting stroma, and adipocytes, and experimental findings have shown the potential of MSCs in differentiating along multiple cell lines—for example, into neuronal, myogenic, and hepatocyte-like cells.[15]

A cell population established from adult male mouse bone marrow[16] has disclosed the morphological and functional characteristics of multipotent mesenchymal progenitor cells that, transplanted into female mice with ARF, have been shown to repair epithelial cell injury and improve renal function. These data suggest a local recruitment of MSCs at the sites of injury and provide evidence that MSCs are involved in the reconstitution of the differentiated tubular epithelium.

RENAL ENDOTHELIUM INJURY AND ENDOTHELIAL PROGENITOR CELLS

Although ischemic and nephrotoxic insult is believed to target mainly the tubular epithelium, renal endothelial cells also suffer early damage and swelling in ARF,[17] causing a narrowing of the vascular lumen followed by impairment of microvascular perfusion.[1,18] The most important consequence of this "no-reflow" phenomenon is a delayed functional recovery of the kidney due to prolonged hypoperfusion. The renal microvasculature thus has a major role in tissue regeneration in ARF.

It was formerly believed that mature endothelial cells in existing vessels proliferate and migrate to form new vessels in a process known as "angiogenesis." Evidence is accumulating, however, to show that specialized endothelial progenitor cells (EPCs), derived from the bone marrow or other sources, take part in the generation of new vessels (*vasculogenesis*). A pioneering study on EPCs and new vessel formation has challenged the view that vasculogenesis occurs only during embryogenesis.[17] In fact, human circulating CD34+ cells (markers of hematopoietic stem cells) were demonstrated to differentiate in vitro into cells with endothelium-like properties.

Acute renal injury probably also leads to a mobilization of the endogenous EPCs, but unfortunately, only a few studies have addressed this topic.

ENDOTHELIAL PROGENITOR CELLS

Characterization and Origin

Mesodermal cell differentiation into angioblasts and ensuing endothelial differentiation were believed to occur only during embryogenesis, but Asahara and colleagues[19] have disproved this belief by demonstrating that CD34+ hematopoietic progenitor cells from adults can differentiate into an endothelial phenotype. These endothelial progenitor cells were shown to become incorporated into neovessels at sites of ischemia. Genetically tagged bone marrow–transplanted cells were also found to cover implanted Dacron grafts like an endothelium.[20] These pioneering studies point to the existence of a pool of circulating hemangioblasts in adults. EPCs have been defined as cells positive for both a hematopoietic stem cell marker (CD34) and an endothelial marker (vascular endothelial growth factor receptor 2 [VEGFR2]). Because CD34 is expressed not only on hematopoietic stem cells but also on mature endothelial cells, subsequent studies used the more immature hematopoietic stem cell marker CD133, which is expressed on hematopoietic stem cells but not on mature endothelial cells or monocytes, and demonstrated that purified CD133+ cells can differentiate into endothelial cells in vitro. CD133+, VEGFR2+ cells are therefore likely to reflect immature progenitor cells, whereas CD34+, VEGFR2+ cells may also represent shed endothelial cells.

There is evidence that more than one endothelial progeny exists in the blood stream, because morphologically and functionally distinct endothelial cell populations can be grown from peripheral blood mononuclear cells.[21] A number of studies have confirmed that other cell populations, as well as hematopoietic stem cells, can give rise to endothelial cells. In fact, non–bone marrow–derived cells have been shown to replace endothelial cells in grafts.[22] Moreover, adult bone marrow–derived stem cells/progenitors, such as side population cells and multipotent adult progenitor cells (which differ from hematopoietic stem cells), have also been shown to differentiate into the endothelial lineage.[23]

Several possible sources of endothelial cells may thus exist in peripheral blood mononuclear cells, as follows[23]:
- Rare hematopoietic stem cells
- Myeloid cells, which may differentiate into endothelial cells under the pressure of cultivation selection
- Other circulating progenitor cells (i.e., side population cells)
- Circulating mature endothelial cells, shed by the vessel wall

Role in Neovascularization

The finding that bone marrow–derived cells can home onto sites of ischemia and express endothelial markers has challenged the use of hematopoietic stem cells or EPCs for therapeutic vasculogenesis and tissue rescue from critical ischemia.[24] The infusion of different cell types isolated from the bone marrow or produced by ex vivo cultivation (expansion) has been shown to increase capillary density and neovascularization in ischemic tissues. In animal models of myocardial infarction, injection of ex vivo–expanded EPCs or progenitor/stem cells significantly improved blood flow and cardiac function and reduced left ventricular scarring.[23] Likewise, the infusion of ex vivo–expanded EPCs deriving from peripheral blood mononuclear cells in nude mice or rats improved the neovascularization in a hind limb ischemia model.[25] Other studies have indicated that progenitor cells derived from bone marrow or circulating blood are useful for improving the blood supply of ischemic tissue. Fully differentiated mature endothelial cells do not improve neovascularization, however, suggesting that as yet undefined functional characteristics are vital to EPC-mediated vasculogenesis after ischemia.[23]

The role of EPCs in neovascularization has been convincingly shown, but the underlying mechanism and the extent to which EPCs improve neovascularization remain to be determined. The basal progenitor cell incorporation rate without tissue injury is extremely low,[26] but in ischemic tissues, it ranges from 0 to 90%.[23] Such a wide variability may be due to an influence of the ischemia model (i.e., the severity and extent of ischemia) on the incorporation rate and to differences in the engraftment efficiency of different progenitor subpopulations. In any case, the number of cells with an endothelial phenotype incorporated in the ischemic tissues is generally quite low. How can such a few cells increase neovascularization? One explanation might be that the efficiency of neovascularization depends not only on the incorporation of EPCs in the new vessels but also on the paracrine activity of proangiogenic factors released by EPCs. Indeed, EPCs cultivated from different sources show a marked synthesis of growth factors, such as VEGF, hepatocyte growth factor, and insulin-like growth factor-1.[23] The release of growth factors would in turn influence angiogenesis by favoring endothelial cell proliferation, migration, and survival.[27] However, both EPC incorporation in newly formed vessels and EPC paracrine activities are needed to improve neovascularization, because the infusion of macrophages (which are known to release growth factors but are not incorporated in vessels) only slightly improves neovascularization after ischemia.[23]

The regenerated endothelium has proved functionally active, as demonstrated by its release of nitric oxide.[28] There are at least two distinct populations of circulating cells capable of contributing to reendothelization: cells mobilized from bone marrow and non–bone marrow–derived cells. The latter may derive from circulating progenitor cells released by non–bone marrow sources (e.g., tissue-resident stem cells) or may represent endothelial cells deriving from the vessel walls.[29]

Whatever their origin, this pool of circulating EPCs may have an important role as an endogenous repair mechanism for preserving the endothelial monolayer by replacing denuded parts of the artery. It is worth noting that risk factors for atherosclerosis, such as diabetes, hypercholesterolemia, hypertension, and smoking, affect the number and functional activity of circulating EPCs.[23]

Mobilization, Homing, and Differentiation

Increasing the number of circulating EPCs may be a smart therapeutic approach to facilitate reendothelization and neovascularization. Stem cells in the bone marrow are mobilized by mobilizing cytokines that affect the local microenvironment, the so-called stem cell niche consisting of fibroblasts, osteoblasts, and endothelial cells.[23] Ischemia is considered the main signal for EPC mobilization via the upregulation of VEGFs,[23] which are released into the circulation and mobilize progenitor cells from the bone marrow via a matrix metalloproteinase-9–dependent mechanism.[23,30,31] Gene therapy studies with plasmids encoding for VEGF have demonstrated an increase in the EPCs circulating in the blood of humans. Other factors that cause the mobilization of EPCs have been discovered by hematologists harvesting hematopoietic stem cells from peripheral blood for bone marrow transplantation. For instance, the granulocyte colony–stimulating factor (G-

CSF), typically used to mobilize CD34[+] cells, is also capable of raising EPC levels in the blood. The granulocyte/monocyte colony–stimulating factor (GM-CSF) also raises EPC levels,[31] and erythropoietin, which stimulates the proliferation and maturation of erythroid precursors, increases peripheral EPC levels.[23,32]

Homing—the recruitment and incorporation of EPCs—demands a coordinated sequence of adhesion and signaling events consisting of chemoattraction, adhesion, and transmigration followed by differentiation into endothelial cells. Given the small numbers of circulating EPCs, chemoattraction is likely to be very important for the recruitment of a sufficient number of progenitor cells in injured tissues. Chemokines and VEGF have been shown to prompt chemoattraction.[23,32]

VEGF also plays a relevant part in EPC differentiation. To become functionally integrated into vessels, it is crucial for EPCs to mature into functional endothelial cells. VEGF and its receptors have a major role in stimulating endothelial differentiation in embryogenesis and in the ex vivo culture of a variety of adult progenitor populations.[23,27]

Endothelial Progenitor Cells and Acute Renal Damage and Ischemia

Few studies are available on EPCs and endothelial regeneration in renal diseases, and in acute ischemic renal failure in particular. The bone marrow–mediated repair of the glomerular endothelium has been reported by Rookmaaker and associates,[33] who observed a more than fourfold rise in the number of bone marrow–derived glomerular endothelial cells in an anti–Thy-1.1 glomerulitis model induced in bone marrow–transplanted rats. Similar findings have been reported in bone marrow–transplanted rats with unilateral nephrectomy and anti–Thy-1.1 glomerulitis.[4,34]

As mentioned previously, the hemodynamic consequences of renal hypoperfusion due to endothelial cell swelling and lumen narrowing have a negative effect on the course of ARF. With a view to containing these consequences, Patschan and coworkers[17] conducted experiments with endothelial cell transplantation. They found that injecting human umbilical vein endothelial cells into athymic nude rats undergoing renal artery clamping dramatically improved their renal function, supporting the conviction that endothelial dysfunction contributes to acute renal injury. These studies were extended to EPCs expanded from a skeletal muscle stem cell pool, the infusion of which was associated with a significantly better-preserved renal function.[4,35,36]

Ischemic preconditioning is an acquired resistance to various stressors after a previous nonlethal stress, studied most extensively in the heart. It is a two-stage process, with an early phase lasting up to 2 hours and a late phase becoming apparent between 24 hours and several days afterwards. Although the mechanisms involved in the acute phase probably vary from organ to organ, the late phase is considered to be a universal response[37] that is dependent on nitric oxide and/or heat shock protein and modulated by protein kinases and nuclear factor-κB. In the murine kidney, ischemic preconditioning peaks 1 to 2 weeks after the initial ischemic episode. Molecular mechanisms of this process in the kidney have been associated with protective changes in tubular function and tissue-infiltrating leukocyte activity; EPCs may also play a part, however.[38] Patschan and associates[4] obtained results suggesting that renal ischemic preconditioning depends partly on the recruitment and engraftment of EPCs, as shown in the myocardium. In their study, numbers of splenic EPCs were significantly higher in renal ischemic mice than in sham-operated or control animals. There was no sign of EPC accumulation in the spleen after ischemic preconditioning, however. A sixfold rise in the number of EPCs localized in the medullopapillary region was observed in ischemically preconditioned mice within 7 days of the initial ischemic episode. These data imply a first, rapid EPC mobilization after acute renal ischemia and a greater medullopapillary EPC accumulation in the late phase of ischemic preconditioning, suggesting a role for EPCs in endothelium maintenance and repair in acute renal ischemia. Ischemic preconditioning thus seems to favor EPC translocation from the transient splenic niche to the ischemic organ.

These ischemia-mobilized EPCs probably have a renoprotective effect in acute renal ischemia. Indeed, transplantation of enriched EPCs in animals with renal ischemia suggests an important biological role for kidney-homed EPCs.[4] These cells were located mainly in the renal medullopapillary region and were associated with a better renal function. Whether such an amelioration is the outcome of a better microvascular function or of paracrine signaling[4] remains to be seen.

CONCLUSION

The data presented in this chapter suggest that bone marrow–derived MSCs can ameliorate ARF, thanks to both paracrine effects and the repair of the injured microvasculature through provision of EPCs. Questions remain to be answered about the source of the stem cells and the stage of their differentiation after ex vivo expansion as well as the methods for enhancing their mobilization, bettering their delivery to the damaged kidney in spite of a severe vasoconstriction, and improving their engraftment, and these issues are being intensively researched. Further progress will also depend on the development of more precise markers of different stem and progenitor cell populations and our understanding of the "stemness" of each cell population.

Key Points

1. Acute renal failure is a complication affecting approximately 5% of all hospitalized patients, with a high related mortality. The most common cause of ARF is a transient drop in regional or total blood flow to the kidneys due to a decrease in the mean arterial blood pressure.

2. Endothelium and tubular epithelium that have become dysfunctional because of longstanding hypoperfusion have a remarkable capacity for recovery: Bone marrow–derived mesenchymal stem cells can ameliorate acute renal failure through paracrine effects and repair of injured microvasculature by provision of endothelial progenitor cells.

3. Endothelial progenitor cells are specialized cells, originating from the bone marrow or other sources, that participate in the generation of new vessels (vasculogenesis).

4. Evidence of a rapid mobilization of endothelial progenitor cells after acute renal ischemia and a subsequent increase in medullopapillary endothelial progenitor cell accumulation suggests a role for these cells in the maintenance and repair of the endothelium.

5. Kidney-homed endothelial progenitor cells are associated with an improvement in renal function after ischemic injury.

Key References

4. Patschan D, Plotkin M, Goligorsky MS: Therapeutic use of stem and endothelial progenitor cells in acute renal injury: Ça ira. Curr Opin Pharmacol 2006;6:176-183.
19. Asahara T, Murohara T, Sullivan A, et al: Isolation of putative progenitor endothelial cells for angiogenesis. Science 1997; 275:964-967.
34. Ikarashi K, Li B, Suwa M, et al: Bone marrow cells contribute to regeneration of damaged glomerular endothelial cells. Kidney Int 2005;67:1925-1933.
35. Brodsky SV, Yamamoto T, Tada T, et al: Endothelial dysfunction in ischemic acute renal failure: Rescue by transplanted endothelial cells. Am J Physiol Renal Physiol 2002;282: F1140-F1149.
38. Fang TC, Alison MR, Cook HT, et al: Proliferation of bone marrow-derived cells contributes to regeneration after folic acid-induced acute tubular injury. J Am Soc Nephrol 2005; 16:1723-1732.

Experimental Models of Acute Renal Failure

CHAPTER 42

Models of Ischemic Renal Injury

Valerie A. Luyckx and Joseph V. Bonventre

OBJECTIVES

This chapter will:
1. Describe experimental models used to study the pathophysiology of ischemic acute kidney injury.
2. Explore the mechanisms of experimental ischemic acute kidney injury.
3. Discuss contributors to reduced glomerular filtration rate in experimental ischemic acute kidney injury.

The utilization of experimental models is critical to furthering the understanding of disease pathogenesis and the development of therapeutic strategies. Human acute renal failure (ARF), now referred to as *acute kidney injury* (AKI) to reflect the importance of the wide spectrum of disease severity to patient outcome, is associated with high morbidity and mortality. Localized or generalized kidney ischemia and toxins are important contributors to AKI. Histologically, AKI due to intrarenal (as opposed to prerenal or postrenal causes) is often associated with scattered tubular necrosis (hence the frequently used descriptor acute tubular necrosis [ATN]), some dilation of the proximal tubules, intratubular casts, and relative preservation of glomerular morphology.[1,2] This observation has directed the major focus of AKI research to the renal tubules. Animal models replicate human ischemic AKI with varying degrees of fidelity, so multiple experimental models with varying strengths and weaknesses have been developed. These models have contributed important insights into the pathophysiology of AKI (Fig. 42-1).[3] In addition to animal models, investigators have utilized proximal tubule cell culture, isolated proximal tubules, and isolated perfused kidneys. The advantages and disadvantages of each of these models are discussed here and are summarized in Table 42-1.

CELL CULTURE

Cultured tubular epithelial cells, whether obtained from primary culture or established cell lines, are the simplest model in which to study tubular epithelial cell physiology. Some aspects of sublethal "ischemic" injury may be mimicked in cultured cells that are subjected to short periods of adenosine triphosphate (ATP) depletion, which is achieved with the use of inhibitors of mitochondrial respiration, such as antamycin A in the setting of glucose deprivation.[3-5] Studies using these models have shown that sublethal tubular epithelial cell injury results in disruption of the actin cytoskeleton, loss of epithelial cell polarity (e.g., localization of Na^+,K^+-ATPase to the apical membrane from the basolateral membrane), and impairment in integrity of the intercellular junctional complex.[6-9] Some of these findings have been confirmed in biopsy specimens with human AKI.[10,11] The study of cultured cells as a model for in vivo responses does, however, have several important caveats. Cells in culture undergo various phenotypical and structural changes in order to survive under the unnatural circumstances.[3,12] For example, cultured cells proliferate more rapidly, and rely more heavily on glycolysis than on mitochondrial metabolism, in contrast to tubular epithelial cells in vivo.[13] As such, cultured cells are much more resistant to hypoxic injury than cells in vivo. In addition, cultured cells represent a single tubular epithelial cell type, which is also not representative of the heterogeneous nature of the renal tubular epithelial cell populations. Despite these limitations, however, cell culture models remain a useful tool for dissecting the molecular pathways of injury and repair, providing insights into and direction for study of more complex models that may be more relevant to human AKI.

ISOLATED PROXIMAL TUBULES

Freshly isolated whole proximal tubules have been widely used to study metabolic and physiological characteristics of the renal tubule in both baseline and ischemic conditions.[3,14,15] The advantages of isolated tubules over cultured cells as an experimental model include that the heterogeneity of the tubular epithelial cell population is maintained and that structural and physiological properties are preserved in the intact tubule. Isolated tubules, however, were initially found to have a greater sensitivity to hypoxia or ATP depletion–induced injury than tubules in vivo.[3,16] Pivotal investigations trying to explain this observation led to the discovery of the cytoprotective effects of acidosis and endogenous glycine in renal tubules in vivo.[16-18] This observation has also permitted identification of other important factors participating in ischemic tubular injury. Refinement of the isolated proximal tubule model, through replacement of glycine and adjustment of pH in the culture medium, restored a degree of resistance to ischemic

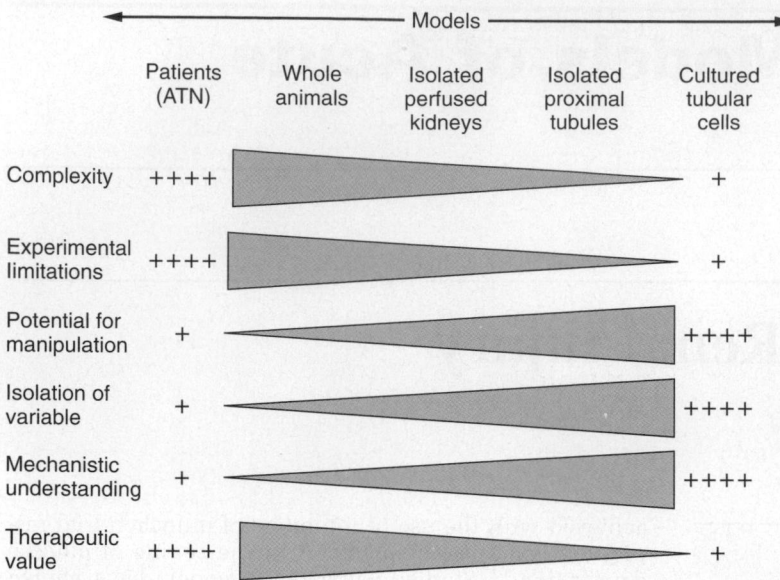

FIGURE 42-1. Experimental models of ischemic acute kidney injury. ATN, acute tubular necrosis. +, minimally applicable; ++++, very applicable. (From Lieberthal W, Nigam SK: Acute renal failure. II: Experimental models of acute renal failure: Imperfect but indispensable. Am J Physiol Renal Physiol 2000;278:F1-F12.)

TABLE 42-1

Advantages and Disadvantages of Experimental Models of Ischemic Acute Renal Failure

	ADVANTAGES	DISADVANTAGES
Cell culture	Easy to obtain Experimental environment easy to control Allows manipulation and study of individual conditions	Not representative of true physiological conditions Single cell type Cells undergo phenotypical changes in culture More resistant to hypoxic injury Loss of cell polarity
Isolated proximal tubule	Differentiated phenotype preserved Structural integrity (polarity) largely preserved Permits full progression of sublethal injury Permits study of early recovery	Isolation injury and necrosis More susceptible to hypoxic injury Does not assess vascular and inflammatory components
Whole animal	Can evaluate tubular, vascular, and inflammatory components simultaneously More closely resembles human acute kidney injury Can test therapeutic strategies Permits observations of whole organ and whole animal physiology	Requires greater resources Usually one-dimensional insult, in contrast to multiple-organ failure that characterizes human acute kidney injury Differences among animal species limit generalizability Positive therapeutic trials have not yet translated into benefit in humans

damage in the isolated tubules, permitting more rigorous study of injury and early recovery events.[3,18] The isolated proximal tubule model system is therefore a powerful method to study epithelial cell responses to injury and recovery, because it lends itself to in vitro experimental manipulations while retaining many characteristics of the proximal tubule in vivo. It is important to recognize, however, that 10% to 15% of tubule cells may be lethally injured during the isolation procedure, suggesting that a greater number may also be sublethally injured, a fact that may confound interpretation of results.[3] Furthermore, tubules do not function in isolation in vivo, because vascular and immunological responses are also critical to the development and recovery of tubular injury; therefore, this isolated tubule model remains useful but limited. Another factor that must be borne in mind with use of cultured cells or isolated tubules is that "ischemia" caused by ATP depletion is usually induced in the setting of normal oxygen tension, and often at physiologic pH. These conditions may result in exaggerated production of harmful

reactive oxygen species in the setting of ATP depletion in vitro compared with in vivo, again potentially confounding observations. While in vitro studies therefore have a significant place on the pathway to understanding ischemic renal injury, observations must be validated more comprehensively at the whole organ or whole animal level to increase the likelihood of true clinical relevance.[3]

ANIMAL MODELS

Ischemic AKI in humans results from a complex interplay between hemodynamic and humoral factors. Isolated perfused whole kidneys are seldom used in studies of ischemic AKI. For investigation of the renal tubule response in the context of the whole kidney and the whole organism, whole animal models are required. Many of the "single insult" models of AKI in whole animals, however, do not accurately replicate the findings in human AKI.[3,18]

For example, prolonged hypotension in the rat does not cause ischemic renal injury. Injury can be induced only after varying periods of total renal artery occlusion, intrarenal infusion of norepinephrine, which reduces renal blood flow to near zero, or significant partial suprarenal aortic ligation, in which renal perfusion pressure is reduced to 20 mm Hg.[19] These observations raise the question whether hypoperfusion alone, even in humans, is enough to cause ischemic ATN. Other models of ATN in animals incorporate multiple simultaneous insults—for instance, gentamicin plus sepsis, or radiocontrast agent plus hypovolemia.

Nonetheless, for study of the pure effects of ischemia, cross-clamping of the renal artery for varying periods (e.g., 30-60 minutes), followed by reperfusion established for minutes to days before kidney harvesting, is a well-established model. Histologically, however, renal artery occlusion in rats results in widespread necrosis of proximal tubule cells, a finding that some researchers have argued is not as common in human ischemic ATN.[2] On the other hand, significant pathological findings that are shared with human ATN are severe proximal tubular injury, loss of proximal tubular brush-border membranes, and intratubular cast formation.[2,3] In addition, the glomerular filtration rate is also severely reduced after renal artery occlusion, which is often followed by recovery of renal function. This model, therefore, although not ideal, does share many features with human ischemic AKI and has been widely used to study both the injury and recovery phases of AKI.[20]

Ischemic renal injury in animals can be modified by preconditioning.[21] In animal models in which mild ischemia is induced, for instance, by renal artery occlusion for 30 minutes, followed by reperfusion, and then ischemia is induced again within days of the initial insult, the kidney subjected to repeated ischemia is more resistant to injury than a kidney subjected to ischemia without preconditioning. The mechanisms conferring this protection appear to be related to upregulation of cytoprotective proteins, reduced expression of adhesion molecules and pro-inflammatory cytokines, altered vascular reactivity, and possible dedifferentiation of recovering cells to make them less susceptible to repeat injury and more resistant to apoptosis.[21] This preconditioning effect is likely to participate on some level in the development of resistance to AKI in humans.

Interestingly, many therapeutic interventions that have proved useful in animal models have not translated to benefit in humans, further emphasizing the need for caution in extrapolation from animal models to human disease.[22-24] Models of AKI in dogs, rabbits, rats, and mice all require procedural modifications to obtain similar levels of renal injury, because of differences in susceptibility to ischemic injury among these animals. Differences between animal species with respect to local and systemic hemodynamic response to injury, medullary vessel anatomy, and urinary concentrating ability may all contribute to observed discrepancies among species.[3] The porcine kidney is structurally the most similar to the human kidney, suggesting that more extensive use of this model is warranted.

MECHANISMS OF ISCHEMIC ACUTE KIDNEY INJURY

The mechanisms contributing to the development of AKI in the setting of ischemia involve vascular, tubular, and inflammatory factors.[1,25,26] In experimental animals, ischemic injury induced either by renal hypoperfusion or by infusion of vasoconstrictors to the kidney has been shown to result in a loss of renal autoregulation and renal vasoconstriction.[1,26] In addition, ischemia and reperfusion lead to renal endothelial cell injury and activation, associated with upregulation of adhesion molecules and leukocyte entrapment in the microvasculature, resulting in congestion of the renal outer medulla and exacerbation of renal ischemia and local tubule dysfunction.[25,28-32] Different properties of renal medullary vessels in humans and various animal species may contribute to the variability in pathophysiology of ischemic AKI among different animals.[3] Structural changes occurring in proximal tubule epithelial cells in response to an ischemic insult lead to impairment of sodium and water reabsorption and other metabolic derangements.[1] Whole cells may be shed into the urine in varying stages of viability, which may contribute to tubular obstruction via their adhesion to other epithelial cells or exposed extracellular matrix or their behavior as casts occluding the distal nephron.[33] In addition, brush-border membranes may be shed, the cytoskeleton may be disrupted, and localization of sodium transporters may be altered, resulting in loss of tubular reabsorptive function.[1,17] Ischemic renal injury also results in a significant inflammatory response, which has been found to play a significant role in the pathophysiology of ischemic AKI.[25] In addition to contributing to medullary congestion, leukocytes may be recruited by pro-inflammatory cytokines elaborated by injured endothelial as well as epithelial cells. Sequestered leukocytes in turn exacerbate injury by generating reactive oxygen species, enhancing inflammation and activation of the complement and coagulation cascades.[25]

FACTORS CONTRIBUTING TO REDUCTION IN GLOMERULAR FILTRATION RATE IN ISCHEMIC ACUTE KIDNEY INJURY

The glomerular filtration rate in patients with established AKI is often less than 10 mL/min.[1,17,34] The severity of uremia apparent in a specific patient therefore depends largely on the duration of AKI. Because the glomeruli in most cases remain relatively intact, this significant reduction in glomerular filtration rate results from several additive processes. First, morphological changes in proximal tubule cells are associated with loss of epithelial cell polarity and redistribution of integrins and transporters from the basolateral to the apical membranes as well as with loss of brush-border membranes into the urine, all of which contribute to tubule dysfunction.[10,34,35] Second, loss of polarity and cellular dysfunction result in reduced proximal tubular sodium reabsorption and increased distal sodium delivery to the macula densa, leading to activation of the tubuloglomerular feedback mechanism and a reduction in single-nephron glomerular filtration rate.[36] Third, increased distal sodium delivery also favors Tamm-Horsfall protein polymerization and cast formation in the distal nephron segments. Shed brush-border membranes, in addition to necrotic, apoptotic or viable proximal tubular cells, may deposit in the casts and contribute to intraluminal tubular obstruction, dilatation of proximal tubule segments, and reduced filtration in affected nephrons.[1,25,37] In addition, viable shed cells may adhere to other tubule cells or denuded basement membrane, via arginine-glycine–aspartic acid (RGD) sequences, and may themselves cause luminal obstruction.[38] Finally, loss of the proximal tubular epithelial cell barrier, or integrity of intercellular junctions, may permit some back-leak of filtrate into the renal interstitium and the circulation, thereby reducing net excretion.[11,39]

CONCLUSION

The study of AKI incorporates experimental models ranging from the most simple (cell culture) to the highly complex (clinical trials). Traveling back and forth between bench and bedside, using models of escalating complexity to identify and test pathophysiological mechanisms, to develop potential therapeutic strategies, and ultimately to test these strategies in humans with AKI, is the ideal continuum of medical research. Despite the complementary nature of experiments in cultured cells, isolated tubules, and whole animals, no therapeutic regimen developed using these models has thus far translated into a successful clinical strategy in humans. It is likely that this fact is not solely related to differences between human AKI and animal models. Human populations are heterogeneous, renal insults are seldom isolated, and detection of AKI is often delayed because of the insensitivity of current diagnostic markers. All of these factors highlight the importance of continued research but also the urgent need for development of early diagnostic biomarkers of AKI as well as better experimental models that more closely resemble the pathophysiology and complexity of human AKI.

Key Points

1. Cell culture does not represent an adequate model of tubular cell physiology.
2. Isolated proximal tubules permit study of tubular epithelial cell response to injury and early recovery.
3. Study of proximal tubules must be carried out with repletion of glycine and maintenance of acid pH.
4. Different animal species have different susceptibility to ischemic renal injury.
5. No single experimental model is adequate to reproduce all aspects of human ischemic acute kidney injury, but existing models are complementary and should be used with results corroborated among models.

Key References

1. Schrier RW, Wang W, Poole B, Mitra A: Acute renal failure: Definitions, diagnosis, pathogenesis, and therapy. J Clin Invest 2004;114:5-14.
3. Lieberthal W, Nigam SK: Acute renal failure. II: Experimental models of acute renal failure: Imperfect but indispensable. Am J Physiol Renal Physiol 2000;278:F1-F12.
17. Bonventre JV, Weinberg JM: Recent advances in the pathophysiology of ischemic acute renal failure. J Am Soc Nephrol 2003;14:2199-2210.
20. Heyman SN, Lieberthal W, Rogiers P, Bonventre JV: Animal models of acute tubular necrosis. Curr Opin Crit Care 2002;8:526-534.
25. Bonventre JV, Zuk A: Ischemic acute renal failure: An inflammatory disease? Kidney Int 2004;66:480-485.
34. Thadhani R, Pascual M, Bonventre JV: Acute renal failure. N Engl J Med 1996;334:1448-1460.

See the companion Expert Consult website for the complete reference list.

CHAPTER 43

Models of Toxic Acute Renal Failure

Wilfred Lieberthal

OBJECTIVES

This chapter will:
1. Discuss the anatomical and physiological features of the kidney that predispose it to toxic injury.
2. Describe how the importance of the kidney in eliminating toxic substances increases its susceptibility to toxic injury.
3. Consider two general models of nephrotoxic acute renal failure in vivo, "single-insult" and "combined-insult."
4. Discuss the use, advantages, and disadvantages of the isolated perfused kidney for the study of nephrotoxins.
5. Describe the role of renal slices, isolated tubules, and cultured renal cells in the study of nephrotoxins.
6. Explain in brief the importance to the field of toxicology of novel techniques derived from advances in molecular biology.

The kidney has unique structural, physiological, and biochemical features that are important contributors to its susceptibility to the adverse effects of toxins. The kidney receives a disproportionately high blood flow so has a higher exposure to blood-borne toxins than other organs. The vascular anatomy of the glomerular capillary is unique in that it is drained by a muscle-walled vessel (the efferent arteriole) rather than a venule. Although the afferent and efferent arterioles provide an efficient mechanism for the control of intraglomerular capillary pressure and glomerular filtration rate, some drugs and toxins can cause a hemodynamic form of acute renal failure (ARF) by inducing either afferent arteriolar vasoconstriction or efferent arteriolar vasodilatation.

The kidney plays an important role in eliminating toxins from the body through both glomerular filtration and the active tubular secretion of anionic and cationic compounds from blood into the tubular lumen. Proximal tubular transport by the organic solute transport system can lead to far higher concentrations of certain toxins in the proximal tubular cells than in any other cell type. The concentrations of toxic substances to which tubular cells are exposed progressively increase along the nephron as water and solute are reabsorbed. Furthermore, the greater acidity of distal luminal fluid can promote the precipitation of some chemicals that are insoluble at low pH. Finally, the processes required to concentrate the urine lead to exposure of the medulla to high concentrations of some toxins that can cause medullary injury and papillary necrosis.

STUDIES OF NEPHROTOXINS IN VIVO

Studies in whole animals are indispensable for demonstrating that the kidney is a target of injury for a particular toxicant and for elucidating the mechanisms involved. Most experimental models of toxic ARF in vivo have relied on the administration of a single nephrotoxic insult (the "single-injury" model). Other toxins induce ARF only when administered together with other renal stresses ("combined-injury" models).

Single-Injury Models of Acute Renal Failure In Vivo

Cisplatin-Induced Acute Renal Failure

Cisplatin, which is usually administered to animals by intraperitoneal injection, reproducibly induces ARF and morphologic changes of tubular injury in rats and mice.[1-8]

Mercury-Induced Acute Renal Failure

While all forms of mercury can induce renal injury, the inorganic form of mercury is more likely than the organic form to induce acute nephrotoxicity. Administration of inorganic mercury induces ARF relatively consistently in animals, with rapid development of renal dysfunction, usually within the first 24 hours after the first dose.[9,10] By contrast, multiple and relatively large doses of organic mercury are required to induce renal injury, which is generally more chronic in nature.

Glycerol-Induced Acute Renal Failure

Another example of a relatively satisfactory "single-injury" model for ATN is induced by intramuscular injection of glycerol, which produces a form of ARF in rats similar to the acute tubular necrosis induced in humans by rhabdomyolysis and/or intravascular hemolysis.[11-13] The tubular damage that results is due to a combination of factors, including severe intrarenal vasoconstriction, heme-mediated oxidant injury to tubular cells, and obstruction of distal tubules by casts of acid hematin.[11-13] The success of the glycerol model in inducing ARF may be partly due to the fact that it induces multiple intrarenal responses that all contribute to the reduction in GFR.

Combined-Injury Models of Acute Renal Failure In Vivo

For many nephrotoxins, the "single-insult" approach does not reproducibly induce ARF. Some investigators have developed models of toxic ARF induced by multiple renal insults and have developed "combined-injury" experimental models in an attempt to "mimic" the process of acute tubular necrosis in humans.

Aminoglycoside-Induced Acute Renal Failure

Gentamicin causes ARF only when administered in very high doses (usually 10 times the therapeutic dose in humans).[14,15] However, Zager[16] has reported that gentamicin toxicity is markedly enhanced in the setting of gram-negative bacteremia.

Radiocontrast Agent–Induced Acute Renal Failure

The administration of radiocontrast agents to animals does not induce ARF. However, Heyman and colleagues[17,18,20,21] have demonstrated that the administration of radiocontrast agents to rats and mice causes ARF when it is combined with other forms of renal "stress," such as volume depletion, uninephrectomy, and inhibition of prostaglandin synthesis. The pathophysiology of ARF in the "combined" model of radiocontrast agent–induced nephropathy in animals[17-21] is consistent with the fact that radiocontrast agent–induced acute tubular necrosis in humans usually does not occur unless other "predisposing factors" (such as volume depletion and preexisting chronic renal insufficiency) are also present. The methods available to evaluate the effect of nephrotoxins on the kidney in vivo—glomerular filtration rate, renal plasma flow, renal blood flow, micropuncture, imaging techniques (scintigrapy, ultrasonography, computed tomography, and magnetic resonance imaging), morphology, and the urinary excretion of albumin, electrolyes, and brush-border enzymes—are all described in detail elsewhere.[22,23]

A concern regarding the use of rodents for toxicological research is that a number of human studies examining the efficacy of interventions demonstrated to ameliorate ARF in rodents have generally been shown to be ineffective in humans.[24] Consideration should be given to the use of other animals that have kidneys physiologically and anatomically more similar to the human kidney than rodent kidneys, such as the pig, as models of ARF in vivo.

STUDIES OF NEPHROTOXINS IN VITRO

The kidney is a complex organ composed of many different cell types. Many nephrotoxic agents target discrete cell types and do not affect other renal cell types. This selectivity has made the in vivo assessment of nephrotoxicity and elucidation of underlying mechanisms difficult. However, a variety of in vitro models have been exploited to study the interactions between nephrotoxic compounds and their target cell(s) (Table 43-1). These include the isolated perfused kidney (IPK), renal slices, freshly isolated tubular fragments, isolated glomeruli, and cultured renal cells.

TABLE 43-1

Advantages and Disadvantages of the Isolated Perfused Kidney When Perfused in the Absence of Red Blood Cells

Advantages	The renal anatomy and the overall vascular-glomerular-tubular anatomic associations are maintained.
	Glomerular function is well maintained.
	The investigator has control over all extrarenal factors.
	The model enables concomitant determination of hemodynamics, function, and morphology.
	Experimental manipulation is relatively easy.
Disadvantages	The model excludes extrarenal factors that could participate in the effects of the toxin being studied (neuroendocrine factors, inflammatory cells, and various plasma factors, e.g., complement).
	The renal vascular resistance of the IPK is very low.*
	Oxygen delivery by the red cell–free perfusate is low.*
	The cells of the medullary thick ascending limb segment undergo necrosis.*
	Fractional sodium excretion is high, and concentrating ability is poor.*

*The addition of red blood cells to the perfusate prevents or ameliorates these problems (see text for additional details).
Data from references 26 and 28.

The Isolated Perfused Kidney

The IPK provides the least-disrupted in vitro model for the study of renal toxicology; it has been described thoroughly in a number of comprehensive reviews.[25,26] In this ex vivo whole-organ model, the kidney is isolated from the animal (dog, rabbit, rat, mouse) and perfused with an oxygenated, albumin-containing, nutrient-rich solution at 37° C at controlled perfusion pressure and perfusate flow rate. The perfusate is driven by a pump that maintains mean intrarenal hydrostatic pressure at about 100 mm Hg. Urine is collected, and glomerular filtration and tubular function are continuously monitored by the sequential determination of electrolyte levels using a marker of glomerular filtration such as inulin. Renal morphology can be assessed subsequently.

In most studies, the IPK has been perfused by a solution that does not contain red blood cells (RBCs).[25-27] The RBC-free perfusate has a low viscosity, which results in a very low renal vascular resistance. The combination of a relatively normal glomerular filtration rate with low renal vascular resistance results in a filtration fraction that is far below normal.[25-27]

The absence of RBCs in the perfusion also leads to the spontaneous necrosis of some tubular cells in the medullary thick ascending limb (mTAL) segment.[25-27] Thus, severe tubular injury occurs in the IPK even in the absence of any toxic exposure. The low filtration fraction of the IPK and injury to mTAL segments of the tubule contributes to an abnormally high fractional excretion of sodium (see Table 43-1). In addition, abnormal mTAL function and "washout" of urea in the medulla impairs the ability of the IPK perfused without RBCs to concentrate the urine.

When the IPK is perfused with a RBC-containing perfusate, many of these problems are ameliorated. The presence

TABLE 43-2

Studies of Nephrotoxins Using the Isolated Perfused Kidney

NEPHROTOXIN	CHAPTER REFERENCE(S)
Contrast-induced nephropathy	19, 67, 68
Cyclosporin	69-71
Paracetamol	72-74
Pentamidine	75
High-energy shock waves	76, 77
Cold injury	78-80
Myoglobinuric acute renal failure	81, 82
Endotoxin	83, 84

of RBCs increases the viscosity of the perfusate so that renal vascular resistance is higher, and closer to normal.[26,28] The presence of RBCs also greatly improves oxygen delivery to all nephron segments, so that necrosis of tubular cells of the mTAL is prevented, the fractional excretion of sodium (FeNa) is reduced, and the concentrating ability is improved.[26,28] However, use of the RBC-perfused IPK has been limited by the inconvenience and expense of the procedure.

The advantages and disadvantages of the IPK as a model of studying toxic injury to the kidney are summarized in Table 43-1. Despite the problems intrinsic to this model, the IPK has been used to elucidate a number of areas of renal toxicology, some examples of which are listed in Table 43-2.

Renal Tissue Slices

Renal tissue slices have been used as experimental models of toxic injury for more than two decades.[29,30] Tissue slices allow the analysis of cellular, molecular, and biochemical endpoints without altering the architecture of the kidney. When first introduced, tissue slices were cut by hand, limiting the ability both to produce slices thin enough to ensure adequate oxygenation and to produce tissue slices of comparable thickness. The usefulness of the model was greatly improved by the introduction of mechanical devices that produce "precision-cut" slices of renal cortex; such slices are thin enough (200-300 μm) to permit adequate oxygen and nutrient diffusion throughout with minimal variation in thickness from slice to slice.[31,32]

A number of methods can be used for maintenance of the tissue slices.[31,32] The most effective system currently available is "dynamic roller culture," in which tissue slices are placed on titanium screens held within cylindrical titanium holders, which are placed in 25-mL liquid scintillation vials. Oxygenated nutrient medium is added to each scintillation vial; the vials are placed in an incubator (37° C; 5%O_2/5%CO_2) that constantly rotates them, facilitating oxygenation and nutrition of the tissue slices.[31,32]

Renal cortical slices have been used to examine the mechanisms of many nephrotoxins and for a wide range of toxicological endpoints (Table 43-3). The major limitation of this model is its finite lifespan, up to 48 hours. Additional information regarding the use of kidney slices for the study of toxicants can be found elsewhere.[32]

TABLE 43-3

The Use of Renal Slices to Study Nephrotoxins

NEPHROTOXIN	ENDPOINT(S) STUDIED	CHAPTER REFERENCE(S)
Gentamicin	Enzyme leakage, organic ion accumulation, lipid peroxidation, glutathione content, toxicant accumulation	85-87
Cephaloridine		87
Cisplatin	Platinum accumulation and biotransformation, histology, cell ATP	3, 88. 89, 90
1,2 Dichloropropane	Morphology, intracellular K^+, cell ATP, toxicant accumulation	91
Cyclosporin	Metabolism	92
Mercury	Lipid peroxidation, glutathione content, toxicant accumulation	87, 93-97
Oxidant injury	LDH release, lipid peroxidation, PAH uptake, intracellular calcium, Na^+, K^+-ATPase activity	98
Carbon tetrachloride	Lipid peroxidation, glutathione content, toxicant accumulation	99, 100
Atractyloside	Membrane dye exclusion, lipid peroxidation, enzyme leakage, glutathione content, gluconeogenesis	101-103
Acetaminophen	Cell viability, covalent binding, PAH accumulation	104, 105
Hexachlorobutadiene	Lipid peroxidation, glutathione content, toxicant accumulation	87
Arsenate	Intracellular K^+, HSP expression, toxicant accumulation, glutathione content, cell signaling, gene expression	93, 106
Chloronitrobenzene	Enzyme leakage, gluconeogenesis, LDH release	107
Benzo(a)pyrene	Intracellular K^+, cell ATP, gene expression	108
Chloroform	Accumulation of organic ions (PAH and tetraethyl ammonium)	99, 100

ATP, adenosine triphosphate; LDH, lactic dehydrogenase; PAH, p-aminohippurate.

NEPHRON COMPONENTS AS MODELS OF TOXIC INJURY

The pathogenesis of toxic ARF is associated with a complex interplay among vascular, tubular, and inflammatory factors. In addition to allowing study of the effects of toxins within the context of the whole animal, models are needed in which the direct effects on toxins on tubular cells can be studied. The use of isolated glomeruli and nephron segments (tubules) has been useful in identifying mechanisms of site-specific toxicity within the kidney.[32] Studies of isolated nephron components complement studies of renal toxicology in vivo by eliminating the effects of extraneous factors, such as blood flow, endocrine effects, and disposition of the toxin.

Suspensions of Isolated Proximal Tubules

In vitro preparations of isolated proximal tubules have been useful for the examination of nephrotoxins because the preparations retain the biochemical properties of the in vivo state as well as the structural integrity of the polarized and normally differentiated proximal tubular epithelium. Freshly isolated proximal tubules provide a powerful system for defining cellular events in response to tubular injury; they completely retain the fully differentiated phenotype as it exists in vivo but are accessible for direct experimental manipulations and measurements.

In vitro preparations of isolated proximal tubules have been widely used for a variety of metabolic and physiological investigations for more than three decades and have also been employed extensively for studies of tubular cell injury for more than two decades.[32] Isolation of proximal tubules from kidneys of rabbits or rats can be achieved by either mechanical or enzymatic disruption of the tissue followed by density-gradient centrifugation using Ficoll or Percoll.[33-35]

Table 43-4 lists examples of studies in which isolated proximal tubular preparations have been used for the study of nephrotoxins.

TABLE 43-4

Studies of Nephrotoxins Using Isolated Proximal Tubular Segments

NEPHROTOXIN	ENDPOINT(S) STUDIED	CHAPTER REFERENCE(S)
Gentamicin	Enzyme leakage, energy metabolism	47, 109
Heavy metals (mercury, cadmium, chromium)	Protein synthesis, lipid peroxidation	110
Oxidant injury	Plasma membrane permeability, mitochondrial function	111
Radiocontrast	Glomerular filtration rate, tubular morphology	19
Hydroquinones	Glutathione, mitochondrial function, cell viability	112, 113
Butadienes	Mitochondrial respiration, lactic dehydrogenase release	114
Bromobenzene	Glutathione levels, mitochondrial respiration, cell viability	115
Dichorovinyl-L-cysteine (DCVC)	Cell viability, sodium transport, oxygen consumption, glucose transport	54
Atractyloside	Enzyme leakage, mitochondrial function, adenosine triphosphate, cell glutathione, p-aminohippurate transport	101, 102

TABLE 43-5

The Use of Isolated Glomeruli for Toxicology Studies

NEPHROTOXIN	ENDPOINT(S) STUDIES	CHAPTER REFERENCE(S)
Gentamicin	Morphology; organic anion transport	116
Cyclosporin	Albumin permeability, ultrafiltration coefficient (Kf), glomerular volume, glomerular contraction	41, 42, 117, 118
Oxidant injury	Albumin permeability, reactive oxygen species, metallothioneins, antioxidants	37-39, 119-123
Metals (mercury, cadmium, copper, zinc, manganese, nickel, cobalt)	Morphology, metabolism, protein and proteoglycan synthesis, glutathione levels, fatty acid synthesis, renin release, enzyme leakage, mitochondrial activity, dye exclusion	110, 124-126
Immunosuppressive drugs	Glomerular contractility	118
Uranyl nitrate	Eicosanoid synthesis	127
Adriamycin	Glucose metabolism, superoxide production	128-130
Irradiation	Arachidonic acid and prostaglandin release, albumin permeability	40

Isolated Glomeruli

Two methods have been used successfully to isolate glomeruli. One relies on the fact that the glomerulus is larger than any other part of the nephron subunit and can be isolated by filtering through screens with pores large enough to allow tubular segments to pass through (and be eliminated) while capturing the glomeruli.[36] An alternative approach is to perfuse the kidney with particles of iron oxide, which become trapped within glomeruli, and then to separate the glomeruli from other tissue fragments by means of a magnetic stir bar.[32,36]

Isolated glomeruli are typically studied in suspension at concentrations of 0.5 to 1.0 μg total protein per mL. The glomeruli are incubated in cell culture medium at 37° C, with gentle agitation. The advantage of using isolated renal glomeruli is that they conserve the architecture of this region of the kidney while being free of any extraneous vascular, nervous, or humoral influences derived from other regions of the kidney.

Several groups have developed methods that allow the assessment of the effect of toxins and other interventions on the permeability of the glomerular basement membrane and on glomerular contractility.[37-43] The effect of toxicants on glomerular contraction (which is induced by mesangial cells) can be assessed by computer-assisted measurements of glomerular volume before and after application of the toxin.[37-45] Examples of studies in which isolated glomeruli have been used to study nephrotoxins are listed in Table 43-5.

CULTURED RENAL TUBULAR CELLS

Cell cultures have been used extensively to study the effects of many nephrotoxins, including gentamicin,[46] cisplatin,[47,48] oxidant injury,[49] S-(1,2-dichlorovinyl)-L-cysteine (DCVC),[50] and cyclosporin.[51]

Primary Cultures

Compared with continuous cell lines, primary cultures in general have been shown to be closer to cells in vivo.[52] Primary cultures are superior to proximal tubular renal cell lines in maintenance of oxidative phosphorylation,

cellular polarity, brush-border enzymes, and the activity of transport functions. In addition, although many renal cell lines are highly resistance to ischemic and toxic injury, the susceptibility of primary cultures to injury has been reported to more closely resemble that of renal tubules in vivo.[53]

The techniques used for primary culture of tubules have been described in detail elsewhere.[54-56] Primary cultured cells usually die after a finite number of cell divisions (passages).[57] In addition, cells in primary culture undergo a number of phenotypic changes, many of which represent adaptations to growth in culture conditions.

Primary cultures of cells have some disadvantages as models of toxic injury. For example, although proximal tubules in vivo depend almost entirely on oxidative phosphorylation for their source of adenosine triphosphate, primary cultures of proximal tubular cells express high activities of glycolytic enzymes. The high glycolytic capacity of proximal tubular cells in culture has been ascribed to adaptation of the cells to the relatively hypoxic conditions of the cell culture system[58] and results in a relative resistance of these cells, compared with proximal cells in vivo, to the effects of ischemic and toxic injury.

Another disadvantage of all primary cultured cells is that they must be prepared repeatedly from fresh tissue each time cells are needed,[52] as opposed to continuous and immortalized cell lines, which can be maintained for many generations and offer the potential for greater convenience and reproducibility.

Continuous and Immortalized Cell Lines

The inconvenience of primary cell culture has led to a search for more suitable cell culture models. Some continuous renal cell lines are available that originated from normal tissue and formed continuous cultures "spontaneously" without any specific intervention. Many of the continuous cell lines used in renal toxicology are available at repositories such as the American Type Culture Collection (ATCC), in Manassas, VA, and the European Collection of Cell Cultures, in the UK.

Two continuous cell lines have been widely used for renal toxicology studies, the LLC-PK1 cell line (derived from the renal cortex of a pig)[59,60] and the MDCK (Madine Darby canine kidney) line.[61] These cell lines are free of microbial and viral contaminants, have retained a diploid number of chromosomes, and do not form tumors in immunosuppressed laboratory animals.[59,61] Both LLC-PK1 and MDCK cell lines grow rapidly and can be passaged easily for many generations in monolayer cultures. LLC-PK1 and MDCK cell lines are epithelial in nature. They are polarized and contain tight junctions.[59] Both cell lines also form "domes," fluid-filled blisters that result from the presence of water and solute transport, the presence of tight junctions, and adhesion of the cells to the substratum.[62]

LLC-PK1 cells share many of characteristics of proximal tubular cells in vivo, including an apical membrane microvilli, high activities of apical membrane enzymes, and expression of parathyroid hormone receptors and sodium-dependent glucose transporters.[59,63] In contrast, MDCK cells have characteristics more typical of distal tubular cells; they express vasopressin, oxytocin, and prostaglandin receptors, which when stimulated activate adenylate cyclase.[52]

However, because cell lines (especially those from humans) rarely arise spontaneously, investigators have developed a number of novel techniques to immortalize cells in culture. The most reliable method currently available for developing immortalized cell lines involves the transfection of cells with genes derived from viruses such as the simian virus (the 40 large T antigen), papilloma viruses, adenoviruses, herpesvirus, and the human T-cell leukemia virus.[64-66]

MOLECULAR BIOLOGICAL TECHNIQUES IN NEPHROTOXICOLOGY RESEARCH

As in most other areas of biological research, the rapid development of molecular biological techniques has been extremely important in advancing the field of toxicology research, a few of which are mentioned here. The availability of "knockout" and transgenic animals provides a powerful tool for examining the roles of specific genes in the effects of nephrotoxins in vivo. For many years, the ability to transfect cultured cells with mutants of DNA that produce "dominant negative" and "constitutively active" proteins has provided a useful technique to study the effect of toxins on kinase cascades and other enzymatic systems. The later development of small interfering RNA (siRNA) has led to specific techniques to "knock down" the expression of genes and to examine the role of genes in the effects of toxicants on the kidney. Finally, the development of the gene microarray allows the examination of the effects of toxicants on global gene expression both in vivo and in vitro.

Key Points

1. The kidney is highly susceptible to the adverse effects of toxic substances as a result of multiple factors, owing to the high exposure of kidneys to potential toxins because of the disproportionate blood flow received by the kidney.
2. High concentrations of toxins can accumulate in proximal tubules, which play an important role in eliminating blood-borne toxins by excreting them into proximal tubular fluid.
3. In vivo models in animals are extremely important in studying the effects of nephrotoxins on the kidney. However, only a few toxins that cause acute tubular necrosis in humans can induce renal injury and dysfunction in animals.
4. Because acute renal failure in humans is often the result of the effects of combined toxins, models of "multiple-insult" acute renal failure should be developed to allow study of nephrotoxins.
5. Interventions that ameliorate acute renal failure in rats or mice have not been effective in ameliorating acute tubular necrosis in humans. Investigators should develop models using animals such as the pig, that have kidneys with anatomical and physiological features closer to those of human kidneys.
6. The isolated perfused kidney is a convenient model for examining effects of toxins on the intact kidney independent of extraneous extrarenal factors. However, the specific advantages and disadvantages of this model as an experimental tool must be understood.
7. Isolated enthrone fragments, such as proximal tubular segments and glomeruli, continue to be useful models for studying the effect of toxins on discrete renal cell types.
8. Renal cells in culture are extremely valuable in toxicological studies. The relative advantages and disadvantages of primary cultures and continuous cell lines should be understood before a model is chosen for a specific experiment.
9. Molecular biological advances—including knockout and transgenic animals, transfection of mutant DNA, knockdown experiments using small interfering RNA, and the availability of the study of gene expression by gene microarray—can be used in multiple models and have contributed greatly to the information gained from in vivo and in vitro studies in renal toxicology.

Key References

See the companion Expert Consult website for the complete reference list.

CHAPTER 44

Animal Models of Septic Acute Renal Failure

Christoph Langenberg, Li Wan, Clive N. May, and Rinaldo Bellomo

---

OBJECTIVES

This chapter will:
1. Review the literature on animal models of sepsis containing information on renal function and on animal models of acute renal failure induced by sepsis.
2. Describe the limitations and clinical relevance of published models.
3. Suggest ways in which animal models can be improved.
4. Discuss the possible lessons that can be derived from such models with regard to septic acute renal failure in humans.

Acute renal failure (ARF) affects approximately 6% of patients admitted to intensive care units.[1] Sepsis and septic shock are the most common predisposing factors for the development of ARF in this setting.[2-6] Furthermore, among septic patients, the incidence of ARF is high,[5,7] as is its mortality.[2,3,8-11] Although little is known about the pathogenesis of ARF in sepsis, it is thought that renal hemodynamics play a key role during the onset of ARF—for example, renal hypoperfusion followed by renal ischemia. At present, however, the assessment of renal blood flow (RBF) in septic patients can be done only by invasive means. Thus, only very few studies, none of them a controlled study, have been performed in humans. The understanding of septic ARF is, therefore, limited. Most of the data relied on for the understanding of septic ARF stem from various animal models. Accordingly, it is vital for clinicians to appreciate the features of septic ARF models, their applicability to the human setting, and their limitations.

INDUCTION OF SEPTIC ACUTE RENAL FAILURE

There are different ways of inducing septic acute renal failure. The most commonly used method is the administration of lipopolysaccharides, also called endotoxins. Lipopolysaccharide (LPS) is a part of the outer membrane of gram-negative bacteria. It consists of three parts: lipid A, a core polysaccharide, and a long O antigen.[12] Probably the most important reasons for the popular use of LPS are that it can be purchased in a standardized form from commercial vendors and that its dose-related effect is almost stable and predictable compared with that of infused live bacteria. LPS can be injected as a bolus or as a continuous infusion, intravenously, subcutaneously, or intraperitone-

ally. Although this method of induction is commonly used, it has major flaws. LPS administration often leads to a hypodynamic circulatory state with low blood pressure and *decreased* cardiac output. In comparison, septic patients in intensive care units around the world have a markedly increased cardiac output and low blood pressure, a so-called hyperdynamic circulatory state.[13] The different hemodynamic profile induced by LPS may be due to a cytokine release pattern different from that seen in septic humans.[14] However, in such hypodynamic models, it might be difficult to determine whether renal dysfunction results from the reduced cardiac output or the effects of sepsis on the kidney per se. Because of this mixing of cardiogenic and septic shock in one model, it may provide misleading information about the pathogenesis of septic acute kidney injury.

Another method to induce sepsis is the administration of live bacteria. Typically, *Escherichia coli* and *Pseudomonas aeruginosa* are used as the bacteria of choice. A standardized preparation of bacteria is more problematic than one of LPS because the concentration and virulence of the organisms must be measured to obtain reproducibility. In addition, only a few conditions in humans (e.g., endocarditis) are associated with almost constant bacteremia. In most other septic states, bacteremia is episodic. However, with this method of induction, it appears more likely that one can induce a hyperdynamic circulatory state, as seen in septic humans, with live bacteria.

The most realistic method to induce sepsis might be the cecal ligation and perforation technique. During a surgical procedure, the cecum is located and ligated just distal to the ileocecal valve so that bowel continuity is preserved. In addition, the cecum is then punctured with a needle, and feces are extracted into the peritoneum. The animal has acute polymicrobial peritonitis leading to sepsis. Although anesthesia and the surgical procedure itself might be strong confounding factors in the development of septic ARF, this model of induction seems closer to the clinical reality.

DIFFERENT ANIMALS

Studies to assess renal function and the development of septic ARF have been undertaken in various kinds of animals, from mice to primates, in small and large animals. Conducting hemodynamic studies in small animals might not be ideal for several reasons; for example, because cardiac output is often difficult to assess and because intravascular volume might already have been decreased by the taking of several blood samples. In addition, organ blood flow, in this case RBF, is very small—7.5 mL/min in rats[15] compared with 250 mL/min in sheep[16]—so the changes occurring in septic ARF might also be very small in a rat.

Accuracy of measurement and ability to detect relatively small changes are diminished. These factors could easily influence the precision and accuracy of measurements and calculations of other variables related to renal function. Therefore, not surprisingly, a systematic review regarding renal vascular resistance in septic ARF showed that vasoconstriction in the renal vascular bed was more likely to occur in small animals, such as mice, rats, and rabbits, than in large animals, such as dogs, sheep, pigs, and primates.[17] Given that the human is a large animal, these observations raise concerns about the applicability and external validity of the observations made in such small animal studies.

CARDIAC OUTPUT CONFOUNDING ACUTE RENAL FAILURE

As mentioned earlier, the most commonly observed systemic hemodynamic state in septic patients is a hyperdynamic circulatory state with a marked increase in cardiac output. To mimic the clinical setting closely, it would therefore be desirable to have animal models with a similar systemic hemodynamic response. Cardiac output is an important confounding factor, at least regarding the renal vascular tone in septic ARF, such that an increase in this parameter predicts decreased or unchanged renal vascular resistance. Accordingly, with decreased cardiac output as in hypodynamic shock, the renal vascular resistance tends to rise, leading to reduced RBF.[17]

RECOVERY BETWEEN PREPARATION SURGERY AND CONDUCTION OF STUDIES

Before the actual experimental study is conducted, animals must undergo a preparation surgical procedure for implantation of flow probes and/or catheters or to prepare the cecal ligation and perforation method. It is well known that anesthesia might have an impact on blood pressure as well as on cardiac output. Because the systemic hemodynamic state is altered, it is difficult to distinguish between effects of the hypodynamic state induced by surgery and anesthesia on renal function and the changes in renal function due to sepsis. Unfortunately, studies vary greatly in having (or not having) a recovery period between surgery and the performance of the study or starting of the assessment of data immediately after the procedure. They also vary in terms of the duration of such recovery periods. This fact makes the already heterogeneous data even more variable. Ideally, experiments should be conducted a week or so after any required surgical procedures, once animals have fully recovered from the operation.

TECHNIQUE OF FUNCTIONAL ASSESSMENT

The outcome of any experimental study depends on the technique used to assess the desired function. As mentioned earlier, there is a paradigm that renal hypoperfu-

sion in septic ARF causes ischemia, which is followed by acute tubular necrosis. Such a paradigm presupposes that measurement of RBF is technically uniform, easy, reproducible, accurate, and precise—which is not true. In fact, there are different ways to measure RBF in animals. The direct measurement, with transit-time flow-probes implanted around the renal arteries, can measure blood flow continuously. In addition, indirect techniques such as the injection of microspheres or the measurement of para-aminohippuric acid clearance are used as well. The advantage of performing the microsphere technique is that the experimental animals do not have to undergo surgery. The method poses the problem, however, that only a few "snapshots" of organ blood flow during the time of injection are available, because continuous assessment is not possible. Not surprisingly, different approaches to measure RBF show different results in septic ARF; for example, studies using direct measurements were more likely to assess a decreased or unchanged renal vascular resistance. Studies using indirect techniques showed a reduced RBF more frequently.[17]

ANIMAL MODELS OF SEPTIC ACUTE RENAL FAILURE

Unfortunately, sepsis is often discovered with delay in patients cared for on general wards because the initial signs can be nonspecific (e.g., elevated temperature, increased heart rate, decreased blood pressure). Usually, it takes a certain time to notice and to completely develop a full septic state. In order to mimic the clinic more closely, it is therefore desirable that animal models involve allowing a longer period for the development of septic ARF instead of observing animals for a short time. Only few studies have been performed over longer periods (>24 hours) in large animals with a hyperdynamic state as seen in humans.

Cumming and associates[18] first induced sepsis in sheep with use of the cecal ligation and perforation method. This group found a marked decrease in GFR (70%) although the renal plasma flow remained stable.[18] The renal plasma flow was indirectly assessed by means of radioactive labeled para-aminohippuric acid clearance. Particularly in the septic setting, this technique has major flaws owing to an inconstant renal excretion rate for para-aminohippuric acid. In addition, this study lacked a control group. Two other studies showed an increase in RBF once a hyperdynamic state developed after 24 hours in the surviving animals.[19,20] These studies were uncontrolled in design as well. A later controlled study demonstrated a fourfold rise in serum creatinine concentration within 2 days, although there was renal hyperemia. In this experimental setting, RBF increased threefold.[16] Actually, these studies provide proof that it is possible to induce development of ARF in the setting of renal hyperemia. This proof contradicts the paradigm that renal ischemia is necessary for ARF followed by acute tubular necrosis to occur in sepsis.

In fact, owing to the complications arising from the performance of biopsies in septic patients, only a few studies have been performed to assess renal histopathology in this setting. However, Hotchkiss and colleagues,[21] performing postmortem examinations of 12 patients with septic ARF, reported that only 1 of the 12 showed signs of acute tubular necrosis. The remaining 11 renal histologic analyses did not reflect the severity of renal injury indi-

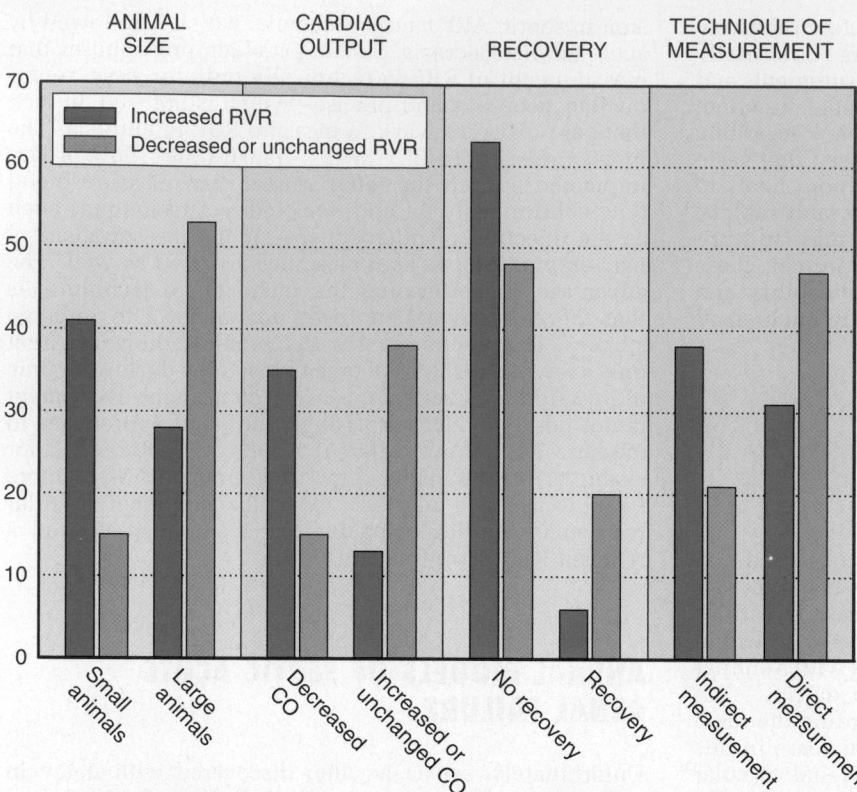

FIGURE 44-1. Bar graph illustrating the confounding effect of variables on renal vascular resistance (RVR) in 137 animal studies. All differences between the corresponding subgroups are significant ($P < .05$). (From Langenberg C, Bellomo R, May CN, et al: Renal vascular resistance in sepsis. Nephron Physiol 2006;104:1-11.)

cated by loss of function.[21] In a second study, 57 biopsies were performed in infectious or hypovolemic patients. Only four of these biopsy specimens showed signs of acute tubular necrosis.[22]

GENERAL CONSIDERATIONS

Our knowledge about the pathogenesis of septic ARF is derived mainly from animal studies because there is almost no information about the pathophysiology of septic ARF in humans. The animal models used to simulate sepsis are extraordinarily heterogeneous in design, techniques of measurement, and execution. Therefore, not surprisingly, there are many unsolved problems and even contradictory results from the use of models with different approaches. Figure 44-1 illustrates the confounding factors in renal vascular resistance in 137 animal studies. It demonstrates how important it is that these confounding factors be taken into account before a study is begun. Figure 44-2 is a comprehensive overview of the confounding factors that can alter RBF. However, the final result in all of those models of septic ARF, whether the RBF is increased or decreased, is impairment of renal function,

As in every animal model, it seems important that it mimic the clinical situation as closely as possible and that investigators be aware of critical confounding factors (animal size, recovery after surgery, cardiac output, technique to assess blood flow; see Figs. 44-1 and 44-2). It seems crucial to take all of these aspects of a given septic model into account when assessing its relevance to human disease. The models developed so far remain highly imperfect and have not yet been shown to predict the response of humans to a particular treatment. Their clinical relevance remains uncertain.

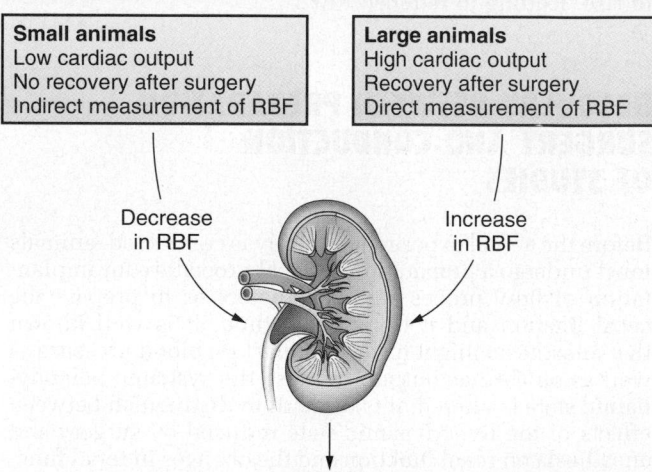

FIGURE 44-2. The confounding effects of certain variables in animal studies on renal blood flow. Although renal blood flow (RBF) is either increased or decreased, renal function is still impaired.

Key Points

1. Animal models of sepsis with acute renal failure are markedly heterogeneous, with great variability in extent of monitoring, animal size, systemic hemodynamics, duration of recovery after surgery, and technique of assessment of renal blood flow.
2. Animal models of true septic acute renal failure with prolonged observation (>24 hours) and clear sustained loss of glomerular filtration rate are

very few and do not show any evidence of acute tubular necrosis.
3. The limitations of published animal models of septic acute renal failure are substantial.
4. The clinical relevance of published models is limited.
5. Animal models can and should be improved with observation lasting at least 48 hours, simultaneous measurement of cardiac output and blood pressure and simulation of the typical clinical scenario of septic ARF.
6. The possible lessons that can be derived from such models with regard to septic acute renal failure in humans are few because no findings from such models have later been shown to predict events or effects in humans.

Key References

13. Parker MM, Shelhamer JH, Natanson C, et al: Serial cardiovascular variables in survivors and nonsurvivors of human septic shock: Heart rate as an early predictor of prognosis. Crit Care Med 1987;15:923-929.
14. Miyaji T, Hu X, Yuen PS, et al: Ethyl pyruvate decreases sepsis-induced acute renal failure and multiple organ damage in aged mice. Kidney Int 2003;64:1620-1631.
16. Langenberg C, Wan L, Egi M, et al: Renal blood flow in experimental septic acute renal failure. Kidney Int 2006;69:1996-2002.
17. Langenberg C, Bellomo R, May CN, et al: Renal vascular resistance in sepsis. Nephron Physiol 2006;104:1-11.
18. Cumming AD, Driedger AA, McDonald JW, et al: Vasoactive hormones in the renal response to systemic sepsis. Am J Kidney Dis 1988;11:23-32.

See the companion Expert Consult website for the complete reference list.

CHAPTER 45

Critical Assessment of Animal Models of Acute Renal Failure

Samuel N. Heyman, Christian Rosenberger, and Seymour Rosen

OBJECTIVES

This chapter will:
1. Underscore the limited data available regarding the pathophysiology and morphological features of the human syndrome of acute kidney injury.
2. Present the general principles for appropriateness of animal models.
3. Outline basic principles of and guidelines for, and describe common pitfalls specifically relevant to, animal models of acute kidney injury.
4. Address specific limitations of different classes of acute kidney injury models—hypoxic, toxic, and septic.

Therapeutic approaches developed in animal models of acute kidney injury (AKI) have repeatedly proved nonapplicable to prevention and treatment of human AKI. These failures serve to illustrate that our understanding of AKI is imperfect and suggest that the animal models used may inadequately represent the human syndrome.

Human AKI is not a single disease. It is a constellation of clinical events that define renal dysfunction of acute onset caused by a multiplicity of ischemic, toxic, and inflammatory factors that may or may not overlap. Furthermore, individuals differ in their propensity to development of AKI under seemingly comparable conditions, indicating the importance of predisposing factors, including genetic propensity and acquired comorbidities.

In human AKI, morphological and functional derangements arc poorly defined. Our understanding of the human syndrome is limited for several reasons. First, the initial clinical presentation of AKI is most often subtle and the disorder is diagnosed later, at its established phase.[1] Second, the renal physiology, including glomerular and tubular functions and the nonhomogeneous pattern of microcirculation and oxygenation, is highly complex and difficult to trace: Whereas current critical care settings allow continuous monitoring of hemodynamics and cardiopulmonary function, technologies that enable repeated, real-time, noninvasive monitoring of such renal physiological parameters are not available. Third, we cannot clearly dissect the effect of true morphological damage from that of pure, nonstructural functional derangement; in other words, we cannot currently identify with certainty evolving renal cell damage and its location at a given time. Last, our knowledge of the human pathology of AKI and its functional correlations is markedly limited: Biopsies are seldom performed; when they are, specimens are of limited volume, most often not containing deep structures, and each represents only one time point along the evolution of AKI. Autopsies also reveal only one stage, usually at the late established or recovery phase of AKI, so that transient or reversible changes are not observable. Furthermore, with the exception of the predialysis era, data regarding the human whole-organ pathology of AKI are limited and based on small series that often lack functional covariants.

Thus, *many of our current concepts are derived not from human data but from experimental AKI and may therefore be erroneous.* For that reason, animal models should

TABLE 45-1

Examples of Advanced Experimental Technologies in the Assessment of Acute Kidney Injury

OBJECTIVES	TECHNOLOGY*	DETAILS	INVASIVENESS	CONTINUOUS REAL-TIME TRACINGS
Determination of renal microcirculation	Laser Doppler needle flow probes[28]	Assessment at selected regions of interest	++	+++
	Dynamic two-photon microscopy[13]	Direct visualization of microcirculation, blood elements, and permeability, restricted to the renal cortex	+++	++
Determination of renal oxygenation	Oxygen microelectrodes[30]	Assessment of selected regions of interest	++	+++
	Dual-wavelength phosphorimetry[14]	Assessment restricted to cortex and outer medulla	+	+++
	Blood oxygenation level–dependent (BOLD) magnetic resonance imaging (MRI)[16]	Spatial assessment of deoxygenated hemoglobin in the kidney. Not applicable for the papilla	0	++
	Immunostaining for hypoxia marker (pimonidazole)[20]	Spatial distribution of severe hypoxia (hypoxia marker pimonidazole), and tissue hypoxia response (hypoxia-inducible factors)	0	0
Determination of renal energy stores	Phosphorus MRI[17]	Detection of renal adenosine triphosphate content	0	++
Determination of glomerular filtration rate and tubular function	Dendrimeric MRI[19]	Detects early changes in contrast agent clearance and urine concentration	0	++
Determination of tubular function	Sodium MRI[18]	Detects early changes in Na$^+$ corticomedullary gradient, reflecting urine-concentrating capacity	0	++
Determination of acute tubular damage	KIM-1 (kidney injury molecule-1), Cyr61 (cysteine-rich angiogenic inducer 61), and other urinary biomarkers	Urinary markers of tubular injury; most markers are selective to proximal tubules	0	0
	ApoSense[21]	Molecular imaging of apoptosis/necrosis	0	0 (+ if radiolabeled)

+, mild; ++, moderate; +++, marked.
*Superscript numbers indicate chapter references.

resemble relevant clinical conditions and must provide both functional and morphological data. However, we should be aware that human and animal kidneys differ functionally and structurally. Furthermore, kidney function evaluated under experimental settings is often restricted to the assessment of the ultimate outcome of glomerular filtration rate, and data on tubular function, intrarenal microcirculation, oxygenation cell metabolism, and morphology are lacking. Some deficiencies are related to technological limitations of real-time functional and structural assessment. Substantial technical progress, briefly presented in Table 45-1, has been introduced in this field, but for the time being, complex functional data are lacking to some extent in the majority of models of AKI. Not surprisingly, limited understanding leads to erroneous conclusions and to misconceptions, ending with frustrating clinical failures of preventive modalities despite their proven effectiveness in probably inadequate animal models.

As shown in Figure 45-1, animal AKI models may consist of an acute hypoxic or toxic insult and additional components that can be controlled for. Inactivation or enhancement of renal defense and adaptive mechanisms, the induction of clinically relevant predisposing condi-

tions, selection of genetically susceptible animals, direct interventions affecting the renal vasculature or cellular injury, and systemic support may all be incorporated in these models.

This chapter addresses various categories of animal- or whole-organ models of AKI. Prerequisites for experimental models of AKI are outlined both generally and specifically for the particular model classes. Many concepts discussed here originate from two expert opinion meetings, held during the second Acute Dialysis Quality Initiative meeting in Vicenza in 2002[2] and the American Society of Nephrology Acute Renal Failure retreat in Washington, DC, in 2004.[3]

MECHANISTIC CLASSIFICATION OF ANIMAL MODELS OF ACUTE KIDNEY INJURY

Like human AKI, animal models have been divided into nephrotoxic (e.g., due to gentamicin or heavy metals), hypoxic AKI (e.g., due to profound hemorrhagic shock),

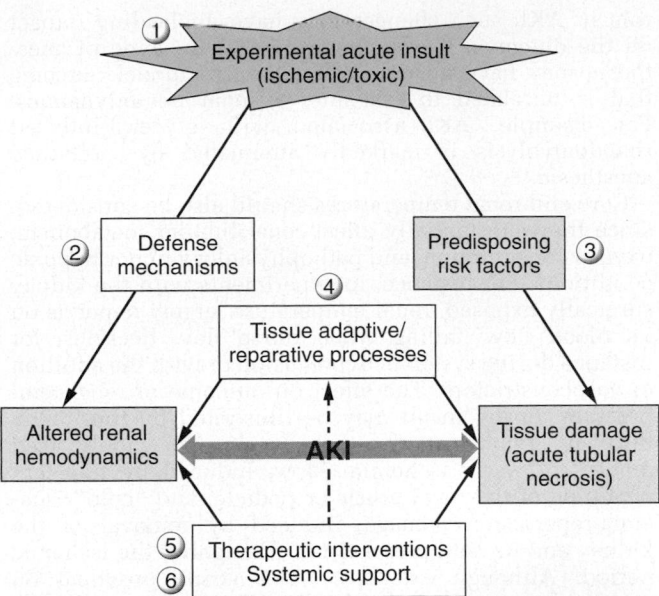

FIGURE 45-1. Determinants of experimental acute kidney injury (AKI). Acute ischemic or toxic insult may lead to AKI by direct cellular injury, via altered renal hemodynamics, or through the integrated association of these two factors. Inherent defense mechanisms and adaptive responses preserve tissue oxygenation and integrity, often at the price of altered hemodynamics and reduced glomerular filtration rate. Predisposing factors for AKI either are characterized by defective defense mechanisms or directly intensify the acute hypoxic or toxic insult.

Experimental AKI models contain one or more of these elements: Some of the acute insults (*1*) may lead to experimental AKI specifically when extreme—for example, prolonged global interruption of renal blood flow (warm ischemia-reflow) or an enormously high dose of a nephrotoxin (gentamicin model). AKI models may be produced with a more modest acute hypoxic or toxic insult if it is combined with the inactivation of defense mechanisms (*2*), such as the inhibition of prostaglandin or nitric oxide synthase. Acute insult may also be combined with a perturbation that directly predisposes to a more pronounced hypoxic or toxic effect (*3*), for instance, cis-platinum toxicity in salt-depleted animals. Experimental AKI may be modulated by interference with or augmentation of intrinsic adaptive or reparative processes (*4*), such as upregulation of hypoxia-inducible factors (HIFs), or by application of other direct interventions (*5*), such as the administration of vasoactive agents (restoring hemodynamics), fluids or alkali (reducing the concentration and retention of the nephrotoxin), or antioxidants (attenuating direct cellular injury and restoring altered microcirculation). Supportive treatment (*6*), such as fluids, antibiotics, and cardiorespiratory assistance, may be needed to extend the viability of the model until AKI develops and to appropriately mimic clinical scenarios.

and septic models. This classification is somewhat artificial, because in humans and animal models, a mixed type of AKI most often exists, in which components of all three mechanisms are involved. Typical toxic AKI, such as cis-platinum, heavy metal, or gentamicin nephropathy, is believed to be mediated primarily through direct tubular cell toxicity, documented principally in in vitro experimental settings. Renal handling of the toxin predominantly determines the distribution pattern of tubular damage. The injury is predictably dose-dependent and consistent, and the contribution of predisposing factors is relatively marginal, with the exception of the state of hydration.

Hypoxic AKI resulting from global renal ischemia and reflow is also highly consistent and reproducible beyond a certain ischemic period.[4] In contrast, hypoxic experimental AKI in more "physiological" models of renal hypoperfusion reflects a clinical spectrum ranging from prerenal azotemia (i.e., reduced glomerular filtration rate [GFR] without overt morphologic damage) to frank AKI. The relative contribution of these pathophysiological problems to the functional derangement is often difficult to assess, as in clinical practice, and the models show marked variability. Furthermore, as in the human syndrome, functional derangement and the induction of tubular damage in these models require the introduction of predisposing factors, such as endothelial dysfunction.

AKI models most often exert both nephrotoxic and hypoxic insults. For instance, amphotericin induces tubular cell membrane injury but at the same time applies profound renal vasoconstriction.[5] AKI in models of pigment nephropathy (myoglobinuria/hemoglobinuria) also consists of direct tubulotoxicity affecting proximal tubules (in which filtered pigment has been reabsorbed and degraded, liberating noxious free iron), together with tubular obstruction (by pigment casts) and hypoxic injury (mediated in part by altered renal microcirculation).[6] Most often, one mechanism of renal injury leads to the other: Radiocontrast agents primarily alter renal parenchymal oxygenation with subsequent hypoxic damage. Subsequent formation of reactive oxygen species leads to both endothelial dysfunction (perpetuating further hypoxic insult) and a secondary tubulotoxic effect. Inversely, primary nephrotoxic injury, as with cis-platinum, may evolve into a secondary hypoxic injury related to disturbance of outer medullary microcirculation.

Extrarenal risk factors also play an important role in AKI. Some, like diabetes, aging, and hyperlipidemia, may predispose to endothelial dysfunction and hypoxic injury.[7] Others, characterized by effective blood volume depletion, may enhance tubular intraluminal concentrations and prolong the transit time of noxious agents, such as myoglobin and radiocontrast agents. Most importantly, a cross-talk based on cytokines and inflammatory cells exists between organs during AKI in models such as rhabdomyolysis and sepsis. The isolated perfused kidney model of AKI may be used to exclude such systemic effects and to explore independent intrarenal processes.

GENERAL PRINCIPLES FOR APPROPRIATENESS OF ANIMAL MODELS

As outlined by Piper and colleagues,[8] some basic principles should be taken into account during the planning, performance, or critical assessment of studies in animal models. There should be a proper randomization of animals into interventional and appropriate control groups. Characteristics such as sex, age, feeding, and baseline kidney function should be similar in the two groups. Studies should be run concurrently with experimental and control groups, so as to exclude confounding factors related to the animals' characteristics or surroundings. The numbers of animals chosen should be appropriate to the reproducibility of outcome measure in the particular model, and mortality should be considered and reported. Assessment of outcome (for instance, morphology) should be performed in a blinded fashion, whenever feasible, and control repeated evaluation by the same investigator or an additional one should be considered. Experiments should be conducted in accord with the National Institutes of

Health *Guide for the Care and Use of Laboratory Animals* and approved by the institutional ethical committee for experiments in animals. Finally, reproducibility in other laboratories is essential before general acceptance of the results.

PRINCIPLES AND GUIDELINES SPECIFICALLY RELEVANT TO ANIMAL MODELS OF ACUTE RENAL FAILURE

Renal structure and function varies significantly between species and even between strains, so caution is needed in extrapolation of experimental data. Indeed, animals differ from humans in their susceptibility to various nephrotoxins. For instance, the gentamicin dose required in animal models of aminoglycoside toxicity is by orders of magnitude higher than the therapeutic dose in humans. These differences may reflect varied modes and rates of metabolism or drug elimination, as a result of different composition of immune responses, dissimilar tubular transport, or, perhaps, the use of healthy rather than diseased animals.

Diversity of the renal morphology and function should also be taken into account. For instance, the rat kidney contains a single pyramid, has a prominent outer stripe of outer medulla (compared with a very shallow one in the human kidney), and has a highly developed papilla that enables double the maximal urinary concentration seen in humans. However, brown Norway rats—which have been shown to be highly resistant to clamp ischemia/reperfusion[9]—like humans, have a less developed outer stripe of the outer medulla than other rat strains and mice and may, therefore, be less susceptible to the characteristic inflammatory low-reflow phenomena that define much of the behavior of this model. Minipigs, with their poorly developed outer medulla, may also suit the purpose of avoiding the strong contribution of outer medullary reflow abnormalities in rodent models. Additional factors that could influence ischemia resistance in brown Norway rats are their unique T cell characteristics and systemic inflammatory response, providing generalized parenchymal cell resistance to injury.

Technological Pitfalls

Potential confounding factors like fluid status, body and kidney temperatures, systemic blood pressure, and anesthesia must be controlled in experimental AKI. Physiological parameters known to affect kidney function or susceptibility to injury—temperature, blood pressure, or fluid status—should be controlled for, measured, and reported. The impact of anesthesia and surgical manipulations should be taken into consideration, because hypotension associated with some anesthetics or surgery-related hypovolemia may markedly affect intrarenal microcirculation, leading to so-called corticomedullary blood redistribution: At mean blood pressure reduction not lower than 70 mm Hg, cortical blood flow substantially declines, but medullary blood flow is maintained. As outlined later (see discussion of physiological background of models of hypoxic AKI), reduced cortical flow leads to diminution of GFR and downstream tubular transport, causing a paradoxical reversal of the physiologic medullary hypoxia, whereas cortical pO_2 (partial pressure of oxygen) declines.[10] Because regional intrarenal hypoxia plays an important

role in AKI, such changes may have misleading impact on the outcome. It is noteworthy that the type of anesthesia may have a direct effect on AKI model outcome that is unrelated to systemic or renal hemodynamics. For example, AKI associated with glycerol-induced rhabdomyolysis is markedly attenuated by isoflurane anesthesia.[11]

Core and renal temperatures should also be considered, since they substantially affect renal tubular metabolism, oxygen consumption, and pathophysiology under hypoxic conditions. For instance, in experiments with the kidney surgically exposed, renal temperature largely depends on its blood flow, falling when blood flow declines, for instance during systemic hypotension or with the addition of vasoconstrictors. The effect on outcome of renal temperature during insult may be illustrated by the totally different injury patterns that develop in widely used models of warm ischemia-reflow, induced by transient clamping of the renal artery or pedicle, and "cold" ischemia-reperfusion damage, induced by removal of the kidney and its cold preservation throughout the ischemic period. Although extensive outer stripe proximal S3 tubular damage occurs in the former model, inner stripe injury pattern predominates in the latter model.[12]

Thus, core temperature and systemic hemodynamics should be checked, controlled, and considered in all animal models of AKI. Furthermore, renal temperature and hemodynamics should be recorded and taken into account under experimental settings of renal exposure to ambient temperature. In these circumstances, renal temperature should be maintained by means of external heating by light, continuous application of warm mineral oil, or renal submersion in warmed fluids. Fluid balance and hematocrit value should be addressed as well so as not to affect systemic and renal hemodynamics, blood viscosity, and renal oxygenation.

Many experimental mechanical interventions directly injure the kidney. Among such technologies are single-nephron functional studies, determination of intrarenal hemodynamics, oxygenation, sampling of efflux, and direct visualization. All such manipulations require the insertion of probes into the renal parenchyma, potentially inflicting damage. The size of the probe and the depth of penetration are especially important, because deep renal structures rely on intact superficial anatomy. Medullary blood supply originates from efferent arterioles, emerging from deep cortical (juxtamedullary) glomeruli, and cortical structures determine the generation and composition of tubular fluids reaching medullary structures. Thus, interference with cortical anatomy may markedly affect the viability and function of deeper structures. Therefore, advanced technologies, such as intravital two-photon microscopy for the visualization of the renal microvasculature,[13] can be applied to the cortex region only, because of the associated tissue damage. Conversely, nonpenetrating probes, such as the renal oxygen determination system described by Johannes and colleagues,[14] which is placed above the renal surface, are better than conventional oxygen microelectrodes inserted into the renal parenchyma. Simple, minimally traumatic extrarenal interventions, such as renal decapsulation, exposure of the papilla, and manipulation of the renal pedicle, may also affect renal physiology by altering renal hydrostatic pressure, urine papillary flow, and renal innervation, respectively.

Noninvasive, real-time functional monitoring: Emerging noninvasive techniques could help to detect functional/structural alterations in experimental and human AKI. The examples described previously illustrate that various technical interventions can adversely affect the renal physiology. They are potential confounders, providing "background noise" that may reduce consistency of the AKI model and blur the outcome. In planning of an experimental design, the use of such invasive procedures should be balanced against the importance of the achieved data. If such procedures are performed, complementary studies, with removal or minimization of such potential confounding factors, may be considered to validate overall results.

New, totally noninvasive technologies are gradually evolving[15] that may replace some of these tissue-destructive procedures (see Table 45-1). Blood oxygen level–dependent magnetic resonance imaging (BOLD MRI) spatially determines the concentration of renal parenchymal deoxygenated hemoglobin.[16] Phosphorus MRI provides data regarding renal energy stores through the determination of renal adenosine triphosphate content.[17] Sodium MRI illustrates the renal corticomedullary sodium gradient, a most sensitive and early marker of the functional derangement in evolving AKI.[18] Polyamine dendrimer–based MRI contrast agents serve as markers of renal perfusion, GFR, and urinary concentration.[19] Labeled molecular imaging probes injected in vivo, such as pimonidazole (HypoxyProbe) and ApoSense, are currently used for the detection of hypoxic and injured tissues, respectively.[20,21] Such molecules, if radiolabeled or bound to residues detected by MRI, may enable in vivo detection of renal tissue alterations. Most importantly, many of these technologies enable real-time repeated observations throughout a dynamic and evolving process, as opposed to the single time-point observations available so far.

Single versus Multiple Insults: The Issue of Model Severity and Complexity

The price paid for reproducibility and homogeneity might be the loss of clinical relevance (Fig. 45-2). Experimental models have traditionally been developed to minimize heterogeneity and improve reproducibility by maximizing the insult—for instance, administration of large doses of the nephrotoxin or induction of ischemia by prolonged clamping of the renal artery. Extensive injury may not mimic the clinical condition, which conceivably contains more focal, intermediate, and reversible phases of tissue damage, and may not include other pathophysiological components, such as the inflammation present in the ischemia-reflow model.

Human AKI frequently occurs in patients of advanced age, with serious comorbidities, or is superimposed on chronic renal failure. By contrast, most experimental AKI models use young and healthy animals, so their results may be less applicable to clinical situations. In other words, the pathogenesis of human AKI is often multifactorial, combining an acute insult with predisposing medical conditions. This association of risk factors and acute insults implies a certain mechanistic link that should be elucidated and manipulated in animal models to successfully simulate clinically relevant human conditions. In some cases, this link may have to do with the renal handling and elimination of the toxin: For instance, salt deficit and effective volume depletion are permissive factors, intensifying clinical and experimental cisplatin, gentamicin, or pigment toxicity, presumably by prolonging the exposure and increasing tubular concentration, transit time, and uptake of the nephrotoxin. In hypoxic/toxic AKI, such as radiocontrast nephropathy, kidney dysfunc-

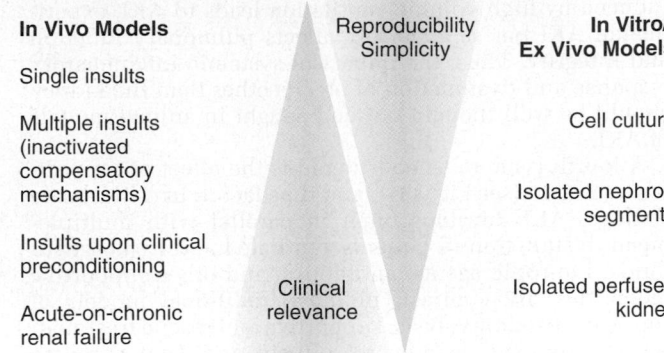

FIGURE 45-2. The spectrum of experimental models of acute kidney injury (AKI) seems to have antagonistic objectives. Simplicity and reproducibility of animal models of AKI, unfortunately, inversely correlate with their clinical relevance. Whole-animal models of AKI as well as in vitro and ex vivo systems are schematically placed along scales of clinical relevance and reproducibility. Single extensively destructive insults in vivo (such as prolonged warm ischemia-reflow) lack immediate clinical relevance to the human situation. Use of multiple insults (such as the administration of radiocontrast agents concomitantly with the inhibition of nitric oxide synthase), however, renders the model more closely akin to the clinical circumstance (because many predisposing factors for radiocontrast nephropathy, for example, are characterized by altered nitrovasodilation). Preconditioning the animal with dehydration or congestive heart failure prior to applying the direct renal insult further strengthens the resemblance to the clinical circumstance. Providing the substrate of acute-on-chronic renal injury is perhaps the most reflective of the circumstances found in clinical practice. Alas, the price for clinical relevance in these complex models is lower consistency, which is in part related to activated compensatory mechanisms and systemic alterations.

Simply manipulated in vitro models such as cell cultures reveal important cellular processes but have limited clinical relevance, because AKI is an integrated process involving cross-talk among various nephron segments and microcirculation at different levels of the renal parenchyma. The ex vivo isolated kidney model, standing halfway on the simplicity/relevance spectrum, has the advantage of maintained structural integrity coupled with a complete control of extrarenal variables and renal function.

tion and damage develops almost exclusively in patients at risk and in preconditioned animals, reflecting acute hypoxic insult in kidneys on top of defective mechanisms designed to maintain parenchymal oxygen sufficiency. Such protective mechanisms may be inhibited pharmacologically (i.e., by inhibition of cyclooxygenase or nitric oxide synthase), by using genetically susceptible strains, or through the induction of the predisposing factor itself, such as heart failure, diabetes, or chronic kidney disease.[7]

Multiple-organ failure reflects a cytokine- and immune-mediated cross-talk between injured organs that markedly affects experimental models of AKI. Zager[22] reported 20 years ago that retained necrotic liver tissue intensifies renal gentamicin uptake and nephrotoxicity. Conceivably, higher renal cortical concentration of the nephrotoxin results from effective volume depletion related to systemic inflammation and, combined with inflammation-mediated alteration in renal microcirculation, leads to increased nephrotoxicity. Later studies by Chien and coworkers[23] illustrate the importance of the extrarenal immune system in mediating AKI and the reciprocal immune/cytokine-mediated modulation of injury between organs. For instance, although experimental lung barotrauma induced by high volume ventilation leads to AKI, experimental AKI per se adversely affects pulmonary function and integrity. Thus, the impact of systemic inflammatory response and dysfunction of organs other than the kidney should be well thought out and sought in animal models of AKI.

A fourth issue to be considered is the effect of supportive treatment (see Fig. 45-1) and time factor: In critical care settings, AKI develops often in parallel with multiple-organ dysfunction in patients ventilated and treated with fluids, inotropic agents, antibiotics, and other supportive modalities. By contrast, in most traditional models of sepsis or rhabdomyolysis, supportive and rescue treatment is not provided, leading to a rapid and fatal outcome without a chance for the development of full-blown functional and morphological characteristics of the renal syndrome.

The aspiration for a simple and reproducible model should be weighed against the drive to use clinically relevant models. The severity of the insult, the inclusion of predisposing factors, and the administration of supportive therapy all deserve consideration in the planning or criticism of animal models of AKI (see Fig. 45-2). There is a place for simple and reproducible models as long as they are complemented by models that explicitly address relevance to clinical situations, with the induction of comorbidities believed to predispose to ARF and its outcome in humans.

The following models, currently hardly available, are critically needed: acute-on-chronic injury and AKI in old animals, diabetic creatures, and pregnant creatures, corresponding to susceptible human groups. Indeed, some newly developed "compound" models of hypoxic[24] and septic AKI[19] adopt this approach and were highly recommended in the 2005 American Society of Nephrology Renal Research Report on AKI.[3] Yet time will tell whether we are truly modeling the human disease with these approaches or merely developing even less well-characterized forms of animal diseases that will be harder to implement, reproduce, and dissect out the features being modified by intervention.

Morphological/Functional Correlations

Morphological damage in both human and experimental AKI ranges from subtle and reversible changes to overt necrosis, is confined to certain renal zones, and may not necessarily correlate with the extent of functional derangement. Therefore, fundamental requirements for a model should include morphology, hemodynamics, oxygenation, and function. Correlations of these variables are of supreme importance in the understanding and interpretation of the outcome. For instance, in some models of AKI, such as sepsis, renal dysfunction occurs almost in the absence of overt morphological findings, underscoring the role of altered renal hemodynamics with a marked decline in GFR. This may reflect renal cortical vasoconstriction with a corticomedullary redistribution of blood, presumably triggered by the so-called tubuloglomerular feedback mechanism[10] or by a yet poorly defined renal parenchymal shunt associated with renal vasodilation.[25] As opposed to the poor functional/morphological association in these models, characterized by rare focal tubular injury,[19,21] in models with widespread damage, the extent of damage seems to correlate more closely with renal dysfunction. Noteworthy, the assessment of tubular injury is limited, principally because it is relevant only to the one time-point of sampling. Transient and reversible injury patterns may disappear,[26] and reparative processes are activated within a short time after the induction of hypoxic insult.[20] Furthermore, apoptotic changes can easily be missed morphologically unless sought via immunostaining.[21]

The importance of functional/morphological correlations is demonstrated by a model of acute-on-chronic renal failure developed by Goldfarb and associates.[24] Their assessment reveals that (1) chronic tubulointerstitial disease may be markedly underdiagnosed if based on GFR only, illustrating that adaptive functional mechanisms such as modified glomerular hemodynamics and hypoxia adaptation are turned on, (2) assessment of tubular function is important in revealing such underlying morphological damage, and (3) AKI in the animals may often reflect disintegration of the adaptive functional mechanisms rather than representing true acute tubular damage.

Colocalization of tissue hypoxia (with pimonidazole adducts), hypoxia sensing (expression of hypoxia-inducible factors [HIFs]), and hypoxia adaptation (HIF-dependent substances, such as heme-oxygenase-1, vascular endothelial growth factor [VEGF] inducible nitric oxide synthase, or erythropoietin), and their correlations with functional derangement further complement the morphological assessment and shed light on pathophysiological processes in AKI.[20,24,27]

The mode of tissue sampling and fixation is extremely important. Samples should be large and should comprise all kidney regions, including cortex, outer medulla, and inner medulla (papilla), because injury may be focal and unevenly distributed and can appear independently at the various levels. Indeed, outer medullary damage may be more pronounced in the fornix region, presumably indicating a more pronounced ambient hypoxia.[28] Furthermore, cortical, outer medullary, and papillary damage may inversely correlate,[6,28,29] possibly illustrating a crosstalk between nephron segments regarding workload and energy expenditure.[10]

Rapid perfusion-fixation of renal tissue improves morphological assessment in experimental AKI and helps avoid potential artifacts related to postmortem processes. We recommend perfusion-fixation in vivo of the kidney for optimal morphological assessment. In rats this procedure consists of intra-aortic placement of a blunted large-caliber needle at the level of the renal arteries, with interruption of the aortic flow above the renal arteries concomitant with the initiation of the perfusion system. Importantly, heparinization is recommended, as is flushing of the kidneys with physiological solution preceding the fixation medium, to avoid plugging of the renal vasculature by blood clots. Notably, ligature of the superior mesenteric artery and the aorta below the renal artery allows for selective renal perfusion-fixation with low volumes of the preservative at physiologic perfusion pressure. Furthermore, the vena cava and ureters should be severed to allow blood/perfusate and urine efflux. With this technique, the kidney remains bloodless and tubular collapse is prevented, markedly improving the detection of fine structural changes. This approach allows for precise identification of tubular segments, accurate quantitation of tubular damage,[24,28,30] and convenient immunostaining.[20,24]

Additional Considerations

Extensive tissue damage, the morphological outcome in most experimental models, is atypical in human acute tubular necrosis. For better understanding of the clinical syndrome and the efficacy of interventional strategies, renal parenchymal response to sublethal injury should be studied with molecular markers to localize the timely stress response in tissue sections.

It is important to exploit models in vitro to gain additional insight into pathophysiological mechanisms as well as to validate observations in isolated cells and organs with confirmation in more complex models in vivo. A potentially important useful tool for such comparisons of in vivo and in vitro models is the identification of comparable altered gene expression pattern by means of microarray techniques.[31]

All animal models may be used for the evaluation of potential pharmacological interventions, including vasodilators, immunomodulatory agents, free radical scavengers, inducers of hypoxia adaptation systems, and growth factors. Despite the great limitations of the warm ischemia-reperfusion model in terms of pathophysiology and clinical relevance, its simplicity and reproducibility make it a practical first step in the assessment of interventions. Important cell biological, pharmacological, and immunopathological information may be gained from this model. Nevertheless, this information need not be translated to applicability to the human situation. Second-step confirmatory studies should be conducted first in more complex, clinically relevant models.

Finally, recovery events occur over several days to weeks after injury, possibly leading to secondary inflammatory damage and chronic and progressive tubulointerstitial disease.[32,33] Thus, evaluation of long-lasting morphological and functional sequelae of AKI should be considered.

MODELS OF HYPOXIC ACUTE KIDNEY INJURY

Models of hypoxic AKI, detailed in Chapter 42, include the in vivo warm and cold ischemia and reperfusion models, the ex vivo isolated perfused kidney model, and complex models of multiple insults that lead to prolonged renal hypoperfusion or intensify physiologic medullary hypoxia (Table 45-2). Those models differ conceptually and physiologically, generating long-standing dispute about their clinical relevance and therapeutic implications.[2,34,35]

Physiological Background

The following three aspects of renal physiology should be acknowledged for adequate assessment of models of hypoxic AKI: The intrarenal gradient of renal parenchymal oxygenation with physiologic low medullary oxygen content, the varied tolerability of different tubular segments to hypoxia, and the polarity of their capacity to mount hypoxia-adaptive response.

1: Physiologic renal oxygen gradients exist along the corticomedullary axis as well as transverse to it. Renal zones with poor oxygenation are medullary rays, the outer medulla, and the papilla. Renal parenchymal oxygenation is not homogeneous: Although cortical pO_2 is about 50 to 70 mm Hg, tissue oxygenation declines to some 25 to 40 mm Hg at the corticomedullary junction,[10,36] and papillary pO_2 is even lower.[37,38] Physiologic medullary hypoxia reflects high regional oxygen consumption for tubular transport, hardly matched by limited regional blood supply.[10] Transport activity, maximal at the outer medulla and related to medullary thick ascending limbs (mTALs), is greatly affected by "preload" of filtered urine reaching the distal nephron. Hence, raised GFR or diminished proximal tubular reabsorption increases distal tubular solute delivery and transport load, whereas diminished GFR or increased proximal tubular reabsorption reduces distal tubular oxygen consumption for transport. Outer medullary oxygen supply is limited because only about 10% of total renal blood flow reaches the medulla. Furthermore, oxygen diffuses from descending to ascending vasa recta, leading to oxygen steal from deeper structures.[37] Thus, medullary hypoxia is the price the mammalian kidney pays for the ability to concentrate urine within the countercurrent system. Very efficient regulatory systems maintain medullary oxygen sufficiency by matching regional blood supply and tubular transport.[10] Major participants in this regulation system are prostaglandins, nitric oxide, and adenosine. With intact regulatory mechanisms, the renal medulla is quite resistant to acute hypoxic stress. By contrast, most risk factors for hypoxic AKI are characterized by altered control of medullary oxygen sufficiency. The potential significance of medullary hypoxia in the development of AKI comes to mind when one considers human pathology. Indeed, historical reports of human AKI during World War II have shown a propensity for medullary hypoxic AKI; hence use of the term "lower nephron nephrosis" in those days.[39] Later electron-microscopic analysis of AKI biopsy specimens also show that most injured and detached cells are of distal tubular origin.[40]

TABLE 45-2

Models of Hypoxic/Ischemic Acute Kidney Injury

MODEL TYPE	SIMPLICITY	REPRODUCIBILITY	MATCH TO HUMAN PATHOLOGY	MATCH TO CLINICAL SCENARIO	USAGE
Warm ischemia-reperfusion	++++	+++	No	–	++++
Cold ischemia-warm reperfusion	–	?	Unclear	++++	+/–
Distal acute tubular necrosis, multiple insults	+	++	Some evidence	+++	+
Prolonged renal hypoperfusion	+	?	?	+++	New model
Cardioplegic whole-body ischemia	++	++	?	+++	New model
Isolated perfused kidney	+/–	+++	No	–	+/–

–, very low; +/–, low; +, mild; ++, moderate; +++, high; ++++, very high.

2: Hypoxia tolerance greatly varies along the nephron. Glomeruli and collecting ducts are much more hypoxia resistant than S3 segments of the proximal tubule or thick ascending limbs of Henle's loop: Various nephron segments differ in their capacity to withstand hypoxic insults. Proximal tubules have little capacity for anaerobic glycolysis and hence are particularly sensitive to total cessation of renal blood flow and oxygen delivery, as occurs in the model of transient clamping of the renal artery (warm ischemia-reflow). By contrast, medullary thick ascending limbs (mTALs) have a greater capacity to generate adenosine triphosphate by glycolysis, and can withstand prolonged ischemia as long as transport is inhibited.[41] This may be the rationale for activation of tubuloglomerular filtration during AKI: Reduced GFR decreases distal tubular transport and diminishes mTAL injury.

3: Although each renal cell holds the potential to mount a transcriptional response to hypoxia (through so-called HIFs), such hypoxic adaptation greatly varies along the nephrons. Hypoxia leads to cellular adaptive response, initiated by the accumulation of HIFs.[10,42] Nephron segments differ also in their capacity to generate HIFs during comparable ambient hypoxia. In collecting ducts, HIF immunostaining is substantial under hypoxic stress, whereas mTAL HIF expression is quite limited in extent and appears only within a narrow window of moderate, nonlethal hypoxic stress.[27] It is conceivable that varied HIF response among tubular segments is in part responsible for their heterogeneous capacity to withstand acute or chronic hypoxia.

Warm Ischemia-Reperfusion

In the most widely used model, warm ischemia-reperfusion (outlined in Chapter 42), the principal preliminary pathophysiological insult is tissue hypoxia. Formation of reactive oxygen species during reperfusion contributes to subsequent endothelial dysfunction, altered outer medullary microcirculation, inflammation, and tubular injury. Damage appears first in the outer stripe of the outer medulla, a region characterized by a relative paucity of intertubular capillaries. S3 segments of proximal tubules are principally affected (Fig. 45-3A). Following 15 to 20 minutes of ischemia, injury is focal and minimal. Prolongation of the ischemic period leads to a more consistent and confluent damage pattern, which spreads to involve S3 segments in medullary rays, and proximal convoluted segments in the cortical labyrinth. Beyond 50 to 60 minutes, damage encompasses most renal parenchyma: The entire outer medulla becomes infarcted, and injury extends to the entire cortical labyrinth, involving proximal and distal convoluted segments.[4] Under such circumstances, focal and limited mTAL injury may expand as well if GFR is maintained.[42a]

This model is simple and reproducible at ischemic periods longer than 45 minutes. A graded response is easily achieved, and a good correlation exists between functional injury and pathology. Characteristic medullary congestion appears in association with sluggish flow, induction of inflammation, and capillary leak. A technical pitfall is a decline in kidney temperature, especially if the kidney is kept exposed, although not to the low range used for renal transplantation. Because hypothermia exerts a marked protective effect, very careful temperature control is important. Delayed reperfusion after the removal of the clamp, related to altered microcirculation,[43] may become a confounding factor in the length of the true ischemic period. This may contribute to different functional and morphological outcomes for each kidney following bilateral ischemia and reperfusion models. Thus, unilateral nephrectomy and ischemia/reperfusion of the remaining kidney seem a preferential option for better functional and morphological correlations.

The warm ischemia-reperfusion model served for years as the source for understanding cellular injury and repair processes, and evolving microvascular depletion during convalescence made it suitable as a model for late and progressive tubulointerstitial disease.[33] Because of its simplicity and predicted reproducibility, it became the most convenient model used for the evaluation of therapeutic interventions. Nevertheless, in expert opinion sessions on AKI animal models sponsored by both the Acute Dialysis Quality Initiative and the American Society of Nephrology, the great deficiencies of this model have been acknowledged.[2,3] First, AKI due to pure ischemia with a total cessation of blood flow seldom happens in the clinical practice. The closest clinical scenarios, transplanted kidneys and surgery of the aorta, are associated with cold rather than warm ischemia and reflow. Indeed, the damage pattern in this model, with predominant S3 segment damage, differs markedly from human pathology. In fact, in most experiments the ischemic period used ends with extensive necrosis of S3 segments, whereas mTAL damage is limited or absent. This injury pattern illustrates the high susceptibility of S3 segments to anoxia and to hypoxia adaptation, and the paucity of peritubular capillaries in the outer stripe of rodents. The relative preservation of mTALs in this model reflects their tolerance to hypoxia as long as tubular transport is inhibited, as happens with total cessation of GFR during clamping, which remains low upon reperfusion. Indeed, studies in the isolated perfusion model[29] and findings in vivo[6] illustrate that proximal tubular damage and reduced GFR protects against distal tubular injury. One other characteristic morphological feature of this model is the intense inflammatory component,[13,44] which is uncharacteristic of human AKI.

Cold Ischemia–Warm Reperfusion

In the cold ischemia–warm reperfusion model, the kidney is removed, flushed, and kept at low temperature under conditions similar to those in cold preservation for transplantation. Kidneys are subsequently reimplanted after variable periods of cold preservation. This model has rarely been used in studies of experimental AKI because of technical difficulties, requiring vascular surgery. Nevertheless, it has high clinical relevance. Importantly, the injury distribution pattern may substantially differ from that of warm ischemia-reperfusion, with a more prominent distal nephron injury,[12] underscoring the marked impact of renal temperature and the major flaw in the warm ischemia-reperfusion model.

The Isolated Perfused Kidney

The isolated perfused kidney model is an ex vivo, whole-organ model. The removed rat kidney is continuously perfused with oxygenated medium through the renal artery under controlled pressure and perfusate flow. Urine is collected, and glomerular filtration and tubular function are continuously monitored by the sequential determination of electrolyte and inulin levels in the perfusate and urine. Renal morphology can be assessed subsequently.[45]

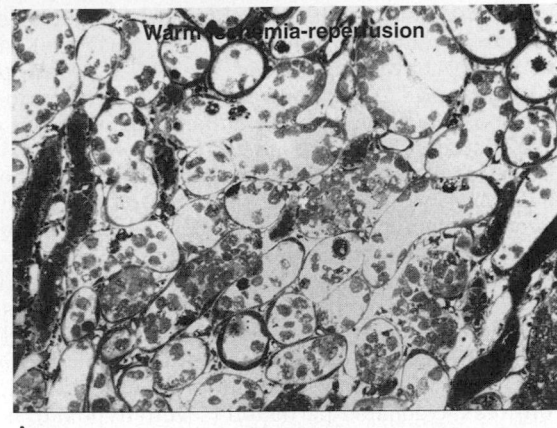

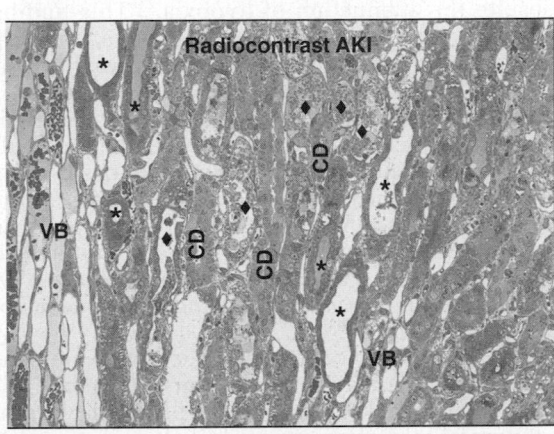

FIGURE 45-3. Morphological hallmarks of hypoxic acute kidney injury (AKI) models in the rat. **A,** Morphology of the outer stripe of the outer medulla 24 hours after a 45-minute clamping of the renal artery. In this convenient and reproducible model, an extensive necrosis is noted, with nearly total destruction of proximal tubules in the outer stripe (S3 segments), with additional variable involvement of cortical parenchyma. Nevertheless, this total cessation of blood flow with the consequent severe injury bears no resemblance to the clinical or pathological findings in the human acute tubular necrosis (ATN), in which limited tubular injury exists in dyssynchrony with severe organ dysfunction.[86] Although admittedly there are relatively few renal biopsy studies in ATN, the extensive injury seen in this experimental model, has rarely, if ever, been demonstrated in human circumstances. Many agents seem to ameliorate the renal failure in the animal, but none of them has been successful in human trials (×250). **B,** Inner stripe injury (predominantly medullary thick ascending limbs [mTALs]) 24 hours after the administration of radiocontrast agents, combined with inhibitors of nitric oxide synthase and prostaglandin synthesis. The basis of this model rests on the aggravation of the medullary hypoxia that has been well documented in multiple species, including humans. The drugs applied (indomethacin, radiocontrast agents) are used in human care, and defective nitric oxide synthase characterizes many predisposing risk factors for radiocontrast nephropathy. Thus, this model is clinically relevant and human driven, actually exploiting and recapitulating known renal vulnerabilities in humans. However, this model is somewhat complicated and suffers inconsistency. There is a typical injury gradient: intact vascular bundles (vasa recta; VBs) with maintenance of adjacent mTALs (*), necrotic mTALs in the mid–interbundle zone (♦), and intact collecting ducts (CDs). This "zonation" of injury is a reflection of the hypoxia gradient characteristic of the renal medulla (see next) (×200). **C,** Cross-section at the level of the outer medulla in the isolated perfused kidney (IPK) model after perfusion with oxygenated cell-free perfusate (i.e., poor renal oxygenation). Oxygenation gradients are illustrated by the hypoxia marker pimonidazole. Pimonidazole adducts (dark-staining) are identified in the mid–interbundle zone, whereas tubules closest to the vasa recta are pimonidazole-negative (i.e., well-oxygenated). VB, vascular bundle (×110).

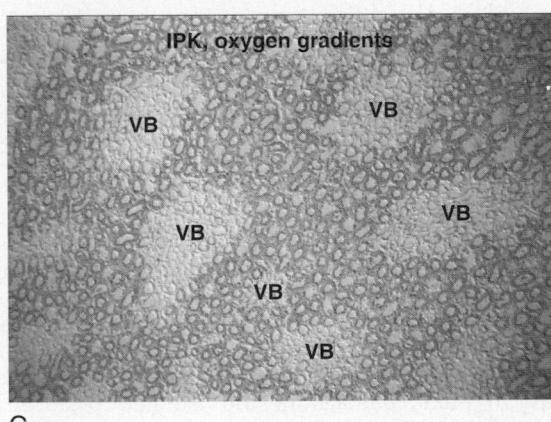

Perfusion with oxygenated erythrocytes yields near-normal morphology and function, whereas cessation of renal perfusion, or perfusion under hypoxic conditions, leads to functional impairment with an injury pattern comparable to that in the warm ischemia-reperfusion model.[46,47] In contrast, perfusion without red cells (i.e., oxygenated cell-free perfusate, which hence has a very low oxygen supply) results in progressive functional impairment associated with predominant outer medullary hypoxic injury.

Medullary TALs are principally affected, showing a reversal injury pattern (mitochondrial swelling and nuclear pyknosis) that progresses to membrane disruption and cell death.[26] A typical gradient of injury is noted, closely related to gradients of tissue oxygenation, beginning at the mid–inner stripe of the outer medulla and spreading inwards and outwards. Medullary TALs located in the mid–interbundle zone, most remote from the vascular bundles and oxygen supply, are predominantly affected, with preservation of tubules adjacent to the vasa recta. The mid–interbundle hypoxic injury zone spreads over time as long as hypoxia is maintained.[26,27] Inhibition of distal tubular transport under these conditions (with loop diuretics or ouabain, or with the abolition of GFR through an increase in albumin content of the perfusate) improves medullary oxygenation (see Fig. 45-3C) and prevents mTAL damage.[27,48] By contrast, measures that reduce medullary oxygenation, such as enhancement of GFR and the administration of contrast media or indomethacin, increase the extent of medullary hypoxia.[49,50] S3 segments, adjacent to mTALs in the outer stripe of the outer medulla, also demonstrate hypoxic injury. S3 damage can be prevented, in parallel with the amelioration of mTAL injury, through improvement of ambient pO_2 with loop diuretics, illustrating how these neighboring tubular segments compete with each other for sparse oxygen supply.[51] Interestingly, medullary HIF expression, which is absent in the red cell–containing perfusion medium and upregulated during cell-free oxygenated perfusion (severe hypoxia), is further upregulated by the inhibition of distal transport activity despite the attenuation of hypoxia.[27] This finding, noted also after use of loop diuretics in vivo,[20] indicates that hypoxia adaptation via HIFs is induced by moderate hypoxia, whereas severe hypoxia turns it off.[42]

The major advantages of the isolated perfused kidney model are the absolute control over all extrarenal factors, the easy experimental manipulation of tissue oxygenation and other variables, and the concomitant determination of hemodynamics, function, and morphology. Furthermore, unlike with isolated tubules and cell culture models of AKI, the renal anatomy and the overall vascular-glomerular-tubular anatomical and functional associations are maintained.

However, this model is complex and time consuming, and factors that may participate in the pathophysiology of AKI, such as leukocytes, various plasma factors, and neurohumoral mediators, are excluded.

Models of Combined Insults with Predominant Distal Nephron Injury: Radiocontrast Nephropathy and Other Models

The physiologic low medullary pO_2 declines under a variety of "nephrotoxic" insults, such as radiocontrast agents, nonsteroidal anti-inflammatory drugs,[30] amphotericin,[5] and myoglobin.[6] The decline in medullary oxygenation reflects enhancement of tubular transport and oxygen consumption, reduction of regional blood flow, or their combination.[10] Indeed, all of these agents increase medullary hypoxic damage in the isolated perfused kidney model, but some (radiocontrast agents, nonsteroidal anti-inflammatory drugs) fail to inflict injury and to reduce kidney function in vivo in intact animals despite a substantial accentuation of medullary hypoxia. Inactivation of defense mechanisms that preserve medullary oxygenation, such as nitric oxide or prostaglandin, further intensifies the decline in medullary hypoxia induced by radiocontrast agents, and a selective outer medullary damage develops.[52] Medullary TALs in the mid–inner stripe are injured predominantly (see Fig. 45-3B), and to a lesser extent adjacent S3 segments in the outer stripe, in a distribution pattern and injury gradients identical to those noted in the isolated perfused kidney model, paralleling the allocation of severe hypoxia.[30,49,52] Papillary tip necrosis may develop as well.[21] Tubular injury appears within 15 minutes and evolves over 24 hours, consisting of both necrosis and apoptosis and associated with reduced GFR and tubular

dysfunction.[30,53] Reduced concentrating capacity, illustrated by sodium MRI as abolished corticomedullary sodium ion gradient, is perhaps the earliest evidence for evolving tubular dysfunction in these models.[18]

Altered nitrovasodilation or prostaglandin synthesis typically characterizes the clinical risk factors for radiocontrast nephropathy, such as diabetes, aging, hypertension, hyperlipidemia, and the concomitant use of nonsteroidal anti-inflammatory drugs, providing clinical relevance for these models.[7] In other AKI models with distal nephron injury from combined multiple insults, AKI has been facilitated by the induction of such clinical risk factors. In addition to their clinical relevance, the logic of the addition of such insults was the potential intensification of medullary hypoxia through enhanced vasoconstrictive stimuli (heart failure, salt depletion, angiotensin II infusion), enhanced tubular transport (prior uninephrectomy with compensatory hypertrophy of the remaining kidney, or acute enhancement of GFR), depletion of medullary microcirculation (chronic tubulointerstitial disease or acute urinary outflow obstruction), or altered nitrovasodilation (diabetes, hypercholesterolemia).[7] Whenever checked in rats, morphology in these models showed intensification of outer medullary hypoxic damage. The principle of combined insults for the generation of radiocontrast nephropathy was found to be applicable also in rabbits and dogs. As in humans, the severity of experimental radiocontrast nephropathy is proportional to the number of concomitantly applied perturbations. The extent of outer medullary tubular necrosis and functional derangement correlates better in the more severe models, whereas in milder forms, reduced GFR is often out of proportion to the extent of tubular necrosis and is associated with low fractional sodium excretion.[7]

All of these models are highly clinically relevant, mimicking human radiocontrast nephropathy and its risk factors. Their disadvantages lie in their complexity and variable reproducibility, requiring large numbers of animals.

In addition to radiocontrast nephropathy, the principle of enhancement of medullary hypoxic injury through the inactivation of defense mechanism or the inclusion of additional clinical risk factors has been adopted in models of endotoxin,[54] myoglobin,[6] amphotericin,[55] cyclosporin,[56] and hypercalcemic nephropathies.[57] Another example of the multiple-insult model is the inhibition of nitric oxide and prostaglandin synthesis in rats with congestive heart failure, which yields focal mTAL necrosis, illustrating the important role of these defense mechanisms in maintenance of medullary oxygen sufficiency in the presence of intense vasoconstrictive stimuli.[58] Notably, mechanisms other than intensified medullary hypoxia may play a role in the genesis of AKI in some of these multiple-insult models, such as enhanced cytotoxicity due to increased intraluminal concentration of the nephrotoxin.

The clinical relevance of these models is obvious, reflecting acute, subacute and chronic insults. Intensification of medullary hypoxia is often indicated by oxygen microelectrodes or pimonidazole adducts, positive responses to medullary HIF immunostaining, and morphological evidence of outer medullary hypoxic damage.[10] In both the acute and chronic models, pathology resembles well-known human morphology, in particular outer cortical "stripped fibrosis" (involving medullary rays) and papillary tip necrosis. All of these models provide data about different types of cellular damage patterns, including reversible injury, apoptosis, and necrosis. However, as with the radiocontrast models, they are quite complicated, are performed almost exclusively in rats, and may require large numbers of animals because of inconsistent reproducibility and endpoint variability.

Newer Models of Hypoxic Acute Kidney Injury

Molitoris and colleagues[59] developed a visceral hypoperfusion model induced by partial suprarenal aortic ligation in rats. The bowel and hindlimbs are also ischemic, and there is some rhabdomyolysis. Altered microcirculation with rouleaux formation of red blood cells and morphological damage are reported to resemble findings in the mild warm ischemia and reflow injury pattern (Bruce Molitoris, personal communication, 2007). This is a compound, clinically relevant model that mimics traumatic scenarios with prolonged hypoperfusion and rhabdomyolysis. Burne-Taney and associates[60] have reported a mice model of whole-body ischemia, induced by 10 minutes of cardioplegia and subsequent resuscitation. Kidney dysfunction is associated with injury at the corticomedullary junction, and gene response is comparable to that in the warm ischemia model, assessed by microarray technique. The elements of generalized tissue ischemia and damage associated with AKI in this model may make it relevant to human ARF.

Summary

The various hypoxic models of AKI range from prolonged total cessation of renal blood flow and GFR, through global renal hypoperfusion, to selective manipulations that alter the control of renal microcirculation and medullary oxygen sufficiency. Different models may be relevant to various clinical scenarios, with markedly different morphological outcome (i.e., proximal vs. distal tubular injury). This difference is not merely semantic, but may have profound impact on therapeutic implications.[2,10] Studies using global ischemia models illustrate beneficial effects of measures that increase renal cortical blood flow and GFR. By contrast, the concept of distal medullary damage implies that diminished GFR may be an adaptive mechanism, designed to reduce medullary damage by restoring medullary oxygenation. According to this concept, increasing GFR may be harmful, intensifying medullary hypoxia, whereas further attenuation of transport activity is warranted, for instance, with loop diuretics. So far, neither approach has been successful in clinical studies, underscoring the limited clinical applicability of these models.

MODELS OF TOXIC ACUTE KIDNEY INJURY

In toxic AKI models, nephrotoxic substances are given, usually to rodents, occasionally with an additional perturbation such as dehydration (Table 45-3). Common clinically relevant models are gentamicin and cisplatin nephropathies. We have classified and discussed radiocontrast nephropathy along with the hypoxic models, because the predominant role of hypoxia in this setup is clearly established.[7] Myoglobin and hemoglobin are clinically important endogenous nephrotoxins that exert some hypoxic injury as well.[6] Nephrotoxins such as amphotericin and cyclosporine induce a more subacute and chronic injury pattern, in part related to evolving renal parenchymal hypoxia, and other agents such as mercury compounds are not clinically relevant. Models applying newly recognized clinically relevant nephrotoxins, such as anti-retroviral and immunosuppressive agents, are lacking.

Gentamicin Nephropathy

In the most widely used models of gentamicin nephropathy, small rodents are given a very high dose of the agent for 3 to 6 consecutive days.[61,62] The gentamicin dose required for consistency of the model is two orders of magnitude higher than human dosages. Direct proximal tubular nephrotoxicity seems to be a predominant pathophysiological process, induced by tubular uptake of the toxin with typical lysosomal swelling (myeloid bodies), disruption, and cell necrosis and the development of acute polyuric renal failure. This simple and highly reproducible model is clinically relevant, and the recovery phase is quite comparable to that in the human syndrome. In accord with the concept of synergic renal insults, experimental gentamicin toxicity is intensified by dehydration, renal hypoperfusion, or transient global ischemia as well as systemic inflammation caused by retained necrotic material or bacteremia.[62-65] By contrast, experimental diabetes seems to attenuate the extent of gentamicin toxicity, possibly through the induction of cellular adaptive response together with solute diuresis and reduced cortical gentamicin uptake.[61] The presence of myeloid bodies noted in these experimental settings is the characteristic morphological feature of gentamicin exposure in humans. However, presence of myeloid bodies should be regarded only as a marker of gentamicin exposure and uptake; it does not necessarily indicate tissue damage and renal dysfunction.[66] Furthermore, in humans, gentamicin nephrotoxicity may appear with only minimal tubular changes

TABLE 45-3

Models of Toxic Acute Kidney Injury

MODEL TYPE	SIMPLICITY	REPRODUCIBILITY	MATCH TO HUMAN PATHOLOGY	MATCH TO CLINICAL SCENARIO	USAGE
Gentamicin*	++++	++++	Unclear	++	+
Cisplatin	++++	++++	Some evidence	++++	+
Pigment:					
Myoglobin	+++	++	Unclear	+/−	+/−
Glycerol rhabdomyolysis	++++	++++	Some evidence	+++	+

+/−, low; +, mild; ++, moderate; +++, high; ++++, very high.
*Huge dose required. Presence of myeloid bodies indicates exposure but is not specific for acute renal failure.

visible on light microscopy, whereas the development of AKI in the rodent model requires extensive tubular necrosis.

Cisplatin Nephropathy

AKI is induced in rodents by a single intraperitoneal injection of cisplatin, with a dose comparable to that used in humans.[67,68] Direct tubular toxicity seems to be a predominant pathophysiological process, with cisplatin being absorbed by and accumulating in the proximal tubule, especially the S3 segment.[69] This is a convenient, simple, and reproducible model, in which outer medullary apoptotic and necrotic tubular damage is comparable to that in human disease. As in humans, tubular dysfunction is prominent, with polyuria, glycosuria, hypomagnesemia, and hypokalemia. The recovery phase is also comparable to that in the human syndrome, as is the predisposition to greater damage with volume depletion. The clinical relevance of this model is somewhat in a decline owing to the introduction of new, less nephrotoxic derivatives such as carboplatin.

Pigment Nephropathy

The pathogenesis of AKI induced by myoglobin and hemoglobin consists of direct nephrotoxicity, as well as hypoxic, obstructive, and prerenal components.[6] These relatively small endogenous molecules are rapidly reabsorbed in proximal tubules (predominantly in S2 segments), and tubular damage develops after their intracellular degradation, release of ferrous atoms, and formation of reactive oxygen species. Vasoconstriction, probably related to nitric oxide consumption by the pigment, leads to decreased medullary oxygenation and may participate in the development of renal dysfunction. Nonreabsorbed pigment binds to Tamm-Horsfall protein and forms pigment casts, leading to tubular obstruction. Finally, in the case of rhabdomyolysis, systemic inflammatory response and hypovolemia related to the formation of third space may further compromise renal function.[70]

Glycerol injection, used predominantly in rats, produces abrupt rhabdomyolysis as well as hemolysis, which is associated with rapidly progressive renal dysfunction. This is a simple, reproducible, and clinically relevant model. It resembles the human crush syndrome, including all pathophysiological processes associated with muscle breakdown. Experimental maneuvers that are predisposing or protective in humans, such as volume depletion or volume repletion, respectively, are also applicable in this model.[4,70]

In myoglobin and hemoglobin infusion models, unlike the glycerol model, the pathophysiological processes do not include dehydration, spillage of other muscle contents such as purines, or the induction of a systemic inflammatory response. Consequently, a milder form of disease is generated than the severe AKI produced by glycerol.[6] These are simple and reproducible models, and their relatively stable systemic hemodynamics enable detection of changes in renal microcirculation and tissue oxygenation during short-term experiments. However, with the exception of acute hemolysis, these models do not represent clinically relevant conditions. Furthermore, myoglobin and hemoglobin may induce systemic vasoconstriction and hypertension, as opposed to what happens in the human crush syndrome. The relatively mild renal damage

in these models can be intensified and transformed from superficial cortical to corticomedullary injury with measures that enhance medullary hypoxia.[6]

SEPSIS MODELS

Sepsis-related renal failure, which is often associated with multiple-organ failure, is a leading cause of ARF in critically ill patients. Yet we are far from reaching a pathophysiologically adequate reproducible animal model that closely resembles the human syndrome. For instance, whereas in human sepsis syndrome renal blood flow increases, it is maintained or declines in the about two thirds of animal sepsis models.[25] Many models fail to reproduce an appropriate rate of multiple-organ dysfunction and death. Others lead to overwhelming and dramatic hemodynamic deterioration with death within 12 hours, a time too short for the development of adaptive systems and a clinically relevant renal deterioration. Moreover, in most models, fluid resuscitation, antibiotics, and vasopressor therapy—the standard care for patients with septic shock—are not given. Finally, many studies do not appropriately define clear endpoints, such as death after 24 or 48 hours, or the occurrence of other organ failure, which is precisely described in scoring systems.

Sepsis models, detailed in Chapter 44, are designed in small rodents[19,71] as well as in large animals, predominantly dogs[72] and sheep.[73] Major advantages of studies in small rodents are their relatively low cost and convenience and the ability to explore the effects of gene manipulation in knockout mice.[71] On the other hand, studies in large animals enable long-term instrumentation, the monitoring of systemic hemodynamics and microcirculation in various organs with the detection of multiorgan functional derangement,[73] and the controlled application of therapeutic interventions such as vasopressors and hemofiltration. Animal models are methodologically divided into four categories (Table 45-4): endotoxin administration, bacterial infusion/injection, single bacterial intraperitoneal inoculation, and continuous intraperitoneal bacterial seeding.

Endotoxin Infusion or Injection

In endotoxin infusion or injection models, lipopolysaccharide is administered by intravenous or intraperitoneal bolus injection or continuous infusion. The primary pathophysiological processes are probably alteration of renal hemodynamics[74] and inflammation[75] with subsequent microvascular damage and obliteration, capillary leak, and tissue hypoxic injury.[76,77]

These are simple models, and the lipopolysaccharide dose is very well standardized. In most cases, however, fluid replacement is insufficient, often leading to generalized vasoconstriction, particularly after repeated administration,[74] as opposed to the generalized vasodilatation seen in humans.[25] Furthermore, AKI requires high doses, which are associated with high mortality. Consequently, these models are short-lived. On the other hand, renal dysfunction is transient with small doses, and renal hypoxic parenchymal injury, predominantly involving medullary structures, appears only with concomitant inhibition of cyclooxygenase or nitric oxide synthase.[54]

It is noteworthy that systemic and renal response varies with different sources of endotoxin, rate of administration, and single or repeated administration as well as among

TABLE 45-4

Models of Septic Acute Kidney Injury*

MODEL TYPE	SIMPLICITY	REPRODUCIBILITY	MATCH TO HUMAN PATHOLOGY	MATCH TO CLINICAL SCENARIO	USAGE
Lipopolysaccharide infusion	++++	+++	Unclear	+/−	+++
Bacteria, infusion/injection[+]	++	++	Unclear	+++	+
Cecal ligation and perforation[+]	+++	++++	Unclear	++++	++
Bacteria, intraperitoneal seeding[+]	+++	++	Unclear	+++	+/−

+/−, low; +, mild; ++, moderate; +++, high; ++++, very high.
*All models are too short-lived.
[+]Additional supportive measures (antibiotics, fluids, etc.) are required for clinical relevance.

species, leading to difficulties in outcome comparisons among laboratories.

Bacterial Infusion

In bacterial infusion models of sepsis, which are used in small and large animals, an intravascular infusion of live bacteria is given. Bacterial dose can be standardized, and the systemic hemodynamic response may be comparable to that in human sepsis. Indeed, in the most-studied model of bacterial infusion in sheep, acute nonlethal hyperdynamic sepsis is produced, with hypotension, lactic academia, and decreased vascular resistance in the renal, coronary, and splanchnic vascular beds, leading to increased cardiac output despite reduced myocardial contractility.[73] Oliguria is observed, in association with decreased GFR. However, multiple-organ failure does not develop in surviving animals in most of these models, and very often, standard supporting measures such as fluid resuscitation, antibiotics, and mechanical ventilation are lacking,

Cecal Ligature and Perforation

Cecal ligature and perforation models of sepsis are created in rodents[19] and sheep.[78] The clinically relevant principle is continuous peritoneal seeding of colonic bacteria. There is a variability of response within and among species, in part in relation to cecal distensibility and variable spontaneous sealing of perforations. Technical aspects are therefore highly important, particularly the mode and size of cecal perforation. For each animal strain, the size of the perforation is adjusted to provide a usable model. In most of the later studies using this model, supportive treatment—antibiotics, fluids, and vasopressors—is provided, enabling extended survival and the development of multisystemic disorder. For example, Dear and associates[10] have developed a well-characterized cecal ligature and perforation model in aged mice that are resuscitated with intraperitoneal fluids and antibiotics.[19]

Using intravital multiphoton microscopy in a comparable model in hydrated rats, Molitoris and colleagues noted a sluggish cortical blood flow consistent with vasoconstriction, associated with microvascular thrombi, tubular cell vacuolization and reduced GFR (Bruce Molitoris, personal communication, 2007). These data appear quite consistent with and complementary to observations by Dear and associates[19] and suggest a sustained global low-flow state. In a comparable cecal ligature and perforation rat model, focal apoptotic tubular cell damage can be identified both in the cortex and in the outer medulla with highly sensitive techniques.[21]

Intraperitoneal Seeding of Bacteria

In the bacterial intraperitoneal seeding model, bacteria are injected directly into the peritoneal cavity or implanted as feces or within a fibrin clot. The last methodology enables complete control over the type and dose of bacteria[79] and a graded, standardized, persistent, and slow release of bacteria over time.[80] Intraperitoneal bacterial seeding models have been utilized principally in large animals such as dogs,[81] pigs,[82] and baboons,[83] but also in rodents.[84] To invoke renal dysfunction, the dose and release rate of bacteria should be adjusted for different animal species so as to produce a prolonged and moderate inflammatory response. A generally applicable rule for all models of AKI is to use highly lethal insult, in this case a large bacterial load, when one is testing potential ameliorating strategies[82] and to apply a mild bacterial burden when one is trying to unmask renal-protective mechanisms through their inactivation.[85]

These models are highly clinically relevant, especially when supportive treatment such as hydration and antibiotics is provided. The animal species used, bacterial type, dose and rate of release, and supportive care provided govern the systemic hemodynamic response. The major disadvantage of the bacterial intraperitoneal seeding models is that, particularly in large animals, the disease is usually severe and systemic derangement is too rapid to produce AKI either clinically or pathologically. Systemic inflammation and disseminated intravascular coagulopathy invariably involve the lungs, liver, and spleen, but the kidneys are often spared.[84] Second, because of the severity of these models, their reproducibility is low, with the animals exhibiting variable clinical course ranging from full recovery to rapid organ dysfunction and death. For these reasons, AKI-focused experiments have not been carried out in sepsis models using bacterial intraperitoneal seeding.

Summary

Although experimental models with lipopolysaccharide infusion may be least appropriate for sepsis-induced AKI, large animal models of bacterial inoculation with concomitant resuscitative maneuvers comparable to standard care in humans (fluids, antibiotics, hemodynamic and respiratory support) seem most appropriate. Considering the complexity and expenses of large animal studies, we should strive to develop comparable models in small animals, such as the cecal ligature and perforation model described by Dear and associates.[19] Control of infectious burden and supportive care should allow enough time for the host response to occur and for the development of systemic inflammatory response. Because of the multisystemic nature of sepsis syndrome, clinical endpoints of sepsis-related AKI studies should extend far beyond renal functional and structural parameters.

CONCLUSION

Animal models are invaluable for our understanding of the pathophysiology of AKI and for the development of effective treatment and preventive strategies. Experiments in cell cultures and isolated nephrons are insufficient, considering the complexity of kidney structure and function and the tightly regulated interaction between renal vasculature, glomerular filtration, and tubular function. Thus, whole-organ and in vivo studies are essential, and the most appropriate ones are those that closely resemble clinical conditions with associated predisposing factors. Experimental outcome should be appraised with the model type taken into account. For the proof of principle, it is reasonable to use first simple and reproducible models such as ischemia and reperfusion and administration of high-dose nephrotoxin. Nevertheless, such studies should be extended and complemented by more clinically relevant models that may be totally different pathophysiologically. Newer noninvasive technologies will enable the detection of evolving changes in intrarenal blood flow, oxygenation, energy stores, glomerular and tubular function, and cellular injury. Implementation of such technologies in experimental studies of AKI will improve our understanding of this disorder and advance assessment of the effects of therapeutic interventions.

Key Points

1. In human acute kidney injury, morphologic and functional derangement is poorly defined. Many of our current concepts are derived not from human data but from experimental disease and may therefore be erroneous.
2. Renal structure and function vary significantly between species and strains, so experimental data should be extrapolated to humans with caution. Furthermore, potential confounding factors in experimental settings, such as fluid status, body

and kidney temperature, systemic blood pressure, and anesthesia, should be controlled for.
3. Acute kidney injury in humans frequently occurs in patients of advanced age with serious comorbidities or is superimposed on chronic renal failure. By contrast, most experimental models use young and healthy animals, so their results may be less applicable to clinical situations.
4. Thus, in the planning or criticism of animal models of acute kidney injury, the aspiration for a simple and reproducible model should be weighed against the drive to use models that are clinically relevant in terms of severity of the insult, inclusion of predisposing factors, and administration of supportive treatment.
5. The complex pathophysiology of acute kidney injury dictates that experimental endpoints should include both renal function (glomerular and tubular) and morphology at different time points along the evolution of acute renal failure, complemented with novel methodologies providing real-time, noninvasive assessment of function, hemodynamics, metabolism, oxygenation, and cellular injury.

Key References

18. Maril N, Margalit R, Rosen S, et al: Detection of evolving acute tubular necrosis with renal ^{23}sodium MRI: Studies in rats. Kidney Int 2006;69:765-768.
19. Dear JW, Kobayashi H, Jo SK, et al: Dendrimer-enhanced MRI as a diagnostic and prognostic biomarker of sepsis-induced acute renal failure in aged mice. Kidney Int 2005;67:2159-2167.
20. Rosenberger C, Heyman SN, Rosen S, et al: Upregulation of HIF in acute renal failure—evidence for a protective transcriptional response to hypoxia. Kidney Int 2005;67:531-542.
21. Damianovich M, Ziv I, Heyman SN, et al: ApoSense: A novel technology for imaging of cell death in acute renal tubular necrosis. Eur J Nucl Med Mol Imaging 2006;33:281-291.
24. Goldfarb M, Rosenberg C, Abassi Z, et al: Acute-on-chronic renal failure in the rat: Functional compensation and hypoxia tolerance. Am J Nephrol 2006;26:22-33.

See the companion Expert Consult website for the complete reference list.

Laboratory Tests and Diagnostic Methods

CHAPTER 46

Kidney Function Tests and Urinalysis in Acute Renal Failure

Sean M. Bagshaw and Rinaldo Bellomo

OBJECTIVES

This chapter will:
1. Provide an overview of kidney function.
2. Discuss the role of serum markers of kidney function in the management of acute renal failure.
3. Identify common urinary biochemical tests used in the diagnosis of acute renal failure.
4. Describe the use of urinary microscopy in the diagnosis of acute renal failure.
5. Evaluate the utility of cystatin C in the estimation of glomerular filtration rate.
6. Summarize emerging knowledge about neutrophil gelatinase-associated lipocalin as an early marker for acute renal failure.
7. Review emerging knowledge about interleukin-18 as an early marker for acute renal failure.

Acute renal failure (ARF) remains a major therapeutic challenge for the modern clinician. Depending on the criteria used to define its presence, ARF has been described in 5% to 25% of critically ill patients.[1-5] Recently, a new consensus definition and classification for ARF have been developed and validated,[6-8] which are considered in more detail in other chapters. To summarize for the purposes of this discussion, this classification, referred to by the acronym RIFLE (*r*isk, *i*njury, *f*ailure, *l*oss of kidney function, *e*nd-stage renal disease), divides acute renal dysfunction into the categories of risk, injury, and failure. The RIFLE classification is likely to be the dominant approach to defining ARF in the intensive care unit (ICU) setting for the foreseeable future.[9] With use of this classification, the incidence of at least some degree of renal dysfunction was shown to be as high as 67% in a recent study of more than 5000 critically ill patients.[8] Moreover, renal dysfunction of maximum RIFLE category of failure was found in up to 28% of critically ill patients and was associated with a several-fold increased risk of hospital death.[7,8] Thus, despite continuing advances in our understanding of the pathophysiology of ARF and application of supportive extracorporeal therapies, the morbidity and mortality attributable to ARF remain excessive. Therefore, the timely and accurate diagnosis of ARF is of paramount prognostic

and therapeutic importance for critically ill patients with ARF.

In this chapter, the common serum measures of kidney function and urinary tests used in ARF are reviewed. In addition, the potential diagnostic and prognostic role for several urinary biomarkers is discussed.

OVERVIEW OF KIDNEY FUNCTION

Before considering the spectrum of serum and urinary tests available to evaluate kidney function for ARF, a logical approach is to begin by reviewing the array of functions performed by the kidney. Of note, many of these functions either are shared with other organs (e.g., acid-base control with lung) or involve complex neurohormonal interactions, which also involve other organ systems (e.g., renin-angiotensin-aldosterone axis). In addition, other functions are not routinely measured (e.g., small peptide excretion, tubular metabolism, hormonal production) in the everyday care of the patient with ARF. The kidney contributes several essential functions for maintaining physiological homeostasis in the body, including the following:

- Maintenance of a constant extracellular milieu (in concert with other body systems) through urinary excretion of water, electrolytes, acids, and metabolic waste products (e.g., creatinine, urea, uric acid)
- Regulation of systemic and renal hemodynamics by production of renin, angiotensin II, endothelin, prostaglandins, and nitric oxide
- Secretion of erythropoietin for regulation of red blood cell production
- Secretion of 1,25-dihydroxyvitamin D_3 for regulation of calcium, phosphate, and bone metabolism
- Participation in metabolism of small peptides
- Participation in gluconeogenesis during fasting or starvation

Thus, in the setting of ARF, some or all of these vital functions may be impaired or absent. The critically ill patient with ARF may have retention of uremic metabolites, decreased capacity for regulation of extracellular volume status, impaired electrolyte and acid-base balance, anemia, or accumulation of exogenous toxins.

ASSESSMENT OF KIDNEY FUNCTION

Generally speaking, ARF is defined by a syndrome characterized by a rapid (hours to days) decrease in the kidney's ability to eliminate waste products, regulate extracellular volume, and maintain electrolyte and acid-base homeostasis. This loss in excretory function may be manifested clinically by an accumulation of end products of metabolism (e.g., creatinine, urea), diminished urine output (not always present), accumulation of nonvolatile acids, or an increased serum potassium concentration.

Clinicians at the bedside have relied on these measurable effects to characterize an acute loss in kidney excretory function and for defining and identifying patients with ARF. As a consequence, various serum and urinary tests have been developed and routinely applied in clinical practice.

In view of the poor prognosis and increased risk of death in critically ill patients with ARF, it is clearly desirable to have tests of kidney function that would allow early diagnosis of ARF and for which results could be correlated with true reductions in kidney function associated with acute injury. Identification of those critically ill patients by such tests would allow early and aggressive intervention, if justified.

Glomerular Filtration Rate

Most tests of kidney function are fashioned to approximate or estimate the *glomerular filtration rate* (GFR). GFR is a global measure of kidney function. The GFR is defined as the sum of the filtration rates for all functioning nephrons in a given patient. GFR is known to vary based on patient age, race, sex, and body mass. In addition, GFR exhibits considerable inter- and intrapatient variation; however, normal values in young healthy adults typically are in the range of 120 ($\pm$25) mL/min/1.73 m^2 of body surface area. ARF, therefore, is regarded as reflecting an acute decrease in GFR. The main difficulty with GFR is that it cannot be measured directly but rather can only be estimated by calculating the clearance of a filtered serum marker:

$$\text{GFR (mL/min)} = (U_a \times V)/P_a$$

where a represents an ideal serum marker of GFR, U_a is the urinary concentration of a, V is the urine flow rate, and P_a is the serum concentration of a; under ideal circumstances, the filtered load of a would equal GFR.

The ideal serum marker to estimate GFR would ideally encompass several characteristics, in particular, such a marker would be endogenous and nontoxic, freely filtered at the glomerulus and excreted unchanged in the urine (i.e., not secreted, metabolized, or reabsorbed by renal tubular cells), and not influenced by exogenous compounds (e.g,. drugs), as well as water soluble, with minimal protein binding. Moreover, this marker would be sensitive to both early and small changes in GFR and could be reliably measured across diverse patient populations with ARF of variable severity. Finally, the ideal marker would be easy, rapid and inexpensive to measure. Regrettably, such an ideal serum marker has yet to be discovered. Although several exogenous serum markers can be used to estimate GFR (i.e., inulin, iothalamate, ethylenediaminetetraacetic acid [EDTA], and iohexol), often their measurement is complex, expensive, and impractical for use in routine clinical practice in critically ill patients.

Serum Markers of Kidney Function in ARF

The most commonly used and practical serum tests to estimate GFR are endogenous markers such as creatinine, urea, cystatin C. Unfortunately, none of these markers is ideal and each has its own limitations. A major limitation with all of these endogenous markers, however, is that none reflect real-time dynamic changes in GFR that occur with acute reductions in kidney function. Rather, each endogenous marker requires time to accumulate before it can be detected as an abnormality, leading to a potential delay in the diagnosis of ARF. In addition, each of these serum markers can potentially be grossly modified by aggressive fluid resuscitation.

Serum Creatinine

Creatinine is an amino acid compound derived from the metabolism of creatine in skeletal muscle and from dietary meat intake. Creatinine has a molecular weight of 113 daltons, is released into the plasma at a relatively constant rate, is freely filtered by the glomerulus, and is not reabsorbed or metabolized by the kidney. Accordingly, the clearance of creatinine is the most widely used means for estimating GFR.[10] Serum creatinine levels generally have an inverse relationship to GFR (Fig. 46-1). Thus, a rise in serum creatinine is associated with corresponding decrease in GFR and generally implies a reduction in kidney function, and vice versa. Limitations to the usefulness of creatinine as a serum marker to estimate GFR are well recognized, however.

First, an estimated 10% to 40% of creatinine clearance occurs by tubular secretion of creatinine into the urine by the organic cation secretory pathways in the proximal renal tubular cells.[11] Although this generally is more important for patients with early chronic kidney disease (CKD), in which serum creatinine levels appear to be stable (i.e., generally in range at less than 133 μmol/L) as a result of compensatory increases in proximal renal tubular secretion. This effect, however, can potentially mask a significant initial decline in GFR. Second, several drugs (e.g., trimethoprim, cimetidine) are known to impair creatinine secretion, which may lead to a transient and reversible increase in serum creatinine. Third, the production and release of creatinine into the serum can be highly variable. Differences in dietary intake (as in vegetarian diets or with use of creatine supplements) or baseline muscle mass (as with neuromuscular disease, malnutri-

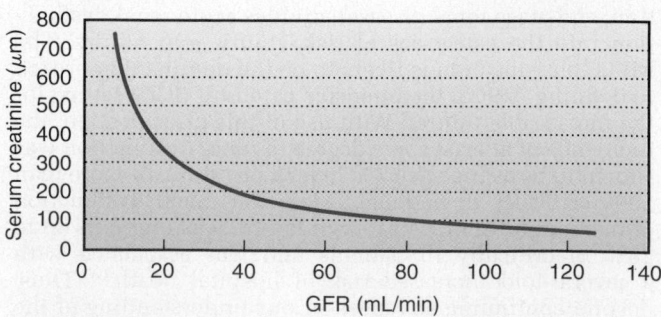

FIGURE 46-1. Relationship between serum creatinine and glomerular filtration rate (GFR). A reduction in GFR decreases clearance of serum creatinine and results in a nonlinear rise in serum creatinine.

tion, or amputation) can result in significant variation in baseline serum creatinine. Likewise, certain pathological states may predispose to variable release of muscle creatinine. For example, in rhabdomyolysis, serum creatinine levels may rise more rapidly owing to release of preformed creatinine from damaged muscle or peripheral metabolism of creatine phosphate to creatinine in extracellular tissue.[12,13] Finally, certain factors can reduce the accuracy of serum creatinine assays and lead to artifactual increases in serum creatinine levels. For example, in diabetic keto-acidosis, increased serum concentration of acetoacetate can cause interference with selected assays (e.g., alkaline picrate method), leading to a falsely elevated serum creatinine value.[14] Some drugs (e.g., cefoxitin, flucytosine) are known to cause similar effects.

Serum Urea Concentration

Urea is a water-soluble, low-molecular-weight by-product of protein metabolism that is recognized to be a useful serum marker of uremic solute retention and elimination. In chronic hemodialysis patients, the degree of urea clearance has clearly shown correlation with clinical outcome and is used to assess the adequacy of hemodialysis over time. Acute and large rises in serum urea concentration are characteristic of development of the uremic syndrome and retention of a large variety of uremic toxins. In addition, the accumulation of urea itself is believed to predispose to adverse metabolic, biochemical, and physiological effects such as increased oxidative stress, altered function of Na^+-K^+-Cl^- cotransport pathways important in regulation of intracellular potassium and water, and alterations in immune function.[15-17]

Similar to serum creatinine, urea exhibits a nonlinear and inverse relationship with GFR. The use of urea to estimate GFR is problematic, however, owing to the numerous potential extrarenal factors, independent of GFR, that can influence its endogenous production and renal clearance.

First, the rate of urea production is not constant (Table 46-1). Urea can increase in response to a high protein intake, critical illness (e.g., sepsis, burns, trauma), gastrointestinal hemorrhage, or drug therapy such as use of corticosteroids or tetracycline.[18] Conversely, patients with chronic liver disease and low protein intake can have lower urea levels without noticeable changes in GFR. In fact, the accurate measurement of kidney function in patients with chronic liver disease can be problematic.[19,20] For example, cirrhotic patients may have near-normal values for urea (e.g., due to decreased production or

protein restriction) and serum creatinine (e.g., decreased production due to decreased hepatic creatine synthesis, increased tubular creatinine secretion, or loss of skeletal muscle mass) despite severely impaired kidney function.

Second, the rate of renal clearance of urea is not constant. An estimated 40% to 50% of filtered urea is passively reabsorbed by proximal renal tubular cells. Moreover, in states of decreased effective circulating volume (e.g., volume depletion, low cardiac output), enhanced reabsorption of sodium and water is seen in the proximal renal tubular cells, along with a corresponding increase in urea reabsorption. Consequently, the serum urea concentration may increase out of proportion to observed changes in serum creatinine and be underrepresentative of GFR. The ratio of serum urea to serum creatinine concentration has, by tradition, been used as an index of discrimination between so-called prerenal ARF and more established ARF (e.g., acute tubular necrosis [ATN]) (Table 46-2).

TABLE 46-1

Reported Factors That May Influence Accuracy of Serum Measures of Kidney Function

SERUM MARKER	FACTOR
Creatinine	Age
	Race
	Sex
	Muscle mass
	Meat ingestion
	Amputation
	Chronic illness
	Neuromuscular diseases
	Vegetarian diet
Urea	Liver disease
	Low protein intake
	Trauma
	Burns
	Sepsis
	Gastrointestinal bleeding
	Corticosteroids
	Tetracycline
Cystatin C	Age
	Sex
	Height
	Weight
	Smoking status
	Inflammation
	Thyroid disease
	Corticosteroids

TABLE 46-2

Traditional Laboratory Tests Used to Help Diagnose "Established" Acute Renal Failure (ARF)

MEASURED PARAMETER	PRERENAL ARF	ESTABLISHED ARF
Urine sediment	Normal	Epithelial casts
Urine specific gravity	High: >1.020	Low: <1.020
Urine sodium (mmol/L)	Low: <10	High: >20
Fractional excretion of sodium	<1%	>1%
Fractional excretion of urea	<35%	>35%
Urine osmolality (mOsmol/kg H_2O)	High: >500	Near serum: <300
Urine-plasma creatinine ratio	High: >40	Low: <10
Plasma urea-creatinine ratio	High	Normal

Adapted from Han WK, Bonventre JV: Biologic markers for the early detection of acute kidney injury. Curr Opin Crit Care 2004;10:476-482.

Serum Cystatin C

Cystatin C is an endogenous cysteine proteinase inhibitor of low molecular weight that possesses many ideal features for use as a surrogate marker of kidney function and an estimate of GFR. Cystatin C is synthesized at a relatively constant rate and is released into plasma by all nucleated cells in the body.[21-23] Cystatin C levels reportedly are not affected by patient age, sex, muscle mass, or changes in diet. Absence of correlation with these parameters, however, has recently been challenged (see Table 46-1). In a large cross-sectional study of 8058 patients, several factors were found to be associated with elevated cystatin C levels, including older age, male sex, greater height, greater weight, current smoking status, and elevated C-reactive protein levels.[24] Cystatin C levels also have been found to be influenced by abnormal thyroid function, use of immunosuppressive therapy (e.g., with corticosteroids), and the presence of systemic inflammation.[24-27]

Nonetheless, the main catabolic site of cystatin C is the kidney, with more than 99% freely filtered by the glomerulus. Cystatin C is not notably secreted or reabsorbed, but it is nearly completely metabolized by proximal renal tubular cells. As a consequence, little to no detectable cystatin C is present in the urine. Thus, although a reduction in GFR correlates well with a rise in serum cystatin C level, true clearance of cystatin C cannot be determined. Nevertheless, serum cystatin C concentrations have demonstrated good inverse correlation with radionuclide scan–derived measurements of GFR.[22,28]

The diagnostic value of cystatin C as an estimate of GFR has now been investigated in multiple clinical studies. Cystatin C has been found to be comparable or superior to serum creatinine for discrimination of normal from impaired kidney function.[22,28] In addition, cystatin C may be more sensitive than creatinine to early and mild changes in kidney function.[29-31]

Recently, estimation equations for GFR based on serum cystatin C levels have been formulated.[32,33] Some evidence suggests that cystatin C–based estimates of GFR may be superior in selected patient populations, particularly those with lower serum creatinine concentrations such as elderly patients, children, renal transplant recipients, cirrhotics, and malnourished persons.[34,35] The main drawback to use of cystatin C, however, is the lack of a widely accepted or available standardized method for its measurement. Thus, whether incorporation of cystatin C assays into routine clinical practice will result in improvement in the diagnosis of ARF and in outcome for critically ill patients requires additional investigations.

Equations to Estimate Glomerular Filtration Rate

Several equations for estimation of GFR have been developed and validated. The most commonly used are the Cockcroft-Gault and Modification of Diet in Renal Disease (MDRD) Study Group equations.[36,37] These equations estimate GFR on the basis of the patient's serum creatinine concentration while at the same time incorporating several recognized demographic and clinical factors that can independently influence serum creatinine concentration such as age, sex, race, and body weight.

The Cockcroft-Gault equation to estimate creatinine clearance is[36]

$$CrCl = (140 - \text{age in years}) \times IBW\ (kg)/SCr\ (\mu mol/L)$$
$$(\times\ 0.85\ \text{for women})$$

where CrCl is creatinine clearance (in mL/min), IBW is ideal body weight (in kg), and SCr is serum creatinine (in $\mu mol/L$).

The abbreviated MDRD equation to estimate GFR (in $mL/min/1.73\ cm^2$) is[37]

$$GFR = 186.3 \times (SCr/88.4)^{-1.154} \times (age)^{-0.203} \times$$
$$(0.742\ \text{if female}) \times (1.21\ \text{if black})$$

where SCr represents serum creatinine (in $\mu mol/L$). The final two terms of the equation are adjustments for patient sex (i.e., female) and race (i.e., black). These formulas can be accessed online at www.kidney.org/professional/kdoqi/gfr_calculator or www.nephron.com, where estimates of GFR can be automatically calculated.

In the end, however, use of these GFR estimation equations is limited, in particular for critically ill patients with ARF, for several reasons. First, these equations have not been validated in certain populations, such as patients with liver disease, kidney transplant recipients, morbidly obese persons, and patients at extremes of age. Second, these equations require stability in kidney function and a stable serum creatinine value. In general, for the critically ill patient with a rapidly changing serum creatinine, data from these equations are not interpretable and would not reflect dynamic changes to GFR. An important point in this context is that in the ICU, exact knowledge of GFR generally is not necessary and provides little supplementary information. Rather, what is vital is to recognize whether kidney function is stable or acutely changing. This determination usually can be made by comparisons of changes in serum creatinine from baseline.[6] As an example, an elderly female who is malnourished may have a baseline creatinine that is well below the lower range of normal (i.e., 35 $\mu mol/L$), and whereby a 2-fold increase would still represent a serum creatinine in the "normal" range. Estimation of GFR in this circumstance would yield a normal value, yet the result would not be valid or interpretable. A change in serum creatinine from baseline, however, would be indicative of a severe reduction in kidney function.

Urinary Tests in Acute Renal Failure
Urine Output

Urine output is a commonly measured parameter of kidney function in ARF. Ongoing monitoring urine output is a dynamic gauge of kidney function. Urine output can be a more sensitive barometer for detection of changes in renal hemodynamics than biochemical markers of solute clearance. Dynamic changes in urine output have been integrated into the RIFLE classification of ARF.[6] Unfortunately, urine output is of limited sensitivity and specificity, with development of severe ARF, as detected by a markedly elevated serum creatinine, seen in patients who maintain normal urine output (i.e., so-called nonoliguric ARF). Because nonoliguric ARF carries a lower mortality rate than that for oliguric ARF, urine output frequently is used to differentiate between these forms of ARF; however, the value of this distinction frequently can be negated by the use of diuretics.[38] Oliguria has classically been defined (approximately) as urine output less than 5 mL/kg per day or 0.5 mL/kg per hour.

Urinary Biochemistry and Derived Indices

Numerous tests of urinary biochemistry and derived indices have been described and traditionally used to aid clinicians in the detection and classification of early ARF into prenatal ARF and so-called ATN or established ARF. These tests and indices are outlined in Table 46-2.

FRACTIONAL EXCRETION OF SODIUM. Traditionally, the fractional excretion of filtered sodium (FeNa) has been advocated for differentiation between prerenal and established ARF.[39-41] Filtered sodium is avidly reabsorbed in the renal tubules from glomerular filtrate in the setting of prerenal ARF, resulting in a FeNa less than 1%, whereas in the setting of renal tubular injury in established ARF, the resulting FeNa is greater than 1%. The diagnostic utility of the FeNa has been questioned, however, and several reports emphasize that the FeNa value mandates careful interpretation.[42,43] For example, the FeNa often is greater than 1% in patients having received diuretic therapy regardless of the fluid status of the patient.[44,45] Furthermore, a FeNa less than 1% has been measured in conditions associated with parenchymal ARF, including sepsis, rhabdomyolysis, and exposure to radiocontrast media, perhaps reflecting nonhomogeneous injury to the renal parenchyma and preservation of tubular function in some regions of kidney.[46-49]

URINARY SODIUM CONCENTRATION. The urinary sodium concentration (UNa) is a widely cited urinary measure for use in the evaluation of patients with ARF, with values less than 10 to 20 mmol/L generally suggestive of a sodium-avid state and prerenal ARF and values greater than 40 mmol/L more consistent with ATN.[40,50-52] Several studies have found that UNa performs poorly for discriminating prerenal ARF from ATN. In one study, only 33% of patients classified as having prerenal ARF had a UNa less than 20 mmol/L, whereas 23% of those classified as having ATN had a UNa less than 20 mmol/L.[53] Even fewer studies have reported changes in UNa over time. Several small reports have found a UNa less than 20 mmol/L in critically ill patients with hyperdynamic septic shock.[49,54,55] Similar data have been reported for a large mammalian model of hyperdynamic septic ARF in which evidence of an early decline in UNa less than 20 mmol/L and FeNa less than 1% was found despite grossly elevated renal blood flow.[46,56] These series of experimental studies challenge the prevailing dogma that low UNa and FeNa reflect a state of prerenal ARF. Moreover, Pru and Kjellstrand suggested that the UNa and FeNa are poor prognostic predictors of the need for renal replacement therapy (RRT) or recovery of renal function after an episode of ARF.[43] The available data suggest that UNa has little diagnostic or prognostic value in critically ill patients with ARF.

FRACTIONAL EXCRETION OF UREA. The fractional excretion of urea (FeU) has been cited as a more precise measure for the detection of early ARF, in particular if concomitant diuretic therapy has been given, with an FeU less than 35% indicating prerenal ARF and an FeU greater than 35% consistent with ATN.[52] In the study by Carvounis and colleagues in which ARF was classified as prerenal ARF by diuretic exposure or ATN, an FeU less than 35% was evident in 90%, 89%, and 4% of patients with prerenal ARF, prerenal ARF with diuretics, and ATN, respectively.[44] This study found that the FeU was superior in sensitivity and specificity to the FeNa for classifying ARF.

URINE-PLASMA CREATININE RATIO. The urine-plasma creatinine ratio has been cited as a measure to aid in the classification of ARF, with values greater than 40 suggestive of prerenal ARF and less than 20 indicative of ATN.[50,51] Although some studies have described the classic pattern in urine-plasma creatinine ratios,[40,44] other studies have shown inconsistent results.[49,54,57] For example, in one series, 83% of ratios were less than 20 in the setting of presumed ATN.[54] Likewise, other studies have found ratios greater than 40 in only 33% to 50% of patients classified as having prerenal ARF.[49,55,57] Moreover, in numerous examples, a ratio less than 20 appears to contradict the relevance of an FeNa less than 1% in classifying ARF.[49,57,58] As a consequence, the value of the urine-plasma creatinine ratio for diagnosing ARF in critically ill patients remains unproved.

SERUM UREA-CREATININE RATIO. A serum urea-creatinine ratio greater than 20 is considered suggestive of prerenal ARF and a ratio less than 10 to 15 reflective of ATN.[51] In one study, a serum urea-creatinine ratio less than 15 was found in 38% of those with presumed prerenal ARF.[57] Likewise, this ratio frequently misclassified ARF in patients in another study.[44] Overall, no studies have evaluated the diagnostic or prognostic value of this ratio in critically ill patients with ARF.

ADDITIONAL BIOCHEMISTRY TESTS AND DERIVED INDICES. Numerous additional urinary biochemistry tests and derived indices have been reported that aim to further improve our capability to discriminate between prerenal ARF and established ARF. These have included urine-plasma urea ratio[40,57,59]; urine uric acid–creatinine ratio[60]; fractional excretion of uric acid[57,60]; fractional excretion of chloride[57]; and the renal failure index (RFI).[40,57,61] Because the available studies are small and few in number, however, the significance of each of these measures for classifying or making predictions about prognosis in critically ill patients with ARF remains unclear.

In summary, in light of the available evidence, the clinical utility of these urinary biochemical tests and derived indices for diagnosis, classification, and prognostication in hospitalized critically ill patients, who often receive massive fluid resuscitation, diuretics, vasopressor infusions, radiocontrast media, and nephrotoxic drugs, remains untested and questionable.[43,62] The significance of these urinary tests and indices in the context of septic ARF was recently reviewed.[62] The study investigators concluded that no single urinary test could be reliably used to diagnose, classify, or predict the clinical course of septic ARF. Moreover, it is imperative to recognize that so-called prerenal ARF and established ATN are part of a continuum, and their separation in diagnostic terms is rather arbitrary, with limited clinical implications or prognostic value. In general, targeted therapeutic interventions would be similar—specifically, to address the underlying cause of ARF while ensuring prompt and adequate resuscitation of the patient.

URINALYSIS AND MICROSCOPY

Urinalysis plus microscopy constitutes an essential and simple noninvasive test that can yield important diagnostic information and patterns suggestive of specific syndromes. Ideally, sterile urine is collected, centrifuged, and separated. The supernatant is then tested for color, pH, specific gravity, protein, and glucose, and the sediment is placed on a slide and examined under a microscope for cells, casts, crystals, and bacteria.

Urinalysis
Color

Urine normally is clear, with a light yellow color that varies with concentration. Several factors can influence the color of urine. Urine appears reddish brown in many pathological states. Red color restricted to the urine sediment is suggestive of hematuria. A red supernatant should prompt assessment for heme pigment, usually due to myoglobinuria or hemoglobinuria. Red supernatant that is heme negative suggests other uncommon causes (e.g., porphyria, drugs, beet ingestion). In addition, the urine may appear white as a result of pyuria; uncommonly, green owing to administration of methylene blue, propofol, or amitriptyline; or blue-black, as a consequence of ochronosis.

Protein

Protein frequently is detected in the urine of critically ill patients.[63] This can result from several factors and may be transient in response to critical illness, physiological stress, fever, or new acute or preexisting kidney disease. An increase in urinary protein excretion commonly is associated with sepsis.[54,61,64-67] The resultant proteinuria generally can be classified into glomerular, tubular, or overflow according to the probable site of origin of the excess protein. Glomerular proteinuria results from leakage and filtration of large-molecular-weight protein (e.g., albumin) across the glomerular capillary wall and implies intrinsic injury to this structure (e.g., glomerulonephritis). Tubular proteinuria, on the other hand, is due to filtration of low-molecular-weight proteins (e.g., immunoglobulin, retinol-binding protein) that are incompletely reabsorbed by proximal renal tubular cells. Overflow proteinuria results from increased ex-cretion of low-molecular-weight proteins that are markedly overproduced (e.g., immunoglobulins in multiple myeloma) and generally exceed the reabsorptive capacity of proximal renal tubular cells. Detecting and quantifying urinary protein in critically ill patients may provide not only data on the etiology of ARF but also important prognostic information.[68-70] Urinary dipstick testing or calculation of a total protein-to-creatinine or albumin-to-creatinine ratio can easily be performed at the bedside. Urinary dipstick testing primarily detects macroalbuminuria only, however, and thus will not detect microalbuminuria (i.e., excretion of less than 300 to 500 mg per day) or the presence of low-molecular-weight proteins. A sulfosalicyclic acid (SSA) test can detect all types of protein in the urine and may alternatively be performed. Radiocontrast media, however, have been shown to cause false-positive results with both urinary dipstick and SSA testing.[71] In the end, in those patients in whom clinically important proteinuria may be present, quantitative assessments of protein excretion should be performed (i.e., by timed urine collection). In addition, serum and urine protein electrophoresis can be done to assess for proteinuria involving low-molecular-weight proteins.

pH

Normal urine pH ranges from 4.5 to 8.0; this value can vary depending on patient acid-base status and therapeutic interventions (e.g., administration of bicarbonate). Routine monitoring of urinary pH in critically ill patients is of little practical importance. Urinary pH can be informative, however, in patients with metabolic acidosis to assess for appropriate urinary acid excretion. In addition, urinary pH monitoring is important during intentional urinary alkalinization (for the treatment of rhabdomyolysis or salicylate poisoning, for example) to monitor

response to sodium bicarbonate loading. Finally, urinary tract infection with urease-splitting pathogens such as *Proteus mirabilis* can be a cause of highly alkaline urine (i.e., pH greater than 7.5).

Urine Specific Gravity and Osmolality

Measurement of the *urine specific gravity* (USG), defined as the ratio of the weight of a given solution compared to that of an equal volume of distilled water, generally is used as a surrogate for urine osmolality. The USG and osmolality usually are well correlated; however, presence of large molecules in the urine, such as glucose or radiocontrast media, can increase USG with no significant change in osmolality. Although serum osmolality generally is regulated within a narrow physiological range (i.e., 280 to 290 mOsmol/kg), the urine osmolality fluctuates widely in response to changes in serum osmolality and the volume status of the patient. Measurement of USG and osmolality is of limited value in critically ill patients.[72] Urine osmolality, however, has traditionally been used as a measure to discriminate between prerenal ARF and established ARF (see Table 46-2).[40,67]

Glucose

Glucose is regularly detected in the urine of critically ill patients and in this setting is of limited clinical value.[67,73] The detection of glucose in the urine can signify surplus filtration due to elevated serum glucose concentrations or dysfunctional reabsorption by the proximal renal tubular cells.

Urine Microscopy

Although small quantities of cells, casts, crystals, and bacteria can be encountered in the urine of healthy patients, in critically ill patients with ARF, assessment of urine sediment by microscopy can yield important diagnostic information.

The cells found in urine sediment include red blood cells (RBCs), white blood cells (WBCs), and epithelial cells. Microscopic hematuria may be commonly encountered in critically ill patients (i.e., severe sepsis); however, evidence of gross hematuria may reflect urogenital trauma or other serious underlying pathology (e.g., bladder cancer), whereas the presence of dysmorphic RBCs or RBC casts is virtually diagnostic of active glomerulonephritis or vasculitis.[61,74,75] Pyuria (presence of WBCs) can arise from several conditions, by far the most common being infection. Sterile (culture-negative) pyuria can occur with active tuberculosis infection, severe sepsis, interstitial nephritis, or nephrolithiasis.[61,74] Although many epithelial cells may appear in the urine, only renal tubular epithelial cells have diagnostic significance.[54,65,74,75] The presence of renal tubular epithelial cells in the urine, particularly in association with casts, indicates a renal source of injury, such as with tubular necrosis, tubular apoptosis, or pyelonephritis.[76]

Several types of casts can be detected in the urine. Casts form as a result of conformation to the renal tubule and appear cylindrical in structure. Hyaline casts are common and can be present under normal circumstances or in concentrated urine specimens. On the other hand, the detection of cellular casts (RBC, WBC, epithelial cell) is abnormal and typically signifies significant kidney injury. RBC casts are virtually pathognomonic for glomerulonephritis or vasculitis. WBC casts are classically seen with acute pyelonephritis or tubulointerstitial diseases.

Epithelial cell casts can be seen in conditions characterized by necrosis or desquamation of epithelial cells, such as ATN, apoptosis, or loss of renal tubular cell basement membrane integrity.[76] Granular and waxy casts generally represent the progressive degeneration of cellular casts. Such descriptions of the urinary sediment represent additional widely accepted criteria for the classification of ARF as prerenal or ATN. The classic urinary sediment description with ATN is evidence of renal tubular epithelial cells with coarse granular, muddy brown or mixed cellular casts, whereas the sediment in prerenal ARF is rather bland in appearance, with occasional hyaline or fine granular casts.[50-52,77] The use of urinary microscopy for classifying ARF is imperfect, however, and findings often fail to correlate with urinary biochemistry values or derived indices. For example, in one small study, no significant differences in microscopy could be found based on a FeNa value either less than or greater than 1%.[74] Moreover, although abnormal sediment has been described in ATN, a normal microscopic appearance also has been described even days after onset of kidney injury.[54,61,64-67,74] In addition, the character of the urinary sediment may be highly variable and dependent more on the timing of measurement, duration, and the underlying pathophysiological condition predisposing to ARF (e.g., ischemic versus septic).[62]

The occurrence of crystals in the urine generally is of little clinical significance in critically ill patients; however, this finding may be important in selected cases. For example, the finding of calcium oxalate crystals in a critically ill patient with a high-anion-gap metabolic acidosis and ARF suggests poisoning with ethylene glycol. Likewise, the presence of uric acid crystalluria and ARF may signify tumor lysis syndrome. Of importance, normal findings on urinalysis also may be of help in the diagnosis, suggesting that ARF is due to factors extrinsic to the kidney (i.e., prerenal) or an obstructive etiology.

URINARY BIOMARKERS

Various proteins, enzymes, antigens, and cytokines, including several novel biomarkers, that can be detected in the urine have been suggested as surrogate markers for acute kidney injury. The rationale for characterization of many of these biomarkers has been to further aid in the early diagnosis of ARF, to help delineate the anatomical site(s) of injury (i.e., proximal tubule, distal tubule, and so on), and to provide potentially important prognostic information about the severity and nature of injury (e.g., septic, toxic, ischemic).[78,79] A summary and classification of currently available biomarkers are presented in Tables 46-3 to 46-5. This section focuses on some of those biomarkers showing early promise for use in routine clinical practice.

Novel Biomarkers
Urinary Na⁺-H⁺ Exchanger Isoform 3

Urinary Na^+-H^+ exchanger isoform 3 (NHE3) is the most abundant sodium transporter in the renal tubule and is responsible for the reabsorption of large amounts of filtered

TABLE 46-3

Urinary Proteins Reported as Potential Indicators of Acute Kidney Injury

URINARY PROTEINS	PROPOSED SITE OF NEPHRON INJURY
Low-Molecular-Weight Proteins	
α_1-Microglobulin	Proximal renal tubule
β_2-Microglobulin	Proximal renal tubule
Retinol-binding protein	Proximal renal tubule
High-Molecular-Weight Proteins	
Albumin	Glomerulus
Immunoglobulin	Glomerulus
Transferrin	Glomerulus
Other	
Tamm-Horsfall glycoprotein	Distal renal tubule–ascending loop of Henle

Adapted from Han WK, Bonventre JV: Biologic markers for the early detection of acute kidney injury. Curr Opin Crit Care 2004;10:476-482.

TABLE 46-4

Urinary Enzymes Reported as Potential Surrogate Markers for Acute Kidney Injury

URINARY ENZYMES	PROPOSED SITE OF NEPHRON INJURY
Brush Border Antigens	
Adenosine deaminase–binding protein	Proximal renal tubule
Proximal renal tubule epithelial antigen (HRTE-1)	Proximal renal tubule
Carbonic anhydrase	Proximal renal tubule
Urinary Enzymes	
Alanine aminopeptidase	Proximal renal tubule
Cathepsin B	Proximal renal tubule
Neutral endopeptidase	Proximal renal tubule
γ-Glutamyl transferase	Proximal renal tubule
Alkaline phosphatase	Proximal, distal renal tubules
β-Glucosidase	Proximal, distal renal tubules
Lactate dehydrogenase	Proximal, distal renal tubules
N-acetyl-β-glucosaminidase	Proximal, distal renal tubules
Kallikrein	Distal renal tubule

Adapted from Han WK, Bonventre JV: Biologic markers for the early detection of acute kidney injury. Curr Opin Crit Care 2004;10:476-482.

TABLE 46-5

Summary of Urinary Biomarkers Reported as Potential Surrogate Markers for Early Acute Kidney Injury

Proteins, Enzymes, and Other/Novel Urinary Biomarkers
Actin
Cysteine-rich protein 61 (Cyr61)
Glutathione-S-transferases
Kidney injury molecule-1 (KIM-1)
Na^+-H^+ exchanger isoform 3 (NHE3)
Neutrophil gelatinase-associated lipocalin (NGAL)
Cytokines
Interleukin-1
Interleukin-6
Interleukin-8
Interleukin-18
Platelet-activating factor (PAF)
Tumor necrosis factor-α

Adapted from Han WK, Bonventre JV: Biologic markers for the early detection of acute kidney injury. Curr Opin Crit Care 2004;10:476-482.

sodium from the urine. NHE3 normally is expressed on the apical membrane of the proximal renal tubule and the thick ascending loop of Henle cells. NHE3 normally is not detectable in the urine. Abnormal elevations of NHE3 in the urine of critically ill patients with ARF have been reported by a small study.[80] In this study, ARF was classified as prerenal azotemia, ATN, or intrinsic ARF other than ATN. The urinary NHE3 was significantly higher in patients whose ARF was designated as ATN than in patients with prerenal azotemia. In addition, urinary NHE3 was not detected in patients with intrinsic ARF other than ATN (e.g., glomerulonephritis, renal transplant rejection). These findings suggest that NHE3 may be a novel early biomarker of acute kidney injury that may aid in discrimination among prerenal azotemia, ATN, and ARF due to other intrinsic renal causes. Further prospective studies are necessary to verify the diagnostic and prognostic value of NHE3.

Neutrophil Gelatinase-Associated Lipocalin

Neutrophil gelatinase-associated lipocalin (NGAL) belongs to the lipocalin superfamily, consisting of more than 20 structurally related secreted proteins that are thought to participate in ligand transport with a β-barreled calyx.[81] Human NGAL originally was isolated as a 25-kD protein covalently bound to gelatinase from human neutrophils and was shown to be markedly upregulated in response to kidney ischemic or nephrotoxic injury.[81,82] The appearance of NGAL in the urine after injury was rapid and preceded the detection of other known urinary biomarkers. These results suggested that NGAL may be an early and sensitive urinary biomarker for ischemic and nephrotoxic acute kidney injury. Elevations in urinary NGAL early (1 to 3 hours) after cardiac surgery with cardiopulmonary bypass have been shown to be highly sensitive, specific, and predictive for delayed acute kidney injury.[83,84] Similarly, early elevations in urinary NGAL after kidney transplantation were predictive of delayed graft failure and of the need for RRT during the first week after transplantation.[85,86]

Kidney Injury Molecule-1

Kidney injury molecule-1 (KIM-1) is a type 1 transmembrane glycoprotein that normally is minimally expressed in kidney tissue but shows marked upregulation in proximal renal tubular cells in response to ischemic or nephrotoxic acute kidney injury.[87-89] The ectodomain segment of KIM-1 is shed from proximal cells and detected in the urine by immunoassay.[90] Kidney biopsy specimens from patients with ATN show increased and significantly greater KIM-1 tissue expression compared with that in other acute and chronic kidney diseases.[90] In addition, urinary levels of KIM-1 were significantly higher in ATN than those in other conditions causing ARF (e.g., prerenal ARF, radiographic contrast–induced nephropathy) or CKD. KIM-1 may represent an early, noninvasive biomarker for proximal tubular acute kidney injury; however, further prospective studies are needed to characterize its usefulness in clinical practice.

Urinary Cytokines

Numerous cytokines have now been detected in the urine of critically ill patients with acute kidney injury, including interleukin-1 (IL-1), IL-6, IL-8, IL-18, tumor necrosis factor-α, and platelet-activating factor (PAF).[21,78,79,91] Inflammatory states characterized by increased production of these cytokines may be both a consequence of and predispose to acute kidney injury. In a series of 40 patients undergoing kidney transplantation, urinary IL-6, IL-8, and actin levels were found to be elevated and were predictive of early and sustained postoperative ARF.[92] In another small series, increased PAF was detected in the urine of patients with septic ARF.[93] Moreover, urinary PAF was correlated with additional serum and urine inflammatory cytokines (e.g., IL-1, IL-6, IL-8, TNF-α), suggesting a possible role for PAF in the pathophysiology of acute kidney injury in sepsis. Experimental studies have shown IL-18 to be a mediator of ischemic acute kidney injury. Urinary IL-18 concentrations were found to be significantly increased in the urine of patients with ATN when compared to urine from those with prerenal azotemia, urinary tract infection, or CKD, or in healthy control subjects.[94] In addition, raised urinary IL-18 concentrations after kidney transplantation have been shown to be predictive of delayed graft failure.[86,94] Early detection (at 4 to 6 hours) of urinary IL-18 after cardiac surgery with cardiopulmonary bypass also has been found to be predictive of late increases (at 48 to 72 hours) in serum creatinine suggestive of acute kidney injury.[95] Recently, in a nested case-control study of critically ill patients with acute respiratory distress syndrome (ARDS), elevated urinary IL-18 values preceded overt clinical manifestations of ARF by 24 to 48 hours.[96] Moreover, in this patient population, a high urinary IL-18 concentration at enrollment was an independent predictor of mortality.

The newer urinary biomarkers generally have only recently been developed and have not been assessed in large prospective studies, and assays are not widely available. Therefore, although early results are encouraging, the value of assays of such biomarkers as early noninvasive tests to diagnose kidney injury, to guide in classifying ARF, or to provide useful prognostic data remains uncertain. Additional investigation can be expected to provide further insight on their role.

CONCLUSION

ARF is a complex and heterogeneous syndrome. This is all the more evident in the context of critical illness. In the critically ill patient with ARF, any of a multitude of factors can predispose to or worsen kidney function, such as the presenting illness (e.g., sepsis, major surgery, liver disease), preexisting comorbid conditions (e.g., CKD), ongoing investigations (e.g., those using radiocontrast media), and therapeutic interventions (e.g., mechanical ventilation, antimicrobials, diuretics). In these circumstances, accurate measures of kidney function and detection of injury are essential. Although many kidney function and urinary tests have been described, it is likely that no one test will ever be considered ideal or have sufficient sensitivity and specificity to be valuable across a broad spectrum of patients with ARF. As a consequence, clinicians generally continue to rely on the measurement of serum creatinine, urea, and urine output as the three pillars of diagnosis and classification of ARF. Future study may clarify the role of cystatin C for routine measurement of kidney function. More traditional tests of urinary biochemistry and derived indices used to differentiate prerenal ARF from ATN appear to have limited value and are expected to be increasingly supplanted by novel noninvasive biomarkers that allow for early detection of kidney injury across a spectrum of ARF severity. Many urinary biomarkers require further investigation to clarify their diagnostic and prognostic utility; for some, however, early results are promising and hold the potential to guide research in critical care nephrology into exciting new directions.

Key Points

1. The assessment of kidney function in the intensive care unit remains limited to estimating glomerular filtration rate by means of serum creatinine.
2. Serum creatinine is an insensitive meaure of glomerular filtration rate.
3. Estimates of glomerular filtration rate that use serum creatinine also are insensitive.
4. Serum cystatin C measurement is emerging as a new way of estimating glomerular filtration rate.
5. The superiority of cystatin C to creatinine is not yet fully established.
6. Biochemical urinalysis is of limited diagnostic and predictive usefulness in acute kidney injury.
7. Urinary microscopy is of limited diagnostic and predictive usefulness in acute kidney injury
8. New markers are emerging (neutrophil gelatinase-associated lipocalin and interleukin-18) that appear to identify patients at risk for acute kidney injury before changes in serum creatinine become evident.

Key References

10. Stevens LA, Levey AS: Measurement of kidney function. Med Clin North Am 2005;89:457-473.
28. Villa P, Jimenez M, Soriano MC, et al: Serum cystatin C concentration as a marker of acute renal dysfunction in critically ill patients. Crit Care 2005;9:R139-R143.
83. Mishra J, Dent C, Tarabishi R, et al: Neutrophil gelatinase-associated lipocalin (NGAL) as a biomarker for acute renal injury after cardiac surgery. Lancet 2005;365:1231-1238.
89. Vaidya VS, Ramirez V, Ichimura T, et al: Urinary kidney injury molecule-1: A sensitive quantitative biomarker for early detection of kidney tubular injury. Am J Physiol Renal Physiol 2006;290:F517-F529.
96. Parikh CR, Abraham E, Ancukiewicz M, Edelstein CL: Urine IL-18 is an early diagnostic marker for acute kidney injury and predicts mortality in the intensive care unit. J Am Soc Nephrol 2005;16:3046-3052.

See the companion Expert Consult website for the complete reference list.

CHAPTER 47

Biomarkers in Acute Kidney Injury

Valerie A. Luyckx and Joseph V. Bonventre

OBJECTIVES

This chapter will:
1. Define characteristics of a useful biomarker in acute kidney injury.
2. Identify known urinary biomarkers of acute kidney injury.
3. Describe serum biomarkers of acute kidney injury as alternatives to serum creatinine.

The classic methods of assessing renal function by measurement of blood urea nitrogen and serum creatinine are insensitive and nonspecific, especially in the setting of kidney injury. Serum creatinine may not rise out of the normal range until more than 50% of renal function has been lost, and the increase becomes apparent several days after the acute kidney injury (AKI) has occurred. In addition, levels of serum creatinine may be affected by other factors, such as muscle mass, age, gender, and hydration status. Identification of sensitive and specific serum and urinary markers that correlate with renal injury would have great practical importance in the management of patients with AKI. Such markers would potentially allow early detection of renal injury, provide prognostic information on the course of AKI, identify the nephron segments most affected, and could be used to screen patients at risk for subclinical renal injury or to assess response to therapy.

An ideal biomarker would be one whose levels are elevated in the urine within minutes to hours of a renal insult, remain elevated as long as the damage persists, and decrease as recovery of renal function takes place. Fluctuations in urinary levels with degree of renal function would be helpful to detect recovery as well as ongoing renal injury. Some researchers would argue that urinary markers are preferable to serum markers because substances present in serum may not necessarily originate from the kidney and therefore may not be specific for renal injury. Absence of a marker in the blood coupled with its presence in the urine is highly suggestive of a renal source. The primary site of injury in most cases of AKI is the renal tubule, with acute tubular necrosis (ATN) a frequent pathological manifestation, so relevant urinary markers should reflect tubular injury or dysfunction. Furthermore, absolute urinary levels may be preferable to normalization of levels of urinary creatinine, because urinary creatinine excretion is not constant in the setting of AKI.

Over the years, urinary markers of renal injury have been evaluated in the study of various forms of AKI.[1-5] Changes in excretion of specific markers in the urine have been found to reflect injury to specific regions of the nephron[4]: High-molecular-weight proteins indicate glomerular injury; low-molecular-weight proteins (retinol-binding protein, Clara cell protein), neutral endopeptidase, brush border antigens, intestinal alkaline phosphatase, and N-acetylglucosaminidase (NAG) indicate damage to individual segments of the proximal tubule; urinary Tamm-Horsfall glycoprotein is a marker of injury to the thick ascending limb of the loop of Henle and distal convoluted tubule; renal kallikrein reflects integrity of the distal tubule; and prostaglandin E_2 and $F_{2\alpha}$ excretion increases with injury to the collecting tubule and medullary interstitium. Different forms of injury, therefore, may be associated with different urinary patterns of excretion of these markers. In most studies, however, these markers have not been found to be clinically useful, in part because of lack of standardized assays and in part because the specificity of patterns of urinary marker excretion has been found to decrease with advancing renal dysfunction.[4,5]

Urinary biomarkers that have shown promise in recent animal and human studies are outlined in Table 47-1 and are described next.

URINARY BIOMARKERS OF ACUTE RENAL FAILURE

Neutrophil gelatinase-associated lipocalin (NGAL) is a small polypeptide found to be significantly induced in experimental ischemic and nephrotoxic AKI.[6,7] NGAL is reabsorbed by renal proximal tubular epithelial cells and participates in recovery from AKI.[8] NGAL is readily detectable in the urine within 3 hours of severe ischemic injury or within 1 day of cisplatin administration in experimental models.[6,7] Urinary NGAL was detectable earlier than other biomarkers of AKI, such as NAG and β_2-microglobulin.[6] Of interest, even after mild ischemia, NGAL was still detectable, although not until later in the postischemic period.[6]

In patients undergoing cardiopulmonary bypass (CPB), urinary NGAL was found to be a highly sensitive early biomarker of postoperative AKI, rising by 2 hours after surgery but declining within 6 hours.[9,10] In children with diarrhea-associated hemolytic uremic syndrome, urinary NGAL levels were found to be predictive of severity of renal dysfunction.[11] Urinary NGAL, therefore, appears to be an early sensitive marker for AKI, and its expression is proportional to the severity of renal injury.[6,11]

Interleukin-18 (IL-18) is associated with AKI in mice.[12] Urinary IL-18 measured in humans was found to be elevated in ATN and delayed graft function, as compared with those with urinary tract infection, nephrotic syndrome, chronic kidney disease (CKD), and volume depletion, having a sensitivity and specificity greater than 90% for established AKI.[13] IL-18 also has been reported to be evaluated in the urine of children undergoing CPB.[14] Among those who developed AKI, serum creatinine rose after 48 to 72 hours, although urinary IL-18 was detectable by 4 to 6 hours after CPB. Levels of urinary IL-18 peaked at 12 hours and remained elevated at 48 hours. In this study, both urinary IL-18 and NGAL were independently associated with the duration of renal dysfunction. Because these two markers are upregulated with different time courses, their measurements may be complementary in diagnosis and prognosis of AKI, as shown in Figure 47-1. In an adult population, urinary IL-18 also was found to be a predictor of subsequent development of AKI, as well as

TABLE 47-1

Biomarkers in Acute Kidney Injury (AKI)

PROPOSED MARKER	SAMPLE	AFFECTED BY GFR/PROTEINURIA?	TIME TO DETECTION	ASSOCIATED INJURY	HUMAN DATA
NGAL	Urine	No	2-3 hours after ischemia, 1 day after cisplatin	↑ after ischemia/nephrotoxic injury	Y
IL-18	Urine	Unlikely	4-6 hours after injury	↑ ischemic ATN; delayed graft function predicts mortality	Y
KIM-1	Urine	No	3-6 hours after ischemia	↑ in ischemic nephrotoxic, protein overload injury	Y
CYR61	Urine	Unlikely	3-6 hours after ischemia	ATN	N
NHE3	Urine	No	?	↑ in AKI vs. prerenal	Y
IGF-1	Urine	Unlikely	?	↑ in AKI	Y
HGF	Urine	No	?	↑ in severe AKI	Y
EGF	Urine	No	↑ with recovery	↑ with recovery of AKI	Y
α-GST	Urine	No	1-2 days before ↑ creatinine	↑ PT injury, cyclosporine toxicity, early CRI	Y
π-GST	Urine	No	1-2 days before ↑ creatinine	↑ DT injury, acute rejection, later CRI	Y
Proteomics	Urine	?	2 hours	↑ 3 proteins 100% predictive of AKI	Y
CXCR3 chemokines	Urine	Unlikely	?	↑ acute allograft dysfunction	Y
Cystatin C	Serum	Yes	Before creatinine	Inconsistent value in AKI	Y
ProANP	Plasma	Yes	?	↑ predicts AKI and mortality	Y
sTNF-R1, sTNF-R2	Serum	Unlikely	?	↑ in patients with AKI	Y

ATN, acute tubular necrosis; CRI, chronic renal insufficiency; DT, distal tubule; EGF, epidermal growth factor; GFR, glomerular filtration rate; α-GST, α-glutathione-S-transferase; π-GST, π-glutathione-S-transferase; HGF, hepatocyte growth factor; IGF, insulin-like growth factor; IL-18, interleukin-18; KIM-1, kidney injury molecule-1; NGAL, neutrophil gelatinase-associated lipocalin; NHE3, sodium-hydrogen exchanger isoform 3; proANP, pro–atrial natriuretic peptide; PT, proximal tubule; sTNF-R, soluble tumor necrosis factor receptor.

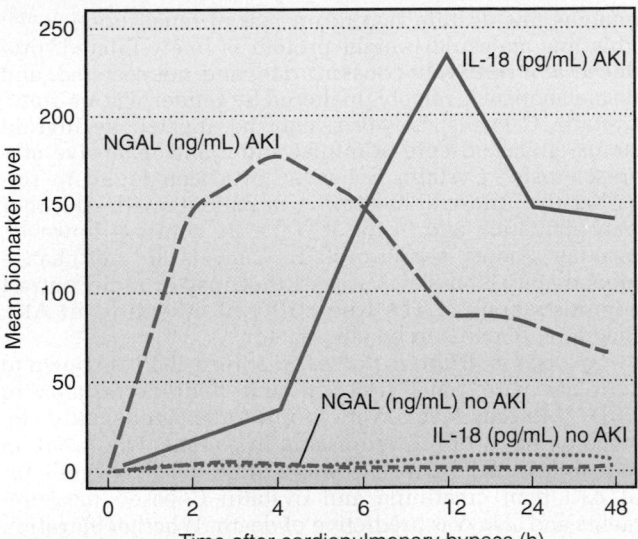

FIGURE 47-1. Pattern of urinary interleukin-18 (IL-18) and neutrophil gelatinase-associated lipocalin (NGAL) levels after cardiopulmonary bypass. Acute kidney injury (AKI), defined as a greater than 50% increase in serum creatinine, developed after 48 to 72 hours in the affected patients. (From Parikh CR, Mishra J, Thiessen-Philbrook H, et al: Urinary IL-18 is an early predictive biomarker of acute kidney injury after cardiac surgery. Kidney Int 2006;70:199-203.)

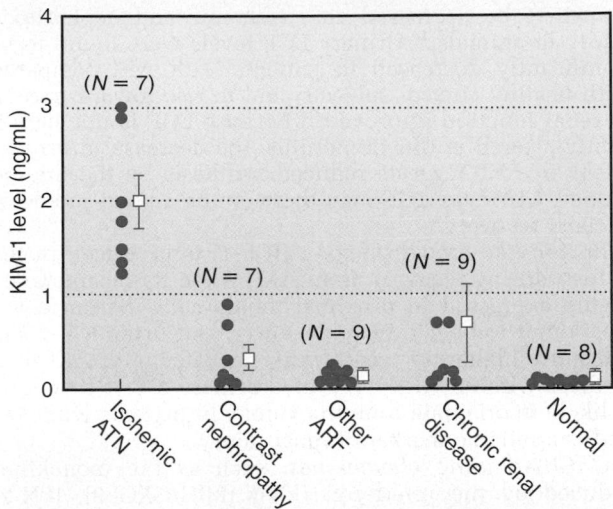

FIGURE 47-2. Urinary kidney injury molecule-1 (KIM-1) concentrations in various forms of renal disease. ATN, acute tubular necrosis; ARF, acute renal failure. (From Han W, Bailly V, Abichandani R, et al: Kidney injury molecule-1 (KIM-1): A novel biomarker for human proximal tubule injury. Kidney Int 2002;62:237-244.)

death, in patients admitted to the intensive care unit (ICU).[15] Urinary IL-18, therefore, has been proposed to be a sensitive and specific marker for presence and severity of AKI.

Kidney injury molecule-1 (KIM-1) is an epithelial cell adhesion molecule that is upregulated in dedifferentiated proximal tubular epithelial cells undergoing replication after AKI.[16] KIM-1 is postulated to play a role in scatter and adhesion of regenerating epithelial cells, as well as in possible protection from injury by formation of a mucinous apical barrier. In animal models, KIM-1 expression increases within 24 hours of ischemic, nephrotoxic, and protein overload–induced AKI.[17-19] A soluble form of KIM-1 is constitutively shed, and urinary levels were most elevated in the presence of ischemic ATN when compared with other types of AKI, CKD, and normal renal function (Fig. 47-2).[20] In addition, absolute urine KIM-1 levels were not affected by proteinuria and were predictive without normalization to serum creatinine. In various animal models of AKI, KIM-1 expression was found to be a highly sensitive and reproducible marker even after mild renal injury.[17,21,22] Urinary KIM-1, therefore, promises to be a reliable marker of renal injury.

Cysteine-rich protein 61 (Cyr61, CCN1) was identified as a potential urinary biomarker in experimental ischemic AKI and is likely to participate in promotion of the healing process.[6,23] Cyr61 is synthesized by the proximal tubule and was detected in the urine 3 to 6 hours after renal ischemia in rodents, but not after volume depletion.[23] Levels peaked at 6 to 9 hours, and Cyr61 was still present 24 hours after AKI. Cyr61 has not yet been evaluated in human AKI but may prove useful in distinguishing early AKI from a prerenal state.

Sodium-hydrogen exchanger isoform 3 (NHE3) is highly expressed in the apical membrane of renal proximal tubule and thick ascending limb epithelial cells.[24] Urinary NHE3 was evaluated in patients with various forms of renal dysfunction on admission to the ICU.[24] Urinary NHE3 was elevated in patients with prerenal azotemia but was six times higher in those with ATN.[24] Levels were not increased in patients with other forms of renal injury. Analysis of NHE3 changes over time was not performed.

Glutathione S-transferases (GSTs) are soluble cytosolic enzymes present in the proximal tubule (α subtype) and distal tubule (π subtype), which participate in detoxifying many compounds. Their presence in the urine correlates with different forms of renal injury. Among renal transplant recipients, urinary levels of π-GST were significantly elevated in those with acute rejection, whereas urinary α-GST was increased in those with cyclosporine toxicity.[25] Transplant recipients with ATN and renal infarction had elevated levels of both isoforms. Absolute GST concentrations were found to correlate well with total amount of enzyme excreted and were not affected by other urinary proteins.[25] Levels of urinary GSTs also were found to be predictive of AKI in a population of critically ill patients.[26] Elevated urinary levels on admission to the ICU predicted serum creatinine elevations 12 to 48 hours later. In patients with glomerular disease and proteinuria, urinary excretion of both GST isoenzymes was found to be independent of blood levels and proteinuria and therefore to reflect loss from damaged renal tubules.[27] In this study, urinary α-GST was more prominent in patients with mild renal dysfunction, and π-GST predominated with advancing renal insufficiency. These findings indicate that the GST enzymes are elevated in CKD but, in patients without known renal disease, may be useful in detecting and discriminating among different types of acute renal injury.

Hepatocyte growth factor (HGF) plays an important role in organogenesis and tissue regeneration in multiple organs. HGF expression is upregulated in animal models of AKI, and short-term HGF administration has been shown to ameliorate renal injury.[28] HGF is not significantly cleared by the kidney, so urinary HGF must originate in the kidney.[29] In humans with AKI, urinary HGF was found to be markedly increased, and levels tended to correlate with severity, especially with oliguria.[30] Urinary HGF levels were significantly higher in patients with AKI than in control subjects and patients with CKD.

Epidermal growth factor (EGF) promotes proliferation and migration of tubular cells in vitro, and its synthesis is known to be decreased after ischemic and nephrotoxic injury in animals.[31] Urinary EGF levels were found to be significantly decreased in patients with AKI compared with healthy control subjects, and to rise toward normal as renal function improved.[32] Because EGF is not significantly cleared at the glomerulus, the decrease in urinary levels in AKI suggests reduced synthesis by the injured kidney.[32] Urinary EGF may therefore be a good predictor of renal recovery.

Insulin-like growth factor-1 (IGF-1) is produced in the kidney during recovery from AKI, when its receptors are highly expressed in proximal tubule cells. Serum IGF-1 was found to be significantly lower, and urine IGF-1 significantly higher, in critically ill neonates with AKI than in those without ARF.[33] Elevated urinary IGF-1, therefore, is likely to originate from the kidney in patients with AKI and is a reliable marker of renal injury.

CXCR3-binding chemokines, such as the monokines induced by the interferon IFN-γ (MIG/CXCL9), IFN-γ–induced protein of 10 kD (IP-10/CXCL10), and IFN-inducible T-cell chemoattractant (I-TAC/CXCL11), determined simultaneously by a triplex assay, all have been shown to be increased in the urine of patients with acute renal allograft dysfunction.[34] The urine assay was more sensitive than determination of serum creatinine in monitoring response to therapy but was not able to discriminate among rejection, ATN, and BK nephropathy. Whether these chemokines have a role in non–transplantation-related AKI has not been investigated.

Other biomarkers that have been investigated in the setting of renal transplantation include urinary intercellular adhesion molecule-1 (ICAM-1), which has been associated with acute rejection but not ATN,[35,36] and urinary actin, IL-6, and IL-8, all of which were elevated in recipients destined to have AKI.[37] In patients with AKI who were not transplant recipients, urinary endothelin-1 (ET) was investigated as a marker of contrast agent–induced renal injury.[38] Urinary ET-creatinine ratio was markedly increased from baseline in patients with CKD but not in those with normal renal function. Of interest, however, contrast agent–induced renal failure did not develop in any of the patients, which raises the question of whether ET is a marker of contrast administration and not renal injury in patients with CKD.

Urinary proteomics has been used to investigate unknown biomarkers as predictors of AKI.[39] Urine from 60 children undergoing CPB was collected at 2 and 6 hours after surgery. AKI developed postoperatively in 15 patients. Analysis of urine samples from these 15 patients consistently showed an increase in four biomarkers of 6.4, 28.5, 43, and 66 kD, respectively. The sensitivity and specificity of the three higher-molecular-mass markers for prediction of subsequent AKI both were 100% at 2 hours after CBP. It is likely that the 28.5-kD protein represents NGAL, and possible that the 66-kD protein may represent albumin, although results of urine dipstick testing were negative.[39] Much more work is required to further develop these promising findings.

SERUM BIOMARKERS OF ACUTE RENAL FAILURE

Cystatin C is an endogenous compound increasingly being recommended as a better measure of GFR than creatinine, especially in early renal disease, when the creatinine

remains low despite significant loss of renal function.[40,41] This low-molecular-weight protein is freely filtered, produced at a relatively constant rate, and not secreted, and its metabolism is largely unaltered by gender, age, or diet.[40] Cystatin C levels, however, may be affected by thyroid status, glucocorticoid administration, and extensive atherosclerosis.[5] Cystatin C levels have been found to rise earlier than those of creatinine in patients with AKI after transplantation and in the ICU.[41-45] By contrast, however, in other studies, serum cystatin C levels did not change immediately after shock wave lithotripsy or radiocontrast administration.[46,47] The true utility of cystatin C in AKI, therefore, remains to be elucidated.

Pro–atrial natriuretic polypeptide (proANP) is known to correlate with renal function and hydration status in CKD.[5,48] Plasma levels were found to be significantly elevated on day 1 of ICU admission in patients who went on to manifest ARF.[48] ProANP was a more sensitive predictor of AKI than creatinine and cystatin C–based measurements and also was predictive of death. Whether elevation of proANP is purely a reflection of degree of renal dysfunction or is confounded by concomitant volume overload in the patient will need to be defined in further studies.

Other predictors in patients with AKI have been recognized: Low plasma fibrinogen was identified as a significant early prognostic marker predictive of death in patients with AKI requiring dialysis.[49] In another cohort, elevated levels of soluble tumor necrosis factor receptors, s-TNF-R1 and s-TNF-R2, in patients with septic shock were independently associated with the development of AKI.[50]

CONCLUSION

Early detection of AKI may be the "missing link" that has hampered significant improvements in outcome in patients with AKI over the past decades. It is likely that no single biomarker will be reflective of all types of renal injury, but the development of a panel of easily detectable urinary and/or serum biomarkers that accurately reflect severity and nature of renal injury will provide a crucial early window of opportunity in which to act to reverse ongoing renal injury. It is possible that with early detection of AKI, specific therapies that have thus far not proved helpful may indeed have benefit if given early enough in the course of disease. Much more study is required to validate and test the biomarkers thus far studied only in small numbers of patients, and to test them in conjunction with each other to maximize diagnostic and prognostic potential.

Key Points

1. Early detection of acute kidney injury is possible using urinary biomarkers.
2. Levels of certain biomarkers (e.g., neutrophil gelatinase-associated lipocalin, kidney injury molecule-1) may reflect severity of renal injury.
3. Biomarkers of acute kidney injury can predict the development of acute kidney injury hours to days before serum creatinine begins to rise.
4. Some biomarkers of acute kidney injury are predictive of mortality.

5. Early detection of acute kidney injury with biomarkers may allow for better stratification of patients for clinical trials and provide an early window for therapy that may revolutionize outcomes in acute kidney injury.

Key References

9. Mishra J, Dent C, Tarabishi R, et al: Neutrophil gelatinase-associated lipocalin (NGAL) as a biomarker for acute renal injury after cardiac surgery. Lancet 2005;365:1231-1238.
13. Parikh CR, Jani A, Melnikov VY, et al: Urinary interleukin-18 is a marker of human acute tubular necrosis. Am J Kidney Dis 2004;43:405-414.
16. Ichimura T, Bonventre J, Bailly V, et al: Kidney injury molecule-1 (KIM-1), a putative epithelial cell adhesion molecule containing a novel immunoglobulin domain, is upregulated in renal cells after injury. J Biol Chem 1998;273:4135-4142.
17. Vaidya VS, Ramirez V, Ichimura T, et al: Urinary kidney injury molecule-1: A sensitive quantitative biomarker for early detection of kidney tubular injury. Am J Physiol Renal Physiol 2006;290:F517-F529.
20. Han W, Bailly V, Abichandani R, et al: Kidney injury molecule-1 (KIM-1): A novel biomarker for human proximal tubule injury. Kidney Int 2002;62:237-244.

See the companion Expert Consult website for the complete reference list.

Imaging of the Kidney in the Critically Ill and Acute Renal Failure

CHAPTER 48

Ultrasonography and Doppler Techniques in Acute Kidney Injury

Lorenzo E. Derchi and Michele Bertolotto

OBJECTIVES

This chapter will:
1. Discuss the role of gray-scale and color Doppler ultrasound in the evaluation of patients with acute renal failure from different causes.
2. Review the ultrasound features of selected conditions manifesting with acute renal failure.
3. Review the limitations of gray-scale and color Doppler ultrasound in patients with acute renal failure.

Acute renal failure (ARF) is a clinical entity characterized by rapid decline in the glomerular filtration rate (GFR) and retention of nitrogenous waste products. It may affect patients with previously normal-functioning kidneys or may develop in those with preexisting chronic renal disease, and may be related to a variety of pathological conditions characterized by renal hypoperfusion (prerenal ARF), intrinsic renal disease (renal ARF), or acute obstruction of the urinary tract (postrenal ARF).

Prerenal ARF is essentially a functional disorder and typically reversible. It is related to renal hypoperfusion due to hypovolemia, low cardiac output, systemic vasodilation, or intrarenal vasoconstriction. Although severe or prolonged renal hypoperfusion may lead to ischemic acute tubular necrosis (ATN), the integrity of renal parenchyma usually is maintained, and renal function normalizes rapidly on restoration of adequate renal perfusion.

Renal ARF (intrinsic renal disease) may be due to a variety of disorders, of which ATN, glomerulopathies, papillary necrosis, and vascular disease are the most common.

Postrenal ARF is due to urinary tract obstruction. To cause impaired function, obstruction must be bilateral or occur in a patient with only one kidney or with preexisting impaired renal function. It may be due to various pathological conditions such as pelvic malignancies or prostatic disease.

ARF often is reversible, with renal replacement therapy ultimately required in less than 20% of patients, and a correct diagnosis is of great importance for proper treatment. The most important diagnostic goals in these patients are (1) identification of correctable causes of renal dysfunction, (2) differentiation between an acute condition affecting previously normal kidneys and a preexisting chronic renal disease that has rapidly worsened, and (3) differentiation among prerenal, renal, and postrenal causes of ARF. In the last instance, the therapeutic approach will differ in accordance with the cause: In prerenal ARF, renal function usually recovers when renal hemodynamics is restored; in instrinsic renal disease, typically ATN, volume changes and optimization of cardiac output are ineffective and can be harmful; and in postrenal ARF, surgical or other intervention is required. The diagnosis is based mainly on patient history and clinical and laboratory findings.

INDICATIONS AND APPLICATIONS FOR ULTRASOUND IMAGING

Appropriate imaging studies are performed to confirm the presence, determine the size, and assess for possible obstruction of the kidneys. Routine administration of iodinated contrast media is not justified, because these agents are potentially nephrotoxic, which will exacerbate the renal dysfunction. Because of its wide availability, portability, and noninvasive nature, ultrasonography—both gray-scale and color Doppler—is regarded as the imaging procedure of choice in these patients and commonly is performed early in the clinical course. Although ultrasound findings usually are nonspecific, they may lead to the right diagnosis and guide the subsequent therapeutic approach, especially when interpreted in light of the clinical findings. Other imaging techniques are rarely needed.

Gray-Scale Ultrasound Imaging

The most important indication for ultrasound imaging in ARF is to exclude obstruction[1] (Fig. 48-1). In clinical practice, this condition accounts for approximately 5% to 25%

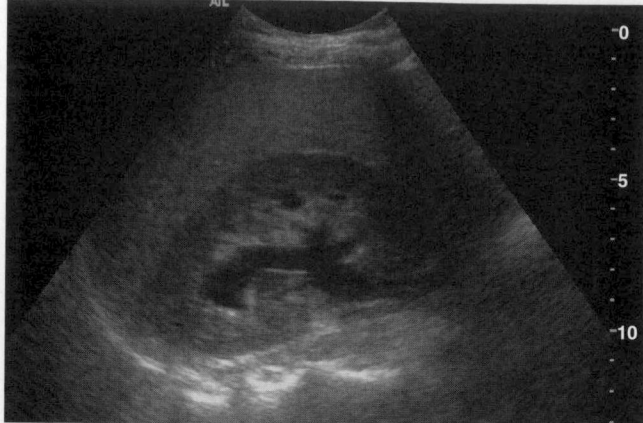

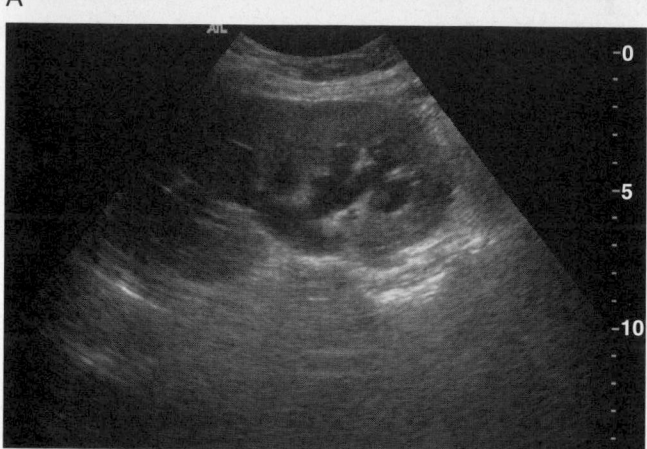

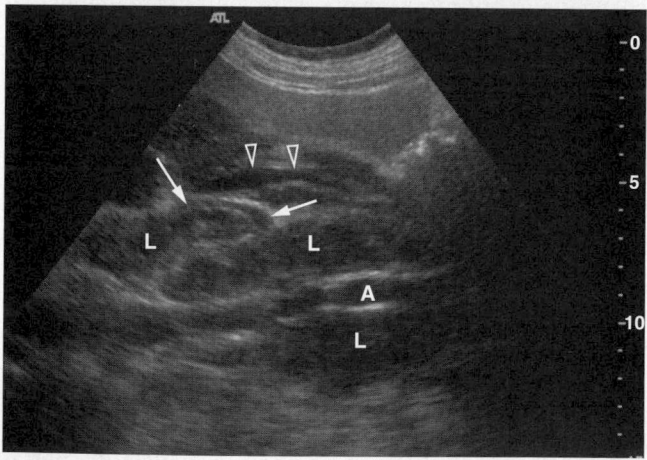

FIGURE 48-1. Ultrasound images of the kidneys in a patient with lymphoma who presented with ARF. **A** and **B,** Coronal views of the right (**A**) and left (**B**) kidneys showing bilateral hydronephrosis. **C,** Coronal view of the right flank demonstrates enlarged lymph nodes (L) surrounding the aorta (A) and inferior vena cava *(small arrows).* The dilated right ureter is compressed and obstructed by the enlarged nodes *(arrowheads).*

of cases of ARF (see Fig. 48-1). Ultrasound imaging is accurate in detecting hydronephrosis, and identification of the dilated urinary tract and of small perirenal urinomas has improved with latest-generation ultrasound equipment, because the recently introduced tissue harmonic

imaging technology allows better signal-to-noise ratio, increased spatial and contrast resolution, and reduced artifact.[2] False-negative results have been reported, however, mostly because of the fact that ARF rarely may result from bilateral obstruction in the absence of urinary tract dilatation.[3]

Because dilatation of the urinary tract also may be present with nonobstructed kidneys, it is important to differentiate obstructive from nonobstructive dilatation, but this can be difficult to resolve by gray-scale ultrasound imaging.[1,4] The accuracy of ultrasound examination in ruling out obstruction increases in patients with a clinical history suggestive of such a condition, such as known pelvic malignancy, palpable abdominal or pelvic mass, or recent pelvic surgery. Patients with urinary tract infection and elevated serum creatinine levels also should undergo ultrasound evaluation to exclude obstruction, because pyonephrosis may quickly result in irreversible renal damage or sepsis.

Size and morphology of the kidneys are important features to evaluate. No specific attributes regarding kidney size are seen in patients with ARF. Of note, however, renal dimensions usually are normal in prerenal ARF, whereas they may be normal or increased in patients with intrinsic renal disease such as ATN, interstitial nephritis, and acute glomerular disease. The finding of large, smooth kidneys with nondilated calices indicates that ARF probably is due to primary acute renal disease, and that the process is likely to be reversible. By contrast, detection of kidneys of reduced size is indicative of preexisting chronic renal disease, with a worse prognosis.

In most patients with ARF, renal echogenicity and parenchymal thickness are normal. With acute and diffuse renal parenchymal disease, however, ultrasound features may include hyperechogenicity, increased parenchymal thickness, and increased corticomedullary differentiation. Reduction in renal parenchymal thickness usually is seen in patients with chronic renal disease (Fig. 48-2).

Duplex Doppler Evaluation

Doppler interrogation of the intrarenal vasculature has proved useful in the evaluation of patients with ARF. In a series of 91 patients with ARF, only 11% showed morphological changes in the renal parenchyma, whereas 69% presented with an elevated renal resistive index (RI).[5] Doppler evaluation of renal hemodynamics provides functional information that can be useful to differentiate among various causes of ARF that are indistinguishable on the basis of morphological features.

Duplex Doppler examination has proved valuable in differentiating between prerenal ARF and ATN.[5-7] Most patients with prerenal ARF demonstrated normal intraparenchymal waveforms, whereas patients with ATN showed abnormal Doppler flow profile, with increased pulsatility and loss of diastolic flow. An RI value of 0.75 was reported as optimal for discrimination between renal and prerenal causes of ARF.[5] The course of ATN may be monitored with duplex Doppler studies using serial measurements of renal RI. Increased RI also can be encountered in other renal pathological conditions causing ARF; follow-up studies during the course of the disease may show improvement of Doppler flow before recovery of renal function[7-9] (Fig. 48-3), as well as complications leading to further deterioration of Doppler waveforms. In clinical practice, however, most cases of ARF are caused by drug abuse or

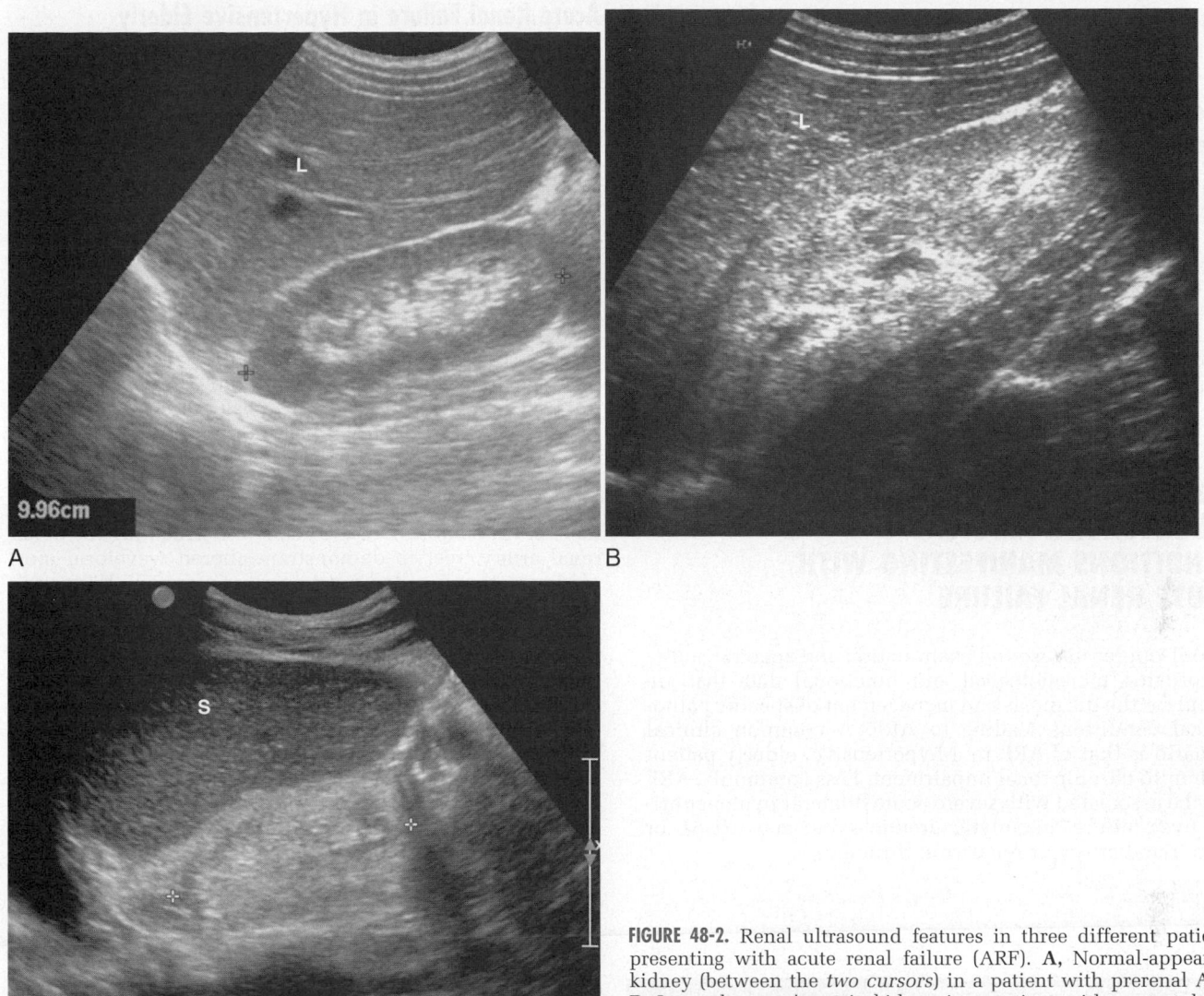

FIGURE 48-2. Renal ultrasound features in three different patients presenting with acute renal failure (ARF). **A,** Normal-appearing kidney (between the *two cursors*) in a patient with prerenal ARF. **B,** Large, hyperechogenic kidney in a patient with acute tubular necrosis. **C,** Small, hyperechogenic kidney in a patient with preexisting chronic renal disease who was experiencing rapid worsening of renal function. L, liver; S, spleen.

are secondary to dehydration in elderly patients with hypertensive intrarenal nephrosclerosis. In these patients, differentiation between renal and prerenal causes of ARF may be difficult, because the RI usually is elevated as a result of preexisting renal parenchymal disease. Furthermore, increased RI also can be appreciated in patients in whom severe and prolonged prerenal ARF leads to ATN. The increased RI is a nonspecific finding, and duplex Doppler ultrasound examination is unable to differentiate among the different causes of ATN. Similar alterations in Doppler waveforms can be encountered in various pathological conditions, including septicemia, rhabdomyolysis, nephrotoxic drug intake, and multiple organ failure.

Renal ARF may be a consequence of a variety of pathologic processes not classified as ATN, such as acute glomerular nephritis, acute interstitial nephritis, severe acute pyelonephritis, systemic lupus erythematosus, and lymphoma. Patients with diseases involving primarily the tubulointerstitial compartment tend to present with abnormal RI values; patients with glomerular disease–based processes often have normal RI values.[5]

Duplex Doppler evaluation also has been reported to be useful in evaluating patients with renal obstruction.[10] A mean RI greater than 0.7, coupled with a difference greater than 0.06 to 0.08 between the average RI of the two kidneys, has been considered to be diagnostic for obstruction. Demonstration of high RI in patients with ARF and hydronephrosis increases the diagnostic confidence for a diagnosis of obstruction. Significant reduction of RI is observed after nephrostomy. The duration of obstruction before its relief is crucial to predict recovery to normal values of the RI. In general, rapid return to normal can be expected if obstruction is relieved within 5 hours, whereas recovery may take days or even weeks if the obstruction was present for at least 18 to 24 hours.[4] An important point is that RI measurements cannot help with identification of patients with obstructed, nondilated kidneys, because many causes other than obstruction may be the origin of the elevated RI.

Color and Power Doppler Ultrasound Imaging

State-of-the-art color and power Doppler ultrasound equipment allows excellent depiction of renal vasculature. In patients with ARF, a significant but nonspecific reduction of intraparenchymal flow signal intensity is usual. More specific information can be obtained in selected cases: Presence of focal avascular areas, either solitary or multiple, can suggest the diagnosis of renal infarction, severe acute pyelonephritis, or embolic disease (see Fig. 48-3).

ULTRASOUND DIAGNOSIS OF SPECIFIC PATHOLOGICAL CONDITIONS MANIFESTING WITH ACUTE RENAL FAILURE

Color Doppler ultrasound examination and spectral analysis provide morphological and functional data that are useful for the diagnosis and management of specific pathological conditions leading to ARF. A common clinical scenario is that of ARF in a hypertensive, elderly patient with mild chronic renal impairment. Less commonly, ARF may be associated with severe acute bilateral pyelonephritis, liver failure, hemolytic uremic syndrome (HUS), or acute renal artery or renal vein thrombosis.

Acute Renal Failure in Hypertensive Elderly Patients with Mild Chronic Renal Impairment

ARF is a relatively common complication of hypertensive nephrosclerosis in elderly patients with mild chronic renal impairment. Worsening of renal function may be precipitated by treatment for hypertension, mainly with angiotensin-converting enzyme (ACE) inhibitors, or by other causes, such as the use of nephrotoxic drugs or dehydration. ARF without an apparent cause or ARF following therapy with ACE inhibitors should suggest renal artery stenosis in well-hydrated elderly patients. Other possible causes are renal artery thrombosis and atheroembolic renal disease.

Because of the nephrotoxic potential of iodinated contrast agents, color Doppler ultrasound examination is the imaging modality of choice in these patients to rule out renal artery stenosis. Identification of kidneys of two different sizes is suggestive of ischemic disease. Doppler studies can be done either directly, interrogating the main renal artery (to demonstrate increased flow velocity at the level of the stenosis), or indirectly, interrogating the distal renal artery tree (to demonstrate altered waveform morphology—the so-called pulsus tardus parvus[11]). Wide variations in the sensitivity and specificity of Doppler ultrasound tests for renal artery stenosis have been reported in the literature, even in the absence of renal insufficiency; indeed, interrogation of the renal artery can be challenging, on account of the difficulties in identification of the vessel in obese patients, related to intervening bowel gas or unusually deep location. Furthermore, accessory renal arteries also are difficult to detect.

State-of-the-art digital ultrasound equipment allows improved evaluation of renal arteries with use of an appropriate scanning technique and performance of the exami-

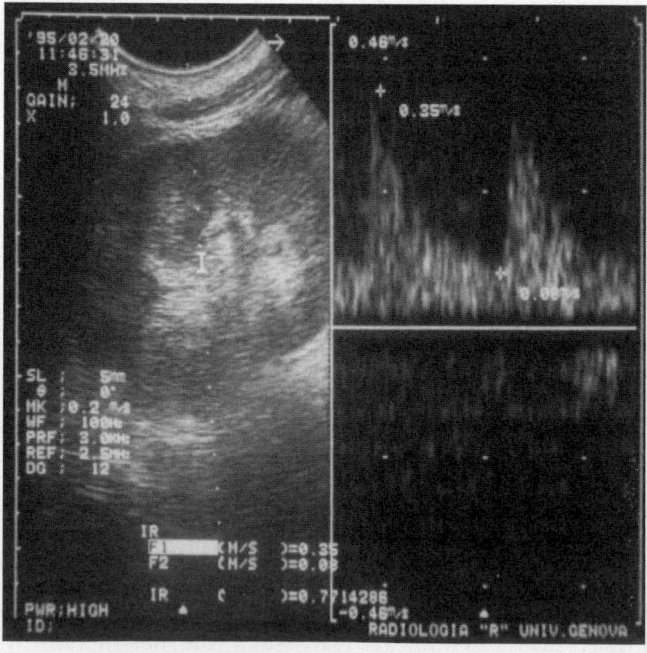
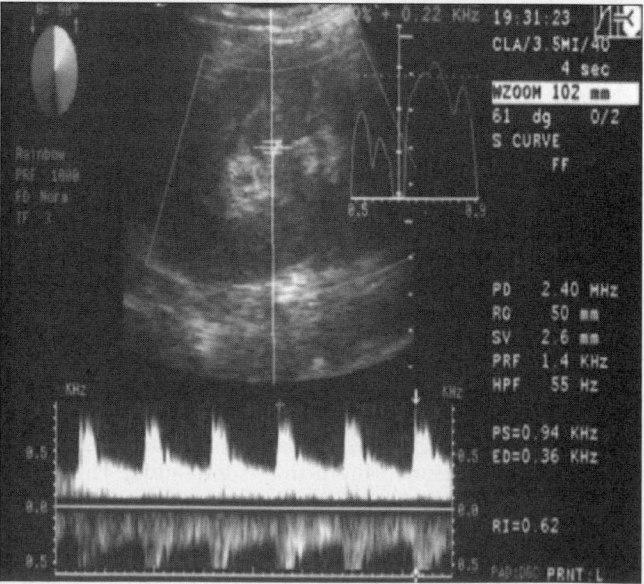

A   B

FIGURE 48-3. Ultrasound studies showing functional recovery in a patient with acute interstitial nephritis. **A,** The first study shows normal-appearing kidney but with elevated resistive index (RI) of 0.77. **B,** Follow-up examination demonstrates return to a normal RI of 0.62. See also color plates.

nation by an experienced and skilled sonologist. When patients at high risk for renal artery stenosis are carefully selected, very high sensitivity and specificity can be attained.[12,13] In general, however, evaluation of elderly patients is more difficult than in the general population, because indirect signs of renal artery stenosis may not be present. These signs, in fact, are produced by interaction between the resistance to flow and arterial compliance and, in elderly patients with decreased arterial wall elasticity, may be reduced or even entirely eliminated, making the diagnosis possible only through demonstration of the velocity increase at the level of the stenosis. Recently, it has been shown that, in these patients, identification of perforating arteries by color Doppler ultrasound examination can be useful to rule out renal artery stenosis even when complete evaluation of the main renal artery cannot be accomplished.[14] Perforating arteries are vessels connecting the capsular plexus with the interlobar and interlobular arteries, which become hypertrophied in pathological processes associated with reduced blood flow through the main renal artery. Perforating arteries with flow directed toward the kidney have been detected and interrogated in 64% of kidneys with renal artery stenosis in hypertensive elderly patients presenting with ARF. By contrast, in kidneys without renal artery stenosis, only perforating arteries with flow directed to the renal capsule could be appreciated on ultrasound examination.[14]

Acute Renal Failure in Patients with Pyelonephritis

Rarely, acute severe and bilateral pyelonephritis can cause ARF. Ultrasound examination has good sensitivity for detection of pyonephrosis. With infected urine or pus within the obstructed collecting system, diffusely dispersed fine echoes will be seen, or the echoes may layer in dependent portions of the dilated pelvis. These features can be difficult to see, especially in obese patients, and are better appreciated with lastest-generation ultrasound equipment, which confers better spatial and contrast resolution and uses tissue harmonic imaging techniques.[2] Renal abscesses may appear as intrarenal fluid collections or as complex lesions, and presence of intralesional air or layering of content can lead to the diagnosis. Color Doppler techniques can increase the sensitivity of ultrasound examination, especially in children and young adults,[15] by detecting single or multiple perfusion defects; however, the technique remains less sensitive than helical (spiral) CT.[16]

Acute Renal Failure in Liver Failure

Hepatorenal failure is a well-recognized cause of ARF in patients with severe liver disease. Although most of these patients have liver cirrhosis, ARF due to fulminant hepatitis or diffuse hepatic tumors may be encountered as well. The hepatorenal syndrome is a clinical situation which is generally regarded as functional in nature, because histopathological changes are absent, ARF reverses with timely liver transplantation, and kidneys can be successfully transplanted in patients with normal livers. Early clinical detection is difficult because the serum creatinine level does not increase until late in the clinical course. The kidney has normal appearance at ultrasound examination in these cases, while duplex Doppler ultrasound imaging

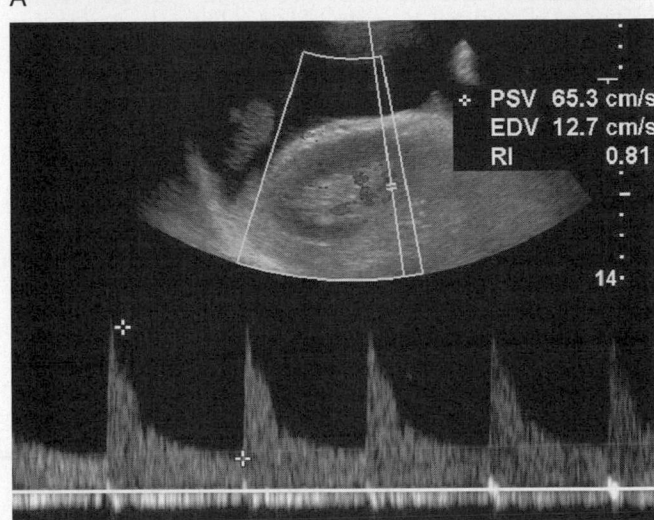

FIGURE 48-4. Doppler imaging may help predict the clinical course, as in this patient with liver cirrhosis and diffuse hepatocellular carcinoma. **A,** Sagittal image of the right flank from a gray-scale ultrasound study. Abundant ascitic fluid is present; the kidney (between the *two cursors*) appears normal. **B,** Duplex Doppler ultrasound image shows an increased resistive index (RI). Hepatorenal syndrome developed subsequently. EDV, end diastolic velocity; L, liver; PSV, peak systolic velocity. See also color plates.

can noninvasively identify a group of normal azotemic patients that is at significantly higher risk for subsequent development of kidney dysfunction and hepatorenal syndrome (Fig. 48-4). The hepatorenal syndrome has been reported, in fact, to develop in 26% of cirrhotic patients with elevated intrarenal RI and in only 1% of those with normal Doppler findings.[17] Virtually all patients with clinically obvious hepatorenal syndrome have markedly elevated RIs.[6,18] Increased renal RI is a negative prognostic factor for patients undergoing liver transplantation. Platt and coworkers found that patients with elevated RIs had a greater chance of subsequent renal dysfunction, need for hemodialysis, and a complicated clinical course after liver transplantation.[19]

Hemolytic Uremic Syndrome

HUS is a form of ARF that occurs mainly in children. It is characterized by thrombotic microangiopathy with resultant small-vessel renal disease. In patients with HUS, the renal cortex typically is hyperechogenic, with sharp delineation of swollen hypoechoic pyramids and increased corticomedullary differentiation. Markedly elevated RIs are found. A decrease in renal RIs can be observed before clinical improvement, and duplex Doppler ultrasound examination can help guide decisions to shorten dialysis sessions or cancel unneeded dialysis treatment.[20]

Acute Renal Artery and Renal Vein Thrombosis

Acute renal artery thrombosis results in lack of intrarenal Doppler signals or in severe tardus-parvus waveform abnormalities distal to the occlusion.[20] In this latter instance, peripheral hypertrophied collateral arteries can be seen on color Doppler ultrasound examination, with flow directed toward the renal parenchyma.[14] In some cases, parenchymal viability may be maintained by means of this accessory supply.

In *acute renal vein thrombosis*, gray-scale and color Doppler ultrasound imaging may aid in the detection of thrombus within the main renal veins. Duplex Doppler evaluation of intrarenal arteries may show increased RIs.[6,21] It has been shown, however, that completely normal arterial waveforms may be seen on ultrasound examination of native kidneys with renal vein thrombosis, possibly because of collateral vessel formation.[22]

Key Points

1. The most important indication for ultrasound evaluation in patients with acute renal failure is to exclude obstruction.
2. Size and morphology of the kidneys are important features to evaluate in patients with acute renal failure. In patients with prerenal and renal acute renal failure, detection of kidneys of reduced size is indicative of preexisting chronic renal disease.
3. Patients with prerenal acute renal failure demonstrate normal intraparenchymal Doppler waveforms, whereas patients with acute tubular necrosis show increased pulsatility and loss of diastolic flow.
4. Presence of focal avascular areas in the renal parenchyma at color Doppler interrogation can suggest renal infarction, severe acute pyelonephritis, or embolic disease.

Key References

3. Canavese C, Mangiarotti G, Pacitti A, et al: The patient with acute renal failure and nondilated urinary tract. Nephrol Dial Transplant 1998;13:203-205.
6. Platt JF: Doppler ultrasound of the kidney. Semin Ultrasound CT MRI 1997;18:22-32.

See the companion Expert Consult website for the complete reference list.

CHAPTER 49

Contrast-Enhanced Renal Ultrasonography

Michele Bertolotto, Giovanni Galli, and Micheline Djouguela Fute

OBJECTIVES

This chapter will:
1. Describe the characteristics of ultrasound contrast agents and contrast-enhanced ultrasound examination techniques for renal imaging.
2. Discuss the role of contrast-enhanced ultrasonography in the evaluation of patients with acute renal failure from vascular causes.
3. Describe the imaging features of various renal vascular diseases visualized with use of ultrasonographic microbubble contrast agents.

The incidence of renal failure due to vascular disease is increasing. Epidemic atherosclerotic vascular disease in the aging population, widespread use of vasoactive drugs, and the increased frequency of invasive vascular procedures have led to a general increase in the incidence of vascular causes of intrinsic acute renal failure (ARF).[1] ARF is particularly common in the intensive care unit (ICU) setting, in which it is characterized by increasing comorbidity, high incidence of sepsis, multiorgan failure, and high mortality rate.[2]

Diagnosis of the underlying cause of ARF relies mainly on the patient's history including signs and symptoms, the clinical findings, and laboratory test results. Gray-scale ultrasonography commonly is performed early in the course of the disease to exclude renal obstruction, and color Doppler imaging is increasingly used to evaluate renal vascular status, especially when vascular disease is clinically suspected.[1,3] In patients with ARF, however, a significant but nonspecific overall reduction in renal perfusion often is appreciable on color Doppler examination,[4] and focal perfusion abnormalities can be difficult to identify. Moreover, it can be very difficult, or even impossible, to differentiate hypoperfused from unperfused areas. Finally, Doppler signal intensity reduces at unfavorable angles in which vessels are targeted at nearly perpendicular angles to the ultrasound beam, in deep renal structures, and with intervening bowel gas.

Other imaging techniques are more sensitive than color Doppler examination for the evaluation of renal perfusion. Angiography and contrast-enhanced computed tomography (CT), in particular, are the imaging modalities of choice, but they often are contraindicated in critically ill patients because the iodinated contrast agents used in these studies are nephrotoxic. Magnetic resonance imaging (MRI) requires a less nephrotoxic contrast agent but may be difficult to perform in critically ill patients, and recently a major concern has been raised about nephrogenic systemic fibrosis associated with the use of gadolinium contrast agents in patients with ARF. Moreover, MRI cannot be done in patients who have an implanted pacemaker.

Recently, microbubble contrast agents have been introduced in the clinical practice to assess vascularity of different organs and lesions. An increasing number of studies are becoming available showing the potential of this technique for depiction of intrarenal blood flow both with normal renal status and in pathological conditions.[5,6] In particular, depiction of focal renal perfusion defects is markedly improved in comparison with Doppler techniques, with a diagnostic performance approaching that of CT. Because microbubbles are not nephrotoxic, contrast-enhanced ultrasound examination may therefore be considered a useful front-line study in the radiologist's armamentarium, especially in critically ill patients and in those with compromised renal function.

MICROBUBBLE CONTRAST AGENTS

Ultrasonographic contrast agents consist of microbubbles of gas, stabilized by a protein, lipid, or polymer shell, that are small and stable enough to traverse the pulmonary circulation after peripheral venous injection. Their typical half-life in blood is a few minutes. Microbubbles remain within the vessels, both large vessels and capillaries, and cannot move through the vascular endothelium into the interstitium. They respond to the ultrasound beam by changing their size, rapidly contracting and expanding in response to the pressure changes induced by the sound wave. As with all oscillating systems, microbubbles of ultrasonographic contrast agents have a natural or resonant frequency at which their response is greatly enhanced. It happens that bubbles of the size range required for transpulmonary passage after intravenous injection resonate at diagnostic ultrasound frequencies.

When properly targeted with an ultrasound beam of appropriate power and frequency, microbubble oscillation becomes nonlinear. As a consequence of a bubble's increased stiffness as the gas within it compresses, the increase of the bubble's diameter in the rarefaction phase of the acoustic cycle exceeds the decrease of the diameter in the compression phase. These asymmetrical oscillations result in nonlinear echoes containing overtones, or harmonics, of the driving frequency. It is this phenomenon that makes possible "nondestructive" contrast-specific imaging in real time. At higher power of the ultrasound beam, microbubble oscillation becomes so pronounced that the bubbles are disrupted and emit a strong, highly nonlinear, transient echo.

A variety of contrast-specific ultrasound modes have been developed by different ultrasound equipment manufacturers, optimized to detect nonlinear signal arising either from microbubble disruption (destructive modes) or from microbubble harmonic oscillation (nondestructive modes). Contrast-specific nondestructive modes, in particular, represent the state of the art in ultrasound imaging with microbubbles and in clinical practice have nearly replaced completely destructive techniques. The major advantage of nondestructive imaging is the possibility to image vascularity of organs and lesions in real time.

Microbubble contrast agents are not nephrotoxic and can be used safely in patients with impaired renal function.

EXAMINATION TECHNIQUE

In our clinical practice we use SonoVue (BR1, Bracco, Milan, Italy), a sulfur hexafluoride–filled microbubble contrast agent licensed for imaging of abdominal organs in most European countries. Other latest-generation microbubbles, however, such as Optison (FSO 69, Amersham Health, Princeton, NJ) and Definity (Lantheus Medical Imaging, North Billerica, MA), have similar uses.

After a preliminary gray-scale and color Doppler evaluation, the ultrasound equipment is set for contrast examination. The power of the ultrasound beam is set to obtain minimum microbubble destruction with the available equipment. Typically, nondestructive contrast-specific imaging is obtained by setting the mechanical index between 0.2 and 0.06, depending on the equipment used. A SonoVue bolus of 1.2 to 2.4 mL is injected to evaluate each kidney using a 20-gauge cannula, followed by a 10-mL normal saline flush. Digital cine-clips should be registered during all contrast-enhanced examinations to allow accurate retrospective evaluation.

CONTRAST-ENHANCED ULTRASOUND FEATURES

Renal Vascular Anatomy

Kidneys enhance quickly and intensively after microbubble administration (Fig. 49-1). First, the arteries enhance, followed within few seconds by complete fill-in of the cortex.[5] Signal from microbubbles is independent from the angle of ultrasound targeting, and visualization of renal perfusion also is excellent at the renal poles.

Unlike with Doppler techniques, medullary vascularization also can be evaluated with contrast-enhanced ultrasonography.[5] The outer medulla enhances first, and then the pyramids gradually fill in. The renal medulla will eventually appear nearly isoechoic, or slightly hypoechogenic relative to cortex.

No significant accumulation of microbubbles is observed in the renal parenchyma. As the microbubble concentration in the general circulation decreases, contrast enhancement fades within 3 to 6 minutes, depending on sensitivity of the equipment used and on the amount of microbubbles injected.

After microbubble administration, adequate evaluation of renal perfusion is obtained with a spatial resolution approaching that of conventional gray-scale ultrasound imaging also in older and obese patients. Kidneys can be successfully evaluated in patients with compromised renal function and in those unable to cooperate as well, since movement artefacts do not significantly affect the study.

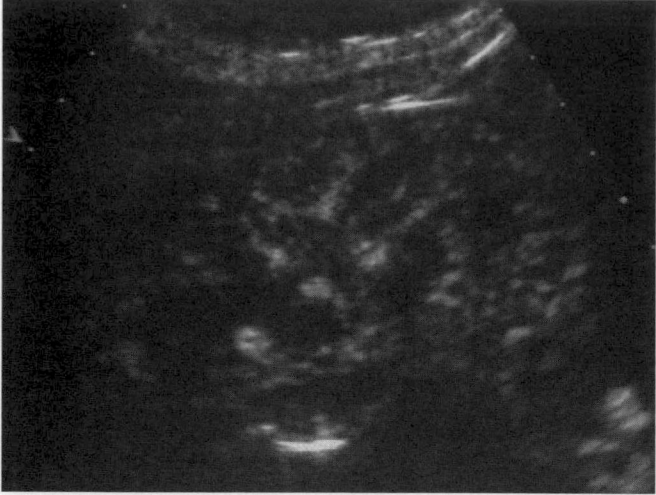

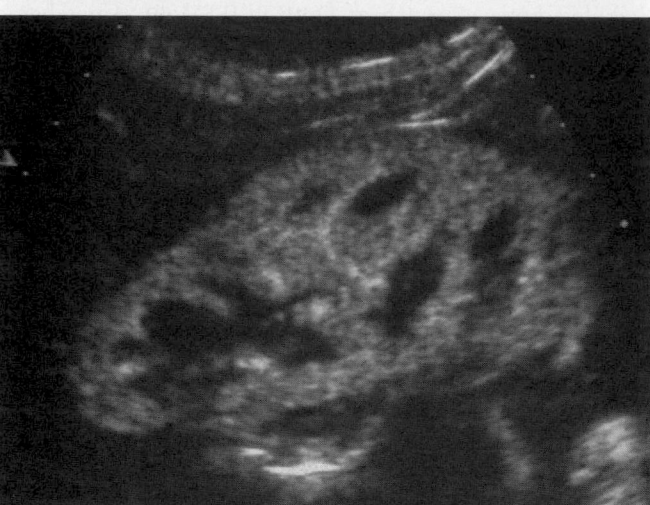

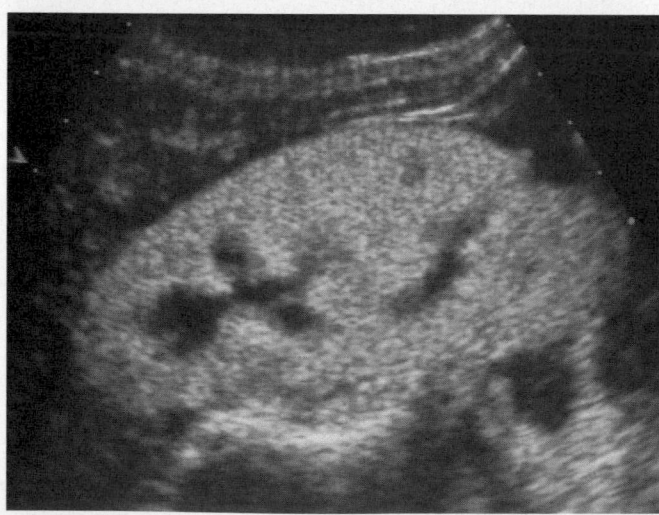

FIGURE 49-1. Normal renal enhancement after microbubble administration for ultrasound examination. Enhancement in the central arteries (**A**) is followed by enhancement of the cortex (**B**) and of the medulla (**C**).

Renal Infarction

Contrast-enhanced ultrasonography should be used to rule out renal infarction in critically ill patients and in patients with compromised renal function. The main risk factor for thromboembolic occlusion of the renal artery is trauma. Nontraumatic causes of renal infarction include aneurysms and pseudoaneurysms of renal artery, vasculitides, antiphospholipid syndromes, nephrotic syndrome, loin-pain hematuria syndrome, and cocaine abuse. Conditions associated with renal artery thromboembolism are previous embolic episodes, atrial fibrillation, valvular heart disease, prosthetic heart valves, bacterial endocarditis, tumor emboli, fat emboli, and vascular manipulation after surgery or endovascular interventional maneuvers.[7]

In patients with renal infarction, contrast-enhanced ultrasound examination readily demonstrates absence of enhancement in the affected renal tissue.[5,8-10] Acute infarcts typically are seen as wedge-shaped nonenhancing areas within an otherwise normal-appearing kidney.[11] Renal shape is preserved. A thin subcapsular rim of viable, enhancing cortex can be preserved as a result of collateral blood supply from the renal capsule, equivalent to the cortical rim sign, frequently described as a sign of renal infarction on CT. Bilateral infarction is expected in patients with ARF (Fig. 49-2), or unilateral infarction in patients with already compromised renal function, in unilateral functioning kidney, or in association with contralateral renal artery stenosis. When unilateral infarction is detected in ARF and the contralateral kidney appears normal after microbubble administration, arteries must be investigated with other imaging techniques to rule out renal artery stenosis.

CT is the standard technique for the assessment of trauma patients because it is panoramic and highly sensitive compared with ultrasound examination; use of ultrasonography, however, predominates in many trauma centers because it is rapid and noninvasive, is easily repeatable, can be used at the bedside of the patient, and does not interrupt resuscitation efforts. The main limitation of ultrasonography is its poor ability to visualize parenchyma lesions. Poletti and associates and Valentino and coworkers showed that contrast-enhanced ultrasonography is effective to evaluate liver and renal traumas, although with lower sensitivity than for contrast-enhanced CT[12,13] (Fig. 49-3). Contrast-enhanced ultrasonography cannot be recommended to replace CT in trauma patients, however, because even under optimal conditions, major solid organ injuries may be missed, vascular injuries can be difficult to detect, and intestinal or mesenteric injuries cannot be identified.

Acute Cortical Necrosis

With prolonged renal ischemia caused by hemorrhage, surgery, or endovascular interventional complications, the resulting necrosis may be restricted to the renal cortex, with sparing of the renal medulla. The process often is bilateral, either multifocal or diffuse. Other causes of acute cortical necrosis are reduced renal artery perfusion secondary to vascular spasm, microvascular injury, and diffuse intravascular coagulation.

Contrast-enhanced ultrasonography allows differentiation between cortical ischemia (Fig. 49-4) and renal infarction, showing enhancing interlobar and arcuate arteries and nonenhancing cortex.[14] A rim of subcapsular cortical

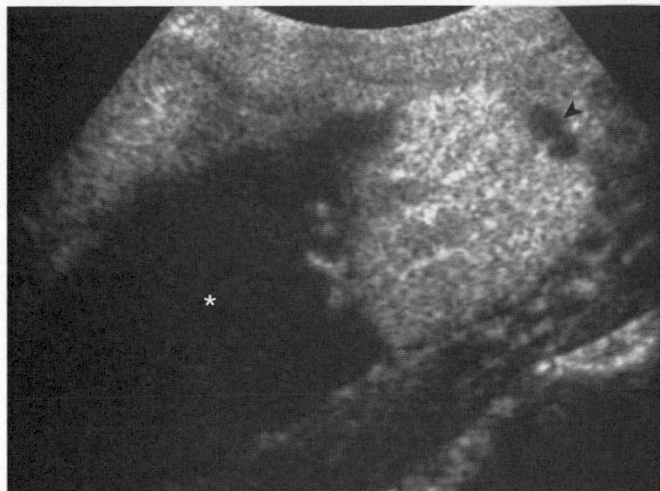

A

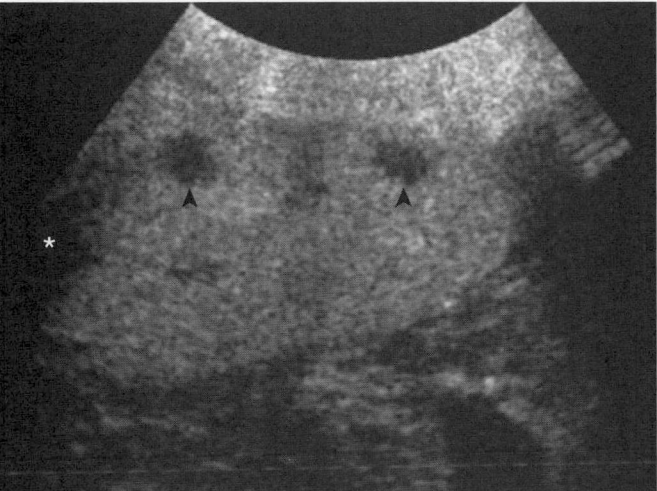

B

FIGURE 49-2. Acute renal failure developed in the postoperative period in a patient who had undergone abdominal surgery. Bilateral renal infarctions can be visualized on these ultrasonographic images. The upper pole and the middle portion of the right kidney (**A**) and the upper pole of the left kidney (**B**) are ischemic *(asterisks)*. Small ischemic areas also are appreciable at the lower pole of the right kidney (**A**, *arrowhead*) and in the middle and lower portions of the left kidney (**B**, *arrowheads*).

enhancement often is apparent owing to collateral flow from the renal capsular vessels.

Atheroembolic Renal Disease

Acute renal failure in the setting of recent intravascular intervention or anticoagulation should prompt consideration of atheroemboli. Clues to this diagnosis include the presence of livedo reticularis and cholesterol crystals on a dilated funduscopic examination. A definitive diagnosis may be made on visualization of cholesterol crystals in a biopsy specimen of the skin or kidney.[1,15]

Imaging can be indicated to rule out renal infarction or other vascular disorders. Color Doppler ultrasound exami-

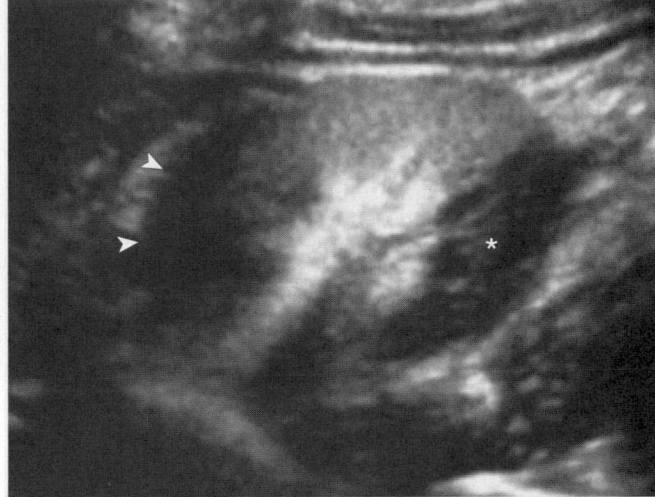

FIGURE 49-3. Post-traumatic renal ischemia. Contrast-enhanced ultrasonography shows a post-traumatic renal infarct *(asterisk)*. Perirenal hematoma *(arrowheads)* is an associated finding.

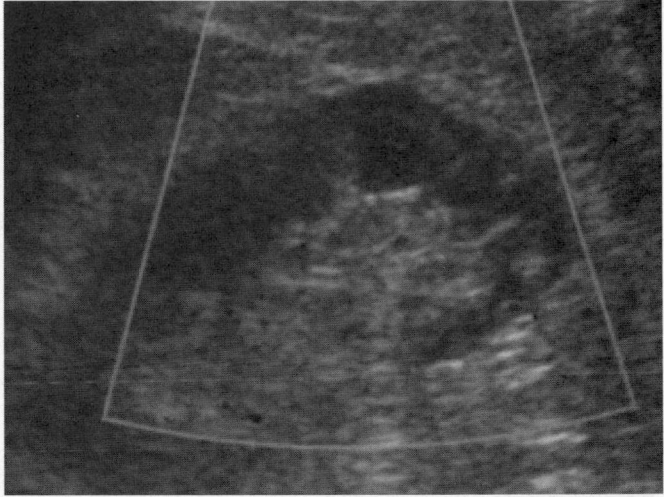

A

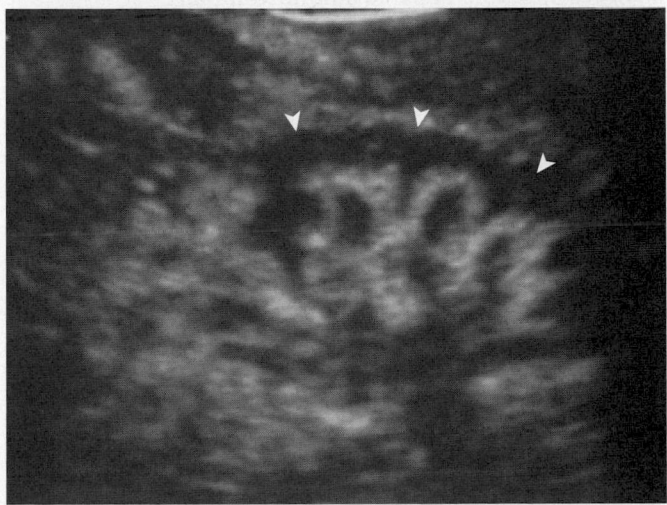

B

FIGURE 49-4. Acute cortical necrosis. **A,** Color Doppler ultrasound examination shows markedly reduced renal perfusion *(outlined area)*. Contrast-enhanced ultrasonography shows enhancing hilar vessels and cortical ischemia *(arrowheads)*.

nation is not specific. After microbubble administration, patients with recent atheroembolic episodes usually present with multiple cortical areas of delayed enhancement (Fig. 49-5). In fact, enhancement is reduced during the early arterial phase and increases in the following vascular phases. In general, no perfusion abnormalities can be appreciated in patients with embolization of several weeks' duration, despite clinically documented irreversible renal parenchymal damage.

Explanation of these findings is speculative. It is conceivable that patchy embolization of small arteries may be detected during the arterial phase as small cortical perfusion abnormalities, which are masked during the following vascular phases by partial volume averaging with patent cortical veins. Progressive disappearance of perfusion defects within some weeks may be due to progressive volume reduction of the cortical ischemic areas.

ACUTE PYELONEPHRITIS

Rarely acute, severe pyelonephritis can complicate with ARF. Regional differences in renal perfusion may be detected in affected patients,[16] but accumulating clinical evidence indicates that microbubble contrast agents do not significantly increase color Doppler sensitivity in diagnosis of pyelonephritis. Poor sensitivity of contrast-enhanced ultrasonography in the evaluation of patients with acute pyelonephritis probably reflects the fact that microbubble contrast agents enhance only the renal vasculature, whereas acute renal infection primarily involves the tubular and interstitial compartments; renal vessels are damaged only later, when formation of parenchymal abscesses leads to destruction of the parenchyma.

In patients with severe pyelonephritis, contrast-enhanced ultrasonography may have a role in selected cases to rule out ischemic changes and abscess formation (Fig. 49-6). In fact, although large abscesses typically are identified at gray-scale ultrasound examination, preabscess lesions and microabscesses usually cannot be detected at baseline examination but are identified as obvious perfusion abnormalities after microbubble administration.[8]

Renal Artery Stenosis

ARF without an apparent cause or with onset after therapy with angiotensin-converting enzyme (ACE) inhibitors strongly suggests renal artery stenosis in elderly patients with hypertensive nephrosclerosis, diabetes mellitus, or peripheral vascular disease.[4] Because of the nephrotoxic potential of iodinated contrast agents, color Doppler ultrasound examination is the first-line imaging modality in these patients. Early clinical studies have demonstrated that the success rate for Doppler visualization of the main renal arteries and of accessory renal arteries improves significantly after microbubble administration,[17] and excellent temporal resolution may allow visualization of segmental renal artery stenosis as areas with delayed enhancement.[18] This finding, however, can be appreciated in other pathologic conditions as well, in particular, in patients with atheroemboli.

In fact, Doppler sensitivity of high-end ultrasound equipment has increased significantly in the last several years, and contrast-enhanced ultrasonography now has a limited role in the diagnosis of renal artery stenosis.

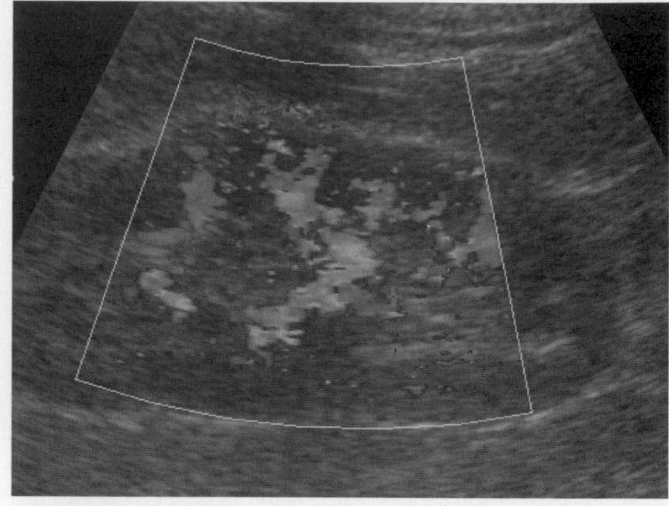

A

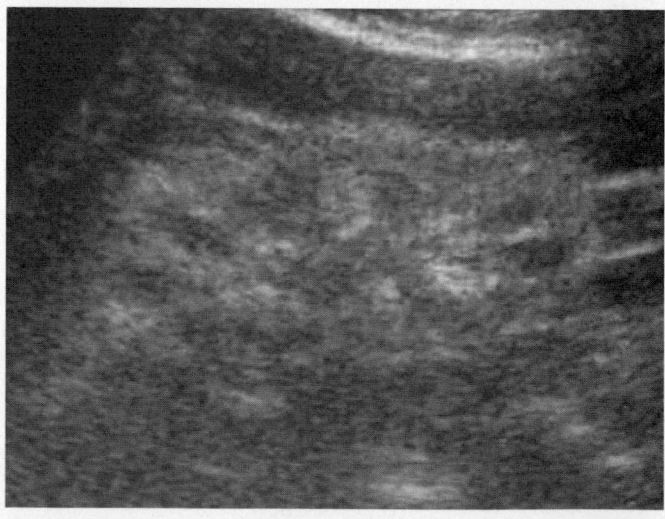

B

C

FIGURE 49-5. Atheroembolic renal disease, right kidney. **A,** Color Doppler ultrasound examination shows reduced renal vascularity *(outlined area).* See also color plates. **B,** Areas with delayed enhancement *(asterisks)* are appreciable on this contrast-enhanced ultrasonographic image 15 seconds after microbubble administration. **C,** No perfusion abnormalities are evident in the following vascular phases.

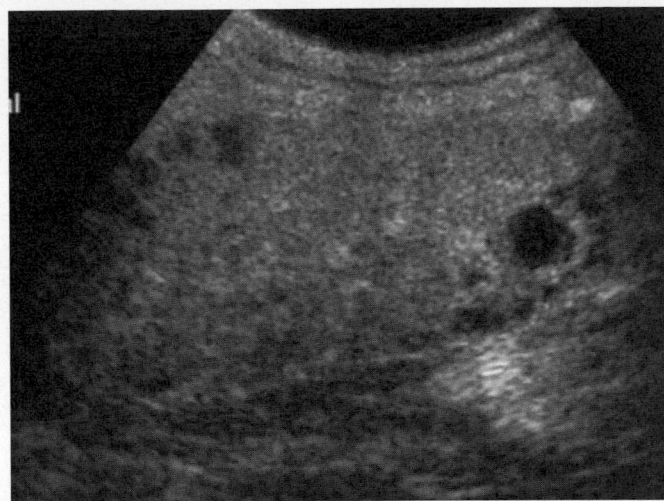

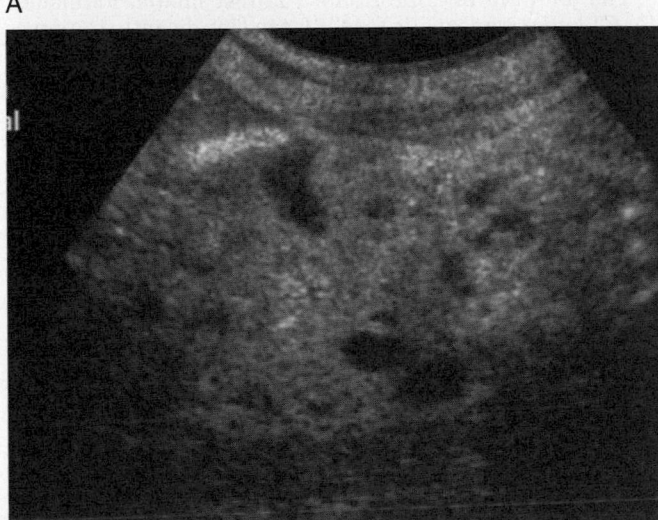

FIGURE 49-6. Severe acute pyelonephritis complicated by acute renal failure. Contrast-enhanced ultrasonography shows multiple microabscesses in both the right (**A**) and the left (**B**) kidneys, manifesting as perfusion defects.

CONCLUSION

A large potential is recognized for the use of intravenous ultrasonographic contrast agents in renal imaging. The intense enhancement of the renal parenchyma makes it easy to detect lesions in which normal parenchyma has been replaced by nonperfused areas, without the use of ionizing radiation. In most hospitals, the standard procedure for the detection of renal perfusion abnormalities is contrast-enhanced CT, but contrast-enhanced ultrasonography is preferred in critically ill patients and in patients with ARF because the bubble contrast agents used are not nephrotoxic, it can be performed in emergency at the bedside, and increasing evidence is accumulating that it is as effective as CT in detection of renal perfusion defects in real time, without the artifacts commonly associated with Doppler methods.

Key Points

1. Ultrasound examination with microbubble contrast is a useful new technique of renal imaging.
2. Ultrasound examination with contrast allows imaging of kidney perfusion without the need for radiation exposure.
3. Nonperfused areas can be easily identified.
4. Contrast-enhanced ultrasound imaging does not require the injection of nephrotoxic radiocontrast material.
5. Ultrasound examination with microbubble contrast can be performed at the bedside.

Key References

4. Pozzi Mucelli R, Bertolotto M, Quaia E: Imaging techniques in acute renal failure. Contrib Nephrol 2001;(132):76-91.
6. Robbin ML, Lockhart ME, Barr RG: Renal imaging with ultrasound contrast: Current status. Radiol Clin North Am 2003;41:963-978.
10. Taylor GA, Barnewolt CE, Claudon M, Dunning PS: Depiction of renal perfusion defects with contrast-enhanced harmonic sonography in a porcine model. AJR Am J Roentgenol 1999;173:757-760.
11. Quaia E, Siracusano S, Palumbo A, et al: Detection of focal renal perfusion defects in rabbits after sulphur hexafluoride–filled microbubble injection at low transmission power ultrasound insonation. Eur Radiol 2006;16:166-172.
13. Valentino M, Serra C, Zironi G, et al: Blunt abdominal trauma: Emergency contrast-enhanced sonography for detection of solid organ injuries. AJR Am J Roentgenol 2006;186:1361-1367.

See the companion Expert Consult website for the complete reference list.

CHAPTER 50

Computed Tomography and Magnetic Resonance Imaging in Acute Renal Failure

Libero Barozzi, Massimo Valentino, Francesco Maria Drudi, and Pietro Pavlica

OBJECTIVES

This chapter will:
1. Describe imaging techniques for computed tomography and magnetic resonance imaging suitable for use in patients with acute renal failure.
2. Identify renal morphological and functional parameters evaluable by computed tomography and magnetic resonance imaging.
3. Review the indications for and diagnostic capabilities of these techniques.
4. Discuss the use of these techniques for evaluation after kidney transplantation.
5. Summarize likely future developments in the use of these imaging modalities for assessing patients with acute renal failure.

COMPUTED TOMOGRAPHY AND MAGNETIC RESONANCE IMAGING TECHNIQUES

The use of computed tomography (CT) and magnetic resonance imaging (MRI) and the choice of specific techniques to investigate acute renal failure (ARF) will depend on the clinical status of the patient, which may range from isolated renal insufficiency to complete multiorgan failure, particularly in patients admitted to the intensive care unit (ICU). The latter instance presents specific management problems related to the need for continuous automated monitoring. Difficulties also may arise in moving such patients to the radiology department. Moreover, with use of CT, the standard radioprotection rules must be respected, especially in children and younger patients, on account of the potential risk for cancer from high doses of ionizing radiation.[1]

Such problems are absent in MRI, in which imaging is achieved with the use of magnetic fields and radiofrequency. Nevertheless, use of nonmagnetic equipment for support of vital functions may be necessary in critically ill patients with renal failure.

Until recently, the use of these imaging tools was limited, but technological advances have led to the design of more streamlined and better-performing devices, with much-improved capabilities. Multislice CT and ultrafast MRI are just two examples of such improved techniques. In addition, more detailed information about morphology and function is now provided by more sophisticated software, making these examinations increasingly useful in critically ill patients.

The addition of appropriate contrast media, iodinated for CT and paramagnetic for MRI, can significantly improve the diagnostic capabilities of these studies by highlighting renal function. The use of contrast agents, however, often is limited by the potential for systemic and renal toxicity.[2]

MORPHOLOGICAL AND FUNCTIONAL PARAMETERS EVALUABLE BY COMPUTED TOMOGRAPHY AND MAGNETIC RESONANCE IMAGING

The new multislice CT scanners take only a few seconds to perform a complete study of the abdomen with high spatial resolution. These studies are characterized by high-resolution anatomical detail, to approximately 400 to 500 μm, and the capability of depicting the passage of contrast through the vasculature (arteries and veins), the cortex and medulla, the tubules, and the excretory system.

The quantity of digital information obtained with state-of-the-art equipment is so great that successive elaborations can give multiplanar reconstructions with use of multiple algorithms (e.g., minimum intensity projection [MIP], multiplanar reformation [MPR], volume vendering [VR]). These reconstructions allow ready access to accurate morphological data (Fig. 50-1), as well as functional information deriving from the analysis of intensity-time curves.

Basal CT scan without contrast often is the only possible examination in patients with ARF, unless immediate dialysis is anticipated. Repeated scans are necessary to evaluate kidney function throughout the vascular and nephrourographic phases. These scans are carried out at well-defined intervals, incurring an increase in radiation dose, which must be considered in terms of potential benefit of these studies to the patient.

In unenhanced studies, morphological features to assess are the long axis (measured on coronal reconstructions) and anteroposterior axis (visible on axial scans) of the kidney, the presence of calcifications (vascular, lithiasis-related, parenchymal), the parenchymal width (mean value calculated from at least three measurements), the presence of masses (solid or cystic), and the condition of the urinary tract. Contrast administration allows delinea-

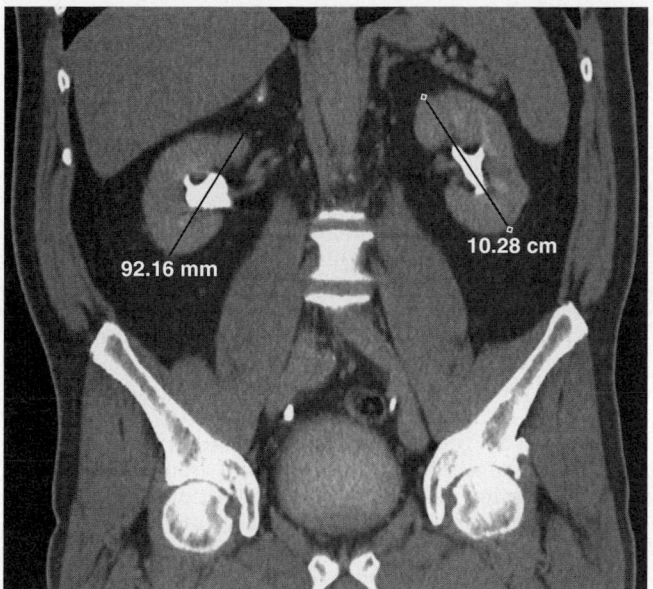

FIGURE 50-1. Renal imaging using contrast-enhanced computed tomography in a patient with acute renal failure. Coronal reconstruction shows normal kidneys, other than a volumetric increase in long axis. Contrast material is still present.

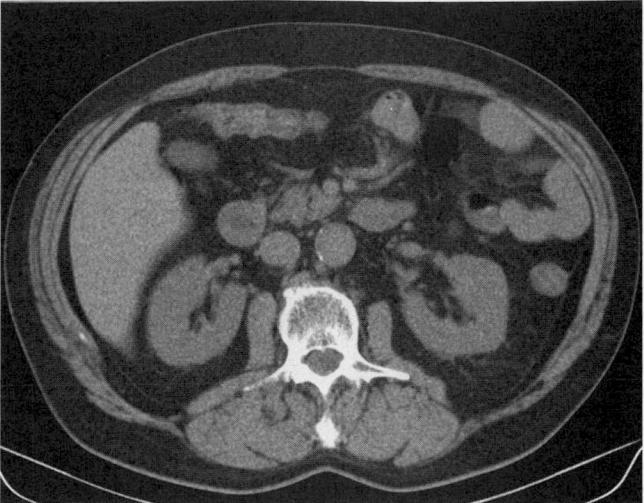

FIGURE 50-2. Renal imaging using computed tomography performed without contrast in a patient with acute renal failure. Enlargement of the kidneys is evident, but no dilatation of the excretory tract is present.

tion of the main renal arteries from the point of origin up to that of secondary branching, in the cortical phase during the passage of contrast within the glomerular and peritubular capillaries (Fig. 50-2), and of the main veins; in the parenchymal phase during the diffusion of contrast within interstitial extracapillary tissue and filtration through the glomerular membrane with opacification of renal tubules; and finally, the excretory system, which is depicted 3 to 4 minutes after contrast administration, the peak being reached after 10 to 15 minutes.[3]

MRI examination of the kidney should include T1- and T2-weighted sequences, with and without contrast. T1 sequences without contrast provide more structurally defined morphological information than that obtainable using unenhanced CT, although spatial resolution is lower with MRI. T2 sequences are used only without contrast. They provide less anatomical detail than is possible with T1 sequences but present better definition, allowing evaluation of the normal and pathological structure of the kidney. With dedicated T2-weighted sequences, it is possible to examine the urinary tract, especially if dilated, allowing the generation of images from static fluid (by means of magnetic resonance urography performed without contrast).[4]

Paramagnetic contrast agents (based on gadolinium) are used with T1-weighted sequences. With use of ultrafast techniques, they allow the acquisition of data to provide high-resolution anatomical detail and functional data. As with CT, it is possible to study the various phases of contrast passage at the vascular, parenchymal, and excretory levels. Fat saturation sequences eliminate the high-intensity signals from fat tissue that interfere with the interpretation of the images, thereby improving the quality of the study.

The basic imaging characteristics are the same as for CT (measurements, profile, and so on). An additional characteristic of MRI is the variation in signal intensity, different in the various sequences and not equivalent to the measurable density of CT. In clinical practice, various T1- and

T2-weighted sequences are used, all of which provide technical parameters that can be selected to maximize detail of the different structures.[5]

INDICATIONS AND DIAGNOSTIC CAPABILITIES

Computed Tomography

CT is rarely used in patients with ARF because the diagnostic information it provides is similar to that obtainable with ultrasonography.

The kidneys usually are of normal dimensions in the prerenal form of kidney disease, unless renal injury of a vascular, inflammatory, or multicystic nature is present.[6] Angiographic CT study (angio-CT) of the main vasculature does not demonstrate any significant variation in diameter; with intraparenchymal vascular constriction, enhancement of both cortex and medulla is reduced.

In ARF from tubular necrosis or other acute renal disease, the CT picture is not substantially different, apart from a subtle volumetric increase in the kidneys, evident on axial scans as an increase in anteroposterior diameter. Intensity-time curves, data for which are obtained by positioning a "region of interest" (ROI) for the study at the corticomedullary level, show a reduced vascularization and a loss of corticomedullary differentiation. Functional recovery is accompanied by the reappearance of this differentiation.

In acute cortical necrosis, the complete absence of contrast in the cortex can be appreciated, although the cortical rim sign may be observed, appearing as a thin line of subcapsular enhancement,[7] because blood flow is ensured by the collateral circle of capsular arteries. Enhancement of the medulla is poor. In all cases of ARF, the excretory phase is essentially absent; contrast does not opacify the urinary tract and remains within the tubules for up 24 to 48 hours, with an intense and prolonged parenchymal effect. In patients with multiorgan failure, CT is indicated not to evaluate the ARF itself but rather to search for the underlying causes of the syndrome.

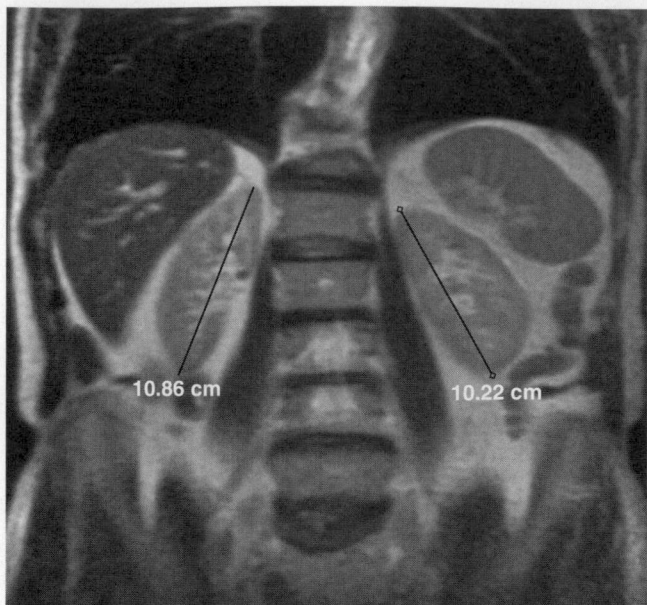

FIGURE 50-3. Coronal T2-weighted magnetic resonance image of the kidneys in a patient with acute renal failure. An appreciable volumetric increase along the long axis of the kidneys is evident.

Magnetic Resonance Imaging

MRI in ARF allows evaluation of both morphological and functional changes and, in contrast with CT, can be performed without contrast or with smaller amounts of contrast with less nephrotoxicity. Of note, however, development of systemic nephrogenic sclerosis after gadolinium administration in a patient with renal failure has recently been reported.[8]

Morphological evaluation consists of definition of the long diameter of both kidneys and of parenchymal width, with visualization of the cortex, as well as corticomedullary differentiation (Fig. 50-3). It also is possible to differentiate peripheral from central cortex. These parameters allow differentiation of a potentially reversible ARF from an exacerbation of chronic renal failure, in which irreversible damage has already occurred.

Functional evaluation includes investigations of renal perfusion and the status of the tubules. In renal failure, paramagnetic contrast material generally does not reach a high enough concentration, so that the enhancement of the signal in the medullary and excretory phases may be completely lost. Moreover, intensity-time curves have demonstrated a delay in the appearance of the medullary phase with a modification of signal intensity in normal kidneys. Dalla Palma and colleagues reported that dynamic MRI may differentiate among glomerular nephropathy, nephroangiosclerosis, and interstitial pathology on the basis of cortical peak value and peak time.[9]

In prerenal ARF from arterial thromboembolism, dissection, or vasculitis, angio-MRI allows depiction of the renal arteries up to the level of the hilum, with the possible demonstration of stenotic and obstructive pathological processes by adding color Doppler investigation, and as an alternative to angiography. Similarly, urographic MRI can readily confirm or exclude acute postrenal failure.

EVALUATION OF TRANSPLANTED KIDNEY

CT generally can detect perfusion deficits in the renal graft parenchyma, but it normally is not used in patients with elevated creatinine values because of the risk of compromising renal function. Today, MRI is gaining popularity in evaluation of the transplanted kidney.

Postgadolinium T1-weighted coronal MR renography assesses renal parenchyma and parenchymal function by acquiring repeated images of the graft in the arterial, venous, and mixed phases of contrast enhancement.

Differences in parenchymal enhancement can indicate the severity of arterial or ureteral stenosis. An abnormal appearance on nephrogram may be seen in acute tubular necrosis (ATN), rejection, or vascular insult[10]; focal abnormalities of the nephrogram may result from infarction. If the transplanted renal artery is widely patent but renal enhancement is minimal, with no excretion of gadolinium seen on the image, then the graft probably has been rejected.[11] Loss of corticomedullary differentiation on MR renography (Fig. 50-4), best assessed in the early cortical phase of enhancement, is found to be the most consistent sign of rejection, with degree corresponding to severity of rejection.[12] It also has been demonstrated that MRI has high accuracy in diagnosing rejection compared with ultrasonography and scintigraphy, although overlap exists among the imaging characteristics of ATN, nephritis, and cyclosporine toxicity.[13] Initial reports that rejection could be accurately diagnosed and differentiated from other parenchymal causes of graft dysfunction have not been substantiated by subsequent studies in which loss of corticomedullary differentiation on MR images was a relatively nonspecific finding.[14]

Szolar and coworkers[15] demonstrated distinct patterns of cortical and medullary enhancement useful in differentiation between ATN and rejection, although the findings were inconclusive because all patients exhibited both histopathological patterns. In both ATN and rejection, poor graft enhancement with little contrast excretion is characteristic.[16] The percentage and pattern of increase in postcontrast signal intensity of the renal parenchyma show a close correlation with serum creatinine levels. Such information is useful in the diagnosis of rejection and in differentiation from ATN.

Some investigators have, with promising results, used angiotensin-converting enzyme inhibitor MR renography to assess cortical signal intensity-time curves and to determine the functional significance of renal artery stenosis.[17]

FUTURE DEVELOPMENTS

Most imaging-focused clinical research today is directed at MRI, on account of the well-known problems linked to radiation exposure and the nephrotoxicity of contrast agents used in CT. In particular, studies are being carried out to investigate the usefulness of *diffusion-weighted MRI* (DW-MRI), *blood oxygen level–dependent MRI* (BOLD-MRI), *arterial spin labeling*, and the newer generation of contrast agents.

DW-MRI investigates the behavior of water molecules in the tissues within a high-intensity magnetic field, by evaluating brownian motion.[18] This phenomenon is quantified by a quantitative parameter, apparent diffusion coefficient (ADC), which reflects the chracteristics of different tissues

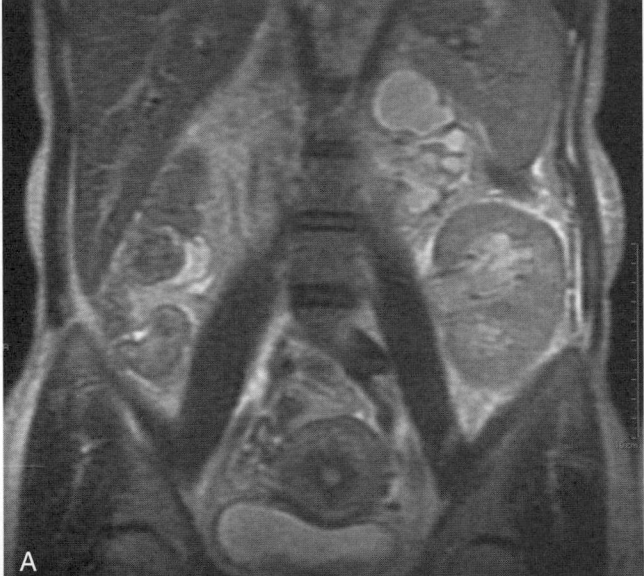

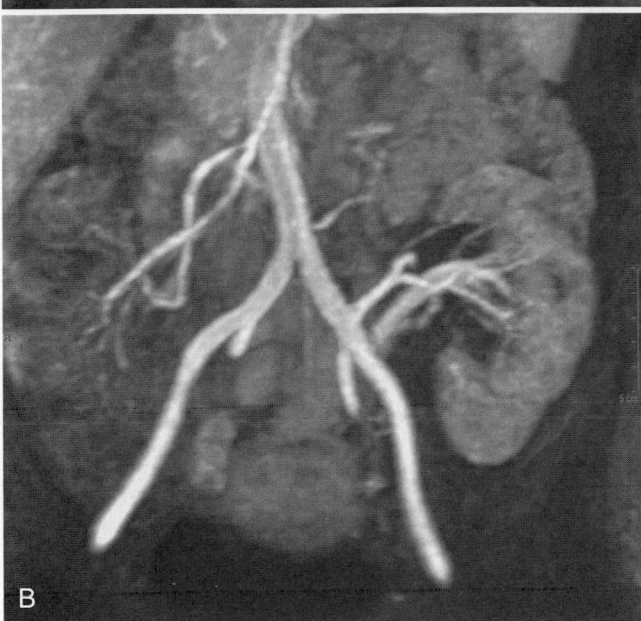

FIGURE 50-4. At 1 week after renal transplantation, biopsy revealed acute rejection in the graft. **A,** Coronal T2-weighted HASTE image. Slight enlargement of the graft in the right pelvic fossa is evident. **B,** Sagittal T1-weighted VIBE fat-suppressed image, nephrographic phase, reveals areas of edema, especially in the lower portion, where the cortical parenchyma appears thinner and hypointense. HASTE, half-Fourier single-shot turbo spin echo; VIBE, volumetric interpolated breath-hold examination.

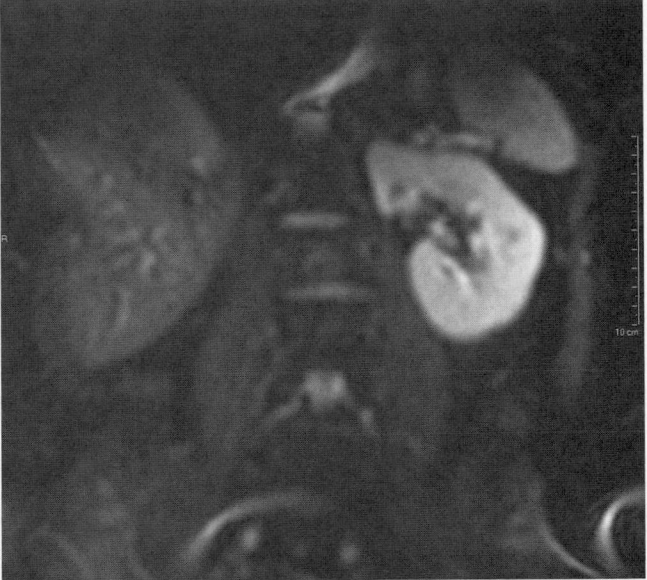

FIGURE 50-5. Diffusion magnetic resonance image from a 47-year-old man with a single kidney. The apparent diffusion coefficient of the kidney is normal.

the medulla of kidneys in patients with ARF, perhaps owing to altered corticomedullary hemodynamics or reduced local O_2 consumption due to decreased tubular function.[22]

Arterial spin labeling allows the noninvasive quantification of renal perfusion and is an alternative to scintigraphic studies.[23]

Among the newer contrast agents, special interest has been shown in ultrasmall superparamagnetic iron oxide (USPIO) particles, which are mostly taken up by infiltrating macrophages in renal grafts undergoing rejection.[24]

Because only preliminary results have thus far been published, further studies are mandatory to evaluate the clinical usefulness of these new imaging techniques.

Key Points

1. The use of multislice computed tomography and ultrafast magnetic resonance imaging is becoming increasingly common in critically ill patients to provide more detailed information about kidney morphology and function.
2. Magnetic resonance techniques are gaining popularity for the evaluation of acute rejection of renal transplants. A comprehensive study is possible, allowing evaluation of changes in both morphology and function. The information obtained appears to be more defined than that from computed tomography, and such studies can be performed without contrast, or with use of a lower amount of contrast with less nephrotoxicity than that from iodinated agents.
3. A complete magnetic resonance imaging investigation should include different sequences

related to structure and viscosity. The technique gives reproducible results in both native (Fig. 50-5) and transplanted kidneys.[19,20] DW-MRI may become a useful noninvasive method for the early diagnosis of acute and chronic rejection.

BOLD-MRI is a rapid, noninvasive method for assessing renal oxygen status in normal and transplanted kidneys. This technique exploits the paramagnetic properties of deoxyhemoglobin to image the local tissue oxygen concentration.[21] This parameter is significantly higher in including T1- and T2-weighted and gadolinium-enhanced T1-weighted sequences. Other magnetic resonance imaging studies that may be useful include diffusion-weighted, blood oxygenation level–dependent, and arterial spin labeling techniques.

4. Magnetic resonance imaging is becoming increasingly important for the evaluation of the transplanted kidney. Postgadolinium T1-weighted sequences in which coronal images of the graft are acquired in the arterial, venous, and mixed phases of enhancement have been shown to be very useful in assessing renal parenchyma and parenchymal function.

5. The new generation of contrast agents used in magnetic resonance imaging, such as ultrasmall superparamagnetic iron oxide particles, may be useful in the evaluation of graft rejection.

Key References

3. Kawashima A, Vrtiska TJ, LeRoy AJ, et al: CT urography. Radiographics 2004;24:S35-S58.
8. Marckmann P, Skov L, Rossen K, et al: Nephrogenic systemic fibrosis: Suspected causative role of Gadodiamide used for contrast-enhanced magnetic resonance. J Am Soc Nephrol 2006;17:2359-2362.
19. Thoeny HC, De Keyzer F, Oyen RH, Peeters RR: Diffusion-weighted MR imaging of kidneys in healthy volunteers and patients with parenchymal diseases: Initial experience. Radiology 2005;235:911-917.
22. Sadowski EA, Fain SB, Alford SK, et al: Assessment of acute renal transplant rejection with blood oxygen level–dependent MR imaging: Initial experience. Radiology 2005;236:911-919.
23. Fenchel M, Martirosian P, Langanke J, et al: Perfusion MR imaging with FAIR true FISP spin labeling in patients with and without renal artery stenosis: Initial experience. Radiology 2006;238:1013-1021.

See the companion Expert Consult website for the complete reference list.

CHAPTER 51

Nephrotoxicity of Contrast Media

Roberto Pozzi Mucelli

OBJECTIVES

This chapter will:
1. Define and clinically characterize contrast agent–induced nephropathy.
2. Identify the risk factors for contrast agent–induced nephropathy.
3. Discuss the incidence of contrast agent–induced nephropathy with different contrast agents and examine pathomechanisms for the greater risk associated with intra-arterial injection.
4. Review strategies to prevent contrast agent–induced nephropathy.

With the increasing use of contrast media in diagnostic and interventional radiology, nephrotoxicity from these contrast agents has become an increasingly common cause of renal impairment.

Contrast agent–induced nephropathy (CIN) is defined as an acute decline in renal function following the administration of intravascular contrast material in the absence of other causes.[1,2] Most study definitions include a 25% increase in serum creatinine or at least a 0.5 mg/dL increase in serum creatinine within 48 to 72 hours of contrast administration. Serum creatinine levels generally return to baseline levels within 1 week of contrast exposure; however, CIN can lead to permanent renal failure and the requirement for ongoing dialysis. In fact, CIN represents an increasingly common cause of hospital-acquired renal failure[3,4] and is associated with an increase in mortality independent of other risk factors.[4]

PATHOGENESIS

CIN can be attributed to either renal medullary ischemia or direct renal tubular epithelial cell toxicity.[1] The injection of contrast results in a biphasic hemodynamic change in the kidney, with a transient, initial increase in renal blood flow followed by a more prolonged decrease in renal blood flow. The direct renal cell toxicity is manifested by histopathological changes and enzymuria.

RISK FACTORS

Major risk factors for CIN include chronic renal insufficiency, diabetes mellitus (especially when accompanied by renal insufficiency), any condition associated with decreased effective circulating volume (e.g., congestive heart failure, dehydration, nephrosis, cirrhosis), and use of large doses of contrast media.[2,5-8] Of course, other causes of acute renal failure, such as atheromatous embolic disease, ischemia, prerenal azotemia, sepsis, or other nephrotoxins, should always be considered, particularly if CIN is suspected in a patient without known risk factors.

CLINICAL FEATURES

Most patients in whom CIN develops have complete recovery of renal function. Dialysis is rarely required. Nevertheless, some degree of residual renal impairment has been reported in approximately 30% of affected patients.[1] Furthermore, the occurrence of acute renal failure can prolong the hospitalization period.

CONTRAST MEDIA AND THE KIDNEY

Contrast agents used in diagnostic radiology can be divided into ionic and nonionic (Table 51-1). Ionic contrast media are no longer used on account of their association with a higher incidence of adverse events. Nonionic contrast media are widely used in radiology in various procedures, such as intravenous urography, computed tomography (CT), and diagnostic and interventional angiography. These types of contrast agents are of low osmolarity relative to plasma (compared with the ionic contrast media) and are characterized by a lower incidence of adverse events. The nonionic contrast agents can be divided into monomeric (having three iodine atoms) and dimeric (having six iodine atoms). The dimeric media also are defined as iso-osmolar because their osmolality is equal to that of plasma.

In the recent literature, different studies have evaluated and compared the contrast media in order to evaluate their nephrotoxicity. Because CIN is observed almost exclusively in "high-risk" patients, this section reviews the available data on use of the newer iodinated agents in patients with preexisting renal failure and assesses whether they perform differently in such patients after *intra-arterial* versus *intravenous* administration.

TABLE 51-1

Ionic and Nonionic Contrast Media

	IODINE CONCENTRATION (mg/mL)	OSMOLALITY (mOsm)*
Ionic Contrast Media		
Monomeric		
Diatrizoate	370	2100
Iothalamate	400	2400
Ioxitalamate	380	2100
Metrizoate	350	1970
Dimeric		
Ioxaglate	320	577
Nonionic Contrast Media		
Monomeric		
Iobitridol	350	915
Iohexol	350	823
Iomeprol	350	610
Iopamidol	370	774
Iopentol	350	810
Iopromide	350	774
Ioversol	350	790
Ioxilan	350	700
Dimeric		
Iodixanol	320	290
Iotrolan	320	290
Plasma		290

*At 37°C, plasma osmolality is 290 mOsm.

Contrast Agent–Induced Nephropathy Developing after Intra-arterial Administration

Several studies have been conducted in patients with mild to moderate renal failure (inclusion criteria: serum creatinine level consistently above 1.5 mg/dL, or creatinine clearance rate of 50 to 60 mL/minute or less, or both; mean baseline serum creatinine of 1.5 to 2.0 mg/dL; mean baseline creatinine clearance of 40 to 60 mL/minute) undergoing diagnostic or interventional angiographic procedures. In all of these studies, the outcome measure was development of CIN as defined by an increase in serum creatinine of 0.5 mg/dL or greater, or by 25% of baseline values or more, 48 to 72 hours after administration of contrast.

Studies with Monomeric Nonionic Contrast Media

Rudnick and colleagues conducted a double-blind, randomized study to compare the incidence of nephrotoxicity with diatrizoate and with iohexol in 1196 patients undergoing cardiac angiography.[6] Patients were divided into four groups based on the presence of renal insufficiency and diabetes mellitus as follows: (1) neither renal insufficiency nor diabetes mellitus, (2) diabetes mellitus but no renal insufficiency, (3) renal insufficiency but no diabetes mellitus, and (4) renal insufficiency and diabetes mellitus present. CIN was defined as an increase in serum creatinine of 1.0 mg/dL or greater at 48 to 72 hours after contrast administration. CIN occurred significantly more frequently with the ionic agent, being reported in 42 patients (7.1%) receiving diatrizoate and in 19 patients (3.2%) receiving iohexol. In both treatment groups, nephrotoxicity was limited almost exclusively to patients with preexisting renal insufficiency, with or without diabetes. A secondary analysis was performed using a more sensitive definition of CIN (an increase in serum creatinine of 0.5 mg/dL or more from baseline within 48 to 72 hours after contrast administration). As would be expected, the overall incidence of CIN increased in both treatment groups (21.1% with diatrizoate, 13.4% with iohexol), but the difference in frequency of nephrotoxicity between diatrizoate and iohexol remained statistically significant. This secondary analysis also showed that nephrotoxicity was most evident in patients with renal insufficiency and diabetes mellitus (47.7% with diatrizoate, 33.3% with iohexol). Among the 61 patients with acute nephrotoxicity, 15 (6 in the iohexol treatment group and 9 in the diatrizoate group) experienced unusually severe nephrotoxicity, and 8 of these patients (5 in the iohexol group and 3 in the diatrizoate group) ultimately required dialysis. All of these 15 patients had preexisting renal insufficiency, and 73% had concomitant diabetes mellitus.

Durham and coworkers[9] conducted a double-blind study assessing the possible preventive effect of N-acetylcysteine in 81 patients with serum creatinine levels of at least 1.7 mg/dL who underwent angiography. Patients were randomized into groups receiving either prophylaxis for CIN with intravenous saline only (the control group) or intravenous saline plus N-acetylcysteine. All patients received iohexol, and contrast nephropathy was defined as an increase in serum creatinine of at least 0.5 mg/dL at 48 hours. Results showed that contrast nephropathy developed in 24% of patients after iohexol administration (26%

in the treatment group and 22% in the control group). In diabetic subjects, the results were even worse, with 42% of the *N*-acetylcysteine group and 28% of the control group experiencing CIN. In all, 5 of 79 patients (6.3%) experienced serum creatinine increases greater than 1.0 mg/dL, and 2 of these 5 patients (2.4% of the patient population) experienced increases over 2.0 mg/dL and required dialysis. The study confirmed a significant nephrotoxic effect of iohexol in patients with preexisting renal compromise.

Studies with Dimeric Nonionic Contrast Media

The Rapid Protocol for the Prevention of Contrast-Induced Renal Dysfunction (RAPPID) study[10] evaluated the efficacy of the use of intravenous acetylcysteine to prevent the nephrotoxic effects of iodixanol in patients with moderate renal failure (mean serum creatinine level, 1.75 ± 0.41 mg/dL; mean creatinine clearance, 44 ± 18 mL/min). The patients who were not randomized to receive the antioxidant had intravenous hydration for 12 hours before receiving iodixanol. The incidence of contrast nephropathy was 21% after iodixanol administration with hydration, but without premedication with acetylcysteine. Premedication with acetylcysteine significantly reduced the incidence of CIN induced by iodixanol.

Boccalandro and coworkers[11] published their findings in a randomized, double-blind trial comparing the renal tolerance of iodixanol-enhanced interventional cardiac angiographic procedures with or without pretreatment with oral acetylcysteine in 181 patients with moderate chronic renal insufficiency. All patients were hydrated for 12 hours before the procedure. Mean baseline serum creatinine level in the study group receiving iodixanol and no premedication was 1 mg/dL. Baseline creatinine clearance was 50 ± 29 mL/minute. The mean increase in serum creatinine after iodixanol administration and hydration was 0.19 ± 0.4 mg/dL. The incidence of contrast nephropathy (defined as an increase in serum creatinine of 0.5 mg/dL or greater at 48 hours after contrast administration) was 12%.

Recently, Stone and associates[12] conducted a randomized, double-blind, placebo-controlled study in 315 patients with moderate to severe renal failure to examine the efficacy of fenoldopam mesylate, a specific agonist of the dopamine D_1 receptor, in preventing contrast nephropathy after invasive cardiovascular procedures. Iodixanol was used in 10% of patients in this trial. CIN occurred in 33.3% of patients who received iodixanol, compared with 25.3% of those who received other contrast agents.

Studies with Both Monomeric and Dimeric Contrast Media

A randomized study by Chalmers and Jackson[13] evaluated the renal tolerance of iodixanol and of iohexol in 102 patients with renal impairment, which was defined as baseline serum creatinine levels greater than 150 µmol/L (1.7 mg/dL). All patients underwent renal or peripheral angiography (or both). Baseline characteristics were similar in both groups. Significantly more patients in the iohexol group experienced an increase in serum creatinine of 20%; the two groups did not significantly differ for serum creatinine increases of 25% or higher. The observed increases in serum creatinine were correlated with the volume of contrast injected in both groups, but no correlation was found between the increase in serum creatinine after contrast injection and its baseline level in either group. According to these data, the differences between the two agents were small and of doubtful clinical significance.

The NEPHRIC study,[8] however, showed that iohexol was significantly more nephrotoxic than iodixanol in patients with preexisting chronic renal failure (serum creatinine concentration between 1.5 and 3.5 mg/dL or serum calculated creatinine clearance of 60 mL/minute or less) undergoing coronary or aortofemoral angiography. All patients were adequately hydrated. The results of the NEPHRIC study showed iohexol caused a significantly higher peak increase in serum creatinine concentration, a significantly higher incidence of CIN (26% of patients with a peak increase in serum creatinine of 0.5 mg/dL or more, 15% of patients with a peak increase of 1.0 mg/dL or greater). Of more importance, six patients (9%) experienced acute renal failure related to the use of iohexol. Three of these patients recovered, two died, and one had persistent renal failure. Iodixanol induced a mean increase in serum creatinine of 0.13 mg/dL. Peak increases greater than 0.5 mg/dL were observed in 3% of patients. None of the patients exhibited a peak increase greater than 1.0 mg/dL.

A publication from the Royal London Hospital[14] reported cases of contrast nephropathy in a total of 267 patients. Of these, 46% had preexisting renal impairment. Two contrast agents were used: iohexol and iodixanol. CIN occurred after 15 procedures. Nine patients died, and 6 recovered. Three deaths occurred directly as a result of the nephropathy. One fatality occurred after the injection of iohexol and two fatalities after injection of iodixanol for angiography.

Studies with Other Nonionic Monomers

In the early 1990s, Taliercio and colleagues[15] compared the nephrotoxicity of diatrizoate and that of iopamidol. In this randomized, double-blind clinical trial, 307 patients with renal impairment undergoing cardiac angiography were enrolled. Renal impairment was defined as serum creatinine 1.5 mg/dL at recruitment; the mean baseline serum creatinine for the entire population was 2.02 mg/dL. At the 24-hour evaluation, mean serum creatinine levels were significantly increased in the diatrizoate group compared with the iopamidol group ($P < 0.001$). The mean maximal rise in serum creatinine was significantly higher in the diatrizoate group than in the iopamidol group. The maximal rise was greater than 0.5 mg/dL in 8% of the patients in the iopamidol group, versus 19% of those in the diatrizoate group. A multivariate analysis that considered contrast agent–specific effects, presence of diabetes mellitus requiring insulin, and presence of severe renal insufficiency (i.e., baseline serum creatinine level greater than 3 mg/dL) revealed that a greater maximal change in serum creatinine was independently related to the use of diatrizoate, the presence of diabetes mellitus requiring insulin, and the presence of severe renal insufficiency. These results indicate that iopamidol is less nephrotoxic than diatrizoate in patients with renal insufficiency.

Huber and associates[16] investigated whether the adenosine antagonist theophylline could prevent or reduce CIN in patients with chronic renal insufficiency. One group of 50 patients received iomeprol and placebo, and 50 additional patients were randomized to receive 200 mg of theophylline intravenously 30 minutes before angiography using iomeprol. High doses of contrast were used for diagnostic or interventional procedures. The vast majority of patients (86% in the iomeprol-placebo group, 88% in the iomeprol-theophylline group) received concomitant nephrotoxic medication (aminoglycoside, vancomycin, nonsteroidal anti-inflammatory drugs, amphotericine B, or nephrotoxic chemotherapy agents). Several patients also suffered from diabetes mellitus (40% in the iomeprol-placebo group, 28% in the iomeprol-theophylline group). The overall incidence of CIN (serum creatinine increase of 0.5 mg/dL or more) was 10% (16% in the placebo group, 4% in the theophylline group). The incidence of CIN in the subset of patients with renal failure and diabetes was 10% in the iomeprol-placebo group. Acute renal failure did not develop in any of the patients in this study.

Kay and coworkers[17] published a randomized, double-blind trial comparing renal tolerance of iopamidol enhanced diagnostic or interventional cardiac angiographic procedures with or without pretreatment with oral acetylcysteine in 200 patients with moderate chronic renal insufficiency. Renal failure did not develop in any of the patients who received iopamidol. In patients who received no premedication, serum creatinine levels showed a decrease 24 hours after the iopamidol-enhanced cardiac angiography procedure and very modest increases (mean increase, 0.02 mg/dL) at days 2 and 7 after contrast administration. An increase in creatinine clearance was observed even in patients receiving iopamidol and no premedication overall, as well as in patients with chronic renal failure and diabetes and in patients with reduced (30% to 50%) left ventricular ejection fraction. These findings indicate that deterioration in renal function in these patients, if any, was minimal or negligible, even in the presence of well-known risk factors for contrast nephropathy. The incidence of contrast nephropathy was 12% without premedication with N-acetylcysteine and 4% with premedication with the antioxidant.

In conclusion, several studies have been conducted to assess the effects of low- and iso-osmolar iodinated contrast agents after intra-arterial administration to patients with preexisting mild to moderate renal failure. Overall, the highest incidence of CIN was observed with iohexol, especially in diabetic patients with renal compromise (26% in NEPHRIC, 33.3% in the Rudnick study,[6] and 42% in the Durham study[9]). Studies conducted with other nonionic monomers showed a lower incidence of CIN than rates of nephrotoxicity reported for iohexol in similar patient populations (8% in the study by Taliercio and colleagues[15] and 12% in that by Kay and coworkers[17]).

Contrast-Induced Nephropathy Developing after Intravenous Administration

Fewer studies have addressed the renal safety of iodinated agents after intravenous administration. Two studies compared two different nonionic monomers with iodixanol. These studies also included patients with impaired renal function.

The first double-blind comparison of the effects of iodixanol and iopromide on renal function in 64 patients with mild to moderate renal insufficiency was conducted by Corraro and associates.[18] Patients with serum creatinine values between 1.5 and 3 mg/dL underwent intravenous urography using one of the two randomly assigned contrast agents. Renal function was assessed before and at 1, 6, 24, and 48 hours and 7 days after urography. Parameters

included serum creatinine and urinary renal tubule enzymes (alanylaminopeptidase and N-acetyl-β-glucosaminidase), α₁-microglobulin, and albumin. Baseline characteristics were similar in the two groups. Serum creatinine levels decreased during the observation period in both groups, but no statistical difference between treatments was noted. CIN developed in one nondiabetic patient in the iodixanol group. Overall, neither alanylaminopeptidase nor N-acetyl-β-glucosaminidase levels changed significantly in the two treatment groups. Levels of α₁-microglobulin and albumin did not change during the observation period, nor did blood pressure or heart rate.

A more recent study[19] was conducted to compare iodixanol and iobitridol in 50 patients undergoing cranial or body contrast-enhanced CT procedures. Both groups received similar volumes of contrast and had similar baseline values for serum creatinine and creatinine clearance. No differences between the two agents were observed. With both agents, the incidence of increase in serum creatinine level of 44 μmol/L or greater (i.e., 0.5 mg/dL or more) was 17%, and a decrease of creatinine clearance of 25% or more was observed in 12.5% of the patients.

In both studies, the renal safety of the nonionic dimeric agent was comparable to that of the nonionic monomeric agents.

Another study[20] evaluated the renal tolerance of iopamidol in pediatric patients (median age, 8.1 years) undergoing contrast-enhanced CT after bone marrow transplantation. These patients received several immunosuppressive and antimicrobial drugs known to be quite nephrotoxic (e.g., cyclosporine, methotrexate, cytarabine, aminoglycosides, amphotericin B, acyclovir). CT is the examination of choice to detect foci of infection and other complications in this patient population. The study assessed the possible potentiation of nephrotoxicity after administration of relatively high doses (2 to 3 mL/kg) of contrast. The nonionic monomer showed no or negligible effects on the kidneys of these children, who were definitely at higher than usual risk for development of acute renal failure after contrast administration.

STRATEGIES TO PREVENT CONTRAST AGENT–INDUCED NEPHROPATHY

The most effective strategy for minimizing the risk for CIN is careful patient assessment. When iodinated contrast-enhanced images are deemed necessary in a "high-risk" patient, a detailed medical history should be obtained and a thorough physical examination should be performed. Identification of risk factors allows the physician to reduce the risk of CIN by proactively addressing these potential problems. For example, prophylactic hydration with saline will correct dehydration. In fact, prophylactic hydration has become a widely accepted means of proactively reducing the incidence of CIN in all patients.[1] Another standard recommendation for reducing the potential for CIN is to use the lowest possible dose of contrast, particularly in patients with reduced renal function. Other prophylactic treatments have been proposed, although the best treatment to prevent CIN remains to be established. The most promising premedication regimen appears to be the use of N-acetylcysteine or theophylline in patients with preexisting renal compromise,[10,16,17] although the results of other studies did not show significant protection of renal function for these agents.[9,11] A meta-analysis[21] of seven randomized controlled trials comparing N-acetylcysteine and hydration with hydration alone showed a significant reduction in the risk for CIN in patients with chronic renal insufficiency. The relative risk of CIN was not related to the amount of contrast given to patients or to the severity of chronic renal insufficiency before the procedure.

Key Points

1. Contrast agent–induced nephropathy manifests as an acute decline in renal function following the administration of intravascular iodinated contrast media.
2. Contrast agent–induced nephropathy is becoming an increasing cause of iatrogenic acute renal impairment.
3. Contrast agent–induced nephropathy is transient, with return to normal renal function within a few days, in the great majority of cases.
4. Contrast agent–induced nephropathy is observed mainly in patients with preexisting renal impairment or diabetes mellitus.

5. Intra-arterial injection of contrast media is associated with a greater risk of contrast nephropathy than that observed with intravenous injection.
6. No significant differences exist in the incidence of contrast nephropathy with monomeric and dimeric nonionic contrast media.
7. Effective means of preventing contrast agent–induced nephropathy include hydration and administration of N-acetylcysteine or theophylline.

Key References

2. Thomsen HS, Morcos SK: Contrast media and the kidney: European Society of Urogenital Radiology (ESUR) Guidelines. Br J Radiol 2003;76:513-518.
6. Rudnick ML, Golfarb S, Wexler L, et al: Nephrotoxicity of ionic and non-ionic contrast media in 1196 patients: A randomized trial. Kidney Int 1995;47:254-261.

See the companion Expert Consult website for the complete reference list.

CHAPTER 52

New Imaging Techniques for Acute Kidney Injury

James W. Dear

OBJECTIVES

This chapter will:
1. Review important new methods for imaging disease processes in vivo.
2. Describe their application in the study of acute kidney injury.
3. Highlight the future clinical applications of novel imaging techniques.

Acute kidney disease (AKD) is a relatively common and significant cause of morbidity, occurring in 5% to 20% of patients in the intensive care unit (ICU) setting.[1-3] Few clinical trials have targeted the prevention or treatment of this disease, and of these studies, only a handful have yielded useful data.[4,5] In part, these limited results reflect the incomplete understanding of the pathogenesis of AKD in vivo and a lack of sensitive biomarkers. Advances in imaging techniques such as magnetic resonance imaging (MRI) promise to provide insights into the mechanisms that lead to acute kidney injury in patients. Multiple pathophysiological processes contribute to loss of renal function in AKD (for example, inflammation); these are covered elsewhere in this book. Novel imaging techniques can quantify these processes in vivo, thereby supporting or refuting observations made possible by invasive means in animal models. This chapter briefly discusses novel imaging techniques and their application in AKD research.

IMAGING THE SITE OF KIDNEY INJURY IN VIVO

The capability of MRI to provide high-quality imaging of kidney tissue in multiple planes with rapid acquisition times makes this imaging modality ideal for studying AKD. The images provided by MRI are of higher quality than those obtained with computed tomography (CT), and novel advances in CT have been limited in relation to AKD. A use for CT in the measurement of glomerular filtration rate (GFR) in AKD has been described,[6] but MRI has the potential to provide many more novel insights.[7]

Functional MRI of the kidneys emerged as a discrete technique with the introduction of gadolinium–diethylaminetriamine-penta-acetic acid (Gd-DTPA). This small molecule (less than 1 kD) is filtered at the glomerulus and

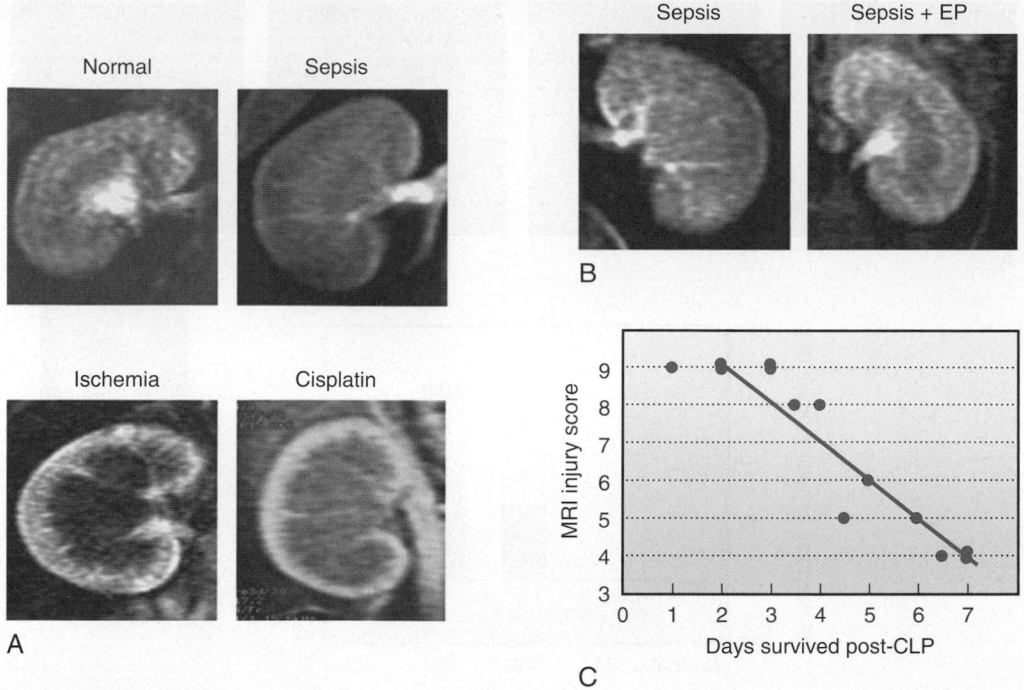

FIGURE 52-1. A, Dendrimer contrast magnetic resonance imaging (MRI) can localize the process leading to an elevation in serum creatinine in clinically relevant mouse models of acute kidney disease (AKD). Shown are images of normal kidney and of kidneys with AKD due to sepsis, ischemia, and cisplatin toxicity. **B,** Dendrimer contrast MRI can track drug therapy in a mouse model of sepsis. Sepsis led to renal abnormalities that were reversed by treatment with ethyl pyruvate (EP). **C,** Dendrimer contrast MRI can predict outcome. At 6 hours after induction of polymicrobial sepsis, the degree of renal injury (MRI injury score) predicts survival. CLP, cecal ligation and puncture.

is neither secreted nor reabsorbed in the tubules, making Gd-DTPA suitable for studying GFR, split renal function, and renal concentrating ability. Over the past two decades, other low-molecular-weight contrast agents have been developed that have imaging properties similar to those of Gd-DTPA.

Recently, macromolecular contrast agents known as *dendrimers* have provided new insights into the pathogenic mechanisms in AKD.[8] Dendrimer particles are branching polymers that can be synthesized to form nanoparticles of precise size. The presence of amino groups on the particle's outer surface allows attachment of gadolinium to form a novel MRI contrast agent. The G4 dendrimer (G4 referring to its size) is excreted rapidly in the urine and accumulates in the outer stripe of the medulla, probably in proximal straight tubular cells. The intrarenal accumulation and excretion of the gadolinium-labeled G4 dendrimer present an opportunity to use this MRI contrast agent as a biomarker to detect and categorize AKD in mouse models. Figure 52-1 demonstrates the different patterns of kidney injury with different insults. These different insults produce different patterns of gene expression and may respond differently to therapeutic intervention.[9] This finding highlights the potential importance of imaging in defining subtypes of AKD. Dendrimer contrast MRI also can detect renal injury before serum creatinine is elevated, but at a time when the novel therapeutic agent ethyl pyruvate is still effective, and can be used to predict outcome in a mouse model of sepsis[10] (see Fig. 52-1). If these advances are translated into clinical application in humans, dendrimer contrast MRI may allow treatment to be targeted to specific AKD subtypes at a time when the therapeutic window is still open.

IMAGING INFLAMMATION IN VIVO

Inflammation plays an important role in the pathogenesis of AKD in certain animal models. Recent advances in MRI have allowed investigators to detect inflammation in a variety of disease models. One such advance is the use of ultra-small superparamagnetic iron oxide (USPIO) particles as an imaging agent. These particles initially remain in the blood pool (being too large to be filtered by the glomerulus) but gradually are internalized by monocytes and macrophages and will locally degrade the MRI signal to produce "black" areas in tissues that correspond to areas of inflammatory cell infiltration. This technique has been applied in various experimental models of AKD. With use of USPIO particle MRI in a murine model of ischemia-reperfusion, for example, Jo and coworkers (2003) were able to demonstrate a black band in the outer stripe of the outer medulla.[11] This imaging feature corresponds to the area of maximal inflammation and the site of proximal tubular injury (Fig. 52-2). Furthermore, the amount of inflammation demonstrated by MRI correlated accurately with the elevation in serum creatinine. Of interest, inflammation was not detected in animals with AKD induced by mercuric chloride, a nephrotoxin that produces minimal renal inflammation. This distinction highlights a possible future application for imaging in the management of patients with AKD: Different etiological causes of AKD have different pathophysiological manifestations, so imaging inflammation in vivo by means of MRI could aid in choosing the correct anti-inflammatory therapy in these patients.

Although ultrasound examination has an established role in the management of patients with acute kidney

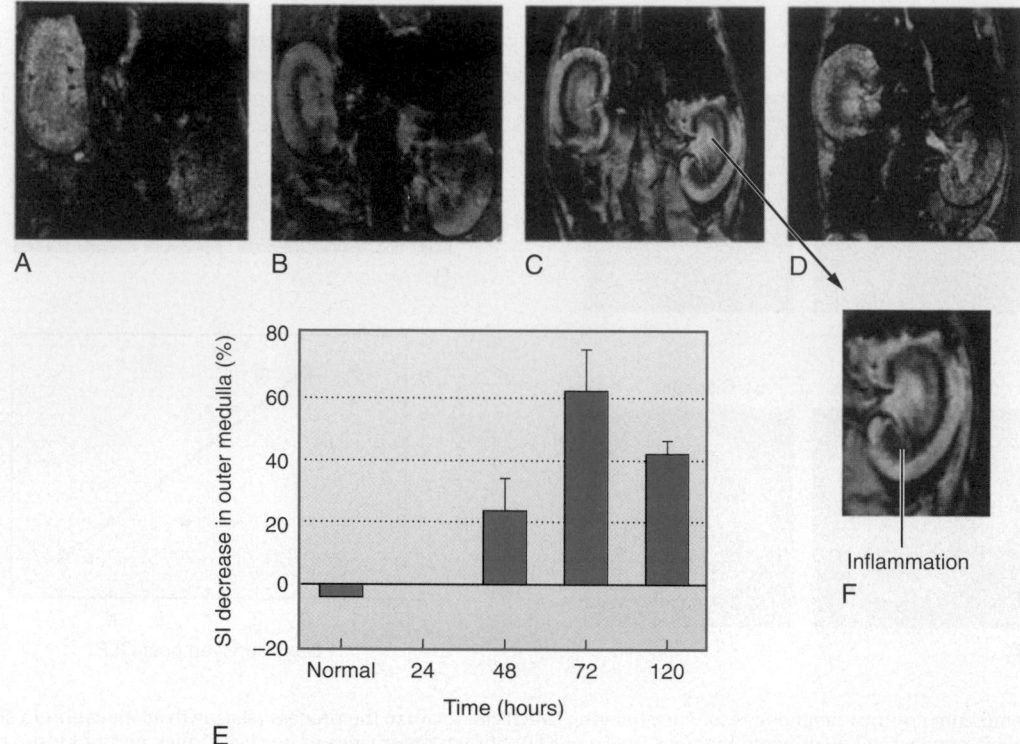

FIGURE 52-2. Time course of magnetic resonance imaging (MRI) changes after injection of ultra-small superparamagnetic iron oxide (USPIO) particles in ischemic acute kidney disease in a rat model. The *black areas* correspond to inflammation. Images were obtained 24 hours after USPIO injection. **A,** Ischemia-reperfusion at 24 hours. **B,** Ischemia-reperfusion at 48 hours. **C,** Ischemia-reperfusion at 72 hours. **D,** Ischemia-reperfusion at 120 hours. **E,** Mean signal intensity (SI) change in the outer medulla was measured at different time points after ischemia. **F,** Close-up view of kidney 72 hours after onset of ischemia-reperfusion changes. Note *black areas* representing inflammation in renal medulla. (From Jo SK, Hu X, Kobayashi H, et al: Detection of inflammation following renal ischemia by magnetic resonance imaging. Kidney Int 2003;64:43-51.)

injury, development of novel techniques with this modality has been less than with MRI. In current clinical practice, ultrasound imaging cannot reliably distinguish among different patterns of acute kidney injury (e.g., sepsis cannot be differentiated from ischemia). The addition of an exogenous contrast agent can increase the information obtained from ultrasonography in AKD. For example, the intravenous administration of microbubble contrast agents improves the detection of vascular insults such as acute cortical necrosis and renal vein thrombosis.[12] As a research tool, modification of the microbubble shell allows measurement of renal inflammation after ischemic injury in mice.[13,14] The great advantage of ultrasonography in clinical practice is that the mobility of the necessary equipment allows imaging to be performed in the critical care setting. Ultrasound contrast agents that quantify disease processes such as inflammation may provide novel insights in critical care nephrology.

IMAGING KIDNEY HYPOXIA IN VIVO

The magnetic properties of hemoglobin change with oxygenation and can be imaged noninvasively with MRI, with deoxyhemoglobin acting as an endogenous contrast agent. Just as capillary blood is considered to be in equilibrium with the surrounding tissue, changes in the oxygenated-deoxygenated state of hemoglobin can be considered to reflect changes in tissue oxygen tension. It is well known that the renal medulla is relatively hypoxic and therefore sensitive to the changes in blood flow that occur with a

number of renal insults. The capability of blood oxygenation level–dependent (BOLD) MRI to noninvasively measure tissue oxygenation has led to its application in the investigation of AKD. One of the strengths of the BOLD technique is that it does not require the administration of exogenous contrast agent, thus allowing early "proof of concept" studies in humans. One of the first studies to apply BOLD MRI for the investigation of renal disease used normal human subjects and demonstrated that well-described, invasively measured observations from animal studies accurately represent human physiology.[15] This correlation demonstrates another important role for imaging in the investigation of AKD—the validation of existing animal models by means of noninvasive human studies.

In animal studies, BOLD MRI has been demonstrated to detect hypoxia induced by experimental renal artery stenosis,[16] acute renal ischemia,[17] ureteral obstruction,[18] and radiocontrast agent–induced nephropathy.[19] In humans, the potential utility of BOLD MRI has been demonstrated by studies investigating the effect of nephrotoxic drugs on renal oxygenation[20] and the effect of age and diabetes on medullary oxygen tension.[21,22] The investigators found that different nephrotoxic agents had different oxygenation effects: Radiocontrast medium decreased oxygenation, but the immunosuppressive agent cyclosporine increased oxygenation. Both older age and diabetes impaired the increase in medullary oxygen tension after water loading—an interesting observation, because age and diabetes are established risk factors for the development of AKD. BOLD MRI has not yet been used to study acute native kidney injury; however, it recently has been applied in the study of acute dysfunction of renal allografts.[23] Not only was BOLD MRI able to distinguish a normal functioning allograft from a nonfunctioning allograft but, of importance, it also distinguished acute tubular necrosis from acute rejection. These findings highlight the potential usefulness of this noninvasive technique, with the strength that it uses deoxyhemoglobin as an endogenous contrast agent.

IMAGING THE KIDNEY CORTICOMEDULLARY SODIUM GRADIENT IN VIVO

The kidney maintains a corticomedullary sodium gradient as an essential mechanism in the process of urine concentration. Sodium MRI (^{23}Na MRI) is a novel MRI technique capable of measuring tissue sodium concentration. In a rat model, this MRI measurement has been used as a biomarker to detect acute tubular necrosis very early in disease pathogenesis, because the corticomedullary sodium gradient is reduced by tubular injury.[24] This technique is now being developed for use in humans[25] and may allow AKD to be distinguished from prerenal failure at a time when the disease process may still be reversible.

IMAGING OXIDATIVE STRESS IN VIVO

Although still purely a research tool, electron paramagnetic resonance (EPR) is an exciting novel imaging technique that can depict the pathological changes that characterize oxidative stress in vivo. EPR uses an exogenous contrast agent ("spin probe") to produce a signal that decays over time. The rate of decay reflects the oxidant-antioxidant balance in the tissue. This technique has been applied to the measurement of renal reducing activity in a mouse model of ischemic AKD and demonstrated reduced activity even after serum creatinine levels had returned to normal.[26]

POTENTIAL CLINICAL APPLICATIONS OF NOVEL IMAGING TECHNIQUES IN ACUTE KIDNEY DISEASE

In the context of basic and clinical research, imaging techniques are very powerful tools because they can provide insight into disease pathogenesis in vivo. Elucidation of the underlying pathophysiology can be expected to galvanize research efforts in both animal models and human studies. Novel imaging techniques also have potential clinical applications, however, and specific imaging findings with such techniques can be considered to represent biomarkers in the same way as that characterized for a serum or urinary protein.

Although certain imaging techniques may not be practical, at least initially, in general clinical practice, they may have an important role in drug development. Imaging may detect AKD earlier in the disease process than is possible with use of existing biomarkers (e.g., serum creatinine). This capability is potentially important for successful drug development, because early kidney dysfunction could be reversible.

In addition, an imaging modality would be useful if it could help localize the pathological process underlying the acute kidney injury. This capability would allow clinical trials to recruit patients with specific types of AKD and would improve the power of a study to detect a drug effect. Imaging also could aid protein biomarker discovery by allowing subgrouping of patients with AKD by pattern of kidney injury. Finally, an imaging technique that can demonstrate a response to intervention would allow phase 2 dose-finding drug studies to be performed with greater sensitivity and specificity.

CONCLUSION

Imaging with techniques such as MRI is a rapidly developing field with enormous potential usefulness in the diagnosis and treatment of disease. Its application to AKD will allow researchers to study the disease in vivo; with increased understanding, much-needed novel therapies may be developed.

Key Points

1. The incidence of acute kidney disease and rates of associated morbidity are high among critically ill patients, and effective treatments are needed. Elucidation of the disease process in humans is therefore needed. Imaging modalities such as magnetic resonance imaging promise to provide essential pathophysiological information.
2. From the researcher's perspective, the techniques discussed in this chapter allow quantification of the relative contributions of different disease processes in models of acute kidney disease and, in certain cases, in human disease.
3. From the clinician's perspective, new imaging techniques may allow earlier detection of renal dysfunction and also help to define subtypes of acute kidney disease. These improvements would increase the likelihood that an effective novel therapy is applied in the correct patient population.

Key References

8. Dear JW, Kobayashi H, Brechbiel MW, Star RA: Imaging acute renal failure with polyamine dendrimer-based MRI contrast agents. Nephron Clin Pract 2006;103:c45-c49.
11. Jo SK, Hu X, Kobayashi H, et al: Detection of inflammation following renal ischemia by magnetic resonance imaging. Kidney Int 2003;64:43-51.
15. Prasad PV, Edelman RR, Epstein FH: Noninvasive evaluation of intrarenal oxygenation with BOLD MRI. Circulation 1996;94:3271-3275.
24. Maril N, Margalit R, Rosen S, et al: Detection of evolving acute tubular necrosis with renal ^{23}Na MRI: Studies in rats. Kidney Int 2006;69:765-768.
26. Hirayama A, Nagase S, Ueda A, et al: In vivo imaging of oxidative stress in ischemia-reperfusion renal injury using electron paramagnetic resonance. Am J Physiol Renal Physiol 2005; 288(3):F597-F603.

See the companion Expert Consult website for the complete reference list.

Light and Electronic Microscopy in Acute Renal Failure

CHAPTER 53

Indications for Renal Biopsy in Acute Renal Failure

Alan D. Salama

OBJECTIVES

This chapter will:
1. Describe the indications for and benefits of performing a renal biopsy in the context of acute renal failure.
2. Identify the main contraindications to renal biopsy, and discuss strategies for prevention of complications and their clinical management.
3. Review other possible approaches to obtaining renal tissue.

Renal biopsy has become an essential tool in the management of acute renal failure. Its development and refinement since the 1960s have been fundamental to the diagnosis and definition of clinical syndromes and the discovery of new pathological entities.[1] Through critical analysis of these findings, certain key pathophysiological features of kidney disease have been discovered that have helped establish new paradigms in nephrology, leading in turn to improvements in patient management. This procedure is extremely useful for assessing native kidneys and even more so for evaluating acute graft deterioration in renal transplants.[2]

The first percutaneous kidney biopsies were performed more than 50 years ago with a liver biopsy needle, using intravenous pyelograms for screening and with the patient sitting or supine. Their success in obtaining renal tissue and in aiding management confirmed the benefit of the procedure.[1] Since those early days, innovations such as the use of real-time ultrasound, spring-loaded needles or needle holders, and careful preoperative evaluation of the patient have improved the rate of obtaining adequate renal tissue while minimizing the risks of the procedure.[3] These advantages have placed percutaneous renal biopsy at the very center of modern clinical nephrology. General criteria for performing a renal biopsy are summarized in Table 53-1, but these will vary from center to center, which in turn will bias the pattern of disease entities found.

COMPLICATIONS OF BIOPSY

Although generally safe, percutaneous renal biopsy carries the risk of some morbidity and measurable mortality, so it is imperative to limit use of this procedure only to those patients for whom the potential benefit will offset those risks. The significant complications related to the procedure are hemorrhage, arteriovenous fistula formation, and sepsis.[4-6] Bleeding with grossly visible hematuria and the development of perinephric hematomas may be minor and self-resolving or more serious, requiring intervention in the form of blood transfusions, embolization, or surgery. Arteriovenous fistulas, if they develop, may be asymptomatic and spontaneously resolve or result in a significant vascular steal syndrome, compromising the rest of the kidney through ischemia. Finally, a risk of sepsis is associated with the procedure through the potential for introduction of a septic focus or its dissemination. The overall complication rates vary from center to center but generally are reported to be between 3.5% and 13%, with a majority of complications being minor (occurring in approximately 3% to 9% of patients undergoing biopsy).[4-6]

Uncommonly, the tissue core obtained at biopsy may be inadequate for diagnosis, either containing too few glomeruli or insufficient cortical material; this complication is reported in up to 5% of biopsy procedures. For confident diagnosis of a focal condition, at least 20 glomeruli in the sample are required,[7] and transplant biopsy studies suggest that obtaining two cores of tissue increases the sensitivity of diagnosis over that attainable with one core.[8]

Mortality associated with the procedure generally is related to undiagnosed bleeding with significant hematoma formation and is reported in up to 0.2% of cases from larger biopsy series.[5,6] Complications appear to be more common in native than in transplanted kidneys, and in patients with more advanced renal impairment (serum creatinine level more than 440 μmol/L) or with lower hemoglobin concentration (12 versus 11 g/dL).[5,6] Careful selection and preparation of the patient for the procedure appear to decrease the overall risk. Certain absolute contraindications that preclude percutaneous biopsy are recognized, as well as a number of relative contraindications (Table 53-2), which may be circumvented depending on

TABLE 53-1

General Indications for Renal Biopsy

- Significant proteinuria (excretion of >1 g of protein/day)
- Microscopic hematuria
- Unexplained renal impairment
- Renal manifestations of systemic disease

TABLE 53-2

Contraindications to Renal Biopsy

ABSOLUTE CONTRAINDICATIONS	RELATIVE CONTRAINDICATIONS
<ul><li>Uncontrolled hypertension</li><li>Bleeding diathesis</li><li>Widespread cystic disease or renal malignancy</li><li>Hydronephrosis</li><li>Inability of the patient to cooperate</li><li>Active urinary sepsis</li></ul>	<ul><li>Single kidney</li><li>Antiplatelet agents</li><li>Anatomical abnormalities</li><li>Small kidneys</li></ul>

the importance of the biopsy, the operator's experience, and the supportive facilities available. Ideally, every effort should be made to compensate for the additional considerations raised by the relative contraindications; however, in the context of acute renal failure, this approach is not always possible. The critical preoperative steps are to ensure that blood pressure is controlled, that the patient does not have a bleeding diathesis or a urinary tract infection, and that the kidneys are suitably imaged, with no evidence of obstruction, generalized cystic disease, or malignant-appearing masses. Careful preoperative assessment should allow those patients unsuitable for percutaneous biopsy to be referred for an alternative approach. In these patients, other means of obtaining renal tissue include open biopsy,[9] laparoscopic biopsy, and transjugular biopsy.[10] Each is associated with certain complications and has particular merits, depending on the clinical scenario (Table 53-3). Overall, these alternative procedures

TABLE 53-3

Alternative Methods for Obtaining Renal Tissue and Their Risks and Benefits Compared with a Percutaneous Approach

METHOD	ADVANTAGE(S)	DISADVANTAGE(S)
Transjugular approach	Can be of use in patients with a bleeding diathesis	Risk of capsular perforation Inadequate material obtained in up to 24% of cases
Open approach	High yield of adequate tissue Hemostasis is more secure	Requires general or spinal anesthesia
Laparoscopic approach	High yield of adequate tissue Hemostasis is more secure	Requires general or spinal anesthesia

generally are required in only a minority of potential biopsy patients.

ACUTE RENAL FAILURE AND RENAL BIOPSY

Acute renal failure is the main indication for renal biopsy in 9% to 13% of the patients undergoing the procedure in large biopsy series but makes up a much greater percentage of the indications in older patients (in up to 27% of those older than 60 years of age),[11-13] whereas it is a relatively uncommon indication in children. Part of the reason for such a relatively low percentage of biopsies being carried out for acute renal failure is the fact that this disorder, especially in the critical care setting, often is secondary to the underlying illness and frequently reversible. Thus, treating the underlying condition, such as sepsis or hypovolemia, and withdrawing nephrotoxic drugs often will result in an improvement in renal function.

A common presumed diagnosis for renal impairment in critical care situations is acute tubular necrosis (ATN). In a series of patients with acute renal failure, however, in whom ATN seemed unlikely, the prebiopsy diagnosis was correct in only 29% of the cases, confirming the requirement for histopathological examination in making an accurate diagnosis.[14] In particular, 89% of cases of tubulointerstitial nephritis were not suspected, and thrombotic microangiopathies were not considered in 80% of the cases. After biopsy, alterations in patient management were possible (for example, withdrawal of drugs with known potential for inducing interstitial nephritis), and overall, 43% of the patients undergoing biopsy achieved renal recovery.

In another series of 250 patients presenting with acute renal failure, 47% of the cases were found to be related to surgery, 2.8% were secondary to obstetrical complications, and the rest were related to a medical condition. In this last group, renal biopsy was required to establish a diagnosis, which was not apparent from the history or routine examination, in 48% of cases.[15] A critical point is that in 35% of these cases, a crescentic or necrotizing glomerulonephritis was found, demonstrating that in the absence of features commonly associated with ATN, a number of important and treatable conditions may be missed without biopsy. Moreover, in the Italian registry series of biopsies for acute renal failure (defined as rapidly deteriorating renal function), the incidence of ATN was only 8%, less than that for necrotizing vasculitis, crescentic glomerulonephritis, and tubulointerstitial nephritis, reinforcing the potential utility of performing a biopsy in this setting (Fig. 53-1).

Other biopsy series have suggested a similar incidence for necrotizing vasculitis and tubulointerstitial nephritis in those patients with more advanced renal impairment (serum creatinine levels greater than 200 µmol/L). In a more recent series of more than 250 biopsies taken from older patients (older than 60 years) with acute renal failure, the histopathological diagnosis confirmed a prebiopsy suspected diagnosis in 67% of the cases and again demonstrated a low frequency of ATN of 14%.[12] In this series, the most common histopathological finding was pauci-immune glomerulonephritis (with or without arteritis) (31.2%), followed by acute tubulointerstitial nephritis (18.6%), ATN with nephrotic syndrome (7.5%) or in isolation (6.7%), atheroemboli (7.1%), and, in lesser frequen-

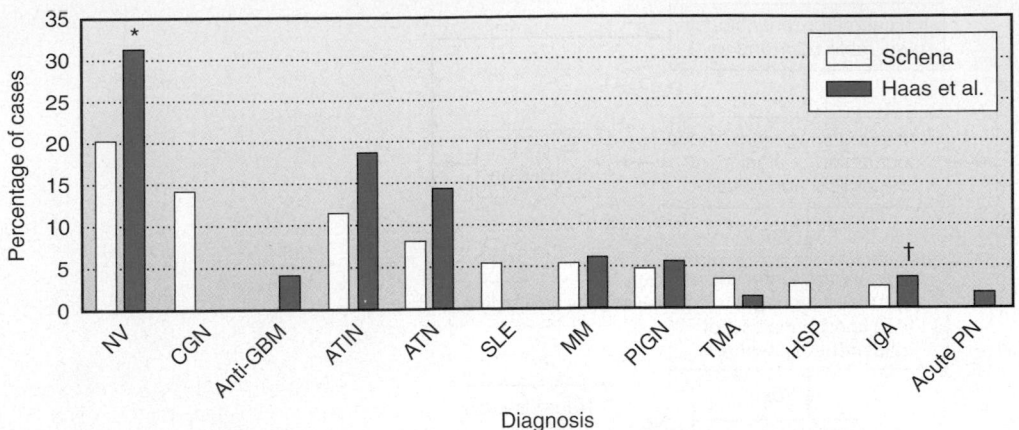

FIGURE 53-1. Frequency of pathological diagnoses recorded for renal biopsy specimens obtained for the diagnosis of acute renal failure. Acute PN, acute pyelonephritis; Anti-GBM, antiglomerular basement membrane disease; ATIN, acute tubulointerstitial nephritis; ATN, acute tubular necrosis; CGN, crescentic glomerulonephritis; HSP, Henoch-Schönlein purpura; IgA, immunoglobulin A nephropathy; MM, multiple myeloma; NV, necrotizing vasculitis; PIGN, postinfectious glomerulonephritis; SLE, systemic lupus erythematosus; TMA, thrombotic microangiopathy. * = pauci-immune GN in the Haas et al. series; † = combined with HSP in the Haas et al. series. (Adapted from Haas M, Spargo BH, Wit EJ, Meehan SM: Etiologies and outcome of acute renal insufficiency in older adults: A renal biopsy study of 259 cases. Am J Kidney Dis 2000;35:433-447; and from Schena FP: Survey of the Italian Registry of Renal Biopsies. Frequency of the renal diseases for 7 consecutive years. The Italian Group of Renal Immunopathology. Nephrol Dial Transplant 1997;12:418-426.)

cies, B cell dyscrasias, postinfectious glomerulonephritis, antiglomerular basement membrane (anti-GBM) disease, and immunoglobulin A (IgA) nephropathy. In 40% of the cases of myeloma kidney, the diagnosis of myeloma was unsuspected until the biopsy result was available. In only 5% of the biopsies was a diagnosis not arrived at, owing to an inadequate tissue sample or a lack of obvious histopathological cause for the acute renal failure. By contrast, data from a large cohort of Indian patients with acute renal failure demonstrated that of 1122 cases, 891 were due to intrinsic renal disease and of these, 705 (79.2%) were due to ischemic or toxic ATN. Thus, intrinsic renal disease other than ATN accounted for only 21% of cases of acute renal failure, attributable to glomerulonephritis in 9.3%, tubulointerstitial nephritis in 7%, and acute cortical necrosis in 4.6% of the cases overall.[16] These marked differences in the frequency of ATN in part reflect local biopsy policies and the threshold for biopsy in the setting of acute renal failure, as well as disease incidence due to geographical and ethnic variations.

In a majority of patients with acute renal insufficiency, prerenal and obstructive causes of ATN will account for most of the cases, as shown in a large series of nearly 750 Spanish patients with acute renal failure, in whom these three conditions were found in 76%.[17] Once these etiologies are excluded clinically, however, a sizable proportion of patients will be found to have acute renal failure, in whom the diagnosis is reached only after biopsy. Thus, in the context of acute renal failure with rapidly deteriorating function, and in the absence of clinical and laboratory features strongly suggestive of ATN (including "bland" findings on urine dipstick testing and presence of hyaline casts), biopsy is indicated. This must obviously be tempered by considering the clinical condition of the patient and the presence of any absolute or relative contraindications (see earlier). A schema detailing the steps required before biopsy is shown in Figure 53-2.

CONCLUSION

Percutaneous renal biopsy generally is safe if care is taken in the selection of candidates for the procedure and in preparation of the patient. It should be considered in any patient with acute renal failure in whom prerenal and obstructive causes are eliminated and in whom ATN is not the most likely diagnosis clinically, or in patients with an abnormal urinary sediment, provided that no contraindications are present.

Key Points

1. Renal biopsy is the only means of establishing certain diagnoses, which may not be suspected from the clinical findings in up to one third of cases.
2. Renal biopsy provides information regarding reversibility of the lesions and hence the likely benefit of therapy.
3. Renal biopsy analysis may change management in more than 40% of cases.
4. With use of real-time ultrasound techniques and small-gauge needles and adherence to strict screening policies, biopsy results in few complications.
5. Close cooperation between nephrologists and pathologists is required for optimal interpretation of the pathological findings on biopsy.
6. Only practitioners at clinical centers with experience in obtaining and processing renal biopsy specimens should perform this procedure.

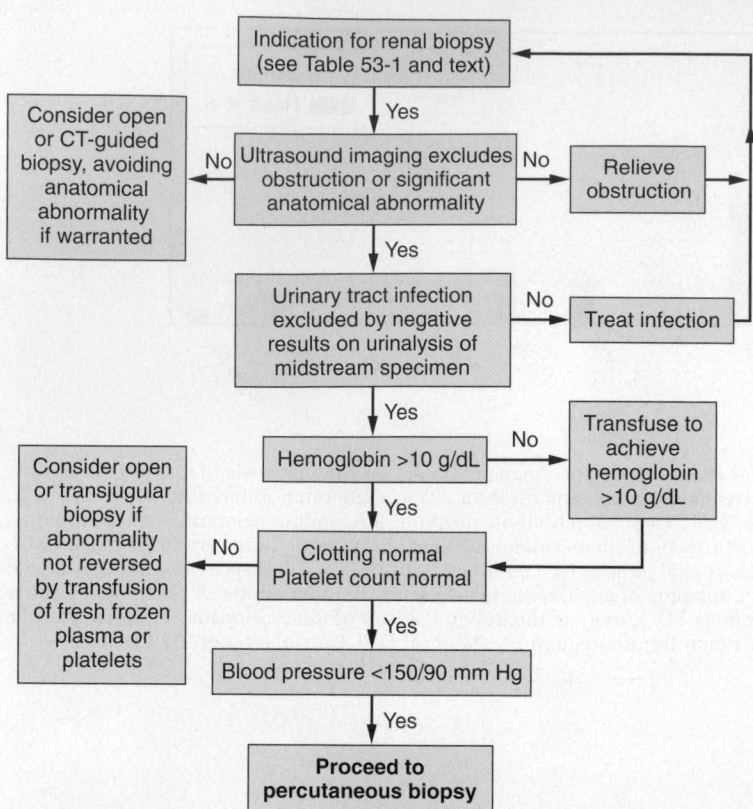

FIGURE 53-2. Proposed schema for proceeding to percutaneous renal biopsy. CT, computed tomography.

Key References

6. Whittier WL, Korbet SM: Timing of complications in percutaneous renal biopsy. J Am Soc Nephrol 2004;15:142-147.
12. Haas M, Spargo BH, Wit EJ, Meehan SM: Etiologies and outcome of acute renal insufficiency in older adults: A renal biopsy study of 259 cases. Am J Kidney Dis 2000;35:433-447.
15. Beaman M, Turney JH, Rodger RS, et al: Changing pattern of acute renal failure. Q J Med 1987;62:15-23.
16. Prakash J, Sen D, Kumar NS, et al: Acute renal failure due to intrinsic renal diseases: Review of 1122 cases. Ren Failure 2003;25:225-223.
17. Liaño F, Pascual J: Epidemiology of acute renal failure: A prospective, multicenter, community-based study. Madrid Acute Renal Failure Study Group. Kidney Int 1996;50:811-818.

See the companion Expert Consult website for the complete reference list.

CHAPTER 54

Histopathological and Electron Microscopy Findings in Acute Renal Failure

Julie Riopel and Kim Solez

OBJECTIVES

This chapter will:
1. Describe the diagnostic morphological features of acute tubular injury (acute tubular necrosis) as seen on light and electron microscopy.
2. Summarize the main features that distinguish transplant-specific and nephrotoxic acute tubular injury from ischemic acute tubular injury in native kidneys.
3. Review the histopathological differential diagnosis for acute tubular injury.

Acute renal failure (ARF) can be prerenal, intrinsic (intrarenal), or postrenal. By definition, prerenal ARF is a functional renal impairment due to hypoperfusion and is not accompanied by renal pathological lesions other than hyperplasia of the juxtaglomerular apparatus.[1] Postrenal ARF results from urinary tract obstruction. Approximately 85% of cases of intrinsic ARF are associated with a constellation of pathological lesions traditionally designated *acute tubular necrosis* (ATN).[2] This term has remained in common use over the years, although it does not accurately reflect actual histopathological findings. Some authors have advocated its replacement by the more accurate term *acute tubular injury* (ATI), which is used in this chapter.[3] A variety of other conditions predominantly affecting glomeruli (e.g., acute glomerulonephritis), tubulointerstitium (e.g., tubulointerstitial nephritis), or vessels (e.g., thrombotic microangiopathy, vasculitis) also can manifest with ARF. The reader is referred to standard renal pathology textbooks for detailed discussion of these entities.

The last few decades have seen a flourishing of publications that have increased our understanding of ATI, yet most studies are based on experimental animal models.[4-11] Human studies have been hindered by the limited availability of biopsy material or the limited quality of autopsy material from ATI patients. A new classification scheme for acute kidney injury based on glomerular filtration rate and urine output criteria is now being used in clinical studies.[12,13] Whether this scheme correlates with morphological features of ATI is not yet known. This chapter focuses on diagnostic features of ATI seen by light microscopy and electron microscopy (EM) and includes some relevant experimental data.

OVERVIEW OF NORMAL TUBULAR HISTOLOGY AND ULTRASTRUCTURE

Various segments of the nephron can be distinguished by light microscopy. Normal tubules have a collapsed lumen. Proximal tubular cells have an abundantly eosinophilic (pink colored on routine hematoxylin-eosin staining) cytoplasm and a prominent apical brush border. This brush border is best visualized as a pink luminal rim with the periodic acid–Schiff (PAS) stain. The thin limb of Henle's loop is lined by a very thin and flat epithelium and can be confused with a capillary. The epithelium of the thick ascending limb of Henle's loop is composed of smaller cuboid cells (in comparison with proximal tubule), with a sparsely eosinophilic cytoplasm and no brush border. Tamm-Horsfall protein (THP), which forms the matrix for tubular cast formation, is synthesized by the thick ascending limb. The epithelium of the distal convoluted tubule is similar to that of the thick ascending loop, but with larger cells and more central nuclei. Cubical cells whose height increases toward the papilla line the collecting ducts. They have a clear cytoplasm and distinct cell borders. More elaborate delineation of tubular subsegments cannot be achieved by routine light microscopy. Cortical tubules are closely apposed to one another, being separated by only a small amount of interstitial space, whereas medullary tubules are farther apart from each other.[14]

EM discloses additional features such as the presence of extensive basolateral infoldings of the cell membrane and abundant organelles (Fig. 54-1), except in the thin limb of Henle's loop and collecting duct principal cells.[14]

ISCHEMIC ACUTE TUBULAR INJURY

Approximately 50% of cases of intrinsic ARF are caused by an ischemic insult.[2,15]

Light Microscopy Findings

The morphological alterations seen by light microscopy usually are mild, contrasting with the degree of dysfunction. The main injury is obviously in the tubular compartment, but the intricate relationships linking glomeruli, vessels, interstitium, and tubules will lead to alterations in each compartment. Although not routinely used in clinical practice, ancillary studies have provided insights into the pathophysiology of ATI and are included in the discussion.

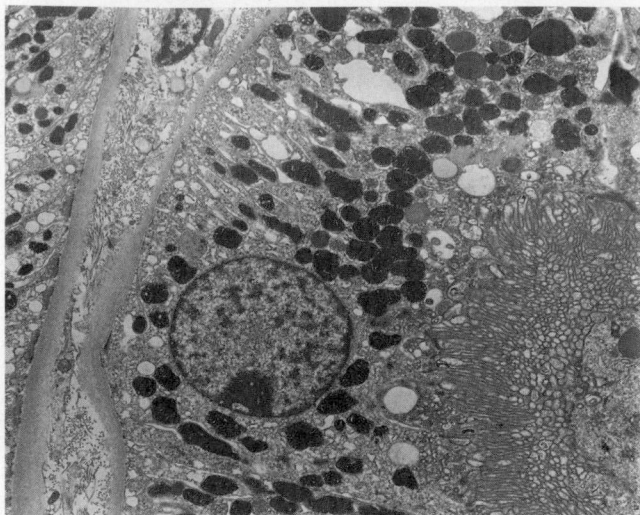

FIGURE 54-1. Electron microscopy appearance of normal proximal tubule.

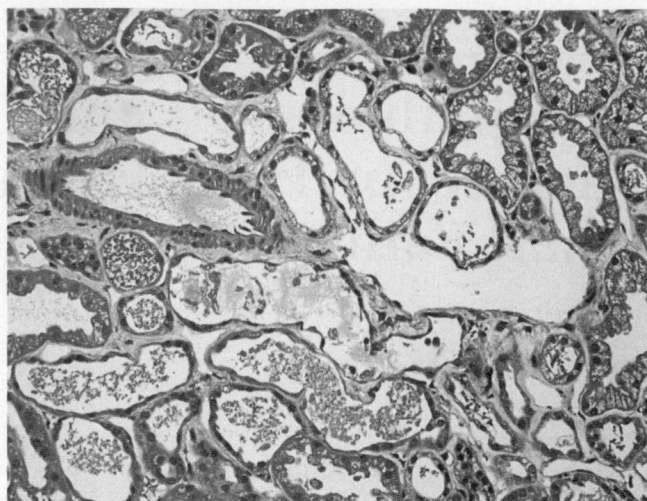

FIGURE 54-2. See also color plates. Histological evidence of acute tubular injury in a native kidney. (Hematoxylin-eosin stain, 200×.) Note the presence of dilated tubules with an attenuated epithelium and granular debris in tubular lumina.

The Tubular Compartment (from Tubular Lumina to Basement Membranes)

Tubular lumina in ATI are dilated, whether or not obstruction by casts or cellular debris is present[16,17] (Figs. 54-2 and 54-3).

Tubular casts are increased in number in ATI. Most are in the distal tubule, especially in the thick ascending loop of Henle, but not infrequently they also can be found in proximal tubules and collecting ducts.[18,19] Three types are recognized:

- Hyaline casts, principally composed of THP and strongly PAS-positive
- Eosinophilic granular casts, composed of THP admixed with proteins from degenerated tubular cells
- Pigmented granular casts, containing heme pigments found in ATI caused by hemolysis or rhabdomyolysis

Sloughed epithelial cells, granular proteinaceous debris, and leukocytes can be seen free floating in tubular lumina (see Fig. 54-3).[20] Some of the cells that are shed in the urine are necrotic or show signs of injury but, surprisingly, approximately 50% are viable and can be cultured in tissue culture. Most of them are of proximal origin.[21] In a recently described case of ATI,[22] sloughed tubular cells were found attached to casts within tubular lumina. On examination by EM, they not only were viable but also demonstrated a differentiated and polarized phenotype, with intercellular junctions, short apical microvilli on the luminal side, and clumps of basement membrane–like material on the side of attachment to the cast. These findings suggest that sloughed epithelial cells can reattach and redifferentiate.[22]

Calcifications can be found within tubular lumina and may represent previous sites of necrosis (Fig. 54-4).[23] Three forms of tubular cell loss are seen:

- True coagulation necrosis (hypereosinophilic cells with hydropic cytoplasm, loss of nuclei) is in fact infrequent in ischemic ATI,[24] justifying the change in terminology from "necrosis" to "injury" (i.e., ATN to ATI). Autofluorescence of hematoxylin-eosin–stained slides of necrotic tubules has been reported.[25] Because true coagulation necrosis is infrequent in ATI, the usefulness of this unusual finding is limited.

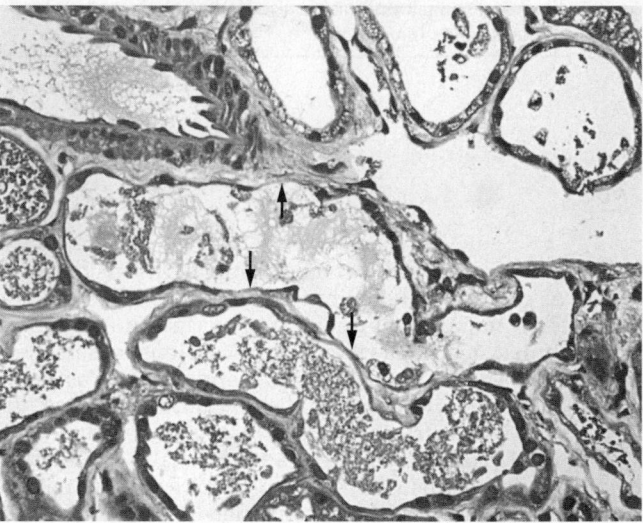

FIGURE 54-3. See also color plates. Portion of same photomicrograph as in Figure 54-2, at higher magnification. (Hematoxylin-eosin stain, 400×.) Tubular lumina are dilated and bordered by a flattened epithelium. Focal tubular cell loss is seen as a portion of denuded basement membrane *(arrows)*. Granular debris and desquamated epithelial cells are present in tubular lumina.

- Condensation of nuclear chromatin, convoluted nuclear membranes, fragmentation of nuclei and shrinkage of the cytoplasm characterize apoptotic cell death. Apoptosis affects a very minor proportion of cells.[24] Because of their small numbers and their presence in normal tissue as well, such cells are of little diagnostic use.
- The *nonreplacement phenomenon* is the presence of denuded segments of tubular basement membrane, indicating that single cell loss has occurred and replacement has not yet taken place (see Fig. 54-3). It is one of the most important lesions of ATI.[24]

Another important lesion is the loss of the PAS-positive brush border of proximal tubules, resulting in thinning or "simplification" of the tubules (Fig. 54-5). The absence of brush border probably is the result of replacement of mature cells by primitive, relatively undifferentiated cells.[26] When the brush border is completely absent, a cortical dilated tubule may be difficult to identify as proximal or distal. A study using immunohistochemical markers specific to proximal and distal tubules showed that tubules with a dilated lumen and attenuated epithelium are in fact predominantly distal.[18] Dilatation of the tubular lumen parallels brush border loss in oliguric patients.[16,24]

Tubular regenerative activity (see Fig. 54-8) is manifested by

- Basophilic staining of the cytoplasm
- Variations in cell size and shape
- Presence of large basophilic hyperchromatic nuclei with prominent nucleoli
- Mitoses

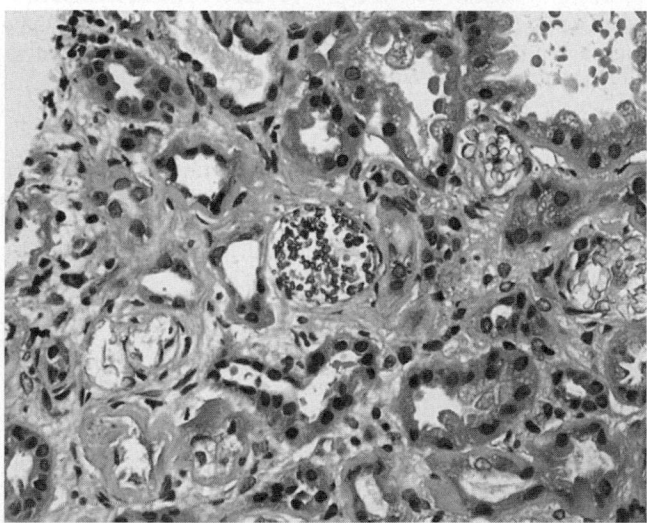

FIGURE 54-4. See also color plates. Histological evidence of acute tubular injury in a native kidney. (Hematoxylin-eosin stain, 400×.) Calcifications are seen replacing tubules.

Collections of macrophages forming nodules within the distal tubular epithelium and protruding into the lumen have been described. The nodules often were associated with THP-positive material and covered by a layer of epithelial cells. They are thought to result from tubular regeneration after cast-induced damage.[18] Extrarenal cells, of possible bone marrow origin, may contribute to a limited degree of tubular cell regeneration after ATI. An experiment involving gender-mismatched transplants has indeed shown that in male patients who had received a kidney from a female donor, a Y chromosome was detectable by fluorescence in situ hybridization (FISH) in approximately 1% of their tubular cells after ATI.[27] On the other hand, animal studies have shown that cells of renal origin are the most important contributors to regeneration after ischemic ATI. Multipotent progenitor cells with a potential for tubule restoration also have been demonstrated in Bowman's capsule epithelium in human kidneys.[28] Proliferation of tubular cells can be evaluated by measuring expression of proliferating cell nuclear antigen (PCNA) using immunohistochemistry techniques. It is increased from less than 0.4% in control preparations to 3.4% in distal tubules and 5.4% in proximal tubules in ATI.[18]

Tubular cells can show cytoplasmic vacuoles of variable size.[3] Inflammatory cells can infiltrate the tubular epithelium, causing tubulitis, especially in the distal tubules.[29]

The tubular basement membrane can be ruptured, leading to a fibrous reaction (the tubulorrhexic lesion) or to a granulomatous reaction to extravasated tubular contents.[16,24] Tubulovenous communications with presence of tubular fluid within veins also have been described.[24] Deposition of small amounts of C3d along tubular basement membrane in ATI suggests that activation of the alternative complement pathway is involved in pathogenesis.[30]

The macula densa shows no significant morphological abnormalities.[18]

Ancillary markers of tubular injury include kidney injury molecule-1 (KIM-1), which was shown to be expressed in proximal tubules by immunohistochemistry studies in 6 of 6 kidney biopsy specimens from patients with ATI. It also has been proposed as a urinary marker

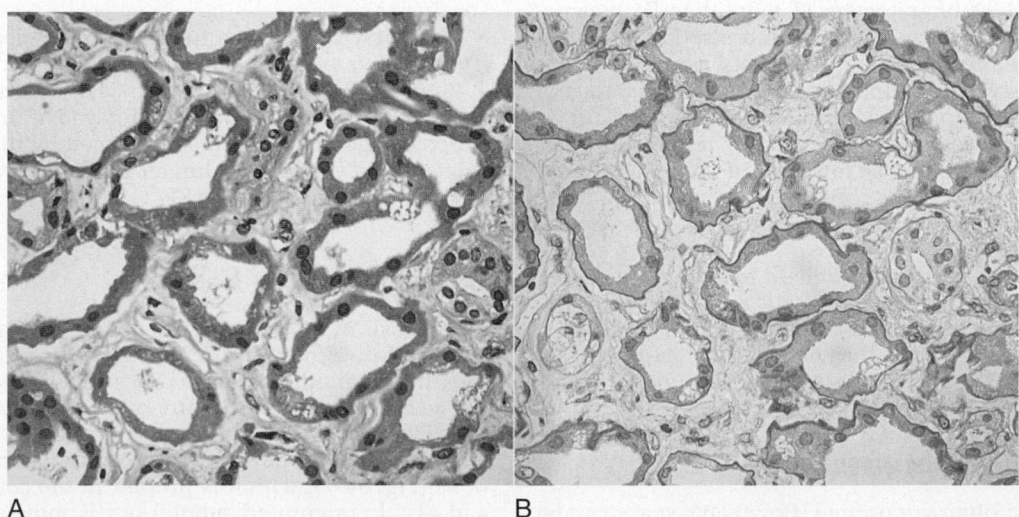

A   B

FIGURE 54-5. See also color plates. Acute tubular injury in a native kidney seen with staining by hematoxylin-eosin (**A**) and periodic acid–Schiff (PAS) (**B**). (400×.) Tubular lumina are dilated. The tubular epithelium is attenuated and shows focal vacuolization. The PAS-positive brush border is lost. Note the presence of interstitial edema.

for early diagnosis of proximal tubule injury.[31] The number of tubules expressing THP seen by immunohistochemistry is decreased in ATI, indicating injury to the thick ascending limb of Henle's loop, which is thought to be particularly sensitive to ischemia.[18]

The Interstitial Compartment

The interstitium is edematous, imparting a pale appearance to the renal cortex on gross examination.[16] Increased water content is responsible for an increase in size and weight of the kidney in ARF.[16] By light microscopy, edema is seen as an increase in spacing between tubules (see Fig. 54-5). Edematous tissue is pale pink on routine hematoxylin-eosin staining and pale blue on Masson's trichrome staining. Dilatation of the tubular lumen accompanies edema in oliguric patients.[16,24]

Edema may be replaced by interstitial fibrosis (strong blue on Masson's trichrome staining) within a few weeks. Both edema and interstitial fibrosis increase the fractional interstitial area. In 11 patients who underwent kidney biopsy an average of 4 days after diagnosis of ARF, the fractional interstitial area of fibrosis was increased from 7.17% to 17.65%.[32] Immunohistochemical staining for components of the cellular fibrogenic machinery (alpha-1 smooth muscle actin, fibronectin, endothelin), pJNK (involved in apoptosis), and NFκB (inducer of inflammation) are increased in the cortical tubulointerstitium in ATI.[32]

Interstitial inflammation usually is scant and seen mostly in the corticomedullary region.[16] The inflammatory infiltrate is composed mainly of B lymphocytes, plasmacytes, and monocytes.[26]

The Vascular Compartment

The medullary vasa recta are congested and the medulla appears dark on gross examination.[33] Nucleated cells accumulate in the medullary vasa recta.[34,35] This accumulation is not caused by a reduction in medullary blood flow, which was shown to be maintained in an animal model.[35] In a study of six cases of ATI by immunohistochemistry, medullary vasa recta were shown to contain mature white blood cells such as lymphocytes (T more than B), plasmacytes, monocytes, and granulocytes but also CD34+ hematopoietic progenitor cells, erythroblasts, and immature megakaryocytes.[36] These findings confirm the presence of intravascular hematopoiesis that had been noted previously on morphological examination,[34] although other possible mechanisms may be involved in the pathogenesis of cell accumulation (e.g., reaction to local damage, increased leukocyte adhesion, accumulation of a chemotactic substance).[35,36]

Although such changes are difficult to evaluate visually, morphometric studies have shown a decrease in the number of cortical peritubular and intertubular capillaries, beyond that expected with the characteristic expansion of the interstitium. The remaining vessels were dilated.[17]

The Glomerular Compartment

Glomeruli most often are normal. Bowman's space can be enlarged, with the degree of enlargement reflecting the degree of tubular lumen dilatation.[16,17,20] Findings may include increased prominence of Bowman's capsular epi-

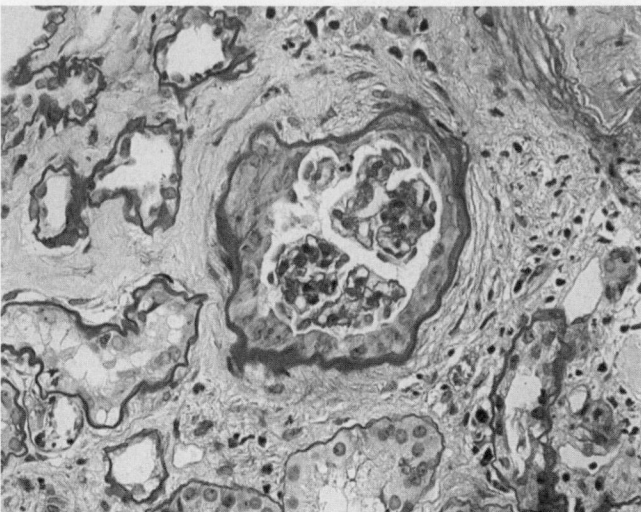

FIGURE 54-6. See also color plates. Tubularization of Bowman's capsular epithelium in a case of acute tubular injury in a native kidney. (Periodic acid–Schiff stain, 400×.)

thelium. Movement of squamocolumnar junction of proximal tubular epithelium into Bowman's space ("tubularization") is thought to result from exuberant tubular regeneration but also can be found to a lesser degree in normal kidneys[20,24] (Fig. 54-6).

Correlation of Morphology and Function

Most of the lesions described are found in the active phase of ATI and persist in the recovery phase when function is restored, with two exceptions[24]: Single cell loss and brush border loss in proximal tubule are more marked in the active than in the recovery phase of ATI,[24] suggesting that they are important morphological correlates of dysfunction. The ratio of brush border–positive tubules to brush border–negative tubules seen by immunohistochemistry also was shown to correlate with renal function in postmortem and biopsy specimens.[37,38] The following also correlate with renal function (in either biopsy or postmortem specimens):

- Ratio of THP-positive tubules to THP-negative tubules (indicative of thick ascending loop integrity)[37,38]
- Ratio of THP-positive casts to THP-negative casts[37]
- 1/ratio of cast-positive to cast-negative tubules[38]
- Percentage of kidney area occupied by tubules[38]

Dilatation of the tubular lumen in oliguric patients is correlated with duration of ARF.[24]

Electron Microscopy Findings

A diagnosis of ATI usually can be reached by light microscopy and does not require EM. EM can help rule out the presence of another disease process. Some features of ATI not seen by light microscopy can be demonstrated using EM. The lesions are mainly in the tubular compartment. They include a simplification of basolateral interdigitations (Fig. 54-7), which is present in the cortex (proximal and distal convoluted tubule) but is most marked in the medulla (straight proximal and thick ascending loops of Henle).[19,39,40] The loss of basolateral interdigitations, as well as brush borders, leads to an important reduction in

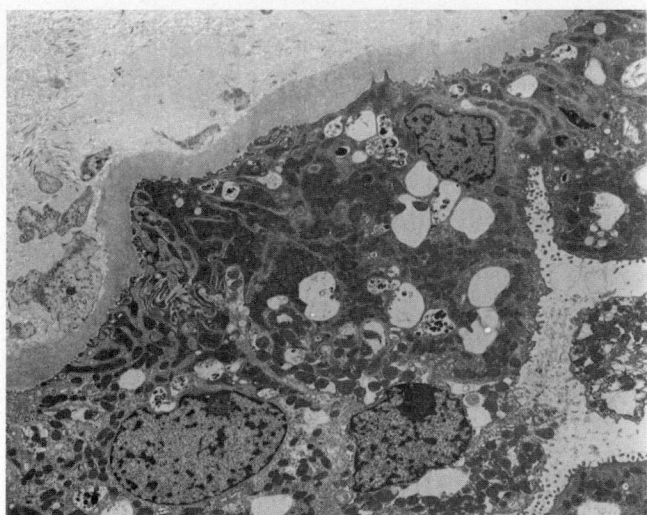

FIGURE 54-7. Electron microscopy of a preparation of native kidney with acute tubular injury. Brush border microvilli are missing or shortened (compare with Fig. 54-1). Basolateral infoldings are simplified. Clear vacuoles are present in the cytoplasm.

TABLE 54-1

Morphological Features of Acute Tubular Injury in Grafts (versus Native Kidneys)

- No predominance of tubular dilatation in distal over proximal tubules
- Less frequent tubular casts (especially THP-positive casts)
- Less frequent brush border loss
- More frequent true tubular cell necrosis
- More frequent distal tubular cell apoptosis
- Less frequent nonreplacement sites
- More frequent calcium oxalate deposition
- Less frequent dilatation of Bowman's capsule
- Relative preservation of basolateral interdigitations in tubular cells (on EM)
- Absence of actin bundle hypertrophy in tubular cells (on EM)

EM, electron microscopy; THP, Tamm-Horsfall protein.

cell surfaces, with significant pathophysiological implications, and is correlated with renal dysfunction.[41]

Microfilamentous attachment bodies composed of actin bundles at the base of tubular cells are abnormally prominent; their volume is doubled in proximal tubule and quadrupled in distal tubule. They may have a role in adjustment of tubular diameter.[40,42]

Other EM features include loss of apical vacuoles in proximal tubule, presence of lipid droplets in distal tubule, presence of large cytoplasmic vacuoles in proximal and distal tubules, and laminar tubular basement membrane thickening in prolonged renal failure.[40]

EM also will confirm diagnostic features of ATI that were seen by light microscopy, such as presence of casts in the distal tubule, loss of brush borders in the proximal tubule (see Fig. 54-7), partial detachment of viable cells in tubular lumens, and tubular cell loss.[19,40,41]

EM studies have attempted to localize cell loss more precisely. The distribution of cell loss is patchy. Although found in both proximal and distal tubules, it appears to be more severe in distal tubules.[43] The three forms of tubular cell loss described previously can be found:

- As seen by light microscopy, negligible numbers of truly necrotic cells are recognized.
- In both ATI and control (normal) preparations, apoptotic cells are present in distal tubules.[26] No significant increase in apoptosis is measured in the distal tubule or in the medulla in ATI.[19,39] Although they are few and isolated, apoptotic cells also are present in the cortical proximal tubules in ATI (1.6% to 2.1%), whereas they are absent in control preparations.[19,39]
- Nonreplacement sites also are significantly increased in ATI. They are more pronounced in the medulla, where they often will affect several adjacent cells. They are found in the straight proximal tubule (3.7% of cells), the thick ascending loop of Henle (10.7%), and the collecting duct (9.3%).[19] In the cortex, such sites constitute 5.2% of cells in distal tubules but not in proximal tubules. In active ARF, these abnormalities are significantly increased above those in control preparations and in recovering ARF.[39]

Glomeruli generally are normal by transmission EM, although some podocyte abnormalities can be seen by scanning EM.[40,44]

ACUTE TUBULAR INJURY IN TRANSPLANTS

In ATI in native kidneys, renal biopsy is rarely performed, because affected patients often are too ill to undergo the procedure.[45] Transplants are more likely to be biopsied, often to rule out rejection. Ischemic damage can manifest clinically as a delay in graft function or as ATI within days after transplantation. In a study presented at the World Transplant Congress in 2006, protocol biopsy specimens taken at 6 weeks and at 3 and 6 months after transplantation were found to exhibit evidence of ATI (mostly focal or mild) in 40%, 34%, and 39% of cases, respectively.[46] ATI was associated with delayed graft function and prolonged cold ischemia time and was inversely correlated with subsequent graft function at 6 months and 1 and 2 years after transplantation.[46]

The pathophysiological basis for ATI in grafts seems to vary and may be related to features unique to transplantation, such as a period of complete cessation of blood flow, cold preservation, uremic environment, pharmaceutical enhancement of diuresis, and potential concomitant nephrotoxicity from immunosuppressive regimens.[47] In general, ATI lesions in grafts are more severe but more focal than those in native kidneys, where they are diffuse and subtle.[48] The main morphological differences between ATI in kidney transplants and in native kidneys are listed in Table 54-1.[18,48,49]

Lesions also differ according to the type of immunosuppressive drug regimen used. For example, in patients receiving cyclosporine, true tubular necrosis is more prominent than in patients receiving azathioprine and involves whole tubular sections in up to 2.4% of tubules.[49] Unlike in native kidney ATI, actin fibril bundles show no abnormality in cyclosporine-treated grafts and are actually decreased in volume in azathioprine-treated transplants.[49] Proliferation index in proximal tubules is significantly increased over that of native kidneys in patients who receive azathioprine.[18] Typical signs of cyclosporine toxicity may be added to features of ATI in patients who receive cyclosporine.

Polarizable calcium oxalate deposits in tubular lumens are more frequent in ATI in grafts than in native kidney ATI. In one study, ATI was of longer duration when calcium oxalate deposits were present.[50] Patients with post-transplant ATI that subsequently progresses to chronic renal failure show a significantly higher fractional interstitial area than those who recover.[32]

Because all transplants are exposed to periods of ischemia during the grafting process, transplant biopsy specimens become an ideal substrate to study early effects of ischemia, for correlation with subsequent graft dysfunction. In cadaveric kidney transplantation, 86% of the kidneys in which delayed graft function subsequently develops will exhibit morphological evidence of tubular injury at the moment of organ procurement, indicating that some damage occurs before the organ is removed from the donor.[51] In general, most grafts (from both dead and living donors) exhibit some degree of tubular injury in biopsy specimens obtained 1 to 3 hours after anastomosis, and no morphological finding is predictive of subsequent function.[44,52-54]

Some potential predictors of graft function have arisen out of ancillary studies. Markers of apoptosis include TUNEL (*t*erminal deoxynucleotidyl transferase–mediated d*U*TP-biotin *n*ick *e*nd *l*abeling) staining, a technique that detects internucleosomal DNA cleavage[55] and staining for the LeY antigen, expressed in apoptotic cells.[56] These markers usually mark more cells than those morphologically identifiable as apoptotic cells.[52,56] TUNEL staining of biopsy specimens performed before engraftment shows that higher numbers of apoptotic tubular cells are found in cases in which ATI subsequently develops.[52] Apoptotic activity seen on TUNEL staining and on morphological examination is sustained after 30 minutes of reperfusion in cadaveric grafts with delayed function.[57] LeY antigen expression also is increased in cadaveric kidneys at 1 hour after transplantation, and the degree of expression is correlated with subsequent delay in graft function.[56] After reperfusion, cadaveric grafts show an increase in apoptosis, with higher proportions of apoptotic cells (6.8% versus 1.8%) and higher expression of proapoptotic molecules (Bax, Bak, tumor necrosis factor receptor-1 [TNFR-1]), compared with grafts from living donors.[55,58] Apoptotic cells are more abundant in distal tubule (2.5%, versus 1% in proximal tubule).[52,58]

A study using antibodies against cytoskeletal proteins and laser confocal microscopy demonstrated redistribution of cytoskeletal proteins (Na$^+$,K$^+$-ATPase, fodrin, and ankyrin) in proximal tubules from the basolateral membrane to the cytoplasm 45 to 60 minutes after transplantation. The extent of misdistribution predicted a subsequent delay in onset of allograft function.[54] In a different study, however, initial loss of polarity for Na$^+$,K$^+$-ATPase distribution persisted at post-transplant day 7 whether or not recovery of renal function had occurred.[45]

NEPHROTOXIC ACUTE TUBULAR INJURY

Isolated nephrotoxic ATI represents approximately 11% of cases of ATI seen in intensive care units.[15] On the other hand, approximately 38% of patients with ATI have mixed ischemic and nephrotoxic ATI.[15] Nephrotoxic ATI can be caused by a variety of agents, including drugs (e.g., cyclosporine, aminoglycosides, cephalosporins, amphotericin

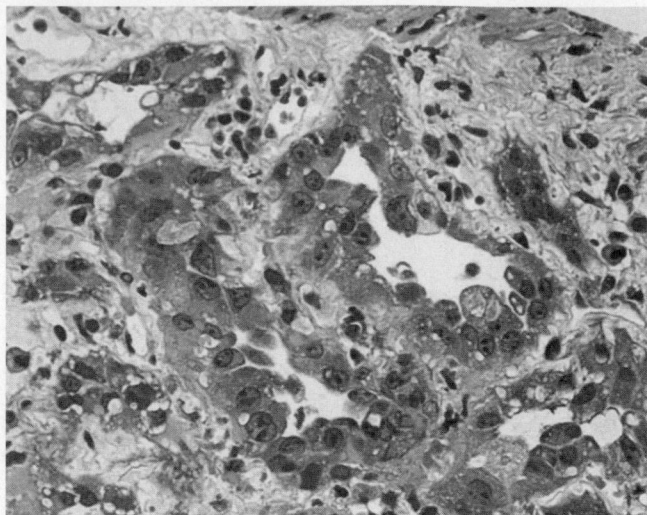

FIGURE 54-8. See also color plates. Nephrotoxic acute tubular injury in a native kidney showing prominent tubular damage with evidence of regeneration (basophilic cytoplasm, nucleoli, variations in cell size and shape). (Hematoxylin-eosin stain, 400×.)

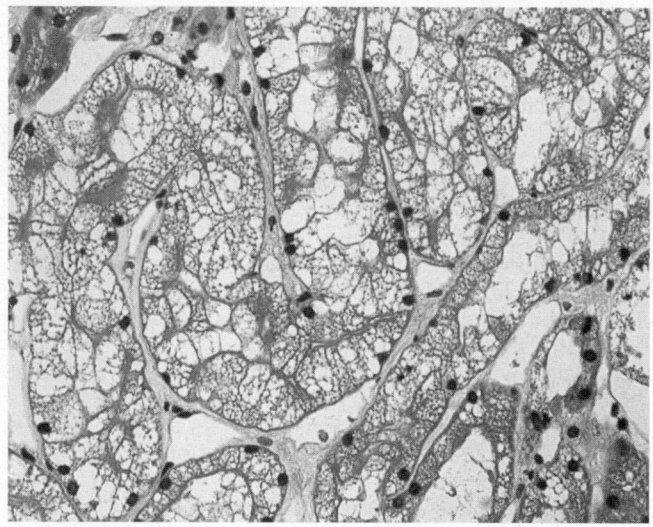

FIGURE 54-9. See also color plates. Nephrotoxic acute tubular injury in a native kidney, showing prominent tubular vacuolization. (Hematoxylin-eosin stain, 400×.) Of note, the vacuoles vary widely in size, unlike the isometric vacuolization caused by cyclosporine toxicity.

B), anesthetic agents (methoxyflurane, halothane), radiocontrast agents, heavy metals (mercury), and natural substances (raw carp bile, snake venom). In recently described cases of biopsy-proven ATI, an association with the following substances has been reported: chromium picolinate–containing dietary supplements,[59] extract of weeping cypress,[60] intravenous acyclovir,[61] tenofovir,[62] cephalexin,[63] vancomycin,[64] phenazopyridine,[65] snake venom,[66] and gadolinium-based contrast media.[67]

Light microscopy and EM findings include those described previously for ischemic ATI (Figs. 54-8 and 54-9). More uniform tubular involvement and more frequent ballooning of the cytoplasm are seen.[3,33] Involvement of proximal tubule is prominent because it often is responsible for excretion of toxic substances.[33] An excep-

TABLE 54-2

Examples of Morphological Lesions Associated with Some Nephrotoxic Agents

| | Characteristic Morphological Features | |
NEPHROTOXIC AGENT	*BY LIGHT MICROSCOPY*	*BY ELECTRON MICROSCOPY*
Acyclovir	Crystal deposition and distal tubule obstruction	
Aminoglycosides		Myeloid bodies in proximal tubule
Amphotericin	Extensive tubular damage and tubular calcifications	Vacuolization of the media of small arteries and arterioles
Carbon tetrachloride	Neutral lipid accumulation in tubular cells	
Chromium		Myeloid bodies
Cocaine	Pigmented casts (rhabdomyolysis)	Electron-dense casts
Diethylene glycol	Cellular atypia	
Ethylene glycol	Marked ballooning of proximal tubular cells	
	Calcium oxalate crystals in the lumen	
Halogenated hydrocarbons	Extensive proximal necrosis	
Halothane	Crystalline casts containing oxalate deposits	
IVIG	Prominent tubular swelling with vacuoles	
Lead	Dark intranuclear inclusions	
Mercuric chloride	Acidophilic inclusions in the pars recta of proximal tubule	
	Extensive tubular necrosis	
Radiocontrast media	Prominent tubular cell vacuolization	Dilated lysosomes
	Casts containing birefringent crystals	

IVIG, intravenous immune globulin.

tion is cisplatin, which primarily affects distal tubules and collecting ducts.[68] Nephrotoxic ATI often is described as showing more severe necrosis than that seen with ischemic ATI. In fact, this feature is mostly associated with heavy metal poisoning (mercury, uranium), which nowadays is much less frequent than drug toxicity.[69] Additional findings on electron microscopy include increase in lipofuscin granules, cytoplasmic vacuolization, and dilation of endoplasmic reticulum.[33] More characteristic light or electron microscopy features can be associated with particular nephrotoxic agents. They are listed in Table 54-2.[3,14,68] Of note, some of these manifestations are not indicative of toxicity but are only secondary to exposure to the toxic agent, such as lysosomal dilatation and tubular crystal formation associated with use of radiocontrast media and myeloid bodies associated with aminoglycoside uptake. Myeloid bodies are membrane-bound, lamellated structures probably corresponding to modified secondary lysosomes.[68]

HISTOPATHOLOGICAL DIFFERENTIAL DIAGNOSIS OF ACUTE TUBULAR INJURY

Changes due to autolysis can be confused with ATI, particularly in autopsy specimens. Nuclei are effaced, cell outlines are vague, and cytoplasmic basophilia is decreased.[70] The interstitium appears loose.[25] Unlike in ATI, alterations caused by autolysis are diffuse and affect glomeruli as well as tubules. Acute tubular damage can be secondary to acute glomerular or vascular diseases (e.g., crescentic glomerulonephritis), for which diagnostic lesions should be readily recognized in the corresponding compartments.

Postrenal obstruction causes histopathological lesions identical with those of ischemic ATI, including tubular

dilatation, loss of proximal tubular brush border, and simplification of basolateral infoldings. In a rat model of ureteral obstruction, medullary tubular necrosis is associated with reduced plasma flow in medullary vessels, presumably due to compression.[71] Postrenal obstruction must be ruled out clinically.[26,40]

Acute interstitial nephritis can show tubular damage similar to ATI but usually will include a more intense inflammatory component, with severe focal degeneration, tubulitis, and destruction of tubules.[19] Eosinophils can be found in ATI but usually are sparse.[3] Their presence is consistent with an allergic interstitial nephritis.[14] Tubular lumina filled with neutrophils suggest acute pyelonephritis.

Tubulitis found in grafts with ATI raises the possibility of acute T cell–mediated rejection. Tubulitis and interstitial inflammation are significantly more severe in acute rejection.[29]

CONCLUSION

Numerous advances in the knowledge of pathophysiological processes involved in ATI have been made in recent years, pertaining to tubular metabolism and cytoskeletal structure, role of endothelial injury, role of inflammatory cells, mechanisms of repair, and modifications in the renal transcriptome, among others. It is hoped that findings from animal models and experimental studies will eventually lead to applications in the interpretation of biopsy findings in patients with ATI.

Key Points

1. The main histological features of ischemic acute tubular injury in native kidneys are tubular dilatation, tubular cell loss (nonreplacement

phenomenon), proximal tubule brush border loss, tubular regenerative changes, and interstitial edema.

2. Additional alterations seen by electron microscopy in tubular cells affected by ischemic acute tubular injury include loss of basolateral interdigitations and an increase in volume of actin bundles.

3. Transplant-specific and nephrotoxic acute tubular injury are characterized by morphological lesions similar to those of ischemic acute tubular injury in native kidneys, with some subtle differences.

4. Studies of early graft biopsy specimens have shown the presence of ischemic changes. Ancillary studies may have predictive value for subsequent graft function.

5. Considerations in the histopathological differential diagnosis of acute tubular injury include autolysis, secondary tubular damage in glomerular or vascular diseases, postrenal obstruction, interstitial nephritis, pyelonephritis, and acute rejection in grafts.

Key References

11. Safirstein RL: Acute renal failure: From renal physiology to the renal transcriptome. Kidney Int Suppl 2004;S62-S66.
12. Bellomo R, Ronco C, Kellum JA, et al: Acute renal failure—definition, outcome measures, animal models, fluid therapy and information technology needs: The Second International Consensus Conference of the Acute Dialysis Quality Initiative (ADQI) Group. Crit Care 2004;8:R204-R212.

See the companion Expert Consult website for the complete reference list.

CHAPTER 55

New Imaging Techniques in Acute Kidney Injury

Asif A. Sharfuddin, Ruben M. Sandoval, and Bruce A. Molitoris

OBJECTIVES

This chapter will:
1. Describe new imaging techniques used to study the kidney.
2. Examine how these techniques help to elucidate disease processes.
3. Review how therapy can be evaluated using these techniques.

Developments in kidney imaging over the past decade have provided researchers with new and tremendously in-depth insights into complex yet highly interdependent processes. A significant advance in these developments has been the emerging technology of studying cells within their natural living environment, rather than in isolated, *ex vivo* controlled settings. Different aspects of cellular pathophysiology and the effects of potential treatments can now be analyzed in the context of an intact, functioning organ interacting within its biological milieu. This capability, coupled with advances in spatial and temporal resolution and sensitivity, has allowed the study of various cellular and subcellular processes, including intra- and intercellular interactions and trafficking of proteins. Rapid determinations can be made over seconds to hours to days, permitting multiple clinical observations of biological status within the same animal.[1] This chapter reviews the major advances in techniques for imaging the kidney in acute kidney injury. The concept, techniques, and applications of multiphoton microscopy are presented first, followed by similar details of other newer techniques in imaging.

MULTIPHOTON MICROSCOPY

Concept

The potential to image more deeply into biological tissue, with far less phototoxicity, was realized with the advent of multiphoton microscopy, in which increased penetration (up to 200 nm) is possible owing to the unique photophysics of multiphoton fluorescence excitation, whereby fluorescence is stimulated by the simultaneous absorption of two low-energy photons by a fluorophore.[2] It also allows for simultaneous use of multiple fluorescent probes, enabling labeling of different physiological compartments. Distinguishing these fluorescent emissions from endogenous or autofluorescence also is easier and enhanced in multiphoton fluorescence microscopy, as compared with confocal microscopy, because the fluorescence excitation occurs only at the focal point of the excitation beam, so out-of-focus fluorescence excitation is eliminated.[2] Of note, an understanding of fluorescent probe characteristics is essential to appropriate interpretation of the data.

Animal Models

Anesthetized rats commonly are used for intravital studies based on two-photon techniques. An inverted microscope or a special "kidney cup" in an upright microscope helps

TABLE 55-1

Applications of Kidney Multiphoton Imaging

STRUCTURAL/FUNCTIONAL/DYNAMIC PATHOPHYSIOLOGY	PHARMACOKINETICS/ THERAPEUTICS/DRUG DELIVERY
Glomerulus • Volume/size • Sclerosis/fibrosis • Filtration fraction • Alterations in permeability • Podocyte changes • Blood flow alterations • Inflammation Microvasculature • Blood flow rate • Vasoconstriction • Endothelial permeability • Leukocyte interactions Tubular • Swelling • Bleb formation • Reabsorption profile • Electrolyte transportation Cellular • Toxicity—necrosis • Apoptosis • Membrane dysfunction • Mitochondrial dysfunction • Ion transportation Subcellular • Endocytosis versus carrier-mediated • Transcytosis • Exocytosis • Metabolism • Organelle distribution • Intracellular trafficking	Glomerulus • Filtration • Protein dissociation Tubules • Site-specific actions • Cellular uptake • Apical versus basolateral uptake • Secretion Cellular • Protein binding • Protein dissociation • Intracellular metabolism Efficacy and safety • Qualitative • Quantitative • Mechanism • Toxicity

minimize distortion secondary to motion and provides optimal resolution. Exteriorization of the left kidney (which has a longer renal pedicle) in an adequately anesthetized animal minimizes body movement. Finally, adequate hydration, maintenance of body temperature with a heated pad and warming blanket, and monitoring of blood pressure and core body temperature are used to reduce the effect of external factors on renal hemodynamics.[3] The fact that animals are anesthetized and the kidneys imaged in a dynamic blood-perfused state, rather than in a fixed post-harvest state, clearly provides a more relevant and physiological model that more closely resembles human acute kidney injury scenarios. Ischemia-reperfusion injury, sepsis-induced acute kidney injury, and other forms of acute kidney injury can be studied in this fashion at different points after injury in the same animal, which reduces subject-to-subject variability.

Applications

Table 55-1 lists the possible types of data that can be acquired using multiphoton imaging of the kidneys. Reviewed next are the techniques used to obtain and analyze data that translate to invaluable structural, dynamic, and functional information. This information can then be correlated with disease states and potential therapeutic targets.

Quantification

To study any state of acute kidney injury, it is very important to accurately define the extent and magnitude of injury along with its mechanism, which in turn provides the opportunity to develop and assess the efficacy of any therapeutic strategy. Yu and coworkers have developed a quantitative ratiometric approach using generalized polarity (GP). This approach was implemented to analyze the multidimensional data obtained from "multi-dextran" infusion experiments, the concept being the comparison of the relative intensities of two fluorescent dyes.[4] Ratiometric imaging methods are relatively independent of the amount of fluorescent probe injected (so long as the ratio remains constant), the excitation power, and the depth of field being imaged. These properties are particularly advantageous for quantitative imaging in animal models in which the quantity of dye injected, appropriate level of laser power used, and imaging depth are variable. In addition, use of ratiometric techniques also minimizes spatial variation in the fluorescence signals across the field of view that results from detector-sample nonuniformity.

Intracellular Uptake, Distribution, and Metabolism

Intracellular uptake, distribution, and metabolism—endocytosis, trafficking, and transcytosis—can be studied and quantified once the fluorescent probe has entered the cell. With multiphoton microscopy, it is now possible to observe and quantify endocytosis occurring across the apical membrane of the proximal tubule cells. To evaluate the reabsorptive properties of the proximal tubules, the change in GP values can be analyzed from a number of different aspects: (1) by directly focusing on the epithelial cells of the proximal tubules; (2) by focusing on the proximal tubule lumens at a given time; (3) by comparing the change in GP values from within the proximal tubule lumens at different time points after infusion; and (4) by comparing the change in GP values from the proximal tubule lumens with those from within Bowman's space.[4] Furthermore, it is possible to follow the intracellular accumulation and subcellular distribution over time in the same animal, and to undertake repeated observations in the same animal at various intervals over days to weeks.[1] Such experiments are particularly useful in elucidating drug delivery for acute kidney injury states (Fig. 55-1).

Intracellular organelles such as mitochondria and lysosomes can be studied in acute injury states by specific labeling of these organelles and then quantifying individual number and fluorescence potential of respective organelles. DNA fluorescent markers can help identify specific cell types based on their nuclear morphology (e.g., nuclei of podocytes are characteristically bean-shaped, whereas endothelial cells have characteristic flattened, elongated morphology). It also permits evaluation of intranuclear uptake of other fluorescent compounds in disease and therapeutic states, as well as analysis of necrosis and apoptosis.[5] The half-life of fluorescent probes and specific biological molecules may vary, however, so these parameters must be carefully correlated and studied.

Glomerular Permeability

Glomerular permeability and filtration of different sized compounds across glomerular capillaries can be quantified

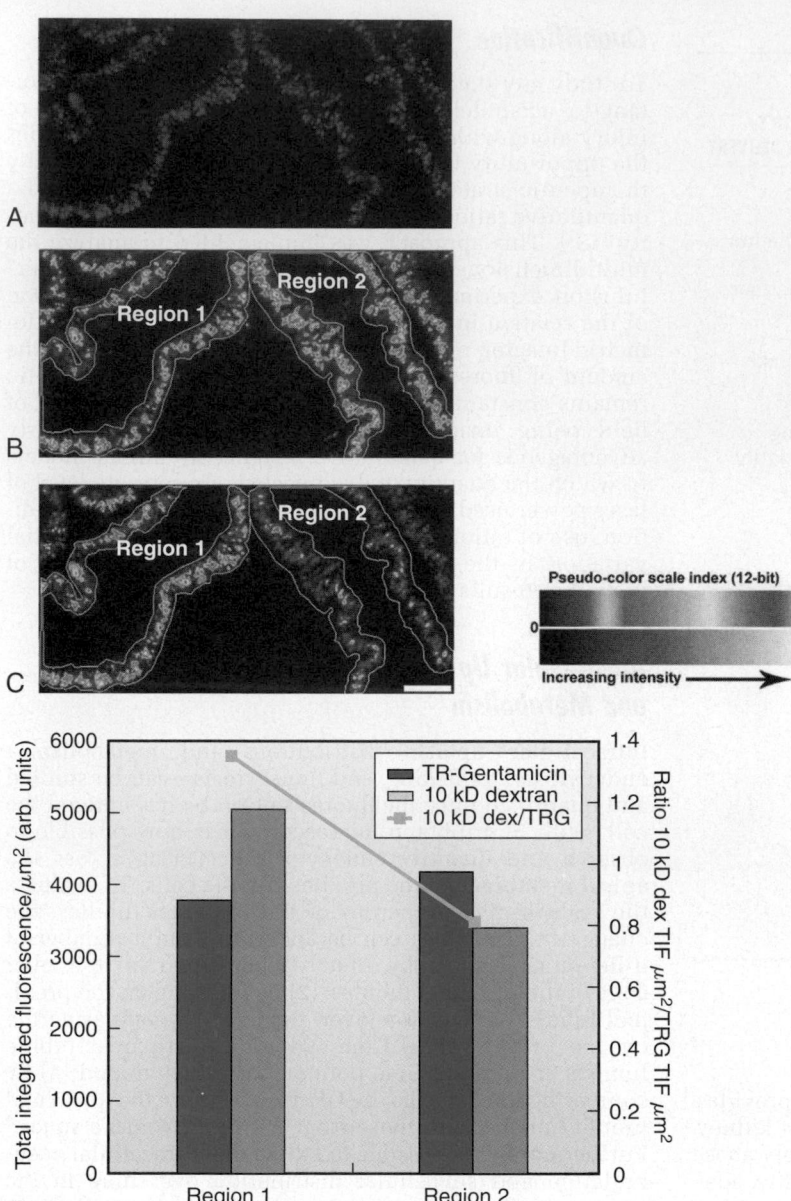

FIGURE 55-1. See also color plates. Texas Red–labeled gentamicin uptake in proximal tubule cells. A Munich-Wistar rat was given an intravenous injection of Texas Red gentamicin (TRG) and a 10-kD fluorescent dextran 24 hours before imaging. In **A,** a 10-μm-thick projection of the two probes (TRG in *red* and the 10-kD dextran in *blue*) shows the accumulation patterns in two different proximal tubule segments. (See color plates.) In **B,** the single channel for TRG accumulation is shown in pseudo-color (see scale index correlating signal intensity and color in **D**). The two tubules are divided into two regions for analysis; note that the overall intensity for TRG is approximately the same in the two regions. In **C,** the single channel for the 10-kD fluorescent dextran is shown in pseudo-color; note the decreased accumulation of this probe in region 2. The graph in **D** shows the total integrated fluorescence per square micrometer for TRG and the 10-kD dextran in regions 1 and 2 *(bars).* Accumulation of TRG is comparable between regions 1 and 2 (3810 and 4177, respectively), whereas region 1 accumulated more of the 10-kD dextran than region 2 (5041 and 3496, respectively). A ratio generated by dividing the intensity of the 10-kD dextran by the more evenly accumulated TRG is shown in the line graph. Relative accumulation between the two probes shows a distinct difference between the two regions. In region 1, 1.3 times more 10-kD dextran was internalized than TRG, whereas in region 2, only 0.8 as much 10-kD dextran was internalized as TRG. Ratios are a valuable tool for analyzing relative abundance of accumulated compounds within different tubule segments. The pseudo-color scale index assigns colors to the different intensities seen in a standard black-and-white image. (Bar = 20 μm.)

and visualized using Munich-Wistar rats with surface glomeruli (100 μm in diameter). Because multiphoton microscopy can visualize up to 200 μm into the kidney, it is possible to record events for an entire glomerulus. Areas of interest can be defined and isolated and fluorescence intensities measured to obtain quantitative data. By using the change in GP or ratiometric methods, it is possible to quantify glomerular permeability by measuring relative change intensities in dyes in the bloodstream or within Bowman's space.[4] Filtration and clearance of smaller molecules typically are faster than for larger molecules. Thus, by using two different-sized fluorescent dextrans, glomerular filtration fraction can be determined by measuring the changes over time in blood concentration of each dextran.

Proximal Tubule Reabsorption

Because many conditions associated with acute kidney injury affect the proximal tubules, it is very important to be able to study the reabsorptive profile of the tubular epithelium and its recovery with or without therapeutic intervention. The reabsorptive properties of the proximal tubule can be evaluated by (1) direct observation of the epithelial cells and lumen of the proximal tubule, (2) luminal GP changes in the proximal tubule, and (3) comparing change in GP values from within proximal tubule lumen with change in GP from within Bowman's capsule.[4]

Red Blood Cell Flow Rates

Multiphoton microscopy also can be used to study and quantify red blood cell (RBC) flow rates in the microvasculature. With sufficiently high temporal resolution (2 ms), the motion of RBCs can be imaged since specific cells can be delineated in the renal cortex microvasculature. RBCs exclude the nonfilterable fluorescent dye used to label the circulating plasma and consequently appear as dark, nonfluorescent objects on the images. The acquisition of repeti-

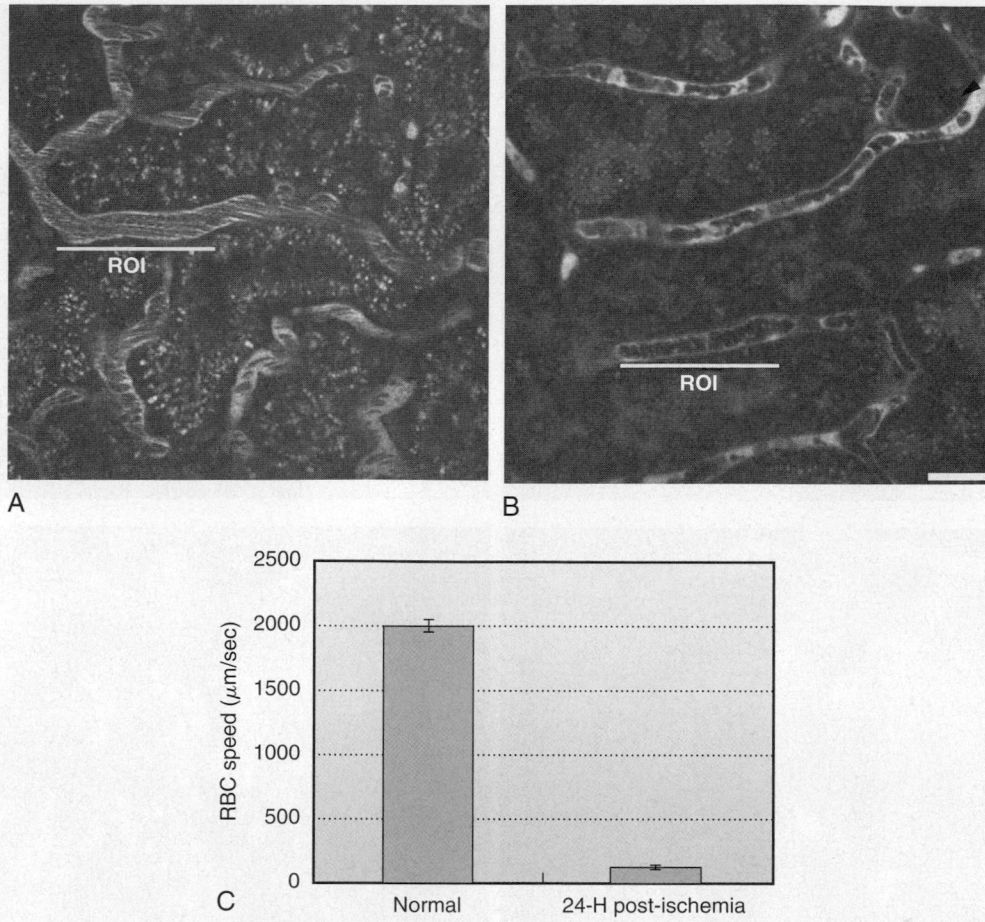

FIGURE 55-2. Microvascular injury 24 hours after acute renal ischemia. White blood cell (WBC) activation induces a reduction in the average speed of red blood cells (RBCs) flowing within the microvasculature. In **A,** an image obtained in a rat under physiological conditions injected with a large fluorescent 500-kD dextran shows the microvasculature and RBCs (which exclude the compound) within the vessels. Because of the speed at which they are traveling, and the acquisition characteristics of the laser scanning microscope, the RBCs appear as *dark streaks* in the region of interest (ROI). In **B,** the RBCs in a postischemic rat, which are flowing much more slowly, display a shape closer to their true morphology. In vessels running horizontally across the image, a line drawn through the center of the cells (in the vertical direction) can be used to determine RBC velocity based on slope, the x-axis being distance and the y-axis being time. The graph in **C** shows the average RBC speed for vessels above the line marking the ROI. In the normal rat, the average velocity was 1996 ± 41 µm/second (standard error of the mean); in the postischemic rat, the RBC velocity was 120 ± 16 µm/second. Aside from alterations in RBC velocity, obstructions can be detected as regions in the vessel filled with the fluorescent plasma but no RBCs (*arrowhead, upper right* in **B**). (Bar = 20 µm.)

tive scans along the central axis of a capillary (the line-scan method) will demonstrate the flow of RBCs, which leaves dark striped bands in the images. The slope of the bands is inversely proportional to the velocity; the more shallow the slope, the faster the flow rate (Fig. 55-2). Using standardized vessel length, diameter, and angles, it is possible to calculate the RBC flow rates in different states, such as ischemia, sepsis, and response to specific treatments.[6,7]

Inflammation and Leukocytes

Inflammation is being increasingly recognized as an important and central process in the initiation, maintenance, and progression of acute and chronic kidney injury. Hence, an understanding of the dynamic roles and functions of different leukocytes and their interactions with soluble and endothelial cell factors is key to the development of preventive and therapeutic strategies. Intravital microscopy provides the opportunity to observe these crucial processes in vivo. The most effective method to image

leukocytes in the kidney involves direct fluorescence labeling of specific WBC lineages. Fluorescent agents such as rhodamine 6G and acridine red or orange are preferentially concentrated in WBCs, allowing intravascular detection. The Hoechst DNA dye, used to label all nuclei, also permits detection of WBCs and differentiation of RBCs in the vascular space. Various markers are available for B lymphocytes, $CD8^+$ T lymphoblasts, macrophages, naive T cells, and others.[8]

Different techniques and methodologies have been devised to study the process and cell of interest. For example, to quantify inflammation in a particular model, dynamic intravital multifluorescence microscopy has been used to differentiate between those leukocytes that are free-flowing in the vascular space from those that are adherent to the endothelium. Continuous time sequence imaging will depict those leukocytes rolling along the endothelial surface[9] (Fig. 55-3). This technique also provides traditional information about location (vascular, glomerular, or tubular), density, and magnitude of inflammation as well. WBC accumulation can then be correlated with

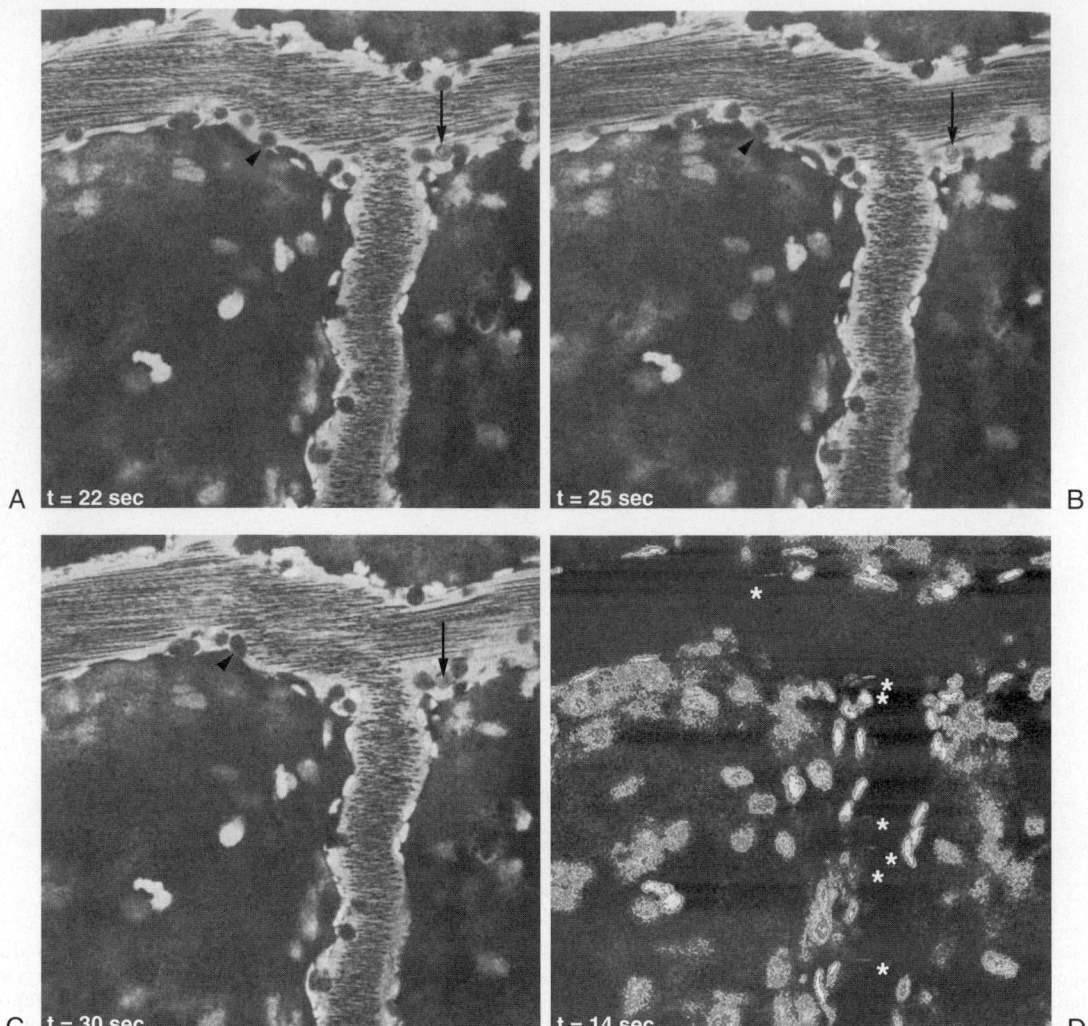

FIGURE 55-3. See also color plates. White blood cell (WBC) movement in the superficial microvasculature of a rat kidney. A Sprague-Dawley rat was injected with a fluorescein dextran with a molecular weight of 500,000 (*green*) along with a nuclear dye (Hoechst 33342, *cyan*), and images were acquired at a rate of 1 frame per second. The dextran fills the plasma in the blood but not the red blood cells (RBCs) or WBCs; hence, RBCs appear as *dark oblong shadows* within the vessel, whereas adherent or rolling WBCs appear as *dark circles* with some nuclear *(cyan)* staining. In **A** to **C,** numerous WBCs can be seen localized to the edge of a large vessel in frames acquired at 22, 25, and 30 seconds, respectively. A rolling WBC *(arrowhead)* moves approximately 15 μm during the elapsed 8-second period for the images in **A** through **C.** An adherent WBC *(arrow)* can be seen localized to the same area for the duration of the imaged sequence. In **D,** a pseudo-color image of the nuclear staining shows rapidly moving WBCs flowing within the vessel. Because the speed at which the WBCs are traveling far exceeds the acquisition rate of the microscope, the well-defined nucleus seen in static or rolling WBCs appears as a *small dash* within the vessel *(yellow asterisks).* In this frame (14 seconds into the sequence), seven WBCs not seen in the previous or following frame appear with the vessel as *faint streaks.* Speeds of RBC/WBC flow within these larger vessels have been documented at well over 1.5 mm/second. See Figure 55-1 for pseudo-color scale index. (Bar = 20 μm.)

regional variations in blood flow, or with adhesion to apoptotic or necrotic cells. Obtaining multiple images of the same site at different time points also will allow delineation of the sequence of events.

Vascular Pathology

Acute kidney injury resulting from ischemia is associated with microvascular permeability defects. Such defects are eventually linked with microvascular dropout.[10] Various other pathological conditions affect the vascular space, especially the glomerular vasculature. Apart from studying flow rates as mentioned earlier, using mixtures of different-sized fluorescence-labeled dextrans, it is now possible to examine the effect of injury on the microvasculature by observing and measuring the extravasation of these dextrans into the interstitium, as elegantly demonstrated by Sutton and associates.[11] Furthermore, multiple fluorescence labeling provides the opportunity to study the effect of injury on the intricate and dynamic interaction of endothelium with matrix proteins such as metalloproteinases.[12] It also allows for correlation and further quantification of the relationship between endothelial permeability and alteration in blood flow rate.

The regulation of glomerular hemodynamics is dependent on the interplay among the microvasculature, the renal tubules, and the juxtaglomerular apparatus. Using quinacrine tagging of renin-secreting granules, Peti-Peterdi and colleagues extended their studies to in vivo quantitation of renin content of the juxtaglomerular apparatus in anesthetized Munich-Wistar rats. These investigators also have been able to measure the diameters of the afferent and efferent arterioles, as well as glomerular volume.[13]

Fluorescence microscopy also has been applied in studies of gene transfer into specific targets such as tubular or endothelial cells. Green fluorescent protein (GFP) linked with the protein of interest, such as actin, which is cloned into an adenovirus vector, can be delivered to the urinary Bowman's space, proximal tubule lumen, or superficial efferent arteriole by micropuncture technique. The expression of these fluorescence-labeled proteins is an invaluable tool in studying dynamic changes in the cell in various disease models.[14]

Image Processing

The advances in computer science and image processing software have enabled further development of applications of multiphoton microscopy. Powerful microscopes and sophisticated imaging programs are now available that provide researchers with systems and applications needed to study an ever-increasing roster of normal and disease states. Imaging involves the following sequence: (1) image acquisition, (2) image processing, (3) volume rendering, (4) image segmentation, and (5) image analysis.

Image acquisition involves programs that control microscopes and associated imaging hardware (light, intensity, and so on) used to collect and store images. Such programs also permit variation in speed of image acquisition, depth, and stacking. Image processing is a critical step in digital microscopy that helps provide improved and more accurate visualization. Unique processing techniques are used to minimize autofluorescence interference and to allow correction for distortion introduced by microscope optics and tissue during image acquisition, enhanced visualization of dim structures, and assessment of co-localization between multiple fluorescent probes. It also allows precise measurement of cellular volume changes and quantification of fluorescence at the subcellular level.

Three-dimensional imaging processing operations such as deconvolution and spherical aberration correction produce high-quality three-dimensional images from closely spaced two-dimensional stacked images. Volume-rendering programs also can display sequences of three-dimensional stacks collected over an extended period that are useful in developmental studies. Image segmentation involves separating an image into discrete regions or isolating particular objects of interest using properties such as pixels, voxels, intensities, intensity gradients, color, shape, orientation, and connectivity. Segmentation can be done automatically or manually if required for complex biological structures, after which ratiometric, photometric, and morphometric analysis can be done.[15]

OTHER NEWER IMAGING TECHNIQUES

Video Microscopy

Recent refinement of intravital video microscopy, combined with sophisticated image analysis, has permitted researchers to monitor microcirculation in vivo with minimal invasion. Yamamoto and coworkers initially used a pencil-lens scope in ischemic rat kidneys to study changes in peritubular capillaries. A 1-mm-tipped video microscope was applied directly to the capsule.[16] Periglomerular microvasculature was evaluated as well, with a small incision in the capsule permitting access to the deeper tissues. The line-shift method of calculation of RBC flow in these capillaries can determine the renal microvascular blood flow in ischemic as well as reperfusion states. These studies were recently extended to the human realm by using high-magnification video endoscopy in a manner similar to that used in renal transplantation. This method demonstrated diminished peritubular flow occurring after reperfusion, which correlated with reductions in creatinine clearance.[17]

Infrared Imaging

Other novel imaging techniques have been investigated for the evaluation of ischemia-reperfusion injury. One such technique is infrared imaging. Kirk and colleagues[18] used an advanced digital infrared camera to image local temperature gradients simultaneously across the entire transplanted kidney by passive detection of infrared radiation emission. Infrared rewarming time was correlated with the subsequent return of renal function; a negative correlation with the regression slope of creatinine and the regression slope of BUN also was observed. The advantages of this method include providing a global whole-kidney image of reperfusion, instead of measurements of a single region, and giving information about regional defects. It also can provide valuable real-time intraoperative data and imaging, which can assist surgeons in executing complicated maneuvers and in making instant therapeutic manipulations.[18]

Dendrimer-Based Magnetic Resonance Imaging in Acute Kidney Injury

Dendrimers are molecules that can be polymerized to form nanoparticles of precise size that can be readily chelated to imaging agents such as gadolinium. Particle size is extremely important because the body handles nanoparticles of various sizes very differently. For instance, 2-nm particles and low-molecular-weight contrast agents are handled very similarly, but the kidney demonstrates significantly decreased excretion of 6-nm particles and virtually no excretion of 11-nm particles.[19] In a rat model of tubular damage caused by cisplatin nephrotoxicity, Kobayashi and associates observed loss of the normal outer stripe in the medulla. The loss of the normal renal architecture after G-4 dendrimer administration was proportional to the degree of renal damage.[20] Thus, dendrimer-based magnetic resonance imaging (MRI) could be used to monitor specific outer medullary damage caused by nephrotoxic events such as drugs, ischemia, infection, and obstruction. Star and colleagues[21] have shown, in a mouse model, that dendrimer-enhanced MRI can distinguish sepsis-induced ARF from prerenal azotemia and renal failure due to ischemia-reperfusion injury or cisplatin toxicity. Furthermore, the injury can be detected as early as 6 hours before serum creatinine is elevated, allowing tracking of the response to therapy and providing prognostic information.[21] Of note, however, the recent link of gadolinium-based contrast agents with nephrogenic systemic fibrosis may limit its use in human clinical studies of AKI.

Ultrasmall Paramagnetic Iron Oxide Particles

In magnetic resonance angiography, contrast is provided by ultrasmall paramagnetic iron oxide (USPIO) particles, which were developed as macromolecular agents based on iron. USPIO particles are 20- to 30-nm dextrans coated in a formulation known as ferumoxtran-10 and are not filterable across the glomerulus. After intravenous injection, these agents circulate intravascularly and may be used to evaluate renal blood volume and flow and to permit dynamic intravascular blood flow measurements. By 24 hours after injection, macrophages and monocytes phagocytose almost all circulating USPIO particles; then they travel to lymph nodes and areas of inflammation.[19]

In acute ischemia-reperfusion injury, USPIO-laden macrophages have been shown to accumulate in the outer medulla, corresponding to an inflammatory infiltrate induced by the ischemia,[22] whereas in renal transplant models of allograft rejection, uptake of USPIO corresponds with the loss of signal in the renal parenchyma and the degree of lymphocytic infiltration. Thus, USPIO uptake could serve as a marker to detect early acute kidney injury.

Blood Oxygen Level–Dependent Magnetic Resonance Imaging

Oxyhemoglobin is a diamagnetic molecule that creates no magnetic moment, because oxygen molecules are bound to iron, whereas deoxyhemoglobin is a paramagnetic molecule that generates magnetic moments by its unpaired iron electrons. Blood oxygen level–dependent (BOLD) MRI is a noninvasive method to assess tissue oxygen bioavailability, using deoxyhemoglobin as an endogenous contrast agent.[23] Higher levels of deoxyhemoglobin result in increased magnetic spin dephasing of blood water protons and decreased signal intensity on T2*-weighted MR imaging sequences. Decreased intensity on T2-weighted images implies increased deoxyhemoglobin (decreased oxyhemoglobin) and decreased partial pressure of oxygen (PO_2) in tissues. This technique can therefore be used to determine intrarenal oxygen bioavailability and has been applied in the investigation of human and experimental models of kidney disease, including radiocontrast nephropathy, acute allograft dysfunction, acute ischemic kidney injury, and unilateral ureteral obstruction.[24] The advantage of this noninvasive imaging modality is its use of an endogenous marker, so that it is free from potentially harmful side effects of exogenous agents.

Other MRI techniques recently studied for imaging ATN and differentiating this entity from other causes of renal failure involve the use of [23]Na. The ability to maintain the corticomedullary sodium gradient, an indicator of normal kidney function, presumably is lost early in the course of ATN. In rat kidneys, at 6 hours after the induction of ATN, [23]Na MRI revealed that the sham-control kidney exhibited a linear increase in sodium concentration along the corticomedullary axis; in the ATN kidney, the cortex–outer medullary sodium gradient was reduced by 21% and the inner medulla–to–cortex sodium ratio was decreased by 40%. This finding was inversely correlated with a small but significant rise in plasma creatinine and very limited outer medullary histological ATN. Thus, it is possible that [23]Na MRI may noninvasively detect corticomedullary sodium gradient abnormalities to allow identification of evolving ATN when morphological tubular injury is still focal and limited.[25]

Electron Paramagnetic Resonance Imaging

Oxidative stress is recognized to play a role in acute kidney injury. As this role is further defined, investigations of the kinetics of reactive oxygen species (ROS) or related substances in vivo will be needed. One method to detect and study oxidative stress is electron paramagnetic resonance (EPR) imaging, which is a technique to detect unpaired electrons. In an ischemia-reperfusion injury model, EPR imaging by Hirayama and colleagues showed significantly impaired renal radical-reducing activity in the early postreperfusion state, with only partial recovery of this activity even after normalization of serum markers. Other models of acute kidney injury such as lipopolysaccharide and puromycin-induced nephrosis also have been investigated using EPR imaging.[26]

Positron Emission Tomography

Positron emission tomography (PET) allows generation of images with higher resolution and absolute quantification of biological processes such as transport activities and enzyme activities and its correlation with renal blood flow and glomerular filtration rate. The value of this study is further enhanced when PET functional information is combined with computed tomography data. With use of new PET tracers, qualitative and quantitative assessments of in vivo hypoxia, apoptosis, endothelial dysfunction, signal transduction, and organic cation transport can be performed.[27]

Contrast-Enhanced Ultrasonography

Sonographic imaging of the kidneys is a routine procedure in clinical practice; however, conventional two-dimensional sonography has drawbacks in the limited sensitivity of color Doppler ultrasonography for the detection of intracortical capillaries and deep pedicular vessels, and in the poor contrast of B-mode imaging for parenchymal disease.[28] The use of microbubble ultrasound contrast agents overcomes these limitations, allowing much-improved assessment of the complete vascular supply of native or transplanted kidneys. After intravenous administration, microbubbles travel through the renal microvasculature but do not pass through Bowman's capsule. Accordingly, they remain in the renal blood pool without sticking to the capillary walls, are not phagocytosed, do not reach the interstitial compartment, and are not excreted into the collecting system. Thus, their pharmacokinetics differs substantially from that of iodinated contrast agents and gadolinium chelates. Unlike most conventional contrast agents, microbubble contrast agents can be administered repeatedly to patients with renal injury; no toxicity has been reported.[28]

Contrast-enhanced sonography has a much higher sensitivity and specificity than conventional ultrasonography and may be considered the technique of choice for the detection of infarction and cortical necrosis, particularly in ischemic renal transplants. This imaging modality provides quantitative information on microvascular perfusion of the renal allografts and, compared with color Doppler ultrasonography, offers improved diagnostic capability for the detection of chronic allograft nephropathy. In contrast with resistance and pulsatility indices obtained by means of color Doppler studies, renal blood flow in kidney allografts estimated by contrast-enhanced sonography has been found to be highly correlated with serum creatinine levels.[29] Perirenal hematoma, ATN, and vascular rejection are associated with characteristic changes in the time-intensity curve for contrast-enhanced sonography. Quantitative determination of time of arterial arrival of an ultrasound contrast medium in the early phase after kidney transplantation has been studied; this approach may allow identification of acute rejection earlier than can be achieved with conventional techniques.[29] In addition to ongoing studies, further research into the role of contrast-enhanced sonography in other disease states is needed to establish its place in the diagnosis of acute kidney injury.

CONCLUSION

In summary, recent advances in imaging techniques, especially intravital multiphoton microscopy, have enabled investigators to develop unique, tailor-made techniques to visualize the functioning kidney. Such improvements also permit the analysis, in dynamic fashion, of the cellular and subcellular processes that occur in various acute kidney injury states, as well as the response to therapy.

Key Points

1. Multiphoton microscopy allows cellular and subcellular analysis in vivo.
2. Multiphoton microscopy can follow, in near-real time, these different processes.
3. Multiphoton microscopy allows for visualization of pathophysiology of disease processes and response to therapy.
4. Advances in magnetic resonance technology, such as blood oxygen level–dependent magnetic resonance imaging, dendrimer-based magnetic resonance imaging, and the use of ultrasmall paramagnetic iron oxide particles for magnetic resonance angiography, has enabled enhanced resolution and allow unique approaches to elucidation of normal physiology and pathophysiology.
5. Contrast-enhanced sonography has enhanced sensitivity and specificity compared with color Doppler ultrasonography.

Key References

3. Dunn KW, Sandoval RM, Kelly KJ, et al: Functional studies of the kidney of living animals using multicolor two-photon microscopy. Am J Physiol Cell Physiol 2002;283:C905-C916.
4. Yu W: Quantitative microscopic approaches for studying kidney functions. Nephron Physiol 2006;103:63-70.
6. Molitoris BA, Sandoval RM: Intravital multiphoton microscopy of dynamic renal processes. Am J Physiol Renal Physiol 2005;288:F1084-F1089.
17. Hattori R, Ono Y, Kato M, et al: Direct visualization of cortical peritubular capillary of transplanted human kidney with reperfusion injury using a magnifying endoscopy. Transplantation 2005;79:1190-1194.

See the companion Expert Consult website for the complete reference list.

Acute Renal Failure: Clinical Aspects

Clinical Syndromes

CHAPTER 56

Multiple Organ Dysfunction Syndrome

Pasquale Piccinni, Claudio Ronco, and Zaccaria Ricci

OBJECTIVES

This chapter will:
1. Review the epidemiology and pathogenesis of multiple organ dysfunction syndrome.
2. Present a modern theory that identifies multiple organ dysfunction syndrome as an adaptive response to systemic inflammation.
3. Describe the pathogenesis of acute renal failure as part of multiple organ dysfunction syndrome and outline its medical management in this context.

A consensus conference in 1992, organized by the American College of Chest Physicians together with the Society of Critical Care Medicine, was held with the aim of establishing a set of definitions that could be applied to a complex cohort of pathological processes that, after that meeting, would be identified as systemic inflammatory response syndrome (SIRS), sepsis, severe sepsis, septic shock, and multiple organ dysfunction syndrome (MODS). In particular, the last term was introduced to describe an evolving clinical syndrome characterized by the development of otherwise unexplained abnormalities of organ function in critically ill patients.[1]

An evolving ability to support vital organ system function during a period of otherwise lethal physiological insufficiency changed the process of hospital care over the latter half of the 20th century. Over a relatively short period, the development of techniques such as positive-pressure ventilation, renal replacement therapies, invasive monitoring, and cardiovascular support transformed life-threatening illness from rapidly lethal events to chronic states that were potentially survivable. In this setting, an entirely unprecedented spectrum of clinical problems arose in the wake of the profound physiological derangements of critical illness and the heroic interventions applied to reverse them. For example, the intensive care unit (ICU) essentially created conditions for the evolution of a range of disorders characterized by a strong association with inflammation and named according to their effects on the function of individual organ systems: acute respiratory distress syndrome, acute renal failure (ARF), disseminated intravascular coagulation, septic shock, and stress-related gastrointestinal bleeding, to name a few. Yet it is not simply that any one of these organ system derangements is the cause of all of the others. Rather, all share common features that justify their consideration as manifestations of a common process, initially described as multiple organ failure (MOF)[2] and then termed *multiple organ dysfunction syndrome* (MODS).[1] Indeed, it is not clear whether MODS is a single pathological process with highly variable clinical expression or is simply the limited phenotypical expression of a large number of pathologically divergent processes.

EPIDEMIOLOGY AND PHYSIOPATHOLOGY OF MULTIPLE ORGAN DYSFUNCTION SYNDROME

The first descriptions of MODS emphasized its common association with occult or poorly controlled infection, frequently either peritonitis or pneumonia.[3] More recent reports, however, indicate that infection, although common in patients with MODS, is not necessarily present and frequently follows, rather than precedes, the development of the syndrome.[4] Indeed, nosocomial infection may be better considered a manifestation of MODS than a cause of it. For this reason, an exact epidemiological estimate of the incidence of the syndrome is virtually impossible. The burden of sepsis-related disease also is rising, however, from 82.7 to 240.4 cases per 100,000 population in the United States and to 51 cases per 100,000 population (1997 figures) in the United Kingdom, where 27.1% of adults admitted to the ICU were found to have severe sepsis in the first 24 hours of hospitalization.[5]

Although infection commonly triggers MODS, the evidence that infection plays an important role in the evolution of the syndrome is not compelling. Meta-analyses of the effects of infection prophylaxis using the techniques of selective digestive tract decontamination show a striking reduction in rates of such infections as pneumonia, wound infection, and bacteremia but a much more modest, albeit statistically significant, reduction in mortality.[6,7] Moreover, peritonitis and pneumonia are frequent causes of MODS, but evidence that successful treatment of either alters outcome is far from definitive.[8,9] Although it is difficult to differentiate the clinical manifestations of inflammation from the infections that commonly are their cause, it can be shown that the severity of the clinical inflammatory response, rather than the presence or absence of infection, is the more important determinant of ICU survival.[10] Other mechanisms, such as tissue hypoxia and microvascular coagulopathy, have raised interest as possible factors in the pathogenesis of MODS and as potential targets of two new therapeutic options: early goal-directed therapy (EGDT)[11] and activated protein C.[12] Nonetheless, MODS is a prototypical example of the application of complex theories to an understanding of the pathophysiology of critical illness.[13] It arises through the interactions of a network of physiological insults including infection, the host inflammatory response, tissue ischemia, injury, and the interventions used to sustain organ function during a time of otherwise lethal insufficiency. Its mediators are many and interdependent, with the activity of one inducing the expression of others that amplify, inhibit, or otherwise modify the expression of the process. The clinical syndrome that emerges reflects the state of dynamic balance that exists among the component mediators and can be considered an evolving disorder.

Strategies directed against specific elements of the process early in the clinical course may be effective as prophylaxis but are unlikely to have a significant effect by the time expression of the targeted entity has become autonomous. For example, although the prevention of infection in critical illness may reduce morbidity and mortality,[7] once such downstream events as pro-inflammatory mediator release have been activated, their persistence is not necessarily dependent on continuing infection. Similar considerations may help to explain the relatively modest impact of neutralization of early pro-inflammatory mediator release in patients with sepsis.[14] By contrast, activation of coagulation is a relatively late consequence of the inflammatory response and, therefore, conceptually a more attractive therapeutic target. In reality, the disparate biological processes that constitute inflammation are intimately interrelated, and strategies directed at one manifestation may have significant and unexpected consequences for others. Unfortunately, these processes are not demonstrated particularly well in small-animal models, and elucidation of the richness of these interactions is emerging only slowly as data from trials of a variety of interventional strategies accumulate.

MULTIPLE ORGAN DYSFUNCTION SYNDROME AS AN ADAPTIVE RESPONSE TO SYSTEMIC INFLAMMATION

A recent hypothesis[15] suggests that if MODS was exclusively ascribed to the effect of inflammatory mediators

with resulting tissue hypoxia and cell damage, then failure should be irreversible, especially in organs such as the liver and kidney, whose constituent cells have poor regenerative capacity. Yet fulminant hepatic failure is exceedingly rare, survivors with so-called acute tubular necrosis seldom require long-term renal replacement therapy, and overall survival rates are roughly 50% to 60%.[16] Especially remarkable is the fact that the failed organs often demonstrate a normal histopathological appearance, with minimum or no apoptosis or necrosis, even in patients who subsequently die.[17] This finding suggests that the defect is principally functional, rather than structural, and potentially reversible. Because increasing severity of sepsis is associated with a progressive fall in tissue oxygen consumption and with a rise in tissue oxygen tension, the underlying problem probably is the reduced cellular use of oxygen, rather than tissue hypoxia per se.[18,19] This notion is compatible with the coexisting decrease in perfused microvessels in sepsis, because similar changes are reported with hyperoxia.[20] Tissue adenosine triphosphate (ATP) concentration represents the balance between local supply and demand. It has been shown that preservation of ATP concentrations in patients with sepsis is associated with subsequent survival, despite concurrent inhibition of mitochondrial complex I of the electron transport chain.[21] The fact that increased glycolytic generation of ATP is unlikely to compensate fully for reduced mitochondrial production suggests that cells are able to reduce their metabolism and, correspondingly, their ATP turnover. Hence, MODS may represent an attempt by the body to ensure cell survival in the face of sustained critical illness, with affected cells entering a dormant state analogous to hibernation or estivation. Such a response can be expected to enhance the chances of recovery of organ function should the patient survive. This state of metabolic dormancy may potentially be induced via cytokine-mediated and hormone-mediated effects on cellular energy production and may be an evolutionary mechanism that increases the chances of survival in the face of a potentially overwhelming external insult.

To provide evidence for the role of mitochondria in the development of multiorgan failure, a temporal relation between rise in ATP concentration, reduction in ATP turnover, and changing clinical status needs to be identified. Clinical improvement and restoration of organ function also should be associated with an increase in bioenergetic and metabolic activity. Proof of principle would be confirmed by use of bioenergetic modulators that hasten recovery. Direct measurement of ATP turnover in vivo is not feasible in the critically ill patient. Incubation of cell lines with endotoxin, cytokines, or both in vitro is not ideal, because their phenotype has altered to predominantly glycolytic ATP production. *Ex vivo* studies assessing changes in ATP turnover and oxygen consumption, however, could be done with freshly isolated cells, tissues, or serum from patients or representative long-term models of critical illness.[22]

The volume of oxygen consumption (Vo_2), a surrogate marker for mitochondrial ATP generation, falls with increasing sepsis severity in renal tubules isolated from a long-term rodent model of sepsis. Vo_2 also is significantly lower in enterocytes isolated from septic animals than in cells taken from control animals 30 minutes after death.[23]

Such temporal relations also would provide evidence that changes in mitochondrial function are the consequence of inflammation acute-phase endocrine and metabolic responses. Animal studies, with subsequent clinical testing, could be devised to investigate the effect of pharmacological manipulation of hormone concentrations and availability on mitochondrial function; assessment data could include quantification of organ function and survival. Although many different mechanisms may underlie any possible link between acute-phase changes and later decreases in mitochondrial function, the induction of insulin resistance—either directly or through an effect on thyroid hormone metabolism—is likely to be important. Because the clinical benefit of returning blood glucose to normal with insulin has been clearly shown by van den Berghe and colleagues,[24] evidence of an effect of high-dose glucose-insulin infusion on the synthesis of ATP through the early and later phases of critical illness would provide strong support for this hypothesis. A similar approach could be considered with early administration of liothyronine (triiodothyronine) to offset any possible pathogenetic effect of the sick euthyroid syndrome on the evolution of multiorgan failure.

PATHOGENESIS AND MANAGEMENT OF RENAL DYSFUNCTION DURING MULTIPLE ORGAN DYSFUNCTION SYNDROME

The importance of maintaining regional perfusion in sepsis is increasingly recognized, not least the hepatosplanchnic circulation. Since the first experiences with use of arteriovenous hemofiltration in anuric patients with fluid overload resistant to diuretics who were managed in the ICU, in the 1970s, ARF in the critically ill has been recognized to be of multifactorial etiology. Hypotension, nephrotoxic drug insults, sepsis, and preceding renal dysfunction all may be relevant. ARF is an independent risk factor for death in the critically ill, with mortality rates ranging from 45% to 70% when associated with sepsis.[25] Factors predicting a poor outcome are advanced age, altered previous health status, later onset of ARF, sepsis, oliguria, and severity of illness.[26] Most animal models that feature the induction of so-called acute tubular necrosis (ATN), however, are based on ischemia-reperfusion (renal artery clamping)—an event with little relevance to human sepsis.

Later research highlighted a new possible and emerging concept for the pathogenesis of septic ARF: acute apoptosis.[27] This concept fits well with the typical paucity of histopathological changes seen in so-called acute tubular necrosis and with growing evidence of a role for apoptosis in organ injury during sepsis and inflammation in general. Furthermore, some evidence suggests that certain treatments shown to decrease the mortality rate in critically ill patients (activated protein C, intensive insulin therapy, and low-volume mechanical ventilation) may have anti-apoptotic activity.[27] The use of low-dose dopamine has been shown to be ineffective in halting progression to ARF in the critically ill.[28] Fenoldopam mesylate is a potent dopamine DA1 receptor agonist that increases blood flow to the renal cortex and outer medulla. A recent meta-analysis of data for a total of 1290 patients from 16 randomized studies concluded that fenoldopam is able to reduce the need for renal replacement and mortality among patients with acute kidney injury.[29] A large prospective, adequately powered, randomized trial is still needed before definitive conclusions can be drawn. N-acetylcysteine (NAC), a drug that has been considered to have an impact in oxidative stress, directly scavenging reactive oxygen species and regenerating the glutathione pool, has been evaluated for the prevention of contrast agent–induced kidney dysfunction, post–cardiopulmonary bypass renal failure, and hypotension- or vasopressor–related ARF.[30-32] Results have been rather disappointing, and the use of NAC is now limited to contrast agent–induced nephropathy. Other recently tested medical strategies (e.g., regimens using atrial natriuretic peptide or levosimendan) are still awaiting confirmation.

The management of renal replacement therapy during MODS is described in detail elsewhere.

CONCLUSION

MODS is a complex syndrome for which the pathophysiological mechanisms are poorly understood; conceivably, multiple pathways lead to organ failure. Organ failure induced by critical illness may be primarily a functional rather than a structural abnormality. Indeed, the central process may not be failure as such but rather a potentially protective, reactive mechanism. By this hypothesis, the decline in organ function is triggered by a decrease in mitochondrial activity and oxidative phosphorylation, leading to reduced cellular metabolism. This effect on mitochondria may be the consequence of acute-phase changes in hormones and inflammatory mediators.

The principles of intensive care medicine are essentially supportive, yet many interventions in the critically ill patient—including sedation, immunonutrition, mechanical ventilation, liberal blood transfusion, inotropes, and endocrine supplementation—have been associated with adverse outcomes. A more sophisticated understanding of the temporal and reactive sequence of hormonal, metabolic, inflammatory, and immunological changes during the acute and later phases of severe illness would promote a more logical basis for therapeutic intervention, which could then be tailored to the individual patient. The timing and degree of any intervention are crucial; the amplification of a response that is primarily protective at the onset of illness may be harmful if it occurs later, or vice versa. This principle is illustrated by the very different outcomes with early and late optimization of oxygen delivery. Similarly, attempts to stimulate metabolism, such as with glucose-insulin or thyroid hormones, may be appropriate as part of early management but may be potentially damaging if the organism has entered a phase of established multiorgan dysfunction in which intracellular metabolism has decreased to improve the chances of cell survival. This mechanism may underlie the increased mortality seen with administration of thyroxine or growth hormone plus insulin-like growth factor-1 to patients with established organ failure.[15]

Key Points

1. Multiple organ dysfunction syndrome is an evolving clinical entity characterized by the development of otherwise unexplained abnormalities of organ function in critically ill patients.
2. Improved intensive care support has brought with it a spectrum of disorders that are characterized by a strong but indefinite association with inflammation and infection: the acute respiratory distress syndrome, acute renal failure, disseminated intravascular coagulation, septic shock, and stress gastrointestinal bleeding.

3. Nonetheless, multiple organ dysfunction syndrome also may represent an attempt by the body to ensure cell survival in the face of sustained critical illness, with affected cells entering a dormant state analogous to hibernation or estivation. This mechanism would increase the chances of survival in subjects in whom an external insult is potentially overwhelming.

Key References

1. Bone RC, Balk R, Cerra F, et al: Definitions for sepsis and organ failure and guidelines for the use of innovative therapies in sepsis. The ACCP/SCCM Consensus Conference Committee. American College of Chest Physicians/Society of Critical Care Medicine. Chest 1992;101:1644-1655.

11. Rivers E, and The Early Goal-Directed Therapy Collaborative Group: Early goal-directed therapy in the treatment of severe sepsis and septic shock. N Engl J Med 2001;345:1368-1377.
15. Singer M, De Santis V, Vitale D, Jeffcoate W: Multiorgan failure is an adaptive, endocrine-mediated, metabolic response to overwhelming systemic inflammation. Lancet 2004;364:545-548.
17. Hotchkiss RS, Swanson PE, Freeman BD, et al: Apoptotic cell death in patients with sepsis, shock, and multiple organ dysfunction. Crit Care Med 1999;27:1230-1251.
27. Wan L, Bellomo R, Di Giantomasso, Ronco C: The pathogenesis of septic acute renal failure. Curr Opin Crit Care 2003;9:496-502.

See the companion Expert Consult website for the complete reference list.

CHAPTER 57

Burns and Acute Renal Failure

Filippo Mariano, Ezio Nicola Gangemi, Maurizio Stella, Luisa Tedeschi, Cesare Gregoretti, and Giorgio Triolo

OBJECTIVES

This chapter will:
1. Review the pathophysiology of burn injury and the major associated changes in renal function.
2. Show how acute renal failure affects burn care.
3. Describe the physiopathology of acute renal failure in burns.
4. Outline the principles of clinical management of the burn-injured patient with renal failure.

A severe burn is a skin injury accompanied by serious systemic illness, with effects on different organs distant from the site of primary injury. Currently, severe burns remain devastating clinical challenges with high mortality rates. Patient age, percentage of total body surface area (TBSA) burned, associated inhalation injury or other traumatic lesions, and preexisting disease are the main factors influencing patient outcome. In large surveys, from one third to two thirds of burn-related deaths are due to a multiorgan dysfunction syndrome (MODS), and the lungs are among the organs invariably affected (100%), followed in frequency by the intestines and kidneys (68%).[1] In a majority of cases, MODS is a consequence of sepsis, which inevitably develops in all patients with extensive burns. In a patient older than 60 years of age, with more than 40% of TBSA burned and inhalation injury, the probability of death is estimated to be higher than 90%.[2]

Fortunately, in the last 20 years, burn-related mortality has decreased in Western countries. This improvement in outcome is due either to primary prevention of all causes of burns or to specific treatment protocols for burn-induced shock, including early fluid resuscitation and immediate hospitalization for care by specialized burn teams.

PHYSIOPATHOLOGY OF BURNS

Burns may be due to thermal, chemical, or electrical injuries. Thermal and chemical injuries cause coagulative necrosis of the skin and underlying subcutaneous tissue. The major determinants of burn severity are extent (as determined by percentage of involved body surface area) and depth (partial- or full-thickness) of the injury. Within a few hours, the injury, in proportion to extent and thickness of the injury, elicits a local and systemic release of inflammatory mediators and changes in hormonal and immunological responses. Circulating and local mediators include cytokines (interleukin [IL]-1, IL-2, IL-6, IL-8, IL-12, tumor necrosis factor [TNF]), growth factors, activation products of coagulation and contact-phase cascades, complement factors, nitric oxide, platelet-activating factor (PAF), prostaglandins, and leukotrienes. This plethora of molecules present at high concentrations for days leads to marked vasodilatation, generalized increased microvascular permeability, extravascular fluid loss, hypotension, and, without appropriate treatment, hypovolemic shock. In the gut, just a few hours after burn injury, increased mesenteric vascular resistance and decreased intestinal perfusion can be observed, leading to bacterial translocation and endotoxemia. Hormonal derangements include increased levels of cortisol, glucagon, and catecholamines, affecting several metabolic functions, such as the observed nitrogen- and calcium-negative balance, lipolysis, massive peripheral muscle wasting, and hepatic fat deposition.

Electrical injury causes tissue destruction at the site of contact and along the current's pathway. The patient may die as a result of cardiac arrhythmia, neurological complications, or musculoskeletal injury. Acute renal failure (ARF) can arise soon after muscle crush injury and rhabdomyolysis.

Inhalation injury due to smoke and associated chemicals causes bronchoconstriction and airway obstruction, leading to lung injury. Both acute lung injury and acute respiratory distress syndrome may occur at any time during the clinical course, however.

RENAL ALTERATIONS IN BURN-INJURED PATIENTS

A wide range of morphological and functional kidney alterations, ranging from transitory contraction of renal function to electrolyte disturbances to severe forms of ARF, have been observed after burns (Table 57-1). Several pathogenic mechanisms such as accumulation of filtered breakdown products, antibiotic toxicity, and sepsis are thought to be involved in these alterations.

In a study of burn-injured patients who were convalescent for more than 2 months, renal blood flow was significantly increased, as was mean kidney weight at autopsy examination of those who subsequently died.[3] Glomerular filtration rate (GFR) may be either decreased or increased in these patients.[4] Serum creatinine level may not be a reliable index of GFR, however, because hyperhydration and reduced muscle mass can lead to overestimation of renal function.

Proteinuria is a constant feature in severely burned patients, starting in the first days after hospital admission and increasing in severity over time. Proteinuria is of a mixed type, reflecting both increased glomerular permeability and decreased tubular reabsorption of filtered proteins such as lysozyme, β_2-microglobulin, and amylase.[5,6] Proteinuria may be in the nephrotic range and peaks at week 2 or 3, when all patients show the clinical signs of severe sepsis (Fig. 57-1). The extent of proteinuria is significantly correlated with indices of inflammatory state and sepsis, suggesting an important pathogenetic role of urinary protein in inducing renal injury.[7]

Hematuria is not common, being present in approximately 5% of burn-injured children. In one study, hematuria was due to urinary tract infection in greater than 50% of the cases, to renal stones in 15%, and in a minority of cases to catheter-related trauma, renal vein thrombosis, or acute tubular necrosis (ATN).[8] In the patients who had ATN, hematuria was considered to represent a fatal prognostic factor.[8]

Metabolic abnormalities involving both proximal and distal tubules have been described. They include increased fractional sodium excretion and uric acid clearance, low

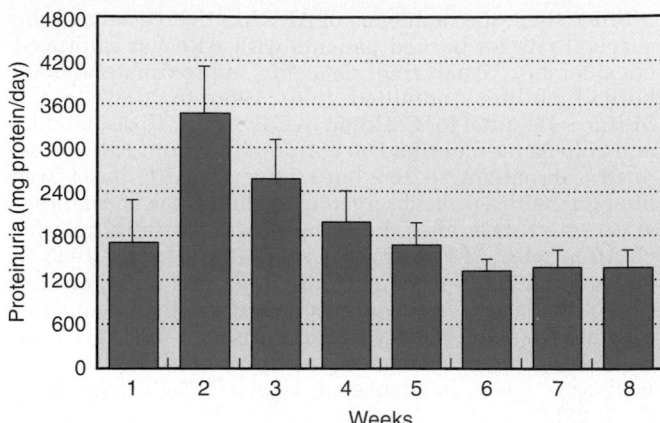

FIGURE 57-1. Severity of proteinuria (measured as mg of urinary protein excreted per 24 hours) observed in 12 severely burned patients from hospitalization to week 8 after injury. (Courtesy of the Burn Center, CTO Hospital, Turin, Italy.)

threshold of phosphate adsorption, glucosuria, and aminoaciduria.[4,5,9] Urinary losses, as well as loss of fluid in burn wound exudates, that are not adequately replaced contribute to blood electrolyte abnormalities, including hypernatremia, hyponatremia, hypokalemia, and decreased calcium and magnesium.[10] Hypercalcemia due to prolonged immobilization also has been described.[11]

ARF in burned patients is not so common as might be expected. Two distinct clinical pictures of ARF can be observed: early ARF, occurring either a few hours after injury or in the first few days, and late ARF, developing approximately 1 or more weeks after burn injury. Early ARF may be due to hypovolemia and hypoperfusion of the kidneys, whereas late ARF is a consequence of infection, endotoxemia, and MODS. Over the past two decades, clinical manifestation of ARF has changed from an early to a late finding, in accordance with the evolution in burn care.

ACUTE RENAL FAILURE

Incidence and Prognosis

The incidence of ARF in burned patients varies widely between 0.5% and 30%, with a mortality rate of 50% to 100%. Different definitions of ARF and, in addition, the nonhomogeneity of the patient populations studied can explain the observed notable variation in epidemiological data.[5,12,13] In older reports from before the end of the 1970s, however, the incidence of ARF as the form of renal injury requiring renal replacement therapy was less than 4%, and survival was very poor, with death of all patients in some series. Indeed, the first report of survival of patients with ARF following burn injury is dated 1965. In an analysis of published data from 1953 to 1979, Davies and colleagues found that ARF developed in 119 of 7126 patients, and only 8 of these survived.[14] Five years later, Sawada and associates published a case report of survival in a severely burned patient with ARF who had been anuric for 20 days and managed with renal replacement therapy for 35 days. On reviewing the literature, these investigators found only 20 survivors from oliguric ARF[15] by 1984.

TABLE 57-1

Renal Alterations in Patients with Burns

Increased mean kidney mass
Increased renal blood flow
Increased/decreased glomerular filtration rate
Proteinuria
Hematuria
Tubular damage with glycosuria, excessive loss of Na^+, K^+, Ca^{2+}, and phosphate
Sodium and water retention, hyponatremia and hypokalemia
Hypocalcemia/hypercalcemia
Hypomagnesemia
Acute renal failure
End-stage renal disease

Since then, the incidence of ARF has decreased and the survival rate for burned patients with ARF has improved considerably. Analyzing data for approximately 5000 burned children admitted from 1966 to 1997 to the Shriners Hospital for Children in Galveston, Texas, Jeschke and colleagues identified 60 children in whom ARF developed subsequent to the burn injury.[16] ARF onset was bimodal, with a peak observed in the first week and another at 19 to 23 days after the burn injury. Mortality rate for children with ARF decreased from 100% before 1983 to 56% after 1984. For patients admitted after 1984, evaluation of the factors involved in survival improvement demonstrated a significantly shorter time to institution of both fluid resuscitation and early wound excision, as well as a lower incidence of sepsis (19% versus 60%; $P < 0.05$).[16]

In a study from the same group of investigators, a clinical picture of ARF developed in 76 of 1404 acutely burned adults (5.4%) with severe burns (involving greater than 30% of TBSA).[17] Diagnostic criteria for ARF were identified as presence of oliguria, serum creatinine level greater than 2 mg/dL, blood urea nitrogen–serum creatinine ratio greater than 20, and requirement for dialysis, with diagnosis confirmed by presence of three of the four criteria. The patients with ARF were divided into two groups: survivors and nonsurvivors. ARF diagnosis in nonsurvivors was bimodal (occurring either within 7 days or during the third week after burn), whereas in survivors it presented a single-peak distribution in the first 7 days. Renal replacement therapy was required in 67% of survivors and 91% of nonsurvivors. Independent risk factors for mortality in patients with ARF were older age (67% of survivors and 25% of nonsurvivors were younger than 40 years; $P < .02$), sepsis (affecting 44% of survivors and 96% of nonsurvivors), ARF as part of MODS (in 96% of nonsurvivors and 11% of survivors; $P < .001$), and time between burn injury and initiation of fluid resuscitation (1.7 ± 1.0 hours in survivors versus 4.4 ± 2.1 hours in nonsurvivors; $P < .001$). In the multivariate analysis, no significant difference between survivors and nonsurvivors was found for percentage of TBSA burned, presence of third-degree burns (%), and presence of inhalation injury. In a comparison of patients with ARF admitted from 1981 to 1989 ($n = 35$) with those admitted from 1990 to 1998 ($n = 41$), no significant differences between the two periods could be seen in the incidence of ARF (5.4% versus 5.1%) or mortality rate (88% versus 87%).[17] From these data, the investigators concluded that "aggressive early fluid resuscitation and the prevention of sepsis may reduce the incidence of ARF in burned adults. This, in turn, may decrease the mortality associated with ARF."[17]

In another series of 147 severely burned patients (mean TBSA, $60\% \pm 21.8\%$), Gheun-Ho and coworkers found that ARF developed in 28 patients (19%), with a mortality rate of 100%, compared with 29.4% among those patients in whom ARF did not occur.[18] Patients with ARF had a significantly larger percentage of TBSA burned ($79.5\% \pm 15.4\%$ versus $55.3\% \pm 20.5\%$) and lower serum albumin concentration on admission (1.92 ± 0.66 g/dL versus 2.48 ± 0.82 g/dL). In a multivariate analysis, burns over greater than 65% of TBSA were associated with a risk for ARF 9.9 times that for patients with burns involving less than 65% of TBSA.[18] Apart from specific causes of mortality related to burns, however, it cannot be ruled out that even in critically ill burn-injured patients with ARF, the untoward consequences of the acutely uremic state constitute an important factor for outcome.[19]

Early Acute Renal Failure

During the first few days after burn injury, renal function frequently is compromised. Several factors are involved, including volume alterations, electrolyte disturbances, hormones, inflammatory mediators, and toxic breakdown products such as myoglobin and hemoglobin.

Additional excessive fluid loss from the burn wound leads to rapid loss and sequestration of large quantities of fluid from the intravascular compartment to the interstitial space, thereby depleting the circulating volume, manifested as both local and generalized edema. Sodium retention in the interstitial space and sodium-potassium pump impairment also contribute to generalized edema. These changes occur mainly in the first 6 to 8 hours after injury. Any delay in fluid resuscitation may exacerbate the volume depletion and decreased renal blood flow.

Burn stresses stimulate the production and release of hormones such as catecholamines, aldosterone, angiotensin II, and vasopressin, which can lead to vasoconstriction and changes in renal blood flow. On the other hand, plasma atrial natriuretic polypeptide (ANP) levels are elevated after burns, counterbalancing the action of the stress-related hormones through vasodilation and natriuresis. Excessively high levels of stress-related hormones or impairment of ANP secretion may contribute to reduced renal function.

Moreover, many inflammatory mediators including cytokines (TNF, IL-1, IL-6), eicosanoids (prostaglandins, thromboxane, leukotrienes), and PAF can affect the kidney in the early postburn period, because they act to variably increase microvascular permeability, as well as to activate circulating inflammatory cells. Inflammatory mediators promote adhesion and migration of activated neutrophils in burned tissue. As a specific prostaglandin in the kidney, the vasodilator prostaglandin E_2 counteracts the aforementioned vasoconstrictor substances, but its production is inhibited in the early phase of a burn injury. In addition, acute burns cause an immediate depression of cardiac output before any detectable reduction in plasma volume. Bacterial translocation and gut-derived factors may be involved in depression of myocardial inotropy.

High-voltage electrical injury may cause muscular damage, massive rhabdomyolysis, and myoglobinuria.[17] Hemoglobinuria may occur after hemolysis in extensive full-thickness burns, when hemoglobin is in excess of haptoglobin-binding capability. Hemoglobin and myoglobin are freely filtered, absorbed by tubular epithelium and degraded into globin and heme; the latter is directly toxic on tubular cells by generating oxygen free radicals through formation of iron ions. This effect could lead to degenerative changes in tubular cells, occlusion of tubules by the formation of hemoglobin casts and eventually renal failure, especially when combined with dehydration, acidosis, shock, or endotoxemia.

Late Acute Renal Failure

Late acute renal dysfunction usually is secondary to hemodynamic changes associated with other burn complications, such as sepsis[2,5,16,17] or MODS with disseminated intravascular coagulopathy. Sepsis is the most life-threatening complication of a severe burn injury; it arises 1 to 2 weeks after burn injury, when incidence of ARF peaks. Sepsis, originating mainly from the burn wound infection, is the most common initiator of MODS and was recognized early on as the primary cause. An impaired gastrointestinal barrier, an open wound, and inadequate delivery of oxygen to peripheral tissues are other potential causes of MODS.

Increasing evidence suggests that bacterial translocation through the damaged intestinal mucosa may lead to repeated episodes of endotoxemia and sepsis. These episodes, lasting several weeks, affect distant organs including the kidney. Endotoxin (the lipopolysaccharide component of gram-negative bacterial cell walls), lipoteichoic acid, and other bacterial wall components are able to induce ARF either directly or by means of synthesis of secondary mediators.[20-22]

ARF also may be due to nephrotoxicity of antibiotics administered during the septic episodes. Antibiotics such as aminoglycosides and certain other drugs are known to lead to renal tubular damage. Acute or chronic intoxication with alcohol, barbiturates, chlorpromazine, toluene, and paint thinner has been reported as a possible associated factor in the etiology of renal failure in burned patients, but early resuscitation therapy was delayed in some of the affected patients.[15]

Prevention of Acute Renal Failure

Prompt and adequate fluid resuscitation as well as monitoring of circulating blood volume has decreased the incidence of early ARF.[16,17] Crystalloids used in the first 48 hours, as either normotonic or hypertonic preparations, are given in accordance with proposed formulas (e.g., Evans,[23] Modified Brooke,[24] Parkland,[25] Slater[26]). Use of colloids in burned patients, mainly frozen plasma, has decreased, because controlled trials have shown no clear advantage. An increased rate of pulmonary complications associated with use of 5% albumin in lactated Ringer's solution has been observed.[27] In addition, the administration of albumin to patients in stable condition after 24 hours of clinically satisfactory crystalloid resuscitation resulted in a significant decrease in the glomerular filtration rate below the normal range despite an increase in plasma volume.[28]

Concomitant inhalation injury necessitates use of even larger volumes of resuscitation fluid. In 51 patients with greater than 25% of TBSA burned and inhalation injury, after initial fluid resuscitation according to the Parkland formula, infusion titration was performed to provide a urine output of 30 to 50 mL/hour. For successful resuscitation, patients with inhalation injuries required a mean infusion rate of 5.76 ml/kg for each % TBSA burned and sodium replacement of 0.94 mEq/kg for each % TBSA burned. Infusion rate and sodium requirement were significantly higher than those observed in the group without inhalation injury (3.98 ml/kg and 0.68 mEq/kg for each % TBSA burned, respectively; $P < 0.05$).[29]

When patients present with prerenal azotemia and rhabdomyolysis with myoglobinuria, enhanced infusion rate, forced diuresis by mannitol or furosemide, and urine alkalinization by sodium bicarbonate to obtain an alkaline urine output higher than 300 mL/hour may be useful in preventing toxic ARF, although data from controlled trials are limited. In patients with deep burns and associated hemolysis, renal damage can arise even from hemoglobinuria. In these patients, administration of haptoglobin may help to prevent hemoglobinuria-induced ARF. In a controlled study of 10 extensively burned patients with overt hemoglobinuria, 5 received fluid resuscitation (control group) and the other 5 patients were given haptoglobin in addition to fluid resuscitation. In the therapy group, free

serum hemoglobin dropped rapidly, whereas its levels in the control group remained unchanged for at least 12 hours. The time required for macroscopic hemoglobinuria to resolve showed a statistically significant difference between the haptoglobin treatment group and the control group.[30]

Sepsis remains the most important cause of death after burn injury and is strongly associated with the development of late ARF. In the past few decades, however, early and aggressive burn wound excision, routine use of topical antimicrobial agents to limit local bacterial colonization, availability of powerful new antibiotics, and early nutritional enteral support to maintain gastrointestinal tropism have been decisive in improving infection control and survival in patients with burn injuries.

RENAL REPLACEMENT THERAPY IN BURN-INJURED PATIENTS

In patients with burn injuries and unequivocal evidence of evolving ARF (incipient oliguria and increasing serum creatinine), early initiation of renal replacement therapy is now recommended.[31]

Standard intermittent hemodialysis was the only technique available until almost the mid-1980s. Usually patients underwent daily hemodialysis procedures to maintain a low level of azotemia and to remove the massive amounts of fluid required for hemodynamic stabilization, parenteral nutrition, and drug administration. Even the use of daily short-duration hemodialysis was not satisfactory, however, because patients often were in septic shock and unable to tolerate a high rate of fluid and solute removal.

For these reasons, over the past 2 decades, extracorporeal continuous techniques became increasingly popular for the management of critically ill burned patients. Although various modalities of continuous renal replacement therapy (CRRT)—including hemodialysis, hemodiafiltration, and hemofiltration—are being used in different burn centers, the available data to guide proactive clinical intervention are quite limited. Even with restriction of data analysis to the past 2 decades, when CRRT routinely achieved good-quality outcomes, results were reported for only 204 burned adults managed with renal replacement therapies, with an overall mortality rate of 70.1%.[14,32-41]

In 1986, continuous arteriovenous hemofiltration was first proved to be an effective tool for removing fluid in severely burned patients with anasarca and ARF. In oliguric patients, continuous arteriovenous hemofiltration allowed maintenance of nutritional support and other fluid intake, leading to effective weight loss.[32]

Holm and coworkers reported their experience with CRRT in 48 severely burned patients with ARF (mean TBSA burned, 48%).[37] Patients received continuous arteriovenous hemofiltration for a mean of 10.5 days, with a dialysis complication rate of 10% (mostly associated with vascular access in the femoral artery). The mortality rate for these patients was 85%, and death was due to MODS in 83% of the cases. When patients were divided into two groups according to whether they had late or early ARF (time of onset, after 5 days or within 5 days after burn injury, respectively), the early ARF group had a significantly higher incidence of myoglobinuria and hypotension during the resuscitation phase, whereas the late ARF group showed a higher frequency of sepsis. Only percentage of TBSA burned and presence of inhalation injury significantly correlated with the development of ARF, whereas age, third-degree burn (%), and presence of electrical injury did not. In a comparison of survivors with nonsurvivors, neither age, % TBSA burned, day of onset of ARF, or duration of CRRT proved to be significantly different.[37]

Two consecutive reports from Leblanc and Tremblay and their associates, spanning the period 1987 to 1998, described outcomes for 28 burned patients with ARF treated with CRRT.[36,38] Overall mortality rate was 67.8% (19 of 28), but survival rate improved from 18% (in the first report, covering the period 1987 to 1994) to 50% (in the second report, covering 1995 to 1998). Comparing the experience with CRRT in burned patients with that in other critically ill patients, these investigators reported that in the burned patients, duration of required CRRT was longer (mean duration, 24.2 ± 9.4 days versus 5.3 ± 0.8 days; $P < .006$), mean fluid intake was higher (8.2 ± 0.7 L versus 3.3 ± 0.2 L/day; $P < .0001$), and total weight loss during the course of the CRRT protocol was lower (12.6 ± 3.6 kg versus 6.8 ± 1.0 kg; $P < .03$). Of note, however, bleeding complications were frequent in burned patients who received CRRT, with an incidence as high as 56%.[35] When the platelet count was lower than 50,000/μL, no heparin was used.[38]

Generally speaking, feasibility of continuous dialysis necessitates continuous anticoagulation, and this requirement remains the main challenge in the application of CRRT. Heparin clearly is contraindicated in patients with active bleeding or in patients with associated injuries (e.g., head trauma), and it can expose patients with extensive open surfaces or surgery to an intolerable risk of hemorrhage.[41]

In severely burned patients at high risk for bleeding, regional anticoagulation with citrate may be an effective alternative for maintaining the patency of the extracorporeal circuit, even with use of sorbent technology.[41,42] In severely burned patients with septic shock–associated ARF, citrate has been used as the sole anticoagulant during coupled plasma filtration absorption–continuous venovenous hemofiltration treatment.[41] In a comparison of data from 58 filtration sessions using systemic anticoagulation with heparin (mean infusion rate, 741 U of heparin/hour) with data from 28 sessions using citrate regional anticoagulation (citrate-containing replacement solutions), no differences in number of spent citrate cartridges were observed, and the number of lost cartridges was significantly lower in the citrate treatment group. These results were obtained at a mean level of citrate in the extracorporeal circuit of 4 mmol/L, with no accumulation of citrate in systemic blood (systemic citratemia; mean citrate level less than 0.5 mmol/L). In one patient suffering from acute kidney and liver failure, a citrate peak level of 2.68 mmol/L in systemic blood at 7 hours was observed; the citrate accumulation was promptly corrected by reduction in blood flow rate and citrate infusion.[41]

Although peritoneal dialysis may be useful for its capability to gradually remove fluid, favorable impact on hemodynamics, lack of need for anticoagulants, and worldwide availability, it has little value in the treatment of ARF in burned patients. In effect, the low efficiency of peritoneal dialysis in severely hypercatabolic patients, any involvement of the abdominal area in the burn injury, and the associated high risk of peritonitis in septic patients have limited its use in the population of burned patients. In addition, without use of this modality, healthy abdominal skin may be saved as a future donor site for skin grafts. Reported experience with peritoneal dialysis in patients with burns is limited, and the procedure is mainly done in children.[43]

CONCLUSION

ARF consequent to burn injury continues to be associated with high morbidity and mortality rates. Aggressive fluid resuscitation in the immediate postburn period has been demonstrated to be effective in reducing the incidence of the early form of ARF; however, improved survival with the late form of ARF is more difficult to achieve because of the associated sepsis and MODS. Use of an early and aggressive excision protocol for burn wound care, new potent antibiotics, and early enteral nutrition for maintaining gastrointestinal trophism has been crucial to improving the control of sepsis, prolonging postburn survival, and preventing the onset of ARF. In established ARF, early and intensive use of CRRT, even for prolonged periods, is effective in ensuring a mean survival rate of 20% to 50% among treated patients.

Key Points

1. Severe burns are characterized by skin injury and serious systemic illness with significant pathophysiological changes in various organs, including the kidneys.
2. Impaired renal function is the rule in burn-injured patients, but acute renal failure requiring renal replacement therapy is fortunately not so common.
3. Two distinct forms of acute renal failure have been described: an early form, due to hypovolemia, and a late form, associated with sepsis and multiple organ dysfunction syndrome.
4. Continuous renal replacement therapy is perhaps more suitable than other modalities for the management of burned patients with sepsis-associated acute renal failure.
5. Despite improved survival in recent years, mortality rates in burned patients with acute renal failure are still as high as 50% to 100%.

Key References

1. Sheridan RL, Ryan CM, Yin LM, et al: Death in the burn unit: Sterile multiple organ failure. Burns 1998;24:307-311.
5. Schiavon M, Di Landro D, Baldo M, et al: A study of renal damage in seriously burned patients. Burns Incl Therm Inj 1988;14:107-112.
37. Holm C, Horbrand F, von Donnersmarck GH, Muhlbauer W: Acute renal failure in severely burned patients. Burns 1999;25:171-178.
38. Tremblay R, Ethier J, Querin S, et al: Veno-venous continuous renal replacement therapy for burned patients with acute renal failure. Burns 2000;26:638-643.
41. Mariano F, Tetta C, Stella M, et al: Regional citrate anticoagulation in critically ill patients managed with plasma filtration and adsorption. Blood Purif 2004;22:313-319.

See the companion Expert Consult website for the complete reference list.

CHAPTER 58

Drug-Induced Acute Renal Failure

Emmanuel A. Burdmann

OBJECTIVES

This chapter will:
1. Explain why the kidneys are especially vulnerable to drugs, delineate the possible mechanisms of drug injury, and describe the renal syndromes caused by drugs.
2. Review the mechanisms of renal injury for the most important drugs, and describe the associated clinical presentation of nephrotoxicity in severely ill patients.
3. Identify the risk factors for nephrotoxicity, along with possible preventive measures, for the most important drugs causing renal injury in severely ill patients.

The epidemiology of acute kidney injury (AKI) has changed remarkably over the last few decades. Nowadays a majority of affected patients are critically ill older persons hospitalized in an intensive care unit (ICU) with comorbid illnesses and multiple organ failure.[1,2] The incidence, frequency, and outcomes statistics for drug-induced AKI fluctuate widely, depending on the definition of renal injury used, experience and expertise of the medical team, available medical facilities, and characteristics of patient populations. In the ICU, nephrotoxicity, either alone or, most commonly, associated with ischemia, has been a related factor in the pathogenesis of AKI in almost half of the cases.[3]

Many factors underlie this renal vulnerability to toxins. The kidneys are responsible for excretion of a number of drugs. The renal concentration mechanisms expose the renal tubule cells to massive intratubular drug concentrations as drug is transported and may be accumulated in the proximal tubule intracellular compartment. The kidneys also metabolize and modify several drugs, inducing the formation of toxic compounds. Finally, high blood renal flow rates and the requirement for energy to keep the tubule transport mechanisms working make the kidneys extremely vulnerable to changes in blood flow or oxygen deprivation, as caused by drug-induced hemodynamic disorders or impaired cellular respiration. Virtually all possible mechanisms or processes leading to renal injury have been associated to drug nephrotoxicity: acute tubular cell injury, changes in renal hemodynamics, intratubular obstruction, acute interstitial nephritis, hypersensitivity vasculitis, thrombotic microangiopathy, osmotic nephrosis, and rhabdomyolysis. The same drug may cause nephrotoxicity by more than one type of mechanism. As an example, nonsteroidal anti-inflammatory drugs (NSAIDs) may induce acute tubular injury, intrarenal vasoconstriction, or acute interstitial nephritis. Drugs also may cause changes in different aspects of renal function; such changes may include decreased glomerular filtration rate, impairment of electrolyte tubular manipulation with consequent

alteration in electrolyte blood concentrations, defects in acid-basic renal homeostasis, impaired dilution and concentration mechanisms, hypertension, and proteinuria, which may reach nephrotic levels. Again, the same drug may cause more than one type of change. Aminoglycosides, for example, can decrease the glomerular filtration rate (GFR), impair electrolyte tubular manipulation, and blunt renal concentrating mechanisms.

Some fundamental principles of management of drug-induced nephrotoxicity should be stressed (Table 58-1). Measurement of serum creatinine should always be performed before administration of potentially nephrotoxic drugs, and creatinine should be monitored for the early detection of renal dysfunction. It should be remembered that even small increments in creatinine are an independent risk factor for increased mortality in hospitalized patients.[4] The use of estimated GFR should be considered to improve detection of renal injury in patients with low muscle mass. Electrolyte and acid-base disorders, that may precede the decrease in GFR, must be monitored. The use of a non-nephrotoxic drug or a procedure that does not use nephrotoxic drugs should be considered for patients at higher risk for renal injury (e.g., older patients; hypotensive, dehydrated, sodium-depleted, or septic patients; those receiving vasoactive drugs; those with abnormal renal function; those already taking potentially nephrotoxic drugs; those with myoglobinuria, hemoglobinuria, or bilirubinuria). Patients must be adequately hydrated and sodium repleted before receiving a nephrotoxic drug. Discontinuation of diuretics should be considered in these patients. The concomitant use of two or more different nephrotoxic drugs must be vigorously avoided. Drugs that promote efferent arteriole vasodilation, such as angiotensin-converting enzyme (ACE) inhibitors or angiotensin receptor blockers, should be used with caution in patients who will receive drugs inducing afferent arteriole vasoconstriction (e.g., calcineurin blockers, contrast agents). Drug dosage should be adjusted in accordance with organ functional status, distribution volume, and specific aspects of drug pharmacokinetics.[5] It should always be checked if a nephrotoxic drug has specific measures to help prevent or attenuate its potential for renal damage.

Currently, numerous drugs have been related to development of AKI. With the increasing complexity of ICU protocols, the development of more efficient life support systems, and the rapid development of new therapeutic and diagnostic compounds, the number of persons exposed to toxic drugs is steadily increasing. Use of the PubMed database to investigate frequency of drug-specific nephrotoxicity shows that contrast agents, NSAIDs, antibiotics, calcineurin inhibitors, and cisplatin account for the highest numbers of "hits" (Fig. 58-1). Discussed in the following section are some of the most important drugs causing nephrotoxicity in patients who are severely ill, or being cared for in an ICU, with regard to mechanism of injury, clinical features, risk factors, and prevention of renal injury. Of the vast array of drugs with potential for nephrotoxicity, those more frequently prescribed for or administered to patients in the ICU are discussed in this chapter: anti-infective agents (aminoglycosides, vancomycin, amphotericin B, polymyxins, and highly active antiretroviral therapy [HAART]), contrast agents, NSAIDs, and drugs blocking the renin-angiotensin-aldosterone system (ACE inhibitors and angiotensin II AT$_1$ receptor blockers). Calcineurin inhibitors and drugs used for cancer treatment are reviewed in other chapters of this book.

ANTI-INFECTIVE AGENTS

Aminoglycosides

Aminoglycosides, a class of antibiotics introduced into clinical practice in the mid-1940s (with the advent of streptomycin), are still widely prescribed owing to their potent bactericidal activity against gram-negative rods,

TABLE 58-1

Important Considerations with Use of Potentially Nephrotoxic Drugs

- Always establish baseline glomerular function before starting the drug (by determination of serum creatinine level or estimated glomerular filtration rate).
- Measure serum creatinine in a timely manner to detect early changes in renal function.
- Measure serum electrolytes and assess acid-base status periodically, because abnormalities can develop before glomerular dysfunction becomes detectable.
- Consider the use of a non-nephrotoxic drug or a diagnostic test that does not require the use of nephrotoxic agents in patients at higher risk for renal injury.
- Ensure adequate hydration and sodium repletion before institution of the nephrotoxic drug.
- Consider the discontinuation of diuretics before institution of the nephrotoxic drug.
- Avoid the simultaneous use of two or more different nephrotoxic drugs.
- Be careful with the use of angiotensin-converting enzyme inhibitors or angiotensin receptor blockers in patients who are taking drugs that induce afferent arteriole vasoconstriction (e.g., contrast agents, calcineurin blockers).
- Adapt drug dosage according to the existence of organ dysfunction, extracellular volume status, and specific aspects of the drug's pharmacokinetics.
- Always check for the existence of specific measures to prevent or attenuate nephrotoxicity from a specific drug.

their positive synergism with other antibiotics against gram-positive organisms, and the infrequent emergence of bacterial resistance with use of these agents. In the mid-1960s and then in the early 1980s, most of the aminoglycosides currently used were launched: gentamicin, tobramycin, amikacin, and netilmicin.

Aminoglycosides are highly water-soluble polycations, with molecular weights ranging from 445 to 600 g/mmol. These characteristics limit distribution of drug to the extracellular space, and these agents do not cross biological membranes, which do not have transport mechanisms. They have very poor oral absorption (less than 1% of a given dose) and must be given by the parenteral route. Their binding to plasma albumin is negligible (10% or less); they are not metabolized and are freely excreted by means of glomerular filtration. They reach peak plasma concentrations 30 to 90 minutes after intramuscular and 30 minutes after intravenous administration and have a serum half-life of approximately 2 to 3 hours in persons with normal renal function. After glomerular filtration, part of the aminoglycoside load (approximately 5% to 10%) binds to proximal tubular cell brush border and is transported into the intracellular compartment by a saturable mechanism. In fact, aminoglycoside cortical concentration may be up to 100 times the plasma concentration. Their half-life in the renal cortex may be up to 700 hours, and urinary excretion of the antibiotic may persist up to 20 to 30 days after the last dose.[6,7]

Aminoglycosides cause tubular and glomerular dysfunction. Tubular injury is characterized by structural changes that may progress to tubular necrosis and by functional changes involving electrolyte and bicarbonate derangements and renal concentrating mechanisms. Although extensively studied for decades, the actual mechanism of the tubular cell lesion is still not well understood.[7] Aminoglycosides also promote glomerular toxicity and cause a decrease in GFR. They affect intraglomerular hemodynamics, with a striking action on mesangial cells, promoting their contraction, with consequent ultrafiltration coefficient (K$_f$) fall.[8]

The reported frequency for aminoglycoside-induced AKI ranges from zero to 50%, depending on the AKI definition used, timing and type of renal tests, and characteristics of the population receiving the drug. In a recent study from a university tertiary care hospital ICU, aminoglycoside therapy was initiated in 360 consecutive patients with baseline GFR greater than 30 mL/minute per 1.73 m^2 of body surface area. AKI, defined as GFR decrease over 20% the baseline value, developed in 58% (209) of the patients. Mortality rate was strikingly higher in the AKI group (44.5% versus 29.1% for the patients in whom AKI did not develop; $P = .0031$).[9] Although in the vast majority

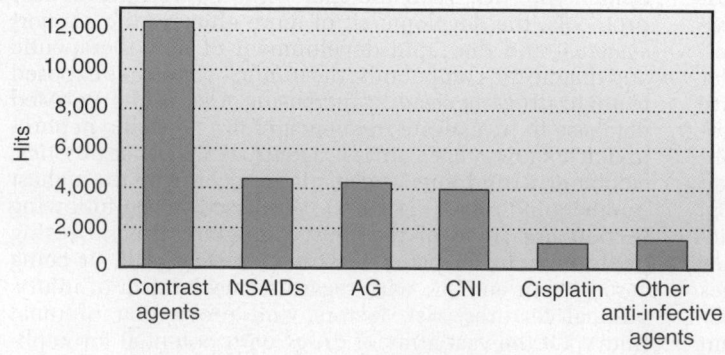

FIGURE 58-1. Drug nephrotoxicity: Frequency of occurrence for various agents by number of PubMed online "hits." AG, aminoglycoside; CNI, calcineurin inhibitor; NSAIDs, nonsteroidal anti-inflammatory drugs.

of instances, aminoglycoside-induced renal injury is related to parenteral administration of the drug, AKI also has been described after the use of inhaled tobramycin[10] or exposure to tobramycin-laden cement in arthroplasty.[11] It is prudent to assume that this class of drugs will always cause some renal toxicity, with minor or major clinical relevance.

Typically, aminoglycoside-induced AKI is nonoliguric and dose- and time-dependent, becoming clinically evident after 5 to 7 days of drug therapy. Besides serum creatinine increase, the drug frequently induces urinary potassium and magnesium wasting, causing hypokalemia, hypomagnesemia, and hypocalcemia. A Fanconi-like syndrome with aminoaciduria, bicarbonaturia, phosphaturia, and glycosuria may rarely occur. Recovery of renal function is the rule for surviving patients with previously normal renal function.[6,7]

Although several risk factors have been related to aminoglycoside renal injury, few studies have been specifically designed to assess this important aspect of the drug's nephrotoxicity. Older age, intravascular volume depletion, shock or hypotension, preexisting renal insufficiency, potassium or magnesium depletion, acidosis, and concomitant liver disease have been described as patient-related risk factors. Larger aminoglycoside doses, duration of therapy (more than 3 days), shorter dose interval, recent aminoglycoside use, concomitant exposure to nephrotoxins, and timing of aminoglycoside administration (between midnight and 7 AM) have been suggested as aminoglycoside- or physician-related risk factors.[6,7] None of these previous studies assessed several factors concomitantly. In a study using the previously described cohort of 209 patients with aminoglycoside-induced AKI, logistic regression analysis was performed to identify independent risk factors for aminoglycoside nephrotoxicity. The initial model (with reference values) included age (younger than 60 years), gender, baseline GFR (greater than 60 mL/minute per 1.73 m^2 of body surface area), days of aminoglycoside use (more than 9.9 days), use of amikacin or gentamicin, presence of previous cardiovascular disease, diabetes, use of other nephrotoxic antibiotics, use of furosemide, use of contrast, presence of acidosis, hypovolemia, hypotension, and jaundice. Diabetes (odds ratio [OR], 2.13), use of other nephrotoxic antibiotic (OR, 1.61), use of contrast (OR, 2.13), and hypotension (OR, 1.83) were identified as statistically significant independent risk factors for aminoglycoside nephrotoxicity in the final model.[9]

In addition to the obvious strategies to avoid or minimize aminoglycoside nephrotoxicity (use of the lowest dose and shortest course for clinical effectiveness, volume and sodium repletion, correction of electrolyte abnormalities and acidosis, avoidance of concomitant use of other nephrotoxins), some specific maneuvers also must be considered. The use of once-daily (OD) regimens versus multiple dosage (MD) for the administration of aminoglycosides is based on the unique characteristics of these drugs, including concentration-dependent bactericidal activity and the fact that the tubular mechanism for cortical uptake of these antibiotics is saturable. Therefore, the administration of a single large dose of the antibiotic would allow higher serum peak levels and less exposure of the tubular cells to the drug. An additional positive feature of OD dosing regimens is an improvement in the post-antibiotic effect: Antibiotic efficacy persists even after the blood level of the drug falls below minimal inhibitory concentration. Of note, the extent of cortical uptake mechanism saturation is different among the different aminoglycosides. It is higher for gentamicin, less saturable for amika-

TABLE 58-2

Maneuvers to Avoid or Minimize Aminoglycoside-Induced Nephrotoxicity

- Use the lowest dose and the shortest course of aminoglycoside treatment that will be clinically effective.
- Ensure adequate hydration and sodium repletion before initiation of drug administration.
- Correct possible electrolyte and acid-base abnormalities.
- Assiduously avoid the concomitant use of other nephrotoxic drugs.
- Use a once-a-day dosing regimen.
- Avoid drug administration in the resting period (midnight to 7:30 AM).
- Adjust drug interval administration in accordance with renal function.

cin and netilmicin, and almost not saturable for tobramycin. Several randomized studies and meta-analyses have compared the efficacy and safety of OD versus MD regimens in adults and children. The results show better or comparable efficacy and decreased or similar nephrotoxicity for the OD schedules, with an overall trend for lower nephrotoxicity and better efficacy in this group.[12-14] The OD approach also is more cost-effective and convenient for hospital administration of the antibiotic. Another potential strategy to minimize aminoglycoside nephrotoxicity is related to its circadian variation. Gentamicin and tobramycin nephrotoxic effects were more intense when the drugs were administered in the resting period (midnight to 7:30 AM) than when they were given during the period ranging from 8 AM to 11:30 PM.[12,15] Finally, pharmacokinetic dosing based on therapeutic drug monitoring also has been advocated as a possible approach to decrease aminoglycoside nephrotoxicity. The efficacy of this maneuver has not been consistently established, however, with different studies generating conflicting results.[12] A summary of recommendations for the prevention of aminoglycoside-induced AKI is presented in Table 58-2.

Vancomycin

Vancomycin is a tricyclic glycopeptide antibiotic extremely effective against gram-positive bacteria, which was introduced into the clinical practice in the 1950s. It is the drug of choice for treatment of methicillin-resistant *Staphylococcus aureus* and coagulase-negative staphylococcal infections and has largely been employed for therapy of endocarditis due to gram-positive organisms and for the empirical treatment of intravascular catheter–induced infections. The increasing nosocomial and community prevalence of gram-positive bacteria has been an important additional indication for its use.

Vancomycin is not absorbed orally and should be given slowly by the intravenous route. It has a complex pharmacokinetics, with a large intraindividual variation in clearance and distribution volume. Approximately 30% of the drug binds to serum protein; its main excretion route is through glomerular filtration as an unchanged drug, and 20% to 30% undergoes nonrenal excretion. Although vancomycin administration must be adjusted in accordance with renal function, failure to account for nonrenal excretion of the drug may lead to underestimation of the dose needed to achieve blood therapeutic levels.[16] Currently, the recommended vancomycin trough level is between 15 and 20 µg/mL.[17] Monitoring of vancomycin serum concentration is recommended in patients with renal impairment, in children, and in the elderly.

The true frequency of vancomycin nephrotoxicity (manifested as elevation in serum creatinine) is in dispute, with reported rates ranging from 5% to approximately 15% when the drug is used alone.[16-18] The mechanisms leading to renal injury have been poorly studied. The drug probably enters the tubular epithelial cells across the basolateral membranes, and acute tubular necrosis in patients receiving this drug has been described.[19] When vancomycin is administered concomitantly with aminoglycosides, the occurrence of nephrotoxicity increases, often reaching frequencies over 20%.[16] Of course, patients receiving this kind of therapy frequently are severely ill, with many concomitant confounding factors that may precipitate AKI. Serum peak levels greater than 40 µg/mL, trough levels greater than 10 µg/mL, prolonged vancomycin therapy (for longer than 21 days), preexisting renal insufficiency, dehydration, and older age also have been related to increased vancomycin-induced nephrotoxicity.[16,17,20] Although the results reported in the literature are not consistent, vancomycin drug monitoring has been shown to decrease vancomycin nephrotoxicity.[21]

Teicoplanin is a glycopeptide antibiotic with an antibacterial profile similar to that of vancomycin. Available studies show that nephrotoxicity is less likely with teicoplanin, even when used in association with an aminoglycoside.[16,18] This drug should be considered as a therapeutic option in patients at risk for the development of vancomycin-induced nephrotoxicity.

Two newer antibiotics have been developed for treatment of resistant gram-positive cocci: linezolid and quinupristin-dalfopristin. Both were not considered nephrotoxic in controlled studies, but they are costly and have other significant side effects. Recently, however, a multivariate analysis suggested that the introduction of linezolid in a surgical ICU was an independent factor for decreasing the risk of severe kidney failure.[22]

Amphotericin B

Since its introduction into clinical practice in 1956, amphotericin B, a polyene antibiotic, remains the most efficient antifungal agent known, and its use continues to have important clinical relevance. In fact, an impressive increase in the number of nosocomial fungal infections was observed after the 1980s, probably reflecting the emergence of acquired immunodeficiency syndrome (AIDS) and the increment of immunosuppressed transplant recipients and patients with cancer.

Amphotericin B is an extremely nephrotoxic antibiotic. It affects the membrane permeability of proximal tubule cells and induces vasoconstriction of intrarenal arteries and afferent arterioles. These effects lead to impaired handling of electrolytes, impaired renal concentrating and acidification mechanisms, and structural tubular epithelial cell injury. Amphotericin B also promotes increases in intrarenal vascular resistance and decreases in renal plasma flow and GFR. Clinically, the tubular lesion manifests as polyuria, hypokalemia, hypomagnesemia, and tubular acidosis occurring 7 to 14 days after the initiation of drug therapy. These changes usually are followed by a decrease in GFR, evidenced as increased serum creatinine. Histologically, the lesion is characterized by acute tubular

TABLE 58-3

Risk Factors for Amphotericin B Nephrotoxicity

MODIFIABLE	NONMODIFIABLE
Elevated daily dose	Older age
Elevated cumulative dose	Male gender
Sodium depletion	Obesity
Dehydration	Previous renal dysfunction
Simultaneous use of diuretics	Sepsis
Simultaneous use of other	Diabetes mellitus
nephrotoxins	Heart failure
Hypokalemia	
Hypomagnesemia	

injury, with tubular dilatation, proximal tubule cell necrosis, and calcification and unspecific vacuolization of medium-sized and small arteries and arterioles. Amphotericin-induced kidney injury is dose- and time-dependent, and nephrotoxicity rates of 33% up to 80% have been reported. Cumulative total doses above 2 to 3 g invariably cause kidney injury. Renal function usually recovers with drug discontinuation, but improvement may take months, especially if amphotericin doses greater than 4 g were used. Chronic renal dysfunction has been described in patients submitted to recurring exposures to amphotericin. Numerous risk factors for amphotericin nephrotoxicity have been described: larger drug dose, older age, male gender, obesity, previous renal dysfunction, diabetes, heart failure, concomitant use of other nephrotoxic drugs, simultaneous use of diuretics, sodium depletion, dehydration, sepsis, hypokalemia, and hypomagnesemia[23-25] (Table 58-3).

Although generally reversible, amphotericin-induced kidney injury is not a benign complication. In fact, it was consistently associated with higher mortality and trends to increased hospital length of stay and costs.[26-28] Several preventive maneuvers to minimize or avoid the nephrotoxicity of this agent have been proposed. The clinical use of mannitol or furosemide in this context was not effective, and the clinical efficacy of calcium channel blockers has not been established. Extracellular volume expansion with intravenous saline administration or generous use of oral rehydration solution was consistently effective in the prevention or minimization of amphotericin-induced creatinine increase but did not prevent drug-induced tubular toxicity.[12,29,30] Amphotericin is an extremely hydrophobic molecule, and deoxycholate, the vehicle used for its solubilization, has nephrotoxic properties. Accordingly, liposomal formulations of amphotericin, which do not include deoxycholate, were developed (amphotericin B lipid complex [ABLC], amphotericin B colloid dispersion, and liposomal amphotericin B [L-AmB]). Several studies have thereafter always shown significantly less nephrotoxicity (hemodynamic and tubular) and at least the same efficacy with the liposomal preparations as compared with the conventional formulation..[12,13,31] Recently, a pharmacology surveillance study in Spain showed that ABLC presented low nephrotoxicity potential even in patients with preexisting renal dysfunction.[32] Finally, new antifungal compounds similar in efficacy to amphotericin but with less nephrotoxicity were developed. Caspofungin and voriconazole have showed prevalence of nephrotoxicity 3 to 6 times lower than amphotericin B in controlled studies,

TABLE 58-4

Potentially Useful Strategies to Prevent Amphotericin B–Induced Nephrotoxicity

- Correct avoidable risk factors, if present.
- Administer up to 1 L of saline intravenously daily, or provide vigorous administration of rehydration solution, in accordance with the clinical limitations of the patient. Always begin this expansion protocol before initiation of amphotericin treatment, and maintain hydration throughout the treatment course.
- In patients with preexisting renal dysfunction or those at high risk for renal injury, use liposomal amphotericin preparations.
- Likewise, consider the use of caspofungin or voriconazole in patients with preexisting renal dysfunction or those at high risk for nephrotoxicity.
- Remember that with amphotericin-induced nephrotoxicity, electrolyte changes frequently precede an increase in serum creatinine level.

and the introduction of these compounds in an ICU was an independent factor for a reduced need for renal replacement therapy in this population of patients.[33] Table 58-4 lists some potentially useful strategies for the prevention of amphotericin B–induced nephrotoxicity.

Polymyxins

Polymyxins constitute a class of antibiotics, discovered in the late 1940s, characterized by their extreme efficiency against gram-negative bacteria. Of the five polymyxins (A, B, C, D, and E), only polymyxin B and polymixin E (colistin) have been introduced into clinical practice. Each of these agents is an amphipathic (having both lipophilic and hydrophilic characteristics), cyclic cationic decapeptide with a molecular weight of approximately 1200 g/mmol. In the 1970s and 1980s, their use was virtually neglected owing to the introduction of new and allegedly safer broad-spectrum antibacterial antibiotics. The 1990s, however, saw a striking emergence of hospital multidrug-resistant gram-negative bacteria (especially *Pseudomonas aeruginosa* and *Acinetobacter baumannii*), which was even more notable in ICUs. This development, coupled with the lack of other efficient options for treatment of these infections, has renewed interest in the polymyxins. They are commercially available for parenteral use in systemic infections as colistimethate sodium (colistin) and polymyxin B sulfate. Their dosage must be corrected in patients with decreased GFR. The role of dialysis in polymyxin excretion needs to be determined. Of note, most of the available clinical data on polymyxins come from studies with colistin.[34,35]

Nephrotoxicity, characterized by decreased creatinine clearance or increased serum creatinine or blood urea nitrogen (BUN), has been reported in both experimental and clinical studies of polymyxins. Oliguria, hematuria, proteinuria, and cylindruria also have been reported. Putatively, the nephrotoxicity has been attributed to changes in cell membrane permeability that ultimately led to cell swelling and lysis. Acute tubular necrosis has been described in polymyxin-induced nephrotoxicity.[34] Early series of patients who received polymyxin treatment revealed high prevalence rates of nephrotoxicity (up to

50%, depending on the definition of renal injury and characteristics of the patients studied), and at this time a relatively high number of polymyxin-induced acute kidney injury case reports were reported in the literature. Many such reports referred to intramuscular administration of colistimethate sodium in daily doses considerably higher than those used in modern practice. Although available data were limited, polymyxin B was reported to be more nephrotoxic than colistin.[34,35] In more recent studies, the prevalence of polymyxin-induced nephrotoxicity was lower than that reported in the older series, and the allegedly greater nephrotoxicity of polymyxin B was not confirmed.[34-36] For instance, acute kidney injury developed in 22% of 114 patients who received polymyxin B for 3 days or longer in a university hospital setting. Abnormal baseline creatinine, need for vasoactive drugs, and abdomen, blood, catheter, or lung as site of infection were identified as independent risk factors for polymyxin B–induced nephrotoxicity in this cohort.[37]

Patients taking polymyxins should undergo baseline and frequent serial measurements of renal function, and drug dosage should be corrected in accordance with the results of such testing. Concomitant use of other nephrotoxic drugs should be carefully avoided, and patients must be adequately hydrated. Specific measures to minimize or prevent polymyxin-induced renal injury are thus far unknown.

Highly Active Antiretroviral Therapy

The combination of drugs used in HAART has become extremely important over the past decade owing to its success in therapy for human immunodeficiency virus (HIV)-infected patients. In general, the HAART regimen includes a combination of two nucleotide reverse transcriptase inhibitors with a protease inhibitor or a combination of three reverse transcriptase inhibitors. Many of these agents may induce clinically significant nephrotoxicity, manifested as acute kidney injury, nephrolithiasis, acute tubular toxicity, Fanconi syndrome, nephrogenic diabetes insipidus, and renal tubular acidosis.[38,39]

Indinavir, first introduced in 1966, is the most widely used protease inhibitor for treatment of HIV infection. Approximately 20% of the drug is excreted in the urine, of which 11% is eliminated as unchanged drug. Indinavir has a very low solubility at physiological urine pH (pH 6), facilitating its intratubular precipitation and the possibility of intrarenal obstruction. The frequency of nephrological or urological signs and symptoms reported with indinavir is 10 times higher than for other protease inhibitors. Asymptomatic crystalluria, hematuria, nephrolithiasis, increases in serum creatinine, oliguric AKI (with or without obstructive renal calculi), chronic kidney disease, and papillary necrosis all have been reported. AKI preceded by persistent sterile leukocyturia has been described in 18% to 33% of patients receiving the drug. The renal dysfunction usually has been mild and reversible on cessation of indinavir therapy. Patients developing renal injury usually received individual doses higher than recommended. Findings on the few available reports of renal biopsy included interstitial inflammation, tubular atrophy, interstitial fibrosis, presence of indinavir crystals in the tubular lumen, and mesangial hypercellularity. The mechanism of renal injury probably is related to drug deposition in renal tissue. Risk factors suggested for indinavir nephrotoxicity include dehydration, low lean body mass, warm environmental temperature, daily indinavir dosages greater than 1 g, and minimal HIV-1 RNA at the beginning of therapy. Although its solubility increases in acid urine, urinary acidification is not recommended in patients receiving this drug.[38-40] At the moment, a reasonable approach is to advise copious fluid ingestion and to avoid daily doses greater than 1 g in patients receiving indinavir.

Early increases in serum creatinine and dialysis-dependent acute kidney injury also were reported with use of another protease inhibitor, ritonavir. Acute tubular necrosis and proximal tubular dysfunction were described with the nucleotide reverse transcriptase inhibitors tenofovir and adefovir.[38,39,41,42]

Iodinated Contrast Media

Intravascular administration of iodinated contrast media for radiodiagnosis is considered one of the most common causes of AKI in the hospital setting. The reported prevalence of contrast agent–induced nephropathy ranges from zero to 90%, depending mainly on the characteristics of the study population, the definition of renal injury and methodology for its assessment, and the interval between contrast administration and renal function evaluation. In an interesting critical literature analysis, Rao and Newhouse[43] reviewed 3081 publications from 1966 to 2004 on contrast agent–induced nephropathy. Only 40 of these reports studied patients after intravenous contrast administration, and all of the others focused on other kinds of procedures involving exposure to contrast, mainly cardiac catheterization. Only 2 of these 40 studies included a control group of patients not receiving contrast. Consequently, much of the available data about contrast nephropathy comes from angiographic cardiac studies in which important factors contributing to potential confusion may be related to creatinine changes (e.g., fluid restriction, arrhythmias, hypotension, hemorrhage) and from studies without appropriate control groups. Data from cardiac catheterization should not be extrapolated to intravenous contrast administration. Nevertheless, because approximately 10 million procedures using intravascular contrast are performed each year in the United States, even a 0.1% incidence would result in 10,000 cases of contrast agent–induced nephropathy each year. Even more important, contrast agent–induced serum creatinine increase has been shown to be an independent factor for increased risk of death.[44,45]

The mechanisms of contrast agent–induced nephropathy are not clearly understood. The injury probably is multifactorial and related to hemodynamic impairment, tubular cell injury, and intraluminal tubular obstruction. After contrast administration, an early and transient vasodilation occurs, followed by vasoconstriction maintained in the renal vasculature and contraction of mesangial cells. This change in vascular tonus has been related to the effects of calcium, prostaglandins, adenosine, endothelin, nitric oxide, and free radicals. Tubular injury has been demonstrated by an increase in urinary enzymes and by the changes of acute tubular necrosis on renal histologic examination. Finally, contrast may cause tubular obstruction by Tamm-Horsfall proteins and oxalate or urate crystal precipitation.[46]

The clinical picture in contrast agent–induced nephropathy may vary, ranging in severity from mild renal dysfunction to dialysis-dependent AKI. Serum creatinine usually increases 48 to 72 hours after contrast administration and returns to baseline around post-exposure day 10, although prolonged renal impairment for up to 2 to 4 weeks is possible. Urinary sediment may show tubular epithelial cells, casts, and calcium oxalate or urate crystals. Fractional excretion of sodium and urinary sodium concentration may be low. Continued visualization of the kidney at 24 to 48 hours after contrast injection is a sensitive indicator of contrast agent–induced nephropathy.[47]

Several risk factors have been correlated with contrast agent–induced nephropathy. Of these, abnormal baseline creatinine is clearly the most important. In patients with diabetes and pre-contrast increased serum creatinine, the risk is considered even higher, whereas results for diabetes alone as a risk factor are not consistent. Other known risk factors for contrast agent–induced nephropathy are increased age, intravascular volume depletion, heart failure, contrast volume greater than 125 mL, repeated contrast exposure, concomitant use of other nephrotoxic drugs, proteinuria, hyperuricemia, liver disease, and multiple myeloma.[48,49]

The first and most obvious preventive strategy is to avoid exposure to contrast agents. In high-risk patients, imaging studies requiring contrast should be replaced if possible by alternative diagnostic methods. Early identification of high-risk patients followed by judicious assessment of the actual need for the test with contrast is essential. Other logical preventive approaches are to use the lowest possible amount of contrast, to avoid repeated exposure to contrast in a short interval of time, to delay performance of an additonal contrast procedure until serum creatinine returns to baseline values, and to cease use of potentially nephrotoxic drugs before contrast administration. Patients at high risk who will receive contrast must be adequately hydrated. Diuretics of any kind should be avoided in these patients. Although mannitol and furosemide have shown protection against contrast agent–induced nephrotoxicity in animal experiments, these results have not been clinically confirmed. In fact, the clinical use of prophylactic furosemide or mannitol worsens contrast agent–induced nephropathy.

Robust evidence suggests that infusion of normal saline started before contrast administration and continued during and after the procedure will minimize the risk of contrast agent–induced nephropathy.[50,51] As an alternative, preventive infusion of sodium bicarbonate also has shown efficacy in prevention of this complication.[51,52] The use of low-osmolality or iso-osmolality nonionic contrast agents was beneficial in diabetic patients with preexisting renal insufficiency.[13,50,53,54] N-acetylcysteine, a free radical scavenger with vasodilating properties, probably is the most studied agent for contrast agent–induced nephropathy prevention. Its reduced cost, safety, and putative efficacy have made N-acetylcysteine administration an increasingly popular prophylaxis strategy. Results of different meta-analyses showed conflicting results, however, and the available data do not allow definitive conclusions about the efficacy of N-acetylcysteine in the prevention of contrast agent–induced nephropathy.[50,55-57]

Two randomized trials showed that preventive hemofiltration started before contrast administration has dramatically decreased the incidence of contrast agent–induced nephropathy and late mortality in patients with impaired renal function undergoing contrast procedures, whereas protocols using prophylactic hemodialysis were inefficient or even harmful.[58,59] Table 58-5 summarizes the recommendations for prevention of contrast agent–induced nephrotoxicity.

TABLE 58-5

Possible Strategies for Prophylaxis of Contrast Agent–Induced Nephropathy

- Evaluate the patient for risk factors for contrast nephropathy.
- Consider the use of an alternative diagnostic procedure in high-risk patients.
- Use the lowest possible amount of contrast, avoid repeated exposures in a short period of time, and wait for serum creatinine to return to baseline values before resubmitting the patient to a new contrasted procedure.
- Discontinue, if feasible, the use of potentially nephrotoxic drugs before contrast administration.
- Do not give diuretics as a prophylactic maneuver; discontinue these agents given for other reasons, if possible, before contrast administration.
- Start infusion of normal saline approximately 12 hours before contrast (*suggested volume*: 1 mL/kg per hour); continue for 6 to 12 hours *after* performance of the contrast procedure.
- Consider infusion of sodium bicarbonate as a possible alternative to saline infusion (intravenous dextrose 5% in water plus sodium bicarbonate, 154 mEq/kg), 3 mL/kg starting 1 hour before and continuing up to 6 hours *after* completion of the procedure.

NONSTEROIDAL ANTI-INFLAMMATORY DRUGS

NSAIDs are widely used for their anti-inflammatory and pain relief properties in different settings, including the ICU. This class of drugs can induce many different kinds of renal injury: hemodynamically mediated AKI, acute interstitial nephritis plus nephrotic syndrome, nephrotic syndrome without AKI, papillary necrosis, cortical necrosis, chronic kidney disease, sodium retention, hyperkalemia, impaired tubular diluting mechanisms, and hypertension.[60]

The most typical nephrotoxic effect seen with NSAIDs is hemodynamically mediated AKI. These drugs act through the blockade of cyclooxygenases. Cyclooxygenase-synthesized vasodilating prostaglandins, however, are crucial for the preservation of renal blood flow and GFR during adverse systemic and renal hemodynamic conditions. Such conditions and disorders include hypovolemia, salt depletion, use of diuretics, hypotension, heart failure, liver injury, nephrotic syndrome, sepsis, postoperative period, chronic kidney disease, hypertension, older age, diabetes, urinary obstruction, concomitant use of other nephrotoxic agents inducing afferent arteriole vasoconstriction (e.g., contrast agents, calcineurin blockers), and drugs that may alter renal hemodynamics, such as ACE inhibitors and angiotension receptor blockers. All of these conditions, and often their combination, may be present in critically ill patients in general, including those in the ICU. NSAID-induced blockade of prostaglandin synthesis in these conditions can cause abrupt and dramatic renal impairment, clinically manifested as AKI. This kind of NSAID-induced nephrotoxicity is characterized by sudden increases in BUN and serum creatinine, oliguria, and low fractional excretion of sodium (less than 1%), but with normal urinary sediment. Disproportional hyperkalemia in relation to the degree of renal insufficiency may occur. NSAID discontinuation usually is followed by rapid recovery of renal function, but progression to irreversible chronic renal disease has been described. NSAID-induced nephrotoxicity can occur after parenteral, oral, and even topical use of these agents.[60,61] Moreover, the newer specific COX-2 inhibitors, such as celecoxib and rofecoxib, promote renal dysfunction by mechanisms similar to those for nonspecific COX inhibitors.[62]

Several effective drugs without the unfavorable renal profile of the NSAIDs are available to promote analgesia. The use of NSAIDs, therefore, should be avoided in critically ill patients at risk for or with already impaired kidney dysfunction.[12]

ANGIOTENSIN-CONVERTING ENZYME INHIBITORS AND ANGIOTENSIN RECEPTOR BLOCKERS

ACE inhibitors and angiotensin receptor blockers are extensively used nowadays owing to their efficacy in the treatment of hypertension and congestive heart failure and in the prevention of diabetic nephropathy and antiproteinuric effects in glomerulopathies. Ironically, although considered renal-protective drugs, ACE inhibitors and angiotensin receptor blockers may cause AKI.[63,64] The true extent of acute renal impairment induced by these drugs is difficult to determine, but many case reports and studies of patients with ACE inhibitor– or angiotensin receptor blocker–induced nephrotoxicity can be found in the literature. Recently, Stirling and coworkers studied 2398 consecutive patients presenting to an acute medical unit. Eighty-nine (3.7%) patients were hospitalized with abnormal serum creatinine. Excluding 9 patients on chronic dialysis, 37.5% of the remaining 80 patients were on ACE inhibitors. Drug withdrawal and fluid replacement returned serum creatinine to baseline values.[65]

These agents cause renal dysfunction in clinical situations in which angiotensin II–dependent efferent arteriole vasoconstriction is essential to maintain the intraglomerular capillary pressure[65-67] (Table 58-6). Blockade of the renin-angiotensin system in such instances may cause a sharp and abrupt decline in GFR. In patients at risk for the development of ACE inhibitor– or angiotensin receptor

TABLE 58-6

Factors Potentially Associated with Angiotensin-Converting Enzyme Inhibitor/Angiotensin Receptor Blocker–Induced Acute Kidney Injury

- Significant renal artery stenosis (>70% occlusion), either bilateral or affecting a single functioning kidney
- Severe congestive heart failure
- Severe intrarenal vasculopathy
- Older age
- Chronic kidney disease with impaired GFR
- Concomitant use of drugs inducing intrarenal vasoconstriction (e.g., cyclosporin, tacrolimus, NSAIDs, contrast agents)
- Hypotension
- Hypovolemia (from hemorrhage, diarrhea, vomiting, other).
- Concomitant use of diuretics
- Salt depletion

GFR, glomerular filtration rate; NSAIDs, nonsteroidal anti-inflammatory drugs.

blocker–induced nephrotoxicity, renal function should be carefully evaluated before initiation of the drug and periodically thereafter, and modifiable risk factors should be managed appropriately. Renal function usually recovers rapidly after drug withdrawal, confirming the functional pattern of the injury. In patients with previous chronic kidney disease, however, renal function loss may be irreversible. Renal artery thrombosis should be suspected in anuric patients or in those with unsatisfactory renal function recovery. ACE inhibitors may cause severe hyperkalemia in patients taking beta-blockers, NSAIDs, or potassium-sparing diuretics.

Key Points

1. The most effective way to prevent drug nephrotoxicity is not to use a potentially offending drug. Always consider use of a non-nephrotoxic drug over one with a known adverse effect on kidney function, or select a diagnostic test that does not require use of a nephrotoxic agent in patients at higher risk for renal injury.
2. Assess renal function before and periodically after the administration of a potentially nephrotoxic drug.
3. Always ensure adequate hydration and sodium repletion before institution of a potentially nephrotoxic drug.

4. Correct drug dosage in accordance with preexisting organ dysfunction, extracellular volume status, and specific aspects of the drug's pharmacokinetics.
5. Always check for the possibility of a specific maneuver to prevent or attenuate a particular drug's nephrotoxicity.

Key References

5. Pea F, Viale P, Furlanut M: Antimicrobial therapy in critically ill patients: A review of pathophysiological conditions responsible for altered disposition and pharmacokinetic variability. Clin Pharmacokinet 2005;44:1009-1034.
12. Schetz M, Dasta J, Goldstein S, Golper T: Drug-induced acute kidney injury. Curr Opin Crit Care 2005;11:555-565.
34. Falagas ME, Kasiakou SK: Toxicity of polymyxins: A systematic review of the evidence from old and recent studies. Crit Care 2006;10:R27.
43. Rao QA, Newhouse JH: Risk of nephropathy after intravenous administration of contrast material: A critical literature analysis. Radiology 2006;239:392-397.
66. Cruz CS, Cruz LS, Silva GR, Marcilio de Souza CA: Incidence and predictors of development of acute renal failure related to treatment of congestive heart failure with ACE inhibitors. Nephron Clin Pract 2007;105:c77-c83.

See the companion Expert Consult website for the complete reference list.

CHAPTER 59

Acute Renal Failure in Pregnancy

Hilary S. Gammill and Arundhathi Jeyabalan

OBJECTIVES

This chapter will:
1. Outline the epidemiology of pregnancy-related acute renal failure.
2. Describe the physiological changes that occur in the kidney secondary to pregnancy.
3. Review fetal considerations in the setting of acute renal failure in the mother.
4. Discuss the etiology of pregnancy-related acute renal failure, including pregnancy-specific diseases such as preeclampsia.
5. Present an evidence-based approach to the diagnosis and therapy of pregnancy-related acute renal failure.

multidisciplinary approach is recommended in the care of these women, including specialists in the fields of maternal-fetal medicine, critical care medicine, nephrology, and neonatology.

Although pregnancy-related ARF has become a rare occurrence in the developed world, it continues to be associated with significant mortality and long-term morbidity. The societal impact of this is particularly pronounced on account of the young and productive status of these women.

EPIDEMIOLOGY OF ACUTE RENAL FAILURE IN PREGNANCY

Acute renal failure (ARF) in the context of pregnancy presents a clinical challenge. The number of diagnostic possibilities increases, and therapeutic options vary. Maternal physiological alterations and fetal implications also must be considered. In view of this complexity, a

In the pregnancy literature, *acute renal failure* has been variably defined, ranging from serum creatinine levels of greater than 0.8 mg/dL to dialysis requirement. This variability renders comparison across epidemiological studies difficult. Furthermore, populations vary significantly in demographics, referral base, and standard of care. Despite these statistical limitations, general epidemiological trends in pregnancy-related ARF can be recognized.

Since the 1960s, the overall incidence of ARF in pregnancy has decreased from 1 case per 3000 to a range of 1 per 15,000 to 1 per 20,000. Similarly, the proportion of total cases of ARF related to pregnancy fell from a range of 20% to 40% in the 1960s to 2% to 10% in the 1980s.[1-3] Coincident with these declines, little change has occurred in the overall mortality and long-term morbidity rates. From the 1950s through the 1990s, overall mortality rates ranged from zero to 30%, with no clear trend over time.[2-5] The consistent mortality rates may be attributable to increased efficiency in the developed world in preventing cases of straightforward ARF, with an associated shift toward higher acuity in the remaining cases. The patients in whom renal failure continues to develop often have multisystem organ dysfunction and a high level of complexity.[3] Long-term prognosis also has remained fairly consistent over time, with reported rates for full recovery of renal function between 60% and 90%.[2,4,5]

The overall decrease in incidence has been attributed to two main trends. First, the legalization of abortion in most developed countries has resulted in a decline in septic abortions. Second, improvements in accessible prenatal care have allowed for improved surveillance for preeclampsia and other obstetrical complications. These causes account for a substantial proportion of cases of pregnancy-related ARF.[2,3]

In the developing world, and in other populations with limited access to health care, pregnancy-related ARF continues to be a major problem, with associated higher mortality and morbidity rates. Epidemiological data from India suggest that pregnancy-related ARF continues to account for 20% of total ARF cases and that mortality rates remain as high as 50%.[6,7] In an inner-city population in Atlanta, a low renal function recovery rate of approximately 50% raises concerns about access to care in certain populations in the United States.[8]

In addition to the estimated impact of pregnancy-related ARF in previously healthy patients, it is well known that in women with underlying chronic renal dysfunction (baseline serum creatinine greater than 1.4 mg/dL), the risk of pregnancy-related loss of renal function is significantly increased at 43%, and an estimated 10% of patients experience rapid deterioration in renal function.[9]

In acute care settings, the primary clinical focus centers on early and optimal intervention to limit renal damage and to minimize both immediate and long-term morbidity and mortality. An evidence-based and scientifically founded approach to the acute management of pregnancy-related ARF is presented later in the chapter.

To optimize acute care for pregnant women, it is crucial to build on an understanding of the physiological changes to the renal system in pregnancy, so the following discussion begins with a consideration of these adaptations. In any acutely ill pregnant patient, one of the most substantial challenges is in caring for both the mother and her fetus. As described in a later section, pregnancy has specific influences on disease processes and on the effect of disease and treatment in the fetus. Also discussed are principles that underlie the balance between what at times may be opposing maternal and fetal goals. A discussion of the common causative disorders associated with pregnancy-related ARF, as well as a review of current evidence regarding efficacy and suitability of diagnostic

and therapeutic options for ARF in pregnancy, also is included.

RENAL PHYSIOLOGY: ALTERATIONS IN PREGNANCY

An understanding of maternal cardiovascular and renal adaptations to pregnancy is fundamental to the appropriate clinical management of normal pregnancy, renal disorders in the gravid patient, and pregnancy-specific conditions such as preeclampsia.

Anatomical Changes of the Upper Urinary Tract

Marked changes occur in the renal vascular and interstitial volume coincident with an increase in total blood volume during normal pregnancy. The renal volume increases by as much as 30%, and the overall dimensions of the kidney increase by approximately 1 cm.[10,11]

In addition, significant dilatation of the renal calyces, pelvis, and ureters is seen. This pregnancy-induced dilatation of the renal collecting system leads to a physiological hydronephrosis and hydroureter in 80% of women by midgestation.[12] Dilatation of the right ureter is more common than on the left during pregnancy.[13] The likely primary etiological disorder is mechanical compression by the enlarging gravid uterus and the ovarian venous plexus.[12] The dextrorotation of the uterus and the presence of the sigmoid colon in the left pelvis may explain the asymmetrical dilatation. The effects of progesterone and other pregnancy hormones on these anatomical changes are unclear. Progesterone may contribute to smooth muscle relaxation and possibly ureteral dilatation[14]; however, some investigators have demonstrated no correlation between the degree of ureteral dilatation and progesterone concentrations.[15]

Systemic Cardiovascular Changes

Normal pregnancy is accompanied by dramatic cardiovascular changes. Because of the relevance of such changes to renal function and dysfunction in pregnancy, a brief review is presented here. (The reader is referred to *Chesley's Hypertension in Pregnancy* for a detailed review of this topic.[16]) During normal pregnancy, systemic vascular resistance is markedly reduced, whereas total blood volume and cardiac output are increased by approximately 50%.[16,17] Both increased plasma volume and, to a lesser degree, red blood cell volume contribute to the expansion in total blood volume. The gradual increase in plasma volume is achieved by a net retention of 900 to 950 mEq of sodium over the course of gestation. This net sodium reabsorption occurs at the level of the renal tubule despite a large filtered load.

A physiological decrease in plasma osmolality also occurs in early pregnancy, reaching its nadir at approximately 10 weeks' gestation and then remaining stable for the remainder of pregnancy. The vasopressin response around this altered threshold is appropriate, suggesting that a "resetting of the osmostat" occurs during pregnancy.[18]

Renal Hemodynamic Alterations during Pregnancy

Both glomerular filtration rate (GFR) and renal plasma flow (RPF) increase markedly in normal pregnancy. As determined by a compilation of data from rigorously selected studies, GFR and effective RPF were increased by 40% to 65% and 50% to 85%, respectively, in the first half of gestation[16] (Fig. 59-1). These studies are notable because (1) GFR and RPF were measured using the gold standard of renal clearance of inulin and para-aminohippurate, respectively; (2) GFR and RPF were compared with pre-pregnant or postpartum values; and (3) effort was made to minimize urinary tract dead space.[16] During pregnancy, RPF rises more substantially than GFR, resulting in a reduced filtration fraction (GFR/RPF). In the late third trimester, RPF declines while GFR is maintained.

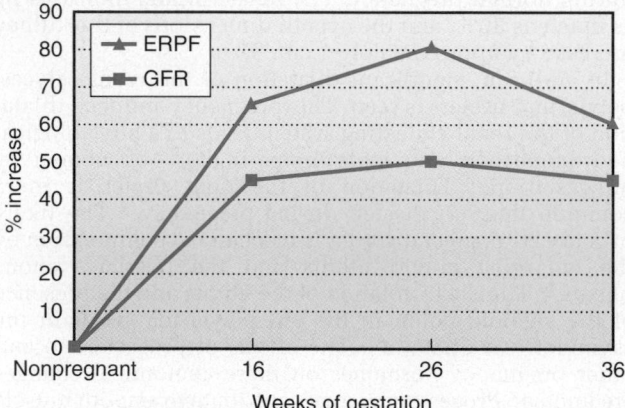

FIGURE 59-1. Glomerular filtration rate (GFR) and effective renal plasma flow (ERPF) during pregnancy. (Data from Conrad KP, Lindheimer MD: Renal and cardiovascular alterations. In Lindheimer MD, Cunningham FG, Roberts JM [eds]: Chesley's Hypertensive Disorders in Pregnancy, 2nd ed. Stamford, Conn, Appleton & Lange, 1999, pp 263-326.)

Creatinine clearance, measured by 24-hour urine collection, is used clinically to assess renal function and estimate GFR during pregnancy. Although endogenous creatinine is both filtered at the level of the glomerulus and secreted by the proximal tubule, creatinine clearance is a reliable measure of GFR during pregnancy.[16,19] The normal creatinine clearance during pregnancy ranges from 100 to 200 mL/minute (Table 59-1). With renal disease and markedly reduced GFR, however, creatinine clearance may overestimate the actual GFR. Using 24-hour urine collection to estimate GFR, Davison and Noble[20] have demonstrated that the GFR increases by 25% by the fourth week after the last menstrual period and by 45% at approximately 9 weeks' gestation. These renal hemodynamic alterations are among the earliest and most dramatic maternal adaptations to pregnancy.

Other commonly used markers for renal function are serum creatinine and blood urea nitrogen (BUN). Both are reduced during pregnancy secondary to the elevated GFR. Average values for serum creatinine and BUN are 0.5 mg/dL and 9.0 mg/dL (see Table 59-1), respectively, in pregnant women, compared with mean values of 0.8 mg/dL and 13.0 mg/dL in nonpregnant women.[16] Circulating creatinine levels are determined by the balance of skeletal muscle production and urinary excretion. In pregnancy, GFR is markedly increased, whereas skeletal muscle production is relatively constant, resulting in reduced serum creatinine levels. Urea also is freely filtered at the glomerulus, and levels are reduced in normal pregnancy, but its handling by the kidney is more complex and discussed in detail later ("Renal Handling of Uric Acid in Pregnancy").

Mechanisms Underlying Renal Hemodynamic Alterations during Pregnancy

The precise mechanisms underlying the renal hemodynamic changes in pregnancy are not completely understood. Reduced renal vascular resistance is likely to be primarily responsible for the increased blood flow to the kidney. The increased blood flow also results in increased

TABLE 59-1

Normal Laboratory Parameters in Pregnancy

VARIABLE	CHANGE COMPARED WITH NONPREGNANT VALUES	NORMAL VALUE IN PREGNANCY
Creatinine	↓	0.5 mg/dL
BUN	↓	9.0 mg/dL
GFR	↑	↑ ~40-65% above baseline
Creatinine clearance	↑	↑ ~25% above baseline
Uric acid	↓	2.0-3.0 mg/dL
Urinary protein excretion	Variable to ↑	<300 mg/24 hours
Urinary albumin excretion	Variable to ↑	<20 mg/24 hours
Sodium retention over pregnancy	↑	900-950 mEq
Plasma osmolality	↓	↓ ~10 mOsm/kg H_2O
P_{CO_2}	↓	↓ ~10 mm Hg below baseline
Serum bicarbonate	↓	18-20 mEq/L
Urinary glucose excretion	Variable to ↑	Variable

BUN, blood urea nitrogen; GFR, glomerular filtration rate; P_{CO_2}, partial pressure of carbon dioxide.
Data from Conrad KP, Lindheimer MD: Renal and cardiovascular alterations. In Lindheimer MD, Cunningham FG, Roberts JM (eds): Chesley's Hypertensive Disorders in Pregnancy, 2nd ed. Stamford, Conn, Appleton & Lange, 1999, pp 263-326; and from Asrat T, Nageotte M: Acute renal failure in pregnancy. In Foley MR, Strong TH Jr, Garite TJ (eds): Obstetric Intensive Care Manual, 2nd ed. New York, McGraw-Hill Professional, 2004, pp 184-195.

GFR. These alterations occur quite early in gestation, even preceding the early gestational changes in plasma volume and cardiac output, thereby anticipating the future needs of the growing fetoplacental unit.[18,21]

Because of ethical and feasibility issues limiting experimental studies in pregnant women, animal models have been used to investigate the mechanisms underlying renal adaptations during pregnancy. The gravid rat has been used extensively, owing to renal, cardiovascular, and endocrine changes that are comparable with those seen in human pregnancy.[22] Micropuncture techniques have been used to study the single nephron in Munich-Wistar rats during midgestation, when renal hemodynamic changes are maximal.[23] Baylis and colleagues demonstrated that the rise in GFR and renal plasma flow was not associated with an increase in intraglomerular hydrostatic pressure, as a result of the concomitant decline in both pre- and post-glomerular arteriolar resistances.[23,24] Indirect evidence using membrane modeling to study the filtration barrier in human pregnancy supports the findings in isolated rat nephrons.[25,26] The conscious, chronically catheterized, gravid rat is another model that has been used by Conrad and others to further define the pregnancy-induced renal hemodynamic changes.[19,21,27]

Hormonal signaling has been proposed as a key factor in initiating these early adaptations. Of note, GFR and RPF rise during the luteal phase of the menstrual cycle, before and perhaps in anticipation of a pregnancy. GFR increases by 20% in the second half of the menstrual cycle and further increases to 40% to 65% above baseline in the early part of gestation.[20] Thus, maternal ovarian hormones and hormones produced by the fetoplacental unit have been implicated in these renal and cardiovascular adaptations.

Various steroid and peptide hormones of ovarian and placental origin have been investigated in this regard (reviewed in detail by Conrad and Lindheimer[16]). Estrogen and progesterone are steroid hormones produced in large quantities during pregnancy. Estrogen has a major role in increasing blood flow to various reproductive and nonreproductive organs during pregnancy but does not appear to influence GFR or RPF.[28,29] Progesterone administration, however, does increase GFR and RPF in animal and human studies, but to a lesser extent than in pregnancy.[30,31] Further investigation is needed to determine the precise role of progesterone and its metabolites in effecting renal hemodynamic changes in human pregnancy.

Various peptide hormones that are markedly increased in pregnancy also have been studied. The role of prolactin in renal adaptations remains unresolved,[32] and human placental lactogens, which are markedly increased in pregnancy, have not been well investigated. The peptide hormone relaxin has been studied extensively using the rat model.[19] Relaxin is a 6-kD peptide that originates from the corpus luteum of the ovary in both rats and humans. Conrad and colleagues have shown that GFR and effective RPF changes comparable with those in midgestation are observed when recombinant human relaxin or porcine relaxin is administered to female, nonpregnant rats.[33] Similar renal hemodynamic changes were demonstrated in ovariectomized female rats,[34] and even in male rats administered relaxin.[35] The increases in GFR and RPF observed in midterm pregnant rats were abolished with administration of relaxin-neutralizing antibodies.[34] This pregnancy- and relaxin-induced renal vasodilation-hyperfiltration in rats has been shown to occur by way of an endothelial endothelin-B receptor and nitric oxide pathway.[35-37] More recently, vascular matrix metallopro-

teinase-2 was shown to be a necessary component of this renal vasodilatory pathway in rats.[38]

Human studies are limited; however, some evidence indicates that relaxin also may play a role in human pregnancies. In women who lack ovarian function, have undetectable levels of serum relaxin, and achieve pregnancy by means of ovum donation, the rise in GFR during pregnancy is less than that observed in women who have normal ovarian function and become pregnant.[39] In nonpregnant healthy subjects, short-term administration of recombinant human relaxin resulted in an increase in RPF by 65% but no increase in GFR.[40] When relaxin was administered chronically to nonpregnant subjects with scleroderma, creatinine clearance was increased by 15% to 20% above predicted levels.[41] Although such findings do not constitute definitive proof, these animal and human studies suggest that relaxin may play an important role in the early renal changes that occur during pregnancy. It also is likely that, at least in humans, more than one pathway exists to achieve the systemic and renal vascular changes of pregnancy, thereby providing some protective redundancy of mechanisms in normal reproductive adaptations.

Renal Handling of Substrates during Pregnancy
Protein

Assessing urinary protein excretion is important in the detection and monitoring of renal disease and of pregnancy-specific pathological conditions such as preeclampsia. Both total protein and urinary albumin excretion are increased in normal pregnancy compared with nonpregnant levels, particularly after 20 weeks' gestation.[16] The average 24-hour total protein excretion and albumin excretion are 200 mg and 12 mg, respectively, with upper limits during normal pregnancy of 300 mg and 20 mg in 24 hours.[42-44] The increased GFR in normal pregnancy and possible alterations in glomerular charge selectivity contribute to the gestational proteinuria and albuminuria. Increased urinary excretion of low-molecular-weight proteins and renal tubular enzymes during pregnancy implicates the physiological impairment of proximal tubular resorptive capacity.[45] No apparent change is observed in glomerular permselectivity based on molecular weight or size during pregnancy.

Glucose

Glucose is freely filtered at the level of the glomerulus and almost completely reabsorbed by a sodium-coupled active transport in the proximal tubule. A lesser amount of glucose also is absorbed in the collecting tubule. In the nonpregnant state, urinary glucose excretion is minimal (less than 125 mg/dL) until the plasma concentrations reach levels above the maximal tubular resorptive capacity or a threshold concentration of 200 to 240 mg/dL.[46]

In pregnancy, the increased GFR and tubular flow rate may limit the ability of the proximal tubule to completely reabsorb glucose, resulting in a physiological glucosuria of pregnancy. Davison and colleagues demonstrated less effective reabsorption of glucose during pregnancy in normal pregnant women, with a return to normal in the postpartum period.[47] Animal studies indicate that glucose reabsorption in the distal nephron may be decreased.[48]

Overall, the amount of urinary glucose excretion in the third trimester increases several-fold above levels in the nonpregnant state. Because of the physiological changes in glucose handling during pregnancy and the normal glucosuria of pregnancy, presence of glucosuria is not a useful screen for renal tubular disorders, glucose intolerance, or diabetes during pregnancy.

Uric Acid

Serum uric acid is decreased by 25% to 35% in normal pregnancy, with a nadir of 2 to 3 mg/dL at 24 weeks' gestation and levels increasing toward nonpregnant-state values in the late third trimester.[16,49] Sources of circulating uric acid are purine breakdown and dietary intake, with clearance effected primarily by renal excretion. Most of the circulating uric acid is unbound and is filtered by the glomerulus. Uric acid is reabsorbed as well as secreted by the proximal tubule of the kidney. Net uric acid reabsorption occurs, with only 7% to 12% of the filtered load undergoing urinary excretion (reviewed by Conrad and Lindheimer[16]). Although multiple factors may play a role in circulating uric acid levels during pregnancy, altered renal handling is the most likely major contributing factor. The mechanisms for increased uric acid clearance include increased GFR and reduced proximal tubular reabsorption, alone or in combination.

Conditions associated with plasma volume contraction, such as preeclampsia, can lead to decreased uric acid clearance and increased circulating levels. Uric acid has gained considerable attention in the obstetrical literature for the prediction, diagnosis, and pathophysiology of preeclampsia.[16,50-53]

Acid-Base Homeostasis

The kidney also plays a unique role in the acid-base homeostasis of pregnancy. The primary alteration in pregnancy is a relative respiratory alkalosis that results from an increase in maternal minute ventilation. This reduces maternal partial pressure of carbon dioxide (PCO_2) as observed on arterial blood gas analysis and serves as an important gradient for gas exchange at the maternal-fetal interface. To compensate for the respiratory alkalosis, bicarbonate excretion is increased by the kidney, resulting in reduced serum bicarbonate levels. This decrease in bicarbonate levels may limit the buffering capacity in pregnancy.

These acid-base alterations and limited buffering capacity are important in interpreting laboratory values and arterial blood gases during pregnancy. These physiological changes are of particular importance in management of the acutely ill gravida.

FETAL CONSIDERATIONS

The normal physiological changes of pregnancy occur to accommodate the growing fetoplacental unit. Although such adaptations have evolved to support fetal growth and development, these alterations can alter maternal compensatory mechanisms, at times to maternal detriment. Therefore, with maternal diseases, it is imperative to have an understanding of the effect of pregnancy on the particular disease condition, as well as the effects of such disease processes on the progression of pregnancy and the implications for fetal development and well-being. Important considerations include viability of the fetus, gestational age, complications of prematurity, and optimization of fetal status.

Uteroplacental hemodynamics, fetal surveillance and monitoring, and interventions that may benefit the fetus in utero and reduce the complications associated with iatrogenic preterm birth warrant specific consideration in the context of pregnancy-related ARF.

Uteroplacental Hemodynamics and Fetal Oxygen Delivery

The adverse perinatal outcomes associated with pregnancy-related ARF most often are due to altered uteroplacental hemodynamics—specifically, reduced uterine blood flow. The fetus depends exclusively on placental gas exchange to maintain oxygenation and to avoid hypoxia and acidosis. The uteroplacental system does not have the capacity to autoregulate; thus, fetal perfusion depends on the maintenance of adequate maternal systemic perfusion. For these reasons, intravascular volume support is a crucial component of management of these patients. Adequate fluid resuscitation not only may preserve uterine blood flow but can also limit renal damage.

In the setting of decreased uteroplacental perfusion, or other causes of limited oxygen delivery to the fetus, multiple protective mechanisms serve to maximize and maintain adequate fetal oxygenation. Fetal hemoglobin, which is composed of two alpha chains and two gamma chains (rather than the two alpha and two beta chains of adult hemoglobin A), has a greater oxygen binding affinity than maternal hemoglobin. This difference allows for higher fetal hemoglobin oxygen saturation at a given partial pressure of oxygen (PO_2).[54] The fetus also has the capacity to alter systemic blood flow by means of autoregulatory mechanisms to ensure preferential oxygen delivery to vital structures such as the brain, adrenals, and heart.[55]

When these mechanisms begin to fail, fetal tissue hypoxia results, and organic acids such as lactate accumulate. Carbonic acid readily diffuses across the placenta, but placental clearance of noncarbonic acids is extremely limited; thus, anaerobic metabolism results in significant fetal metabolic acidosis. Maternal oxygen supplementation can significantly improve fetal oxygen content.[56]

In addition to volume support, uteroplacental perfusion can be altered by maternal positioning. Direct supine positioning causes compression of the maternal inferior vena cava by the gravid uterus and can lead to impaired venous return, inadequate uterine perfusion and generalized hypotension. This can be avoided with simple measures such as lateral positioning or placement of a support under the left hip in order to shift the uterus away from the aortocaval system.

In an acutely ill population, fluid resuscitation, supplemental oxygen, and anatomical maneuvers may not be sufficient to maintain adequate systemic blood pressure. In such situations, a potential role for vasopressor medications has been recognized. Knowledge of the effects of these agents on uteroplacental blood flow is limited. Dopamine, a norepinephrine precursor, has been shown to reduce uterine blood flow in animal models, including the baboon and sheep. Animal studies investigating the uteroplacental effects of epinephrine and norepinephrine have demonstrated significant decreases in placental perfusion with intravenous bolus administration of pressors, an effect that is not seen with continuous infusion of lower doses (reviewed by Leonardi and Gonik[57]).

Fetal Surveillance and Monitoring

Fetal heart rate monitoring allows continuous, real-time evaluation of fetal status and placental oxygen delivery. In viable gestations (beyond 23 to 24 weeks of gestation), fairly frequent fetal heart rate monitoring may be indicated for fetal evaluation. Before the stage of viability, fetal monitoring may provide an indirect means to assess overall maternal systemic perfusion, even though fetal considerations are substantially different. The frequency of fetal monitoring should follow the acuity of the clinical situation, with particularly close surveillance in women with hemodynamic instability.

Intermittent monitoring using the non-stress test is a noninvasive method of assessing fetal health utilizing fetal heart rate and maternal uterine contraction patterns. A normal fetal heart rate pattern reflects both fetal neurological maturity and normal acid-base status. The positive predictive value of a nonreassuring non-stress test result in the prediction of hypoxia is less than ideal, with a stillbirth rate after a nonreassuring test result of 26 per 1000.[58] For this reason, other tests such as the biophysical profile may be helpful.

The biophysical profile uses ultrasonography to assess fetal well-being by quantifying normal fetal behavior. Fetal gross movements, tone, breathing movements, and amniotic fluid volume are assessed; the non-stress test may also be incorporated into this scoring system. In observational studies the biophysical profile has decreased perinatal mortality; however, despite its excellent negative predictive value, similar to non-stress testing, the biophysical profile has a limited positive predictive value.[59] The utility of the non-stress test and biophysical profile have not been tested directly in the intensive care unit (ICU) setting.

Owing to the limitations of periodic fetal assessment in an acutely ill pregnant woman, fetal well-being often is best assessed with continuous fetal monitoring. Continuous assessment allows serial interpretation, which improves the predictive value of fetal heart rate pattern interpretation and enables real-time titration of blood pressure support and supplemental oxygen.

Fetal Interventions and the Maternal-Fetal Balance

With any seriously ill pregnant woman and her fetus, an intervention that may benefit one of the two involved patients may be detrimental to the other. These scenarios may present ethically troubling conflicts. What remains clear is that maternal stability must be ensured before an intervention specifically for fetal benefit should be undertaken. In general, the acute maternal condition must take precedence; once it is stabilized, the fetal situation can be considered. The most extreme example is the need for emergency delivery of the fetus in order to provide effective cardiopulmonary resuscitation for a pregnant woman. In less extreme situations, when the maternal condition is relatively stable, delivery may be delayed until optimization of the fetal condition can occur. The most common example of this clinical scenario is the short-term delay of delivery for glucocorticoid (betamethasone or dexamethasone) administration to accelerate fetal lung maturity before planned induced preterm birth.[60] With nonreassuring fetal status that does not improve with treatment of the mother, immediate delivery may be necessary for fetal benefit.

Other in utero treatments to optimize the fetal condition include careful attention to maternal intravascular volume status, stringent glucose control in patients with diabetes or glucose intolerance, and supplemental oxygen administration. In addition to the complications associated with prematurity, neonatal management also is important, because these infants may have high intravascular solute loads, which puts them at risk for osmotic diuresis and dehydration. In anticipation of these problems, specialized neonatologists and a tertiary care neonatal ICU are crucial components of the multidisciplinary team approach. The team also should include specialists in maternal-fetal medicine, critical care medicine, and nephrology. Patient care should be approached comprehensively, involving family members; in particularly difficult situations, incorporating medical ethicists may be helpful.

ETIOLOGY OF PREGNANCY-RELATED ACUTE RENAL FAILURE

In caring for the gravid woman with ARF, it is helpful to divide the disorder into two types: (1) pregnancy-specific ARF and (2) ARF affecting reproductive-age women that may occur coincident with pregnancy. Pregnancy-specific cases of ARF often are improved—or cured—by conclusion of the pregnancy. Furthermore, treatment strategies other than delivery typically are lacking. The classic example is preeclampsia, a disease of endothelial dysfunction that is unique to pregnancy, can cause multiorgan system dysfunction, and generally is reversible on delivery of the fetus and placenta. Clinical decision making in such conditions depends on the gestational age and hinges on a balance of the risks of ongoing disease to the mother and the fetus with the risks of prematurity to the neonate associated with delivery.

Pregnancy-Specific Acute Renal Failure Diagnoses

Several general categories of pregnancy-specific ARF are recognized: hypertensive, thrombotic microangiopathic, infectious, hypovolemic, and obstructive. These categories and their component disease processes are reviewed next, with a focus on pathophysiology, prognosis, and specific therapies.

Hypertension and Thrombotic Microangiopathy

PREECLAMPSIA AND HELLP SYNDROME. One of the most important contributors to pregnancy-related ARF is preeclampsia. Clinically, the diagnosis of preeclampsia is made using criteria involving the development of hypertension and proteinuria in the latter half of pregnancy.[61] The disease can manifest as dysfunction of multiple organ systems, including renal failure. The underlying pathophysiological processes that contribute to the development of preeclampsia include endothelial dysfunction and disruptions in immune, thrombotic, and metabolic function.[62,63] Renal histological effects of preeclampsia include the classic lesion of glomeruloendotheliosis and decreased glomerular size. Glomerular endothelial cells accumulate electron-dense material, resulting in increased cytoplasmic volume and a decrease in capillary lumen diameter, sometimes with complete capillary obliteration. Glomeruloendotheliosis occurs in up to 70% of patients with preeclampsia and persists immediately post partum,[64] but it appears to reverse completely in the vast majority of cases.[65,66] Coincident with these histopathological changes, overall decreases in GFR and effective renal plasma flow (ERPF) are seen in preeclampsia in comparison with normal pregnancy. These decrements are approximately 32% and 24%, respectively, from normal late-pregnancy levels.[16]

Secondary consequences of preeclampsia superimposed on intrinsic renal compromise can dramatically increase the degree of renal failure. Examples of such secondary effects include relative intravascular volume depletion, vasoconstriction, and activation of the inflammatory and coagulation cascades. Hemorrhage (e.g., placental abruption, postpartum hemorrhage) can have a profound effect on renal perfusion, thereby increasing risk of renal deterioration. Several studies have found that patients with pregnancy complications superimposed on preeclampsia are at increased risk for the development of ARF, suggesting that processes that further reduce intravascular volume or that predispose to thrombotic microangiopathy may be pivotal.[67] Entities specifically associated with preeclampsia-related ARF include placental abruption, disseminated intravascular coagulation (DIC), HELLP syndrome (a variant of severe preeclampsia involving hemolysis, elevated liver enzymes, and low platelets, which occurs in 4% to 14% of cases of preeclampsia),[68,69] and antiphospholipid antibody syndrome.[70-73] It follows that in preeclampsia-related ARF, the primary pathological process is acute tubular necrosis (ATN), with the most severe cases at risk for renal cortical necrosis.[74]

Two of the most comprehensive recent studies regarding pregnancy-related ARF related to preeclampsia suggest an overall incidence of 1.5% to 2%, although studies are limited and definitions have varied.[70,71] In another study, this incidence was significantly higher, with more than 7% of cases of preeclampsia in patients with HELLP syndrome.[72] Maternal mortality rates in these studies were zero to 10%, and perinatal mortality rates were 34% to 41%. In terms of renal prognosis, short-term dialysis rates were 10% to 50%. In these three studies, long-term follow-up evaluation spanned an average of 4 years, and the need for long-term renal replacement therapy depended on renal and hypertensive status entering pregnancy; none of the previously healthy preeclamptic patients required therapy. By contrast, of women with preexisting hypertension or renal disease, 40% to 80% required long-term dialysis, and several of these patients ultimately died of end-stage renal disease.[70-72]

As with any case of ARF, treatment must first address underlying disorders. As discussed, preeclampsia is a progressive, multisystem disease process without effective treatment strategies aside from delivery of the fetus and placenta. Therefore, in preeclampsia-related ARF, delivery is indicated. The mode of delivery (vaginal versus cesarean) depends on the combination of obstetrical and other clinical factors; beyond this, the principles of management are primarily supportive and include replacement of blood products as indicated, maintenance of intravascular volume, and renal replacement therapy as needed.

ACUTE FATTY LIVER OF PREGNANCY. Acute fatty liver of pregnancy (AFLP) is a disorder characterized by rapidly progressive hepatic failure in late gestation. It initially was described by Stander and Cadden in 1934[75] and was considered to be extremely rare and frequently fatal for both mother and baby. The incidence of AFLP has increased (to possibly as high as 1 in 7000 births), and maternal and perinatal mortality rates have decreased to approximately 1% to 12.5% and 7% to 9%, respectively.[76-78] This decline probably is the result of earlier diagnosis and intervention. Patients typically present with nausea, vomiting, malaise, and occasionally mental status changes. Laboratory evaluation frequently demonstrates hyperbilirubinemia, moderate elevations in transaminases, elevated ammonia levels, and moderate hypoglycemia.[74,78]

The diagnosis of AFLP is made after excluding other etiological possibilities such as gallbladder disease and acute hepatitis. The clinical manifestations of AFLP resemble those of preeclampsia and HELLP syndrome, and the metabolic abnormalities of AFLP can help make this differentiation.[76] Rarely, liver biopsy is needed to confirm the diagnosis, although the potential for significant clotting abnormalities in these patients should factor into the decision to biopsy. Other manifestations of AFLP include disseminated intravascular coagulation (associated with decreased antithrombin III levels), major intra-abdominal bleeding, central diabetes insipidus, pancreatitis, and renal abnormalities.[74,76-78]

The renal dysfunction seen in AFLP probably is multifactorial. One study suggests that modest elevations in serum creatinine levels indicative of mild insufficiency precede many of the clinical manifestations of the disease.[76] Microvesicular fatty infiltration of hepatocytes occurs in some patients due to inherited defects in mitochondrial β-oxidation of fatty acids. A mutation in long-chain 3-hydroxyacyl–CoA dehydrogenase (LCHAD) causing an enzyme deficiency in both mother and fetus predisposes to AFLP.[79] It is hypothesized that this abnormal fatty acid oxidation may lead to fatty infiltration of tissues other than the liver, including the kidney. Hepatorenal syndrome also may contribute, and in patients who experience hemorrhage and significant volume depletion, acute tubular necrosis can result. In published series, renal recovery in survivors of AFLP was complete.[74,76,77]

As with preeclampsia, the only curative intervention for AFLP is delivery. Recovery tends to be prolonged for AFLP; however, long-term sequelae are rare. Additional supportive measures, including correction of coagulopathy, maintenance of intravascular volume, and treatment of superimposed infections, are crucial. Renal replacement therapy is rarely indicated.[74,76-78]

AMNIOTIC FLUID EMBOLISM. Amniotic fluid embolism (AFE), more recently referred to as "anaphylactoid syndrome of pregnancy," is a rare but dramatic clinical entity. AFE manifests clinically as the acute onset of hypoxia, respiratory failure, cardiogenic shock, and DIC in pregnancy.[80] In 70% of cases, the cardiorespiratory collapse occurs during labor. The maternal mortality rate for AFE is estimated to be more than 60%, with a similar perinatal mortality rate. Approximately 85% of survivors suffer neurological sequelae.[81] Owing to the associated

TABLE 59-2

General Principles in the Differential Diagnosis for Preeclampsia, TTP, HUS, and AFLP

PARAMETER	PREECLAMPSIA/HELLP	TTP	HUS	AFLP
Onset	Usually third trimester	Median of 23 weeks	Often postpartum	Close to term
Primary/unique clinical manifestation	Hypertension and proteinuria	Neurological symptoms	Renal involvement	Nausea, vomiting, malaise
Purpura	Absent	Present	Absent	Absent
Fever	Absent	Present	Absent	Absent
Hemolysis	Mild	Severe	Severe	Mild
Coagulation studies	Variable	Normal	Normal	Prolonged abnormal
Hypoglycemia	Absent	Absent	Absent	Present
vWF multimers	Absent	Present	Present	Absent

AFLP, acute fatty liver of pregnancy; HELLP, hemolysis, elevated liver enzymes, low platelets; HUS, hemolytic uremic syndrome; TTP, thrombotic thrombocytopenic purpura; vWF, von Willebrand factor.
Data from references 82 through 85, 90, and 94.

DIC, cardiac dysfunction, and hemorrhage contributing to intravascular volume depletion, ARF is a factor to consider in all immediate survivors, and careful attention to volume resuscitation is crucial.

THROMBOTIC THROMBOCYTOPENIC PURPURA AND HEMOLYTIC UREMIC SYNDROME. Thrombotic thrombocytopenic purpura (TTP) and hemolytic uremic syndrome (HUS) are disorders characterized by microangiopathic hemolytic anemia, thrombocytopenia, systemic ischemia, and multiorgan failure.[82-85] Although not specific to pregnancy, these disorders often are included in the microangiopathic differential diagnosis of pregnancy-related ARF. Classically, TTP is identified by a pentad of clinical findings: thrombocytopenia, hemolytic anemia, fever, neurological abnormalities, and renal dysfunction.[86] HUS can have similar components, but with a shift away from neurological involvement and toward more significant renal manifestations. Often difficult to differentiate from severe preeclampsia or HELLP[87] (Table 59-2), these disorders occur in pregnancy at least as frequently as in the general population,[82] and some authors report that pregnancy-related TTP or HUS accounts for 10% to 25% of cases overall.[83,84] The incidence of TTP or HUS in pregnancy has been estimated to be 1 case per 25,000 births.[82]

From a histopathological perspective, TTP and HUS are thought to result from intravascular thrombi, which cause consumption of platelets, fragmentation of red blood cells, and variable systemic ischemia.[83] Large, multimeric forms of von Willebrand factor are found in these patients, and some evidence suggests that a plasma protease that normally cleaves these multimers may be genetically absent or deficient or may be inhibited by an acquired autoantibody.[88,89]

ARF occurs in two thirds of these patients.[84] A number of retrospective reviews of TTP and HUS in pregnancy have been conducted. The maternal mortality rate has decreased over time and ranges between 8% and 44%; similarly, the perinatal mortality rate also has decreased but remains substantial, between 30% and 80%.[82,87,90] In a report from Parkland Hospital of 13 cases occurring between 1972 and 1997, the overall mortality rate was fairly low; however, long-term morbidity and mortality were quite significant in the follow-up period (mean, 9 years). A majority of these patients had persistent renal insufficiency and hypertension. Over the long term, many of them required dialysis and transplantation, and one death from end-stage renal disease has been reported.[82] Long-term neurological sequelae also are possible with

TTP and HUS.[90] Other pregnancy-specific complications include fetal growth restriction, fetal distress, and intrauterine demise.[82-84,90] The magnitude of risk for recurrence with future pregnancies remains unresolved.[82,91] Although TTP or HUS can occur at any time during pregnancy or the postpartum period, the median gestational age at onset is approximately 23 weeks, with a tendency to occur earlier than in preeclampsia.[83]

Plasmapheresis is the cornerstone of therapy for TTP and HUS and is associated with a decrease in mortality rate from 90% to between 10% and 20%.[92] Other modalities, albeit with less demonstrated benefit, include glucocorticoids, antiplatelet agents, and for refractory cases, splenectomy or vincristine.[83,84] No clear benefit has been recognized for early delivery,[82] and anticoagulation with heparin is potentially harmful.[84] Supportive measures including intravenous fluid, blood transfusion (with caution in administration of platelets, because this can exacerbate intravascular occlusion), and renal replacement therapy also are essential components of therapy.[83,84]

The differentiation of TTP and HUS from preeclampsia and its variants can be challenging; often, the diagnosis is delayed until the postpartum period. Typically, these patients will be given an initial diagnosis of severe preeclampsia, and subsequent to delivery they will demonstrate worsening renal dysfunction, further hematological decompensation, or multisystemic ischemia, rather than an improvement in renal functional status.[84]

POSTPARTUM IDIOPATHIC ACUTE RENAL FAILURE. Cases of pregnancy-related ARF confined to the postpartum period that do not meet specific criteria for TTP, HUS, preeclampsia, or AFLP have been grouped into a category of idiopathic postpartum ARF.[74,93] Recently, it has become clear that these cases fall along the spectrum of thrombotic microangiopathy with predominantly renal manifestations. No specific therapeutic principles regarding this entity are recognized; rather, treatment should be given according to the likely underlying causative disorder, with supportive care and plasmapheresis if indicated.[82,94]

Infection and Sepsis

Sepsis from any cause can lead to hypotension and decreased renal perfusion, with the associated risks for prerenal ischemia and acute tubular necrosis (ATN). The most common sources of sepsis in pregnancy include pyelonephritis, chorioamnionitis, and pneumonia.

Pyelonephritis is the most common serious infectious complication of pregnancy. Although the incidence of asymptomatic bacteriuria remains unchanged in pregnancy, the consequences of asymptomatic bacteriuria are substantial—specifically, a higher likelihood of ascending infection and pyelonephritis.[95] In addition, pyelonephritis is associated with a higher risk of systemic inflammation and sepsis in the pregnant versus the nonpregnant state. These elevated risks can be attributed to several of the physiological adaptations of the renal system to pregnancy, including ureteral dilation, bladder wall flaccidity, and increased sensitivity to bacterial endotoxin–induced tissue damage. Although pyelonephritis can lead to sepsis and ARF in both the pregnant and nonpregnant host, the risk of ARF due to pyelonephritis in pregnancy is increased independent of the presence or absence of sepsis. One historical study showed that 25% of women with nonseptic pyelonephritis in pregnancy demonstrated a significant decrement in GFR.[96] The most common organisms involved in pyelonephritis in pregnancy are *Escherichia coli*, *Proteus mirabilis*, *Klebsiella* species, *Enterobacter*, and *Enterococcus*. *Staphylococcus saprophyticus* and group B streptococci also are potential pathogens.[97]

As mentioned, septic abortion was once a significant contributor to ARF in pregnancy. With the legalization of abortion and subsequent decrease in the incidence of related infections, this has become a less important contributor. Nevertheless, cases of septic abortion associated with spontaneous and therapeutic abortion persist. In our own institution, a recent case of sepsis with ARF in a septic spontaneous abortion was possibly associated with chorionic villus sampling (an invasive procedure used for chromosomal assessment in cases of increased risk of fetal aneuploidy). There is some suggestion of a higher incidence of renal cortical necrosis in sepsis associated with septic abortion than would be expected with sepsis in general.[98] These infections tend to be polymicrobial, often involving anaerobic species. The most common organisms implicated in bacteremia due to ascending infection are *Escherichia coli*, group B streptococci, and anaerobic streptococci; *Bacteroides* species, *Clostridium* species, and *Enterococcus* also may be involved.[99,100]

In terms of therapeutic considerations for all of these cases, general supportive measures, including hydration and blood pressure support, should be accompanied by antibiotic therapy. The choice of antibiotic coverage should be governed by the organisms involved, either based on epidemiological data or documented culture results. For polymicrobial ascending infections of the genital tract, including septic abortion, antibiotic selection should be broad-spectrum, ensuring adequate anaerobic coverage. For cases of septic abortion or chorioamnionitis, it should be noted that antibiotic penetration of the uterine cavity is suboptimal and that evacuation of the uterine contents is necessary for effective treatment, regardless of gestational age and fetal viability or gestational age considerations.

Volume Depletion

Volume depletion can lead to ARF by causing prerenal ischemia. In pregnancy, the most common cause of volume depletion of this magnitude is obstetrical hemorrhage, which can occur at any gestational age. Severe cases of hyperemesis gravidarum leading to refractory nausea and vomiting, if insufficiently treated, also could result in poor renal perfusion.

Obstetrical hemorrhage can occur early in pregnancy due to spontaneous or induced abortion. More commonly, third trimester hemorrhage from placenta previa, placental abruption, or postpartum hemorrhage are contributors to significant blood loss, putting patients at risk of ARF. These processes also can be associated with consumptive coagulopathy, which can exacerbate the process, or disseminated intravascular coagulation, which can additionally cause direct intrarenal damage. Treatment of hemorrhage sufficient to cause prerenal ischemia includes volume support, replacement of blood products, and correction of coagulopathy. In the antepartum setting, delivery is indicated, either vaginally or by cesarean section, depending on the obstetrical indications. In the postpartum setting, the underlying problem must be addressed. For surgical bleeding, exploratory laparotomy and repair may be indicated. In cases of uterine atony leading to hemorrhage, medical therapy with uterotonics or surgical intervention for refractory cases may be necessary.

Hyperemesis gravidarum is a common complication of pregnancy, with 70% to 85% of pregnant women experiencing some degree of nausea and vomiting[101]; in 1% to 2% of women, signs and symptoms can be severe, often including a loss of 5% of body weight.[102] In general, hyperemesis can be managed with oral antiemetic medications. In a small subset of patients, aggressive management with enteral or parenteral nutrition, or both, and hydration may be required. In rare cases in which access to such supportive care may be limited, severe hypovolemia can result in prerenal ischemia and ARF. A case report describes a good outcome for one such patient, who required short-term renal replacement therapy and supportive care and subsequently went on to recover full renal function.[103]

Obstruction

The gravid uterus can significantly compress the maternal urinary system, particularly in conditions characterized by uterine overdistention, such as polyhydramnios, multiple gestation, or uterine fibroids. Although rare, obstructive pregnancy-related ARF has been described in association with such conditions in several case reports.[104-115] Maternal genitourinary anomalies or previous surgery also can increase susceptibility to such processes, particularly in patients with a unilateral kidney or collecting system.[107] Nephrolithiasis is another potential obstructive cause of ARF, because the incidence of stones is similar to that in a population of nonpregnant reproductive-age women.[116]

Approaches to treatment of obstructive pregnancy-related ARF include cystoscopy and retrograde ureteral stent placement or percutaneous nephrostomy.[106,107,110] If the clinical situation suggests that delivery would be appropriate, this may relieve the urinary obstruction.[104,105,111,112,114,115] Published case reports indicate excellent prognosis for general recovery and restoration of renal function once the obstruction is relieved.[104,105,107,108,110-115] Rarely, hemodialysis has been suggested as a temporizing measure until more definitive treatment of the obstruction can be achieved.[115]

Other Intrinsic Renal Dysfunction in Pregnancy

As mentioned, the evaluation of a pregnant patient with ARF must take into consideration those etiologic disorders

TABLE 59-3

Differential Diagnosis of Intrinsic Renal Disease in Reproductive-Age Women

CATEGORY/LOCATION	MECHANISM/SUBTYPE	SPECIFIC DIAGNOSES
Tubular necrosis	Continuum with prerenal ischemia	Ischemia Toxins
Vasculitis	Systemic vascular inflammation with renal involvement	Wegener's granulomatosis Thromboembolic disease Scleroderma
Acute glomerulonephritis	Focal glomerulonephritis	IgA nephropathy Thin basement membrane disease Lupus nephropathy Hereditary nephritis Mesangial proliferative glomerulonephritis
	Diffuse glomerulonephritis	Postinfectious glomerulonephritis Lupus nephropathy Rapidly progressive glomerulonephritis Fibrillary glomerulonephritis Membranoproliferative glomerulonephritis
	Nephrotic syndrome	Focal glomerulosclerosis Minimal change disease Membranous nephropathy (including lupus) Diabetic nephropathy Late-stage postinfectious glomerulonephritis
Acute interstitial nephritis	Hypersensitivity response	Drug/toxin (e.g., penicillins, cephalosporins, sulfonamides, rifampin, ciprofloxacin, NSAIDs, thiazide diuretics, furosemide, cimetidine, phenytoin, allopurinol) Autoimmune disease (e.g., lupus) Infiltrative disease (e.g., sarcoidosis) Infectious disease (e.g., legionnaire's disease, hantavirus infection)

NSAIDs, nonsteroidal anti-inflammatory drugs.
Data from references 125 and 152 through 154.

that may occur coincident with gestation but may not be specific to pregnancy. Table 59-3 outlines this differential diagnosis in detail, with a focus on those diseases that are more common in reproductive-age women. Differentiating glomerular disease from preeclampsia and other forms of pregnancy-related ARF can be challenging. Some of the distinguishing characteristics are summarized in Table 59-4.

AN EVIDENCE-BASED APPROACH TO DIAGNOSIS AND THERAPY OF PREGNANCY-RELATED ACUTE RENAL FAILURE

The Role of Renal Biopsy

In nonpregnant patients with ARF, renal biopsy can be diagnostic and help direct management. Histological findings have been shown to alter diagnosis in up to 70% of cases of ARF.[117] In this population, the serious complication rate for renal biopsy also is reassuringly low, at less than 1%.[118]

In pregnancy, specific disorders tend to be clinically discernible in the large majority of cases; therefore, the role of renal biopsy may be less prominent. Furthermore, theoretical concerns have been raised regarding the possibility of increased morbidity associated with the procedure in pregnancy. In this population, renal biopsy functions primarily to identify causative disorders other

than preeclampsia when patients present with renal failure before term. As noted earlier, this differentiation is crucial because ARF related to preeclampsia necessitates delivery. The discovery of lesions not associated with preeclampsia has the potential to identify patients who can be managed by therapies other than delivery, thereby minimizing iatrogenic preterm birth and its attendant complications.

A review of the literature on renal biopsy in pregnancy reveals complication rates of approximately 1.6% to 4.4%, including perirenal bleeding necessitating nephrectomy and perirenal hematoma; as many as 17% of women had gross hematuria.[119] Most studies reported mortality rates of zero, but one study did describe a maternal death.[120] Packham and colleagues, in 1987, addressed the safety and utility of renal biopsy in pregnancy; their indications for biopsy included new-onset hematuria, proteinuria, and impaired renal function in the first or second trimester.[121] In a series of 111 biopsies in 104 women, they reported a 97% tissue procurement rate; a serious perirenal hematoma developed in 1 patient, and 4 patients experienced transient hematuria or pain that resolved spontaneously. In 80% of the pregnant women undergoing biopsy, a specific glomerulonephritis was identified.[121] Lindheimer reviewed these conflicting findings and suggested that although the overall safety profile of renal biopsy in pregnancy probably is not significantly less favorable than outside of pregnancy, the procedure does have associated risks, and the indications for biopsy should be limited to situations in which "there is sudden deterioration in renal function before 32 weeks gestation and no obvious cause is apparent."[122] This philosophy, which intends to maximize the clinical relevance of biopsy results, has since become the standard of care.

TABLE 59-4

Differentiation of Acute Glomerulonephritis and Preeclampsia

PARAMETER	ACUTE GLOMERULONEPHRITIS	PREECLAMPSIA
Gestational age	Any	Mostly third trimester
Hypertension	Present	Present
Systemic manifestations	Collagen vascular disease, preceding infection	Neurological, hematological, or hepatic involvement
Urine sediment	Hematuria, red blood cell casts, oval fat bodies	Isolated proteinuria or findings of acute tubular necrosis (brown granular casts, renal tubular cells)
Proteinuria	>2 g/24 hours	>300 mg/24 hours (mild), >5 g/24 hours (severe)
Complement levels	↓	↔
Antinuclear antibodies (ANA)	↑	↔
Antistreptolysin-O titers	↑	↔
Other autoantibodies	↑	↔

↓, decreases; ↑, increases; ↔, no apparent change.
Data from Deering S, Seiken G: Acute renal failure. In Dildy GA III, Belfort MA, Saade GR (eds): Critical Care Obstetrics, 4th ed. Malden, Mass, Blackwell Science, 2004, pp 372-379.

More recent series of renal biopsies, performed using the current method of ultrasound guidance, suggest that in a well-selected population, histological findings specifically direct management in 66% to 100% of patients. Complication rates in these studies ranged from zero to 40% for perirenal hematoma, with up to 25% of affected patients requiring transfusion; no maternal deaths were reported.[123,124] These recent studies substantiate the suggestion that renal biopsy has a role in pregnancy and that the invasiveness of the procedure should be factored into the decision whether to biopsy. The current state of neonatal care, with excellent outcomes beyond 30 weeks, should lead to a reassessment of the gestational age threshold for biopsy, taking into consideration the time frame within which the implications of iatrogenic prematurity are most significant.

Medical Management of Acute Renal Failure in Pregnancy

General management of ARF begins with correction of underlying etiological factors and removal of renal toxins (most commonly, aminoglycoside antibiotics and radiocontrast agents). Care also must be taken to adjust the dosing of medications that are renally cleared; one such agent commonly used in pregnancy is magnesium sulfate, which is used for seizure prophylaxis in preeclampsia and occasionally for inhibition of preterm labor. Prevention and treatment of infection are crucial in this population, because sepsis is the most common cause of death in ARF. After these measures, the single most important intervention is fluid management. The goal is to restore and maintain renal perfusion in order to reverse preischemic changes. Even after tubular necrosis has developed, the extent of further damage can be limited by adequate perfusion. In most instances, clinical assessment can guide this therapy; however, in more complicated cases, invasive hemodynamic monitoring may be necessary.[125] Central venous pressure monitoring and pulmonary artery catheterization should be considered for use in obstetrical populations in which noninvasive assessment is inadequate. Maternal physiological cardiovascular adaptations must be accounted for in the interpretation of the data derived from these assessments. For a detailed review of this subject, the reader is referred to the article by Fujitani and Baldisseri.[126]

Pharmacological measures remain secondary therapies for the treatment or amelioration of ARF. Low-dose dopamine infusion has traditionally been used because of its vasodilatory effect on renal arterioles, with resultant increase in renal blood flow. The current evidence, however, suggests that this beneficial effect does not translate into any difference in clinical outcome, at least in the nonpregnant population. A large placebo-controlled trial comparing low-dose dopamine and placebo showed no differences in serum creatinine, need for renal replacement therapy, or duration of ICU or hospital stay.[127] Meta-analyses of smaller studies have found similar results.[128,129] Dopamine can trigger tachyarrhythmias, pulmonary shunting, or gastrointestinal or digital necrosis.[125] A particular concern in pregnancy is the effect of vasoactive medications on uterine blood flow and thus the fetoplacental unit. Evidence from animal models suggests that dopamine infusion reduces uterine artery blood flow in both normotensive and hypotensive settings. Furthermore, dopamine also may inhibit prolactin release and therefore has the potential to negatively affect lactation.[130] As supported by the lack of clinical benefit and recognition of associated risks, no clear role for dopamine infusion in the treatment of pregnancy-related ARF has been identified.

Loop diuretics increase renal intratubular flow rates, which may decrease intratubular obstruction and ameliorate resulting cellular damage. This has been the rationale for the use of loop diuretics in ARF. Furthermore, because the overall prognosis is better for nonoliguric ARF than for the oliguric type, a plausible approach is to convert an oliguric state to a nonoliguric one with the use of pharmacological diuresis, with expected positive effect on prognosis.[125] The published evidence in this regard is conflicting. Some data suggest that diuretic therapy does not decrease the need for renal replacement therapy or reduce mortality rates. As pointed out in a recent review, although several observational cohort studies suggest that diuretics may be associated with an increased risk of death or renal death, these results are difficult to interpret owing to their lack of randomization.[131] In a large, multicenter international cohort study, multivariate analyses showed no difference in mortality rates among those patients who received diuretic therapy.[132] On the basis of this evidence, the use of loop diuretics in the treatment of ARF in a

TABLE 59-5

Other Pharmacotherapeutics in Acute Renal Failure (ARF)

AGENT	MECHANISM	CLINICAL UTILITY	PREGNANCY CONCERNS
Calcium channel blockers	Renal vasodilation	No clinical benefit; may cause hypotension and worsen ARF	Hypotension, decreased uteroplacental blood flow (UPBF)
Dopamine receptor agonists	Renal vasodilation	No clinical benefit; may cause hypotension and worsen ARF	No data; theoretical concern for hypotension and decreased UPBF
Atrial natriuretic peptide (ANP)	Renal vasodilation	No clear clinical benefit; there may be subsets of patients that would benefit	No data; hemodynamically active, need to watch for hypotension and decreased UPBF
Theophylline	Adenosine antagonist	May help prevent renal damage from radiocontrast agents in patients at risk	Transient neonatal jitteriness and tachycardia immediately after delivery with recent exposure; no long-term risks
N-Acetylcysteine (NAC)	Free radical scavenger	May help prevent renal damage from radiocontrast agents in patients at risk	Very limited data; appears to be safe
Osmotic agents (e.g., mannitol)	Diuresis	Effective in the prevention of early myoglobinuric renal failure	Very limited data; hemodynamically active, need to watch for hypotension and decreased UPBF

Data from Thadhani R, Pascual M, Bonventre J: Acute renal failure. N Engl J Med 1996;334:1448-1460; and from Reprotox: Dopamine. 2006. Available at www.reprotox.org (subscription required).

general medical population is reserved for treatment of volume overload, in an attempt to avoid renal replacement therapy. Specific fetal risks of diuretic use have not been reported; however, any agent that alters maternal hemodynamics and has potential to affect uteroplacental perfusion must be used with caution in pregnancy.

Other agents that have been considered for use in ARF are listed in Table 59-5.[125]

Hyperkalemia, metabolic acidosis, and anemia are downstream effects of ARF that may require specific treatment short of renal replacement therapy. Hyperkalemia can be treated with potassium-binding resins (polystyrene sulfonate) or glucose plus insulin.[125] Published data on polystyrene sulfonate in pregnancy are lacking, but because of its mode of action and lack of absorption, a reasonable conclusion is that on physiological grounds, it is not likely to be harmful.[133] Metabolic acidosis in the setting of ARF can be treated with sodium bicarbonate.[125] No specific pregnancy-related contraindications to the use of glucose-insulin or bicarbonate have been recognized; however, the physiological compensatory metabolic acidosis of pregnancy must be accounted for in the use of bicarbonate.

Anemia related to ARF is due to both hemolysis (from uremia-induced red blood cell membrane fragility) and decreased hematopoiesis (from decreased erythropoietin levels).[134] Acute therapy generally consists of transfusion; however, erythropoietin supplementation may play a role if the process is prolonged. Exogenous erythropoietin can be associated with hypertension,[135] and increased dosing often is needed in pregnancy in order to attain therapeutic response.[136-140] Experience with erythropoietin in pregnancy is limited, but the available evidence suggests that placental transfer is negligible and that this agent is not teratogenic.[141]

Renal Replacement Therapy in Pregnancy

As with nonpregnant patients, if supportive measures are insufficient in the management of pregnancy-related ARF, the next step in treatment is the initiation of renal replacement therapy. Whether the threshold for initiation of such therapy in pregnancy should be lower than that in non-

pregnant populations remains undetermined. Effects on the fetus and uteroplacental blood flow should be accounted for in this decision. Published outcomes of dialysis in pregnancy are limited to retrospective reviews and case reports. The vast majority of this data is from patients with chronic renal disease. Thus, current ability to translate the existing medical evidence to the bedside of the pregnant patient with acute renal failure remains primarily extrapolative.

The past three decades have seen substantial improvements in both fertility and successful pregnancy rates in women with chronic renal failure. Since the first case report of a successful pregnancy on dialysis in 1971,[142] and an initial case series in the 1980s that suggested high rates of preterm birth, low birth weight, and refractory hypertension,[143] the overall prognosis for these patients has improved significantly. These pregnancies continue to be high-risk, however, and outcomes remain quite variable.

Some evidence suggests that these improvements may be due to the recognition that a more intensive dialysis regimen may be beneficial. Okundaye and colleagues in 1998 noted that an increase in the number of hours of dialysis per week (beyond a threshold of 20 hours per week) led to increasing survival and decreasing prematurity.[140] Bagon and coworkers found similar trends in their national survey of dialysis centers in Belgium.[144] To minimize the effects of uremia on pregnancy outcomes, dialysis regimens were adjusted with the goal of attaining maximum dialysis urea levels of 100 mg/dL or less. In doing so, a positive correlation was noted between birth weight and "excess dialysis hours" (the number of hours of dialysis delivered minus the hours that would have been given if the patient were not pregnant).[144] These two publications have influenced the prescription of dialysis for pregnant women with chronic kidney disease internationally, with the recommendation that an increased dialysis dose be the standard of care for pregnant women.[145]

Subsequent case reports have described improved perinatal outcome with intensive dialysis.[137,146] A majority of these studies assessed the role of hemodialysis; however, peritoneal dialysis also has been evaluated in the setting of chronic renal failure in pregnancy. This modality of dialysis remains a viable option and may have the bene-

TABLE 59-6

Specific Considerations for Dialysis in Pregnancy

PARAMETER	PREGNANCY-SPECIFIC CONCERN
Hemodynamics	Careful attention to avoiding hypotension, fluid fluctuations, and volume changes in pregnancy; hypertension also should be treated if severe
Blood urea nitrogen	Try to maintain lower than 60 mg/dL
Maternal weight	Weight gain in pregnancy (baseline normal BMI) should be 1-2.5 kg total in the first trimester and 0.3-0.5 kg/week in the second and third trimesters
Serum bicarbonate levels	Remember physiological metabolic acidosis (compensatory for respiratory alkalosis) in pregnancy; bicarbonate normally is decreased 4-5 mEq/L
Contractions	Scrutinize closely for preterm contractions and preterm labor associated with dialysis
Vitamin and folate supplementation	Required in pregnancy and removed by dialysis; need to increase supplementation
Anemia/erythropoietin levels	If exogenous erythropoietin is needed, therapeutic dosing generally is higher in pregnancy
Serum calcium levels	Avoid hypercalcemia; calciferol doses often must be reduced

BMI, body mass index.
Data from references 136, 138, 139, and 156.

ficial effect of minimizing maternal hemodynamic changes.[147,148] Other considerations for dialysis in pregnancy are summarized in Table 59-6.[136,138,139]

In an attempt to minimize the stress of dialysis on the patient, a great deal of interest has arisen in the use of continuous renal replacement therapy (CRRT). This may be particularly applicable to certain populations, including pregnant women, who may benefit from minimization of hemodynamic and solute fluctuations.[149]

The theoretical benefits of CRRT in women with pregnancy-related ARF are substantiated by improved outcomes with more intensive dialysis in the pregnant woman with chronic renal failure. In pregnancy, the hemodynamic shifts inherent in intermittent dialysis may negatively affect uteroplacental perfusion, thereby increasing the risk of placental oxidative stress with cyclical placental hypoperfusion and reperfusion. This effect has the potential to impair fetal growth and well-being. An additional concern is that uremia, which results in increased delivery of urea to the fetus and increases fetal solute load, may lead to fetal diuresis and resultant polyhydramnios, thereby increasing risks of preterm birth and preterm rupture of membranes.[136,138,139,150] Furthermore, an "azotemic intrauterine environment" may contribute to the increased risk of developmental delay seen in patients with chronic renal failure.[140] Although it is impossible to separate out the relative contributions of underlying disease and specific treatments in the causality of these adverse outcomes, a reasonable speculation is that CRRT could ameliorate these risks by minimizing volume and solute fluctuations. Published data directly substantiating any benefit of CRRT in pregnancy are lacking, however.

Clearly, aggressive dialysis appears to be safe and beneficial in a pregnant population in general, and this must be considered while assessing the risks and benefits of early and intensive dialysis in pregnancies complicated by ARF.

CONCLUSION

Pregnancy alters maternal physiology. It confounds the status of one patient with the needs of another, sometimes with conflicting goals. Although many of the maternal physiological adaptations to pregnancy are understood, the underlying mechanisms remain incompletely elucidated. The etiology of some pathological processes unique to pregnancy also remains elusive. The diagnosis, classification, and treatment of women with pregnancy-related ARF can be challenging and require a multidisciplinary clinical team, a systematic approach guided by the available literature, and careful attention to the balance between the needs of a mother and those of her fetus.

Key Points

1. Although the incidence of pregnancy-related acute renal failure has declined in the developed world, it is not uncommon in the developing world. Furthermore, mortality and the risk of long-term renal failure remain quite significant in such cases.
2. An approach to the management of pregnancy-related acute renal failure must be informed by a thorough understanding of maternal renal adaptations to pregnancy, including alterations in renal hemodynamics and substrate handling.
3. Management strategies should incorporate an understanding of fetal considerations, including the importance of maintaining uteroplacental blood flow and interventions that may ameliorate the effects of prematurity.
4. In addition to causes of acute renal failure that may occur coincident with pregnancy, several disease processes unique to pregnancy should be considered in the pregnant patient. The most common of these is preeclampsia.
5. The determination of the specific cause of pregnancy-related acute renal failure can allow for the differentiation of conditions that require delivery for treatment from those that would not be altered by delivery. This distinction allows for minimization of iatrogenic prematurity and its associated complications. In making this distinction, prudent use of renal biopsy may be indicated.
6. When indicated, renal replacement therapy can be administered to pregnant women, and care should be taken to minimize hemodynamic and solute fluctuations. Frequent or continuous therapy may be helpful in these patients.
7. A multidisciplinary team approach is imperative for optimal management of the pregnant woman with acute renal failure.

Key References

16. Conrad KP, Lindheimer MD: Renal and cardiovascular alterations. In Lindheimer MD, Cunningham FG, Roberts JM (eds): Chesley's Hypertensive Disorders in Pregnancy, 2nd ed. Stamford, Conn, Appleton & Lange, 1999, pp 263-326.
19. Conrad KP, Novak J, Danielson LA, et al: Mechanisms of renal vasodilation and hyperfiltration during pregnancy: Current perspectives and potential implications for preeclampsia. Endothelium 2005;12:57-62.
94. Sibai BM, Kustermann L, Velasco J: Current understanding of severe preeclampsia, pregnancy-associated hemolytic uremic syndrome, thrombotic thrombocytopenic purpura, hemolysis, elevated liver enzymes, and low platelet syndrome, and postpartum acute renal failure: Different clinical syndromes or just different names? Curr Opin Nephrol Hypertens 1994;3:436-445.
151. Asrat T, Nageotte M: Acute renal failure in pregnancy. In Foley MR, Strong TH Jr, Garite TJ (eds): Obstetric Intensive Care Manual, 2nd ed. New York, McGraw-Hill Professional, 2004, pp 184-195.
156. Davison J, Lindheimer M: Renal disorders. In Creasy RK, Reznik R, Iams J (eds): Maternal-Fetal Medicine: Principles and Practice, 5th ed. Philadelphia, Saunders, 2003, pp 901-923.

See the companion Expert Consult website for the complete reference list.

CHAPTER 60

Diagnosis and Management of the HELLP Syndrome

Pasquale Piccinni and Giampiero Gallo

OBJECTIVES

This chapter will:
1. Review the main pathophysiological features of the HELLP syndrome.
2. Outline the diagnosis and treatment of the HELLP syndrome and characterize the prognosis, especially in patients with renal failure.
3. Describe the role of continuous renal replacement therapy in the management of patients with the HELLP syndrome.

The HELLP syndrome—characterized by *h*emolysis, *el*evated *l*iver enzymes, and *l*ow *p*latelets—is a severe, life-threatening pregnancy-related disorder that occurs in 0.2% to 0.8% of all pregnancies and in approximately 10% (range, 2% to 20%) of pregnancies complicated by severe preeclampsia. Together, HELLP syndrome, preeclampsia, and acute fatty liver of pregnancy (AFLP) constitute a spectrum of disease that ranges from involving mild symptoms to severe, life-threatening multiorgan system dysfunction.

From a pathophysiological standpoint, HELLP syndrome is a thrombotic microangiopathy that usually resolves after delivery of the baby.[1] Serious maternal complicating factors include acute renal failure (ARF), disseminated intravascular coagulation (DIC), pulmonary edema, severe ascites, pleural effusion, and acute respiratory distress syndrome (ARDS). HELLP syndrome probably is the most frequent disorder leading to ARF in pregnancy.[2] If complicated by oliguric ARF, HELLP syndrome carries relatively higher maternal and perinatal mortality rates.[3,4] In women with chronic renal disease, pregnancy may accelerate decline in renal function and worsen hypertension and proteinuria, with increases in maternal (preeclampsia) and fetal (intrauterine growth retardation, intrauterine death) complications.[5] Pregnancy success rates vary, ranging from 20% to 95%, depending on baseline creatinine levels.

RISK FACTORS

In recent years, few advances have accrued regarding the understanding of the underlying pathophysiology and possible effective prevention of preeclampsia.[6] Many women with a history of preeclampsia have either a thrombophilic or a vascular or hemostasis disorder, which is associated with advanced maternal age but not with gestational age or blood pressure on hospital admission or at the time of convulsions.[7,8] The risk of vasculoplacental disease increases with age, body mass index, insulin resistance, hypertriglyceridemia, primiparity, stressful working conditions, and personal history of vascular events during pregnancy.[9,10]

PATHOGENESIS

HELLP syndrome is a complex preeclamptic condition characterized by intravascular platelet activation, resulting in thrombocytopenia, and by microangiopathic hemolytic anemia, responsible for the increase in total bilirubin and lactate dehydrogenase (LDH). The etiology and pathogenesis are not completely understood.[11] Most probably, at approximately week 16 of gestation, an inadequate trophoblastic invasion of the spiral arteries of the myometrium causes a secondary placental ischemia, which subsequently leads to preeclampsia. The HELLP syndrome represents a group of clinical and pathological manifesta-

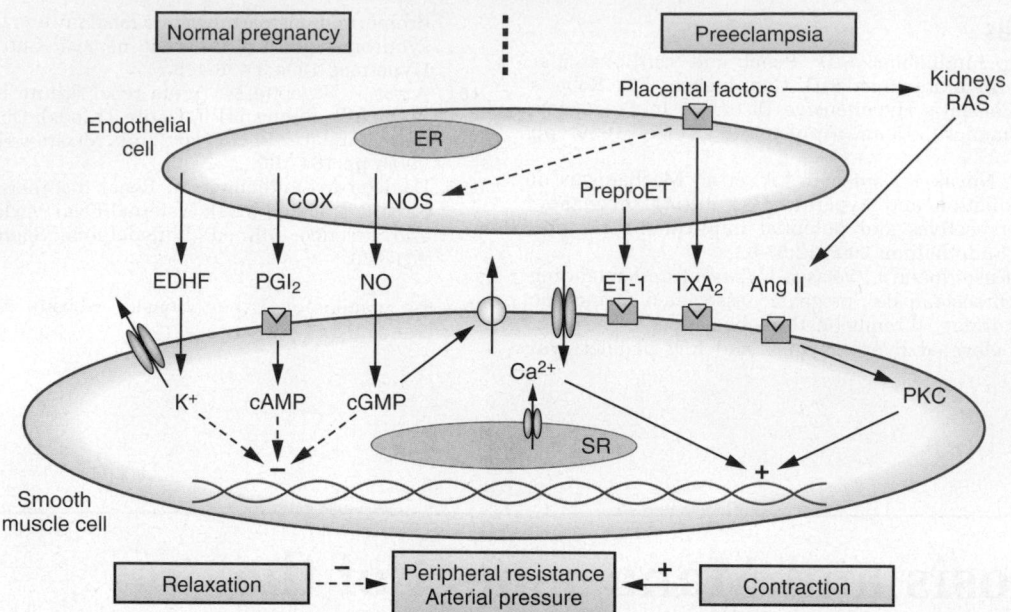

FIGURE 60-1. Vascular changes during normal pregnancy and preeclampsia. During normal pregnancy there is an increase in the activity of endothelial nitric oxide synthase (NOS) and cyclooxygenase (COX) and increased production of nitric oxide (NO), prostacyclin (i.e., prostaglandin I_2 [PGI_2]), and endothelium-derived hyperpolarizing factor (EDHF). NO increases cyclic guanosine monophosphate (cGMP), and PGI_2 increases cyclic adenosine monophosphate (cAMP) in smooth muscle, which decreases intracellular Ca^{2+} and the myofilament sensitivity to Ca^{2+}. Also, EDHF opens K^+ channels in smooth muscle, leading to membrane hyperpolarization, with consequent smooth muscle relaxation and decreased peripheral resistance and arterial pressure. In preeclampsia there is increased release of placental cytokines that inhibit the production of endothelium-derived relaxing factors and thereby decrease smooth muscle relaxation. Cytokines also stimulate the release of endothelium-derived contracting factors such as endothelin (ET-1) and thromboxane (TXA_2) and may activate the renin-angiotensin system (RAS) in the kidney, leading to increased angiotensin II (ANG II) secretion. ET-1, TXA_2, and ANG II stimulate specific receptors in smooth muscle, contributing to increased intracellular Ca^{2+}, protein kinase C (PKC) activity, and smooth muscle contraction, as well as increased peripheral resistance and arterial pressure. ER, endoplasmic reticulum; SR, sarcoplasmic reticulum. (From Khalil RA, Granger JP: Vascular mechanism of increased arterial pressure in preeclampsia: Lessons from animal models. Am J Physiol Regul Integr Comp Physiol 2002;283:R29-R45.)

tions due to an imbalance in prostanoid metabolism (perhaps due to placental ischemia) and consequent alteration in the release of nitric oxide cyclic guanosine monophosphate (cGMP) and prostacyclin (i.e., prostaglandin I_2 [PGI_2]) cyclic adenosine monophosphate (cAMP)[12] (Fig. 60-1). These changes lead in turn to generalized vasospasm and subsequent endothelial damage. Organ hypoperfusion typically results in liver damage, which is responsible for the clinical signs and symptoms. Intravascular coagulation also plays a significant part in the pathophysiology of the preeclamptic syndrome, and it has been suggested that antithrombin III (AT III) concentrates may have potential for the treatment of this condition.[13] In addition, an early rise in serum of atrial natriuretic peptide (ANP) suggests a pathogenetic role for such a factor, which could be related not directly to hypertension but rather to the regulation or normalization of blood volume and vascular reactivity[8,14,15] (Fig. 60-2).

Other potentially involved molecules include the metabolites of prostacyclin (6-keto-$PGF_{1\alpha}$) and thromboxane A_2.[16] Both of these factors can increase intracellular Ca^{2+} concentration and stimulate Ca^{2+} contraction pathways in vascular smooth muscle. These endothelial abnormalities, in turn, cause hypertension by impairing renal pressure natriuresis and increasing total vascular resistance.[17]

Once the syndrome is established, volume contraction, reduced cardiac output, enhanced vascular reactivity, increased vascular permeability, and platelet consumption follow.

DIAGNOSIS

HELLP typically develops in the third trimester of pregnancy. Sometimes it can occur in the second trimester of pregnancy, and very rarely it may develop within 48 to 72 hours after delivery.

Diagnosis is complicated by the lack of specific clinical signs. Other diagnostic possibilities to be ruled out include AFLP, idiopathic thrombocytopenia, hemolytic uremic syndrome, and appendicitis.[18]

Diagnostic criteria are the following:
- Pregnancy-induced hypertension (PIH), defined as blood pressure levels above 140/90 mm Hg on two successive measurements at 4-hour intervals or isolated diastolic pressure above 90 mm Hg in serial measurements. Both systolic and diastolic pressure have circadian regularity, with an elevation (acrophase) in early afternoon and a nadir during the night.[9]
- Proteinuria, defined as urinary protein excretion of more than 0.3 g/day. Microscopic examination of urine is important, particularly for the presence of red blood cells and casts. In gestational hypertension, the presence of proteinuria is associated with a 3.8-fold increase in the incidence of severe maternal disease.[19]
- Microalbuminuria, an early index of glomerular function impairment. Urinary albumin excretion of more than 25 mg/day constitutes a significant risk factor for the development of hypertension.

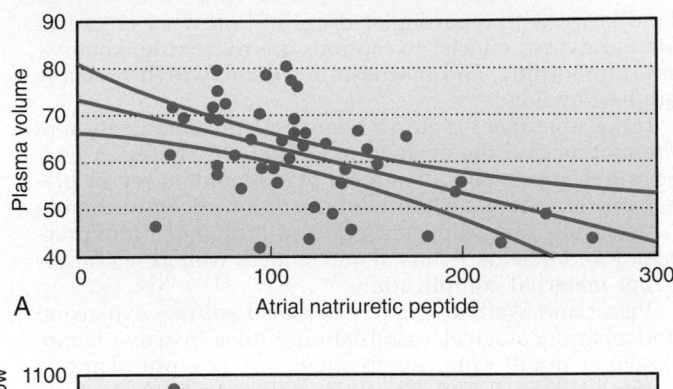

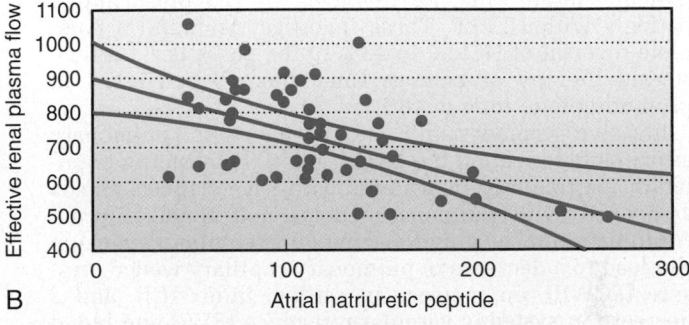

FIGURE 60-2. Atrial natriuretic peptide (ANP) in monitoring for preeclampsia. **A,** Linear regression analysis of plasma volume (mL·kg^{-1} lean body mass) as a function of α-ANP (nmol·L^{-1}) at 7 weeks of gestation ($y = -0.11x + 74$, $P < .001$). **B,** Linear regression analysis of effective renal plasma flow (mL·min^{-1}· 1.73 m^{-2}) as a function of α-ANP (nmol·L^{-1}) at 7 weeks of gestation ($y = -1.5x + 903$, $P < .001$). **C,** Linear regression analysis of stroke volume (mL) as a function of α-ANP (nmol·L^{-1}) at 7 weeks of gestation ($y = 0.11x + 70$, $P < .0001$). (From Spaandreman M, Ekhart T, van Eyck J, et al: Preeclampsia and maladaptation to pregnancy: A role for atrial natriuretic peptide? Kidney Int 2001;60:1397-1406.)

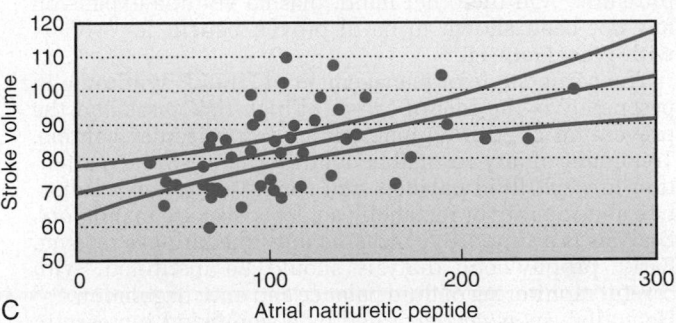

- Edema
- Oliguria
- Increased blood urea nitrogen (BUN) and serum creatinine

Because most of the associated clinical signs are non-specific, astute clinical judgment and careful laboratory evaluation are vital to appropriate diagnosis. Diagnostic errors are more frequent when the syndrome is not associated with preeclampsia (10.9%) or occurs in the middle trimester (15%) or in the postpartum period (30%).[20]

The disease manifests itself on average at 32.6 ± 4.8 weeks of gestation. A recent study demonstrated that ARF develops in 36% of patients with HELLP, and that 50% of these patients were given hemodialysis.[21] The cardinal symptom of the disease is right upper quadrant or epigastric pain accompanied by nausea, vomiting, and malaise. In 20% of cases, hypertension is absent, and 5% to 15% of the pregnant patients present with a low level of proteinuria or no proteinuria at all. The early recognition of hemolysis is achieved by the measurement of serum haptoglobin. The increases in serum aspartate aminotransferase (AST) and alanine aminotransferase (ALT) often precede a decrease in platelet count.[22]

In one series, the most common reason for ICU admission was respiratory insufficiency. The need for invasive mechanical ventilation was described in 45% of the patients.[23]

MANAGEMENT

Because the HELLP syndrome can cause severe DIC, the treatment of choice remains early delivery, when possible. This therapeutic decision, however, must take into account fetal age, maternal signs and symptoms, and fetal condition, as well as pregnancy status, in order to ensure the best overall outcome. A conservative approach is acceptable before 32 weeks but requires ongoing and careful maternofetal follow-up evaluation.

Treatment includes corticosteroids, hydroxychloroquine, azathioprine, and nonsteroidal anti-inflammatory drugs. Blood pressure must be controlled with methyldopa, nifedipine or dihydralazine, or prazosin.[6] Nifedipine and prazosin are used as second-line antihypertensive agents in pregnancy and recent studies show that nicardipine and labetalol can also be used in severe, early onset preeclampsia when other antihypertensive drugs have failed.[24-26] Because no antihypertensive drug has clearly been demonstrated to be more effective, the therapeutic choice should depend on the clinician's experience and familiarity with a particular drug, and on what is known about adverse effects. Exceptions are diazoxide, ketanserin, nimodipine, and magnesium sulfate, which probably are best avoided.[27]

Initial treatment requires hemodynamic stabilization of the mother and the evaluation of fetal well-being. A conservative approach to treatment of moderate to severe preeclampsia, based on the administration of antithrombin concentrate, may allow a significant prolongation of pregnancy and a better neonatal outcome, as well as leading to fewer maternal complications.[28]

Visser and Wallemburg in 1995 used volume expansion and pharmacological vasodilation, under invasive hemodynamic monitoring, for treatment in 128 preeclamptic patients with HELLP. These investigators found a complete reversal of HELLP in 43% of the patients.[29] Corticosteroid therapy or hemodynamic therapy can assist in promoting fetal lung maturity.

Invasive hemodynamic monitoring with pulmonary artery catheterization has been used in the obstetric population, particularly in patients with severe preeclampsia associated with pulmonary edema and renal failure.[30] Administration of dihydralazine after volume expansion can lead to a decrease in pulmonary capillary wedge pressure (PCWP), an increase in cardiac index (CI), and a decrease in systemic vascular resistance (SVR) and blood pressure.[31] On the other hand, plasma volume expansion has not been shown to be of proven benefit for women with preeclampsia.[32]

The cornerstone of management of HELLP syndrome in pregnancy is the identification of high-risk cases and the prevention of ARF by maintaining intravascular volume. Treatment of any reversible contributing disorders, attention to strict fluid balance, and correction of any electrolyte abnormality or metabolic acidosis also are mandatory. Dialysis is a supportive measure until the kidneys recover. Early, prophylactic dialysis should be instituted, with careful monitoring of fluid balance and anticoagulation.[33,34] Hemodialysis is accompanied by a significant increase in the systolic-diastolic ratio measured in the proximal uterine artery in these women.[35]

Postpartum early plasma exchange therapy has been used in selected patients with HELLP who have organ failure or in whom the syndrome appears to be refractory to treatment. This treatment has been reported to lead to rapid improvement in platelet count and serum AST, ALT, and LDH levels.[36]

Proposed theories of the cause and pathogenesis of the HELLP syndrome appear to have the common link of endothelial cell injury and exaggerated inflammatory response. Accordingly, continuous renal replacement therapy (CRRT) appears to be an appealing therapeutic option. Indeed, CRRT has been reported to exert a beneficial effect on the clinical course and outcome in critically ill patients with shock resulting from the systemic inflammatory response syndrome (SIRS). Such an effect could not be explained by fluid removal; convective elimination of toxic media and high-molecular-weight substances has been claimed to be an important mechanism contributing to these nonrenal effects of CRRT.

Decreasing serum levels of thromboxane A_2 and PGE_2, for instance, also were observed both in endotoxemic pigs and in patients with treatment-refractory shock after CRRT. Piccinni and colleagues used CRRT in four preeclamptic women (of whom three were primigravidas at 33 weeks)[37] in response to worsening renal, pulmonary, hematological, and coagulation parameters (Table 60-1). The early start of the continuous (5 to 10 days) extracorporeal treatment,

TABLE 60-1

Laboratory and Hemodynamic Profiles in Patients with HELLP Syndrome before and after Continuous Venovenous Hemofiltration (CVVH)

PARAMETER	MEAN VALUE*	
	PRE-CVVH	POST-CVVH[†]
Weight (kg)	66 ± 19	60 ± 15
BUN (mg/dL)	106 ± 30	88 ± 49
Creatinine (mg/dL)	2.9 ± 2	3.2 ± 2
Urine output (mL/day)	600 ± 200	1200 ± 250
Total bilirubin (mg/dL)	4 ± 2	5 ± 2
Hemoglobin (g/dL)	6 ± 2	8 ± 2
Platelets (×1000/mm³)	40 ± 20	60 ± 30
AT III (%)	20 ± 10	60 ± 20
Serum AST (IU/L)	250 ± 50	100 ± 20
Serum ALT (IU/L)	220 ± 40	80 ± 30
Blood LDH (IU/L)	1200 ± 300	400 ± 100
CVP (mm Hg)	10 ± 3.1	11 ± 2.8
PCWP (mm Hg)	9.8 ± 2.7	10 ± 3.7
PaO₂/FiO₂ ratio	130 ± 80	250 ± 80
PEEP (cm H₂O)	15 ± 3	11 ± 5

*With standard deviation.
[†]Measured after 96 hours of CVVH.
ALT, alanine aminotransferase; AST, aspartate aminotransferase; AT III, angiotensin III; BUN, blood urea nitrogen; CVP, central venous pressure; FiO₂, fraction of inspired oxygen; HELLP, hemolysis, elevated liver enzymes, low platelets; LDH, lactate dehydrogenase; PaO₂, arterial partial pressure of oxygen; PEEP, positive end-expiratory pressure; PCWP, pulmonary capillary wedge pressure.
Data from Piccinni P, Dan M, Marafon S, et al: Continuous renal replacement therapy in patients with HELLP syndrome. Curr Opin Crit Care 1998,4:384-388.

which used convective solute transport with elevated ultrafiltration rates, appeared to promote recovery of organ function. All four patients survived to hospital discharge.

PROGNOSIS

The overall mortality rate as reported by a major study is approximately 13%; the perinatal mortality rate is 34%, with 72% of births being preterm. Residual renal damage is a rare sequela, but women who have a history of preeclampsia and are relatively hypovolemic tend to have lower effective renal plasma flow and higher renal vascular resistance and filtration fraction.[38,39]

The mortality rate increases with increased impairment of organ function. APACHE II scores overestimate the risk of mortality in these patients. Lack of prenatal care and delay in intensive care unit referral adversely affect outcome and are easily preventable.[40]

CONCLUSION

HELLP syndrome is a severe, life-threatening, pregnancy-related thrombotic microangiopathy. Early diagnosis is difficult because only nonspecific signs may be present. A high index of clinical suspicion is useful, together with careful laboratory assessment. Early CRRT should be considered in cases of renal impairment.

Key Points

1. HELLP syndrome is a thrombotic microangiopathy due to an imbalance in prostanoid metabolism with consequent generalized vasospasm, subsequent endothelial damage, and intravascular coagulation

2. Diagnosis is complicated because specific clinical signs are lacking. Accordingly, clinical judgment and laboratory evaluation of the patient are vital to appropriate diagnosis.

3. The cornerstone of management of HELLP syndrome in pregnancy is the identification of high-risk cases and the prevention of acute renal failure by maintaining intravascular volume, treatment of any reversible causes, attention to strict fluid balance, and correction of any electrolyte abnormality or metabolic acidosis.

4. The choice of antihypertensive drugs depends on the clinician's experience and familiarity with a particular drug. Exceptions are diazoxide, ketanserin, nimodipine, and magnesium sulfate, which probably are best avoided.

5. Continuous renal replacement therapy has been reported to exert a beneficial effect on the clinical course and outcome in critically ill patients with shock resulting from the systemic inflammatory response syndrome. Early institution of such therapy appears to promote recovery of organ function.

Key References

1. Del Fante C, Perotti C, Viarengo G, et al: Daily plasma exchange for life threatening class I HELLP syndrome with prevalent pulmonary involvement. Transfus Apher Sci 2006;34:7-9.
2. Selcuk NY, Odabas AR, Cetinkaya R, et al: Outcome of pregnancies with HELLP syndrome complicated by acute renal failure (1989-1999). Ren Fail 2000;22:319-327.
3. Drakeley AJ, Le Roux PA, Anthony J, et al: Acute renal failure complicating severe preeclampsia requiring admission to an obstetric intensive care unit. Am J Obstet Gynecol 2002;186: 253-256.
39. Sibai BM, Ramadan MK: Acute renal failure in pregnancies complicated by hemolysis, elevated liver enzyme and low platelets. Am J Obstet Gynecol 1993;168:1682-1687.

See the companion Expert Consult website for the complete reference list.

CHAPTER 61

Oliguria

Sanjay Subramanian, John A. Kellum, and Claudio Ronco

OBJECTIVES

This chapter will:
1. Review the current definitions and epidemiology of oliguria.
2. Discuss the pathophysiology and clinical significance of oliguria in the setting of critical illness.
3. Outline a diagnostic approach to oliguria in the critically ill patient.
4. Review current evidence for treatment of oliguria, and define the basic principles for a therapeutic approach.

DEFINITIONS AND EPIDEMIOLOGY

A number of definitions for oliguria can be found in the literature, generally ranging from a urine output of less than 200 to 500 mL in 24 hours. To standardize the use of the term across different studies and populations, the Acute Dialysis Quality Initiative (ADQI) has in 2004 adopted a definition of oliguria as urine output less than 0.3 mL/kg per hour for at least 24 hours (www.ADQI.net).

In view of the lack of consensus over definitions until now, it is difficult to determine the incidence of oliguria. Some studies have estimated that up to 18% of patients with intact renal function in a medical-surgical intensive care unit (ICU) setting exhibit episodes of oliguria.[1] Furthermore, of those patients in whom acute renal failure (ARF) subsequently develops, 69% will be oliguric.[2]

Overall, ARF in the ICU carries a poor prognosis (mortality rates range from 30% to 70%), which has remained unchanged despite advances in critical care and nephrology. In general, oliguric ARF is associated with worse outcomes than those for nonoliguric ARF. Thus, it is essential to understand the physiological derangements leading to this exceedingly common problem.

PATHOPHYSIOLOGY

Urine output is a function of glomerular filtration and tubular secretion and reabsorption. The former is directly dependent on renal perfusion. Adequate perfusion in turn is a function of arterial pressure and renal vascular resistance. The intrarenal vasculature is capable of preserving glomerular filtration rate (GFR) in the face of varying systemic pressure through important neurohumoral autoregulating mechanisms that affect the afferent and efferent arterioles, of which the renin-angiotensin-aldosterone system is perhaps most significant (Fig. 61-1). Oliguria indicates either a dramatic reduction in GFR or a mechanical obstruction to urine flow.

Reduction in Glomerular Filtration Rate

Oliguria secondary to a decrease in GFR usually is related to one of the following conditions:

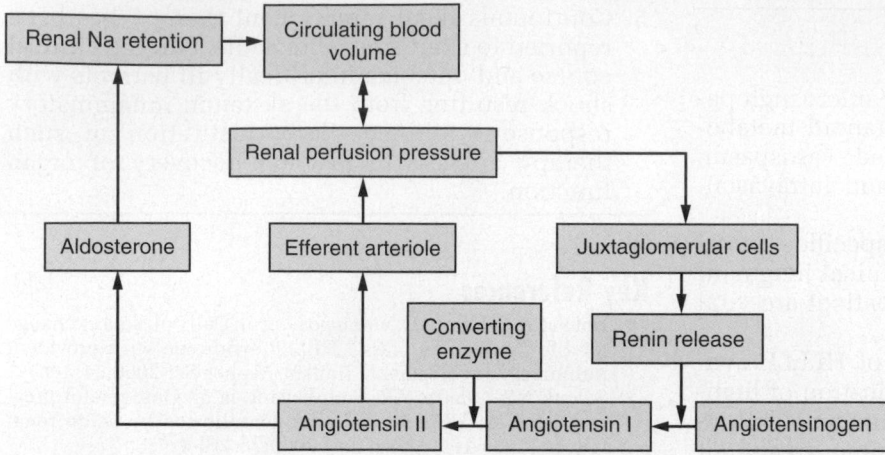

FIGURE 61-1. Network of effects and feedback loop for the renin-angiotensin-aldosterone system. As circulating blood volume or renal perfusion changes, renin secretion changes, resulting in downstream effects that ultimately influence renal resistance and sodium handling by the kidney. Changes in urine output are a direct result of these changes.

- *Absolute decrease in intravascular volume* (as with trauma, hemorrhage, burns, diarrhea, or sequestration of fluid as in pancreatitis or abdominal surgery).
- *A relative decrease in blood volume* in which the primary disturbance is an alteration in the capacitance of the vasculature due to vasodilatation. This is commonly encountered in sepsis, hepatic failure, nephrotic syndrome, and use of vasodilatory drugs including anesthetic agents.
- *Decreased renal perfusion.* This may be due to structural causes such as thromboembolism, atherosclerosis, dissection, inflammation (vasculitis especially scleroderma) affecting either the intra- or extrarenal circulation. Although renal arterial stenosis manifests as subacute or chronic renal insufficiency, renal atheroembolic disease can manifest as ARF with acute oliguria. Renal atheroemboli (usually due to cholesterol emboli) usually affect older patients with a diffusive erosive atherosclerotic disease. It most often is seen after manipulation of the aorta or other large arteries during arteriography, angioplasty, or surgery.[3] This condition also may occur spontaneously or after treatment with heparin or warfarin or thrombolytic agents. Drugs such as cyclosporine, tacrolimus, and angiotensin-converting enzyme (ACE) inhibitors cause intrarenal vasoconstriction, resulting in reduced renal plasma flow and consequent oliguria. Rarely, decreased renal perfusion may occur as a result in an outflow problem such as renal vein thrombosis or, more commonly, abdominal compartment syndrome.
- *Acute tubular necrosis* (ATN). Although this often is an end result of the foregoing factors, it also may be due to direct nephrotoxicity of various agents including antibiotics, heavy metals, solvents, radiocontrast agents, and crystals such as uric acid or oxalate.

Mechanical Obstruction

Oliguria secondary to mechanical obstruction can be further subclassified according to the anatomic site of the obstruction:

- Tubular-ureteral obstruction, which may be caused by stones, papillary sloughing, crystals, or pigment
- Urethra or bladder neck obstruction, which usually is more common and typically is due to prostatic hypertrophy or malignancy
- A malpositioned or obstructed urinary catheter

DIAGNOSTIC APPROACH TO OLIGURIA

Oliguria is associated with considerable morbidity and mortality. Of note, however, merely reversing oliguria, particularly by use of diuretic agents, does not improve outcome. Thus, rapidly determining the cause of oliguria is essential.

Rule Out Urinary Tract Obstruction

The initial step in diagnosis is to rule out urinary tract obstruction before embarking on a lengthy workup for prerenal versus intrarenal causes of oliguria. A history of prostatic hypertrophy may provide some clues to the presence of distal obstruction. In the ICU setting, however, distal obstruction manifesting as oliguria commonly is due to obstruction of the urinary catheter (especially in male patients). Hence, in patients with new-onset oliguria, the urinary catheter must be flushed or changed in order to rule out obstruction. Although uncommon in the acute setting, complete or severe partial bilateral ureteral obstruction also may lead to acute, "acute on chronic," or chronic renal failure. Early diagnosis of urinary tract obstruction is important, because many cases can be corrected and a delay in therapy can lead to irreversible renal injury. Renal ultrasonography usually is the test of choice to exclude obstruction.[4] It is noninvasive, can be performed by the bedside, and also carries the advantage of avoiding the potential allergic and toxic complications of exposure to radiocontrast media. It can, in a majority of affected patients, diagnose hydronephrosis and establish its cause; it also can detect other causes of renal disease such as polycystic kidney disease. Under some circumstances, however, renal ultrasound examination may not yield good results. For example, in early obstruction or obstruction associated with severe dehydration, evidence of hydronephrosis may not be seen on initial ultrasound imaging but may appear on an ultrasound scan later in the course of the disease. Computed tomography (CT) scanning should be performed if the ultrasound results are equivocal or if the kidneys cannot be well visualized, or if the cause of the obstruction cannot be identified.

TABLE 61-1

Biochemical Indices Useful to Distinguish Prerenal from Renal (Intrinsic) Causes of Acute Renal Failure

MEASUREMENT	PRERENAL	RENAL
Urine osmolality (mOsm/kg)	>500	<400
Urinary sodium concentration (mmol/L *or* mEq/L)	<20	>40
Serum urea-creatinine ratio	>0.1	<0.05
Urine-serum creatinine	>40	<20
Urine-serum osmolality	>1.5	>1
Fractional excretion of sodium (%)*	<1	>2
Fractional excretion of urea (%)	<25	>25

*Calculated as FeNa = [(u Na/s Na)/(u creatinine/s creatinine)] × 100, where u is urine, Na is sodium (concentration), and s is serum.

Laboratory Indices

Some authorities advocate examining the urine sediment; others do not. Because hyaline and fine granular casts are common in prerenal disease, ATN usually is associated with coarse granular casts and tubular epithelial casts. The discriminating ability of these findings is of limited practical value, however, especially in the ICU setting. A systematic review of studies describing urinary biochemistry, indices, and microscopy in septic ARF demonstrated significant variability and inconsistency in these measures.[5] The main utility of examining the urine sediment is in the detection of red blood cell casts, which indicates glomerular disease. The urine sediment in postrenal failure often is very bland in appearance. No casts or sediments generally are seen. Occasionally a few red cells and white cells (e.g., in renal calculi with urinary tract infection) may be seen. Eosinophilia, eosinophiluria, and hypocomplementemia, if present, point to an atheroembolic cause for acute oliguria.[6]

Table 61-1 lists laboratory values of use in distinguishing prerenal from intrarenal causes of ARF. A fractional excretion of sodium of less than 1 traditionally has been used as a marker for a prerenal cause of oliguria. Of importance, these indices are unreliable once the patient has received diuretic or natriuretic agents (including dopamine and mannitol) and also may be confounded by endogenous osmolar substances such as glucose or urea.

Clinical Parameters

Traditional indicators of hydration status and tissue perfusion such as systemic blood pressure, heart rate, body weight, jugular venous pulsation (JVP), and peripheral edema may provide important information to determine appropriate interventions. In the ICU, however, some of these indicators are less useful, for a variety of reasons.

The JVP is not an accurate surrogate for right ventricular filling pressures in the presence of positive-pressure ventilation and positive end-expiratory pressure (PEEP). Similarly, peripheral edema often is due to coexistent hypoalbuminemia and decreased oncotic pressure in critically ill patients. Thus, patients may be total body water overloaded and yet intravascularly volume depleted. Blood pressure and heart rate are affected by numerous physiological and treatment variables in the ICU and are unreliable measures of volume status.

In the ICU, it is common to assume that a more accurate assessment of preload can be obtained by measuring the central venous pressure (CVP) or pulmonary artery occlusion pressure (PAOP). This is the case, however, only when these pressures are low (less than 10 mm Hg). An increased CVP or PAOP does not ensure adequate filling pressures. Response to a single fluid challenge or even multiple fluid challenges may not detect hypovolemia depending on the degree of hypovolemia and myocardial compliance. A cardiac index greater than 3.0 L/minute per m² of body surface generally suggests *adequate* preload but may not reflect *optimal* preload. The mixed venous oxygen saturation ($S\bar{v}O_2$) can serve as a surrogate for cardiac output but again does not define optimal filling. In sedated patients on mechanical ventilation, a pulse pressure variation threshold of less than 13% (and, to a lesser extent, systolic pressure variation) provides a robust indicator of adequacy of fluid loading as described by Michard and coworkers.[7] In other cases, echocardiography may provide the only reliable evidence of fluid optimization (see Chapter 95).

Abdominal Compartment Syndrome

Another important and often overlooked reason for acute oliguria is *abdominal compartment syndrome*, defined as symptomatic organ dysfunction that results from an increase in intra-abdominal pressure (see Chapter 62). Although this condition initially was described in trauma patients, it occurs in a wide variety of medical and surgical patients. Abdominal compartment syndrome sometimes is seen after major abdominal surgery necessitating large-volume resuscitation, emergency laparotomies with tight abdominal wall closures, and abdominal wall burns with edema, among other causes. Abdominal compartment syndrome causes ARF and acute oliguria mainly by directly increasing renal outflow pressure, thereby reducing renal perfusion. Other mechanisms include direct parenchymal compression and arterial vasoconstriction mediated by stimulation of the sympathetic nervous and renin-angiotensin systems by the fall in cardiac output related to decreased venous return. These factors lead to decreased renal and glomerular perfusion and hence manifest as acute oliguria. Intra-abdominal pressures higher than 15 mm Hg can lead to oliguria, and pressures greater than 30 mm Hg can cause anuria.[8]

Abdominal compartment syndrome should be suspected in any patient with a tensely distended abdomen, progressive oliguria, and increased airway pressures (transmitted across the diaphragm). The mainstay of diagnosis is measurement of intra-abdominal pressure. The most common measure of intra-abdominal pressure is bladder pressure, because it is easily obtained. Bladder pressure has been shown to correlate well with intra-abdominal pressure over a wide range of pressures. Decompression of the abdomen with laparotomy, sometimes requiring that the abdomen be left open for a time, is the only definitive treatment for oliguria from abdominal compartment syndrome.

TREATMENT OF OLIGURIA

Ensuring Adequate Renal Perfusion

Optimal treatment of oliguria requires identification and correction of the precipitating factors, supportive measures such as avoidance of nephrotoxic agents and dose adjustment of renally excreted drugs, and ensuring adequate renal perfusion. The last involves correction of hypotension and appropriate intravascular volume expansion. Correction of hypotension is especially crucial because in sepsis and ischemic ARF, some of the important autoregulating mechanisms that help preserve GFR in the face of fluctuating blood pressures are disrupted. Hence, in these patients, renal blood flow is directly related to systemic arterial pressure, and vasoactive drugs may be necessary in the ICU setting to raise the mean arterial pressure (MAP) to higher than usual values to maintain adequate renal perfusion pressures and adequate urine output.[9] In patients with chronic hypertension and renal vascular disease, the autoregulation curves are shifted to the right, so a higher MAP may be required to ensure adequate renal perfusion. It is essential, however, to ensure adequate volume resuscitation before administration of these vasoactive drugs, and in many instances initial treatment consists of fluid challenges in the hope of correcting unrecognized volume depletion. The ideal blood pressure to aim for must be individualized in accordance with factors such as the patient's premorbid blood pressure, presence of vascular disease, and so on. Hemodynamic monitoring devices may provide important clues to the intravascular volume status that may enable a more streamlined, "goal-directed" approach to therapy.

Role of Diuretic Agents

The use of diuretic agents in oliguric renal failure is widespread despite the lack of convincing evidence supporting their efficacy. Diuretics traditionally have been used in the early phases of oliguria to "jump start" the kidney and establish urine flow. Presumably, the absence of oliguria makes it easier to regulate volume status, and because nonoliguric renal failure generally has a better prognosis, clinicians frequently use diuretics in this setting.[10] A study by Anderson and colleagues in 1977 claimed a reduction in mortality rate from 50% to 26% with use of high-dose loop diuretics to convert oliguric to nonoliguric renal failure.[11] This study excluded patients with shock and perioperative renal failure. These results have not been reproduced in more recent trials.

A study in 1997 by Shilliday and coworkers examined the effect of loop diuretics in patients with ARF on the incidence of renal recovery, dialysis, and death. Although loop diuretics did result in a diuresis, no difference was observed in the aforementioned outcomes compared with placebo in these patients.[12] Two other randomized controlled trials by Brown and associates and Kleinknecht and colleagues also have not shown any benefit on survival with the use of loop diuretics in oliguric renal failure.[13,14]

The PICARD study group reported the results of a large cohort study of critically ill patients with ARF from 1989 to 1995.[15,16] The study showed that diuretic use was in fact associated with an increased risk of death or nonrecovery of renal function. Although this factor may or may not be causal, it is unlikely that use of diuretics in the setting of oliguric ARF affords any benefit to the kidney. The use of diuretics in this setting should therefore be restricted to the treatment of volume overload, and, even then, caution is advised.

Vasoactive Agents

Other agents have been used to "treat" oliguria, including dopamine and related compounds. Because urine output often increases with the addition of low-dose dopamine,

many intensivists assume that it has a beneficial effect. Indeed, low-dose dopamine has been advocated for nearly 30 years as therapy for oliguric renal failure on the basis of its action on dopamine DA1 receptors in doses less than 5 µg/kg per minute. As supported by abundant evidence, however, low-dose dopamine does not afford any renal protection in oliguria. Most evidence in favor of low-dose dopamine comes from uncontrolled trials or anecdotal studies. A comprehensive meta-analysis of dopamine in critically ill patients by Kellum and Decker showed that dopamine did not prevent the onset of ARF or decrease mortality or the need for dialysis.[17]

Furthermore, important physiological considerations argue against a protective role for dopamine or any other dopamine receptor agonists such as fenoldopam or dopexamine in the oliguric state. First, the effect of dopamine agonists on urine output may be merely the natriuretic response mediated by inhibition of Na^+,K^+-ATPase at the tubular epithelial cell level[18]; therefore, dopamine increases urine output because it is essentially a diuretic. Second, dopamine antagonists such as metoclopramide, which essentially negate any dopaminergic activity peripherally, have not been shown to result in any loss of renal function. Third, the effect of dopamine may be counteracted by increased plasma renin activity in the critically ill, and furthermore, a significant hysteresis effect has been shown for the action of dopamine on renal blood flow. Finally, although dopamine increases renal blood flow, it does not increase medullary oxygenation,[19] and in fact, by increasing solute delivery to the distal tubule, dopamine agonists actually worsen medullary oxygen balance.[20] Fenoldopam, a pure DA1 agonist, is thought to cause greater degree of medullary vasodilatation, and limited data suggest that it can augment renal blood flow. This possibility has generated enthusiasm for studying this drug as a prophylactic and therapeutic agent. A recent comparative trial of fenoldopam and low-dose dopamine demonstrated a greater degree of reduction in creatinine levels with fenoldopam. Whether this difference translated into decreased mortality or need for renal replacement therapy was not addressed in this non–placebo-controlled, underpowered trial.[21] Until results from further large randomized trials are available, the use of newer dopamine agonists such as fenoldopam and dopexamine should be considered experimental and non–evidence-based.

Key Points

1. Oliguria is a sign, not a diagnosis. It should alert the clinician to look for correctable underlying causes.
2. The mainstay of treatment of oliguria is to ensure adequate renal perfusion through optimization of cardiac output and volume status.
3. The use of renovasodilating agents is not supported by current evidence and may cause harm.
4. Diuretics are never a treatment for oliguria, although they often are necessary to manage volume overload.
5. Oliguria is an exceedingly common diagnostic challenge facing the critical care practitioner. A practical, physiology-based approach is needed in diagnosing and treating oliguria.

Key References

1. Zaloga GP, Highes SS: Oliguria in patients with normal renal function. Anesthesiology 1990;72:598-602.
5. Bagshaw SM, Langenberg C, Bellomo R: Urinary biochemistry and microscopy in septic acute renal failure: A systematic review. Am J Kidney Dis 2006;48:695-705.
8. Bailey J, Shapiro MJ: Abdominal compartment syndrome. Crit Care 2000;4:23-29.

16. Uchino S, Doig GS, Bellomo R, et al: Beginning and Ending Supportive Therapy for the Kidney (B.E.S.T. Kidney) Investigators. Diuretics and mortality in acute renal failure. Crit Care Med 2004;32:1669-1677.

See the companion Expert Consult website for the complete reference list.

CHAPTER 62

Abdominal Compartment Syndrome

Gerard A. Betro and Lewis J. Kaplan

OBJECTIVES

This chapter will:
1. Define intra-abdominal hypertension, abdominal compartment syndrome, and abdominal perfusion pressure.
2. Identify key indicators of increased risk for intra-abdominal hypertension and abdominal compartment syndrome.
3. Review appropriate monitoring techniques for intra-abdominal hypertension and abdominal compartment syndrome.
4. Discuss therapeutic interventions for intra-abdominal hypertension and abdominal compartment syndrome.

In 1993 Rotondo and colleagues introduced the term "damage control" to describe a therapeutic strategy to manage injuries accompanied by near-exsanguinating hemorrhage.[1] Along with the concept of staged laparotomy for managing these life-threatening intra-abdominal injuries came recognition of the consequences of increased intra-abdominal pressure. In the trauma patient, intra-abdominal hypertension (IAH) principally reflected ongoing hemorrhage or solid organ and visceral wall edema. Accordingly, a plethora of techniques arose to manage the sequelae of the increased intraperitoneal pressure. These organ system–devastating consequences were termed the *abdominal compartment syndrome* (ACS).[2] It is likely that recognition of the ACS represents one of the most important life-saving concepts introduced into trauma care in the past 2 decades.

Recently, critical care has aggressively focused on managing sepsis and its associated syndromes. Today, ICUs across the world readily embrace "sepsis bundles," and emergency medicine practitioners adopt early goal-directed therapy (EGDT) to rapidly resuscitate patients presenting with sepsis.[3] The end result of EGDT is a vigorous crystalloid volume resuscitation of the vascular space, as well as the interstitium, in a patient with vasodysregulation and capillary leak, leading to significant organ edema and, in particular, pulmonary complications during resuscitation.[4] Thus, rapid volume resuscitation may lead to tense ascites even in a patient whose initial presentation did not include intra-abdominal pathology. This clinical condition has been termed *secondary abdominal compartment syndrome* and often occurs in patients without surgical disease.[5]

Finally, emergency general surgery increasingly is undertaken by trauma surgeons as the U.S. model of emergency surgery moves toward the new paradigm of acute care surgery.[6] Borrowing from the success of damage control techniques in trauma, many surgeons have applied this approach in management of general surgery catastrophes including intestinal ischemia, gastrointestinal perforation with feculent peritonitis, and intestinal obstruction. The patients requiring surgical intervention for these conditions are no different from their medical counterparts just described except that they suffer from intra-abdominal pathology. IAH and ACS may develop in patients in whom the peritoneal space is initially closed before vigorous resuscitation, or in those with an open peritoneal space managed with a temporary abdominal wall closure leading to an unplanned relaparotomy. An important point is that despite the different pathophysiological processes leading to IAH and ACS, the therapeutic goals and interventions remain identical and are universally applicable. The pathomechanisms for developing ACS and its consequences are not universally understood across different medical specialties, leading to disparate rates of recognition and therapy.[7]

INTRA-ABDOMINAL HYPERTENSION

A normal intra-abdominal pressure (IAP) is accepted to be less than 5 to 7 mm Hg by consensus arrived at by the World Society of Abdominal Compartment Syndrome (WSACS) (www.wsacs.org).[8] Some variation in this baseline occurs with conditions that increase the pressure exerted on the peritoneal space and its contents, including clinically severe obesity.[9] The upper limit of nonpathological IAP generally is accepted to be 12 mm Hg by the WSACS, and sustained increases above 12 mm Hg constitute *intra-abdominal hypertension*, four grades of which are recognized, as outlined in Table 62-1. IAH may be

TABLE 62-1

Grading of Intra-abdominal Hypertension

GRADE	INTRA-ABDOMINAL PRESSURE
I	12-15 mm Hg
II	16-20 mm Hg
III	21-25 mm Hg
IV	>25 mm Hg

further classified by duration of increased pressure as chronic (clinically severe obesity, chronic ambulatory peritoneal dialysis [CAPD]), acute (postoperative ongoing hemorrhage, visceral and bowel wall edema—i.e., primary ACS), subacute (ascites from massive volume resuscitation—i.e., secondary ACS), and hyperacute (ruptured acute aortic aneurysm, massive postoperative hemorrhage, resuscitation from extra-abdominal injury).[10] On account of the individual variation in baseline pressure, and the possibility that IAH may be an individually contextually sensitive measurement, a more clinically useful measure may be the abdominal perfusion pressure (APP).[11]

The APP is calculated in a fashion similar to that for intracranial pressure and represents the difference between the inflow pressure, which is the mean arterial pressure (MAP), and the pressure limiting egress, which is IAP. Thus, APP = MAP − IAP. A normal abdominal perfusion pressure is defined as 60 mm Hg. Thus, an MAP of 65 mm Hg minus an IAP of 10 mm Hg gives an APP of 55 mm Hg. Accordingly, some controversy exists regarding the diagnosis of IAH in a patient with an IAP of 10 mm Hg. Ongoing clinical trials will help define the usefulness of these parameters as indications for therapy. As a practical matter, clinicians commonly use the transition from Grade II to Grade III IAH (IAP greater than 20 mm Hg) or the presence of the ACS as the trigger for initiating therapy.

ABDOMINAL COMPARTMENT SYNDROME

The diagnosis of ACS is based on a sustained IAP greater than 20 mm Hg or an APP less than 60 mm Hg that occurs in association with new-onset organ dysfunction or failure.[8] The commonly identified constellation of signs and symptoms outlined in Table 62-2 represent the typical manifestations of organ dysfunction and failure that constitute the ACS. Regardless of cause, the increased IAP diminishes venous return and distorts cardiac performance. The decreased cardiac output is further embarrassed by limited diaphragmatic excursions due to visceral displacement. Reduced thoracic cage space increases the reflected endobronchial pressures, increasing intrathoracic and intrapleural pressures still further, thereby further limiting venous return. Additionally, pulmonary artery pressures increase, limiting right ventricular ejection fraction on the basis of a relative increase in afterload. As a result, cerebral oxygen delivery falls and mentation is compromised. Indeed, intractable intracranial hypertension has been directly related to and resolved by treating the ACS.[12] Other important clinical correlates include oliguria secondary to renal vein compression and diminished renal blood flow from inadequate cardiac output. At the bedside,

TABLE 62-2

Common Signs and Symptoms of Abdominal Compartment Syndrome Associated with Organ Dysfunction or Failure

- Hypotension
- Oliguria
- Increased peak airway pressures (volume-cycled ventilation)
- Decreased resultant tidal volumes (pressure-cycled ventilation)
- Decreased release volumes (airway pressure–release ventilation)
- Hypoxia and decreased CO_2 clearance
- Lactic acidosis
- Increased core to peripheral temperature gradient
- Disordered mentation

the triad of oliguria, hypotension, and increased peak airway pressures (on volume-cycled ventilation) or resultant decreased tidal volumes (on pressure-cycled ventilation) or decreased release volumes (on airway pressure–release ventilation) should enjoin the clinician to consider a diagnosis of ACS in at-risk patients (see later and Table 62-3). An increased IAP in isolation or in combination with a decreased APP will then establish the diagnosis and should prompt urgent surgical consultation for therapy. In one multicenter, prospective study of 265 patients admitted to a critical care unit, IAH was present in 32% (85 patients); of these, 4% (11) were hospitalized with ACS, and 68% of the overall series (140) had a normal IAP.[13] IAH on admission was associated with multiple organ dysfunction and failure. Moreover, IAH during the ICU stay served as an independent outcome predictor, but mean IAP at admission failed to surface as a marker of mortality.

At-Risk Patient Populations

As noted earlier, at-risk patient populations fall into three discrete categories (Table 62-3):
- Trauma patients who have undergone a damage control laparotomy or thoracotomy for near-exsanguinating hemorrhage

TABLE 62-3

Risk Factors for Intra-abdominal Hypertension and Abdominal Compartment Syndrome

- Massive-volume resuscitation (>10 L crystalloid or 5 L colloid over 24 hours)
- Massive-volume transfusion protocol (>10 units packed RBCs over 24 hours)
- Management with an open body cavity (chest or abdomen)
- Core hypothermia (temperature <33°C)
- Coagulopathy requiring blood component therapy (aPTT >2× normal; INR >1.5)
- Sepsis, severe sepsis, or septic shock regardless of cause
- Critical illness in the setting of cirrhosis or other form of liver failure accompanied by ascites
- Mechanical ventilation
- PEEP at >10 cm H_2O pressure (extrinsic or intrinsic)

aPTT, activated partial thromboplastin time; INR, international normalized ratio; PEEP, positive end-expiratory pressure; RBCs, red blood cells.

TABLE 62-4

Common Operative or Postoperative Interventions with Increased Risk for Intra-abdominal Hypertension and Abdominal Compartment Syndrome

- Repair of giant ventral hernia with a tight abdominal closure
- Postoperative abdominal binder
- Ileus
- Peritonitis of any cause
- Preoperative deliberate pneumoperitoneum for giant ventral hernia management
- Colonic gaseous distention (colonoscopy, Ogilvie's syndrome)
- Postoperative hemorrhage
- Open body cavity with or without cavitary packing for hemorrhage control

---

- Medical patients suffering from severe sepsis or septic shock who have undergone massive crystalloid or colloid resuscitation
- General surgery patients requiring massive volume resuscitation for an intra-abdominal catastrophe

Of note, any of these patient populations may receive massive crystalloid resuscitation directed at the intravascular space, but they commonly require massive resuscitation directed at the interstitium as well.[14] Coagulopathy is not an uncommon accompaniment to massive volume loading, and trauma patients in particular may be managed with a massive transfusion protocol as well. However, patients suffering from esophageal variceal hemorrhage, spontaneous retroperitoneal hemorrhage, or massive upper or lower gastrointestinal hemorrhage (non–portal hypertension–associated) may be similarly managed. Thus, IAH and ACS may develop within hours of initiating resuscitation. Some data suggest that volume resuscitation with colloids instead of crystalloids may minimize risk of IAH and ACS,[15] but the current U.S. standard remains crystalloid infusion for plasma volume expansion; colloid resuscitation more commonly is used in the European Union, the United Kingdom, and Australia. Certain operative maneuvers or postoperative interventions also increase the risk of IAH and ACS (Table 62-4). Nonetheless, at-risk patients should be monitored for development of these entities to achieve early detection.

Monitoring Techniques

The most widely utilized monitoring technique to assess intraperitoneal pressure is measurement of intravesical pressure (bladder pressure). This technique is safe, reproducible, and readily accomplished by the bedside nurse using simple instrumentation that is routinely available in the critical care unit. A sample protocol for bladder pressure monitoring is presented in Table 62-5. Figure 62-1 shows a diagram of an assembled bladder pressure monitoring apparatus. Some controversy exists regarding how much volume to infuse into the empty bladder to obtain the most accurate measurement. Currently, volumes between 25 and 50 mL of 0.9% saline solution (normal saline solution [NSS]) are regularly used; the WSACS suggests using no more than 25 mL of NSS to eliminate coaptation of the bladder walls around the measuring catheter. Greater than 50 mL increases the risk of overestimation of IAP.[16] It is important to use a consistent volume to reduce

TABLE 62-5

Bladder Pressure Monitoring Guideline

Purpose
Measuring bladder pressure has been demonstrated to correlate well with intra-abdominal pressure (IAP). Progressive increases in IAP have been shown to lead to the abdominal compartment syndrome (ACS). ACS results in decreased perfusion to the kidneys and the gut, while decreasing cardiac output and impeding respiratory excursion. ACS confers increased mortality and morbidity risk to patients with increased IAP. Recognition of a developing ACS allows the opportunity for early intervention before onset of complications from ACS.

Patients Covered by Guideline
All SICU patients at risk for intra-abdominal hypertension

Risk Identifiers for Increased IAP
- Damage control laparotomy
- Intra-abdominal procedure *in conjunction with*
  - Large-volume resuscitation (>10 L crystalloid equivalent) *or*
  - Coagulopathy requiring correction with the massive transfusion protocol *or*
  - Large-volume blood component therapy (packed RBCs >10 units *or* FFP >8 units)
- Severe sepsis or septic shock
- Open body cavity
- Core hypothermia
- Sepsis, severe sepsis, or septic shock
- Cirrhosis or liver failure with ascites
- Mechanical ventilation with PEEP at >10 cm H_2O pressure (intrinsic or extrinsic)
- Physician discretion

Definitions
1. *Intra-abdominal hypertension*: IAP >12 mm Hg
2. *Abdominal compartment syndrome*: a clinical syndrome resulting from increased IAP manifested as increased peak airway pressure, oliguria, metabolic acidosis, decreased cardiac performance (mean arterial pressure, cardiac output, $S\bar{v}O_2$), decreased abdominal perfusion pressure, and decreased mentation. ACS commonly is associated with IAP >20 mm Hg but may occur at lower pressures, as well as with specific patient characteristics.
3. *Abdominal perfusion pressure* (APP)
   APP = mean arterial pressure (MAP) – IAP
   Normal APP: ≥60 mm Hg

Guideline
1. On admission to the SICU, patients will be evaluated by the bedside nurse and the physician team for risk identifiers for increased IAP.
2. Patients who are identified as at risk will be monitored by bladder pressure measurements according to the following schedule, and using the Yale–New Haven Hospital bladder measurement methodology (nursing procedure).
   a. On arrival at the SICU
   b. Every 2 hours for the first 8 hours
   c. Every 4 hours for the next 8 hours
   d. Every 8 hours for the next 24 hours
3. The physician team will be notified of all bladder pressure measurements >12 mm Hg and abdominal perfusion pressures <60 mm Hg.
4. These values will be recorded on the nursing bedside flowsheet.

FFP, fresh frozen plasma; PEEP, positive end-expiratory pressure; RBCs, red blood cells; SICU, surgical intensive care unit; $S\bar{v}O_2$, mixed venous oxygen saturation.

variability in measurement among clinicians. Additionally, IAP should be recorded at end expiration, with the patient supine and the transducer secured at the phlebostatic axis, to obtain the most accurate reading. Ideally, significant muscular activity should be absent; a tempo-

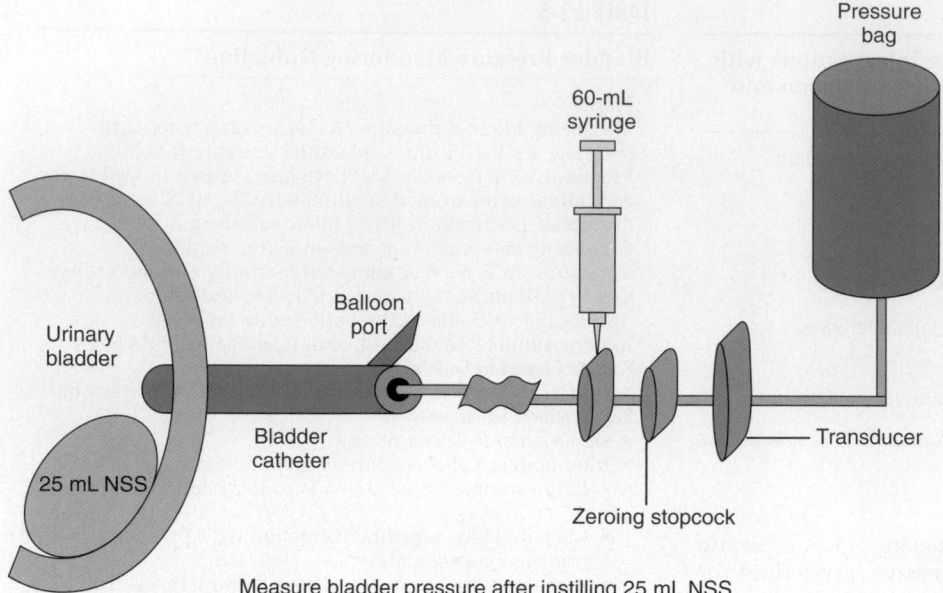

Measure bladder pressure after instilling 25 mL NSS

FIGURE 62-1. A standard bladder pressure monitoring set-up.

rary increase in sedation may be needed to achieve optimal conditions. Neuromuscular blockade generally is not needed or recommended to obtain satisfactory measurements.

A variety of other locations and techniques have been proposed to record intraperitoneal pressure, including but not limited to the inferior vena cava and stomach[17] and use of a continuous pressure monitor for the peritoneal space.[18] Gastric tonometry also has been proposed as a sensitive means of detecting the end result of decreased cardiac performance—intestinal ischemia.[19] However, the same technique has been demonstrated to be insensitive to up to a 50% mesenteric flow reduction, casting clinically relevant doubt on the usefulness of this technique, regardless of whether the CO_2 gap or the calculated intramucosal pH (pH_i) is selected as the delimiter of choice.[20] Of importance, none of the cited methods demonstrates the durability and ease of intravesical monitoring.

Therapeutic Interventions

The standard of care for IAH leading to the ACS is decompressive laparotomy, which follows the same principles as those for managing an extremity compartment syndrome or a thoracic compartment syndrome.[21] Although reoperative therapy has been widely accepted in the trauma community, some reticence remains in the medical community to readily embrace surgical therapy for patients without abdominal disease. Similarly, the nontrauma surgical community less readily welcomes relaparotomy and open abdominal management than do their trauma counterparts. Instead, a variety of nonsurgical remedies have been explored as surgical alternatives. Of note, none of the alternatives has been subjected to prospective, randomized controlled trial analysis to substantiate their efficacy compared with the gold standard of decompressive laparotomy.

Nonsurgical Interventions

Proposed alternative modalities include neuromuscular blockade, percutaneous catheter fluid decompression (ascites management only),[22] gastrointestinal content reduction, volume reduction strategies (diuretic therapy, continuous renal replacement therapy),[23] and laparoscopic fasciotomy or component separation of parts (to eliminate or reduce fascial constraints while preserving skin integrity). Neuromuscular blockade is thought to reduce the measured pressure by eliminating muscular resistance of the abdominal and chest walls. Although use of this strategy may result in reduction in the measured value, in clinical practice, little physiological benefit is realized, because the mean IAP change rarely exceeds 5 mm Hg. At least one animal model and one clinical trial of catheter management of secondary compartment syndrome due to ascites have been described.[24] Although attractive, the technique may not be applied to compartment syndrome from blood and is subject to catheter dysfunction (kinking, malposition, obstruction), which may allow recurrent IAH and ACS at a time when the clinical picture is falsely benign (owing to decreased drainage).

Reduction in luminal gastrointestinal contents may be accomplished by means of nasogastric suctioning, rectal lavage, or prokinetic therapy. These maneuvers are useful in small bowel obstruction, colonic distention after colonoscopy, and Ogilvie's syndrome but have little to no therapeutic effectiveness with other causes of IAH or ACS. Volume reduction strategies may be intuitively attractive but must be applied after the patient's resuscitation has been completed. Attempts at volume reduction earlier than that may be fraught with hypoperfusion, unintentionally reestablishing the pathophysiologic process abrogated by the initial volume reduction therapy. Because many affected patients suffer from organ dysfunction, commonly, acute kidney injury with oliguria despite appropriate effective circulating volume restoration (i.e., acute tubular necrosis), renal replacement therapy, especially ultrafiltration, may provide the sole means of volume reduction. Several retrospective reviews have interrogated the success of this modality to repair intra-abdominal hypertension, with reports of limited success at best, so this therapy cannot be recommended as treatment for IAH or ACS.

Surgical Interventions

Minimally invasive approaches enjoy great success in managing appendicitis, cholecystitis, and inguinal and ventral hernias. Their application to ACS is relatively new but appears to be reasonably logical for secondary ACS. Clearly, these approaches are not appropriate for the trauma patient requiring damage control laparotomy, nor for relaparotomy in that patient population, because an intact anterior abdominal wall is absent. The general surgery patient in whom IAH or ACS develops in the postoperative period, as well as the medical patient with extra-abdominal disease, may be well served by these techniques. The most promising of these appears to be use of a laparoscopic but subcutaneous approach to performing multiple fascial releases without violating the peritoneal space.[25] An important point is that the driving forces that generate ascites will not abate with decompression of the ascites. Moreover, any passage that connects the peritoneal space with the skin will provide a ready conduit for flow of ascitic fluid. Thus, maintaining an intact peritoneum or anterior abdominal wall (albeit an expanded one) will reduce the risk of uncontrolled volume loss and inoculation of ascitic fluid leading to infection and peritonitis.

Decompressive laparotomy simply enlarges the available space for the solid organs and viscera while evacuating fluid, blood, or clot from the peritoneal space. The peritoneal envelope is not reestablished in any way other than with temporary abdominal wall closure. In one animal model, IAH and the ACS have been demonstrated to create venous hypertension and to diminish mesenteric lymph flow as a mechanism of gut edema formation. Thus, early decompression provides one means of limiting further hollow viscus wall edema.[26] Of importance, traditional temporizing interventions such as fluid loading have been demonstrated to be ineffective in patients with IAH and impending ACS; immediate decompression is the treatment of choice.[27] The temporary closure uses an impermeable barrier that covers a suction system positioned over some protective cover placed on top of the intestines (Figs. 62-2 and 62-3). A proprietary system, the Vacuum Assisted Closure (VAC) device (Kinetic Concepts Incorporated, Langford Locks, UK), is available commercially, in addition to "home-grown" versions using Jackson-Pratt drains and wall suction. The value of these systems is that fluid losses may be quantified, heat and evaporative losses minimized, and patient and bed soilage from fluid drainage controlled, leading to improved skin integrity. These devices are changed every 48 to 72 hours; peritoneal lavage and débridement, as appropriate, are common supportive measures. The procedures may be performed at the bedside or in the operating room with equal safety and efficacy, with only 5.8% of bedside laparotomy patients requiring urgent transport to the operating room for additional therapy.[28]

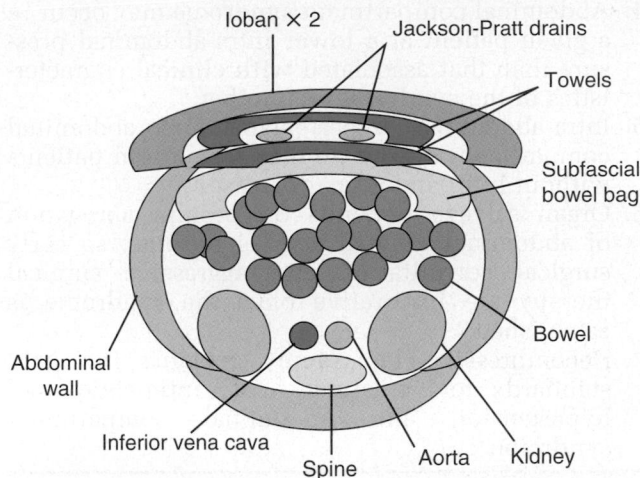

FIGURE 62-2. One method of securing a temporary abdominal wall closure using an impermeable bowel bag, sterile towels, two No. 10 flat Jackson-Pratt drains, and two sheets of Ioban secured to the skin.

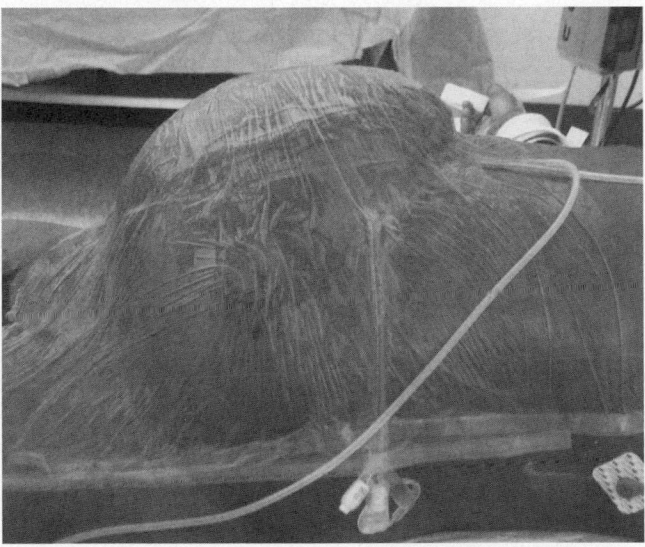

FIGURE 62-3. A patient with a temporary abdominal wall closure using the method outlined in Figure 62-2.

Key Points

1. Routine screening and monitoring for intra-abdominal hypertension and abdominal compartment syndrome are indicated in patients at risk for the development of these conditions.
2. Colloid resuscitation may be considered in at-risk patients as one strategy to reduce the incidence of intra-abdominal hypertension and abdominal compartment syndrome in this population.
3. A standardized monitoring protocol is used to ensure accuracy and reproducibility.

4. Abdominal compartment syndrome may occur in a given patient at a lower intra-abdominal pressure than that associated with clinical characteristics of the syndrome in another.

5. Intra-abdominal hypertension and abdominal compartment syndrome may develop in patients without intra-abdominal disease.

6. Organ salvage depends on prompt abrogation of abdominal compartment syndrome, so early surgical consultation and aggressive surgical therapy are imperative once the syndrome is established.

7. Decompressive laparotomy remains the gold standard for treatment of intra-abdominal hypertension and abdominal compartment syndrome.

Key References

1. Rotondo MF, Schwab CW, McGonigal MD, et al: "Damage control": An approach for improved survival in exsanguinating penetrating abdominal injury. J Trauma 1993;35:375-382.

4. Cotton BA, Guy JS, Morris JA, Abrumad NN: The cellular, metabolic, and systemic consequences of aggressive fluid resuscitation strategies. Shock 2006;26:115-121.

11. Cheatham M, White MW, Sagraves SG, et al: Abdominal perfusion pressure: A superior parameter in the assessment of intra-abdominal hypertension. J Trauma 2000;49:621-626.

14. Lucas CE, Ledgerwood AM, Rachwal WJ, et al: Colloid oncotic pressure and body water dynamics in septic and injured patients. J Trauma 1991;31:927-931.

28. Diaz JJ, Mejia V, Subhawong AP, et al: Protocol for bedside laparotomy in trauma and emergency general surgery: A low return to the operating room. Am Surg 2005;71:986-991.

See the companion Expert Consult website for the complete reference list.

Specific Disorders

CHAPTER 63

Acute Tubular Necrosis

Kevin W. Finkel

OBJECTIVES

This chapter will:
1. Define and clinically characterize acute tubular necrosis.
2. Discuss the use and pitfalls of the clinical, laboratory, and radiographic diagnosis of acute tubular necrosis.
3. Review the effects of the development of acute tubular necrosis on prognosis
4. Summarize the factors underlying the current lack of effective therapy in acute tubular necrosis.

Acute kidney injury (AKI) is a common condition, affecting 5% to 7% of all hospitalized patients, particularly those in the intensive care unit (ICU) with sepsis.[1,2] The most common presentation of AKI in hospitalized patients is acute tubular necrosis (ATN) from ischemia-reperfusion injury, nephrotoxic injury, or inflammation (e.g., sepsis). In a significant number of patients, the etiology is multifactorial.[6] Quite often the pathological process includes a component of renal hypoperfusion from vasoconstrictor agents, sepsis-induced capillary leak, positive-pressure ventilation, or cardiac or hepatic dysfunction. In ICU patients with ATN, the mortality rate approaches 60% when renal replacement therapy (RRT) is required and has remained relatively stable over the past 3 decades. ATN significantly increases hospital length of stay and cost of care.[4,5] Additional morbidity and cost result from chronic dialysis therapy, needed by 5% to 30% of surviving patients.

DEFINITION

AKI is characterized by deterioration in the glomerular filtration rate (GFR) over a period of hours or days, resulting in accumulation of nitrogenous waste products and a variety of fluid and electrolyte disorders. Its presence is manifested by a decline in urine output or a rise in the serum creatinine level, or both. ATN designates any form of AKI not due to obstruction, a vascular disorder, or glomerular or interstitial disease. Because accurate measurement of tubular function or anatomy is not readily available in the clinical setting, a precise definition of ATN remains elusive. This element of uncertainty explains in part why trials of agents proven to be beneficial in animal studies of ATN have failed in humans.

Renal biopsy is rarely performed in the evaluation of patients with ATN. Of note, the word *necrosis* as used to name this entity is misleading because frank tubular necrosis is rarely seen.[6] Prominent findings on examination of biopsy specimens include tubular simplification, patchy loss of tubular cells, focal areas of proximal tubular dilatation, distal tubular casts, areas of regeneration, and evidence of apoptosis. Additional features are vascular congestion and leukocyte accumulation in peritubular capillaries.[7-9]

DIAGNOSIS

The diagnosis of ATN is suggested by the presence of known inciting conditions and is made by the exclusion of other disorders such as a prerenal azotemia, tubulointerstitial nephritis, vascular disorders (thrombotic microangiopathy, cholesterol emboli syndrome), and obstructive nephropathy. No gold standard diagnostic procedure exists. Evaluation begins with a thorough physical examination and history and proceeds to analysis of laboratory and radiographic data, particularly the urinary sediment and electrolytes.

The salient point in the historical evaluation of a patient with AKI pertains to the timing of potential insults. For example, radiocontrast agent–induced nephropathy typically develops within 72 hours, whereas drug-induced tubulointerstitial nephritis requires several days of drug exposure before a rise in creatinine occurs. Because hospitalized patients often are exposed to multiple potential insults, an accurate time line for the hospital course should be constructed in evaluating a patient with AKI.

The physical examination of a patient with AKI often is unrevealing except for signs of volume overload or uremia (pericardial friction rub, asterixis). Certain examination findings, however, will argue against the diagnosis of ATN (Table 63-1). For example, conjunctival hemorrhages and punctate purpura of the toes suggest cholesterol emboli syndrome, rather than ATN from radiocontrast. Fever and rash are more consistent with tubulointerstitial nephritis. The laboratory evaluation for the patient with AKI to determine etiology is discussed in greater detail in Chapters 46 and 47.

Monitoring Serum Creatinine Levels

The pitfalls of using changes in serum creatinine as a marker of changes in GFR are well described. As GFR falls,

TABLE 63-1

Clinical Findings in Acute Kidney Injury

DISORDER	CLINICAL FINDINGS
Prerenal azotemia	Dry mucous membranes
	Orthostatic blood pressure
	Flat neck veins
Atheroembolic disease	Hypertension
	Livedo reticularis
	Purple toes
	Pancreatitis
	Splinter hemorrhages
	Conjunctival hemorrhages
Tubulointerstitial nephritis	Fever
	Drug rash
Glomerulonephritis	Rash
	Arthritis
	Oral ulcers
	Pleural/pericardial rub
	Neuropathy
Obstruction	Palpable bladder
	Prostatic hypertrophy

TABLE 63-2

Urinary Findings in Acute Kidney Injury

CLINICAL DISORDER	URINARY FINDING(S)
Glomerulonephritis	Red blood cell casts
Vasculitis	
Atheroembolic disease	
Tubulointerstitial nephritis	White blood cells
Pyelonephritis	White blood cell casts
Tubulointerstitial nephritis	Eosinophils
Atheroembolic disease	
Acute tubular necrosis	Renal tubular epithelial cells and casts
Ethylene glycol	"Muddy brown" granular cast
Myoglobinuria	Oxalate crystals
Hemoglobinuria	2+ blood on dipstick testing; no red cells
Prerenal obstruction	Bland

tubular secretion increases, thereby maintaining the serum level of creatinine at near-normal levels until late in the course of ATN. The increase in serum creatinine also may be blunted by the vigorous administration of intravenous fluids in the critically ill patient. Therefore, the diagnosis of ATN often is delayed and the severity of injury underestimated. Conversely, the rise in serum creatinine level may overestimate the change in GFR whenever creatinine production is markedly increased (as in rhabdomyolysis) or when its secretion is blocked by medications such as trimethoprim or cimetidine.

Urinalysis

Urinalysis and examination of the urinary sediment can help identify the underlying etiology of AKI. Prerenal azotemia typically is associated with normal urinalysis findings. Nevertheless, patients with prerenal azotemia can have abnormal sediment if they have a preexisting renal disorder, bilirubin in the urine (causing granular casts), or microscopic hematuria and bacteriuria from an indwelling bladder catheter. In ATN, tubular epithelial cells, epithelial cell casts, and coarse granular casts often are seen. Pyuria and white blood cell casts are indicative of glomerulonephritis, infection, or acute tubulointerstitial nephritis (TIN). Staining for the presence of urine eosino-

phils can help identify TIN, although their presence is not diagnostic. Eosinophils have been seen in patients with rapidly progressive glomerulonephritis, bacterial prostatitis, acute cystitis, and postinfectious glomerulonephritis.[10] Red blood cell casts indicate acute or rapidly progressive glomerulonephritis. Nephrotic-range proteinuria suggests intrinsic glomerular disease. In hemoglobinuria and myoglobinuria, the urine dipstick is positive for large blood in the absence of red blood cells on microscopic analysis. The classification of AKI and the typical urinary findings are listed in Table 63-2. Of note, however, two recent systematic reviews of the urinary findings in sepsis-related AKI (one human and one experimental animal study) demonstrated substantial heterogeneity between studies, suggesting that the scientific basis for the use of urinary microscopy in septic AKI is weak.[11,12]

Urinary Electrolytes

The measurement of urinary sodium concentration (UNa) and calculation of the fractional excretion of sodium (FeNa) has been routinely recommended as a means to differentiate oliguria secondary to volume depletion from oliguric ATN, as shown in Table 63-3. In the study reported by Miller and colleagues, a UNa of less than 20 mEq/L had an 80% sensitivity and specificity for differentiating prerenal oliguria from ATN.[13] The FeNa performed even better, with a sensitivity and specificity of 98% and 95%,

TABLE 63-3

Urinary Indices in Acute Renal Failure: Distribution of Values

INDEX	PRERENAL FAILURE	OLIGURIC ATN	NONOLIGURIC ATN
Urine Sodium Concentration			
<20 mEq/L	18/30 (60%)	0/24 (0%)	2/13 (6%)
20-40 mEq/L	12/30 (40%)	14/24 (59%)	11/31 (35%)
>40 mEq/L	0/30 (0%)	10/24 (41%)	18/31 (59%)
FeNa			
<1%	27/30 (90%)	1/24 (4%)	4/31 (12%)

ATN, acute tubular necrosis; FeNa, fractional excretion of sodium.
Adapted from Miller TR, Anderson RJ, Linas SL, et al: Urinary diagnostic indices in acute renal failure: A prospective study. Ann Intern Med 1978;89:47-50.

respectively. The utility of either measurement was significantly less in the absence of oliguria. Numerous exceptions to the general rule are recognized, however.[14-16] Both UNa and FeNa can be low, suggestive of prerenal azotemia with ATN from sepsis, hepatorenal syndrome, rhabdomyolysis, radiocontrast agent–induced nephropathy, transplant rejection, and amphotericin B. In addition, in the Miller group study, patients were excluded if they had an elevated baseline creatinine (greater than 1.6 mg/dL), had received any diuretic within the preceding 24 hours, exhibited evidence of underlying adrenal or liver disease, or had glucosuria or bicarbonaturia. Also, the percentage of patients with sepsis was not described, nor was the actual cause of ATN provided. With only 85 patients included in this study, it is probable that ICU patients were not well represented and that these indices have lower predictive ability in this population.

The use of diuretics can increase urinary sodium loss even in the face of prerenal oliguria, thus negating the utility of the FeNa in differentiating this entity from ATN. Because the fractional excretion of urea (FeUN) is dependent primarily on passive forces, it is less influenced by the administration of diuretics and may be more useful in such circumstances. A series of 102 patients with AKI were divided into three groups: those with prerenal oliguria, those with prerenal oliguria treated with diuretics, and those with ATN.[17] FeNa was low in 92% of patients with prerenal oliguria and in 48% of patients with prerenal oliguria treated with diuretics. Both groups had similar and significantly lower FeUN values compared with those measured in the patients with ATN.

Ultrasound

Ultrasonography is the preferred imaging modality for screening patients suspected to have urinary tract obstruction on the basis of clinical findings. Its role in the evaluation of patients with a high probability of ATN based on history and physical examination, however, is not defined. Because ATN is a frequent complication in hospitalized patients, the practice of routine ultrasonography to "rule out" hydronephrosis in patients without a history suggestive of obstruction is costly and probably is unwarranted. Keyserling and colleagues reviewed the results of 105 renal sonograms obtained in ICU patients with AKI and no signs or symptoms of obstructive nephropathy.[18] Only a single study showed hydronephrosis, which was graded as mild. Incidental findings, most commonly cysts, were noted in 91 sonograms but did not affect patient care.

PROGNOSIS

ATN once was considered to be merely a marker of illness severity, rather than an independent predictor of mortality, because patients could be supported if necessary by means of dialysis. It is now clear, however, that ATN, as the most common presentation of AKI, is an independent predictor of death in hospitalized patients.[4,19-21] In patients with ATN and no other significant comorbid illness, mortality rates range between 5% and 25%. Various risk factors associated with increased mortality rates in patients with ATN include male gender, oliguria, sepsis, presence of malignancy, mechanical ventilation, older age, multiple organ dysfunction, and increased severity-of-illness scores.[22,23]

Traditionally, ATN is categorized as oliguric or nonoliguric on the basis of a 24-hour urine output of more or less, respectively, than 480 mL per day. By the newer RIFLE (i.e., risk, injury, failure, loss of kidney function, end-stage disease) criteria, AKI also is defined by a urinary output less than 0.3 mL/kg per hour for longer than 6 hours. This amount of urine output is the lowest quantity of maximally concentrated urine that can be produced by a person on a normal diet without retaining solute. Urine output is prognostic in the evaluation of patients with ATN; patients with oliguria are more likely to require renal replacement therapy (RRT) and have a higher mortality rate compared with those who do not. This observation probably reflects the degree of renal injury. Oliguric patients whose urine output responds to loop diuretics have a better outcome than that for patients who remain oliguric. Of importance, this observation does not mean that loop diuretics improve outcome; rather, it implies that those patients with less renal injury who can respond to diuretics will do better overall. It also is not an indication for the routine use of diuretics in the face of ATN in the ICU. In fact, one retrospective trial of loop diuretics in ICU patients with ATN suggested that diuretic use was associated with an increased mortality rate.[24]

PREDICTION/EARLY DETECTION

Numerous predictive scores have been developed for different populations. The clinical characteristics of patients in whom ATN developed in the setting of systemic inflammatory response or sepsis were evaluated in 257 patients at a single center.[25] In a multivariate analysis, high baseline creatinine level, liver dysfunction, older age, and increased central venous pressure were associated with the development of ATN. Another scoring model to predict ATN requiring dialysis after cardiac surgery was developed at the Cleveland Clinic Foundation.[26] Using a randomly selected test set of patients from a total cohort of 33,217 subjects, a scoring model was devised and then validated on the remaining patients. Four risk categories of increasing severity were defined. The frequency of ATN across these categories ranged between 0.5% and 22.1%. The score also was valid in predicting ATN across all risk categories. Although such studies improve our predictive power, the generalizability of such information to other populations in other centers may be limited.

Earlier detection of ATN with the use of serum or urinary biomarkers also is of considerable interest. Kidney injury molecule-1 (KIM-1) is a transmembrane receptor of unknown function that is produced in very high levels in the proximal tubule after ischemic or nephrotoxic injury. In small trials, urinary KIM-1 level can distinguish ATN from chronic kidney disease and prerenal failure and increases well before the serum creatinine after cardiac surgery with cardiopulmonary bypass.[27,28] Neutrophil gelatinase-associated lipocalin (NGAL) is a 25-kD protein that is filtered and reabsorbed by the proximal tubule. Urinary NGAL significantly increases in patients with ischemic ATN, and high urinary NGAL levels predict the onset of ATN 2 hours after cardiopulmonary bypass in children, 2 to 4 days before a rise in serum creatinine.[29,30] Urinary NGAL also is increased in patients with urinary tract and systemic infections; therefore, further studies will be needed in more seriously ill patients to elucidate its utility in this population. Interleukin-18 (IL-18) is a pro-inflammatory cytokine that is released into the urine by proximal tubules injured by ischemia.[31] Urinary IL-18 elevation predicts ATN 1 day earlier than serum creatinine in patients with acute respiratory distress syndrome and was an independent predictor of death in one series.[32] Several other potential biomarkers are in various stages of development.[33] Although early results are promising, the use of ATN biomarkers remains under investigation.

PREVENTION

Prevention strategies are limited by an inability to identify those patients with an increased risk for development of ATN. A variety of renal vasodilators (dopamine, fenoldopam, and atrial natriuretic peptide [ANP]) have proved ineffective in the prevention of ATN. In a randomized, controlled trial of 315 patients undergoing coronary artery angiography, low-dose fenoldopam had no effect on urine output, creatinine level for up to 96 hours, or the need for dialysis.[34]

TREATMENT

Currently, no effective therapy for ATN in humans is available. This lack of efficacy results from numerous factors: the multifactorial nature of ATN, reliance on changes in serum creatinine levels to detect changes in GFR, variability in definitions of ATN, the high mortality rate among patients with ATN, and a lack of consensus on the timing and appropriate form of acute dialysis. Although a wide variety of agents, including loop diuretics, low-dose dopamine, ANP, thyroid hormone, and insulin-like growth factor-1 (IGF-1), are effective in animal models, they have not been effective in the treatment of ATN in the clinical setting.[24,35-39]

CONCLUSION

ATN is the most common cause of AKI in hospitalized patients and is associated with significant morbidity and mortality. Despite improvement in medical care and dialysis techniques, little improvement in mortality rates has been realized over the past 3 decades. The diagnosis of ATN still relies on clinical features that are imprecise, particularly changes in serum creatinine levels, leading to both underestimation of the degree of injury and delay in diagnosis. Although no established treatments for ATN are currently available, earlier detection through the use of biomarkers or application of the RIFLE criteria for diagnosis of AKI may lead to more rapid intervention than in previous trials. Finally, the role of dialysis in the treatment of ATN, whether based on timing of initiation or on dosing, is still undefined and awaits the results of ongoing clinical trials.

Key Points

1. Acute tubular necrosis is common in hospitalized patients.
2. The development of acute tubular necrosis is an independent risk factor for death.
3. The diagnosis of acute tubular necrosis often is delayed and its severity underestimated.
4. The diagnosis of acute tubular necrosis is clinical; laboratory and radiographic findings often are nonspecific.
5. Currently, no effective means to treat or reverse acute tubular necrosis are available.

Key References

2. Nash K, Hafeez A, Hou S: Hospital-acquired renal insufficiency. Am J Kidney Dis 2002;39:930-936.
4. Chertow GM, Burdick E, Honour M, et al: Acute kidney injury, mortality, length of stay, and costs in hospitalized patients. J Am Soc Nephrol 2005;16:3365-3370.
7. Bonventre JV, Zuk A: Ischemic acute renal failure: An inflammatory disease? Kidney Int 2004;66:480-485.
20. Lassnigg A, Schmidlin D, Mouhieddine M, et al: Minimal changes of serum creatinine predict prognosis in patients after cardiothoracic surgery: A prospective cohort study. J Am Soc Nephrol 2004;15:1597-1605.
33. Han WK, Bonventre JV: Biologic markers for the early detection of acute kidney injury. Curr Opin Crit Care 2004; 10:476-482.

See the companion Expert Consult website for the complete reference list.

CHAPTER 64

Acute Interstitial Nephritis

Michele Andreucci, Teresa Faga, and Vittorio E. Andreucci

OBJECTIVES

This chapter will:
1. Present an overview of the etiology of acute interstitial nephritis.
2. Review the pathogenesis and pathophysiology of acute interstitial nephritis.
3. Describe the clinical presentation of acute interstitial nephritis, with common and less common signs and symptoms.
4. Suggest how to obtain the diagnosis of acute interstitial nephritis by differentiating it from other forms of acute renal failure.
5. Indicate the prognosis of acute interstitial nephritis.

Acute interstitial nephritis (AIN) defines a pattern of renal injury that frequently is associated with an abrupt deterioration in renal function.[1] It is an important cause of acute renal failure (ARF) resulting from immune-mediated tubulointerstitial injury, initiated by medications, infection, and other causes. It may be implicated in up to 15% of patients hospitalized for ARF.

AIN has become a frequent cause of ARF, as a consequence of drug hypersensitivity reactions, with the increasing use of antibiotics and other drugs capable of inducing an allergic response in the renal interstitium. The renal tubules and interstitium are affected, with sparing of the glomeruli. This rapidly developing inflammatory process is characterized histopathologically by inflammation and edema of the renal interstitium with mild abnormalities of the tubules, such as necrosis, degeneration, or atrophy. A variety of clinical signs and symptoms are possible, depending on the severity and extent of kidney involvement. AIN usually is induced by exposure to drugs or other nephrotoxic agents such as heavy metals. Other, less common causes include autoimmune disorders and, rarely, infections.[2-4]

Because both renal tubules and renal interstitium are involved, the term *acute tubulointerstitial nephritis*, rather than "acute interstitial nephritis," more accurately describes this disease entity, although the latter remains in common use.

ETIOLOGY

AIN most often is induced by drug therapy, although infection or immunological disease also can be the precipitating factor.[4] Of interest, in as many as 25% of patients with chronic renal failure, evidence of injury as a long-term sequela of acute interstitial inflammation can be demonstrated.[5]

Drug-Induced Acute Interstitial Nephritis

The number of drugs potentially associated with AIN is impressive, but few of them have been reported frequently in the literature or have been implicated on the basis of a renal biopsy. The drug-induced inflammatory process in AIN is not dose-dependent; it can occur again with a new exposure to the same drug or to a related drug.

In the past, the classic etiological agent of AIN was methicillin, which is no longer used in clinical practice.[5] Nowadays, AIN usually is the consequence of a hypersensitivity reaction to the following drugs: nonsteroidal anti-inflammatory drugs (NSAIDs), penicillin-like compounds, cephalosporins, rifampicin, and sulfonamides, including trimethoprim-sulfamethoxazole. In addition, ciprofloxacin, allopurinol, diuretics, interferon, quinolones, cimetidine, and omeprazole, among others, have been reported to be responsible for AIN[4-12] (Table 64-1).

Infection-Associated Acute Interstitial Nephritis

Infections due to *Legionella pneumophila*, *Leptospira*, streptococci, cytomegalovirus, human immunodeficiency virus (HIV), or hepatitis B may cause AIN. The pathological changes may result from chemokine release by the pathogen, leading to an interstitial infiltration of leukocytes[13] (Table 64-2).

Autoimmune Disorders and Acute Interstitial Nephritis

Autoimmune disorders are the most common causes of inflammation of the glomeruli, but tubules also can be affected. Some types of autoimmune inflammation can in fact lead to AIN. Autoimmune AIN may represent solely a nephropathy or may occur together with inflammation of the eyes in the TINU (*tubulointerstitial nephritis and uveitis*) syndrome. AIN also may occur as part of Sjögren's syndrome, consisting of eye dryness leading to eye irritation, decreased tear production, "gritty" sensation, infection, and abrasion of the cornea; inflammation of the salivary glands leading to mouth dryness, swallowing difficulties, dental decay, gum disease, mouth sores and swelling, stones (sialoliths), or infection of the parotid gland; extraglandular problems including arthritis, Raynaud's phenomenon, lung inflammation, lymph node

TABLE 64-1

Drugs Reported as Responsible for Acute Interstitial Nephritis

CLASS	SPECIFIC DRUGS
NSAIDs	Most of these drugs (e.g., acetaminophen, ibuprofen, naproxen, aspirin)
Antibiotics	Cephalosporins, ciprofloxacin, ethambutol, isoniazid, macrolides, penicillin-like compounds, rifampicin, sulfonamides (including trimethoprim-sulfamethoxazole), tetracycline, vancomycin
Diuretics	Thiazides, furosemide, triamterene
Others	Acyclovir, allopurinol, amlodipine, azathioprine, captopril, carbamazepine, cimetidine, clofibrate, cocaine, diltiazem, famotidine, indinavir, interferon, omeprazole, phenytoin, propylthiouracil, quinine, quinolones, ranitidine

NSAIDs, nonsteroidal anti-inflammatory drugs.
Data from Conte G, Bellizzi V, De Nicola L, Andreucci V: Drug-induced acute renal failure. In Ronco C, Bellomo R (eds): Critical Care Nephrology. Dordrecht, The Netherlands, Kluwer Academic Publishers, 1998, pp 669-681; and from Rose B, Appel G: Clinical manifestations and diagnosis of acute interstitial nephritis. UptoDate 2007;14:3.

TABLE 64-2

Diseases Associated with Acute Interstitial Nephritis

CLASS	SPECIFIC DISEASES
Bacterial infections	*Corynebacterium diphtheriae* infection, *Legionella pneumophila* infection, staphylococcal infections, streptococcal infections
Viral infections	Cytomegalovirus, Epstein-Barr virus, hantaviruses, hepatitis virus C, herpes simplex virus, human immunodeficiency virus (HIV), and polyomavirus infections
Other infections	Leptospirosis, mycobacterial infection, mycoplasmal infection, rickettsiosis, syphilis, toxoplasmosis
Immune and neoplastic disorders	Acute rejection of a renal transplant, glomerulonephritis, Goodpasture's syndrome, lymphoproliferative diseases, necrotizing vasculitis, plasmacell dyscrasias, Sjögren's syndrome, systemic lupus erythematosus, TINU syndrome, Wegener's granulomatosis

TINU, tubulointerstitial nephritis and uveitis.
Data from Conte G, Bellizzi V, De Nicola L, Andreucci V: Drug-induced acute renal failure. In Ronco C, Bellomo R (eds): Critical Care Nephrology. Dordrecht, The Netherlands, Kluwer Academic Publishers, 1998, pp 669-681; and from Rose B, Appel G: Clinical manifestations and diagnosis of acute interstitial nephritis. UptoDate 2007;14:3.

enlargement, and kidney, nerve, and muscle disease and even vasculitis. Sometimes AIN occurs with autoimmune disorders affecting other parts of the body, such as lupus and Goodpasture's syndrome (see Table 64-2).[5,14]

PATHOGENESIS

Some evidence suggests that AIN is immunologically mediated. Although pathomechanisms are not clear as yet, an antigen-driven immunopathologic process seems to be key. The presence of helper inducer and suppressor cytotoxic T lymphocytes in the inflammatory infiltrate suggests that T cell–mediated hypersensitivity reactions and cytotoxic T cell injury are involved in pathogenesis of AIN.[15] In some cases, humoral mechanisms are involved, because complement proteins, immunoglobulins, and anti–tubular basement membrane antibodies are found in the interstitium.[16]

PATHOPHYSIOLOGY

Lethal or sublethal injury to renal cells causes the expression of new local antigens and infiltration by inflammatory cells, thereby leading to activation of pro-inflammatory and chemoattractant cytokines. The cytokines are in fact produced by the inflammatory cells (i.e. macrophages and lymphocytes) and by the damaged renal cells (i.e., proximal tubular cells, vascular endothelial cells, and renal interstitial cells), resulting in acute interstitial inflammation.

CLINICAL PRESENTATION

The clinical features of AIN are essentially those of ARF resulting from any cause. Signs and symptoms include

oliguria, hypertension, sometimes gross hematuria, malaise, anorexia, and nausea and vomiting, of acute or subacute onset (Table 64-3). No specific history, physical examination, or laboratory findings can distinguish AIN from other causes of ARF. Only a history of a new illness or a new drug exposure is an indicator in favor of AIN. The initial manifestation of AIN may be an asymptomatic increase in serum creatinine and blood urea nitrogen

TABLE 64-3

Signs and Symptoms of Acute Interstitial Nephritis (AIN)

- Acute increase in serum creatinine (0.3 to 0.5 mg/dL per day) temporally related to exposure to a drug never taken before
- Fever (in 70% of patients with AIN)
- Skin rash (in 30% to 50% of patients with AIN)
- Eosinophilia (less than 30%); more often associated with β-lactam antibiotic–induced AIN
- Urinalysis
  - Mild or moderate proteinuria (excretion of less than 1 g of protein/day)
  - Red and white cells
  - White blood cell casts
  - Eosinophiluria (80% of cases; uncommon in AIN as a result of use of NSAIDs)
- Unilateral or bilateral flank pain (uncommon)
- Positivity to radioactive gallium citrate scanning

Data from Conte G, Bellizzi V, De Nicola L, Andreucci V: Drug-induced acute renal failure. In Ronco C, Bellomo R (eds): Critical Care Nephrology. Dordrecht, The Netherlands, Kluwer Academic Publishers, 1998, pp 669-681; and from Rose B, Appel G: Clinical manifestations and diagnosis of acute interstitial nephritis. UptoDate 2007;14:3.

(BUN) levels or the finding of abnormal urinary sediment. Sometimes the clinical presentation is that of a generalized hypersensitivity syndrome with fever (present in 20% to 30% of cases), skin rash (in 30% to 50%), eosinophilia (in 25%), generalized aches, bilateral or unilateral flank pain (probably due to distention of the renal capsule caused by a diffuse swelling of the kidney), arthralgias (present in 15% to 20% of cases), and oliguric renal failure. The classic triad of fever, skin rash, and arthralgias is present in only 5% to 10% of cases of AIN.[4,5,16] A rapid decrease in renal function, as mirrored by the increase in serum creatinine and BUN, is quite frequent. All of these signs and symptoms, however, may be absent in up to two thirds of patients.

Urinalysis reveals mild to moderate proteinuria (excretion of less than 1 g of protein/day), with moderate amounts of red or white blood cells and white cell casts, hematuria (rarely, with red cell casts), renal tubular epithelial cells or casts, and eosinophiluria (in 80% of the cases).[5,16]

Serum chemistry will show an increase in serum creatinine and BUN, hyperkalemia (due to ARF), and signs of tubulointerstitial damage, such as Fanconi syndrome and renal tubular acidosis, although more frequent in chronic interstitial nephropathy.[17]

Most patients with AIN have a fractional excretion of sodium (FE_{Na}) greater than 1%, which is suggestive of the presence of tubular damage. Nevertheless, lower values of FE_{Na} can be associated with concurrent volume depletion.[18] In the presence of the characteristic findings and after exclusion of prerenal and postrenal causes, the diagnosis of AIN becomes highly probable.

The blood cell count will show anemia and eosinophilia, particularly with β-lactam antibiotic–induced AIN. In the case of associated drug-induced liver injury, serum transaminase levels will be elevated. Increased plasma immunoglobulin E levels occasionally have been reported in patients with AIN.[16,19]

The onset usually occurs within a few days to as long as 2 weeks, on average, after administration or longer, in the case of first exposure to the drug. The recurrence or the exacerbation can be detected after a second exposure to the same drug or to a related drug, usually within 3 to 5 days.[4,7] The latent period may be as short as 1 day with rifampicin[7] or as long as 18 months with an NSAID.[20]

DIAGNOSIS

Urinalysis often reveals the presence of eosinophils that are typical of allergic reactions. The demonstration of eosinophils in the urine can be best documented by Hansel's stain, rather than Wright's stain. Indeed, the former is associated with a sensitivity of 100%, whereas the sensitivity of the latter stain is only 18%.[21] False-positive reactions (e.g., from acute prostatitis or rapidly progressive glomerulonephritis) decrease the specificity and the predictive value of Hansel's stain.[21] Alkalinization of the urine also may be helpful in detecting eosinophilic granules. Other conditions such as cystitis and prostatitis also can be associated with eosinophiluria. Thus, the diagnostic value of eosinophils in the urine is still unclear.[5,16,21,22] An increase in eosinophils often is detected in the blood.

Renal ultrasonography may show kidneys that are normal to enlarged in size but does not help in confirming or excluding AIN versus other causes of ARF.[16] Gallium 67 scanning, a nuclear medicine imaging technique, has been proposed as a test to diagnose AIN. For this procedure, a radiologist injects the patient with gallium 67, which will accumulate in the areas of infection or malignancy and can be viewed with a special camera. Results on radioactive gallium citrate scanning generally are positive in interstitial nephritis owing to the presence of an inflammatory cell infiltrate.[23] This test, more useful early in the course of the disease, is relatively specific. Of note, a poor uptake is seen in the presence of acute tubular necrosis (ATN), which is the condition that usually must be differentiated from AIN. Thus, a positive gallium scan is highly suggestive for AIN; a negative scan, however, does not exclude the diagnosis of AIN, because a false-negative result is possible.

After discontinuation of the suspected drug, if renal function begins to improve within several days, no further evaluation or therapy is required. Otherwise, renal biopsy becomes necessary. In fact, for a definitive diagnosis of AIN, a kidney biopsy is necessary because it can reveal inflammation of the renal interstitium. This procedure usually is undertaken when the diagnosis is unclear and when the patient does not improve clinically after discontinuation of the drug suspected as the cause of the ARF.

Renal biopsy shows glomeruli and blood vessels as normal, whereas the tubules show patchy and mild abnormalities such as necrosis, degeneration, and atrophy. The major histological changes are interstitial edema and marked infiltration of inflammatory cells within the renal interstitium, consisting mainly of polymorphonuclear leukocytes, mononuclear cells, and T lymphocytes, with a variable number of plasma cells and eosinophils. Of note, eosinophils may be totally absent from the infiltrate, however, or may concentrate in small foci, forming eosinophilic microabscesses. Fibrotic lesions may be diffuse or patchy. Renal biopsy may be able to differentiate AIN from ATN; the latter is characterized by extensive tubular damage and absence of significant inflammatory cell reaction.

An alternative approach for patients thought to have drug-induced AIN, particularly in those who are poor candidates for renal biopsy, is to initiate a trial of corticosteroids (such as 1 mg/kg of prednisone per day).[14] Only patients with drug-induced AIN will show, within 1 to 2 weeks, improvement in renal function, which thereafter will rapidly return to baseline values.[4,24]

PROGNOSIS

Usually patients with AIN in whom offending drugs are withdrawn within 2 weeks of the onset of AIN can recover normal or near-normal renal function in a few weeks. Recovery is less likely in patients who remain on the offending drug therapy for 3 or more weeks. The evidence suggests that after an initial rapid phase (6 to 8 weeks) of improvement, a phase of slower improvement follows, leading to the previous value of renal function or to a new baseline renal function in approximately 1 year.[16,25] As indicated by findings on renal biopsy, adverse prognostic factors in recovery are diffuse inflammation, great number of neutrophils in the renal interstitium, and extensive or severe interstitial fibrosis.[25]

The disorder may be more severe and is more likely to lead to permanent chronic renal failure in the elderly.

Key References

3. Cooper K, Bennett WM: Nephrotoxicity of common drugs used in clinical practice. Arch Intern Med 1987;147:1213-1218.
4. Neilson EG: Pathogenesis and therapy of interstitial nephritis. Kidney Int 1989;35:1257-1270.
5. Conte G, Bellizi V, De Nicola L, Andreucci V: Drug-induced acute renal failure. In Ronco C, Bellomo R (eds): Critical Care Nephrology. Dordrecht, The Netherlands, Kluwer Academic Publishers, 1998, pp 669-681.
16. Kodner CM, Kudrimoti A: Diagnosis and management of acute interstitial nephritis. Am Fam Physician 2003;67: 2527-2534.

See the companion Expert Consult website for the complete reference list.

CHAPTER 65

Acute Obstructive Nephropathy

Dorella Del Prete and Angela D'Angelo

OBJECTIVES

This chapter will:

1. Present an overview of the epidemiology and causes of obstructive nephropathy.
2. Describe renal function in obstructive nephropathy.
3. Review the major pathophysiological mechanisms involved in obstructive nephropathy.
4. Outline the molecular mechanisms of renal damage in obstructive nephropathy.
5. Report on a novel therapeutic approach for management of acute obstructive nephropathy.

The recognition of obstructive nephropathy should be a fundamental skill for clinicians because it is a common condition at all ages that is potentially amenable to treatment and often reversible. Among adults, its incidence is 1 per 1000 population. Patients with obstructive nephropathy may be asymptomatic or may exhibit a variety of clinical syndromes (Table 65-1).[1] *Obstructive uropathy* refers to the presence of structural or functional changes in the urinary tract, between the renal pelvis and the urethra, that interfere with the normal flow of urine and lead to the development of hydronephrosis and associated renal impairment. The obstruction may be congenital or acquired, partial or complete, in the upper or lower urinary tract, unilateral or bilateral. When the obstruction is short-lived, the condition is said to be acute, and this is most often due to stones.

Upper urinary tract obstructions (above the ureterovesical junction) usually are unilateral, whereas lower urinary tract obstructions are, by definition, bilateral. The etiology varies according to patient age and gender. In young and middle-aged males, acute obstruction due to renal stones is common but temporary, whereas pelvic cancer is an important cause of obstructive uropathy in females of this age group. In older age groups, urinary tract obstruction is more common in the male, resulting from prostatic hypertrophy or malignancy.[1] Congenital obstructive nephropathy almost always is concurrent with ureter, bladder, or urethra abnormalities. The most common of these disorders is obstruction at the ureteropelvic junction,[2,3] followed by obstruction at the ureterovesical junction and at the bladder outlet. When the urinary tract becomes obstructed during early development, kidney morphogenesis, maturation, and growth also are profoundly affected.[4]

Obstructive nephropathy is classified according to its cause, duration, degree, and level, and further distinguished according to whether it is intraluminal, intramural (intrinsic), or extramural (extrinsic). The obstruction is said to be high-grade when it is complete and low-grade when partial.[1]

CLINICAL SIGNS AND DIAGNOSIS

Urinary tract obstruction is a common cause of renal dysfunction and one of the most frequent causes of reversible renal failure. The clinical signs of urinary tract obstruction of acute onset are shown in Table 65-2. They depend mainly on the level and degree of obstruction, the consequent rate of distention of the collecting system, whether the obstruction is unilateral or bilateral, and whether it is accompanied by complications, particularly infection.

Urinary tract obstruction may be completely asymptomatic. Much more commonly, however, signs and symptoms are more or less evident (particularly abnormal micturition, altered urine volume, or pain, alone or in combination). Altered micturition is a predictable consequence of mechanical or functional obstruction of the bladder outlet. Signs and symptoms may include a reduction in the caliber or velocity of the urine stream, difficulty

TABLE 65-1

Most Frequent Causes of Ureteral Obstruction by Age Group

AGE GROUP	CAUSE(S)
Adults	Stones
	Retroperitoneal fibrosis/malignancy
	Local tumor extension
	Vesical tumor (involving ureteral orifice)
	Iatrogenic
	Ureteral stricture (following infection or injury)
Children	Ureteropelvic junction obstruction

TABLE 65-2

Clinical Presentations in Acute Urinary Tract Obstruction

Acute renal failure
Tubular disorders
Renal pain
Urinary sepsis

in initiating urination, intermittency of the stream, hesitancy, urgency, frequent urination, nocturia, and overflow incontinence. Urine output may range from anuria (in complete obstruction) to rather impressive degrees of polyuria.

The main feature of the postobstructive phase is sustained polyuria with urine concentration and acidification defects. In fact, direct renal tubule injury is followed by nephrogenic diabetes insipidus with water and sodium depletion and metabolic acidosis (salt-losing nephritis).

Urinary tract obstruction may interfere with the kidney's ability to concentrate urine through several mechanisms. An increase in urine volume also is quite characteristic of chronic partial obstruction. Obstruction-induced pain is caused by distention of the collecting system. The intensity of the pain usually reflects the rapidity, rather than the degree, of the distention. Acute ureter blockage by a stone, for example, characteristically is associated with excruciating pain, whereas a slow-onset but massive dilation of the urinary tract may be painless. Particularly when acute, ureteral obstruction typically results in flank pain radiating to the lower abdomen, suprapubic area, or genitalia.

Depending on the level of renal function affected, different approaches are used for diagnostic purposes. Imaging typically is accomplished with ultrasonography; if renal function is normal or only mildly or moderately reduced, then excretory urography with tomography may be necessary, with antegrade pyelography in selected cases.

RENAL FUNCTION IN OBSTRUCTED NEPHROPATHY

In experimental animal models, acute ureteral obstruction causes a transient increase in blood flow to the affected kidney, followed by progressive vasoconstriction. The local production of eicosanoids, particularly prostacyclin and prostaglandin E_2, may account for the greater renal blood flow observed transiently after the obstruction has developed. Usually 3 to 5 hours after the onset of the obstruction, an increase in intrarenal resistance is observed. Vasoconstriction is mediated by several vasoactive compounds, including angiotensin II (AT II), thromboxane A_2, and vasopressin. A decline in the production of nitric oxide (NO) also seems to have a role in increasing vascular resistance. The single-kidney glomerular filtration rate (GFR) progressively declines once the ureteral obstruction has become complete, because the rising intraluminal pressure in the proximal tubule results in a drop in the net hydraulic pressure gradient across the glomerular capillaries. The decrease in whole-kidney GFR after ureteral ligation is due to a reduction in both single-nephron GFR and the number of filtering nephrons.

Tubular concentration function also is affected. Studies in animal models suggest that the pathophysiology underlying the loss of urine-concentrating capacity is complex and involves different tubular segments. These studies have shown an impaired water reabsorption at collecting duct level during bilateral ureteral obstruction and massive vasopressin-insensitive polyuria after removal of the obstruction, suggesting that bilateral obstruction can be considered a form of nephrogenic diabetes insipidus.[5] A decrease in the solute content of the papillary interstitium may be the main factor behind this anomaly, although a limited expression of aquaporins in the distal tubule also may play a part.[1] The vasopressin-sensitive water channel aquaporin 2 (AQP2) is the chief target for collecting duct water permeability regulation.[6-7] AQP2 is translocated from intracellular vesicles to the apical membrane of collecting duct cells after vasopressin stimulation and is downregulated in multiple forms of acquired nephrogenic diabetes insipidus characterized by severe polyuria.

In a model of bilateral ureteral obstruction in the rat, postobstructive polyuria with a urine-concentrating defect was found to be associated with reduced trafficking and expression of AQP2 measured after removing the obstruction. Moreover, in an animal model of unilateral ureteral obstruction, a reduced AQP2 expression was demonstrated not only in the obstructed kidney but also in the contralateral unobstructed kidney, associated with a 150% increase in urine production, suggesting that AQP2 regulation depends on both intrarenal and systemic factors.[5]

The fractional excretion of potassium may drop in obstructive uropathy, so hyperkalemic or hyperchloremic acidosis may develop in patients with this disorder, especially in the case of chronic obstruction.[1]

The evolution of renal structural changes after urinary tract obstruction has been well described. Early renal hemodynamic changes are followed by an interstitial inflammatory response initially characterized by macrophage infiltration, tubular dilation, extravasation of tubular cast material (Fig. 65-1), and renal tubular apoptosis, leading to tubular atrophy. Some tubular cells undergo epithelial-mesenchymal transdifferentiation, acquiring mesenchymal markers and even migrating across the damaged tubular basement membrane to the interstitial space, where they can become activated myofibroblasts. Along with damaged tubular cells and interstitial macrophages, myofibroblasts produce cytokines and growth factors that promote the deposition of extracellular matrix and hinder its degradation.

The renal cell response to urinary tract obstruction can be divided into three broad categories: interstitial inflammation, tubular apoptosis, and interstitial fibrosis. Numerous interconnections have been disclosed between these processes that progress in an overlapping sequence.[4] Most

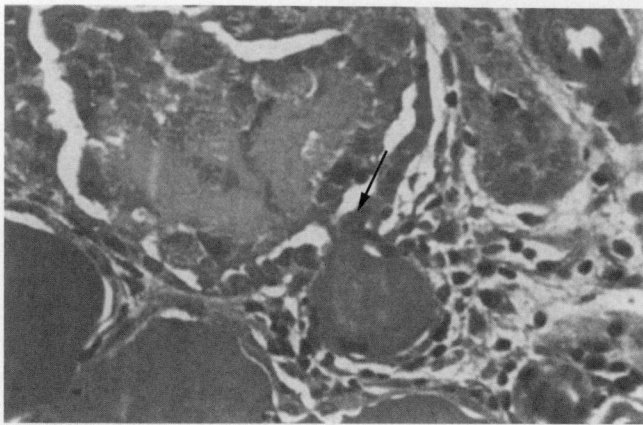

FIGURE 65-1. See also color plates. Ruptured tubular basement membrane. Periodic acid–Schiff (PAS)–positive cast-like material flows from the tubular lumen into the adjacent interstitium (*arrow*). This extravasation of tubular cast material often is noted in patients with renal obstruction (intrarenal or extrarenal). (From D'Agati VD, Jennette JC, Silva FG [eds]: Atlas of Nontumor Pathology: Non-Neoplastic Kidney Diseases, Vol 4. Washington, DC, ARP Press, 2005.)

of the information has been generated in the past several years using models of unilateral ureteral obstruction in rats and mice, and findings in cell cultures have provided complementary data.

PATHOPHYSIOLOGICAL MECHANISMS

In response to a number of cellular stresses, alterations in renal cell death and proliferation, and the development of renal inflammation combine to give rise to tubulointerstitial lesions.

The principal stresses affecting the tubular epithelium during unilateral ureteral obstruction are described as mechanical stretching and desquamation of the tubular epithelium; these early events occur as a consequence of peristaltic retrograde pressure transfer and urinary stasis in the obstructed ureter. An early increment in intratubular pressure is likely to be further promoted by early increases in renal perfusion and filtration after the local rise in NO generation. Felsen and colleagues[8] demonstrated an increase in NO generation and in inducible NO synthase (iNOS) expression in tubular epithelial cell cultures within 60 minutes of the initiation of pressure transfer. Both iNOS and constitutive NO synthase (eNOS) enzyme activity are increased in the injured tubular epithelium, however.[9] Increasing NO dose promotes relaxation of the afferent arterioles, leading to a higher GFR, thereby compounding the urine-pooling effect.[10]

Histological examination of the kidney soon after obstruction shows tubule dilatation, confirming the importance of the urine-pooling effect. The transferred pressure gives the epithelial cells lining the nephron a flattened appearance. The interruption of this primary insult relies on an increased compliance in the ureteropelvic region and the shunting of pooled urine to local lymphatics during the first 24 hours after the obstruction has developed. Later in the course of obstruction, renal blood flow becomes markedly decreased, preventing further increases in the volume of pooled urine by causing a reduction in the GFR.

These initial stressful stimuli in the tubular compartment are known to cause cell injury and death. The affected cells prompt the generation of an inflammatory response. Tubular cell death during unilateral ureteral obstruction has been shown to occur principally by way of programmed cell death or apoptosis.

MOLECULAR MECHANISMS OF RENAL DAMAGE

A number of studies have demonstrated that obstructive nephropathy leads to activation of the intrarenal renin-angiotensin system.[11-12] AT II has a central role in the initiation and progression of obstructive nephropathy, both directly and indirectly, by stimulating the production of molecules that contribute to renal injury.

It has been demonstrated that during unilateral ureteral obstruction, AT II activates nuclear factor kappa B (NFκB), a transcriptional factor that promotes the expression of pro-inflammatory genes. The angiotensinogen gene is stimulated in turn by the activation of NFκB.[13] Inhibiting NFκB activation, by inhibiting or inactivating the angiotensin I (AT I) receptors, reduces apoptosis and interstitial fibrosis in rats with unilateral ureteral obstruction. An alternative strategy is to administer a proteosome inhibitor to maintain the levels of IκB (an endogenous NFκB inhibitor), thereby reducing the macrophage influx after unilateral ureteral obstruction.

In mice with unilateral ureteral obstruction, it also has been shown that AT II stimulates the activation of the small guanosine triphosphatase (GTPase) Rho, which subsequently activates the Rho-associated coiled-coil–forming protein kinase (ROCK) that leads to macrophage infiltration and interstitial fibrosis. Inhibiting ROCK significantly reduces these phenomena.

Studies of osteopontin (OPN) also have helped explain some of the features of the renal damage observed after obstruction. OPN is a glycosylated phosphoprotein produced by bone, macrophages, and endothelial and epithelial cells that mediates cell adhesion and migration. OPN receptors comprise two families: integrins and CD44. The many regulatory functions of OPN include wound repair and the promotion of cell survival. Renal tubular epithelial cells have been shown to synthesize OPN, and its expression is upregulated in glomerulonephritis, hypertension, ischemic acute renal failure, renal ablation, and unilateral ureteral obstruction. The role of OPN in modulating renal injury is still not clear, but available evidence suggests that it has both inflammatory and anti-inflammatory actions.[14] Targeted *OPN* gene deletion reduces macrophage infiltration and interstitial fibrosis in mice with unilateral ureteral obstruction, but *OPN* deletion also enhances tubular cell apoptosis, suggesting that although it contributes to renal interstitial injury, it may have a protective role for the tubules.

OPN and CD44 receptor interaction seems to be important in this respect. In mice with unilateral ureteral obstruction, Rouschop and associates[15] recently demonstrated that CD44 expression reduces tubular injury as a consequence of increased tubular proliferation and decreased tubular apoptosis. In vitro, CD44 has been implicated in cell proliferation and apoptosis. Its expression may help to maintain tubular cell viability in response to renal injury, because CD44 facilitates cell-cell and cell-matrix interactions. Ligand-receptor interaction between

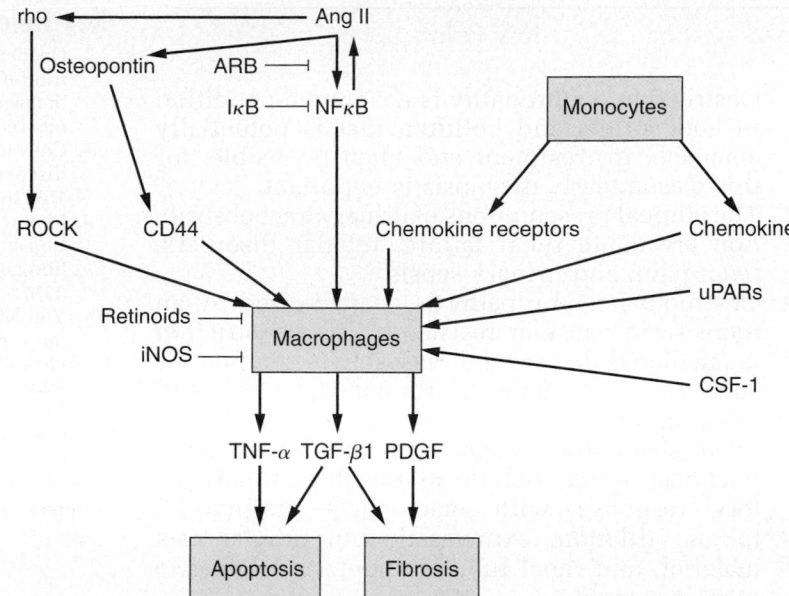

FIGURE 65-2. Pathogenesis of renal interstitial inflammation in obstructive nephropathy. Ang II, angiotensin II; ARB, angiotensin receptor blocker; IκB, endogenous inhibitor; iNOS, inducible nitric oxide synthase; NFκB, nuclear factor kappa B; PDGF, platelet-derived growth factor; ROCK, rho-associated coiled-coil–forming protein kinase; TGF-β1, transforming growth factor-β1; TNF-α, tumor necrosis factor-α; uPARs, urokinase receptors; CSF-1, colony-stimulating factor-1.

OPN and CD44 induces tubular epithelial cell proliferation and reduces their apoptosis in culture.

The role of tubular apoptosis in the genesis of tubular atrophy in obstructive nephropathy was first described in 1987. It is now clear that a mechanical stretching of the epithelial cells is a powerful apoptotic stimulus in the dilated tubules of the hydronephrotic kidney effected through transforming growth factor-β1 (TGF-β1) overexpression, which triggers a p38 MAP kinase–dependent mechanism. It is by means of this same signaling cascade that AT II induces apoptosis in renal tubular cells.

Mechanisms of macrophage infiltration of the obstructed kidney have been investigated. Resident renal cells (glomerular mesangial cells and tubular epithelial cells) are sources of tumor necrosis factor-α (TNF-α) in renal injury, particularly during unilateral ureteral obstruction. In an animal model, Kaneto and colleagues[16] measured TNF-α messenger RNA (mRNA) in the renal cortex of rats at different time points after the onset of unilateral ureteral obstruction and studied whether AT II inhibition or total body irradiation affected the level of TNF-α expression. The authors showed that TNF-α upregulation was restricted to the renal tubular cells of the obstructed kidney. TNF-α mRNA levels increased significantly in the kidney as early as 1 hour after ureteral ligation when compared with the contralateral kidney of the same rats. Angiotensin-converting enzyme (ACE) inhibition with enalapril before and during unilateral ureteral obstruction reduces TNF-α mRNA levels in the obstructed kidney by approximately 40% at 4 hours after the onset of obstruction. Conversely, total body irradiation (which prevents the migration of macrophages to the obstructed kidney) did not affect the TNF-α mRNA upregulation.[16] As indicated by these data, TNF-α may have a role in initiating tubulointerstitial injury in the obstructed kidney, and AT II seems to contribute to the early increase in this cytokine's expression. TNF-α then plays a part in increasing macrophage migration to the renal interstitium of the affected kidney as early as 4 hours after the onset of unilateral ureteral obstruction.

The early increase in renal TNF-α after ureteral obstruction thus upregulates the production of monocyte chemoattractants and contributes to macrophage infiltration of the obstructed kidney. Figure 65-2 is a schematic drawing of the pathogenic pathways involved in kidney damage after obstruction.

In experimental models of unilateral ureteral obstruction, Moon and coworkers[17] demonstrated that 7 days after ureteral ligation, the kidney showed the typical features of obstructive nephropathy, with myofibroblasts and inflammatory cells in the interstitium, tubular degeneration and atrophy, and interstitial fibrosis. The tubulointerstitial damage progressed up to day 14. The morphological changes were accompanied by an increase in the amounts of alpha-smooth muscle actin (αSMA), hydroxyproline, collagen, and fibronectin, which are specific biochemical markers of fibrosis.[17] These investigators synthesized an inhibitor of activin receptor–like kinase 5 (ALK5), IN-1130, that specifically inhibits Smad3 phosphorylation. They showed that IN-1130 almost completely suppresses the expression of αSMA, collagen, and fibronectin in obstructed kidneys at an early stage (day 7), accompanied by an attenuation of the tubulointerstitial fibrosis. IN-1130 does not provide complete protection against renal fibrosis at a later stage, however (day 14).

If the stimulus is transient, all changes can reportedly lead either to remodeling or to regeneration of the tubular epithelium. If the insult is severe or prolonged, however, a maladaptive response is activated, resulting in attraction of inflammatory cells to the interstitium with resultant further damage to the tubules, leading to an increased deposition of extracellular matrix.[18]

The major clinical challenges of evaluating and managing patients with obstructive nephropathy relate to the indication for and timing of surgery, and to the definition of prognostic indicators of progression. Identifying suitable biomarkers of renal injury resulting from urinary tract obstruction could help track the progression of the disorder, or monitor response to new therapies.

1. Obstructive nephropathy is a common condition in both adults and children that is potentially amenable to treatment and often reversible; for this reason, early diagnosis is important.
2. The clinical presentations of urinary tract obstruction are acute renal failure, tubular disorders, renal pain, and urinary sepsis.
3. Obstructive nephropathy is characterized by an increase in vascular resistance; vasoconstriction is mediated by several vasoactive compounds such as angiotensin II, thromboxane A_2, and vasopressin.
4. Renal structural changes occurring after urinary tract obstruction include an interstitial inflammatory response with macrophage infiltration, tubular dilation, extravasation of tubular cast material, and renal tubular apoptosis leading to tubular atrophy.
5. Molecular mechanisms of renal damage involve the renin-angiotensin system and nuclear factor κB, which promotes the expression of pro-inflammatory genes.

Key References

2. Docherty NG, O'Sullivan OE, Healy DA, et al: Evidence that inhibition of tubular cell apoptosis protects against renal damage and development of fibrosis following ureteric obstruction. Am J Physiol Renal Physiol 2006;290:F4-F13.
4. Chevalier RL: Obstructive nephropathy: Towards biomarker discovery and gene therapy. Nat Clin Pract Nephrol 2006;2: 157-168.
9. Manucha W, Oliveros L, Carrizzo L, et al: Losartan modulation on NOS isoforms and COX-2 expression in early renal fibrogenesis in unilateral obstruction. Kidney Int 2004;64:2091-2107.
14. Yoo KH, Thornhill BA, Forbes MS, et al: Osteopontin regulates renal apoptosis and interstitial fibrosis in neonatal chronic unilateral ureteral obstruction. Kidney Int 2006;70:1735-1741.
18. Chevalier RL: Specific molecular targeting of renal injury in obstructive nephropathy. Kidney Int 2006;70:1200-1201.

See the companion Expert Consult website for the complete reference list.

CHAPTER 66

Glomerulonephritis

Judy Savige and Graeme Duke

OBJECTIVES

This chapter will:
1. Describe the clinical features and investigations that indicate rapidly progressive glomerulonephritis as the cause of acute renal failure.
2. Define the features that distinguish between different causes of rapidly progressive glomerulonephritis.
3. Review the principles of treatment for the common forms of rapidly progressive glomerulonephritis.

Glomerulonephritis is the cause of acute renal failure in fewer than 10% of all affected patients and is even less common in those patients admitted to the intensive care unit (ICU), most of whom have acute tubular necrosis. Of note, however, some patients admitted to the ICU for respiratory support also have acute renal failure from small-vessel vasculitis or anti–glomerular basement membrane (anti-GBM) disease.[1]

Acute renal failure in glomerular disease usually is due to *rapidly progressive glomerulonephritis*, in which renal function deteriorates over days or weeks. The most common causes are Wegener's granulomatosis, microscopic polyangitiis, anti-GBM disease, and, less often, diffuse proliferative lupus nephritis, immunoglobulin A (IgA) disease, and poststreptococcal glomerulonephritis. Acute renal failure also may be a feature of mixed cryoglobulinemia, mesangiocapillary glomerulonephritis, membranous nephropathy, hemolytic uremic syndrome–thrombotic thrombocytopenic purpura (HUS-TTP), and scleroderma.

In addition, acute renal failure in glomerulonephritis also results from nonglomerular complications such as acute tubular necrosis from renal hypoperfusion or the nephrotic syndrome, drug- or radiocontrast agent–induced interstitial nephritis, macroscopic hematuria–associated cast nephropathy,[2] renal vein thrombosis, and malignant hypertension.

Early recognition of rapidly progressive glomerulonephritis as the cause of acute renal failure or of respiratory failure is critical because kidney and lung function do not recover spontaneously, and specific and aggressive treatment greatly improves patient outcome.

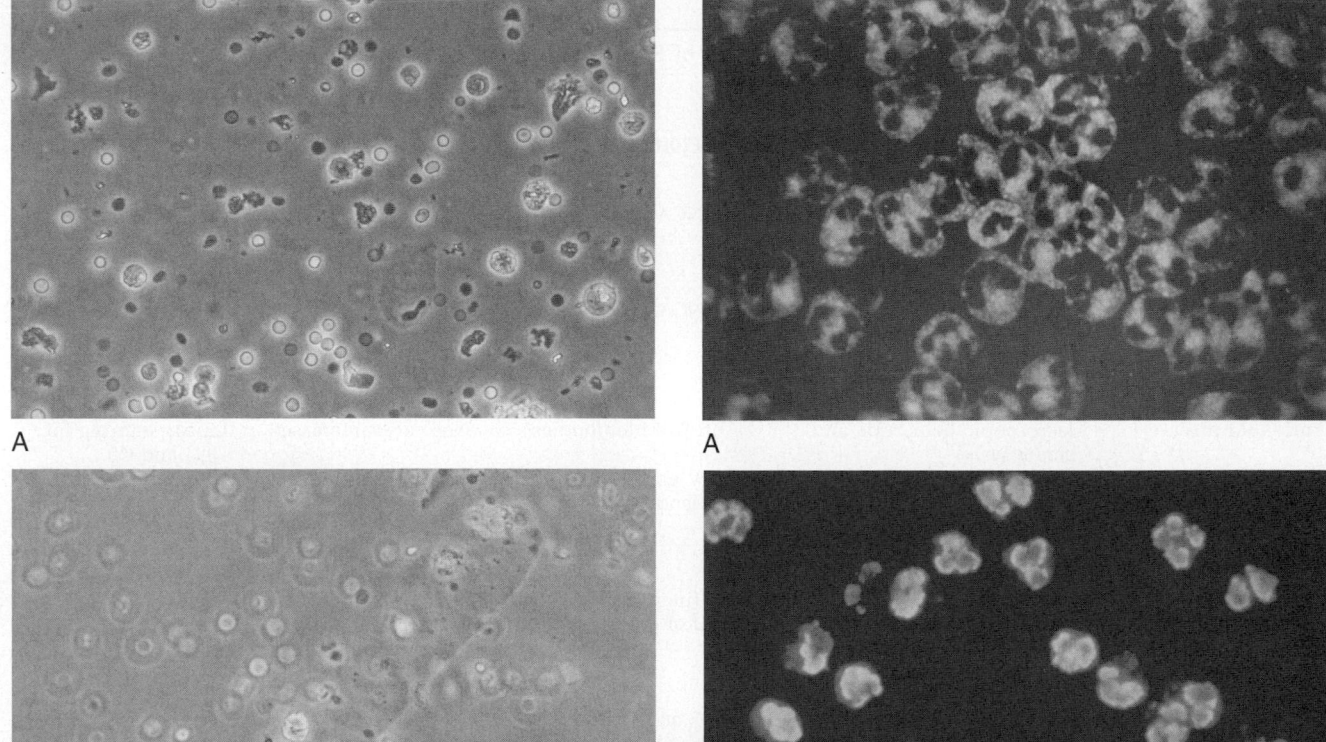

FIGURE 66-1. See also color plates. Phase contrast microscopy of the urinary sediment showing a mixed population of dysmorphic or "glomerular" red blood cells with fragments of varying size, shape, and hemoglobin content (**A**) and a cast containing red blood cells and red cell debris (**B**).

FIGURE 66-2. See also color plates. **A,** Cytoplasmic ANCA (C-ANCA) with coarse granular fluorescence of the neutrophil cytoplasm and interlobular accentuation. **B,** Perinuclear ANCA (P-ANCA) with perinuclear staining with nuclear extension. ANCA, antineutrophil cytoplasmic antibodies.

APPROACH TO MANAGEMENT OF RAPIDLY PROGRESSIVE GLOMERULONEPHRITIS

Diagnosis

With rapidly progressive glomerulonephritis, a prodrome of fever, malaise, arthralgia, and loin pain is characteristic. All patients have microscopic hematuria, but macroscopic hematuria, proteinuria, and oliguria are common too. Phase contrast microscopy of the urinary sediment confirms the glomerular origin of bleeding,[3] together with presence of red cell and granular casts (Fig. 66-1A and B). Urinary red blood cell (RBC) counts are at least 500,000/mL, and an additional isomorphic population may be present.[4] Other clinical features depend on the underlying disease, but pulmonary hemorrhage occurs in Wegener's granulomatosis, microscopic polyangiitis, anti-GBM disease, and sometimes systemic lupus erythematosus (SLE). Anemia, neutrophilia, and thrombocytosis are common. Inflammatory markers such as C-reactive protein are elevated, and the serum creatinine is increased.

A number of assays for autoantibodies (and antibodies) are helpful diagnostically. These include tests for antineutrophil cytoplasmic antibodies (ANCA) in Wegener's granulomatosis and microscopic polyangiitis (Fig. 66-2A and B)[5,6] anti-GBM antibodies (in anti-GBM disease or Goodpasture's syndrome), antinuclear antibodies (ANA) and anti–double-stranded DNA (anti-dsDNA) antibodies (in SLE), serum IgA levels (in IgA glomerulonephritis), antistreptolysin O and anti-DNase B antibodies (in poststreptococcal glomerulonephritis), and rheumatoid factor, cryoglobulins, and serologic hepatitis C markers (in mixed cryoglobulinemia and mesangiocapillary glomerulonephritis) (Table 66-1). Antiphospholipid antibodies (anticardiolipin, anti–β_2-glycoprotein 1 antibodies, lupus anticoagulant) can be detected in some of these diseases (especially SLE and microscopic polyangiitis) and are associated with an increased risk of venous thrombosis.[7] In patients with suspected rapidly progressive glomerulonephritis, assays for ANCA and anti-GBM antibodies are requested urgently, and new technologies test for both antibodies simultaneously.

Complement levels also are helpful diagnostically. These are normal or elevated in Wegener's granulomatosis,

TABLE 66-1

Clinical and Laboratory Features in the Different Causes of Rapidly Progressive Glomerulonephritis

DISEASE	TYPICAL CLINICAL FEATURES	SEROLOGIC FINDINGS	COMPLEMENT LEVELS	IMMUNE DEPOSITS IN GLOMERULUS ON RENAL BIOPSY
Vasculitis				Few/pauci-immune
Wegener's granulomatosis	Prodrome of nasal stuffiness, blocked ears, arthralgia; then onset of hemoptysis, purpura, peripheral neuropathy	C-ANCA	Normal or increased	
Microscopic polyangiitis	Similar to Wegener's granulomatosis or affecting the kidneys only (renal-limited) or overlap with polyarteritis nodosa	P-ANCA	Normal or increased	
Anti-GBM disease	Macroscopic hematuria and hemoptysis	Anti-GBM antibodies	Normal or increased	Linear staining for IgG and C3
SLE (diffuse proliferative, WHO class IV)	Previous history of SLE, marked hematuria and proteinuria, hypertension "telescoping" urinary sediment	ANA, anti-dsDNA antibodies	Low C3, low C4	Granular immune deposits
IgA disease	Persistent microscopic hematuria with episodes of synpharyngitic macroscopic hematuria, with proteinuria, hypertension	IgA (increased in about half of cases)	Normal or increased	
Poststreptococcal glomerulonephritis	At 1 to 3 weeks after streptococcal pharyngitis or impetigo, macroscopic hematuria, edema, hypertension, oliguria	ASO, anti-DNase B antibodies	Low C3, normal C4	

ANA, antinuclear antibodies; anti-dsDNA, anti–double-stranded DNA; ASO, antistreptolysin O; C-ANCA, cytoplasmic antineutrophil cytoplasmic antibodies; GBM, glomerular basement membrane; P-ANCA, perinuclear antineutrophil cytoplasmic antibodies; SLE, systemic lupus erythematosus.

microscopic polyangiitis, anti-GBM disease and IgA glomerulonephritis but are low in conditions in which complement is consumed: SLE (low C3 and C4), poststreptococcal glomerulonephritis (low C3 and normal C4), HUS-TTP, mixed cryoglobulinemia, and mesangiocapillary glomerulonephritis.

Chest radiography demonstrates lung nodules and the alveolar opacities seen with hemorrhage (Fig. 66-3A). Chest computed tomography (CT) scans indicate cavitation of the lung nodules and air bronchograms in the alveolar shadows (see Fig. 66-3B). Abdominal ultrasound examination confirms normal kidney size and excludes some of the other causes of acute renal failure.

The underlying histological diagnosis usually is obvious on urgent renal biopsy. The biopsy specimen also demonstrates the activity and reversibility of the glomerular lesion and the presence of any coincidental acute tubular necrosis (Fig. 66-4A to C). Crescents with epithelial cells and inflammatory cell infiltrates are seen in Bowman's space. Immune deposits are present in one of three patterns: *few or none* ("pauci-immune") in Wegener's granulomatosis and microscopic polyarteritis[8]; *linear* in anti-GBM disease; and *granular* in SLE, IgA, and poststreptococcal glomerulonephritis.

Specific Treatment

The institution of urgent therapy with high-dose corticosteroids and cyclophosphamide is the mainstay of treatment for rapidly progressive glomerulonephritis due to small-vessel vasculitis, anti-GBM disease, and many cases of lupus and IgA nephropathy. A typical protocol begins with daily intravenous methylprednisolone (1 g) for 3 days followed by oral prednisolone (1 mg/kg), together with oral cyclophosphamide (50 to 150 mg/day). An every-other-day regimen is associated with fewer side effects but is less effective, and a lower dose of cyclophosphamide must be used in the elderly and other patients with impaired renal function. Regimens vary slightly for the different types of glomerulonephritis, but the general principle is, as always, to use the smallest effective dose for the shortest duration to minimize toxicity without compromising efficacy. Plasma exchange is helpful in anti-GBM disease and in some cases of small-vessel vasculitis.

Complications of Treatment

The most severe complications of treatment are due to the use of cyclophosphamide.[9,10] If neutropenia or thrombocytopenia develops after 2 or 3 weeks, the cyclophosphamide should be stopped and then reinstituted at a lower dose after counts have recovered. Cyclophosphamide predisposes the patient to infection even when white cell counts are normal, and in one study, nearly half of the patients with vasculitis treated with cyclophosphamide required hospitalization for infection. Infections are particularly common with nosocomial bacteria, cytomegalovirus, *Pneumocystis*, and fungi, and all patients should

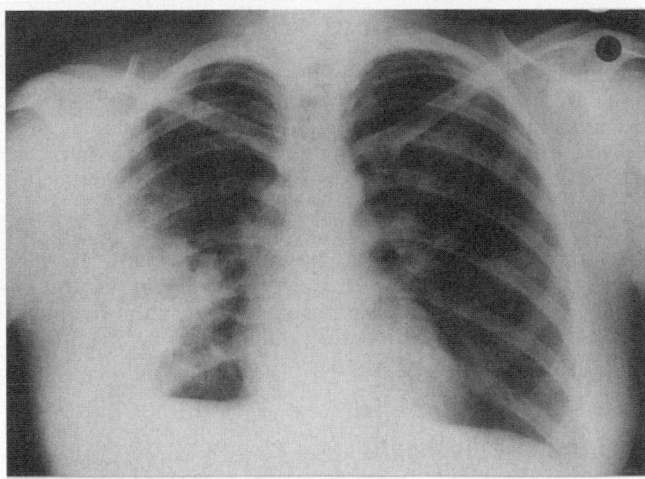

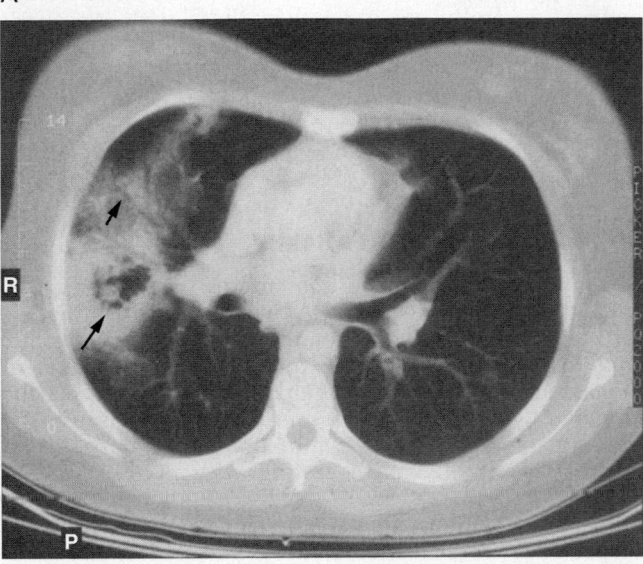

FIGURE 66-3. A, Chest x-ray film showing alveolar hemorrhage in the right (R) lung in a patient with Wegener's granulomatosis. **B,** Chest computed tomography scan taken at about the same time showing an air bronchogram *(long arrow)*, typical of alveolar hemorrhage, and cavitation in a nodule *(short arrow).*

receive prophylaxis for *Pneumocystis* infection. A common clinical difficulty is in determining whether a new abnormality on the chest radiograph is due to infection or to active vasculitis. In general, new vasculitic lesions are not seen when patients are on high-dose immunosuppressants and the disease is resolving elsewhere, but if doubt persists, an open lung biopsy is the most useful investigation.

Prolonged use of cyclophosphamide is associated with an increased risk of cancer, especially transitional cell bladder cancer, myelodysplasia, and lymphoma.[9,10] Approximately half of the patients who receive cyclophosphamide for more than 1 year have hematuria 8 years later, and 16% have bladder cancer after 15 years. The risk of bladder complications from cyclophosphamide is reduced

with morning administration and a lower total dose, but all patients should be monitored for hematuria regularly and for life. A year's treatment with cyclophosphamide induces infertility in most patients, both male and female, as well as early menopause and low testosterone levels and impotence. When relevant, embryo, ovum, and sperm storage should be offered before treatment is started.

High-dose steroids may cause disturbed sleep and altered mood, hypertension, hyperglycemia, gastrointestinal bleeding, and predisposition to infections. Long-term complications include osteoporosis (contributed to by the low estrogen and testosterone), weight gain, increased skin fragility, cataracts, and myopathy. The bone loss is greatest in the first 6 months of steroid treatment,[11] and patients require calcium, vitamin D, or bisphosphonates from the initiation of therapy.

Management in the Intensive Care Unit

Patients with rapidly progressive glomerulonephritis usually are managed on the renal ward but may be admitted to the ICU for treatment of acute renal failure, or for respiratory support in cases of alveolar hemorrhage, pulmonary edema, or severe underlying lung disease. Patients also may be hospitalized for the management of complications such as pneumonia or overwhelming sepsis.[12] Other challenges in the ICU include the need for vigilance for alveolar hemorrhage, anemia and hypoxemia, gastrointestinal hemorrhage, hyperglycemia, and sepsis, and the treatment of subglottic tracheal stenosis in patients with Wegener's granulomatosis.

Prognosis

Patients with glomerulonephritis admitted to the ICU with a high Acute Physiology and Chronic Health Evaluation (APACHE) II score have an increased mortality rate and a 5-year survival rate of only 25% to 50%.[13] Most deaths in these patients are due to sepsis and other adverse effects of treatment.

CLINICAL PRESENTATION AND MANAGEMENT OF RAPIDLY PROGRESSIVE GLOMERULONEPHRITIS

Small-Vessel Vasculitis

Wegener's granulomatosis and microscopic polyangiitis account for the majority of cases of rapidly progressive glomerulonephritis. Microscopic polyangiitis includes a renal-limited form,[14] consisting of glomerular disease only, as well as the overlap syndrome with polyarteritis nodosa, which affects medium-sized vessels and results in renal, mesenteric, and coronary artery aneurysms and ischemia.[15] Renal-limited microscopic polyangiitis is the most common presentation of small-vessel vasculitis.

All forms of small-vessel vasculitis are characterized histologically by a pauci-immune segmental necrotizing glomerulonephritis (see Fig. 66-4A) and necrotizing vasculitis of the other capillaries, venules, arterioles, and arteries within the kidney. Granulomas typically are present in Wegener's granulomatosis.

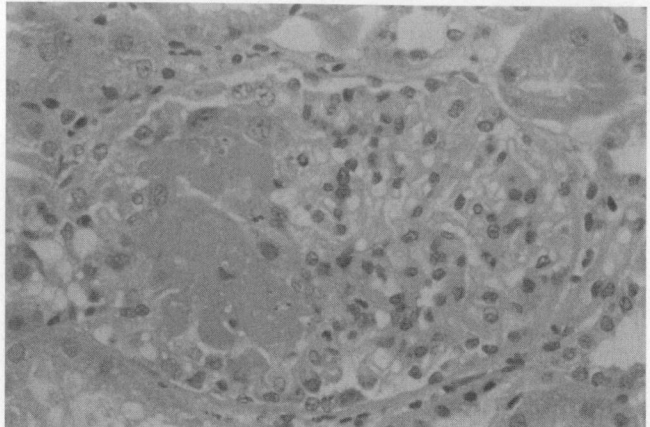

A

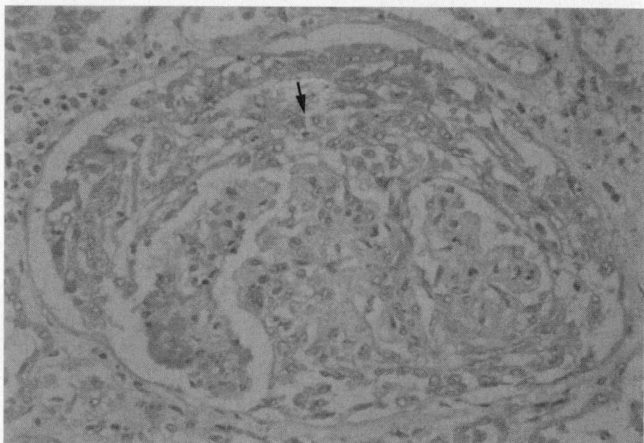

B

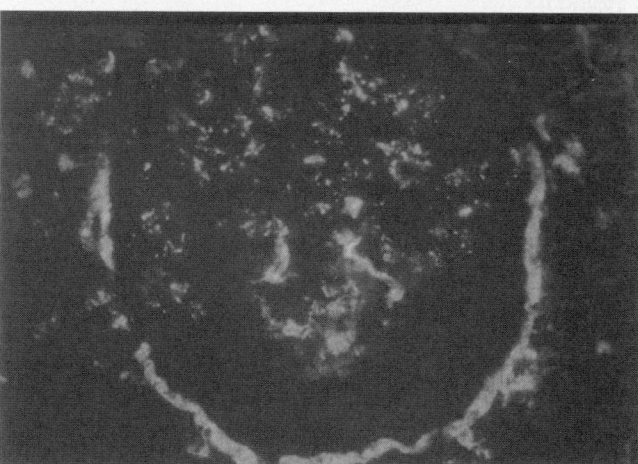

C

FIGURE 66-4. See also color plates. **A,** Segmental necrotizing lesion typical of that seen in Wegener's granulomatosis and microscopic polyangiitis. **B,** Cellular crescent *(arrow)* in Bowman's space, enveloping the glomerular tuft. **C,** "Pauci-immune" pattern, with only a few scattered C3 deposits in the glomerulus.

Wegener's Granulomatosis

Wegener's granulomatosis affects males more often than females, and all age groups are involved, but the average age at presentation is 50 years. The prodrome may be prolonged, and the diagnosis may be overlooked for months. Presenting features include rapidly progressive glomerulonephritis, pulmonary hemorrhage, episcleritis, persistent sinusitis, hearing loss, rhinorrhea, purpura, peripheral neuropathy, and subglottic tracheal stenosis.[16-18] Sometimes disease is limited to the ear, nose, or respiratory tract. Wegener's granulomatosis is a chronic relapsing disease that often recurs within the first few years after the initial presentation and remission.

Microscopic Polyangiitis

Males are again affected more often than females, but patients generally are older than those with Wegener's granulomatosis. Presenting features are similar except that all patients have glomerulonephritis, and respiratory tract and ear and nose disease is less common.[17,18] Microscopic polyangiitis is less likely to relapse than Wegener's granulomatosis and may resolve permanently after several years.

ANCA in Small-Vessel Vasculitis

Wegener's granulomatosis and microscopic polyangiitis are both associated with ANCA, which are autoantibodies directed against enzymes found within the cytoplasmic granules of neutrophils and monocytes. Recognition of the association with ANCA has greatly increased the clinician's ability to diagnose small-vessel vasculitis,[5,6] but no patient should receive treatment on the basis of a positive result on ANCA testing without independent confirmation.

Sera from patients in whom small-vessel vasculitis is suspected are screened for ANCA by indirect immunofluorescence of normal peripheral blood neutrophils,[19] and all fluorescence-positive sera are confirmed by enzyme-linked immunosorbent assays (ELISAs) for the major ANCA specificities, proteinase 3 (PR3) and myeloperoxidase (MPO).[20,21] Ninety percent of patients with active generalized Wegener's granulomatosis and 60% of those without kidney involvement have cytoplasmic ANCA (C-ANCA) directed against PR3. Nearly 80% of patients with active microscopic polyangiitis have perinuclear ANCA (P-ANCA) directed against MPO, and the few with P-ANCA and specificity for PR3 have disease that more closely resembles Wegener's granulomatosis with increased respiratory tract, ear, and nose disease and an increased tendency to relapse. In small-vessel vasculitis, ANCA levels usually are high at presentation, fall with treatment, and, in approximately half of the patients, increase just before relapse. These antibodies also are found in inflammatory bowel disease, autoimmune liver disease, rheumatoid arthritis, and chronic infections, but in such cases, the diagnosis usually is obvious, ANCA levels are low, and the major antigens are not PR3 and MPO.[18]

ANCA and Disease Pathogenesis

The development of ANCA is more likely in persons with certain α_1-antitrypsin and neutrophil FcγR111 receptor genotypes,[22,23] but infections have a role in disease initiation too. Experimental models and evidence of disease transmission in utero indicate that MPO-ANCA and probably PR3-ANCA are pathogenetic.[24-26] The mechanism is as follows: Infections increase levels of circulating tumor necrosis factor (TNF),[27,28] which induces neutrophils to express surface PR3 and MPO.[29] ANCA bind to these molecules, and activate the neutrophils, which degranulate and release cytokines, reactive oxygen species, and lytic enzymes. These damage the vascular endothelium. The activated neutrophils also release PR3 and MPO, which adhere to the endothelial cells, allowing further ANCA to bind, resulting in increased inflammation. Patients with Wegener's granulomatosis appear to have more neutrophils that constitutively express membrane PR3 and can be stimulated by ANCA without priming by infection.[30]

Treatment

The major aim of treatment is to prevent renal involvement in Wegener's granulomatosis, and to delay renal failure in cases in which kidney involvement is already present in Wegener's granulomatosis and microscopic polyangiitis. Less than 20% of patients with small-vessel vasculitis and kidney disease survive without treatment for 1 year, and those given steroids alone exhibit a transient and incomplete response. Thus, all patients, including the elderly, should have at least a trial of steroids and immunosuppressants if the intent is to salvage renal function.

Induction therapy for patients with small-vessel vasculitis and rapidly progressive glomerulonephritis, pulmonary hemorrhage, inflammatory tracheal stenosis, and other serious manifestations is high-dose corticosteroids and cyclophosphamide.[28] The most commonly used regimens continue cyclophosphamide for either 3 or 12 months after remission has been induced, and the shorter course results in more relapses. Newer regimens often use regular repeated pulse intravenous cyclophosphamide. Methotrexate is as effective as cyclophosphamide at inducing remission in patients with normal renal function but also is associated with a higher relapse rate.[28]

Plasma exchange is indicated in patients with small-vessel vasculitis and rapidly progressive glomerulonephritis or severe pulmonary hemorrhage. With use of this therapy, fewer patients require dialysis at 1 year.[28]

Disease that is resistant to these regimens is rare but responds to rituximab and certain TNF antagonists such as infliximab.[31,32]

Response to Treatment

Patients should be monitored for general well-being and specific symptoms, as well as urinary RBC counts, FBE, C-reactive protein, serum creatinine, and ANCA. A rapid response to treatment is typical.[18] Hemoptysis resolves in days, and radiological evidence of pulmonary hemorrhage and nodules clears within 1 week and 1 month, respectively. Urinary RBC counts and C-reactive protein levels stabilize and begin to fall within days. Maximal improvement in serum creatinine occurs between 10 days and 2 months. Deafness and neuropathy resolve more slowly, and recovery may be incomplete. Proteinuria decreases gradually and does not necessarily return to baseline. ANCA persist for at least 4 months.

Clinical Course

After the initial course of therapy, cyclophosphamide typically is substituted with another agent, usually azathioprine, but sometimes methotrexate, mycophenolate, or tacrolimus; this regimen is continued for 3 years in Wegener's granulomatosis and 2 years in microscopic polyangiitis if no relapses occur. Relapses are common, however, and often occur when the medication dose is reduced too quickly. Relapses tend to be less severe than the initial disease and to respond more rapidly to increased medication, but sometimes a further short course of cyclophosphamide is necessary.

When renal transplantation is required, it is delayed for at least 6 months after the initial presentation or the most recent relapse to prevent disease recurrence in the graft.[33] Elective surgery such as nasal reconstruction should be delayed for a year after presentation, but a tracheal stricture that predisposes the patient to infections should be corrected immediately with surgery or, if necessary, a tracheostomy.

Disease-Associated Morbidity

Disease-related morbidity occurs in possibly 90% of patients with small-vessel vasculitis and arises from delays in instituting treatment, progression of subclinical disease, and relapse. Nearly half of all patients have some degree of renal impairment at presentation, and 20% have moderate to severe respiratory disease. Overall, the single most important determinant of outcome in these patients is the presence of renal disease, and the strongest predictor of renal outcome is the serum creatinine level at presentation.[34]

Anti–Glomerular Basement Membrane Disease

Anti-GBM disease[35] accounts for less than 5% of all cases of rapidly progressive glomerulonephritis. It affects patients of all ages, but especially young males and the elderly. Anti-GBM disease is associated with human leukocyte antigen (HLA)-DR2 and is seen occasionally after renal injury—for example, with lithotripsy and after pyelonephritis.[36,37]

Clinical Features

The prodrome usually is mild, and patients often present late in the clinical course with hemoptysis, macroscopic hematuria, or acute renal failure. One third have dyspnea or hemoptysis (Goodpasture's syndrome), which may be precipitated by cigarette smoking, hydrocarbon exposure, pulmonary infection, or fluid overload.[38] The severity of hemoptysis is a poor indicator of the extent of alveolar hemorrhage. Hypertension is uncommon.

Anti-GBM disease may be differentiated from small-vessel vasculitis by the paucity of systemic features, the presence of a very active urinary sediment (often with RBC counts higher than 1 million/mL, with many red cell casts and marked proteinuria), and the rapidity of the deterioration in renal function. Patients often require dialysis at presentation.

Diagnosis

The diagnosis of anti-GBM disease is confirmed with the demonstration of circulating anti-GBM antibodies or linear IgG bound to the glomerular basement membrane in a renal biopsy specimen. Anti-GBM antibodies usually are detected in a sensitive and specific ELISA, but antibody levels do not correlate with disease activity and are undetectable in 10% of patients. Anti-GBM antibodies also are found occasionally in patients with small-vessel vasculitis.[39]

A renal biopsy is critical in determining the severity and reversibility of the glomerular disease, and the presence of tubular damage. The glomerular lesion varies, ranging from mild mesangial hypercellularity to a diffuse proliferative glomerulonephritis with extensive crescent formation. Acute tubular necrosis and interstitial inflammation often are present. Linear IgG and C3 are found in the glomerular basement membrane, Bowman's capsule, and the distal tubular membrane within the kidney, and in the alveolar membrane in the lung.

Disease Pathogenesis

The adult glomerular and alveolar basement membranes comprise mainly type IV collagen heterotrimers with $\alpha 1(IV)$-$\alpha 5(IV)$ collagen chains, and the Goodpasture antigen target is found within the $\alpha 3(IV)$ chain.[40] Antibody binding, complement activation, phagocyte accumulation, and T cells all contribute to glomerular damage.

Treatment and Outcome

Renal function declines more rapidly in anti-GBM disease than in any other form of rapidly progressive glomerulonephritis; without treatment, affected patients die of renal failure or pulmonary hemorrhage. Thus, all patients with anti-GBM disease, except those with minimal renal involvement or irreversible renal damage, should undergo treatment. The aim is to remove circulating anti-GBM antibodies and inflammatory mediators[41,42] using plasma exchange together with high-dose cyclophosphamide and prednisolone. Some physicians do not perform plasma exchange in patients with a creatinine level greater than 600 µmol/L with oliguria,[41] but acute renal failure in patients with anti-GBM disease often is at least partly due to acute tubular necrosis, which is reversible.

With this treatment, the urinary glomerular RBC counts stabilize and fall, and the creatinine begins to improve within a week. The response is slower in patients who require dialysis. Hemoptysis ceases within a few days, and alveolar hemorrhage clears radiologically within a week. Oral prednisolone and cyclophosphamide are reduced over 3 months and then ceased if the disease is inactive and anti-GBM antibodies are undetectable.

Anti-GBM disease rarely recurs,[35] and any subsequent deterioration in renal function is due to an inexorable decline or superimposed membranous glomerulonephritis.[43] Renal transplantation should be delayed until anti-GBM antibodies are undetectable at least 6 months after the initial presentation, to prevent disease recurrence in the graft.

OTHER TYPES OF GLOMERULONEPHRITIS THAT CAUSE ACUTE RENAL FAILURE

Less common causes of glomerulonephritis account for less than 40% of all cases of rapidly progressive glomerulonephritis.

Systemic Lupus Erythematosus

Systemic lupus erythematosus (SLE) is associated with a variety of renal histological patterns, but rapidly progressive glomerulonephritis in this disorder most often is associated with diffuse proliferative glomerulonephritis (class IV in the World Health Organization [WHO] classification). This occurs in less than 10% of all patients with lupus nephritis.

The diagnosis of diffuse proliferative lupus glomerulonephritis is suspected in patients who fulfil the American Rheumatology Association criteria for SLE and who have high urinary RBC counts and marked proteinuria. Renal function usually is impaired, and hypertension is common. Other findings include anti-dsDNA antibodies and low complement levels. In the renal biopsy specimen, more than 50% of the glomeruli demonstrate a proliferative lesion, crescents are common, and the capillary walls are thickened with "wireloop" subendothelial deposits. A "full hand" of IgG, IgM, IgA, C3, and C1q immune deposits is characteristic.

High-dose corticosteroids and immunosuppressants are indicated when urinary RBC counts are markedly elevated, proteinuria with excretion of greater than 2 g of protein/day is present, or renal function is impaired.[44] Pulse cyclophosphamide often is used, but some physicians prefer oral azathioprine for the initial regimen. Again, patients respond quickly, and urinary RBC counts and renal function normalize over weeks. Urinary protein levels fall more slowly. Monthly pulse cyclophosphamide may be used for maintenance. A repeat renal biopsy may be necessary to assess the amount of scarring.

Immunoglobulin A Glomerulonephritis

Most patients with IgA glomerulonephritis have a benign disease with persistent microscopic hematuria, mild proteinuria, and episodes of infection-associated macroscopic hematuria, but one third progress to renal failure over years.[45] In a small group of patients, a rapidly progressive glomerulonephritis with crescentic change and tubulointerstitial inflammation develops. High-dose corticosteroids and immunosuppressants are useful in these patients.[46]

Poststreptococcal Glomerulonephritis

Poststreptococcal glomerulonephritis is common in children in developing countries 1 to 3 weeks after pharyngitis or impetigo. Most cases are asymptomatic, but in 20% of affected patients, the nephritic syndrome develops, manifesting as hematuria, hypertension, oliguria, and an elevated serum creatinine. Antistreptolysin O and anti-DNase B antibodies are detectable after throat and skin infections, respectively, and C3 levels are low. The prognosis usually is excellent, and no specific treatment is needed. In up to 1% of patients, however, acute renal failure with a crescentic glomerulonephritis develops, sometimes associated with ANCA.[47] The role of corticosteroids and immunosuppressants in these patients is controversial.

Key Points

1. Glomerulonephritis is a rare cause of acute renal failure, especially in the intensive care unit, and may be misdiagnosed as acute tubular necrosis.
2. Rapidly progressive glomerulonephritis constitutes a medical emergency, and an urgent renal biopsy is indicated both to make an accurate diagnosis and to determine the extent of irreversible renal damage.
3. An urgent diagnosis is critical because renal function does not recover spontaneously, and because aggressive treatment improves function and delays the onset of end-stage renal failure.

Acknowledgments

I thank the following colleagues for providing illustrations: Dr. Ian Forbes (urinary sediment); Dr. Roger Sinclair (renal histology and immunofluorescence); and Professor Don Campbell (chest radiology).

Key References

4. Fairley KF, Birch DF: Haematuria: A simple method for identifying glomerular bleeding. Kidney Int 1982;21:105-108.
18. Savige J, Davies D, Falk RJ, et al: Antineutrophil cytoplasmic antibodies and associated diseases: A review of the clinical and laboratory features. Kidney Int 2000;57:846-862.
19. Savige J, Gillis D, Benson E, et al: International consensus statement on testing and reporting of antineutrophil cytoplasmic antibodies (ANCA). Am J Clin Pathol 1999;111:507-513.
24. Xiao H, Heeringa P, Hu P, et al: Antineutrophil cytoplasmic autoantibodies specific for myeloperoxidase cause glomerulonephitis and vasculitis in mice. J Clin Invest 2002;110:955-963.
43. Walker RG, Scheinkestel C, Becker GJ, et al: Clinical and morphological aspects of the management of crescentic antiglomerular basement membrane antibody (antiGBM nephritis/Goodpasture's syndrome). Q J Med 1985;54:75-89.

See the companion Expert Consult website for the complete reference list.

CHAPTER 67

Acute Lupus Nephritis

Geoffrey R. Bihl

OBJECTIVES

This chapter will:
1. Describe the histopathological and clinical features of lupus nephritis.
2. Outline the clinicopathological diagnosis of lupus nephritis.
3. Review the current treatment strategies for this condition.
4. Summarize expected short- and long-term outcomes for patients with lupus.

Systemic lupus erythematosus (SLE) is a syndrome of multifactorial etiology, characterized by widespread inflammation, most commonly affecting women during the childbearing years and being more severe in African Americans. SLE is a disease of great clinical diversity, and virtually every organ of the body may be involved. Patients with lupus nephritis (LN) do not constitute a clear subset with regard to other manifestations, although statistically they tend to have a lower frequency of rashes, arthritis, and Raynaud's syndrome and a higher frequency of alopecia and oral ulceration. Lupus may first manifest as LN, which not only may be life-threatening in itself but will require the use of aggressive immunosuppressive agents, with their inherent risks of infection. Consequently, patients with SLE admitted to the intensive care unit (ICU) will tend to have a poor outcome. Despite progress in the approach to diagnosis, categorization of histological lesions, and treatment, optimal therapy remains an unresolved issue. Mycophenolate mofetil, an agent used in organ transplantation, is an attractive option for the treatment of severe LN, in light of the inherent toxicities of cyclophosphamide, previously considered a panacea.

PATHOGENESIS AND HISTOPATHOLOGY OF LUPUS NEPHRITIS

Systemic lupus and LN develop in people with a genetic predisposition following exposure to environmental triggers for immune responses (e.g., ultraviolet light and Epstein-Barr virus).[1,2]

The pathogenesis of systemic lupus is complex and involves many components of the immune system. A brief summary follows: Innate immunity (first-line defense, such as that mediated by phagocytes and dendritic cells) and adaptive immunity (antigen-specific immune response) both participate in this process. More specifically, DNA and RNA are present in infectious agents complex with proteins responsible for activating dendritic cells and B lymphocytes by way of Toll-like receptors 7 and 9.[3]

Dendritic cells and other antigen-presenting cells then activate T lymphocytes, which further stimulate B lymphocytes[4] to produce autoantibodies against human glomerular mesangial cells. Together with immune complexes, these autoantibodies become affixed to tissues in the kidney, where they cause inflammation by upregulating pro-inflammatory cytokines (TNF-α and IL-6).[5,6]

Furthermore, T and B lymphocytes are intrinsically abnormal in SLE, with T lymphocytes unable to make anti-inflammatory IL-2 and autoreactive B lymphocytes failing to be eliminated, especially during active disease.[7] Prolactin and estradiol alter B lymphocyte selection, resulting in an increase in the number of autoreactive B lymphocytes, with increased autoantibodies; this association may partly explain why lupus is nine times more common in women than in men.

Cardinal histopathological features of lupus nephritis include mesangial proliferation, elevated levels of anti-DNA antibodies and the aforementioned deposition of immune complexes in the tissue of the kidney.

With regard to lupus glomerulonephritis, the International Society of Nephrology (ISN)/Renal Pathology Society (RPS) classification suggests six histopathological categories.[8] Essentially, class I and class II demonstrate purely mesangial involvement; class III is for focal glomerulonephritis, either active and sclerotic lesions; class IV is for diffuse glomerulonephritis, with either segmental (class IV-S) or global (class IV-G) involvement, and also with subdivisions for active and sclerotic lesions; and class V is for membranous lupus nephritis. Class VI is reserved for advanced sclerosing lesions or end-stage kidney disease. Furthermore, histopathological diagnosis also should include evidence for any vascular or tubulointerstitial lesions. With rigorous diagnosis and classification of the histopathological subtype, judicious treatment planning can be instituted, and more accurate prognostic indicators can be entertained, including markers of activity and chronicity.

CLINICAL PRESENTATION OF ACUTE LUPUS NEPHRITIS

Although chronic fatigue, skin rashes, and arthralgias are prominent among the clinical symptoms and signs of SLE, major visceral disease, especially renal involvement, often is associated with fewer and less imposing signs and symptoms. A detailed urinalysis should form part of the basic examination in all patients with lupus, especially those with a history of renal involvement, in whom a renal biopsy also is indicated.

The dominant feature in almost every patient with LN is proteinuria with levels reaching the nephrotic range (greater than $3.5 \text{ g}/1.73 \text{ m}^2$ of body surface per 24 hours) in 45% to 65% (Table 67-1). Asymptomatic proteinuria or hematuria may be overlooked as evidence of minor abnormalities in the genitourinary tract, although aggressive management directed at correction of these abnormalities

TABLE 67-1

Distribution of Clinical Features of Lupus Nephritis

FEATURE	FREQUENCY
Peripheral signs of SLE	
Alopecia/oral ulceration	60-70%
Arthritis/rash	30-40%
Proteinuria	100%
Proteinuria in nephrotic range	45-60%
Hematuria	
Microscopic	80%
Macroscopic	<5%
Granular/red cell casts	10-30%
Renal function	
Reduced function	40-80%
Rapidly declining function	30%
Acute renal failure	<5%
Hypertension	15-50%

SLE, systemic lupus erythematosus.
Adapted from Cameron JS: Clinical manifestations of lupus nephritis. In Lewis EJ, Swartz MM, Korbet SM (eds): Lupus Nephritis. Oxford, Oxford University Press, 1999, pp 159-184.

early on may prevent or at least delay the onset of overt nephrosis (including nephritic and nephrotic syndromes). Patients with heavy proteinuria and renal impairment are likely to demonstrate more severe renal histopathological changes, although this association is not predictable, and a renal biopsy is certainly suggested in most patients with suspected LN, even if their level of proteinuria is very low.[9,10]

Patients with a nephritic urinary sediment (dysmorphic red blood cells, red blood cell casts) with or without proteinuria and hypertension, in combination with a deterioration in renal function, require urgent and aggressive immunosuppressive therapy. Of importance, approximately half of the patients with acute LN will have mild derangement in renal function and occasionally acute renal failure. The use of anti-inflammatory agents for the treatment of articular lupus also may be associated with acute renal failure.

The pulmonary-renal syndrome associated with SLE and, in this scenario, a rapidly progressive glomerulonephritis with deteriorating renal function and a nephritic urinary sediment is associated with diffuse alveolar hemorrhage and severely compromised pulmonary function. A small-vessel vasculitis seems to explain the pathological changes, exacerbated by a thrombotic microangiopathy. Expedient and aggressive treatment, preferably in an ICU, will improve the outcome in such clinical circumstances.

Patients with more severe forms of nephritis are more commonly hypertensive, and in fact, malignant hypertension may develop, especially in those patients with concomitant antiphospholipid syndrome.[11] The presence of poorly controlled hypertension portends a worse long-term outcome in these patients and requires therapy in its own right.[12]

Recently, the development of distal renal tubular acidosis has been suggested to be a manifestation of lupus nephritis and may be an indicator of more severe interstitial disease.[13]

It is important to make an accurate clinicopathological correlation in the patient with LN to plan treatment, prognosticate outcome, and keep the patient informed regarding the course of the disease.

Acute LN in the pregnant patient poses a particularly difficult diagnostic conundrum, especially when a suspicion of preeclampsia is entertained. In this setting, the presence of new-onset hypertension, development of proteinuria in the third trimester with a bland urinary sediment, a rising serum uric acid, normal complement, and negative results on lupus serologic tests would suggest preeclampsia rather than active lupus nephritis.[14] Also of importance, however, is the fact that hypertension and preeclampsia are more common in those pregnant patients with preexisting proliferative LN.

MANAGEMENT OF ACUTE LUPUS NEPHRITIS

Aims of therapy should be to bring about remission, control extrarenal disease adequately, and minimize toxicity. Of interest, as of 2004, medications approved by the U.S. Food and Drug Administration (FDA) for the treatment of SLE included only aspirin, hydroxychloroquine, and corticosteroids. Although not on the FDA approval list, standard therapy for severe lupus nephritis for nearly 3 decades has been the National Institutes of Health (NIH) regimen.[15] This consists of intravenous-pulse cyclophosphamide, 1.0 g/m², monthly for 6 consecutive months and then every 3 months, in conjunction with high-dose prednisone (initially, then tapered) for 2 more years. Such treatment was based on studies comparing intravenous and oral cyclophosphamide, azathioprine (AZA), and prednisone alone. The outcome measure of the NIH studies was doubling of serum creatinine, not end-stage renal failure, and overall survival (as opposed to renal survival) did not differ among the treatment groups. Furthermore, patients in the AZA plus prednisone treatment group and those in the intravenous cyclophosphamide plus prednisone treatment group fared similarly. Such differences in outcomes were not seen at 2 or 5 years but took more than 10 years to be demonstrated. It is this 10-year outcome that has justified adoption of the NIH regimen.

Because of toxicity and because, in the real world outside NIH, treatment failures are much more common than might be expected, nephrologists have sought alternatives to intravenous cyclophosphamide for some time. Investigators from the United Kingdom and Europe have been exploring lower-dose, shorter cyclophosphamide regimens and have claimed equivalence of outcome, and less toxicity, than with the NIH regimen.[16]

Mycophenolate Mofetil

Mycophenolate mofetil (MMF) is a potent immunosuppressant that has a good safety profile. It inhibits the de novo pathway of purine synthesis and therefore lymphocyte proliferation.[17] Several case reports and case series have described the use of MMF together with steroids in treating LN in patients in whom the disease was relapsing or resistant to cyclosporin.

Data from three randomized trials have recently come to the fore. Chan and coworkers reported a controlled trial in 42 patients with class IV LN and mild renal impairment that compared the effect of MMF administered for induction (1 g twice daily for 6 months, then 0.5 g twice daily for 6 months) plus prednisone with oral cyclophosphamide (2.5 mg/kg per day for 6 months, followed by AZA 1.5 mg/kg per day) plus prednisone.[18] Both drug regimens led to comparable rates of complete response, partial response, death, and relapse. Infections, alopecia, amenor-

rhea, and leukopenia were more common in patients receiving cyclophosphamide. Comparing MMF, cyclophosphamide, and AZA for maintenance therapy, Contreras reported a prospective controlled trial involving three maintenance regimens: quarterly intravenous injections of cyclophosphamide (pulse cyclophosphamide), oral MMF, and oral AZA.[19] Randomization took place after patients had received 4- to 6-monthly intravenous doses of cyclophosphamide given for induction therapy. Of the 59 patients with proliferative or mixed membranous and proliferative LN who were enrolled in the study, 46% were black, 49% were Hispanic, and 5% were white. As expected from previous data, remission of nephritis during the pulse cyclophosphamide induction phase occurred in more than 80% of patients. The proportions of patients who met the criteria for remission were evenly distributed among the three maintenance therapy groups. Overall survival among patients was significantly higher with AZA than with cyclophosphamide given for maintenance therapy. No significant differences in actuarial renal survival were found, but event-free survival (based on a composite endpoint of death and renal failure) was significantly better in both the azathioprine and MMF treatment groups than in the cyclophosphamide treatment group. Relapse-free survival was significantly better with MMF than with cyclophosphamide. Of importance, the rate of hospital admissions and the number of infectious episodes were significantly higher in the cyclophosphamide treatment group. This finding confirmed that the dosage of corticosteroids is the overriding independent determinant of the risk of infection among patients with SLE.

Ginzler and associates recently reported results for an American study comparing MMF and intravenous cyclophosphamide for induction of renal response in patients with severe LN.[20] The 24-week study recruited 140 patients from 19 separate centers. Fourteen of 71 patients who received MMF and 4 of 69 patients who received cyclophosphamide achieved complete remission; 21 additional patients in the MMF treatment group achieved partial remission, versus 10 patients in the cyclophosphamide treatment group.

These data suggest that MMF treatment can be considered as an alternative to the NIH regimen. Obstacles to recommending first-line use of MMF in LN have been recognized, however, including the lack of long-term data, lack of separate information on different ethnic groups, and lack of separate information on the more severe forms of class IV LN. Although prospective long-term data are awaited, MMF may be recommended in those patients with disease refractory to the NIH regimen, those intolerant of cyclophosphamide, and those concerned about gonadal toxicity.[21] From the limited data available, a 12-month course of MMF induction therapy, followed by MMF or AZA maintenance therapy, appears to be safe, well tolerated, and effective in stabilizing renal function for up to 36 months after completion of therapy.[22]

Other Agents and Modalities

Emerging data for those patients with resistant LN suggest that the use of monoclonal antibodies against CD20 (rituximab) may be effective in reducing both clinical and pathological parameters of active lupus nephritis, although randomized trials are awaited.[23,24]

Boumpas advocated a possible role for the use of monoclonal anti-CD40 ligand antibody in the therapy of LN. This particular study was terminated after an inordinate number of thrombotic events was reported.[25] The use of autologous hematopoietic stem cell transplantation after immunoablative chemotherapy is a newer therapy for autoimmune disease that is of potential use in severe SLE including LN. Registry data and some small studies suggest efficacy of stem cell transplantation for remission induction of refractory SLE, although mortality remains unacceptably high. As patient selection and choice of immunosuppression are improved, the favorable safety profile and outcome of this procedure may afford its more widespread usage. Biological agents that block co-stimulatory pathways (e.g., CTLA4-Ig) show promise in murine models, although human data are awaited.[26,27] Tumor necrosis factor-α (TNF-α) is a pro-inflammatory cytokine with various roles in inflammatory processes. The role TNF-α plays in human SLE is controversial, although TNF is increased in the blood and in the inflamed kidneys of patients with SLE.[28] Several TNF blockers currently are approved for use in rheumatoid arthritis, although clinical data on SLE are lacking.

LUPUS IN THE INTENSIVE CARE UNIT

Lupus is a highly variable disease characterized by episodic exacerbations, some of which are severe enough to require admission to the ICU. The presence of infection, disease activity including rapidly progressive glomerulonephritis, and cardiovascular complications are among the major reasons for ICU admission.

The use of high-dose immunosuppressants in the treatment of LN predisposes the patient to serious infection, especially in combination with corticosteroids and cyclophosphamide-containing regimens. Also of importance is the fact that infections are more common in patients with untreated lupus.[29] Both viral infections, including cytomegalovirus and varicella-zoster virus infections, and bacterial infections (especially those due to gram-negative bacteria) can result in septicemia, acute respiratory distress syndrome, and admission to the ICU.[30]

Aggressive antimicrobial and antiviral therapy, together with a reduction in immunosuppression, may improve outcome, although at the risk of an acute exacerbation of the illness. An acute infection may well precipitate a lupus flare, including LN, and this possibility must be taken into consideration when patients with lupus are admitted to the ICU. In this clinical setting, an elevated CRP or procalcitonin may be more suggestive of infection rather than a lupus flare.

Outcomes for patients with lupus admitted to the ICU are poor, with reported mortality rates of more than 45%. Survival seems worse in those patients with renal involvement including renal failure or with an Acute Physiology and Chronic Health Evaluation (APACHE) score higher than 20, in the elderly, and in African Americans.[31,32]

Superimposed pulmonary hemorrhage in the setting of rapidly progressive glomerulonephritis portends a particularly poor outcome.[33]

LONG-TERM OUTCOMES WITH ACUTE LUPUS NEPHRITIS

Overall outcome for patients with LN has improved, with more than 90% surviving more than 10 years. Complete renal remission—the absence of nephritic flares and their complete reversibility after therapy—has a favorable impact on survival; in those patients who progress to end-stage renal disease, dialysis and renal transplantation offer an adequate alternative.[34,35]

Preventing flares of the condition and preventing evolution of LN to more severe forms of disease remain a challenge, and some investigators have tried hydroxychloroquine and low-dose steroids with this aim. Such low-dose steroids also may impart an anti-inflammatory role with regard to endothelial inflammation, thus offering some reduction in cardiovascular risk. Of interest, high-density lipoproteins (HDLs) are pro-inflammatory in a significant proportion of patients with SLE and may impair the body's ability to prevent low-density lipoprotein (LDL) oxidation, thereby predisposing the patient to development of atherosclerosis.[36]

Decreasing overall cardiovascular risk by optimizing blood pressure and lipid profiles, exercise, and weight reduction, together with control of LN disease activity, will improve long-term survival in the patient with LN.

Key Points

1. Lupus nephritis is a sinister manifestation of systemic lupus erythematosus, and the possibility of this complication must be entertained in all affected patients.
2. Early and accurate diagnosis will afford the patient the best chance of reversal of the pathological and clinical abnormalities and will encourage better short- and long-term outcomes.
3. Although recommended therapeutic regimens will effect improvement in most patients, uncertainty remains regarding the optimal treatment. Therapy should be individualized and adjusted to the patient's clinical response.
4. Patients with systemic lupus erythematosus who are admitted to the intensive care unit have a poor prognosis and may require a reduction in immunosuppression at the risk of a lupus flare. Patients with lupus in whom nephritis develops have an added mortality risk.

Key References

8. Weening JJ, D'Agati VD, Schwartz MM, et al: The classification of glomerulonephritis in systemic lupus erythematosus revisited. J Am Soc Nephrol 2004;15:241-250.
12. Contreras G, Pardo V, Cely C, et al: Factors associated with poor outcomes in patients with lupus nephritis. Lupus 2005;14:890-895.
19. Contreras G, Pardo V, Leclercq B: Sequential therapies for proliferative lupus nephritis. N Engl J Med 2004;350:971-980.
20. Ginzler EM, Aranow C, Buyon J: A multicenter study of mycophenolate mofetil (MMF) vs. intravenous cyclophosphamide (IVC) as induction therapy for severe lupus nephritis (LN). Presented at the 7th International Congress on SLE and Related Conditions, New York, April 2004.
29. Williams FM, Chinn S, Hughes GR, Leach RM: Critical illness in systemic lupus erythematosus and the antiphospholipid syndrome. Ann Rheum Dis 2002;61:414-421.

See the companion Expert Consult website for the complete reference list.

CHAPTER 68

Hemolytic Uremic Syndrome

Caterina Mele and Giuseppe Remuzzi

OBJECTIVES

This chapter will:
1. Define and clinically characterize the hemolytic uremic syndrome.
2. Delineate the differences between Shiga-like toxin–associated and non–Shiga toxin–associated forms of hemolytic uremic syndrome.
3. Describe hemolytic uremic syndrome as a disease of complement dysregulation.
4. Review today's perspectives on treatment for hemolytic uremic syndrome.

DEFINITION

Hemolytic uremic syndrome (HUS) is a rare disease characterized by microangiopathic hemolytic anemia, thrombocytopenia, and acute renal failure due to occlusion of kidney microvessels by platelet thrombi. Anemia is marked by high serum levels of lactate dehydrogenase (LDH), circulating free hemoglobin, and the presence of reticulocytes and fragmented red blood cells (schistocytes) in the peripheral blood smear. Platelet trapping within thrombi results in a remarkable reduction in the platelet count (to less than 60,000/mm³).[1]

The common microvascular lesion of HUS, thrombotic microangiopathy, consists of vessel wall thickening with endothelial swelling, which allows accumulation of proteins and cell debris in the subendothelial layer, creating a space between endothelial cells and the underlying basement membrane of affected microvessels.[1,2] Together, the widening of the subendothelial space and the formation of intraluminal platelet thrombi lead to a partial or complete obstruction of the vessel lumina. It probably is because of the partial occlusion of the lumen that erythrocytes are disrupted by mechanical trauma, which explains the hemolysis and fragmented and distorted erythrocytes present in the blood smear.

In children younger than 2 years of age, the lesion is confined mainly to the glomerular tuft and is noted in an early phase of the disease. Glomerular capillary lumina are partly or completely occluded. In patent glomerular capillaries packed with red blood cells and fibrin, thrombi occasionally are seen. Examination of biopsy specimens taken several months after disease onset shows that although most glomeruli are normal, 20% eventually became sclerotic. Arterial thrombosis does occur but is uncommon and appears to represent a proximal extension of the glomerular lesion.[3,4] In the acute phase, tubular changes include foci of necrosis of proximal tubular cells and the finding of red blood cells and eosinophilic casts in the lumina of distal tubules. Occasionally, fragmented red blood cells can be detected in the distal tubular lumina. In adults and older children, glomerular changes are dif-

ferent from those in infants, and more heterogeneous. The classic pattern of thrombotic microangiopathy is less evident.

HUS most commonly is triggered by Shiga-like toxin (Stx)–producing *Escherichia coli* (Stx *E. coli*) and manifests with diarrhea, often bloody. In this Stx-associated form of HUS (Stx-HUS), acute renal failure manifests in 55% to 70% of the cases[5]; however, renal function subsequently is recovered in up to 70% of affected patients in various series.[1,2,6]

Non–Shiga toxin–associated HUS (non-Stx-HUS) is rarer, affecting a heterogeneous group of patients in whom an infection by Stx-producing bacteria can be excluded as a cause of the disease. Non-Stx-HUS can be sporadic or familial. Collectively, non-Stx-HUS forms have a poor outcome. Up to 50% of cases progress to end-stage renal disease (ESRD), and 25% of affected patients may die during the acute phase of the disease.[7,8]

SHIGA-LIKE TOXIN–ASSOCIATED HEMOLYTIC UREMIC SYNDROME

Epidemiology

Stx-HUS is more common than non-Stx-HUS and affects especially children, male and female in equal proportions. The overall annual incidence of Stx-HUS is estimated to be 2.1 cases per 100,000 persons, with a peak incidence in children younger than 5 years of age (6.1 per 100,000) and the lowest rate in adults 50 to 59 years of age (0.5 per 100,000).[1] The incidence of the disease parallels the seasonal fluctuation of Stx *E. coli* infections, with a peak in warmer months.

Stx-HUS generally manifests in sporadic form, but epidemics have been described with a common source of Stx *E. coli* infection.

In the United States, approximately 70,000 illness and 60 deaths have been attributed annually to Stx-HUS.[9] In Argentina and Uruguay, Stx *E. coli* infections are endemic, and Stx-HUS is a common cause of acute renal failure in children, with an estimated annual incidence of 10.5 per 100,000 population. An association between traditional extensive production of cattle with endemic HUS in Argentina has been proposed, as supported by detection of Stx *E. coli* strains in stool samples from 39% of Argentine healthy young beef steers.[10,11]

Etiology

Shiga-like toxins have been identified as triggering factors for Stx-HUS: They are powerful, harmful exotoxins for endothelial cells, produced by certain strains of *E. coli*. In 70% of cases in North America and western Europe, Stx-

HUS is secondary to infection with the *E. coli* serotype O157:H7.[12,13] This serotype has a unique biochemical property—lack of sorbitol fermentation—that renders it readily distinguishable from other fecal strains of *E. coli*.[14] Many other *E. coli* serotypes (O111:H8, O103:H2, O121, O145, O26, and O113[12,15]), however, have been shown to cause Stx-HUS. Infection by Stx-producing *Shigella dysenteriae* serotype 1 has been commonly linked to Stx-HUS in developing countries of Asia[16] and Africa,[17] but an association with this pathogen rarely has been reported from industrialized countries.[18]

Stx *E. coli* strains colonize healthy cattle intestine but also have been isolated from deer, sheep, goats, horses, dogs, birds, and flies.[1] People become infected after ingestion of contaminated milk, meat, or water or from contact with infected animals or other people, or with their excreta, and occasionally through environmental contamination. Fruits and vegetables also may be contaminated; radish sprouts, lettuce, and apple cider all have been implicated.[19,20]

Person-to person transmission has been reported in day care and chronic care facilities.[21]

Pathogenesis

After ingestion, Stx *E. coli* reaches the gut and closely adheres to the epithelial cells of the gastrointestinal mucosa through intimin, an outer membrane protein. Stx is then picked up by polarized gastrointestinal cells and moved into the circulation. Circulating human blood cells, such as erythrocytes, platelets, and monocytes, express Stx receptors on their surface, and a role for these cells in Stx transport has been hypothesized. When Stx reaches the kidney, it binds to the receptor expressed on glomerular endothelial cells, which possess higher affinity for the toxin. Here, by inducing endothelial apoptosis and increasing chemokines expression, Stx determines leukocyte attraction and triggers inflammatory reactions, which culminates in formation of thrombi,[13] causing the clinical manifestations of HUS.

Two types of Shiga-like toxin exist: Stx-1 and Stx-2. Despite their similar sequences, Stx-1 and Stx-2 cause different degrees and types of tissue damage, as documented by the higher pathogenicity of strains of *E. coli* producing only Stx-2 than that of strains producing Stx-1.[22]

Both Stx-1 and Stx-2 are 70-kD AB5 holotoxins—comprising a single A subunit and 5 B subunits. Binding of Stx molecules to target cells is dependent on B subunits and occurs by way of the glycolipid cell surface receptor globotriaosylceramide (Gb3). After internalization by receptor-mediated endocytosis, the toxins are carried to the endoplasmic reticulum, where the A and B subunits probably dissociate. Then the A subunit is translocated to the cytosol and nuclear envelope, where it enzymatically blocks cellular protein synthesis[13] (Fig. 68-1).

Clinical Manifestations

After exposure to Stx *E. coli*, hemorrhagic colitis develops in 38% to 61% of exposed persons, with progression to overt HUS in 3% to 20%.[20] The average interval between Stx *E. coli* exposure and onset of symptoms is 3 days. Illness typically begins with abdominal cramps and non-bloody diarrhea, which becomes hemorrhagic in 70% of the cases, usually within 1 or 2 days.[23] Vomiting occurs in 30% to 60% of cases, and fever in 30%.

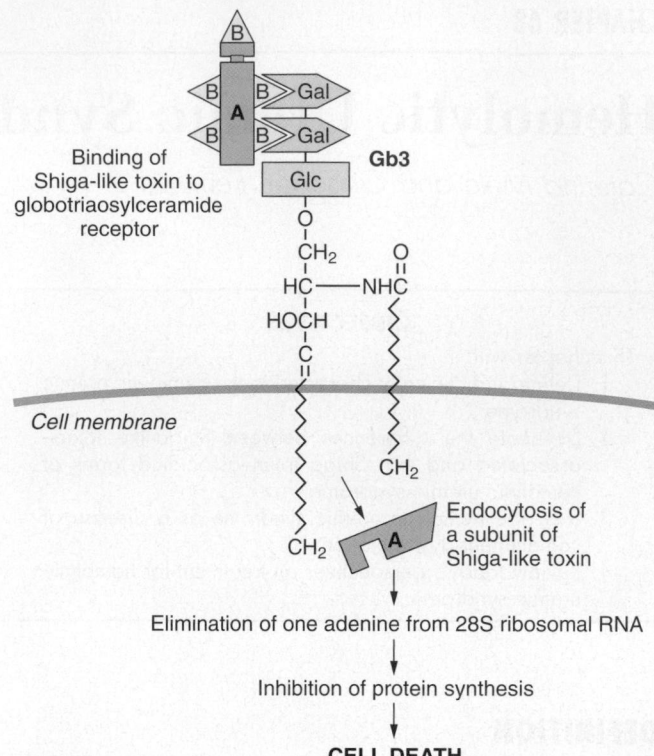

FIGURE 68-1. Binding and mechanism of action of Shiga-like toxin (Stx). The B subunits of Stx molecules attach to galactose (Gal) disaccharides of globotriaosylceramide (Gb3) receptors on the membrane of monocytes, polymorphonuclear cells, platelets, glomerular endothelial cells, and tubular epithelial cells. The toxin is internalized by means of retrograde transport through the Golgi complex. Then the A and B subunits dissociate, and the A subunit is translocated to the cytosol. The A subunit blocks peptide chain elongation by eliminating one adenine from the 28S ribosomal RNA.

Stx-HUS signs and symptoms appear 2 to 14 days after the first manifestations of Stx *E. coli* infection. Clinical findings include signs and symptoms of renal failure (such as macro- and microhematuria, proteinuria, and occasionally polyuria and oliguria), acute anemia, and thrombocytopenia. Twenty-five percent of patients exhibit neurological involvement, including stroke, seizure, and coma. Although mortality rates in industrialized countries decreased when dialysis became available, 3% to 5% of patients still die during the acute phase of the disease.[24]

HUS usually is diagnosed 6 days after the onset of diarrhea. Diagnosis rests on detection of Stx *E. coli* in stool cultures. Serological tests for antibodies to Stx and O157 lipopolysaccharide can be done in research laboratories, and tests are being developed for rapid detection of Stx *E. coli* O157:H7 and Stx in stool samples.

NON–SHIGA TOXIN–ASSOCIATED HEMOLYTIC UREMIC SYNDROME

Epidemiology

Non-Stx-HUS is significantly less common than Stx-HUS and accounts for approximately 5% of all cases of the disease.[13] According to a recent U.S. study, the incidence of non-Stx-HUS in children is approximately one-tenth that of Stx-HUS, corresponding to 2 cases per 1 million persons per year.[25]

Both familial and sporadic forms of non-Stx-HUS have been described. Non-Stx-HUS is defined as familial when the disease occurs in two or more members of the same family at least 6 months apart. It is defined as sporadic when one or more episodes of the disease manifest in an individual patient for whom a family history of the disease is excluded.

In contrast with Stx-HUS, no clear-cut causative agent or seasonal pattern has been recognized. A wide variety of triggers have been identified, including various nonenteric infections, drugs, malignancies, transplantation, and pregnancy. A thrombotic microangiopathy indistinguishable from that typical of non-Stx-HUS also is seen in association with multisystem diseases such as scleroderma, systemic lupus erythematosus, and antiphospholipid antibody syndrome. *Streptococcus pneumoniae* infection has been reported to be responsible for approximately 40% of cases of non-Stx-HUS in children in the United States.[25] Neuraminidase produced by S. *pneumoniae* cleaves sialic acid residues from cell surface glycoproteins, exposing the Thomsen-Freidenreich antigen (T antigen). Binding of naturally occurring immunoglobulin M (IgM) antibodies to the exposed T antigen on platelets and endothelial cells may then predispose to a thrombotic microangiopathy.[26] In approximately 13% of female patients with non-Stx-HUS, the disease is associated with pregnancy,[27] with most episodes occurring at term or post partum. Changes in pregnancy that may predispose affected women to non-Stx-HUS included increased concentrations of pro-coagulant factors, decreased fibrinolytic activity, and reduced expression of endothelial thrombomodulin. Previously, non-Stx-HUS occurred often in advanced HIV infection. With the advent of highly active antiretroviral therapy (HAART), however, the incidence of this complication has decreased.[28] Many drugs have been associated with non-Stx-HUS, including cytotoxics, immunosuppressants, and antiplatelet agents.[29] The mechanism of action is either one of direct toxicity or immune-mediated. An example of a drug with the former pathomechanism is quinine, which is associated with the development of autoantibodies reactive with platelet glycoproteins.[29] An example of a drug with the latter pathomechanism is mitomycin C, with an incidence of HUS between 4% and 15% in patients receiving this drug in combination chemotherapy.[30] De novo non-Stx-HUS is seen after renal transplantation in association with the use of calcineurin inhibitors.[31] The risk is increased by acute rejection and cytomegalovirus (CMV) infection.

Of note, in approximately 50% of cases of non-Stx-HUS, no clear-cut triggering condition has been identified. These cases are termed idiopathic HUS.[1]

Genetic Factors Associated with Non–Shiga Toxin–Associated Hemolytic Uremic Syndrome

The existence of familial forms suggested that the etiology of non-Stx-HUS may include a genetic component. Moreover, complement abnormalities associated with non-Stx-HUS have been recognized for many years. In particular, both low levels of C3 and glomerular deposition of C3 have been reported.[32] Recent studies have documented that the familial form is associated with genetic abnormali-

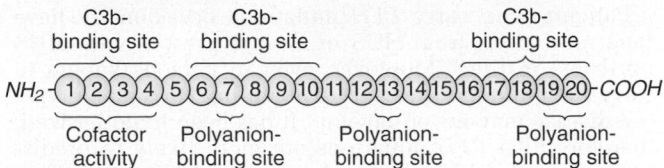

FIGURE 68-2. Complement factor H (CFH) functions and their localization within the polypeptide chain. The basic CFH structure consists of 20 short consensus repeats (SCRs). C3b-binding site localization, cofactor activity domains (at the amino-terminal [NH2] end of the chain), and the SCRs involved in polyanion binding are shown.

ties of complement regulatory protein, and evidence is now emerging that similar genetic alterations can predispose affected persons to the development of sporadic cases of non-Stx-HUS as well.

In 1998, Warwicker and colleagues[33] studied three families with non-Stx-HUS and found a co-segregation of the disease with chromosomal region 1q32, where a cluster of genes important in the regulation of complement activation (RCA) is contained. The first candidate gene to be screened in the RCA cluster was that encoding complement factor H (CFH), because previous reports had shown an association between CFH deficiency and non-Stx-HUS.[34]

Complement Factor H

CFH plays an important role in the regulation of the alternative pathway of complement. It serves as a cofactor for the C3b-cleaving enzyme complement factor I (CFI) in the degradation of C3b molecules.[35] Synthesized mainly by the liver, CFH is a 150-kD single-chain plasma glycoprotein and consists of 20 homologous structural domains called short consensus repeats (SCRs), each comprising approximately 60 amino acids (Fig. 68-2).

The complement regulatory domains that are needed to prevent alternative pathway amplification have been localized within SCRs 1 to 4, 6 to 10, and 16 to 20, which correspond to C3b-binding sites. Other CFH domains are able to interact with polyanionic molecules; these increase CFH affinity for C3b, which in this way is inactivated more efficiently. The most important of these domains have been mapped to SCRs 19 and 20 of CFH. Human glomerular endothelial cells and kidney glomerular basement membrane are rich in polyanionic molecules, so CFH deposited on their surface presumably provides an efficient shield against complement attack.

Mutations in *CFH* in persons with non-Stx-HUS have been widely described and are found in approximately 30% of affected patients.[36] These include patients with both sporadic and with familial forms. A majority of the genetic changes are heterozygous missense mutations that cluster in the exons that code for the carboxyl-terminal portion of CFH (SCRs 19 and 20) and are associated with normal CFH levels. A minority are deletions or missense mutations that result in either a severely truncated protein or impaired secretion.

Functional studies showed that mutated CFH has a low binding affinity for polyanionic molecules and C3b deposited on endothelial cell surfaces. Consequently, control of complement system activation on endothelial cells is reduced, while the function of CFH remains unaltered in fluid phase.[37]

Patients who carry *CFH* mutations occasionally have long remissions from HUS or do not present with HUS until late in life.[38] Moreover, even in persons known to carry such mutations as part of a familial HUS phenotype, the disease may never develop. It has been hypothesized, therefore, that *CFH* mutations are more likely to predispose affected persons to development of HUS, rather than directly causing the syndrome. In fact, in approximately 60% of patients with mutated *CFH*, the acute event is precipitated by conditions that trigger complement activation, either directly (from bacterial and viral infections) or indirectly by causing endothelial insult (from drugs, systemic diseases, or pregnancy).[39]

All of the foregoing observations can be reconciled by reasoning that in these patients, the suboptimal CFH activity is enough to protect the host from complement activation in physiological conditions. On exposure to an agent that activates complement, however, C3b is formed in higher-than-normal amounts, and its deposition on vascular endothelial cells cannot be fully prevented.

Such a scenario applies particularly to the glomerular capillary bed, which has a fenestrated endothelium and a basement membrane that supplies a surface rich in polyanions for CFH binding. This conducive environment could explain the preferential renal localization of microvascular injury of HUS.

Non-Stx-HUS characterized by an acquired autoimmune CFH defect has recently been described.[40] The existence of autoantibodies against CFH could explain those cases in which genetic alterations have not been noted.

Membrane Cofactor Protein

In only one of the three original families reported by Warwicker and coworkers[33] was a mutation in *CFH* found. In one of the two remaining families, three siblings who all had received a renal transplant did not experience recurrence of HUS in the allograft. This finding suggested that abnormalities in transmembrane proteins might be implicated in this family. Accordingly, the second candidate gene contained in the RCA cluster to be screened was *MCP*, encoding membrane cofactor protein (MCP) (i.e., CD46).

MCP is a widely expressed transmembrane glycoprotein that inhibits complement activation, serving as a cofactor for CFI to cleave C3b and C4b deposited on host cell surfaces. MCP has four extracellular SCRs important for its inhibitory activity; they are followed by a serine-threonine-proline–rich region (the STP region), a transmembrane domain (TM), and a cytoplasmic tail (Cyt) (Fig. 68-3).

MCP is highly expressed in the kidney. It probably exerts a main role in protecting glomerular endothelial cells against C3 activation, as indicated by data showing that cofactor activity was completely blocked by anti-MCP antibody.[41]

Mutations in *MCP* have been identified in approximately 12% of patients with non-Stx HUS.[36,42] Functional studies have shown that these mutations result in reduced cell surface expression and reduced C3b binding and cofactor activity.

As has been hypothesized for CFH, it is likely that mutations in MCP constitute a predisposing factor, rather than directly causing HUS. On exposure to conditions that lead to activation of the complement cascade, reduced MCP levels or defective C3b-binding capability and cofactor activity of mutated MCP on glomerular endothelial cells

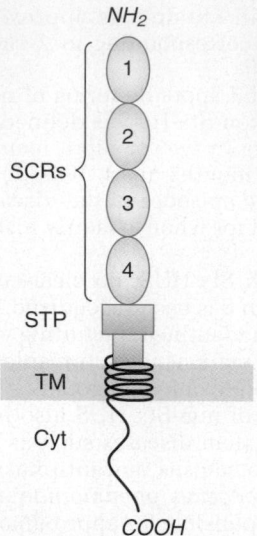

FIGURE 68-3. Membrane cofactor protein (MCP) (i.e., CD46) structure. MCP consists of four short consensus repeats (SCRs), a serine-threonine-proline (STP)-rich region, a hydrophobic transmembrane domain (TM), and a cytoplasmic tail (Cyt). Each SCR can bind C3b or C4b, thereby making it accessible for cleavage by complement factor I (CFI), in this manner conferring the protein's capability of inhibiting complement activation on host cells.

presumably result in insufficient protection of these cells from complement activation (Fig. 68-4).

Complement Factor I

Besides abnormalities of soluble and membrane-bound regulators of complement activation, mutations in the gene coding for complement factor I (CFI) recently have been described in patients with non-Stx HUS.[36]

CFI is a soluble regulatory serine protease of the complement system that cleaves C3b and C4b, thereby inactivating them. It is encoded by a gene localized to chromosomal region 4q25. Produced mainly by the liver, CFI is a 88-kD plasma glycoprotein with a modular structure, like that of many other complement proteins. It is a heterodimer and consists of a noncatalytic 50-kD heavy chain linked to a catalytic 38-kD light chain by a disulfide bond (Fig. 68-5).

Mutations described until now in *CFI* account for 5% to 10% of the cases of non-Stx-HUS.[36,43] A majority of these mutations cluster in the exons that encode the serine-protease domain. Approximately 40% of the mutations result in partial CFI deficiency. The functional significance of the remaining mutations remains to be determined.

PERSPECTIVES ON TREATMENT: FUTURE DIRECTIONS

Today, research efforts are aimed at identifying more specific approaches that may interfere with the primary pathomechanism of microangiopathy in the different forms of HUS (Table 68-1).

In Stx-HUS, new agents that are targeted at preventing organ exposure to Stx are currently under evaluation.

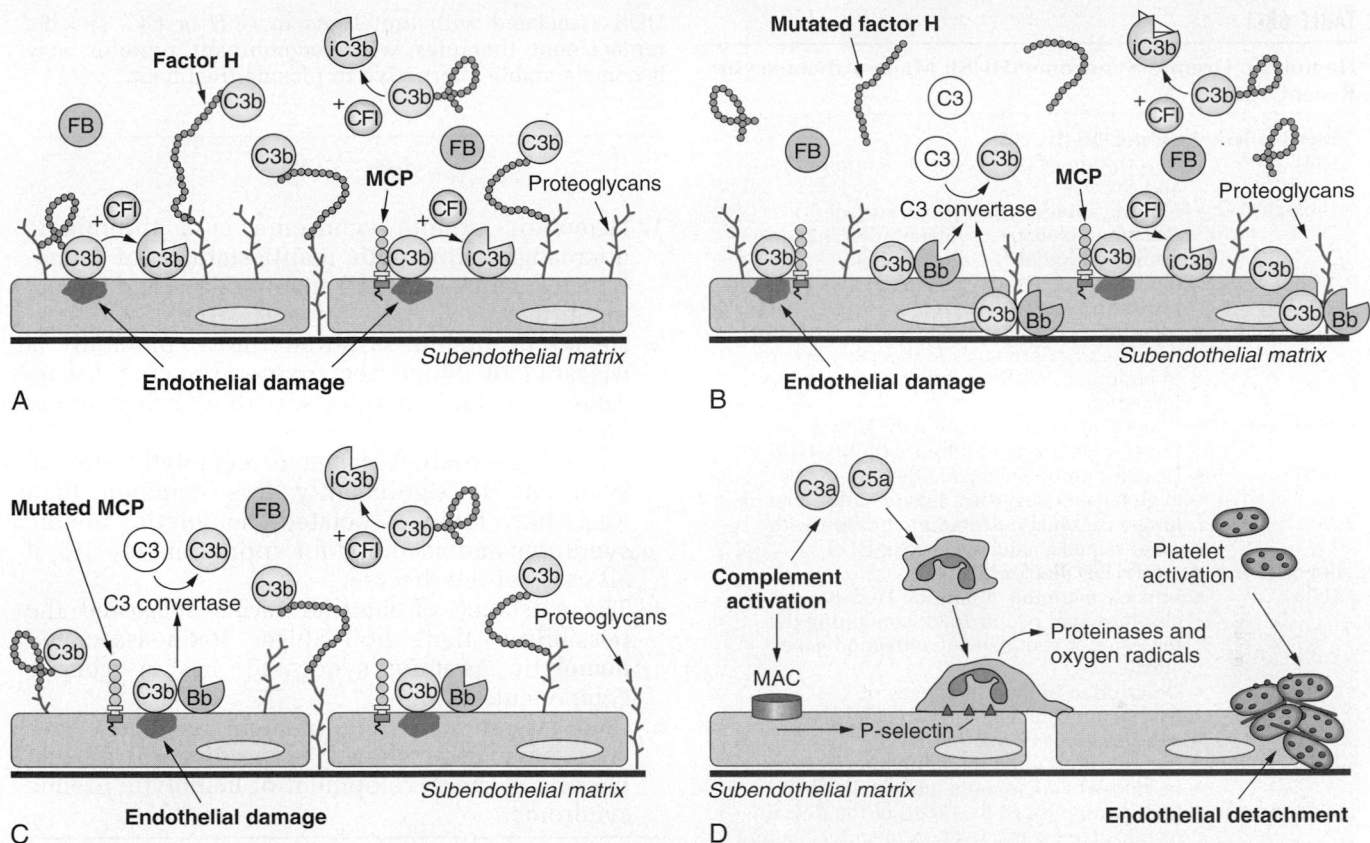

FIGURE 68-4. Proposed model for the pathological consequences of complement factor H (CFH) and membrane cofactor protein (MCP) mutations. **A,** After viral or bacterial infection or endothelial insult, complement is activated and C3b is formed. In the presence of normal CFH, C3b is rapidly inactivated to inactive C3b (iC3b). CFH in the circulation binds fluid-phase C3b and favors its degradation by complement factor I (CFI). In addition, it binds to polyanionic proteoglycans that are present on the endothelial cell surface and in the subendothelial matrix, where, because of its high affinity for C3b, it entraps fluid-phase C3b, thereby preventing its deposition on host surfaces and its binding with factor B (FB) to form the C3 convertase complex (C3bBb). The subendothelial matrix lacks endogenous complement regulators and is completely dependent on CFH to control complement activation. MCP also inactivates C3b deposited on endothelial cells by favoring its cleavage to iC3b by CFI. **B,** Proposed consequences of CFH mutations found in patients with hemolytic uremic syndrome (HUS). Mutant CFH has a normal cofactor activity in fluid phase. However, the mutations affect the polyanion inter-action site at the carboxyl terminus of CFH, so that it shows reduced binding to proteoglycans on the endothelial cell surface and in the subendothelial matrix. Consequently, more C3b reaches the endothelial cell surface so that MCP is not enough to adequately control complement activation on the cell membrane. In addition, C3b deposited on exposed extracellular matrix is not degraded and forms the C3 convertase of the alternative pathway of complement, which further cleaves C3 to C3b. **C,** MCP deficiency also predisposed to HUS. MCP mutations found in patients with HUS result in a reduced surface expression of the protein or in a reduced capability of MCP to bind C3b. In both cases, membrane-bound C3b is not efficiently inactivated, which leads to undesirable amplification of C3b formation and deposition on damaged endothelial cells through the formation of C3 convertase. **D,** The sequence of events leading to microvascular thrombosis. The proteolysis of C3 and C5 by convertases causes the release of the chemotactic anaphylatoxins C3a and C5a, which bind to receptors on inflammatory cells and attract them toward the endothelial layer. The deposition of C3b on endothelial cells is followed by the formation of the membrane attack complex (MAC), which leads to cellular injury and detachment and to sublytic membrane perturbation, leading in turn to endothelial activation and expression of adhesion molecules (P-selectin). The latter favor leukocyte attachment and activation with the release of oxygen radicals and proteinases that further damage the endothelium. After endothelial damage, cell detachment ensues, exposing basement membrane. Under these conditions, platelets from the microcirculation adhere and aggregate to the exposed matrix.

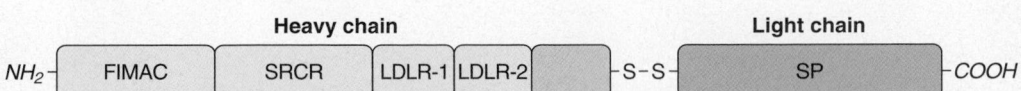

FIGURE 68-5. Complement factor I (CFI) structure. At the amino-terminal (NH$_2$) end of the molecule, the heavy chain contains a CFI membrane attack complex (FIMAC) domain, a scavenger receptor cysteine-rich (SRCR) domain, two class A low-density lipoprotein receptor (LDLR) domains (i.e., LDLR-1 and LDLR-2), and a region of unknown function. The light chain is made up entirely of the serine-protease domain (SP). The heavy and light chains are covalently linked by a disulfide bond.

TABLE 68-1

Hemolytic Uremic Syndrome (HUS): Major Advances in Recent Years

Shiga–Like Toxin–Associated HUS (Stx-HUS)

1994-2004	• Description of the crystal structure of Stx-1 and Stx-2
1993-2001	• Identification of specific Stx surface receptors (globotriaosylceramide, Gb3) on human endothelial cells, platelets, monocytes, erythrocytes, and polymorphonuclear cells
1995-2003	• Identification of the molecular mechanisms by which Stx promotes leukocyte adhesion to endothelial cells and induces thrombus formation
2002-2003	• Reports of good outcome with kidney transplantation in children with Stx-HUS
2004	• Description of beneficial effect of angiotensin-converting enzyme inhibitors on long-term renal outcome in children with renal sequelae after severe Stx-HUS

Non–Shiga Toxin–Associated HUS (Non-Stx-HUS)

1998	• Linkage mapping of familial HUS to chromosomal region 1q32, containing the regulator of complement activation gene cluster
1999	• Description of high incidence of hypocomplementemia (low C3 levels) in familial forms of non-Stx-HUS
1998-2004	• Identification of 50 mutations in *CFH* gene in familial and sporadic non-Stx-HUS
2002-2004	• Localization (in SCRs 19-20) of the domain responsible for inactivation of surface-bound C3b by factor H • Demonstration that mutations found in patients with non-Stx-HUS cause loss of the capability of factor H to bind polyanions on endothelial cells and extracellular matrix and to bind C3b
2003	• Identification of mutations in another complement regulatory gene, *MCP*, in non-Stx-HUS
1997-2003	• Description of high incidence of recurrence in the kidney graft in patients with non-Stx-HUS
2004	• Mutations in *CFI* in non-Stx-HUS

Thus far, three genes—*CFH*, *MCP*, and *CFI*—have been found to account for approximately 50% of cases of non-Stx-HUS. It follows that other genes involved in the pathogenesis of this form of the disorder need to be identified.

The increased knowledge of the role of complement in non-Stx-HUS suggests that complement inhibition may represent a valuable therapeutic approach. It is hoped that complement inhibitors will be useful to block complement-mediated kidney damage during the acute episode or to prevent recurrence after kidney transplantation. For HUS associated with mutations in *CFH* or *CFI*, specific replacement therapies with recombinant proteins may become a viable alternative to plasma treatment.

Key Points

1. Hemolytic uremic syndrome is a thrombotic microangiopathy with manifestations of hemolytic anemia, thrombocytopenia, and renal impairment.
2. Hemolytic uremic syndrome most commonly is triggered by Shiga-like toxin–producing *Escherichia coli* and manifests with diarrhea, often bloody.
3. Non–Shiga toxin–associated hemolytic uremic syndrome is significantly less common than Shiga-like toxin–associated hemolytic uremic syndrome and accounts for approximately 5% of all cases of the disease.
4. The existence of familial forms suggested the possibility that non–Shiga toxin–associated hemolytic uremic syndrome has a genetic component.
5. Gene alterations in complement regulatory proteins have been shown to predispose affected persons to the development of hemolytic uremic syndrome.

Acknowledgments

Research on hemolytic uremic syndrome on which this chapter is based was supported by the Associazione Ricerca Trapianto (ART), the Fondazione Aiuto Ricerca Malattie Rare (ARMR), the Associazione ALICE, and the National Institutes of Health (NIH) grant DK071221-01A1.

Key References

1. Ruggenenti P, Noris M, Remuzzi G: Thrombotic microangiopathy, haemolytic uremic syndrome and thrombotic thrombocytopenic purpura. Kidney Int 2001;60:831-846.
12. Thorpe CM: Shiga toxin–producing *Escherichia coli* infection. Clin Infect Dis 2004;38:1298-1303.
13. Noris M, Remuzzi G: Hemolytic uremic syndrome. J Am Soc Nephrol 2005;16:1035-1050.
36. Caprioli J, Noris M, Brioschi S, et al: Genetics of HUS: The impact of MCP, CFH and IF mutations on clinical presentation, response to treatment and outcome. Blood 2006; 108:1267-1279.
37. Maneulian T, Hellwage J, Meri S, et al: Mutations in factor H reduce binding affinity to C3b and heparin and surface attachment to endothelial cells in hemolytic uremic syndrome. J Clin Invest 2003;111:1181-1190.

See the companion Expert Consult website for the complete reference list.

CHAPTER 69

Acute Renal Failure in Oncological Disorders and Tumor Lysis Syndrome

Monica Bonello and Claudio Ronco

OBJECTIVES

This chapter will:
1. Examine specific considerations relative to renal disease in the patient with cancer.
2. Review the causes of acute renal failure in the setting of oncological diseases.
3. Describe the pathogenesis of acute renal failure in specific settings such as myeloma, bone marrow transplantation, and tumor lysis syndrome.
4. Summarize recommendations on how to prevent acute renal failure in oncological disorders and how to treat the condition when it develops.

Acute renal failure (ARF) is a serious complication of cancer and constitutes a major source of morbidity and mortality. Moreover, ARF may preclude optimal cancer treatment by requiring a decrease in chemotherapy dosage or by contraindicating potentially curative treatment.

In general, the initial pathways leading to ARF in patients with cancer are common to its development in other conditions. In these patients, however, etiological factors for ARF also may include those related to treatment of cancer or the disease itself. Multiple causes of ARF in critically ill patients with cancer often are present in combination (Table 69-1). Although some of these causes are common to the general intensive care unit (ICU) population (sepsis, shock, aminoglycosides), others are related to the malignancy itself or to its treatment. Elucidation of the pathomechanisms of organ failure related to malignant disease may potentially lead to an improvement in these patients' outcomes.

ACUTE RENAL FAILURE AND PROGNOSIS IN ONCOLOGICAL DISEASE

Although ARF is a frequent occurrence in patients with cancer, little is known about its impact on morbidity and mortality in this population. Nevertheless, currently available data on ARF and its consequences suggest that this disorder has the potential to substantially alter the outcome for patients with cancer and jeopardize their chances of receiving optimal cancer treatment and a potential cure. Data on global ARF-related mortality rates in patients with cancer are scarce, and physicians have no choice but to rely on data generally extrapolated from studies on the general ICU population. The risk for ARF seems higher in critically ill patients with cancer than in other critically ill patients. Of those with cancer, 12% to 49% experience ARF, and 9% to 32% require renal replacement therapy during their ICU stay. In critically ill patients with cancer, acute renal dysfunction usually occurs in the context of multiple organ dysfunction and is associated with mortality rates ranging from 72% to 85% when renal replacement therapy is needed.[1-3]

Managing chemotherapy is delicate because the pharmacokinetics of most cytotoxic agents have not been adequately studied in patients with altered renal function. The necessary dose adjustments may therefore be approximate, or adjustments in dosing may be inappropriate or even omitted. Consequently, patients may be either underdosed, with a decreased chance of remission, or overdosed, with an increased risk of systemic toxicity leading to potentially severe and unexpected complications in the course of chemotherapy. Furthermore, it may be necessary to repeatedly increase doses of supportive therapies, which carries some additional risk of treatment-related toxicity to the patient, with potentially dramatic consequences. Underdosing drugs also is unacceptable; pain may not be relieved and immunosuppression becomes insufficient or anti-infective treatment ineffective, especially in neutropenic patients, with the risk of emergence of antibiotic-resistant organisms.

CAUSES OF ACUTE RENAL FAILURE IN PATIENTS WITH CANCER

Nephrotoxic Chemotherapy Agents

Currently, the five primary agents most commonly responsible for chemotherapy-induced nephrotoxicity are mitomycin C, gemcitabine, platinum compounds, methotrexate, and ifosfamide. These agents produce subacute or chronic renal insufficiency, except for cisplatin and methotrexate (when given in high doses), which can cause ARF. In addition, the development of nephrotic syndrome and a form of "collapsing glomerulopathy" have been described in patients receiving repeated high doses of bisphosphonates, such as pamidronate.[4] Most recently, zoledronate has been reported to produce acute tubular necrosis. Interferons also have the potential to cause nephrotoxicity, including the development of thrombotic microangiopathy. Pentostatin, a drug used to treat some hematological malignancies, also can produce ARF when given at doses higher than 4 mg/m². The nitrosoureas, semustine, carmustine, and lomustine, can cause chronic renal insufficiency after prolonged use. Streptozotocin causes proximal

TABLE 69-1

Causes of Acute Renal Failure in Patients with Cancer

Prerenal Failure
Sepsis
Extracellular dehydration (diarrhea, mucositis, vomiting)
Sinusoidal obstruction syndrome (formerly called hepatic veno-occlusive disease)
Drugs (e.g., calcineurin inhibitors, ACE inhibitors, NSAIDs)
Capillary leak syndrome (IL-2)
Intrinsic Failure
Acute tubular necrosis
• Ischemia (shock, severe sepsis)
• Nephrotoxic agents (contrast agents, aminoglycosides, amphotericin, ifosfamide, cisplatin)
• Disseminated intravascular coagulation
• Intravascular hemolysis
Acute interstitial nephritis
• Immunoallergic nephritis
• Pyelonephritis
• Cancer infiltration (e.g., lymphoma, metastasis)
• Nephrocalcinosis
Vascular nephritis
• Thrombotic microangiopathy
• Vascular obstruction
Glomerulonephritis
• Amyloidosis (with AL type of amyloid: myeloma; with AA type: renal carcinoma or Hodgkin's disease)
• Immunotactoid glomerulopathy
• Membranous glomerulonephritis (pulmonary, breast or gastric carcinoma)
• IgA glomerulonephritis, focal glomerulosclerosis
Postrenal Failure
Intrarenal obstruction (e.g., urate crystals, light chain disease, acyclovir, methotrexate)
Extrarenal obstruction (retroperitonal fibrosis, ureteral or bladder outlet obstruction)

ACE, angiotensin-converting enzyme; IgA, immunoglobulin A; IL-2, interleukin-2; NSAIDs, nonsteroidal anti-inflammatory drugs.

tubular toxicity and in rare cases can lead to the development of ARF.[5-7]

Mitomycin C

Mitomycin C–induced nephrotoxicity carries significant mortality, with associated pulmonary and neurological manifestations being the most common signs of poor prognosis. Long-term treatment with mitomycin C can lead to progressive renal insufficiency and subacute renal failure. In most cases, mitomycin C nephrotoxicity manifests as hemolytic-uremic syndrome (HUS) caused by thrombotic microangiopathy. The pathophysiological changes are due to the direct toxic effects of mitomycin C on the endothelium. Patients experience gradual onset of anemia and thrombocytopenia, with high lactate dehydrogenase levels and undetectable haptoglobin levels. Progressive renal insufficiency is accompanied by increasing blood urea nitrogen (BUN) and creatinine levels, as well as severe hypertension. The urinalysis shows microhematuria and proteinuria. A clear-cut relationship exists between the cumulative dose of mitomycin C and risk of HUS: The incidence of nephrotoxicity rises markedly after total doses higher than 40 to 60 mg/m² are given over several months. Current practice therefore restricts mitomycin C treatment to 2 to 3 months. Nevertheless, some patients are still seen who have received mitomycin C for 4 or 5 months, and these usually present with a slow rise in BUN and creatinine levels, hypertension, thrombocytopenia, and anemia.[8,9]

Gemcitabine

Gemcitabine-induced HUS is increasingly common in clinical practice.[10] The pathogenesis is the same as that for mitomycin C, with concomitant features of anemia, thrombocytopenia, hypertension, and raised BUN and creatinine levels. In HUS from gemcitabine, the urinalysis also shows blood and protein. Unlike in mitomycin C–related HUS, no clear-cut relationship has been established between the cumulative dose of gemcitabine and risk of HUS. Most affected patients, however, have received gemcitabine for at least 3 to 5 months before the onset of HUS. The hematological abnormalities often regress spontaneously, and renal function also may improve with time.

Platinum Compounds

Cisplatin probably is the most extensively studied nephrotoxic anticancer agent. Although direct tubular toxicity may cause ARF, cisplatin also has been associated with chronic, dose-dependent reduction of the glomerular filtration rate.[11] Cisplatin usually induces only mild renal failure that does not require dialysis, and patients typically recover renal function. Patients usually are nonoliguric, and hyponatremia may be observed, which probably is related to a salt-losing nephropathy. Hypomagnesemia, which can be long-lasting, is much more common than ARF and is related to urinary magnesium losses.

The maximum dose of cisplatin should not exceed 120 mg/m² of body surface area, and renal dysfunction may require a dosage reduction. Repeated administration up to a cumulative dose of 850 mg was associated with a 9% reduction in glomerular filtration rate over a 5-year period, compared with a 40% reduction in patients given more than 850 mg.[11] The most widely used protective measure is saline infusion to induce solute diuresis. Amifostine (inorganic thiophosphate) has been found to be effective in preventing renal failure, even after repeated exposure. Accordingly, the American Society of Clinical Oncology has stated that amifostine (910 mg/m²) may be considered for the prevention of nephrotoxicity in patients receiving cisplatin-based chemotherapy (grade of recommendation A).[12] Stevens-Johnson syndrome and toxic epidermic necrolysis have been reported in patients given amifostine.

Methotrexate

Methotrexate is a widely used anticancer drug. High doses of methotrexate (>1 g/m²) are used to treat osteosarcoma and Burkitt's lymphoma and to facilitate brain penetration in central nervous system lymphoma. These high doses are associated with a high risk of ARF due to precipitation of methotrexate or its metabolite, 7-hydroxymethotrexate, within the renal tubules. When ARF occurs, the resulting decrease in methotrexate clearance leads to extrarenal toxicity (neutropenia, hepatitis, orointestinal mucositis, or neurological impairment). Thus, methotrexate toxicity may manifest as multiorgan failure.[13]

Prevention of nephrotoxicity, together with methotrexate level monitoring, is crucial to prevent extrarenal methotrexate toxicity. During methotrexate infusion and elimination, fluids should be given to maintain a high urinary output, and urinary alkalinization should be performed to keep the urinary pH above 7.5. Rescue with folinic acid (50 mg four times a day) should be started 24 hours after completion of each high-dose methotrexate infusion, and serum methotrexate concentrations should be measured daily. Patients are considered to be at high risk for methotrexate toxicity when serum drug levels are greater than 15 µmol/L at 24 hours, 1.5 µmol/L at 48 hours, or 0.5 µmol/L at 72 hours. Unless such agents are absolutely necessary, patients should not be given medications that inhibit folate metabolism (e.g., trimethoprim-sulfamethoxazole), exhibit intrinsic renal toxicity (e.g., nonsteroidal anti-inflammatory agents, contrast agents), or decrease the fraction of methotrexate bound to albumin (e.g., aspirin).[13-15]

When all of these measures were taken, the incidence of ARF was 1.8% in patients with sarcoma.[13] Because methotrexate is highly protein bound, regular dialysis will not clear the drug efficiently, and high doses of leucovorin are needed to prevent systemic toxicity. Hemoperfusion and daily high-flux hemodialysis also have been used to remove methotrexate.[14,15]

Carboxypeptidase-G2 is a bacterial enzyme that converts methotrexate into an inactive metabolite (2,4-diamino-N-10-methylpteroic acid), thus providing an alternative route of elimination. Its use lowered plasma methotrexate concentrations to nontoxic levels (by 98% in 15 minutes), although rebounds (with an increase no greater than 10% in plasma methotrexate concentrations) occurred in 60% of the patients. Carboxypeptidase-G2 and high-dose leucovorin have been tested in patients with methotrexate intoxication and ARF, with similar results.[16] Therefore, no recommendations can be made concerning renal replacement therapy or carboxypeptidase-G2 in this population.

Alkylating Agents

The main anticancer agents responsible for hemorrhagic cystitis are alkylating agents, such as cyclophosphamide and ifosfamide. Maintaining a high urinary output and concomitantly administering the bladder epithelium protectant mesna have virtually eliminated hemorrhagic cystitis related to the toxicity of anticancer agents. Several other toxic effects of these drugs, however, have been described, including emesis, alopecia, myelosuppression, and neurotoxicity. Moreover, ifosfamide has been associated with ARF or acute tubular dysfunction Ifosfamide causes proximal tubular defects (Fanconi's syndrome) and chronic renal insufficiency but rarely ARF.[17] Hypokalemia, hyperchloremic metabolic acidosis, hypophosphatemia (despite concomitant renal insufficiency), and renal glucosuria are characteristic of ifosfamide-induced nephrotoxicity. Fanconi's syndrome should therefore be considered if a clinical picture consisting of phosphaturia, glucosuria with normal glucose levels, aminoaciduria, and a proximal tubular metabolic acidosis develops in a patient receiving ifosfamide.

Urinary Tract Obstruction or Infiltration of the Kidney by Tumors

Cancer can damage the kidneys in a variety of ways. Renal compression or urinary tract obstruction by a tumor close to the kidney, such as ovarian or bladder tumor, frequently is seen in patients with cancer. Metastatic disease also is observed in the kidneys, but it is rare for lung, breast, or colon cancer metastases to cause ARF. Metastatic solid tumors usually result in ARF through involvement of the lymph nodes, causing ureteric obstruction and vascular occlusion. Lymphomas, particularly high-grade lymphomas, and acute lymphoblastic leukemia often infiltrate the kidneys; although usually clinically silent, such neoplastic extension can lead to ARF. Chemotherapy, however, usually produces a prompt reduction in tumor mass and control of infiltration. Unfortunately, a rapid decrease in tumor size can induce tumor lysis syndrome, which in turn increases the risk of ARF.

Tumor Lysis Syndrome

Tumor lysis syndrome is a potentially life-threatening condition that frequently occurs after the rapid degradation of tumors. It is particularly common in patients with a large tumor burden with a high rate of cellular turnover after cytotoxic therapy (including steroids in steroid-sensitive hematological malignancies) but also can occur spontaneously, especially in patients with lymphoid malignancies, as a result of rapid cell turnover and an increased rate of purine metabolism.

The release of large volumes of intracellular contents into the systemic circulation leads to the accumulation of purine-derived metabolites such as uric acid, and of cytoplasmic ionic content (mainly, phosphorus and potassium), overwhelming the renal excretion capacity. Renal dysfunction in tumor lysis syndrome results principally from acute uric acid accumulation, hyperkalemia, hyperphosphatemia, and hypocalcemia. Tumor lysis syndrome–related ARF is believed to be the consequence of tubular obstruction secondary to intratubular precipitation of several compounds, such as uric acid and xanthine, whose concentrations in urine exceed their solubility threshold. Although still not completely understood, the exact pathophysiology of tumor lysis syndrome probably is more complex, resulting from the combination of several phenomena, including acute urate nephropathy and acute nephrocalcinosis, one aggravating the other.

Animal models have shown that hyperuricemia leads to urate nephropathy through both intratubular and parenchymatous uric acid precipitations, with further renal injury being caused by a granulomatous reaction and necrosis of the distal tubule epithelium. In addition to urate nephropathy, acute nephrocalcinosis caused by hyperphosphatemia can play a pivotal role in tumor lysis syndrome–related ARF, with diffuse parenchymatous depositions of calcium-phosphate complexes, explaining why ARF develops in some patients despite adequate treatment of hyperuricemia. Finally, tumor lysis syndrome–related ARF frequently is precipitated by volume depletion, which has repeatedly been observed as a major aggravating factor over the past 3 decades.[17]

Tumor lysis syndrome occurs primarily in patients with hematological malignancies; those with a high tumor burden and rapidly proliferating diseases are particularly at risk The incidence of tumor lysis syndrome ranges between 20% and 50% in high-risk groups (Burkitt's lymphoma, aggressive non-Hodgkin's lymphoma, acute lymphoid leukemia, acute myeloid leukemia [mainly types 4 and 5], and chronic lymphocytic leukemia [mainly aggressive lymphoma and childhood acute lymphoid leukemia]). With the exception of small cell lung cancer, neuroblastoma, and breast cancer, occurrence of ARF in patients with solid malignancies is rare.

Prevention of tumor lysis syndrome–related ARF is a cornerstone in the care of patients with hematological malignancies since the introduction of allopurinol, a xanthine oxidase inhibitor, and urate oxidase more than 25 years ago (in France and Italy). Allopurinol specifically inhibits xanthine oxidase, which catalyzes the metabolism of xanthine to uric acid, thereby preventing uric acid formation. Uric acid formation is thus stopped, and the existing uric acid is slowly excreted over 2 to 3 days. In patients with impaired renal function, however, the uric acid load may not be eliminated. Allopurinol also may lead to accumulation of poorly soluble xanthine in the kidney, which is less soluble than uric acid, and occasional cases of xanthine nephropathy and calculi have been reported.

In most mammals, uric acid is oxidized to allantoin by way of the urate oxidase enzymatic pathway. Urate oxidase is not present in humans, however, because of a nonsense mutation of the encoding gene.[18] Nonrecombinant urate oxidase can be extracted from *Aspergillus flavus*, although the yield is low. Injection of urate oxidase reduces plasma uric acid levels by catalyzing the breakdown of uric acid to allantoin, which is a readily excreted metabolite that is 5 to 10 times more soluble than uric acid.[19] Nonrecombinant urate oxidase has been shown to reduce the risk of ARF from tumor lysis syndrome when compared with allopurinol, and can reduce the need for dialysis in patients with aggressive lymphoma at high risk for tumor lysis syndrome.[18] Less than 2% of patients who received urate oxidase–based therapy in France and Italy required dialysis, whereas 16% to 20% of patients who had allopurinol-based therapy in England and the United States needed dialysis. Nevertheless, approximately 4.5% of patients experience allergic reactions to this preparation, with serious events such as bronchospasm and hypoxemia being rare. Recently, a recombinant form of urate oxide, rasburicase, has been engineered.[20] Clinical studies have demonstrated that rasburicase is a highly effective drug for the prevention and treatment of tumor lysis syndrome–related hyperuricemia.[20]

Vigorous hydration increases elimination of uric acid, and urinary alkalinization increases the solubility of uric acid in urine. The formerly widespread use of urinary alkalinization is now a controversial practice, however, because an alkaline urine pH favors calcium phosphate crystal precipitation. Sodium bicarbonate administration, therefore, increases the risk of acute nephrocalcinosis, which may contribute to rapid alteration of renal function. Rasburicase lowers uric acid levels so quickly that the need for urinary alkalinization no longer exists, thereby reducing the risk of acute nephrocalcinosis.

Uric Acid

Uric acid can be considered a new potential factor in the pathogenesis of ARF. Uric acid can cause both mechanical obstruction due to intratubular precipitation of urate crystals and direct glomerular and tubular cell toxicity as a result of endothelial dysfunction, oxidant stress, cell disruption, and platelet activation. Uric acid also serves as a mediator in the local inflammatory response and the progression to systemic inflammation, by stimulating production of cytokines (interleukin-1β and tumor necrosis factor-α) and chemoattractants (Table 69-2). Hyperuricemia commonly is associated with hypertension, and elevated uric acid levels may be a risk factor for cardiovascular

TABLE 69-2

Uric Acid: A New Pathogenetic Factor in Acute Renal Failure

TUBULAR OBSTRUCTION	TISSUE DAMAGE	ACUTE INFLAMMATION
Uric acid crystals	Endothelial dysfunction— nitric oxide mediated	Correlates with circulating cytokines
Mechanical obstruction	Platelet activation	Stimulates synthesis of MCP-1
Tubular nephropathy	Oxidant stress and cell disruption	Stimulates monocyte production of interleukin-1β and tumor necrosis factor-α

MCP-1, monocyte chemoattractant protein-1.

and renal disease.[21] In preclinical studies in the rat, reducing uric acid levels prevented the development of hypertension, vascular disease, and renal disease. These findings raise the possibility that lowering uric acid levels may be similarly beneficial in reducing the incidence of cardiovascular disease in people.[21]

Acute Renal Failure in Patients with Multiple Myeloma

Multiple myeloma is the hematological neoplasia most frequently associated with acute or chronic renal failure. Renal failure predates the diagnosis of myeloma in half of those patients in whom renal dysfunction will occur and develops in most of the remaining patients within 1 month of the diagnosis of myeloma. Of the 50% of patients with multiple myeloma who experience renal impairment, 10% will require dialysis. Patients with multiple myeloma and renal failure have a significantly worse survival compared with all patients with multiple myeloma.

Myeloma is characterized by the uncontrolled proliferation of a B cell clone. The aberrant B lymphocyte population secretes a paraprotein: either an intact monoclonal immunoglobulin or a derived fragment (usually a light chain fragment). Production of this nephrotoxic paraprotein by the abnormal B cells is primarily responsible for ARF in multiple myeloma. The light chains normally are found together with heavy chains in the immunoglobulin molecule and are detected by urine protein electrophoresis and immunofixation. Renally excreted light chains cause nephrotoxicity by two main mechanisms: Free light chains are directly nephrotoxic, and they also contribute to the formation of casts in the distal tubules. Myeloma casts are composed principally of monoclonal light chains and Tamm-Horsfall glycoprotein (THP), a major constituent of normal urine synthesized exclusively by cells of the thick ascending limb of the loop of Henle. THP is able to form high-molecular-weight aggregates at high (but physiological) concentrations of sodium and calcium, and at low urinary pH. Accordingly, precipitating factors leading to an acute fall in GFR will increase the intratubular concentration of light chains and consequently their precipitation.

Renal dysfunction may develop in patients with multiple myeloma for a number of reasons. Specific mechanisms of renal injury include myeloma cast nephropathy, amyloid deposition, and glomerular infiltration with light chains. ARF frequently is triggered by an event such as treatment with nonsteroidal anti-inflammatory agents for pain control, use of intravenous contrast agents, development of hypercalcemia, volume depletion (diuretic treatment, septicemia), or cryoglobulinemia-associated renal failure. Furthermore, water, electrolyte, and acid-base disturbances are common in patients with myeloma; such abnormalities also may affect renal load.

In addition to the avoidance of precipitating factors, including the treatment of hyperuricemia, active management of ARF associated with multiple myeloma includes maintaining sufficient urine flow by volume expansion and administration of loop diuretics and, in selected cases, alkalinizing the urine. Reports also describe the benefits of plasma exchange with myeloma and renal failure. Furthermore, although response to chemotherapy is the major factor determining overall survival, recovery of renal function also is associated with improved survival. Specific treatment for multiple myeloma may improve renal function; in patients on chronic dialysis, improvement can be sufficient to allow discontinuation of dialysis. Nevertheless, chronic renal failure is common in many of the patients who present with severe alteration of renal function. Therefore, prevention of further renal damage is imperative, and particular attention must be paid to the avoidance of nephrotoxic drugs and hypovolemia. The prognosis for patients with multiple myeloma and chronic renal failure has improved considerably over the past 2 decades, with recovery of normal function with appropriate treatment in more than 50% of the patients. Renal failure alone should therefore no longer be considered to be an absolute contraindication to intensive treatment of myeloma if appropriate dose reduction is applied.[22,23]

Acute Renal Failure in Hematopoietic Stem Cell Transplant Recipients

ARF is extremely common in patients undergoing hematopoietic stem cell transplantation (HSCT), with studies reporting incidence rates ranging from 6.5% in some autologous HSCT series, to 26% to 64% in most series, and up to 81% in allogeneic transplantation settings.[24] Identified risk factors include use of allogeneic transplants, presence of veno-occlusive disease, and patient age older than 25 years. ARF in patients undergoing HSCT is associated with severe prognosis. Mortality rates are dependent primarily on the severity of renal failure, the need for dialysis, and the type of transplant (autologous versus allogeneic).

Patients who undergo HSCT are exposed to a number of factors that contribute to their worsening renal function. In the "conditioning" phase of transplantation, two rare conditions can cause rapidly progressive ARF. First, acute tumor lysis syndrome is a rare occurrence in patients undergoing transplantation, because candidates for HSCT are given routine prophylaxis for this syndrome. Second, marrow infusion toxicity is another complication that is now rare. ARF is caused by massive hemoglobinuria due to both intravascular hemolysis secondary to use of dimethyl sulfoxide (DMSO) as a cryoprotectant and release of free hemoglobin by red cells disrupted during the thawing of the graft.[24] This complication has become infrequent because lower DMSO concentrations are now used

and marrow grafts are "rinsed" after thawing and before infusion.

During the month after transplantation, patients are at risk of developing ARF from acute tubular necrosis of various causes, as discussed earlier. The most frequent of these etiologic disorders is sepsis, followed by exposure to nephrotoxic drugs, especially antimicrobials; volume depletion caused by vomiting and diarrhea; and more rarely, hemorrhage. The role of cyclosporine in the pathogenesis of ARF after allogeneic transplantation has been the subject of debate. The major dose-limiting toxicity of cyclosporine is nephrotoxicity, although the ARF it induces usually responds to dose reduction and is reversible on drug discontinuation. The risk of acute cyclosporine-related renal dysfunction generally correlates with plasma concentrations but, of note, is markedly increased by concomitant administration of other nephrotoxic drugs, especially amphotericin B.[25]

Of greatest importance in this setting, a complication known as veno-occlusive disease of the liver develops in most patients with severe forms of ARF. Liver damage is a common complication of cytoreductive therapy and develops in 20% to 40% of bone marrow transplant recipients.[26] The main site of liver damage in these patients is the hepatic sinusoid, and the resulting clinical syndrome is called sinusoidal obstruction syndrome (SOS). Most cases of SOS are clinically obvious, with jaundice, liver pain, edema, and ascites. These clinical manifestations may be associated with ARF mimicking hepatorenal syndrome, with normal histologic appearance of renal biopsy specimens. SOS can be classified as mild (i.e., clinically obvious, requires no treatment, and resolves completely), moderate (i.e., requires treatment but resolves completely), or severe (i.e., requires treatment but does not resolve before death or day 100). Severe SOS carries a bleak prognosis, with a 98% mortality rate in a cohort study.[27] ARF, as would be expected with any form of organ failure, influences the prognosis for SOS. In patients with moderate SOS, diuretic therapy and analgesics are usually sufficient. In patients with severe SOS, treatment rests on supportive care. No satisfactory specific therapies are available. Defibrotide (a polydeoxyribonucleotide with anti-ischemic, antithrombotic, and thrombolytic properties) produced promising results in an open-label study but has not yet been investigated in randomized studies. Thrombolytic therapy is of uncertain efficacy and carries a risk of fatal bleeding.

Viral Infections

Viral infections are an emergent cause of ARF in bone marrow transplant recipients. Several studies confirm an association between ARF and adenovirus, polyomavirus (BK virus or JC virus), and simian polyomavirus. The well-documented association between the BK virus and hemorrhagic cystitis may explain not only the high incidence of hemorrhagic cystitis after bone marrow transplantation (20% to 25%) but also the occurrence of nephropathy. The simian 40 virus was recently found to exhibit an association with ARF and hemorrhagic cystitis.[28] Finally, adenovirus is associated with disseminated infections, encephalitis, pneumonitis, and ARF. To allow either a prompt reduction in immunosuppression or the initiation of antiviral therapy, the diagnosis of adenoviral disease must be made early. Polymerase chain reaction testing or enzyme-linked immunosorbent assay may help to achieve this goal.[28]

CONCLUSION

ARF is a serious complication in patients who have cancer that causes additional morbidity and mortality. The renal dysfunction results from various causes, including metabolic disturbances, renal infiltration by malignant cells, sepsis, and drug-induced toxicity. Prevention of ARF is mandatory in critically ill patients with cancer. Protecting against ARF involves identifying those patients most at risk and, when applicable, timely intervention with preventive strategies. ARF from a number of causes, particularly contrast agent–induced nephropathy and tumor lysis syndrome, can be avoided. Fluid expansion and uricolytic treatment in patients with a high risk of acute tumor lysis syndrome, prevention of contrast agent–induced nephropathy, scrupulous avoidance of nephrotoxic drugs in high-risk patients, and monitoring of serum methotrexate concentrations are among the measures that may reduce the risk of ARF. Further studies are needed to improve the prognosis for these patients, to determine optimal treatments, and to identify additional causative factors. A multidisciplinary approach that incorporates adequate assessment, use of appropriate preventive measures, and early intervention is essential to reduce the incidence of life-threatening ARF in patients with cancer.

Key Points

1. Acute renal failure is a serious but, in certain cases, preventable complication of cancer.
2. Acute renal failure in patients with cancer is associated with increased morbidity and mortality.
3. A multidisciplinary approach and early intervention are needed to ensure adequate assessment and to reduce the incidence of life-threatening acute renal failure in patients with cancer.

Key References

1. Benoit DD, Depuydt PO, Vandewoude KH, et al: Outcome in critically ill medical patients treated with renal replacement therapy for acute renal failure: Comparison between patients with and those without haematological malignancies. Nephrol Dial Transplant 2005;20:552-558.
2. Darmon M, Thiery G, Ciroldi M, et al: Intensive care in patients with newly diagnosed malignancies and a need for cancer chemotherapy. Crit Care Med 2005;33:2488-2493.
3. Bagshaw SM, Laupland KB, Doig CJ, et al: Prognosis for long-term survival and renal recovery in critically ill patients with severe acute renal failure: A population-based study. Crit Care 2005;9:R700-R709.
9. Valavaara R, Nordman E: Renal complications of mitomycin C therapy with special reference to the total dose. Cancer 1985;55:47-50.
11. Arany I, Safirstein RL: Cisplatin nephrotoxicity. Semin Nephrol 2003;23:460-464.

See the companion Expert Consult website for the complete reference list.

Physiological Consequences of Acute Renal Failure: Clinical Syndromes

CHAPTER 70

Bleeding and Hemostasis in Acute Renal Failure

Miriam Galbusera and Giuseppe Remuzzi

OBJECTIVES

This chapter will:
1. Review the physiology of hemostasis.
2. Characterize platelet abnormalities in uremia.
3. Examine abnormalities of coagulation and fibrinolysis in renal failure.
4. Delineate the impact of dialysis on uremic bleeding.
5. Describe the role of anemia in uremic bleeding.

Bleeding is a common and potentially serious complication of acute and chronic renal failure.[1] The clinical manifestations vary, ranging from ecchymoses, epistaxis, and bleeding from gums and venipuncture site to overt gastrointestinal bleeding, which has been observed in up to one third of uremic patients. Low-grade gastrointestinal bleeding may be even more common. The advent of modern dialysis techniques has reduced but not eliminated the risk of hemorrhage. The pathogenesis of uremic bleeding is multifactorial; however, a major role is played by abnormalities in platelet-platelet and platelet–vessel wall interaction. On the other hand, abnormalities of blood coagulation and fibrinolysis may predispose the uremic patient to a hypercoagulable state, rather than bleeding.

In acute renal failure (ARF), hemostatic abnormalities are not due to the effect of uremia alone. In fact, the frequently accompanying pathological conditions, such as disseminated intravascular coagulation (DIC), sepsis, major surgery, severe trauma, thrombotic microangiopathies, and hypovolemic and cardiogenic shock, are associated with changes in the hemostatic system. These conditions constitute the most common causes of ARF and multiple organ dysfunction syndrome (MODS), which, particularly when the liver is involved, contribute to the hemostatic derangement in affected patients.

In patients with ARF, anticoagulation regimens for renal replacement therapy may further contribute to the hemostatic abnormalities.

NORMAL HEMOSTASIS

Physiological hemostasis is a complex process that controls blood fluidity and rapidly induces hemostatic plug formation at the site of vascular injury (Fig. 70-1). Hemostasis consists of three phases—primary hemostasis, coagulation, and fibrinolysis—that are closely linked to one another.

Primary Hemostasis

Primary hemostasis is due to interactions between platelets and adhesive proteins and the vessel wall. Normal vascular endothelium is a thromboresistant surface that possesses antiplatelet, anticoagulant, and profibrinolytic properties, but after vascular injury, platelets are rapidly recruited to form the hemostatic plug. Normal platelet adhesion requires initial platelet contact, followed by platelet spreading at the site of vascular injury. This complex process is mediated mainly by the interaction of two platelet receptors, the glycoprotein GPIb and the activation-dependent receptor $\alpha_{IIb}\beta_3$ complex, with the adhesive molecules von Willebrand factor (VWF) and fibrinogen.

In flowing blood, the initial contact of platelet with the vessel wall is dependent on the binding of VWF (bound to collagen on the exposed subendothelium or to P-selectin on activated endothelial cells) with the GPIb on platelets. This interaction promotes the rolling of platelets on the endothelial surface, initiating platelet activation. In activated platelets, the $\alpha_{IIb}\beta_3$ complex undergoes conformational change that allows the binding of this receptor with fibrinogen and VWF, leading to further platelet adhesion. Subsequent to this conformational change, platelets release the contents of the granules, liberating substances such as adenosine diphosphate (ADP), thromboxane, VWF, fibrinogen, thrombin, serotonin, and epinephrine, leading to further platelet activation and aggregation, as well as vasoconstriction. The process of platelet adhesion is counteracted by cleaving of the VWF molecule by the protease ADAMTS13, thereby blocking initial thrombus formation.

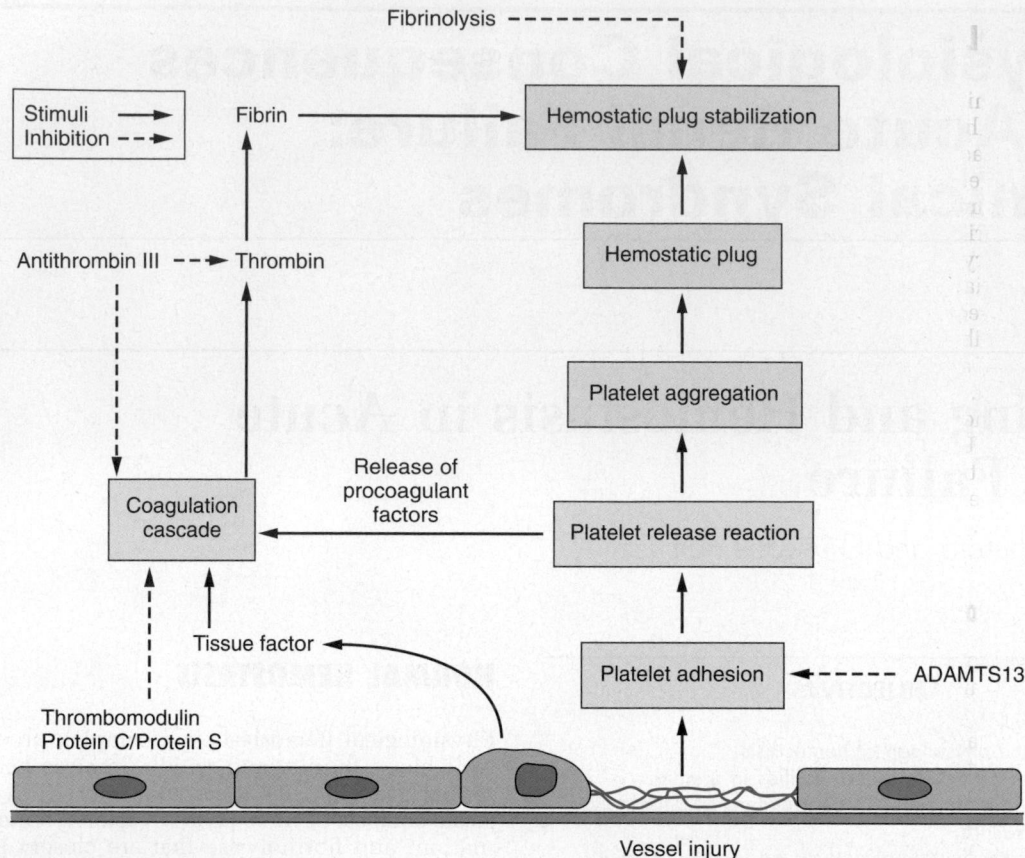

FIGURE 70-1. Overview of hemostasis.

Coagulation

Coagulation is divided into the *intrinsic pathway*, initiated by contact with negatively charged surfaces, and the *extrinsic pathway*, initiated by tissue factor (TF). The contact system probably plays a minor role in in vivo activation of blood coagulation. The coagulation cascade is promoted by TF, a cell membrane protein that is exposed at the site of vascular injury, leading to formation of TF–factor VIIa complex, which, in turn, may activate both factor IX and factor X. Factor Xa activates factor V to factor Va, leading to formation of factor Xa–factor Va complex, which is capable of converting prothrombin to thrombin. At this point, thrombin may activate factors VIII, V, and XI and separate factor VIII from VWF. Once formed, thrombin converts fibrinogen to fibrin by cleaving the fibrinogen molecule to create fibrin monomers that are cross-linked to form fibrin polymers by the action of thrombin-activated factor XIIIa.

Thrombin stimulates positive feedback that activates platelets and produces thrombin burst, leading to maintenance of fibrin formation. In addition, thrombin activates endothelial cells and leukocytes.

Natural Anticoagulants

Several plasma and endothelial anticoagulatory mechanisms exist for controlling the coagulation cascade, including antithrombin, the protein C system, the TF pathway inhibitor, and glycosaminoglycans. Antithrom-

bin III (ATIII) inhibits thrombin, factor Xa, and factor IXa. The capacity of ATIII to block thrombin is greatly accelerated by heparin and heparin-like glycosaminoglycans present on the endothelial cell surface. Thrombin also is inhibited by thrombomodulin, a thrombin receptor expressed by endothelial cells. The thrombin-thrombomodulin complex activates protein C, which, together with its cofactor protein S, inactivates both factor Va and factor VIIIa. On endothelium is localized another anticoagulant, the TF pathway inhibitor that inhibits factor Xa and the TF–factor VIIa complex.

Fibrinolysis

Fibrinolysis is a regulated mechanism that leads to fibrin dissolution through the proteolytic degradation exerted by plasmin. Activation of fibrinolysis is achieved by conversion of plasminogen to plasmin through the action of tissue plasminogen activator (tPA) or urokinase or by the contact system. TPA is released by activated endothelium. Fibrinolysis is controlled by plasminogen activator inhibitors (i.e., PAI-1 and PAI-2), plasmin inhibitors (α_1-antiplasmin, α_2-macroglobulin), and the thrombin-activatable fibrinolysis inhibitor (TAFI). Once produced, plasmin cleaves factor V, factor VIII, fibrinogen, and the GPIb receptor on platelets. Finally, fibrin and fibrinogen degradation products (FDPs) interfere with fibrin formation and impair platelet function by $\alpha_{IIb}\beta_3$ complex occupancy.

PATHOPHYSIOLOGY

The cause of uremic bleeding has been the subject of the major debate in the last 35 years. The pathogenesis is considered multifactorial (Table 70-1); however, platelet-platelet and platelet–vessel wall interactions appear to be of crucial importance. In uremia, the bleeding tendency initially was attributed to vascular defects, because increased capillary fragility has been reported to be common in uremia; however, this finding has not been confirmed in subsequent studies. Abnormalities of blood coagulation and fibrinolysis are less consistent and are more indicative of a hypercoagulable state than of a hemorrhagic condition.

Bleeding tendency in uremic patients has been extensively evaluated. Unfortunately, the studies have been done mainly in patients with chronic renal failure, and it is not clear whether these findings can be extrapolated to acute renal failure.

Thrombocytopenia

Moderate thrombocytopenia is a common finding in uremic patients[2-4] and may be caused by inadequate platelet production or overconsumption.[5] Nevertheless, the platelet count is rarely less than $80 \times 10^9/L$,[2,6] a number considered adequate for normal hemostasis.

The interaction of blood with hemodialysis membranes that may cause complement activation (e.g., cuprophane) leads to transient neutropenia and significant thrombocytopenia during dialysis.[7,8] This phenomenon does not occur with biocompatible membranes that do not activate complement.[7,8] Thrombocytopenia in uremic patients also may derive from the anticoagulation regimen used to inhibit clotting in the extracorporeal circuit; in fact, heparin occasionally may activate platelets and induce thrombocytopenia by an immunologic mechanism.[9]

A major decrease in platelet count is detected in patients with renal failure associated with hemolytic uremic syndrome–thrombotic thrombocytopenic purpura, disseminated intravascular coagulation, eclampsia, or renal allograft rejection. In uremia, the mean platelet volume

TABLE 70-1

Mechanisms Affecting Hemostasis in Uremia

Thrombocytopenia
Platelet abnormalities
Defects in platelet–vessel wall interaction
- Abnormal platelet adhesion
- Altered von Willebrand factor
- Increased formation of vascular PGI_2
Uremic toxins
Abnormal production of nitric oxide
Anemia
- Altered blood rheology
- Defective platelet diffusivity
- Decreased release of ADP by erythrocytes
- Erythropoietin deficiency
Drug treatment
- Anticoagulants
- Antiplatelet agents
- Nonsteroidal anti-inflammatory drugs
- β-Lactam antibiotics
- Third-generation cephalosporins

ADP, adenosine diphosphate; PGI_2, prostacyclin (prostaglandin I_2).

TABLE 70-2

Platelet Abnormalities in Renal Failure

Subnormal dense granule content
Reduction in intracellular ADP and serotonin
Impaired release of the platelet α-granule proteins and β-thromboglobulin
Enhanced intracellular cAMP
Abnormal mobilization of platelet Ca^{2+}
Abnormal platelet arachidonic acid metabolism
Abnormal ex vivo platelet aggregation in response to different stimuli
Defective cyclooxygenase activity
Abnormality of the activation-dependent binding activity of $\alpha_{IIb}\beta_3$ complex

ADP, adenosine diphosphate; cAMP, cyclic adenosine monophosphate.

also may be decreased, causing a reduction in the circulating platelet mass that is inversely related to the bleeding time.

Platelet Abnormalities

A variety of platelet abnormalities have been described in uremia (Table 70-2), including subnormal dense granule content and impaired release of the platelet α-granule proteins and β-thromboglobulin. Reduced capacity to form thromboxane A_2, reduction in serotonin and ADP, and elevation of cyclic AMP have been reported. Platelet dysfunction also has been attributed to the prostaglandin-forming enzyme cyclooxygenase and to abnormal Ca^{2+} mobilization in platelets, leading to an impairment of Ca^{2+}-dependent platelet function. Because the platelet defect is partially corrected by dialysis, uremic toxins such as urea, phenol, and guanidinosuccinic acid (GSA) have been causally related to uremic platelet dysfunction.

Several studies have pointed out that the platelet–vessel wall interaction is impaired in uremic patients.[10-12] This abnormality is attributable to impaired function of the platelet $\alpha_{IIb}\beta_3$ complex receptor, accounting for the decreased binding of the two main adhesive proteins circulating in human blood, VWF and fibrinogen, to stimulated uremic platelets.[13] In one study, removal of substances present in uremic plasma improved the binding capacity of $\alpha_{IIb}\beta_3$ complex, suggesting that the defective function may be attributable to uremic toxins or may be due to receptor occupancy by fibrinogen fragments present in uremic blood.[13] The impaired $\alpha_{IIb}\beta_3$ complex activation in uremia may explain aggregation defects, as well as reduced VWF-dependent adhesion and thrombus formation.[10-12] Although quantitative and qualitative abnormalities of VWF have not been consistently observed in uremia,[11,14,15] a functional defect in the VWF-platelet interaction may indeed play a role, because in these patients, cryoprecipitate (a plasma derivative rich in VWF) and desmopressin (a synthetic derivative of antidiuretic hormone that releases autologous VWF from storage sites) significantly shorten the bleeding time.

In addition, molecules such as prostacyclin (PGI_2) and nitric oxide (NO) that inhibit platelet function and modulate vascular tone, affecting platelet–vessel wall interaction, are increased in uremia.[16,17] The guanidino compound related to arginine guanidinosuccinate accumulates in the plasma of patients with uremia and is involved in the generation of NO.[17] GSA's effect of stimulating NO release provides a biological explanation for early data showing that among uremic toxins, GSA was the only one that consistently inhibited platelet function to such a degree that it was defined as the "x factor" in uremic bleeding.

The effect of estrogen therapy to prevent bleeding in uremic patients rests on the capacity of estrogens to counteract the excessive production of NO. The anecdotal observation of diminished gastrointestinal bleeding in uremic patients who received conjugated estrogens and the improved hemostasis in von Willebrand's disease during pregnancy led to investigations of the effect of estrogens on bleeding tendency in uremia.[15,18] In an experimental model of chronic uremia, the effect of estrogens on bleeding time was completely reversed by the NO precursor L-arginine,[19] suggesting that the effect of estrogens on primary hemostasis in uremia may be mediated by changes in the NO synthesis pathway.

Abnormalities of Coagulation and Fibrinolysis

Despite the hemorrhagic tendency, activation of coagulation has been demonstrated in uremic patients, and it is more prominent in those who undergo hemodialysis. Risk factors[4] include enhanced platelet aggregability, increased plasma fibrinogen, factor VIII:C and VWF, decreased protein C anticoagulant activity and protein S, impaired fibrinolytic system activity, raised plasma lipoprotein(a), increased plasma concentration of homocysteine, and the presence of lupus anticoagulant. Thrombin is continuously formed, as demonstrated by the increased levels of thrombin–antithrombin III levels,[20-23] D-dimers[21,22] and fibrinopeptide A.[21,22,24] Conflicting results have been obtained regarding the fibrinolytic system. Initial reports noted decreased fibrinolytic activity in uremia, either absolute or relative to the extent of activation of the coagulation[5,24]; this finding has been used as an explanation for the hypercoagulable state. Later reports, however, described activation of fibrinolysis in uremia, with an increase in plasmin-antiplasmin complexes[20,25] and fibrinogen and fibrin degradation products,[20,21] together with a decrease in plasminogen activator inhibitor activity[20] after hemodialysis sessions.[23,26] These later findings probably reflect a fibrinolytic response secondary to fibrin deposition that also takes place if overall fibrinolytic activity is depressed. Dialysis partially corrects the coagulation and fibrinolytic abnormalities associated with uremia.

Thrombotic Tendency

Uremic patients are at higher risk for thrombotic complications of vascular access as a consequence of hemodialysis. Percutaneous cannulas, arteriovenous shunts, and native vein or prosthetic arteriovenous fistulas, or fistulas made of artificial polymers, are particularly prone to thrombotic occlusion.

Because platelet aggregation plays a major role in thrombus formation, antiplatelet agents have been used, with encouraging results. Aspirin, dipyridamole, ticlopidine, and sulfinpyrazone have been proved useful in several studies. Fibrinolytic agents, such as streptokinase or urokinase, as well as recombinant tissue plasminogen activator, have produced conflicting results.

In the nephrotic syndrome, an association with renal vein thrombosis has been long recognized.[27,28] In this syndrome, a hypercoagulable state caused by increased levels of coagulation factors, reduced levels of antithrombin, and

an increased platelet response to various stimuli plays an important role in the development of renal vein thrombosis and other venous and arterial thromboembolic complications (reviewed by Joist and colleagues[4]).

The activity of the protease ADAMTS13 is reduced in uremia, as well as in acute inflammation and cirrhosis, and levels also fall in the postoperative period.[29] A complete loss of ADAMTS13 activity—as a result of congenital or immune-mediated deficiency—is the main cause of thrombotic occlusion of arterioles and capillaries in a majority of patients with thrombotic thrombocytopenic purpura.[30] A complete ADAMTS13 deficiency also has been found in a subgroup of patients with the atypical form of hemolytic uremic syndrome.[30] Replacement of the deficient activity with plasma is the treatment of choice for congenital cases, and clearance of the autoantibodies by plasma exchange, or inhibition of their production by immunosuppressive agents, is the key component of treatment in the immune-mediated form of the disease.

Dialysis

Dialysis improves platelet functional abnormalities and decreases, but does not eliminate, the risk of hemorrhage. In addition, hemodialysis per se can contribute to the hemostatic abnormalities because the interaction between blood and artificial surfaces may induce chronic activation of platelets. The consequent release of platelet-derived proteins can induce platelet exhaustion, leading to their dysfunction. It has been documented that plasma levels of the potent NO inducers tumor necrosis factor-α (TNF-α) and interleukin-1β (IL-1β) rise during dialysis.[31,32] IL-1β and TNF-α are generated in vivo by circulating monocytes during hemodialysis with complement-activating membranes. Production of increased cytokines also may be triggered by intact endotoxin, endotoxin fragments, and other bacterial toxins that may cross dialysis membranes, as well as by acetate-containing dialysate. As a result of massive release of cytokines during dialysis, NO synthesis increases. Thus, the capacity of the dialysis procedure to remove uremic toxins is counterbalanced by its effects on platelet activation and NO synthesis. On the other hand, some evidence suggests that NO synthesis does not increase during the course of a dialysis session; instead, it decreases. This finding indicates that under optimal hemodialysis conditions with no or minimal cytokine activation, hemodialysis corrects the exaggerated NO synthesis, possibly by removing from uremic plasma some dialyzable NO-releasing substances.

Heparin, used to obtain systemic anticoagulation, can occasionally induce platelet activation and thrombocytopenia.[9] In patients at risk for bleeding, alternative means to routine heparinization can be used to prevent clotting in the extracorporeal circulation during hemodialysis. Alternative strategies, developed specifically for anticoagulation in patients at high risk for bleeding, include regional anticoagulation with heparin and protamine, use of low-dose heparin, hemodialysis without anticoagulation, regional anticoagulation with citrate, and the use of low-molecular-weight heparin. The use of anticoagulants during renal replacement therapy is discussed in other chapters.

Role of Anemia

Anemia, initially mild, is a constant feature of acute and chronic renal failure and is the main determinant of the prolonged bleeding time in uremic patients. Some evidence suggests that bleeding time is inversely related to the hematocrit in uremia,[33,34] as well as in other types of anemia.

An important function of red blood cells within the normal circulation is to increase platelet–vessel wall contact by displacing platelets away from the axial flow and toward the vessel wall; they also enhance platelet function by releasing ADP[35] and inactivating PGI_2. This erythrocyte activity explains the shortening of the bleeding time seen in uremic patients after partial correction of anemia by red blood cell transfusions[34] or with administration of recombinant human erythropoietin (rhEPO).[36,37] Many factors contribute to the anemia of uremic patients, including shortened survival of the red cell, failure of the erythroid marrow, repeated blood loss during dialysis, and, perhaps of greatest importance, defective secretion of erythropoietin. The role of erythropoietin deficiency as the primary underlying defect in the anemia of renal failure is supported by data showing that partial correction of anemia by rhEPO was sufficient to correct defective primary hemostasis in uremia. Good evidence indicates that substances present in uremic serum, including polyamines, parathyroid hormone, and various cytokines, can inhibit erythropoiesis.[38]

The cloning of the human erythropoietin gene followed by the production of rhEPO has provided clinicians with a powerful tool to correct the anemia associated with renal failure, thereby eliminating the dependency on transfusion. No consistent changes are found in platelet number, platelet aggregation, or platelet thromboxane A_2 formation.[36] The hematocrit levels during rhEPO treatment should be controlled carefully because a complete correction of renal anemia carries the risk of hypertension, encephalopathy, thrombosis, and hyperkalemia. A controlled study established the minimum hematocrit necessary to achieve with rhEPO to correct the prolonged bleeding time in uremic patients.[37] A threshold hematocrit between 27% and 32% has to be reached for the bleeding time to become normal, or nearly normal, indicating that a partial correction of renal anemia is sufficient for this purpose.

Drugs

Uremic patients may be at an increased risk for bleeding complications caused by drug treatment. The risk of bleeding associated with the accumulation of β-lactam antibiotics in uremia has been highlighted.[39] β-Lactam antibiotics apparently act by perturbing platelet membrane function and interfering with ADP receptors. The prolonged bleeding time and the abnormal platelet aggregation are related to the dose and duration of treatment and are promptly reversible on discontinuation of the drug. Third-generation cephalosporins also may inhibit platelet function, which may lead to marked disturbance in blood coagulation.[40]

CLINICAL AND LABORATORY FINDINGS

The most common bleeding complications in uremia are petechial hemorrhages, blood blisters, and ecchymoses at the site of fistula access puncture or temporary venous access insertion. Gatrointestinal bleeding occurs with greater frequency and higher mortality in uremic patients than in the general population,[41] and upper gastrointestinal tract bleeding is the second leading cause of death in ARF.[42] The causes of bleeding usually are peptic ulcer, hemorrhagic esophagitis, gastritis, duodenitis, and gastric telangiectasias.[43-46] Other bleeding complications reported in chronic uremia are subdural hematoma, spontaneous retroperitoneal bleeding, spontaneous subcapsular hematoma of the liver, intraocular hemorrhage, and though now rare, hemorrhagic pericarditis with cardiac tamponade.

The advent of modern dialysis techniques and the correction of anemia have definitively reduced the incidence of severe bleeding, but hemorrhage is still a potentially fatal complication in patients with renal failure who are undergoing major surgery or invasive procedures, including kidney and liver biopsy. In the ICU setting, serious complications may develop, such as prolonged bleeding from the site of central venous line insertion or associated with surgery or other invasive procedures. Patients with ARF are at increased risk for bleeding; however, the results of coagulation screening tests (activated partial thromboplastin time, prothrombin time, and thrombin time) generally are normal, unless the uremia is associated with other disorders such as liver disease, vitamin K deficiency, presence of lupus anticoagulant, or disseminated intravascular coagulation.

To identify patients at risk for hemorrhagic complications, efforts have been aimed at establishing which abnormal laboratory findings in uremia correlate most specifically with an increased likelihood of clinically significant bleeding. The best laboratory indicator of clinical bleeding caused by uremia is believed to be the cutaneous bleeding time,[47] a test measuring the primary phase of hemostasis—that is, the interaction of the platelet with the blood vessel wall—and formation of the hemostatic plug.

CONCLUSION

The association between a bleeding tendency and uremia has been demonstrated repeatedly. Although modern dialysis techniques and the use of erythropoietin to correct anemia have reduced its frequency, bleeding is still a potentially life-threatening complication in uremic patients and may preclude therapeutic interventions including surgery and other invasive procedures.

The pathogenesis of uremic bleeding is multifactorial; however, it has been attributed mainly to abnormalities of primary hemostasis, particularly platelet dysfunction, and impaired platelet–vessel wall interaction. Despite the hemorrhagic tendency, abnormalities of coagulation and fibrinolysis predispose uremic patients to a hypercoagulable state.

In ARF, hemostatic abnormalities also may be due to accompanying disorders that, particularly when the liver is involved, contribute to the hemostatic derangement in these patients. Anticoagulation regimens for renal replacement therapy may further contribute to the hemostatic abnormalities.

Key Points

1. The pathogenesis of uremic bleeding is multifactorial; however, a major role is played by abnormalities of platelet-platelet and platelet–vessel wall interaction.

2. Dialysis decreases but does not eliminate the risk of bleeding.
3. Anticoagulation regimens used for renal replacement therapy may further contribute to the hemostatic abnormalities.
4. Correction of anemia improves hemostasis in uremic patients.
5. Abnormalities of blood coagulation and fibrinolysis may predispose the uremic patient to a hypercoagulable state, rather than bleeding.

Key References

4. Joist JH, Remuzzi G, Mannucci PM: Abnormal bleeding and thrombosis in renal disease. In Colman RW, Hirsh J, Marde

VJ, Salzmann EW (eds): Hemostasis and Thrombosis: Basic Principles and Clinical Practice. Philadelphia, JB Lippincott, 1994, pp 921-935.
17. Noris M, Remuzzi G: Uremic bleeding: Closing the circle after 30 years of controversies? Blood 1999;94:2569-2574.
20. Mezzano D, Tagle R, Panes O, et al: Hemostatic disorder of uremia: The platelet defect, main determinant of the prolonged bleeding time, is correlated with indices of activation of coagulation and fibrinolysis. Thromb Haemost 1996;76:312-321.
34. Livio M, Marchesi D, Remuzzi G, et al: Uraemic bleeding: Role of anemia and beneficial effect of red cell transfusions. Lancet 1982;2:1013-1015.
39. Andrassy K, Ritz E: Uremia as a cause of bleeding. Am J Nephrol 1985;5:313-319.

See the companion Expert Consult website for the complete reference list.

CHAPTER 71

Gastrointestinal Problems in Acute Renal Failure

Ramin Sam, Orly F. Kohn, May T. Chow, and Todd S. Ing

OBJECTIVES

This chapter will:
1. Present an overview of the epidemiology, pathogenesis, and clinical features of common gastrointestinal problems associated with acute renal failure.
2. Describe the management of common gastrointestinal problems associated with acute renal failure.

The second half of the 20th century saw remarkable changes in the clinical presentation of patients suffering from acute renal failure (ARF). These changes relate to the emergence of new nephrotoxic agents, the change in pattern of ARF-inducing diseases, and improvement of medical care through use of more effective drugs and the earlier application of efficient renal replacement therapies. Because patients with untreated terminal ARF are rarely encountered these days, some of the advanced gastrointestinal (GI) complications of uremia, such as stomatitis and colitis, for example, are seen less frequently than in years past. Nevertheless, certain other GI complications such as bleeding still warrant close attention. Furthermore, uremia-induced GI symptoms such as anorexia, dysgeusia, nausea, and vomiting continue to plague patients and often herald the need for prompt renal replacement therapy.

PATHOGENESIS OF UREMIC LESIONS IN THE GASTROINTESTINAL TRACT

The entire GI tract may be involved in advanced uremia, with the stomach and the small and large intestines being most commonly affected. Jaffe and Laing[1] found the earliest pathologic changes in the GI tract of uremic patients to be in the form of capillary hyperemia, dilatation of submucosal veins, edema, hemorrhage, and subsequent bacterial invasion of the devitalized areas, accompanied by fibrinous exudates and necrosis.

Urea retention can alter gastric defense against autolysis. Edward and Skoryna demonstrated that an increase in gastric juice urea level may lead to dissolution of gastric mucus.[2] In addition, by investigating ionic fluxes across the stomach of experimental animals, Davenport[3] found that intraluminal urea in high concentrations could raise gastric permeability. A consequence of this gastric hyperpermeability is an augmented back-diffusion of hydrogen ions from the gastric lumen to the mucosa. Fisher and colleagues[4] observed that gastrin could cause pyloric incompetence by antagonizing the effects of cholecystokinin and secretin on the pyloric sphincter. Gastrin is catabolized by the normal kidneys. With ARF, gastrin catabolism is impaired and plasma gastrin level commonly rises.

Wesdorp and associates observed a nearly six-fold increase in the mean plasma gastrin level in patients with ARF as compared with control subjects, with levels in approximately half of the patients reaching levels in the Zollinger-Ellison range.[5] Although an elevated plasma gastrin level may foster GI bleeding and gastritis, intragastric pH is not lower in patients with renal failure. Indeed, a low basal acid output with a high basal intragastric pH, but with a significant peak acid output, has been found in patients with ARF.[5] Moreover, pentagastrin-stimulated gastric acid secretion is normal in patients with ARF.[5] The high basal intragastric pH may reflect the neutralizing effect of a high gastric ammonia concentration. Lieber and Lefevre detected higher gastric ammonia values and lower acid levels in uremic patients as compared with normal control subjects.[6] Gastric ammonia levels are higher as a result of the splitting of the available higher-than-normal amounts of urea by urease-rich bacteria in the stomach. Impairment of cell renewal and cell division in ARF may reduce the competence of the mucosal barrier, contributing to the initiation and persistence of a uremic lesion by impairing epithelial wound healing.[7]

GASTROINTESTINAL PROBLEMS COMMONLY ASSOCIATED WITH ACUTE RENAL FAILURE

Dysgeusia, Anorexia, Dyspepsia, Hiccups, Nausea, and Vomiting

In uremic patients, dysgeusia commonly manifests as a metallic or a foul taste in the mouth. Additionally, anorexia, dyspepsia, hiccups, nausea, and vomiting are frequent components of the uremic syndrome. Persistent vomiting may bring about dehydration (with associated dryness of the tongue and of the mouth), electrolyte disturbances, and wasting.[8] With regard to therapy for nausea and vomiting, apart from dialysis, symptomatic improvement can be obtained with phenothiazines or metoclopramide, given either parenterally or rectally.

Of note is the fact that in hemodialysis patients, maintaining a blood urea level above 50 mmol/L (300 mg/dL) for periods of 7 to 90 days through the use of a urea-enriched dialysis solution can bring about vomiting.[9] A rapid reduction of a very high blood urea level can lead to a constellation of manifestations known as the *dialysis disequilibrium syndrome* (DDS). Salient features of the syndrome include nausea and vomiting. DDS is believed to be the consequence of cerebral edema engendered by either the entry of water into brain cells during dialysis, secondary to the rapid decline in extracellular fluid osmolality, or by the induction of a dialysis-induced acidosis of the cerebrospinal fluid and of the brain.[10]

Stomatitis, Uremic Fetor, and Inflammation of Salivary Glands

In advanced uremia, uremic stomatitis, characterized by a red, thickened buccal mucosa with a superimposed gray, thick, and gluey exudate, can occur.[11] Ulcerations also are a prominent feature in some patients. Stomatitis and glossitis, often accompanied by a dry burning mouth, commonly are associated with poor dental hygiene. Patients with advanced uremia may exhibit the fetor of uremia (uremic odor) in addition to uremic stomatitis. The fetor of uremia is an ammoniacal odor, reminiscent of that of stale urine.[8] The suggestion has been made that large amounts of ammonia are formed as a result of the action of bacterial urease on urea, present in high levels in the saliva of uremic patients. The ammonia so produced is suspected to be the cause of the stomatitis.[8] Inflammation of the salivary glands (e.g., parotitis) also may occur in uremic patients, often in association with stomatitis.[8]

Gastrointestinal Hemorrhage

In the early part of the last century, acute GI hemorrhage was a dreaded complication in patients with ARF. Indeed,

before the 1970s, GI bleeding, occurring in as many as a third of these patients, was the second leading cause of death.[12-15] Subsequent reports indicate a fall in the incidence of such bleeding. For example, in a 1978 study involving 276 patients with ARF, GI bleeding was seen in 90 patients (33%). The bleeding was mild and readily controlled in 75 of these patients, however, and only 4 patients died from the GI bleeding (1.5%).[16] In addition, in a series of 636 patients with ARF treated between 1980 and 1989, only one of 214 deaths was attributed to GI bleeding.[17] The dearth of GI hemorrhage as a cause of death in ARF in more recent years may be related to prophylactic therapy with effective acid-lowering regimens,[18] as well as to the better control of uremic bleeding by prompt and effective renal replacement therapies.[17,19,20]

Although many earlier-published reports apparently supported the notion that a fall in the incidence of GI bleeding among patients with ARF had occurred in the recent past,[17,19,20] a 1997 investigation nevertheless described an 8% to 13% incidence of GI bleeding among patients with ARF.[21] Furthermore, a 2001 study also reported a 13% incidence of acute GI bleeding as a complication of ARF. In this prospective study, involving 514 patients with ARF, GI bleeding occurred despite prophylaxis with ranitidine therapy. In most cases, the bleeding was the result of upper GI disease. In 48 endoscopic procedures performed, gastric erosions or ulcers were found in 42% of the patients, duodenal ulcers in 12%, esophageal varices in 11%, and gastric neoplasia in 6%. The severity of the underlying illness, the intensity of the uremia, a low blood platelet count, and the presence of hepatic disease were found to be significant risk factors.[22] According to the study investigators, acute GI bleeding in patients with ARF is a risk indicator of increased health resource utilization and death.[22] The aforementioned gastric erosions and ulcers, along with duodenal ulcers, are likely to be the manifestations of stress-related mucosal disease (SRMD), a continuum of conditions spanning stress-related injury (superficial mucosal damage) to stress ulcers (focal deep mucosal damage).[18] Whether an element of concomitant uremic gastritis also was present, leading to bleeding from the gastric erosions, however, has not been ruled out.

Noteworthy is the fact that both stress ulcer and gastritis are common among patients with ARF.[23] Myriad studies have suggested that patients suffering from ARF do not belong to a homogeneous group,[24] and bleeding-prone GI (including hepatic) diseases that occur in patients who do not have ARF also can afflict patients with ARF.[22] The difference in disease mix and a host of other variables such as age, gender, ethnicity, nutrition status, ARF etiology (nephrotoxic, hypoperfusion-related, or a combination of both),[24] severity of bleeding, disease acuity, severity of uremia, comorbidity (such as sepsis, disseminated intravascular coagulation, hepatic failure, diabetes, hypertension, or cardiac disease), and treatment regimens, are likely to be the reasons why the incidence of GI bleeding varies widely among studies involving patients with ARF. Finally, it should be noted that bleeding originating from the lower intestinal tract is not an infrequent terminal event in uremic patients.[8] Under such circumstances, it is likely that uremic enterocolitis is the main cause of the bleeding episode.

Presumed to be a result of a variety of factors including those of gastric acid, mucosal ischemia and bile reflux, SRMD most often is seen in critically ill patients in the intensive care unit (ICU) setting.[18,25] Although the cost-effectiveness[26] or even the necessity[27] of SRMD prophylaxis in all critically ill patients in general is uncertain, such an approach using antacids (see later), sucralfate (see later), histamine H₂ blockers, or proton pump inhibitors often has been practiced.[18,25-29] In this regard, most authorities are of the opinion that prophylaxis against SRMD may reduce major bleeding but has not yet been shown to improve survival.[18] Patients at very high risk for the development of SRMD are those with prolonged mechanical ventilation and coagulopathy. Additional risk factors include sepsis, renal failure, hepatic failure, hypotension, trauma, burns, and myocardial infarction. Therefore, it has been suggested that ARF patients, especially those who also suffer from coagulopathy or are mechanically ventilated, should certainly receive SRMD prophylaxis to prevent GI bleeding.[18,26]

H₂ receptor antagonists can be used for prophylaxis of SRMD but are not all equally potent. Some of these agents (e.g., cimetidine) have a long list of drug interactions and can cause neurological and hematological side effects.[30] A potent H₂ receptor antagonist with minimal drug interactions such as famotidine may be used, but the development of tolerance to H₂ receptor antagonists remains a concern.[30] Garnering increasing popularity, proton pump inhibitors are the most potent antisecretory agents, inhibiting the gastric H^+,K^+-ATPase in the parietal cells and capable of raising gastric pH to above 6.[29,30] Pantoprazole, lansoprazole, and esomeprazole are available in many countries in intravenous formulations. Such intravenous formulations with long-lasting antisecretory effect and little risk of drug interactions are ideally suited for use in the ICU. Finally, when H₂ receptor antagonists and proton pump inhibitors are discontinued, the dosage should be tapered gradually, or the drugs should be substituted with alternatives (e.g., antacids) in order to prevent acid rebound.[30]

Chromium labeling studies have indicated that even in the absence of overt bleeding, uremic patients have increased GI blood loss when compared with control subjects.[31] Such minor blood loss in the absence of any demonstrable histopathological lesions may be the consequence of a generalized bleeding tendency secondary to a uremia-induced defect in platelet aggregability and in platelet–vessel wall interaction.[32] This bleeding tendency is reflected in the presence of a prolonged bleeding time.[32]

GI bleeding appears to increase during the hemodialysis procedure and may be compounded by several factors in addition to the use of anticoagulants. During hemodialysis, gastric acid secretion rises whenever blood pressure falls, and this gastric acid hypersecretion may contribute to the higher incidence of GI bleeding.[33] Moreover, intradialytic hypotension due to excessive ultrafiltration or other causes can precipitate bowel infarction with resultant GI bleeding.[34] GI bleeding can worsen preexisting azotemia by engendering a hypovolemia-induced reduction in renal perfusion and, hence, in glomerular filtration.[35] Absorption of blood proteins from the GI tract, followed by the catabolism of those absorbed proteins by the liver to form urea, probably also plays a role in aggravating azotemia.[36]

Conventional treatment for patients with ARF-related upper GI bleeding has included nasogastric suction, blood transfusion, and the administration of an antacid, sucralfate (see later), an H₂ receptor antagonist, or a proton pump inhibitor. The use of antacids is labor-intensive and not popular because of the large amounts required[18] and because of the generally inadequate results.[30] Also, the administration of aluminum-based sucralfate to patients with renal dysfunction can lead to hyperaluminumemia.[37] Although therapy with aluminum-containing drugs (such as aluminum-based antacids and sucralfate) in these

patients at conventionally given doses and for a short duration has not been reported to be overtly detrimental, it would seem prudent to avoid the use of such agents because of the risk of hyperaluminumemia. With regard to other antacids, use of magnesium-based preparations is discouraged because of the possibility of hypermagnesemia. Administration of desmopressin,[38] cryoprecipitate,[39] or conjugated estrogen[40,41] can help to reduce GI blood loss in uremic patients with a prolonged bleeding time. Raising the hematocrit level by blood transfusion can shorten bleeding time,[42] probably by enhancing the ability of platelets to adhere to the vascular endothelium.

Dialytic therapy also can shorten the prolonged bleeding time and curtail the bleeding.[43] Kleinknecht and coworkers were among the first to suggest that dialysis could curb uremic bleeding.[14] Of note, in a controlled prospective study of intensive versus nonintensive dialysis in patients with ARF, although overall morbidity and mortality were not different, intensively dialyzed patients suffered fewer hemorrhagic complications.[44]

Finally, a consultation with a gastroenterology specialist who is conversant with diagnostic and hemostatic endoscopic procedures should be promptly obtained for the uremic patient with active GI bleeding.

Hemodialysis treatment in the presence of GI bleeding should be performed without systemic anticoagulation (e.g., up to 7 L of saline introduced into the arterial blood line over a dialysis session in the case of a heparin-free protocol[45-47] or a regional citrate anticoagulation regimen using either a calcium-free or a calcium-containing dialysis solution).[45,46,48,49] Similar anticoagulation techniques also have been used for continuous renal replacement therapies (CRRTs).[46,49] With respect to anticoagulant-free dialysis, the use of saline flushes, 100 mL every 30 minutes, along with the administration of reduced doses of dalteparin has not been found to be effective.[50] The recently introduced method of using low-dose citric acid (on the order of 0.8 mM [2.4 mEq/L]) of citrate in the final dialysis solution) as an acidifying agent for the "acid concentrate" in a dual-concentrate, bicarbonate-based dialysate delivery system may help to reduce the extracorporeal circuit requirement for anticoagulants.[45,51,52]

Patients receiving total parenteral nutrition (TPN) and those requiring broad-spectrum antibiotic therapy are at risk for the development of vitamin K deficiency, hypoprothrombinemia, and resultant bleeding. Prophylactic vitamin K therapy often is indicated, especially in high-risk patients with ARF receiving TPN or broad-spectrum antibiotic therapy.[53-56] In general, the optimal dose of vitamin K has not been established. For TPN, an intravenous dose of 1 mg/day was found to be effective.[54] For antibiotic therapy, most patients will require a dose of 5 to 10 mg orally or subcutaneously once to three times weekly, although as much as 10 mg/day may be necessary.[55] It is preferable to administer vitamin K subcutaneously or intramuscularly, because intravenous administration has been associated with severe reactions resembling anaphylaxis.[56]

Gastritis, Duodenitis, and Peptic Ulcer Disease

In patients with ARF, apart from the SRMD involving the stomach and the duodenum mentioned previously, a progressively diffuse erosive gastritis with thinning of the mucosa and bleeding also has been described.[8] Gastritis and duodenitis presenting as superficial mucosal lesions also can be associated with the use of ulcerogenic drugs such as salicylates, corticosteroids, nonsteroidal anti-inflammatory drugs, and iron.[57] Fatal hemorrhage may result from these lesions. It is unclear whether peptic ulcer disease is more common among patients with ARF.[58] Noteworthy is the fact that the raised blood urea levels in uremic patients have not been found to interfere with the urease-based tests used in the detection of *Helicobacter pylori*.[59]

Treatment of gastritis, duodenitis, and peptic ulcer disease is similar to that described previously for the prophylaxis of SRMD. In patients with ARF who have active gastritis, duodenitis, or peptic ulcer disease, the anticoagulation methods used for renal replacement therapy in the face of GI bleeding, as described, also should be applied.

Pancreatitis

The pancreas, like the kidney, is susceptible to ischemic necrosis.[60] Autopsies of patients dying from oligemic shock showed a 50% incidence of major pancreatic injury in those with concomitant ARF, but only a 9% incidence in those without. Similarly, patients dying after nonoligemic shock had a 35% incidence of major pancreatic injury if acute tubular necrosis also was present but only a 12% incidence of pancreatic ischemic injury in the absence of acute renal lesions.[60]

The serum total amylase concentration (a summation of amylases produced by the pancreas, the salivary glands, and other tissues) rises in renal failure, but the value usually does not exceed three times the upper limit of normal.[61] Serum lipase activity is elevated (as high as twice the upper limit of normal) in approximately 50% of patients undergoing dialysis in the absence of pancreatitis.[61] Serum lipase activity increases after hemodialysis as a result of a heparin-induced release of endothelium-bound lipoprotein lipase. Consequently, only predialysis serum samples should be used for the determination of the enzyme.[61] In patients with pancreatitis, with or without renal failure, the serum levels of total amylase, pancreatic P3 isoamylase (P refers to pancreatic), total lipase, and pancreatic lipase levels frequently are markedly elevated. Because P3 isoamylase and pancreatic lipase are of solely pancreatic origin, the magnitude of their levels serves as a more valuable diagnostic pointer. Nonelevated serum levels of these two enzymes often suggest that the diagnosis of pancreatitis is less likely.[62] In patients with renal failure and acute pancreatitis, both the total amylase and the pancreatic P3 isoamylase levels in the serum often are markedly elevated. If, however, a substantial amount of pancreatic tissue has been destroyed from prior disease, serum pancreatic enzymes may not be elevated at all in spite of current acute pancreatitis. The diagnosis of acute pancreatitis in the setting of ARF should be based on a combination of clinical evidence as well as elevated lipase and amylase values. Finally, serum amylase activity may be spuriously low in peritoneal dialysis patients using icodextrin-based dialysis solutions, on account of the interference of icodextrin with amylase measurement.[63]

Cholecystitis

A high incidence of acute acalculous cholecystitis in critically ill patients with ARF has been reported.[64] Some of these patients may suffer from biliary peritonitis, a complication of gallbladder rupture. The diagnosis can be difficult and requires a high index of suspicion in addition to ultrasonography. Biliary drainage often is necessary for treatment.

Enterocolitis and Other Colonic Problems

Uremic enterocolitis has been described in the form of necrotizing ulcers in the lower part of the small bowel and the large bowel, particularly in the lymphoid tissue. Severe diarrhea with purulent or bloody stools may be a feature.[65] Apart from uremia, whether such intestinal pathology is related to a secondary bacterial infection also is unknown.[8] Uremic "colitis," characterized by diarrhea that cannot be attributed to other causes, is one of the terminal complications of uremia (but is a rare event in ARF).[66] Patients with uremic enterocolitis may present with an acute abdomen[67] with pain, rigidity, and tenderness, as well as nausea, vomiting, and weight loss. Commonly, the presence of positive fecal occult blood or of even frank hematochezia is evident. Because patients with ARF often receive renal replacement therapies early in the disease course (or perhaps also because of more frequent exposure to antibiotics), uremic enterocolitis is rarely encountered in clinical practice these days. On account of the frequent need to use antibiotic therapy combined with the presence of an impaired immune system and the reduction of gastrointestinal motility, patients with ARF suffer from an increased incidence of *Clostridium difficile*–associated pseudomembranous colitis.[68] Although patients afflicted by this form of colitis usually have severe symptoms, some may be asymptomatic. A high index of suspicion for this serious ailment is required. Its eradication has become more difficult with the emergence of increasingly resistant organisms.

Constipation in ARF patients can result from the administration of aluminum-based antacids, sucralfate, iron, calcium carbonate,[69] or analgesic narcotics, as well as from a restricted fluid intake. During hemodialysis, the splanchnic blood flow is reduced even if blood pressure remains within normal limits.[70] Often transient, this reduction may be more marked and more persistent in patients with hypotension. It has been suggested that episodes of hypotension from any cause (such as those from volume depletion due to vomiting, diarrhea, or excessive ultrafiltration) may precipitate bowel infarction.[71] On account of a variety of complicating factors such as old age, chronic hypertension, hyperlipidemia, diabetes, and elevated serum calcium-phosphorus product, many ARF patients suffer from atherosclerosis, arteriosclerosis, and calcification of blood vessels. When these patients experience hypotension, bowel ischemia and infarction can occur as a result of the failure of the damaged mesenteric blood vessels to respond to the hypotension through vasodilatation (failure of autoregulation). Prevention of mesenteric ischemia entails the maintenance of a proper blood volume and the avoidance of hypotension. In cardiovascularly unstable patients requiring renal replacement treatment, the use of techniques that can lessen the precipitation of hypotension such as slow, low-efficiency daily dialysis or CRRTs is preferred. Bowel infarction requires emergency surgery and carries a high morbidity and mortality.

Uremia is a common cause of metabolic ("paralytic") ileus. The ileus is of the overactive or spastic type, and its manifestations are similar to those of mechanical ileus or of intestinal obstruction.[8] Metabolic ileus occurs most frequently in post-traumatic ARF and crush syndrome, in which the ileus often is confused with the primary pathological features of injury.[8] Thus, the decision whether or not to perform exploratory surgery can be difficult.

In some reports, mucosal injury or necrosis of the large intestines developed in uremic patients after rectal administration of a mixture of sodium polystyrene sulfonate (SPS) and sorbitol.[72] Similar lesions also have been found, albeit less frequently, in the upper gastrointestinal tract after oral administration of the mixture.[73] In severe cases, bowel perforation has occurred. Studies in experimental animals have suggested that sorbitol alone was the culprit in this bowel complication.[72] Similar data for humans are lacking, however. At this stage of incomplete knowledge, it seems prudent to use instead another laxative in the case of oral SPS administration and another liquid vehicle in the case of rectal administration. Finally, it should be noted that SPS, when given orally alone, can bring about fecal impaction, especially in the face of dehydration and in the elderly. Because the serious complication of intestinal necrosis is often associated with a high mortality rate, some authors have suggested that it would seem wise to avoid the use of SPS to treat hyperkalemia unless such use is absolutely necessary and no other means of treatment are available.

Hepatic Disease

ARF often is associated with the concomitant failure of other organs—that is, multiorgan system failure (MOSF).[74] Hypoxic hepatic injury ("shock liver"), frequently due to hypotension, is seen commonly in this setting. There is usually an early and sometimes transient elevation in serum hepatic enzyme values followed by a steady rise in serum bilirubin levels and frank jaundice. Histological changes in the liver include centrilobular necrosis, bile stasis, and fatty infiltration.[74] The risk of infection is heightened by a combination of hepatic failure and renal failure. Azotemia is a predisposing factor for hepatic encephalopathy in patients with concomitant liver failure. This predisposition is believed to be due to the absorption of ammonia produced in the gut lumen in quantities much larger than usual because of the increased amount of available urea,[75] as well as to the accumulation of other toxic nitrogenous products. A higher blood pH can bring about a higher NH_3/NH_4^+ ratio, thereby augmenting the transport of the easily diffusible NH_3 across the blood-brain barrier and worsening the encephalopathy.[76] Intermittent modes of renal replacement therapy have been shown to lead to an increase in intracranial pressure and cardiovascular instability in susceptible patients with concomitant acute liver failure and renal failure.[46,77,78] Such changes are the result of a combination of (1) adverse effects on cerebral oxygen delivery or cerebral perfusion pressure, or both[77]; (2) the generation of an osmotic gradient between plasma on the one hand and cerebral and other tissues on the other; and (3) possibly too-rapid removal of excess fluid from the vascular space in a patient in a malnourished and weakened state. With CRRTs, these cardiovascular and cerebrovascular changes generally are much amelio-rated.[46,77,78] Patients with hepatic failure are at risk for intracranial hemorrhage. Conventional heparin administration during renal replacement therapies may more readily precipitate bleeding. Consequently, heparin-free or regional citrate administration approaches are preferred.[45,46]

Because of all of the aforementioned concerns, when a patient with combined liver dysfunction and ARF requires renal replacement therapy, the use of an appropriate (commonly lower than normal) bicarbonate level in the dialysis solution or replacement fluid (e.g., 30 mM or lower) to ensure that metabolic alkalosis does not occur, the use of a slightly higher-than-normal sodium level in the dialysis solution or replacement fluid (e.g., greater than 140 mM) to discourage entry of water into the brain during treatment, and the use of a treatment technique that avoids or minimizes bleeding should receive careful consideration.[45,46,79] Because patients with liver dysfunction may not be able to metabolize lactate or citrate readily,[80] it seems prudent to use a bicarbonate-based dialysis or replacement solution for all patients with concomitant hepatic and renal dysfunction and to monitor plasma bicarbonate level often when regional citrate anticoagulation is practiced. Finally, in severe cases of uncontrolled intracranial pressure, cooling of the dialysis or replacement solution may be helpful, in addition to other measures to cool the patient to 32° to 33°C. At these temperatures, oxygen demands of the brain are reduced.[46]

GASTROINTESTINAL TRACT–RELATED ACID-BASE AND ELECTROLYTE DISTURBANCES ASSOCIATED WITH ACUTE RENAL FAILURE

Metabolic alkalosis can readily develop in patients with ARF suffering from vomiting or undergoing nasogastric suction if the resultant loss of hydrogen ions is greater than the gain as a result of renal dysfunction. In this clinical setting, the hydrogen cation that is derived from carbonic acid and secreted by the gastric parietal cells along with the chloride anion in the form of hydrochloric acid, is removed from the body, and the bicarbonate anion left behind is retained because of failure of renal excretion. Prophylactic use of H_2 blockers or proton pump inhibitors in patients undergoing nasogastric suction or suffering from vomiting is effective in the prevention of metabolic alkalosis, but such agents will not correct any existing metabolic alkalosis once it has been generated.[69] In the presence of renal failure, any nonprogressing metabolic alkalosis will be gradually corrected by the metabolic acidosis secondary to renal failure (unless the patient receives renal replacement therapy using low buffer-base dialysis solution or replacement fluid for the correction of the metabolic alkalosis).

Administration of excessive quantities of absorbable alkali, such as sodium bicarbonate and calcium carbonate, in patients with renal dysfunction also can result in metabolic alkalosis. Although the use of nonabsorbable antacids in the form of aluminum- or magnesium-containing compounds ordinarily does not cause metabolic alkalosis, combined administration of these agents and sodium polystyrene sulfonate can produce metabolic alkalosis. In patients with ARF, severe metabolic alkalosis can be treated with hemodialysis, peritoneal dialysis, hemofiltration or hemodiafiltration using buffer base–poor and chloride-rich dialysis solutions, or replacement fluids.[80-82]

Hypernatremia can result from the diarrhea induced by lactulose therapy given for the treatment of hepatic encephalopathy.[83] The administration of sodium phosphate salts as oral laxatives or as enemas is not advised in ARF because of the frequent occurrence of hyperphosphatemia and hypocalcemia.[84] Worsening of renal function can also occur. In its extreme, hyperphosphatemia induced by the administration of sodium phosphate by the foregoing mechanisms can be accompanied by hypernatremia and an increased anion gap in the plasma.[84] On the other hand, at times, hypophosphatemia may develop in certain patients with ARF, as a result of, for example, reduced oral phosphorus intake, excessive phosphate binder ingestion, parenteral nutrition, administration of glucose, or intensive renal replacement therapy.[84] With true phosphate depletion, soluble sodium phosphate salts can be given judiciously by the oral or intravenous route or in the dialysis solution or replacement fluid.[79,84-86]

DRUG-PRESCRIBING GUIDELINES IN ACUTE RENAL FAILURE

The drug-dosing guidelines for drugs that are excreted by the kidney are mostly derived from studies carried out in patients with stable, chronic renal dysfunction. An important point in this regard is that the equations of Cockcroft and Gault,[87] as well as those of the Modification of Diet in Renal Disease (MDRD) study,[88] were derived from data for patients with steady-state chronic renal functional impairment. Hence, unless the patient with ARF has stable renal function, these equations should not be applied to estimate creatinine clearance (in the case of the Cockcroft-Gault equations) and glomerular filtration rate (in the case of the MDRD equations). Finally, it should be noted that in patients who retain some degree of renal function, cimetidine reduces the secretion of creatinine into the proximal tubule, leading to an elevation in serum creatinine concentration.[89] By contrast, ranitidine has no effect on tubular secretion of creatinine.[90]

With regard to drugs that are metabolized by the liver, an important consideration is that many ARF patients also suffer from concomitant liver dysfunction and therefore also may require a reduction in dosages of such drugs.

Key Points

1. Gastrointestinal bleeding, often the result of stress-related mucosal disease, is still frequently encountered in patients with acute renal failure.
2. Histamine H_2 receptor antagonists and proton pump inhibitors often are used in the prophylaxis and management of gastrointestinal bleeding that is secondary to stress-related mucosal disease.
3. Problems involving other aspects of the alimentary tract in the form of, for example, colonic ulceration, pancreatitis, cholecystitis, liver ailments, and gastrointestinal tract–related acid-base and electrolyte disorders, all deserve emphasis.

Key References

18. Spirt MJ: Stress-related mucosal disease: Risk factors and prophylactic therapy. Clin Ther 2004;26:197-213.
19. Woodrow G, Turney JH: Causes of death in acute renal failure. Nephrol Dial Transplant 1992;7:230-234.
22. Fiaccadori E, Maggiore U, Clima B, et al: Incidence, risk factors, and prognosis of gastrointestinal hemorrhage complicating acute renal failure. Kidney Int 2001;59:1510-1519.
71. John AS, Tuerff SD, Kerstein MD: Nonocclusive mesenteric infarction in hemodialysis patients. J Am Coll Surg 2000;190:84-88.
73. Abraham SC, Bhagavan BS, Lee LA, et al: Upper gastrointestinal tract injury in patients using kayexalate (sodium polystyrene sulfonate) in sorbitol: Clinical, endoscopic, and histopathologic findings. Am J Surg Pathol 2001;25:637-644.

See the companion Expert Consult website for the complete reference list.

CHAPTER 72

Cardiovascular Problems in Acute Renal Failure

Martin K. Kuhlmann

OBJECTIVES

This chapter will:
1. Delineate the differences between cardiovascular problems in acute renal failure and those in chronic renal failure.
2. Characterize the typical cardiovascular problems occurring in acute renal failure and their consequences for patient outcome.
3. Review the basic pathophysiological concepts underlying the development of cardiovascular problems in acute renal failure.

CARDIOVASCULAR PROBLEMS IN CHRONIC RENAL FAILURE

It is well appreciated that the cardiovascular mortality rate is excessively high in end-stage renal disease (ESRD) as a result of accelerated arteriosclerosis and vascular calcifications.[1] The disease process leading to these complications, however, starts during much earlier stages of chronic kidney disease, and even mild to moderate chronic renal failure is associated with increased cardiovascular morbidity and mortality.[2] The evidence is becoming increasingly clear that renal dysfunction not only carries the risk for development of cardiovascular diseases but also is a significant independent risk factor for adverse events in patients with acute illnesses such as myocardial infarction. It has been demonstrated that the presence of mild to moderate renal impairment in these patients increases the rate of adverse outcomes and that the mortality risk increases with declining renal function. For patients with a glomerular filtration rate (GFR) below 81.0 mL/minute per 1.73 m^2 of body surface, each 10-unit reduction in baseline estimated GFR is associated with a 10% increase in the relative risk of death or nonfatal cardiovascular complications. Furthermore, rates of reinfarction, congestive heart failure, stroke, and resuscitation all are significantly higher in patients with GFRs less than 45 mL/minute per 1.73 m^2 than in those with better renal function.[3] Therefore, among patients who have had a myocardial infarction, which frequently is treated in the intensive care unit (ICU), any degree of preexisting renal impairment has to be considered a potent and independent risk factor for cardiovascular complications.

The typical cardiovascular problems associated with *chronic* renal failure include vascular and valvular calcifications, left ventricular hypertrophy, left ventricular dilatation, arrhythmias, and sudden cardiac death. The exact mechanisms by which renal dysfunction increases the cardiovascular risk are currently under investigation. The progressive increase in cardiovascular risk with worsening GFR is at least partly explained by factors associated with the decline in renal function, such as anemia, oxidative stress, disturbances of calcium-phosphate homeostasis, inflammation, and conditions promoting coagulation. All of these factors are associated with accelerated atherosclerosis and endothelial dysfunction.[4]

CARDIOVASCULAR PROBLEMS IN ACUTE RENAL FAILURE

Even in patients without preexisting renal dysfunction, the occurrence of *acute* renal failure increases the risk for cardiovascular complications and in-hospital death.[5] For a long time it was assumed that the high mortality rate in septic patients with ARF was due mainly to the consequences of sepsis alone, and that ARF was only an expression of an aggravated course of the disease. Today, however, the higher mortality rates reported for patients with ARF and sepsis than for septic patients with similar disease severity but without ARF suggest that the relationship between sepsis and ARF may be more complex than has been previously appreciated.[6] Furthermore, the prognosis for patients in whom ARF develops during an ICU stay is worse than that for patients with ESRD referred to ICUs. These differences in outcome between patients with these two forms of kidney disease are not explained by differences in disease severity, but rather reflect a higher incidence of hemodynamic instability and leukocytosis in the group of patients with ARF.[5]

Hemodynamic instability is one of the most common cardiovascular problems seen in patients with ARF. Other problems include the wide spectrum of conditions and disorders leading to cardiac and pulmonary dysfunction, which are among the most common causes of death in patients with ARF[7] (Table 72-1). Patients with ARF more frequently require vasoactive medication, mechanical ventilation, cardiopulmonary resuscitation, and treatment of

TABLE 72-1

Spectrum of Cardiovascular Problems in Acute Renal Failure

- Hypotension
- Hemodynamic instability
- Congestive heart failure
- Decreased cardiac contractility
- Myocardial ischemia
- Cardiac arrhythmias
- Pulmonary edema
- Respiratory failure
- Acute respiratory distress syndrome (ARDS)

acid-base disturbances, and hypotension, congestive heart failure, respiratory failure, plasma potassium levels, and plasma bicarbonate levels all have been shown to be of significant prognostic value for in-hospital death.[8] From several studies examining outcomes and prognostic factors in ARF, it can be concluded that the development of cardiovascular dysfunction in patients with ARF has an important impact on survival in the ICU.[5,9] This complex array of cardiovascular problems in patients with ARF may not necessarily reflect an increased severity of the underlying illness but rather may be mediated by cardiovascular side effects of ARF itself.

PATHOPHYSIOLOGY OF CARDIOPULMONARY DYSFUNCTION IN ACUTE RENAL FAILURE

In health, a strong physiologic interaction between renal and cardiovascular function operates to control extracellular fluid volume and arterial blood pressure. Renal failure modifies most of the factors regulating cardiovascular function through direct hemodynamic effects, neurogenic reflexes, and circulating hormones. The main players involved in these interactions are the renin-angiotensin system (RAS), nitric oxide (NO), and the sympathetic nervous system. ARF affects each of these systems separately, with consequences for cardiovascular function.

Renin-angiotensin-system: In ARF, a decrease in renal perfusion pressure results in the activation of the RAS with favorable effects on systemic vasoconstriction and volume retention. At the same time, RAS activation also has some unfavorable effects, such as the formation of reactive oxygen species (ROS) due to activation of reduced nicotinamide-adenine dinucleotide phosphate (NADPH) oxidase, an increase in gene expression of pro-inflammatory substances, and activation of the sympathetic nervous system.[10]

NO/ROS system: NO contributes to the renal control of extracellular fluid volume and arterial blood pressure by causing vasodilatation, natriuresis, and desensitization of the tubuloglomerular feedback.[11] Superoxide, the most aggressive ROS, on the other hand, may have the opposite effect on extracellular fluid volume control and may increase blood pressure. Although NO and ROS are balanced in health, the balance in ARF is shifted toward an increased production of ROS, with a depletion of antioxidants and reduced availability of NO. The resulting oxidative stress has been shown to increase sympathetic nervous system activity, shifting the inflammatory response toward production of pro-inflammatory cytokines.[10]

Sympathetic nervous system: Peripheral and central sympathetic nerve activity is known to be increased in chronic renal failure. Data from several experimental studies indicate that the sympathetic nervous system stimulates RAS activation, increases the production of ROS, and induces pro-inflammatory cytokine production.[10]

Taken together, disturbances in the heart-kidney axis in ARF lead to a dysbalance between oxidants and antioxidants with consequent activation of the RAS and sympathetic nervous system. Eventually, each of these alterations by itself and, even more, the combination of these disturbances result in a common pathway—the enhanced release of inflammatory mediators. Accumulating evidence from clinical and experimental studies suggests that the sudden activation of the body's cytokine machinery may in fact be the pathophysiological driving force for cardiovascular problems in ARF.

The kidney seems to play an important role as an inflammatory focus or mediator in ARF. A sudden reduction in renal function due to renal ischemia or other injury results in an increase in systemic cytokine levels.[12] Critically ill patients with ARF have levels of pro-inflammatory and anti-inflammatory cytokines much higher than those measured in anuric patients with ESRD.[13] The induction of a pro-inflammatory environment, however, is not explained by the loss of the renal cytokine-degrading activity alone. The volume overload resulting from diminished urine output may itself also be a significant mediator of plasma cytokine elevation in ARF—a scenario similar to that observed in patients with congestive heart failure.[14]

The presence of myocardial depressant substances in the plasma of patients with chronic as well as acute renal failure, which can be removed by hemofiltration, has been long recognized.[15,16] Although for many years the origin of these myocardial depressant substances was obscure, many indications now point to substances that resemble pro-inflammatory cytokines, including tumor necrosis factor-α (TNF-α) and interleukin-1β (IL-1β), which exert distinct effects on cardiac function.

Cytokine-Mediated Effects of Acute Renal Failure on Cardiac Function

In recent animal studies, renal ischemia induced a systemic inflammatory response as shown by increased serum levels of TNF-α. It was further demonstrated in those excellent studies that the inflammatory process triggered by ARF led to increased cardiac intercellular adhesion molecule-1 (ICAM-1) expression, infiltration of cardiac tissue by inflammatory cells, and enhanced apoptosis of cardiac myocytes. These changes were accompanied by distinct changes in cardiac function, such as a decrease in cardiac contractility, left ventricular dilatation, and a decrease in fractional shortening.[17] Because cardiac changes were not related to the magnitude of azotemia but increased progressively with duration of renal ischemia, a logical conclusion is that renal ischemic injury, rather than the loss in GFR, is the cause of the associated cardiac dysfunction. Elegant studies in heart failure models have revealed the pathophysiological basis for the damaging effects of cytokines on cardiac function.

Cytokines may exert an impact on myocardial function through direct effects on myocyte contractility. Pro-inflammatory cytokines such as TNF-α, IL-1β, and IL-6 and the immunomodulatory cytokine IL-2 typically are considered to impart negative inotropic effects. In vivo as well as in vitro studies have demonstrated that the nature and pattern of the inotropic response is complex, consisting of an immediate response within minutes that can be either stimulatory or depressant, depending on the experimental conditions and physiological milieu, and a delayed response lasting hours to days that is uniformly cardiodepressant and dependent on the production of secondary mediators. This delayed response may be mainly responsible for the cardiac dysfunction observed during ARF.[18]

Several studies have evaluated the in vivo effects of cytokines on cardiac function. For example, a single infusion of TNF-α in conscious dogs resulted in a delayed (2 hours to 2 days after infusion) appearance of left ventricular systolic dysfunction that persisted for up to 10 days. The decline in left ventricular ejection fraction was not normalized by volume resuscitation, suggesting intrinsic cardiac dysfunction rather than a pre-load-dependent response.[19] Reduced left ventricular performance has also been associated with several diastolic abnormalities including slowing of relaxation, left ventricular dilatation without changes in end-diastolic pressure, and a leftward shift of the end-diastolic pressure-strain relation, indicating increased diastolic stiffness. Generally, cytokine-mediated contractile dysfunction was found to be reversible over an extended time period of several days.[18] Corresponding to these experimental findings, dose-dependent cardiovascular depression and negative inotropy also have been observed in human studies in which TNF-α and IL-2 were used for immunomodulatory therapy in patients with cancer.[20]

The cellular mechanisms underlying the delayed cardiodepressant effects of pro-inflammatory cytokines are multiple. It is currently believed that these effects are primarily the result of the combined influence of NO generated from inducible nitric oxide synthase (iNOS), the production of ROS, and impaired β-adrenergic receptor (β-AR) sensitivity (Fig. 72-1). The delayed onset and prolonged duration of the cardiodepressant response suggest indirect effects requiring the induction of de novo gene expression and protein synthesis and the activation of secondary mediators.[21] Although ARF alone can be viewed as a state of sustained chronic augmentation of pro-inflammatory cytokine expression, such increased expression will be even more pronounced in cases in which ARF complicates other diseases with increased cytokine production, such as sepsis. Generally, pro-inflammatory cytokines can be considered to impart negative inotropic and cardiodepressant effects, thereby contributing to the occurrence of any of the wide spectrum of cardiovascular problems in ARF.

Sympathetic Activity in Acute Renal Failure

Catecholamines control heart rate, myocardial contractility, and the tone of resistance vessels and thus play an important role in maintaining blood pressure. Whereas sudden, excessive sympathetic activity may induce cardiomyocyte apoptosis, with subsequent hypertrophy and focal myocardial necrosis, chronic sympathetic overactivity may cause β-adrenoceptor insensitivity, a reduction in heart rate variability, and increased susceptibility to arrhythmias. Although chronic renal failure is known to

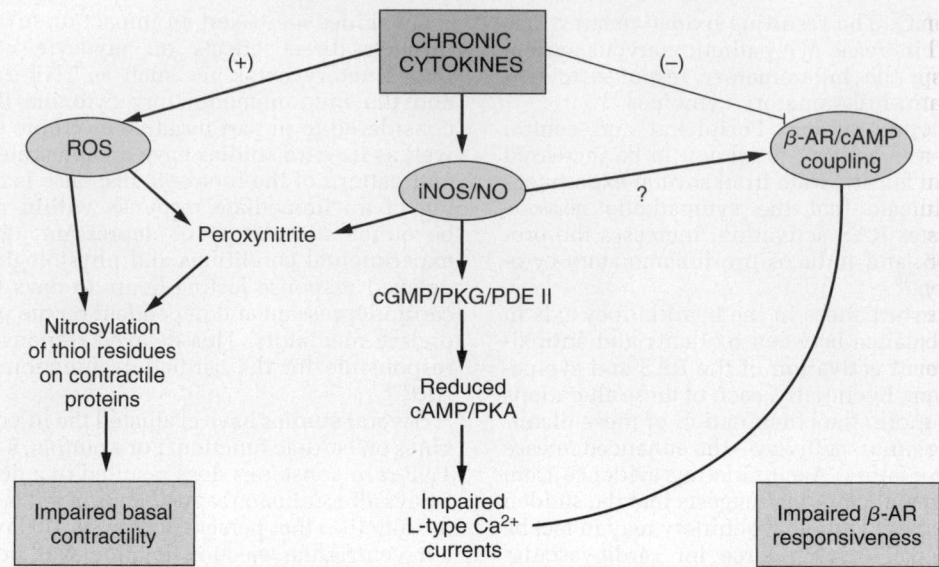

FIGURE 72-1. Negative effects of sustained presence of cytokines on cardiac contractility. Impaired β-adrenergic receptor (β-AR) responsiveness results from stimulation of iNOS-mediated NO production which leads to inhibition of cAMP/PKA-mediated effects on Ca^{2+} homeostasis and to inhibitory effects on β-adrenergic activation-cAMP coupling. Basal contractility is impaired through increased ROS production, enhanced generation of superoxide-peroxynitrite by way of the iNOS pathway and through nitrosylation of contractile protein thiol residues. cAMP, cyclic adenosine monophosphate; cGMP, cyclic guanosine monophosphate; iNOS, inducible nitric oxide; NO, nitric oxide; PDE II, phosphodiesterase II; PKA, protein kinase A; PKG, protein kinase G; ROS, reactive oxygen species. (Adapted from Mehra VC, Ramgolam VS, Bender JR: Cytokines and cardiovascular disease. J Leuk Biol 2005;78:805-818.)

be associated with increased sympathetic activity, available clinical data on sympathetic activity in pure ARF are limited. Experimental studies have yielded evidence that both induction and repression of sympathetic activity may occur in ARF.

Sympathetic overactivity may be due to diminished degradation of catecholamines directly related to the loss of renal function. Only recently, a new peptide, renalase, has been described that is produced and secreted into the blood by the human kidney. Renalase is a flavin adenine dinucleotide (FAD)-dependent amine oxidase that metabolizes circulating catecholamines and lowers blood pressure by decreasing cardiac contractility and heart rate and preventing a compensatory increase in peripheral vascular tone. In humans, *renalase* gene expression is highest in the kidney but also is detectable in the heart, skeletal muscle, and small intestine. Plasma concentrations of renalase are markedly reduced in patients with ESRD, as compared with healthy subjects, suggesting a causal link to the increased plasma catecholamine levels in ESRD.[22] In ARF, production and secretion of renalase may be significantly reduced, favoring a state of increased sympathetic hyperactivity and the resultant cardiovascular consequences. Thus far, clinical data supporting this hypothesis are lacking.

Alternatively, depression of the sympathetic nervous system may occur during ARF. In animal studies, ARF induced in hypertensive or normotensive rats was associated with significantly lower mean arterial blood pressure and heart rate, while at the same time the pressor responses to norepinephrine and the chronotropic responses to right cervical sympathetic and vagal nerve stimulation were diminished. It was concluded from these studies that ARF induces cardiovascular depression.[23] This acquired "resistance" to norepinephrine may be responsible for the higher doses of adrenergic substances required in patients with ARF complicating sepsis.

Coronary Vasoregulation in Acute Renal Failure

Myocardial ischemia frequently complicates ARF. Coronary vasoregulation is important for preservation of coronary blood flow and myocardial oxygen supply during sudden changes in blood pressure. Coronary reserve may be reduced as a result of increases in left ventricular mass, circulating neurohumoral factors, and anemia. A recent study in dogs demonstrated that coronary vascular tone, coronary reserve, and vessel reactivity are markedly diminished in ARF, indicating an impaired function of the coronary vasculature. Consequently, during ARF, small increases in myocardial oxygen demand presumably will induce subendocardial ischemia as a result of a limited capacity to increase oxygen supply. These factors will contribute to the higher risk for adverse coronary events and the increased cardiovascular mortality risk in patients with acute renal failure if increases in myocardial oxygen demand cannot be met because of limited coronary vascular reserve.[24]

Pulmonary Injury in Acute Renal Failure

Pulmonary complications, particularly noncardiogenic acute lung injury, acute respiratory distress syndrome (ARDS), and respiratory failure, commonly are associated with ARF and contribute to mortality.[25,26] The traditional paradigm suggests that lung injury is caused by volume overload due to impaired renal fluid excretion accompanied by increased capillary hydrostatic pressure and pulmonary edema. Circulating macrophages and cytokines have been shown to be implicated in the pathogenesis of acute lung injury in various settings. In experimental studies, renal ischemia-reperfusion injury increases pulmonary vascular permeability and induces interstitial edema, alveolar hemorrhage, and red blood cell sludging.[27] Because the lung has the largest microcapillary network in the body, it responds to circulating pro-inflammatory signals with activation of lung macrophages, secretion of pro-inflammatory cytokines, recruitment of neutrophils and macrophages, and resultant lung injury.[26]

Acute renal failure may directly promote lung injury independent of volume retention either by affecting plasma levels of mediators of lung injury, such as pro-inflammatory cytokines,[28] or by directly or indirectly downregulating the pulmonary expression of sodium channels and aquaporins.[29] These molecular derangements may have detrimental effects on lung fluid balance, especially in the settings of antecedent or concurrent structural injury of the lung. Impaired pulmonary fluid handling may impair lung function, increasing the susceptibility of the lung to injury, particularly during mechanical ventilation.

CONCLUSION

Acute renal failure is associated with a wide array of cardiovascular problems that are assumed to be related mainly to elevated circulating levels of pro-inflammatory cytokines. These mediators of acute and chronic inflammation exert unfavorable effects on cardiac contractility, coronary perfusion, and, last but not least, pulmonary vascular permeability. The onset of acute renal failure, with or without concomitant severe illness, has to be regarded as an additional risk factor for increased cardiovascular morbidity and mortality.

Key Points

1. Acute renal failure promotes cardiovascular instability and cardiac dysfunction.
2. The occurrence of cardiovascular dysfunction in patients with acute renal failure increases in-hospital mortality rates.
3. Elevation in levels of circulating proinflammatory cytokines is viewed as the pathophysiological mechanism for cardiovascular dysfunction in acute renal failure.
4. Pro-inflammatory cytokines exert distinct cardiodepressant effects.
5. Acute renal failure may lead to an increase in pulmonary vascular permeability, most likely mediated by pro-inflammatory cytokines.

Key References

2. Go AS, Chertow GM, Fan D, et al: Chronic kidney disease and the risks of death, cardiovascular events, and hospitalization. N Engl J Med 2004;351:1296-1305.
3. Anavekar NS, McMurray JJ, Velazquez EJ, et al: Relation between renal dysfunction and cardiovascular outcomes after myocardial infarction. N Engl J Med 2004;351:1285-1295.
8. Behrend T, Miller SB: Acute renal failure in the cardiac unit: Etiologies, outcomes, and prognostic factors. Kidney Int 1999;56:238-243.
18. Prabhu SD: Cytokine-induced modulation of cardiac function. Circ Res 2004;95:1140-1145.
26. Rabb H, Chamoun F, Hotchkiss J: Molecular mechanisms underlying combined kidney-lung dysfunction during acute renal failure. Contrib Nephrol 2001;132:41-52.

CHAPTER 73

Water and Electrolyte Disturbances in Acute Renal Failure

Robert C. Albright, Jr.

OBJECTIVES

This chapter will:
1. Describe the common electrolyte disturbances seen in patients with acute renal failure.
2. Review the diagnosis and treatment of hyperkalemia.
3. Review the diagnosis and treatment of hyponatremia and hypernatremia.

Water and electrolyte disturbances are among the most common complications of acute renal failure. Imbalances in plasma sodium, potassium, calcium, and phosphate are the most common electrolyte disturbances and require a comprehensive approach to management.

HYPERKALEMIA

Hyperkalemia is arguably the most dramatic, and certainly most life-threatening, of the metabolic consequences of acute renal failure in the intensive care unit (ICU) setting. Estimates for mortality associated with hyperkalemia are difficult to determine for the ICU population. The 1996 U.S. Renal Data System survey, however, estimated a mortality rate of 1.9% for 1993.[1] The incidence of hyperkalemia among all hospitalized patients has been reported to range between 1.1 and 10 patients per 100 hospitalized.[2-5] The severity of hyperkalemia most often is determined by the concomitant severity of the pathophysiologic derangements leading to acute renal failure, and certainly, because acute renal failure typically is a multifactorial process, the distinct pathophysiology of hyperkalemia in association with this disorder often is also multifactorial.

In general, factors mediating potassium balance may be separated into external factors and internal factors. External factors refer to the renal and extrarenal factors controlling potassium balance in the serum. Internal factors are those that mediate the transcellular distribution of potassium. The body loses minimal potassium in sweat. The main extrarenal site of potassium elimination is in the colon, where mineralocorticoid may affect potassium secretion. This source of potassium loss is negligible during acute renal failure but may account for up to 10% of dietary potassium elimination among patients with chronic renal failure under the direct stimulation of increased aldosterone.[6] By contrast, the kidneys are extremely efficient at excreting potassium loads. It is difficult to induce hyperkalemia among patients with normal renal function strictly by increasing ingestion of potassium. In patients who have persistent hyperkalemia, particularly those who are critically ill with associated acute renal failure, hyperkalemia is nearly always associated with a decreased glomerular filtration rate (GFR), a defect in tubular flow, or inadequate aldosterone activity.

Acidosis, also a prominent feature of acute renal failure, promotes potassium exit from the cells. Maintaining normal serum potassium concentration between 3.5 and 5 mEq/L depends on the balance of potassium ingestion and potassium excretion, as well as the distribution of potassium into its usual intracellular location. Because 98% of total body potassium is located intracellularly, small shifts of even as little as 1% to 2% can cause increases in serum potassium that indeed can be life-threatening. These disorders are dramatically exacerbated in acute renal failure, in which ability to excrete this potassium load is decreased.

In acute renal failure, hyperkalemia results from either exogenous or endogenous sources. Medications including potassium and penicillin VK and some multivitamins, and potassium chloride administration, are common sources of exogenous intake among patients in the intensive care unit (ICU) (Table 73-1). Endogenous sources are more common, however. Pathomechanisms of endogenous potassium accumulation such as tissue hypoxemia, specifically from skeletal muscle necrosis or red cell lysis, resorption of hematoma, or tumor lysis, often result in a dramatic shift of potassium from the intracellular to the extracellular space, with resultant life-threatening hyperkalemia.

Treatment of Hyperkalemia in Acute Renal Failure

Surprisingly, despite the dogmatic approach that has been advocated, actual evidence-based evaluation of treatment for life-threatening hyperkalemia is fairly scant. A cursory review of the available literature reveals the woeful inadequacy of current knowledge about effective treatments for hyperkalemia.[7-9] In general, treatment of hyperkalemia is guided by three major tenets. Initially, antagonism of the membrane effects of the increased potassium should be facilitated with the administration of calcium and, potentially, the use of hypertonic sodium if the patient is notably hyponatremic in association with the hyperkalemia. Thereafter, the administration of glucose plus insulin and sodium bicarbonate, to induce shifting of potassium from the extracellular to the intracellular space, should be the next step. Finally, removal of the excess potassium needs to be facilitated by either renal or extrarenal mechanisms.

TABLE 73-1

Drugs Associated with Hyperkalemia by Pathomechanism

Increased Potassium Intake
- KCl
- Salt substitutes
- Blood transfusion
- Penicillin (K formulation)
- Rarely multivitamin preparations

Transmembrane Shifting
- Succinylcholine
- β-Blockade
- Digitalis intoxication
- Mannitol

Cellular Lysis
- Radiation
- Chemotherapy

Decreased Potassium Excretion
- NSAIDs
- COX-2 inhibitors
- ARBs, ACE inhibitors
- Heparin
- Ketoconazole
- Aldactone
- Triamterene
- Calcineurin inhibitors
- Trimethoprim
- Amiloride

ACE, angiotensin-converting enzyme; ARBs, angiotensin receptor blockers; COX-2, cyclooxygenase-2; KCl, potassium chloride; NSAIDs, nonsteroidal anti-inflammatory drugs.

Specifically, in diuretic-responsive states, use of diuretics is indicated. Among patients who are oliguric, cation exchange resins such as sodium polystyrene sulfonate (Kayexalate) or extracorporeal therapy with dialysis, or both, also is indicated. Figure 73-1 shows recommended specific therapies for hyperkalemia.

Much evidence exists regarding the danger of colonic administration of cation exchange resins such as Kayexalate. Particularly among patients who are critically ill, colonic necrosis associated with use of this preparation has been widely reported.[10-14] Furthermore, the sodium content of Kayexalate is only 4 mEq/g. Because sodium ions exchange theoretically one for one with potassium ions, a 30-g dose of Kayexalate would maximally remove only 120 mEq of potassium. This degree of exchange does not occur physiologically in the gastrointestinal tract, however. The limited exchange becomes obvious on evaluation of the potassium concentration in the lumen of the bowel: At no point in the bowel lumen does the potassium concentration reach 120 mEq/L. Actual data reporting the degree of serum potassium decrease with the use of Kayexalate are virtually nonexistent. Thus, particularly among critically ill patients, Kayexalate enemas are likely to be ineffective and are potentially dangerous.

Optimally, dialysis should be considered the primary modality for removal of potassium during an episode of acute renal failure and critical illness–associated hyperkalemia. Obviously, this protocol will require mobilization of resources for placement of intravenous access safely and expeditiously, and the availability of urgent dialysis. The most effective route of potassium removal for decreasing serum potassium in patients with acute renal failure is dialysis. Peritoneal dialysis, intermittent hemodialysis

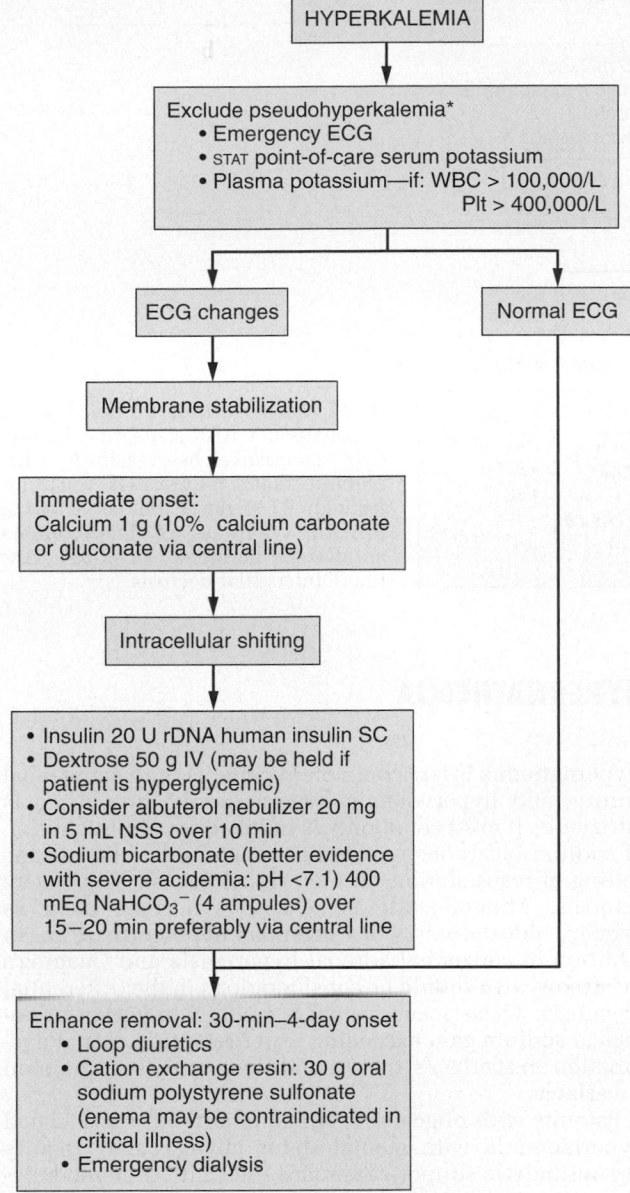

HYPERKALEMIA

Exclude pseudohyperkalemia*
- Emergency ECG
- STAT point-of-care serum potassium
- Plasma potassium—if: WBC > 100,000/L
  Plt > 400,000/L

ECG changes

Normal ECG

Membrane stabilization

Immediate onset:
Calcium 1 g (10% calcium carbonate or gluconate via central line)

Intracellular shifting

- Insulin 20 U rDNA human insulin SC
- Dextrose 50 g IV (may be held if patient is hyperglycemic)
- Consider albuterol nebulizer 20 mg in 5 mL NSS over 10 min
- Sodium bicarbonate (better evidence with severe acidemia: pH <7.1) 400 mEq NaHCO$_3^-$ (4 ampules) over 15–20 min preferably via central line

Enhance removal: 30-min–4-day onset
- Loop diuretics
- Cation exchange resin: 30 g oral sodium polystyrene sulfonate (enema may be contraindicated in critical illness)
- Emergency dialysis

*May be unnecessary in appropriate clinical situation

FIGURE 73-1. Algorithm for treatment of hyperkalemia. ECG, electrocardiogram; IV, intravenously; NSS, normal saline solution; Plt, platelet count; WBC, white blood cell count.

(IHD), and continuous venovenous hemodialysis (CVVHD) may be considered.

Peritoneal dialysis yields variable results with respect to control of emergent hyperkalemia, particularly among patients with acute renal failure. Complications arising from placement of a temporary peritoneal dialysis access are common. Reliable control of potassium with peritoneal dialysis is difficult to achieve. Removal of potassium with peritoneal dialysis is related to the relative size of the fluid-membrane contact surface area, as well as the blood flow to the peritoneal surface. These factors often are extraordinarily variable among critically ill patients. Peritoneal fluid generally has a zero potassium bath, so exchange should be conducted roughly on an hourly basis for life-threatening hyperkalemia. With the possible exception of pediatric patients and patients in whom intra-

venous access cannot be achieved, peritoneal dialysis has a very limited role in the management of acute renal failure–associated hyperkalemia in the ICU.

The preferred method for control of hyperkalemia in acute renal failure is use of blood-based dialytic techniques. Very little evidence is available, however, regarding the reliable decrement of plasma potassium with respect to dialysis potassium baths. Several concerns must be addressed with respect to rapid shifts in potassium among critically ill patients. One study evaluated the use of a 1-mEq/L potassium bath for 1 hour. A decrease in serum potassium by 1.34 mEq/L was noted.[9] Stepwise approach to management of acute hyperkalemia may be reasonable. In fact, a study performed in 1996 showed better tolerance from the perspective of decreasing ventricular dysrhythmias by means of a stepwise potassium modeling approach to dialytic potassium concentration.[15] In general, a reasonable recommendation would be a dialytic potassium concentration of approximately 2 to 3 mEq below the current plasma potassium (depending on the current situation) for approximately 1 hour, with stepwise hourly increases in dialysate potassium concentration as treatment progresses.

Continuous therapies (continuous venovenous hemofiltration, CVVHD, continuous venovenous hemodiafiltration) have been used effectively for treatment of hyperkalemia. In severe acute hyperkalemia, however, continuous therapies may not remove the potassium quickly enough. Hence, a combination approach of dialytic modalities has been advocated. An initial session of intermittent hemodialysis, followed by institution of continuous therapies, has been used with success in many centers, including our own. This approach may be particularly advantageous among critically ill patients with hypoperfusion and ongoing shock.

HYPONATREMIA

Patients with acute renal failure typically present with hypervolemic hyponatremia. As in patients without renal failure, however, a systematic approach to diagnosis is recommended. A rational stepwise approach is shown in Figure 73-2. Patients who clinically appear to be hypervolemic have accumulated an excess of sodium but proportionately more water. These patients most often are edematous and hyponatremic. Commonly, these patients are those suffering from severe congestive heart failure, hepatic dysfunction, and renal failure.

Fortunately, cellular mechanisms directed at rectifying the movement of water from the extracellular to the intracellular space are stimulated by hypo-osmolality—most often caused by hyponatremia. Initially, cells combat this swelling by exporting potassium, sodium, and chloride. The decrease in these "osmolytes" may be seen within minutes to hours after induction of hyponatremia.[16] At a certain point, however, the cells have exhausted their capacity to quickly decrease intracellular tonicity, and the exporting of other organic osmolytes is affected. These substances include glutamine, creatine, taurine, myoinositol, glutamine, and glycerol phosphorylcholine. Their export requires a carrier-mediated process that can take days to weeks.[17] These acute and chronic processes lead to adaptation whereby neuromuscular homeostasis is maintained and catastrophic herniation and decrease in cerebral blood flow is avoided. These processes—particularly the organic ion transport pathways—are reversed

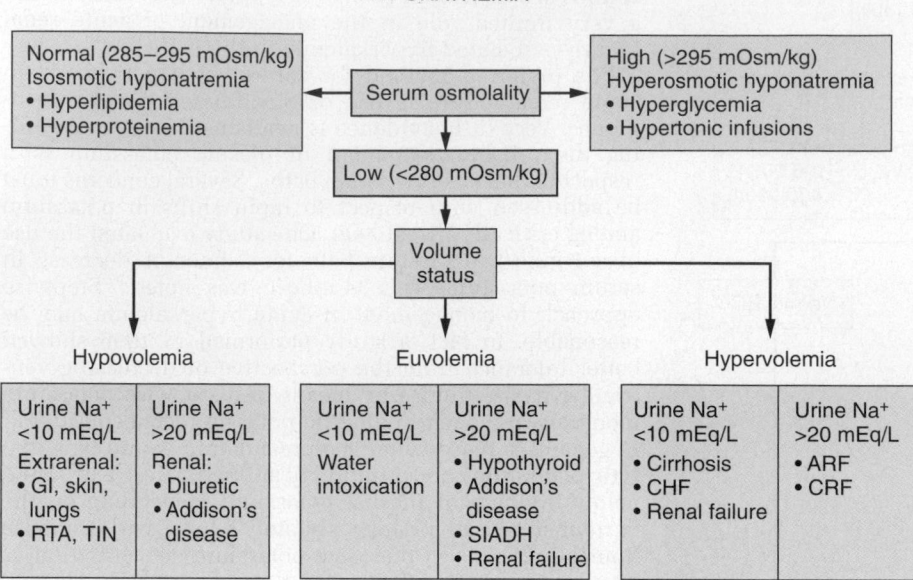

FIGURE 73-2. Algorithm for diagnosis of hyponatremia. ARF, acute renal failure; CHF, congestive heart failure; CRF, chronic renal failure; GI, gastrointestinal; RTA, renal tubular acidosis; SIADH, syndrome of inappropriate antidiuretic hormone (secretion); TIN, tubulointerstitial necrosis.

slowly, however. Therefore, correction of hyponatremia needs to be accomplished with extraordinary care to avoid rapid increases in serum tonicity.

Cellular contraction due to osmotic movement of water from the intracellular to the extracellular space may result from overly rapid correction of hyponatremia. The theoretical sudden decrease in cellular volume may be a leading cause of mechanical shear stress causing disruption of myelin and leading to the radiologically and apparent manifestations of central pontine myelinolysis. Often, these lesions are not apparent for weeks after the hyponatremic event.[18,19] Certain patient groups seem to be at particular risk for brain damage and pontine myelinolysis: patients with hypokalemia, malnutrition, alcoholism, or cirrhosis of the liver; perhaps young menstruant female patients; and burn-injured patients.[20]

Correction and Therapy of Hyponatremia

A guiding tenet in therapy for hyponatremia beyond the laboratory assessment of osmolality and clinically effective tissue perfusion is that of symptomatic presentation. The severity of symptoms will dictate the aggressiveness of therapy. Another guiding tenet needs to be the overarching goal of conservative correction: keeping the actual increase in serum sodium concentration to 12 mEq/L or less in 24 hours and approximately 20 mEq/L over 48 hours. These conservative correction rates are guided by retrospective clinical studies evaluating the occurrence of permanent neurological sequelae among patients with severe hyponatremia.[21] In general, the more rapid the development and more severe the degree of hyponatremia, the more likely this condition is to prove symptomatic.

Renal failure rarely results in severe hyponatremia except in combination with exogenous water loading. Correction of the underlying pathophysiology usually will help correct the hyponatremia. Among patients with hypervolemic hypotonic hyponatremia with renal failure—a very common scenario in the ICU—often the sole option available may be extracorporeal therapy (dialysis or hemofiltration).

HYPERNATREMIA

Hypernatremia is less common in patients with acute renal failure, and hypervolemic hypernatremia most often is iatrogenic. It most commonly is induced by administration of sodium bicarbonate in intravenous fluids, often in the setting of resuscitation during critical illness with severe acidosis. Mineralocorticoid excess syndrome such as primary aldosteronism or exogenous hypercortisolism, in addition to congenital adrenal hyperplasia and Cushing's syndrome, also should be considerations in the differential diagnosis. These scenarios share a common pathophysiological sodium gain exceeding water retention. Renal dysfunction exacerbates these conditions and is a common covariable.

Patients with oligoanuric acute renal failure–associated hypernatremia with mental status changes may require urgent dialytic support. Standard intermittent hemodialysis may correct sodium too rapidly in these situations. Prescribing an increased dialysate sodium to target less dramatic changes in serum sodium level seems to be a reasonable approach. Alternatively, continuous renal replacement therapy (CRRT) may offer a less dramatic change in the rate of serum sodium correction and may be warranted among critically ill patients.[22]

DISORDERS OF CALCIUM AND PHOSPHATE BALANCE

Calcium and phosphate imbalances are extremely common in patients with acute renal failure. These disorders are discussed in detail in Chapter 91.

Acknowledgment

I am greatly indebted to the expert editorial and administrative assistance of Kathy Mandery for the preparation of the manuscript for this chapter.

Suggested Reading

Gross P, Reimann D, Neidel J, et al: The treatment of severe hyponatremia. Kidney Int 1998;53(Suppl):S6-S11.

Faber MD, Kupin WL, Heilig CW, Narins RG: Common fluid-electrolyte and acid-base problems in the intensive care unit: Selected issues. Semin Nephrol 1994;14:8-22.

Mandal AK, Wirnsberger GH, Saklayen MG, Puchalski J: Hospital-acquired hypernatremia: Strategies of fluid therapy. Kidney 1998;7:91-96.

Key References

5. Acker CG, Johnson JP, Palevsky PM, Greenberg A: Hyperkalemia in hospitalized patients: Causes, adequacy of treatment, and results of an attempt to improve physician compliance with published therapy guidelines. Arch Intern Med 1998; 158:917-924.
8. Iqbal V, Friedman EA: Preferred therapy of hyperkalemia in renal insufficiency: Survey of Nephrology Training-Program Directors. N Eng J Med 1989;320:60-61.
19. Sterns RH, Cappuccio JD, Silver SM, Cohen EP: Neurologic sequelae after treatment of severe hyponatremia: A multi-center perspective. J Am Soc Nephrol 1994;4:1522-1530.
22. Morimatsu H, Uchino S, Bellomo R, Ronco C: Continuous renal replacement therapy: Does technique influence electrolyte and bicarbonate control? Int J Artif Organs 2003;26:289-296.

See the companion Expert Consult website for the complete reference list.

CHAPTER 74

Neurological Problems in Acute Renal Failure

Andrew Davenport

OBJECTIVES

This chapter will:
1. Outline the basic pathophysiology of the brain in acute renal failure.
2. Identify the infections known to be associated with the development of acute renal failure and cerebral dysfunction.
3. Describe the role of vascular disease in the pathogenesis of acute renal failure and cerebral dysfunction.
4. Delineate the mechanisms by which electrolyte disorders may cause or potentiate acute renal failure leading to cerebral dysfunction.
5. Examine the metabolic disorders that may result in or exacerbate acute renal failure and cerebral dysfunction.
6. Review those drugs implicated in the pathogenesis of acute renal failure and cerebral dysfunction.

BASIC PATHOPHYSIOLOGY OF THE BRAIN IN ACUTE RENAL FAILURE

In the intensive care unit (ICU) setting, the patient may be admitted with acute renal failure (ARF), or ARF may develop during the course of the patient's stay in the ICU.

A majority of patients will experience additional aspects of organ failure other than ARF, and sepsis, trauma, and surgery also will have an impact on cerebral function. In ARF, cerebral blood flow often is reduced, with alterations in the blood-brain barrier leading to localized areas of increased permeability, with astrocyte swelling. In part, these changes are compensatory as a result of the changes in plasma osmolality, owing to the retention of urea and other osmolytes, and accompanying acidosis. Neurotransmitter regulation is affected, with inhibition of the GABA-ergic inhibitory system, and activation of the excitatory *N*-methyl-D-aspartate system.[1] These changes can be exacerbated by other conditions; for example, in severe sepsis without direct central nervous system infection, cerebral perfusion is decreased, with increased blood-brain barrier permeability and an influx of glutamate and other amino acids, resulting in increased elaboration of neurotransmitters.[2] Postmortem examination has shown various anatomical changes including astrocyte and glial cell swelling in the cortex, cerebral micro- and macroinfarcts, multiple small white matter hemorrhages, central pontine myelinosis, and disseminated microabscesses.[3]

In clinical practice, neurological assessment may be difficult, especially when patients are sedated and paralyzed. More recently, S-100β protein, a calcium-binding protein found predominantly in astrocytes, and neuron-specific enolase, an intracytoplasmic glycolytic enolase located in neurons and Schwann cells, have been proposed as bio-markers of brain injury, with increasing levels when the blood-brain barrier is disrupted with underlying brain injury.[4]

INFECTIONS CAUSING ACUTE RENAL FAILURE AND CEREBRAL DYSFUNCTION

Both acute uremia and systemic sepsis can cause delirium. With ARF due to sepsis, it often is difficult to exclude underlying structural brain abnormalities, such as abscesses, in patients who are confused and unable to fully cooperate in the acute setting. All patients admitted to the ICU with renal failure and sepsis should have an ultrasound examination of the urinary tract to exclude renal obstruction.

Although ARF can develop in patients admitted to the ICU with severe sepsis of any cause, some infections typically cause acute cerebral involvement and renal dysfunction. Cerebral involvement may be due to direct infection of the brain and meninges, causing encephalitis and meningitis, or confusion due to toxin release or a vasculopathy due to infection-induced vasculitis or local thrombosis (Table 74-1). The key to clinical management is to recognize when ARF is not due to simple renal hypoperfusion consequent to sepsis—for example, acute proliferative or crescentic nephritis following staphylococcal infection resolves more quickly with steroid therapy once the infection has been appropriately treated with antibiotics. Thus, an essential component of evaluation is dipstick testing of urine for blood and protein, along with both standard microscopy and culture, as well as cytological examination, of the urine.[5]

In immunocompromised patients such as renal transplant recipients and other patients who have received solid organ transplants, ARF may readily occur in systemic sepsis. The scope of the differential diagnosis widens, owing to the possibility of *Listeria monocytogenes* meningitis, cerebral toxoplasmosis, fungal meningitis, viral encephalitis, and cerebral lymphoma due to post-transplantation lymphoproliferative disease.[6]

VASCULAR DISEASES CAUSING ACUTE RENAL FAILURE CAUSING CEREBRAL DYSFUNCTION

Vascular disease includes a spectrum of conditions ranging from vascular hemorrhage to thrombosis of large and small blood vessels, with subsequent tissue infarction, to occlusion and local inflammation or thrombosis. Of note, in patients with atheroembolic stroke, ARF may develop as a result of myoglobinuria secondary to a fall and muscle necrosis from hypostasis.

In confused patients, for whom the differential diagnosis often is wide in scope, it is important to obtain an accurate medical history, which often may require the help of relatives and other witnesses, so that uncommon conditions are not overlooked. Table 74-2 lists some conditions that typically cause both acute renal dysfunction and cerebrovascular disease[6] (Fig. 74-1). If an underlying vasculitis is suspected, then appropriate immunological investigations

TABLE 74-1

Infections Causing Acute Cerebral Dysfunction and Renal Failure

INFECTION	CEREBRAL DYSFUNCTION	RENAL LESION
Bacterial Infections		
SBE	Cerebral abscess/infarct	Acute proliferative MPGN
Ventriculoatrial shunt	Cerebral abscess	Acute proliferative MPGN
Visceral abscess	Toxin-induced confusion	Acute proliferative MPGN
E. coli infection	Cerebral vasculitis	HUS
Streptococcal infection	Chorea/meningitis	Acute DPGN/DIC
Staphylococcal infection	Toxin-induced confusion	Acute DPGN/CGN
Legionella infection	Hypoxia-induced confusion	AIN
Leptospirosis	Cerebral vasculitis	AIN
Yersinia infection	Cerebral vasculitis	AIN
Rickettsia rickettsii infection	Cerebral vasculitis	AIN/DPGN/vasculitis
Mycoplasma infection	Meningitis	AIN/DPGN
Protozoal Infections		
Malaria	Encephalopathy/seizures	AIN/vascular occlusion
Viral Infections		
Epstein-Barr virus infection	Encephalitis	AIN
HIV infection	Encephalitis	Collapsing FSGS/HUS
	Secondary infections	
Dengue fever	Cerebral vasculitis	HUS
Hanta virus infection	Cerebral vasculitis/hypoxia	AIN
Hepatitis B	Hepatic encephalopathy	HRS/MCGN/vasculitis
Hepatitis C	Hepatic encephalopathy	HRS/MCGN/vasculitis
Other Conditions		
Sarcoidosis	Lymphocytic meningitis	AIN

AIN, acute interstitial nephritis; CGN, (acute) crescentic glomerulonephritis; DIC, disseminated intravascular coagulopathy; DPGN, (acute) diffuse proliferative glomerulonephritis; FSGS, focal segmental glomerulosclerosis; GN, glomerulonephritis; HIV, human immunodeficiency virus; HRS, hepatorenal syndrome; HUS, hemolytic uremic syndrome; MCGN, mesangiocapillary glomerulonephritis; MPGN, mesangioproliferative glomerulonephritis; SBE, subacute bacterial endocarditis.

TABLE 74-2

Differential Diagnosis for Vascular Diseases Causing Acute Renal Failure and Cerebral Dysfunction

DISEASE/CONDITION	CEREBRAL DYSFUNCTION	RENAL LESION
Intracranial Infection/SAH		
Malignant hypertension	Intracranial aneurysm	HUS
Polycystic kidney disease	Intracranial aneurysm	Renal cystic disease
Polyarteritis nodosa	Intracranial aneurysm	Vasculitis
Kawasaki's disease	Intracranial aneurysm	Vasculitis
Cerebral Infarction		
Cholesterol emboli	Multiple cerebral emboli	Renovascular disease
Atrial myxoma	Multiple cerebral emboli	Renal infarction
Cardiac valve vegetation	Multiple cerebral emboli	Renal infarction
Antiphospholipid syndrome	Multiple cerebral infarcts	Multiple renal infarcts
Behçet's syndrome	Multiple cerebral infarcts	AIN/renal vasculitis
TTP	Multiple cerebral infarcts	HUS
HUS	Multiple cerebral infarcts	HUS
Malignant hypertension	Seizures/cerebral infarction	HUS
Scleroderma	Seizures/cerebral infarction	HUS
Eclampsia	Seizures/cerebral infarction	HUS
Fatty liver of pregnancy	Hepatic encephalopathy	HUS
Cryoglobulinemia	Small-vessel cerebral infarction	MCGN
Sickle cell disease	Multiple cerebral infarcts	FSGS
Waldenström's disease	Hyperviscosity syndrome	AIN
SLE	Cerebral vasculitis	RPGN/renal vasculitis
Microscopic polyangiitis	Cerebral vasculitis	RPGN/renal vasculitis
Wegener's granulomatosis	Cerebral vasculitis	RPGN/renal vasculitis
Churg-Strauss syndrome	Cerebral vasculitis	RPGN/renal vasculitis
Henoch-Schönlein purpura	Cerebral vasculitis	RPGN/renal vasculitis
Other Conditions		
Sarcoidosis	Lymphocytic meningitis	AIN

AIN, acute interstitial nephritis; FSGS, focal segmental glomerulosclerosis; HUS, hemolytic uremic syndrome; MCGN, mesangiocapillary glomerulonephritis; RPGN, rapidly progressive glomerulonephritis; SAH, subarachnoid hemorrhage; TTP, thrombotic thrombocytopenic purpura.

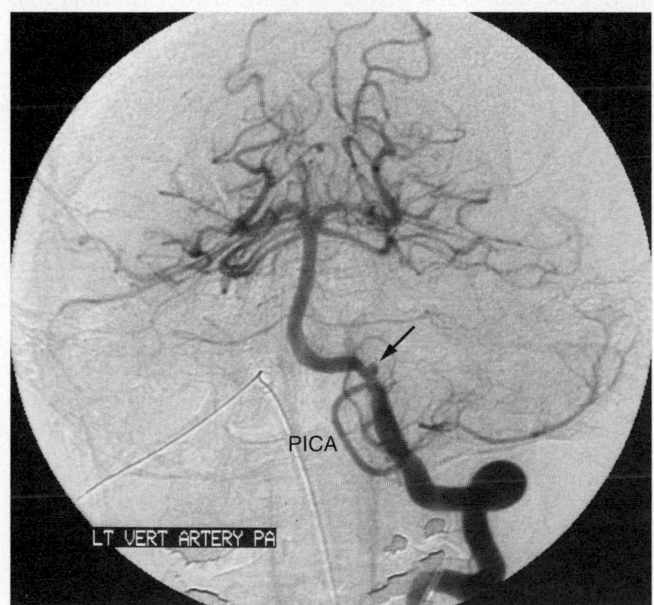

FIGURE 74-1. Intracranial aneurysm *(arrow)* in a patient with polyarteritis nodosa. PICA, posterior internal communicating artery.

should be requested, including screening for antineutrophil cytoplasmic antibodies and the more specific enzyme-linked immunosorbent assays (ELISAs) for myeloperoxidase and proteinase 3. Similarly, in suspected systemic lupus erythematosus, assays for complement proteins, antinuclear antibodies, and double-stranded DNA antibodies may help substantiate the diagnosis. In cases of scleroderma, extractable nuclear antigens should be requested, and for cryoglobulinemia, complement proteins, rheumatoid factor, and cryoglobulin should be measured. In Waldenström's disease, elevated plasma immunoglobulin M (IgM), with increased plasma viscosity, is characteristic. Patients with hemolytic uremic syndrome (HUS) and thrombotic thrombocytopenic purpura (TTP) typically have fragmented red blood cells on the blood film, with an increased reticulocyte count, thrombocytopenia, anemia, minimally deranged clotting in comparison with disseminated intravascular coagulopathy, with elevated lactate dehydrogenase and reduced haptoglobins. In some patients with HUS, especially those with a family history of the disease or without an antecedent diarrheal illness, complement protein H, or membrane complement protein may be reduced or phenotypically abnormal; particularly in TTP, ADAMNTS13 may be reduced.

ELECTROLYTE IMBALANCE IN ACUTE RENAL FAILURE CAUSING CEREBRAL DYSFUNCTION

Marked hyponatremia may occur in patients with acute kidney injury due to severe volume depletion. Although other causes include excess water intake, which may occur in "fun runners" taking part in half-marathons, in whom ARF typically develops secondary to heat stroke, ARF also may occur in "all-night-rave" participants who take ecstasy

(3,4-methylenedioxymethamphetamine [MDMA]), which causes rhabdomyolysis (see Chapter 58). Hypernatremia may occur in diabetic hyperosmolar coma, and a delay in obtaining appropriate treatment may lead to ARF as a result of hypovolemia.

Severe hypokalemia may lead to muscle paralysis but only rarely causes rhabdomyolysis and renal impairment. Hypercalcemia may result in neurological sequelae ranging from irritability to confusion and convulsions, and marked renal impairment. In clinical practice, malignancy is the most common cause of hypercalcemia in patients with previously normal renal function.

Electrolyte imbalances may occur in the patient with ARF treated by dialysis. Typically, such derangements have occurred with failures in treatment of the domestic water supply, particularly in hard water areas, resulting in a high-calcium dialysate, or from compositional errors in the preparation of the final dialysate, leading to marked hypernatremia. Similarly, hyponatremia has been reported with errors in the preparation of dialysis fluids for continuous renal replacement therapy.[7]

METABOLIC DISORDERS CAUSING CEREBRAL DYSFUNCTION WITH ACUTE RENAL FAILURE

The clinical presentation in pathological conditions due to environmental insults, such as heat stroke, typically includes confusion and evidence of acute kidney injury secondary to muscle breakdown and dehydration. Unfortunately, many survivors are left with permanent neurological deficit. Snakebite, particularly from Australian elapids, and bites from venomous fish can manifest with neurotoxicity, with a characteristic sequence of paralysis followed by rhabdomyolysis and acute kidney injury.

Inherited defects of mitochondrial function may manifest with an acute encephalomyopathy, particularly after stress such as sepsis and surgery, and more commonly seen in patients given supplemental feeding. Such defects include mitochondrial encephalomyopathy with lactic acidosis and stroke-like episodes (MELAS) and myoclonic epilepsy with ragged red fibers (MERRF). Renal tubular defects are common in these conditions, and renal failure may ensue as a result of interstitial renal disease. Wilson's disease is now known to include a mitochondrial defect. In this condition, patients can present with an acute crisis with hepatic encephalopathy and red cell hemolysis, resulting in acute kidney injury. Other inborn errors of metabolism associated with intermittent encephalopathy due to hyperammonemia include defects of the urea cycle, including the organic acidemias, typified by methylmalonic acidemia. Now that affected infants are surviving childhood into their teens, renal failure develops as a consequence of renal tubular damage with interstitial fibrosis. Myoglobinuric renal damage also may occur in the glycogen storage diseases and with carnitine palmitoyl transferase deficiency. Acute intermittent porphyria can manifest with hallucinations, frank paranoia, and seizures. Renal impairment may be secondary to the combination of hypertensive nephrosclerosis with acute myoglobinuric injury. In the lysosomal storage condition Anderson-Fabry disease, chronic kidney failure often develops in later life, and patients can present with acute thrombotic stroke in the fifth decade. Other metabolic conditions associated with cerebral disease and renal impairment include cysti-

nosis, a lysosomal disorder that leads to cystine crystal accumulation leading to a Fanconi syndrome and chronic kidney failure, and the Lesch-Nyhan syndrome, which leads to intellectual deterioration in later childhood and is complicated by urate nephropathy.

ARF often develops in patients with hepatocellular failure due to hepatorenal syndrome, both in patients with acute hepatic failure and in those with advanced cirrhosis. In addition, ARF may be due to prerenal hypovolemia from sepsis, hemorrhage, or overdiuresis, or may be secondary to toxin-induced renal tubular damage after acetaminophen overdose, mushroom poisoning, exposure to carbon tetrachloride and other dry cleaning solvents, or phosgene poisoning, or to the presence of free hemoglobin in cases of acute hemolysis, including those due to chromium, copper, and propylene glycol poisoning.

DRUGS CAUSING ACUTE BRAIN AND KIDNEY INJURY

Many drugs taken for deliberate self-poisoning can cause a depressed level of consciousness and hypotension, sometimes complicated by seizures, resulting in acute myoglobinuric kidney injury.

Both malignant hyperpyrexia and the neuroleptic malignant syndrome can be precipitated by anesthetic agents (including halothane, ketamine, and suxamethonium), which, along with antidopaminergic drugs—typically, phenothiazines and butyrophenones—can cause muscle breakdown and acute kidney injury. Nightclub "ravers" who take ecstasy (MDMA) and other amphetamines are at risk of heat stroke from drug-induced hyperthermia, seizures, and hypertension. Similarly, cocaine causes hypertension, seizures, and muscle breakdown, as does self-poisoning with monoamine oxidase inhibitors and strychnine. Other agents occasionally are ingested, such as rodenticides containing α-chloralose, which cause seizures and myoglobinuric acute kidney injury. Dapsone poisoning causes methemoglobinemia but also hemolysis, leading to renal injury, coma, and seizures. Phenol ingestion also causes coma and rhabdomyolysis with acute kidney injury. Ethylene glycol ingestion can lead to seizures, coma, and ARF.

Lead toxicity can lead to encephalopathy, and chronic exposure results in interstitial fibrosis and renal failure. Arsenic poisoning causes acute hepatorenal dysfunction, seizures, and encephalopathy. Bismuth is a direct renal tubular toxin, and self-poisoning can result in ARF and encephalopathy. Exposure to other toxic agents, such as hydrogen fluoride, and accidental self-poisoning with oral iron can result in acute hepatorenal failure and coma. Some Chinese herbal remedies and bush teas have been reported to cause acute hepatic and renal failure. Lithium intoxication may result in coma in severe cases, and patients may have underlying renal interstitial fibrosis secondary to previous lithium therapy.

Other drugs that can acutely affect both the kidney and the brain include cyclosporine, tacrolimus, mitomycin C, gemcitabine, quinine, and cocaine, which all have been reported to cause a hemolytic uremic syndrome. In addition, the calcineuron inhibitors (cyclosporine and tacrolimus) can cause an acute encephalomyelitis with cerebral white matter changes and seizures, particularly in association with hypomagnesemia.[8] Depending on its glucose load and cytokine content, intravenous immunoglobulin

TABLE 74-3

Effect of Renal Function on Sedatives, Analgesics, and Muscle Relaxants Commonly Used in the Intensive Care Unit

DRUG	METABOLISM	ACCUMULATION IN RENAL FAILURE	ACTIVE OR TOXIC METABOLITE
Sedatives			
Midazolam	Hepatic	Yes	α-Hydroxymidazolam
Propofol	Hepatic	Minimal	Glucuronide/sulfate conjugates
Thiopental	Hepatic	Minimal	No
Analgesics			
Fentanyl	Hepatic	No	No
Alfentanil	Hepatic	No	No
Remifentanil	Plasma breakdown	No	No
Morphine	Hepatic	Yes	Morphine 6-glucuronide
Muscle Relaxants			
Atracurium	Plasma breakdown	Yes	Laudanosine
Cisatracurium	Plasma breakdown	Much less than with atracurium	Laudanosine
Rocuronium	Hepatic and renal	Yes	30% excreted unchanged in urine
Vecuronium	Hepatic and renal	Yes	20% excreted unchanged in urine

can cause both acute tubular toxicity and encephalopathy. Occasionally, the newer monoclonal and polyclonal agents used in treating hematopoietic cancers, rheumatoid arthritis, and other immunological diseases (e.g., anti-CD25 antibody, antilymphocyte globulin [ALG], orthoclone anti-human lymphocyte [OKT3] globulin, etanercept, rituximab, adalimumab) can result in an acute capillary leak–like syndrome, resulting in prerenal ischemia and an acute encephalopathy.

In patients with traumatic head injury, or after neurosurgery, drugs that can potentially suppress renal function or cause nephrotoxicity should be avoided. Such drugs include nonsteroidal anti-inflammatory drugs, aminoglycoside antibiotics, angiotensin-converting enzyme inhibitors, and sartanes (e.g., losartan). Other drugs such as cyclosporine and tacrolimus should be carefully monitored with trough levels. Radiocontrast media are nephrotoxic, and although the risk can be reduced by using hypo-osmolar contrast agents, along with volume expansion with isotonic bicarbonate, use of other imaging modalities such as ultrasonography and magnetic resonance imaging, if at all possible, is preferable to multislice three-dimensional computed tomography (CT) scanning.

Other drugs when given to patients with renal impairment can lead to acute confusion, coma, or seizures. These include the penicillin and cephalosporin antibiotics and the antiviral agents acyclovir and ganciclovir.

Similarly, patients in the ICU typically are given sedative drugs, analgesics, and muscle relaxants. Many of these agents have prolonged half-lives in ARF, so several days may be required for their effects to dissipate (Table 74-3). This has to be taken into account in assessing neurological status in patients in the ICU.

CONCLUSION

A majority of patients admitted to the ICU with acute kidney injury and confusion, delirium, or unconsciousness have underlying sepsis or drug-induced self-poisoning and require supportive management. The key to effective management is recognizing when patients have other conditions that require additional investigation and active treatment (Table 74-4). As a baseline screening approach, therefore, simple urine dipstick testing is important to detect blood and protein that may signify underly-

TABLE 74-4

Summary of Investigations for Conditions Causing Acute Kidney Injury

LOCATION OF DEFECT	EVIDENCE OF	INVESTIGATE FOR
Kidney	Renal obstruction	Bladder/prostate/cervical tumor
	Cholesterol emboli	Renal artery stenosis
	Hematuria/proteinuria	Intrinsic renal disease
		Vasculitis
		Bacterial endocarditis
	Myoglobin	Drug overdose
	Red cell fragments	Hemolytic uremic syndrome
	Severe hypertension	Scleroderma
Brain	Intracranial hemorrhage	Polycystic kidney disease
		Polyarteritis nodosa
	Ischemic stroke	Anticardiolipin syndrome
		Anderson-Fabry disease
	Encephalopathy	Drug overdose
		Metabolic disorder

ing intrinsic renal disease. This test should be performed not only on admission but also periodically throughout the course of the ICU stay, because in patients with initial prerenal ischemic injury, a later interstitial nephritis may potentially develop secondary to the administration of antibiotics or other drugs. A renal biopsy is indicated in patients who have not recovered renal function after 3 weeks. Similarly, careful examination of the stuporous or comatose patient, including funduscopy and auroscopy, is warranted to exclude localizing neurological signs. Many patients undergo simple CT brain scanning, without contrast, and it must be remembered that unenhanced scans, typically performed outside of normal working hours and without the benefit of interpretation by an experienced specialist, are designed to look for intracranial hemor-

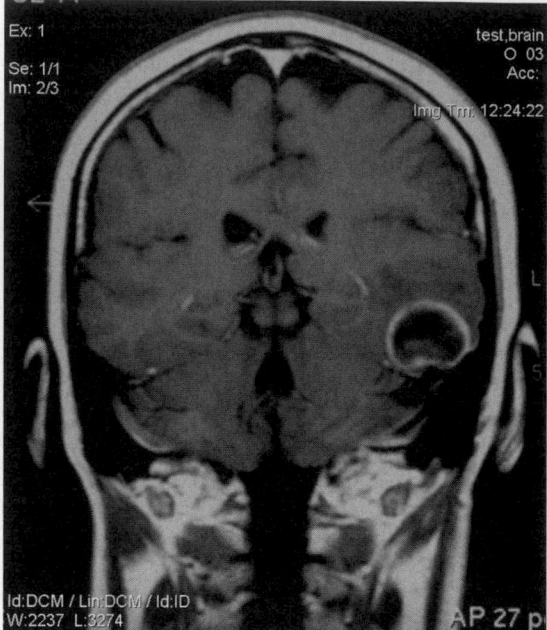

FIGURE 74-2. Cerebral abscess in a patient with bacterial endocarditis, secondary to infection of a central venous access catheter inserted for treatment of acute renal failure.

rhage, large masses, and hydrocephalus, whereas other pathologic processes may well be missed (Fig. 74-2). Cerebral function also can be affected by electrolyte imbalances, which should be corrected, and by prescribed drugs. In patients with acute kidney injury, drug doses may well need to be adjusted, and similarly, nephrotoxins should be avoided.

Key Points

1. Both acute uremia and the systemic inflammatory response can cause an encephalopathy that may be difficult to distinguish from primary cerebral infections and other pathological processes.
2. Atypical infections and post-transplantation lymphoproliferative disorders need to be considered in renal transplant recipients with neurological symptoms and signs.
3. Preexisting vascular disease is common in the elderly and in patients with underlying chronic kidney disease.
4. Subarachnoid hemorrhage is more common in patients with malignant hypertension and in those with polycystic kidney disease.
5. Drug metabolism is altered in acute kidney injury, and patients are more prone to the development of neurological side effects.

Key References

1. Battaglia F, Quartarone A, Bagnato S, et al: Brain dysfunction in uraemia: A question of cortical hyperexcitability? Clin Neurophys 2005;116:1507-1514.
2. Green R, Scott L, Minger A, et al: Sepsis associated encephalopathy (SAE): A review. Front Biosci 2004;9:1637-1641.
3. Jackson AC, Gilbert JJ, Young GB, Bolton CF: The encephalopathy of sepsis. Can J Neurol Sci 1985;12:303-307.
4. Nguyen DM, Spapen H, Fuhong S, et al: Elevated serum levels of S-100β protein and neuron specific enolase are associated with brain injury in patients with severe sepsis and septic shock. Crit Care Med 2006;34:1967-1974.
8. Davenport A: Neuropsychiatric disorders. In Davison AM, Cameron JS, Grunfeld JP, Ponticelli C (eds): Oxford Textbook of Clinical Nephrology, 3rd ed. Oxford, Oxford University Press, 2005, pp 1886-1895.

CHAPTER 75

Immunological and Infectious Complications of Acute Kidney Injury

Eric A. J. Hoste, Dominique M. Vandijck, Jan J. De Waele, and Stijn I. Blot

OBJECTIVES

This chapter will:
1. Provide an overview of the epidemiology of infection in patients with acute kidney injury.
2. Describe the diverse pathophysiological mechanisms that may explain the increased risk for infection in patients with acute kidney injury.

EPIDEMIOLOGY OF INFECTION IN PATIENTS WITH ACUTE KIDNEY INJURY

Infection is among the most important causes of morbidity, hospitalization, costs, and mortality in patients with end-stage renal disease. After cardiovascular disease, infection is the second most frequent cause of hospitalization among chronic hemodialysis patients, as reported by the United States Renal Data System (USRDS) (www.usrds.org).[1-3] Moreover, in the United States alone, an estimated 450,000 cases of sepsis per year are responsible for more than 100,000 deaths annually. Consequently, sepsis is, after acute myocardial infarction, the most frequent cause of mortality, also as reported by the USRDS. The Centers for Disease Control and Prevention has warned that incidence of sepsis is still increasing.[2,4] Furthermore, the subgroup of patients diagnosed with end-stage renal disease managed with renal replacement therapy have an approximate annual sepsis-attributed mortality rate up to 45 times higher than in the general population.[5] With regard to infectious complications in patients with acute kidney injury (AKI), considerably fewer data are available. To date, several studies demonstrated that infection and sepsis are nowadays the most important etiologic factors in the development of severe AKI.[6-9] In the Beginning and Ending of Supportive Therapy (B.E.S.T.) Kidney trial, including almost 30,000 critically ill patients from 54 centers in 23 different countries, septic shock was present in approximately half of the affected patients and was the main contributing factor in the development of severe AKI.[7]

In comparison with patients hospitalized on a general ward, increasing evidence indicates that patients with AKI are more susceptible to infection, as in patients with chronic kidney disease. In our own institution, of all patients with acute disease undergoing renal replacement therapy, 87% experienced an episode of infection during their ICU course. Of these infections, 41% developed during and 59% developed before or after renal replacement therapy, respectively.[10] In another study of our group, we found that critically ill patients with AKI treated with renal replacement therapy had a two-fold higher risk for development of nosocomial bloodstream infection compared with those without AKI.[11] In addition, in two thirds of patients, bloodstream infection was caused by an antimicrobial-resistant microorganism.[12,13] In a single-center study, performed in the Cleveland Clinic Foundation, Thakar and colleagues found that the postoperative course of patients who had undergone open heart surgery in whom AKI developed and was treated with renal replacement therapy, was complicated with infection in 58.5%, compared with 23.7% and 1.6% in patients with AKI not treated with renal replacement therapy, and patients without AKI, respectively (both, $P < .001$).[14] Finally, in the multicenter prospective observational trial on the epidemiology of AKI conducted in Madrid during 1991 and 1992, infection was identified as the cause of death in 40% of ICU patients with severe AKI.[15]

PATHOGENESIS OF INFECTION IN PATIENTS WITH ACUTE KIDNEY INJURY

As noted earlier, infection is a dreaded complication, in both chronic and acute kidney disease, because of its associated worse outcome. In patients maintained on chronic dialysis, several pathophysiological factors have been proposed that enhance the risk for infection.[16] Relevant data in the medical literature for patients with AKI are far more limited. However, many of the factors that may contribute

to the development of infection in patients with chronic kidney disease also are present in patients with AKI. These factors are highlighted and discussed in detail in this section (Table 75-1; Fig. 75-1).

Increased Inflammation

Increasing evidence suggests that AKI is caused, at least in part, by an inflammatory cascade resulting in a deterioration of organ function.[17-21] This response occurs as the release of cytokines and other inflammatory mediators and is seldom localized to one single organ system but will also negatively affect other organ systems as well.[22] Accordingly, this systemic inflammatory response also is likely to cause generalized inflammation and organ dysfunction. An enhanced inflammatory response reaction is particularly evident in patients with AKI treated with renal

TABLE 75-1

Factors Contributing to Increased Risk for Infection in Patients with Acute Kidney Injury (AKI)

Factors Associated with AKI
Volume overload
Metabolic acidosis
Malnutrition
Uremia
RRT Procedure–Related Factors
Presence of intravascular catheter
Loss of micronutrients—malnutrition
Inadequate dosing of antimicrobial agents
- Dose
- Dosing interval

RRT, renal replacement therapy.

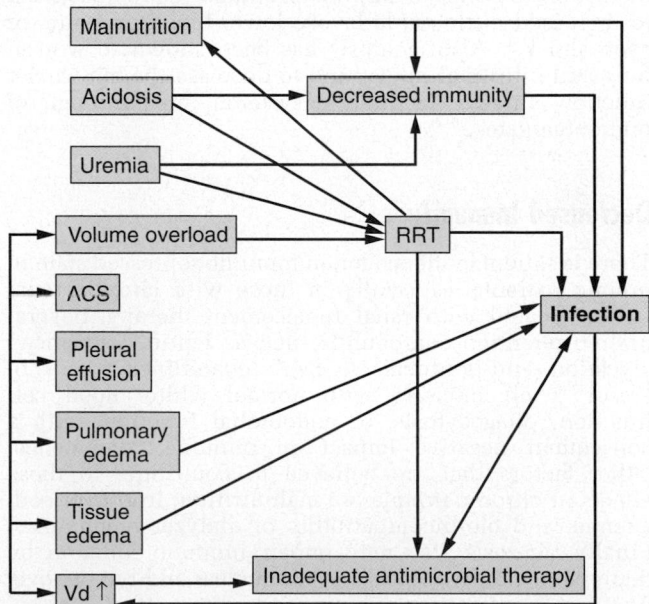

FIGURE 75-1. Interactions among various pathogenetic factors that contribute to increased risk for infection in patients with acute renal failure. ACS, abdominal compartment syndrome; RRT, renal replacement therapy; Vd, volume of distribution.

replacement therapy.[23,24] Despite decreased monocyte cytokine production,[25] patients with AKI have increased levels of pro-inflammatory mediators such as tumor necrosis factor-α (TNF-α), interleukin (IL)-1β, IL-6, and IL-8, compared with patients with end-stage renal disease and with normal subjects.[23,24,26] Furthermore, patients with AKI experience a *compensatory anti-inflammatory response syndrome* (CARS), resulting in increased levels of the anti-inflammatory mediator IL-10. It has also been demonstrated that there is increased oxidative stress in AKI patients.[27] Finally, evidence is growing for what is called "organ cross-talk," by which infection may lead to AKI, which may lead in turn to decreased functioning of other organs, as has been clearly demonstrated for the lungs. After ischemia-reperfusion injury of the kidneys, deregulation of the salt and water channels will occur, resulting in increased vascular permeability in the lungs, leading secondarily to interstitial edema.[28,29] In contrast with sepsis-induced acute respiratory distress syndrome (ARDS), AKI-induced ARDS generally is characterized by an induction of cytokine-induced neutrophil chemoattractant 2, a distinct expression of various heat shock proteins, and a low level of cellular infiltration.[30]

The underlying etiology for this deregulated inflammatory response is not entirely clear. Deregulation of the lung salt and water channels is related to the severity of AKI, suggesting that uremia may be responsible.[28] Increased cytokine levels and oxidative stress in patients with end-stage renal disease additionally suggests that uremia may play a crucial role in the development of a deregulated inflammation state.[31-33] Next, acidosis may also contribute to the degree of the inflammatory status in patients with acute renal failure (ARF). The effects on inflammation appear to vary according to the type of acidosis— respiratory versus metabolic and hyperchloremic versus lactic acidosis, respectively. Hyperchloremic acidosis is more pro-inflammatory than lactic acidosis. In vitro experiments demonstrated that hyperchloremic acidosis increased the ratio of IL-6 to IL-10 and the extent of nuclear factor-κB (NF-κB) DNA binding.[34] In vivo experiments, on the other hand, demonstrated that acidosis led to increased nitric oxide levels, lower blood pressure, or even shock.[35] Also, acidosis has been shown to worsen lung and intestinal injury, and to decrease the gut barrier function, thereby facilitating systemic breakthrough of microorganisms.[36-39]

Decreased Immunity

There is salient evidence for an immunodepressed state in uremic patients, especially in those with chronic renal failure treated with renal replacement therapy. Several uremic retention compounds such as leptin,[40] advanced glycation end-products (AGEs),[41] guanidines,[42] and *p*-cresol[43-45] all interfere with normal white blood cell function, phagocytosis, or endothelial function, with a consequent negative impact on immune competence. Other factors that are believed to contribute to these effects in chronic uremia are malnutrition, iron overload, anemia, and bio-incompatibility of dialyzer membranes. Finally, acidosis also may impair immune function by depressant effects on polymorphonuclear and lymphocyte function.[46,47] Because uremia and many of the aforementioned factors also are present in patients with ARF, immune suppression seems plausible in this population.[16,33]

Loss of Protective Barriers against Invading Microorganisms

In view of the acute setting, renal replacement therapy in a majority of patients with AKI usually is performed by the use of an indwelling intravascular catheter with a large diameter, and not by means of surgically constructed arteriovenous fistula or by peritoneal dialysis. To ascertain sufficient blood flow through the catheter, insertion into the femoral vein is preferred above, respectively, the internal jugular and the subclavian vein. Nevertheless, in same order of appearance the risk for developing an intravascular device—related bacteremia increases substantially, as a result of increased microbial skin colonization at these sites.[48-50] Because of all of these specific conditions related to hemodialysis treatment (e.g., temporary use of a dialysis catheter, frequent manipulation of the catheter, use of an extracorporeal circuit or multiple infusates), whereby various protective barriers are affected, infection heralds a major problem in dialyzed patients.

Volume Overload and Altered Permeability of Tissue Membranes

In critically ill patients, especially those with severe systemic infection, large amounts of fluids are administered during resuscitation. The subsequent fluid retention, which also may be due to AKI, will result in changes in total body water and in the characteristic distribution of many drugs.[51] Fluid imbalance resulting in tissue edema negatively influences wound healing because of compromised tissue perfusion,[52] with consequent increase in length of hospital stay and use of health care resources. Moreover, massive tissue edema puts the patient at greater risk for infection and other complications such as pulmonary edema and bedsores. Volume overload may result in intra-abdominal hypertension and, subsequently, in a secondary abdominal compartment syndrome, which in turn promotes bacterial translocation through the intestinal mucosa.[53,54] In sepsis-induced AKI, endothelial damage may be promoted by polymorphonuclear white blood cells, prostaglandins, or leukotrienes or by way of an activated complement cascade.[55] Because of the secondary capillary leak, large amounts of fluids will shift from the intracellular space to the interstitium, leading to prolonged water accumulation, necessitating hemofiltration.[56] All of these factors may contribute to hampering the patient's recovery.

Pulmonary Function

Volume overload may cause pulmonary vascular congestion, formation of pleural effusions, or intra-abdominal hypertension, leading to decreased gas exchange between the alveolar and capillary membranes. Compared with the general population, patients with ARF more often experience interstitial edema by deregulation of the inflammatory cascade and increased vascular permeability.[28,29,37] As noted earlier, AKI may affect the lung by way of increased renal production or impaired clearance of mediators of lung injury, such as pro-inflammatory cytokines.[57] Decreased immune function, in combination with all of the previously mentioned factors, and paralleled by an increase in baseline activity, may lead to inflammation, infection, or pneumonia. As well, loss of muscle mass, due to the patient's being confined to bed for a long periods or to decreased mobility, and oversedation secondary to retention of sedative and anesthetic drugs may prolong the duration of required mechanical ventilation and hence the period of increased risk for infection or other life-threatening complications.

Malnutrition

Malnutrition is an important problem in hospitalized patients, being particularly prevalent among severely ill patients. It has been established that a significant proportion of patients with AKI suffer from malnutrition. Fiaccadori and coworkers found that approximately 42% of patients who were referred to the renal intermediate care unit were severely malnourished.[58] Malnourished patients had impaired immunological function, as illustrated by lower total lymphocyte count, and lower levels of IgG, IgA, and IgM. In addition, severely malnourished patients with accompanying AKI had increased odds for developing severe sepsis as compared to patients without. Patients with AKI are at greater risk for preexisting malnourishment on admission to the ICU but probably are also at greater risk for development of malnourishment or suboptimal feeding during their ICU stay. The same investigators found that patients with AKI are at greater risk for gastroparesis and consequent withdrawal of enteral nutrition.[59] Finally, renal replacement therapy in these patients may be associated with loss of important amounts of micronutrients such as vitamin C, folate, magnesium, calcium, selenium, and thiamine, which should therefore be supplemented.[60]

Glucose Metabolism

The increased incidence of infection in patients with ARF can be explained by decreased immunity and deregulation of inflammation, and possibly by an altered glucose metabolism. Systemic infection provokes a stress-induced hypermetabolic response through the activation of the hypothalamic-adrenal axis, which in turn increases hepatic glucose production and inhibits insulin-mediated glucose uptake into skeletal muscles.[61] Acidosis has untoward effects on glucose metabolism, causing induction of insulin resistance and inhibition of anaerobic glycolysis.[62] Hyperglycemia secondary to this altered glucose metabolism has been associated with immune dysfunction and increased susceptibility to infection,[63] probably by pro-inflammatory effects and decreased phagocytosis.[64] It is well known that critical illness contributes to the release of inflammatory mediators, which in turn are associated with pronounced insulin resistance in affected patients.[65] Hyperglycemia is now recognized as an important risk factor for multiple organ dysfunction and death in critically ill patients; therefore, a protocol of strict glucose control should be implemented with the aim of improving outcome in this patient population.[66-68]

Pharmacokinetics of Antimicrobial Agents

Suboptimal dosing of antibiotic agents is an important cause of failure to eradicate microorganisms. Most antimicrobial agents are eliminated through the kidneys, and dose and dosing interval should be adjusted to kidney function as necessary. Of note, however, kidney function is seldom a steady state in patients with AKI. Moreover, it is very difficult, if not impossible, to assess kidney function in a non–steady state situation, as is the case in patients with AKI being managed in the ICU.[69] Adjustments of antimicrobial dose or interval in accordance with renal changes are therefore frequently based on incorrect or less accurate assessment of kidney function. Also, distribution volumes may increase considerably in severely ill patients with AKI, which may in turn result in decreased, possibly nontherapeutic levels of antimicrobial agents. Finally, correct dosing of antimicrobial agents in patients with AKI on renal replacement therapy is a challenge. Although recommendations concerning dosing and interval frequencies are available for most antibiotic agents, these may not necessarily be correct in a specific situation. For instance, dosage adjustment recommendations for antibiotics may be based on observations in patients maintained on chronic dialysis. Large variation between different renal replacement therapy strategies used in clinical practice is characteristic. For instance, CVVH protocols may differ in many aspects: Substitution fluid may be administered in predilution or postdilution mode, or the "dose" of CVVH or ultrafiltration volume may vary considerably: Some dialysis units use 20 mL/kg per hour, whereas others use 35 or even 50 mL/kg per hour or still other doses.[70] All of these factors may lead to inadequate antimicrobial therapy and therapeutic failure in patients with AKI and infection, thereby increasing the risk for antimicrobial resistance.

CONCLUSION

Infection remains a frequent and major problem in patients with ARF treated with renal replacement therapy. To date, data on the effect of immunological changes on the increased susceptibility to infection in this specific cohort of patients are rather limited. To treat ARF more effectively, however, improved knowledge regarding the underlying immunological changes in these patients is essential. Also, better insight into the epidemiology of infection in these patients is warranted. Future studies should be conducted in well-defined populations with special emphasis on both immunological and infectious factors.

Key Points

1. Infection is an important cause of acute kidney injury, and in turn, patients with acute kidney injury are at increased risk for infection.
2. Acute kidney injury is associated with increased inflammation, which in turn may decrease the immune response.
3. Volume overload may, through diverse mechanisms, contribute to the pathogenesis of infection.
4. Malnutrition probably is a frequent and less well-appreciated complication that also contributes to impaired immune status and increased risk for infection.

5. Finally, inappropriate dosing of antimicrobial agents may lead to inadequate eradication of microorganisms.

Key References

11. Hoste EA, Blot SI, Lameire NH, et al: Effect of nosocomial bloodstream infection on the outcome of critically ill patients with acute renal failure treated with renal replacement therapy. J Am Soc Nephrol 2004;15:454-462.
14. Thakar CV, Yared JP, Worley S, et al: Renal dysfunction and serious infections after open-heart surgery. Kidney Int 2003; 64:239-246.
16. Vanholder R, Van Biesen W: Incidence of infectious morbidity and mortality in dialysis patients. Blood Purif 2002;20:477-480.
28. Rabb H, Wang Z, Nemoto T, et al: Acute renal failure leads to dysregulation of lung salt and water channels. Kidney Int 2003;63:600-606.
47. Kellum JA, Song M, Li J: Science review: Extracellular acidosis and the immune response: Clinical and physiologic implications. Crit Care 2004;8:331-336.

See the companion Expert Consult website for the complete reference list.

CHAPTER 76

Nonpharmacological Management of Acute Renal Failure

Vijay Karajala-Subramanyam, Ramesh Venkataraman, and John A. Kellum

---

OBJECTIVES

This chapter will:
1. Review nonpharmacological strategies for the prevention and management of acute kidney injury.
2. Describe the role of fluid in preventing acute kidney injury.
3. Review the importance of renal perfusion pressure and nephrotoxicity in the pathophysiology of acute kidney injury.

The epidemiology and management of acute renal failure (ARF) have changed dramatically over the past 3 decades.[1-4] ARF that is severe enough to require renal replacement therapy affects nearly 6% of all critically ill patients, with a hospital mortality rate of 60%.[2] The etiology of severe ARF in the intensive care unit (ICU) is multifactorial. In a multinational, multicenter study by Uchino and colleagues,[2] the most common etiological factor in the development of ARF in the ICU was septic shock (reported in 47.5% of the cases).

Recently, focus on renal dysfunction has expanded to include milder or early forms of the syndrome, and consensus criteria for diagnosis and classification have been proposed[3] and subsequently validated.[5] The term *acute kidney injury* (AKI) has been proposed to describe the renal lesion in these patients.[6] Of interest, AKI appears to be quite common in the ICU (occurring in more than 65% of patients),[5] and even outside the ICU the condition is not rare (seen in 18% of all hospitalized patients).[2]

Surgery is believed to contribute to 20% to 25% of all cases of hospital-acquired AKI, and exposure to radiocontrast agents is another important cause.[7] Nephrotoxic drugs such as antineoplastics, antifungals, antibiotics, and recreational drugs also contribute significantly to AKI.[8] An important point is that most affected patients have more than one antecedent contributing factor.

Based on the pathophysiology of AKI, a plethora of therapeutic nondrug and drug interventions have been proposed. Of note, strategies that improve survival in critically ill patients (e.g., glucose control, nutrition) also may reduce the incidence of organ injury, including AKI.[9] This chapter presents some important nonpharmacologic strategies that may help to prevent or attenuate renal injury. Three main treatment strategies are described in detail: hydration, maintenance of mean arterial pressure, and minimizing nephrotoxin exposure.

IMPORTANCE OF EARLY DIAGNOSIS

For any treatment strategy to work its best, early initiation is a must. Not infrequently, AKI develops in critically ill patients under predictable clinical circumstances (e.g., septic shock, major vascular surgery); appropriate steps for prevention are therefore indicated.[10] Certain uncommon but easily reversible causes (such as urinary obstruction or abdominal compartment syndrome) should always be ruled out in the management of these patients (see Chapters 65 and 62, respectively). Early recognition however, may be difficult because of several reasons. First, reliable early kidney injury biomarkers are lacking. Serum creatinine has significant limitations—it is an inaccurate measure of GFR in an non–steady state, can be affected by other factors such as muscle mass, and often does not rise for a day or two after injury.[8,11,12] Several early biomarkers have been described, and several studies are underway to validate these markers for clinical use[13] (see Chapter 47). It is hoped that in the future, more sensitive means of detecting renal injury will result in better application of existing therapies and the ability to test new therapies more efficiently.

ADEQUATE HYDRATION AND CIRCULATING PLASMA VOLUME

Volume status is critical in maintaining hemodynamic stability, tissue perfusion, and organ function, and inadequate volume is an important risk factor for development of AKI.[1,9,14] It is increasingly being recognized that accurate assessment of volume status and the appropriate use of fluid replacement is associated with better outcomes.[15] Although volume expansion has been shown not to linearly increase glomerular filtration or consistently improve renal function in acute tubular necrosis (ATN), hypovolemia still remains a leading risk factor for and contributor to the onset of AKI.[16]

No randomized controlled trials (RCTs) have been conducted to directly evaluate the role of fluids versus placebo in the prevention of AKI.[14] Isotonic, intravenous fluids, however, have been studied for the prevention of ATN associated with radiocontrast media, amphotericin B, and the intrarenal tubular precipitation of crystals after high doses of methotrexate, sulfonamides, acyclovir, and various chemotherapeutic agents.[17] In certain conditions such as traumatic rhabdomyolysis and the postsurgical state after certain types of procedures, pretreatment with fluids has been associated with better outcomes.[8] Treatment and prevention of dehydration also may reduce the risk of AKI, and even when circulating blood volume is adequate, fluids may reduce the risk of nephrotoxicity from a wide variety of agents.

Choice of Fluids for Prevention of Acute Kidney Injury

Although no RCTs have compared fluids with no intervention, some trials have combined fluid administration (especially 0.45% sodium chloride infusion) with other active treatments and have compared different types of fluid and different routes of administration. One small RCT[18] comprising 53 patients who underwent nonemergency cardiac catheterization compared intravenous 0.9% saline solution (1 mg/kg per hour for 24 hours), begun 12 hours before cardiac catheterization, with unrestricted oral fluids. In the intravenous saline group, 3.7% of patients had contrast nephropathy, compared with 34.6% of patients in the unrestricted oral fluid group (relative risk, 0.11; 95% confidence interval [CI], 0.015 to 0.79). These data suggest that isotonic intravenous fluids clearly help to prevent radiocontrast agent–induced nephropathy; the type of fluid that is most protective is still under debate, however.

Mueller and associates[19] compared hydration using 0.9% saline solution infusion with 0.45% saline solution in dextrose for prevention of radiocontrast-induced nephropathy in 1620 patients undergoing coronary angiography. In this study, 0.9% saline solution infusion significantly reduced the frequency of contrast nephropathy compared with 0.45% saline solution in dextrose (occurring in 0.7% of patients who received the 0.9% solution versus 2% of the patients who received the 0.45% solution; $P = .04$). In a recent single-center RCT,[20] however, 119 patients with stable serum creatinine of at least 1.1 mg/dL received infusion of either isotonic sodium chloride ($n = 59$) or isotonic sodium bicarbonate ($n = 60$) before and after radiocontrast (iopamidol) administration. Radiocontrast-induced nephropathy, defined as a greater than 25% increase in creatinine from baseline within 48 hours, developed in 1 of 60 patients (1.7%) in the bicarbonate group, compared with 8 of 59 patients (13.6%) in the saline solution group ($P = .02$). This study had several limitations, including a high incidence of radiocontrast-induced nephropathy in the isotonic saline group and a high rate of dropout in both groups. It also was stopped early without a predefined statistical stopping rule. In summary, intravenous isotonic fluids should be used to expand intravascular volume to prevent AKI in patients receiving contrast media. Use of intravenous isotonic bicarbonate solution does not carry any significant additional risks in most patients, so this infusate is a reasonable alternative to 0.9% saline, especially in high-risk patients.

Urine alkalinization with sodium bicarbonate infusion also has been used to alleviate heme pigment–induced AKI (e.g., rhabdomyolysis). Ward[21] examined 157 patients with both traumatic and nontraumatic rhabdomyolysis and analyzed factors predictive for the development of AKI. Multivariate analysis revealed that the presence of dehydration on presentation was an independent risk factor for AKI. The traditional approach to manage pigment-induced ARF is saline resuscitation followed by forced diuresis with mannitol alkalinization to maintain pH higher than 6.5. Theoretically, urine alkalinization helps prevent tubular pigment cast formation and also may reduce the conversion of hemoglobin to methemoglobin and the release of iron from myoglobin. This approach is controversial, however, because evidence is lacking that mannitol or bicarbonate is more effective than saline solution alone.[22] Furthermore, use of bicarbonate therapy carries potential risks, including precipitation of calcium phosphate and inducing or exacerbating hypocalcemia. Furthermore, mannitol should be used with great caution, if at all, because it may result in a hyperosmolar state, particularly when renal failure has already occurred.[23]

Sort and colleagues[24] examined the effect of albumin administration on renal function in 126 patients with spontaneous bacterial peritonitis. In this randomized study, patients were given either cefotaxime and intravenous albumin or cefotaxime alone. The patients in the cefotaxime plus albumin group received albumin at a dose of 1.5 g/kg at the time of diagnosis and 1 g/kg on treatment day 3. Renal impairment, defined by the study investigators as a greater than 50% rise in blood urea nitrogen or creatinine, occurred in 33% of the patients receiving cefotaxime alone, but in only 10% of the patients receiving both cefotaxime and albumin. The administration of albumin also was associated with a significant reduction in mortality.

On the basis of the foregoing evidence, we recommend that isotonic intravenous fluids be used for prevention of AKI. The ideal composition of such a fluid and the optimal rate of infusion remain unclear and should be individualized. Of note, just as intravenous fluids may be beneficial in preventing radiocontrast-induced nephropathy, prevention of volume depletion also is important. Hence, diuretics should be viewed as potentiating the nephrotoxicity of radiocontrast agents and possibly other toxins as well.

MAINTENANCE OF ADEQUATE MEAN ARTERIAL PRESSURE

In the acute setting, the two most significant threats to renal perfusion pressure are systemic arterial hypotension and increased intra-abdominal pressure (including so-called abdominal compartment syndrome). Intra-abdominal hypertension is associated with decreased renal perfusion and may result in AKI.[25] Prompt recognition, often guided by urinary bladder pressure measurement, followed by surgical treatment offers the best potential for recovery[25] (see Chapter 62 for a more detailed discussion).

Specific recommendations to maintain renal perfusion pressure are difficult to make in light of the available evidence. Of note, however, vasopressors should be initiated only after (or concurrently with) adequate restoration of intravascular volume. Specific arterial pressure targets for titration of therapy to avoid renal hypoperfusion are not known. For example, in sepsis and ischemic AKI, some of the important autoregulating mechanisms that help preserve renal blood flow (RBF) and glomerular filtration rate (GFR) in the face of fluctuating blood pressures are disrupted. Hence, in these patients, RBF is directly related to systemic arterial pressure, and vasoactive drugs may be necessary in the ICU setting to raise the mean arterial pressure to more than usual values to maintain adequate renal perfusion pressures and adequate urine output.[26] Patients with chronic hypertension and renal vascular disease may have autoregulation curves that are shifted to the right; in these patients, a higher mean arterial pressure may be required to ensure adequate renal perfusion even when autoregulation remains intact.

Although norepinephrine has been shown to reduce RBF in healthy animals and humans, no evidence exists to indicate that reversing systemic hypotension with norepinephrine compromises mesenteric or renal blood flow.[9,14] Of interest, one study of septic patients demonstrated that norepinephrine increased urine output and GFR.[27] Another prospective, observational study of 97 patients with septic shock found lower mortality in patients treated with norepinephrine than with other vasopressors (high-dose dopamine).[28] (See Chapter 77 for a more complete discussion of vasoactive medications and AKI.)

MINIMIZING NEPHROTOXIN EXPOSURE

Minimizing nephrotoxin exposure is an important strategy in AKI prevention. Primary preventive strategies require knowledge of patients' risk factors for nephrotoxicity, alternative therapies for drugs with significant nephrotoxic potential, appropriate dosing and vigilant monitoring of renal function, continued reassessment of concomitant medications for possible interactions, and maintaining adequate hydration and volume status. Radiocontrast agents, aminoglycosides, and amphotericin are the most studied nephrotoxins in the ICU. In addition to intravenous fluid administration as discussed previously, specific strategies for minimizing nephrotoxicity have been developed and are discussed in detail in Chapter 58.

Aminoglycosides

Aminoglycosides are well-recognized nephrotoxins that often are used in the treatment of serious gram-negative sepsis. Aminoglycoside toxicity develops in approximately 10% to 15% of patients receiving these agents.[1] The accumulation of drug in renal tubular epithelial cells, with alteration in renal blood flow, appears to be the pathophysiological mechanism.[23] Aminoglycosides are excreted entirely by glomerular filtration. Although drug levels traditionally have been monitored, trough levels do not rise until substantial renal injury has occurred. A standard per kg dosing may be excessive in obese patients.[23]

Prins and colleagues[29] found that, compared with conventional thrice-daily dosing, once-daily aminoglycoside dosing resulted in a marked reduction in the incidence of AKI (defined as an increase in serum creatinine of 0.5 mg/dL) from 24% to only 5%. Two meta-analyses[30,31] and one systematic review[32] have been performed comparing the efficacy and toxicity of multiple-daily and once-daily aminoglycoside dosing schedules. In all three studies, no differences were found in the efficacy of aminoglycosides with once-daily dosing, and a trend toward lower nephrotoxicity was identified in the once-daily-dosing groups.

Amphotericin

The incidence of AKI associated with amphotericin administration may be as high as 30%.[33] Nephrotoxicity from this drug is related to renal vasoconstriction and direct tubular injury by deoxycholate, used as a solubilizing agent.[23] Sodium administration is suggested to reduce nephrotoxicity in one trial,[34] but significant nephrotoxicity may still occur. Evidence indicates that the risk of nephrotoxicity is lower with liposomal formulations of amphotericin.[35] One study[36] of patients with neutropenic fever found that amphotericin B colloid dispersion was equal in therapeutic efficacy to conventional amphotericin B but was associated with reduced nephrotoxicity (55% in the conventional group versus 36% in the colloid dispersion group; $P < .001$). A phase II trial of a lipid formulation of amphotericin B ($n = 556$) found an incidence of renal toxicity of 24%, compared with 60% to 80% incidence reported with standard formulations of amphotericin B. In addition, patients with baseline serum creatinine greater than 2.5 mg/dL on standard amphotericin B showed a significant decrease in serum creatinine when transferred to the lipid formulations ($P < .0001$). Another study[37] compared liposomal amphotericin B with conventional amphotericin B for empirical antifungal therapy in patients with persistent neutropenic fever. Although liposomal amphotericin B was as effective as the conventional type, it was associated with less nephrotoxicity (19% with A lipid complex versus 34% with the conventional B; $P < .001$). On the basis of these data, we recommend that lipid forms of amphotericin be used preferentially in patients with renal insufficiency or other risks for AKI or with evidence of renal tubular dysfunction.

CONCLUSION

Adequate volume and hydration status, maintenance of mean arterial pressure, and minimizing nephrotoxin exposure remain the most effective strategies to prevent AKI. Hypotension should be prevented and treated promptly. Vasopressors should be initiated to maintain mean arterial pressure, but restoration of intravascular volume must be achieved promptly. Intravenous isotonic fluids should be used to prevent nephrotoxic AKI. Use of sodium bicarbonate may be warranted in selected high-risk patients to prevent radiocontrast-induced AKI. Nephrotoxic medications should be avoided when possible, and if needed, careful dosing and monitoring are required. Once-daily dosing of aminoglycosides, lipid formulations of amphotericin B, and iso-osmotic contrast media should be used in preference to older regimens or agents in all high-risk patients.

Key Points

1. For intravenous fluid therapy, isotonic fluids are better than hypotonic fluids; no advantage of colloids over crystalloids has been established, and no benefit of blood transfusion is recognized.
2. "Adequate" mean arterial pressure should be ensured; precise pressure depends on the individual patient.
3. In order to minimize exposure to nephrotoxins, iso-osmolar nonionic contrast agents should be used, in the lowest volume necessary; lipid formulations of amphotericin B should be used, and aminoglycosides should be dosed daily or by levels.

Key References

1. Venkataraman R, Kellum JA: Prevention of acute renal failure. Chest 2007;131:300-308.
2. Uchino S, Kellum JA, Bellomo R, et al: Acute renal failure in critically ill patients: A multinational, multicenter study. JAMA 2005;294:813-818.
8. Lameire N, Van Biesen W, Vanholder R: Acute renal failure. Lancet 2005;365:417-430.
9. Kellum JA, Leblanc M, Gibney RT, et al: Primary prevention of acute renal failure in the critically ill. Curr Opin Crit Care 2005;11:537-541.

See the companion Expert Consult website for the complete reference list.

CHAPTER 77

Vasoactive Drugs and Acute Renal Failure

Rinaldo Bellomo, Li Wan, and Clive N. May

OBJECTIVES

This chapter will:
1. Present an overview of the rationale for the use of vasoactive drugs in critically ill patients.
2. Describe the effects of vasoactive drugs on the systemic and renal circulations.
3. Identify the adverse effects of vasoactive drugs.
4. Review the experimental evidence on the effect of vasoactive drugs on the renal circulation.
5. Summarize the available evidence on the effect of vasoactive drugs in humans.

Septic shock, systemic inflammation (from trauma, major surgery, cardiopulmonary bypass, and the like), and pharmacological vasodilatation (from phosphodiesterase inhibitors, sedative drugs, or epidural or spinal block) usually are associated with systemic hypotension despite normal or increased cardiac output.[1] Under these circumstances, hypotension may persist despite vigorous volume expansion. Potent systemic vasopressor agents, such as norepinephrine (noradrenaline outside of North America) or so-called high-dose dopamine or epinephrine (adrenaline) or phenylephrine or low-dose vasopressin or terlipressin, can then be used to restore an acceptable mean arterial blood pressure.[2-5]

Under these conditions, renal dysfunction is common (manifested as oliguria or a rising serum creatinine level, or both), and the use of vasopressors typically is fraught with controversy. This chapter reviews the evidence on the renal effects of the use of such drugs in critically ill patients. Vasoactive drugs that induce vasodilatation (nitroprusside, glyceryl trinitrate) or drugs that, although vasodilating, are predominantly inotropic in nature (phosphodiesterase inhibitors) are not discussed here; so-called low-dose dopamine is discussed in Chapter 79.

WHY USE VASOPRESSORS?

The rationale for vasopressor therapy in hypotensive states is based on the physiological principle that in all regional circulations, including the renal, splanchnic, cerebral and coronary beds, blood flow is autoregulated. This means that, if cardiac output is preserved, so long as blood pressure is maintained at a sufficient value, organ blood flow also is preserved. When blood pressure falls below a given value (the autoregulatory threshold), however, such autoregulation is lost. Then, as blood pressure falls, organ blood flow also decreases in an almost linear fashion. Decreased blood flow may induce organ ischemia, which in turn may contribute to organ failure. This decrease in blood flow may be particularly marked in those patients with critical renal, mesenteric, carotid, or coronary artery lesions (as with atheroma, fibroplasia, and the like). Furthermore, this fall in renal blood flow is likely to occur at higher blood pressures in these patients, as well as in those with long-standing hypertension. Of note, different vascular beds will lose autoregulation at different blood pressure values. For example, the mammalian kidney appears to do so at a mean arterial pressure (MAP) of approximately 80 mm Hg, whereas the brain and coronary circulations require a MAP of somewhere between 30 and 50 mm Hg (Fig. 77-1). In addition, the pressure-flow rela-

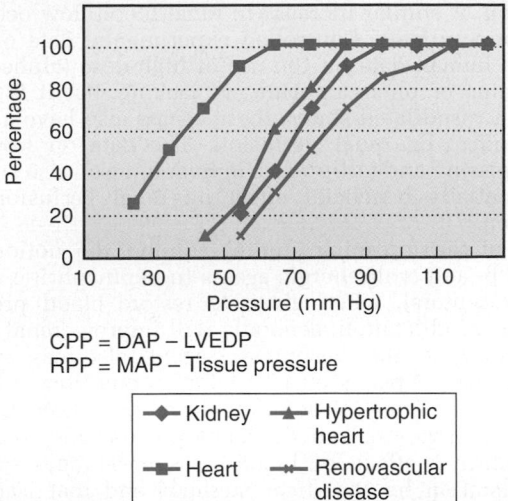

CPP = DAP – LVEDP
RPP = MAP – Tissue pressure

◆ Kidney   ▲ Hypertrophic heart

■ Heart   ✻ Renovascular disease

FIGURE 77-1. Graph illustrating the pressure-flow relationship for the kidney and heart under normal and pathophysiological conditions. Flow is expressed as percent of normal, and pressure is in mm Hg. The equation for renal perfusion pressure (RPP) indicates the importance of mean arterial pressure (MAP) and tissue pressure. Similarly, coronary perfusion pressure (CPP) depends on diastolic arterial pressure (DAP) and left ventricular end-diastolic pressure (LVEDP).

tionship for the kidney appears to follow a relatively steeper slope than that of other regional beds. Thus, for a given fall in blood pressure, the proportional fall in blood flow would be expected to be particularly sharp for the kidney.

The foregoing physiological observations suggest that the restoration of blood pressure is a logical and desirable therapeutic goal in the pursuit of renal protection, particularly if a patient remains hypotensive and oliguric after adequate fluid resuscitation. Unfortunately, the drugs necessary to restore a higher MAP have properties that raise concerns about their use.

Norepinephrine

Norepinephrine is very effective in raising arterial blood pressure and, under almost all circumstances, can be titrated to achieve the desired MAP in a given patient. Because norepinephrine induces vasoconstriction by means of α-adrenergic stimulation, however, a concern is that it also may decrease organ blood flow if regional vascular beds constrict in excess. In such a scenario, intra-organ vascular resistance would increase proportionately more than perfusion pressure, and overall blood flow would decrease, particularly for the kidney. In fact, norepinephrine infusions have been reported to decrease splanchnic[6,7] and renal blood flow[8-10] under normal circulatory conditions, as well as during essential hypertension and hypovolemic hypotension. These reports have significantly inhibited the clinical use of norepinephrine.

The studies that suggest that norepinephrine may induce splanchnic or renal ischemia, however, are open to several criticisms. An important point is that they do not address the effects of norepinephrine in vasodilated, hypotensive states and may not even accurately reflect the longer-term effect of norepinephrine infusion in normal subjects. On

the other hand, if norepinephrine infusion induces visceral organ hypoperfusion in the vasodilated patient, then it could induce multiple organ dysfunction, loss of gut mucosal integrity,[11] renal ischemia, and the development of acute renal failure (ARF). In the light of such considerations, concern remains regarding the advisability of sustained vasopressor infusions in the hypotensive patient.

It is not clear, however, if the hypothetical scenario of vasopressor-induced renal hypoperfusion actually occurs in sepsis or other vasodilated states. Such clinical states are characterized by profound alterations in vascular tone. Downregulation of vascular smooth muscle through α-adrenergic receptor responsiveness[12] and active vasodilation occur as a result of massive nitric oxide release.[13] In addition, microvascular obstruction by aggregation of platelets and white blood cells, formed by adhesion to the activated vascular endothelium, can disrupt local blood flow distribution independent of α-adrenergic tone.[14] Finally, increased cyclic AMP concentrations in the smooth muscle cells of blood vessels, induced by the administration of phosphodiesterase inhibitors, also will decrease vessel tone, as will the loss of sympathetic outflow from epidural blockade.

Under circumstances of marked vasodilatation, it makes physiological sense that the restoration of normal or near-normal vascular tone and adequate renal perfusion pressure should improve renal blood flow and glomerular filtration rate. Whether norepinephrine can achieve these goals safely, however, remains a matter of controversy.

Experimental Data

Norepinephrine can be used to induce a reversible model of ARF[15,16] when infused into the renal artery. Such ARF is induced by marked renal vasoconstriction. Once again, such observations make the physician wary of using norepinephrine in the clinical setting of renal dysfunction, in case it may induce or contribute to ARF. However, a more accurate analysis of the available data is warranted. Norepinephrine-induced intense vasoconstriction has been seen to occur only with infusion of the drug directly into the renal artery, not by way of the systemic route at clinically relevant doses.[15,16] In addition, the dose of drug used in models of norepinephrine-induced acute renal failure was twice to three times that used in appropriate animal studies and *well beyond* the mean dose usually administered in clinical practice. The relevance of these investigations to clinical practice is, at best, negligible.

Schaer and coworkers also have reported the renal effects of norepinephrine infusion at different doses with or without the addition of low-dose dopamine.[17] These investigators measured renal blood flow with the technique of regional thermodilution (an unvalidated approach). They found that although renal vascular resistance appeared to increase from baseline (the study did not include a placebo arm), total renal blood flow progressively increased with increasing doses of intravenous norepinephrine up to 1.6 μg/kg per minute. In their study, any adverse effects of norepinephrine infusion on renal vascular resistance (of note, total renal blood flow actually increased) were seen in animals with a baseline mean arterial blood pressure of 151 mm Hg. No sane clinician would prescribe norepinephrine to a patient with an MAP of 150 mm Hg!

On the other hand, a study by Anderson and colleagues[18] appears to mimic clinical practice more closely. These

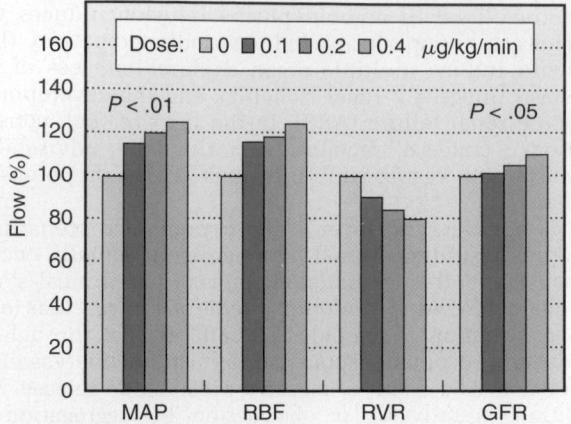

FIGURE 77-2. Histogram illustrating the effect of different doses (from 0 to 0.4 μg/kg per minute) of norepinephrine (noradrenaline) on mean arterial pressure (MAP), renal blood flow (RBF), renal vascular resistance (RVR), and glomerular filtration rate (GFR) in the dog. Flow is presented as percentage, with 100% being flow in control subjects receiving placebo. Both MAP and GFR are significantly increased by norepinephrine at clinically relevant doses.

investigators infused norepinephrine intravenously at 0.2 to 0.4 μg/kg per minute (a clinically relevant dose) in conscious dogs and, using an electromagnetic flow probe, evaluated renal blood flow, renal vascular resistance, and glomerular filtration rate. They found that renal blood flow *increased* and renal vascular resistance *decreased* in response to short-term norepinephrine infusion (Fig. 77-2). Such norepinephrine-induced renal vasodilatation was unaffected by pretreatment with indomethacin, propranolol, or angiotensin-converting enzyme (ACE) inhibitors. Therefore, renal vasodilatation was not prostaglandin-mediated and was independent of β-receptor stimulation or of angiotensin-derived changes in vascular tone. Efferent autonomic sympathetic nerve blockade with pentolinium before norepinephrine infusion, however, completely abrogated norepinephrine-induced renal vasodilatation. These investigators logically concluded that, in keeping with previous experimental data,[19] most of the renal vasodilating effect of intravenous norepinephrine could be attributed to an increase in systemic blood pressure, which decreased renal sympathetic tone through a baroreceptor response, leading to vasodilatation.

The effect of norepinephrine infusion on regional blood flow in the dog has also been recently explored by Zhang and coworkers.[20] These investigators demonstrated that, in the endotoxemic dog, norepinephrine did not induce any decrease in renal or hepatic blood flow.

The effects of norepinephrine infusion on renal blood flow may not be unique to this vasopressor; rather, such effects may be representative of those of a group of potent vasoconstrictor agents. For example, Bersten, working with Rutten and other investigators, studied the renal effects of epinephrine, another potent vasopressor agent, with a strong mixed β- and α-adrenergic effect.[21,22] These researchers administered epinephrine by continuous infusion at clinically relevant doses in normal and septic sheep. After a short-lived (minutes) and small decrease in renal blood flow at the highest doses tested (0.4 to 0.8 μg/kg per minute), renal blood flow progressively increased. It remained elevated for up to 6 hours of norepinephrine

infusion. A similar increase in renal blood flow occurred in septic animals. Controlled experimental data or controlled human data on the use of high-dose (alpha-dose) dopamine or phenylephrine are lacking, but it is likely that, in vasodilated states, these agents also have a beneficial effect on renal perfusion. The data on low-dose vasopressin[23] and terlipressin in liver failure[24] also support a potentially beneficial effect on renal perfusion and function.

All of the foregoing studies support the notion that mixed β- and α-adrenergic agents (norepinephrine affects both receptors), when given to restore blood pressure during vasodilatation, generally will improve renal blood flow and that other vasopressor agents also may achieve similar goals. A persisting physiological question, however, concerns the effect of norepinephrine per se on the tone of the renal vasculature. Such analysis demands that norepinephrine's effects on blood pressure be removed from consideration by statistical methods and that issues of preload also be eliminated by experimental methods. To address this issue, Bellomo and coworkers conducted a complex and highly invasive physiological study in the dog.[25] Although a discussion of the methodology is not warranted here, a few points merit emphasis. First, the vascular occlusion technique for the inferior vena cava was used. Such occlusion induces a fall in preload that allows differences in preload between different hemodynamic states to be essentially eliminated from the assessment of the effect of the drug itself on the renal vasculature. Second, both the pressure-flow relationship (dynamic resistance) and the point of zero flow (Pzf) were defined. The Pzf represents precapillary sphincter tone. Finally, these investigators studied the animal in the septic and the normal state with repeated control observations and a crossover design.

Norepinephrine infusion, at clinically relevant dosages, affected renal blood flow differentially during basal and acute endotoxemic conditions. When normal circulatory controls existed in the otherwise unstressed circulation, norepinephrine infusion failed to proportionately increase dynamic renal blood flow despite increasing arterial pressure. By contrast, once the circulation had been perturbed by the insult of acute endotoxemia (and probably any other state inducing a major degree of vasodilatation), identical dosages of norepinephrine increased both dynamic renal blood flow and perfusion pressure. Of importance, the methodology used allowed the investigators to isolate the effect of the intravenous infusion of norepinephrine on the determinants of steady-state renal blood flow independent of perfusion pressure. Under normal conditions, norepinephrine, infused intravenously at a rate capable of increasing MAP by approximately 15 mm Hg, induced a decrease in renal vascular ohmic resistance but an increase in vascular critical closing pressure. This change was such that, in the aggregate, these combined renal vasoactive effects reduced renal blood flow for a constant perfusion pressure. During acute endotoxemic conditions, however, the initial state of the renal vasculature was altered, reflecting the profound effects that endotoxemia has on vascular smooth muscle tone and vascular responsiveness. Under these conditions, the addition of norepinephrine infusion further decreased renal vascular ohmic resistance. It also decreased the vascular critical closing pressure, such that overall, these combined renal vascular effects served to increase renal blood flow for a constant perfusion pressure. Thus, norepinephrine infusion in acute endotoxemia appears to reverse systemic hypotension and to improve renal blood flow independent of perfusion pressure. These findings, in association with those from other reports in the literature, provide a physiological basis for the administration of norepinephrine during septic shock and other vasodilated states.

WHICH VASOPRESSOR?

Studies that directly measure renal blood flow and resistance in humans are not available. Many clinical reports, however, support the notion that the continuous infusion of norepinephrine may increase urine output and improve creatinine clearance in hyperdynamic septic shock.[26-31] Of particular interest is a study by Martin and coworkers because it is the only randomized controlled study available.[3] These investigators randomized 32 patients with hyperdynamic and hypotensive septic shock to receive either *high-dose dopamine* (up to 50 μg/kg per minute) or *norepinephrine* up to 1 μg/kg per minute in order to achieve a predetermined arterial blood pressure (greater than 80 mm Hg). They evaluated the overall hemodynamic response as well as lactate and urinary output after 1 and 6 hours of therapy. They found that high-dose dopamine failed to restore normotension in one third of patients, while norepinephrine succeeded in all patients. In addition, in those patients whose hypotension could not be corrected with dopamine, norepinephrine restored an MAP to more than 80 mm Hg. Urinary output was significantly improved from baseline once blood pressure was increased. This controlled study strongly suggests that norepinephrine is superior to alpha-dose dopamine in restoring blood pressure in septic, vasodilated patients and that such correction of blood pressure induces an improvement in urine output.

More recently, Martin and colleagues also reported on outcomes for 97 adult patients with septic shock, of whom 57 received treatment with norepinephrine. Patients treated with norepinephrine had a lower mortality than those treated with other pressor drugs,[31] and norepinephrine use was identified as a predictor of survival on multivariate logistic regression analysis. These findings support the argument that norepinephrine is safe and effective in hypotensive vasodilated states and that its renal effects under those circumstances are likely to be beneficial.

No controlled studies have been conducted to compare other vasopressor drugs like phenylephrine or epinephrine with norepinephrine. Phenylephrine and epinephrine are not recommended as first-line agents,[32] however, because of concern regarding unbalanced α-adrenergic vasoconstriction with phenylephrine and lack of sufficient human data and, in the case of epinephrine, concern about its ability to induce hyperlactatemia, acidosis, hyperglycemia, and tachycardia. On the other hand, low-dose vasopressin (10 international units/hour) has been proposed as an adjunct to decrease the dose of norepinephrine in the treatment of septic shock.[33] A large international multicenter trial, the Vasopressin in Septic Shock Trial (VASST), sought to address this issue by comparing low-dose vasopressin plus norepinephrine and norepinephrine alone in the vasopressor treatment of septic shock and found no significant difference in clinical outcomes.[34]

CONCLUSION

The use of norepinephrine (and probably vasopressor therapy in general) in patients with hypotensive vasodilatation and evidence of renal dysfunction in an ICU setting remains the subject of much debate and controversy. Although concern about the use of these drugs remains, the data suggest otherwise. It may indeed be that restoration of blood pressure with norepinephrine has a nephroprotective effect and that in vasodilated states, use of other vasopressor drugs to restore blood pressure to acceptable levels is similarly safe. Much work remains to be done on the renal effects of hemodynamic manipulation with catecholamines, however, before clinical decisions can be based on level I evidence.

Key Points

1. The rationale for the use of vasoactive drugs in critically ill patients is based on the concept that vasodilatory shock is best treated with vasoconstrictive drugs.
2. The effect of vasoactive drugs on the systemic circulation is one of vasoconstriction. Their effect on the renal circulation, however, is variable, reflecting local vasomotor changes, changing perfusion pressure, and the intrarenal sympathetic response.
3. The adverse effects of vasoactive drugs may differ from agent to agent, with epinephrine having significant metabolic effects and other agents having limited metabolic effects. All can be dangerous if given to inadequately resuscitated patients with a low cardiac output.
4. Experimental evidence on the effect of vasoactive drugs (especially norepinephrine) on the renal circulation suggests that renal blood flow is preserved.
5. All evidence available on the effect of vasoactive drugs in humans suggests no deleterious effect on renal function, provided that these drugs are used in vasodilated, high-cardiac-output states.

Key References

3. Martin C, Papazian L, Perrin G, et al: Norepinephrine or dopamine for the treatment of hyperdynamic septic shock? Chest 1993;103:1826-1831.
18. Anderson WP, Korner PI, Selig SE: Mechanisms involved in the renal responses to intravenous and renal artery infusions of noradrenaline in conscious dogs. J Physiol 1981;321:21-30.
26. Martin C, Eon B, Saux P, et al: Renal effects of norepinephrine used to treat septic shock patients. Crit Care Med 1990;18:282-285.
31. Martin C, Viviand X, Leone M, Thirion X: Effect of norepinephrine on the outcome of septic shock. Crit Care Med 2000;28:2758-2765.
32. Beale RJ, Hollenberg SM, Vincent JL, Parrillo JE: Vasopressor and inotropic support in septic shock: An evidence-based review. Crit Care Med 2004;32(11 Suppl):S455-S465.

See the companion Expert Consult website for the complete reference list.

CHAPTER 78

Use of Diuretics in Acute Renal Failure

Vijay Karajala-Subramanyam, Ramesh Venkataraman, Miet Schetz, and John A. Kellum

---

OBJECTIVES

This chapter will:
1. Review the actions of the commonly used diuretic agents.
2. Describe the rationale for use of loop diuretics in patients with or at risk for acute kidney injury.
3. Discuss the relevant clinical studies on the prophylactic or therapeutic use of loop diuretics in acute kidney injury.
4. Present recommendations for clinical use of diuretics in patients with or at risk for acute kidney injury.

Intravenous diuretics frequently are used in acute care settings to facilitate fluid management.[1-4] Although many classes of diuretics initially were used in acute fluid management, agents such as acetazolamide and spironolactone have been replaced by more efficacious diuretics—"high-ceiling" or potent loop diuretics. This chapter provides a brief overview of these other diuretic agents; the focus, however, is on the most commonly used intravenous diuretics (i.e., loop diuretics). The current state of the evidence for use of loop diuretics in patients with, or at risk for, acute kidney injury (AKI), particularly in a setting of critical illness, is reviewed. A summary of the role of different classes of diuretics is provided in Table 78-1.

OSMOTIC DIURETICS: MANNITOL

Osmotic diuretics are freely filtered at the glomerulus, undergo limited reabsorption by the renal tubule, and are relatively inert pharmacologically. They act primarily at the loop of Henle, and also on the proximal tubule, by extracting water from intracellular compartments. Osmotic diuretics expand the extracellular fluid volume, decrease blood viscosity, and inhibit renin release. These effects generally result in an increase in renal blood flow and a reduction in medullary tonicity.

Animal models have shown that mannitol is effective in attenuating the reduction in glomerular filtration rate associated with acute tubular necrosis (ATN) when administered before the ischemic insult or offending nephrotoxin.[5] The renal protection afforded by mannitol may be due to removal of obstructing tubular casts, dilution of nephrotoxic substances in the tubular fluid, or reduction in swelling of tubular elements by means of osmotic extraction of water. In addition, mannitol also has been shown to increase renal blood flow and to act as a free radical scavenger during reperfusion of the kidney. Although prophylactic mannitol is effective in animal models of ATN, the clinical efficacy of mannitol is less well established. Most published clinical studies have been underpowered and uncontrolled, with conflicting results.[6-9] Solomon and colleagues randomized 78 patients with mild to moderate renal insufficiency to receive either 0.45% saline alone, saline plus mannitol, or saline plus furosemide; compared with saline alone, both diuretics were associated with greater risk of renal injury.[10]

Although the use of osmotic diuretics in the setting of rhabdomyolysis and myoglobinuric renal failure is common clinical practice in many centers, no large randomized controlled trials have studied the effect of mannitol in this setting. In one study, Homsi and associates[11] performed a retrospective analysis on 24 patients admitted to the intensive care unit (ICU) with rhabdomyolysis. A treatment regimen of saline, bicarbonate, and mannitol was used in 15 of the patients; the rest of the patients received saline alone. No additional benefit to aggressive hydration was found with mannitol use in this study. In summary, despite the presence of animal and anecdotal human evidence of the beneficial effects of mannitol, no adequately powered prospective, randomized clinical trials have been conducted to compare these effects with those of saline alone. Thus, no basis for the use of mannitol in the prevention or management of ARF has been established.

LOOP DIURETICS

Loop diuretics inhibit the $Na^+-K^+-2Cl^-$ cotransporter in the apical membrane of the ascending loop of Henle. Their potency can be explained by the high salt reabsorption that normally takes place in this nephron segment (25% to 40% of the filtered load).[12] In a survey by the European Workgroup of Cardio-thoracic Intensivists, 11 of 38 centers used furosemide continuously for "renal protection," and 34 centers used furosemide bolus injections when diuresis decreased.[13] Despite this common use, no data have established that loop diuretics have a beneficial effect on renal function.

Rationale for Use of Loop Diuretics in Patients with or at Risk for Acute Kidney Injury

Two recent large observational studies reported that 59% to 70% of the patients with AKI received diuretics at the time of nephrology consultation or before the start of renal replacement therapy.[14,15] It is commonly held that the oli-

TABLE 78-1

Summary of the Role of Different Diuretics in Acute Renal Failure (ARF)

CLASS	THERAPEUTIC ROLE	COMMENT(S)
Loop diuretics • Furosemide • Torsemide • Bumetanide • Ethacrynic acid	No role in prevention of ARF; however, makes patient management easier in the ICU by avoiding excessive fluid overload	No impact on mortality rate, or need for dialysis or renal recovery. A short trial of loop diuretics, preferably as an infusion, may be reasonable before initiation of dialysis in the ICU.
Osmotic diuretics • Mannitol	No role in the prevention or treatment of ARF from any cause	Use of saline hydration alone was shown to be superior to saline with mannitol administration in radiocontrast agent–induced nephropathy.
Carbonic anhydrase inhibitors • Acetazolamide	No role in the prevention or treatment of ARF from any cause	Natriuretic response is not as profound.

ICU, intensive care unit.

guria accompanying ATN is due, at least in part, to tubular obstruction caused by debris including denuded epithelium. This tubular obstruction leads to back-leakage of glomerular filtrate into the renal interstitium, further perpetuating the renal injury, and to a further decrease in glomerular filtration rate. Loop diuretics may wash out the tubules, which are partially blocked with necrotic debris. Furthermore, because some studies have shown that oliguric ARF carries a worse prognosis than nonoliguric renal failure,[1,2] many clinicians treat oliguria with diuretics. This line of reasoning has led to the idea that maintaining a greater urinary flow in the setting of a renal insult is desirable. Loop diuretics also decrease the metabolic demand of the renal tubular cells with a corresponding reduction in local oxygen demand,[16,17] thereby theoretically protecting the renal tubular cell from ischemia. Inhibition of the Na^+-K^+-$2Cl^-$ cotransporter by loop diuretics reduces active sodium transport and thus also O_2 consumption and ischemic damage of the most vulnerable outer medullary tubular segments.[18,19] Furosemide indeed has been shown to decrease renal O_2 consumption and extraction in critically ill patients,[20] thereby conferring potential protection against ischemic or nephrotoxic injury. Loop diuretics also reduce renal vascular resistance and may therefore increase renal blood flow,[18] possibly by the inhibition of prostaglandin dehydrogenase. This inhibition leads to decreased degradation of prostaglandin E_2 (PGE_2), a potent renal vasodilator, and contributes to the increased renal blood flow. Another mechanism through which loop diuretics may potentially improve renal blood flow is inhibition of the tubuloglomerular feedback, which involves afferent vasoconstriction elicited by increased solute delivery at the macula densa.

All of these theoretical advantages of loop diuretics, along with the prospect of easier maintenance of fluid and electrolyte balance in patients with ARF, has prompted the use of these agents in the management of ARF. (An algorithm for protocols currently in use is presented in Fig. 78-1.) Unfortunately, despite these promising experimental results and theoretical advantages, clinical trials using diuretics have failed to show benefit, and some studies suggest harm.

Clinical Studies in Prevention

Radiocontrast agent administration is a leading cause of acute changes in renal function in hospitalized patients.[10] Pathogenesis of AKI in this setting is not completely

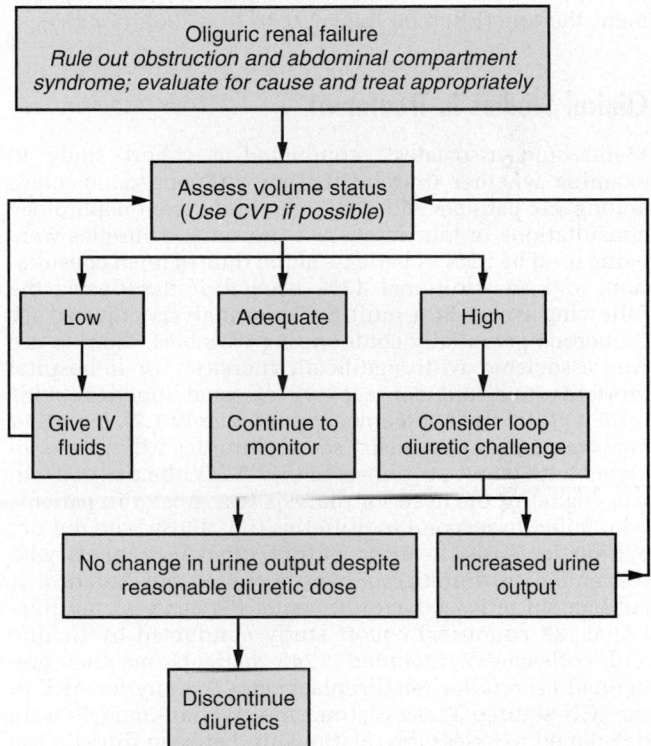

FIGURE 78-1. Use of diuretics in acute renal failure. CVP, central venous pressure; IV, intravenous.

understood (see Chapter 51). Animal studies have suggested that diuretics may be of benefit in this setting,[16] and four prospective randomized clinical studies have evaluated the potential protective effects of loop diuretics in patients recieving radiocontrast media.[10,21-23] Most of these studies compare fluids alone with the combination of fluids and furosemide. Reported postprocedural increases in serum creatinine were either not significantly different[22] or more pronounced[10,22,23] in the patients receiving furosemide. The incidence of *radiocontrast agent–induced nephropathy*, defined as an increase in serum creatinine level of 0.5 mg/dL or greater, was higher in the furosemide group[10] or was not affected.[21]

ARF is a common and serious complication in the setting of cardiac surgery.[24] Hager and coworkers compared low-dose furosemide (1 mg/hour) with placebo in 121 patients admitted to the ICU after major surgery (raising the question of whether this regimen constitutes true prevention or early treatment) and found no difference in postoperative serum creatinine or creatinine clearance.[25] The most convincing study was performed in 126 cardiac surgery patients, randomized to receive either furosemide (0.5 µg/kg per minute), dopamine, or placebo, started at anesthesia induction. Compared with placebo, furosemide resulted in a significantly higher urine output but also in a more pronounced postoperative increase of serum creatinine.[13] The investigators concluded that furosemide was "detrimental" and that their use was "not superior to placebo (isotonic saline) in protection of renal dysfunction after cardiac surgery."

A recent meta-analysis[26] and several small studies[10,13,25] could not find a beneficial effect of furosemide on in-hospital mortality rate (relative risk [RR], 2.33 [range, 0.75 to 7.25]; $n = 202$) or on the requirement for renal replacement therapy (RR, 4.06 [range, 0.46 to 35.96]; $n = 255$).

Clinical Studies in Treatment

Mehta and associates[14] conducted a cohort study to examine whether diuretic therapy influenced outcomes among 552 patients with ARF who underwent nephrology consultations in four intensive care units. Diuretics were being used by 59% of patients at the time of renal consultation, and an additional 12% used diuretics during the following week. In a multivariable analysis adjusted for numerous potentially confounding variables, diuretic use was associated with significant increases in in-hospital mortality rate and nonrecovery of renal function (odds ratio [OR] for each outcome, approximately 1.7). In further analyses using a propensity score, diuretics still were associated with worse outcomes. In this study, the risk of death was higher or the need for dialysis was greater in patients who failed to respond to diuretics (i.e., those who did not exhibit increases in urine output) than in patients who responded to diuretics or who received no diuretics. A subsequent prospective multicenter (54 centers), multinational (23 countries) cohort study conducted by Uchino and colleagues[15] included 1743 patients meeting predefined criteria for renal replacement therapy for ARF in the ICU setting. Three distinct multivariate models were developed to assess the relationship between diuretic use and subsequent mortality. None demonstrated a significant difference between subjects who did and those who did not receive diuretics. Evidence of benefit was lacking, however, and the point estimates from all three models were on the side of harm (OR for death, 1.2).

Randomized controlled clinical trials evaluating the effect of loop diuretics in patients with established AKI demonstrate an increase of urine output[27-32] without alteration in patient-centered clinical outcomes (e.g., death, renal recovery or need for dialysis). Older (not placebo-controlled) trials report contradictory effects on the duration of the oliguric period and the required number of dialysis sessions.[28,29,32] Recently, two prospective, randomized, placebo-controlled clinical trials have been performed. In the first study, 92 patients with serum creatinine levels above 2.0 mg/dL who were not obstructed, and who did not respond to fluid administration, received either furosemide, torsemide, or placebo. Although the loop diuretics increased urine output, no significant effect on renal recovery, need for dialysis, or mortality rate at day 21 was observed. Patients remaining oliguric had a worse

outcome but were sicker at randomization.[27] The second study included 330 patients requiring renal replacement therapy (mean serum creatinine level of 4.5 mg/dL or greater). The daily administration of 25 mg/kg of intravenous furosemide shortened the time to achieve a diuresis of 2 L/day but did not affect mortality rate, time on dialysis, and number of dialysis sessions or time to achieve a creatinine level below 2.6 mg/dL. Patients in the furosemide group had higher baseline creatinine, more diabetes, and more sepsis.[31] A meta-analysis of clinical studies on loop diuretics in the treatment of AKI[26] could not establish a reduction of in-hospital mortality rate (RR, 1.09 [range, 0.90 to 1.31]; $n = 474$)[27,29-32] or in the requirement for renal replacement therapy (RR, 0.94 [range, 0.71 to 1.26]; $n = 204$).[27,32] The number of dialysis sessions and the proportion of patients with persistent oliguria also were unaffected.[26]

Thus, although most clinical studies report an increased urine output with diuretics, evidence for a beneficial effect on renal function is lacking. Critically ill patients in the ICU who have ARF, however, often receive large volumes of fluids for provision of nutrition, vasopressors, and antibiotics. Diuresis using loop diuretics in such patients minimizes fluid overload and may make clinical management easier. Nevertheless, the preponderance of current evidence suggests that the use of diuretics should be limited to management of volume overload and not for AKI or oliguria per se.

Why Do Diuretics Not Work?

Several putative explanations have been put forward to account for the absence of a beneficial effect of loop diuretics on renal function in humans, despite experimental data suggesting such benefit. First, loop diuretics decrease effective circulating volume, either through prostaglandin-mediated venodilation[33] or through increased urinary losses, potentially resulting in reduced renal blood flow and decreased glomerular filtration rate. Diuresis may deceive physicians and prevent them from taking other necessary measures such as improving volume status or increasing cardiac output or perfusion pressure. Also, reductions in the effective arterial volume, as occurs in hypovolemia, low cardiac output, heart failure, or liver failure, for example, provoke stimulation of the adrenergic and renin-angiotensin systems. Both systems cause a preferential vasoconstriction in the renal cortex, resulting in corticomedullary redistribution of renal blood flow (redistributing the blood flow to the deeper salt-retaining nephrons and the vulnerable medulla).[34,35] The absence of a beneficial effect of loop diuretics on renal function also could be explained by an adverse effect on this intrarenal blood flow distribution and abolition of the beneficial tubuloglomerular feedback system (a protective adaptive mechanism that autoregulates the medullary oxygen balance).[36] This differential effect of furosemide on cortical and medullary blood flow may endanger the medullary oxygen balance, thereby worsening the renal injury. Using laser Doppler flowmetry, Dobrowolski and Sadowski[37] indeed demonstrated a more pronounced decrease in medullary compared with cortical blood flow after furosemide administration.

A second possible reason for lack of benefit of loop diuretics is that they may promote the aggregation of Tamm-Horsfall proteins in the tubular lumen,[38] so tubular obstruction may not be prevented or may even be worsened, contrary to popular belief. Because of tubular obstruction, loop diuretics may not reach their site of action (the luminal Na⁺-K⁺-2Cl⁻ cotransporter in the ascending loop of Henle) in sufficient concentration and thus may not be pharmacologically active in many patients.

Third, because the binding of loop diuretics to plasma proteins generally is high, proximal tubular secretion is the main route of urinary excretion. Hence, reductions in renal function or renal blood flow impair the delivery of loop diuretics into the tubular fluid. Tubular secretion is further impaired by increased concentrations of endogenous and exogenous organic acids that compete for the organic anion transporter in the proximal tubule. Moreover, hypoalbuminemia increases the volume of distribution of furosemide, augmenting the drug's extrarenal clearance, thereby decreasing urinary excretion. In other words, albumin is required as a vehicle to deliver the loop diuretic to the site of tubular secretion. On the other hand, albuminuria will result in urinary drug binding, decreasing the amount of free drug reaching its target.[12]

Finally, loop diuretics do not improve renal blood flow.[20,39-41] This lack of effect may be related to the inability of prostaglandins to counteract strong vasoconstrictive effects of the furosemide-induced stimulation of renin release. Loop diuretics stimulate renin release[42-44] through different mechanisms: a decrease in renal perfusion pressure, adrenergic stimulation, and a direct effect at the macula densa, where they diminish the NaCl transport–dependent renin-inhibitory signal to the granular cells.[45]

These physiological arguments and lack of clinical evidence challenge the wisdom of routine clinical use of diuretics in patients with or at risk for AKI. Therefore, the initial care of such patients should focus on optimizing systemic and renal perfusion, reversing underlying causes of renal injury, and correcting hypovolemia and electrolyte abnormalities. The decision to administer or remove fluids often is difficult for the intensivist, because both strategies can have detrimental consequences if pursued inappropriately.[1] Once AKI is established, volume resuscitation may be ineffective. "Optimal" hemodynamics in critically ill patients with or without AKI is still largely undefined, however.[46]

The Fluid and Catheter Treatment Trial (FACTT)[47] involving 1000 patients from the Acute Respiratory Distress Syndrome (ARDS) network provided important information concerning fluid management in ARDS. This trial tried to determine if conservative fluid management was better than liberal fluid management and if the pulmonary artery catheter was better than the central venous catheter. The prerandomization fluid balance data showed that these patients were already fluid positive: The mean total fluid balance was +2700 mL, mean central venous pressure (CVP) was 12.1 mm Hg, and mean pulmonary artery occlusive pressure (PAOP) was 15.6 mm Hg. Patients in whom fluids were restricted and diuretics administered to maintain a CVP less than 4 mm Hg or PAOP less than 8 mm Hg and who were in net even fluid balance (i.e., the conservative group) did better than patients in whom fluids were used to maintain CVP between 10 and 14 mm Hg or PAOP at 14 to 18 mm Hg or who were maintained in positive fluid balance (i.e., the liberal fluid group). Although the 60-day mortality rate was not affected by this fluid strategy, the conservative strategy was associated with significant improvement in lung function, decreased ICU stay and ventilator dependency. The conservative strategy also was associated with a small but significant increase in creatinine, blood urea nitrogen, and bicarbonate, but these changes were not associated with an increase in the use of dialysis to day 60 (10% of conservative group versus 14%

of liberal group; $P = .0642$). Although this study concluded "less is better" in ARDS, both study arms used explicit rules for fluid management. Parameters that specifically guided fluid therapy were: urine output (target greater than 0.5 mL/kg per hour), blood pressure (target of 60 mm Hg for the mean arterial pressure), and "tissue perfusion" (target cardiac index in the pulmonary artery catheter group was greater than 2.5 L/minute/m²; targets in the central venous catheter group included capillary refill and other physical signs). Although the CVP target in the conservative group was supposed to be less than 4 mm Hg, this was rarely achieved.

CONCLUSION

If volume status is monitored closely and optimized, use of diuretics can be useful in conversion of ARF to nonoliguric renal failure, possibly making patient management easier in the ICU. None of the available evidence, however, suggests that the use of loop diuretics in AKI reduces mortality, reduces the need for dialysis, reduces the number of dialysis sessions, reduces length of ICU or hospital stay, or increases the recovery of renal function. Moreover, limited data point to the potential for harm from use of these agents. Accordingly, diuretics should not be used in the prevention or treatment of AKI. The role of diuretics in management of volume overload in critically ill patients deserves further investigation.

Key Points

1. Although diuretic use is not associated with increased mortality, routine use of diuretics is not recommended for either prevention or management of acute kidney injury or oliguria and is associated with some harm.
2. If volume status is monitored closely, diuretics may be indicated in conversion of oliguric acute kidney injury to nonoliguric acute kidney injury only to facilitate fluid management.
3. Optimal physiological fluid resuscitation should be the prime goal in the initial management of acute kidney injury; if intravascular volume status is difficult to assess clinically, placement of a central venous line may be required for monitoring.

Key References

4. Kellum JA: Use of diuretics in the acute care setting. Kidney Int Suppl 1998;66:S67-S70.
10. Solomon R, Werner C, Mann D, et al: Effects of saline, mannitol, and furosemide to prevent acute decreases in renal function induced by radiocontrast agents. N Engl J Med 1994;331:1416-1420.
12. Shankar SS, Brater DC: Loop diuretics: From the Na-K-2Cl transporter to clinical use. Am J Physiol Renal Physiol 2003;284:F11-F21.
15. Uchino S, Doig GS, Bellomo R, et al: Diuretics and mortality in acute renal failure. Crit Care Med 2004;32:1669-1677.
26. Ho KM, Sheridan DJ: Meta-analysis of frusemide to prevent or treat acute renal failure. BMJ 2006;333:420.

See the companion Expert Consult website for the complete reference list.

CHAPTER 79

Dopamine Receptor Agonists

Paolo Calzavacca, Elisa Licari, and Rinaldo Bellomo

OBJECTIVES

This chapter will:
1. Present an overview of the physiology of dopamine receptor subfamilies.
2. Describe the effects of low-dose dopamine on the kidney.
3. Identify the side effects of low-dose dopamine.
4. Review current evidence concerning the pharmacology of fenoldopam and its potential clinical use.

Sodium and water handling by the kidney is a complex process that is not completely understood. Many mediators regulate it at endocrine, paracrine, and autocrine levels.[1] Such a complicated system is needed to maintain water balance and tonicity. Although many receptors at different levels of the nephron are involved in this process, sodium handling seems to be related mainly, at least in the renal proximal tubule, to the effect of two local hormonal subsystems: the dopaminergic system and the renin-angiotensin system.[2] These two hormonal systems are likely to have opposite effects on natriuresis. The renin-angiotensin system increases Na^+ transport across the cell from the lumen into the interstitial space in the renal proximal tubule through enhancement of the Na^+-H^+ exchanger-3 (NHE-3) and Na^+,K^+-ATPase activity, thereby decreasing natriuresis.[3] Conversely, dopamine inhibits NHE-3 and Na^+,K^+-ATPase activity, facilitating natriuresis.[4]

This chapter reviews the role of dopaminergic receptors in regulating natriuresis and summarizes the available evidence on two drugs that act as dopamine receptor agonists: dopamine and fenoldopam. The targets of these drugs are the dopamine receptors. Thus far, five different dopaminergic subtypes have been described, with different distribution and different actions in the glomerulus. Selective agonists and antagonists for each receptor (Table 79-1) are known; of the dopamine D_1-like receptor agonists, only fenoldopam has been introduced into clinical use.

A molecular-level description of dopamine receptors is presented next, followed by a review of the clinical evidence available on dopamine and fenoldopam use in the intensive care unit (ICU).

DOPAMINE RECEPTOR SUBTYPES

Dopamine is an endogenous catecholamine. It is present in the kidney, where it is produced at tubular and neuronal sites. It acts as an autocrine and paracrine substance[5] on at least five different dopamine receptor subtypes. Dopamine synthesis begins from L-dopa, which is taken up by the bloodstream by means of a sodium transporter in the apical membrane of proximal tubular cells.[6] L-Dopa is then decarboxylated to dopamine by aromatic amino acid decarboxylase. The activity of this enzyme is upregulated by a high-sodium diet and downregulated by a low-salt diet.[7] Essentially nothing is known about storage of dopamine in tubular cells. Renal catabolism is due mainly to catechol-O-methyl-transferase[8] and monoamine oxidase A.[9]

Dopamine behaves in a compartmentalized fashion within the kidney[10]: Outward transport of this substance from the proximal tubule cell is directed mainly to the tubular lumen. Dopamine production seems to rely chiefly on local stimuli. Sympathetic nerve activity has been shown to have no role in intrarenal dopamine production.[11,12]

Dopamine activity is mediated by different peripheral receptors. These receptors are all members of the G protein–coupled superfamily.[13] The five dopamine receptor subtypes that have been described so far are classified into two major groups, or subfamilies: the D_1-like family and the dopamine-2 (D_2)–like family.[13] D_1-like subfamily receptors stimulate adenylyl cyclase.[13] D_1 and D_5 (also known as D_{1A} and D_{1B} in rodents) are grouped in this subfamily. The other subfamily, D_2-like, comprises the D_2, D_3, and D_4 receptors. The common feature of the receptors of this second subfamily is the inhibition they exert on adenylyl cyclase.[13]

The localization and action of the five receptors are briefly reviewed next.

DOPAMINE RECEPTORS AND NATRIURESIS

The D_1-like family plays a major role in the regulation of sodium tubular reabsorption.[14] In conditions of normal or elevated sodium dietary intake, dopamine, on stimulating D_1 and D_5 receptors, promotes natriuresis. In a situation of normal sodium balance,[15,16] endogenous dopamine is a major physiological determinant of natriuresis, being responsible for up to 50% of basal sodium excretion.[1,17,18] This action is achieved by inhibition of sodium reabsorption in both proximal and distal tubules.[16,19,20] At the molecular level, natriuresis seems to be achieved through inhibition of Na^+,K^+-ATPase activity[4,14,21-25] throughout the whole nephron. Na^+-H^+ exchange inhibition[14,26] and Na^+-P_i (inorganic phosphate) cotransport activation[27] also contribute to the natriuresis due to dopamine.

D_1-like receptors have been localized to the medial layer of renal blood vessels and both the luminal and basolateral layers of the proximal convoluted tubule and the cortical collecting duct.[14] Interaction with angiotensin II type 1 receptors has been shown.[28] In experimental models,[19] the response to stimulation of D_1-like receptors is not sustained for more than 12 hours, suggesting that some form

TABLE 79-1

Agonist and Antagonist Substances for Dopamine Receptor Subtypes

RECEPTOR FAMILY	D₁-LIKE RECEPTORS	D₂-LIKE RECEPTORS		
Group-selective agonist	SKF 38393 Fenoldopam	Bromocriptine Apomorphine		
Group-selective antagonist	SCH 23390	YM-09151		

SUBTYPE	D_1	D_5	D_2	D_3	D_4
Subtype-selective agonist	None	None	U91356A PHNO	Quineralone Pramixole PD128907 7-OH-DPAT	N-Propyl-noramorphine PD-1680777
Subtype-selective antagonist	None	None	L741,626 Raclopride	Nafadotride U-99194A SB-277011	Mesoridazine L-745, L-879 NGD-94 RBI-257 U-101958
Predominant effect	↑ cAMP	↑ cAMP	↓ cAMP and Ca^{2+} and K^+ channel	↓ cAMP and Ca^{2+} and K^+ channel	↓ cAMP and Ca^{2+} and K^+ channel

cAMP, cyclic adenosine monophosphate.

of downregulation or tachyphylaxis of D_1 receptors must exist for protracted stimulation.

The D_2-like family action is less well known. D_2-like family receptors probably interact with D_1-like family receptors modulating Na^+,K^+-ATPase, Na^+-H^+ exchange, and Na^+-P_i cotransport[2,29,30] function. D_2-like receptors have been identified presynaptically on sympathetic nerve terminals, in the adventitia of the renal vasculature, throughout the glomerulus,[14,19] and on the basolateral aspect of the cortical collecting duct.[31-35]

DOPAMINE AGONIST RECEPTORS IN CLINICAL USE

Of the many different agonists and antagonists of dopamine receptors (see Table 79-1), only two have been introduced into clinical use so far: dopamine and fenoldopam. Fenoldopam is a D_1-like receptor selective agonist, whereas dopamine acts on all receptor subtypes.

Dopamine

Reports in 1963 and 1964[36,37] were the first to describe the use of low-dose dopamine ("renal dopamine") to increase renal blood flow in both humans and animals and to sustain diuresis and natriuresis. Since then, many published studies have attempted to demonstrate that low-dose dopamine can increase renal blood flow[38-41] and that this drug can be associated with a degree of prevention of the development of acute kidney injury (AKI) and with a better outcome in patients with AKI as a result of its ability to increase diuresis and natriuresis (see previous discussion).

Unfortunately, many of the studies performed in the 1970s and 1980s looking at clinical outcomes were uncontrolled or underpowered. In the 1990s, published editorials advocated large RCTs to determine whether low-dose dopamine is indeed beneficial in the clinical setting.[42]

Many authors began discouraging its use because of lack of supportive evidence.[43-45]

Since 2000, four meta-analyses,[46-49] several reviews,[50-52] and the first and, so far, the only large multicenter, double-blind, placebo-controlled RCT[53] have been published. Table 79-2 shows the design of the meta-analyses and their major findings. Extrapolation from the findings of the meta-analyses and the large RCT points to the following conclusions:

- A majority of studies in humans are underpowered.
- Only two randomized controlled trials[53,54] have been performed, and of these, only one is large and multicentric and compares low-dose dopamine with placebo.
- Evidence that low-dose dopamine can reduce mortality or prevent renal dysfunction is lacking.
- If low-dose dopamine provides any beneficial effect, it consists of an increase in urine output. This effect, however, is not sustained.
- Concerns exist regarding the safety of low-dose dopamine.

The concerns about the predictability of action and the safety of low-dose dopamine are related to the following findings:

1. *Use of low-dose dopamine does not lead to predictable dopamine levels in the critically ill.* The concept of low-dose probably is invalid in critically ill patients, because a great interindividual variation has been shown in dopamine clearance and plasma dopamine levels[55,56] among patients in an ICU setting.
2. *Increased plasma renin activity counteracts the effects of dopamine in the critically ill.* Marik[57] showed a significant inverse correlation between plasma renin activity and increased urine output. It was concluded that the response to renal dopamine in critically ill patients probably was negated in those with high plasma renin activity.
3. *Tachyphylaxis exists in the effect of dopamine on renal blood flow in severe sepsis.* Although some studies have shown a transient improvement in renal function due to low-dose dopamine, in all of these studies, tolerance has been shown to occur after 2 to 48 hours.[58,59] This tolerance has been attributed to

TABLE 79-2

Major Trials and Meta-analyses of Low-Dose Dopamine

STUDY	STUDY DESIGN	MAJOR FINDING(S)	RENAL EFFECT(S)
ANZICS Clinical Trials Group[53]	Randomized controlled, double-blind trial in 328 patients with 2 or more criteria for SIRS and evidence of early renal dysfunction	No difference between treatment group and control group in peak levels of and change in creatinine, need for RRT, hospital and ICU length of stay, number of deaths	No difference
Kellum and Decker, 2001[46]	Screening of 58 studies (comprising 2149 patients); outcomes reported in 24 studies (in 1019 patients); included in the analysis of 17 RCTs (854 patients)	Use of LDD for treatment or prevention of AKI cannot be justified on the basis of evidence and should be eliminated from routine clinical practice.	No renoprotective effect
Marik, 2002[47]	Screening of 122 studies; 21 RCTs identified; included in the analysis of 15 RCTs (970 patients)	No significant difference was found between the absolute change in serum creatinine and the incidence of AKI.	No renoprotective effect
Friedrich et al, 2005[48]	61 RCTs identified (3359 patients)	LDD offers transient (24-hour) improvement in urine output, but good evidence for clinical benefit in patients with or at risk for AKI is lacking.	No renoprotective effect
Zacharias et al, 2005[49]	37 RCTs (1227 patients) studying renal protection (dopamine and fenoldopam, diuretics, hydration, ACE inhibitors, calcium channel blockers) in patients undergoing surgery	No reliable evidence is available suggesting that interventions during surgery can protect the kidneys from damage.	No renoprotective effect in the perioperative period for all strategies used thus far

ACE, angiotensin-converting enzyme; AKI, acute kidney injury; ICU, intensive care unit; LDD, low-dose dopamine; RCT, randomized controlled trial; RRT, renal replacement therapy; SIRS, systemic inflammatory response syndrome.

desensitization or downregulation of low-dose dopamine receptors.[58-60]

4. *Medullary dysoxia is a "demand-side" problem, not a renal blood flow problem.* The renal medulla has an oxygen extraction efficiency that approaches 90%.[61,62] Dopamine can increase medullary oxygen demand,[63] thereby increasing the delivery of solute load to the distal tubular cells by inhibition of proximal solute reabsorption.

5. *Increasing diuresis seems to have no apparent benefit on important clinical outcomes.*[48,53,58]

6. *Low-dose dopamine blunts ventilatory drive.* Dopamine has been shown both to reduce sensitivity of the fast chemoreflex loop to carbon dioxide[64,65] and to depress hypoxic ventilatory responses.[66] It also increases pulmonary shunt fraction.[67]

7. *Dopamine may have proarrhythmic and ischemic effects.* Although dopamine's potential to produce tachycardia and arrhythmic events is a well-known side effect,[68-70] the large aforementioned RCT[53] failed to demonstrate any significant difference in the incidence of arrhythmia between the placebo and the dopamine groups.

8. *Low-dose dopamine harms the splanchnic circulation in the critically ill.* Many studies have demonstrated in both animals and humans that dopamine increases splanchnic blood flow.[71-73] Nevertheless, dopamine paradoxically increases gastrointestinal mucosal ischemia. This effect, in turn, may cause translocation of endotoxin and decreased hepatic clearance of pro-inflammatory cytokines.

9. *Low-dose dopamine harms the endocrine system.* Dopamine is an endogenous hormone. When low-dose dopamine infusion is instituted, a 40- to 100-fold

higher plasma level than normal is achieved.[74] Such a high level of dopamine has been shown to interact with many hormonal systems. In particular, it can cause hypopituitarism,[75] leading to additional hormonal effects:

- Lower prolactin levels,[76] which in turn can affect the immune system[77]
- Lower growth hormone,[76,78] which in turn can cause a negative nitrogen balance
- Decreased luteinizing hormone[79]
- Decreased secretion of thyrotropin,[80] thereby aggravating the sick euthyroid syndrome in critical illness

10. *Low-dose dopamine harms the immunologic system in the critically ill.* Dopamine both directly decreases T cell function and responsiveness[81] and indirectly affects these attributes through a decrease in prolactin.[76]

In light of the absence of demonstrable advantage and some doubts and concerns about safety, use of low-dose dopamine should now be avoided.

Fenoldopam

Fenoldopam mesylate is the only drug with selective action on dopamine receptors that has been introduced into clinical practice. Fenoldopam is a selective D_1-like family receptor agonist (see earlier) with no effect on D_2-like family receptors. It produces systemic and renal vasodilation.[82-84] Recently, it also has been shown to increase natriuresis by means of an angiotensin type 2 receptor mechanism.[2] Fenoldopam decreases systemic vascular resistance and also increases renal blood flow[85,86] in healthy

TABLE 79-3

Randomized Controlled Trials of Fenoldopam

CLINICAL ENVIRONMENT	STUDY	STUDY DESIGN	STUDY INTERVENTION	MAJOR FINDING(S)
Major surgery	Halpenny et al, 2001[88]	31 patients undergoing cardiac surgery; single-center RCT	Fenoldopam 0.1 µg/kg/min versus placebo	Fenoldopam showed a renoprotective effect in the placebo but not the fenoldopam group; mean (SD) creatinine clearance decreased after separation from cardiopulmonary bypass, from 107 (36) to 71 (22) mL/min ($P < .01$) and from 107 (36) to 79 (26) mL/min ($P < .01$) for the 0- to 4-hr and 4- to 8-hr intervals after cardiopulmonary bypass, respectively.
	Halpenny et al, 2002[89]	28 patients undergoing infrarenal aortic surgery; double-blind RCT	Fenoldopam 0.1 µg/kg/min versus placebo	Fenoldopam showed a renoprotective effect without hemodynamic instability. After aortic cross-clamping, creatinine clearance significantly decreased from 83 ± 20 to 42 ± 29 mL/min in placebo group but not in fenoldopam group.
	Caimmi et al, 2003[91]	160 patients with CKD undergoing cardiac surgery; single-center, unblinded RCT	Fenoldopam 0.1 to 0.3 µg/kg/min (group B) versus standard management (group A)	Fenoldopam was effective in protecting kidney. *Group B*: preoperative serum creatinine 1.82 ± 0.2 versus 1.43 ± 0.73 mg/dL postoperatively ($P < .001$), preoperative creatinine clearance 51.34 ± 22.26 versus 67.14 ± 18.55 mL/min postoperatively ($P < .001$). *Group A*: preoperative serum creatinine 1.78 ± 0.3 versus postoperative 1.94 ± 0.41 ($P = .02$) and preoperative creatinine clearance 50.3 ± 21 versus postoperative 44.9 ± 9.9 mL/min ($P - .02$).
	Bove et al, 2005[90]	80 patients undergoing cardiac surgery with increased risk for AKI; single-center, double-blind RCT	Fenoldopam 0.05 µg/kg/min versus LDD (dopamine 2.5 µg/kg/min) after induction for first 24 postoperative hours	No difference in clinical outcome was observed between the two groups. Incidence of intraoperative hypotension was higher in the fenoldopam group.
Radiocontrast agent–induced nephropathy	Stone et al, 2003[92]	Double-blind, multicenter RCT in 315 patients with creatinine clearance <60 mL/min	Prehydration; fenoldopam 0.05 µg/kg/min versus placebo (saline 0.45%) starting 1 hour before and continuing for 12 hours after procedure	No difference was observed in clinical outcome or in the incidence of radiocontrast-induced nephropathy. A trend toward hypotension and tachycardia was noted in the fenoldopam group.
ICU	Morelli et al, 2005[97]	Double-blind, multicenter RCT in 300 ICU septic patients with normal renal function (preventive treatment)	Fenoldopam (group F) 0.09 µg/kg/min versus placebo (group P) infusion for the period in ICU	Lower incidence of AKI was found in the F group. No complications of fenoldopam infusion were reported.
	Tumlin et al, 2005[96]	Double-blind multicenter RCT, 155 ICU patients with early renal dysfunction	Fenoldopam (group F) 0.05 to 0.02 µg/kg/min versus placebo (group P, saline 0.45%) infusion for 72 hours	Fenoldopam failed to decrease death or dialysis therapy; subgroup analysis in nondiabetic patiens and post cardiovascular surgery showed a better outcome for group F.
	Brienza et al, 2006[94]	Unblinded multicenter RCT in 100 ICU patients with early renal dysfunction	LDD (dopamine 2 µg/kg/min): group D; or fenoldopam (0.1 µg/kg/min): group F; for 4 days	Fenoldopam does not cause hemodynamic impairment. Reduction in creatinine values in group F was more than in group D from day 2 to day 4; no difference was noted in urine output after day 1 (day 1 output was higher in group D).

AKI, acute kidney injury; CKD, chronic kidney disease; ICU, intensive care unit; LLD, low-dose dopamine; RCT, randomized controlled trial; SD, standard deviation.

volunteers in a dose-dependent manner, with the greatest effect with use of infusion rates in the range of 0.03 and 0.1 µg/kg per minute.[87] In this range, no concomitant significant reduction in systemic blood pressure has been shown.

During the past decade, fenoldopam has been studied in many different situations associated with renal dysfunction or as a prophylactic nephroprotective drug in different clinical settings (Table 79-3).[88-92] Unfortunately, thus far, only underpowered studies have been performed. Recently, Landoni and associates published a meta-analysis[93] in which a total of 16 RCTs (in a total of 1290 patients) in different clinical settings were analyzed. These investigators concluded that fenoldopam may reduce the need for renal replacement therapy and mortality rate in patients with AKI. Unfortunately, the meta-analysis included both RCTs comparing fenoldopam with placebo and RCTs comparing fenoldopam with other drugs. The investigators noted that all of the studies available so far are underpowered. Moreover, this meta-analysis included data on a comparison of the use of fenoldopam for treatment or prevention of AKI in different patient populations (e.g., ICU patients, postoperative patients, transplant recipients). The pathogenesis of AKI is poorly understood, but an easy comparison in such a wide range of clinical situations is unlikely. Moreover, concerns can be raised regarding the validity of comparing a treatment with a specific drug with its use as an option to prevent that derangement. Indeed, another recent meta-analysis[49] on perioperative use of renal-protective strategies failed to show any advantage with the use of fenoldopam.

Only four RCTs have been performed in critically ill patients only.[94-97] Of these four RCTs, one compared fenoldopam with low-dose dopamine in 100 patients[94] with early renal dysfunction in the ICU setting and was unblinded; one studied the effect of fenoldopam on gastric mucosal perfusion in 40[95] patients, also in the ICU. Only two studies were double-blind, placebo-controlled RCTs.[96,97] The first of these, by Tumlin and colleagues,[96] enrolled 160 patients with early acute tubular necrosis, and the second,[97] by Morelli and coworkers, enrolled 300 patients with sepsis; both used fenoldopam as a protective prophylactic drug.

In the study by Tumlin and colleagues,[96] fenoldopam failed to reduce the incidence of death or dialysis therapy in ICU patients with an early (before 24 hours) diagnosis of acute tubular necrosis. The study population included 160 patients in a mixed medical-surgical ICU, of whom nearly 60% were postoperative. The infusion dosage for fenoldopam ranged from 0.05 to 0.2 µg/kg per minute; the placebo group received 0.45% saline. The infusion lasted 72 hours. Although the study failed to show any difference in the two groups, a trend to a lower increase in serum creatine in the fenoldopam group was found, raising the possibility that the study might have been underpowered. Moreover, in a post-hoc subgroup analysis, a better outcome was found in the fenoldopam group for patients without diabetes and in post–cardiac surgery patients. In this study, the infusion of fenoldopam was well tolerated by the patients.

On the other hand, Morelli and coworkers[97] found that fenoldopam, administered at an infusion rate of 0.09 µg/kg per minute, showed a significant beneficial effect in septic patients for the prevention of AKI. This study enrolled 300 patients in the ICU setting. Findings included a reduction in the incidence of AKI in the fenoldopam group, as well as a trend toward a reduction in severe AKI and in ICU and hospital length of stay. An effect of fenoldopam different from the increase in renal blood flow that affected the outcome was suggested; in this context, a possible anti-inflammatory effect of fenoldopam has been proposed. Of interest, some evidence is available on the interaction of fenoldopam with inducible nitric oxide synthase.[98,99] Moreover, fenoldopam recently was shown in an animal model to inhibit the nuclear translocation of nuclear factor-κB,[100] the cellular promoter of cytokine production.

CONCLUSION

The available evidence suggests that the clinical use of fenoldopam may be indicated in selected cases[101] after careful consideration of the possible benefits and the potential side effects (hypotension) of this drug. The effect of fenoldopam may be independent of its dopaminergic stimulation. Further investigation in a large, multicenter RCT is warranted.

Key Points

1. Dopamine receptors have been extensively studied. Although much information is available from animal studies on the effect of different receptors on renal blood flow regulation and natriuresis, the applicability of these findings to humans in the clinical setting is not clear.
2. Dopamine at low doses should not be used in an attempt to prevent or treat acute kidney injury, because the evidence is against its utility and some concerns exist about its safety.[102]
3. Fenoldopam is a complex drug with effects on dopaminergic receptors, nitric oxide synthase, and nuclear factor-κB.
4. The prophylactic use of fenoldopam for nephroprotection in sepsis deserves further investigation; clinical use for this indication should await evidence from suitably powered clinical studies.

Key References

2. Jones D, Bellomo R: Renal-dose dopamine: From hypothesis to paradigm to dogma to myth and, finally, superstition? J Intensive Care Med 2005;20:199-211.
53. The Australian and New Zealand Intensive Care Society (ANZICS) Clinical Trials Group: A multicenter, randomised, double-blind, placebo-controlled trial of low dose dopamine in patients with early renal dysfunction. Lancet 2000;356: 2139-2143.
94. Brienza N, Malcangi V, Dalfino L, et al: A comparison between fenoldopam and low-dose dopamine in early renal dysfunction of critically ill patients. Crit Care Med 2006;34:707-714.
95. Morelli A, Rocco M, Conti G, et al: Effects of short-term fenoldopam infusion on gastric mucosal blood flow in septic shock. Anesthesiology 2004;101:576-582.
96. Morelli A, Ricci Z, Bellomo R, et al: Prophylactic fenoldopam for renal protection in sepsis: A randomised, double-blind, placebo-controlled pilot trial. Crit Care Med 2005;33:2451-2456.

See the companion Expert Consult website for the complete reference list.

Atrial Natriuretic Peptide in Acute Renal Failure

Sven-Erik Ricksten and Kristina Swärd

OBJECTIVES

This chapter will:
1. Review the effects of atrial natriuretic peptide on renal hemodynamics and function in humans.
2. Describe the effects of atrial natriuretic peptide on renal blood flow, glomerular filtration rate, and renal oxygen consumption in patients with normal renal function.
3. Describe the effects of atrial natriuretic peptide on renal blood flow and glomerular filtration rate in patients with ischemic acute renal failure.
4. Describe the renal vasodilator effects of atrial natriuretic peptide during long-term infusion in clinical ischemic acute renal failure.
5. Describe the effects of long-term infusion of atrial natriuretic peptide on renal outcome in clinical ischemic acute renal failure.

In 1956, Bruno Kisch[1] published electron microscopic investigations demonstrating that guinea pig atrial cardiocytes contained numerous small electron-dense granules. In the same year, Henry and colleagues found that distention of the left atrium in anesthetized dogs resulted in increased urine flow.[2] Other morphological studies indicated that the atrial granules contained polypeptide hormones. In 1964, Jamieson and Palade[3] described granules in the human atria similar to those found by Kisch. It was not until 1981 that de Bold and coworkers[4] demonstrated a "rapid and potent natriuretic response to intravenous injection of atrial myocardial extract in rats." These investigators observed a 30-fold increase in sodium and chloride excretion, with a 10-fold increase in urine volume. Two years later, Flynn and colleagues[5] identified the amino acid structure of the atrial natriuretic factor from rat atrial muscle as a 28-amino-acid peptide with diuretic and natriuretic activity, which was named *atrial natriuretic peptide* (ANP). This sequence is highly homologous among species. In 1984, Kangawa and Matsuo described the complete amino acid sequence of human ANP.[6]

The natriuretic peptide system is primarily an endocrine system that maintains fluid and pressure homeostasis by modulating cardiac and renal function. ANP and brain natriuretic peptide (BNP) are released continuously from the heart, and the rate of release increases in response to atrial and ventricular stretch, respectively, and will cause vasodilation in both the arterial and the venous systems, natriuresis, and inhibition of the sympathetic nervous system and the renin-angiotensin-aldosterone axis.[7] The natriuretic peptides are ligands to high-affinity natriuretic peptide receptors, and the vasodilatory action of ANP is mediated by cellular accumulation of cyclic guanosine monophosphate (cGMP) through the activation of membrane-bound particulate guanylyl cyclase.[7]

RENAL ACTIONS OF ATRIAL NATRIURETIC PEPTIDE IN HUMANS

Renal Blood Flow

In humans, variable effects of ANP on renal blood flow have been demonstrated. This variability is not surprising because the dilatory effects of ANP on venous capacitance vessels and resistance vessels may to a variable degree decrease cardiac output and systemic vascular resistance, with a consequent fall in renal perfusion pressure, which in turn may modify a potential renal vasodilatory effect of ANP. The effects of ANP on renal hemodynamics and function in humans have been studied both in healthy volunteers[8-11] and in patients with normal renal function after cardiovascular surgery.[12-14] Investigators reported that no change[8,12,13] or a decrease[9-11,14] in renal blood flow occurred when plasma levels of ANP were increased 5- to 10-fold by ANP infusion at a rate of 25 to 75 ng/kg per minute. In a majority of these studies, renal vascular resistance was calculated and was found not to change after ANP infusion[12-14]; one study found an increase in renal vascular resistance with ANP infusion.[11]

Glomerular Filtration Rate

In healthy volunteers and in post–cardiovascular surgery patients with normal renal function, a majority of studies have shown that the natriuretic response to ANP is associated with an increase in glomerular filtration rate.[8,11-14] At the infusion rates mentioned earlier, glomerular filtration rate and filtration fraction increased by 5% to 35% and 20% to 60%, respectively.[8,11-14] Taken together, these data suggest that in humans with normal renal function, ANP causes a decrease in preglomerular vascular resistance and an increase in postglomerular vascular resistance. These findings in humans are in line with results from previous animal studies showing that ANP dilates preglomerular (afferent) arterioles and constricts postglomerular (efferent) arterioles, leading to increased hydraulic pressure within glomerular capillaries.[15]

Tubular Effects of Atrial Natriuretic Peptide

The increase in glomerular filtration rate alone cannot account for the pronounced natriuresis and diuresis induced by ANP in humans. The finding that ANP increases fractional sodium excretion by 50% to 200% in healthy volunteers and in patients who have just undergone cardiovascular surgery strongly suggests that ANP also directly alters tubular sodium and water reabsorption.[8,9,11-14] Extensive evidence from experimental studies indicates that ANP inhibits sodium transport in the inner medullary collecting duct by means of binding to natriuretic receptors and production of cGMP, and that ANP exerts an inhibitory action on angiotensin II–induced antinatriuresis at the proximal tubules.[7] Furthermore, ANP inhibits tubular actions of arginine, vasopressin, and aldosterone.[7]

Effects of Atrial Natriuretic Peptide on Renal Oxygen Consumption

It is well known that tubular sodium reabsorption is a major determinant of renal oxygen consumption (RVO_2).[16] A recent study showed a positive correlation between tubular reabsorption and RVO_2 in humans, with a positive correlation between glomerular filtration rate and both tubular sodium reabsorption and RVO_2.[14] In other words, an increase in glomerular filtration rate will increase the tubular sodium load, which in turn will increase tubular sodium reabsorption and RVO_2. ANP promotes a preglomerular vasodilatation and postglomerular vasoconstriction, thereby increasing glomerular filtration rate, which would increase the renal oxygen demand. On the other hand, experimental data suggest that ANP inhibits tubular sodium reabsorption in the medullary collecting duct, which would decrease RVO_2.[17] In patients with cirrhosis and treatment-refractory ascites, human ANP (hANP) induces an increase in glomerular filtration rate, which is accompanied by a natriuresis and a decrease in RVO_2, attributable to an inhibitory effect of hANP on the elevated levels of antinatriuretic substances in this condition.[18] Conversely, Swärd and associates demonstrated that the ANP-induced increase in glomerular filtration rate and filtration fraction in postoperative patients with normal renal function was accompanied by a 26% increase in RVO_2, in contrast with furosemide, which decreased RVO_2 by 23%.[14] Thus, the potential energy-conserving, tubular effect of ANP was offset by the increase in glomerular filtration rate and tubular sodium reabsorption in patients with normal renal function.

EFFECTS OF ATRIAL NATRIURETIC PEPTIDE IN ISCHEMIC ACUTE RENAL FAILURE

Acute renal failure (ARF) occurring after cardiovascular surgery is associated with significant morbidity and mortality.[19] The pathogenesis of postoperative ARF is believed to predominantly involve renal hypoperfusion and ischemia, particularly of the renal medulla.[20,21] The renal medullary concentrating mechanism, requiring large amounts of oxygen, in combination with the relatively low medullary blood flow, renders the renal medulla hypoxic, with already low tissue PO_2 levels under normal conditions.[20] The renal medulla, particularly the outer portion, is therefore sensitive to acute renal ischemia. A logical approach in the management of clinical ischemic ARF, therefore, would be to improve the renal oxygen supply-demand relationship by augmenting renal blood flow or to reduce oxygen consumption of the renal medulla.

In 1986, Schafferhans and coworkers were the first to demonstrate that ANP improves glomerular filtration rate after ischemic injury in a model of norepinephrine-induced ARF in rats.[22] Later studies reported similar findings using different experimental models of ARF.[23] A recently published study in dogs showed that ANP infusion improved renal blood flow and creatinine clearance after suprarenal abdominal aortic cross-clamping, compared with the control group.[24]

In clinical ARF, Rahman and associates studied the effects of intrarenal ($n = 10$) or intravenous ($n = 20$) infusion of ANP versus diuretics ($n = 23$) on creatinine clearance in patients with ARF caused by various disorders.[25] These investigators demonstrated that the short-term (24-hour) infusion of ANP improved creatinine clearance by 70% and reduced the need for dialysis. In a pharmacodynamic dose-finding study, Valsson and colleagues studied 12 patients with early ischemic ARF caused by postcardiac surgical heart failure, requiring inotropic and vasoactive agents and intra-aortic balloon counterpulsation.[26] The infusion of ANP at a rate of 50 to 100 ng/kg per minute caused a 30% to 40% increase in renal blood flow and glomerular filtration rate, with no change in filtration fraction, and a 30% reduction in renal vascular resistance (Fig. 80-1). In other words, in ischemic ARF, ANP preferentially induces a reduction in preglomerular resistance, as also reflected by a minimal change in the filtration fraction, in contrast with the effects of ANP in patients with normal renal function. The ANP-induced increase in glomerular filtration rate in these patients would increase RVO_2, which would potentially be balanced by the proportional increase in renal blood flow, due to the dilation of the afferent arterioles. The effects of ANP on RVO_2 and the renal oxygen supply-demand relationship in patients with ischemic ARF remain, however, to be determined.

ARE THE RENAL VASODILATOR EFFECTS OF ATRIAL NATRIURETIC PEPTIDE MAINTAINED DURING LONG-TERM INFUSION IN CLINICAL ISCHEMIC ACUTE RENAL FAILURE?

The renal vasodilatory effect of ANP on the afferent arterioles in clinical ischemic ARF was demonstrated during a short-term infusion (over hours) of ANP. Swärd and coworkers studied the effects of ANP withdrawal on renal blood flow and glomerular filtration rate after long-term treatment (for 2 to 9 days) of patients with ischemic ARF after complicated cardiac surgery, requiring inotropic and vasoactive agents and intra-aortic balloon counterpulsation.[27] Discontinuation of a long-term infusion of ANP at a rate of 50 ng/kg per minute substantially reduced glomerular filtration rate (−32%) and renal blood flow (−31%) and increased renal vascular resistance (+93%). In this situation, the reinstitution of ANP increased renal blood flow and glomerular filtration rate by 30% to 40% and reduced renal vascular resistance by 40%, with no change in filtration fraction. These effects of ANP were almost identical to those described by Valsson and colleagues[26] during acute administration in a similar group of patients and further support the findings of an ANP-induced renal vasodilation of the afferent arterioles. Thus, the acute renal vasodilatory effects of ANP are maintained during long-term infusion, suggesting that tachyphylaxis in response

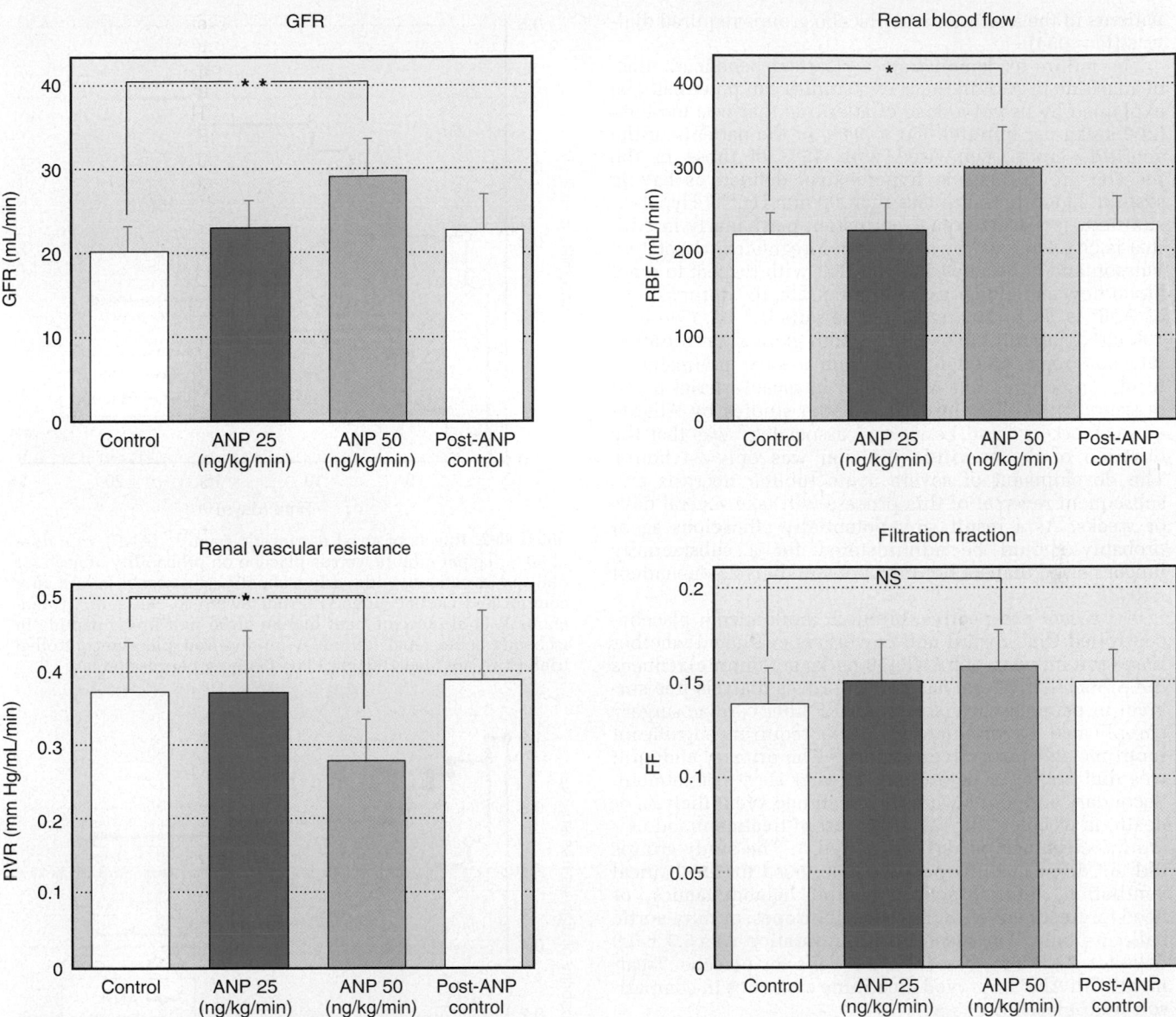

FIGURE 80-1. Renal effects of atrial natriuretic peptide (ANP) infusion, in doses of 25 and 50 ng/kg per minute, in patients with early ischemic acute renal failure after complicated cardiac surgery. ANP induced a renal vasodilatation preferentially of the afferent arterioles, because both glomerular filtration rate (GFR) and renal blood flow (RBF) increased with no change in filtration fraction (FF). NS, not significant. (Modified from Valsson F, Ricksten SE, Hedner T, Lundin S: Effects of atrial natriuretic peptide on acute renal impairment in patients with heart failure after cardiac surgery. Intensive Care Med 1996;22:230-236, by permission.)

to ANP does not develop during a prolonged administration of ANP. This is in striking contrast with the recently described renal tolerance to low-dose dopamine in patients with early acute renal dysfunction in the ICU setting.[28]

EFFECTS OF LONG-TERM INFUSION OF ATRIAL NATRIURETIC PEPTIDE ON RENAL OUTCOME IN CLINICAL ISCHEMIC ACUTE RENAL FAILURE

Despite encouraging results relating to the beneficial effects of ANP in experimental ARF, two recent multi-center, prospective, randomized trials in patients with ARF of various causes treated with the ANP analogue anaritide[29,30] failed to show any significant beneficial effect on renal outcome. Anaritide did not reduce the need for dialysis or improve dialysis-free survival in this heterogeneous group of patients with ARF.[29] In a subgroup of patients with oliguria, however, anaritide administration was associated with an improvement in dialysis-free survival rates from 8% in the placebo group to 27% in the anaritide group.[29] The same researchers then conducted a prospective, randomized, double-blind, placebo-controlled study of anaritide in patients with oliguric ARF of various causes.[30] In this later study, no difference in the primary outcome variable, dialysis-free survival through day 21, was observed between the two groups. At day 14 of the study, however, 64% and 77%, respectively, of the patients in the anaritide and placebo groups required dialysis ($P = .054$).

The failure to demonstrate a clear-cut beneficial effect of anaritide in ARF in these two studies can potentially be explained by use of a dose of anaritide that was too high (200 ng/kg per minute). Up to 94% of the patients in the anaritide group, compared with 45% of those in the placebo group, became hypotensive, defined as having systolic blood pressure less than 90 mm Hg.[29,30] Hypotension may jeopardize renal perfusion, particularly in ARF that is characterized by a loss of autoregulatory capacity.[31] Valsson and colleagues showed that with respect to renal blood flow and glomerular filtration rate, the optimal dose of ANP is 50 to 100 ng/kg per minute.[12,26] At a dose of 100 ng/kg per minute or higher, both glomerular filtration rate and renal blood flow decline toward pretreatment levels, in conjunction with a fall in mean arterial blood pressure.[12] Another limitation in the studies by Allgren and coworkers[29] and Lewis and associates[30] was that the duration of the anaritide infusion was only 24 hours. The development of severe acute tubular necrosis and subsequent reversal of this process will take several days or weeks. As a result, any potentially efficacious agent probably should be administered for a substantially longer period than 24 hours to prevent dialysis-dependent ARF.

In a recent prospective, blinded, randomized, placebo-controlled trial, Swärd and coworkers evaluated whether long-term infusion of hANP (50 ng/kg per minute) reduces the probability of dialysis and improves dialysis-free survival in patients with ischemic ARF after cardiac surgery complicated by circulatory shock, requiring significant inotropic and vasoactive support.[32] The primary endpoint was dialysis on or before day 21 after start of treatment. Secondary endpoints were the combined event dialysis or death on or before day 21 after start of treatment and creatinine clearance on days 1, 2, and 3. The study groups did not differ in intraoperative data, need for mechanical ventilation, renal function, central hemodynamics, or need for treatment with diuretics, inotropes, or intra-aortic balloon pump. The mean infusion duration was 5.3 ± 0.8 days for ANP and was 4.3 ± 0.7 days for placebo. Treatment with ANP improved creatinine clearance in comparison with placebo.

The Kaplan-Meier estimates of the probability of dialysis and dialysis-free survival are shown in Figures 80-2 and 80-3, respectively. Six (21%) patients in the ANP group, compared with 13 (47%) in the placebo group, needed dialysis before or at day 21 (hazard ratio, 0.28 [95% CI, 0.10 to 0.73]; $P = .009$). Eight (28%) patients in the ANP group, compared with 17 (53%) in the placebo group, suffered from the combined endpoint dialysis or death before or at day 21 (hazard ratio, 0.35 [95% CI, 0.14 to 0.82]; $P = .017$). Administration of ANP was not stopped prematurely in any of the patients, and no differences were observed between groups with respect to the incidence of hypotension during the first 24 hours after start of treatment or the number of hypotensive episodes. Creatinine clearance was approximately 30 mL/minute at patient enrollment in the study by Sward and coworkers. Thus, renal dysfunction was much less severe than in the studies by Allgren and coworkers[29] and Lewis and associates,[30] suggesting that the beneficial effects of ANP on renal function and outcome are seen in patients with moderately depressed early renal dysfunction.

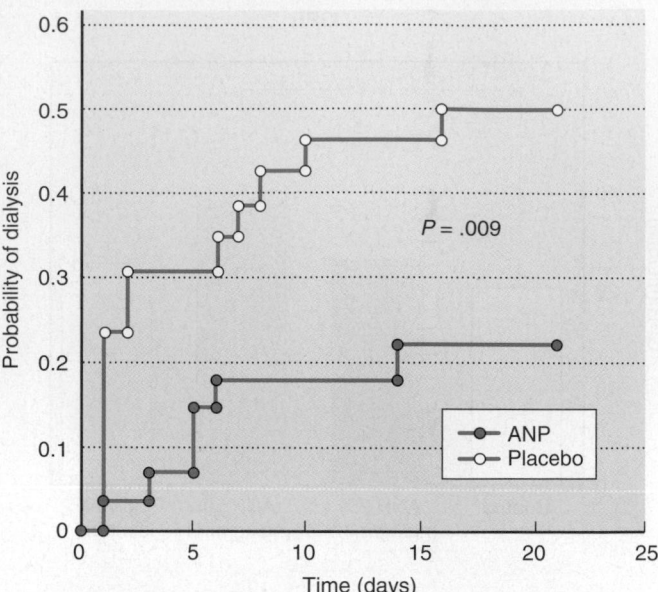

FIGURE 80-2. Effects of atrial natriuretic peptide (ANP), in a dose of 50 ng/kg per minute, versus placebo on probability of need for dialysis in patients with early ischemic acute renal failure after complicated cardiac surgery. (From Swärd K, Valsson F, Odencrants P, et al: Recombinant human atrial natriuretic peptide in ischemic acute renal failure: A randomized placebo-controlled trial. Crit Care Med 2004;32:1310-1315, by permission.)

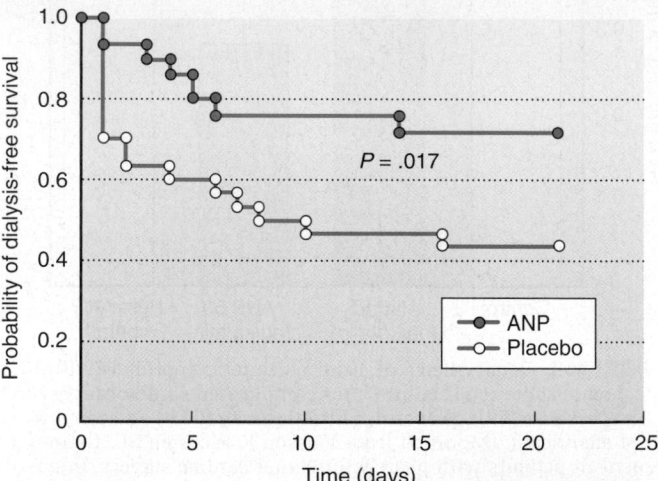

FIGURE 80-3. Effects of atrial natriuretic peptide (ANP), in a dose of 50 ng/kg per minute, versus placebo on dialysis-free survival in patients with early ischemic acute renal failure after complicated cardiac surgery. (From Swärd K, Valsson F, Odencrants P, et al: Recombinant human atrial natriuretic peptide in ischemic acute renal failure: A randomized placebo-controlled trial. Crit Care Med 2004;32:1310-1315, by permission.)

EFFECTS OF ATRIAL NATRIURETIC PEPTIDE IN OTHER FORMS OF CLINICAL ACUTE RENAL FAILURE

Cyclosporine-Induced Acute Renal Failure

Immunosuppression after transplantation with cyclosporine is complicated by nephrotoxicity. Cyclosporine induces a renal vasoconstriction with a fall in both renal blood flow and glomerular filtration rate, suggesting a vasoconstriction of preferentially the renal afferent arterioles.[33] Valsson and colleagues studied the effects of ANP (50 to 100 ng/kg per minute) in heart transplant recipients with early, cyclosporine-induced ARF. In these patients, ANP infusion produced a marked increase in renal blood flow (+53%) and glomerular filtration rate (+69%) and a decrease in renal vascular resistance (−45%), with no change in filtration fraction.[12] This partial or complete reversal of cyclosporine-induced renal vasoconstriction may thus be explained by the opposite effects of ANP and cyclosporine on preglomerular resistance vessels.

Liver Transplantation

ARF occurring immediately after liver transplantation is a major problem resulting in a poor prognosis. Akamatsu and coworkers[34] studied the efficacy of ANP in preventing ARF after liver transplantation. Thirty-seven patients who underwent living donor liver transplantation were prospectively randomized into two groups: patients who received ANP ($n = 19$), at a dose of 50 to 100 ng/kg per minute for 5 days, and those who received conventional diuretics ($n = 18$). The perioperative and postoperative changes in hemodynamic status and renal function were compared between the two groups. No statistical differences were noted in the changes in hemodynamic status between groups. The incidence of hemodialysis was 11% in the ANP group and 39% in the diuretic group ($P = .04$). Postoperative creatinine clearance was significantly higher in the ANP group.

Radiocontrast Agent–Induced Nephropathy

In a multicenter, prospective, randomized controlled trial, Kurnik and colleagues evaluated the efficacy of the intravenous ANP analogue anaritide (ANP 4-28) to prevent radiocontrast agent–induced nephropathy.[35] Patients with stable chronic renal failure were assigned to receive either placebo or one of three doses of anaritide (10, 50, or 100 ng/kg per minute) for 30 minutes before and continuing for 30 minutes after radiocontrast administration. This short-term administration of intravenous anaritide before and during a radiocontrast study did not reduce the incidence of subsequent nephropathy in patients with preexisting chronic renal failure.

CONCLUSION

ANP increases glomerular filtration rate and renal blood flow in both ischemic and cyclosporine-induced ARF by a preglomerular vasodilation. It also has been shown to decrease the need for dialysis in early ischemic ARF after cardiac surgery and to prevent ARF requiring dialysis after liver transplantation.

Key Points

1. In patients with normal renal function, atrial natriuretic peptide increases glomerular filtration rate, fractional excretion of sodium, and urine flow, with no changes in renal blood flow or renal vascular resistance. These findings suggest that atrial natriuretic peptide decreases preglomerular and increases postglomerular vascular resistance and directly inhibits tubular sodium reabsorption.
2. In patients with normal renal function, atrial natriuretic peptide increases renal oxygen consumption by means of the increase in glomerular filtration rate, caused by an increase in the filtered load of sodium to the tubules.
3. In patients with early ischemic or cyclosporine-induced acute renal failure, atrial natriuretic peptide improves both glomerular filtration rate and renal blood flow by way of renal vasodilation of the afferent arterioles.
4. The renal vasodilatory effects of atrial natriuretic peptide in ischemic acute renal failure are maintained during long-term infusion (over longer than 48 hours). Renal tolerance to atrial natriuretic peptide does not appear to develop.
5. A small two-center study suggests that low-dose atrial natriuretic peptide infusion reduces the probability of dialysis and improves dialysis-free survival in early ischemic acute renal failure after cardiac surgery complicated by circulatory shock. A similar study shows that atrial natriuretic peptide may decrease the need for dialysis after liver transplantation.

Key References

4. de Bold AJ, Borenstein HB, Veress AT, Sonnenberg H: A rapid and potent natriuretic response to intravenous injection of atrial myocardial extract in rats. Life Sci 1981;28:89-94.
24. Mitaka C, Hirata Y, Habuka K, et al: Atrial natriuretic peptide infusion improves ischemic renal failure after suprarenal abdominal aortic cross-clamping in dogs. Crit Care Med 2003;31:2205-2210.
26. Valsson F, Ricksten SE, Hedner T, Lundin S: Effects of atrial natriuretic peptide on acute renal impairment in patients with heart failure after cardiac surgery. Intensive Care Med 1996;22:230-236.
32. Swärd K, Valsson F, Odencrants P, et al: Recombinant human atrial natriuretic peptide in ischemic acute renal failure: A randomized placebo-controlled trial. Crit Care Med 2004;32:1310-1315.
34. Akamatsu N, Sugawara Y, Tamura S, et al: Prevention of renal impairment by continuous infusion of human atrial natriuretic peptide after liver transplantation. Transplantation 2005;80:1093-1098.

See the companion Expert Consult website for the complete reference list.

CHAPTER 81

Adenosine Antagonists

Ramesh Venkataraman and John A. Kellum

OBJECTIVES

This chapter will:
1. Present an overview of the rationale for use of adenosine antagonists for the prevention and treatment of acute renal failure.
2. Review the literature on the use of adenosine antagonists for the prevention and treatment of acute renal failure.

RATIONALE FOR USE OF ADENOSINE ANTAGONISTS

Adenosine, in contrast with its general systemic effect as a vasodilator, is a renal arterial vasoconstrictor.[1] This unique effect has been implicated as part of the tubuloglomerular feedback mechanism,[2] which increases afferent arteriolar tone in response to increased distal tubular solute delivery. Adenosine also acts synergistically with angiotensin II to constrict afferent arterioles.[3] Adenosine has now been shown to be a possible mediator, by means of A_1 receptors, of the intrarenal hemodynamic changes that lead to acute kidney injury (AKI) after radiocontrast agent administration[4] and other insults. With onset of AKI, the depletion of adenosine triphosphate within the kidney is thought to lead to local accumulation of adenosine, resulting in prolonged vasoconstriction.[5] A number of factors such as extracellular volume contraction, angiotensin II, and cyclooxygenase inhibitors all enhance the renal vascular response of adenosine.[2] Animal studies of radiocontrast administration, using an adenosine antagonist (theophylline or aminophylline) before treatment, have demonstrated attenuation of this intrarenal vasoconstriction.[6-8] Moreover, it has been shown that adenosine A_1 receptor knockout mice are protected against radiocontrast agent–induced AKI.[6] Nevertheless, inhibiting tubuloglomerular feedback as a preventive strategy for AKI has limited physiological support. Indeed, increasing renal blood flow and consequently renal medullary oxygen demand in the setting of nephrotoxic injury may potentially be harmful.

CLINICAL STUDIES

Theophylline and aminophylline have been specifically evaluated in two particular clinical settings for the prevention of AKI: after vascular surgery and after radiocontrast agent administration.

Prevention of Acute Kidney Injury after Vascular Surgery

In the first pilot open, within-patient, controlled clinical study, Parker and colleagues enrolled 20 patients who underwent major abdominal surgery requiring admission to the intensive care unit (ICU) for postoperative management.[9] These patients were studied in three phases of 6 hours each. During the first period, the *control period*, the patients received no active medication. At the start of the second period, the *aminophylline infusion period*, a 5.6-mg/kg bolus of aminophylline was infused over 20 minutes, followed by an infusion of 0.5 mg/kg per hour. During the third period, the *post-aminophylline period*, no active medication was given. Creatinine clearance corrected to a body surface area of 1.73 m^2; sodium, free water, and osmolar clearance; and fractional sodium excretion all were calculated using standard formulas. The study showed a significant increase in osmolar clearance and sodium clearance ($P < .05$) after administration of aminophylline that appears to return toward baseline after cessation of therapy. No change in creatinine clearance, however, was observed during the entire study. Of note, this study was severely underpowered and was nonrandomized. Furthermore, it did not report any clinically relevant outcome measures such as need for dialysis or mortality.

Subsequently, Kramer and associates performed a double-blind randomized controlled trial (RCT) evaluating the effectiveness of theophylline for prevention of renal impairment after elective coronary artery bypass surgery.[10] In this small study, 56 patients with normal renal function received a bolus of 4 mg/kg and a subsequent continuous infusion of 0.25 mg/kg per hour of theophylline ($n = 28$) or isotonic saline ($n = 28$) for up to 96 hours. Renal impairment (defined as an increase in serum creatinine level of 0.4 mg/dL or greater from baseline at postsurgery day 5) was not significantly different between the two groups.

Theophylline for the Prevention of Radiocontrast Agent–Induced Acute Kidney Injury

Several clinical studies have evaluated the role of theophylline or aminophylline in the prevention of radiocontrast agent–induced AKI.[11-16] Several of these studies, however, were either underpowered or nonrandomized or did not evaluate clinically relevant endpoints. These studies varied in their definition of AKI and dose, administration route, and timing of theophylline and provided conflicting results. A recent meta-analysis included randomized controlled trials of theophylline or aminophylline in hospitalized patients receiving radiocontrast media (7 of the 11 published clinical trials; $N = 480$).[17] This analysis showed that patients who received theophylline had a smaller increase in serum creatinine compared with those who received placebo. The difference in mean change in serum creatinine was 11.5 μmol/L (95% confidence interval, 5.3 to 19.4 μmol/L; $P = .004$) lower in the theophylline/aminophylline group than in the control subjects. Only one subject required dialysis for AKI in the entire cohort. This study excluded 3 trials, each for a different reason: Relevant clinical endpoints were not reported; a case-control study design was used; or the subjects were included in another RCT. Of note, however, this meta-analysis included studies that did not control for hydration status and that used as their endpoint changes in creatinine, as opposed to predefined criteria for AKI. One RCT showed that administration of theophylline with adequate intravenous hydration did not bring any additional benefit.[12] Accordingly, it remains unclear if theophylline may be useful in preventing radiocontrast-induced nephropathy in some patients. Moreover, theophylline has a narrow therapeutic index, and potential benefits should be weighed against its serious side effects (arrhythmias, gastrointestinal, and neurological).

In theory, in high-risk patients in whom aggressive hydration may not be possible, careful administration of theophylline may reduce the occurrence of AKI after administration of radiocontrast media. Larger multicenter RCTs examining valid clinical outcomes (e.g., dialysis requirement, mortality rates), however, will be necessary to adequately address this issue before routine use of theophylline to prevent contrast nephropathy can be recommended.

CONCLUSION

Although limited physiological rationale exists for the use of theophylline or aminophylline in AKI, clinical studies have not produced convincing results. As of now, adequate hydration, minimizing the amount of contrast medium, and the use of nonionic, iso-osmolar contrast agents are key to the prevention of radiocontrast agent–induced AKI. Routine use of theophylline to prevent AKI cannot be recommended on the basis of current data. Use of theophylline in certain high-risk patients in whom adequate hydration is not possible (e.g., patients in heart failure) may represent an important point of study, however.

Key Points

1. Adenosine causes constriction of the renal vasculature, unlike in the systemic circulation, in which it causes vasodilation.
2. Adenosine is thought to mediate the tubuloglomerular feedback.
3. Adenosine antagonists have not been convincingly shown to prevent acute kidney injury after vascular surgery.
4. One large meta-analysis revealed that adenosine antagonists decreased the degree of change in serum creatinine after radiocontrast administration, without influencing other clinically relevant outcomes.
5. Adenosine antagonists may be of value in selected patients in whom hydration adequate to prevent radiocontrast agent–induced nephropathy may not be possible.

Key References

10. Kramer BK, Preuner J, Ebenburger A, et al: Lack of renoprotective effect of theophylline during aortocoronary bypass surgery. Nephrol Dial Transplant 2002;17:910-915.
17. Ix JH, McCulloch CE, Chertow GM: Theophylline for the prevention of radiocontrast nephropathy: A meta-analysis. Nephrol Dial Transplant 2004;19:2747-2753.

See the companion Expert Consult website for the complete reference list.

CHAPTER 82

Antioxidants

Kai Singbartl and Alexander Zarbock

OBJECTIVES

This chapter will:
1. Describe the role of reactive oxygen species in acute kidney injury and acute renal failure.
2. Review existing data on the use of antioxidants (N-acetylcysteine, ascorbic acid, statins) in clinical practice.
3. Discuss experimental antioxidant agents (edaravone, iron chelation, and transport agents) as potential agents for treatment of acute kidney injury.

The critical role of reactive oxygen species (ROS) in the pathogenesis of acute renal failure (ARF) has become increasingly evident over the past decade. Although the kidney can generate ROS, it also is extremely vulnerable to the destructive effects of ROS.[1] The most prevalent such species are superoxide (O_2^-), hydrogen peroxide (H_2O_2), and hydroxyl radical (OH^-). O_2^- and OH^- are more reactive than H_2O_2, which is not a radical but rather a generator of oxidants. ROS profoundly affect cellular function and viability by altering basic cellular constituents such as lipids, carbohydrates, proteins, and nuclear acids. Loss of structural integrity of membranes, lysosomes, and

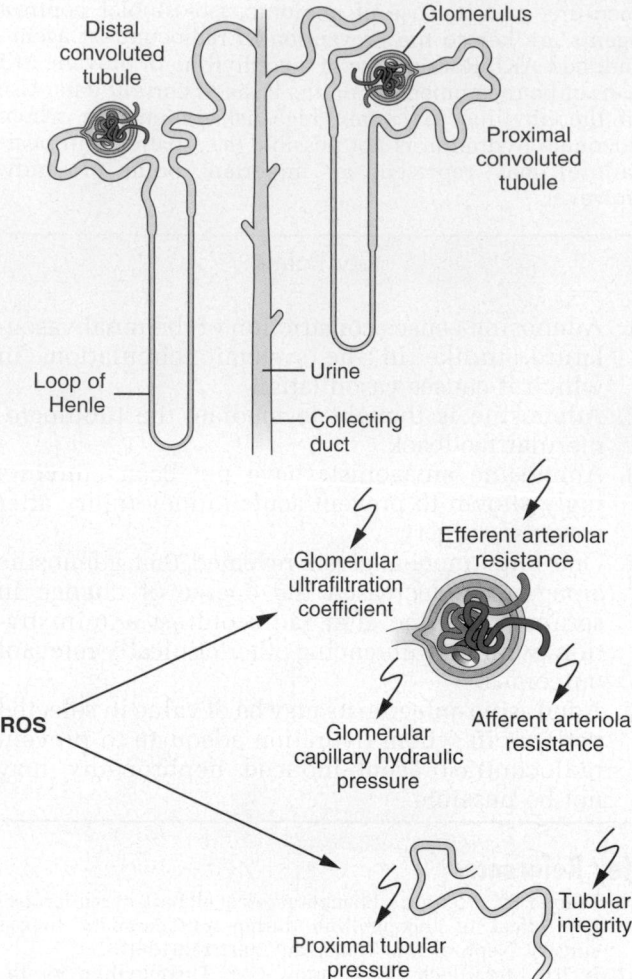

FIGURE 82-1. Various sites at the single-nephron level that can be affected by reactive oxygen species (ROS): afferent arteriolar resistance, efferent arteriolar resistance, glomerular plasma flow rate, glomerular capillary hydraulic pressure, glomerular ultrafiltration coefficient, proximal tubular pressure, and the integrity of tubular structures. Overall, ROS-induced injury of the kidney leads to decreased glomerular filtration rate and effective urine excretion.

mitochondria subsequently occurs, which in turn leads to alterations in cellular function, such as ion transport and membrane permeability. Although H_2O_2 itself lacks such reactivity, it can freely diffuse across cell membranes and thereby exert its effect distant from the site of generation. O_2^- also scavenges nitric oxide (NO) and thereby blunts the effect of NO on the renal microcirculation. ROS-induced injury of the kidney leads to decreased glomerular filtration rate and effective urine excretion. At the single-nephron level (Fig. 82-1), ROS can affect afferent arteriolar resistance, efferent arteriolar resistance, glomerular plasma flow rate, glomerular capillary hydraulic pressure, glomerular ultrafiltration coefficient, proximal tubular pressure, and the integrity of tubular structures. These effects, together with the observation that oxidative stress is markedly elevated during ARF,[2,3] have made ROS an attractive target for strategies to prevent ARF, particularly in critically ill patients. Currently, no evidence from clinical studies indicates that antioxidants are effective for the treatment of ARF. Adequately powered studies are lacking, however.

CLINICALLY AVAILABLE ANTIOXIDANTS

N-Acetylcysteine

Originally developed as a mucolytic agent for treatment of a variety of pulmonary diseases, and later used as an antidote for acetaminophen poisoning, *N*-acetylcysteine (NAC) also is the best-studied antioxidant in the context of ARF, especially for the prevention of radiocontrast agent–induced nephropathy. NAC is a synthetic derivative of cysteine, which is one of three amino acids that make up glutathione. Glutathione is a cellular thiol that is essential for antioxidant defense. NAC itself also is capable of scavenging ROS by providing sulfhydryl groups.[4] Animal as well as human clinical studies have identified potential mechanisms by which NAC may potentially confer renal protection. These mechanisms include attenuation of tubular necrosis and medullary hypoperfusion during renal ischemia-reperfusion,[5] as well as reduction of leukocyte apoptosis and blunted oxidative stress response in patients undergoing hemodialysis.[6,7] Clinical studies examining the efficacy of NAC have focused on the prevention of radiocontrast-induced nephropathy or ARF after vascular or cardiac surgery.

Although numerous clinical trial studies as well as several meta-analyses have evaluated the potential for NAC to prevent radiocontrast-induced nephropathy, substantial controversy remains regarding its beneficial effect on preservation of renal function (recently reviewed by Stacul and colleagues[8]). Moreover, the effects of NAC on "hard" outcome parameters, such as morbidity, mortality, and need for chronic hemodialysis, are still unknown. Several aspects of study design have contributed to this confusion. Although a majority of studies have included patients undergoing (interventional) coronary angiography, patient populations have been very heterogeneous, especially with respect to risk stratification. Great variability also has been noted in dose (ranging from 300 to 1200 mg), duration (for up to 48 hours after the procedure), and mode (enteral versus intravenous) of NAC administration; concomitant hydration has been inconsistent as well. Furthermore, a recent study in healthy volunteers has provided evidence that NAC itself has a direct effect on serum creatinine concentrations[9]: NAC induced a decrease in serum creatinine concentrations without any changes in cystatin C, an independent measure of glomerular filtration rate. It is possible, then, that after administration of NAC for the prevention of radiocontrast-induced nephropathy, serum creatinine concentrations may have falsely indicated preserved or even improved glomerular filtration rate.

Because of its low cost and excellent safety and tolerance, prophylaxis of radiocontrast-induced nephropathy with NAC is still very popular. Nonetheless, recent consensus statements[8] and a meta-analysis[10] do not support the routine use of NAC for this purpose. Instead, they recommend new randomized trials of large sample size and with the inclusion of "hard" outcome data, as well as a more cautious interpretation of existing data (see Chapter 51).

Randomized clinical studies examining the effectiveness of NAC in preventing ARF after cardiac or major vascular surgery have yielded negative results. Even with high-dose NAC administration or selection of high-risk patients, such as those with preexisting renal dysfunction, no benefit of NAC over placebo has been demonstrated.[11,12]

Although some studies revealed a trend toward lower serum creatinine concentrations after NAC administration, it remains unclear whether this change actually reflected better renal function or NAC-specific effects on serum creatinine concentrations. At present, the prophylactic use of NAC before major vascular or cardiac surgery cannot be recommended.

Ascorbic Acid

Administration of ascorbic acid has conferred protection from oxidative stress in animal models of postischemic ARF and drug-induced nephrotoxicity. Current belief holds that ascorbic acid acts through an increase in antioxidant activity and elimination of oxidation reactions. Ascorbic acid also can regenerate other antioxidants and act thereby as a co-antioxidant. It significantly affects the antioxidant status 2 hours after oral ingestion.[13] Because of its excellent safety record in humans and attractive pharmacoeconomic profile, ascorbic acid also has become of interest for the prevention of drug-induced nephropathy.

Data from only one double-blind, placebo-controlled trial are currently available.[13] Compared with placebo treatment, oral administration of 3 g of ascorbic acid before injection of radiocontrast agents, followed by two additional 2-g doses after the procedure, provided a significant reduction in radiocontrast-induced nephropathy, defined by a transient increase in serum creatinine. Despite these promising results, further randomized, controlled trials, including large-scale, multi-institutional studies, are necessary to confirm these findings.

3-Hydroxy-3-Methylglutaryl–Coenzyme A Reductase Inhibitors

3-Hydroxy-3-methylglutaryl–coenzyme A (HMG-CoA) reductase inhibitors, or statins, have demonstrated a variety of pleiotropic effects in addition to their cholesterol-lowering potency.[14] The main feature of these pleiotropic or cholesterol-independent effects of statins appears to be restoration or improvement of endothelial function. Statins improve endothelial function by increasing the bioavailability of nitric oxide, promoting reendothelialization, inhibiting inflammatory responses, and reducing oxidative stress.[15] Statins have been shown to lower ROS production by inhibition of nicotinamide adenine dinucleotide phosphate oxidase activity.[15] In addition to endothelial cells, these effects also have been demonstrated in smooth muscle cells and leukocytes.

Clinical data supporting the broad application of statins for their antioxidative properties are rather limited. A retrospective study,[16] which included more than 1000 patients undergoing coronary angiography, indicated that the risk for radiocontrast-induced nephropathy was lower in patients who had received statins before the procedure. Initiation of treatment with statins, however, had no effect on survival or need for dialysis. Review of data from a prospective, multicenter regional registry of patients undergoing percutaneous coronary interventions showed that patients who had been on statin therapy before the procedure had a lower incidence of radiocontrast-induced nephropathy.[17] Although these data emphasize the need for initiation of statin therapy before coronary angiography, if indicated, they do not provide enough evidence to support the broad use of statins in patients who otherwise lack indications for therapy with such agents.

Although treatment with statins improved the lipid profile in patients after renal transplantation, as expected, such agents had no short-term effect on renal function.[18]

EXPERIMENTAL ANTIOXIDANTS

Because of limited, inconclusive, or even disappointing results from clinical trials, current research activities also aim at discovering and evaluating new, alternative antioxidants.

Edaravone

Edaravone (3-methyl-1-phenyl-2-pyrazolin-5-one) is a potent scavenger of free radicals and inhibitor of lipid peroxidation. Edaravone exerts its protective effects within or adjacent to ischemic areas by transferring electrons to radicals. As a result of the electron transfer, edaravone itself is converted to 2-oxo-3-(phenylhydrazono) butanoic acid. In addition to myocardial and cerebral ischemia, experimental studies also have demonstrated protective effects of edaravone in animal models of renal ischemia-reperfusion and drug-induced nephropathy.[19,20] Edaravone ameliorated renal dysfunction, renal tubular damage, mitochondrial damage, renal protein oxidation, ROS production in tubular cells, and tubular apoptosis. Edaravone has been approved for human use in the treatment of cerebral ischemia in Japan. Current trials also are exploring a potential benefit of edaravone in myocardial ischemia.

Iron Chelation and Transport

Free iron, which is released from injured cells, is believed to be one of the most potent generators of ROS. Unbound iron can catalyze the conversion of H_2O_2 to OH and OH^- (Haber-Weiss reaction), as well as forming reactive ferryl or perferryl species. These ions have the potential to induce mutation in several types of molecules, including lipids, nucleotides, and DNA. Moreover, catalytic iron in urine or blood and peroxidized lipids occur in various forms of ARF, such as that caused by free hemoglobin-myoglobin, chemotherapy, ischemia-reperfusion, transplant-related ischemia, or proteinuria-induced tubular damage. Pretreatment of animals with iron worsened renal injury. Current belief holds that iron-catalyzed damage is one of the earliest events in kidney dysfunction; it also appears to be crucial in the mechanism of injury to other organs, such as the heart and liver.[21]

Conversely, experimental studies have demonstrated that iron chelation drastically reduces oxidative stress and subsequent renal injury in animal models of renal ischemia-reperfusion and glycerol-induced nephropathy. Iron chelation also appears to be more effective in preventing postischemic renal injury than an increase in intracellular free radical scavengers, as seen with administration of NAC.[22] In contrast with deferoxamine, administration of NAC did not improve renal microcirculation and prevent lipid peroxidation. Deferoxamine mesylate, the only iron chelator currently available for clinical application, is not suitable for acute care situations because it carries a risk for significant toxicity (hypotension), especially when given at high intravenous doses.[23]

Apotransferrin, an endogenous iron-binding protein, exhibits great efficacy in reducing free "redox-active" iron, and it also lacks significant adverse effects in humans. Reductions in circulating redox-active iron by treatment with apotransferrin abolished renal ischemia-reperfusion injury in mice through inhibition of oxidative stress, inflammation, and subsequent loss of function.[24]

Neutrophil gelatinase-associated lipocalin (NGAL) is a major endogenous iron transport protein. NGAL and NGAL also are among the most upregulated genes and overexpressed proteins, respectively, in the kidney after renal ischemia-reperfusion. Both animal and clinical studies have shown that NGAL is present in urine and serum after acute renal injury and can therefore serve as a biomarker.[25] Injection of NGAL in murine models of postischemic ARF resulted in preservation of proximal tubule N-cadherin, inhibition of cell death, increase in proliferation of proximal tubule cells, and improved renal function.[21,26]

CONCLUSION

Despite a convincing pathophysiological rationale and sound experimental evidence, the efficacy of currently available antioxidants in preventing ARF under clinical conditions remains uncertain. Although some evidence indicates that NAC may help to prevent radiocontrast agent–induced nephropathy, no role for NAC in prevention of ARF after major vascular or cardiac surgery has been established. Because of the low incidence of adverse effects and favorable pharmacoeconomic profile for this agent, widespread belief holds that the potential benefit of avoiding radiocontrast-induced nephropathy by means of NAC greatly outweighs the risks of its administration. Together with sufficient hydration, administration of 600 to 1200 mg of NAC, twice daily, on the day before and the day of the procedure represents a frequently used regimen. Similar considerations hold for the use of ascorbic acid. Nonetheless, the available evidence is insufficient to endorse routine administration of ascorbic acid to prevent radiocontrast-induced nephropathy. Even greater caution and accumulation of more data are warranted before statins can become part of protocols to prevent (or treat) ARF.

To overcome this uncertainty with currently used antioxidants, the following steps appear to be necessary: In addition to adequate power, future studies need to include patient-centered outcomes, such as survival or need for hemodialysis, and they need to define patient populations more carefully regarding procedures and risk factors. Clinical trials with new antioxidants, which are anxiously awaited, must adhere to the same principles. Last, but not least, the role of antioxidants in the treatment of ARF remains completely unknown and needs to be explored by means of both experimental studies and clinical trials.

Key Points

1. N-acetylcysteine may confer some protection from radiocontrast agent–induced nephropathy but not from acute renal failure after cardiac or major vascular surgery.
2. Prophylactic application of vitamin C appears to attenuate renal dysfunction after radiocontrast agent administration.
3. Currently, no indication is recognized for antioxidants in the treatment of acute renal failure.
4. Future clinical trials for both current and new antioxidants must focus on patient-centered outcome data (e.g., survival, need for and duration of renal replacement therapy).

Key References

8. Stacul F, Adam A, Becker CR, et al: Strategies to reduce the risk of contrast-induced nephropathy. Am J Cardiol 2006;98:59K-77K.
10. Zagler A, Azadpour M, Mercado C, Hennekens CH: N-acetylcysteine and contrast-induced nephropathy: A meta-analysis of 13 randomized trials. Am Heart J 2006;151:140-145.
12. Ristikankare A, Kuitunen T, Kuitunen A, et al: Lack of renoprotective effect of i.v. N-acetylcysteine in patients with chronic renal failure undergoing cardiac surgery. Br J Anaesth 2006;97:611-616.

See the companion Expert Consult website for the complete reference list.

CHAPTER 83

Antiapoptotic Agents

Gur P. Kaushal, Didier Portilla, and Sudhir V. Shah

OBJECTIVES

This chapter will:
1. Present an overview of the molecular pathways of apoptosis.
2. Summarize preclinical studies on various antiapoptotic agents including caspase inhibitors, p53 inhibitors, inhibitors and activators of members of the Bcl-2 family, and others.
3. Review the findings of clinical studies on some antiapoptotic agents.
4. Consider the relevance of antiapoptotic agents for the prevention of kidney injury.

The apoptotic mode of cell death is an evolutionarily conserved and highly regulated physiological process that is crucial for maintaining tissue homeostasis in multicellular organisms.[1,2] Under normal conditions, it is involved in embryogenesis, development, tissue remodeling, and regulation of the immune response. Under pathological conditions, derangement of apoptosis results in a wide variety of diseases including ischemic and toxic injury, autoimmune and immunodeficiency diseases, and neurodegenerative disorders, as well as injury due to oxidants, ultraviolet or γ-irradiation, or growth factor withdrawal, all leading to dysregulation of tissue homeostasis. Many signaling transduction pathways (as described later) regulate the mechanisms of cell death. The principal molecular

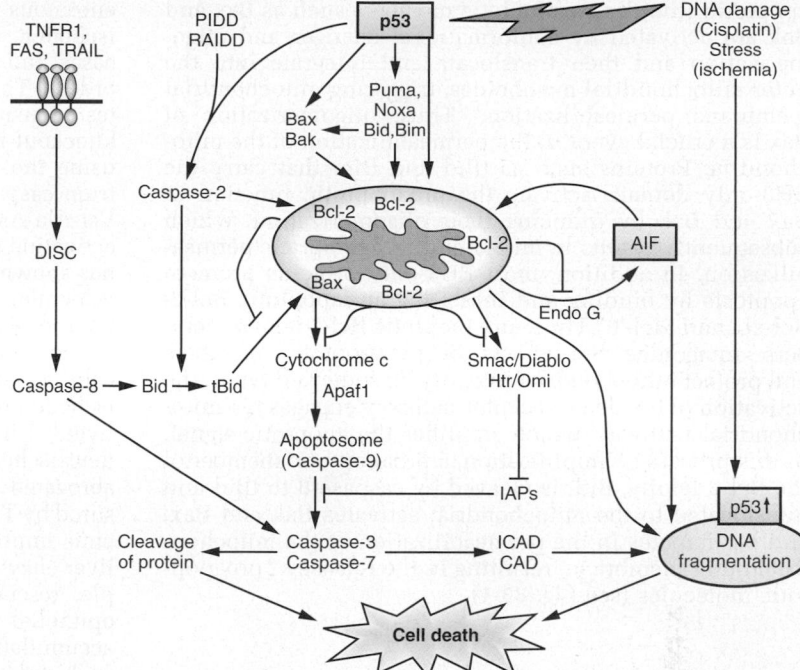

FIGURE 83-1. Extrinsic and intrinsic apoptotic pathways of cell death. Both death receptor (extrinsic) and mitochondrial-dependent (intrinsic) pathways of cell death and their regulation are depicted. AIF, apoptosis-inducing factor; CAD, caspase-activated DNase; DISC, death-inducing signaling complex; Endo G, endonuclease G; IAPs, inhibitors of apoptosis proteins; ICAD, inhibitors of caspase-activated DNase; PIDD, p53-induced protein with a death domain; RAIDD, receptor-interacting protein–associated ICH-1/CED-3 homologous protein with a death domain; TNFR, tumor necrosis factor receptor; TRAIL, TNF-related apoptosis-inducing ligand.

components of these pathways recently have been considered as therapeutic targets for cytoprotection in preclinical and clinical studies. Several inhibitors of the apoptotic molecules have been designed and explored as effective therapeutic antiapoptotic agents. Many encouraging results have been obtained using experimental models of human diseases, and some of these antiapoptotic agents are being tested in clinical trials.

Apoptosis is regulated by many signaling pathways that in most cases converge into the activation of caspases. Although caspases play a central role in the execution of most of the apoptotic pathways, caspase-independent cell death pathways also have been documented.[3] Among the 14 caspases encoded by distinct genes in mammalian cells, caspase-2, -8, -9, and -10 have long N-terminal prodomains and are termed *initiator caspases*. On receiving a proapoptotic stimulus, the initiator caspases activate the downstream *executioner caspases*, caspase-3, -6, and -7, with short N-terminal prodomains. The activation of executioner caspases involves proteolytic processing to the active form from their normally synthesized inactive proenzyme form. Activated caspases mediate the execution of apoptosis by cleaving cellular proteins that are essential for cell survival and proliferation.

Multiple pathways can result in the activation of executioner caspases. Two well-characterized pathways (Fig. 83-1), the *death receptor pathway* and the *mitochondrial pathway*, participate in the activation of the executioner caspases caspase-3, -6, and -7 by the initiator caspases caspase-8, -9, and -10. The death receptor pathway is initiated by activation of cell death receptors such as Fas/CD95/APO1, tumor necrosis factor receptor-1 (TNFR1), TNF-related apoptosis–inducing ligand receptors -1 and -2 (TRAIL-R1 and -R2), DR3, and DR6 on binding to their corresponding ligands. These receptors are characterized by the presence of intracellular conserved death domains (DDs). The homophilic interactions between the conserved DD of the receptor and an adaptor molecule such as Fas-associated death domain or TNF receptor–associated death domain form the receptor-adaptor complex that, on oligomerization, recruits the initiator caspases, procaspase-8 or

-10, resulting in the formation of a death-inducing signaling complex (DISC). The DISC then facilitates dimerization and activation of procaspase-8 or -10 to its active form. Active caspase-8 in turn cleaves and activates the downstream executioner caspases caspase-3, -6, and -7.[4]

The other pathway of caspase activation is mitochondrial-dependent and also is known as the intrinsic pathway of cell death. A majority of the apoptotic signals induced by stress and genotoxic agents engage this intrinsic pathway for activation of the executioner caspases. This pathway is triggered by the permeabilization of the mitochondrial outer membrane, resulting in the release of many mitochondrial intermembrane proteins, including cytochrome *c*, Smac/Diablo, Omi/HtrA2, endonuclease G (Endo G), and apoptosis-inducing factor (AIF). Cytochrome *c* released from the mitochondria recruits an apoptotic protease-activating factor-1 (Apaf-1) in the cytosol, allowing Apaf-1 to bind to the nucleotide deoxyadenosine triphosphate (dATP). The binding of dATP to the Apaf-1–cytochrome *c* complex induces its oligomerization to form a high-molecular-weight, caspase-activating complex termed the *apoptosome*. The apoptosome recruits procaspase-9 by caspase recruitment domain (CARD) interactions that facilitate dimerization and activation of procaspase-9 to its active form. Activated caspase-9 then cleaves and activates downstream procaspase-3.[5] Other proapoptotic molecules such as AIF, Endo G, and Htr/Omi, once released from the mitochondria, cause caspase-independent cell death. AIF and Endo G are translocated to the nucleus, where they cause DNA fragmentation. Omi/HtrA2, once released into the cytosol, can induce cell death in a caspase-independent manner, owing to its serine protease activity,[6] or it can induce cell death in a caspase-dependent manner by inactivating the inhibitor of apoptosis proteins (IAP), subsequently releasing active caspases from IAP-bound caspases.[7] Thus, in the intrinsic pathway, mitochondrial outer membrane permeabilization plays a crucial role in the activation of caspases.

Permeabilization of the mitochondrial outer membrane is regulated by interplay between the proapoptotic and antiapoptotic Bcl-2 family of proteins.[1,8] In response to apoptotic stimuli, proapoptotic members such as Bax and Bak are activated by conformational changes and oligomerization and then translocate and integrate into the outer mitochondrial membranes, triggering mitochondrial membrane permeabilization.[8] Thus, oligomerization of Bax is a crucial event in the permeabilization of the mitochondria. Proteins such as tBid and Bim that carry the BH3-only domain activate the proapoptotic function of Bax and Bak by inducing their oligomerization, which subsequently results in mitochondrial membrane permeabilization. In addition, most BH3-only proteins promote apoptosis by binding and inhibiting antiapoptotic Bcl-2, Bcl-xL, and Mcl-1.[9] Thus, antiapoptotic Bcl-2 family members antagonize the effects of proapoptotic members and protect mitochondrial integrity. In some cell types, the activation of the death receptor pathway engages the mitochondrial pathway, which amplifies the apoptotic signal. In this process of amplification, a proapoptotic member of the Bcl-2 family, Bid, is cleaved by caspase-8 to tBid and translocated to the mitochondria, activates Bak and Bax, and participates in the permeabilization of the mitochondrial outer membrane, resulting in the release of proapoptotic molecules (see Fig. 83-1).

CASPASE INHIBITORS

Since caspases are activated in pathological conditions and are essential components of many apoptotic pathways, they are potential targets for intervention to control cell death. Thus development of caspase inhibitors has enormous therapeutic potential in diseases ranging from ischemia, sepsis, rheumatoid arthritis, autoimmune diseases, and myocardial infarction to neurodegenerative disorders. The animal models of these diseases have been tested using peptide inhibitors of caspases or caspase knockout mice. Most of the experiments were performed using the active site mimetic peptide-based broad-spectrum caspase inhibitor zVAD-fmk (N-benzyloxycarbonyl-Val-Ala-Asp-fluoromethyl-ketone). Blocking caspase activation and other components of the cell death pathway has shown striking efficacy in different animal models of ischemia, sepsis, hepatitis, and other diseases including neurodegenerative disorders (Table 83-1).[10-12]

The pancaspase inhibitor zVAD-fmk conferred significant functional protection in the experimental models of ischemia-reperfusion injury of the kidney,[13] heart,[14] liver,[15,16] intestine,[17] and brain (focal, transient and permanent ischemia).[18,19] In these studies, pancaspase inhibitor abrogated caspase activity, decreased apoptosis as measured by TUNEL staining, increased survival (in liver ischemia improved survival by at least threefold and reduced liver enzyme release), improved organ function (for example, rescued renal function and reduced renal tubular epithelial cell apoptosis and neutrophil infiltration and accumulation), and significantly decreased infarct size (reduced infarct area at least 50% in both cardiac and focal cerebral ischemia). In an endotoxin model of acute kidney injury, the pancaspase inhibitor zVAD-fmk prevented apoptotic cell death, decreased neutrophil accumulation, and ameliorated an inflammatory response.[20,21] zVAD-fmk prevented cell apoptosis and improved myocardial contractility in a rat endotoxin model,[22] prevented epithelial

TABLE 83-1

Caspase Inhibitors as Therapeutic Targets of Cell Death in Experimental Models

CASPASE INHIBITOR	EXPERIMENTAL MODEL(S)	EFFECT(S)
zVAD-fmk	Ischemia-reperfusion in kidney,[13] heart,[14] liver,[15,16] intestine,[17] and brain (focal, transient, and permanent ischemia)[18,19]	Functional protection; reduced inflammation and apoptosis
	Sepsis/endotoxemic injury in kidney,[20,21] heart,[22] lung,[23] and lymphocyte[10]	Ameliorated AKI, improved myocardial contractility, reduced survival and apoptosis
	Death receptor Fas–mediated liver injury[2]	Reduced liver transaminases and hepatocellular apoptosis
	Spinal cord injury[26] and neurodegenerative diseases[27]	Neuroprotection; reduced toxicity of neurotoxins
	Organ transplantation–related ischemia-reperfusion injury of pancreas[28]	Reduced ischemia-reperfusion and graft injury
	Liver graft injury[15] and graft coronary artery injury[29]	
Q-VD-OPH	Renal ischemia-reperfusion injury[32]	Reduced necrosis and AKI
	Virus-induced myocardial injury[30] and myocardial apoptosis and injury	
	Neurodegenerative diseases (Parkinson's and Huntington's diseases)[3]	Prevented MPTP-induced loss of dopaminergic neurons in the substantia nigra and in Huntington's disease model reduced the size of striatal lesion
IDN-6556	Fas-induced[43] and bile duct ligation–induced[44] liver damage	Reduced liver transaminases, hepatocyte apoptosis, and liver inflammation and fibrosis
	Neonatal ischemic brain injury in rat model[4]	Neuroprotection
M-826	Huntington's disease[4]	Prevented striatal neuron cell death
M-791 or M-920	Cecal ligation puncture model of sepsis[1]	Prevented lymphocyte apoptosis, improved animal survival.
MX1013	Ischemia-reperfusion in brain and heart and Fas-mediated liver damage[4]	Neuroprotection; reduced infarction and liver damage
VX765	Rat model of seizure[1]	Delay in seizure
Ad-XIAP	Transient ischemia in rat forebrain[51] and in retina[52]	Neuroprotection in brain, functional protection of retina

AKI, acute kidney injury; MPTP, 1-methyl-4-phenyl-1,2,3,6-tetrahydropyridine.

and endothelial apoptosis in endotoxin-induced lung injury and improved animal survival,[23] and reduced lymphocyte apoptosis in an experimental model of sepsis.[10] In other disease models, pancaspase inhibitor has provided efficient protection in death-receptor-mediated liver injury,[24] blocked progression of type II collagen-induced arthritis,[25] and afforded protection from post-traumatic tissue damage and neurological injury in a rat model of spinal cord injury[26] and in neurodegenerative diseases including amyotrophic lateral sclerosis (ALS).[27] In organ transplantation models, pancaspase inhibitor was effective in reducing ischemia-reperfusion injury in pancreas transplantation,[28] early graft injury after ischemia-reperfusion in a rat liver,[15] and in preventing the development of graft coronary artery disease.[29] Thus, these studies demonstrate that caspase inhibition is of potential therapeutic benefit in organ transplantation, cardiac arrest, liver injury, and stroke. A new broad-spectrum caspase inhibitor, Q-VD-OPH (quinolyl-Val-Asp-(OMe)-[2,6-difluorophenoxy)]-methyl ketone (developed by ICN/Enzyme Systems Products, Livermore, CA), is highly potent, stable, and has reduced toxicity compared with the widely used inhibitor zVAD-fmk. In a murine model of reovirus viral myocarditis, Q-VD-OPH reduced virus-induced myocardial apoptosis and injury[30] and provided neuroprotection in a 1-methyl-4-phenyl-1,2,3,6-tetrahydropyridine (MPTP)-induced mouse model of Parkinson's disease and in a 3-nitropropionic acid (3NP)- and malonate-induced mouse model of Huntington's disease,[31] and provided functional protection in a mouse model of renal ischemia-reperfusion injury.[32]

Caspase knockout mice have also provided insight into the role of caspase depletion in various experimental models. There is a limitation using these mice for experimental models because the KO mice may develop compensatory mechanisms that may confound the effect of depletion of the targeted caspase. However, some studies have shown efficacy of depletion in some disease models. Mice deficient in caspase 1 were resistant to ischemia-reperfusion injury in the kidney, heart, and brain.[33] Caspase-1 knockout mice were resistant to endotoxemic and cisplatin-induced acute kidney injury[33]; in the sepsis model of lung injury, knockout mice delayed neutrophil apoptosis and prolonged inflammatory response.[34] Expression of a dominant-negative caspase-1 mutant extended survival and delayed disease progression in a model of Huntington's disease[35] and prevented neuronal cell death induced by trophic factor withdrawal and ischemic brain injury.[33] Mice with caspase-1 gene deletion showed a 70% reduction in seizures and an approximate fourfold delay in their onset.[33] Mice deficient in caspase-1,[33] -11,[36] and -12[37] are resistant to endotoxic shock.

However, there are some problems and caveats associated with the use of peptide-based irreversible inhibitors of caspases. The irreversible inhibitor z-VAD-fmk, in some instances, is promiscuous and less specific for caspases and also can inhibit other proteases such as cathepsin and calpains.[38,39] In addition, the peptide and hydrophobic nature of the inhibitors reduce the efficacy of the inhibitor due to the poor cell permeability. There are also concerns that z-VAD-fmk may just inhibit apoptotic morphology but not cell death, or may delay cell death or, in some cells, promote alternative cell death pathway, whereby cells die due to autophagy or necrosis.[11,40] Also, other recent studies have also suggested some nonapoptotic function of caspases.[41]

Compelling evidence for the beneficial role of caspase inhibitors in animal studies has nevertheless provided an impetus for designing pharmaceutical drugs to caspase inhibitors. Clinically relevant potent nonpeptidyl small-molecule inhibitors for caspases are being developed by several pharmaceutical companies.[42] The first broad-spectrum caspase inhibitor, IDN-6556, has entered into clinical trials as a therapeutic drug by IDUN, which has now been acquired by Pfizer. IDN-6556 is an irreversible inhibitor based on oxamyl dipeptides that target the catalytic site of caspases.[43] In preclinical studies using a mouse model of Fas-induced liver injury, IDN-6556 was quite effective in reducing serum levels of liver transaminases, decreasing hepatocellular apoptosis, and exhibiting marked post-insult efficacy.[43] In the mouse bile duct ligation model, IDN-6556 reduced not only hepatocyte apoptosis but also liver inflammation and fibrosis.[44] The result of the first clinical trial in patients with hepatic impairment showed a significant reduction in serum transaminase enzymes.[45] IDN-6556 also was effective in normalizing transaminase levels in patients infected with the hepatitis C virus.[12] In another study in an animal model of liver transplantation, IDN-6556 significantly reduced tissue injury due to cold-ischemia/warm-reperfusion.[12] The U.S. Food and Drug Administration (FDA) recently has granted orphan drug status to IDN-6556 for administration to patients undergoing liver transplantation and other solid organ transplantation. Phase 2 clinical trials currently are under way in transplantation centers in the United States and Europe.[42]

Administration of pralnacasan (intracerebroventricular) or VX-765 (intraperitoneal, 25 to 200 mg/kg) to rats blocked seizure-induced production of interleukin (IL)-1β in the hippocampus and resulted in a twofold delay in seizure onset and 50% reduction in seizure duration.[12]

Merck has developed a small reversible caspase-3 inhibitor, M-826, that prevented brain tissue loss and provided neuroprotection in a neonatal rat model of ischemic brain injury.[46] M-826 also prevented cell death of striatal neurons in a melonate-induced rat model of Huntington's disease.[47] In a cecal ligation mouse model of sepsis, broad-spectrum caspase inhibitor M-920 or M791 prevented lymphocyte apoptosis and improved animal survival.[10] MX1013, a dipeptide caspase inhibitor developed by Maxim Pharmaceuticals (San Diego, CA), was effective in reducing apoptosis in Fas-mediated liver damage, neuronal cell death in brain ischemia-reperfusion injury, and acute myocardial infarction.[48]

In addition to the synthetic inhibitors of caspases, highly conserved natural or endogenous inhibitors of apoptosis (IAPs) are recognized as important intrinsic regulators of apoptosis. Members of the IAP family characterized by discrete one to three baculovirus IAP repeat (BIR) domains mediate antiapoptotic function because they are involved in the inhibition of activated caspase-3, -7, and -9.[49] Thus, IAPs are important potential tools for gene therapy because of their impressive ability to inhibit the final caspase cascade. Use of IAPs recently has been considered for so-called rescue strategies in several neurodegenerative diseases. Among the mammalian IAP members, XIAP is well characterized and the most potent inhibitor.[49] After transient ischemia in the rat forebrain, neuronal apoptosis was rescued by adenoviral delivery of XIAP or the neuronal inhibitory protein.[50] Recent studies also have examined retinal neurons after ischemia-induced cell death. Delivery of adeno-associated viral vector expressing XIAP by intravitreal injections afforded both functional and structural protection to the retina after a retinal transient ischemic injury.[51] Overexpression of the *XIAP* gene in islet cells by ex vivo adenoviral transduction of isolated islets provided protection of these cells from allograft rejection

TABLE 83-2

Calpain Protease and Omi/HtrA2 Protease Inhibitors as Antiapoptotic Therapeutic Targets of Cell Death in Experimental Models

CALPAIN INHIBITOR	EXPERIMENTAL MODEL(S)	EFFECT(S)
Calpain inhibitor 1	Renal ischemia-reperfusion[54,55]	Functional protection from AKI;
	Hemorrhagic shock in ischemia[55]	ameliorated multiple organ failure
PD150606 or E-64	Renal ischemia-reperfusion in rat[54]	Attenuated renal dysfunction and reduced
	Rat cerebral ischemia[56]	histological renal damage; reduced neuronal cell death
	AMPA-induced toxicity to cerebellar Purkinje neurons[57]	Attenuated AMPA-induced dark cell degeneration
MDL28170	Focal cerebral ischemia[5]	Reduced infarction and neuronal injury
	TAA-induced acute liver failure[55]	Attenuated TAA-induced acute liver failure and hepatocyte apoptosis
	Spinal cord injury in rodents[5]	Prevented neuronal cell death and ameliorated motor disturbances
	MPTP-induced Parkinson's disease[6]	Protected nigral dopamine neuronal loss and motor function
Cbz-LLY-CHN$_2$	Liver ischemia-reperfusion injury[5]	Reduced sinusoidal endothelial cell apoptosis
	Reperfusion in liver transplantation[5]	Decreased aspartate aminotransferase
AK-295	Focal brain ischemia[54]	Neuroprotection
	Paclitaxel-induced neuropathy[54]	Prevented axonal degeneration and clinical neuropathy
Inhibitor XI	Adult spinal cord injury in mice[5]	Inhibited apoptosis in motor neurons
Serine Protease Omi/HtrA2 Inhibition		
Ucf-101	Cisplatin-induced nephrotoxicity[6]	Ameliorated AKI and reduced apoptosis
	Myocardial ischemia-reperfusion[6]	Reduced cardiomyocyte apoptosis and infarct size
	Focal cerebral ischemia[6]	Provided neuroprotection

AKI, acute kidney injury; AMPA, α-amino-3-hydroxy-5-methyl-4-isoxazolepropionic acid; MPTP, 1-methyl-4-phenyl-1,2,3,6-tetrahydropyridine; TAA, thioacetamide.

without impairing β cell function.[52] Thus, long-term protection of islet allografts by XIAP overexpression may enhance the survival of islet transplants in diabetes.

Calpain Inhibitors

Calpains, like caspases, are well-conserved members of cysteine proteases but require calcium for their activity.[53] The members of the calpain family are upregulated in a wide variety of biological processes and diseases including muscular dystrophy, cancer, Alzheimer's disease, neurological injury, ischemia-reperfusion injury, atherosclerosis, diabetes, and cataract formation.[54] Because calpains are involved in pathogenic cell death,[54,55] their inhibitors are potentially important therapeutic agents for blocking cell death. Most of the calpain inhibitors are promiscuous because many of them also inhibit other cysteine proteases, serine proteases, and even the proteosome. The naturally occurring calpain inhibitor calpastatin is the only specific inhibitor of the calpain family discovered to date that controls calpain activity in vivo. Different kinds of calpain inhibitors, including peptidyl epoxide, aldehyde, and ketoamide inhibitors, are capable of inhibiting calpains and are being evaluated in animal models of human disease (Table 83-2). The lack of specificity toward cysteine proteases and other proteolytic enzymes is the major limitation of calpain inhibitors. A variety of calpain inhibitors including Z-Leu-Abu-CONHEt (AK275), E64 analogues, 27-mer calpastatin peptide, leupeptin, calpain inhibitor I, calpain inhibitor II, calpeptin, Cbz-Val-Phe-H (MDL28170), and 3-(4-iodophenyl)-2-mercapto-(Z)-2-propenoic acid (PD150606, a Ca^{2+}-binding site inhibitor) afforded protection from ischemic and toxicant-induced cell death in various in vitro models.[55]

The involvement of calpain has been documented in ischemia-reperfusion and toxic injury in the kidney, brain, liver, and myocardium (reviewed by Carragher[54] and Liu and colleagues[55]). Calpain inhibitor I conferred significant functional protection in a rodent model of ischemia-reperfusion injury of the kidney and ameliorated multiple organ failure produced by hemorrhagic shock during ischemia-reperfusion injury (reviewed by Liu and colleagues[55]). Structurally different calpain inhibitors have shown promising protective effects in various experimental studies in vivo. For example, the calpain inhibitor Cbz-Leu-Leu-Tyr-CHN$_2$ afforded protection from ischemic-reperfusion liver injury and from preservation-reperfusion injury in rat liver transplantation (both reviewed by Liu and colleagues[55]). Another calpain inhibitor (Cbz-Val-Phe-H; MDL28170) conferred protection against hippocampus neuron injury and death, reduced focal cerebral ischemia (also reviewed by Liu and colleagues[55]), and attenuated thioacetamide (TAA)-induced acute liver failure and hepatocyte apoptosis.[54] PD150606 attenuated renal ischemia-reperfusion[54] and reduced neuronal cell death in rat cerebral ischemia[56] and α-amino-3-hydroxy-5-methyl-4-isoxazolepropionic acid (AMPA)-induced toxicity.[57] AK295 protected neurons from focal brain ischemia (reviewed by Carragher[54]), prevented paclitaxel-induced axonal degeneration and clinical neuropathy in mice, and prevented traumatic brain injury (also reviewed by Carragher[54]). Leupeptin and calpain inhibitor XI inhibited apoptosis in the motor neurons of adult spinal cord injury.[58] Calpain inhibitors also prevented neuronal cell death and ameliorated motor disturbances after compression-induced spinal cord injury in rodents[59] and was protective in muscular dystrophies,[60] Alzheimer's disease,[61] and optic nerve degeneration.[62] Calpain inhibitor MDL28170 or adenovirus-mediated overexpression of the endogenous calpain inhibitor protein calpastatin also attenuated loss of nigral dopamine neurons in an MPTP-induced mouse model of Parkinson's disease. The inhibition of calpains prevented reduced motor function in this model.[63]

Serine Protease Omi/HtrA2 Inhibitor

Serine protease Omi/HtrA2 is a nucleus-encoded mitochondrial-resident protein in healthy cells which in response to an apoptotic signal is released to the cytoplasm. Once in the cytosol, Omi/HtrA2 can induce cell death in a caspase-independent manner owing to its protease activity,[6] or it can induce cell death in a caspase-dependent manner by inactivating the IAPs and subsequently releasing active caspases from IAP-bound caspases.[7] Omi is markedly upregulated in the mouse kidney after ischemia-reperfusion. A nonpeptidyl inhibitor, Ucf-101, entered mammalian cells and specifically inhibited Omi's proteolytic activity both in vitro and in vivo.[64] Thus, this specific inhibitor has enabled delineation of the function of Omi in cell injury and apoptosis in experimental models. In mouse and larval zebrafish models of cisplatin-induced acute kidney injury, Ucf-101 improved renal function and blocked proteolytic activity of Omi/HtrA2.[65] Ucf-101 ameliorated ischemia-reperfusion injury in a rat heart,[66] provided neuroprotection in focal cerebral ischemia,[67] and prevented renal failure and increased animal survival. Pre-ischemia treatment of animals with ucf-101, the specific inhibitor of Omi/HtrA2, reduced the number of TUNEL-positive cells, attenuated XIAP breakdown, and reduced infarct size.

p53 Inhibitors

The p53 protein is a transcription factor that is activated in response to intrinsic and extrinsic stress signals including DNA damage, telomere attrition, oncogene activation, hypoxia, and loss of normal growth and survival signals.[68] The activation of p53 involves protein modification including phosphorylation, acetylation, methylation, and ubiquitination, depending on the nature of the stress signal. Thus, signal-specific activation of p53 controls either cell cycle arrest, senescence, differentiation, or apoptosis.[68] Many DNA-damaging agents such as radiation, chemotherapeutic agents, hypoxia, and oxidative stress generally activate p53-dependent apoptosis.[69] This apoptosis involves direct transcriptional control of a multitude of proapoptotic genes that code for BH-3–only proteins of the Bcl-2 family, death receptors, and other factors involved in various steps of the apoptotic pathway[68] (see Fig. 83-1). In addition to transcriptional regulation, extranuclear transcriptionally independent activities of p53 play a role in mediating the induction of apoptosis.[70] The extranuclear p53 that accumulates in the cytoplasm after stabilization can directly activate Bax[70] or directly bind to Bcl-xL and Bcl-2 proteins to induce mitochondrial permeabilization and cytochrome c release.[71] Thus, as p53 activation plays a key role in the permeabilization of the outer mitochondrial membrane, it can be an important target for interruption upstream of caspase activation.

The p53 protein is activated in a variety of pathological conditions including ischemic acute kidney injury[72] as well as ischemic damage from strokes or cardiac arrest,[73] degenerative diseases such as arthritis, multiple sclerosis,[74] and neuropathies such as Alzheimer's and Parkinson's diseases.[75] In addition, the side effect of cancer treatment with radiation and chemotherapeutic agents results in p53-dependent apoptosis of normal cells. Acute p53 activation contributes to the side effects of cancer chemotherapy, whereas chronic p53 activation can contribute to aging.[73] The discovery of pifithrin-α, a pharmacological inhibitor of p53, and the availability of p53-deficient mice have enabled exploration of the role of p53 in experimental models that involve genotoxic stress (Table 83-3).

Pifithrin-α ameliorated renal dysfunction in renal ischemia-reperfusion injury,[75] provided neuroprotection from ischemic brain damage in both transient focal cerebral ischemia[75,76] and transient global cerebral ischemia,[75,76] and significantly decreased infarct size and provided cardioprotection in an ischemic heart model.[77] Pifithrin-α also protected dopaminergic neurons in a classic mouse model of Parkinson's disease, wherein selective dopaminergic cell death was induced by the mitochondrial poison MPTP.[75] In a model of Alzheimer's disease induced by administration of the excitotoxin kainite (an analogue of glutamate), pifithrin-α prevented the degeneration and death of pyramidal neurons.[75]

Gamma irradiation, which results in activation of p53, increases Huntington's gene expression in the striatum and cortex of the mouse brain, the major pathological sites for Huntington's disease, in p53[+/+] but not isogenic p53[−/−] mice. These results demonstrate that p53 protein can regulate Huntington's expression at the transcriptional level and suggest that a p53 stress response may be a modulator of the pathogenesis of Huntington's disease.[78] Pifithrin-α protected healthy cells from treatment with DNA-damaging agents or exposure to γ-radiation without a detectable increase in tumor incidence.[79] Another p53 inhibitor, pifithrin-μ, recently was discovered that inhibits p53 binding to the mitochondria by reducing its affinity for antiapoptotic proteins Bcl-2 and Bclx. This inhibitor protected the mouse thymocyte from p53-mediated apoptosis caused by radiation.[79]

TABLE 83-3

p53 Inhibitors as Antiapoptotic Therapeutic Targets of Cell Death in Experimental Models

p53 INHIBITOR	EXPERIMENTAL MODEL(S)	EFFECT(S)
Pifithrin-α	Renal ischemia-reperfusion injury[75]	Prevented apoptosis and renal dysfunction
	Focal and global cerebral ischemia[75,76]	Neuroprotection from brain damage
	Myocardial ischemia-reperfusion[7]	Reduced infarct size; cardioprotection
	MPTP-induced Parkinson's disease[7]	Prevented dopaminergic neuronal apoptosis
	Kainite-induced Alzheimer's disease[7]	Prevented cell death of pyramidal neurons
	DNA-damaging agents and γ-radiation treatments for tumors[7]	Protected healthy cells from apoptosis
Pifithrin-μ	Radiation-induced thymocyte injury[7]	Prevented thymocyte apoptosis

MPTP, 1-methyl-4-phenyl-1,2,3,6-tetrahydropyridine.

PARP Inhibitors

Poly(ADP)-ribose polymerase (PARP), the most abundant enzyme in the nucleus, plays an important role in DNA repair, depletion of cellular ATP pools, and transcriptional control of pro-inflammatory genes.[80] PARP is activated by means of single- and double-stranded DNA breaks and subsequently cleaves NAD+ to transfer the ADP-ribose moiety of nicotinamide adenine dinucleotide (NAD) to nuclear proteins associated in DNA repair. Under conditions of excessive DNA breakage, overactivation of PARP results in depletion of its substrate NAD+ and eventually ATP, leading to cell death. PARP is one of the first substrates of caspase-3 to be identified and generally is recognized as the "death substrate." Caspase-3–mediated cleavage of PARP has been used extensively as a biochemical marker of apoptosis. The role of this cleavage was determined using PARP-1 knockin mice in which the caspase cleavage site of PARP-1 was mutated to render the protein resistant to caspase cleavage. PARP-1 knockin mice developed normally; however, they were highly resistant to endotoxic shock and to renal and intestinal ischemia-reperfusion injury. This protection was associated with reduced inflammatory responses.[81]

A variety of PARP inhibitors have been used in animal models of human diseases, including shock, ischemia-reperfusion, and diabetes (Table 83-4). The most effective and potent inhibitors have been derived from the benzamide pharmacophore.[81] PARP inhibitors such as 3-aminobenzamide and PARP knockout mice preserved the decline in ATP levels and renal function and attenuated an inflammatory response in ischemia-reperfusion injury in the mouse model.[81,82] In addition, PARP inhibitors afforded protection in ischemia-reperfusion damage in a wide variety of models including brain, heart, liver, eye, bowel, and skin.[81,82] PARP inhibitors such as nicotinamide; 3-aminobenzamide, 4-amino-1,8-naphthalimide, and 1,5-isoquinolinediol have been demonstrated in cerebral ischemia-reperfusion injury.[83] The novel and highly potent PARP inhibitor FR247304 was more effective in attenuating cerebral brain ischemia[84] than the other widely used PARP inhibitors 3-aminobenzamide and PJ34. Similarly another PARP inhibitor, NU1025, is more potent than conventional PARP inhibitors such as nicotinamide, benzamide, and 3-aminobenzamide in that it was neuroprotective and reversed NAD depletion and DNA fragmentation in a rat model of cerebral ischemia.[85] Administration of various pharmacologic PARP inhibitors or PARP knockout genotypes afforded resistance to septic shock.[82] Details of the cytoprotective effect of PARP inhibitors have been reviewed.[82]

One of the potent PARP inhibitors (developed by Inotek Pharmaceuticals, Beverly, MA) is the isoindolinone-based PARP inhibitor INO-1001, which afforded protection from stroke in preclinical studies, myocardial infarction, and chronic heart failure.[86-88] Also, INO-1001 reduced vascular permeability and inflammatory response in lung ischemia-reperfusion injury.[82] In a rat model of diabetic nephropathy of Lepr(db/db), INO-1001 ameliorated albumin excretion and mesangial expansion.[89] INO-1001 has entered into phase 2 clinical trials for the treatment of reperfusion injury in myocardial infarction, cardiopulmonary bypass, and thoracoabdominal aortic aneurysm surgery.[80,82] Another PARP inhibitor, AG140699 (developed by Pfizer and University of Newcastle, United Kingdom), is undergoing clinical trials, in combination with temozolomide, for the treatment of malignant melanoma.

Bcl-2 Family Members
Targeting Antiapoptotic Bcl-2 Overexpression

In a mouse model of renal ischemia-reperfusion injury, intrarenal arterial administration of the adenovirus vector–expressing Bcl-2 (Ad-Bcl-2) gene inhibited proximal and distal tubular apoptosis, reduced ROS production, and improved renal function.[90] Transgenic mice overexpressing Bcl-2 ameliorated ischemia-reperfusion injury in the myocardium[11] and provided neuroprotection from focal cerebral ischemic injury.[11,91] Cardiomyoblast grafts expressing human Bcl-2 were more resistant to apoptosis, which led to enhanced graft survival in the ischemic rat myocardium.[92] Bcl-2 overexpression also improved survival of newly generated neurons in the hippocampal dentate gyrus under normal and ischemic conditions.[93]

TABLE 83-4

PARP Inhibitors as Antiapoptotic Therapeutic Targets of Cell Death in Experimental Models

PARP INHIBITOR	EXPERIMENTAL MODEL	EFFECT(S)
BGP-15	Cisplatin-induced nephrotoxicity[8]	Preserved ATP levels, renal function
FR247304	Cerebral ischemia-reperfusion[84]	Decreased ischemic brain damage
PJ34	Experimental model of cardiopulmonary bypass[8]	Recovery of myocardial and endothelial function
3-AB	Myocardial ischemia-reperfusion[8]	Diminished infarct size and preserved ATP pools
	Renal ischemia-reperfusion injury[8]	Reduced renal dysfunction, decline in ATP and inflammatory response
NU1025	Rat model of cerebral ischemia[8]	Neuroprotection
INO-1001	Experimental model of cardioplegic arrest and extracorporeal circulation[8]	Recovery of myocardial and endothelial function
	Heart failure by coronary ligation[8]	Improved both cardiac function and vascular relaxation
	Lung ischemia-reperfusion injury[81]	Reduced vascular permeability and alveolar leukocyte accumulation
	Rat cardiac transplantation[8]	Improved cardiac function and survival
	Diabetic nephropathy of Lepr(db/db)[8]	Ameliorated albumin excretion and mesangial expansion
	Traumatic brain injury[8]	Improved recovery from traumatic brain injury

ATP, adenosine triphosphate; PARP, poly(ADP)-ribose polymerase.

Targeting Depletion of Proapoptotic Members of the Bcl-2 Family

Conversely, depletion of Bid or Bax, the proapoptotic members of the Bcl-2 family, ameliorated ischemia-reperfusion injury in the kidney, brain, and heart.[94,91] These results indicate that modulation of Bcl-2 levels may have implications for therapeutic intervention in ischemia-reperfusion injury in these organs. In an effort for therapeutic intervention, the Bax channel inhibitor was tested in an animal model of global brain ischemia.[11,91] Ku70, a new Bax suppressor protein, blocked the mitochondrial translocation of Bax in response to an apoptotic stimulus.[91] Peptides based on the amino acid sequence of Bax-binding domain of human Ku70 demonstrated that these peptides bind Bax and inhibit Bax-dependent apoptosis in human cell lines.[91] Using a nuclear magnetic resonance (NMR) spectroscopy approach, a class of small molecules were identified that specifically bind to tBid, preventing its translocation to the mitochondrial membrane and the subsequent release of proapoptotic stimuli and inhibiting neuronal apoptosis.[95] On the basis of their chemical-biological features, antiapoptotic compounds hold great promise for the treatment of disorders associated with Bid activation, such as ischemic injury, neurodegenerative diseases, or brain trauma.

Fas and Tumor Necrosis Factor

Increasing evidence has implicated Fas-mediated apoptosis in ischemia-reperfusion injury in multiple tissues including the brain, heart, kidney, and gut.[11,12] Injection of small interfering RNA–targeting Fas protected mice against renal ischemia-reperfusion injury.[11] Mice lacking functional CD95 (lpr) displayed a marked reduction in cell death in a model of myocardial ischemia-reperfusion.[11] Neutralization of the CD95 ligand (CD95L) using CD95L-specific antibodies or FasL-mutant mice or mice lacking a functional Fas receptor reduced cell death and promoted axonal regeneration and functional recovery in a model of spinal cord injury.[96] Several studies have documented that

a soluble Fas receptor (sFasR) can prevent Fas and FasL binding.[11,12] Thus, administration of sFasR attenuated post-traumatic apoptosis and improved functional outcome (neuroprotection and oligodendrocyte survival) in traumatic spinal cord injury.[97] Neutralization of CD95L and TNF-α by administration of their specific antibodies led to a marked decrease in both infarct volume and mortality rate in a mouse model of stroke[11,12] (Table 83-5). *Fas* or *TNFR1* gene ablation ameliorated cell death and renal dysfunction in toxic acute kidney injury induced by cisplatin.[98]

Mice deficient in TNFR1 were resistant to lipopolysaccharide (LPS)-induced renal failure.[99] However, TNFR2-deficient mice developed less severe renal dysfunction and showed reduced necrosis and apoptosis and leukocyte infiltration into the kidney compared with either TNFR1-deficient or wild-type mice.[100] In addition, the TNF-α inhibitors GM6001 and pentoxifylline or lack of a functional TNF-α gene in a mouse model also ameliorated cisplatin-induced renal dysfunction and reduced cisplatin-induced structural damage.[101] Inhibition of TNF-α action, whether with a TNF-binding protein,[102] pentoxifylline,[103] or neutralizing antobodies,[104] reduced renal dysfunction in ischemia-reperfusion injury. Because TNF is involved in the pathogenesis of rheumatoid arthritis and inflammatory bowel disease, anti-TNF antibodies were studied for possible benefit in this setting and were found to prevent the development of clinical disease.[105] Treatment of these arthritic mice[106] and mice with Crohn's disease[107] with a monoclonal antibody against human TNF completely prevented development of this disease. Chimeric neutralizing antibodies have been approved by the FDA for the treatment of inflammatory arthritis and inflammatory bowel disease in patients.[108]

CONCLUSION

Limited information exists on the details of signal transduction pathways of cell death, which are predominant in the pathophysiology of renal injury. More research is needed to delineate both caspase-dependent and caspase-

TABLE 83-5

CD95L, CD95/Fas, TNF-α, and TNFR as Antiapoptotic Therapeutic Targets of Cell Death in Experimental Models and Clinical Therapy

TARGET/REAGENT	EXPERIMENTAL MODEL(S)	EFFECT(S)
Fas siRNA	Ischemia-reperfusion in mouse kidney[11]	Protected from AKI and apoptosis
Fas	Myocardial ischemia-reperfusion in Fas-deficient lpr mice[11,12]	Reduced myocardial cell death
CD95L Ab	Mouse model of spinal cord injury[96]	Functional recovery, reduced cell death
sFasR	Traumatic spinal cord injury[12,96]	Neuroprotection; survival of oligodendrocyte
CD95LAb or TNFAb	Mouse model of stroke[11,12]	Reduced infarct size and improved animal survival
Fas or TNFR1	LPS model of renal injury in TNFR1−/− mice[9]	Functional protection; reduced apoptosis and neutrophil infiltration
TNFR1 and TNFR2	Cisplatin nephrotoxicity in TNFR1−/− mice and in TNFR2−/− mice[98,10]	Reduced apoptosis, necrosis, and leukocyte infiltration
TNF-α Inhibitors		
GM6001, pentoxifylline	Renal ischemia-reperfusion[103,104] and cisplatin nephrotoxicity[101]	Ameliorated renal dysfunction and structural damage
TNF monoclonal Ab	Animal models of rheumatoid arthritis[106] and inflammatory bowel disease[107]	Prevented development of the disease

Ab, antibody; AKI, acute kidney injury; LPS; lipopolysaccharide; siRNA, small interfering ribonucleic acid; TNF, tumor necrosis factor; TNFR, tumor necrosis factor receptor.

independent pathways of cell death in this context. Nonetheless, initial preclinical studies with certain antiapoptotic agents have yielded preliminary results indicating some degree of cytoprotection in renal injury. Many new tissue-permeable and more stable therapeutic agents are being designed and developed by pharmaceutical companies that target both caspase-dependent and -independent pathways of cell death that are involved in a wide variety of human diseases. Most of these agents, however, have not been tested in preclinical studies related to kidney disease. Future studies of these pharmaceutical agents, either alone or in combination therapy, are warranted to explore their potential for the treatment or prevention of renal diseases.

Key Points

1. Apoptosis is regulated by many signaling transduction pathways and in most but not all cases these pathways converge into activation of caspases.
2. Antiapoptotic agents include not only caspase inhibitors but in many cases inhibitors of calpain, serine proteases, p53, poly(ADP)-ribose polymerase, and members of the proapoptotic Bcl-2 family.
3. Many new cell-permeable antiapoptotic agents have been designed that should be considered for use in preclinical trials involving experimental models of kidney diseases.
4. Future clinical trials for inhibition of cell death should consider combination therapy for inhibition of both caspase-dependent and caspase-independent pathways.

Key References

11. Green DR, Kroemer G: Pharmacological manipulation of cell death: Clinical applications in sight? J Clin Invest 2005;115:2610-2617.
12. Fischer U, Schulze-Osthoff K: New approaches and therapeutics targeting apoptosis in disease. Pharmacol Rev 2005;57:187-215.
27. Waldmeier PC, Tatton WG: Interrupting apoptosis in neurodegenerative disease: Potential for effective therapy? Drug Discov Today 2004;9:210-218.

See the companion Expert Consult website for the complete reference list.

CHAPTER 84

Growth Factors

Antonio Dal Canton, Ciro Esposito, Filippo Mangione, and Teresa Rampino

OBJECTIVES

This chapter will:
1. Present an overview of the rationale for use of growth factors in prevention and treatment of acute tubular necrosis.
2. Describe the effects of exogenously administered growth factors in experimental models of acute tubular necrosis.
3. Review the clinical trials in which patients with acute tubular necrosis have been treated with growth factors.

Treatment with growth factors is restricted to acute renal failure caused by ischemic or toxic injury—that is, acute tubular necrosis (ATN). Therefore, this chapter deals only with ATN.

RATIONALE FOR USE OF GROWTH FACTORS IN ACUTE TUBULAR NECROSIS

Three basic pathophysiological concepts support the therapeutic use of growth factors in ATN:

In ATN, tubular cell death is the main cause of renal dysfunction. Replacement of died cells with new ones regenerated from surviving cells is fundamental to recovery of tubular integrity and function. Regeneration implies cell *proliferation* and differentiation, processes that are driven by growth factors.

By definition, in ATN, tubular cells die from necrosis—that is, they are directly killed by the lethal ischemic or toxic injury. In ATN, however, overt necrosis is not as widespread and is usually limited to the last segment of the proximal tubule. Apoptosis is another cause of death that predominates in cells of the distal nephron. Apoptosis is a form of programmed cell death that results from an active process. Normal cells constitutively express the machinery necessary for apoptosis but are prevented from undergoing apoptosis by survival factors. Loss of these factors triggers apoptosis by way of a default pathway. Growth factors can *prevent apoptosis* by working as or inducing survival factors.[1]

Cells that are exposed to a nonlethal ischemic injury resist subsequent ischemic attack more effectively. This kind of protection is called *preconditioning*. Several mediators of preconditioning have been identified, including enzymes of the mitogen-activated protein kinase/extracellular signal-regulated kinase (MAPK/ERK) cascade. The MAPK/ERK system typically is activated by growth factors; thus, growth factors can afford protection against ischemia by evoking preconditioning.

A prerequisite for the therapeutic use of a growth factor in ATN is that it bring about one or more of the aforementioned effects—proliferation, protection from apoptosis, preconditioning—in tubular cells. In addition, any growth factor that participates in the spontaneous process of healing may be presumed to be therapeutic when administered exogenously. Growth factors that possess these requisites are discussed next.

CANDIDATE GROWTH FACTORS FOR EXOGENOUS USE

Epidermal Growth Factor

Epidermal growth factor (EGF) is a 6045-D protein belonging to a family of molecules that includes transforming growth factor-α and heparin-binding EGF-like growth factor (HB-EGF). The receptor of EGF is part of the family of the *erb* tyrosine kinase receptors. In vitro, EGF stimulates the proliferation of several types of renal tubular cells, either of proximal or of distal origin, and protects tubular cells from apoptosis. Furthermore, in confluent cultures EGF accelerates the repair of a mechanical injury by stimulating cell migration, and inhibits the release of endothelin-1, a vasoconstrictor with a pathogenic role in ischemic ATN. Of interest, in tubular cells mechanically injured in vitro, the EGF receptor is activated even in the absence of exogenous EGF, suggesting an autocrine loop in which HB-EGF is the probable ligand; in fact, HB-EGF is constitutively expressed in cultured proximal tubular cells (PTCs).[2] In PTCs, the EGF-induced proliferation requires the activation of the phosphoinositide-3 kinase (PI3K)/Akt, MAPK, and ERK1/2 signal transduction pathways and is mediated by the trascription factor nuclear factor (NF)-κB; EGF protects from apoptosis by inhibiting dephosphorylation of BAD (a Bcl-2 agonist of cell death)—that is, the reaction that allows BAD to move to the mitochondrial membrane and initiate apoptosis.[3]

In the normal kidney EGF is moderately expressed in the distal tubule, whereas its receptor is localized to both distal and proximal tubules. In experimental models of ATN, total renal EGF and EGF messenger RNA (mRNA) decrease, and the total amount of EGF receptor is markedly reduced. In patients with ATN, urinary levels of EGF are significantly decreased. These findings argue against a role for EGF in renal repair; however, recovery from ATN was markedly impaired in mice with a mutation of the EGF receptor, causing its functional failure.[4] In addition, in the regeneration phase of ATN, tubular expression of EGF trails the expression of the antiapoptotic protein Bcl-2, and the number of EGF receptors localized to the basolateral membrane of the proximal tubule is increased, suggesting that EGF of systemic origin or released from inflammatory cells may enhance cell proliferation.[5]

Insulin-like Growth Factor-1

Insulin-like growth factor-1 (IGF-1) is a peptide of 7650 D. The IGF-1 receptor has tyrosine kinase activity. In both serum and tissues, IGF-1 is bound to a series of binding proteins (IGFBPs) that regulate its bioavailability. IGF-1 increases protein synthesis, is mitogenic, and reduces anoxia-induced apoptosis in PTCs. PI3K, MAPK, and ERK activation is required for IGF-1–induced protein synthesis, and inhibition of BAD accounts for IGF-1 antiapoptotic activity.[6] IGF-1 is minimally expressed in the adult kidney, whereas its receptor is abundant in the proximal tubule. The synthesis of IGF-1 in the kidney is regulated by the growth hormone. In the early phase of experimental

ATN, the levels of total kidney IGF-1 peptide and IGF-1 mRNA decrease. At 2 to 7 days after injury, however, both IGF-I mRNA and peptide are clearly detectable in the regenerating cells, as well as in infiltrating macrophages. In ATN, the number of renal IGF-1 receptors increases, and this abundance of receptors is associated with increased availability of free IGF-1 resulting from a decrease in tissue IGFBP levels.[7]

Hepatocyte Growth Factor

Hepatocyte growth factor (HGF), known also as scatter factor, is a 75- to 100-kD protein. HGF receptor is the product of the *Met* proto-oncogene, is expressed in tubular cells both in vitro and in vivo, and has tyrosine kinase activity. HGF is a pleiotropic agent that induces proliferation, resistance against apoptosis, movement, and formation of tubules in cultured tubular cells. HGF is much more effective than EGF or IGF-1 in stimulating tubular cell growth and differentiation, and in protecting tubular cells from damage caused by hypoxia or glucose deprivation.[8] The multiple activities of HGF result from recruitment of a complex network of intracellular signal transducers. In particular, the most notable and complicated biological event induced by HGF—tubulogenesis—is mediated by Gab 1 adaptor protein, SHP2 phosphatase downstream of Gab 1, the PI3 kinase pathway, and the ERK/MAPK pathway. Recent studies demonstrate that the potassium channel KCNA1, the calcium channel TRPC6, and the sodium-proton exchanger NHE1 are cell machineries that are exploited by HGF to effect its biological outcome in renal tubular cells.[9] HGF is synthesized in the kidney by interstitial fibroblasts, and its renal production increases in ATN.[10] After experimental ischemic, toxic, or mechanical renal injury, HGF is released as an inactive profactor not only in the kidney but also in distant organs such as the liver, lung, and spleen, and pro-HGF is transformed into active HGF by enzymes released in the injured renal tissue. A systemic release of HGF and a marked rise of HGF serum levels also occur in human ATN. In ATN, renal Met expression increases.[11] These observations indicate that HGF is both a paracrine and an endocrine effector of renal tissue repair.

Erythropoietin

The finding that erythropoietin (EPO) receptors are expressed throughout the kidney, particularly in tubular cells, underscored a potential paracrine role for EPO other than the regulation of erythropoiesis. Because EPO production is controlled by hypoxia, it was logical to suppose a protective role for EPO in ischemic-hypoxic injury. In fact, in vitro EPO affects survival of PTCs exposed to serum deprivation or hypoxia. Furthermore, EPO stimulates proliferation of PTCs in a dose-dependent manner.[12] The signals that mediate EPO-regulated cell survival include JAK2 and transcription factors of the STAT family, which activate the antiapoptotic protein Bcl-X$_L$, and the PI3/AKT cascade, which inhibits the proapoptotic proteins BAD and caspase-9. Of interest, endothelial cells also express the EPO receptor, and EPO antagonizes apoptosis of endothelial cells subjected to hypoxic stress in vitro.[13] Thus, EPO may protect from endothelial dysfunction, which has been recognized to play a major role in the extension and maintenance phase of ATN.

Other Growth Factors

Parathormone (PTH)-related protein (PTHrP) is a protein homologous to PTH that binds to type 1 PTH receptor. PTHrP is mitogenic for distal tubule–like MDCK (Madin-Darby canine kidney) cells and subconfluent PTCs. PTHrP mRNA and protein increase in the renal cortex during the recovery phase after ischemia- or toxin (folic acid)-induced injury. On the basis of these findings, suggesting that PTHrP participates in the renal regenerative process as an autocrine factor, exogenous PTHrP has been tested in ATN.[14]

Some growth factors, such as basic fibroblast growth factor (bFGF) and bone morphogenic protein-7 (BMP-7), participate as morphogens in early kidney development and are expressed in the kidney in the regeneration phase of acute renal failure. These observations have suggested that renal regeneration recapitulates part of the organogenic process and have led to use of these morphogens to accelerate the repair process in ATN.[1]

Growth hormone is the hormone that induces the release of IGF-1, a growth factor of potential therapeutic utility in ATN, as discussed earlier. Because renal expression of IGF-1 falls in ATN, it seems rational to administer exogenous growth hormone to increase circulating and local renal levels of IGF-1. Ghrelin is a stomach-derived growth hormone secretagogue that has been tested in ATN with the aim of stimulating growth hormone and therefore IGF-1 release.[15]

Thyroid hormones are not growth factors but are mentioned here because they have been used in ATN as enhancers of endogenous EGF activity. In fact, T_3 increases the expression of EGF receptor, EGF-induced cell growth, and DNA synthesis in PTCs in vitro.[2]

TREATMENT WITH GROWTH FACTORS IN EXPERIMENTAL ACUTE TUBULAR NECROSIS

Treatment with exogenous growth factors has been investigated in a variety of ischemic-toxic models of ATN. Growth factors have been administered either before inducing the injury, to prevent renal failure, or at different stages after the injury has been established. The reproducibility of the clinicopathological picture and the possibility of administering growth factors at specific intervals, at different stages of the disease, have made experimental models an invaluable tool for elucidating growth factor pharmacodynamics.

Epidermal Growth Factor

Humes and colleagues[16] first reported that EGF administered to rats soon after release of bilateral renal artery clamp enhanced tubular cell regeneration and accelerated renal functional recovery. It was then demonstrated that EGF also reduced the mortality rate among rats with postischemic ATN. The beneficial effects of EGF were confirmed in toxin-induced ATN: Administration of EGF before injection of a toxic dose of gentamicin lowered peak blood urea nitrogen (BUN) and serum creatinine levels and increased renal DNA synthesis in the recovery phase. Similar results were observed when EGF was given 2 to 4 days after induction of ATN with mercuric chloride.[1] In contrast with these results in rats, administration of EGF directly into the artery of an autotransplanted pig kidney after 120 minutes of warm ischemia had no beneficial effect on renal function.[17]

Insulin-like Growth Factor-1

The pilot study by Miller and coworkers[18] showing a beneficial effect of IGF-1 in postischemic ATN in rats was followed by a considerable number of experimental studies in the same animal model. IGF-1 was given either before or after ischemia, and in the latter case either as bolus injection or by continued subcutaneous administration for up to 7 days after the ischemic insult. Most of the studies were confirmatory, showing that IGF-1 reduced the fall in glomerular filtration rate and the rise in BUN, decreased the score of histological damage and the number of tubular cells undergoing apoptosis, increased DNA synthesis, accelerated functional and anatomical recovery, and decreased mortality. Some voices did not join in the chorus, however, indicating no benefit or even a worse outcome in rats that received IGF-1.[19] Treatment with IGF-1 also was investigated in toxic models of ATN and was found effective in mercuric chloride– and cisplatin-induced but not in radiocontrast agent–induced renal failure.

It is thought that the therapeutic efficacy of IGF-1 does not depend only on its mitogenic activity. Part of the protective action of IGF-1 has been attributed to its renal vasodilating effect, resulting from nitric oxide (NO) and prostaglandin release. Actually, it has been shown that IGF-1 increases renal blood flow and glomerular filtration rate in rats as well as in normal human volunteers.[20] In addition, IGF-1 may promote tissue regeneration and reduce mortality by promoting anabolism and protein synthesis. In the case of pretreatment, the mechanism of action of IGF-1 is thought to be similar to the preconditioning effect of sublethal hypoxia-ischemia, which induces cellular proteins that protect against successive injury. A downstream target of IGF-1 relevant to ischemic preconditioning has been proposed: osteopontin, a protein that contains an R-G-D peptide (arginine-glycine-aspartate) sequence that binds to integrins. Osteopontin induced by IGF-1 would serve as a source of R-G-D that binds to integrins expressed on the surface of tubular cells, preventing integrin-mediated cell aggregation and tubular plugging.[21] An interesting clue to how IGF-1 works as a cell survival factor has been provided by the observation that in cisplatin-induced ATN, IGF-1 enhanced p21 expression and suppressed cyclin D_1 expression in damaged tubular cells. The protein p21 is a cyclin-dependent kinase inhibitor that is responsible for controlling the G_1-S phase checkpoint. In the event of DNA damage, enhanced p21 and suppressed cyclin D_1 would arrest cisplatin-exposed cells in the G_1 phase, allowing DNA repair before the start of DNA replication.[22]

Hepatocyte Growth Factor

The protean effects of HGF observed in vitro and the identification of HGF as a powerful endocrine and paracrine effector of renal tissue regeneration prompted Kawaida and coworkers to administer exogenous HGF in mice given nephrotoxic doses of cisplatin or mercuric chloride, or subjected to partial nephrectomy.[23] The remarkable suppression of renal dysfunction and the reconstruction of normal renal tissue effected by HGF induced these investigators to conclude that the long-sought renotropic factor had been found. Successive studies confirmed the renoprotective capacity of HGF in other models of toxic ATN—ATN induced by glycerol, cyclosporine, and folic acid and postischemic ATN, in both mice and rats. The beneficial effects of HGF included a decrease in tubular necrosis and apoptosis scores, an increase in DNA synthesis, and a fall in mortality rate. Of interest, HGF also reduced the number of infiltrating inflammatory cells, an effect that was explained by a suppression of tubular adhesion molecules and chemokines such as intercellular adhesion molecule-1 (ICAM-1) and RANTES. The protective effect of HGF was particularly impressive when its production was induced in the kidney by direct transfer of a plasmid vector encoding HGF, or in transgenic mice overexpressing HGF in proximal tubular cells.[24]

Erythropoietin

An impressive capacity of EPO to prevent ischemic damage was first shown in animal models of ischemic brain injury and was thought to depend on induction of preconditioning by EPO. Yang and coworkers then showed the protective effect of a preconditioning regimen of EPO in the rat model of renal ischemia-reperfusion.[25] Similar results were obtained in successive studies in rats and mice, not only in the ischemic model but also in cisplatin- and radiocontrast-induced ATN. In most of these studies, the administration of EPO preceded the injury and the dose was high, on the order of thousands of units per kilogram. A protective effect also was shown with lower doses, however, and when the treatment was started soon before ischemia or at reperfusion. The most striking finding in treated animals was a marked suppression of tubular cell apoptosis associated with a reduction in caspase activity and an increase in Bcl-2 expression. An increased renal expression of heat shock protein-70 and a reduced recruitment of leukocytes also were observed.

Other Growth Factors

In transgenic mice overexpressing PTHrP in the proximal tubule, the severity of postischemic or folic acid–induced renal damage was similar to that observed in control mice.[14] Rats with ischemic ATN treated with bFGF had better renal function and more normal morphology than control animals. In treated rats, apoptotic tubular cells and infiltrating monocytes were decreased, and the renal expression of nephrogenic proteins that participate in early kidney development was increased.[1]

In 1998, a promising study performed in rats with ischemic renal failure showed that BMP-7 given 10 minutes before or at different times up to 72 hours after reperfusion preserved renal function, minimized cell necrosis, decreased the number of plugged tubules, and suppressed neutrophil accumulation.[2] Unfortunately, no further study with BMP-7 has been done since then.

Growth hormone administered to rats with ischemic ATN did not modify the course of the disease. By contrast, ghrelin ameliorated renal function and increased renal injury score and survival in mice with ischemic ATN.[15]

A limited number of studies have yielded evidence that thyroxine can preserve renal function in rats given nephrotoxic salts (potassium dichromate and uranyl nitrate) or subjected to renal ischemia. Of interest, in the ischemia model, thyroxine was more effective when administered 24 hours after the ischemic insult.[2]

CLINICAL USE OF GROWTH FACTORS IN ACUTE RENAL FAILURE

The unavailability of preparations designed and licensed for administration in humans has hindered the clinical use of some growth factors, such as HGF. The endogenous production of HGF is markedly increased by hemodialysis, a phenomenon that is independent of the type of dialyzer and of anticoagulation, and lasts for 24 hours after the end of treatment.[26] Serum levels of HGF also are increased by heparin administration. These observations raise the question of whether hemodialysis or heparin treatment may potentially accelerate renal recovery by stimulating HGF release. This question will be difficult to answer in view of the multiple effects of both treatments and of the complexity of the clinical picture in human ATN.

Another major obstacle to use of growth factors in patients is the potential tumorigenic effect of these agents. This consideration is especially important in the case of EGF, which is thought to sustain growth in several cancers—so much so that its receptor is the target of therapeutic neutralizing antibodies or inhibitors currently under clinical experimentation.[27] Similarly, bFGF, PTHrP, and HGF are suspected of being involved in tumor cell growth.

Insulin-like Growth Factor-1

Franklin and colleagues[28] enrolled 54 patients who underwent surgery of the suprarenal aorta or the renal arteries requiring 60- to 70-minute renal ischemia in a double-blind, randomized, placebo-controlled trial. IGF-1 (100 μg/kg) was administered subcutaneously every 12 hours for 6 doses. The primary endpoint was the incidence of renal dysfunction. None of the patients required dialysis, and a smaller proportion of patients in the IGF-1 treatment group experienced a postoperative decline in renal function (22%) than in the placebo group (33%). The rise in serum creatinine was mild, however, and no significant differences in levels of serum creatinine at discharge were found. This study was underpowered to provide evidence of the utility of IGF-1 and merely established the feasibility of administration of IGF-1 in humans.

Hirschberg and associates performed a multicenter randomized, double-blind, placebo-controlled clinical trial in intensive care units in 20 teaching hospitals.[29] Seventy-two patients with acute renal failure were recruited, in whom the most common causes of renal failure were sepsis and hypotension or hemodynamic shock. IGF-1 was administered subcutaneously (100 μg/kg) every 12 hours starting within 6 days of the onset of renal failure, for up to 14 days. The primary endpoint was a change in glomerular filtration rate from baseline. Other endpoints included changes from baseline in urine volume, serum urea, serum albumin, frequency of dialysis, and death. The study was terminated at a predetermined interim evaluation owing to lack of effect of IGF-1 on renal function or any other clinical outcome.[29]

Several possible explanations have been suggested for such failure of IGF-1 treatment, in contrast with the beneficial effects of IGF-1 in experimental models. First, in animals, acute renal failure is created as an isolated disorder, whereas the patients were very ill and had many comorbid conditions potentially associated with reinjury to nephrons or release of cytokines antagonizing IGF-1. Second, throughout the period of study, patients received medicines, such as antibiotics or vasoactive agents, that were potentially nephrotoxic, thereby slowing the healing process. Third, IGF-1 was administered as late as 6 days after the onset of renal failure, whereas in experimental models, IGF-1 was given before or early after the induction of ATN. To circumvent these confounding factors, a further study was performed in a selected population of patients that served as a human model of postischemic ATN: These patients were recipients of cadaveric renal allograft with delayed graft function.[30] Once again, the results were disappointing, and it was concluded that IGF-1 treatment does not benefit patients with acute renal failure.

Erythropoietin

Despite the widespread use of EPO for treatment of anemia in renal and nonrenal patients, as well as the exciting results obtained in experimental models, no clinical trial of EPO in patients at risk for ischemic ATN has yet been performed. A preconditioning EPO regimen seems especially applicable in selected clinical scenarios such as elective cardiac surgery or with the programmed use of radiocontrast media or other nephrotoxic agents. The high doses of EPO used in experimental models suggest that the dose of EPO for humans should be much higher than that used to treat anemia. This consideration adds argument for caution in view of the dose-dependent side effects of EPO.

Other Growth Factors

Growth hormone was administered to patients with acute renal failure with the objective of studying its effects on metabolic and nutritional parameters. It was found that growth hormone improved nitrogen balance and reduced total nitrogen appearance rate. No significant effect on renal function was reported.

A prospective, randomized, placebo-controlled, double-blind trial investigated the effects of treatment with thyroxine in patients with acute renal failure. Endpoints were dialysis requirement, time to renal recovery, and death. Thyroxine had no effect on the course of the renal disease.[31] Similar disappointing results were obtained in a controlled study in which triiodothyronine was administered to recipients of cadaveric renal transplants with delayed graft function.[32]

CONCLUSION

Experimental studies, both in vitro and in vivo, provide a firm rationale for the therapeutic use of some growth factors in acute renal failure. Nonetheless, the results of clinical trials performed until now have been disappointing. Two promising therapeutic candidates, HGF and EPO, have not yet been investigated in humans. Because HGF is not yet available for clinical use, EPO probably will be the next protagonist in a randomized, double-blind, placebo-controlled study.

Key Points

1. Acute tubular necrosis is a reversible process characterized by tubular cell death followed by a phase of cell regeneration with recovery of renal function.
2. Growth factors play a central role in defense against and recovery from acute tubular necrosis: protection of tubular cells from necrosis and apoptosis. In addition, they drive cell regeneration, inducing proliferation and differentiation.
3. Experimental evidence suggests that among the several growth factors identified thus far, epidermal growth factor, hepatocyte growth factor, insulin-like growth factor-1, and epoietin may facilitate recovery from acute tubular necrosis as endogenous factors, suggesting therapeutic potential.
4. The clinical use of some growth factors has been limited by major obstacles such as their tumorigenic effect, unavailability of preparations, and lack of approval for administration in humans.
5. Once the relevant obstacles have been overcome, some growth factors are likely to be effective agents for the treatment of acute tubular necrosis.

Key References

1. Hammerman MR: Growth factors and apoptosis in acute renal failure. Curr Opin Nephrol Hypertens 1998;7:14-19.
2. Liu KD: Molecular mechanisms of recovery from acute renal failure. Crit Care Med 2003;31:S572-S581.
23. Kawaida K, Matsumoto K, Shimazu H, et al: Hepatocyte growth factor prevents acute renal failure and accelerates renal regeneration in mice. Proc Natl Acad Sci U S A 1994;91:4357-4361.
30. Hladunewich M, Corrigan G, Derby GC, et al: A randomized, placebo controlled trial of IGF-l for delayed graft function: A human model to study postischemic ARF. Kidney Int 2003;64:593-602.

See the companion Expert Consult website for the complete reference list.

CHAPTER 85

Other Experimental Interventions for the Management of Acute Renal Failure

Laurent Mesnard, Jean-Philippe Haymann, and Eric Rondeau

OBJECTIVES

This chapter will:
1. Present an overview of the current knowledge regarding the prevention and treatment of acute renal failure.
2. Summarize the principles of three specific and still experimental approaches: RNA interference, stem cell therapy, and preconditioning.

KIDNEY INJURY AND RNA INTERFERENCE THERAPY

Historical Overview

In 1998, the discovery of a new mode of post-transcriptional regulation mediated by small double-stranded RNA (dsRNA), as seen in the flatworm *Caenorhabditis elegans*, opened up a whole new therapeutic field known as *RNA interference* (RNAi).[1] Indeed, the current development of RNAi holds promise for successful treatment of a wide variety of human diseases.[2] The huge therapeutic and experimental potential of RNAi is illustrated by the 2006 Nobel Prize in Medicine awarded to Craig Mello (at the University of Massachusetts Medical School) and Andrew Fire (at Stanford University School of Medicine) for their contributions to the discovery of RNAi. So long as a morbid process leads to the overexpression of a pathological protein, whether directly or indirectly implicated, a therapeutic approach based on RNAi is suitable.[2] This is particularly true for disorders caused by mutant gene expression, including dominant pathological proteins, aberrant isoform splicing, and gene overexpression leading to accelerated pathological evolution. An overview of the RNA interference machinery is presented in Figure 85-1.

RNA Interference and Double-Stranded RNA Formation

The RNAi Galaxy and the Sound of Gene Silence

Multiple cellular post-transcriptional regulation pathways are mediated by tiny RNA molecules called small interfering RNA (siRNA) and microRNA (miRNA). Use of these pathways in medicine with a therapeutic objective is known as *RNA interference* (RNAi) or *RNA silencing*. Both siRNA and miRNA are functionally equivalent when mediating RNAi but differ in their biogenesis. MiRNAs, or small hairpin RNAs (shRNAs), are produced from transcripts that form a stem-loop structure by means of complementary base pairing at the ends.[2] By contrast, siRNAs are produced from double-stranded RNA (dsRNA) precursors, which can be either endogenously produced or exogenously provided. Both the endogenous and exogenous dsRNA molecules (miRNA and siRNA) are processed through cleavage by the cytoplasmic ribonuclease Dicer.[3] Dicer activity leads to the formation of short 21- to 26-nucleotide duplexes with a symmetrical two-nucleotide overhang at the 3′ end plus a 5′-phosphate and 3′-hydroxy group; such complexes are called siRNA.

The resulting siRNA is incorporated into a nuclease-containing multiprotein complex, RISC (for *R*NA-*i*nduced *s*ilencing *c*omplex), which becomes activated after the loss of one strand of the siRNA duplex, as a result of helicase activity. By binding the now single-stranded siRNA to a complementary target messenger RNA (mRNA) molecule, its sequence specifically guides RISC to this target mRNA and induces endonucleolytic cleavage of the mRNA strand within the target site, thereby generating unprotected RNA ends and rapidly degrading the entire mRNA molecule (by the same enzymes that degrade bulk cellular mRNA), whereas RISC is recovered for further cleavage cycles. For the moment, the best-understood RNAi route is degradation of targeted mRNA by RISC.[3]

Nonspecific Small Interfering RNA Side Effect

Another possible nonspecific siRNA side effect is exportin-5 transport enzyme saturation, leading to liver toxicity. This effect recently was demonstrated in vivo in rodents; however, concomitant adenoviral vector toxicity has not been formally eliminated.

Potential Applications of miRNA/siRNA in Kidney Disease and Characteristics of Renal Cells in Vivo

RNAi techniques have already revolutionized biomedical research. By transfecting shRNAs or siRNAs into cells in vitro, expression of a target gene can be specifically reduced 10-fold. Thus, RNAi now represents an important tool for defining the roles of specific genes in cellular processes. For example, the injection of siRNAs targeting the death receptor Fas has led to the first successful inhibition of

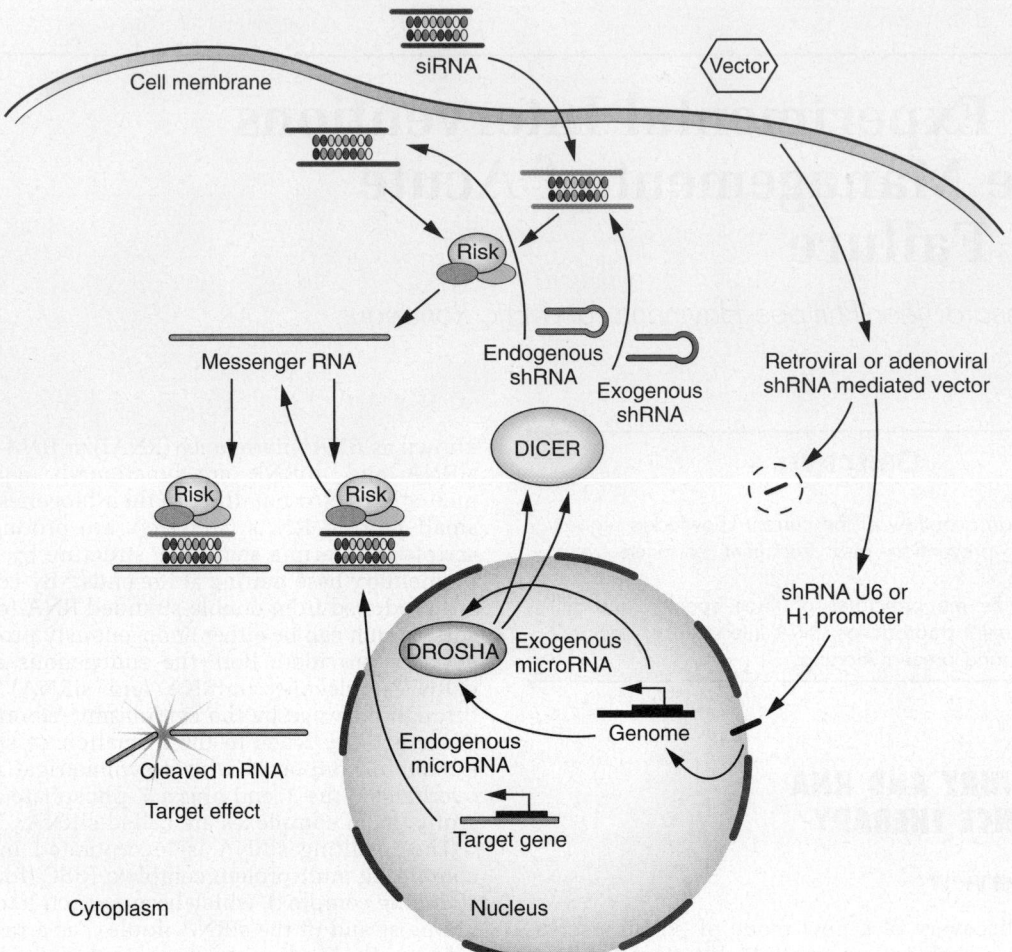

FIGURE 85-1. Overview of RNA interference machinery. See text for details. mRNA, messenger RNA; shRNA, small hairpin RNA; siRNA, small interfering RNA.

experimental autoimmune hepatitis in mice.[4] The potential for RNAi to control overactivation of certain cytokines during the host response also has been confirmed by in vivo studies in sepsis, in which blocking downstream disease mediators such as caspase 8 and tumor necrosis factor-α (TNF-α) may be beneficial.[1] For such systemic and therapeutic use in vivo, the greatest challenge lies in the difficulty of delivery.[1]

A review of published literature regarding the use of RNAi in animal models applicable to the field of kidney disease is presented next, along with an overview of methods currently available for in vivo siRNA application, with particular emphasis on viral delivery.

Viral Delivery: Focus on Adenoviral Vectors

Selection or design of appropriate transfer vectors may turn out to be the rate-limiting step in the development of RNAi based therapeutic strategies. To solve these problems, a promising approach is the use of DNA vectors encoding dsRNA. In this approach, a partially palindromic hairpin loop mRNA with the required sequence is expressed using a plasmid incorporated into the vector designed for a target delivery. The ability of viral vectors

to efficiently transduce cells in vivo coupled with the efficacy of virally expressed siRNA extends the application of siRNA to virus-based therapies and in vivo targeting experiments defining the function of specific genes for further therapeutic implications. With use of currently available viral vectors, however, transduction of the kidneys has been quite difficult.[5] When viral transduction occurs, it often is heterogeneous and transient and sometimes is associated with immune and toxic side effects.[5] A complete evaluation of the efficacy of recombinant adeno-associated virus (AAV) and lentiviral vectors in the kidney remains to be performed, however. The former is small enough to filter through the glomerular basement membrane.[6] This attribute may be critical, because glomerular filtration is required for DNA complex–mediated transduction of tubular cells.

An alternative to in situ renal gene transfer is production of a therapeutic siRNA from a distant site, such as skeletal muscle or liver. Several examples indicate the clinical relevance of this approach for sustained delivery of siRNA in vivo. In addition, it could enable accurate elucidation of the pathophysiological mechanisms implicated in the establishment and maintenance of experimental models of glomerulonephritis or acute renal injury.[5]

Nevertheless, several in vivo studies in rodents have used high-pressure, large-volume tail vein injections to deliver siRNAs either systemically or locally. After intravenous siRNA injection, the liver is the primary site of siRNA uptake, followed by the proximal tubule. Virally mediated siRNAs are promising vectors for RNAi in vivo, and they specifically reduce expression of targeted genes in various cell types, including proximal tubular cells. At present, five types of viral vectors are used for RNAi: retrovirus, lentivirus, baculovirus, AAV, and adenovirus vectors.

Several advantages over other possible vectors make AAV the most promising vector for siRNA delivery. First, AAV is not known to be pathogenic and has a broad range of possible target cells, including nondividing cells and kidney cells. Some experiments have described the use of AAV for in vivo transfection of siRNA, all of them using local injection methods. Thus, the use of AAV for RNAi-based treatment in vivo, for renal disease in particular, still needs to be explored.

Nonviral Delivery

Delivery of RNAi without viral vectors has been attempted with a wide variety of agents, including pure unmodified siRNA or chemically stabilized or modified RNA, siRNA encapsulated in microparticles or liposomes, and siRNA bound to cationic or other particulate carriers.

UNMODIFIED OR "NAKED" siRNA: PARTICULARITY OF HYDRODYNAMIC METHODS. Activity of RNAses in serum led to the use of stabilized or packaged RNA molecules. In mice, if the liver is the only target organ, the problem of distribution of siRNAs for treatment can be successfully addressed. In this setting, siRNAs can be delivered using the so-called hydrodynamic method. Using this method, successful silencing of marker genes in hepatocytes was demonstrated after injection of naked siRNA30 and of hairpin RNA encoding DNA plasmids. With this approach, described only in mice, relatively high volumes ranging from 500 to 2000 µL were injected into the tail vein at high pressures within seconds.

The uptake mechanism is not entirely clear but may involve endothelial leakage through liver sinusoids combined with transient formation of membrane pores in hepatocytes. Direct local delivery of a low volume of Fas naked siRNA by renal vein injection and hydrodynamic injection into the tail vein are equally efficient in protecting mice from renal ischemia-reperfusion injury induced by clamping the renal artery. In this type of experiment, protective effects were shown for siRNA directed against Fas ligand (FasL) proteins.[7] Indeed, 24 hours later, Fas mRNA in the kidneys decreased by 74% ± 8% without ischemia and was four- to fivefold lower at 1 day after the renal ischemic insult. Of note, however, it was not possible to exclude a indirect anti-inflammatory effect of silencing Fas ex-pression elsewhere that contributed to the protective outcome.[7]

Obviously, systemic delivery by hydrodynamic methods may be an option for delivery into renal cells, but this approach is now used for RNAi-targeted proximal tubular cells. Indeed, naked siRNA uptake is most prevalent in the proximal tubule after a single-tail vein injection.[6] In the rat, van de Water and associates demonstrated that radiolabeled siRNA is delivered spontaneously to the kidney and can effectively silence a transporter gene in the renal proximal tubule. Even after intravenous administration of small amounts, siRNA preferentially accumulates in the kidney. At 1 hour after injection, the amount of siRNA present in the kidneys was approximately 40 times higher than in other organs. This siRNA accumulation is safe and causes no dysfunction of proximal tubular cells.[6]

To date, hydrodynamic delivery is an elegant method for use in the mouse, with appreciable delivery efficacy and relatively few side effects, but its applicability is limited to murine models.

CHEMICALLY MODIFIED siRNA MOLECULES. In serum, dsRNA is more stable than single-strand RNA (ssRNA) but will be degraded within a few hours as a result of RNAse activity. Chemical modifications of siRNAs that may increase their stability are possible without affecting RNAi. Furthermore, these chemical modifications also may contribute to increasing cellular tropism and silencing activity. For example, chemical modifications with the use of a locked nucleic acid residue are now being tested in vivo.

Conclusion

Several delivery methods for siRNAs are currently under investigation. The principal pitfalls are transfection efficacy and potential toxicity. Promising results with delivery of siRNA to proximal tubular cells after intravenous injection, with or without hydrodynamic pressure, are currently under examination for particular genes implicated in tubular injury.

ADULT STEM CELLS

Regeneration of Renal Cells

The concept of regenerative medicine using adult stem cells for renal regeneration after injury has been the focus of several groups of investigators for the last several years. At the same time, the search for the "pure" plastic stem cell was undertaken, and the debate of which stem cell for which lineage commitment was raging. The scientific debate since 2000 highlights some unsolved issues regarding kidney regeneration and thus provides valuable data for a prospective overview.

The story of bone marrow stem cells within kidneys was first described in 1978 by Schiffer and Michael[8] using Y chromosome staining and was revisited by Grimm and colleagues in 2001.[9] These latter investigators showed that in male transplant recipients who received a renal graft from a female donor, mesenchymal cells from the recipient (positive for the Y chromosome) were present within the kidney. The number of these cells was correlated with the degree of chronic rejection. These investigators also found that 4% of tubules were positive for Y chromosome staining as well, suggesting that some cells, presumably from the recipient's bone marrow, could account for tubule regeneration.[9] These findings were confirmed by Poulsom and coworkers,[10] in both human biopsy specimens and mice after renal ischemic injury. Several subsequent studies suggested that an increasing number of bone marrow stem cells (up to 30% of renal cells in some studies) could "home" within the kidney, engraft, and differentiate into tubular cells. In subsequent studies, much more modest engraftment percentages have been cited, with a general consensus of less than 5% and sometimes less than 1%, raising the question of the biological relevance of those bone marrow stem cells after renal injury.[11,12] Indeed, if bone marrow stem cells do not participate (or do so only marginally) in tubule regeneration, several groups of investigators agree that stem cell infusion may be beneficial to renal function. Such benefit has been reported in both cisplatin-induced nephropathy and ischemia-reperfusion renal injury.[12-14] The harvesting of stem cells before infusion to the injured animals gave striking differences between mesenchymal and hematopoietic lineage, with a beneficial effect on renal function only for mesenchymal stem cells.[14] These data have been confirmed by other studies showing a potential benefit of mesenchymal stem cell infusion for renal function in different models of renal injury.[15,16] Of note, the explanation for such renal improvement was enhanced endothelial regeneration and enhanced tubular regeneration, but with decreased renal lesions[11-13,16] with less apoptosis and, of interest, less inflammation.

On the other hand, the presence of resident renal progenitors, whether or not they are multipotent (i.e., capable of differentiating into several cell lineages), has been confirmed in all reported studies. Their isolation and characterization are still under debate, with some evidence for scattered tubular cells,[17] Bowman's capsule cells,[18] interstitial cells,[19] or cells located in the papilla.[20] They probably can proliferate at a high rate, accounting for the impressive proliferation index seen after most insults leading to acute tubular necrosis lesions.[17] To date, no functional studies have been reported. Nevertheless, the targeting of renal cell progenitors for proliferation in acute renal failure (ARF) seems indeed a reasonable hope for future trials.

Prevention of Lesions

Of interest, in the experimental models of renal injury, mesenchymal stem cells were found to exert a beneficial effect when infusion was given at the time of the injury, or no later than day 1, for ischemia-reperfusion injury or cisplatin-induced nephropathy.[12-14,16] These data suggest that although regeneration was enhanced, the decrease in renal lesions probably is the main explanation for the improvement achieved by means of angiogenesis.[21] It raises the possibility of a systemic or paracrine effect of infused mesenchymal stem cells.[11] Indeed, several lines of evidence suggest that both lesion and repair phenomena are taking place at the same time, although not at the same location within the kidney. Development of some lesions may even be delayed, especially those related to an inflammatory process,[22] explaining why even on day 1 or 2 after the initial insult, some preconditioning treatment may be of benefit. Among such preconditioning agents, growth factors such as granulocyte colony-stimulating factor (GCSF) has been shown to be beneficial when given before or at the time of the renal insult.[13,23] This issue gives rise to a potential therapeutic hope in clinical practice, because pharmacological agents are less expensive and easier to administer than stem cell preparations. From this perspective, all pharmacological candidates that have shown a benefit in preconditioning studies should be considered to be of potential interest even within the next few days after the time of injury. Caution is required before translation of these findings to clinical studies, however, because unexpected deleterious effects may occur. As was noted in the GCSF-treated rat model, the time of infusion is critical, with the potential to worsen the lesions through an increased inflammatory response,

rather than protecting renal function.[24] It is presumably more difficult to assess a gain of function for molecules involved in cell proliferation (such as different fibroblast growth factors, ligands of epidermal growth factor [EGF] receptors and vascular endothelial growth factor [VEGF] receptors, among potential candidates), because renal failure without dialysis carries a high mortality rate, so that a time window for detection of a benefit for renal function seems out of reach.

A Secret Hope: Prevention of Renal Fibrosis

To date, no long-term data supporting the possibility of prevention of renal fibrosis are available. Therapeutic interventions during ARF seem indeed meaningless if renal function is not ultimately preserved. The general belief, however, is that if the initial insult induces fewer lesions and less inflammation, as is observed after injection of mesenchymal stem cells,[16,22,25,26] better outcomes can be achieved, unless mesenchymal cell engraftment is inherently fibrogenic. Obviously, the only available data today support a deleterious effect of mesenchymal cells from bone marrow origin, as suggested in the original paper of Grimm and colleagues.[9] These data are collected from studies of renal allografts, however, rather than from work with autologous tissue, raising the question of whether it is the primary events that lead to mesenchymal cell infiltrates, rather than potential primary deleterious effects.

PRECONDITIONING AND PREVENTION OF ACUTE RENAL FAILURE

Historical Overview

ARF is associated with high morbidity and mortality rates. In most of the cases, ARF is due to ischemic or toxic kidney injury, leading to so-called acute tubular necrosis (ATN). Several lines of evidence suggest that after a first exposure to a toxin or an ischemic insult, the kidney, like some other organs, may develop some intrinsic mechanisms that protect it against a subsequent exposure to the toxin or ischemia. This phenomenon is not specific to the kidney and has been called "ischemic preconditioning" in the dog heart. A recent review indicates that preconditioning in the kidney was actually first described at the beginning of the 20th century.[27] Uranium injection may induce renal injury but also protects against injury from a subsequent injection. Similar results were obtained with glycerol-, mercuric chloride–, and ischemia-induced ARF. Both the delay between the two insults and the type of injury are important to demonstrate the protective effect of preconditioning.

In a mouse model, Bonventre demonstrated that prior exposure to ischemia protects against a second ischemic insult 8 or 15 days later.[27] A short period of initial ischemia (15 minutes) is less protective than a longer period (30 minutes) if a subsequent 30-minute period of ischemia is induced 8 days later. Of interest, unilateral ischemia also is protective against a subsequent ischemic insult to that kidney but not to the contralateral kidney, revealing that systemic uremia is not necessary for protection and that the first ischemic insult induces local tissue changes responsible for further kidney resistance to ischemia.[27]

Molecular and Cellular Mechanisms Involved in Kidney Preconditioning

Dedifferentiation of Tubular Epithelial Cells

Ischemic injury may induce ATN, and regenerating epithelial cells are less differentiated and less sensitive to ischemia than fully differentiated tubular cells. Similarly, mild ischemia may induce such dedifferentiation without necrosis of epithelial cells and resistance to further hypoxic injury.[27]

Park and coworkers reported that ischemic preconditioning of the rat kidney inhibits further activation by ischemia of the jun N-terminal kinase (JNK) and p38 but not that of signal-regulated kinase (ERK)1/2.[28] The balance between ERK and JNK-p38 pathways seems to determine whether kidney cells survive or undergo apoptosis. These investigators also demonstrated that preconditioning ischemia reduced the phosphorylation of MAPK kinase (MMK)7, MKK4, and MKK3/6, the upstream activators of JNK and p38, but not that of MEK1/2, the upstream activator of ERK1/2. In addition, heat shock protein (HSP)-25 levels were shown to be increased by ischemic preconditioning, suggesting that it may regulate the expression of the kinases and stabilize the actin cytoskeleton after ischemic injury.[28]

After ischemic insult, preconditioned kidneys have no significant outer medullary congestion, the hallmark of the nonpreconditioned postischemic kidney. This finding suggests that the kidney protection is in part related to a decreased expression of adhesion molecules involved in leukocyte–endothelial cell interactions. JNK and p38 activation enhance the expression of adhesion molecules and cytokine production and may be involved in the increased adhesion of circulating leukocytes and platelets to the small vessels of the outer medulla. The reduced expression of these kinases in the preconditioned kidney may potentially explain the lack of medullary congestion after the second ischemic insult.[27]

Adenosine, which is released after a short period of ischemia, may protect the kidney from a second ischemic insult by decreasing endothelial cell P-selectin and intercellular adhesion molecule-1 (ICAM-1) expression and consequent leukocyte adhesion.[29]

More recently, preconditioning activation of hypoxia-inducible factors (HIFs) has been shown to ameliorate ischemic acute renal failure.[30] Normoxic degradation of HIFs is mediated by oxygen-dependent hydroxylation of specific prolyl residues of the regulative α subunits by HIF prolyl hydroxylases (PHDs). In the rat, ARF secondary to renal ischemia is significantly ameliorated by pretreatment with either carbon monoxide, which leads to tissue hypoxia, or a PHD inhibitor, FG-4487. Both of these pretreatment regimens were associated with a marked accumulation of HIF-1α and HIF-2α in tubular and peritubular cells, respectively, as well as HIF target gene expression. Tissue injury and apoptosis were less severe in preconditioned kidneys.[30]

Similar results have been reported with FG-0041, which also protects against myocardial ischemia reperfusion injury. In isolated hearts of heterozygously HIF-1α–deficient[+/−] mice, the effect of delayed hypoxic preconditioning was abolished in comparison with hearts of HIF-1α[+/+] mice. In the kidney, pretreatment with cobalt, which also activates HIF, induces protection against ischemia-reperfusion injury. By contrast, HIF-1α deficiency in the brain was shown to protect against severe ischemia, but the prolyl hydroxylase PHD inhibitors have

been reported to provide protection. Thus, the role of HIF may not be uniform in different models of injury.

The target genes of HIF activation are likely to be the main factors contributing to the renal protection induced by preconditioning. In particular, preischemic EPO treatment was shown to reduce ischemia-reperfusion injury in rodent kidneys.[31] Very high doses were required to obtain these effects, well above those that could be induced by endogenous HIF activation. It is likely, however, that ischemia induces HIF-2α expression and EPO synthesis in interstitial fibroblasts, the major source of renal EPO expression, with potentially paracrine protective effects on the adjacent tubular cells.

Preconditioning activation of heme oxygenase-1 (HO-1) by means of heat preconditioning, cobalt chloride pretreatment, or gene transfer also has been shown to attenuate ischemia-reperfusion injury of the kidney. Accordingly, ischemic ARF is enhanced in HO-1–deficient mice or with inhibition of HO-1 by tin mesoporphyrin. It is not clear to date which target gene of HIF is the most important in the protective role against ischemia, but probably several such genes cooperate to promote metabolic pathways and inhibit cell death and apoptosis after ischemia.[30]

Heat preconditioning has been shown to attenuate renal injury in ischemic ARF in rats, with marked functional protection and reduced histological evidence of tubular necrosis.[32] Heat shock has both anti-inflammatory and antiapoptotic effects and inhibits NF-κB activation. It also suppresses the accumulation of phosphorylated inhibitory κBa (IκBa), with a resultant depletion in cytoplasmic IκBa, indicating that heat preconditioning blocks the activation of the IκB kinase complex. Ischemia-induced tubular cell apoptosis also is decreased by heat preconditioning, along with decreased caspase 3 activation. HSP-70 is induced primarily by heat preconditioning, and inhibition of HSP-70 by quercetin has been shown to reverse almost completely the functional protection provided by heat preconditioning. Several reports have indicated that the protective effect of HSP-70 is partly mediated through inhibition of NF-κB pathway–related inflammation, as well as modulation of cell necrosis or apoptosis.

Key Points

1. Several delivery methods for small interfering RNAs are currently under investigation for particular genes involved in tubular injury.
2. Stem cells may protect from ischemia-reperfusion injury, but the mechanisms at play are still debated: a paracrine role versus repopulation of tubular epithelial cells.
3. Preconditioning by either ischemic or toxic stimulators can protect the kidney from further injury.
4. Several new experimental approaches have proved to be effective in the prevention of acute renal injury, but it remains to be demonstrated whether these results apply to human disease.

Key References

9. Grimm PC, Nickerson P, Jeffery J, et al: Neointimal and tubulointerstitial infiltration by recipient mesenchymal cells in chronic renal allograft rejection. N Engl J Med 2001;345:93-97.

12. Duffield JS, Park KM, Hsiao LL, et al: Restoration of tubular epithelial cells during repair of the postischemic kidney occurs independently of bone marrow–derived stem cells. J Clin Invest 2005;115:1743-1755.

16. Tögel F, Hu Z, Weiss K, et al: Administered mesenchymal stem cells protect against ischemic acute renal failure through differentiation-independent mechanisms. Am J Physiol Renal Physiol 2005:289:F31-F42.

30. Bernhardt WM, Câmpean V, Kany S, et al: Preconditional activation of hypoxia-inducible factors ameliorates ischemic acute renal failure. J Am Soc Nephrol 2006;17:1970-1978.

32. Jo SK, Ko GJ, Boo CS, et al: Heat preconditioning attenuates renal injury in ischemic ARF in rats: Role of heat-shock protein 70 on NF-κB–mediated inflammation and on tubular cell injury. J Am Soc Nephrol 2006;17:3082-3092.

See the companion Expert Consult website for the complete reference list.

CHAPTER 86

Adenosine 2A Receptor Agonists in Acute Kidney Injury

Mark D. Okusa

OBJECTIVES

This chapter will:
1. Identify barriers to the successful treatment of acute kidney injury.
2. Present the pharmacology classification of adenosine receptors.
3. Describe the role of adenosine 2A receptors on kidney function.
4. Summarize the mechanisms by which adenosine 2A receptor activation blocks inflammation.
5. Review the potential use of adenosine 2A receptor agonists for the treatment of acute kidney injury.

Acute kidney injury (AKI) often complicates critical illness, and despite advances in medical technology, AKI is an independent risk factor for death in the intensive care unit (ICU) setting.[1,2] The incidence of AKI has increased over the past 3 decades, and the mortality rate is in excess of 50% to 70%,[3] although recent evidence points to an apparent decrease.[4,5] This encouraging trend notwithstanding, AKI-associated mortality and morbidity rates remain unacceptably high. Today, the changing spectrum of AKI in the critically ill is characterized by a high incidence of comorbid disease and extensive extrarenal complications.[4-6]

ACUTE KIDNEY INJURY AND INFLAMMATION: CONSIDERATIONS IN THERAPEUTIC INTERVENTION

For improved clinical outcomes, a multidisciplinary effort is necessary to elucidate the pathogenesis of AKI and to develop and implement newer compounds in well-designed clinical trials. Inflammation has been established as an early event in the pathogenesis of AKI and is therefore a potential target for therapeutic intervention. Accord-ingly, a current approach to AKI aims at limiting inflammation through the use of compounds that stimulate adenosine 2A receptors ($A_{2A}Rs$). $A_{2A}Rs$ are members of a family of guanine nucleotide–binding protein receptors that have become a focus of interest primarily because of their ability to broadly attenuate the inflammatory cascade.

Except for a few isolated studies, the vast majority of clinical studies have yet to conclusively demonstrate the benefit of pharmacological treatment of AKI. A number of barriers to successful clinical trials are recognized: (1) a high rate of comorbid illness in patients with AKI; (2) the complexity of AKI, including pathogenic factors such as vasoconstriction, leukostasis, vascular congestion, apopto-sis, and abnormalities in immune modulators and growth factors; (3) the multisystem nature of the underlying disturbance in AKI; and (4) design issues related to past clinical trials.[7] These factors necessitate continued emphasis on elucidating the pathogenesis of AKI and rapid translation of novel compounds in well-designed clinical trials.

Ischemia remains a major cause of AKI, and its pathogenesis is reviewed elsewhere. Of particular importance are the role of inflammation and the systemic nature of AKI in critically ill patients. In several studies, either congestive heart failure[8] or noncardiogenic acute respiratory distress syndrome (ARDS)[9] has been associated with AKI. Thus, a consequence of AKI is the involvement of multiple organs, leading to a high mortality rate. This chapter focuses on $A_{2A}R$ agonists as promising therapeutic drugs that are aimed at broadly attenuating inflammation and preventing and treating AKI.

ADENOSINE 2A RECEPTORS

Adenosine and Adenosine Receptor Subtypes

Locally produced adenosine in the kidney controls renal circulation and metabolic cellular activity.[10] Microdialysis experiments have shown that adenosine concentrations in

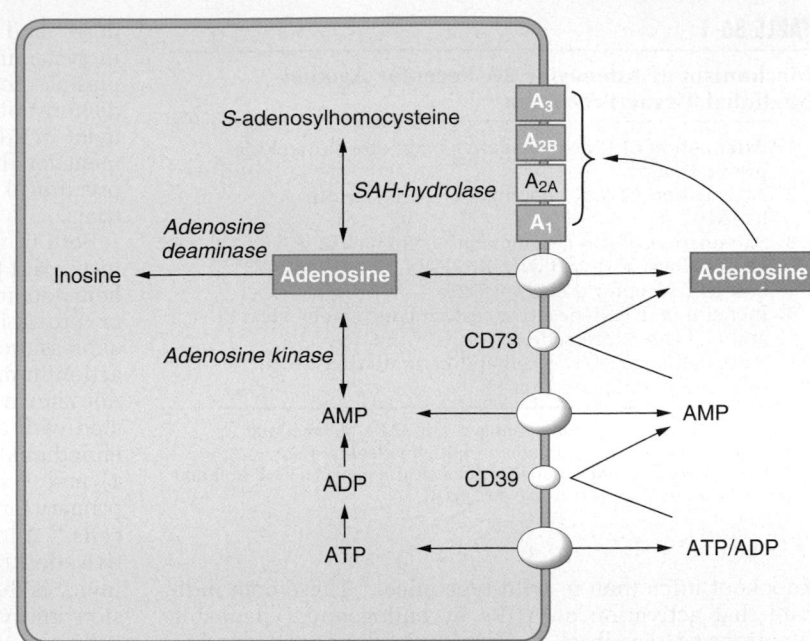

FIGURE 86-1. Pathways and enzymes in the formation of intracellular and extracellular adenosine. CD73 is ecto-5′-nucleotidase; CD39 is vascular nucleoside triphosphate diphosphohydrolase (NTPDase). ADP, adenosine diphosphate; AMP, adenosine monophosphate; ATP, adenosine triphosphate.

kidneys of anesthetized rat,[11] dog,[12] and rabbit[13] range between 0.1 and 1 µM. Kidney ischemia for 2 minutes increases tissue adenosine concentration more than 6-fold and the concentration of its metabolite hypoxanthine 300-fold. Extracellular adenosine is derived from cellular stores or from the extracellular metabolism of ATP (Fig. 86-1). Adenosine is released from cellular stores through nucleoside transporters, whereas extracellular adenosine is produced through ecto-5′-nucleotidase (CD73).[10] ATP and ADP serve as substrates for CD39, a transmembrane protein that belongs to the family of proteins with ecto-nucleoside triphosphate diphosphohydrolase (NTPDase) activity and originally was defined as an activation marker for leukocytes and endothelial cells.[14] CD39 produces AMP, which in turn is a substrate for CD73. Adenosine and adenine nucleotides bind to P_1 and P_2 purinergic receptors, respectively.[15] Adenosine binds to P_1 purinergic receptors, which are members of the G protein–coupled receptor family.

Four subtypes of adenosine receptors—A_1, A_{2A}, A_{2B}, and A_3—are characterized by seven putative transmembrane-spanning domains; together, they mediate a multitude of physiological responses.[16] Adenosine acts on these receptors in organs such as brain, heart, and skeletal muscle and induces vasodilatation to allow matching of oxygen delivery and work.[10] Adenosine can increase or decrease neurotransmitter release, depending on the adenosine receptor subtype.[10] A_{2A}Rs stimulate adenylyl cyclase and increase the production of cyclic AMP by coupling to cholera toxin–sensitive stimulatory G protein (G_s).[16]

Adenosine 2A Receptor Function in Kidney

Understanding the biological role of A_{2A}Rs has been aided by development of subtype-selective reagents. Recently, the use of selective pharmacological agents,[15] development of a monoclonal antibody,[17] molecular cloning of A_{2A}Rs,[15] and generation of the A_{2A} knockout mouse[18] have shed light on the broad functional role of A_{2A}Rs in a variety of

organs. Furthermore, the development of small molecules that bind to A_{2A}Rs allows the potential for clinical investigations that target these receptors. CGS21680[19] and ATL146 ester (ATL146e),[20] selective A_{2A} agonists, have been used principally to examine the effect of A_{2A}R activation.

A_{2A}Rs are widely distributed in renal and nonrenal tissue.[15,21-23] In the kidney, A_{2A}R mRNA is expressed in cells of the outer medullary descending vasa recta[22] and the glomerulus,[21] whereas immunohistochemical studies have localized A_{2A}Rs to the cortical collecting duct of kidneys.[23] A_{2A}R activation controls glomerular filtration rate[10,24] through effects on afferent and efferent arterioles[25] and medullary blood flow through effects on the descending vasa recta.[26]

In nonrenal tissue, A_{2A}Rs are abundantly expressed in hematopoietic tissues and cells, including spleen, thymus, leukocytes, and platelets and, to a lesser extent, in heart, lung, and blood vessels.[15] A_{2A}Rs are expressed in a variety of bone marrow–derived leukocytes, including monocytes, lymphocytes, neutrophils, basophils, and mast cells.[27]

Endogenous Adenosine Activates Adenosine 2A Receptor to Attenuate Immune-Mediated Injury

Adenosine is released from ischemic or hypoxic tissue and acts on A_{2A}Rs to attenuate inflammation and collateral damage.[28] Because A_{2A}Rs are expressed on immune cells, they are in fact poised to carry out this function. After infection, the pro-inflammatory process contributes to the eradication of the pathogen, but the sustained and unregulated inflammation injures tissue.[29] After ischemia-reperfusion injury, endogenous adenosine accumulates in response to hypoxia and has a crucial role in terminating an overactive, unregulated immune system.[30] Concanavalin A–induced liver injury, mediated by T cells, macrophages, and cytokines, is markedly worse in A_{2A}R knockout mice than in their wild-type counterparts.[31] Renal ischemia-reperfusion injury also is more pronounced in A_{2A}R

TABLE 86-1

Mechanism of Adenosine 2A Receptor Agonist–Mediated Tissue Protection

1. Attenuation of PMNs: oxidative burst and superoxide production[36,37]
2. Attenuation of $\alpha_4\beta_1$ integrin, VLA-4, P-selectin, ICAM-1[34,38]
3. Attenuation of pro-inflammatory cytokines and chemokines: TNF-α, IFN-γ, RANTES, IL-12P$_{70}$, IL-2[39-42,45] and IL-2 receptor α chain (CD25)[39-42,44,45]
4. Increase in T cell–negative costimulatory molecules: PD-1 and CTLA-4 expressed on T cells[45]
5. Attenuation of CD4$^+$ T cell and natural killer T cell infiltration and activation[51,52]

CTLA-4, cytotoxic T-lymphocyte antigen-4; ICAM-1, intercellular adhesion molecule-1; IFN-γ, interferon-γ; IL, interleukin; PD-1, programmed death-1; PMN, polymorphonuclear leukocyte; TNF-α, tumor necrosis factor-α; VLA-4, very late antigen-4.

knockout mice than in wild-type mice.[32] These data indicate that activation of A$_{2A}$Rs by endogenous adenosine functions as a feedback mechanism leading to attenuation of inflammation and tissue injury.

In vitro studies have generated insight into the mechanism by which A$_{2A}$R agonists block inflammation.[33-35] Immune cells abundantly express A$_{2A}$Rs,[15] and the activation of these receptors is central to abrogating the inflammatory response. Activation of A$_{2A}$Rs expressed on neutrophils attenuates oxidative burst and superoxide anion production[36,37] and adhesion of neutrophils to endothelial cells by blocking very late antigen (VLA)-4.[38] Macrophages produce tumor necrosis factor-α (TNF-α) and interleukin (IL)-12, an effect blocked by A$_{2A}$Rs.[39-42] Thus, A$_{2A}$R agonists broadly attenuate the actions of mediators of inflammation.

Cognate immunity requires interaction among the T cell receptor, major histocompatibility complex (MHC), and antigenic peptide on antigen-presenting cells, plus positive and negative costimulatory signals.[43] T cell activation is associated with enhanced secretion of interferon-γ (IFN-γ) and IL-2 and expression of IL-2 receptor α chain (CD25), an effect that is blocked by A$_{2A}$R agonists.[44] A$_{2A}$R agonists block allogenic recognition by attenuating the release of release of inflammatory cytokines IFN-γ, RANTES, IL-12P$_{70}$, and IL-2 and increasing the expression of negative costimulatory molecules (molecules that block costimulation) programmed death-1 (PD-1) and cytotoxic T-lymphocyte antigen-4 (CTLA-4) expressed on T cells.[45] These results indicate that A$_{2A}$R agonists attenuate allogenic recognition by action on both T lymphocytes and antigen-presenting cells in vitro and delayed acute rejection in vivo. Table 86-1 summarizes the mechanisms by which A$_{2A}$R agonists block inflammation and immune-mediated tissue injury.

Adenosine 2A Receptor Activation Attenuates Acute Kidney Injury

A$_{2A}$R activation ameliorated renal ischemia-reperfusion injury in rat kidneys[46,47] by approximately 70% when infusion was initiated before, or at the time of, ischemia-reperfusion injury and was continued for 24 hours.[34,46] Dose-dependent studies in mice indicated that infusion rates of 1 to 10 ng/kg per minute deliver the most effective

dose[34] and that protection is independent of any change in systemic hemodynamic parameters.[46] Measurement of plasma creatinine at 24 hours after ischemia-reperfusion demonstrated that treatment for 6 hours produced improvement in kidney function that was comparable with treatment for the entire 24 hours of reperfusion. Thus, these preclinical data provide the foundation for future clinical trials.

Both in vivo and in vitro data suggested that A$_{2A}$R agonists exert their protective effects through direct action on hematopoietic cells (as reviewed earlier), endothelial cells, or proximal tubule cells.[48] In view of the ubiquitous expression of A$_{2A}$Rs, the precise target of A$_{2A}$R agonist action in mediating tissue protection in vivo initially was not known. A$_{2A}$R agonist–induced protection was associated with a reduction in neutrophil accumulation and in endothelial cell intracellular adhesion molecule-1 (ICAM-1) and P-selectin.[49] Subsequent studies found that the primary target of A$_{2A}$R agonists was bone marrow–derived cells.[32] Additional experiments indicated that the protective effect of A$_{2A}$R agonists in kidney ischemia-reperfusion injury is due to effects on CD4$^+$ T cells.[50] In liver, reperfusion injury is initiated by activation of natural killer T cells, and the activation of these cells is inhibited by A$_{2A}$R activation.[51] In a similar manner, natural killer T cells have been found to play a critical role in renal ischemia-reperfusion injury,[52] and A$_{2A}$R agonists block natural killer T cell activation in renal ischemia-reperfusion injury (unpublished data). These studies highlight the pronounced degree of protection conferred on renal tissue by ATL146e administered before or at the onset of ischemia-reperfusion insult. These characteristics may potentially allow intervention to prevent or treat human AKI.

A$_{2A}$R agonists also have been shown to reduce injury in other organs, including the heart,[53] lung,[54] liver,[42] spinal cord,[55] and gut.[56,57] These findings suggest that common mechanisms appear to initiate and maintain ischemia-reperfusion injury associated with different organs. Furthermore, the observation that A$_{2A}$R agonists mediate protection in multiple organs suggests potential clinical value in the treatment of AKI in critically ill patients characterized by multiorgan dysfunction.

CONCLUSION

Both cellular and humoral immunity are key mediators of AKI. Activation of A$_{2A}$Rs has been demonstrated to interrupt innate and adaptive immunity. The potent inhibitory effect on these pathways is not limited to the kidney but appears to block similar pathways in other organs. Thus, the use of A$_2$R agonists for the prevention and treatment of AKI and subsequent systemic derangements is appealing.

The A$_{2A}$R agonist ATL146e is currently being tested in a phase III clinical trial as a pharmacological stress agent in cardiac perfusion imaging studies. This study, together with extensively published preclinical data, will facilitate performance of clinical trials of ATL146e for AKI in critically ill patients.

Key Points

1. To improve therapeutic interventions in the prevention or treatment of AKI, well-designed clinical trials are needed to study the efficacy of novel

therapeutic agents, either alone or in combination, that target multiple pathogenic pathways.

2. Adenosine 2A receptor agonists block innate and adaptive immunity and have potent effects to reduce experimental ischemia-reperfusion injury to kidney, heart, lung, liver, and spinal cord.

3. Adenosine 2A receptor agonist–mediated protection in multiple organs suggests potential clinical value for such agents in the treatment of acute kidney injury in critically ill patients characterized by multiorgan dysfunction.

Acknowledgments

The author is grateful to Ms. Liping Huang and Hong Ye (Department of Medicine, University of Virginia, Charlottesville, Virginia) for expert technical assistance and Drs. Joel Linden (Department of Medicine, University of Virginia), Diane Rosin (Department of Pharmacology, University of Virginia), and Yuan Ji Day (Department of Anesthesiology, Chang Gung Memorial Hospital, Taipei, Taiwan) for fruitful collaborations. This work was supported in part by National Institutes of Health (NIH) grants RO1DK56223, RO1DK62324, and RO1DK065957.

Competing Interests

Mark D. Okusa is a Scientific Advisor for Adenosine Therapeutics, LLC, Charlottesville, Virginia. Adenosine Therapeutics, LLC, provided ATL146e for studies reported in this chapter.

Key References

3. Star RA: Treatment of acute renal failure. Kidney Int 1998;54:1817-1831.
31. Ohta A, Sitkovsky M: Role of G-protein–coupled adenosine receptors in downregulation of inflammation and protection from tissue damage. Nature 2001;414:916-920.
32. Day YJ, Huang L, McDuffie MJ, et al: Renal protection from ischemia mediated by A2A adenosine receptors on bone marrow–derived cells. J Clin Invest 2003;112:883-891.
36. Cronstein BN, Rosenstein ED, Kramer SB, et al: Adenosine; a physiological modulator of superoxide anion generation by human neutrophils. Adenosine acts via an A2 receptor on human neutrophils. J Immunol 1985;135:1366-1371.
46. Okusa MD, Linden J, Macdonald T, Huang L: Selective A2A-adenosine receptor activation during reperfusion reduces ischemia-reperfusion injury in rat kidney. Am J Physiol 1999;277:F404-F412.

See the companion Expert Consult website for the complete reference list.

CHAPTER 87

Biochemical and Clinical Indications to Initiate Renal Replacement Therapy

Andrew Davenport

OBJECTIVES

This chapter will:
1. Review biochemical indications to start renal replacement therapy.
2. Review clinical indications to start renal replacement therapy.
3. Present an overview of the rationale for early versus late initiation of renal replacement therapy.
4. Identify biomarkers of acute kidney injury to help initiate renal replacement therapy.
5. Review nonrenal indications to start renal replacement therapy.

Acute kidney injury (AKI) is increasingly recognized as a secondary complication in hospitalized patients, particularly those in the intensive care unit (ICU). In addition, AKI is a primary risk factor for death.[1,2]

Interventions designed to prevent or minimize the development of AKI are limited to those aimed at a small number of clinical conditions including prerenal azotemia, radiocontrast agent–induced nephropathy, rhabdomyolysis, tumor lysis syndrome, and cadaveric renal transplantation. Similarly, in only a few situations are specific therapies for intrinsic AKI available, such as in acute proliferative and crescentic glomerulonephritis, acute interstitial nephritis, and hemolytic uremic syndrome and the thrombotic microangiopathies. Thus, renal replacement therapy (RRT) is the mainstay of supportive care for patients with AKI. Whereas the options for RRT some 25 years ago were limited to intermittent hemodialysis and peritoneal dialysis, an array of techniques are now available, ranging from various modalities of continuous renal replacement therapy (CRRT) to the more recently introduced so-called hybrid therapies, such as extended-duration dialysis (EDD), sustained low-efficiency dialysis (SLED), and the Genius system for intermittent hemodialysis, hemofiltration, or hemodiafiltration. Despite the increasing technological sophistication of RRT, criteria for the key clinical management decisions, such as when to initiate RRT and which modality and regimen are most effective, remain to be determined.

Current practice suggests that RRT is indicated for patients with AKI who demonstrate an abrupt and sustained fall in glomerular filtration rate (GFR), with or at risk for clinically significant solute imbalance or toxicity and volume overload.

BIOCHEMICAL PARAMETERS TO INITIATE RENAL REPLACEMENT THERAPY

The traditional biochemical markers of renal function, urea and creatinine levels, vary with age, being lower in neonates and other infants than in older children and adults (Table 87-1). Newer markers of renal function, such as cystatin C, also vary with age, increasing in the older patient; as yet, no normal reference range has been established for the very young. In addition, urea and creatinine not only are dependent on renal function but also can be affected by the underlying clinical condition and basal metabolic rate[3] (Table 87-2). To overcome the inherent problems in creatinine measurement, the concept of an *estimated glomerular filtration rate* (eGFR) has been introduced to help detect early stages of chronic kidney disease in the community. A simplified form of the Modification of Diet in Renal Disease equation (sMDRD formula) is used for this purpose[4]:

$$\text{eGFR mL/min/1.73 m}^2 = 175 \times (\text{serum creatinine in mg/dL})^{-1.154} \times (\text{age in years})^{-0.203} \times 0.742 \text{ (if subject is female)} \times 1.212 \text{ (if subject is black)}$$

$$\text{eGFR mL/min/1.73 m}^2 = 175 \times ((\text{serum creatinine in } \mu\text{mol/L} - 3)/1.004 \times 0.011312)^{-1.154} \times (\text{age in years})^{-0.203} \times 0.742 \text{ (if subject is female)} \times 1.212 \text{ (if subject is black)}$$

Because the sMDRD equation has now been introduced into standard clinical practice in the United States, the United Kingdom, and Australia, many laboratories now automatically report eGFR when serum creatinine is requested.[5] As yet, a role for eGFR in the management of AKI has not been validated, although daily changes in eGFR may prove helpful, and prospective studies are required. Absolute biochemical values have different clinical implications in patients with true AKI, in those with AKI on a background of chronic kidney disease (CKD), and in patients with CKD stage 5 (dialysis-dependent).

TABLE 87-1

Normal Renal Function in Neonates and Children

AGE	GFR	SCr (μmol/L)*
26 weeks' gestation	0.7 mL/min/kg	
33 weeks' gestation	0.8 mL/min/kg	
Full term	1.0 mL/min/kg	73 (17-188)
1 month	10 mL/min	35 (20-65)
1 year		45 (25-65)
2 years	80 mL/min	48 (25-70)
12 years		60 (40-95)

*Mean serum creatinine ± 95% confidence limits. At birth, the serum creatinine reflects maternal values; in premature babies, it initially rises to a mean of 221 μmol/L within 48 hours and then falls over the next 2 weeks.
GFR, glomerular filtration rate; SCr, serum creatinine.

TABLE 87-2

Common Clinical Conditions and Drugs That Affect Serum Urea and Creatinine

ALTERATION	CAUSE
Serum Urea	
Increased	Cardiac failure
	Dehydration
	Gastrointestinal hemorrhage
	Severe burns
	Systemic sepsis
	Tumor lysis
	Hematoma
	Hyperalimentation
	Steroid therapy
Decreased	Liver disease
	Starvation
	Pregnancy
Serum Creatinine	
Increased	Rhabdomyolysis
	Hypothyroidism
	African ethnicity
	Cephalosporins (in infants)
	Trimethoprim
	Cimetidine
	Unconjugated bilirubin
Reduced	Muscle wasting
	Amputation
	Chronic organ disease
	Liver disease
	Obesity
	Vegetarian diet
	Infants/young children
	Elderly

Thus, the decision to initiate RRT cannot necessarily be based solely on absolute urea and creatinine values, and the more recent scoring systems for acute kidney failure, such as the RIFLE[6] (risk, injury, failure, loss, end-stage renal disease) and Acute Kidney Injury Network[7] (AKIN) classifications, use changes in baseline creatinine to define acute renal failure (threefold increase in creatinine) or GFR (decrease in GFR by greater than 75%) and, to encompass patients with preexisting CKD and those for whom no baseline values are available, both an absolute serum creatinine value and an acute rise in creatinine[8] (Tables 87-3 and 87-4). The RIFLE classification uses changes in GFR, although traditionally GFR is calculated on the basis of a steady-state system. Therefore, in the dynamic setting of the ICU, assessment of GFR based on creatinine clearances has not been validated in AKI. This limitation is due in part to the inherent error in measuring creatinine with use of the standard modified Jaffe method. Proponents of measuring GFR in AKI have suggested performing timed urinary collections—for example, between 4 and 8 hours with a midpoint serum creatinine. Possibly owing to the inaccuracies in determining GFR in the critically ill patient, the more recently introduced AKIN classification has dispensed with changes in GFR. Since the widespread introduction of the eGFR in many countries, however, future classifications of AKI probably will be modified to include a change in eGFR criteria.

Although these classification and staging systems define renal failure, which by definition warrants consideration of RRT, they cannot be used to predict which patients will require support with RRT and those who will spontaneously recover renal function with conservative support alone. Thus, the decision to initiate RRT cannot be made simply on the basis that the patient has reached RIFLE stage F or AKIN stage 3.

Traditional biochemical values to initiate RRT in adults with AKI, other than urea and creatinine, include a severe metabolic acidosis with pH of 7.1 or less (because acidosis decreases the strength of myocardial contraction), urea greater than 30 mmol/L, creatinine 500 to 700 μmol/L, and hyperkalemia, defined as serum potassium greater than 6.5 mmol/L, or accompanied by electrocardiographic changes unresponsive to standard medical management. In clinical practice, however, the decision to initiate RRT usually is based on findings on clinical assessment of the patient and the biochemical parameters.[9,10]

Occasionally, in adult patients, RRT has been used to control refractory hypercalcemia in cases of AKI due to intrarenal calcium deposition that has failed to respond to conventional medical therapy. In pediatric patients, electrolyte abnormalities that fail to respond to standard medical therapy, such as severe hyponatremia and hypernatremia, hypocalcemia, and hyperphosphatemia, particularly associated with the tumor lysis syndrome, have been used as indications to start RRT. The recent introduction of rasburicase has now reduced RRT requirement for the tumor lysis syndrome.

CLINICAL PARAMETERS TO INITIATE RENAL REPLACEMENT THERAPY

In nonobstructive AKI, oliguria is used in both RIFLE and AKIN classifications as a criterion for acute renal failure, defined as a urine output less than 0.3 mL/kg for 24 hours or absolute anuria for 12 hours.[7,8] In routine medical practice, the decision to initiate RRT often is made on the basis of oliguria and the clinical scenario, and on whether or not renal function is anticipated to rapidly improve.[10] Traditional clinical scenarios for starting RRT include pulmonary edema, or severe peripheral edema unresponsive to diuretics, and AKI with evidence of end-organ damage due to azotemia, such as uremic pericarditis, encephalopathy, bleeding, neuropathy, and myopathy. In other instances, RRT may be used to remove fluid to allow for nutrition or other fluids to be administered, such as plasma infusions during plasma exchange or intravenous immunoglobulin.

TABLE 87-3

RIFLE Classification of Acute Kidney Injury

RIFLE GRADE	GFR	SCr*	URINE OUTPUT
Risk	>25% ↓	1.5 × ↑	<0.5 mL/g/hr for 6 hr
Injury	>50% ↓	2.0 × ↑	<0.5 mL/g/hr for 12 hr
Failure	>75% ↓	3.0 × ↑ or	<0.3 mL/kg/hr for 24 hr
		SCr > 355 μmol/L with	*or* anuria for 12 hr
		acute ↑ >44 μmol/L	
Loss	Persistent loss of kidney function for >4 wk		
ESRD	Dialysis dependent for >3 mo		

*Conversion factor, μmol/L to mg/dL: 0.11 (e.g., SCr 355 μmol/L = 3.9 mg/dL and 44 μmol/L = 4.8 mg/dL).
GFR, glomerular filtration rate; RIFLE, *r*isk, *i*njury, *f*ailure, *l*oss, end-stage renal disease (ESRD); SCr, serum creatinine.
From Bellomo R, Ronco C, Kellum JA, et al: Acute renal failure—definition, outcome measures, animal models, fluid therapy, and information technology needs: The Second International Consensus Conference of the Acute Dialysis Quality Initiative (ADQI) Group. Crit Care 2004;8: R204-R212.

TABLE 87-4

AKIN Classification/Staging of Acute Kidney Injury

AKIN STAGE	SERUM CREATININE (SCr) CRITERIA*	URINE OUTPUT CRITERIA
1	↑ SCr ≥3.0 mg/dL *or* ↑ SCr ≥150-200% above baseline	< 0.5 mL/kg/hr for >6 hr
2	↑ SCr > 200-300% above baseline	< 0.5 mL/kg/hr for >12 hr
3	↑ SCr > 300% above baseline *or* SCr ≥0.4 mg/dL with an acute rise of ≥0.5 mg/dL	< 0.3 mL/kg/hr for 24 hr *or* anuria for 12 hr

*Conversion factor, mg/dL to μmol/L: 90.9 (e.g., SCr 0.4 mg/dL = 36 μmol/L and 0.5 mg/dL = 45 μmol/L).
AKIN, Acute Kidney Injury Network.
From Mehta RL, Kellum JA, Shah SV, et al: Acute Kidney Injury Network: Report of an initiative to improve outcomes in acute kidney injury. Crit Care 2007;11:R31.

In clinical practice, the decision to initiate or withhold RRT will depend on whether the patient has AKI, rather than AKI on a background of CKD, or was already dialysis-dependent with CKD stage 5, and similarly whether the patient has single organ or multiple organ failure. RRT usually is started earlier in patients with multiple organ failure in the ICU setting than in those with renal failure alone on the general medical ward.

In selected cases that meet recognized criteria for initiation of RRT on biochemical or clinical grounds, such therapy may nevertheless be withheld because of the clinical condition of the patient, with respect to preexisting comorbidity, quality of life, and life expectancy.[9]

EARLY VERSUS LATE INITIATION OF RENAL REPLACEMENT THERAPY

The decision to initiate RRT is straightforward in those patients with AKI complicated by refractory hyperkalemia, metabolic acidosis and volume overload, or overt uremic symptoms. In the absence of these overt manifestations, however, debate continues regarding the optimal time to initiate renal support. On one hand, early introduction of RRT as soon as the patient enters RIFLE stage F, or AKIN stage 3,[7,8] may be of benefit, to prevent exposure to the potential deleterious effects of metabolic abnormalities and volume overload. On the other hand, with early initiation of RRT, some patients will suffer the adverse conse-

quences of treatment, such as venous thrombosis and bacteremia secondary to vascular access catheters, hemorrhage from anticoagulants, and other treatment-related complications. In addition, some patients with AKI, especially those with single organ failure, may recover renal function without ever manifesting an "absolute" indication for RRT.

Initial reports, some dating back 50 years, suggested a clinical benefit of early initiation of RRT.[11,12] These and other studies formed the basis for the standard clinical practice of instituting dialytic support when the serum urea reaches 28 mmol/L (or BUN, 100 mg/dL). In the past decade, several retrospective studies have reported improved clinical outcomes with early institution of dialysis at a serum urea level less than 21.5 mmol/L (BUN 60 mg/dL),[13] or CRRT in post–cardiac surgery patients with a urine output less than 100 mL/8 hours,[14,15] and a recent observational study reported that starting RRT at higher urea values was associated with a twofold increased risk of death.[16] A prospective randomized study, however, did not show any survival advantage with early initiation, although this study probably was underpowered.[17]

More recent studies have focused on the timing of initiation of CRRT. Gettings and colleagues retrospectively assessed outcomes among 100 consecutive adults with post-traumatic AKI treated with continuous venovenous hemofiltration and reported improved survival when CRRT was initiated earlier at a BUN of 42.6 mg/dL compared with 94.5 mg/dL.[13]

Thus, the current consensus from retrospective and observational studies suggests that "early" initiation of

RRT in AKI is associated with improved survival, although this benefit remains to be confirmed by adequately powered prospective, randomized trials. In everyday clinical practice, RRT typically is started earlier in patients with multiple organ failure than in those with AKI alone.

BIOMARKERS TO INITIATE RENAL REPLACEMENT THERAPY

Biomarkers may potentially be of value in differentiating AKI from CKD, and also in predicting at an early stage which patients would require RRT and, equally important, which ones would recover residual renal function with conservative management. One of the first biomarkers was carbamylated hemoglobin, because urea dissociation in plasma and binding to hemoglobin is readily reversible, contrasting with glycated hemoglobin in diabetics. Early studies showed that carbamylated hemoglobin can help to differentiate AKI from AKI on a background of CKD,[18] but no commercially available assays have been developed.

Cystatin C has been advocated for assessing renal function in AKI, because its generation is less variable than that of creatinine between individual patients, and rapid, fully automated immunonephelometric assays are now available. Although it is now recognized that cystatin C is affected by several factors, including sex, age, weight, height, smoking status, proteinuric states, chronic liver disease, malignancy, C-reactive protein, renal transplantation, thyroid disease, malignancy, and some drugs, such as steroids and chemotherapeutic agents, changes in daily serum cystatin C concentration predicted progression to RIFLE grade F some 2 days earlier than corresponding serum creatinine measurements.[19] Cystatin C measurements could not differentiate between those patients who then required RRT and those who recovered with conservative support alone.

Urinary markers such as kidney injury molecule-1 (KIM-1), neutrophil gelatinase-associated lipocalin (NGAL), and interleukin-18 also have been shown to be early markers of ischemic AKI in children and adults, after cardiac bypass surgery, but again could not predict which patients subsequently required RRT and those who did not.[20]

Thus, the currently available biomarkers are not robust enough to predict the subsequent need for RRT. Development of biomarkers of AKI that more accurately predict the need for CRRT would allow major trials to assess the effect of early versus late initiation of RRT.

NONRENAL INDICATIONS TO INITIATE RENAL REPLACEMENT THERAPY

Renal replacement therapy has been used to remove fluid from patients with severe fluid retention, refractory to diuretics, in cases of congestive cardiac failure and nephrotic syndrome. RRT has similarly been used to aid in tight control of fluid balance in patients with adult respiratory disease.[21]

Both dialysates and replacement solutions can be heated to help rewarming in patients with severe hypothermia; conversely, deliberately cooling solutions can aid in reducing body core temperature in patients with hyperthermia and those with cerebral edema or other brain injury.

RRT can be very effective in removing small, biologically active compounds that are retained in acquired disorders of intermediary metabolism. In children with urea cycle defects, due to transport defects of urea cycle intermediates, or the organic acidurias, encephalopathy may rapidly develop after infections and other precipitant factors, as a result of the rapid accumulation of ammonia, methylmalonic acid, and other potentially toxic compounds. Similarly, hyperammonemia-induced encephalopathy also can develop in childhood Reye's syndrome and as a complication of valproate therapy.

Similarly, RRT has been used in severe cases of poisoning that have not responded to forced diuresis and other conservative management modalities. Drugs and poisons that can be removed by RRT include methanol (usually at plasma concentrations greater than 500 mg/L), long-acting barbiturates, boric acid, bromide, carbromal, choral hydrate, dichlorophenazone, ethchlorvynol, ethylene glycol, fluoride, lithium (at plasma concentrations greater than 3 mEq/L), methylsalicylate, salicylate (at plasma concentrations greater than 80 mg/dL), sodium chlorate, ethylene glycol (at plasma concentrations greater than 500 mg/L), and sodium valproate (at plasma concentrations greater than 1000 mg/L).[22]

No indications for RRT outside AKI have been clearly established. Nevertheless, several case series and small studies advocate a role for RRT in patients with severe sepsis and after cardiac arrest (see Chapter 208).

CONCLUSION

AKI resulting in an abrupt and sustained fall in GFR that does not respond to standard resuscitation and supportive management, leading to volume overload or accumulation of potentially deleterious metabolites or severe metabolic acidosis, will necessitate RRT. As yet, evidence is lacking regarding the optimal level of renal function at which to initiate RRT,[23] and the absolute values of urea and creatinine have different connotations for management in patients with AKI and those with CKD. On the basis of historic studies, it generally is accepted in clinical practice to start RRT in patients with a serum urea of 30 mmol/L or greater (or BUN of 50 mg/dL), or with persistent severe oliguria or absolute anuria. In recent years, new classification and scoring systems have been introduced in an attempt to standardize the definition of AKI and the degree of renal impairment potentially requiring RRT. The introduction of these staging and scoring systems may potentially be expected to facilitate future studies of the optimal time to initiate RRT in patients with AKI, and such investigations may be aided by finding biomarkers that not only predict AKI but also differentiate between patients who will recover quickly with conservative management alone and those who will require support with RRT.

In day-to-day clinical practice, however, the decision to initiate RRT usually is based on a review of the patient's clinical condition in conjunction with both absolute values and trends in biochemical results. Thus, patients with multiple organ failure typically start RTT at much lower absolute values on serum laboratory studies than those with AKI alone or with preexisting CKD.

Indications generally used to start renal replacement therapy in standard clinical practice in patients with AKI are summarized in Table 87-5.

TABLE 87-5

Indications for Initiation of Renal Replacement Therapy in Standard Clinical Management of Patients with Acute Kidney Injury (AKI)

Biochemical Indications

Refractory hyperkalemia >6.5 mmol/L

Serum urea >30 mmol/L *or* BUN >50 mg/dL

$3.0 \times \uparrow$ baseline serum creatinine *or* absolute SCr > 355 μmol/L (0.4 mg/dL), *or* with acute $\uparrow$ in SCr >44 μmol (0.5 mg/dL)

Refractory metabolic acidosis with pH $\leq$ 7.1

Other refractory electrolyte abnormalities: hypo- or hypernatremia and hypercalcemia

Tumor lysis syndrome with hyperuricemia and hyperphosphatemia

Urea cycle defects and organic acidurias, resulting in hyperammonemia, methylmalonic acidemia

Clinical Indications

Urine output <0.3 mL/kg for 24 hours or absolute anuria for 12 hours

AKI with multiple organ failure

Refractory volume overload

End-organ damage: pericarditis, encephalopathy, neuropathy, myopathy, uremic bleeding

Need to create intravascular space for plasma and other blood product infusions and nutrition

Severe poisoning or drug overdose

Severe hypothermia or hyperthermia

BUN, blood urea nitrogen; SCr, serum creatinine.

Key Points

1. After the introduction of the estimated glomerular filtration rate, a background of preexisting chronic kidney disease was recognized in many adult patients in whom acute kidney injury develops.

2. Although prerenal acute kidney injury is the most common form of acute kidney injury in the intensive care unit setting, other causes should always be considered and investigated when appropriate.

3. A rise in serum creatinine typically occurs 24 to 72 hours after acute kidney injury; similarly, once kidney function recovers, a fall in creatinine is likewise delayed.

4. Apart from cases of life-threatening electrolyte abnormalities, the decision to initiate renal replacement therapy remains a clinical decision based on preexisting renal function, the setting of acute kidney injury, and assessment of the patient in combination with review of biochemical and other laboratory data.

5. In cases of poisoning or drug overdose, renal replacement therapy may have a role in patients with potentially toxic drug concentrations and also in those who are deteriorating despite maximal supportive medical management.

Key References

5. Stevens LA, Coresh J, Greene T, Levey AS: Assessing kidney function—measured and estimated glomerular filtration rate. N Engl J Med 2006;354:2473-2483.

16. Liu KD Himmelfarb J, Paganini E, et al: Timing of initiation of dialysis in critically ill patients with acute kidney injury. Clin J Am Soc Nephrol 2006;1:915-919.

19. Herget-Rosenthal S, Marggraf G, Husing J, et al: Early detection of acute renal failure by serum cystatin C. Kidney Int 2004;66:1115-1122.

20. Parikh CR, Mishra J, Thiessen-Philbrook H, et al: Urinary IL-18 is an early predictive biomarker of acute kidney injury after cardiac surgery. Kidney Int 2006;70:199-203.

23. Strazdins V, Watson AR, Harvey B: Renal replacement therapy for acute renal failure in children: European guidelines. Pediatr Nephrol 2004;19:1999-207.

See the companion Expert Consult website for the complete reference list.

CHAPTER 88

Proteomics and Acute Renal Failure

John M. Arthur, Milos N. Budisavljevic, Sanju A. Varghese, and T. Brian Powell

OBJECTIVES

This chapter will:

1. Describe the proteomic methodologies used to study acute renal failure.

2. Review the advantages and limitations of proteomic techniques.

3. Summarize proteomic studies in acute renal failure.

4. Present an overview of future directions in research on acute renal failure using proteomics.

The word *proteome* was coined in 1994 to describe the set of proteins encoded by the genome. *Proteomics* is the group of methods that seeks to characterize this global set of proteins. The feature that distinguishes proteomics from other protein identification methods such as Western blotting is large-scale identification of proteins. Whereas Western blot or enzyme-linked immunosorbent assay (ELISA) measures a single protein at a time, proteomic methods identify and quantitate hundreds or thousands of proteins simultaneously. In addition, most proteomics tools are "unbiased" because it is not necessary to have

TABLE 88-1

Summary of Methods Used for Proteomics

TECHNIQUE	DESCRIPTION	USES IN ARF	REFERENCE(S)
Liquid chromatography–mass spectrometry	Proteins are digested and peptides are separated by chromatography. Generates a list of proteins. Proteins can be quantified by isotopes or using "tagless" approaches.	Identification of candidate biomarkers present in urine. Identification of proteins in tissue to be used as biomarkers or to help elucidate pathophysiology.	6, 16
SELDI/MALDI polypeptide analysis	Polypeptides are ionized from target and mass spectra are analyzed. Peak height correlates with polypeptide abundance, and peak position correlates with polypeptide mass.	Good for rapid assessment of polypeptides in biological fluids. These polypeptides can be used as biomarkers of diagnosis or prognosis or as markers of early injury.	12
Capillary electrophoresis–mass spectrometry	Separation of polypeptides by capillary electrophoresis followed by measurement of size and abundance by mass spectrometry.	Studies in several diseases have identified biomarkers. The technique should be useful for urine biomarker discovery in ARF.	4, 14
Two-dimensional gel electrophoresis/difference gel electrophoresis	Separation of proteins in two dimensions by isoelectric point and size. Protein abundance is determined from staining intensity. Proteins are identified by mass spectrometric analysis of spots after tryptic digestion.	Two-dimensional gel electrophoresis has been used in several studies to identify candidate biomarkers in acute renal failure. Also useful for investigation of pathophysiological process in ARF.	5, 18, 19
MALDI tissue imaging	Tissue section is placed on MALDI target. Rastering of the laser across a tissue sample produces an image of proteins in the sample for every mass.	Will be an outstanding technique for imaging the proteins in a tissue sample. The resolution of current instruments (10 µm) is approaching the level at which nephron features can be observed.	3, 24

ARF, acute renal failure; MALDI, matrix-assisted laser desorption-ionization; SELDI, surface-enhanced laser desorption-ionization–mass spectrometry.

a priori knowledge that the protein is present. Unbiased proteomic analyses use methods that identify a spot or a protein sequence without requiring a protein-specific reagent such as an antibody. By contrast, to perform a Western blot analysis, the investigator must know that the protein exists, have enough information about the protein to hypothesize that the protein is expressed differently in a given condition, and obtain an antibody to measure the protein. Proteomic methodologies do not require a preexisting hypothesis regarding what protein will be altered. For instance, urine from patients who are known to have a disease can be examined to identify diagnostic protein markers specific for that disease. Proteomic techniques can be applied to tissue or body fluids and have been widely used in nephrology.[1,8] This chapter reviews some of the proteomic techniques available, discusses their advantages and disadvantages, and describes their uses in the field of acute renal failure.

METHODS USED IN PROTEOMICS STUDIES

Proteomic analyses typically use one or more separation techniques, together with a method to identify or quantify the proteins. Combinations of methods used for proteomics include liquid chromatography–mass spectrometry, surface-enhanced laser desorption–ionization (SELDI)

mass spectrometry, matrix-assisted laser desorption-ionization (MALDI) polypeptide analysis, capillary electrophoresis–mass spectrometry, two-dimensional gel electrophoresis, MALDI tissue imaging, and other methodologies (Table 88-1).

Mass Spectrometry

The use of mass spectrometry is fundamental to most types of proteomic analysis. A mass spectrometer measures the mass, or mass-to-charge ratio (m/z), of polypeptide ions. These ions are introduced into the mass analyzer of mass spectrometers, which use magnetic or electrical fields to alter the flight of the ions and also detectors to determine the mass-to-charge ratio of the ion. A spectrum is generated that describes the abundance of polypeptide ions at each mass-to-charge ratio. An example of mass spectra from four patients with acute renal failure is shown in Figure 88-1.

Tandem mass spectrometers use two consecutive mass analyzers to obtain information about the sequence of the polypeptide. The identity of the original protein is ascertained according to peptide sizes or peptide sequence determined using computer programs. The polypeptides typically are ionized for introduction into the mass spectrometer by one of two methods: electrospray ionization (ESI) or MALDI. ESI injects droplets of polypeptides dissolved in a liquid through a small capillary. The solute evaporates, thereby bringing the charged polypeptides

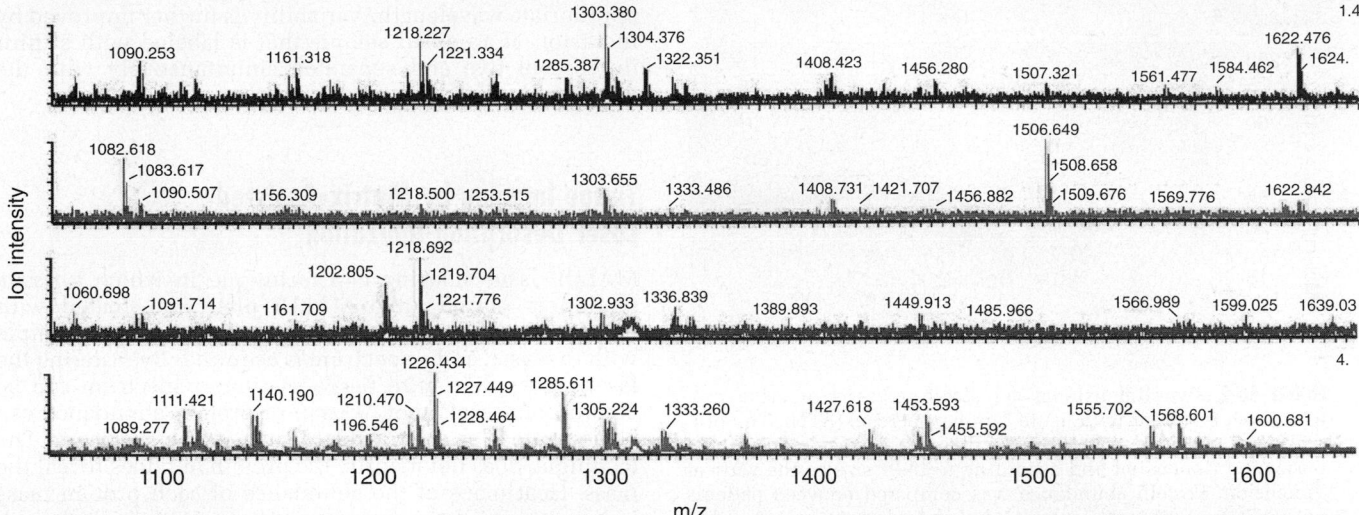

FIGURE 88-1. MALDI mass spectrometer spectra from urine of four patients with acute kidney injury. A small portion of the total spectrum, from 1050 to 1650 daltons, is shown. The *m/z* values on the *x*-axis correspond to peptide sizes. A large number of peptides can be seen in urine. Patterns of these peptides and their relative abundances can potentially be used as biomarkers to identify the disease the patient has, to identify acute kidney injury in its early stages, or to predict whether a patient will require dialysis.

closer to each other, which causes the droplets to break up further before entering the mass analyzer.

When a MALDI ion source is used, the polypeptide is mixed with crystallized matrix on a metal plate. A laser is fired at the polypeptide on the plate, and the energy from the laser is transferred through the matrix to the polypeptide. The polypeptide is ionized and desorbed from the metal surface and enters the mass analyzer.

Liquid Chromatography–Mass Spectrometry

When liquid chromatography–mass spectrometry is used for proteomic analysis, proteins are enzymatically digested before separation by liquid chromatography. The peptides are eluted from the column, ionized by ESI, and analyzed by mass spectrometry. Software is used to identify the proteins by comparison with database sequences. A list of proteins in the sample is generated. A large number of proteins have been identified in urine using this approach.[16] Abundance differences between samples can be compared by labeling individual samples with isotopic tags and mixing the samples before analysis.[6] These tags are chemically identical but contain isotopically different forms of atoms (such as ^{12}C and ^{13}C), so that the peak intensity can be compared between samples in the same spectrum. By contrast, "tagless" quantification methods do not require an isotopic label to determine the abundance of the protein. Instead, they directly compare the peak intensities of ions to determine abundance differences between samples. Liquid chromatography–mass spectrometry has a high sensitivity and can be automated but requires additional techniques to identify post-translational modifications.

Surface-Enhanced Laser Desorption-Ionization Mass Spectrometry

SELDI is a form of MALDI wherein the metal plate is enhanced by coating it with a substance that has affinity

for a subset of the proteins.[11] The protein sample is incubated on the plate, where only a portion of the proteins are bound to the surface. The unbound proteins are washed off. The bound polypeptides are ionized with a laser, and a spectrum is obtained that shows the masses of proteins. The spectrum can be compared with others to determine the relative abundance of proteins between samples.

Polypeptide Analysis by Matrix-Assisted Laser Desorption-Ionization

A similar technique is MALDI polypeptide analysis. In this approach, polypeptides are concentrated and purified before being put on the MALDI target plate. In the example shown in Figure 88-1, a combination of reverse phase and size exclusion separation on a solid phase support was used before samples were spotted on the MALDI target. The figure shows a portion of the spectrum, from 1050 to 1650 daltons, for 4 of the 64 patients with acute renal failure for whom data were analyzed. The goal of this study was to find patterns of peaks that could predict which patients would require dialysis. Several peaks are present in all patients, although many are unique. Analysis of these data to identify biomarkers requires informatic approaches such as use of artificial neural networks (ANNs) in order to find patterns of peaks that can be used as markers. Preliminary data indicate that a combination of eight peaks from the spectrum can predict which patients will require dialysis. These results need to be validated but demonstrate a promising approach to prognostic biomarker discovery in acute kidney injury.

Capillary Electrophoresis–Mass Spectrometry

Capillary electrophoresis coupled to mass spectrometry has been used for biomarker discovery. This technique separates proteins using capillary electrophoresis followed by ESI and injection directly into a mass spectrometer.[10]

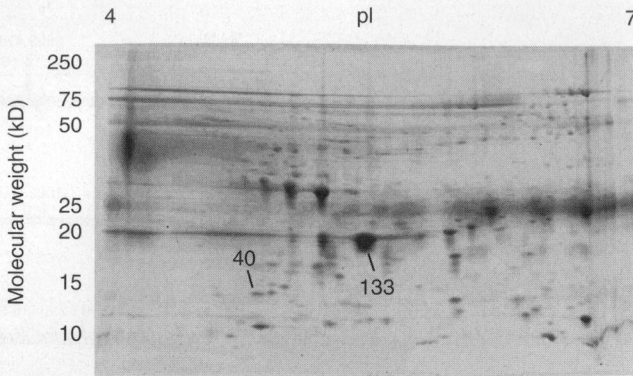

FIGURE 88-2. Two-dimensional gel electrophoresis of urine proteins from a patient with acute tubular necrosis (ATN). The proteins are separated according to their isoelectric point in the horizontal dimension and according to their size in the vertical dimension. Protein abundance was compared between patients with ATN and prerenal azotemia. Numbered spots were found to be necessary to differentiate ATN from prerenal azotemia (PRA). Spot number 133 was identified as plasma retinol-binding protein, and spot number 40 contains fragments of albumin and plasma retinol-binding protein.

A spectrum is obtained at each elution time point from the mass spectrometer. The protein mass is determined from the spectrum and is plotted against the elution time. The ion intensity is used as a measure of polypeptide abundance. Capillary electrophoresis–mass spectrometry is reproducible and sensitive but does not directly identify proteins, and its use typically is limited to proteins smaller than 20 kD. This technique has not yet been applied to look for biomarkers in acute renal failure but has been used to look for urinary biomarkers of diabetes[14] and congenital ureteropelvic junction obstruction.[4]

Two-Dimensional Gel Electrophoresis

Two-dimensional gel electrophoresis is used to separate proteins according to isoelectric point and size.[5] The gels are stained to visualize individual protein spots. The spots on each gel are aligned across the gels to identify spots that represent the same protein in each sample. The total intensity of the pixels for each spot can be compared between samples to determine the relative abundance of the proteins. An example of urine proteins from a patient with acute tubular necrosis (ATN) is seen in Figure 88-2. Spots can be cut from the gel, enzymatically digested, and identified by mass spectrometry. The technique is widely available and is an excellent tool to visualize post-translationally modified proteins but performs poorly for high-molecular-weight or hydrophobic proteins and is not easily automated. Two-dimensional gel electrophoresis has been used to identify urine biomarkers that can predict the cause of disease.[13,18]

Difference Gel Electrophoresis

The use of difference gel electrophoresis, in which two samples are fluorescently stained with different dyes, combined, and separated in the same gel, has improved reproducibility. The abundance of the individual samples can be measured by excitation of the individual dyes at the appropriate wavelength. Variability is further improved by inclusion of a pooled sample that is labeled with a third fluorescent dye and separated simultaneously with the two samples.[17]

Tissue Imaging by Matrix-Assisted Laser Desorption-Ionization

MALDI tissue imaging is a technique in which a tissue section is placed on a MALDI plate and coated with matrix.[3] Proteins are ionized directly out of the sample with the laser, and a spectrum is acquired. By rastering the laser across the entire tissue section, a spectrum can be obtained for each spot. A map of protein abundance can be generated for every protein seen in the spectrum. The technique does not identify the protein but does reveal the mass. Heat maps of the abundance of each protein mass in every area of the image are made. With high-enough resolution, the approach could be used to map proteins within kidney biopsy samples. For example, an image showing proteins at the molecular weight of nephrin would be expected to highlight the glomerular basement membranes and an image at the molecular weight of the Na^+-K^+-$2Cl^-$ cotransporter would show primarily thick ascending limbs. Scanning through other molecular weights can reveal unexpected changes in protein expression. The technique has been used in combination with laser capture microscopy to identify changes in expression of renal proteins[24] but has not been used on renal biopsy samples.

CLINICAL STUDIES USING PROTEOMICS IN ACUTE RENAL FAILURE

Proteomic analysis has been used in two ways for acute renal failure studies: (1) It has been used to analyze kidney tissue to help elucidate the pathophysiology of renal injury and the response to injury. (2) It also has been used to identify biomarkers in tissue, blood, or urine that can provide information about the cause of renal failure, improve early diagnosis, or predict the course of the disease. Relatively few studies have used proteomics to evaluate acute renal failure. Several studies have looked at changes associated with toxins. The effects of gentamicin,[2] lead,[9,15,22,23] jet fuel,[20,21] and fluoride[25] on renal protein expression have been examined using two-dimensional gel electrophoresis.

Holly and colleagues used a rat model of cecal ligation and puncture to study sepsis-induced acute renal failure.[7] They used two-dimensional gel electrophoresis–difference gel electrophoresis to investigate changes in urinary proteins. The rats developed multi-organ injury. Thirty urinary proteins were identified that demonstrated changes in levels in the acute renal failure model, including the brush border membrane protein meprin 1-alpha. Because meprin 1-alpha was increased in the model and previous studies had shown that it was important in ischemic injury, the investigators tested the effects of actinonin, an inhibitor of brush border membranes. The inhibitor reduced the rise in serum creatinine. This study demonstrates the potential of proteomic techniques to identify therapeutic targets in acute renal failure.

Analysis of urinary exosomes by two-dimensional gel electrophoresis–difference gel electrophoresis in cisplatin and ischemia-reperfusion models of renal injury demonstrated changes in levels of specific protein.[26] Exosomes are apical membrane vesicles that are secreted into the urine. The investigators showed that fetuin-A was increased in both the cisplatin and the ischemia-reperfusion injury models. Fetuin A also was increased in three patients with acute kidney injury in an ICU setting compared with patients without. This study demonstrated the ability of proteomic analysis to identify new candidate markers. Markers identified in this way will need to be validated in larger numbers of patients and using techniques that can be used clinically.

Early diagnosis of kidney injury is difficult because the most commonly used marker, serum creatinine, is unreliable during acute changes. An early marker of injury that can be used in the same way that troponins are measured—that is, to indicate cardiac ischemic injury—would be valuable both for diagnosis and to facilitate research. Nguyen and colleagues used SELDI to search for early markers of acute kidney injury in urine.[12] Urine was collected from 60 patients at 2 and 6 hours after they underwent cardiopulmonary bypass. Mass peaks that correlated with a 50% increase in serum creatinine within 3 days after cardiopulmonary bypass were found at 6.4, 28.5, 43, and 66 kD. The identity of these peaks was not determined. This study shows the potential for an unbiased approach to biomarker discovery. In order to be useful for diagnostic or research purposes, the peaks should be identified and the findings validated in a different and larger set of patients, preferably using a methodology that is widely available.

These studies identified individual proteins that may be useful biomarkers in uncomplicated situations. The proteins have not yet been tested in groups of patients with related or confounding diseases. Other studies that have looked at complex clinical situations have not been able to find individual proteins that can differentiate a single disease from a group of diseases. It is becoming more apparent that panels of biomarkers will be necessary to differentiate diseases with a high degree of accuracy.

A recent study using two-dimensional gel electrophoresis was performed to differentiate between patients with increases in serum creatinine caused by ATN or prerenal azotemia (PRA).[19] Urine samples from 19 patients with ATN and from 19 patients with PRA were obtained. Proteins were separated by two-dimensional electrophoresis, and 231 spots were aligned across the gels from the 38 patients. Analysis by ANNs was used to identify sets of protein markers that could predict the disease. The 38 patients in the set were randomly assigned to one of three groups: training (with internal testing), internal testing (used for variable selection but not made directly available to the ANN), and external testing (a true test of the predictability of the ANN). The first set was used to "train" the network, and the second set was used to test the output. The third set was kept completely separate to serve as an independent test for the accuracy of the algorithm. The urine protein abundance data for the third group of 10 patients were analyzed using the ANN algorithm created using the first set and initially tested in the second. All 5

of the patients with ATN in the external set were correctly identified, and 4 of 5 patients with PRA were correctly identified. These findings correspond to 90% accuracy, 100% sensitivity, and 80% specificity for the diagnosis of ATN in this novel sample. A receiver operating characteristic (ROC) curve was generated for the external set, with a total area under the curve (AUC) of 0.88. Because the data from these patients were not used to train the network, this study constitutes an independent assessment of predictability. A nonlinear relationship (called an XOR interdependency) of two proteins was found to be responsible for the accuracy of the test. The two protein spots were identified by mass spectrometry as plasma retinol-binding protein and a spot that contained fragments of both albumin and plasma retinol-binding protein (see Fig. 88-2).

Only a small number of studies using proteomics have been done in the area of ARF. Discovery of new biomarkers that can diagnose the source of the injury, diagnose the injury earlier, or predict the outcome of the kidney injury is urgently needed. Proteomic analysis can identify novel candidates that will be useful to include in biomarker assays. Proteomic methodologies also can be used to help identify pathophysiological processes in ARF, which may lead to new therapies. The application of these tools to problems in ARF will help speed testing and introduction of new therapies.

Key Points

1. Proteomic techniques are useful to identify biomarkers or to elucidate pathophysiological processes in acute renal failure.
2. Many proteomic techniques are available, with different advantages and disadvantages.
3. Single proteins are not good markers for complex diseases.
4. Results of informatic analysis of proteomic studies must be confirmed in future trials.

Acknowledgments

The authors are grateful for support from the Department of Veterans Affairs and the NHLBI Proteomics Initiative from the National Heart, Lung, and Blood Institute, National Institutes of Health, under Contract No. N01-HV-28181.

Key References

1. Arthur JM: Proteomics. Curr Opin Nephrol Hypertens 2003;12: 423-430.
3. Chaurand P, Norris JL, Cornett DS, et al: New developments in profiling and imaging of proteins from tissue sections by MALDI mass spectrometry. J Proteome Res 2006;5:2889-2900.
8. Janech MG, Raymond JR, Arthur JM: Proteomics in renal research. Am J Physiol Renal Physiol 2007;292:F501-F512.

See the companion Expert Consult website for the complete reference list.

SECTION 6

Fluid and Electrolyte Problems

Basic Physiology

CHAPTER 89

Regulatory Mechanisms of Water and Sodium Balance

Kamel S. Kamel, Manjula Gowrishankar, and Mitchell L. Halperin

OBJECTIVES

This chapter will:
1. Illustrate that the content of sodium ion in the body is the major determinant of the extracellular fluid volume and that the plasma sodium concentration reflects the intracellular fluid volume in an inverse fashion. Given time (≈48 hours), brain cells are the critical cells that regulate their volume.
2. Emphasize that regulation of renal excretion of sodium ion is mediated via signals related to the "effective" arterial blood volume (i.e., induce a pressure natriuresis).
3. Stress that changes in the release of vasopressin control the excretion of water. When vasopressin fails to act, the urine flow rate is determined by the distal delivery of filtrate minus basal water permeability.
4. Underscore that acute dysnatremias are associated with large changes in brain cell volume and they require urgent therapy to return their volume toward the normal range. In contrast, a rapid rise in the plasma sodium concentration in patients with chronic hyponatremia may lead to osmotic demyelination.

It is not our intention to provide a comprehensive review of the physiology of sodium ion (Na^+) and water. Rather, because of space limitations, we elected to emphasize the "big picture" in each area and use physiological principles to develop key concepts that the reader can use to improve clinical decision-making. We also highlight the clinical implications of this physiology, which are of particular interest to the critical care setting.

PERTINENT PHYSIOLOGY OF SODIUM

Traditional View of Regulation of the Excretion of Sodium Ion: A Focus on Extracellular Fluid Volume

Na^+ and its attending anions (chloride [Cl^-] and bicarbonate [HCO_3^-]) are the major effective osmoles in the extracellular fluid (ECF) compartment. Therefore, the content of Na^+ in the body largely determines ECF volume (Fig. 89-1). Each day, the kidney must excrete all the Na^+ that is ingested, absorbed, and not lost by nonrenal routes (e.g., in sweat). The most important site of regulation of Na^+ balance is control of its rate of excretion—an expanded ECF volume generates the signals to excrete the extra Na^+. It is common to rely on physical findings to reflect the ECF volume.

Alternative View of Regulation of the Excretion of Sodium Ion: A Focus on "Pressure" Rationale

Because venous capacitance vessels undergo contraction and dilation, the control system must recognize changes in pressure (i.e., changes in the effective arterial blood volume).

Control System

The majority of the sensors in the control system that maintains Na^+ balance are in the large arterial blood vessels (the carotid sinus and the aortic arch), the afferent glo-

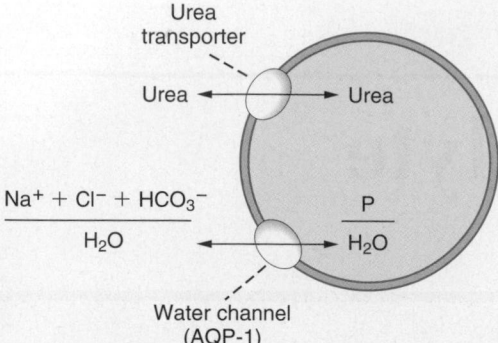

FIGURE 89-1. Factors regulating water distribution across cell membranes. The circle represents the cell membrane. Water crosses this membrane rapidly through specific channels (AQP-1) to achieve osmotic equilibrium. Particles such as urea also cross this membrane rapidly via urea transporters; hence urea does not play a role in water distribution. The major particles restricted largely to the extracellular fluid compartment are sodium ion (Na^+) and the anions chloride (Cl^-) plus bicarbonate (HCO_3^-); the particles (P) restricted primarily to the intracellular fluid compartment are predominantly potassium ion (K^+), organic phosphates, and amino acids.

TABLE 89-1

Use of the Hematocrit to Estimate Plasma Volume*

HEMATOCRIT (%)	HEMOGLOBIN (G/L)	% DROP IN PLASMA VOLUME
40	140	0
50	175	33
60	210	60

*The assumptions made when one uses this calculation are that the patient did not have anemia or erythrocytosis, the red blood cell (RBC) volume is 2 L, and the plasma volume is 3 L (blood volume 5 L). Hematocrit = RBC volume (2 L)/Blood volume (2 L RBC + 3 L plasma) = 0.40 (40%) in normal subjects. When the hematocrit is 60% and there is no change in the RBC volume, the equation becomes, $0.60 = 2$ L RBC/X L blood volume; rearranging: $0.6X = 2.0$ L; hence, $X = 3.3$ L blood volume. Subtracting the 2 L of RBC from the blood volume of 3.3 L yields a plasma volume of 1.3 L.

merular arterioles, and the large central veins. Because it is so important to defend the "effective" arterial blood volume, these sensors send a number of signals that act in concert to promote the excretion of NaCl, largely by inhibiting its reabsorption (i.e., changes in renal sympathetic stimulation and in hormone levels that may act directly or via modulation of renal hemodynamics). Although 99.5% of filtered Na^+ is reabsorbed in the human consuming a typical Western diet, filtration and reabsorption of Na^+ are linked so that the right amount is excreted no matter what the glomerular filtration rate is (within reason).

Defense of the Vascular Volume

Hydrostatic and colloid osmotic pressures (largely due to the concentration of albumin in plasma (40 g/L [4.0 g/dL]) are the major Starling forces that determine the distribution of the ECF between its vascular and interstitial compartments. Interstitial fluid is returned to the venous system via the lymphatics. The negative net charge on albumin causes ions to redistribute so that the vascular space will have a slightly larger number of ionic species (≈ 0.4 mmol/L). Although this difference is small, its contribution to the colloid osmotic pressure is appreciable relative to the concentration of albumin in plasma (0.6 mmol/L).

Clinical Implications
Normal Values for the Extracellular Fluid Volume

Because there is a large daily intake of Na^+, a "normal" ECF volume in modern times is in fact an expanded ECF volume in comparison with Paleolithic times, when regulatory mechanisms developed because the primitive diet had a very low NaCl content.[1] In fact, there are no pressures in modern times that have enough control strength to override these primitive mechanisms.

Bedside Assessment of the Effective Arterial Blood Volume

The physical examination is useful to detect the presence of a very low effective arterial blood volume, but it cannot detect mild or modest changes or, moreover, provide a quantitative estimate of the degree of volume contraction. The best way to detect a contracted plasma volume is to measure the hematocrit and/or the total protein concentration (Table 89-1).[2] Although still a measure of volume, the plasma volume is directly related to the effective arterial blood pressure in most settings (an exception is during congestive heart failure, in which the venous plasma volume is expanded but the arterial plasma volume is low). There are two caveats for this method of assessment. First, since the normal range for the hematocrit is relatively wide, the hematocrit may not be useful to detect mild or modest changes. Second, if a patient is anemic or hypoproteinemic, one must use serial measurements of these parameters to obtain quantitative information about changes in this volume.

Use of Concentrations of Sodium Ion and Chloride Ion in the Urine to Detect a Low Effective Arterial Blood Volume

The expected renal response in a patient with a low effective arterial blood volume is the excretion of urine that is virtually free of Na^+ and Cl^-. If the urinary concentrations of sodium (U_{Na}) and chloride (U_{Cl}) are both high despite a low effective arterial volume, the cause may be a lack of actions of a stimulator for the reabsorption of Na^+ (e.g., aldosterone), inhibition of a transporter for the reabsorption of Na^+ (e.g., a diuretic), inborn errors affecting the reabsorption of Na^+ and Cl^- (e.g., Bartter's syndrome), or diseases affecting the renal parenchyma. At times, the U_{Cl} may be low while the U_{Na} is high (e.g., the excretion of Na^+ is obligated by a high rate of excretion of HCO_3^- or organic anions (e.g., prolonged vomiting), or certain drug anions (e.g., penicillin, salicylate anions). On the other hand, the U_{Na} may be low while the U_{Cl} is high (e.g., due to a high rate of excretion of ammonium [NH_4^+] in the patient who has metabolic acidosis due to loss of $NaHCO_3$ in diarrhea fluid).[3]

Use of the Fractional Excretion of Sodium Ion

It is common to use the fractional excretion of Na^+ (FE_{Na}) and the fractional excretion of Cl^- (FE_{Cl}) to assess the renal response to a low effective arterial blood volume. They are used most often to try to distinguish between prerenal failure ($FE_{Na} < 1\%$) and acute tubular necrosis ($FE_{Na} > 1\%$). The problem with these fractional excretions is that they must be adjusted for the glomerular filtration rate. If the patient has been given diuretics, however, the fractional excretion of urea is a more useful index.

Cerebral Salt Wasting: A Reinterpretation

Although the presence of a cerebral lesion is obvious, the definition of salt wasting is not clear. When there is an adrenergic surge that constricts the major capacitance vessels,[4] the cardiac filling pressure rises. As a result, the kidney receives messages to excrete Na^+ even if the ECF volume is contracted. Whether this situation should be considered cerebral salt "wasting" depends on the use of the ECF or the effective arterial blood volume to define wasting. An excellent example of this conundrum was described by Cort and Yale,[5] who placed a patient with cerebral salt "wasting" on a very low intake of NaCl for 9 days. As a result, a very large deficit of Na^+ plus K^+ developed, but there was little change in the patient's arterial hemodynamics.

- In the neurosurgical intensive care unit, the clinical picture of cerebral salt wasting is complicated by infusion of a very large quantity of saline to patients who have undergone neurosurgery for a subarachnoid hemorrhage or a brain tumor, because this infusion causes downregulation of transporters for the reabsorption of Na^+ through the increase in pressure created by the greatly expanded effective arterial blood volume.[6]
- If the higher effective arterial blood volume is deemed to be important to improve outcome in these patients, the physician must ensure that the composition of the urine is equal to that of the infusate to avoid the development of hyponatremia in this setting (i.e., must create a tonicity balance (Fig. 89-2).[7] The physician must decrease the extent of expansion of the ECF volume later, and do so slowly owing to the downregulation of transporters for the reabsorption of Na^+.

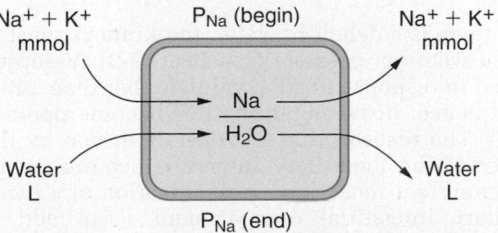

FIGURE 89-2. Calculation of a tonicity balance. The values needed to calculate a tonicity balance are the composition and volumes infused, the volumes excreted, and measurements of the urinary concentrations of sodium (U_{Na}) and potassium (U_K). If the body weight is known, one can explain why the plasma sodium concentration (P_{Na}) changed and design the appropriate therapy.

Risk of Cerebral Edema in Children with Diabetic Ketoacidosis

When treating children with diabetic ketoacidosis (DKA), if saline is infused too rapidly, the Starling forces will be altered in favor of the movement of an ultrafiltrate of plasma across the blood-brain barrier, thereby expanding the ECF volume in the skull (the hydrostatic pressure rises while the colloid osmotic pressure falls when saline is infused too rapidly). Therefore saline should be infused rapidly only if there is a hemodynamic emergency. The venous PCO_2 and the hematocrit are used to guide the rate of infusion of saline in these patients.

Edema States

Elastic stockings may improve hemodynamics in the edematous patient with a low "effective" arterial blood volume. Application of such stockings helps move fluid from the interstitial space to the intravascular space.

PERTINENT PHYSIOLOGY OF WATER

Water Control System

The three components of the water control system, which adjusts body tonicity, are shown in Figure 89-3. The goal of this system is to return the P_{Na} to 140 mmol/L. Its sensor, located in the hypothalamus, is called the osmostat or tonicity receptor; it is linked to both the thirst center and the vasopressin release center.

The three types of stimuli for the release of vasopressin are a high P_{Na}, a very low effective arterial blood volume ($\approx 10\%$ reduction), and nonosmotic stimuli such as anxiety, pain, nausea, and vomiting (Table 89-2).[8] After release, vasopressin binds to its V_2 receptor on the basolateral membrane of the late distal nephron,[8] which causes the insertion of aquaporin-2 (AQP-2) water channels in the luminal membranes of these nephron segments via a mechanism mediated by cyclic adenosine monophosphate.[9] As a result, these nephron segments become permeable to water, and the osmolality values in the luminal fluid and in the medullary interstitial compartment equalize.

Control of Water Intake

Thirst is stimulated by an increased plasma tonicity (high P_{Na}).[10] A low "effective" arterial blood volume also stimulates thirst; elevated levels of angiotensin II may be the mediator.

Excretion of Dilute Urine

When water is ingested without electrolytes, the kidney must excrete as much water as possible. Hence, the late distal nephron sites must become impermeable to water (Fig. 89-4).[9] For this impermeability to happen, vasopressin must be absent; the signal is a low P_{Na}.[8] Accordingly, the distal portions of the nephron lack AQP-2 water channels.[9] In this setting, the volume of dilute urine excreted depends on the distal delivery of filtrate minus the volume

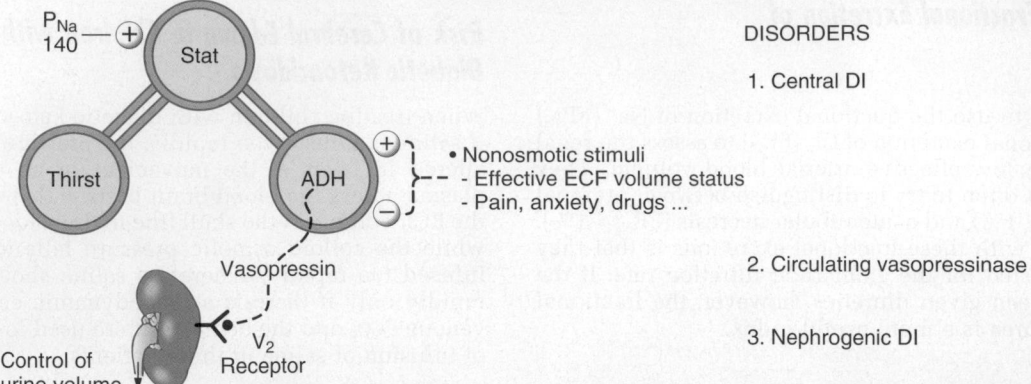

FIGURE 89-3. Water control system. The primary sensor (Stat, *top circle*) detects a change in plasma sodium concentration (P_{Na}) via an effect on its cell's volume. This "stat" is linked to the thirst center (*lower left circle*) and to the vasopressin (ADH [antidiuretic hormone]) release center (*lower right circle*). Nonosmotic stimuli (e.g., nausea, pain, anxiety) also influence the release of vasopressin. If the extracellular fluid (ECF) volume is expanded, release of vasopressin may be diminished; the converse is also true. DI, diabetes insipidus.

TABLE 89-2

Causes of a Lower Rate of Excretion of Water than "Expected"

Low water excretion due to low distal delivery of filtrate (trickle-down hyponatremia):
  Thiazide diuretic given to an edematous patient or one with a low salt intake
  Marathon runner with large deficit of sodium ion due to large sweat loss
  Beer potomania with low salt intake
  Infant with diarrhea and ingesting water with sugar
  Patient with cystic fibrosis in a hot environment
Vasopressin release due to physiologic stimuli (e.g., low "effective" arterial blood volume)
Nonosmotic stimuli for vasopressin release (e.g., pain, nausea, vomiting, anxiety)
Central stimulation of vasopressin release by drugs:
  Ecstasy
  Nicotine
  Morphine
  Clofibrate
  Tricyclic antidepressants
  Antineoplastic agents such as vincristine, cyclophosphamide (probably via nausea and emesis)
Vasopressin release without a physiologic stimulus:
  Central nervous system or lung lesions (e.g., neoplasms, granulomas such as tuberculosis)
  Exogenous administration of dDAVP (desmopressin acetate) (e.g., in a nursing home for urinary incontinence, as treatment for diabetes insipidus)
  Absence of glucocorticoids increasing the release of corticotropin-releasing factor and thus vasopressin
  Possibly, administration of oxytocin for labor induction

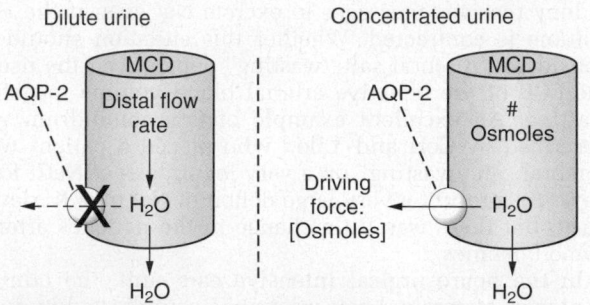

FIGURE 89-4. Excretion of dilute or concentrated urine. The barrel-shaped structure represents the late distal nephron; luminal fluid delivered here is hypotonic. To excrete dilute urine (*left*), these nephron segments must not respond to vasopressin (AQP-2 water channels are absent). In this setting, the volume of dilute urine depends on the distal delivery of filtrate minus basal water permeability in the inner medullary collecting duct (MCD). In contrast, to excrete concentrated urine (*right*), these nephron segments must respond to vasopressin and must contain AQP-2 water channels in their luminal membranes. Hence, the volume of concentrated urine is now influenced by the delivery of osmoles and the osmolality in the medullary interstitial compartment.

of water that is reabsorbed in the inner medullary collecting duct owing to its basal water permeability.

Arterial versus Venous Plasma Sodium after Large Water Intake

When normal subjects consumed a standard water load (20 mL/kg) rapidly (i.e., <30 minutes), their arterial P_{Na} was 4 mmol/L lower than the simultaneously obtained brachial venous P_{Na} (Fig. 89-5).[11] As a result, the P_{Na} delivered to the brain is much lower than the steady state value

after equilibrium of water in all body compartments occurs. The arterial P_{Na} is the one that is "seen" by the brain, whereas the brachial venous P_{Na} is the one that is evaluated by the physician.

Conservation of Water

When there is a deficit of water, the kidneys must excrete as little water as possible (see Fig. 89-3). Vasopressin is released in response to a P_{Na} value higher than 140 mmol/L, and hence, distal nephron sites become permeable to water.[12] The reabsorption of water is driven by the high tonicity of the medullary interstitial compartment. The most important renal step in the creation of a hypertonic medullary interstitial compartment is to add solutes (Na^+ and Cl^-) without water from the water-impermeable medullary thick ascending limb of the loop of Henle.[12] In this setting, the minimum urine volume is directly proportional to the number of "effective" osmoles delivered and the tonicity in the medullary interstitial compartment.[13]

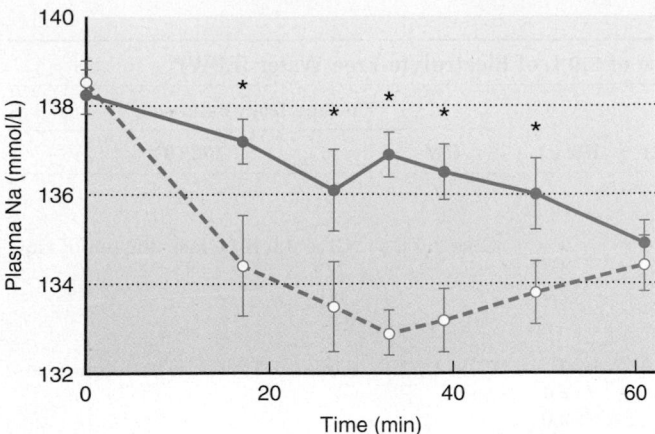

FIGURE 89-5. Fall in plasma sodium concentration (P_{Na}) in arterialized and venous plasma during a 20-mL/kg water load. The time in minutes after consumption of 20 mL of water in <15 minutes is shown on the x axis, and the P_{Na} in mmol/L on the y axis. The *dashed line* represents the arterialized P_{Na}, and the *solid line* the P_{Na} in the antecubital vein. All P_{Na} values except the 0-time and the 60-minute time values were significantly lower in the arterialized blood than the venous P_{Na} values by paired value analysis ($*P < .01$).[11]

Clinical Implications
Thirst

When assessing a conscious patient with a high P_{Na}, the physician must ask whether the patient is thirsty in order to evaluate the function of the osmostat and thirst center (see Fig. 89-3).

Differential Diagnosis of Polyuria

The two major causes of polyuria are a water diuresis and an osmotic diuresis. Both cannot be present at the same time because the late distal nephron must be impermeable to water in the former setting and permeable to water in the latter setting.

Response to Desmopressin Acetate

Because a prior water diuresis washes out the renal medulla, the expected maximum urine osmolality when desmopressin acetate (dDAVP) is administered to the patient with central diabetes insipidus and a very recent water diuresis is close to 400 mOsm/kg H_2O.

Once dDAVP is given to treat a water diuresis, an osmotic diuresis may ensue if there is a high rate of excretion of osmoles. Hence, it is important to calculate the osmole excretion rate in a patient with polyuria.

If the osmole excretion rate is high, the physician may deduce the nature of osmoles (electrolytes and/or organic compounds) by examining the concentrations of "likely suspects" in plasma and determine their source (e.g., a high rate of excretion of urea may be a catabolic state).[14]

The physician must be aware that a decrease in the urine flow rate after dDAVP is administered to a patient with polyuria it may be due to an effect of dDAVP that causes a decrease in the glomerular filtration rate and, thereby, in the distal delivery of filtrate rather than an effect on reabsorption of water in distal nephron.

Water Diuresis

The minimum urinary osmolality in the absence of actions of vasopressin (30 to 80 mOsm/kg H_2O) depends on the number of osmoles excreted and the maximum urine flow rate ($\approx$15 mL/min).

The three major groups of causes of water diuresis are central diabetes insipidus, nephrogenic diabetes insipidus, and the presence of a circulating vasopressinase.[15] These diagnostic categories can be distinguished by the presence of renal response to vasopressin (central diabetes insipidus), the presence of a response to dDAVP but not to vasopressin (circulating vasopressinase), or the absence of response to both (nephrogenic diabetes insipidus).

Trickle-Down Hyponatremia

We use the term trickle-down hyponatremia to create a mental picture of hyponatremia that is due to a low distal delivery of filtrate.[16] The prototype of this clinical picture is an elderly woman who produces very few osmoles as a result of her dietary intake (tea and toast type of diet) and is started on hydrochlorothiazide to treat hypertension, for example. Although a mild degree of decreased "effective" arterial blood volume may be present, water reabsorption in the distal nephron may be enhanced because of the low distal delivery of filtrate and the presence of basal water permeability.[17] It is important to recognize this situation, because an infusion of isotonic saline may increase the distal delivery of filtrate and cause a large water diuresis, leading to the possible development of a too-rapid rise in the P_{Na} and, thereby, osmotic demyelination.

Importance of a Tonicity Balance

In a critical care patient with an acute dysnatremia, the physician must know the volume and composition of the fluids administered and excreted to determine why the P_{Na} has changed and what the goals for therapy should be (i.e., calculate a tonicity balance; see Fig. 89-2).[7]

It is common to use a calculation of electrolyte-free water balance for this purpose.[18] However, this calculation can indicate why the P_{Na} has changed but cannot reveal what the goals of therapy should be, because it makes a surplus of 150 mmol of Na^+ equivalent to a deficit of 1 L of pure water. Moreover, there are a number of ways to achieve a negative balance of 2 L of electrolyte-free water; hence, many options for therapy are possible, but only one is correct in a given setting (Table 89-3).

DISTRIBUTION OF WATER ACROSS CELL MEMBRANES

Synopsis of the Pertinent Physiology
Water Distribution

The physiology for distribution of water across cell membranes is based on the following five facts (see Fig. 89-1); the concept is that the P_{Na} reflects the intracellular fluid (ICF) volume in an inverse fashion:

- Almost all cell membranes are permeable to water because they have open water channels (AQP-1)[19];

TABLE 89-3

Three Situations with Hypernatremia and a Negative Balance of 2.0 L of Electrolyte-Free Water (EFW)*

	NA⁺ + K⁺ (mmol)	WATER (L)	EFW (L)	Therapy from Balances	
				EFW	*TONICITY*
If IV is 3 L of isotonic saline and the output is 3 L with 50 mmol/L NaCl:					
Input	450	3	0	Give 2.0 L	Give 0 L H₂O, lose 300 mmol Na
Output	150	3	2.0		
Balance	+300	0	−2.0		
If IV is 4 L of isotonic saline and the output is unchanged:					
Input	600	4	0	Give 2.0 L	Give 1 L H₂O, lose 450-mmol Na
Output	150	3	2.0		
Balance	+450	−1	−2.0		
If no IV treatment is given and the output is unchanged:					
Input	0	0	0	Give 2.0 L	Give 3 L H₂O and 150 mmol Na
Output	150	3	2.0		
Balance	−150	−3	−2.0		

*The plasma sodium concentration (P_{Na}) rises from 140 to 150 mmol/L in each setting. The only difference is the volume of isotonic saline infused over the period of observation. In all three settings, there is a negative balance of 2.0 L of EFW. Nevertheless, the goals of therapy to correct the hypernatremia are clear only after a tonicity balance has been calculated.

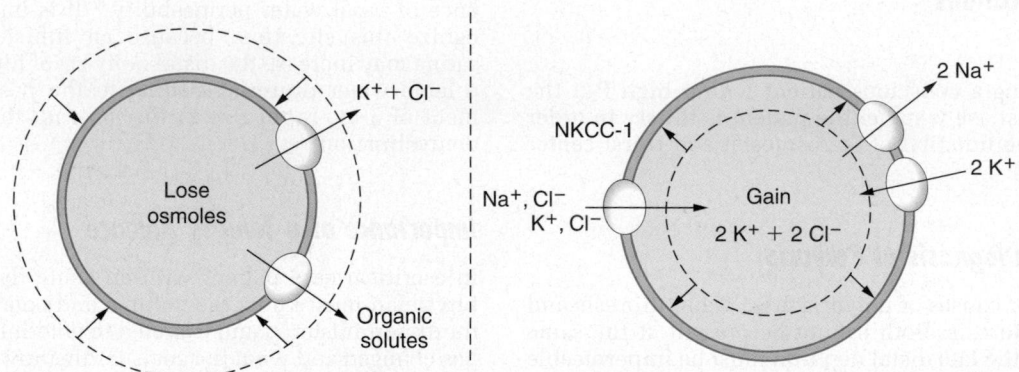

FIGURE 89-6. Regulation of brain cell volume. The *solid circle* represents the normal volume of a cell. *Left,* Brain cells have enlarged (acute hyponatremia is present [*dashed circle*]). To return their volume toward normal (*solid circle*), these cells export "effective" osmoles; about half are potassium ions (K⁺) and, perhaps chloride (Cl⁻), and half are organic osmoles. *Right,* Brain cells have decreased in size (hypernatremia is present [*dashed circle*]). To return their volume toward normal (*solid circle*), these cells must import "effective" osmoles—sodium (Na⁺), potassium K⁺, and Cl⁻—and some organic osmoles as well (*not shown*).

accordingly, water moves rapidly to osmotic equilibrium.[9]

- "Effective" osmoles are restricted to one compartment and hence determine the distribution of water between it and other compartments. Particles like urea and ethanol diffuse rapidly to achieve equal concentration between the ECF and the ICF compartments, so they are not "effective" osmoles.
- The "effective" osmoles in the ECF compartment that keep water out of cells are Na⁺ and its attendant anions, Cl⁻ and HCO_3^-.
- The "effective" osmoles in the ICF compartment are potassium ions (K⁺) and a number of smaller organic compounds, for the most part.
- Intracellular osmoles rarely change in amount, except in brain cells (Fig. 89-6).[20]

Defense of Brain Cell Volume

Because water cannot be compressed, a gain of water inside the rigid skull causes a rise in intracranial pressure unless this water gain can force other water to exit from the skull. Therefore, as the "effective" plasma osmolality declines and water enters brain cells, this rise in volume can be accommodated initially without an appreciable rise in intracranial pressure if the volume of cerebrospinal fluid within the brain falls (e.g., by diminishing the volume of cerebral ventricles). The patient may experience only mild symptoms while the P_{Na} declines rapidly toward 125 mmol/L. With a further fall in the P_{Na}, even a small rise in intracranial volume can become very dangerous: As the cerebral cortex is forced downwards on the bony margin of the foramen magnum, veins become compressed and venous outflow declines. Because the arterial pressure is high enough to permit an inflow of blood to continue, the intracranial pressure rises abruptly, leading to serious symptoms (seizures, coma) and quickly thereafter to respiratory arrest and irreversible brain damage unless a sufficient volume of water is removed from the skull to lower intracranial pressure. On the other hand, an acute rise in P_{Na} causes brain cells to shrink; accordingly, blood vessels may rupture and cause a cerebral hemorrhage.

When brain cells have an altered volume, there is a response to return this volume toward normal values. This means that "effective" osmoles must be lost from brain cells when they are swollen and gained when brain cells have shrunk (see Fig. 89-6).[20] In experimental animals, these mechanisms are well on their way to restore brain volume toward normal if the dysnatremia persists for more than 48 hours.

Clinical Implications
Treatment of Patients with Acute Hyponatremia

If hyponatremia is acute, the P_{Na} is less than 130 mmol/L, and even if symptoms are mild, this is a medical emergency. Therefore, the P_{Na} must be rapidly increased by at least 5 mmol/L. The physician must be aware of "hidden" water that may cause further lowering of P_{Na} and the risk of brain cell swelling. Examples of "hidden" water are as follows:

- Water that shifted into muscle cells because of seizures may return later to the ECF compartment.
- Patients in whom a large volume of water is retained in the stomach may be at greater risk of brain herniation if it is absorbed rapidly once gastrointestinal motility increases.[21] This is particularly dangerous because it will lower the arterial P_{Na} to a level at which the brain is exposed more than the observed decline in the brachial venous P_{Na}, which is evaluated by the physician.
- Ingested water or ice chips.
- The patient with a small muscle mass is at risk from a given water load.

Treatment of Patients with Chronic Hyponatremia

Targets for the rate of rise of the P_{Na} in a patient with chronic hyponatremia are not goals to be achieved but levels not to be exceeded. In a patient with chronic hyponatremia in whom actions of vasopressin may disappear or the volume of filtrate delivered to the distal nephron may increase and hence a water diuresis may ensue, DDAVP should be administered to prevent a rapid rise in P_{Na}.

In a patient with chronic hyponatremia, the rate of rise in P_{Na} should not exceed 8 mmol/L over a 24-hour period. The rate of correction of chronic hyponatremia must be much slower when the body has a deficit of "effective" osmoles that were lost from brain cells. The two categories are ions (e.g., K^+)[22,23] and organic osmoles. The latter or their precursors must be supplied from diet; hence, patients with malnutrition are at higher risk.[24] The rate of rise of P_{Na} in these patients should not exceed 4 mmol/L over 24 hours.[25]

Treatment of Hypernatremia

Rapid correction of chronic hypernatremia may not allow brain cells to export their "gained" osmoles, so swelling of brain cells may develop. The rate of correction in patients with this disorder has not been defined, but it rarely occurs rapidly unless too much water is given.

Risk of Cerebral Edema in Children with Diabetic Ketoacidosis

A rise in the brain cell volume must not be created in a child with DKA.[26] The "effective" plasma osmolality ($2 P_{Na}$ + $P_{Glucose}$ in mmol/L) must not be permitted to fall through infusion of hypotonic fluids during therapy of DKA.[27] A bolus of insulin must not be given to the child with DKA because it would cause a gain of osmoles inside brain cells through activation of the Na^+,H^+ exchanger in brain cell membranes.[28]

Key Points

1. The content of sodium in the body is the major determinant of the extracellular fluid volume, and the plasma sodium concentration reflects the intracellular fluid volume in an inverse fashion. After about 48 hours, brain cells regulate their volume.
2. The physical examination is not sensitive enough, nor can it provide quantitative information about the extracellular fluid volume. Even when one uses changes in the hematocrit or total protein in plasma values to mirror changes in the plasma volume, there are settings in which one must deduce what the "effective" arterial blood volume might be.
3. The volume of urine depends on the volume of filtrate delivered distally when vasopressin does not act. In this setting, the osmole excretion rate influences the urine osmolality, but not its volume. In contrast, when vasopressin acts, the urine volume depends on the number of "effective" osmoles excreted and the medullary interstitial osmolality.
4. Urgent therapy is needed to return brain cell volume toward the normal range in a patient with acute hyponatremia, whereas a rapid rise in the plasma sodium concentration is contraindicated in patients with chronic hyponatremia because it may lead to osmotic demyelination. To prevent the latter, desmopressin acetate should be administered to avoid a water diuresis if the actions of vasopressin are likely to disappear, and distal delivery of filtrate will rise.

Key References

2. Kamel KS, Davids MR, Lin S-H, Halperin ML: Interpretation of urinary electrolyte and acid-base parameters. In Brenner BM (ed): Brenner and Rector's The Kidney, 8th ed, vol 1. Philadelphia, WB Saunders, 2007, pp 749-774.
7. Carlotti APCP, Bohn D, Mallie J-P, Halperin ML: Tonicity balance and not electrolyte-free water calculations more accu-

rately guide therapy for acute changes in natremia. Intensive Care Med 2001;27:921-924.

11. Shafiee MA, Charest AF, Cheema-Dhadli S, et al: Defining conditions that lead to the retention of water: The importance of the arterial sodium concentration. Kidney Int 2005;67:613-621.

25. Halperin ML, Kamel K: A new look into an old problem: Therapy of chronic hyponatremia. Nat Clin Pract Nephrol 2007;3:2-3.

27. Carlotti APCP, Gohn D, Jankiewica N, et al: A hyperglycaemic hyperosmolar state in a young child: Diagnostic insights from a quantitative analysis. Q J Med 2007;100:125-137.

See the companion Expert Consult website for the complete reference list.

CHAPTER 90

Potassium and Magnesium Physiology

Markus J. Kemper

> ## OBJECTIVES
>
> This chapter will:
> 1. Summarize the renal physiology of potassium and magnesium handling.
> 2. Describe the pathophysiology of renal potassium and magnesium handling.
> 3. Discuss specific genetic disorders of altered potassium and magnesium metabolism.

In humans, a narrow range of low extracellular potassium concentration must be maintained by extrarenal and renal mechanisms. Although extrarenal mechanisms are able to rapidly shift K^+ intracelluarly, the kidney is mainly responsible for elimination of potassium from the body, using a complex pump-leak system involving both active and passive transport mechanisms. Extracellular magnesium levels are also tightly controlled; however, intestinal transporters and ion channels also play a role. A dramatic increase in the knowledge of molecular mechanisms relating to renal ion transporters and channels as well as their receptors has allowed comprehension of specific physiological functions and the identification of several molecular defects of long-known genetic disorders of potassium and magnesium homeostasis.

POTASSIUM PHYSIOLOGY

Potassium (K^+) is the major intracellular solute and is critical for many physiological functions. In total, the human body contains 50 to 55 mEq of K^+ per kg of body weight, of which 95% to 98% is found intracellularly, mainly in muscles. The normal intracellular K^+ level is around 140 mEq/L (range 100-150 mEq/L), and the extracellular levels are maintained at 4 to 5 mEq/L. Even small fluctuations of extracellular K^+ may be fatal, and cardiac arrhythmias may occur when levels are less than 3.5 mEq/L or more than 5 to 5.5 mEq/L.

Depending on the diet, the normal potassium intake can vary between 50 and 500 mEq/day. Intake is high in fruits, vegetables, and grain, and conversely, high-fat diets contain small amounts of potassium. Absorption of K^+ from the gastrointestinal tract is rapid, so tight control of potassium distribution between intracellular and extracellular compartments must be maintained; this control is facilitated by the energy-consuming enzyme Na^+,K^+-ATPase, which pumps Na^+ out of and K^+ into the cell in a $3:2$ ratio.[1]

Na^+,K^+-ATPase is also present in nonrenal tissues and is important for the rapid control of high extrarenal potassium concentrations, because it shifts K^+ into the cells. This enzyme is influenced by several hormones, of which insulin and catecholamines are the most important. Insulin binding hyperpolarizes the cell membrane, facilitating potassium uptake; it also activates the Na^+,K^+-ATPase directly. Catecholamines and methylxanthines can stimulate the β_2-adrenergic receptors, leading to the generation of cyclic adenosine monophosphate (cAMP), which then activates the Na^+,K^+-ATPase, resulting in intracellular uptake of potassium.[2]

Renal Handling

Excretion of the vast majority of the daily potassium intake ($\approx 90\%$) occurs in the kidney, only about 10% being cleared by the gastrointestinal tract. Nevertheless, the latter route should not be forgotten in situations of acute or chronic hyperkalemia, in which constipation can even worsen the problem.[3] Conversely, hypokalemia can become a significant problem in diarrheal states. Renal excretion correlates with dietary intake, but extreme adjustments cannot be achieved. In humans there is a minimum K^+ excretion of 5 to 15 mEq/day; thus, a minimum intake of potassium is recommended to prevent potassium depletion.

Renal potassium handling in the nephron depends on two mechanisms, reabsorption and secretion. Renal reabsorption of potassium is closely linked to that of sodium and water, with the *proximal tubule* being a site of extensive reabsorption. Active renal secretion of potassium occurs mainly in the distal tubule and accounts for most of net urinary potassium excretion. It should be noted that reabsorption and secretion of potassium occur simultaneously and that many modulators are important, such as diet, adrenal steroids, and acid-base balance–related factors. Furthermore, distinct differences in electrolyte

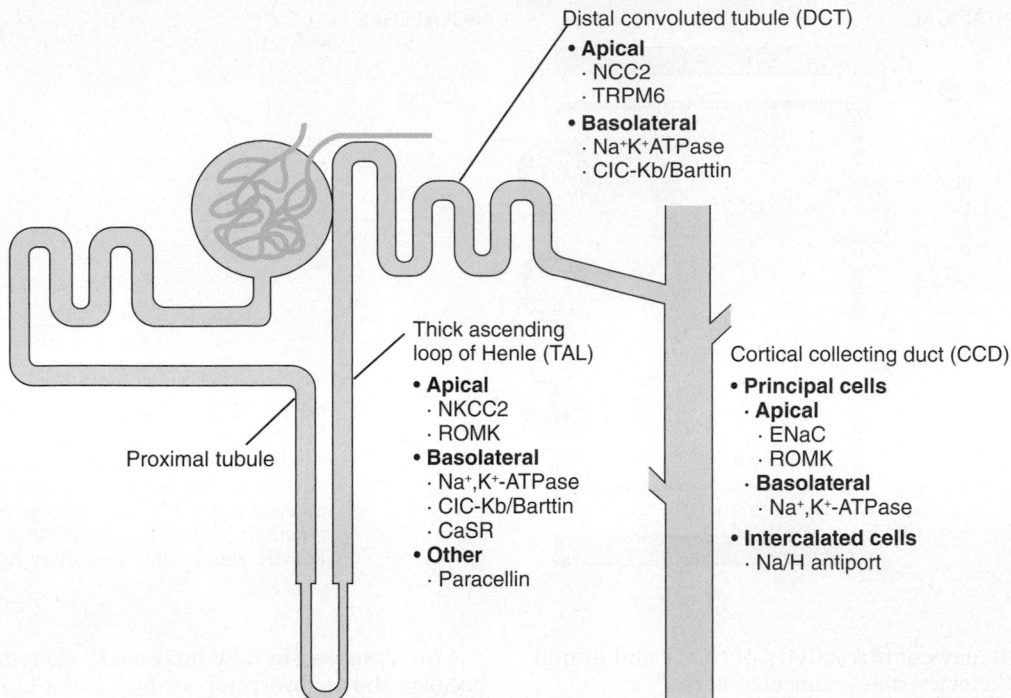

FIGURE 90-1. Distribution and types of tubular transporters. CaSR, calcium-sensing receptor; ClCKb, a kidney-specific chloride channel; ENaC, epithelial Na$^+$ channel; NKCC2, Na$^+$-K$^+$-2Cl$^-$ cotransporter; ROMK, renal outer medullary K$^+$ channel; TRPM6, a long transient receptor potential channel protein.

handling in general are present in the various nephron segments (Fig. 90-1).[4]

Renal Reabsorption of Potassium
Proximal Tubule

Most of the filtered K$^+$ is reabsorbed in the proximal tubule, so that less than 10% is delivered to the early distal convoluted tubule (DCT). The two absorptive mechanisms of relevance are diffusion and solvent drag. Reabsorption by solvent drag coupled to Na$^+$ transport is the most important mechanism in the proximal tubule. The Na$^+$/H$^+$ antiporter is the most important system in this respect, other examples being sodium cotransport with glucose, phosphate, and amino acids. Paracellular shunt-pathways are also present, and diffusion is driven by lumen-negative electrical potential created by the Na$^+$,K$^+$-ATPase in the second half of the proximal tubule, which creates high Cl$^-$ concentrations in the lumen. Specific regulatory mechanisms do not seem to be present in the proximal tubule. K$^+$ channels are present but seem to be activated only by cell swelling.[5]

Reabsorption in the Thick Ascending Limb of the Loop of Henle

The thick ascending limb of the loop of Henle (TAL) is the next important site of sodium, chloride, and potassium reabsorption. In this segment, several cotransporters and ion channels are involved in a complex regulatory system (Fig. 90-2). First, reabsorption from the lumen depends on transcellular electroneutral cotransport of K$^+$ tightly coupled to one sodium ion and two chloride

ions. This apical Na$^+$-K$^+$-2Cl$^-$ (NKCC2) cotransporter is inhibited by loop diuretics (furosemide and ethacrynic acid) and is driven by the lumen-positive potential created by the basolateral Na$^+$,K$^+$-ATPase. Activity of the NKCC2 requires recycling of potassium into the lumen, which is facilitated by an apical, inwardly rectifying K$^+$ channel called the renal outer medullary K$^+$ channel (ROMK).

The basolateral systems in the TAL are more complex and include chloride channels, mainly the ClCKb. Excretion of Cl$^-$ into the interstitium creates an electrochemical voltage that allows a paracellular reabsorption of calcium and magnesium involving paracellin-1 (see later). Further basolateral transporting systems for chloride and potassium include the KCl cotransporter and other chloride channels such as ClC5 and CFTR (cystic fibrosis transmembrane regulator). The multitude of these channels and transporters may be one explanation for the heterogeneity of chloride- and potassium-losing tubulopathies.[6,7]

Distal Convoluted Tubule

The distal convoluted tubule (Fig. 90-3) is the site of the apical sodium chloride cotransporter (NCCT), which can be blocked by thiazides. A defect in this transporting system leads to salt loss and, via secondary hyperaldosteronism, to significant hypokalemia. It also modulates final excretion of potassium, calcium, and, even more, magnesium; such modulation is exemplified by long-term thiazide administration. Studies now indicate that NCCT and ROMK channels regulate potassium excretion under the strong influence of serine/threonine kinases, especially lysine-deficient protein kinase-4 (WNK-4 [with no lysine

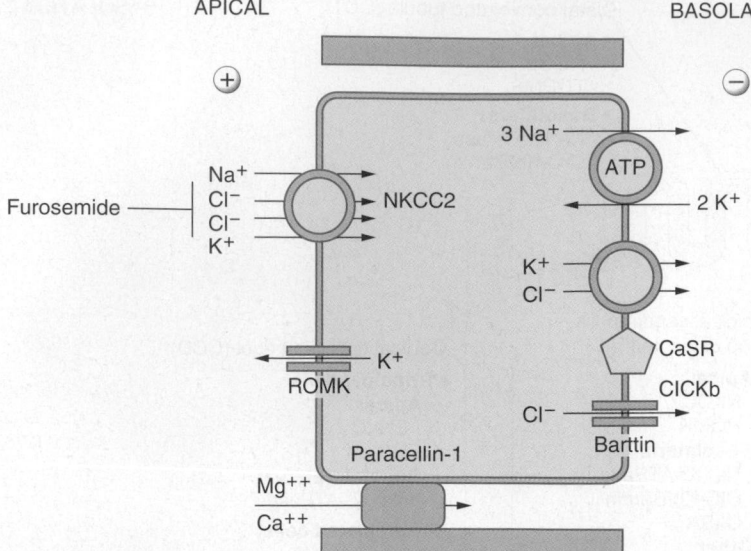

APICAL

BASOLATERAL

FIGURE 90-2. Cotransporters and ion channels involved in a complex regulatory system of the thick ascending limb of the loop of Henle. ATP, adenosine triphosphate; CaSR, calcium-sensing receptor; ClCKb, a kidney-specific chloride channel; NKCC2, Na^+-K^+-$2Cl^-$ cotransporter; ROMK, renal outer medullary K^+ channel.

kinases]), which may control activity of NCCT and inhibit ROMK in hypokalemic states, and vice versa.[8]

Potassium Secretion in the Cortical Collecting Duct

Potassium secretion mainly takes place in the cortical collecting duct (CCD), which contains two cell types, the principal cells and the intercalated cells. The principal cells line the initial, cortical, and outer medullary connecting tubules and are the main site of K^+ secretion and Na^+ reabsorption. The Na^+,K^+-ATPase transports K^+ intracellularly and promotes further luminal Na^+ reabsorption, creating a lumen-negative voltage, which then leads to secretion of K^+ down an electrochemical gradient through luminal K^+ channels (ROMK isoforms).[9] Absorption of Na^+ also occurs via epithelial Na^+ channels (ENaCs) in the luminal membrane of principal cells. Aldosterone is a strong regulator of these processes, because it increases the activity of the Na^+,K^+-ATPase as well as the number of open Na^+ and K^+ channels in the luminal membrane.[10]

The final adaptation of K^+ excretion then occurs in the distal CCD owing to potassium reabsorption in intercalated cells. This process is mediated by H^+,K^+-ATPase and is closely related to acid-base regulation. Evidence now also underlines the role of the calcium-sensing receptor (CaSR) in inhibiting the activity of the ROMK.[11]

Extrarenal Control of Renal Potassium Handling in the Cortical Collecting Duct

As already mentioned, aldosterone is the most important regulatory hormone, affecting not only absorption of Na^+ but also kaliuresis. Activation occurs directly by two mechanisms, hyponatremia/hypovolemia and hyperkalemia. Aldosterone increases the Na^+ flux through ENaCs, which can be blocked by potassium-sparing diuretics such as amiloride. Aldosterone also influences the electrochemical gradient by increasing Na^+ uptake, leading to a lumen-negative charge that promotes potassium excretion.[12]

Also, vasopressin may increase K^+ excretion in animals, because the reabsorption of Na^+ and Cl^- in the loop of Henle is stimulated by vasopressin, with appropriate effects on potassium secretion.[13] A further modulator of active K^+ secretion is diet; high K^+ intake is able to modulate a specific K^+-sensitive phosphorylation site in the apical K^+ channels.[5] Lastly, in metabolic acidosis, reciprocal H^+ and K^+ shifts occur in the extracellular space. K^+ is exported from cells during acidosis, resulting in decreased tubular secretion, and the opposite occurs during alkalosis. The effect of chronic acid-base disturbances on K^+ secretion is more complex, however.[14]

MAGNESIUM PHYSIOLOGY

Most of the magnesium in the human body is stored in the bones and intracellularly in muscles and soft tissues. Only a minimal fraction (<1%) of total body Mg^{++} circulates in the blood.[15] As with potassium, magnesium levels in serum are kept in a narrow range, typically between 0.7 and 1.2 mmol/L. The magnesium homeostasis depends on the balance between renal excretion and intestinal uptake: If intake is low, intestinal absorption is enhanced and will be counteracted by reduced renal excretion. These transport processes are regulated by metabolic and hormonal influences.[16] Most of the intestinal Mg^{++} absorption takes place in the small intestine, and only a fraction in the colon. Two different pathways are involved, a saturable active transcellular transport and a nonsaturable paracellular passive transport. Saturation kinetics of the transcellular transport system are explained by the limited transport capacity of active transport. At low intraluminal concentrations, magnesium is absorbed primarily via the active transcellular route and, with rising concentrations, via the paracellular pathway, yielding a curvilinear function for total absorption.

Magnesium Handling in the Proximal Tubule

About 80% of total serum magnesium is filtered in the kidney via the glomeruli, but more than 95% is reabsorbed

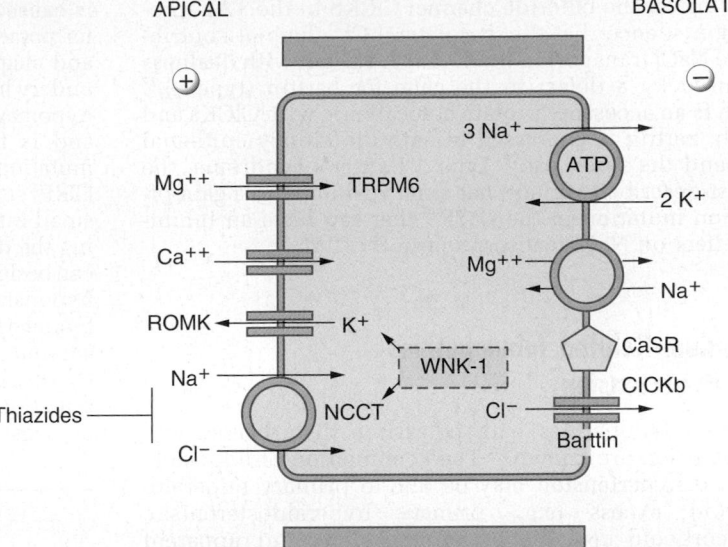

FIGURE 90-3. Cotransporters and ion channels involved in the complex regulatory system of the distal convoluted tubule. ATP, adenosine triphosphate; CaSR, calcium-sensing receptor; ClCKb, a kidney-specific chloride channel; NCCT, apical sodium chloride cotransporter; ROMK, renal outer medullary K+ channel; TRPM6, long transient receptor potential channel protein; WNK-1, lysine-deficient protein kinase-1.

by the tubular system. As with potassium, different nephron segments display different reabsorption and kinetics profiles. For instance 15% to 20% of filtered Mg^{++} is reabsorbed in the proximal tubule of the adult kidney, but this amount can be much higher in immature neonates, in whom up to 70% of the filtered magnesium can be absorbed in the proximal tubule.[17] Later in life, the major site of reabsorption is in the loop of Henle, especially the TAL, where about two thirds of magnesium is absorbed. This transport is passive and paracellular, driven by the lumen-positive transepithelial voltage that is created by the NKCC2. Paracellular transport of calcium and magnesium in the TAL is regulated by paracellin-1, which contributes to a paracellular conductance through the creation of a pore permitting Ca^{++} and Mg^{++} flux down their electrochemical gradients (see Fig. 90-2).[18,19]

Magnesium Handling in the Distal Convoluted Tubule

In the DCT, 5% to 10% of the filtered magnesium is reabsorbed. Although this amount is only a fraction of filtered Mg^{++}, this part of the nephron is important in the fine adjustment of renal magnesium excretion. Apical entry is facilitated by an Mg^{++}-cation channel that is coded by the transient receptor potential gene family (TRPM6), which is also expressed in the intestine. Furthermore, a basolateral exit through an Mg^{++}/Na^+ interchange mechanism[20] is present (see Fig. 90-3). Interestingly, there is no significant reabsorption of magnesium in the collecting duct, so the reabsorption rate in the DCT defines the final urinary magnesium excretion. In contrast to transport mechanisms in the TAL, magnesium transport in the DCT is active and transcellular in nature and is closely related to the lumen-positive voltage created by the NCCT. Mutations in the NCCT lead to hypokalemia via salt loss, although the exact mechanisms of hypocalciuria and hypermagnesiuria are not yet completely understood. As already mentioned, the expression of NCCT (and the function of ROMK) are under the control of WNK-1 and especially WNK-4, further regulators of the trafficking of Na^+, Cl^-, and K^+ and possibly of

Mg^{++}.[8] Finally, 3% to 5% of the filtered magnesium is excreted in the urine.

GENETIC DISORDERS OF POTASSIUM AND MAGNESIUM HOMEOSTASIS

Advances in the understanding of and knowledge about the complex tubular regulation of potassium and magnesium absorption and secretion have led to better comprehension of clinically known disorders of potassium and magnesium homeostasis, and vice versa. One example is Bartter's syndrome; described more than 30 years ago, this disorder is characterized clinically by hyperkalemia, metabolic alkalosis, hyperreninemia, and hyperaldosteronism. Originally it was thought to be one disorder of macula densa hypertrophy; now, however, several clinical subtypes are known—the neonatal variant, the classic variant, the Gitelman variant with hypomagnesemina,[21] and a variant with deafness.

All of these disorders can now be specifically explained by molecular defects involving specific tubular cotransporters or ion channels previously described. Also, genetically determined functional alterations of ion channel receptors, such as the ENaC and CaSR, as well as molecular modulators of receptors are known and further explain specific potassium and magnesium disturbances. In the future, drug-related electrolyte disturbances beyond the diuretic effect may also be understood as resulting from specific effects on renal ion transporters and channels.[22,23]

Bartter's Syndromes

Currently, five types of the Bartter's syndrome leading to hypokalemia are known. Type 1 (antenatal variant) is most often due to inactivating mutations of the gene encoding for NKCC2; mutations in the gene encoding for the apical K^+ channel ROMK explain type 2.[24,25] The classic Bartter's syndrome (type 3) is caused by mutations in the gene encoding for the chloride channel ClCKb in the TAL, providing evidence that this basolateral Cl⁻ channel contributes to NaCl transport in the TAL.[26] A variant with deafness is caused by a defect in the gene for barttin (type 4),[27] which is an accessory protein colocalizing with ClCKa and ClCKb; barttin is expressed in both the kidney epithelial cells and the inner ear.[28] Type 5 Bartter's syndrome, the newest-described variant, has been attributed to a gain-of-function mutation in the CaSR[29] that can have an inhibitory effect on NaCl reabsorption in the TAL.

Potassium-Related Tubulopathies with Hypertension

Several tubulopathies with potassium disturbances and hypertension are known.[30] The combination of hypokalemia and hypertension may be due to primary mineralocorticoid excess (e.g., primary hyperaldosteronism, glucocorticoid remediable hypertension, and apparent mineralocorticoid excess). Specific disorders relating to defective tubular sodium exchange have to be considered, such as mutations of the ENaC. Gain-of-function mutations in the ENaC cause Liddle's syndrome, which leads to volume expansion and secondary potassium depletion by the activation of ROMK. Liddle's syndrome responds to amiloride, which blocks the ENaC.

The combination of hyperkalemia, acidosis, and hypertension may be due to type I pseudohyperaldosteronism, which is either caused by loss-of-function mutations in the ENaC (autosomal recessive, leading to a severe phenotype) or due to mutations in the mineralocorticoid receptor, usually autosomal dominant with a milder phenotype.[31] In autosomal dominant Gordon's syndrome (pseudohypoalderosteronism type 2), mutations in WNK-4 and WNK-1 result in activation of the (thiazide-sensitive) NCCT, giving rise to clinical symptoms opposite to those of Gitelman's syndrome. Gordon's syndrome can be easily treated with thiazides, which block the NCCT.

Hypomagnesemia

Molecular events in hypomagnesemic states have also been unraveled. For example, the Gitelman variant of Bartter's syndrome, which is clinically characterized by hypokalemia, hypomagnesemia, and hypocalciuria, has been shown to be caused by mutations in the gene encoding for the (thiazide-sensitive) NCCT in the DCT,[32] although a variant due to mutations in ClCKb ion channel has been described. Another disorder with clinically overt hypomagnesemia is the syndrome of familial hypomagnesemia with hypercalciuria and nephrocalcinosis (FHHNC), which is caused by a mutation in the claudin 16 gene encoding for paracellin-1 in the TAL,[33] leading to defective calcium and magnesium reabsorption. Hypomagnesemia with secondary hypocalcemia (HSH), a severe disorder of profound hypomagnesemia that leads to neurological complications and is fatal if untreated, is caused by loss-of-function mutations in the gene for the transient receptor potential (TRP) superfamily.[34] TRPM6 protein is expressed along the small intestine and the apical membrane of DCT, explaining the defects in intestinal resorption and renal leak that can be demonstrated after Mg loading. Inherited or acquired hypoparathyroidism can also be an important cause of hypomagnesemia. Lastly, trafficking mutations in the y-subunit of the Na⁺,K⁺-ATPase cause isolated dominant hypomagnesemia,[35] and activating and inactivating mutations in the CaSR can cause disturbances of Mg homeostasis.

Key Points

1. The regulation of potassium and magnesium physiology involves complex tubular interactions of reabsorption and secretion.
2. Knowledge of specific ion channels and transporters has enabled the understanding and mapping of specific clinical disorders, and vice versa.
3. Detailed description of distinct clinical entities has helped to identify candidate genes for tubular transporting systems and, thus, diseases.
4. Comprehensive understanding of the physiology of potassium and magnesium handling will enable clinicians to translate this information into diagnostic and potentially therapeutic strategies.

Key References

5. Giebisch G, Hebert SC, Wang WH: New aspects of renal potassium transport. Pflugers Arch 2003;446:289-297.
16. Quamme GA: Renal magnesium handling: New insights in understanding old problems. Kidney Int 1997;52:1180-1195.
17. Konrad M, Schlingmann KP, Gudermann T: Insights into the molecular nature of magnesium homeostasis. Am J Physiol Renal Physiol 2004;286:F599-F605.
21. Simon DB, Lifton RP: The molecular basis of inherited hypokalemic alkalosis: Bartter's and Gitelman's syndromes. Am J Physiol 1996;271:F961-F966.
31. Landau D: Potassium-related inherited tubulopathies. Cell Mol Life Sci 2006;63:1962-1968.

See the companion Expert Consult website for the complete reference list.

CHAPTER 91

Calcium and Phosphate Physiology

*Mario Cozzolino, Maurizio Gallieni, Andrea Galassi,
and Diego Brancaccio*

OBJECTIVES

This chapter will:
1. Analyze calcium homeostasis, absorption, and excretion in healthy adult subjects.
2. Discuss phosphate homeostasis, absorption, and excretion in healthy adult subjects.
3. Describe the physiology of vitamin D and its central role in regulating calcium and phosphate physiology.

CALCIUM METABOLISM AND HANDLING

The calcium content in a healthy adult body is 1000 to 2000 g (25,000 to 50,000 mmol). In particular, less than 2% of calcium is present in the extracellular fluid (ECF), and more than 98% is part of the mineral component of bone.[1] The calcium of the mineral phase at the surface of the crystals is in equilibrium with ECF calcium, even if only a minor fraction of the total pool (0.5%) is really exchangeable. In a given healthy individual, this value is remarkably stable over time, never deviating by more than 2% from its set point. Under normal conditions, both ECF calcium concentration and body calcium content are maintained at fixed values; however, under pathological conditions, the maintenance of ECF calcium concentration may require an alteration in calcium balance and body calcium content.[2] Furthermore, the calcium in ECF is critical for different functions, and calcium ions inside the cell play a variety of cellular functions. Most intracellular calcium is found in insoluble complexes. In addition, intracellular calcium levels are very low (0.1 mmol/L). The gradient between intracellular and plasma free calcium levels is constantly regulated, playing a critical role in the functional regulation of the single cell. These tightly regulated processes keep a constant gradient between ECF and intracellular calcium ions (10,000:1).[3]

Extracellular calcium activates the extracellular calcium sensing receptor (CaSR), which is a plasma membrane-bound G protein–coupled receptor.[4] This receptor is present in different tissues, such as parathyroid glands, thyroid, intestine, kidney, bone, bone marrow, brain, skin, lung, pancreas, and heart. Once the calcium-sensing receptor is activated by calcium, it couples to a complex array of intracellular signal transduction cascades.[4]

The normal plasma levels of calcium in healthy adults range from 8.8 to 10.4 mg/dL (2.2 to 2.6 mmol/L). Plasma calcium is present in three forms: free ions, ions bound to plasmatic proteins, and diffusible complexes. Importantly, free calcium ion concentrations might influence many cellular functions, subjecting them to tight parathyroid hormone (PTH) and vitamin D $(1,25[OH]_2D_3)$ control.[5] Because most calcium ions are bound to albumin, plasma protein concentration is a very important factor when calcium ion concentration is investigated. The pH of plasma influences the percent of protein-bound calcium.[6] In particular, to distinguish ionized calcium from the protein-bound calcium fraction, the National Kidney Foundation's Kidney Disease Outcomes Quality Initiative (K/DOQI) guidelines state that total calcium levels have to be adjusted for serum albumin concentration in order to better describe the free calcium.[7] Usually, the following formula is used:

Corrected calcium (mg/dl, mmol/L) = Total calcium (mg/dL, mmol/L) + 0.02 × [40 − Serum albumin (g/L)]

Figure 91-1 shows a schematic of calcium homeostasis in healthy adults. First, calcium goes into the plasma via absorption from the intestinal tract and resorption from the bone. Second, it leaves the ECF via secretion into the gastrointestinal tract, urinary excretion, deposition in bone, and losses in sweat.

Three organs create calcium flux into or outside the ECF: the intestine, the bone, and the kidney.

Calcium Handling in the Gastrointestinal Tract

The average daily dietary calcium intake for most healthy adults in Western countries is about 0.6 to 0.8 g. Unfortunately, less than 50% of dietary calcium is absorbed, and an even smaller proportion with advancing age. In contrast, children and women during either pregnancy or breastfeeding usually have higher calcium absorption. However, intestinal calcium absorption after a meal does not contribute to maintenance of the serum calcium value at its set point. Nevertheless, adequate dietary calcium intake and normal intestinal calcium absorption are essential to maintaining normal calcium balance and normal bone metabolism.[8]

In the intestine, absorption efficiency can vary inversely with dietary calcium intake (chronic adaptation). Clearly, with 0.5 g of calcium intake, 50% absorption means 0.25 g; in contrast, with 1.5 g of calcium intake, the intestinal absorption will be 0.5 g (30%). Moreover, 0.1 to 0.2 g of calcium is secreted each day into the intestinal lumen constantly and independently by calcium intake and absorption. Thus, although intestinal calcium absorption cannot regulate serum calcium levels, it provides the calcium needed to keep bone calcium mass within the normal range.[3]

Calcium Handling in the Bone

Bone, a dynamic tissue that is constantly remodeled throughout life, controls serum calcium levels in the

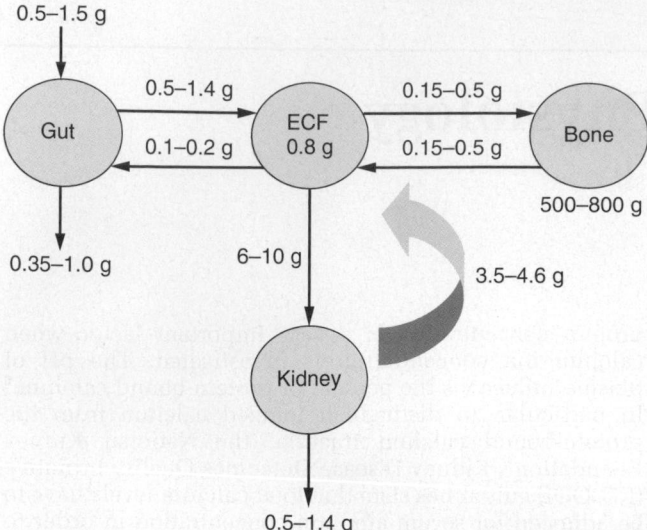

FIGURE 91-1. Calcium homeostasis. ECF, extracellular fluid.

happens in uremia, an extraskeletal process of mineralization occurs.[11,12]

Importantly, the bone system corrects deviations from the calcium set point. In the fasting state, the urinary calcium level increases and the serum calcium concentration decreases. The parathyroid cells enter in the cell cycle and immediately secrete great amounts of PTH, which stimulate release of calcium from bone tissue and resorption of calcium from the kidney, allowing the serum calcium value to return to the set point. Even if bone calcium release is so rapid that it creates a fast correction of serum calcium levels, bone remodeling is a slow process because it involves the entire skeleton.[13,14]

Calcium Handling in the Kidney

Urinary calcium excretion in healthy adults with a normal calcium intake is 0.1 to 0.4 g daily. Different amounts of calcium are filtered, reabsorbed, and excreted by the kidney, and in all situations, renal calcium reabsorption is more than 95% of filtered load. When the calcium intake is less than 0.2 g daily, urinary calcium excretion is less than 0.2 g daily.[15] Moreover, the amount of calcium in the urine is usually very small compared with the quantity of calcium filtered by the glomeruli (from 6 to 10 g daily), because the rate of proximal tubular calcium reabsorption is generally high.[16]

The majority of calcium reabsorption takes place along the proximal tubule (60%) and thick ascending limb of the loop of Henle (25%). In addition, 15% of the filtered load of calcium is reabsorbed in the distal convoluted tubule, the connecting tubule, and the initial part of the cortical collecting duct. Importantly, in this distal portion of the nephron, calcium reabsorption actively opposes the natural electrochemical gradient. This active transcellular transport is regulated by PTH, 1,25(OH)$_2$D$_3$, calcium intake, estrogens, and calcitonin. Different genes have been found to be involved in transepithelial calcium transport, of which *TRPV5* and *TRPV6* seem to play a central role.[17]

The concentration of ECF calcium depends on the balance between the amount of calcium entering into the ECF (mainly from bone) and the amount of calcium leaving the ECF (in the urine). Clearly, an increase in the ECF calcium value may result from two processes, a decrease in the renal excretion of calcium entering into the ECF or an increase in the calcium flow into the ECF.

Table 91-1 summarizes renal calcium handling in a healthy subject.

fasting state. In fact, to keep serum calcium levels constant, bone releases an amount of calcium identical to the amount excreted in the urine. The calcium set point is the value for which the net calcium inflow, from the bone pool to the ECF, matches the net outflow, from the ECF to the urine. This mechanism is regulated primarily by PTH, which increases the release of calcium from the bone and limits the renal loss of calcium through increased tubular resorption of filtered calcium in the ascending loop of Henle and the distal tubule.[9]

In addition, bone provides storage for calcium and other ions necessary for homeostatic functions. In bone, the deposition of inorganic mineral is controlled by an orderly organic matrix. Importantly, the mineral phase is composed of calcium phosphate, so the serum concentration of calcium and phosphate regulate the bone formation rate.[10] Nevertheless, bone mineralization does not occur when ECF concentrations of these two ions reach a limit value and a solubility product for bone formation reaches a steady state that depends on proteins that promote or inhibit calcification. In fact, when serum calcium and phosphate values are elevated and levels of inhibitory proteins, such as fetuin-A, matrix Gla protein, osteoprotegerin, osteopontin, and pyrophosphate, are reduced, as

TABLE 91-1

Renal Calcium Handling

SEGMENT	TRANSPORT MECHANISMS	REGULATION
Glomerulus	Free filtration	Glomerulotubular feedback
Proximal tubule	Na$^+$,K$^+$-ATPase; Na$^+$/calcium symport	ECF variations cause changes in Na$^+$ and calcium reabsorption
Loop of Henle:		
Thin loop	Permeable to calcium only in thin ascending limb, with no active transport	In thin descending limb, calcium depends on water and urea reabsorption
Thick ascending limb	On basolateral membrane: Na$^+$ reabsorption On apical membrane: Calcium links to Na+ reabsorption	Na$^+$,K$^+$-ATPase Na$^+$-K$^+$-2Cl$^-$ symport
Distal tubule	On apical membrane, calcium does not link to Na$^+$ reabsorption	PTH increases and acidosis reduces calcium reabsorption
Collecting tubule	On apical membrane, calcium does not link to Na$^+$ reabsorption	PTH increases and acidosis reduces calcium reabsorption

ATPase, adenosine triphosphatase; ECF, extracellular fluid; PTH, parathyroid hormone.

TABLE 91-2

Renal Phosphorus Handling

SEGMENT	TRANSPORT MECHANISMS	REGULATION
Glomerulus	Free filtration	Glomerulotubular feedback
Proximal tubule	Na^+,K^+-ATPase; Na^+ and PO_4^- reabsorption	ECF variations cause changes in Na^+ and PO_4^- reabsorption PTH induces PO_4^- excretion
Loop of Henle		
Thin loop	Permeable to PO_4^- only in thin ascending limb, with no active transport	In thin descending limb, PO_4^- depends on water and urea reabsorption
Thick ascending limb	Extremely low PO_4^- reabsorption	—
Distal tubule	On apical membrane, PO_4^- reabsorption depends on PTH but does not link to Na^+ reabsorption	Increased PTH inhibits PO_4^- reabsorption and enhances PO_4^- excretion Reduced serum PO_4^- levels suppress PTH and increase PO_4^- reabsorption
Collecting tubule	On apical membrane, PO_4^- reabsorption depends on PTH but does not link to Na^+ reabsorption	Increased PTH inhibits PO_4^- reabsorption and enhances PO_4^- excretion Reduced serum PO_4^- levels suppress PTH and increase PO_4^- reabsorption

ATPase, adenosine triphosphatase; ECF, extracellular fluid; PO_4^-, phosphate; PTH, parathyroid hormone.

PHOSPHORUS METABOLISM AND HANDLING

In healthy adult subjects, phosphorus represents a key component not only of bone tissue but also of many other tissues, being involved in many cellular processes. About 1000 g (32 mol) of phosphorus is maintained in the body of a healthy adult, of which 850 g are usually stored into bone tissue.[1]

In a fasting plasma specimen, most of the phosphorus is present as inorganic orthophosphate in concentrations from 2.8 to 4.0 mg/dL (0.9 to 2.3 mmol/L). Contrary to calcium, of which approximately 50% is bound, only about 12% of phosphorus is bound to plasma proteins. Free dihydrogen phosphate ($H_2PO_4^-$) normally accounts for about 10% of the total phosphorus, whereas free hydrogen phosphate (HPO_4^{2-}) and sodium phosphate ($NaPO_4^-$) account for 75%. Phosphate has a pKa of 6.8, but at normal physiologic pH (7.4), it primarily exists as a divalent ion.[2] Different forms of phosphorus are present in plasma, depending on pH and other factors. In fact, children and postmenopausal women have higher phosphorus levels than the general population. Importantly, elevated total phosphorus values do not seem to depend on higher intake of phosphorus with meals. In addition, a circadian variation in levels of phosphorus during a 24-hour fast, in part mediated by the adrenal cortex, has been demonstrated. A low-phosphorus diet clearly decreases the morning fasting levels and probably reduces the enhancement and the plateau typically seen in the afternoon. Serum ionized calcium levels do not change even when serum phosphorus increases two-fold.[3]

A low phosphate intake promotes a reduction in renal phosphate excretion, preventing hypophosphatemia. Clearly, renal tubular cells retain the ability to increase the phosphate tubular transport, with variability among different portions of the proximal tubules. Hypophosphatemia stimulates 25(OH)D-1α-hydroxylase, which is critically modulated by renal tubular phosphate fluxes.[18] Contrarily, hyperphosphatemia and increased renal tubular fluxes result in reduced phosphate reabsorption, increased clearance of phosphate, and suppressed activity of 25(OH)D-1α-hydroxylase.

The kidney is the major organ for control of phosphate losses. Phosphorus filtered through the glomerulus is usually reabsorbed in the proximal tubule, resulting in only 10% to 15% excretion of the filtered load. Physiologically, the proximal tubular reabsorption increases if the filtered phosphate load decreases. In contrast, both phosphate clearance and renal tubular reabsorption increase if the filtered phosphate load increases. Basically, urinary phosphate excretion reflects dietary phosphate intake (Table 91-2).

In contrast to intestinal calcium absorption, phosphate is greatly reabsorbed by the gut. In fact, at levels of phosphate intake of about 2 mg per kg of body weight daily, 85% of ingested phosphorus is absorbed. Furthermore, phosphate is a key regulatory factor in parathyroid function. In fact, elevated serum phosphorus levels induce secondary hyperparathyroidism through direct (inhibition of 1,25[OH]$_2$D$_3$ production) and indirect (subsequent reduction of calcium levels) mechanisms. Furthermore, phosphorus regulates PTH messenger RNA stability, controlling parathyroid function at a post-transcriptional level.[13] Finally, the physiological role of phosphorus in regulating parathyroid cell growth has been well demonstrated.[14]

PHYSIOLOGY OF VITAMIN D

Vitamin D is not a "vitamin" but rather a hormone. Classically, the metabolic control for activation of vitamin D is regulated by liver and kidney, and the target tissues for vitamin D are the bone and the gut. Calcium, phosphate, PTH, and other peptides regulate renal vitamin D handling (Fig. 91-2).

The vitamin D precursors, cholecalciferol (vitamin D_3) and ergocalciferol (vitamin D_2), derive from dietary sources (animal and fish liver, eggs, fish oils). However, cholecalciferol is also produced in the skin from 7-dehydrocholesterol (pre-vitamin D_3), through the nonenzymatic effect of the ultraviolet B rays of sunlight (UVB; wavelengths 295-305 nm). Both cholecalciferol and ergocalciferol are enzymatically hydroxylated at carbon 25 in the liver and at carbon 1 in renal tubules.[18]

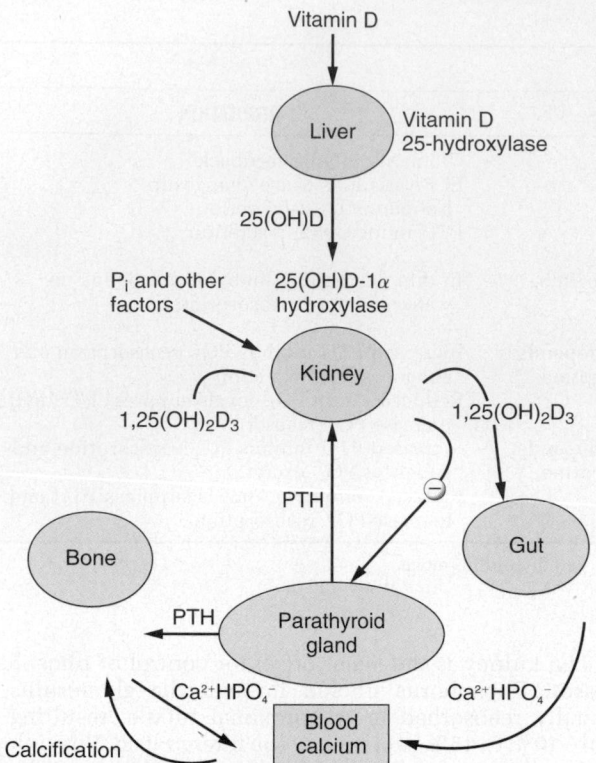

FIGURE 91-2. Vitamin D physiology. P_i, inorganic phosphate; PTH, parathyroid hormone.

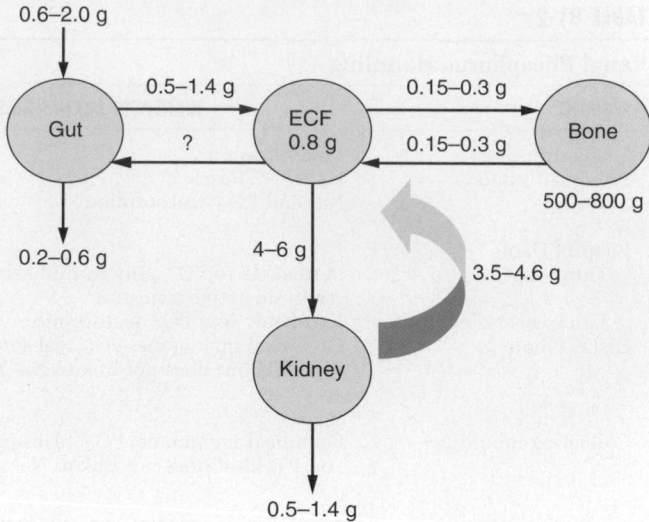

FIGURE 91-3. Phosphate homeostasis.

The monohydroxylated metabolite, 25-hydroxycholecalciferol (25[OH]D_3), is 500 times less active than 1,25(OH)$_2$$D_3$, but its serum concentration is the best indicator of vitamin D body stores. In spite of its low affinity for the vitamin D receptor (VDR), 25(OH)D_3 maintains some biological effects, because its serum concentrations are 1000 times higher than those of 1,25(OH)$_2$$D_3$, thus compensating for the low affinity for VDR.[2] Furthermore, lower 25(OH)D_3 serum concentrations are associated with higher risk of fracture and low bone mineral density at different bone sites in young and elderly healthy individuals of both genders. Conversely, excessively high 25(OH)D_3 levels are associated with low bone turnover. The need to maintain normal vitamin D stores suggests that an unknown vitamin D metabolite in addition to 1,25(OH)$_2$$D_3$ may have a beneficial effect on bone and parathyroid metabolism.[19]

The final product, 1,25-dihydroxycholecalciferol (1,25[OH]$_2$$D_3$), is the active metabolite of vitamin D, although its serum concentration does not correlate with vitamin D stores. It has been demonstrated that 1,25(OH)$_2$$D_3$ promotes active and passive intestinal absorption of calcium and phosphate and, consequently, bone mineralization. Conversely, 1,25(OH)$_2$$D_3$ suppresses PTH synthesis and parathyroid cell proliferation through a genomic activity.[20] The genomic effect of 1,25(OH)$_2$$D_3$ is modulated by specific cytosolic VDRs in target cells. VDR forms a heterodimer with the retinoid X receptor that enables the complex 1,25(OH)$_2$$D_3$–VDR to bind with high affinity to the vitamin D response element (VDRE) on the transcription promoters of vitamin D–sensitive genes. VDR has been detected in vitamin D–sensitive tissues (bone, intestine, kidney and parathyroid glands) and even in tissues in which vitamin D activity is still unclear (myocardium,

brain, pancreas, and testis). In addition to the genomic effect, a rapid nongenomic effect of 1,25(OH)$_2$$D_3$ has been found in intestinal cells.[2]

Vitamin D receptors are diffusely present in the intestine, bone, kidney, skin, breast, parathyroid gland, brain, gonads, pituitary gland, skeletal muscle, circulating monocytes, and activated lymphocytes of healthy adults. Clearly, 1,25(OH)$_2$$D_3$ controls the proliferation of fibroblasts and keratinocytes, stimulates keratinocyte differentiation, and enhances interleukin-1 synthesis by monocytes. Importantly, 1,25(OH)$_2$$D_3$ suppresses PTH synthesis and secretion and controls parathyroid cell proliferation in renal insufficiency, maintaining a central role in the pathogenesis and treatment of secondary hyperparathyroidism.[1]

Modification of serum calcium levels is the major physiological mechanism that regulates 1,25(OH)$_2$$D_3$ production, PTH secretion, and phosphate homeostasis (Fig. 91-3).

CONCLUSIONS

In healthy subjects, the calcium and phosphate balance may be positive, normal, or negative in the absence of any overt abnormality in either serum calcium or phosphate concentration. Therefore, simply measuring serum calcium and phosphate concentrations is of poor help in predicting calcium and phosphate balance. Anyway, if treatment is initiated assuming an initial condition of low serum calcium or high serum phosphate levels, a subsequent increase in PTH synthesis and secretion, accompanied by a rapid parathyroid gland hyperplasia, occurs. Target tissues for PTH are bone, kidney, and gut. The effects on bone are to enhance bone resorption in order to increase serum calcium and phosphate levels. The effects on kidney are to increase calcium reabsorption but produce phosphate excretion, with an enhancement in active vitamin D. Active vitamin D increases calcium and phosphate reabsorption from the gut. Finally, higher calcium levels suppress PTH secretion through negative feedback.

Key Points

1. Calcium and phosphate physiology is regulated by the intestine, bone, kidney, and the parathyroid gland.
2. Parathyroid hormone and vitamin D are the two key hormones that control calcium and phosphate handling.
3. Renal calcium and phosphate transport is regulated differently along the proximal and distal tubules.
4. Serum calcium and phosphate concentrations poorly predict calcium and phosphate balance.
5. Vitamin D receptors and calcium-sensing receptors are widely expressed in the body, and both types of receptors biologically regulate calcium and phosphate homeostasis.

Key References

4. Kos CH, Karaplis AC, Peng J-B, et al: The calcium-sensing receptor is required for normal calcium homeostasis independent of parathyroid hormone. J Clin Invest 2003;111:1021-1028.
8. Heaney RP: Thinking straight about calcium. N Engl J Med 1993;l328:503-505.
12. Cozzolino M, Brancaccio D, Gallieni M, Slatopolsky E: Pathogenesis of vascular calcification in chronic kidney disease. Kidney Int 2005;68:429-436.
15. Kurokawa H: The kidney and calcium homeostasis. Kidney Int 1994;45:S97-S105.
20. Darwish H, DeLuca H: Vitamin D-regulated gene expression. Crit Rev Eukaryotic Gene Expression 1993;3:89-96.

See the companion Expert Consult website for the complete reference list.

CHAPTER 92

Colloid Osmotic Pressure

Maximilian Ragaller and Hermann Theilen

OBJECTIVES

This chapter will:
1. Explain the physiological effect of colloid osmotic pressure.
2. Describe the physiological regulation of colloid osmotic pressure.
3. Discuss the physiological effect of derangements in colloid osmotic pressure.
4. Consider the consequences of abnormal colloid osmotic pressure in critically ill patients.

Trauma, surgery with substantial blood loss, and specific diseases like renal or heart failure either acutely or chronically alter the volumes and the composition of different fluid compartments. Subsequently, therapeutic interventions such as infusion of fluids, primarily intended to resuscitate intravascular volume and maintain cardiac output, or the application of drugs like diuretics may further derange the compartments and may cause hazards to the organism. Whereas the intracellular compartment is relatively constant regarding fluid amount and composition, the extracellular compartment is characterized by a permanent exchange of fluids and substrates that is vital for tissue survival. The fluid shift occurs at the microvascular level across the capillary walls. Only 5% of the circulating blood is permanently in the capillaries, representing the amount of the blood volume that crosses the endothelial barrier. Oxygen, water, and nutrients enter the interstitial space, whereas carbon dioxide and waste products of the metabolism enter the bloodstream. The hydrostatic pressure is the main driving force shifting fluids out of the vessels, and the plasma colloid osmotic pressure (COP) is the only force acting to maintain fluid in the intravascular space. Therefore, the COP plays a substantial role in the appropriate regulation of fluid flux across the microvascular wall to maintain intravascular volume and avoid edema, so it might influence patient's outcome subsequently.

For example, an early observational study of 99 critically ill patients demonstrated a close relationship between COP and patient survival time.[1] A lower incidence of pulmonary edema was observed in 128 critically ill patients with a higher level of plasma COP.[2] Drummond and colleagues[3] showed that COP reduction per se aggravates brain edema after traumatic head injury. A reduction of COP levels increases the occurrence of cerebral vasospasm following subarachnoidal hemorrhage, as demonstrated in a study by Ikeda and associates.[4] However, Eid and coworkers[5] could not find a relationship between serum albumin level and pleural effusion in critically ill patients.

Accordingly, it is apparent that the monitoring of COP may be advocated in critically ill patients to improve therapeutic strategies and clinical outcome. Furthermore, there is a long and ongoing debate about use of colloids (usually increasing the COP) or crystalloids (usually lowering the COP by dilution) for fluid resuscitation in the critically ill and their effects on outcome.[6-8]

The following chapter discusses the basic biochemical principles of COP, the classic physiological view of COP, and methods of COP measurement and presents some new insights in the understanding of COP's effects on the microcirculatory level.

DEFINITIONS

Osmosis

Osmosis is a biophysical phenomenon that usually occurs in biological systems, where cells or fluid compartments are separated by semipermeable membranes. *Osmosis* describes the diffusion of the solvent through a semipermeable membrane. The driving force of the solvent shift is the concentration difference of solutes in the solutions separated by the semipermeable membrane. In contrast to the solvent, the solutes such as Na^+, K^+, glucose and macromolecules cannot pass this barrier. Water, the usual solvent in biological systems, migrates from the side of the lower concentration to the side of the higher concentration of solutes. The net fluid flux ends when the concentration of osmotic active molecules is equal on the two sides of the membrane. Therefore, the distribution of water is a matter of osmosis and not transport of solutes. The principle behind osmosis is the thermodynamic quest to reach lower energy levels or an increase in entropy.

Osmolarity and Osmolality

The two terms osmolarity and osmolality describe the concentration (number of molecules) of a specific substance related to the volume or mass of a given solvent (usually water). *Osmolarity* is the number of molecules per liter of solvent (Osmol/L), and *osmolality* is the concentration of molecules per kg of solvent (Osmol/kg). The regular osmolality of human plasma is about 290 ± 5 mOsm/kg.[9,10]

Osmotic Pressure

The osmotic movement of the solvent (e.g., water) can be prevented by the application of a pressure in opposition to the force generated by the water gradient. For a given solution, the pressure required to inhibit the fluid shift into a solution is called the *osmotic pressure* (P) of the solution. The osmotic pressure of an ideal solution can be calculated by the van't Hoff equation, as follows:

$$P = n \cdot \left(\frac{c}{M}\right) \cdot RT$$

where P is osmotic pressure in mm Hg; n is the number of solute particles; c/M is the molar concentration of the substance in mOsmol/kg; R is the universal gas constant; and T is the absolute temperature (° K).

When this equation is used to calculate the plasma osmotic pressure at ideal physiological conditions (Osmolality = 280 mOsm/kg; T = 310° K; R = 0.082), the total osmotic pressure of plasma is about 5409 mm Hg (i.e., about 7.1 atmospheres). This result indicates further that each mOsm/kg of solute contributes approximately 19.3 mm Hg to the osmotic pressure.

Colloids

The term *colloid* is used collectively for high-molecular-weight particles (nominally, a molecular weight > 30,000 Da) in a given solution. In normal plasma, proteins like albumin and globulins are the major colloids present. In clinical practice, artificial colloids such as hydroxyethyl starch, gelatin, and dextran are used to achieve plasma expansion by raising COP.[6,7,11,12] Because the colloids dissolve in aqueous solutions like plasma, they contribute to the total osmotic pressure. Their contribution or fraction of pressure is referred to as the *colloid osmotic pressure*. In plasma, the colloid osmotic pressure averages about 25 mm Hg, which represents approximately 0.5% of the total osmotic pressure.

Donnan Equilibrium

The Donnan equilibrium takes into account that COP's effect on plasma proteins not only depends on their number of molecules but also on their electrical charge. As an amphophilic molecule, albumin has negatively and positively charged areas, which affect the concentrations of osmotically active particles on both sides of the membrane. The negatively charged parts of proteins restrict an equivalent number of cations (mostly Na^+) to the intravascular space. Through this effect, these cations are osmotically effective across the capillary membrane and raise the protein oncotic pressure. Therefore the measured plasma colloid osmotic pressure may be as much as 30% to 50% higher than that calculated from plasma protein concentration only. The net charge of the plasma proteins depends on temperature, pH, and distribution of albumin and globulins.[10,13]

PHYSIOLOGY OF THE FLUID COMPARTMENTS

Total body water is distributed to the intracellular (60%) and extracellular (40%) compartments. The intracellular compartment is usually constant, and fluid changes in it are relatively slow. The extracellular compartment is divided into the intravascular space (25% of the 40%) and the interstitial space (75% of the total 40%). Thus only a small part of whole body water, approximately 12%, is located intravascularly.

Although water is almost freely diffusible from one compartment to the other and through all membranes, the movement of all other molecules is more or less strictly controlled. The intracellular fluid is characterized by a high concentration of potassium, with a concentration of approximately 150 mmol/L. The predominant extracellular cation is sodium, with a concentration of approximately 140 mmol/L in the intravascular and interstitial spaces. Sodium is restricted to the extracellular compartment because the cell membrane is nearly impermeable to it. In fact, sodium crosses the cell membrane very slowly in most tissues, but very rapidly and locally limited during excitation in muscle and nerve. The distribution of electrolytes is sustained by energy-dependent Na^+,K^+-ATPase, which transports Na^+ out of the cells and K^+ into the cells to keep electric neutrality. The high concentration of sodium in the interstitial fluid, which compasses all body cells, generates a high osmotic pressure gradient over the cell membrane and is compensated mostly by the K^+ concentration. Fluid shifts between intracellular and extracellular spaces are usually regulated by changes in the sodium concentration. Under physiological conditions, the *principle of iso-osmolarity* is realized.[10,14]

The regulation of the permanent fluid flux from intravascular space to interstitial space and back is located in the small capillaries and depends physiologically on the ultrastructure of the capillary walls and on a fine balance between outwardly and inwardly directed forces. Capillaries are classified according to their ultrastructure, as follows:

- Capillaries with continuous membranes (skeletal muscle or lungs)
- Capillaries with fenestrated membranes (glomeruli of the kidney, gut mucosa)
- Capillaries with discontinuous membranes (liver sinusoids, bone marrow, spleen)

Furthermore, large pores for the convective transport of macromolecules have been suggested by experimental data. The importance of the endothelial surface layer and the endothelial glycocalyx to the fluid exchange have been described.[15-20]

The permeability of molecules depends on the relation between the dimension of the molecules and the size of the membrane pores. The velocity of diffusion of water is so high (40 times per capillary passage) that there is a continuous intermixture of plasma water and interstitial fluid. This implies a diffusion capacity of approximately 60 L/min, or 80,000 L per 24 hours, for the whole capillary surface of the human organism.[10]

The second major mechanism of fluid interchange between the intravascular space and interstitial space is represented by filtration and reabsorption. This mechanism was firstly described by E. H. Starling.[21]

STARLING'S HYPOTHESIS

The capillary fluid exchange, the balance of filtration and reabsorption, is attributed to the interactions among four different forces (two hydrostatic pressures and two colloid osmotic pressures, as follows[14,21]:

$$J_v/A = K_f \times [(P_c + \pi_i) - \sigma \times (P_i + \pi_c)]$$

where J_v/A is the volume flux of fluid (J_v) per unit area (A), in mL/min/cm^2; K_f is the capillary filtration coefficient, in cm $\times$ min^{-1} $\times$ mm Hg^{-1}; σ is the osmotic reflection coefficient; P_c is the capillary hydrostatic pressure, in mm Hg; P_i is the interstitial hydrostatic pressure, in mm Hg; π_c is the capillary colloid osmotic pressure, in mm Hg; and π_i is the interstitial colloid osmotic pressure, in mm Hg.

The capillary filtration coefficient (K_f) takes into account the permeability of the capillary wall and the area available for filtration and varies in different tissues.

The capillary hydrostatic pressure (P_c), the driving force of filtration, is generated by the systemic blood pressure and ranges from 30 to 35 mm Hg at the arterial end to 10 to 15 mm Hg at the venous end of the capillary. The second hydrostatic pressure, the interstitial fluid pressure (P_i), varies from organ to organ and is usually negative (−2 to −3 mm Hg) in subcutaneous tissues (outward force). However, in solid organs such as the liver and kidneys, it is positive, being as high as 6 mm Hg in the brain, and provides a small counterpressure to the hydraulic forces. The third outward force is the interstitial fluid osmotic pressure (π_i) generated by osmotic active macromolecules, which ranges from 14 mm Hg in the lungs to approximately 4.5 mm Hg in other tissues.[10,14,22]

COLLOID OSMOTIC PRESSURE

The colloid osmotic pressure in plasma is generated by all plasma proteins in the intravascular space and depends on whether or not they can pass through the capillary walls. The colloid osmotic pressure of plasma is about 25 mm Hg at a plasma protein concentration of 7.3 g/dL. Representing only 60% of the total mass of the plasma proteins, albumin (67 kDa) is responsible for approximately 80% of the colloid osmotic pressure. The other 40% of plasma protein mass consists of plasma globulins, which have very high molecular mass (170 kDa) but a much lower number of molecules and consequently a much lower contribution to COP. About two thirds of the COP generated by albumin is the simple van't Hoff pressure, whereas one third arises from the Donnan equilibrium, which is due mainly to albumin and its low electrical charge at physiological pH.[10,13,14]

The Starling equation roughly estimates the movement of fluids between the intravascular and interstitial spaces. Distal of the precapillary arterial sphincters, there is an outward force of about 39.5 mm Hg (P_c = 32.5 mm Hg + π_i = 4.5 mm Hg – P_i = −2.5 mm Hg), which is opposed by the colloid osmotic pressure (π_c) of 25 mm Hg, resulting in an effective filtration pressure of 14.5 mm Hg. At the venous end, the outward pressure is reduced to 19.5 mm Hg (P_c = 12.5 mm Hg + π_i = 4.5 mm Hg – P_i = −2.5 mm Hg). At a constant COP this results in an effective inward pressure of 5.5 mm Hg.

Under the simplified condition of a linear pressure drop along the capillary vessel and stability of all other conditions, filtration forces slightly overcome reabsorption forces. Thus, approximately 10% of the filtrated fluid must be removed from the interstitial space by the lymphatic circulation. The mean filtration rate of all capillaries is about 14 mL/min, or 20 L per 24 hours, whereas the reabsorption rate is about 12.5 mL/min, or 18 L per 24 hours. The excess of 2 L must be eliminated from the interstitial space via the lymphatic vessels (Fig. 92-1).[10,14]

It must be noted, however, that the process of fluid exchange is not as static as proposed by the Starling equation. In the single capillary, protein permeability rises from the arterial to the venous end owing to the increase in number of large pores toward the venous ends, which gives rise to a variable interstitial oncotic pressure. Depending on the ultrastructure of the capillaries in specific organs, different amounts of proteins (albumin) cross into the interstitial fluid. The protein concentrations in the interstitial spaces as well as in the lymph are: 6 g/dL in the liver, 3 g/dL in the heart, 1 g/dL in the dermis, and 2 g/dL in the skeletal muscles. Another physiological condition that deviates from the Starling model is exercise or mechanical stress.[14,23] In active tissues (skeletal muscles), capillary filtration pressure exceeds the COP throughout the length of the capillary, and additionally, osmotic active metabolites temporarily accumulate in the interstitial space. The amount of fluid leaving the vascular space is markedly increased. Despite the increase in lymphatic flow to compensate, the volume of an exercising muscle is nearly 25% larger.[14]

Gravity is another outward force not considered in Starling's equation. With a body in the upright position, gravity tends to increase interstitial fluid in the capillary circulation of the legs because of the high venous pressure transmitted through them by the venules. Usually the contraction of the skeletal muscles reduces the venous hydrostatic backpressure, but in situations involving prolonged

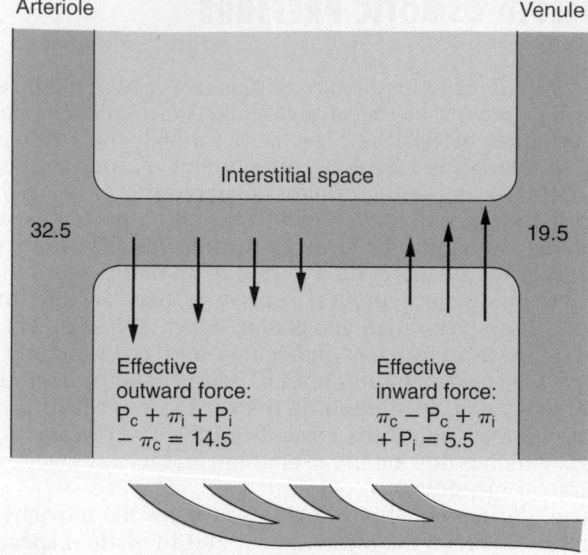

Arteriole   Venule

Interstitial space

32.5   19.5

Effective   Effective
outward force: inward force:
$P_c + \pi_i + P_i$ $\pi_c - P_c + \pi_i$
$- \pi_c = 14.5$ $+ P_i = 5.5$

Lymphatic drainage

FIGURE 92-1. Simplified schematic graph of the pressure gradients across the capillary walls, as described by the Starling equation. This model estimates a linear reduction of the hydrostatic pressure (P_c) from 32.5 mm Hg at the arterial end to 12.5 mm Hg at the venular end of the capillary unit. With the interstitial oncotic pressure (π_i) at 4.5 mm Hg and the interstitial hydraulic pressure (P_i) at −2.5 mm Hg (for subcutaneous or muscle tissue). These outward forces are opposed by an estimated constant colloid osmotic pressure (π_c) of 25 mm Hg. These conditions result in an effective filtration pressure of 14.5 mm Hg at the arterial side and an effective inward pressure of 5.5 mm Hg at the venular side of the capillary vessel. The excess of fluid filtration compared with reabsorption is compensated by the lymphatic drainage. (Modified from Schmidt RF, Thews G: Kreislauf. In Schmidt RF, Lang F, Thews G [eds]: Physiologie des Menschen. Heidelberg, Springer Verlag, 2005, pp 603-666; and Ganong WL: Dynamics of blood & lymph flow. In Ganong WL [ed]: Review of Medical Physiology. New York, McGraw-Hill, 2001, pp 556-573.)

periods of feet in dependent positions (e.g., long trip by airplane), gravity contributes substantially to edema.

MEASUREMENT OF COLLOID OSMOTIC PRESSURE

In contrast to the other forces regulating filtration and reabsorption, the COP can be calculated or measured easily. Theoretical and empirical formulas considering plasma protein or albumin concentrations have been used to determine COP.[24] Landis and Pappenheimer[25] proposed an empirical model to predict COP in human plasma on the basis of total protein concentrations (TP), the law of van't Hoff (term 1), and the Gibbs-Donnan effect (terms 2 and 3):

$$COP = 2.1 \times TP + 0.16TP2 + 0.009TP3$$

However, such calculations are only approximations, and a COP calculation from total protein concentration is reasonable only in healthy subjects.[24,26] In critically ill patients, not only total protein concentration but also albumin-to-globulin ratio must be considered.[24]

Therefore, the direct measurement of the COP at the bedside with a membrane osmometer is advocated in critically ill patients.[24,26,27] A membrane osmometer consists of a reference chamber filled with normal saline solution (0.9%) directly connected to a pressure transducer. The measurement chamber is clamped to this reference chamber via a semipermeable membrane with a cutoff point of usually 10 to 20 kDa. When a colloid-containing fluid such as a sample of the patient's blood is placed in the measurement chamber, water shifts from the reference chamber into the measurement chamber, and this pressure drop in the reference chamber is directly proportional to the COP of the colloid-containing fluid.[24,28] In clinical practice, COP measurement seems to be useful for the risk of assessing peripheral or pulmonary edema during fluid resuscitation. COP measurement can furthermore serve as a guide for selection of colloids or crystalloids in severely ill patients.

NEW INSIGHTS INTO CAPILLARY FLUID REGULATION

Role of the Endothelial Glycocalyx

The endothelium-blood interface in humans, estimated to be about 350 m², is known as an actively involved structure with many functions, such as regulation of fluid exchange, vascular tone, hemostasis, coagulation, and inflammatory response. Early theoretical considerations, results from later electron microscopic studies, and knowledge of the molecular composition led to the general acceptance of an endothelial surface layer (ESL). This macromolecular network at the luminal side of the endothelial cells, with a thickness of about 0.4 to 0.5 µm, consists of membrane-bound proteoglycans and glycoproteins representing the glycocalyx in the strict sense, which covers the surface of nearly all cells to a thickness between 0.05 and 0.1 µm. Further structures, such as filaments of a length of about 0.35 µm that are bound into the glycocalyx and interacting with plasma proteins in a dynamic equilibrium, build a gel-like ESL that impedes plasma flow.[15,18,19,29,30] The glycocalyx consists of glycoproteins (selectins, integrins, immunoglobulin superfamily), proteoglycans (heparan sulfate proteoglycans), proteins (antithrombin, factor Xa inhibitor) and glypicans. Despite the specific functions of these molecules (inflammatory response, coagulation) the composition as well as the physical properties of the ESL lead to a dynamic equilibrium with plasma proteins, first of all albumin. A strong but transient binding of albumin to the stationary molecules of the glycocalyx can be demonstrated (Fig. 92-2).[15,30] This is probably mediated by the electrostatic interaction between positive charges of the amphophilic albumin molecule (arginine, lysine) and the negative charges carried by sulfate groups (heparan, dermatan, and chondroitin sulfates) in the glycocalyx.[15,31] Adamson and colleagues[17] found, in an isolated vessel preparation, that the colloid osmotic pressure balancing the filtration pressure across the capillaries is developed across the endothelial glycocalyx. In the capillaries, the ESL has several functions, such as sensing and withstanding the mechanical shear stress of blood flow, regulation of oxygen transport, coagulation, immunologic response, and the very important modulation of the capillary barrier function relating to fluid exchange.[15,17,19,22]

A new model of the capillary barrier based on these findings suggests that the ESL acts like a sponge in the

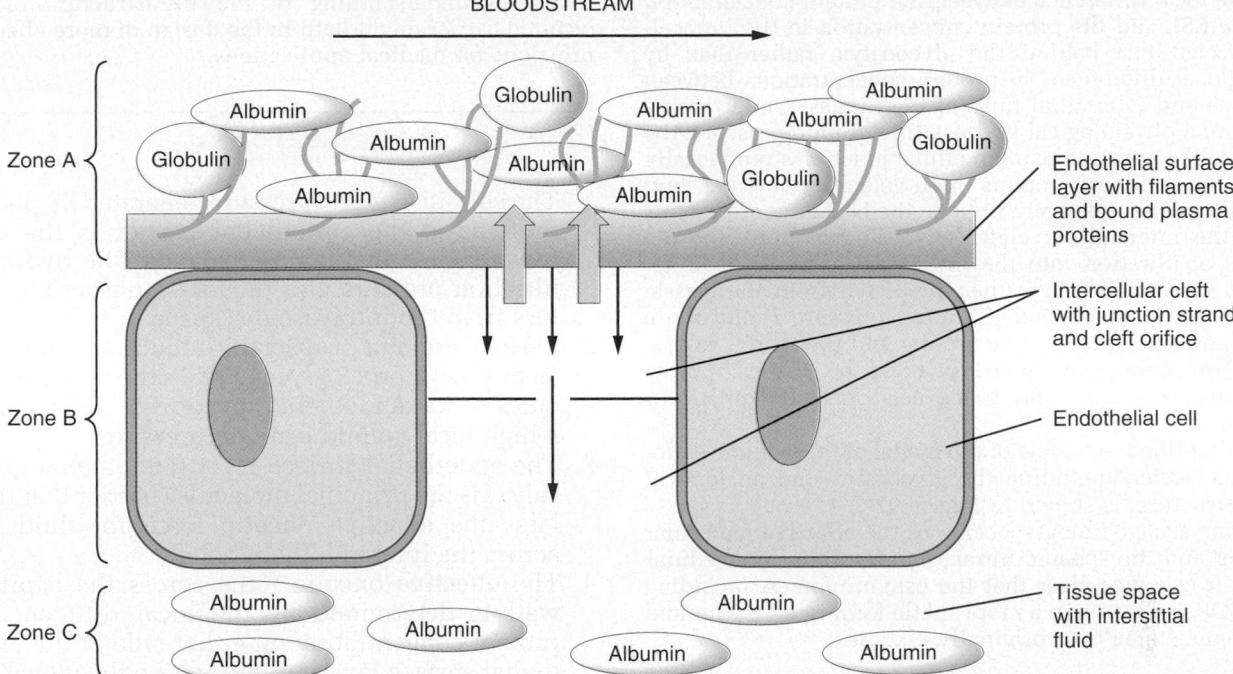

FIGURE 92-2. This figure shows a schematic model of the fluid flux across the capillary wall as proposed on the basis of new insights from animal experiments into the complex and dynamic ultrastructure of the capillary vessel.[15,17,22,32] Zone A represents the dynamic interaction of the plasma proteins on the plasmatic side and the negatively charged endothelial glycocalyx (proteoglycans, etc.) at the endothelial surface matrix. The transient binding of albumin generates a high local osmotic pressure at the luminal side of the endothelial cleft (*blue arrows*). This functional area has a thickness of about 300 to 500 nm, depending on the amount of albumin bound to the endothelial surface layer. Zone B represents the ultrastructure just behind the glycocalyx, in the intercellular cleft with the junction strand and cleft space. At high hydraulic pressure (*black arrows*), the orifice of the cleft acts like a throat, clearing the cleft space from interstitial osmotic active molecules. The fluid exchange across the endothelial barrier takes place in this very local area. Zone C represents the zone of interstitial fluid with a colloid concentration and composition nearly those of blood plasma. This area represents the homogeneous interstitial fluid that encompasses all tissue cells.

outward fluid stream, permeable to fluids but nearly impermeable to proteins or charged molecules. Because of this sieving effect of the ESL, a high concentration of proteins (colloids) in the ESL generates a high local oncotic force. In combination with the very low concentration of proteins in the intracellular clefts due to the high clearing flow at physiological filtration pressure, as described by several studies,[17,22,32] this process leads to an effective COP that prevents substantial fluid loss from the intravascular space (see Fig. 92-2). According to this model, the local Starling forces that determine water flux across the capillary endothelium are due to the local differences between hydrostatic and oncotic pressures across the ESL at the intracellular clefts rather than the global difference in P_c and π_c, as proposed by Starling's law.[17,22,32] According to this model of the capillary barrier, the transient binding of plasma proteins, especially albumin to the ESL, is essential to generate an effective COP.

When fluid resuscitation is achieved with artificial colloids, the interaction of these colloids with the ESL might be of substantial interest in terms of their plasma volume effect. Results from a trauma model have demonstrated significantly greater long-term (3 hours) volume-expanding effects for albumin and dextran than for hydroxyethyl starch and gelatin.[33] In the model of an isolated perfused heart, Jacob and colleagues[16] found that albumin more effectively prevented fluid extravasation from the intact capillaries of the heart than crystalloid or a hydroxyethyl starch solution (HES 130,000/0.4, 6%). Because this effect

was partly independent from the measured COP, these researchers suggested that this effect was linked to a different interaction of albumin and hydroxyethyl starch with the endothelial glycocalyx. Although the positively charged albumin molecule binds to the negatively charged glycocalyx, the negatively charged hydroxyethyl starch does not.[34,35]

The conclusion from these results is that not only the number and size of the molecules of artificial colloids but also their interaction with the capillary barrier are of clinical relevance. These new insights into physiology will further stimulate the debate on albumin as a volume replacement fluid.[7,15,16,36,37]

Role of the Ultrastructure of the Capillary

There is growing evidence from ultrastructural studies that the classic Starling model is a strong oversimplification of the effective oncotic barrier acting across the capillary endothelium. On the basis of data from animal experiments, a number of investigators developed a new and detailed hypothesis that qualitatively and quantitatively describes the fluid flux across the capillary barrier. In this spatial and heterogeneous microstructural model, the endothelial surface layer (glycocalyx) serves as the primary molecular barrier for plasma proteins and represents the principal barrier determining the oncotic forces for water flux. Therefore, the effective oncotic force is determined by the local difference between the protein concentration in the ESL and the protein concentration in the intracellular cleft just behind the glycocalyx, rather than by the global differences in protein concentrations between plasma and interstitial fluid of the tissues. Under conditions of a physiological hydrostatic filtration pressure, the orifice-like pores at the intercellular junction strand locally clear the region of proteins (high velocities of water flux) and therefore effectively impede the backflow of proteins into the intercellular cleft.[17,22,32,38] Furthermore, the net result of filtration into the interstitial space is quantitatively distinctively less than predicted from the classic equation, in which both filtration pressure P and π are based on their global intravascular and interstitial values. This low amount of water flux along the whole capillary indicates that there may be no need for end-capillary or venous reabsorption.[22,32]

A simplified overview of the model of the osmotic endothelial barrier, including the glycocalyx and anatomical ultrastructure, is shown in Figure 92-2.

If one accepts the glycocalyx as the effective molecular barrier and the specific ultrastructure of the intercellular cleft, it becomes clear that the osmotic forces, including the COP, are acting in a more subtle form in a very limited anatomical area than originally assumed.

CONCLUSION

The colloid osmotic pressure of plasma is physiologically generated by plasma proteins, especially by albumin. This pressure counteracts the capillary filtration pressure, is the main force preventing fluid extravasation, and therefore has fundamental importance in the regulation of water flux between the intravascular and interstitial spaces. In contrast to the capillary filtration pressure, the COP can be measured easily in plasma (osmometer). However, as indicated from newer models of the endothelial barrier, the balance of hydraulic and osmotic forces is regulated in more subtle ways. COP is determined not only by the measured COP but also by the interaction of osmotically active colloids with the endothelial surface layer. Because of the given conditions of ultrastructure and the very local balance of outward and inward forces of water flux at the endothelial cleft, net fluid flux is much smaller than predicted by the conventional Starling model.

Although this new model of the capillary barrier describes the physiological conditions, the situation during pathological conditions needs further elucidation. In case of sepsis, traumatic shock, or acute lung injury, in which the endothelial barrier is impaired and permeability is increased, the role of the glycocalyx and local COP has yet to be determined more clearly in further studies. The improved understanding of the ultrastructure of the osmotic barrier might help in the design of more effective infusions for medical applications.

Key Points

1. The colloid osmotic pressure generated by plasma proteins at the endothelial barrier is the only inward force that counterbalances the hydraulic filtration pressure and prevents substantial fluid loss from the intravascular space.
2. Plasma proteins, especially albumin, bind transiently with proteoglycans and other macromolecules of the endothelial glycocalyx and generate a high local colloid osmotic pressure.
3. The endothelial surface layer (endothelial glycocalyx) is the principal molecular barrier that regulates the effective oncotic force for fluid flux across the interendothelial cleft.
4. The effective oncotic force across the capillary wall is determined by the local difference in protein concentration on either side of the endothelial surface layer rather than by the global difference in concentration between plasma and the interstitial fluid of the tissue.
5. The role of the glycocalyx and the changes of the ultrastructure of the microvessels must be elucidated further in humans, especially in the state of shock, trauma, and during general inflammation or sepsis.

Key References

7. Finfer S, Bellomo R, Boyce N, et al: A comparison of albumin and saline for fluid resuscitation in intensive care unit. N Engl J Med 2004;350:2247-2256.
15. Pries AR, Secomb TW, Gaehtgens P: The endothelial surface layer. Pflugers Arch 2000;440:653-666.
16. Jacob M, Bruegger D, Rehm M, et al: Contrasting effects of colloid and crystalloid resuscitation fluids on cardiac vascular permeability. Anesthesiology 2006;104:1223-1231.
24. Nematbakhsh M, Moradi A, Khazaei M, Jafari S: Mathematical model for determination of colloid osmotic pressure: The role of the albumin-globulin ratio. J Research Med Sciences 2006;11:364-369.
32. Hu X, Adamson B, Liu F, et al: Starling forces that oppose filtration after tissue oncotic pressure is increased. Am J Physiol Heart Circ Physiol 2000;279:1724-1736.

See the companion Expert Consult website for the complete reference list.

CHAPTER 93

Blood Biochemistry: Measuring Major Plasma Electrolytes

David A. Story

OBJECTIVES

This chapter will:
1. Outline relevant principles of physical chemistry.
2. Describe the assays used to measure sodium chloride and potassium in blood.
3. Examine the reliability of such assays.

In clinical work, the most commonly measured electrolytes in plasma are sodium, potassium, and chloride. These variables are assessed in their own right and are used to derive other variables, such as tonicity, water balance, anion gap, strong ion difference, and strong ion gap.[1] The plasma concentrations of sodium, potassium, and chloride are measured by ion-specific electrodes[2]—electrodes designed to measure specific ions. Sodium and potassium are positive ions (*cations*), while chloride is a negative ion (*anion*).[3] The results for these electrodes are reported as mmol/L of total plasma, although the electrodes actually measure a different quantity, known as the activity.[3] To understand the fundamentals of these electrodes and some of their shortcomings, one must examine some of the underlying physical chemistry.

Ion-specific electrodes are involved with electrochemical reactions with their designated ions—for this discussion, one of sodium, potassium, or chloride. When an ion interacts with its ion-specific electrode, not all of the ions present can take part. The reason is the interactions between the measured ion and other ions in the solution; in the clinical situation, the solution is plasma.[3] These interactions depend on both the types of other ions present and their concentrations. For example, less sodium interacts with a sodium ion-specific electrode if more chloride is present.[4] This type of interaction results in an effective concentration known as the *activity*. The electrical potential of the ion-specific electrode is directly related to the activity (effective concentration) of the electrolyte rather than to the actual concentration.

For estimating the total plasma concentration of an electrolyte, the first step is to convert the measured activity to the concentration in plasma water.[5] The activity is related to the concentration of the electrolyte by means of the activity coefficient of that electrolyte, as follows:

$$\text{Activity} = \text{Concentration} \times \text{Activity coefficient}$$

The value of the activity coefficient depends on several factors, including the specific ion, the chemistry of the surrounding solution, and the temperature. Clinical assays measure at 37° C. One variable for the activity coefficient is the *ionic strength*, the sum of the charge effects of the electrolytes in the solution. Plasma has particularly complex chemistry with many types of ions, both fully dissociated ions and partly dissociated ions such as phosphate.[6] In addition are other very complex charged molecules, such as albumin.[7] Furthermore, particularly in critical illness, the concentrations of many of these constituents may change. Because of these factors, the variation of activity coefficients for electrolytes in plasma is unclear. The final step in converting the activity to the concentration in total plasma is to account for the proportion of plasma volume that is solid rather than water. The solid phase, usually about 7% of plasma volume, is a combination of lipids and proteins with much of the protein being albumin.[2,3] Therefore 93% of plasma volume is usually water (Fig. 93-1). Unlike calcium and magnesium, sodium, potassium, and chloride do not form significant bonds with plasma proteins.[3,6,8] Therefore, the solid phase is assumed not to contain sodium, potassium, or chloride.[3] It follows that the total plasma concentration of an electrolyte is about 93% of the plasma water concentration.

For example, the measured activity for sodium is 112 (no units). The activity coefficient for sodium in plasma at 37° C is 0.737. The plasma concentration is calculated as follows:

$$\text{Concentration} = \text{Activity} \div \text{Activity coefficient}$$

Therefore, the plasma water concentration is 112 ÷ 0.737, or 150 mmol/L. Multiplying the plasma water concentration by the proportion of plasma that is water (93% × 150 mmol/L) yields the total sodium plasma concentration, 140 mmol/L.

The physicochemical activity of an ion is also the best measure of the biological activity of an ion.[3] Clinical chemists accept, however, that clinicians are unlikely to ever use chemical activities.[2] If possible, clinical chemists would prefer that clinicians use the concentration of an ion in plasma water rather than in total plasma. This is because changes in plasma solids may lead clinicians to misinterpret changes in total plasma concentration for parallel changes in the plasma water concentration. The plasma water concentration of an ion has a stronger rela-

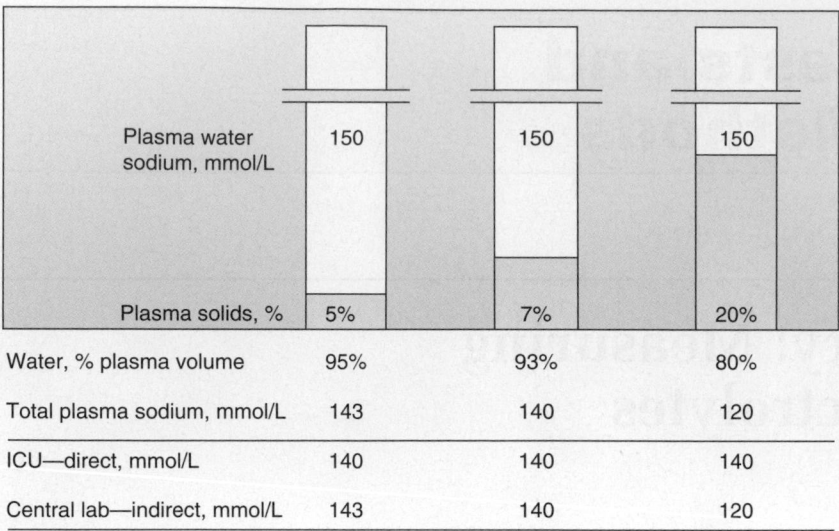

Plasma water sodium, mmol/L	150	150	150
Plasma solids, %	5%	7%	20%
Water, % plasma volume	95%	93%	80%
Total plasma sodium, mmol/L	143	140	120
ICU—direct, mmol/L	140	140	140
Central lab—indirect, mmol/L	143	140	120

FIGURE 93-1. Effect of plasma solids on sodium estimates. ICU, intensive care unit.

tionship to the physiological effect of an ion than the total plasma concentration.[3] Again, clinical chemists recognize that clinicians are unlikely to change from using total plasma concentrations, so the methods used by different assays for determining total plasma concentration are important.

When a blood sample is processed by a blood gas machine such as those in intensive care unit (ICU) laboratories, the software process is identical to the calculations just described.[3] The ion-specific electrodes are known as *direct electrodes* because there is no predilution of the sample. However, central laboratories often use *indirect assays*.[3] The indirect assays use ion-specific electrodes, but before analysis the sample is diluted with a solution with high ionic strength. The high ionic strength means that the activity coefficient for each electrolyte is 1. Therefore the measured activity effectively equals the concentration of the electrolyte (Concentration = Activity/Activity coefficient) in total plasma. The indirect assays use smaller volumes of plasma than direct assays, allowing more assays per sample in multicomponent analyzers and faster automated processing of multiple samples.

For the clinician, it is possible that electrolyte measurements in plasma could be derived from either direct or indirect assays, or both, depending on the equipment used at a given site in a given hospital. Because of differences in the methodology between direct and indirect ion-specific electrodes, the reported electrolyte concentrations in total plasma can differ considerably even with paired samples from the same patient.[9] The desirable and maximum acceptable errors (Table 93-1) in the assays are related to biological variation and instrument error.[10,11]

Morimatsu and colleagues[9] examined the agreement for plasma electrolyte measurements between indirect hospital (central laboratory) assays and direct ICU laboratory blood gas machine (ICU) assays. They found that the limits of agreement for sodium, potassium, and chloride exceeded both the desired and maximum acceptable error limits (see Table 93-1).

One phenomenon associated with the disagreement between direct and indirect sodium assays is pseudohyponatremia.[12] In this situation, increased plasma solids (see Fig. 93-1) lead to a decreased total plasma sodium estimate from the indirect sodium assay (central laboratory) when plasma water sodium is unchanged.[12] This is called pseudohyponatremia because there is hyponatremia without hypotonicity.[11] In contrast, because direct (ICU) assays use a fixed value for plasma solids, the direct assays maintain a fixed relationship with plasma water concentration in the presence of increased plasma solids (see Fig. 93-1). What is little recognized is that decreases in plasma solids should also alter the relationship between the total plasma concentration and plasma water concentration of sodium with indirect assays, leading to possible pseudonormonatremia and pseudohypernatremia.[13] Because of reported morbidity with psuedohyponatremia,[11] much of the published research and commentary has focused on sodium assays, with far less attention on other ion assays.

In a 2007 study, my colleagues and I[1] examined possible causes for these differences between indirect (central laboratory) and direct (ICU laboratory) sodium and chloride assay results. In theory, changes in plasma solids should affect differences between direct and indirect assays for

TABLE 93-1

Plasma Analytes and Measurement Error(s)*

ANALYTE	REFERENCE RANGE[3]	DESIRABLE TOTAL ERROR[10]	MAXIMUM ACCEPTABLE ERROR[11]
Sodium (mmol/L)	136-145	1.3	4
Potassium (mmol/L)	3.5-4.5	0.2	0.5
Chloride (mmol/L)	98-107	1.5	5

*Superscript numbers in column headings indicate chapter references.

sodium and chloride in a similar manner.[3] In line with expectations, we found that as the plasma albumin (a plasma solid) value fell, the direct estimate for sodium was increasingly greater than the direct estimate. Among 300 critically ill patients 13% had pseudonormonatremia and 7% had pseudohypernatremia. Contrary to expectations, the indirect chloride estimate was on average 1 mmol/L *less* than the direct estimate. Further, the difference bore no relationship to changes in albumin or other plasma constituents, including pH, bicarbonate, and lactate. Importantly, changes in albumin are likely to be only one of several causes for the differences between direct and indirect sodium assay results.[1] These findings also highlight the complexity of plasma chemistry and its measurement.

When a clinician assesses plasma chemistry, it is important to know what kind of assay has been used and the reference range for that electrolyte. The frequently used indirect assays for sodium represent plasma water sodium concentration in critically ill patients less reliably than the direct assay. Previously, clinical chemists have recommended that direct assays should be used to measure plasma sodium in patients with increased plasma solids to avoid the risk of pseudohyponatremia.[3,12] This recommendation should be extended to patients with decreased plasma solids so as to avoid the risk of pseudonormonatremia and pseudohypernatremia. In critically ill patients, decreased plasma albumin is almost universal[14,15]; therefore direct sodium assays are preferred for critically ill patients. If only indirect sodium estimates are available, the value can be corrected by subtracting 1.6 mmol/L from the reported sodium value for every 10-g/L decrease in albumin value.[1] The situation for potassium and chloride is less clear, but purely for convenience, the easiest path is to use the direct assay results available with sodium.

Key Points

1. Plasma physical chemistry is complex.
2. Assays measure activities but report concentration in total plasma.
3. Direct and indirect assays can have important differences.
4. Indirect estimates of electrolyte concentrations may be unreliable in the critically ill.
5. Direct assays are preferable to indirect assays.

Key References

1. Story DA, Morimatsu H, Egi M, Bellomo R: The effect of albumin concentration on plasma sodium and chloride measurements in critically ill patients. Anaesth Analg 2007;104:893-897.
3. Scott MG, Klutts JS: Electrolytes and blood gasses. In Burtis CA, Ashwood ER, Bruns DE (eds): Tietz Textbook of Clinical Chemistry and Molecular Diagnostics, 4th ed. Philadelphia, Elsevier, 2005, pp 983-1018.
5. Lewenstam A: Electric potential measured, concentration reported: How to get mmols from mV. Scand J Clin Lab Invest Suppl 1996;224:135-139.
9. Morimatsu H, Rocktaschel J, Bellomo R, et al: Comparison of point-of-care versus central laboratory measurement of electrolyte concentrations on calculations of the anion gap and the strong ion difference. Anesthesiology 2003;98:1077-1084.
12. Weisberg LS: Pseudohyponatremia: A reappraisal. Am J Med 1989;86:315-318.

See the companion Expert Consult website for the complete reference list.

CHAPTER 94

Assessment of Fluid and Electrolyte Problems: Urine Biochemistry

Shane Rowan and Robert J. Anderson

OBJECTIVES

This chapter will:
1. Discuss the use of urinary sodium concentration and fractional excretion of sodium to assess extracellular fluid volume and responsiveness to diuretic agents.
2. Describe the appropriate use of urinary chloride concentration to assess extracellular fluid volume and the cause of metabolic alkalosis.
3. Explain the use of urine osmolality measurements to assess the cause and therapy of water excess and deficiency and the cause of polyuric states.
4. Consider the urine electrolyte–to–plasma electrolyte ratio as a predictive guide to therapy of hyponatremia.

5. Describe the use of urinary potassium concentration and transtubular potassium gradient in the evaluation of hypokalemia and hyperkalemic states.
6. Discuss the interpretation of the urinary anion gap to facilitate the diagnosis of non–anion gap metabolic acidosis.
7. Review the analysis of urinary calcium measurements as a diagnostic aid in hypercalcemic disorders.
8. Discuss use of the fractional excretion of magnesium to determine presence or absence of a renal cause of hypomagnesemia.

The kidney is exquisitely sensitive to alterations of the volume and composition of extracellular fluid and usually responds quickly and appropriately to restore body fluid volume and content to normal. Therefore, analysis of urine electrolyte, acid, and water excretion can provide diagnostically helpful clues in patients in whom body fluid homeostasis is altered. It is important to acknowledge that there are no "normal" values for urinary content of electrolytes and water, only ranges. Thoughtful analysis of urinary electrolyte and water content depends on recognition of the expected renal response to abnormalities of the extracellular fluid volume and composition. This chapter reviews the use of urinary indices of electrolyte, water, and acid excretion in disorders of fluid and electrolyte balance encountered in the intensive care unit.

URINARY SODIUM AND CHLORIDE CONCENTRATIONS AND FRACTIONAL EXCRETION OF SODIUM TO ASSESS EXTRACELLULAR FLUID VOLUME STATUS AND RESPONSE TO DIURETICS

The kidney responds to actual or perceived decreases in circulating volume by quickly enhancing tubular sodium and chloride reabsorption in an effort to restore circulating volume.[1-8] This response results in relatively low (less than 30 mEq/L and usually less than 20 mEq/L) concentrations of sodium and chloride in single or "spot" urine samples. Although the concentrations of urine sodium and chloride usually fall in parallel, a significant percentage of patients with extracellular fluid volume depletion show a "disparity" between urine sodium and chloride concentrations. This finding can be due to the presence of anion such as bicarbonate in cases of metabolic alkalosis, in which excretion of sodium bicarbonate results in a relatively high urinary sodium concentration and low urine chloride concentration despite extracellular fluid volume depletion. Conversely, the presence of a cation can be associated with a rise in urine chloride concentration despite extracellular fluid volume depletion. For example, in patients with diarrhea and metabolic acidosis, urinary excretion of ammonium chloride can lead to a relatively high urine chloride concentration despite volume depletion. In this case, the urine sodium concentration is low. In a patient who appears to be volume depleted but in whom a spot urine sodium concentration is relatively high, measurement of a spot urine chloride concentration can be helpful.

Fractional excretion of sodium (FENa) is calculated as follows:

$$FENa = \frac{(U_{Na}/P_{Na})}{(U_{Cr}/P_{Cr})} \times 100$$

where U_{Na} is urine sodium concentration, P_{Na} is plasma sodium concentration, U_{Cr} is urine creatinine concentration, and P_{Cr} is plasma creatinine concentration. An FENa value significantly less than 1.0% almost always indicates avid tubular sodium reabsorption and decreased renal perfusion. The FENa value may be more sensitive than the spot urinary sodium value in determining the presence of volume depletion. Spot urine sodium and chloride determinations and FENa values can be especially useful for

TABLE 94-1

Conditions of Extracellular Fluid Volume Depletion That May Be Associated with a High Spot Urine Sodium Concentration

Glycosuria
Recent diuretic use
Bicarbonaturia (urine pH > 7)
Primary adrenal insufficiency
Chronic kidney disease (usually tubulointerstitial in nature)
Nonoliguric acute kidney failure

assessing renal perfusion in acute renal failure and extracellular fluid volume in hyponatremic states.

There are two caveats about the clinical use of spot urine sodium and chloride determinations and FENa calculation to assess the status of the extracellular volume. First, a low urine sodium or chloride concentration or low FENa value does not differentiate between extracellular fluid loss/sequestration (e.g., gastrointestinal loss, pancreatitis, muscle crush injury, early sepsis) and decreased effective circulating volume (e.g., congestive heart failure, cirrhosis, marked hypoalbuminemia). The disorders of decreased effective circulating volume are accompanied by edema and other clinical manifestations of the primary disorder. Second, the kidney may be the source of sodium chloride loss and, thus, diminished extracellular fluid volume. In these cases, spot urine sodium and chloride determinations may be high despite volume depletion (Table 94-1).

In some patients with edematous states and refractoriness to diuretic therapy, analysis of urinary excretion of sodium and potassium may be helpful.[6-8] In diuretic-resistant patients, the presence of concomitant low spot urine sodium and potassium concentrations (<10 mEq/L) predicts no diuretic response to adding a distally acting diuretic agent (e.g., spironolactone, eplerenone, amiloride) to more proximally acting agents (e.g., loop diuretics), because delivery of sodium to the distal sodium-potassium exchange site is not sufficient for an additive diuretic effect. Conversely, if the spot urine concentration of sodium is low (<10 mEq/L) and that of potassium high (>30 mEq/L), sodium is being exchanged for potassium distally, and an agent that acts on distal tubules would be effective. As a goal of diuretic therapy in edematous patients with cirrhosis, daily elimination of more than 78 mEq of sodium is desirable. A ratio of spot urine sodium to spot potassium determination greater than 1 predicts excretion of more than 78 mEq/day of sodium.[8]

URINE CHLORIDE IN METABOLIC ALKALOSIS

Most forms of metabolic alkalosis are responsive to sodium chloride and are associated with a low spot urine chloride concentration (<25 mEq/L).[9] There are less common causes of metabolic alkalosis (primary aldosteronism, adrenocorticotropic hormone–producing tumors, profound hypokalemia, unusual syndromes like Bartter's and Gitelman's) that are not corrected by sodium chloride therapy. These non–sodium chloride–responsive forms of metabolic alkalosis are characterized by relatively high urinary chloride concentrations (>40 mEq/L).

URINE OSMOLALITY AND URINE ELECTROLYTE–TO–PLASMA ELECTROLYTE RATIO IN DISORDERS OF WATER BALANCE AND POLYURIC STATES

Positive water balance (intake/input in excess of elimination) results in hyponatremia, and negative water balance (intake/input less than elimination) in hypernatremia. The kidney is usually the primary source of water elimination from the body. The presence of normal glomerular filtration rate, normal delivery of tubular fluid to the distal nephron, and normal suppression of antidiuretic hormone allows elimination of substantial amounts of water. Conversely, the presence of a hypertonic renal medulla and antidiuretic hormone allows for maximal water conservation.[1,4]

Renal water elimination can be grossly estimated from the concentration of the urine, which is most precisely determined by measurement of urine osmolality. A measure of the number of osmotically active articles in the urine, urine osmolality ranges from 50 mOsm/kg (maximally dilute) to about 1200 mOsm/kg (maximally concentrated). When urine osmolality is less than plasma osmolality, some free water is being eliminated by the kidney. When urine osmolality exceeds plasma osmolality, water is being retained. Urine specific gravity is a measure of not only the number but also the size of the particles in the urine. Although urine osmolality and urine specific gravity are generally correlated (specific gravity value of 0.001 is approximately equal to urine osmolality of 40 mOsm/kg), specific gravity can be disproportionately high when large particles (e.g., radiocontrast agents, glucose) are present.

Measurement of urine osmolality can be diagnostically helpful in three conditions. First, in hypernatremic patients, a urine-to-plasma osmolality ratio less than 1 suggests central diabetes insipidus as a cause of the water deficit. Second, polyuria (>3 L of urine per day) can be due to either a water diuresis or a solute diuresis. If the urine osmolality is less than 200 mOsm/kg, a water diuresis is present and the patient most likely has polydipsia, has received excess free water, or has central diabetes insipidus. If the urine osmolality is greater than 300 mOsm/kg, a solute diuresis is operative, and the presence of glucosuria, mannitol, other osmotic agents and diuretics should be sought. Occasionally, a patient with these findings could have nephrogenic diabetes insipidus. Third, in hyponatremic patients, a urine osmolality between 100 and 150 mOsm/kg suggests either primary polydipsia (in which massive ingestion of water temporarily overwhelms the kidney's ability to excrete the water) or beer-drinker's potomania (which can also be seen in malnourished patients in whom dietary solute intake and excretion is so low that renal water excretion is impaired even though urinary diluting mechanisms are intact). The urine osmolality may also be relatively low if it is measured after the cause of hyponatremia has been reversed and renal water elimination has begun to correct it. The urine osmolality in most hyponatremic states is greater than the plasma osmolality and usually ranges between 300 and 600 mOsm/kg. The magnitude of increase has no diagnostic value.

In the treatment of hyponatremia, inducing negative water balance is the goal. Urine volume and urine osmolality are often poor predictors of the amount of free water

the kidney is eliminating.[10-12] A better bedside estimate of renal free water clearance can be determined from the urine electrolyte–to–plasma electrolyte ratio, as follows:

$$\frac{U_{Na} + U_K}{P_{Na} + P_K}$$

where U_K is urine potassium concentration and P_K is plasma potassium concentration. When this ratio is greater than 1, no free water is being eliminated by the kidney, and water restriction of the hyponatremic patient will not raise the plasma sodium concentration. When this ratio is less than 0.5, significant free water clearance is occurring, and restriction of water intake to 500 to 750 mL/day would increase plasma sodium concentration.[10-12]

URINARY POTASSIUM CONCENTRATION AND THE TRANSTUBULAR POTASSIUM GRADIENT IN HYPOKALEMIC AND HYPERKALEMIC STATES

In many patients with disorders of serum potassium concentration, the cause is readily apparent from review of the clinical course and medication list. In patients with hypokalemia, the kidney attempts to conserve potassium by enhancing tubular potassium reabsorption. Thus, a renal cause of hypokalemia (e.g., diuretics, enhanced aldosterone action, renal tubular acidosis, hypomagnesemia) is suggested by (1) a urine potassium concentration higher than 15 to 20 mEq/L, (2) a 24-hour urine potassium excretion greater than 15 mEq/L, or (3) a ratio of spot urine potassium determination (mEq/L) to spot urine creatinine concentration determination (mmol) greater than 1. Conversely, in the setting of hypokalemia, a spot urine potassium of less than 15 to 20 mEq/L suggests a nonrenal source of potassium loss.[13-15]

Calculation of the transtubular potassium gradient (TTKG) may be diagnostically helpful in some cases of hyperkalemia and, sometimes, of hypokalemia. The TTKG provides a quantitative approximation of the potassium secretory process in the distal nephron. It is calculated as follows:

$$TTKG = \frac{[U_k/(U_{Osm}/P_{Osm})]}{P_k}$$

where U_{Osm} is urine osmolality and P_{Osm} is plasma osmolality. The TTKG value varies in normal individuals between 6 and 12. In hypokalemic patients, nonrenal causes of potassium depletion are associated with a TTKG usually less than 3. If a value higher than 3 is seen in a hypokalemic patient, a renal source of potassium depletion is likely. In hyperkalemic states, the TTKG would be anticipated to be greater than 10, and certainly greater than 7. Causes of an inappropriately low TTKG in hyperkalemia include use of potassium-sparing diuretics, aldosterone deficiency, tubular resistance to aldosterone, and use of drugs that can block sodium channels (trimethoprim, pentamidine). Either measurement of plasma aldosterone or assessment of the response of TTKG to exogenous aldosterone is necessary to determine whether either aldosterone deficiency or end-organ nonresponsiveness is operational. Sometimes hyperkalemia can be due to

TABLE 94-2

Transtubular Potassium Gradient (TTKG) in Hyperkalemic and Hypokalemic Disorders

TYPE OF DISORDER	TTKG VALUE	CAUSE(S)

Hyperkalemia	<7	Potassium-sparing diuretics
		Aldosterone deficiency
		Tubular unresponsiveness to aldosterone
		Medications that block sodium channels:
		  Trimethoprim
		  Pentamidine

	>7	Marked volume depletion or marked effective volume depletion
Hypokalemia	<3	Gastrointestinal loss of potassium
	>3	Hyperaldosteronism Diuretics

marked extracellular volume depletion and impaired delivery of sodium to the distal sodium-potassium exchange site. In this setting, the TTKG is usually higher than 7 (Table 94-2).

URINE ANION GAP IN HYPERCHLOREMIC METABOLIC ACIDOSIS

A non–anion gap metabolic acidosis is usually due to loss of base from the bowel (diarrhea) or kidney (renal tubular acidosis) or from a gain of mineral acid (hydrochloric acid). Often, the cause is apparent from the clinical setting. Sometimes it is useful to calculate the urine anion gap (urine sodium and potassium concentrations minus urine chloride concentration) in defining the cause of non–anion gap metabolic acidosis; the calculation is as follows:

$$\text{Urine anion gap} = (U_{Na} + U_K) - U_{Cl}$$

where U_{Cl} is urine chloride concentration. With metabolic acidosis, the kidney excretes acid in the form of ammonium (NH_4^+). When this occurs, the urine anion gap becomes negative (average of −20) because urine chloride excretion increases to maintain electroneutrality as NH_4Cl is eliminated in the urine and exceeds the urine sodium plus potassium concentration (negative urine anion gap). With renal tubular acidosis, low levels of urine acid excretion occur, and the urine anion gap remains positive (average 20-30).[16]

URINE CALCIUM IN HYPERCALCEMIC DISORDERS

Urine calcium excretion is most commonly assessed to evaluate an individual with kidney stones. In the intensive care setting, evaluation of urine calcium excretion is less frequently performed. In patients with hypercalcemia, measurement of urine calcium may be done to help determine the cause. Many causes of hypercalcemia are associated with hypercalciuria. Typically, hypercalcemia without hypercalciuria is seen with familial hypocalciuric hypercalcemia, with use of thiazide diuretics, and in the milk-alkali syndrome. Screening test results for hypercalciuria are (1) spot urine calcium concentration–to–urine osmolality ratio of 0.14 mg/L/mOsm/kg or greater and (2) a urine calcium–to–urine creatinine ratio of 0.18 mg/mg or greater. A 24-hour urine with a calcium concentration more than 4 mg/kg also represents hypercalciuria.[17]

URINE MAGNESIUM IN HYPOMAGNESEMIA

Hypomagnesemia can be due to nutritional deficiency, gastrointestinal losses, renal loss, and multiple other factors (chronic alcohol ingestion). Often, hypomagnesemia comes to the attention of the clinician because of the associated renal potassium wasting with hypokalemia or because of the presence of hypocalcemia due to impaired parathyroid hormone secretion and effect. The fractional excretion of magnesium (FEMg) is calculated as follows:

$$FEMg = \frac{(U_{Mg} \times P_{Cr}) \times 100}{0.7 \times P_{Mg} \times U_{Cr}}$$

where U_{Mg} is urine magnesium concentration and P_{Mg} is plasma magnesium concentration. In hypomagnesemia due to nonrenal loss or nutritional deficiency, the fractional excretion of magnesium is less than 4%, whereas renal losses are associated with FEMg values higher than 4%.[18]

Key Points

1. The kidney is sensitive to alterations in body fluid volume and composition and reacts appropriately to restore body fluid and composition to normal. Therefore, examination of the urinary excretion of electrolytes and water can be diagnostically helpful in states of altered body fluid volume and composition.
2. The finding of low spot urinary sodium and chloride concentrations (<15-20 mEq/L) and low fractional excretion of sodium (<1.0%) indicates either extracellular fluid volume loss/sequestration or a decrease in effective extracellular fluid volume, as is commonly seen in edematous disorders.
3. Relatively low values for spot urinary sodium concentration and fractional excretion of sodium in the setting of an abrupt decline in renal function suggest diminished kidney perfusion with intact renal tubular function and potentially reversible renal failure. Conversely, relatively high values for these measurements in the setting of an abrupt decline in kidney function suggests impaired tubular function and the possibility of more prolonged renal failure with tubular necrosis.

4. Urine osmolality measurements can be diagnostically helpful in cases of abnormal plasma sodium concentration and polyuric states. In hyponatremia, a urine osmolality less than 200 mOsm/kg suggests psychogenic polydipsia, beer-drinker's potomania, or spontaneous correction of the cause of hyponatremia. In hypernatremia, a urine osmolality–to–plasma osmolality ratio less than 1 suggests central diabetes insipidus as the cause of the water deficit. In polyuric states, a urine osmolality value lower than 200 mOsm/kg suggests polydipsia or central diabetes mellitus, whereas a urine osmolality value greater than 300 mOsm/kg suggests solute diuresis.

5. Measurement of the urinary excretion of potassium and calculation of the transtubular potassium gradient can be diagnostically helpful in determining the cause of hypokalemia and hyperkalemic disorders.

Key References

1. Miller TR, Anderson RJ, Linas SL, et al: Urinary diagnostic indices in acute renal failure. Ann Intern Med 1978;89:47-50.
3. Sherman RA, Eisinger RP: The use and misuse of urinary sodium and chloride measurements. JAMA 1982;247:3121-4124.
8. Steihm AJ, Mendler MH, Runyon BA: Detection of diuretic-resistance or diuretic sensitivity by the spot urine Na/K ratio in 729 specimens from cirrhotics with ascites: Approximately 90% accuracy as compared to 24 hour urine excretion. Hepatology 2002;36:222A.
10. Rose BD: New approach to disturbances in the plasma sodium concentration. Am J Med 1986;81:1033-1041.
15. Joo KW, Chang SH, Lee JG, et al: Transtubular potassium concentration gradient (TTKG) and urine ammonium in differential diagnosis of hypokalemia. J Nephrol 2000;13:120-125.

See the companion Expert Consult website for the complete reference list.

CHAPTER 95

Assessment of Volume Status

Miet Schetz

OBJECTIVES

This chapter will:
1. Discuss the importance of volume assessment in critically ill patients.
2. Clarify the difference between preload and preload responsiveness.
3. Describe the limitations of static preload parameters.
4. Explain the physiological basis and clinical use of dynamic preload parameters (parameters of fluid responsiveness).

Many disease states encountered in the intensive care unit are associated with a decreased effective blood volume that, alone or in conjunction with other factors, has the potential to jeopardize tissue perfusion and accelerate the risk of multiple-organ failure. Bedside assessment of volume status is perhaps one of the most difficult clinical problems in critical care medicine. Hypovolemia can be *absolute* (external or internal losses of circulating volume) or *relative* (diminished peripheral vascular resistance with pooling of blood in peripheral regions). This distributive form of circulatory failure is seen in sepsis and liver failure or may be caused by drugs. Appropriate and, most importantly, timely resuscitation of critically ill patients, including adequate fluid replacement, can improve outcome.[1,2]

Maintaining volume status is not a purpose in itself. The aims of fluid management are to preserve adequate blood pressure and tissue perfusion ("goal-directed"). Hence, any sign of tissue hypoperfusion, however subtle, should

prompt an assessment of volume status to determine whether fluids are a treatment option. These signs of tissue hypoperfusion may be clinically overt, such as low blood pressure, vasopressor requirement, tachycardia, oliguria, mottled skin, slow capillary refill, or central-peripheral temperature gradients, or may require more invasive monitoring, such as low cardiac output (CO), low mixed venous oxygen saturation (SvO_2), high arteriovenous CO_2 gradient, increased lactate level or base excess, high gastric or sublingual CO_2 (gastric or sublingual tonometry), impaired microcirculation (orthogonal polarization spectral imaging), or impaired local tissue oxygenation (near-infrared spectroscopy)). A further discussion of these parameters of tissue perfusion is beyond the scope of this chapter; see reviews by Ward and colleagues[3] and Gunn and associates.[4]

It is obvious that hypotension, tachycardia, oliguria, mental confusion, and poor peripheral perfusion in the setting of acute blood or fluid loss or in early sepsis will prompt fluid administration. In patients with such problems, no sophisticated parameters are needed. Far more difficult is to define at which point further fluid administration becomes useless or even dangerous. In addition, outside the setting of resuscitation of overt decompensated hypovolemia, many critically ill patients have persistent signs of tissue hypoperfusion that may or may not be remedied by further volume expansion. The recognition of this covert compensated hypovolemia is far more difficult, as its clinical signs lack both sensitivity and specificity.[5-7] Physicians therefore often have to rely on more sophisticated and/or invasive methods to detect hypovolemia in critically ill patients. The detection of volume overload and avoidance of unnecessary volume replacement are equally important to prevent the development of pulmonary edema, RV overload, intra-abdominal hypertension, and fluid overload in general that are associated with increased morbidity and mortality.[8-12] This chapter focuses mainly on the assessment of hypovolemia and fluid overload in the critical care setting. Methods for the assessment of fluid status in patients undergoing long-term dialysis are not discussed.

PRELOAD VERSUS PRELOAD RESPONSIVENESS

According to the Frank-Starling principle, for a given level of contractile function, the greater the heart muscle is stretched, the greater the force of cardiac contraction and the greater the quantity of blood pumped into the aorta. This presystolic fiber stretch, or ventricular wall stress at end diastole, is called *preload* and is determined by end-diastolic volume, end-diastolic pressure, and wall thickness. Although we do not have a true gold standard for preload estimation, the left ventricular end-diastolic volume (LVEDV) is often regarded as the clinical gold standard. The Frank-Starling curve, plotting stroke volume (SV) or CO against LVEDV, reaches a plateau level expressing the maximal amount of venous return a heart can pump (Fig. 95-1). It is evident that in patients with reduced myocardial contractility, this plateau is reached at lower SVs.[13,14]

The literature on preload assessment contains two types of studies that answer two different questions. The first question is What is the preload of my patient, or, otherwise stated, how can I measure the end-diastolic ventricular filling in my patient? These studies evaluate *static preload parameters*. The second, and clinically more relevant, question is How can I detect whether my patient's fluid status is on the ascending limb of the Starling curve, so that fluid administration can improve SV or CO (and thus tissue perfusion)—or in other words, whether my patient is preload-dependent or fluid-responsive?[15,16] This question can be answered by *dynamic preload parameters* that allow prediction of a patient's response to fluid administration, thus avoiding needless or even deleterious volume expansion. The importance of these predictive parameters is illustrated by the fact that only about 50% of critically ill patients with suspected hypovolemia actually show favorable response to fluid administration.[17]

It should be emphasized that preload and preload dependence or fluid responsiveness are two different physiological entities and that dynamic preload parameters predict the response to volume expansion, not whether the patient actually needs fluids. The actual need for fluid should be determined on the basis of a set of clinical and other criteria, reflecting the adequacy of tissue perfusion.[18] In addition, determining that the patient is preload-responsive does not always mean that giving fluids is the right approach. In some patients, another treatment option might be more appropriate, such as the administration of low-dose norepinephrine for a patient with vasodilatory shock.

STATIC PRELOAD PARAMETERS

The validity of static preload parameters can be assessed by their correlation with end-diastolic volume (not easy to measure), SV, or CO. It is evident that the latter correlation exists only in fluid-responsive patients whose fluid status is on the ascending portion of the Starling curve. In addition, different levels of ventricular function result in different slopes, which might obscure this correlation in a heterogeneous group of patients or if too much time elapses between two measurements in the same patient.

Filling Pressures

Filling pressures—central venous pressure (CVP) and pulmonary artery occlusion pressure—are the most popular surrogate markers of preload. CVP, determined by the interaction of cardiac function and venous return, reflects both the filling pressure of the right ventricle and the back-pressure to venous return.[19] Pulmonary artery occlusion pressure, obtained after inflation of the distal balloon of a pulmonary artery catheter, is thought to reflect the LV end-diastolic pressure, although high alveolar pressures, pulmonary venous obstruction, and mitral valve abnormalities may disturb this relationship.[20-22]

Filling pressures show a poor correlation with LVEDV, SV, and CO in normal subjects[23] as well as in critically ill patients.[24-27] This can be explained by the curvilinear, often abnormal and changing ventricular compliance and by the effect of changes in intrathoracic or pericardial pressure (Fig. 95-2).[19-22] Indeed, the clinically measured pressure is the intracavitary pressure, whereas the true filling pressure is the transmural pressure, or the difference between the intracavitary and extracavitary pressures. This situation complicates the interpretation of filling pressure values in patients undergoing positive-pressure or positive end-expiratory pressure (PEEP) ventilation, especially because the transmission of airway pressure to the pleural space depends on both lung and

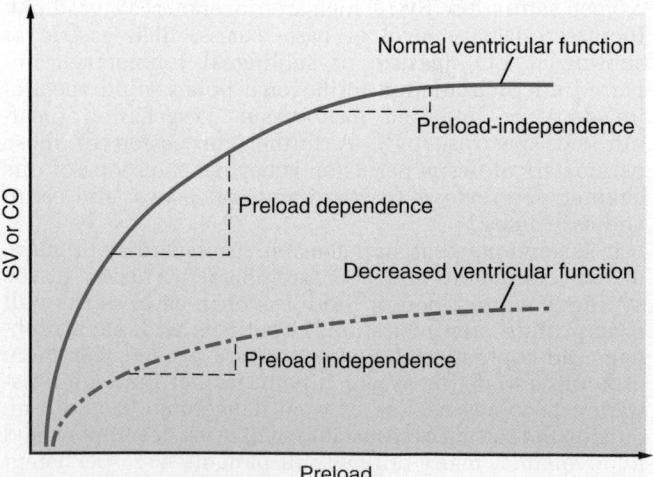

FIGURE 95-1. The Starling curve, relating preload to stroke volume (SV) or cardiac output (CO), reaches a plateau that, in patients with decreased ventricular function, is situated at a lower level of SV or CO. If the ventricle is operating on the steep portion of the curve, a given increase in preload is associated with an increase in SV or CO (preload dependence). If the ventricle operates on the plateau, such an increase is not observed (preload independence).

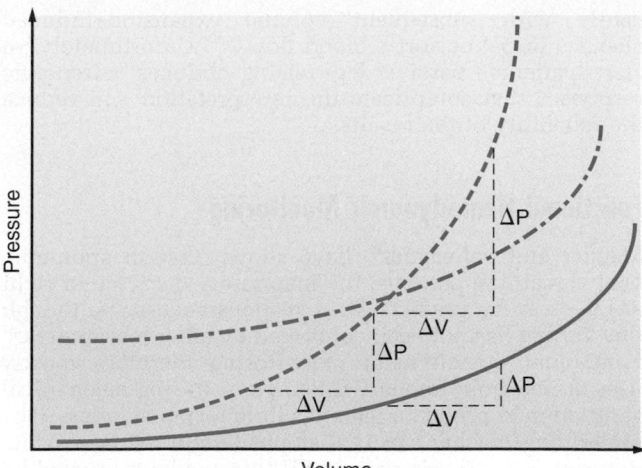

FIGURE 95-2. Different diastolic pressure-volume curves (compliance curves) for the left ventricle, indicating how the same change in left ventricular end-diastolic volume (ΔV) may cause different changes in end-diastolic pressure (ΔP). An increase in intrathoracic or pericardial pressure causes an upward shift of the compliance curve. *Solid line* indicates normal compliance, *dashed line* indicates decreased compliance, and *dash-dotted line* indicates increased intrathoracic or pericardial pressure.

chest wall compliance. An increased intra-abdominal pressure may also result in falsely elevated filling pressure values.[28] In addition, the measurement and interpretation of both the CVP[19] and the pulmonary artery pressure tracings[21] appear to be susceptible to error and interobserver variability. A 2006 Cochrane review showed no benefit from the use of the pulmonary artery catheter in high-risk surgical or intensive care unit patients,[29] and similar results were obtained in patients with acute respiratory distress syndrome.[30]

Despite this poor performance, CVP and pulmonary artery occlusion pressure are commonly used, and guidelines for the hemodynamic management of critically ill patients continue to promote the inclusion of filling pressures in treatment algorithms.[31,32] A randomized trial comparing different fluid management strategies in patients with acute lung injury also included filling pressure in the algorithms,[33] and the algorithm of the early goal-directed therapy for the treatment of sepsis included the CVP.[1] Indeed, filling pressure measurements are not completely useless. The chance that a patient's fluid status is on the ascending limb of the Frank-Starling curve is much higher with low filling pressures than with high filling pressures. Only intermediate readings give very little useful information. In addition, filling pressures are safety factors and are more important than volume if the major concern is the development of pulmonary edema.[32] The threshold pressure above which interstitial and, ultimately, alveolar edema occurs depends on the other determinants of the Starling equation and is lower in patients with increased capillary permeability. In this regard, it is important to realize that the hydrostatic force driving fluid out of the pulmonary capillaries into the interstitium is not the pulmonary artery occlusion pressure but the pulmonary capillary pressure, the difference between the two depending on postcapillary venous resistance and CO. Pulmonary capillary pressure can be determined by analyzing a pressure tracing after an acute pulmonary artery occlusion with the balloon of a Swan-Ganz catheter.[21,34]

Volumetric Preload Parameters

Several volumetric preload parameters show a better correlation with changes in SV or CO than filling pressures; they are right ventricular end-diastolic volume (RVEDV) measured with a pulmonary artery catheter equipped with a fast thermistor,[25-27] LV end-diastolic area (LVEDA) measured with echocardiography,[23,35-37] and global end-diastolic volume (GEDV) or intrathoracic blood volume (ITBV) measured with transpulmonary thermodilution.[38-41]

RVEDV might become a poor reflector of LV preload when the RV is the limiting factor in circulatory failure and can be erroneous in the case of tricuspid insufficiency. Although echocardiography can provide an excellent estimate of preload and LVEDA is considered the gold standard, this technique is limited by problems such as costs, patient discomfort, the requirements for a high level of operator training and skill, and the inability to monitor many patients simultaneously or one patient for a long period.

In addition to volumetric preload assessment, transpulmonary thermodilution allows one to determine extravascular lung water, which might be of special value in the fluid management of patients with systemic inflammatory response syndrome or acute respiratory failure. Although transpulmonary thermodilution overestimates extravascular lung water,[42] is influenced by changes in perfusion and ventilation,[43] and shows a moderate correlation with clinical parameters such as oxygenation and lung compliance,[44,45] it might be useful to monitor changes in extravascular lung water over time and, when used to direct therapy, might improve outcome.[46] However, the experience with this method is still limited, and further studies are required.

Other Static Preload Parameters
Radiographic Measurement of Preload

Vascular pedicle width and other radiographic features, such as the cardiothoracic ratio,[47] are undoubtedly useful to distinguish cardiogenic edema or volume overload from noncardiogenic pulmonary edema but can hardly be used as monitoring tools during fluid resuscitation.

Bioimpedance

Bioelectrical impedance analysis (BIA) is a noninvasive method based on the electrical current conductance properties of tissues. It has been used to detect perioperative fluid accumulation and appears to be better than daily fluid balances at detecting changes in body weight.[48,49] Thoracic BIA has proved useful for early identification of an increase in lung water in patients at risk for pulmonary edema[50,51] and may detect pulmonary fluid not apparent on a chest radiograph.[52] However, the clinical application of BIA in intensive care medicine is still limited, and its place remains to be established.

Hormones

B-type natriuretic peptide (BNP) and its amino-terminal prohormone (NT-proBNP), in contrast to what their names would suggest, are synthesized and stored primarily by the ventricular myocardium. BNP is released in response to myocyte stretch, so its measurement could be useful in identifying systolic dysfunction or volume overload. In the emergency department, BNP values may distinguish heart failure from other causes of dyspnea[53] and transfusion-related acute lung injury from transfusion-associated circulatory overload.[54] In critically ill patients, BNP and NT-proBNP appear to be more markers of (systolic) myocardial dysfunction than of volume status, and because of multiple confounding factors, the correlation of BNP value with filling pressures is often poor.[55-58] A small study in cardiac surgery patients showed no difference in BNP levels between patients who did and those who did not respond to a volume load.[59]

DYNAMIC PRELOAD ASSESSMENT EQUALS FLUID RESPONSIVENESS

No matter how exactly we can measure LVEDV, static preload parameters remain of limited clinical value. Starling curves vary so considerably among patients that a given preload may be associated with a positive response to fluid challenge (preload dependency) or with no response (preload independency). Indeed, several clinical studies could not find a threshold value for static preload parameters that can be used to predict fluid responsiveness.[17,60,61] The three methods of evaluating a patient's fluid responsiveness are exogenous fluid administration (fluid challenge), endogenous fluid administration (passive leg raising), and functional hemodynamic monitoring that takes advantage of heart-lung interactions during mechanical ventilation.

Fluid Challenge

The oldest and most widely used approach to test a patient's fluid responsiveness (and still considered the gold standard) is the administration of a fluid challenge, already suggested by Baek and associates[62] in 1975 and later "revisited" in 2006.[63] It consists of the administration of a defined amount of fluid within a defined interval and evaluation of its effect on CO or a surrogate of tissue perfusion adequacy while the patient is monitored for potential fluid overload. In general, there is little consensus about how much fluid should be given, how fast it should be administered, when the effect should be measured, and how much effect is significant. Although simple and attractive at first sight, and certainly advisable in a patient who has sufficient cardiopulmonary reserve capacity, this fluid challenge approach remains a retrospective evaluation that may lead to inappropriate volume expansion in an unresponsive patient. In other words, the fluid challenge approach is least useful and safe in the most vulnerable patients.

Passive Leg Raising

An alternative method for detecting fluid responsiveness without actually administering fluid is passive leg raising. When the patient's legs are raised by care providers, a transient and readily reversible "self-fluid challenge" occurs from the capacitance veins of the legs. Changes in arterial pulse pressure or in aortic blood flow induced by passive leg raising have been shown to correlate signifi-

cantly with subsequent volume expansion–induced changes in SV or aortic blood flow.[64,65] Unfortunately, in alert patients, passive leg raising induces adrenergic responses that complicate the interpretation and reduce the reliability of the results.

Functional Hemodynamic Monitoring

Magder and colleagues[66] have shown that in spontaneously breathing patients, the inspiratory decrease in right atrial pressure predicts fluid responsiveness,[66] although this finding has not been confirmed by other researchers.[67] Functional hemodynamic monitoring therefore mostly uses the cardiopulmonary interactions during mechanical ventilation to predict a patient's fluid responsiveness. The underlying mechanism is that positive-pressure ventilation causes cyclic changes in SV that can be evaluated by direct measurement of SV or measurement of one of its surrogates—systolic blood pressure, pulse pressure (PP) (systolic minus diastolic pressure), or aortic blood flow. These changes, which can be quantified in absolute or relative terms, are minimal in hypervolemic conditions and are exaggerated in the presence of hypovolemia, so they can be used as indicators of fluid responsiveness.

Correct interpretation of dynamic preload parameters requires an understanding of the underlying mechanisms (Figs. 95-3 and 95-4).[68-70] The mechanical ventilation–induced changes in SV have "delta down" (ΔDown) and "delta up" (ΔUp) components. The ΔDown component relates to the inspiratory increase in pleural pressure that reduces venous return because of an increase in right atrial pressure and compression of the vena cava. If the RV operates on the steep part of the Starling curve, the early

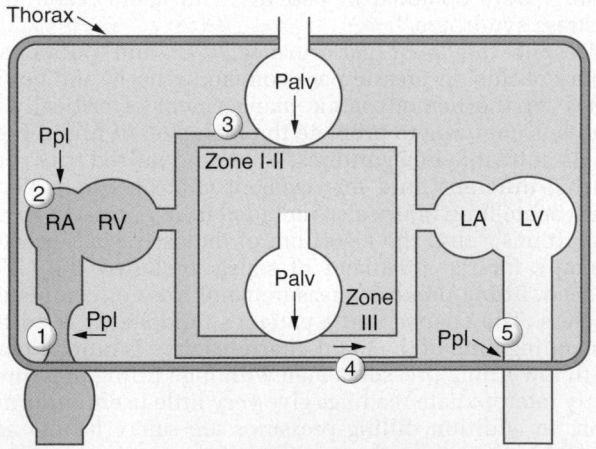

FIGURE 95-3. Physiological effects of mechanical ventilation in hypovolemic conditions. Right ventricular (RV) preload decreases because the increase in pleural pressure (Ppl) induces a compression of the superior vena cava (1) and an increase in intramural right atrial (RA) pressure (2), but the transmural RA pressure decreases. In West zones I (pulmonary artery pressure < alveolar pressure) and II (pulmonary venous pressure < alveolar pressure), RV afterload increases because pulmonary capillaries are compressed (3). In West zone III (alveolar pressure < pulmonary venous pressure), the increase in alveolar pressure (Palv) squeezes out the blood contained in the capillaries toward the left side of the heart (4). The increase in Ppl induces a decrease in left ventricular (LV) afterload (5). LA, left atrium. (Redrawn from Michard F: Changes in arterial pressure during mechanical ventilation. Anesthesiology 2005;103:419-428.)

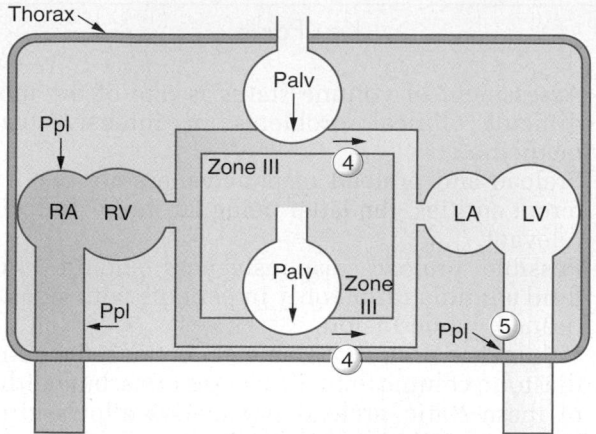

FIGURE 95-4. Physiological effects of mechanical ventilation in hypervolemic conditions. The vena cava and right atrium (RA) are poorly compliant and poorly compressible, so they are relatively insensitive to changes in pleural pressure (Ppl). West zones III (alveolar pressure < pulmonary venous pressure) are predominant in the lungs such that each mechanical breath increases pulmonary venous flow and left ventricular (LV) preload (4). The increase in pleural pressure (Ppl) induces a decrease in LV afterload (5). LA, left atrium; Palv, alveolar pressure. RV, right ventricle. (Redrawn from Michard F: Changes in arterial pressure during mechanical ventilation. Anesthesiology 2005;103:419-428.)

inspiratory decrease in preload is accompanied by a decrease in RVSV, in turn causing a late inspiratory or early expiratory decrease in LV preload. If the left LV also operates on the ascending limb of the Starling curve, cyclic changes in LVSV will result. Both ventricles need to be preload responsive for this ΔDown component to be observed. The steeper the slope of the Starling curve, the more pronounced is the ΔDown of the SV. On the other hand, the disappearance of the ΔDown component is a sign of LV failure. An alternative explanation for the ΔDown is a transient increase in RV afterload, which in patients with RV dysfunction impairs RV output and, thus, LV preload. The ΔUp is explained by an early inspiratory squeezing of pulmonary vessels, which, depending on the predominating zone conditions in the lung, increases (in hypervolemic patients) or decreases (in hypovolemic patients) pulmonary venous flow and, thus, LV preload. An alternative physiological mechanism underlying the early inspiratory increase of LVSV is a transient reduction in afterload due to the direct compression of the heart and a decreased transmural aortic diastolic pressure. In other words, a large ΔUp rather reflects hypervolemia and LV failure.

SV variation can be measured with arterial pulse contour analysis (computation of the area under the systolic portion of the arterial pressure curve), transesophageal echocardiography, or an esophageal Doppler probe. When direct measurement of SV variation is not possible, one of its surrogates—systolic pressure variation (SPV) or pulse pressure variation—can be used, provided that arterial compliance remains constant over one respiration. The ΔDown component of SPV, which is more preload-dependent than SPV itself, is the difference between the minimal value and the value found during a short apnea or end-expiratory pause (Fig. 95-5). In contrast to pulse pressure variation, SPV is influenced by intrathoracic pressure-induced changes in both systolic and diastolic pressures. Theoretically, therefore, SV variation is more reliable than pulse pressure variation, which in turn is more reliable than ΔDown SPV.[70]

The investigations evaluating functional hemodynamic monitoring relate the baseline values and the changes in the investigated parameters to the extent of blood loss or to the changes in CO or SV induced by volume expansion. Other studies, in addition, compare the baseline parameters in patients who do respond (defined as showing 5%-15% increase in SV or CO) and those who do not respond to a fluid load and investigate whether these parameters can predict responsiveness and whether the magnitude of the cyclic changes predicts the extent of response. With a few exceptions, most of these investigations show that the dynamic preload parameters better predict fluid responsiveness that static parameters.[17,60] Proposed threshold values that distinguish fluid-responsive from fluid-nonresponsive patients vary between 12% and 15% for SPV, 10% and 12% for pulse pressure variation, and 9.5% to 12% for SV variation. There are, however, no randomized trials with prospective testing of the proposed thresholds.

Other dynamic preload parameters are pulse oximetry plethysmographic waveform variability (threshold 13%),[71] the inferior vena cava distensibility index (threshold 12% or 18%),[72,73] and the superior vena cava collapsibility index (threshold 36%).[74]

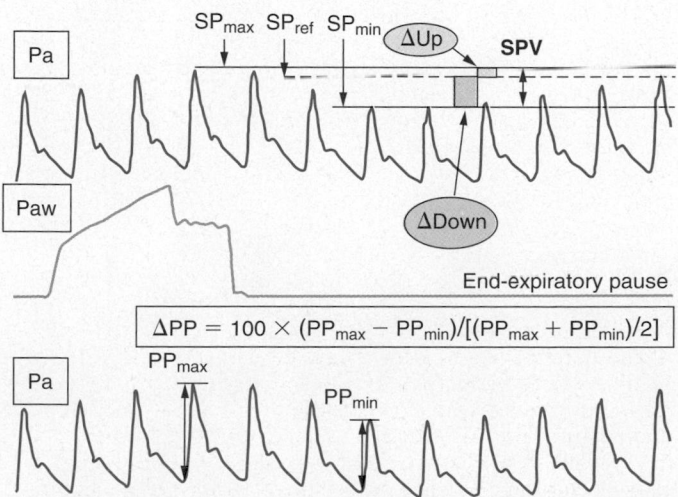

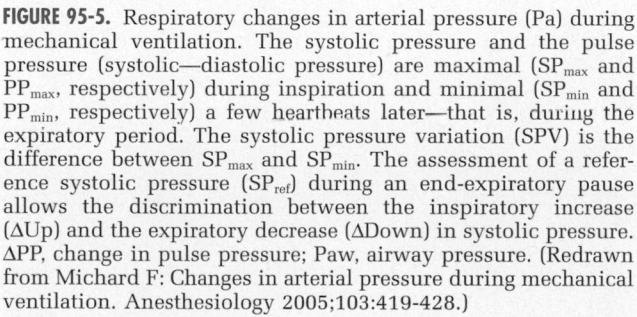

FIGURE 95-5. Respiratory changes in arterial pressure (Pa) during mechanical ventilation. The systolic pressure and the pulse pressure (systolic—diastolic pressure) are maximal (SP_{max} and PP_{max}, respectively) during inspiration and minimal (SP_{min} and PP_{min}, respectively) a few heartbeats later—that is, during the expiratory period. The systolic pressure variation (SPV) is the difference between SP_{max} and SP_{min}. The assessment of a reference systolic pressure (SP_{ref}) during an end-expiratory pause allows the discrimination between the inspiratory increase (ΔUp) and the expiratory decrease (ΔDown) in systolic pressure. ΔPP, change in pulse pressure; Paw, airway pressure. (Redrawn from Michard F: Changes in arterial pressure during mechanical ventilation. Anesthesiology 2005;103:419-428.)

Dynamic preload assessment has several limitations.[70,75] It can be used only in patients undergoing mechanical ventilation who make no active breathing efforts and have no arrhythmias. The magnitude of the changes in SV depends on tidal volume, the dynamic preload parameters being more accurate with higher tidal volumes. A clear dissociation between responders and nonresponders has been established only in patients who are ventilated with relatively high tidal volumes (higher than those that currently advocated for the mechanical ventilation of patients with acute respiratory distress syndrome). In addition, dynamic preload parameters are influenced by chest wall compliance. The determination of SPV, ΔDown, and pulse pressure variation requires invasive monitoring of arterial pressure, with measurement on a recorded waveform and, for ΔDown, the introduction of a short apnea.

CONCLUSION

The determination of adequate intravascular volume (preload) continues to present major difficulties in the care of critically ill or injured patients. As Rivers[76] observes, "fluid may be a friend when appropriately titrated during the resuscitation, or ebb, phase. . . . Excess fluid becomes an enemy when it is no longer physiologically needed." Unfortunately, assessment of volume status is most problematic in patients who are more susceptible to the deleterious effects of fluid loading (those with acute respiratory distress syndrome or LV failure). In contrast to static preload parameters, dynamic preload parameters (functional hemodynamic monitoring) allow the prediction of volume responsiveness. Unfortunately, this method can be used only in mechanically ventilated patients who have relatively high tidal volumes and no respiratory movements. Valuable alternatives are the fluid challenge approach and passive leg raising. Experience with the use of bioimpedance and hormone levels to assess volume status is limited.

1. Assessment of volume status is one of the most difficult clinical problems in intensive care medicine.
2. Preload and preload responsiveness are two different entities, the latter being far more clinically relevant.
3. Possible preload responsiveness should elicit fluid administration only in patients with signs of tissue hypoperfusion.
4. Volumetric preload parameters better reflect end-diastolic volume than filling pressures, but neither of these static preload parameters allows clinicians to predict a patient's fluid responsiveness.
5. Functional hemodynamic monitoring uses cardiopulmonary interactions during mechanical ventilation to predict fluid responsiveness and allows clinicians to better distinguish "responders" from "nonresponders" to fluid administration.

Key References
17. Michard F, Teboul JL: Predicting fluid responsiveness in ICU patients: A critical analysis of the evidence. Chest 2002;121: 2000-2008.
21. Pinsky MR: Pulmonary artery occlusion pressure. Intensive Care Med 2003;29:19-22.
22. Pinsky MR: Clinical significance of pulmonary artery occlusion pressure. Intensive Care Med 2003;29:175-178.
60. Bendjelid K, Romand JA: Fluid responsiveness in mechanically ventilated patients: A review of indices used in intensive care. Intensive Care Med 2003;29:352-360.
61. Coudray A, Romand JA, Treggiari M, Bendjelid K: Fluid responsiveness in spontaneously breathing patients: A review of indexes used in intensive care. Crit Care Med 2005;33: 2757-2762.

See the companion Expert Consult website for the complete reference list.

Clinical Syndromes

CHAPTER 96

Nephrotic Syndrome

Carla Sala

> ## OBJECTIVES
>
> This chapter will:
> 1. Explore the pathogenesis of proteinuria and of sodium/water retention.
> 2. Describe the clinical complications of the nephrotic syndrome.
> 3. Discuss the underfilling and overfilling hypotheses.
> 4. Consider the proposed unifying hypothesis.

Nephrotic syndrome is a pathological condition characterized by severe proteinuria (>3.5 g/24 hr) as a result of the increased flux of albumin and plasma proteins across the glomerular filtration barrier.

In adults, diabetic nephropathy is the major cause of proteinuria in the nephrotic range.[1] In approximately 80% of cases in nondiabetic subjects, nephrotic syndrome, the annual incidence of which has been estimated at 3 cases per million, is related to a primary glomerular disease, membranous glomerulonephritis being the most common histological variety (Table 96-1). Secondary causes of nephrotic syndrome in the remaining 20% of adult cases include multiple systemic diseases. In children, the incidence of nephrotic syndrome is tenfold higher than that in adults (3 cases per 100,000/year); primary forms account for more than 90% of cases, and minimal change disease is the most common variety.[2]

PATHOGENESIS OF GLOMERULAR PROTEINURIA

In idiopathic nephrotic syndrome, the etiological factor causing increased glomerular permeability to proteins is still undefined. A circulating factor produced by lymphocytes has been hypothesized on the basis of multiple observations, such as the induction of proteinuria in rats injected with plasma from patients with idiopathic nephrotic syndrome,[3] the relapse of the disease after renal transplantation,[4] and the decreased proteinuria in transplant recipients after adsorption of plasma proteins.[5] A defect of both the charge-selective and size-selective barrier to the passage of proteins across the glomerular membrane has been involved in the increased permselectivity.[6,7] Genetic studies in congenital nephrosis have partially clarified the role of a single gene defect in the

pathogenesis of the disease; however, the contribution of the three major components of the glomerular filter—endothelium, basement membrane, and podocytes—to the increased permeability to proteins has not been completely clarified by molecular and physiological studies.

CLINICAL COMPLICATIONS

Sodium/water retention and edema are common clinical complications of the nephrotic syndrome (Table 96-2); controversies about the mechanism(s) of sodium/water retention are discussed later.

Thromboembolic events occur in about 50% of nephrotic patients; the venous compartment is more commonly involved by the thrombotic process than the arterial compartment. Renal vein thrombosis occurs in 20% to 30% of cases associated with membranous glomerulonephritis.[8] Symptoms (hematuria, flank pain, loss of renal function) may be absent in the majority of cases. Deep venous thrombosis is also a common complication in nephrotic patients. Pulmonary embolism may be clinically manifested in less than 30% of cases.[2] The conditions more frequently associated with thromboembolic complications are a low serum albumin concentration (<2.5 gr/dL), severe proteinuria (>10 g/24 hr), hypovolemia, high fibrinogen level, and low antithrombin III level.

Nephrotic dyslipidemia is variably represented by hypercholesterolemia alone or by the combined elevation of serum cholesterol and triglycerides. Dyslipidemia probably results from an increased production and a reduced catabolism of lipoproteins due to the altered glomerular permeability. Nephrotic syndrome, in addition to diabetes mellitus and hypothyroidism, should be routinely excluded during the clinical assessment of hypercholesterolemic patients.

Infectious diseases at present are relevant complications in patients receiving immunosuppressive drugs.

PATHOGENESIS OF SODIUM/WATER RETENTION

Two mutually exclusive hypotheses, the underfilling hypothesis and the overfilling hypothesis, have been classically proposed to explain sodium/water retention in nephrotic syndrome; both hypotheses are supported by experimental and clinical evidence.[2,9]

TABLE 96-1

Causes of Nephrotic Syndrome in Adults

Idiopathic (primary glomerular disease)	Membranous glomerulonephritis
	Minimal changes glomerulopathy
	Focal glomerulosclerosis
	Membranoproliferative glomerulonephritis
Secondary	Diabetic nephropathy
	Neoplasia: carcinoma, lymphoma, leukemia
	Systemic lupus erythematosus
	Amyloidosis
	Infectious diseases: bacterial endocarditis, hepatitis B and C
	Drugs: penicillamine, nonsteroidal anti-inflammatory drugs; illicit drugs (e.g., heroin)

TABLE 96-2

Major Clinical Complications of Nephrotic Syndrome

Sodium/water retention and edema formation
Thromboembolic events:
 Renal vein thrombosis
 Deep venous thrombosis
 Pulmonary embolism
Hyperlipoproteinemia
Infectious diseases

Underfilling Hypothesis

The underfilling hypothesis explains sodium/water retention as a consequence of the neurohumoral activation in response to hypovolemia induced by protein losses.[9-12] The findings supporting this hypothesis are as follows:
1. Intravascular volume is reduced in approximately 30% of nephrotic patients.[11]
2. A neurohumoral profile compatible with hypovolemia and characterized by low levels of plasma atrial natriuretic peptide (ANP)[13] and high levels of plasma norepinephrine,[14] renin, aldosterone,[15] and vasopressin[16] has been described in approximately 50% of nephrotic patients.
3. A hemodynamic profile characterized by low cardiac output and increased vascular resistance described in nephrotic animals is compatible with hypovolemia.[17]

Overfilling Hypothesis

According to the overfilling hypothesis, the retention of sodium and water is the result of a primary renal defect causing hypervolemia.[2,18] The findings in support of this hypothesis are as follows:
1. Intravascular volume is normal or increased in the majority of nephrotic patients.[12] Although plasma volume measurement in nephrosis is beset by methodological limitations,[19] the distribution of plasma volume in hundreds of nephrotic patients has been described to fit a gaussian curve; in particular, 33%, 42%, and 25% of patients, respectively, have reduced, normal, and increased plasma volumes.[9]
2. A neurohumoral profile compatible with hypervolemia is observed in a large percentage of nephrotic patients; this profile is characterized by high plasma ANP levels, as a result of atrial wall distention and suppressed plasma renin activity.[20,21]
3. Multiple renal defects have been alternatively proposed as causes of sodium/water retention and hypervolemia. A tubular defect has been documented in experimental nephrosis induced by toxic agents[22]; this experimental evidence, however, should be extrapolated with caution to the human condition. In nephrotic patients, a transient functional impairment of glomerular filtration rate (GFR) has been described during the sodium retentive

TABLE 96-3

Renal, Hemodynamic, and Clinical Data in Nephrotic Patients*

PARAMETER	POSITIVE SODIUM BALANCE ($n = 8$)	P VALUE	NEGATIVE SODIUM BALANCE ($n = 5$)
Renal			
Urinary protein (g/24 hr)	14.6 ± 2.4	NS	10.9 ± 1.4
Creatinine clearance (mL/min)	83 ± 9	<.05	137 ± 18
Urine volume (mL/24 hr)	841 ± 84	<.01	1547 ± 258
Sodium balance (mEq)	$+242 \pm 24$	<.05	-35 ± 38
Hemodynamic			
Arterial pressure (mm Hg)	$138/83 \pm 7/3$	NS	$135/80 \pm 9/5$
Heart rate (beats/min)	71 ± 3	NS	67 ± 4
Stroke volume index (mL/m^2)	35 ± 3	<.05	56 ± 4
Total peripheral resistance index (dyne/sec/cm^5/m^2)	3490 ± 418	<.01	2171 ± 184
Clinical			
Serum albumin (g/dL)	2.4 ± 0.1	NS	2.5 ± 0.2
Serum cholesterol (mg/dL)	429 ± 36	NS	373 ± 37
Serum sodium (mEq/L)	142 ± 0.9	NS	143 ± 1.1
Erythrocyte sedimentation rate (%)	61.9 ± 11	NS	35.2 ± 15

*Sodium balance was assessed during a 5-day trial of controlled salt intake. Values given are mean ± SEM.
NS, not significant.
Modified from Sala C, Bedogna V, Gammaro L, et al: Central role of vasopressin in sodium/water retention in hypo- and hyper-volemic nephrotic patients: A unifying hypothesis. J Nephrol 2004;17:653-657.

phase.[23] A relationship between the impairment of GFR in nephrotic forms associated with chronic glomerulonephritis and volume status has been proposed by some researchers,[11] but has not been confirmed by others.[12,24] Thus, the site and the nature of the renal defect causing sodium/water retention are still undefined.

A Unifying Hypothesis for Sodium/Water Retention in Nephrosis

The underfilling and overfilling hypotheses may each explain sodium/water retention in less than 50% of nephrotic patients, at best. A unifying hypothesis for sodium/water retention has been proposed on the basis of the renal, hemodynamic, and humoral parameters simultaneously measured in a group of nephrotic patients.[25]

In 13 untreated patients with idiopathic nephrotic syndrome in the proteinuric-edematous phase, sodium balance during a 5-day trial of controlled salt intake was positive in 60% of patients and negative in the other 40% (Table 96-3). In sodium-retentive patients, the neurohumoral profile was compatible with a condition of either hypovolemia or hypervolemia, because supine plasma ANP levels were low in half of the patients and high in the other half; an opposite trend was observed for plasma renin activity and aldosterone (Fig. 96-1A-C). In patients with negative sodium balance, ANP, plasma renin activity, and aldosterone values were within normal ranges. Plasma vasopressin was elevated in hypovolemic and even more in hypervolemic nephrotic patients, and tended to normalize in sodium excretors (Fig. 96-1D).

GFR (determined by creatinine clearance) was 40% lower in sodium-retentive patients than in sodium excretors, although still within the normal range (see Table 96-3); the inverse relationship between GFR and sodium balance (Fig. 96-2A) suggests that GFR impairment plays a major role in sodium/water retention, as previously reported.[23] The functional impairment of GFR may be related to the involvement of renal vasculature in the systemic vasoconstriction characterizing the hemodynamic profile of sodium-retentive patients (see Table 96-3), because GFR was found to be inversely related to systemic vascular resistances (Fig. 96-2B).

The systemic and renal vasoconstriction in sodium-retentive patients is likely sustained by multiple vasoconstrictor agents in hypovolemic patients, namely catecholamines, angiotensin II, and vasopressin and mostly by vasopressin in the hypervolemic patients; the central role of vasopressin in sustaining vasoconstriction in both volume conditions is supported by its direct relationship

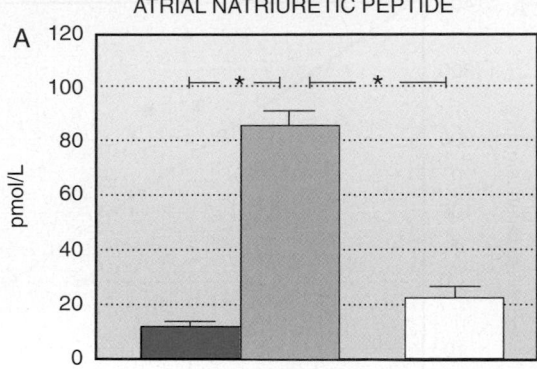

ATRIAL NATRIURETIC PEPTIDE

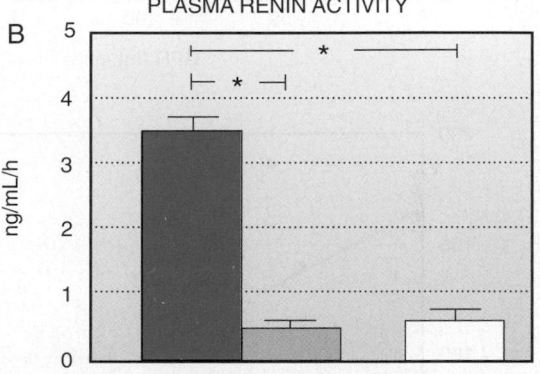

PLASMA RENIN ACTIVITY

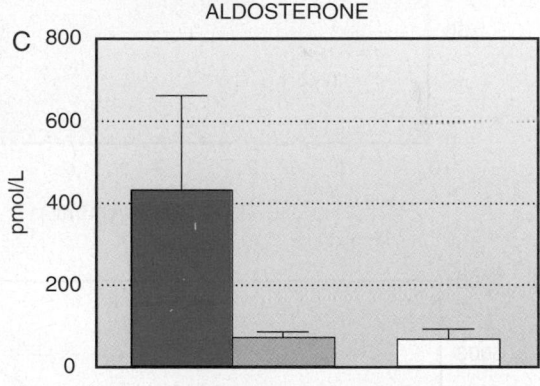

ALDOSTERONE

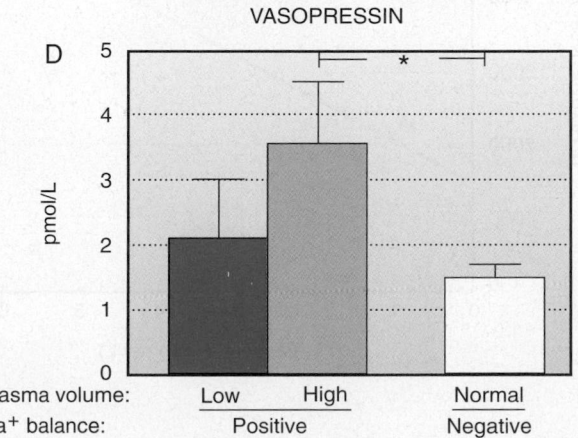

VASOPRESSIN

FIGURE 96-1. Humoral data in patients with idiopathic nephrotic syndrome (*n* = 13). **A,** In patients with positive sodium balance, the supine plasma atrial natriuretic peptide (ANP) value was either low (*dark bar, n* = 4) or high (*light bar, n* = 4); this pattern is compatible with a condition of low or high intravascular volume, respectively. Plasma renin activity (PRA; **B**) and aldosterone concentration (**C**) showed opposite trends. **D,** The plasma vasopressin value was high in both hypovolemic and hypervolemic patients. Normal values for ANP level, PRA, and aldosterone and vasopressin levels were observed in patients with negative sodium balance (*white bars, n* = 5). *, *P* < .05. (From Sala C, Bedogna V, Gammaro L, et al: Central role of vasopressin in sodium/water retention in hypo- and hyper-volemic nephrotic patients: A unifying hypothesis. J Nephrol 2004;17:653-657.)

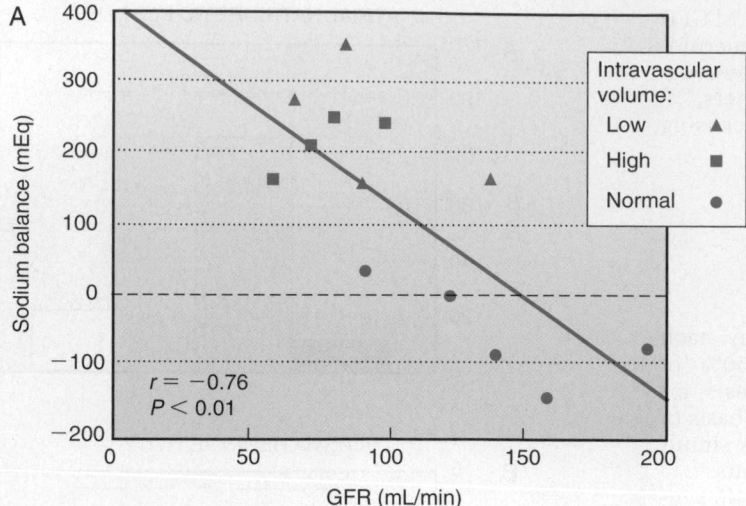

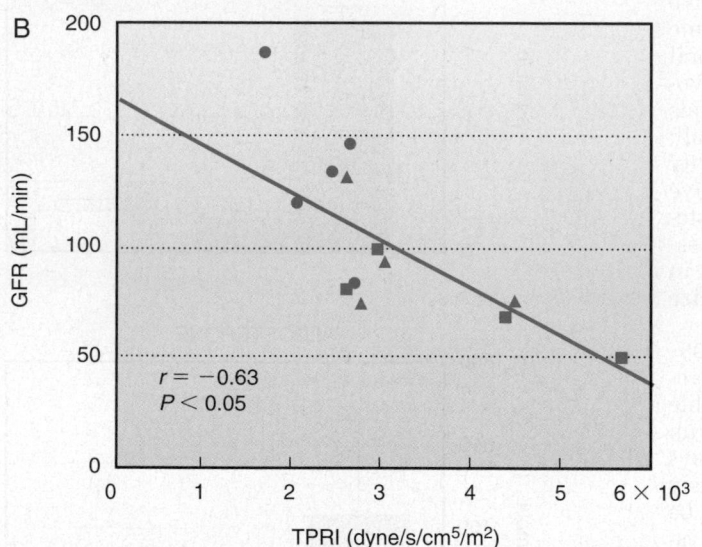

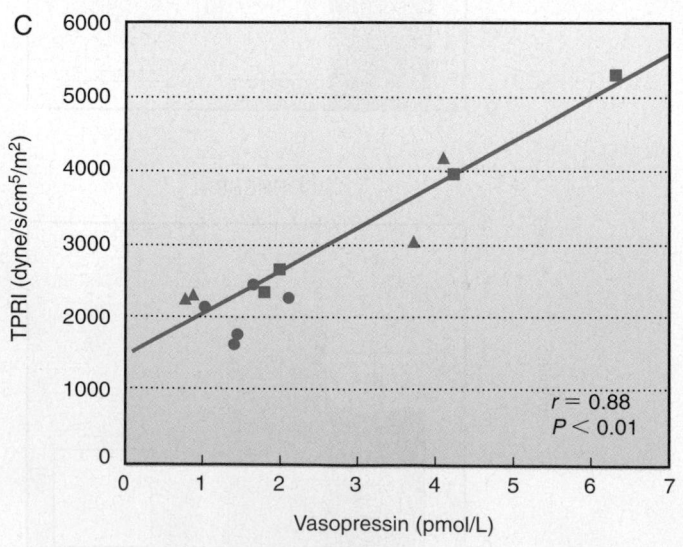

FIGURE 96-2. Relationship between renal, hemodynamic, and hormonal variables in nephrotic patients. **A,** The inverse relationship between glomerular filtration rate (GFR, from creatinine clearance) and sodium balance favors a major role for GFR impairment in sodium retention in both hypovolemic and hypervolemic patients. **B,** The inverse relationship between systemic vascular resistances (shown as TPRI [total peripheral resistance index]) and GFR suggests that the functional impairment of GFR in hypovolemic and hypervolemic sodium-retentive patients may be related to the involvement of the renal vasculature in the systemic vasoconstriction characterizing their hemodynamic profile. **C,** The direct relationship between plasma vasopressin value and systemic vascular resistances suggests a major role for vasopressin in the vasoconstriction characterizing either hypovolemic or hypervolemic patients. (From Sala C, Bedogna V, Gammaro L, et al: Central role of vasopressin in sodium/water retention in hypo- and hyper-volemic nephrotic patients: A unifying hypothesis. J Nephrol 2004;17:653-657.)

FIGURE 96-3. Hypothesized clinical stages of nephrotic syndrome. First stage (1): The neurohumoral activation induced by hypovolemia is responsible for the systemic/renal vasoconstriction and sodium/water retention via the vascular and tubular effects of the sympathetic nervous system (SNS), renin-angiotensin-aldosterone system (RAAS), and vasopressin (VP). Second stage (2): Once hypovolemia has been corrected, the persistence of an osmotic stimulus for VP release causes a further expansion of extracellular volume; in this stage, the SNS and RAAS are suppressed by hypervolemia. Third stage (3): Once the osmotic stimulus for vasopressin release has waned, sodium/water excretion finally occurs and blood volume returns to normal. (From Sala C, Bedogna V, Gammaro L, et al: Central role of vasopressin in sodium/water retention in hypo- and hypervolemic nephrotic patients: A unifying hypothesis. J Nephrol 2004;17:653-657.)

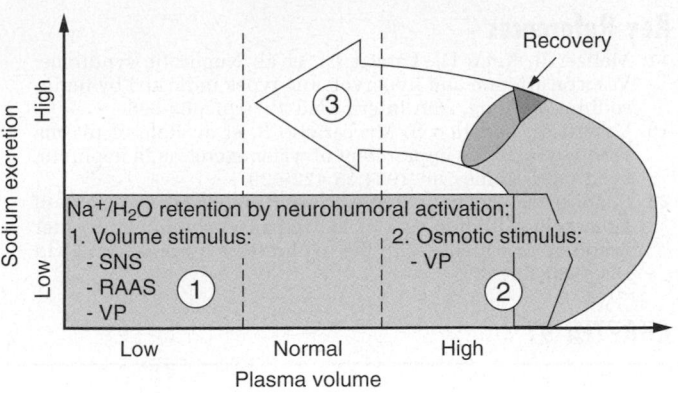

to systemic vascular resistances in the whole group of patients (Fig. 96-2C). From the observation that levels of inflammatory markers and dyslipidemia progressively tend to decrease from hypovolemic to hypervolemic to normovolemic patients, in spite of the persistence of severe proteinuria (see Table 96-3), it was hypothesized that the three volume conditions are subsequent stages of nephrotic syndrome (Fig. 96-3).

Thus, according to the unifying hypothesis, hypovolemia in the first stage of nephrotic syndrome activates the neurohumoral systems, which are responsible for sodium/water retention, via the intrarenal vascular and tubular effects of catecholamines, angiotensin II, and vasopressin. The contribution of multiple systems to sodium/water retention in this stage of the disease may explain the failure of the selective blockade of the renin system to restore sodium/water excretion in hypovolemic nephrotic patients.[26]

In the second stage, once hypovolemia has been corrected, persistence of an osmotic stimulus for vasopressin release causes a further expansion of intravascular volume via the renal vascular and tubular effects of vasopressin. Experimental and clinical evidence shows that the osmotic stimulus may overcome the volume stimulus in the control of vasopressin secretion.[27] The expansion of intravascular volume tends to suppress the activity of the sympathetic nervous system and renin-angiotensin system and to stimulate ANP secretion; it is conceivable that in this stage of the nephrotic syndrome, the capillary-permeabilizing effect of ANP may contribute to edema formation.[28] The functional impairment of GFR in sodium-retentive patients may be related to vasoconstriction of the afferent arterioles sustained by the combined effect of catecholamines, angiotensin II, and vasopressin in hypovolemic patients and by vasopressin alone in hypervolemic patients; a similar pathogenetic mechanism is supported by the observation that GFR is similarly reduced in both hypovolemic and hypervolemic patients.

Thus, hypovolemia and hypervolemia may represent subsequent stages of the nephrotic syndrome, in which the neurohumoral activation subsequently induced by a volume and an osmotic stimulus is responsible for sodium/water retention. In the third stage, remission finally occurs when the osmotic stimulus for vasopressin release fades. This stage is characterized by systemic and renal vasodilation, sodium/water excretion, and normalization of plasma volume. It is interesting to note that resolution of salt retention may occur in spite of the persistence of severe proteinuria and hypoalbuminemia, as previously reported during steroid treatment.[26]

Pharmacological interventions with vasopressin receptor antagonists may clarify the role of this peptide in sodium/water retention in nephrotic patients. In congestive heart failure, another clinical condition characterized by sodium/water retention, the blockade of vasopressin receptors has been shown to exert multiple beneficial effects—a decrease in systemic vascular resistance and increases in stroke volume,[29] GFR, renal blood flow, and diuresis.[30] In nephrotic patients, maximal beneficial effects from vasopressin V1 (vascular) receptor and V2 (renal) receptor antagonists should be expected, according to the unifying hypothesis, in hypervolemic patients. Vasopressin antagonists may be superior to loop diuretics in volume control, because the former increase diuresis without adversely affecting renal hemodynamics, serum electrolyte levels, and the neurohumoral system.[30] These agents should also prevent a reduction in GFR due to an excessive renal vasconstriction that characterizes the cardiorenal syndrome, an adverse renal effect that is often precipitated by an excessive use of loop diuretics.

Key Points

1. A major clinical complication of nephrotic syndrome is sodium/water retention with edema formation.
2. The pathogenesis of sodium/water retention is hypothesized by two opposite mechanisms: the neurohumoral activation in response to hypovolemia (underfilling) and a primary renal defect causing hypervolemia (overfilling). Both hypotheses are supported by the clinical and experimental evidence that plasma volume is either decreased or increased in nephrosis.
3. A unifying hypothesis is proposed, according to which hypovolemia and hypervolemia are subsequent stages of the nephrotic syndrome. Sodium/water retention is the consequence of the renal vascular and tubular effects of multiple volume-controlled systems in hypovolemic patients and of osmotically controlled vasopressin in hypervolemic patients.

Key References

11. Meltzer JI, Keim HJ, Laragh JH, et al: Nephrotic syndrome: Vasoconstriction and hypervolemic types indicated by renin-sodium profiling. Ann Intern Med 1979;92:688-696.
16. Usberti M, Federico S, Meccariello S, et al: Role of plasma vasopressin in the impairment of water excretion in nephrotic syndrome. Kidney Int 1984;25:422-429.
23. Shapiro MD, Nicholls KM, Groves BM, Schrier RW: Role of glomerular filtration rate in the impaired sodium and water excretion of patients with the nephrotic syndrome. Am J Kid Dis 1986;8:81-87.

25. Sala C, Bedogna V, Gammaro L, et al: Central role of vasopressin in sodium/water retention in hypo- and hyper-volemic nephrotic patients: A unifying hypothesis. J Nephrol 2004;17: 653-657.
27. Schrier RW, Berl T, Anderson RJ: Osmotic and nonosmotic control of vasopressin release. Am J Physiol 1979;234: F321-F332.

See the companion Expert Consult website for the complete reference list.

CHAPTER 97

Intravascular Volume Depletion

Jonathan Buckmaster

OBJECTIVES

This chapter will:
1. Describe the complexity of physiological responses to intravascular volume depletion.
2. Explain the pathological processes by which intravascular volume depletion may occur.
3. Define the risks and effects of sedation and intermittent positive-pressure ventilation on the response to intravascular volume depletion in critically patients.

Intravascular volume depletion is a pathophysiological state that is defined by a reduction in stressed blood volume. Prior to discussion of this condition, a review of the conceptual basis of the distribution of blood volume within the circulation and the pressures therein is provided.

CAPACITANCE AND COMPLIANCE

Capacitance is the relationship between the blood volume and transmural pressure within a given segment of the circulation.[1] For most parts of the circulation, there is a finite volume of blood within each segment at zero distending pressure. This volume is referred to as the *unstressed blood volume*, because it does not contribute to the generation of pressure within that vessel.[2] To describe the capacitance of a segment, one must know both the magnitude of the unstressed blood volume and the compliance of the segment with additional filling. Compliance is defined as the ratio of change in volume within a segment to the resulting change in distending pressure ($\Delta V/\Delta P$). It is important to recognize that compliance depends not only on the elastic properties of a segment but also on the volume of that segment. Vascular distensibility, which is independent of the volume of a segment, is the ratio of fractional change in volume to change in pressure, as follows:

$$\Delta V/V_o\Delta P$$

where V_o is the initial volume of the segment.

Total blood capacity is the sum of stressed blood volume and unstressed blood volume; it normally amounts to approximately 70 mL/kg.[1-4] Stressed blood volume is the component of total blood capacity that stretches the elastic parts of the vascular tree and, thus, generates mean circulatory filling pressure (P_{mcf}).[1] It accounts for approximately 20% to 25% of the total blood capacity under normal circumstances.[3,4] From the preceding considerations, it can be seen that a decrease in stressed blood volume may arise either from an absolute reduction in blood volume or from a redistribution of blood from the stressed blood volume to the unstressed blood volume—a condition often referred to as *relative hypovolemia* (Fig. 97-1).

The remainder of this chapter describes the pathophysiological changes that ensue from a reduction in stressed blood volume and the medical conditions that cause intravascular hypovolemia (Table 97-1).

THE RESPONSE TO HYPOVOLEMIA

The prototypical cause of absolute intravascular volume depletion is hemorrhage. This involves the loss of all elements of circulating blood from the circulation, including blood cells, plasma proteins, water, and electrolytes. It has been known for centuries that progressive loss of blood from the circulation leads to a sequence of changes in the otherwise intact animal that is characterized by an initial, compensated phase (phase I) followed by a second, decompensated phase (phase II).[5-7] Finally, unless treated, ongoing hemorrhage leads to a third phase, irreversible shock. At this point, no amount of resuscitation can lead to recovery from the insult. Hypovolemic shock has been studied extensively in animals and humans, using both hemorrhage and models that simulate hemorrhage.[8-11] Because of the difficulty of obtaining controlled data in hemorrhagic shock in human subjects, lower body negative pressure has been developed as a model of simulated hemorrhage.[8]

Phase I of the Hypovolemic Response

A reduction in stressed blood volume causes a decrease in P_{mcf}. This leads to a short-term reduction in venous return,

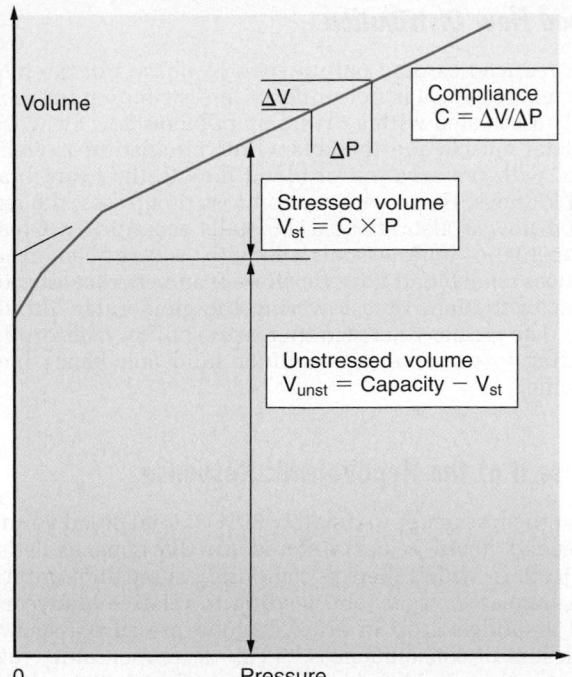

FIGURE 97-1. Diagram illustrating the principles of vascular capacitance. Vascular capacity is made up of stressed (V_{st}) and unstressed (V_{unst}) blood volume. Note that the curve relating intravascular pressure (P) to volume (V) becomes nonlinear as pressure approaches zero. Unstressed blood volume is estimated by extrapolation. C, compliance.

In the figure:

Volume

ΔV

ΔP

Compliance
$C = \Delta V / \Delta P$

Stressed volume
$V_{st} = C \times P$

Unstressed volume
$V_{unst} = Capacity - V_{st}$

0   Pressure

TABLE 97-1

Causes of Intravascular Volume Depletion

Loss of whole blood	
External	Trauma
	Surgery
	Gastrointestinal bleeding
Internal	Intrathoracic
	Intraperitoneal
	Retroperitoneal
Loss of plasma	Burns
	Extensive skin loss
	Abdominal paracentesis
	Nephrotic syndrome
Loss of extracellular fluid	
Nonrenal	Third space losses
	Diarrhea and vomiting
	Sweat loss
Renal	Diabetes mellitus
	Diabetes insipidus
	Polyuric renal failure
Increased circulatory capacitance	Neurogenic shock
	Sepsis
	Neuraxial anesthesia

which is driven by the difference between P_{mcf} and right atrial pressure (P_{ra}). Hence, cardiac output starts to fall.[1] As a consequence, arterial blood pressure initially tends to fall, but this tendency is rapidly compensated by neural feedback from the carotid sinus and aortic baroreceptors, which mediate increased sympathetic tone and decreased

vagal tone in the brainstem.[7] Arterial baroreceptors are fundamentally involved in the adaptive response to hypovolemia as well as volume excess. Their output changes markedly with small changes in blood pressure, facilitating rapid and effective autonomic changes to keep blood pressure in a narrow operating range.[12] In addition to the major role played by the arterial baroreceptors, there may also be a component of unloading of cardiac baroreceptors in the observed sympathetic response to hemorrhage.[5] In general, however, cardiac baroreceptors appear to be involved more in the defense against hypervolemia.[7,13]

Increased sympathetic tone leads to arteriolar vasoconstriction, which increases total peripheral resistance and hence restores arterial blood pressure to normal or near-normal levels. Arteriolar vasoconstriction occurs in skeletal muscle, splanchnic, and renal beds.[14] Increased sympathetic tone also causes active vasoconstriction of venous capacitance vessels. Consequently, unstressed blood volume drops, leading to a rise in stressed blood volume and partial restoration of P_{mcf} and cardiac output.[1,15-17] It is important to note that this recruitment of stressed volume from a reservoir of unstressed volume is not accompanied by a significant change in venous compliance.[1] The sympathetic reflexes are vital in the adaptive response to acute intravascular volume depletion because they are rapid in onset, reaching a maximum output within a minute.[3,5] In addition to the effects on peripheral resistance, sympathetic arteriolar vasoconstriction causes a decrease in capillary pressure in tissue beds, which results in increased transcapillary absorption of interstitial fluid into the circulation, further tending to restore the stressed blood volume, over a period of minutes to hours.[3,10] This process is inevitably accompanied by a decrease in hematocrit, which may be helpful from a diagnostic point of view. Interstitial fluid absorption is an important component of the compensation for acute volume loss, although full recovery depends on the mobilization of behavioral mechanisms, such as thirst and salt appetite, to replace the interstitial fluid volume over a longer period.[3]

There is considerable debate about the relative importance of active and passive venoconstriction in the redistribution of blood volume in humans under differing circumstances. Passive venoconstriction occurs through reduction in transmural venous pressure and causes a decrease in venous blood volume in accordance with venous compliance, thus making more blood available to other parts of the circulation. A major part of this passive venoconstriction mechanism derives from upstream arteriolar vasoconstriction, which reduces blood flow through an organ.[2,15-17] A further contribution to the stressed blood volume comes about from the reverse stress-relaxation mechanism that may be observed in every blood vessel as a consequence of reduced pressure within the vessel. This phenomenon allows smooth muscle–lined organs to maintain a relatively constant transmural pressure in the face of changes in volume. The reverse stress-relaxation mechanism occurs over a span of minutes to hours.[3] However, there is also evidence that a significant role is played by active, sympathetically mediated venoconstriction within the gut and liver, although, unlike in dogs, there is no significant contribution from the spleen in human subjects. The liver is known to contain about 15% of the total blood volume, including about half the stressed blood volume.[18,19] Sympathetic stimulation of the heart causes tachycardia and increased contractility, leading to a decrease in P_{ra}. Up to a point, this decrease in

P_{ra} allows increased venous return, despite the reduction in P_{mcf}.

Cardiac output is maintained up to a loss of about 10% of blood volume but thereafter declines progressively with further blood loss.[3] Although the cardiac output is only partly restored by the sympathetic reflexes described previously, arterial blood pressure is well preserved in the presence of falling cardiac output during phase I.[5-7,9] In addition to the sympathetic vascular and cardiac responses already described, activity of sympathetic preganglionic neurons innervating adrenal medullary chromaffin cells increases, leading to greater secretion of norepinephrine but not epinephrine. Renal sympathetic nerve activity also increases.[14]

Hormonal Responses to Intravascular Volume Depletion

Other, hormonal mechanisms that contribute to the maintenance of blood pressure with progressive hemorrhage are angiotensin II and vasopressin. Angiotensin II is formed peripherally by the action of renin, which is released from the juxtaglomerular cells of the afferent and efferent arterioles of the kidney in response to sympathetic stimulation and decreased blood pressure.[3,7] It is a potent, relatively rapidly acting arteriolar vasoconstrictor, with less effect on veins. Therefore, its early effects on arterial blood pressure are achieved through greater peripheral resistance, which occurs over 10 to 20 minutes. In addition, angiotensin II decreases renal water and salt losses, both directly and indirectly, by regulating aldosterone release from the adrenal cortex. Angiotensin II causes predominantly renal efferent arteriolar vasoconstriction, which decreases renal blood flow but tends to preserve the glomerular filtration rate by raising glomerular hydrostatic pressure. It also promotes salt and water reabsorption from renal tubules. These actions come into play over a period of minutes to hours.[3] Angiotensin II stimulates thirst and salt appetite centrally and is thus important in the longer-term compensation for acute blood loss.[7] Angiotensin II is a potent stimulus to aldosterone secretion by the adrenal glands. Aldosterone acts on renal tubules to increase sodium reabsorption and consequently to reexpand extracellular fluid volume over hours to days. Angiotensin II has the added property of increasing vasopressin release in hypovolemia and hypotension.

Oxytocin is another hormone known to be released from the posterior pituitary during hemorrhage. Its adaptive role in the hormonal response to intravascular volume depletion has only been partially elucidated. It is now known that oxytocin stimulates renin release through a β-adrenergic receptor–mediated sympathetic mechanism.[20,21] It also increases heart rate in hypovolemia and hypotension, possibly through modulation of the baroreceptor reflex response. Like angiotensin II, oxytocin increases vasopressin release in response to hypotension.[7]

Vasopressin levels rise in hemorrhagic shock, and this rise has been shown to be mediated primarily by the arterial baroreceptors in response to severe hypotension. By contrast, unloading of atrial receptors does not increase vasopressin secretion.[22] Because blood pressure is well preserved during phase I, vasopressin levels rise little. However, even a very small increase in vasopressin release leads to a marked decrease in renal water loss in urine,[3] which may play a role in longer-term recovery from hypovolemia.

Blood Flow Distribution

The reduced cardiac output seen in phase I of the hypovolemic response is not uniform in distribution but is initially associated with a diversion of blood flow away from skeletal muscle and the splanchnic circulation as well as skin, with preservation of blood flow to the heart, brain, and kidneys. However, as blood loss progresses, the renal blood flow is also affected and falls accordingly. Greater sympathetic tone associated with severe hemorrhage reduces renal blood flow via afferent and efferent arteriolar vasoconstriction, thus lowering the glomerular filtration rate. The greater tone also increases sodium reabsorption, tending to preserve extracellular fluid and hence blood volume.[3]

Phase II of the Hypovolemic Response

After the loss of approximately 30% of total blood volume, a second phase is encountered (in the nonanesthetized subject), in which there is temporary sympathoinhibition and increased vagal tone leading to relative bradycardia and a sudden drop in arterial blood pressure associated with loss of consciousness.[5-7] The decompensatory reflex appears to be mediated by neurons within the lateral parabrachial nucleus of the pons and may involve serotoninergic and opioidergic pathways.[5,6,23] In many species, the afferent input to this reflex appears to originate from a paradoxical increased output of cardiac baroreceptors with decreased chamber pressures, although there is evidence for alternative pathways in humans.[5] The sudden decrease in sympathetic tone of systemic blood vessels and the heart contrasts with a marked increase in sympathetically mediated adrenal epinephrine secretion[14] in addition to increased hormonal responses. These help prevent immediate and irreversible cardiovascular collapse.

Unlike the observed responses in phase I of the hypovolemic response, there is also a marked change in vasopressin release from the posterior pituitary in phase II, which increases exponentially with progressive hypotension.[22] Vasopressin is a potent vasoconstrictor with rapid onset, so it acts to lessen the magnitude of the hypotensive response. Although vasopressin also reduces renal water loss, this effect is of little immediate consequence in the adaptive response to hemorrhage. The onset of phase II may be delayed or prevented by μ-opioid receptor agonists such as fentanyl[5,23] and may be modified by the presence of other central mechanisms. It is important to appreciate that recovery from this state can occur. If further blood loss is prevented, normalization of blood pressure due to circulating catecholamines and vasopressin precedes recovery from the loss of vascular and cardiac sympathetic tone itself.[23]

Irreversible Shock

Acute loss of more than about 40% of the total blood volume, left untreated, leads to a spiral of shock that inevitably leads to death. When this state is established, although there may be temporary responses to volume replacement and inotropic support, there is a subsequent inexorable and progressive decline in cardiac output and blood pressure over several hours.[24] Decreased blood flow to the heart causes a positive feedback loop whereby a reduction in blood flow leads to reduced cardiac performance, which then further reduces blood flow, culminating in cardiac arrest. Substantial reduction in cerebral blood flow is known to cause an initial, maximal sympathetic response, but further, prolonged decrease in cerebral blood flow subsequently leads to total vasomotor failure and circulatory collapse. The major changes that are thought to lead to irreversible shock occur at a cellular level in multiple organs, although the obvious clinical consequence of irreversible shock is circulatory failure.

Hemorrhage

Hemorrhage is a common problem, especially within the surgical intensive care unit (ICU). Overt, external hemorrhage is easily recognized, leading to prompt treatment and correction of hypovolemia. On the other hand, hemorrhage may be occult, resulting in potentially delayed resuscitation. Common sites of concealed bleeding are gastrointestinal, retroperitoneal, pelvic and intrathoracic compartments. If hemorrhage occurs subacutely, the compensatory pathophysiological mechanisms previously described may lead to delay in recognition of the problem. Tachycardia may be ascribed to other causes, such as pain and anxiety, because arterial blood pressure tends to be well preserved.

Unexplained agitation in a surgical patient should always lead to consideration of concealed hemorrhage as a possible cause. Once hemorrhage is diagnosed, the next problem is to estimate the severity of the condition. In dogs, arterial base deficit was found to be the best predictor, among common clinical parameters, of the severity of hemorrhage.[11] A drop in hemoglobin concentration or hematocrit is also a relatively delayed response to hemorrhage and is not immediately helpful in the assessment of a patient who may be bleeding. On the other hand, tachycardia, tachypnea, decreased central venous pressure, low urine output, cold extremities, restlessness, and increasing acidemia, taken as a constellation of symptoms and signs, all point to acute severe hypovolemia. Except in situations in which the compensatory mechanisms of the phase I hypovolemic response are blocked, such as by general anesthesia, hypotension is a late feature of acute blood loss.

OTHER CAUSES OF INTRAVASCULAR VOLUME DEPLETION

Plasma loss from the circulation, without accompanying red blood cell loss, may be a cause of absolute intravascular volume depletion.[3] This phenomenon is seen frequently with severe burns or very rarely with extensive skin loss secondary to dermatological conditions such as toxic epidermal necrolysis. The major clinical difference from hemorrhage is that the hematocrit is *increased* rather than decreased. This increase leads to the additional problem of greater viscosity and, hence, reduced microvascular perfusion as well as all the other effects of hypovolemia. Other potential causes of plasma loss are traumatic crush injury and bowel obstruction.

Dehydration, or loss of water and electrolytes from the body, is a common cause of intravascular volume depletion. Massive fluid losses may occur through the gastrointestinal tract, with vomiting or diarrhea due to viral gastroenteritis or cholera; this is one of the major causes of infant death throughout the world. Glycosuria associated with diabetic ketoacidosis frequently causes severe dehydration at the time of presentation. Similarly, polyuric nephropathy may readily cause hypovolemia, the circulatory consequences of which may lead to further renal injury. In the postoperative setting, third space losses of isotonic fluids associated with major operations may lead to hypovolemia, which is easily overlooked. Increased sweating and other insensible losses in the setting of inadequate fluid replacement constitute another potential cause.

Neurogenic shock is a condition characterized by sudden vasomotor failure, the causes of which include acute spinal cord injury and brainstem injury. It is a common cause of relative hypovolemia. Complete loss of sympathetic tone in an otherwise normal individual leads to a decrease in stressed blood volume of approximately 5 mL/kg and a drop in P_{mcf} from about 7 to 4 mm Hg.[3] Consequently, there is a decrease in venous return. Arterial blood pressure falls not only because of decreased cardiac output but also as a result of arteriolar vasodilatation and a consequent decrease in total peripheral resistance. In addition, the increased capillary pressure that occurs in the setting of arteriolar vasodilatation leads to a higher gradient for transcapillary fluid movement into the tissues, potentiating the tendency for edema.[3] Restoration of blood pressure can be achieved through the judicious use of vasoconstrictor agents such as norepinephrine. Administration of volume replacement alone can restore the stressed blood volume and, hence, venous return but, because of arteriolar vasodilatation, does not fully compensate the hypotension. In practice, most clinicians use a combination of fluid replacement and vasoconstrictor agents to restore the decreases in cardiac output and blood pressure caused by vasomotor failure.

SIGNIFICANCE OF RELATIVE HYPOVOLEMIA IN THE INTENSIVE CARE UNIT

Many patients in ICUs have features of sepsis or systemic inflammatory response syndrome. These patients characteristically experience circulatory changes related to both uncontrolled vasodilatation and increased vascular permeability. The consequent reduction in stressed blood volume would be expected to compromise cardiac output. However, patients with sepsis treated in the ICU undergo very generous fluid resuscitation, as witnessed by the fluid balance charts at the ends of their beds and the prevalence of significant edema in medical ICU patients. As with neurogenic shock, restoration of vasomotor tone with exogenously administered vasopressor medications is an important part of resuscitation in sepsis, although it does not obviate the need for appropriate volume replacement.

There is no doubt that unrecognized hypovolemia can compromise the management of many ICU patients, potentially leading to inadequate cardiac output and progressive renal impairment.[25-27] The difficulty in clinical practice lies in the assessment of volume status, which is inherently flawed by the inconsistency of changes in physiological parameters such as central venous pressure (CVP) and pulmonary artery occlusion pressure (PAOP). Much evidence suggests that changes in these parameters are unreliable in the assessment of volume status not only in critically ill patients but also in normal subjects.[28,29] The reason is that the relationship between chamber pressure and chamber volume is nonlinear in practice, even in an individual. In other words, cardiac chamber compliance varies over time. For example, in the case of a patient with demonstrably normal or above-normal cardiac output with normal values for heart rate, blood pressure, and urine output, and with normal peripheral circulation, a CVP measurement of 4 to 6 mm Hg is evidence not of intravascular volume depletion but of normal cardiac function. On the other hand, in the presence of a low cardiac output state, with clinical evidence of inadequate circulation and compromised organ blood flow, including hypotension, tachycardia, oliguria, and lactic acidosis, a CVP of 8 to 10 mm Hg may warrant careful volume challenge.

The best guide to the effectiveness of such a volume challenge is an observed change in cardiac output and, ultimately, organ function after treatment. Baseline static pressure measurements as well as echocardiographic end-diastolic volume measurements fail to predict response to volume challenge, even in normal subjects with normal cardiac performance.[29] In addition, the entire clinical paradigm of the administration of intravenous crystalloid solutions to achieve greater cardiac output by means of an increase in cardiac preload has been called into question.[30] Evidence is growing that transpulmonary thermodilution measurements, such as intrathoracic blood volume index, correlate well with echocardiographic measurements of preload, allowing much more convenient assessment of clinical response to volume replacement.[28] Transpulmonary thermodilution measurements may be performed by PiCCO (Pulsion Medical Systems AG, Munich).

Intensive Care Unit Procedures in the Hypovolemic Patient

A common problem in the resuscitation of patients with intravascular volume depletion is that it may be necessary to perform procedures, such as line insertion and intubation, that require administration of sedative or anesthetic medications. In the setting of reduced circulating blood volume and maximal sympathetic tone, anesthesia is extremely hazardous, because sedative and induction agents block many of the compensatory mechanisms that are staving off circulatory collapse.[5]

Thus, it is vital to restore volume as much as possible prior to the administration of sedative agents. If the administration of sedative agents to the under-resuscitated patient is unavoidable, concomitant administration of vasopressor agents is essential. Positive-pressure ventilation in the setting of hypovolemia leads to the additional problem of increased P_{ra} secondary to the change in mean intrathoracic pressure from subatmospheric to positive. Venous return is therefore reduced both by lower P_{mcf} and increased P_{ra}. This effect is especially marked in the setting of decreased chest wall compliance (and hence greater transmission of airway pressures to pleural pressures and intrathoracic vessels), so is a major problem in pregnancy, morbid obesity, or exacerbations of asthma or chronic obstructive pulmonary disease. Hypovolemia in these conditions must be corrected before intubation.

Key Points

1. Intravascular volume depletion is defined by a decrease in the stressed blood volume.
2. Hemorrhage, plasma loss, and salt/water loss cause absolute volume deficit.
3. Vasodilatation causes relative volume deficit with manifestations similar to those of absolute intravascular volume depletion.
4. Physiological responses to intravascular volume depletion are complex.
5. Initiation of positive-pressure ventilation or administration of sedation can cause significant hemodynamic instability in patients with absolute or relative intravascular volume depletion. Preventive measures such as administration of vasoconstrictors and/or fluids are typically needed.

Key References

1. Rothe CF: Mean circulatory filling pressure: Its meaning and measurement. J Appl Physiol 1993;74:499-509.
4. Magder S, De Varennes B: Clinical death and the measurement of stressed vascular volume. Crit Care Med 1998;26:1061-1064.
10. Rothe CF, Drees JA: Vascular capacitance and fluid shifts in dogs during prolonged hemorrhagic hypotension. Circ Res 1976;38:347-356.
18. Rothe CF, Maass-Moreno R: Hepatic venular resistance responses to norepinephrine, isoproterenol, adenosine, histamine and ACh in rabbits. Am J Physiol Heart Circ Physiol 1998;274:H777-H785.
29. Kumar A, Anel R, Bunnell E, et al: Pulmonary artery occlusion pressure and central venous pressure fail to predict ventricular filling volume, cardiac performance, or the response to volume infusion in normal subjects. Crit Care Med 2004;32:691-699.

See the companion Expert Consult website for the complete reference list.

Specific Disorders

CHAPTER 98

Disorders of Sodium and Water Balance

Sean M. Bagshaw and Rinaldo Bellomo

OBJECTIVE

This chapter will:
1. Present a brief overview of normal water metabolism.
2. Discuss the diagnosis of and approach to hyponatremia.
3. Discuss the diagnosis of and approach to hypernatremia.

Disorders of sodium (Na⁺) and water balance are commonly encountered in critically ill patients.[1] Critical illness, multiple-organ dysfunction, fluid resuscitation, and the numerous additional interventions applied in the routine care of patients admitted to the intensive care unit can interfere with the complex mechanisms that maintain total body sodium and water homeostasis.[2]

Disorders of sodium and water balance are generally categorized as hypo-osmolar or hyperosmolar depending on the balance (i.e., excess or deficit, respectively) of total body water relative to total body sodium content. Because sodium is the primary extracellular constituent of serum osmolality, disorders of sodium and water balance can classically be recognized as hyponatremia and hypernatremia. Both of these disorders can contribute to significant morbidity and mortality, and given their prevalence in critically ill patients, clinicians must have a solid understanding of their pathophysiology, diagnosis, and management.

OVERVIEW OF SODIUM AND NORMAL WATER BALANCE

Under normal circumstances, the serum sodium concentration is preserved within a fine physiologic range despite large variations in daily sodium and water intake.

Sodium is the major extracellular cation in the body and the most important osmotically active solute. Sodium metabolism is narrowly regulated by the kidney through the interaction of numerous neurohormonal mechanisms, including the renin-angiotensin-aldosterone system, the sympathetic nervous system, and the presence of atrial natriuretic peptide and brain natriuretic peptide. In addition, sodium regulation is closely correlated with the body's *effective circulating volume* (ECV), defined as the

intravascular volume needed to provide adequate tissue perfusion. As a result, the major determinant of serum sodium is in fact the serum water content. Thus, disturbances in sodium balance most often reflect abnormalities in the ECV and serum water content.

Water metabolism, on the other hand, is regulated predominantly by arginine vasopressin (AVP) and strongly influenced by water intake and output. AVP is produced in the supraoptic and paraventricular hypothalamic nuclei and stored in the posterior pituitary. AVP secretion is tightly regulated by (1) changes in serum osmolality (as little as 1%-2%) that are detected by osmoreceptors in the anterior hypothalamus and (2) changes in mean arterial pressure and/or blood volume detected by baroreceptors in the aortic arch and carotid bodies. AVP controls the water permeability of the kidney by directing the insertion of aquaporin-2 (AQP-2) channels on the luminal surfaces of the distal tubules and collecting duct. AVP induces an increase in AQP-2 channels and acts to stimulate free water reabsorption and antidiuresis.

HYPONATREMIA

Hyponatremia is commonly defined as a serum sodium concentration less than 135 mmol/L; however, this definition may vary with different institutional laboratories. The presence of hyponatremia, for the most part, indicates an underlying disorder of an excess in body water relative to body sodium content, yet, less commonly, may result from a depletion of body sodium content in excess of concurrent body water losses.

Epidemiology

Hyponatremia is recognized as the most common electrolyte abnormality encountered in clinical medicine. Its prevalence in the United States is estimated between 3.2 and 6.1 million patients per year.[3] Of these, approximately 1% of cases are classified as acute and symptomatic, 4% as acute and asymptomatic, 15% to 20% as chronic and symptomatic, and 75% to 80% as chronic and asymptomatic. Moreover, an estimated 75% of patients with hyponatremia require treatment in the hospital, translating into a considerable burden on health resources.[3]

Epidemiological studies have found that hyponatremia occurs in approximately 1% to 2% of hospitalized patients.[4] However, the incidence varies according to the threshold for diagnosis and the population assessed. For example, hyponatremia (serum Na$^+$ ≤ 130 mmol/L) has been described in 4.4% of patients after surgery[5] and in nearly 30% of patients admitted to intensive care (serum Na$^+$ ≤ 134 mmol/L).[6] A variety of risk factors have been reported for hospital-acquired hyponatremia, including older age, diabetes mellitus with or without insulin therapy, chronic kidney disease, surgery, pulmonary infection, diuretic therapy, administration of antibiotics, opioid analgesia, and the use of hypotonic intravenous fluids.[7-9]

It is important also to recognize that hyponatremia, although common, is not a banal diagnosis and is associated with serious complications that have been linked to increased morbidity and mortality.[1,8,10-13] The presence of hyponatremia after an acute ST-elevation myocardial infarction, in congestive heart failure, and in cirrhosis has been found to predict mortality.[10-13] Similarly, in critically ill patients, severe hyponatremia (serum Na$^+$ < 125 mmol/L) has been found to be an independent predictor of hospital mortality, with an estimated risk for death approaching 40%.[1] The mortality rate has also been reported higher for patients in whom hyponatremia initially worsens after hospital admission.[8]

Clinical Presentation

Symptoms attributable to hyponatremia correlate both with the severity and rate of decline in serum sodium value and generally reflect neurological dysfunction induced by cerebral edema. A reduction in serum sodium creates an osmotic gradient that favors water movement into the brain. This increase in brain intracellular volume contributes to cerebral edema and raised intracranial pressure and leads to the appearance of neurological manifestations.

Mild hyponatremia (serum Na$^+$ 130-135 mmol/L) can often be asymptomatic; with further acute declines in serum sodium, however, overt symptoms become more apparent. Nonspecific symptoms, such as fatigue, malaise, nausea and unsteadiness, may occur with a serum sodium value in the range of 125 to 130 mmol/L. Rapid declines to a serum sodium value less than 115 to 120 mmol/L can provoke headache, restlessness, lethargy, and obtundation that may progress to seizures, coma, brainstem herniation, respiratory arrest, and death.[14]

Alternatively, in hyponatremia that evolves more gradually (i.e., over days or weeks), the serum sodium value may be much lower prior to the development of overt symptoms. This occurs because the brain undergoes a process of intracellular adaptation to preserve osmotic balance and prevent edema. Over hours to days, the brain transports osmoles (i.e. sodium, potassium, chloride) from the intracellular to the extracellular space, and later actively transports organic solutes (i.e., osmolytes), such as glutamine, glutamate, taurine, and myo-inositol. These activities help maintain osmotic balance by contributing to early water loss from the brain so as to attenuate subsequent hyponatremia-induced brain edema and, hence, lead to a greater threshold decline in serum sodium value before symptoms appear.

Diagnostic Approach

Hyponatremia can broadly be classified on the basis of serum osmolality into hypo-osmolar, iso-osmolar, and hyper-osmolar. The underlying cause of hyponatremia is usually evident after a thorough medical history, physical examination, and performance of selected serum and urinary tests, in particular the determinations of serum osmolality, urine osmolality, and urine sodium value. The medical history should be focused on presence of comorbid illnesses, acute illnesses, medications, and other therapies or interventions that have been applied that may predispose to the development of hyponatremia (Table 98-1). A focused physical examination should provide an estimate of volume status. A reduction in ECV may be suggested by orthostatic changes in heart rate and blood pressure, large variations in pulse pressure, low jugular or central venous pressure, and other surrogates such as reduced skin turgor, furrowed tongue, and dry mucous membranes or axilla. On the other hand, an expansion in ECV would be suggested by increased jugular or central venous pressure, pleural effusions, ascites, and peripheral edema.

Hypo-Osmolar Hyponatremia

Hypo-osmolar hyponatremia, which is most commonly encountered in critically ill patients, can generally be classified, according to an assessment of ECV, as hypovolemic, isovolemic, or hypervolemic.

HYPOVOLEMIC HYPO-OSMOLAR HYPONATREMIA. The simultaneous loss of solute and water from the extracellular space results in a reduced ECV and triggers the nonosmotic release of AVP in an attempt to restore vascular volume and attenuate free water loss. Subsequent intake of hypotonic fluids or free water by ingestion or infusion leads to hyponatremia. There are numerous conditions that contribute to true volume depletion, such as insensible fluid loss, gastrointestinal losses, hemorrhage, and renal fluid and solute losses (i.e., diuretics, mineralocorticoid deficiency, chronic nephropathies) (see Table 98-1). This form of hyponatremia has emerged as an important cause of morbidity in endurance athletes (i.e., marathon, ultramarathon, triathlon). One study found that an estimated 13% of runners in the 2002 Boston Marathon had serum sodium concentration values lower than 135 mmol/L, and approximately 1% had critical values lower than 120 mmol/L.[15] Moreover, the frequent use of nonsteroidal anti-inflammatory drugs may further compound hyponatremia in these athletes. In the absence of exposure to diuretics, true hypovolemia in such patients may be corroborated by demonstration of a urine sodium concentration less than 10 to 20 mmol/L.

Cerebral salt-wasting syndrome is a unique disorder of the hypothalamic-renal axis characterized by natriuresis and volume depletion followed by AVP-induced water retention. The resulting hyponatremia is typified by an inappropriately high urine osmolality, a high urine sodium (generally >40 mEq/L), and, if measured, an increased serum AVP level. Although the pathogenesis is not completely understood, increased sympathetic nervous system outflow along with raised levels of atrial and brain natriuretic peptides may, in part, mediate the inciting natriuresis and volume depletion. This syndrome typically occurs in critically ill patients with intracranial injury, often in association with subarachnoid hemorrhage or traumatic brain injury and less commonly after neurosurgical procedures, with glioma or with tuberculous or carcinomatous meningitis.[16] Cerebral salt-wasting syndrome is often difficult to differentiate from syndrome of inappropriate antidiuretic hormone (secretion) (SIADH), which is also

TABLE 98-1

Major Causes of Hyponatremia

Disorders causing hyponatremia associated with elevated arginine vasopressin (AVP)	Decreased effective circulating volume: True volume depletion Congestive heart failure Cirrhosis Diuretic therapy (e.g., thiazides) Syndrome of inappropriate antidiuretic hormone secretion Resetting of osmostat Endocrinological: Adrenal insufficiency Hypothyroidism Pregnancy
Disorders causing hyponatremia in which AVP may be appropriately suppressed	Advanced renal failure Primary polydipsia (i.e., associated with psychiatric illness or use of ecstasy) Malnutrition Beer-drinker's potomania
Disorders causing hyponatremia with normal or elevated plasma osmolality	High plasma osmolality: Hyperglycemia Mannitol Maltose (i.e., intravenous immune globulin) Normal plasma osmolality: pseudohyponatremia due to hyperlipidemia or hyperproteinemia Glycine or sorbitol solution: Transurethral prostate resection Hysterectomy

TABLE 98-2

Criteria for the Diagnosis of Syndrome of Inappropriate Antidiuretic Hormone Secretion

Major	Decreased extracellular fluid osmolality (<275 mOsm/kg H_2O) Inappropriately elevated urine osmolality (>100 and usually > 300 mOsm/kg H_2O) in context of normal kidney function Clinical euvolemia Urine Na^+ > 40 mEq/L Absence of hypothyroidism, hypocortisolism (primary or secondary), and diuretic use Relatively normal serum creatinine value Normal acid-base and potassium balances Low serum urea and serum uric acid levels
Minor	Abnormal water load test result Inappropriately elevated plasma arginine vasopressin level relative to plasma osmolality No significant correction of plasma Na^+ with volume expansion, but improvement after fluid restriction

Adapted from Adler SM, Verbalis JG: Disorders of body water homeostasis in critical illness. Endocrinol Metab Clin North Am 2006;35:873-894, xi.

common after neurologic injury; however, the key differentiation is that in cerebral salt-wasting syndrome, there is clear evidence of volume depletion and increased urine sodium excretion prior to development of hyponatremia, whereas in SIADH, patients are typically euvolemic or have mild volume expansion.[17]

ISOVOLEMIC HYPO-OSMOLAR HYPONATREMIA. There are several important causes of isovolemic hypo-osmolar hyponatremia, including SIADH, endocrinopathies such as adrenal insufficiency or hypothyroidism, and pregnancy.

SIADH is characterized by an inappropriate or persistent release of AVP that results in a decreased capacity for free water excretion. This syndrome is the most common cause of acquired hyponatremia in hospitalized patients.[4] The diagnostic criteria for SIADH are shown in Table 98-2. The major criteria for the diagnosis of SIADH are evidence of serum hypo-osmolality (<275 mOsm/kg) and a less than maximally dilute urine osmolality greater than 100 mOsm/kg. In addition, patients are euvolemic, have normal acid-base and potassium balances, and typically have urine sodium concentrations higher than 40 mmol/L. In general, SIADH is a diagnosis of exclusion and can be confirmed only in the context of normal kidney, thyroid, and adrenal function. Several conditions encountered in critically ill patients can lead to this syndrome. SIADH can be broadly categorized into disorders of the central nervous system, pulmonary disorders, disorders associated with medications or tumors, and a variety of miscellaneous causes (Table 98-3). Interestingly, in an estimated one third of patients with SIADH, the inappropriately elevated AVP is countered by a downward resetting of the osmostat to a serum sodium value typically in the range 125 to 130 mmol/L. These patients are often asymptomatic and achieve relative stability of serum sodium concentration.

As such, confirmation of the diagnosis is important and can have significant implications for subsequent therapy.

Adrenal insufficiency generally leads to hyponatremia because of an increased release of AVP and subsequent diminished water excretion. Cortisol deficiency may contribute to reductions in cardiac output and blood pressure, thus stimulating a nonosmotic release of AVP. In addition, AVP is an adrenocorticotropic hormone (ACTH) secretagogue, so AVP release may be stimulated as a result of an increased release of ACTH due to the lack of negative feedback from absent serum cortisol.[10] Similarly, aldosterone deficiency leads to sodium wasting and reductions in ECV, stimulating AVP release.

The pathophysiology of hyponatremia in hypothyroidism remains incompletely understood. Studies have suggested these patients have impairment of free water excretion due to inability to maximally suppress AVP secretion; however, this problem may be aggravated by declines in cardiac output that stimulate the nonosmotic release of AVP and by reductions in glomerular filtration that further impair free water clearance.[19]

During pregnancy, increased serum levels of human chorionic gonadotropin released from the placenta are believed to be associated with a downward-reset osmostat (≥5 mmol/L), leading to mild asymptomatic hyponatremia.[20]

HYPERVOLEMIC HYPO-OSMOLAR HYPONATREMIA. Several conditions can predispose to hypo-osmolar hyponatremia in the context of an excess of total body water and sodium. Congestive heart failure, cirrhosis, and chronic kidney disease (i.e., nephrotic syndrome) involve similar pathophysiology for the development of hyponatremia in edematous states.

Congestive heart failure is classically associated with extracellular fluid overload, but the reductions in cardiac output (and blood pressure) cause a relative reduction in ECV. These hemodynamic changes activate carotid baroreceptors that stimulate the nonosmotic release of AVP. Additionally, the impaired cardiac output contributes to reduced renal perfusion, which in turn activates the renin-angiotensin-aldosterone and sympathetic nervous

TABLE 98-3

Common Causes of Syndrome of Inappropriate Antidiuretic Hormone Secretion

Central nervous system disorders	Mass lesions (tumors, brain abscess, subdural hematoma)
	Inflammatory disorders (encephalitis, meningitis, systemic lupus erythematosus)
	Degenerative/demyelinative disorders (multiple sclerosis, Guillain-Barré syndrome)
	Other (subarachnoid hemorrhage, delirium tremens, traumatic brain injury, acute psychosis, postoperative pituitary stalk section, hydrocephalus)
Pulmonary disorders	Infections (bacterial/viral pneumonia, tuberculosis, empyema, aspergillosis)
	Mechanical/ventilatory problems (mechanical ventilation, noninvasive positive-pressure ventilation, chronic obstructive pulmonary disease, asthma, acute respiratory failure, pneumothorax, hypercapnia)
Medication-related causes	Stimulation of arginine vasopressin (AVP) release (nicotine, phenothiazines, tricyclic antidepressants)
	Direct renal effects or potentiation of AVP (desmopressin acetate, oxytocin, prostaglandin synthesis inhibitors)
	Mixed effects (angiotensin-converting enzyme inhibitors, carbamazepine, chlorpropamide, clozapine, cyclophosphamide, ecstasy, omeprazole, selective serotonin reuptake inhibitors, vincristine)
Tumor-related/paraneoplastic causes	Pulmonary/mediastinal disorders (bronchogenic carcinoma, mesothelioma, thymoma, lymphoma)
	Non-chest disorders (pancreatic carcinoma, nasopharyngeal carcinoma, leukemia)
Other causes	Acquired immunodeficiency syndrome
	Prolonged strenuous activity (e.g., marathon running)
	Senile atrophy
	Postoperative pain

systems. These mechanisms, along with concomitant diuretic therapy, all contribute to amplified renal sodium retention and a secondary decrease in free water excretion to restore intravascular ECV to normal. However, this maladaptive positive feedback leads to dilutional hyponatremia associated with progressive hypervolemia.[21]

Advanced cirrhosis is typically characterized by significant splanchnic and systemic vasodilatation. This leads to relative reductions in ECV, nonosmotic release of AVP, and diminished capacity for free water excretion, leading to serum sodium values less than 125 to 130 mmol/L in up to 50% of patients. The increase in AVP secretion and, thus, the level of hyponatremia, is often proportional to the underlying progression and severity of cirrhosis.[22] Diuretic therapy, often used to treat ascites, can worsen hyponatremia in cirrhotic patients by reducing ECV, stimulating compensatory increases in AVP release, and further impairing free water excretion.

In advanced chronic kidney disease (stage IV and beyond), the reduction in nephron mass and glomerular filtration are associated with progressive impairments in capacity for maximal urine dilution and free water excretion such that water retention commonly predisposes to hyponatremia.

Primary polydipsia is characterized by an abnormal thirst stimulus leading to an increase and/or excess of free water intake. It is often found in psychiatric illness or with prescription of antipsychotic medications that cause a dry mouth.[23] Infrequently, primary polydipsia can occur from infiltrative diseases of the hypothalamus (e.g., sarcoidosis) that disrupt the normal sensation of thirst.[24] Severe hyponatremia has also been described after acute water intoxication in workers undergoing urine drug testing.[25] In these circumstances, water intake exceeds the renal capacity for excretion despite a maximally dilute urine (i.e., osmolality < 100 mOsm/kg). Ingestion of the recreation drug ecstasy (3,4-methyldioxymethamphetamine [MDMA]) has also been associated with severe acute hyponatremia.[26] The underlying pathophysiology is thought to result from a large free water intake coupled with SIADH.

Poor dietary intake of solute can directly impair capacity for free water excretion and lead to dilutional hyponatremia. This may be encountered in patients with chronic alcoholism (i.e., beer potomania) or malnutrition.[27,28] These patients have appropriately dilute urine, but because of a low intake of solute (i.e., sodium and potassium), the daily solute excretion decreases to less than 200 to 250 mOsm/kg (normal, 600-900 mOsm/kg) and leads to a reduction in the maximal achievable urine output.

Hyperosmolar Hyponatremia

The accumulation of osmotically active particles in the plasma induces an osmotic efflux of water from the intracellular space to the extracellular space, resulting in both hyponatremia and hyperosmolality. This condition is often encountered with marked hyperglycemia (i.e., diabetic ketoacidosis, hyperosmolar nonketotic hyperglycemia), and less commonly with use of mannitol, glycerol, or sorbitol and the administration of radiocontrast media. Similarly, hyperosmolar hyponatremia has also been described with the use of intravenous immune globulin suspended in 10% maltose solution.[29]

The calculation to correct the serum sodium concentration for hyperglycemia was shown on average as a decrease of 2.4 mmol/L in serum sodium concentration per 5.6-mmol/L increase in serum glucose concentration; however, this relationship was nonlinear and could vary.[30] In addition, this calculation is not ideal but, rather, at best an estimate, because of its failure to consider ongoing water loss from osmotic diuresis and the influence of insulin administration, both of which contribute to the increase in serum sodium concentration.

Iso-Osmolar Hyponatremia

Iso-osmolar hyponatremia can occur with the accumulation of isotonic non–sodium-containing fluid in the extracellular space or with marked elevations in serum compounds such as proteins and lipids (i.e., pseudohyponatremia).

Transurethral resections of prostate or bladder tumors often require use of large volumes of glycine or sorbitol-containing flushing solutions. As a consequence, variable amounts of such fluids can be absorbed either directly through large prostatic veins or indirectly via leaked fluid into the retroperitoneal space, leading to a significant dilutional reduction in serum sodium concentration.[31] Postoperative declines in serum sodium to less than 100 to 110 mmol/L have been described and have been associated with serious neurological sequelae and death.[31] Similar problems have been described with the use of large-volume glycine irrigation during hysterectomy.[32] This diagnosis is supported by the finding of a large serum osmolal gap (≥30-40 mOsm/kg). A normal serum osmolal gap, 5 to 10 mOsm/kg, is determined by the laboratory measured serum osmolality minus the calculated serum osmolality. The serum osmolality can be estimated by the following equation:

$$\text{Serum osmolality} = (2 \times \text{serum Na}^+) + \text{serum glucose} + \text{serum urea}$$

The normal content of serum is approximately 93% water and 7% nonaqueous substances, principally proteins and lipids. In general, the nonaqueous proportion of serum does not influence osmolality. However, in disorders causing marked elevations in serum proteins (e.g., multiple myeloma, hypergammaglobulinemia) or lipid content (e.g., hypertriglyceridemia, elevated chylomicrons), the nonaqueous proportion of serum is increased relative to the aqueous portion, leading to an artifactual decrease in serum sodium concentration (i.e., pseudohyponatremia) despite there having been no actual change to serum sodium or serum osmolality. This problem has largely been overcome by the use of ion-selective electrodes that directly measure serum sodium concentration.

HYPERNATREMIA

Hypernatremia is typically defined as a serum sodium concentration higher than 145 mmol/L; like hyponatremia, however, this definition may vary with different laboratories. The presence of hypernatremia, by and large, indicates a relative deficit of body water in relation to body sodium content; less commonly, however, it can also be induced by the administration of an excess sodium load relative to water.

Epidemiology

Hypernatremia (serum Na$^+$ > 148 mmol/L) has been reported to occur in an estimated 1% of hospitalized elderly patients.[33,34] This incidence will fluctuate, however, depending on the threshold serum sodium concentration and the population being evaluated. Of critically ill patients, hypernatremia (serum Na$^+$ ≥ 150 mmol/L) has been reported in an approximately 9% at the time of admission and has developed in an additional 5.7% during the course of intensive care.[35]

Several factors have been associated with an increased risk of hypernatremia, including older age, prior brain injury, diabetes mellitus, surgery, diuretic therapy, and altered mental status.[33-35] Most hypernatremia is hospital-acquired (iatrogenic) and can be attributed to inadequate or inappropriate prescription of fluid therapy to patients with identifiable water losses, impaired thirst, or reduced access to free water.[34]

As with hyponatremia, a diagnosis of hypernatremia has been associated with an increased risk of hospital death.[33,34,36] However, it may be difficult to separate the contribution to mortality of hypernatremia alone from that of the underlying disease process and overall illness severity. Nonetheless, mortality has been shown to be higher for critically ill patients with hypernatremia (serum Na$^+$ ≥ 150 mmol/L). In addition, the risk of hospital death was greater for patients with hospital-acquired than for those who had hypernatremia at the time of admission to the intensive care unit.[35] The prognosis for patients presenting with more extreme hypernatremia (serum Na$^+$ > 180-200 mmol/L) may be poor.[37] Survival has been described,[38-40] particularly in children,[41] although survivors may have residual and permanent neurological disability.[42]

Clinical Presentation

The clinical manifestations of hypernatremia are principally neurological and correlate with both the severity and the rapidity of onset of the change in serum sodium concentration. The rise in serum sodium concentration leads to movement of water from the brain intracellular space to the extracellular compartment. Large shifts in brain water content can decrease brain volume and predispose to vascular damage and intracerebral and/or subarachnoid hemorrhage, and can potentially lead to irreversible neurological injury. Although typically described as a late complication after rapid correction of hyponatremia, osmotic myelinolysis has infrequently been described with acute severe hypernatremia.[43]

Initial symptoms may be subtle and nonspecific; they include anorexia, restlessness, irritability, lethargy, muscle weakness, and nausea. These can progress to more serious manifestations such as hyperreflexia, seizures, and coma. Severe symptoms are generally seen after sudden and large elevations of serum sodium concentration to 158 to 160 mmol/L.[44]

Elevations in serum sodium concentration typically generate an intense sensation of thirst that acts to protect against the neurological injury associated with severe hypernatremia. This normal physiological response, however, may be impaired in patients with an altered mental status or with hypothalamic lesions attenuating their sense of thirst (i.e., hypodipsia/adipsia). Older age is also associated with a diminished osmotic stimulation for thirst that may further predispose to reduced capability to replace water loss.[45,46]

Diagnostic Approach

Hypernatremia can be broadly categorized according to the etiological factors involved, including free water depletion that is unreplaced (i.e., reduced ECV or dehydration), hypodipsia, and an excess intake sodium or hypertonic solution (i.e., expanded ECV) (Table 98-4).

The cause of hypernatremia is typically evident from routine history and physical findings, although additional diagnostic tests of the AVP-renal axis may be needed to establish the diagnosis. In general, an increase in serum

TABLE 98-4

Major Causes of Hypernatremia

Unreplaced water depletion (in excess of body sodium)	Insufficient water intake:
	    Water unavailable
	    Impaired thirst (hypodipsia/adipsia, age-related)
	    Neurologic deficit (impaired mental status, hypothalamic lesion)
	Hypotonic fluid depletion:
	    Diabetes insipidus:
	        Central (impaired arginine vasopressin [AVP] secretion)
	        Nephrogenic (impaired renal effect AVP)
	    Renal losses:
	        Osmotic diuresis (glucose, mannitol, urea, intravenous immune globulin)
	        Diuretics (furosemide, thiazides)
	        Postobstructive diuresis
	    Nonrenal losses:
	        Insensible losses (dermal, respiratory)
	        Gastrointestinal losses (diarrhea, vomiting, nasogastric suction)
	        Peritoneal dialysis

Transient water shift into cells	Severe exercise Seizures

Sodium overload (in excess of body water)	Hypertonic sodium solutions:
	    Excess sodium administration (3% NaCl, 0.9% NaCl, sodium bicarbonate)
	    Ingestion of seawater
	Other hypertonic solutions: hyperalimentation (intravenous, parenteral)
	Primary hyperaldosteronism
	Cushing's syndrome

sodium concentration to more than 145 mmol/L or serum osmolality to more than 295 mOsm/kg H$_2$O represents a potent stimulus for sufficient AVP secretion to cause maximal concentration of urine to more than 700 to 800 mOsm/kg H$_2$O. Exogenous administration of more AVP would likely result in no further increase in urine osmolality. Hypernatremia in the context of maximally concentrated urine generally suggests that insufficient water intake, hypotonic insensible or gastrointestinal losses, or sodium overload is responsible. The measurement of urinary sodium may further aid in discriminating between reduced ECV and sodium overload. In conditions of reduced ECV, the urinary sodium concentration is typically less than 25 mEq/L, whereas in circumstances of sodium overload, urinary sodium concentration is often more than 100 mEq/L.

Alternatively, a serum sodium concentration above 145 mmol/L or serum osmolality value exceeding 295 mOsm/kg H$_2$O associated with a urine osmolality value less than 700 to 800 mOsm/kg H$_2$O suggests a defect in the capability for urine concentration. More specifically, if the urine osmolality is less than the serum osmolality, a diagnosis of either central (AVP deficiency) or nephrogenic (AVP insensitivity) diabetes insipidus (DI) is confirmed. These conditions can be distinguished by administration of exogenous AVP (i.e., DDAVP, 10 µg intranasally or vasopressin 5 µg subcutaneously). In central DI, urine osmolality increases by 50% or more, whereas no significant change occurs in nephrogenic DI.

Insufficient Water Intake

Hypernatremia due to inadequate water intake is usually a consequence of insufficient access to free water, impairment or alteration of the sensation of thirst, or neurological injury with alterations in mental status. Inadequate access to free water, particularly in hospitalized patients, is probably more common than appreciated. For instance, in one observational study, 86% of hospitalized, mostly elderly patients with hypernatremia were shown to have inadequate access to water.[34]

In addition, there are likely age-related declines in thirst (i.e., hypodipsia/adipsia). For example, in response to a study involving 24 hours of water deprivation, and despite increases in serum osmolality, serum sodium, and vasopressin levels, elderly men experienced less thirst and lower water intake than younger adults.[45,46]

True deficits in thirst and osmoregulation, however, are more likely to occur in patients with acquired hypothalamic structural lesions from conditions such as traumatic brain injury, tumors, granulomatous infiltration (i.e., sarcoid), and vascular disease.[47]

Certainly, age-related declines in thirst and hypodipsia from hypothalamic lesions would be aggravated in patients with any condition causing an alteration in mental status (e.g., delirium) or with significant neurologic injury (e.g., stroke).

Diabetes Insipidus

In general, a urine osmolality value lower than 800 mOsm/kg in the setting of an elevated serum osmolality (>295 mOsm/kg) or hypernatremia (serum sodium ≥145 mol/L) indicates a renal concentrating defect. In the absence of another cause to account for the high urine osmolality, such as osmotic diuresis, this finding generally reflects the presence of DI.

Central diabetes insipidus refers to polyuria and a urine concentration defect as a consequence of a deficiency of AVP secretion from the hypothalamic-pituitary axis. True central DI is uncommon, and most cases can be linked to lesions or to injury to the hypothalamus such as after pituitary surgery, traumatic brain injury, aneurysmal subarachnoid hemorrhage, brain death, or, with tumors, granulomatous infiltration or autoimmune disease (Table 98-5). Damage to the neurohypophyseal stalk during neurosurgery or by trauma can result in a classic triphasic response.[48] This syndrome typically manifests as early (<24 hours) postoperative polyuria lasting 3 to 5 days that reflects inhibition of AVP release due to hypothalamic dysfunction. The second phase is characterized by release of stored AVP from the posterior pituitary, which often results in hyponatremia. Finally, the third phase can again be characterized by central DI as a result of hypothalamic dysfunction; it can be permanent and usually occurs in 5 to 10 days once stored AVP is completely depleted from the posterior pituitary gland.

Nephrogenic diabetes insipidus refers to polyuria and a urine concentration defect due to renal resistance to the antidiuretic effects of AVP. There are hereditary forms of nephrogenic DI, but they are usually encountered in children and less commonly in critically ill patients. Hereditary nephrogenic DI can result from either gene mutations to the AVP-2 receptor or to the AQP-2 water channels. Acquired nephrogenic DI is typically related either to AVP resistance at the site of action in the distal tubule or collecting ducts or to interference in the medullary

TABLE 98-5

Differential Diagnosis of Central Diabetes Insipidus

Idiopathic/autoimmune
Primary neurologic:
  Neurosurgery (usually transsphenoidal)
  Traumatic brain injury
  Aneurysmal subarachnoid hemorrhage
  Hypoxic/ischemic encephalopathy
  Brain death
Tumors:
  Leukemia
  Lymphoma
  Metastatic lung cancer
Infiltrative disorders:
  Histiocytosis X/eosinophilic granuloma
  Sarcoidosis
  Wegener's granulomatosis
  Autoimmune lymphocytic hypophysitis
Other:
  Anorexia nervosa
  Acute fatty liver of pregnancy
  Postsupraventricular tachycardia
  Familial/Wolfram's syndrome

TABLE 98-6

Differential Diagnosis of Nephrogenic Diabetes Insipidus

Drug-related causes	Lithium
	Antibiotic agents:
	Demeclocycline
	Ofloxacin
	Rifampin
	Netilmicin
	Antifungal agent: amphotericin B
	Antiviral agents:
	Cidofovir
	Foscarnet
	Indinavir
	Tenofovir
	Antineoplastic agents:
	Cyclophosphamide
	Ifosfamide
	Methotrexate
	Other drugs:
	Radiocontrast agents
	Colchicine
	Ethanol
	Orlistat
Metabolic abnormalities	Hypokalemia
	Hypercalcemia
Other conditions	Sjögren's syndrome
	Sickle cell disease
	Release of urinary tract obstruction
	Amyloidosis
	Pregnancy

Modified from Garofeanu CG, Weir M, Rosas-Arellano MP, et al: Causes of reversible nephrogenic diabetes insipidus: A systematic review. Am J Kidney Dis 2005;45:626-637.

countercurrent mechanism causing impairment of renal concentrating capacity. Lithium toxicity and metabolic abnormalities, particularly hypokalemia and hypercalcemia, are the most common causes of acquired nephrogenic DI, although numerous other causes have been implicated (Table 98-6).[49] Long-term lithium therapy can lead to polyuria and impairment of renal concentrating defects in an estimated 20% to 30% and to DI in 10% to 12% of patients due to the downregulation of AVP-2 receptors and/or reduced expression of AQP-2 channels.[50,51] Hypercalcemia (serum Ca^+ > 2.75 mmol/L) can impair maximal urine-concentrating capacity by causing a reversible defect in sodium and chloride reabsorption in the ascending loop of Henle and by decreased expression and/or function of AQP-2 channels. As with lithium and hypercalcemia, persistent hypokalemia (serum potassium < 2.5 mmol/L) can decrease the renal responsiveness to AVP through reduced AQP-2 expression and/or function and diminished reabsorption of sodium and chloride in the thick ascending loop of Henle.

Other Renal Hypotonic Fluid Losses

There are several additional renal causes of hypotonic fluid losses.

Osmotic diuresis is caused by an excess of urinary solute, typically nonreabsorbable, that induces polyuria and hypotonic fluid loss. Osmotic diuresis can result from hyperglycemia (i.e., diabetic ketoacidosis), use of mannitol, increased serum urea, or administration of other hypertonic therapies.

The use of diuretics (i.e., loop or thiazide diuretics) is also common in critically ill patients and can contribute to hypotonic urinary fluid losses.

The relief of complete postrenal urinary obstruction can initially be associated with a large diuresis. Although much of this diuresis may be appropriate, there may also be a mild urine-concentrating defect due to downregulation of AQP-2 channels that can predispose to significant hypotonic fluid loss.

Nonrenal Hypotonic Fluid Losses

Insensible fluid losses from the skin (i.e., sweat) and respiratory tract (i.e., evaporation) are generally hypotonic to serum. Hence, hypernatremia will ensue in circumstances of increased insensible fluid loss such as fever, diaphoresis or tachypnea if losses are not replaced. Critically ill patients with burns or post-operative patients with open abdominal or other surgical wounds may be at risk for greater insensible fluid loss and need to be monitored accordingly.

Fluid losses from the gastrointestinal tract are also generally hypotonic to serum, and thus, if not replaced, will lead to hypernatremia. These losses can occur from vomiting, nasogastric drainage, enterocutaneous fistulas, or diarrhea. The use of osmotic cathartic agents (i.e., lactulose) or various oral medication suspensions (i.e., sorbitol) can also lead to hypotonic fluid losses.

Water Shift into Cells

Transient hypernatremia can be induced by intense exercise or during prolonged seizure activity.[52,53] This phenomenon typically occurs in the context of marked lactic acidosis and can transiently raise serum sodium concentration by 10 to 15 mmol/L. The breakdown of glycogen into osmotically more active solutes acutely raises intracellular osmolality and as a consequence induces a shift of hypotonic fluid from the extracellular to the intracellular compartment. The serum sodium generally returns to normal within 10 to 15 minutes and is not associated with any apparent sequelae.

Sodium Overload

Acute and often severe hypernatremia can be induced by administration of hypertonic sodium-containing solutions or by a massive ingestion of salt.

In critically ill patients, the administration of sodium bicarbonate for a range of conditions, such as metabolic acidosis, tricyclic antidepressant overdose, and rhabdomyolysis, can potentially lead to hypervolemic hypernatremia. Similarly, hypernatremia can occur with use of hypertonic saline to manage, for instance, intracranial hypertension in traumatic brain injury.

Enteral nutrition with hyperosmolar or high-protein feeds accompanied by insufficient free water may lead to hypernatremia, particularly in patients receiving long-term nutritional support.

Numerous reports of severe hypernatremia in patients after surgery with hypertonic saline irrigation for hydatid cysts (*Echinococcus granulosus*) have been reported.[54-56] Iatrogenic hospital-acquired hypernatremia has also been reported with the use of hypertonic saline in gastric lavage and of hypertonic saline-soaked wound packs for gas gangrene.[57,58]

There are also numerous reports of accidental or nonaccidental acute salt poisoning and extreme hypernatremia due to massive ingestion of table salt or the use of salt or hypertonic saline as an emetic.[59,60]

CONCLUSIONS

Critically ill patients commonly have disorders of sodium and water balance that are often iatrogenic. These disorders are generally categorized as hypo-osmolar or hyperosmolar, depending on the balance (i.e., excess or deficit) of total body water relative to total body sodium content and more classically recognized as hyponatremia and hypernatremia. These disorders may represent a surrogate for increased neurohormonal activation, organ dysfunction, and worsening severity of illness or progression of underlying chronic disease. Hyponatremia and hypernatremia both require timely recognition and appropriate intervention to prevent increases in the morbidity and mortality that accompany these disorders.

Key Points

1. Disorders of sodium and water balance are common in hospitalized and critically ill patients.
2. Disorders of sodium and water balance may represent a surrogate for underlying illness severity or progression of chronic disease.
3. Hyponatremia and hypernatremia are associated with an increase in morbidity and mortality.
4. SIADH is the most common cause of hyponatremia in hospitalized patients.
5. Most cases of hypernatremia are iatrogenic and often attributed to inappropriately prescribed fluid therapy.

Key References

2. Adler SM, Verbalis JG: Disorders of body water homeostasis in critical illness. Endocrinol Metab Clin North Am 2006;35:873-894, xi.
6. DeVita MV, Gardenswartz MH, Konecky A, Zabetakis PM: Incidence and etiology of hyponatremia in an intensive care unit. Clin Nephrol 1990;34:163-166.
9. Hoorn EJ, Lindemans J, Zietse R: Development of severe hyponatremia in hospitalized patients: Treatment-related risk factors and inadequate management. Nephrol Dial Transplant 2006;21:70-76.
34. Palevsky PM, Bhagrath R, Greenberg A: Hypernatremia in hospitalized patients. Ann Intern Med 1996;124:197-203.
35. Polderman KH, Schreuder WO, Strack van Schijndel RJ, Thijs LG: Hypernatremia in the intensive care unit: An indicator of quality of care? Crit Care Med 1999;27:1105-1108.

See the companion Expert Consult website for the complete reference list.

CHAPTER 99

Disorders of Potassium Balance

Isabelle Plamondon and Martine Leblanc

OBJECTIVES

This chapter will:
1. Identify factors affecting intracellular and extracellular potassium balance and explain the mechanisms of potassium excretion.
2. Describe the clinical manifestations of hypokalemia and hyperkalemia.
3. Classify main causes of hypokalemia and hyperkalemia in acutely ill patients.
4. Briefly summarize the treatment of hypokalemia and hyperkalemia.

DISTRIBUTION AND FUNCTION OF POTASSIUM

Potassium, the most abundant cation in the intracellular fluid, serves several functions crucial to the normal working of cells. More than 98% of body potassium is intracellular ($\approx$3000 mEq), whereas less than 2% is contained in the extracellular fluid ($\approx$60 mEq). The intracellular potassium concentration is approximately 140 to 150 mmol/L (140-150 mEq/L), whereas the normal serum potassium concentration is near 4 mmol/L. In order to maintain an intracellular concentration of 140 mmol/L and an extracellular concentration of 4 mmol/L, the Na^+,K^+-ATPase pumps sodium out of the cells and potassium into the cells. Thus, the entry of potassium in the cell is an active transport via the Na^+,K^+-ATPase, whereas exit from the cell occurs by passive diffusion. Insulin and aldosterone, both catecholamines, can stimulate the activity of Na^+,K^+-ATPase and therefore promote an intracellular potassium shift.

The potassium concentration gradient across cell membranes—the ratio of intracellular potassium ($[K]_i$) to extracellular potassium ($[K]_e$) is about 35—is the major determinant of the resting membrane potential, which is near −90 millivolts. Potassium is essential for conductance in excitable fibers in neural, cardiac, and muscular cells; it is also essential for cell metabolism and contributes to the synthesis of structural proteins, enzymes, and hormones. Furthermore, potassium is involved in cell volume adjustments and in intracellular pH regulation.

The extracellular potassium concentration is kept within physiologic limits by the maintenance of the internal and the external balance. Normally, the daily potassium intake (≈100 mEq) is excreted mainly via the renal route, because less than 10% is eliminated via stools and sudation. If the intake varies widely, kidneys adapt their excretion, but not as rapidly as for sodium and water.

FACTORS INFLUENCING INTRACELLULAR AND EXTRACELLULAR POTASSIUM BALANCE

Several mechanisms exist to maintain the total body potassium content and the distribution of potassium between intracellular and extracellular compartments. Table 99-1 summarizes the major factors involved in regulation of potassium balance.

In chronic renal failure, the activity of the Na^+,K^+-ATPase pump is impaired, leading to the potential development of hyperkalemia. Maintenance of basal epinephrine and insulin activity is necessary for normal potassium homeostasis. Stimulation of β_2-adrenergic receptors by epinephrine and other β_2 agonists enhances the Na^+,K^+-ATPase pump, whereas α-adrenergic receptor stimulation impairs the cellular entry of potassium. Insulin has the ability to promote potassium uptake by muscle and liver cells; this effect is independent of the hypoglycemic activity of insulin. After a meal, insulin stimulates Na^+,K^+-ATPase activity, allowing a shift of the absorbed potassium into

the cells to avoid hyperkalemia. This transcellular redistribution is achieved a few minutes after a potassium load to avoid dangerous increases in plasma potassium concentrations, because renal excretion takes several hours. Insulin deficiency can induce hyperkalemia, and hyperkalemia can develop during hyperglycemia in diabetic patients.

Aldosterone is essential for potassium excretion by the kidney. However, mineralocorticoid stimulation can enhance cellular uptake of potassium and increase potassium secretion in the colon.[1] Glucocorticoids increase the number of Na^+,K^+-ATPase in muscle, and high-dose glucocorticoids also have a small mineralocorticoid effect.[2]

Serum potassium concentration by itself has an impact on distribution of potassium. In situations of hyperkalemia, potassium tends to enter the cell, probably by a passive mechanism, whereas in situations of hypokalemia, potassium tends to exit the cell. There is an inverse relationship between extracellular fluid pH and potassium serum concentration. In metabolic acidosis, potassium shifts from the intracellular compartment to the extracellular compartment as the hydrogen ion enters the cells to be buffered. In metabolic alkalosis, the process is reversed. Respiratory acidosis and alkalosis have little impact on potassium distribution. Even small changes in plasma osmolality can induce major changes in the internal potassium balance by relatively simple mechanisms. As water flows out of the cell in conditions of hyperosmolality, potassium follows the convective current (solvent-drag effect). Moreover, because potassium exits less readily than water, the intracellular concentration of potassium rises. This higher intracellular potassium concentration will favor the exit of potassium via potassium channels.

Finally, the rate of cell production and breakdown can affect the transcellular balance of potassium; a rapid cell production can cause potassium shift into the cells, whereas cell breakdown may lead to potassium efflux to the extracellular fluid.

POTASSIUM EXCRETION

The kidney is the main elimination pathway for the daily potassium intake. Almost 90% of the filtered potassium load is reabsorbed, passively in the proximal tubule and by the Na^+-K^+-$2Cl^-$ cotransporter in the loop of Henle. Most of urinary potassium excretion occurs through secretion in the distal nephron (connecting segment, cortical collecting tubule, and outer medullary collecting tubule) after aldosterone activity and is influenced by both distal sodium and water delivery and plasma potassium concentration. Indeed, distal sodium and water delivery is crucial; rapid distal tubular flow increases the potassium concentration gradient between tubular and intracellular fluid as the potassium secreted is washed away and replaced by potassium-depleted fluid. Increased distal sodium delivery enhances absorption of sodium in the distal nephron, promoting potassium secretion to maintain electroneutrality.

The Na^+,K^+-ATPase pump induces a potassium and sodium concentration gradient between the tubular fluid and the cell; sodium entry into the cells via sodium channels creates an electrical gradient favorable to potassium efflux from the cell into tubular fluid (Fig. 99-1). Sodium reabsorption creates a lumen-negative electrical gradient that is partially counteracted by chloride passive absorption via the paracellular route. The time lag between

TABLE 99-1

Majors Factors Involved in Regulation of Potassium Balance

Intracellular to extracellular shift	Epinephrine (via β_2-adrenergic receptors)
	Insulin
	Serum potassium concentration
	Metabolic acid-base status
Renal secretion by collecting tubule	Aldosterone
	Serum potassium concentration
	Distal water and sodium delivery

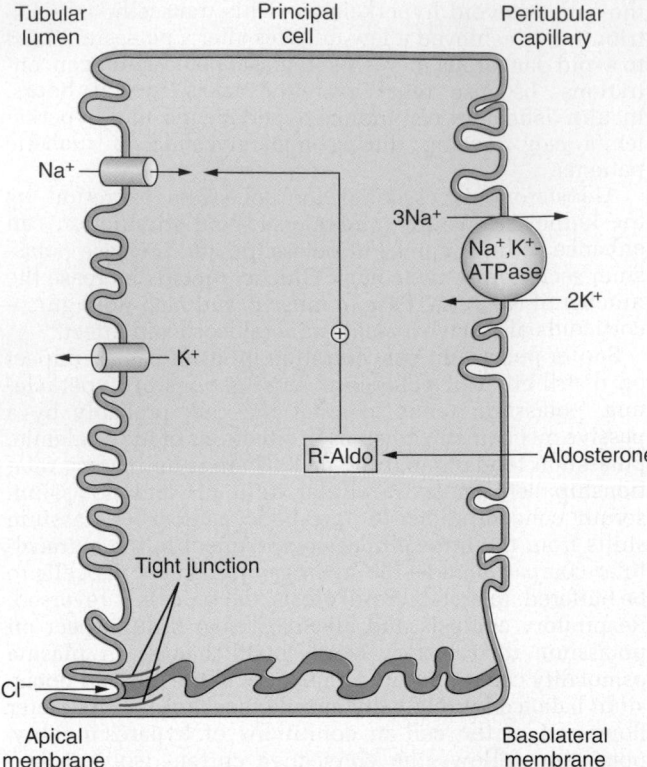

FIGURE 99-1. Transport pathways for potassium secretion in the principal cell in the collecting tubule. R-Aldo, cytosolic receptor for aldosterone.

sodium reabsorption and chloride reabsorption is responsible for the transepithelial potential difference that favors potassium secretion.

The acid-base status has also a significant effect on renal potassium excretion. Extracellular pH alters potassium uptake at the basolateral border of potassium-secretory cells, hence influencing intracellular potassium concentration and the driving force for secretion. In acidosis, activity of the basolateral Na^+,K^+-ATPase is decreased, leading to a reduction in cell potassium and secretion of potassium. Acid-secreting type A intercalated cells can actively reabsorb potassium via the H^+,K^+-ATPase pump in conditions of potassium depletion. The activity of the pump is decreased after a potassium load. Alkalosis favors potassium secretion.

ALTERATIONS OF SERUM POTASSIUM

Alterations of serum potassium are relatively common in hospitalized patients; 20% of patients have hypokalemia, whereas 1% to 10% experience hyperkalemia.[3-6] Disorders of serum potassium level are more often the consequences of an abnormal external balance—for instance, positive balance from an increased intake or reduced excretion or negative balance from a reduced intake or increased excretion. However, the internal balance may be disturbed in the following circumstances during critical illness: by potassium release following cell destruction, by metabolic acid-base disorders, and by hormonal influence.

Hypokalemia

Hypokalemia is defined as a serum concentration below 3.5 mmol/L.

Causes of Hypokalemia

The three different mechanisms that may be responsible for the development of hypokalemia are (1) reduction in potassium intake, (2) increase in renal or digestive losses, and (3) redistribution of potassium from the extracellular to the intracellular compartment (without changing overall body content). Increased renal losses remain the most common cause of hypokalemia.

DECREASED POTASSIUM INTAKE. Decreased potassium intake is rarely the sole cause of hypokalemia; it usually may be a contributing component with other causes, such as diuretic use.

POTASSIUM SHIFT INTO CELLS. The Na^+,K^+-ATPase pump maintains potassium distribution between the different compartments. An increase in the activity of the pump can cause transient hypokalemia without a decrease in total body potassium. Insulin promotes Na^+,K^+-ATPase activity, thus inducing potassium movement into the cells. In diabetic ketoacidosis and a nonketoacidosis hyperosmolar state, plasma potassium concentration rapidly falls after the administration of insulin. A glucose load stimulates insulin secretion and may predispose to hypokalemia, as in the refeeding syndrome. When potassium supplements are administered in dextrose solutions, they may not correct hypokalemia as optimally and may transiently reduce serum potassium concentration.

Since β_2-adrenergic receptor stimulation increases Na^+, K^+-ATPase pump activity, stressful situations, such as coronary ischemia, alcohol withdrawal, and acute illness, associated with an increase in endogenous catecholamines may induce a drop in serum potassium level, usually by 0.5 to 0.6 mmol/L. β-Adrenergic agonists given for treatment of asthma or heart failure or for the prevention of premature labor can induce a reduction in serum potassium level of 0.5 to 1 mmol/L. Augmentation in adrenaline not only stimulates β_2-adrenergic receptors but also promotes insulin secretion through a direct effect on the pancreas and glycolysis.

During alkalosis, there is an efflux of hydrogen ion out of the cell to buffer the extracellular pH. As hydrogen leaves a cell, potassium moves into the cell to maintain its electroneutrality. Extracellular pH has also an effect on renal potassium handling; alkalosis favors potassium excretion.

Hypokalemic periodic paralysis is a rare genetic disease characterized by severe hypokalemia secondary to transcellular shift. Precipitating events include a high carbohydrate intake, rest after strenuous exercise, alcohol consumption, obstetric delivery, infection, trauma, cold exposure, and emotional stress, all situations that may induce a release in insulin and/or epinephrine. Between transient episodes, serum potassium level remains normal. The clinical picture is muscle weakness and even total flaccid paralysis that initially involves proximal muscles before spreading distally but spares the muscles responsible for ventilation, deglutition, and ocular movements. Rare variants exist—thyrotoxic periodic paralysis, which affects mostly Asian men in the third and fourth decades, and Andersen's syndrome, an autosomal dominant disorder characterized by dysmorphic features, prolonged QT interval, ventricular arrhythmias, and periodic paralysis.

Rapid cell production after administration of vitamin B_{12} (folic acid) or granulocyte-macrophage colony-stimulating factor can induce hypokalemia. A false-positive hypokalemia in people with acute myeloid leukemia has been reported in which very active cells can capture the extracellular potassium after blood sampling.

Barium intoxication produces a clinical picture of flaccid skeletal paralysis, hypertension, vomiting, diarrhea, cardiac arrhythmias, and, potentially, respiratory paralysis.[7] Hypothermia and chloroquine intoxication are other rare causes of hypokalemia induced by potassium redistribution.[8,9]

INCREASED RENAL EXCRETION. Potassium wasting is due to exaggerated secretion in the distal nephron. The main factors are hyperaldosteronism with maintained distal flow and increased distal flow with normal or high aldosterone levels.

INCREASED EXTRARENAL LOSS. Secretions of the lower gastrointestinal tract are relatively high in potassium (20 to 50 mmol/L), whereas gastric secretions contain less potassium (concentrations between 5 and 10 mmol/L). In diarrhea, the potassium concentration in stool decreases as water content increases, but the enlarged volume explains the ensuing hypokalemia. Hypokalemia during vomiting or tube drainage is subsequent to increased renal losses. Profuse sudation during heat stress can result in potassium depletion with secondary hyperaldosteronism from hypovolemia and, thus, further potassium loss via increased renal excretion. Plasmapheresis with albumin replacement may cause hypokalemia through a dilution effect, because plasma is not substituted by a solution with an equivalent potassium concentration.

Clinical Manifestations

True total body potassium depletion is more often responsible for pathological consequences than low serum concentration due to a shift effect. Muscular weakness, general malaise, restless leg syndrome, cramps, and myalgias are common complaints with a serum potassium concentration below 3.0 mmol/L.

When the serum potassium level is less than 2.5 mmol/L, muscle enzyme levels begin to rise; rhabdomyolysis and myoglobinuria may develop when serum potassium falls below 2 mmol/L. Muscle weakness is secondary to a change in transmembrane ion transport, absence of the increase in blood flow normally seen in exercising muscle, lack of energy production, and loss of cellular integrity leading eventually to muscle necrosis. It may result in total paralysis and respiratory arrest. Gastrointestinal and urinary bladder hypomotility are often seen in potassium depletion states.

Potassium depletion can induce electrical and contractile cardiac problems. Consequences of hyperpolarization of the membrane potential at the end of repolarization are enhanced automaticity, decreased conduction velocity, and shortened refractory period. The most common arrhythmias are atrial tachycardia with or without block, atrioventricular dissociation, ventricular tachycardia, and ventricular fibrillation. Patients who have ischemic heart disease or are taking digitalis are particularly at risk[10]; cardiac sensitivity to digitalis is increased with hypokalemia. Electrocardiographic manifestations of hypokalemia include flattening or inverting of the T wave, depression of the ST segment, prominent U waves, diminished QRS voltage, and increased AV conduction time (Fig. 99-2).

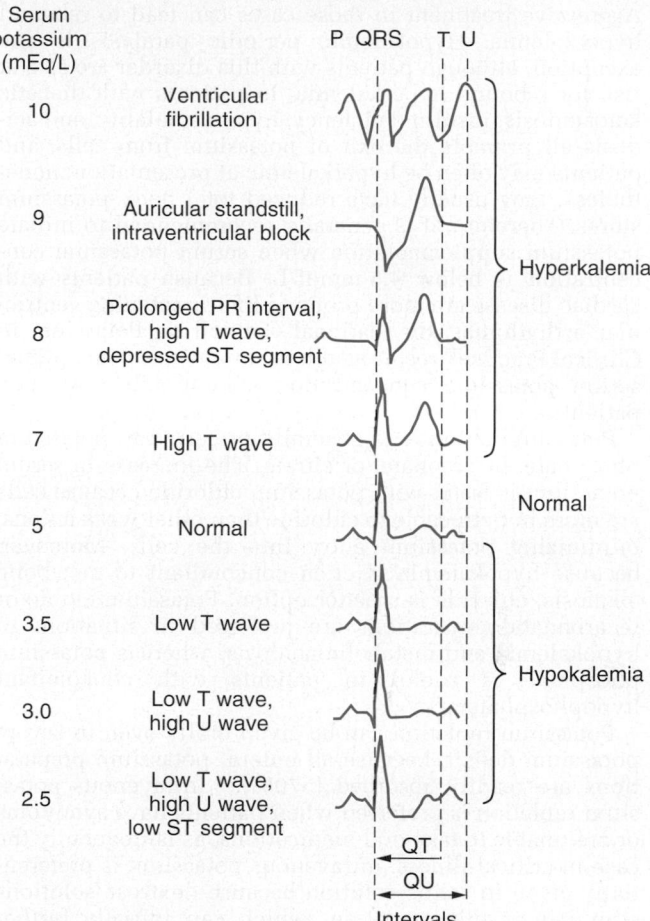

FIGURE 99-2. Expected electrocardiographic changes with abnormal serum potassium concentrations.

Potassium depletion can induce impairments of glomerular filtration rate, renal blood flow, and renal acidification as well as several tubular defects, alteration of renal sodium handling, and increased plasma renin activity. A mild nephrogenic diabetes insipidus secondary to polydipsia and impairment of urine concentration has been described.

Treatment of Hypokalemia

The objectives of potassium repletion are to prevent or cease life-threatening cardiac arrhythmias, to reverse paralysis, and ultimately to replenish total potassium body stores. A rapid repletion is desirable in symptomatic patients, in patients taking digitalis, and when serum potassium is below 3 mmol/L, especially in patients taking diuretics. The magnitude of potassium deficit is difficult to estimate because the correlation between plasma potassium concentration and total potassium deficit is poor and because only 2% of body potassium is extracellular. The following guide may be used: In the absence of abnormalities in internal balance, the potassium deficit is nearly 100 mEq per 0.3-mmol/L decrease in serum potassium value.

In cases of hypokalemia secondary to potassium redistribution, it is generally advisable not to give potassium supplements, the hypokalemia being typically transient.

Aggressive treatment in those cases can lead to rebound hyperkalemia. Hypokalemic periodic paralysis is one exception, although patients with this disorder are also at risk for rebound hyperkalemia. In patients with diabetic ketoacidosis, insulin deficiency, hyperosmolality, and acidosis all promote the exit of potassium from cells, and patients may often be hyperkalemic at presentation; nonetheless, they usually have reduced total body potassium stores. Therefore, it is generally recommended to initiate potassium supplementation when serum potassium concentration is below 4.5 mmol/L. Because patients with cardiac disease are more prone to life-threatening ventricular arrhythmias, the National Council on Potassium in Clinical Practice[11] recommends maintenance of an optimal serum potassium concentration (>4.0 mmol/L) in such patients.

Potassium chloride is generally preferred to potassium phosphate, bicarbonate, or citrate. The increase in serum potassium is faster with potassium chloride because cells are more impermeable to chloride than other weak anions, minimizing potassium entry into the cells. Moreover, because hypokalemia is often concomitant to metabolic alkalosis, chloride is a better option. Potassium citrate or bicarbonate preparations are preferred in situations of hypokalemia and metabolic acidosis, whereas potassium phosphate is useful in patients with concomitant hypophosphatemia.[12]

Potassium repletion can be given orally even in severe potassium deficit, because all enteral potassium preparations are readily absorbed (>70%).[13] Intravenous potassium repletion is preferred when patients have symptoms or are unable to take oral medications, as is frequently the case in critical illness. Intravenous potassium is preferentially given in saline solution because dextrose solutions stimulate insulin secretion, which can initially further reduce extracellular potassium concentration. However, using saline with very diluted concentrations of potassium carries the risk of volume overload if significant amounts of potassium are required. The fear of inducing arrhythmias from local hyperkalemia near the infusion site seems unjustified. Studies have shown that potassium infusions with high concentrations are safe; a 200-mmol/L potassium chloride solution given at a rate of 20 mmol/hr can be safely infused via a peripheral vein, despite a burning sensation reported in less than 3% of cases.[14,15]

Coexisting potassium and magnesium depletions can lead to refractory hypokalemia.[16] In patients with resistance to potassium supplementation, first measuring the magnesium concentration, and giving magnesium repletion if the value is low, is recommended. In patients with hypokalemia associated with gastric suction, decreasing the loss of hydrogen chloride with proton pump inhibitors can ameliorate the hypokalemia.[17]

Hyperkalemia

Hyperkalemia is defined as a serum concentration more than 5.5 mmol/L.

Causes of Hyperkalemia

Hyperkalemia may result from the following mechanisms: (1) increased potassium intake, (2) reduction in renal excretion of potassium, and (3) redistribution of potassium from the intracellular to the extracellular compartment. Reduced renal potassium excretion is the most common cause.

INCREASED POTASSIUM INTAKE. Increased potassium intake is normally not a cause of hyperkalemia unless it is an acute phenomenon or the patient has impaired renal excretion, as with renal failure. The potassium concentration of plasma in transfused blood rises with storage duration as potassium diffuses out of red blood cells. Stored blood can be a significant source of potassium, because one unit of blood stored for 10 days contains as much as 30 mmol/L of potassium. Renal allograft preservation solution contains potassium and can contribute to post-transplantation hyperkalemia. Solutions used for cardioplegia during cardiac surgery also have high potassium content. Potassium citrate used to alkalinize urine can induce hyperkalemia in the patient with renal insufficiency. Penicillin can also be prepared as a potassium salt: A 1 million unit dose contains 1.7 mmol/L of potassium. Enteral nutrition solutions generally contain between 26 and 54 mmol/L of potassium; they may also become significant sources of potassium intake.

INCREASED POTASSIUM RELEASE FROM CELLS. Transient hyperkalemia is often due to increased release of potassium from cells. Pseudohyperkalemia, a relatively common event, can be induced by difficult blood sampling and the tourniquet technique. In metabolic acidosis, excess hydrogen ion buffering in the cell and potassium efflux into the extracellular fluid to maintain electroneutrality induce an increase in extracellular potassium concentration. Metabolic acidosis causes a greater shift of potassium than respiratory acidosis. The nature of the accompanying anion is important because mineral acids or strong anions (e.g., chloride) cause a greater shift of potassium than organic acids (e.g., ketoacids, lactate), the membrane being more impermeable to nonorganic acids. The duration of the acidosis and the change in plasma bicarbonate concentration per se are also important factors in the change in serum potassium concentration.

Because insulin promotes potassium uptake by the cell, insulin deficiency and insulin antagonists (such as somatostatin and diazoxide) promote hyperkalemia. Hyperosmolality induced by hyperglycemia, mannitol, or hypernatremia may also cause hyperkalemia; the osmotic force drives a water movement out of the cell, and some potassium is carried along with water by solvent drag. Also, the higher intracellular potassium concentration induced by the intracellular water loss favors potassium exit.

Direct cell destruction, as in tumor lysis syndrome, hematoma reabsorption, hemolysis, rhabdomyolysis, burns, or crush syndrome, result in the release of potassium into the extracellular fluid. Massive amounts can be released but cannot be precisely estimated. During gastrointestinal bleeding, the intestinal tract can absorb large amounts of potassium. Exercise can cause hyperkalemia via two different mechanisms: First, there is a delay between the exit of potassium during the depolarizing phase of muscle contraction and the reuptake of potassium; second, reduction of adenosine triphosphate (ATP) increases the number of open ATP K^+ channels, promoting potassium exit from the cell.

As noted previously, β_2-adrenergic receptor stimulation leads to cellular potassium uptake. Thus, nonselective β_2-adrenergic blockers interfere with transcellular potassium shift; β_1-specific blockers interfere much less. Digoxin overdose blocks the Na^+,K^+-ATPase pump in skeletal muscles, impairing transcellular potassium redistribution, an effect not seen at therapeutic doses. Utilization of depolarizing agents (such as succinylcholine and suxamethonium) can induce hyperkalemia, although the molecular mechanism has not yet been completely elucidated.[18,19]

DECREASED SECRETION. Chronic hyperkalemia is due to a defect in potassium secretion at the distal nephron. The main causes are hypoaldosteronism and decreased distal delivery of sodium and water (by volume depletion or renal failure). Aldosterone stimulates potassium secretion by enhancing the basolateral Na^+,K^+-ATPase and by increasing the number of open Na^+ and K^+ channels in the luminal membrane. All conditions inducing hypoaldosteronism can cause hyperkalemia. In critical illness, a relative reduction in adrenal hormone production is more common than thought before and does not necessarily lead to florid adrenal insufficiency. However, hypoaldosteronism may occur in such conditions. Also, increased production of adrenocorticotropic hormone in very sick patients may reduce aldosterone synthesis, because substrates are preferably used for cortisol production.[20]

Hyporeninemic hypoaldosteronism is a condition seen in diabetic patients or in patients with chronic interstitial nephritis with moderate kidney failure. Nonsteroidal anti-inflammatory drugs (NSAIDs), cyclooxygenase-2 inhibitors, angiotensin-converting enzyme inhibitors, angiotensin II receptor blockers (ARBs), cyclosporine, tacrolimus, ketoconazole, and human immunodeficiency virus infection are other causes of low values for plasma renin activity and aldosterone concentration. Angiotensin-converting enzyme inhibitors raise the serum potassium level by 0.4 to 0.6 mmol/L, whereas ARBs are associated with more modest increases, reported in the range of 0.05 to 0.3 mmol/L. Less than 2% of patients receiving angiotensin-converting enzyme inhibitors or ARBs demonstrate a potassium concentration above 5.6 mmol/L.[21]

Unfractionated heparin and low-molecular-weight heparins may induce a reversible reduction in the number of adrenal angiotensin II receptors in the zona glomerulosa with heparin dosages as low as 5000 units twice daily. It has been reported that nearly 7% of patients receiving heparin demonstrate a modest hyperkalemia.[22]

Potassium-sparing diuretics are frequently associated with the development of hyperkalemia. Spironolactone and eplerenone decrease aldosterone binding to its receptor. Triamterene and amiloride act as blockers of the apical sodium channel in the cortical collecting duct, thereby directly inhibiting potassium secretion. Trimethoprim and pentamidine induce hyperkalemia by a mechanism similar to that of potassium-sparing diuretics.[23,24] Trimethoprim in both high and low doses has been shown to raise the serum potassium level by 0.3 to 1.1 mmol/L after 7 to 10 days of treatment in 75% of patients.[25,26]

Hypovolemia and effective circulating volume depletion may contribute to hyperkalemia because distal water delivery is reduced. In renal insufficiency, hyperkalemia develops generally in situations of decreased glomerular filtration rate and distal flow or when other hyperkalemia-inducing factors are present. Hyperkalemia in advanced uremia occurs from a diminution of Na^+,K^+-ATPase activity that results in defective extrarenal potassium handling.[27]

Clinical Manifestations

Membrane excitability depends on the resting membrane potential and on activation of membrane sodium channels. As the extracellular concentration of potassium rises, the ratio of intracellular to extracellular potassium decreases.

Because this ratio is the major determinant of the resting potential, depolarization is easier and excitability is increased. However, persistent depolarization inactivates sodium channels, producing a diminution in membrane excitability.

Hyperkalemia shortens the refractory period (and hence speeds the repolarization) and induces a reduction in conduction velocity. The former is the first abnormality to appear and can be seen with a serum potassium level of 5.5 to 6.0 mmol/L. Electrocardiographic changes include increased T wave amplitude with ST segment shortening, followed by P wave flattening and QRS complex widening (see Fig. 99-2). Ultimately, the electrocardiogram takes a sinusoidal form. Nevertheless, different types of arrhythmias and conduction disturbances can be seen even before any electrocardiographic changes. Hyperkalemia-induced hyperexcitability is determined by the rate of change in serum potassium level; a rapid onset of hyperkalemia and a combination of hyperkalemia with hyponatremia, hypocalcemia, hypomagnesemia, and disturbed extracellular pH are factors that may enhance arrhythmias. Concomitant use of drugs can also influence the occurrence of such arrhythmias.

Paresthesia, muscular weakness, and ascending paralysis are seen with severe hyperkalemia (>7 mmol/L, or near 9 mmol/L in patients with chronic renal failure). Respiratory musculature can be involved, but cranial nerves are generally spared. Endogenous release of insulin, glucagon, aldosterone, and catecholamines is enhanced in hyperkalemia.

Treatment

Treatment of hyperkalemia must be adjusted according to the cause, the physical signs, or the complications and severity of elevation in serum concentration. Tolerance of hyperkalemia is diminished when hypocalcemia and/or metabolic acidosis is also present and in patients with heart disease. Chronic elevation is better tolerated than a rapid rise in serum potassium. Patients with serum potassium levels above 6.5 to 7.0 mmol/L, with severe muscular weakness, or with electrographic changes require immediate treatment. A more conservative approach can be used for those with lower serum concentrations and without symptoms and signs. The objectives of treatment are threefold: to antagonize membrane actions of potassium, drive potassium into cells, and remove excess potassium from the body. At first, it is logical to discontinue all potassium sources, including potassium supplements and medications containing potassium, or to restrict potassium elimination, transfusions (if possible), and potassium content in food.

ANTAGONIZE THE MEMBRANE ACTIONS OF POTASSIUM. Calcium is given to patients with hyperkalemia-induced electrocardiographic changes. Calcium gluconate and calcium chloride are both effective, but the former is generally preferred because it irritates the veins less. The cardioprotective effect of calcium against potassium is immediate and lasts for approximately 1 hour. The usual dose is one ampule (1 gram in 10 mL) of 10% calcium gluconate solution given over 3 minutes with cardiac monitoring. The dose can be repeated once if there is no electrocardiographic improvement after 5 minutes. There is a relative contraindication to using calcium in digoxin toxicity. Digoxin Fab antibodies must be given to patients with hyperkalemia secondary to digoxin toxicity. Calcium reverses the effects of hyperkalemia at the membrane level but has no effect on serum potassium level.

DRIVE POTASSIUM INTO CELLS

Glucose-Insulin. Insulin enhances the entry of extracellular potassium into the cells by increasing the activity of the Na^+,K^+-ATPase pump. Because insulin alone can induce hypoglycemia, it is preferable to give glucose simultaneously with the intravenous insulin (except in hyperglycemic patients, who may initially receive only insulin). Generally 10 to 20 units of fast-acting insulin are given intravenously with 50 to 100 g of glucose.

β_2 Agonists. β_2-Adrenergic receptor agonists decrease serum potassium concentrations by inducing a transcellular shift. Intravenous, subcutaneous, nebulized, or inhaled forms have all been shown to be effective. A mild tachycardia is often observed without a significant rise in blood pressure; however, clinicians should be careful about the use of these agents in coronary patients. Tremor, vasomotor flushing, and palpitations have also been reported. A transient rise in serum potassium level of 0.15 mmol/L can happen 1 minute after the completion of the treatment; afterwards, potassium concentration falls progressively.[28] Moreover, the combination of intravenous insulin-glucose and a β_2 agonist seems to be more effective than either alone.[29]

Sodium Bicarbonate. Results of studies on the beneficial effect of sodium bicarbonate for hyperkalemia treatment are equivocal, and those of studies on possible superiority of sodium bicarbonate over β agonists or insulin are conflicting.[29] For patients with end-stage renal disease, it has been shown that intravenous sodium bicarbonate alone is ineffective in lowering plasma potassium, except in patients with significant acidosis.[30,31] Hypernatremia, sodium retention, carbon dioxide retention, and hypocalcemia are adverse effects associated with administration of excessive sodium bicarbonate.

REMOVE EXCESS POTASSIUM

Digestive Elimination. There is no randomized evidence for the efficacy of cation exchange resins in an emergency setting to reduce serum potassium concentration.[29,32] However, potassium excretion from the gastrointestinal tract can be forced by these agents. Their effect usually occurs after a few hours (>2 hrs). Sodium polystyrene sulfonate can be given orally (20-30 g with sorbitol) or by enema (50-100 g diluted in 200 mL of water). However, their use can also have serious complications.[33]

Renal Elimination. Restoring diuresis is helpful for potassium elimination and the use of diuretics of the loop of Henle enhance renal potassium excretion; however, patients with advanced renal failure may show little response. In case of hypoaldosteronism or resistance to aldosterone, an exogenous mineralocorticoid such as fludrocortisone is useful to increase potassium excretion.

Extracorporeal Elimination. For severe cases, hemodialysis is the fastest way to correct hyperkalemia, because 25 to 50 mEq (and probably more than that with very efficient dialysis) of potassium can be removed hourly. However, with a low potassium dialysate bath (0 or 1 mmol/L), cardiac arrhythmias can occur. A close monitoring of serum potassium concentration is advisable, and the dialysate potassium concentration should be increased once hyperkalemia is no longer life-threatening. If therapies inducing intracellular potassium shift have been used previously, the effectiveness of dialysis decreases, and the patient may demonstrate a higher post-dialysis potassium rebound (usually after 3 to 4 hours). Continuous renal replacement therapies can be effectively used to treat hyperkalemia; depending on the effluent flow rate obtained, more than 15 to 20 mmol/hr can be eliminated.

Key Points

1. The potassium concentration gradient across cell membranes is the major determinant of the resting membrane potential.
2. Insulin, aldosterone, and catecholamines stimulate the activity of Na^+,K^+-ATPase and promote an intracellular potassium shift.
3. In metabolic acidosis, potassium shifts from the intracellular compartment to the extracellular compartment; in metabolic alkalosis, the process is reversed. Respiratory acidosis and alkalosis have little impact on potassium distribution.
4. The daily potassium intake is excreted mainly via the renal route; most of urinary potassium excretion occurs by secretion in the distal nephron after aldosterone activity.
5. Alterations of serum potassium are common in hospitalized patients; 20% of patients have hypokalemia, and 1% to 10% experience hyperkalemia. Disorders of serum potassium concentration are more often the consequences of an abnormal external balance; for instance, positive balance from an increased intake or reduced excretion or negative balance from a reduced intake or increased excretion.

Key References

5. Stevens MS, Dunlay RW: Hyperkalemia in hospitalized patients. Int Urol Nephrol 2000;32:177-180.
11. Cohn JN, Kowey PR, Whelton PK, Prisant LM: New guidelines for potassium replacement in clinical practice: A contemporary review by the National Council on Potassium in Clinical Practice. Arch Intern Med 2000;160:2429-2436.
15. Kruse JA, Clark VL, Carlson RW, Geheb MA: Concentrated potassium chloride infusions in critically ill patients with hypokalemia. J Clin Pharmacol 1994;34:1077-1082.
18. Jeevendra Martyn JA: Succinylcholine-induced hyperkalemia in acquired pathologic states: Etiologic factors and molecular mechanisms. Anesthesiology 2006;104:158-169.
20. Braley LM, Adler GK, Mortensen RM, et al: Dose effect of adrenocorticotropin on aldosterone and cortisol biosynthesis in cultured bovine adrenal glomerulosa cells: In vitro correlate of hyperreninemic hypoaldosteronism. Endocrinology 1992;131:187-194.

See the companion Expert Consult website for the complete reference list.

CHAPTER 100

Alterations in Calcium and Phosphorus Metabolism in Critically Ill Patients

Piergiorgio Messa, Roberta Cerutti, and Brigida Brezzi

OBJECTIVES

This chapter will:
1. Explain the major epidemiological, pathophysiological, and clinical aspects of hypocalcemia and of hypercalcemia in critically ill patients.
2. Explain the major epidemiological, pathophysiological, and clinical aspects of hypophosphatemia and of hyperphosphatemia in critically ill patients.

CALCIUM

Pathophysiological Background

Calcium (Ca) is essential for normal cellular functions and for extracellular processes. Extracellular calcium ion concentration is kept within a relatively narrow range (total calcium, 8.4-10.4 mg/dL or 2.1-2.6 mmol/L; ionized calcium, 1.1-1.3 mmol/L). Extracellular calcium levels are controlled by the combined activity of parathyroid and C thyroid cells, bone cells, and renal tubular cells. At all these sites, the activity and/or expression level of the calcium-sensing receptor (CaSR) work to couple small changes in circulating calcium concentration with intracellular pathways that modify parathyroid hormone (PTH) and calcitonin secretion as well as bone and renal handling of calcium.

Intracellular calcium concentration is by far (about 10,000 times) lower than the extracellular calcium concentration and even more tightly controlled. The narrow limits of intracellular calcium concentration are maintained at the expense of energy-requiring processes. Changes in intracellular calcium can induce cellular damage by lipase, protease, and nuclease activation, free radical generation, and prostanoid release.

Alterations in calcium homeostasis are common in critically ill patients.

Evaluation of Serum Calcium Concentration

Calcium levels can be evaluated by different methods. Although the direct ionized calcium (i-Ca) measurement is the most correct method for assessing the active concentration of this electrolyte,[1,2] total serum calcium, "normalized" through the use of different variables (serum albumin, arterial pH, anion gap, or a combination of all), is also used. The most commonly utilized formulas for total calcium correction are reported in Table 100-1. Most cor-

rections take into account that changes in either serum albumin or pH can alter the ratio between the protein-bound and free fractions of calcium.

It should be kept in mind that serum calcium concentration, however measured, is a poor indicator of calcium status in critically ill patients.

Hypocalcemia in Critically Ill Patients
Definition and Prevalence

Although different definitions of hypocalcemia have been utilized in the literature, major agreement exists in defining the limits of both corrected total calcium (lower than 7-7.5 mg/dL) and i-Ca (lower than 0.7-0.9 mmol/L) that require treatment.

The overall prevalence of hypocalcemia (i-Ca levels between 0.9 and 1.15 mmol/L) has been variably reported in different series of critically ill patients, ranging from 15% to 88% in adults[3] and from 12% to 75% in the pediatric population.[4-6] Lower prevalence has been reported for severe hypocalcemia (10%-12%).

Hypocalcemia has been more commonly found in patients affected by sepsis, pancreatitis, severe burns, and major trauma.

Pathogenesis of Hypocalcemia

Mechanisms underlying hypocalcemia in critically ill patients are not fully understood. Several factors may be involved, including decreased secretion of PTH, increased procalcitonin/calcitonin levels, reduced vitamin D bioavailability, peripheral resistance to either PTH or vitamin D action, increased renal loss and/or reduced intestinal absorption of calcium, impaired bone resorption, elevated inflammatory cytokines, and drug effects. Increased urinary calcium excretion does not seem to be a prominent causal factor of hypocalcemia in patients with acute disease.

Reduction in both secretion and bioactivity of PTH has been claimed to play a pivotal role in hypocalcemia in critically ill patients. Relatively low levels of PTH have been found, particularly in patients with sepsis, multiple-organ failure, pancreatitis, rhabdomyolysis, hypermagnesemia, and severe hypomagnesemia.[7]

In experimental models of sepsis or severe burn injury, both hypocalcemia and hypoparathyroidism have been observed. These findings have been related to an upregulation of parathyroid gland CaSR expression, probably mediated by proinflammatory cytokines. In fact, interleukin-1β can upregulate parathyroid, thyroid, and kidney CaSR mRNA levels as a consequence of increased CaSR gene

TABLE 100-1

Formulas for Total Calcium Correction

FORMULA	SOURCE
Corrected calcium = total calcium + 0.8(1 − albumin)	Modified from Orell (1971)[29]
Corrected calcium = total calcium − 0.675(total protein − 7.2)	Dent (1962)[30]
Corrected calcium = total calcium − $4[(0.0019 \times$ albumin)$(0.12 \times \frac{albumin}{173})$ $(7.42 - pH)] + 0.0001[(total protein - albumin)(0.42 \times$ $\frac{total\ protein - albumin}{250})$ $(7.42 - pH)]$	Moore (1970)[31]
Calculated ionized calcium concentration = $\frac{total\ calcium}{4} - (0.0613 \times total$ calcium $\times$ albumin) $- [0.0244 \times total$ calcium $\times$ (total protein − albumin)] $- (0.0043 \times$ total calcium $\times$ anion gap) $- (0.00375 \times$ total calcium $\times$ total CO_2)	Nordin (1989)[32]

TABLE 100-2

Most Relevant Symptoms of Hypocalcemia

Neuromuscular symptoms	Muscle weakness
	Myalgia
	Paresthesia
	Cramps
	Tetany
	Dysphagia
	Laryngospasm
	Bronchospasm
	Biliary colics
	Intestinal colics
	Focal and general seizures
	Papilledema
Behavioral symptoms	Anxiety
	Irritability
	Psychosis
	Dementia
	Confusion
Cardiovascular symptoms	Impaired myocardial contractility
	Bradycardia
	Hypotension
	Ventricular dysrhythmias
	Prolongation of QT interval and ST segment on electrocardiography

transcription mediated by nuclear factor-kappaB (NF-κB). Upregulation of CaSRs present in the proximal tubule probably contributes to hypocalcemia by reducing 25-hydroxyvitamin D 1α-hydroxylase activity, thereby accounting for the low 1,25-dihydroxyvitamin D levels frequently observed in the critically ill.

Overall, the upregulation of CaSRs by interleukin-1 induces a concurrent reduction of serum PTH, 1,25(OH)$_2$D levels, and calcium.

However, it is worth noting that increased PTH levels have also been occasionally reported in critically ill patients.[8,9] Muller and associates[10] found high levels of PTH associated with hypocalcemia in patients with sepsis, suggesting an intact response of the parathyroid gland to hypocalcemia. These researchers suggested that hypocalcemia might be due to the hypocalcemic effect of calcitonin precursor(s), levels of which are frequently found to be increased in critically ill patients.[10]

Impaired vitamin D bioavailability is another important cause of hypocalcemia. Vitamin D deficiency in critically ill patients may occur by a reduction of either intestinal absorption or synthesis. The former may be secondary to impaired biliary and pancreatic secretion or to altered intestinal mucosal integrity, which is frequently observed in critically ill patients. The reduction in vitamin D synthesis may be secondary to impaired hydroxylation at both liver (25-OHase) and kidney (1,25-OHase) levels, due either to reduced function of both organs or to an indirect effect of cytokine release and growth hormone/insulin-like growth factor-1 deficiency, which may contribute to impairment of 1α-hydroxylase activity.[11]

PTH and/or vitamin D end-organ resistance has been observed in critically ill patients, in whom it was also related to severe hypomagnesemia or to drugs that decrease calcium mobilization from bone (calcitonin, cisplatin, diphosphonates, mithramycin). Hypomagnesemia is a common feature in critically ill patients, with an incidence as high as 60% to 65%, and is frequently associated with hypocalcemia. The mechanisms of this association are not completely clear.[12]

Other factors that can occasionally induce hypocalcemia in critically ill patients and that should be mentioned are as follows: calcium chelation secondary to citrate administration during intensive transfusional therapy or extracorporeal circulation; ethylene glycol intoxication; use of ethylenediaminetetraacetic acid; pancreatitis; hyperphosphatemia secondary to rhabdomyolysis or tumor lysis syndrome; and increased calcium uptake by bone after the removal of overactive parathyroid glands or after treatment of bone metastasis. Hypocalcemia has been also occasionally reported during resuscitation in patients with severe trauma who have been overhydrated with colloid infusion or lactate-containing solutions.[13]

Clinical Presentation of Hypocalcemia

Symptoms of hypocalcemia depend on both the severity and rapidity of calcium reduction, mostly of the biologically active ionized fraction. However, symptoms are not evident until the serum i-Ca level drops below 0.7 mmol/L. Acute hypocalcemia is characterized by neuromuscular, cardiovascular, and behavioral clinical signs. The most relevant symptoms of hypocalcemia are listed in Table 100-2.

In critically ill patients, disease severity and mortality have been found to be inversely correlated with ionized calcium levels.[3,7,14] The lowest calcium levels have been reported in patients with sepsis, particularly nonsurvivors. However, the possible cause-and-effect relationship between hypocalcemia and mortality has still to be demonstrated. Probably, low calcium levels simply mark the severity of the global clinical condition and have no independent predictability for death from any cause in this clinical setting.[6]

Therefore, there is no clear evidence of the need to treat asymptomatic hypocalcemia. Furthermore, the effect of calcium administration on survival in the critically ill has not been fully investigated, and this treatment may even adversely affect outcome.

Hypercalcemia in Critically Ill Patients
Definition and Prevalence

There is no general agreement on the definition of hypercalcemia in critically ill patients. In our opinion, *moderate hypercalcemia* can be defined as total corrected serum calcium level from more than 2.6 to 3.0 mmol/L (10.5 to 12 mg/dL), and *severe hypercalcemia* as serum calcium greater than 3.0 mmol/L (>12 mg/dL). When i-Ca is taken into account, hypercalcemia can be defined as i-Ca level higher than 1.33 mmol/L. Hypercalcemia occurs when calcium influx into blood from bone and/or the intestine exceeds the efflux to bone, intestine, and/or kidney.

The prevalence of hypercalcemia in intensive care units varies considerably in different reports, ranging from 2.1% to 32%.[1,15] Some investigators report that the higher the number of failing organs at patient presentation, the more frequent the occurrence of hypercalcemia later in the course of disease.[15,16]

Pathogenesis

Many conditions can be associated with hypercalcemia in the general population. Even though any of these conditions can also be present in critically ill patients, the most common causes of increased calcium levels in this clinical set are malignancies, acute endocrine disturbances, and prolonged immobilization.

Critically ill patients with hypercalcemia often have malignancies. Any type of tumor can produce hypercalcemia, although breast and lung carcinoma and multiple myeloma are the most common causes. Neoplastic diseases can induce hypercalcemia through either direct bone destruction or secretion of calcemic factors by malignant cells.

Usually, cancer-associated hypercalcemia is due to skeletal metastases. When skeletal metastases are present, tumor cells secrete soluble factors (hormones, cytokines, growth factors) that stimulate osteoclastic bone resorption by inducing production of receptor activator for nuclear factor-κB ligand (RANKL) by osteoblastic stromal cells or by tumor cells themselves. On the other hand, osteoblast activity is often inhibited by tumor-produced cytokines (interleukin-6, tumor growth factor-β). This uncoupling between bone resorption and bone formation contributes to the rapid rise in serum calcium concentration and to a weakened bone structure, which can facilitate occurrence of fractures.[17,18]

Hypercalcemia can also occur without bone metastases. This finding may depend on production by cancer cells of a PTH-related peptide, which shares the PTH receptor and has considerable overlapping effects on target organs. It is worth emphasizing that PTH-related peptide cannot be detected by standard PTH assay (specific assays for parathyroid-related protein [PTHrP] are available).

In all the conditions described so far, serum PTH levels are greatly reduced.

Less frequently, hypercalcemia in critically ill patients can be secondary to some acute endocrine disturbances.

Even though tertiary hyperparathyroidism is usually recognized to occur in patients with long-lasting secondary hyperparathyroidism, this disorder has been also described after recovery from multiple-organ failure with a prolonged acute oliguric renal failure. Occasionally, after renal function is restored, the increased PTH level and the consequent hypercalcemia can represent a life-threatening problem because they can induce cardiac arrhythmias.[15,19]

Hyperthyroidism secondary to subacute thyroiditis can occasionally cause hypercalcemia in critically ill patients. The increased calcium levels are due to osteoclast stimulation by thyroid hormones. Another endocrine disease that can cause hypercalcemia in critically ill patients is acute Addison's disease. Hypercalcemia in this disorder is due to a combination of increased calcium release from bone and reduced calcium removal by the kidney. The factors responsible for calcium mobilization from bone are not completely clear; on the other hand, decreased glomerular filtration and increased tubular reabsorption of calcium, secondary to volume depletion, are identified causal mechanisms for reduced renal calcium excretion.

Increased bone resorption due to prolonged immobilization, usually longer than 4 weeks, is one of the most common causes of hypercalcemia in critically ill patients. Long-lasting immobilization in patients with intact renal function induces hypercalciuria, usually without hypercalcemia. However, when renal failure is present and skeletal mineral losses exceed the renal ability to eliminate calcium, hypercalcemia can ensue. Hypercalcemia due to immobilization is more commonly observed in conditions in which preexisting bone turnover is high, such as in children, adolescents, and patients with Paget's disease, fractures, malignancy, or primary or secondary hyperparathyroidism. The pathogenesis of hypercalcemia during immobilization is not completely clear. Suppression of osteoblastic activity and increased bone resorption, apparently not related to calcium-regulating hormones, has been suggested by results of bone biopsy studies.[20]

Up to 30% of patients with rhabdomyolysis experience hypercalcemia during the recovery phase of rhabdomyolysis-induced renal insufficiency. In some patients, hypercalcemia develops during the diuretic phase, when serum PTH levels are undetectable but 1,25-dihydroxyvitamin D levels are significantly increased, suggesting a pathogenetic role for vitamin D in this clinical setting. In other cases, levels of both PTH and vitamin D are suppressed, indicating a causal role for calcium mobilization from tissue deposits.[21] Among the different causes of rhabdomyolysis in critically ill patients, it is worth mentioning malignant hyperthermia, a genetic disorder that affects skeletal muscle and is characterized by severe muscle catabolism when prone subjects are exposed to anesthetic or myorelaxant drugs (succinylcholine, phenothiazine, haloperidol).

Figure 100-1 is a simplified diagnostic flow chart for the most common forms of hypercalcemia.

Clinical Presentation

Symptoms of hypercalcemia correlate with the value and the rapidity in the rise of calcium; mild hypercalcemia is generally asymptomatic. Severe hypercalcemia is associ-

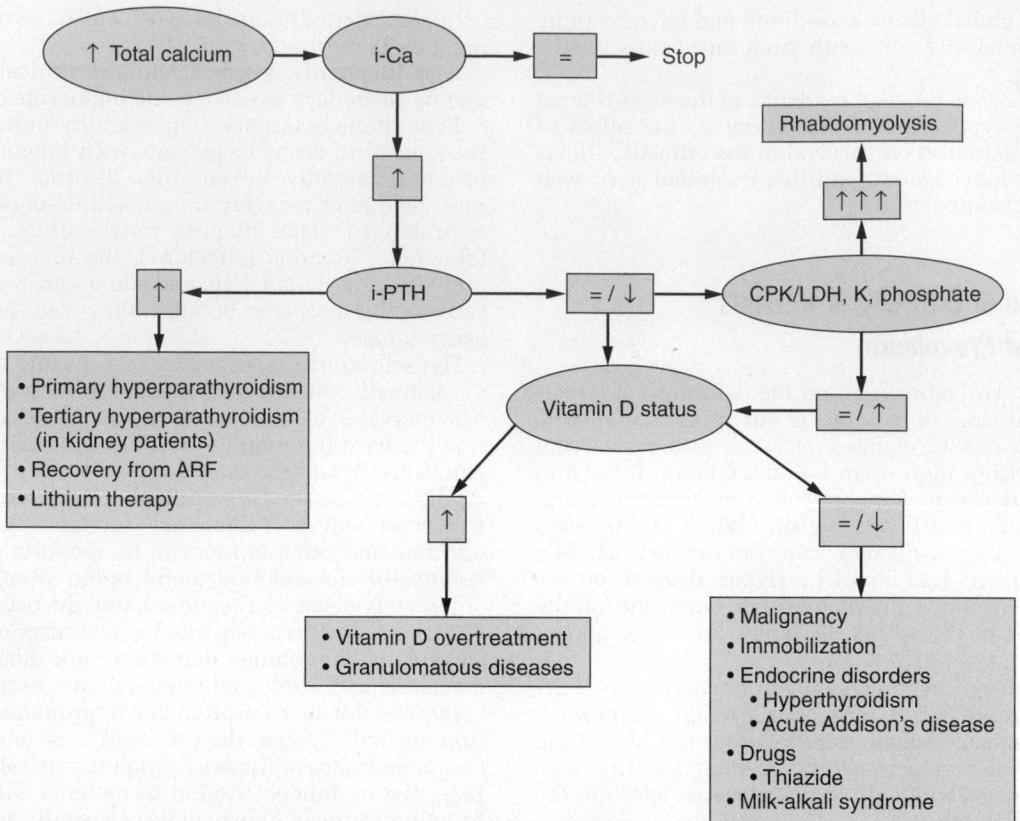

FIGURE 100-1. Simplified diagnostic flow chart for hypercalcemia. ARF, acute renal failure; Ca, calcium; CPK, creatine phosphokinase; i-, ionized; K, potassium; PTH, parathyroid hormone; =, normal; ↑, increased; ↓, decreased.

ated with neurological, cardiac, gastrointestinal, and renal symptoms (Table 100-3).

PHOSPHATE

Pathophysiological Background

Phosphate is the major intracellular anion, mainly bound to lipids, carbohydrates, and proteins; less than 1% is present in plasma. It is involved in almost all metabolic processes, such as generation of adenosine monophosphate and triphosphate, coagulation process and platelet aggregation, activity of many coenzymes, and formation of 2,3-diphosphoglyceric acid.

Normal phosphate serum concentration ranges between 2.5 and 4.5 mg/dL (0.81 and 1.45 mmol/L), with only 12% of phosphate being bound to proteins. Phosphate serum levels are controlled mainly by the kidney (through both glomerular filtration and tubular reabsorption) and to a minor extent by bone (through both resorption and exchange). The gut contributes significantly to maintenance of phosphate balance by modulating dietary phosphate absorption through both active sodium-dependent transport and passive diffusion. Some of the factors regulating all these processes are PTH, vitamin D, calcitonin, phosphatonin(s), diet phosphate content, diuretics, steroids, and hypokalemia.

TABLE 100-3

Major Symptoms of Hypercalcemia

Neurological symptoms	Depression
	Mental confusion
	Psychosis
	Weakness
	Drowsiness
	Lethargy to coma
Cardiac symptoms	Prolonged PR interval
	Shortened QT interval
	Bradycardia or atrioventricular block
	Increased sensitivity to digitalis
	Severe arrhythmias through cardiac arrest
Gastrointestinal symptoms	Anorexia
	Nausea
	Vomiting
	Constipation
	Peptic ulcer disease
	Acute pancreatitis
Renal symptoms	Marked polyuria
	Dehydration
	Nephrolithiasis
	Nephrocalcinosis

Hypophosphatemia in Critically Ill Patients
Definition and Prevalence

Moderate hypophosphatemia is defined as serum phosphate values between 1.0 and 2.0 mg/dL (0.32 and 0.65 mmol/L), and *severe hypophosphatemia* as serum phosphate value less than 1.0 mg/dL (<0.32 mmol/L).

Hypophosphatemia is relatively rare in the general hospitalized patient population, but its prevalence rises in critically ill patients, ranging from 8.8% to 80%.[22] It is more common in patients with chronic pulmonary obstructive disease, malignancy, or diabetic ketoacidosis and in those undergoing long-term treatment with total parenteral nutrition. Patients in intensive care units, especially those with sepsis, have higher prevalence of hypophosphatemia (60%-80%). Patients who have multiple trauma or have suffered burn injury are at high risk of severe hypophosphatemia.[23]

Pathogenesis

Hypophosphatemia can occur with either low-normal or increased total body phosphate concentration, depending on different pathogenic mechanisms. When hypophosphatemia occurs with reduced total body pool, decreased intestinal absorption and increased urinary loss can variably contribute to its development.

Reduced intestinal absorption and increased renal excretion of phosphate can be induced by endogenous or exogenous glucocorticoids. Administration of high amounts of magnesium- or aluminium-containing drugs, which bind phosphate in the intestine, reduce its absorption, resulting in hypophosphatemia. Urinary loss can occur during volume overexpansion or as a consequence of acquired renal tubular defects, which can be related to the causal factors in concomitant acute renal failure. Phosphatonin(s), including fibroblast growth factor (FGF-23), frizzled-related protein-4, and matrix extracellular phosphoglycoprotein, have been described as factors promoting phosphorus renal excretion independent of PTH activity.[23a]

The major pathogenic mechanism of hypophosphatemia in critically ill patients, however, is shift from the extracellular to the intracellular compartment. Hyperventilation, with subsequent alkalosis, has the most relevant effect, acutely lowering phosphate values by 1.5 to 3.0 mg/dL. The mechanism is stimulation of glycolysis due to elevated pH and leading to an accelerated production of phosphorylated metabolites.

Another common cause of intracellular phosphate shift is the intravenous administration of insulin, which increases cellular uptake of glucose and phosphorus. This phenomenon is particularly evident during refeeding procedures, when insulin-stimulated glucose consumption superimposes on preexisting phosphate deficiency, further lowering phosphate levels by 0.2 to 0.5 mg/dL. Insulin therapy for diabetic ketoacidosis also reduces phosphate levels a few hours after the initiation of treatment.[24,25]

During cardiopulmonary bypass, inflammatory cytokines (interleukin-6) and hypothermia can induce severe hypophosphatemia through an enhanced intracellular phosphate shift secondary to sympathetic activation, hyperglycemia, and insulin release.[26]

However, a combination of factors responsible for hypophosphatemia is commonly observed in critically ill patients. In patients who have undergone surgery (mainly hepatic, cardiac, and major vascular procedures) or who are septic, the coexistence of phosphate depletion, glucose and saline infusion, high levels of catecholamines, and respiratory alkalosis may contribute to hypophosphatemia. Alcoholic patients, who are frequently malnourished with vitamin D depletion, often have hypophosphatemia due to both renal phosphate wasting and intracellular shift if they are treated with glucose infusion.

Clinical Presentation

Correlation between moderate phosphate deficiency and symptoms is weak; symptoms occur with phosphate values below 1.5 mg/dL and are typically neurological (paresthesias, tremor, confusion, hyporeflexia, seizures, coma). Structural and functional disturbances of skeletal muscle membrane and erythrocyte membrane can cause rhabdomyolysis and hemolysis, respectively. Another described consequence of hypophosphatemia is insulin resistance, which can be responsible for the hyperglycemia frequently observed in critically ill patients. Alteration in muscle cell activity may also induce ventricular tachycardia, congestive heart failure, hypotension, and respiratory failure. The decreased production of 2,3-diphosphoglyceric acid secondary to reduced phosphate levels can further impair tissue oxygenation.

Hyperphosphatemia in Critically Ill Patients
Definition and Prevalence

Hyperphosphatemia is considered significant when phosphate levels are higher than 1.6 mmol/L (5 mg/dL). There are no reliable data in the literature about the prevalence of hyperphosphatemia in critically ill patients. This lack is probably due to the relatively low clinical impact of this electrolyte disturbance compared with others.

Pathogenesis

Hyperphosphatemia occurs when the phosphate load exceeds renal excretion and tissue uptake; patients at highest risk for hyperphosphatemia are those with preexisting chronic or superimposed acute renal failure.

Hyperphosphatemia can be related to an increase in endogenous sources (because of either cell lysis or a shift from the intracellular to the extracellular compartment), to increased exogenous sources, or to reduced urinary excretion (Table 100-4).

The emergency physician must be aware of the presence of pseudohyperphosphatemia, which can be due to interference with biochemical assay results in patients with hyperglobulinemia, extreme hypertriglyceridemia, or hyperbilirubinemia, or because of in vitro hemolysis.[27]

Clinical Presentation

Symptoms of hyperphosphatemia can theoretically involve many organs (Table 100-5). However, the symptoms seem related less to the phosphate elevation itself than to more relevant electrolyte-associated disturbances, such as hyperkalemia and hypocalcemia. It has also been claimed that, when the calcium × phosphate product exceeds 70 mg²/mL², soft tissue deposition of calcium-phosphate salts can occur, with possible severe peripheral ischemic disorders.[28]

TABLE 100-4

Main Causal Factors for Hyperphosphatemia

Increased endogenous sources	Rhabdomyolysis Malignant hyperthermia Tumor lysis syndrome Hemolysis Bowel infarction Lactic acidosis and ketoacidosis
Increased exogenous sources	Large amounts of phosphate salts (intravenous infusion, oral supplements, enemas, oral or rectal laxatives) Vitamin D intoxication Cow's milk (in infants)
Reduced urinary excretion	Renal failure Hypoparathyroidism Vitamin D intoxication Acromegaly Bisphosphonate therapy

TABLE 100-5

Major Symptoms of Hyperphosphatemia

Neurological symptoms	Decreased mental status Seizures
Cardiac symptoms	Dysrhythmias Prolongation of the QT interval on electrocardiography
Musculoskeletal symptoms	Weakness Cramps Hyperreflexia Tetany
Gastrointestinal symptoms	Anorexia Nausea Vomiting
Eye symptoms	Conjunctivitis Decreased visual acuity
Renal symptom	Renal failure
Skin symptom	Papular eruption

Key Points

1. Among disturbances of calcium and phosphate metabolism in critically ill patients, hypocalcemia and hypophosphatemia are the most common.
2. Disturbances of calcium and phosphate metabolism in critically ill patients are clinically relevant.
3. Only the most severe of these calcium and phosphate disturbances must be corrected.
4. There is no evidence that any of these disturbances per se affects clinical outcome in critically ill patients.

Key References

3. Zivin J, Gooley T, Zager R, Ryan M: Hypocalcemia: A pervasive metabolic abnormality in the critically ill. Am J Kidney Dis 2001;374:689-698.
10. Muller B, Becker KL, Kranzlin M, et al: Disordered calcium homeostasis of sepsis: Association with calcitonin precursors. Eur J Clin Invest 2000;30:823-831.
19. Jeffries C, Ledgerwood AM, Lucas CE: Life-threatening tertiary hyperparathyroidism in the critically ill. Am J Surg 2005;189:369-372.
22. Charron T, Bernard F, Skrobik Y, et al: Intravenous phosphate in the intensive care unit: More aggressive repletion regimens for moderate and severe hypophosphatemia. Intensive Care Med 2003;29:1273-1278.
25. Brown G, Greenwood J. Drug and nutrition-induced hypophosphatemia: mechanisms and relevance in the critically ill. Ann Pharmacother 1994;28:626-632.

See the companion Expert Consult website for the complete reference list.

CHAPTER 101

Disorders of Magnesium Balance

Isabelle Plamondon and Martine Leblanc

OBJECTIVES

This chapter will:
1. Discuss mechanisms of magnesium absorption and excretion.
2. Review main causes of altered serum magnesium concentrations.
3. Describe clinical manifestations of hypomagnesemia and hypermagnesemia.
4. Summarize modalities of treatment of altered serum magnesium.

Magnesium (Mg^{++}) is the second most abundant intracellular cation and the fourth most prevalent cation in the body. The human body normally contains 21 to 28 g (or 1750 to 2400 mEq) of magnesium; 1 mEq of Mg^{++} is equivalent to 0.5 mmol of Mg^{++} or 12.3 mg of magnesium. Magnesium is concentrated in bone (67%), muscles (20%), and nonmuscle soft tissues (11%). Only 1.3% of the total magnesium pool is extracellular.[1] Magnesium is present in three fractions: ionized, which is the active form (65%), protein-bound (27%), and complexed with anions such as phosphate and citrate (8%) (Fig. 101-1).

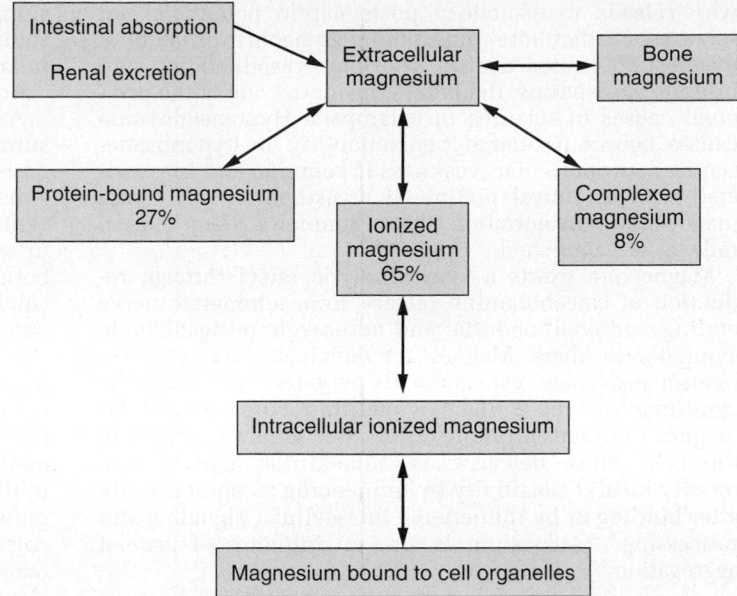

FIGURE 101-1. Magnesium homeostasis.

Magnesium disorders are common in intensive care: In a prospective study, 52.5% of patients had total hypomagnesemia at admission to intensive care units, and 13.5% had total hypermagnesemia.[2] Hypoalbuminemic patients may demonstrate low total serum magnesium concentrations, although biologically active ionized magnesium levels are normal. The ionized magnesium fraction is not routinely measured, and correlation between ionized magnesium and bound fraction in critical illnesses seems variable and controversial. Development of ionized hypermagnesemia has been associated with a higher mortality.

ROLE OF MAGNESIUM AT THE CELLULAR LEVEL

Magnesium is a cofactor in a wide spectrum of enzymatic reactions required for DNA and RNA synthesis and nucleic acid polymerization. Various phosphokinases and phosphatases involved in energy metabolism also need magnesium. Magnesium is essential for the activation of adenosine triphosphatases (ATPases) involved in maintaining adequate intracellular electrolyte content and in many other ATPases distributed in all cell compartments. The generation of cyclic adenosine monophosphate (cAMP), the intracellular second messenger, comes from the conversion of Mg^{++}-ATP in the presence of adenylate cyclase.

Mg^{++} competes with calcium (Ca^{++}) for membrane-binding sites and affects Ca^{++} binding with and release from the sarcoplasmic reticulum. Magnesium is a physiological antagonist of calcium, acting as a calcium channel blocker and a modulator of calcium channel activity. Also, hypomagnesemia impairs secretion and action of parathyroid hormone (PTH), leading to hypocalcemia.

Membrane Na^+,K^+-ATPase requires magnesium to regulate sodium (Na^+) and potassium (K^+) fluxes, which determine the electrical potential across the cell membrane. Mg^{++} has a critical role in maintaining intracellular K^+ concentrations, because a low intracellular magnesium concentration causes an outward movement of K^+ from the cells, inducing depolarization.

CLINICAL EFFECTS OF MAGNESIUM

Magnesium's actions on the cardiovascular system derive from its effects on calcium channels and pumps to regulate transmembrane and intracellular ionic flows. Magnesium has recognized vasodilatory effects, predominantly on the arteriolar vasculature, and modulates calcium fluxes, causing smooth muscle cell contraction. Magnesium exerts a "calcium antagonist" effect on myocytes by inhibiting calcium uptake and reducing cardiac contractility. Magnesium depletion is associated with coronary spasm and vasospastic angina: Magnesium infusion produces non–site-specific basal coronary dilatation and has a beneficial effect in patients with variant angina.[3]

Cardiac rhythm disorders are often associated with disturbances in cellular ionic movement of K^+, Ca^{++}, and Na^+, disturbances that may be induced by dysmagnesemia. Antiarrhythmic properties of magnesium are associated with its direct action on membrane permeability for potassium, with its capacity to block slow channels for sodium movement and its calcium antagonist effects. During perfusion of magnesium in humans, prolongation of the PR interval and an atrioventricular nodal effective refractory period, with no significant effect on QRS duration, QT interval, or atrial and ventricular refractory periods, have been observed on electrocardiography.[4]

Neuromuscular transmission is altered in magnesium disorders. Magnesium competes with entry of Ca^{++} into presynaptic endings, reducing acetylcholine release. Magnesium also decreases the effects of acetylcholine on postsynaptic muscle receptors, raising the axonal excitation threshold. The action of nondepolarizing neuromuscular blockers is potentiated by magnesium. Magnesium has a depressant effect on the synapses in the nervous system by competing with calcium in transmitter release. The anticonvulsant effect of magnesium is controversial but could be induced by a noncompetitive blockade of N-methyl-D-aspartate (NMDA) receptors, stimulation of which leads to excitatory postsynaptic potentials and seizures. Furthermore, the calcium antagonist property of magnesium causes central arteriolar vasodilatation and inhibits vasospasms, the latter considered one of the principal causes of seizures in eclampsia. Hypomagnesemia causes neuromuscular hyperexcitability. In hypermagnesemia, neuromuscular weakness is common and is associated with a clinical picture of myasthenia; with serum magnesium concentration above 9 mmol/L, deep tendon reflexes are abolished.

Magnesium exerts a sympatholytic effect through reduction of catecholamine release from adrenergic nerve endings, adrenal medulla, and adrenergic postganglionic sympathetic fibers. Magnesium deficiency may increase insulin resistance, especially in patients with metabolic syndrome or type 2 diabetes mellitus. Low intracellular magnesium concentrations may alter glucose entry into the cell, cause defective tyrosine-kinase activity, and modify insulin sensitivity by influencing receptor activity after binding or by influencing intracellular signaling and processing.[5] Magnesium is also an inhibitor of platelet aggregation.[6]

REGULATION OF MAGNESIUM

Absorption

The average daily intake of magnesium is 250 to 370 mg (10-15 mmol). One third is absorbed mainly in the distal portion of the small bowel through paracellular pathways and a saturable transport system. Intestinal absorption may vary according to the dietary magnesium content and total body magnesium level. Vitamin D metabolites, PTH, and intraluminal complexing agents have an effect on magnesium absorption. Magnesium absorption is also influenced by water movement: Diarrhea can induce intestinal malabsorption of magnesium. Approximately 40 mg of magnesium is usually lost through intestinal secretions, and the large bowel absorbs 20 mg. Changes in magnesium intake are counterbalanced by changes in magnesium reabsorption and excretion by the kidney.

Excretion

Seventy percent to 80% of total plasma magnesium is ultrafiltered by the glomerulus, and 15% to 25% is reabsorbed at the proximal tubule through passive diffusion down a favorable concentration gradient, because the concentration of magnesium rises to 1.5 times that of the glomerular filtrate.

The thick ascending limb of the loop of Henle is the principal site of magnesium reabsorption. Paracellular diffusion of magnesium is passive and depends on the sodium chloride–generated transmembrane potential. Passive diffusion is facilitated by paracellin-1, a protein present in renal tight junctions. Changes in paracellular permeability and transmembrane potential affect magnesium reabsorption. Loop diuretics reduce magnesium reabsorption by blocking sodium chloride reabsorption and inhibiting the creation of an electrical gradient.

Magnesium transport in the cortical collecting tubule is active and transcellular. Magnesium channels in the apical membrane allow entry of Mg^{++} into the distal tubular cells via a favorable transmembrane voltage and a low intracellular free magnesium concentration (0.5 mmol/L). Magne-

sium exit from the basolateral side could occur via sodium-magnesium exchange favored by a lower intracellular (10-15 mmol/L) than extracellular fluid sodium concentration.

An inverse relationship exists between serum magnesium concentration and magnesium transport: Hypermagnesemia enhances magnesuria, and hypomagnesemia enhances magnesium reabsorption. Serum calcium concentration also affects magnesium excretion. An elevation in serum calcium concentration inhibits reabsorption of both calcium and magnesium, whereas an elevation in calcium or magnesium concentration in the tubular fluid enhances magnesium reabsorption.

In hypercalcemia or hypermagnesemia (defined according to the serum divalent cation concentration sensed by extracellular Ca^{++}/Mg^{++}–sensing receptors present in the basolateral membrane of the thick ascending loop and the distal collecting tubule), a series of intracellular signals inhibits apical potassium channel. The consequence is a reduction in the amount of K^+ available for the Na^+-K^+-2Cl^- cotransporter, thereby diminishing Na^+ and Cl^- (chloride) reabsorption. Also, it inhibits the creation of the favorable electrical current induced by potassium secretion and permits the passive paracellular reabsorption of Ca^{++} and Mg^{++}.

In cases of negative magnesium balance, the earliest change is a drop in extracellular magnesium concentration, because several weeks are needed for magnesium mobilization from bones (the main reservoir) to occur. The only mechanism to reduce magnesium loss in hypomagnesemia is the increased reabsorption occurring principally in the thick ascending limb of the loop of Henle. The fractional magnesium excretion rate in normal subjects is 3% to 5% but can decrease to 0.5% in hypomagnesemia induced by extrarenal losses. In chronic renal failure, the reduction in glomerular filtration rate has the effect of raising the fractional magnesium excretion by a magnitude similar to the rise in calcium and sodium excretion. However, in end-stage renal failure, retention of magnesium occurs because the number of nephrons is not sufficient to excrete the ingested magnesium load.

Metabolic alkalosis enhances magnesium reabsorption by increasing magnesium permeability across the paracellular pathway in the thick ascending limb of the loop of Henle and by stimulating Mg^{++} entry into the distal tubular cells. Metabolic acidosis results in an increase in urinary magnesium excretion, because magnesium absorption in the distal tubule cells is diminished by protonation of the Mg^{++} entry pathway.[7] Hypokalemia inhibits magnesium transport in the loop of Henle, but the cellular mechanisms responsible for magnesium wasting in potassium deficiency remain unclear. In phosphate depletion, renal magnesium wasting can lead to overt hypomagnesemia. The means by which phosphate alters magnesium handling are also unclear. Administration of PTH or infusion of neutral phosphate can correct the situation. In experimental studies, several hormones have demonstrated the ability to modulate magnesium reabsorption, but at this time, the importance of those effects is unknown.

HYPOMAGNESEMIA

A serum total magnesium concentration less than 0.75 mmol/L is usually considered abnormally low (Fig. 101-2). However, serum total magnesium concentrations

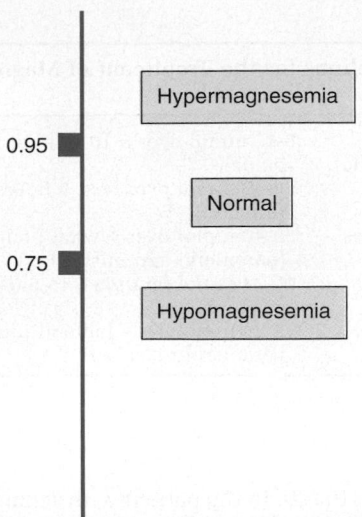

FIGURE 101-2. Normal range for total serum magnesium concentration, in mmol/L (1 mmol/L = 2 mEq/L = 2.43 mg/dL).

TABLE 101-1

Principal Causes of Magnesium Deficiency

Gastrointestinal	Diarrhea
	Malabsorption syndromes
	Prolonged nasogastric suction
	Inadequate intake
	Malnutrition
	Refeeding syndrome
	Intestinal and biliary fistulas
Renal	Osmotic diuresis
	Diuretic (loop or thiazides)
	Volume expansion
	Hypercalcemia and hypercalciuria
	Post-transplantation
	Polyuric phase (after acute tubular necrosis or obstruction)
	Drugs (cyclosporine, amphotericin B, cisplatin, foscarnet, pentamidine, aminoglycosides)
	Hypophosphatemia
Redistribution	Acute pancreatitis
	Hungry bone disease
	Correction of chronic systemic acidosis
	Severe burns
	Massive blood transfusion

are not well correlated with serum ionized concentrations in acutely ill patients because of alterations in serum proteins, acid-base disturbances, and the potential influence of concomitantly administered drugs on magnesium balance. A low serum total magnesium concentration may well represent pseudohypomagnesemia in a severely hypoalbuminemic patient. The normal serum ionized magnesium concentration is between 0.52 and 0.60 mmol/L. Despite experimental studies showing the superiority of extracellular ionized magnesium concentration measure over serum total concentration to accurately assess total body magnesium, there is no consensus on the use of the former method in the critical care setting. In critically ill patients, serum total magnesium concentration has been found to be sensitive (75%) but not specific (<40%) in predicting ionized hypomagnesemia; on the other hand, studies have found serum ionized magnesium concentrations to be normal in more than 70% of patients who had low total serum magnesium concentrations.[8,9] The potential consequences of various magnesium measures for the outcome of different subpopulations of critically ill patients are undefined at present.

Low serum magnesium concentration usually indicates significant magnesium deficiency. However, the serum magnesium concentration may be normal in the presence of intracellular magnesium depletion. A significant proportion of critically ill patients are magnesium depleted. Mortality has been shown to be increased in acutely ill patients who have hypomagnesemia at admission.[10] Magnesium depletion is often associated with hypokalemia, hypocalcemia, and metabolic alkalosis. Because the exchange between the extracellular and intracellular magnesium reserves (into cells and bones) is slow, hypomagnesemia occurs rapidly with magnesium deficit.

Causes

Hypomagnesemia can be induced by gastrointestinal losses, renal losses, or cellular redistribution of magnesium (Table 101-1). Distinction between renal and extrarenal losses can be made by measuring the 24-hour urinary magnesium excretion or the fractional magnesium excre-

tion (FE_{Mg}) on a urinary spot specimen, which is calculated as follows:

$$FE_{Mg} = U_{Mg} \times P_{Mg} \times \frac{100}{0.7} \times P_{Mg} \times U_{creat}$$

where U_{Mg} is urinary magnesium concentration, P_{Mg} is plasma or serum magnesium concentration, and U_{creat} is urinary creatinine concentration. Moreover, the magnesium-loading test appears to be valid for detection of normomagnesemic magnesium depletion (isolated cellular depletion) in critical care patients.[11]

Gastrointestinal losses are not regulated and are more important with small bowel disease (diarrhea, malabsorption, short-bowel syndrome, small bowel bypass surgery). Diarrheal fluids and fistula drainage contain as much as 7 to 8 mmol/L total magnesium ions (or 15 mEq/L). Losses via nasogastric suctioning are not large but are associated with poor magnesium intake, contributing to progressive depletion. Magnesium content of upper gastrointestinal fluids is about 0.5 mmol/L (or 1 mEq/L).

The fractional urinary excretion of filtered magnesium is normally 5%; in the initial phase of magnesium deficiency, the kidneys can normally reduce urinary magnesium excretion to less than 1 mmol without a drop in plasma magnesium concentration.[12] Two mechanisms may cause renal losses of magnesium: an intrinsic defect in tubular magnesium reabsorption and an extrinsic defect that causes renal magnesium wasting. Tubular dysfunction in the recovery phase of acute tubular necrosis is not unusual and may be associated with magnesium wastage. Tubular dysfunction with hypomagnesemia may also be present in acute interstitial nephropathy and postobstructive diuresis as well as after renal transplantation. In alcoholics, hypomagnesemia is not unusual because magnesium intake is often decreased and an alcohol-induced (but reversible) tubular dysfunction increases magnesium excretion.

Loop diuretics and long-term administration of thiazide diuretics and mannitol may induce hypomagnesemia. The other most common therapeutic agents that cause hypomagnesemia by increasing renal magnesium losses are aminoglycosides, antibiotics, cisplatin, amphotericin B, cyclosporine, pentamidine, insulin, carbenicillins, and digoxin.

Because calcium and magnesium compete in the thick ascending limb of the loop of Henle for paracellular diffusion, increased intratubular calcium concentration, as found in hypercalcemia or hypercalciuria, favors calcium reabsorption over magnesium reabsorption.

In volume expansion, sodium reabsorption is decreased, leading to diminished passive diffusion of magnesium. In patients with severe head injury, particularly those with hypothermia, severe electrolyte depletion, including hypomagnesemia, is common and is related in part to the greater urinary excretion through polyuria.[13,14] Increased magnesuria has been observed in severe phosphate depletion and thyrotoxicosis.

Greater uptake of magnesium by bone occurs in hungry bone syndrome and after correction of chronic acidosis. The infusion of citrate with massive tranfusions, particularly during liver transplantation or apheresis, may affect levels of ionized magnesium.[15,16] During acute pancreatitis or after pancreatic surgery, saponification of magnesium in necrotic fat and by free fatty acids can occur, resulting in hypomagnesemia. Hypomagnesemia, due to large cutaneous magnesium losses, is also observed after severe burns.[17]

Signs and Symptoms

Concurrent hypokalemia is present in 60% to 65% of hypomagnesemic patients, because the underlying cause frequently induces both potassium and magnesium wastage. Hypomagnesemia can also cause hypokalemia secondary to increased tubular secretion of potassium; this hypokalemia is refractory to supplementation unless hypomagnesemia is also corrected. Hypocalcemia is also common and is induced by a suppressive effect of hypomagnesemia on PTH secretion, a resistance to vitamin D, and end-organ resistance to PTH action.

Central neuronal excitability and neuromuscular transmission are increased in situations of magnesium depletion. Clinical manifestations include tremor, myoclonic jerks, seizures, Chvostek's and Trousseau's signs, spontaneous carpopedal spasm, ataxia, nystagmus, and dysphagia. Various psychiatric abnormalities may manifest, from delirium to apathy to coma.[18]

In severe hypomagnesemia, PR and QT intervals are prolonged, predisposing to ventricular arrhythmias, tachycardia, and abnormal T wave. Cardiac effects of hypomagnesemia are probably due to an interaction of magnesium with calcium channels. Increased arteriolar tone is also common when extracellular magnesium is low, because calcium uptake is enhanced and intracellular calcium concentration is increased. Digoxin sensitivity is increased in hypomagnesemia. Many patients with symptomatic mitral valve prolapse are hypomagnesemic, and magnesium supplementation has been shown to improve symptoms.[19] Hypomagnesemia may rarely cause pseudogout by inducing deposition of calcium pyrophosphate dihydrate crystals in articular structures.[20]

Treatment

The modality and rapidity of magnesium repletion are functions of the symptoms and serum magnesium concen-

TABLE 101-2

Broad Guidelines for the Treatment of Magnesium Deficiency

Emergency (symptomatic)	8-12 mmol over 5-10 minutes (parenteral bolus)
	20-40 mmol over next 5 hours (parenteral infusion)
Critical illness	20-40 mmol over several hours on day 1 (parenteral administration)
	16-24 mmol on days 2 to 5 (can be enteral or parenteral)
Maintenance	12-24 mmol daily (enteral route or via parenteral nutrition)

tration (Table 101-2). In the patient with seizures or cardiac arrhythmias, 8 to 12 mmol of magnesium should be rapidly given in 5 to 10 minutes, followed by a perfusion over several hours. Because renal magnesium reabsorption is slow and inversely proportional to serum magnesium concentration, rapid magnesium infusion will result in excretion of up to 50% of the dose given. Thus, oral supplementation may be preferred over intravenous supplementation for asymptomatic patients. However, several magnesium salts induce diarrhea when given by the enteral route. Patients with hypomagnesemia induced by renal wastage may benefit from the use of a potassium-sparing diuretic (amiloride, triamterene) to improve magnesium reabsorption at the collecting tubule.

Before initiation of magnesium supplementation, the patient's renal function should be assessed, and doses reduced by 25% to 50% in patients with moderate to severe renal failure. Moreover, because magnesium has a calcium antagonist effect, with a potential for severe heart block and cardiac conduction defects, caution is mandatory.

Magnesium has also been used as a therapeutic agent, in the absence of hypomagnesemia, in patients with preeclampsia/eclampsia, cardiac arrhythmias, ischemic heart disease, bronchial asthma, and urolithiasis. Despite the remaining controversy for some of these indications, it can be a useful adjunct when other therapeutic modalities are insufficient.[21-23]

HYPERMAGNESEMIA

Hypermagnesemia corresponds to a serum concentration in excess of 0.95 mmol/L (see Fig. 101-1). Because the efficacy of the kidneys to excrete a magnesium load is very good, more than 250 mmol/day or nearly 100% of the filtered load can be eliminated by the person with increased plasma magnesium concentration, and hypermagnesemia is rarely seen.

Clinically significant hypermagnesemia is rare in the absence of acute or chronic renal failure and/or administration of a massive magnesium load. In chronic renal failure, urinary magnesium excretion falls but plasma magnesium concentration usually stabilizes at approximately 1 to 1.5 mmol/L. Because there is no regulatory system other than renal excretion and also no protection mechanism against hypermagnesemia with loss of renal function, magnesium-containing antacids and cathartics, as well as large doses of magnesium salts supplementation, are contraindicated in the patient with renal failure.

The prevalence of hypermagnesemia has been reported as 0.8% to 9.3% among hospitalized patients, and 13.5% at admission to intensive care.[2,24,25] Severe hypermagnesemia may occur after multiple doses of a magnesium-containing cathartic for treatment of drug overdose. The usual total average dose of magnesium citrate (9.22 g magnesium) induces an increment in serum magnesium concentration.[26] Forty-seven percent of patients experience hypermagnesemia (>1.2 mmol/L), and 12% severe hypermagnesemia (>1.5 mmol/L), although there is no correlation between the total amount of magnesium citrate administered and the rise in serum magnesium concentration. Magnesium enemas may also induce hypermagnesemia. Laxative abuse and accidental ingestion of Epsom salts are other reported causes. Elderly patients and patients with bowel disorders associated with enhanced absorption (active ulcer disease, gastritis, colitis, perforated viscus or massive gastric dilatation) are particularly at risk for hypermagnesemia with oral ingestion of magnesium-containing antacids and cathartics even though the amount of magnesium ingested is not excessive.[27]

Hypermagnesemia is one of the metabolic complications of tumor lysis syndrome, massive tissue damage from seizure, and ischemia. Some cases of hypermagnesemia associated with diabetic ketoacidosis have been documented.

Intravenous magnesium sulfate is widely used in obstetrics to decrease neuromuscular excitability in women with preeclampsia/eclampsia and as a tocolytic drug for preterm labor. Target serum magnesium concentrations suggested for treatment of eclamptic convulsions are between 1.8 and 3.0 mmol/L.[28] Maternal toxicity associated with this regimen is rare, although adequate monitoring is recommended. Rare reported causes of mild hypermagnesemia are Addison's disease, lithium treatment and intoxication, and hypothyroidism.[29]

Clinical Manifestations

Symptoms of hypermagnesemia are uncommon when serum magnesium levels are less than 2 mmol/L. The first symptoms to appear are nausea, vomiting, and flushing with reduced tendon reflexes. Neurological manifestations include flaccid paralysis, lethargy, coma, and respiratory depression. Cardiovascular effects of hypermagnesemia occur with serum magnesium concentrations above 2 to 2.5 mmol/L. Calcium antagonist properties of magnesium induce bradycardia and hypotension. Prolongation of PR interval, QRS complex, and QT interval may be seen at higher concentrations, between 2.5 and 5 mmol/L. With further increases in magnesemia, evolution toward complete heart block and cardiac arrest is possible.

Asymptomatic hypocalcemia—although electrocardiographic abnormalities may be present—can be induced by hypermagnesemia. Magnesium excess produces calcium wasting, inhibits PTH secretion, and reduces bone responsiveness to PTH.

Magnesium infusion may prolong the action of nondepolarizing muscle relaxants.[30] Because citrate and sulfate are the most common anions in magnesium-containing salts and are unmeasured anions, the serum anion gap can be increased in hypermagnesemia associated with ingestion or infusion of those salts.[31]

Treatment

Discontinuation of magnesium intake (supplementation, medication, parenteral nutrition) is the first step in management of hypermagnesemia. In patients with normal kidney function, discontinuing magnesium intake allows hypermagnesemia to correct itself; in patients with renal failure or with severe symptomatic hypermagnesemia, renal replacement therapy may be necessary. Hemodialysis is preferable to hemofiltration because the decline in magnesium serum concentration occurs faster with the former. When severe symptoms are present, calcium may be given as a magnesium antagonist to reverse cardiac arrhythmias, hypotension, and respiratory depression. The usual dose is 50 to 100 mg elemental calcium over 5 to 10 minutes, but larger amounts may be required.

CONCLUSION

Magnesium metabolism has not been as well defined as metabolism of other ions, and interest in further research should be encouraged. Therapeutic doses of magnesium are actually given in several clinical situations, mostly when hypomagnesemia is present, but more studies are needed to demonstrate the advantages of supplementation in patients without hypomagnesemia.

Key Points

1. Magnesium is the second most abundant intracellular cation.
2. Magnesium has several important physiological roles.
3. Serum total magnesium concentration currently remains the most frequently used tool for diagnosis and repletion of suspected deficiency, despite its potential limitations.
4. Hypomagnesemia usually results from increased gastrointestinal or renal losses.
5. Hypermagnesemia occurs rarely, with the exception of renal failure and iatrogenic overdosing.

Key References

2. Escuela MP, Guerra M, Añón JM, et al: Total and ionized serum magnesium in critically ill patients. Intensive Care Med 2005;31:151-156.
8. Noronha JL, Matuschak GM: Magnesium in critical illness: Metabolism, assessment, and treatment. Intensive Care Med 2002;28:667-679.
9. Huijgen HJ, Soesan M, Sanders R, et al: Magnesium levels in critically ill patients: What should we measure? Am J Clin Pathol 2000;114:688-695.
21. Dubé L, Granry JC: The therapeutic use of magnesium in anesthesiology, intensive care and emergency medicine: A review. Can J Anaesth 2003;50:732-746.
28. Lu JF, Nightingale CH: Magnesium sulfate in eclampsia and pre-eclampsia: Pharmacokinetic principles. Clin Pharmacokinet 2000;38:305-14.

See the companion Expert Consult website for the complete reference list.

CHAPTER 102

Disorders of Trace Elements and Vitamins

Anthony J. Hennessy and Andrew R. Davies

OBJECTIVES

This chapter will:
1. Describe what trace elements and vitamins are and which are most important.
2. Discuss each major trace element in terms of its main roles and the effects on it of critical illness and acute renal failure (including continuous renal replacement therapy).
3. Discuss each vitamin in terms of its main roles and the effects on it of critical illness and acute renal failure (including continuous renal replacement therapy).
4. Discuss the known benefits and risks of supplementation of those trace elements and vitamins for which the issue has been studied.

Trace elements and vitamins are micronutrients that are not usually synthesized in the human body but are required in small, sometimes minute, amounts for the various physiological functions of the body. *Trace elements* are inorganic minerals, and *vitamins* are a heterogeneous group of organic compounds. Trace elements can be further divided into (1) those known to be essential to humans for health and cellular function and (2) ultra-trace elements, which have been found to be essential in experimental animals but for which the role in human health remains unclear. Although the association between micronutrient deficiency and illness has long been known, the recognition of the low endogenous antioxidant capacity in critical illness and the possible role of trace elements and vitamins as supplemental antioxidants have added new impetus to micronutrient research.[1-3]

The principal aims of this chapter are (1) to delineate the role of these micronutrients in the body, (2) to collate the evidence for the behavior of these substances in both critical illness and critical illness–related acute renal failure (ARF) (including the use of continuous renal replacement therapy [CRRT]), and (3) to discuss the known benefits and risks of supplementation if studied.

One of the most important concepts is that critically ill patients suffer from oxidative stress caused by reactive oxygen species and reactive nitrogen species.[4] These species can damage most cellular structures, including DNA, proteins, and lipids. Although these species are also produced in healthy states, they are dealt with by adequate levels of endogenous antioxidants. Sepsis is associated with reduced circulating antioxidants and an alteration in the pro-oxidant/antioxidant balance that may have a role in the progression to multiple-organ failure.[5,6]

This process has led to the hypothesis that supplementation of trace elements and vitamins in critical illness will bolster endogenous antioxidant function and, therefore, will combat oxidative damage.[2,7] Such supplementation has led to clinical improvements in several studies[8-11]; however, combinations of various trace elements and vitamins have been used in these studies, making it difficult to tell whether a specific micronutrient, rather than all of them, should be supplemented.

Given that the critically ill patients who receive the lowest amounts of the recommended dietary allowance (RDA) of vitamins and trace elements have the greatest oxidative stress,[12] it is also not clear whether the predominant rationale for the administration of trace elements and vitamins in patients in intensive care units (ICUs) is to just replace what the patient would have been eating or to give large doses of one or more micronutrients as a so-called pharmaconutrient.

A 2005 meta-analysis found that antioxidants reduced mortality and that the effect was stronger in trials using a single micronutrient, trials using parenteral administration, and trials in which selenium was administered.[13] This finding has certainly brought a focus to research on which micronutrients are the most important to replace.

TRACE ELEMENTS

Trace elements known to be essential to humans are zinc, iron, copper, selenium, manganese, chromium, and iodine (Table 102-1). Deficiency of these trace elements has given rise to specific clinical states that are often improved with supplementation of the same trace element.

Ultra-trace elements are other minerals present in tissues in minute quantities, such as arsenic, boron, fluorine, tin, silicon, vanadium, nickel, bromine, and cadmium. The role of these elements in critical illness and ARF is unclear, requires further investigation, and is not discussed further here.

Trace elements circulate as protein-bound complexes that are not necessarily in equilibrium with tissue stores in critical illness. Levels are affected by altered protein binding, third space losses, redistribution, the acute-phase response, extracorporeal circuit losses, and both wound and drain losses.[14,15] All of the essential trace elements except for chromium are excreted predominantly via the gastrointestinal tract, so abnormalities of gastrointestinal function and motility may also alter trace element requirements. Although some trace elements may accumulate in chronic renal failure, levels are more likely to fall in critical illness–associated ARF,[16] raising the specific question whether individual trace element supplementation should be performed in patients with critical illness in general and in those with critical illness–associated ARF.

TABLE 102-1

Daily Trace Element Requirements for Generally Healthy People

TRACE ELEMENT	ENTERAL	PARENTERAL
Chromium (μg)	30	10-15
Copper (mg)	0.9	0.3-0.5
Fluoride (mg)	4	Not well defined
Iodine (μg)	150	Not well defined
Iron (mg)	18	Not routinely added
Manganese (mg)	2.3	60-100
Molybdenum (μg)	45	Not routinely added
Selenium (μg)	55	20-60
Zinc (mg)	11	2.5-5

Adapted from ASPEN Board of Directors and the Clinical Guidelines Task Force: Guidelines for the use of parenteral and enteral nutrition in adult and pediatric patients [erratum in: JPEN J Parenter Enteral Nutr 2002;26:144]. JPEN J Parenter Enteral Nutr 2002;26(Suppl):1SA-138SA.

Zinc

Zinc, an essential trace element, is recognized as being a cofactor in numerous enzyme systems. It is an important component of gene regulatory proteins.[17] Zinc deficiency, which can lead to growth problems, hypogonadism, and abnormalities of cellular immunity, hair growth, and wound healing, is a large public health problem in Third World countries, and many detailed reviews of the cellular functions of zinc and associated problems of zinc deficiency have been published.[18]

Serum zinc levels in an ICU patient are difficult to interpret accurately because they may decrease during the acute phase of the inflammatory response and they are also affected by protein binding. In animals, the principal zinc transport system has been found to be cytokine dependent, and thus, zinc levels alter in inflammation.[19] Metallothionein proteins participate in the uptake, transport, and regulation of zinc in biological systems; this fact may be important in some patients, such as those with major burns, in whom the initial fall in zinc level is followed by a rebound rise in levels with enhancement of metallothionein expression.[20] Some studies have shown increased urinary losses of zinc during critical illness,[15] and patients with burns would be expected to have greater losses due to tissue injury.[21]

A number of studies have measured zinc levels in patients receiving CRRT.[22-24] In the first two of these studies,[22,23] zinc did not appear in the ultrafiltrate, but in the third study,[24] zinc was detected in the ultrafiltrate at low levels—however, these were lower than the amounts in the replacement fluid. Zinc levels in patients receiving CRRT seem comparable to those in critically ill patients not receiving CRRT.[22,23]

Increased body losses and low plasma levels suggest that zinc becomes deficient at the tissue level in critical illness because plasma zinc balance is maintained tightly. Even when zinc levels seem normal, zinc-related dermatological conditions have arisen and have responded to zinc supplementation, perhaps because homeostatic regulatory mechanisms can maintain plasma zinc concentrations during zinc restriction.[25] Given the difficulty in assessing serum zinc levels, other approaches have been taken to diagnosis of zinc deficiency states—including the measurement of the activity of zinc-dependent enzymes such as alkaline phosphatase, copper-zinc superoxide dismutase, and lymphocyte 5'-nucleotidase[26]—although there seems a reasonable rationale to supplement zinc regardless.

Zinc supplementation may have a place in patients with traumatic brain injury in light of the results of a moderately sized clinical trial demonstrating an improvement in clinical outcomes in association with biochemical improvements.[27] Studies in other subgroups of patients, however, are not available. Although serum zinc levels may be low in critically ill patients and the clinician is tempted to supplement zinc, further research is required before zinc supplementation can be recommended as routine in patients with critical illness with or without renal failure.

Iron

Anemia is a common problem in the critically ill. Causes for its development are multiple, including hemorrhage, recurrent blood sampling, decreased synthesis of endogenous erythropoietin, and alterations of iron metabolism. With the inflammatory process, iron distribution is altered, with decreased serum iron levels and increased iron stores. The reduction in serum iron levels may be a protective mechanism because iron is essential for bacterial growth. Functional iron deficiency, measured by red cell hypochromasia on flow cytometry, was present in about one third of patients at admission to the intensive care unit in one study and was associated with a longer stay and more pronounced systemic inflammatory response syndrome.[28]

This issue raises the question whether iron supplementation may be useful, because it has been controversial in the past owing to a perceived association with higher infection rates. Although intravenous iron supplementation may not be associated with an increased risk of bacteremia in patients with chronic renal failure,[29] this may not be the case when iron supplementation is combined with administration of erythropoietin,[29] and concerns are raised by experimental data demonstrating exacerbation of sepsis by iron therapy.[30]

Corwin and associates[31] showed that administration of erythropoietin was a useful transfusion-sparing strategy in critically ill patients,[31] although it must be noted that these researchers used oral iron supplementation concurrently with erythropoietin to optimize the erythropoietic response. Whether the iron supplementation was truly necessary is still not known, but in view of the lack of research supporting iron supplementation and the risk of harm, it seems wise to await further studies.[32]

Copper

Copper is widely distributed in human tissues and is required for the function of more than 30 proteins, including superoxide dismutase, ceruloplasmin, lysyl oxidase, cytochrome c oxidase, tyrosinase, and dopamine-β-hydroxylase. Deficiency of copper can cause leukopenia, neutropenia, bone demineralization, and decreased immune function.

The majority (90%) of plasma copper is in the form of ceruloplasmin, and although copper is known to be an acute-phase reactant,[33] there is little understanding of the effects of general critical illness on copper levels in the body. The fact that the cuproenzyme lysyl oxidase is essential for the pathway involving cross-linking of collagen suggests that copper has a major role in wound healing.

In the specific population with burn injury, copper and ceruloplasmin levels have been shown to be low with elevations of urinary copper excretion[34] and exudative losses, leading to a copper deficiency state.[21] In the same population, copper supplementation (when given in combination with zinc and selenium) has been shown to decrease nosocomial pneumonia.[3]

Information pertaining to copper in ARF is limited. However, this element has been shown to be lost via the ultrafiltrate in patients receiving CRRT.[23,24] Although moderate amounts are lost through this mechanism, the risk/benefit ratio for copper supplementation in patients with renal failure and in other critically ill patients remains unknown.

Selenium

Selenium is an essential trace element, and low levels are often found when selenium is measured in critically ill patients, particularly those suffering from sepsis, trauma, and burns. Low levels are partly due to redistribution and movement of selenium to tissues and organs involved in protein synthesis and immune cell production, although selenium losses can also occur through drains, wounds, and urinary excretion. It also appears that selenium is lost through the ultrafiltrate of CRRT.[24] Whether low selenium levels lead to a reduction in available endogenous antioxidant activity is unclear, but because the antioxidant system requires selenium (for the enzymes glutathione-peroxidase and thioredoxin reductase), allowing selenium deficiency to develop or persist would seem to be counterproductive, especially when sepsis is present.

The hypothesis that selenium supplementation might improve antioxidant potential in critically ill patients has led to clinical trials investigating the issue. Supplementation was found in one trial to increase glutathione peroxidase activity,[35] and intravenous administration of selenium at 1000 µg per day in another trial improved survival in the subgroup of the most severely unwell patients with septic shock.[1] A meta-analysis has demonstrated clinical outcome improvements with selenium,[13] and another large trial is under way.[36]

Selenium toxicity is also well described, particularly in areas of high soil selenium content. Fortunately, toxicity usually occurs from years of high intake, and administration of high-dose supplementation for short periods to previously deficient patients is unlikely to have adverse effects.

Extra selenium supplementation should be considered for all critically ill patients who may have increased losses. Careful attention must be given to interpretation of selenium levels in critically ill patients, however, and definitive markers of benefit must be confirmed before widespread selenium supplementation can be recommended for all patients with critical illness.

Manganese

The data available on manganese in intensive care patients is extremely limited. Deficiency of this element gives rise to growth retardation, skeletal muscle abnormalities, impaired reproductive function, and impaired glucose tolerance in experimental animals, although documentation of manganese levels and manganese deficiency in humans is sparse.

However, there have been reports of manganese toxicity in patients receiving long-term parenteral nutrition, with manganese deposition having been noted in the basal ganglia on magnetic resonance imaging.[37] This toxicity

may occur more quickly in patients with cholestasis, because biliary excretion of excess manganese is the usual method of excretion.[38]

The effects of renal failure and CRRT on manganese levels are not known, and all that can be currently recommended is to avoid excess manganese in the administration of parenteral nutrition.

Chromium

Chromium deficiency in animals causes a syndrome of glucose intolerance similar to diabetes in adults. Chromium has been detected in the ultrafiltrate of patients receiving CRRT,[23] but because chromium is renally excreted, it accumulates in patients with renal failure even when they are receiving CRRT. The clinical significance of this fact is unclear and needs further clarification before any recommendations can be made.

Iodine

Iodine is an essential trace element involved in thyroid hormone production and is necessary in quantities for thyroid hormone synthesis. This topic is covered in other texts elsewhere and is beyond the scope of this chapter.

VITAMINS

Vitamins are a group of heterogeneous organic compounds that are essential micronutrients. They are present in most foodstuffs and are routinely provided in nearly all enteral and parenteral nutrition formulations (Table 102-2).

Daily requirements are based on the amounts required to avoid acute or chronic illness in healthy subjects eating average diets, and the adequacy of supplementation of amounts in critically ill patients has not been extensively studied. Many critically ill patients have demonstrated acute deterioration from a preexisting chronic

TABLE 102-2

Daily Vitamin Requirements for Generally Healthy People

VITAMIN	ENTERAL	PARENTERAL
Thiamine (mg)	1.2	3
Riboflavin (mg)	1.3	3.6
Niacin (mg)	16	40
Folic acid (µg)	400	400
Pantothenic acid (mg)	5	15
Vitamin B_6 (mg)	1.7	4
Vitamin B_{12} (µg)	2.4	5
Biotin (µg)	30	60
Choline (mg)	550	Not defined
Ascorbic acid (mg)	90	100
Vitamin A (µg)	900	1000
Vitamin D (µg)	15	5
Vitamin E (mg)	15	10
Vitamin K (µg)	120	1

Adapted from ASPEN Board of Directors and the Clinical Guidelines Task Force: Guidelines for the use of parenteral and enteral nutrition in adult and pediatric patients [erratum in: JPEN J Parenter Enteral Nutr 2002;26:144]. JPEN J Parenter Enteral Nutr 2002;26(Suppl):1SA-138SA.

illness and may have lower vitamin levels on admission. Whether acute illness–related redistribution reduces vitamin availability for cellular activity is also unclear. A rationale is therefore developing that larger doses of many vitamins may be required in critically ill patients, not only for their antioxidant effects but also because patients can have vitamin deficiencies despite "adequate" supplementation.[39]

Vitamin A

Vitamin A is a lipid-soluble vitamin comprising a family of compounds called the *retinoids*. It occurs in nature in three forms, but in humans, retinol is the predominant form and 11-*cis*-retinol is the active form. Vitamin A is essential for vision, immune response, epithelial cell growth and repair, bone growth, and reproduction. The effects of vitamin A on immunity are diverse, with most research having been performed in children with measles, diarrhea-related illness, and human immunodeficiency virus infection.[40]

Carotenoids are absorbed in the ileum and are detectable in various tissues, but unlike vitamin A, they do not combine with specific transport proteins and are transported mainly as nonpolar lipids.[41] Levels can be measured by checking plasma β-carotene and serum retinol levels. Serum retinol levels tend to remain constant until liver stores are severely depleted or in excess. Plasma β-carotene levels tend to reflect current intake, decrease rapidly with restriction of intake, and have been shown to be reduced in multiple-organ failure and further diminished in patients with both multiple-organ failure and renal failure.[42] Because vitamin A is lipid soluble, it is not found in the ultrafiltrate in patients receiving CRRT.[23]

Supplementation of vitamin A (with other vitamins) has been shown to increase β-carotene levels as well as markers of lipid peroxidation,[2] but further research on the benefits for clinical outcome is clearly required. Excess vitamin A is usually well tolerated over the short term, but it may accumulate in the tissues, and long-term ingestion of excess amounts may lead to portal hypertension and cirrhosis.[43]

Vitamin B

The B vitamins are made up of eight different, chemically distinct water-soluble compounds historically thought to be the same substance. They were later found to be different substances all found in the same foods. Supplements containing all eight compounds are known as *vitamin B complex*. They generally function as coenzymes that catalyze chemical processes.

Thiamine (Vitamin B₁)

Thiamine deficiency, known as beriberi, occurs in the following three forms: (1) dry beriberi, involving the nervous system, (2) wet beriberi, referring to the cardiovascular effects, and (3) Wernicke's encephalopathy. Thiamine pyrophosphate acts as a coenzyme in carbohydrate metabolism through the decarboxylation of alpha-ketoacids and in the formation of glucose by acting as a coenzyme for the transketolase in the pentose monophosphate pathway.

Up to 20% of patients in ICUs have been found to be thiamine deficient, and these patients had a much higher mortality rate.[44] In a prospective study of thiamine status, patients with severe injuries showed signs of thiamine deficiency (based on transketolase activity) within the first week of their injuries despite routine enteral or parenteral vitamin supplementation.[45]

Thiamine has been detected in the ultrafiltrate of patients receiving CRRT,[24] with daily losses amounting to about 4 mg. Given that the thiamine RDA is approximately 1 mg, body stores would be depleted in about a week of such losses without supplementation. Fortunately, thiamine replacement seems unlikely to be harmful in ICU patients, so adequate supplementation should be given. The optimal dose in critically ill patients, especially those with ARF, remains unknown.

Riboflavin (Vitamin B₂)

Riboflavin is important for energy production, enzyme function, and normal fatty acid and amino acid synthesis and is necessary for the reproduction of glutathione, a free radical scavenger. Data on isolated riboflavin deficiency in ICU patients are very limited. Because the vitamin is water soluble, larger amounts of riboflavin may be lost during continuous venovenous hemofiltration.

Niacin (Vitamin B₃)

Dietary niacin deficiency (causing pellagra) is uncommon. Clinical manifestations include the "three Ds": diffuse pigmented rash (dermatitis), gastroenteritis (diarrhea), and widespread neurologic deficits, including cognitive decline (dementia). Little is known about niacin levels in critical illness.

Pantothenic Acid (Vitamin B₅)

Pantothenic acid deficiency is exceptionally rare and has not been thoroughly studied. Evidence is insufficient for any recommendations for vitamin B₅ supplementation to be made for critically ill patients.

Pyridoxine (Vitamin B₆)

Pyridoxal 5′-phosphate, the active coenzyme form of pyridoxine, is an essential cofactor in decarboxylation, hydrolysis, and synthesis pathways involving carbohydrate, sphingolipid, amino acid, heme, and neurotransmitter metabolism. Isolated pyridoxine deficiency is rare, and data on its occurrence in critical illness are scant. Levels decrease by approximately 14% per day in patients receiving CRRT,[46] but excess replacement of pyridoxine over long periods has been associated with painful sensory neuropathy. Caution in pyridoxine replacement is required until research is undertaken into its function in critical illness.

Biotin (Vitamin B₇)

Biotin is synthesized in the intestine. Optimal levels and their interpretation in critically ill patients are unclear.

Folates and Folic Acid (Vitamin B₉)

Folate deficiency is relatively common in ICU patients, rates of around 2% having been reported.[47] Adults are believed to require 3 µg/kg/day of folates. Patients at higher risk of deficiency include those undergoing therapy with erythropoietin, sulfasalazine, phenytoin, trimethoprim, and methotrexate. These require increased supplementation. Patients receiving CRRT have also been shown to be at risk, with folate levels decreasing daily by 12%.[46]

Vitamin B₁₂

Vitamin B12 is unique among the vitamins in that it contains cobalt. Hence *cobalamin* is the term used to refer to compounds having vitamin B_{12} activity. The rate of vitamin B_{12} deficiency in critical illness was found to be 2% in a general intensive care population.[47]

Vitamin C

Vitamin C is also known as ascorbic acid. It has numerous functions, but its role as an antioxidant and its potential to reduce the effects of free radical damage have received a large proportion of research. Vitamin C is also required for collagen synthesis, neurotransmitter function, coagulation, and the metabolism of cholesterol and bile salts. Vitamin C assays are prone to interference, and levels may be falsely low with aspirin therapy,[48] but levels of vitamin C have been shown to be consistently low in critically ill patients at admission to ICUs.[49,50] Lower concentrations are associated with more severe illness, and although there is some redistribution effect, it is likely that the inflammatory process and the generation of free radicals cause greater oxidation of ascorbic acid and its removal from plasma.

Vitamin C appears in the ultrafiltrate in patients receiving CRRT in significant amounts.[23] Calculated daily ultrafiltrate from continuous venovenous hemofiltration losses are 68 mg, so an RDA of 90 to 100 mg is likely to be inadequate in patients receiving CRRT. Patients with ARF have more depressed antioxidative systems than those without it,[42] so perhaps there should be a low threshold to supplement vitamin C in these patients. This approach should be tempered with the knowledge that massive doses of vitamin C may lead to secondary oxalosis and ARF.[51]

Studies of antioxidant supplementation that have included vitamin C have shown moderate clinical benefits. Repletion of vitamin C at RDA amounts seems inadequate to normalize vitamin C levels,[50] but when vitamin C is given at a larger than standard dose, albeit when in combination with vitamin E, other antioxidants, and lipids, it seems to have a powerful effect on clinical outcomes in patients with acute lung injury.[9,10] Vitamin C may also be useful when combined with other antioxidants for other groups of critically ill patients.[8,11] However, it seems fairly unlikely that vitamin C supplementation alone might lead to such improvements, so further studies are needed.

Vitamin D

Vitamin D, which is lipid soluble, is essential for maintaining normal calcium metabolism. Vitamin D_3 (cholecal-ciferol) can be synthesized by humans in the skin upon exposure to ultraviolet B radiation from sunlight or can be obtained from diet. When exposure to ultraviolet radiation is insufficient for the synthesis of adequate amounts of vitamin D_3 in the skin, adequate intake of vitamin D from the diet is essential for health. The RDA for vitamin D is difficult to estimate because the skin synthesizes a large amount. The current American Society for Parenteral and Enteral Nutrition's recommendation in parenteral nutrition is for 200 IU/day for ICU patients,[52] although other groups have recommended up to 400 IU/day[53] because of concerns about the rising incidence of fractures in an aging population.

Very low serum concentrations of 25-hydroxyvitamin D and 1,25-dihydroxyvitamin D_3 have been documented in patients with prolonged critical illness[54]; also, because of the catabolic nature of critical illness, a very large increase in bone resorption occurs in patients receiving intensive care.[55] Whether this increase translates into slower healing of fractures in the ICU or predisposes patients to fractures after discharge from the ICU has not been established, but it has led to renewed interest in vitamin D studies in critically ill patients.

One study comparing the effect of two doses of vitamin D (200 IU and 500 IU daily) in patients with prolonged critical illness found that both doses failed to normalize vitamin D levels, although the higher dose caused a greater reduction in systemic inflammatory markers, suggesting a potential anti-inflammatory role for vitamin D.[56]

Excessive vitamin D can cause hypercalcemia, and although metabolic bone disease has been reported in patients receiving long-term total parenteral nutrition,[57] acute toxicity seems rare. Nevertheless, what the real benefits and risks are for vitamin D supplementation in critically ill patients remains to be seen.

Vitamin E

Vitamin E is a lipid-soluble vitamin that exists in eight different forms, four tocopherols and four tocotrienols. Alpha-tocopherol (α-tocopherol), the most active form of vitamin E in humans, is the form found in the largest quantities in the blood and tissue. Its main function is as an antioxidant, and vitamin E supplementation has been tested in patients with ischemia-reperfusion injury and sepsis. Vitamin E belongs to the most powerful group of lipid-soluble chain-breaking antioxidants that prevent lipid peroxidation and disruption of membrane integrity,[58] and its levels are reduced in critically ill patients with sepsis for various reasons, including redistribution, altered lipid levels, and protein binding.[5]

In ARF, vitamin E levels have been shown to be profoundly depressed.[59] This depression does not appear to be due to losses through CRRT.[23]

Clinical trials of vitamin E supplementation have been conducted in patients who have undergone liver[60] and cardiac surgery[61] for its effects on ischemia-reperfusion injury. In patients undergoing liver resection, 600 IU of parenteral vitamin E given the day before surgery ameliorated the drop in vitamin E levels and improved liver function test values, leading to a shorter ICU stay.[60] In the patients undergoing cardiac surgery, supplementation maintained vitamin E levels throughout the perioperative period but failed to demonstrate a clinical effect,[61] perhaps because of the lack of co-supplementation with vitamin C, which is known to maximize the antioxidant effect of vitamin E.[62] Certainly vitamin E combined with both vitamin C and allopurinol may be beneficial in patients undergoing cardiac surgery.[63]

Trials of antioxidants in sepsis have also involved multiple antioxidants, making it difficult to ascribe an effect to vitamin E alone. Enteral vitamin A, C, and E supplements in ICU patients seem to be adequately absorbed and to improve biochemical markers of sepsis,[2] but isolated vitamin E trials are clearly required. Fortunately, vitamin E toxicity seems very rare.

Vitamin K

Vitamin K is a lipid-soluble vitamin essential for coagulation, with several vitamin K–dependent clotting factors being vital to the human coagulation cascade. The three main forms are phylloquinone (also known as vitamin K_1), vitamin K_2 (of microbial origin), and the synthetic parent compound vitamin K_3. Vitamin K levels have been found to be low in critically ill patients,[64] even at admission to the ICU,[65] leading to prolongation of clotting times.

Vitamin K seems to be the best-preserved vitamin in patients with renal failure,[59] and because vitamin K is lipid soluble, it is unlikely to be lost in great amounts through CRRT.[23]

There is very little prospective information on clinical outcomes with vitamin K supplementation in either general ICU patients or targeted high-risk groups (such as those receiving warfarin), so it cannot be recommended at present.

CONCLUSION

Trace elements and vitamins deserve careful attention in the critically ill patient with or without renal failure. Serum levels of the more important trace elements, such as zinc, iron, copper, and selenium, are often very low, and the fact that they are not commonly measured in clinical practice may lead to an underemphasis on these deficiencies. Vitamin deficiencies are also common, and although deficiencies of thiamine, folate, vitamin B_{12}, and vitamin K are more often considered in clinical practice, disorders of the other vitamins, specifically A, C, D, and E, may well be more important than commonly thought.

Restoring "normal" levels of trace elements and vitamins with supplementation makes theoretical sense, but evidence of clinical outcome benefits to support this practice is sparse. Therefore, clinicians should remain alert for the known clinical syndromes of the various vitamin deficiencies. What seems more appealing than merely replacing micronutrient deficiencies is the rationale that giving supranormal doses of the well-recognized antioxidant micronutrients, such as selenium, vitamin A, vitamin C, and vitamin E, might have clinical outcome benefits, an issue that is just starting to emerge from the literature.

Key Points

1. Trace elements are micronutrients that are not usually synthesized in the body but are consumed in healthy diets and are required for various physiological functions.
2. Serum levels of the trace elements, such as zinc, iron, copper, and selenium, are often very low in critical illness because of losses from various mechanisms.
3. Several well-understood clinical syndromes of the various vitamin deficiencies occur, but levels of most vitamins are also moderately deficient in critical illness.
4. Trace element and vitamin levels are rarely measured in clinical practice, possibly leading to underemphasis on the potential issues of these deficiency states.
5. Restoration of "normal" levels of trace elements and vitamins with supplementation makes theoretical sense, but evidence to support this practice is lacking.
6. Given endogenous antioxidant systems are commonly dysfunctional in critical illness (particularly sepsis), exogenous administration of selenium, vitamin A, vitamin C, and/or vitamin E might improve outcomes; however, more research is clearly required before this practice should be routine.

Key References

1. Angstwurm MWA, Engelmann L, Zimmermann T, et al: Selenium in Intensive Care (SIC) study: Results of a prospective randomized, placebo-controlled, multiple-center study in patients with severe systemic inflammatory response syndrome, sepsis, and septic shock. Crit Care Med 2007;35: 118-126.
3. Berger MM, Eggimann P, Heyland DK, et al: Reduction of nosocomial pneumonia after major burns by trace element supplementation: Aggregation of two randomised trials. Crit Care 2006;10:R153.
11. Pontes-Arruda A, Aragao AM, Albuquerque JD: Effects of enteral feeding with eicosapentaenoic acid, gamma-linolenic acid, and antioxidants in mechanically ventilated patients with severe sepsis and septic shock. Crit Care Med 2006;34: 2325-2333.
13. Heyland DK, Dhaliwal R, Suchner U, Berger MM: Antioxidant nutrients: A systematic review of trace elements and vitamins in the critically ill patient. Intensive Care Med 2005;31: 327-337.
23. Story DA, Ronco C, Bellomo R: Trace element and vitamin concentrations and losses in critically ill patients treated with continuous venovenous hemofiltration. Crit Care Med 1999;27:220-223.

See the companion Expert Consult website for the complete reference list.

CHAPTER 103

Loop Diuretics

Miet Schetz

OBJECTIVES

This chapter will:
1. Explain the mechanism of action of loop diuretics.
2. Discuss pharmacokinetic and pharmacodynamic factors underlying resistance to loop diuretics in edematous disorders.
3. Discuss the adverse effects and toxicity of loop diuretics.

In critically ill patients, both the underlying disease and its treatment often result in the development of edema. Edema is seen in patients with decreased ability to excrete water and solutes (kidney disease) and in conditions associated with arterial underfilling, such as congestive heart failure (CHF), liver cirrhosis, and nephrotic syndrome, in which a complex interplay between hemodynamic forces and neurohumoral factors results in fluid retention.[1] In many patients receiving intensive care, edema is a consequence of aggressive fluid resuscitation in conditions associated with an increased capillary permeability, such as sepsis, trauma, burns, and major surgery. The excess volume can lead to peripheral edema or increased extravascular lung water with associated impairment of pulmonary function. Although no causal relationship has been established, positive fluid balances in critically ill patients have been associated with poor outcome.[2-4] A restrictive fluid regimen, including the use of diuretics, though not improving mortality, has been shown to result in shorter duration of mechanical ventilation and intensive care in patients with acute respiratory distress syndrome.[5] Of all the various classes of diuretics, loop diuretics are the most powerful and are often first-line treatment for these edematous conditions in critically ill patients.[6] This chapter reviews the clinical use of loop diuretics in critically ill patients. It mostly refers to review articles; for more details, the reader should consult the references given in these articles.

MECHANISMS OF ACTION

Different classes of diuretics act on different nephron segments, in relation to the different mechanism of sodium reabsorption in each segment. Different tubular segments also reabsorb different fractions of the filtered sodium (Na^+) load, accounting for the difference in potency among diuretics (Table 103-1). The loop diuretics, acting pre-dominantly on the thick ascending limb (TAL) of the loop of Henle, have the highest potency because this nephron segment normally reabsorbs 25% to 30% of the filtered sodium load.[7,8] The inhibition of sodium chloride (NaCl) reabsorption in the TAL also abolishes the hypertonicity of the interstitium and so inhibits water reabsorption in the collecting duct.

Loop diuretics are weak inhibitors of carbonic anhydrase, but their main action is to inhibit sodium reabsorption by inhibiting the Na^+-K^+-$2Cl^-$ cotransporter (NKCC2) in the apical membrane of the TAL. Chloride delivery is the rate-limiting step of NKCC2, and loop diuretics bind to the chloride-binding site. The Na^+,K^+-ATPase, localized in the basolateral membrane of epithelial cells throughout the nephron, reduces the cytosolic Na concentration and provides the driving force for the operation of the apical NKCC2. The low luminal potassium concentration might limit NKCC2 transport, which is overcome by potassium recycling via the luminal membrane. The chloride that enters the cell leaves across the basolateral membrane through selective chloride channels and perhaps also via potassium-chloride cotransporters. Both the back-leakage of potassium and the basolateral chloride transport are electrogenic and create a lumen-positive transepithelial gradient, driving the passive paracellular reabsorption of cations such as sodium, calcium, and magnesium (Fig. 103-1). Loop diuretics thus increase the fractional excretion of water, sodium, potassium, chloride, calcium, and magnesium.[9]

PHARMACOKINETICS

The most commonly used loop diuretics are furosemide, bumetanide, and torasemide. Ethacrynic acid has important ototoxicity and is therefore used only in patients with allergic reactions to the other loop diuretics. The adsorption of oral furosemide is highly variable, with bioavailability ranging from 10% to 90%. The oral dose should therefore always be higher than the intravenous dose, and in critically ill patients, the intravenous route is preferred. The bioavailability of bumetanide and torasemide is almost complete.

Loop diuretics have a rapid onset but relatively short duration of action. Only the fraction of the drug that is eliminated in the urine as unchanged drug can interact with the NKCC2 receptor at the luminal site of the tubular cells in the TAL. Because all loop diuretics are highly bound (>95%) to serum albumin, only a minimal fraction is filtered at the glomerulus. Loop diuretics reach their

TABLE 103-1

Site and Mechanism of Action of Different Classes of Diuretics

NEPHRON SEGMENT	% Na REABSORBED	MECHANISM OF ACTION	DRUG(S)
Proximal tubule	40-60	Carbonic anhydrase inhibitors	Acetazolamide
Loop of Henle	25-30	Na^+-K^+-$2Cl^-$ inhibitors	Loop diuretics
Distal tubule	5-10	Na-Cl cotransporter inhibitors	Thiazides
Collecting duct	3-5	Aldosterone antagonists	Spironolactone
		Na channel blockers	Amiloride, triamterene

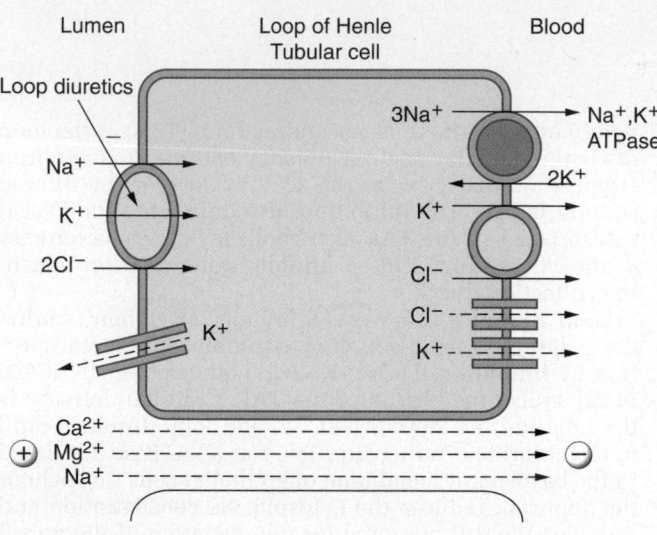

FIGURE 103-1. Mechanism of NaCl reabsorption in the loop of Henle. The Na^+,K^+-ATPase, localized in the basolateral membrane, reduces the cytosolic Na concentration and provides the driving force for the operation of the apical NKCC2 transporter—the site of action of loop diuretics. *Dashed lines* denote passive transport. See text for more details. (Adapted from Reeves WB, Molony DA: The physiology of loop diuretic action. Semin Nephrol 1988;8:225-233.)

target site by being actively secreted into the proximal tubule, using the organic acid transporter (OAT) that is found predominantly in the S2 segment. This transporter has a very high affinity for loop diuretics that are stripped from the albumin and transported into the tubular lumen. Increased concentrations of endogenous and exogenous organic acids may compete for this transporter and impair both the entry of diuretics into the luminal fluid and the associated diuretic response. Hypoalbuminemia increases the volume of distribution of loop diuretics and reduces their delivery to the OAT.[7,8]

Furosemide is the loop diuretic with the lowest extrarenal clearance. About 50% of a dose of furosemide is excreted as unchanged active drug in the urine, the remaining 50% being metabolized in the kidney through conjugation with glucuronic acid. Its normal half-life is 1.5 to 2 hours. Bumetanide and torasemide undergo substantial hepatic metabolism (40% and 80%, respectively) and have half-lives of 1 hour and 3 to 4 hours, respectively.[8] The pharmacokinetics of the loop diuretics are summarized in Table 103-2.

DIURETIC RESPONSIVENESS AND RESISTANCE

The more diuretic that reaches the target site (NKCC2), the greater the diuretic response, with a sigmoidal dose-response curve (Fig. 103-2). The excretion rate causing a half-maximal response is lowest for bumetanide (the most potent loop diuretic), intermediate for torasemide, and

highest for furosemide (see Table 103-2). The maximal response, which occurs when all receptors are occupied, is a fractional sodium excretion of 25% to 30%—the amount that is normally reabsorbed at the TAL. Both the threshold dose (the minimal dose required to elicit a response) and the ceiling dose (the lowest dose eliciting a maximal response) may differ among patients, thus requiring individual titration. In healthy volunteers, the ceiling dose is usually 40 mg for furosemide, 10-20 mg for torasemide, and 1 mg for bumetanide.[8]

Many patients, especially those with renal failure, heart failure, cirrhosis, and/or nephrotic syndrome, are or become resistant to the effect of loop diuretics. This diuretic resistance may be due to short-term tolerance, known as the *braking phenomenon* and characterized by avid sodium retention at the end of the dosing interval, when the diuretic plasma concentration has decreased below the effective level. This effect is more pronounced for diuretics with short half-lives, occurs in response to decreases in effective arterial blood volume, and is mediated by a complex of interrelated factors, including baroreceptors and greater activity of the renin-angiotensin-aldosterone axis, increased sympathetic outflow, enhanced release of antidiuretic hormone, reduced release of atrial natriuretic peptide, and changes in peritubular hemodynamics that lead to enhanced proximal sodium reabsorption.[7,8] Combining loop diuretics with restricted sodium intake is therefore extremely important. Another approach to overcoming this short-term tolerance is more frequent diuretic administration or the use of continuous infusions.

Long-term diuretic resistance can occur because of either *pharmacokinetic* factors (not enough drug being delivered

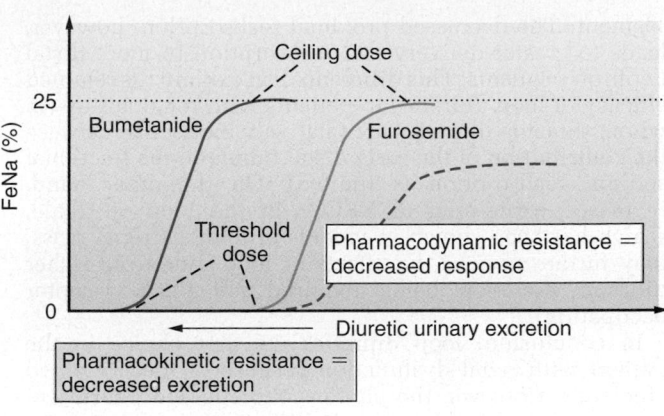

FIGURE 103-2. Sigmoidal dose-response curve of loop diuretics: fractional sodium excretion (FeNa) is plotted against the diuretic delivery at the site of action. Threshold dose = lowest dose that elicits a diuretic response; ceiling dose = lowest dose that elicits a maximal diuretic response. Compared with furosemide, the dose-response curve of bumetanide, which is a more potent diuretic, is shifted to the left. Pharmacokinetic resistance results from decreased urinary excretion (decrease on the x-axis), whereas pharmacodynamic resistance results in shift of the dose-response curve to the right and downwards.

TABLE 103-2

Pharmacokinetics of Loop Diuretics

	FUROSEMIDE	BUMETANIDE	TORASEMIDE
Relative potency	1	40	3
Bioavailability (%)	10-90	80-100	80-100
Protein binding (%)	>95	>95	>95
Elimination (%):			
Renal	90*	60	20
Hepatic	10	40	80
Half-life (hrs)	1.5-2	1	3-4
Maximal effective intravenous dose (mg)	40	1	10-20

*50% of a dose is excreted as unchanged active drug in the urine, and 50% is metabolized in the kidney through conjugation with glucuronic acid.

TABLE 103-3

Causes of Resistance to Loop Diuretics

Pharmacokinetic resistance	Reduced bioavailability
	Reduced renal blood flow
	Reduced number of functioning nephrons
	Competition at organic acid transporter
	Hypoalbuminemia
	Albuminuria
Pharmacodynamic resistance	Reduced total fractional sodium reabsorption
	Increased proximal sodium reabsorption
	Increased Na⁺-K⁺-2Cl⁻ cotransporter expression
	Distal tubular hypertrophy
	Increased distal sodium reabsorption

to the site of action) or *pharmacodynamic* mechanisms (decreased response or increased activity of the receptor or compensatory reabsorption at other nephron segments) (see Fig. 103-2). The causes of this diuretic resistance (Table 103-3) may differ according to the clinical situation and are discussed here.

Renal Failure

The discussion on whether diuretics may protect against the development of acute renal failure can be found in Chapter 78. The focus in this chapter is on the use of diuretics for the treatment of fluid overload in patients with reduced renal function (reviewed in references 7, 8, and 10). The bioavailability of loop diuretics is not affected by renal insufficiency. Renal failure prolongs the half-life of furosemide (because both excretion and metabolism are reduced), whereas the half-lives of bumetanide and torasemide are only minimally prolonged. When equipotent doses (based on studies in healthy volunteers) are used in patients with renal dysfunction, furosemide produces more natriuresis than bumetanide, because the former achieves a greater serum concentration. In other words, the relative potency of furosemide and bumetanide changes from 40 : 1 in healthy volunteers to 20 : 1 in patients with renal dysfunction.[11]

On the other hand, diminished renal blood flow reduces the delivery of all loop diuretics to the tubular fluid, and larger doses are needed to attain an effective level at the target site. The OAT is responsible for the peritubular uptake and secretion of loop diuretics. At this transporter, there is competition with other organic acids that accumulate in renal failure. Furthermore, metabolic acidosis depolarizes the proximal tubular cells, thus decreasing organic acid secretion. Both of these factors contribute to impairment of the delivery of loop diuretics into the tubular fluid.

The remaining nephrons retain their responsiveness to the diuretic.[12] However, the reduced number of functioning nephrons results in a decrease in the filtered load of NaCl and fluid. In order to maintain Na and fluid balance, the fractional reabsorption of NaCl is reduced in proportion to the fall in glomerular filtration rate. The reduction limits the maximal effect of diuretics, which is determined by the maximal fractional reabsorption in the target segment. The decreased proximal reabsorption, however, leads to greater delivery and reabsorption in more distal nephron segments. This difference can explain the retained efficacy of loop diuretics in patients with renal failure (in whom thiazide diuretics are relatively ineffective because the contribution of the early distal tubule to the fractional sodium reabsorption is limited). On the other hand, increased expression of NKCC2 in the loop of Henle, which has been shown in models of reduced renal mass, may further oppose the effects of loop diuretics (higher diuretic excretion being required for 100% receptor occupation).

In conclusion, loop diuretics are first choice in the patient with renal dysfunction because of their retained efficiency. However, the pharmacokinetic and pharmacodynamic alterations resulting in diuretic resistance require higher doses. In patients with chronic renal insufficiency, ceiling doses of 160 to 200 mg for furosemide, 6 to 8 mg for bumetanide, and 80 to 100 mg for torasemide have been reported. Such larger doses of furosemide result in increased plasma concentrations and the risk of extrarenal toxicity, whereas the substantial nonrenal clearance of torasemide prevents accumulation in patients with renal insufficiency even with larger doses. In addition, continuous infusions of loop diuretics have been shown to be more efficacious in patients with chronic renal failure[13] and allow better titration to the maximally effective dose. Diuretic responsiveness in patients with renal failure can be further improved through optimization of blood pressure and body fluids to restore renal blood flow, correction of the uremic milieu and acidosis, and avoidance of other drugs competing for the OAT. Combining loop diuretics with thiazides can solve the problem of enhanced NaCl reabsorption in downstream nephron segments.

Congestive Heart Failure

CHF is associated with avid sodium and water retention due to arterial underfilling, resulting in alterations in the sympathetic nervous system, the renin-angiotensin system, the vasopressin axis, and the vasodilatory natriuretic pathway.[1] Although diuretics used to be the mainstay in the treatment of CHF, they have now become secondary to beta-blockers, angiotensin-converting enzyme inhibitors, angiotensin receptor blockers, and mineralocorticoid antagonists. Adequately powered, prospective, placebo-controlled, randomized trials of diuretics in CHF have not been performed. However, a 2006 Cochrane review still concludes that "conventional diuretics appear to reduce the risk of death and worsening heart failure compared to placebo."[14] In addition to their diuretic effect, loop diuretics induce prostaglandin-mediated venodilation, explaining the rapid clinical benefit in patients with pulmonary edema.[15,16] On the other hand, excessive diuresis may activate the same hemodynamic and neurohumoral forces that modern therapy of chronic heart failure is designed to inhibit.[17]

With the exception of a delayed intestinal reabsorption, the delivery of loop diuretics to the site of action is normal in the patient with CHF, and normal doses result in adequate urinary excretion of the diuretic unless the patient also has associated renal dysfunction. However, the relationship between urinary diuretic excretion and urinary sodium excretion is blunted (pharmacodynamic resistance),[18-20] for the following reasons:

- The previously described acute tolerance or braking phenomenon.

- The neurohumoral alterations induced by chronic heart failure, which result in excess sodium and water reabsorption in the proximal tubule with reduced sodium delivery to the TAL, thus decreasing the maximal effect of loop diuretics.
- Vasopressin-mediated increase in expression of NKCC2, which may amplify the defect in water excretion and contribute to diuretic resistance.[7]
- Functional and structural adaptations in downstream nephron segments, which increase distal sodium reabsorption. In animals, long-term administration of loop diuretics induces hypertrophy and hyperplasia in epithelial cells of the distal convoluted tubule, with increased expression of the NaCl cotransporter in the luminal membrane and of the Na+,K+-ATPase in the basolateral membrane.[21] This leads to increased reabsorption in this segment, thereby blunting the natriuretic effect and shifting the dose-response curve downward and to the right. Combining loop diuretics with thiazides not only has a synergistic effect on NaCl excretion but also prevents adaptive changes in the distal nephron.
- Increased aldosterone levels, which mediate sodium reabsorption in the collecting duct.

In conclusion, diuretic resistance in patients with CHF may be overcome through the use of the intravenous route or the administration of higher doses (if associated with renal dysfunction), continuous infusions, and combinations with other classes of diuretics (sequential nephron blockade). A 2005 Cochrane analysis on the use of continuous infusions of loop diuretics in patients with CHF concludes that although greater diuresis and a better safety profile are suggested by small and heterogeneous studies, definitive recommendations for clinical practice cannot be given.[22] Compared with furosemide, torasemide has better bioavailability and a longer duration of action, reducing the braking phenomenon. A few comparative studies have indeed shown improved outcome with torasemide.[23,24]

Liver Cirrhosis

Cirrhosis of the liver is also associated with an apparent decrease in arterial filling, resulting in the development of edema.[1] Because secondary hyperaldosteronism is an important cause of water and sodium retention in patients with cirrhosis of the liver, aldosterone antagonists (spironolactone) are first-line treatment for this condition,[25] and the use of loop diuretics is limited mostly to patients whose cirrhosis is resistant to spironolactone and thiazide diuretics. Whereas the presence of liver disease will not appreciably alter the kinetics of furosemide, the plasma half-lives of bumetanide and torasemide are prolonged, so theoretically, more of those drugs can reach the tubular fluid.[26] However, the response to a maximal effective dose is substantially reduced.[7,8] This reduction is largely unexplained, although competition of bile salts for the OAT and greater distal sodium reabsorption via aldosterone might contribute.

Hypoalbuminemia

The addition of albumin to furosemide has been shown to improve oxygenation, with greater net negative fluid balance and better maintenance of hemodynamic stability in hypoproteinemic patients with acute respiratory distress syndrome.[6] This response may be related to the oncotic effect of albumin, which reduces depletion of the intravascular compartment. However, albumin also has an effect on the pharmacokinetics of loop diuretics. Low albumin levels increase the distribution volume and lead to insufficient delivery of drug to the tubular fluid.[7,8] Whether this phenomenon has important clinical implication remains a matter of debate.[7] The presence of large amounts of albumin in the filtrate (as occurs in nephrotic syndrome) may also prevent interaction with its receptor.

CONTINUOUS VERSUS INTERMITTENT ADMINISTRATION

In patients with renal insufficiency, continuous infusion of bumetanide has been shown to be more effective and less toxic than intermittent boluses.[13] A review of clinical studies in critically ill patients shows decreased dosage requirements, improved diuretic response, and fewer adverse effects with continuous infusions,[27] and a 2005 meta-analysis showed a greater diuretic response and less ototoxicity, but no difference in electrolyte disturbances in patients with CHF.[22] Continuous infusion also allows better titration to the required effect. To enable the drug to reach effective plasma levels in a timely manner, one must start with a loading dose.

Adverse Effects and Toxicity

The major adverse consequences of loop diuretics result from their alterations of fluid, electrolyte, and acid-base balance. The most frequently observed electrolyte disorders are hypokalemia and hypomagnesemia, both of which predispose patients to serious cardiac arrhythmias, particularly in the presence of digitalis. Frequent electrolyte monitoring is therefore essential. Loop diuretics block solute reabsorption at nephron sites that are important for concentrating the urine, leading to water excretion in excess of sodium excretion. Hypernatremia can therefore result. Loop diuretics increase urinary calcium excretion and are used in hypercalcemia. On the other hand, chronic hypercalciuria may lead to metabolic bone disease. Therapy with loop diuretics is one of the most common causes of metabolic alkalosis, which occurs because of

volume depletion, hypokalemia, and secondary hyperaldosteronism.[28] For more details on electrolyte and acid-base disorders, the reader is referred to other chapters in this book.

High doses of loop diuretics are associated with a higher risk of temporary deafness and tinnitus.[29] Other, less commonly reported side effects are acute interstitial nephritis, loss of water-soluble vitamins (e.g., thiamine deficiency[30]), skin reactions, and even anaphylaxis.[31]

Key Points

1. Loop diuretics are the most potent diuretics.
2. Renal failure, congestive heart failure, liver cirrhosis, and hypoalbuminemia are associated with resistance to diuretics.
3. Strategies to overcome diuretic resistance include sodium and fluid restriction, increased diuretic doses, increased frequency of administration, continuous infusions, and/or combination therapy.
4. Continuous infusion of loop diuretics results in a greater and more controlled diuretic response and an improved safety profile.
5. Adverse effects of loop diuretics include hypokalemia, hypomagnesemia, hypocalcemia, metabolic alkalosis, ototoxicity, and interstitial nephritis.

Key References

7. Shankar SS, Brater DC: Loop diuretics: From the Na-K-2Cl transporter to clinical use. Am J Physiol Renal Physiol 2003;284:F11 F21.
8. Brater DG: Diuretic therapy. N Engl J Med 1998;339:387-395.
10. Wilcox CS: New insights into diuretic use in patients with chronic renal disease. J Am Soc Nephrol 2002;13:798-805.
14. Faris R, Flather MD, Purcell H, et al: Diuretics for heart failure. Cochrane Database Syst Rev 2006;(1):CD003838.
27. Martin SJ, Danziger LH: Continuous infusion of loop diuretics in the critically ill: A review of the literature. Crit Care Med 1994;22:1323-1329.

See the companion Expert Consult website for the complete reference list.

CHAPTER 104

Osmotic Diuretics

Susan Garwood

OBJECTIVES

This chapter will:
1. Explain the mechanisms of action of osmotically active agents as diuretics.
2. Explore the other, nondiuretic actions of the prototype osmotic diuretic mannitol.
3. Review the literature and summarize the evidence regarding the current uses of mannitol as a renal protection agent.

OSMOTIC DIURETICS

The proximal tubule and descending limb of Henle's loop are freely permeable to water, and any osmotically active agent that is filtered by the glomerulus but is not reabsorbed causes water to be retained in these segments and promotes a water diuresis. Such agents are termed *osmotic diuretics*. Four osmotic diuretics are available (Table 104-1), glycerin, isosorbide, mannitol, and urea; mannitol is the most commonly used in clinical practice and the most extensively studied.

Osmotic diuretics are classified as pregnancy category B (isosorbide) and C (glycerin, mannitol, and urea).

Pharmacokinetics of Mannitol

Mannitol, a six-carbon alcohol with a molecular weight of 182, is prepared commercially by the reduction of dextrose. A metabolically inert, obligate extracellular solute, mannitol is freely filtered by the glomerulus, poorly absorbed throughout the tubule, and mostly excreted unchanged in the urine. Its distribution and elimination follow a two-compartment open model, with elimination from the central compartment by first-order kinetics.[1] In a study of four human adult subjects (two healthy subjects and two with increased intracranial pressure but without clinical evidence of inappropriate antidiuretic hormone secretion or diabetes insipidus), the distribution half-life of mannitol was 2.11 ± 2.67 minutes, and the elimination half-life was 71.15 ± 27.02 minutes; the volume of distribution was approximately 0.5 L/kg, and the clearance was independent of dose.[1] There was a strong positive correlation ($r = 0.90$) between maximum serum mannitol concentration and serum osmolality, but neither increased proportionally with dose. In a study of 15 patients who underwent surgery for intracranial tumors under general anesthesia and who were given mannitol (1 g per kg body weight) over 30 minutes, the plasma half-life for the distribution phase was approximately 10 minutes, and that for the elimination phase was just under 2.5 hours.[2] The variability seen in plasma clearances for mannitol depends on renal function and can be as long as 30 hours in patients with renal failure.

Because mannitol is poorly absorbed, it must be given parenterally; if administered orally, it would cause osmotic diarrhea. Clinical protocols recommend intravenous infusion of mannitol as a 15% or 20% solution in the dosage range of 0.5 to 2.0 mg/kg over 30 to 60 minutes to a daily maximum of 200 g (see later).

Pharmacodynamics of Mannitol

Mannitol is thought to have its major effect in the proximal tubule and the descending limb of Henle's loop. The concentration of mannitol increases as water is reabsorbed along the tubule; the osmolality in the tubule increases, inhibiting further water reabsorption. The concentration of tubular sodium is thereby reduced, creating a gradient for back-flux of reabsorbed sodium into the tubule, and a natriuresis (albeit of lower magnitude) accompanies the diuresis.

Earlier studies have attributed a number of other mechanisms to mannitol to explain the diuresis and excretion of electrolytes (sodium, chloride, potassium, inorganic phosphate, and calcium but not magnesium), urea, and uric acid, as follows:
- Increased extracellular volume and cardiac output,[2] associated with increased renal plasma flow.[3]
- Afferent renal vasodilation via release of prostaglandins (PGI_2) and natriuretic peptides.[4,5]
- Washout of the medullary hypertonicity.[6]
- Inhibition of tubuloglomerular feedback mechanism secondary to enhanced distal flow.[7]
- Reduced renin secretion.[8]
- Antagonism of antidiuretic hormone (ADH) secretion in the collecting tubule.

However, some inconsistencies exist within the literature, and some of the listed findings have been challenged by researchers citing differences in micropuncture techniques and volume expansion as some of the reasons.[9] For example, in a rat experiment of osmotic diuresis induced by 10% mannitol, Leyssac and colleagues[9] determined that although urine flow increased tenfold and sodium excretion increased 177%, plasma renin concentration *increased* by 58% and early distal sodium chloride concentration decreased; these investigators concluded that the natriuresis associated with osmotic diuresis is a result of impaired sodium reabsorption in the distal tubules and collecting ducts.[9]

In general, mannitol produces a diuresis in excess of a natriuresis, and if free water losses are excessive, hypernatremia and hyperkalemia may ensue.

Pharmacology of Glycerin

Glycerin may be given both orally and parenterally as a 10% solution. Although administration of intravenous solutions with higher concentrations can lead to hemoly-

TABLE 104-1

Pharmacokinetics of Commonly Used Osmotic Diuretics

DRUG	STRUCTURE	ORAL BIOAVAILABILITY	HALF-LIFE (HR)	ROUTE OF ELIMINATION
Glycerin (Osmoglyn)		Orally active	0.5-0.75	80% by metabolism 20% unknown
Isosorbide (Ismotic)		Orally active	5.0-9.5	Renal excretion of unchanged drug
Mannitol (Osmitrol)		Negligible	0.27-1.7	80% renal 20% bile/metabolized
Urea (Ureaphil)		Negligible	Insufficient data	Renal excretion of unchanged drug

sis, oral administration of glycerin at concentrations of 50% or greater does not appear to be associated with this adverse event. Glycerin is extensively (80%-90%) metabolized by the liver after both oral and intravenous administration and is excreted to a lesser extent by the kidneys. Elimination by the liver follows zero-order kinetics, and renal excretion follows first-order kinetics. The serum half-life of glycerin varies from 10 minutes to an hour, with high doses lengthening the half-life further. Glycerol treatment may be complicated by profound hyperglycemia requiring insulin therapy and may interfere with the measurement of triglycerides by engendering falsely elevated triglyceride levels.

Glycerin is used primarily for the treatment of glaucoma.

Pharmacology of Isosorbide

Isosorbide (trade name Ismotic) is available in a 45% weight-to-volume solution in a flavored vehicle for oral administration only. Rapidly absorbed after oral administration, isosorbide is essentially nonmetabolized and is eliminated by the kidney unchanged. The recommended initial dose of isosorbide is 1.5 gm per kg body weight. The onset of action is usually within 30 minutes, and the maximum effect is expected at 1 to 1.5 hours. The useful dose range is 1 to 3 gm/kg, and the drug effect persists up to 5 to 6 hours.

Isosorbide is used primarily for the treatment of glaucoma.

Pharmacology of Urea

The commercial product Ureaphil is reconstituted directly before use as a 30% solution of synthetic urea in dextrose. The usual dose is 1 to 1.5 g/kg (3.3-5 mL/kg of a 30% solution), not to exceed a daily dose of 120 g. Rapid infusion of Ureaphil results in intravascular hemolysis, so its rates

of administration should not exceed 4 mL/min. Headaches, nausea and vomiting, disorientation, and confusional states have also been reported with rapid infusion rates. Urea is excreted in the urine of a patient who has received Ureaphil, with an elimination half-life of approximately 75 minutes. A portion of an intravenous dose of urea is hydrolyzed in the gastrointestinal tract by the bacterial enzyme urease, but the products of this reaction may be resynthesized into urea. Approximately 50% is reabsorbed by the kidney. Urea distributes into the intracellular and extracellular fluids in equal proportions and apparently also crosses the placenta and penetrates the eye. It is also found in the breast milk of lactating women.

Ureaphil is used in the treatment of glaucoma and raised intracranial pressure.

Clinical Uses of Mannitol

Mannitol has been in clinical use since the 1960s, and much of its current popularity is a result of its long history of anecdotal successes, which have become clinical dogma. Mannitol is not used as a diuretic in generalized volume overload (congestive heart failure, liver failure, renal failure) as are other diuretics, such as the loop diuretics. It is used, however, as a diuretic in more specific situations, such as cerebral edema.[10,11] Other properties not directly related to its pharmacological activity as an osmotic diuretic have rendered mannitol attractive, at least in theory, for renal protection. In vitro and animal models of renal injury have shown that mannitol reduces the production of oxygen radicals associated with ischemia-reperfusion injury,[12] diminishes endothelial and epithelial cell swelling,[13-15] and, by virtue of increased luminal diameter and urine flow, removes tubular cell debris.[13]

These laboratory findings have translated into the clinical use of mannitol as a renal protectant, with varying success. It is now used almost invariably to protect against the renal toxicity of myoglobin in rhabdomyolysis, crush injuries, or extensive soft tissue trauma and compartment syndrome. In these situations, it is mostly used in combination with bicarbonate to produce a forced alkaline diuresis. Despite its widespread use in rhabdomyolysis, mannitol's actual effectiveness has been questioned; for example, a retrospective study of patients with rhabdomyolysis found that the combination of mannitol and bicarbonate was no different from fluid resuscitation with saline alone.[16] However, until prospective, randomized controlled trials of mannitol-bicarbonate are performed, it is likely that mannitol will remain part of the standard of care for the treatment of rhabdomyolysis.

Other clinical situations in which mannitol is used liberally without category 1 evidence for its effectiveness as a renal protection agent are vascular surgery and cardiopulmonary bypass. In a prospective, randomized controlled trial of either mannitol or saline given before cross-clamping of the aorta in infrarenal aortic surgery in 28 patients, there were no differences in serum creatinine concentration or creatinine clearance rate between the mannitol group and the saline group at 6 hours or at 1, 3, or 7 days after operation. Urinary albumin-to-creatinine and N-acetyl glucosaminidase–to-creatinine ratios were lower in the mannitol group throughout the study period, and the researchers claimed that mannitol reduced subclinical renal injury.[17] Other groups found higher second-day creatinine clearance rates when mannitol was used as part of a multi-antioxidant supplementation during aortic surgery,[18] but not when mannitol was used alone in similar patients.[19] Similarly, mannitol used during cardiopulmonary bypass in adult cardiac surgery has not been shown to make any difference in a number of renal parameters, including serum creatinine concentration, creatinine clearance rate, proteinuria, or excretion of N-acetyl glucos-

aminidase or β_2-microglobulin.[20,21] However, one study, a randomized prospective controlled study of prophylactic administration of mannitol, 0.5 g per kg body weight, in 40 children undergoing cardiopulmonary bypass surgery, showed significantly lower serum creatinine concentration and urinary albumin excretion rate in those receiving mannitol than in the control group.[22] A 2005 review of the use of pharmacological adjuvants in major surgery (excluding organ transplant surgery) concluded that there was no evidence to support the notion that mannitol is a renal protectant in the perioperative period.[23]

In the setting of radiocontrast agent–induced nephropathy in high-risk patients, a forced diuresis with mannitol has proved to be less beneficial than saline alone in one study,[24] and no different from saline hydration in another study as long as an optimal diuresis is maintained.[25]

The only setting in which mannitol is thought to be a useful renal protectant is in renal transplantation,[26-28] when given intravenously to the recipient and/or a living donor intraoperatively or used as a constituent of the flush solution after excision of the graft. As with other uses of mannitol, much of the work in this area was completed in the 1980s and early 1990s, so that most studies lack scientific rigor. Although a prospective, observational, multicenter study of more than 500 transplanted kidney allografts from 54 European centers showed that the use of mannitol during recipient surgery significantly lowered the rate of delayed graft function, this effect had no significance in multivariate analysis (Table 104-2).[28] A Medline search of English language publications of renal or kidney transplant or allograft or transplantation and mannitol produced only one prospective randomized trial of mannitol used in adult renal transplantation within the last 10 to 15 years.[28]

TABLE 104-2

Studies of Mannitol Given to Patients Intraoperatively during Human Kidney Transplantation

STUDY (YEAR)*	NO. PATIENTS IN STUDY	TYPE OF DONOR KIDNEY	STUDY DESIGN	TREATMENT GROUPS	OUTCOME (PERCENTAGE OF PATIENTS)
Weimar (1983)[32]	50	Cadaver	Prospective, randomized; blinding not reported	Saline Mannitol 50 g	ATN (54%[†]) ATN (14%)
Tiggeler et al (1985)[27]	61	Cadaver	Historical controls followed by 2 consecutive treatment groups	Restricted fluids Restricted fluids + mannitol 50 g Moderate hydration + mannitol 50 g	ATN (43%[†]) ATN (53%[†]) ATN (4.8%)
Van Valenberg (1987)[33]	131	Cadaver	Prospective, randomized; blinding not reported	Hydration + 5% dextrose Hydration + mannitol	ARF (33%[†]) ARF (18%)
Richards (1989)[34]	261	Cadaver	Historical controls	Hydration Hydration + mannitol 100 g	ATN (47%[†]) ATN (20%)
Salahi (1995)[26]	240	Unrelated donor	Historical controls	Hydration Hydration + mannitol 50 g (donor)	ATN (26%[†]) ATN (17%)
Koning (1997)[28]	547	Cadaver	Multicenter, observational	Patients not receiving mannitol intraoperatively Patients receiving mannitol intraoperatively	DGF (30%[†]) DGF (21%)

*Superscript numbers indicate chapter references.
[†]Significantly different from the mannitol treatment group ($P < .05$).
ATN, acute tubular necrosis; ARF, acute renal failure; DGF, delayed graft function.

ADVERSE EFFECTS OF OSMOTIC DIURETICS

Osmotic diuretics are rapidly distributed in the extracellular compartment, extracting water from the intracellular space. Before the diuresis, this can lead to expansion of the extracellular volume and hypervolemia. Consequently, headache, nausea, and vomiting are common transient side effects observed in patients treated with osmotic diuretics, but in patients with cardiac disease, this condition may be clinically seen as heart failure and pulmonary edema.

Excessive use of mannitol without adequate water replacement can ultimately lead to severe dehydration, free water losses, and hypernatremia. As water is extracted from cells, intracellular K^+ and H^+ concentrations rise, leading to cellular losses and hyperkalemic acidosis.

There are a number of reports in the literature of acute renal failure caused by mannitol, predominantly in patients with renal failure or in patients given doses exceeding 200 g/day.[29] The pathophysiology is thought to be hyperosmolar nephrosis and is manifested on biopsy as proximal tubular vacuolization with tubular lumen obliteration.[30] Furthermore, mannitol has been shown to induce endothelial cell apoptosis, which is accompanied by activation of stress kinases and elevation of intracellular free calcium.[31] Although the clinical implications of these findings are still unclear, the current understanding that the renal endothelial cell plays a pivotal role in the maintenance phase during renal injury might explain in some small part why mannitol is unsuccessful as a renal protectant under these circumstances.

Key Points

1. Osmotically active agents cause a diuresis secondary to improved hemodynamic changes as well as tubular effects.

2. A number of nondiuretic actions of mannitol, such as free radical scavenging, have proved to be effective in laboratory models of renal failure.
3. Mannitol is an old drug that has passed into clinical use as a renal protection agent with little category 1 evidence of its effectiveness.
4. Renal transplantation is the only clinical scenario in which mannitol has been shown to improve renal outcome.
5. The use of mannitol is associated with a number of adverse events, including acute renal failure, volume overload, electrolyte abnormalities, and severe dehydration.

Key References

9. Leyssac PP, Holstein-Rathlou NH, Skott O: Renal blood flow, early distal sodium, and plasma renin concentrations during osmotic diuresis. Am J Physiol 2000;279:R1268-R1276.
13. Lindstrom KE, Ronnstedt L, Jaremko G, Haraldsson B: Physiological and morphological effects of perfusing isolated rat kidneys with hyperosmolal mannitol solutions. Acta Physiol Scand 1999;166:231-238.
28. Koning OH, Ploeg RJ, van Bockel JH, et al: Risk factors for delayed graft function in cadaveric kidney transplantation: A prospective study of renal function and graft survival after preservation with University of Wisconsin solution in multiorgan donors. European Multicenter Study Group. Transplantation 1997;63:1620-1628.
30. Visweswaran P, Massin EK, Dubose TD Jr: Mannitol-induced acute renal failure. J Am Soc Nephrol 1997;8:1028-1033.
31. Malek AM, Goss GG, Jiang L, et al: Mannitol at clinical concentrations activates multiple signaling pathways and induces apoptosis in endothelial cells. Stroke 1998;29:2631-2640.

See the companion Expert Consult website for the complete reference list.

CHAPTER 105

Thiazide Diuretics

Alun D. Hughes

OBJECTIVES

This chapter will:
1. Describe the history and chemistry of thiazide and thiazide-like diuretics.
2. Summarize the fundamental pharmacology and molecular mechanism of action of thiazide diuretics.
3. Discuss the pharmacokinetics and pharmacodynamics of thiazide diuretics.
4. Outline the uses, adverse effects, and major drug interactions of thiazides.

DEVELOPMENT AND CHEMISTRY OF THE THIAZIDES

Thiazide (benzothiadiazine) diuretics were originally developed more than 50 years ago as a result of chemical modification of sulfanilamide, a sulfonamide inhibitor of carbonic anhydrase.[1] Unlike inhibitors of carbonic anhydrase, however, thiazides were found to be associated with higher excretion of sodium and chloride with minimal loss of bicarbonate. Chlorothiazide was the first thiazide to be

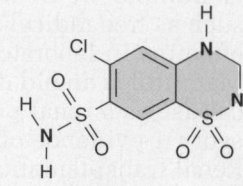

Bendroflumethiazide
1,1-dioxo-3-(phenylmethyl)-6-
(trifluoromethyl)-3,4-dihydro-
2H-benzo[e] [1,2,4]
thiadiazine-7-sulfonamide

Chlorothiazide
6-chloro-1,1-dioxo-4H-benzo[e]
[1,2,4] thiadiazine-
7-sulfonamide

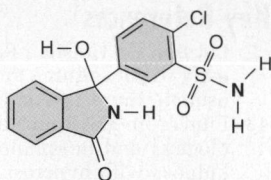

Hydrochlorothiazide
6-chloro-1,1-dioxo-3,4-dihydro-
2H-benzo[e] [1,2,4]
thiadiazine-7-sulfonamide

Chlortalidone
2-chloro-5-(1-hydroxy-3-oxo-
2H-isoindol-1-yl)
benzenesulfonamide

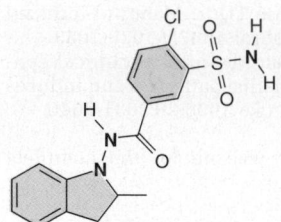

Indapamide
4-chloro-N-(2-methyl-2,3-
dihydroindol-1-yl)-3-
sulfamoyl-benzamide

Metolazone
7-chloro-2-methyl-3-
(2-methylphenyl)-4-oxo-
1,2-dihydroquinazoline-6-
sulfonamide

FIGURE 105-1. The chemical structures of some of the more commonly used thiazides. (Data from Wishart DS, Knox C, Guo AC, et al: DrugBank: A comprehensive resource for in silico drug discovery and exploration. Nucleic Acids Res 2006;34:D668-D672.)

marketed, in 1957. It quickly found use as both a diuretic and an antihypertensive agent, and subsequently, a range of thiazide and thiazide-like diuretics were developed.[2] Thiazide-like diuretics differ chemically from thiazides but share identical primary modes of action; in this review, these agents are referred to collectively as *thiazides*.

The chemical structures of some of the more commonly used thiazides are shown in Figure 105-1. Most thiazides possess a sulfamyl side group on the benzene ring that accounts for some additional inhibitory effects on carbonic anhydrase. This property contributes little to the overall diuretic action of this class of drugs but may underlie pharmacodynamic and pharmacokinetic differences between thiazides and between their effects unrelated to inhibition of Na$^+$ reabsorption by the distal tubule. Carbonic anhydrase inhibitory activity is most marked for chlortalidone, whereas bendroflumethiazide and metolazone lack inhibitory effects on carbonic anhydrase at clinically used doses.

FUNDAMENTAL PHARMACOLOGY AND MOLECULAR MECHANISM OF ACTION

All thiazides inhibit Na$^+$ reabsorption in the early distal convoluted tubule. This effect is due to inhibition of the NaCl cotransporter (NCC).[3] This transporter is a major mechanism of sodium reabsorption in the distal collecting tubule and is responsible for reuptake of 5% to 8% of the Na$^+$ load under normal conditions (Fig. 105-2).

The rank order of potency of commonly used thiazides is as follows[4]:

indapamide > bendroflumethiazide = metolazone > chlorthalidone = hydrochlorothiazide > chlorothiazide

Despite these differences in potency, however, the maximum efficacy of different thiazides does not differ significantly.

Inhibition of Na$^+$ reabsorption by thiazides is accompanied by hypocalciuria and hypomagnesemia. Thiazides have been shown to cause activation of a transcellular Ca^{2+} transport system with upregulation of an apical Ca^{2+} channel, TRPV5, and the calcium-binding proteins, calbindin-D(28k), and calbindin-D(9k).[5] However, Na$^+$ loss, and a reduction in extracellular volume that triggers a compensatory increase in proximal tubular Na$^+$ reabsorption, is probably more important in thiazide-induced hypocalciuria in vivo. The effect of the greater Na$^+$ reabsorption on the electrochemical gradient in proximal tubular cells leads to enhanced passive Ca^{2+} transport from the tubule.[6] The mechanism of hypomagnesemia remains less well

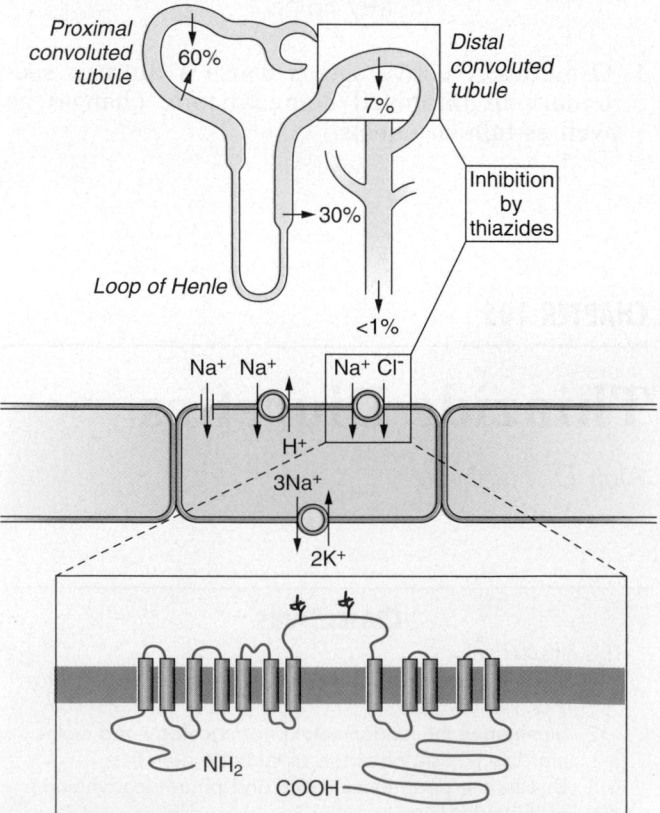

FIGURE 105-2. The NaCl cotransporter: the target of thiazides in the distal convoluted tubule.

understood but may result from downregulation of an epithelial Mg^{2+} channel, transient receptor potential channel subfamily M, member 6 (Trpm6), after long-term treatment with thiazides.[6]

The NCC is a 1021–amino acid protein (120-180 kDa when glycosylated). It consists of 12 membrane-spanning domains with a short intracellular amino-terminus and a long carboxy-terminus (see Fig. 105-2) and may function as a homodimer.[7] A member of the SLC12 gene family (SLC12A3) of electroneutral cation-coupled Cl^- cotransporters,[8] NCC is closely related to the NaCl transporter found in the urinary bladder of the winter flounder, *Pseudopleuronectes americanus*. Other, more distantly related members of this family are the Na^+,K^+-2Cl^- cotransporters NKCC1 and NKCC2, which share about 50% identity, and the KCl cotransporters KCC1 to KCC4, which share about 25% homology.[8] Despite their similarities, thiazides have no therapeutic action on these transporters.[9] The NCC is found almost exclusively in the apical membrane of distal convoluted tubular cells,[10] although it has been described in peripheral blood mononuclear cells[11] and an osteoblast-derived cell line.[12]

Levels of NCC in the distal tubule are regulated by a variety of physiological processes. Metabolic acidosis and K^- depletion decrease NCC expression[13]; aldosterone raises NCC levels, although this effect does not seem to involve changes in levels of messenger RNA.[13] Vasopressin also increases NCC,[13] and this effect may at least partially account for the increase seen after water deprivation.[14] Insulin also increases NCC,[13] possibly contributing to the elevations of NCC seen in obesity. Estrogen may also raise NCC levels in the distal collecting tubule.[13]

The binding sites in NCC for Na^+ and Cl^- ions and thiazides have not been identified. Thiazide ($[^3H]$metolazone) binding was inhibited by elimination of extracellular glycosylation sites from rat NCC in one study,[15] but a similar dependence on glycosylation was not seen in flounder NCC.[16] Although Cl^- inhibits the binding and action of thiazides,[17] data now suggest that thiazides bind to a site located within the transmembrane 8-12 region of NCC, whereas Cl^- binds to a different site in the transmembrane 1-7 region.[16]

The identification of gene defects affecting NCC has shed some additional light on its physiological role. Gitelman's syndrome (OMIM 263800) is an autosomal recessive salt-wasting condition characterized by hypocalciuria, hypomagnesemia, and hypokalemic alkalosis and a tendency to low blood pressure,[10] although hypertension has been described in one patient with Gitelman's syndrome.[18] This syndrome is due to a loss-of-function mutation in the SLC12A3 gene,[19] and deletion of the SLC12A3 gene in

mice leads to a similar phenotype. Loss of NCC is also associated with a reduction in number of distal convoluted tubular cells in renal cortical epithelium, suggesting a role for NCC in survival or development of distal convoluted tubular cells.[20]

In contrast to Gitelman's syndrome, pseudohypoaldosteronism type II (PHAII [Gordon's syndrome], OMIM 145260) is an autosomal dominant condition characterized by salt-sensitive hypertension that is highly sensitive to thiazide diuretics.[21] PHAII is caused by mutations in WNK1 or WNK4,[22,23] both of which are serine-threonine protein kinases that normally act as negative regulators of membrane trafficking of NCC, resulting in overexpression of NCC in distal collecting tubule cells.[24] Data now suggest that WNK4 is the key regulator and that mutations in WNK1 influence NCC via effects on WNK4.[23]

PHARMACOKINETICS AND PHARMACODYNAMICS

The clinical pharmacology of thiazide diuretics has not been as extensively studied as that of loop diuretics. Most thiazides are administered orally, although chlorothiazide is available as an intravenous preparation. After oral dosing with thiazides, the onset of diuresis is usually relatively rapid (1-4 hours), with the possible exception of chlortalidone and metolazone, which may have delayed peak effects.[25] Individual thiazides differ markedly in terms of plasma half-life ($t_{1/2}$) (Table 105-1). Drugs with a short half-life include bendroflumethiazide and hydrochlorothiazide, whereas that of chlortalidone is relatively long. Published values for the half-life of hydrochlorothiazide are quite variable, and discrepancies may relate to a complex polyexponential disposition function.[26] Whether this possibility applies to all thiazides is not known. Thiazides are generally highly bound to plasma proteins, such as albumin, and the apparent volume of distribution is usually high. For some agents, such as indapamide and chlortalidone, the high volume of distribution may also be due to extensive accumulation in erythrocytes, possibly as a result of binding to carbonic anhydrase.[27] The majority of thiazides are excreted by the kidney, but bendroflumethiazide and indapamide are metabolized by the liver. It has been suggested that a major metabolite of indapamide (5-OH indapamide) contributes to its vasodilator action.[28]

Because many thiazides are excreted by the kidney, impaired renal function leads to slowed elimination, but in practice, the consequence of this slowing is often out-

TABLE 105-1

Pharmacokinetics of Thiazides

DIURETIC	ORAL BIOAVAILABILITY (%)	HALF-LIFE	ELIMINATION	VOLUME OF DISTRIBUTION (L/KG)
Bendroflumethiazide	≈100	2-5	≈70% hepatic (metabolism), ≈30% renal	0.9-1.5
Chlorothiazide	9-56	0.75-2	Renal	
Hydrochlorothiazide	65-75	2.5-14.8	Renal	1.5-7.8
Hydroflumethiazide	≈75	6-25	Renal	?
Chlortalidone	≈65	24-55	Largely renal	3-13
Indapamide	≈93	14-24	Hepatic and renal metabolism	25-60
Metolazone	40-65%	8-14	Largely renal	113

Data from Jackson EJ: Diuretics. In Brunton LL, Lazo JS, Parker J, et al (eds): Goodman and Gilman's The Pharmacological Basis of Therapeutics, 11th ed. New York, McGraw-Hill, 2006, pp 737-769; and Brater DC: Diuretic therapy. N Engl J Med 1998;339:387-395.

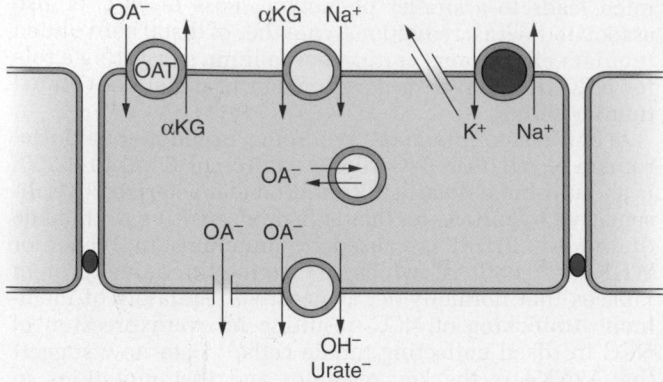

FIGURE 105-3. Secretion of thiazides into the tubular fluid by an organic anion transporter (OAT). OA⁻, organic anions; αKG, α-ketoglutarate. (Modified from Wilcox CS: New insights into diuretic use in patients with chronic renal disease. J Am Soc Nephrol 2002;13:798-805.)

weighed by the reduced effect of thiazides in renal impairment.[25] The increased plasma levels of thiazides in renal impairment, however, may increase the adverse effects.[29] Unlike with loop diuretics, congestive heart failure does not affect the pharmacokinetics of thiazides in a patient without impaired renal function.[25] The clinical importance of differences in pharmacokinetics between thiazides is uncertain, because response in terms of diuresis and particularly blood pressure–lowering relate poorly with drug concentration in plasma.

In order to act on the NCC, thiazides must enter the tubular fluid. Plasma concentrations of unbound thiazides achieved during therapeutic use are considerably less than the concentration for 50% inhibition (IC_{50}) of NCC activity; for example, the IC_{50} for NCC of hydrochlorothiazide is 7×10^{-5} M NCC,[17] and the plasma free concentration is 2.6×10^{-6} M.[4] Urinary concentrations of thiazide have rarely been measured, although one would expect that they should be of more relevance. It is known that urinary levels of thiazides may exceed plasma levels by 10- to 20-fold,[30] and the limited data available suggest that there is considerable variability between agents in terms of the amount of drug reaching the urine (ranging from about 5% for indapamide to about 80% for hydrochlorothiazide). Factors accounting for this variation are not fully understood. The high degree of plasma protein binding means that very little thiazide is filtered: thiazides gain access to the tubular fluid as a result of secretion by proximal tubular cells in the S2 segment.[31] Secretion occurs via an organic anion transporter (OAT-1) that transports a variety of organic anions, including loop diuretics (Fig. 105-3). Agents that inhibit OAT-1, such as probenecid, reduce the acute natriuretic effect of thiazides but also prolong their action and ultimately result in greater cumulative diuresis.[30] It has been suggested that competition for basolateral anion transport by uremic toxins and bilirubin may, in part, account for the reduced effects of thiazides in chronic renal insufficiency and jaundice.[30] In principle, other anionic drugs—aspirin, nonsteroidal anti-inflammatory drugs (NSAIDs), β-lactam antibiotics, and some radiographic contrast agents—could also interfere with secretion of thiazides, but there are few reports of diuretic resistance linked to this mechanism.

USES OF THIAZIDES

An extensive description of the clinical uses of thiazides is beyond the scope of this chapter, but the major indications for thiazide use are outlined.

Hypertension

Ever since their introduction, thiazides have been used to treat elevated blood pressure, and large-scale clinical trials have reinforced their role as a first-line therapy in hypertension.[32] Despite the widespread use of these agents, their mechanism of action in hypertension is obscure. Over the long term, thiazides are associated with vasodilation rather than volume depletion, but whether this feature is a consequence of renal adaptation or some other mechanism is unclear.[33]

Congestive Heart Failure and Other Causes of Edema

Thiazides are occasionally used alone in mild congestive heart failure, but more commonly, they are used in combination with loop diuretics. With long-term use, the effectiveness of diuretics in heart failure can wane as a result of the braking phenomenon (short-term tolerance), which prevents excessive losses of salt and fluid and impaired efficacy of diuretics as a result of renal insufficiency. This "diuretic resistance" is sometimes alleviated by sequential nephron blockade using a combination of loop diuretics and thiazides.[34]

Although they are less effective than aldosterone antagonists in edema associated with hepatic cirrhosis, thiazides may be used as adjunctive therapy.[25] They can also be used to treat edema associated with corticosteroid or estrogen therapy. Thiazides may also be used usually in combination with other diuretics in edema due to various forms of renal dysfunction, such as nephrotic syndrome, acute glomerulonephritis, and chronic renal failure.[35]

Use of Thiazides in Renal Impairment

Patients with chronic renal insufficiency have reductions in both glomerular filtration rate and filtered load of NaCl and fluid. Consequently, fractional reabsorption of NaCl and fluid is reduced to maintain salt and water balance.[31] These effects, along with reduced secretion into the tubular lumen, limit the efficacy of thiazides and other diuretics in severe renal insufficiency.[36] Nevertheless, high-dose thiazides may retain some efficacy even in advanced renal disease.[31] Thiazides tend to lower glomerular filtration rate even in normal subjects,[37] and this effect can be marked in chronic renal insufficiency.[31] High-dose thiazides in combination with loop diuretics are effective in promoting diuresis and reducing blood pressure in patients with mild and moderate azotemia, but often at the expense of large elevations in serum creatinine and blood urea nitrogen concentrations in addition to hypokalemia and electrolyte disorders.[31] Thiazide use is therefore generally reserved for highly resistant cases. A benefit of combining thiazides with loop diuretics is that thiazides may attenuate the hypercalciuria that occurs with loop diuretics.

Other Uses of Thiazides

Thiazides are also of benefit in calcium nephrolithiasis because they can decrease urinary Ca^{2+} excretion by 20% to 50%.[38] Their effectiveness is reduced by high dietary sodium intake. The hypocalciuric action of thiazide diuretics is useful in the treatment of idiopathic hypercalciuria[39] and Dent's disease.[40] Thiazides are also useful as adjunctive therapy to maintain serum Ca^{2+} concentration and reduce hypercalciuria in some patients with hypoparathyroidism.[41] Paradoxically, thiazides can diminish urine flow markedly in patients with central or nephrogenic diabetes insipidus,[42] possibly as a result of their ability to modulate expression of channels and transporter important for water and sodium reabsorption in the collecting system.[43] Long-term thiazide use is associated with increased bone mineralization.[44] The effect is modest,[45] but use of thiazides seems to protect against hip fractures.[46] Thiazides have also been used to treat Ménière's disease, but their usefulness is uncertain.[47]

ADVERSE EFFECTS OF THIAZIDES

Thiazide use can be associated with a number of adverse effects, including disturbances of electrolytes, metabolic abnormalities, and impotence. Unlike the blood pressure–lowering effects of thiazides, which show a relatively flat dose-response relationship, complications of thiazide use are usually highly dose-related and occur much more commonly with high doses. Adverse effects are also thought to be more likely with longer-acting compounds, such as chlortalidone and metolazone.[36,48] It has been suggested that metabolic disturbances are less common with the thiazide-like agent indapamide, but this difference may reflect the comparatively weak diuretic properties of indapamide at the doses used to treat hypertension.

Hyponatremia

Hyponatremia is a relatively infrequent but serious complication of thiazide therapy. In one study, 13.7% of patients receiving low-dose thiazide therapy in a primary care setting were found to have hyponatremia, which was severe (serum Na concentration <125 mmol/L) in 1%.[49] Because they do not interfere with the ability of the kidney to concentrate the urine, thiazide diuretics are more prone than loop diuretics to induce hyponatremia. Risk factors predisposing to thiazide-induced hyponatremia are old age, low serum potassium concentration, reduced body mass, physical immobility, concurrent use of other medications that impair water excretion, and behavioral disturbances that may increase thirst and water intake. It has been suggested that women are more at risk, but the higher risk could reflect the preponderance of women in the thiazide-treated population or sex imbalance in distribution of risk factors.

Thiazide-induced hyponatremia typically develops over days, usually shortly after commencement of therapy, but it can occur at any time during long-term treatment.[50] Thiazide-induced hyponatremia is a potentially serious adverse effect because it may cause severe central nervous system symptoms and can lead to permanent brain damage or death. A prior history of thiazide-induced hyponatremia is a strong predisposing factor for subsequent episodes; in a patient with such a history, thiazides should be used with great caution, if at all.[48]

Hypokalemia

Hypokalemia is a well-recognized complication of thiazide therapy. Estimates of its frequency range from 7% to 56%, but its prevalence is probably similar to that of mild hyponatremia.[49] Hypokalemia results from the increased Na^+ delivery to the distal segment of the distal tubule and collecting duct, where there is increased Na^+ reabsorption in exchange for K^+ and H^+. Further loss of K^+ is also attributable to activation of the renin-angiotensin-aldosterone system secondary to extracellular volume depletion. Plasma K^+ concentration usually falls rapidly after administration of thiazides, the typical drop being about 0.6 mmol/L, largely irrespective of dose or duration of treatment.[51] Although it is relatively rare for plasma K^+ concentration to fall below 3 mmol/L, there have been persistent concerns about the arrhythmogenic potential of even modest hypokalemia, and it has been suggested that thiazide use may be associated with an increase in the rate of sudden death.[52] This issue is unresolved[48]; at present, there is no consensus about either whom to treat with potassium supplementation or the coadministration of a potassium-sparing diuretic. Interestingly, hypokalemia may fail to respond to potassium supplementation if Mg^{2+} depletion is not corrected.[53]

Hypercalcemia

Thiazides reduce renal Ca^{2+} excretion and may also directly stimulate bone resorption.[48] In healthy people, these effects do not lead to hypercalcemia, but serum Ca^{2+} concentration can rise in people with immobilization hypercalciuria or those with hyperparathyroidism or vitamin D–treated hypoparathyroidism who cannot reduce parathyroid secretion in response to a rise in serum Ca^{2+} concentration. If hypercalcemia develops in response to thiazide treatment, an underlying disorder of calcium metabolism should be suspected.

Hypomagnesemia

Thiazides increase urinary Mg^{2+} excretion, and prolonged therapy reduces serum Mg^{2+} concentration by 5% to 10%.[54] Hypomagnesemia occurs more frequently in the elderly and often coexists with hyponatremia and hypokalemia. Secondary hyperaldosteronism from congestive heart failure, poor dietary magnesium intake, and high alcohol intake also raise the risk of hypomagnesemia. The main consequence of hypomagnesemia is increased risk of cardiac arrhythmias, but routine monitoring of serum Mg^{2+} concentration is not widely advocated.[48]

Acid-Base Disturbances

Mild metabolic alkalosis is a common feature of thiazide diuretic therapy, particularly with higher doses, but severe metabolic alkalosis is much less frequent. Classically, treatment with thiazides can produce hypokalemic, hypochloremic metabolic alkalosis, which responds to replacement of potassium and chloride deficits. The metabolic alkalosis is initially a result of volume depletion, which elevates aldosterone levels and stimulates proton secretion in the distal nephron. As chloride availability for proximal reabsorption with Na^+ diminishes, Na^+ reabsorption by the Na^+/H^+ exchanger increases, maintaining the metabolic alkalosis. Lack of chloride may also impair distal bicarbonate secretion in exchange for chloride or may promote distal bicarbonate reabsorption.

Hyperuricemia

Thiazides raise serum urate concentrations in a dose-dependent manner. An increase in urate after thiazide administration is common, and rises of about 30% have been reported after high-dose thiazide therapy.[48] The effect of thiazides on serum urate occurs rapidly and persists, but asymptomatic hyperuricemia is probably not harmful,[55] and development of gout is infrequent.[56] The increase in urate is due to greater reabsorption secondary to depletion of extracellular fluid volume and competition for tubular secretion of urate by thiazides.[48] Coadministration of angiotensin-converting enzyme inhibitors or angiotensin receptor blockers attenuates the rise in urate seen with thiazides.[57,58]

Altered Glucose Metabolism (Hyperglycemia/Insulin Resistance/Diabetes)

Thiazide use is associated with elevated fasting glucose value, impaired glucose tolerance, insulin resistance, and increased risk of development of type 2 diabetes mellitus. The significance of this impairment of glucose metabolism is disputed, and it is not clear that the increase in blood glucose resulting from thiazide use has the same long-term health impact as such an increase occurring in other circumstances.[59] The development of glucose intolerance appears to be related to the degree of hypokalemia,[60] and this relationship has been proposed as a mechanism of impaired glucose tolerance. Increased sympathetic activation secondary to volume depletion probably also contributes. Rarely, thiazides can induce a severe hyperosmolar nonketotic syndrome.[61]

Dyslipidemia

In the short term (less than 1 year), treatment with thiazides is associated with increases in serum total cholesterol (≈6.5%), low-density-lipoprotein cholesterol (15%), and triglycerides (23%).[48] Longer-term studies show less marked changes in lipid levels.[62] The mechanism responsible for dyslipidemia is uncertain. Both activation of the sympathetic nervous system secondary to volume depletion and hypokalemia have been suggested as causes.[63]

Impotence

Thiazides are associated with increased impotence and male sexual dysfunction.[48] For example, in the Treatment of Mild Hypertension Study (TOMHS),[64] male participants randomly assigned to receive chlorthalidone reported a significantly higher incidence of erection problems through 24 months of therapy than participants who received placebo (17.1% vs. 8.1%, respectively). The mechanism of this effect is not known, and it seems unrelated to hypokalemia or blood pressure lowering.

Rare Adverse Effects of Thiazides
Interstitial Nephritis

Interstitial nephritis, occasionally with granulomas, is a rare complication of thiazides. It may develop either abruptly or some months after therapy is initiated. Interstitial nephritis usually resolves after thiazide treatment is stopped, but the presence of granulomas may be an indication for treatment with corticosteroids.[65]

Pancreatitis

Reversible hyperamylasemia has also been noted after chlorothiazide administration, and clinical pancreatitis has been reported in association with chlorothiazide and chlortalidone use.[48]

Pulmonary Edema

Occasional cases of noncardiogenic pulmonary edema have been reported after administration of thiazides.[66] Symptoms can occur after first exposure or in patients taking thiazides intermittently. The majority of cases have occurred in women, and the mechanism is not known.

Renal Cell Carcinoma

A meta-analysis of nine case-control and three large cohort studies has indicated that diuretic use is associated with increased risk of renal cell carcinoma (odds ratio = 1.54; 95% confidence interval, 1.41-1.68]. The risk was higher in women and was increased with high doses of diuretics. At present, whether the higher risk is due to diuretic use per se or is related to concurrent diseases such as hypertension or obesity is uncertain.[67]

Allergic Reactions and Photosensitivity

Allergic reactions, including rashes, eosinophilia, purpura, and blood dyscrasias, have been reported in association with thiazide use.[48,62] Hydrochlorothiazide seems to cause photosensitivity more commonly than other thiazides.[62]

DRUG INTERACTIONS

Thiazides interact with many drugs. They may diminish the effects of anticoagulants, uricosuric agents, sulfonylureas, and insulin. They may increase the effects of anesthetics, diazoxide, and vitamin D. Bile acid sequestrants may reduce absorption of thiazides from the gut, and methenamines reduce their effects due to alkalinization of the urine. Some other important drug interactions are listed in more detail here.

Nonsteroidal Anti-Inflammatory Drugs

NSAIDs reduce the natriuretic effect of thiazides, induce weight gain, and can cause loss of blood pressure control in hypertensive patients.[68] These effects are probably a consequence of the inhibition of renal eicosanoid synthesis, but whether they are due to the hemodynamic or tubular effects of NSAIDs is unclear.[68]

Cardiac Glycosides and Antiarrhythmic Agents

Thiazides can enhance the risk of cardiac arrhythmias in patients receiving cardiac glycosides through the enhancement of action of cardiac glycosides by hypokalemia. Hypokalemia is also responsible for the increased risk of torsades de pointes and ventricular fibrillation when thiazides are used in conjunction with quinidine.

Angiotensin-Converting Enzyme Inhibitors

Acute renal failure is an occasional complication of the combination of angiotensin-converting enzyme inhibitors and thiazides. It may occur irrespective of the presence of renal artery stenosis and is probably due to Na^+ depletion. In many cases, renal function improves after correction of Na^+ depletion and cessation of therapy with the two types of agents.

Lithium

Thiazide diuretics can increase serum lithium concentrations quite markedly,[69] but a large study did not identify thiazide use as a major factor in hospital admission for lithium intoxication.[70] This latter fact may reflect the current use of low-dose thiazides in hypertension. The specific thiazide used may also be important, because some evidence suggests that inhibition of lithium clearance is due to inhibition of carbonic anhydrase in the proximal tubule,[71] a property not shared by all thiazides.

Key Points

1. Thiazide and thiazide-like diuretics (thiazides) increase salt and water excretion by the kidney.
2. Thiazides cause natriuresis by inhibiting the NaCl cotransporter in the distal convoluted tubule.
3. Thiazides are secreted into the tubular fluid by an organic anion transporter and act from the luminal side of the tubule to inhibit the NaCl cotransporter.
4. Individual thiazides differ considerably in terms of their pharmacokinetics, but all induce a rapid diuresis.
5. Thiazides are widely used in the treatment of hypertension and are also used as adjunctive therapy in congestive heart failure and chronic renal insufficiency.

Key References

10. Reilly RF, Ellison DH: Mammalian distal tubule: Physiology, pathophysiology, and molecular anatomy. Physiol Rev 2000;80:277-313.
23. Yang CL, Angell J, Mitchell R, Ellison DH: WNK kinases regulate thiazide-sensitive Na-Cl cotransport. J Clin Invest 2003;111:1039-1045.
34. Hughes AD: How do thiazide and thiazide-like diuretics lower blood pressure? J Renin Angiotensin Aldosterone Syst 2004;5:155-160.
35. Kramer BK, Schweda F, Riegger GA: Diuretic treatment and diuretic resistance in heart failure. Am J Med 1999;106:90-96.
49. Greenberg A: Diuretic complications. Am J Med Sci 2000;319:10-24.

See the companion Expert Consult website for the complete reference list.

CHAPTER 106

Aldosterone Antagonists, Amiloride, and Triamterene

Stephen Warrillow

OBJECTIVES

This chapter will:
1. Review the structure, mechanism of action, and biological effects of aldosterone antagonists, amiloride, and triamterene (the potassium-sparing diuretics).
2. Contrast the properties of the potassium-sparing diuretics with other diuretic drugs.
3. Discuss the renal and extrarenal effects of aldosterone antagonism.
4. Review the use of aldosterone antagonists, amiloride, and triamterene in clinical practice.

The aldosterone antagonists as well as amiloride and triamterene are often collectively referred to as the *potassium-sparing diuretics* (Table 106-1) to distinguish them from the thiazides and loop diuretics, which cause kaliuresis. As a group, the potassium-sparing diuretics are relatively weak diuretics, but their distinctly different site and mechanism of action result in quite a different influence on renal electrolyte handling and metabolic effects, including a tendency to greater serum potassium and mild metabolic acidosis. These drugs are usually used in combination with more potent diuretic agents to treat hypertension and conditions of fluid overload and to treat specific disorders of the renin-angiotensin-aldosterone system.

ALDOSTERONE ANTAGONISTS

Aldosterone is a steroid hormone secreted by the zona glomerulosa of the adrenal cortex. It binds to the mineralocorticoid receptor within the cytoplasm of tubular epithelium, causing an increase in the expression of Na^+,K^+-ATPase sodium pumps on the interstitial sides of the late distal convoluted tubule and collecting duct. This results in active sodium (and hence water) reabsorption from, and potassium excretion into, the urine. Net effects of aldosterone therefore include sodium retention, potassium excretion, and an overall expansion of the extracellular fluid volume. Nonrenal sites of aldosterone-mediated sodium and potassium exchange are of minor clinical significance but include other epithelialized tissues, such as the salivary glands and gastrointestinal tract. Aldosterone synthesis in the adrenal cortex is regulated mainly by angiotensin II, serum potassium and, to a lesser extent, serum sodium and adrenocorticotrophic hormone. Circulating plasma concentrations of aldosterone are markedly elevated through the neurohormonal processes associated with congestive heart failure and contribute to the perpet-

uation of cardiovascular injury.[1] It is also increasingly appreciated that aldosterone has important actions beyond the kidney and ion transport, including participation in inflammatory processes, collagen formation, and organ fibrosis.[2-4] The known pathological effects attributable to aldosterone excess continue to accumulate; currently they include atherosclerosis, cardiac fibrosis, endothelial dysfunction, arrhythmias, and cardiac hypertrophy.[5]

Although the renin-angiotensin-aldosterone system has been previously regarded as a salt-, blood pressure–, and fluid-regulating system centered on the kidney, it is increasingly appreciated that some or all of the constituents of the system are synthesized in vascular structures such as the heart and in vessel walls, where concentrations can greatly exceed circulating levels.[6] In addition, the mineralocorticoid receptors can be found in nonepithelial tissues, including the brain, heart, and vascular tissue.[5] The possibility that aldosterone has effects that are not mediated through the classic intracellular mineralocorticoid receptors has been raised, but clear evidence to clarify the exact mechanisms responsible remains elusive.[5,7] This situation, in part, explains why the full effects of aldosterone blockade on the cardiovascular system cannot be completely explained solely through its effect on the renal tubule. The renal effects of aldosterone antagonists may not manifest for several days, and full cardiovascular effects may take weeks. Several drugs of varying specificity have been developed to interfere with aldosterone's binding at the mineralocorticoid receptor within renal tissue and at other sites.

Spironolactone

Spironolactone, a synthetic 17-lactone steroid aldosterone antagonist developed more than 50 years ago, competitively binds at the mineralocorticoid receptor (Fig. 106-1). Blocking the mineralocorticoid receptor inhibits production of Na^+,K^+-ATPase, effectively reducing the number of Na^+ pumps present on the interstitial side of target tubular epithelial cells. Impeding the action of aldosterone thus causes renal retention of potassium, excretion of sodium (natriuresis), and modestly increased urine volume (diuresis). Secondarily, there is a tendency to increased urinary chloride and calcium excretion and for magnesium and hydrogen ions to be retained. Although mineralocorticoid antagonism has been shown to produce sustained increases in plasma renin and serum aldosterone levels that are consistent with interference with the negative regulatory feedback of aldosterone on renin secretion, these changes do not overcome the effects of spironolactone on the kidney. Spironolactone also has moderate antiandrogenic effects owing to its antagonistic binding at peripheral androgen receptors and inhibition of ovarian testosterone synthesis.[8]

TABLE 106-1

Comparisons of the Potassium-Sparing Diuretics

PROPERTY	SPIRONOLACTONE	EPLERENONE	AMILORIDE	TRIAMTERENE
Class/action	Mineralocorticoid and androgen receptor antagonist	Selective mineralocorticoid receptor antagonist	Inhibition of amiloride-sensitive sodium channels in the distal convoluted tubule (DCT) and collecting ducts	Inhibition of Na^+-K^+-$2Cl^-$ cotransporter in the DCT and collecting ducts
Absorption	Readily absorbed; absorption increased with food	Probably well absorbed	Readily absorbed	Readily absorbed
Onset and duration of effect	Days	Days	Hours	Hours
Protein binding (%)	90	50	23	67
Metabolism	Liver	Liver	Not metabolized	Liver
Active metabolites?	Yes	No	No	Yes
Route of excretion (in order of importance)	Renal Bile-feces	Renal Bile-feces	Renal Bile-feces	Renal Bile-feces
Usual starting dose	25 mg twice daily	25 mg daily	2.5-5.0 mg twice daily	50 mg daily
Usual maintenance dose	25-100 mg twice daily	50 mg daily	5-10 mg twice daily	50-100 mg twice daily

Data from Wishart DS, Knox C, Guo AC, et al: DrugBank: A comprehensive resource for in silico drug discovery and exploration. Nucleic Acids Res 2006;34;D668-D672. Available at http://redpoll.pharmacy.ualberta.ca/drugbank.index.html/; Caswell A, Harvey A, Bellantonio J (eds): eMIMS. Available at http://mims.hcn.net.au/; and Barnes BJ, Howard PA: Eplerenone: A selective aldosterone receptor antagonist for patients with heart failure. Ann Pharmacother 2005;39:68-76.

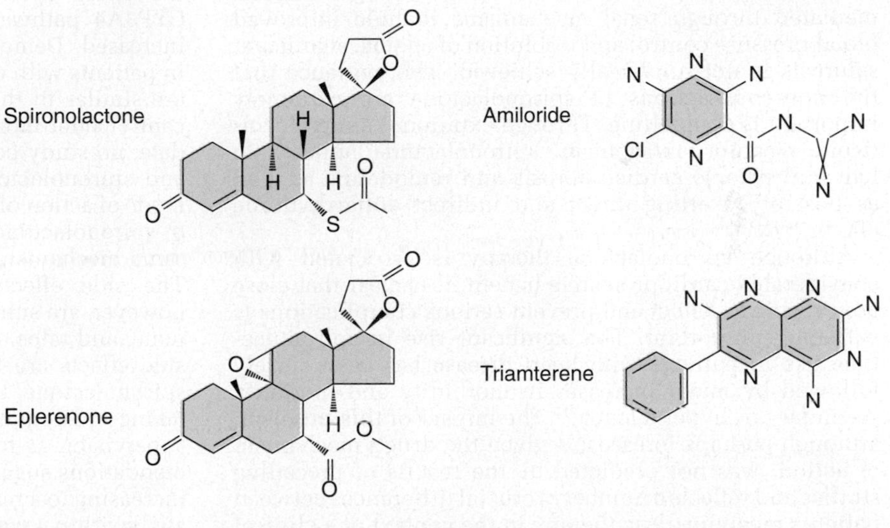

FIGURE 106-1. Structure of potassium-sparing diuretics.

Spironolactone is well absorbed from the gastrointestinal tract, especially when coadministered with food, and undergoes rapid and extensive metabolism. Its mainly sulfur-containing active metabolites are highly bound to plasma proteins and undergo predominantly renal excretion. Approximately a quarter of the administered dose is metabolized to canrenone, which also exerts significant mineralocorticoid receptor blockade and antiandrogenic effects. Adverse effects attributable to spironolactone can be largely predicted from its mode of action. Hyperkalemia is a potentially serious problem that is especially likely to occur in patients who have impaired renal function or are receiving other drugs that can raise serum potassium levels. Although spironolactone would be expected to accumulate in patients with significant hepatic dysfunction, dose reduction is not generally necessary in such patients. The antiandrogenic properties of spironolactone,

although exploited in the treatment of conditions involving androgen excess, can also have undesirable effects, particularly in men, who may experience gynecomastia and sexual dysfunction.

An obvious clinical role for spironolactone is primary hyperaldosteronism (Conn's syndrome), in which unregulated aldosterone excess results in potassium depletion, hypertension, and expansion of the extracellular fluid volume. Consistent with its mechanism of action, spironolactone appears effective and well tolerated for this disorder and can be used as preoperative therapy for the patient with a secreting adenoma or as medical therapy for such a patient in whom surgery is inappropriate.[9] Another longstanding use for spironolactone is in medical management of patients with ascites due to chronic liver disease. In this clinical situation, spironolactone as a single agent or in combination with loop diuretics has been demonstrated to be more effective and better tolerated than other regimens.[10] The antiandrogenic properties of spironolactone have been utilized as first-line treatment for hirsutism, in which it is as effective as cyproterone acetate and flutamide.[11] Combination therapy incorporating spironolactone and another of these hormonal therapies is common practice for idiopathic hirsutism.

The most common use for spironolactone, however, is in treatment of cardiac failure, for which it has become established therapy as an adjunct to other agents, such as angiotensin-converting enzyme (ACE) inhibitors, loop diuretics, and β-blockers. Spironolactone's major use had previously been to counteract the kaliuretic action of loop and thiazide diuretics, which are frequently used as first-line therapy for cardiac failure and hypertension. The widespread use of ACE inhibitors as standard therapy for cardiac failure also contributed to past low use of aldosterone antagonists, which was based on concerns (that have subsequently been validated) about the potential for serious hyperkalemia. Cumulative evidence for the cardiovascular benefits of mineralocorticoid receptor blockade, however, has resulted in a significant resurgence in the use of spironolactone.[12] The administration of relatively low doses of spironolactone (25 mg daily) has been demonstrated to improve symptoms and reduce mortality for patients with severe left ventricular systolic dysfunction who are already receiving loop diuretics and ACE inhibitors.[13] It is likely that several mechanisms contribute to these cardioprotective effects. Although predicted effects mediated through renal mechanisms include improved blood pressure control and resolution of edema, significant saluresis is not universally achieved. The evidence that the nonrenal actions of spironolactone are extremely important is compelling. Through extrarenal mineralocorticoid receptor antagonism, spironolactone appears to halt and reverse cardiac fibrosis and remodeling as well as possibly exerting direct and indirect antiarrhythmic effects.[13,14]

Although spironolactone therapy is associated with considerable cardioprotective benefit, it is clear that close monitoring to detect and prevent serious complications is extremely important. The significant rise in spironolactone use in patients with heart disease has been closely followed by major increases in morbidity and mortality secondary to hyperkalemia.[12] The impact of this problem, although perhaps foreseeable given the drug's mechanism of action, was not predicted by the results of preceding studies and reflects a number of crucial differences between patients receiving drug therapy in the context of a clinical trial and those managed in the broader context of day-to-day clinical practice. Therefore, the importance of giving careful consideration to comorbid medical conditions (such as renal impairment, especially diabetic nephropathy), coadministered drugs (particularly ACE inhibitors, angiotensin II blockers, nonsteroidal anti-inflammatory drugs, and potassium supplements), and drug dosing is readily apparent. Recommended doses vary from 50 to 200 mg per day, along with regular monitoring of serum electrolyte values. The level of renal dysfunction at which the risks of dangerous hyperkalemia outweigh the cardioprotective benefits of spironolactone is not clear. Avoiding spironolactone therapy in patients with serum creatinine values greater than 221 µmol/L is prudent, because patients with poorer renal function were excluded by the major study in which benefit was demonstrated.[13] Such an approach cannot completely prevent hyperkalemia, however, which can still occur in patients with more normal renal function.[15] Baseline potassium measurement

should be undertaken in all patients; a serum potassium concentration greater than 5 mmol/L is a contraindication to the use of spironolactone. Vigilant monitoring and downward dose adjustment are advised for the use of this agent in patients with serum potassium levels exceeding 5.5 mmol/L.

Eplerenone

The incidence of undesirable effects relating to spironolactone's antiandrogenic properties leads to discontinuation of this agent in a significant number of patients. Painful breast enlargement and erectile dysfunction in men are particularly common complaints, even with relatively low doses. Eplerenone is substantially more specific to the mineralocorticoid receptor than spironolactone, with a chemical structure that differs by replacement of the 17-α thioacetyl group with a carboxymethoxy group (see Fig. 106-1). Although it is a competitive antagonist of the mineralocorticoid receptor, eplerenone binds only very weakly to androgen, glucocorticoid, and progesterone receptors and is therefore essentially devoid of the feminizing side effects characteristic of spironolactone.[16] Other important differences of eplerenone from spironolactone are a lack of active metabolites, only modest protein binding, and a lack of change in bioavailability when administered with food.

Because eplerenone is metabolized via the hepatic CYP3A4 pathway, its potential for drug interactions is increased. Demonstrable beneficial effects of eplerenone in patients with cardiac failure after myocardial infarction are similar to those of spironolactone, including significantly better mortality and hospitalization outcomes.[17] To date, no study comparing the effectiveness of eplerenone and spironolactone has been conducted. Given that the mode of action of eplerenone is essentially identical to that of spironolactone (aside from antiandrogenic effects), the same mechanisms leading to benefit would be expected. The side effects associated with androgen blockade, however, are substantially lower in patients taking eplerenone, and rates of discontinuation of therapy due to such side effects are the same as those for placebo. As with spironolactone, the tendency to hyperkalemia in patients taking eplerenone is a serious problem mandating close supervision as long as therapy continues. Dosing recommendations suggest commencing at a dose of 25 mg daily, increasing to a maximal target dose of 50 mg daily (if tolerated) within 4 weeks. Baseline evaluation of renal function is useful to assess the potential for hazardous hyperkalemia. Patients with baseline serum creatinine concentrations greater than 221 mmol/L were excluded from the largest clinical trial of eplerenone, and a creatinine clearance less than 50 mL/min was found to confer a significant risk of elevated serum potassium concentration.[17] Regular monitoring is important with eplerenone therapy, even in patients with apparently preserved renal function, and dose reduction should occur with serum potassium levels exceeding 5.5 mmol/L.

NON–ALDOSTERONE ANTAGONIST POTASSIUM-SPARING DIURETICS

Non–aldosterone antagonist potassium-sparing diuretics have net effects on renal electrolyte handling very similar to those of the mineralocorticoid antagonists, but their mechanisms of action are quite distinct.

Amiloride

Amiloride hydrochloride, a pyrazine-carbonyl-guanidine, is chemically unrelated to other known diuretics (see Fig. 106-1). By binding to sodium channels in the distal convoluted tubule and collecting ducts, amiloride inhibits sodium reabsorption, producing a mild natriuresis and diuresis. Sodium channel blockade also leads to a decrease in the net negative potential of the tubular lumen, reducing the secretion of potassium and hydrogen ions into the urine.[18] Compared with thiazides and loop diuretics, amiloride is therefore potassium sparing and may be used to offset potential kaliuresis in patients taking these more potent potassium-wasting diuretics.[19] Improved adherence to therapy may be achieved through fixed-dose combination preparations, which incorporate thiazide diuretics, as treatment for conditions leading to edema and for ascites and hypertension. Amiloride is readily absorbed from the gastrointestinal tract and is predominantly excreted unchanged by the kidneys. It does not undergo any hepatic metabolism. Recommended dose ranges from 2.5 to 5.0 mg daily.[19] Monitoring of serum electrolyte values and careful assessment for additional factors that could potentiate hyperkalemia are important.

Triamterene

Triamterene is a potassium-sparing, weak diuretic with a mode of action similar to that of amiloride. Through inhibition of the Na^+-K^+-$2Cl^-$ cotransporter, triamterene reduces sodium reabsorption from the tubule, creating an electrical potential difference unfavorable to passive excretion of potassium by the distal tubule. This agent is often used in combination with thiazides and loop diuretics to reduce urinary potassium and magnesium losses and so obviate the need for supplementation of these electrolytes.[20] Triamterene is metabolized mainly to the sulfate conjugate hydroxy-triamterene, which possesses activity similar to that of the parent drug. Patients with significant liver dysfunction are at risk for drug accumulation owing to increased bioavailability from alterations in first-pass metabolism and decreased clearance. Apart from hyperkalemia, adverse effects relating to triamterene include triamterene-containing renal calculi.[21] Recommended dosing for triamterene ranges from 50 to 100 mg up to twice daily.[19]

CONCLUSION

Aldosterone antagonists, amiloride, and triamterene have a distinctive niche role in clinical practice because of their specific effects on electrolyte handling. Their potassium-sparing properties make them useful adjunct therapies to more potent diuretic drugs given for edema and hypertension. The aldosterone antagonists spironolactone and eplerenone also have an important role as components of cardiac failure management, partly by virtue of their extrarenal beneficial cardiovascular effects. The safe use of these agents, however, requires consideration of factors that may contribute to hyperkalemia and careful monitoring of serum electrolyte values.

Key Points

1. The potassium-sparing diuretics act via mechanisms in the renal tubule that are distinct from those of other diuretic agents.
2. These unique properties result in biological effects specific to drugs within the class that can be complementary to other diuretics, especially kaliuretic agents such as loop diuretics and thiazides.
3. These agents may be useful therapies for hypertension and clinical disorders causing edema.
4. The aldosterone antagonists have clinically important cardioprotective effects in patients with cardiac failure mediated via both renal and nonrenal mechanisms.
5. Consistent with their effect on renal tubule electrolyte handling, the potassium-sparing diuretics can cause hyperkalemia, especially in patients with renal impairment or during co-administration of other agents that can lead to elevations in serum potassium concentration (e.g., ACE inhibitors, angiotensin II blockers).

Key References

2. Williams JS, Williams GH: 50th anniversary of aldosterone. J Clin Endocrinol Metab 2003;88:2364-2372.

4. Sica DA: Pharmacokinetics and pharmacodynamics of mineralocorticoid blocking agents and their effects on potassium homeostasis. Heart Fail Rev 2005;10:23-29.

13. Pitt B, Zannad F, Remme WJ, et al: The effect of spironolactone on morbidity and mortality in patients with severe heart failure. Randomized Aldactone Evaluation Study Investigators. N Engl J Med 1999;341:709-717.

15. Svensson M, Gustafsson F, Galatius S, et al: How prevalent is hyperkalemia and renal dysfunction during treatment with spironolactone in patients with congestive heart failure? J Card Fail 2004;10:297-303.

17. Pitt B, Remme W, Zannad F, et al: Eplerenone, a selective aldosterone blocker, in patients with left ventricular dysfunction after myocardial infarction. N Engl J Med 2003;348:1309-1321.

See the companion Expert Consult website for the complete reference list.

CHAPTER 107

Carbonic Anhydrase Inhibitors

Stephen Warrillow

OBJECTIVES

This chapter will:
1. Review the structure, mechanism of action, and biological effects of the carbonic anhydrase inhibitors.
2. Contrast the properties of the carbonic anhydrase inhibitors with those of other diuretic drugs.
3. Discuss the renal and extrarenal effects of carbonic anhydrase.
4. Review the use of the carbonic anhydrase inhibitors in clinical practice.

Carbonic anhydrase is a zinc-complexed enzyme found in tissues of all animal species and photosynthesizing organisms, in which it catalyzes the reversible hydration of carbon dioxide (CO_2). In solution, carbon dioxide exists in equilibrium with bicarbonate; however, the rate of conversion is extremely slow at physiologic pH. Carbonic anhydrase dramatically increases the speed of this reaction (Fig. 107-1) and is one of the fastest-known enzymatically catalyzed biological processes. In most situations, the times required for diffusion of CO_2 and bicarbonate are the rate-limiting steps. Carbon dioxide can freely diffuse across cell membranes, whereas bicarbonate must be transported. Carbonic anhydrase therefore has an essential role in facilitating transport of CO_2, bicarbonate, and hydrogen ions across the following cell membranes for a variety of processes:

- Erythrocytes, where carbonic anhydrase contributes to carriage of CO_2 transport from the tissues to the lungs
- Stomach, pancreas, and salivary glands, where carbonic anhydrase participates in the production of acidic and alkaline enteral secretions
- Kidneys, where carbonic anhydrase in the proximal renal tubule participates directly and indirectly in determining the concentration of hydrogen ions, bicarbonate, and other electrolytes in the urine
- Eyes, where carbonic anhydrase contributes to the formation of the aqueous humor
- Brain, where carbonic anhydrase is involved in production of cerebrospinal fluid

The human forms of carbonic anhydrase have a molecular weight of around 30,000 kDa, with seven distinct isoenzymes identified. These various forms of the enzyme exhibit differing tissue distributions, cellular locations, grades of activity, and susceptibility to inhibition. Carbonic anhydrase II, the most widely distributed, is particularly important for processes within the kidney, brain, and bone.[1]

The wide variety of tissues utilizing carbonic anhydrase to effect changes in ion transport has resulted in the therapeutic use of blocking agents for a range of otherwise unrelated medical conditions. Interference with the normal action of carbonic anhydrase has been used to treat patients with heart failure and subsequent edema, hypertension, glaucoma, childhood seizure disorders, periodic paralysis, metabolic alkalemia, and acute mountain sickness. Within the proximal tubule of the kidney, carbonic anhydrase catalyzes the formation of carbonic acid and, thus, is responsible for creating hydrogen ions to exchange for sodium via the Na^+-H^+ antiport situated on the membrane on the luminal side of the tubular epithelium (Fig. 107-2). This permits the creation of acidic urine and the retention of bicarbonate, which diffuses back into the interstitial fluid.

CARBONIC ANHYDRASE INHIBITORS

Acetazolamide

Acetazolamide is a nonbacteriostatic sulfonamide structurally quite different from the antimicrobial sulfonamides (Fig. 107-3).[2] A powerful, but reversible, noncompetitive inhibitor of carbonic anhydrase, acetazolamide has effects at all sites with significant amounts and activity of this enzyme. Like other sulfonamides, acetazolamide can cause adverse reactions, including gastrointestinal upset, rashes, and rare but serious idiosyncratic disruption of blood cell formation. Nephrolithiasis with calcium oxalate and phosphate stones can also occur. The drug is very well absorbed from the gastrointestinal tract and can also be administered intravenously.

Acetazolamide is highly protein bound and is eliminated unmetabolized, predominantly by the kidneys.[3] In the kidney, acetazolamide reduces the availability of hydrogen ions for excretion into the urine at the proximal tubule and reduces bicarbonate reabsorption by up to 80%. This reduction results in production of alkaline urine, owing to increased bicarbonate losses, and promotes a normal anion gap metabolic acidosis. In addition, because acetazolamide decreases the availability of hydrogen ions that can be exchanged for sodium ions in the proximal and distal renal tubule, both sodium and bicarbonate remain in the tubule and cause a mild diuresis. Acetazolamide-mediated inhibition of carbonic anhydrase facilitates bicarbonate loss in the urine and, indirectly, results in chloride retention, causing elevations of this strong ion in the serum. As sodium excretion is maintained, a reduced strong ion difference results, and a normal-anion-gap, hyperchloremic metabolic acidosis occurs.[4] These effects, mediated through the drug's action on the renal tubule, lead to most of the important clinical manifestations of acetazolamide administration and have been used to treat edema states as well as cases of metabolic alkalemia as can occur with loop diuretic therapy.

Acute mountain sickness is a clinical syndrome occurring at altitudes of more than 2000 m above sea level as a result of failure to adapt to acute hypobaric hypoxia. Acetazolamide is the most commonly used and best-studied agent for this disorder.[5,6] Characteristic features of acute mountain sickness are headache, nausea, dyspnea, lethargy, and insomnia, and severe cases can progress to fatal cerebral and/or pulmonary edema. Acetazolamide's efficacy has been previously attributed to its action on the proximal renal tubule and resultant metabolic acidosis causing a compensatory increase in minute ventilation. Several other factors are likely to also contribute, however, including effects on central and peripheral chemoreceptors and diuresis.[7] Chronic mountain sickness, a condition in which long-term residents of high-altitude locations experience polycythemia, cardiac failure, and neurological problems, has been less well studied, although acetazolamide appears to be effective treatment for it.[8] Efforts to demonstrate benefits of acetazolamide for obstructive sleep apnea and chronic obstructive pulmonary disease have not been convincing.[9,10]

Another use for acetazolamide is in pediatric seizure disorders, particularly absence and localization-related epilepsy, in which it is used in conjunction with conventional anticonvulsant therapies.[11] The exact mechanism whereby carbonic anhydrase inhibition has an anticonvulsant effect has not been fully elucidated, but there is evidence of a direct effect within the central nervous system, causing a local rise in tissue CO_2 tension that inhibits conduction of excitatory impulses. Within the eye, acetazolamide reduces the production of aqueous humor by a significant volume and substantially reduces the intraocular pressure in glaucomatous eyes. Effective carbonic anhydrase inhibition within the eye markedly lowers the flow of sodium, bicarbonate, and water into the posterior chamber, making acetazolamide an effective adjunct therapy for glaucoma. However, newer topical carbonic anhydrase inhibitors, use of which avoids many of the side effects related to systemic carbonic anhydrase inhibition, are better tolerated by patients.[12] Dosing recommendations for the various indications for acetazolamide are detailed in Table 107-1.

Other Carbonic Anhydrase Inhibitors

Methazolamide and dorzolamide, sulfonamide derivative carbonic anhydrase inhibitors similar to acetazolamide, were developed to treat chronic open-angle glaucoma. Dorzolamide may be administered as a topical preparation in the eye, thus avoiding many of the side effects caused by systemically administered carbonic anhydrase inhibitors. Dichlorphenamide is another carbonic anhydrase inhibitor that may be used as systemic therapy for glaucoma. It has also been used to treat primary periodic paralysis syndromes, for which it appears to be more effective and better tolerated than acetazolamide.[13]

$$H_2O + CO_2 \rightleftharpoons H_2CO_3 \rightleftharpoons H^+ + HCO_3^-$$

Carbonic acid

FIGURE 107-1. Reactions catalyzed by carbonic anhydrase.

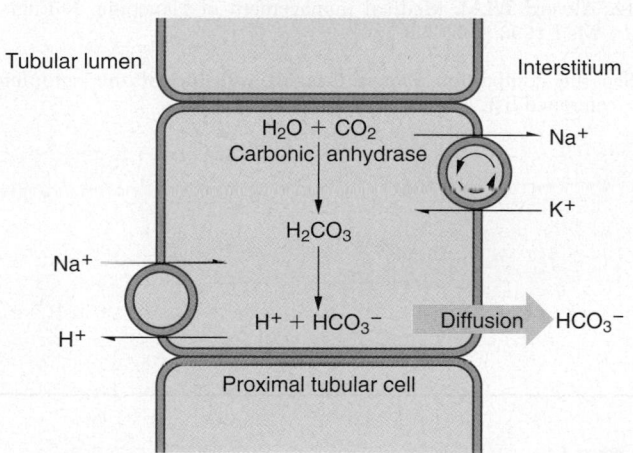

FIGURE 107-2 Role of carbonic anhydrase within the proximal renal tubule.

CONCLUSION

Apart from their topical use for glaucoma, the carbonic anhydrase inhibitors can be regarded as essentially niche therapies for specific disorders that are uncommon in the day-to-day practice of most clinicians. Their utility as diuretics is limited by their relatively low potency and frequent tendency to induce undesirable metabolic acidosis. More effective diuretic agents possessing fewer clinically significant side effects have largely usurped this role. As prophylaxis for and treatment of acute mountain sickness, however, carbonic anhydrase inhibition is extremely useful. For this and other disorders in which the induction of a metabolic acidosis may be useful, carbonic anhydrase inhibitors continue to play an important role. Their action at specific sites such as the brain also remains important for treating some forms of pediatric epilepsy.

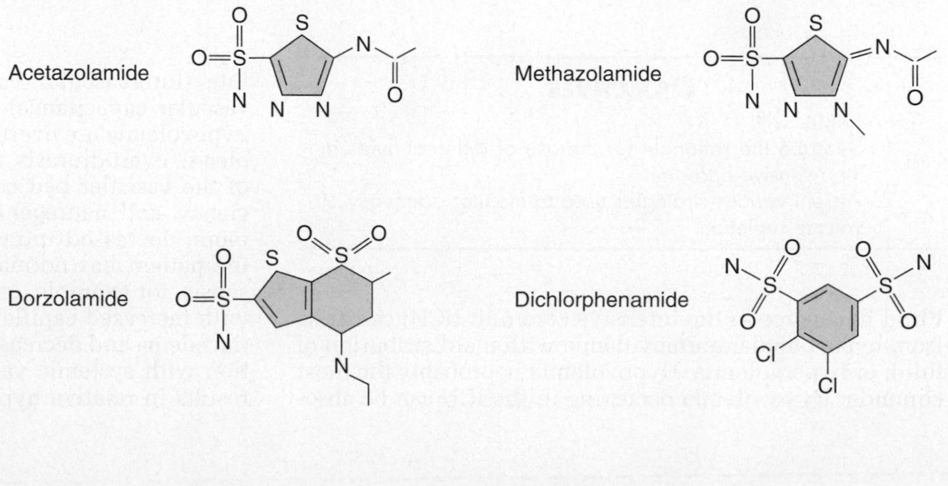

Acetazolamide

Methazolamide

Dorzolamide

Dichlorphenamide

FIGURE 107-3. Structures of the carbonic anhydrase inhibitors.

TABLE 107-1

Dosing Recommendations for Acetazolamide*

INDICATION	USUAL STARTING DOSE	USUAL MAINTENANCE DOSE
Glaucoma	250 mg daily	250 mg qid
Childhood epilepsy	8 mg/kg/day	30 mg/kg/day (maximum daily dose 750 mg)
Epilepsy in adults	250 mg daily	250 mg qid
Edema states	250-375 mg IV or orally daily	250 mg IV or orally twice daily
Acute mountain sickness	375 mg IV or orally twice daily for prophylaxis and treatment	
Severe metabolic alkalosis	250-500 mg IV or orally tid for 2 days	

*Significant dose reduction is necessary in patients with renal failure.
Data from Dumont L, Mardirosoff C, Tramèr MR: Efficacy and harm of pharmacological prevention of acute mountain sickness: Quantitative systematic review. BMJ 2000;321:267-272; and Caswell A, Harvey A, Bellantonio J (eds): eMIMS. Available at http://mims.hcn.net.au/

Key Points

1. Carbonic anhydrase is found in most tissues and contributes to a wide range of biological processes involving ion transfer across cellular membranes.
2. Its activity in the proximal renal tubule is especially important for acid-base physiology and can be impeded by various drugs.
3. The mild diuresis and metabolic acidosis induced by carbonic anhydrase inhibitors can be used to treat disorders in which such responses are beneficial, such as acute mountain sickness and serious metabolic alkalemia.
4. With the advent of more potent diuretic drugs that possess fewer metabolic side effects, the role of the carbonic anhydrase inhibitors as treatment for hypertension and edema is limited.
5. As topical agents for glaucoma, carbonic anhydrase inhibitors are very effective.

Key References

1. Lindskog S: Structure and mechanism of carbonic anhydrase. Pharmacol Ther 1997;74:1-20.
3. Warden CR, Burgess JL: Acetazolamide. In International Programme on Chemical Safety: Poison Information Monographs. Available at www.inchem.org/documents/pims/pharm/acetazol.htm/
7. Leaf DE, Goldfarb DS: Mechanisms of action of acetazolamide in the prophylaxis and treatment of acute mountain sickness. J Appl Physiol 2006;102:1313-1322.
11. Katayama F, Miura H, Takanashi S: Long-term effectiveness and side effects of acetazolamide as an adjunct to other anticonvulsants in the treatment of refractory epilepsies. Brain Dev 2002;24:150-154.
12. Alward WLM: Medical management of glaucoma. N Engl J Med 1998;339:1298-1307.

See the companion Expert Consult website for the complete reference list.

CHAPTER 108

Principles of Fluid Therapy

Ramesh Venkataraman and John A. Kellum

OBJECTIVES

This chapter will:
1. Describe the rationale for the use of different fluids in the intensive care unit.
2. Present various strategies used to monitor adequacy of volume repletion.

Fluid imbalance in the intensive care unit (ICU) can arise from hypovolemia, normovolemia with maldistribution of fluid, or hypervolemia. Hypovolemia is probably the most common. Hypovolemia occurring in the ICU can be abso-lute (intravascular volume loss) or relative (increased vascular capacitance). Some common causes of absolute hypovolemia are overt blood loss (trauma, gastrointestinal bleed), overt diuresis, and diarrhea. Increased capacitance of the vascular bed can occur in sepsis, adrenal insufficiency, and neurogenic shock, and from drugs. Furthermore, decreased intravascular volume can occur even if the patient has normal or increased total body water. In sepsis, for example, endothelial dysfunction is associated with increased capillary permeability,[1] leading to interstitial edema and decreased intravascular volume; in association with systemic vasodilatation, the decreased volume results in relative hypovolemia and shock. The extent of intravascular fluid depletion, the associated signs and symptoms, and the presence or absence of hemodynamic instability determine how fast the fluid deficit must be corrected. This chapter discusses the rationale for fluid therapy in the ICU, the choice of fluids, and the effective assessment of the adequacy of volume repletion.

CONSEQUENCES OF HYPOVOLEMIA

The main consequence of hypovolemia is reduction in effective circulating blood volume. Compensatory systemic release of catecholamines causes peripheral vasoconstriction, increased cardiac contractility, and tachycardia. Systemic blood pressure can remain normal during early phases of hypovolemia. However, as the hypovolemia worsens, these compensatory mechanisms are inadequate to maintain a normal blood pressure, and the patient becomes hypotensive. In general, blood pressure does not change as long as the volume loss is less than 20% of the total intravascular volume. Compensatory tachycardia can give rise to increased oxygen demand on the heart, leading to myocardial failure. Finally, reduced perfusion and increased catecholamines may produce acidosis and, together with myocardial dysfunction, precipitate multiple-organ failure.

Vital organs autoregulate their blood flow to some degree, although autoregulation for many organs (e.g., the kidney) is often lost in various disease states (e.g., sepsis). The human body tends to compensate for hypovolemia-induced hypoperfusion by redistributing blood flow to vital organs at the expense of the skin and adipose tissue. With more progressive shock, the splanchnic bed also becomes underperfused. Activation of the sympathetic, renin-angiotensin, and antidiuretic hormone systems helps maintain peripheral circulation.[2] However, in ICU patients, these regulatory mechanisms can become blunted from various causes (e.g., sepsis)[3] and are ineffective in maintaining adequate blood flow under hypovolemic conditions. Hence, the splanchnic organs are particularly susceptible to the deleterious effects of hypotension, and these effects, depending on their duration and severity, may be irreversible despite restoration of normovolemia by fluid administration. Gut mucosal ischemia occurs relatively early with hypovolemia and, if not corrected in a timely manner, can lead to mucosal necrosis. Mucosal ischemia impairs gut barrier function, which in turn allows translocation of bacteria and endotoxins into the systemic circulation. Similarly, organs such as the kidneys, brain, and myocardium depend to a large extent on perfusion pressure for adequate blood flow, and a drop in these pressures contributes to worsening organ function and multisystem organ failure. Therefore, rapid volume repletion is indicated in patients with severe hypovolemia or hypovolemic shock to minimize and possibly avert these potentially fatal consequences.

RATE OF VOLUME REPLETION

It is often not possible to precisely predict the total fluid deficit in a given patient with hypovolemic shock, particularly if fluid loss continues because of, for example, bleeding or third space sequestration. In general, at least 1 to 2 L of isotonic saline is given as rapidly as possible in an attempt to restore tissue perfusion. Subsequent fluid reple-

tion should continue at a similar rate as long as hypotension persists, and further monitoring should be performed to assess preload (e.g., measurement of central venous pressure), cardiac function (e.g., via pulmonary artery catheter or echocardiogram), blood pressure, and preload responsiveness (e.g., with fluid challenge or measurement of pulse-pressure variation). In addition to repletion of the initial volume loss in a patient with chronic volume losses, such as with high ileostomy output, a maintenance fluid regimen must be initiated to prevent worsening volume depletion. In general, a 1:1 replacement of the volume lost can be given every 4 to 6 hours with a solution similar in composition to the fluid that is being lost.

WHAT FLUID TO GIVE

The ideal fluid of choice for resuscitation is still debatable. Although several studies have focused on various volume replacement strategies, there is no persuasive evidence regarding the choice of fluid for volume replacement in critically ill patients. Most experts would agree, however, that in a patient who is hypovolemic, any fluid is better than none, and timely administration of "adequate" volume is more important than the specific type of fluid given. However, the following issues must be considered in the choice of a fluid for resuscitation.

Colloids versus Crystalloids

Colloids and crystalloids are addressed in detail in Chapter 109. However, some basic considerations must be made before a colloid or a crystalloid is chosen, as follows:
1. A larger volume of fluid is required when a crystalloid is used than when a colloid is used for intravascular volume repletion. The larger volume obviously may not be desirable in patients with impaired renal or cardiac function.
2. Colloid resuscitation can theoretically restore intravascular volume status faster than crystalloid resuscitation.
3. Patient characteristics must be taken into account; for example, patients with liver failure and spontaneous bacterial peritonitis might benefit from albumin administration.
4. Although this issue is controversial, some studies have shown increased risk of acute renal failure with the use of colloids, specifically certain preparations of hydroxyethyl starch.
5. Crystalloid solutions are significantly cheaper than colloid solutions.

A meta-analysis of 24 studies (1419 patients) published by the Cochrane Injuries Group Albumin Reviewers[4] concluded that the administration of albumin-containing fluids resulted in higher risk of death than the administration of crystalloid solutions. However, a second meta-analysis did not find evidence for harm; neither did it find better outcomes with albumin.[5] A later multicenter, randomized controlled study of nearly 7000 patients (Saline versus Albumin Fluid Evaluation [SAFE] study) did not find any differences between 4% albumin in saline and 0.9% saline in terms of 28-day mortality, ICU length of stay, hospital length of stay, days of mechanical ventilation, or days of renal replacement therapy.[6]

On the basis of these studies, the choice of colloid versus crystalloid should be made according to specific patient characteristics. There is currently no evidence to suggest that one type of solution is always superior to the other.

Crystalloid Solutions

Crystalloids are freely permeable across the vascular membrane and hence are distributed into plasma and the interstitial fluid. Owing to their limited volume-stabilizing effect,[7] repeated boluses of crystalloids are often necessary in the unstable ICU patient. The two solutions commonly used for resuscitation are 0.9% saline and lactated Ringer's solution. The 0.9% saline solution is isotonic and is very effective in improving intravascular volume status. However, using large volumes of 0.9% saline leads to hyperchloremic acidosis, which can then contribute to worsening of hypotension and inflammatory load in patients with sepsis.[8] No clinical studies have so far shown that one crystalloid solution is superior to another for resuscitation in a patient with shock.

Hypertonic Saline

Data from animals have shown that small-volume hypertonic saline is as effective as large-volume crystalloids in expanding plasma volume and improving cardiac output.[9] Other theoretical advantages of hypertonic saline resuscitation are decreased swelling of endothelium and red blood cells and better microcirculatory perfusion. In addition, the resuscitative effectiveness of hypertonic saline was found to be enhanced when it was combined with dextran.[10] Although several animal studies and small clinical studies have been performed over the past two decades, no large clinical trial has compared hypertonic saline with 0.9% saline and/or lactated Ringer's solution. In one meta-analysis, subgroup analysis revealed that the use of hypertonic saline dextran benefited most of the patients with closed-head injury and shock who received it.[11] Therefore, despite several theoretical advantages of hypertonic saline for resuscitation, especially in the trauma setting, no definite data exist to recommend its routine use.

ASSESSMENT OF VOLUME REPLETION

Traditional parameters used to estimate intravascular volume status have important limitations. Clinical parameters such as heart rate, blood pressure, capillary refill, and urine output are all very insensitive markers of hypovolemia. They may not be altered until hypovolemia is very severe and are often affected by factors other than intravascular volume status. Importantly, in the ICU setting, peripheral edema is often due to hypoalbuminemia and should not be used as a marker for adequate fluid resuscitation or fluid overload. Similarly, biochemical parameters such as fractional excretion of sodium and blood urea nitrogen–to-creatinine ratio are very nonspecific and can be affected by factors other than intravascular volume status. Finally, it is also important to understand that monitoring intravascular volume status alone may not be helpful, because size of the intravascular space, cardiac function, and mean perfusion pressure also determine adequacy of organ or tissue perfusion.

In general, if the patient remains hypotensive after the initial fluid bolus, attempts to accurately evaluate intravascular volume should be undertaken. Placement of a central venous catheter should be considered for monitoring of preload. A low central venous pressure value in a hypotensive patient strongly suggests hypovolemia. However, a normal or a high central venous pressure value in a hypotensive patient does not guarantee adequate preload. It is also important to remember that the relationship between filling pressures and ventricular end-diastolic volume can be obscured by changes in ventricular compliance. A bedside transthoracic echocardiogram gives a good estimate of ventricular filling and function and may be used to guide fluid resuscitation.

Once resuscitation has been initiated, adequate volume replacement must be recognized. One useful measure in this regard is preload responsiveness—the increase in stroke volume related to the increase in preload. In other words, the absence of preload responsiveness suggests that further fluid administration will not result in increases in stroke volume (hence cardiac output and blood pressure). Determining preload responsiveness therefore helps guide the decision to terminate fluid administration and initiate or continue assessment and management of cardiac contractility. Preload responsiveness can be predicted from the presence of respiratory variations in systolic pressure, pulse pressure, or aortic flow velocity in mechanically ventilated patients.[12,13] Currently, various commercially available devices (e.g., LiDCO Cardiac Sensor System, LiDCO, Cambridge, United Kingdom) accurately measure pulse pressure variation, and other measures of preload responsiveness (aortic flow velocity, USCOM Ultrasonic Cardiac Output Monitor, USCOM, Sydney, Australia) are emerging as useful tools to guide resuscitation. Of course, the "tried and true" fluid challenge may also be used, with the disadvantage that it shows only after the fact whether the patient is fluid responsive. Given that the volume of fluid used is small (e.g., 250-500 mL), however, it is usually not a significant problem.

The ultimate goal of resuscitation is to improve organ perfusion. Hence, it is important to monitor organ perfusion in some way. Unfortunately, markers such as serum lactate, pH, and base excess are insensitive and nonspecific. The existing measures of regional perfusion, such as gastric tonometry, although more sensitive in detecting early hypovolemia,[14] may be overly sensitive, and specific guidelines for their use in clinical practice are absent. Studies evaluating other measures of regional perfusion, such as sublingual tonometry, are currently under investigation but are not routinely used in the clinical setting. Mixed venous oxygen saturation ($S\bar{v}O_2$) under conditions of relatively stable oxygen comsumption is a good surrogate for global oxygen delivery and cardiac output. In a single-center randomized controlled study, 263 patients with severe sepsis or septic shock were randomly assigned in the emergency department to receive either 6 hours of early goal-directed therapy (EGDT) or standard therapy (as a control) before admission to the ICU.[15] The patients assigned to EGDT received a central venous catheter capable of measuring central venous oxygen saturation continuously. An $S\bar{v}O_2$ value higher than 70% was targeted in the EGDT group, with the use of a standardized protocol. Intravenous fluids, packed red blood cells, and/or inotropic support was initiated on the basis of the protocol to achieve and maintain the $S\bar{v}O_2$ target during the first 6 hours. The investigators reported that in-hospital mortality was 30.5% in the group assigned to EGDT, compared with 46.5% in the standard therapy group ($P = .009$).

Because this study was conducted in a single center and the mortality rate in the control group was unexpectedly high, further study of this approach is needed.

On the basis of the preceding studies, early repletion of volume is more important than the actual type of fluid used. Efforts must be undertaken to constantly monitor adequacy of resuscitation with a multitude of measures. No one clinical, laboratory, or technological measure adequately estimates adequacy of volume repletion.

CONCLUSION

Early aggressive volume repletion should be undertaken with an isotonic fluid in critically ill patients with hypovolemia. Intravenous hydration is clearly superior to oral hydration. If hypotension is not corrected by initial intravenous hydration, aggressive monitoring of preload, cardiac function, preload responsiveness, and, possibly, global oxygen delivery should be undertaken to accurately and rapidly improve organ perfusion. There is currently no evidence that the choice of fluid affects clinical outcomes. However, to avoid undesired effects of a particular fluid (e.g., saline-induced acidosis), a strategy of using different kinds of isotonic fluids (e.g., 0.9% saline, albumin, lactated Ringer's solution) for resuscitation in a given patient may be advisable. The endpoint for resuscitation should be establishment of organ and tissue perfusion, which should be assessed via a combination of clinical, laboratory, and hemodynamic measures.

Key Points

1. Early intravenous volume repletion should be performed in hypovolemic critically ill patients.
2. Isotonic fluids are preferred over hypotonic fluids.
3. Choice of fluid (colloid vs. crystalloid) does not affect clinical outcome.
4. The endpoint of resuscitation is the establishment of organ perfusion.
5. Multiple modes of monitoring for adequate volume repletion should be used to guide resuscitation.
6. Resuscitation strategy must be individualized according to patient need.

Key References

6. Finfer S, Bellomo R, Boyce N, et al: A comparison of albumin and saline for fluid resuscitation in the intensive care unit. N Engl J Med 2004;350:2247-2256.
13. Michard F, Teboul JL: Predicting fluid responsiveness in ICU patients: a critical analysis of the evidence. Chest 2002;121:2000-2008.
15. Rivers E, Nguyen B, Havstad S, et al: Early goal-directed therapy in the treatment of severe sepsis and septic shock. N Engl J Med 2001;345:1368-1377.

See the companion Expert Consult website for the complete reference list.

CHAPTER 109

Crystalloids and Colloids

Simon Finfer and Daryl A. Jones

OBJECTIVES

This chapter will:
1. Summarize the properties of crystalloid and colloid solutions.
2. Describe the evidence on clinician preferences for resuscitation fluids.
3. Discuss the evidence for the safety and efficacy of crystalloid and colloid solutions.

Administration of intravenous fluids to expand or maintain intravascular fluid volume is one of the commonest therapeutic interventions undertaken in the intensive care unit (ICU). Nevertheless, there is a long-running debate over the type of fluid that should be given to the critically ill.[1,2]

Fluids can be divided into two broad classes, crystalloids and colloids. A *crystalloid* is a solution of a substance that can pass through a semipermeable membrane and be crystallized; examples are the various concentrations of saline, glucose solutions that may also be combined with saline, and the balanced salt solutions. Crystalloid solutions may be isotonic or hypertonic; isotonic crystalloids are largely distributed into the extracellular space, so approximately one third of the administered volume remains in the intravascular space. In the medical context, a *colloid* is a fluid containing small, osmotically active particles in emulsion or in suspension that do not settle out. Colloids are designed to stay in the intravascular compartment; examples are human albumin solutions, starch solutions, dextrans, and gelatins. Properties of a selection of crystalloid and colloid solutions are summarized in Tables 109-1 and 109-2.[3]

CURRENT DATA ON CLINICIANS' PREFERENCES AND FLUIDS USED FOR RESUSCITATION

A number of surveys have been conducted to assess clinicians' preferences for fluids used for resuscitation in the ICU. In 1989, the Victorian Drug Advisory Committee

TABLE 109-1

Comparison of Contents, Osmolarity, and pH of Crystalloid Solutions for Intravenous Administration

SOLUTION	OSMOLARITY (mOsmol/L)	pH	Na⁺ (mm)	Cl⁻ (mm)	K⁺ (mm)	Ca²⁺ (mm)	GLUCOSE (mg/L)	HCO₃⁻ (mm)	LACTATE (mm)
Glucose 5%	252		—	—	—	—	50	—	—
Glucose 50%	2520		—	—	—	—	500	—	—
Sodium chloride 0.9%	300	5	154.0	154.0	—	—	—	—	—
Sodium chloride and glucose	262		30.0	30.0	—	—	40	—	—
Lactated Ringer's solution	309		147.0	156.0	4.0	2.2	—	—	—
Compound sodium lactate*	278		131.0	111.0	5.0	2.0	—	—	29.0
Plasmalyte B	298.5	5.5	140	98	5	—	—	50	—

*Hartmann's solution or lactated Ringer's solution.
Modified from Grocott MP, Hamilton MA: Resuscitation fluids. Vox Sang 2002;82:1-8.

TABLE 109-2

Comparison of Contents of Some Colloid Solutions for Intravenous Administration

SOLUTION	COLLOID	MOLECULAR WEIGHT (Da)	DEGREE OF SUBSTITUTION	Na⁺ (mmol/L)	Cl⁻ (mm)	K⁺ (mm)	Ca²⁺ (mm)	GLUCOSE (mg/L)
Albumex 4%	Human albumin	66,000	—	140	128	—	—	—
Albumex 20%	Human albumin	66,000	—	140	128	—	—	—
Gelofusin (4%)	Succinylated gelatin	30,000	—	150	150	—	—	—
Haemacel (3.5%)	Polygeline	30,000	—	145	145	5.1	6.25	—
EloHaes 6%	Hetastarch	60,000	—	150	150	—	—	—
HAES-steril 6% or 10%	Hetastarch	70,000	0.5	150	150	—	—	—
Hespan 6%	Hetastarch	70,000	0.7	150	150	—	—	—
Pentaspan 6% or 10%	Pentastarch	63,000	0.45	150	150	—	—	—
Gentran 40	Dextran 40	40,000	—	150	150	—	—	—
Gentran 40	Dextran 40	40,000	—	—	—	—	—	50
Gentran 70	Dextran 70	70,000	—	150	150	—	—	—
Gentran 70	Dextran 70	70,000	—	—	—	—	—	50
Macrodex	Dextran 70	70,000	—	150	150	—	—	—
Macrodex	Dextran 70	70,000	—	—	—	—	—	50

Modified from Grocott MP, Hamilton MA: Resuscitation fluids. Vox Sang 2002;82:1-8.

conducted a 3-month survey of albumin use in three teaching hospitals in Victoria, Australia.[4] The three most commonly reported indications for albumin administration were hypovolemia, hypoalbuminemia, and plasmapheresis. The patients most likely to receive albumin were those undergoing cardiac surgery, those in ICUs, and those undergoing hemodialysis.

In 1994, a 1-month inception cohort study to assess "the appropriateness of albumin use" was conducted in 15 centers in the United States.[5] Albumin was most commonly used in the ICU and operating room. In 76% of cases, albumin was administered for indications not in keeping with guidelines current at the time. Boldt and coworkers[6] surveyed 451 ICUs in Germany by means of a questionnaire.[6] Forty-three percent of respondents reported that they used exclusively colloids for volume resuscitation. Hydroxyethyl starch (HES) was the colloid most commonly used, and albumin-containing solutions were rarely used as a first choice. Albumin-based fluids were preferred primarily in patients with hypoalbuminemia.

In 2002, Miletin and colleagues[7] published the results of a survey of 364 clinicians from medical and surgical specialties in Ontario, Canada.[7] The majority (70%) of respondents reported using crystalloids for volume expansion more than 90% of the time. Albumin was the colloid most commonly used, followed by HES. Factors influencing the choice of colloid included the type of clinician's

practice, the practice location, and clinician exposure to a drug detailer in the previous 12 months. Albumin was most commonly administered to patients with burns or hypoalbuminemia. Two years later, Schortgen and associates[8] reported results of a survey of more than 2400 ICU doctors from the European and French intensive care societies.[8] The majority (65%) of clinicians reported using a mixture of crystalloids and colloids for volume resuscitation. The fluids most commonly used were isotonic crystalloids, HES, and gelatins.

In addition, Schortgen and colleagues conducted a 4-week inception cohort study of fluid resuscitation in 115 predominantly European ICUs. Of 687 patients whose status satisfied the definition of shock, 17% received crystalloid resuscitation alone, 67% a mixture of colloid and crystalloid fluids, 16% colloids alone, 48% starch, 38% gelatin, 28% plasma, 15% albumin, and 3% dextran (F. Schortgen, personal communication, 2007).

In an ongoing randomized controlled trial in Europe (The CRISTAL study), patients requiring fluid resuscitation for any indication are randomly assigned to receive crystalloid or colloid for all fluid resuscitation in the ICU.[9] The choice of colloid fluid in patients assigned to colloid resuscitation is left to the preference of the treating clinicians, although an individual patient may receive no more than 30 mL/kg of starch in 24 hours.[9] In the early stages of the study, 85% of patients assigned to colloid resuscitation had received starch, with only 3% receiving albumin (D. Annane, personal communication, 2006).

These studies indicate that there is wide variation in clinicians' preferences for resuscitation fluids, which translates into wide variation in the type of fluid administered to patients.

CURRENT EVIDENCE ON THE SAFETY AND EFFICACY OF RESUSCITATION FLUIDS

Colloid versus Crystalloid

Pending completion of the CRISTAL study,[9] there are no individual studies adequately powered to directly compare the safety and efficacy of colloids in general and those of crystalloids in general. In the absence of such trials, the best current evidence comes from meta-analyses of a number of heterogeneous trials, most of which recruited relatively few participants.[10-12] Velanovich,[10] reporting on a meta-analysis of eight trials involving a total of 826 patients, concluded that crystalloid should be preferred in trauma patients and colloid in non-trauma patients. However, the 95% confidence intervals (95% CIs) of the estimates of mortality difference associated with administration of fluid types assessed were wide in this study. In the studies enrolling trauma patients, the crystalloid administration was associated with a 12.3% reduction in risk of death; however, the 95% CI varied between a 20.8% reduction in mortality to a 4.6% increase. Similarly, in non-trauma patients, colloid administration was associated with a 7.8% reduction in mortality, with the 95% CI ranging between 19.0% and –3.4%).

Choi and colleagues[11] reported on a meta-analysis of 17 trials involving a total of 814 patients; they concluded that overall there was no apparent difference between isotonic crystalloid and colloid but that the power of the aggregated data was insufficient to exclude small but important differences in outcome. Like Velanovich, Choi and colleagues[11] noted an effect favoring crystalloid in trauma patients. In 1998, Schierhout and Roberts[13] published a meta-analysis on behalf of the Cochrane Collaboration. In 26 trials with 1662 participants in which colloid resuscitation was compared with isotonic crystalloid, these investigators found that resuscitation with colloids was associated with an increased absolute risk of mortality of 4% (95% CI, 0% to 8%). In contrast with the Velanovich and Choi studies, Schierhout and Roberts[13] found no evidence for differences in effect in trauma patients.

In 2004, The Cochrane Collaboration published an updated meta-analysis using the data from the Saline versus Albumin Fluid Evaluation (SAFE study) (see later).[12,14] The researchers reported the results by colloid type: 19 trials reported data on mortality for trials of albumin or plasma protein fraction; the relative risk of death (RR) versus crystalloids was 1.02 (95% CI, 0.93 to 1.11), on the basis of data from 7576 participants and 1547 deaths, of which data for 6933 participants (91.5%) and 1455 (94.1%) deaths were from the SAFE Study. Ten trials involving 374 participants compared HES with crystalloids; the pooled RR was 1.16 (95% CI, 0.68 to 1.96). Seven trials involving 346 participants compared modified gelatin with crystalloid, the pooled RR being 0.54 (95% CI, 0.16 to 1.85). Nine trials involving 834 participants compared dextran with a crystalloid; the pooled RR was 1.24 (95% CI, 0.94 to 1.65). The results illustrate that with the exception of the SAFE study, there are few reliable data to guide clinicians' choice of resuscitation fluids (Fig. 109-1).

The Safety of Albumin

In July 1998, the Cochrane Injuries Group Albumin Reviewers published a meta-analysis of 24 studies involving 1419 patients resuscitated with either albumin or crystalloid for the treatment of hypovolemia, hypoalbuminemia or burns.[15] These investigators reported that the administration of albumin-containing fluids resulted in a 6% increase in the absolute risk of death compared with administration of crystalloid solutions. A subsequent meta-analysis in a broader patient population, covering 55 trials and 3504 patients, did not find an increased risk of death with albumin-containing fluids; the pooled RR for albumin versus crystalloids was 1.11 (95% CI, 0.95 to

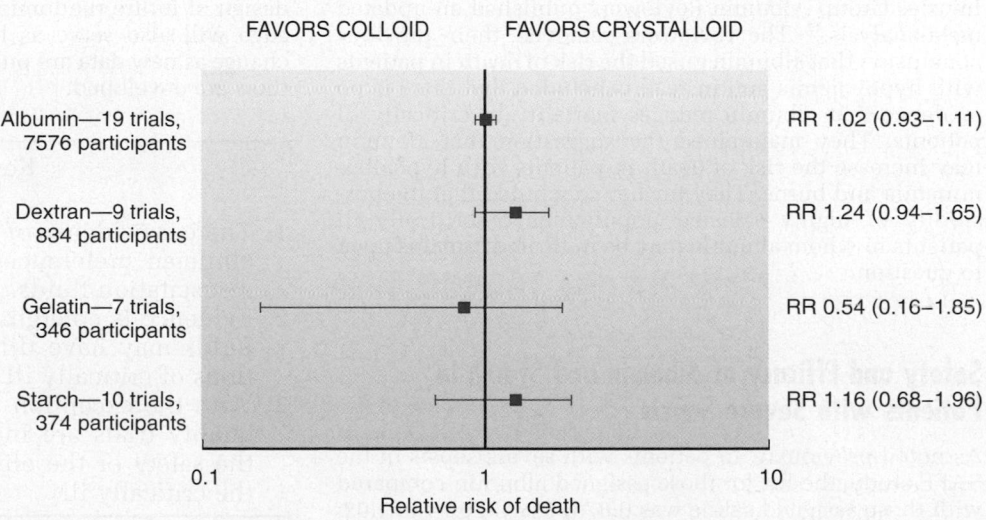

FAVORS COLLOID   FAVORS CRYSTALLOID

Albumin—19 trials, 7576 participants — RR 1.02 (0.93–1.11)

Dextran—9 trials, 834 participants — RR 1.24 (0.94–1.65)

Gelatin—7 trials, 346 participants — RR 0.54 (0.16–1.85)

Starch—10 trials, 374 participants — RR 1.16 (0.68–1.96)

Relative risk of death

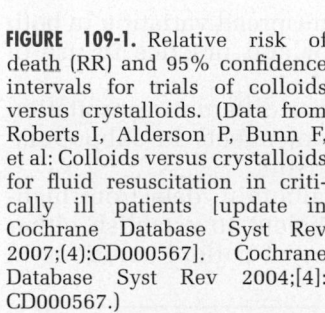

FIGURE 109-1. Relative risk of death (RR) and 95% confidence intervals for trials of colloids versus crystalloids. (Data from Roberts I, Alderson P, Bunn F, et al: Colloids versus crystalloids for fluid resuscitation in critically ill patients [update in Cochrane Database Syst Rev 2007;(4):CD000567]. Cochrane Database Syst Rev 2004;[4]: CD000567.)

574 Section 6 / Fluid and Electrolyte Problems

1.28).[16] The conflicting results of such meta-analyses left many clinicians unsure about the effect of albumin-containing fluids on the survival of critically ill patients.

To address this uncertainty, the Australian and New Zealand Intensive Care Society Clinical Trials Group (ANZICS CTG), in collaboration with the Australian Red Cross Blood Service (ARCBS) and The George Institute for International Health, conducted the SAFE study in 16 ICUs in Australia and New Zealand.[14] The study enrolled 6997 participants and to date is the only adequately powered trial on fluid resuscitation published. The investigators reported that there were 726 deaths in the patients assigned to receive albumin and 729 in patients assigned to receive saline; the RR for those assigned albumin compared with saline was 0.99 (95% CI, 0.91 to 1.09; P = .87).

In addition to similar overall mortality rates, the SAFE study investigators reported that patients receiving saline and albumin had similar incidences of new organ failures, similar lengths of stay in ICU and hospital, and similar duration of mechanical ventilation and renal replacement therapy. There were no conclusive differences in the predefined subgroups; in patients with severe sepsis, the RR for albumin administration compared with saline administration was 0.87 (95% CI, 0.74 to 1.02; P = .09), and in patients with trauma, the RR was 1.36 (95% CI, 0.99 to 1.86; P = .06).

In patients with trauma and brain injury in the SAFE study, the RR for those assigned albumin compared with those assigned saline was 1.62 (95% CI, 1.12 to 2.34; P = .009). This cohort has been the subject of a long-term follow-up study. Although the results have not yet been published, they have been presented at scientific meetings and are now in the public domain. The follow-up study demonstrated that patients with trauma and brain injury who were resuscitated with albumin had a significantly higher mortality rate that persisted to 2 years after study randomization; the difference was not due to imbalance in prognostic factors at baseline, and the functional neurological outcome of survivors was the same (i.e., the additional survivors in the saline group were not profoundly disabled). The mechanism for the difference in mortality is as yet unknown, but unless contradictory evidence is forthcoming, it seems prudent to avoid albumin during the acute injury phase in patients with traumatic brain injury (SAFE Study Investigators, personal communication, 2007).

After publication of the SAFE study, the Cochrane Injuries Group Albumin Reviewers published an updated meta-analysis.[17] The reviewers removed their previous conclusion that albumin raised the risk of death in patients with hypovolemia and instead concluded that there is no evidence that albumin reduces mortality in critically ill patients. They maintained the suggestion that albumin may increase the risk of death in patients with hypoalbuminemia and burns. They further concluded that the possibility of highly selected populations of critically ill patients in whom albumin may be indicated remains open to question.

Safety and Efficacy of Albumin and Starch in Patients with Severe Sepsis

As noted previously, in patients with severe sepsis in the SAFE study, the RR for those assigned albumin compared with those assigned saline was 0.87 (95% CI, 0.74 to 1.02;

P = .09). In the comparison of the RR for albumin versus saline in those with severe sepsis and those without severe sepsis, the test for a common relative risk yielded a P value of 0.06, suggesting that the treatment effect in patients with severe sepsis might be different from that in the overall population.

Support for the suggestion that albumin might have a beneficial effect in patients with severe sepsis comes from studies in children with severe falciparum malaria.[18,19] In two pilot studies, Maitland and colleagues[19] demonstrated a significantly lower mortality for children resuscitated with albumin than in those resuscitated with saline. Comparison of albumin with a Gelofusine (succinylated modified fluid gelatin 4% intravenous infusion) showed similar reductions in mortality for children resuscitated with albumin, suggesting a specific effect of albumin rather than a generic effect due to better volume expansion when a colloid was used.[18] These results are by no means definitive, and a larger phase III study is now planned. In addition, albumin may have a beneficial effect on renal function in patients with cirrhosis and spontaneous bacterial peritonitis.[20]

In contrast, however, two studies have suggested that HES may be harmful in patients with severe sepsis. Schortgen and colleagues[21] published the results of a prospective, randomized controlled trial comparing gelatins and HES in 129 patients with severe sepsis or septic shock. Patients who received HES had significantly higher risks for acute renal failure (42% vs. 23%; P = .028), oliguria (56% vs. 37%; P = .025) and peak creatinine value (225 vs. 169 µmol/L; P = .04) than patients who received gelatins.[21] In a later study, Reinhart and associates[22] reported on a randomized controlled trial of HES and lactated Ringer's solution in patients with severe sepsis or septic shock; use of HES resulted in a higher risk of acute renal failure and greater requirement for renal replacement therapy.[22]

CONCLUSION

There is evidence of widespread practice variation in the prescription of resuscitation fluids. New data suggest that specific fluids may have beneficial or harmful effects in specific subpopulations of critically ill patients. A more detailed knowledge of current fluid use and the factors that influence choice of resuscitation fluids will assist the design of future randomized controlled trials; the knowledge will also serve as baseline data to study practice change as new data are published and international guidelines are developed.

Key Points

1. There is evidence of widespread variation in both clinician preferences for and practice in use of resuscitation fluids.
2. Evidence is emerging that different resuscitation fluids may have different effects in subpopulations of critically ill patients.
3. With the exception of albumin, data from high-quality trials are insufficient to establish either the safety or the efficacy of colloid solutions in the critically ill.

Key References

11. Choi PT, Yip G, Quinonez LG, Cook DJ: Crystalloids vs. colloids in fluid resuscitation: A systematic review. Crit Care Med 1999;27:200-210.
12. Roberts I, Alderson P, Bunn F, et al: Colloids versus crystalloids for fluid resuscitation in critically ill patients [update in Cochrane Database Syst Rev 2007;(4):CD000567]. Cochrane Database Syst Rev 2004;(4):CD000567.
14. Finfer S, Bellomo R, Boyce N, et al; SAFE Study Investigators: A comparison of albumin and saline for fluid resuscitation in the intensive care unit. N Engl J Med 2004;350:2247-2256.

17. Alderson P, Bunn F, Lefebvre C, et al; Albumin Reviewers: Human albumin solution for resuscitation and volume expansion in critically ill patients. Cochrane Database Syst Rev 2004;(4):CD001208.
21. Schortgen F, Lacherade JC, Bruneel F, et al: Effects of hydroxyethylstarch and gelatin on renal function in severe sepsis: A multicentre randomised study. Lancet 2001;357:911-916.

See the companion Expert Consult website for the complete reference list.

CHAPTER 110

Blood and Blood Products

Craig French

OBJECTIVES

This chapter will:
1. Outline the principles of blood component therapy in the patient with acute bleeding.
2. Provide an overview of indications for the elective administration of allogeneic red blood cells, platelets, fresh-frozen plasma, and cryoprecipitate in critically ill patients.
3. Discuss the use of this information in the clinical setting.

In the last decade, clinical research has improved the understanding of the epidemiology and pathophysiology of the anemia of critical illness and of the use of blood transfusion in critically ill patients.[1-5] On the basis of this research, many jurisdictions have developed guidelines for the use of red blood cells (RBCs).[6-12] Guidelines for the administration of other blood components, including platelets and plasma, have also been developed.[9,10,13-17] The evidence base for guidelines other than RBCs, both within and outside the critical care environment, is frequently limited to expert opinion. This chapter provides an overview of current guidelines and recommendations for the transfusion of RBCs, platelets, fresh-frozen plasma (FFP), and cryoprecipitate to both acutely bleeding and nonbleeding critically ill adult patients. An overarching principle is that blood component therapy should be given only when the expected benefits to the patient are likely to outweigh the potential hazards. The recommendations made in this chapter attempt to achieve this balance.

MASSIVE TRANSFUSION AND ACUTE BLOOD LOSS

Massive transfusion is most commonly defined as the transfusion of 10 or more units of RBCs in less than 24 hours. A 2006 review of massive transfusion practices demonstrated that few institutions have protocols.[18] The researchers of this study summarize results of the literature on massive transfusion, in addition to the importance of controlling the source of bleeding, as follows: (1) coagulopathy is common, (2) once present, coagulopathy is difficult to correct, (3) early and intensive therapy with plasma and platelets appears to be associated with better outcomes, and (4) keeping plasma coagulation factor activity at 40% or more of normal and platelet counts in the range of 50 to 100×10^9/L usually provides adequate coagulation.[18] The prevention and treatment of hypothermia, acidosis, and organ dysfunction are also crucial in obtaining hemostasis. Most data have been derived from, and guidelines developed for, trauma patients with acute blood loss. Massive nontraumatic bleeding is also managed in the critical care environment; in the absence of any specific guidelines for patients with this condition, it is reasonable to utilize those developed for trauma resuscitation.

The only "national" guideline for acute blood loss was developed by the United Kingdom National Blood Service and published in 2000.[19] Importantly, the authors of this guideline stress that successful patient outcomes require not only the restoration of blood volume and hemostasis but also effective and rapid communication lines among clinicians, laboratory staff, and central blood banks. Hospital transfusion committees can develop these processes within institutions. The UK template guideline is shown in Table 110-1. It is similar to that of other published guidelines.[20,21] In the resuscitation phase, group O Rh-negative blood or non–cross-matched, group-specific blood is administered. A target hemoglobin concentration of between 70 and 100 g/L is recommended. Even in hospitals with efficient systems, this type of therapy may continue for 30 to 45 minutes—the minimum time required to type blood and prepare and issue compatible plasma products and platelets.[22] In recognition of this need, the early use of blood component therapy during initial resuscitation, prior to the availability of laboratory results, is advocated because the plasma of the most severely injured and rapidly bleeding patients will have been diluted[16]; recommendations are as follows:
- Administration of platelets when the estimated blood loss is approximately two or more blood volumes, at

TABLE 110-1

Template Guideline for Treatment of Acute Massive Blood Loss

GOAL	PROCEDURE	COMMENTS
Restore circulating volume	Insert wide-bore peripheral cannulas	14G cannulas or larger
	Give adequate volumes of warmed crystalloid, ?colloid, blood	Monitor central venous pressure
		Blood loss is often underestimated
	Aim to maintain blood pressure at normal level and urine output >30 mL/hr^{-1}	Refer to Advanced Trauma Life Support guidelines
		Keep patient warm
Contact key personnel	Clinician in charge	Nominated coordinator should take responsibility for communication and documentation
	Duty anesthetist	
	Blood bank	
	Duty hematologist	
Arrest bleeding	Early surgical or obstetric intervention	
	Interventional radiology	
Request laboratory investigations	CBC	Take samples at earliest opportunity because results may be affected by colloid infusion
	PT	
	aPTT	
	Fibrinogen measurement	
	Blood-bank sample	
	Biochemical profile	
	Blood gas analysis or pulse oximetry	
	Ensure correct sample identity	Misidentification is most common transfusion risk
	Repeat CBC, PT, aPTT, and fibrinogen measurement every 4 hrs or after $\frac{1}{3}$ of blood volume replaced	Components may have to be given before results are available
	Repeat tests after blood component infusion	

Request suitable red blood cells	Non–cross-matched, group O, Rh-negative blood:
	    In extreme emergency
	    No more than 2 units
		Rh-positive blood is acceptable if patient is male or a postmenopausal female

	Non–cross-matched blood specific for ABO group: When blood group known	Laboratory will complete cross-match after issue

	Fully cross-matched blood:
	    If irregular antibodies present
	    When time permits
		Further cross-match not required after replacement of 1 blood volume (8-10 units)

	Use blood warmer and/or rapid infusion device	Blood warmer indicated if flow rate >50 mL/kg/hr in adult
	Employ blood salvage if available and appropriate	Salvage contraindicated if wound is heavily contaminated
Request platelets	Allow for delivery time from blood center	Target platelet count:
	Anticipate platelet count <50 × 10^9/L after 2 × blood volume replacement	>100 × 10^9/L for multiple/central nervous system trauma or if platelet function abnormal
		>50 × 10^9/L for other situations
Request FFP (12-15 mL per kg body weight = 1 L or 4 units for an adult)	Aim for PT and aPTT < 1.5 × control mean	PT and aPTT values >1.5 × control means correlate with increased surgical bleeding
	Allow for 30-min thawing time	
Request cryoprecipitate (1-1.5 packs per 10 kg body weight)	Replace fibrinogen and factor VIII	Fibrinogen level <0.5 g/L strongly associated with microvascular bleeding
	Aim for fibrinogen >1.0 g/L Allow for delivery time plus 30-min thawing time	Fibrinogen deficiency develops early when plasma-poor red blood cells are used for replacement
Suspect DIC	Treat underlying cause if possible	Shock, hypothermia, acidosis leading to risk of DIC
		Mortality from DIC is high

aPTT, activated partial thromboplastin time; CBC, complete blood count; DIC, disseminated intravascular coagulation; FFP, fresh-frozen plasma; PT, prothrombin time.
Modified from Stainsby D, MacLennan S, Hamilton PJ: Management of massive blood loss: A template guideline. Brit J Anaesth 2000;85:487-491.

which point the measured platelet count is likely to be less than 50 × 10^9/L.
- Administration of FFP, 12 to 15 mL/kg or roughly 4 units for an adult, after transfusion of 6 to 8 units of RBCs, at which point the prothrombin time (PT) and activated partial thromboplastin time (aPTT) are likely to be greater than 1.5 × control values).

- Administration of cryoprecipitate, 1 to 1.5 units per 10 kg of body weight, if the fibrinogen level is less than 1 g/L.

Guidelines for patients with ongoing bleeding who have already received the preceding blood component therapy have been published.[18] In this group of patients, who in one series represent less than 2% of all trauma patients,

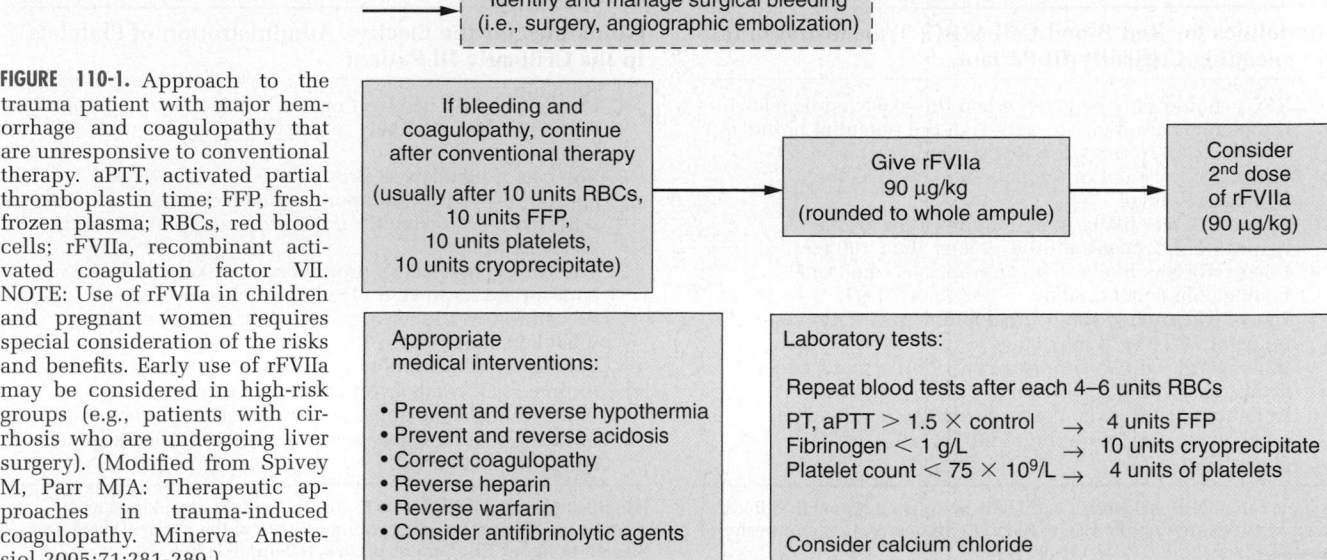

FIGURE 110-1. Approach to the trauma patient with major hemorrhage and coagulopathy that are unresponsive to conventional therapy. aPTT, activated partial thromboplastin time; FFP, fresh-frozen plasma; RBCs, red blood cells; rFVIIa, recombinant activated coagulation factor VII. NOTE: Use of rFVIIa in children and pregnant women requires special consideration of the risks and benefits. Early use of rFVIIa may be considered in high-risk groups (e.g., patients with cirrhosis who are undergoing liver surgery). (Modified from Spivey M, Parr MJA: Therapeutic approaches in trauma-induced coagulopathy. Minerva Anestesiol 2005;71:281-289.)

the consensus view is that RBCs, platelets, and plasma are administered in a 1:1:1 ratio. This ratio probably represents the limits of what can be achieved in patients with uncontrolled hemorrhage who are receiving massive transfusion; otherwise, the administration of one component may occur at the expense of another. Apheresis platelets and pooled platelets are equivalent to 6 to 11 units of conventional platelets. When the former are administered, the ratio of RBCs to apheresis or pooled platelets to plasma is 10:1:10.

Two protocols also advocate the use of recombinant activated coagulation factor VII (rFVIIa) in massive transfusion.[20,21] The role of rFVIIa in the management of hemorrhage has not been fully established. In their protocol, Spivey and Parr[21] advocate the use of rFVIIa if bleeding and coagulopathy continue after a minimum of 10 units of RBCs have been administered, early use of other blood components has been performed, and surgical bleeding has been identified and managed (Fig. 110-1). Numerous case reports demonstrate an association between the administration of rFVIIa and hemostasis; however, in the absence of data from well-designed clinical trials, the administration of this agent should be restricted to situations in which conventional management has been ineffective.

ELECTIVE TRANSFUSION OF BLOOD COMPONENTS IN THE CRITICALLY ILL

Allogeneic Red Blood Cell Transfusion

Anemia is common in critically ill patients, and between 20% and 53% of such patients receive RBC transfusion.[1,2,4,5] Many such transfusions are administered electively rather than for acute bleeding, with the aim of improving oxygen delivery and reducing or limiting tissue damage secondary to hypoxia. At extremely low hemoglobin concentrations (<50 g/L), it is clear that allogeneic RBC transfusions can be lifesaving: Prospective randomized controlled studies of transfusion in patients with such hemoglobin concentrations would be unethical and are not required. Unfor-

tunately compelling research demonstrating the benefits of transfusion at moderate levels of anemia (hemoglobin 70-90 g/L) is lacking. In addition, in the last decade, the risks associated with transfusion, including infectious disease transmission, transfusion-related immunomodulation, transfusion-related acute lung injury, and procedural errors, have been increasingly reported. These risks together with a reducing donor pool have forced clinicians to reevaluate traditional indications for RBC transfusion.

Two 1999 studies have influenced the recommendations for RBC transfusion in the critically ill[3,23] and heavily affected meta-analyses of transfusion triggers.[24,25] In a single-center prospective study involving 428 patients undergoing cardiac surgery, Bracey and colleagues[23] compared two transfusion triggers, hemoglobin concentrations of 80 g/L and 90 g/L. The researchers demonstrated no difference in morbidity or mortality between the two triggers. In a larger, multicenter study, Hebert and associates[3] compared a restrictive transfusion strategy (hemoglobin concentration maintained at 70-90 g/L) with a liberal one (hemoglobin concentration maintained at 100-120 g/L). There was no difference between groups in the primary outcome measure, 28-day all-cause mortality. The restrictive strategy group had lower hospital mortality (22% vs. 28%; P = .05) and two post hoc subgroups, those with Acute Physiology and Chronic Health Evaluation II (APACHE II) scores of less than 20 and those younger than 55 years. The researchers concluded that in a heterogeneous population of critically ill patients, a restrictive transfusion strategy is safe and efficacious. These data, together with those from prospective cohort studies that suggest greater mortality in critically patients who receive an RBC transfusion,[1,5] have led to the widespread adoption of a restrictive transfusion strategy in critical care medicine. The implementation of restrictive transfusion practice in patients with acute coronary syndromes, however, remains controversial because of conflicting evidence; a hemoglobin concentration of 100 g/L has been recommended as the level for transfusion in this patient group.[26]

Table 110-2 outlines guidelines for RBC transfusion in nonbleeding critically ill patients. These have been adapted from those published by the Australian National Health

TABLE 110-2

Guidelines for Red Blood Cell (RBC) Transfusion in the Nonbleeding Critically Ill Patient

1. RBCs should only be given when the expected benefits to the patients are likely to outweigh the potential hazards.
2. The decision to transfuse RBCs should be based on clinical assessment of the patient as well as the hemoglobin level.
3. Use of RBCs is likely to be inappropriate when hemoglobin concentration is greater than 100 g/L.
4. Use of RBCs is likely to be appropriate when the hemoglobin concentration is less than 70 g/L.
5. Use of RBCs when the hemoglobin concentration is in the range of 70-100 g/L may be appropriate. The decision to transfuse should be supported by clinical signs and symptoms.
6. In patients with acute coronary syndromes, a target hemoglobin concentration of 90-100 g/L may be appropriate.

Adapted from National Health and Medical Research Council: Clinical Practice Guidelines on the Use of Blood Components. Commonwealth of Australia, 2002 (ISBN Print:1864961449).

TABLE 110-3

Guidelines for the Elective Administration of Platelets in the Critically Ill Patient

1. Platelets should be given only when the expected benefits to the patients are likely to outweigh the potential hazards.
2. The use of platelets as prophylaxis is likely to be appropriate to prevent spontaneous bleeding in the setting of very severe thrombocytopenia (platelet count $<20 \times 10^9$/L).
3. The use of platelets as prophylaxis is likely to be appropriate to prevent bleeding prior to invasive procedures in the setting of severe thrombocytopenia (platelet count $<50 \times 10^9$/L).
4. Platelet transfusion is not indicated for the treatment of thrombotic thrombocytopenic purpura and heparin-induced thrombocytopenia or to prevent spontaneous bleeding in moderately severe thrombocytopenia (platelet count $10\text{-}50 \times 10^9$/L).

Modified from Gajic O, Dzik WH, Toy P: Fresh frozen plasma and platelet transfusion for nonbleeding patients in the intensive care unit: Benefit or harm? Crit Care Med 2006;34(Suppl):S170-S173.

and Medical Research Council.[9] The general principles are consistent with those published in other jurisdictions.[11,12] The decision to administer a transfusion to an individual patient is complex and depends on the patient's ability to tolerate an existing hemoglobin concentration, the likelihood of any further reduction in hemoglobin concentration, and the patient's reserve before perceived or actual tissue hypoxia. The published guidelines and recommendations provide general statements designed to help clinicians determine whether the benefits of RBC transfusion outweigh the risks. The 70 g/L hemoglobin concentration trigger has been challenged.[27] It is postulated that many of the immunomodulatory effects of RBC transfusion are related to the age and presence of leukocytes in RBCs. The worse outcomes demonstrated in epidemiological studies of RBC transfusion may be eliminated or reduced by the administration of fresh, leukocyte-depleted blood. In most jurisdictions, the availability of such a product is not assured. Therefore, for the majority of critically ill patients, a transfusion threshold of 70 g/L is indicated until the results of further research become available.

Elective Platelet Transfusion

Platelets are presented as either single units, apheresis units, or pooled units.[28] One whole blood–derived platelet unit contains at least 5.5×10^{10} platelets. It is generally believed that this content will raise the platelet count in a patient without antibodies by about 10,000 per μL. A unit of apheresis platelets contains approximately 2.4×10^{11} platelets derived from a single donor. A unit of pooled platelets contains at least 2.4×10^{11} platelets and is derived from approximately five donors.

Few data exist to determine the indications for platelet transfusion to the nonbleeding critically ill patient. There is also a lack of data regarding the incidence of thrombocytopenia or the use of platelet transfusion in this population.[4,29] Elective administration of platelets when the level of thrombocytopenia is high significantly increases the risk of spontaneous hemorrhage or prior to an invasive procedure. The critically ill patient may also demonstrate platelet dysfunction owing to uremia and/or antiplatelet drugs; transfusion with apparently "normal" platelet numbers may be indicated in such a patient, particularly

before an invasive procedure. Guidelines have been developed for transfusion in oncology patients.[30] The etiology of thrombocytopenia in the critically ill is multifactorial, involving both immune and non-immune mechanisms. How applicable these mechanisms are to the critically ill is unclear. Suggested guidelines for elective platelet transfusion in the critically ill are presented in Table 110-3. Data from oncology trials recommend the elective administration of platelets to prevent spontaneous bleeding at a platelet count less than 10×10^9/L.[30] Most intensive care patients have additional risk factors for spontaneous bleeding, such as sepsis and concomitant drug therapy. This patient group has not been included in trials evaluating platelet transfusion to prevent spontaneous bleeding in moderately severe thrombocytopenia ($10\text{-}50 \times 10^9$/L). Thus, guidelines in the critically ill are based on expert opinion combined with extrapolation of data from other clinical environments. The elective administration of platelets to prevent spontaneous bleeding in critically ill patients is therefore generally recommended when the platelet count is less than 20×10^9/L and is "not indicated" for a higher platelet count.

There are also few data to support platelet transfusion prior to an invasive procedure, and none from randomized controlled trials. The British Committee for Standards in Haematology's Blood Transfusion Task Force recommends that the platelet count be raised to at least 50×10^9/L prior to "lumbar puncture, epidural anaesthesia, gastroscopy and biopsy, insertion of indwelling lines, transbronchial biopsy, liver biopsy, laparotomy or similar procedures."[13] This policy is consistent with other published guidelines.[9,20] For all invasive intensive care procedures, a platelet count higher than 50×10^9/L is indicated.

Fresh-Frozen Plasma and Cryoprecipitate

Table 110-4 provides an overview of the indications for FFP and cryoprecipitate in the critically ill. FFP is separated and frozen within 18 hours after collection of whole blood. A bag of FFP contains all coagulation factors, including approximately 200 units of factor VIII as well as the other labile plasma coagulation factors and factor V.[31] Abnormal coagulation results occur commonly in the critically ill. No clear evidence exists to support the routine

TABLE 110-4

Guidelines for the Elective Transfusion of Fresh-Frozen Plasma (FFP) and Cryoprecipitate to Critically Ill Patients

1. FFP transfusion is likely to be indicated for the treatment of thrombotic thrombocytopenic purpura.
2. FFP transfusion is likely to be indicated for the reversal of warfarin anticoagulation in patients who are at high risk of bleeding, in combination with prothrombin complex concentrates where available.
3. FFP transfusion may be indicated in patients with multiple coagulation deficiencies prior to invasive procedures when the International Normalized Ratio value is greater than 2.
4. Cryoprecipitate transfusion may be indicated in patients with multiple coagulation deficiencies prior to invasive procedures when the fibrinogen level is less than 1.0 g/L.
5. FFP is not indicated for the treatment of hypovolemia, plasma exchange procedures, or the treatment of patients with supratherapeutic warfarin effect who have a low risk of bleeding.

administration of FFP to reduce the risk of spontaneous bleeding. The side effects of FFP are well described and include allergic reactions and transfusion-related acute lung injury.[14] In the nonbleeding patient, the routine administration of FFP to normalize the coagulation profile is not recommended, nor should it be used to correct hypovolemia. Methylene blue- and light-treated preparations may reduce the incidence of transfusion-related acute lung injury.[13]

Traditionally, FFP has been used to treat over therapeutic warfarin effect. Guidelines now advocate the use of prothrombin complex concentrates (25-50 IU/kg) for bleeding patients or those with an International Normalized Ratio (INR) value higher than 9 and a high risk of bleeding.[32] Such concentrates have low levels of factor VII, so some FFP (150-300 mL) is still indicated. If prothrombin complex concentrates are not available, then large volumes of FFP (12-15 mL/kg) are required.

The administration of FFP to normalize coagulation prior to invasive procedures remains controversial, with a wide variation in practice. Its uses in a number of procedures, including central venous catheterization, thoracocentesis, and liver biopsy, have been evaluated.[14] No clear correlation between coagulation abnormality and bleeding has been demonstrated. Australian and British guidelines do not recommend the routine use of FFP to normalize coagulation prior to invasive procedures.[9,17] Others "recommend" its use in this setting but do not specify a target INR value.[14] In the absence of clear evidence, it is suggested that skilled operators could safely perform most ICU procedures in the setting of mildly abnormal INR (<2).

Cryoprecipitate is available as a single-unit or apheresis preparation. It is prepared through the thawing of FFP between 1° and 6° C and recovering the precipitate,[33] which is then refrozen. The precipitate contains most of the factor VIII, fibrinogen, factor XIII, von Willebrand factor, and fibronectin from the FFP. A standard 10- to 40-mL unit has more than 140 mg/mL of fibrinogen and 70 IU of factor VIIIc. It has been recommended for use in fibrinogen deficiency (fibrinogen concentration <1.0 g/L) prior to the performance of an invasive procedure.[9] One small study comparing the effects of administering cryoprecipitate and FFP on INR in patients with fulminant hepatic failure found a significant reduction in INR with the administration of 10 units of cryoprecipitate.[34]

CONCLUSION

Intensive care medicine requires the safe and effective use of blood components. Guidelines have been developed from the results of prospective, randomized controlled trials for the elective administration of allogeneic packed RBCs. As a result of the high-level evidence, these guidelines have been successfully adopted. The evidence supporting transfusion guidelines in acutely bleeding patients and for plasma components is less impressive. There is a wide variation in practice. The recommendations made in this chapter constitute a conservative approach to plasma component therapy that balances the benefits with the risks of what is, but often not considered, a transplantation.

Key Points

1. Blood component therapy should be given only when the expected benefits to the patient are likely to outweigh the potential hazards.
2. In acutely bleeding patients with massive transfusion requirements, the early administration of plasma and platelets to patients is associated with better outcomes. After transfusion of approximately 20 units of RBCs, RBCs, platelets, and fresh-frozen plasma should be administered in a 1:1:1 ratio.
3. The use of recombinant activated factor VIIa in acutely bleeding patients remains controversial but may be considered when conventional therapy is ineffective.
4. Guidelines for allogeneic RBC transfusion in the critically ill are heavily influenced by results of a single prospective, randomized controlled trial.
5. Guidelines for platelets and plasma products are heavily influenced by expert opinion. Further research on their use in critically ill patients is indicated.

Key References

3. Hebert PC, Wells G, Blajchman MA, et al: A multicenter, randomized, controlled clinical trial of transfusion requirements in critical care. Transfusion Requirements in Critical Care Investigators, Canadian Critical Care Trials Group. N Engl J Med 1999;340:409-417.
6. American Society of Anesthesiologists Task Force on Perioperative Blood Transfusion and Adjuvant Therapies: Practice guidelines for perioperative blood transfusion and adjuvant therapies: An updated report by the American Society of Anesthesiologists Task Force on Perioperative Blood Transfusion and Adjuvant Therapies. Anesthesiology 2006;105:198-208.
13. British Committee for Standards in Haematology, Blood Transfusion Task Force: Guidelines for the use of platelet transfusions. Brit J Haematol 2003;122:10-23.
17. O'Shaughnessy DF, Atterbury C, Bolton Maggs P, et al: Guidelines for the use of fresh-frozen plasma, cryoprecipitate and cryosupernatant. Brit J Haematol 2004;126:11-28.
32. Baker RI, Coughlin PB, Gallus AS, et al: Warfarin reversal: Consensus guidelines, on behalf of the Australasian Society of Thrombosis and Haemostasis. Med J Austral 2004;181:492-497.

See the companion Expert Consult website for the complete reference list.

Acid-Base Problems

Basic Physiology

CHAPTER 111

Clinical Acid-Base Chemistry

Peter Constable

OBJECTIVES

This chapter will:
1. Explain acids and acidity.
2. Describe the difference between pH and hydrogen ion concentration as well as why blood pH is regulated.
3. Discuss buffering, buffer capacity, pK_a, and pK_a' as they relate to clinical acid-base chemistry.
4. Explain the derivation and anomalies of the Henderson-Hasselbalch equation as a description of clinical acid-base balance.
5. Introduce strong ion difference theory.

ACIDS AND THEIR DEFINITION IN CLINICAL ACID-BASE CHEMISTRY

Acids have been defined by means of a number of different approaches, such as Brønsted acids, Lewis acids (electron acceptor), and Arrhenius acid. The choice of definition for an acid is determined primarily by the milieu being investigated. The Brønsted-Lowry system is the most useful method for describing acids in aqueous systems, in which the solvent is water; for this reason, the Brønsted-Lowry system is the most widely used method of defining an acid in clinical acid-base chemistry.

The Brønsted-Lowry classification system defines an *acid* (HA) as a molecule that consists of a *proton donor* (H^+) and its *conjugate base* (A^-):

$$HA \rightarrow H^+ + A^-$$

Conversely, a *base* (B) is defined as a proton acceptor:

$$B + H^+ \rightarrow BH^+$$

With this approach, hydrochloric acid (HCl) is a Brønsted-Lowry acid because it donates a proton (HCl $\rightarrow$ H^+ + Cl^-) and ammonia (NH_3) is a Brønsted-Lowry base because it accepts a proton ($NH_3 + H^+ \rightarrow NH_4^+$); obviously, NH_4^+ could act as an acid if the direction of the reaction were reversed.

When the solvent is water, as in plasma, extracellular fluid, cerebrospinal fluid, synovial fluid, amniotic/allan-toic fluid, aqueous humor, saliva, gastric fluid, and urine, the acid HA is in equilibrium with A^- in water (H_2O), as described by the following equilibrium equation, in which *aq* indicates aqueous phase:

$$HA(aq) + H_2O \leftrightarrow H_3O^+(aq) + A^-(aq)$$

In water, the acid-conjugate base pair remains the same as in the general case described previously. However, it is important to note that the proton (H^+) does not exist in a solution of water. Instead, the proton exists predominantly in a hydrated form called the *hydronium ion* (H_3O^+), although other hydrated forms, such as $H_5O_2^+$, and more complex forms are also present.[1]

Henderson[2] noted in 1908 that the ratio of the *activity* of products to reactants is constant when equilibrium is reached between an acid-conjugate base pair in water. He designated this equilibrium constant K. Accordingly, the following equation can be developed relating K to the activity (*a*) of the hydronium ion, conjugate base, acid, and water:

$$K = \frac{a(H_3O^+)a(A^-)}{a(HA)a(H_2O)}$$

When water is the diluent, the value for $a(H_2O)$ is extremely large relative to those for the activity of HA, H_3O^+, and A^-. For this reason, both sides of this equation can be multiplied by $a(H_2O)$ in order to provide the general form of the Brønsted equilibrium equation, as follows, with K_a being used instead of K to indicate that the subject is an acid:

$$K_a = \frac{a(H_3O^+)a(A^-)}{a(HA)}$$

It is very cumbersome to write the value for K_a in this format, because in biological systems, the value for K_a can range from more than 0.1 to less than 10^{-10} (<0.0000000001). It is therefore much more convenient to take the negative logarithm to the base 10 of the K_a value (termed pK_a), as follows:

$$pK_a = -\log K_a$$

in which a lower value for pK_a indicates a stronger acid. This result may appear counterintuitive for some clinicians, because a higher number usually means more (and therefore a larger number for pK_a should seem to indicate a stronger acid). As a result, some clinicians prefer to express the equilibrium constant as K_a instead of pK_a. However, pK_a is more biologically meaningful than K_a because the pK_a value is linearly related to the Gibbs energy of the proton donation reaction that produces the hydronium ion. Use of pK_a instead of K_a is therefore not a sleazy chemical logarithmic trick but based on sound thermodynamic principles.

pH

Water is an interesting fluid because it can act as both an acid and a base, as demonstrated by the following equilibrium equation:

$$H_2O + H_2O \leftrightarrow H_3O^+(aq) + OH^-(aq)$$

which produces the following equation for the equilibrium constant K:

$$K = \frac{a(H_3O^+)a(OH^-)}{a(H_2O)a(H_2O)}$$

Multiplying both sides of the preceding equation by $a(H_2O)a(H_2O)$ produces an equation for the equilibrium constant for water (K_w) as follows:

$$K_w = a(H_3O^+)a(OH^-)$$

The negative logarithm to base 10 of $a(H_3O^+)$ was defined by Sørenson[3] as a dimensionless quantity called *pH*, with *p* indicating a logarithmic value and *H* indicating the proton, whereby $pH = -\log a(H_3O^+)$. Likewise, the negative logarithm of $a(OH^-)$ is defined as *pOH* (the *p* indicating a logarithmic value and the *OH* indicating the hydroxyl ion), whereby $pH = -\log a(OH^-)$. Taking the negative logarithm of both sides of the equilibrium constant equation for water and applying the rule for the logarithm of quotients provides the following equation:

$$pK_w = pH + pOH$$

At room temperature, the value for K_w is $\approx 1 \times 10^{-14}$, and $pK_w = 14.0$. A pH value of 7.0 is regarded as being neutral at room temperature because in pure distilled water $a(H_3O^+) = a(OH^-)$; it therefore follows that for pure distilled water at room temperature:

$$pH = pOH = \frac{pK_w}{2} = 7.0$$

The operative definition of *pH* is hydronium ion activity, which is most commonly measured from the electromotive force developed by a hydrogen ion–selective glass electrode and a saturated KCl solution as a salt bridge. The hydronium ion activity is usually less than the hydronium ion concentration in nondilute ionic solutions; however, the concentration approximates the activity in very dilute solutions (total ion concentration <1 mmol per kg of solution). Because the total ion concentration approximates 280 mmol per kg of solution in vertebrate fluids, the activity of any ion in solution is always less than its concentration but approaches its concentration as the concentration becomes more dilute. In other words, the activity of an ion

(a_i) is equal to the product of the activity coefficient (γ_i) and the concentration of the ion (C_i), such that:

$$a_i = \gamma_i \times C_i$$

and γ_i approaches 1 as C_i approaches 0.

HYDROGEN ION CONCENTRATION

The standard Brønsted equilibrium constant can be expressed in terms of concentrations instead of activities. Under these circumstances:

$$K_a' = \frac{a(H_3O^+)[A^-]}{[HA]}$$

with the convention being that *square brackets* indicate concentrations instead of activities; the prime symbol in K_a' indicates an apparent equilibrium constant based on concentrations. Hydrogen ions are expressed as activity because they are measured with an electrochemical system. It is important to realize that the value for K_a' can be altered by changes in temperature or ionic strength (concentration of ions in solution) but that the value for K_a (indicating activities) is altered only by changes in temperature.

The term "hydrogen ion concentration" has infuriated some chemists for a variety of reasons. First, although it is biologically meaningful to talk about the concentration of large molecules such as serum albumin (molecular weight of 65,000 g) that have a measurable dimension, it does not appear to be useful to express hydrogen ion as a concentration. The reason is that the hydrogen ion is unique, in that it consists only of a proton without an accompanying electron shell and is therefore orders of magnitude smaller than other ions in plasma. Second, the proton does not exist as its own entity in water; instead the hydronium ion (H_3O^+) is its most prevalent form. In other words, even if it were biologically meaningful to express protons in terms of concentration, the term "hydrogen ion concentration" would be a misnomer, and "hydronium ion concentration" more correct. Third, pH is measured as an activity through measurement of the electromotive force. Converting the measured quantity (activity) to concentration requires knowledge of the value of the activity coefficient under the conditions of measurement. Accurate values for the activity coefficient of the hydrogen ion are unavailable, although the value is commonly assumed to be 1 in biological solutions. Fourth, statistical comparison between groups usually requires an assumption of similar variances. Perusal of many articles presenting data as both pH and hydrogen ion concentration indicates that mean values for pH, but not hydrogen ion concentration, meet this assumption. Fifth, the implication that hydrogen ion concentration has clinical significance is nonsense, in that it is the activity of the proton (pH) that has clinical significance. For these reasons, it remains preferable to use *pH* instead of "hydrogen ion concentration" in clinical acid-base discussions. If clinicians prefer to not use a logarithmic scale to characterize acidity, "hydrogen ion activity" is preferred over "hydrogen ion concentration."

WHY IS BLOOD pH REGULATED?

The normal blood pH for adult humans is 7.40, and this pH value is vigorously defended at normal body temperature. At first glance, acid-base regulation in poikilothermic (cold-blooded) animals appears to differ from that of homoiothermic (warm-blooded) animals, such as mammals, marsupials, and monotremes, because at cold ambient temperatures, the blood pH of a poikilothermic animal is considerably higher than that of a mammal. This phenomenon was first reported in 1927 by Austin and colleagues,[4] who recorded a blood pH of 7.70 in alligators kept at 7° to 11° C, a value considerably different from that of mammals kept in the same environment or alligators kept at 33° to 38° C.[4] Later studies have indicated that many fish species swimming in cold water in the Arctic and Antarctic regions have blood pH values greater than 8.00. Subsequent studies demonstrated that acid-base regulation in poikilothermic animals is not fundamentally different from that in mammals but, rather, blood pH varies inversely with the temperature.[5-10] Two hypotheses have been proposed for the marked effect of temperature on blood pH: the constant relative alkalinity model[5] and the alphastat or constant net protein charge model,[11] with the latter model being preferred.

The constant net protein charge model for acid-base regulation hypothesizes that net protein charge is driven by the degree of dissociation of the imidazole group on histidine, and that acid-base regulation in vertebrates is aimed at keeping the imidazole charge and, consequently, net protein charge, constant. A constant protein charge state ensures that protein function is preserved during changes in body temperature. Reeves[6] called this theory the "alphastat hypothesis," in which *alpha* represents the fractional dissociation of histidine imidazole groups. This amino acid group was selected because of the presence of a significant number of titratable groups in plasma, and because its pK_a was within the limits of an effective buffer (pH ± 1.5) at physiologic pH. Another reason for the selection of imidazole as the major plasma buffer was that its enthalpy of ionization is approximately 7 kcal/mol, providing a $\Delta pH/\Delta T$, where T is temperature, of −0.016 units per degree Centigrade, which is virtually identical to that for plasma in most, but not all, air breathers (−0.015 to −0.020 units/° C).[6]

The constant net protein charge model has biological plausibility, in that it is consistent with current belief that many biological reactions are sensitive to changes in acidity and the distribution of protein charge.[11] In other words, pH is regulated to ensure constant net protein charge at different temperatures, in turn maintaining constant protein structure and, therefore, function at different temperatures. Any deviation from the optimal pH for a given temperature is energetically unfavorable and leads to reduced performance. An excellent example of the effect that changes in pK_a have on protein structure and function is provided by hemoglobin. The mean pK_a values of imidazole groups in reduced hemoglobin and oxygenated hemoglobin are different,[12] with the change being associated with a large and reversible change in hemoglobin conformation and oxygen-binding affinity.

Knowledge of the effect of temperature on blood pH facilitates the understanding that the normal blood pH at 34° C is 7.45, at 37° C is 7.40, and at 40° C is 7.35. The effect of temperature on blood pH is rarely recognized clinically because the blood sample is always equilibrated to a temperature of 37° C in modern blood gas analyzers before pH is measured, regardless of the original temperature of the patient.

BUFFERS AND BUFFER CAPACITY

A solution is a *buffer* if it resists change in pH even when acid or alkali is added to it. Acids can be defined as strong acids (which are completely dissociated) or weak acids (which are partially dissociated). In general, an acid is called a *weak acid* or a *buffer* when its pK_a lies within the range of pH ± 1.5, with maximal buffering occurring when pH = pK_a. Because normal plasma pH in healthy adult humans is 7.40, substances in plasma that act as weak acids at physiologic pH possess a pK_a between 5.9 and 8.9. The quantitatively important buffers in blood are bicarbonate, imidazole (histidine) amino acid groups on hemoglobin, albumin, and globulin, and phosphate. For comparison, the quantitatively important buffers in urine are bicarbonate, phosphate, and creatinine.

Buffers can be compared by their buffer capacity (β), measured in units of (mEq/L)/pH unit, which was defined by van Slyke[13] in 1922 as follows:

$$\beta = \Delta B/\Delta pH = 2.303 \times \frac{[HA][A^-]}{([HA]+[A^-])}$$

The buffer capacity equation indicates that β is maximal when [HA] = [A$^-$] (i.e., pH = pK_a') and that at a specific pH, the buffer capacity is proportional to the total buffer concentration. In essence, a higher value for buffer capacity reflects a greater capacity of the system to resist changes in pH.

Application of acid-base buffer theory to blood is most easily conceptualized if buffer ions are categorized as being volatile buffer ions (bicarbonate) or nonvolatile buffer ions (hemoglobin, albumin, globulin, phosphate). Bicarbonate is considered separately from the nonvolatile buffers because the bicarbonate buffer system is an open system in blood; rapid changes in CO_2 tension and hence arterial plasma bicarbonate concentration can be readily induced through alterations in respiratory activity—in other words, bicarbonate is an effective buffer beyond the limits of pH = pK_a ± 1.5. Bicarbonate and phosphate are effective buffers in erythrocytes, plasma, and interstitial fluid, hemoglobin is an effective buffer in erythrocytes, and albumin and globulin are effective buffers in plasma. However, even though buffering is an important role of hemoglobin, plasma protein, and phosphate, the primary purpose of these three buffers is different from that of pH homeostasis, whereas the primary purpose of bicarbonate is to buffer extracellular fluid. It is for these reasons, as well as historical reasons related to development of acid-base theory and ease of laboratory measurement, that the emphasis has been traditionally and correctly placed on bicarbonate as the most important buffer in extracellular fluid. This concept is best demonstrated in the Henderson-Hasselbalch equation.

THE HENDERSON-HASSELBALCH EQUATION

Every clinician dealing with acid-base abnormalities is familiar with the Henderson-Hasselbalch equation, probably the most famous equation in biology. Unfortunately, most clinicians are not aware of the limitations of this equation: It contains a number of anomalies and is more descriptive than mechanistic.

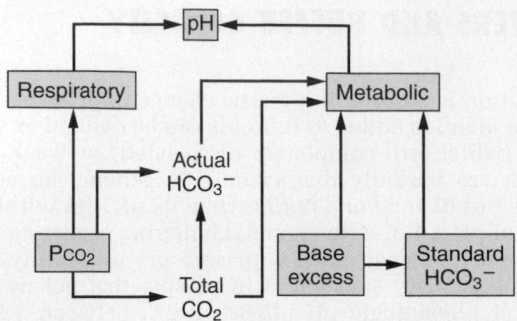

FIGURE 111-1. Determinants of plasma pH, as assessed by the Henderson-Hasselbalch equation. Note that only the extracellular base excess and the standard HCO_3^- provide an independent measure of the nonrespiratory (metabolic) component of plasma pH.

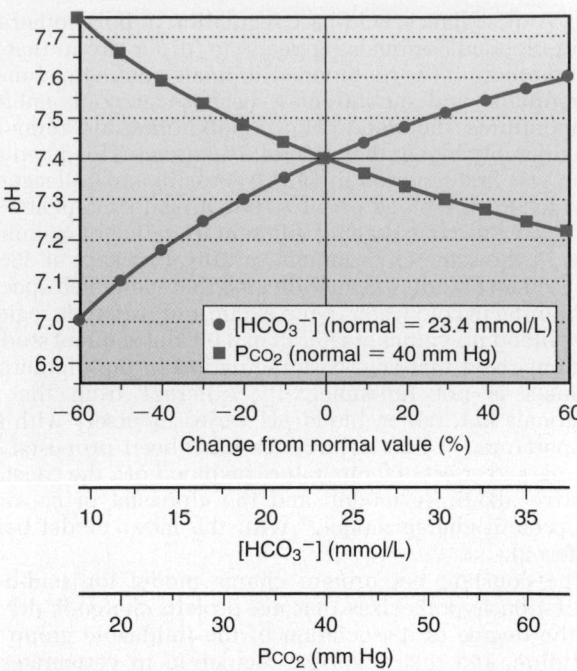

FIGURE 111-2. Spider plot revealing the dependence of plasma pH in humans on changes in two variables—plasma bicarbonate concentration (HCO_3^-) and partial pressure of CO_2 (Pco_2)—identified by the Henderson-Hasselbalch equation. The spider plot was obtained by systematically varying one variable while holding the other variable at the normal values for human plasma. pH was calculated using the Henderson-Hasselbalch equation[14]; pK_1' was 6.12[19,22] and S was 0.0307 mm Hg^{-1}.[23] Note that pH = 7.40 when bicarbonate concentration and Pco_2 are at their normal values.

The traditional approach for assessing acid-base balance focuses on how plasma carbon dioxide tension (Pco_2), plasma bicarbonate concentration ($[HCO_3^-]$), the negative logarithm of the apparent dissociation constant (pK_1') for carbonic acid (H_2CO_3) in plasma, and the solubility (S) of CO_2 in plasma interact to determine plasma pH. The equilibrium reaction is as follows:

$$Pco_2 \leftrightarrow CO_2(aq) + H_2O \leftrightarrow H_2CO_3 \leftrightarrow H^+ + HCO_3^-$$

At equilibrium, the relationship can be expressed as the Henderson-Hasselbalch equation, as follows[2,14]:

$$pH = pK_1' + \log \frac{HCO_3^-}{(S\,Pco_2)}$$

The Henderson-Hasselbalch equation has proved invaluable in aiding the understanding of mammalian acid-base physiology and is routinely used in the treatment of acid-base abnormalities. With the traditional Henderson-Hasselbalch approach, the following primary acid-base disturbances have been defined (Figs. 111-1 and 111-2)[15]:
- Respiratory acidosis (increased Pco_2)
- Respiratory alkalosis (decreased Pco_2)
- Metabolic acidosis (decreased extracellular base excess, actual HCO_3^- concentration, or standard HCO_3^- [bicarbonate concentration under standard conditions])
- Metabolic alkalosis (increased extracellular base excess, actual HCO_3^- concentration, or standard HCO_3^-)

It was evident as early as 1922 that factors other than Pco_2, $[HCO_3^-]$, pK_1', and S influence plasma pH.[16] In 1925, pK_1' (and therefore pH) was shown to be influenced by ionic strength (μ)[17] and temperature,[18] the $\Delta pK_1'/\Delta T$ being -0.005 units/° C over a temperature range of 20° to 38° C. It had been expected that pK_1', like all equilibrium constants based on molalities, would be altered by changes in ionic strength and temperature. It was unexpectedly found, however, that the measured $\Delta pH/\Delta T$ of plasma was -0.015 to -0.020 units/° C, a value three to four times the -0.005 units/° C predicted by pK_1'.[6] This finding shows that the Henderson-Hasselbalch equation cannot be accurately applied to mammalian blood cooled in vitro or to poikilothermic animals.

Determination of accurate pK_1' values for plasma has been more problematic, because the experimental value for pK_1' (the apparent dissociation constant) in plasma differs marginally from the value obtained in aqueous nonplasma solutions. A number of studies have demonstrated that the value for pK_1' in plasma is influenced by pH, protein concentration, and sodium concentration.[19-22] Although these observations troubled most investigators, the value for pK_1' in plasma is routinely adjusted through the use of nomograms, tables, or polynomial equations to account for changes in plasma pH, protein concentration, and sodium concentration. The mechanistic basis for these adjustments is currently unknown.

The value for pK_1' at an ionic strength of 0.16 (mammalian extracellular fluid) is obtained from the sum of pK_s (the apparent dissociation constant) (6.029 at 37° C)[19] and the negative logarithm of the activity coefficient of the hydrogen ion (0.091),[22] producing a value of 6.120 at 37° C. The value for pK_1' should be corrected for temperature and ionic strength only when applied to biological fluids. The value used for S in plasma at 37° C is 0.0307 mm Hg^{-1}; S varies with ionic strength, temperature, and protein concentration, and accurate values are available for mammalian plasma.[23]

Because the Henderson-Hasselbalch equation does not satisfactorily account for the temperature dependence of plasma pH or for the apparent dependence of pK_1' in plasma on pH, protein concentration, and sodium concentration, the approach can be accurately applied to only mammalian blood at normal body temperatures and approximately normal pH, protein concentration, and sodium concentration. The empirical nature of the adjustments to the value of pK_1' in plasma suggests that the Henderson-Hasselbalch equation is more descriptive than mechanistic. A more mechanistic approach is therefore desirable, and strong ion difference theory provides such a model.

STRONG ION DIFFERENCE THEORY

Strong ion difference theory focuses on chemical reactions in plasma that involve simple ions in solution.[24] This is a valid simplification, because the quantitatively important plasma cations (Na^+, K^+, Ca^{2+}, Mg^{2+}) and anions (Cl^-, HCO_3^-, protein, lactate, sulfate, ketoacids) bind each other in a saltlike manner. Plasma ions (such as Cu^{2+}, Fe^{2+}, Fe^{3+}, Zn^{2+}, Co^{2+}, and Mn^{2+}) that enter into oxidation-reduction reactions, complex ion interactions, and precipitation reactions are not categorized as simple ions but are quantitatively unimportant in determining plasma pH, primarily because their plasma concentrations are low. Simple ions in plasma can be differentiated into two main types, non-buffer ions (*strong ions* or strong electrolytes) and *buffer ions*.[24] Strong ions are fully dissociated at physiologic pH and therefore exert no buffering effect. Strong ions do, however, exert an electrical effect, because the sum of completely dissociated cations does not equal the sum of completely dissociated anions. Stewart[25] called this difference the *strong ion difference* (SID), which has a mean value of +28 to +42 mEq/L for plasma from healthy humans and domestic animals.[26-28] Because strong ions do not participate in chemical reactions in plasma at physiologic pH, they are regarded as a collective unit of charge (SID), the unit of measure being mEq/L.

Singer and Hastings[29] proposed in 1948 that plasma pH was determined by two independent factors, Pco_2 and net strong ion charge, which is equivalent to the strong ion difference (SID).[29] Stewart[25] suggested in 1983 that a third variable, the total concentration of nonvolatile weak buffers in plasma (A_{tot}), such as albumin, globulins, phosphate, also exerted an independent effect on plasma pH. One of Stewart's major contributions to clinical acid-base physiology was his proposal that plasma pH is determined by three independent factors: Pco_2, net strong ion charge (equivalent to the strong ion difference, SID, the difference in charge between fully dissociated strong cations and anions in plasma), and the total plasma concentration of nonvolatile weak buffers (A_{tot}) (Fig. 111-3).[25]

Strong ion difference theory assumes that plasma ions act as either strong ions, volatile buffer ions (HCO_3^-), or nonvolatile buffer ions (A^-).[24] Plasma therefore contains three types of charged entities; SID, HCO_3^-, and A^-. The requirement for electroneutrality dictates that at all times the SID equal the sum of bicarbonate buffer ion activity (HCO_3^-) and nonvolatile buffer ion activity (A^-), such that[23]:

$$SID - HCO_3^- - A^- = 0$$

A second assumption of the strong ion approach is that the acid-conjugate base pair HA and A^- do not take part in plasma reactions that result in the net destruction or creation of HA or A^-. The sum of [HA] and [A^-] (called A_{tot}) therefore remains constant through conservation of mass[25], as follows:

$$A_{tot} = [HA] + [A^-]$$

Through the combination of equations consisting of the electroneutrality equation for plasma, an equation for conservation of mass, and two dissociation equations (K_1' for H_2CO_3 and K_a for plasma weak acids), the following logarithmic equation, called the *simplified strong ion equation*, relating plasma pH to three independent variables (Pco_2, SID, A_{tot}) and three constants (K_a, K_1', S), was developed[24]:

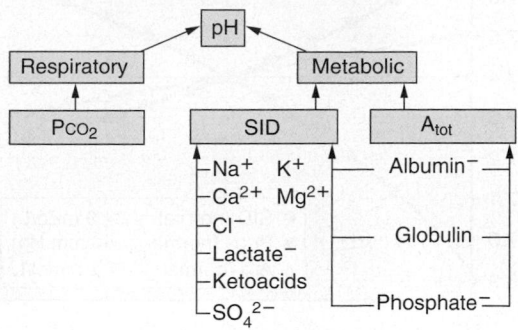

FIGURE 111-3. Schematic of the effects of the three independent variables—strong ion difference (SID), partial pressure of CO_2 (Pco_2), and total concentration of nonvolatile weak buffers in plasma (A_{tot})—on the pH of human plasma, as assessed by the simplified strong ion model. Note that SID and A_{tot} provide independent measures of the metabolic (nonrespiratory) component of plasma pH and that albumin, globulin, and phosphate contribute to SID and A_{tot}.

$$pH = \log(2SID/\{K_1'S\,Pco_2 + K_aA_{tot} - K_aSID\} + \sqrt{\{(K_1'S\,Pco_2 + K_aSID + K_aA_{tot})^2 - 4K_a^2SIDA_{tot}\}})$$

A number of clinical ramifications arise from the simplified strong ion equation. Because clinically important acid-base derangements result from changes in Pco_2, SID, and concentrations of individual nonvolatile plasma buffers (albumin, globulins, phosphate), six primary acid-base disturbances can be distinguished (Fig. 111-4): respiratory acidosis, respiratory alkalosis, strong ion acidosis, strong ion alkalosis, nonvolatile buffer ion acidosis, and nonvolatile buffer ion alkalosis.[24] Acidemia results from an increase in Pco_2 and nonvolatile buffer concentration or from a decrease in SID. Alkalemia results from a decrease in Pco_2 and nonvolatile buffer concentration or from an increase in SID.

The strong ion model offers a novel insight into the pathophysiology of mixed acid-base disorders and is mechanistic. It also explains how hypoproteinemia and hyperproteinemia alter pH (through alterations in A_{tot}; see Figs. 111-3 and 111-4), whereas the Henderson-Hasselbalch approach provides no such explanation (see Figs. 111-1 and 111-2).[24] The change in SID from normal is equivalent to the base excess value, assuming a normal nonvolatile buffer ion concentration (normal albumin, globulins, and phosphate concentration). This means that clinicians who have used the traditional Henderson-Hasselbalch approach with base excess to indicate the metabolic component of the derangement have also been using the strong ion approach to evaluate acid-base status, because albumin, globulin, and phosphate concentrations are often normal.

The simplified strong ion equation provides a quantitative mechanistic acid-base model that simplifies to the Henderson-Hasselbalch equation when applied to aqueous nonprotein solutions (in which $A_{tot} = 0$ mEq/L, and SID = HCO_3^-),[24] as indicated by the following algebraic rearrangement:

$$pH = pK_1' + \frac{\log\left\{\dfrac{SID - A_{tot}}{(1 + 10^{pK_a - pH})}\right\}}{SPco_2}$$

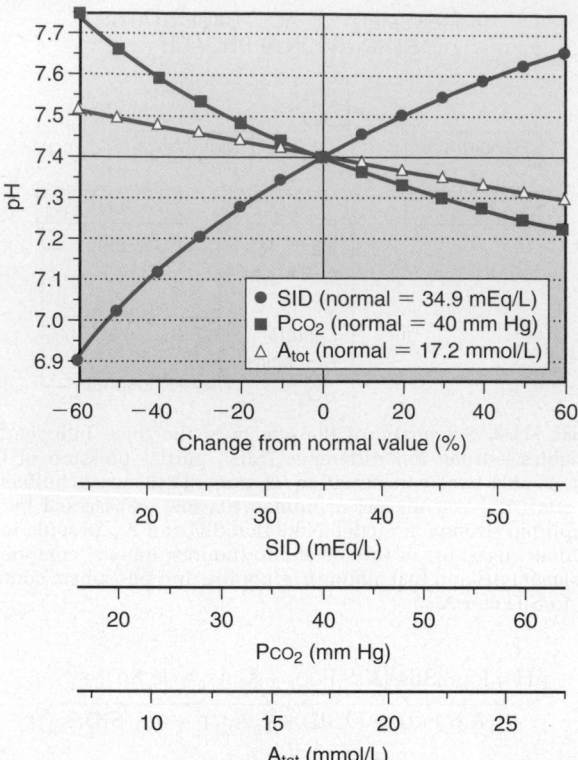

FIGURE 111-4. Spider plot revealing the dependence of plasma pH in humans on changes in the three independent variables—strong ion difference (SID), partial pressure of CO_2 (PCO_2), and the total concentration of nonvolatile weak acids (A_{tot})—identified by the strong ion difference theory. The spider plot was obtained by systematically varying one independent variable while holding the other two independent variables at the normal values for human plasma. The pH was calculated with the simplified strong ion difference equation and experimentally determined values for SID (34.9 mEq/L),[26] A_{tot} (17.2 mmol/L),[26] pK_a' (7.10),[26] pK_1' (6.12),[19,22] and S (0.0307 mm Hg^{-1}).[23] Note that pH = 7.40 when SID, PCO_2, and A_{tot} are at their normal values, and that pH is more sensitive to changes in plasma electrolyte concentrations (SID) than in PCO_2. Note also that changes in plasma protein concentration (the major contributor to A_{tot}) change plasma pH; the Henderson-Hasselbalch equation does not provide a mechanism for this observation.

A comparison of this equation with the Henderson-Hasselbalch equation shows that strong ion difference theory produces a general equation for clinical acid-base equilibrium that simplifies to the Henderson-Hasselbalch equation when $A_{tot} = 0$, because under these circumstances, SID = HCO_3^-. The simplified strong ion model therefore unites the Henderson-Hasselbalch equation[2,14] and Stewart's strong ion model[25] when applied to protein- and phosphate-free solutions. Wooten[30] has elegantly shown how the base excess value in the Henderson-Hasselbalch approach to acid-base balance is derived by extending strong ion difference theory from plasma to blood.

CONCLUSION

Clinical acid-base chemistry has evolved over the past century. The development and application of strong ion difference theory to the evaluation of complex clinical acid-base disorders has given a new insight into the mechanism for acid-base derangement and will lead to more focused treatment of critically ill patients.

Key Points

1. Acids in clinical acid-base chemistry are best described through the use of the Brønsted-Lowry system, whereby an acid is a proton donor and a base is a proton acceptor.
2. The degree of acidity is best described as pH rather than hydrogen ion concentration.
3. Blood pH is regulated in order to keep protein structure constant at different temperatures.
4. Buffers resist a change in pH when acid or alkali is added to the solution. The most important buffers in extracellular fluid are bicarbonate, hemoglobin, plasma proteins, and phosphate.
5. The Henderson-Hasselbalch equation is a simplified version of strong ion difference theory. Development and application of strong ion difference theory promises to provide a new and mechanistic insight into complex acid-base disorders.

Key References

6. Reeves RB: An imadazole alphastat hypothesis for vertebrate acid-base regulation: Tissue carbon dioxide content and body temperature in bullfrogs. Resp Physiol 1972;14:219-236.
11. Cameron JN: Acid-base homeostasis: Past and present perspectives. Physiol Zool 1989;62:845-865.
24. Constable PD: A simplified strong ion model for acid-base equilibria: Application to horse plasma. J Appl Physiol 1997;83:297-311.
25. Stewart PA: Modern quantitative acid-base chemistry. Can J Physiol Pharmacol 1983;61:1444-1461.
26. Staempfli HR, Constable PD: Experimental determination of net protein charge and A_{tot} and K_a of nonvolatile buffers in human plasma. J Appl Physiol 2003;95:620-630.

See the companion Expert Consult website for the complete reference list.

CHAPTER 112

Renal Acid-Base Physiology

Howard E. Corey

OBJECTIVES

This chapter will:
1. Explain the distribution, function, and regulation of renal epithelial acid-base transporters.
2. Relate the abundance and expression of renal epithelial acid-base transporters to systemic acid-base balance.
3. Describe the homeostatic control mechanisms that integrate the bicarbonate transporter family (SLC-encoded proteins), the plasma strong ion difference, and PCO_2.

To maintain plasma hydrogen ion homeostasis, renal transport proteins excrete acid and regenerate plasma bicarbonate buffer. However, changes in proton balance do not translate easily to corresponding changes in plasma pH. In a now classic investigation, Lemann and associates[1,2] fed NH_4Cl to human volunteers on a fixed diet and studied hydrogen ion balance over three 6-day observation periods followed by two recovery periods. Hydrogen ion balance was determined by subtracting absorbed dietary alkali {urine-stool {$[Na^+ + K^+ + Ca^{2+} + Mg^+] - [Cl^- + 1.8 PO_4^{2-}]$}} and net acid excretion {urine $[HCO_3^- - (NH4^+ + titratable\ acid + H^+)]$} from exogenous and endogenous acid production {urine $[NH_4^+ + organic\ acids + SO_4^{2-}]$}. Although net acid excretion increased in parallel with NH_4Cl administration, acid loading resulted in a positive proton balance and a negative calcium ion balance. These findings suggest that bone was recruited to buffer protons that escaped the renal response. As the apparent volume of distribution of protons exceeds the inulin (extracellular) space, hydrogen ion balance did not correlate with plasma $[H^+]$ in any observation period. As a consequence, the "bone buffer" theory has garnered criticism owing to the intangibility of the key variables.

A potentially useful solution to this quandary is to tally electrical charges rather than protons. Models of acid-base balance are based on the colligative properties of plasma, such as the proton number, the proton acceptor site density, or electrical charge. Although these approaches are equivalent mathematically, models based on the proton number or acceptor site density may fail because these properties are dispersed throughout the total body water. The apparent volume of distribution of Na^+ and Cl^- approximates the inulin space, so a model predicated upon the conservation of charge is more likely to be successful in clarifying acid-base balance.

Equations of state based on this approach reveal that plasma pH is determined by three independent variables, the strong ion difference (SID $\approx Na^+ - Cl^-$), the PCO_2, and the total plasma weak acids (A_{tot}).[3] Metabolic acidosis is due either to retention of chloride or to loss of sodium (low

SID), and conversely, metabolic alkalosis is due either to loss of chloride or to retention of sodium (high SID). The role of the kidney is to regulate plasma SID and, in turn, to be regulated by plasma SID and PCO_2.

The original data collected by Lemann and associates[1,2] may be reanalyzed on the basis of these physiochemical principles. If one assumes that the chloride space is equal to approximately 25% of the total body weight (a mean of ≈68 kg in this study), the measured positive cumulative chloride balance of 185 mEq would account for the observed 11-mEq/L increase in plasma chloride.[4,5] As predicted, plasma [H+] rose in direct proportion to the increase in plasma chloride concentration (decrease in SID) ($r = 0.98$; $P < .05$) (Fig. 112-1). These observations suggest that SID balance yields a more tractable analysis of NH_4Cl-induced acidosis than proton balance.

The purpose of this chapter is to integrate the biology of renal transport proteins with a quantitative, physiochemical model of plasma acid-base balance. The human solute carrier superfamily of bicarbonate transporters and anion exchangers consists of two structurally distinct groups. The bicarbonate transport group, the SLC4 or AE family, consists of 10 genes. Four genes (SLCA1, SLCA2, SLCA3, and SLACA9) encode proteins (AE1, AE2, AE3, and AE4, respectively) that are expressed by the kidney and function as $Cl^--HCO_3^-$ exchangers. The best described member of this group, SLC4A1, encodes AE1 (band 3 protein), which is expressed by red blood cell membranes, the colon, the heart, and the basolateral membrane of type B intercalated cells. The remaining six genes of the SLC4 family encode proteins that appear to function as sodium-bicarbonate ($Na^+-HCO_3^-$) cotransporters (NBCs). The best described is SLC4A4, which encodes the electrogenic NBCe1 (NBC1) found in renal proximal tubule cells. In renal epithelium, SLC4 family members are expressed mostly on the basolateral domain and promote net sodium reabsorption or chloride excretion, thereby increasing plasma SID.

The anion transport group, the SLC26 or sulfate exchange family, consists of chloride-anion exchangers SLC26A1 through SLC26A11. Some members of this family are expressed in the kidney and play an important role in acid-base balance. In the proximal tubule, SLC26A6 (CFEX, PAT-1) mediates apical chloride-anion exchange, permitting separate regulation of NaCl (by SLC26A family members) and $NaHCO_3$ (by SLC4 family members) reabsorption. In the distal nephron, SLC26A4 (pendrin) mediates Cl^--anion exchange across the luminal membrane of type B intercalated cells, whereas SLC4A mediates $Cl^--HCO_3^-$ exchange across the basolateral domain of type A intercalated cells. In renal epithelium, SLC26 family members are expressed mostly on the apical surface and promote chloride reabsorption, thereby decreasing plasma SID.

A simple but powerful model of acid-base balance may be constructed on the basis of the interaction of renal epithelial SLC transporter proteins and plasma SID.

PROXIMAL CONVOLUTED TUBULE

NaHCO₃ Reabsorption

Mechanism

The majority of the Na^+, Cl^-, and HCO_3^- filtered by the kidney is reabsorbed in the proximal convoluted tubule (PCT). The components of the PCT acid-base transport system, which have been identified with the use of isolated perfused tubules, microvesicles, and expression cloning, include a Na^+-HCO_3^- cotransporter (NBC), an Na^+,H^+ exchanger (NHE), and the aquaporin-1 gas channel (Table 112-1). In brief, apical NHE3 secretes H^+ into the tubular lumen, in a process that also reclaims about 80% of filtered bicarbonate. In a reaction mediated by apical carbonic anhydrase IV, luminal H^+ is catalyzed along with filtered HCO_3^- to form CO_2 and H_2O. Luminal CO_2 and H_2O may enter the cytosol via apical aquaporin-1 gas channels, whereupon they are recombined by carbonic anhydrase II to form H^+ and HCO_3^-. HCO_3^- is reabsorbed into the circulation by basolateral NBCs.[6] The net result of these processes is reabsorption of NaHCO₃, thereby increasing plasma SID.

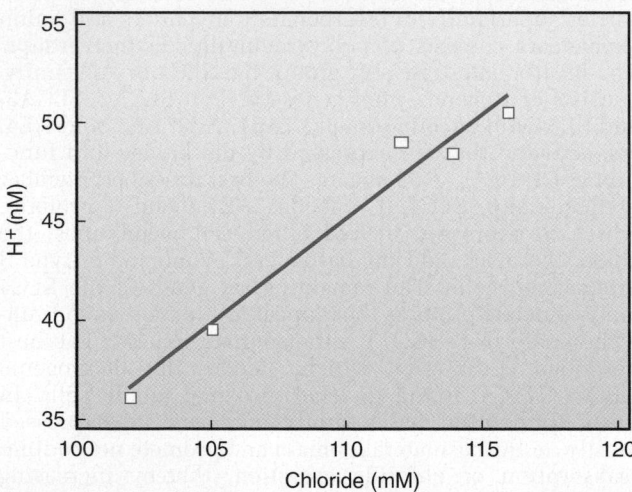

FIGURE 112-1. Correlation of plasma chloride concentration (in mM) and plasma [H⁺] (in nM) in human volunteers fed NH₄Cl. (Data from Lemann J Jr, Litzow JR, Lennon EJ: The effects of chronic acid load in normal man: Further evidence for the participation of bone mineral in the defense against chronic metabolic acidosis. J Clin Invest 1966;45:1608-1614.)

Regulation

Apart from local factors such as phosphokinases and cyclic adenosine monophosphate, bicarbonate flux is regulated by systemic acid-base balance. For example, respiratory acidosis rapidly elicits an increase in renal H^+ secretion and HCO_3^- reabsorption.[7,8] In chronically hypercapnic rats, studies using immunoblotting reveal upregulation of NBC expression. To unravel the mechanism, Chen and Boron[9] perfused the apical and basolateral surfaces of isolated rabbit tubules with solutions that contained CO_2/HCO_3^-. Apical Na^+-H^+ exchange was stimulated by the addition of CO_2/HCO_3^- to the bath but not to the luminal perfusate, suggesting a pH-independent sensor for CO_2 and/or HCO_3^- on or near the basolateral surface.

To determine the sensor, Zhao and associates[10] also perfused isolated proximal tubules, but with "out of equilibrium" solutions that contained either CO_2 or HCO_3^- (but not both) at various pH levels. Apical NHEs and basolateral NBCs were stimulated by basolateral CO_2, inhibited by basolateral HCO_3^-, and unaffected by [H+]. These findings suggest that CO_2 and HCO_3^- regulate transcellular HCO_3^- flux by binding to specific basolateral receptor sites, perhaps triggering tyrosine kinase- or angiotensin II–dependent mechanisms.[6] These observations suggest that both plasma proton concentration and transcellular bicarbonate flux depend on plasma SID and PCO_2 as part of a homeostatic mechanism.

NaCl Reabsorption

Mechanism

In rats, micropuncture studies have revealed that about 25% of filtered chloride is reabsorbed by passive transport through "leaky" epithelium, and another 20% by active transport through chloride channels.[11] The remaining 40% to 50% of chloride reabsorption is mediated by apical chloride-anion (formate, oxalate, bicarbonate) exchangers that work in parallel with NHE3 (Table 112-2).

In brief, apical chloride-anion recycling loads proximal tubule cells with chloride. Chloride-formate exchange, Na^+-H^+ exchange, and H^+-formate symport occur in parallel with chloride-oxalate exchange, oxalate-sulfate exchange, and Na^+-sulfate cotransport. Chloride exits the opposite side of the cell via basolateral chloride-bicarbonate exchangers and/or chloride channels.[11-15]

Regulation

In the PCT, both respiratory and metabolic acidosis induce NaHCO₃ absorption and inhibit NaCl reabsorption.[16] In chronically hypercapnic rats, micropuncture studies

TABLE 112-1

Acid-Base Transport Proteins of the PCT

TRANSPORTER	GENE	DISTRIBUTION	FUNCTION	REGULATION
NBCe1	SLC4A4	Basolateral	Electrogenic Na-bicarbonate cotransport	Strong ion difference, CO_2, angiotensin II
NHE3	SLC9A3	Apical	Electroneutral Na^+-H^+ countertransport	Parathyroid hormone, cyclic adenosine monophosphate, protein kinase, aldosterone
Aquaporin-1	7p14	Apical	Gas channel for CO_2 Water permeability	Osmolarity

TABLE 112-2

Chloride Reabsorption by the Renal Proximal Tubule

	PASSIVE TRANSPORT	CONDUCTANCE	COUPLED TRANSPORT
Component	Paracellular	Cl⁻ channel and channel–like structures	SLC26A6 (CFEX, PAT-1) apical Cl⁻-anion exchanger
Mechanism	Electrochemical concentration gradient (passive), Starling's forces	Chloride conductance	Active transport
Percentage of reabsorption	20%-25%	40%-50%	30%
Regulation	Extracellular volume	Intracellular volume Angiotensin II	HCO_3^-, P_{CO_2}, PKC

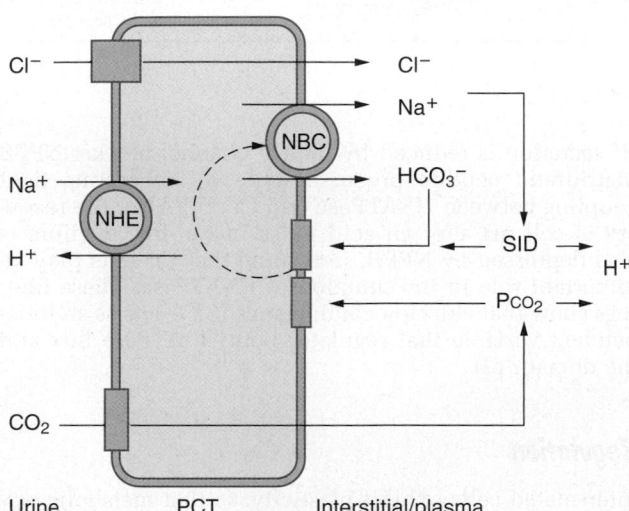

Urine   PCT   Interstitial/plasma

FIGURE 112-2. Strong ion difference (SID) and P_{CO_2} regulate the proximal convoluted tubule (PCT) and plasma [H+]. The PCT reabsorbs HCO_3^- (through the coordinated activity of Na^+-H^+ exchanger [NHE] and Na-bicarbonate cotransporter [NBC] proteins), chloride (by passive paracellular transport and active transcellular mechanisms), and CO_2 (via apical aquaporin-1 gas channels). Plasma CO_2 and HCO_3^- occupy basolateral PCT receptors, upregulating or downregulating NHE and NBC activity. Plasma SID and P_{CO_2} determine plasma HCO_3^- and pH.

reveal blunted PCT chloride flux, chloriduria, and hypochloremia.[8] These observations suggest that P_{CO_2} directly regulates chloride transport.

In normal rats, microperfusion of proximal tubule segments with oxalate- or formate-containing solutions stimulates chloride flux. After ammonium chloride loading, the low PCT chloride transport may be restored by the provision of $NaHCO_3$, but not by NaCl, formate, or oxalate.[16-18] These findings suggest that metabolic acidosis downregulates and $NaHCO_3$ upregulates apical chloride–organic anion countertransport. It appears that SLC family members act as "regulons," adjusting their function to maintain systemic acid-base homeostasis. A picture of acid-base balance emerges that integrates SLC family transport protein mechanisms with strong ion difference theory (Fig. 112-2).

DISTAL CONVOLUTED TUBULE

In the distal nephron, intercalated (acid-base–secreting) cells mediate H^+ and HCO_3^- transport. Three types of inter-

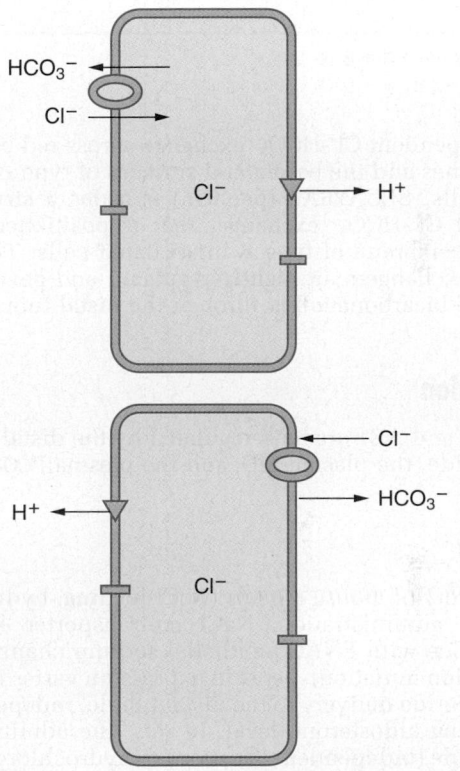

FIGURE 112-3. Type A (*top*) and type B (*bottom*) intercalated cells.

calated cell have been identified, type A (proton-secreting) cells, type B (bicarbonate-secreting) cells, and non-A, non-B cells. The components of the distal convoluted tubule (DCT) acid-base transport system are H^+-ATPase, H^+-K^+ exchangers, and Cl⁻-HCO_3^- exchangers (Fig. 112-3 and Table 112-3).

CHLORIDE, PROTON, AND BICARBONATE HANDLING BY PENDRIN, BAND 3 PROTEIN, H⁺-ATPase, AND H⁺,K⁺-ATPase

As in the proximal tubule, members of the SLC family play an important role in chloride, proton, and bicarbonate handling. SLC4A1, or band 3 protein, mediates

TABLE 112-3

Acid-Base Transport Proteins of the Distal Tubule

TRANSPORTER(S)	GENE	DISTRIBUTION	FUNCTION	REGULATION
ATP6V0A4, ATP6B1	ATP6N1B	Apical surfaces of type A intercalated cells and endocytotic vesicles	Proton secretion (H^+-ATPase)	Aldosterone, metabolic acidosis, chloride conductance
P-type cation-transporting ATPases, which also include Ca^{2+}-ATPase and Na^+,K^+-ATPase (EC.3.6.1.36)	ATP4B	Apical surfaces of type A intercalated cells	Proton secretion (H^+-K^+-ATPase)	Hypokalemia, metabolic acidosis
AE1	SLC4A	Basolateral surfaces of type A intercalated cells	Chloride-bicarbonate exchange	SID, PCO_2
Pendrin	SLC26A4	Apical surfaces of type B intercalated cells	Chloride-bicarbonate exchange	SID, PCO_2, distal chloride delivery, angiotensin II, desmopressin acetate

SID, strong ion difference.

Na-independent Cl^--HCO_3^- exchange across red blood cell membranes and the basolateral surfaces of type A intercalated cells. SLCA26A9 (pendrin) encodes a structurally different Cl^--HCO_3^- exchanger that is positioned on the apical membrane of type B intercalated cells. These Cl^--HCO_3^- exchangers are tightly regulated and govern chloride and bicarbonate flux through the distal tubule.[19-23]

Regulation

Pendrin and AE1 are both regulated by the distal delivery of chloride, the plasma SID, and the plasma PCO_2.

Pendrin

In a variety of mouse models (NaCl loading, hydrochlorothiazide administration, NaCl co-transporter knockout mice, mice with ENAC [epithelial sodium channel] gain-of-function mutation), pendrin expression varies inversely with chloride delivery to the distal tubule, independent of circulating aldosterone level. In rats, the administration of chloride (independent of cation) or hydrochlorothiazide downregulates pendrin expression, whereas NaCl restriction or the long-term administration of $NaHCO_3$ or furosemide (chronically) upregulates pendrin expression.[24-28]

Hypercapnia in rats is associated with low values for arterial blood pH and plasma chloride concentration and high values for plasma PCO_2 and HCO_3^- concentration. Immunoblot analysis and immunocytochemistry reveal an increase in proximal tubule NBCe1 expression, no change in proximal tubule NHE3 expression, and a decrease in distal tubule pendrin expression, independent of chloride load or aldosterone level.[29]

Pendrin expression is also upregulated by angiotensin II.[30] In Brattleboro rats, the long-term administration of desmopressin acetate (DDAVP) increases pendrin expression and downregulates the expression of AE1 and H^+-ATPase. Because kidney renin messenger RNA and plasma aldosterone levels are raised, the effect of desmopressin acetate is probably mediated by stimulation of the renin-angiotensin-aldosterone system.[31]

H^+-ATPase and H^+,K^+-ATPase

H^+-ATPase activity depends on chloride conductance.[32-34] In MDCK (Madin-Darby canine kidney) cells, the rate of

H^+ secretion is reduced by the Cl^- channel blocker NPPB (natriuretic peptide precursor type B), suggesting tight coupling between H^+-ATPase and Cl^-.[32,33] Also, the recovery of cell pH after an acid pulse in Na^+-free medium is also depressed by NPPB, indicating that Cl^- ions play an important role in the function of H^+-ATPase. These findings show that chloride conductance (SID) acts as an independent variable that regulates both H^+-ATPase flux and the domain pH.

Regulation

Intercalated cells exhibit plasticity, so that metabolic acidosis induces a reversal of the polarity of HCO_3^- flux. In cortical collecting duct cells incubated in vitro in acid media, type B intercalated cells are remodeled so that H^+-ATPase is expressed apically rather than basolaterally.[35]

AE1 (Band 3 Protein)

In rats given either NH_4Cl or $NAHCO_3$, Sabolic and colleagues[36] used confocal microscopy and immunocytochemistry to study the expression of AE1 and H^+-ATPase by type A and type B intercalated cells. Metabolic acidosis increased the immunostaining of AE1 on type A cells and was accompanied by a redistribution of H^+-ATPase immunostaining from the basolateral surface toward the apical surface. Metabolic alkalosis decreased the immunostaining of AE1 and was accompanied by a redistribution of H^+-ATPase immunostaining from the apical surface toward the basolateral surface. These findings suggest that the chloride conductance of intercalated cells is oriented to keep plasma SID within normal values. As expected, hyperchloremic metabolic acidosis develops in knockout mice deficient in band 3 protein.[37]

SUMMARY

One goal of renal acid-base physiology is to relate the expression of renal epithelial transport proteins to colligative properties of plasma, such as proton number and charge. As protons are dispersed throughout the whole body water and are consumed in chemical reactions, the abundance of H^+-OH^- transporter proteins expressed by each segment of the nephron does not correlate directly

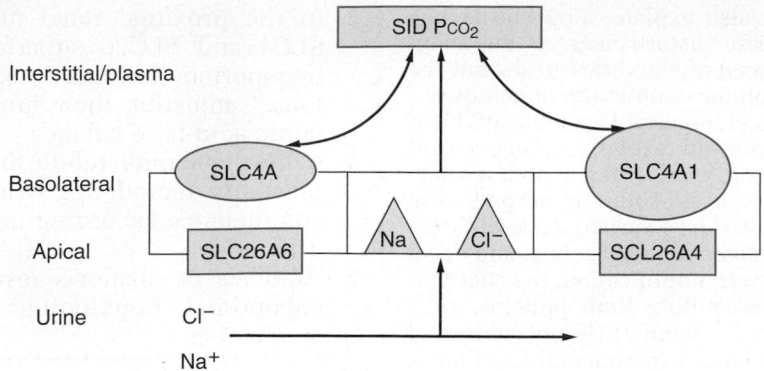

FIGURE 112-4. A proposed model of renal epithelial acid-base transport proteins, plasma strong ion difference (SID), and P_{CO_2}. Defending against volume contraction, proteins encoded by SLC26 (solute carrier family 2 member 6) genes as well as other strong ion transporters reabsorb chloride, sodium, and water. Defending against acidosis, the proteins encoded by SLC4 (solute carrier family 4) genes reabsorb sodium and bicarbonate. The function of the proximal tubule transporters is regulated by plasma SID and P_{CO_2}, whereas the activity of the distal tubule transporters also depends on the distal delivery of chloride. The renal tubule, in association with local paracrine hormones (e.g., cyclic adenosine monophosphate, phosphokinase) and systemic circulating factors (e.g., angiotensin II, aldosterone), functions as a "regulon" of acid-base homeostasis.

with net acid excretion or proton balance. On the other hand, strong ions have a relatively small apparent volume of distribution and do not irreversibly combine with other reactive species. Therefore, a strong ion model may be suitable for exploring the interaction of plasma SID and renal SLC family members.

This leads to the conjecture that homeostasis of the organism is maintained by an equilibrium between two domains, an apical domain that retains acid, expresses proteins encoded by SLC26, and has evolved to conserve salt and water and a basolateral domain that retains base, expresses proteins encoded by SLC4, and has evolved to defend against acidosis.

SLC proteins are regulated by plasma SID and P_{CO_2}, as are plasma pH and HCO_3. Low SID (metabolic acidosis) and high P_{CO_2} (respiratory acidosis) downregulate apically expressed, chloride-retaining SLC26 transporters such as CFEX and pendrin and upregulate basolaterally expressed, Na^+-retaining but Cl^--losing SLC4 transporters such as NBCe1 and AE1. The net effect of these processes maintains plasma pH (Fig. 112-4).

This model is consistent with what is known about the terminal differentiation of embryonic to adult renal epithelium. Minuth and colleagues[38] and Schumacher and coworkers[39] incubated embryonic collecting duct cells obtained from explants of neonatal rabbit kidney in standard Iscove-modified Dulbecco's medium on the basal side, with additional NaCl on the luminal side. Cells cultured under isotonic conditions did not differentiate, but epithelial cells cultured in a luminal-basal gradient developed features of principal and intercalated cells. These observations suggest that differentiation is regulated at least in part by the electrolyte environment.

This model is also consistent with data obtained from knockout mice and human gene mutations.[37,40] Mutations in SLC4A4 are associated with proximal renal tubular acidosis, and those in SLC4A1 with distal renal tubular acidosis, Southeast Asian ovalocytosis, and hereditary spherocytosis.

Mutations in genes encoding proteins that transport strong ions are also associated with acid-base disorders. Metabolic alkalosis (high plasma SID) is observed in gain-of-function mutations of the epithelial Na^+ channel (Liddle's syndrome), due to a disproportionately high rate of Na^+ reabsorption. Metabolic alkalosis is also seen in loss-of-function mutations of the Na^+-K^+-$2Cl^-$ cotransporter (Bartter's syndrome) or Na^+-Cl^- cotransporter (Gitelman's syndrome), owing to a low distal fractional reabsorption of chloride. Metabolic acidosis (low plasma SID) is observed in loss-of-function mutations of the mineralocorticoid receptor or epithelial Na^+ channel (pseudohypoaldosteronism type I), as a result of sodium wasting.

This model lends itself to "back of the envelope" calculations relating plasma pH to renal transport protein expression and function. In the patients investigated by Lemann and associates,[1] one can assume that low SID downregulates the expression of SLC26-encoded CFEX by 25% (despite compensatory hypocapnia), that plasma chloride concentration is raised to 116 mM, and that glomerular filtration rate remains at 100 mL/min. In the initial recovery period, the mean filtered chloride load is ≈16704 mEq/day and the proximal reabsorption of chloride by CFEX is reduced from the expected value of about 4000 mEq/day to about 3000 mEq/day. As a result, the distal delivery of chloride is increased by about 1000 mEq/day. If one then assumes normal fractional distal reabsorption of chloride of 85%, an additional 150 mEq of chloride would appear in the urine (negative balance) accompanied by a decrease in plasma chloride concentration of 9 mM. These approximations are very close to the actual values found in the balance study.

This model also helps explain the phenomenon of chloride-depletion metabolic alkalosis, originally described as a "contraction alkalosis." Galla and coworkers[41] infused either albumin or non–sodium chloride salts to rats that had been dialyzed against 0.15 M $NaHCO_3^-$. Only the administration of chloride corrected the alkalosis, despite a persisting volume contraction. One hypothesis to explain these findings is that metabolic alkalosis stimulated proteins encoded by SLC26 (CFEX in the proximal tubule and pendrin in the distal tubule) and downregulated proteins encoded by SLCA (NBCe1 in the proximal tubule and AE1 in the distal tubule). The tubule, now "primed" to defend against volume contraction, would avidly reabsorb chloride and thereby restore homeostasis.

In summary, analysis of SLC proteins and the strong ion difference leads to a simple model of the renal control mechanisms that govern plasma acid-base balance. The model is consistent with the molecular biology of renal transport proteins, observations made in knockout mice, and human mutations. It also explains how the kidney "compensates" for acid-base disturbances, as the abundance of SLC-encoded transporters varies to defend the organism against either volume contraction or acidosis.

The model also has several important weaknesses. First, the understanding of the role and regulation of many renal transport proteins is evolving, and knockout models sometimes do not provide the expected solution. Second, as in traditional paradigms, the model's variables are SLC (H^+- or HCO_3^--transporting) proteins of the proximal and distal tubule. This is clearly an oversimplification; the contribution of important thick ascending limb proteins, such as ENAC (epithelial sodium channel), is not addressed explicitly. Third, in other than experimental conditions, the interplay of local paracrine and circulating hormones remains poorly understood. For example, by stimulating ENAC and vacuolar H^+-ATPase while simultaneously inhibiting NHE3, aldosterone evokes a disparate affect on renal tubular handling of Na^+ and Cl^- and, thereby, on plasma SID as well as HCO_3^- and H^+ concentrations.[42] Further studies are needed to validate any model that attempts to integrate the action, abundance, and regulation of renal tubular transport proteins with the metrics of systemic acid-base balance.

3. In the proximal renal tubule, members of the SLC4 and SLC26 superfamilies of bicarbonate transporters and anion exchangers act as "regulons," adjusting their function to maintain systemic acid-base balance.
4. In the distal renal tubule, intercalated cells exhibit plasticity, remodeling so as to orient net chloride conductance according to the plasma strong ion difference.
5. Acidosis or alkalosis results from improper or suboptimal functioning of these homeostatic mechanisms.

Key References

6. Boron WF: Acid-base transport by the renal proximal tubule. J Am Soc Nephrol 2006;17:2368-2382.
10. Zhao J, Zhou Y, Boron WF: Effect of isolated removal of either basolateral HCO_3^- or basolateral CO_2 on HCO_3^- reabsorption by rabbit S2 proximal tubule. Am J Physiol Renal Physiol 2003;285:F359-F369.
13. Aronson PS: Ion exchangers mediating Na^+, HCO_3^- and Cl^- transport in the renal proximal tubule. J Nephrol 2006;(Suppl 9):S3-S10.
21. Mount DB, Romero MF: The SLC26 gene family of multifunctional anion exchangers. Pflugers Arch 2003;447:710-721.
33. Fernandez R, Bosqueiro JR, Cassola AC, Malnic G: Role of Cl^- in electrogenic H^+ secretion by cortical distal tubule. J Membr Biol 1997;157:193-201.

See the companion Expert Consult website for the complete reference list.

Key Points

1. Plasma pH is determined by three independent variables: the strong ion difference (SID) value, PCO_2, and the plasma weak acids (A_{tot}).
2. The strong ion difference and PCO_2 values, along with various hormones, paracrine hormones, and other intermediaries, act to regulate renal tubule transport proteins.

CHAPTER 113

Respiratory Acid-Base Physiology

Michael C. Reade and David A. Story

OBJECTIVES

This chapter will:
1. Demonstrate the role of CO_2 as an acid and the role of ventilation in acid-base status.
2. Describe the mechanisms of production, transport, and elimination of CO_2.
3. Outline the physiological mechanisms that maintain CO_2 within a constant range.
4. Compare the effect of net gain or loss of CO_2 in terms of the Stewart and the Henderson-Hasselbalch approaches to acid-base physiology.
5. Outline the mechanisms of compensation for chronic respiratory acid-base changes.

As explained in Chapter 120, respiratory acid-base disorders involve abnormalities in the regulation of carbon dioxide (CO_2).[1] Increased alveolar ventilation decreases the partial pressure of CO_2 (PCO_2) in both the alveolus ($PACO_2$) and arterial blood ($PaCO_2$), causing a respiratory alkalosis. Conversely, reduced alveolar ventilation raises the PCO_2, leading to respiratory acidosis. Changes in CO_2 production can add to these phenomena.

For the last 50 years, clinicians have assumed that the metabolic (nonrespiratory) component of acid-base physiology is determined by bicarbonate.[2] This bicarbonate-centered approach is largely derived from the Henderson-Hasselbalch equation. Like the bicarbonate-centered approach, Stewart's approach to acid-base disorders uses PCO_2 as both the marker and the mechanism for the respiratory side of acid-base physiology.[3,4] In the Stewart approach, however, bicarbonate is a useful marker for assessment of acid-base disorders but is not the mechanism.[2] This means that in the consideration of metabolic compensation for changes in P_{CO_2}, particularly the renal response, changes in the strong ion difference (SID) and weak acids should be examined. One difficulty in this is that much of the underlying research has a bicarbonate-centered approach[5] and must be reassessed.

The Stewart approach uses a definition of *acid* that differs from the Brønsted-Lowry definition of acid as a proton (hydrogen ion) donor.[2] In the Brønsted-Lowry approach, CO_2 is not an acid, but carbonic acid is. Stewart[3] defined an acid as a substance that, when added to a solution, increases the hydrogen ion concentration. With this definition, CO_2 itself is an acid. Another important difference is the view of the role of "buffers," such as hemoglobin and albumin,[3] which with the Stewart approach are considered weak acids. Because of the influence on pH of SID and weak acids (and P_{CO_2}), all three must be analyzed simultaneously.[4] For example, when a solution has more weak acid, the weak acid will exert a greater influence for a given SID or change in SID.

CARBON DIOXIDE PRODUCTION AND TRANSPORT

CO_2 is produced by every human cell as part of the aerobic metabolism of carbohydrate, protein, and fat. CO_2 production is often increased in critical illness because of a higher metabolic rate[6] and with overfeeding.[7] In healthy humans, CO_2 production is approximately 15,000 mmol/day and Pa_{CO_2} is highly dependent on alveolar ventilation.[8] In an average human, if ventilation ceased for 20 minutes, Pa_{CO_2} would rise to 110 mm Hg and pH would fall to 7.03. If renal function ceased for the same period, arterial pH would remain unchanged.[9]

CO_2 tension is highest in the mitochondria, where it is produced, and progresses down a series of gradients to the lungs, where it is excreted. A robust set of mechanisms has evolved to transport CO_2 produced by the tissues to the lungs, and these mechanisms are fundamental to respiratory acid-base physiology (Fig. 113-1).[5]

Almost 90% of CO_2 is transported as bicarbonate ion, formed in the following reaction:

$$CO_2 + H_2O \leftrightarrow H_2CO_3 \leftrightarrow H^+ + HCO_3^-$$

A simplified version is as follows:

$$CO_2 + H_2O \leftrightarrow H^+ + HCO_3^-$$

At equilibrium, at pH 7.40, plasma contains 20 times more HCO_3^- ions than dissolved CO_2.[10] Therefore, about 5% of the carbon dioxide is transported as dissolved gas. The rapid equilibration required during transit of red blood cells through systemic and pulmonary capillaries would not be possible without carbonic anhydrase, which reduces the time to equilibrium between CO_2 and HCO_3^- from more than 1 minute to only a few milliseconds.[11] Carbonic anhydrase is present in red blood cells and pulmonary capillary endothelium but not in plasma.

CO_2 is also carried in blood as carbamino compounds. CO_2 can combine with some amino (NH_2) groups on hemoglobin and, to a much lesser extent, on plasma proteins. About 5% of the arterial CO_2 is in the carbamino form. Deoxygenated hemoglobin more readily forms

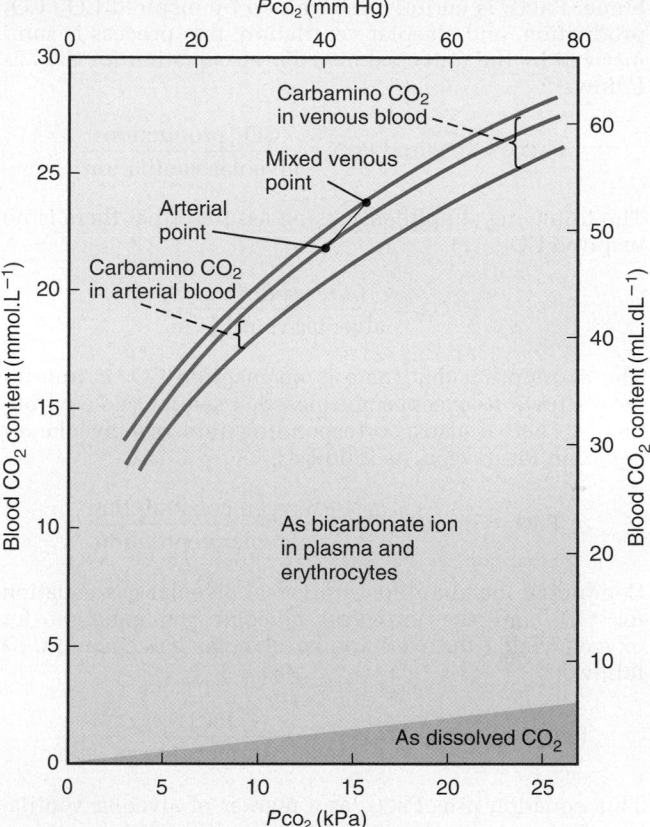

FIGURE 113-1. Components of the CO_2 dissociation curve for whole blood. Dissolved CO_2 and bicarbonate ion vary with P_{CO_2} but are little affected by the state of oxygenation of the hemoglobin (Reduced hemoglobin, being more basic, does cause a slight increase in formation of bicarbonate ion). Carbamino carriage of CO_2 is strongly influenced by the state of oxygenation of hemoglobin but hardly at all by P_{CO_2}. (Redrawn from Lumb AB: Nunn's Applied Respiratory Physiology, 6th ed. Philadelphia, Elsevier, 2005.)

carbamino compounds. These compounds account for the majority of the Haldane effect: For a certain P_{CO_2}, the CO_2 content of deoxygenated hemoglobin is higher than that of oxyhemoglobin. Although carbamino carriage accounts for a relatively small proportion of the total CO_2 in arterial and venous blood, the effect of deoxygenation is such that one third of the extra CO_2 carried by venous blood is due to carbamino compounds (see Fig. 113-1).[5]

Because carbonic anhydrase is not present in plasma, and because plasma proteins are quantitatively much less important than hemoglobin in CO_2 transport, almost all CO_2 is processed in red blood cells. Therefore, most of the CO_2 must diffuse into red blood cells to be processed. Bicarbonate anions are transferred out of red blood cells in exchange for chloride anions. This process alkalinizes the plasma by decreasing plasma chloride and increasing plasma SID.

Carbon Dioxide Elimination and the Carbon Dioxide Steady State

CO_2 is delivered by blood vessels to the lung, where rapid equilibration of gases occurs across the thin alveolar membrane. $PaCO_2$ is entirely determined by inspired CO_2, CO_2 production, and alveolar ventilation; this process is summarized by the universal alveolar air equation for CO_2, as follows[12]:

$$PaCO_2 = \text{inspired } PCO_2 + \frac{CO_2 \text{ production}}{\text{alveolar ventilation}}$$

The following simplified version assumes that there is no inspired CO_2:

$$PaCO_2 = \frac{CO_2 \text{ production}}{\text{alveolar ventilation}}$$

The assumption that there is no inspired CO_2 is true for most situations except some closed or semiclosed environments. There is also a corresponding universal alveolar air equation for oxygen, as follows[12]:

$$PaO_2 = \text{inspired } PO_2 - \frac{\text{oxygen consumption}}{\text{alveolar ventilation}}$$

Combining the simplified universal alveolar gas equation for CO_2 and the universal alveolar gas equation for oxygen yields the well-known alveolar gas equation, as follows:

$$PaO_2 = \text{inspired } PO_2 - \frac{PaCO_2}{\text{respiratory exchange ratio}}$$

This equation uses $PaCO_2$ as a marker of alveolar ventilation because alveolar ventilation is difficult to measure. Unfortunately, this equation also gives the false impression that changes in oxygen due to changes in alveolar ventilation are secondary to changes in CO_2.[13]

Normal values at steady state are shown in Figure 113-2. Equilibration of CO_2 across the alveolar membrane is so rapid that the CO_2 contents of arterial blood and alveolar gas are considered equal. In contrast to the effect of pulmonary shunt on arterial oxygen, even a substantial shunt of blood through the lungs without exposure to alveolar gas has only a minimal effect on arterial CO_2 content. For example, a 30% shunt causes a CO_2 gradient of only 2 mm Hg between alveolar gas and arterial blood.[5]

When considering the effect of a sudden alteration of ventilation on the CO_2 content of the body, one must realize that the body's CO_2 is conceptually contained in three separate compartments that are affected by alveolar ventilation at different rates. CO_2 in the lungs and central circulation equilibrates rapidly with alveolar gas. A sudden rise in alveolar ventilation produces an equally rapid fall in the CO_2 concentration of the central compartment. However, CO_2 in skeletal muscle falls less rapidly, and CO_2 in fat and other poorly perfused tissues falls least rapidly of all. In contrast, a sudden reduction in alveolar ventilation does not cause an equally rapid rise in the CO_2 concentration in the central compartment, because the rate of CO_2 production is unchanged. Even in complete apnea, when all CO_2 is retained, the rate of rise of arterial PCO_2 is only 3 mm Hg/min.[5]

Ventilation-Perfusion Matching

In both healthy and diseased lungs, alveolar ventilation and perfusion are not matched across the lung. The ideal ventilation-perfusion ratio is 1 but ranges from 0 (perfused

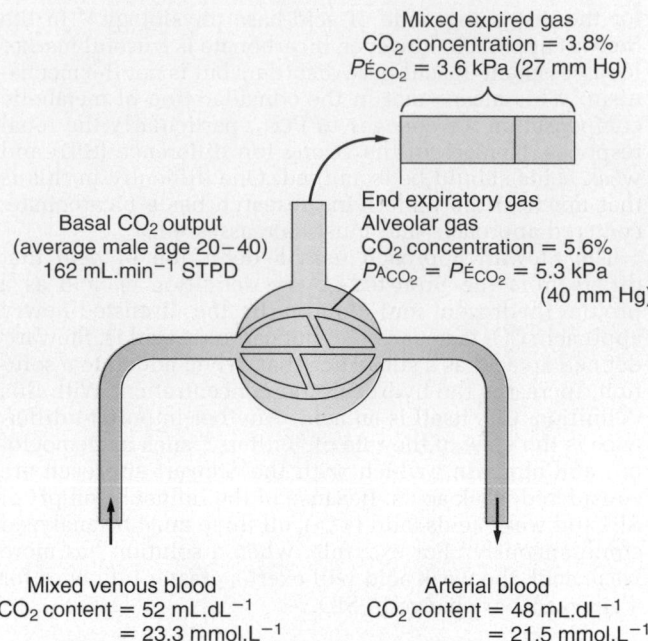

FIGURE 113-2. Normal values of CO_2 levels. These normal values are rounded off, with the small differences in PCO_2 among end-expiratory gas, alveolar gas, and arterial blood ignored. Actual values of PCO_2 depend mainly on alveolar ventilation, but the differences depend on maldistribution; the alveolar/end-tidal expiratory PCO_2 difference depends on alveolar dead space, and the very small arterial-alveolar PCO_2 difference on shunt. Scatter of $\dot{V}/\dot{Q}$ ratios makes a small contribution to both alveolar/end-expiratory and arterial-alveolar PCO_2 gradients. The arterial/mixed venous CO_2 content difference is directly proportional to CO_2 output and inversely proportional to cardiac output. A, alveolar; a, arterial; $\bar{E}$, mixed expired; E', end-expiratory; STPD, standard temperature and pressure, dry; $\bar{v}$, mixed venous. (Redrawn from Lumb AB: Nunn's Applied Respiratory Physiology, 6th ed. Philadelphia, Elsevier, 2005.)

but not ventilated) to infinity (ventilated but not perfused). In the healthy lung, this ventilation-perfusion mismatch is often due to gravitational effects. In disease (see Chapter 131) there is often much greater mismatch. Various strategies attempt to quantify the extent and type of mismatch. One of the most sophisticated is the multiple inert gas elimination technique (MIGET), which reduces the continuous spectrum of ventilation-perfusion matching to 50 compartments of varying ventilation-perfusion matching. MIGET allows detailed quantitative analysis of ventilation-perfusion matching in a variety of physiological and pathological settings.[5]

Another approach used clinically is to reduce the ventilation-perfusion spectrum to three compartments. The first compartment is the "ideal compartment," where ventilation and perfusion are matched, a ratio of 1. A second compartment compresses all lung units with ventilation-perfusion less than 1 into the shunt group, as if all the units were perfused but had no ventilation. The third compartment compresses all units with ventilation-perfusion ratios greater than 1 into the dead space group, as if all the units were ventilated but not perfused. The Bohr equation allows us to calculate the proportion of tidal volume that goes to "unventilated" dead space units.

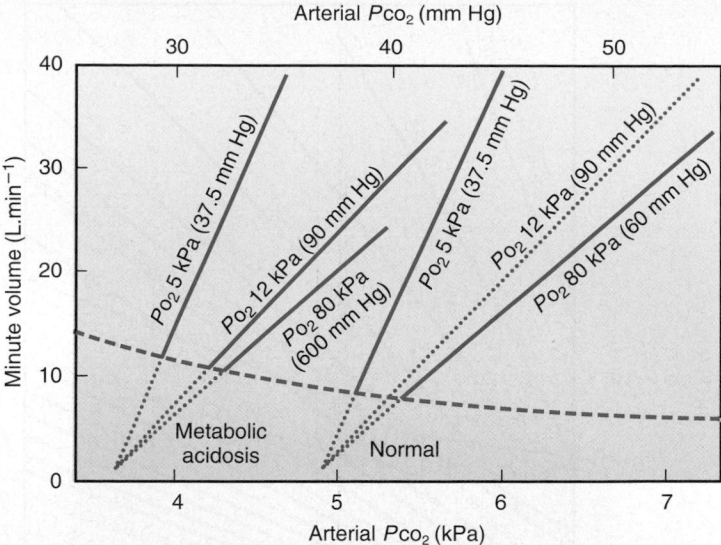

FIGURE 113-3. Two fan plots of the $PaCO_2$/ventilation response at different values of PaO_2. The X axis represents the arterial PCO_2 in either kilopascals (*bottom*) or mm Hg (*top*). The Y axis represents the minute ventilation in liters per minute. The right-hand fan represents the normal metabolic acid-base state (base excess = 0). The left-hand fan represents metabolic acidosis. Each line of the fan represents the response to a particular PaO_2 as shown in parentheses. The *dotted line* represents the $PaCO_2$ that would be seen at rest and at a basal metabolic rate for that given ventilation expressed as minute volume. The intersection between the *dashed line curve* and any of the fan lines indicates the resting $PaCO_2$ and the ventilation that would be seen for that relevant metabolic state and PaO_2. This figure shows that, in metabolic acidosis, for a given ventilation, the $PaCO_2$ is markedly lower and that the response to hypoxemia is maintained. (Redrawn from Lumb AB: Nunn's Applied Respiratory Physiology, 6th ed. Philadelphia, Elsevier, 2005.)

Therefore, even with tidal volume fixed, as the dead space increases, the effective alveolar ventilation falls. This effective decrease in alveolar ventilation raises the $PaCO_2$. For restoration of the usual $PaCO_2$, the minute ventilation must rise.

Control of Carbon Dioxide Elimination

Highly soluble CO_2 crosses the blood-brain barrier and dissociates in the cerebrospinal fluid to form HCO_3^- and H^+. The H^+ is sensed by central chemoreceptor in the medulla,[14] which responds to an increase in H^+ concentration by stimulating an increase in alveolar ventilation. An increase in arterial CO_2 thus stimulates an increase in CO_2 elimination by the lung, completing the feedback loop. A rise in arterial H^+ concentration (as in metabolic acidosis) has less effect on ventilation than a rise in CO_2, because the blood-brain barrier is relatively impermeable to H^+.[15] Metabolic acidosis does increase alveolar ventilation, but by a peripheral rather than central effect (see later). Factors other than CO_2 can cause isolated changes in cerebrospinal fluid pH. For example, the reduction in cerebrospinal fluid pH after intracranial hemorrhage stimulates hyperventilation.[16]

If alveolar ventilation does not increase in response to raised arterial CO_2 (if, for example, the patient is mechanically ventilated), the cerebrospinal fluid H^+ concentration gradually returns to normal (reviewed by Lumb[5]). In the past this phenomenon has been explained with bicarbonate mechanisms, but the actual mechanism is an increased SID. The ventilatory response to arterial CO_2 is thus reset to a new level.

Arterial CO_2 is not the only influence on alveolar ventilation. Peripheral chemoreceptors in the carotid bodies stimulate an increase in alveolar ventilation in response to hypoxia, acidemia, raised temperature, and drugs such as nicotine and doxapram (reviewed by Lumb[5]). In terms of the control of CO_2, these peripherally sensed influences change the slope of the $PaCO_2$/alveolar ventilation curve, shown in Figure 113-3. Of note in this figure is the divergence from the straight line as $PaCO_2$ falls, illustrating one further influence on the control of $PaCO_2$. Although receptor-mediated influences might demand very low alveolar ventilation (even apnea), a conscious subject's higher cortical centers prevent ventilation from falling below a certain point. When cortical input is abolished (as, for example, under anesthesia), this effect is not present. Hyperventilated, hyperoxic anesthetized patients are often apneic—a state that does not occur during consciousness. At the other extreme, cortical input is an important factor in the control of ventilation during exercise, in which $PaCO_2$ falls despite increased production.[5] The net effect of these control mechanisms is to keep the arterial CO_2 tension between 35 and 45 mm Hg in the conscious, healthy person. Numerous disorders can interfere with this control mechanism; they are discussed in Chapter 136.

One further point is worthy of comment. CO_2 easily crosses cell membranes. Changes in plasma CO_2 are rapidly reflected in intracellular pH. This is not true of changes in A_{tot} (the total concentration of nonvolatile weak acids in plasma) or SID. Respiratory acid-base disorders thus have a more rapid effect on intracellular pH than do changes in A_{tot} and SID. Additionally, regulation of $PaCO_2$ cannot be a physiological mechanism for inducing a differential pH between adjacent body compartments.

MECHANISMS OF COMPENSATION FOR RESPIRATORY ACID-BASE DISORDERS

In the bicarbonate-centered Henderson-Hasselbalch approach to acid-base chemistry, a persistently increased H^+ due to raised CO_2 is buffered by increased HCO_3^- production and resorption by the kidney. The Stewart approach to acid-base chemistry deals with compensation for persistently elevated CO_2 and H^+/HCO_3^- differently. According to this approach, the independent influences on plasma pH and HCO_3^- are PCO_2, A_{tot}, and SID. Chronic elevation of PCO_2 causes a rise in the SID (Fig. 113-4) brought about by the kidney, which excretes chloride and retains sodium. The mechanisms for this process are discussed in detail in Chapter 121, but a summary should suffice here: Basically, excretion of

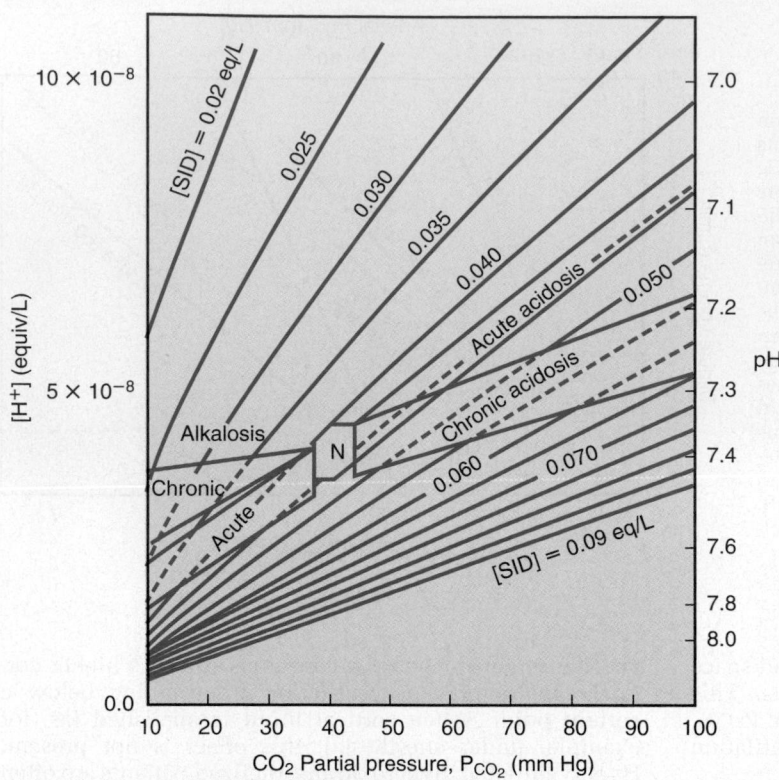

FIGURE 113-4. The H^+ concentration–P_{CO_2} diagram for plasma, with superimposed areas to indicate normal values (N) and common ranges of values for patients with acute or chronic P_{CO_2} abnormalities, labeled *acidosis* and *alkalosis*. SID, strong ion difference. (Redrawn from Stewart PA: How to Understand Acid-Base: A Quantitative Acid-Base Primer for Biology and Medicine. New York, Elsevier, 1981.)

chloride with ammonium cations (NH_4^+) is accomplished, allowing sodium to be retained while electroneutrality is maintained.[17] This process is associated with, but not caused by, an increase in HCO_3^-. Patients with renal disease are not able to compensate as well for respiratory acidosis. When renal function is intact, the compensation takes a few days to occur. It is unclear whether this delay is a necessary consequence of the cellular changes required or whether it exists as a control mechanism to avoid excessive sensitivity to transient changes in alveolar ventilation.

A number of studies have investigated the adaptations of the kidney to chronic respiratory acidosis and alkalosis from an enzyme and gene expression perspective. Ruiz and colleagues[18] found that the maximal transport velocity of the proximal tubule basolateral Na^+-HCO_3^- and luminal Na^+-H^+ transporters (responsible for Na^+ retention) were highly correlated with plasma (H^+) in hypercapnia and hypocapnia in rabbits. Eiam-ong and coworkers[19] reported similar results after examining the H^+,K^+-ATPase and H^+-ATPase in the rat collecting duct.

CONCLUSION

The metabolic production of CO_2 represents the largest acid load with which the body must deal. CO_2 is rapidly eliminated by ventilation. Any interference with the control or mechanism of ventilation rapidly alters the acid-base balance of all cells in the body. The mechanism of this alteration and that of renal compensation for prolonged respiratory acid-base abnormalities have been discussed. Chapter 136 explores the pathophysiology of respiratory acidosis and alkalosis in more detail.

Key Points

1. CO_2 is one of the three independent determinants of plasma pH (the others being strong ion difference and the total concentration of nonvolatile weak acids in plasma [A_{tot}]).
2. CO_2 is a product of metabolism, and its effect on pH would be much larger than that of any other metabolic acid in the absence of highly efficient mechanisms of sensing, control, transport, and elimination.
3. Carbonic anhydrase is essential to the carriage of CO_2 in the blood as well as the renal handling of acid-base chemistry.
4. Physiological mechanisms involving the strong ion difference partially correct pH in response to chronically abnormal levels of CO_2.

Key References

2. Story DA: Bench-to-bedside review: A brief history of clinical acid-base. Crit Care 2004;8:253-258.
3. Stewart PA: How to Understand Acid-Base: A Quantitative Acid-Base Primer for Biology and Medicine. New York, Elsevier, 1981.
5. Lumb AB: Nunn's Applied Respiratory Physiology, 6th ed. Philadelphia, Elsevier, 2005.
8. Kellum JA: Determinants of blood pH in health and disease. Crit Care 2000;4:6-14.
13. Story DA: Alveolar oxygen partial pressure, alveolar carbon dioxide partial pressure, and the alveolar gas equation. Anesthesiology 1996;84:1011.

See the companion Expert Consult website for the complete reference list.

CHAPTER 114

Pathophysiology of Hyperlactatemia

Barry A. Mizock

> **OBJECTIVES**
>
> This chapter will:
> 1. Discuss the major factors that modulate lactate production and utilization during critical illness.
> 2. Review acid-base aspects of lactic acidosis (LA).

Lactate has traditionally been viewed as a toxic metabolic byproduct of excessive anaerobic glycolysis. This view in turn has engendered therapeutic approaches to hyperlactatemia directed at enhancing lactate removal (e.g., dialysis, dichloroacetate). However, this view has been challenged, and lactate is now recognized to play an important role in maintaining cellular bioenergetics. The pathogenesis of acidosis in hyperlactatemic states is also controversial.

PATHOPHYSIOLOGY

An increase in blood lactate ultimately reflects an imbalance between production and utilization. Lactate may be viewed as a metabolic "dead end," because its generation and removal both require transition through pyruvate as catalyzed by lactate dehydrogenase (LDH). Any condition raising the concentration of pyruvate further enhances lactate production by virtue of mass action[1,2]—that is, greater availability of pyruvate augments lactate production without altering the kinetic rates between substrates. All tissues produce lactate, but skeletal muscle, because of its large mass, has the greatest potential.[2] The most important determinant of pyruvate (and lactate) production is glycolytic flux.[1-3] Pyruvate production may also be increased by transamination of alanine to pyruvate.[4] This mechanism plays a significant role in enhancing lactate production during sepsis.[5] The major factors that increase glycolytic flux during critical illness are (1) a decrease in the tissue phosphorylation state, (2) hormones (especially epinephrine), (3) inflammatory cytokines (e.g., tumor necrosis factor [TNF]), and (4) alkalemia (Fig. 114-1). The *phosphorylation state* is expressed by the following ratio:

$$\frac{ADP + ATP}{AMP + ADP + ATP}$$

where ADP is adenosine diphosphate. The phosphorylation state may be reduced by either a decrease in synthesis of adenosine triphosphate (ATP) (e.g., secondary to tissue hypoperfusion) or an increase in energy demand.

It had previously been thought that LA during shock resulted from increased "anaerobic" glycolysis consequent to global oxygen delivery below the critical oxygen delivery threshold. Connett and associates[6] proposed that the term *dysoxia* be used to describe conditions in which cytochrome turnover is limited by oxygen delivery. However, the clinical significance of a dysoxic stimulus for lactate production is questionable, given the results of a study finding that the critical delivery threshold in septic and nonseptic humans was approximately 4 mL/kg/min, a value 50% lower than previously thought and that would be very uncommon in patients who were actively treated.[7] In this context, hyperlactatemia can be viewed as an unreliable indicator of dysoxia.

According to Connett and associates,[6] the state of tissue oxygenation in the majority of patients with shock is best described by the term *adapted cell hypoxia*. In this physiological state, tissue oxygenation is less than that in the absence of stress but sufficient to maintain oxygen and ATP flux because of adaptive changes in cellular metabolism. These changes can be briefly summarized. A drop in the phosphorylation state enhances aerobic glycolysis in skeletal muscle by stimulating the rate-limiting enzyme phosphofructokinase. This stimulus in turn raises the concentration of lactate in the cytosol. Lactate is then "shuttled" into the mitochondria, where it supports ATP synthesis by (1) supplying reducing equivalents for the respiratory chain and (2) converting to pyruvate by means of mitochondrial LDH, with subsequent oxidation. Aerobic formation of lactate is thus a mechanism by which the cytosol and mitochondria interact to maintain adequate oxidative synthesis of ATP in skeletal muscle.[8] Evidence supporting the presence of a lactate shuttle in cardiac muscle and liver has also been reported.[9] As stated by Leverve,[10] "hyperlactatemia in patients with circulatory compromise may be best viewed as a sentinel that signals the upper limit for metabolic adaptation that is not necessarily linked to inadequate oxygen delivery."

Lactate production in skeletal muscle may also be enhanced by hormones (e.g., epinephrine, insulin). James and colleagues[11] observed that in septic or hemorrhagic animal models, lactate production in muscle was markedly increased by virtue of a β_2-adrenergic receptor–mediated increase in activity of Na^+-K^+ membrane pumps.[11] The resultant activation of Na^+,K^+-ATPase generated ADP, which in turn augmented aerobic glycolytic flux. This mechanism has been confirmed in humans with septic shock.[12] Inflammatory cytokines (e.g., tumor necrosis factor) promote an increase in lactate production by stimulating glucose uptake and glycolytic flux in tissue macrophages.[2,13] This mechanism is important in the pathogenesis of hyperlactatemia accompanying systemic inflammatory states. Alkalemia enhances glycolysis through stimulation of phosphofructokinase; however, the resultant increase in blood lactate is generally mild.

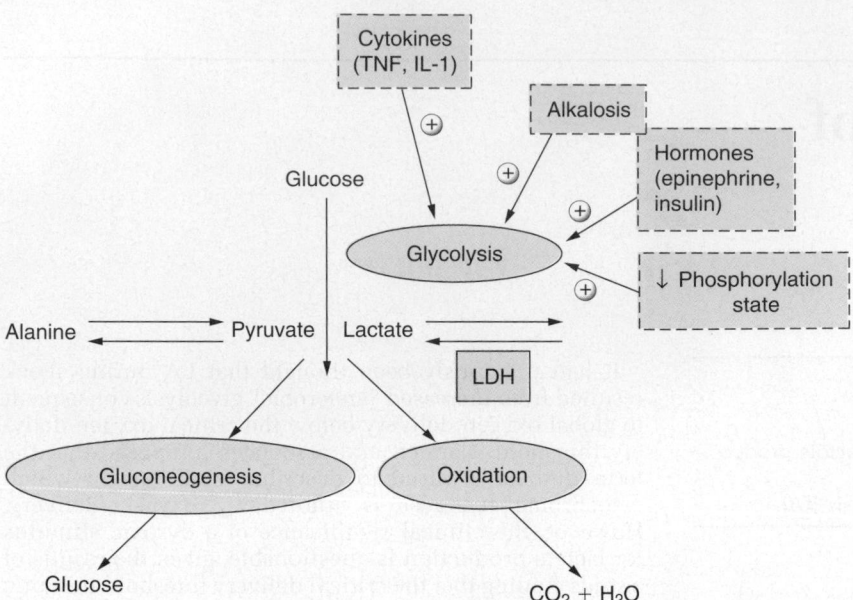

FIGURE 114-1. Production and utilization of lactate. IL-1, interleukin-1; LDH, lactate dehydrogenase; TNF, tumor necrosis factor.

The liver is the major organ of lactate clearance, metabolizing approximately 40% to 50% of daily lactate production. Uptake (and egress) of lactate in liver and other organs occurs as the consequence of facilitated transport by a family of monocarboxylate transporters.[14] This process is saturable and involves cotransport of H$^+$.[14] Lactate is metabolized in liver through oxidation and gluconeogenesis; the relative importance of these processes varies according to the underlying physiological state. Gluconeogenesis appears to predominate during health, whereas oxidation assumes a more important role in the setting of critical illness. The liver has substantial functional reserve, and hepatic dysfunction per se does not generally result in significant hyperlactatemia unless concomitant factors increase lactate production. In addition, other organs also participate in the metabolism of lactate. A human study performed during the anhepatic phase of liver transplantation showed that the steady-state concentration of lactate in blood increased by only 1 mm/L after the liver was removed.[15] The kidney metabolizes lactate through oxidation and gluconeogenesis. An animal study indicated that approximately 30% of infused lactate was removed by the kidneys.[16] The relative contributions of oxidation and gluconeogenesis are influenced by physiological state and pH. Acidosis decreases renal lactate oxidation but increases its conversion to glucose. Hypoglycemia enhances renal gluconeogenesis from lactate (presumably mediated by epinephrine). Although lactate is freely filtered by the glomerulus, more than 95% is reabsorbed. Urinary loss of lactate may occur during severe hyperlactatemia, but the total amount is relatively small ($\geq$2% of total lactate removal).[17] The heart takes up lactate for oxidation, especially during hyperlactatemia. Oxidation of lactate may satisfy up to 60% of myocardial energy needs and, because it may be directly oxidized, is a more efficient energy source than glucose.[9] Lactate has a positive inotropic effect, and removal of lactate via dichloroacetate has been shown to reduce cardiac performance.[18] Wounds have also been shown to oxidize lactate in preference to glucose.[19]

In summary, critical illness is commonly accompanied by enhanced glycolytic flux and lactate production. An increase in blood lactate in this setting is best viewed as the manifestation of an adaptive stress response rather than as a reflection of cellular dysoxia.

ACID-BASE ASPECTS OF HYPERLACTATEMIA

The mechanism by which acidosis accompanies increased glycolytic production of lactate is controversial. In 1978, Zilva[20] proposed that anaerobic glycolysis was not acidifying[20]; that is, that glycolytic flux generates lactate, ATP, and water but does not directly produce lactic acid. This researcher postulated that the acidosis accompanying hyperlactatemia occurred as the consequence of increased H$^+$ production resulting from unreversed cytoplasmic ATP hydrolysis, as follows:

$$ATP \rightarrow ADP + P + H^+$$

In this view, a decrease in oxidative regeneration of ATP consequent to tissue hypoperfusion results in an accumulation of H$^+$ and a fall in pH. Conversely, in the setting of maintained oxidative metabolism, H$^+$ is buffered when ATP is reconstituted (providing a potential explanation for the occurrence of hyperlactatemia in the absence of acidosis). However, Bellomo and Ronco[21] questioned the concept of unreversed ATP hydrolysis. In reality, ATP is converted to ADP and orthophosphate (a very weak acid; pK_a = 6.8). If unreversed ATP hydrolysis were occurring, one would also expect to see increased plasma phosphate, which is not the case. In addition, severe septic shock would result in profound ATP depletion, which has not been documented.[22] Finally, the rise in acidity would be small because the total amount of ATP in the body is less than 0.1 mol. A more likely explanation is provided by Stewart's physicochemical theory of acid-base.[23] In this view, an increase in concentration of a strong anion such as lactate results in a relative excess in anionic charge in the blood. Electroneutrality is maintained by an increase in [H$^+$] consequent to enhanced dissociation of water, which in turn promotes a fall in pH (see Chapter 111).

Although severe hyperlactatemia (e.g., serum lactate > 10 mM/L) is generally accompanied by acidemia, the correlation between lactate and pH may not be tight with less severe hyperlactatemia. Critically ill patients with hypermetabolic stress (e.g., sepsis, burn, trauma) commonly display a modest elevation in lactate (e.g., serum lactate 2-5 mM/L), which can occur in the absence of acidemia. The term *stress hyperlactatemia* has been proposed to describe this state.[24] As described previously, it was postulated that greater lactate production is not necessarily acidifying provided that oxidative metabolism is maintained, because H^+ ions are consumed when ATP is regenerated. However, it is more plausible that a normal pH is preserved because of intracellular buffering of H^+ or, more likely, as the consequence of an intracellular shift of chloride, thereby maintaining the strong ion difference.[25] In addition, increased production of unmeasured cations has been described during critical illness and could also serve to counterbalance excess anionic charge.[26] It is therefore unlikely that the lack of acidosis during hyperlactatemic stress reflects a distinct pathogenesis.[27]

CONCLUSION

All tissues produce lactate, but skeletal muscle has the greatest capacity to increase lactate in the blood. Hyperlactatemia results from enhanced aerobic glycolytic flux as the consequence of a decrease in the phosphorylation state and/or a β_2-adrenergic receptor–mediated increase in membrane pump activity. Lactate is an important metabolic intermediate that helps maintain mitochondrial ATP production during critical illness. Significant disturbances in the bioenergetic state are signaled by an increase in lactate in the blood. Lactate can therefore be viewed as a sentinel that monitors cellular energy charge in muscle. The presence of hyperlactatemia is an important indicator of a potentially serious disorder and should prompt further evaluation by the clinician.

Key Points

1. An increase in blood lactate level has poor specificity as an indicator of tissue dysoxia.
2. Increased lactate production during circulatory shock results from enhanced aerobic glycolysis in skeletal muscle secondary to a β_2-adrenergic receptor–mediated stimulation of membrane Na^+-K^+ pumps.
3. Lactate production by tissue macrophages also plays a significant role in the pathogenesis of hyperlactatemia in patients with a systemic inflammatory response (e.g., sepsis, burn, trauma).
4. Acidosis accompanying hyperlactatemia is not the result of unreversed hydrolysis of adenosine triphosphate. It is best explained by the physicochemical theory of acid-base balance.

Key References

6. Connett RJ, Honig CR, Gayeski TEJ, Brooks GA: Defining hypoxia: A systems view of VO_2, glycolysis, energetics, and intracellular PO_2. J Appl Physiol 1990;68:833-842.
9. Brooks GA, Dubouchaud H, Brown M, et al: Role of mitochondrial lactate dehydrogenase and lactate oxidation in the intracellular lactate shuttle. Proc Nat Acad Sci U S A 1999;96:1129-1134.
10. Leverve XM: Lactic acidosis: A new insight? Minerva Anestesiol 1999;65:205-209.
11. James JH, Luchette FA, McCarter FD, Fischer JE: Lactate is an unreliable indicator of tissue hypoxia in injury or sepsis. Lancet 1999;354:505-508.
12. Levy B, Gibot S, Franck P, et al: Relation between muscle Na^+K^+ ATPase activity and raised lactate concentrations in septic shock: A prospective study. Lancet 2005;365:871-875.

See the companion Expert Consult website for the complete reference list.

CHAPTER 115

Impact of Acid-Base Disorders on Different Organ Systems

Kyle J. Gunnerson

OBJECTIVES

This chapter will:
1. Describe the unique organ system effects of different acid-base disorders.
2. Discuss the effects of hypercapnia with potential use of CO_2 as a therapeutic strategy in acute respiratory distress syndrome and ischemic reperfusion injury.
3. Emphasize that metabolic acidosis affects virtually all organ systems and different etiologies of metabolic acidosis have different effects.
4. Explain that intracellular pH appears to be the major force affecting cellular and organ function.
5. Explain that the role of extracellular pH on organ function usually depends on how it affects intracellular pH.

It is not uncommon for critically ill patients to have disturbances in acid-base equilibrium. Extracellular acid-base disorders have been recognized for many years and form the historical base of the understanding of the body's regulation of pH. New findings have led to an appreciation of the complexity and tight regulation of intracellular pH (pH_i). It is becoming apparent that pH_i may be more important in cellular function. Observations of the effects that extracellular pH has on organ systems may be a representation of their effect on pH_i. The etiology (respiratory vs. metabolic) and duration of acid-base alterations also determine how they affect organ function.

Conventional thought holds that acid-base imbalance is more a result, or marker, of organ dysfunction than a cause. The association of organ dysfunction with worsening metabolic acidosis has been known for some time in a variety of states—burns,[1] trauma,[2,3] advanced age,[4] vascular injury,[5] and sepsis.[6] However, a growing body of literature suggests that acid-base disturbances, most commonly metabolic acidosis, not only may be a consequence of but also may contribute to organ, tissue, and cellular dysfunction. This chapter reviews how acute acid-base disturbances may affect various organ systems.

ALKALOSIS

Metabolic Alkalosis

Metabolic alkalosis is a commonly encountered acid-base disturbance in hospitalized patients, accounting for up to 50% of all acid-base disturbances in one study.[7] The causes of metabolic alkalosis are commonly iatrogenic and result in "chloride responsive" alkalosis (diuretics, hypokalemia, nasogastric suctioning, and vomiting). Other, less common forms are hyperaldosteronism, inborn errors of metabolism, and cationic excess (otherwise known as bicarbonate excess). Mild metabolic alkalosis is well tolerated, and symptoms are usually not apparent until the pH exceeds 7.50. In this mild stage, most signs and symptoms are related to the underlying pathology, such as diuretic-induced hypovolemia. However, severe metabolic alkalosis has been associated with mortality as high as 80% if the pH is greater than 7.65.[8] Although the relationship is not causal, this mortality association should be viewed with concern. Table 115-1 summarizes the effects of metabolic alkalosis.

Cardiovascular Effects

Metabolic alkalosis affects the cardiovascular system mostly through conduction disturbances. Hypokalemia-induced cardiac arrhythmias can be observed during alkalotic states. Severe alkalosis has also been associated with decreased coronary blood flow and increased myocardial oxygen demand.[9,10] However, this alkalosis-mediated myocardial ischemia appears to be more common in respiratory alkalosis.

Renal and Electrolyte Effects

Electrolyte abnormalities are common with disturbances in physiological pH and are associated with a wide range of symptoms. Severe alkalemia increases protein binding of ionized calcium, thus leading to hypocalcemia. Hypocalcemia is the most likely explanation for the central nervous system (CNS) alterations associated with metabolic alkalosis, such as lethargy, headache, delirium, seizures, and coma.[11] Hypokalemia, which is an almost invariable consequence of metabolic alkalosis, can itself also cause metabolic alkalosis. In chloride-responsive metabolic alkalosis due to the most common causes, potassium loss is largely due to increased renal excretion. Actually, any condition that elevates serum aldosterone levels (i.e., hypovolemia) enhances sodium reabsorption at the expense of potassium and hydrogen ion excretion.[12]

Metabolic alkalosis can also stimulate anaerobic glycolysis and increase the production of lactic acid and ketones.[13] Ammoniagenesis also increases owing to greater renal ammonium (NH_4) uptake in the setting of hypokalemia. This situation may contribute to mental status alterations in patients with hepatic encephalopathy.[14]

TABLE 115-1

The Effects of Metabolic Alkalosis on Various Organ Systems

Cardiovascular	Impaired coronary artery blood flow—severe alkalosis
	Increased myocardial oxygen consumption
	Myocardial ischemia—more common in respiratory alkalosis
	Dysrhythmias—QT prolongation
	Coronary artery vasoconstriction
	Decreased inotropy—decreased cytosolic calcium
Pulmonary	Hypoventilation
	Respiratory depression
	Increased 2,3-diphosphoglyceric acid (late)
	Increased hemoglobin O_2 affinity
Central nervous	Cerebral vasculature vasoconstriction
	Decreased cerebral blood flow
	Altered mental status—may be due to hypocalcemia
	Coma—severe alkalosis
	Seizures—severe alkalosis and hypocalcemia
	Neuromuscular irritability—hypocalcemia
Endocrine—metabolic	Increased anaerobic glycolysis
	Increased lactic acid
	Increased ketone production
	Increased protein binding to calcium
Renal—electrolyte	Hypokalemia
	Hypocalcemia
	Hypernatremia
	Increased renal absorption of ammonium
	Hypophosphatemia
	Hypomagnesemia

Alkalemia has been shown to alter cardiovascular and cerebral perfusion by causing arteriolar vasoconstriction.[9,15] Clinical CNS abnormalities observed include headache, lethargy, delirium, seizures, and coma. Alkalemia can also depress respiration, resulting in hypercapnia and hypoxemia, which may contribute to difficulty in weaning a patient from mechanical ventilation.

To a large extent, the observed clinical findings in alkalemia can be attributed to metabolic and electrolyte disturbances, such as hypokalemia. Hypokalemia is commonly associated with alkalemia, more so with metabolic etiologies. Hypokalemia itself has several adverse effects, such as arrhythmias, neuromuscular weakness, polyuria, rhabdomyolysis, and increased ammoniagenesis.[16]

Respiratory Alkalosis

Respiratory alkalosis, or hypocapnic alkalosis, is a result of increased minute ventilation and is usually well tolerated with few apparent effects. Hypocapnia is often a physiological response to underlying problems (e.g., hypoxia, increased metabolic demands, metabolic acidosis). Other causes, such as pain, anxiety, and some CNS disorders, increase minute ventilation without a specific physiological need. Hypocapnia may cause some mild immediate symptoms, such as confusion, dizziness, par-

TABLE 115-2

The Effects of Respiratory Alkalosis on Various Organ Systems

Cardiovascular	Increased cardiac contractility—increased myocardial oxygen consumption
	Increased systemic vascular resistance
	Increased risk of thrombosis—platelet aggregation
	Dysrhythmias—supraventricular tachydysrhythmias
	Cardiac ischemia
Pulmonary	Increased airway resistance
	Increased microvasculature permeability
	Decreased lung compliance
	Direct parenchymal lung injury
	Altered surfactant function
	Attenuated hypoxic pulmonary vasoconstriction
	Increased intrapulmonary shunting
	Associated with poor outcomes in ALI and acute respiratory distress syndrome
	Increased hemoglobin O_2 affinity
	Decreased systemic oxygen delivery
Central nervous	Cerebral vasculature vasoconstriction
	Decreased cerebral blood flow
	Decreased intracranial pressure
	Improved cerebral vasculature autoregulation
	Increased cerebral oxygen demand
	Increased anaerobic metabolism and lactate
	Potential to cause cerebral ischemia
Ischemia-reperfusion (IR)	Increased oxidative stress in IR cardiomyocytes
	Accentuates cerebral IR injury in cardiac arrest
	May attenuate IR small bowel injury (controversial)
	May cause direct hepatocellular injury—decreased blood flow

esthesesias, and muscle cramps or spasms. Chronic hypocapnia is usually asymptomatic. Organ systems affected by respiratory alkalosis are mainly the CNS, cardiovascular system, and pulmonary system (Table 115-2).

Central Nervous System Effects

The CNS response to carbon dioxide has been extensively studied, specifically in regard to cerebral blood flow (CBF) and perfusion. Nitric oxide is a well-known cerebrovascular modulator, but carbon dioxide can also be a very potent modulator of CBF. For every 1–mm Hg change in PCO_2, there is a 3% to 5% change in CBF. Basically, hypercapnia causes cerebral vessels to dilate, whereas hypocapnia causes them to constrict. This fact is reflected in the improvement of the autoregulatory capacity of the cerebral vasculature during states of hypocapnia and its worsening during hypercapnia. This vascular tone modulation effect is mostly due to carbon dioxide's effect on extracellular pH.[17] The effects of carbon dioxide are mediated through adenosine triphosphate (ATP)–sensitive potassium (K_{ATP}) channels.[18] This response to CO_2 is actually a continuum,

so hypercapnic acidosis triggers K_{ATP} channel opening and hypocapnic alkalosis triggers K_{ATP} channel closing.[19]

CBF is well documented to decrease in hypercapnia, with a resultant reduction in potentially life-threatening intracranial hypertension. This acute, transient change in CBF may be lifesaving during the wait for definitive care. However, these potentially beneficial effects of hypocapnia on intracranial pressure may be outweighed by reduced oxygen delivery. If the reduction in CBF is disproportionately greater than that in intracranial blood volume, cerebral ischemia may occur.[20,21] Additionally, it has been demonstrated that hypocapnia increases neuronal excitability and seizure activity.[22] Hypocapnia also raises cerebral oxygen demand, anaerobic metabolism, and the cerebral lactate production associated with ischemia.[23] Furthermore, there is evidence that hypocapnia during cardiopulmonary resuscitation may exacerbate brain injury and worsen neurological outcome.[24]

Pulmonary Effects

The effect of hypocapnia on pulmonary physiology is observed in the airway resistance, alveolar-capillary permeability, lung compliance, and the pulmonary vasculature. Although hypocapnia is a common component of asthma, whether it has a pathological role is not clear. Hypocapnia has been shown to cause bronchospasm and increasing microvasculature permeability, resulting in an increase in airway resistance.[25] This demonstration supports more than 30 years of clinical observations that hyperventilating during an acute asthma exacerbation would exacerbate a patient's bronchospasm. This hypocapnia-induced bronchospasm appears to be associated with adverse outcomes.[26] Interestingly, alveolar hypocapnia occurs during cardiopulmonary bypass, which can increase airway resistance and decrease lung compliance.; these changes are reversed by the addition of inspired CO_2.[27]

Acute lung injury is another entity commonly associated with both hyperventilation and hypocapnic alkalosis. The deleterious affects initially appeared to be associated primarily with excessive mechanical lung stretch. Historically, hypocapnia has been thought to have been a result rather than a cause of this process. However, in 1971, a small study of patients with post-traumatic acute lung injury showed that hypocapnia was associated with worsened pulmonary function that resolved upon the administration of inhaled CO_2. This early, small study has been the genesis for several subsequent investigations into the pathological nature of hypocapnic alkalosis and how it affects pulmonary physiology. Hypocapnia causes direct parenchymal injury,[20] depletion of lamellar bodies,[29] and greater pulmonary capillary permeability.[30] Surfactant function is altered, reducing overall lung compliance in humans.[31] It also appears that hypocapnia attenuates hypoxic pulmonary vasoconstriction, thereby worsening intrapulmonary shunting and systemic oxygenation.[32] Many of these negative effects are reversed with the administration of inhaled CO_2. It is becoming more apparent that hypocapnia has some causative role in acute lung injury and that hypercapnia may actually be protective.[33]

Cardiovascular Effects

The cardiovascular effects of hypocapnic alkalosis include alterations in vascular tone, cardiac contractility, and dysrhythmias. Systemic vascular resistance and myocardial contractility are both increased during acute episodes of hypocapnia, leading to a decrease in myocardial oxygen delivery in the setting of growing myocardial oxygen demand.[34] Hypocapnia may also induce coronary thrombosis secondary to increased platelet aggregation.[35] The combination of these effects contributes to the angina reported with hypocapnia and may actually have a role in clinically relevant acute coronary syndromes. Dysrhythmias associated with hypocapnia have been observed in critically ill patients as well as those with panic disorder. The dysrhythmias may be due to myocardial ischemia or to direct myocardial effects. Ironically, hypocapnia may actually attenuate dysrhythmias induced by tricyclic antidepressant toxicity or from local anesthetics. In these cases, the alkalosis itself appears to be causal. Lavani and colleagues[36] have reported that in a hypocapnic reperfusion environment, cardiomyocyte cell death occurs faster than in a normocapnia or hypercapnia reperfusion environment. These researchers also found that cardiomyocytes in the hypocapnic environment demonstrated a much larger associated oxidant burst during the first 10 minutes of reperfusion compared with cardiomyocytes in the hypercapnic environment. These findings in an ischemia-reperfusion model suggest that a hypocapnic environment is associated with increased oxidative stress and cell death, whereas a hypercapnic environment attenuates this oxidant burst, improving cardiomyocyte function and survival.[36]

ACIDOSIS

Respiratory Acidosis

Respiratory acidosis, or hypercapnic acidosis, is common in mechanically ventilated patients. It has been known for several years that patients tolerate hypercapnia well. In severe lung disease states, such as acute lung injury, there is an associated mortality benefit for those who are treated with permissive hypercapnia.[37] The mortality benefit has been attributed mostly to a decrease in mechanical lung stretch through the use of lower tidal volumes and pulmonary pressures.[38] A growing body of literature has supported the hypothesis that hypercapnia itself may have some beneficial effect on cellular and organ functions. Table 115-3 summarizes the effects of respiratory acidosis.

Central Nervous System Effects

Neurological consequences of hypercapnia are among the most commonly encountered; in the extreme, they are collectively often referred to as CO_2 narcosis. The severity of the clinical presentation depends on the severity of acidosis, rapidity of the changes in P_{CO_2} and pH, and the presence of concomitant hypoxemia. In acute cases, CO_2 rapidly diffuses across the blood-brain barrier and lowers the cerebrospinal fluid pH. These changes last only about 24 hours because the cerebrospinal fluid bicarbonate concentration rises to normalize the pH. The cerebral vasculature is very sensitive to changes in pH, and acute acidosis results in vasodilation, which increases CBF and cerebral blood volume. The results are a rise in intracranial pressure and a decrease in cerebral compliance.[39,40] These effects appear to be mediated by acute changes in pH,

TABLE 115-3

The Effects of Respiratory Acidosis on Various Organ Systems

Cardiovascular	Myocardial depression—severe acidosis with hypoxia
	Increased inotropy—mild acidosis secondary to increased catecholamine
	Systemic arterial vascular smooth muscle relaxation
	Dysrhythmias—supraventricular tachydysrhythmias
Pulmonary	Hypoxic pulmonary vasoconstriction
	Acute pulmonary hypertension
	Hyperventilation
	Dyspnea—independent of accompanying tachypnea
	Alveolar and arterial hypoxemia
	Decreased 2,3-diphosphoglyceric acid (late)
	Decreased hemoglobin O_2 affinity (Bohr effect)
	Improved survival in acute respiratory distress syndrome—permissive hypercapnia
Central nervous	Cerebral vasculature vasodilation
	Increased cerebral blood flow
	Increased intracranial pressure
	Decreased cerebral compliance
	Stimulation of increased ventilation
	CO_2 narcosis—varying degrees of mental status
Endocrine—metabolic	Sympathetic nervous system stimulation
	Increased cortisol secretion
	Increased epinephrine secretion
	Insulin resistance
Renal—electrolyte	Increased renovascular resistance
	Hypernatremia
	Hyperphosphatemia—release of phosphate from tissue
	Hyperkalemia
Gastrointestinal	Gastroparesis—emesis
	Decreased splanchnic blood flow (controversial)
	Increased splanchnic blood flow (controversial)
Ischemia-reperfusion (IR)	Avoids the "pH paradox"
	Protects cardiomyocytes from IR injury
	Attenuates lipopolysaccharide-induced nuclear factor-κB
	Suppression of interleukin-8
	Reduction in oxidative nitrogen species

because the concomitant use of bicarbonate (titrated to pH 7.4) blocks the response.[41] Some of the clinical CNS manifestations of hypercapnia are altered mental status, headache, irritability, confusion, somnolence, lethargy, and coma. Stupor and coma are seen at high levels of P_{CO_2}, usually exceeding 70 to 100 mm Hg.

Cardiovascular Effects

Hypercapnia appears to affect the cardiovascular system mostly through a greater release of circulating catecholamines (epinephrine and norepinephrine) and by direct peripheral vasodilation through inhibition of vascular smooth muscle.[42-44] Severe hypercapnia is associated with direct myocardial depression, especially if hypoxemia also occurs.[45] An increase in dysrhythmias has been noted (mostly supraventricular tachydysrhythmias), which may be due to concomitant hypoxia, rapid fluctuations in electrolyte levels, and increases in catecholamine levels. Acidosis itself causes a rightward shift of the hemoglobin dissociation curve, favoring unloading of oxygen at the tissue level and thereby improving oxygen delivery.

The hemodynamic effects of permissive hypercapnia vary from direct tissue effects, to local vascular bed reactions, to autonomic nervous system control. In health, it appears that the increased cardiac output that is associated with hypercapnia is due to the rise in circulating catecholamines. The concentration of these catecholamines overcomes the direct depressant effects on the vascular smooth muscle and the myocardium.[43,44] The addition of sodium bicarbonate to correct blood pH has been shown to attenuate the greater catecholamine release.[46]

Pulmonary Effects

Hypercapnia can cause an increase in inspiratory effort sensation independent of the simultaneous rise in minute ventilation that may accompany it. Hypercapnia also leads to reductions in alveolar and arterial partial pressures of oxygen, as predicted by the alveolar air equation. These reductions result in hypoxic pulmonary vasoconstriction and acute pulmonary hypertension.[47] Controversy exists as to what effect hypercapnia truly has in healthy patients, even though there is evidence to support the increases in pulmonary artery pressures and pulmonary vascular resistance. The direct pulmonary vasoconstriction effect of hypercapnia appears to be mediated more by the hydrogen ion concentration than by PCO_2.[48] Hypercapnia does substantially potentiate the vasoconstrictive effects of hypoxia, as seen in patients with acute lung injury. Patients being treated with permissive hypercapnia have higher pulmonary artery pressures even though pulmonary vascular resistance may not have been increased; this effect may be due to increased flow across the pulmonary circulation as a result of a rise in cardiac output.

Renal Effects

Renal hemodynamics appear to be affected by changes in both oxygen and carbon dioxide levels. Patients with hypoxia and chronic obstructive pulmonary disease patients both have a decreased renovascular resistance when hyperoxemia is induced. In contrast, hypercapnia causes a rise in renovascular resistance and appears to override the vasodilating effects of hyperoxemia.[49] The overall effect of renal blood flow in the hypercapnic patient is still unclear. Larrieu and colleagues demonstrated increased cortical and medullary blood flow rates when the hypercapnia increased cardiac output. However, other investigators have shown an actual decrease in total and effective renal blood flow rates upon an increase in renal vascular resistance, resulting in a reduction in glomerular filtration rate during hypercapnia.[50] The higher renal vascular resistance appears to be secondary to an increase in local sympathetic nerve activity, as mediated by peripheral chemoreceptors[51] or higher concentrations of catecholamines and renin.[50]

Gastrointestinal Effects

The effect of hypercapnic acidosis on the gastrointestinal tract, specifically the splanchnic circulation, has been unclear. Investigators have demonstrated an increase in superior mesenteric artery flow during a graded hypercapnic experiment.[52] In contrast, others have shown decreases in splanchnic blood flow during hypercapnia or a vasoconstrictive response leading to ulcerative gastrointestinal hemorrhage.[53,54] Using an ischemic gut model for acute lung injury, Laffey and associates[55] found that therapeutic hypercapnia, while protecting the lung from reperfusion injury, had no effect on the extent of gut reperfusion injury. Other gastrointestinal manifestations attributed to respiratory (and metabolic) acidosis pertain to the stomach. Acidosis in general has negative effects on gastric antral rhythms and fundic tone, thereby contributing to gastroparesis.[56]

Hypercapnia and Reperfusion Injury

Interest in the potential beneficial effect of hypercapnia has grown, fueled by the numerous studies showing the beneficial effects of permissive hypercapnia in acute lung injury. However, it appears that the beneficial effects of hypercapnia extend beyond pulmonary protection. Multiple organ systems have demonstrated a "pH paradox" during ischemia reperfusion. This paradox can best be described as a rapid normalization of pH during normoxic reperfusion of previously hypoxic-acidotic cells, resulting in reduced cell survival compared with an acidotic reperfusion through either a hypercapnic environment (cardiomyocytes)[57] or a metabolic acidotic environment (liver).[58]

Vanden Hoek and coworkers[59,60] have demonstrated, through an ischemia-reperfusion model, that after prolonged hypercapnic ischemia, significant injury and cell death occur at an accelerated rate immediately after reperfusion, when oxygen and CO_2 are normalized and substrates are reintroduced. In contrast, these cardiomyocytes can remain remarkably intact without membrane damage or caspase activation if allowed to remain hypercapnic and ischemic for much longer without reperfusion. Taking the thinking a step further, Lavani and colleagues[36] have shown, in a similar ischemia-reperfusion injury model, that hypercapnia appears to be protective of cardiomyocytes whereas eucapnia or hypocapnia appears to be harmful. Finally, carbon dioxide is now being recognized as a mediator of multiple endothelial and immunologic functions, such as attenuating lipopolysaccharide-induced activation of nuclear factor-κB, suppression of intracellular adhesion molecule-1, suppression of interleukin-8, and a reduction in oxidative nitrogen species.[55,61]

Metabolic Acidosis

Metabolic acidosis can arise from a variety of organic or inorganic fixed acids. There appears to be a difference in physiological variables and clinical outcomes between metabolic acidosis and respiratory acidosis. There is also evidence that the different types of metabolic acidosis differ in outcome.[62] These findings give credence to the hypothesis that the etiology of the acidosis, rather than the acidosis itself, is the determining factor in outcome. Because metabolic acidosis is a common finding in critically ill patients, it is very difficult to establish a pure

TABLE 115-4

The Effects of Metabolic Acidosis on Various Organ Systems

Cardiovascular	Myocardial depression
	Systemic arterial vascular smooth muscle relaxation
	Systemic venoconstriction with central blood pooling
	Dysrhythmias—lower threshold for ventricular fibrillation
	Resistance to vasopressors
Pulmonary	Pulmonary vasoconstriction
	Hyperventilation
	Dyspnea
	Improved $\dot{V}/\dot{Q}$ matching
	Decreased 2,3-diphosphoglyceric acid (late)
	Decreased hemoglobin O_2 affinity (Bohr effect)
Central nervous	Increased cerebral blood flow
	Increased ventilation
Endocrine—metabolic	Sympathetic nervous system stimulation
	Increased cortisol secretion
	Increased epinephrine secretion
	Protein wasting
	Bone demineralization
	Parathyroid hormone and aldosterone stimulation
	Insulin resistance
	Decreased glycolysis
Renal—electrolyte	Hyperkalemia
	Hypercalcemia
	Hyperuricemia
Coagulation	Reduction in thrombin formation
	Thrombocytopenia
	Reduction in fibrinogen
	Impairment of:
	Factor VIIa
	Factor VIIa/tissue factor complex
	Factor Va complex
Gastrointestinal	Emesis

causal effect of acidosis on outcome. Regardless of the etiology, metabolic acidosis continues to remain a strong marker of poor prognosis in critically ill patients.[37,63-65]

Cardiovascular Effects

Metabolic acidosis can affect numerous organ systems (Table 115-4), but its impact on the cardiovascular system is most critical to survival in the acute setting. Thus, the effect of metabolic acidosis on the cardiovascular system has been most extensively studied. The lethality associated with severe forms of metabolic acidosis is typically attributed to some form of cardiac dysfunction; however, complication-free survival has been observed in previously healthy adults in whom a lactic acidosis–induced pH of 6.8 after strenuous exercise has been tolerated without sequela.[66] Common adverse cardiac effects of metabolic acidosis include myocardial depression, dysrhythmias, hypotension, vasopressor resistance, and venoconstriction with the centralization of blood volume. Myocardial depression has been the subject of numerous experiments, some with conflicting results. However, it

does appear that a decrease in the pH_i of myocytes plays a major role in the negative inotropy observed in ischemia. The mechanisms responsible for this decrease in pH_i are still under debate, but it is evident that acidosis inhibits most if not all of the steps in the excitation-contraction coupling process. Some of the processes implicated are alterations in intracellular calcium levels,[67] changes in calcium binding to the troponin-myosin complex,[68] and impairment of actin-myosin cross-bridge cycling by monovalent phosphate.[69]

The role that extracellular pH plays is not quite as clear. There appears to be an association between severity of extracellular pH and contractility. This finding was semiquantitated by Steenbergen and colleagues[70] in a rat heart model 30 years ago. They reported that left ventricular pressure decreased minimally (5% to 10%) as the pH was lowered from 7.4 to 7.2 in a bicarbonate-titrated solution. As the pH was lowered to less than 7.2, a greater decrease was observed (15%). When the pH was lowered to 6.7, there was a further decrease in left ventricular pressure of about 30%. Interestingly, a mixed respiratory and metabolic acidosis caused an even greater reduction in contractile forces for the same pH, supporting the observations that pH_i is most likely more important in myocardial contractility.[70]

Other studies have correlated the severity of metabolic acidosis with ventricular function. In animal experiments, detectable cardiac depression was apparent only when blood pH was decreased below 7.2. There was actually a small positive inotropic effect as the pH was decreased from 7.4 to 7.2, which was maintained as long as the pH did not go below 7.2. The greater contractility appears to be mediated by a rise in circulating catecholamines, because blockade of the adrenergic response with propranolol eliminated any positive inotropy. There is also evidence of various responses in cardiac contractility with different causes of metabolic acidosis. Lactic acidosis has been shown to reduce contractility by up to 50% through similar pH ranges.[71] This finding suggests that lactic acid may have a more profound negative inotropic effect on the heart than other forms of metabolic acidosis.

Thus, both in vitro and in vivo studies have demonstrated substantial reductions in cardiac contractility when the extracellular pH is reduced below 7.2. However, it appears that pH_i may be the most important factor determining myocardial depression in acute acidosis, given that respiratory acidosis has a more profound impact on cardiac function than metabolic acidosis, especially when the pH is below 7.2.

Conduction abnormalities can be caused by extracellular acidosis in both the presence and absence of myocardial ischemia. In metabolic acidosis, even small reductions in blood pH to 7.3 have been shown to decrease the ventricular fibrillation threshold with a subsequent drop in pH to 7.1, reducing the threshold even further.[72] Interestingly, respiratory acidosis causes repolarization abnormalities but has no impact on the ventricular fibrillation threshold. Metabolic acidosis–induced cardiac dysrhythmias are thought to be caused in part by a rise in the diastolic depolarization rate.[73] Other causes are changes in blood and intracellular potassium, calcium, and magnesium concentrations and the associated increase in sympathetic discharge noted with acidosis.[73,74]

Acute metabolic acidosis also affects vascular tone. It has a direct vasodilatory effect, causing a decrease in peripheral vascular resistance. However, an increase in sympathetic discharge is also associated with acidosis; therefore, the ultimate vascular effect depends on the individual contributions of these two opposing forces.[74] Patients receiving beta-blockers can experience a more profound decrease in blood pressure because of the loss of compensatory mechanisms necessary for the direct vasodilatory effects. Vascular response to both α- and β-adrenergic stimulation is decreased with metabolic acidosis, vasopressor resistance being seen with low pH (<7.1). This blunted vascular response is most evident with the combination of low pH and high lactate levels.[75]

Not all vascular beds are uniform in their responses to metabolic acidosis. The cerebral circulation is very sensitive to acute changes in blood pH, and metabolic and respiratory acidosis both cause a decrease in cerebral vascular resistance, resulting in increased cerebral blood flow. Renal vascular resistance is increased in some experiments and decreased in others. Myocardial blood flow is complicated by a direct effect of metabolic acidosis and an indirect effect that causes a rise in myocardial oxygen consumption.[76] Both a decrease and an increase in coronary blood flow have been demonstrated in metabolic acidosis. Venoconstriction is also associated with metabolic acidosis, owing to the increased sympathetic discharge. The resulting effect displaces blood volume into the central circulation, raising both pulmonary vascular volume and pressure. Thus, in patients with severe metabolic acidosis, the associated myocardial depression along with the increase in central circulating volume due to venoconstriction results in a predisposition to congestive heart failure.

Pulmonary Effects

Pulmonary manifestations of metabolic acidosis are mostly compensatory in nature. Metabolic acidosis stimulates both central and peripheral chemoreceptors controlling ventilation, resulting in alveolar hyperventilation. The subsequent decrease in PCO_2 raises extracellular and intracellular pH values close to a normal range. The increase in minute ventilation occurs within minutes, but pH correction may take several hours. The increase in minute ventilation is primarily an increase in tidal volume rather than a rise in respiratory rate. This pattern of respiration, often noted on physical examination, is described as Kussmaul's respiration and may be a cause of dyspnea. An acidotic pH also reduces the affinity of hemoglobin for oxygen, usually within minutes, thus improving the delivery of oxygen to the tissues. This has been described as the Bohr effect. However, glycolysis is reduced over the next 36 hours, depleting red blood cells of 2,3-diphosphoglyceric acid. Because 2,3-diphosphoglyceric acid decreases the affinity of hemoglobin for oxygen, a reduction in its content leads to greater oxygen binding to hemoglobin. The resulting effect is a decrease in oxygen delivery. Thus, acute acidosis can increase oxygen delivery, whereas chronic acidosis can impair oxygen delivery.[77]

Renal and Electrolyte Effects

Electrolyte disturbances are common in metabolic acidosis. Acute acidemia has complex effects on various electrolyte levels. These electrolyte imbalances in turn have a profound impact on the cardiovascular system during severe metabolic acidosis. Hyperkalemia is present during metabolic acidosis as a result of enhanced cellular potassium efflux. This efflux has been noted to be more prevalent in hyperchloremic acidosis than in lactate acidosis.[12]

Initially, urinary excretion of potassium is reduced, so prolonged metabolic acidosis can result in a kaliuresis resulting in a net loss of potassium. Thus, acute metabolic acidosis can cause hyperkalemia, whereas prolonged metabolic acidosis can cause hypokalemia.[12] Changes in calcium levels are regulated by several mechanisms in metabolic acidosis. Ionized calcium levels may initially increase owing to a pH-related decrease in calcium-albumin binding. Also, total and ionized calcium levels can be altered by the influence of vitamin D and parathyroid hormone, which stimulate the release of calcium from bone and enhance urinary calcium excretion. Thus, the resulting impact of metabolic acidosis on total and ionized calcium concentrations depends on the severity and duration of metabolic acidosis as well as renal function. Calcium levels are essential in cardiovascular function; a higher level of ionized calcium increases contractility, and a lower level decreases contractility.[78,79]

Effects on Coagulation

Metabolic acidosis can severely impair coagulation to the extent that it can be life-threatening. This impairment is most evident when a large amount of blood loss occurs, such as in trauma.[80] Metabolic acidosis is thought to cause a coagulopathy from several mechanisms: (1) impairment of factor VIIa, factor VIIa/tissue factor complex, and factor Va complex, (2) a reduction in the formation of thrombin, (3) a decrease in fibrinogen levels, and (4) a reduction in platelet count. The coagulopathy of metabolic acidosis is even more pronounced if the patient is hypothermic.[81] In one study, induction of hyperchloremic metabolic acidosis to a pH of 7.1 caused a 30% reduction in plasma fibrinogen level and a 50% drop in the platelet count. Normalization of the pH with tris-hydroxymethyl aminomethane (THAM) did not affect the fibrinogen level or platelet count.[82] Similar irreversible fibrinogen and platelet losses were noted when bicarbonate was used to correct the pH.[83] It appears that decreased fibrinogen levels can be attributed to greater proteolysis, which may be amplified in a metabolic acidotic state.[84] However, the etiology of the decrease in platelets in a metabolic acidosis environment is currently unknown.

Effects on Cellular Function

The cellular response to extracellular metabolic acidosis is a complicated, multifactorial process. Cells of many organs have an extremely effective capacity to regulate their pH_i. Virtually all intracellular processes are sensitive to changes in pH_i.[85] With the exception of erythrocytes, all cells appear to function at a pH_i appreciably higher than would be predicted if hydrogen ions and bicarbonate were passively distributed across the plasma membrane. Transmembrane pH differences vary among tissues but range between 0.2 and 0.5 units, compared with the expected 0.8- to 1.5-unit difference if there were no intracellular pH regulation.[86] The same transmembrane ion exchanges that occur during health can be stimulated to maintain pH_i in states of extracellular acidosis. These include the exchange of extracellular Na^+ for intracellular H^+ via the Na^+-H^+ membrane antiporter, and active H^+ extrusion via the ATPase-driven proton pumps. In metabolic acidosis, these transmembrane ion exchangers can become overwhelmed or dysfunctional, leading to cellular injuries such as increases in intracellular calcium, intracellular sodium, and apoptosis and loss of potassium flux regulation.

CONCLUSION

The acid-base status of critically ill patients has generally been viewed as an end product of a specific disease process. Attention usually is given to the underlying disorder, with the assumption that changes in pH are the result, rather than the cause, of organ injury. With a better understanding of intracellular mechanisms and how they are affected by small changes in pH_i as well as how the extracellular environment can affect pH_i, there is a growing appreciation of how extracellular pH can affect organ function directly. Evidence now shows that different forms of acid-base dysequilibrium affect cells in different ways. An example is the observation that different causes of metabolic acidosis have different cellular effects, which may ultimately translate into observed differences in patient outcomes. Paradoxically, in some disease states, creating a mild acidosis in the form of hypercarbia may actually improve cellular function and patient survival.

Many different cells and organ systems are affected by changes in extracellular acid-base disturbances. Changes in extracellular pH have different effects on different organ systems. Cellular function and survival depends on a very precise pH_i. Homeostatic control of a narrow pH_i range is tightly regulated through several, not completely known, transmembrane mechanisms. This interorgan variability limits broad generalizations; however, it appears that extracellular acidosis, specifically metabolic acidosis, has more detrimental effects on organ function. Adverse organ effects are most likely attributed to altering pH_i, which appears to be more important in cellular function than extracellular pH.

Key Points

1. Complex transmembrane mechanisms allow cells to tolerate fluctuations in extracellular pH.
2. Each organ system may respond differently to different acid-base disorders.
3. Ischemia-reperfusion injury may be attenuated with hypercapnic acidosis.
4. The effects of extracellular acid-base disturbances on organ systems are most likely due to their effect on intracellular pH.

Key References

33. Kregenow DA, Rubenfeld GD, Hudson LD, Swenson ER: Hypercapnic acidosis and mortality in acute lung injury. Crit Care Med 2006;34:1-7.
36. Lavani R, Chang WT, Anderson T, et al: Altering CO_2 during reperfusion of ischemic cardiomyocytes modifies mitochondrial oxidant injury. Crit Care Med 2007;35:1709-1716.
49. Sharkey RA, Mulloy EM, O'Neill SJ: The acute effects of oxygen and carbon dioxide on renal vascular resistance in patients with an acute exacerbation of COPD. Chest 1999;115:1588-1592.
58. Currin RT, Gores GJ, Thurman RG, Lemasters JJ: Protection by acidotic pH against anoxic cell killing in perfused rat liver: Evidence for a pH paradox. FASEB J 1991;5:207-210.
81. Martini WZ, Pusateri AE, Uscilowicz JM, et al: Independent contributions of hypothermia and acidosis to coagulopathy in swine. J Trauma 2005;58:1002-1009.

CHAPTER 116

Arterial and Venous Blood Gases

Luciano Gattinoni and Eleonora Carlesso

OBJECTIVES

This chapter will:
1. Explain the differences between the measured and the computed acid-base variables and their limitations.
2. Describe the differences between arterial and mixed venous/central venous samplings in the assessment of respiratory and acid base equilibrium.
3. Emphasize the greater importance of mixed venous/central venous blood gases compared with the arterial gases for monitoring and targeting the resuscitation of critically ill patients.

Blood gas analysis is likely the most common diagnostic tool used in critically ill patients. Blood gases are primarily assessed in arterial blood samples and much less in venous blood samples, either central or mixed venous (pulmonary artery catheter). This chapter discusses the diagnostic utility of blood gas analysis, its limits, and, more important, the value of venous blood assessment, either alone or in association with arterial sampling. Before the discussion of the relative value of arterial and venous blood gas assessment, the chapter presents a brief description of the variables, measured or computed, and their use in the framework of acute illness.

THE MEASURED VARIABLES

Hydrogen Ion Concentration: pH

The *pH*, usually measured by glass electrode, expresses the activity of protons free in the plasma according to the following relationship:

$$pH = -\log_{10}[H^+]$$

where $[H^+]$ denotes the concentration of protons, expressed in mol/L. As an example, a pH value of 7.4 corresponds to $[H^+]$ of 39.8×10^{-9} mol/L, or 39.8 nanomoles per liter. It is worthwhile to stress that this order of magnitude is 1 million times lower than CO_2 and O_2 concentrations, which are on the order of millimoles per liter.

Oxygen Tension (Arterial Partial Pressure of Oxygen)

Oxygen tension, or arterial partial pressure of oxygen (PaO_2), is the activity of the molecules of oxygen dissolved in the plasma. PaO_2 is measured by the Clark's electrode[1] at a temperature of 37°C. The normal values[2] of PaO_2, in a person breathing room air, range from 80 to 100 mm Hg and decline with age according to the following formula[3]:

$$PaO_2 = 100 - 0.3 \times age\ (yrs)$$

The PaO_2 and the related amount of oxygen dissolved into the plasma are linked by the solubility coefficient which, at 37° C, equals 0.0036 mL/mm Hg/dL. Indeed, at 100 mm Hg PaO_2, the corresponding amount of oxygen dissolved is 0.36 mL per dL of plasma or 0.16 mmol/L (1 mmol = 22.4 mL).

Carbon Dioxide Tension (Arterial Partial Pressure of Carbon Dioxide)

The *partial pressure of carbon dioxide* ($PaCO_2$) measures the activity of the carbon dioxide molecules dissolved into the plasma. The $PaCO_2$ is measured by the Stow-Severinghaus electrode. The normal values of $PaCO_2$ range from 35 to 45 mm Hg.[2] The solubility coefficient is 0.0306 mmoL/mm Hg/L.[4] Indeed, at a $PaCO_2$ of 40 mm Hg, the CO_2 molecules dissolved into the plasma amount to 1.224 mmol/L, corresponding to 27.4 mL of CO_2 per dL of plasma.

Hemoglobin Oxygen Saturation

Hemoglobin oxygen saturation (SatHb), measured by infrared spectroscopy, is the statistical average of all oxygen bound to hemoglobin molecules relative to the total amount that could be bound. Indeed, a saturation of 90% HbO_2 indicates that 90% of the binding sites of hemoglobin are actually bound to oxygen molecules. Such a saturation value implies that most of the hemoglobin molecules carry four molecules of oxygen each, some three, and a few others two or one. The relationship between the oxygen tension (PO_2) and hemoglobin saturation is the *oxygen dissociation curve.* The S shape of this curve indicates that the affinity of hemoglobin for oxygen increases with rising O_2 saturation (*cooperative oxygen binding*). However, under physiological conditions, the PO_2-SatHb relationship depends largely on heterotropic molecules.[5] The major regulators of O_2 affinity are protons (Bohr effect); an increase in proton concentration decreases oxygen affinity. 2,3-Diphosphoglyceric acid, a metabolite of the glycolytic pathway, as well as chloride ion (Cl^-) shift, reduce the O_2 affinity with human hemoglobin. A minor role in oxygen affinity is played by carbon dioxide, which shares binding sites with 2,3-diphosphoglyceric acid. Several attempts to compute oxygen saturation from PO_2 have been performed, first by Hill,[6] later by Adair[7]; subsequently, several models have been proposed and implemented in blood gas machines.[8] However, owing to the large number of covariables that may affect the oxygen dissociation curve, the direct measurement of hemoglobin oxygen saturation is highly recommended.

THE COMPUTED VARIABLES

Oxygen Content

The *oxygen content* of whole blood is the plasma-dissolved oxygen plus the oxygen bound to the hemoglobin in the red blood cells. The maximal binding capacity of oxygen to hemoglobin (100% saturation) is 4 moles of oxygen (89.6 L) for each mole of hemoglobin tetramer (molecular weight 64,500 Da). Accordingly, the oxygen-carrying capacity coefficient for hemoglobin should be 1.389 mL O_2 per gram hemoglobin. Quite surprisingly, this coefficient in the literature ranges from 1.32 to 1.39, with 1.36 mL O_2/g being most commonly used. This range reflects the different molecular weights attributed to the hemoglobin, which varies from about 64,000 to about 67,000 Da.

It must also be noted that 22.4 L is the volume of 1 mole of oxygen in standard pressure/temperature conditions (STP)—760 mm Hg and 0° C. The actual volume occupied by 1 mole of oxygen at body temperature 37° C (BTP) is therefore 25.455 L, according to the general equation of gases, PV = nRT, in which R = 0.08207 L per atm per mole per ° K. Indeed, the hemoglobin oxygen-carrying capacity coefficient 1.36 becomes 1.54 at 37° C.

The oxygen content at STP is computed according to the following formula, which may be applied to either the arterial or the venous blood:

$$Ca/vO_2 = Pa/vO_2 \times 0.003 + 1.36 \times Hb \times SatHb$$

where Hb is the hemoglobin concentration. This formula allows estimation of the oxygen content of arterial (CaO_2) and venous (CvO_2) blood. Ideal capillary blood oxygen content (CcO_2) can be calculated, assuming that the value of oxygen tension is the same as the alveolar oxygen tension and the SatHb 100%. These values, in turn, are used to compute other variables, as follows[9]:

- Oxygen transport (DO_2)
- Arteriovenous difference (ΔavO_2)
- Oxygen consumption by reverse Fick's method (where CO is cardiac output in L/min × 10):

$$\dot{V}O_2 = \Delta avO_2 \times CO$$

- Riley's shunt fraction (where Qs is shunt flow and Qt is cardiac output):

$$\frac{Q_s}{Q_t} = \frac{(CcO_2 - CaO_2)}{(CcO_2 - CvO_2)}$$

Riley's fraction measurements are minimally affected by the use of different hemoglobin oxygen-carrying capacity coefficients at either STP or BTP conditions. More attention has to be paid, however, to the consideration of ΔavO_2 and more important, $\dot{V}O_2$ when measured by reverse Fick's method. In fact, this computed $\dot{V}O_2$ is the amount of oxygen at 0° C. If this value is compared with the $\dot{V}CO_2$, which is usually measured in expired gases either at ambient or at body temperature, an artifactual difference may rise simply owing to the fact that the gas volumes do not refer to the same condition, either STP or BTP. Great attention was devoted to these corrections decades ago, but nowadays they are usually ignored.

Carbon Dioxide Content

The total CO_2 content (tCO_2) in the plasma includes various species in which CO_2 is present, as follows:

$$tCO_2 = dCO_2 + HCO_3^- + CO_3^{2-} + PrNHCOO^- + NaCO_3^-$$

in which dCO_2 is dissolved CO_2, HCO_3^- is bicarbonate, CO_3^{2-} is carbonate, $PrNHCOO^-$ is carbamino compound, and $NaCO_3^-$ is sodium carbonate. The last three species are usually ignored in human plasma, and the tCO_2 provided by the blood gas machine is the sum of the dCO_2 and HCO_3^-. This amount in normal plasma at pH 7.40 is 1.224 + 24.8, or 26.02 mmol/L, which is equivalent to 58.28 mL of CO_2 per dL. It is worth remembering that the total CO_2 given by the blood gas machine refers to the CO_2 content of plasma only, and not of whole blood. In fact, for the same PCO_2, the content of CO_2 in the red blood cells is lower than that in plasma because the red blood cell pH is lower. The order of magnitude of the total CO_2 difference at the same PCO_2, between 1 L of plasma and 1 L of blood with a normal hematocrit, is 5 to 10 mmol/L, depending on PCO_2 and pH.

The primary variable derived from PCO_2 and pH measurement is bicarbonate, with the Henderson-Hasselbalch equation rearranged as follows:

$$HCO_3^- \, [mmol/L] = 10^{pH-pK} \times 0.0306 \times PCO_2$$

The problem is the pK. In some blood gas machines, the algorithm for HCO_3^- computation includes the pK variations with pH. Some others use slightly different pK values. It is beyond the purpose of this chapter to discuss the biochemistry of the carbon dioxide hydration (see Siggaard-Andersen[4]); here, it is sufficient to say that different blood gas machines measuring exactly the same pH and PCO_2 may provide different values of HCO_3^- owing to the differences of the implemented algorithms. The differences are minimal at physiological pH and PCO_2 but may be as high as 2 mmol/L in case of severe alkalosis or acidosis. As in the intensive care unit, what is important is the trend of the variables with time, and if only one blood gas machine is used, this problem is irrelevant. It may become important if two blood gas machines with different implemented algorithms are used to follow the clinical course of a given patient.

Base Excess

The base excess (BE) is a way to quantify the presence of strong acid (metabolic acidosis) or strong base (metabolic

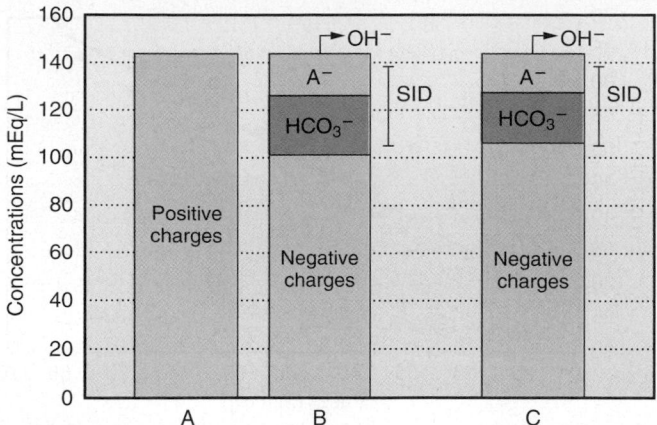

FIGURE 116-1. Gamblegram (graphic display of the ionic environment). Columns A and B indicate plasma electroneutrality. SID (strong ion difference; difference between strong positive ions and the strong negative ions) is "balanced" by the sum of bicarbonate (HCO_3^-), A^- (concentration of dissociated weak acids), and OH^- (hydroxyl concentration). When the strong ion lactates increase (column C), the space of HCO_3^- and A^- is reduced, as well as the OH^-. Because the product of OH^- and H^+ concentration is constant (called the ion product of water), any decrease of OH^- implies an increase in H^+ and, consequently, a decrease in pH.

alkalosis), either (1) in the whole blood, called blood base excess, BE(B), or actual base excess, ABE, or (2) in the extracellular fluid, called extracellular BE (BEecf) or standard BE (SBE). The difference is due to the presence of hemoglobin in the whole blood (a component of total weak acids concentration [A_{tot}]). The buffer base (BB; see later) of the whole blood, indeed, is higher than the BB of the extracellular fluid, in which by convention the hemoglobin contribution to the BB is assumed to be equal to 6 g/dL.

Conceptually, the meaning of base excess is relatively simple, referring to the strong ion difference (SID) approach.[10] As shown in Figure 116-1, the positively charged strong ions (primarily Na^+) exceed the negatively charged ions (primarily Cl^-) by about 42 mEq/L in normal conditions. The additional negative charges required to reach electroneutrality (i.e., the number of electrons lost by a compound must be gained by another compound and their sum, lost *plus* gained, must be equal to 0) are provided by the negatively charged "weak acids," both carbonic (HCO_3^-) and noncarbonic (A^- [concentration of dissociated weak acids, primarily the negatively charged albumin and phosphates]), otherwise known as "buffers," and by OH^-, which comes from water dissociation and the concentration of which is 1 million times lower than concentrations of HCO_3^- and A^-. In other words, SID (owing to ions that are always negatively or positively charged, as they are "strong") equals the sum of the negatively charged forms of the weak acids—HCO_3^- and A^-—and OH^-. If an abnormal strong ion, such as lactate (almost completely dissociated), is added to the system, SID decreases, and as a consequence, the sum of HCO_3^-, A^-, and OH^- must decrease by the same amount. Of note, the sum of the negatively charged "weak" ions is called the buffer base (BB). Indeed SID = BB.

BE (positive and negative) is a measure of how much, *compared with normal*, the BB and SID are increased (alkalosis) or decreased (acidosis). The concept of BE implies the knowledge of a "normal reference state," that is the value of SID (BB) in standard conditions. The refer-

ence state is the BB when $PaCO_2$ is 40 mm Hg, the pH is 7.4, and the temperature is 37° C and the values of A_{tot} (i.e., protein) is normal (70 gr/L). It follows that:

$$BE = actual\ BB - normal\ BB\ (42\ mEq/L)$$

or:

$$BE = actual\ SID - normal\ SID\ (42\ mEq/L)$$

Note that the preceding equations do not apply when A_{tot} is abnormal (see Chapters 117 and 121).

Two methods are available for the computation of BE. The first refers to empirical equations derived by Siggaard-Andersen[4]; the second uses the following formula:

$$BEecf = (actual\ HCO_3^- - 24.8) + 16.2 \times (actual\ pH - 7.4)$$

Both methods imply several assumptions. First, the BE/pH relationship is normally curvilinear, but for simplicity, both methods use a straight-line approximation. Second, both methods assume a "normal" protein content. The two methods provide similar results around pH 7.4 and disagree at higher or lower pH values.

CLINICAL USE

The measured and computed variables derived from blood gas analysis are used primarily to assess a patient's respiratory and metabolic acid-base status. In general, arterial blood samples are analyzed more frequently than central venous blood samples. This chapter discusses the relative importance of arterial blood analysis and venous blood analysis in gathering clinical relevant information. The least amount of information is obtained from arterial samples; more data may be acquired from central venous sampling, and complete information may be obtained through the analysis of arterial and venous blood samples drawn simultaneously.

Arterial Sampling

Arterial sampling allows the precise assessment of oxygenation (PaO_2 and SatHb, either computed or measured directly by oximetry), of ventilatory status ($PaCO_2$), and of acid-base equilibrium (BE and pH). It is important to emphasize, however, that oxygenation status may be, at least in part, assessed by pulse oximetry, which is well related to the directly measured SatHb. Pulse oximetry, obviously, cannot discriminate the very high levels of PaO_2, for example, greater than 100 mm Hg, because at that level the hemoglobin is usually 100% saturated. However, for clinical purposes, what matters is that a normal oxygenation status and a pulse oximetry reading greater than 90% to 95% is clinically adequate. Moreover, what is clinically relevant is the oxygenation trend, which is more adequately described by a continuous recording of arterial saturation as derived from pulse oximetry.

Central Venous Sampling

Central venous blood is inadequate to assess the arterial oxygenation, because venous oxygen partial pressure (PvO_2) primarily reflects tissue oxygenation. As discussed previously, however, arterial oxygenation status may be assessed from pulse oximetry. If this value is available, as in most critically ill patients, central venous blood analysis provides further relevant clinical information. Central venous oxygen saturation (SatvO₂) is an extremely sensitive indicator of respiratory hemodynamic and metabolic status, as expressed in the following equation:

$$\text{SatvO}_2 = \text{SataO}_2 - \frac{\dot{\text{V}}\text{O}_2(\text{mL/min})}{\dot{\text{Q}}(\text{L/min})} \times \frac{1}{\text{Hb} \times 1.36}$$

or:

$$\text{SatvO}_2 = \text{Lung} - \frac{\text{Metabolism}}{\text{Hemodynamics}} \times \frac{1}{\text{Anemia}}$$

As shown by this equation, any change in lung function, metabolism, hemodynamics, or anemia affects SatvO₂. Indeed, SatvO₂ is an extremely sensitive (not specific) monitor of basic vital functions. Moreover, it may be used as a target of therapy during resuscitation. In an unselected population of critically ill patients, Gattinoni and colleagues[11] have shown that an SatvO₂ target equal to or greater than 70% is equivalent to a normal cardiac output target.[11] In septic patients, keeping SatvO₂ equal to or greater than 70% has been shown to confer survival benefit.[12] Sampling central venous blood in patients in whom pulse oximetry is available provides information on tissue oxygenation and hemodynamic status not derivable from arterial sampling.

For ventilatory status and the acid-base equilibrium, it is important to emphasize that central venous blood may provide the same information as arterial blood. As shown in Figure 116-2A, PaCO₂ and central venous carbon dioxide tension (PvCO₂) are strongly correlated (at least in patients in a steady state). Obviously, normal PvCO₂ is not 40 mm Hg but 3 to 3.5 mm Hg higher. The same applies, as shown in Figure 116-2B, for BE. It is important to note that normal BE in the venous blood is about 1.5 mmol greater than that in arterial blood. To compute venous BE exactly, the reference normal values should be for venous and not arterial blood; for example, pH value about 7.38 and HCO₃⁻ about 25.7 mmol/L. If one keeps the normal values for central venous blood in mind, it is easy to quantify both ventilatory status and acid-base equilibrium. Indeed, central venous blood provides not only the same information on ventilation and acid-base equilibrium as arterial blood but also information about tissue oxygenation and hemodynamic adequacy.

Arterial and Central Venous Sampling

The most complete information, however, is provided by the simultaneous sampling of arterial and central venous blood. The cause of the oxygenation defect may be measured by measuring the shunt fraction. The venous-arterial difference allows a better assessment of hemodynamic status. The PvCO₂-to-PaCO₂ difference, owing to an unsteady-state period, may give insights about tissue acidosis, which sharply increases PvCO₂, before a new equilibrium is reached.

CONCLUSION

Blood gas analysis is widely used in the assessment of respiratory and acid-base status in critically ill patients. For this purpose, the blood gases are usually measured in an arterial sample. Actually, the mixed venous/central

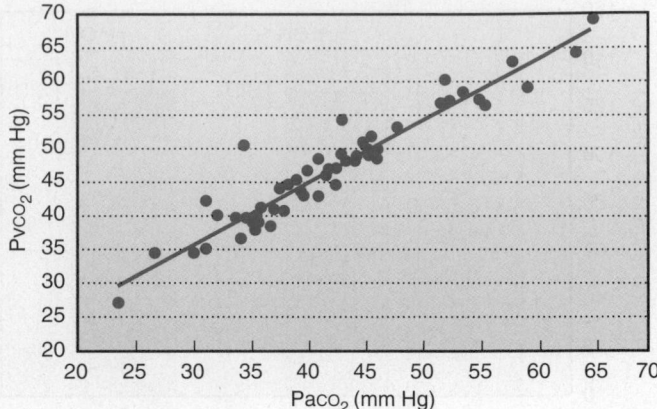

A

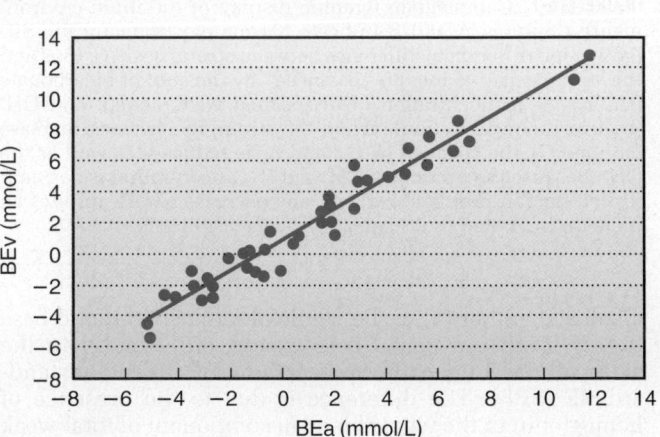

B

FIGURE 116-2. A, Relationship of PvCO₂ vs. PaCO₂ in 62 patients with acute lung injury or acute respiratory distress syndrome. *Solid line* represents linear regression (PvCO₂ = 8.18 + 0.92 × PaCO₂; $r^2 = 0.91$, $P < .0001$). **B,** Central venous access (BEv) vs. arterial base excess (BEa) in 45 patients with acute lung injury or acute respiratory distress syndrome. *Solid line* represents linear regression (BEv = 0.66 + 0.99 × BEa; $r^2 = 0.96$, $P < .0001$). PaCO₂, arterial carbon dioxide tension; PvCO₂, central venous carbon dioxide tension.

venous blood gases, if measured along with pulse oximetry, may provide the same information about ventilatory and acid-base status (base excess and PCO₂) as arterial blood gases. However, venous sampling may provide better insight about tissue oxygenation by assessing the venous hemoglobin oxygen saturation. In turn, this variable may be also used as a resuscitation target for critically ill patients with sepsis.

Key Points

1. Blood gas values are essential diagnostic tools in critically ill patients, allowing the assessment of oxygenation, tissue perfusion, and hemodynamic and acid-base equilibrium.
2. In ascending order, the information acquired is least from arterial sampling, higher from central venous pulse oximetry, and most complete from simultaneous arterial and central venous sampling.

Key References

4. Siggaard-Andersen O: Acid-Base Biochemistry: The Acid-Base Status of the Blood, 4th ed. Oxford, Alden & Mowbray Ltd at the Alden Press, 1963, pp 29-91.
5. Baumann R, Bartels H, Bauer C: Blood oxygen transport. In Fahri LE, Tenney SM (eds): Handbook of Physiology: Section 3: the Respiratory System: Volume IV: Gas Exchange. Bethesda, MD, American Physiology Society, 1987, pp 147-172.
10. Stewart PA: How to Understand Acid-Base: A Quantitative Acid-Base Primer for Biology and Medicine. New York, Elsevier, 1981.

See the companion Expert Consult website for the complete reference list.

CHAPTER 117

Anion Gap and Strong Ion Gap

John A. Kellum and Raghavan Murugan

OBJECTIVES

This chapter will:
1. Define anion gap and strong ion gap.
2. Explain why these terms are used.
3. Illustrate how to use them.
4. Discuss the interpretation of anion gap and strong ion gap.

Syndromes resulting in metabolic acidosis occur as a result of either loss of base from or addition of acid to the plasma. Acids and bases are ionic compounds, meaning that they are composed of negatively charged anions and positively charged cations. Plasma anions and cations include abundant electrolytes such as Na^+ and Cl^- and less abundant molecules such as lactate and albumin. Whereas the electrolytes are routinely measured, the less common ions are not. In order to satisfy electroneutrality (see Chapter 111), the total charges on cations and anions, added together, must equal zero.

THE ANION GAP

For more than 30 years, the anion gap (AG) has been used by clinicians to exploit the principle of electroneutrality, and it has evolved into a major tool for evaluating acid-base disorders.[1] Simply speaking, the *anion gap* is the difference between the sum of charges from plasma anions and cations. The AG is calculated, or rather estimated, from the differences between the routinely measured concentrations of serum cations (Na^+ and K^+) and anions (Cl^- and HCO_3^-). Because there can be no actual difference (electroneutrality must be preserved), the measured difference reflects the missing or "unmeasured" ions. Normally, this difference, or "gap," is filled primarily by the ionized portion of the weak acids (A^-) (see Chapter 111). A^- comprises principally albumin and, to a lesser extent, phosphate. Sulfate and lactate also contribute a small amount to the normal AG, typically less than 2 mEq/L. However, there are also unmeasured cations, such as Ca^{2+} and Mg^{2+}, which tend to offset the effects of sulfate and lactate except

when either is abnormally increased (Fig. 117-1). Plasma proteins other than albumin can be either positively or negatively charged but, in the aggregate, tend to be neutral,[2] except in rare cases of abnormal paraproteins, such as in multiple myeloma.

When the anion gap is greater than that produced by albumin and phosphate, other anions (e.g., lactate, ketones) must be present in higher than normal concentrations. For this reason, the AG can be used to narrow the differential diagnosis of a metabolic acidosis. Futhermore, the magnitude of the anion gap reflects the concentration of the offending acid and can therefore provide a means of monitoring when measurement of the acid is difficult (e.g., in ketoacidosis). Finally, the AG may provide a clue to the presence of life-threatening conditions, such as poisonings (see Chapter 130).

Calculating the Anion Gap

In practice, the AG is calculated as follows:

$$AG = (Na^+ + K^+) - (Cl^- + HCO_3^-)$$

Because of its low and narrow extracellular concentration, K^+ is often omitted from the calculation. Respective normal values with relatively wide ranges reported by most laboratories are 12 ± 4 (if K^+ is considered) and 8 ± 4 mEq/L (if K^+ is not considered). The value of a "normal AG" has decreased after the introduction of more accurate methods for measuring Cl^- concentration.[3,4] However, the various measurement techniques available mandate that each institution report its own expected "normal AG."

Furthermore, the concept of a "normal AG" is based on the premise that A^- is normal, a premise that requires albumin and phosphate, the two major constituents of the A^-, to be normal both in concentration and in charge. As it turns out, this premise is usually the case in healthy subjects but rarely so in critically ill patients.[5,6] Dehydration may induce a parallel increment in the apparent AG by raising the concentrations of all the ions. Conversely, severe hypoalbuminemia causes a decrease in the AG, and "correction" of the AG for the prevailing albumin concentration has been recommended because each (1 g/dL) decline in serum albumin reduces the apparent AG by 2.5 to 3 mEq/L.[7]

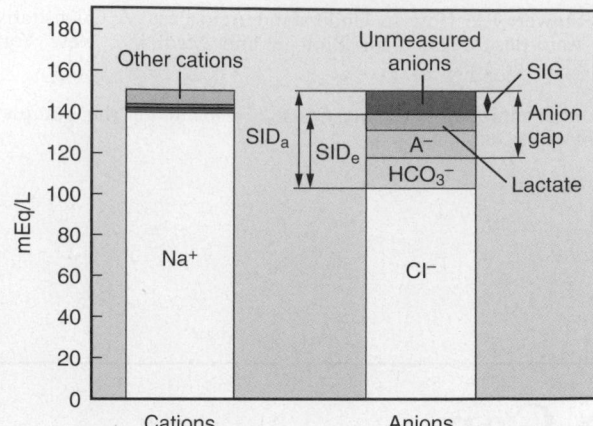

FIGURE 117-1. Charge balance in blood plasma. "Other cations" include Ca^{2+} and Mg^{2+}. The strong ion difference (SID) is always positive (in plasma) and SID minus effective SID (SIDe) must equal 0. Any difference between SID apparent (SIDa) and SIDe is the strong ion gap (SIG) and must represent unmeasured anions. A^-, concentration of dissociated weak acids; HCO_3^-, bicarbonate.

Correcting the Anion Gap

Some investigators have cast doubt on the diagnostic value of the AG in certain situations.[5,8] Salem and Mujais,[5] for example, found routine reliance on the AG to be "fraught with numerous pitfalls." The primary problem with the AG is its reliance on the use of a normal range produced by albumin and, to a lesser extent, phosphate, as discussed previously. Levels of these constituents may be grossly abnormal in patients with critical illness, leading to a change in the normal range for these patients. This problem has prompted some investigators to adjust the "normal range" for the AG by the patient's albumin[7] or even phosphate[9] concentration. Because these anions are not strong anions, their charge will be altered by changes in pH. Each g/dL of albumin has a charge of 2.8 mEq/L at pH 7.4 (2.3 mEq/L at 7.0, and 3.0 mEq/L at 7.6), and each mg/dL of phosphate has a charge of 0.59 mEq/L at pH 7.4 (0.55 mEq/L at 7.0, and 0.61 mEq/L at 7.6). Thus, under physiological conditions, the variance is reasonably small. A convenient way to estimate the "normal" AG for a given patient is by use of the following formula[9]:

"Normal" AG = 2(albumin [g/L]) + 0.5(phosphate [mg/dL])

Or, for international units:

$$\text{"Normal" AG} = 0.2(\text{albumin [g/L]}) +$$
$$1.5(\text{phosphate [mmol/L]})$$

When Kellum[9] used this patient-specific normal range to examine the presence of unmeasured anions in the blood of critically ill patients, the accuracy of the method improved from 33% with the routine AG (normal range = 12 mEq/L) to 96%.[9]

Alternatively, the estimated charge coming from albumin and phosphate can be added in with Cl^- and HCO_3^- as total anions. Lactate can also be considered. The resultant "corrected AG" (cAG) should be close to zero, as follows:

$$cAG = (Na^+ + K^+) - [Cl^- + HCO_3^- + 2(\text{albumin}) +$$
$$0.5(\text{phosphate}) + \text{lactate}]$$

Or, for international units:

$$cAG = (Na^+ + K^+) - [Cl^- + HCO_3^- + 0.2(\text{albumin}) +$$
$$1.5(\text{phosphate}) + \text{lactate}]$$

Either technique is accurate only within 5 mEq/L. It is important to note that the presence of an increased anion gap after correction for albumin and phosphate indicates the presence of unmeasured anions and therefore acidosis irrespective of pH or HCO_3^-. Therefore, it is imperative that the anion gap be estimated in all patients with suspected acid-base disorder even in the absence of obvious acidemia. Because patients with mixed acid-base disorders often have apparently normal pH, an increased anion gap may be the only clue to an underlying mixed acid-base disorder.

THE STRONG ION GAP

Another alternative to using the traditional AG is to use the strong ion difference (SID). By definition, the SID must be equal and opposite to the negative charges contributed by A^- and total CO_2. This latter value, the sum of charges from A^- and total CO_2, has been called the effective SID (SID_e).[2] The apparent SID (SID_a) is obtained through individual measurement of each strong ion (Na^+, K^+, Cl^-, Ca^{2+}, Mg^{2+}, lactate). SID_a and the SID_e should both equal the true SID. If SID_a and SID_e differ, unmeasured ions must exist. If SID_a is greater than SID_e, these ions are anions, and if SID_a is less than SID_e, they are cations. This difference has been termed the *strong ion gap* (SIG) to distinguish it from the AG.[10] Unlike the AG, the SIG is normally 0 and does not change with changes in pH or albumin concentration as does the AG, as the following equations show:

$$SID_a = (Na^+ + K^+ + Ca^{2+} + Mg^{2+}) - (Cl^- + \text{lactate})$$

$$SID_e = 2.46 \times 10^{-8} \times \frac{P_{CO_2}}{10^{-pH}} + [\text{albumin}] \times (0.123 \times pH -$$
$$0.631) + [PO_4^{2-}] \times (0.39 \times pH - 0.469)$$

$$SIG = SID_a - SID_e$$

The term strong ion gap is somewhat misleading, because it may not reflect an abnormality in strong ions. Weak ions such as proteins can also increase the SIG. The SIG is a "gap" in the strong ion balance equations but it may be due to either strong or weak ions.

INTERPRETING THE GAPS

The utility of the anion and strong ion gaps comes primarily from their ability to quickly and easily limit the differential diagnosis in a patient with metabolic acidosis. If increased AG or SIG is present, the explanation will almost invariably be found among five disorders: ketosis, lactic acidosis, poisoning, renal failure, and sepsis. Table 117-1 lists all disorders associated with increased AG and SIG.

A number of factors may influence the AG apart from those corrected for in the previous discussion. Respiratory alkalosis and metabolic alkalosis are associated with an increase of up to 3 to 10 mEq/L in the apparent AG due to enhanced lactate production (from stimulated phosphofructokinase enzymatic activity), a reduction in the ionized

TABLE 117-1

Causes of Increased Anion Gap and Strong Ion Gap

Common causes	Renal failure
	Ketoacidosis:
	Diabetic
	Alcoholic
	Starvation
	Metabolic errors
	Lactic acidosis*
	Toxins:
	Methanol
	Ethylene glycol
	Salicylates
	Paraldehyde
	Toluene
Rare causes	Dehydration
	Severe liver disease
	Sodium salts:
	Sodium lactate*
	Sodium citrate
	Sodium acetate
	Sodium penicillin (>50 million units/day)
	Carbenicillin (>30 g/day)
	Decreased unmeasured cations:
	Hypomagnesemia*
	Hypocalcemia*
	Alkalemia

*Already accounted for by strong ion gap.

weak acids (A^-), and, possibly, the additional effect of dehydration (with its own impact on AG calculation). Low Mg^{2+} concentration with associated low K^+ and Ca^{2+} concentrations, as well as the administration of sodium salts of poorly reabsorbable anions (such as beta-lactam antibiotics) are known causes of increased AG.[11] Certain parenteral nutrition formulations, such as those containing acetate, may increase both the AG and the SIG, and citrate may rarely have the same effect in the setting of multiple blood transfusions, particularly if massive doses of banked blood are used, such as during liver transplantation.[12] It is important to emphasize that because both strong and weak ions alter SIG and AG, the exact chemical makeup of the SIG may vary significantly from patient to patient. None of these rare causes increases the AG or SIG significantly,[13] however, and they are usually easily identified.

Some additional causes of an increased AG have been reported. In the nonketotic hyperosmolar state of diabetes, an AG has been found that remains unexplained.[14] Unmeasured anions have been reported in the blood of patients with sepsis[8,15] or with liver disease[10,16] and in experimental animals given endotoxin.[17] These anions may be the source of much of the unexplained acidosis seen in patients with critical illness (See Chapter 124).[18]

THE SIZE OF THE GAP

AG, cAG, and SIG are all expressed in mEq/L because they quantify the amount of charge, not molecules. Therefore, whenever the AG is increased, the putative anion should be sought and its concentration expressed in mEq/L, compared with the change in the AG. When the gap is due completely to a strong ion (e.g., lactate) there is a 1-for-1 effect on the base excess (e.g., 1 mEq/L increase in lactate will increase the AG or SIG by 1 mEq/L, which will

TABLE 117-2

Causes of Normal Anion Gap

Nonrenal causes: urine SID (Na + KCl) < 0	Diarrhea or other intestinal Cl^- losses
	Saline infusion
	Toluene ingestion
	Carbonic anhydrase inhibitors
	Ureteral diversion
Renal causes: urine SID (Na + KCl) > 0	Type 1 (distal) RTA
	Type 2 (proximal) RTA
	Type 4 RTA (hypoaldosteronism)

RTA, renal tubular acidosis; SID, strong ion difference.

decrease the standard base excess by 1 mEq/L). This relationship has prompted many researchers to devise ways of comparing the AG or SIG to the base excess or (with more difficulty) the HCO_3^- concentration in order to detect the presence of mixed metabolic acidosis (see Chapter 121). The techniques have various names but all do the same thing. If a patient has a metabolic acidosis that is due in part to unmeasured anions (e.g., ketones) and in part to hyperchloremia, the increase in AG or SIG will be smaller than the decrease in base excess. Similarly, the change in HCO_3^- concentration, in the context of CO_2, will be greater than the AG or SIG. In this way, a mixed disorder can be revealed.

Furthermore, when the increase in AG cannot be explained by lactate or ketones, other acids must be present; the calculation of an osmolar gap can, as follows, be useful:

$$Osmolar\ gap = Measured\ osmolality -$$
$$\left[(1.86 \times Na^+) + \frac{glucose}{18} + \frac{BUN}{2.8} + \frac{ethanol}{4.6} \right]$$

where glucose and BUN are given in mg/dL. An osmolar gap greater than 10 mOsm/L is abnormal and indicates the presence of osmotically active unmeasured anions in poisoning syndromes (e.g., methanol, ethanol, ethylene glycol) (see also Chapter 130). Note that ethanol also contributes to the osmolar gap; this contribution can be taken into account through subtraction of the ethanol level, in mg/dL, after it has been divided by 4.6.

If a normal AG (hyperchloremic) metabolic acidosis is present, its cause can be determined through examination of the urine SID. If the kidneys are functioning normally in a metabolic acidosis, the urine SID should be negative, because the kidney excretes strong anions in excess of strong cations (Table 117-2).

It is important to recognize that determination of cAG and SIG has important prognostic implications in critically ill patients. For instance, increased SIG prior to resuscitation has been found to be associated with higher risk of death in various critically ill patients, such as those with trauma,[19] those who have undergone cardiac surgery,[20] and those with severe malaria.[21]

Key Points

1. Although few unmeasured ions are normally found in healthy plasma, the plasma of the critically ill or injured patient has increased concentrations of both anions and cations. These ions are

not normally measured by standard chemistry profiles.

2. Estimates of the amount of unmeasured anions in the blood are affected by the assay technology used to measure electrolytes as well as by the technique used to calculate unmeasured anions (e.g., anion gap, strong ion gap). In particular, the measurement of Cl^- is more accurate with modern, ion-specific electrodes.

3. The anion gap is affected by albumin and phosphate concentrations; thus, the expected range should be corrected for abnormalities in these values.

4. Unmeasured anions (e.g., strong ion gap) appear to predict poor prognosis in critically ill patients.

5. Lactate should always be measured, rather than estimated from the anion gap.

Key References

8. Mecher C, Rackow EC, Astiz ME, Weil MH: Unaccounted for anion in metabolic acidosis during severe sepsis in humans. Crit Care Med 1991;19:705-711.
9. Kellum JA: Determinants of blood pH in health and disease. Crit Care 2000;4:6-14.
10. Kellum JA, Kramer DJ, Pinsky MR: Strong ion gap: A methodology for exploring unexplained anions. J Crit Care 1995;10:51-55.
20. Kaplan L, Kellum JA: Initial pH, base deficit, lactate, anion gap, strong ion difference, and strong ion gap predict outcome from major vascular injury. Crit Care Med 2004;32:1120-1124.
21. Dondorp AM, Chau TT, Phu NH, et al: Unidentified acids of strong prognostic significance in severe malaria. Crit Care Med 2004;32:1683-1688.

See the companion Expert Consult website for the complete reference list.

Clinical Syndromes

CHAPTER 118

Metabolic Acidosis

Howard E. Corey

OBJECTIVES

This chapter will:
1. Describe how to determine the magnitude, cause, and prognosis of metabolic acidosis using a physiochemical model.
2. Relate physiochemical parameters to intracellular energetics and metabolism.
3. Offer a targeted, physiological approach to the treatment of metabolic acidosis.

In the critically ill patient, significant metabolic acidosis is associated with a poor prognosis.[1] In this setting, metabolic acidosis is not only a marker of extreme illness but also a central mediator in the matrix of trauma, burns, and sepsis. In studies of critically ill adults with peritonitis due to perforation of the colon, severe burns, placement of a ventricular assist device, penetrating or blunt trauma, pancreatitis, or severe malaria, multiple logistic regression analysis has shown that base excess (BE) is a significant variable in predicting mortality, independent of Acute Physiological and Chronic Health Evaluation II (APACHE II) or other clinical scoring systems.[1-10] Similar observations have been made in children.[11-13]

In addition to mortality, BE may also predict the onset of abdominal compartment syndrome[14] and the need for blood products.[15] In aggregate, these studies suggest that clinically "sicker" but less acidotic patients may in some cases fare better than patients who are less severely injured but have a higher level of acidosis.

This seeming paradox does not hold true for all causes of acidosis, because there are differences in outcome between respiratory acidosis and metabolic acidosis in similar pH ranges.[16] Although severe acidemia predisposes to cardiac arrhythmias, causes venoconstriction, and impairs oxygen delivery, some studies suggest that BE is superior to pH in predicting mortality in the intensive care unit.[17] These observations suggest that the "metabolic" aspect of metabolic acidosis is more significant than the perturbation in plasma hydrogen ion concentration [H+] per se.

Furthermore, the outcome of critical illness may be influenced not only by the *magnitude* of a metabolic disorder but also by its specific *cause*. For example, the accumulation of "unmeasured" anions (lactate, ketoacids, byproducts of intermediate metabolism, and intoxicants) in the setting of trauma or sepsis may portend a dire consequence, whereas acidosis secondary to the accumulation of chloride anion in the same setting may be relatively benign.[16,18,19]

"Unmeasured" anions may serve as markers (if not determinants) of degraded cellular energetics.[20-23] In clinical practice, the plasma lactate-to-pyruvate (L/P) ratio and the arterial ketone body ratio (acetoacetate-to-3-hydroxybutyrate ratio [AKBR]) are used as markers of the cytoplasmic state and the mitochondrial redox state (ratio of the reduced form of nicotinamide adenine dinucleotide [NADH] to the oxidized form of nicotinamide adenine dinucleotide ion [NAD+]), respectively. In patients with lactic anion acidosis and hemodynamic instability, Levy and associates[24] found an especially poor prognosis among those with an elevated plasma L/P ratio, a low AKBR, and an inability to clear lactate rapidly.

These observations reiterate that acid-base physiology and intracellular metabolism are coupled closely. In order to guide treatment successfully, a model of acid-base balance must account for, consider, and unravel these multiple, divergent processes.

THE PHYSIOCHEMICAL MODEL OF ACID-BASE BALANCE

One may assume that human plasma consists of fully dissociated ions ("strong ions" such as Na+, K+, Cl-, and lactate), partially dissociated "weak" acids (mostly albumin and phosphorus), and volatile buffers (carbonate species).[25] This system, constrained by the laws of mass action, the conservation of mass, and the conservation of charge, may be completely described by six thermodynamic equilibrium equations, which are listed in Table 118-1.

If we ignore the contribution of the smaller terms in the electrical neutrality equation, solving for pH yields the following:

$$pH = pK' + \log \frac{[SID^+] - K_a[A_{tot}]/K_a + 10^{-pH}}{SP_{CO_2}}$$

The implications of these simple equations are startling. First, plasma pH is presented as a function of three independent variables, strong ion difference (SID), the total concentration of weak acids (A_{tot}), and carbon dioxide tension (P_{CO_2}), rather than the quantity of [H+] added or subtracted. As a corollary, the transcellular ionic flux that regulates these three variables must also ground clinical acid-base physiology.

TABLE 118-1

Thermodynamic Equations that Describe Human Plasma

THERMODYNAMIC PRINCIPLE	EQUATION	VARIABLES AND CONSTANTS
Water dissociation equilibrium	$[H^+] \times [OH^-] = K_w$	K_w' is the auto-ionization constant for water
Electrical neutrality equation	$[SID^+] + [H^+] = [HCO_3^-] + [A^-] + [CO_3^{2-}] + [OH^-]$	SID (strong ion difference) $= Na^+ + K^+ - Cl^-$ – fully dissociated "unmeasured" anions
Weak acid dissociation equilibrium	$[H^+] \times [A^-] = K_a \times [HA]$	K_a is the weak acid dissociation constant for HA
Conservation of mass for "A"	$[A_{tot}] = [HA] + [A^-]$	A_{tot} is the total concentration of weak acids A^- is the concentration of dissociated weak acids
Bicarbonate ion formation equilibrium	$[H^+] \times [HCO_3^-] = K_1' \times S \times P_{CO_2}$	K_1' is apparent equilibrium constant for the Henderson-Hasselbalch equation, and S is the solubility of CO_2 in plasma
Carbonate ion formation equilibrium	$[H^+] \times [CO_3^{2-}] = K_3 \times [HCO_3^-]$	K_3 is the apparent equilibrium dissociation constant for bicarbonate

Second, the Henderson-Hasselbalch equation is unmasked as a limiting case of the more general equation shown previously, and is obtained when the contribution of weak acids is ignored by setting $[A_{tot}]$ to 0. This simplification may be especially misleading in the intensive care setting, where hypoalbuminemia is commonplace.

Third, the curvilinear relationship of pH and P_{CO_2} (the "buffer curve") is explained by the explicit inclusion of an A_{tot} term. The slope of the curve generated by plotting SID against pH is the buffer value (β) of blood (β_{blood}) or separated plasma (β_{plasma}), where β is the change in noncarbonate base divided by the change in pH, as follows[26]:

$$\beta = (1 - Hct)1.2 \times [albumin \ g/dL] + (1 - Hct)0.097 \times$$
$$[phosphate \ mg/dL] + 1.58 \ [Hgb \ mg/dL] + 4.2 \ (Hct)$$

where Hct is hematocrit. If we define a physiological state with hemoglobin [Hgb] at 12 mg/dL, [albumin] at 4.2 g/dL, and [phosphate] at 4.3 mg/dL, then β_{blood} is 24 mEq/L. If we set [Hgb] to 0, then β_{plasma} is 5.4 mEq/L.

Fourth, when weak acids are held constant, the *magnitude* of the metabolic disturbance (base excess) is equal to the change in SID (ΔSID).[27] The *cause* of the metabolic acidosis may be due either to retention of chloride or to accumulation of "unmeasured" anions.

Finally, from the electrical neutrality equation, the familiar anion gap (AG) which is equal to $Na^+ + K^+ - Cl^- - HCO_3^-$, is revealed as a metric of the charge not only of "unmeasured" anions but also of weak acids (A^-). To achieve clinical utility, the AG must be "corrected" for A^-.[28-33]

THE STRONG ION GAP

If one considers the charge of weak acids, such as albumin and phosphorus, then "unmeasured" anions may be obtained from the strong ion gap (SIG), defined as follows:

$$SIG = Na^+ + K^+ - Cl^- - HCO_3^- - A^-$$

SIG is obtained by subtracting the "effective" strong ion difference (SID_e = bicarbonate + A^-) from the "apparent" strong ion difference ($SID_a = Na^+ + K^+ - Cl^- -$ "unmeasured" anions). To calculate A^-, Figge and colleagues[34] used electrolyte solutions that contained albumin as the sole protein moiety and computed the individual charges of each of albumin's constituent amino acid groups along with their individual pK_a values, as follows:

$$SIG = AG - \{[albumin \ g/dL](1.2 \times pH - 6.15) -$$
$$[phosphate \ mg/dL](0.097 \times pH - 0.13)\}$$

Unlike the AG, the SIG (normal range 0-5 mM) conforms to the laws of conservation of mass and charge (the physiochemical approach) and accurately reflects lactate and other "unmeasured" anions.[35,36] For example, lactate anion acidosis is an important prognostic indicator in hepatic cirrhosis.[37] Because it ignores the alkalinizing effect of hypoalbuminemia, the AG approach may fail to arrive at a diagnosis.[38]

In shock, nonlactate "unmeasured" anions may also be clinically relevant. For example, in patients with sepsis, the activity of mitochondrial electron chain transport enzymes (citrate synthetase, respiratory chain complexes I and IV) are attenuated markedly so that tricarboxylic acid cycle intermediates may accumulate in the plasma.[39-43] In patients with lactate anion acidosis due to anaerobic glycolysis, Forni and colleagues[40] observed a significant increase in isocitrate, alpha-ketoglutarate, malate, and D-lactate. In 30 patients with sepsis and hypoperfusion, Mecher and associates[42] found that "unmeasured" anions other than lactate contributed significantly to acidosis. In patients with severe malaria, Dondorp and coworkers[43] observed that "unidentified anions" other than lactate were the most important contributors to metabolic acidosis. In this investigation, SIG was highly predictive of mortality (area under the receiver operating characteristic curve, 0.73), independent of plasma lactate and creatinine concentrations. A reflection of hypoxia-induced mitochondrial dysfunction, these "unmeasured" anions may be approximated if one subtracts the plasma lactate concentration from SIG.

In several investigations, SIG appears to be superior to BE and AG in the diagnosis of metabolic acidosis.[16,44] These findings suggest a classification scheme of metabolic acidosis (SID < 38 mM) based on the physiochemical parameter of SIG.

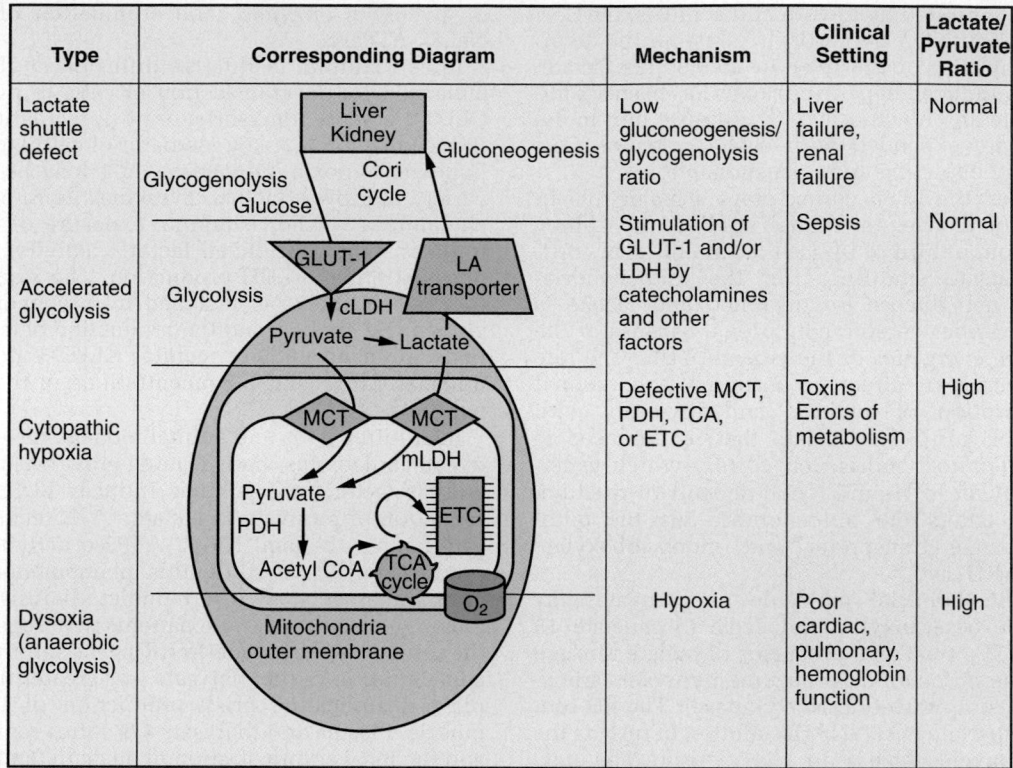

Type	Corresponding Diagram	Mechanism	Clinical Setting	Lactate/Pyruvate Ratio
Lactate shuttle defect		Low gluconeogenesis/ glycogenolysis ratio	Liver failure, renal failure	Normal
Accelerated glycolysis		Stimulation of GLUT-1 and/or LDH by catecholamines and other factors	Sepsis	Normal
Cytopathic hypoxia		Defective MCT, PDH, TCA, or ETC	Toxins Errors of metabolism	High
Dysoxia (anaerobic glycolysis)		Hypoxia	Poor cardiac, pulmonary, hemoglobin function	High

FIGURE 118-1. Lactic anion acidosis. cLDH, cytoplasmic lactate dehydrogenase; CoA, coenzyme A; ETC, electron transport chain; GLUT-1, facilitative glucose transporter; LA transporter, lactate/H^+ cotransporter; MCT, monocarboxylic acid transporter; mLDH, mitochondrial lactate dehydrogenase; PDH, pyruvate dehydrogenase; TCA, tricarboxylic acid.

METABOLIC ACIDOSIS ASSOCIATED WITH A HIGH STRONG ION GAP

Lactate Anion Acidosis

Generated by hepatic glycogenolysis, glucose enters the cytosol by facilitative diffusion through glucose transporter GLUT-1, whereupon it is oxidized by a sequence of enzymatic reactions to form two molecules each of pyruvate, NADH, adenosine triphosphate (ATP), and H^+. Cytosolic NADH may traverse the mitochondria, where oxidation yields an additional four to six molecules of ATP, depending on the pathway (the glycerol phosphate shuttle or the malate-aspartate shuttle).[45-49]

In an H^+-consuming but free energy–favorable step ($\Delta G = -6$ kcal/mol), pyruvate is reduced by the cytosolic enzyme lactate dehydrogenase (LDH) to form lactate anion. Lactate anion, along with H^+ derived from the hydrolysis of ATP, may enter the circulation by way of the membrane-bound lactate-H^+ cotransporter.[50] The flux of lactate anion from the cell lowers plasma SID and causes metabolic acidosis. Because lactic acid is not formed (a conundrum for proponents of the "lactic acid" theory of muscle fatigue), "lactic acidosis" is a misnomer and should be replaced by the physiochemical term *lactate anion acidosis*.

Traditionally, lactate anion acidosis (plasma concentration >1 mM) has been divided into two categories. Type A is associated with ischemia and tissue hypoxia, and type B is due to other causes, such as drug intoxication and errors of metabolism. Later investigations have shown that lactate anion acidosis arises from four commingled and interrelated mechanisms, as follows (Fig. 118-1)[45-49]:

- Poor lactate "shuttling," which in patients with severe liver and/or renal failure promotes a high plasma lactate concentration (>1 mM) despite normal values for lactate production rate (1 mEq/k/hr or 1400 mEq/day), mitochondrial function, and plasma L/P ratio (normally 4:1 to 20:1).
- Accelerated glycolysis, which in patients with sepsis but without tissue hypoxia results in a high lactate production rate (>1400 mEq/day) and hyperlactatemia.
- "Cytopathic hypoxia," an inability of pyruvate to enter the tricarboxylic acid cycle or the electron transport chain because of drugs (biguanides, isoniazid, salicylates), toxins (ethanol, methanol, ethylene glycol), or errors of metabolism (inborn, thymine deficiency).
- Dysoxia, which is the inability of cells to generate sufficient ATP to meet metabolic demand when mitochondrial PO_2 drops to less than 1 mm Hg (normal 4-20 mm Hg), is due to pulmonary disease, cardiac disease, or hemoglobin deficiency.

Poor Lactate Shuttling

Lactate plays a central role in cellular energetics, in part via the mechanism of interorgan and intraorgan lactate shuttling. In normal muscle, glycolysis produces lactate at a rate of about 0.15 mg/min/kg. In a muscle-to-liver interorgan shuttle known as the Cori cycle, lactate is consumed as a carbon source and is recycled to form glucose (gluconeogenesis) at a rate of about 0.83 mg/min/kg.[51] From glycogenolysis and gluconeogenesis, the liver produces glucose at a rate of about 2.4 mg/minute/kg, with the Cori cycle accounting for about 20% ($\approx$ 0.48 mg/min/

kg) of the total. Inhibited by insulin and acidosis, the Cori cycle may be stimulated by cortisol.[52] Despite the abundant reserve capacity of the liver to metabolize lactate, acetaminophen-induced hepatic cirrhosis has been associated with lactate anion acidosis.[38,53-56] Because four molecules of ATP are expended with each cycle, the Cori shuttle is energy-depleting and unsustainable.

After the liver, the renal cortex plays a major role in the clearance of lactate. In animal studies, the kidney metabolizes about a third of infused lactate through corticomedullary lactate shuttling.[57] In the mitochondria-poor medulla, net glucose is consumed and lactate is produced even under aerobic conditions, because of the highly favorable energetics of the enzyme LDH. The rate of glycolysis varies in direct proportion with proximal tubular reabsorption of sodium, and inversely with intracellular pH (pH_i). The lactate that is produced is shuttled to the mitochondria-rich cortex, which generates pyruvate by an LDH- and NAD^+-dependent reaction. Pyruvate then enters the mitochondria via the mitochondrial pyruvate transporter and monocarboxylate transporter-1 (MCT-1).[58-62]

Each intramitochondrial molecule of pyruvate may either enter the tricarboxylic acid cycle to generate 15 molecules of ATP or act as a precursor of malate through the action of the mitochondrial enzyme pyruvate carboxylase (phosphoenolpyruvate carboxykinase). The pH-sensitive malate-aspartate NAD^+/NADH shuttle, in turn, is the pathway to gluconeogenesis in the cytosol. The new glucose formed may be shuttled back to medulla, where it is again consumed to produce lactate.

Investigating L6 cells by laser scanning confocal microscopy, Hashimoto and colleagues[63] identified each of the intracellular components of the corticomedullary lactate shuttle and observed the co-localization of MCT-1, CD147, and LDH in mitochondrial inner membrane reticulum. Western blot analysis showed that cytochrome oxidase, NADH dehydrogenase, LDH, MCT-1, and CD147 are abundant in mitochondrial fractions. Interactions among cytochrome oxidase, MCT-1, and CD147 in mitochondria were confirmed by immunoblot analysis after immunoprecipitation. These findings are consistent with a mitochondrial lactate oxidation complex.

Lactate may be an important source of energy for other organs. For example, although glucose is the preferred substrate in normal brain, lactate improves mitochondrial respiration after traumatic brain injury.[64,65] This finding suggests that lactate anion plays a dual role, by functioning both as the cause of metabolic acidosis and as a consumable source of cellular energy.

In the critically ill, poor lactate clearance, severe anemia, and hypoalbuminemia are each associated with a poor outcome.[66-73] The buffer value, which links these markers together in a single equation, as shown earlier, is a measure of the blood's capacity to adsorb an acid load. If we define a disease state with [Hgb] at 8 mg/dL, [albumin] at 2 g/dL and [phosphate] at 4.3 mg/dL, then β_{blood} is 18.4 mEq/L, a loss of almost one quarter of the normal buffer value.

Accelerated Aerobic (Oxygen-Dependent) Glycolysis

Glycolytic enzymes such as phosphofructokinase are induced by alkalosis and inhibited by acidosis. Despite this feedback control, accelerated glycolysis under aerobic conditions may occur via several mechanisms, including facilitated cellular uptake of glucose, induction of glycolytic enzymes, and stimulation of sarcolemmal Na^+,K^+-ATPase.

In cell culture, facilitative diffusion of glucose may be enhanced by the transfection of cells to overexpress the GLUT-1 glucose transporter or by upregulation of hypoxia-induced factor-1. A key mediator of cellular adaptation to hypoxia, hypoxia-induced factor-1 may be induced by a variety of growth factors, cytokines, hormones, and catecholamines.[74-79] For example, exposure of cells to $CoCl_2$ induces hypoxia-induced factor-1 activity, glucose phosphorylation, and LDH production. The resulting increase in glucose uptake is matched by a concomitant rise in glucose metabolism and the production of lactate. Interestingly, humans with congenital GLUT-1 deficiency have unusually low lactate concentrations in their cerebrospinal fluid.[79]

In cultured cells and animal models, the administration of catecholamines, transforming growth factor, epidermal growth factor, or cytokines induces LDH, favoring the reduction of pyruvate to lactate.[76-79] Catecholamines raise cellular metabolism, Na^+,K^+-ATPase activity, and lactate production.[80-87] To study this phenomenon in humans, Levy and associates[88] inserted microdialysis catheters into the thigh muscles of seven patients with sepsis and infused the catheters with lactate-free Ringer's solution. The lactate concentration in the dialysate was greater than that in the plasma, indicating brisk production of lactate by the muscle. Plasma and dialysate L/P ratios remained normal, and the local administration of ouabain (an Na^+,K^+-ATPase inhibitor) significantly reduced the production of lactate. Similar findings have been observed after adrenergic blockade with propranolol and phenoxybenzamine.[87]

Findings of these studies suggest that lactate anion is produced abundantly under aerobic conditions owing to accelerated glycolysis, in parallel with high ATP turnover.[89-91] Cytosolic lactate anion may join the circulation by way of the lactate-H^+ cotransporter or enter the mitochondria via MCT-1 as a substrate for oxidative phosphorylation.

Cytopathic Hypoxia

As previously discussed, *cytopathic hypoxia* refers to disruption of normal mitochondrial function under aerobic conditions as a result of drugs, toxins, or inborn errors of metabolism. For example, propofol, inhibitors of viral reverse transcriptase, and metformin may degrade mitochondrial function by interfering with the synthesis of respiratory chain enzymes.[92-94] Congenital lactate anion acidosis is characterized by progressive neuromuscular deterioration and often results in early death. More than 100 different disorders have been reported, most of which are due to a defect in the pyruvate dehydrogenase complex or in one or more enzymes of the respiration chain. For example, mutations in the transfer RNA genes of mitochondrial DNA cause MELAS (mitochondrial myopathy, encephalopathy, and lactate anion acidosis due to low complex I activity syndrome) and MERRF (myoclonic epilepsy and ragged red fiber disease due to deficiency in complex I and complex IV) syndrome.[95] Characterized by a high plasma L/P ratio, these disorders mimic dysoxia under stressful but still aerobic conditions.

The pathophysiology of some of these disorders has been partly clarified. The oxidation of mitochondrial NADH is coupled to the proton motive force, a chemostatic potential gradient of H^+ across the inner and outer mitochondrial membranes that varies in response to cellular energy charge. As demand for intracellular energy increases (high intracellular ADP), the proton motive force gradient is discharged through membrane-bound ATP synthase (complex V), regenerating the ATP pool.[96,97] In fibroblasts obtained from patients with MELAS and MERRF, James and associates[98] found that stimulating ATP demand by incubation with the Na^+,K^+-ATPase ionophore gramicidin did not increase intracellular ATP. This finding suggests that some forms of cytopathic hypoxia may be due to degeneration of the proton motive force, so that energy supply cannot meet energy demand under conditions of stress.

In pyruvate dehydrogenase complex deficiency, carbohydrate-rich meals may exacerbate or precipitate lactate anion acidosis. Treatment may consist of a ketogenic diet, carnitine, thiamine, biotin, lipoate, riboflavin, coenzyme Q, or dichloroacetate. Dichloroacetate induces the pyruvate dehydrogenase complex, thereby favoring the oxidation of pyruvate to acetyl coenzyme A rather than reduction to lactate.[99] Although the concentration of plasma lactate is lowered reliably, the safety and efficacy of dichloroacetate treatment remain controversial.[100-103]

Lactate anion acidosis may also result from ethanol intoxication, especially in patients who are deficient in thiamine. In ethanol intoxication, the oxidation of ethanol to acetyl aldehyde is coupled by the $NADH/NAD^+$ reaction to the reduction of pyruvate to lactate. In thiamine deficiency, pyruvate dehydrogenase cannot efficiently oxidize pyruvate to acetyl coenzyme A so as to precipitate lactic anion acidosis.

Dysoxia

The first stage of oxidative phosphorylation, the conversion of glucose to pyruvate, yields a net of 2 ATP molecules. Under aerobic conditions, mitochondrial pyruvate dehydrogenase oxidizes pyruvate to acetyl coenzyme A, which enters the tricarboxylic acid cycle to yield 36 more ATP molecules. When oxygen is unavailable, pyruvate is reduced to lactate by cytosolic LDH, resulting in a high plasma L/P ratio (>20:1) and a low cytoplasmic redox state. In groups of domestic pigs fitted with splanchnic intravasal microdialysis catheters, Backstrom and colleagues[104] simulated mesenteric ischemia and reperfusion, endotoxic shock, or hemorrhagic shock. In the mesenteric ischemia and reperfusion group, a high dialysate L/P ratio correlated with dysoxia.

As ATP supply fails to meet ATP demand, the ratio of intracellular ATP to ADP and Pi falls, membrane Na^+,K^+-ATPase becomes depleted, and intramembrane Na^+ and K^+ channels fail to maintain normal ionic gradients. This process leads inexorably to cell swelling and death. The mitochondrial redox state may be estimated from the AKBR (normal ratio ≈ 1). In patients with hemorrhagic shock, Nakatani and associates[105] observed a high mortality rate in those patients with AKBR values less than 1. Shime and coworkers[106] made similar observations in patients who had undergone cardiac bypass surgery. These findings suggest that plasma SIG, lactate anion concentration, L/P ratio, and AKBR are important indicators of systemic acid-base balance precisely because they provide insight into cellular energetics.

The insight gained from the application of physiochemical parameters may be translated into a targeted approach to therapy. For instance, lactate anion acidosis due to poor lactate shuttling, accelerated glycolysis, cytopathic hypoxia, or dysoxia, may respond differently to organ replacement therapy/hemofiltration, a reduction of metabolic demand, induction of pyruvate dehydrogenase, or improvement in oxygen delivery. The use of base to increase SID (with $NaHCO_3^-$ [Carbicarb]) or buffer value (with THAM [tris-hydroxymethyl aminomethane]) remains controversial.[107-110]

Other Causes of High–Strong Ion Gap Metabolic Acidosis

Other causes of high-SIG metabolic acidosis are inborn errors of metabolism, diabetic ketoacidosis, alcoholic ketoacidosis, methanol ingestion, ethylene glycol poisoning, and salicylate ingestion.[111,112] Because their treatments differ markedly, the determination of the root cause of the acidosis in the individual patient is essential. The differentiation may be made through calculation of the anion gap and osmol gap (see later), specific toxicological or other testing, and urine microscopy to detect calcium oxalate crystals. In some settings, SIG may be more accurate than AG for the diagnosis.[113]

METABOLIC ACIDOSIS ASSOCIATED WITH A NORMAL SIG

Hyperchloremic metabolic acidosis arises from a blunted renal response to chloride loading whether it is due to renal failure, a diet with low "cation minus anion difference," renal tubular acidosis, or unbalanced crystalloid solutions.[16,19,25,27,114,115,116] Acidosis with a normal SIG may also result from renal sodium wasting, as in mineralocorticoid deficiency. Because cellular energetics are preserved, the prognosis of hyperchloremic acidosis is relatively good. In 75 consecutive surgical intensive care patients in whom BE value exceeded −2.0 mM, Brill and associates[117] observed 4 deaths (10.8%) in the patients with hyperchloremic metabolic acidosis and 13 deaths (34.2%) in the remaining patients ($P = .03$). Demographic and other clinical features were similar in the two groups. In 18 (48.6%) of the patients with hyperchloremia, metabolic acidosis resulted from fluid resuscitation with lactated Ringer's solution. Other investigators have made similar observations.[118]

DIAGNOSIS OF METABOLIC ACIDOSIS

Some of the causes of metabolic acidosis are listed in Table 118-2. An algorithm for the diagnosis of three common clinical presentations (shock, stupor, and diabetes) that may be associated with metabolic acidosis is presented in Figure 118-2. The bedside calculation of SIG and osmol gap (OG = measured plasma osmolarity − calculated plasma osmolarity) will suggest more specific investigations that lead to the correct diagnosis—which in this example could be unbalanced crystalloid administration, dysoxia, intoxication, diabetic ketoacidosis, or the hyperglycemic hyperosmotic state.

CONCLUSION

A successful model of acid-base balance must determine the magnitude and cause of a metabolic acidosis and relate them to the intracellular energy charge, the capacity of the

TABLE 118-2

Causes of Metabolic Acidosis According to Strong Ion Gap

	Strong Ion Gap	
	<5 mM	**>5 mM**
Children	Renal tubular acidosis Salt-wasting forms of congenital adrenal hyperplasia Corticosterone methyloxidase deficiency Pseudohypoaldosteronism Improper formula preparation Diarrhea	Inborn errors of metabolism Congenital lactate anion acidosis
Adults	Dilutional acidosis Unbalanced crystalloids Sjögren's syndrome Mineralocorticoid deficiency Chronic renal failure Total parenteral nutrition	Ketoacidosis (starvation, ethanol, diabetes) Salicylate toxicity Ethanol, methanol, isopropyl, propylene glycol toxicity Renal failure Toluene Cyanide Isoniazid Lactic anion

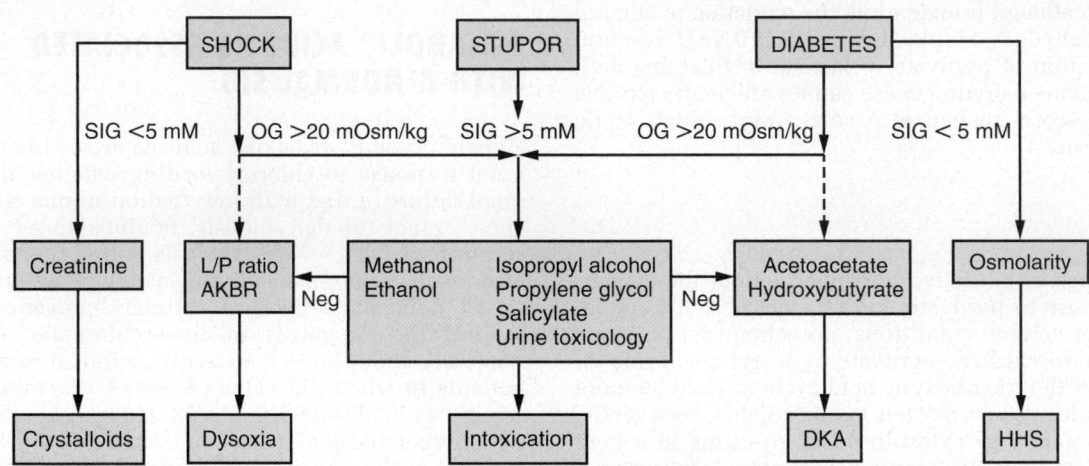

FIGURE 118-2. Diagnostic algorithm in patients with shock, stupor or diabetes, and base excess (BE) > −2 mM. Presentation with shock, stupor, or diabetes always warrants investigation for metabolic acidosis. In the patient with BE > −2 mM, the strong ion gap (SIG) and OG (osmol gap; OG = measured osmolarity − calculated osmolarity) suggest further studies to assign the case to a specific diagnostic category. AKBR, acetoacetate/3-hydroxybutyrate ratio; DKA, diabetic ketoacidosis; HHS, hyperglycemic hyperosmotic state; L/P, lactate/pyruvate.

blood to resist changes in pH, the most efficacious treatment, and the likely outcome. Although overly simple approaches are likely to fail, overly detailed formulations are unlikely to be useful at the bedside.

Based on standard thermodynamic principles, the physiochemical model avoids both of these pitfalls. As shown earlier in the equation solving for pH, which may be thought of as a more elaborate version of the familiar Henderson-Hasselbalch equation, pH is determined by SID, A_{tot}, and PCO_2. The manipulation of SID according to the conservation of charge yields the SIG, a sensitive and specific indicator of "unmeasured" anions, including lactate anion. The physiochemical parameters SID and SIG, which may be computed readily, reveal the magnitude, cause, and impact of metabolic acidosis.

The physiochemical paradigm does not rescind other models of acid-base balance, but rather transcends them, because SIG may serve as a rough guide to the proton motive force. In sepsis and shock, metabolic acidosis associated with a high SIG is a harbinger of a poor outcome. In this setting, plasma L/P ratio and AKBR may provide insight into the cellular redox potential. The physiochemical approach unites these variables in a single framework, thereby unraveling the mechanism (see Fig. 118-1). In the diagnosis of ketosis, intoxication, or error of metabolism, SIG may be more accurate than BE or AG.

Hyperchloremic acidosis carries a better prognosis, perhaps because cellular energetics are generally preserved. SID may be useful in the understanding and correction of hyperchloremic acidosis associated with "dilution," renal failure, and renal tubular disorders, thereby avoiding overly aggressive treatment.

Key Points

1. Metabolic acidosis may contribute to the poor prognosis of some critically ill patients.
2. Physiochemical parameters may be superior to base excess for the diagnosis of metabolic acidosis.

3. A physiochemical approach may determine the magnitude and reveal the underlying cause of metabolic acidosis.

4. In some cases, physiochemical parameters may correlate with the level of intracellular stress.

5. The plasma osmol gap and the urine anion gap are also useful for the diagnosis of metabolic acidosis.

Key References

16. Kaplan LJ, Kellum JA: Initial pH, base deficit, lactate, anion gap, strong ion difference, and strong ion gap predict outcome from major vascular injury. Crit Care Med 2004;32:1120-1124.
27. Corey HE: Stewart and beyond: New models of acid-base balance. Kidney Int 2003;64:777-787.
36. Kellum JA, Kramer DJ, Pinsky MR: Strong ion gap: A methodology for exploring unexplained anions. J Crit Care 1995;10:51-55.
47. Levy B: Lactate and shock state: The metabolic view. Curr Opin Crit Care 2006;12:315-321.
50. Robergs RA, Ghiasvand F, Daryl Parker D: Biochemistry of exercise-induced metabolic acidosis. Am J Physiol Regul Integr Comp Physiol 2004;287:R502-R516.

See the companion Expert Consult website for the complete reference list.

CHAPTER 119

Diagnosis and Therapy of Metabolic Alkalosis

Alan C. Heffner, Raghavan Murugan, Nicholas Madden, and John A. Kellum

---

OBJECTIVES

This chapter will:
1. Review the physiochemical mechanisms underlying metabolic alkalosis.
2. Explain the differential diagnosis of metabolic alkalosis.
3. Describe the treatment principles of chloride and strong ion difference manipulation to correct metabolic alkalosis.

Metabolic alkalosis is the most common acid-base abnormality encountered in the hospital setting, affecting more than 50% of patients with acid-base imbalance.[1-3] The disorder carries substantial morbidity and mortality that correlate with the severity and duration of alkalosis.[4,5] Patients with metabolic alkalosis have limited physiological compensation compared with patients with metabolic acidosis and therefore more readily sustain adverse cardiovascular and neurologic effects.[6,7] Patients with metabolic alkalosis experience longer duration of mechanical ventilation and longer intensive care unit stay than patients without the disorder.[2] Compensatory hypoventilation to limit alkalemia produces respiratory insufficiency and delays weaning from mechanical ventilation.[8]

PHYSIOLOGICAL REGULATION OF STRONG ION BALANCE

Aqueous solutions contain an inexhaustible source of hydrogen ion (H^+) in the form of water (H_2O). Although pure water dissociates only slightly, biological solutions contain electrolytes and carbon dioxide (CO_2) with powerful electrochemical forces that influence water dissociation. Quantitative physiochemical principles demonstrate that only three mathematically independent variables determine water dissociation and hence the H^+ concentration of body fluids—strong ion difference (SID), total concentration of nonvolatile weak acids (A_{tot}), and carbon dioxide tension (P_{CO_2}).[9,10] Increases in SID or diminutions in A_{tot} cause metabolic alkalosis by decreasing the dissociation of H_2O, thereby raising pH. Importantly, serum bicarbonate (HCO_3^-) reflects but does not determine pH, because serum bicarbonate is a dependent variable and its concentration is determined by the interplay of SID, A_{tot}, and P_{CO_2}. Physiological compensatory mechanisms regulate pH through manipulation of SID, P_{CO_2}, and A_{tot}. The kidney exerts a major influence on SID through regulation of chloride ion (Cl^-) balance.[11] In metabolic alkalosis, the kidney retains Cl^- to correct the SID. However, renal compensation is slow and requires intact function and solute load. Respiratory compensation for alkalemia occurs by alveolar hypoventilation leading to CO_2 retention.

Under normal physiological conditions, the body regulates the strong ions and P_{CO_2} to maintain a normal arterial pH. For instance, in the gastrointestinal tract, Cl^- is removed from the plasma and enters the stomach during gastric acid production. This process lowers the SID in the gastric juice, resulting in greater water dissociation and thereby raising H^+ concentration and lowering the pH. In plasma, the loss of Cl^- into the stomach creates an increase in SID, resulting in alkalosis, also known as the "alkaline tide." Subsequently, however, the reabsorption of Cl^- from the duodenum returns the plasma pH to normal under physiological circumstances. Working in conjunction with the duodenum is the pancreas, which secretes a fluid with high SID and low Cl^- into the small intestine. Thus, the

SID of the plasma that perfuses the pancreas is decreased, a phenomenon that peaks approximately an hour after a meal. The depletion of plasma Cl^- in the alkaline tide formation and the subsequent reabsorption in the duodenum offset each other, allowing for the maintenance of physiological pH. If large amounts of pancreatic fluids are lost (e.g., from surgical drainage), acidosis results as a consequence of the reduced plasma SID.

The colon also contributes to electrolyte homeostasis. Water absorption, a major physiological function of the colon, involves the reabsorption of Na^+ and K^+ ions (as most of the Cl^- has already been removed from the duodenum). Strong ions that are not absorbed in the colon are excreted. The role of the liver in acid-base homeostasis must also be acknowledged. Sensitive to plasma pH and stimulated by acidosis, hepatic glutaminogenesis contributes to overall pH balance.[4] Under normal conditions, the liver releases only a small amount of ammonium (NH_4^+), and the vast majority of the nitrogen is incorporated during the synthesis of glutamate and urea in the liver. Glutamate is transported to the kidney, where it is used to synthesize NH_4^+, which is then used by the kidney to co-excrete Cl^-, exerting an alkalinizing effect on plasma pH.[5] The liver is also responsible for the synthesis of albumin, a weak acid with a role in acid-base disorders discussed later.

Along with the gastrointestinal tract and the liver, the kidneys function to counterbalance the changes in plasma electrolyte concentrations. The goal of the kidney is to maintain a normal pH by altering SID. The SID of the plasma enables the clinician to predict the response of a healthy kidney. If the SID is elevated (e.g., in cases of metabolic alkalosis induced by prolonged vomiting), the kidney responds by increasing reabsorption of Cl^- ions and in turn contributing to a rise in plasma H^+ concentration. Conversely, when plasma SID is below the normal physiological level (e.g., in metabolic acidosis), the kidneys respond by decreasing reabsorption of Cl^-. It is through the selective reabsorption of Cl^- that kidneys are able to contribute to the overall maintenance of physiological pH.

EVOLUTION OF METABOLIC ALKALOSIS

Metabolic alkaloses evolve as a consequence of an inappropriately large SID or a decrease in A_{tot}. Sodium ion (Na^+) and Cl^- are the principal extracellular strong ions that determine SID. Pathophysiological disorders and compensatory mechanisms change pH through alterations in these strong ions. Five primary mechanisms increase the SID to generate metabolic alkalosis. First, *depletion of free water* induces a parallel increase in Na^+ and Cl^-. Because the relative plasma concentration of Na^+ is greater than that of Cl^-, the difference between them increases, subsequently widening the SID.

Second, any disorder that leads to *Cl^- loss in excess of Na^+* causes a similar increase in SID and is the most common cause of metabolic alkalosis. Common sources of Cl^- loss are the kidney, gastrointestinal tract, and skin. Disproportionate loss of Cl^- from the urine occurs as a consequence of loop and thiazide diuretics. Absolute or apparent mineralocorticoid excess and Bartter's and Gitelman's syndromes also produce urine Cl^- wasting.[12-14] Gastrointestinal fluids proximal to the duodenum are chloride-rich, and vomiting or nasogastric drainage can lead to Cl^- depletion. Less commonly, chloride-rich stool

TABLE 119-1

Physiochemical Mechanisms of Metabolic Alkalosis

PHYSIOCHEMICAL ALTERATION	PATHOPHYSIOLOGICAL MECHANISM
Increased strong ion difference (SID)	Loss of electrolyte free water
	Loss of chloride in excess of sodium
	Gain of sodium in excess of chloride
	Post-hypercapnic metabolic alkalosis
	Intracellular cation deficiency (K^+, Mg^+)
Decreased total weak acids (A_{tot})	Hypoalbuminemia
	Hypophosphatemia

may occur from colonic villous adenoma, congenital chloridorrhea, or laxative abuse.[15] Chronic respiratory acidosis induces renal Cl^- wasting.[16,17] This compensation is particularly potent and normalizes the pH over an extended period. The equilibrium of hypochloremia and hypercarbia is often disrupted by iatrogenic normalization of PCO_2. Aggressive ventilation of a patient with compensated chronic respiratory failure exposes the unopposed large SID to produce posthypercapnic metabolic alkalosis.

Third, metabolic alkalosis occurs with *Na^+ gain in excess of Cl^-*. Administration of nonchloride sodium salts occurs with blood transfusions (sodium citrate), parenteral nutrition (sodium acetate), plasma volume expanders (sodium lactate in Ringer's solution), and sodium bicarbonate. Sodium bicarbonate treatment of organic acidosis may also produce delayed "overshoot" alkalosis after metabolism of the organic ions (e.g., ketones and lactate).[18,19] Penicillins are administered as sodium salts and represent an often overlooked source of excess Na^+.[20]

Fourth, *severe deficiency of intracellular cations such as magnesium or potassium* produces alkalosis. Cation deficiency decreases intracellular Cl^- and, secondarily, total body Cl^-; the net result is increased SID. Fifth, metabolic alkalosis can also occur from a *decrease in A_{tot}* (Table 119-1). Proteins are the preponderant nonvolatile weak acid in plasma, followed by a negligible contribution from inorganic phosphate. Globulins play little role as weak acids, leaving albumin as the chief contributor to acid-base equilibrium.[21] Primary hypoproteinemic alkalosis is common in clinical practice owing to the high prevalence of hypoalbuminemia.[1,22] A 1–gm/dL drop in serum albumin drives a 3–mEq/L increase in serum bicarbonate and raises the standard base excess value by 3.5 mEq/L.[23] However, it is important to note that hypoalbuminemia is usually a slow process, providing the kidney ample time to compensate. Thus, so-called primary hypoproteinemic alkalosis can occur only if it is acute or occurs in conjunction with another of the causes of metabolic alkalosis described previously.

GENERATION AND MAINTENANCE OF METABOLIC ALKALOSIS

Transient metabolic alkalosis occurs in many clinical and iatrogenic situations. Normal kidneys exhibit marked capacity to reabsorb Cl^- and restore the SID to avoid persistent alkalosis.[24] Urine alkalinization strategies use this capacity to therapeutic advantage. However, withdrawal of an inciting precipitant does not always resolve metabolic alkalosis. Alkalosis persists when it occurs in conjunction with a factor that sustains the increased SID. Therefore, contributing sources of metabolic alkalosis are divided into generation factors and maintenance factors. Depending on the clinical situation, these factors may be the same, dissimilar, or a consequence of one another. Inadequate effective circulating volume and aldosterone excess represent the most important maintenance factors. For example, Cl^- loss from diuretic use or nasogastric drainage initiates metabolic alkalosis and simultaneously induces volume depletion, and compensatory mineralocorticoid stimulation sustains the disorder. In contrast, autonomous hyperaldosteronism is sufficient to generate and sustain chronic metabolic alkalosis. Although Cl^- repletion corrects the SID and alkalosis, generation and maintenance factors require specific attention to sustain normal balance.

Clinical Features

Adverse neurological and cardiopulmonary effects of alkalemia are well documented. Mental status change, coma, and seizures are associated with severe alkalemia.[7,25] Peripheral neuromuscular irritability manifested as paresthesias, myoclonus, and tetany are also well described but are not completely explained by the hypocalcemic effects of alkalemia as previously believed.[26] Alkalemia is implicated in supraventricular and ventricular dysrhythmias, which can be refractory to standard antiarrhythmic agents until pH is corrected.[27]

Compensatory hypoventilation and hypercapnia are associated with hypoxemia, pulmonary atelectasis, and infection, all of which contribute to arterial hypoxemia, respiratory failure, and cardiac arrest.[28] Reversible ventilation-perfusion mismatch arises from altered hypoxic vasoconstriction during alkalemia.[29,30] The combination of hypoxemia and hypoventilation contributes to prolonged mechanical ventilation.[2] Lastly, leftward shifting of the oxygen-hemoglobin dissociation curve caused by the Bohr effect contributes to tissue hypoxia by diminishing peripheral oxygen unloading.[31,32] Concomitant electrolyte and acid-base abnormalities are common in metabolic alkalosis and may mask typical laboratory findings. Metabolic or respiratory alkalosis may even overshadow organic acidosis (e.g., diabetic or alcoholic ketoacidosis) to produce neutral to alkaline pH.[33,34] Compensation for metabolic alkalosis occurs through CO_2 retention, which is achieved by hypoventilation. The capacity for respiratory compensation in metabolic alkalosis is limited compared with that in metabolic acidosis and may precipitate or prolong respiratory failure.[8]

DIAGNOSTIC EVALUATION

A careful history and physical examination demonstrate most causes of metabolic alkalosis. Gastric drainage, diuretic use, steroid treatment, and alkali administration are important historical points. Chronic hypertension and hypercapnic pulmonary disease are noteworthy previous medical conditions. Arterial blood pressure and intravascular volume status should be assessed at the bedside. Clinical evidence of hypovolemia is helpful because it

TABLE 119-2

Differential Diagnosis of Metabolic Alkalosis Based on Urine Chloride Concentration

High urine chloride ($\geq$20 mmol/L)	Primary hyperaldosteronism
	Apparent mineralocorticoid excess
	Bartter's syndrome
	Gitelman's syndrome
	Acute diuretic use
Low urine chloride ($\leq$10 mmol/L)	Renal: after diuretic use
	Gastrointestinal causes:
	Upper:
	Vomiting
	Bulimia
	Nasogastric drainage
	Lower:
	Villous adenoma
	Laxative abuse
	Congenital chloridorrhea
	Skin: cystic fibrosis
	Administration of non–chloride-containing sodium salts:
	Bicarbonate
	Acetate (parenteral nutrition)
	Citrate (blood products)
	Lactate (Ringer's solution)
	Penicillins
	Miscellaneous:
	Post-hypercapnia
	Hypoalbuminemia

represents the most prevalent maintenance factor of metabolic alkalosis. Effective circulating volume should be distinguished from total body fluid status, because the two may not correlate.

Except when part of a complex (mixed) disorder, metabolic alkalosis manifests as alkalemia (arterial pH > 7.45), hyperbicarbonatemia ($HCO_3^- > 26$ mmol/L), hypercarbia ($PCO_2 > 40$ mm Hg) and an increased standard base excess value (> 2 mEq/L). Importantly, the patient with elevated bicarbonate may have primary metabolic alkalosis or renal compensation for chronic respiratory acidosis. Arterial pH discriminates the two disorders; in the absence of a secondary acid-base disorder, pH is elevated in primary metabolic alkalosis and decreased in chronic respiratory acidosis. The urine Cl^- concentration reflects the renal response to metabolic alkalosis and is the most important discriminator for narrowing the differential diagnosis (Table 119-2). Chloride is intensely conserved through enhanced renal tubule reabsorption until hypochloremia is corrected.[35,36] Chloride avidity, reflected by a urine Cl^- value less than 10 mmol/L, identifies *chloride-responsive* (formerly known as saline- or volume-responsive) alkalosis, which is amenable to Cl^- repletion. A urine Cl^- value greater than 20 mmol/L indicates inappropriate renal Cl^- wasting. *Chloride-resistant* alkaloses constitute 5% of cases and largely comprise syndromes marked by absolute or apparent mineralocorticoid excess. Active diuretic use disables compensatory renal Cl^- retention and stands as an important exception.

Treatment

As in all acid-base disorders, the first priority of clinical management is to prevent death or injury. Arterial pH greater than 7.60 requires rapid corrective action even in the absence of immediate end-organ dysfunction. Modest but not full correction is the goal of immediate therapy. Lesser degrees of alkalemia should be expeditiously addressed to avoid worsening. Restoration of the SID is the cornerstone of treatment and is accomplished by administration of Cl^-.[19,37] The safest therapeutic cation to accompany the Cl^-—sodium, potassium, or hydrogen—is determined by the patient's volume status and potassium deficit. Alkalosis can be reversed by the administration of Cl^- without volume expansion, but many patients suffer associated volume depletion with this approach.[38] Isotonic saline (0.9% NaCl), which simultaneously repairs the Cl^- and volume deficits, is a mainstay of therapy. In stable patients, accompanying free water deficits may be better served with use of 0.45% saline. Patients with volume overload, renal failure, or intolerance to fluid loading require alternatives to NaCl therapy. Potassium chloride (KCl) may be used alone or in conjunction with loop diuretics. Alternatively, potassium-sparing diuretics and acetazolamide induce urinary excretion of Na^+ in excess of Cl^- to reduce SID.[39-41] Hydrochloric acid (0.1-0.2 N) administered via central access is well described but its use is still accompanied by a significant volume load.[30] In patients with renal insufficiency, hemodialysis or continuous renal replacement therapy may also be used to achieve rapid acid-base correction with or without the previously mentioned adjuncts.[42,43]

Secondary treatment is aimed at removing the stimulus of alkalosis generation and restoring the kidney's ability to reabsorb Cl^-. Discontinuation or modification of gastric drainage, diuretic regimen, and alkalinizing salts prevent continued Cl^- depletion. Slow, controlled correction of hypercarbia in patients with chronic respiratory failure avoids post-hypercapnic metabolic alkalosis. Chloride-resistant cases are more difficult to manage. Mineralocorticoid excess may be ameliorated via potassium-sparing diuretics, hormone antagonism, or steroid suppression. Surgical resection or medical ablation of the adrenal glands may be required for definitive cure.

Key Points

1. Metabolic alkalosis is the most common acid-base disorder in hospitalized patients and is associated with increased morbidity and mortality.
2. Metabolic alkalosis occurs from an increase in the strong ion difference or a decrease in the total concentration of weak acids.
3. Generation and maintenance factors in metabolic alkalosis each require specific therapeutic attention.
4. Clinical estimation of fluid status and urine chloride measurement are important diagnostic and therapeutic discriminators in metabolic alkalosis.
5. Chloride repletion is the mainstay of therapy for correction of most metabolic alkaloses.

Key References

1. Hodgkin JE, Soeprono FF, Chan DM: Incidence of metabolic alkalemia in hospitalized patients. Crit Care Med 1980;8:725-728.
11. Kellum JA: Determinants of plasma acid-base balance. Crit Care Clin 2005;21:329-346.
35. Galla JH, Bonduris DN, Dumbauld SL, Luke RG: Segmental chloride and fluid handling during correction of chloride-depletion alkalosis without volume expansion in the rat. J Clin Invest 1984;73:96-106.
36. Galla JH, Bonduris DN, Sanders PW, Luke RG: Volume-independent reductions in glomerular filtration rate in acute chloride-depletion alkalosis in the rat: Evidence for mediation by tubuloglomerular feedback. J Clin Invest 1984;74:2002-2008.
39. Moviat M, Pickkers P, van der Voort PH, van der Hoeven JG: Acetazolamide-mediated decrease in strong ion difference accounts for the correction of metabolic alkalosis in critically ill patients. Crit Care 2006;10:R14.

See the companion Expert Consult website for the complete reference list.

Respiratory Acid-Base Disorders

Michael C. Reade and David A. Story

OBJECTIVES

This chapter will:
1. List the common causes of respiratory acidosis and alkalosis.
2. Describe ways to determine whether nonrespiratory changes are expected physiological compensation or secondary metabolic disorders.
3. Summarize the pathological effects of respiratory acid-base disorders.
4. Briefly discuss management strategies for respiratory acid-base disorders.
5. Describe the features of two particularly common respiratory conditions: hypercapnic chronic obstructive pulmonary disease and altitude sickness.

In the 1950s, during the Copenhagen polio epidemic, the only available clinical acid-base tool was measurement of total plasma carbon dioxide, which is 95% bicarbonate (see Chapter 113).[1] During the initial phase of the epidemic, patients were diagnosed with metabolic alkalosis on the basis of greatly increased total carbon dioxide values.[2] Mortality was very high until Ibsen, an anesthesiologist, correctly interpreted the problem as severe respiratory acidosis and instituted tracheotomy and positive-pressure ventilation as lifesaving management.[2] These events led clinicians to improve the clinical chemistry analysis of acid-base disorders and to pursue methods to separate respiratory and metabolic disorders. The Copenhagen epidemic also led to the development of the intensive care unit.[2]

Alveolar partial pressure of carbon dioxide ($Paco_2$), and therefore arterial partial pressure of carbon dioxide ($Paco_2$),[1] are determined by the inspired CO_2, CO_2 production, and alveolar ventilation (see Chapter 113). The extent of respiratory acid-base disturbance is reflected in the $Paco_2$ and pH. Unlike for metabolic acid-base disturbances, determining the etiology for primary respiratory acidosis or alkalosis is usually not difficult. It is more difficult to determine whether there is an appropriate metabolic (largely renal) compensation in the context of a primary respiratory abnormality or appropriate respiratory compensation in a primary metabolic disorder. Determining whether a respiratory abnormality is a primary or compensatory process requires prediction of the expected $Paco_2$. This chapter uses the terms *respiratory acidosis* and *hypercapnia* and *respiratory alkalosis* and *hypocapnia* interchangeably. This practice relies on the understanding that respiratory "acidoses" or "alkaloses" are processes that contribute to acidemia or alkalemia and that may be caused by processes affecting CO_2.

CAUSES OF RESPIRATORY ACIDOSIS

Table 120-1 lists the major causes of respiratory acidosis. $Paco_2$ may rise as a result of increased production. If the mechanisms for sensing and eliminating CO_2 are intact, the alveolar ventilation will increase in concert with CO_2 production, and $Paco_2$ will remain unchanged. For example, during vigorous exercise, CO_2 production rises from 200 mL/min to 2000 to 4000 mL/min, but alveolar ventilation also increases, so that $Paco_2$ actually falls somewhat.[1] A patient with respiratory disease may not be able to increase the alveolar ventilation sufficiently to compensate for the increase in CO_2 production. These compensatory mechanisms also do not function during controlled mechanical ventilation. For example, the first sign of malignant hyperthermia in a patient under general anesthesia is often a raised $Paco_2$, reflected in the end-tidal CO_2 capnograph.[3]

$Paco_2$ may also rise if the concentration of CO_2 in the inspired air is raised. Anesthetic machines in the past often incorporated a CO_2 cylinder. The purpose was to stimulate respiration during emergence from anesthesia and occasionally to make use of the cardiovascular effects of the higher sympathetic tone caused by a raised CO_2. As recently as 1997, 75% of anesthetic machines in the United Kingdom had attached CO_2 cylinders,[4] although the practice has now been discontinued. In some countries it remains possible to remove the CO_2 absorber from the anesthetic breathing circuit, achieving the same effect. Although accurate end-tidal CO_2 monitoring makes the addition of CO_2 to inspired gas safer than in the past, in practice the same monitoring along with advances in pharmacology has removed the need for such a technique. Use of inspired CO_2 may, however, make a comeback. Some new studies have suggested that increased inspired CO_2 and mild respiratory acidosis during colonic surgery may enhance blood flow to the skin and gut and may play a future role in reducing wound infections and anastomotic breakdown.[5]

One accepted clinical indication for adding CO_2 to the inspired gas is pediatric congenital heart disease, in which respiratory acidosis augments hypoxic pulmonary vasoconstriction and so decreases pulmonary blood flow in single-ventricle circulations.[6] Another is the use of supplemental CO_2 during cardiopulmonary bypass to overcome temperature-related alkalemia when the "pH stat" approach is used.[7] However, during most clinical situations, the use of raised CO_2 in the inspired gas is now almost always an unwanted effect of apparatus dead space. Modern ventilator and airway connector design ensures that this effect rarely occurs in the intensive care unit. However, a patient ventilated by means of an anesthetic circuit with an inadequate fresh gas flow can easily be exposed to a high inspired fraction of CO_2 ($Fico_2$). Common examples are the use of a Mapleson A circuit during controlled ventilation

TABLE 120-1

Causes of Respiratory Acidosis

Increased CO_2 in inspired gas	Rebreathing in a ventilator circuit due to apparatus deadspace
	Soda lime exhaustion in a circle breathing system
	Closed environment; e.g., spacecraft.
Increased CO_2 production*	Fever
	Seizures
	Hypermetabolic state—trauma, sepsis, burns
	Overfeeding
	Malignant hyperthermia
	CO_2 insufflation during laparoscopy
	Bicarbonate administration
Reduced alveolar ventilation—either reduced minute ventilation or increased dead space or both	Impaired lung mechanics:
	ARDS
	Pneumothorax
	Pulmonary edema
	Interstitial lung disease
	Asthma
	$\dot{V}/\dot{Q}$ mismatch—increased dead space:
	Pulmonary embolus
	Many lung disorders
	Impaired neuromuscular strength:
	Pharmacological neuromuscular blockade
	Toxins: elapid snake venom, organophosphates
	High central neuraxial anesthetic block
	Myasthenia gravis
	Guillain-Barré syndrome
	Phrenic nerve palsy
	Cervical cord damage (at or above C4)
	Muscular dystrophy
	Impaired CO_2 control mechanism:
	Obesity—hypoventilation syndrome
	Drugs: opioids, benzodiazepines, inhaled anesthetic agents
	CNS disease: encephalitis, meningitis, trauma, hemorrhage, ischemia
	Iatrogenic
	Inadequate mechanical ventilation
	Spontaneous ventilation general anaesthesia

*This will not cause a respiratory acidosis unless alveolar ventilation is not increased in parallel

TABLE 120-2

Causes of Respiratory Alkalosis

Decreased CO_2 production*	Hypothermia
Increased alveolar ventilation	Due to hypoxia
	High altitude
	Severe anemia
	Shock
	Right to left shunt
	Lung disease
Abnormal CNS respiratory drive	Voluntary
	Pain
	Anxiety
	Cerebral irritation—infection, bleeding, tumor, stroke
	Drug effects: salicylates; progesterone; paraldehyde; catecholamines; doxapram
	Extreme exercise
Iatrogenic hyperventilation	Accidental
	Treatment of raised ICP
Miscellaneous	Hyperthyroidism
	Liver failure
	Sepsis
	Pregnancy

*This will not cause a respiratory alkalosis unless alveolar ventilation is not reduced in parallel, as during mechnical ventilation.

ingly common in the intensive care unit after the finding that ventilation with smaller tidal volumes and "permissive hypercapnia" improves outcome in patients with the acute respiratory distress syndrome (ARDS).[9] Although this practice is conventionally thought to reflect the beneficial effect of reduced repetitive lung stretching, a subsequent analysis found that patients in the control arm of the study (who received the higher lung volumes) who were hypercapnic had a lower 28-day mortality than those who were not hypercapnic, after adjustment of the data for comorbidities and severity of lung injury.[10] An earlier animal model had demonstrated a similar protective effect of raised inspired CO_2,[11] perhaps due to an anti-inflammatory effect.

CAUSES OF RESPIRATORY ALKALOSIS

Respiratory alkalosis has many causes (Table 120-2). It is said to be the most common acid-base disorder in critical illness because multiple psychological and pathophysiological mechanisms can stimulate respiration.[12] Hypocapnia is significantly correlated with adverse outcome in a variety of critical illnesses.[13] However, in contrast to respiratory acidosis, in which pH can decrease markedly, it is unusual for respiratory alkalosis to cause a pH greater than 7.6, except at extremes of altitude.[1]

Respiratory Pseudoalkalosis

When cardiac output is markedly reduced (as, for example, during resuscitation in cardiac arrest), the blood that does reach the lung transits more slowly. If ventilation is maintained, CO_2 in this blood falls even further than normal, so blood returning to the left heart (and the arterial circulation) is relatively alkalotic. This arterial blood may also be relatively well oxygenated. In contrast, venous blood

or of a Mapleson B or C circuit, such as may be used during resuscitation in intensive care units. In the non-intubated patient, an oxygen mask with inadequate oxygen flow can quickly cause respiratory acidosis.[8] In other closed environments, such as hyperbaric chambers, submarines, and spacecraft, accumulation of expired CO_2 can lead to increased inspired CO_2. One of the best-known examples was in the ill-fated Apollo 13 spacecraft flight, during which the astronauts had to rig up a lithium carbonate system, similar to a CO_2 absorber on an anesthetic machine, to prevent life-threatening respiratory acidosis.

The most common causes of respiratory acidosis are those that reduce the alveolar ventilation. Some may be transient (such as spontaneous ventilation under general anesthesia), but most are chronic. Chronic respiratory acidosis usually stimulates a metabolic compensation (see Chapter 129). Respiratory acidosis has become increas-

TABLE 120-3

Rules for Predicting Appropriate Acid-Base Compensation

ACID-BASE PROBLEM	USING THE "BOSTON APPROACH"[†]	USING BASE EXCESS[†]
Respiratory acidosis Acute	The expected $[HCO_3^-] = 24 + \dfrac{PaCO_2 - 40}{10}$ *or* the $[HCO_3^-]$ increases 1 mmol/L for every 10-mm Hg elevation in $PaCO_2$ above 40 mm Hg	The expected base-excess change is zero
Chronic	The expected $[HCO_3^-] = 24 + \left(4 \times \dfrac{PaCO_2 - 40}{10}\right)$ *or* the $[HCO_3^-]$ increases 4 mmol/L for every 10-mm Hg elevation in $PaCO_2$ above 40 mm Hg	The expected change in base excess = 0.4 × change in CO_2
Respiratory alkalosis Acute	The expected $[HCO_3^-] = 24 - \left(2 \times \dfrac{40 - PaCO_2}{10}\right)$ *or* the $[HCO_3^-]$ decreases 2 mmol/L for every 10-mm Hg decrease in $PaCO_2$ below 40 mm Hg	The expected base-excess change is zero
Chronic	The expected $[HCO_3^-] = 24 - \left(5 \times \dfrac{40 - PaCO_2}{10}\right)$ *or* the $[HCO_3^-]$ decreases 5 mmol/L for every 10-mm Hg decrease in $PaCO_2$ below 40 mm Hg NOTE: The limit of compensation is around 12-15 mm Hg	The expected change in base excess = 0.4 × change in CO_2
Metabolic acidosis	The expected $PaCO_2 = 1.5 \times [HCO_3^-] + 8*$	The expected change in CO_2 = change in base excess
Metabolic alkalosis	The expected $PaCO_2 = 0.7 \times [HCO_3^-] + 20*$	The expected change in $CO_2 = 0.6 \times$ change in base excess

*A less accurate, but more easily recalled, rule of thumb is that in a metabolic acid-base disorder, the $PaCO_2$ is approximately equal to the last two digits of the pH; e.g., in a metabolic acidosis with a pH = 7.25, the $PaCO_2$ should be approximately 25.
[†]Units for $PaCO_2$ are mm Hg and for HCO_3 and base excess mmol/L.

reflects the metabolic state of the tissues, where there is marked respiratory and metabolic acidosis and hypoxia due to hypoperfusion. Respiratory pseudoalkalosis is an unsustainable state that rapidly progresses to death unless the circulation is restored.

ASSESSING THE NATURE OF RESPIRATORY ACID-BASE DISORDERS

To adequately assess the severity of a respiratory acid-base disorder from the $PaCO_2$ value, one must determine from the patient's history whether the disorder is acute or chronic. Additionally, a simultaneous metabolic acid-base abnormality is also sometimes present, and identification of this fact is often diagnostically useful. An apparent respiratory acidosis or alkalosis is sometimes entirely a compensatory process for a metabolic acid-base abnormality. It is important to determine whether a primary respiratory abnormality is also present. A number of approaches to this problem can be taken, and which is selected often depends on geography. The first of the two broad approaches (Table 120-3) is the CO_2/bicarbonate rules of thumb known as the "Boston approach." These rules are particularly popular in the United States. In the rest of the world, the base-excess approach developed in Copenhagen is widely (but not universally) used (see Table 120-3). For many years there has been dispute between the rules-of-thumb and base-excess camps, also known as the "Great TransAtlantic Acid-Base Debate."[14] Importantly, both

approaches are compatible with the Stewart approach, although the base-excess approach lends itself better to quantitative assessment.[15] However, although both approaches help assess the acid-base status, neither identifies the underlying mechanisms, which depend on the combined effects of the PCO_2, strong ion difference, and total concentration of weak acids.[7]

The utility of these rules is frequently demonstrated in acute asthma. Many asthmatic patients present with a metabolic acidosis (28% in one series)[16] caused by hyperchloremia (associated with hyperventilation) and hyperlactatemia (associated with tissue hypoxia and the effect of β_2 agonists). A typical blood gas sample might have the following parameters: PaO_2 (arterial pressure of oxygen) 60 mm Hg, pH 7.27, $PaCO_2$ 40 mm Hg, HCO_3^- 18 mmol/L, and base excess −8.9 mmol/L. The CO_2 value is "normal," but this fact is not as reassuring as it should be. The predicted CO_2 value (from Table 120-3) is 30 to 35 mm Hg, so in fact, a respiratory acidosis is present as well. The PaO_2 would be expected to drive a respiratory alkalosis, so a patient with such readings is likely to be tiring and possibly has impending respiratory failure.

ADVERSE EFFECTS OF RESPIRATORY ACID-BASE DISORDERS

The signs and symptoms of respiratory acidosis and alkalosis are listed in Table 120-4. Because any alteration in $PaCO_2$ is quickly mirrored by the PCO_2 inside cells, the

TABLE 120-4

Effects of Respiratory Acidosis and Alkalosis

Respiratory acidosis	Cyanosis
	Vasodilation
	Diaphoresis
	Somnolence
	Headache
	Raised cerebral blood flow and ICP
	Stimulation of ventilation, or apnea
	Hypoxia
	Increased myocardial contractility, vessel tone and blood pressure (unless at the limit of sympathetic drive)
	Shift of oxyhemoglobin dissociation curve to the right
Respiratory alkalosis	Lightheadedness
	Visual disturbance
	Dizziness
	Paresthesia and tetany
	Transiently reduced ICP
	Cerebral vasoconstriction and ischemia
	Reduced myocardial contractility
	Cardiac arrhythmia
	Mildly reduced extracellular K^+ and ionized Ca^{2+}
	Inhibition of respiratory drive
	Shift of oxyhemoglobin dissociation curve to the left

effects of respiratory acid-base disorders occur more rapidly than those of metabolic disorders in which the pH is changed to the same extent. Nonetheless, most of the effects of respiratory acid-base disturbances are the consequence of altered pH rather than of the abnormal PCO_2 per se.[12]

If a respiratory acid-base disturbance becomes chronic, many of the adverse effects are minimized by compensatory mechanisms in the kidney, gut, and central nervous system, as described later. Compensation also occurs at a widespread cellular level: for example, respiratory alkalosis stimulates phosphofructokinase, which increases glycolysis and lactate production,[17] inducing an intracellular acidosis.

CO_2 has numerous effects on the neurological system. Hypocapnia causes dizziness and lightheadedness, probably through cerebral vasoconstriction and consequent ischemia. Conversely, patients with hypercapnic respiratory failure become somnolent or even unconscious when $PaCO_2$ reaches 90 to 120 mm Hg.[1] Inspired CO_2 is still used as a veterinary anesthetic, but its use in humans is precluded by its tendency to cause convulsions. CO_2 causes dilatation of the resistance vessels in the cerebral circulation, with a linear relationship between $PaCO_2$ and cerebral blood flow over the physiological range. The cerebral blood volume in part determines intracerebral pressure, so this phenomenon is sometimes used to transiently reduce intracerebral pressure in cases of expanding space-occupying lesions and brain swelling.[18] The utility of this technique is limited by the ischemia produced by excessive vasoconstriction,[19] and also by the loss of the vasoconstrictor effect after a few hours of hyperventilation.[20] Additionally, localized disease may abolish the usual vascular response to CO_2. The many adverse effects of hypocapnia in a variety of neurological conditions have been

reviewed,[12] and current recommendations are to maintain normocapnia in all circumstances other than to temporize an acutely raised intracerebral pressure prior to definitive therapy.

Many of the cardiovascular effects of hypercapnia are mediated by increased sympathetic tone. In the healthy patient, this mediation outweighs the direct effect of raised CO_2 on the heart and blood vessels. For example, although CO_2 is a direct vasodilator and myocardial depressant, the sympathetic effect of CO_2 is such that hypercapnia during anesthesia usually raises the blood pressure.[21] In critical illness, the capacity for increased sympathetic output may be limited, and so the direct effects of hypercarbia unmasked.[10] Hypocapnia reduces myocardial oxygen delivery while raising oxygen demand, effects that may explain the higher incidence of cardiac dysrhythmias in hypocarbic patients.[12]

Raised $PaCO_2$ increases pulmonary vascular resistance in a manner analogous to, but quantitatively less than, hypoxic pulmonary vasoconstriction,[1] explained as another means of minimizing $\dot{V}/\dot{Q}$ mismatch. Conversely, lowered $PaCO_2$ blunts hypoxic pulmonary vasoconstriction, causing shunting and a reduction in the PaO_2.[22] Lowered $PaCO_2$ also causes bronchoconstriction, and possibly worsens acute lung injury.[12] $PaCO_2$ affects the position of the oxyhemoglobin dissociation curve. Alkalosis shifts the curve to the left, and the greater affinity of hemoglobin for oxygen reduces oxygen offloading in the tissues. Because hypercapnia is often the result of hypoventilation, a parallel event can be hypoventilation-related hypoxia. The alveolar gas equation uses $PaCO_2$ as a marker of alveolar ventilation, as follows:

$$PAO_2 = FIO_2(P_B - 47) - \frac{PaCO_2}{R}$$

where P_B is barometric pressure and R is the respiratory quotient (normally about 0.8). However, many clinicians incorrectly believe, on the basis of the alveolar gas equation, that the mechanism for decreased alveolar oxygen during hypoventilation is displacement by CO_2. The actual mechanism is a direct effect of hypoventilation on oxygen, as shown in the universal alveolar air equation for oxygen (see also Chapter 113), as follows[7]:

$$PAO_2 = \text{inspired } PO_2 - \frac{\text{oxygen consumption}}{\text{alveolar ventilation}}$$

Patients with severe respiratory acidosis always require supplemental oxygen as alveolar ventilation falls. When $PaCO_2$ rises to 90 mm Hg (as may happen in severe chronic obstructive pulmonary disease) at atmospheric pressure (760 mm Hg) in a patient breathing room air, the PAO_2 would be only 42 mm Hg. Furthermore, hypercapnia associated with dead space may also be associated with hypoxia due to shunt.[1] If not breathing supplemental oxygen, patients never die of respiratory acidosis: Hypoxia is lethal first.

The putative beneficial effect of hypercapnia in acute respiratory distress syndrome has already been discussed. Hypercapnia appears to induce a generally anti-inflammatory state, with reductions in activation of nuclear factor-κb and release of pro-inflammatory mediators, perhaps by interference with Toll-like receptor 4 signaling mechanisms.[10] Hypercapnia may also diminish the toxicity of reactive nitrogen metabolites.[10]

Alterations in $PaCO_2$ cause rapid changes in the distribution of electrolytes. Plasma K^+ is increased as $PaCO_2$ rises and extracellular H^+ is exchanged for intracellular K^+. Raised $PaCO_2$ causes a reduction in the ionized fraction of calcium, a finding that has been used to explain the peripheral neurological symptoms of hypercarbia listed in Table 120-4, although quantitative analysis suggests this may not be the case.[1]

TREATMENT OF RESPIRATORY ACID-BASE DISORDERS

The best treatment for any respiratory acid-base disorder is to address the underlying cause. It will be appreciated from the information in Tables 120-1 and 120-2 that doing so is not always possible. Respiratory alkalosis is often mild and, if transient, is not in itself problematic. Treatment is usually treatment of the cause. Exceptions are the use of rebreathing for anxiety-induced hyperventilation (having the patient breath into and from a paper bag) and opiates for hyperventilation due to cerebral irritation during mechanically assisted ventilation. Acetazolamide induces a renal tubular acidosis, which can accelerate or augment the renal response to more prolonged respiratory alkalosis such as that seen at altitude or in spontaneously breathing mechanically ventilated patients with cerebral irritation.

Respiratory acidosis is more often problematic, because the pH may fall to the point of interfering with cellular metabolism and $PaCO_2$ can rise far enough to cause coma. Sedation, intubation, and mechanical ventilation constitute the only effective treatment when hypercapnia has impaired consciousness, but at earlier stages, noninvasive positive-pressure ventilation via a tightly fitting face mask has been shown to lead to improved outcomes.[23] Spontaneously breathing patients with both hypoxia and respiratory acidosis must be given oxygen therapy with caution, because this measure can worsen the acidosis by removing hypoxic pulmonary vasoconstriction and thus worsening shunt. This problem appears to be quantitatively more important than the blunting of the hypoxic respiratory drive[24] and the decreased binding affinity of oxygen for carbon dioxide, the explanations usually advanced for this common clinical phenomenon. Nonetheless, patients with severe respiratory acidosis always require supplemental oxygen, as predicted by the alveolar gas equation already presented.

Sometimes it is not possible or desirable to correct the pH entirely by normalizing the $PaCO_2$, as, for example, in the mechanical ventilation of patients with severe lung disease. The level of acidosis that should be tolerated is unknown. It has been suggested that if the pH in patients undergoing permissive hypercapnia ventilation becomes too acidemic, an appropriate treatment is sodium bicarbonate. Such a strategy was used in the ARDSNet trial of low tidal volumes.[25] Adding HCO_3^- moves the CO_2/HCO_3^- equilibrium to the left, which although reducing (H^+) only produces more CO_2, worsening the hypercapnia. The strategy is effective only if alveolar ventilation can be increased to keep $PaCO_2$ constant—and because elimination of CO_2 is the primary problem, this measure is illogical and indeed ineffective.[26]

In many cases of respiratory acidosis it *is* possible to rapidly return the $PaCO_2$ to "normal" with mechanical ventilation, but it is often not desirable. The rapid reduction in $PaCO_2$ commonly removes the heightened sympathetic drive, contributing to cardiovascular collapse. Patients

with chronic respiratory acidosis will have developed a metabolic compensation. This was previously ascribed to increased bicarbonate but is better viewed as due to changes in the strong ion difference. Driving $PaCO_2$ into the normal range ("normal" for the population, not the patient) would leave an unopposed metabolic alkalosis, which among other adverse consequences would reduce respiratory drive, making it more difficult to wean the patient from artificial ventilation.

A number of pharmacological agents may have some use in respiratory acid-base disorders. Doxapram increases the sensitivity of peripheral chemoreceptors to oxygen and so acts as a respiratory stimulant. The major side effect is generalized central nervous system stimulation, which along with the requirement for intravenous administration limits its utility.[1] Naloxone is highly effective in reversing the respiratory depressant effects of opioids, as is flumazenil for benzodiazepines, although each must be used with caution if withdrawal symptoms are to be avoided. The carbonic anhydrase inhibitor acetazolamide has been extensively used in the treatment of acute mountain sickness (see later). The effect has traditionally been attributed to the induction of a renal metabolic acidosis, which allows alveolar ventilation to be increased beyond the usual limit imposed by respiratory alkalosis. Acetazolamide also affects the central chemoreceptors, inducing an intracellular acidosis that permits higher alveolar ventilation. This respiratory stimulant action is also beneficial in hypercapnic chronic obstructive pulmonary disease.[27] Although these explanations remain true, it seems that acetazolamide also has other beneficial effects, as reviewed by Leaf and Goldfarb.[28]

Common Clinical Situations

Of all the disorders listed in Tables 120-1 and 120-2, two warrant particular mention here.

Chronic Obstructive Pulmonary Disease

Discussed in great detail in Chapter 129, chronic obstructive pulmonary disease is very common, and presents in two distinct patterns. Type I respiratory failure exists where the CO_2 sensitivity has not been reset. Patients are often distressed by the effort required to keep the $PaCO_2$ at normal levels. In type II respiratory failure, patients tolerate abnormally high levels of $PaCO_2$ because of the reduced sensitivity in the central chemoreceptors. The prognosis is better in type I respiratory failure than in chronic type II, although hypercapnia associated only with an acute deterioration does not worsen outcome.[29] The problems with oxygen therapy and overly aggressive mechanical ventilation in type II respiratory failure have been discussed. Also worth mentioning is the tendency for a mixed acid-base status in such patients. Commonly, these patients are prescribed corticosteroids to influence the progression of their lung disease and diuretics to reduce the effect of the heart failure often coexistent with the pulmonary problem. Both corticosteroids and diuretics can cause metabolic alkalosis, which may augment the level of hypercapnia.

Altitude Sickness

Although the proportion of oxygen in the atmosphere is always 21%, the barometric pressure falls at altitude, and so does the partial pressure of oxygen. At 10,000 feet above sea level, the partial pressure of oxygen is the equivalent of breathing 14% oxygen at sea level.[1] Hypoxia on abrupt exposure to high altitude causes hyperventilation, the magnitude of which is limited by the resultant respiratory alkalosis. Ventilatory drive falls somewhat after about 30 minutes owing to rapid changes in the hypoxic response.[1] However, ventilation increases again over the subsequent days due to "acclimatization."[30] This increase was originally thought to be due to buffering of the pH change in the cerebrospinal fluid; although this buffering does occur, its time course is inconsistent with the observed respiratory effects. In reality, changes in central and peripheral chemoreceptor sensitivity as well as renal compensation for respiratory alkalosis are also involved.[1] *Altitude sickness* is a syndrome comprising both respiratory and central nervous system effects, affecting 42% of people who rapidly travel to 10,000 feet.[31] Symptoms caused by hypoxia, hyperventilation, and respiratory alkalosis include headache, nausea, insomnia, dizziness, and fatigue. Severe cases can progress to cerebral and pulmonary edema. The clinical features of this condition have been comprehensively reviewed.[31] Of interest is a finding that the metabolic response to chronic hyperventilation and hypocapnia at altitude may, in part, be due to an increase in concentration of weak acids (albumin).[30]

CONCLUSION

Respiratory acid-base disorders are usually given less attention in textbooks than acid-base disorders due to renal and gastrointestinal disease. Nonetheless, respiratory disorders are very common. A sound understanding of the physiology and pathophysiology involved facilitates their diagnosis and management.

Key References

1. Lumb AB: Nunn's Applied Respiratory Physiology, 6th ed. Philadelphia, Elsevier, 2005.
12. Laffey JG, Kavanagh BP: Hypocapnia. N Engl J Med 2002;347: 43-53.
21. Cullen DJ, Eger EI: Cardiovascular effects of carbon dioxide in man. Anesthesiology 1974;41:345-349.
24. Aubier M, Murciano D, Milic-Emili J, et al: Effects of the administration of O_2 on ventilation and blood gases in patients with chronic obstructive pulmonary disease during acute respiratory failure. Am Rev Respir Dis 1980;122:747-754.
25. Gehlbach BK, Schmidt GA: Bench-to-bedside review: Treating acid-base abnormalities in the intensive care unit—the role of buffers. Crit Care 2004;8:259-265.

See the companion Expert Consult website for the complete reference list.

CHAPTER 121

Complex (Mixed) Acid-Base Disorders

Raghavan Murugan and John A. Kellum

OBJECTIVES

This chapter will:
1. Describe complex acid-base disorders.
2. Present a step-by-step approach to identification of these disorders.
3. Discuss the principles of management of complex acid-base disorders.

Over the last century, acid-base chemistry has played an important role in acute medicine. Although virtually every physician would agree that acid-base disorders are important, there has been a tremendous amount of confusion and controversy regarding how best to approach an understanding of acid-base disorders, especially if these disorders are complex. Complex acid-base disorders arise frequently in critically ill patients, especially in those with multiple-system organ failure. To diagnose, to treat, and to avoid acid-base disorders, the clinician must recognize complex acid-base disturbances and understand how and why they occur. Advances in the understanding of acid-base physiology have resulted from the application of basic physicochemical principles of aqueous solutions. This application involves a systematic and quantitative approach to analysis of the determinants of complex acid-base disorders. In blood plasma, only three independent variables determine the H^+ concentration: PCO_2, strong ion difference (SID), and the total weak acid concentration (A_{tot}).[1]

Normally, arterial plasma pH is maintained between 7.35 and 7.45. Because blood plasma is an aqueous solution containing both volatile (carbon dioxide) and fixed acids, its pH is determined by the net effects of all of these components on the dissociation of water. The determinants of blood pH can be grouped into two broad categories, respiratory and metabolic. Respiratory acid-base disorders are disorders of carbon dioxide (CO_2) tension, whereas metabolic acid-base disorders comprise *all* other conditions affecting the pH. This latter category includes disorders of both strong acids and bases (including both organic and inorganic acids) and weak acids and bases (e.g., albumin and phosphate). *Acidemia* and *alkalemia* relate only to blood pH (relative to 7.40), whereas *acidosis* and *alkalosis* refer to the actual physiological (or pathophysiological) processes.

COMMON MIXED ACID-BASE DISTURBANCES

Some of the common forms of mixed acid-base disorders and their causes are listed in Table 121-1. Knowledge of common clinical conditions that are likely to be associated with mixed disturbances often provides valuable clues to the diagnosis. For instance, in patients presenting with status asthmaticus and acute respiratory acidosis, a subset of patients often experience superimposed lactic acidosis due to hypoxemia and a combination of hyperinflation and hypoperfusion. Similarly, patients who have experienced cardiopulmonary arrest often demonstrate lactic acidosis due to hypoperfusion and respiratory acidosis due to inadequate ventilation. A hypercapnic patient with chronic obstructive lung disease who is taking diuretics may present with compensated respiratory acidosis and metabolic alkalosis. If this patient then has a pulmonary infection, he or she is likely to have acute-on-chronic respiratory acidosis against a background of chronic metabolic alkalosis. The characteristic feature of salicylate toxicity is metabolic acidosis and respiratory alkalosis. Similarly, early sepsis may cause lactic and/or strong ion gap (SIG) metabolic acidosis owing to a combination of hypoperfusion, increased aerobic metabolism, and respiratory alkalosis due to the stimulatory effect of endotoxin on the brainstem respiratory center. Chronic hepatic failure is often associated with respiratory alkalosis and metabolic alkalosis as a result of diuretic-induced volume depletion.

IDENTIFICATION OF COMPLEX ACID-BASE DISORDERS

Acid-base disorders can be suspected from either the clinical presentation or the plasma electrolyte levels, but blood

TABLE 121-1

Common Mixed Acid-Base Disorders

DISORDER	ETIOLOGY
Metabolic acidosis and respiratory alkalosis	Severe sepsis and septic shock
	Salicylate toxicity
	Congestive heart failure and renal failure
Metabolic acidosis and respiratory acidosis	Cardiorespiratory arrest
	Hypoxemic respiratory failure
Metabolic alkalosis and metabolic acidosis	Diuretic therapy and ketoacidosis
	Vomiting and renal failure
	Vomiting and lactic acidosis/ ketoacidosis
Metabolic alkalosis and respiratory alkalosis	Diuretic therapy and chronic hepatic failure
	Diuretic therapy and sepsis
Metabolic alkalosis and respiratory acidosis	Diuretic therapy and chronic obstructive pulmonary disease
	Vomiting and chronic obstructive pulmonary disease
Mixed hyperchloremic and high–anion gap acidosis	Early chronic renal failure
	Diarrhea and lactic acidosis/ ketoacidosis
	Renal tubular acidosis and uremic acidosis
	Hyporeninemic hypoaldosteronism and diabetic ketoacidosis
Multiple acid-base disorders	Mixed metabolic acidosis + metabolic alkalosis + respiratory alkalosis and/or acidosis
	Increased anion gap acidosis + non–anion gap acidosis + strong ion gap acidosis
	Any combination of the above

gas measurement is required to confirm or help exclude the disorders. Evaluation of any acid-base disorder can then be approached in a stepwise manner, as discussed here.

Step 1: History and Physical Examination

Comprehensive history taking and physical examination can often give clues as to the underlying acid-base disorder. For example, patients who present with gastroenteritis manifested as diarrhea typically have non–anion gap metabolic acidosis from loss of cations such as Na^+ and K^+. Patients who present with chronic obstructive lung disease may have underlying chronic respiratory acidosis from retention of CO_2. Patients with diabetic ketoacidosis who present with shock due to severe dehydration secondary to vomiting and polyuria often present with mixed metabolic acidosis (increased anion gap acidosis due to ketoacids, and lactic acidosis due to shock) and metabolic alkalosis (due to vomiting). If this patient then receives large volumes of saline for resuscitation, a fourth, iatrogenic, acid-base disorder arises—hyperchloremic non–anion gap metabolic acidosis superimposed on preexisting ketoacidosis, lactic acidosis, and metabolic alkalosis.

TABLE 121-2

Acid-Base Patterns Observed in Humans

DISORDER	HCO₃⁻ (mEq/L)	Pco₂ (mm Hg)	SBE (mEq/L)
Metabolic acidosis	<22	$= (1.5 \times HCO_3^-) + 8$ $= 40 + SBE$	<−5
Metabolic alkalosis	>26	$= (0.7 \times HCO_3^-) + 21$ $= 40 + (0.6 \times SBE)$	>+5
Respiratory acidosis			
Acute	$= (P_{CO_2} - \dfrac{40}{10}) + 24$	>45	= 0
Chronic	$= (P_{CO_2} - \dfrac{40}{3}) + 24$	>45	$= 0.4 \times (P_{CO_2} - 40)$
Respiratory alkalosis			
Acute	$= 24 - (40 - \dfrac{P_{CO_2}}{5})$	<35	= 0
Chronic	$= 24 - (40 - \dfrac{P_{CO_2}}{2})$	<35	$= 0.4 \times (P_{CO_2} - 40)$

SBE, standard base excess.
From Kellum JA: Determinants of blood pH in health and disease. Crit Care 2000;4:6-14.

Step 2: Order Simultaneous Arterial and Venous Blood Gas Analysis and Complete Biochemical Profile, Including Lactate Measurement

The next step is to obtain simultaneous arterial and mixed (or central venous) blood gas measurements for pH, PO_2, and PCO_2 as well as a biochemistry profile. Measurement of all strong ions (including Ca^{2+}, Mg^{2+}) and of weak acids (albumin and phosphate) provides a more quantitative and precise characterization of the acid-base abnormality. The blood lactate level should always be directly measured whenever metabolic acidosis is suspected rather than estimated from the anion gap. The arterial PO_2 (PaO_2) allows the clinician to exclude arterial hypoxemia, and the venous oxygenation parameters, particularly the mixed venous O_2 saturation level, provides important information on tissue oxygenation. The two together allow the clinician to evaluate tissue perfusion as well (see Chapter 116).

Acid-base imbalances are usually recognized from abnormalities in the venous plasma electrolyte concentrations. Although HCO_3^- is a dependent variable, the venous HCO_3^- concentration is the easiest way to screen for acid-base disorders. However, a normal HCO_3^- concentration does not exclude the presence of serious, especially mixed acid-base derangements. Therefore, if the history and physical examination lead to suspicion of a disease process that results in an acid-base imbalance, more investigation is required. The HCO_3^- concentration is normally 22 to 26 mEq/L. Increases in HCO_3^- concentration occur with primary and compensatory metabolic alkaloses, and decreases occur with primary or compensatory metabolic acidoses. Regrettably, in mixed disorders, the HCO_3^- concentration may be misleading, and the presence of any abnormality in HCO_3^- concentration requires further investigation.

Step 3: Identify the Primary Disturbance

The next step is to determine whether the patient is acidemic (pH < 7.35) or alkalemic (pH > 7.45) and whether the primary process is metabolic (initiated by a change in strong ions or weak acids) or respiratory (initiated by a change in PCO_2). It is important to remember that normal values for pH, PCO_2, and HCO_3^- do not exclude an acid-base abnormality, because mixed acid-base disorders often manifest as apparently normal pH due to balancing of opposing forces that determine the pH.[2] Therefore, it is imperative that the clinician follow all the subsequent steps involved in delineating or excluding the disorder in all acid-base analyses.

Acid-base disorders are divided into *simple* (or pure), denoting a single process, and *complex* (or mixed), denoting a condition in which two or more processes are occurring simultaneously. Simple acid-base disorders result in predictable patterns both in terms of carbonic acid equilibrium and physiological compensation. When measured acid-base variables fall outside the parameters described in Table 121-2, the patient has a complex acid-base disorder.[3] Classification of a complex acid-base disorder is accomplished first through determination of the pH. If the pH is less than 7.35, at least one type of acidosis is present; if the pH is more than 7.45, at least one type of alkalosis is present. It is generally unwise to assume that the disorder that is changing the pH most is the primary or most important disorder. The most life-threatening condition may not be the one with the greatest effect on the pH. Finally, it is possible for two or more acid-base disorders to exist simultaneously, with the result that the pH is normal; it is even possible for the pH, PCO_2, and HCO_3^- to be normal. Only an astute clinician avoids missing such a disorder.

Step 4: Calculate the Expected Compensation

Well-recognized and well-characterized patterns of acid-base compensation (see Table 121-2) can be used to determine whether a complex disorder is present and to help diagnose it.

For instance, a simple metabolic acidosis gives rise to the following findings:

- Standard base excess (SBE) value <−2 mEq/L
- Plasma bicarbonate concentration lower than 22 mmol/L

- PCO_2 value 1.5 × the bicarbonate level + 8 *or* 40 + the SBE value (either formula has a range of ± 2)

If the arterial PCO_2 value is outside this range, a secondary respiratory acid-base disorder is present—respiratory alkalosis if the PCO_2 is lower than expected, and respiratory acidosis if the PCO_2 is higher than expected.

A simple chronic respiratory acidosis gives rise to the following findings:

- pH < 7.35
- PCO_2 > 45 mm Hg
- Plasma bicarbonate concentration = $PCO_2 - \dfrac{40}{3} + 24$ (range ± 2)
- SBE = 0.4 × (PCO_2 − 40) (range ± 2)

Chronic respiratory acid-base disorders are those that have been present long enough to permit metabolic (primarily renal) compensation. This process generally takes 2 to 5 days. In general, the decrease in pH with chronic respiratory acidosis is approximately half that seen with acute respiratory acidosis. Of course, a given patient may present at a point between the acute and chronic stages of the acidosis, making classification difficult.

Step 5: Calculate the "Gaps"

Because patients with mixed acid-base disorders often have an apparently normal pH, an increased anion gap may be the only clue to the underlying mixed acid-base disorders.[3] Thus, the anion gap should always be evaluated for the diagnosis of an acid-base disorder. Of course, as discussed in Chapter 117, it is not enough merely to calculate the anion gap in most critically ill patients. The anion gap must be corrected for the patient's serum albumin and sometimes even phosphate concentrations.

Corrected Anion Gap

The corrected anion gap (AGc) is calculated as follows:

$$AGc = (Na^+ + K^+) - (Cl^- + HCO_3^-) - (2.0 \times Alb\,[g/dL]) - (0.5 \times Phos\,[mg/dL])$$

A normal AGc is close to 0. An increased AGc indicates the presence of unmeasured anions and hence a metabolic acidosis irrespective of the pH or HCO_3^-. Clues to existence of a balanced complex disorder include the emergence of imbalance on repeated measurements and the presence of an abnormal corrected anion gap. Importantly, the AGc has several limitations. First, the AGc is near 0 because the sum of normal unmeasured anions (e.g., lactate, sulfate) equals the sum of unmeasured cations (e.g., Mg^{2+}, Ca^{2+}). If unmeasured cations are markedly reduced (only the ionized portion contributes to the charge balance), a small increase in AGc occurs. Secondly and more importantly, the AGc calculation assumes acidemia. In the presence of alkalemia, the charges on albumin and phosphate increase. Therefore, if the AGc is calculated from an alkalemic blood sample, only significant departures from normal (>5 mEq/L) should be considered abnormal.

Strong Ion Gap

When greater accuracy is desired, a slightly more complicated method of estimating unmeasured anions is required—the strong ion gap (SIG) (see Chapter 117).[4] Like the AGc, the SIG is normally near 0, and is usually less than 2 mEq/L in health. Unlike the AGc, the SIG is not influenced by abnormities in Ca^{2+} or Mg^{2+} or by changes in pH.

Step 6: Compare the Strong Ion Gap or Corrected Anion Gap with the Standard Base Excess

When the SIG or AGc is completely due to a strong ion (e.g., lactate), there is a one-for-one effect on the base excess. For instance, a 1 mmol/L increase in lactate raises the AGc/SIG by 1 mEq/L, which decreases the SBE by 1 mEq/L. This relationship has prompted multiple investigators to devise ways of comparing the AGc/SIG with the base excess or (with more difficulty) with the HCO_3^- concentration, in order to detect the presence of mixed metabolic acidosis. If a patient has a metabolic acidosis that in part is due to unmeasured anions (e.g., ketones) and in part is hyperchloremic, the increase in AGc/SIG will be smaller than the decrease in base excess. Similarly, the change in HCO_3^- concentration, in the context of PCO_2, will be greater than the AG/SIG. In this way, a mixed disorder can be revealed. Similarly, if the increase in AGc is significantly larger than the change in SBE, a metabolic alkalosis is present and partially offsetting the metabolic acidosis. Finally, a high SIG or AGc should always prompt consideration of the differential diagnosis for a positive–anion gap metabolic acidosis (see Chapter 117), including various toxic ingestions (see Chapter 130). (For an example of a complex acid-base disorder, see the case tutorials available on the companion Expert Consult website.)

TREATMENT OF MIXED ACID-BASE DISORDERS

Therapy of a mixed acid-base disorder primarily consists of treating the components that cause the disorder. Whenever possible, the treatment should be directed at the primary pathophysiological mechanism that resulted in the disorder. If prudence dictates that symptomatic therapy is to be provided, consideration should be given to the likely duration of the disorder. If it is expected to be short-lived (e.g., diabetic ketoacidosis), maximizing respiratory compensation is usually the safest approach. Once the disorder resolves, ventilation can be quickly reduced to normal, with no lingering effects of therapy.

In certain circumstances, however, acid-base derangements are dangerous and life-threatening. For instance, when both the primary disorders move the pH in the same direction quickly (e.g., metabolic acidosis and respiratory acidosis), they are likely to cause extreme changes in pH (e.g., pH < 7.0 or > 7.7) and to be life-threatening. Under these circumstances, the goal of therapy is emergency correction of pH, although correction is usually only partial. It can be accomplished most quickly through treatment of both the metabolic and the respiratory component. Correction of PCO_2 can sometimes be achieved rapidly and should usually be attempted first. This is accomplished by institution of mechanical ventilation or by making a change in the rate or tidal volume setting on the ventilator in the appropriate direction. Next, the metabolic component of the acid-base disorder should be treated. For metabolic acidosis, a sodium bicarbonate infusion can be used, and for metabolic alkalosis, sodium chloride or HCl infusion can be used (see Chapters 118 and 119).

It should be remembered, however, that correction of the pH may often result in creation of a new iatrogenic acid-base abnormality. For instance, if the SID is increased, for example through the use of sodium bicarbonate infusion, there is a risk of alkalosis when the underlying disorder resolves. Therefore, every effort should be made to prevent "overshoot" acid-base disorders. In cases of metabolic disorders, the therapeutic target can be quite accurately determined from the SBE. The SBE corresponds to the amount the SID must change in order to restore the pH to 7.4, assuming a PCO_2 of 40 mm Hg. Thus, if the SID is 30 mEq/L and the SBE is –10 mEq/L, the target SID is 40 mEq/L. Accordingly, the plasma Na^+ concentration would have to rise by 10 mEq/L for sodium bicarbonate administration to completely repair the acidosis. If increasing the plasma Na^+ concentration is inadvisable for other reasons (e.g., hypernatremia), administration of sodium bicarbonate would be inadvisable.

When the primary disorders move pH in the opposite direction (e.g., metabolic acidosis and respiratory alkalosis), acidemia or alkalemia is relatively mild and therapy can be more leisurely. However, treating one of the disorders can unmask the pH-altering effect of the other. It is therefore often desirable to treat both disorders simultaneously. If one disorder is easily treatable, the clinician may face a dilemma: treat one and have a marked pH abnormality, or treat neither and have a normal pH. Such dilemmas must be resolved on a case-by-case basis.

Key Points

1. Mixed acid-base disorders are common in the modern intensive care unit.
2. A stepwise approach to analysis of all acid-base disorders helps unravel most complex entities.
3. Treatment of complex disorders must be directed at treating the underlying pathophysiological mechanism whenever possible.
4. Every effort must be made to avoid iatrogenic acid-base disorders during treatment.

Key References

1. Stewart PA: Modern quantitative acid-base chemistry. Can J Physiol Pharmacol 1983;61:1444-1461.
2. Schlichtig R, Grogono AW, Severinghaus JW: Human PaCO$_2$ and standard base excess compensation for acid-base imbalance. Crit Care Med 1998;26:1173-1179.
3. Kellum JA: Determinants of blood pH in health and disease. Crit Care 2000;4:6-14.
4. Kellum JA, Kramer DJ, Pinsky MR: Strong ion gap: A methodology for exploring unexplained anions. J Crit Care 1995;10:51-55.

See the companion Expert Consult website for the complete reference list.

Specific Disorders

CHAPTER 122

Lactic Acidosis—Clinical Syndrome

Barry A. Mizock

OBJECTIVES

This chapter will:
1. Review etiologies of lactic acidosis that have particular relevance to critical care practitioners.
2. Provide a framework for the approach to patients with lactic acidosis of unknown etiology.

Lactic acidosis is one of the more common metabolic disorders observed in critically ill patients. However, the precise incidence of lactic acidosis in this population is unknown. A study of 50 intensive care unit patients with metabolic acidosis found that almost two thirds had increased blood lactate levels.[1] Lactic acidosis accompanies a wide variety of clinical disorders, and its manifestations are often protean.

CLASSIFICATION OF LACTIC ACIDOSIS

In 1976, Cohen and Woods[1a] proposed a system that is most widely used to classify lactic acidosis. They divided lactic acidosis into two categories: *Type A* lactic acidosis occurs in *association with clinical evidence* of poor tissue perfusion or oxygenation of the blood (e.g., hypotension, cyanosis, cool or clammy extremities). Cardiogenic and hypovolemic shock are the prototypes of type A lactic acidosis. *Type B* is lactic acidosis occurring in the *absence of clinical evidence* of poor tissue perfusion. Type B is subdivided into B_1 (lactic acidosis occurring in association with an underlying disease), B_2 (lactic acidosis due to drugs or toxins), and B_3 (lactic acidosis due to inborn errors of metabolism). This system has limited utility in classifying lactic acidosis on a mechanistic basis, because of substantial overlap in underlying pathophysiology. Nevertheless, it provides a structure that facilitates organization of the various etiologies (Table 122-1).

TYPE A LACTIC ACIDOSIS: TISSUE HYPOPERFUSION

Circulatory Shock

Circulatory shock is best viewed as a profound and widespread reduction in *effective* tissue perfusion leading to cellular dysfunction and organ failure. Its pathogenesis is multifactorial and includes inadequate cardiac performance, maldistribution of cardiac output, alterations in microcirculatory blood flow, and abnormalities in cellular bioenergetic function. Lactic acidosis, a cardinal manifestation of circulatory shock, has traditionally been viewed as resulting from a combination of increased anaerobic lactate production and impaired hepatic lactate clearance. However, this view has been called into question by Revelly and colleagues,[2] who studied lactate and glucose metabolism in patients with severe sepsis and cardiogenic shock. These investigators observed that lactate clearance in the patients was similar to that in healthy controls. In addition, no defects in lactate oxidation were found. The investigators concluded that hyperlactatemia during severe sepsis and cardiogenic shock occurred mainly as the consequence of increased lactate production.

Circulatory shock results in a profound activation of the hypothalamic-pituitary-adrenal axis. The ensuing sympathetic outflow from brain stimulates the secretion of epinephrine from the adrenal glands. James and colleagues[3] postulated that hyperlactatemia during circulatory shock results in large part from the β_2-adrenergic effects of epinephrine on glycolytic flux in skeletal muscle.[3] Glycolysis in muscle is compartmentalized with two separate sets of glycolytic enzymes in the cytosol. One pathway is channeled into oxidative metabolism, and the other provides energy to enable Na^+-K^+ exchange at the cell membrane. Epinephrine stimulates β_2-adrenergic receptors that in turn increase the activity of Na^+,K^+-ATPase. The resultant increase in adenosine diphosphate (ADP) enhances glycolytic flux and lactate production. Levy and associates[4] documented this process in humans with septic shock. They also noted that lactate output from muscle was totally inhibited by ouabain, thereby confirming a Na^+,K^+-ATPase–dependent mechanism and providing further proof that muscle lactate production during sepsis is not mediated by tissue hypoxia. Nevertheless, certain differences exist between shock states. Reduction in tissue perfusion is more likely to be a pathogenic mechanism in cardiogenic shock than in septic shock. In contrast, lactic acidosis accompanying septic shock is mediated to a greater degree by systemic inflammation. A study found that blood levels of tumor necrosis factor-α (TNF-α) were significantly higher in septic shock than in cardiogenic shock.[5] In addition, nitric oxide production was markedly increased in septic shock but not in cardiogenic shock. Nitric oxide interacts with superoxide to form peroxynitrite, which in turn activates poly(ADP-ribose) polymerase.[6] This enzyme depletes cellular stores of NAD^+, thereby inhibiting glycolysis, the Krebs cycle, and mitochondrial respiration. This process ("cytopathic hypoxia") may play a role in the

TABLE 122-1

Causes of Lactic Acidosis

Type A	Tissue hypoperfusion:
	    Circulatory shock
	    Mesenteric ischemia

Type B_1	Underlying disease:
	    Systemic inflammatory response
	      syndrome
	    Asthma
	    Liver failure
	    Malignancy
	    Thiamine deficiency
	    Cardiopulmonary bypass
	    Severe hypophosphatemia

Type B_2	Drugs/toxins:
	    Metformin
	    Alcohols (ethanol, methanol, ethylene
	      glycol, propylene glycol)
	    β_2-adrenergic receptor agonists
	    Salicylates
	    Cyanide/nitroprusside
	    Carbon monoxide
	    Antiretroviral agents
	    Propofol
	    Dialysis

Type B_3 Miscellaneous	Congenital D-lactic acidosis Hypoglycemia

pathogenesis of lactic acidosis in patients with sepsis-associated multiple-organ dysfunction syndrome.[7]

Mesenteric Ischemia

The presence of lactic acidosis in the setting of acute abdominal disease has been proposed as an indicator of mesenteric ischemia or infarction. However, lactic acidosis is often a late finding in bowel ischemia and has poor specificity (e.g., thiamine deficiency may also manifest as acute abdominal pain and lactic acidosis). An elevation of the D-lactate isomer in serum has been promoted as a diagnostic tool for acute mesenteric ischemia, but the assay has only limited availability.[8]

TYPE B₁ LACTIC ACIDOSIS: UNDERLYING DISEASE

Systemic Inflammatory Response Syndrome

Any acute condition that elicits a significant systemic inflammatory response may promote an increase in blood lactate, and the level of hyperlactatemia reflects the severity of stress. Tumor necrosis factor-α and interleukin-1 have been shown to increase cellular glucose uptake, glycolytic flux, and lactate production in tissue macrophages.[9] This process is directed toward providing energy for the "respiratory burst" and is therefore most prominent in organs or tissues that are rich in macrophages (e.g., lung, intestine, wound).[10] Hepatic macrophages (Kupffer cells) also produce significant amounts of lactate during systemic inflammatory states. However, net lactate production from liver usually does not occur because of efficient local metabolism by hepatocytes. A study in patients with sepsis-related multiple-organ failure compared the local

production of cytokines and lactate from patients with lung involvement (acute respiratory distress syndrome) with that in patients with predominant hepatic dysfunction.[11] Net release of cytokines and lactate from the lung was found in patients with acute respiratory distress syndrome, whereas increased efflux of these substances was found in hepatic venous blood (reflecting the net contribution of liver and gut) in patients with predominant hepatic dysfunction. Therefore, local production of lactate depends on the severity of organ involvement.

Release of alanine from muscle is increased during sepsis, and alanine serves as a substrate for gluconeogenesis. Alanine is also transaminated in the bloodstream to pyruvate and ultimately converted to lactate.[12] Siegel and coworkers[13] proposed that alanine-pyruvate transamination is the major mechanism accounting for hyperlactatemia during sepsis.

As mentioned previously, lactate utilization appears to be maintained during septic shock.[2] This finding contrasts with the findings from a study of patients with stable sepsis in whom mild hyperlactatemia was attributed to impaired hepatic lactate clearance.[14] However, the results of the second study may have been confounded by methodological problems (e.g., use of the rate of concentration decay of a lactate bolus as an index of clearance).

Asthma

Hyperlactatemia is common in patients with acute severe asthma. The pathogenesis has been attributed to increased lactate production from respiratory muscles. However, the peak elevation in lactate often occurs at the point at which the patient is improving and showing little signs of respiratory dysfunction.[15] It is more likely that the mechanism relates to the stimulatory effect of β_2 agonists (e.g., albuterol) on glycolytic flux, as previously discussed.[3] Although lactic acidosis accompanying status asthmaticus was thought to be a bad prognostic sign, one study found that initial or delayed hyperlactatemia had little prognostic value.[16] The reason that lactic acidosis develops from β_2 agonists in only certain asthmatic patients is unclear but might relate to the presence of polymorphisms in the β_2 receptor gene.[17]

Liver Failure

Lactic acidosis is unusual during *chronic* liver disease in the absence of conditions that enhance lactate production. In contrast, hyperlactatemia is very common in patients with *acute* liver failure, consequent to an associated systemic inflammatory response resulting from hepatocellular necrosis.[18] It is likely that the mechanism involves both an increase in lactate production by activated Kupffer cells and impairment of lactate clearance by hepatocytes. The lung has also been shown to produce lactate during acute liver failure, even in the absence of obvious pulmonary injury.[19]

Malignancy

Malignancy-associated lactic acidosis is most commonly seen with underlying leukemia or lymphoma. It has also been described with solid tumors, usually in the presence of liver or bone marrow metastases. The pathogenesis is thought to involve a cytokine-mediated stimulation of glycolytic flux in neoplastic cells. Although lactic acidosis generally occurs in patients with established malignancies, leukemia or lymphoma may rarely manifest as lactic acidosis. Malignancy-associated lactic acidosis may also be accompanied by hypoglycemia.[20] Although hypoglycemia may *cause* lactic acidosis in patients with chronic hepatic or renal failure (see later), it does not appear to have a causal relationship with underlying malignancy, because lactic acidosis persists even after the low blood glucose concentration has been treated. The mechanism may involve increased glucose utilization by neoplastic cells or may represent a paraneoplastic syndrome.[21]

Thiamine Deficiency

Thiamine pyrophosphate is an essential cofactor for pyruvate dehydrogenase. Deficiency of thiamine therefore impairs oxidative metabolism of pyruvate in the Krebs cycle. The resultant reduction of oxidative phosphorylation stimulates glycolytic flux, leading to lactic acidosis. Thiamine deficiency can develop rapidly (within days) in critically ill patients as the consequence of decreased thiamine intake and/or increased urinary or intestinal losses. The associated clinical manifestations are varied; they include Shoshin beriberi and Wernicke's encephalopathy. One report described thiamine deficiency manifesting as a primary gastrointestinal syndrome in which lactic acidosis occurred concurrently with acute abdominal pain.[22] This presentation could easily be misdiagnosed as that of acute mesenteric ischemia, resulting in unnecessary surgery.

Cardiopulmonary Bypass

Development of lactic acidosis in association with cardiopulmonary bypass (CPB) is well recognized; however, the precise pathophysiology is not clear. A 2001 study found that lactate elevation after CPB was most strongly related to two factors, the duration of CPB and the occurrence of episodes of hypotension during the commencement of CPB.[23] The investigators in this study hypothesized that lactic acidosis may have been caused by a CPB-induced impairment of tissue oxygen utilization, perhaps as the consequence of sludging of microvascular flow. Other studies have attributed post-CPB lactic acidosis to perioperative administration of epinephrine or to a cytokine-mediated activation of a systemic inflammatory response resulting from exposure of blood to the extracorporeal circuit.[24,25] An inflammatory etiology is supported by a report that the development of lactic acidosis after cardiac surgery was influenced by genetic factors; all patients in this study who had polymorphisms in either tumor necrosis factor-β or interleukin-10 genes experienced postoperative lactic acidosis.[26]

Severe Hypophosphatemia

Severe hypophosphatemia (e.g., serum phosphate concentration <1.5 mg/dL) has been described as a cause of lactic acidosis.[27] The mechanism appears to involve depletion of intracellular adenosine triphosphate and decreased red blood cell 2,3-diphosphoglyceric acid. Severe hypophosphatemia may also be associated with a non–anion gap metabolic acidosis on the basis of impaired tubular reabsorption of bicarbonate.[27]

TYPE B₂ LACTIC ACIDOSIS: DRUGS/TOXINS

Metformin

Although diabetes mellitus is often listed as a cause of lactic acidosis, whether diabetes per se predisposes to lactic acidosis is unclear. The initial recognition of the association between lactic acidosis and diabetes followed the introduction of the biguanide oral hypoglycemic agent phenformin and led to the agent's withdrawal from the U.S. market in 1977 (although it has reappeared in Asia as a "traditional Chinese herbal medicine"). Metformin was subsequently shown to be associated with a markedly lower incidence of lactic acidosis (approximately 9 cases per 100,000). The vast majority of cases occurred in patients who were prescribed the drug despite the presence of contraindications (e.g., renal impairment, heart failure requiring pharmacological treatment, advanced age) or in the setting of accidental or suicidal overdose. The underlying pathogenesis is not entirely clear but may relate to the ability of the drug to bind to complex 1 of the mitochondrial respiratory chain.[28]

Alcohols (Ethanol, Methanol, Ethylene Glycol, Propylene Glycol)

Ethanol, methanol, and ethylene glycol are all metabolized in the liver by alcohol dehydrogenase and cytochrome P-450 systems to end products that have toxic effects on cellular metabolism. Ethanol is metabolized to acetaldehyde, which can potentially depress electron transport. However, acute ethanol intoxication is not generally associated with lactic acidosis in the absence of other concomitant factors that enhance lactate production (e.g., thiamine deficiency, salicylates).[29] Lactic acidosis more commonly occurs in patients with methanol or ethylene glycol poisoning. The pathogenesis relates to the metabolic end products of methanol (formate) and ethylene glycol (glycolate) that are potent inhibitors of oxidative phosphorylation. Ethylene glycol poisoning may also be associated with spurious hyperlactatemia because glycolate cross-reacts with lactate in certain blood chemistry analyzers.[30]

Numerous case reports have documented the occurrence of lactic acidosis in patients receiving parenteral drugs that contain propylene glycol as a vehicle (e.g., lorazepam, diazepam, diphenylhydantoin, trimethoprim-sulfamethoxazole). Propylene glycol is cleared predominantly by the kidney and liver, and consequently, lactic acidosis is most common in patients with dysfunction of these organs. Commercial preparations of propylene glycol are a 50:50 mixture of D and L isomers. The D isomer of PG is metabolized to D⁻ lactate, which is cleared more slowly than L⁺ lactate. The resultant accumulation of D-lactate in the brain has been implicated as the cause of the central nervous system manifestations of propylene glycol toxicity. Periodic monitoring of serum osmolarity has been recommended as a means to detect potentially toxic levels of propylene glycol.[31]

β₂-Adrenergic Receptor Agonists

Beta agonists promote increases in blood lactate by stimulating Na⁺,K⁺-ATPase in skeletal muscle.[3,16] Lactic acidosis was initially reported in pregnant patients who were given parenteral ritodrine or terbutaline for tocolysis. Lactic acidosis was subsequently described in asthmatic patients who were receiving β_2-adrenergic receptor agonists by intermittent or continuous nebulization (see previous discussion).[16]

Salicylates

Lactic acidosis secondary to salicylate toxicity occurs as the consequence of uncoupling of oxidative phosphorylation and inhibition of Krebs cycle enzymes. The development of metabolic acidosis further enhances toxicity by decreasing the renal elimination of the drug as well as by increasing the un-ionized fraction, thereby augmenting passage into brain and other tissues. A study of salicylate poisoning in adults found that 20% had blood lactate concentrations above 2 mmol/L; however, 90% of those patients had mixed salicylate/ethanol ingestion.[32] This latter fact suggests that ethanol and salicylates may have synergistic effects in promoting lactic acidosis.

Cyanide and Nitroprusside

Cyanide poisoning usually occurs as the result of smoke inhalation or with suicidal attempt. Cyanide produces lactic acidosis by combining with cytochrome c and inhibiting oxidative phosphorylation. Blood cyanide levels have limited clinical utility in diagnosis of cyanide poisoning because of the associated delay in processing the specimen. The diagnosis may be suspected in patients with a suggestive history who present with lactic acidosis accompanied by neurological and/or cardiovascular manifestations (e.g., confusion, seizures, coma, hypotension). One study found that in patients with a history suggestive of poisoning, a plasma lactate concentration higher than 8 mmol/L had good sensitivity and specificity as an indicator of a toxic blood cyanide concentration.[33]

Nitroprusside infusion may also cause cyanide toxicity, which is typically heralded by the appearance of hyperlactatemia. Toxicity is most common with prolonged infusion (i.e., more than 72 hours), particularly when infusion rates exceed 2 μg/kg/min. Lactic acidosis may also occur with short-term infusion of nitroprusside at doses high enough to deplete thiosulfate stores (most healthy adults can usually detoxify approximately 50 mg of the drug). Nitroprusside toxicity correlates best with measurements of cyanide in plasma. However, most clinical laboratories perform cyanide analysis on whole blood, which is a less reliable predictor of toxicity.[34] Patients are best evaluated for toxicity by means of clinical assessment (e.g., presence of tachycardia, agitation, seizures) and measurement of blood lactate concentration. Lactic acidosis can be virtually eliminated by the routine addition of sodium thiosulfate to the infusion bag.

Carbon Monoxide

Lactic acidosis may occur as a complication of severe carbon monoxide poisoning.[35] Carboxyhemoglobinemia causes tissue dysoxia, which occurs with diminished ability of hemoglobin to transport oxygen as well as through induction of a leftward shift of the oxyhemoglobin dissociation curve.

Antiretroviral Agents

Mild to moderate hyperlactatemia (e.g., serum lactate level 2.5-5 mmol/L) occurs in up to 25% of patients with human immunodeficiency virus who are taking nucleoside reverse transcriptase inhibitors (especially stavudine).[36] Low-grade elevations in lactate concentrations are not predictive of subsequent lactic acidosis, and most of these patients remain asymptomatic. However, some have symptoms (e.g., dyspnea, abdominal pain, dysesthesias), usually in the first 3 to 4 months after commencing therapy. Prompt recognition and withdrawal of antiretroviral agents at this stage usually leads to recovery. Rarely, severe lactic acidosis (lactate level >10 mmol/L) can ensue, which is associated with high mortality. The mechanisms underlying symptomatic hyperlactatemia and lactic acidosis have not been fully elucidated but appear to involve mitochondrial toxicity secondary to inhibition of DNA polymerase-γ, which uncouples oxidative phosphorylation.[36] Uncommonly, lactic acidosis can develop in patients with acquired immunodeficiency syndrome in the absence of antiretroviral drugs or other precipitating causes; this condition may reflect virally induced mitochondrial dysfunction.[37]

Propofol

Reports of the association between propofol and lactic acidosis were initially described in children. This association is now also well recognized in adults and has come to be known as the propofol infusion syndrome (PIS).[38] It consists of lactic acidosis, cardiac failure, rhabdomyolysis, and renal failure. This syndrome is usually seen in ventilator-dependent patients who are receiving continuous infusion of propofol (usually at rates exceeding 5 mg/kg/hr for more than 2 days). The syndrome has also been noted with short-term infusion of propofol at high doses for general anesthesia. The pathogenesis may involve uncoupling of oxidative phosphorylation and impaired oxidation of free fatty acids.

Dialysis-Associated Hyperlactatemia

Hyperlactatemia has been reported in patients undergoing intermittent or continuous hemofiltration with lactate-containing replacement solutions. It is most likely to occur in patients with underlying liver dysfunction.[39] This phenomenon is discussed in greater detail elsewhere in the book (see Chapters 87, 133, 210).

TYPE B₃ LACTIC ACIDOSIS: CONGENITAL

Most cases of congenital lactic acidosis result from mutations or deletions in respiratory chain genes or in the pyruvate dehydrogenase complex.[37] The manifestations of congenital lactic acidosis, which usually appear during infancy or early childhood, consist of episodes of lactic acidosis accompanied by various neurological and developmental abnormalities. However, some forms of congenital lactic acidosis may manifest during adulthood. A mitochondrial cause of lactic acidosis should be suspected in patients with no evidence of hypoxia or sepsis who demonstrate muscle weakness or in whom weaning from mechanical ventilation is difficult.[40] Other neurological manifestations of congenital lactic acidosis are stroke, seizures, dementia, migraines, and ophthalmoplegia.

MISCELLANEOUS CAUSES OF LACTIC ACIDOSIS

D-Lactic Acidosis

D-Lactic acidosis usually occurs in patients either with short-bowel syndrome secondary to bowel resection or bypass surgery or with chronic pancreatic insufficiency. Patients typically present with metabolic acidosis and neurological manifestations (e.g., slurred speech, confusion, ataxia) that are triggered by ingestion of large amounts of carbohydrate. These symptoms may last from a few hours to several days. The pathophysiology involves carbohydrate malabsorption in the shortened or bypassed loop of bowel. The carbohydrates reach the colon in undigested form, where they are fermented to organic acids that in turn decrease colonic pH. The resultant acidic colonic milieu promotes overgrowth of gut flora with acid-tolerant organisms that produce D-lactate. The mechanism for the neurological manifestations involves either the direct effect of D-lactate on the brain or toxins produced simultaneously with D-lactate.[41] Suggestive laboratory findings include anion gap metabolic acidosis, increased strong ion gap, and a normal serum lactate level (analyzers detect only L-lactate). The diagnosis is confirmed by finding a serum D-lactate level higher than 3 mmol/L.[41]

Hypoglycemia

Patients with chronic renal or hepatic disease are at risk for hypoglycemia because of a reduced capacity for gluconeogenesis. Low blood glucose concentration in turn is a potent stimulant of the sympathetic nervous system; the resultant release of epinephrine enhances lactate production from skeletal muscle via mechanisms previously discussed. It has also been theorized that in patients with hepatic dysfunction, a critical amount of glucose is needed as an energy source to enable gluconeogenic conversion of lactate.[42] Hypoglycemia-associated lactic acidosis usually responds promptly to administration of glucose. This response contrasts with hypoglycemia occurring in patients with underlying malignancy, in which lactic acidosis persists even after blood glucose concentrations are normalized.

DIAGNOSTIC CONSIDERATIONS

Diagnostic Criteria for Lactic Acidosis

The generally accepted diagnostic criteria for lactic acidosis are blood lactate level higher than 5 mmol/L and pH lower than 7.35.[43] These criteria were selected to minimize false-negative and false-positive classifications. However, critically ill patients commonly manifest subdiagnostic elevations of blood lactate (e.g., lactate level >2 mmol/L but <5 mmol/L) that may not be accompanied by a low pH.[43,44] Although this phenomenon usually occurs as the consequence of the underlying stress response, it may also be an early indicator of a potentially correctable distur-

bance (e.g., tissue dysoxia, drug toxicity) and should prompt further evaluation.

Anion Gap and Lactic Acidosis

The anion gap cannot be used as a surrogate in the diagnosis of lactic acidosis because the association between hyperlactatemia and the anion gap is poor.[45] Furthermore, correcting the anion gap for hypoalbuminemia does not appear to improve detection of hyperlactatemia.[46] The lack of tight correlation between lactate concentration and the anion gap may be due to the fact that metabolic acidosis in critically ill patients is commonly multifactorial; hyperchloremia and/or an increase in unidentified anions often accompanies hyperlactatemia.[1] Gunnerson and colleagues,[47] comparing lactate acidosis with non-lactate metabolic acidosis in 548 critically ill patients, noted that patients with lactic acidosis had the highest mortality rate (56%), whereas mortality was lower in those with strong ion gap (unmeasured anion) acidosis (39%) and hyperchloremic acidosis (29%).

The pathogenesis of strong ion gap acidosis is not completely understood. Forni and associates[48] proposed that these "unmeasured" anions were negatively charged intermediates of the Krebs cycle. However, other investigators have provided data suggesting that strong ion gap acidosis is probably multifactorial in nature.[49]

Lactate as an Index of Tissue Perfusion

As previously discussed, hyperlactatemia is not a specific indicator of tissue hypoperfusion. Concomitant measurement of pyruvate in blood was proposed as a means to improve the specificity of lactate as an index of tissue perfusion. Low-output states typically involve an increased lactate-to-pyruvate (L/P) ratio [>10-15:1]), whereas the ratio is normal in the setting of persistent hyperlactatemia after adequate resuscitation of sepsis, burn, or trauma patients.[3] However, the diagnostic value of the lactate-to-pyruvate ratio is limited by poor specificity as well as lack of availability of pyruvate analysis in most hospitals. Nevertheless, measurement of blood lactate level may be used to guide therapy in patients with circulatory shock. This approach involves sequential measurements of blood lactate level during resuscitation, with normalization of the level (i.e., <2 mmol/L) serving as the therapeutic end point. A study in postoperative cardiac patients demonstrated that those in whom resuscitation using lactate as an end point was successful had shorter hospital stays and lower morbidity.[50] In another study, trauma patients in whom blood lactate level returned to normal within 24 hours of resuscitation had better survival and a lower incidence of multiple-organ dysfunction when compared with those in whom lactate failed to normalize within 24 hours.[51] Larger confirmatory studies are therefore required before this method can be more widely adopted. It should be kept in mind that normalization of blood lactate level may not be possible in patients in whom greater lactate production is mediated by inflammatory cytokines (e.g., burn, sepsis).

Blood Lactate Level and Prognosis

Measurement of blood lactate level may also be used as a means to assess prognosis. Early research in patients with circulatory shock suggested that a single–time point measurement of lactate at presentation was useful in predicting mortality. Weil and Afifi[52] found that in patients with circulatory shock, an increase in blood lactate level from 2 to 8 mmol/L was associated with a decrease in the estimated probability of survival from 90% to 10%. However, the prognosis of lactic acidosis accompanying circulatory shock also varies according to the etiology. Hyperlactatemia resulting from hemorrhagic shock has a better prognosis than that due to either cardiogenic or septic shock, because there is a greater chance of reversing the hyperlactatemia due to hemorrhagic shock. In addition, the extent of elevation in blood lactate concentration is also influenced by the patient's ability to clear lactate. Compared with patients with normal liver function, patients with chronic liver disease would be expected to have a higher level of hyperlactatemia after a similar insult. For those reasons, sequential measurements of blood lactate during resuscitation from circulatory shock have been shown to provide more useful prognostic information than single-point measurements. Failure to clear lactate over time (e.g., within 24 to 48 hours) is associated with greater likelihood of multiple-organ failure and higher mortality.[53]

Approach to Lactic Acidosis of Uncertain Etiology

Clinicians occasionally encounter patients with lactic acidosis in whom the etiology is not obvious. Transient lactic acidosis may result from a period of occult hypoglycemia or an unrecognized seizure. In patients with persistent lactic acidosis, the following approach is suggested:
- Consider the possibility of thiamine deficiency. Empirical administration of thiamine carries little risk, and a prompt response strongly supports the diagnosis.
- Discontinue potentially causative drugs (e.g., antiretroviral agents, β_2 agonists, nitroprusside, propofol, parenteral lorazepam, metformin).
- Consider the possibility of poisoning (e.g., toxic alcohol, cyanide) and evaluate the need for empirical therapy.
- Congenital mitochondrial dysfunction may occasionally manifest in adults and should be considered in patients with unexplained weakness or difficulty weaning from mechanical ventilation.

CONCLUSION

Lactic acidosis is a cardinal manifestation of circulatory shock. However, lactic acidosis also may occur as the consequence of an underlying chronic disease or may be the presenting manifestation of significant drug toxicity or poisoning. The presence of hyperlactatemia is therefore an important indicator of a potentially serious disorder and should prompt further clinical evaluation.[54]

Key Points

1. Lactic acidosis during circulatory shock results from increased lactate production secondary to enhanced aerobic glycolysis in skeletal muscle. This in turn is the consequence of a β_2-adrenergic receptor–mediated stimulation of membrane Na^+-K^+ pumps.
2. A cytokine-mediated increase in lactate production by tissue macrophages plays a significant role in the pathogenesis of hyperlactatemia in patients with a systemic inflammatory response (e.g., sepsis, burn).
3. Sequential determinations of lactate concentration may be useful in guiding resuscitation from circulatory shock as well as in assessing prognosis.
4. Occult thiamine deficiency or poisoning should be considered in patients with lactic acidosis of unclear etiology.

Key References

1. Moviat M, van Haren F, van der Hoeven H: Conventional or physiochemical approach in intensive care unit patients with metabolic acidosis. Crit Care 2003;7:R41-R45.
2. Revelly JP, Tappy L, Martinez A, et al: Lactate and glucose metabolism in severe sepsis and cardiogenic shock. Crit Care Med 2005;33:2235-2240.
4. Levy B, Gibot S, Franck P, et al: Relation between muscle Na^+K^+-ATPase activity and raised lactate concentrations in septic shock: A prospective study. Lancet 2005;365:871-875.
11. Douzinas EE, Tsidemiadou PD, Pitaridis MT, et al: The regional production of cytokines and lactate in sepsis-related multiple organ failure. Am J Respir Crit Care Med 1997;155:53-59.
36. Arenas-Pinto A, Grant AD, Edwards S, Weller IVD: Lactic acidosis in HIV infected patients: A systematic review of published cases. Sex Transm Infect 2003;79:340-344.

See the companion Expert Consult website for the complete reference list.

CHAPTER 123

Diabetic Ketoacidosis

Andrew Durward

OBJECTIVES

This chapter will:
1. Discuss the pathophysiology of diabetic ketoacidosis.
2. Describe the diagnosis of diabetic ketoacidosis.
3. Detail the management of diabetic ketoacidosis.
4. Discuss other disorders of ketosis.

Diabetic ketoacidosis (DKA) is a metabolic derangement secondary to a deficiency of insulin, which results in a triad of biochemical abnormalities: hyperglycemia, excessive ketone formation (metabolic ketoacidosis), and polyuria accompanied by fluid and electrolyte depletion. Although the mortality rate associated with DKA is less than 5%, this disorder may rarely be complicated by permanent neurological injury or death if cerebral edema develops during its treatment.[1] This complication is more common in children, but numerous risk factors have been identified that may predispose to its development. Insights into acid-base and fluid physiology have highlighted issues that may have important implications in the treatment of DKA.

PATHOPHYSIOLOGY

The lack of insulin, either relative or absolute, results in the unopposed action of counter-regulatory hormones such as glucagon, cortisol, and catecholamines, which promote glycolysis and gluconeogenesis (Fig. 123-1). In conjunction with a decrease in peripheral glucose utilization, hyperglycemia occurs, leading to an osmotic diuresis, dehydration, and depletion of electrolytes, including sodium, potassium, and phosphate.[2] Intracellular dehydration occurs as a consequence of the osmolarity-induced shift of intracellular fluid into the extracellular compartment secondary to hyperglycemia. Failure of insulin to inhibit lipolysis causes breakdown of adipose tissue to free fatty acids, which are metabolized by the liver to the ketone bodies β-hydroxybutyrate (β-OHB), and acetoacetate. These ketone bodies are normally in equilibrium (1:1 ratio, respectively), but a higher ratio (≈5:1) occurs in DKA because of a reduction-oxidation (redox) shift favoring β-OHB production, typically with blood β-OHB levels of 10 mmol/L and blood acetoacetate levels of 3 mmol/L. By contrast, acetone (about 5 mmol/L) is produced from nonenzymatic decarboxylation of acetoacetate and is excreted via the lungs or kidneys. Total ketoanion levels can exceed 25 mmol/L in severe DKA, with levels of β-OHB normalizing within 8 hours after treatment, in parallel with its maximal urinary excretion.[2-4] A similar time profile occurs for brain β-OHB levels; ketoacidosis develops as hepatic production of β-OHB in the absence of insulin far exceeds its metabolism or renal excretion.

Oliguric renal failure is rare in uncomplicated DKA and is usually associated with other precipitating causes, such as sepsis and rhabdomyolysis. Elevation of the plasma urea concentration is not uncommon and may be a marker of disease severity and a risk factor for cerebral edema.[5] The kidneys work at maximal capacity in DKA, with urine acidification excreting about 40% of the hydrogen load produced via hepatic ketone production; hence the importance of maintaining adequate urine output as an effective means of ketoacid removal.[3] Evidence for a renal tubular defect is lacking, because hyperchloremic acidosis may be a physiological consequence of preferential excretion of ketones over the chloride anion[2] or may result from volume loading with saline.

DIAGNOSIS

Criteria for the diagnosis of DKA are glycosuria with elevated blood glucose concentration (>11 mmol/L), metabolic acidosis (pH < 7.3 or blood bicarbonate <15 mmol/L), and blood ketonemia with a raised anion gap.[6] Occasionally in infancy, in pregnancy, or after partial insulin treatment, the blood glucose concentration can be normal in a patient with DKA. Severe DKA is characterized by metabolic acidosis with pH less than 7.1 or bicarbonate concentration less than 5 mmol/L, but severity of acidosis does not always correlate with the extent of dehydration, which may vary from mild (1%) to extreme (20%).[7-9]

Urine ketone tests do not detect the predominant ketoanion β-OHB and therefore do not correlate with plasma ketone levels, of which the majority is β-OHB. A strongly positive urine test result for ketones (nitroprusside reaction) indicates high levels of acetoacetate and by inference is suggestive of plasma ketosis.[4] Severe ketoacidosis with a disproportionate increase in β-OHB and low levels of acetoacetate can occur with negative or weakly positive urine ketone test results; nevertheless, the anion gap is usually higher. Other causes of ketosis, such as starvation, sepsis, and alcohol-related disease, may also manifest as acidosis, but typically, hyperglycemia is absent in such conditions. They are explained in more detail at the end of the chapter. Rapid bedside tests to measure plasma β-OHB levels are available but have not been universally adopted.

MANAGEMENT

The bulk of evidence for the safe and effective treatment of DKA has been extrapolated from animal models or based on analysis of large pediatric or adult case series and is hence driven by expert consensus.[6] Details for the exact mechanisms of cerebral edema are not known, but sufficient knowledge is available to formulate workable prin-

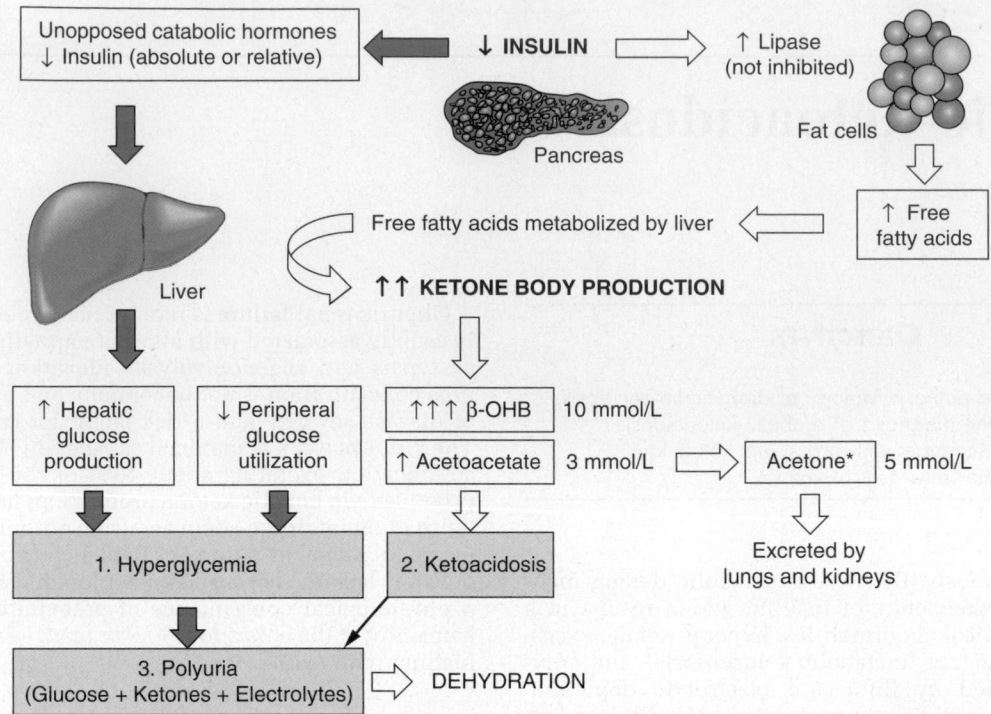

FIGURE 123-1. The pathophysiology of diabetic ketoacidosis. *Nonionized (no contribution to anion gap). Normal levels of β-hydroxybutyrate (β-OHB) + acetoacetate <1 mmol/L.

ciples to minimize the risks of this devastating complication. The most important aspect of treatment is the careful and meticulous monitoring of the individual patient.

Treatment of DKA involves the following broad principles:
- Rapid correction of shock
- Slow rehydration over 48 hours
- Insulin therapy
- Treatment of precipitating causes
- Prevention and early treatment of cerebral edema
- Monitoring of the resolution of acidosis

Rapid Correction of Shock

Hypovolemic shock should be rapidly corrected with isotonic resuscitation fluid (10-20 mL/kg), particularly if hypotension is present.[6] However, it is important not to overtreat patients with excessive quantities of fluid, because Kussmaul's breathing with cold and mottled peripheral areas and poor capillary refill are not reliable indicators of shock in DKA.[8] Hypotension is rare in pediatric DKA. Administration of large volumes of fluid (>40-50 mL/kg) in the first 4 hours of treatment is a risk factor for cerebral edema.[1,10,11,12] A low threshold for use of inotropic agents should be adopted if shock is refractory to fluid resuscitation or other diagnoses are present, such as septic shock (e.g., coexistent lactic acidosis). It is not known whether small-volume resuscitation with hypertonic saline to avoid large fluid volumes reduces the risk of cerebral edema, although there is a suggestion that creation of hypernatremia to prevent a drop in effective osmolality may be an effective strategy.[12] There is no evidence to support the use of colloids in preference to crystalloids for fluid resuscitation in DKA. Normal saline (0.9%) is the most widely used resuscitation fluid, and although it may promote hyperchloremic acidosis, there is no evidence that this is detrimental in DKA.

Slow Rehydration Over 48 Hours

Detailed fluid balance studies in two adult diabetic patients in 1933 demonstrated fluid losses of about 5 L and a 20% depletion of plasma sodium and potassium concentrations when ketoacidosis was induced by withholding of insulin.[13] Estimating the severity of dehydration in DKA is notoriously unreliable and inaccurate.[6-8] Such an estimation may lead to errors in the calculation of rehydration volumes and may contribute to overzealous fluid administration rates, because many fluid regimens are based on percentage of dehydration and "deficit therapy." There is supportive evidence in adults and children that slow rehydration rates lead to earlier resolution of acidosis.[14,15] Although a subject of heated debate, studies have failed to show any fluid regimen capable of minimizing the risk of cerebral edema, with some researchers strongly advocating physiological regimens with careful patient monitoring.[16-18] Bohn and Daneman[17] have suggested a reasonable approach for children in which the aim is to use "no more than 7.5 to 10 mL/kg during the first hour of treatment of 0.9% saline with a reduction to 3.5 to 5 mL/kg/hr thereafter," with no replacement of urine losses.[17]

Over the last decade, the dangers of hypotonic pediatric maintenance fluid (0.45% saline or less) have been highlighted as causal factors in iatrogenic hyponatremia, cerebral edema, and death.[19,20] These fluids had been widely advocated as appropriate for use in DKA. Given the fact that hypotonic fluids increase intracranial pressure in DKA,[21] it is prudent to avoid them—a statement supported by the 2004 American European expert consensus group.[6] Careful monitoring of the patient is essential and should include identification of a drop in effective osmolality or corrected sodium as a warning of the possibility of cerebral edema, particularly if associated with a decline in neurological status.[5,12] Table 123-1 contains examples of how effective osmolality and corrected sodium are calculated and used for this purpose. In the absence of hyperkalemia,

TABLE 123-1

Theoretical Illustrations of Changes in Corrected Plasma Sodium and Effective Osmolality after a 15 mmol/L Fall in Blood Glucose Level

PARAMETER	STARTING VALUES	SCENARIO A	SCENARIO B
Measured plasma sodium (mmol/l)	133	142	137
Blood glucose (mmol/L)	30	15	15
Difference in glucose from 5.6 mmol/L	24.5	9.5	9.5
Change in plasma sodium due to glucose (mmol/L)*	7.1	2.8	2.8
Corrected plasma sodiumn (mmol/L)	140.1	144.8 ($\uparrow$)	137.8 ($\downarrow$)
Effective osmolality (mOsm/kg H_2O))	296	299 ($\uparrow$)	289 ($\downarrow$)
Risk of cerebral edema	—	No	Yes

*Plasma sodium will fall by 0.29 mmol/L for every mmol/L rise in glucose above a reference value of 5.6 mol/L, according to the formula of Katz. The corrected plasma sodium on admission is therefore $[133 + 0.29 \times (30 - 5.6)] = 133 + 7.1 = 140.1$ mmol/L.

In Scenario A, the corrected plasma soidum has risen from 140 mmol/L (start) to 144.8 mmol/L $[142 + 0.29 \times (15 - 5.6)]$. The effective osmolality has also increased from 296 (start) to 299 mOsm/kg. The patient therefore should be at low risk for development of cerebral edema.

In Scenario B, with the identical fall in glucose of 15 mmol/L, the corrected plasma sodium has fallen from 140 mmol/L at the start to 137.8 mmol/L. Together with a fall in effective osmolality (296 to 289 mOsm/kg), this suggests that the patient in Scenario B is at higher risk for development of cerebral edema. This is despite the apparent increase in measured plasma sodium in Scenario B from 133 mmol/L to 137 mmol/L.

potassium should be routinely replaced (20-40 mmol/L), but evidence for correction of mild to moderate hypophosphatemia is lacking.[6]

Insulin Therapy

The primary aims of insulin therapy are to inhibit lipolysis and prevent the ongoing production of ketones. Low-dose insulin (0.05 to 0.1 U/kg/hr) achieves this goal without the risk of rapid changes in blood glucose concentration.[22] Ultra-low-dose insulin infusion rates as low as 0.01 U/kg/hr have been used in adult patients with good results.[22] Correction of hyperglycemia should occur over 8 to 12 hours, in parallel with resolution of ketosis; however, the extent of hyperglycemia does not always correlate with the severity of ketoacidosis. For example, patients who ingest glucose-rich drinks may have marked hyperglycemia without severe acidosis yet may be at risk for cerebral edema if they ingest large quantities of electrolyte-free water. Because of the risks of major transcellular fluid shifts with rapid changes in blood glucose concentration (osmotic dysequilibrium), a precipitous fall in glucose concentration—more than 5 mmol per hour—should be avoided. Insulin should be continued as long as blood ketones are present, and additional glucose provided intravenously if the blood glucose concentration drops rapidly. Results of urine ketone tests, which detect acetoacetate rather than β-OHB, may remain positive despite resolution of systemic ketoacidosis. The wider use of the bedside β-OHB test would avoid this problem because it provides reliable quantification of blood ketosis.

There is no evidence to support high-dose insulin therapy (>0.1 U/kg/hr) in adults or children, although clinicians are often tempted to use it for persisting acidosis. In this scenario, it is important to quantify the acidifying effect of hyperchloremia or to look for other causes of acidosis (e.g., septic shock with lactic acidosis). The early use of insulin has been documented as a risk factor for cerebral edema in children,[10] possibly owing to its role as a sodium-proton exchanger that regulates brain electrolyte and fluid flux, a finding also shown in animal models of DKA.[23]

Treatment of Precipitating Causes

Infection is the most common precipitating factor in DKA, especially in adults, with the site of infection typically the

TABLE 123-2

Risk Factors for the Development of Cerebral Edema in Children with Diabetic Ketoacidosis

Younger age
PCO_2 < 15 mm Hg at presentation
pH < 7.1 at presentation
More than 40 mL/kg intravenous fluids given in first 4 hours
Rapid drop in corrected plasma Na value
Bicarbonate therapy
Raised plasma urea concentration
Hyperventilation after intubation
Early use of insulin (first hour)

urinary or respiratory tract. Sepsis may manifest as a persisting acidosis despite insulin, frequently with the accompanying elevation of the blood lactate concentration.

Prevention and Early Treatment of Cerebral Edema

Cerebral edema is more common in pediatric patients than in adults but is reported in less than 1% of cases.[6] This figure may well be an underestimation, because many children are referred for intensive care with neurological deterioration 2 to 4 hours after commencement of therapy and have received large quantities of intravenous fluids (>40 mL/kg) for weak indications such as failure of rapid resolution of acidosis or poor capillary refill. Cerebral edema should be suspected in patients with unexplained alteration in mental status (obtundation or disorientation), which typically occurs during the first 6 hours of therapy in patients with known risk factors (Table 123-2).[5,8-12] Although there are many proposed mechanisms for cerebral edema (Table 123-3), there is as yet no single, well-defined, unifying explanation.[6] Failure to identify and treat cerebral edema with osmotherapy can be devastating, death or permanent neurological injury having been reported in up to 50% of cases.[24,25] Failure to treat cerebral edema early, before a respiratory arrest, increases the chances of a poor outcome.[24] An improvement in neurological status after osmotherapy should be regarded as clinical evidence of cerebral edema. Early treatment of suspected cerebral edema should not be delayed by the need for neuro-imaging, which is nevertheless important because the cause of coma in DKA may vary from edema to ischemia, infarction, cerebral thrombosis, and infection.

Traditionally, mannitol (0.5 to 1 g/kg) has been used as the preferred agent to reduce brain swelling; however, the use of 3% hypertonic saline (2-3 mL/kg) has a number of advantages: It increases blood pressure via intravascular volume expansion and is not a dehydrating obligate osmole like mannitol. Use of hypertonic saline also allows for easy calculation of effective plasma osmolality, unlike use of mannitol, which as an unmeasured osmole requires calculation of an osmole gap for its quantification.[26,27] The protective effect of hypernatremia in preventing a fall in effective osmolality has been described in children with DKA (Fig. 123-2),[12] suggesting that monitoring changes in effective osmolality is a clinically useful tool. Raising the plasma sodium level with boluses of hypertonic saline may be necessary to avoid progression to cerebral edema in patients who initially show response to osmotherapy but require further management.

Unfortunately, most expert texts and consensus statements either do not describe what a clinician should do after giving the first dose of mannitol for cerebral edema or merely suggest repeating a dose after 2 hours.[6]

The question of intubation and at what level to target arterial P_{CO_2} remains uncertain. If respiratory drive is adequate (an appropriately low P_{CO_2} for the degree of acidosis) and a response to osmotherapy is achieved, it is reasonable not to institute mechanical ventilation provided that close and careful monitoring is possible. Tasker and colleagues[28] have hypothesized that hyperventilation after intubation is a necessary target to avoid rapid changes in cerebral blood volume that would occur if P_{CO_2} were normalized. Conversely, hyperventilation after intubation has been reported as a risk factor for cerebral edema.[29] However, the brain is capable of remarkably rapid adaptation to hypocapnia that buffers cerebrospinal fluid and brain tissue acidosis via changes in brain electrolytes coupled to the regulation of cell volume.[30] Clarification of the response and reactivity of the brain to carbon dioxide in DKA is essential to answer these questions. Doppler ultrasonographic studies have shown abnormalities in cerebral autoregulation but no increase in blood flow with normalization of P_{CO_2}.[31] Magnetic resonance imaging findings suggest a vasogenic rather than cytotoxic mechanism of edema.[32] My preference is to maintain normal P_{CO_2} after intubation.[33,34] There is no evidence for intracranial pressure monitoring in DKA.

Monitoring of the Resolution of Metabolic Acidosis

In the absence of routine bedside blood ketone measurement, clinicians rely on pH, the anion gap, or base excess value to monitor resolution of ketoacidosis. In 1982, the value of the anion gap in DKA was questioned by Adrogue and colleagues,[2] who demonstrated that bicarbonate does not rise with a 1:1 equimolar fall in ketones during recovery from ketoacidosis—in other words, that the anion gap decreased at a faster rate than bicarbonate increased. Explanations for this discrepancy included different apparent distributions of bicarbonate and ketones. Taylor and associates,[35] in a 2006 study of 18 children with DKA,

TABLE 123-3

Theoretical Mechanisms of Cerebral Edema in Diabetic Ketoacidosis

Over-zealous rehydration with hypotonic intravenous fluids
Rapid changes in blood glucose level with administration of insulin (osmotic dysequilibrium)
Movement of sodium and water into cells via insulin-mediated activation of the Na^+-H^+ transporter
Increased permeability of the blood-brain barrier (vasogenic edema)
Abnormalities of cerebral autoregulation and blood flow
Cytotoxicity of idiogenic osmoles
Dysregulation of cerebral vasopressin

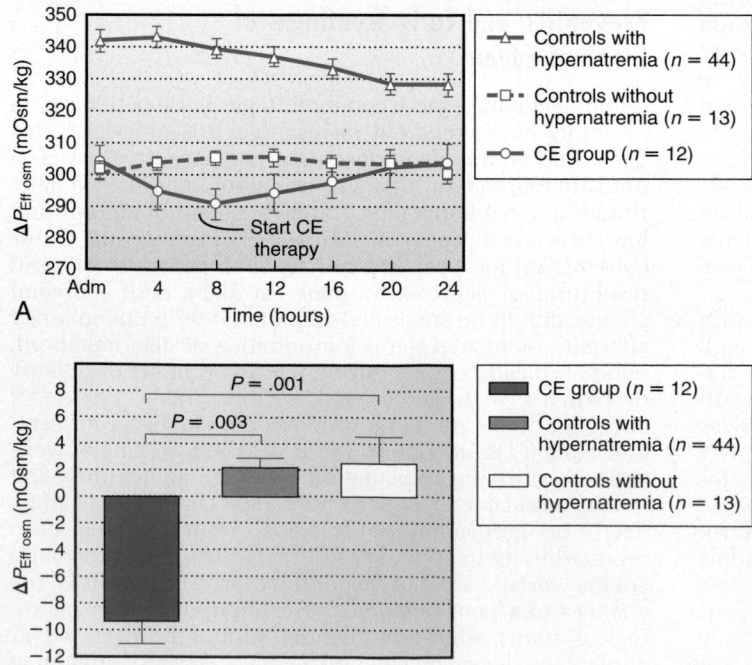

FIGURE 123-2. A, Temporal profile for effective osmolality (ΔP Eff osm) in patients with cerebral edema (CE) (*circles*; n = 44), controls (*squares*; n = 13), and hypernatremia (*triangles*; n = 12). B, Changes in effective plasma osmolality during the first 4 hours of therapy. *Dark blue bar*, cerebral edema group (n = 12); *gray bar*, controls with hypernatremia (n = 44); *white bar*, controls without hypernatremia (n = 13). Group comparisons were performed using analysis of variance and post hoc tests. P values from the post hoc tests are shown.

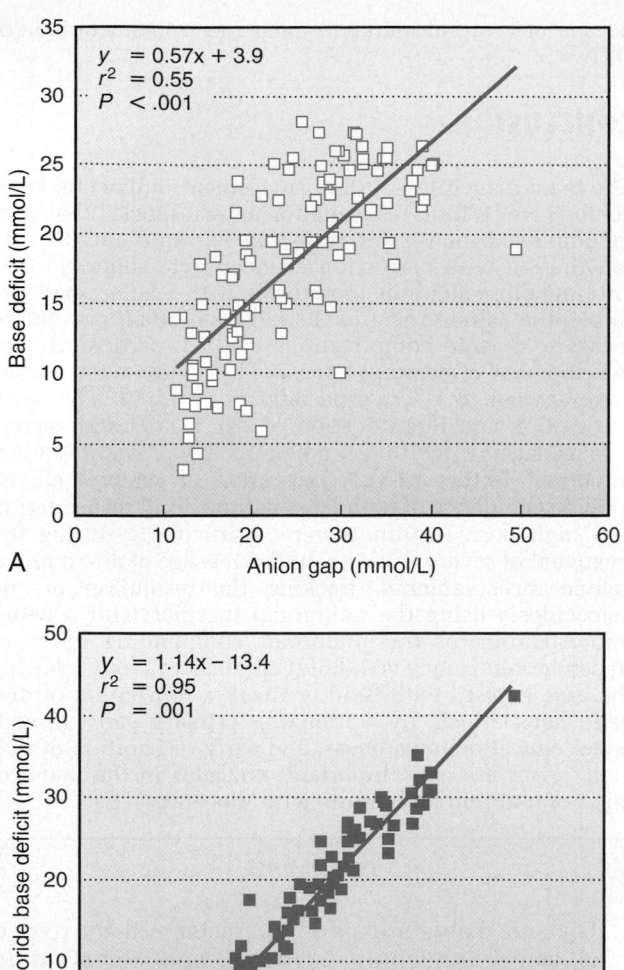

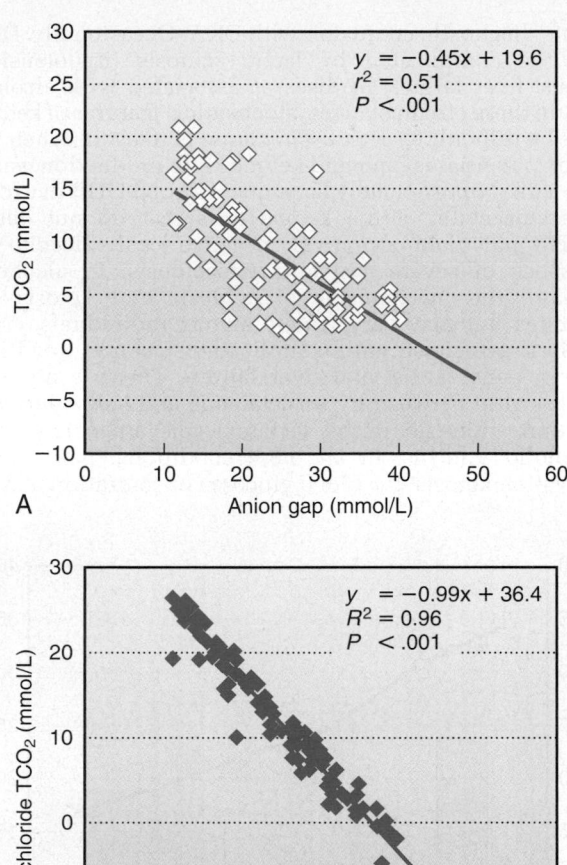

FIGURE 123-3. Regression plots for albumin corrected anion gap versus base deficit before (**A**) and after correction for chloride (**B**).

FIGURE 123-4. Regression plots for albumin corrected anion gap versus bicarbonate before (**A**) and after correction for chloride (**B**). Plasma bicarbonate is represented by the total carbon dioxide content (TCO_2). Note the equimolar relationship of bicarbonate with the anion gap after chloride has been accounted for (slope of regression = 0.99).

demonstrated that this discrepancy is due to the acidifying effect of hyperchloremia and that an equimolar relationship between anion gap and bicarbonate (and base excess) is in fact present when this factor is accounted for (Figs. 123-3 and 123-4). This study revalidates the accuracy of the anion gap in DKA as a useful tool to track resolution of ketosis. Furthermore, if the base deficit is partitioned to separate chloride, the effect of hyperchloremia during treatment is evident (Fig. 123-5), increasing from 6% at the start of treatment to 94% at 20 hours.

Although there is a paucity of fluid and electrolyte balance studies in DKA, Adrogue and colleagues[2] demonstrated that the retention of chloride by the kidneys in preference to excretion of negatively charged ketones was an important mechanism of hyperchloremia. There is also an apparent compensatory drop in plasma chloride concentration early in DKA, as shown by Funk and co-workers[36] where plasma chloride was only 67% of sodium

(normal value 72% to 79%), the mechanism of which remains unknown. This finding may partly explain the low incidence of hyperchloremia in the early phase of DKA, i.e., chloride anions need to make way for negatively changed ketoanions in order to preserve electroneutrality, resulting in a hypochloremic state. Given the limitations of the base deficit in DKA, clinicians should either correct the base deficit for chloride or use the albumin-corrected anion gap. No acid-base studies have examined the impact of solutions with physiological concentrations of chloride on DKA. There are, however, no data to support bolus bicarbonate therapy to rapidly correct acidosis in DKA but some evidence that ketone metabolism is itself inhibited by administration of bicarbonate to correct pH.[37]

OTHER DISORDERS OF KETOSIS

Table 123-4 lists the key features of disorders associated with abnormal ketone production and acidosis that may create diagnostic confusion with DKA. Occasionally, DKA may be complicated by lactic acidosis (hypotension, sepsis, liver failure) or diseases associated with alcoholism. In these circumstances, biochemical features of ketosis may be difficult to detect. This issue is relevant when the redox potential is high and ketone body production generates a disproportionately large quantity of β-OHB in excess of acetoacetate.[5] Urine ketone tests that do not detect β-OHB may yield deceptively negative results despite the presence of severe systemic ketoacidosis. In alcoholic disease, the mechanisms of acidosis and ketosis are complex but may vary widely among individuals, especially if associated with complications such as vomiting, sepsis, pancreatitis, and liver failure. There is no clear relationship between hyperlactatemia and ketoanion production, although raised lactate levels are common in alcoholic acidosis. In all these conditions, particularly starvation ketosis, the blood glucose concentration may be normal or low, not markedly raised as is characteristic of DKA.

CONCLUSION

The main principles in the management of diabetic ketoacidosis are (1) fluid resuscitation to treat shock, (2) insulin to inhibit ketogenesis and restore euglycemia, and (3) slow rehydration with correction of electrolyte abnormalities. Careful and meticulous monitoring with regular reevlauation of the patient remains the most important preventive measure to avoid complications in DKA, particularly the development of cerebral edema. This is the most serious complication of DKA, especially in children. The early recognition and identification of risk factors and aggressive management with osmotherapy may prove lifesaving. Important factors in the prevention of cerebral edema include avoidance of both large volume fluid resuscitation and high dose insulin therapy, particularly during the treatment of severe acidosis. In the absence of direct blood ketone measurements, tracking the resolution of the ketoacidosis using the anion gap together with a better understanding of the important confounding effect of hyperchloremia may be helpful adjuncts to avoid "chasing the base excess" with fluid or insulin. Prevention of diabetic ketoacidosis by optimizing primary care through better education, awareness, and early recognition of diabetic crises are also important strategies in the management of children and adults with diabetes.

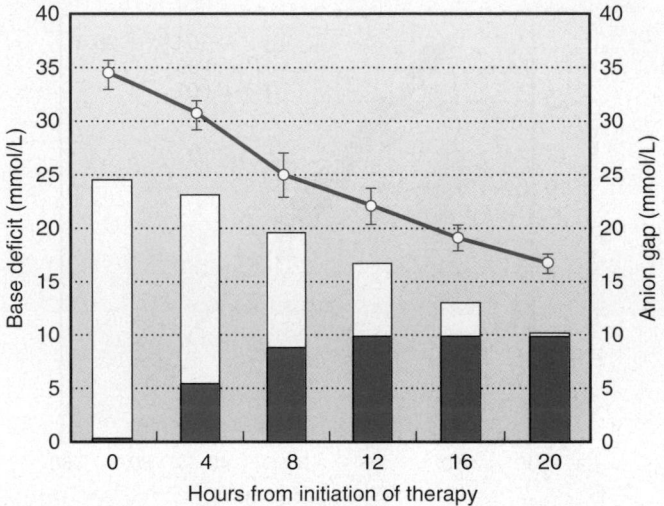

FIGURE 123-5. Temporal profiles of the base deficit and anion gap. The base deficit is partitioned into chloride (*blue bars*) and non-chloride (*white bars*) components. Values are mean; error bars = standard of mean. Temporal profile for the anion gap is on the secondary left axis (*circles*).

Key Points

1. Diabetic ketoacidosis is characterized by hyperglycemia, metabolic acidosis, and elevation in blood ketone levels with depletion of body water and electrolyte levels.
2. Careful and meticulous individual monitoring is the most important goal of therapy, the major principles being the rapid correction of hypovolemia or shock, slow rehydration, and low-dose insulin.

TABLE 123-4

Main Characteristics of Starvation Ketosis, β-Hydroxybutyric Acidosis, and Alcoholic Acidosis

VARIABLE	STARVATION KETOSIS	β-HYDROXYBUTYRIC ACIDOSIS	ALCOHOLIC ACIDOSIS
Clinical scenario	Chronic starvation	DKA complicated by lactic acidosis	Alcoholic patients after binge drinking
Mechanism	Insulopenia with lipolysis	Increased redox potential, with excess β-OHB formation relative to acetoacetate	Multifactorial: accelerated ketosis
Association with DKA?	No	Yes	Yes
Blood glucose level	Normal or low	Normal or low	Normal, raised, or low
Acidosis	Mild to moderate	Moderate to severe	Variable (acidosis or alkalosis)*
Lactic acidosis	Rare	Frequently coexists	Frequently coexists
Blood ketone levels	Raised (mild or moderate)	Can be very high	Can be very high
Ratio of β-OHB to acetoacetate	Raised 3:1 (similar to that in DKA)	High: can exceed 10:1	Variable: 3:1 to 5:1
Urine ketone test results	Strongly positive	Weakly positive or negative	Weakly positive or negative

β-OHB, β-hydroxybutyrate; DKA, diabetic ketoacidosis.
*Alkalosis may be respiratory (from hyperventilation) or metabolic (e.g., from vomiting).

3. Rapid changes in plasma osmolality should be avoided by ensuring that effective plasma osmolality does not fall with therapy. This goal can be achieved by raising the plasma sodium concentration with hypertonic saline.

4. Excessive fluid administration should be avoided, particularly the use of hypotonic intravenous fluids (0.45% saline).

5. The anion gap should be used to quantify resolution of ketosis rather than of the base deficit, which is strongly influenced by hyperchloremia, a universal finding in diabetic ketoacidosis.

Key References

5. Glaser N, Barnett P, McCaslin I, et al: Risk factors for cerebral edema in children with diabetic ketoacidosis. N Engl J Med 2001;25:344:264-269.

6. Dunger DB, Sperling MA, Acerini CL, et al; European Society for Paediatric Endocrinology; Lawson Wilkins Pediatric Endocrine Society: European Society for Paediatric Endocrinology/Lawson Wilkins Pediatric Endocrine Society consensus statement on diabetic ketoacidosis in children and adolescents. Arch Dis Child 2004;89:188-194.

10. Edge JA, Jakes RW, Roy Y, et al: The UK case-control study of cerebral oedema complicating diabetic ketoacidosis in children. Diabetologia 2006;49:2002-2009.

35. Taylor D, Durward A, Tibby SM, et al: The influence of hyperchloraemia on acid base interpretation in diabetic ketoacidosis. Intensive Care Med 2006;3:295-301.

See the companion Expert Consult website for the complete reference list.

CHAPTER 124

Unmeasured Anions in Metabolic Acidosis

Lui G. Forni and Philip J. Hilton

OBJECTIVES

This chapter will:

1. Outline the often multifactorial origin of metabolic acidosis, especially in the critically ill patient.

2. Describe how the use of simple tools, such as calculation of the anion gap, can alert the clinician to the presence of unmeasured anions.

3. Discuss the organic acids that have been proposed as potential causative agents for the genesis of unmeasured anion acidosis in both animal models and patients.

4. Demonstrate that the concentrations of unmeasured anions may in themselves have an impact on survival in the critically ill patient.

As has been discussed in previous chapters, metabolic acidosis remains a commonly encountered problem in both acute medical practice and the intensive care units (ICUs).[1,2] The "classical" causes of metabolic acidosis are diabetic ketoacidosis, lactic acidosis, the ingestion of acid-generating poisons, and, more rarely, congenital enzyme deficiencies. However, in many cases, the acidosis cannot be ascribed solely to one of these causes or, indeed, to any single causative anion. In such cases, the origin is often multifactorial, and the source of the acidosis remains unidentified or unmeasured. Diabetic ketoacidosis is a commonly encountered example of an acidosis associated with large quantities of unmeasured anions. In the patient with this disorder, the ketoacids responsible are unmeasured, although in practice their concentrations are inferred.

The presence of an unmeasured anion contributing to a metabolic acidosis is often highlighted by that most simple of tools, the anion gap. However, in the critically ill patient with metabolic acidosis, this simple categorization is often an inadequate description of the underlying metabolic state. For example, in lactic acidosis, a significant discrepancy between the blood lactate concentration and the base deficit is often observed, and this fact has given rise to the concept of the "unmeasured anions" as an important component of human metabolic acidosis. Indeed, at times, these appear to be quantitatively much more important than the measured lactic acid, as highlighted by studies examining the issue in patients with trauma, in those in ICUs, and in those who have experienced cardiac arrest.[3-6] The nature of these unmeasured anions has proved difficult to elucidate, but work has now provided some insights as to their composition and clinical relevance.

IDENTIFYING UNMEASURED ANIONS

The presence of unmeasured anions contributing to metabolic acidosis is not a new phenomenon. More than 40 years ago, in discussing lactic acidosis, Waters and colleagues[7] hypothesized that, under certain conditions, disturbances in acid-base balance may be "characterised by the accumulation of an organic acid other than lactate." Subsequently, a case was reported in which hydroxybutyrate contributed significantly to an observed metabolic

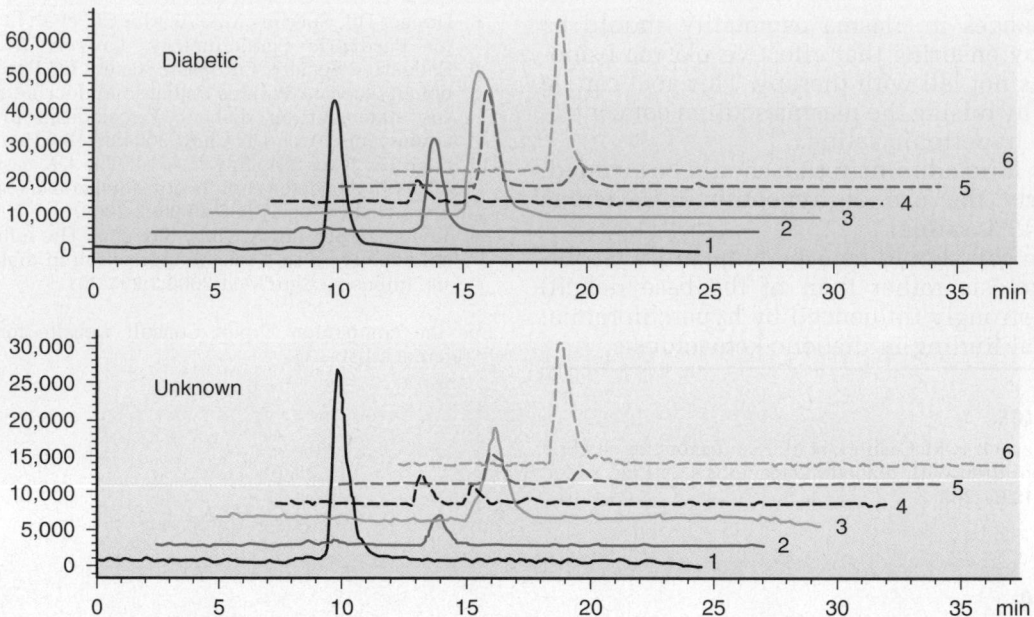

FIGURE 124-1. Ion exchange chromatograms/negative ion mass spectra of plasma from a patient with diabetic ketoacidosis (*top*) and a patient with acidosis of unknown etiology (*bottom*). Liquid chromatography/electrospray ionization mass spectrometry was performed on a Hewlett-Packard Series 1100 liquid chromatography system directly coupled to a Series 1100 Mass Spectrometer fitted with electrospray ionization and operating in "negative ion" mode (Agilent Technologies UK Ltd, Wokingham, Berkshire, UK). The extracted ion currents are shown: 1, lactate; 2, acetoacetate; 3, hydroxybutyrate; 4, malate; 5, ketoglutarate; 6, citrate/isocitrate. (From Forni LG, McKinnon W, Hilton PJ: Unmeasured anions in metabolic acidosis: Unravelling the mystery. Crit Care 2006;10:220-225; BioMed Central Ltd.)

acidosis of a nondiabetic patient, and further studies demonstrated elevated succinate levels in the plasma of both hypoxic patients and animal models.[8,9] The proposed mechanism for this observed rise was a disturbance in the oxidation of succinate to oxaloacetate. Later studies in critically ill patients demonstrated elevations in the observed anion gap that could not be accounted for solely by increased lactate levels, implying the presence of unmeasured anions.[10,11] Quantification of the hitherto unmeasured ions, such as urate and phosphate, as well as plasma proteins could not account for the observed anion gap.[12,13]

Animal Studies

In an attempt to elucidate these ionic species, several investigators have employed animal models to study unmeasured anions. One of the earliest studies examined critically ill horses with an acidosis associated with an increase in the anion gap. This unexplained anion gap could not be accounted for by the determination of pyruvate, β-hydroxybutyrate, acetoacetate, phosphate, or albumin concentrations.[14] Later studies addressed the contribution of unmeasured anions to the anion gap observed in a rat model of sepsis after cecal perforation.[15] The septic animals demonstrated a metabolic acidosis with higher plasma lactate and lower bicarbonate concentrations than found in control animals. Only 15% of the observed anion gap could be explained by lactate, and measurement of a variety of small acids, including pyruvate, β-hydroxybutyrate, acetoacetate, citrate, and amino acids, did not explain the observed differences. Moreover, no differences in these anions could be detected between the control

group and study animals. It should be noted, however, that no precise detail as to the handling of these samples was provided. In another animal study on diarrheic calves, the observed anion gap was explained in part, but not completely, by the accumulation of D-lactate.[16] Yet another study employing a canine model of sepsis demonstrated that the liver released anions into the circulation at a rate of 0.12 mEq/min, and the investigators observed that the gut became a "consumer" of anions after development of endotoxemia.[17] Impaired hepatic extraction of lactate coupled with increased splanchnic production of lactate in lactic acidosis has been implied in canine models, but studies in humans do not support this view.[18] To date, animal studies have therefore provided little information as to the nature of the unmeasured anions.

Human Studies
Pyroglutamic Acidemia

Pyroglutamic acidemia is typically an inherited disorder that manifests in infancy because of deficiency of either 5-oxoprolinase or glutathione synthetase. Several case reports have described the occurrence of this phenomenon in adults and a resultant elevated anion gap acidosis, often in association with drug administration, particularly paracetamol.[19,20] Pyroglutamic acid concentrations were noted to be elevated in four patients in an early study of patients in an ICU.[21] Mizcock and associates,[22] in another study on 23 ICU patients with metabolic acidosis and unexplained increases in ion gap, found no correlation between the ion gap and pyroglutamic acid levels and concluded that in their population, pyroglutamic acid could not account for the unmeasured anions.

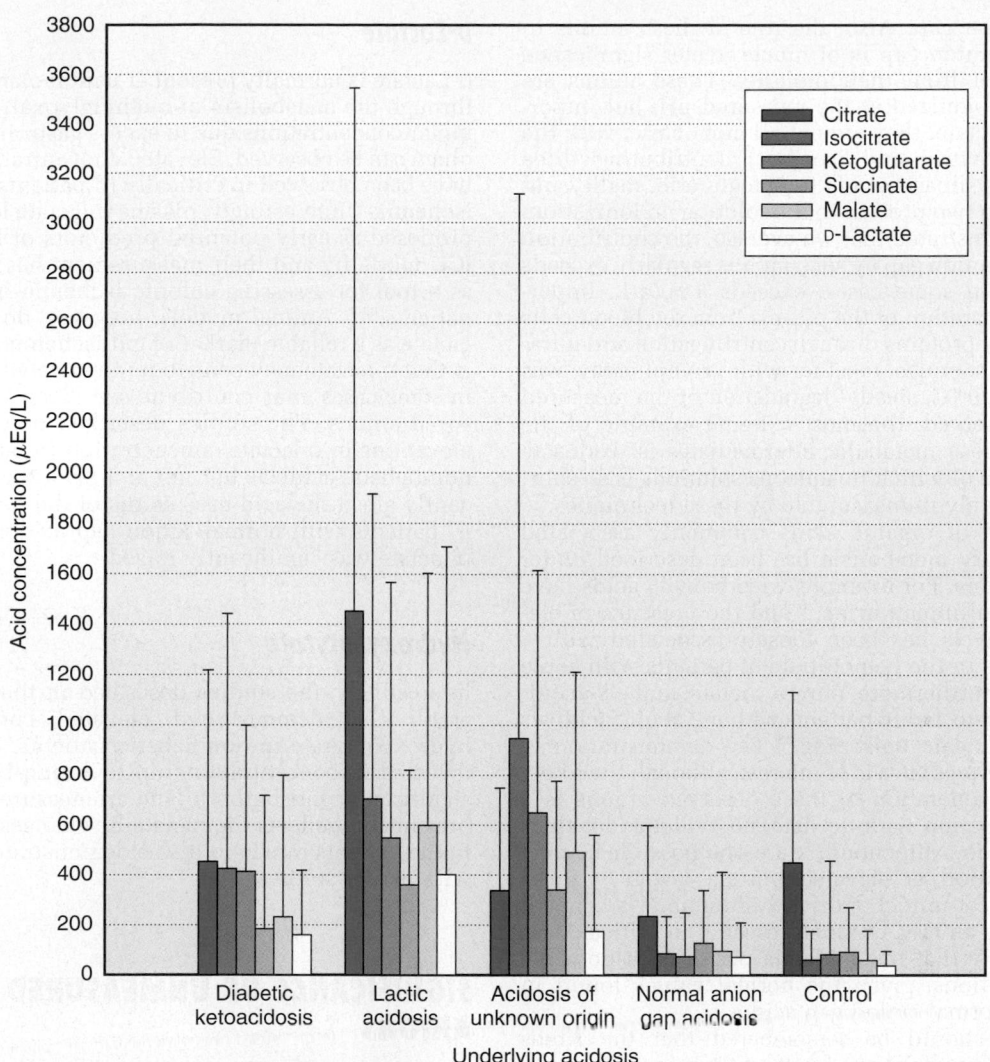

FIGURE 124-2. The concentrations of various weak acids measured in patients with metabolic acidosis. The results are grouped according to underlying etiology (mean ± upper range). (From Forni LG, McKinnon W, Lord GA, et al: Circulating anions usually associated with the Krebs cycle in patients with metabolic acidosis. Crit Care 2005;9:R591-R595; BioMed Central Ltd.)

Krebs Cycle Intermediates

Later, more detailed attempts to identify the unknown anions employed negative ion mass spectrometry coupled with ion exchange chromatography.[23] Plasma samples from acidotic patients with various forms of metabolic acidosis were examined and demonstrated the presence of ions of relatively low mass equivalent to those of the known Krebs cycle components. Standards of these tricarboxylic acid intermediates proved to have retention times identical to the plasma-derived peaks, and no ions attributable to other substances could be seen apart from urate, which was also demonstrated in control samples. Figure 124-1 shows two typical ion exchange chromatograms/negative ion mass spectra, one obtained from the plasma extract of a patient with metabolic acidosis of unknown etiology and the other of a patient with diabetic ketoacidosis. Furthermore, enzyme studies confirmed the presence of Krebs cycle intermediates in the plasma of these patients together with D-lactate.

Figure 124-2 shows the mean results together with the maximal value for each anion measured in each type of acidosis.[24]

Plasma from patients with diabetic ketoacidosis showed significant increases relative to the control values in citrate, isocitrate, α-ketoglutarate, malate, and D-lactate levels, whereas citrate and succinate concentrations were not elevated. In patients with lactic acidosis, higher concentrations of citrate, isocitrate, α-ketoglutarate, succinate, malate, and D-lactate were observed. In patients with an acidosis of unknown origin (acidosis disproportionate to the blood lactate concentration or unmeasured anion acidosis), elevations in the concentrations of isocitrate, α-ketoglutarate, succinate, malate, and D-lactate were seen. This observation—that plasma concentrations of acids usually associated with the Krebs tricarboxylic acid cycle are significantly increased in patients with lactic acidosis as well as those with "unexplained acidosis" with normal or near normal blood lactate concentrations—may go some way to addressing the "imbalance" in the anion gap or strong ion gap. Also, the role of these anions in generating the anion gap is of much greater significance than is apparent from their molarity. These anions are effectively fully ionized at the measured pH, but importantly, unlike lactate, they are not all monobasic, with the tribasic acids (citric and isocitric) contributing three protons and the dibasic acids (α-ketoglutaric, malic, and succinic) adding two protons to the solution on ionization. This work demonstrated that, on average, the contribution to the observed anion gap by such anions regularly exceeds 3 mEq/L, and, in some cases, exceeds 5 mEq/L. Importantly, rapid separation of the plasma from red blood cells and also from its proteins through centrifugation and ultrafiltration of the samples, together with prompt assay, was vital. Even at $-20°$ C, steady degradation of the measured anions was observed; the most extreme example of the instability of these metabolic intermediates is oxaloacetate, the half-life of which in aqueous solutions is so short that it is effectively unmeasurable by these techniques.[25]

The presence of organic acids commonly associated with intermediary metabolism has been described under various conditions. For example, tricarboxylic acids have been detected in human urine,[26] and the presence of elevated citrate levels has been loosely associated with a worse prognosis in the hemofiltrate of patients with acute renal failure.[27] Furthermore, citrate, malate, and cis-aconitate have been detected in patients with metabolic acidosis ascribed to salicylate poisoning.[28] The demonstration of Krebs cycle intermediates is of interest, although the likely source for the generation of these observed anions is a matter of speculation with, to date, no evidence for their site of production. Mitochondria are one possible source, and the generation of elevated plasma levels of these anions may reflect mitochondrial dysfunction—a concept that is currently an area of much research in critical care. It seems unlikely that the acidemia per se is responsible for the observations, given the normal values found in patients with normal–anion gap acidosis.

However, it should be remembered that the Krebs cycle functions not only as a "catalytic" process in intermediary metabolism but also as a source of substrates for other metabolic pathways. During protein synthesis, α-ketoglutarate and oxaloacetate are removed from the cycle to become aminated to glutamate and aspartate (cataplerosis). This process inevitably results in anaplerotic reactions, ensuring continued function by replenishing tricarboxylic acid intermediates.[29] In gluconeogenesis, oxaloacetate is converted to phosphoenolpyruvate and is lost to the Krebs cycle. Lipogenesis requires the transfer of citrate from the mitochondria to the cytosol, the site of the synthetic process. In disease, the opposite applies. Anaplerotic reactions—that is, those that generate rather than consume Krebs cycle ketoacids—are likely to predominate. Excess protein catabolism in particular gives rise to the component amino acids. These approximately neutral compounds are rapidly transaminated and/or deaminated to form oxaloacetic acid, α-ketoglutaric acid, and succinyl coenzyme A (effectively, succinic acid), thereby potentially providing an excess of acidic Krebs cycle components. Few data on these processes in the critically ill patient are available. However, under other conditions of stress, such as prolonged starvation and extreme exercise,[30] tricarboxylic acid concentration has been measured and shown to be elevated. It has also been shown that glutamine, for example, undergoes deamination (an anaplerotic process) to form α-ketoglutarate, which enters the Krebs cycle and is sequentially converted to malate which then leaves the mitochondria.[30]

D-Lactate

D-Lactate is normally present at nanomolar concentrations through the metabolism of methylglyoxal, although millimolar concentrations due to excess gastrointestinal metabolism can be observed. Elevated concentrations of D-lactate have been observed in critically ill patients with intestinal ischemia.[31] Interestingly, plasma D-lactate levels have been proposed as early potential predictors of reduced 28-day ICU mortality and their measurement has been suggested as a tool for assessing colonic ischemia in postoperative patients.[32,33] Animal models, however, do not confirm D-lactate as a reliable marker of gut ischemia.[34] What is clear is that D-lactate may contribute to metabolic acidosis and, in some cases, may contribute significantly to the unmeasured anions. The studies described here showed slight elevations in D-lactate concentration in both diabetic and nondiabetic acidosis but not at a level that would significantly affect the acid-base status of the patient. However, in patients with normal–anion gap acidosis, the level of D-lactate was significantly raised.

Hydroxybutyrate

Interestingly, the studies described in the previous paragraph also demonstrated elevated concentrations of hydroxybutyrate in nondiabetic patients. This anion was detected in concentrations up to 4 mEq/L, so it can be a significant contributor to the unmeasured anions. This presumably reflects the metabolic changes of "starvation" in the patients in whom it was demonstrated in agreement with earlier studies.[8]

SIGNIFICANCE OF UNMEASURED ANIONS

Although many studies have highlighted the presence of unmeasured anions in critically ill patients with metabolic acidosis, few have been successful in addressing the potential chemical nature of these anions. The prognostic significance of unmeasured anions, however, has proved a source of much debate. For example, in a pediatric ICU population, the presence of unmeasured anions was an important predictor of mortality.[35] Two studies in adult ICU populations did not find such a relationship,[36,37] but later studies seem to suggest some predictive ability.[38,39] Certainly in patients with metabolic acidosis secondary to malarial infection, unidentified anions other than lactate were the most important contributors to the observed metabolic acidosis. Studies on the primary pathophysiological events of malarial infection in animals reveal upregulation of gene transcription, which controls host glycolysis, and one may speculate that the unmeasured anions are related to changes in intermediary metabolism.[40]

CONCLUSIONS

The phenomenon of unexplained metabolic acidosis is well recognized, as is the generation of "unexplained" anions. Little is known about the nature of these species, although studies suggest that anions usually associated with the Krebs cycle may contribute to the observed anion or strong ion gap. These observations may provide the first glimpse of the underlying derangement in the metabolic acidosis associated with unmeasured anions.

Key Points

1. Classic causes of metabolic acidosis are diabetic ketoacidosis, lactic acidosis, the ingestion of acid-generating poisons, and, more rarely, congenital enzyme deficiencies.
2. In critically ill patients with metabolic acidosis, simple categorization with tools such as the anion gap is often an inadequate description of the underlying metabolic state but may indicate the presence of unmeasured anions.
3. Under certain conditions, including trauma and critical illness, and after cardiac arrest, unmeasured anions may be quantitatively more important than commonly measured anions such as lactic acid.

4. Studies now suggest that anions usually associated with the Krebs cycle may contribute to the observed anion or strong ion gap.

Key References

15. Rackow EC, Mecher C, Astiz ME, et al: Unmeasured anion during severe sepsis with metabolic acidosis. Circ Shock 1990;30:107-115.
24. Forni LG, McKinnon W, Lord GA, et al: Circulating anions usually associated with the Krebs cycle in patients with metabolic acidosis. Crit Care 2005;9:R591-R595.
35. Balasubramanyan N, Havens PL, Hoffman GM: Unmeasured anions identified by the Fencl-Stewart method predict mortality better than base excess, anion gap, and lactate in patients in the pediatric intensive care unit. Crit Care Med 1999;27:1577-1581.
38. Dondorp AM, Chau TTH, Phu NH, et al: Unidentified ions of strong prognostic significance in severe malaria. Crit Care Med 2004;32:1683-1688.
39. Kaplan LJ, Kellum JA: Initial pH, base deficit, lactate, anion gap, strong ion difference and strong ion gap predict outcome from major vascular injury. Crit Care Med 2004;32:1120-1124.

See the companion Expert Consult website for the complete reference list.

CHAPTER 125

Iatrogenic Hyperchloremic Metabolic Acidosis

Thomas John Morgan

OBJECTIVES

This chapter will:
1. Confirm that metabolic acidosis can result from large volume saline and colloid infusions.
2. Explore the harm that might arise from such an outcome.
3. Provide a physicochemical explanation for the phenomenon.
4. Explain why "hyperchloremic acidosis" is a misleading description.
5. Identify the essential design characteristics of balanced crystalloids and colloids.

For years medical practitioners have known that replacing large fluid deficits with intravenous saline can cause a metabolic acidosis.[1-6] Similar disturbances are encountered after normovolemic hemodilution[7] and cardiopulmonary bypass.[8-10] Colloid plasma expanders containing albumin,[11] gelatin,[12] or starch[11] can also cause this phenomenon.

The questions this chapter aims to answer are as follows:
- Is this iatrogenic saline-induced metabolic acidosis harmful?
- What is its mechanism?
- How can it be prevented?

IS IATROGENIC SALINE-INDUCED METABOLIC ACIDOSIS HARMFUL?

There are no data from adequately powered clinical mortality studies comparing volume replacement using saline with replacement using more balanced fluids. To date, the only reported clinical problems arising from saline infusions, apart from the acidosis itself, have been an elevated perioperative gastric CO_2 gap[13] and increased postoperative bleeding.[14] Further human data are confined to volunteers; they experienced mental changes, abdominal discomfort, and relative oliguria when given 50 mL/kg normal saline over 1 hour, but not after receiving the same volume of Hartmann's solution.[15]

Results of animal studies are more convincing. In two models of hemorrhagic shock, Ringer's lactate outperformed saline in terms of morbidity and survival.[16,17] Similar findings were obtained in endotoxemia, although the balanced fluid under investigation in this study was actually a colloid (a hetastarch preparation), and the non-balanced fluid was a crystalloid (saline).[18]

Is there less direct evidence that saline-induced acidosis might cause harm? Acidemia per se has adverse effects. Severe acidemia reduces myocardial contractility, stimulates tachydysrhythmias and bradydysrhythmias, and causes systemic arteriolar dilatation, venoconstriction, and pulmonary vasoconstriction. The respiratory drive is increased and the diaphragmatic function depressed. There are also adverse effects on the brain, splanchnic circulation, and musculoskeletal system. Cell membrane pump disturbances, hyperglycemia, and hyperkalemia complete the picture.[19]

More specific evidence is based on experimental hyperchloremia and its associated acidosis. In rats, hyperchloremia reduces renal blood flow and glomerular filtration rate.[20] In other rodent models, HCl infusion causes activation of inducible nitric oxide synthase, hypotension, and acute lung injury or intestinal dysfunction.[21-23] HCl is pro-inflammatory both in vitro[24] and in vivo.[25]

However, such findings should be interpreted with caution, because the toxicity profile of HCl differs from that of saline. For example, HCl has specific effects on the pulmonary circulation[26] and on platelet production of thromboxane A_2.[27] Moreover, the acidemia from saline infusions is relatively mild,[1,2,6] unlike that of HCl injury models. Standard base excess rarely falls below −10 mEq/L, so that with appropriate respiratory compensation, plasma pH should remain above 7.3.

Acidemia even has some advantages. The Bohr effect increases tissue oxygen availability,[28] although the rightward shift of the oxyhemoglobin dissociation curve disappears within hours as 2,3-diphosphoglycerate production decreases.[29] Lowering pH can protect against hypoxic stress,[30,31] and lactic acidosis itself is arguably a protective adaptation.[32] Respiratory acidosis may also be beneficial in a range of scenarios.[33]

Therefore, at present, there is limited clinical evidence that saline-induced acidosis causes harm, backed up by stronger direct and indirect experimental evidence. It would take a large multicenter project along the lines of the Saline versus Albumin Fluid Evaluation (SAFE study) to provide the definitive answer.[34]

WHAT IS THE MECHANISM OF THIS ACIDOSIS?

The normal anion gap in saline-induced acidosis means that lactate or the more exotic anions of critical illness[35] are unlikely culprits. Coincident hyperchloremia is common, prompting the traditional classification of this condition as a "hyperchloremic" acidosis. Many researchers regard hyperchloremia as an association rather than a cause and explain the phenomenon as simple dilution of plasma bicarbonate by bicarbonate-free fluids.[36] Others blame excessive proton activity in the administered fluid and advocate "pH-balanced" fluids.[37]

Proponents of the Stewart approach,[38,39] of which I am one, regard saline-induced acidosis as a classic illustration of physicochemical principles. This approach not only

yields a logical explanation for the underlying mechanism but also provides a platform on which to design fluids for specific acid-base outcomes. It also calls into question the "hyperchloremic" designation itself.

From the Stewart perspective, two physicochemical properties of extracellular fluid together determine its metabolic acid-base status. These are the strong ion difference (SID) and the total concentration of nonvolatile weak acids (A_{tot}). (See Chapter 111 for a detailed description of the Stewart approach to acid-base physiology.) A metabolic acidosis arises from an increase in A_{tot} and/or a decrease in SID; the converse applies in metabolic alkalosis. When both are abnormal, the outcome is determined by the net effect.

The acid-base effects of fluids are generated when they mix and equilibrate with extracellular fluid. In the case of crystalloid, large volumes of infused fluid force extracellular SID toward the SID of the crystalloid, at the same time causing a metabolic alkalosis by diluting A_{tot}. The SID of saline is 0 (equal concentrations of the strong cation Na^+ and the strong anion Cl^-). High-volume saline infusion causes extracellular SID to fall so precipitously that the resultant metabolic acidosis outstrips the A_{tot} effect.

Of note, the extent of SID reduction, not the extent of hyperchloremia, is the important outcome determinant, in concert with the final A_{tot}. The same phenomenon can occur with hypotonic NaCl solutions as well as with dextrose and mannitol.[40] In all cases, extracellular SID is forced downwards by equilibration with a fluid SID of 0. During this process, hypotonic solutions can actually cause a fall in the chloride concentration. Here it is the even larger fall in sodium that narrows the SID. This is why "hyperchloremic acidosis" is a misleading term.

HOW CAN IATROGENIC SALINE-INDUCED ACIDOSIS BE PREVENTED?

For prevention of crystalloid-induced acid-base disturbances, extracellular SID must fall during the infusion only enough to counteract the progressive A_{tot} dilutional alkalosis. The SID of balanced crystalloids therefore lies somewhere between extracellular SID (42 mEq/L) and 0. From experimental hemodilution data, the balance point appears to be 24 mEq/L (Fig. 125-1).[7,41,42] In other words, saline can be "balanced" through the replacement of 24 mEq/L of Cl^- with HCO_3^-.

There is a problem with using HCO_3^-. Unless the fluid is stored in an impermeable container, CO_2 is gradually lost to the atmosphere (atmospheric P_{CO_2} = 0.3 mm Hg). The fluid becomes more alkaline, and about 5 mEq/L of the HCO_3^- progressively dissociates to CO_3^{2-}. The concern with the use of alkaline intravenous fluids is a resulting intravascular hemolysis plus the possibility of local endothelial damage and phlebitis. On atmospheric equilibration, the fluid pH is unlikely to exceed 9.4; it is unclear whether this is high enough to cause harm.[43]

To eliminate the whole question of CO_2 loss, commercial suppliers have substituted various organic anions, such as L-lactate, acetate, gluconate and citrate, for HCO_3^- (Table 125-1). Provided that these strong anions disappear by rapid metabolism, the in vivo or "effective" SID can be calculated as though they were not present.[43]

Hartmann's solution (see Table 125-1), otherwise known as compound sodium lactate solution, contains 29 mmol/L of L-lactate, of which all but about 1 to 2 mmol/L rapidly disappears on infusion in the absence of severe liver dysfunction. Hence Hartmann's solution should be slightly alkalinizing. Although slight alkalinization is difficult to demonstrate, even experimentally, there is little doubt that Hartmann's solution can reduce or eliminate infusion-related metabolic acidosis.[6,14,17,44] Unfortunately, the fluid has design flaws, including hypotonicity, the presence of reactive divalent cations, and the need for efficient lactate metabolism.

Several commercial fluids have much higher effective SID values (see Table 125-1). Perhaps best known is Plasma-Lyte 148 (Baxter Worldwide, Deerfield, IL). With efficient metabolism of the infused organic anions, these crystalloids should correct preexisting acidosis more rapidly. Over-correction, however, will cause "breakthrough" metabolic alkalosis.[9] At times of impaired tissue

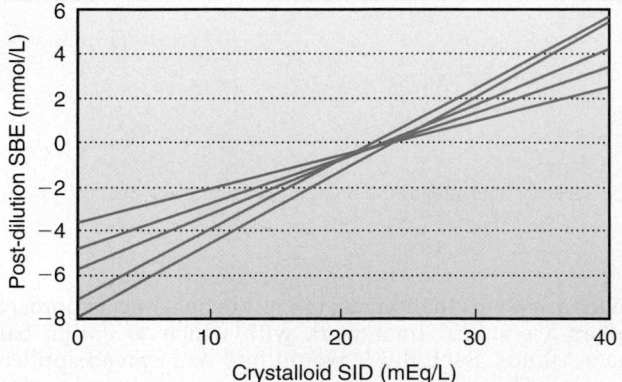

FIGURE 125-1. Normovolemic hemodilution in rats. Regression lines of standard base excess (SBE) versus crystalloid strong ion difference (SID) are shown. They represent progressive hemodilutions to a final hemoglobin concentration ([Hb]) of approximately 50 g/L. Although the increasing slopes indicate escalating acid-base effects, the balance point (SBE = 0) at each dilution is consistently close to 24 mEq/L. (From Morgan TJ, Venkatesh B, Hall J: Crystalloid strong ion difference determines metabolic acid-base change during acute normovolaemic haemodilution. Intensive Care Med 2004;30:1432-1437.)

oxygen delivery, fluid-induced metabolic alkalosis may exacerbate bioenergetic dysfunction.[42]

Colloids

With colloids, the effective SID remains a fundamental property. Extracellular dilution is less, because the same hemodynamic effect can be achieved with lower infusion volumes.[34] More importantly, some colloids, such as albumin and gelatin preparations, contain physiologic or supraphysiologic concentrations of A_{tot} (Table 125-2).[45] A_{tot} dilutional alkalosis should thus be eliminated when these fluids are infused, at least while the colloid remains in the extracellular space.

If the colloid A_{tot} is present in physiologic concentrations, a SID similar to that of extracellular fluid (42 mEq/L) should provide balance. If the contained A_{tot} is supraphysiologic, the balancing SID must exceed the normal extracellular SID. This was nicely illustrated in a study in which volunteers receiving an intravenously administered 5% albumin solution remained free of acid-base disturbances; when given the same volume of hetastarch 4 weeks later, the same volunteers demonstrated metabolic acidosis.[46] Five percent albumin represents a supraphysiologic concentration of A_{tot}. The SID of this albumin preparation was also supraphysiologic, at 57 mEq/L.[46] The net result was a balanced fluid.

However, SID values of other commercial albumin and gelatin preparations vary considerably (see Table 125-2) and are generally not high enough to prevent infusion-associated metabolic acidosis.[8,11,47] In this context, another important lesson can be learned from a subgroup analysis of the SAFE study.[48] As might have been predicted, the acid-base outcomes of patients receiving 4% albumin over 28 days as the default resuscitation fluid were largely indistinguishable from those who received saline. However, there was a strong trend away from metabolic acidosis over time in those receiving albumin,[48] highlighting the weakness of the acidifying fluid signal in the complex milieu of critical illness.

Starch preparations are not known to have weak acid activity. With one exception, the SID of these preparations is 0 (see Table 125-2). Their acid-base effects are therefore

TABLE 125-1

Four Commercial Crystalloid Solutions*

	COMPOUND SODIUM LACTATE[†]	PLASMA-LYTE 148 INJECTION[‡]	ISOLYTE S pH 7.4[§]	ISOLYTE E[‖]
Electrolytes (mEq/L):				
Sodium	129	140	141	140
Chloride	109	98	98	103
Potassium	5	5	5	10
Calcium	4			5
Magnesium		3	3	3
Lactate	29			
Acetate		27	27	49
Gluconate		23	23	
Citrate				8
Phosphate			1	
Effective SID*	27	50	50	57

*SID values assume stable plasma lactate concentrations of 2 mmol/L.
[†]Baxter, Toongabbie, Australia.
[‡]Baxter Worldwide, Deerfield, IL.
[§]B. Braun Medical Inc., Bethlehem, PA.
[‖]B. Braun Medical Inc., Bethlehem, PA.
Modified from Morgan TJ: The meaning of acid-base abnormalities in ICU. Part III: Effects of fluid administration. Crit Care 2005;9:204-211.

TABLE 125-2

Six Colloid Solutions

	ALBUMEX[‡]	HAEMACCEL[§]	GELOFUSINE[‖]	PENTASPAN[¶]	HE SPAN[**]	HEXTEND[††]
Albumin (g/L)*	40 g/L					
Gelatin,						
Urea-linked (g/L)*		35				
Succinylated (g/L)*	4		40			
Pentastarch (g/L)				100		
Hetastarch (g/L)	29				60	60
Sodium (mEq/L)	140	145	154	154	154	143
Potassium (mEq/L)		5.1				3
Calcium (mEq/L)		12.5				5
Magnesium (mEq/L)						0.8
Chloride (mEq/L)	128.0	145	120	154	154	124
Lactate (mEq/L)						28
Glucose (mEq/L)						5.5
Octanoate (mEq/L)	6.4					
Effective SID[†]	12	17.6	34	0	0	26

*Weak acid.
[†]SID values assume stable plasma lactate concentrations of 2 mmol/L.
[‡]CSL Bioplasma, Melbourne, Australia.
[§]DeltaSelect GmbH, Dreieich, Germany.
[‖]B. Braun Medical Inc., Bethlehem, PA.
[¶]B. Braun Medical Inc., Bethlehem, PA.
[**]B. Braun Medical Inc., Irvine, CA.
[††]Abbott, Chicago.
Modified from Morgan TJ: The meaning of acid-base abnormalities in ICU. Part III: Effects of fluid administration. Crit Care 2005;9:204-211.

probably similar to those of saline. The exception is Hextend (Abbott, Chicago), a balanced hetastarch preparation containing 28 mEq/L of L-lactate (see Table 125-2).[49] In the absence of weak acid activity, this balance should be sufficient to eliminate infusion-related metabolic acidosis. The higher tonicity of Hextend compared with Hartmann's solution is also an advance.

On available evidence, Hextend does appear to be balanced.[13] It has other advantages, perhaps related to this attribute. For example, the tendency for starch preparations to cause bleeding in higher volume[50] appears to be less with this solution.[49] Findings on gastric tonometry suggest better mucosal blood flow if Hextend is used perioperatively for volume replacement.[13] Experimentally, the colloid also offers a survival advantage in endotoxemia.[18]

On the other hand, in certain situations there may be a basis for switching to balanced albumin-based colloids. Unbalanced albumin preparations already have possible advantages when used for volume expansion in sepsis[34] and in severe liver dysfunction.[51,52] To balance the colloid Albumex (CSL Bioplasma, Melbourne, Australia), which currently has a SID of 12 mEq/L (see Table 125-1), a further chloride reduction of approximately 30 mEq/L is required. As with crystalloids, this reduction could be achieved through replacement of this amount of chloride with HCO_3^- or with organic anions rapidly metabolized on infusion, such as L-lactate, acetate, gluconate, or citrate.

CONCLUSION

Peter Stewart's legacy continues to bear fruit. The physicochemical approach to acid-base physiology provides the simplest and most logical explanation for the phenomenon of saline-induced metabolic acidosis. If harm can indeed arise from fluid-induced acid-base disturbances, as current evidence seems to indicate, the physicochemical approach offers a practical framework with which to design balanced fluids. Such fluids would find widespread application in hypovolemic resuscitation, cardiopulmonary bypass, and normovolemic hemodilution.

Key Points

1. Metabolic acidosis is a consequence of large-volume saline and colloid infusions.
2. There is limited clinical evidence that saline-induced acidosis causes harm, supported by stronger direct and indirect experimental evidence.
3. The phenomenon is best understood via the Stewart approach. The key property of an infused crystalloid is its effective strong ion difference, which when less than 24 mEq/L overwhelms the metabolic alkalosis caused by dilution of extracellular weak acid.
4. In resuscitation with hypotonic fluids, the resulting metabolic acidosis may be hypochloremic.
5. Balanced crystalloids require an effective strong ion difference (SID) of 24 mEq/L. This should also apply to colloids without weak acid activity (A_{tot}) such as hetastarch. With weak acid preparations such as the albumin and gelatin colloids, the SID required for balance depends on their A_{tot} activity.

Key References

7. Morgan TJ, Venkatesh B, Hall J: Crystalloid strong ion difference determines metabolic acid-base change during acute

normovolaemic haemodilution. Intensive Care Med 2004;30: 1432-1437.

8. Hayhoe M, Bellomo R, Lin G, et al: The aetiology and pathogenesis of cardiopulmonary bypass-associated metabolic acidosis using polygeline pump prime. Intensive Care Med 1999;25:680-685.

25. Kellum JA, Song M, Venkataraman R: Effects of hyperchloremic acidosis on arterial pressure and circulating inflammatory molecules in experimental sepsis. Chest 2004;125:243-248.

43. Morgan TJ: The meaning of acid-base abnormalities in ICU. Part III: Effects of fluid administration. Crit Care 2005;9:204-211.

45. Liskaser F, Story DA: The acid-base physiology of colloid solutions. Curr Opin Crit Care 1999;5:440-442.

See the companion Expert Consult website for the complete reference list.

CHAPTER 126

Renal Tubular Acidosis

Troels Ring

OBJECTIVES

This chapter will:
1. Define renal tubular acidosis.
2. Review the types of this disorder.
3. Present clinical methods of diagnosis and differential diagnosis.
4. Analyze contrasting acid-base discourses with a view to renal tubular acidosis.

DEFINITION

Renal tubular acidosis (RTA) is a group of hyperchloremic (non–anion gap) metabolic acidoses caused by impaired renal acid excretion that is not explained by reduced glomerular filtration rate (GFR) alone. RTA may be isolated or it may be a component of mixed disorders, including states with reduced GFR. Also, RTA may manifest only under imposed acidosis.

Although not necessary in the ordinary case of RTA occurring in the "otherwise well" and stable patient, a comprehensive analysis of the renal participation of acid-base balance is required in the patient with a complicating disease (including low GFR). This requirement is already evident from the fact that although the acidosis under RTA is often defined as a hyperchloremic acidosis (compared with anion gap acidosis), hyperchloremia per se is certainly not required for the diagnosis of RTA in the complicated patient. Only increased chloride ion (Cl^-) concentration compared with sodium ion (Na^+) and, ultimately, a decrease in plasma strong ionic difference (SID) are required to cause RTA in this circumstance.[1] The opposing discourses of acid-base physiology are presented in more detail by Ring and colleagues.[2]

As discussed in Chapters 111 and 112, the pH of plasma is a function solely of the independent determinants SID, weak acids, and PCO_2. Hence, the role of the kidneys with regard to acid-base homeostasis is to influence plasma Na^+ and Cl^- concentrations and thereby alter the SID. In addition, adjusting potassium ion (K^+) excretion similarly influences the SID of *intracellular compartment*. A number of observations indicate that this approach is constructive and necessary in renal acid-base physiology.[3] First, studies of perturbations in whole body potassium balance strongly indicate that the plasma homeostasis and intracellular homeostasis can be separately regulated.[4] Second, detailed analyses of proximal tubule bicarbonate reabsorption show that regulation occurs neither from intracellular nor basolateral pH, but from PCO_2 and bicarbonate, which are stoichiometrically equivalent to SID.[5] Third, it has been difficult to establish a direct relationship between conventional plasma acid-base parameters and renal responses.[6]

In the classic approach to acid-base balance, the renal component is measured as net acid excretion (NAE), which is computed as urine titratable acidity plus ammonium minus excreted bicarbonate. The equivalence between this method and SID-based methods is discussed at the end of this chapter, but the technical problems in using the NAE approach have been well exposed by Cohen and associates.[6]

TYPES OF RENAL TUBULAR ACIDOSIS

Four types of RTA are described. Table 126-1 lists the characteristics of well-defined forms of RTA among these types.

- Type 1 or distal RTA involves impaired distal acidification of urine.
- Type 2 or proximal RTA is related to decreased reclamation of filtered bicarbonate in the proximal tubules in the presence of unimpaired distal tubule function.
- Type 3 shows both impaired proximal and distal function and is caused by dysfunction of carbonic anhydrases.
- Type 4 is a heterogeneous group of RTAs accompanied by hyperkalemia.

Type 1: Distal Renal Tubular Acidosis

Type 1 RTA may be overt or covert; in either case, if left untreated it may cause bone demineralization and nephrolithiasis because of hypercalciuria or decreased excretion of citrate. A characteristic finding in RTA type 1 is that urine pH does not fall in spite of systemic acidosis. Importantly, there is no simple relationship between urine

TABLE 126-1

Types of Renal Tubular Acidosis (RTA)

TYPE	MUTATION TYPE; SITE	CONVENTIONAL MECHANISM OF ACIDIFICATION DEFECT	PHYSICOCHEMICAL MECHANISM	GENE
1: Distal RTA	Dominant; anion exchanger-1 (AE-1)	HCO_3^- absorption inhibited; NH_4^+ excretion/trapping decreased	Cl^- secretion inhibited and Na^+ excretion increased, thus increasing urine SID	17q21-22
	Recessive; H^+-ATPase	H^+ secretion inhibited; NH_4^+ excretion/trapping decreased	Lumen-positive potential obviated, decreasing drive for Na^+ absorption and Cl^- secretion, thus increasing urine SID	7q33-34, 2cen-q13
2: Proximal RTA	Recessive; basolateral electrogenic sodium bicarbonate cotransporter kNBC1	HCO_3^- absorption inhibited	Cl^- secretion inhibited and Na^+ absorption inhibited, thus increasing urine SID	4q21
	X-linked; phosphatidylinositol 4,5-bisphosphate 5-phosphatase OCRL1 (aka Lowe's syndrome)	Intracellular trafficking of transporters HCO_3^- absorption inhibited	Probably as above	Xq26.1
3: Combined RTA	Recessive; carbonic anhydrase II	Proximal HCO_3^- reclamation and distal H^+ secretion inhibited	Urine Cl^- decreases relative to Na^+, increasing urine SID	8q22
4: Hyperkalemic RTA	Dominant; serine-threonine kinase WNK1	Hyperkalemia—decreases NH_4^+ secretion/trapping	Urine Na^+ and Cl^- reabsorption enhanced via NCC, urine K^+ decreases (ROMK) and urine Cl^- decreases (paracellular), all leading to increased urine SID and decreased body SID	12p.13.3
	Dominant; serine-threonine kinase WNK4	As above	As above	17q21-22

pH and renal excretion of acid, because it depends on the content of buffer. A most characteristic feature of RTA type 1 is that it is easy to treat with 1 to 2 mEq of base per kg per day in spite of the alkaline urine.

The physiological problems causing RTA type 1 are manifest in the collecting duct, although evidence shows that—as is the case for sodium and potassium balance—the connecting tubule assumes an expanding role.[7] Some of the factors are portrayed in Figure 126-1. The architecture and differentiation of cell types and constituents in the distal nephron, which is necessary for acidification, are coordinated, for instance by transcription factor Foxi1.[8] Also, acid-base status may dynamically influence the cell population, as evidenced by recruitment of acid-secreting type A intercalated cells in the collecting duct from type B intercalated cells (i.e., type B cells become type A cells). This finding constitutes an explanation for RTA type 1 during treatment with cyclosporin A, which inhibits this process.[9] It is possible that similar mechanisms might explain other forms of acquired RTA type 1.

The best-understood cases of RTA type 1 occur with inherited malfunction of the apical vacuolar H^+-ATPase or of anion exchanger-1 (AE-1), the basolateral Cl^--HCO_3^- exchanger. The diseases are very rare, but it is hoped that an understanding of their mechanisms will elucidate more common problems.

Mutations of vacuolar H^+-ATPase are recessive and affect the a4 or B1 subunit of the proton pump.[10] In fami-

lies with the B1 mutation, progressive sensorineural deafness is often found.[11] The effects tend to be early in onset and severe, with nephrocalcinosis, growth delay, and bone problems. The AE-1 mutations are most often dominant, although recessive forms are found in Asia.[12] Because the same protein has a vital effect in red blood cell and whole-body CO_2 transport, the mutations causing RTA type 1 are related to mistargeting of the dimer AE-1 molecules.[12] AE-1 mutations may cause late-onset and milder diseases.[13] Incomplete disease has been identified in patients with bone problems or nephrolithiasis who apparently have normal acid-base balance in the unstressed state but who do not acidify urine if they have imposed acidosis.[14]

The vacuolar H^+-ATPase is strongly electrogenic.[15] Hence, the lumen-negative potential generated by Na^+ absorption by the epithelial sodium channel (ENaC) may accentuate the H^+ secretion, as is seen, for example, after administration of a loop diuretic.[7] There does not seem to be an apical membrane Cl^- conductance, and the generated charge is balanced by basolateral Cl^- conductance, while the produced lumen-positive potential drives Na^+ and K^+ absorption or Cl^- (paracellular) secretion.[16] Likewise, the acidosis that has been described in mice without basolateral K^+-Cl^- cotransporter KCC4 may be related to indirect inhibition of the vacuolar H^+-ATPase.[17]

These two well-defined forms of RTA type 1 correspond to a *secretory* defect in analysis of pathophysiology and contrast with states in which proton secretory capacity is

FIGURE 126-1. Renal tubular acidosis type 1: distal renal tubular acidosis (dRTA). Type A and type B intercalated cells in the collecting tubule are shown. In the normal state, acid extrusion occurs via the vacuolar H^+-ATPase (H-pump), which is strongly electrogenic, resulting in a lumen-positive potential that drives efflux of cations or influx of Cl^- to decrease the urine strong ion difference (SID). With mutations, for example in a4 or B1 components of the pump, this extrusion does not occur, and urine SID increases. Amphotericin B may short-circuit the potential instead, by increasing permeability. In the basolateral membrane, dominant mutations in anion exchanger AE-1 may interrupt Cl^- and HCO_3^- exchange, also leading to hyperchloremic acidosis. In acidosis, type B intercalated cells may transform to type A intercalated cells, a process inhibited by cyclosporin A. ATP, adenosine triphosphate; CA-II, carbonic anhydrase II; Foxi1, a forkhead transcription factor; KCC4, potassium-chloride exchanger 4.

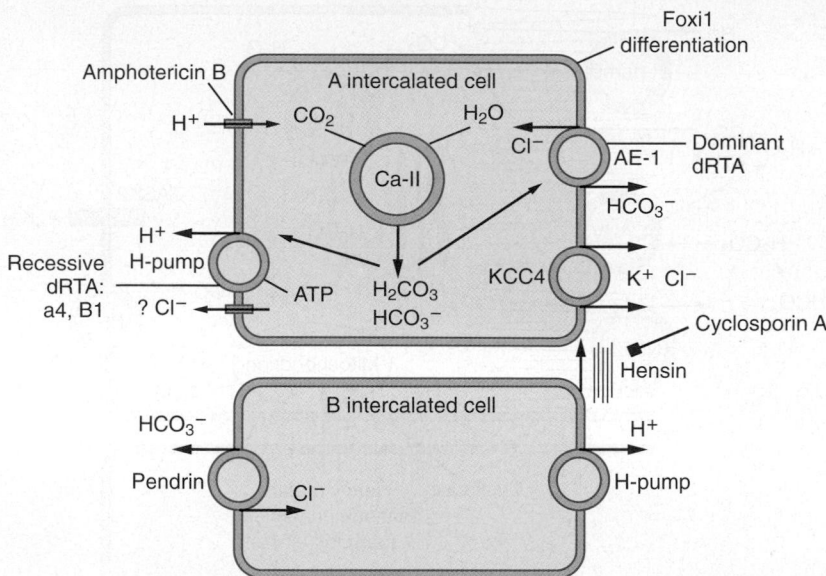

Type 2: Proximal Renal Tubular Acidosis

In the proximal tubules, about 80% of filtered bicarbonate is reclaimed by a saturable process. Characteristically in RTA type 2, fractional absorption of bicarbonate is reduced in the proximal tubules but maintained in the distal secretory pathways. Hence, when the filtered bicarbonate level drops, total reclamation may be obtained in the distal

thought to be primarily intact but only secondarily impaired.[18] The reason could be an inability either to maintain a steep H^+ gradient over the apical cell membrane (classically termed a *gradient* defect) or to generate lumen-negative potential to support H^+ secretion (*voltage-dependent* defect).

Acquired diseases may also impinge on the function of vacuolar H^+-ATPase and AE-1, as occurs in Sjögren's syndrome or systemic lupus erythematosus, and behave as secretory defects.[19] Laing and coworkers[20] described a case of RTA type 1 in an untreated patient with human immunodeficiency virus infection and suggested that the accompanying hypergammaglobulinemia was the reason for the RTA.[20] Laing and Unwin[21] have proposed that hypergammaglobulinemia is involved in the pathogenesis of RTA type 1 in a number of autoimmune or inflammatory diseases, but details of the mechanism are unavailable.[21] A gradient defect has been suggested to explain RTA induced by amphotericin B,[22,23] and a number of diseases are thought to lead to RTA type 1 through a voltage-dependent defect (obstructive nephropathy or lithium, amiloride, or methicillin treatment).[18,24,25] In contrast to typical RTA type 1 with hypokalemia, this voltage-dependent defect is often accompanied by normal or high levels of potassium. In contrast to patients with hyperkalemic (type 4) RTA, however, the typical patient with RTA type 1 is unable to acidify urine maximally.

The status of the voltage-dependent defect in RTA type 1, however, is debated, and direct effects of lithium or urinary obstruction, for example, on the vacuolar H^+-ATPase, have been suggested as more important factors in the acidosis.[26,27]

nephron and a normal low pH may result. However, distal transport is overwhelmed and fractional excretion of bicarbonate is more than 10% when bicarbonate is administered to attain a plasma bicarbonate value of 20 mmol/L. Hence, a distinguishing feature for RTA type 2 is that normalization of plasma bicarbonate concentration is very difficult to attain with normal GFR.

Most of the bicarbonate is absorbed as CO_2 over the apical membrane, possibly through aquaporin-1, but leaves the tubule cell through basolateral electrogenic sodium bicarbonate cotransporter kNBC1.[5] The arrangement of key enzymes and transporters is shown in Figure 126-2. Included is the TASK2 potassium channel short-circuiting the potential generated by kNBC1 to sustain transport of bicarbonate.[28] This demonstration continues the theme that dominant factors in acid transport are directly linked to transport of SID components (in this case, potassium).

RTA type 2 occurs as an isolated disorder or as part of a generalized tubular syndrome.

Inherited isolated RTA type 2 occurs in three forms. A very rare autosomal dominant form, the genetic mechanism of which has not been identified (a plasma membrane Na^+/H^+ exchanger [NHE] is a candidate) is typically lifelong.[29] A more common, also permanent, recessive form accompanied by eye abnormalities is caused by mutations in kNBC1, which may cause mistargeting or absence of the transporter.[30] Finally, a sporadic, transient form that requires treatment only in early infancy has been described; the cause is unknown but immaturity of NHE3 has been suggested.[18]

Inherited syndromic RTA type 2 occurs as part of generalized proximal disorder, Fanconi's syndrome, which consists of aminoaciduria, (renal) glucosuria, phosphaturia, and low-molecular-weight proteinuria (LMWP). An autosomal dominant syndrome has been located to 15q15.3, but the gene and protein have not been identified.[21]

A number of diseases thought to impair integrative metabolic functions in the proximal tubule are causes of Fanconi's syndrome, often involving RTA type 2. Dent's disease, an X-linked proximal tubulopathy with LMWP,

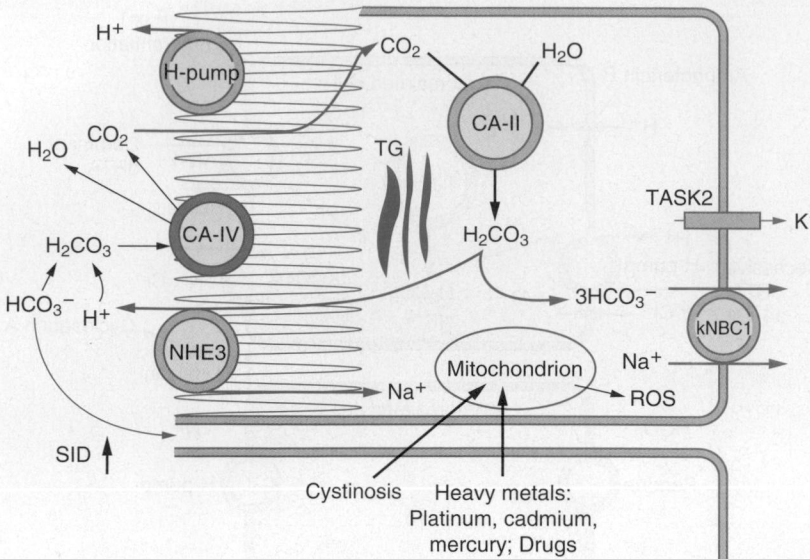

FIGURE 126-2. Renal tubular acidosis (RTA) type 2. Proximal tubule cell is shown. Rare inherited recessive diseases inhibits HCO_3^- reabsorption by perturbing function or localization of the basolateral electrogenic sodium bicarbonate cotransporter kNBC1; most diseases causing RTA type 2, however, are acquired and lead to proximal tubule cell distress by influencing mitochondrial function to exacerbate oxidative stress. Also in cystinosis, mitochondrial function may be inhibited, causing proximal cell apoptosis. In Lowe's syndrome and Dent's disease, Golgi apparatus function is inhibited, causing widespread disarray in proximal tubule cell function. With rising urine bicarbonate concentration, urine Cl^- concentration must drop, and thereby the urine strong ion difference (SID) invariably increases in RTA type 2. CA-II, carbonic anhydrase II; CA-IV, carbonic anhydrase IV; H-pump, hydrogen pump; NHE3, Na^+/H^+ exchanger 3; ROS, reactive oxygen species; TASK2, a potassium channel; TG, trans golgi.

often with phosphaturia, hypercalciuria, and nephrocalcinosis, is classically related to a mutation in the gene for Cl^- channel CLCN5. Interest focuses on how impairment of this Cl^- channel, which mediates acidification of lysosomes, can explain the variety of features noted in Dent's diseases.[31] In Lowe's syndrome, X-linked Fanconi's syndrome, often with RTA type 2, mental impairment, and cataracts, is due to mutation in OCRL1, a phosphatidylinositol 4,5-bisphosphate 5-phosphatase found in the Golgi apparatus that seems to influence trafficking between endosomes and the trans-Golgi network.[32] Mutations in this same gene may also cause a phenotype resembling Dent's disease.[31]

In Wilson's disease, Fanconi's syndrome is thought to be caused by copper deposition in the proximal tubule, although in both cystinosis and tyrosinemia, mitochondrial dysfunction may be the underlying mechanism in proximal tubule cell disarray.[33]

Acquired RTA type 2 also often appears as a general proximal tubule cell problem. Many important acute and probably chronic cases occur with poisoning due to a (heavy) metal—cadmium, cobalt, copper, lead, platinum, vanadium, chromium, mercury, iron, or uranium. The mechanisms putting proximal tube cells in jeopardy seem to center on oxidative stress and mitochondrial dysfunction.[33,34] A great number of drugs cause proximal tubule disease because of their constituent metal (cisplatin, carboplatin); inhibition of mitochondrial functions by antiviral agents used to treat human immunodeficiency virus may also be contributory.[35] Also, aminoglycosides, valproate, ifosfamide, and suramin are suggested to influence mitochondrial metabolism and thereby the functions of the proximal tubule cell so as to cause Fanconi syndrome.[33]

A well-investigated case of RTA type 2 with Fanconi's syndrome and osteomalacia has been reported as a reversible result of vitamin D and calcium deficiency.[36] Also, a patient with renal glucosuria, aminoaciduria, phosphaturia, severe bone problems, and hyperchloremic metabolic acidosis against the background of Sjögren's syndrome was reported to have Fanconi's syndrome and RTA type 2. However, the urine SID in this patient was +33 mmol/L,

and in spite of acidosis, the urine pH was 8.5, indicating at least additional distal tubule dysfunction.[37]

Fanconi's syndrome with RTA type 2 is well described with plasma cell dyscrasias. One central mechanism appears to be light chains, which are absorbed by endocytosis in the proximal tubule cell and, if overproduced, stress the cell by a variety of mechanisms.[38]

Type 3: Combined Renal Tubular Acidosis

As shown in Figure 126-2, carbonic anhydrases II and IV (CA-II and CA-IV, respectively) are involved in reabsorption of bicarbonate in the proximal tubule. Inhibition of these enzymes is therefore expected to affect proximal bicarbonate transport; as shown in Figure 126-1, however, CA-II is also necessary for distal acidification, so the resulting clinical picture is that of a combined proximal and distal acidosis. This picture has been described in patients undergoing treatment with acetazolamide but also in those treated with the antiepileptic drug topiramate.[39] In immunological diseases, deficiency of distal transporters was noticed together with deficiency of CA-II; also, autoantibodies against CA-II were found in patients with Sjögren's syndrome, and more frequently in those who also had RTA.[19,40] A rare recessive syndrome with CA-II deficiency producing osteopetrosis, RTA type 3, cerebral calcification, short stature, and cognitive defects has been described.[18]

Type 4: Hyperkalemic Renal Tubular Acidosis

RTA type 4 is a heterogeneous disorder wherein hyperkalemia in combination with aldosterone deficiency or resistance causes impaired renal excretion of ammonium (shown in Fig. 126-3).[18,27] Characteristically, and in contrast to voltage-dependent RTA type 1, patients with RTA type 4 are able to lower urine pH normally in the presence of acidosis. There is, however, overlap between RTA types 1 and 4, and some arbitrariness in determining that urinary pH target that must be reached, especially in the presence

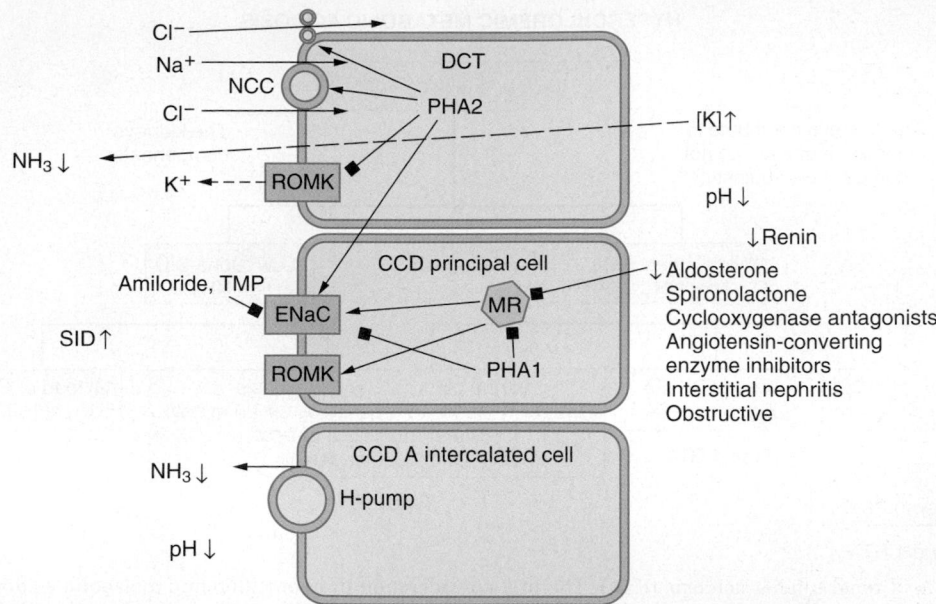

FIGURE 126-3. Renal tubular acidosis (RTA) type 4. Distal nephron cells are shown. The main problems in RTA type 4 are hyperkalemia and lack of ammonium, which occur with direct and indirect obstruction in the renin-angiotensin-aldosterone pathway by multiple mechanisms, respectively, including mutation in mineralocorticoid receptor or epithelial Na channel (ENaC) in pseudohypoaldosteronism (PHA) type 1. Mutations in WNK1 and WNK4 have been shown to cause PHA type 2 (PHA2), a condition comprising metabolic acidosis, hyperkalemia, and hypertension. Directly increased absorption of Cl⁻ in these disorders invariably increases urine SID (strong ion difference) and causes acidosis. ACE, angiotensin-converting enzyme; CCD, cortical collecting duct; COX, cyclooxygenase; DCT, distal collecting duct; MR, mineralocorticoid receptor; NCC, thiazide-sensitive Na chloride cotransporters; ROMK, renal outer medullary K channel; TMP, trimethoprim.

of underlying renal impairment, which is commonly found in RTA type 4. Aldosterone deficiency, besides causing low ammonium concentration, is also directly expected to inhibit activity of vacuolar H⁺-ATPase in type A intercalated cells.[41]

Mineralocorticoid deficiency occurs in primary forms with Addison's disease and congenital adrenal hyperplasia and in a selective aldosterone deficiency found in critically ill patients or in congenital syndromes. Secondary forms of aldosterone deficiency occur with hyporeninemic hypoaldosteronism or drugs inhibiting aldosterone synthesis.

Mineralocorticoid resistance may be congenital or acquired. Most severe is pseudohypoaldosteronism type 1 (PHA1), which is characterized by salt wasting, hyperkalemia, and metabolic acidosis. PHA1 occurs in a dominant form, caused by mutations in the mineralocorticoid receptor, and in a recessive form, due to deficiency in the epithelial Na channel ENaC.[42] In contrast, pseudohypoaldosteronism type 2 (PHA2) is characterized by hyperkalemia, metabolic acidosis, and age-related hypertension. Studies now indicate that these findings are explained by hyperabsorption of Na⁺ and Cl⁻ through the thiazide-sensitive cotransporter in the distal convoluted tubule combined with paracellular Cl⁻ absorption (shunt) and declining function of (or drive for) potassium secretion in the renal outer medullary K (ROMK) channel—all of which are secondary to dominant mutations in two newly described serine-threonine kinases, WNK1 and WNK4.[43] The RTA in PHA2 is particularly interesting from the physicochemical point of view because no direct involvement of renal acid-base transporters has been identified.

Acquired mineralocorticoid resistance occurs with interstitial nephropathies of many kinds (sickle cell disease, human immunodeficiency virus nephropathy,

medullary cystic disease, analgesic abuse nephropathy). A number of drugs causing hyperkalemia work by inhibiting the renin-angiotensin-aldosterone axis or its effects. They include cyclooxygenase-1 (COX1) and COX2 inhibitors, angiotensin-converting enzyme (ACE) inhibitors, potassium-sparing diuretics, trimethoprim, and pentamidine.[27]

DIAGNOSIS OF RENAL TUBULAR ACIDOSIS

The diagnosis of RTA is entertained in a patient with non–anion gap ("hyperchloremic") metabolic acidosis or in a patient with unexplained nephrolithiasis or hypokalemia. An approach to such a patient is shown in Figure 126-4. When a clinician is looking for gastrointestinal losses of bicarbonate or direct acid loads, the first step is to investigate the renal compensation. Urine is therefore examined for pH (pH electrode), Na⁺, K⁺, Cl⁻, urea, creatinine, glucose, phosphate, and tubular protein content as well as its osmolality.

Normally, urine charge balance results in urine net charge, as follows[44]:

$$\text{Net charge} = \text{SID} = Na^+ + K^+ - Cl^- = 80 - NH_4^+$$

Hence, if urine net charge is negative, the NH₄⁺ concentration is greater than 80 mEq/L. This response is seen with imposed acidosis under normal circumstances and with intact distal acidification. According to the classic approach to acid-base balance, these findings indicate that ammonium excretion has been increased; from the physicochemical (Stewart) point of view, however, there is no doubt that excretion of a urine with negative SID must

HYPERCHLOREMIC METABOLIC ACIDOSIS

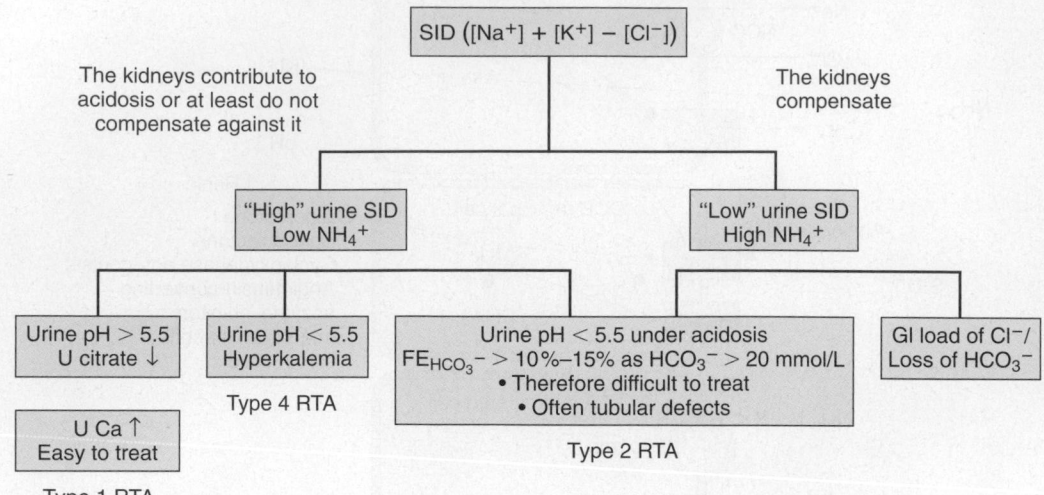

FIGURE 126-4. Diagnosis of renal tubular acidosis (RTA). The first consideration in hyperchloremic metabolic acidosis is assessment of urine SID. If this is low, urine will not decrease bodily SID, but if it is high, urine will contain minimal ammonium and result in perturbation of acidosis or initial precipitation. GI, gastrointestinal; SID, strong ion difference; U, urine.

necessarily increase whole-body SID and combat metabolic acidosis.

If urine net charge (SID) is positive, ammonium excretion is low, and differential diagnosis can frequently be made from urine pH and potassium values. Urine ($[K]u$) and plasma potassium concentrations ($[K]p$) can possibly be used to compute the transtubular potassium gradient (TTKG) as follows:

$$TTKG = \frac{[K]_u/[K]_p}{OSM_u/OSM_p}$$

where OSM_u is urine osmolality and OSM_p is plasma osmolality. With hyperkalemia, a TTKG value less than about 6 would indicate a cause renal, such as RTA type 4.[27]

If there is no spontaneous acidosis when the patient is examined, acidification tests can be performed with ammonium chloride or calcium chloride or, more simply, with furosemide (40 mg) and fludrocortisone (1 mg) given orally, with urine pH monitored for 6 hours. A normal response is pH less than 5.3.[21] The principles of this test were explored in detail by Wagner and coworkers.[7] The mineralocorticoid ensures activity of epithelial sodium channel (ENaC), which generates a strong lumen-negative potential when the distal nephron is reached by a rich amount of Na^+. This in turn accentuates the vacuolar H^+-pump—if present and functioning.

Loading with bicarbonate has had two purposes. One is to verify that fractional excretion of bicarbonate ($FE_{HCO_3^-}$) is more than 10% when plasma bicarbonate is more than 20 mmol/L, so as to diagnose RTA type 2. Fractional excretion of bicarbonate is calculated as follows:

$$FE_{HCO_3^-} = \frac{\dfrac{[HCO_3^-]_u}{[Crea]_p}}{\dfrac{[HCO_3^-]_p}{[Crea]_u}}$$

The other purpose is to investigate distal acidification, in which a PCO_2 gradient between urine and arterial blood of 30 mm Hg is a normal response to loading with bicarbonate.[27,45]

Both the assessment of NH_4^+ excretion and the urine PCO_2 response have been controversial in characterizing the renal response, and the diagnosis of RTA type 1 from urine pH has also had defects.[46,47] Formal assessment of net acid excretion (NAE) has rarely been performed in clinical practice. A single study showed that NAE was not significantly lower in patients with metabolic acidosis after renal transplantation.[48] These problems in diagnosing and characterizing acidosis as RTA are bound to worsen in the presence of additional renal failure[46] or in the unstable patient.

CONTRASTING VIEWS ON ACID-BASE PHYSIOLOGY

To enhance the understanding of RTA, a direct measurement of what the urine excretion does to body acid-base homeostasis should be of interest. This requires an explicit model of acid-base homeostasis. Much has been written about this controversial subject, but to inspire experimentation and help analyze existing data, an attempt is made here to bring the physicochemical and conventional treatises into a common approach with regard to renal acid-base homeostasis to see what is at stake.[2,49,50]

As Uribarri and colleagues[51] suggest, total charge balance in urine may be presented in the following way, in which TA is titratable acidity and OA is organic anions[51]:

Ion balance = all cations − all anions

Ion balance = $Na^+ + K^+ + Mg^{2+} + Ca^{2+} + NH_4^+ + TA^+ -$

$(Cl^- + 1.8P + SO_4^{2-} + OA^{x-} + HCO_3^-)$

from which it follows that, if ion balance is zero, then:

$$SID = (Na^+ + K^+ + Mg^{2+} + Ca^{2+} - Cl^-) = (NH_4^+ + TA^+ - HCO_3^-) + (SO_4^{2-} + OA^{x-}) + 1.8P$$

or

$$SID - 1.8P = -NAE + EAP$$

where *EAP* is endogenous acid production and *1.8P* represents the overall valence of phosphate at pH 7.4.

Hence, the urine loss of SID—in the mindset of conventional acid-base physiology—is expected to be equivalent to "acid balance," apart from the term including P (which will be analyzed shortly). Importantly, this derivation by Uribarri and colleagues[51] shows that the term SID − 1.8P includes estimates of the acid-base equivalents absorbed from the gastrointestinal tract in steady state (and possible bone buffering). Because the result of urine SID − 1.8P is positive under general conditions, the metabolic situation is such that endogenous acid production must balance the net intake of an alkaline diet.[52] This requirement seems to be the case currently, and was even more so when humans adhered to a diet rich in fruit and vegetables, as was prevalent during the evolutionary development of the mammalian kidney.[53] Therefore, one of the major problems in renal acid-base physiology may be that the kidneys were, in fact, not primarily designed for excreting acid.[50,54]

It is quite clear that from a physicochemical approach, the only way the kidneys could influence acid-base homeostasis would be by affecting the independent determinants of acid-base *in specified compartments*. This process could, in principle, involve inactivation of active factors, as has been described for Na[+] in relation to dysnatremia, but otherwise would be expected to be reflected directly in the urine.[55] For the smaller extracellular volume, this process would quantitatively be reflected in a conventional SID, although neither weak acids nor P_{CO_2} in that compartment is normally expected to be changed by urinary excretion. However, for the larger intracellular compartment, the situation must be different. Cl[−] is not abundant in the cell cytoplasm, and the anions balancing the dominant cation (K[+]) are probably (more or less) fixed charges on polyphosphates in organic molecules. Hence, the effect of phosphate excretion, which surfaces in the algebraic derivation of Uribarri and colleagues,[51] could be understood as a measure of intracellular balance.[51] If phosphate is high, the result of SID − 1.8P drops, causing intracellular alkalosis or repairing of intracellular acidosis. In balance, endogenous acid production minus net acid excretion then also declines. This analysis also fits with the results of hyponatremia from a single study on fasting rats.[56]

The prominence of the Stewart-based approach now rests on its possible theoretical advantage,[2] but certainly also on its much more straightforward applicability in clinical practice: The result of urine SID − 1.8P will be directly informative with regard to the renal effect on whole-body acid-base balance. The theoretical problems in the conventional acid-base discourse were discussed forcefully by Cohen and associates,[6] who, referring to the work by Uribarri and colleagues,[51] stressed the practical difficulties in actually measuring, for example titratable acidity. It is noteworthy that in later accounts, proponents of the classic discourse have given up actually titrating urine but instead propose computing TA from phosphate concentration and pH.[49] This approach still leaves the problem of defining the reference pH: arterial, mixed venous, or intracellular—and then where? It may be a major advantage that this problem is nonexistent in the physicochemical approach, wherein pH is only a dependent variable. As a corollary, in relation to RTA, Kamel and associates[57] discussed the necessity for understanding the incorporation of urinary excretion of organic anions; in a later study, Corey and coworkers[58] ventured to demonstrate that a Stewart-based approach explained the findings in RTA better than conventional analysis.

The use of urine SID to qualitatively calculate the expected changes in whole-body acid-base balance has been described in the amelioration of metabolic alkalosis by acetazolamide.[59] Also, an attempt to model changes in whole-body SID from urine SID has been reported.[60] Further development along these lines is expected, including the necessity to account for individual SID components with reference to volume and compartment of distribution. Individual components of SID, for example, in plasma, as they change with interventions must be modeled and understood along the lines suggested for intracellular plasma concentration [Na], as follows:

$$[Na]_2 = \frac{TBW_1 \times [Na]_1 + \Delta(Na + K)}{TBW_2 + \Delta TBW}$$

where *TBW* is total body water, subscript *1* denotes initial value, and subscript *2* denotes final value, and which also shows the interdependence between K and Na.[61]

RTAs are important causes of hypokalemia and hyperkalemia, both of which can be very dangerous. Incomplete RTA may be an important cause of bone disease and nephrolithiasis. RTA gives several important insights into renal physiology. Attempts at explicit modeling are still being pursued.

CONCLUSION

Renal tubular acidosis is easy to spot, and a differential diagnosis is easily made in the outpatient setting. It is probably much more difficult to think about and to diagnose an RTA in the hospitalized patient, in whom acute and/or chronic disease complicates the presentation, and even more difficult in the patient receiving intensive care. Under all circumstances, understanding RTA requires a solid understanding of renal physiology, and the controversies in the literature expose the problems still present in acid-base physiology. This chapter attempted to make explicit the relationship between conventional and Stewart-based approaches to acid-base homeostasis. A much more quantitative and explicit approach is needed to exploit the potentials therein.

Key Points

1. Renal tubular acidosis is a hyperchloremic metabolic acidosis diagnosed and classified on the basis of urinary findings.
2. The differential diagnosis between type 2 and other types of renal tubular acidosis is often easy if based on the amount of base needed to normalize the plasma.
3. Diagnoses become difficult in the presence of renal failure.

Key References

5. Boron WF: Acid-base transport by the renal proximal tubule. J Am Soc Nephrol 2006;17:2368-2382.
6. Cohen RM, Feldman GM, Fernandez PC: The balance of acid, base and charge in health and disease. Kidney Int 1997;52:287-293.
7. Kovacikova J, Winter C, Loffing-Cueni D, et al: The connecting tubule is the main site of furosemide-induced urinary acidi-

fication by the vacuolar H$^+$-ATPase. Kidney Int 2006;70:1706-1716.
18. Soriano JR: Renal tubular acidosis: The clinical entity. J Am Soc Nephrol 2002;13:2160-2170.
49. Lemann J Jr, Bushinsky DA, Hamm LL: Bone buffering of acid and base in humans. Am J Physiol 2003;285:F811-F832.

See the companion Expert Consult website for the complete reference list.

CHAPTER 127

Acid-Base Disorders Secondary to Renal Failure

Paolo Calzavacca, Elisa Licari, and Rinaldo Bellomo

OBJECTIVES

This chapter will:
1. Explore the derangements leading to metabolic acidosis in acute kidney injury and chronic kidney disease.
2. Describe the effect of renal replacement therapy on acid-base balance.

MECHANISMS BY WHICH THE KIDNEY AFFECTS THE STRONG ION DIFFERENCE

As discussed in Chapter 112, under normal circumstances, the kidney is the primary organ controlling the relative concentrations of strong ions (i.e., the strong ion difference [SID]).[1-3] However, the kidney can excrete only very small amount of strong ions over time, so it usually requires hours to significantly alter the SID.

The chloride ion (Cl$^-$), a strong anion,[4,5] appears to be the ion that the kidney mainly regulates to alter the SID,[6] because more complex pathways are involved in the handling of cations (Na$^+$ is related to intravascular volume and water homeostasis, K$^+$ to the plasma homeostasis of resting electric potential). Accordingly, renal control of acid-base status is mostly mediated through Cl$^-$ balance. This occurs because every Cl$^-$ ion that is filtered but not reabsorbed increases plasma SID (alkalosis).

To achieve chloride excretion unaccompanied by Na$^+$ or K$^+$ excretion, the kidney excretes another cation, typically ammonium (NH$_4^+$), a cation obtained from the ammonia cycle. This step allows the concomitant excretion of Cl$^-$, a strong anion, while sparing the strong cations Na$^+$ and K$^+$ and thus increasing the SID.

NH$_4^+$ is a product of nitrogen metabolism, which is crucial for metabolic acid-base handling. The components of nitrogen metabolism are nutritional intake (gut metabolism), hepatic nitrogen metabolism,[7] by which the liver can manage nitrogen to produce either urea or glutamine and NH$_4^+$, and finally, the renal ammonia production cycle (Fig. 127-1).

Acidosis has been shown to stimulate the liver to release a larger amount of glutamine.[8] Such a release may facilitate the excretion of chloride without sodium or potassium losses.

ACID-BASE DISORDERS IN ACUTE KIDNEY INJURY

The nature of acid-base disorders (mainly metabolic acidosis[9]) in critically ill patients with acute kidney injury (AKI) is complex.[10,11] It is the result of the balance between the acidifying effect of unmeasured anions, hyperphosphatemia, hyperlactatemia, and hypocalcemia and the lesser alkalinizing forces, hypoalbuminemia and hyperkalemia.

Quantitative acid-base assessment reveals multiple metabolic acid-base processes, which contribute to the preceding overall net metabolic acid-base disorder.[12-15] Typically, the following four main sources of acidosis can be identified:
- Unmeasured anions
- Hyperphosphatemia
- Hyperlactatemia
- Hypocalcemia

These acidifying changes are usually attenuated by metabolic alkalosis due to hypoalbuminemia and hyperkalemia. In the early stages of AKI, hyperchloremia may be the main cause of a decreased SID leading to acidosis.[16] In the later stages, unmeasured anions,[17] like keto-acids, intermediate members of the Krebs cycle[18] (such as citrate, acetate, and fumarate), sulfate, urate, hydroxypropionate, oxalate,

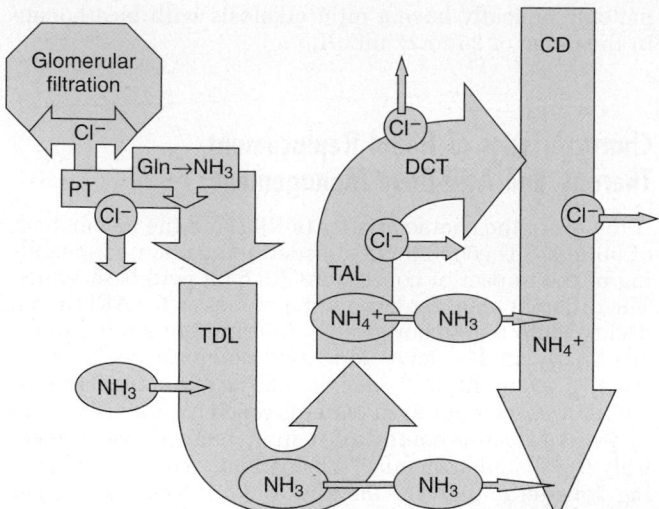

FIGURE 127-1. Movement of ammonia ion (NH_3) and chloride ions (Cl^-) in the nephron. The ammonia cycle in the nephron starts from glutamine (Gln) metabolism in the mitochondria of proximal tubular cells, where NH_3 is produced along the metabolic pathway that leads to deamination of glutamine to glutamate. The nephron membrane is highly permeable to NH_3, which moves across it, but is impermeable to ammonium (NH_4^+). NH_4^+ is generated from NH_3 through water hydrolysis and deprotonation. A gradient develops along the medullary space, leading to a final concentration of NH_3 in the urine that can range from 0.3 to 30 mmol/L. Cl^- is freely filtered in the glomerulus from the blood and reabsorbed, 60% in the proximal tubule (PT), 30% in the thick ascending limb of Henle's loop (TAL), 7% in the distal convoluted tubule (DCT), and 2% to 3% in the collecting duct (CD). TDL, thin descending limb of Henle's loop.

furanpropionate and the like, appear to be the major contributors to acidosis of acute renal failure. It has been shown that unmeasured anions can contribute to 50% to 60% of this acidosis.[19]

Hyperphosphatemia is a common finding in patients with AKI. It is likely due to loss of glomerular filtration rate with a related decrease in filtration of phosphate and also to secondary hyperparathyroidism. The rise in serum phosphate concentration can be responsible for up to 30% of the acidosis. Critically ill patients are often hyperlactatemic. Nevertheless, normally less than 15% of acidosis in patients with AKI is due to lactate. Hypocalcemia is probably a response to hyperphosphatemia and can account for a small part of the acidemia encountered in patients with AKI.

ACID-BASE DISORDERS IN CHRONIC KIDNEY DISEASE

Acid-base derangements are perhaps even more complicated in the setting of chronic kidney disease (CKD).[20,21] This complexity is related mainly to the wide spectrum of pathophysiological alterations associated with CKD, ranging from mild renal impairment to end-stage renal failure with the need for dialysis.[12] Impaired urinary excretion, intercurrent disease processes, long-term medication therapy, and renal replacement therapy (RRT) all contribute to acid-base derangement in patients with CKD.[22]

The most common feature noted in CKD, as already discussed in relation to AKI, is metabolic acidosis.[6] Acidosis usually develops when the glomerular filtration rate is less than 20% to 25% of normal.[23-25] The acidosis observed is usually mild to moderate, with serum bicarbonate concentration in the range of 12 to 22 mEq/L. The type of renal disease (i.e., diseases affecting different parts of the glomerulus) as well as aldosterone production derangement can affect the onset and severity of metabolic acidosis.[26,27] Patients with hypoaldosteronism,[16] prominent interstitial disease, or diseases affecting the collecting duct[28] are more likely to have a more severe acidosis or to have acidosis at higher levels of glomerular filtration rate than patients with diseases affecting the more proximal part of the glomerulus.

Diet is another factor playing a major role in acid-base derangements in patients with CKD, whose ability to manage acidic load (proteins) is decreased.[29] Historically, patients with metabolic acidosis due to CKD have been divided into those with high–anion gap acidosis and those with normal–anion gap (hyperchloremic) acidosis.[23,30] However, Story and colleagues[19] performed a study in 40 patients with CKD and mild to moderate metabolic acidosis. Analyzing the results using the Stewart model, these researchers found that in patients with CKD, metabolic acidosis is due mainly to a strong ion acidosis. Unmeasured ions seemed to play only a minor role. These researchers found that such strong ion acidosis is a consequence of a decrease in the Na^+-Cl^- effect on base excess (BE). In this study, Story and colleagues[19] used the following definitions, in which brackets ([]) indicate concentration:

- Na^+-Cl^- effect on BE = $[Na^+]$ − $[Cl^-]$ − 38
- Albumin effect on BE (mmol/L) = 0.25 × (42 − albumin in g/L)
- Unmeasured ions effect on BE = BE − (Na^+ − Cl^- effect) − (albumin effect)
- Phosphate effect = [phosphate in mmol/L] × 1.8

They found the following abnormalities:

1. The metabolic acidosis in patients with CKD is due mainly to a Na^+-Cl^- effect, with both an increase in chloride and a decrease in sodium.
2. The plasma concentration of phosphate (a weak acid) is increased because of a reduced excretion of phosphate in the urine and contributes to acidosis.
3. However, the concentration of albumin (another weak acid) is decreased.

All of these abnormalities lead to no overall variation in the unmeasured ion effect. This finding shows an important difference in the patterns of metabolic acidosis in AKI and CKD. Only at a very late stage of CKD do unmeasured acids contribute to plasma acidification.

Metabolic acidosis in CKD has the following consequences:

- *Bone disease:* Although this issue is controversial,[31] metabolic acidosis due to CKD seems to stimulate bone reabsorption and inhibit bone formation, leading to osteoporosis.[32-35] It also inhibits vitamin D production and affects parathyroid hormone balance.
- *Muscle wasting and reduced albumin synthesis:* A progressive decline in muscle mass in patients with CKD has been extensively reported.[36-38] It is caused by protein catabolism through the adenosine triphosphate–dependent ubiquitin-proteosome system. Acidosis has been found to increase the transcription of genes of this system,[2] and albumin levels are decreased because of a reduction in liver synthesis.[26,39,40]
- *Cardiac disease:* No definitive data are available on CKD-related acidosis and myocardial function.[41]

- *Impaired glucose homeostasis:* An acidic milieu impairs insulin sensitivity.[42]
- *Accumulation of β_2-microglobulin:* Acidosis may play a role in the development of amyloid.[43] Also, patients undergoing acetate-based dialysis have been shown to be more prone to development of amyloid than those undergoing bicarbonate-based dialysis.[44]
- *Growth hormone and thyroid function:* Metabolic acidosis seems to reduce triiodothyronine (T_3) and thyroxine (T_4) levels and to raise thyroid-stimulating hormone (TSH) levels.[45] Growth hormone–induced increments in levels of insulin-like growth factor-1 are blunted by metabolic acidosis.[46]
- *Inflammation:* Data on a possible contribution of metabolic acidosis and CKD to chronic inflammatory status are conflicting.[47] This is an interesting field of research in which more study is needed to better determine whether there is any relation between inflammation and CKD.

ACID-BASE STATUS AND RENAL REPLACEMENT THERAPY

As previously described, metabolic acid-base disorders are particularly common and complex in patients requiring renal replacement therapy.[19] Once instituted, RRT in turn causes modifications of acid-base status.[19,48]

Metabolic acidosis is the most common derangement both in AKI and CKD and is multifactorial in origin.[49,50] Once continuous hemofiltration is started, profound changes in acid-base status are rapidly achieved. They result in the progressive resolution of acidemia and acidosis with a lowering of the concentrations of phosphate and of unmeasured anions. The discussion that follows reviews the evidence currently available about the effect of RRT on acid-base status.

The exchange of approximately 30 L of plasma water per day is necessary to achieve adequate control of uremia and acid-base disorders in AKI.[51] During RRT, according to conventional acid-base thinking, there is a substantial loss of endogenous bicarbonate, which must be substituted by the addition of "buffer" substances. Quantitative acid-base analysis explains acid-base management during RRT as follows: There is loss of a fluid with an SID of approximately 30 to 40 mEq/L, which must be replaced by a fluid with a similar or greater SID value (SID generator, according to the Stewart approach) to restore acid-base balance.

The nature and extent of these acid-base changes are governed by the intensity of plasma water exchange/dialysis and by the buffer/SID generator content of the replacement fluid/dialysate, with different effects depending on the choice and amount of lactate, acetate, citrate, or bicarbonate as the SID generator(s) in the replacement fluid. These effects can be achieved in any patient, with AKI, with CKD, or with no renal derangement, because of the overwhelming effect of plasma water exchange on nonvolatile acid balance. In the end, these effects are usually achieved in AKI through the correction of hyperphosphatemia and hyperchloremia, and a decrease in unmeasured anions.[19] These processes eventually lead to the development of metabolic alkalosis (usually over 48 to 72 hours).

In patients with end-stage kidney disease, hemodialysis rapidly corrects the mild acidosis that usually develops in the interdialysis period.[52] By the end of the dialysis session, patients typically have a mild alkalosis with bicarbonate in the range of 26 to 27 mEq/L.

Characteristics of Renal Replacement Therapy and Acid-Base Management

A review of the characteristics of RRT and the metabolism of buffers/SID generators is needed to enable understanding of the impact of continuous RRT on acid-base status. The different renal replacement techniques for AKI can be divided into two major groups, intermittent and continuous. Many studies have addressed comparisons between the two techniques,[53-57] demonstrating the advantages of continuous techniques in patients receiving intensive care in terms of better control of hemodynamics, water, electrolytes,[58,59] and azotemia.[60] For patients with CKD requiring long-term dialysis therapy, only intermittent renal replacement techniques are typically used.

Whether intermittent or continuous, RRT can be performed in two ways,[61] hemodialysis and hemofiltration. The two techniques can be combined into hemodiafiltration (HDF). Unfortunately, only a few studies have specifically addressed the differences in acid-base effects of these different therapies.[62,63] Continuous venovenous hemodiafiltration appears to be superior to intermittent hemodialysis in the correction of metabolic acidosis in patients with AKI who are receiving intensive care. Finally, the technique of high-volume hemofiltration can exchange more than 6 liters of plasma per hour.[64] It has been described as a useful technique in the management of patients with sepsis.[44,65,66]

Buffers/SID generators have been extensively used to correct the acidemia related to AKI and CKD. Bicarbonate (the physiologic buffer/SID generator) as well as lactate and acetate (multicarbon anions) have been used as SID generators during RRT. Citrate (another multicarbon anion) has been used as both an SID generator and an anticoagulant. When oxidizable anions are used in the replacement fluids, the anion (acetate, lactate, or citrate) must be taken up from the circulation and metabolized to CO_2 and H_2O in order to generate an SID difference. If the metabolic conversion of nonbicarbonate anions proceeds without accumulation, their buffering capacity is equal to that of bicarbonate. Thus, the effect on acid-base status depends on the final concentration of SID generator(s) in plasma rather than on the kind of SID generator used. When metabolic conversion is impaired, however, the higher blood concentration of the anions leads to an increased strong anion concentration, which lowers the effective SID (SIDe) and, to some extent, acidifies blood.[67]

Bicarbonate has the major advantage of being the most physiologic anion equivalent.[68] However, the production of a commercially available bicarbonate-based solution is not easy because of the formation of calcium and magnesium salts during long-term storage. Furthermore, the cost of this solution is approximately three times higher than that of other replacement solutions. Accordingly, acetate and lactate have been used widely for RRT. Many studies have compared bicarbonate-buffered solutions with other buffers, above all lactate.[69-73] Overall, bicarbonate solutions appear to be equivalent to lactate solutions in correcting acidosis. The major indication for the use of a bicarbonate-buffered solution is in patients with lactic acidosis, shock, or hepatic failure, because lactate in these patients is best avoided, especially in the setting of high-volume hemofiltration.

Lactate is the most commonly used buffer. It is metabolized mainly by the liver,[61] but up to 30% of lactate metabolism can occur in the kidney in a healthy subject.[74] The advantages of lactate over bicarbonate are related to the greater stability of the solution and a lower cost.

Acetate is converted on a 1:1 basis to bicarbonate in the liver and in the skeletal muscle. It is less widely used because of a negative effect on hemodynamics[60,75] and because it has been demonstrated to be inferior in managing acidosis[76] compared with bicarbonate- and lactate-buffered solutions.

Citrate has been used in patients with coagulation disorders to provide regional anticoagulation.[62,77] Under normal conditions, citrate metabolism is rapid and occurs mainly in the liver and, to a lesser extent, in skeletal muscle and renal cortex. Once citrate enters the circulation, it is taken up by the liver and metabolized to CO_2 on a 1:3 basis. At low dose, citrate-buffered solution has been shown to cause a mild metabolic acidosis owing to a decrease in SID (due to a rise in Cl^- concentration and a drop in ionized Ca^{2+} concentration) and an increase in strong ion gap. The acidosis caused by citrate-buffered solutions is mild and is completely reversed when the treatment is stopped. In any case, if the dose of citrate is increased so that the SID of replacement fluid is increased, the acidosis normally caused by citrate is instead a metabolic alkalosis,[78] unless clearance of citrate by the liver is decreased because of hepatic failure.[79] The composition of replacement fluids is given in Table 127-1.

TABLE 127-1

Dialysate/Replacement Fluid Solutions in Studies Using Different Strong Ion Difference (SID) Generator Solutions

STUDY (YEAR)*	ELECTROLYTE COMPONENTS	SID GENERATOR
Thomas et al (1997)[80]	Lactate replacement fluid: Na^+ 142 mmol/L Cl^- 103 mmol/L K^+ 0-6 mmol/L Ca^{2+} 2 mmol/L Mg^{2+} 0.75 mmol/L	Lactate 44.5 mmol/L
	Bicarbonate replacement fluid: Na^+ 155 mmol/L Cl^- 120 mmol/L K^+ 0-6 mmol/L Ca^{2+} 1.8 mmol/L Mg^{2+} 0.77 mmol/L	Bicarbonate 40 mmol/L + lactate 3 mmol/L
Cole et al (2001)[81]	Na^+ 140 mmol/L K^+ 1 mmol/L Cl^- 100 mmol/L Ca^{2+} 1.6 mmol/L Mg^{2+} 0.8 mmol/L Glucose 10.8 mmol/L	Lactate 46 mmol/L
Naka et al (2005)[62]	Na^+ 140 mmol/L Cl^- 108 mmol/L K^+ 1 mmol/L	Citrate 11 mmol/L
Tan et al (2004)[88]	Bicarbonate replacement fluid: Na^+ 140 mmol/L K^+ 3.7 mmol/L Cl^- 113.2 mmol/L Ca^{2+} 1.75 mmol/L Mg^{2+} 0.5 mmol/L	Bicarbonate 32 mmol/L + lactate 3 mmol/L
	Lactate replacement fluid: Na^+ 140 mmol/L K^+ 3.7 mmol/L Cl^- 102.7 mmol/L Ca^{2+} 1.6 mmol/L Mg^{2+} 0.8 mmol/L	Lactate 46 mmol/L + glucose 10.8 mmol/L
Kierdorf et al (1999)[71]	Lactate replacement fluid: Na^+ 142 mmol/L Cl^- 103 mmol/L Ca^{2+} 2.0 mmol/L Mg^{2+} 0.75 mmol/L Glucose 5.6 mmol/L	Lactate fluid: lactate 44.5 mmol/L
	Bicarbonate I replacement fluid: Na^+ 140 mmol/L Cl^- 110 mmol/L Ca^{2+} 1.75 mmol/L Mg^{2+} 0.5 mmol/L Glucose 5.6 mmol/L	Bicarbonate 34.5 mmol/L + lactate 3 mmol/L

TABLE 127-1

Dialysate/Replacement Fluid Solutions in Studies Using Different Strong Ion Difference (SID) Generator Solutions—cont'd

STUDY (YEAR)*	ELECTROLYTE COMPONENTS	SID GENERATOR
Heering et al (1999)[75]	Bicarbonate II replacement fluid: Na$^+$ 142 mmol/L Cl$^-$ 104.5 mmol/L Ca^{2+} 1.75 mmol/L Mg^{2+} 0.5 mmol/L Glucose 5.6 mmol/L	Bicarbonate 40 mmol/L + lactate 3 mmol/L
	Lactate replacement fluid: Na$^+$ 142 mmol/L Cl$^-$ 103 mmol/L Ca^{2+} 2 mmol/L Mg^{2+} 0.75 mmol/L	Lactate 44.5 mmol/L
	Bicarbonate replacement fluid: Na$^+$ 140 mmol/L Cl$^-$ 109 mmol/L Ca^{2+} 1.5 mmol/L Mg^{2+} 0.5 mmol/L	Bicarbonate 35 mmol/L
	Acetate replacement fluid: Na$^+$ 140 mmol/L Cl$^-$ 111 mmol/L Ca^{2+} 2 mmol/L Mg^{2+} 1 mmol/L	Acetate 35 mmol/L

*Superscript numbers indicate chapter references.

Key Points

1. The most common acid-base imbalance found in patients with both acute kidney injury and chronic kidney disease is metabolic acidosis.
2. This acidosis is multifactorial in origin. In acute kidney injury, acidosis is due to (in decreasing order of importance): unmeasured anions, hyperphosphatemia, hyperlactatemia, and hypocalcemia.
3. In patients with chronic kidney disease, metabolic acidosis results from: decreased strong ion difference, due to the Na$^+$-Cl$^-$ effect with both an increase in chloride and a decrease in sodium; increased plasma phosphate (a weak acid) levels, due to a reduced excretion of phosphate in the urine; and late (with advanced chronic kidney disease) accumulation of unmeasured acids/anions.
4. All of these changes in chronic kidney disease lead to no overall variation in the unmeasured ion effect until late in the course of disease, this feature representing the main difference between acidosis in chronic kidney disease and that in acute kidney injury.
5. Despite the different techniques that can be applied to the treatment of acute kidney injury or chronic kidney disease, renal replacement therapy rapidly corrects acidosis in both acute kidney injury and chronic kidney disease, usually leading to (sometimes transient) metabolic alkalosis.

Key References

10. Rocktaeschel J, Morimatsu H, Uchino S, et al: Acid-base status of critically ill patients with acute renal failure: analysis based on Stewart-Figge methodology. Crit Care 2003;7(4):R60.
18. Forni LG, McKinnon W, Lord GA, et al: Circulating anions usually associated with the Krebs cycle in patients with metabolic acidosis. Crit Care 2005;9:R591-R595.
19. Story DA, Tosolini A, Bellomo R, et al: Plasma acid-base changes in chronic renal failure: A Stewart analysis. Int J Artif Organs 2005;28:961-965.
48. Naka T, Bellomo R: Bench-to-bedside review: Treating acid-base abnormalities in the intensive care unit—the role of renal replacement therapy. Crit Care 2004;8:108-114.

See the companion Expert Consult website for the complete reference list.

CHAPTER 128

Acute Metabolic Alkalosis

Nicholas Madden, Raghavan Murugan, Matthew A. Butkus, and John A. Kellum

OBJECTIVES

This chapter will:
1. Describe the generation and maintenance of acute metabolic alkalosis.
2. Discuss syndromes and complications associated with acute metabolic alkalosis.
3. Outline management and treatment strategies for acute metabolic alkalosis.

Most syndromes of acute metabolic alkalosis result from a sudden loss of chloride (Cl^-) leading to increased strong ion difference (SID) in extracellular fluid. Acute metabolic alkalosis, except when part of a mixed acid-base disorder, is perceptible as the presence of alkalemia (arterial pH > 7.45), and a standard base excess (SBE) higher than 2 mEq/L.[1] In critically ill patients, metabolic alkalosis accounts for up to 50% of all acid-base disorders[2] and is associated with a 45% mortality rate in patients with an arterial pH higher than 7.55 and with an 80% mortality rate in patients with an arterial pH higher than 7.65.[3] Given the clinical severity and frequency of this disorder, it is imperative that intensive care clinicians correctly recognize and treat this condition. This chapter discusses the pathophysiology, diagnosis, and management of acute metabolic alkalosis.

GENERATION OF ACUTE METABOLIC ALKALOSIS

Role of Strong Ions

Acute metabolic alkalosis can be generated from a change in strong ion concentration or, less commonly, a change in weak acid concentration. A change in strong ion concentration is accountable for the onset of most cases of metabolic alkalosis. It is important to note that the concentrations of H^+ and HCO_3 (dependent variables, concentrations of which fluctuate with pH) are determined primarily by the strong ions and PCO_2 (independent variables, concentrations of which are independent of changes in pH).

Syndromes resulting in acute loss of anions, such as chloride (e.g., vomiting, nasogastric suction), lead to increased strong ion difference (SID), which in turn decreases the dissociation of water, thereby lowering H^+ concentrations and elevating pH. There are three common mechanisms for an acute increase in SID.

First, in normal physiological conditions, serum Na^+ concentration is greater than serum Cl^- concentration. That being said, depletion in free water concentration yields increases in both Na^+ and Cl^- concentrations. Owing to the higher baseline value of serum Na^+ in comparison with Cl^-, free water depletion causes increases in Na^+ relative to Cl^- concentrations, thereby leading to a net increase in SID. Critically ill patients often succumb to free water depletion because of depressed level of consciousness and diminished response to thirst stimuli.

Second, chloride loss from the gastrointestinal tract (e.g., from vomiting or gastric drainage) or from urine (e.g., in diuretic use) is greater than the corresponding Na^+ loss. For instance, if gastric secretions are removed from the patient, through either continuous suction catheter or vomiting, Cl^- is lost progressively and the SID increases steadily. The Cl^- loss, not the H^+ loss, is the determinant of plasma pH. Although H^+ is lost as HCl, it also is lost with every molecule of water removed from the body. When Cl^- (a strong anion) is lost without the loss of a strong cation, the SID is increased, and therefore, the plasma H^+ concentration is decreased. When H^+ is lost as water, rather than as HCl, there is no change in the SID and, hence, no change in the plasma H^+ concentration. Similarly, the loss of chloride-rich fluid in the stool in diarrhea leads to contraction of extracellular fluid volume as well as metabolic alkalosis. Alternatively, Cl^- depletion can have a renal origin, as when loop diuretics are being administered. The mechanism involves increased stimulation of the renin-angiotensin-aldosterone pathway. The end result of the pathway, aldosterone, is associated with an increase in Na^+ reabsorption and a loss of K^+ and Cl^-. The excretion of K^+ and Cl^- results not only from increased aldosterone concentrations but also from the diuretic itself. The movement of these ions due to the diuretic leads to a more rapid onset of metabolic alkalosis.

Third, although less common, an increase in SID due to cation administration rather than anion depletion can also generate metabolic alkalosis (Table 128-1). Acute metabolic alkalosis results when Na^+ is administered in excess of Cl^-, for instance with blood transfusions (sodium citrate), parenteral nutrition (sodium acetate), plasma volume expanders (acetate or citrate), or lactated Ringer's solution (sodium lactate), when an antibiotic (e.g., penicillins) is administered as a sodium salt, or with use of excessive sodium bicarbonate. During blood transfusions, Na^+ is given with citrate rather than Cl^-. As citrate is metabolized, SID rises.

Role of Total Weak Acid Concentration

The second mechanism for the generation of acute metabolic alkalosis is a change in weak acid concentration. Weak acids, unlike strong ions, can exist in an ionized $[A^-]$ or protonated $[AH]$ state in normal physiological conditions, such that:

$$A_{tot} = [AH] + [A^-]$$

A_{tot} represents the total concentration of nonvolatile weak acids (most commonly albumin and phosphate). All else

TABLE 128-1

Etiologies of Acute Metabolic Alkalosis

Anion depletion	Gastric losses (e.g., vomiting, mechanical drainage, bulimia)
	Use of a chloruretic diuretic (e.g., bumetanide, chlorothiazide, metolazone)
	Diarrheal states (e.g., villous adenoma, congenital chloridorrhea)
	Posthypercapnic state
	Gastrocystoplasty
Cation excess	Acute milk-alkali syndrome
	Sodium salt administration (acetate, citrate)
	Blood transfusions
	Plasma volume expanders
	Sodium lactate
	Parenteral nutrition
Disorders of total concentration of non-volatile weak acids (A_{tot})	Hypoalbuminemia Hypophosphatemia

being constant, a decrease in A_{tot} also has the potential, albeit less significant, to yield acute metabolic alkalosis (e.g., hypoalbuminemia and hypophosphatemia). Hypoalbuminemia is commonly found in critically ill patients. Although albumin synthesis is regulated largely by osmolality of the extravascular hepatic space and colloid osmotic levels, low concentrations of albumin not only result from hepatic irregularities but also can be induced by conditions such as sepsis and nephrotic syndrome. The charge on the surface of albumin, primarily the function of histidine moieties, fluctuates with changes in pH. Thus, albumin acts as a plasma weak acid, and the albumin concentration must be considered in determination of the underlying cause of alkalosis. Likewise, phosphate serves as a nonvolatile weak acid. Its representation in A_{tot}, although less pronounced than that of albumin, can have significant clinical implications in cases of hypophosphatemia. Generally this disorder manifests as an intracellular shift of phosphate, increased urinary excretion, or dietary deficiencies.

COMPLICATIONS

The metabolic nature of the alkalosis generates a response from the respiratory system that manifests as hypoventilation. The result in this instance is a subsequent increase in P_{CO_2} that, in metabolic alkalosis, is typically higher than 40 mm Hg. In severe alkalosis, the consequences of decreased levels of oxygen delivery throughout the system can be quite serious (pH > 7.60). Severe metabolic alkalosis can result in appreciable respiratory, metabolic, cardiovascular, and neurological complications. Less severe cases may cause few symptoms that are unique to the alkalosis. Respiratory complications generally include a decrease in oxygen delivery (increased P_{CO_2}). The Bohr effect, which is enhanced by elevations of HCO_3^-, is the associated mechanism. An increase in hemoglobin affinity for oxygen ultimately results. In severe metabolic alkalosis, hypoxia may result. Hypokalemia, hypophosphatemia, decreased Ca^{2+} ionization, and hypomagnesemia may also be present.

The cardiovascular responses are primarily vasoconstriction and a subsequent decrease in coronary blood flow. Increased inotropy and digoxin toxicity may also result. In some cases of more pronounced metabolic alkalosis, cardiac arrhythmias may be detectable. Neurological symptoms of metabolic acidosis include delirium, apathy, neuromuscular excitability, and, in more severe instances, seizures.

MANAGEMENT

The primary goal of management of a patient in whom acute metabolic alkalosis is suspected should be to treat the underlying etiology. The recognition of the disorder and the subsequent differential diagnosis (chloride-responsive or chloride-resistant) that can be made are essential first steps. Obtaining a thorough history and physical examination will most likely demonstrate the underlying etiology. In cases of acute metabolic alkalosis, losses from the gastrointestinal tract, volume contraction, or administration of nonchloride sodium salts are the most common causes. Serum electrolyte levels and arterial blood gas values should be reviewed. Additionally, measuring the urine Cl^- concentration is useful in differentiating between chloride-responsive and chloride-resistant alkalosis (see Chapter 119). Additional consideration must be given to the possibility of a concomitant respiratory component of the acid-base disorder. The expected arterial P_{CO_2} value associated with metabolic alkalosis should be calculated through the use of the HCO_3^- concentration or the SBE value, as follows:

$$P_{CO_2} \text{ (mm Hg)} = (0.7 \times HCO_3^-) + 21$$

$$P_{CO_2} \text{ (mm Hg)} = 40 + (0.6 \times SBE)$$

A measured P_{CO_2} value that is more than 2 mm Hg higher than the derived expected value indicates respiratory acidosis, whereas a P_{CO_2} value less than 2 mm Hg higher indicates respiratory alkalosis.

The successful treatment of acute metabolic alkalosis depends largely on the ability to treat the underlying cause. Depending on that cause, attention should be given to the reversal of Cl^- and K^+ depletion, restoration of volume, and prevention of additional losses (Table 128-2). Diuretic use is the most common cause of acute metabolic alkalosis. Isotonic saline should be administered in this instance. In patients with diuretic-induced alkalosis, treatment with nonsodium chloride salts (e.g., KCl) is often sucessful in reversing the alkalosis, whereas the condition often persists without Cl^- replacement. A 0.9% saline solution is effective at reversing the free water deficit and chloride depletion. Several liters may be required throughout the first day of treatment. If hypokalemia is present with volume depletion, maintenance doses of 20 mEq/L of KCl can be given in normal saline to normalize K^+ levels and provide an additional source of Cl^-. Additionally, diuretics should be discontinued when possible. In patients with underlying renal failure or risk for volume overload, 0.1 M hydrochloric acid (HCl; 100 mmol Cl^- per liter) can be administered via a central venous line to treat the Cl^- depletion. Another evaluation of the metabolic alkalosis after each liter is infused is recommended (see Table 128-2).

Metabolic alkalosis in the presence of volume overload (e.g., in the presence of congestive heart failure) is best treated with potassium chloride solutions. If diuresis is

TABLE 128-2

General Treatment Strategies for Acute Metabolic Alkalosis

Reversal of Cl^- and K^+ depletion
Volume restoration
Prevention of additional strong ion losses
Administration of isotonic saline solution (0.9%)
Correct hypokalemia
Discontinuation of inciting agents (e.g., diuretics) as soon as possible

necessary, K^+-sparing diuretics (e.g., spironolactone), which also spare Cl^- concentrations, can be used. Alternatively, in patients with adequate renal function, a carbonic anhydrase inhibitor such as acetazolamide can be administered at a dose of 250 to 500 mg twice daily. Acetazolamide is associated with Na^+ excretion in excess of Cl^- excretion, and thus a net increase in SID.[4] Acetazolamide also increases K^+ secretion, making it useful in conjunction with KCl. Complications of acetazolamide use are hypokalemia and metabolic acidosis.

In patients actively losing gastric fluid, histamine H_2 blockers and/or proton pump inhibitors are useful in treatment because these agents appear to be associated with a decrease in gastric Cl^- loss.

Although the previously outlined medical treatments are highly successful for mild to moderate cases of metabolic alkalosis, additional interventions, such as renal replacement therapy, may be required. Renal failure and acetazolamide-resistant volume overload are common indications for dialysis. Normal saline should be used in peritoneal dialysis, with electrolyte concentrations as

indicated. In hemodialysis, the dialysate should have a low HCO_3^- concentration. Additionally, HCl can be administered in cases of severe metabolic alkalosis. HCl therapy is typically preferred over dialysis in severe cases in which the patient is symptomatic (e.g., presence of arrhythmia or hepatic encephalopathy). The infusion rate over a 24-hour period should not exceed 25 mEq/hr.

Key Points

1. Changes in strong ion concentration generally underlie acute metabolic alkalosis.
2. The treatment of metabolic alkalosis requires identification and correction of the underlying cause of the acid-base disturbance.
3. Additional treatment focuses on restoring Cl^- through supplementation or renal replacement therapy.

Key References

1. Kellum JA: Determinants of blood pH in health and disease. Crit Care 2000;4:6-14.
2. Hodgkin JE, Soeprono FF, Chan DM: Incidence of metabolic alkalemia in hospitalized patients. Crit Care Med 1980;8:725-728.
3. Anderson LE, Henrich WL: Alkalemia-associated morbidity and mortality in medical and surgical patients. South Med J 1987;80:729-733.
4. Moviat M, Pickkers P, van der Voort PH, van der Hoeven JG: Acetazolamide-mediated decrease in strong ion difference accounts for the correction of metabolic alkalosis in critically ill patients. Crit Care 2006;10:R14.

See the companion Expert Consult website for the complete reference list.

CHAPTER 129

Disorders of Chronic Metabolic Alkalosis

Matthew A. Butkus, Raghavan Murugan, Nicholas Madden, and John A. Kellum

OBJECTIVES

This chapter will:
1. Briefly review the mechanisms of metabolic alkalosis.
2. Identify specific disorders that produce chronic metabolic alkaloses.
3. Discuss management strategies for chronic metabolic alkaloses.

Chronic metabolic alkalosis is rare, accounting for only about 5% of metabolic alkaloses. This disorder usually manifests as alkalemia (arterial pH > 7.45), hyperbicarbonatemia (HCO_3^- > 26 mmol/L), hypercarbia (PCO_2 > 40 mm Hg), and an increased standard base excess (SBE)

(>2 mEq/L).[1] The alkalemia observed in chronic metabolic alkalosis may be quite pronounced, especially in comparison with that in chronic metabolic acidosis (e.g., renal failure); although the respiratory system can decrease PCO_2 through hyperventilation, it cannot reduce minute ventilation enough to match the increased alkali with CO_2 during alkalosis. The physical symptoms of metabolic alkalosis include changes in central and peripheral nervous system function (e.g., confusion, obtundation, seizures, paresthesias), muscular cramping and/or tetany, arrhythmias, and hypoxemia. Clues to the underlying etiology of the disorder can be obtained through evaluation of the urine chloride ion (Cl^-) concentration. Chronic metabolic alkalosis tends to involve urine Cl^- values higher than 20 mmol/L (i.e., chloride-resistant metabolic alkalosis).

TABLE 129-1

Disorders and Mechanisms of Chronic Metabolic Alkalosis

CONDITION	MECHANISM
Bartter's syndrome	Causes chronic hyperaldosteronism and hypokalemia; renal salt excretion and volume depletion
Gitelman's syndrome	Similar mechanism to Bartter's syndrome; characterized by hypomagnesemia and hypocalciuria
Liddle's syndrome	Chronic K^+ over-excretion produces hypokalemia, causing intracellular H^+ shift and increasing extracellular pH.
Cushing's syndrome	Causes mineralocorticoid activity with high Na^+, hypokalemia, and alkalosis
Hyperaldosteronism (primary and secondary)	Produces K^+ depletion, chloride loss, and alkalosis
Strong ion imbalances (hypokalemia, hypomagnesemia)	Ion deficiencies stimulate reabsorption of the missing ions and produce intracellular H^+ shifts
Use of antineoplastic drugs	Many of these agents cause tubular toxicity and can produce a hypokalemic chronic metabolic alkalosis
Long-term use of glycyrrhizin-containing compounds (e.g., licorice)	Glycyrrhizin inhibits conversion of cortisol to less active metabolites (cortisone); cortisol increases the activity of the epithelial sodium channel and competes with aldosterone in mineralocorticoid binding
Long-term use of diuretics	Has multiple mechanisms—can produce either secondary hyperaldosteronism due to volume or Cl^- depletion or concomitant hypokalemia
Long-term use of laxatives	Unclear mechanism, but likely due to K^+ or Cl^- excretion in feces (uncommon)

ETIOLOGY OF CHRONIC METABOLIC ALKALOSIS

Chronic metabolic alkalosis is rare and generally is due to congenital defects and/or mineralocorticoid excess (Table 129-1). Congenital causes of metabolic alkalosis tend to involve malformation of the renal tubule or dysfunction of ion exchangers, both of which produce imbalances in strong ion concentrations.

Hyperaldosteronism (Primary and Secondary)

The classic example of chloride-resistant metabolic alkalosis is primary hyperaldosteronism, a condition in which an intrinsic adrenal defect, such as an adenoma or hyperplasia, leads to an oversecretion of aldosterone. Aldosterone is a key element of the renin-angiotensin-aldosterone pathway in fluid volume maintenance. In hyperaldosteronism—whether due to an adenoma or malignant neoplasm (primary) or due to renal artery stenosis (secondary)—the renal epithelial cells retain an excess of sodium and excrete potassium and chloride, producing hypokalemia and hypochloremia. This chloride wasting produces greater loss of anions than of cations (especially in the extracellular compartment), increasing the strong ion difference (SID) and producing alkalemia.

Cushing's Syndrome

Cushing's syndrome results from overexposure to cortisol, whether through a neoplasm affecting the adrenal glands or through overexposure to corticosteroids. Cortisol acts as a mineralocorticoid, increasing the activity of epithelial cells and producing ion imbalances like hypokalemia/hypochloremia (sodium and water are retained, increasing blood pressure, while potassium is lost as a result). The renal Cl^- wasting produces an increase in SID and metabolic alkalosis.

Bartter's, Gitelman's, and Liddle's Syndromes

Bartter's syndrome is a set of related autosomal recessive disorders of the renal tubule that produce chronic hyperaldosteronism, hypokalemia, hypochloremia, and hyperreninemia.[2] In this syndrome there are significant urinary losses of sodium, chloride, calcium, and potassium. Gitelman's syndrome, also an autosomal recessive disorder of the renal tubule, causes chronic hypokalemia, hypomagnesemia, and hypocalciuria.

Liddle's syndrome is due to an autosomal dominant disorder resulting in chronic hypokalemia and hyporeninemia. In addition to the cation and renin deficiencies, it is marked by severe hypertension and suppressed aldosterone secretion. These cation losses are more than offset by chloride loss, producing a net strong anion loss greater than the net strong cation loss, which increases the SID, thereby inducing alkalemia.

Antineoplastic Drugs

Certain antineoplastic agents (e.g., cisplatin) cause nephrotoxicity. Renal injury can prevent proper or adequate ion reabsorption or elimination and is often associated with potassium deficiencies (chronic hypokalemic metabolic alkalosis) as well as chloride wasting that parallels that seen in other disorders.[3] This chloride loss increases the SID, producing alkalemia.

Long-Term Use of Glycyrrhizin-Containing Compounds

Glycyrrhizin, the active compound in licorice, is used as a flavoring in foods and medications; it inhibits enzymatic conversion of cortisol to its less active metabolites (cortisone). As in Cushing's syndrome, cortisol acts as a mineralocorticoid, increasing sodium and fluid retention while producing other ion deficiencies (e.g., hypokalemia, hypochloremia).[4] These changes directly affect the SID because potassium losses tend to be balanced with sodium retention but chloride losses are unbalanced with other strong anions. This imbalance increases the SID, thereby raising the pH.

Long-Term Use of Diuretics or Laxatives

Long-term use of diuretics is the most common cause of metabolic alkaloses. There are multiple mechanisms by which diuretics produce pH imbalances. First, they can produce a so-called contraction alkalosis because of free water loss; this occurs because plasma SID is positive and concentration of plasma (removal of free water) raises the concentrations of both strong cations and anions proportionally. Thus, SID increases as free water is removed—a 10% loss of water results in a 10% increase in SID. However, the effect on plasma pH is moderated by a proportional rise in the concentration of weak acids (e.g., albumin, phosphate). For example, a 10% free water loss from normal plasma leads to a rise in pH from 7.40 to 7.44. Second, diuretics may produce secondary hyperaldosteronism through intravascular volume depletion. This condition mimics the effects of primary hyperaldosteronism discussed previously and results in renal Cl⁻ losses and, thus, increased SID. Third, diuretics reduce the ability of the patient to respond to chloride salt administration, because of ongoing Cl⁻ losses and concomitant hypokalemia.

The specific mechanisms by which laxative abuse produces metabolic alkalosis are less clear. The available evidence suggests mechanisms comparable to the mechanisms involved in potassium-wasting and chloride-wasting diarrhea.

DIAGNOSIS AND TREATMENT

The first essential aspect of management is diagnosis of the underlying disorder causing the chronic metabolic alkalosis. Most causes of chronic metabolic alkalosis manifest as elevated blood pressure due to volume expansion from excess aldosterone. In contrast, Bartter's syndrome causes urinary salt wasting and therefore does not cause hypertension or manifest as volume expansion. Thus, a patient with metabolic alkalosis who has a normal or elevated urinary Cl⁻ value and normal or low blood pressure is likely to be surreptitiously abusing diuretics or to have Bartter's syndrome. If results of a urinary diuretic screen are negative, Bartter's syndrome should be suspected. Among the hypertension-associated causes, broad categories can be distinguished by plasma levels of renin and aldosterone: Primary defect of renin secretion causes high plasma levels of both renin and aldosterone; primary defect of high aldosterone secretion causes low plasma renin level and high plasma aldosterone level; and primary increases in aldosterone agonists, such as deoxycorticosterone, cause low plasma levels of both renin and aldosterone.

In general, chloride-resistant alkaloses are more difficult to manage than chloride-responsive alkaloses. When the underlying cause is a congenital disorder, symptom management and correction of recurrent ion imbalances are necessary. Cushing's syndrome and hyperaldosteronism may respond to spironolactone (an aldosterone receptor antagonist that induces sodium and fluid loss while reducing potassium excretion); typically, these disorders require surgery. Angiotensin-converting enzyme inhibitors may be effective in the management of secondary hyperaldosteronism. Triamterene (a potassium-conserving diuretic) may be useful in Bartter's or Liddle's syndrome, but the success rate of its use is variable.

Key Points

1. Chronic metabolic alkalosis is rare, accounting for only about 5% of cases of metabolic alkalosis.
2. Chronic metabolic alkaloses are often difficult to treat, and therapy of the underlying disorder is often required to correct the acid-base imbalance.

Key References

1. Kellum JA: Determinants of blood pH in health and disease. Crit Care 2000;4:6-14.
2. Zaffanello M, Taranta A, Palma A, et al: Type IV Bartter syndrome: Report of two new cases. Pediatr Nephrol 2006;21:766-770.
3. Panichpisal K, Angulo-Pernett F, Selhi S, Nugent KM: Gitelman-like syndrome after cisplatin therapy: A case report and literature review. BMC Nephrol 2006;7:10.
4. Lin SH, Yang SS, Chau T, Halperin ML: An unusual cause of hypokalemic paralysis: chronic licorice ingestion. Am J Med Sci 2003;325:153-156.

See the companion Expert Consult website for the complete reference list.

CHAPTER 130

Acid-Base Disorders Secondary to Poisoning

Kenneth Scott Whitlow and Kyle J. Gunnerson

OBJECTIVES

This chapter will:
1. Explain the significance of acid-base disturbances in the setting of the critically ill, poisoned patient.
2. Discuss acetaminophen as a common toxin and cause of metabolic acidosis.
3. Describe the importance of both alcohol dehydrogenase inhibition and extracorporeal removal of toxic alcohols in the treatment and prevention of profound metabolic acidosis.
4. Discuss the mechanism and possible significant morbidity and mortality associated with metformin-induced lactic acidosis.
5. Review the significance of metabolic disturbances in the setting of salicylate, theophylline, or lithium poisoning and how such disturbances may guide therapy.

Systemic toxins are a common cause of serious and sometimes fatal acid-base disturbances. Toxin-induced acid-base disorders occur through a variety of distinct metabolic pathways. Individual toxins also exert their effects at different stages during a poisoning. Some of these mechanisms are production of organic acids through metabolic pathways, the direct addition of exogenous ions, mitochondrial dysfunction, direct impairment of renal function, impairment of oxygen delivery, tissue hypoperfusion, and altered ventilation.[1] In a critically ill patient, these toxin-induced disturbances may be compounded by non–toxin-related sources of acid-base dysequilibrium (e.g., hyperchloremia, chronic renal failure). These compounding circumstances make the management of the critically ill poisoned patient challenging. Nephrologists and intensive care clinicians must be aware of both the toxin-induced and non–toxin-induced causes of acid-base dysequilibrium and must be familiar with the mechanisms and treatments of each. Consultations with a regional poison center and a clinical or medical toxicologist are strongly recommended in the care of all critically ill poisoned patients.

The differential diagnosis list for toxin-induced acid-base disturbances is quite long. Many xenobiotics, pharmaceuticals, chemicals, and other substances have been implicated in acid-base disturbances. This chapter discusses the most frequently encountered and most widely recognized substances, as well as a few of the uncommon but particularly interesting or historical poisons with metabolic acid-base effects. The discussion follows a "toxin-based" format, detailing mechanisms within each class or specific toxin mentioned. Some toxicants may cause separate and distinct disturbances, depending on the setting, and are discussed in each section as needed, to avoid combining and confusing the mechanisms.

The issue of toxin-induced respiratory acid-base disturbances, although interesting, pales in comparison with the metabolic issues surrounding poisonings, and is usually due to hyperventilation or hypoventilation. The vast majority of toxin-induced respiratory acidoses are secondary to substances that cause respiratory depression either centrally or via respiratory muscle dysfunction (e.g., opiates).[2] The opposite is also true, in that most poison-related respiratory alkaloses are related to respiratory stimulants (e.g., salicylates, methylxanthines, and nicotine) or are compensatory in nature.[3-5] These respiratory acid-base changes are briefly mentioned in the general context of the substances discussed and their relationship to the overall metabolic picture.

SPECIFIC DISTURBANCES

Metabolic Acidosis

Metabolic acidosis is commonly encountered in the setting of systemic poisoning associated with many toxicants. Toxicants can cause a metabolic acidosis via numerous mechanisms, which may manifest as one of three distinct types based on the anion gap. The first and foremost type in this section are poisons that cause a high–anion gap metabolic acidosis. The toxins discussed are the most well known, most frequently discussed, and most serious or concerning, and their treatment may require both the intervention of a critical care–trained nephrologist and hemodialysis. A comprehensive list of toxins that cause metabolic disturbances is shown in Tables 130-1 and 130-2.

High–Anion Gap Metabolic Acidosis

ACETAMINOPHEN. Acetaminophen (amide of acetic acid and *p*-aminophenol [APAP]; known as paracetamol outside the United States) is an over-the-counter analgesic. It is one of the most commonly used, misused, and abused drugs, and now also the most common cause of acute liver failure, in the United States. It is available in combination with many prescription narcotic analgesics, such as codeine and oxycodone. Overdose of this drug can be acute with suicidal intent, can be secondary to therapeutic misadventures, or can occur with long-term use. Most patients are usually unaware of its toxic properties and perceive it as a "safe" drug. Acetaminophen is contained in many over-the-counter cold preparations or "non-aspirin" pain relievers, and it is quite common for patients to ingest multiple APAP-containing pharmaceuticals

TABLE 130-1

Toxins Causing Anion Gap Metabolic Acidosis

TOXINS	ANION GAP	CLASS	MECHANISM(S)	CHAPTER REFERENCE(S)
"CATMDPILES" Toxins				
Carbon monoxide	High	Asphyxiant	Lactate	53, 54
Carbenicillin	High	Antimicrobial	Unmeasured anions	55
Catecholamines	High	Neurotransmitter	Lactate	56
Chlorine	High	Chemical	Lactate/high chloride	57
Cholestyramine	Normal	Binder	High chloride	58
Citric acid	High	Fungicide	Metabolized to organic acids	59
Cocaine	High	Stimulant	Lactate	60-62
Cyanide	High	Asphyxiant	Lactate	63-68
Acetaminophen	High	Analgesic	Lactate	69-75
Acetazolamide	Normal	Carbonic anhydrase inhib	Enzyme inhibition/renal tubular acidosis	76-78
Acetonitrile	High	Solvent	Metabolized to organic acids/lactate	79-81
Aminocaproic acid	High	Hemostatic agent	Metabolized to organic acids	82
Ammonium chloride	Normal	Algaecide	High chloride	
Theophylline	High	Methylxanthine	Lactate	83-85
Toluene	High/normal	Solvent	Metabolized to organic acids/high chloride/renal tubular acidosis	86-89
Topiramate	Normal	Anticonvulsant	Enzyme inhibition	90
Triethylene glycol	High	Solvent	Metabolized to organic acids	91, 92
Metformin	High	Biguanide	Lactate	93, 94
Methamphetamine	High	Stimulant	Lactate	95
Methanol	High	Solvent	Metabolized to organic acids/lactate	96, 97
Didanosine	High	Antiviral	Lactate	98
Diethylene glycol	High	Solvent	Metabolized to organic acids/lactate	91, 92
Paraldehyde	High	Sedative	Metabolized to organic acids	99
Phenformin	High	Biguanide	Lactate	100, 101
Propofol	High	Sedative	Unknown	102-107
Propylene glycol	High	Diluent/solvent	Lactate	108-121
Ibuprofen	High	Nonsteroidal	Unknown/lactate	122
Iron	High	Metal/supplement	Lactate	123
Isoniazid	High	Antimicrobial	Lactate	124, 125
Lithium	Low	Salt	Unmeasured cations/renal tubular acidosis	126
Ethanol	High	Solvent	Lactate	127-135
Ethylene glycol	High	Solvent	Metabolized to organic acids/lactate	136-139
Salicylates	High	Nonsteroidal	Metabolized to organic acids/lactate	140-145
Sodium chloride	Low	Electrolyte	High chloride	146
Stavudine	High	Antiviral	Lactate	147
Sympathomimetics	High	Stimulants	Lactate	56
Other Important Toxins				
Benzene	High	Solvent	Metabolized to organic acids	
Bromide	Low	Salt	Overestimation of chloride	
Hydrogen sulfide	High	Byproduct	Lactate	148
Nalidixic acid	High	Antimicrobial	Lactate	149
Niacin	High	Vitamin	Lactate	150
Nitroprusside	High	Vasodilator	Lactate	151
Valproic acid	High	Anticonvulsant	Metabolized to organic acids	152, 153
Zidovudine	High	Antiviral	Lactate	154

concurrently without being aware of the higher concentrations of the active drug.[6,7] The major toxicity associated with APAP is fulminant hepatic failure secondary to the formation of its toxic metabolite, N-acetyl-p-benzylquinoneimine (NAPQI), via metabolism of APAP through cytochrome P-450 (CYP450; through its forms 2E1, 1A2, and 3A4) and depletion of hepatic glutathione stores.[8-10] NAPQI causes necrotic injury most notably in the central lobular area or zone 3 of the liver owing to the greater concentration of CYP450 pathways in this specific anatomical location.[11] Acute renal failure in the setting of APAP toxicity is by far most commonly seen in conjunction with fulminant hepatic failure and secondary to that process. However, acute renal failure alone in this setting does occur; possibly the direct effect of NAPQI on the renal

tubule, it manifests in about 5% of patients exposed to toxic levels of APAP. APAP-induced renal failure may require immediate hemodialysis as a bridge until normal renal function returns, but most patients do not need this treatment.[12]

The acid-base disturbances seen in the setting of APAP toxicity are associated with the preceding processes and their contribution to the development of lactic acidosis and uremia. Historically, APAP has not been included in the differential diagnosis of a high–anion gap metabolic acidosis. In severe poisonings, a lactic acid elevation is present and is the primary cause of the high anion gap. The cause of the lactic acidosis in this setting is still unclear and may be related to direct mitochondrial toxicity, inhibition of mitochondrial respiration, organ failure,

TABLE 130-2

Toxins Causing Metabolic Alkalosis

TOXIN	CLASS	CHAPTER REFERENCE(S)
Antacids	Alkali	39, 40
Carbenicillin	Antimicrobial	41
Carbenoxolone	Antiulcer/licorice derivative	42
Capreomycin	Antimicrobial	43
Chewing tobacco	Plant	44
Diuretics	Diuretic	45
Gentamicin	Antimicrobial	46
Licorice	Plant	47-51
Penicillin	Antimicrobial	45
Sodium bicarbonate	Alkali	52
Ticarcillin	Antimicrobial	45

hypoperfusion, or some combination of these processes.[13] Treatment of the underlying fulminant hepatic failure consists of administration of the antidote *N*-acetylcysteine (a precursor of glutathione that inhibits formation of NAPQI), aggressive symptomatic and supportive care, and, possibly, immediate hemodialysis for the anuric patient with worsening acidosis.

DIETHYLENE GLYCOL. Diethylene glycol (DEG) is a commonly used agent but a less common toxin than ethylene glycol. DEG causes an anion gap metabolic acidosis that has been associated with significant historical poison outbreaks. It was the toxin implicated in the Massengill antibiotic poison epidemic in 1937 that was responsible for the first drug and pharmaceutical regulation in the United States. That regulation was the precursor to what has today become the U.S. Food and Drug Administration (FDA). DEG was also implicated in other mass outbreaks from contaminated over-the-counter pharmaceuticals in Haiti (1995-1996), Bangladesh (1990), and Panama (2006).[14-16] This substance is used in the formulation of brake fluid and was once thought to be a nontoxic, less expensive diluent. DEG is a potent renal toxin that can cause a progressive and profound anion gap metabolic acidosis.

The poison epidemics previously listed have also been associated with liver toxicity, respiratory failure, and seizures. The exact mechanism of renal toxicity, acidosis, and other aspects of the poisoning are unknown. Whether the toxicity is a result of direct injury from DEG or a metabolite is still unclear.[17,18] A DEG metabolite, 2-hydroxyethoxyacetic acid, has been identified in an animal model but has not subsequently been seen in humans.[19] The treatment of DEG toxicity is aggressive symptomatic and supportive care and early hemodialysis. The initiation of fomepizole therapy may also be a useful therapeutic adjunct.[20]

ETHYLENE GLYCOL. Ethylene glycol (EG), a common toxicant, has been associated in the United States with multiple high-profile murder cases. It is found most commonly in automobile antifreeze. Patients who are poisoned with it present with severe, delayed metabolic acidosis, hypocalcemia, oxaluria, central nervous system damage, cardiovascular instability, and renal failure.[21] EG intoxication may manifest in early stages as lethargy and altered mental status resembling that in alcohol intoxication. EG, like all alcohols, is rapidly absorbed and reaches peak serum levels 1 to 2 hours after ingestion. Severe toxicity is rare with peak serum EG levels less than 20 mg/dL.

The mechanism for the metabolic acidosis is well defined (Fig. 130-1), being related to the accumulation of glycolic

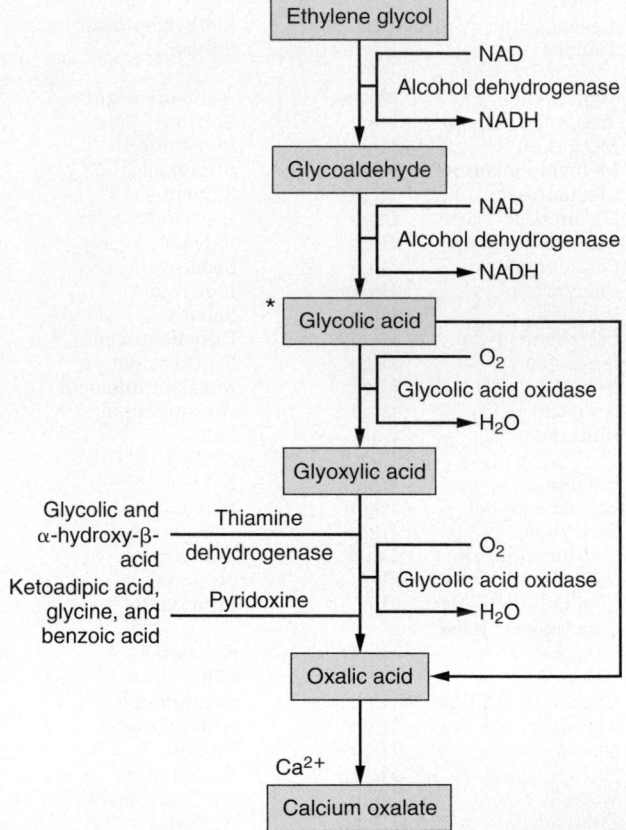

FIGURE 130-1. Metabolic cascade for ethylene glycol. Notice that the cascade is initiated by the enzyme alcohol dehydrogenase. *Cause of metabolic acidosis. NAD, nicotinamide adenine dinucleotide; NADH, reduced form of nicotinamide adenine dinucleotide.

acid as an intermediate metabolite.[22] The first step in the metabolism of EG is initiated by the enzyme alcohol dehydrogenase, which begins the cascade for the development of anion gap metabolic acidosis and eventual renal failure. The delayed renal failure is secondary to the formation of oxalic acid and its precipitation with calcium (as calcium oxalate crystals) in the proximal renal tubule.[23] Understanding the first step in this metabolism is the key to successful treatment of EG intoxication. Administration of an alcohol dehydrogenase competitive inhibitor, such as fomepizole or ethanol, early in the intoxication (or until the serum EG level is <20 mg/dL) prevents the metabolite cascade.[24] In a patient with elevated serum EG, hemodialysis should also be started early, even in the setting of normal acid-base balance and normal renal function. Hemodialysis (HD) shortens the half-life of EG to less than 4 hours, eliminates the parent EG compound, and expedites disposition of the patient. If the acidosis and acute renal failure have already appeared and the serum EG level is higher than 20 mg/dL, both fomepizole therapy and hemodialysis should be instituted. However, if the serum EG level is less than 20 mg/dL and the patient has renal failure with acidosis, hemodialysis alone is sufficient, because the serum concentration of EG is at a point at which prevention of future toxic metabolites is clinically insignificant.

METFORMIN. Metformin is an antihyperglycemic agent in the biguanide class. Its mechanism of action involves raising peripheral glucose uptake by increasing both the binding capacity of insulin to its receptor and the translocation and synthesis of glucose transporters. Metformin also inhibits gluconeogenesis in the liver, which is responsible for the metformin-induced lactic acidosis.[25] This agent decreases the conversion of pyruvate to glucose via inhibition of pyruvate carboxylase, which is involved in the first step of gluconeogenesis. The inhibition occurs at higher serum levels and results in the accumulation of lactate. Lactic acidosis is divided into two types, anaerobic (type A) and aerobic (type B), with the latter occurring in the absence of tissue hypoxia. Type B lactic acidosis is associated with metformin accumulation and is the result of impairment of lactate metabolism.[26] Several factors predispose a patient to metformin-induced lactic acidosis, including renal insufficiency, dehydration, liver disease, advanced age, excessive alcohol consumption, supratherapeutic dosing, and drug-drug interactions.

Severe lactic acidosis associated with metformin is rare but can be serious and possibly fatal. It may manifest as generalized symptoms, such as nausea, vomiting, abdominal pain, and malaise.[27] Maintaining a high index of suspicion is of utmost importance to the diagnosis. Patients with metformin-induced lactic acidosis may progress to a critically ill state, with hypotension, altered mental status, respiratory failure, and hypothermia that may mimic septic shock. These patients need aggressive symptomatic and supportive care, including intravenous volume expansion and, occasionally, the use of vasopressors. Some patients may benefit from emergency hemodialysis or venovenous hemofiltration with a bicarbonate buffer.[28]

METHANOL. A common ingredient in automotive products such as windshield wiper fluid, methanol is a frequent agent in toxic exposure. It has much historical significance in medical toxicology, because it was an agent implicated in mass poisonings due to contamination of illicit alcohol or "moonshine."[29] It is a toxic alcohol much like ethylene glycol and is, in fact, metabolized via the same pathways to a metabolite that causes its toxicity. The enzyme alcohol dehydrogenase initiates this metabolic cascade. The pathway eventually yields formic acid, the compound responsible for the target organ damage to the optic nerve (Fig. 130-2).[30] Formic acid also inhibits mitochondrial cytochrome c oxidase and prevents oxidative metabolism, leading to a profound anion gap metabolic acidosis mostly from lactate accumulation.[31] Methanol poisoning has the clinical appearance of poisoning from other toxic alcohols, ranging from little or no sign of intoxication to overt obtundation. The hallmark is the development of a severe and worsening anion gap metabolic acidosis and eventual "snow blindness." The treatment of

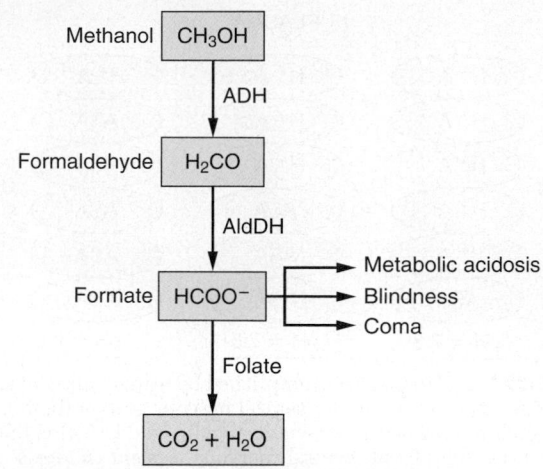

FIGURE 130-2. The metabolic cascade for methanol. The initiation of this cascade, like that of the ethylene glycol cascade, is initiated by the enzyme alcohol dehydrogenase (ADH). Note formate and its contribution to methanol toxicity. AldDH, aldehyde dehydrogenase.

methanol intoxication also requires an alcohol dehydrogenase competitive inhibitor (fomepizole) and hemodialysis if the blood methanol level is higher than 50 mg/dL. In contemporary toxicology management, specific alcohol assays with rapid "turnaround" times are now commonplace. Timely serum alcohol identification has all but relegated the use of an elevated serum osmolar gap in the diagnosis of toxic alcohol poisoning to that of a historical finding.

SALICYLATES. Salicylates are commonly encountered as over-the-counter substances such as aspirin, Goody's Powder, Pepto-Bismol, and oil of wintergreen. They are hydrolyzed in the stomach to salicylic acid and then rapidly absorbed. Salicylates are weak acids and can change chemical states according to the pH of the ambient environment. As the pH of the ambient environment (blood) becomes more acidic, the salicylic acid is driven into its un-ionized or HA state, which renders it more amenable to crossing cell membranes and the blood-brain barrier. As its pH rises, the blood "ion traps" the salicylic acid into its ionic or charged form, preventing it from passing easily into cells and crossing the blood-brain barrier. This behavior enables the use of alkalinization as a therapy to decrease cellular absorption and increase renal excretion of H^+ and A^- (Fig. 130-3). Primarily mitochondrial toxins, salicylates exert their effect via uncoupling of oxidative phosphorylation that contributes to an incomplete production of adenosine triphosphate. The associated metabolic acidosis is a result of the hydrolysis of adenosine triphosphate with the accumulation of lactate and ketones and a dissipation of heat, which is observed clinically as hyperpyrexia. Salicylates also directly stimulate the respiratory centers in the medulla, resulting in the classic clinical signs of tachypnea, hyperpnea, and respiratory alkalosis.[32]

Salicylism is divided into acute, acute-on-chronic, and chronic intoxication. Patients may present with tinnitus, nausea, vomiting, fever, tachypnea, and profound mental status changes with shock. Salicylate-exposed patients may have a metabolic acidosis with a compensatory respiratory alkalosis early in the course and, without adequate therapy, may progress to an overwhelming uncompensated metabolic acidosis. The mainstay of treatment is

PLASMA

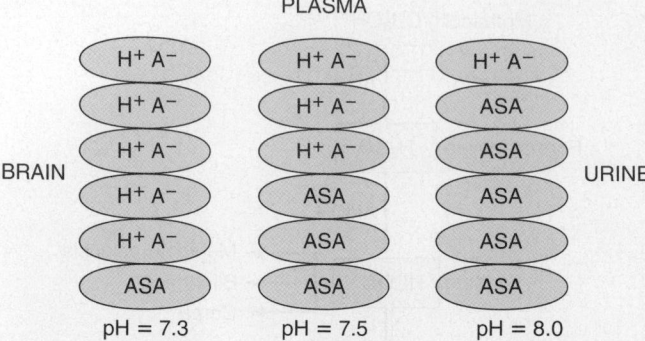

FIGURE 130-3. Ion trapping accomplished by urinary alkalinization. Notice the neutral pH in the central nervous system (brain). One main goal in elimination of acetylsalicylic acid (ASA) is the prevention of significant central nervous system acidosis. This diagram shows the relative concentrations of ionized ASA ($H^+ A^-$) to salicylate in its un-ionized form in each of the three fluid compartments at the target urinary pH of 8.0. With proper urinary alkalinization, much more un-ionized salicylate is excreted in the urine.

alkalinization and, in certain instances, hemodialysis. The indications for hemodialysis are well delineated and are based on clinical criteria and plasma salicylate levels. An absolute level of 60 mg/dL in chronic intoxication and 100 mg/dL in acute intoxication usually requires hemodialysis. The clinical signs that should trigger extracorporeal removal of salicylates are altered mental status or seizures, pulmonary edema, rising salicylate level despite adequate decontamination and urinary alkalinization (urine pH 7.5-8), worsening metabolic acidosis despite adequate therapy, inability to tolerate hydration or alkalinization, and acute renal failure.

THEOPHYLLINE. Like caffeine, theophylline is a derivative of xanthine and resembles adenosine in chemical structure. It is used as a bronchodilator and respiratory stimulant for the management of asthma and emphysema. Theophylline is absorbed completely via the oral route and has a small volume of distribution except in the extremely young or extremely old patients; in these populations, theophylline has a prolonged half-life and a larger volume of distribution. Theophylline undergoes Michaelis-Menten kinetics, and in an overdose, the pharmacokinetics is unpredictable. Patients may have chronic or acute theophylline toxicity, chronic being more common. Theophylline's toxic effects are usually secondary to its activity at the adenosine receptors, which result in an indirect increase in catecholamines and subsequent stimulation of α- and β-adrenergic receptors. It also is a phosphodiesterase inhibitor, increasing cyclic adenosine monophosphate and, therefore, possibly affecting intracellular calcium.

Toxicity from xanthines primarily affects the gastrointestinal, cardiovascular, and central nervous systems. Theophylline also has classic metabolic effects, including hypokalemia, hyperglycemia, and metabolic acidosis. The most common form of acidosis generated by xanthine toxicity is lactic acidosis, which occasionally causes profound alterations in serum pH. Fortunately, most of the metabolic changes associated with xanthine toxicity are of minor clinical significance.[33] Treatment of theophylline toxicity consists of appropriate symptomatic and supportive care, decontamination, and extracorporeal removal of the drug via hemodialysis or charcoal hemoperfusion. The indications for hemodialysis are related to the severity of

clinical manifestations, comorbidity, and absolute plasma theophylline levels.

Low–Anion Gap Metabolic Acidosis

LITHIUM. Lithium (Li^+) intoxication initially manifests as gastrointestinal and neurological findings that can progress to seizures and cardiovascular collapse. Renal dysfunction, including nephrogenic diabetes insipidus, may also be associated with Li^+ intoxication. There is a grading scheme to characterize Li^+ intoxication, modified to include four progressive grades of intoxication. Grade 0 intoxication is asymptomatic, and grade 4 intoxication may manifest as seizures, coma, myoclonus, and/or cardiovascular dysfunction.[34] Li^+ intoxication may also manifest as a normal–anion gap metabolic acidosis, primarily from unmeasured cations and a type 4 renal tubular acidosis.[35] Treatment generally comprises symptomatic and supportive care with additional decontamination or enhanced elimination via aggressive intravenous hydration to increase renal clearance. Hemodialysis has been used in severe cases, although the use of extracorporeal removal of lithium remains controversial. The indications for dialysis reported in the literature rely heavily on the clinical condition of the patient, the plasma Li^+ level, and renal function; however, there are no widely accepted guidelines for its use. The only well-supported indication for dialysis is in the patient with significant renal dysfunction that would not support aggressive hydration and fluid resuscitation. Most clinicians would also use dialysis in lithium-intoxicated patients with grade 3 or severe Li^+ intoxication.[36]

Metabolic Alkalosis

Metabolic alkalosis is typically related to an underlying cause of the abnormality, and rarely related to poisoning. It may occur as an unintentional sequela to fluid loss associated with certain toxic exposures. Metabolic alkalosis requires two distinct factors, a bicarbonate source and a renal tubule stimulus to reabsorb bicarbonate. It is usually associated with a decrease in extracellular fluid volume and an increase in aldosterone excretion.

The most common cause of toxigenic metabolic alkalosis is the use or abuse of diuretics and intractable vomiting.[37] This chapter discusses a rare but potentially serious cause of metabolic alkalosis due to the overconsumption of calcium and alkali substances from antacids. The other toxic causes of metabolic alkalosis are listed in Table 130-2.

MILK-ALKALI SYNDROME. Milk-alkali syndrome is rare and is usually due to the use of high doses of calcium and an absorbable alkali (particularly calcium carbonate) for antacid relief. It has become almost nonexistent with modern nonabsorbable antacid therapy such as histamine H_2 receptor blockade and proton pump inhibition. Milk-alkali syndrome is seen in patients who are unaware of the potential toxicity of over-the-counter absorbable antacids. It can manifest in acute, subacute, or chronic form. The precise mechanism is not known but seems to be related to an interaction between the calcium and alkali that prevents the renal excretion of calcium and bicarbonate. Presenting symptoms of milk-alkali symptoms are those of the classic triad of hypercalcemia, metabolic alkalosis, and acute renal failure. In severe cases, the associated renal failure may require emergency hemodialysis.[38]

CONCLUSION

Acid-base disturbances are common in critically ill poisoned patients. Metabolic acidosis, the most common and concerning of these, carries a long differential diagnosis list. Historically, clinicians have relied heavily on the anion gap to differentiate categories of toxins. In critically ill patients, comorbidities such as hypoalbuminemia may falsely lower the anion gap. The quantitative acid-base analysis approach may be helpful in identifying unmeasured ions in the form of an elevated strong ion gap. Unfortunately, this approach is infrequently used in toxicology. Many xenobiotics and chemicals have been implicated in metabolic changes. Metabolic changes occur via multiple, well-described, or virtually unknown mechanisms. Understanding of these mechanisms may help guide the recognition and possible therapy of poisoning-induced critical illness. If not recognized, poisoning-induced metabolic disorders can significantly contribute to morbidity and mortality.

Key Points

1. Metabolic acidosis is by far the most common and most concerning acid-base disturbance in toxin-induced critical illness.
2. Toxin-induced acidosis may be caused by many different mechanisms.

3. Recognition and maintenance of a high index of suspicion for the important toxin-induced causes of metabolic disturbances is paramount.
4. Lactic acidosis due to metformin can be fatal.
5. Extracorporeal removal of toxin via hemodialysis and aggressive supportive care are essential in treatment of many acid-base disturbances due to toxins.

Key References

1. Boron S: Acid-base disorders. In Brent J, Wallace K, Burkhart K (eds): Critical Care Toxicology: Diagnosis and Management of the Critically Poisoned Patient. Philadelphia, Elsevier, 2005.
13. Koulouris Z, Tierney MG, Jones G: Metabolic acidosis and coma following a severe acetaminophen overdose. Ann Pharmacother 1999;33:1191-1194.
24. Brent J, McMartin K, Phillips S, et al: Fomepizole for the treatment of ethylene glycol poisoning. Methylpyrazole for Toxic Alcohols Study Group. N Engl J Med 1999;340:832-838.
32. Curry SC: Salicylates. In Brent J, Wallace K, Burkhart K (eds): Critical Care Toxicology: Diagnosis and Management of the Critically Poisoned Patient. Philadelphia, Elsevier, 2005, pp 621-629.
34. Hansen HE, Amdisen A: Lithium intoxication: Report of 23 cases and review of 100 cases from the literature. Q J Med 1978;47:123-144.

See the companion Expert Consult website for the complete reference list.

CHAPTER 131

Acid-Base Disorders in Chronic Lung Diseases

Vicente Alfaro

OBJECTIVES

This chapter will:
1. Introduce basic concepts of acid-base physiology and blood gas measurement.
2. Explain differences between acute and chronic respiratory acidosis.
3. Illustrate the renal compensatory mechanisms for respiratory acidosis.
4. Summarize the main acid-base disorders found in patients with chronic lung diseases.

Arterial pH must be maintained within a narrow range of values (Table 131-1). The pH is actually the $-(\log [H^+])$; therefore, problems with acid-base balance occur as a result of changes in $[H^+]$. According to the Henderson-Hasselbalch equation—as follows:

$$pH = pK(6.1) \times \log\left(\frac{HCO_3^-}{0.03 \times PaCO_2}\right)$$

The pH may be changed by alterations in either arterial carbon dioxide tension ($PaCO_2$) or bicarbonate concentration ($[HCO_3^-]$), the latter being the most important buffer in blood. However, buffering has a limited capacity, and ultimately, other changes (e.g., excretion of strong anions) must take place in order to maintain acid-base homeostasis. Although CO_2 control occurs both in the lungs and in the kidneys in a manner described by the following equation, the kidneys have an exclusive role in strong ion regulation:

$$\text{(renal regulation) } H^+ + HCO_3^- \leftrightarrow H_2CO_3 \leftrightarrow H_2O +$$
$$CO_2 \text{ (ventilatory regulation)}$$

In both cases, the reaction is catalyzed by the enzyme carbonic anhydrase. The lungs may blow off excess CO_2 in the presence of an acid load, whereas the kidney's role in regulating H^+ ion activity involves regulation of strong ions, as described in detail in Chapters 111 and 112. Renal regulation is always slower than ventilatory regulation.[1,2]

Asthma and chronic obstructive pulmonary disease (COPD, a term that comprises the two common diseases

TABLE 131-1

Arterial Acid-Base Values: Normal Range and Changes in Blood Gases during Acute Respiratory Failure

PARAMETER	NORMAL RANGE	RESPIRATORY FAILURE
PaO$_2$	90-95 mm Hg	Normal Lungs PO$_2$ →; PCO$_2$ → ↓ e.g., PO$_2$ = 90 mm Hg; PCO$_2$ = 40 mm Hg
PaCO$_2$	35-45 mm Hg	Lung Disease; V̇/Q̇ Inequality PO$_2$ ↓↓; PCO$_2$ ↑ ↓ e.g., PO$_2$ = 45 mm Hg; PCO$_2$ = 52 mm Hg
pH	7.35-7.44	Response of Chemoreceptors
HCO$_3^-$ concentration	24 mEq/L	Increased Ventilation PO$_2$ ↓; PCO$_2$ → e.g., PO$_2$ = 50 mm Hg; PCO$_2$ = 40 mm Hg

chronic bronchitis and emphysema) are two chronic diseases affecting lung function. They are pulmonary disorders in which persistent inflammation and alterations in lung structure contribute to a progressive loss of lung function, including airflow limitation and inefficient alveolar gas exchange, changes in blood gas levels and acid-base status, and respiratory failure.[3] The primary pulmonary disease or process responsible for the disorder is usually known from the patient's history and physical findings, but the abnormality of either PaCO$_2$ or other acid-base balance–related indices (e.g., base excess or strong ion difference) is used to evaluate the magnitude of the primary impairment and further compensations.[3]

MEASUREMENT OF ARTERIAL BLOOD GASES AND ACID-BASE STATUS

Gas exchange and resultant acid-base status are measured via measurement of arterial blood gases (ABGs), and changes from baseline values may elucidate requirements for interventions and predictions for appropriate compensation. The methodology for sampling of arterial blood is standardized and safe, and complications are uncommon and relatively minor. Sources of error in ABG measurements include improper sample site (vein rather than artery), inadequate blood handling techniques (e.g., contamination with room air), and poor instrument calibration.[4] ABG analyzers directly measure arterial oxygen tension (PaO$_2$), PaCO$_2$, and pH. The bicarbonate concentration is calculated through the use of algorithms based on the Henderson-Hasselbalch equation.[5] Several derived indices are used to separate the respiratory from the nonrespiratory components; examples are standard bicarbonate (i.e., the plasma bicarbonate concentration in fully oxygenated blood and equilibrated to a carbon dioxide tension [PCO$_2$] value of 40 mm Hg at 37°C), buffer base (i.e., the sum of the concentrations of all the buffer anions in the blood—hemoglobin, bicarbonate, protein, and phosphate), base excess or deficit (i.e., the titratable base or acid needed to titrate blood in vitro to a pH of 7.4 at a PCO$_2$ of 40 mm Hg at 37° C), and standard base excess (i.e., in vivo

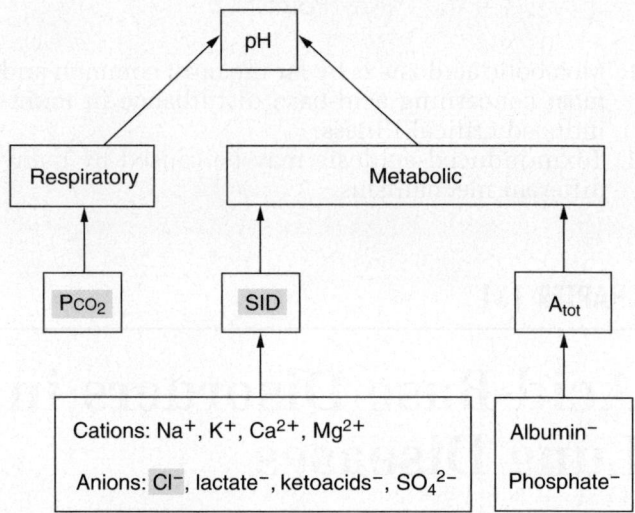

FIGURE 131-1. Determinants of blood pH, as assessed by the quantitative physicochemical acid-base approach of Stewart[7]). For a particular acid-base disorder and resulting pH change, PCO$_2$ provides an independent measure of the respiratory component, whereas the strong ion difference (SID) and the total weak acid concentration (A$_{tot}$) provide independent measures of the nonrespiratory (metabolic) component. Variables shown with shading are expected to be changed in the blood of patients with stable chronic lung disease: Increased PCO$_2$ as a primary respiratory disorder and decreased SID (due to decrease in chloride) as a compensatory metabolic change mediated by kidney.

base excess in which correction factors are used to estimate the buffering effect of the extracellular fluid).[6]

In fact, buffer base is conceptually identical to the strong ion difference (SID), a quantitative, physicochemical approach introduced in 1983 by Stewart.[7] The SID approach involves complex equations related to both chemical equilibrium and electrical neutrality, but it has become useful thanks to the greater availability of ion analyzers and computers. Briefly, the three independent determinants of pH in whole blood are the "respiratory" component (PaCO$_2$) and two "metabolic" components, SID and the nonvolatile weak acid buffer component (A$_{tot}$) (Fig. 131-1). This quantitative acid-base approach allows the establishment of physicochemical predictions that have generally proved accurate in several experimental and clinical conditions.[8-11]

RESPIRATORY FAILURE AND HYPERCAPNIA

A widely used working definition of respiratory failure is given as a PaO_2 less than 60 mm Hg, with or without an elevated $PaCO_2$ value, when the subject is at rest and breathing room air at sea level. In chronic lung diseases, respiratory failure may be acute (as in exacerbations) or chronic (due to progression of the underlying pulmonary disease). Alveolar ventilation-perfusion ($\dot{V}/\dot{Q}$) mismatching and load/capacity imbalance are the major physiological determinants of chronic respiratory failure. When ventilation and blood flow to various regions of the lung are mismatched, gas transfer becomes inefficient, and as a result, hypoxemia develops and the alveolar-arterial gradient for oxygen increases. The load/capacity imbalance causes chronic ventilatory failure and hypercapnia as a consequence of an inefficient breathing pattern, with lower tidal volume and higher respiratory rate that increase the physiological dead space. Some researchers postulate that alveolar hypoventilation may be a protective strategy to prevent excessive respiratory effort and eventual respiratory muscle fatigue and failure.[12,13] Airflow obstruction resulting from intrinsic airways disease and reduced lung elastic recoil (which increases airways resistance) also leads to air trapping and hyperinflation. Both air trapping and hyperinflation place the diaphragm and other inspiratory muscles at severe mechanical disadvantage, producing alveolar hypoventilation and hypercapnia. In chronic lung disorders, particularly in COPD, $\dot{V}/\dot{Q}$ mismatching and the load/capacity imbalance coexist at the most advanced stage of the disease. In other lung disorders, one of the two mechanisms prevails: For instance, $\dot{V}/\dot{Q}$ in pure lung diseases, and chest wall mechanics in thoracic disorders. This fact has important therapeutic implications, because oxygen administration may relieve hypoxemia, and mechanical ventilation may prevent excessive hypercapnia and respiratory acidosis.[14]

Another factor that may cause alveolar hypoventilation and hypercapnia is impaired chemical responsiveness to rising levels of hypoxia or hypercapnia. Alveolar ventilation is under the control of central respiratory centers located in the pons and the medulla. Thus, ventilation is influenced and regulated by chemoreceptors for $PaCO_2$, PaO_2, and H^+ ions located in the brainstem or peripherally, as well as by neural impulses from lung stretch receptors. However, inadequate chemoresponsiveness has been found to be a minor factor responsible for CO_2 retention compared with mechanical impairment in patients with COPD, with or without chronic hypercapnia, during a CO_2 rebreathing test.[15]

Hypercapnia is produced by a failure of the respiratory system.[16] Three physiological reasons explain why elevated $PaCO_2$ is potentially dangerous. First, as $PaCO_2$ increases, the pH falls and acidemia appears, although renal compensation will temper this effect in time. Second, as $PaCO_2$ rises, the alveolar pressure of oxygen and therefore the PaO_2 falls concomitantly unless inspired oxygen is supplemented. Third, the higher the $PaCO_2$, the less defended the patient is against any further decline in alveolar ventilation or against conditions implying a higher

CO_2 production (exercise, carbohydrate loading, etc.). The blood CO_2 transport capacity may be diminished in patients with respiratory acidosis. The CO_2 dissociation curve represents the relation between blood PCO_2 and whole blood CO_2 content. This curve is less steep at higher PCO_2 levels: thus, high PCO_2 levels make CO_2 transport less effective than with low PCO_2 levels.[17] Furthermore, as described later, CO_2 retention may be tolerable only for the patient with chronic lung disease who has an intact renal system, who is therefore capable of reabsorbing enough bicarbonate to maintain acid-base balance. As mentioned previously, the ability of the patient with chronic lung disease to tolerate CO_2 retention (so-called permissive hypercapnia) is thought to be an adaptive mechanism that lessens the effort of breathing[13] and presumably is less injurious to the lungs in the setting of acute lung injury.

ACUTE AND CHRONIC RESPIRATORY ACIDOSIS IN CHRONIC LUNG DISEASES

Metabolism in tissues rapidly generates a large quantity of volatile acid (CO_2) and nonvolatile acids (e.g., lactate), with a normal CO_2 production per day of about 13,000 mmol. In a healthy condition, the lungs excrete the volatile fraction (CO_2) through ventilation, and acid accumulation does not occur. However, a failure of alveolar ventilation (hypoventilation) reduces pulmonary CO_2 elimination, quickly raises $PaCO_2$, and finally leads to respiratory acidosis. For instance, if pulmonary ventilation were to cease for 20 minutes in a human, $PaCO_2$ would rise to 110 mm Hg and arterial pH would fall to 7.03. In contrast, if renal function were to cease for a similar period, no changes in arterial pH would occur.[1] The reference range for $PaCO_2$ is 35 to 45 mm Hg (see Table 131-1). However, $PaCO_2$ values between 80 and 100 mm Hg have been reported in patients with COPD breathing air at sea level.[18] Higher $PaCO_2$ values in patients breathing room air are incompatible with life, because the corresponding PaO_2 values would be 20 to 40 mm Hg.[1]

Respiratory acidosis may be acute or chronic. In acute respiratory acidosis, $PaCO_2$ is elevated above the upper limit of the reference range (i.e., >45 mm Hg) with an associated acidemia (i.e., pH < 7.35). Acute hypercapnia elicits an immediate increase in plasma HCO_3^-, which has nothing to do with adaptation but emanates directly from mass action law: As $PaCO_2$ rises, so does HCO_3^-. In the presence of carbonic anhydrase, this effect is completed within 5 to 10 minutes from the rise in $PaCO_2$,[19] and assuming a stable level of hypercapnia, no further changes in blood acid-base equilibrium are detectable for a few hours, at which point adaptation begins to be exhibited. Adaptation to chronic hypercapnia originates from the kidneys[20] and entails adjustments in the renal ion handling. In chronic respiratory acidosis, the $PaCO_2$ is elevated above the upper limit of the reference range, with a normal or near-normal pH value secondary to renal compensation. In such conditions, plasma SID is elevated, as is bicarbonate (i.e., $HCO_3^- > 30$ mmol/L) (Fig. 131-2). Secondary adjustments of plasma SID help ameliorate the impact on acidity of the primary changes in $PaCO_2$, and these adjustments should be viewed as an integral part of the respiratory disorder.[21]

In chronic lung disease, sudden failure in ventilation may be caused by airway obstruction during disease exac-

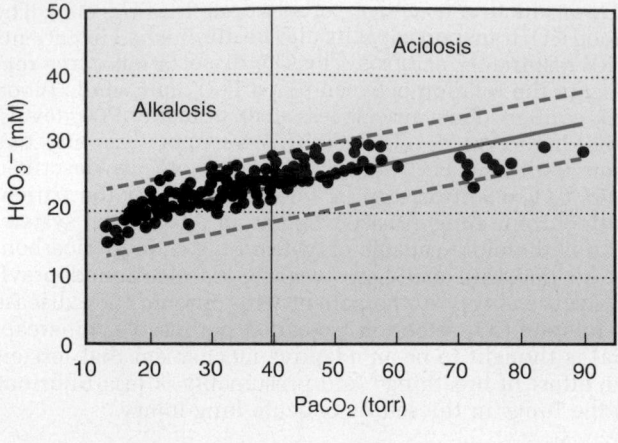

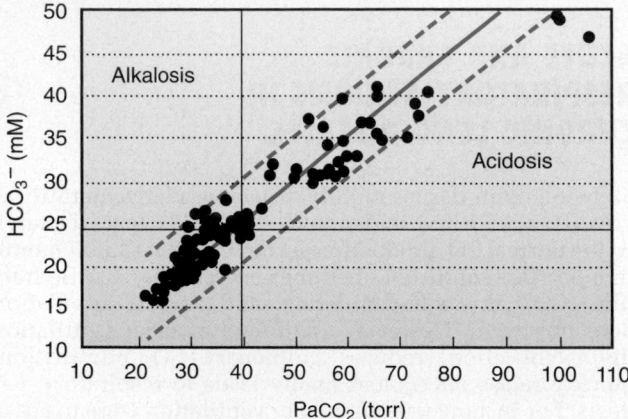

FIGURE 131-2. Relation between plasma (HCO_3^-) and $PaCO_2$ in acute and respiratory chronic respiratory disturbances. Arterial pH, $PaCO_2$, and/or HCO_3^- data sets were obtained from 21 published reports of patients considered to have purely acute (*top*) or chronic (*bottom*) respiratory acid-base problems. (From Schlichtig R, Grogono AW, Severinghaus JW: Human $PaCO_2$ and standard base excess compensation for acid-base imbalance. Crit Care Med 1998;26:1173-1179.)

erbation.[16] Chronic, sustained respiratory acidosis is also reported in chronic lung disease and is particularly severe and uncompensated in end-stage disease. As mentioned previously, hypoventilation in COPD involves multiple mechanisms, including ventilation-perfusion mismatch, leading to greater dead space ventilation, and reduced diaphragm force secondary to fatigue and hyperinflation. Lung diseases that primarily cause abnormalities in alveolar gas exchange usually do not cause hypoventilation in earlier stages but tend to cause stimulation of ventilation and hypocapnia secondary to hypoxemia. Hypercapnia occurs only if severe disease or respiratory muscle fatigue occurs. In such cases of chronic hypercapnia, pulmonary arterial hypertension and further complications often occur.[22] For instance, dysregulation of airway pH control has been reported as a new aspect of asthma pathophysiology, because changes in the acid-base equilibrium of airway lining fluid may stimulate neurogenic reflexes leading to cough, bronchospasm, and airway reactivity.[23] The morbidity and mortality of respiratory acidosis would depend on the underlying cause and associated conditions as well as the patient's compensatory mechanisms and ease of access to medical care.

Renal Compensation for Respiratory Acidosis

In acute respiratory acidosis, compensation occurs over 3 to 5 days. With renal compensation, chloride is excreted and sodium is reabsorbed, resulting in a rise in plasma SID. Plasma bicarbonate also rises about 3.5 to 4.0 mEq/L for each 10–mm Hg increase in $PaCO_2$ as a result of the new equilibrium that occurs with an increase in $PaCO_2$ and SID. The expected changes in arterial bicarbonate concentration and pH in acute and chronic respiratory acidosis are summarized in Table 131-2. A graphic depiction of expected changes in pH, pCO_2, and bicarbonate in acute and respiratory acidoses is also shown in Figure 131-3. Nevertheless, later data suggest that in patients with chronic stable hypercapnia, acid-base compensatory mechanisms might be more effective than predicted from

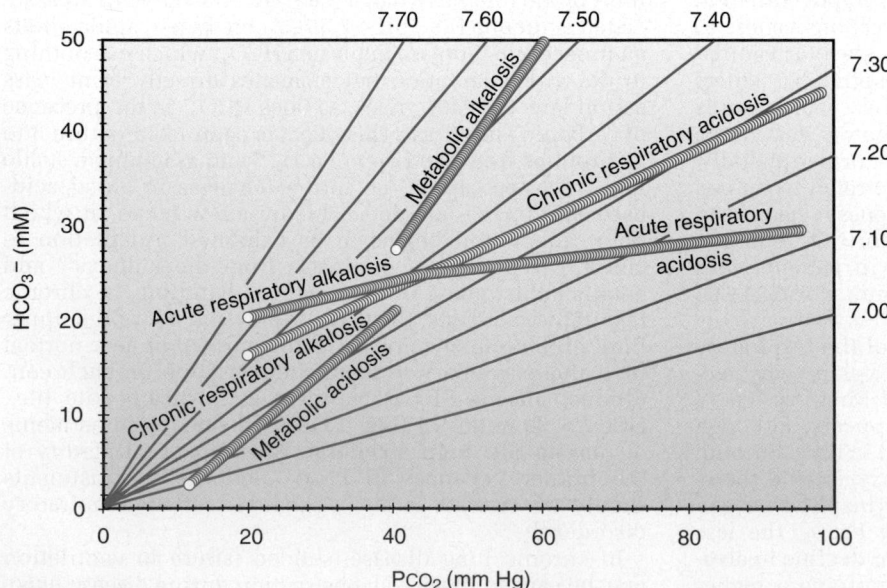

FIGURE 131-3. Acid-base map of main acid-base disorders, including acute and chronic respiratory acidosis. The different trend shown by the chronic respiratory disorder is due to compensatory renal mechanisms that raise plasma bicarbonate to restore pH to normal values. (From Schlichtig R, Grogono AW, Severinghaus JW: Current status of acid-base quantitation in physiology and medicine. Anesthesiol Clin North Am 1998;16:211-233.)

TABLE 131-2

Expected Changes in Arterial Bicarbonate and pH in Patients with Respiratory Acidosis

	HCO_3^- INCREASE PER 10-mm Hg RISE IN $PaCO_2$	pH DECREASE PER 20-mm Hg RISE IN $PaCO_2$
Acute respiratory acidosis (exacerbations or respiratory decompensation)	1 mEq/L	0.1
Chronic respiratory acidosis (stable, compensated disease)	3.5-4.0 mEq/L	0.05

use of the classic rules described previously—that is, pH decreased by 0.014 and HCO_3^- increased by 5.1 mEq/L for each 10–mm Hg increase in $PaCO_2$.[24]

ACID-BASE DISORDERS IN STABLE CHRONIC LUNG DISEASE

Patients with chronic lung disease have CO_2 retention owing to inadequate alveolar ventilation for the amount of CO_2 delivered to the lungs. $PaCO_2$ is the so-called respiratory component of acid-base balance (see Fig. 131-1) and, therefore, primary respiratory acid-base disorders are expected to be found in patients with chronic pulmonary disorders. $\dot{V}/\dot{Q}$ mismatch is typically present in chronic lung diseases like COPD.[25] The effects of $\dot{V}/\dot{Q}$ mismatch in lung disease are not easily separated from the reflex ventilatory responses to abnormal blood gas values (i.e., the ventilatory responses to hypercapnia mediated by central chemoreceptors, and to hypoxia mediated by peripheral chemoreceptors). $\dot{V}/\dot{Q}$ mismatch always causes hypoxemia (low PaO_2) and hypercapnia. However, provided that the chemoreceptor responses are normal, these abnormal blood gas values will in turn cause reflex adjustments to ventilation that will return the CO_2 to normal levels.

Meanwhile, the alveolar-arterial gradient for oxygen delivery (A-aDO_2) is not returned to normal by these ventilatory adjustments (see Table 131-1) because oxygen diffusion is poor, being limited by the carboxyhemoglobin dissociation curve. Therefore, hypoxemia may be more severe than hypercapnia in the initial stages of the disease. In fact, patients in the earlier stages often breathe faster than normal to maintain PaO_2 and thus usually have low $PaCO_2$ and normal pH values or even a slight respiratory alkalosis. However, advanced stages of chronic lung disease become severe enough to limit CO_2 exchange, and at that point, the patients begin to demonstrate chronic respiratory acidosis. Moreover, severe episodes of acute respiratory acidosis may be found transiently during exacerbations of the disease in both the earlier and later stages of disease. Acute increases in $PaCO_2$ raise the concentration of HCO_3^- according to the chemical equilibrium defined by the carbonic acid–bicarbonate buffer system. In these cases, the higher HCO_3^- does not buffer the higher H^+ concentration, so renal compensation and increased SID are required, and acidosis develops. Nevertheless, other acid-base profiles have also been reported in some cases of acute asthma, ranging from respiratory alkalosis in the most hypoxemic patients to metabolic acidosis in patients with more severe airflow obstruction.[26]

An acid-base disturbance commonly seen in patients with stable, mild to moderate COPD is fully compensated respiratory acidosis.[27-29] This fully compensated status consists of pH within normal limits with values of respiratory ($PaCO_2$) and metabolic (SID) acid-base components outside their normal ranges although in opposite directions with respect to their effect on H^+ concentration. In other words, these patients with stable chronic lung disease remain in an abnormal steady state of "acid-base unbalance." In chronic lung disease, sustained elevation of $PaCO_2$ results in a compensatory response mediated by renal mechanisms that increase plasma SID. A new chronic steady state emerges despite ventilatory limitation.[2] Because plasma SID is gradually being increased by a greater renal chloride excretion,[21,30,31] hypochloremia is sustained by a persistently depressed renal chloride reabsorption rate that accompanies chronic respiratory acidosis. Low plasma chloride levels have been reported in patients with COPD.[29] As a consequence of chloride decrease, with minor contributions from other anions such as lactate, SID (i.e., the difference between strongly dissociated cations and anions) is increased in the arterial plasma of hypercapnic patients with COPD (Fig. 131-4). The rise in plasma HCO_3^- is due to a shift in the equilibrium of H^+–HCO_3^- relationship in the arterial plasma compartment because of changes in SID. Accordingly, similar quantitative changes (in mEq/L) have been reported for HCO_3^- (dependent variable according to the Stewart physicochemical approach) and SID (independent variable) in hypercapnic patients with COPD.[29] Therefore, SID increase is a metabolic compensation that helps keep the H^+ concentration within the normal range (i.e., pH values at least higher than 7.35).

The renal response to chronic hypercapnia is not altered appreciably by moderate hypoxemia (PaO_2 45-55 mm Hg), dietary sodium or chloride restriction, moderate potassium depletion, alkali loading, or adrenalectomy.[21,32] If $PaCO_2$ is lower than 60 mm Hg, pH may be restored to normal. However, renal compensation is usually incomplete, especially with $PaCO_2$ values greater than 60 mm Hg.[1] Furthermore, renal insufficiency obviously compromises the compensation of respiratory acidosis found in chronic lung disease.

CONCLUSION

Patients with chronic lung disease have CO_2 retention owing to inadequate alveolar ventilation for the amount of CO_2 delivered to the lungs. $PaCO_2$ is the so-called respiratory component of acid-base balance, and therefore, primary respiratory acidosis is expected to be found in these patients. Respiratory acidosis associated with respiratory failure may be acute (in disease exacerbations) or chronic. In chronic respiratory acidosis, sustained elevation of $PaCO_2$ results in a compensatory response mediated

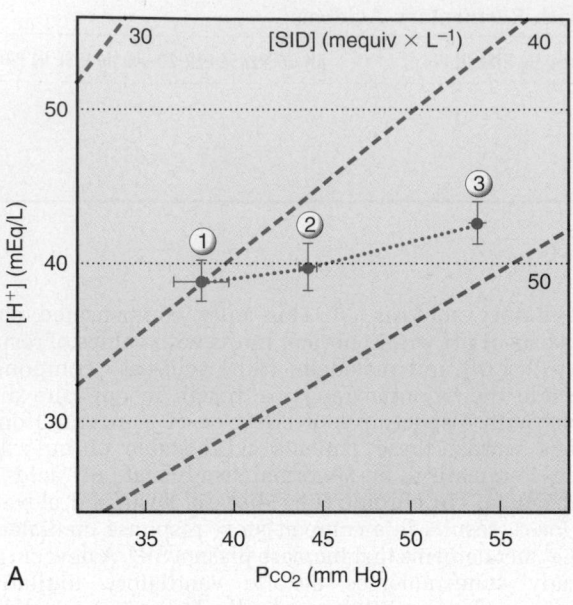

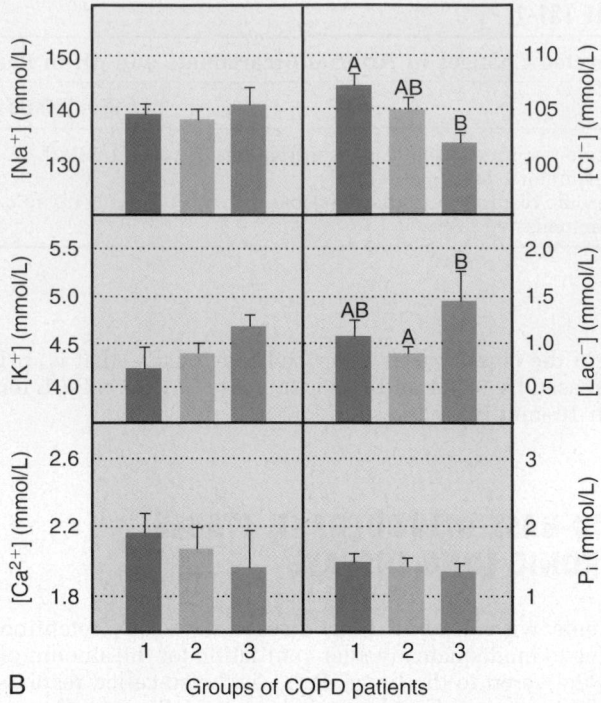

FIGURE 131-4. A, Physicochemical diagram of Stewart,[7] showing almost constant plasma H$^+$ despite changes in PaCO$_2$, through an increase in strong ion difference (SID), in three groups of patients with chronic obstructive pulmonary disease (COPD) and different levels of hypercapnia: group 1, PaCO$_2$ < 40 mm Hg; group 2, PaCO$_2$ 40-50 mm Hg; group 3, PaCO$_2$ > 50 mm Hg. In this graph, the weak acids buffer (A$_{tot}$) was assumed to be constant at 15 mEq/L. Isopleths are for different values of SID in mEq/L, and results are mean ± standard error of mean (SEM). **B,** Changes in plasma strong ions in the same patient population. *Left,* main cations; *right,* main anions and inorganic phosphate (P$_i$). The main change reported with hypercapnia was a decrease in plasma chloride. Results are mean ± SEM. (From Alfaro V, Torras R, Ibanez J, Palacios L: A physical-chemical analysis of the acid-base response to chronic obstructive pulmonary disease. Can J Physiol Pharmacol 1996;74:1229-1235.)

by renal mechanisms, including chloride excretion resulting in an increased SID. A new chronic steady state emerges when the changes in SID reach the level required to offset daily endogenous acid production despite ventilatory limitation. From a quantitative point of view, the rise in plasma HCO$_3^-$ is due to a shift in the equilibrium of H$^+$–HCO$_3^-$ relationship in the arterial plasma compartment because of changes in SID. Therefore, SID increase is a metabolic compensation that helps keep the H$^+$ concentration within the normal range (i.e., pH values at least higher than 7.35).

Key Points

1. Respiratory failure associated with chronic lung disease causes altered alveolar ventilation and resultant abnormal acid-base balance owing to primary respiratory acid-base disorders.
2. Alveolar hypoventilation may be a protective strategy that prevents excessive respiratory effort and eventual respiratory muscle fatigue and failure but reduces pulmonary CO$_2$ elimination, quickly increases PaCO$_2$ (hypercapnia), and finally may result in respiratory acidosis.
3. Respiratory acidosis may be acute or chronic. In acute respiratory acidosis, PaCO$_2$ is elevated above the upper limit of the reference range

(i.e., > 45 mm Hg) with associated acidemia (i.e., pH < 7.35).
4. In chronic respiratory acidosis, PaCO$_2$ rises above the upper limit of the reference range, with a normal or almost normal pH secondary to renal compensation and an elevated plasma bicarbonate value (i.e., HCO$_3^-$ > 30 mmol/L). The secondary adjustments in plasma SID serve to ameliorate the impact on acidity of the primary changes in PaCO$_2$, and these adjustments should be viewed as an integral part of the respiratory disorder.
5. An acid-base disturbance commonly seen in patients with stable, mild to moderate COPD is a fully compensated respiratory acidosis, consisting of pH within normal limits but values of the respiratory (PaCO$_2$) and metabolic (strong ion difference) acid-base components outside their normal ranges although in opposite directions with respect to their effect on H$^+$ concentration. The rise in plasma HCO$_3^-$ is due to a shift in the equilibrium of H$^+$–HCO$_3^-$ relationship in the arterial plasma compartment because of increased SID (due to reduced renal chloride reabsorption). The SID increase is a metabolic compensation that helps keep the H$^+$ concentration within the normal range (i.e., pH values at least higher than 7.35).

Key References

7. Stewart PA: Modern quantitative acid-base chemistry. Can J Physiol Pharmacol 1983;61:1444-1461.
10. Kellum JA: Clinical review: Reunification of acid-base physiology. Crit Care 2005;9:500-507.
21. Madias NE, Adrogue HJ: Cross-talk between two organs: How the kidney responds to disruption of acid-base balance by the lung. Nephron Physiol 2003;93:p61-p66.
29. Alfaro V, Torras R, Ibanez J, Palacios L: A physical-chemical analysis of the acid-base response to chronic obstructive pulmonary disease. Can J Physiol Pharmacol 1996;74:1229-1235.
33. Schlichtig R, Grogono AW, Severinghaus JW: Human PaCO$_2$ and standard base excess compensation for acid-base imbalance. Crit Care Med 1998;26:1173-1179.

See the companion Expert Consult website for the complete reference list.

General Treatment Concepts

CHAPTER 132

Alkalinizing Therapy in the Management of Acid-Base Disorders

Karl W. Thomas and Gregory A. Schmidt

OBJECTIVES

This chapter will:
1. Discuss the effect of alkali therapy on arterial hydrogen ion concentration, hemodynamic responses, and ventilatory requirements
2. Offer an approach to the clinical evaluation and therapeutic monitoring of patients being considered for alkalinizing treatments.
3. Describe the strengths and limitations of data on the use of alkali therapy in the treatment of acid-base disorders
4. Discuss the effect and expected result of sodium bicarbonate, tromethamine, and carbicarb treatment for patients with acid-base disorders.

The acid-base status of the critically ill patient serves as a marker for severity of illness and provides clinically relevant prognostic information.[1-3] The use of alkalinizing solutions to normalize arterial hydrogen ion concentration ([H+]) has therefore become a therapeutic option, with the rationale that correction of the acid-base disorder will improve clinical outcome. Although the use of sodium bicarbonate or other alkalinizing solutions has been established by this empirical approach, there is limited and often conflicting experimental evidence to justify this practice. Alkali therapies may either improve or worsen clinically relevant endpoints such as arterial [H+], partial pressure of carbon dioxide (PCO_2), lactate concentration, strong ion difference (SID), and cardiac output. The variability in effects of alkali therapy has contributed to a wide range of clinical practices and expert recommendations regarding these treatments.[4-6] This chapter reviews the clinical evidence regarding the effects of alkali therapy for critically ill patients, including the physiological rationale for treatment, the effects of treatment, the categorization and recognition of patients likely to benefit from alkalinizing treatments, and monitoring of the effects of treatment.

PHYSIOLOGICAL RATIONALE FOR ALKALI THERAPY

Both acidemia and alkalemia have been associated with deterioration in the function of virtually all organ systems. In particular, acidemia has been associated with clinically significant decreases in cardiovascular, respiratory, metabolic, and cerebral functions.[6] The underlying rationale for administration of bicarbonate or alkalinizing solutions to patients with acidemia can be summarized within the framework of the following four related clinical hypotheses[5,7]:
- An elevation in arterial [H+] in and of itself contributes to the observed pathology (organ dysfunction, hemodynamic instability, death).
- Administering alkali intravenously lowers the arterial [H+].
- Lowering arterial [H+] mitigates pathology or reduces the risk of deterioration.
- The benefits of alkali administration outweigh any adverse effects.

The physiological rationale for the use of alkali therapy depends upon the validity of these four main hypotheses.

Arterial Hydrogen Ion Concentration, Organ Dysfunction, and Cell Viability

Investigations using isolated cardiac preparations, whole animal models, and human tissue have consistently demonstrated depressed myocardial contractility when [H+] is raised.[8-12] However, the overall effect of increased extracellular [H+] on cellular function depends on a large number of variables, limiting generalizations about these effects. For example, in the myocardium as well as other organ systems, the end result of increased extracellular [H+] on intracellular [H+] and cellular function is related to the disease state producing the acidosis, the organ and cell type in question, catecholamine response, intracellular energy stores, and other extracellular conditions such as oxygen tension and the concentrations of sodium, chloride, and lactate.[5,13-15] Furthermore, it is likely that diseases that cause acidosis (such as sepsis) also produce profound changes in cellular energy metabolism and local microcirculatory regulation that contribute to organ dysfunction and confound the understanding of the effect of increased [H⁺]. Thus, it is little surprise that in experimental whole animal preparations, acidosis causes a wide range of myocardial consequences—no change in contractility, a marginal decrease, or a transient increase followed by decrease (despite controlled heart rate, preload, and afterload).[8,10,16]

In contrast to early assumptions that elevated [H⁺] is surely harmful, many protective or beneficial effects have also been described. In a wide variety of cell preparations and experimental conditions, raising extracellular [H⁺] has been shown to protect cells against the effects of hypoxia and energy depletion.[17-20] Furthermore, acidosis limits myocardial infarction size, stroke volume, hepatocyte death, and lung damage in models of ischemia-reperfusion injury.[21] Many potential salutary effects of acidemia have been described with regard to inflammation, free radical generation, and regulation of gene expression to suppress injury pathways. In conclusion, it is not clear that the association of acidemia with organ dysfunction or cell death is causal.

Effect of Alkalinizing Therapy on Arterial Hydrogen Ion Concentration

Bicarbonate is not one of the fundamental determinants of the acid-base state. Rather, the independent determinants of the blood [H⁺] are SID, total concentration of weak acids ([A_{tot}]), and $PaCO_2$. Sodium bicarbonate and other alkalinizing solutions affect arterial [H⁺] by changing these quantities. Administration of sodium bicarbonate increases the SID because sodium is a strong cation (whereas HCO_3^- is not a strong anion), but at the same time raises $PaCO_2$ (Fig. 132-1). The net effect of the increase in SID (which tends

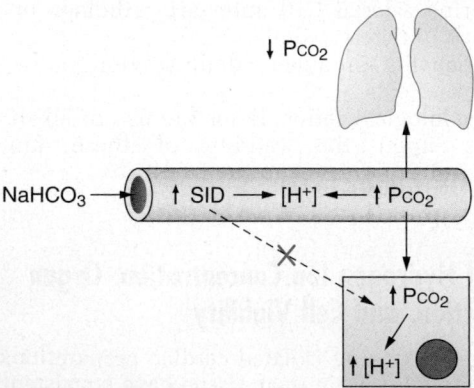

FIGURE 132-1. Sodium bicarbonate raises the blood strong ion difference (SID) (tending to lower hydrogen ion concentration [H⁺]) but also raises the $PaCO_2$ (tending to raise [H⁺]). The lungs tend to lower $PaCO_2$, modulating the effect of bicarbonate, but this effect may be limited when ventilation is limited, as in chronic obstructive pulmonary disease or during lung-protective ventilation. Because CO_2 diffuses readily into cells, raising the intracellular PCO_2, and strong ions generally equilibrate more slowly, the intracellular [H⁺] tends to rise even when the arterial [H⁺] falls. The effect of the total concentration of weak acids (A_{tot}) on arterial [H⁺] is modest and has been omitted from this figure.

to lower [H⁺]) and the increase in $PaCO_2$ (which tends to raise [H⁺]) may be to counteract each other (i.e., no change in [H⁺]) or to raise or lower the [H⁺]. The effect in an individual patient depends on other factors, such as ventilatory response and the patient's ability to exhale the generated CO_2. Thus, although most clinical studies have demonstrated that bicarbonate lowers [H⁺] in acidemic conditions, the effect is modest and in some instances (most notably during lung-protective ventilation), [H⁺] may remain constant or may even rise after bicarbonate infusion.[8,22-24]

Effect of Alkalinizing Therapy on Critical Organ Function

Several alkalinizing treatments have been evaluated for clinical use, including sodium bicarbonate, dichloroacetate, carbicarb, and tromethamine (THAM). Data for the efficacy of each of these agents are from animal models as well as clinical trials. Clinical data have been obtained in diverse patient groups, including those with lactic acidosis, cardiac arrest, or heart disease, those undergoing permissive hypercapnia ventilatory strategy, those in the postoperative state, and women who have delivered preterm babies. Generalization of these data to the typical clinical setting (adult sepsis) should take into account the specific patient characteristics as well as the dose and timing of the experimental treatments. In general, the data for alkalinizing therapy either have been developed in animal models or rest upon observational and small randomized clinical trials. In total, the available clinical evidence for the effect of alkali therapy on critical organ function should be interpreted and applied cautiously, given the limitations of these experimental methods and the results of these studies.

Sodium bicarbonate administered in animal models of lactic acidosis, hemorrhagic shock, and respiratory acidosis consistently demonstrates improvements in arterial [H⁺] but no significant effects on myocardial function or hemodynamic parameters.[8,23,25-30] Two small clinical trials of sodium bicarbonate in patients with lactic acidosis did not demonstrate any significant hemodynamic effects after administration of a bicarbonate dose of 1 to 2 mmol per kg body weight.[22,31] Animal studies in dogs and one clinical study in humans with intraoperative metabolic acidosis have reported negative effects of bicarbonate on myocardial contractility and cardiac function.[23,24,30,32] In comparison with saline or dextrose solutions, bicarbonate therapy in other clinical situations, including neonatal resuscitation and cardiopulmonary resuscitation, has no consistent beneficial effect on hemodynamic endpoints.[33,34] Bicarbonate also has not been shown to be significantly better than saline and dextrose solutions for the metabolic recovery of patients with diabetic ketoacidosis.[35] Finally, despite the inclusion of options for bicarbonate treatment in patients undergoing permissive hypercapnia and low–tidal volume ventilation protocols in the acute respiratory distress syndrome (ARDS), there are data to suggest that arterial [H⁺] may actually rise after bicarbonate therapy in this group.[36,37]

Dichloroacetate has been studied in a placebo-controlled, randomized trial of 252 subjects with lactic acidosis, most of whom were being ventilated and given vasoactive drugs.[38] Despite highly significant effects on [H⁺] and lactate, dichloroacetate had no effect on hemodynamics or survival.

TABLE 132-1

Observed Clinical Effects of Alkalinizing Therapy

TREATMENT	EXPECTED AND BENEFICIAL EFFECTS	POTENTIALLY DELETERIOUS OR ADVERSE EFFECTS
Sodium bicarbonate	Decrease in arterial hydrogen ion concentration ($[H^+]$) Increase in serum HCO_3^-	Increased arterial PCO_2 Increased $[H+]$ Hypernatremia Decreased ionized calcium Intravascular volume overload Increased serum lactate Paradoxical increased intracellular $[H^+]$
Tromethamine	Decreased arterial $[H^+]$ Constant or decreased arterial PCO_2	Hypoglycemia Hyperkalemia Extravasation-related skin necrosis Hepatic necrosis in neonates
Carbicarb	Decreased arterial $[H^+]$	Increased arterial PCO_2 (less than with bicarbonate)

Carbicarb, an equimolar solution of sodium carbonate and sodium bicarbonate, has less osmolality and lower $[H^+]$ than sodium bicarbonate. Carbicarb produces decreases in arterial $[H^+]$ similar to those for bicarbonate infusion but also causes a predictable drop in arterial $PaCO_2$. Despite these results, there are no consistent data on the effects of carbicarb on hemodynamic endpoints,[25,26,29,32] and this agent is not available for use in humans.

Tromethamine, or tris-hydroxymethyl aminomethane (THAM), is a weak base that is excreted in urine after protonation. Thus, the effect of THAM on $[H^+]$, unlike that of sodium bicarbonate, does not depend on respiratory function to excrete CO_2. THAM has shown favorable effects on normalization of $[H^+]$ and improvement in myocardial contractility in an animal heart model.[39] Small clinical trials in patients with metabolic acidosis, ARDS, or acute lung injury have demonstrated improvements in $[H^+]$, no change or decreases in arterial PCO_2, and improvements in myocardial contractility after administration of THAM.[37,40,41] Whether these physiological effects confer clinical benefit is unknown.

To briefly summarize: Alkalinizing therapies are generally effective in lowering $[H^+]$ in arterial blood in most, but not all situations (especially for sodium bicarbonate). Much less is known about the effect in tissues or at the cellular level. Moreover, despite the ability of such therapies to lower $[H^+]$, no clinically relevant benefits have been conclusively demonstrated by animal or clinical studies. In particular, the hoped-for hemodynamic effects of treating acidemia have not been confirmed in human subjects, although the trials examining this issue have generally been limited in scope. Other hypotheses have been advanced that could provide a rationale for alkalinizing treatment. For example, acidemia may negatively affect immune function or contribute to systemic inflammation.[42]

Potential Adverse Effects of Alkalinizing Therapy

In the treatment of patients with unproved medications, safety concerns are paramount. Alkalinizing therapies have generally been subjected to little scrutiny in this regard, perhaps because most severely acidemic patients who receive such treatment are expected to die. Both animal and human data have shown the potential of this therapy to reduce cardiac function and cardiac output.[23,24,30,32] Other potential adverse effects of these treatments may result from effects on $PaCO_2$, concentrations of sodium and ionized calcium, and intravascular volume. Of particular concern is the generation of carbon dioxide by bicarbonate infusion.[22,30,31,43] Although the rise in arterial PCO_2 is modest in most patients and the carbon dioxide is generally excreted with time, there may be greater effects on intracellular PCO_2 (and, therefore, on intracellular $[H^+]$) (see Fig. 132-1). Such effects on many tissues have been shown in both animal and human studies, although it is not clear that any of them is clinically meaningful. Other adverse effects of bicarbonate treatment for acidosis are hypernatremia, hyperosmolality, hypervolemia, increases in lactate concentration, decreases in ionized calcium concentration, and heightened risk of cerebral edema.[6,7,31,41,44] Reported adverse effects of THAM include hypoglycemia, hyperkalemia, extravasation-related skin necrosis, and (in neonates) hepatic necrosis (Table 132-1).[6]

CLINICAL APPROACH TO ADMINISTRATION OF ALKALINIZING THERAPY

The complexity and diversity of acid-base disorders in critically ill patients, combined with the lack of definitive evidence of benefit in human clinical trials, has produced significant variability in the use of alkali therapy. A survey of nephrology and pulmonary/critical care training directors has confirmed the absence of a standard approach to treatment recommendations for treatment of acute metabolic acidosis.[4] Surveys of published literature, including systematic reviews and meta-analyses, demonstrate controversy and the absence of consistent recommendations.[5-7,33] Given the absence of clinical data demonstrating improvements in mortality, length of stay, or other clinical outcome variables, the decision to use alkali therapy remains empirical and cannot be directly supported by robust experimental data. Clinical decision-making for or against alkali therapy thus should depend on (1) treating the underlying condition, (2) determining whether the patient is likely to benefit or suffer from the treatment, and (3) monitoring the effects of treatment.

TABLE 132-2

Patient Populations Likely to Benefit or Suffer from Alkalinizing Therapy

Groups with potential for benefit from bicarbonate or alkalinizing therapy	Patients with: Classic distal (type 1) renal tubular acidosis Severe hyperchloremic metabolic acidosis secondary to diarrhea or surgical ureteral diversion Specific poisonings and intoxications including salicylate overdose with metabolic acidosis
Groups with potential for harm from bicarbonate or alkalinizing therapy	Patients with: Hypernatremia Hypervolemia Acute renal failure Congestive heart failure or acute cardiac disease Pulmonary disease or insufficient ventilation Acute lung injury or acute respiratory distress syndrome with lung-protective ventilation Diabetic ketoacidosis

Treating the Underlying Condition

Patients with lactic acidosis due to hypoxemia, hypoperfusion, or sepsis, especially those who are hemodynamically unstable despite vasoactive drug infusions, are commonly considered for bicarbonate or other alkalinizing therapy. No published, clinical experimental evidence demonstrates improvement in hemodynamic parameters, vasopressor requirements, or clinical outcome when bicarbonate is given to these patients.[22,31] On the other hand, effective resuscitation both repairs acidosis and improves outcome.[45] Effort should be directed primarily to timely administration of antibiotics, early initiation of hemodynamic monitoring, intravascular volume repletion, lung-protective mechanical ventilation, and prophylaxis for common intensive care complications, including pneumonia, deep venous thrombosis, gastric ulceration, and skin breakdown.

Determining Whether Patient Is Likely to Benefit or Suffer from Alkali Therapy

Specific populations of critically ill patients are most likely to benefit or suffer harm from alkali treatment (Table 132-2). In general, most clinicians agree that alkali therapy may be beneficial in the management of classic distal (type 1) renal tubular acidosis, severe hyperchloremic metabolic acidosis secondary to diarrhea or surgical ureteral diversion, and specific poisonings, intoxication, and toxic ingestions, such as salicylate poisoning with metabolic acidosis. With the exception of acute toxic ingestions, most of these conditions are chronic or subacute and may be managed with oral sodium bicarbonate. For acutely ill patients in whom oral intake is not possible, intravenous bicarbonate may be indicated.

For unstable patients with septic lactic acidosis, clinicians should exhaust all effective treatment strategies before considering salvage therapy with alkali. It is important that alkali therapy not interfere with nor distract from

TABLE 132-3

Alkalinizing Drug Regimens

DRUG	HOW SUPPLIED	DOSE
Sodium bicarbonate	1 mEq/mL (generally)	1-mEq/kg bolus over 1-2 min *or* 2-5 mEq/kg/hr continuously
Tromethamine (THAM)	0.3 M solution	1 mmol/kg/hr continuously; adjust from 0.2 to 4 mmol/kg/hr to target hydrogen ion concentration

proven interventions. Lacking data on effectiveness, the clinical use of alkalinizing treatments, no matter the degree of acidemia, is discouraged. Nevertheless, because clinical studies are lacking in scope, some intensivists will choose to give bicarbonate or other treatments. Guidelines are provided in Table 132-3, with the emphasis that doses and regimens lack any evidence base. Furthermore, even calculations of dose based on, for example, volume of bicarbonate distribution, rely on outmoded concepts of acid-base physiology.

There are specific patients in whom administration of sodium bicarbonate is contraindicated or may result in clinical deterioration. Such patients include those with hypernatremia, hypervolemia, or hyperosmolality, because treatment may worsen these conditions in the absence of clear benefit. Acutely ill patients with renal failure and acidemia may not tolerate the sodium and water necessary to deliver bicarbonate and thus should be considered for hemodialysis. Similarly, patients with congestive heart failure, unstable cardiac disease, or cardiac arrest may experience clinical deterioration as the result of intravascular volume changes or deleterious effects on cardiac function.[23,24,34,43] Given the consistently demonstrated effects in both animal and human investigations on elevations of $PaCO_2$ after sodium bicarbonate therapy, patients with limited pulmonary function or inability to increase alveolar ventilation should also not receive bicarbonate-based alkali therapy. Finally, patients with diabetic ketoacidosis should not receive bicarbonate therapy, given the consistent results of clinical trials showing no clinically significant benefit.[35]

Monitoring the Effects of Alkali Treatment

Given the diversity in both the diseases and patients with metabolic acidosis who may be considered for alkali treatment, no uniform recommendations on therapeutic endpoints can be made. These decisions depend on the underlying disease state, comorbid conditions, and available treatment options. Carbicarb is not available for patient use in the United States, and THAM may not be consistently available or routinely supplied by hospital pharmacies. If the clinician determines that the patient is likely to benefit from alkalinizing therapy, a rational framework for treatment decisions should include careful attention to physiological parameters that can be frequently and easily measured. The clinician should actively determine the primary variables that will function as indicators of therapeutic effect (global perfusion, work of breathing, stability of cardiac rhythm) and the frequency of clinical monitoring. Therapeutic monitoring variables should include arterial [H^+], $PaCO_2$, hemodynamic status, intravascular volume, patient-ventilator interaction, and concentrations of serum sodium, calcium, and potassium. Further clinical studies are needed to resolve uncertain aspects of alkalinizing therapy, such as dosage calculations, bolus or continuous dosing regimens, and meaningful endpoints such as the target [H^+].

CONCLUSION

Available evidence from animal and human studies does not show consistent benefit of administration of bicarbonate, carbicarb, or THAM. Although a limited number of patients may benefit from sodium bicarbonate treatment, the majority of patients with metabolic and respiratory acidosis do not. As a result of effects on intravascular volume, serum sodium concentration, and arterial $PaCO_2$, a large number of critically ill patients have contraindications to bicarbonate treatment. The clinician should focus therapeutic interventions for patients with acute acid-base disorders on the timely initiation of treatments known to be effective for the underlying disease.

Key Points

1. No consistent experimental results in animal or human studies support the routine use of alkali therapy for critically ill patients with acidemia.
2. Alkali therapy has been shown to result in both favorable and unfavorable effects on arterial [H^+], $PaCO_2$, and organ system function.
3. The routine use of alkali therapy in critically ill patients has been established through empirical and historical practice patterns, but there is little

experimental evidence demonstrating clinically useful effects of these treatments, such as hemodynamic stability, duration of mechanical ventilation, organ failures, length of stay, or mortality.

4. Despite a paucity of supportive evidence, the alkalinizing solution most commonly in clinical use is sodium bicarbonate. An additional option with limited evidence for efficacy is tromethamine.
5. Bicarbonate treatment may be contraindicated in patients with evidence of volume overload, hypernatremia, hyperosmolality, severe cardiac disease, congestive heart failure, or limited pulmonary function.

Key References

3. Stacpoole PW, Wright EC, Baumgartner TG, et al: Natural history and course of acquired lactic acidosis in adults. DCA-Lactic Acidosis Study Group. Am J Med 1994;97:47-54.
7. Forsythe SM, Schmidt GA: Sodium bicarbonate for the treatment of lactic acidosis. Chest 2000;117:260-267.
22. Mathieu D, Neviere R, Billard V, et al: Effects of bicarbonate therapy on hemodynamics and tissue oxygenation in patients with lactic acidosis: A prospective, controlled clinical study. Crit Care Med 1991;19:1352-1356.
31. Cooper DJ, Walley KR, Wiggs BR, Russell JA: Bicarbonate does not improve hemodynamics in critically ill patients who have lactic acidosis: A prospective, controlled clinical study. Ann Intern Med 1990;112:492-498.
37. Kallet RH, Jasmer RM, Luce JM, et al: The treatment of acidosis in acute lung injury with tris-hydroxymethyl aminomethane (THAM). Am J Respir Crit Care Med 2000;161:1149-1153.

See the companion Expert Consult website for the complete reference list.

CHAPTER 133

The Role of Renal Replacement Therapy in the Management of Acid-Base Disorders

Karl Reiter

OBJECTIVES

This chapter will:
1. Present the indications for and goals of acid-base control by renal replacement therapy.
2. Describe mechanisms at work in renal replacement therapy that influence acid-base state.
3. Discuss the clinical factors that should be considered in the choice of buffer in replacement fluids—liver dysfunction, lactate intolerance, and hemodynamic instability.

Renal replacement therapy (RRT) is a powerful tool in the management of acid-base disorders. In a 70-kg adult undergoing hemofiltration with 1.5 L/hr ultrafiltrate, eight to ten times the total amount of plasma water can be filtered within 24 hours (including mineral acids and bases dissolved in plasma water, which are lost in the ultrafiltrate) and replaced by a solution containing specific buffers. Buffer type and concentration can be chosen according to specific goals and administered without major volume restrictions because fluid balance can be maintained and regulated by adjustments in ultrafiltration rate.

Rarely, an acid-base disorder is a primary or exclusive indication for RRT. In the critically ill patient, this modality is initiated more commonly for other reasons, but concomitant consequences for a patient's acid-base state must be considered in every procedure performed. Therefore, mechanisms of acid-base control during RRT are important to understand and have been the subject of investigations.

Acidoses caused by mineral acids, by virtue of their low molecular weight and high diffusibility, are amenable to treatment by hemofiltration, hemodialysis, and peritoneal dialysis. Depending on molecular weight, organic acids can be removed by RRT as well, but only to a variable extent. Hemofiltration is superior to peritoneal dialysis and hemodialysis in removal of substances of middle molecular range.

RRT almost always is a symptomatic therapy of acid-base disorders, so treatment of the underlying disease is essential. Exceptions are some rare intoxications.

AIMS OF ACID-BASE INTERVENTION

Under most circumstances, RRT can correct abnormal blood pH within 12 to 24 hours, and a balanced acid-base milieu can be maintained for 24 hours a day with use of a continuous technique. The goal and extent of correcting acid-base disorders in the critically ill patient have become matters of debate. Severe metabolic acidosis has a plethora of adverse effects.[1] Nevertheless, the benefit of correction of acidosis through administration of buffer has been strongly questioned.[2,3] Bicarbonate administration in metabolic acidosis raises lactate production,[1] does not improve hemodynamics,[4] and may even be detrimental.[5] Complete or too rapid correction of blood pH therefore may not be indicated in most if not all critically ill patients. Specific physiological endpoints of acid-base intervention via RRT in the critically ill population have not been defined.

On the other hand, metabolic acidosis may be more a marker of severity of illness than a major causative factor in morbidity or mortality in the acutely ill patient, and refractoriness of acidosis to RRT appears to define a subpopulation with very high mortality.[6,7]

ACID-BASE INDICATIONS FOR RENAL REPLACEMENT THERAPY

Severe metabolic acidosis caused or aggravated by ARF is considered a standard indication for RRT, because intravenous buffering rarely suffices when kidney function is compromised. Severe acidosis is arbitrarily defined by most authorities as a pH value less than 7.10 or 7.15. Most often metabolic acidosis occurs in the context of further ARF-induced disturbances, such as hypervolemia, electrolyte disturbances, and intolerable nutritional restriction, and serves as an adjunctive indication.

Rarely, RRT is indicated for the treatment of an acid-base disorder in the absence of ARF. This may be the case with certain intoxications producing a severe lactic acidosis, in which RRT serves the goal of eliminating the toxin as well as ameliorating the acidosis. Examples are intoxications with metformin,[8] methanol, and ethylene glycol. In the neonatal and pediatric age group, some inborn errors of metabolism (organic acidemias) may manifest as severe acidosis, often accompanied by hyperammonemia. When conservative measures fail, continuous venovenous hemofiltration or intermittent hemodialysis is indicated to rapidly remove both ammonia and the offending organic acid. Maple syrup urine disease may manifest as severe acidemia, necessitating RRT.[9] Peritoneal dialysis is not sufficiently effective in patients with these disorders.

Another rare indication for continuous RRT may be the oliguric patient with cardiac failure and severe metabolic alkalosis due to diuretic-induced chloride depletion.[10] In such a patient, a delicate volume balance must be maintained, and less invasive therapies, such as addition of acetazolamide, may not suffice.

Many critically ill patients with and without ARF experience lactic acidosis because of severe sepsis or hemodynamic compromise. Decreased lactate metabolism has been shown to be the underlying mechanism.[11] Only minor amounts (<3%-5%) of lactate are removed by continuous RRT.[12] Treatment of lactic acidosis must always address the underlying disease.

MECHANISMS OF ACID-BASE CONTROL IN RENAL REPLACEMENT THERAPY

The precise mechanisms of the acid-base effects of RRT are complex and still incompletely understood. New insights into the pathophysiology of acid-base disorders in critically ill patients have been gained through applications of physiochemical principles.[13,14] These efforts have led to a broader understanding of the acid-base changes exerted by RRT as well.

Acid-Base Disturbances in Acute Renal Failure

Metabolic acidosis of ARF has conventionally been regarded as a high–anion gap acidosis caused by the accumulation of urate, phosphate, sulfate, hippuric acid, and diverse acids of intermediary metabolism. The major role of strong ions (most importantly Na^+, Cl^-, and lactate) and weak acids (predominantly albumin and phosphate) in determining acid-base status has been underappreciated. Important acid-base effects are exerted by increasing plasma sodium concentration or decreasing plasma chloride or albumin, for instance, all of which have alkalinizing effects. According to this concept, calculation of the charge differences between measured strong cations and anions, including carbon dioxide and the weak acids phosphate and albumin, allows the quantification of the amount of further unmeasured substances with acidifying effect (unmeasured anions) (the strong ion gap).

Several investigators have analyzed acid-base changes in the critically ill population with ARF according to these more comprehensive principles.[15-17] In one study, patients with ARF being treated in an intensive care unit (ICU) showed a higher degree of metabolic acidosis, due to higher plasma levels of lactate, phosphate, and unmeasured anions, than ICU patients (matched for severity of illness) with normal renal function (Fig. 133-1). An incomplete compensation by the alkalinizing effect of hypoalbuminemia occurred in the patients with ARF. Interestingly,

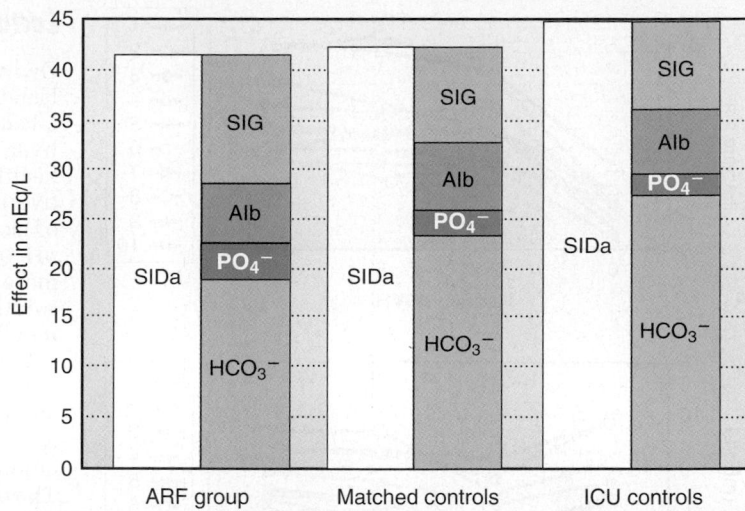

FIGURE 133-1. Physiochemical analysis of anionic and cationic charges in patients with acute renal failure (ARF group), a control group without ARF matched for severity of illness (matched controls), and a control group treated in an intensive care unit (ICU controls) who did not have ARF. The ARF group was associated with a high strong ion gap (SIG) and a high phosphate concentration compared with the other groups. SIDa, mean apparent strong ion difference; SIDe, mean effective strong ion difference, which is equal to the sum of Alb (albumin effect), PO_4^- (phosphate effect) and HCO_3^- (CO_2 effect). (Modified from Rocktaeschel J, Morimatsu H, Uchino S, et al: Acid-base status of critically ill patients with acute renal failure: Analysis based on Stewart-Figge methodology. Crit Care 2003;7:R60-R66.)

this effect led to a normal anion gap in half of the patients with ARF despite elevations of unmeasured anions, revealed only by an analysis of strong ion differences (SIDs).[15]

Acid-Base Mass Balances in Renal Replacement Therapy

The acidifying substances removed by RRT are phosphate and unmeasured anions. Concurrently, during standard continuous venovenous hemofiltration (CVVH), up to 800 to 1000 mmol per day bicarbonate is lost in the ultrafiltrate. Convective bicarbonate and electrolyte losses are generally equivalent to plasma levels of these solutes multiplied by the ultrafiltration rate. Lactate removal is significantly less because of lower plasma concentrations and contributes to total lactate clearance by less than 3% to 5%[12,18] when an ultrafiltration rate of 1 L/hr is applied. Conversely, net lactate gain during continuous RRT may amount to about 50 to 65 mmol/hr at a rate up to 2 L/hr of lactate-buffered replacement fluid, compared with an endogenous lactate production during sepsis of 60 mmol/hr[11] to 90 mmol/hr[18] and a capacity to metabolize lactate of about 100 mmol/hr in a normal adult.

Mass balances of electrolytes are greatly influenced by the site of replacement fluid infusion, even in isovolemic—that is, zero-balance—CVVH. This finding was reported in a study applying ultrafiltration rates higher than 35 mL/kg/hr with a stepwise decrease in the amount of predilution fluid from 6 L/hr to 0 L/hr and concomitant increase in postdilution fluid rates.[19] Significant changes in mass transfer were noted for sodium, calcium, magnesium, chloride, and total CO_2. With decreasing predilution rates, sodium gains increased, whereas chloride mass transfer changed from massive gains with high predilution rates to significant losses with increasing postdilution rates.

In several replacement fluids, chloride levels may be high and SID therefore low, a combination that may lead to a chloride gain with possible acidifying and volume effects. On the other hand, serum chloride changes are not directly predictable from chloride concentrations in the replacement fluid. The sieving coefficient may be greater than 1, and the serum chloride level may fall below the

replacement fluid level, exerting an alkalinizing effect.[17] However, clinically relevant effects may be seen only in high-volume continuous RRT.

In an analysis of acid-base changes during high-volume hemofiltration using lactate-buffered solutions, iatrogenic hyperlactatemia with a mean increase of about 5 mmol/L developed, but the pH and base excess changes associated with this increase were only minor and transient. This finding was due to a decrease in chloride, unmeasured anions, albumin, and phosphate, which fully compensated for possible acidifying effects of lactate (Fig. 133-2).[17]

High-volume continuous RRT and intermittent hemodialysis are the fastest ways to ameliorate acid-base disturbances, although continuous RRT may confer superior acid-base control on a day-to-day basis.[20] An outcome benefit favoring one technique has not been shown.

REPLACEMENT SOLUTIONS

During RRT, buffer must be administered because of losses in the ultrafiltrate and to compensate for an accumulated base deficit as well as ongoing buffer consumption. Most centers use commercial replacement solutions (Table 133-1). It is worth noting that solute concentrations differ widely. Custom-made solutions carry substantial risk of contamination, and errors in solute concentration have led to death.

The site of buffer administration, whether infused as predilution or postdilution fluid, added to the dialysate, or given intravenously, may be chosen according to local preferences. Important caveats are as follows:
- Acid-base effects will differ according to site of administration.[19]
- Utmost caution must be applied in the use of the intravenous route, because there is no automatic coupling of ultrafiltration or dialysate flow rates to buffer administration rates.

Type of Buffer

Biochemical and metabolic considerations are important in the choice of buffers in RRT in critically ill patients. Possible substances are bicarbonate, lactate, acetate, and

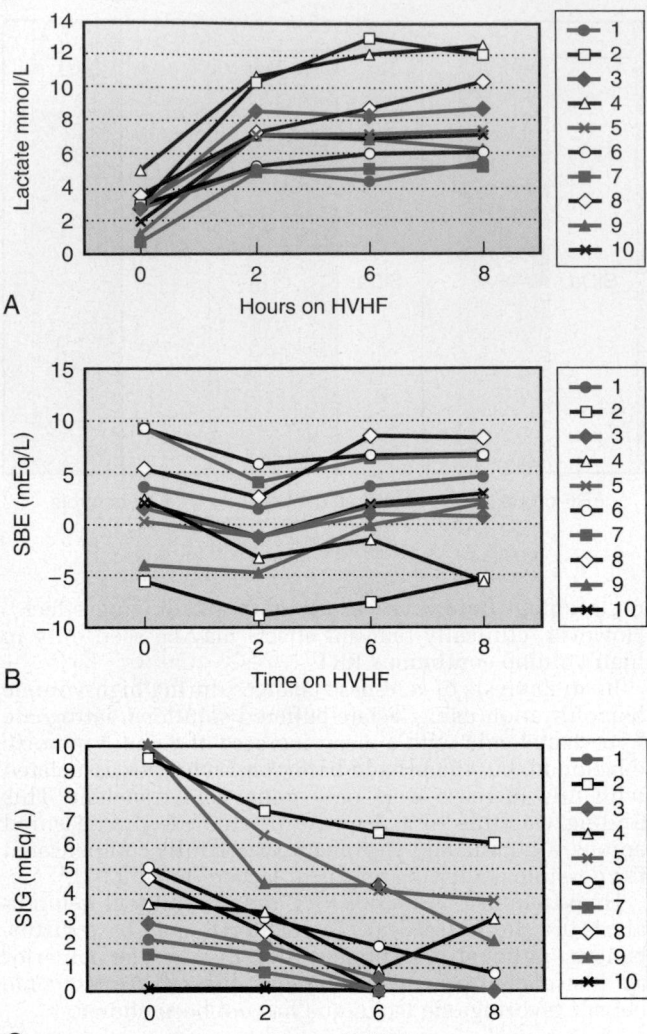

FIGURE 133-2. Acid-base changes during high-volume hemofiltration (HVHF). Diagrams illustrate individual changes in lactate concentration (**A**), standard base excess (SBE) (**B**), and strong ion gap (SIG) (**C**) from baseline during HVHF ($n = 10$ patients in septic shock). SBE is only transiently decreased in spite of rising lactate levels. Unmeasured (acidifying) anions best quantified by strong ion gap (SIG) are removed by HVHF and compensate for rising lactate concentration to an important extent. (Modified from Cole L, Bellomo R, Baldwin I, et al: The impact of lactate-buffered high-volume hemofiltration on acid-base balance. Intensive Care Med 2003;29:1113-1120.)

citrate. Acetate has been abandoned because of inferior efficiency and well-known untoward side effects.[21,22]

Bicarbonate

A bicarbonate-based solution may seem to be the most physiological choice, but issues of stability and cost hinder its use in many parts of the world. Because of possible calcium (and magnesium) precipitation, Ca-containing or Mg-containing replacement solutions cannot be mixed until shortly before use. Moreover, CO_2 may be lost by diffusion from plastic containers, thereby decreasing bicarbonate concentration. Massive application of bicarbonate carries a risk of raising blood P_{CO_2}, an effect that may be undesirable in patients with acute respiratory distress syndrome.

Lactate

Owing to its availability, high stability, and low cost, lactate has been most commonly used as buffer in CRRT. L-Lactate, the physiological isomer, is metabolized by liver, heart and skeletal muscle as well as the kidney in healthy humans. Either the gluconeogenetic or the oxidative pathway may be used, and one proton per molecule of lactate is consumed in either reaction, thereby reducing pH. D-Lactate, the isomer of L-lactate, is metabolized much more slowly. Unfortunately, some lactate replacement solutions still contain small amounts of D-lactate, which may have adverse neuropsychiatric effects.

In critically ill patients, lactate production is increased but lactate utilization may be impaired. This has been shown in septic patients.[11] Use of lactate-based RRT administers an additional lactate load. Lactate is a strong anion that has acidifying effects when not metabolized. The endogenous production of lactate is enhanced by ischemia, endotoxin, and other inflammatory mediators, including epinephrine. On the other hand, lactate metabolism is significantly decreased by reduced liver blood flow or hepatic insufficiency. Nevertheless, an exogenous lactate load has been shown to be rapidly metabolized even in cardiogenic shock[23] and after extensive liver resection.[24]

The metabolic fate of lactate administered in amounts exceeding the capacity of metabolizing pathways is incompletely understood. Bollmann and colleagues[18] have shown that in severely ill patients with increased plasma lactate concentrations, an exogenous lactate load may lead to higher glucose turnover without aggravating acidosis or causing hemodynamic compromise. These investigators found that gluconeogenesis was increased and that hyperglycemia frequently occurred.[18]

Iatrogenic hyperlactatemia induced by lactate-containing solutions may impede the interpretation of blood gas measurements.

Citrate

Regional anticoagulation of the extracorporeal circuit with citrate instead of systemic heparinization is being used increasingly in order to avoid iatrogenic bleeding complications. Citrate is metabolized by the liver, whereby three protons are consumed per molecule of citrate. Routinely, 18 to 28 mmol/hr of citrate must be infused during CVVH.[25] No further buffer should be administered, and rigorous monitoring of pH is required. If anticoagulation is deemed necessary at all, citrate must be used with utmost caution in patients with septic shock and hepatic failure; citrate metabolism may be impaired in such patients, and aggravation of metabolic acidosis has been described.[26] The latter effect occurs because citrate is a negatively charged strong ion and therefore has acidifying effects. Metabolic alkalosis may occur when citrate is fully metabolized. HCl infusion may be necessary for correction.

Amount of Buffer Required

The amount of buffer needed is defined by the accumulated deficit as well as by ongoing consumption and losses (including ultrafiltrate losses). Therefore, supraphysiologic concentrations should routinely be used.

With use of a buffer concentration of at least 35 mmol/L in replacement or dialysis solutions and ultrafiltration rates exceeding 1 L/hr, pH normalization can be achieved

TABLE 133-1

Composition of Typical Replacement Solutions

CONSTITUENT (mmol/L)	LACTATE-BASED SOLUTION[‡]	BICARBONATE-BASED SOLUTION[§]
Na^+	140	140
K^+	1	2
Cl^-	100	105
Ca^{2+}	1.6	0
Mg^{2+}	0.8	1.5
Lactate	46	—
Bicarbonate	—	35
Glucose	10.8	0
SID*[†]	43 (when lactate is fully metabolized)	39

*Normal value for SID (strong ion difference) in plasma is 39 ± 1 mmol/L.
[†]Effect on blood pH of different replacement solutions is affected by the value for SID. High values have alkalinizing effects, low values have acidifying effects. Lactate has to be metabolized fully for the replacement fluid to exert an alkalinizing effect. High chloride concentrations in replacement solutions have an acidifying effect because of low SID, and vice versa. According to manufacturer, concentrations differ markedly. With Ca^{2+} or K^+ supplements, chloride concentration will be increased and SID lowered.
[‡]Baxter Pharmaceuticals, Deerfield, IL.
[§]Dialysis Solutions Inc., Whitby, ON, Canada.

by continuous RRT within 24 hours in most patients with ARF. Not infrequently, metabolic alkalosis may be induced in these patients after the second or third day of continuous RRT, when deficits are corrected and sources of acidosis have been treated. In a large retrospective study, metabolic alkalemia developing during CRRT was not associated with increased mortality.[40]

CLINICAL TRIALS

The choice of buffers for replacement solutions or dialysate in continuous RRT has been the subject of several clinical studies in critically ill patients. Lactate- and bicarbonate-containing solutions have been shown to convey better acidosis control and hemodynamic stability than acetate-based solutions.[22] The evidence for or against lactate or bicarbonate as replacement buffer is less clearcut. The outcome parameters that have been investigated are acidosis control, hemodynamic tolerance, and mortality. Case series and retrospective cohort studies predominate, and few prospective, randomized, controlled studies have been performed.[18,27-29]

Effectiveness of Bicarbonate and Lactate Replacement Solutions in Acid-Base Control

Early uncontrolled case series reported better acidosis control in severely ill patients when lactate was replaced by bicarbonate in replacement fluids.[30] Controlled studies showed controversial results,[18,27-29,31,32] however, the majority reported equal efficacy for the two solutions.[18,27,29,31] All but one study[18] used continuous RRT with ultrafiltration rates of 1 to 1.5 L/hr.

Iatrogenic Hyperlactatemia

Hyperlactatemia often occurs in the patient receiving lactate-buffered replacement fluids. With replacement fluid rates of 1 to 2 L/hr, plasma lactate rarely rises more than 2 or 3 mmol/L, although it typically increases more

than 5 mmol/L in high-volume hemofiltration (HVHF). In only a minority of cases is iatrogenic hyperlactatemia accompanied by lactic acidosis (see later). Whether hyperlactatemia without ensuing acidosis increases morbidity is unclear. One study reported hyperglycemia with very high lactate loads.[18]

In two studies conducted in critically ill patients with ARF but without severe acidosis at the start of RRT, the administration of up to 210 mmol/hr of lactate replacement fluid led to only modest changes in pH.[33,34] Only one study noted hemodynamic deterioration.[33] On the other hand, in a randomized study comparing lactate-based HVHF with standard CVVH about 270 mmol/hr lactate was administered in the high-volume hemofiltration arm.[17] Mean lactate levels rose from 2.5 to 7.3 mmol/L, but pH and base excess values decreased only mildly and were restored to normal within 6 hours. Patients with hepatic dysfunction or high initial lactate levels were not included in these studies.

Lactic Acidosis at Initiation of Renal Replacement Therapy

An important clinical subgroup are patients with high initial blood lactate levels, who are the most severely ill. Most investigators have excluded such patients from studies comparing lactate-buffered with bicarbonate-buffered solutions for continuous RRT. With regard to this subgroup, Zimmerman and colleagues[27] reported only a trend toward better acidosis control with the use of bicarbonate dialysis solutions. Mortality trended higher when lactate levels showed a further increase during lactate dialysis (so-called lactate intolerance). In an uncontrolled case series, lactate-intolerant patients (defined as demonstrating an increase in plasma lactate value of more than 5 mmol/L after 90 minutes of lactate-buffered hemofiltration) had better acid-base control after a switch to bicarbonate-based solutions.[35]

Persistent lactic acidosis should always incite efforts to identify hidden causes of lactate overproduction (suboptimal hemodynamic state, septic or necrotic focus). Acidosis refractory to HVHF or continuous venovenous hemodiafiltration (ultrafiltration 2 L/hr plus dialysis 1 L/hr) using bicarbonate replacement fluid has been shown to define a subgroup of patients with septic shock who have high mortality.[6,7]

Concomitant Hepatic Dysfunction

When hepatic dysfunction accompanies ARF, acid-base disturbances are aggravated. Plasma lactate and unmeasured anion values may be higher than the levels seen in isolated ARF. These elevations may persist even during CVVH using bicarbonate replacement at 2 L/hr,[36] necessitating higher ultrafiltration volumes in patients with hepatic insufficiency. Lactate metabolism is impaired in hepatic insufficiency. Therefore, lactate-buffered RRT must be used with caution in patients with hepatic dysfunction and ARF.

In an early study, patients with combined liver failure and renal failure, lactate-based continuous RRT led to hyperlactatemia with ensuing lactic acidosis and hemodynamic compromise.[30] Other studies could not confirm this finding, however. A prospective study reported significantly higher lactate levels in patients with hepatic dysfunction during lactate dialysis than during bicarbonate dialysis, but because of the low number of patients studied, the investigators were unable to demonstrate a significant effect on acid-base control, hemodynamic parameters, or mortality.[27] In a nonrandomized crossover trial, patients with multiple-organ failure with and without hepatic dysfunction showed no differences in pH or hemodynamic effects with either lactate dialysis or bicarbonate dialysis.[32]

Although data are not conclusive and the level of hepatic dysfunction leading to intolerance of a lactate load has not been defined, it is probably wise to avoid lactate replacement solutions in patients with all grades of hepatic insufficiency. At a minimum, lactate levels must be monitored closely if lactate replacement is used in a patient with hepatic disease.

Lactate versus Bicarbonate: Hemodynamic and Mortality Effects

Whether hemodynamic adverse effects are more common with lactate than with bicarbonate replacement solutions in patients without liver dysfunction is controversial. Studies have shown contradictory results without clear explanation. Barenbrock and associates,[28] in the largest study (117 patients), demonstrated significantly more cardiovascular adverse events in patients treated with lactate replacement solutions. Previous cardiovascular disease was a prominent risk factor. In a retrospective study conducted in 54 patients with multiple-organ failure, continuous RRT with bicarbonate solutions led to lower requirements for inotropic agents than continuous RRT using lactate solutions.[32] On the other hand, Thomas and colleagues[29] found equal results for lactate-based and bicarbonate-based replacement fluids with respect to hemodynamic and oxygen transport variables. In a larger prospective study in 132 patients, no difference was found between bicarbonate-based and lactate-based fluids in terms of acidosis control and hemodynamic variables.[31] A prospective crossover trial in 8 patients with severe multiple-organ failure could not identify differences in acid-base control or hemodynamic parameters between lactate-based and bicarbonate-based solutions.[18] No study

has been able to demonstrate that bicarbonate-based and lactate-based replacement solutions have different effects on mortality, but patient numbers in all studies were generally limited.

Recommendations by a working group of the Acute Dialysis Quality Initiative published in 2002 stated, after analysis of then-available evidence, that lactate and bicarbonate solutions are able to correct metabolic acidosis with similar efficacy in most patients undergoing continuous RRT.[37] The group recommended that bicarbonate be used for patients with lactic acidosis or liver failure and when HVHF is used.

Effect of Ultrafiltration Rate

The application of high ultrafiltration rates allows the administration of higher amounts of buffer. Moreover, and probably more important, more substances causing acidosis are removed with such rates. Brause and coworkers[38] demonstrated a significantly more rapid pH normalization with an ultrafiltration rate of 1.5 L/hr than with 1 L/hr. Patients with ARF and hepatic insufficiency often need higher ultrafiltration rates, 2 L/hr or higher, for correction of acidosis.

Honore and associates[6] reported impressive clinical results for HVHF with bicarbonate replacement fluid in patients with severe refractory shock. Eleven of the 20 patients in their study showed improvement in metabolic acidosis and hemodynamic state, which translated into a significantly better survival rate.[6] In another study, a significant decrease in vasopressor requirements was achieved with the use of lactate-based HVHF in patients with septic shock.[39] This decrease probably represents the beneficial effect of high ultrafiltration rates. Therefore, the choice of buffers may influence prognosis less than the rate of ultrafiltration.

CONCLUSIONS

RRT is a unique and powerful tool in the management of metabolic acid-base disturbances. Amenable to treatment by RRT are acid-base disorders caused by highly water-soluble mineral acids and low-molecular-weight organic acids. ARF is the most common underlying disease in patients in whom RRT is indicated. Control of pH can be achieved in less than 24 hours in the majority of cases, and a constant acid-base milieu can be maintained 24 hours a day, by continuous RRT.

Lactic acidosis frequently develops in critically ill patients. Despite a high sieving coefficient, lactate removal by RRT is relatively insignificant, given the high endogenous production rates, for instance, in sepsis. Therefore, RRT is not a primary treatment for lactic acidosis.

The principal mechanism of action of RRT is the removal of acids by ultrafiltration or diffusion. Concomitant losses of base by ultrafiltration must be accounted for by infusion of replacement solutions containing buffer. Buffer must be administered in supraphysiologic concentration to compensate for preexisting or ongoing deficits. Gain or loss of strong ions (e.g., major blood electrolytes and lactate) plays a significant role in acid-base changes and differs according to RRT technique. Ultrafiltration rate may be more important than buffer type in severely ill patients.

Probably the best choice for replacement or dialysis fluids in RRT is a bicarbonate-based solution. Lactate exerts incompletely understood metabolic effects, and lactate metabolism may be impaired in hepatic insufficiency. When availability, stability, or cost imposes constraints on the use of bicarbonate solutions, most patients—except those who are in overt liver failure or have severe lactic acidosis (arbitrarily defined as a blood lactate level >5 mmol/L)—can probably be safely managed with lactate solutions. Bicarbonate solutions should be used in liver failure, with HVHF, and in patients with deteriorating lactic acidosis or hemodynamic state during lactate RRT.

Key Points

1. Renal replacement therapy is a therapeutic modality by which, under most circumstances, abnormal blood pH can be corrected within 12 to 24 hours.
2. The most common indication is acute renal failure, but renal replacement therapy may be indicated in severe acid-base disturbances without acute renal failure, for example, intoxication and the refractory acidosis due to severe shock.
3. Mechanisms at work in acid-base control by renal replacement therapy include acid removal and replacement of buffer but extend to changes in strong ions (e.g., sodium and chloride) and weak anions. These mechanisms are best explained by a physiochemical analysis.
4. Hepatic insufficiency and severe lactic acidosis may lead to intolerance of lactate-buffered replacement solutions with deterioration of acidosis and hemodynamic compromise.

5. Higher ultrafiltration rates confer better acidosis control. The rate of ultrafiltration may be more important than the choice of buffer.
6. Bicarbonate-based replacement fluids are the preferred choice for renal replacement therapy in critically ill patients. When availability, stability, or cost imposes constraints on the use of bicarbonate solutions, most patients (except those in overt liver failure or with severe lactic acidosis) can probably be safely managed with lactate solutions. In high-volume hemofiltration, use of bicarbonate replacement solutions is recommended.

Key References

17. Cole L, Bellomo R, Baldwin I, et al: The impact of lactate-buffered high-volume hemofiltration on acid-base balance. Intensive Care Med 2003;29:1113-1120.
19. Uchino S, Cole L, Morimatsu H, et al: Solute mass balance during isovolaemic high volume haemofiltration. Intensive Care Med 2003;29:1541-1546.
28. Barenbrock M, Hausberg M, Matzkies F, et al: Effects of bicarbonate- and lactate-buffered replacement fluids on cardiovascular outcome in CVVH patients. Kidney Int 2000;58:1751-1757.
31. Heering P, Ivens K, Thümer O, et al: The use of different buffers during continuous hemofiltration in critically ill patients with acute renal failure. Intensive Care Med 1999;25:1244-1251.
37. Schetz M, Leblanc M, Murray PT: The Acute Dialysis Quality Initiative. Part VII: Fluid composition and management in CRRT. Adv Renal Replacement Ther 2002;9:282-289.

See the companion Expert Consult website for the complete reference list.

Aspects of Metabolisms, Endocrinology, and Hematology in Critical Illness and Acute Renal Injury

Basic Physiology

CHAPTER 134

Energy Requirement and Consumption in the Critically Ill Patient

Lindsay D. Plank and Graham L. Hill

OBJECTIVES

This chapter will:
1. Describe the pathogenesis of hypermetabolism in critical illness.
2. Delineate the components of total energy expenditure.
3. Review techniques for the measurement of energy expenditure in critically ill patients.
4. Explain how to estimate energy expenditure in the critically ill.
5. Highlight the distinction between energy requirement and energy consumption in critical illness.

INTRODUCTION: THE METABOLIC RESPONSE TO CRITICAL ILLNESS

In 1932, Cuthbertson[1] was the first to describe the metabolic response to traumatic injury. Later, he divided the response to such injury into two distinct phases.[2] Characteristics of these phases are listed in Table 134-1. The short-lived "ebb," or hypometabolic, phase immediately following injury is manifested clinically by cold, clammy extremities and a thready pulse. After adequate resuscitation, the patient warms up and cardiac output increases. The flow, or hypermetabolic, phase is characterized by a rise in energy expenditure which peaks at 5% to 60% above normal, depending on the magnitude of the injury. The duration of this phase depends on the severity of injury and the development of complications. Profound metabolic changes occur during this phase, and the increased oxygen consumption serves to support these interorgan substrate exchanges.

Metabolism in serious sepsis is similar to that in major traumatic injury.[3] A systemic inflammatory response is induced in patients with sepsis as well as in patients with major traumatic injury, and the two groups of patients also experience similar metabolic sequelae. This generalized response is evident in patients with major burn injury,[4] who may exhibit oxygen consumption rates far in excess of those seen in patients with severe sepsis and major trauma.[5] A high percentage of patients with so-called systemic inflammatory response syndrome (SIRS) develop dysfunction of one or more organ systems. A major cause of acute renal failure in critically ill patients is SIRS with associated organ dysfunction. The hypermetabolism associated with sepsis and the inflammatory response is shown in Figure 134-1 for patients with and without acute renal failure. These data, derived from Uehara and colleagues,[6] illustrate the similarity in response for both groups of patients, peaking approximately 10 days after admission to an intensive care unit (ICU). The onset of SIRS is the predominant determinant of the degree of hypermetabolism, whereas the development of organ failure portends a prolonged hyperdynamic phase.

TABLE 134-1

Characteristics of the Ebb and Flow Phases of Cuthbertson

EBB PHASE	FLOW PHASE
Hypometabolic	Hypermetabolic
Low core temperature	Raised core temperature
Decreased energy expenditure	Increased energy expenditure
Normal glucose production	Increased glucose production
Mild protein catabolism	Profound protein catabolism
Raised blood glucose	Raised or normal blood glucose
Raised catecholamines	Raised or normal catecholamines
Raised glucocorticoids	Raised or normal glucocorticoids
Low insulin	Raised insulin
Raised glucagon	Raised or normal glucagon
Low cardiac output	Increased cardiac output
Poor tissue perfusion	Normal tissue perfusion
Patient cold and clammy	Patient warm and pink
Preresuscitation phase	Recovery phase

From Cuthbertson DP: Post-shock metabolic response. Lancet 1942;1:433-437.

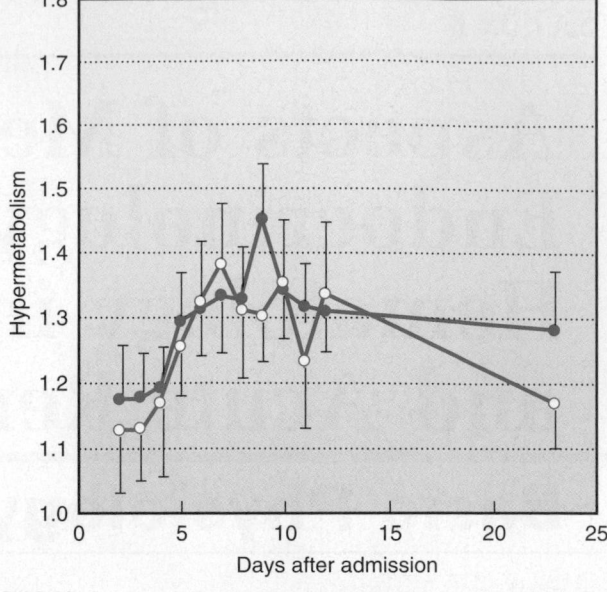

FIGURE 134-1. Hypermetabolism (expressed as the ratio of measured resting energy expenditure [REE] to predicted energy expenditure) for patients with serious sepsis with ($n = 5$, *closed circles*) or without ($n = 7$, *open circles*) early acute renal failure from 2 days after admission to the intensive care unit through day 12, with subsequent measurements at day 23.

Reprioritization of the normal nutritional homeostasis of the body occurs in response to the hypermetabolism and catabolism of the systemic inflammatory response. Marked alterations in carbohydrate, fat, and protein metabolism occur (see Chapters 135, 136, and 138). Hyperglycemia, hypertriglyceridemia, high lactate levels, and high free fatty acid concentrations are characteristic of the critically ill patient and indicate major derangements in intermediary metabolism. Optimal nutritional management of these patients requires an understanding of fuel utilization and the control of energy balance in the flow phase of critical illness.

Physiological Aspects of Energy Metabolism

The human body can be considered as a continuous energy exchange device in which energy is taken in as food and released as heat (Fig. 134-2). The energy conversion occurs through the oxidation of ingested macronutrients, carbohydrates, fats, and proteins. Oxygen is consumed, carbon dioxide is produced, and heat is generated in proportion to the quantity of substrate oxidized. The heat production, that is, the energy expenditure, of the body can be measured by *direct calorimetry* in which a sealed, insulated chamber is used to isolate the subject. In steady-state conditions, respiratory gas exchange (measured by *indirect calorimetry*) reflects cellular gas exchange, and under these conditions a close correspondence is found between the direct and indirect calorimetric techniques for determining energy expenditure.[7]

Oxidation of a given substrate is associated with production of a particular quantity of heat for a given quantity of oxygen consumption and a unique ratio of carbon dioxide production (VCO_2) to oxygen consumption (VO_2) (respiratory quotient [RQ]). For instance, the combustion of one mole of glucose requires 6 moles of O_2 with release of 6 moles of CO_2 and an RQ of 1.0:

$$C_6H_{12}O_6 + 6\ O_2 \rightarrow 6\ CO_2 + 6\ H_2O,$$

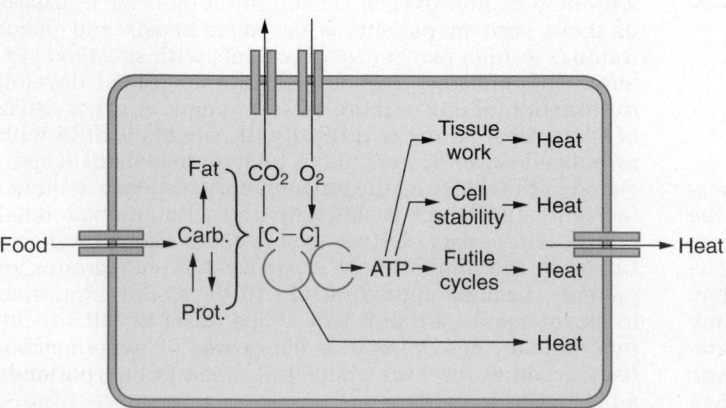

FIGURE 134-2. The human body viewed as an "engine" in which macronutrients are metabolized with associated oxygen consumption and carbon dioxide (CO_2) production and the ultimate generation of heat. (Adapted from Kinney JM: Energy metabolism: Heat, fuel and life. In Kinney JM, Jeejeebhoy KN, Hill GL, Owen OE [eds]: Nutrition and Metabolism in Patient Care. Philadelphia, WB Saunders, 1988, pp 3-34.)

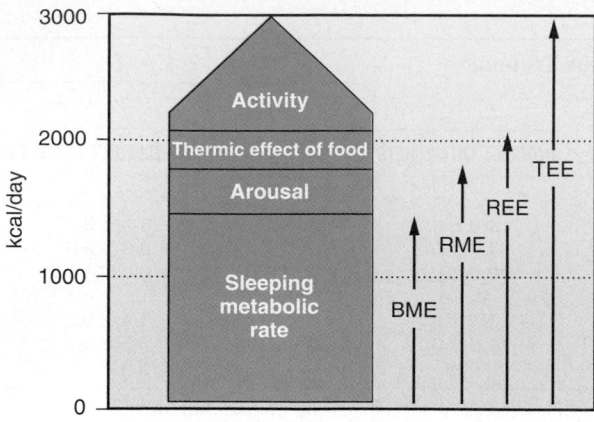

FIGURE 134-3. The components of total energy expenditure (TEE) with typical values for a male with a body weight of 70 kg and 10% body fat. BME, basal metabolic expenditure; REE, resting energy expenditure; RME, resting metabolic expenditure.

whereas combustion of a typical fat (triglyceride of palmitic acid) yields an RQ of 0.703:

$$2\ C_{51}H_{98}O_6 + 145\ O_2 \rightarrow 102\ CO_2 + 98\ H_2O.$$

The calculation for protein oxidation must account for the incomplete combustion of protein in the body where some of the oxygen and carbon remain combined with nitrogen and are excreted as nitrogenous products. Livesey and Elia[8] have published constants for heat release and gas exchange for typical macronutrients.

Components of Energy Expenditure

It is useful to distinguish between the basal metabolic rate, also called the basal metabolic expenditure (BME), and the resting metabolic expenditure (RME). BME refers to the basal requirement occurring in deep sleep and is generally of little clinical relevance. RME applies to the fasted, rested patient in a thermoneutral environment and may be 5% to 10% higher than BME. The thermic effect of food is the energy expended in the assimilation of nutrients which, in the critical care situation, may be provided enterally or parenterally in a continuous manner. It varies depending on the type of diet consumed and the metabolic state of the patient but approximates 10% of RME. The term *resting energy expenditure* (REE) refers to the energy expenditure of the patient receiving continuous enteral or parenteral nutrition and is the sum of the RME and the thermic effect of food. The remaining component contributing to the total energy expenditure (TEE) is activity energy expenditure. In health, REE typically comprises 60% to 70% of TEE (Fig. 134-3).

MEASUREMENT METHODS

The measurement of TEE in the critically ill patient raises formidable problems. Continuous whole-body calorimetry[9] is the most accurate means of assessing TEE, but for obvious reasons this technique is not applicable to hospital patients. The doubly labeled water technique for measuring total free-living energy expenditure has been widely applied in healthy individuals.[10] The assumptions underlying this

method[11] may be seriously violated in critically ill populations and the approach relies on measurements over an extended period (typically 10 to 14 days), which renders it of limited value in the intensive care setting. TEE has also been measured over defined periods of time by measuring the changes in body composition that occur so that changes in the energy stores of fat, carbohydrate, and protein can be derived.[12] The total change in energy stores, or energy balance, is the difference between TEE and energy intake. In practice, this method is not applicable to individual patients because of the limited precision with which the energy balance can be measured.

In principle, continuous indirect calorimetry could be used to measure TEE in critically ill patients.[13,14] This technique measures O_2 consumption and CO_2 production rates from which energy expenditure can be calculated if the urinary nitrogen excretion rate is known.[8] The classic formula of Weir[15] is generally used:

$$\text{Energy Expenditure (kcal/day)} = 3.94\ \text{V}_{O_2}\ (\text{L/day}) +$$
$$1.11\ \text{V}_{CO_2}\ (\text{L/day}) - 2.17\ U_N\ (\text{g/day})$$

where U_N is urinary nitrogen excretion which corrects for the incomplete oxidation of protein in vivo. Ignoring this correction results in less than 2% error on average in energy expenditure even with the higher than normal protein oxidation in critically ill patients.[16]

Although it has the advantage of providing estimates of TEE over periods of a day or less, the indirect calorimetry approach is problematic in patients in the early flow phase of their illness. It is suitable for patients on mechanical ventilation, but the errors in oxygen consumption measurement increase markedly with inspired oxygen fraction (FIO_2), particularly above 60%.[17] Recent commercial developments have improved performance in the 60% to 80% range of FIO_2. Conditions such as changing metabolic acid-base status and the use of extracorporeal CO_2 removal or oxygenation devices effectively rule out the indirect calorimetry method.[17,18] These situations commonly apply in the intensive care setting.

Typically, indirect calorimetry measurements are carried out over short periods of time (less than 1 hour) on patients in a steady-state condition. The latter ensures that the respiratory gas exchange measurements reflect the metabolic gas exchanges. In mechanically ventilated patients, a steady-state measurement of REE closely approximates TEE.[13]

ESTIMATION OF ENERGY EXPENDITURE

In many hospitals, limited access to equipment for measuring energy expenditure necessitates estimation by equations, usually based on prediction of RME that would apply in health, with allowances made for the thermal effect of food, degree of injury or stress, and activity. The principal determinant of RME in health is body size (e.g., weight, fat-free mass, or body surface area). Age and gender are also important factors by virtue of the covariation among RME, age, gender, and fat-free mass. The Harris-Benedict equations,[19] which relate RME measured by indirect calorimetry in healthy adults to weight, age, and gender, were developed in the early 1900s and remain the most widely used equations for estimating energy expenditure. Substantial uncertainty results when applying such equations to individual patients. In particular, use of body

TABLE 134-2

Estimation of Total Energy Expenditure in Patients with Sepsis or Trauma*

| | TOTAL ENERGY EXPENDITURE | | TEE/REE | |
	TEE (kcal/day)	TEE/Bwt (kcal/kg/day)	INDIRECT CALORIMETRY[†]	HARRIS–BENEDICT EQUATION[‡]
Sepsis				
Week 1	1927 ± 370	25 ± 5	1.0 ± 0.2	1.3 ± 0.2
Week 2	3257 ± 370	47 ± 6	1.7 ± 0.2	2.3 ± 0.3
P[§]	0.046	0.021	0.042	0.027
Trauma				
Week 1	2380 ± 422	31 ± 6	1.1 ± 0.2	1.4 ± 0.3
Week 2	4123 ± 518	59 ± 7	1.8 ± 0.2	2.5 ± 0.3
P[§]	0.049	0.029	0.089	0.039

*Data are calculated from 5-day study periods in 12 sepsis and 12 trauma patients. Values are mean ± standard error of mean (SEM).
[†]REE measured by indirect calorimetry.
[‡]REE (men) = 66.5 + 13.8 × Bwt + 5.0 × height − 6.8 × age; REE (women) = 655.1 + 9.6 × Bwt + 1.9 × height − 4.7 × age.
[§]Comparison of weeks 1 and 2 by paired t-test.
Bwt, averaged measured body weight over the 5-day study period; REE, resting energy expenditure; TEE, total energy expenditure.
From Uehara M, Plank LD, Hill GL: Components of energy expenditure in patients with severe sepsis and major trauma: A basis for clinical care. Crit Care Med 1999;27:1295-1302.

weight for patients with fluid retention may be misleading. Use of a pre-illness weight,[20] an adjusted weight,[14] or a "dry" weight (correcting for fluid excess)[21,22] have been advocated. Furthermore, application of a stress factor may not be straightforward given the interindividual variation in the effect of the injury or insult on metabolic expenditure. Coupled with this, the stage of the patient in the typical stress response to illness must be considered. Figure 134-4 suggests an adjustment to RME between 20% and 50% for a ventilated patient with severe sepsis. When patients are taken off ventilation, their energy consumption may increase significantly. This is illustrated in Table 134-2 where, in sepsis and post-trauma patients, REE approximated TEE during the first week of admission while the patients were ventilated, but over the second week, when many were taken off mechanical ventilation, TEE rose to 170% to 180% of REE.

Equations have been developed from indirect calorimetry measurements in mechanically ventilated critically ill patients where less reliance is placed on the use of stress categories. These equations use dynamic physiological variables, which allow daily recalculation of energy expenditure (Table 134-3). The Swinamer equation[23] was based on REE measurements in 108 (48 trauma, 60 non-trauma) patients on day 1 or day 2 of their ICU admission. The effect of the inflammatory response on metabolic rate is represented by the body temperature, respiration rate, and tidal volume variables, and there is no factor representing type of insult. No nutritional support was provided (except for IV dextrose in some patients). Ireton-Jones and colleagues[24] developed an equation from 65 (52% burn, 31% trauma) patients requiring nutritional support and subsequently published an amended version based on the same data.[25] Frankenfield and coworkers[26-28] produced a series of equations, which included an RME prediction in health with a "stress multiplier" in addition to terms reflecting the inflammatory response. The first of these equations[26] was based on 423 measurements over a maximum of 10 days in 56 multiple-trauma patients (30 of whom developed SIRS). Subsequently, three forms of the "Penn State equations" were constructed from retrospective analysis of 169 measurements in a mix of trauma, surgical, and medical ICU patients (see Table 134-3). All three equations involved similar adjustments to RME as estimated by

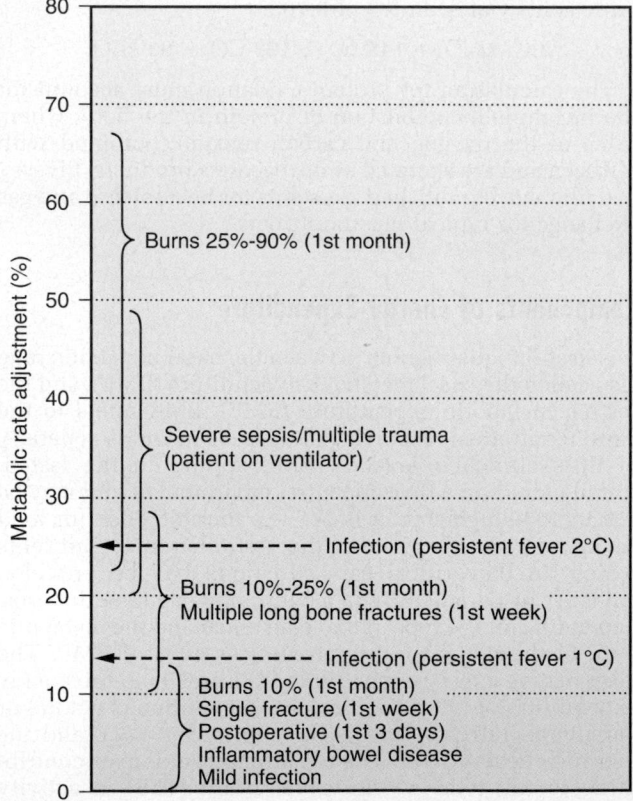

FIGURE 134-4. Approximate adjustments to resting metabolic expenditure (RME) for the effects of disease and injury. (Adapted from Elia M: Organ and tissue contribution to metabolic rate. In Kinney JM, Tucker HN [eds]: Energy Metabolism: Tissue Determinants and Cellular Corollaries. New York, Raven Press, 1992, pp 61-79.)

either the Harris-Benedict equations[19] or the equations developed by Mifflin and colleagues.[29] The Faisy and colleagues[30] equation, developed from measurement in 70 patients, was shown to better predict energy expenditure in this group than was the use of the Harris-Benedict equations with factors for severity of insult.

TABLE 134-3

Equations for Prediction of Resting Energy Expenditure in Mechanically Ventilated Critically Ill Patients

EQUATION	REFERENCE	PREDICTED ENERGY EXPENDITURE (KCAL/DAY)	R^2
Swinamer	23	RME = 945 (BSA) − 6.4 (A) + 108 (T) + 24.2 (RR) + 817 (V_T) − 4349	0.75
Ireton-Jones 1992[a]	24	REE = 5 (W) − 10 (A) + 281 (sex) + 292 (trauma) + 851 (burns) + 1925	0.34
Ireton-Jones 2002[a]	25	REE = 5 (W) − 11 (A) + 244 (sex) + 239 (trauma) + 804 (burns) + 1784	0.34
Frankenfield[b]	26	REE = 1.5 (RME_{HB}) + 250 (T) + 100 (V_E) + 40 (dobut) + 300 (sepsis) − 11000	0.77
Penn State 1998[c]	27	REE = 1.1 (RME_{HB}) + 32 (V_E) + 140 (T_{max}) − 5340	0.70
Penn State 2003a[d]	28	REE = 0.85 (RME_{HB}) + 33 (V_E) + 175 (T_{max}) − 6433	0.67
Penn State 2003b[e]	28	REE = 0.96 ($RME_{Mifflin}$) + 31(V_E) + 167 (T_{max}) − 6212	0.69
Faisy	30	RME = 8 (W) + 14 (H) + 32 (V_E) + 94 (T) − 4834	0.61

[a]For sex, 1 = male, 0 = female; for trauma, 1 = present, 0 = absent; for burns, 1 = present, 0 = absent.
[b]RME_{HB} calculated using actual or adjusted (if greater than 120% of ideal) body weight. For sepsis, 1 = present, 0 = absent based on clinical evidence of presumed infection, systemic inflammation, and organ dysfunction.
[c]RME_{HB} calculated using actual or adjusted (if greater than 120% of ideal) body weight.
[d]RME_{HB} calculated using actual body weight if less than or equal to admission weight, otherwise admission weight. RME_{HB} is calculated using the Harris-Benedict equations (see Table 134-2).
[e]$RME_{Mifflin}$ calculated using actual body weight if less than or equal to admission weight, otherwise admission weight. $RME_{Mifflin}$ is calculated using the Mifflin-St Jeor equations[29]:
   RME (men) = 10 (W) + 6.25 (H) − 5 (A) − 161
   RME (women) = 10 (W) + 6.25 (H) − 5 (A) + 5
A, age; BSA, body surface area (m²); dobut, dobutamine dose (μg/kg/min); H, height (cm); R^2, coefficient of determination; REE, resting energy expenditure; RME_{HB}, resting metabolic expenditure by Harris-Benedict equations[19]; $RME_{Mifflin}$, resting metabolic expenditure by Mifflin-St Jeor equations[29]; RR, respiratory rate (breaths/min); T, temperature (°C); T_{max}, maximum temperature (°C); V_E, minute ventilation (L/min); V_T, tidal volume (L); W, weight (kg).

Validation studies of these equations are limited and have been summarized by Frankenfield.[31] Flancbaum and colleagues[32] found a poor correlation between energy expenditure predicted by the Ireton-Jones 1992[24] and Frankenfield and colleagues[26-28] equations and that measured by indirect calorimetry in a group of surgical intensive care patients on mechanical ventilation and nutritional support. MacDonald and Hildebrandt[33] compared 24-hour indirect calorimetry measurements in a heterogeneous group of 76 patients on nutritional support with the predictions from the Harris-Benedict,[19] Ireton-Jones 1992,[24] Swinamer,[23] Frankenfield,[26] and Penn State 1998[27] equations. The Swinamer and Harris-Benedict equations (using a 1.6 stress factor) performed better than the others and predicted energy expenditure within 20% of measured values approximately 88% of the time. The two Ireton-Jones[24,25] and three Penn State equations[27,28] were compared by Frankenfield and colleagues[28] against resting indirect calorimetry measurements in 47 patients (trauma, surgical, and medical) on mechanical ventilation. The Penn State 2003a equation[28] predicted energy expenditure within 10% of measured values 72% of the time compared to 60% for the Ireton-Jones 1992 equation. The former equation predicted energy expenditure more than 15% above or below measured values 11% of the time versus 32% for the latter. The Ireton-Jones 2002 equation performed less well for this patient group than its predecessor, with predicted energy expenditure within 10% of measured values 36% of the time and outside 15% of measured values 40% of the time.

ENERGY REQUIREMENT VERSUS ENERGY CONSUMPTION

Measurement of energy expenditure in a critically ill patient provides an estimate of energy consumption or energy use rather than energy requirement or need. It cannot be assumed that providing energy intake to match energy expenditure is optimal for the management of critically ill patients.[34,35] A typical indirect calorimetric measurement of RME or REE in a sedated, ventilated critically ill patient provides a "snapshot" measure of energy consumption, assumed to approximate TEE, which reflects metabolism of endogenous (and possibly exogenous) nutrient substrates. The effect of brief nursing interventions, such as chest physiotherapy and dressing changes, may increase TEE by little more than 5%.[13] Energy requirement encompasses this objective measure of energy use but also includes other aspects, such as the effect of the route of feeding, problems with nutrient tolerance and assimilation, and whether energy intake should be adjusted to promote tissue gain or loss.

In critically ill patients with multiple injury, Frankenfield and colleagues[36] found that achievement of energy balance, compared with moderate energy deficit, led to fat deposition but did not improve nitrogen balance. Nitrogen loss did not correlate with energy balance. In these mechanically ventilated patients, energy intake was matched to REE to achieve energy balance. They concluded that high protein, hypocaloric nutrition support is preferable for these patients. Underfeeding for a period of time may result in improved clinical outcome.[37,38] However, large cumulative energy deficits are associated with adverse outcomes.[39] With enteral feeding, gastrointestinal intolerance is the primary mechanism for protecting the patient from substrate excess. Mechanically ventilated patients receiving narcotic sedation, muscle relaxants, or both, will have reduced splanchnic circulation and, as a consequence, compromised gut motility, which will limit effectiveness of nutrition by this route.

Overfeeding exacerbates the hyperglycemia that accompanies the catabolic stress response, causes excess CO_2 production that potentially prolongs the need for mechanical ventilation, may result in hepatic steatosis and hypertriglyceridemia, and, with excessive protein intake, may produce azotemia and metabolic acidosis.[40] Increased ventilator dependence and length of ICU stay have been associated with high-energy intake.[41] Critically ill patients fed parenterally are vulnerable to overfeeding because of fewer impediments to the delivery of substantial energy loads by this mode of administration compared with enteral delivery. The patient receiving parenteral nutrition has no protective mechanism for dealing with overfeeding and must assimilate substrate. Increased sepsis complication rates in patients with major trauma have been attributed to overfeeding by the parenteral route.[42] Hypocaloric support for critically ill patients who are not malnourished has been suggested as a means to prevent overfeeding-related complications.[43] The question of hypocaloric or hypercaloric nutritional support for critically ill patients continues to receive much attention.

In view of the difficulties associated with estimation of energy requirements in the critically ill, many centers, without access to indirect calorimetry equipment, adopt the simple approach of providing 25 to 30 kcal/kg body weight. The American College of Chest Physicians consensus statement[44] recommends 25 kcal/kg usual body weight for ICU patients, with the additional caveats that caloric requirements may need to be increased 10% to 20% in such patients with SIRS and, for overweight (i.e., body mass index greater than 25) patients, usual body weight should be replaced by ideal body weight. It can be seen from Table 134-2 that over the first week of intensive care for sepsis and post-trauma patients on mechanical ventilation, TEE was 25 to 30 kcal/kg measured body weight, which increased to approximately 50 to 60 kcal/kg in the second week when many of the patients were taken off ventilation. For these patients, it remains to be determined whether provision of more than 25 to 30 kcal/kg is of benefit.[45]

Key Points

1. Hypermetabolism is a characteristic feature of critical illness.
2. Wide variation is seen in the degree and duration of hypermetabolism among individual patients.
3. Predicting energy expenditure for individual patients is difficult.
4. Indirect calorimetry is the preferred approach for assessing energy expenditure in individual patients.
5. Matching energy requirement to energy expenditure may not be optimal for nutritional management.

Key References

8. Livesey G, Elia M: Estimation of energy expenditure, net carbohydrate utilization, and net fat oxidation and synthesis by indirect calorimetry: Evaluation of errors with special reference to the detailed composition of fuels. Am J Clin Nutr 1988;47:608-628.
13. Frankenfield DC, Wiles CE, Bagley S, et al: Relationships between resting and total energy expenditure in injured and septic patients. Crit Care Med 1994;22:1796-1804.
18. Brandi LS, Bertolini R, Calafà M: Indirect calorimetry in critically ill patients: Clinical applications and practical advice. Nutrition 1997;13:349-358.
28. Frankenfield D, Smith JS, Cooney RN: Validation of 2 approaches to predicting resting metabolic rate in critically ill patients. JPEN J Parenter Enteral Nutr 2004;28:259-264.
31. Frankenfield D: Energy requirements in the critically ill patient. In Cresci G (ed): Nutrition Support for the Critically Ill Patient: A Guide to Practice. Boca Raton, Fla, CRC Press, 2005, 83-98.

See the companion Expert Consult website for the complete reference list.

CHAPTER 135

Carbohydrates and Lipids

Bruno Cianciaruso and Lucia Di Micco

OBJECTIVES

This chapter will:
1. Describe the main alterations in carbohydrate and lipid metabolism in isolated and complicated acute renal failure.
2. Elucidate the mechanisms of carbohydrate and lipid metabolic dysfunctions.
3. Highlight the therapeutic implications of the metabolic alterations.

Patients with acute renal failure (ARF) may present with a widely varying hormonal and metabolic status. The isolated acute loss of excretory renal function causes metabolic alterations that are similar to those encountered in chronic renal failure. More often, however, ARF is associated with conditions such as sepsis, trauma, and multiple-organ failure and is seen in 10% to 30% of patients in the intensive care unit (ICU).[1] These latter patients usually sustain profound hormonal dysfunction which results in impairment of protein, carbohydrate, and lipid metabolisms.

The metabolic response to stress in critically ill patients is characterized by the increased production of stress mediators, such as counterregulatory hormones (catecholamines, cortisol, glucagon, growth hormone), cytokines (interleukin-1, interleukin-6, tumor necrosis factor-α), and other immune mediators (thromboxane A2, prostaglandins). These stress mediators are responsible for insulin resistance, enhanced proteolysis, glycogenolysis, gluconeogenesis, and lipolysis and ultimately lead to negative nitrogen balance, hyperglycemia, and hypertriglyceridemia.

CARBOHYDRATE METABOLISM

Hyperglycemia is the most significant manifestation of altered carbohydrate metabolism in critically ill patients with ARF. It has been shown that poor glucose control may result in significant complications in critically ill patients,[2] and hyperglycemia has been found to be an independent predictor of death in patients admitted to ICUs with ARF.[3] Furthermore, recent randomized prospective data have demonstrated that the administration of intensive insulin therapy may play an important role in reducing morbidity and mortality in surgical and medical ICU patients.[4,5] There are four major causes of elevated blood glucose concentrations in this condition: insulin resistance, augmented hepatic glucose output, inadequate insulin secretion, and impaired metabolic clearance of insulin.

Elevated plasma insulin levels have been reported in acutely uremic patients,[6] anephric subjects,[7] and in rats induced with acute uremia.[8-10] The importance of the kidney in removing insulin from the bloodstream has been shown in humans and in experimental animals[11,12] and, in fact, many diabetic patients, once they develop renal insufficiency, register a decreased requirement for exogenous insulin.[13] The lack of renal tissue, however, is not the only mechanism responsible for the decrease in insulin degradation. Cianciaruso and colleagues[14] studied endogenous insulin production and degradation in a model of acutely uremic dogs. Conscious, and with catheters in the portal vein, the femoral artery, and the main left hepatic vein, the animals were studied in both the postabsorptive state and during a combined hyperinsulinemic and hyperglycemic state induced by the exogenous infusion of insulin and glucose. The study showed that, in the basal (fasting) state, the endogenous production and hepatic removal of insulin in uremic dogs were not different from those in controls. Thus, the hyperinsulinemia observed in the postabsorptive state in ARF is not related to altered splanchnic insulin kinetics; rather, other factors (extrasplanchnic), such as decreased degradation of insulin by the kidney and the muscle, appear to be responsible for the higher insulin levels in this condition. These findings are in accordance with in vitro data, where, in nephrectomized rats, a decreased degradation of insulin by the muscle has been observed.[15] During the combined infusion of insulin and glucose, plasma insulin levels rose much higher in uremic dogs than in controls, as was expected because of the lack of renal tissue, but also observed was the consistently reduced insulin removal by uremic dogs' livers. This study[14] also found a lower endogenous secretion in acute uremia, probably because the markedly higher plasma insulin concentration in the uremic animals prevented endogenous insulin production from being activated by hyperglycemia. Thus, reduced hepatic insulin degradation contributes to the hyperinsulinemia observed in acutely uremic patients following exogenous insulin infusion.

Several studies have shown that sensitivity to the action of insulin, with respect to glucose metabolism, is markedly impaired in patients with renal failure[16] and in critically ill patients.[17,18] Insulin resistance is a condition characterized by impaired glucose disposal in the presence of either normal or elevated serum insulin concentrations. The clinical manifestation of insulin resistance is often a state of hyperglycemia in the setting of hyperinsulinemia. The major glycoregulatory functions are impaired, including stimulation of glucose transport, inhibition of gluconeogenesis, and stimulation of net glycogen synthesis and glucose oxidation.[19] Along with alterations in glucose metabolism, the anti-lipolytic effect of insulin is impaired in these conditions, with fatty acids being the major oxidative fuel for energy requirements. The metabolic changes induced by insulin resistance, however, may be a natural response to starvation or injury. In fact, in a condition of lack of food, insulin resistance may ensure that the limited stores of carbohydrates are used for glucose-dependent and insulin-insensitive tissues such as the brain. Insulin-sensitive tissues will use fat instead of glucose as a source for energy.

The presence of insulin resistance can be detected and quantified by the technique of hyperinsulinemic euglycemic clamp,[20] by which exogenous insulin is infused at a fixed rate to increase plasma insulin concentration and maintain it at a constant level. Variable amounts of glucose are delivered, with an infusion pump, to avoid hypoglycemia and maintain euglycemia. Hence, in this condition, glucose disposal is primarily dependent upon the dose of exogenous insulin administered, and dose-response curves may be constructed between glucose disposal and plasma insulin concentration. The severity of insulin resistance in patients with ARF has never been tested with this technique; however, data are available in critically ill medical patients, studied with the hyperinsulinemic euglycemic clamp, 1 day after their admission to a medical ICU.[21] Admission diagnoses of these patients included respiratory insufficiency, sepsis, primary multiple-organ failure, neurological disorders, and cardiogenic shock. These data show that, in critically ill patients, insulin sensitivity is reduced by 70% compared to healthy controls, indicating severe impairment of insulin-mediated glucose uptake by all body tissues. In this study, the development of insulin resistance and its severity were not related to the underlying causes for ICU admission but to the severity of illness as assessed by the APACHE score, thereby indicating that insulin resistance is mainly a response to critical illness.

Basi and colleagues[3] studied insulin resistance in 90 critically ill patients with ARF. These patients were participants in the Program to Improve Care in Acute Renal Disease (PICARD),[22] an observational study of 618 adult ICU patients with ARF. In this study, the homeostasis model of insulin resistance (HOMA-R) index was used as a measure of insulin resistance,[23] wherein HOMA-R index = serum insulin (μIU/mL) $\times$ plasma glucose (mmol/L)/22.5; normal value is assumed 1.0 in healthy subjects, aged 35 or younger, with normal body weight. The median value of HOMA-R in the population studied was 9.47 (interquartile range 4.10 to 18.81), indicating that insulin resistance was, in fact, highly prevalent in ARF.

The development of insulin resistance with renal failure has two main causes: the loss of the homeostatic and metabolic functions of the kidney and the metabolic conditions caused by the critical illness. Studies employing a combination of isotopic and net balance techniques[24] have shown in conscious dogs and in healthy, postabsorptive (overnight fasted state) humans[25] that renal glucose release accounts for about 25% of all glucose released into the circulation and its uptake of glucose accounts for almost 20% of all glucose removed from the circulation. Since the normal human kidney does not contain appreciable glycogen stores, it is likely that the release of glucose by the kidney is due exclusively to gluconeogenesis. Renal glucose production is regulated by hormonal influence, with insulin inhibiting and catecholamines stimulating this process. Observations in humans have shown that, during euglycemic hyperinsulinemic clamp experiments, systemic glucose (i.e., the sum of hepatic and renal glucose) appearance decreases to zero[26] and that renal glucose production in humans is not irrelevant; therefore, the loss of a major target organ for insulin could result in insulin resistance.

Site and possible mechanisms of insulin resistance in renal failure have been extensively studied. However, most of the research conducted in humans refers to chronic rather than acute renal failure,[16] whereas ARF has been studied in experimental models, in vitro and in vivo.[27] Using a combined technique (the hyperinsulinemic euglycemic clamp with the arterial-venous femoral catheterization for the measurement of leg glucose exchange), De Fronzo and colleagues[28] found that the major site of insulin resistance in chronic renal failure resides in peripheral tissues. Since muscle tissue accounts for more than 90% of the disposal of the infused glucose load, the authors conclude that skeletal muscle is the primary site of insulin resistance in uremia.

Data on peripheral glucose uptake in ARF have been obtained in conscious dogs, studied 24 to 30 hours after bilateral nephrectomy and undergoing a mild hyperglycemic (160 to 180 mg/dL) glucose clamp.[27] The results (Figure 135-1) indicate that the rate of non–hepatic glucose uptake was significantly reduced in uremic dogs as compared with sham-operated normal dogs. The average values were 737 ± 341 µmol/min in the acutely uremic dogs and 1337 ± 393 µmol/min in the control animals ($P < 0.01$). The data suggest that the ability of insulin to direct the disposal of glucose into oxidative metabolism or glycogen synthesis, in acute uremia, is markedly reduced as is the ability of insulin to reduce the proteolysis and the release of lactate. These findings are consistent with the observations of other investigators that determined the responsiveness to insulin of skeletal muscle from acutely uremic rats.[29]

Studies conducted in patients with advanced chronic renal failure, using the hyperinsulinemic euglycemic clamp technique, in combination with hepatic vein catheterization and H-3 glucose, have shown normal basal hepatic glucose production, normal splanchnic glucose balance, and normal splanchnic glucose uptake. In response to insulin infusion, glucose production was similarly suppressed in uremic and control subjects, whereas the splanchnic glucose uptake was unchanged.[28] In dogs experimentally induced with ARF,[27] in the basal period, the hepatic release of glucose was greater in the control dogs as compared with the uremic animals (Figure 135-2). This result is likely the consequence of higher insulin levels in the uremic dogs. However, during the hyperglycemic clamp procedure (0 to 90 min), net hepatic uptake occurred in the control dogs, whereas in the uremic animals, hepatic glucose output fell but never switched to uptake. The response of hepatic lactate metabolism to the glucose and insulin infusion was also altered: The uremic dog liver continued to take up lactate, whereas in control dogs there was net hepatic output of lactate. This experiment indicates that, even during glucose infusion, there is persistent gluconeogenesis and an increased hepatic glucose output, mainly from conversion of amino acids released during protein catabolism.

The data confirm that in ARF the resistance to insulin-stimulated glucose uptake occurs mainly in peripheral tissues, but the liver contributes to glucose intolerance and insulin resistance, mainly during a glucose load as occurs with parenteral nutrition.

LIPID METABOLISM

In contrast to the abundance of studies on chronic renal failure, few data are available on lipid metabolism in patients with ARF. The most frequent alterations of plasma lipids in ARF are hypertriglyceridemia and low cholesterol levels.[30] In fact, in ARF patients, the lipoprotein composition usually shows an increased triglycerides concentration, especially of low-density lipoprotein and very low–density lipoprotein, while total cholesterol and, in particular, high-density lipoprotein cholesterol levels are decreased. The leading cause of lipid abnormalities in ARF is impaired lipolysis. The enzyme that hydrolyzes triglycerides, contained in the circulating chylomicrons and very low–density lipoprotein, is lipoprotein lipase. In adipose tissue, the activity of lipoprotein lipase is increased by administration of insulin. When heparin is given intravenously, lipoprotein lipase activity is released into the blood plasma. This is a pharmacological action of heparin, and heparin is not a physiological cofactor of the enzyme. The lipolytic activity that is released is made up of two different enzymes that hydrolyze triglycerides. One of the lipases is derived from the liver and is resistant to inactivation by protamine. The second enzyme is of extrahepatic origin and is inhibited by protamine; it is primarily responsible for the hydrolysis of the triglycerides taken into the

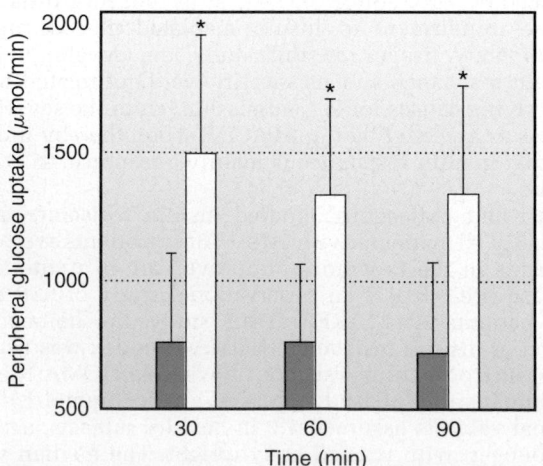

FIGURE 135-1. Calculated peripheral uptake of glucose after 30, 60, and 90 minutes of glucose and insulin infusion in acutely uremic dogs (*blue bars*) as compared with control dogs (*white bars*). (From Cianciaruso B, Bellizzi V, Napoli R, et al: Hepatic uptake and release of glucose, lactate, and amino acids in acutely uremic dogs. Metabolism 1991;40(3):261-269, with permission.)

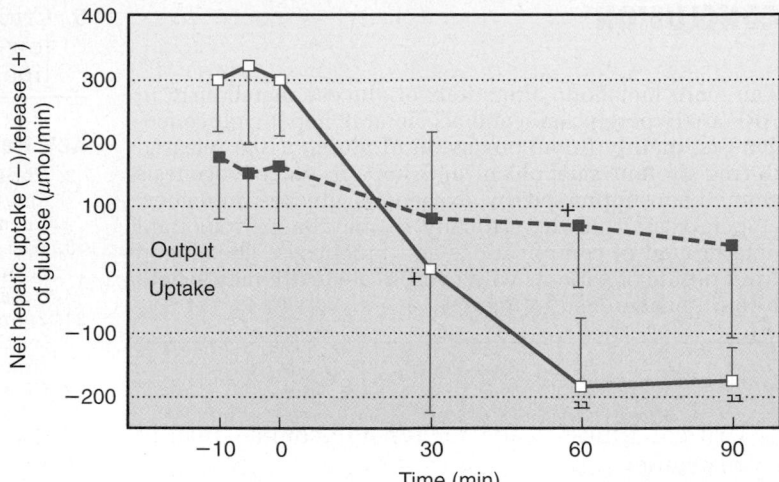

FIGURE 135-2. Net hepatic uptake or release of glucose during baseline and during a 90-minute infusion of glucose and insulin in acutely uremic dogs (*closed squares*) as compared with control dogs (*open squares*). (From Cianciaruso B, Bellizzi V, Napoli R, et al: Hepatic uptake and release of glucose, lactate, and amino acids in acutely uremic dogs. Metabolism 1991;40(3):261-269, with permission.)

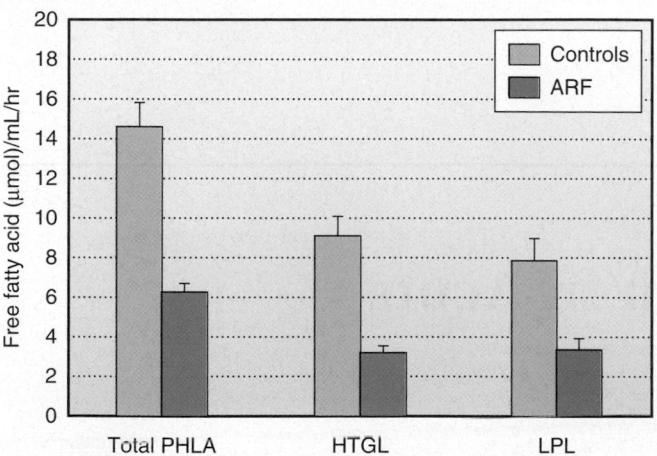

FIGURE 135-3. Maximal postheparin lipolytic activity (PHLA), hepatic triglyceride lipase (HTGL), and peripheral lipoprotein lipase (LPL) in 10 controls and 8 subjects with acute renal failure (ARF). (Adapted from Druml W, Zechner R, Magometschnigg D, et al: Postheparin lipolytic activity in acute renal failure. Clin Nephrol 1985;23:289-293, with permission.)

body in the form of chylomicrons. After heparin injection, from 45% to 95% of the lipolytic activity that appears in the blood plasma is protamine resistant; that is, it is the liver lipase. Maximal postheparin lipolytic activity, hepatic triglyceride lipase, and peripheral (protamine-inactivated) lipoprotein lipase were studied by Druml and colleagues[31] in 10 controls and 8 subjects with ARF (Figure 135-3). The activities of both lipolytic systems, peripheral lipoprotein lipase, and hepatic triglyceride lipase were decreased in patients with ARF to less than 50% of normal. However, in contrast to this impairment of lipolysis, oxidation of fatty acids was not affected by ARF. During infusion of labeled long-chain fatty acids, carbon dioxide production from lipids was comparable between healthy subjects and patients with ARF.[32] Metabolic acidosis can contribute to the impaired lipolysis of ARF by inhibiting lipoprotein lipase.

Alternatively to impaired lipolysis, there may be in ARF an increase in hepatic triglyceride secretion, due to the elevated concentrations of insulin, free fatty acids, or both.

Data obtained in studies of animals experimentally induced with ARF show increased, normal, or decreased plasma fatty acids and very low–density lipoprotein secretion.[33] In patients with ARF, plasma triglyceride levels do not correlate with triglyceride clearance or postheparin lipolytic activity; these results suggest that lipid secretion is increased in patients with ARF.[31]

Changes in lipid metabolism develop rapidly in patients with ARF; impaired fat elimination is evident already at 48 to 96 hours from the start of renal failure, and the threshold below which these metabolic alterations are activated is a creatinine clearance of 50 to 30 mL/min.[33]

Changes in lipid metabolism in patients with ARF are characteristic of the metabolic response to severe stress and are promoted by catecholamines and inflammatory cytokines and exaggerated by the decreased insulin sensitivity of adipose tissue. The plasma cholesterol concentration is decreased in stress conditions, with decreased concentration of both low- and high-density lipoproteins. The mechanism for the hypocholesterolemia in acute illness is most likely multifactorial, where both decreased synthesis and enhanced catabolism occur. Giovannini and coworkers[34] demonstrated that, in critically ill surgical patients, cholesterol levels correlate with decreased plasma proteins and hepatic protein synthesis, suggesting that hypocholesterolemia may be part of the negative acute phase response to acute illness. Several lines of evidence indicate that increased levels of pro-inflammatory cytokines may explain the hypocholesterolemia of acute illness. The parenteral administration of pro-inflammatory cytokines has been demonstrated to lower lipid levels[35,36] and show an inverse correlation between interleukin-6 and apolipoprotein A-1 levels in surgical ICU patients.[37]

The degree of hypocholesterolemia appears to correlate with the severity of the acute illness, morbidity, and mortality. Obialo and colleagues[38] reported that cholesterol levels below 150 mg/dL and serum albumin below 3.5 g/dL were independent predictors of mortality in patients with ARF. Emerging data show that tight glycemic control can result in an increase in both high-density lipoprotein and low-density lipoprotein levels[39]; furthermore, a multivariate analysis of survival in surgical ICU patients by Van den Berghe and colleagues[40] suggests that the improvement in the lipid profile independently determined that insulin therapy contributed to a decrease in both morbidity and mortality.

CONCLUSION

The main metabolic alterations of glucose metabolism in ARF are hyperglycemia and accelerated hepatic gluconeogenesis, mainly from conversion of amino acids released during protein catabolism, and hepatic gluconeogenesis cannot be suppressed by exogenous glucose infusions. Hyperglycemia in the critically ill may be an important determinant of complications and prognoses. The altered lipid profile of patients with complicated ARF may benefit from intensive insulin therapy.

Key Points

1. Critical illness leads to hyperglycemia—insulin resistance.
2. Critical illness leads to accelerated gluconeogenesis.
3. Critical illness leads to low cholesterol and high-density lipoprotein levels.
4. Critical illness leads to impaired lipolysis.

5. Critical illness leads to increased triglycerides, low-density lipoprotein, and very low–density lipoprotein levels.

Key References

2. Christiansen C, Toft P, Jørgensen HS, et al: Hyperglycaemia and mortality in critically ill patients: A prospective study. Intensive Care Med 2004;30:1685-1688.
3. Basi S, Pupim LB, Simmons EM, et al: Insulin resistance in critically ill patients with acute renal failure. Am J Physiol Renal Physiol 2005;289:F259-F264.
21. Zauner A, Nimmerrichter P, Anderwald C, et al: Severity of insulin resistance in critically ill medical patients. Metabolism 2007;56:1-5.
27. Cianciaruso B, Bellizzi V, Napoli R, et al: Hepatic uptake and release of glucose, lactate, and amino acids in acutely uremic dogs. Metabolism 1991;40(3):261-269.
38. Obialo CI, Okonofua EC, Nzerue MC, et al: Role of hypoalbuminemia and hypocholesterolemia as copredictors of mortality in acute renal failure. Kidney Int 1999;56:1058-1063.

See the companion Expert Consult website for the complete reference list.

CHAPTER 136

Amino Acid and Protein Turnover and Metabolism in Acute Renal Failure

Wilfred Druml

OBJECTIVES

This chapter will:
1. Discuss the complex factors affecting amino acid and protein metabolism in a patient with acute renal failure.
2. Identify the specific factors induced by acute uremia.
3. Discuss the impact of renal replacement therapy on protein metabolism.
4. Explore the potential consequences of nutrition therapy for patients with acute renal failure.

INTRODUCTION

Amino acid and protein metabolism in patients with acute renal failure (ARF) is affected by a broad pattern of various factors: the presence of an acute disease state (systemic inflammatory response syndrome, acute phase reaction), that is, the underlying disease process leading to ARF; and associated complications, especially infections and sepsis (Table 136-1). However, the acute uremic state exerts fundamental and specific alterations of metabolism, and

metabolic and nutritional balances are affected also by renal replacement therapy. Both the type and the intensity of renal replacement therapy are relevant in this respect, and, in particular, modern continuous renal replacement therapies (CRRTs), with high fluid turnover rates, have significant effects on nutritional requirements.[1]

PROTEIN METABOLISM IN ACUTE DISEASE STATES

Any acute disease process is accompanied by a characteristic metabolic response syndrome, affecting protein, lipid, and carbohydrate metabolisms. This syndrome presents a uniform reaction of the organism to various exogenous and endogenous insults, independent of the type of the insult or underlying disease, and can also be seen during intense pain or—to a mitigated extent—even during emotional stress. The extent of this metabolic response, however, is dependent on the severity or duration of the precipitating event, or both.

A predominant characteristic of this well-orchestrated metabolic response syndrome is the activation of muscular (peripheral) protein catabolism. Amino acids are released

TABLE 136-1

Metabolic Environment of Acute Renal Failure

- Renal failure (acute uremic state)
- SIRS, acute phase reaction (acute disease state)
- Underlying illness (type, severity, duration)
- Associated complications (infections)
- General effects of extracorporeal circulation (bio-incompatibility, etc.)
- Specific effects of CRRT (nutrient losses, etc.)

CRRT, continuous renal replacement therapy; SIRS, systemic inflammatory response syndrome.

from muscle tissue into the circulation and are taken up by the liver, and hepatic metabolic functions are upregulated (such functions can be more than doubled in patients with sepsis).[2]

The primary stimulus for this activation of proteolysis is located in the liver. The scenario is not that muscle-liberated amino acids are concentration dependent and absorbed by the liver, but the liver "drags" amino acids from the circulation and from the periphery, and hepatic extraction of amino acids is augmented. Because of this enhanced uptake, the plasma concentrations of most amino acids are decreased despite the augmented release from the peripheral tissues.[3]

These reactions facilitate various synthetic functions of the liver to support the organism to cope with an acute disease process. Hepatic gluconeogenesis is augmented, hepatic synthesis of various proteins is increased, and fatty acid synthesis and triglyceride formation are upregulated. Classic acute phase reactants, such as C-reactive protein or coagulation factors, are activated and the synthesis of numerous other proteins is enhanced. On the other hand, hepatic albumin synthesis as a "negative" acute phase reactant is inhibited.

In terms of energy, by far the most relevant reaction is gluconeogenesis. To understand proteolysis in acute disease states, it is important to note that activation of protein catabolism and augmentation of hepatic gluconeogenesis can be mitigated but not completely suppressed by exogenous substrates or nutrition.[4] Thus, acute disease states, in general, represent "obligatory catabolic" events.

The underlying mechanisms for these metabolic alterations are manifold and not fully elucidated. A complex network of catabolic hormones and inflammatory mediators is involved, and both humoral and cellular events participate in this process, which nowadays are subsumed under the term *inflammation* (see later). Especially, tumor necrosis factor-α (TNF-α) has been shown both to stimulate peripheral proteolysis and activate hepatic cellular amino acid transport.[5] The final pathway of protein catabolism is uniform and independent of the underlying disease process. The ubiquitin-proteasome system has been identified as a main pathway.[6] Moreover, lysosomal factors and, as recently elucidated, a calpain-dependent pathway are involved.[2]

AMINO ACID AND PROTEIN METABOLISM IN ACUTE RENAL FAILURE

In ARF, protein metabolism shares characteristics with that observed in other acute disease states. ARF presents a hypercatabolic, inflammatory, and pro-oxidative state, and in patients with ARF several mechanisms can aggravate this metabolic response syndrome.

The main characteristic of metabolic alterations in ARF is the augmented activation of protein catabolism with excessive release of amino acids from skeletal muscle and sustained negative nitrogen balance. Muscular protein degradation and amino acid catabolism are activated. Not only is protein breakdown accelerated, muscular utilization of amino acids for protein synthesis is defective. Amino acid transport into skeletal muscle is impaired in ARF. This abnormality can be linked to insulin resistance and to a generalized defect in ion transport in uremia; both the activity and receptor density of the sodium pump are abnormal in adipose cells and muscle tissue.[7]

Amino acids are redistributed from muscle tissue to the liver. Hepatic extraction of amino acids from the circulation, hepatic gluconeogenesis, and ureagenesis are increased. In the liver, protein synthesis and secretion of acute phase proteins are stimulated.

Amino Acid Pools and Amino Acid Utilization in Acute Renal Failure

As a consequence of these metabolic alterations, imbalances in amino acid pools in plasma and in the intracellular compartment occur in ARF, and a typical plasma amino acid pattern is induced. In patients with ARF, plasma concentrations of cystine, taurine, methionine, and phenylalanine are elevated, whereas levels of valine and leucine are decreased.[8]

Moreover, the elimination of amino acids from the intravascular space is altered. As expected from the stimulation of hepatic extraction of amino acids observed in animal experiments, overall amino acid clearance and clearance of most glucoplastic amino acids are enhanced.[8] In contrast, the clearance of phenylalanine, proline, and valine is decreased in patients with ARF.

Causes of Protein Catabolism in Acute Renal Failure

The causes of hypercatabolism in ARF are complex and manifold and, as detailed earlier, present a combination of nonspecific mechanisms induced by the acute disease process, systemic inflammatory response syndrome, acidosis, underlying illness and associated complications, specific effects induced by the acute loss of renal function, and type and intensity of renal replacement therapy (Table 136-2).[9]

A dominating mechanism of accelerated protein breakdown is the stimulation of hepatic gluconeogenesis from amino acids. In healthy subjects, but also in patients with chronic renal failure, hepatic gluconeogenesis from amino acids is readily and completely suppressed by exogenous glucose infusion. In contrast, in patients with ARF, hepatic glucose formation is decreased but not halted by exogenous substrate supply: Even during glucose infusion, gluconeogenesis from amino acids persists.[10]

These findings have important implications for nutritional support in patients with ARF, because it is impossible to achieve a positive nitrogen balance in such patients during the acute phase of disease. Protein catabolism cannot be suppressed by the provision of conventional

TABLE 136-2

Factors Contributing to Protein Catabolism in Acute Renal Failure

Impairment of metabolic functions by uremic toxins
Endocrine factors
    Insulin resistance
    Increased secretion of catabolic hormones (catecholamines, glucagon, glucocorticoids)
    Hyperparathyroidism
    Suppression of release of, or resistance to, growth factors
Acidosis
Acute disease state (e.g., acute phase reaction, systemic inflammatory response syndrome) (activation of cytokine network)
Release of proteases
Inadequate supply of nutritional substrates
Renal replacement therapy
    Loss of nutritional substrates
    Activation of protein catabolism

nutritional substrates alone; to effectively suppress protein catabolism, alternative means for preserving lean body mass must be identified.

The stimulation of muscular protein catabolism and enhanced hepatic gluconeogenesis is mediated by the glucocorticoid-dependent ubiquitin-proteasome pathway.[6] Experiments have shown that increased protein catabolism from animals with ARF can be normalized either by adrenalectomy or by pre-treatment with glucocorticoid receptor blocking agents.[11]

An important stimulus of muscle protein catabolism in ARF is insulin resistance. In muscle, the maximal rate of insulin-stimulated protein synthesis is depressed by ARF and protein degradation is increased, even in the presence of insulin. An inefficient intracellular energy metabolism stimulates protein breakdown and interrupts the normal control of protein turnover.[12]

Acidosis was identified as a major factor in muscle protein breakdown. Metabolic acidosis activates catabolism of protein and oxidation of amino acids independently of azotemia.[13] Although the exact role of acidosis on protein metabolism in patients with ARF has not yet been evaluated systematically, there is evidence that increased muscle protein degradation and amino acid catabolism can be mitigated by correcting metabolic acidosis in ARF.[13a]

Several additional catabolic factors are operative in ARF. The secretion of catabolic hormones (catecholamines, glucagon, glucocorticoids); hyperparathyroidism (which is also frequently present in ARF); suppression or decreased sensitivity of growth factors; and the release of proteases from activated leukocytes all can stimulate protein breakdown.[1]

As in other acute disease processes, inflammatory mediators such as TNF-α and interleukins play a role in ARF. However, in comparison to other acute disease states, in ARF this inflammatory reaction is augmented, because the kidneys play an important role in the catabolism of cytokines.[14]

Also specific to patients with ARF is the fact that type and frequency of renal replacement therapy can affect protein metabolism and nutritional balances profoundly. Aggravation of protein catabolism, in part, is mediated by the loss of nutritional substrates, but findings suggest that, in addition, both an activation of protein breakdown and

inhibition of muscular protein synthesis can be induced by hemodialysis (see later).

Last but not least, of major relevance for the clinical situation is the fact that inadequate nutrition contributes to the loss of lean body mass in patients with ARF. In experimental animals, starvation potentiates the catabolic response of ARF, and in patients with ARF, malnutrition has been identified as a major determinant of further complications and of prognosis.[15]

Metabolic Functions of the Kidney and Protein and Amino Acid Metabolism in Acute Renal Failure

Protein and amino acid metabolism in ARF is also affected by impairment of multiple metabolic functions of the kidney itself: Various amino acids are synthesized or converted by the kidneys and released into the circulation: arginine, tyrosine, cysteine, methionine (from homocysteine), or serine. Thus, loss of renal functions can contribute to the altered amino acid pools in ARF; as a result, several amino acids, which conventionally are termed nonessential, such as arginine, tyrosine, or cysteine, might become conditionally indispensable in ARF.[16]

In addition, the kidney is an important organ of protein degradation. Multiple peptides are filtered and catabolized at the tubular brush border with the constituent amino acids being reabsorbed and recycled into the metabolic pool. In renal failure, catabolism of peptides such as peptide hormones is retarded as is degradation of proinflammatory cytokines, which contributes to the proinflammatory state. This is also the case with insulin, so insulin requirements may decrease in diabetic patients after development of ARF.

With the increased use of dipeptides as a source of amino acids (such as glutamine or tyrosine) in parenteral nutrition, the metabolic function of the kidney may also gain importance in the utilization of nutritional substrates. However, most dipeptides currently evaluated as sources of glutamine or tyrosine contain alanine or glycine in N-terminal position and are rapidly hydrolyzed in the presence of renal dysfunction.[17]

THE IMPACT OF EXTRACORPOREAL THERAPY

The impact of hemodialysis therapy on protein metabolism is manifold. Hemodialysis per se is a catabolic event.[18,19] There is a relevant loss of small water-soluble molecules and, thus, also of amino acids, which accounts for about 2 g/hour dialysis session. Protein catabolism during dialysis is caused by amino acid losses; by the activation of protein breakdown, mediated by release of leukocyte-derived proteases and inflammatory mediators (TNF-α and interleukins) induced by blood membrane interactions; or by endotoxin.[20] Potentially, dialysis also induces an inhibition of muscular protein synthesis. Moreover, it has been suggested that generation of reactive oxygen species is augmented during treatment.[20a]

CRRTs also are associated with a broad pattern of metabolic consequences (Table 136-3). The continuous mode of therapy and the recommended high fluid turnover has

TABLE 136-3

Metabolic Effects of Continuous Renal Replacement Therapy

Amelioration of uremic intoxication ("renal replacement")
plus
1. Heat loss
2. Excessive load of substrates (lactate, citrate, glucose)
3. Loss of nutrients (amino acids, vitamins)
4. Loss of electrolytes (phosphate, magnesium)
5. Elimination of short-chain proteins (hormones, mediators)
6. Loss of proteins
7. Metabolic consequences of bio-incompatibility (induction or activation of mediator-cascades, stimulation of protein catabolism)

a pronounced impact on nutritional balances.[21] One major effect is the elimination of small- and medium-sized molecules. The sieving coefficient of amino acids is within the range of 0.8 to 1.0, so amino acid losses can be estimated from the volume of the filtrate and the average plasma concentrations. Usually, this will account for a loss of approximately 0.2 g/L filtrate and, depending on the filtered volume, will result in a total loss of 10 to 15 g amino acid per day, representing about 10% to 15% of amino acid intake. Amino acid losses during continuous hemofiltration and continuous hemodialysis are of a comparable magnitude.

Patients with ARF who are treated by CRRT must be given nutrition solutions during extracorporeal therapy. Nutrition should also be provided during intermittent therapeutic modalities. The endogenous clearance of amino acids is in the range of 80 to 1800 mL/min and thus exceeds dialytic clearance 10 to 100 times, so infusion results in minimal increases in plasma amino acid concentrations. Thus, nutrition infused during hemodialysis or CRRT does not augment amino acid losses substantially, and about 10% to 15% of amino acids given are lost in the dialysate/hemofiltrate.

With the high molecular size cutoff of membranes used in hemofiltration, small proteins, such as peptide hormones (insulin, catecholamines, potentially also cytokines and mediators) are also filtered. In view of their short plasma half-life, hormone losses are probably not of pathophysiologic importance. However, CRRTs are associated with protein loss, which—depending on the type of therapy and the membrane material used—can vary between 1.2 and 7.5 g/day.[22] The use of high cutoff membranes will even augment this protein loss, making it clinically relevant.[23]

CLINICAL STUDIES ON PROTEIN CATABOLISM IN ACUTE RENAL FAILURE

Several studies evaluated protein catabolism, mostly to define the optimal intake of amino acids and protein, in critically ill patients with ARF on CRRT. Kierdorf[24] measured a protein catabolism of about 1.5 g per kg body weight (BW) per day and found that provision of 1.5 g amino acids per kg BW/day was more effective in reducing

nitrogen (N) loss than was infusion of 0.7 g (−3.4 vs. −8.1 gN/day). However, a further increase in amino acid intake to 1.74 g/kg BW/day had no additional effect on nitrogen balance (−3.2 gN/day). Chima and colleagues[25] evaluated the protein catabolic rate (PCR), urea nitrogen appearance, and total nitrogen appearance in 19 critically ill patients on CRRT. A mean PCR of 1.7 g/kg BW/day was observed, and it was concluded that protein needs in these patients range from 1.4 to 1.7 g/kg BW/day. In a similar patient group, Macias and coworkers[26] evaluated a protein catabolic rate of 1.4 g/kg BW/day. There was an inverse relationship between protein and energy provision, and protein catabolic rate and nitrogen deficit was less in those patients receiving nutritional support. Again, a protein intake of 1.5 to 1.8 g/kg BW/day was recommended. In agreement with these studies, Leblanc and colleagues[27] found a PCR of 1.75 + 0.82 g/kg BW/day with wide variations in 38 ARF patients on CRRT.

Australian working groups have assessed higher protein intakes on nitrogen balance in ARF patients on CRRT. In a nonrandomized study, Bellomo and colleagues[28] compared a protein intake of 1.2 g/kg BW/day with an intake of 2.5 g/kg BW/day in critically ill patients with ARF on CRRT. This excessive protein intake improved nitrogen balance (−5.5 g/day vs. −1.92 g/day) but at the cost of an augmented urea generation rate and the need for more aggressive renal replacement therapy. Similarly, in an inadequately randomized manner, Scheinkestel and coworkers[29,30] evaluated the impact of three levels of protein and amino acid intake (1.5, 2.0, and 2.5 g/kg BW/day) on nitrogen balance and outcome. PCR was not reported, but nitrogen balance was inversely related to energy expenditure and positively related to protein intake and, not surprisingly, was associated with ICU and hospital outcome.

Hypercatabolism certainly cannot be overcome by simply increasing protein or amino acid intake. Even in patients with normal kidney function who are suffering from sepsis or burns, the provision of more than 1.5 g protein or amino acids per kg BW per day does not abolish catabolism. More excessive intakes have no proven benefits. Moreover, they increase the accumulation of waste products, aggravate uremic complications, induce hyperammonemic states, and lead to an increased need for dialysis, which in turn stimulates muscle protein degradation and increases nutrient losses. Moreover, improving nitrogen balance is not necessarily an adequate end point for nutritional interventions (see later discussion).

POTENTIAL INTERVENTIONS FOR CONTROLLING CATABOLISM

Excessive mortality in ARF is tightly correlated with the extent of hypercatabolism. Unfortunately, no effective methods have been identified to reduce or stop catabolism in the clinical situation. It must be stressed that inhibiting the final pathway of protein catabolism cannot be the primary target of therapy; more "upstream" therapeutic interventions aimed at mitigating the underlying inflammatory response are required. Principally, hypercatabolism can be modified at four levels of metabolic interventions (Table 136-4):

Substrate level: As discussed earlier, it is impossible to halt hypercatabolism and persisting hepatic

TABLE 136-4

Potential Interventions for Controlling Catabolism

Substrate Level
  Nonspecific: energy substrates, amino acids, protein
  Specific ("pharmaconutrients," "immunonutrients"):
    glutamine, fish oil, anti-inflammatory nutrients
Endocrine Level
  Insulin, growth factors (hGHr, IGF-1, anabolic steroids)
  Anti-glucocorticoids, β-blockers
Mediator Level
  Anti-inflammatory nutrients (ω-3 fatty acids, glutamine)
  Anti-cytokines
Direct Inhibitors
  Proteolytic enzyme inhibitors
  Proteasome inhibitors

hGHr, human growth hormone recombinant; IGF-1, insulin growth factor-1.

gluconeogenesis in patients with ARF simply by providing conventional nutritional substrates. However, several nutrients ("pharmaconutrients," "immunonutrients") can interfere with the inflammatory status, and it remains to be demonstrated whether these novel nutritional substrates, such as glutamine, fish oil, or structured triglycerides, will exert a more pronounced anti-catabolic effect in patients with ARF.

Endocrine level: Endocrine interventions include therapy with hormones (insulin, insulin-like growth factor-1 (IGF-1), human growth hormone recombinant (hGHr), and hormone antagonists (such as anti-glucocorticoids). In rats with ischemic ARF, IGF-1 not only accelerated recovery from renal failure but also improved nitrogen balance. However, available clinical results are rather disappointing. A multicenter study using IGF-1 in patients with ARF was terminated prematurely because of a lack of effect. hGHr should not be used in the treatment of critical illness, because an increase in mortality became apparent during hGHr therapy of critically ill patients, many of whom also had ARF.

Mediator level: Cytokines, such as interleukins and TNF-α, mediate excessive release of amino acids from skeletal muscle and activation of hepatic amino acid extraction in acute disease states. Therapies to limit overwhelming release or action of inflammatory mediators (antagonists of thromboxane, of platelet activating factor, of interleukins, antibodies to TNF-α, soluble TNF-α receptors, etc.) are under experimental evaluation. It should be recognized that nutritional elements, such as amino acids (glutamine, glycine, arginine) or ω-3 fatty acids, can modify the inflammatory response and the release of mediators.

Direct inhibitors: Experimentally, several interventions aimed at inhibiting the final pathway of protein catabolism, such as inhibition of nonspecific proteolytic enzymes or of the ubiquitin-proteasome pathway, have been assessed.[31,32] It remains highly questionable whether this presents a reasonable target of therapy.

Some of these novel therapeutic strategies offer promising perspectives, but few have entered clinical routine. It is highly improbable that a single factor is responsible for hypercatabolism in ARF or that a single agent will reverse inflammatory states and accelerated protein degradation.

Key Points

1. Acute renal failure is a catabolic, pro-oxidative, and pro-inflammatory syndrome characterized by a pronounced increase in protein catabolism.
2. Both nonspecific factors (acute disease state [e.g., systemic inflammatory response syndrome, acute phase reaction]), the underlying disease process, associated complications (especially infections, sepsis), acute renal failure per se, and the type and intensity of renal replacement therapy contribute to metabolic alterations.
3. Loss of metabolic kidney function contributes to the altered amino acid pools in ARF, so several amino acids conventionally referred to as "nonessential" may become conditionally indispensable. Moreover, tubular degradation of peptides (hormones, cytokines) is retarded in acute renal failure.
4. Continuous renal replacement therapies exert a profound effect on protein metabolism mainly by inducing relevant losses of amino acids but also of peptides and protein.
5. Those designing nutrition therapy for patients with acute renal failure must consider these metabolic alterations.

Key References

1. Druml W: Nutritional support in patients with acute renal failure. In Molitoris B, Finn W (eds): Acute Renal Failure. A Companion to Brenner & Rector's The Kidney. Philadelphia, WB Saunders, 2001, pp 465-489.
2. Hasselgren PO, Menconi MJ, Fareed MU, et al: Novel aspects on the regulation of muscle wasting in sepsis. Int J Biochem Cell Biol 2005;37:2156-2168.
6. Lecker SH, Goldberg AL, Mitch WE: Protein degradation by the ubiquitin-proteasome pathway in normal and disease states. J Am Soc Nephrol 2006;17:1807-1819.
9. Mitch WE: Mechanisms causing loss of muscle in acute uremia. Ren Fail 1996;18:389-394.
13. Mitch WE: Metabolic and clinical consequences of metabolic acidosis. J Nephrol 2006;19(Suppl 9):S70-S75.

See the companion Expert Consult website for the complete reference list.

CHAPTER 137

Endocrinology of the Stress Response during Critical Illness

Paul E. Marik

> ## OBJECTIVES
>
> This chapter will:
> 1. Provide an overview of the stress response.
> 2. Review changes in the hypothalamic-pituitary-adrenal axis during critical illness.
> 3. Describe the sick euthyroid syndrome.
> 4. Discuss stress hyperglycemia.

The stress system receives and integrates a diversity of cognitive, emotional, neurosensory, and peripheral somatic signals that arrive through distinct pathways. Activation of the stress system leads to behavioral and physical changes that are remarkably consistent in their qualitative presentation (Table 137-1). This observation was first noted by Hans Selye, who in 1936 reported that biological, physical, or psychological stressors generally precipitate a similar response which he named the "general adaption syndrome" or stress response.[1] The stress response is normally adaptive and time limited and improves the chances of the individual for survival.

Behavioral adaptation during stress includes increased arousal, alertness, and vigilance; improved cognition; and inhibition of vegetative functions, such as appetite, feeding, and reproduction. A concomitant physical adaption also occurs mainly to promote an adaptive redirection of energy. Oxygen and nutrients are shunted to the central nervous system and the stressed body sites where they are most needed. Increases in cardiovascular tone, respiratory rate, and intermediate metabolism (gluconeogenesis, lipolysis) work in concert with these alterations to promote availability of vital substrates. The stress response was "designed" to be of short or limited duration. The time-limited nature of this process renders its accompanying antigrowth, anti-reproductive, catabolic, and immunosuppressive effects temporarily beneficial, of no adverse consequence to the individual, or both. However, chronic activation of the stress system may lead to a number of disorders that are the result of increased secretion of corticotropin-releasing hormone (CRH) and changes in the hypothalamic-pituitary end-organ axes. In essence, critical illness is a state characterized by a pathologically prolonged stress response; indeed, these are patients with profound activation of the stress response in whom modern technology is used to cheat "programmed death" of the organism.

The stress response is mediated largely by the hypothalamic-pituitary-adrenal (HPA) axis and the sympathoadrenal system, which includes the sympathetic nervous system and the adrenal medulla.[2-4] The HPA axis is essential for the adaption and maintenance of homeostasis during critical illness, and the adrenal gland—through cortisol as the primary glucocorticoid secreted from the adrenal gland—has long been recognized as a requirement for survival in critical illness. If, however, the stress is prolonged or the homeostatic response is inadequate, the HPA axis can contribute to a worsened clinical state. The HPA axis and the sympathoadrenal system are functionally related. Activation of the sympathoadrenal system results in the secretion of epinephrine and norepinephrine from the adrenal medulla and to an increased production of inflammatory cytokines such as interleukin-6 (IL-6). Pro-inflammatory mediators such as IL-6 and leukemia inhibitory factor increase transcription of the pro-opiomelanocortin gene, resulting in increased production of adrenocorticotropic hormone (ACTH).

Activation of the HPA axis results in increased secretion from the paraventricular nucleus of the hypothalamus of CRH, a 41–amino acid peptide, and arginine vasopressin. CRH plays a pivotal integrative role in the response to stress. Arginine vasopressin is a weak corticotropin (ACTH) secretagogue but has a synergistic role with CRH in the secretion of corticotropin. In animal models, administration of CRH will produce most of the signs associated with exposure to a stressor.[5] In addition, CRH serves as a gatekeeper of the stress response as it is subject to negative feedback on several fronts. CRH stimulates the production of ACTH by the anterior pituitary, causing the zona fasciculata of the adrenal cortex to produce more glucocorticoids (cortisol in humans). The increase in cortisol production results in multiple effects (metabolic, cardiovascular, and anti-inflammatory) that serve to maintain homeostasis during stress.

CRH has multiple integrative actions: It activates the sympathoadrenal system and sympathetic nervous system; increases somatostatin production, thereby inhibiting growth hormone secretion; and inhibits the production of thyroid-stimulating hormone (TSH) and gonadotropin-releasing hormone, thus suppressing thyroid and gonadal functions, respectively.[6] Cytokines (e.g., IL-1β, IL-6, tumor necrosis factor-α) are released not only in response to injurious/immune/inflammatory insults but also during acute physical or psychological stress. The mechanisms by which cytokines stimulate cortisol include primarily centrally mediated actions (e.g., stimulation of CRH secretion), as well as actions at the level of the pituitary gland, the adrenal cortex, or both.[7-9] During acute stress, the rise in cytokine levels lags behind plasma ACTH responses. However, cytokines seem to play an important role in conditions of prolonged stress, during which CRH and ACTH are inhibited, but circulating cortisol levels remain high (Fig. 137-1). During nonstressful periods, the production of ACTH, CRH, and arginine vasopressin follows a pulsatile pattern with a circadian rhythm highest in the morning with cortisol exerting a negative feedback on CRH, ACTH, and arginine vasopressin production. In prolonged stress, the circadian rhythm of cortisol production is abolished, and the negative feedback from cortisol is attenuated. Failure to terminate a response to acute stress can result in the chronic stress syndrome, which causes endocrine, metabolic, psychiatric, and immunological alterations.

CORTISOL PHYSIOLOGY DURING ACUTE ILLNESS

In general, there is a graded cortisol response to the degree of stress, such as the type of surgery. Cortisol levels also correlate with the severity of injury, the Glasgow Coma Scale, and the APACHE score.[10-12] There is often a wide, bimodal spectrum of cortisol concentrations in critically ill patients, with patients at either extreme faring the worst.[13] Over 90% of circulating cortisol is bound to corticosteroid-binding globulin, with less than 10% in the free, biologically active form. The adrenal gland does not store cortisol; increased secretion arises as a result of increased synthesis under the control of ACTH.[14] Cholesterol is the principal precursor for steroid biosynthesis in steroidogenic tissue. In a number of sequential enzymatic steps, cholesterol is metabolized by p450 cytochromes to aldosterone, dehydroepiandrosterone (DHEA), androstenedione, and cortisol.[14] The first and rate-limiting step is the formation of pregnenolone from cholesterol. At rest and during stress, about 80% of circulating cortisol is derived from plasma cholesterol, the remaining 20% being synthesized in situ from acetate and other precursors.[15] Experimental studies suggest that high-density lipoprotein is the preferred cholesterol source of steroidogenic substrate in the adrenal gland.[16] Recently, mouse SR-B1 (scavenger receptor, class B, type 1) and its human homolog (Cla-1) have been identified as the high-affinity, high-density lipoprotein receptor mediating selective cholesterol uptake.[17-19]

Cortisol exerts its effects following uptake from the circulation by binding to intracellular glucocorticoid receptors (GRs).[20] The binding of cortisol to GR in the cytoplasm results in the activation of the steroid receptor complex via a process involving the dissociation of heat shock proteins (HSP 90 and HSP 70) and the binding to FK binding protein 52 (FKBP52).[21-23] Intracellularly, the cortisol-GR complex moves to the nucleus where it binds as a homodimer to DNA sequences called glucocorticoid-responsive elements, located in the promoter regions of target genes, and then activates or represses transcription of the associated genes. By this mechanism, glucocorticoids affect the transcription of thousands of genes in every cell of the body. It has been estimated that glucocorticoids effect 20% of the genome of mononuclear blood cells.[24] In addition, the cortisol-GR complex may affect cellular function by nontranscriptional mechanisms.

Cortisol has several important physiological actions on metabolism, cardiovascular function, and the immune system.[25,26] The metabolic effects of cortisol include the increase in blood glucose concentrations through the activation of key enzymes involved in hepatic gluconeogenesis and inhibition of glucose uptake in adipose tissue. Additionally, in adipose tissue, lipolysis is activated and its activation results in the release of free fatty acids into the circulation. Cortisol also has a permissive effect on other hormones, including catecholamines and glucagon, with resultant development of insulin resistance and hyperglycemia, at the expense of protein and lipid catabolism.

TABLE 137-1

Behavioral and Physical Adaptation during Stress

Behavioral Adaptation
Increased arousal and alertness
Increased cognition, vigilance, and attention
Heightened analgesia
Suppression of reproductive axis

Physical Adaptation
Increased heart rate
Increased blood pressure
Increased cardiac output
Blood flow directed to brain and skeletal muscle
Increased temperature
Increased respiratory rate
Increased gluconeogenesis (stress hyperglycemia)
Increased lipolysis
Inhibition of digestion
Stimulation of colonic motility
Containment of inflammatory/immune response

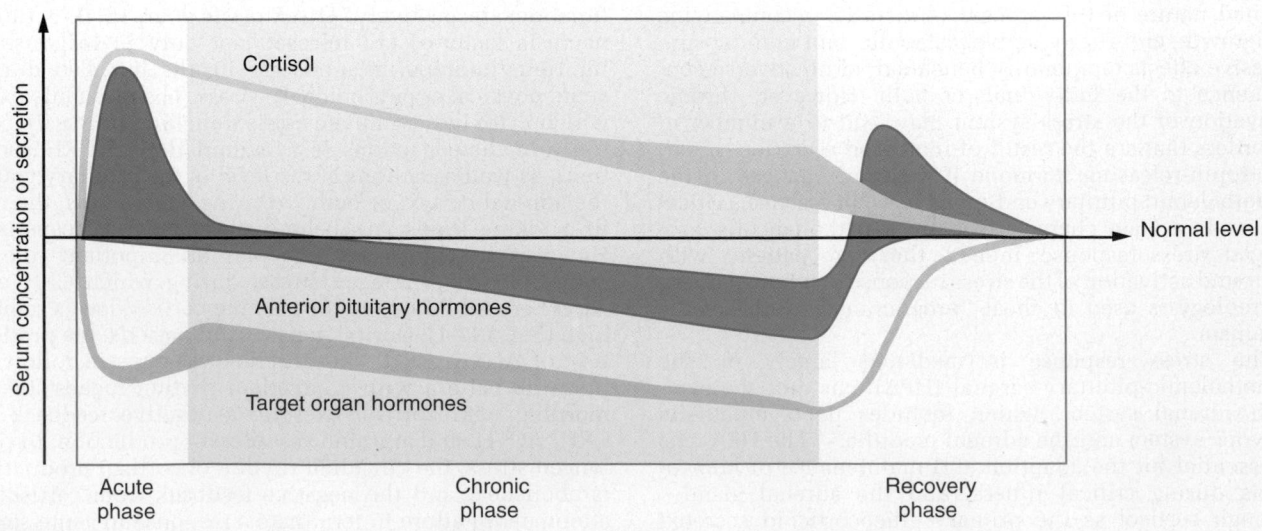

FIGURE 137-1. The neuroendocrine response to chronic critical illness.

Glucocorticoids are required for normal cardiovascular reactivity to angiotensin II, epinephrine, and norepinephrine, contributing to the maintenance of cardiac contractility, vascular tone, and blood pressure. These effects are mediated partly by the increased transcription and expression of the receptors for these hormones.[27,28] Glucocorticoids are required for the synthesis of Na^+,K^+-ATPase and catecholamines. Glucocorticoid effects on synthesis of catecholamines and catecholamine receptors are partially responsible for the positive inotropic effects of these hormones.[29] Cortisol has potent anti-inflammatory actions, including the reduction in number and function of various immune cells, such as T and B lymphocytes, monocytes, neutrophils, and eosinophils, at sites of inflammation. Glucocorticoids play a major role in regulating the activity of nuclear factor kappa B (NF-κB), which plays a crucial and generalized role in inducing cytokine gene transcription.[30-32]

DHEA and dehydroepiandrosterone sulfate (DHEAS) are the most abundant steroids secreted by the adrenal cortex and are under CRH control. Only DHEA is considered biologically active, mediating its action mainly indirectly via downstream conversion to sex steroids. DHEA is a pleiotropic adrenal hormone with pro-immune and pro-inflammatory effects, opposing the immunosuppressive effects of glucocorticoids. DHEA and DHEAS levels may be depressed in the acute phase of severe illness.[33] The implications of these findings are unclear; however, a high cortisol-to-DHEA ratio has been suggested to be a poor prognostic marker in patients with severe sepsis.[33,34]

DYSFUNCTION OF THE HYPOTHALAMIC-PITUITARY-ADRENAL AXIS DURING ACUTE ILLNESS

While the acute stress response is characterized by activation of the HPA and sympathoadrenal system axis with increased secretion of cortisol, an increase in the percentage of free cortisol, and increased translocation of the glucocorticoid receptor complex into the nucleus, there is increasing evidence that in many critically ill patients this pathway may be impaired.[35-37] The incidence of glucocorticoid deficiency in critically ill patients is variable and depends upon the underlying disease and severity of the illness. The reported incidence varies widely (from 0 to 77%) depending upon the population of patients studied and the diagnostic criteria used to diagnose adrenal insufficiency.[38-49] However, the overall incidence of adrenal insufficiency in critically ill medical patients approximates 10% to 20%, with an incidence as high as 60% in patients with septic shock.[13,26,41,50-52] The major impact of adrenal insufficiency in the critically ill is on the systemic inflammatory response and cardiovascular function.[53-55]

The mechanisms leading to dysfunction of the HPA axis during critical illness are complex and poorly understood and likely include decreased production of CRH, ACTH, and cortisol as well as their receptors. A subset of patients may suffer structural damage to the adrenal gland from either hemorrhage or infarction, and this may result in long-term adrenal dysfunction. Adrenal hemorrhage has been described with blunt abdominal trauma, following major surgery, in disseminated intravascular coagulation associated with sepsis, and in patients with burns, heparin-induced thrombocytopenia, and the anti-phospholipid syndrome.[20,56-61] However, it appears that the majority of

critically ill patients develop reversible dysfunction of the HPA axis. Tissue resistance to cortisol also may occur, as a result of abnormalities of the glucocorticoid receptor or increased tissue conversion of cortisol to cortisone. In addition, patients who have been treated with "long-term" corticosteroids are likely to have secondary adrenal insufficiency, which may increase the risk of developing adrenal insufficiency.[20,26]

Tumor necrosis factor-α (TNF-α) and interleukin-1 (IL-1) have been implicated in the reversible dysfunction of the HPA axis during critical illness. TNF-α impairs CRH-stimulated ACTH release, and a number of clinical studies have reported inappropriately low ACTH levels in patients with severe sepsis and the systemic inflammatory response syndrome.[49,62-64] TNF-α has been shown to reduce adrenal cortisol synthesis by inhibiting the stimulatory actions of ACTH and angiotensin II on adrenal cells.[65-67] Pro-inflammatory cytokines have also been shown to influence the number, expression, and function of the GR.[68-70] Meduri and colleagues[71,72] have demonstrated tissue resistance to glucocorticoids with decreased nuclear translocation of the GR complex in patients dying from acute respiratory distress syndrome. Decreased production of cortisol during acute illness may occur due to substrate deficiency. High-density lipoprotein is substantially reduced in patients with many acute illnesses, including sepsis and burns, following myocardial infarction and in patients undergoing surgical interventions.[73-81] For the diagnoses and management of glucocorticoid deficiency in critical illness see Chapter 139.

THE GROWTH HORMONE AXIS IN CRITICAL ILLNESS

Growth hormone (GH) is a polypeptide hormone with anabolic, immunomodulatory, and lipolytic properties. Its action is partly mediated via insulin growth factor-1 (IGF-1), which is synthesized in the liver as well as the kidneys and pituitary gland. GH secretion is stimulated by GH-releasing hormone and inhibited by somatostatin. It is noteworthy that the pulsatile secretion of GH seems to be particularly important for its action. During the first hours or days after an acute insult, such as surgery, trauma, or infection, circulating GH levels become elevated, and the normal GH profile, consisting of peaks alternating with virtually undetectable troughs, is altered; peak GH and interpulse concentrations are high and the GH pulse frequency is elevated.[82-84] However, serum concentration of IGF-1 and the GH-dependent binding protein—IGF binding protein-3—decreases. This reflects reduced GH-receptor expression in peripheral tissues and results in acquired peripheral resistance to GH. It has been suggested that the pro-inflammatory mediators reduce GH expression which, in turn, through negative feedback inhibition, induces the abundant release of GH, exerting direct lipolytic, insulin-antagonizing, and immune-stimulating actions, while the indirect IGF-mediated effects of GH are attenuated.[85-87] In prolonged critical illness, lowered GH levels and a reduced pulsatile fraction have been found. As a result of this low pulsatility, levels of IGF-1 and IGF binding protein-3 are low.[84,88-90] Low levels of IGF-1 are associated with muscle wasting.

To investigate the effect of administration of (high doses) of GH in critically ill patients, Takala and colleagues[91] carried out two parallel randomized controlled trials. A total of 532 patients who had been in the intensive care unit (ICU) for 5 to 7 days and who were expected to require intensive care for at least 10 days were enrolled. The in-hospital mortality rate was significantly higher in patients who received GH in both studies. Among the survivors, length of stay in the ICU was prolonged in the GH group. The study has been criticized for the very high dose of GH used, which may have (1) been associated with insulin resistance and hyperglycemia, (2) aggravated concealed hypoadrenalism and hypothyroidism, and (3) promoted apoptosis in compromised tissue. Furthermore, it does not appear logical to treat patients with prolonged critical illness, who have normal to moderately decreased GH, with high doses of GH. Attempts to restore GH pulsatility with GH secretagogues may be more physiological.

THYROID HORMONES DURING CRITICAL ILLNESS

TSH is released from the anterior pituitary gland and stimulates the thyroid gland. Thyroxine (T_4) is released into the circulation predominantly by the thyroid gland. Approximately 80% of the circulating triiodothyronine (T_3) is produced in peripheral tissues by 5′-deiodination of free T_4, while the remainder is secreted by the thyroid itself. T_3 is the active hormone; free T_4 is considered the pro-hormone. The function of T_3 is to maintain metabolic stability; this hormone affects the function of every organ system.

Serum thyroid hormone levels undergo predictable changes in systemic nonthyroidal illness and critical illness. The initial change in the HPT axis during a mild illness is a decrease in T_3 production caused by inhibition of the conversion of T_4 to T_3, with a reciprocal increase in reverse T_3 (rT_3), the so-called low T_3 syndrome or sick euthyroid syndrome (SES).[92-97] This decrease can occur very rapidly, and both the decrease in serum T_3 and the rise in rT_3 have been reported to correlate with severity of illness. Thyroxine-binding globulin levels are usually decreased as is the total T_4; however, free T_4 is usually normal, as are the TSH levels. With severe disease and in patients with chronic illness, the free T_4 (T_4 syndrome) and TSH may decrease. These changes in thyroid function are considered adaptive—an attempt to decrease catabolism and energy expenditure at a time of need. Although the cause of the SES is poorly understood, cytokines, most notably IL-1 and IL-6, may play a role by decreasing hepatic 5′-deiodinase type 1 expression.[98-100]

The role of thyroid hormone replacement in patients with SES is controversial.[97,101] Brent and Hershman[102] randomized medical ICU patients with severe SES (low free T_4) to receive T_4 (1.5 µg/kg) daily for 2 weeks or placebo. In the treatment group, total T_4 and free T_4 concentrations increased significantly by day 3 and were normalized by day 5. A significant rise in the T_3 occurred in the control group on day 7 but was delayed until day 10 in the treatment group. Mortality was equivalent in the two groups (75% control versus 73% treatment).

In a study of severely burned patents given 200 µg T_3 daily, there was no evidence of benefit from thyroid replacement.[103] In a randomized controlled study of patients with acute renal failure, treatment with thyroxine (150 µg four times daily over 2 days) was associated with an increase in mortality compared to the control group (43% versus 13%).[104] Van den Berghe and coworkers[105]

investigated the effects of a continuous infusion of TRH alone and in combination with GH-releasing hormone and GH-releasing peptide-2. Twenty adult patients who remained critically ill for several weeks were studied. Reduced pulsatile fractions of TSH, GH, and prolactin secretion and low concentrations of T_4, T_3, and IGF-1 were found in the untreated state. With TRH infusion alone, the thyroid axis could be reactivated, with TSH secretion and increases in T_4 and T_3. Infusion of TRH in combination with GH secretagogues augmented the pulsatility of the TSH release and avoided an increase in rT_3. These data suggest that in patients with SES, treatment with T_4 or T_3 alone may not be beneficial.[97,101] The administration of TSH secretagogues seems to have a more "physiological" effect; however, additional studies are required before this therapy can be recommended.

STRESS HYPERGLYCEMIA

The prevalence of stress hyperglycemia in critical illness is difficult to establish because of limited data and variations in the definition of hyperglycemia. Stress hyperglycemia has been defined as a plasma glucose above 200 mg/dL.[106] However, in view of the results of the Leuven Intensive Insulin Therapy Trial, stress hyperglycemia should now be considered in any critically ill patient with a blood glucose in excess of 110 mg/dL.[107] In a study of septic nondiabetic ICU patients, 75% had a baseline blood glucose level above 110 mg/dL.[108] In the Leuven Intensive Insulin Therapy Trial, 12% of patients had a baseline blood glucose above 200 mg/dL. However, 74.5% of patients had a baseline blood glucose above 110 mg/dL, with 97.5% having a recorded blood glucose level above 110 mg/dL sometime during their ICU stay.[107]

The metabolic milieu in which stress-induced hyperglycemia develops in the critically ill in the absence of pre-existing diabetes mellitus is complex and reflects activation of the stress response. A combination of several factors, including the presence of excessive counterregulatory hormones such as glucagon, GH, catecholamines, glucocorticoids, and cytokines such as IL-1, IL-6, and TNF-α, combined with exogenous administration of catecholamines, dextrose, and nutritional support, together with relative insulin deficiency play an important role.[106] However, increased gluconeogenesis and hepatic insulin resistance are the major factors leading to hyperglycemia.[109] Recent human data suggest that hepatic insulin resistance (and phosphoenylpyruvate carboxykinase suppression) remains refractory to intensive insulin therapy.[110] Increased hepatic output of glucose may therefore be more important than peripheral insulin resistance in the genesis of stress hyperglycemia.[111] Gluconeogenic substrates released during stress include lactate, alanine, and glycerol, with exogenous glucose failing to suppress gluconeogenesis.[112,113] Glucagon is the primary hormonal mediator of gluconeogenesis, with critically ill patients having a significant increase in serum glucagon levels.[113] This effect is mediated by adrenergic stimulation by catecholamines and by cytokines.[114] In addition, cytokines such as TNF-α and IL-1 and catecholamines independently and synergistically promote hepatic glucose production.[115,116]

In patients with sepsis, insulin resistance contributes to the development of stress hyperglycemia.[117-122] During sepsis, insulin-induced tyrosine phosphorylation of insulin receptor substrate-1 and subsequent activation of phosphatidylinositol 3-kinase is impaired, resulting in defective glucose transporter (GLUT)-4 receptor translocation, diminished glucose uptake with skeletal muscle and hepatic insulin resistance.[123] The mechanisms whereby sepsis induces these alterations are unknown, but increased levels of TNF-α may play a key role. Recently Gao and colleagues[124] have demonstrated that activation of the inhibitor κB kinase (IKK) complex is associated with serine phosphorylation of insulin receptor substrate-1. IKK is activated by endotoxin via Toll-like receptor 4 as well as by TNF-α and IL-1.[125-127] The serine phosphorylation of insulin receptor substrate-1 and I κB by IKK may partly explain the insulin resistance noted with activation of the pro-inflammatory cascade.

Catecholamines have also been shown to inhibit insulin binding, tyrosine kinase activity, and translocation of GLUT-4 either directly through a receptor or a postreceptor mechanism.[128,129] Glucocorticoids impair insulin-mediated glucose uptake in skeletal muscle, by downregulating various signaling proteins with resulting inhibition of translocation of GLUT-4 glucose transporter from its internal membrane stores to the plasma membrane.[130] Growth hormone inhibits the insulin pathway by reducing insulin receptors and impairing its activation through phosphorylation on tyrosine residues.[131,132]

Hyperglycemia and insulin resistance are common in patients receiving parenteral nutrition. In a meta-analysis that compared enteral with parenteral nutrition in postoperative patients, Moore and colleagues[133] reported the mean blood glucose to be 130 mg/dL with enteral nutrition as compared to 224 mg/dL with parenteral nutrition (a difference of 94 mg/dL!). O'Keefe and colleagues demonstrated significantly higher blood glucose levels with insulin resistance in healthy volunteers who received intravenous glucose as compared to the same glucose load given enterally.[134] The increased risk of infections in patients receiving standard parenteral nutrition may be related to the presence of hyperglycemia. Bustamante[135] has demonstrated that in patients receiving parenteral nutrition, a blood glucose greater than 120 mg/dL increased the risk of developing *Candida* bloodstream infection (OR 2.6). In a retrospective analysis of 111 hospitalized patients receiving parenteral nutrition, Cheung and coworkers[136] reported that hyperglycemia was independently associated with an increased risk of cardiac complications, sepsis, acute renal failure, and death.

Until recently, stress hyperglycemia was considered a beneficial adaptive response, providing a ready source of fuel during a time of increased demand. However, both short- and long-term hyperglycemia (diabetes) is now recognized to have significant deleterious effects. Hyperglycemia potentiates the pro-inflammatory response, increases oxidative injury, and is pro-thrombotic, whereas insulin has the opposite effect.[137-143] Glucose increases the expression and plasma concentration of matrix metalloproteinase-2 and matrix metalloproteinase-9, which aid in the spread of inflammation.[144] Hyperglycemia predisposes patients to infections.[107,145-147] The in vitro responsiveness of leukocytes stimulated by inflammatory mediators is inversely correlated with glucose levels.[148,149] Acute hyperglycemia reduces endothelial nitric oxide levels, causing abnormal vascular reactivity and organ perfusion.[150] Indeed, glucose appears to be a toxic molecule in acutely ill and injured patients in ways similar to its toxicity in the diabetic patient.[137,140,151]

Stress hyperglycemia has been shown to be associated with a worse outcome following acute myocardial infarction, stroke, and congestive heart failure.[152-159] In patients with diabetics undergoing cardiac surgery, glucose control reduces the risk of wound infection and reduces mortality.[147,160] Recent provocative data suggest that tight glycemic control improves the outcome of critically ill patients.[107,161,162] In a landmark study, Van den Berghe and colleagues[107] randomized 1548 surgical ICU patients to an intensive insulin therapy regimen aimed at maintaining blood glucose between 80 mg/dL to 110 mg/dL or a control group in which an insulin infusion was only initiated when glucose level was greater than 215 mg/dL with the maintenance of glucose between 180 and 200 mg/dL. At 12 months, the mortality was 4.6% with the intensive insulin regimen compared to 8.0% in the control group. The benefit was most apparent in patients with more than 5 days of stay in the ICU. In a follow-up study in medical ICU patients, these authors demonstrated a reduction in hospital mortality from 52% to 43% in patients randomized to the intensive insulin group who had an ICU length of stay more than 3 days.[161] In both these studies, patients with preexistent diabetes did not demonstrate an improved outcome. This suggests that in diabetes a higher threshold may be preferable (this remains to be tested). In both the studies performed by Van den Berghe and colleagues, 60% of the caloric intake was provided by intravenous glucose. Tight glycemic control may therefore act primarily to reduce the toxicity of parenteral glucose, that is, parenteral nutrition.[163] Van der Voort and colleagues[151] demonstrated that the ICU and hospital mortality of critically ill patients was independently related to the mean amount of infused glucose. It is therefore likely that both hyperglycemia and the glucose load increase insulin-independent cellular glucose uptake with subsequent toxic intracellular effects. The benefits of tight glycemic control in patients who receive hypocaloric nutrition remain to be determined; it is possible that in such patients, "less tight" glycemic control may outweigh the benefits of tight glycemic control.

CONCLUSION

The HPA peripheral-hormone axes are uniformly dysregulated in critical illness (Table 137-2). The dysregulation of

TABLE 137-2

Hormonal Changes during the Acute Stress Response

Hypothalamic-Pituitary-Adrenal (HPA) Axis
    Increased corticotropin (ACTH)
    Decrease in cortisol binding globulin (CBG)
    Increase in total and free cortisol
    Increase in glucocorticoid receptor expression
    Decrease in dehydroepiandrosterone
    Decreased androgen synthesis
    Decreased aldosterone synthesis
Sympathoadrenal System Activation
    Increased epinephrine
    Increased norepinephrine
Growth Hormone Axis
    Increased growth hormone (GH)
    Decreased GH receptor
    Decreased insulin growth factor-1 (IGF-1)
Thyroid hormone axis
    Decreased triiodothyronine (T_3)
    Increased reverse triiodothyronine (rT_3)
Increased Prolactin
Increased Glucagon
Increased Pro-inflammatory Cytokines

these axes is related to the severity of illness and is a dynamic process that changes over time. The acute stress response is characterized by increased serum catecholamines, GH and cortisol levels, blunted GH pulsatility, low T_3, insulin resistance, and hyperglycemia. In prolonged critical illness, catecholamine and cortisol levels decrease compared to the acute phase, with a decrease in the levels of GH, TSH, and thyroid hormone. Treatment with hydrocortisone may be beneficial in selected patients with glucocorticoid deficiency. Replacement of GH or thyroxine has not been demonstrated to improve outcome in critically ill patients. Glycemic control improves the outcome of critically ill patients; however, the optimal regimen remains to be determined.

Key Points

1. Corticotropin-releasing hormone plays a pivotal role in integrating the stress response
2. Adrenal insufficiency and glucocorticoid resistance are common in critically ill patients, particularly those with severe sepsis.
3. Critical illness causes a decrease in T_3 with an increase in rT_3 with a normal TSH. There is no evidence that treatment with thyroid hormone is beneficial in this situation.

4. Stress hyperglycemia is almost universal in critically ill patients. Hyperglycemia is pro-inflammatory and pro-thrombic and increases oxidant injury. Glycemic control improves outcome of critically ill patients.

Key References

52. Annane D, Maxime V, Ibrahim F, et al: Diagnosis of adrenal insufficiency in severe sepsis and septic shock. Am J Respir Crit Care Med 2006;174:1319-1326.
55. Keh D, Boehnke T, Weber-Cartens S, et al: Immunologic and hemodynamic effects of "low-dose" hydrocortisone in septic shock: A double-blind, randomized, placebo-controlled, crossover study. Am J Respir Crit Care Med 2003;167:512-520.
91. Takala J, Ruokonen E, Webster NR, et al: Increased mortality associated with growth hormone treatment in critically ill adults. N Engl J Med 1999;341:785-792.
107. Van den Berghe G, Wouters P, Weekers F, et al: Intensive insulin therapy in critically ill patients. N Engl J Med 2001;345:1359-1367.
151. van der Voort PH, Feenstra RA, Bakker AJ, et al: Intravenous glucose intake independently related to intensive care unit and hospital mortality: An argument for glucose toxicity in critically ill patients. Clin Endocrinol 2006;64:141-145.

See the companion Expert Consult website for the complete reference list.

CHAPTER 138

Nitrogen Balance and Nutritional Assessment

Xavier M. Leverve and Noël J. M. Cano

OBJECTIVES

This chapter will:
1. Discuss nutritional status assessment in acute renal failure by examining its history, anthropometric, and biological parameters.
2. Describe the specificity of acute renal failure, especially regarding hydration status, in interpreting clinical and biological data.
3. Consider the risks of glucose dysregulation and protein depletion in patients with acute renal failure.

INTRODUCTION

The prevalence of protein-energy malnutrition in patients in intensive care units (ICUs) in Western countries is high (30%). This is related to the clinical characteristics of these patients with various co-morbidities and prior history of sickness before admission to the ICU. In addition, the severity of the metabolic derangement linked to the severity of the disease induces an acute malnutrition, potentially worsened by inadequate nutrient supply. Depending on the cause of renal failure and its clinical presentation, two types of patients with acute renal failure must be considered: those with isolated renal disease, characterized by a high rate of recovery and a low prevalence of malnutrition, and those with acute renal failure complicating a severe disease.[1]

The first step required for determining nutrient needs is assessment. Nutritional assessment is based on three groups of parameters: anthropometric variables, biological variables, and composite scores. Similar approaches and tools are used for acutely ill patients regardless of the occurrence of acute renal failure. However, because of specific metabolic features, the presence of renal deficiency complicates the interpretation of findings.[2] The reference data pertaining to patients with acute renal failure are often different from those of patients without renal failure, and they are less available as well. Finally, because of the close metabolic relationships between renal function and protein metabolism and because of the particularly high risk of protein hypercatabolism, specific

tools are necessary for investigating protein metabolism in patients with renal failure. Evaluation of nutritional status and body composition (when available) should be recorded at the time of admission and monitored over time, in order to obtain a dynamic nutritional assessment.

ANTHROPOMETRIC MEASUREMENTS AND BODY COMPOSITION

Monitoring body weight or body mass index (BMI, weight [kg]/height^2 [m^2]) is a well-established practice for evaluating nutritional status in patients with moderate diseases and without renal disease. However, it is less appropriate for patients with renal failure, especially for those in ICUs. Indeed, patients with renal failure have limitations related to the frequent large changes in fluid status, for instance, due to large volumes of fluid for resuscitation and other supportive measures. Loss of lean body mass in these catabolic patients may not be apparent in daily weight measurements because of fluid retention. Hence, caution must be taken in using BMI since its accuracy is uncertain in the context of acute renal failure.[3,4] The most functional way for using these parameters is allowing the patient to evaluate the changes in his or her body in time rather than relying on an absolute value in a given situation. Normal values of BMI are between 18.5 and 25 kg/m^2. Values lower than 18.5 kg/m^2 indicate undernutrition: 18.5-17 mild grade I, 17-16 moderate grade II, 16-13 moderate grade III, 13-10 severe grade IV, 10 and below very severe grade V.

Evaluation of the different body compartments, particularly lean body mass, is important but difficult, especially in patients in the ICU. Body composition can be considered at different levels (Fig. 138-1), and several methods have been proposed in the literature for assessing these different levels. However, the methods currently available in ICU practice have limitations. Anthropometric triceps skinfold and mid upper arm circumference measurements have been used in the past to estimate body fat and lean mass in healthy subjects and chronically ill patients. However, these determinations have very little use, if any, in acutely ill patients because standards have not been established.

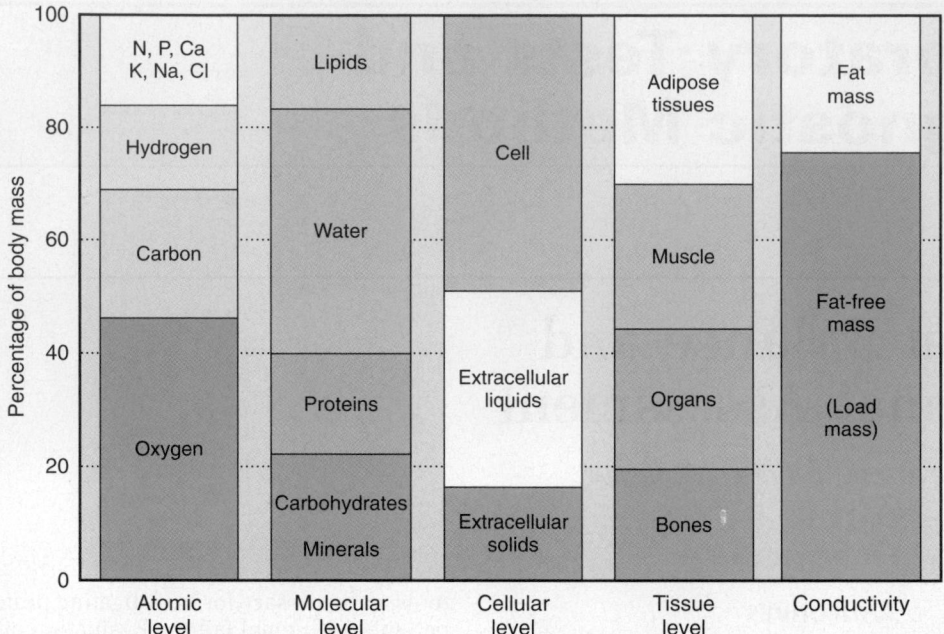

FIGURE 138-1. Body compartment at different levels.

Bioelectrical impedance analysis, a noninvasive technique, has been proposed for measuring fat-free mass, total body water, percent fat, body cell mass, intracellular water, and extracellular water, but its use is not well established in the critically ill.[3]

BIOLOGICAL PARAMETERS

Although several biological parameters have been validated in patients with protein-energy malnutrition, their significance is more complicated in acutely ill patients, especially those with acute renal failure.

Several plasma proteins have been widely recognized as markers of protein status and therefore have been proposed to detect protein malnutrition. However, the plasma proteins currently proposed for this purpose—albumin, transthyretin, and transferrin—are also influenced by other factors beyond undernutrition, such as inflammatory conditions, liver function, and renal failure. Hence, as it was already mentioned for the anthropometric markers, caution should be taken with the use of biological markers in ICU patients with acute renal failure.

Albumin is the oldest and most widely used plasma protein for assessing protein status. Its normal value is 35 to 50 g/L; a value below 30 g/L is considered as an indication of protein malnutrition. Because of its long half-life (20 days), it is not accurate for evaluating acute changes. Moreover, acute metabolic response in ICU patients leads to a fall in serum albumin by several mechanisms besides a nutritional effect: (1) a shift of fluid from intravascular to extravascular spaces,[2] (2) an increased degradation, and (3) changes in hydration status.

Transthyretin (also known as prealbumin, thyroxin binding protein, or retinol binding protein) is also used as a marker of protein malnutrition. It is also affected by inflammation and liver failure. Its value as an indicator of protein status has been well validated in the general population and, in particular, in patients with chronic renal

failure.[5] However, one must be aware that due to renal degradation, its normal value (i.e., in the absence of malnutrition) is higher in patients with chronic renal failure as compared to patients with normal renal function.[6] Transthyretin represents a better indicator of acute changes in protein status than does albumin because it has a shorter half-life (48 hours).

Transferrin has also been proposed as a protein indicator because its concentration is sensitive to nutritional status; however, it is not very specific, depending on inflammation, iron status, liver function, and so forth. Therefore, it has no real advantage despite its half-life of 10 days.

Creatinine is the final metabolite of creatine, a key intermediate in muscle energy metabolism, and both plasma concentration and urine excretion have been proposed as indicators of muscle mass. Plasma concentration of creatinine is not a good reflection of the muscular mass in renal failure because its level also depends on the degree of renal function.

Renal failure is responsible for several other metabolic alterations, which may affect the course of the disease and its management. Hence, some other metabolic parameters should be included for assessing the nutritional and metabolic state of these patients.

Glucose metabolism is altered in acutely ill patients because of insulin resistance leading to hyperglycemia and its related effects on co-morbidities and outcome.[7] However, renal failure also affects glucose metabolism. The kidney is a prominent site of low-molecular-weight protein and polypeptide breakdown.[8] Thus, acute renal failure is associated with a decrease in insulin degradation, which contributes to the pathogenesis of hyperinsulinemia and insulin resistance. In addition, the kidney is the second most important organ, after the liver, for gluconeogenesis from lactate and amino acids[9]; this is especially important in patients potentially subjected to liver failure. It is important to consider that renal failure is the second most common cause of hypoglycemia in the ICU after insulin therapy. Hence, careful monitoring of blood glucose is recommended in ICU patients with renal failure.

Lipid Metabolism

Disorders of lipid and fatty acid metabolism are also present during acute renal failure. They are characterized by hypertriglyceridemia and a low level of high-density lipoprotein cholesterol secondary to a defect in lipoprotein lipase activity.[10] Long- and medium-chain triglyceride clearances are typically lessened during acute renal failure.[11-13]

A depressed total lymphocyte count ($<1200/mm^2$) or delayed cutaneous sensitivity (abolished) to skin test antigens has been proposed as indicators of protein energy malnutrition. Accumulation of toxins during renal failure may be responsible for impairing the immune response.[14]

NITROGEN METABOLISM AND NITROGEN BALANCE IN PATIENTS WITH ACUTE RENAL FAILURE

Because of the renal dysfunction, most of the urinary parameters used to assess the magnitude of protein catabolism in acutely ill patients cannot be proposed in patients with acute renal failure. Hence 24-hour excretion of creatinine (evaluating muscle mass), urea (evaluating oxidized proteins), total nitrogen (evaluating total protein breakdown) and 3-methylhistidine (an amino acid specific of actin and myosin chains and reflecting muscle protein catabolism) cannot be performed. As presented in Table 138-1, it is possible to assess the protein catabolic rate in patients with renal failure.[14,15] Urea nitrogen appearance (i.e., daily urea production) can be calculated from the sum of urinary urea nitrogen and dialysate urea nitrogen in the case of intermittent hemodialysis and persistent urine production. In the case of anuria and continuous renal replacement therapy, urea nitrogen appearance is obtained by the sum of ultrafiltrate urea nitrogen and the change in body urea nitrogen, which can be calculated from the difference in serum urea nitrogen and the dilution space of urea, estimated to be 60% of body weight. Hence, total nitrogen appearance and protein net catabolism can be derived, allowing estimation of the needs for protein (enteral nutrition) or amino acid (parenteral nutrition) administration.

FUNCTIONAL PARAMETERS AND COMPOSITE SCORES

Several functional tests have been proposed to evaluate muscular strength, which represents a valuable parameter for assessing nutritional status in clinical practice. However, its use in ICU patients is difficult, and therefore its practical value is negligible in these patients.

Because of the low specificity and sensitivity of these different tests in patients with acute renal failure, no single factor properly reflects nutritional status, which can be described only by integrating biochemical markers, anthropometric measurements, and functional parameters with the subjective well-being of the patient. Different nutritional indexes have been proposed in order to define an integrated way for assessing nutritional status. None of these indexes has been evaluated specifically in ICU patients with acute renal failure. However, even if their prognostic value in this particular clinical condition is uncertain, they can be used safely as reliable guides for the implementation of the nutritional support.

The Subjective Global Assessment (SGA), introduced by Detsky and colleagues,[16] is based on patients' medical history, functional symptoms, and clinical evaluation. With use of this assessment tool, patients are classified into three groups: well nourished, moderately malnourished, and severely malnourished. This SGA index was used in a prospective cohort study,[17] which demonstrated that severe malnutrition was present in 42% of patients with acute renal failure. Hospital length of stay and in-hospital mortality were increased in malnourished patients while malnutrition appeared as a predictor of in-hospital mortality independently of complications and co-morbidities.[17]

Another well-recognized nutritional index, the Nutritional Risk Index (NRI), was introduced by Buzby and colleagues.[18] This composite score includes the time course of weight changes and the concentration of albumin ($=1.519 \times$ [albumin] $+ 0.417 \times$ [percentage of weight change]).

TABLE 138-1

Nitrogen Excretion and Protein Catabolism in Acute Renal Failure

PROTEIN/NITROGEN PARAMETER (g/day)	EQUATIONS
Urea nitrogen appearance (UNA)	= Urinary urea nitrogen (g/day) + dialysate urea nitrogen (g/day) or Ultrafiltrate urea nitrogen (g/day) + CBUN (g/day)
Change in body urea nitrogen	= (SUNf − SUNi [g/L]) × BWi × 0.6 + (BWf − BWi [kg/day]) × SUNf (g/L)
Total nitrogen appearance (TNA)	= 1.27 + 1.19 UNA (g/day)
Protein equivalent of total nitrogen appearance = net protein catabolism	= TNA (g/day) × 6.25

BWf, body weight (final); BWi, body weight (initial); SUNf, serum urea nitrogen (final value); SUNi, serum urea nitrogen (initial value).

CONCLUSION

Assessing the nutritional status of ICU patients with acute renal failure is not very specific when compared with assessing the nutritional status of similar patients without renal impairment. The step of clinical and biological evaluation is important not only for guiding nutritional support but also for anticipating the risk of co-morbidities and complications classically related to the undernourished status. The specificity of the metabolic alterations related to acute renal failure is related to (1) the sensitivity of almost all parameters to the patients' hydration state, (2) the particular risk of protein hypercatabolism, (3) the management of glycemia with the risk of both hyperglycemia (insulin resistance) and hypoglycemia (impairment of renal gluconeogenesis), and (4) the frequent deficit in micronutrients.

Key Points

1. Nutritional depletion is an independent risk factor for patients with acute renal failure.
2. Assessing nutrition status in patients with acute renal failure is similar to assessing nutrition status in other patients in the intensive care unit, in that the same tools are used and the same limitations exist. One difference is the scarcity of reference data pertaining to patients with acute renal failure.
3. Assessing nutritional status is always a multiparametric approach, which should be recorded at the beginning and regularly to obtain follow-up data.
4. Carbohydrate management in patients with acute renal failure is difficult because of the increased risk of hyperglycemia due to insulin resistance

and increased risk of hypoglycemia due to renal failure.
5. Patients with acute renal failure are at risk of protein depletion; protein catabolic rate can be assessed in anuric patients.

Key References

3. Bistrian BR, McCowen KC, Chan S: Protein-energy malnutrition in dialysis patients. Am J Kidney Dis 1999;33:172-175.
5. Cano N, Fernandez JP, Lacombe P, et al: Statistical selection of nutritional parameters in hemodialyzed patients. Kidney Int Suppl 1987;22:S178-S180.
10. Kopple JD: The nutrition management of the patient with acute renal failure. JPEN J Parenter Enteral Nutr 1996;20: 3-12.
13. Plauth M, Merli M, Kondrup J, et al: ESPEN guidelines for nutrition in liver disease and transplantation. Clin Nutr 1997;16:43-55.
17. Fiaccadori E, Lombardi M, Leonardi S, et al: Prevalence and clinical outcome associated with preexisting malnutrition in acute renal failure: a prospective cohort study. J Am Soc Nephrol 1999;10:581-593.

See the companion Expert Consult website for the complete reference list.

CHAPTER 139

Diagnosis and Management of Critical Illness–Related Corticosteroid Insufficiency

Paul E. Marik

OBJECTIVES

This chapter will:
1. Review the concept of critical illness–related corticosteroid insufficiency.
2. Discuss the difficulties in diagnosing adrenal insufficiency in the critically ill.
3. Define that population of patients most likely to benefit from treatment with corticosteroids.

Interest in the assessment of adrenal function and the indications for adrenal replacement therapy in critically ill patients has increased in recent years. Once considered a rare diagnosis in the intensive care unit (ICU), "adrenal insufficiency" is being reported with increased frequency in critically ill patients. The incidence of adrenal failure varies widely depending on the criteria used to make the diagnosis and the patient population studied. It is important to distinguish between patients presenting to hospital with evidence of chronic adrenal insufficiency (Addison's disease) and those with acute adrenal insufficiency. The

latter condition is best referred to as critical illness–related corticosteroid insufficiency (CIRCI). CIRCI is defined as inadequate corticosteroid activity for the severity of the patient's illness. The terms *absolute adrenal insufficiency* and *relative adrenal insufficiency* are best avoided in the context of critical illness. CIRCI may arise due to adrenal insufficiency or tissue resistance to corticosteroids (see Chapter 137). CIRCI may occur in patients with underlying disease of the hypothalamic-pituitary-adrenal (HPA) axis (primary or secondary adrenal insufficiency) who are unable to increase production of cortisol in the face of stress, or it may develop acutely due to infarction or hemorrhage of the pituitary or adrenal gland (Table 139-1). However, reversible corticosteroid insufficiency is increasingly being recognized in critically ill patients with sepsis and patients with systemic inflammatory response syndrome associated with burns, pancreatitis, trauma, cardiopulmonary bypass, and liver disease. The overall incidence of corticosteroid insufficiency in critically ill patients is 10% to 20%, with an incidence as high as 60% in patients with septic shock.[1-6]

The major impact of corticosteroid insufficiency in the critically ill is on the systemic inflammatory response. Glucocorticoids play a central role in modulating the

TABLE 139-1

Causes of Adrenal Insufficiency

Reversible Dysfunction of the Hypothalamic-Pituitary-
  Adrenal Axis
  Sepsis, systemic inflammatory response syndrome
  Drugs
    Corticosteroids (secondary AI)
    Ketoconazole (primary AI)
    Etomidate (primary AI)
    Megestrol acetate (secondary AI)
    Rifampin (increased cortisol metabolism)
    Phenytoin (increased cortisol metabolism)
    Metyrapone (primary AI)
    Mitotane (primary AI)
  Hypothermia (primary AI)
Primary Adrenal Insufficiency
  Autoimmune adrenalitis
  HIV infection
    HIV
    Drugs
  Cytomegalovirus infection
    Metastatic carcinoma
    Lung
    Breast
    Kidney
  Systemic fungal infections
    Histoplasmosis
    Cryptococcosis
    Blastomycosis
  Tuberculosis
  Acute hemorrhage or infarction
    Disseminated intravascular coagulation
    Meningococcemia
    Anti-coagulation
    Anti-phospholipid syndrome
    Heparin-induced thrombocytopenia (HIT)
    Trauma
Secondary Adrenal Insufficiency
  Chronic steroid use
  Pituitary or metastatic tumor
  Pituitary surgery or radiation
  Empty-sella syndrome
  Craniopharyngioma
  Sarcoidosis, histiocytosis
  Post-partum pituitary necrosis
  HIV infection
  Head trauma

AI, adrenal insufficiency.

TABLE 139-2

Symptoms and Signs of Critical Illness–Related Corticosteroid Insufficiency

Specific Features
  Hypotension resistant to volume resuscitation
  Eosinophilia
  Hypoglycemia (usually mild)
  Hyponatremia and hyperkalemia (rare and usually mild)
  Pituitary deficiencies (gonadotrophin, thyroid, diabetes
    insipidus)
Nonspecific Features
  Unexplained fever
  Unexplained mental status changes
  Hyperdynamic circulation
  Anemia
  Metabolic acidosis
  Nausea, vomiting
  Diarrhea

Clinical signs include orthostatic hypotension and hyperpigmentation (primary adrenal insufficiency). Laboratory testing may demonstrate hyponatremia, hyperkalemia, hypoglycemia, and a normocytic anemia.[11] This presentation contrasts with the features of CIRCI (Table 139-2). Hypotension refractory to fluids and requiring vasopressors is the most common feature of acute adrenal insufficiency.[11,12] CIRCI should be considered in all ICU patients requiring vasopressor support. Patients usually have a hyperdynamic circulation, which may compound the hyperdynamic profile of the patient with sepsis or systemic inflammatory response syndrome.[12] However, the systemic vascular resistance, cardiac output, and pulmonary capillary wedge pressure can be low, normal, or high.[2] The variability in hemodynamics reflects the combination of CIRCI and the underlying disease. Central nervous system dysfunction is common, frequently compounded by the underlying disease. Individuals with CIRCI may present with altered mental status, particularly unexplained confusion, as the major clinical finding. In addition, CIRCI should be considered in critically ill patients with unexplained fever. Laboratory assessment may demonstrate eosinophilia and hypoglycemia. Hyponatremia and hyperkalemia are uncommon.

activation of NF-κB, the major nuclear transcription factor responsible for the production of pro-inflammatory mediators.[7,8] Diminished glucocorticoid activity results in excessive production of these mediators.[7,9,10] Patients with CIRCI (severe sepsis, septic shock, acute respiratory distress syndrome, etc.) are characterized by insufficient glucocorticoid activity with excessive production of pro-inflammatory mediators (Fig. 139-1). The clinical manifestations of CIRCI, therefore, are those of an exaggerated inflammatory response (hypotension, fever, increased tissue injury).

CLINICAL PRESENTATION

Patients with chronic adrenal insufficiency (Addison's disease) usually present with a history of weakness, weight loss, anorexia, and lethargy; some patients will complain of nausea, vomiting, abdominal pain, and diarrhea.

DIAGNOSIS OF ADRENAL INSUFFICIENCY AND CRITICAL ILLNESS–RELATED CORTICOSTEROID INSUFFICIENCY

The diagnosis of adrenal insufficiency in the critically ill has been based on the measurement of a random total serum cortisol ("stress" cortisol level) or the change in the serum cortisol in response to 250 μg of synthetic adrenocorticotropic hormone (cosyntropin), the so-called delta cortisol.[1,4] Both of these tests have significant limitations in the critically ill.[13] Assays for serum total cortisol measure the total hormone concentration (serum free cortisol plus the protein-bound fraction). The current consensus is that the free cortisol, rather than protein-bound fraction, is responsible for the physiological function of the hormone.[1,14,15] In critically ill patients cortisol-binding

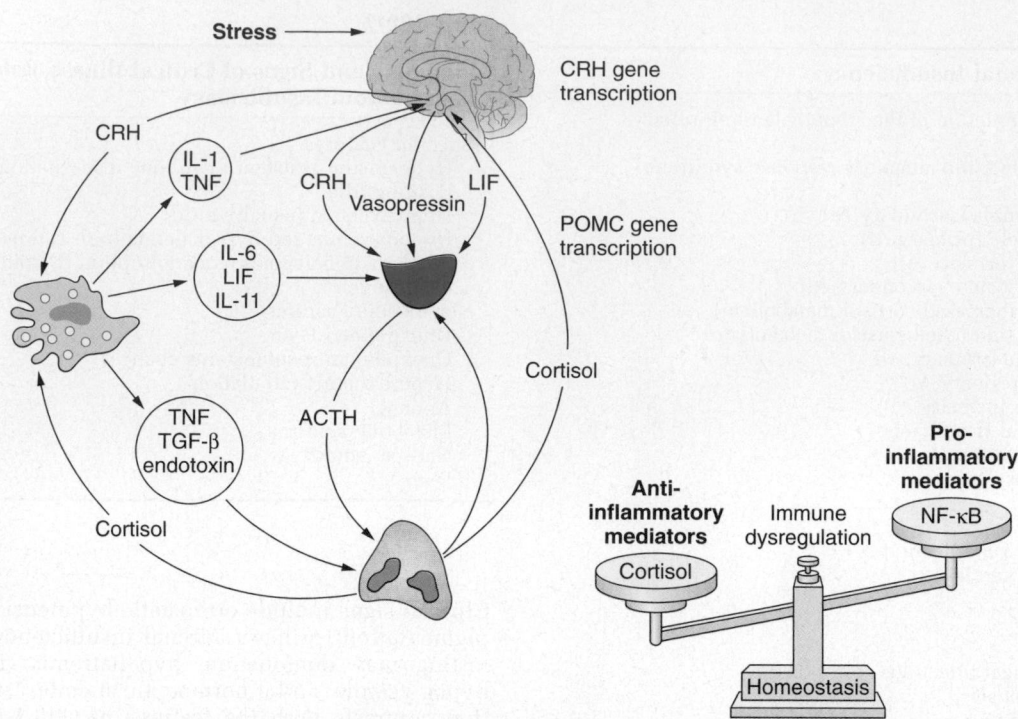

FIGURE 139-1. Cortisol inhibits production of pro-inflammatory mediators and suppresses adrenocorticotropic hormone (ACTH) and corticotropin releasing hormone (CRH) production. Failure to produce adequate amounts of cortisol or cortisol resistance results in excessive production of cytokines such as interleukin-6 (IL-6), interleukin-1 (IL-1), and tumor necrosis factor (TNF). LIF, leukocyte inhibitory factor; POMC, proopiomelanocortin; TGF-β, transforming growth factor-beta.

globulin levels are decreased.[15-19] Furthermore, with acute stimulation of the adrenal gland, the relative increase of the free bioactive cortisol concentration is substantially more pronounced than the increase of total cortisol concentration.[15-20] Consequently, the total serum cortisol may not accurately reflect the free cortisol. This dissociation between the total and free cortisol level is most marked in patients with a serum albumin less than 2.5 mg/dL.[13,16] The threshold total cortisol level (15, 20, or 25 µg/dL) that defines adrenal insufficiency has not been accurately determined.[1,4,14] While measurement of the free cortisol may therefore be preferable, this is a laborious and expensive test that is not widely available. To complicate the issue further, recent data suggest that the commercially available cortisol immunoassays may not be accurate, particularly in patients with sepsis. Using mass spectrometry as the gold standard, Vogeser and colleagues[21] have demonstrated that the different commercial cortisol immunoassays may over- or underestimate the actual cortisol value and the delta cortisol. The 95% confidence level of the variation in the cortisol may be as high as 20 µg/dL for a random level and 10 µg/dL for the delta response (personal communication; Corticosteroid Therapy of Septic Shock [(CORTICUS] Trial Data). Furthermore, these authors have demonstrated a higher variation in serum cortisol from septic shock patients compared to nonseptic ICU controls. The presence of interfering heterophile antibodies may account for this observation.[22,23]

While a delta cortisol of less than 9 µg/dL has proven to be an important prognostic marker,[5,24-26] and a marker of response to treatment with corticosteroids,[3,27] this test has a number of limitations. Most notably, the delta cortisol is a measure of adrenal reserve and adrenal responsiveness to adrenocorticotropic hormone; it does not assess the integrity of the HPA axis and is not a measure of adrenal function. Indeed, over 50% of healthy volunteers and patients with no evidence of HPA disease have been reported to have a delta cortisol of less than 9 mg/dL.[10,13,16,28] In addition, the adrenocorticotropic hormone stimulation test may be poorly reproducible in patients with septic shock.[29,30] Furthermore, this test may not allow for the recognition of secondary adrenal insufficiency.

As there are no clinically useful tests available to assess the cellular actions of cortisol, the accurate diagnosis of adrenal insufficiency and CIRCI remains elusive. At this time, the diagnosis of adrenal insufficiency may be made based on the free cortisol level or the total cortisol level stratified by serum albumin (Table 139-3).[5,13] As these criteria are based on limited data, it is likely that these diagnostic thresholds will be refined with time. It is important to stress that the diagnosis of adrenal insufficiency, or CIRCI, should not be made on the basis of laboratory criteria alone. An otherwise asymptomatic patient with one or more of the criteria listed in Table 139-3 should not be considered to have CIRCI. CIRCI should be considered in all patients with vasopressor-dependent septic shock as well as in patients with unexplained hemodynamic instability. This diagnosis should also be considered in patients with unexplained fever, confusion, or both. Eosinophilia may be a useful marker to screen for adrenal insufficiency in the ICU.[31-34]

Who to Treat?

The benefit of low-dose (200 to 300 mg/day) hydrocortisone in patients with septic shock has been evaluated in

TABLE 139-3

Diagnostic Criteria for Adrenal Insufficiency

	ALBUMIN >2.5 g/dL	ALBUMIN <2.5 g/dL
Total cortisol (mg/dL)		
Baseline	15	10
Stimulated	20	15
Free cortisol (mg/dL)		
Baseline	—	1.8
Stimulated	—	3.0

seven randomized controlled trials.[3,35-40] Although many of the studies were statistically underpowered, two published meta-analyses—which included five of the studies—demonstrated a reduction in mortality and greater shock reversal in those patients who received low-dose hydrocortisone.[41,42] A meta-analysis of all seven studies (including the recently completed CORTICUS study) demonstrates greater shock reversal with low-dose steroids but no benefit in terms of mortality.[43]

The French Multicenter study performed by Annane and colleagues[3] and the recently completed European Multicenter study (CORTICUS)[40] were more adequately powered to allow further analysis. Annane and colleagues[3] randomized 300 patients with refractory septic shock to treatment with hydrocortisone (50 mg intravenously every 6 hours) and oral fludrocortisone (50 μg daily) or matching placebo. All patients underwent a 250-μg cosyntropin stimulation test. There was a 30% decrease in 28-day mortality in the hydrocortisone-fludrocortisone group (hazard ratio 0.67; 95% confidence interval of 0.47 to 0.95; $P = .02$).[3] This benefit was confined to the group of nonresponders (delta cortisol of less than 9 mg/dL).

The recently completed CORTICUS study was a double-blind, randomized, placebo-controlled study performed in 52 centers throughout Europe.[40] Five hundred patients (499 analyzable) were enrolled between March 2002 and November 2005. Inclusion criteria included septic shock (systolic blood pressure less than 90 mm Hg despite adequate fluid resuscitation or need for pressors) and evidence of organ dysfunction attributable to sepsis. Patients were randomized to hydrocortisone (50 mg every 6 hours for 5 days; then 50 mg every 12 hours for 3 days, followed by 50 mg daily for 3 days) or matching placebo. Patients did not receive fludrocortisone. Although the baseline characteristics of the patients were similar, only 35% of the cohort were medical patients, with the abdomen being the most common source of infection (42%). There was no difference in the 28-day all-cause mortality between those patients who received hydrocortisone as compared to those who received the placebo. Furthermore, there was no difference in mortality between the groups when stratified as responders (delta cortisol of greater than 9 mg/dL) or nonresponders. However, the patients who received hydrocortisone (both responders and nonresponder) had significantly more rapid resolution of shock ($P = 0.003$ for log rank test). The incidence of adverse events, including critical illness polyneuropathy and complicating infections, was similar between groups. It is not clear why greater shock reversal did not translate into a better survival in the hydrocortisone group. It is possible that improvements in the supportive care of critically ill patients with septic shock over the past decade have contributed to the survival of patients with CIRCI who

otherwise would have died. Furthermore, there may be a number of reasons why hydrocortisone improved outcome in the French Multicenter study and not in the CORTICUS study. The patients enrolled in the Annane study had refractory septic shock and were therefore sicker than those enrolled in the CORTICUS study. The demographics and clinical characteristics of the patients enrolled in the two studies were quite different. Furthermore, the use of etomidate in a large number of patients in the Annane study was an important confounding variable.

Given the different outcome of these two studies, what should the clinician do? Considering the central role of cortisol in mediating the stress response and recognizing the effect of sepsis on the HPA axis and on cellular glucocorticoid activity, the use of supplemental "stress" doses of hydrocortisone appears logical in patients with septic shock. The best available clinical evidence suggests that stress doses of hydrocortisone result in significantly more rapid shock resolution without an increase in steroid-related adverse effects. The effects of low-dose hydrocortisone on mortality is less clear. Based on the data from the French Multicenter study and the CORTICUS study, low-dose hydrocortisone should be considered in the management strategy of patients with septic shock, particularly those patients with refractory septic shock requiring high doses of vasopressor agents. At this time, it appears that the decision to treat patients with septic shock should not be based on the results of a stress serum cortisol level or the response to cosyntropin. In addition, the administration of hydrocortisone during septic shock was found to reduce the incidence of post-traumatic stress disorder and improve the emotional well-being of septic shock survivors.[44]

The role of stress doses of corticosteroids has been investigated in other clinical settings. Confalonieri and colleagues[45] randomized 46 patients with severe community-acquired pneumonia to receive hydrocortisone or a placebo. Inclusion in this study required the presence of severe pneumonia but not septic shock. Hydrocortisone was given as an initial bolus of 200 mg followed by an infusion at a rate of 10 mg/hr for 7 days. Treatment with corticosteroids was associated with a more rapid improvement in oxygenation, a lower incidence of multiple-organ failure and delayed septic shock, a reduction in the length of ICU stay, and a marked reduction in 28-day mortality (70% vs. 100%; $P = 0.009$). This study suggests that treatment with corticosteroids may be beneficial in patients with severe community-acquired pneumonia who are not in shock. Additional studies are required to confirm this finding.

Sepsis and end-stage liver disease have a number of pathophysiological mechanisms in common (endotoxemia, increased levels of pro-inflammatory mediators, decreased levels of high density lipoprotein), and it is therefore not surprising that adrenal insufficiency is common in patients with end-stage liver disease.[46-48] Tsai and colleagues[24] performed a corticotropin stimulation test in 101 patients with cirrhosis and sepsis. In this study, 51.4% of the patients were diagnosed with adrenal insufficiency; survival at 90 days was 15.3% in these patients compared to 63.2% in those patients with normal adrenal function. None of the patients was treated with corticosteroids. The results of the Hepatic Cortisol Research and Adrenal Pathophysiology Study (HeCRAPS), in which 245 of 340 (72%) patients with liver disease were diagnosed with adrenal insufficiency (the hepato-adrenal syndrome), were reported in 2005.[49] Although this was not a randomized study designed to test the benefit of treatment with corticosteroids, an escalation of pressors over 24 hours was reported in those patients with adrenal insufficiency who were not treated with corticosteroids, whereas the dose of pressors was reduced in the group treated with corticosteroids. Furthermore, the mortality was significantly lower in the group treated with corticosteroids. Treatment with corticosteroids should therefore be considered in critically ill patients with cirrhosis who are hemodynamically unstable.

In summary, the benefit of treatment with low-dose corticosteroids at this time appears to be limited to patients with refractory septic shock. Adrenal function testing is not required in these patients. Preliminary data suggest that corticosteroids may be of benefit in patients with severe pneumonia (without shock), early in the course of acute respiratory distress syndrome, in patients with liver failure and during weaning from mechanical ventilation.[27,45,49-52] The role of corticosteroids in patients with adrenal insufficiency who have pancreatitis, burns, head injury, or sub-arachnoid hemorrhage has not been investigated. The potential benefits of treatment with hydrocortisone in these and other critically ill patients deserves further investigation.

How to Treat?

The optimal dose and duration of treatment with hydrocortisone remains to be determined in well-controlled and powered studies. However, recommendations can be made based on the results of previously published studies. A number of randomized clinical trials have investigated the use of a high-dose short course treatment with corticosteroids in patients with acute respiratory distress syndrome and sepsis. Doses of methylprednisolone as high as 20 to 30 mg per kg of body weight (total of 10,000 to 40,000 mg of hydrocortisone) over 24 hours were investigated.[41,42,53] These studies were unable to demonstrate an improved outcome, and a higher risk of complications was found in patients who received high-dose corticosteroids.[41,42,53] The literature therefore does not support the use of high-dose corticosteroids in critically ill patients (except to prevent or treat rejection in transplant patients). Furthermore, although widely used, high-dose corticosteroids are not considered the standard of care for patients with acute spinal cord injuries.[54-57] Indeed, according to the most recent Neurosurgical Guidelines, the "evidence suggesting harmful side effects (of high dose methylprednisolone) is more consistent than any suggestion of clinical benefit."[58]

Myopathy and an increased risk of superinfections have been reported in patients receiving in excess of 300 mg/hydrocortisone equivalents per day; however, these complications have not been reported in patients receiving 300 mg or less hydrocortisone equivalents per day.[41,42,59] Furthermore, while suppressing an exaggerated pro-inflammatory response a dose of 200 to 300 mg hydrocortisone per day does not appear to have immunosuppressive effects.[60] Based on these data, treatment with 50 mg hydrocortisone intravenously every 6 hours is recommended. Full-dose hydrocortisone treatment should continue for 5 to 7 days before tapering, assuming that there is no recurrence of signs of shock. The role of an abbreviated course (3 to 5 days) of hydrocortisone in patients with septic shock who are weaned off pressors within 24 to 48 hours remains to be determined. Hydrocortisone should be tapered slowly and not stopped abruptly. The hydrocortisone dose should be reduced every 2 to 3 days by 50%

unless there is clinical deterioration, which would then require an increase in hydrocortisone dose. Abruptly stopping hydrocortisone will likely result in a rebound of pro-inflammatory mediators and recurrence of the features of shock.[59,60] At the time of this writing, the addition of fludrocortisone to hydrocortisone is considered optional.

ADRENAL EXHAUSTION SYNDROME

Adrenal function in the critically ill is a dynamic process. Normal "adrenal function" testing on admission to the ICU does not preclude the development of adrenal insufficiency later in the patients' ICU course. This development is referred to as the adrenal exhaustion syndrome."[1,61,62] Van der Voort and Koopman[63] measured the baseline and cortisol response 30 and 60 minutes after a high-dose (250 µg) tetracosactide (Synacthen) test in 38 consecutive ICU patients on days 1, 4, 7, 10, 14, and 21 of their ICU stay. On day 1, 26% and 0% were diagnosed with adrenal and HPA axis failure, respectively, while the incidence rose to 100% and 11%, respectively, by day 4. Similarly, Beishuizen and colleagues[33] measured the eosinophil count (a marker of adrenal failure) daily in 612 consecutive patients admitted to a medical-surgical ICU. During their ICU stay, 40 (7%) of these patients developed an eosinophil count of greater than 3%. Low-dose (1 µg) Synacthen testing revealed adrenal failure in 10 of these 40 patients. In this study, adrenal insufficiency was diagnosed a mean of 7.3 ± 4.2 days after admission to the ICU. In the HeCRAPs study, 16% of patients with liver disease who, on admission to the ICU, had normal adrenal function were subsequently diagnosed with adrenal insufficiency.[62] In this study, the only factor that was predictive of the development of adrenal insufficiency was the high-density lipoprotein, which was 11.7 ± 7.0 in patients who developed syndrome compared to 28.4 ± 14.4 in the control group. The finding that a low level of high-density lipoprotein was predictive of the subsequent development of adrenal failure strongly supports the concept of adrenal exhaustion and the role of altered lipoprotein metabolism in the pathophysiology of CIRCI.[43,61,64-66] Adrenal function in the critically ill should therefore be considered a dynamic process; repeat adrenal function testing is indicated in patients who, on initial testing, have appropriate cortisol levels and who remain hemodynamically unstable or who fail to improve with aggressive supportive treatment.

Key Points

1. Acute adrenal insufficiency in critically ill patients is best referred to as critical illness–related corticosteroid insufficiency.
2. Critical illness–related corticosteroid insufficiency may arise due to adrenal insufficiency or tissue resistance to cortisol.
3. The stress total cortisol level and the cortisol response to 250 µg cosyntropin have been used to diagnose adrenal insufficiency. Both these tests have significant limitations in the critically ill.
4. The diagnosis of adrenal insufficiency, or critical illness–related corticosteroid insufficiency,

should not be made on the basis of laboratory criteria alone.

5. Treatment with low-dose hydrocortisone (200 mg/day) should be considered in patients with refractory septic shock. The role of low-dose hydrocortisone in patients with severe sepsis and other clinical situations in the intensive care unit remains to be determined.

Key References

5. Annane D, Maxime V, Ibrahim F, et al: Diagnosis of adrenal insufficiency in severe sepsis and septic shock. Am J Respir Crit Care Med 2006;174(12):1319-1326.

16. Hamrahian AH, Oseni TS, Arafah BM: Measurement of serum free cortisol in critically ill patients. N Engl J Med 2004; 350:1629-1638.

27. Huang CJ, Lin HC: Association between adrenal insufficiency and ventilator weaning. Am J Respir Crit Care Med 2006;173: 276-280.

41. Annane D, Bellissant E, Bollaert PE, et al: Corticosteroids for severe sepsis and septic shock: A systematic review and meta-analysis. BMJ 2004;329:480-489.

60. Keh D, Boehnke T, Weber-Cartens S, et al: Immunologic and hemodynamic effects of "low-dose" hydrocortisone in septic shock: A double-blind, randomized, placebo-controlled, crossover study. Am J Respir Crit Care Med 2003;167:512-520.

See the companion Expert Consult website for the complete reference list.

CHAPTER 140

Nutritional Support in the Critically Ill with Acute Renal Failure

Wilfred Druml

OBJECTIVES

This chapter will:
1. Describe the complex metabolic environment in critically ill patients with acute renal failure.
2. Illuminate the specific metabolic consequences induced by acute renal failure.
3. Explain the impact of renal replacement therapy on metabolism and nutrient balances.
4. Outline the relevant information necessary for tailoring nutrition programs to the individual needs of critically ill patients with acute renal failure.

INTRODUCTION

In critically ill patients, acute renal failure (ARF) presents a pro-oxidative, pro-inflammatory, and hypermetabolic state which has a profound impact on the course of disease and the evolution of complications and which is associated with a high attributable mortality.[1,2] Nutritional and metabolic management is a cornerstone in the care of these patients. Metabolic and nutritional requirements are affected not only by the acutely uremic condition of patients with ARF but also by the underlying disease process and associated complications (as related to metabolic management) and by the type and intensity of renal replacement therapy (RRT) (as related to nutritional requirements).

A nutritional program for a patient with ARF is not fundamentally different from that for other critically ill patients, but the complex metabolic alterations have to be taken into consideration and nutrition must be coordinated with RRT. Moreover, nutritional requirements may differ vastly between individual patients and also during the course of disease.[3]

Modern nutritional support has left behind a merely quantitative approach to providing energy to critically ill patients and has become a more qualitative type of metabolic intervention aimed at modulating the inflammatory state, the oxygen radical scavenger system, and immunocompetence and at taking advantage of specific pharmacological effects of various nutrients. Metabolic factors also play a crucial role in the prevention and treatment of ARF.

METABOLIC ENVIRONMENT AND NUTRITIONAL REQUIREMENTS IN PATIENTS WITH ACUTE RENAL FAILURE

Clinical presentation of a patient with ARF may range from uncomplicated mono-organ failure in a noncatabolic patient to a critically ill patient with multiple-organ dysfunction syndrome. Thus, metabolic changes will be determined not only by ARF but also by the underlying disease process, associated complications, organ dysfunction, and other factors (see Table 136-1).[3] In addition to the obvious effects on water, electrolyte, and acid-base metabolism, ARF affects all metabolic pathways of the body with specific alterations in protein and amino acid, carbohydrate, and lipid metabolisms (Table 140-1). Moreover, the type and intensity of RRT have a profound effect on nutritional balances.

The optimal intake of nutrients in patients with ARF is mainly influenced by the nature of the illness causing ARF, the extent of catabolism, and the type and frequency of RRT.

Energy Metabolism and Energy Requirements

In patients with uncomplicated ARF, energy expenditure is within the range of that of healthy subjects. In the presence of sepsis or multiple-organ dysfunction syndrome, oxygen consumption may increase by approximately 25%.[4] Thus, energy expenditure in patients with ARF is determined by the underlying disease and its associated complications rather than by renal failure.

Energy intake for nutritional support in the critically ill patient should never exceed actual energy requirements. Complications from slightly underfeeding are less deleterious than from overfeeding. Increasing energy intake from 30 kcal/kg body weight (BW)/day to 40 kcal/kg BW/day in patients with ARF increased the frequency of metabolic complications, such as hyperglycemia and hypertriglyceridemia, and had no beneficial effects.[5]

TABLE 140-1

Metabolic Alterations Induced by Acute
Renal Failure

- Activation of protein catabolism
- Peripheral glucose intolerance/increased gluconeogenesis
- Inhibition of lipolysis and altered fat clearance
- Depletion of the antioxidant system
- Induction of a pro-inflammatory state
- Impairment of immunocompetence
- Endocrine abnormalities: hyperparathyroidism, insulin resistance, erythropoietin resistance, resistance to growth factors

Patients with ARF should receive 20 to 30 kcal/kg BW/day. Even in hypermetabolic conditions such as sepsis or multiple-organ dysfunction syndrome, energy expenditure rarely is higher than 130% of calculated basic energy expenditure, and energy intake should not exceed 30 kcal/kg BW/day.[3,4]

Carbohydrate Metabolism

Frequently, ARF is associated with hyperglycemia. The major cause of elevated blood glucose concentrations is insulin resistance. Plasma insulin concentration is elevated; maximal insulin-stimulated glucose uptake by skeletal muscle is decreased.[6]

A second feature of glucose metabolism in ARF is accelerated hepatic gluconeogenesis—stemming mainly from conversion of amino acids released during protein catabolism—that cannot be suppressed by exogenous glucose infusions.[7]

Hyperglycemia in the critically ill is an important determinant in the evolution of complications (such as infections or organ failures) and of prognosis.[8] Thus, maintaining normoglycemia during nutritional support is essential, as insulin requirements are higher in patients with ARF (see also Chapter 136).

Lipid Metabolism

Profound alterations of lipid metabolism occur in patients with ARF. The triglyceride content of plasma lipoproteins, especially of very-low-density lipoprotein, is increased, and total cholesterol and, in particular, high-density lipoprotein cholesterol are decreased.[9] The major cause of lipid abnormalities in ARF is an impairment of lipolysis; this is in sharp contrast to other acute disease states in which lipolysis usually is augmented.[10]

Fat particles of artificial lipid emulsions for parenteral nutrition are degraded similarly to endogenous very-low-density lipoproteins, and thus, impaired lipolysis in ARF also slows down the elimination of intravenously infused lipids containing both long- and medium-chain triglycerides. Intestinal lipid absorption also is retarded in renal failure.[11]

Protein and Amino Acid Metabolism and Protein Requirements in Acute Renal Failure

Amino acid and protein metabolism in ARF are detailed in Chapter 136. In short, the hallmark of metabolic alterations in ARF is activation of protein catabolism with excessive release of amino acids from skeletal muscle and sustained negative nitrogen balance.[12] In critically ill patients on continuous renal replacement therapy (CRRT), protein catabolic rate accounts, on average, for 1.4 to 1.7 g/kg BW/day. Moreover, hepatic protein synthesis and secretion of acute-phase proteins are stimulated.

The causes of accelerated protein breakdown are manifold; the dominating mechanism is the stimulation of hepatic gluconeogenesis from amino acids, which, in contrast to both healthy subjects and patients with chronic renal failure, can be decreased but not halted by exogenous substrate supply (see Table 136-2).[1]

The most controversial question relating to nutritional support in critically ill patients with ARF is the optimal intake of amino acids and protein. This topic is discussed in Chapter 136. In conclusion, an amino acid/protein intake of 1.2 to a maximum of 1.7 g/kg BW/day is recommended.[13] These calculations include amino acid/protein losses induced by RRT. Although an even higher amino acid intake of up to 2.5 g/kg BW/day has been recommended,[14] there are no proven advantages of such excessive intakes, and the disadvantages are that they can increase uremic toxicity and provoke metabolic complications.

METABOLISM AND REQUIREMENTS OF MICRONUTRIENTS

Disorders of vitamins and trace elements are reviewed in Chapter 102. Serum levels of water-soluble vitamins usually are low in ARF patients, mainly because of losses induced by RRT; thus, requirements are increased.[12] Intake of ascorbic acid should be kept below 250 mg/day because any excessive supply may precipitate secondary oxalosis.

Despite the fact that there are minimal losses during RRT, plasma concentrations of lipid-soluble vitamins A, D, and E, but not of vitamin K, are decreased in patients with ARF.[15]

Alterations of trace-element homeostasis are a reflection of a nonspecific acute phase response. Selenium levels are profoundly decreased, and CRRTs are associated with relevant selenium losses.[16]

Several micronutrients are important components of the organism's defense mechanisms against oxygen free radical–induced injury. A profound depression in antioxidant status has been documented in patients with ARF, and an adequate supplementation of micronutrients to meet the increased requirements must be strictly observed.[17]

Electrolytes

Derangements in electrolyte balance in patients with ARF are affected by a broad spectrum of factors in addition to renal failure, including the type of underlying disease and degree of hypercatabolism, type and intensity of RRT, drug

TABLE 140-2

Metabolic Impact of Continuous Renal Replacement Therapy

- Heat loss
- Excessive load of substrates (lactate, citrate, glucose)
- Loss of nutrients (amino acids, vitamins, selenium)
- Loss of electrolytes (phosphate, magnesium)
- Elimination of (short-chain) proteins (hormones, mediators, but also of albumin)
- Metabolic consequences of bio-incompatibility (induction/ activation of mediator-cascades, of an inflammatory reaction, stimulation of protein catabolism)

therapy, and timing, type, and composition of nutritional support.[3]

Electrolyte requirements vary considerably not only between patients but also during the course of the disease in any given patient. In non-oliguric patients, in subjects on CRRT, and during the polyuric phase of ARF, electrolyte requirements can be increased considerably. Nutritional support, especially parenteral nutrition with low electrolyte contents, can induce hypophosphatemia and hypokalemia ("refeeding syndrome"). Thus, electrolyte requirements must be evaluated in patients with ARF on a day-to-day basis and intake has to be adjusted frequently.

Metabolic Impact of Extracorporeal Therapy

The impact of intermittent hemodialysis on metabolism is manifold. Several water-soluble substances, such as amino acids, vitamins, and carnitine, are lost during hemodialysis. Protein catabolism is caused not only by amino acid losses but also by activation of protein breakdown. Moreover, the generation of reactive oxygen species is augmented during hemodialysis.

The treatment of critically ill patients with ARF with CRRT is also associated with a broad pattern of metabolic consequences, which may become relevant because of the continuous mode of therapy and associated high fluid turnover of up to more than 60 L/day (Table 140-2).[18]

A major effect of CRRT is the elimination of small- and medium-sized molecules. In the case of amino acids, the sieving coefficient is within the range of 0.8 to 1.0, so the loss of amino acids can be estimated from the volume of the filtrate and the average plasma concentrations. This amounts to a loss of approximately 0.2 g/L filtrate and, depending on the filtered volume, results in a total of 5 to 15 g amino acid/day loss representing about 10% to 15% of amino acid intake. Amino acid losses during continuous hemofiltration and continuous hemodialysis are of a comparable magnitude. Depending on the type of therapy and the membrane material used, additional losses of protein can account for up to 10 g/day.

Water-soluble vitamins, such as folic acid, vitamin B6, and vitamin C, are also eliminated during CRRT, and an intake above the recommended daily allowance is required to maintain plasma concentrations of these vitamins in patients with ARF. Moreover, selenium losses during CRRT can account for twice the recommended daily allowance.[16]

Glucose balance during CRRT is dependent on the glucose concentration of the substitution fluid. Solutions designed for peritoneal dialysis should no longer be used for CRRT because they promote excessive glucose uptake. Dialysate glucose concentrations should range between 1 and 2 g/dL to maintain a zero glucose balance.

NUTRIENT ADMINISTRATION

General Considerations

- **Who needs nutritional support?** The decision to initiate nutritional support is influenced by the following factors:
  a. The patient's ability to eat.
  b. The nutritional status of the patient. In any patient with evidence of malnourishment, nutritional therapy should be initiated regardless whether the patient will be likely to eat. If a well-nourished patient will resume a normal diet within 5 days, no specific nutritional support is necessary.
  c. The severity of disease and degree of accompanying catabolism. In patients with underlying diseases associated with excess protein catabolism, nutritional support should be initiated early.
  d. Specific risks (e.g., immunosuppression, chemotherapy, or agranulocytosis).
- **When should nutritional support be started?** As previously mentioned, the timing of nutritional support will be determined by the nutritional status and the severity of disease. The more severe the malnutrition is and the more pronounced the degree of catabolism, the earlier nutrition should be initiated ("early [enteral] nutrition"). The decision should be made early in the course of disease to avoid the development of deficiencies.
- **At what degree of renal dysfunction should the nutritional regimen be adapted to renal failure?** Specific metabolic derangements of renal dysfunction occur when renal function falls below 30% of normal. Thus, at a serum creatinine above 3 mg/dL, a creatinine clearance below 40 mL/min, or both, nutritional regimens should take into account the specific metabolic abnormalities caused by ARF.
- **Is enteral or parenteral nutrition the most appropriate means of providing nutritional support in patients with ARF?** Enteral feeding is the preferred type of nutritional support for all critically ill patients, including those with ARF. Nevertheless, in many patients with ARF parenteral nutrition, total or supplementary nutrition may become necessary to meet nutritional requirements.
- **How should nutritional support be started?** Because of the broad spectrum of derangements in substrate utilization and patient intolerance to various nutrients, both enteral and parenteral nutrition should be started at a low rate and be gradually increased over several days until requirements are met.

The practice of nutrition support in critically ill patients with ARF is not fundamentally different from that in patients without renal dysfunction. For more discussion of enteral and parenteral nutrition in patients with ARF, see Chapters 144 and 145. Nutrient requirements in patients with ARF are summarized in Table 140-3. Again, requirements may differ considerably between individual patients and may vary fundamentally during the course of disease.

TABLE 140-3

Nutrient Requirements in Patients with Acute Renal Failure*

Energy Intake 20-30 (max. 35) kcal/kg BW/day
   Glucose 3-5 g/kg BW/day
   Lipids 0.8-1.2 (max. 1.5) g/kg BW/day
Amino Acids/Protein
   Conservative therapy 0.6-1.2 g/kg BW/day
   RRT 1.2-1.5 g/kg BW/day
   Hypercatabolism (max. 1.7) g/kg BW/day
Vitamins (Combination products providing RDA)
   Water-soluble 2 × RDA/day
     (Cave: Vitamin C < 250 mg/day)
   Lipid-soluble 1-2 × RDA/day
     (Higher for vitamin E)
Trace Elements (Combination products providing RDA)
   1 × RDA/day
   (Selenium 300 µg/day)
Electrolytes (Requirements must be assessed individually)
   (Cave: Hypokaliemia, hypophosphatemia, or both)

*Note: Requirements differ between individual patients and may vary considerably during the course of disease.
BW, body weight; RDA, recommended dietary allowance.

Oral Feeding

In all patients who can tolerate them, oral feedings should be used. However, oral feedings generally are restricted to non–critically ill, non-hypercatabolic patients. An initial dose of 40 g of high-quality protein per day is given (0.6 g/kg BW/day) and subsequently increased gradually to 1.0 to 1.2 g/kg BW/day as long as blood urea nitrogen (BUN) remains below 100 mg/dL. For patients treated by hemodialysis or peritoneal dialysis, protein intake should be increased to 1.0 to 1.4 g/kg BW/day. A supplement of water-soluble vitamins is recommended.

Enteral Nutrition (Tube Feeding)

In the past, parenteral nutrition was the preferred route of nutritional support in patients with ARF. During recent years, enteral nutrition has become the primary type of nutritional support for all critically ill patients, including those with ARF.[19] Even small amounts of luminally provided diets can help to support intestinal defense functions, support the intestinal immune system, and reduce infectious complications.

Moreover, enteral nutrition might exert specific advantages in ARF. In experimental ARF, enteral nutrition can augment renal plasma flow and improve renal function.[20] Enteral nutrition was a factor associated with an improved prognosis in critically ill patients with ARF.[21]

Nevertheless, gastrointestinal motility is impaired in many patients with ARF, and frequently it is not possible to meet requirements by the enteral route alone; in these cases, supplementary or temporary parenteral nutrition may be necessary.[11,22]

Few systematic studies on enteral nutrition have been conducted in patients with ARF. In the largest study to date, the nutritional effects, feasibility, and tolerance of enteral nutrition were examined in 182 patients with ARF.[23] Patients were administered either a conventional diet or a preparation adapted to the metabolic needs of hemodialysis patients. The incidence of side effects was higher and the amount of nutrients provided was lower in patients with ARF as compared to patients with normal renal function, but in general enteral nutrition was well tolerated and proved to be safe and effective.

For further discussion on the practice of enteral nutrition, tube placement, and enteral formulas, see Chapter 144.

Parenteral Nutrition

In critically ill patients with ARF, it is frequently impossible to cover nutrient requirements by the enteral route alone, and supplementary or even total parenteral nutrition may become necessary. Parenteral and enteral nutrition should not be viewed as conflicting but rather as complementary types of nutrition support, a combination resulting in an optimal nutrient provision in many critically ill patients.[22]

For further discussion on the practice of parenteral nutrition, tube placement, and parenteral formulas, see Chapter 145.

Complications of Nutritional Support

Technical problems and infectious complications originating from central venous catheters or enteral feeding tubes, metabolic complications of artificial nutrition, and gastrointestinal side effects of enteral nutrition in ARF patients are similar to those in non-uremic subjects. However, both metabolic and gastrointestinal complications are far more pronounced and occur more frequently in ARF because the utilization of various nutrients is impaired and the tolerance to electrolytes and volume load is limited; moreover, gastrointestinal motility is impaired in ARF.[3]

By gradually increasing the infusion rate and avoiding any infusion above requirements, many of the side effects can be minimized. Moreover, nutrition therapy must be closely monitored in patients with ARF.

CONCLUSIONS

Nutritional support must be viewed as a cornerstone in the treatment of patients with ARF, a specific type of metabolic intervention that must be planned together with RRT and fluid and electrolyte management. Modified by the clinical context in which it occurs, ARF presents a catabolic, pro-oxidative, and pro-inflammatory syndrome.

Modern CRRTs—because of the continuous mode of therapy and the high fluid turnover associated with the recommended dose—exert a massive impact on electrolyte and nutrient balances.

A nutritional program for a patient with ARF is not fundamentally different from that for a patient without ARF. However, in a patient with ARF who needs nutritional support, the nutritional regimen must take into account the multiple metabolic consequences of ARF, of RRT, and of the underlying disease process and associated complications. In the critically ill patient with ARF, nutritional support must be initiated early and must be both qualitatively and quantitatively sufficient.

Enteral nutrition has become the preferred type of nutritional support in patients with ARF. Nevertheless, many patients have severe limitations to enteral nutrition and will require supplementary or even total parenteral nutrition.

Modern nutrition therapy has evolved from a merely quantitative approach, covering nitrogen and energy requirements, to a more qualitative metabolic intervention aimed at modulating the inflammatory state, the oxygen radical scavenger system, immunocompetence, and endothelial functions and taking advantage of specific pharmacological effects of various nutrients (such as glutamine, fish oil, selenium, antioxidants). A reduction of the high mortality rate of patients with ARF will depend largely on further improvements in metabolic care.

Key Points

1. The metabolic environment in a patient with acute renal failure is complex: Nonspecific factors (such as the acute disease state [e.g., systemic inflammatory response syndrome, acute phase reaction]), the underlying disease process and its associated complications (especially infections and sepsis), acute renal failure per se, and the type and intensity of renal replacement therapy contribute to metabolic alterations.
2. Because of the prolonged duration of therapy and the required treatment dose and fluid turnover, continuous renal replacement therapy exerts a profound effect on metabolism and nutrient balances.
3. Understanding of all these metabolic alterations is mandatory for designing an appropriate nutritional protocol for patients with acute renal failure.
4. Patients with acute renal failure present an extremely heterogeneous group with differing nutrient requirements, which also can vary considerably during the course of disease.
5. Enteral nutrition has become the preferred type of nutrition support in patients with acute renal failure. Nevertheless, many patients will require supplementary or even total parenteral nutrition.

Key References

3. Druml W: Nutritional support in patients with acute renal failure. In Molitoris B, Finn W (eds): Acute Renal Failure. A Companion to Brenner & Rector's *The Kidney*. Philadelphia, WB Saunders, 2001, 465-489.
11. Druml W, Mitch W: Enteral nutrition in renal disease. In Rolandelli RH (ed): Clinical Nutrition: Enteral and Tube Feeding. Philadelphia, WB Saunders, 2004.
12. Druml W: Nutritional management of acute renal failure. J Ren Nutr 2005;15:63-70.
18. Druml W: Metabolic aspects of continuous renal replacement therapies. Kidney Int Suppl 1999;72:S56-S61.
19. Cano N, Fiaccadori E, Tesinsky P, et al: ESPEN Guidelines on Enteral Nutrition: Adult renal failure. Clin Nutr 2006;25:295-310.

See the companion Expert Consult website for the complete reference list.

CHAPTER 141

Hematological Malignancies and Critical Illness

Angelo F. Perego and Andrea De Gasperi

OBJECTIVES

This chapter will:
1. Present the clinical picture of critical illness and hematological malignancies.
2. Review recent scientific literature outlining outcome and prognostic parameters of intensive care unit treatment of patients with hematological malignancies.
3. Describe the various severity-of-illness scoring systems used to assess and reassess the condition of critically ill patients with hematological malignancies admitted to the intensive care unit.
4. Elucidate the relationship between intensive care unit admission policy for critically ill patients with hematological malignancies and the survival rate of these patients.

In recent years, aggressive and more appropriate treatments for patients suffering from hematological malignancies (HMs) have markedly improved prognosis and life expectancy for these patients.[1,2]

Patients with HMs, or even solid tumors, may require admission to the intensive care unit (ICU) before chemotherapy is initiated. The main reasons for admitting such patients are if they have severe infections or multiple-organ dysfunction. Most acute events are potentially reversible and chemotherapy, despite severe and life-threatening therapy-related complications,[3,4] may improve the patients' prognosis, so admission to the ICU to treat critical conditions or severe organ dysfunctions may be appropriate.[3] In fact, HM patients suffering from acute organ dysfunction and in severe clinical conditions requiring admission to the ICU usually are considered to have poor short-term and long-term survival.[4-6]

This assumption is largely derived from studies carried out in the late 1980s, which documented—for hematological patients admitted to the ICU—that the short-term mortality rate was 70% to 80% when patients were suffering from life-threatening conditions such as critical hypotension requiring vasopressors, acute renal and hepatic failure, and acute respiratory failure requiring mechanical ventilation (MV).[7]

Mortality rate figures were even worse in bone marrow recipients who required MV. In this subset of critically ill patients, short-term mortality was reported to be as high as 85%.[4,7] In 1989, commenting on mortality in MV patients undergoing bone marrow transplantation, Carlon,[8] in a 1989 editorial in *Critical Care Medicine*, gave this laconic advice to these patients: "Just say no" to being admitted to the ICU.

Based on this early literature, in many hospitals, cancer patients and particularly patients with HM, because of their assumed dismal prognoses, are frequently not considered suitable candidates for ICU admission and intensive therapies.[5,7] However, recent European and U.S. published series showed a rather different picture, with progressive improvement in the prognosis for hematologic patients admitted to the ICU.[9-18]

Rubenfeld and colleagues[19] found an increased survival rate from 5% to 16% in the period between 1988 and 1992 in allogenic bone marrow transplant recipients requiring MV.

Azoulay and colleagues[20] found a ten-fold lower risk of death in patients with multiple myeloma who required ICU support between 1996 and 1998 as compared to those in the period from 1992 to 1995. The same group reported a four-fold lower risk of death in cancer patients who required MV between 1996 and 1998 as compared to the period 1990 to 1995.[21]

Over the past decade, substantial improvements have occurred in the prognosis of critically ill cancer patients aggressively treated in the ICU for septic shock, acute respiratory failure, acute renal failure, or artificial support of acutely failing organs.[3,16,22] Thus, particularly in France, ICU admission is being increasingly offered to selected critically ill cancer or HM patients with good chronic health status and a well-defined treatment plan. Better patient selection, new insights into hematologic treatments, optimal management of failing organs, and the use of noninvasive MV have been cited as the most probable reasons for this tremendous improvement in results.[10,11,21]

This improved hematologic and intensive care management of patients, leading to improved survival rates, drives the reevaluation of the eligibility of HM patients for admission to the ICU. Ideally, the admission criteria for patients with malignancy (solid or hematologic) should be the same as for patients with severe congestive heart failure, acute pancreatitis, severe burns, cirrhosis, chronic obstructive pulmonary disease with acute respiratory failure due to pneumonia, and acute renal failure requiring renal replacement therapy, all conditions long known to be at high risk of mortality but rarely under contention as far as concerns about the appropriateness of ICU admission.[11,16,18,22]

The decision to admit oncohematologic patients to ICU is, thus, very complex. Specific, prospectively validated tools (such as the severity of illness scoring systems (Acute Physiology and Chronic Health Evaluation II and III [APACHE II, APACHE III], Simplified Acute Physiology Score II [SAPS II], Organ System Failure [OSF], and Sequential Organ Failure Assessment [SOFA]), long used to assist ICU physicians in estimating survival, do not

seem to be suitable for these patients. In this specific subset of patients, these scoring systems grossly correlate with outcome, but their accuracy is not such that they can be confidently used for decision making, especially when decisions about an individual patient need to be taken.[7,9,10,23-25]

Benoit and coworkers[11] suggested that urea levels, leukopenia, need for vasopressors, and presence of bacterial infection may represent more reliable prognostic indicators than the APACHE II score and the SAPS II in discriminating future survivors from nonsurvivors at the time of admission to the ICU. Their results confirm the limited use of the available scoring system for the assessment of prognosis in critically ill patients with HMs and underline the need for developing and validating alternative scoring systems specifically designed for this patient population and easily applicable at the bedside.

An alternative way of using available scoring systems was presented by Guiguet and colleagues.[26] They proposed a so-called multiple assessment of the severity scores (SAPS II and OSF), with assessment of the scores on admission and reassessment 48 to 72 hours after ICU admission. This new modality of assessment could provide information on neutropenic patients, allowing the patients to be allocated into homogeneous subgroups according to the mortality risk.[26] In this multiple assessment by Guiguet and colleagues,[26] the mean number of acute organ failures decreased in survivors over the first 72 hours. In contrast, no changes or worsening in a patient's clinical profile was associated with a deteriorating prognosis. The pattern of change in the scores between ICU admission and 72 hours later was also considered of value for assessing a patient's chance of recovery. In this setting, life support measures can be offered to all patients for whom the approach is indicated, a new assessment being performed on day 3 or day 4. In the opinion of Guiguet and colleagues, the "aggressive treatment can be reasonably withdrawn if the number of OSFs has not decreased or is more than 3 on the third day in ICU."[26]

A similar approach has been proposed by Rubenfeld and Crawford,[19] for bone marrow recipients undergoing MV; by Blot and colleagues,[27] for febrile neutropenic patients evaluated while still in the hematology ward; and recently by Azoulay and Afessa.[15]

Such tools of clinical assessment and prognosis were further completed with the observations of Soares and colleagues[28] about the impact of comorbidities on the 6-month mortality of these critically ill patients and with the results of Lecuyer and colleagues' new admission policy: the ICU Trial.[2]

Persistently high ICU mortality rates render admission policies a pivotal point of discussion: Both excessive obstructionism to admission (the "Just say no" policy) and emotional, aggressive but useless consumption of resources (so-called futile treatment) should be avoided. For HM patients, becoming critically ill or frankly unstable during their clinical course, directives for intensive caring in the hematology ward must be developed[27]: early, close physiological monitoring of critical patients, more aggressive treatment of potentially but not yet full blown failing organs, frequent consultation with the ICU specialists, and reassessment should become everyday practice.

The time has come for a high dependency unit within the hematology ward, a sort of step-up unit, where semi-invasive monitoring and treatments such as noninvasive MV are available. Early treatment of the unstable HM patient in this semi-intensive unit should precede (and sometimes, eventually, avoid) admission to the ICU.

Implementation of such directives, locally developed, with a daily assessment of score systems as suggested by Guiguet and colleagues,[26] Rubenfeld,[19] and Blot and colleagues,[27] might become a valuable tool to standardize a correct approach to the management of the acute HM patient.

While the optimal timing for ICU referral has yet to be defined, it might be effectively preceded by efforts to reverse initial organ failures while the patient is still on the hematology ward.[27] As underlined before, proper indications for ICU admission of HM patients rely upon both physiological and hematologic parameters.

Massion and coworkers[5] were able to demonstrate that severity of the underlying hematological malignancy does not influence ICU or hospital mortality, the short-term prognosis (mainly hospital mortality) being exclusively predicted by acute organ failures, aggressiveness of pathogens (fungi), and transplant status.[3]

Among risk factors that influence short- and long-term prognosis in hematological patients, neutropenia is under great debate, and the importance of leukopenia as a risk factor for mortality is controversial. Many studies have reported a higher mortality in patients with (prolonged) neutropenia, particularly when mechanically ventilated; however, this has not been confirmed by other studies.[4]

In a study by Benoit and colleagues,[11] leukopenia on admission—which was, in most cases, related to chemotherapy—was an independent risk factor for adverse outcome. However, the higher mortality in this subgroup of patients was not related to the duration of leukopenia before or during ICU admission.

A good selection of patients likely to benefit from ICU admission seems to have played a role in the relatively good outcomes reported in most studies.[3,10,11,15,20,21] Admission criteria should be discussed and shared between primary care physicians (hematologists) and intensive care specialists, keeping two points in mind. First, admission to the ICU must be considered only for patients who have a potential long-term survival or a treatable relapse.[11,15] This policy was proposed by Massion,[5] Rubenfeld and Crawford,[19] and Guiguet and coworkers,[26] whose admission criteria were life expectancy exceeding 6 months or, in the case of progressive disease, chemotherapy expected to allow partial or complete remission; it is the responsibility of the hematologist to determine this expectancy. Second, the criteria for an ICU consultation (e.g., simple preemptive consultation, use of noninvasive MV in the ward, or call for urgent admission) must be clearly planned,[6] discussed, shared, and implemented. The requested consultation by the hematologist should be neither early (useless) nor late (futile).

Directions to care for patients with HMs whose clinical course worsens and for whom ICU consultation is warranted are cornerstones of the program of quality of care.[27] The intensivists must be able to select, together with the hematologist, cancer patients for ICU admission. As stated by Azoulay and Afessa,[15] unlimited management of critically ill patients with HMs must be delivered promptly and for a limited period of time. Clinical progress must then be properly reassessed before further decisions about care are made (e.g., decisions such as forgoing life-sustaining therapies or maximizing vital supporting measures including chemotherapy).

An earlier ICU referral during the critical illness evolution and advanced ICU management will reduce the number of failing organs and preserve these patients from irreversible organ failure (severe hemodynamic, respiratory, or neurological impairment). As reported in several studies, multiple-organ failure and the combined need for ventilation and renal replacement therapy have a profound adverse effect on survival in both the general ICU population and in patients with HM.[12,16,26]

Reductions in morbidity and mortality in critically ill HM patients admitted to intensive care treatments may result from two more factors: (1) the very early detection of worsening clinical conditions, as assessed by daily evaluation of OSF score[27]; and (2) better tuning and tailoring of the supportive care. These could be the rationales for early noninvasive monitoring or the application of noninvasive MV while in the ward (or, better, still in a high dependency unit) or admission to the intensive care setting in a quasi preemptive treatment.

As emphasized by Benoit and colleagues,[11] commenting on their crude ICU and in-hospital mortality rates of 42% and 54%, "the reluctance to admit patients with hematologic malignancy to the ICU may be unjustified" in spite of the severe clinical conditions of their patients as based on ICU length of stay, the high prevalence and long duration of artificial ventilation, use of vasopressors, and the need for renal replacement therapy. Using a well-planned ICU admission policy and providing advanced and, in some cases, prolonged supportive care to these patients, Benoit and colleagues[11] were able to achieve a 6-month survival rate that was superior to the 6-month survival rate of 20% observed in the same institution in a general ICU population with acute renal failure who needed renal replacement therapy. ICU management cannot and should not be routinely considered futile in critically ill HM patients.[13]

A brand new item proposed by Benoit and colleagues[14] is the ICU admission for critically ill patients requiring cancer chemotherapy along with aggressive life support or invasive monitoring. In the study by Benoit and colleagues, most patients received MV (62%) or extracorporeal renal support (24%). Mortality was associated with the need for MV: In-hospital mortality was 14% in nonventilated patients and 61% in ventilated patients. Using the "preemptive consultation and admission philosophy," Benoit and colleagues concluded that starting chemotherapy in the ICU for a life-threatening malignancy-related complication could be lifesaving even when infection or organ failure is present.[14]

According to the results recently presented by Darmon,[3] concomitant life-sustaining treatment and chemotherapy led to a 40% mortality rate after 30 days and a 51% mortality rate after 180 days in cancer patients with advanced disease (even in the presence of an uncertain prognosis and undefined treatment goals), and a 30-day mortality rate close to 30% in patients with acute leukemia undergoing full-dose chemotherapy regimens.

Early ICU admission corresponds with the recently documented improved survival rates among critically ill patients with cancer, regardless of the characteristics of their malignancies,[14,17,18,25,28-30] pointing out that organ failure before cancer chemotherapy initiation should not be interpreted, by default, as a futile treatment. These studies confirm that patient survival is strongly dependent on the number of organ failures. Acute cardiorespiratory failure carries the greatest risk of death, and earlier ICU admission can prevent the development of multiple-organ failure.[25,26]

Patient selection, advances in the understanding of the pathophysiological profile, and the use of noninvasive diagnostic and therapeutic strategies are the mainstay of the improved prognosis of cancer patients admitted to the ICU.

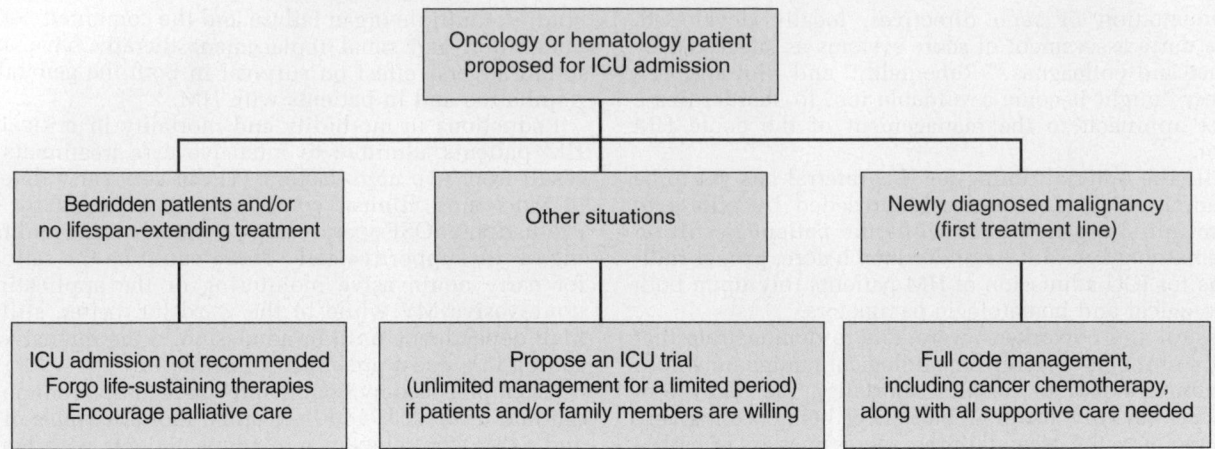

FIGURE 141-1. How to decide intensive care unit (ICU) admission and status of patients with cancer. (Redrawn from Azoulay E, Afessa B: The intensive care support of patients with malignancy: Do everything that can be done. Intensive Care Med 2006;32:3-5).

As assessed by Azoulay and Afessa,[15] all these arguments represent a good reason for readdressing ICU admission criteria in patients with cancer who require life-sustaining therapies: "Do everything that can be done" (Fig. 141-1). According to the results presented by Azoulay and colleagues[20] in patients with both HMs and acute respiratory failure who are undergoing noninvasive MV, "improvements in ICU treatments and oncohematologic management have stripped classic predictors of ICU mortality of much of their value."

In conclusion, as proposed by Groeger and Bach[9] commenting on Benoit's study[11] and more recently by Azoulay and Afessa[15] dealing with a similar item, the old statement made by Carlon[8] ("Just say no") is to be rewritten as "Consider saying yes."

Key Points

1. The prognosis and life expectancy of patients with hematological malignancies are improving.
2. Chemotherapy for hematological malignancies, although improving patients' survival, accounts for a number of related life-threatening complications.
3. Survival rates of critically ill patients with hematological malignancies admitted to intensive care are improving and are pivotal to eligibility criteria for admission to the intensive care unit.
4. Admission to the intensive care unit should be considered only for patients with hematological

malignancies who have potential long-term survival or a treatable relapse.
5. Unlimited and prompt management of critically ill patients with hematological malignancies should be delivered for a limited period and then reassessed according to clinical progress.

Key References

2. Lecuyer L,Chevret S, Thiery G, et al: The ICU Trial: A new admission policy for cancer patients requiring mechanical ventilation. Crit Care Med 2007;Jan 16 (Epub ahead of print).
3. Darmon M, Thiery G, Ciroldi M, et al: Intensive care in patients with newly diagnosed malignancies and a need for cancer chemotherapy. Crit Care Med 2005;33:2488-2493.
23. Benoit D, Depuydt P, Vandewoude K, et al: Outcome in severely ill patients with haematological malignancies who received intravenous chemotherapy in the intensive care unit. Intensive Care Med 2006;32:93-99.
24. Azoulay E, Afessa B: The intensive care support of patients with malignancy: Do everything that can be done. Intensive Care Med 2006;32:3-5.
28. Lim Z, Pagliuca A, Simpson S: Outcomes of patients with haematological malignancies admitted to intensive care unit. A comparative review of allogeneic haematopoietic stem cell transplantation data. Br J Haematol 2007;136(3):448-450.
30. Darmon M, Thiery G, Ciroldi M, et al: Should dialysis be offered to cancer patients with acute kidney injury? Intensive Care Med 2007;Mar 7 (Epub ahead of print).

See the companion Expert Consult website for the complete reference list.

CHAPTER 142

Anemia of Critical Illness

Craig French

OBJECTIVES

This chapter will:
1. Elucidate the limitations of current definitions of anemia.
2. Describe the relationship of the anemias of inflammation and critical illness.
3. Review recent literature outlining the epidemiology of the anemia of critical illness.
4. Outline the proposed mechanisms of the anemia of critical illness.

In the past decade, significant advances in our understanding of the anemia found in critically ill patients have been made. Emerging evidence suggesting allogenic red cell transfusion might be harmful[1] along with the possibility of supply restrictions (due to fewer donors), and the availability of transfusion alternatives (such as human recombinant erythropoietin) has driven research in this area.[2] The anemia of critical illness has been described as an acute variant of the anemia of chronic disease.[3] Indeed, there appears to be significant overlap in the pathogenesis of the anemia of chronic disease, renal failure, and critical illness (Fig. 142-1). Two recent reviews of this condition exist.[4,5] This chapter provides an overview of the epidemiology and pathogenesis of this clinical syndrome.

DEFINITION OF ANEMIA

Anemia may be defined as a reduction in circulating red cell mass with an associated decrease in the oxygen carrying capacity of blood.[6] In clinical practice, this is determined by measurement of the hemoglobin concentration; hematocrit or red cell count with hemoglobin concentration and hematocrit are most commonly used. In 1968 a World Health Organization report outlined criteria required for the diagnosis of anemia: a hemoglobin concentration of 140 g/L in adult males and 120 g/L for (nonpregnant) adult females.[7] Despite being derived from very limited data, these definitions were widely promulgated and adopted by the medical profession. Recently their validity has been challenged with several alternate definitions derived from large population–based studies.[6] Given the lack of consensus regarding the definition of anemia, it is not surprising that no definition or grades severity exists for anemia observed in critically ill patients. Developing a specific grading system for the critically ill is difficult because both the underlying illness and the therapies provided influence red cell mass and plasma volume. In addition, despite the publication of randomized controlled trials of transfusion strategies and guidelines for transfusion, variation in practice will inevitably still exist. Such

variation will influence epidemiological studies of anemia in the critically ill.

EPIDEMIOLOGY

Numerous studies have demonstrated that anemia is a common problem in the intensive care unit (ICU).[1,8-11] In 1995 Corwin and colleagues[9] demonstrated that more than 90% of critically ill patients have a subnormal hemoglobin level within 72 hours after ICU admission. In any individual ICU, the case mix, severity of illness, and local transfusion practice influence the prevalence of anemia. Accordingly, the most robust data come from multicenter observational cohort studies. In the past decade five such studies have been published.[1,5,8,12,13] These studies demonstrate the prevalence of anemia on admission to ICU and also the development of anemia during stay in the ICU. These two subsets of the epidemiology of anemia of critical illness will be addressed separately in this chapter.

The Anemia and Blood Transfusion in Critical Care (ABC) study,[1] published in 2002, is an observational cohort study of 3534 patients admitted to 146 European ICUs. Consecutive patients admitted to the participating ICUs during a 2-week period in 1999 were enrolled. The researchers' objective was to define the incidence of anemia in this group of patients. The mean (SD) hemoglobin concentration on admission to ICU was 113 (2.3) g/L, with 63% having a hemoglobin level of less than 120 g/L and 29% less than 100 g/L. The study enrolled a broad cross section of elective surgical (41.4%), medical (32.6%), emergency surgical (16.6%), and trauma patients (7.6%) with a mean APACHE II score of 14.8 (7.9), mean SOFA score of 5.2 (3.8), and length of stay of 4.5 (6.7) days. In this study only 13% of patients had a recent history of anemia. Of all patients admitted with a hemoglobin concentration of less than 100 g/L (36.6%), only 50% had a history of either acute bleeding or documented cause for their anemia. A weak negative correlation between hemoglobin concentration on ICU admission, severity of illness, and ICU length of stay was observed.

A similar study was performed in the United States. The CRIT study[8] enrolled 4892 patients from 284 ICUs during a 9-month period from August 2000 to April 2001. It is not reported what proportion of total admissions this represents. The risk of selection bias and the potential for an overestimation of the prevalence of anemia exist. There were fewer elective postoperative admissions in this cohort of patients (20% vs. 41.4%). The mean hemoglobin level on admission was similar—110 (2.4) g/L, with just less than two thirds having a hemoglobin concentration less than 120 g/L. In contrast to the ABC study, the patient cohort was sicker, with a median APACHE II score of 19.7 (8.2), SOFA score of 6.2 (3.7), and ICU length of stay of 7.4 (7.3) days. These differences are most likely explained by

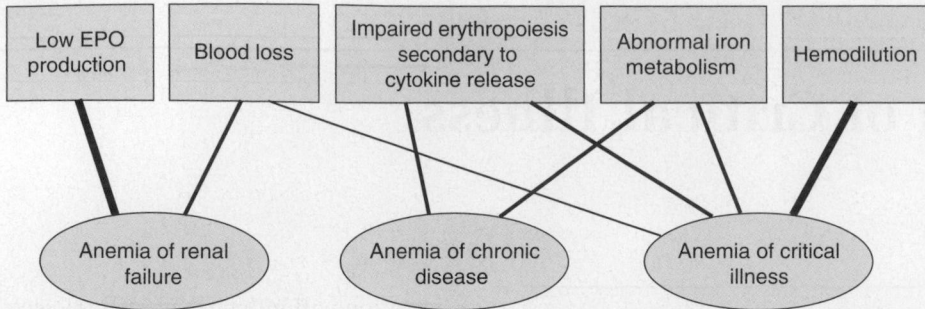

FIGURE 142-1. Schematic presentation of overlap between the anemias of renal failure, chronic illness, and critical illness. The size of the lines indicates the relative contributions of contributing factors. EPO, erythropoietin. (Modified from Eckardt KU: Anemia of critical illness—implications for understanding and treating rHuEPO resistance. Nephrol Dial Transplant 2002;[Suppl 17]:S48-S55.)

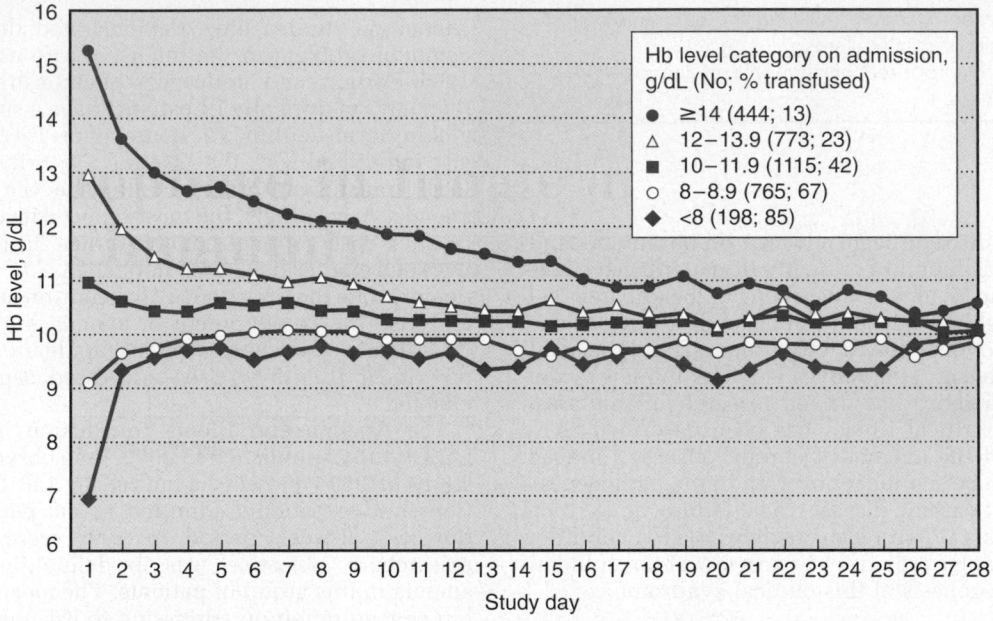

FIGURE 142-2. Course of hemoglobin (Hb) patterns over 28 days by Hb level on admission to the ICU. (From Vincent JL, Baron JF, Reinhart K, et al: Anemia and blood transfusion in critically ill patients. JAMA 2002;288:1499-1507.)

selection bias. Despite the CRIT study having a sicker patient cohort, the mean admission hemoglobin and the distribution are remarkably similar. This suggests that severity of illness may not be associated with a higher prevalence of anemia on admission to the ICU. Observational cohort studies reporting the hemoglobin concentration on admission have also been done in Scotland[5] and Australia,[12] where the median hemoglobin concentrations on admission were 105 g/L and 98 g/L, respectively.

Differences in methodology limit the generalizability of the previously mentioned data. Nevertheless, it appears that in Western ICUs, up to 25% of patients will have a hemoglobin concentration of 90 g/L or less. As such, anemia is one of the most frequently encountered clinical syndromes that intensive care physicians must manage.

The ABC[1] and CRIT[8] studies also describe the development and severity of anemia during ICU stay. In contrast, hemoglobin concentrations measured during ICU stay are obviously associated with transfusion practice. These will vary between institutions and jurisdictions. The TRICC[14] trial demonstrated the equivalence of restrictive and liberal transfusion strategies in a heterogeneous group of criti-

cally ill patients. Improved outcome in patients randomized to the restrictive strategy (transfusion trigger hemoglobin concentration 70 g/L) was demonstrated in a secondary endpoint (hospital mortality) and a subgroup of less severely ill patients (APACHE II score of less than 25). Observational studies suggest that this study has had a significant impact on transfusion practice.[1,5,8,12,13] In Western ICUs, the observed transfusion trigger is approximately 80 g/L. This is in contrast to clinicians' attitudes toward transfusion practice as published prior to the TRICC study.[15] Although there will inevitably be variation in transfusion practice, it seems that the TRICC study has improved uniformity among jurisdictions.

Figure 142-2 displays ABC[1] study data that demonstrate the time course of hemoglobin concentrations according to day 1 hemoglobin level. A convergence of hemoglobin levels over time, irrespective of the hemoglobin level on admission, is observed. The evolution of the hemoglobin concentration over 30 days was similar for the cohort of patients without acute bleeding and those with acute bleeding. These data, however, were not presented in the paper. The study did not present comparative data of

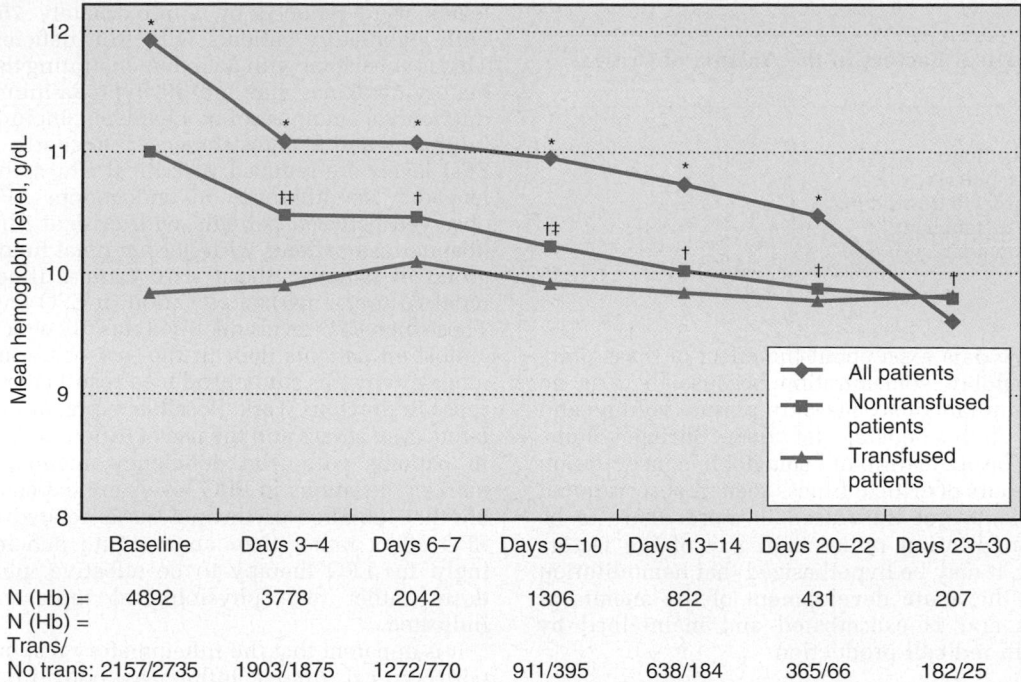

N (Hb) =

	Baseline	Days 3–4	Days 6–7	Days 9–10	Days 13–14	Days 20–22	Days 23–30
N (Hb) =	4892	3778	2042	1306	822	431	207
N (Hb) = Trans/ No trans:	2157/2735	1903/1875	1272/770	911/395	638/184	365/66	182/25

*The difference across groups (transfused vs. nontransfused) is significant at $p<0.007$ (using Bonferonni adjustment).

†The difference is significant at $p<0.0045$ (using ANOVA and Bonferonni adjustment) compared with baseline (all patients sample).

‡The difference is significant at $p<0.0045$ (using ANOVA and Bonferonni adjustment) compared with previous period (all patients sample).

FIGURE 142-3. Hemoglobin (Hb) levels day 1 through day 30. ANOVA, analysis of variance; Trans/No trans, ratio of patients who received transfusions to those who did not.

transfused patients versus nontransfused patients. The CRIT[8] study is the only observational study to report longitudinal hemoglobin concentration data of transfused compared with nontransfused patients (Fig. 142-3). Figure 142-3 shows the hemoglobin concentration levels from day 1 through day 30 in all patients, those transfused, and those not transfused. In the nontransfused group, the mean admission hemoglobin concentration was approximately 120 g/L. This decreased acutely to approximately 110 g/L after 3 to 4 days. After this, only a slow decline in mean hemoglobin in concentration is observed.

In a single center observational study, Nguyen and colleagues[10] also investigated the time course of hemoglobin concentration in critically ill patients who were not transfused. This study excluded patients with recent evidence of bleeding, the majority of postsurgical patients, those with either acute or chronic renal failure, and those with an ICU length of stay less than 24 hours. Follow-up was for 7 days. Despite the differences in methodology, their results are similar to those of the CRIT study: a rapid decrease in hemoglobin (about 50 g/L) for the first 3 days followed by a slow decline in hemoglobin concentration (12 g/L).

The previously mentioned studies demonstrate that anemia is frequently present on admission to ICU. If not present, anemia develops rapidly within the first 72 hours in the majority of patients. Thereafter, a slow decline in hemoglobin concentration is observed. The available data also suggest that the majority of patients with an ICU length of stay greater than 7 days have a hemoglobin concentration less than 90 g/L at some time during their ICU stay.

ETIOLOGY OF THE ANEMIA OF CRITICAL ILLNESS

The etiology of the anemia of critical illness is multifactorial and complex. Many of the etiological factors are shared with the anemia of chronic disease; it is their relative contribution that differs.[16] Contributing factors include hemodilution, overt or occult blood loss (including iatrogenic blood loss secondary to phlebotomy), abnormal red cell production, and decreased red cell survival due to increased uptake by the reticuloendothelial system (Table 142-1). More recently the role of alterations in iron metabolism in the development of the anemias of critical illness and inflammation[17,18] has been investigated.

Hemodilution

Fluid resuscitation is a cornerstone of intensive care practice.[19] It is recommended not only when replacing absolute fluid deficits, such as those observed in trauma, but also for relative intravascular volume depletion believed to occur in other critical illnesses, such as sepsis.[20] Fluid resuscitation usually commences with a crystalloid or colloid solution rather than with transfusion of packed red

TABLE 142-1

Potential Etiological Factors in the Anemia of Critical Illness

Phlebotomy
Pathological bleeding
Impaired erythropoiesis
Increased erythrocyte destruction
Abnormal iron metabolism
Blunted erythropoietin response

blood cells. Few data exist about the effect of these practices on hemoglobin concentration because there is no easy way to simultaneously measure plasma volume and red cell mass at the bedside, let alone during volume resuscitation. The acute drop in hemoglobin concentration in the first 72 hours of critical illness seen in observational studies in patients not transfused is more likely to be caused by hemodilution rather than any of the factors discussed later. It may be hypothesized that hemodilution contributes to the acute development of the anemia of critical illness and is exacerbated and maintained by abnormalities in red cell production.

Blood Loss

The role of phlebotomy in the development of anemia has been debated over the years. Once thought to play a dominant role, its significance has been challenged,[3,9] and the belief that anemia in the critically ill is simply the result of excess phlebotomy has been debunked.[1] The influence of phlebotomy was best evaluated in a substudy of the ABC[1] study. The ABC investigators collected 24-hour sampling data on 1136 patients. The mean number of draws per patient was 4.6 (3.2) with a mean volume of 10.3 (6.6) mL. The average total volume for the 24-hour period was 41.1 (39.7) mL. Not unexpectedly, increased severity of illness correlated positively with increased number of draws and volume of blood removed. Although the amount of blood drawn is relatively small, and clearly other factors have a greater role in the pathogenesis of anemia, clinicians should still ensure that only necessary investigations are requested and, in patients who require more frequent tests, should consider the use of blood-conserving devices.

Impaired Erythropoiesis

Erythropoiesis is the development of mature red blood cells. Critical illness and inflammation interfere with both the formation of erythroblasts and their subsequent maturation. The mechanisms for this have been reviewed recently.[21] The kidney plays a central role in red blood cell production in adults. In response to low arterial oxygen tension, red blood cells release erythropoietin (EPO), a glycoprotein hormone produced primarily by the cells of the peritubular capillary endothelium. This acts upon the bone marrow to stimulate red blood cell production by a mechanism that is not completely understood. In healthy individuals the normal serum concentration is 5 to 10 international units (IU) per liter.[22] Studies performed during the 1990s demonstrated that endogenous EPO levels were inappropriately low in critically ill patients.[23-25] After controlling for hemoglobin levels, EPO levels were reduced by approximately 75% compared with ambulatory patients with iron deficiency anemia.[25] This is consistent with data demonstrating that pro-inflammatory cytokines may inhibit hypoxia-induced EPO production via a number of mechanisms, including EPO gene inhibition and EPO resistance.[26,27] Recently, the belief that EPO levels are reduced in critical illness has been challenged.[28] No difference in endogenous EPO levels was observed between patients with critical illness and non-hospitalized patients with normal renal function. In a subgroup of patients, those with critical illness and acute renal failure, a marked elevation in EPO level was noted. These high EPO levels declined rapidly over 72 hours with almost all patients then in the low or normal range. It is unclear why this study produced results that differed from those in previous work. Possible explanations include differences in assays and the use of different control groups—in patients with iron deficiency anemia, for example, marked elevations in EPO levels are expected. It is possible that impaired erythropoiesis is related to a failure of EPO effect rather than an absolute deficiency. Accordingly, for EPO therapy to be effective, pharmacological doses rather than physiological replacement may be indicated.

It is apparent that the inflammatory response associated with critical illness influences both iron metabolism and erythropoiesis and that alteration in iron metabolism plays a major role in the maintenance of the anemia of chronic disease.[18,29] Iron metabolism in critical illness has recently been reviewed.[17] Diagnosis and management of iron-related anemia are difficult and require an understanding of the measures of iron deficiency in critical illness and the mechanisms of the anemia of critical illness.[30] In general it is believed that acute inflammation decreases iron available for erythropoiesis. Under normal circumstances, most iron is recycled following the catabolism of red cells by the reticuloendothelial system. Iron is transported by transferrin, which in turn binds to either the surface of erythroblasts or to apoferritin. Erythroblasts then internalize the iron and mature to become erythrocytes, and apoferritin stores iron in the form of ferritin.[17]

Acute inflammation initiates a series of events that result in iron misdistribution: a decrease in serum iron, decrease in transferrin, and normal or elevated ferritin levels. Teleologically these mechanisms appear to have evolved to deprive bacteria of iron.[18] Iron overload can also impair polymorphonuclear leukocyte function with impaired phagocytosis and bacterial killing;[31] however, data regarding iron and its effects on immune function are conflicting.[32] As part of the acute phase response, the synthesis of ferritin is increased principally in response to the cytokines interleukin-1 (IL-1) and interleukin-6 (IL-6) and to tumor necrosis factor.[21,33] These medicators lead to increased iron storage with an associated decrease in the mobilization of iron. Accordingly, a decrease in serum iron is observed, and a correlation between the severity of inflammation and reduction in serum iron concentration exists. In addition, IL-1 stimulates lactoferrin synthesis.[33] Lactoferrin has greater affinity for iron than does transferrin. Iron bound to lactoferrin is not available for erythropoiesis; it may only be stored as ferritin. In addition, the pro-inflammatory cytokines influence the binding affinity of iron regulatory proteins and decrease expression of the transferrin receptor.

Researchers have recently begun to elucidate the essential role of hepcidin antimicrobial peptide (HAMP) in iron metabolism. HAMP was first identified in 2001.[34] It is a

TABLE 142-2

Admitting Clinical Data*

	NO. (%)	MEAN ADMITTING APACHE II SCORE	MEAN ADMITTING SOFA SCORE[†]	MEAN ADMITTING HB LEVEL (g/dL)	PRIOR TRANSFUSION[‡] (%)
Admission Type					
Elective surgery	1464 (41.4)	11.6	4.2	11.0	26.1
Medical	1151 (32.6)	17.9	5.9	11.9	6.6
Emergency surgery	586 (16.6)	16.3	6.1	10.8	34.2
Trauma	269 (7.6)	15.1	5.6	11.5	19.6
Other	58 (1.6)	14.5	4.0	12.0	17.2
Shock at ICU Admission[†§]	705 (20.2)	21.8	8.8	10.5	28.0
Sepsis/septic	271 (38.4)	22.1	9.0	10.4	6.6
Cardiogenic	205 (29.1)	23.4	9.4	11.1	12.1
Hemorrhagic	180 (25.5)	21.0	8.4	9.2	68.4
Other	94 (13.3)	21.8	8.3	11.8	12.9
Primary Admission Diagnosis					
Coronary ischemic heart disease	637 (18.2)	13.6	5.6	11.2	20.8
Circulatory	579 (16.5)	15.6	5.8	11.0	29.9
Respiratory	549 (15.6)	16.2	5.3	11.5	12.8
Neurologic	397 (11.3)	15.3	5.1	12.3	6.3
Gastrointestinal	353 (10.1)	14.0	4.6	10.8	30.5
Trauma	237 (6.8)	14.9	5.4	11.5	24.6
Kidney/urinary tract	126 (3.6)	14.4	4.9	10.6	27.2
Infectious	115 (3.3)	18.2	6.6	10.7	10.4
Hepatobiliary/pancreatic	94 (2.7)	15.0	5.6	10.8	34.4
Poisoning	88 (2.5)	11.6	3.8	13.3	0
Endocrine/metabolic	52 (1.5)	15.1	3.1	12.7	5.8
Orthopedic	51 (1.5)	10.5	2.5	10.7	35.3
Obstetric/gynecologic	46 (1.3)	9.2	2.6	10.4	26.1
Hematologic/immunologic	18 (0.5)	23.4	8.5	9.0	52.9
Other	166 (4.7)	11.6	3.2	11.3	16.4

*Numbers do not total 3534 because of missing data (some forms incomplete).
[†]Range of scores for APACHE II, 0-71; for SOFA, 0-24.
[‡]Within 24 hours prior to ICU admission.
[§]Types were not mutually exclusive; total percentage exceeds 100%.
APACHE II, Acute Physiology and Chronic Health Evaluation II; Hb, hemoglobin; ICU, intensive care unit; SOFA, Sequential Organ Failure Assessment.
From Weiss G, Goodnough LT: Anemia of chronic disease. N Engl J Med 2005;352(10):1011-1023.

small (25–amino acid) peptide whose production by the liver is modulated in response to anemia, hypoxia, or inflammation. It has dual roles: It is an effector of the innate immune system, and it is a negative regulator of iron transport, so it exerts an inhibitory effect on iron absorption by duodenal enterocytes and on iron release from the reticuloendothelial system. Its expression is induced by inflammation but is decreased by anemia and hypoxia. It has been described as a molecular link between inflammation and anemia.[35] As IL-6 is a strong stimulus for human HAMP production, it has been proposed that HAMP could be the medicator ultimately responsible for functional iron deficiency and inadequate erythropoiesis in the anemia of inflammation.[36] Further investigation into the role of HAMP in the pathogenesis of the anemia of inflammation is indicated.

The inflammatory state has also been shown to interfere with erythroblast maturation. Tumor necrosis factor-alpha, IL-1, and IL-6 directly inhibit red cell formation.[37,38] Interferon gamma has been demonstrated experimentally to induce apoptosis in red cell precursors. Data of changes in bone marrow cell lines in the critically ill are limited. Some evidence to support erythrocyte precursor in this population exists.

In summary, for critically ill patients without acute bleeding, the reduction in the hemoglobin concentration observed in the first 72 hours of hospital stay is probably related to fluid resuscitation. There does not appear to be any other biologically plausible explanation. There is no evidence to suggest that this acute reduction of up to 5 g/L/day occurs in the early phases of related anemias (chronic disease and renal failure). Table 142-2 summarizes the pathophysiological factors in the anemia of chronic disease.[21] It is probable that many of these factors are shared with the anemia of critical illness. The onset of inflammation rapidly induces changes in iron homeostasis, the proliferation of erythroid progenitor cells, erythropoietin production, and red cell life span that contribute to the maintenance of anemia. In the majority of patients, phlebotomy contributes to the condition but is not the dominant cause.

CONCLUSION

Anemia in the critically ill is common. Despite the lack of a clear definition, recent well-conducted observational studies have demonstrated the condition's epidemiology in Western populations. It shares many of its etiological factors with the anemia of chronic disease and renal failure. As our understanding of the epidemiology and pathophysiology improves, clinicians will be able to make more informed choices about whom they transfuse and to whom they prescribe adjuvant therapies, such as recombinant human erythropoietin and iron.

1. Anemia is one of the most common clinical syndromes encountered by intensive care physicians.
2. Observational studies indicate that only a small percentage of patients have a preexisting cause for their anemia.
3. On average, the hemoglobin concentration decreases by approximately 5 g/L for the first 3 days following intensive care unit admission.
4. In nonbleeding patients, hemodilution is likely to be the cause of this initial rapid decrease in hemoglobin.
5. Pro-inflammatory cytokines initiate a cascade that results in impaired erythropoiesis, abnormal iron homeostasis, and a blunted erythropoietin response.

Key References

14. Hébert PC, Wells G, Blajchman MA, et al, for the Transfusion Requirements in Critical Care Investigators, Canadian Critical Care Trials Group: A multicenter, randomized, controlled clinical trial of transfusion requirements in critical care. N Engl J Med 1999;340(6):409-417.
16. Eckardt KU: Anemia of critical illness—implications for understanding and treating rHuEPO resistance. Nephrol Dial Transplant 2002;17(Suppl 5):S48-S55.
17. Darveau M, Denault AY, Blais N, Notebaert E: Bench-to-bedside review: Iron metabolism in critically ill patients. Crit Care 2004;8(5):356-362.
29. Walsh TS, Saleh EE: Anemia during critical illness. Br J Anaesth 2006;97(3):278-291.
36. Roy CN, Andrews NC: Anemia of inflammation: The hepcidin link. Curr Opin Hematol 2005;12(2):107-111.

See the companion Expert Consult website for the complete reference list.

CHAPTER 143

Adrenal Dysfunction in the Critically Ill: Doubts and Controversies

Daryl A. Jones, Bala Venkatesh, and Steve Webb

This chapter will:
1. Discuss the role of cortisol in the stress response associated with critical illness.
2. Elucidate the etiology and diagnosis of adrenal insufficiency in the non–critically ill patient.
3. Explain the concept of relative adrenal insufficiency in septic shock.
4. Describe the features of adrenal insufficiency in the critically ill.
5. Identify diagnostic criteria for relative adrenal insufficiency in critical illness.
6. Provide evidence supporting the role of steroid therapy to treat relative adrenal insufficiency associated with septic shock.
7. Discuss doubts and controversies in the area of adrenal insufficiency in critical illness.

Cortisol is a glucocorticoid hormone secreted from the adrenal cortex in response to corticotropin produced in the anterior pituitary. In healthy humans, the normal daily output of cortisol is estimated to be 15 to 30 mg/day, producing a peak plasma cortisol level of 110 to 520 nmol/L (4-19 µg/dL) at 8 to 9 AM and a nadir cortisol level of less than 140 nmol/L (less than 5 µg/dL) after midnight.[1] The majority (90%) of secreted cortisol circulates bound to cortisol-binding globulin.[2] The polymorphonuclear enzyme neutrophil elastase cleaves cortisol-binding globulin, markedly decreasing its affinity for cortisol.[3] This enzymatic cleavage results in the liberation of free cortisol, especially at sites of inflammation.[1]

It is the free (unbound) fraction of cortisol that diffuses into cells to cause biological effects.[1] Cortisol has a plasma half-life of 70 to 120 minutes and is eliminated primarily by hepatic metabolism and glomerular filtration. The excretion of free cortisol through the kidney represents 1% of the total excretion rate.

Cortisol has several metabolic actions, including induction of gluconeogenesis, lipolysis, and proteolysis. In addition, it has anti-inflammatory properties, such as inhibition of phagocyte migration and inflammatory cytokine production, as well as induction of leukocyte apoptosis.[4] Finally, cortisol upregulates production of adrenergic receptors in vascular smooth muscle to increase responsiveness to endogenous and exogenous vasopressors.[1]

ROLE OF CORTISOL IN STRESS RESPONSE OF CRITICAL ILLNESS

Critical illness is associated with acute inflammation secondary to inflammatory cytokines leading to organ injury, arteriolar vasodilation, and multiple-organ dysfunction syndrome. Critical illness is associated with increased production of total cortisol of up to six-fold, most likely in response to endotoxin and the inflammatory cytokines tumor necrosis factor-α (TNF-α), interleukin-1 (IL-1), and interleukin-6 (IL-6).[5] The increase in total cortisol level is roughly proportional to the severity of illness.[6,7] Although attenuated compared with healthy subjects, diurnal variation of cortisol release is still present in critical illness.[8] In addition, production of cortisol-binding globulin is reduced, and its cleavage at sites of inflammation (by neutrophil elastase) is increased.[1] This results in increased levels of free cortisol in the critically ill patient, especially at the tissue level.

The increased production of cortisol in response to critical illness is likely to be adaptive and may reduce the severity of the inflammatory response, as well as increase vaso-motor responsiveness to endogenous and exogenous vasoconstrictors.[1]

DIAGNOSIS OF ADRENAL INSUFFICIENCY IN THE NON–CRITICALLY ILL PATIENT

Adrenal insufficiency in the non–critically ill may occur secondary to one of three mechanisms. First, reduced production of cortisol may result from primary adrenal insufficiency due to auto-immune destruction of the gland or invasion by metastatic cancer. Second, chronic administration of therapeutic doses of glucocorticoids (more than 7.5 mg of prednisolone or equivalent for more than 30 days)[1] results in inhibition of corticotropin production, adrenal atrophy, and reduced secretion of cortisol by the adrenal gland. Consequently, sudden cessation of therapeutic glucocorticoid therapy may result in acute adrenal insufficiency. Third, although it is rare, adrenal insufficiency may occur secondary to hypopituitarism.

Historically, the diagnosis of adrenal insufficiency in the non–critically ill patient has been made using a corticotropin stimulation test. The test was first described in 1948 by Thorn and colleagues[9] using hog pituitary extract.

It was further established that 25 International Units of pituitary extract was the dose required to test the maximal secretory capacity of the adrenal cortex.[10]

The allergic reactions to animal pituitary extracts were reduced considerably by the development of synthetic corticotropin (Synacthen). The current recommendation for performing the stimulation test using Synacthen is administering a dose of 250 µg intravenously or intramuscularly. This dose, designed to test the maximal secretory capacity of the cortex, was derived from equivalence studies comparing animal extracts with synthetic corticotropin in bioassays (1 International Unit of extract = 10 µg of Synacthen).[11]

The short Synacthen test is conventionally performed by measurement of a baseline serum cortisol level followed by parenteral administration of 250 µg of Synacthen. Further serum cortisol levels are obtained at 30 and 60 minutes thereafter. There is controversy both about the

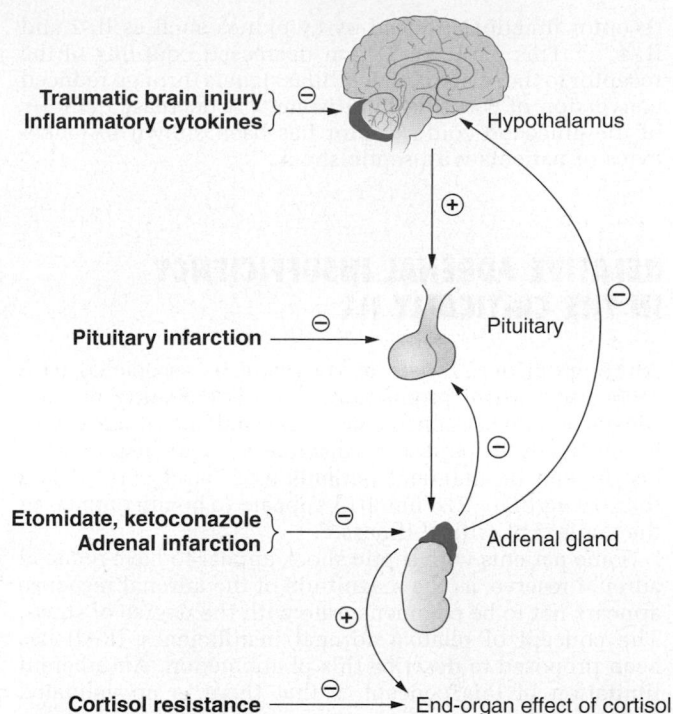

FIGURE 143-1. Disease states and site of action for induction of relative adrenal insufficiency in the critically ill.

levels of cortisol that indicate a normal response and about the appropriate dose of Synacthen to test adrenal reserve. The commonly quoted reference ranges for peak cortisol response at 30 and 60 minutes of levels more than 500 to 550 nmol/L (18-20 µg/dL) have been derived from studies in unstressed healthy volunteers.[12] The applicability of these levels to stressed critically ill patients has been questioned.

MECHANISMS AND ETIOLOGY OF ADRENAL INSUFFICIENCY IN THE CRITICALLY ILL

The mechanisms and causes of adrenal insufficiency in the critically ill differ from those in the ambulant patient, and in many cases the etiology is multifactorial (Fig. 143-1). Impairment of corticotropin production may be seen in association with traumatic brain injury.[13] Although it is rare, frank adrenal infarction (Waterhouse-Friderichsen syndrome) may occur in the context of disseminated intravascular coagulation, particularly in association with meningococcal infection.[1] Infections such as cytomegalovirus or fungi may cause destruction of the adrenal gland, particularly in patients with HIV infection.[14] Cortisol synthesis may be impaired by medications that inhibit the enzymes responsible for its synthesis, including the anesthetic agent etomidate[15,16] and the imidazole antifungals, especially ketoconazole.[1] High levels of pro-inflammatory cytokines also may impair cortisol production.[17] Increased hepatic catabolism of cortisol may be seen in patients on medications such as rifampicin and phenytoin.[1]

Finally, a condition of tissue-specific corticosteroid resistance may exist as a result of altered glucocorticoid receptor function induced by cytokines such as IL-2 and IL-4.[17,18] This may result from decreased coupling of the receptor to the related intracellular signals through reduced conversion of cortisol to cortisone.[19] A decreased affinity of the glucocorticoid receptor has been shown in leukocytes of patients with septic shock.[20]

RELATIVE ADRENAL INSUFFICIENCY IN THE CRITICALLY ILL

Although critical illness is known to be associated with increased cortisol production, there is currently no consensus as to what constitutes a "normal" basal cortisol in the critically ill patient.[1,5] Absolute adrenal insufficiency (as defined in ambulant patients as a basal cortisol less than 10 µg/dL or 278 nmol/L) appears to be uncommon in the context of critical illness.[21]

Some patients with septic shock appear to have reduced adrenal reserve, as the magnitude of the adrenal response appears not to be commensurate with the degree of stress. The concept of relative adrenal insufficiency (RAI) has been proposed to describe this phenomenon. An inherent limitation of this concept is that there is no validated measure of stress against which the magnitude of the adrenal response can be compared. In addition, any single test of adrenal function fails to consider dynamic changes in function with time. Similar transitory changes are seen for thyroid function in association with critical illness (so-called sick-euthyroid disease).

Reduced adrenal reserve has been associated with increased patient mortality. In a study of 189 patients with septic shock, Annane and colleagues[22] developed a 3-level prognostic classification system based on the adrenal response to septic shock. The study considered both the basal cortisol and the maximum increment in response to the high-dose Synacthen stimulation test (HDSST). The highest risk of death at 28 days was seen in patients with a high basal cortisol (more than 34 µg/dL or 944 nmol/L) who also had an inadequate response to the HDSST (defined as an increase in plasma cortisol of less than 9 µg/dL or 250 nmol/L). Increased risk of death in association with impaired response to the HDSST has also been seen in at least two other studies.[23,24] These studies assume that the level of adrenal function is insufficient for the degree of stress and that the increased risk of mortality is attributable to the inability of the gland to respond further. However, an alternative explanation could be that in these patients, very high basal cortisol levels are merely a marker of severe disease and are associated with, rather than responsible for, the observed increased risk of death. Furthermore, there is currently no evidence that the prognosis of the patient would improve if the adrenal gland "worked better."

FEATURES OF ADRENAL INSUFFICIENCY IN THE CRITICALLY ILL

Recognition of adrenal insufficiency in critical illness remains extremely difficult,[1] even in cases of absolute adrenal insufficiency. Many of the classic symptoms of adrenal insufficiency, such as weakness, fatigue, nausea

TABLE 143-1

Diagnostic Features of Adrenal Insufficiency and Other Aspects of Critical Illness that Mimic Them*

DIAGNOSTIC FEATURE SUGGESTING ADRENAL INSUFFICIENCY	DISEASE STATES OR TREATMENTS THAT MAY MIMIC FEATURE
Weakness and fatigue	Any critical illness
Hypotension	Hypovolemia
	Septic shock
	Cardiogenic shock
Tachycardia, fever	Sepsis and SIRS
Hypoglycemia	Hepatic failure
Hyponatremia, hyperkalemia	Fluid and electrolyte administration
	Renal failure
Constipation/diarrhea	Morphine, antibiotics, enteral feeds, use of laxatives
Eosinophilia	Drug reactions

*Adapted from Cooper MS, Stewart PM: Corticosteroid insufficiency in acutely ill patients. N Engl J Med 2003;348(8):727-734; Hamrahian AH, Oseni TS, Arafah BM: Measurements of serum free cortisol in critically ill patients. N Engl J Med 2004;350(16):1629-1638.
SIRS, systemic inflammatory response syndrome.

and vomiting, myalgias, and memory impairment, are not ascertainable in the critically ill. Similarly, the short time course of acute adrenal insufficiency in the critically ill does not allow pigmentation, decreased body hair, or weight loss to occur. Many of the other manifestations of adrenal insufficiency may not be present. Alternatively, the features may be masked by, or may mimic, other aspects of critical illness or the therapies used to treat it (Table 143-1). Cooper and Stewart[1] suggest that RAI should be suspected in instances where there is hemodynamic instability despite adequate fluid replacement, and in cases when there is ongoing evidence of inflammation without an obvious source.

DIAGNOSTIC CRITERIA FOR RELATIVE ADRENAL INSUFFICIENCY IN CRITICAL ILLNESS

Currently, there are no consensus criteria for diagnosis of RAI in critical illness.[1,25] Proposed criteria for the laboratory diagnosis of RAI are based on either a low baseline total cortisol level or an inadequate total cortisol response to the HDSST.

Cooper and Stewart[1] state that adrenal insufficiency is present when a random cortisol of less than 15 µg/dL (416 nmol/L) is detected but is unlikely when it is more than 34 µg/dL (944 nmol/L). Such demarcations are arbitrary and lack rigorous validation. Thus, a random cortisol of 412 is considered to indicate adrenal insufficiency, but a value of 418 is not, regardless of the severity of the patient's illness or the time of day that the sample was drawn.

The criteria proposed by Annane and colleagues[22,25] are the most widely used. These criteria state that an increase of less than 9 µg/dL (250 nmol/L) following a HDSST is indicative of RAI, irrespective of the baseline cortisol value. This definition is based on observations that an increase of cortisol of less than 9 µg/dL in patients with septic shock is independently associated with impaired vascular responsiveness to catecholamines and increased risk of death.[22,26-28] This definition, in part, theorizes that septic shock patients with highest baseline cortisol levels fare worst, possibly because their glands are maximally stressed with little reserve.[28] A low baseline cortisol in association with an inadequate total cortisol response to the HDSST should raise the possibility of absolute adrenal insufficiency.[1] Again, there are a number of limitations to the criteria proposed by Annane and colleagues. First, it is unlikely that a cut-off of 9 μg/dL will dichotomously indicate adrenal insufficiency and adequate adrenal reserve. It is more likely that there would be a graduated increased risk in mortality with increased severity of adrenal insufficiency, assuming that the syndrome exists. Second, high basal cortisol levels may be a marker of disease severity and may not be responsible for the increased mortality risk. Finally, improved catecholamine responsiveness in association with steroid therapy does not necessarily guarantee reduced patient mortality.

Limitations and controversies associated with diagnostic testing for adrenal insufficiency are discussed later in the chapter.

EVIDENCE FOR THE ROLE OF STEROID THERAPY IN TREATING RELATIVE ADRENAL INSUFFICIENCY ASSOCIATED WITH SEPTIC SHOCK

There are at least two theoretical reasons why steroid supplementation may benefit patients with critical illness. First, glucocorticoid therapy may reduce excessive production of pro-inflammatory cytokines associated with the systemic inflammatory response syndrome.[1,29] (Note: By 24 hours, most critically ill patients are actually in the anti-inflammatory phase with immunosuppression.[30]) Second, steroid therapy may reverse the adrenergic receptor downregulation that occurs in conjunction with prolonged exogenous catecholamine administration.[31]

Meta-analyses of trials conducted in the 1980s indicate that high-dose corticosteroids do not improve 28-day or hospital mortality when used to treat patients with septic shock.[32,33] More recently, there has been enthusiasm for the use of low-dose steroids in the treatment of septic shock, particularly in those who have RAI.

In 2002 a multicenter randomized trial of low-dose hydrocortisone (50 mg every 6 hours) and fludrocortisone (50 μg daily) in 299 patients with septic shock was published.[34] In patients who failed to respond to the HDSST (defined as a maximal increase of less than 9 μg/dL or 250 nmol/L), low-dose steroid supplementation was associated with more frequent withdrawal of vasopressor therapy. Improved survival at 28 days was also demonstrated, but only after adjustment for basal cortisol, cortisol response, McCabe classification, logistic organ dysfunction, arterial lactate, and PaO_2/FIO_2 ratio.[34] The study did not report on the effect of low-dose steroid supplementation on the incidence of organ dysfunctions (including renal failure). A number of concerns have been raised about the findings of this randomized trial. In particular, almost a quarter of patients (72 of 299) had been exposed to etomidate before undergoing the HDSST and the patients studied were exceedingly unwell, experiencing a mortality of 61% in the placebo group. Etomidate has been shown to impair the responsiveness of the adrenal gland to adreno-

corticotropic hormone for at least 24 hours.[15] The applicability of the reduced mortality observed in this study to a more heterogeneous population of patients with septic shock who have not been exposed to etomidate remains to be tested.[24,35] More fundamentally, the criteria used to diagnose adrenal insufficiency continue to generate debate.

A recently concluded multicenter trial (CORTICUS) using low-dose corticosteroid therapy in septic shock did not demonstrate any mortality benefit with the use of steroids.

A recent meta-analysis assessed the effect of corticosteroid dose on outcomes of severe sepsis and septic shock.[36] In the eight trials (conducted between 1971 and 1996) in which short courses of high-dose corticosteroids were used to treat patients with septic shock, there was no difference in mortality at either 28 days or hospital discharge. In contrast, the pooled analysis of the five studies of long courses of low-dose hydrocortisone (including the 2002 study by Annane and colleagues)[34] demonstrated improved survival at 28 days and hospital discharge.

DOUBTS AND CONTROVERSIES CONCERNING ADRENAL INSUFFICIENCY IN THE CRITICALLY ILL

There are several controversies in the area of adrenal insufficiency in the critically ill (Table 143-2). As there is no clinical gold standard for what constitutes adrenal insufficiency in the critically ill, there are no validated labora-

TABLE 143-2

Doubts and Controversies in the Diagnosis of Adrenal Insufficiency in the Critically Ill

1. Diagnosis Using Random Cortisol
   a. Even in the critically ill, there is a marked fluctuation in plasma cortisol concentration, thus limiting the utility of a random cortisol.
   b. The "normal" range of cortisol in critical illness is not defined.
   c. There is no consensus "cut-off" value below which adrenal insufficiency is present.
2. Diagnosis Using Adrenal Response to HDSST
   a. The HDSST results in Synacthen levels that are highly supra-physiological.
   b. An inadequate response to the HDSST does not take into account the basal cortisol.
   c. Published data may have overestimated the incidence of adrenal insufficiency, as many studies have not excluded patients who received etomidate.
   d. The low-dose SST may be a better predictor of outcome.
3. Diagnosis Using Any Total Cortisol Level
   a. There is large variation in results when the same specimen is tested in different laboratories and using different assays.
   b. Peripheral tissue-specific glucocorticoid resistance is not tested.
   c. Free cortisol is the biologically active fraction of cortisol.

Note: The external validity of the study by Annane and colleagues[34] remains untested.
HDSST, high-dose Synacthen stimulation test; SST, Synacthen stimulation test.

tory diagnostic criteria. In addition, the majority of literature has focused on RAI in septic shock. Few studies have investigated adrenal function in other forms of shock.[14]

Although it is known that cortisol production increases in response to critical illness, there is no consensus on what constitutes a "normal" cortisol level in critically ill patients.[1] Accordingly, multiple levels for a minimum cortisol have been proposed, ranging from 10 µg/dL (276 nmol/L)[1] to 34 µg/dL (414 nmol/L).[22] Even if a consensus on criteria for adrenal insufficiency based on basal cortisol existed, there is a diurnal variation of cortisol secretion even in the critically ill patient. Thus, it is conceivable that a patient's adrenal status may depend on the time of day that the specimen was taken. In addition, cortisol levels and adrenal function may vary according to the phase of illness.[37,38] Most studies have assessed adrenal function at a single time point. There is little information on the longitudinal function of the adrenal gland throughout the course of critical illness.

A further problem with diagnosing RAI is the increasing evidence of substantial interlaboratory variation in the results of testing for total serum cortisol.[38] Hence, a given patient may or may not be diagnosed with adrenal insufficiency depending on the assay and the laboratory where testing is done.

Diagnostic criteria using the HDSST often fail to take into account the basal cortisol level. Also, it is possible that RAI in critical illness can result from suboptimal corticotropin production (e.g., in individuals with traumatic brain injury).[13] In such patients, a normal adrenal response to administration of exogenous Synacthen in the HDSST would miss the diagnosis of secondary adrenal insufficiency.[14]

The administration of 250 µg of Synacthen results in serum levels of Synacthen that are markedly supra-physiological (up to 200-fold greater than maximal stress levels of corticotropin)[14] and may override adrenal resistance to corticotropin. Accordingly, other investigators have proposed that the low-dose (1 µg) Synacthen stimulation test (SST) may be more sensitive in the diagnosis of adrenal insufficiency in the critically ill.[39] The 1 to 2 µg dose of corticotropin is more physiological, better approximating the adrenocorticotropic hormone levels found in severe stress and results in concentrations similar to those seen in the insulin hypoglycemia and the metyrapone tests.[40]

A recent study has suggested that adrenal response to a low-dose SST may be more predictive of mortality than the HDSST in critical illness.[41]

Finally, studies reporting the incidence of adrenal insufficiency in septic shock often do not exclude patients who have received drugs such as etomidate, which has been associated with life-threatening adrenal insufficiency in the critically ill.[42] Such studies may lead to an overestimation of the "true incidence" of adrenal insufficiency attributable to the critical illness. Thus, in the randomized trial of steroid replacement therapy by Annane and coworkers,[36] 77% of the 299 patients enrolled had adrenal insufficiency. Importantly, 72 enrolled patients received the drug etomidate before undergoing the HDSST; 68 of these patients failed to adequately respond (29.7% of all nonresponders). In a recent retrospective study conducted in three intensive care units in Australia (where etomidate is not licensed for use), the incidence of adrenal insufficiency in a group of ventilated patients with septic shock was only 34.2%, less than half that seen in the study by Annane and coworkers.[24]

A further limitation of current tests using either a low basal cortisol or a reduced increment following Synacthen administration is that they measure total rather than the biologically active free cortisol. In critically ill patients, the presence of hypoproteinemia (and low cortisol-binding globulin levels) may lead to misdiagnosis of adrenal insufficiency based on total cortisol levels. In such patients, free cortisol levels are preserved or may be increased.[2] Currently, measurement of free cortisol is not widely available, and its significance in the critically ill requires further assessment. Finally, no current laboratory test is able to take into account the syndrome of tissue-specific glucocorticoid resistance.

CONCLUSION

Cortisol is a hormone with multiple actions in regulating metabolism, the immune system, and vascular responsiveness to circulating catecholamines. Critical illness is associated with increased cortisol production that is roughly proportional to the severity of the underlying disease. Critical illness may be associated with a syndrome of RAI, although there is considerable controversy as to how this syndrome should be defined. The largest trial investigating the role of low-dose steroid supplementation in septic shock failed to exclude those who had been exposed to etomidate in the previous 24 hours. A recent multicenter trial (CORTICUS) using low-dose corticosteroid therapy in septic shock did not demonstrate any mortality benefit with the use of steroids. There continues to be clinical equipoise regarding the issues of cortisol testing, the administration of corticotropin, and the use of hydrocortisone in septic shock.[43] Further research in this field is urgently needed.

Key Points

1. Critical illness is associated with a stress response, part of which involves increased production of cortisol.
2. Cortisol has anti-inflammatory properties that may be of benefit in modulating the inflammatory response to critical illness.
3. Absolute adrenal insufficiency is an uncommon entity in critical illness. Relative adrenal insufficiency may be seen in 30% to 77% of patients with septic shock, depending on the diagnostic criteria used. Controversy still exists as to the existence of relative adrenal insufficiency and the criteria used for diagnosing this entity.
4. High-dose glucocorticoid therapy has not been associated with improved outcome in patients with septic shock. Low-dose steroid therapy has been consistently shown to improve vasopressor responsiveness in septic shock. Its role in improving mortality in patients with septic shock continues to be debated.
5. Further research is needed to establish the role of cortisol testing, administration of corticotropin, and the use of hydrocortisone in septic shock.

Key References

1. Cooper MS, Stewart PM: Corticosteroid insufficiency in acutely ill patients. N Engl J Med 2003;348(8):727-734.
19. Annane D: Time for a consensus definition of corticosteroid insufficiency in critically ill patients. Crit Care Med 2003;31(6):1868-1869.
21. Lamberts SW, Bruining HA, de Jong FH: Corticosteroid therapy in severe illness. N Engl J Med 1997;337(18): 1285-1292.

32. Cronin L, Cook DJ, Carlet J, et al: Corticosteroid treatment for sepsis: A critical appraisal and meta-analysis of the literature. Crit Care Med 1995;23(8):1430-1439.
34. Annane D, Sébille V, Charpentier C, et al: Effect of treatment with low doses of hydrocortisone and fludrocortisone on mortality in patients with septic shock. JAMA 2002;288(7): 862-871.

See the companion Expert Consult website for the complete reference list.

General Treatment Concepts

CHAPTER 144

Enteral Nutrition

Andrew R. Davies and Anthony J. Hennessy

OBJECTIVES

This chapter will:
1. Describe the benefits that nutritional support can provide in the critically ill.
2. Explain the reasons why enteral nutrition should be preferred.
3. Discuss the risks associated with gastric feeding.
4. Outline three alternative strategies for patients with enteral feeding intolerance.
5. Discuss how to optimize the choice of substrates (particularly glutamine and omega-3 fatty acids) in the composition of enteral nutrition.

INTRODUCTION

Nutritional support is considered to be the standard of care for critically ill patients based on the rationale that malnutrition is associated with increased morbidity and mortality[1] and that administration of nutritional support will improve wound healing,[2] reduce complication rates,[3] and reduce the duration of hospitalization.[4,5] In fact, optimal management of nutritional support may well be as important as the management of renal, cardiovascular, ventilatory, or other organ system support.

Three high-quality evidence-based clinical practice guidelines have recently been published,[6,7,8] and the use of one of these guidelines is strongly advised in clinical practice. Several of the specific recommendations are consistent across all three guidelines (Table 144-1) with a strong preference for enteral nutrition.

WHY SHOULD ENTERAL NUTRITION BE PREFERRED?

Enteral nutrition is preferred to parenteral nutrition as there seems little controversy that delivering nutrition into the gut is more physiological and less expensive.[9] In comparison to parenteral nutrition, enteral nutrition has also been associated with improved gut function in the critically ill,[10] reduced inflammatory cytokine levels,[11] and reduced rates of infectious complications.[3,6,12]

Parenteral nutrition appears to increase the risk of infectious complications when compared to no nutritional intake,[13] so it has often been maligned in critically ill patients as a harmful intervention.[14] Such views have been challenged,[15,16] and a recent meta-analysis found that parenteral nutrition may in fact be advantageous if given early when enteral nutrition would otherwise be delayed.[17] It may also be the case that parenteral nutrition is safer when used in a lower-energy formulation than it was previously,[18] particularly now that greater attention to glycemic control seems warranted.[19]

Nevertheless, there is general consensus that when the gut is considered to be functioning adequately, enteral nutrition should be preferred to parenteral nutrition, and it should be started within 24 to 48 hours of admission.[6,7,8] Parenteral nutrition should be saved for those patients about whom there is a good clinical reason for not beginning enteral nutrition in this time frame. The most likely such reason is a condition where the gut is expected to be dysfunctional for many days, although it is worth noting that patients with esophageal surgery,[20] intestinal perforation and peritonitis,[21] colorectal surgery,[22,23] abdominal aortic aneurysm surgery,[24] and acute pancreatitis[25,26] can all be readily enterally fed with few complications.

POTENTIAL RISKS ASSOCIATED WITH ENTERAL FEEDING

Enteral nutrition is typically delivered into the stomach with a nasogastric tube,[27-29] and in many cases this leads to satisfactory delivery of nutrition. However, gastric motility (particularly gastric emptying) and absorption are impaired in critical illness,[30-32] and this may lead to enteral feeding intolerance.[33]

Enteral feeding intolerance has been reported to occur in 31% to 46% of patients with gastric feeding[33,34] and is usually manifest by large gastric residual volumes and vomiting.[27,33,35] It leads to a large number of patients not achieving their expected energy delivery requirements[36] and appears to place patients at a higher risk of pneumonia and possibly mortality.[33] This is often exacerbated in critically ill patients when their enteral nutrition is withheld for diagnostic and therapeutic procedures.

Managing potential enteral feeding intolerance by delaying the initiation of nasogastric feeding is illogical, as it will reduce the chance of the patient's meeting energy requirements, may worsen intestinal permeability,[37] and may lead to increased infectious complications and hospital length of stay.[4] There is therefore a much greater rationale for more proactive strategies such as the use of an evidence-based feeding guideline that includes the use

TABLE 144-1

Recommendations Based on Consistent Statements from Recent Evidence-Based Guidelines for Feeding of the Critically Ill

Early gastric feeding (started within 24-48 hours) should be used in preference to parenteral nutrition in patients with no major gut dysfunction.

Promotility drugs should be used if gastric feeding is not tolerated.

Small bowel feeding should be used if gastric feeding is not tolerated.

Enteral nutrition should be supplemented with parenteral nutrition if nutritional goals are not met but only after attempts at a promotility drug and a small bowel feeding tube.

When enteral nutrition is used:
- It SHOULD NOT be supplemented with arginine or other select nutrients (immunonutrition) in patients with severe sepsis.
- It SHOULD be supplemented with omega-3 fatty acids and antioxidants in patients with acute lung injury.
- It SHOULD be supplemented with glutamine in burn and trauma patients.

When parenteral nutrition is used:
- It SHOULD be supplemented with glutamine.
- It SHOULD be limited in energy to avoid complications such as hyperglycemia.

of promotility drugs and small bowel feeding when patients develop features of intolerance.[5]

REDUCING THE RISKS OF ENTERAL NUTRITION

Promotility Drugs

Since it was discovered that critical illness leads to significant gastrointestinal dysmotility,[30] promotility drugs have been considered a sensible option. Both metoclopramide and erythromycin improve gastric emptying,[38,39] and erythromycin seems the superior agent because of its ability to improve short-term tolerance in patients with enteral feeding intolerance[40,41] and also when administered routinely with gastric feeding.[42] While the dose of erythromycin for this indication is often recommended as 200 to 250 mg four times daily, 70 mg seems equally effective.[43] Naloxone also reduces gastric residual volume,[44] but its effect on feeding tolerance has not been established. Cisapride accelerates gastric emptying and lowers gastric residual volume[45,46] but is unfortunately no longer commercially available because of the risk of cardiac dysrhythmia.[47] Several other novel promotility drugs are being investigated, but none is yet commercially available.[48]

Metoclopramide is the only promotility drug that has been subjected to a study large enough to determine its efficacy on clinically meaningful outcomes and despite its useful gastric emptying effect, it had no effect on nosocomial pneumonia or mortality rate.[38] Given also that erythromycin may increase the risk of antibiotic resistance[49] and naloxone seems likely to be more effective only in the presence of large narcotic doses, it is difficult to make strong treatment recommendations about promotility drugs. Nevertheless, careful use of either erythromycin or metoclopramide seems warranted when the first signs of

enteral feeding intolerance develop. Erythromycin is more likely to be effective, although if intolerance persists with the use of either drug, the combination of both seems reasonable practice.[50]

Small Bowel Feeding

Small bowel feeding has some inherent advantages over gastric feeding, as the small bowel has a greater absorptive capacity than the stomach,[51] has less impaired motility in critical illness,[52] and is further away from the pharynx and respiratory tree, thereby potentially reducing the risk of pneumonia caused by gastroesophageal reflux.[53] Clinical studies comparing small bowel and gastric feeding have shown that small bowel feeding lowers gastric residual volume,[34,54] and although this has sometimes led to improved nutritional intake,[55,56] this has not been a consistent finding.[34,54,57] One meta-analysis found that small bowel feeding was associated with a reduced risk of pneumonia,[6] although others have not been as conclusive.[58,59]

Gastric feeding should therefore be regarded as the initial method of enteral feeding for critically ill patients, but small bowel feeding is recommended when patients develop feeding intolerance. Whether a promotility drug should be tried before a small bowel feeding tube is placed is not well established at the present time, but recent clinical practice surveys have suggested that clinicians prefer promotility drugs to small bowel feeding,[60,61] seemingly because of the logistical and technical concerns that are associated with nasojejunal tube placement. Numerous insertion techniques have been described,[62] and while "blind" placement at the bedside is certainly the least logistically challenging, this is time consuming and less successful than the placement of a nasogastric tube.[57] Erythromycin used specifically to assist insertion appears to improve success rates,[63] and specific mechanical maneuvers have also been described.[64] Fluoroscopy and endoscopy improve the success rates,[34,65] but logistical concerns remain a deterrent in many institutions. "Self-migrating" tubes such as the frictional NJ tube (Tiger Tube, Cook Critical Care, Bloomington, IN) may improve the insertion success and can be used safely and easily in clinical practice.[66,67]

Patients in the intensive care unit (ICU) who develop feeding intolerance during gastric feeding should therefore have a small bowel feeding tube placed. Institutional considerations should determine which insertion technique is chosen, and because gastric residual volumes often remain large (placing the patient at risk of pneumonia), a promotility drug, such as metoclopramide or erythromycin, is recommended, as is the use of a supplementary nasogastric tube to drain this gastric fluid.

Supplementary Parenteral Nutrition

Parenteral nutrition has often been considered an easy option for enteral feeding intolerance (especially when it is severe), as most critically ill patients already have central venous access. Although two recent clinical practice guidelines[7,8] recommend supplementary parenteral nutrition to assist meeting nutritional goals in the presence of enteral feeding intolerance, caution is advised, as supplementary parenteral nutrition has been shown to lead to excess mortality in burn patients[68] and has not been shown to improve clinical outcomes over enteral nutrition alone

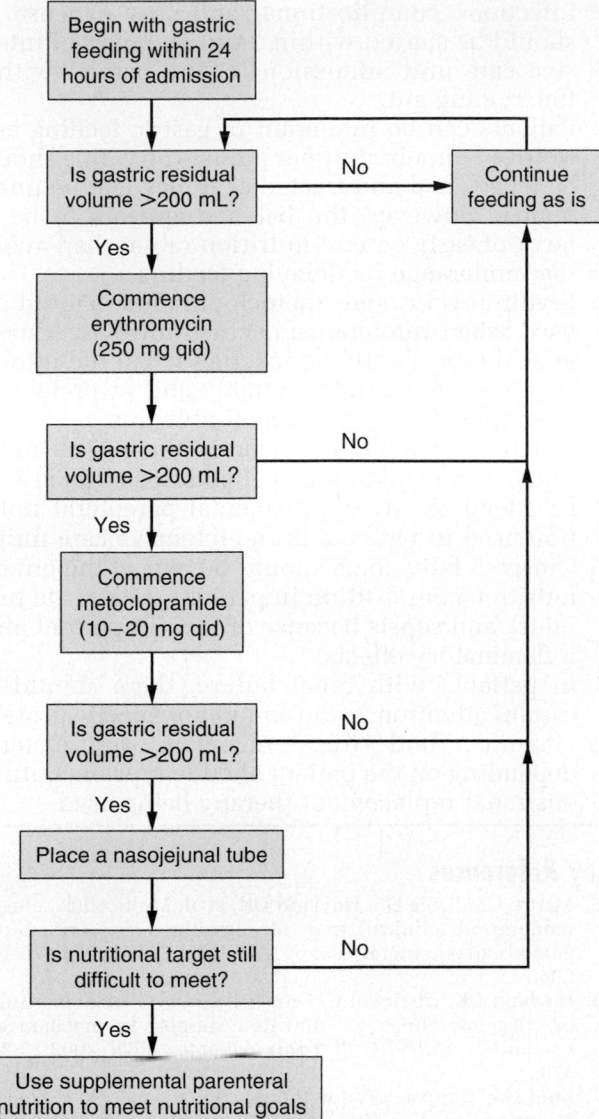

FIGURE 144-1. Simple algorithm for nutritional support in the critically ill patient.

in meta-analyses.[6,7] It therefore seems prudent that parenteral nutrition should not be used to supplement enteral nutrition in critically ill patients until all other strategies to maximize enteral nutrition (including promotility drugs and small bowel feeding) have been attempted (Fig. 144-1).

CHOOSING THE OPTIMAL ENTERAL NUTRITION PRODUCT

The optimal macronutrient composition (i.e., carbohydrate, lipid, and protein content) of enteral nutrition for the heterogeneous critically ill patient remains largely unknown, and consequently there are dozens of commercially prepared enteral nutrition products with specific variations in the combination of carbohydrate, lipid, and protein.

All three recently published evidence-based guidelines have suggested that a standard polymeric enteral formula should be administered,[6,7,8] and this seems reasonable for most critically ill patients. Estimation of both energy and protein requirements should be performed using standardized equations leading to an hourly goal rate being established. In some specific patient groups, evidence is accumulating that varying the nutrient composition with the aims of either replacing important deficiencies or modulating immune function may be useful, although controversy in this area continues.

Glutamine

There is recent consensus that glutamine-supplemented parenteral nutrition should be used in the ICU patient who requires parenteral nutrition[6,7,8]; this consensus is based on studies in ICU and abdominal surgical patients.[69-71] This is in contrast with enteral nutrition where glutamine has not been shown to improve clinical outcomes when administered enterally to heterogeneous groups of critically ill patients.[72,73]

However, glutamine-supplemented enteral nutrition may be efficacious in two homogeneous groups of patients: those with burns and those with trauma.[74,75] Glutamine should therefore be strongly considered in all ICU patients having parenteral nutrition and all burn and trauma patients having enteral nutrition, and although the exact dose remains controversial, a dose in the range of 0.4 to 0.5 g/kg body weight seems reasonable.

Immunonutrition

Enteral nutrition products with a mixture of arginine, nucleotides, and omega-3 fatty acids have been considered to modulate immune function and therefore considered "immunonutrition." Despite more than a decade of research, these products still remain controversial in critical care practice as they appear to elicit harmful effects in patients with sepsis and septic shock.[6] Of the various substrates, arginine appears to be the sole culprit of the substrates, as a recent study in animals demonstrated the scientific rationale for the potential lethality of arginine in septic shock.[76]

Given immunonutrition had no effect in the largest of all the heterogeneous ICU patient studies,[77] the pragmatic view is that if immunonutrition causes harm in septic patients (presumably due to arginine), it may therefore have a beneficial effect in nonseptic patients (presumably due to omega-3 fatty acids). The way of the future must be to study the individual nutrients in specific disease states rather than the immunonutrition package in heterogeneous populations,[78] and the present recommendation is not to administer immunonutrition products containing arginine to ICU patients.

Omega-3 Fatty Acids

There have now been two recent studies[79,80] where enteral nutrition products containing fish oil (eicosapentaenoic acid), borage oil (gamma-linolenic acid), and antioxidants led to beneficial clinical outcomes in patients with acute lung injury and septic shock. Given a previous study demonstrated similar effects in patients with acute lung injury,[81] it appears that an enteral nutrition product containing these omega-3 fatty acids should be used when patients with acute lung injury and septic shock are treated in the ICU.

ISSUES SPECIFIC TO THE CRITICALLY ILL RENAL FAILURE PATIENT

The principles of nutritional support in critically ill patients with acute renal failure are similar to those in critically ill patients without renal failure. While some clinicians feel that restriction of fluid and protein may be required when renal failure is present, there is little evidence to support this notion and there seems a greater rationale to use either earlier or more effective continuous renal replacement therapy to improve outcomes.

What is known is that amino acids (including glutamine), vitamins, and trace elements are often lost from the body through the filter in continuous renal replacement therapy, although the exact amount in individual patients varies.[82] Making sure that the nutritional prescription does not have inadequate amounts of energy, protein, vitamins, and trace elements is therefore extremely important, especially as gastric emptying can also be more significantly impaired in patients with renal failure. The threshold to use promotility drugs, small bowel feeding tubes, and supplemental parenteral nutrition should therefore be lowered so as to maximize nutritional intake.

CONCLUSION

Evidence-based guidelines for nutritional support in the ICU should be followed where possible, meaning that enteral nutrition should be preferred to parenteral nutrition, and that when intolerance occurs, both small bowel feeding and promotility drugs should be attempted before supplementary parenteral nutrition is used (see Fig. 144-1). Clinicians should carefully consider the composition of the enteral nutrition with regard to lipid content, antioxidants, and glutamine as clinical outcomes are improved in some specific groups of patients.

Key Points

1. Nutritional support leads to a reduction in complication rates and shorter hospitalization in critically ill patients, especially when evidence-based guidelines are followed.
2. Enteral nutrition should be preferred to parenteral because of improved gut function, reduced

infectious complications, and less expense. It should be started within 24 to 48 hours of intensive care unit admission in any patient with a functioning gut.
3. Patients can be intolerant of gastric feeding as a result of impaired upper gut motility; this should be recognized and treated as it may lead to pneumonia. However, the balance appears to be in favor of early enteral nutrition rather than avoiding intolerance by delaying feeding.
4. Erythromycin and metoclopramide should be used when intolerance occurs; however, a nasojejunal tube should be inserted when the intolerance does not resolve quickly and in preference to supplementary parenteral nutrition.
5. Glutamine should be added to the enteral nutrition in burn and trauma patients. It should always be added to any supplemental parenteral nutrition used in patients in the intensive care unit.
6. Omega-3 fatty acids should be part of the enteral nutrition composition in patients with acute lung injury and sepsis because of their important anti-inflammatory effects.
7. In patients with renal failure, there should be careful attention to the amount of energy, protein, vitamins, and trace elements administered depending on the patient and the type of continuous renal replacement therapy being used.

Key References

5. Martin CM, Doig GS, Heyland DK, et al: Multicentre, cluster-randomized clinical trial of algorithms for critical-care enteral and parenteral therapy (ACCEPT). CMAJ 2004;170:197-204.
6. Heyland DK, Dhaliwal R, Drover JW, et al: Canadian clinical practice guidelines for nutrition support in mechanically ventilated, critically ill adult patients. JPEN 2003;27:355-373.
7. Doig GS, Simpson F, for the Australian and New Zealand Intensive Care Society Clinical Trials Group: Evidence-based guidelines for nutritional support of the critically ill: Results of a bi-national guideline development conference. 2005. Downloadable from www.evidencebased.net
69. Novak F, Heyland DK, Avenell A, et al: Glutamine supplementation in serious illness: A systematic review of the evidence. Crit Care Med 2002;30:2022-2029.
80. Pontes-Arruda A, Aragao AM, Albuquerque JD: Effects of enteral feeding with eicosapentaenoic acid, gamma-linolenic acid, and antioxidants in mechanically ventilated patients with severe sepsis and septic shock. Crit Care Med 2006;34:2325-2333.

See the companion Expert Consult website for the complete reference list.

CHAPTER 145

Parenteral Nutrition

Gordon S. Doig and Fiona Simpson

OBJECTIVES

This chapter will:
1. Explain the benefits, risks, and indications for parenteral nutrition use in the critically ill, with emphasis on patients with renal injury.
2. Discuss timing of start, energy and protein goals, composition, and monitoring of parenteral nutrition.
3. Address issues relevant to parenteral nutrition use in patients who are receiving renal replacement therapy.

BACKGROUND

The provision of adequate nutritional support to the hospitalized patient is widely accepted as a standard of care. Mounting evidence suggests that the provision of *early* nutritional support to the critically ill patient may impart significant benefits to patient-oriented outcomes, although it is not yet considered a standard of care.

Independent evidence-based guideline initiatives, which reviewed all available clinical trials evaluating nutritional support interventions in critical illness, agree that mortality can be reduced by 8% to 12% through the provision of early enteral nutrition (EN).[1,2] Unfortunately, observational studies demonstrate that only 50% of eligible patients receive EN within 48 hours of intensive care unit (ICU) admission.[3] Based on the implementation of evidence-based guidelines for nutritional support in ICUs throughout Australia, New Zealand, and Canada, it is estimated that 75% of patients who are expected to stay longer than 2 days may be eligible to receive EN within 48 hours of ICU admission. The remaining 25% of patients are likely to benefit from receiving early parenteral nutrition (PN).[2]

It is widely accepted that "parenteral nutrition clearly has a role in the critically ill patient with an absolute contraindication to EN" (Table 145-1).[4] Indeed, a recent meta-analysis of high-quality clinical trials demonstrated that, in patients who cannot receive early EN, mortality can be reduced by 13% if PN is started within 24 hours of ICU admission.[5] In addition to this meta-analysis, a Canadian cluster randomized trial that evaluated the impact of evidence-based guidelines for nutrition support, which included a recommendation for the provision of early PN to patients who could not receive early EN (Fig. 145-1), demonstrated an overall mortality reduction of 10%.[6] Based on the strength of the meta-analysis and guidelines validation trial, the current recommendation is to start PN within 24 hours of ICU admission in all critically ill patients who cannot receive early EN.[5] As long as the patient has timely access to renal replacement therapy (RRT), this recommendation for early PN also applies to critically ill patients with acute renal injury.

This chapter focuses primarily on the use of PN in critically ill patients, with particular reference to its use in those with acute renal injury. Acute renal injury tends to affect the most severely ill subgroup of critically ill patients and mortality remains high. For this reason, the discussion focuses on treatment concepts that are supported by research that has demonstrated improvements in patient-oriented outcomes.

GENERAL PRINCIPLES OF NUTRITIONAL SUPPORT FOR CRITICALLY ILL PATIENTS WITH RENAL DISEASE

In general, critically ill patients with renal injury should be fed in a proactive manner to that applied to other critically ill patients in intensive care.[7] The following principles should guide the clinician:
1. The presence of renal injury in a critically ill patient should never lead to restrictions in nutritional support. For example, nutritional support should not be compromised to reduce uremia. RRT should be commenced to prevent uremia and allow continuation of nutritional support.
2. Nutritional support for critically ill patients with renal injury should be the same as for those with multiple-organ dysfunction. Nitrogen catabolism induced by multiple-organ dysfunction is far greater than that induced by renal dysfunction alone.
3. Concerns regarding nutritional support should not compromise early and aggressive RRT. RRT has only a small effect on patient catabolism, so the application of RRT does not significantly compromise nutritional support.

INDICATIONS FOR PARENTERAL NUTRITION

Early PN should be considered in all patients admitted to the ICU who are unlikely to receive early EN (Table 145-2). Patients with absolute contraindications to EN are easy to identify at admission to the ICU and should receive PN within 24 hours of admission. Some absolute contraindications to EN include gut obstruction, high-output fistula (greater than 0.5 L/hr), severe non-hypovolemic gut ischemia or gut failure due to extensive resection or absorption impairment. Patients with relative contraindications to early EN also may be easy to identify. For example, although the literature suggests that gut anastomoses may heal faster with enteral feeding, some surgeons are reluctant to provide early EN to certain patients. Likewise, a patient may be admitted to the ICU with the expectation that they are likely to receive multiple surgical interventions, and thus EN is not scheduled to begin until after the final procedure. Early PN is recommended in both of these cases.

Previous systematic reviews have suggested that malnourished patients who receive PN may have significantly fewer major complications.[8] More recent systematic reviews of high-quality trials conducted in critically ill patients failed to find that this benefit was restricted to malnourished patients. Indeed, it is likely that well-nourished critically ill patients also benefit from early

PN.[5] Therefore, early PN for both adequately nourished and malnourished patients is recommended. Although it is advisable that obese (body mass index greater than 30) patients be fed to their ideal body weight, there is no good evidence that feeding should be delayed in obese patients.

As a general rule, shock should be stabilized before PN is begun; this usually is possible within hours of ICU admission. The most important contraindication to PN in a patient with acute renal injury is the inability to provide the patient with RRT.

TABLE 145-1

Summary Points: Background

- There is good evidence that *early* nutritional support improves survival in the critically ill. This includes good evidence for the use of *early* parenteral nutrition.
- In patients expected to remain in the intensive care unit longer than 2 days, if it is anticipated that enteral nutrition or oral nutrition cannot be started within 48 hours of admission to the intensive care unit, parenteral nutrition should be initiated within 24 hours of admission.
- With timely access to renal replacement therapy, there is no reason to delay parenteral nutrition in critically ill patients with renal injury.

TABLE 145-2

Summary Points: Indications

- Patients with absolute or relative contraindications to enteral nutrition should receive parenteral nutrition *early* during their stay in the intensive care unit.
- Malnourished patients may have fewer major complications if provided with parenteral nutrition.
- Both malnourished and well-nourished patients are likely to benefit from a mortality reduction due to early parenteral nutrition.
- Stabilize shock before beginning parenteral nutrition.
- Early renal replacement therapy facilitates the provision of early parenteral nutrition.

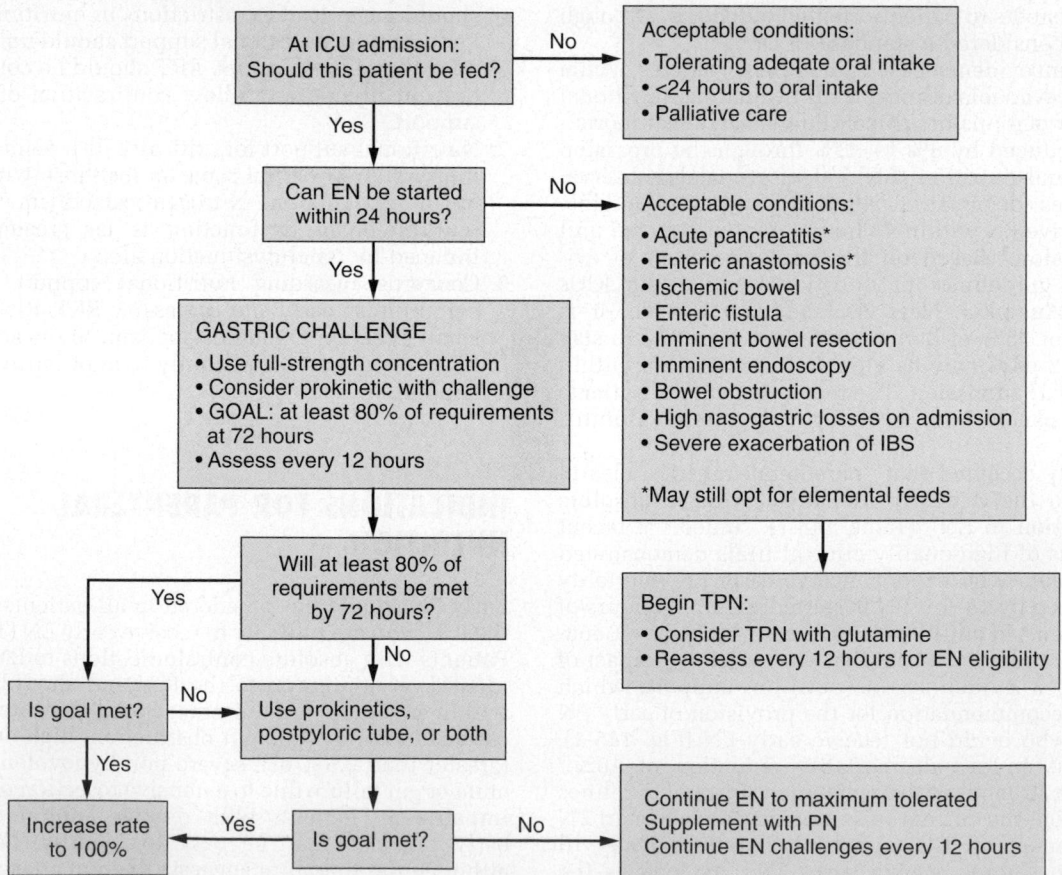

FIGURE 145-1. Example of intensive care unit (ICU) evidence-based feeding guideline. EN, enteral nutrition; IBS, irritable bowel syndrome; PN, parenteral nutrition; TPN, total parenteral nutrition. (Evidence updated by the ANZICS CTG Feeding Investigators Group October 28, 2003. Chief investigator: Dr. Gordon S. Doig, University of Sydney.)

PARENTERAL NUTRITION AND INFECTIOUS COMPLICATIONS

An increase in infectious complications is often cited as the main reason to avoid the use of PN in the critically ill. In many previous trials and meta-analyses, urinary tract infections, surgical wound infections, catheter-related infections, and full-blown sepsis were treated as equally serious complications and added together to demonstrate an increase in composite "infectious complications."[1,8] Recent meta-analyses have attempted to examine each type of infection separately.

Of all the infections listed in the previous paragraph, the most comprehensive systematic review conducted on the topic shows that PN use was associated with a significant increase in catheter-related bloodstream (CRB) infections only (absolute increase 3.5%, 95% confidence interval [CI] from 1.2% to 5.8%) (Table 145-3), compared to patients receiving EN.[9] Unfortunately, each individual trial reviewed in this meta-analysis used vastly different definitions of infection and, with the recent emphasis on tighter blood glucose control in critically ill patients, the authors of the meta-analysis acknowledged that the impact of PN on infectious complications may be much *lower* than they estimated.[9]

Although CRB infections have been associated with an increased length of stay, there is no good evidence to suggest that they increase mortality.[10,11] CRB infections are often caused by less pathogenic organisms (e.g., coagulase-negative *Staphylococcus*) and may be easier to identify, manage, and treat compared to bloodstream infections from other sources.[10] Appropriate antibiotic treatment and prompt catheter removal are known to be associated with a shorter duration of bloodstream infection, fewer recurrent infections, and improved patient outcomes.[12] Given that critically ill patients with renal injury who require RRT have an underlying mortality rate as high as 60%,[13] an increase in CRB infections may be of lesser clinical importance when considered in the context of the mortality benefit attributable to early PN use.

PN has been used in humans with chronic nonfunctioning gastrointestinal tracts since the 1960s[14] and is a lifesaving intervention for these patients. High-quality evidence suggests that *early* PN may be lifesaving in critically ill patients as well.[5] To minimize potential harm associated with CRB infections, the recommended intervention is aseptic catheter insertion combined with heightened vigilance to detect catheter infections, treat the infections with appropriate antibiotics, and replace catheters whenever the appearance of an infection is found.

ENERGY GOALS FOR THE CRITICALLY ILL PATIENT FED PARENTERAL NUTRITION

The energy needs of critically ill patients are determined by the underlying disease state. In general, the caloric expenditure of critically ill patients with any form of renal dysfunction is similar to that of patients with other forms of multiple-organ dysfunction, ranging between 30 and 35 kcal/kg/day.[7] Unfortunately, there is no gold standard evidence that demonstrates patient outcomes can be improved by meeting energy expenditures, but there is general consensus that overfeeding should be avoided.

Over time, the recommended energy intakes for critically ill patients with renal dysfunction have been progressively lowered (Table 145-4). A recent small cross-over trial[15] that included ICU patients with renal failure who required RRT provides some insight as to why intakes have been reduced. In this randomized trial, patients received isonitrogenous (1.5 g/kg/day) PN solutions targeted to deliver either 40 kcal/kg/day or 30 kcal/kg/day total calories. No positive benefits of the higher caloric goal were found, and there were no improvements in nitrogen balance, protein catabolism, or urea generation between the patient groups. However, the higher calorie intake did result in significantly higher glucose levels and insulin requirements. Although clinicians should exercise caution and not overinterpret results from small clinical trials with surrogate outcomes, this trial does serve as an example of the type of research that is being used to guide current clinical recommendations.

Current recommendations for total energy goals in critical illness range between 20 and 25 kcal/kg/day during the early or initial phase of critical illness followed by between 25 and 30 kcal/kg/day during the anabolic phase.[16-18] Table 145-5 provides an example of a protocol for the early delivery of PN that gradually increases intake to achieve calculated goals by day 3.

TABLE 145-3

Summary Points: Infectious Complications

- Parenteral nutrition use is associated with an increase in catheter-related bloodstream (CRB) infections.
- CRB infections may increase length of stay but are not known to increase mortality.
- In the context of decreased mortality from early parenteral nutrition use in critically ill patients, the clinical importance of increased CRB infections must be questioned.
- The clinician should closely monitor the patient for signs of line infections.
- If a central line appears infected on clinical grounds, appropriate antibiotic therapy should be implemented and the line must be removed, replaced, or repositioned as soon as possible.
- If the patient is hemodynamically stable, a new bag of parenteral nutrition can be restarted through the new line.

TABLE 145-4

Summary Points: Energy Goals

- Avoid overfeeding in the critically ill patient.
- A reasonable target range for critically ill patients with renal injury is 25 to 30 kcal/kg/day.
- When determining the energy content of various parenteral nutrition solutions, total energy (not nonprotein energy) should be considered.
- Obese patients (body mass index greater than 30) should be fed to their ideal body weight.

TABLE 145-5

Example of Parenteral Nutrition Protocol for Well-Nourished Patients in the Intensive Care Unit

Feeding Day 1 (first 24 hours of parenteral nutrition)
Commence parenteral nutrition at 60 mL/hr (or goal rate,* whichever is lower).
Consider trace element, mineral, and vitamin needs as clinically appropriate.
Feeding Day 2 (second 24 hours of parenteral nutrition)
Increase parenteral nutrition to 80 mL/hr (or goal rate, whichever is lower).
Consider trace element, mineral, and vitamin needs as clinically appropriate.
Feeding Day 3 (next 24 hours)
Increase parenteral nutrition to goal rate, as appropriate.
Consider trace element, mineral, and vitamin needs, as clinically appropriate.
Recommend trialing enteral nutrition, oral nutrition, or both, if clinically appropriate.
Once the patient tolerates up to 475 kcal/day enteral nutrition, complete remainder of 24-hour parenteral nutrition infusion and do not hang another bag.
If patient tolerates any oral caloric intake from food, complete remainder of 24-hour parenteral nutrition infusion and do not hang another bag.
Feeding Day 4 (next 24 hours plus all additional days after day 4)
Consider long-term needs regarding trace element, mineral, and vitamins as clinically appropriate.
Recommend trialing enteral nutrition, oral nutrition, or both, if clinically appropriate.
Once the patient tolerates up to 475 kcal/day enteral nutrition, complete remainder of 24-hour parenteral nutrition infusion and do not hang another bag.
If patient tolerates any oral caloric intake from food, complete remainder of 24-hour parenteral nutrition infusion and do not hang another bag.

*Goals set at 25 to 35 total kcal/kg body weight and 1.0 to 1.5 g protein/kg body weight.

PROTEIN NEEDS IN THE CRITICALLY ILL PATIENT FED PARENTERAL NUTRITION

On average, the critically ill patient can lose up to 150 g of protein per day[7] and loses between 5% and 10% of lean body mass per week of stay in the ICU.[19] Although recent research has suggested there may be some benefit from increased protein intake in patients undergoing dialysis, these benefits are not convincing enough to initiate large-scale changes to current practice. Current guidelines recommend a daily protein intake of between 1.0 and 1.5 g/kg (Table 145-6).[16,17]

It is recognized that during PN administration, RRT may remove between 10% and 17% of individual amino acids, and some clinicians recommend that an additional 0.2 g/kg/day of protein be administered to compensate for this loss.[20] Because it is not known whether a higher intake might simply worsen losses, increase costs, exacerbate uremia, and result in little improvement in nitrogen balance, it is not considered standard practice to correct for this loss. Small nonrandomized studies involving critically ill, anuric, ventilated patients requiring PN have evaluated the impact of increasing protein intake during RRT.[21,22] These studies suggest that an intake of 2.5 g

TABLE 145-6

Summary Points: Protein

- Protein loss in critically ill patients with renal injury is not appreciably higher than protein loss in critically ill patients without renal injury.
- Renal replacement therapy may remove between 10% and 17% of circulating individual amino acids.
- The recommended daily protein intake for other hospitalized and critically ill patients (1.0 to 1.5 g/kg) is also appropriate for critically ill patients with renal disease.

protein/kg/day can maintain near-normal values of most amino acid levels and can maintain an acceptable nitrogen balance in up to 50% of patients.[7] Unfortunately, other evidence from observational studies conducted in critically ill patients with trauma or sepsis contradicts these results. Using in vivo neutron activation analysis to measure changes in total body protein over 10 days, Ishibashi and colleagues[23] failed to find any difference in actual protein loss between patients receiving either 1.5 or 1.9 g protein/kg/day. Because the clinical relevance of treating amino acid levels can be questioned, randomized clinical trials are needed to demonstrate the benefits of higher protein intake using clinically meaningful patient-oriented outcomes.[7,22]

LIPIDS AND THE CRITICALLY ILL PATIENT FED PARENTERAL NUTRITION

There is much discussion regarding the different types of parenteral lipids and their role in specific clinical situations in critical illness. Lipids provide essential fatty acids, calories with less carbon dioxide production, and fat-soluble vitamins. Lipids are also known to influence the structure and function of cell membranes, cytokine production, membrane receptor activities, and gene expression. Unfortunately, because of major differences in trial design and the absence of patient-oriented outcomes in many trials, it remains difficult to recommend one specific type of lipid over any other.[2,24]

Overall, lipids are powerful nutrients that may improve outcomes in critically ill patients. One recommendation is that PN solutions should contain approximately 30% of total calories from some form of commercially available lipid (Table 145-7). Lipids should be provided daily, except when lipid profiles are severely elevated (e.g., total cholesterol greater than 6 mmol/L or triglycerides greater than 3 mmol/L).

TABLE 145-7

Summary Points: Lipids

- Approximately 30% of total calories should come from lipids.
- Unless contraindicated, patients should receive lipids daily.

TABLE 145-8

Summary Points: Trace Elements and Vitamins

- Daily supplementation of all vitamins and trace elements at the recommended dietary intake (RDI) level may prevent acute micronutrient deficiencies in patients with renal disease.
- Patients requiring continuous renal replacement therapy should receive twice the RDI of folate, vitamin B_6, and vitamin C.

TABLE 145-9

Summary Points: Supplementing Enteral Nutrition Intake with Parenteral Nutrition

- If 80% of caloric goals are not achieved within 72 hours of beginning enteral nutrition, use prokinetics, postpyloric feeding tubes, or both, to increase enteral nutrition intake. If 80% of goals still cannot be met, parenteral nutrition should be used as a supplement to enteral nutrition intake.

TRACE ELEMENTS AND VITAMINS

At time of admission to the ICU, if there is no history of malnutrition or acute reduction of intake, micronutrient deficiencies are expected to be rare. However, deficiencies may develop rapidly in patients with burns, trauma, or those receiving RRT.[25]

Testing of blood levels in ICU patients may be of limited value, and supplementation should occur without reliance on laboratory tests.[25] Administering at least the recommended dietary intake for all vitamins and trace elements for patients with renal injury is recommended (Table 145-8). Patients on continuous RRT should receive at least twice the recommended dietary intake for the water-soluble vitamins folate, vitamin B_6, and vitamin C. Additional zinc and selenium may also be considered.[17,7]

GLUTAMINE IN THE CRITICALLY ILL

Glutamine is the most abundant amino acid in the body and plays an important role as an energy source for enterocytes and the immune system. Glutamine contributes to the body's antioxidant defenses through the production of glutathione, enhances the expression of heat shock protein, and may help maintain the integrity of the gut's barrier function.

Despite promising results from one clinical trial,[26] the most recent comprehensive systematic review of all available trials failed to find a significant reduction in mortality, or infectious complications, attributable to glutamine supplementation in critical illness.[27] Although the meta-analysis reveals a slight mortality benefit from glutamine supplementation, the finding is not statistically significant. There is a clear need for a well-conducted Level I trial that would evaluate the impact of glutamine on patient-oriented outcomes before wide-scale supplementation can be recommended in critically ill patients.

ACHIEVING CALORIC GOALS BY SUPPLEMENTING ENTERALLY FED PATIENTS WITH PARENTERAL NUTRITION

Meta-analysis of trials that compared EN alone to EN supplemented with PN failed to find any evidence of benefit and actually suggested the practice may increase mortality when PN supplementation occurs early.[2] Because of the possibility of increased mortality, supplementing enterally fed patients with PN to achieve their caloric goals is not recommended within 72 hours of ICU admission.

If a patient is not achieving 80% of caloric goals within 72 hours of EN commencement, prokinetics and the placement of a postpyloric feeding tube should be considered (Table 145-9). If these two interventions are not successful, the next step should be supplementing intake with PN to achieve the patient's caloric requirements.[2] This sequence of actions was recommended by the evidence-based guideline evaluated in a recent Canadian cluster randomized trial, which resulted in a overall mortality reduction of 10%.[6]

REFEEDING SYNDROME/ ELECTROLYTE MONITORING

Malnourished patients are at risk of developing refeeding syndrome when they receive increased nutritional support. Refeeding syndrome is life threatening and is characterized by severe hypophosphatemia, hypokalemia, hypomagnesemia, abnormal blood glucose levels, and vitamin deficiencies, especially thiamine deficiency.[28] Although many believe that refeeding syndrome is rare in ICU patients, a prospective observational study[29] suggests that up to 34% of all ICU patients who are unfed for at least 48 hours may develop the syndrome (Table 145-10).

In addition to daily monitoring of serum potassium, magnesium, and calcium, it is extremely important to recognize changes in phosphates as refeeding syndrome. A decrease of more than 0.16 mmol/L to below 0.65 mmol/L after initiation of nutritional support can be considered characteristic of refeeding syndrome in those without renal injury. Immediate replacement and correction of

TABLE 145-10

Summary Points: Refeeding Syndrome and Electrolyte Monitoring

- Up to 34% of all critically ill patients who are unfed for 48 hours may develop refeeding syndrome. Malnourished patients are at high risk of developing refeeding syndrome.
- Thiamine may be administered prophylactically to patients at high risk of refeeding (i.e., patients who are malnourished, alcoholic, unfed, or have a decreased intake for more than 48 hours).
- Electrolytes, especially phosphates and potassium, should be monitored closely and replaced when needed.
- Intake may be reduced to 20 kcal/kg/day and increased slowly over 3 to 5 days to achieve goals.

electrolytes, with the addition of 100 mg thiamine daily, should be undertaken. Although some clinicians recommend reducing the caloric intake to approximately 20 kcal/kg/day and gradually rebuilding intake to achieve the appropriate nutritional goal over 3 to 5 days, many patients in a *closely monitored environment*, such as the ICU, respond satisfactorily to electrolyte, mineral, and vitamin replacement alone.

Because this text deals specifically with patients with renal injury, it is important to note that phosphate additions should be used with extreme caution in these patients. Refeeding syndrome may be more difficult to identify in patients with renal injury who have elevated phosphate. Attention to other changes associated with the syndrome is warranted in these patients.

CONCLUSION

Mounting evidence supports the presence of a reduction in the risk of mortality attributable to the provision of early nutritional support in critical illness. This evidence extends to include the use of early PN if there are absolute or relative contraindications to early EN.

The need for RRT in the critically ill should not delay the provision of nutritional support. Indeed, timely early RRT may facilitate the early provision of nutritional support.

Key Points

1. In patients expected to remain in the intensive care unit longer than 2 days, if it is anticipated that enteral nutrition or oral nutrition cannot be started within 48 hours of intensive care unit admission, parenteral nutrition should be initiated within 24 hours of admission. The use of early parenteral nutrition is associated with a 13% reduction in mortality.
2. The presence of renal injury in a critically ill patient should never lead to restrictions in nutritional support. Early renal replacement therapy facilitates the provision of early parenteral nutrition.
3. Concerns regarding nutritional support should not compromise early and aggressive renal replacement therapy.
4. Nutritional support for critically ill patients with renal injury should be the same as for those with multiple-organ dysfunction: energy goals between 25 and 30 kcal/kg/day (avoid overfeeding), protein goals between 1.0 to 1.5 g/kg, and 30% of energy

from daily lipids. Obese patients (body mass index greater than 30) should be fed to their ideal body weight.
5. Use total calories when determining the energy content of a parenteral nutrition solution to avoid overfeeding.
6. Parenteral nutrition use is associated with an increase in catheter-related bloodstream infections. Catheter-related bloodstream infections may increase length of stay but are not known to increase mortality. Signs of line infections should be detected, and if a central line appears infected on clinical grounds, appropriate antibiotic therapy should be implemented and the line should be removed, replaced, or repositioned as soon as possible.
7. Daily supplementation of all vitamins and trace elements at the recommended dietary intake level may prevent acute micronutrient deficiencies in patients with renal injury. Patients requiring continuous renal replacement therapy should receive twice the recommended dietary intake of folate, vitamin B_6, and vitamin C.
8. Up to 34% of all critically ill patients who are unfed for 48 hours may develop refeeding syndrome; malnourished patients are at higher risk. Thiamine may be administered prophylactically to patients at high risk (i.e., those who are malnourished, alcoholic, unfed, or have a decreased intake after 48 hours). Electrolytes, especially phosphates and potassium, should be monitored closely and replaced, where needed.

Key References

2. Doig GS, Simpson F: Evidence-Based Guidelines for Nutritional Support of the Critically Ill: Results of a Bi-National Guideline Development Conference, Sydney, 2005. Available at www.evidencebased.net/files
5. Simpson F, Doig GS: Parenteral vs. enteral nutrition in the critically ill patient: A meta-analysis of trials using the intention to treat principle. Intensive Care Med 2005;31:12-23.
7. Bellomo R: How to feed patients with renal dysfunction. Blood Purif 2002;20:296-303.
16. National Collaborating Centre for Acute Care: Nutrition support in adults: Oral nutrition support, enteral tube feeding and parenteral nutrition. National Collaborating Centre for Acute Care, London, 2006. Available at www.rcseng.ac.uk
17. Cano N, Fiaccadori E, Tesinsky P, et al: ESPEN Guidelines on Enteral Nutrition: Adult renal failure. Clin Nutr 2006;25:295-310.

See the companion Expert Consult website for the complete reference list.

CHAPTER 146

Blood Glucose Control in Critical Care

Moritoki Egi and Rinaldo Bellomo

OBJECTIVES

This chapter will:
1. Describe the nature of stress-induced hyperglycemia.
2. Explore the possible significance of normoglycemia in critically ill patients.
3. Discuss the importance of blood glucose control and nutritional support.
4. Describe the risk and incidence of hypoglycemia in relation to pursuing tighter blood glucose control.
5. Review recent recommendations for blood glucose control in critically ill patients.

INTRODUCTION

Acute hyperglycemia is common in critically ill patients. Approximately 90% of all patients develop blood glucose concentrations more than 110 mg/dL during critical illness.[1] Until recently, this "acute hyperglycemia" related to physiological stress was believed to represent a beneficial adaptive response by promoting cellular glucose uptake. However, recent studies have suggested that treating this hyperglycemia using intensive insulin therapy (IIT) might reduce mortality and morbidity in critically ill patients. Thus, lowering blood glucose control has moved to center stage of critical care.

STRESS-INDUCED HYPERGLYCEMIA

Stress-induced hyperglycemia is common in critically ill patients.[2] There are no accepted criteria to define this acute hyperglycemia, unlike "chronic diabetes mellitus." In acute illness, "stress" in response to tissue injury or infection can have profound effects on carbohydrate metabolism. This type of hyperglycemia occurs despite elevation in insulin levels (insulin resistance). It is assumed that several mechanisms contribute to this stress-induced hyperglycemia.

Decreased glucose uptake and utilization: Insulin-stimulated glucose uptake and utilization is achieved by skeletal muscle for 80% to 85% of all peripheral glucose uptake and by adipose tissues for 5%. In skeletal muscle, exercise is an important stimulating factor for glucose uptake and utilization. However, in critical illness, this exercise-stimulated glucose uptake is decreased, because patients are typically bed-bound. Furthermore, in critically ill patients, glucose transporter-4 (GLUT-4)-dependent insulin-stimulated glucose uptake is inhibited.[3]

Increased glucose production: The liver is the dominant organ for glucose production from glycogen (gluconeogenesis). In the fasting phase, the liver can produce 2 mg/kg/min of glucose, which represents 85% of whole body gluconeogenesis in healthy subjects. In critically ill patients, this hepatic gluconeogenesis increases because of increased levels of glucagon, cortisol, growth hormone, and cytokines.[4]

Depressed glycogen production: The production of glycogen from glucose (glycogenesis) is one of the key roles of the liver. In critically ill patients, increases in the level of glucagon, epinephrine, and cytokines inhibit glycogenesis by inactivation of glycogen synthase through increased glycogen synthase-kinase.[5]

Increased free fatty acids: In critically ill patients, free fatty acid and triglyceride production from adipose tissue increases secondary to increased activity of hormone-sensitive lipase. The increase in the blood level of glucagon and adrenalin enhance such activity, which in turn decreases peripheral glucose uptake.

It is well known that stress-induced hyperglycemia reflects severity of illness and is associated with mortality and morbidity in various patient groups, such as those with acute myocardial ischemia, cerebral infarction and hemorrhage, and multiple trauma and burns. Until recently, it was suggested that stress-induced hyperglycemia may be an adaptive response, promoting glucose uptake into brain and red cells and facilitating wound healing. Even relative hypoglycemia was considered dangerous and was to be avoided. Thus, "optimal" blood glucose concentrations were considered to be in the range of 160 to 200 mg/dL (8.8-11.1 mmol/L).[6] Insulin administration was only appropriate when blood glucose exceeded 215 mg/dL (12 mmol/L), because at such levels it might induce osmotic diuresis and fluid shifts that might be clinically undesirable.

NORMOGLYCEMIA IN CRITICALLY ILL PATIENTS

In 2001, in a single-center randomized controlled study, Van den Berghe and colleagues[1] found that IIT reduced mortality and morbidity in selected surgical patients. In this trial, 1548 mechanically ventilated surgical patients requiring intensive care were randomly allocated to the IIT group (target glucose: 80-110 mg/dL [4.4-6.1 mmol/L]), starting insulin administration when blood glucose levels exceeded 110 mg/dL (6.1 mmol/L), or to a conventional treatment group (target glucose range: 180-200 mg/dL [10.0-11.1 mmol/L]), starting insulin administration when blood glucose levels exceeded 215 mg/dL (11.9 mmol/L).

In this trial, ventilated postoperative intensive care unit (ICU) patients allocated to IIT had a 43% risk reduction for ICU mortality (8.0% vs. 4.6%, $P = 0.04$), when compared with patients receiving conventional glucose control. The benefit of IIT occurred particularly in the patients receiving intensive care for more than 5 days (ICU mortality: 20.2% vs. 10.6%, $P = 0.005$) and with multiple-organ failure with proven septic focus. IIT also decreased the duration of ventilatory support and ICU stay; reduced the need for blood transfusions; and reduced the incidence of bloodstream infections, critical illness polyneuropathy, and acute renal injury. Logistic regression analysis indicated that the reduction of blood glucose levels, not the administration of insulin, explained the clinical benefit.[7] However, because more than 60% of patients in this trial were post–cardiac surgery patients, the benefit of IIT might be altered in other ICUs with a different case mix.[8]

In 2006, the same research group assessed the benefit of IIT in a medical ICU.[9] The protocol of blood glucose management was the same as previously reported in the IIT trial in the surgical ICU.[1] In the intention-to-treat analysis of 1200 patients, IIT did not significantly reduce hospital mortality (40.0% in the conventional treatment group vs. 37.3% in the intensive treatment group, $P = 0.33$). However, morbidity was significantly reduced by the prevention of newly acquired renal injury, accelerated weaning from mechanical ventilation, and accelerated discharge from the ICU and the hospital. However, in a post-hoc analysis, among 433 patients who stayed in the ICU for less than 3 days, mortality was greater among those receiving IIT. In contrast, among 767 patients who stayed in the ICU for 3 or more days, mortality was reduced in the IIT group from 52.5 to 43.0% ($P = 0.009$); morbidity was also reduced (Table 146-1).

OTHER KEY STUDIES OF GLUCOSE CONTROL AND INSULIN THERAPY

Chronic Diabetes Mellitus

In 1993 in the Diabetes Control and Complications Trial of 1441 type 1 diabetes patients, strict blood glucose control (mean blood glucose 155 mg/dL [8.6 mmol/L]) was shown to reduce the rate of progression in retinopathy, nephropathy, and peripheral and autonomic neuropathy over a 6-year follow-up in comparison with conventional treatment (mean blood glucose 230 mg/dL [12.8 mmol/L]).[10] Furthermore, strict blood glucose control was later shown to reduce the risk of any cardiovascular event and the risk of nonfatal myocardial infarction, stroke, or death from cardiovascular disease over a 17-year follow-up.[11] In 1998 the United Kingdom Prospective Diabetes Study showed that strict blood glucose control in type 2 diabetics decreased hemoglobin A1C by 0.7% and reduced the incidence of retinopathy, microalbuminuria, cataracts, and myocardial infarction.[12] Thus, improving blood glucose control in chronic diabetic mellitus appears to be effective in preventing complications and is considered desirable for the chronic management of diabetes.

Acute Glucose Control

In 1995 the Diabetes and Insulin Glucose Infusion in Acute Myocardial Infarction study assessed the benefit of lowering blood glucose from 277 to 173 mg/dL (from 15.4 to 9.6 mmol/L) in diabetic patients with an acute myocardial infarction. Patients with the intensive treatment had improved 1-year survival but no change in short-term survival (in hospital and 3 months).[13]

In 2004 Grey and colleagues[14] showed that strict glucose control (targeted blood glucose less than 140 mg/dL [7.8 mmol/L]) reduced nosocomial infection significantly when compared with standard glucose control (targeted blood glucose: 180-220 mg/dL [10-12.2 mmol/L]) in 61 predominantly nondiabetic, general surgical ICU patients. Unfortunately, this trial did not have enough power to detect any benefit of IIT on mortality.

In 2005, the Diabetes Mellitus Insulin Glucose Infusion in Acute Myocardial Infarction 2 study randomized more than 1000 patients with myocardial infarction to receive either insulin infusion or routine metabolic treatment; the study failed to show any benefit on mortality.[15]

In 2005 the Clinical Trial of Reviparin and Metabolic Modulation in Acute Myocardial Infarction Treatment Evaluation/Estudios Cardiológicas Latin America Study Group study randomized 20,201 patients with acute ST-segment elevation myocardial infarction to a glucose-insulin potassium infusion regimen or usual care.[16] The trial found no benefit in morbidity and mortality from the intervention despite a reduction in blood glucose levels.

The VISEP (Efficacy of Volume Substitution and Insulin Therapy in Severe Sepsis) trial is the first multicenter randomized control trial to evaluate the quality of blood glucose adjustment by insulin treatment on mortality and organ dysfunction in patients with severe sepsis or septic shock (see Table 146-1).[17] In this trial, IIT (target blood glucose: 80-110 mg/dL [4.4-6.1 mmol/L]) was associated with a significantly increased incidence of hypoglycemia, defined as less than 40 mg/dL (2.2 mmol/L). This study found that there were no differences in 28-day (21.9 vs. 21.6%, $P = 1.0$) and 90-day mortality rates (32.8% vs. 29.5%, $P = 0.43$), respectively, when comparing IIT with conventional treatment (target blood glucose: 180-200 mg/dL [10.0-11.1 mmol/L]). Because the observed rate of hypoglycemia was considered unacceptably high, the data safety monitoring committee strongly recommended stopping the insulin arm of the trial. The investigators concluded that IIT was associated with an increased rate of hypoglycemia without any beneficial effect on outcome in patients with severe sepsis and septic shock.

BLOOD GLUCOSE CONTROL AND ACUTE KIDNEY INJURY

In the IIT trial in the surgical ICU,[1] IIT was shown to reduce acute kidney injury as defined by (1) a peak plasma creatinine concentration more than 2.5 mg/dL (12.3% to 9.0%, $P = 0.04$), (2) a peak plasma urea nitrogen concentration more than 54 mg/dL (11.2% to 7.7%, $P = 0.02$), and (3) the need for renal replacement therapy (8.2% to 4.8%, $P = 0.007$). Similarly, in the medical ICU, IIT was shown to reduce acute kidney injury as defined by either a level of serum creatinine twice that present on admission to the ICU or a peak level of serum creatinine of greater than 2.5 mg/dL (8.9% to 5.9%, $P = 0.04$).[9]

In contrast with chronic diabetic nephropathy (where injury is mostly glomerular), the pathophysiology of kidney injury in critically ill patients is not clearly iden-

TABLE 146-1

Three Randomized Control Trials to Assess the Benefit of Normoglycemia

	DEATH DURING INTENSIVE CARE*			INCIDENCE OF HYPOGLYCEMIA†			
	CONVENTIONAL TREATMENT	*INTENSIVE INSULIN TREATMENT*	*P-VALUE*	*CONVENTIONAL TREATMENT*	*INTENSIVE INSULIN TREATMENT*	*P-VALUE*	*RELATIVE RISK*
IIT trial in surgical ICU[1]	63/783 (8.0%)	35/765 (4.6%)	<0.04	6/783 (0.8%)	39/765 (5.1%)	<0.001	6.65
IIT trial in medical ICU (ICU stay >3 days)[9]	145/381 (38.1%)	121/386 (31.3%)	0.05	15/381 (3.9%)	97/386 (25.1%)	<0.001	6.38
IIT trial in medical ICU (all patients)[9]	162/605 (26.8%)	144/595 (24.2%)	0.3	19/605 (3.1%)	111/595 (18.7%)	<0.001	5.94
VISEP trial[17]	53/241 (21.9%)	53/247 (21.6%)	1.0	5/241 (2.1%)	30/247 (12.1%)	<0.001	6.38

*In the VISEP trial, short-term mortality was assessed with 28-day mortality, ICU mortality.
†Hypoglycemia was defined as a glucose concentration less than 40 mg/dL (2.2 mmol/L).
ICU, intensive care unit; IIT, intensive insulin therapy; VISEP, Efficacy of Volume Substitution and Insulin Therapy in Severe Sepsis.

tified. Thus, the mechanism by which IIT might prevent acute renal injury is also unclear.

BLOOD GLUCOSE CONTROL AND INFECTIONS

It is well known that diabetic patients are at greater risk of infection. Even acute short-term hyperglycemia might affect the immune response and impair the ability of patients to deal with infection. For example, hyperglycemia impairs (1) neutrophil activity (chemotaxis, formation of reactive oxygen species, phagocytosis of bacteria), (2) microvascular reactivity to dilating agents such as bradykinin, and (3) complement function (opsonization, chemotaxis), despite elevations of complement factors.

In critically ill patients, poor glycemic control defined as more than 200 mg/dL (11.1 mmol/L) is associated with increasing wound infection.[18,19] Introducing stricter blood glucose control reduces wound complication.[20,21] In the IIT trial in surgical patients,[1] IIT reduced the incidence of septicemia by 46% and also reduced the mortality of patients with a proven septic focus. In another small randomized control trial, strict glucose control reduced nosocomial infection significantly when compared with standard glucose control.[14] However, in the VISEP trial,[17] which specifically targeted septic critically ill patients, IIT had no benefit on mortality in comparison with conventional treatment.

Thus, some evidence suggests that better glycemic control might be able to reduce the incidence of infection and mortality from sepsis. However, the degree and generalizability of this benefit of stricter blood glucose concentration is still unclear, and the findings of the VISEP study raise concerns about the robustness of findings from single-center studies.

BLOOD GLUCOSE CONTROL AND NUTRITIONAL SUPPORT

Nutritional support should affect blood glucose control. In the IIT trial, nutritional support in both IIT and conventional treatment groups was scheduled in the form of continuous intravenous glucose (800-1200 kcal/day) on admission day, and then 20 to 30 nonprotein kcal/kg/day as total parenteral nutrition, enteral feeding or both combined In some countries, nutritional support was quite different. For example, in Canadian ICUs, only 20 to 200 kcal/day of continuous intravenous glucose was administered on the first day[22] and even less was used in Australian and New Zealand ICUs.[23]

Although there is little information about "optimal" caloric intake in critically ill patients, hypercaloric nutrition (35 to 40 kcal/kg/day) to critically ill patients might be associated with increased rates of infection and metabolic complications.[24] Furthermore, der Voort and coworkers[25] reported that, in critically ill patients requiring intensive care more than 7 days, the amount of intravenous glucose infusion, not mean blood glucose control, was associated with greater ICU and hospital mortality.

The benefit of a targeted blood glucose strategy might be different with different approaches to nutritional support, and a high amount of intravenous glucose administration might be harmful. Physicians might need to pay attention to their nutritional strategy as much as to blood glucose control in critically ill patients.

INCIDENCE OF HYPOGLYCEMIA RELATED TO LOWERING BLOOD GLUCOSE CONTROL

Although much evidence exists to suggest a benefit from stricter blood glucose control, no evidence has so far shown that lowering blood glucose levels is harmful. Additionally the cost of lowering blood glucose control appears low, because it only seems to require more frequent glucose measurements and greater insulin dose. Such observations would invite clinicians to simply apply IIT to their patients even if no multicenter randomized controlled trials have yet proven it effective. However, another important "cost" of IIT is the increased incidence of hypoglycemia and the workload associated with maintaining normoglycemia in the ICU (see Table 146-1).

In the IIT trial,[1] hypoglycemia, defined as a blood glucose less than 40 mg/dL (2.2 mmol/L), was seen in 5.2% of patients in the IIT group and in 0.8% in the conventional group. This six-fold increase in the incidence of hypoglycemia associated with introducing normoglycemia was also seen in medical ICU[9] (18.7% vs. 3.1%) and the VISEP trial[17] (12.1% vs. 2.1%). These observations raise the issue of safety with IIT.

To minimize the incidence of hypoglycemia during IIT, physicians need to (1) develop a nutritional and insulin administration protocol that is easy to follow, (2) train nurses to achieve targeted blood glucose control, and (3) measure blood glucose concentration frequently. If continuous blood glucose measurements could be developed and used as a reliable tool, it should reduce the "cost" of IIT.

VARIABILITY (FLUCTUATION) OF BLOOD GLUCOSE CONTROL IN CRITICALLY ILL PATIENTS

In the IIT trial in the surgical ICU, IIT reduced mean blood glucose concentration and mortality. It also reduced the standard deviation of blood glucose concentration, an accepted measure of variability, from 19 mg/dL (1.05 mmol/L) in the IIT group to 33 mg/dL (1.83 mmol/L) in the conventional control group—a relative reduction of 42%. However, the benefit of IIT was ascribed to a reduction in the mean glucose concentration rather than minimization of its variability. Fluctuations in glucose concentration might be pathophysiologically important, especially from a neurological perspective, and possibly as important as sustained hyperglycemia.

Egi and colleagues[26] reported data from a large multi-center cohort of patients and set of glucose measurements and found that the standard deviation and coefficient of variability of glucose were independent predictors of ICU and hospital mortality and that their predictive ability was greater than that of the mean blood glucose concentration (Figs. 146-1 and 146-2). This finding is consistent with data on acute hyperglycemia in pediatric critically ill patients[27] and chronic type 2 diabetes mellitus patients.[28]

Decreasing the variability of blood glucose concentration might be an important dimension of glucose management, a possible mechanism by which IIT exerts its beneficial effects and an important goal of glucose management in ICU. Continuous glucose measurements might assist in achieving less variability (higher quality) of blood glucose control in critically ill patients.

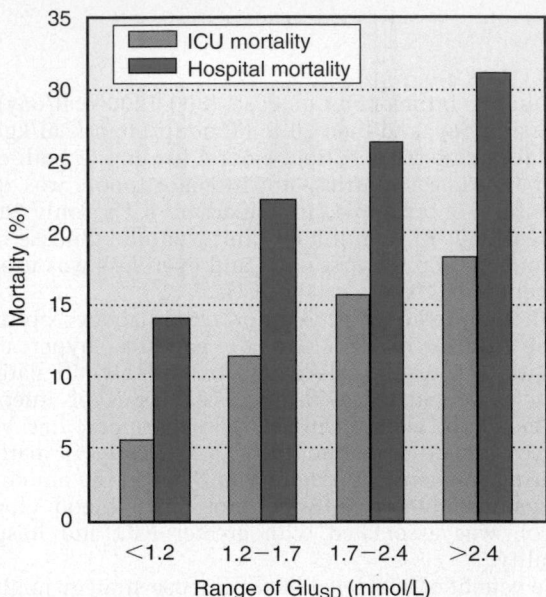

FIGURE 146-1. The relationship between mortality and variability of blood glucose control in critically ill patients. The standard deviation of blood glucose control during stay in intensive care unit (ICU) was used as a marker of variability of blood glucose control. Glu_{SD}, standard deviation of blood glucose concentration.

RECENT RECOMMENDATIONS FOR BLOOD GLUCOSE CONTROL IN THE CRITICALLY ILL

In a post-hoc analysis, Van den Berghe and colleagues[29] suggested that with blood glucose levels of 110 to 150 mg/dL, mortality was higher than with blood glucose greater

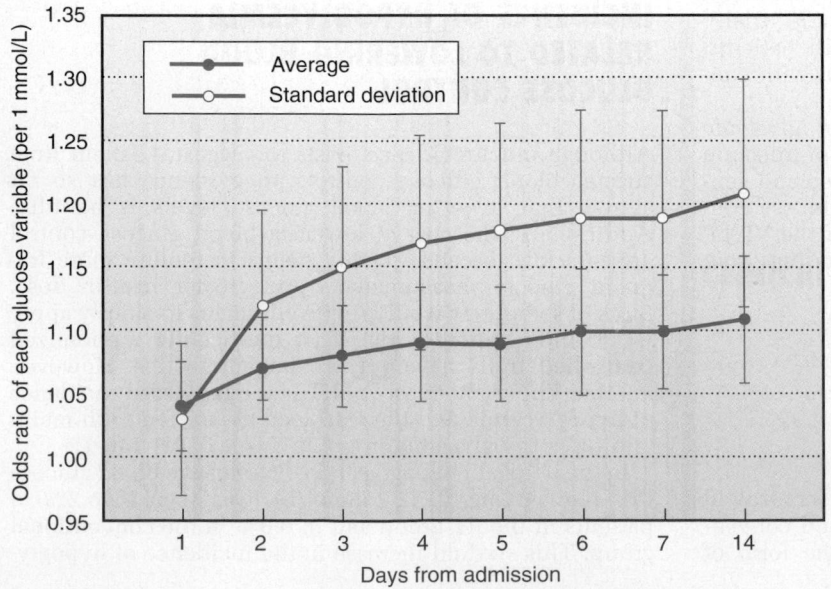

FIGURE 146-2. The time course of the predictive ability of average and standard deviation of blood glucose. Odds ratio (expressed with 95% confidential interval) for glucose indices indicate the risk change of ICU mortality per 1 mmol change in each index. For example, average of blood glucose on 7 days from admission means average of entire glucose measurements during 7 days from admission. As time in intensive care unit increased so did the ability of glucose control indices to predict outcome.

than 150 mg/dL (odds ratio 1.38, $P = 0.007$) and lower than with less than 110 mg/dL (odds ratio 0.77, $P = 0.02$). While prevention of renal injury and critical illness polyneuropathy required blood glucose to be kept strictly at less than 110 mg/dL, this level carried the highest risk of hypoglycemia. The investigators concluded that the "best results" were obtained when blood glucose concentration was maintained between 80 and 110 mg/dL (4.4 and 6.1 mmol/L). However, achieving a goal of less than 150 mg/dL (8.3 mmol/L) also improved outcome when compared with higher concentrations. This goal would likely reduce the risk of hypoglycemia.

In the Surviving Sepsis Campaign guidelines,[30] maintenance of blood glucose levels less than 150 mg/dL (8.3 mmol/L) using continuous infusion of insulin and glucose was recommended with a Grade D recommendation. Using this approach, measuring glucose frequently—after introducing lowering blood glucose (every 30 to 60 minutes) and on a regular basis (every 4 hours) once the blood glucose concentration has stabilized—was also recommended.

CONCLUSIONS

Acute hyperglycemia is a common condition in critically ill patients. Lowering blood glucose control might reduce mortality and morbidity in critically ill patients. Normoglycemia might also prevent acute kidney injury in critically ill patients. Although recent recommendations for blood glucose control support maintaining blood glucose levels below 150 mg/dL (8.3 mmol/L), physicians should be aware that the benefit of lowering blood glucose concentration might change according to different case-mix and nutritional support. More importantly, these recommendations will almost certainly be updated after the results of a multinational multicenter randomized control trial currently being conducted by a consortium of Australian, New Zealand, and Canadian ICUs become available. This trial, called NICE (Normoglycemia in Intensive Care Evaluation), has already randomized close to 3000 patients (as of December 2006) and is likely to be completed by 2008. It will deliver the highest possible level of evidence in this field and will further inform physicians on the best approach to glucose management in the critically ill.

Key Points

1. Acute hyperglycemia is common in critically ill patients. This "stress-induced hyperglycemia" is not yet defined by specific diagnostic criteria.

2. Stress-induced hyperglycemia, up to 215 mg/dL (12 mmol/L), was believed to be a beneficial physiological response that promoted cellular glucose uptake.

3. A single-center prospective randomized control trial has shown that ventilated postoperative intensive care unit patients allocated to intensive insulin therapy (target glucose: 80-110 mg/dL [4.4-6.1 mmol/L]) had a 43% risk reduction in mortality when compared with patients receiving conventional glucose control (mean glucose level: 152 mg/dL [8.49 mmol/L]). This study has led to the widespread adoption of protocols aimed at achieving and maintaining normoglycemia in patients in intensive care.

4. Normoglycemia might help prevent or attenuate acute renal injury in critically ill patients. This beneficial effect of intensive insulin therapy has now been shown in two single-center randomized controlled studies.

5. Recent recommendations suggest that blood glucose should be kept at less than 150 mg/dL (8.3 mmol/L) using continuous infusion of insulin and glucose (Grade D).

6. Because of the lack of multicenter randomized control trials, the generalizability of intensive insulin therapy is unknown.

7. Physicians should be aware that the benefit of intensive insulin therapy might be altered by different case-mix and nutritional support.

Key References

1. Van den Berghe G, Wouters P, Weekers F, et al: Intensive insulin therapy in the critically ill patients. N Engl J Med 2001;345:1359-1307.
9. Van den Berghe G, Wilmer A, Hermans G, et al: Intensive insulin therapy in the medical ICU. N Engl J Med 2006;354:449-461.
17. VISEP Study: http://webanae.med.uni-jena.de/WebObjects/DSGPortal.woa/WebServerResources/sepnet/visep.html
26. Egi M, Bellomo R, Stachowski E, et al: Variability of blood glucose concentration and short-term mortality in critically ill patients. Anesthesiology 2006;105:244-252.
29. Van den Berghe G, Wilmer A, Milants I, et al: Intensive insulin therapy in mixed medical/surgical intensive care units: benefit versus harm. Diabetes 2006;55:3151-3159.

See the companion Expert Consult website for the complete reference list.

Infectious Diseases

Basic Physiology

CHAPTER 147

Microbiological Considerations in the Intensive Care Patient

Peter K. Linden

OBJECTIVES

This chapter will:
1. Discuss the general prevalence and risk factors for major nosocomial infections occurring in the intensive care unit.
2. Review the important epidemiological trends and risk factors for antimicrobial resistance among nosocomial acquired pathogens.
3. Describe the basic pathophysiology and risk factors culminating in infections commonly acquired in the intensive care unit.

EPIDEMIOLOGY OF INFECTION IN THE INTENSIVE CARE UNIT

Infections that are either community- or health care–associated are a frequent complication culminating in intensive care unit (ICU) admission, and nosocomial infections occurring in the ICU continue to be a leading cause of morbidity and mortality. Nosocomial infections complicate the ICU course in approximately 30% of patients, although there is a wide dispersion of incidence ranges based on the case mix of the ICU population.[1]

A 1-day point prevalence study in Europe (European Prevalence of Infection in Intensive Care), which assayed more than 10,000 patients in 1417 ICUs, demonstrated infections in 4501 (44.8%) with slightly less than half (20.6%) classified as ICU-acquired infection. Pneumonia (46.9%), lower respiratory tract infection (17.8%), urinary tract infection (17.6%), and bloodstream infection (12%) were the most frequent types of ICU infection reported.[2] The effect of iatrogenic intervention on nosocomial infection in all types of general medical, surgical, and specialty ICUs is illustrated by data from ICUs participating in the National Nosocomial Infection Surveillance system in the United States between the years 1986 and 1990, which indexed the site incidence (respiratory, urinary tract, and bloodstream) to the number of "device days" (duration of bladder catheterization or central venous catheterization and days of mechanical ventilation) or non-device days (Table 147-1).[3] Another significant modifier of nosocomial infection incidence is the ICU population type. For instance, burn patients have the highest rates of bacteremia whereas trauma and neurosurgical patients have a higher incidence of ventilator-associated pneumonias.[4] Increasingly the higher prevalence of multiple-drug resistant organisms in some units (e.g., methicillin-resistant *S. aureus*, vancomycin-resistant enterococci [VRE], *P. aeruginosa*, extended-spectrum beta-lactamase–producing *E. coli,* and *K. pneumoniae*) may increase the risk for certain types of infection as well as add substantially to morbidity, mortality, and hospital costs.[5-9] Selection and amplification of drug-resistant strains via appropriate or inappropriate antimicrobial exposure and horizontal cross transmission due to inadequate enforcement of infection control policies are undoubtedly the two major forces behind this last trend.

COLONIZATION OF THE CRITICALLY ILL PATIENT

The vast majority of all infections in the critically ill patient arise from an endogenous reservoir of colonizing microorganisms present in the gastrointestinal tract, skin, and mucosal surfaces.[10] The microbial composition of such flora may represent typical community-acquired organisms and antimicrobial susceptibility patterns or become "modified" within days of admission to the hospital or ICU setting as a result of exposure to health care workers, the inanimate nosocomial environment, and antimicrobials. However, many patients admitted from the community may already have an antimicrobial-modified

TABLE 147-1

Median Incidence Range of Common Intensive Care Unit Infection Rates from National Nosocomial Infection Surveillance*

	Incidence Range	
SITE OF INFECTION	PER 1000 DEVICE DAYS	PER 1000 NON-DEVICE DAYS
Urinary tract[†]	5.8-15.6	0-2.5
Pneumonia[‡]	4.7-34.4	0-3.2
Bloodstream infection[§]	2.1-30.2	0-2.0

*Surveillance data from 79 NNIS system ICUs from October 1986 to December 1990. ICU types included respiratory, neurosurgical, medical/surgical, medical, surgical, coronary, pediatric, and burn units.
[†]Number of urinary catheter–associated UTIs and number of urinary catheter days or number of non–urinary catheter days.
[‡]Number of ventilator-associated pneumonias and number of ventilator days or number of nonventilator days.
[§]Number of central line–associated bloodstream infections and number of central line days or number of non–central line days.
ICU, intensive care unit; NNIS, National Nosocomial Infection Surveillance; UTI, urinary tract infection.

and thus more resistant colonizing flora due to protracted outpatient antimicrobial therapy, prior admission to a para-hospital or skilled nursing facility, or recent hospitalizations. The upper and lower gastrointestinal tracts are colonized with a variable microbial inoculum, with less dense concentrations in the proximal anatomy, that is, the stomach (10^2 to 10^3 organisms per milliliter), and as high as 10^{12} organisms per gram in the colon. Although anaerobes comprise more than 99% of the colonizing gut flora and may be a very significant cause of infection in intra-abdominal abscess or aspiration-related empyema, they exert a beneficial ecological effect by competing against intrusive nosocomial pathogens such as multiresistant enteric or nonfermenting gram-negative or gram-positive pathogens. This process has been termed *colonization resistance*.[11] Important pathogens in this realm to consider are VRE, enteric gram-negative, bacilli, nonfermenting gram-negative pathogens (*Acinetobacter baumannii, P. aeruginosa*), *Clostridium difficile*, and *Candida* spp. The nasopharynx and oropharynx, which should be viewed as a proximal extension of the gut reservoir, may harbor either methicillin-susceptible or methicillin-resistant strains of *S. aureus*, the most common cause of ventilator-associated pneumonia and a common cause of catheter-related infection and wound infection. Anticipating what pathogens comprise the colonizing flora when the patient becomes symptomatic is a key piece of information that an astute ICU clinician must consider in order to enhance the empirical accuracy of antimicrobial selection when a patient presents with a clinical syndrome suggestive of infection. Surrogate measures may include length of hospital or ICU stay, knowledge of the unit- or hospital-wide antimicrobial susceptibilities or recent epidemic outbreaks, and most certainly prior inpatient or outpatient antimicrobial exposure which may select or induce for the presence of more virulent organisms, resistant organisms, or both. More direct supportive evidence can come from surveillance cultures, which many centers now perform for both epidemiological infection control tracking and to direct enhanced isolation precautions or review the patient's prior clinical isolates in the microbiological archive. For instance, knowledge that a recent nasal swab

detected methicillin-resistant strains of *S. aureus* helps direct empirical coverage in patients presenting with a clinical syndrome commonly caused by *S. aureus* (ventilator-associated pneumonia, catheter-related sepsis, or wound infection).

Similarly, patients presenting with an intra-abdominal abscess, hepatobiliary sepsis due to cholangitis, or other sites of infection commonly associated with enterococci, and a positive rectal swab for VRE would merit empirical therapy with an antimicrobial that has VRE activity, for example, linezolid or quinupristin-dalfopristin.

Two other pathogens that also arise from perturbations in the colonizing flora and merit emphasis are *C. difficile* and *Candida* spp. Non-toxigenic strains of *C. difficile* may be found in 3% of people with no recent antibiotic exposure.[12] However, acquisition and induction of *C. difficile* due to cross transmission via *C. difficile* spores contaminating the ICU environment and antimicrobial use may culminate in toxigenic *C. difficile* strains and colitis, which increasingly is associated with frequent symptomatic relapses and a malignant treatment–refractory course characterized by fulminant colitis leading to significant morbidity and mortality.[13,14] Such emerging strains appear closely related to quinolone exposure and production of much higher quantities of toxin.

Candida has now risen to be fourth most common cause of nosocomial bloodstream infection, which is usually secondary to infected indwelling catheters or tissue-invasive infection often in the setting of long-standing antibacterial therapy and local or systemic compromise of host defenses.[15] Clinical discrimination is still required for appropriate interpretation and action. Isolation of any *Candida* spp. from a blood culture or sterile body site, such as ascites, joint fluid, or surgical specimens, should always be considered as a true pathogen until proven otherwise.[16] Conversely, *Candida* isolated from sputum, bronchoalveolar lavage, and other respiratory specimens usually reflects saprophytic colonization and does not merit antifungal therapy.[17]

SYSTEMIC PRESENTATION OF ICU-ACQUIRED INFECTION

Although a diverse spectrum of infections may occur in the critically ill patient, five sites of infection comprise the vast majority of experience even in specialized ICUs managing immunocompromised hosts. These include pneumonia, urinary tract infection (discussed in Chapter 163), bacteremia, catheter-related infection, and surgical site infection. It is important to emphasize that critically ill patients do not present in such predesignated fashion and may lack discernible or typical localizing signs and symptoms due to a poor host response, iatrogenic sedation, limitations of radiographic imaging, and confounding noninfectious conditions that mimic infection, such as drug-induced fever, sterile inflammatory states (pancreatitis), ileo-femoral thrombosis, or pulmonary emboli and other conditions. Although the presence of fever (T > 38.0-38.3°C core or core equivalent) is the most common clinical prompt to initiate a diagnostic evaluation for infection, more complex presentations, which may not include fever, need to be as seriously evaluated. The definition of *sepsis* based on the consensus of the Society of Critical Care Medicine, European Society of Intensive Care Medicine, American College of Chest Physicians, American Thoracic Society, and Surgical Infection Society is a more inclusive and realistic menu of physiological and laboratory alterations that may indicate serious infection even in the absence of localizing signs and symptoms.[18] A partial listing of this definition includes unexplained mental status deterioration, hyperglycemia, lactic acidosis, new onset oliguria, coagulopathy, or thrombocytopenia.

WHAT FACTORS LEAD TO COMMON INFECTIONS IN CRITICALLY ILL PATIENTS?

Becoming colonized in the hospital or ICU setting with potential pathogens that are more treatment resistant will not, in and of itself, necessarily culminate in infection.

Breaches in anatomical integrity or normal physiological function, which may or may not be accompanied by immunological defects in local or systemic host response, are the catalyst for the clinical progression to the majority of ICU-acquired infections (Fig. 147-1). These infections are summarized in Table 147-2. For instance, 90% of bloodstream infections in the ICU are related to infected intravascular access devices, primarily short-term, non-tunneled multilumen, central venous catheters (CVCs).[19] The top four pathogens in this category (coagulase-negative staphylococci, *S. aureus*, enterococci, and *Candida*) are common commensals that can be found on the cutaneous surface. However, only the minority of CVCs lead to bloodstream infection. The critical circumstances leading to catheter-related infection and bloodstream infection are called "risk factors," which have been elucidated in epidemiological studies that have examined the progression from colonization to infection. In the case of catheter-related infection, cited risk factors include the type of catheter, adequacy of skin preparation, duration of catheterization, more manipulations of the catheter, type of dressing, and anatomical location of the catheter.[20] It is noteworthy that all of these risk factors are remediable to modifications of physician and nursing interventions.

TABLE 147-2

Predisposing Risk Factors for Common Intensive Care Unit–Acquired and Nosocomial Infections

	Risk Factors	
SITE OF INFECTION	*IATROGENIC*	*HOST*
Pneumonia	Duration MV >2 days	Hypoalbuminemia
	Inadequate cuff volume	Age >60 yr
	Reintubation	ARDS
	Supine head positioning	COPD
	Nasogastric tube	Burns, trauma
	Paralytics or continuous sedation	Impaired consciousness
	H2 blockers or antacids	Illness severity
	Prior antibiotics	Large volume aspiration
		Sinusitis
Catheter	Duration of catheterization	Illness severity
	Noncuffed, nontunneled CVCs	Burns
	Internal jugular, femoral site	
	Multilumen catheter	
Urinary tract	Duration of catheterization	Renal transplantation
	Improper insertion technique	Upper tract pathology
	Open drainage system	

ARDS, acute respiratory distress syndrome; COPD, chronic obstructive pulmonary disease; CVC, central venous catheter; MV, mechanical ventilation.

Indeed strict evidence-based protocol for CVC insertion and maintenance techniques has yielded a reduction in CVC-related bloodstream infections in recent years.[21]

Lower respiratory tract infection is the second most common nosocomial ICU infection, the leading reason for antimicrobial prescription, and associated with a 30% to 70% mortality, which is the highest among all ICU-acquired infections.[22] Risk factors for pneumonia can be deduced from the pathophysiological circumstances leading to its development. Oropharyngeal colonization with potential pathogens, which may derive from the proximal gastrointestinal tract, or less commonly exogenous pathogens, which can originate from contaminated respiratory equipment or hospital air. Pathogenic colonization may be enhanced both by acquired achlorhydria due to H2 blocker or proton pump inhibitor therapy for gastric ulcer prophylaxis; however, its causal link to ventilator-associated pneumonia remains controversial.[23] In addition, changes in the surface mucosal receptors have been demonstrated with concomitant critical illness, which facilitates binding and protracted colonization with potential pathogens in the oropharynx and upper respiratory passages. Introduction of pathogens occurs primarily due to micro-aspiration of flora which, coupled with reduced pulmonary clearance mechanisms and compromised lower airway host defense, may progress to pneumonia. As this process is partially gravity-driven there is a predisposition for ventilator-associated pneumonia to occur in the inferior and posterior dependent regions of the lungs. Risk factor modifications are aimed at reducing the bacterial

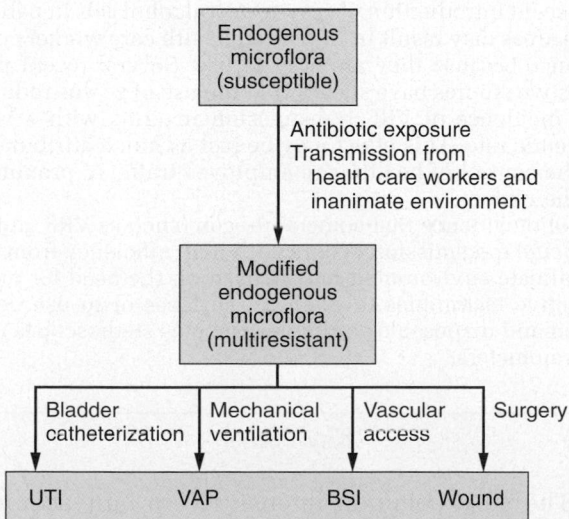

FIGURE 147-1. Progression from colonization with susceptible to resistant microflora and subsequent infection with iatrogenic interventions. BSI, bloodstream infection; UTI, urinary tract infection; VAP, ventilator-associated pneumonia.

inoculum and the amount of micro-aspiration. These include avoiding excessive acid-reduction therapy, topical oropharyngeal antisepsis (e.g., chlorhexidine), positioning patients to at least 30 degrees upright, ensuring adequate cuff inflation, avoiding unnecessary sedation, and proactive ventilatory weaning to minimize the duration of mechanical ventilation.[24]

Risk factors for urinary tract infection are almost completely linked to the insertion, manipulation, and maintenance of indwelling urinary catheters and are related to colonizing microflora in the periurethral and perineal areas.[25] Although these are often necessary devices to monitor urinary output and control urinary stream in sedated or encephalopathic patients, such devices are often maintained for excessive durations or become contaminated as a result of improper maintenance. Asymptomatic bacteriuria may occur in up to 5% of patients per catheter day and is the usual precursor to either lower or occasionally ascending upper urinary tract infection.

It is remarkable that given the same pathogen(s), site of infection, and similar hosts, a wide variation in both illness severity and outcome may exist. The variation in severity is only partially understood but may be due to a number of factors, including the inoculum and virulence of the infecting pathogen(s), site of infection, comorbidities, and host response parameters, which may either be immunosuppressive or hyper-inflammatory, such as tumor necrosis factor hyper-responders as recently shown by genetic polymorphic markers.[26,27]

SPECIAL PATHOGENS IN SPECIAL HOSTS

Patients in the ICU with preexisting or de novo immunosuppression due to native illnesses, iatrogenic interventions, or both, are prone to a broader array of opportunistic pathogens which need to be considered for both the diagnostic evaluation and empirical treatment strategies.[28-30] Patients with HIV-1 infection, solid organ transplantation, bone marrow or stem cell transplantation during the engraftment phase, and oncology patients with or without neutropenia are common ICU patients in these categories, although this spectrum needs to be considered in less immunocompromised hosts as well.

Opportunistic pathogens in such hosts fundamentally originate from several sources. Latent or dormant organisms have been acquired from distant past exposure but may become reactivated as a result of the failure of previously intact cellular immune defenses. A partial list of such organisms include *M. tuberculosis*, the Herpesviridae family (cytomegalovirus, varicella zoster virus, herpes simplex virus, Epstein-Barr virus, human herpesvirus 6 and 7), geographical mycoses (*Histoplasma capsulatum, Coccidioides immitis*), *Pneumocystis jiroveci, Toxoplasma gondii*, and parasites (*Strongyloides stercoralis*). Exogenous environmental exposures either in the community or nosocomial setting via air, water, or food ingestion are a second important category. Examples include *Aspergillus, Zygomycoses,* and other mycelial fungi, *Nocardia, Legionella, Listeria,* among others. A unique category of such primary exposures are pathogens transmitted via organ or blood transfusion, particularly cytomegalovirus, which is more likely to cause symptomatic disease in recipients who test seronegative for cytomegalovirus.

TABLE 147-3

Conventional Infection Control Policies in Intensive Care Units

Identify Reservoirs
  Surveillance for colonized or infected patients
  Environmental surveillance and routine decontamination
Reduce Transmission
  Hand hygiene
  Signage for colonized or infected patients
  Barrier precautions (gloves, gowns)
  Environmental disinfection
  Isolation rooms
  Cohort colonized or infected patients
  Dedicated equipment
  Source control (i.e., rectal bags in patients with diarrhea)
Reduce Progression from Colonization to Infection
  Aseptic techniques for catheterization (full coverage, chlorhexidine skin preparation)
  Minimizing duration of mechanical ventilation, bladder catheterization, or vascular catheterization
  Antibiotic-coated or antiseptic-coated catheters
  Head of bed elevation
  Oral antisepsis (chlorhexidine)
  Minimize ventilatory circuit changes
  Avoid gastric alkalinization

CONTROL OF INFECTION IN THE INTENSIVE CARE UNIT

Infection control measures are aimed both at controlling the introduction and transmission of colonizing resistant organisms and reducing progression to infection (Table 147-3).

Reducing the burden of pathogen colonization and infection among critically ill patients requires an active surveillance program, sound and evidence-based policies, and monitoring and enforcement of compliance.[31] Hand hygiene and the use of gloves are simple ways of controlling the transmission of potential pathogens among patients in the ICU; however, candid observational studies show disappointingly poor compliance rates.

Recent introduction of easy-to-use alcohol gels in patient care areas may result in improved health care worker compliance because they are easy to use. Several recent prospective studies have shown that the use of gowns reduces the incidence of VRE transmission in units with a high endemic rate. This effect may be just as much attributable to the control of health care employee traffic in proximity to the patient.

Solid evidence that some pathogen (such as VRE and *C. difficile*) transmission occurs with high efficiency from the inanimate environment has focused on the need for more effective techniques to disinfect surfaces or to use dedicated and disposable equipment such as stethoscopes and thermometers.

Key Points

1. The most common intensive care unit–acquired infections are closely linked to iatrogenic interventions, such as mechanical ventilation, vascular catheterization, and bladder drainage catheters.

2. Most infections arise from the endogenous colonizing microbial flora of which the major reservoirs are the gastrointestinal tract, skin, and mucosal surfaces.

3. Modification of the endogenous flora due to nosocomial cross transmission and antimicrobial selection and amplification invariably leads to the acquisition of more antimicrobial-resistant microorganisms and increases the risk for superinfection and poor outcome.

4. Progression to infection is secondary to breaches of local and systemic host defenses.

Key References
1. Vincent JL: Nosocomial infections in adult intensive-care units. Lancet 2003;361:2068-2077.

9. Cosgrove SE: The relationship between antimicrobial resistance and patient outcomes: Mortality, length of hospital stay, and health care costs. Clin Infect Dis 2006;42(Suppl 2): S82-S89.
10. Donskey CJ: The role of the intestinal tract as a reservoir and source for transmission of nosocomial pathogens. Clin Infect Dis 2004;39:219-226.
19. Maki DG, Lluger DM, Crnich CJ: The risk of bloodstream infection in adults with different intravascular devices: A systematic review of 200 published prospective studies. Mayo Clin Proc 2006;81:1159-1171.
31. Muto CJ, Jernigan JA, Ostrowsky BE, et al: SHEA guideline for preventing nosocomial transmission of multidrug resistant strains of *Staphylococcus aureus* and *Enterococcus*. Infect Control Hosp Epidemiol 2003;24:362-386.

See the companion Expert Consult website for the complete reference list.

CHAPTER 148

Endotoxin Recognition

Najam Zaidi and Steven M. Opal

OBJECTIVES
This chapter will:
1. Explain the role of endotoxin as a key activator of host innate immunity.
2. Enumerate the extracellular events that may modify the biological effects of endotoxin.
3. Explain the intracellular mechanisms by which endotoxin recognition leads to synthesis of inflammatory mediators.
4. Elaborate how endotoxin induces tissue injury, and delineate protective strategies that target key areas of lipopolysaccharide signaling.

In the critically ill patient there is an apparent immunological "dissonance." A discordant, activated immune system triggers a series of biochemical reactions, which cause uncontrolled inflammation and inadvertent tissue damage. These complex biochemical networks have evolved from phylogenetically ancient, simpler defense mechanisms, developed originally to maintain the internal milieu of a living organism and protect its integrity. Endotoxin, itself an ancient "archetypal" foreign molecule, is a potent trigger of several such reaction cascades, which cause inflammation and tissue damage in patients who are critically ill or have sepsis. These reactions not only continue to exist but are often bottlenecks in the broader tapestry of diffuse inflammation and offer strategic targets in modern therapeutic interventions. The molecular interactions of endotoxin are also important in the study and understanding of the innate immune system, which is based on repetition of similar motifs. Historically, the core

understanding and gradual unraveling of the mechanisms of tissue injury in sepsis arguably began with the preclinical studies into the nature of endotoxin more than a century ago.

EARLY STUDY

Pfeiffer in 1892[1] and, independently, Centanni in 1894[2] isolated a heat-stable, lipid-soluble compound from gram-negative bacteria, which produced fever, shock, and tissue injury when injected into laboratory animals. This "toxic" biochemical was quite distinct from secreted *exotoxins*, such as diphtheria and pertussis toxins. It was not a protein and was apparently a structural component of the gram-negative outer membrane. Almost a century of further research has revealed the precise structure of the macromolecule. The major component of endotoxin is now known to be lipopolysaccharide (LPS), and the two terms are used interchangeably. LPS is a complex amphipathic, macromolecule common to virtually all clinically significant, gram-negative bacteria. There are between 3 and 4 million LPS molecules per bacterial cell accounting for approximately 75% of the outer leaflet. Its presence is essential for viability of all gram-negative organisms with only one known exception: *Neisseria meningitidis* lipid A–deficient bacteria.[3]

ENDOTOXIN AND THE TOLL-LIKE RECEPTORS

Biochemical evidence suggests that endotoxin evolved and was expressed in cyanobacteria that existed on earth

TABLE 148-1

Mammalian Toll-Like Receptors and Their Ligands

RECEPTORS	CURRENTLY RECOGNIZED LIGANDS	KNOWN ACTIONS
TLR1	Bacterial lipoproteins (tri-acylated) Outer surface proteins of *Borrelia* spp.	Fusion partner with TLR2 in recognition of bacterial lipopeptide
TLR2	Peptidoglycan Bacterial lipoproteins Lipoteichoic acid Fungal cell wall components Lipoarabinomannan from *Mycobacteria* *Leptospira* lipopolysaccharide	Broad spectrum pattern recognition molecule Forms heterodimers with TLR1 and TLR6 in recognition of bacterial and *Mycoplasma* lipopeptide
TLR3	Double-stranded RNA	Recognizes double-stranded RNA viruses
TLR4	Lipopolysaccharide (LPS) Heat shock proteins (HSPs) Respiratory syncytial virus proteins High mobility group box-1 (HMGB-1)	The endotoxin receptor; also recognizes endogenous "danger" signals (e.g., HMGB-1, HSP)
TLR5	Bacterial flagellin	Binds flagellin (gram-negative and gram-positive) and induces pro-inflammatory cytokines
TLR6	Lipoteichoic acid	Forms heterodimers with TLR2 in recognition of di-acylated *Mycoplasma* lipopeptide and zymosan
TLR7	ssRNA (viral)	Recognizes single-stranded RNA viruses (in mice)
TLR8	ssRNA (viral)	Recognizes single-stranded RNA viruses (in humans).
TLR9	Unmethylated CpG motifs found in microbial DNA (viral and bacterial)	Bacterial DNA receptor
TLR10	Unknown	Structural homology with TLR6 May interact with TLR2 and play a role in asthma

Modified from Cristofaro P, Opal SM: Role of Toll-like receptors in infection and immunity: Clinical implications. Drugs 2006;66(1):15-29. Review.

at least 2 billion years ago.[4] The innate immune system evolved to recognize such highly conserved, simple but essential structures that are widely expressed within members of the Archea and Bacteria kingdoms but are not found in multicellular, eukaryotic organisms. Molecules such as bacterial flagellin, peptidoglycan, and unmethylated CpG motifs of bacterial DNA are some of the other structural elements ubiquitous in prokaryotes. The ability to discriminate rapidly between these non-self–molecules and self-molecules has an obvious survival advantage and forms the fundamental molecular basis for the innate immune defense strategy.[5,6] Toll-like receptors (TLRs) are a family of pattern recognition receptor molecules that perform an essential function in the innate immune system and have evolved to interact with endotoxin and other such pathogen-associated molecular patterns. The common endogenous and microbial ligands recognized by the human TLRs are enumerated in Table 148-1.[7]

COMMON ORIGINS OF BIOLOGICAL CASCADES

An early rapid response to endotoxin might have contributed to the evolutionary origin of the clotting system. Host defenses of the horseshoe crab (*Limulus polyphemus*) perhaps best exemplify the evolutionary linkage between coagulation and inflammation.[8] The fossil remains of this invertebrate species have remained largely unchanged for almost 1 billion years. Like other arthropods, the horseshoe crab possesses an open circulatory system (the *hemolymph*) and a single circulating blood element (the *hemocyte* or *amebocyte).* Any exoskeletal injury not only poses a threat of loss of the internal milieu but may be a portal of entry to pathogenic microorganisms. In response, the amebocyte behaves both as a platelet and a phagocytic

cell. It detects endotoxin via its Toll homologue and attempts to clear the microbes by phagocytosis. LPS also induces release of a complex series of soluble proteins from granules within amebocytes. These proteins react as a cascade system that terminates in the formation of an insoluble extracellular clot that rapidly seals up the breach in the exoskeleton. This reaction occurs with such speed and reliability that it forms the basis for the widely used *Limulus* amebocyte lysate gelation reaction for endotoxin detection.[9]

Such host cascades with often-redundant catalytic pathways offer an evolutionary advantage, providing diversity for the natural selection process and hence "evolvability." Alternative backup pathways permit mutational variation to be tolerated in the human genome.[8]

Paradoxically, the same systems that provided a significant survival advantage in human phylogenetic ancestors may actually prove to be deleterious to the severely injured host in the critical care unit. Humans are considered exceptionally sensitive to the pathophysiological effects of bacterial endotoxin.[10,11] Throughout much of the history of the human species, a vigorous inflammatory response to microbial infection likely provided a major survival advantage. However, the availability of antibiotics, blood transfusions, and aggressive supportive care over the past few human generations now make this hyperinflammatory reaction to endotoxin a significant liability.[8]

STRUCTURE OF LIPOPOLYSACCHARIDE

Although multiple variations of biosynthetic elements exist among LPS structures in microbial pathogens (Fig. 148-1), three conserved components of LPS make up the essential building blocks of endotoxin structure throughout myriad genera of gram-negative bacteria (Fig. 148-2):

1. The hydrophobic and diphosphorylated lipid A
2. The core glycolipid central region
3. The highly variable and serotype-specific polysaccharide side chain

Lipid A

Lipid for essentially all the toxigenic properties is ascribed to endotoxin itself and is the most highly conserved region of LPS. In most enteric gram-negative bacilli, it consists of six or seven asymmetrically placed C-12 or C-14 fatty acids linked by amide or ester bonds to a β 1-6 linked di-glycosamine backbone. This lipid structure is buried deep into the outer membrane of bacterial cell membranes, largely sequestered from antibodies. Lipid A usually contains two

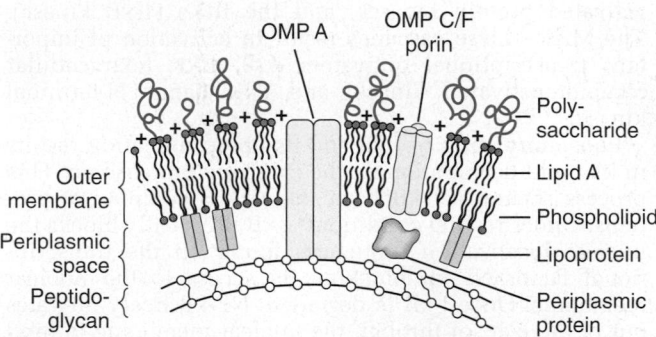

FIGURE 148-1. Structure of the cell surface of a gram-negative bacterium. Lipopolysaccharide (LPS) is an essential component of the outer membrane of gram-negative bacteria. LPS is oriented with the lipid structure buried deep into the cell membrane, whereas the polysaccharide O-antigen specific portion of LPS is exposed on the outer surface of the bacterium. OMP, outer membrane protein.

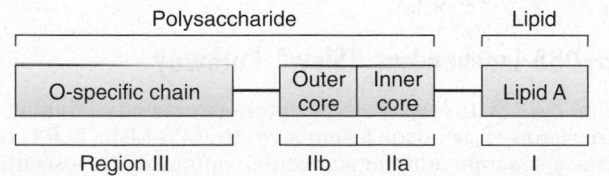

FIGURE 148-2. General architecture of lipopolysaccharide (LPS). The polysaccharide O side chain generates serotype-specific antibodies (*region III*) while the toxic principle of the molecule resides in the hydrophobic lipid A portion of the molecule (*region I*).

covalently linked phosphate groups. The loss of either phosphate group, hydrolysis of two or more fatty acids, or alteration in the size of the C-12- or C-14-containing fatty acid moieties greatly reduces the toxic potential of the LPS structure. Some gram-negative bacteria, like the common, enteric anaerobe *Bacteroides fragilis,* have exploited these tight physiochemical requirements for immune recognition of LPS by altering their lipid A. *Extraordinarily* long fatty acid moieties and a monophosphorylated lipid A make this organism's LPS unusual and much less immunologically active than the LPS for *Escherichia coli.*[12]

Core Oligosaccharide

The core oligosaccharide is a highly conserved, central structural component of LPS. Its inner core is made up of several characteristic, hexose and heptose monosaccharide moieties arranged in a specific sequence. One such component is 2-keto-3-deoxyoctonic acid, which is covalently linked to lipid A. The other is L-glycero-D-mannoheptose. The outer core region contains covalently linked hexoses, such as glucose, galactose, and glycosamine, arranged in eight different chemotype-specific sequences.[13] This core glycolipid structure, consisting of lipid A plus the core oligosaccharide region, has been targeted as a vaccine candidate and for immunotherapy by monoclonal antibodies (Fig. 148-3).[14]

Serotype-specific Polysaccharide Side Chain

The outer core oligosaccharide structure is attached to repeating units of five to eight hexose monosaccharides of variable chain lengths. These polysaccharide sequences are linked in unique order and different combinations of glycosidic cross-links. This variation gives each polysaccharide molecule its serotype specificity. This hydrophilic potion of the molecule projects out onto the external exposed surface of the bacterial outer leaflet. It provides the principal immunodominant epitopes of endotoxin. The O antigen of the bacterial cell wall is determined by the primary and conformational linkage of the polysaccharide component of LPS. Serotype-specific antibodies are generated upon exposure of LPS to the immune system. More than 170 O-antigen serotypes are described for *E. coli* alone. A variety of other bacterial species, including *Haemophilus* and *Neisseria* spp., express O-side chains with single or short sequences of repeating hexose moieties rather than multiple repeating sequences seen in most enteric bacteria. For this reason, they are often referred to as *lipooligosaccharides* rather than LPSs.[15]

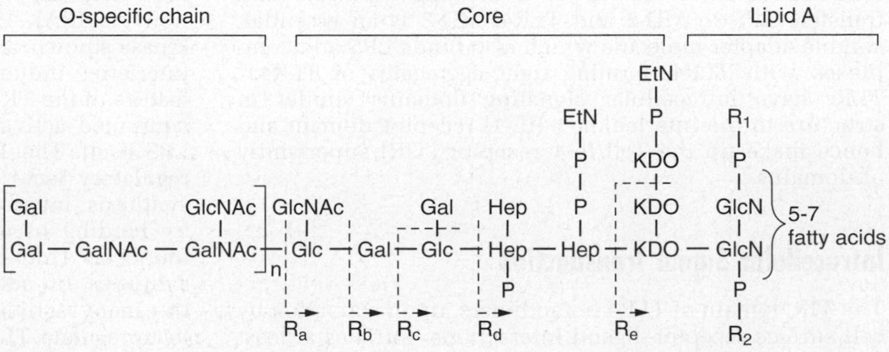

FIGURE 148-3. General structure of *Salmonella* lipopolysaccharide (LPS). EtN, ethanolamine; Gal, galactose; GalNAc, N-acetyl-galactose; Glc, glucose; GlcN, glucosamine; Hep, heptose; KDO, 2-keto-3-deoxyoctonate; P, phosphate; R_1 and R_2, phosphoethonolomine or amino arabinose. R_a to R_e show variations in incomplete forms of LPS with missing side groups or sugars.

INTERACTIONS OF ENDOTOXIN

Extracellular Interactions

Key molecules in the serum that interact with endotoxin are albumin, LPS-binding protein (LBP), soluble CD14 (sCD14), low-density lipoprotein, and high-density lipoprotein.[10,16] Bacterial cell wall or whole bacteria may bind to LBP. This hepatically synthesized acute-phase reactant binds to polymeric LPS aggregates and transfers LPS monomers to membrane-bound CD14 (mCD14) on immune effector cells.[14] The physiological and pathophysiological role of sCD14 is concentration dependent and rather complex. Cells not expressing mCD14 may be unresponsive to LPS and can be activated by sCD14. In mice sCD14 reduced mortality after LPS injection even if given minutes after LPS injection.[17] Yet, several studies show associations of higher sCD14 levels and mortality.[14,18] Soluble CD14 can transfer LPS to non-myeloid cells and may also transfer it into high-density lipoprotein.[19] It also binds peptidoglycan and lipopeptides, delivering them to TLR2. High-density lipoprotein readily complexes with LPS and removes its endotoxic activity from the circulation. Low high-density lipoprotein levels are associated with a higher mortality in sepsis.[20]

Bacterial permeability–increasing protein (BPI) is also an acute-phase reactant produced by granulocytes. This 456–amino acid cationic peptide has antibacterial properties and competes with LBP for LPS binding. In contrast to LBP, BPI neutralizes LPS activity upon binding its biologically active amino-terminal 21 κDa domain.[21] In human plasma, the concentration of LBP is two to three orders of magnitude higher than BPI. The opposite occurs in abscess cavities. This favors LPS activating activity in plasma and LPS inhibitory activity in abscesses.[22] In the plasma, alkaline phosphatase may dephosphorylate lipid A and thereby detoxify LPS at physiological pH levels.[23,24]

Interactions with Receptors at the Cell Membrane

At the cell surface of immune effector cells, endotoxin interacts with several key molecules, which include mCD14, MD-2, TLR4, and CD11/CD18 molecules (β2 integrins). This reaction is facilitated by LBP, and perhaps sCD14, acting as shuttle molecules. The receptors mCD14, TLR4 and MD-2 co-localize on the surface of immune effector cells to form a functional receptor complex for LPS along the cell membrane.[25,26] Membrane-bound CD14 is attached to the cell membrane by a glycosyl-phosphatidyl-inositol anchor but lacks transmembrane or intracellular domains.[5] It serves as a docking molecule and transfers LPS to MD-2 and TLR4. MD-2 is an essential, soluble adapter molecule which also binds LPS and complexes with TLR4, forming tight aggregates of TLR4.[27] TLRs have intracellular signaling domains similar in structure to the interleukin-1 (IL-1) receptor domain and hence make up the Toll/IL-1 receptor (TIR) superfamily of domains.[5]

Intracellular Signal Transduction

The TIR domain of TLR4 homodimers, upon activation by cell surface receptor–ligand interactions, initiates at least two known cytoplasmic signal transduction pathways. These include the MyD88-dependent "fast pathway" of NF-κB activation and the MyD88-independent Toll receptor–associated activator of interferon-γ (TRIF) or "slow pathway" of NF-κB activation (Fig. 148-4).

MyD88-Dependant "Fast" Pathway

The MyD88 (myeloid differentiation factor-88) pathway uses an adaptor molecule Mal (MyD88 adaptor-like) that also has a TIR domain homologous to the TIR domain of TLR4. MyD88 activates IRAK-4 and IRAK-1 (IL-1R-associated kinases) by a series of phosphorylation reactions. IRAK-1 subsequently activates TRAF-6 (TNF receptor-associated factor-6). Activated and ubiquitinylated TRAF-6 activates TAK-1 (transforming growth factor β–associated kinase) and a related binding protein TAB-1. This reaction is followed by a set of phosphorylation reactions that include a series of MAPKs (mitogen-activated protein kinases) and the IKKs (1-κB kinase). The MAK kinase cascades result in activation of important transcriptional activators p38, ERK (extracellular receptor–activated kinase) and JNK (janus N-terminal kinase).[5,7,28,29]

Phosphorylation of I κB and its ubiquitinylation results in its rapid degradation by the cytosolic proteosome. This process separates I κB from the NF-κB complex of proteins. Under resting conditions, I κB physically blocks the nuclear localization sequences found on the transcriptional factor NF-κB blocking its access to the nuclear membrane. Once I-κB is degraded, NF-κB freely migrates out of the cytosol through the nuclear membrane to bind to a large number of NF-κB–responsive promoter sites. This results in an outpouring of transcripts directing the synthesis of an array of acute-phase proteins, cytokines, chemokines, complement factors, coagulation elements, differentiation factors and nitric oxide synthase. This gene transcript profile is highly characteristic and a well-known signature expression pattern seen in severe sepsis.[30-32]

MyD88-Independent "Slow" Pathway

The TRIF pathway (Toll receptor–associated activator of interferon-γ) is also responsive to LPS-MD2-TLR4 but uses a separate adaptor molecule containing the essential TIR domain (see Fig. 148-4). TRAM (TRIF-related adaptor molecule) links TLR4 homodimers to TRIF, resulting in intracellular signal transduction. This pathway shares many of the essential components of the MyD88 pathway and although significantly slower is likely to be quantitatively more important.[33] TRIF can activate TAK-1 and the later elements of the signaling pathway for NF-κB activation via IRAK-1: TRAF-6 or through another signaling kinase known as RIP-1 (receptor interacting protein-1). Interferon induction is a specific, critically important feature of the TRIF pathway in antiviral host defense and continued activation of the innate immune response to LPS itself. The TRIF pathway activates IRF-3 (interferon regulatory factor), a transcriptional factor for interferon synthesis. Interferon-β generates a positive feedback loop by binding to extracellular type-1 interferon receptors found on TLR4-bearing myeloid cells. This induces the synthesis of additional interferon production. One of the many activities ascribed to interferon is its ability to upregulate TLR4 expression on effector cells, thereby

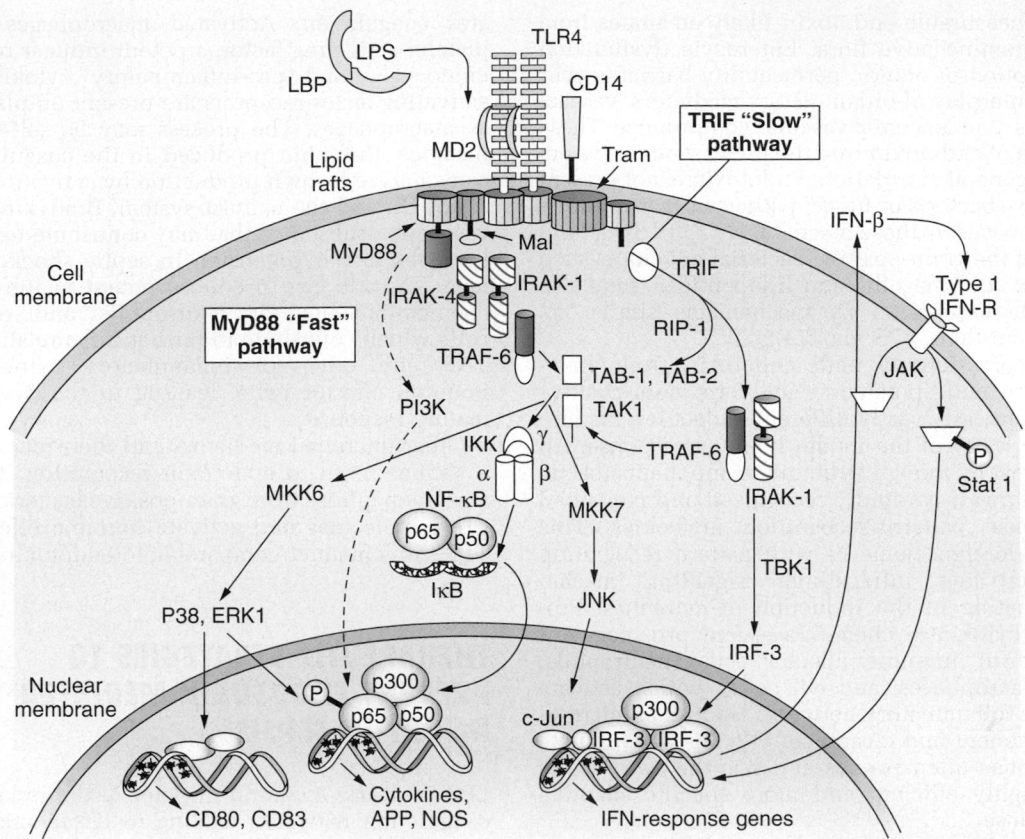

FIGURE 148-4. The intracellular signaling pathways of the Toll-like receptor 4 (TLR4) complex. APP, acute-phase proteins; ERK, extracellular receptor–activated kinase; IFN, interferon; IKB, inhibitory subunit κB; IKK, I κB kinase; IRAK, interleukin-1 receptor–associated kinase; IRF, interferon regulatory factor; JAK, janus-associated kinase; JNK, janus N-terminal kinase; LBP, lipopolysaccharide-binding protein; LPS, lipopolysaccharide; Mal, myeloid differentiation factor adaptor-like; MKK, mitogen-activated protein kinase; MyD88, myeloid differentiation factor; NF-κB, nuclear factor-κB; NOS, nitric oxide synthase; PI3K, phosphatidylinositol-3-hydroxyl kinase; RIP, receptor-interacting protein; STAT, signal transduction and transcription; TAB, transforming growth factor–associated binding protein; TAK, transforming growth factor–associated kinase; TBK1, TRAF binding kinase; TRAF-6, TNF receptor–associated factor-6; TRAM, TRIF-related adaptor molecule; TRIF, Toll receptor–associated activator of interferon-γ.

counteracting the full expression of LPS tolerance (or reprogramming).[7]

Important bottlenecks in the signaling pathway follow LPS to mCD14 to gene activation by the nuclear factors and offer intriguing therapeutic targets.[25,28,34] Lipoteichoic acid from gram-positive bacteria interacts via heterodimerization of TLR2 and TLR1. TLR2-dependant NF-κB activation also requires a TIR-MyD88-IRAK complex that induces TRAF-6.[7] Similar pathways used by different pathogens also use the TLRs (see Table 148-1).

PATHOGENESIS OF TISSUE INJURY

Administration of minute quantities (2 to 4 ng/kg) of *Escherichia coli* endotoxin to humans leads to signs and symptoms of clinical sepsis, activates the complement and coagulation cascades, and triggers the release of pro-inflammatory cytokines and chemokines like IL-1, TNF, and IL-8.[15,35] LPS is the major pathogen-associated molecular pattern molecule recognized by the innate immune system. LPS within the systemic circulation is immediately recognized by the early warning system of innate immunity to represent an apparent bacterial invasion. A vigorous defensive response is called upon to rapidly

respond to this immediate threat to survival of the host.[5] The transcriptional frequency of nearly 4000 human genes is altered within 2 hours upon exposure to bacterial endotoxin.[30] IL-1 or TNF may in themselves induce a syndrome that resembles fulminant septic shock, if introduced into laboratory animals or volunteers in appropriate concentrations.[36] Higher doses of endotoxin may cause septic shock, multiple-organ failure, or mortality in a dose-related pattern.[37-39] The clinical features of sepsis caused by the LPS of *E. coli* are no different than those caused by the LPS of *Vibrio cholerae* or *Salmonella typhi* initially described by Pfeiffer and Centanni.[1,2]

Septic shock may occur in the absence of endotoxin, but endotoxin remains its most potent mediator. The endotoxin-deficient strain of *Neisseria meningitidis* elicits a 100-fold less TNF than the wild-type strain.[3] Endotoxin may enter the human circulation bound to cell walls of live bacteria or in its free form shed from viable bacteria or released from dead organisms. In patients with meningococcemia, higher levels of endotoxin correlate with high levels of pro-inflammatory cytokines and pro-coagulant factors that can terminate in overt disseminated intravascular coagulation.[15] Endotoxin levels tend to be higher in the early phases of gram-negative bacterial infection, but the presence of high endotoxin concentrations in severe sepsis seems independent of the provoking organism.

Much of the measurable endotoxin likely emanates from endogenous gram-negative flora. Enterocyte dysfunction and the disruption of enteric permeability barriers occur secondary to interplay of inflammatory mediators, vasoactive substances, and ischemic vascular compromise. These allow entrance of endotoxin into the portal venous system and then into general circulation. Endotoxin is not present in gram-positive bacteria or fungal pathogens, yet endotoxemia may still occur by these mechanisms.[10,38,39] Structural components of the gram-positive bacterial envelope, such as lipoteichoic acid, flagella, and lipopeptides, may also cause cytokine expression by mechanisms similar to, albeit less potent than, LPS via TLR2.[11,28,29]

Cytokine expression by both endotoxin from gram-negative bacteria and lipoteichoic acid form gram-positive organisms, chemically vastly different molecules, fits into the broader tapestry of the innate immune response: An immediate threat by foreign structural components (bacterial, viral, or fungal) is rapidly recognized and contained by host defense pattern recognition molecules. This interaction of foreign elements with pattern recognition molecules activates intracellular signaling mechanisms, culminating in the induction of cytokines. Pro-inflammatory cytokines, chemokines, and pro-coagulant molecules recruit immune effector cells (neutrophils, monocytes, macrophages, and NK cells), which activate multiple other inflammatory networks leading to microorganism containment and clearance.[5,40-42] The early, innate immune response often primes and sets the pace of the slower but highly efficient and more specific adaptive immune response.

Triggering of Complement, Kinin, and Clotting Cascades by Endotoxin

Endotoxin may activate other enzyme cascades simultaneous to its recognition receptor mechanisms. The contact factors of the intrinsic clotting system are activated directly by the negatively charged LPS. Contact factor activation is a potent stimulator of the release of bradykinin from high-molecular-weight kininogen. Although the extrinsic (tissue factor) pathway is the dominant pathway for thrombin and fibrin generation in sepsis, the intrinsic pathway is secondarily activated by thrombin and serves as an accessory amplification pathway for disseminated intravascular coagulation. Pro-inflammatory cytokines induce tissue factor expression by monocytes/macrophages and endothelial cells and initiate the extrinsic pathways. The fibrinolytic system is similarly activated by pro-inflammatory cytokines but, in later stages of sepsis, may be inhibited by tissue plasminogen activator inhibitor.[8] Complement activation can be triggered by lipid A of LPSs or by whole bacteria via the mannan-binding lectin pathway or the alternative pathway.[43,44]

Endotoxin Recognition Consequences

Clotting elements, acute-phase proteins, cytokines, and nitric oxide synthase genes have NF-κB binding sites in their regulatory elements. Markedly elevated levels of cytokines like IL-1 and TNF can be found 30 to 90 minutes after interaction with microbial mediators like endotoxin.[45] Tissue factor is not normally expressed on endovascular cells and is exposed and released only after injury or cytokine induction. Tissue factor activates factor VII and initi-

ates coagulation. Activated macrophages also release platelet-activating factor, a potent inducer of neutrophils, monocytes, and pro-inflammatory cytokines. Platelet-activating factor receptors are present on platelets as well as macrophages. The process may be self-sustained; for instance, thrombin produced in the coagulation cascade can catalyze its own production by activation of factor XI, factor IX, and the contact system. Bradykinin is a potent vasoactive substance that may contribute to diffuse capillary leak and hypotension in septic shock. The complement cascade also produces potent anaphylotoxins and chemoattractants for neutrophils and other effector cells which contribute to further inflammation.[44] IL-1 and TNF and other pro-inflammatory cytokines activate immune effector cells, leading to the systemic inflammatory response.

Other microbial mediators and their recognition follow a similar motif to endotoxin recognition. Peptidoglycan and lipopeptides from gram-positive bacteria interact with CD14 molecules and activate immune effector cells via TLR2 in a manner comparable to endotoxin and TLR4.[7]

THERAPEUTIC STRATEGIES TO PREVENT ENDOTOXIN-MEDIATED INJURY IN SEPSIS

LPS is clearly a central initiator of the inflammatory and coagulation networks leading to tissue injury in sepsis. In severe sepsis these networks are uncontrolled and dysregulated and lead to severe end-organ damage.[32] It is reasonable to attempt to remove LPS from the circulation or subsequent triggers after LPS reaches its cellular targets as early as possible to halt these destructive cascades.[25] Several approaches have been proposed, and numerous preventive and therapeutic strategies directed at endotoxin are in clinical development (Table 148-2).[46-52] Key potential targets in LPS signaling include inhibition or clearance of LPS from the extracellular fluid; LPS interactions with CD14-MD2-TLR4 at the cell surface; and intracellular signaling pathways. TLRs are exceptionally promising as targets of therapeutic intervention. Analysis of the human genome has revealed 10 TLRs. Because the search has been thorough, there are unlikely to be more TLRs. They offer a unique opportunity to target both LPS and non–LPS-mediated tissue injury pathways.

CONCLUSION

Sepsis is a disease of medical progress and its incidence is rising.[32] Successful management of a variety of medical and surgical conditions has led to a large population with advanced age, multiple medical problems, critical illness, and impaired host defenses. Innovations in chemotherapy, organ transplantation, prosthetic devices, and long-term vascular access devices are contributing to the expansion of this population. The increasing prevalence of antimicrobial resistance may also contribute to the increasing cases of sepsis by virtue of delayed appropriate antibiotic therapy. The conceptual understanding of complex molecular events[10] that underlie sepsis pathophysiology is essential for further innovations in sepsis therapy and management. An alarmingly long list of failed clinical trials with promising therapeutic interventions over the

TABLE 148-2

Anti-endotoxin Therapeutic Strategies

TARGET	AGENT	COMMENTS
LPS clearance or inhibition in plasma	Lipid emulsion	In phase II trials
	BPI	Limited success in phase III trials in meningococcal sepsis[46]
	Anti–core glycolipid LPS antibodies	Preclinical work[47]
	Anti-LPS vaccines	Preclinical work[48]
	LPS removal devices by hemoperfusion	Used clinically in Asia; in phase II clinical trials in North America and Europe[49]
	Alkaline phosphatase to inactivate LPS	Early clinical testing[24]
Inhibition of LPS signaling at the cell membrane	MD-2-TLR4 inhibitors (E5564)	Phase III testing[25]
	Anti-CD14 monoclonal antibody	Phase II studies complete[14]
	Monophosphoryl lipid A	Induces cellular hyporesponsiveness to LPS[50]
	Stain compounds	Decreases TLR4 expression[51]
LPS signaling pathway inhibitors within the intracellular space	TAK242	Small molecule inhibitor of early events in LPS signaling in phase II testing[14]
	TRIF inhibitors	Preclinical work[28,33,34]
	MyD88 inhibitors	
	IKAK4 inhibitors	
Other signaling inhibitors	Stress-dose steroids to limit NF-κB nuclear translocation	In phase III trials[52]

BPI, bacterial permeability–increasing protein; IKAK, IL-1 receptor–associated kinase; LPS, lipopolysaccharide; NF-κB, nuclear factor-κB; MD-2, cell surface molecule; MyD88, myeloid differentiation factor; TAK, transforming growth factor–associated kinase; TLR, Toll-like receptor; TRIF, Toll receptor–associated activator of interferon-γ.

past two decades underscores the complexity of these molecular events. Despite early disappointments with anti-endotoxin monoclonal antibody treatments, therapeutic agents that target endotoxin remain potentially viable intervention strategies in severely septic patients. A number of current clinical trials now under way will confirm or refute the therapeutic value of LPS inhibition in sepsis.

Key Points

1. Lipopolysaccharide is the most potent and most highly conserved pathogen-associated molecular pattern molecule found in gram-negative bacterial pathogens.
2. Early recognition of lipopolysaccharide is a major survival advantage for humans as an indicator of bacterial invasion and the need to activate host defensive measures to rapidly eliminate the potential pathogen.
3. Lipopolysaccharide signaling is initiated by linkage of the molecule to the cell surface receptor Toll-like receptor 4 in association with MD-2 and CD14.
4. Two major intracellular signaling pathways exist to induce host response genes after lipopolysaccharide engages the TLR4-MD-2-CD14 receptor complex: the MyD88-dependent pathway and the MyD88-independent of TRIF pathway.

5. A number of lipopolysaccharide inhibitors are in clinical trials at the present time, which are designed to block the deleterious consequences of excess lipopolysaccharide signaling in severe sepsis.

Key References

4. Rietschel ET, Westphal O: Endotoxin: Historical perspectives. In Brade H, Opal SM, Vogel SN, Morrison D (eds): Endotoxin in Health and Disease. New York, Marcel Dekker, 1999, pp 1-30.
6. O'Neill LA, Greene C: Signal transduction pathway is activated by the IL-1 receptor family: Ancient signaling machinery in mammals, insects, and plants. J Leukoc Biol 1998;63:650-657.
7. Cristofaro P, Opal SM: Role of Toll-like receptors in infection and immunity: Clinical implications. Drugs 2006;66(1):15-29. Review.
8. Opal SM, Esmon CT: Bench-to-bedside review: Functional relationships between coagulation and the innate immune response and their respective roles in the pathogenesis of sepsis. Crit Care 2003;7(1):23-38.
10. Opal SM: The clinical relevance of endotoxin in human sepsis: A critical analysis. J Endotoxin Res 2002;8(6):473-476.
32. Hotchkiss RS, Karl IE: The pathophysiology and treatment of sepsis. N Engl J Med 2003;348:138-150.

See the companion Expert Consult website for the complete reference list.

CHAPTER 149

Innate Mechanisms of Host Defense

Russell L. Delude

OBJECTIVES

This chapter will:
1. Briefly review early studies that established the germ theory of disease and the cellular and humoral schools of immune function.
2. Describe strategies used by the innate immune system to kill and control growth of microbes, with particular emphasis on mechanisms utilized in the urinary system.
3. Describe the molecular mechanisms underlying pathogen recognition by, and subsequent activation of, innate immune effector cells.

BRIEF REVIEW OF INFECTIOUS DISEASE AND IMMUNITY THROUGH THE TURN OF THE TWENTIETH CENTURY

In the early 1700s the process of variolation or inoculation with material from active smallpox pustules had made its way from the Far East to Europe. While it effectively decreased mortality, the procedure carried a high risk of fatal infection. In 1798, Edwin Jenner reported that inoculation with material from cowpox pustules established immunity to smallpox infection. Remarkably, this gigantic advance in medical practice yielded only limited insight into the underlying infectious disease process. Well into the end of the 19th century, dogma held that disease was spread by "bad air" or "miasma" brought about by atmospheric disturbances or divine justice. In 1854 John Snow applied statistical analysis to trace the source of a cholera outbreak to a single contaminated water source. However, the scientific and medical implications of this research were again largely overlooked because of the lack of rudimentary knowledge of the etiologic agent itself, the microbe. In 1862 Louis Pasteur proposed his germ theory to refute spontaneous generation. In 1875 Robert Koch reported his postulates that firmly established the germ theory of infectious disease.

FEUD BETWEEN THE FRENCH CELLULAR AND GERMAN HUMORAL SCHOOLS OF IMMUNITY

The first step toward understanding immunity is credited to Ilya (Élie) Ilyich Metchnikoff, who identified cells in the starfish that locomote in response to, and quickly ingest, foreign particles. He was also the first to report that cells in human blood engaged in what he called "phagocytosis," which he argued was required for clearing pathogens from the body. From these studies at the close of the 19th century, Metchnikoff gained the support of Louis Pasteur and spent the rest of his career at the Pasteur Institute in Paris investigating the role of phagocytic cells in acquired immunity. Whereas the modern observer would find the conclusion of Metchnikoff to be obvious, it was considered near heretical at the time.[1] White blood cells were known to accumulate at sites of traumatic injury and were thought to damage tissue and be associated with poor prognosis. Scientists also argued that phagocytes may be responsible for disseminating infection, since no evidence had yet been presented for a microbicidal function of phagocytes.

The competing school of humoral immunity was championed by individuals with strong training in the new empirical methods of biochemistry. Soon after George Nuttall reported in 1888 that cell-free serum from immunized animals could kill *Bacillus anthracis*, Behring and Kitasato of the Koch Institute in Berlin showed that similar immune serum could passively immunize nonimmune animals. More importantly, passive immune transfer required serum that could be prepared devoid of cells. Add to this the fact that the newly discovered antibodies in immune serum could aggregate, precipitate, and kill (with complement) bacteria in the complete absence of cells. These early studies quickly established the dominance of humoral immunology, which was evident for many decades as research would be directed largely at understanding antibody function and antibody formation at the expense of studying innate immune function.

The true role of the phagocytic leukocyte in innate and acquired immune function was not described in detail until the end of the 20th century. The advent of advanced molecular and cellular biology techniques has facilitated investigations into the functional roles of proteins and cells involved in this ancient and indispensable arm of the immune system.

CELLS OF THE INNATE IMMUNE SYSTEM

The macrophage is classically used to introduce the concept of an innate immune cell. These cells include their circulating progenitor monocytes and tissue resident cells, including hepatic Kupffer cells, lymph-associated macrophages in spleen and lymph nodes, Langerhans cells, alveolar macrophages, and highly specialized dendritic cells. Polymorphonuclear cells, or neutrophils, would constitute the other cell type that is classically characterized as an innate immune cell. At this point the discussion gets a bit complicated because the characteristics that make these cells members of the innate immune system are also shared by a variety of cell lineages depending on the local environment and the functional role of the cell at any given time. For example, M cells differentiate from the epithelial lineage in response to cues from lymphocytes and are found in specialized gut-associated lymphoid tissues called Peyer's patches.[2] These cells continuously sample the gut luminal environment through active endocytosis. Endosomes fuse with specialized organelles containing machinery required to digest the ingested material and present pieces of it bound to major histocompatibility complex (MHC) molecules on the cell surface. T lymphocytes recognize and respond to the presented antigens as part of the tightly orchestrated acquired (adaptive) immune response to antigen. This process is more often associated with the innate immune response of "dedicated phagocytes" like macrophages and dendritic cells and not epithelial cells. B lymphocytes phagocytose antibody or complement opsonized microbes, and they possess mechanisms that make them efficient antigen-processing and antigen-presenting cells. Infected and activated T lymphocytes also present antigen on class I or II MHC molecules and release pro-inflammatory cytokines in the process. Thus, most cells in the human body possess the capacity to recognize microbes and their toxins at the innate level and initiate and modulate various aspects of the immune response.

MOLECULES OF THE INNATE IMMUNE ARSENAL THAT ARE EXPRESSED IN THE URINARY TRACT

Defensins

Unlike the gastrointestinal tract and pulmonary airways, the urinary tract lacks a thick unstirred mucous layer and microvillus-rich epithelium. Alternative strategies are used to maintain a sterile environment in the upper urinary tract. The secretions of the renal system are rich with antibacterial substances, including a group of cationic antimicrobial peptides called β-defensins.[3] The first defensin identified was an essential element of the *dipteran* immune system.[4] Homologous proteins have since been identified in plants, insects, fungi, reptiles, and birds.[5] Thus, these genes have been coevolving with pathogenic microbes for millennia, and as such, microbes have evolved a wide array of effective countermeasures to thwart these peptides. For example, in *Drosophila,* which lacks the adaptive immune lymphocytic systems of higher vertebrates, there are three distinct families of small antimicrobial peptides directed against gram-positive bacteria (defensin), gram-negative bacteria (cecropins, drosocin, attacins, diptericin, MPAC [maturated pro-domain of attacin C]), or fungi (drosomycin, metchnikowin).

In humans, the defensins are divided functionally into two groups: a group called α-defensins (six gene products including four proteins stored in neutrophil granules and two proteins stored in Paneth cell granules) and a group of at least five β-defensins.[6] β-defensins are produced by activated epithelial cells that line the pulmonary, gastrointestinal, and genitourinary tracts. Numerous studies have documented a role for defensins in immune defense. Both α- and β-defensins have been shown to induce degranulation of mast cells.[7,8] Mice lacking α-defensins have decreased resistance to orally administered bacteria compared to wild-type litter mates.[9] α-Defensin secretion

by Paneth cells is thought to maintain a sterile environment in the intestinal crypt.[10] Mice lacking the *Defb1* β-defensin 1 gene show delayed clearance of *Haemophilus influenzae* from the lung[11] and increased incidence of *Staphylococcus* sp. in the bladder[12] compared to normal litter mates. Mice lacking matrilysin, a metalloproteinase that is required for the processing of defensin precursors, are susceptible to microbial invasion of the intestinal mucosa.[9]

Defensins act by binding strongly to the surface of microbes where they are proposed to perturb lipid ordering in the outer bacterial membrane. This interferes with membrane barrier properties and enzymatic activities of various transport proteins, with subsequent loss of transmembrane potential and eventual death of the cell. Defensins also act as opsonins through interactions with chemokine receptors.[13] β-defensins are produced by epithelial cells in the loop of Henle, distal convoluted tubule, and the collecting duct.[14] β-defensin 1 is produced constitutively at very high levels, and β-defensins 2 and 3 are induced in renal epithelia in response to infection or pro-inflammatory cytokines.[15]

Tamm-Horsfall Protein

Tamm-Horsfall protein (THP) is a glycoprotein produced exclusively by renal tubular epithelial cells within the distal loop of Henle, and it is one of the most abundant urine proteins in mammals.[16,17] THP function remained unclear for many years until recent reports that THP binds to type 1[18] and type S[19] fimbriated *Escherichia coli* and impedes microbe interaction with the uroepithelium. THP also appears to activate cells via direct signaling through Toll-like receptor (TLR) 4.[16,20] THP was shown to induce tumor necrosis factor-α (TNF-α) and tissue factor production via TLR4 in monocytes.[21,22] These findings were supported by reports that intravenous injection with THP rapidly induces systemic TNF-α production in control TLR2$^{-/-}$ mice and TLR9$^{-/-}$ mice but not in TLR4$^{-/-}$ or MyD88$^{-/-}$ mice (MyD88 protein is required for TLR4-dependent signaling).[21] C3H/HeJ mice are homozygous for a nonconservative mutation in the gene encoding TLR4.[23] These mice show decreased responsiveness to gram-negative bacterial endotoxin and decreased recruitment of neutrophils and monocytes in response to gram-negative bacterial infection, two defects that help explain the increased incidence and severity of urinary tract infection in the mice.[20] The relative contribution of lost THP signaling through TLR4 to the development of the urinary tract infection in these mice needs to be further investigated.

Other Proteins

Bactericidal/permeability-increasing protein (BPI), lipopolysaccharide (LPS)-binding protein, and a growing number of homologous mammalian proteins[24] play an important role in controlling systemic dissemination with blood-borne bacteria and colonization of epithelial surfaces with microbes.[25-27] BPI was originally described in neutrophil and eosinophil granules, and it is known to be actively secreted by nasolacrimal, oral, and intestinal epithelial cells.[28,29] There are no reports of studies of BPI expression in other epithelia, but this is probably because it has not been assayed for. Urine from normal volunteers contains BPI at 0.2 to 1.2 ng/mL, in the absence of apparent white blood cells monitored using microscopy.[30] These levels are greatly increased in patients with active infection and renal disease. The majority of urinary BPI is believed to be made locally, and this is most likely the result of production of the bactericidal protein in the uroepithelium. A comparative microarray analysis of mRNA expressed in various organs has detected levels approaching that of myeloid cells in total RNA preparations from kidney, lung, and liver (NCBI Accession number GDS1087).[31] Thus, further studies of the role of BPI in the innate immune defense of the urinary tract seem warranted.

Like the cationic defensins, BPI is directly bactericidal and possesses opsonic properties. Cytotoxicity is due to the high affinity of BPI for the lipid core of endotoxin in the outer leaflet of the gram-negative bacterial outer membrane.[32] The binding receptor for microbe-bound BPI has not been described. Binding of BPI to endotoxins disrupts the membrane leading to bacterial death. The actions of BPI and the defensins are amplified by other factors that are actively secreted from immunostimulated epithelial cells, including phospholipase A2 and complement proteins.[33,34] While BPI activity is usually associated with its effects on gram-negative bacteria, BPI also has activity against gram-positive bacteria with a compromised cell wall and some fungi.[27]

Complement Activation

Complement activation represents another powerful mechanism for controlling microorganisms and their toxins. In humans, there are currently three distinct mechanisms that activate the complement cascade. The classic pathway involves binding of at least one IgM or two IgG antibodies to a surface-associated antigen. This complex recruits complement protein C1, which cleaves C2 and C4 to C2a and C4b, which assemble to form an active C3 convertase on the surface of the microbe. C3b fragments generated can bind with C2aC4b complexes to form the C5 convertase. The alternative activation pathway is initiated as follows. Serum C3 is continuously activated by reaction with water to form what is referred to as $C3(H_2O)$. Some microbial carbohydrate structures can activate C3 directly. Once activated, C3 binds factor B, triggering its cleavage by factor D. Factor Bb remains bound to $C3(H_2O)$ and functions as a soluble C3 convertase. This protein complex can covalently react with any surface in blood or body fluids including urine, where it generates C3b at the surface of target cells and additional convertases are assembled. Binding of an additional C3b fragment to the C3bBb complex forms a functional C5 convertase. The lectin pathway of complement activation is initiated when lectin-like proteins, including mannose-binding protein and ficollins, bind to saccharide units found specifically on the surface of microbes and recruit mannose-binding protein-associated serine proteases (MASPs) to the cell surface. These MASPs cleave C4 to C4b, which cleaves C2 to form C2a, which forms the C3 convertase that culminates in formation of the C5 convertase. Assembly of the C5 convertase initiates the first common step of the complement pathway. At this point, the cells are opsonized for complement receptor 2 on any white blood cells that are nearby. Alternatively, recruitment of complement proteins 5 thru 9 leads to the formation of mature membrane attack complexes that form large pores in the microbial membrane leading to osmotic rupture of the cell. The smaller fragments generated during complement action, particularly the C3a, C4b, and C5a fragments, function as anaphylatox-

ins, recruiting lymphocytes and leukocytes to the site of infection. Signaling through specific receptors also modulates the immune activity of recruited and resident leukocytes.

The majority of complement protein production occurs in the liver, but surface epithelia and endothelial cells have also been shown to produce complement proteins.[35] Glomerular epithelia[36] and mesangial cells[37,38] release complement proteins locally. Tubular epithelial cells also synthesize complement proteins in normal and diseased states.[39,40]

Genes encoding complement proteins have been identified in organisms as evolutionarily distant as horseshoe crabs, in which a C3 convertase activity and lectin-like nucleating activity have been identified.[41] Given that antigen-specific antibodies that are generated through somatic recombination of highly polymorphic alleles are not present in the vertebrate lineage until the appearance of the bony jaw fish, the absence of the classic complement activation system in this animal was not surprising. Thus, the initial selective advantage of the complement system was to opsonize invading organisms for destruction inside specialized phagocytes. Receptors on dedicated arthropod phagocytes called *hemocytes* bind complement-coated microbes and rapidly trigger their phagocytosis. This is critical because unlike higher vertebrates, most antimicrobial peptides and enzymes are located within these specialized immune effector cells.

CONCLUSION

It is essential to remember that at every stage of the host–pathogen interaction, all the cells in the vicinity of the infection, including T cells and B cells and endothelial cells that are not immediately thought of as *innate* immune cells, can release cytokines and present antigenic substances to other cells, processes usually relegated to myeloid cells and other "dedicated" antigen-presenting cells. Therefore, it may be simpler to consider T and B cells as members of the acquired immune cell lineages and assume that all cell types are capable of functioning in an innate immune capacity to some extent. For example, the specialized epithelia that line the urinary tract and comprise the parenchyma of the kidney can function as innate immune effector cells.

As microbes are attacked by complement or other opsonizing and bactericidal factors, small amounts of the microbe can be released. The *Toll* gene was originally identified using a saturation mutagenesis strategy to identify developmental mutants in *Drosophila*. It was subsequently found that Toll mutant larvae were susceptible to fungal infection.[42] Humans express at least 11 unique TLRs, each one with its own ligand specificity due to primary structural differences in the extracellular domains. The intracellular portions of TLRs are highly conserved within the group and are highly homologous to the cytoplasmic domain of the interleukin-1β receptor. Because of this, similar signal transduction pathways are engaged following engagement of these receptors with their distinct ligands.

The relatively recent advances in the TLR field have only recently been directed at studying the uroepithelium. Evidence for an important role for epithelial TLR-dependent recognition of bacteria has been presented. Secretion of C-C chemokines by tubular epithelial cells was shown to be dependent on their expressing TLR2 and TLR4.[43]

TLR4-deficient C3H/HeJ mice demonstrate reduced polymorphonuclear cell recruitment and impaired bacterial clearance in experimental pyelonephritis.[20] TLR11 is expressed on urinary tract epithelial cells, and it protects mice against uropathogenic bacterial infection.[44] These findings represent some of the earliest insights into the potential importance of the innate functions of the urinary epithelium itself in maintaining immune homeostasis in the urinary tract. The finding that epithelial cells themselves can sense and respond specifically to different bacteria is quite revolutionary, as pathogen-specific responses were thought to be reserved for cells of the lymphocyte lineage.

Key Points

1. A variety of general and kidney-specific innate immune mechanisms are continuously operating in normal health and disease to control microbial growth in the urinary tract.
2. Early advances in the field of immunology favored research into antibody-dependent responses at the cost of research advances in the field of innate immunity.

3. The identification of pathogen-sensing systems that are present on most mammalian cells has greatly increased the number of cells that can be considered innate immune effector cells.
4. The uroepithelium is well equipped to function in the sensing and elimination of potentially pathogenic microbes.

Key References

1. Silverstein AM: A History of Immunology. San Diego, Academic Press, 1989.
3. Nitschke M, Wiehl S, Baer PC, Kreft B: Bactericidal activity of renal tubular cells: The putative role of human beta-defensins. Exp Nephrol 2002;10(5-6):332-337.
9. Wilson CL, Ouellette AJ, Satchell DP, et al: Regulation of intestinal alpha-defensin activation by the metalloproteinase matrilysin in innate host defense. Science 1999;286(5437):113-117.
13. Klotman ME, Chang TL: Defensins in innate antiviral immunity. Nat Rev Immunol 2006;6(6):447-456.

See the companion Expert Consult website for the complete reference list.

CHAPTER 150

The Neutrophil and Inflammation

Jennifer L. Y. Tsang and John C. Marshall

OBJECTIVES

This chapter will:
1. Describe the biological features of the polymorphonuclear leukocyte (neutrophil) that support its role as a key early cellular effector of innate immunity.
2. Discuss the process of constitutive neutrophil apoptosis and its modulation by the inflammatory microenvironment.
3. Review the role of the activated neutrophil in the pathogenesis of organ injury involving the lung and kidney.

INTRODUCTION

Sepsis is a syndrome caused by a systemic inflammatory response to infection. Severe sepsis—sepsis of sufficient severity to result in life-threatening organ dysfunction—affects approximately 750,000 patients in the United States annually[1] and portends a mortality rate of 30% to 50% over the first month.[2,3] Severe sepsis and septic shock (sepsis associated with cardiovascular failure that is non-responsive to fluid replacement) have become the most common cause of death in patients admitted to an intensive care unit (ICU) and account for more than 210,000 deaths annually.[1,4]

Neutrophils, recognized histologically by their multilobed nuclei and abundant cytoplasmic granules, were first described by Metchnikoff in the 19th century.[5] They are derived from hematopoietic stem cells in the bone marrow and mature to terminally differentiated phagocytes that are incapable of cell division.[5] Neutrophils are the first cells of the innate immune response to migrate to the sites of inflammatory challenge.[6] Their functions include the recognition and phagocytosis of pathogens, elaboration of oxidative and nonoxidative degradative enzymes and release of chemotactic factors to recruit other inflammatory cells, and, ultimately, to activate an adaptive immune response.[6] After ingesting, killing, and eliminating pathogens, neutrophils undergo apoptosis (programmed cell death), with the result that inadvertent bystander tissue damage is minimized.

Neutrophils are activated during sepsis and accumulate in tissues such as the lung, liver, and kidney. Their anti-infectious arsenals are nonspecific, targeting microorganisms and healthy host tissues with equal ferocity. Bystander injury is common and is an important contributing factor to the pathogenesis of sepsis-related organ dysfunction.

NEUTROPHIL STRUCTURE

Neutrophils have a characteristic histological appearance on a blood film, with multilobed nuclei and abundant cytoplasmic granules (Fig. 150-1). Their specific biochemical features reflect a central role in the early recognition of, and immediate response to, danger (Fig. 150-2).

Cell Surface Receptors

Neutrophils express multiple-cell surface receptors that are involved in pathogen recognition, adhesion to endothelium, transendothelial migration, cell activation, and

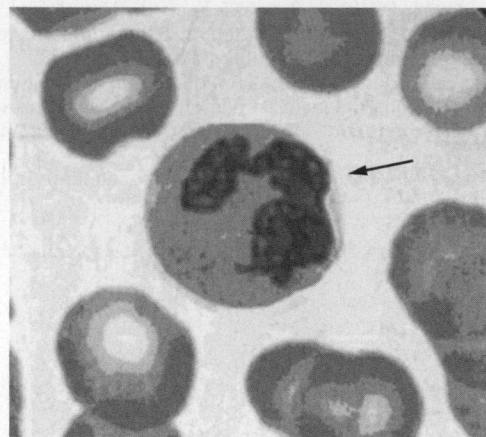

FIGURE 150-1. Neutrophil on a peripheral blood smear. Note the characteristic multilobed nucleus and the granular cytoplasm.

apoptosis. Toll-like receptors recognize danger by binding conserved biochemical patterns in microbial pathogens or host proteins, such as elastase or heparin sulfate, exposed during tissue injury.[7] Sialyl Lewis[x] (CD15)[7-9] and L-selectin[10] are important in the initial rolling of neutrophils along endothelial cells, while CD11/CD18 β_2 integrins (Mac-1 [CD11b/CD18] and leukocyte function–associated molecule-1 [LFA-1] [CD11a/CD18]) mediate the firm adhesion of neutrophils to endothelial cells.[11] Other surface receptors are activated by inflammatory mediators of host origin, including platelet-activating factor, granulocyte-macrophage colony-stimulating factor (GM-CSF), granulocyte colony-stimulating factor (G-CSF), and interferon-γ (IFN-γ). Neutrophils recognize and bind to opsonized bacteria through complement receptors and receptors for the Fc chain of immunoglobulin.[12] Finally, Fas and tumor necrosis factor (TNF) receptors play an integral role in initiating neutrophil apoptosis.[13,14]

Granules

Neutrophils employ a repertoire of proteins contained in cytoplasmic granules to kill pathogens. There are four types of intracellular granules—azurophilic (primary) granules, specific (secondary) granules, gelatinase (tertiary) granules, and secretory vesicles[15]—containing a diverse array of proteases (elastase, cathepsin G, proteinase 3, collagenase, gelatinase), microbicidal enzymes (myeloperoxidase, lysozyme, neuraminidases), and other proteins involved in the acute inflammatory response.[15]

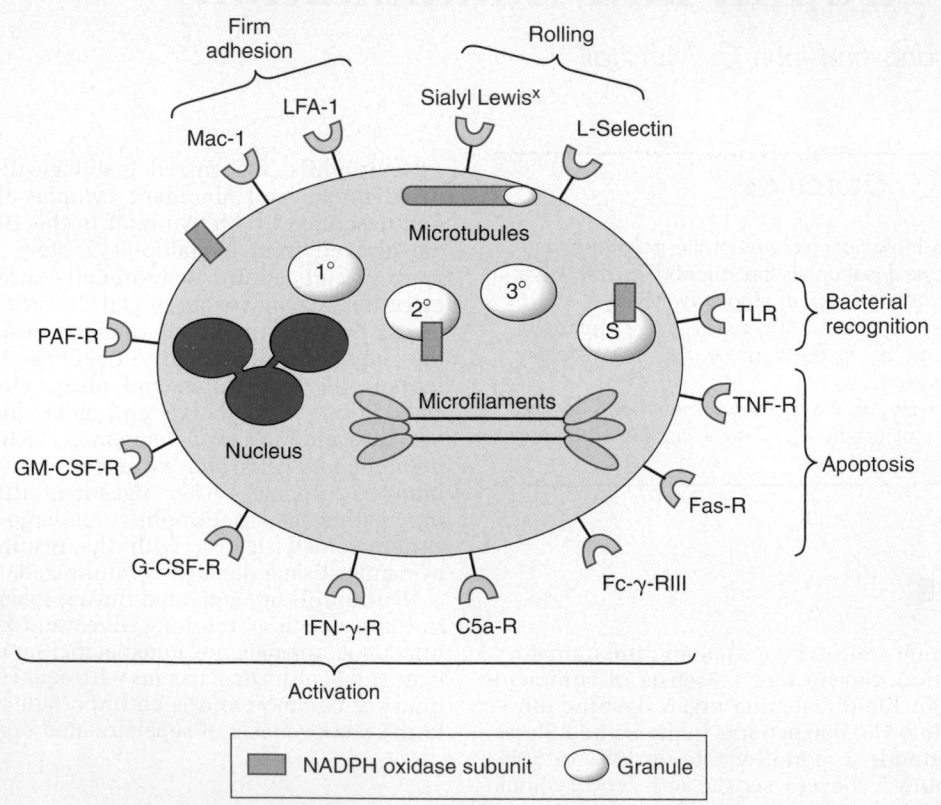

FIGURE 150-2. Schematic diagram of a neutrophil illustrating the important cell surface receptors, granules, and cytoskeleton. Granules: 1°, azurophilic (primary) granule; 2°, specific (secondary) granule; 3°, gelatinase (tertiary) granule; S, secretory vesicle. Fas-R, Fas receptor; G-CSF-R, granulocyte colony-stimulating factor receptor; GM-CSF-R, granulocyte-macrophage colony-stimulating factor receptor; IFN-γ-R, interferon-γ receptor; LFA-1, leukocyte function–associated molecule-1; PAF-R, platelet-activating factor receptor; TLR, Toll-like receptor; TNF-R, tumor necrosis factor receptor.

Nicotinamide Adenine Dinucleotide Phosphate (NADPH) Oxidase Subunits

The capacity to generate reactive oxygen intermediates through the NADPH oxidase is central to the antimicrobial arsenal of the neutrophil. Subunits of the NADPH oxidase are in the cell membrane, cytosol, and granules (specific granules and secretory vesicles) and assembled in response to inflammatory stimuli to create the active complex.

Cytoskeleton

The neutrophil cytoskeleton is composed of microtubules and microfilaments that move symmetrically toward the membrane when the cells are activated. These coordinated movements enable neutrophils to migrate in a directed fashion toward inflammatory stimuli in response to chemokines such as interleukin-8 (IL-8) and complement-5a (C5a).[16]

NEUTROPHIL FUNCTION

Neutrophils are the first cells recruited in response to an inflammatory stimulus. An efficient antimicrobial response requires the coordinated expression of multiple steps, including migration to the site of inflammation, pathogen recognition by specific receptors, priming and activation, phagocytosis, respiratory burst with the production of reactive oxygen species, release of microbicidal enzymes, and production of pro-inflammatory mediators.

Migration

Local release of IL-8 creates a concentration gradient that results in the influx of neutrophils into the site of inflammation. The interaction of sialyl Lewis^x on the neutrophils with E-selectin on the endothelial cells, and of neutrophil L-selectin with glycosylated cell adhesion molecules and P-selectin glycoprotein ligand-1 on the endothelial cells, causes the circulating neutrophil to roll along the endothelium and to slow down in preparation for firmer adhesion.[17] Firm adhesion of neutrophils to endothelial cells occurs through the interaction of Mac-1 and LFA-1 on the neutrophil with intracellular adhesion molecule 1 (ICAM-1) on the endothelial cells. Once firm adhesion has occurred, diapedesis of the neutrophil between endothelial cells delivers the neutrophil to the extravascular site of inflammation where the process of pathogen recognition begins. Transmigration of neutrophils through activated endothelial cells occurs by both IL-8–dependent and IL-8–independent pathways.[18] IL-8 release can be inhibited by transforming growth factor (TGF)-β, thus inhibiting neutrophil transmigration.[19] Neutrophils become activated during the process of endothelial transmigration.

The biological processes involved in neutrophil recruitment have been studied in a rodent lung model.[20] Gram-negative bacteria induce the local expression of proteins involved in trafficking, including KC, macrophage inflammatory protein-2 (MIP-2), and ICAM-1 by a nuclear factor-κB (NF-κB)–dependent mechanism. KC and MIP-2 bind to CXC chemokine receptor 2 (CXCR2) on neutrophils, whereas ICAM-1 binds to CD11/CD18 β$_2$ integrins. These interactions induce cytoskeletal reorganizations, with localization of actin in the front end of neutrophil and myosin in the rear, leading to suppression of lateral pseudopod formation and to retraction of uropod in the rear.[16] Pseudopod formation is biased by the gradient of chemoattractant, and polarization arises because the leading edge of the neutrophil is more sensitive to chemokines.[16] These changes in cytoskeletal organization support chemotaxis and lead to recruitment of neutrophils to site of inflammation.

Pathogen Recognition

The recognition of danger by the innate immune system is effected through an evolutionarily conserved family of proteins, known as the Toll-like receptors (TLRs).[21] TLRs are type 1 transmembrane receptors that recognize and bind to danger-associated molecular patterns—conserved molecular patterns that are unique to microbes and host proteins that are normally intracellular.[22] Human cells express 10 different TLRs, and all except TLR3 are present in the neutrophil; engagement leads to neutrophil activation.[23,24] TLRs recognize distinct ligands. For example, TLR2 binds to gram-positive products such as lipoteichoic acid, TLR4 binds to lipopolysaccharide from gram-negative bacteria, TLR5 binds to flagellin, and TLR9 binds to CpG sequences in bacterial DNA.

The binding of a ligand to a neutrophil TLR results in the production of IL-8, triggers the shedding of L-selectin, primes for N-formulated-methionine-leucine-phenylalanine peptide–mediated superoxide production, increases the rate of phagocytosis, and decreases IL-8–induced chemotaxis.[23]

Phagocytosis

Neutrophils can phagocytose both opsonized and nonopsonized particles and express two principal opsonin receptors—the Fc receptors (FcγRIIA, FcγRIIIB, and FcγRI) that bind to immunoglobulin and a subgroup of β2 integrins that bind to complement-coated particles.[25,26] Phagocytosis results in internalization of the pathogen, setting the stage for its degradation and disposal.

Ligand binding induces receptor clustering, which in turn promotes receptor phosphorylation[27] and the recruitment of intracellular proteins,[28,29] actin polymerization,[30,31] changes in membrane structure, and particle ingestion. Ingested particles are confined in a membrane-bound structure called the *phagosome*.

The nascent phagosome undergoes "phagosome maturation" to acquire the appropriate cellular machinery necessary for the degradation and disposal of pathogenic particles,[26] a process that involves sequential interactions with cellular granules[32,33] and that is initiated by cytosolic calcium increase.[34] Phagosome maturation typically results in increased phagosomal acidity—a key factor in particle degradation.[35]

Oxidative Mechanisms of Pathogen Killing

A key mechanism of neutrophil killing of pathogens involves the production of reactive oxygen species via two pathways—the nicotinamide adenine dinucleotide phosphate (NADPH) oxidase and inducible nitric oxide synthase (iNOS).[36]

The NADPH oxidase is a multimolecular complex of seven subunits. Before activation, each exists in an inactive form in the cell membrane and cytoplasm. Activation induces translocation of cytoplasmic subunits to the plasma membrane, to form a multimeric complex that is capable of oxidizing activity.[37,38] The first step in producing oxygen radicals involves the addition of single electrons to oxygen to form superoxide anion (O^{2-}), a very weak oxygen radical.[39-41] Superoxide anion can reduce intracellular iron, converting ferric (Fe^{3+}) to ferrous state (Fe^{2+}). The addition of a hydrogen ion produces hydrogen peroxide (H_2O_2).[41] Further reduction by iron (Fe) creates hydroxyl radical (HO•), the most reactive oxygen species.[42-44] Hydroxyl radical causes DNA strand breaks, enzyme inactivation, and lipid peroxidation.[45] In the presence of halide (Cl^-), the release of myeloperoxidase from the azurophilic granules converts H_2O_2 to hypochlorous acid (HClO),[46] another potent oxidant (Fig. 150-3).

Reactive intermediates are also created through the action of inducible nitric oxide synthase (iNOS).[47] iNOS expressed in activated neutrophils catalyzes the conversion of arginine to citrulline, releasing a molecule of nitric oxide (·NO). Nitric oxide is mildly reactive with aromatic amino acids, forming stable adducts such as nitrotyrosine. It is further converted to peroxynitrite anion, which reacts strongly with thiol groups (Fig. 150-4).[48]

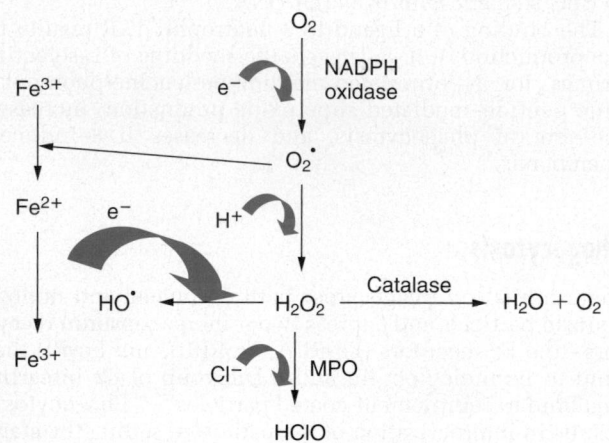

FIGURE 150-3. Respiratory burst sequence (NADPH oxidase pathway). Cl^-, chloride ion; Fe^{3+}, ferric state; Fe^{2+}, ferrous state; H_2O, water; H_2O_2, hydrogen peroxide; HClO, hypochlorous acid; MPO, myeloperoxidase; NADPH, nicotinamide adenine dinucleotide phosphate; O_2, oxygen; O_2•, superoxide anion; OH•, hydroxyl radical.

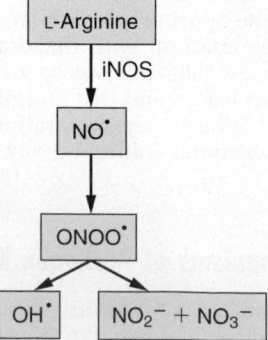

FIGURE 150-4. Respiratory burst sequence (iNOS pathway). iNOS, inducible nitric oxide synthase; NO•, nitric oxide; OH•, hydroxyl radical; ONOO•, peroxynitrite ion.

The NADPH oxidase is a powerful enzyme, able to generate large amounts of reactive oxygen species. Its importance in antimicrobial immunity is illustrated by chronic granulomatous disease, a genetic disease in which the NADPH oxidase is inactive. Patients with chronic granulomatous disease suffer recurrent and often fatal infections (lung, gastrointestinal, and skin) caused by *Staphylococcus aureus*, *Aspergillus*, enteric gram-negative bacteria, and *Burkholderia cepacia*.[49,50]

Pathogen Killing by Granular Enzymes

Neutrophils contain four different types of granules which are classically divided into granules that contain myeloperoxidase and those that do not. Granules that do not contain myeloperoxidase are further classified into early-appearing peroxidase-positive granules (azurophilic granules) and later-appearing peroxidase-negative granules, composed of the secondary (specific) granules and the tertiary (gelatinase) granules.[51] Delivery of granule-associated proteins to the cell surface facilitates cell adhesion and locomotion to the site of infection while delivery to the phagosome aids in microbial killing.[15]

Neutrophils kill ingested pathogens by two nonoxidative methods: increasing bacterial permeability by disrupting anionic surfaces (defensins, lysozymes, bactericidal permeability-increasing protein) and degrading bacterial proteins through the activity of enzymes such as elastase and cathepsin G. Other granule proteins contribute to phagosomal acidification, activating hydrolytic enzymes that function optimally under conditions of low pH (4.5 to 6.0).

Neutrophil granules contain more than 20 enzymes; serine proteinase, elastase, and two metalloproteinases (collagenase and gelatinase) are the most important mediators of tissue destruction.[52] Their toxicity to the host is regulated by anti-proteinases such as alpha$_1$-proteinase inhibitor.[53]

Production of Pro-inflammatory Mediators by Neutrophils

Mature neutrophils produce a variety of different cytokines including IL-8, IL-1β, IL-6, TNF-α, MIP-1α, G-CSF, and GM-CSF.[12] In addition to pro-inflammatory mediators, they also produce anti-inflammatory cytokines, such as IL-1 receptor antagonist (IL-1ra) and TGF-β,[54,55] which can act on neutrophils themselves and inhibit the inflammation locally.[12]

APOPTOSIS AND THE REGULATION OF NEUTROPHILIC INFLAMMATION

Neutrophils mature in the bone marrow over approximately 2 weeks and then are released into the circulation; approximately 10^{11} neutrophils are released each day. They circulate for only 6 to 10 hours before migrating into tissues where, in the absence of any inflammatory stimulus, they undergo spontaneous apoptosis over the ensuing several days.[56]

Apoptosis, or programmed cell death, is a conserved cellular process that is fundamental for tissue remodeling

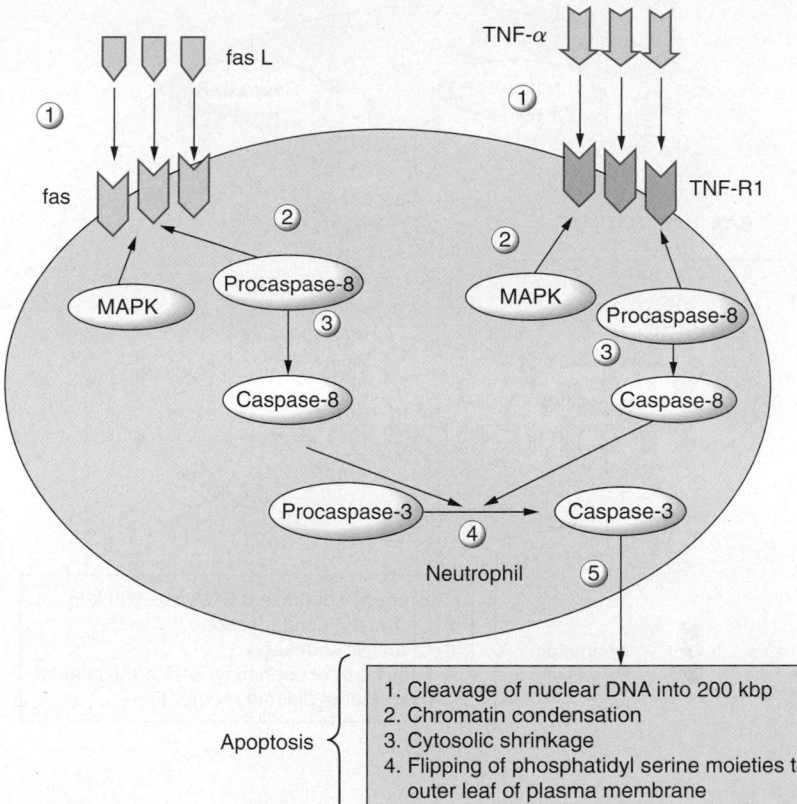

FIGURE 150-5. Extrinsic apoptosis pathway. fas-L, fas ligand; MAPK, mitogen-activating protein kinase; TNF, tumor necrosis factor; TNF-R, tumor necrosis factor receptor.

Text within figure:

fas L

TNF-α

fas

TNF-R1

MAPK   Procaspase-8

Caspase-8

MAPK

Procaspase-8

Caspase-8

Procaspase-3   Caspase-3

Neutrophil

Apoptosis
1. Cleavage of nuclear DNA into 200 kbp
2. Chromatin condensation
3. Cytosolic shrinkage
4. Flipping of phosphatidyl serine moieties to outer leaf of plasma membrane

and development. Apoptosis is a highly organized process that requires the expenditure of energy in the form of adenosine triphosphate; it differs from necrosis in that cell death occurs without inflammation or damage to tissues. The multiple facets of the apoptotic process include cell shrinkage, cleaving of nuclear DNA, chromatin condensation, and membrane blebbing.[57]

Apoptosis can be initiated by an extrinsic pathway in response to stimuli in the cellular environment or by an intrinsic pathway in response to stimuli that alter mitochondrial membrane permeability.[6] Both pathways are effected through a family of proteases known as caspases. All caspases have a conserved cysteine residue at their active sites and cleave target proteins adjacent to aspartate residues (cysteine aspartate proteases). They exist within the cytoplasm as zymogens (inactive procaspases). "Initiator" caspases triggered by extrinsic or intrinsic pathways cleave further "executor" caspases, which effect the characteristic morphological changes of apoptosis.[56]

The extrinsic pathway is activated when death receptors such as Fas or the receptors for TNF are bound by their respective ligands. Death receptor clustering leads to auto-activation and recruitment of key intracellular regulators of the caspase cascade.[58,59] Caspase-8 cleaves and activates caspase-3, which, in turn, results in cleavage of nuclear DNA into oligonucleosomal fragments of multiples of 200 kilo-base pair, condensation of chromatin, cytosolic shrinkage, and flipping of phosphatidyl serine moieties to the outer leaf of plasma membrane.[60] The distinctive phosphatidyl serine residues promote recognition and efficient removal of apoptotic cells by local phagocytes (Fig. 150-5).[61]

Activation of the intrinsic pathway is initiated by loss of potential of the inner mitochondrial membrane, increas-

ing its permeability to molecules up to 1500 daltons in size.[61] Opening of the mitochondrial transition pore leads to efflux of calcium and redistribution of cytochrome c to the cytoplasm. Cytochrome c binds to apoptosis protease-activating factor-1 and caspase-9 to form a ternary complex called the *apoptosome*. Caspase-9 is cleaved and activated in the process and, in turn, activates caspase-3 (Fig. 150-6).[62]

Whether the cell survives or dies also depends on the expression of antiapoptotic proteins, including members of the Bcl-2 family.[63] Some Bcl-2 family members are antiapoptotic (Bcl-x_L, Bcl-w, A-1, MCL-1), whereas others are proapoptotic (Bax, Bak, BAD, Bid). These proapoptotic proteins localized to outer mitochondrial membrane facilitate the release of cytochrome c. In the absence of survival signals and de novo synthesis of antiapoptotic proteins, levels of MCL-1[64] and A-1[65] fall, and neutrophils undergo spontaneous apoptosis. Control of cell survival or apoptosis is regulated by modulation of mitochondrial membrane permeability[66,67]; in septic patients, for example, MCL-1 mRNA was increased, promoting neutrophil survival.[68]

Many studies have demonstrated that redox imbalance can alter neutrophil apoptosis.[69-71] Endogenously produced reactive oxygen species are important in activating apoptosis in response to both Fas[72,73] and TNF-α.[74] Death receptor clustering and subsequent activation of caspase-8 are reactive oxygen species–dependent and can occur in the absence of Fas ligation.[73,75] Moreover, exogenous H_2O_2 induces apoptosis in neutrophils.[76] Neutrophils from patients with chronic granulomatous disease have decreased rates of spontaneous, or Fas/TNF-α–induced apoptosis, a defect that can be restored by exogenous

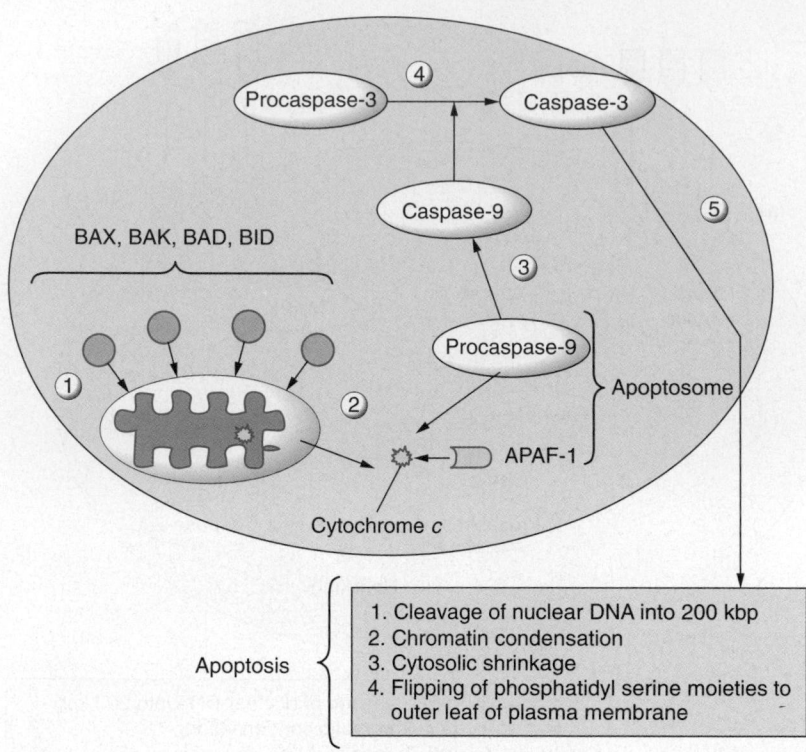

1. Cleavage of nuclear DNA into 200 kbp
2. Chromatin condensation
3. Cytosolic shrinkage
4. Flipping of phosphatidyl serine moieties to outer leaf of plasma membrane

Apoptosis

FIGURE 150-6. Intrinsic (spontaneous) apoptosis pathway. APAF-1, apoptosis protease–activating factor-1.

H_2O_2.[72] The induction of apoptosis by reactive oxygen species may therefore be of fundamental importance to neutrophil removal from a site of inflammation, a potential mechanism of negative feedback in the inflammatory response.[56]

Phagocytosis of Apoptotic Neutrophils by Macrophages

After neutrophils have phagocytosed and killed pathogens, they undergo apoptosis. Macrophages recognize the apoptotic neutrophil while the cell membrane is structurally and functionally intact, before granule enzymes have been disgorged; as a result, tissue injury in inflammation is limited.[77] The phagocytosis of apoptotic neutrophils inhibits the release of pro-inflammatory cytokines from macrophages,[78] but promotes release of the anti-inflammatory cytokine, IL-10.[79]

ROLE OF THE NEUTROPHIL IN SEPSIS

The multiple-organ dysfunction syndrome is a common, and frequently fatal, complication of sepsis, affecting many organs, including the lung, liver, and kidney, and leading to acute respiratory distress syndrome (ARDS), hepatic dysfunction, and renal dysfunction.[80-82]

Delayed Apoptosis during Systemic Inflammation

Under normal circumstances, neutrophils undergo apoptosis after less than a day in the systemic circulation.

However, during sepsis, apoptosis of neutrophils is delayed,[83] leading to accumulation of neutrophils in tissues and neutrophil-mediated organ injury. Hoesel and colleagues[84] demonstrated that when neutrophils are depleted in mice 12 hours after cecal ligation and puncture, there was evidence of reduced hepatic and renal dysfunction. If neutrophils are depleted too early, however, hepatic dysfunction is greater, likely a consequence of reduced bacterial clearance.[84]

Delayed neutrophil apoptosis is a hallmark of severe systemic inflammatory conditions, evident, for example, in neutrophils exposed to superantigen,[85] in patients suffering from systemic inflammatory response syndrome,[83,86] in trauma patients units with septic complications[87] and in patients in intensive care units with severe sepsis.[88] Suppression of neutrophil apoptosis in sepsis is accompanied by evidence of increased neutrophil activation, as measured by spontaneous respiratory burst activity, but a reduced capacity to respond to further stimulation.

Delayed neutrophil apoptosis may be caused by a soluble mediator.[83,85-87] Serum from patients suffering from systemic inflammatory response syndrome, sepsis, and trauma with septic complications delays the apoptosis of neutrophils from healthy volunteers.[83,85-87] Candidate soluble antiapoptotic mediators include GM-CSF,[85,86] G-CSF,[87] TNF-α,[89] and IFN-γ.[85,89] The relative importance of each mediator may depend on the intensity and type of the injury stimulus or the type of antigen.[61] GM-CSF delays neutrophil apoptosis through a phophoinositide-3-kinase and extracellular signal regulating–dependent pathway.[90] IL-10, on the other hand, reverses the inhibition of human neutrophil apoptosis induced by lipopolysaccharide by inhibition of tyrosine phosphorylation.[89]

Inhibition of neutrophil apoptosis is an active process. Antiapoptotic cytokines lead to activation of NF-κB, reduced activity of caspases-3 and -9, maintenance of mitochondrial transmembrane potential, and retention of intramitochondrial cytochrome *c*.[88,91,92] Inhibition of

NF-κB suppresses acute inflammation and reduces organ dysfunction.[93]

Central to the antiapoptotic activity of a number of inflammatory mediators is a novel cytokine-like molecule, pre-B cell colony-enhancing factor (PBEF), originally isolated as a secreted factor that synergized with IL-7 and stem cell factor to promote the differentiation of B cell precursors. PBEF decreases the activity of caspase-8 and caspase-3, but not of caspase-9. Neutrophils from septic patients show markedly increased expression of PBEF.[94]

Other work suggests that delayed neutrophil apoptosis in sepsis involves complex interactions of neutrophils with monocytes and macrophages through both TLR4 and TLR2 pattern recognition receptor molecules.[95,96] Other factors associated with delayed apoptosis include cellular calcium overload, tissue hypoxia, and ischemia reperfusion–type injury.[96]

ROLE OF THE NEUTROPHIL IN ACUTE RESPIRATORY DISTRESS SYNDROME

Neutrophils play an important role in the development of the ARDS during sepsis. Endotoxin from gram-negative bacteria exerts potent pro-inflammatory activity[97] and primes neutrophils for an augmented respiratory burst with increased release of superoxide and elastase.[98] Following endotoxin administration, neutrophils rapidly enter the pulmonary parenchyma,[99,100] where they contribute to oxidant-induced injury and loss of epithelial integrity.[101,102] Neutrophil elastase is particularly important in increased vasopermeability, accumulation of leukocytes, pulmonary hemorrhage, and parenchymal injury.[103] Elastases can also cleave surfactant-specific proteins and impair surfactant function.[104] Neutrophil matrix metalloproteinases such as collagenase have been identified in the bronchoalvoolar lavage fluid of patients with ARDS[105] and are thought to be involved in the subsequent development of lung fibrosis.[48] Phospholipase A$_2$ is increased in the bronchoalveolar lavage fluid of animals with chemically induced ARDS[106] and in the plasma of patients with sepsis or pancreatitis.[107-109] Intratracheal phospholipase A$_2$ can induce lung injury with interstitial and alveolar edema, accumulation of inflammatory cells, and alveolar wall thickening, all typical features of ARDS.[110,111] Lysophosphatidylcholine damages alveolar type I cellular membranes,[112] increases capillary permeability,[113] and inactivates surfactant.[114] Platelet-activating factor causes margination of neutrophils, formation of toxic oxygen metabolites, and lung endothelial damage.[115,116]

ROLE OF THE NEUTROPHIL IN ACUTE RENAL FAILURE

Acute renal failure can occur as a consequence of trauma, hemorrhage, sepsis, and ischemia-reperfusion injury.[117-119] There is evidence that neutrophils play a key role in the development of acute renal failure.[120-122] Cytokines such as IL-1β, TNF-α, and IL-8 that recruit neutrophils to end-organ have been implicated in acute renal failure,[123,124] and upregulation of adhesion molecules such as ICAM-1 on endothelial cells in glomerular or peritubular capillaries contributes to acute renal failure.[52,125] The importance of reactive oxygen intermediates in renal failure was demonstrated in studies in which the reperfusion of ischemic kidneys with neutrophils from a patient with granulomatous disease attenuated renal injury.[123] Scavenging H$_2$O$_2$ with catalase also minimized neutrophil-mediated renal injury during reperfusion.[123] Neutrophil elastase has been shown to contribute to degradation of the glomerular basement membrane.[126] Oxygen intermediates inactivate antiproteinases and so enable proteases to degrade extracellular matrix.[127] Neutrophils are also capable of producing lipo-oxygenase products such as platelet-activating factor, which has been implicated in renal injury through a reduction in glomerular filtration rates and renal blood pressure leading to decreased urine output and sodium excretion.[128-130]

CONCLUSION

Neutrophils play a fundamental role in innate immunity by virtue of their capacity for pathogen recognition, chemotaxis, phagocytosis, respiratory burst, degranulation, and production of pro-inflammatory cytokines. After ingesting, killing, degrading, and disposing of pathogens, neutrophils undergo apoptosis, with the result that tissue injury in the host is minimized. Apoptotic neutrophils are recognized and phagocytosed by macrophages and, through this process, trigger the production of anti-inflammatory cytokines which further protect host tissue from inflammatory damage. Dysregulation of the normal kinetics of neutrophil activation and removal contributes to inflammatory organ injury and represents a still-unproven avenue for anti-inflammatory therapy.

During sepsis, there is a delay in apoptosis of neutrophils and an increase in activation of neutrophils. This combination leads to accumulation of activated neutrophils in various tissues, leading to multiple-organ failure and ARDS.

Key Points

1. Neutrophils are highly mobile cells that are recruited to sites of tissue injury or infectious challenge through interactions between chemokines, receptors on the neutrophil and endothelium, and the intrinsic capacity of the neutrophil for directed locomotion.
2. Neutrophils exert potent antimicrobial immunity through both oxidative and nonoxidative mechanisms. Oxidative mechanisms involve the generation of reactive oxygen intermediates through the activity of the NADPH oxidase, producing damage to DNA, lipids, and proteins. Nonoxidative mechanisms involve the activity of a large number of granule proteins with proteolytic and antibacterial activity.
3. Defects in neutrophil innate defense systems predispose the host to infection, but overactivity of the neutrophil is equally harmful, producing nonspecific bystander injury to host tissues.
4. Regulation of neutrophil inflammatory function is effected through the capacity of the neutrophil to undergo constitutive apoptosis. Apoptosis limits

neutrophil-mediated injury and activates host transcriptional programs that are anti-inflammatory and reparative. In response to inflammatory stimuli, this constitutive apoptotic program can be inhibited, prolonging neutrophil functional activity, but at the cost of increased bystander injury.

5. Dysregulated neutrophil-mediated inflammation contributes to tissue injury in sepsis, particularly injury of the lung and kidney.

Key References

7. Takeda K, Akira S: Microbial recognition by Toll-like receptors. J Dermatol Sci 2004;34(2):73-82.

15. Moraes TJ, Zurawska JH, Downey GP: Neutrophil granule contents in the pathogenesis of lung injury. Curr Opin Hematol 2006;13(1):21-27.
26. Lee WL, Harrison RE, Grinstein S: Phagocytosis by neutrophils. Microbes Infect 2003;5(14):1299-1306.
94. Jia SH, Ly Y, Parodo J: Pre-B cell colony-enhancing factor inhibits neutrophil apoptosis in experimental inflammation and clinical sepsis. J Clin Invest 2004;113(9):1318-1327.
95. Sabroe I, Dower SK, Whyte MK: The role of Toll-like receptors in the regulation of neutrophil migration, activation, and apoptosis. Clin Infect Dis 2005;41(Suppl 7):S421-S426.

See the companion Expert Consult website for the complete reference list.

CHAPTER 151

The Macrophage in Innate and Adaptive Immunity

Sarah Doernberg and Richard Bucala

OBJECTIVES

This chapter will:
1. Define the basis and function of innate and adaptive immunity.
2. Define the importance of the macrophage in innate and adaptive immune responses.
3. Describe the macrophage-derived products that mediate the innate, inflammatory response.

The human immune system has evolved to protect against tissue invasion by infectious pathogens. The host response to these threats comprises two arms: the innate and the adaptive immune systems.[1] The innate immune system is the first line of defense, which relies on a limited number of germline gene products to respond to a broad variety of threats. The adaptive immune system becomes activated more gradually and relies on gene rearrangement, selection, and clonal expansion to produce both a tailored response and immunological memory. The adaptive response thus takes time to develop, and the innate response must be sufficiently effective so as to ensure host survival in the acute phase. The innate and the adaptive systems also are closely linked, and many elements of the immune response play roles in both arms.[1,2]

Inflammation is a direct consequence of the innate response and acts to control threats to the host by bringing molecules and cells to the site of invasion, walling off infection, and repairing the injury.[3,4] Macrophages are central cellular elements in this well-orchestrated response and serve important purposes in both the innate and adaptive arms of the immune response. These cells recognize foreign molecules, phagocytize debris, produce inflammatory mediators, interact with other immune cells, coordinate the transition from innate to adaptive immunity, and help to resolve inflammation.[5] Derived from circulating monocytes, macrophages terminally differentiate in the tissues to form heterogeneous populations of related cells. These populations include Langerhans cells of the epidermis, osteoclasts, alveolar macrophages, microglia and other central nervous system macrophages, splenic macrophages, Kupffer cells of the liver, and inflammatory-derived monocytes. These cells remain in the tissues to help mobilize a response to threat.[6]

RECOGNITION OF FOREIGN MOLECULES

To execute a rapid response to foreign molecules, the innate immune system, especially the sentinel macrophage population, has evolved nonspecific, germline-encoded mechanisms to recognize threat. As described by Medzhitov and colleagues,[7] pattern recognition receptors, which are well conserved among plants, invertebrates, and vertebrates, are designed to serve this purpose by recognizing non-self molecules (also called pathogen-associated molecular patterns [PAMPs]). PAMPs are distinguished from self molecules by their unique structures, which are not found in host cells.[8,9] A classic example of a PAMP is lipopolysaccharide (LPS), a sugar that comprises part of the gram-negative bacterial cell wall.[10] The engagement of a pattern recognition receptor by a PAMP indicates the presence of a pathogen and leads to a series of downstream events resulting in a coordinated innate and adaptive immune response.[11] The receptors can function to promote phagocytosis, stimulate chemotaxis, or induce effector mechanisms important in the innate and adaptive immune responses. Because macrophages are among the first immune cells exposed to these PAMPs, they contain many cell surface and intracellular receptors that aid in detection of foreign molecules.[12]

Toll-Like Receptors

Perhaps the best-studied pattern recognition receptors on macrophages are the Toll-like receptors (TLRs) (see Chapter 148).[9,11] These molecules were first identified in *Drosophila* fruit flies, which rarely contract microbial infections despite lacking adaptive immunity. In the late 1990s, Medzhitov and colleagues[7] identified a human homologue of the *Drosophila* Toll receptor and showed that activation of this receptor resulted in induction of inflammatory cytokines and co-stimulatory molecules, which are necessary for the transition to adaptive immunity. Ensuing work demonstrated the existence of several other members of the human TLR family, which contained structural similarities to *Drosophila* Toll receptors and vertebrate interleukin-1 receptors.[11] Subsequent studies revealed the importance of the TLRs in activating the immune response to foreign material.

Much of what is known about TLRs comes from studies of gram-negative bacterial infections, and specifically, LPS. Prior to the discovery of human TLRs, several experiments had revealed that LPS exerts its cellular response only after being opsonized by LPS-binding protein (LBP) and CD14, a soluble or membrane-bound receptor.[13] However, the exact mechanism of signal transduction leading to the clinical development of septic shock after LPS binding remained unidentified until researchers delved into the molecular basis for LPS unresponsiveness that had been observed in certain strains of mice. Positional cloning studies demonstrated that these mice had mutations in their *TLR4* genes, leading to the LPS-resistant phenotype.[14] The LBP-CD14-LPS complex later was shown to bind to TLR4, which leads to a robust downstream inflammatory response.[15]

TLRs signal through several well-conserved molecular pathways that ultimately result in the translocation of nuclear factor-κB (NF-κB) into the nucleus and activation of many pro-inflammatory genes, including those for cytokines and co-stimulatory molecules.[9,11] TLRs exist as both membrane-bound and cytosolic receptors. Thus far, 10 different human TLRs have been described that recognize various PAMPs, including the components of bacteria, yeast, and viruses (Table 151-1). When an individual is exposed to specific bacteria, it is likely that different structural aspects of the pathogen (e.g., LPS, certain DNA patterns) activate several TLRs. As central cellular elements of the immune system, macrophages utilize these receptors to recognize an invasive threat and activate downstream immune events. Emerging evidence also points to a role for the TLRs in sterile inflammation and autoimmunity as well as infectious diseases.

Intracellular Pattern Recognition Molecules

Although the TLRs undoubtedly play a crucial role in detection of pathogens, particular microbes can enter cells undetected. Recent work has uncovered a group of intracellular pattern recognition receptors known as nucleotide-binding oligomerization domains (NODs) that have

TABLE 151-1

Human Toll-like Receptor Ligands

TLR1	Triacyl lipopeptides
TLR2	Lipoproteins
	Peptidoglycan
	Lipoteichoic acid
	Lipoarabinomannan
	Porins
	Zymosan
TLR3	Viral double-stranded DNA
TLR4	Lipopolysaccharide
	Respiratory syncytial virus fusion protein
TLR5	Flagellin
TLR6	Diacyl lipopeptides
	Lipoteichoic acid
	Zymosan
TLR7/8	Viral single-stranded RNA
	Synthetic materials (imidazoquinoline, bropirimine, loxoribine)
TLR9	Unmethylated CpG-containing DNA, hemozoin
TLR10	Unknown

Adapted from Warren HS: Toll-like receptors. Crit Care Med 2005;33: S457-S459.

been implicated in activating an immune response against intracellular microbes. More than 20 related human proteins have been described, which are homologous to human apoptotic regulatory proteins and a group of plant disease-resistant gene products. Specifically, NOD1 and NOD2 appear to mediate responsiveness to peptidoglycan (PDG) moieties, including muramyl dipeptide MurNAc-L-Ala-D-isoGln and diaminopimelic acid.[16,17] Although the pathways have not been well elucidated, there are two hypotheses for how the PDG products activate NOD-dependant pathways. First, the bacterial products could be phagocytized and presented directly to the NOD proteins. Alternatively, the products could activate a yet-to-be determined extracellular domain, which in turn triggers the NOD pathways.[18,19]

Mutations in the NOD family have been linked to several inflammatory diseases. For instance, certain patients with Crohn's disease possess a frameshift mutation in *NOD2*, which also lowers responsiveness to LPS.[20] Similar to the TLR family, several of the NOD proteins lead to downstream activation of NF-κB via a signal transduction cascade leading ultimately to inflammatory cytokine production, albeit at lower levels than described with TLRs. Why macrophages contain both the TLR family, some of which recognize PDG, and NOD1 and NOD2 is not clear, but this may represent a redundant mechanism for the cellular recognition and response to invasive pathogens.[21]

ANTIGEN UPTAKE AND PROCESSING

Besides interacting with pathogens via TLRs and NODs, macrophages also can recognize foreign patterns and altered self-patterns of apoptotic cells through the macrophage mannose receptor, scavenger receptors, or complement receptors.[5] Often the PAMPs do not bind directly to these receptors. Rather, opsonization, or alteration of the molecule via complement or antibody occurs to allow for more efficient and specific receptor binding. Once engaged, each of these receptors aids in phagocytosis of

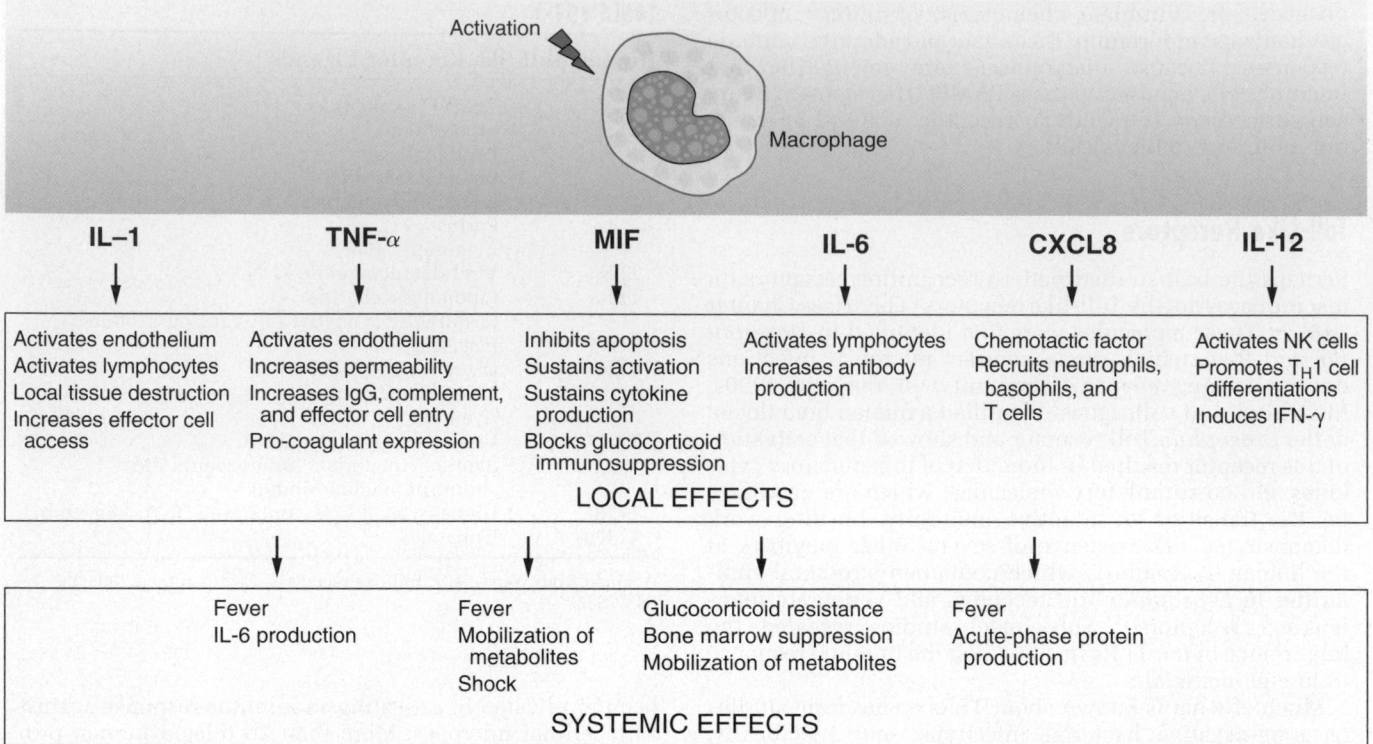

FIGURE 151-1. Selected effector cytokines secreted in response to bacterial peptides include interleukin-1 (IL-1), IL-6, CXCL8, IL-12, and tumor necrosis factor-α (TNF-α). CXCL8, CXC ligand 8; IFN-γ, interferon-γ; IgG, immunoglobulin G; MIF, migration inhibitory factor; NK, natural killer. (Adapted from Janeway CA, Travers P, Walport M, Shlomchik M: Immunobiology: The Immune System in Health and Disease, 6th ed. New York, Garland, 2005.)

the pathogen in addition to activating an inflammatory response.

Phagocytosis plays an essential role in clearance of dying cells, tissue remodeling, embryonal development, and host defense. Along with neutrophils, macrophages serve as one of the main phagocytic cell populations. Phagocytosis is a diverse and complex event that requires many coordinated events. Following binding to specific receptors, the actin membrane rearranges to allow the cell membrane to surround the pathogen and form a phagosome. This phagosome subsequently becomes acidified and fuses with a lysosome to form a phagolysosome, which contains enzymes and other bactericidal mediators that aid in pathogen destruction. Specifically, the lysosomal nicotinamide adenine dinucleotide phosphate oxidases function to produce toxic molecules, such as hydrogen peroxide, superoxide, and nitric oxide, in respiratory burst. Pathogenic organisms often have evolved mechanisms to avoid phagocytosis. A considerable number of signaling pathways help to coordinate the multistep process of phagocytosis. Examples include cascades involving protein kinase C, phosphoinositide-3 kinase, and the Rho GTPases. These signaling pathways not only allow for the mechanics of phagocytosis to occur but also lead to the innate release of inflammatory mediators and the activation of adaptive immunity.[4,5]

INNATE RESPONSE

Once a pathogen has been detected or internalized by a host cell, the innate immune response is induced. This series of events can result either in elimination of the invasive agent or transition to the more precise adaptive immune response. Macrophage mediators of the innate response include pro-inflammatory cytokines, chemokines, prostaglandin products, and reactive oxygen and nitrogen species. Although these molecules are crucial for normal immune function and clearance of pathogens, sustained production and mediator entry into the circulation produces endothelial dysfunction and microvascular injury that characterize septic shock.

Macrophages secrete many cytokines, including interleukin-1 (IL-1), tumor necrosis factor-α (TNF-α), IL-6, macrophage migration inhibitory factor (MIF), IL-8, and IL-12 (Fig. 151-1). These cytokines play diverse and overlapping roles to produce a robust response to infectious threat. Both IL-1 and TNF-α activate the vascular endothelium and increase vascular permeability, which allows access of cells and mediators to the site of injury. When released into systemic circulation in sepsis, however, these cytokines result in vasodilation, systemic edema, and shock. TNF-α, in particular, is injurious to endothelium because it leads to the expression of pro-coagulant on the endothelial surface. IL-1, TNF-α, and IL-6, which is produced in response to IL-1 release, together lead to the systemic febrile response. IL-6 also promotes the activation of lymphocytes and induces acute-phase reactant protein production by hepatocytes. IL-12 induces the generation of a T_H1 adaptive immune response and recruits natural killer (NK) cells, which play an important role in intracellular infection.[1]

Chemokines are a specific group of low-molecular-weight cytokines that serve to induce chemotaxis of immune cells by changing integrin structure and creating a gradient to direct cellular migration. Important macrophage chemokines include IL-8, which recruits neutrophils, basophils, and T cells; macrophage inflammatory protein-1α; and macrophage chemoattractant protein-1. Together with macrophage cytokine-mediated increase in endothelial adhesion molecules, such as intracellular adhesion molecule-1, intracellular adhesion molecule-2, P-selectin, and E-selectin, these chemokines lead to recruitment and infiltration of tissues with a variety of inflammatory cells. Macrophages contain cytokine and chemokine receptors, which lead to amplification of the inflammatory response. In addition, the pro-inflammatory cytokines released by macrophages have a pro-coagulant effect by promoting tissue factor, platelet-activating factor, and plasminogen-activator inhibitor-1 release, and by decreasing production of activated protein C. Arachidonic acid–derived prostaglandins result in further recruitment of leukocytes and vascular permeability while reactive oxygen and nitrogen species aid in microbial killing.

TRANSITION TO ADAPTIVE IMMUNITY

Although the innate immune system can clear some pathogens, others survive these defenses and, as a result, trigger the induction of an adaptive immune response. This arm takes several days to activate but results in an antigen-specific, targeted response that also establishes long-lasting immunity. The innate and adaptive immune systems are tightly linked, and activation of the adaptive response relies on innate immunity. T cells are activated by antigen-presenting cells, which include dendritic cells, macrophages, and B cells. Binding and recognition of PAMPs by receptors on macrophages results in increased expression of both major histocompatibility class (MHC) II and co-stimulatory B7 molecules, allowing them to serve as antigen-presenting cells. Following phagocytosis, microorganisms are degraded, which allows for presentation of constituent peptides by MHC II molecules on macrophages to T-cell receptors in the presence of appropriate co-stimulation. The B7 molecule binds to T cell CD28, allowing for production of IL-2, which is necessary for T-cell growth and the development of an adaptive immune response. This response results in both cell-mediated and humoral immunity. Macrophages remain crucial to this response by shaping T-cell differentiation and acting as effector cells. Certain macrophage cytokines also participate in directing the adaptive response. For instance, IL-12 favors the T_H1 response of CD4$^+$ T cells, which in turn activates more macrophages.

MACROPHAGES AS EFFECTOR CELLS OF THE ADAPTIVE RESPONSE

While macrophages are often considered as important initiators of the host response, they also serve as key effectors of the ensuing adaptive response. For example, intracellular pathogens such as mycobacteria are able to avoid cytotoxic T cells and antigens produced by B cells and some extracellular organisms have adaptations that allow them to survive within macrophages despite phagocytosis and cytotoxic mechanisms. To defend against such pathogens, the adaptive immune response recruits and activates macrophages to act as targeted effector cells. Macrophages can be activated by interferon-γ (IFN-γ) produced by T or NK cells, and by a variety of other signals. For instance, CD4$^+$ T_H1 cells secrete IFN-γ and express CD40 ligand (CD40L), which contacts the macrophage CD40 receptor, leading to activation. CD8$^+$ T cells also secrete IFN-γ and activate macrophages that are already presenting antigens from cytosolic proteins or LPS. The activated macrophages augment secretion of TNF-α and expression of TNF receptors, which results in autocrine intensification of the activation response. Activated macrophages have more efficient phagocytotic mechanisms, increased production of antimicrobial radicals and peptides, and higher expression of co-stimulatory and MHC molecules. These macrophage products are toxic to host cells as well as pathogens, and thus, the activation of macrophages by T_H1 cells is tightly regulated.[3,5]

RESOLUTION OF INFLAMMATION

Inflammation itself is not harmful, and typically, the inflammatory response appropriately removes the threat and helps to resolve tissue injury. However, without resolution, persistent inflammation can lead to further tissue damage and organ dysfunction. As with the initiation of the inflammatory process, macrophages also play a role in termination.[22] Neutrophils, which have invaded the inflamed area, undergo programmed apoptosis, and macrophages respond by phagocytizing these dead cells. Phagocytosis of neutrophils likely signals to the macrophages to migrate to the lymphatic system and to release anti-inflammatory cytokines, such as TGF-β and IL-10. Other molecular mechanisms, such as suppressors of cytokine signaling proteins and arachidonic acid products, are likely involved in resolution as well.[23]

UNRESOLVED INFLAMMATION

As discussed earlier in this chapter, inflammation generally resolves once the stimulus has been removed. This normally useful response, however, can become pathologic if it remains ongoing. Several forms of chronic inflammation exist, and macrophages play a role in a number of these disorders.

Granuloma Formation

Granulomatous inflammation is one form of chronic inflammation that occurs in response to a wide variety of agents, including persistent infectious pathogens and certain foreign bodies. It is likely that granulomas evolved as a mechanism to wall off chronic infection with intracellular pathogens that are able to evade acute host defense mechanisms. Granulomas are composed mainly of macrophages that have fused into multinucleated giant cells with a surrounding edge of T lymphocytes. These are active sites of dynamic, ongoing inflammation with continuing influx of effector and secretory cells, such as macrophages, NK cells, and T cells. Together, these cells interact with each other via direct contact and cytokine release to destroy the pathogen or foreign body. Granulomas serve to limit injury or infection, but as with all other inflammatory responses, granulomatous inflammation can be excessive and result in tissue and organ damage. In certain types of granulomas, such as those that form in tuberculosis, the core becomes necrotic from lack of oxygen and cytotoxic effects of macrophages, a process known as caseation necrosis. Certain diseases such as sarcoidosis result in widespread granuloma formation and resultant tissue damage. A lack of effective granuloma formation, such as with visceral leishmaniasis in patients with advanced HIV and low CD4[+] T-cell counts, can result in extensive infection.[4]

Fibrosis

Unresolved inflammation can lead to a tissue remodeling response that contributes significantly to end-organ damage. This response is especially evident in many commonly occurring, chronic diseases. Prolonged or repeated inflammation of the airways, as in asthma; the liver, as in chronic hepatitis; the kidney, as in glomerulonephritis; and the arterial wall, as in atherosclerosis, results in an impaired or dysregulated repair response. Tissue remodeling thus describes the replacement of normal tissue components and organ architecture by cellular changes produced by chronic inflammation: fibrosis, angiogenesis, and fibroproliferation. Tissue remodeling is often progressive and irreversible. Sustained activation of macrophages and the excessive release of matrix metalloproteases, fibrogenic growth factors (TGF-β, PDGF, FGF), and vascular endothelium growth factor (VEGF) are responsible for remodeling. Adaptive immunity, once activated in response to a persistent antigen, is believed to contribute to the sustained, unresolved activation of macrophages in many conditions. In a classic example, T-cell activation to persistent parasite antigens leads to hepatic fibrosis and the obliteration of normal liver function in chronic schistosomiasis.[4] Activation of the adaptive immune response also is considered to underlie inflammatory tissue damage in different autoimmune disorders.

Atherogenesis

Coronary artery disease causes substantial morbidity and mortality among populations of developed nations, and the problem continues to escalate. Atherosclerosis is an inflammatory process that begins with injury to the vessel endothelium and progresses from fatty streak to stable and then to vulnerable plaque.[24] Ultimately, plaque rupture can occur, which limits blood flow and leads to cardiac ischemia. As with all other inflammatory processes, macrophages play a large role in atherogenesis. Once activated by injury, the endothelium expresses adhesion molecules and macrophage chemotactic factors, such as oxidized low-density lipoprotein and macrophage chemoattractant protein-1, which attract monocytes to differentiate and become activated as tissue macrophages in the subendothelium. These activated macrophages express a host of pro-inflammatory cytokines and take up modified lipoproteins via scavenger receptors on the cell surface. The TLR pathway also plays an important role in lipoprotein uptake and macrophage activation. The fatty streak develops as these lipoprotein-laden macrophages, or foam cells, become engorged. At the same time, the activated macrophages present antigens to lymphocytes within the atheroma and express enzymes that function in lipoprotein metabolism, extracellular matrix degradation, and the

coagulation cascade. Though the macrophages initially enter the injured subendothelium to phagocytize lipoproteins and other foreign material, these cells eventually contribute to lesion expansion and vessel wall injury. The central role for macrophages in inflammation points to possible targets of specific macrophage-activating molecules for prevention of atheroma formation.[25]

CONCLUSION

Macrophages are essential cells for both the innate and the adaptive immune responses. These versatile cells act in all stages of the inflammatory response to defend against foreign molecules.

Key Points

1. The host response to infection comprises two major pathways: the innate response, which provides for the initial recognition of the invasive stimulus and is mediated by cells such as monocytes/macrophages, and the adaptive pathway, which comprises B and T lymphocytes and leads to the production of specific antibody and T-cell memory.
2. Initial microbial recognition proceeds by a family of evolutionarily conserved pattern recognition receptors. These include the Toll-like receptors and nucleotide-binding oligomerization domain proteins, which recognize pathogen-associated molecular patterns that access the endocytic and intracellular compartments of innate cells.
3. The macrophage is a versatile innate cell that functions to recognize pathogen-associated molecular patterns, mount the initial antimicrobial effector response, and coordinate the ensuing adaptive response.
4. The macrophage is a rich source of cytokines, or immunological hormones, that act at both local and systemic levels to regulate the host inflammatory response.
5. An excessive or dysregulated macrophage activation response can lead to diverse inflammatory sequelae, which include not only acute complications such as septic shock but also chronic conditions such as atherosclerosis.

Key References

1. Janeway CA, Travers P, Walport M, Shlomchik M: Immunobiology: The Immune System in Health and Disease, 6th ed. New York, Garland, 2005.
6. Gordon S, Taylor PR: Monocyte and macrophage heterogeneity. Nat Rev Immunol 2005;5:953-964.
19. Inohara N, Nuñez G: NODs: intracellular proteins involved in inflammation and apoptosis. Nat Rev Immunol 2003;3:371-382.
22. Serhan CN, Savill J: Resolution of inflammation: The beginning programs the end. Nat Immunol 2005;6:1191-1197.
25. Hansson GK: Inflammation, atherosclerosis, and coronary artery disease. N Engl J Med 2005;352:1685-1695.

See the companion Expert Consult website for the complete reference list.

CHAPTER 152

Alarm Phase Cytokines

Raghavan Murugan and Michael R. Pinsky

OBJECTIVES

This chapter will:
1. Describe interrelated pathways that underlie sepsis recognition by the host.
2. Characterize the link between various cytokines and sepsis syndromes.
3. Illustrate the mechanisms and networks of activation, function, and downregulation of various pro-inflammatory and anti-inflammatory cytokines during sepsis.

Sepsis, a systemic inflammatory response to infection, is currently the leading cause of death among critically ill patients. In the United States alone, approximately 750,000 cases of sepsis occur each year, at least 225,000 of which are fatal.[1] Despite the use of antimicrobial agents and advanced life-support care, the case fatality rate for patients with sepsis has remained between 30% and 40% for the past 3 decades. Several billions of dollars have been spent in efforts to improve the survival of patients with sepsis. However, results have been disappointing, and many observers argue that knowledge of the underlying pathophysiology of this syndrome is grossly insufficient.

Sepsis triggers an inflammatory response that involves an expression of a complex network of cytokines, coagulation factors, and other mediators. Nonsurvivors of sepsis exhibit a persistent elevation of cytokines that correlates with the development and sustenance of multiple-system organ failure.[2] However, attempts at downregulating the inflammatory response with novel agents directed at specific pro-inflammatory cytokines during early stages of severe sepsis have been associated with increased mortality.[3] This underscores the critical importance of cytokines for survival during early stages of severe sepsis. However, the increased expression of cytokines during sepsis is only part of this evolving immunological picture. In patients with severe sepsis, pro-inflammatory and anti-inflammatory stimuli coexist in the circulation in markedly increased amounts, and this paradoxical expression of mediator cytokines, when sustained, results in unregulated immune response, organ dysfunction, and death. Therefore, therapeutic strategies that uniformly modulate the induction of pro-inflammatory and anti-inflammatory cytokines at different time intervals of severe sepsis are current avenues of intense research. Obviously the success of such strategy would involve the understanding of the mechanisms of cytokine activation, such as genetic polymorphisms, timing of activation, their concentrations, their local and systemic effects, as well as their downregulation. This review explores some of the networks of various cytokines during sepsis as well as their role in the stressed host.

INFECTION RECOGNITION IN THE HOST

Microbial products that activate the innate immune system include both cell wall components and secreted proteins. Lipopolysaccharide (LPS), or bacterial endotoxin, forms a major portion of all gram-negative cell walls and is the most important product implicated in sepsis.[4] LPS binds to an acute-phase plasma protein known as LPS-binding protein (LBP), which transfers LPS to the cell surface receptor (CD14) found on the surface of monocytes, macrophages, and neutrophils.[5] LPS activity is modulated to a degree by a number of proteins, including bactericidal-permeability-increasing protein (BPI). BPI is produced by neutrophils and prevents LPS from binding to LBP. LPS-induced signal transduction begins with CD14-mediated activation of Toll-like receptor 4 (TLR4) (Fig. 152-1).[5] The sequence of the cytoplasmic domain of the Toll proteins is similar to that of the mammalian interleukin-1 (IL-1) receptor.[6] Both the IL-1 and Toll-like receptors induce signal-transduction pathways that lead to the activation of the major pro-inflammatory transcription factor, namely, nuclear factor-κB (NF-κB). The binding of LPS to CD14 leads to the association of CD14 with the TLR4-MD-2 complex with the activation of TLR4. TLR4 then activates a number of internal membrane–associated kinases, which leads to the activation of I κB kinase-1 and I κB kinase-2, which phosphorylate the inhibitory component of NF-κB, called I κBα, with the release of the active p50-p65 dimer of NF-κB. This p50-p65 NF-κB moiety translocates to the nucleus where it binds to multiple target promoter sites inducing transcriptional activation of a wide variety of inflammatory and immune response genes (see Fig. 152-1).[4] Sustained immune effector cell activation leads to a shedding of CD14, which can then bind to previously immune silent cell types. For example, LPS activation of cells such as endothelia, which do not express the membrane-bound CD14, can take place via soluble CD14. In addition, LPS activates both the classical and the alternative complement pathways, leading to the production of anaphylatoxins C3a and C5a and terminal C5b-9 complexes.

The cell wall of gram-positive bacteria contains a thick layer of peptidoglycan, which lies directly over the plasma membrane. Embedded in the peptidoglycan are molecules of lipoteichoic acid. In vitro studies have demonstrated that the structural components of the gram-positive cell walls are able to activate monocytes by the CD14 receptor–mediated NF-κB activation and the subsequent release of pro-inflammatory mediators.[7] Peptidoglycan and lipoteichoic acid may act synergistically in this process.[8] TLR2 has been implicated as the receptor for gram-positive and fungal cell-wall components and for bacterial, mycobacterial, and spirochetal lipoproteins.[9] Even though peptidoglycan is considerably less potent than LPS, the similarity of clinical response to invasive infection by

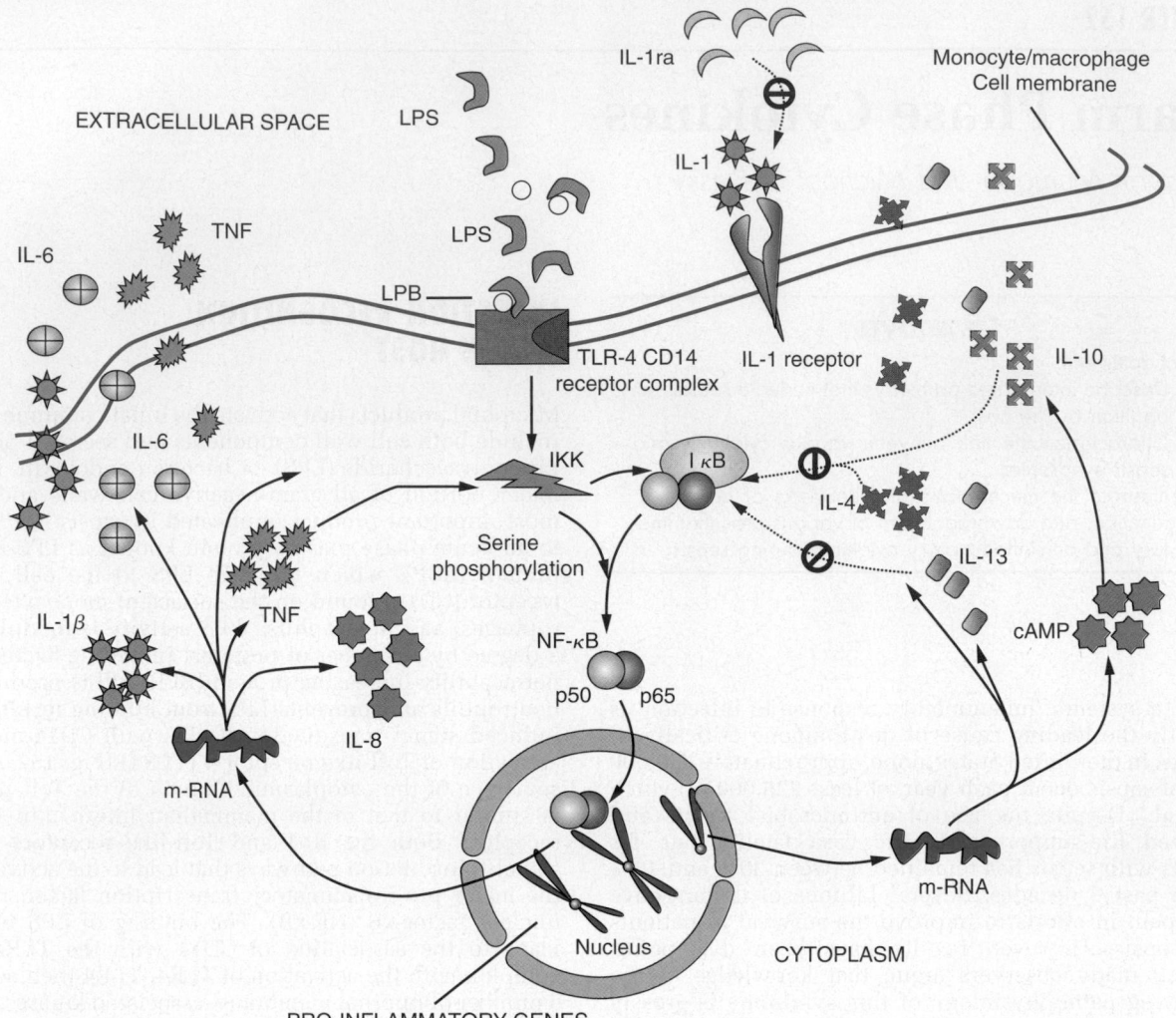

FIGURE 152-1. Schematic illustration of various cytokine networks in sepsis syndrome linked through nuclear factor-κB. cAMP, cyclic adenosine monophosphate; I κB, inhibitory κB; IKK, inhibitory κ kinase; IL, interleukin; IL-1ra, interleukin-1 receptor antagonist; LBP, lipopolysaccharide-binding protein; LPS, lipopolysaccharide; mRNA, messenger ribonucleic acid; NF-κB, nuclear factor-κB; TLR4, Toll-like receptor 4; TNF, tumor necrosis factor.

gram-positive and gram-negative bacteria is due to bacterial recognition via similar Toll-like receptors (TLR2 and TLR4, respectively).

ROLE OF NUCLEAR FACTOR-κB

Although many interrelated pathways and promoters induce intracellular signal transduction from external stimuli, including STAT, JNK, and AKT (Fig. 152-2), the primary promoter of the pro-inflammatory response is the transcription factor NF-κB. NF-κB activation is central to immune effector cell activation. Endotoxin LPS can induce the initial steps of signal transduction up to NF-κB, but NF-κB activation is required for subsequent intracellular signaling. The NF-κB family is composed of various members, p50 (NF-κB1), p52 (NF-κB2), p65 (RelA), RelB, and c-Rel, which can form homodimers and heterodimers.[10] The p65 subunit has the most variability, with a common variation being the RelA subunit substitution for p65. The phosphorylation of the inhibitory IκB-α subunit of the NF-κB complex following intracellular oxidative stress frees the dimer to translocate into the nucleus.[11] LPS induces IκB-α phosphorylation through activation of the inhibitory κ kinase (IKK).[12] The phosphorylated IκB-α is rapidly degraded by proteasomes. Processes that inhibit IκB-α phosphorylation, such as 4-hydroxynoneal, prevent NF-κB activation.[13] The p65 moiety has a DNA-binding domain that allows it to bind to numerous specific DNA sites throughout the genome, regulating gene transcription for most, if not all, of the pro-inflammatory species, including TNF, IL-1β, inducible nitric oxide synthase,[14] lipoxygenase, and cyclooxygenase 2 (see Fig. 152-1).[15] IκB-α is a heat shock protein, and its increased synthesis also downregulates NF-κB activation by dissociating the p50-p65 heterodimer from its responsive elements on the genome and keeping it in an inactive form in the cytoplasm.[16] The pro-inflammatory nuclear regulatory protein NF-κB is thus a major player in the previously mentioned innate immune response and a potential target for modulation.

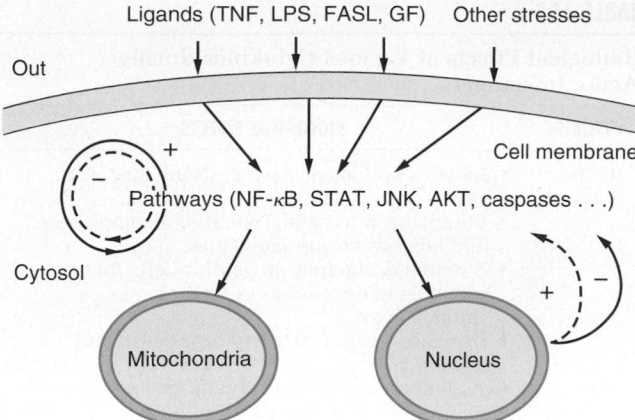

FIGURE 152-2. Sample pathways currently induced in a parallel fashion by inflammation, which induce pro-inflammatory responses, anti-inflammatory responses, and apoptosis. FASL, fas ligand; GF, growth factor; JNK, Jun kinase; LPS, lipopolysaccharide; NF-κB, nuclear factor-κB; STAT, signal transducers and activators of transcription; TNF, tumor necrosis factor.

TABLE 152-1

Proteins Induced by Tumor Necrosis Factor and Interleukin-1β Activation through Nuclear Factor-κB

- Intercellular adhesion molecule-1
- Endothelial leukocyte adhesion molecule
- Tissue factor
- Urokinase-type plasminogen activator
- Plasminogen activator inhibitor-1
- Pro-inflammatory cyokines
- IL-6 and IL-8
- Anti-inflammatory cytokines
- IL-4, IL-10, IL-1 receptor antagonist
- Secretory phospholipase A2
- Inducible nitric oxide synthase
- Cyclooxygenase 2

IL, interleukin.

CYTOKINE INDUCTION

Cytokines are low-molecular-weight proteins that are synthesized de novo in response to a specific external stimulus such as infection or tissue injury. Cytokines act in an autocrine, paracrine, and/or endocrine fashion to influence a broad range of cellular functions. These proteins are very potent, with biological effects observed in the picomolar–nanomolar range. Because of their temporal appearance and physiological consequences, cytokines have been generally classified as pro-inflammatory or anti-inflammatory. This categorization is unfortunate because many cytokines demonstrate both pro-inflammatory and anti-inflammatory effects. Cytokine signaling appears to function in most conditions as a local process, wherein local injury or infection induces a local inflammatory response. However, once these cytokines gain access to the bloodstream in levels capable of inducing a systemic response, their specific adaptive inflammatory response may be lost since the response is not compartmentalized or specific to the initiating site. Similarly, since cytokine activation and action occur on a cell-to-cell signaling level, blood levels of these cytokines may not reflect tissue levels or tissue effects. During critical illness, small changes in the inflammatory response have important clinical effects in patients. Development of organ failure and mortality have been shown to correlate more with the duration of inflammation rather than the peak concentrations of mediators in patients with sepsis.[2] On the contrary, a rapid downregulation and clearance of inflammatory mediators are associated with increased survival.[2]

THE PRO-INFLAMMATORY AND ANTI-INFLAMMATORY CYTOKINES

Cytokines activate and regulate T and B lymphocytes and mediate many of the manifestations of the inflammatory response (Table 152-1). They are produced by a wide variety of hematopoietic and nonhematopoietic cells. The cytokines are conveniently divided into three groups: (1) immunoregulatory cytokines that are involved in the activation, growth, and differentiation of lymphocytes, monocytes, and leukocytes (e.g., interleukin-2 [IL-2], interleukin-3 [IL-3], and interleukin-4 [IL-4]); (2) pro-inflammatory cytokines that are produced predominantly by mononuclear phagocytes in response to infectious agents (e.g., interleukin-1β [IL-1β], tumor necrosis factor-α [TNF-α], interleukin-6 [IL-6], and interleukin-8 [IL-8]); and (3) the anti-inflammatory cytokines (e.g., IL-4, IL-6, interleukin-10 [IL-10], interleukin-13 [IL-13], and transforming growth factor-β). Some cytokines, such as IL-4 and IL-6, have overlapping actions.

Cytokines exert their effects at low concentrations via highly specific interactions with cell surface receptors. Cytokine receptor molecules are predominantly integral plasma membrane glycoproteins with up to three distinct domains. First, there is a recognition domain that protrudes from the plasma membrane and confers specificity with regard to ligand binding. Second, there is a hydrophobic region that spans the plasma lipid bilayer. Third is the cytoplasmic domain, which is located on the inner surface of the plasma membrane and has intrinsic enzyme activity. All the cytokine receptors are associated with one or more members of the Janus kinases. These kinases couple ligand binding to tyrosine phosphorylation of various known signaling proteins and a unique family of transcription factors termed the *signal transducers and activators of transcription (STATs)* (see Fig. 152-2).[17]

LINK BETWEEN CYTOKINE RESPONSE AND SEPSIS SYNDROME

The concept that cytokines play a pivotal role in the pathogenesis of sepsis is made on the basis of several lines of evidence. First, intravenous administration of cytokines (TNF-α, IL-1) induces a septic shock–like syndrome in animals or human beings. Second, inhibition of the effects of some cytokines (TNF-α, IL-1) by administration of neutralizing antibodies, soluble cytokine receptors, or receptor antagonists attenuates sepsis in animal models. Third, administration of anti-inflammatory cytokines, such as IL-10, mitigates severe sepsis in animals. And fourth, plasma levels of cytokines (TNF-α, IL-1, IL-6, IL-8, and macrophage migration inhibition factor), both in experimental models of sepsis and in human beings, generally reflect the severity of the septic insult. Further evidence that cytokines are essential for the manifestations of sepsis is evident from genetic knockout models. TNF-deficient mice are resistant to the lethality of LPS.[18] Transgenic TNF-R55 knockout mice do not display hemodynamic or systemic immune alterations to intravenous LPS.[19]

Monocytes, macrophages, and CD4+ helper T (T_H) cells are the most important sources of cytokines. CD4+ T_H cells develop into two distinct subsets: T_H1 and T_H2 cells. T_H1 cells (type 1 helper T cells) secrete IL-2, TNF-β, and interferon-γ (IFN-γ) and are the principal effectors of cell-mediated immunity against intracellular microbes. T_H2 cells (type 2 helper T cells), on the other hand, secrete IL-4, IL-5, IL-10, and IL-13, which largely inhibit macrophage function.[20] A number of factors play a role in driving native CD4+ T cells toward T_H1 or T_H2 cells, including antigen-presenting cells, hormones, and cytokines. Glucocorticoids enhance T_H2 activity and synergize with IL-4, whereas dehydroepiandrosterone and IFN-γ enhance T_H1 activity.[21]

THE CYTOKINE RESPONSE

Tumor Necrosis Factor

In patients with sepsis, TNF is the first pro-inflammatory cytokine that is released, followed by IL-1β, IL-6, and IL-8 (see Fig. 152-1).[22] TNF and IL-1β are the most important pro-inflammatory cytokines; they are biologically closely related, act synergistically, and are largely responsible for the clinical manifestations of sepsis such as capillary leak, hypotension, acute respiratory distress syndrome, and multiple-organ failure.[23] Binding of TNF and IL-1 to their cellular receptors induces activation and generation of a number of secondary messengers, such as G proteins, adenyl cyclase, phospholipase A_2 and C, and oxygen-free radicals. In addition, a number of genes are transcribed, including those that code for most if not all of the known inflammatory processes (Table 152-2). The production of TNF is tightly controlled to prevent excessive activity of this potentially toxic molecule. Transcription of TNF is regulated by nuclear transcription factors such as NF-κB and is suppressed by short-lived repressors. Furthermore, the messenger ribonucleic acid (mRNA) transcripts of the TNF gene have a relatively short half-life compared to other transcripts. Differences in the regulatory sequences of the TNF gene may potentially influence the response of TNF after a microbial challenge.

In patients with severe sepsis, genomic polymorphism within the TNF locus has been found to be associated with TNF production and patient outcome.[24] A variety of agents are known to modulate the biosynthesis of TNF by macrophages. Norepinephrine, platelet-activating factor, granulocyte-monocyte colony-stimulating factor, C5a, engagement of CD11b/CD18, and nitric oxide may enhance the synthesis of TNF, whereas agents that increase intracellular cyclic adenosine monophosphate, such as β-agonists, prostaglandin E_2 (PGE_2), and phosphodiesterase inhibitors, decrease TNF mRNA in response to LPS.[25]

As described earlier, several single nucleotide polymorphisms within the regulatory region of the gene coding for TNF have been identified that are associated with both spontaneous and stimulated TNF production in vitro, in vivo, or both.[26] These include a G-to-A transition at -308

TABLE 152-2

Biological Effects of Various Cytokines during Acute Infections

CYTOKINE	BIOLOGICAL EFFECTS
IL-1β	• Induces cyclooxygenase 2, iNOS, and PGE_2 expression • Stimulates release of TNF, IL-6, chemokines, and other adhesion molecules • Stimulates myeloid progenitor cells thereby inducing neutrophilia, as well as thrombocytosis • Decreases response to erythropoietin and anemia
TNF	• Activates macrophages, lymphocytes, neutrophils, eosinophils, fibroblasts, osteoclasts, chondrocytes, endothelial cells, and nerve cells • Induces the expression of ICAM-1, ELAM, VACAM-1 • Activates cyclooxygenase 2, phospholipase A2, NO synthase, PAF, PGE_2, PGI_2, NO • Activates complements • Induces release of IL-1, IL-6, IL-8, MCP-1, IL-4, IL-10, IL-1ra, PDGF, IL2, Endothelin-1, PAI • Downregulates thrombomodulin • Increases the expression of surface adhesion molecules, C3bi receptors, L-selectin, superoxide production, and phagocytosis
IL-6	• Regulates synthesis of ACTH in pituitary gland and neuronal growth factor • Activates Janus kinase/signal transducer and mitogen-activated protein kinase cascades through binding of gp130 receptor molecules • Induces thrombosis by enhancing the release of von Willebrand's factor fragments, and inhibiting its cleaving protease • Induces gut barrier dysfunction
IL-10	• Downregulates TNF and other pro-inflammatory cytokines • Causes T cell anergy, suppresses T-cell and T_H1 proliferation • Induced T- and B-cell apoptosis • Causes defects in antigen presentation and induces macrophage "paralysis"

ACTH, adrenocorticotropic hormone; ELAM, endothelial leukocyte adhesion molecule; ICAM-1, intercellular adhesion molecule-1; IL, interleukin; IL-1ra, interleukin-1 receptor antagonist; iNOS, inducible nitric oxide synthase; MCP-1, membrane cofactor protein-1; NO, nitric oxide; PAF, platelet-activating factor; PAI, plasminogen activator inhibitor; PDGF, platelet-derived growth factor; PGE_2, prostaglandin E_2; PGI_2, prostaglandin I_2; T_H1, type 1 helper T cell; TNF, tumor necrosis factor; VACAM-1, vascular cell adhesion molecule-1.

(upstream from the transcriptional start site for the TNF gene). A strong association also has been made between the TNF polymorphisms and clinical presentation, outcome, or both, in a variety of infectious diseases. These include cerebral malaria,[27] human immunodeficiency virus dementia in adults,[28] septic shock in adults,[29] and community-acquired pneumonia in adults.[30]

Interleukin-1 and Interleukin-1 Receptor Antagonist

The IL-1 family consists of three structurally related polypeptides: IL-1α, IL-β, and the interleukin receptor antagonist (IL-1ra). IL-1α and IL-1β are the key pro-inflammatory cytokines secreted early in the response to a bacterial challenge and play an important role in the pathogenesis of sepsis and septic shock. These molecules stimulate the production of prostaglandins and nitric oxide, two mediators of the vasodilation observed in sepsis.[31] IL-1β also increases the expression of nearly all other cytokines, including TNF, IL-6, and the chemokines, as well as adhesion molecules. In contrast, IL-1ra is an inhibitor that acts via competing with IL-1 for binding to its receptor (see Fig. 152-1).[32] Serum levels of IL-1β and IL-1ra are elevated in patients with meningococcal disease and appear to be higher in those with more severe disease.[33]

The genes coding for IL-1α, IL-1β, and IL-1ra are clustered together on chromosome 2, and several polymorphisms have been described in this locus.[34] Several of these polymorphisms have been examined for association with susceptibility to and outcome from sepsis, and the polymorphism most studied is the A2 allele in the IL-1ra gene. A higher frequency of the A2 allele in Caucasian adults with severe sepsis places these patients at a greater risk for mortality once sepsis has developed.[35,36]

Interleukin-6

IL-6 is a key pro-inflammatory cytokine that is stimulated by TNF and IL-1 in response to endotoxin by the monocytes and fibroblasts. Various viruses (including HIV) and a variety of other molecules, such as IL-2, interferon-γ, platelet-derived growth factor, protein kinase C, and agents that increase intracellular cyclic adenosine monophosphate levels, induce IL-6 production (see Fig. 152-1). Molecules such as IL-1, TNF, and IL-2 induce IL-6 expression. In contrast, IL-4 and IL-13 inhibit IL-6 production. Since IL-6 persists in the plasma much longer than any other cytokine, it is a useful marker of pro-inflammatory cytokine activation. Numerous studies have shown an association between mean plasma IL-6 concentrations over time and mortality rate. Persistent elevations in IL-6 appear to be more important than initial or peak levels in terms of outcome associations.[2] Plasma IL-6 concentrations have been directly correlated with risk of death in intra-abdominal sepsis, and measurements of this single variable predicted outcome in these cases with remarkable (82.9%) accuracy.[37] There is mounting evidence that neutralizing anti-IL-6 antibody is beneficial in various experimental models of sepsis, including nonhuman primates. However, although anti-IL-6 monoclonal antibody attenuated coagulation activation in experimental endotoxemia in chimpanzees, it had no impact on (low-dose) endotoxin-induced coagulation activation in humans.[38] Therefore, it is currently unknown whether anti-IL-6 monoclonal antibody would be useful in human sepsis.

The promoter region for IL-6 has been shown to have several single nucleotide polymorphisms.[39] The best studied of these polymorphisms is a relatively common regulatory polymorphism comprising a G-to-C substitution at position -174 in the promoter region. In healthy adults, the G allele is associated with higher basal serum levels of IL-6.[40] However, in septic adult surgical patients, there was no association between the genotypes and serum levels of IL-6, nor was there a significant difference in genotype distribution between critically ill patients and healthy controls or between patients with sepsis and patients without sepsis.[41] This would suggest that the IL-6 G-174C polymorphism is not associated with an increased susceptibility to sepsis.

Interleukin-10

IL-10 is a key anti-inflammatory cytokine that is expressed and secreted by a variety of cell types, including T cells, monocytes/macrophages, dendritic cells, and epithelial cells, usually after an activation stimulus, but its expression is differentially regulated by the various cell types that secrete it.[42] Functionally, IL-10 acts on a wide variety of cells, including B cells, natural killer cells, cytotoxic and helper T cells, mast cells, granulocytes, dendritic cells, keratinocytes, and endothelial cells. More recent evidence suggests that IL-10 plays a role in the generation and action of regulatory dendritic cells and T cells.[43] Experimental studies of bacteremic or endotoxemic shock in rodents and primates have revealed that the primary inducers of systemic IL-10 release are proximal pro-inflammatory cytokines, such as TNF and IL-1. When administered to healthy adults, TNF induces a monophasic IL-10 response, which is characterized by a peak in the IL-10 level 45 minutes after the administration of TNF.[44] Thus, IL-10 production can be a direct consequence of the more proximal pro-inflammatory cytokine response, predominantly the release of TNF, and the subsequent endogenous production of IL-10 acts as an endogenous counterregulatory mechanism to suppress endogenous TNF production.[45] Because of this feedback loop involving IL-10 and more proximal pro-inflammatory cytokines, it was suggested that pretreatment with IL-10 might prevent the pro-inflammatory response and subsequent endogenous IL-10 production.

The potent anti-inflammatory effects of IL-10 suggest that this cytokine might play a crucial role in both the resolution and pathogenesis of acute illnesses in critical care settings. Similar reasoning also provided the justification for administering IL-10 to patients early in the propagation of an inflammatory response. However, IL-10 is endogenously expressed in animals and patients with sepsis syndrome, and concentrations of IL-10 often indicate the magnitude of the inflammatory response. Several studies characterized the IL-10 response in patients with sepsis syndromes.[46,47] These studies showed that IL-10 concentrations in the blood vary greatly, typically being between 12 and 2400 pg/mL, but sometimes exceeding 20,000 pg/mL. The concentration of IL-10 is higher in patients with septic shock than in patients with sepsis and correlates strongly with concentrations of circulating TNF in septic patients.[46,47]

CYTOKINE EFFECTS AND DOWNREGULATION

After the release of IL-1 and TNF, the anti-inflammatory cytokines IL-4, IL-10, and IL-13, and transforming growth factor-β are released into the circulation. The production of anti-inflammatory cytokines is associated with a switch from T_H1 to T_H2 activation. The anti-inflammatory cytokines suppress the expression of the genes for IL-1 and TNF-α. In addition, these cytokines inhibit antigen presentation by monocytes as well as T- and B-lymphocyte function. The role of the anti-inflammatory cytokines is to keep the inflammatory response in check. In most infected persons, the body is able to achieve a balance between pro-inflammatory and anti-inflammatory mediators, and homeostasis is restored. In some patients, however, this balance is upset, resulting in systemic inflammatory response syndrome and multiple-organ dysfunction syndrome if the pro-inflammatory process is excessive.[48] If the compensatory anti-inflammatory response is excessive, it will manifest clinically as anergy with an increased susceptibility to infection. Bone[48] has called this the "compensatory anti-inflammatory response syndrome," as it probably represents the normal balance of response to any initial pro-inflammatory stimulus. In addition to activating a pro-inflammatory cytokine cascade, inflammatory stimuli activate the production of specific cytokine-neutralizing molecules, which include cytokine receptors and cytokine receptor antagonists. Soluble cytokine receptors result from proteolytic cleavage of the extracellular binding domain of the receptors, which are then released into the circulation.[49] Soluble cytokine receptors have been identified for both the p75 and p55 TNF receptors and the IL-1 and IL-6 receptors. The release of surface receptors may downregulate the receptors, reducing cell responsiveness, with circulating receptors acting as a buffer for the free cytokines in circulation

CONCLUSIONS

Sepsis triggers a local inflammatory response that is proportional to the severity of the insult. This local inflammatory response is then propagated systemically by induction of a network of cytokines. Some of these cytokines, in turn, inhibit the inflammatory response, which is modulated by a variety of factors such as the genetic susceptibility of the host. Duration of cytokine response is therefore instrumental in determining critical illness severity, duration, and recovery. In this regard, altered levels of some of these mediators are associated with development of organ failure and death. Clearly, the interrelated stimuli, causing selective and time-dependent pro-inflammatory or anti-inflammatory responses and the multiple parallel, reciprocating, and redundant pathways make specific pharmacological blockade of one or a series of specific cytokines of questionable clinical significance. Restoration of the normal cellular and metabolic processes rather than either blockade or stimuli of specific pathways

represents a proven and logical therapeutic approach. It is still unknown whether cytokines are a marker, a cause, or a cure for sepsis.

Key Points

1. An initial inflammatory response is essential for survival during early stages of sepsis.
2. However, persistence of both pro-inflammatory and anti-inflammatory cytokines over time is associated with increased organ dysfunction and mortality.
3. Relationship between cytokine activation, persistence, and downregulation is complex and depends on a number of factors, including genetic control.
4. Modulation of specific cytokines by either pharmacological blockade or stimulation during sepsis is not associated with improved survival.

Key References

2. Pinsky MR, Vincent JL, Deviere J, et al: Serum cytokine levels in human septic shock. Relation to multiple-system organ failure and mortality. Chest 1993;103(2):565-575.
4. Medzhitov R, Janeway C Jr: Innate Immunity. N Engl J Med 2000;343(5):338-344.
14. Taylor BS, de Vera ME, Ganster RW, et al: Multiple NF-kappaB enhancer elements regulate cytokine induction of the human inducible nitric oxide synthase gene. J Biol Chem 1998;273(24):15148-15156.
30. Waterer GW, Quasney MW, Cantor RM, Wunderink RG: Septic shock and respiratory failure in community-acquired pneumonia have different TNF polymorphism associations. Am J Respir Crit Care Med 2001;163(7):1599-1604.
44. van der Poll T, Jansen J, Levi M, et al: Regulation of interleukin-10 release by tumor necrosis factor in humans and chimpanzees. J Exp Med 1994;180(5):1985-1988.

See the companion Expert Consult website for the complete reference list.

CHAPTER 153

The Role of Complement in Sepsis

J. Vidya Sarma and Peter A. Ward

OBJECTIVES

This chapter will:
1. Discuss the derangements in innate immunity that occur as a consequence of excessive complement activation during sepsis.
2. Discuss the role that C5a-C5aR signaling pathways play in sepsis.
3. Discuss how the cecal ligation and puncture rodent model of sepsis has helped uncover the C5a-induced pathophysiology of sepsis.

The complement system consists of more than 30 soluble and cell membrane–bound proteins and is integral to the host defense arsenal as part of the innate immune system. The name *complement* was first used when it was initially identified as a heat-sensitive serum factor that complemented or augmented bactericidal activity of heat-stable antibodies also present in the serum.[1-2] It appears to be evolutionarily conserved, since many of the components of the complement system or their homologues are found in invertebrates and vertebrates, including mammals, suggesting that complement evolved long ago as part of the

COMPLEMENT ACTIVATION PATHWAYS

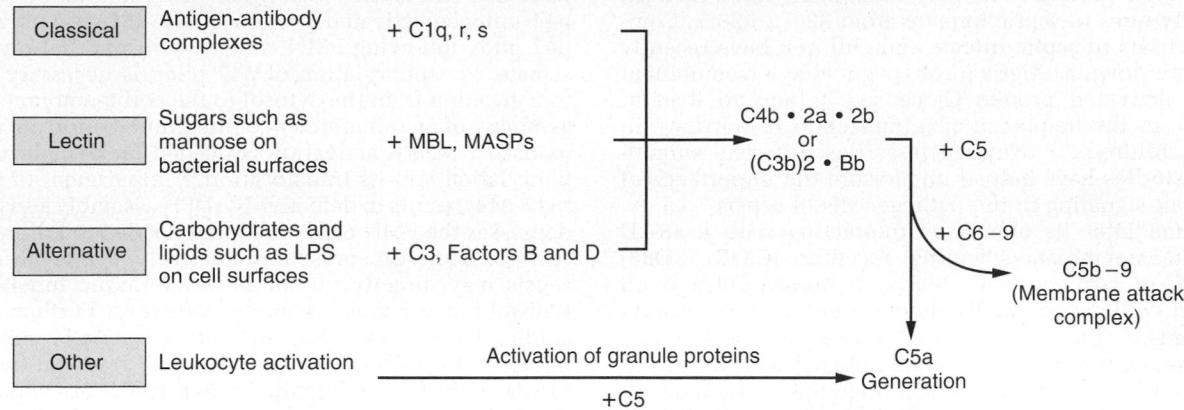

FIGURE 153-1. Generation of the anaphylatoxin C5a. C5a generation occurs via three complement activation pathways: the classical, lectin, and alternate pathways. In addition, C5a can also be generated by other proteases that can cleave complement components such as C5. LPS, lipopolysaccharide; MBL, mannose-binding lectin; MASPs, MBL-associated serine proteases.

host defense system to help maintain homeostasis.[3] As a response to triggering stimuli, the complement system is activated and, similar to other systems such as the coagulation or clotting system, an amplified cascade of sequentially acting proteases is initiated, culminating in the formation of the powerful phlogistic anaphylatoxins C3a and C5a and the membrane attack complex that causes bacterial lysis. C3a and C5a are generated via three different activation pathways: the classical, the alternative and the mannose-binding lectin (MBL) pathways[1-2] (Fig. 153-1). In addition, C5a can be generated by a protease released from activated macrophages or neutrophils (polymorphonuclear leukocyte [PMN]).[4] C5 chemotactic fragments can also be generated by trypsin and trypsin-like enzymes.[5]

The classical pathway was one of the first to be discovered and is activated by antigen-antibody complexes containing either IgG or IgM.[1] The alternate pathway is activated by lipid- and carbohydrate-containing molecules derived from cell surfaces. The lectin pathway was the most recent to be discovered and is initiated upon recognition of sugars found on the bacterial cell surface, such as mannose. This results in activation of MBL-associated serine proteases (MASPs), which can then generate C3a and C5a. C3a and C5a exert myriad functions, including chemotaxis of leukocytes, histamine release from mast cells, and smooth muscle contraction.[6] As a rule, the generation of C3a and C5a is tightly regulated, but when dysregulation occurs in conditions such as sepsis, these anaphylatoxins are persistently elevated[7] to the detriment of the patient, who then is at risk of developing multiple-organ failure (MOF) and a poor prognosis of survival. Although C5a has been implicated in playing a significant role in many inflammatory disorders (including asthma, acute respiratory distress syndrome, and ischemia-reperfusion injury), the role of C5a in the particularly insidious problem of sepsis is the subject of this review.

Sepsis is rapidly becoming a major health burden in North America. More than 700,000 cases occur each year in the United States,[8] with the numbers continuously increasing, probably due to the fact that the population is aging (with concomitant immunosuppression), and with better medical care many patients are subjected to invasive surgical procedures. There are also many more patients

TABLE 153-1

Human Sepsis Definitions

SIRS	Hyperresponsive state due to release of pro-inflammatory mediators in the absence of obvious infection
Sepsis	SIRS with infection
Severe sepsis	Sepsis with MOF
Septic shock	Severe sepsis with hypotension

MOF, multiple-organ failure; SIRS, systemic inflammatory response syndrome.

who are immune compromised as a result of cancer immunotherapy. In many instances, sepsis results in death associated with MOF, especially renal failure and cardiac and lung dysfunction. Sepsis is a complex clinical syndrome that develops in response to insult or infection related to intact bacteria or their breakdown products such as lipopolysaccharide (LPS), lipoteichoic acid, or peptidoglycan containing gram-positive bacteria that can release exotoxins (as in toxic shock syndrome related to *Staphylococcus aureus*) and fungal infections, often resulting in an uncontrolled inflammatory response with the release of pro-inflammatory mediators such as C3a, C5a, interleukin-1 (IL-1), interleukin-6 (IL-6), tumor necrosis factor-α (TNF-α), and others. Debatable is the issue of the release of anti-inflammatory mediators such as IL-4 and IL-10 as an anti-compensatory mechanism at a later time point in sepsis. However, in many patients, presence of microorganisms (bacteremia) and LPS in the blood (endotoxemia) cannot be detected.[9] Therefore, the term *systemic inflammatory response syndrome* (SIRS) was agreed upon when a hyperresponsive state due to release of pro-inflammatory mediators was seen in patients in the absence of obvious infection. Further, as shown in Table 153-1, SIRS with infection is referred to as *sepsis*; sepsis with MOF as *severe sepsis*; and severe sepsis with hypotension as *septic shock*.

Various animal models of sepsis have been utilized to help elucidate the derangements of inflammatory responses that occur during sepsis.[10] However, these findings have not translated into efficacious therapeutic interventions in human clinical trials except for one, where administration of activated protein C or its recombinant form reduced mortality rates in septic humans from 38% to 28%. Companion trials in septic infants and children have recently been shut down as Xigris (drotrecogin alfa, a recombinant human activated protein C) caused a four- to fivefold increase in the frequency of intracerebral hemorrhage in septic children.[11-12] Nevertheless, the different animal-model studies have helped underscore the importance of C5a-C5aR signaling in the pathogenesis of sepsis.

C5a mediates its effects by interacting with a 45-kD seven-transmembrane-spanning receptor (C5aR, CD88) that is G-protein coupled. C5aR is expressed not only on myeloid cells (as originally thought) but also on nonmyeloid cells.[13] The recently described C5L2 receptor for C5a is also seven-transmembrane-spanning but does not signal via G-proteins because of a mutation in one of the intracellular loops.[14-15] Because of this lack of signaling, it is thought to be a default receptor, although its function has yet to be determined. C5L2 is expressed on a wide variety of cells including neutrophils (PMNs) and dendritic cells.

BLOCKADE OF C5a-C5aR INTERACTION IN SEPSIS

Early studies relying on a primate model of sepsis gave the first hint of the importance of C5a-C5aR signaling in sepsis. Septic shock and acute respiratory distress syndrome induced in monkeys by massive infusions of live *Escherichia coli* could be attenuated by the administration of anti-C5a antibodies.[16] C5a infusion into rats can mimic LPS-induced shock.[17] Anti-C5a antibodies can reduce the development of LPS-induced shock in both rodents and monkeys. The cecal ligation and puncture (CLP) model in rodents (with its limitations[10]) to study sepsis closely mimics the pathophysiology of human sepsis. In this model, studies have shown that blockade of C5a with anti-C5a antibodies[18] or blockade of C5aR with a C5aR antagonist (C5aRa)[19] significantly improved survival rates. At the same time, anti-C5a treatment prevented development of MOF and preserved the H_2O_2-producing capacity of blood PMNs.[20] Further, blockade of C5aR with antibodies resulted in reduction in blood TNF-α and IL-6 levels when compared to animals that had undergone sham surgery.[21] In the same study, C5aR expression was found to be upregulated in many organs (heart, kidney, liver, and lung) during the early phase of sepsis. Blockade of C5aR also dramatically improved survival with significant reduction in the colony-forming units of bacteria in the kidneys and lung.

SEPSIS-INDUCED IMPAIRED SIGNALING IN POLYMORPHONUCLEAR LEUKOCYTES

Recent studies have shown that blood PMNs obtained from CLP rats exhibited profound defects in innate immune responses.[22] There was a markedly decreased ability to generate H_2O_2, the phagocytic ability was lowered, and the cells were unable to chemotactically respond to either C5a or fMLP, suggesting a global impairment in signaling pathways. Interestingly, similar impairment was seen when normal PMNs were exposed in vitro to C5a levels found

in the blood of septic patients. Pre-incubation of PMNs with C5a results in blocking of phosphorylation of p42-p44 mitogen-activated protein kinase (MAPK) as well as p47 phox following PMN contact with phorbol myristate acetate. Phosphorylation of p47 phox is necessary for its translocation from the cytosol to the cell membrane in the assembly of nicotinamide adenine dinucleotide phosphate oxidase.[23] MAPK activation is needed for p47 phox phosphorylation and its translocation.[22] Impairment of MAPK (p42-p44) results in defective NADPH assembly and greatly depresses the PMN oxidative burst needed to kill ingested bacteria. Thus, C5a present in relatively high levels during sepsis may directly impair innate immune functions of PMNs by paralyzing signaling pathways. Further, recent studies have shown that not only is p42-p44 activation impaired in PMNs obtained from CLP rats, but also p38 MAPK activation is impaired when PMNs are exposed to C5a.[24] In contrast, alveolar macrophages obtained from CLP rats exhibit enhanced activation of both p42-p44 and p38 MAPKs. Thus, in experimental sepsis blood, PMNs have defective innate immune functions while tissue macrophages have enhanced immune functions. The impaired activation of the MAPKs seen in CLP PMNs affects their ability to produce the CXC chemokine, macrophage inflammatory protein-2 (MIP-2), which is a powerful PMN chemoattractant, whereas alveolar macrophages from CLP rodents are unaffected in MIP-2 production.[24] As a result, increased MIP-2 in lungs enhances lung PMN accumulation, setting the stage for PMN-mediated lung tissue injury during sepsis with C5a playing a pivotal role in this process.

EXPRESSION OF RECEPTORS FOR C5a DURING SEPSIS

In the CLP model of sepsis, C5aR expression on PMNs dramatically drops, reaching a nadir at 24 hours and slowly returning to normal levels thereafter in surviving rats.[25] This drop in expression can be linked to the increased systemic levels of C5a, in which C5aR on PMNs bind C5a, followed by internalization of C5a-C5aR complexes before being recycled to the cell surface. Blockade of C5a within CLP rats preserved C5aR expression on blood PMNs. Interestingly, the level of C5aR expression on PMN correlated with survival. Those animals that had higher overall expression survived longer, whereas 67% of the animals that had expression levels below the median did not survive. Thus, C5aR expression on blood PMNs could serve as a prognostic marker in the clinical setting. A recent examination of the expression of the second C5a receptor C5L2 on blood PMNs revealed that after CLP, there was an initial decrease followed by a gradual restoration of C5L2.[26] On the other hand, PMN expression of C5L2 in patients with septic shock was found to be virtually abolished, whereas survivors showed retained C5L2 expression on blood PMNs. It remains to be seen if C5L2 expression on PMNs can be used as a prognostic marker.

EFFECT OF C5a ON CELL APOPTOSIS DURING SEPSIS

Recent studies show that apoptosis has a significant role in sepsis.[27] Apoptosis helps to remove unwanted activated

PMNs from tissues and organs, reducing release of harmful products from PMNs that would injure organs. Significant decreases in PMN apoptosis have been observed in patients with SIRS when compared to PMNs from healthy patients.[28] Delayed apoptosis in lung PMNs has been observed after endotoxemia.[29] Recent studies showed that in CLP-induced septic rat PMNs, susceptibility to apoptosis could be restored by anti-C5a treatment of rats at the start of CLP.[30] Further, PMNs from CLP rats showed increased protein expression of the anti-apoptotic gene, *Bcl-xL.* In striking contrast, there were significantly reduced levels of Bcl-xL in thymocytes from CLP rats. Extensive thymocyte apoptosis is known to occur in rodents with sepsis, which may help explain the massive reduction in thymic mass. Bcl-xL levels were restored with blockade of C5a, suggesting that C5a effects on apoptosis may be cell specific depending upon the extent of C5aR expression on the cells. Studies in septic mice also suggest a relationship between lymphocyte apoptosis and development of immunosuppression.

C5a-MEDIATED CARDIAC DYSFUNCTION DURING SEPSIS

Cardiac dysfunction ("septic cardiomyopathy") often develops in patients with sepsis. This dysfunction puts septic patients at high risk of heart failure and death. MOF results from impaired cardiac function and decreased cardiac output, which leads to compromised tissue or organ perfusion, decreased oxygen and nutrient supply, ischemia, organ dysfunction, and a hyporeactive immune system. The degree of cardiac dysfunction is often decisive in determining survival or death during sepsis. Although altered Ca^{2+} homeostasis may contribute to defective cardiomyocyte contractility, the mechanisms underlying this dysfunction are poorly understood. The finding that C5aR expression increases in heart homogenates of CLP rats[21] prompted an investigation into the role of C5a in septic cardiomyopathy. The findings showed significant reductions in left ventricular pressures in vivo during sepsis and reduced cardiomyocyte contractility in vitro when individual cardiomyocytes were evaluated. Cardiac function was restored to levels found in sham animals when anti-C5a antibodies were administered at the beginning of CLP.[31] Further, increased expression of C5aR mRNA and protein was seen on single cardiomyocytes during the course of CLP-induced sepsis. When cardiomyocytes obtained from either sham or CLP rats were incubated with C5a in vitro, there was a profound decrease in contractility. Thus, these studies suggest a link between the interaction of C5a and C5aR on cardiomyocytes and the subsequent cardiac dysfunction that develops during sepsis. However, how C5a mediates this dysfunction remains to be determined.

C5a AND COAGULATION DURING SEPSIS

Sepsis is often accompanied by disseminated intravascular coagulation with thrombin formation and fibrin deposition in the microvasculature. The success with the anticoagulant, activated protein C (as described earlier in this chapter), in clinical trials suggests the importance of the coagulation pathway in the septic syndrome. In the CLP model, it has been shown that increased procoagulant activity and reduced platelet counts in blood, together with increased plasma fibrinogen levels and presence of fibrin split products, are significantly reduced in rats that had been given anti-C5a antibodies at the start of CLP as compared to animals that were administered irrelevant IgG.[32] Recently, it has been shown that C5a-C5aR interaction can induce tissue factor generation by PMNs. Tissue factor can activate the coagulation cascade by binding to factor VIIa, initiating the extrinsic coagulation pathway cascade.[33] Therefore, C5a production during sepsis may indirectly or directly lead to the disseminated intravascular coagulation that is often seen in sepsis.

CONCLUSION

Complement, especially C5a-C5aR interaction, appears to play a significant role in the pathophysiology of sepsis. Normally, complement maintains homeostasis and bacterial killing (and removal) as part of the innate host defense system. It is this attribute that bacteria like *Staphylococcus aureus* attempt to subvert by secreting proteins such as chemotaxis inhibitory protein of staphylococci (CHIPS) and staphylococcal complement inhibitor (SCIN) that prevent complement-mediated enhancement of host defenses.[34] CHIPS is a C5a receptor antagonist that can prevent chemotaxis. SCIN, on the other hand, can bind C4b2a and C3bBb and help stabilize C3 convertases, thereby preventing further C3b deposition and phagocytosis. However, when overexuberant complement activation occurs, as in sepsis, the resultant overproduction of C5a can harm the host with grave consequences (as described earlier). Although animal models have helped elucidate the complex pathophysiology of sepsis, more studies are needed to obtain clinically efficacious therapeutic interventions for the treatment of human sepsis.

Key Points

1. Excessive complement activation in sepsis results in elevated levels of the anaphylatoxins, especially C5a.
2. Excessive C5a-C5aR interaction occurring in sepsis, especially on neutrophils, can paralyze neutrophil innate immune functions, affect neutrophil and thymocyte apoptosis, induce cardiomyopathy, and directly or indirectly affect coagulation pathways.
3. Blockade of either C5a or C5aR in the cecal ligation and puncture model of sepsis in rodents largely abrogates results of C5a-C5aR interactions that impair innate immune functions (including neutrophil phagocytosis, chemotaxis, and the oxidative burst), induce neutrophil resistance to apoptosis, improve cardiomyocyte contractility, reduce disseminated intravascular coagulation, and dramatically improve survival in experimental sepsis.

Key References

1. Walport MJ: Complement. First of two parts. N Engl J Med 2001;344:1058-1066.

2. Guo RF, Ward PA: Role of C5a in inflammatory responses. Annu Rev Immunol 2005;23:821-852.
6. Ward PA: The dark side of C5a in sepsis. Nat Rev Immunol 2004;4:133-142.
10. Rittirsch D, Hoesel LM, Ward PA: The disconnect between animal models of sepsis and human sepsis. J Leukoc Biol 2007;81:137-143.

22. Huber-Lang MS, Younkin EM, Sarma JV, et al: Complement-induced impairment of innate immunity during sepsis. J Immunol 2002;169(6):3223-3231.

See the companion Expert Consult website for the complete reference list.

CHAPTER 154

Oxidative Stress in Acute Kidney Injury

Jonathan Himmelfarb and T. Alp Ikizler

OBJECTIVES

This chapter will:
1. Explain how increased oxidative stress contributes to the pathogenesis of renal tubular epithelial cell injury in ischemic and toxic animal models.
2. Review principles of biomarkers of oxidative stress status in human studies.
3. Review clinical data indicating increased renal and systemic oxidative stress in patients with acute kidney injury.
4. Elucidate the potential role of antioxidant therapy in preventing complications associated with acute kidney injury.

During normal physiological conditions, cellular metabolism results in the continuous formation of reactive oxygen species, a phenomenon that is counterbalanced by their detoxification and decomposition through endogenous antioxidant compounds. Antioxidants are a varied group of molecules with diverse functions, including proteins with specific catalytic properties, small water- and lipid-soluble chemical moieties with relatively nonspecific scavenging capacity, and metal chelating agents that inhibit oxidant production. As a rule, antioxidants control the prevailing relationship between reducing and oxidizing (redox) conditions and biological systems. In pathophysiological states, increased oxidative stress occurs when an imbalance develops between oxidant production and antioxidant defense. Reactive oxygen species were once regarded as virtually a medical curiosity; however, a large body of evidence now implicates them as important mediators of ischemic and toxic tissue injury.

Considerable experimental data point to increased oxidative stress as a contributor to renal tubular epithelial cell injury and resulting acute kidney injury (AKI). Furthermore, as uremia has now been unequivocally established as an increased oxidative stress state,[1] the resulting loss of kidney function in AKI may exacerbate systemic oxidative stress. Finally, increased systemic oxidative stress may contribute to the development and maintenance of the multiple-organ failure syndrome, thereby directly contributing to adverse outcomes in critically ill patients with AKI. This chapter reviews available data pointing to a critical role for increased oxidative stress in the pathogenesis and pathobiology of AKI.

WHAT IS OXIDATIVE STRESS?

Oxidative stress can be viewed as a disturbance in the balance between oxidant production and antioxidant defense. An imbalance in favor of prooxidants can lead to the oxidation of macromolecules, thereby resulting in tissue injury. Oxygen is ubiquitous in the environment, and the prooxidant status of an organism is at least partly dependent on the state of oxygenation of the organism or cell. In eukaryotes, oxidative processes occur predominantly within the mitochondria, and the mitochondrial cytochrome oxidase enzyme complex accounts for the majority of the oxygen humans metabolize. The cytochrome oxidase enzyme complex transfers four electrons to oxygen in a coordinated reaction that produces two molecules of water as a by-product. The enzyme complex contains four redox centers, each of which stores a single electron. The simultaneous reduction of the four redox centers results in the transfer of results in no detectable reactive oxygen intermediates and thereby limits the production of reactive oxygen species (Fig. 154-1A). Nevertheless, mitochondrial oxygen can leak through the electron transport chain, resulting in the formation of reactive oxygen intermediates and free radicals, which can then diffuse out of the mitochondria and be a source of oxidant stress (Fig. 154-1B).[2,3]

An additional important in vivo source of excess oxidants occurs through the action of another enzyme complex, nicotinamide adenine dinucleotide phosphate (NADPH) oxidase. NADPH oxidase is important within the endothelium and in phagocytic cells in the generation of reactive oxygen intermediates.[4,5] During an inflammatory response, phagocytes deliberately use high levels of oxygen and the generation of reactive oxygen intermediates for a host defense against pathogens via the respiratory burst. Phagocytes contain other enzymes (including superoxide

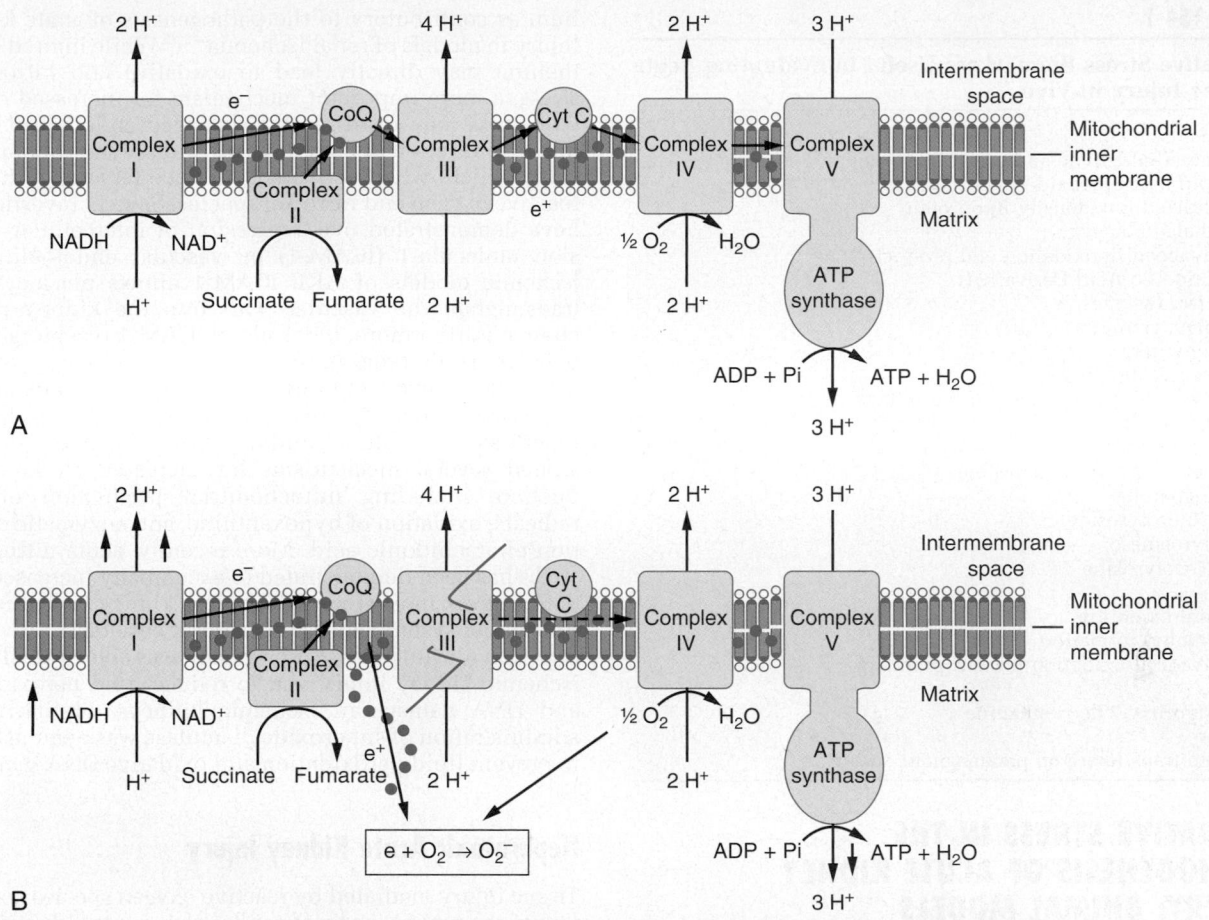

A

B

FIGURE 154-1. A, Coupled electron transport and oxidative phosphorylation in the mitochondria. **B,** Mitochondrial uncoupled electron transplant and reactive oxygen species leak. (**A** and **B,** Redrawn from Chew GT, Watts GF: Coenzyme Q10 and diabetic endotheliopathy: Oxidative stress and the "recoupling hypothesis." QJM 2004;97:537-548.)

dismutase, nitric oxide synthase, and myeloperoxidase), which also contribute to the production of hydrogen peroxide, nitric oxide, peroxynitrite, and hypochlorous acid, respectively (Fig. 154-2).[6,7] Recently a novel additional oxidative pathway within phagocytes has been described, whereby nitrite is converted to nitryl chloride and nitrogen dioxide via the myeloperoxidase enzyme or via hypochlorous acid.[8] Ozone derived from singlet oxygen in inflammatory cells may also be a by-product of oxidative stress that contributes to atherosclerosis.[9]

Although the definition and pathophysiological processes leading to an increase in oxidative stress may seem clear-cut, the use of the terms *oxidative stress* and *oxidant stress* are relatively nonspecific. Whereas oxidants are continuously being produced in living organisms, a multitude of antioxidant defense mechanisms are also constantly at work, and few biological systems are at redox equilibrium. In most biological systems, reducing equivalents are constantly being generated and converted and interconverted, indicating that a major component of "antioxidant balance" has to do with how extensively fed the cell or organism is at any moment. This limitation on the definition of oxidative stress requires that mechanisms thought to contribute to oxidative stress be investigated in vivo with a series of detailed biochemical assays (Table 154-1).

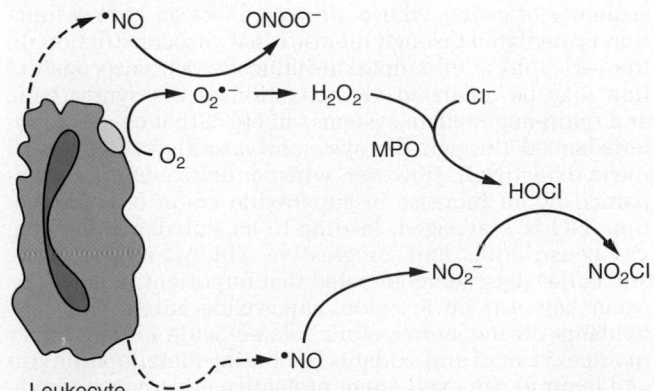

FIGURE 154-2. Pathways of reactive oxygen species generation by activated leukocytes. Cl$^-$, chloride; HOCl, hypochlorous acid; H$_2$O$_2$, hydrogen peroxide; MPO, myeloperoxidase; •NO, nitric oxide; NO$_2^-$, nitrite; NO$_2$Cl, nitryl chloride; O$_2$•$^-$, superoxide anion; ONOO$^-$, peroxynitrite. (Redrawn from Himmelfarb J, Stenvinkel P, Ikizler TA, Hakim RM: The elephant in uremia: Oxidant stress as a unifying concept of cardiovascular disease in uremia. Kidney Int 2002;62:1524-1538.)

TABLE 154-1

Oxidative Stress Biomarkers Useful in Evaluating Acute Kidney Injury in Vivo

Lipids
    Malondialdehyde and other aldehydes
    Lipid hydroperoxides
    Oxidized low-density lipoprotein
    Exhaled alkanes
    Advanced lipoxidation end products
Arachidonic Acid Derivatives
    F_2 isoprostanes
    Isolevuglandins
Carbohydrates
    Reactive aldehydes
    Advanced glycosylation end products
Amino Acids
    Cysteine/cystine
    Homocysteine/homocystine
    Isoaspartate
    3-Chlorotyrosine
    Dityrosine
    3-Nitrotyrosine
Proteins
    Thiol oxidation
    Carbonyl formation
    Advanced oxidation protein products
DNA
    8-Hydroxy-2′deoxyguanine
Other
    Spin traps (electron paramagnetic resonance)

OXIDATIVE STRESS IN THE PATHOGENESIS OF ACUTE KIDNEY INJURY: ANIMAL MODELS

Sepsis and Endotoxemia

Sepsis has been identified as the most common cause of acute kidney injury.[10] Increased production of reactive oxygen species has been demonstrated in animal models,[11] as well as in patients with septic shock.[12] Acute kidney injury during sepsis is known to involve a complex sequence of events whose ultimate effect on kidney function is mediated through intense renal vasoconstriction. In the early phase of endotoxin-induced AKI, vasoconstriction may be mediated via activation of the sympathetic and renin-angiotensin systems, an effect that can be counterbalanced through the systemic vasodilatory effects of nitric oxide (NO). However, when endotoxemia is accompanied by an increase in superoxide anion (O_2^-) production, NO is scavenged, leading to an imbalance favoring vasoconstriction and progressive kidney injury. Wang and colleagues[13] demonstrated that important interactions occur between nitric oxide, superoxide anion, and antioxidants during endotoxemia-related acute kidney injury in mice. Several antioxidants (including metalloporphyrin and tempol) can exert a renoprotective effect via potentiation of NO function. In this model, antioxidant protection was associated with a significant decrease in mortality 24 hours after exposure to lipopolysaccharide. Increased tissue levels of peroxynitrite, the end product of the reaction between superoxide anion and nitric oxide, have also been detected in animal models of acute kidney injury.[14]

Ischemic Acute Kidney Injury

More than 3 decades ago, Alexander Leaf, Rex Jamison, and their colleagues first incriminated damaged endothe-lium as contributory to the pathogenesis of acute kidney injury in models of renal ischemia.[15,16] While injured endothelium may directly lead to oxidative and nitrosative stress, a more important mechanism for increased oxidative stress may result as the damaged endothelium promotes infiltration of macrophages and polymorphonuclear cells, which, when activated, produce large quantities of reactive oxygen and nitrogen species. Several investigators have demonstrated overexpression of intercellular adhesion molecule-1 (ICAM-1) by vascular endothelium in ischemic models of AKI. ICAM-1 allows phagocytes to transmigrate the vascular wall into the kidney parenchyma. Furthermore, blockade of ICAM-1 receptors attenuates ischemic renal injury.

Studies have reported on the development of increased oxidative stress during acute renal ischemia-reperfusion.[17-19] These studies have collectively demonstrated several mechanisms for increased oxidant production, including mitochondrial production of free radicals, oxidation of hypoxanthine, and enzymatic oxidation of arachidonic acid. More recently, acute nitrosative stress has been demonstrated to accompany increased oxidative stress in a rat model of acute kidney ischemia.[20] In this model system, administration of ebselen (a scavenger of peroxynitrite) prior to reperfusion was able to ameliorate ischemic kidney injury and to reduce lipid peroxidation and DNA damage in ischemic kidneys. Similarly, the administration of superoxide dismutase was demonstrated to prevent lipid peroxidation and oxidative DNA damage.

Nephrotoxic Acute Kidney Injury

Tissue injury mediated by reactive oxygen species contributes to the pathogenesis of nephrotoxic acute kidney injury with a wide variety of agents, including gentamicin, glycerol, cisplatin, and cyclosporine A.[21,22] In the glycerol model of myohemoglobinuric acute kidney injury, the resulting rhabdomyolysis and hemolysis led to the release and tubular cell absorption of heme proteins. Heme-loaded cells produce excess hydrogen peroxide, which can subsequently increase the release of iron from porphyrin compounds, thereby amplifying iron-dependent free radical injury. The result of these processes is massive lipid peroxidation that leads to cell death, a process that can be attenuated both in vitro and in vivo with the use of iron chelators such as deferoxamine.

Baliga and colleagues[21] demonstrated that increased oxidative stress also contributes to gentamicin-induced nephrotoxicity. While the precise mechanisms of gentamicin nephrotoxicity remain unclear, it is known that gentamicin alters mitochondrial respiration and increases hydrogen peroxide generation. Gentamicin also induces superoxide anion and hydroxyl radical formation in renal cortical tissue. Gentamicin may also mobilize iron from mitochondria, and several iron chelators have been shown to be beneficial in animal models of gentamicin-induced nephrotoxicity. Reactive oxygen species also are active in cisplatin-induced and cyclosporine A–induced nephrotoxicity.

Biomarkers of Oxidative Stress in Clinical Acute Kidney Injury

In vivo, oxygen intermediates are produced in minute quantities and have very short biological half-lives. The combination of low concentration and extreme reactivity

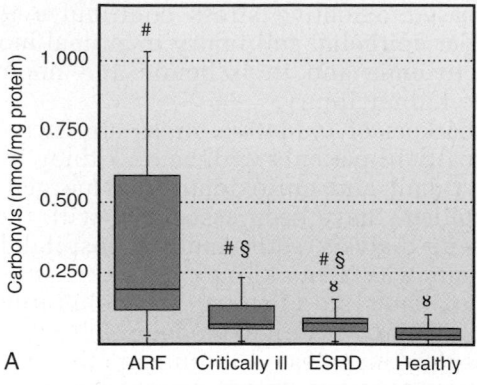

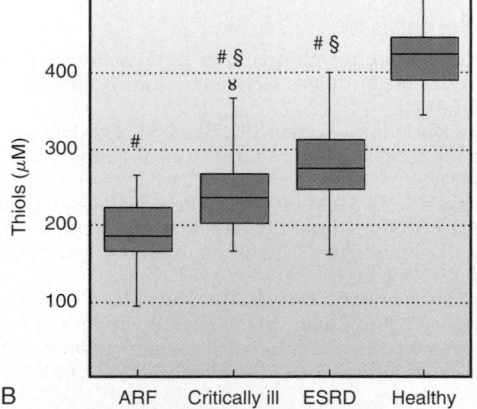

FIGURE 154-3. A, Increased oxidative stress in human acute kidney injury (acute renal failure [ARF]): Plasma protein carbonyl content in four study groups. Box plots show the median, interquartile range, and outliers. **B,** Increased oxidative stress in human acute kidney injury (ARF): Plasma protein thiol content in four study groups. Box plots show the median, interquartile range, and outliers. [#]$P < .001$ vs. healthy, [§]$P < .001$ vs. ARF. ESRD, end-stage renal disease. (**A** and **B,** Redrawn from Himmelfarb J, McMonagle E, Freedman S, et al, for the PICARD Study Group: Oxidative stress is increased in critically ill patients with acute renal failure. J Am Soc Nephrol 2004;15:2449-2456.)

makes the in vivo detection of reactive oxygen species extremely technically difficult. In response to these difficulties, a powerful strategy has emerged for understanding the underlying in vivo mechanisms of oxidative injury by detecting stable end products of oxidative chemistry produced by different reaction pathways. These biomarkers of increased oxidative stress measure the oxidation of important macromolecules, including lipids, carbohydrates, proteins, amino acids, and DNA. The application of these biomarkers of increased oxidative stress have now unequivocally demonstrated that AKI is an increased oxidative stress state (Fig. 154-3).[23]

Reactive aldehydes can be formed as the end products of a variety of oxidative reactions, including the oxidation of alcohol groups, amino groups, and via the addition of oxygen to unsaturated double bonds. In particular, the formation of α,β-unsaturated aldehydes are important oxidation products in that the formation of two sites of reactivity frequently leads to the formation of cyclic adducts or cross-links with other macromolecules.[24] α,β-Unsaturated aldehydes are capable of reacting with protein nucleophiles to form advanced glycation end products.[25] Several groups have demonstrated that many reactive aldehyde compounds—including glyoxal, methylglyoxal, malondialdehyde, acrolein, and 4-hydroxynonenal—are detectable at concentrations up to 10-fold higher in uremic plasma than in the plasma of healthy individuals.[25,26] In acute kidney injury, reactive aldehydes accumulate as a result of diminished renal catabolism and through increased production, largely via myeloperoxidase-catalyzed phagocytic cell activation (see Fig. 154-3A).[23]

Thiol groups have an important antioxidant function as redox buffers.[27] Intracellular thiols, including glutathione and thioredoxin, are predominant in maintaining the highly reduced environment within the cell, as glutathione is found in millimolar concentrations.[28] In addition, extracellular thiols constitute an important component of antioxidant defense.[29] The plasma protein–reduced thiols (located primarily on the albumin molecule) are depleted in AKI patients and thus are not able to participate in antioxidant defense.[23] Furthermore, although protective reduced thiols are depleted in AKI, oxidized thiols that include homocysteine and cysteine accumulate and may have toxic effects on the endothelium (see Fig. 154-3B).

Prooxidant and Antioxidant Enzyme Gene Polymorphisms in Acute Kidney Injury

In ischemic AKI, toxic AKI, or both, there are a number of potential sources of excess reactive oxygen species production, including mitochondrial dysfunction, xanthine oxidase activation, and endothelial- and phagocyte-associated respiratory burst through activation of $NADP^+$. Several gene polymorphisms have been described in key prooxidant and antioxidant enzymes that could potentially account for interindividual variability in the response to AKI. Perianayagam and colleagues[30] examined gene polymorphisms associated with the prooxidant enzyme $NADP^+$ and the antioxidant enzyme catalase in a cohort of 200 patients with established AKI. A genotype-phenotype association was demonstrable between the $NADP^+$ genotype and plasma nitro tyrosine levels as a measure of increased oxidative and nitrosative stress. Furthermore, a genotype-phenotype association was also demonstrable between catalase genotypes and whole blood catalase activity. Of considerable potential importance, the inheritance of an $NADP^+$ allele was associated with a 2.1-fold higher odd for dialysis requirement or hospital death. These data suggest that propensity to increased oxidative stress may contribute to adverse outcomes in patients with established AKI; however, these results need to be confirmed in larger, multi-institutional studies.

Antioxidant Therapy in Acute Kidney Injury

Current data indicate that increased oxidative stress may play a pathogenetic role in the progression of AKI and may contribute to adverse outcomes in patients with established AKI. Furthermore, in a small, single-center observational study, Metnitz and colleagues[31] demonstrated that plasma levels of the antioxidants ascorbic acid, β-carotene, and selenium are depleted in critically ill patients with multiple-organ failure syndrome with and without acute kidney injury in comparison to healthy subjects. These investigators also demonstrated that plasma levels of these antioxidants were further depleted in patients with AKI in comparison to patients with preserved kidney function. Thus, the hypothesis that administration of appropriate antioxidants may be beneficial in patients with early or well-established AKI is attractive. However, at the present time, there are no carefully controlled trials in the literature reporting the results of antioxidant administration in patients with AKI.

The use of several antioxidants has been evaluated in the intensive care unit setting for treatment of increased oxidative stress associated with critical illness. N-acetylcysteine, a thiol-containing antioxidant, is known to be a safe agent with a relatively wide toxic-to-therapeutic window. Several small trials evaluating the use of n-acetylcysteine therapy for the treatment of acute lung injury in critically ill patients have been performed, with somewhat mixed results.[32] Similarly, parenteral nutrition with a diet containing eicosapentaenoic acid and antioxidants has been shown to reduce pulmonary inflammation and improve clinical outcomes in a small prospective randomized double-blind controlled trial in patients with acute respiratory distress syndrome.[33] In a single center study, Kirov and colleagues[34] randomized patients in septic shock to receive placebo or methylene blue, an inhibitor of the nitric oxide pathway. Patients receiving methylene blue had improved oxygen delivery, reduced body temperature, and reduced requirements for pressor support. In animal models of ischemic AKI, both edaravone (a potent free radical scavenger developed for clinical use) and mesna (a potent thiol-containing antioxidant) have been demonstrated to have renoprotective effects and may be suitable for clinical trials in patients with AKI.[35,36]

Key Points

1. Multiple pathways contribute to increased oxidative stress in acute kidney injury.

2. Increased oxidative stress contributes to renal tubular epithelial cell injury in animal models of endotoxemia and in ischemic and nephrotoxic acute kidney injury.
3. Biomarkers of oxidative stress are increased in critically ill patients with acute kidney injury.
4. Prooxidant and antioxidant enzyme gene polymorphisms have been associated with increased odds for dialysis requirement or hospital death in patients with acute kidney injury.
5. Antioxidants are effective in ameliorating acute kidney injury in animal models, but they have not been rigorously tested in human clinical trials.

Key References

20. Noiri E, Nakao A, Uchidna K, et al: Oxidative and nitrosative stress in acute renal ischemia. Am J Physiol 2001;281: F948-F957.
21. Baliga R, Ueda N, Walker PD, Shah SV: Oxidant mechanisms in toxic acute renal failure. Am J Kidney Dis 1997;29: 465-477.
23. Himmelfarb J, McMonagle E, Freedman S, et al, for the PICARD Study Group: Oxidative stress is increased in critically ill patients with acute renal failure. J Am Soc Nephrol 2004;15:2449-2456.
30. Perianayagam MC, Liangos O, Kolyada AY, et al: NADPH oxidase p22phox and catalase gene variants are associated with biomarkers of oxidative stress and adverse outcomes in acute renal failure. J Am Soc Nephrol 2007;18:7-9.

See the companion Expert Consult website for the complete reference list.

CHAPTER 155

High Mobility Group Box 1 Protein

Russell L. Delude

OBJECTIVES

This chapter will:
1. Review the many roles high mobility group box 1 protein plays in biology.
2. Review studies directed at elucidating the mechanisms underlying regulated high mobility group box 1 protein subcellular compartmentalization and release from activated cells.
3. Present the results of tissue culture and animal studies that form the basis for the hypothesis that high mobility group box 1 protein plays a causative role in critical illness.
4. Review recent clinical studies of high mobility group box 1 protein in patients with severe sepsis.
5. Outline major challenges in contemporary research on high mobility group box 1 protein and highlight potential directions for continued exploration in this rapidly progressing field.

THE DISCOVERY OF HIGH MOBILITY GROUP BOX 1 PROTEIN AS A LATE-ACTING MEDIATOR OF SEPSIS

An underlying hypothesis driving critical care research is that soluble mediators released by stimulated cells may be responsible for much of the morbidity and mortality associated with severe sepsis. Sepsis is classically associated with an underlying infectious process, even in the absence of undefined focal or systemic infection. Therefore, it should come as no surprise that tumor necrosis factor-α (TNF-α) was hailed as an obvious target for treating sepsis in humans. After all, it could be shown convincingly that TNF-α fulfilled a molecular permutation of Koch's postulate: (1) TNF-α is found at elevated levels in septic humans and experimental animals compared to healthy controls, (2) TNF-α can be purified from septic animals and humans, (3) injection of TNF-α into laboratory animals and human volunteers recapitulates many aspects of the septic process, and (4) blocking TNF-α action in animal and human models was shown to be protective. In spite of the tremendous amount of work associating TNF-α with severity of sepsis, clinical trials based on decreasing or eliminating TNF-α in critically ill patients were not only unsuccessful, but the results suggested that blocking TNF-α activity may be detrimental.[1]

It is generally accepted that monocytes are an important source of small-soluble molecular mediators of the sepsis process. Mediators like TNF-α and interleukin 1β (IL-1β) are released within the first few hours following activation. However, most patients presenting with severe sepsis have resolved this early inflammatory cascade, and targeting these low levels of pro-inflammatory cytokines would not be expected to improve outcome.[2,3] Though other inflammatory mediators had been described that appeared late in experimental models of the systemic inflammatory response, none of the "late" sepsis markers known in the late 20th century proved to be useful interventional targets. In 1999, Wang and colleagues[4] reported the results of an intriguing series of studies designed to identify novel "late-acting mediators of endotoxemia." They began by exposing a mouse macrophage-like cell line to gram-negative bacterial lipopolysaccharide (LPS). Supernatants were removed from the cells at various times and analyzed using reducing sodium dodecyl sulfate–polyacrylamide gel electrophoresis (SDS-PAGE). They identified a 30-kD protein band that was present in culture supernatants at later and not earlier time points. Mass spectroscopy identified this protein as high mobility group box 1 protein (HMGB1). Wang and colleagues showed that HMGB1 was detectable in plasma of mice 8 hours after injecting them with LPS. Sequestration of circulating HMGB1 with an antigen-specific antibody improved survival after LPS injection, and administration of recombinant HMGB1 was lethal. Thus, HMGB1 appeared with delayed kinetics and remained in the circulation for extended periods of time, fulfilling the requirements of the hypothesized "late-acting mediator of endotoxemia." The strong results presented by Wang and colleagues, together with those culled from numerous subsequent cell-based and animal-based studies, would suggest that this was true for human sepsis as well. This question is considered later in the chapter after discussion of HMGB1 studies published before 1999.

THE TWO IDENTITIES OF HIGH MOBILITY GROUP BOX 1 PROTEIN

HMGB1 made its début in a 1973 study of nonhistone components of calf-thymus chromatin.[5] Differential protein precipitation with trichloroacetic acid was used to isolate a group of approximately 16 proteins that migrate with high mobility on SDS-PAGE. The member of this "high mobility" group with the highest relative molecular weight was designated *high mobility group 1 protein*, or HMG-1. In independent studies, a 30-kD brain-derived heparin-binding polypeptide was identified that promoted outgrowth of cultured neurons.[6] Sequencing the gene that encoded the 30-kD protein revealed that approximately 85% of the protein was enriched in positively charged basic amino acids, whereas the extreme carboxyl end of the protein (approximately 15% of the protein sequence) consisted entirely of negatively charged aspartate and glutamate residues. This polar structure earned it the name

amphoterin[7] (amphoteric molecules behave as both acids and bases). In 1993, it became apparent that HMG-1 and amphoterin were identical proteins encoded by the same gene.[8] The HMG chromosomal proteins were consequently renamed to better reflect structural and functional differences between the members, and proteins of the HMG group that contained at least one "B box" protein–folding motif were delegated to high mobility group box. Thus, HMG-1 was designated *high mobility group box 1 (HMGB1) protein*.[9]

HIGH MOBILITY GROUP BOX 1 PROTEIN STRUCTURE AND FUNCTION

HMGB1 is encoded on human chromosome 15, and the protein is expressed in most nucleated cells. HMGB1 consists of two structurally conserved HMG domains referred to as an A box and B box (Fig. 155-1A). The gene encoding HMGB1 differs by only one or two typically conservative amino acid substitutions when comparing mammalian HMGB1 protein sequences. For comparison, mouse TNF-α contains only 79% amino acid identity when compared to the human protein. This apparently high rate of sequence conservation suggests that there is intense selective pressure against any gene mutations that would cause HMGB1 protein sequence changes. This is further supported by the fact that targeted HMGB1 gene deletion is lethal in mice.[10]

Any discussion of HMGB1 function would be remiss without at least mentioning its role in regulating nucleosome spacing, gene transcription, and deoxyribonucleic acid (DNA) repair.[11] The primary sequence of HMGB1 contains two conserved domains called the A box and B box, whose secondary structures are essentially super imposable. HMG box protein–folding domains are present in a wide range of proteins where they are known to direct binding to the minor groove of double-stranded DNA (Fig. 155-1B). HMGB1 has a preference for binding to bent and single-stranded DNA, and it has been shown to induce bending in double-stranded DNA.[11]

HIGH MOBILITY GROUP BOX 1 PROTEIN IS RELEASED FROM A WIDE VARIETY OF CELL TYPES

Studies of the role of HMGB1 in enhancing neuronal development were the first to show that this protein is released passively by resting cells, but more importantly, that cells can be stimulated to release large amounts of the protein.[12] However, the actions of HMGB1 in neuronal growth and development were largely regarded as autocrine and paracrine in nature. This was because HMGB1 release was considered to be tightly controlled, and its affinity for heparin, a constituent of the extracellular matrix, would greatly restrict its diffusion from the site of production.[13] Studies of the induced release of HMGB1 by activated macrophages were the first to suggest that HMGB1 can also act in a systemic manner.[4] Additional cell types reported to release HMGB1 in response to infectious, immune, or endocrine stimuli include dendritic cells,[14] natural killer cells,[15] endothelial cells,[16] epithelial cells,[17] and bone cells.[18]

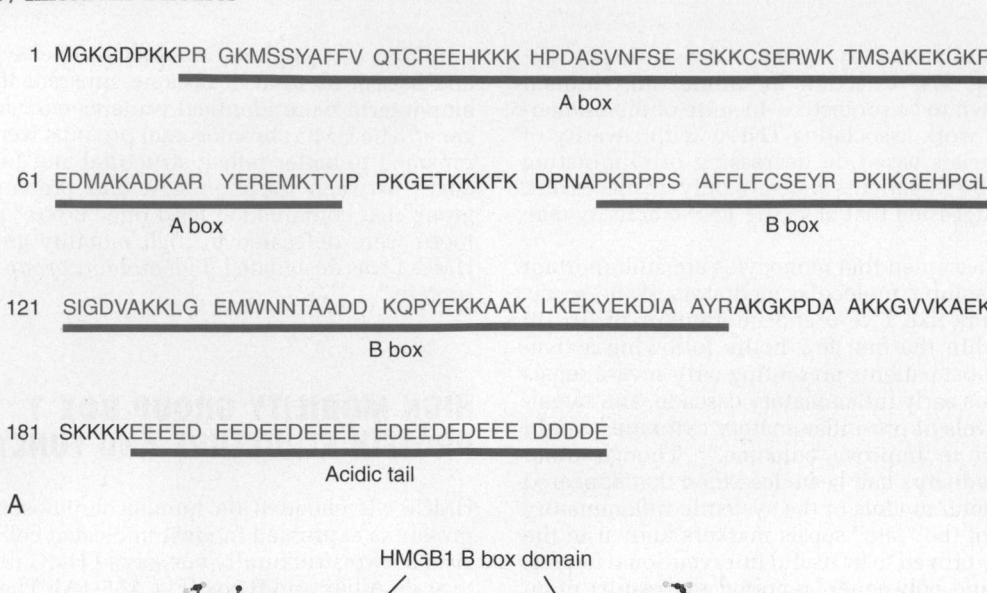

1   MGKGDPKKPR GKMSSYAFFV QTCREEHKKK HPDASVNFSE FSKKCSERWK TMSAKEKGKF

A box

61   EDMAKADKAR YEREMKTYIP PKGETKKKFK DPNAPKRPPS AFFLFCSEYR PKIKGEHPGL

A box   B box

121 SIGDVAKKLG EMWNNTAADD KQPYEKKAAK LKEKYEKDIA AYRAKGKPDA AKKGVVKAEK

B box

181 SKKKKEEEED EEDEEDEEEE EDEEDEDEEE DDDDE

Acidic tail

A

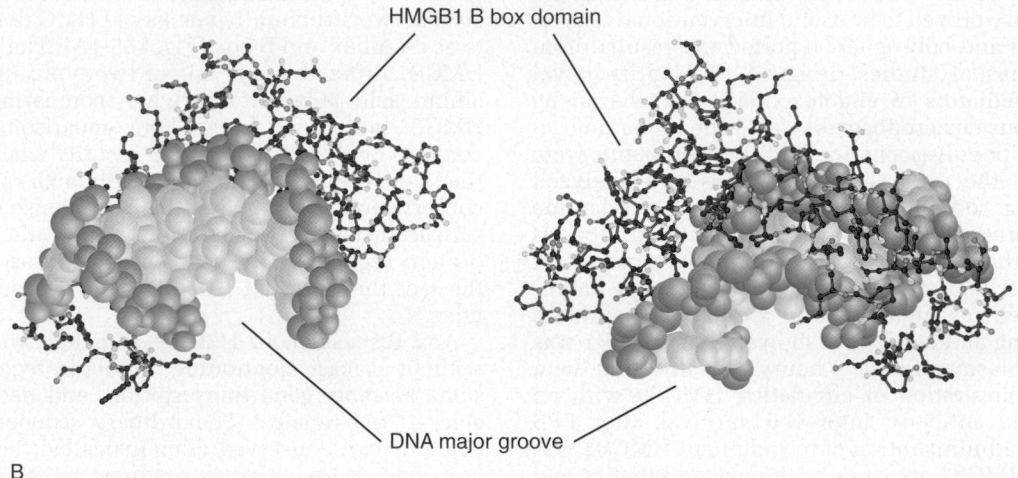

HMGB1 B box domain

DNA major groove

B

FIGURE 155-1. High mobility group box 1 (HMGB1) primary structure and its interaction with deoxyribonucleic acid (DNA). **A,** Amino acid sequence of human HMGB1. Amino acids that form the A and B box domains and the acidic tail are underlined. **B,** Interaction of B box domain with a sequence of DNA. The DNA helix is shown as a space-filling model with nucleotide bases shown in *light blue* and the phosphate backbone shown in *dark blue.* The HMGB1 B box peptide is shown as a tube model with carbon atoms in *black,* oxygen in *light gray,* nitrogen in *dark gray,* and sulfur in *blue.* Hydrogen atoms are not shown. The image on the right was formed by rotating the image on the left approximately 200 degrees out of the page.

REGULATION OF HIGH MOBILITY GROUP BOX 1 GENE EXPRESSION

Relatively high copy numbers of HMGB1 messenger ribonucleic acid (mRNA) are present in most nucleated cells, and several groups report that a two- to threefold increase in steady-state HMGB1 mRNA occurs in response to various pro-inflammatory stimuli.[19-21] This increase appears to involve increased transcription of the HMGB1 gene following binding of the Sp1 transcription factor to its promoter.[21] Given the high basal level of HMGB1 mRNA in cells, a requirement for increased HMGB1 gene transcription in the induced release of HMGB1 from activated cells remains to be established.

STUDIES ON THE MECHANISM OF INDUCED HIGH MOBILITY GROUP BOX 1 RELEASE FROM CELLS

HMGB1 is synthesized as a leaderless protein on cytosolic ribosomes and is not secreted from cells through the clas-

sical secretory pathway. Consistent with this, the majority of HMGB1 is located in the nucleus of resting cultures of human monocytes and most other cells, and HMGB1 is detected in both the nuclear and cytosolic compartments following cell activation.[22] ζ-N-acetylation of lysine residues within the HMGB1 nuclear localization sequence is associated with its accumulation in late endosomal vesicles in activated macrophages.[22,23] Acetylation appears to be required but not sufficient for this process, since mono- or bi-ADP-ribosylation by poly(ADP) ribose polymerase may also be required for release of HMGB1 from DNA.[24]

The question remains: How does cytosolic HMGB1 get packaged into vesicles? Acetyl-lysine residues of histones bind to highly conserved bromo domains. These domains are found in proteins involved in transcription, yet they are also present in many proteins that reside outside the nucleus. Hyperacetylation of HMGB1 may increase its affinity for bromo domain–containing proteins that target HMGB1 to the endosomal compartment. Likewise, a number of proteins with affinity for ADP-ribosylated proteins are residents of the late secretory pathway, and this could theoretically target ADP-ribosylated HMGB1 to the late endosomal pathway. It is also conceivable that hyperacetylation increases the affinity of HMGB1 for membrane subdomains (i.e., lipid rafts) that are enriched in budding endosomal membranes.[13,23,25] Further studies are needed to better understand the molecular basis of this nonclassical secretory pathway as it relates to the packaging and export of HMGB1.

Cultured enterocytes direct HMGB1 release toward the apical compartment following exposure to pro-inflammatory cytokines.[17] The released HMGB1 is, at least in part, associated with small 50- to 100-nm membrane vesicles called *exosomes*. Exosomes are released following fusion of multivesicular bodies with the plasma membrane and were first described as a means used by reticulocytes to shed unnecessary components of their plasma membrane.[26] Exosomes form by inward budding of membrane vesicles into organelles called *multivesicular bodies* (MVBs). These vesicles contain exosomes that are destined for release from the cell following fusion of the MVB with the plasma membrane. MVBs play a sorting role and should be thought of as dynamic structures that fuse with incoming early endosomes and other vesicles in the late secretory compartment. Proteins are actively sorted either back to the membrane for recycling or toward the lyso-somal compartment for additional sorting, degradation, or both, or they are packaged into endosomes.

Targeting of proteins to exosomes appears to be a highly regulated process. It is now appreciated that exosomes are released from many cell types into the extracellular compartment. For example, antigen-presenting cells were reported to release major histocompatibility complex with bound antigenic peptides to nearby cells in vitro and in vivo.[27] Surprisingly, mast cells appear to sequester mRNA and microRNA in exosomes and release them after activation.[28] The released exosomes work in a paracrine fashion, delivering functional RNA to target cells.

It remains to be established whether the vesicles described in macrophages represent intermediates in exosome release or if HMGB1 is released from the endosomal compartment by targeting to exocytic vesicles. Furthermore, it has not been established that HMGB1 is hyperacetylated in cultured enterocytes, so the question of whether vesicular compartmentalization and exosomal export of HMGB1 requires protein acetylation remains to be determined. The answers to these questions are important if one is to understand the physical nature and, thus, the biological significance of HMGB1 that is released from cells during infection, severe sepsis, and other diseases associated with the inflammatory response.

HIGH MOBILITY GROUP BOX 1 RELEASE FROM NECROTIC AND APOPTOTIC CELLS

Cells undergoing necrosis appear to release HMGB1 in contrast to apoptotic cells that do not release HMGB1 to their surroundings.[29] Interestingly, necrosis-associated release of HMGB1 in animal models was associated with inflammation in surrounding tissue, but this effect was greatly ameliorated in mice engineered to lack the HMGB1 gene. These findings resulted in the inclusion of HMGB1 in a growing family of "danger associated molecules" together with such molecules as heat shock protein 70 and calreticulin. These molecules have been implicated in the pathogenesis of renal ischemic disease and severe sepsis.[30,31] These studies have a teleological appeal in that necrosis is associated with poor resolution of infection, while apoptosis is thought of as a highly orchestrated

process that removes dead cells and potentially immunogenic debris efficiently. However, this simple picture was challenged by a report of HMGB1 release from cultured apoptotic T lymphocytes and HeLa cells.[32]

CONSEQUENCES OF FREELY SOLUBLE VERSUS EXOSOMAL RELEASE OF HIGH MOBILITY GROUP BOX 1

Gardella and colleagues[22] and Bonaldi and coworkers[23] both report that mononuclear cells redistribute HMGB1 from the nuclear to the cytosolic compartment in response to various stimuli. This HMGB1 is detected in lysosomal endosomes and is presumably released to the extracellular space. The images in these manuscripts cannot distinguish whether HMGB1 is exclusively in secretory lysosomal/endosomes or whether it is also associated with exosomes within MVBs or some combination of the two compartments. Activated endothelial cells also release HMGB1 in culture and presumably during human sepsis, but the mechanism of HMGB1 release from these cells has not been reported.[16,33] In contrast to macrophages, a considerable proportion of the HMGB1 released from activated enterocytes is associated with exosomes.[17] The distinction between free and membrane-associated HMGB1 seems to be fairly important, as HMGB1 released within exosomes may not be available for binding to receptors on the surface of nearby cells. By analogy to other systems, one would expect that exosomal HMGB1 may actually be targeted to the cytoplasmic compartment of nearby cells; however this concept needs to be supported with experimental evidence. Alternatively, packaging of protein like HMGB1 into exosomes may serve as a method for releasing damaged or excess cellular constituents from cells to the extracellular space. The physical nature of HMGB1 (i.e., soluble or membrane-associated) released from mononuclear or endothelial cells has not been reported. Furthermore, it remains to be determined whether circulating HMBG1 exists free in plasma or is sequestered by exosomes, or if it exists in both forms.

CURRENT CONCEPTS IN HMGB1-MEDIATED SIGNAL TRANSDUCTION

The mechanism used by cells to sense and respond to extracellular HMGB1 remains unclear. This is due to a variety of technical issues making HMGB1 difficult to purify and study. The ability of highly purified HMGB1 to unequivocally evoke pro-inflammatory responses has been questioned in the literature.[30,34] With that said, numerous transmembrane proteins have been reported to bind HMGB1 and effect subsequent signal transduction. Theses include the receptor for advanced glycation end products (RAGE)[35] and Toll-like receptors 2 and 4.[36] Major downstream mediators activated in response to ligation of these receptors appear to include activation of the mitogen-activated protein kinase pathway and nuclear translocation of nuclear factor-κB. This results in increased cell motility, upregulation of genes that encode pro-inflammatory proteins, and proteins that generate reactive oxygen and nitrogen species in immunostimulated cells. The involvement of RAGE in these processes is supported, at least in part, by a variety of studies showing that strategies that decrease

RAGE expression or provision of a RAGE decoy or binding protein (e.g., soluble RAGE or RAGE-specific HMGB1 antibodies) decreased morbidity and mortality associated with systemic release of HMGB1.[25]

CELL AND ANIMAL STUDIES OF HIGH MOBILITY GROUP BOX 1 SUPPORT ITS ROLE AS A LATE MEDIATOR OF SEPSIS

HMGB1 promotes the release of pro-inflammatory and procoagulant factors and increases expression of intercellular adhesion molecules by myeloid[37] and endothelial[38,39] cells. Enterocytes and hepatocytes exposed to HMGB1 increase inducible nitric oxide synthase—dependent nitric oxide production and show a concomitant decrease in metabolic activity and epithelial barrier function.[17,40,41] Consistent with these observations, administration of HMGB1 antagonists decreased organ damage and mortality in animal models of systemic inflammation.[4,42-44] More importantly, several groups reported that delayed treatment with HMGB1 decoys afforded significant protection in animal models of severe sepsis.[4,42,44] Thus, strong evidence from numerous in vitro and in vivo studies implicates HMGB1 as an important mediator of the systemic inflammatory response in critically ill patients.

CLINICAL STUDIES OF HIGH MOBILITY GROUP BOX 1 PRODUCTION IN CRITICALLY ILL PATIENTS

In their initial publication, Wang and colleagues[4] reported that HMGB1 was undetectable in the plasma of 8 healthy subjects and detectable in the plasma of 25 patients with severe sepsis and present at even higher concentrations in nonsurvivors. Yang and colleagues[45] reported that serum concentrations of HMGB1 were higher in blood samples obtained from 25 trauma victims with hemorrhagic shock compared to 9 normal volunteers. Ueno and colleagues[46] reported increased HMGB1 concentrations in the plasma of 21 patients with severe sepsis, and Sunden-Cullberg and colleagues[47] demonstrated persistently elevated HMGB1 concentrations in 59 patients with severe sepsis. In contrast to the findings reported by Wang and colleagues,[4] these authors reported lower concentrations of HMGB1 in nonsurvivors. Each of these studies used a case-control design, comparing patients with severe sepsis to healthy controls. None assessed the role of HMGB1 in subjects who developed infection but did not progress to organ dysfunction, and only Sunden-Cullberg and colleagues[47] measured HMGB1 concentrations over time.

PLASMA HIGH MOBILITY GROUP BOX 1 LEVELS IN PATIENTS WITH DIFFUSE INTRAVASCULAR COAGULATION

Hatada and colleagues[48] reported the results of a study of 201 patients in the intensive care unit with suspected disseminated intravascular coagulation (DIC). HMGB1 levels were measured using an "in-house" enzyme-linked immunosorbent assay (ELISA). Plasma HMGB1 was not detected in normal controls, but mean concentrations were 4.54 ng/mL in infected patients, 2.15 ng/mL in patients with malignancies, and 6.47 ng/mL in trauma patients. Subgroup analysis revealed that patients with DIC, patients with organ failure, and patients who died had a mean plasma HMGB1 concentration of 14.05, 8.29, and 16.58 ng/mL, respectively. These authors concluded that circulating HMGB1 levels may be a useful indicator of severity of DIC and organ dysfunction.

HIGH MOBILITY GROUP BOX 1 IN COMMUNITY-ACQUIRED PNEUMONIA–ASSOCIATED SEVERE SEPSIS

Angus and colleagues constructed an outcome-dependent stratified random sample of 122 subjects[49] from a larger, prospective in-patient community-acquired pneumonia (CAP) study cohort.[3] The subjects included 43 who never developed severe sepsis and survived to hospital discharge, 49 who developed severe sepsis and survived to discharge, and 30 who developed severe sepsis and died in the hospital. A quantitative Western blot was used to measure HMGB1 concentration in plasma. Median HMGB1 concentration on the day of admission was elevated compared to healthy controls (190 vs. 0 ng/mL, $P < 0.0001$; 93.7% of all CAP sample measurements were elevated). Circulating HMGB1 was elevated throughout the hospital course and remained elevated at discharge. In contrast, 64% and 63% of CAP subjects had normal concentrations of TNF-α and IL-10, respectively, and the mean concentrations of both cytokines declined rapidly over the first week.[3] Importantly, HMGB1 was elevated not only in subjects who developed severe sepsis but also in those who had an uncomplicated response to infection. Whereas those subjects with severe sepsis who died had higher HMGB1 levels than those who survived, HMGB1 concentrations were similar to those with an uncomplicated course and recovery.

HIGH MOBILITY GROUP BOX 1 IN COMMUNITY-ACQUIRED INFECTION– ASSOCIATED SEVERE SEPSIS

Gaïni and colleagues[50] reported the results of a prospective randomized study of severe sepsis. Groups were composed of 32 healthy controls, 67 noninfected patients, 32 infected patients with no evidence of systemic inflammatory response syndrome, 47 patients with sepsis, and 27 patients with severe sepsis. A commercially available ELISA was used to measure HMGB1 concentration in plasma. Although this study included a significant number of patients with CAP, it also included a significant proportion of non-CAP patients that were diagnosed with and without other types of viral and bacterial infection. The median concentration of HMGB1 in healthy controls was 0.77 ng/mL, 1.54 ng/mL in noninfected patients, 2.41 ng/mL in infected patients without systemic inflammatory response syndrome, 2.24 ng/mL in patients with sepsis, and 2.18 ng/mL in patients with severe sepsis. No analysis was provided concerning the relationship between HMGB1 concentration and survival. Gaïni and colleagues[50] concluded that the levels of HMGB1 were significantly higher in all patient groups compared to healthy controls. Interestingly, HMGB1 levels were not significantly different in noninfected patients compared to infected patients.

THE ROLE OF HIGH MOBILITY GROUP BOX 1 IN CLINICAL ILLNESS

The finding of persistent HMGB1 elevation in CAP patients that survived CAP is incongruous with previous observations reported for tissue culture and animal models[4,16,17,43,44,46,51,52] and human clinical studies[4,47,53] that support a causative role for circulating HMGB1 in the development of severe sepsis and progression to death. The finding that HMGB1 was elevated in infected patients compared to healthy controls was common to most of these studies. The study of Gaïni and colleagues[50] includes a noninfected patient population, which appeared to have lower levels of HMGB1 in plasma compared to infected patients but higher HMGB1 levels when compared to healthy controls.

Several other issues become apparent when these studies are compared. HMGB1 levels are essentially the same in normal controls regardless of the method used to measure HMGB1 concentration. However, the levels of HMGB1 detected in plasma from patients with infection, severe sepsis, or both, are significantly higher (>150 ng/mL) when assayed using quantitative Western blotting compared to the ELISA (<10 ng/mL). The reasons for this discrepancy remain unclear. Another issue to consider is that cell culture studies typically employ HMGB1 concentrations greater than 1 μg/mL, which exceeds the highest levels of HMGB1 measured using either assay procedure. One explanation for this difference may be that only a portion of purified HMGB1 is active in these assays, thus requiring "higher" concentrations to achieve an effect. Another explanation may be that the HMGB1 released by cells in vivo is more potent due to modification during cell export in comparison to recombinant sources or calf thymus extract, which is primarily of nuclear origin. Two recent reports by Zimmermann and colleagues[34] and Rouhiainen

and colleagues[54] have addressed this issue in some detail, but additional studies are needed before definitive conclusions can be drawn on this important issue. Clearly, considerable research is still needed to answer the many questions that remain concerning the role of HMGB1 in the pathophysiology of systemic inflammatory diseases and critical illness.

Key Points

1. High mobility group box 1 plays a role in gene expression and DNA recombination and repair.
2. While high mobility group box 1 was first described as a DNA-binding protein, myriad roles have been suggested for outside of the cell.
3. High mobility group box 1 appears to act in both an autocrine-paracrine and exocrine manner.
4. Strong evidence suggests that high mobility group box 1 plays an important, possibly causative, role in the pathogenesis of what may be loosely defined as severe sepsis in many animal models.
5. The importance of high mobility group box 1 in the pathogenesis of human sepsis and its role in the infectious disease process in humans remains to be fully elucidated.

Key References

4. Wang H, Bloom O, Zhang M, et al: HMG-1 as a late mediator of endotoxin lethality in mice. Science 1999;285:248-251.
23. Bonaldi T, Talamo F, Scaffidi P, et al: Monocytic cells hyperacetylate chromatin protein HMGB1 to redirect it towards secretion. EMBO J 2003;22:5551-5560.
36. Park JS, Svetkauskaite D, He Q, et al: Involvement of toll-like receptors 2 and 4 in cellular activation by high mobility group box 1 protein. J Biol Chem 2004;279:7370-7377.
49. Angus DC, Yang L, Kong L, et al: Circulating high mobility group box 1 (HMGB1) concentrations are elevated in both uncomplicated pneumonia and pneumonia with severe sepsis. Crit Care Med 2007;35:1061-1067.
54. Rouhiainen A, Tumova S, Valmu L, et al: Pivotal advance: analysis of proinflammatory activity of highly purified eukaryotic recombinant HMGB1 (amphoterin). J Leukoc Biol 2007;81:49-58.

See the companion Expert Consult website for the complete reference list.

CHAPTER 156

Epithelial Barrier Dysfunction as a Mechanism Underlying the Pathogenesis of Multiple-Organ Dysfunction

Mitchell P. Fink, Donna Beer-Stolz, Shiguang Liu, Penny L. Sappington, and Russell L. Delude

OBJECTIVES

This chapter will:
1. Review various competing models of multiple-organ dysfunction, including cytopathic hypoxia, cellular apoptosis, and epithelial barrier dysfunction.
2. Describe the roles of tight junctions in the maintenance of epithelial polarity and barrier function.
3. Discuss the relationship between nitric oxide and tight junction assembly and function.
4. Discuss the relationship between lipopolysaccharide and tight junction expression.
5. Review the evidence in support of epithelial dysfunction as a cause of liver, kidney, and lung dysfunction.

There is widespread agreement that the multiple-organ dysfunction syndrome (MODS) is the clinical manifestation of a dysregulated inflammatory response (Fig. 156-1). Indeed, most of the published research regarding the pathogenesis of MODS has focused on the various signaling pathways that lead to the activation of the innate immune system and the elaboration of cytokines, oxidants, tissue-destructive enzymes, and other pro-inflammatory mediators. Interestingly, however, the biochemical and cell-biological basis for organ dysfunction per se remains poorly understood. It is clear, however, that the histopathology of MODS in humans is remarkably bland; massive cell death, whether due to necrosis or apoptosis, is almost certainly not the cause of MODS. Rather, the final step in the development of MODS is probably the widespread *dysfunction* of parenchymal cells in multiple organs as a result of the deleterious effects of a poorly controlled systemic inflammatory response. In particular, derangements in the formation, function, or both, of specialized structures in epithelial cells—tight junctions and adherens junctions—may be a key factor leading to lung, liver, gut, and kidney dysfunction associated with conditions, such as sepsis and trauma, that are associated with dysregulated inflammatory processes.

POSSIBLE UNDERLYING MECHANISMS OF ORGAN DYSFUNCTION

Cytopathic Hypoxia

One possible explanation for cellular dysfunction in sepsis and MODS is an acquired intrinsic derangement in mitochondrial function leading to inadequate production of adenosine triphosphate (ATP)—a pathological state, which has been termed *cytopathic hypoxia*.[1,2] Although a number of subsequent clinical studies have confirmed that cellular respiration is deranged in patients with sepsis,[3-5] data obtained by Berg and colleagues[6] raise the possibility that mitochondrial dysfunction is more likely to be an epiphenomenon rather than a fundamental factor contributing to organ dysfunction in MODS. Berg and colleagues[6] carried out a study using cytomix-stimulated IEC-6 (nontransformed rat) enterocyte-like cells as a reductionist in vitro model of sepsis; results showed that the rate of ATP turnover actually increases in immunostimulated as compared to control monolayers. The increase in ATP utilization (and production) is maintained by a marked increase in the rate of glycolysis. In related studies, Scharte and colleagues[7] and Bertges and co-workers[8] showed that incubating Caco-2 (human enterocyte-like) or IEC-6 (nontransformed but immortalized rat enterocyte-like) cells with cytomix increases DNA binding by hypoxia-inducible factor (HIF)-1, the key transcription factor responsible for acute cellular adaptation to hypoxic conditions. Moreover, Scharte and colleagues[7] showed that incubating IEC-6 cells with cytomix leads to the transcriptional activation of two key HIF-1 responsive genes, aldolase A and enolase-1, that encode proteins important in the glycolytic pathway. Other results from both animal[9,10] and clinical studies[11,12] also support the view that sepsis is associated with a shift toward increased ATP production via glycolysis and away from oxidative phosphorylation.

Increased Cellular Apoptosis

Certainly, massive apoptosis among lymphoid cells is a prominent feature of sepsis in both human patients and mice.[13-16] Moreover, using pharmacological or genetic

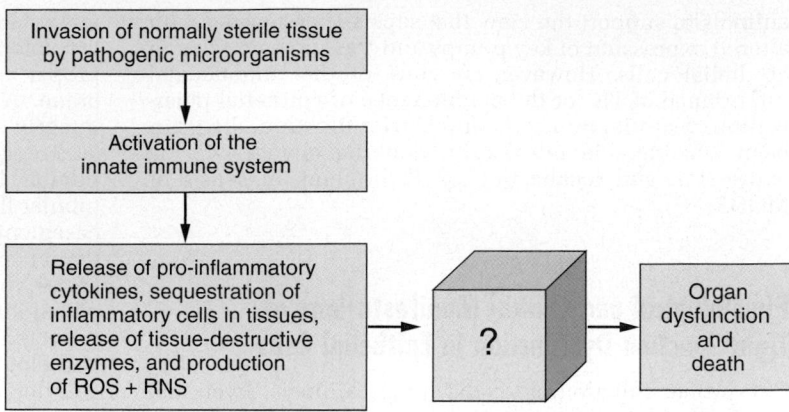

FIGURE 156-1. Current model for the pathogenesis of multiple organ dysfunction syndrome (MODS) due to sepsis. Although there is little controversy that dysregulated elaboration of pro-inflammatory mediators, reactive oxygen species (ROS), and reactive nitrogen species (RNS) is crucial for the development of MODS, the actual process involved remains a mystery. In the case of hepatic, intestinal, pulmonary, and renal failure due to sepsis, the "black box" in the pathway from inflammation to organ dysfunction may relate to alterations in the epithelial components of these organs.

approaches to limit lymphoid cell apoptosis improves survival in mice with bacterial peritonitis,[13,15] a finding that supports the view that increased programmed cell death of lymphocytes is significant in the pathogenesis of sepsis. Presumably, blocking lymphocytic apoptosis improves survival in experimental sepsis by improving host defenses against infection.[17] Alternatively, however, phagocytosis of apoptotic lymphocytes by macrophages may trigger the secretion of a pro-inflammatory cytokine-like protein, high mobility group box (HMGB)-1, exacerbating the deleterious systemic inflammatory response to infection and further promoting organ system injury.[18]

Intestinal epithelial apoptosis also occurs in both patients and animals with sepsis,[14,19] although most cells in the epithelial sheet are not affected. Despite these observations, neither apoptosis nor necrosis are prominent features in other organs, notably the lungs, liver, or kidneys, that are commonly involved in cases of MODS.[14,20] Thus, it is highly improbable that loss of cell mass per se can account for the development of lung, liver, gut, or kidney dysfunction in patients with MODS.

TIGHT JUNCTIONS

Role of Tight Junctions in Maintaining Epithelial Polarity and Barrier Function

The normal functioning of the lungs, liver, kidneys, and intestine, among other organs, depends on the establishment and maintenance of compositionally distinct compartments that are lined by sheets of epithelial cells. An essential element in this process is the formation of tight junctions (TJs) between adjacent cells making up the epithelial sheet. The TJ serves as a fence that differentiates the cytosolic membrane into apical and basolateral domains. This fence function preserves cellular polarity and, in combination with transcellular vectorial transport processes, generates distinct internal environments in the opposing compartments that are formed by the epithelial sheet. In addition, the TJ acts as a regulated semi-permeable barrier that limits the passive diffusion of solutes across the paracellular pathway between adjacent cells. Thus, the barrier function of the TJ is necessary to prevent dissipation of the concentration gradients that exist between the two compartments defined by the epithelium. In some organs, notably the gut and the lung, this barrier

function is also important to prevent systemic contamination by microbes and toxins that are present in the external environment.[21]

Situated immediately basal to the TJ is the adherens junction (AJ), which also is a continuous, circumferential belt-like structure and location for cell-cell interactions. The molecular architecture of the AJ is similar to that of the TJ. Importantly, the TJ is evolved from and stabilized by the AJ and is structurally and functionally interrelated to the AJ.[22]

Role of Multiple Proteins in the Assembly and Functioning of Tight Junctions

The formation of TJs involves the assembly of at least nine different peripheral membrane proteins and at least three different integral membrane proteins.[23] Among the peripheral membrane proteins associated with TJs are the membrane-associated guanylate kinase-like proteins, ZO-1, ZO-2, and ZO-3. The integral membrane proteins involved in TJ formation include, but are not limited to, occludin and members of a large class of proteins called claudins. Both occludin and the claudins contain four transmembrane domains and are thought to be the actual points of cell-cell contact within the TJ.[24] ZO-1 has been shown to interact with the cytoplasmic tails of occludin and the claudins.[25] In addition, ZO-1 interacts with ZO-2 and ZO-3, which then interact with various actin-binding proteins, such as pp120 CAS,[26,27] thereby linking the TJ with the cytoskeleton. Studies of mouse embryos indicate that ZO-1 localizes in plasma membrane plaques well before occludin is incorporated,[28,29] suggesting that ZO-1 probably plays a central role in the assembly of mature TJs.

Organ dysfunction due to systemic inflammation may be the aggregate "macroscopic" manifestation of derangements in cellular physiology that are not necessarily sufficient to cause cell death. Since many of the organs commonly affected in MODS (e.g., the lungs, liver, kidneys, and gut) depend on the proper functioning of an epithelial component, it is reasonable to hypothesize that epithelial cell dysfunction is important in this syndrome. Of course, the proper functioning of epithelia depends not only on the formation of TJs and AJs but also on the appropriate expression, localization, and activity of many other cellular constituents (e.g., membrane pumps, cytoskeletal proteins, and cell-surface integrins and receptors). Indeed, data have accumulated from studies using experimental animals to support the view that sepsis is associated with altered expression of key pumps and transport proteins in epithelial cells. However, in view of the fundamental importance of TJs for the maintenance of epithelial polarization, vectorial transport, and barrier function, there has been considerable interest in studying changes in the expression and localization of TJ proteins in sepsis or MODS.

Physiological and Clinical Manifestations of Tight Junction Dysfunction in Epithelial Cells

The proper functioning of the lungs, kidneys, liver, and gut depends on the generation and maintenance of compositionally distinct compartments. In the lungs, failure to maintain normal TJ formation would be expected to promote alveolar flooding, and hence pulmonary edema, on the basis of back-leakage of salt and water that is pumped from the apical side of the alveolar epithelium to the basolateral side. Of course, TJ dysfunction is not the only potential cause of impaired alveolar fluid clearance. Another cause might be decreased expression of Na^+,K^+-ATPase, the pump responsible for the vectorial transport of sodium ions,[30,31] or the epithelial sodium channel.[31]

Cholestatic jaundice is a fairly common clinical manifestation of MODS and is associated with an increased risk of mortality.[32,33] Efforts to understand the pathophysiological mechanisms responsible for cholestatic jaundice due to sepsis have largely focused on alterations in the function and expression of various bile acid transporters.[34-37] Nevertheless, another factor that could contribute to the development of intrahepatic cholestasis is back-leakage of bile from the canalicular spaces into the sinusoids.[38,39]

Alterations in the barrier function of the intestinal epithelium could permit the leakage of bacterial or microbial products, such as lipopolysaccharide (LPS), bacterial (CpG rich) DNA, or flagellin, from the lumen of the gut into the systemic compartment, leading to the initiation or amplification of a deleterious inflammatory response. The notion that this process actually occurs in patients with MODS is supported by results from a number of clinical studies, which have documented increases in intestinal epithelial permeability in a variety of acute conditions that are associated with systemic inflammation.[40-43] Moreover, in several recent studies, increased intestinal permeability in critically ill patients has been shown to be associated with an increased risk of complications, MODS, or even mortality.[42-46]

Acute renal failure in patients with sepsis or MODS is manifested by the development of azotemia and often also oliguria. The mechanisms underlying development of acute renal failure due to sepsis are likely multiple and remain poorly understood. Important factors are thought to be excessive renal vasoconstriction,[47] glomerular thrombin deposition,[48] and decreased expression of urea transporters in renal epithelial cells.[49] Without minimizing the importance of these and other mechanisms, it is reasonable to postulate that another factor might be back-leakage of tubular fluid as a result of TJ dysfunction in the tubular epithelium. Certainly, evidence from both animal[50] and human studies[51-53] supports the concept of back-leakage of glomerular filtrate during acute renal failure.

Additionally, loss of "fence function" (i.e., disruption of renal epithelial polarization) as a consequence of TJ and AJ dysfunction can lead to aberrant apical localization of membrane proteins, such as the integrins, which are normally localized to the basolateral aspect of the cells.[22] The basolateral localization of integrins is important for the proper anchoring of tubular cells to the basement membrane. ATP depletion results in the redistribution of β_1-integrin subunits to the apical membrane, and the loss of anchorage allows the exfoliation of viable cells into the tubular lumen,[54] potentially promoting back-leakage of tubular fluid via two mechanisms. First, denudation of the basement membrane on the basis of the detachment epithelial cells would be expected to expose a greater surface area for back-leakage of tubular fluid. Second, the presence of exfoliated cells within the tubular lumen would be expected to increase back-pressure, further exacerbating pathological back-leakage of glomerular filtrate. Tubular cell detachment[55,56] and obstruction[50] have been reported in studies of acute renal failure.

Role of Nitric Oxide and Peroxynitrite in the Regulation of Tight Junction Protein Expression and Function

The permeability of cultured epithelial monolayers increases when the cells are incubated with various pro-inflammatory cytokines.[57-62] The mechanisms responsible for cytokine-induced epithelial hyperpermeability are not completely understood. It is known, however, that compounds that spontaneously release nitric oxide (NO•) increase the permeability of cultured intestinal epithelial cell monolayers.[63,64] This observation is pertinent, since incubating Caco-2 human enterocyte-like cells with either the pro-inflammatory cytokine, interferon (IFN)-γ, or a mixture of the pro-inflammatory cytokines, IFN-γ + tumor necrosis factor (TNF) and interleukin (IL)-1β, leads to increased expression of inducible NO• synthase (iNOS) and increased production of NO•.[58,65,66] Moreover, compounds that inhibit the enzymatic activity of iNOS have been shown to ameliorate the development of hyperpermeability induced by exposing Caco-2 cells to IFN-γ[58] or "cytomix" (IFN-γ + TNF + IL-1β).[66] Similarly, L-N^6 (1-iminoethyl)lysine (L-NIL), an isoform-selective iNOS inhibitor, blocks the development of hyperpermeability when Calu-3 (human alveolar epithelial) monolayers are incubated with cytomix.[67] Thus, IFN-γ or cytomix appears to increase intestinal epithelial permeability, at least in part, by increasing the production of NO• by enterocytes.

NO• reacts rapidly with superoxide (O_2•⁻) to form the potent oxidizing and nitrating species, peroxynitrite (ONOO⁻).[68,69] Several lines of evidence support the view that ONOO⁻ (or some related species) rather than NO• per se is responsible for the deleterious effects of NO• on intestinal epithelial barrier function. Thus, when Caco-2 monolayers are incubated with the NO• donor, sensory nerve action potential (SNAP), permeability is significantly increased, but the magnitude of the effect is small.[64] Furthermore, the permeability of Caco-2 monolayers is not affected when the cells are incubated with pyrogallol, a compound that spontaneously generates O_2•⁻ in aqueous solutions.[64] However, if Caco-2 cells are co-incubated with both SNAP and pyrogallol, then epithelial permeability is dramatically increased.[64] SNAP-induced hyperpermeability is also markedly enhanced by co-incubating the cells with diethyldithiocarbamate, a compound that is known to inactivate Cu-Zn superoxide dismutase and would thereby be expected to increase the concentration of endogenously generated O_2•⁻.[64] Taken together, these findings support the view that NO•-induced hyperpermeability is enhanced by the simultaneous availability of $O_2\bullet^-$, that is, conditions favoring the formation of $ONOO^-$. Because ONOOH is a weak acid (pKa~6.8) and many of the effects of $ONOO^-$ are thought to be mediated by an unstable form of the protonated species, studies showing that NO•-induced hyperpermeability is enhanced under mildly acidic conditions further support the notion that $ONOO^-$/ONOOH is the responsible moiety.[70,57]

The mechanism(s) responsible for NO•- or $ONOO^-$-mediated intestinal epithelial hyperpermeability remain to be elucidated. However, it is known that NO• generated endogenously as the result of iNOS expression induced by incubating Caco-2 cells with cytomix or exogenously from the NO• donor DETA-NONOate ((Z)-1-(2(2-aminoethyl)-N-(2-ammonioethyl)amino)diazen-1-ium-1,2-diolate)) decreases the expression and impaired proper localization of the TJ proteins, ZO-1, ZO-3, and occludin.[59] Furthermore, incubating Caco-2 cells with either DETA-NONOate or cytomix increases the expression of another key TJ protein, claudin-1, and promotes the accumulation of this protein in what appear to be vesicles within the cells. These findings support the view that NO• (or a related reactive species) increases epithelial permeability by causing derangements in the expression, localization, or both, of several key TJ proteins.

Effect of NO•-Dependent Changes in Na$^+$,K$^+$-ATPase Activity on Tight Junction Assembly and Function

Sugi and colleagues[71] proposed that one way that NO• might alter the expression or localization of various TJ proteins is by modulating the activity of the membrane pump, Na$^+$,K$^+$-ATPase. In a series of studies using monolayers of T84 enterocyte-like cells, these investigators reported that intracellular sodium concentration and cell volume increase following exposure to the pro-inflammatory cytokine, IFN-γ. Additionally, Sugi and colleagues showed that incubating T84 cells with either NO• or IFN-γ decreases the expression and activity of Na$^+$,K$^+$-ATPase. Remarkably, growing the monolayers in medium with low sodium concentration inhibits the development of hyperpermeability following exposure to IFN-γ and also prevents IFN-γ-induced alterations in occludin expression. These findings suggest a pathway that involves the following steps: IFN-γ (and/or other pro-inflammatory cytokines) → iNOS induction → NO• production → inhibition of Na$^+$,K$^+$-ATPase expression and function → cell swelling → altered expression and/or targeting of TJ proteins (e.g., occludin) → hyperpermeability.

Qayyum and colleagues[72] reported that treatment of rat brain membranes with $ONOO^-$ in vitro decreases the activity of the Na$^+$,K$^+$-ATPase, and they hypothesized that this effect may be caused by nitration of the Na$^+$,K$^+$-ATPase. However, these authors did not demonstrate that $ONOO^-$ actually modifies the Na$^+$,K$^+$-ATPase. Mishra and colleagues implicated lipid peroxidation in the inactivation of the Na$^+$,K$^+$-ATPase in a previous report,[73] but only showed an association between lipid peroxidation and altered Na$^+$,K$^+$-ATPase activity in their studies. However, these authors convincingly showed that reactive oxygen species decrease the affinity of the Na$^+$,K$^+$-ATPase for Na$^+$ and K$^+$, inhibiting transport of these ions.[72,73] Taken together, these results support the notion that oxidative or nitrosative post-translational modifications of the Na$^+$,K$^+$-ATPase can lead to decreased epithelial barrier function.

FUNCTIONAL INDUCIBLE NITRIC OXIDE SYNTHASE EXPRESSION

Functional iNOS expression is essential for lipopolysaccharide-induced alterations in intestinal permeability in mice. When Han and colleagues[67] injected C57Bl/6J mice with a small sublethal (2 mg/kg) dose of *Escherichia coli* LPS, intestinal mucosal permeability to the permeability probe, fluorescein isothiocyanate-labeled dextran (molecular mass, 4 kD; FD4), increased significantly. Treatment of endotoxemic mice with L-NIL, an isoform-selective iNOS inhibitor,[74] ameliorated LPS-induced ileal mucosal hyperpermeability. Basal ileal mucosal permeability in control (PBS-treated) iNOS knockout (iNOS$^{-/-}$) mice on a C57Bl/6J background was greater than that measured in control (wild-type) iNOS$^{+/+}$ mice, a finding that is consistent with reports that basal levels of NO• are required for normal gut homeostasis.[75,76] Despite a basal defect in intestinal barrier function in iNOS$^{-/-}$ mice, permeability to FD4 failed to increase further when these mice were challenged with LPS.

Functional iNOS expression is essential also for lipopolysaccharide-induced bacterial translocation in mice. Bacterial translocation from the gut lumen to mesenteric lymph nodes is another measure of in vivo mucosal barrier function. In a recent study, endotoxemia increased the number of bacteria that were recovered from mesenteric lymph nodes from wild-type (iNOS$^{+/+}$) mice.[77] Treatment of endotoxemic iNOS$^{+/+}$ mice with L-NIL to block iNOS-dependent NO• production decreased LPS-induced bacterial translocation. Similarly, LPS failed to induce bacterial translocation in iNOS$^{-/-}$ mice. These findings are consistent with data reported by other investigators.[78]

LIPOPOLYSACCHARIDE DECREASES THE EXPRESSION OF SEVERAL TIGHT JUNCTION PROTEINS IN MICE

Han and colleagues used a portion of ileal tissue to prepare total and NP-40 (detergent)-insoluble protein extracts, the latter being enriched for TJ-associated and other cytoskeletal proteins.[77] Total protein extracts were subjected to immunoblotting. NP-40 insoluble proteins were first solubilized with detergent-containing buffer and concentrated by immunoprecipitation before immunoblotting. The expression of occludin in NP-40 insoluble extracts was decreased in samples obtained 6 hours after injecting mice with LPS.[77] Occludin expression in NP-40 insoluble extracts decreased still further at 12 hours, but was starting to return toward normal 18 hours after LPS challenge. In total protein extracts, changes in occludin levels were less dramatic, and the maximal decrease was observed at 12 hours. ZO-1 expression decreased slightly in total protein extracts from ileal mucosa of mice exposed to LPS. However, there was a large decrease in ZO-1 levels in the NP-40 insoluble fraction. This finding suggests that the ZO-1 that is present in the cells of endotoxemic animals is unable to assemble into TJs. Consistent with observations obtained using the Caco-2 system,[59] claudin-1 expression increased in total protein extracts prepared from ileal mucosa. Immunoblotting total protein extracts for actin revealed equivalent loading of the samples in these gels. As expected, iNOS protein expression increased in total protein extracts from ileal mucosa of LPS-treated mice.

ENDOTOXEMIA IS ASSOCIATED WITH DERANGEMENTS IN ILEAL MUCOSAL PROTEIN LOCALIZATION

Immunohistochemical studies of ileal tissue from endotoxemic mice were performed using samples harvested 12 hours after injection of LPS. ZO-1 formed a continuous staining pattern around the enterocyte layer near the apical region of the lateral membrane of crypt and villous cells of the epithelium and the endothelium of the lamina propria from normal mice. Following injection of mice with LPS, ZO-1 staining was maintained in the crypts, but staining progressively decreased over the tips of the villi. In sections from endotoxemic mice, the staining patterns for ZO-1 were disrupted only in focal regions of the ileum; approximately 60% of the villi in a given section stained normally. If the endotoxemic mice were treated with L-NIL to pharmacologically block iNOS-dependent NO• production, then the correct targeting of ZO-1 in the ileal mucosa was preserved. Similar findings were obtained when staining was carried out for occludin instead of ZO-1.

Parallel experiments were performed using iNOS$^{-/-}$ mice. The levels of occludin and ZO-1 in ileal mucosa from control iNOS$^{-/-}$ mice (i.e., those not challenged with LPS) were reproducibly lower than the levels of these proteins in control iNOS$^{+/+}$ mice. To some extent, these basal differences in occludin and ZO-1 expression confounded interpretation of the results obtained in LPS-challenged animals. Nevertheless, it was apparent that injecting iNOS$^{-/-}$ mice with LPS failed to cause a further decrease in the expression of ZO-1 or occludin in ileal mucosa. The localization of ZO-1 and occludin was preserved in ileal sections prepared from LPS-treated iNOS$^{-/-}$ mice, being essentially unchanged from what was observed in sections from iNOS$^{-/-}$ animals injected with vehicle.

LIPOPOLYSACCHARIDE IMPAIRS HEPATOBILIARY BARRIER FUNCTION VIA AN iNOS-DEPENDENT MECHANISM

Lora and colleagues[80] reported that hepatic TJ function can be assessed by measuring serum concentrations of bile acids and conjugated bilirubin. Han and associates[81] showed that circulating levels of both of these bile components were increased in mice injected 12 hours earlier with LPS. However, when endotoxemic mice were treated with L-NIL, serum levels of bile acids and conjugated bilirubin were not different from normal. Although basal serum and conjugated bilirubin levels were somewhat higher in vehicle-treated iNOS$^{-/-}$ as compared to iNOS$^{+/+}$ mice, LPS-induced changes in circulating bile acid and conjugated bilirubin levels were prevented by genetic ablation of iNOS function. Collectively, these data support the view that systemic inflammation in mice (induced by injecting LPS) is associated with hepatobiliary epithelial barrier dysfunction via an iNOS-dependent mechanism.

To further confirm these findings, Han and colleagues[81] employed another approach for assessing hepatobiliary tight junctional integrity. They cannulated the common bile duct of mice and assayed bile for the appearance of fluorescein isothiocyanate–labeled dextran (mol mass 40 kD; FD40) following intravenous injection of the tracer.

In control mice, biliary FD40 concentration increased only very slowly following injection of the tracer.[81] However, in mice injected with LPS (2 mg/kg) 12 hours earlier, the concentration of FD40 in bile increased rapidly after intravenous injection of the tracer. The LPS-induced increase in biliary FD40 concentration was prevented if the endotoxemic animals were treated with L-NIL. The rate of bile flow was about 50% lower in endotoxemic mice as compared to control mice, a finding that is consistent with other studies.[36] While decreased bile flow rate would tend to increase the measured concentration in bile of a marker like FD40, the approximately 50% decrease in bile flow rate observed in the endotoxemic mice is insufficient to account for the nearly 10-fold increase in FD40 concentration in bile that was detected in LPS-challenged as compared to control animals. Accordingly, the marked increase in biliary FD40 concentration was evidence of deranged hepatobiliary TJ function.

LIPOPOLYSACCHARIDE INDUCES HEPATIC iNOS EXPRESSION AND ALTERATIONS IN HEPATIC TJ PROTEIN EXPRESSION

In the studies carried out by Han and colleagues[81] of the effects of endotoxemia on hepatobiliary epithelial barrier function in mice, immunoreactive iNOS was not detectable by Western blotting of hepatic protein extracts from control mice. However, within 6 hours after the injection of LPS, hepatic iNOS expression was clearly evident. Levels of iNOS protein in liver increased still further 12 and 18 hours after the injection of LPS. Following the induction of endotoxemia, occludin and ZO-1 expression decreased in NP-40 insoluble (cytoskeletal fraction with associated TJ proteins) extracts of hepatic tissue. Decreased expression of these TJ proteins was also observed in total protein extracts, but the change in occludin expression occurred more gradually. ZO-2 and ZO-3 levels also decreased in total protein extracts. Claudin-1 expression did not change reproducibly in total protein extracts.

ENDOTOXEMIA IS ASSOCIATED WITH DERANGEMENTS IN HEPATIC TJ PROTEIN LOCALIZATION

Han and colleagues found minimal evidence of hepatic inflammation or necrosis when they examined hematoxylin- and eosin-stained thin sections of liver tissue from mice injected 12 hours earlier with LPS, irrespective of whether the animals were treated with L-NIL.[81] In control specimens, occludin and ZO-1 were largely detected as parallel strands of staining representing the outlines of canaliculi. Consistent with previously reported data,[82] staining of occludin and ZO-1 in normal liver tissue was predominantly limited to focal regions of hepatocyte-hepatocyte contact and endothelial cell-cell junctions. Hepatic tissue from endotoxemic mice showed a widespread decrease in occludin staining. The remaining areas of occludin staining were tortuous and discontinuous. Similarly, ZO-1 staining was greatly reduced following injection of LPS, and the residual ZO-1 staining was distorted. In contrast to the dramatic decrease of immunostaining for ZO-1 and occludin in hepatocytes of the LPS group, there was obvious preservation of occludin and ZO-1 staining along the outlines of canaliculi in endotoxemic mice treated with L-NIL. Similar protection against LPS-induced alterations in ZO-1 and occludin staining were observed when hepatic sections from LPS-challenged iNOS$^{+/+}$ and iNOS$^{-/-}$ mice were compared.

A PRO-INFLAMMATORY MILIEU DECREASES PULMONARY EPITHELIAL BARRIER FUNCTION

Prompted by the findings noted in the previous section supporting the notion that systemic inflammation induced by injecting LPS causes alterations in epithelial TJ formation in two organs (liver and intestine), Han and colleagues[67] extended these observations by examining the effect of LPS (2 mg/kg) on the leakage of FD4 from plasma into the alveolar space in C57Bl/6J mice. At various time points after injection of LPS (or PBS), mice were injected intravenously with FD4 in saline. Within 6 hours after the induction of endotoxemia, the bronchoalveolar lavage fluid (BALF)/serum FD4 ratio had increased significantly. At 12 hours, the BALF/serum FD4 ratio had increased still further. However, by 18 hours, the BALF/serum FD4 ratio had normalized. Delayed treatment with L-NIL significantly ameliorated the increase in lung permeability caused by LPS. These findings indicate that injecting mice with LPS transiently impairs bronchoalveolar epithelial barrier function and support the view that LPS-induced bronchoalveolar barrier dysfunction is mediated, at least in part, by iNOS-dependent NO• synthesis.

Injecting mice with LPS significantly increased the concentration of the NO• breakdown products, NO_2^- and NO_3^-, in BALF and serum (data not shown). Treatment with L-NIL only partially inhibited the accumulation of NO_2^- and NO_3^- in serum, whereas treatment with the iNOS inhibitor almost completely blocked accumulation of these NO• metabolites in BALF.

NP-40 insoluble occludin and ZO-1 levels decreased in lung tissue within 6 hours after injecting mice with a sublethal dose of LPS and were maximally decreased at 12 hours. By 18 hours, NP-40 insoluble occludin and ZO-1 levels were starting to normalize. In lung tissue specimens from normal mice, ZO-1 was localized as a continuous line along the boundaries between neighboring bronchial and alveolar epithelial cells. The intensity of this staining was markedly reduced in lung tissue harvested from mice that were challenged with LPS 12 hours earlier.

HMGB1 IS A MEDIATOR OF EPITHELIAL DYSFUNCTION

Mammalian high mobility group (HMG) proteins are grouped into three distinct families—the HMGB family, the HMGN family, and the HMGA family—on the basis of characteristic functional sequences.[83-85] Originally identified in the early 1960s,[86] HMG proteins have been isolated and characterized from a wide variety of species, ranging from yeast to humans.[87] All HMG proteins bind DNA and are soluble in 5% perchloric acid.[87] HMG proteins all have an unusual amino acid composition characterized by a high content of charged amino acids and a high content of proline.[83]

The HMGB family proteins—namely, HMGB1 (previously called HMG1) and HMGB2 (previously called HMG2)—have molecular masses of about 28 kD and share greater than 80% amino acid sequence identity.[83,88] The HMGB proteins bend DNA by virtue of a conserved DNA binding domain, the so-called HMG1 box.[85] Each HMG1 box contains a string of 70 to 80 amino acid residues, which is folded into a characteristic, twisted, L-shaped structure.[85,89] HMGB1 facilitates the binding of several regulatory protein complexes to DNA, particularly members of the nuclear hormone–receptor family,[90,91] V(D)J recombinases,[92] and the tumor suppressor proteins p53 and p73.[93]

In 1999, HMGB1 was identified as a cytokine-like mediator of LPS-induced mortality in mice.[94] Subsequently, these findings were extended by Yang and colleagues,[95] who showed that HMGB1 is also a mediator of lethality in mice rendered septic by the induction of polymicrobial bacterial peritonitis. Additional studies have documented that extracellular HMGB1 can promote TNF release from mononuclear cells[96] and increase the permeability of Caco-2 monolayers.[97] Interestingly, HMGB1 released by immunostimulated Caco-2 cells (discussed later in this section) seems to be capable of further amplifying derangements in TJ function initially triggered by other pro-inflammatory cytokines.[98] Furthermore, treatment with a polyclonal anti-HMGB1 neutralizing antibody has been shown to ameliorate gut mucosal hyperpermeability and improve survival in mice subjected to hemorrhagic shock.[99]

HMGB1 also has been implicated in the pathogenesis of human diseases. In the original report describing HMGB1 as a mediator of LPS-induced lethality, Wang and colleagues[94] reported that circulating levels of this protein are increased in patients with severe sepsis. Shortly thereafter, Ombrellino and co-workers[100] described a patient with high circulating levels of HMGB1 following an episode of hemorrhagic shock. More recently, increased levels of HMGB1 mRNA have been detected in whole blood samples from patients with septic shock, particularly among nonsurvivors.[101] Similarly, persistently high serum levels of HMGB1 protein have been detected in patients with septic shock and sepsis.[102] Elevated circulating levels of HMGB1 also have been documented and shown to correlate with severity of injury in victims of multiple trauma.[99,103]

One of the most interesting features of HMGB1 as a cytokine-like mediator of inflammation is that this protein is released much later in the inflammatory process than are the classical "alarm-phase" cytokines, such as TNF and IL-1β. For example, in mice, injection of a bolus dose of LPS elicits a monophasic spike in circulating TNF that peaks within 60 to 90 minutes of the pro-inflammatory challenge and is finished within 4 hours.[104] The peak in IL-1β concentration occurs somewhat later, that is, 4 to 6 hours after the injection of LPS.[105] In contrast, after injecting mice with LPS, circulating levels of HMGB1 are not elevated until 16 hours after the pro-inflammatory stimulus but remain elevated for more than 30 hours.[94] Furthermore, treatment with neutralizing anti-HMGB1 antibodies[94,95] or various pharmacological agents that block HMGB1 secretion, such as nicotine[106] or ethyl pyruvate,[107] is effective in preventing LPS- or sepsis-induced lethality, even when treatment is started 4 to 24 hours after the initiation of the disease process. Because of the delayed kinetics for release, HMGB1 is a very attractive drug target for acute, often lethal, syndromes, such as severe sepsis and hemorrhagic shock, because the "treatment window" for anti-HMGB1 therapies should be longer than is the case for therapeutic agents directed at more proximal mediators of the inflammatory cascade (e.g., TNF or IL-1β).

HMGB1 is passively released by necrotic, but not apoptotic, cells.[108] In this fashion, the release of HMGB1 from tissue damaged by trauma or ischemia may serve as an endogenous "danger signal" that alerts the immune system to the presence of injured cells.[109,110]

HMGB1 is actively secreted by immunostimulated macrophages,[94,111-113] natural killer cells,[114] plasmacytoid dendritic cells,[115] and pituicytes.[116] Like members of the IL-1 family of cytokines, the primary amino acid sequence of HMGB1 lacks a signal peptide. Accordingly, secretion of HMGB1 presumably occurs via a nonclassical secretory pathway. Indeed, when monocytes are activated by exposure to LPS, HMGB1 relocalizes from the nucleus into cytoplasmic organelles that belong to the endolysosomal compartment.[112] Gardella and colleagues[112] reported that 65% of HMGB1 is confined to the nucleus in resting monocytes, but only 26% of HMGB1 is nuclear and 74% is associated with cytoplasmic organelles in LPS-stimulated monocytes. In activated monocytes, the transfer of HMGB1 from the nucleus to the cytoplasm is mediated by hyperacetylation of critical lysine clusters that are components of nuclear localization signals.[113] This acetylation prevents HMGB1 from interacting with the nuclear-importer protein complex, so re-entry to the nucleus is blocked. Acetylated, cytosolic HMGB1 subsequently migrates to cytoplasmic secretory vesicles. It is currently not known how cellular activation leads to acetylation of HMGB1.

Epithelial cells, including enterocytes, also secrete HMGB1 following immune stimulation. Kuniyasu and colleagues[117] recently reported that WiDr human colon cancer cells constitutively release HMGB1 into culture supernatants. In contrast, Liu and colleagues[98] observed only very low levels of HMGB1 in the media of unstimulated Caco-2 cells. However, following stimulation of the cells with cytomix, Liu and colleagues observed a large increase in the amount of HMGB1 released into the culture media. These investigators also showed that incubating Caco-2 cells with the synthetic Toll-like receptor (TLR) 2 ligand, FSL-1, or the TLR5 ligand, flagellin, caused a large increase in the amount of HMGB1 released into the media. Interestingly, the TLR4 agonist, LPS, failed to stimulate HGMB1 secretion by Caco-2 cells.

Since it is known that HMGB1 is released by necrotic cells,[108] it was important to document that incubating Caco-2 cells with cytomix for 48 hours was associated with neither an increase in the number of cells taking up the vital dye (trypan blue) nor increased release of the intracellular enzyme, lactate dehydrogenase (LDH). These observations confirm findings previously reported, which showed that incubation of Caco-2 cells with cytomix fails to increase staining with the fluorescent dye ethidium homodimer-1, which only penetrates into dead cells.[118] Because Kuniyasu and colleagues[117] showed that colon cancer cells release HMGB1 and Caco-2 cells are cancer cells, it is noteworthy that it was also shown that cytomix-stimulated (but not resting) *primary* murine enterocyte cultures release HMGB1. Thus, these findings support the view that immunostimulated enterocytes (and not just colon cancer cells) secrete HMGB1, and the release of this protein by these cells is the result of an active process rather than a process secondary to cell death.

CONCLUSION

Collectively, the results from more than a decade of work by scientists around the world support the view that an inflammatory milieu leads to marked alterations in the structure and function of TJs in the epithelia of multiple organs. These data have been obtained using both reductionist in vitro models, such as Caco-2 enterocyte-like cells growing as monolayers in diffusion chambers, and in vivo models, such as mice injected with the pro-inflammatory bacterial product LPS. Although the mechanism(s) responsible for TJ dysfunction associated with acute inflammation are likely to be complex, and in any case remain poorly delineated, findings suggest that induction of iNOS and increased production of NO• are almost certainly important. Determining how NO• production leads to alterations in the expression and targeting of TJ proteins currently is the focus of a major research program at the Delude Laboratory at the University of Pittsburgh. In addition to determining how NO• and pro-inflammatory cytokines (and, possibly, other mediators) cause epithelial barrier dysfunction, another important goal of this research program is to move beyond studies using just cultured cells or rodent models of sepsis and begin obtaining data to support (or refute) the notion that the expression and targeting of TJ proteins is impaired in the pulmonary, hepatic, renal, or intestinal epithelia of patients with sepsis and MODS. Finally, it is obviously important to seek therapeutic strategies that can prevent or even reverse TJ dysfunction in patients with MODS.

Key Points

1. Results from work by scientists around the world support the view that an inflammatory milieu leads to marked alterations in the structure and function of epithelial tight junctions in multiple organs.
2. While the mechanisms responsible for tight junction dysfunction associated with acute inflammation are complex and poorly delineated, available data suggest that induction of inducible nitric oxide synthase and increased production of nitric oxide are key steps.
3. Efforts to find therapeutic strategies that can prevent or even reverse tight junction dysfunction in patients with multiple-organ dysfunction are currently under way.

Key References

67. Han X, Fink MP, Uchiyama T, Delude RL: Increased iNOS activity is essential for the development of pulmonary epithelial tight junction dysfunction in endotoxemic mice. Am J Physiol Lung Cell Mol Physiol 2004;286:L259-L267.
77. Han X, Fink MP, Yang R, Delude RL: Increased iNOS activity is essential for intestinal epithelial tight junction dysfunction in endotoxemic mice. Shock 2004;21:261-270.
81. Han X, Fink MP, Uchiyama T, et al: Increased iNOS activity is essential for the development of hepatic epithelial tight junction dysfunction in endotoxemic mice. Am J Physiol Gastrointest Liver Physiol 2004;286:G126-G136.
94. Wang H, Bloom O, Zhang M, et al: HMG-1 as a late mediator of endotoxin lethality in mice. Science 1999;285:248-251.
97. Sappington PL, Yang R, Yang H, et al: HMGB1 B box increases the permeability of Caco-2 enterocytic monolayers and impairs intestinal barrier function in mice. Gastroenterology 2002;123:790-802.

See the companion Expert Consult website for the complete reference list.

CHAPTER 157

The Coagulation System in Inflammation

Yann-Erick Claessens, Christophe Vinsonneau, Jean-Christophe Allo, and Jean-François Dhainaut

---

OBJECTIVES

This chapter will:
1. Explain the contribution of the coagulation pathway in innate immunity.
2. Discuss the role of coagulation in the pathophysiology of sepsis.
3. Describe the network that links coagulation and inflammation in sepsis.

A consensus conference defined *sepsis* as "the systemic inflammatory response syndrome that occurs during infection."[1] This definition suggests that the host must develop mechanisms for fighting off the microorganism responsible for the infection; these mechanisms include inflammation driven by endothelium and mononuclear cells that cooperate to produce various responses. The process of fighting off infection also involves the activation of the coagulation pathway, mainly through the production of tissue factor, with generation of thrombin that leads to clotting.

It was initially suggested that sepsis represents an uncontrolled inflammatory response. Lewis Thomas popularized this notion when he wrote that "the microorganisms that seem to have it in for us turn out to be rather more like bystanders. It is our response to their presence that makes the disease. Our arsenals for fighting off bacteria are so powerful that we are more in danger from them than the invaders."[2] This notion applies perfectly to the coagulation activation that may provide more harm than benefit when uncontrolled. For instance, disseminated intravascular coagulation is regarded as a cornerstone of sepsis pathophysiology and results in microvasculature thrombosis leading to ischemia of organs whose impairment may lead to multiple-organ failure and death. This chapter summarizes the current knowledge about coagulation and the intricate network it shares with inflammation during sepsis.

THE EVOLUTIONARY POINT OF VIEW

Coagulation was initially recognized as a separate mechanism involved in clotting, which limited blood loss after blood barrier injury. However, data from archaic invertebrates have underscored the intimate relationship between innate immunity and coagulation. For instance, the horseshoe crab *Limulus* has developed a specialized blood cell called an *amebocyte* that has both phagocyte and clotting capacities.[3] After exposure to endotoxin (lipopolysaccharide [LPS]), the amebocyte undergoes aggregation, adhe-

sion, and degranulation at the site of injury after recognition through the Toll-like receptor pathway, inducing microorganism engulfment. Degranulation results in release of proteins involved in antimicrobial defenses but also in a proteolytic cascade that leads to clotting after processing of the coagulable coagulogen. This clotting system, initiated by pathogens, is important not only in the prevention of potential leakage hemolymph (the horseshoe crab blood) after exoskeletal injury but also in the immobilization of invaders as part of the defense system. Additionally, *Limulus* anti-LPS factor, a protein involved in the clot, neutralizes gram-negative bacterial invasions.[4] This underscores that arthropods have summarized in a single cell the fundamental components of the innate immune system that is refined in more evolved organisms such as mammals.

COAGULATION IN HUMANS

Procoagulant Systems

The triggering of coagulation after exposure to LPS has been conserved and emphasized throughout evolution, as it ubiquitously activates clotting pathways in animals, especially in humans who are among the most sensitive species who enhance the innate anti-infectious response.[5] LPS is responsible for vascular wall injury and thereby activates the intrinsic coagulation pathway[6]: factors XII and XI, prekallikrein, and high-molecular-weight kininogen Fig. 157-1. The downstream pathway is not specific to activation by sepsis and is shared by other triggers. It involves the generation of a multimolecular complex with the activated form of factors IX and VIII and promotes activation of factor X. Association of activated factors X and V with calcium and phospholipids allows activating cleavage of prothrombin. Thrombin generation facilitates production and polymerization of fibrin and subsequent stabilization by factor XIII. However, the intrinsic coagulation pathway is thought to be secondary during response to sepsis. The activation of the intrinsic coagulation pathway is not constant, even in the presence of LPS, and it may be produced by an amplification loop during sepsis-related disseminated intravascular coagulation,[7] especially due to activation by thrombin,[8] and may play a role in sepsis-induced hemodynamic failure by way of kininogen products.[9] Thus the procoagulant contribution of intrinsic pathway is limited in septic-related coagulopathy and does not contribute much to thrombin generation.[10]

The extrinsic coagulation pathway depends on tissue factor (TF) expression and its combination with activated factor VII. As in the intrinsic pathway, this complex allows thrombin generation after activation of factor X. Activating coagulation by TF is the prevailing mechanism in sepsis.[11]

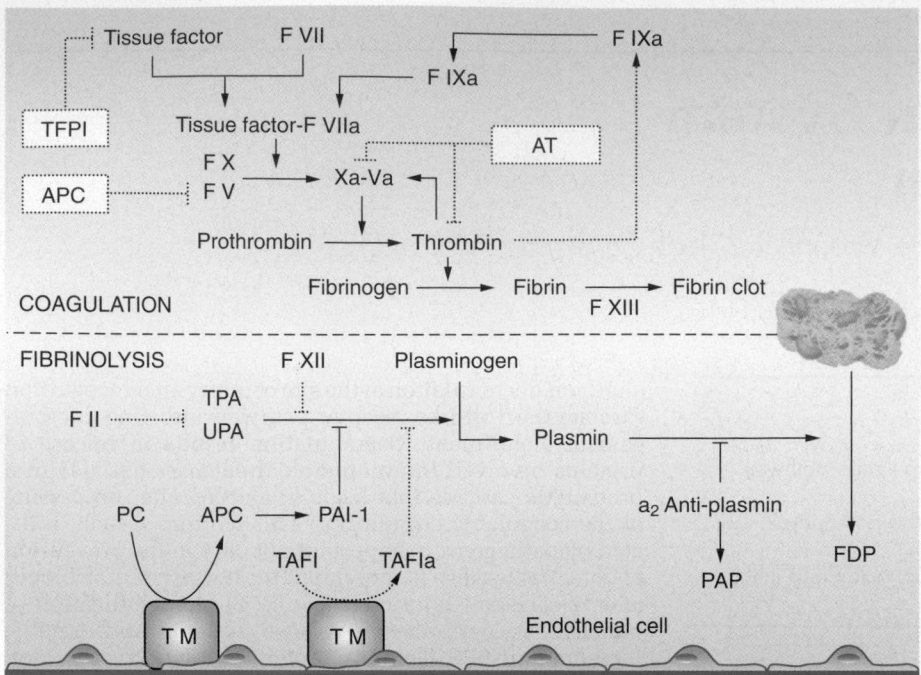

FIGURE 157-1. Global scheme of coagulation and mechanisms of regulation. APC, activated protein C; AT, antithrombin; F, factor; FDP, fibrin degradation product; PAI-1, plasminogen activator inhibitor 1; PAP, plasmin-antiplasmin complex; PC, protein C; TAFI, thrombin-activatable fibrinolysis inhibitor; TAFIa, activated thrombin-activatable fibrinolysis inhibitor; TFPI, tissue factor–pathway inhibitor; TPA, tissue plasminogen activator; UPA, urokinase plasminogen activator; Xa-Va, factor Xa-factor Va complex.

At steady state, TF is expressed on cells surrounding the vascular bed, especially myoblasts and fibroblasts, to activate fibrin clotting in case of blood vessel–wall injury. Systemic inflammatory stimuli are responsible for soluble TF activity. This is the consequence of membrane TF overexpression on monocyte/macrophage and endothelial cells after exposure to LPS, C reactive protein, and interleukins 1 (IL-1) and 6 (IL-6)[12]; during sepsis, these cells produce microparticles that can spread along the bloodstream[13] and carry TF.[14] TF associates with factor VII in a molecular complex that activates coagulation through factors X and IX. Thrombin generation feeds back the procoagulant mechanism at the level of factor XI and, to a lesser degree, factors VIII and V, to promote factor X conversion and thrombin generation via the contact factor system.[15]

Anticoagulant Systems

Clotting can be counteracted by means of several mechanisms: fibrinolysis, anticoagulation proteins (protein C, protein S, thrombomodulin), and TF pathway inhibitor (TFPI). Impairment in these systems contributes to defective clot removal and microvasculature disseminated intravascular coagulation.

Fibrinolysis is physiologically activated once a clot has been generated. The contact factor pathway also functions to activate the fibrinolytic system, along with the pro-inflammatory cytokine tumor necrosis factor (TNF).[16] Fibrinolysis functions efficiently after the activating cleavage of plasminogen into plasmin. Plasmin counteracts clotting by degradation of fibrin and factors V and VIII. Plasmin itself is downregulated by specific inhibitors. Plasminogen activator inhibitors 1 (PAI-1) and 2 (PAI-2) counteract intravascular clotting, while extravascular fibrinolysis is primarily driven by PAI-2. Systems that decrease thrombin formation, like activated protein C–protein S

complex, favor fibrinolysis by inhibiting the generation of thrombin-activatable fibrinolysis inhibitor (TAFI), which decreases susceptibility of fibrin to plasminogen and plasminogen activator.[16,17]

TFPI uses a single mechanism to inhibit coagulation. This molecule, stored in endothelial cells, combines with the activated form of factor X to bind to TF-VIIa. This condition is responsible for a shift that privileges the factor IX pathway. Then TF–factor VIIa complex becomes critical for thrombin generation and hemostasis.[18] In the setting of sepsis proteases induce an inhibiting cleavage of TFPI resulting in the generation of a less active form of the enzyme. TFPI may have a key role during sepsis.[19] *TFPI* knock-out mice present an embryonic lethality related to microvascular thrombi. Antibodies that inhibit TFPI are responsible for exacerbation of the effects of LPS. Addition of exogenous TFPI decreases coagulation and inflammation in sepsis models.[20] Since those effects were observed, TFPI was considered a suitable target for adjunctive therapy in sepsis. However, a multicenter phase III study has been unable to find a benefit of this compound to improve prognosis.[21]

A number of proteins involved in the coagulation pathway are enzymes with serine protease activity, such as thrombin, factor X, and many others. Antithrombin counteracts the activity of these factors. Antithrombin is activated by conformational changes after binding to specific motifs of heparans (linear polysaccharides whose structure is very similar to heparin), especially on endothelium, and acquires the capacity to inhibit serine proteases. Additionally, antithrombin has an anti-inflammatory role through endothelial production of prostacyclin, a potent agent that inhibits endothelial attachment of platelets and neutrophils and decreases endothelial and monocytic ability to produce IL-6, IL-8, and TNF, especially after LPS exposure.[22,23] In cell lineages, it decreases the activity of nuclear factor-κB (NF-κB). These experimental findings have also been observed in vivo in animal models.[24] The addition of antithrombin after LPS challenge decreases interaction between endothelium and cells involved in inflammation in rodents. It further limits capillary leakage, cell damage, and subsequent organ dysfunction usually prompted by their interaction. These vessel-protective effects of antithrombin are reversed in the presence of circulating heparin, probably because of the competitive binding to inadequate motifs out of the endothelium.[25] This might partly explain the failure of a human, phase III clinical trial that tested antithrombin administered during 4 days as an adjunctive therapy in 2314 septic patients.[26] In patients receiving heparin during the trial, a significant risk of hemorrhage was observed as compared to the control group (10.9% vs. 6.2%; $P < 0.01$). In the remaining population that did not receive heparin, a 15% benefit on 90-day mortality was observed. Although a minor effect was observed in the heparin-free subgroup, the use of heparin that suppressed circulating antithrombin could have been responsible for a detrimental effect, limiting the anti-inflammatory and vascular protective effects of antithrombin and providing a greater risk for clinically relevant hemorrhage. Finally, this can partly support absence of benefit on the overall treated group.[27] During sepsis, antithrombin activity is impaired by rapid consumption on activated factors and inactivating cleavage operated by neutrophil elastase, and its liver production decreases. This contributes to the procoagulant condition observed during sepsis. Inhibition by antithrombin of IL-8-related neutrophil chemotaxis is blocked by the addition of exogenous heparins that compete with antithrombin's endothelial binding.[28]

Protein C is a vitamin K–dependent anticoagulant generated in a thrombin-dependent manner, which gives birth to activated protein C (APC), a long plasma half-life protease. When thrombin binds to its membrane receptor thrombomodulin, it loses its ability to bind fibrin and platelets and enables the formation of APC after an activating proteolytic cleavage. APC limits the formation of new thrombin by degradation of factors Va and VIIIa. Its activity is increased by association to protein S. Additionally APC favors fibrinolysis, inhibiting two major fibrinolytic inhibitors. It binds to PAI-1 and inhibits its enzyme activity.[16] It also interacts with TAFI, as described earlier.

The interference of APC with fibrinolysis is enhanced by its interaction with proteins released by platelets, contributing to the successful treatment with its recombinant human counterpart.

TAFI is activated through thrombin; it controls thrombin itself but also controls complement activation by inactivating C5a and then decreasing endothelium changes and neutrophil recruitment.[6]

Apart from anticoagulation, APC has anti-inflammatory properties after binding to the specific endothelial protein C receptor (EPCR) to activate downstream intracellular pathways.[29] The mechanisms might be driven through cleavage of protease-activated receptor (PAR) type 1.[30] A number of phenomena that sustain APC's anti-inflammatory functions have been described. In a murine model, animals pretreated with rHuAPC did not experience hemodynamic changes usually observed after LPS challenge.[31] This was also noticed in a human phase II trial in which blood pressure was preserved by the use of drotrecogin alpha (activated).[32] Analyses of these models revealed that APC decreased TNF levels and leukocyte activation. In vitro data confirm the protective effect of APC. APC diminishes the level of inflammation[33] after various injuries by lowering the transcription level of NF-κB, which plays a major role in inflammation.[34] The result is a decrease in pro-inflammatory circulating factors and an imbalance of gene transcription in favor of anti-apoptotic signal. For instance, in various models of endothelial cell lineage, genes encoding for proteins involved in cell survival like Bcl-2 are upregulated, and expression of proapoptotic factors is significantly diminished, once again decreasing NF-κB transcriptional activity.[35] It is currently unclear if these findings have clinical relevance for septic patients.

Experimental sepsis animal models and human septic patients develop a deficit in natural anticoagulants. More precisely the levels of circulating antithrombin, protein S, and protein C decrease dramatically, especially in the more severe conditions.[36-38] The abnormal levels of thrombomodulin and functional EPCR in the microvasculature of septic patients also result in a defect of the cleavage of protein C into its activated form.[39,40] Altogether these findings lead to a strong rationale for supplementation of circulating APC levels as a valuable strategy to fight against consequences of coagulopathy in septic patients.

On behalf of the signals driven through the activation of protein C, both thrombomodulin and EPCR bear intrinsic anti-inflammatory capacities. The lectin domain of thrombomodulin reduces membrane expression of adhesion molecules and subsequently decreases blood leukocyte ability to bind to activated endothelium.[41] EPCR is released in the blood circulation after endothelium activation by thrombin. Soluble EPCR combines with proteases to inhibit neutrophil binding proteins.[42] These data suggest that protein C receptors could be potential targets for adjunctive therapy in sepsis.

INFLAMMATION ACTIVATES COAGULATION

Inflammation and coagulation interact to modulate global innate immunity response. This section describes some of the tight regulation of the inflammatory system on the coagulation network.

Pro-inflammatory Molecules

Sepsis leads to increased levels of circulating pro-inflammatory cytokines like IL-6.[43] These have been described to enhance the expression of TF at the membrane of endothelial cells and monocytes, leading to a subsequent activation of the extrinsic coagulation pathway. EPCR and thrombomodulin, the protein C receptors, have a decreased expression in the presence of the pro-inflammatory TNF-α and IL-1β, and then impair generation of thrombin.[44] Paradoxically, TNF-α induces development of a sustained fibrinolysis simultaneously to its procoagulant activity. However, the overproduction of tissue plasminogen activator is counteracted by PAI-1 and maintains the imbalance between pro- and anticoagulation mechanisms with overproduction of thrombin.[45]

Complement Factors and Acute Phase Proteins

A synergistic association of acute phase proteins participates in the procoagulant state in septic patients by direct or indirect pathways. C reactive protein activates the complement system that also plays a critical role in the coagulation balance. It also favors neutrophil activation, chemotaxis, and cytokine production. C reactive protein increases TF while α1 antitrypsin C4-binding protein induces inhibition of the activated form of anticoagulant protein C and protein S, respectively.[15,46]

An original mechanism that regulates coagulation involves catalytic immunoglobulins. Immunoglobulins that acquire enzyme functions were first described in autoimmune circumstances. It is now supposed that such proteins also exist during sepsis and may contribute to the inactivating cleavage of coagulation factors and counterbalance the deleterious effect of the uncontrolled procoagulant state.[47]

Cells: Neutrophils, Monocytes, Endothelium

The impact of inflammation on coagulation cascade is best represented by the study of neutropenic patients with infection. Septic patients with normal white blood cell count have activation of the fibrinolytic system involving an increased level of tissue plasminogen activator and PAI-1 that are subsequently combined, and thrombin formation is enhanced. A decreased production of tissue plasminogen activator and thrombin is observed in patients with neutropenia.[48,49] However, higher levels of PAI-1 are observed in the more severely septic patients whatever the white blood cell count. Activated neutrophils, mononuclear cells, and endothelium are involved in the procoagulant spiral. Especially activated neutrophils release elastase that induces proteolysis of antithrombin and then impairs anticoagulant properties.[50] As mentioned earlier, the septic coagulation relies mainly on TF and its downstream network. However, the intrinsic pathway also plays a role and amplifies coagulation. C1 esterase inhibitor is a key regulator of this latter pathway.[51] It also undergoes an inactivating cleavage after exposure to elastase released by activated neutrophils.

COAGULATION MODULATES INFLAMMATION

Procoagulant System

An important part of the coagulation-related inflammatory response depends on protein G coupled receptors named PARs, located on platelets, white blood cells, and endothelium.[51] Signals driven by PARs include production of pro-inflammatory cytokines, nitric oxide, and intracellular calcium flux. Several coagulation components have the capacity to activate PARs, including the TF–factor VIIa complex and factor Xa.[52] Thrombin generation promotes a high level of inflammatory response through the activation of PARs after cleavage of the amino-terminal extremity leading to the autoactivation of the receptors.[53] Thrombin also allows production of platelet-activating factor that favors neutrophil adhesion.[54]

Clotting can also promote inflammation through platelets. Activated platelets induce production of cytokines, including IL-1,[55] and activation of circulating mononuclear cells and their adhesion to endothelium through CD40 ligand[56] and P-selectin.[57] P-selectin production also depends on thrombin. The subsequent neutrophil activation results in the release of elastase that, as mentioned

earlier, induces degradation of antithrombin, C1 esterase, and TFPI.

Besides the disruption of anticoagulant mechanism, thrombin has the ability to promote IL-6 overexpression, which leads to TF overexpression and then enters an amplification loop of the coagulopathy.[23]

CLINICAL RELEVANCE OF COAGULATION SYSTEM IN HUMAN SEPSIS AND THERAPEUTIC INSIGHTS

Evidence now exists to support the clinical relevance of coagulation abnormalities in sepsis. Consequently several compounds that modulate clotting have been tested as adjunctive therapies in severe sepsis and septic shock.

A multicenter controlled double blind trial tested the effect of antithrombin in this setting. In spite of promising preclinical data, the results of this study showed no benefit of the use of antithrombin.[26] Despite a discussion about the potential negative role of low-molecular-weight heparin that could suppress antithrombin activation, the development of this strategy has ceased since the results of the study were published. TFPI was considered a suitable target for the treatment of sepsis-related coagulopathy. A multicenter phase III study named OPTIMIST tested tifacogin (recombinant TFPI) without benefit for the treatment group.[21]

One single-trial testing modulation of coagulation in sepsis has brought positive results.[58] The PROWESS phase III study reported a relative risk reduction of death of 19.4% in the intervention group. Initially designed to fight off coagulopathy, drotrecogin alpha (activated) has shown evidence of having several other beneficial effects, especially regarding inflammation, apoptosis, and microvasculature.[59,60]

This illustrates the difficulties of physicians in charge of severely ill septic patients. Besides the specific treatment of sepsis, targeting a coagulation or inflammation pathway leads to a cascade of modifications in a tightly regulated network. Reversing an imbalance may provoke impairment of the overall host defense.[61]

However, the experience of the recombinant activated protein C reopens a field of hope for development of strategies to modulate the host response in septic patients.

CONCLUSION

Coagulation is the cornerstone of the pathophysiology of sepsis. It relies on an imbalance between impaired fibrinolysis and an enhanced procoagulation state, whose key factor is TF which allows the overproduction of thrombin through the intrinsic pathway. Besides its main role, coagulation is part of a complex network that involves pro-inflammatory factors with bidirectional interactions that synergistically lead to an efficient innate immunity. When imbalanced, this tightly regulated system contributes to tissue ischemia and apoptosis. This complex pathomechanism has been only partially described, and further research in this area is essential to the successful treatment of sepsis.

Key Points

1. The coagulation pathway in sepsis relies mainly on thrombin formation.
2. The imbalance between coagulation and fibrinolysis induces a procoagulation state.
3. Coagulation and inflammation are tightly associated and provoke an activating loop.

Key References

6. Opal SM, Esmon CT: Bench-to-bedside review: Functional relationships between coagulation and the innate immune response and their respective roles in the pathogenesis of sepsis. Crit Care 2003;7:23-38.
7. Levi M, ten Cate H: Disseminated intravascular coagulation. N Engl J Med 1999;341:586-592.
12. Johnson K, Choi Y, DeGroot E, et al: Potential mechanisms for a proinflammatory vascular cytokine response to coagulation activation. J Immunol 1998;160:5130-5135.
53. Riewald M, Ruf W: Mechanistic coupling of protease signaling and initiation of coagulation by tissue factor. Proc Natl Acad Sci U S A 2001;98:7742-7747.
60. Cheng T, Liu D, Griffin JH, et al: Activated protein C blocks p53-mediated apoptosis in ischemic human brain endothelium and is neuroprotective. Nat Med 2003;9:338-342.

See the companion Expert Consult website for the complete reference list.

Laboratory Tests and Diagnostic Methods

CHAPTER 158

Laboratory Testing in Infectious Diseases

Peter K. Linden

OBJECTIVES

This chapter will:
1. Describe the routine indications for ordering a laboratory workup for infection and common stain and cultures for usual sites of suspected intensive care unit–acquired infection.
2. Outline the limitations of laboratory techniques for infection, including sensitivity, specificity, and predictive value.
3. Elucidate the advantages and limits of quantitative culture methodology for respiratory, urine, and catheter infections.

Critically ill patients presenting with signs or symptoms suggestive of infection require a prompt and clinically directed diagnostic evaluation to determine whether infection is present and what is its source(s) and microbial etiology. The most common clinical prompt to initiate such an evaluation is fever, most commonly defined as a temperature greater than 38.3° C and most reliably detected by core thermistor, bladder thermistor, oral, rectal, or tympanic methods. Laboratory evaluation for the presence of infection may also be appropriate for a much broader constellation of signs and symptoms encompassed by the Society for Critical Care Medicine and American College of Chest Physicians consensus definition for sepsis, which includes unexplained alterations in mental status, lactic acidosis, new onset oliguria, and hypotension, among others.

Since microbiological diagnostics incur expense, carry some risk, and may only yield data with a low specificity, they should be tailored to the patient's clinical presentation and epidemiological history. Thus "automatic" orders of blood, urine, and sputum cultures for a fever, which are not coupled with an individual contemporaneous assessment for localizing signs and symptoms, are inherently less effective from both a clinical and a cost perspective. This chapter concentrates on conventional microbiological diagnostic approaches in the critically ill patient. Clinical practitioners are encouraged to refer to the com-

prehensive evidence-based guidelines for the diagnostic evaluation of fever in critically ill patients, endorsed by the Society for Critical Care Medicine and Infectious Disease Society of America.[1]

DIAGNOSTIC METHODS

Laboratory tests to evaluate for infection are best divided into those that will yield information within a brief interval (minutes to hours) and methods that require a period of at least 1 to 2 days before results are available. Rapid data such as a leukocyte count and differential, routine stains, and newer, direct antigen–detection methods are particularly valuable in directing other diagnostic modalities, including radiological methods, and the empirical antimicrobial choices. Moreover, such techniques are less affected by prior or ongoing antimicrobial therapy. While culture methods are considered a gold standard, prior antimicrobial therapy may reduce their sensitivity and negative predictive value or, at the least, delay a positive result.

LABORATORY EVALUATION FOR BLOODSTREAM INFECTION

The bloodstream is normally a sterile body fluid compartment. Thus, demonstrating that a patient has bloodstream infection (BSI)–circulating organism(s) has significant diagnostic and prognostic import. Conversely, the absence of bacteremia or fungemia has a low negative predictive value for the presence of serious infection, as only the minority of patients with sepsis have documented bloodstream infection. Notably, the incidence of BSI increases sharply with progression from systemic inflammatory response syndrome (sepsis) to severe sepsis and shock.[2] Proper blood-culturing technique will maximize their sensitivity and reduce the number of false positives (contaminants). The rudiments of obtaining and interpreting blood cultures are summarized in Table 158-1.

Ideally after adequate skin preparation with chlorhexidine, two separate venipunctures are performed with 20

TABLE 158-1

Important Features for the Performance and Interpretation of Blood Cultures

PARAMETER	RECOMMENDATION	COMMENT
Site	Peripheral venipuncture	
Catheter-obtained	Distal lumen newest catheter	Coupled with 1-2 peripheral sets
Preparation	Chlorhexidine preferred	Alternative—iodine tincture
Number of cultures	2 for one culturing episode	
	2-3 for a 24-hour period	
Volume per set	20-30 mL per set	
On antimicrobial treatment	Resin bottles	Incremental yield usually contaminants
Mycobacteria, fungi	Isolator tubes	

to 30 mL of blood per culture set (aerobic and anaerobic bottle).[3]

From a recent study of 37,568 blood cultures, the cumulative diagnostic yield for detecting bacteremia or fungemia in patients without endocarditis was 80.6% for the first blood culture set, 95.7% for two sets, and 99% for three sets.[3] Thus, obtaining more than three blood culture sets within a 24-hour period is rarely justified. Conversely, obtaining only a single blood-culture set during a blood-culturing episode makes clinical interpretation difficult, particularly when coagulase-negative staphylococci are isolated, as these represent contaminants in 70% to 90% of instances and may lead to unneeded diagnostics, therapy, and costs.[4] The practice of drawing blood cultures through indwelling venous or arterial catheters to avoid a venipuncture is common but controversial since some studies have shown a high rate of false positives when compared to simultaneously drawn peripheral venipuncture cultures due to hub contaminants or colonizing organisms on the catheter's luminal surface.[5] Such practice should always be accompanied by at least one peripheral venipuncture culture and ideally should be obtained from the most recently placed vascular access device. Ongoing antimicrobial therapy may reduce the sensitivity of blood cultures. Routine blood-culture broth media contain sodium polyanethol sulfonate, which inactivates some antimicrobials. Although resin-containing blood-culture systems are commercially available, their value in boosting diagnostic yield in antimicrobial-treated patients appears minimal (less than 10%).[6] Special blood collection tube systems (Isolator, Inverness Medical Professional Diagnostics, Princeton, NJ), which employ a cell lysis–centrifugation processing method are available for intracellular bacteria, fungi, or mycobacteria, can be requested. Such systems are more commonly employed for immunocompromised hosts or patients from areas with endemic mycoses (histoplasmosis, coccidioidomycosis).

LABORATORY EVALUATION OF RESPIRATORY TRACT INFECTION

Infections of the upper and lower respiratory tract are the second most common nosocomial infection and most frequent reason for antimicrobial prescription and thus frequently require laboratory evaluation. Microbial colonization of the oropharynx, artificial airway surface, and upper airways complicates the performance and interpretation of respiratory stains and cultures. The patient's symptoms, physical findings, quantity and appearance of the sputum, and radiologic findings indicate respiratory tract cultures should be requested. The initial evaluation specimen may be an expectorated or saline-induced sputum, endotracheal aspirate, or blind or bronchoscopic washing or bronchoalveolar lavage sample.

Although strong advocates for each approach exist, current practice guidelines still emphasize that there is insufficient evidence to advocate bronchoscopic methods over less invasive methods.[7] Laboratory techniques for the processing of respiratory specimens, including those that may only be indicated in immunocompromised patients and other select epidemiological scenarios, are summarized in Table 158-2. A Gram stain should be performed to demonstrate the adequacy of the specimen as representative of lower respiratory origin with more than 25 polymorphonuclear neutrophils and fewer than 25 squamous epithelial cells per high-powered field. The dominant bacterial morphology on the Gram stain is valuable in guiding empirical antimicrobial selection. Several studies have shown that the presence of intracellular organisms in more than 2% to 5% of cells on Giemsa-stained lavage specimens correlated with quantitative proof of lower respiratory tract infection; however, this technique depends on the services and expertise of the local microbiological laboratory.[8]

In some circumstances other stains should be requested: Calcofluor white (for fungi), acid-fast stains (for *Mycobacterium tuberculosis* and atypical mycobacteria), wet mount (for parasites), and silver, Giemsa, or toluidine-blue stains (for *Pneumocystis jiroveci*).

Routine respiratory cultures can be performed in a semi-quantitative or quantitative fashion. Quantitative methodology may be performed on endotracheal, mini-bronchoscopic, or nonbronchoscopic bronchoalveolar lavage, bronchoscopic, and protected specimen brush specimens and has been a better discriminator for the presence of true lower respiratory tract infection than have nonquantitative methods in some but not all studies.[9-12] Despite the more prevalent use of quantitative methods in recent years, there has not yet been uniform standardization of either quantitative methodology or the diagnostic quantitative threshold of importance.[13] Viral pathogens of significance include influenza A or B, parainfluenza, Herpes simplex virus, cytomegalovirus, metapneumovirus, respiratory syncytial virus, adenovirus, and *Coxsackie*. Significant advances in the laboratory detection of viral respiratory pathogens with rapid detection methods, including fluorescent antibody, enzyme immunoassays, and polymerase chain reaction (PCR) techniques, are commercially available although their availability

TABLE 158-2

Laboratory Techniques for the Diagnosis of Respiratory Pathogens

PATHOGEN	STAINING—RAPID DETECTIONS METHOD(S)	CULTURE METHOD(S)	COMMENTS
Legionella	Urinary antigen for *L. pneumophila*, serogroup 1	Selective media	Nucleic acid tests
Nocardia	Gram stain Modified acid-fast stain	Selective media	Nucleic acid tests
M. tuberculosis	Acid-fast stain Fluorochrome stain	Culture in liquid and solid media	Nucleic acid tests
M. avium complex	Acid-fast stain	Culture in liquid and solid media	Nucleic acid tests
Mycobacteria spp.	Acid-fast stain	Culture in liquid and solid media	Nucleic acid tests
Rhodococcus equi	Gram stain	Routine media	May be reported as "diphtheroids"
P. jiroveci	Fluorescent-labeled antibody Grocott stain Giemsa stain Gomori stain Toluidine-blue stain		
Aspergillus Other mycelia	KOH wet mount Calcofluor white Silver stains	Fungal-selective media	Serum ELISA for detection of galactomannan or 1,3β-glucan has variable sensitivity for invasive aspergillosis
Herpes simplex virus	Direct fluorescent antibody Wright or Giemsa stain for intranuclear inclusions or multinucleated giant cells	Viral culture	BAL cytology for inclusion bodies Nucleic acid tests
Cytomegalovirus	Shell vial Antigen detection Nucleic acid tests	Viral culture (very slow growth)	BAL cytology for inclusions Blood assay for antigenemia
Human herpesvirus 6, human herpesvirus 7	Nucleic acid tests	Viral culture	
Adenovirus	Rapid antigen detection	Viral culture	Nucleic acid tests
Influenza A/B	Direct fluorescent antibody Enzyme immunoassay Rapid antigen-detection kit RT-PCR	Viral culture-EIA	
Respiratory syncytial virus	Enzyme immunoassay Nucleic acid tests	Viral culture	
Strongyloides stercoralis	Wet mount		Serum ELISA
Toxoplasma gondii	Giemsa stain Nucleic acid tests		

BAL, bronchoalveolar lavage; EIA, enzyme immunoassay; ELISA, enzyme-linked immunosorbent assay; KOH, potassium hydroxide; RT-PCR, reverse transcriptase–polymerase chain reaction.

will vary significantly across different microbiology laboratories.

Tests from specimens other than the respiratory tract may identify the etiology of pneumonia. These include serum antigenemia or PCR for cytomegalovirus, serum galactomannan for invasive aspergillosis, and urinary enzyme-linked immunosorbent assay (ELISA) for *Legionella pneumophila*.

LABORATORY EVALUATION OF URINARY TRACT INFECTION

Urinary tract infection is the most common intensive care unit (ICU)–acquired infection. Asymptomatic bacteriuria or candiduria also is quite common in bladder-catheterized patients in the ICU setting. Laboratory analysis of urine to discriminate infection from colonization still remains rather limited and thus requires clinical acumen to interpret. Urinanalysis for the presence of leukocytes (pyuria) is indicative of mucosal inflammation, although not necessarily urinary tract infection, and may be absent in the presence of true infection.[15] Leukocyte casts from a sediment are almost always indicative of upper tract infection. Leukocyte esterase and nitrite dipstick testing have not been shown to be reliable detectors of catheter-associated urinary tract infection.[16]

Urine should be collected from the aspiration port of the catheter tubing and sent quickly (<1 hour) to the laboratory for processing to avoid overgrowth of organisms. Urine Gram stain of a centrifuged specimen is a valuable and readily available tool used to demonstrate the predominant microbial morphology as well as the presence of leukocytes, indicative of an inflammatory response.

Quantitative methods are standardly performed and reported as the number of colonies per milliliter of urine.

Although 10⁵ organisms per milliliter of urine remains an accepted quantitative threshold for clean-catch specimens from noncatheterized patients, a similar threshold for catheterized patients is not established, as quantities as low as 10³ organisms per milliliter may be significant.[17]

LABORATORY EVALUATION OF CATHETER INFECTION

Since local evidence of infection at the entrance site (purulence, erythema, warmth, or tenderness) is notoriously absent in catheter-related infection, laboratory evaluation is often the only determinant for diagnosis.[18] The majority of catheter-related BSIs and local infections are due to noncuffed, short-term, multilumen central venous catheters; there are significantly lower rates of BSI in tunneled, peripheral, and arterial catheters.[19]

Patients with suspected catheter infection should have at least two peripheral blood cultures from separate venipunctures. If the catheter is removed, it should be performed in an aseptic manner. The intradermal segment, the catheter tip, or both, may be sent for culture. The most common laboratory method is the "roll technique," whereby the catheter segment is rolled along the agar surface several times and a quantitative count is reported. Some laboratories will also perform a broth culture by immersing the segment in a liquid culture medium which appears more sensitive for the detection of intraluminal pathogens; however, this is reported only as a semiquantitative result. An alternative approach, particularly in patients with long-term catheters who are not septic and lack local signs of catheter or tunnel infection, is to obtain one set of blood cultures through the catheter and a second set peripherally and record the "time-to-detection" of each specimen in the laboratory. In vitro growth of the same organism in the catheter-obtained blood specimen more than 120 minutes before the peripheral specimen is indicative that the catheter is the source of BSI.[21,22] The positive predictive value of catheter cultures is predicated on performing cultures only on removed catheters when there is reasonable clinical suspicion of catheter-related infection. Routine culturing of all removed catheters will yield a lower predictive value due to detecting incidental colonization of the catheter surface.[23]

LABORATORY EVALUATION OF SURGICAL SITE INFECTION

Surgical site infection is usually suspected based upon local findings such as tenderness, fluctuance, erythema, or purulence. Cultures of superficial wound swabs in patients without such local findings are likely to grow colonizing skin flora or mucosal flora and are not recommended. Removal of sutures or staples to allow staining and culture of expressed fluid or pus should be performed in postoperative infections. Tissue specimens are preferable to simple swabs. Anaerobic cultures need to be sent to the laboratory in a closed system or syringe. Quantitative wound cultures have principally been utilized in burn patients and are otherwise not considered routine practice.

LABORATORY EVALUATION OF CENTRAL NERVOUS SYSTEM INFECTION

Although the diagnostic yield of lumbar puncture is extremely low in the ICU setting, analysis of cerebrospinal fluid (CSF) to evaluate patients with unexplained mental status changes and other neurological signs and symptoms is the most common evaluation for central nervous system infection.[24] CSF is usually obtained by lumbar puncture, although it may be obtained via a ventriculostomy drain in neurosurgical or trauma patients with such drains. CSF obtained from patients with suspected central nervous system infection should be submitted to the laboratory for cell counts and leukocyte differential, glucose and protein concentrations, Gram stain, and bacterial cultures. Additional tests, such as latex agglutination for *Cryptococcus*, fungal stains and cultures, acid-fast stains and cultures, PCR for herpes simplex virus, syphilis testing, and viral cultures, depend upon the epidemiological history and presentation of the patient.

The immunocompromised patient may require additional tests, such as PCR, for herpes simplex virus, cytomegalovirus, Epstein-Barr virus, human herpesvirus 6, JC-papovavirus, West Nile virus, adenovirus, and enterovirus. Patients with bacterial meningitis usually have a hypoglycorrachia (CSF glucose <35 mg/dL), a CSF to blood glucose ratio less than 0.23, an elevated CSF protein level concentration higher than 220 mg/dL, and a neutrophilic pleocytosis (>2000 total white cells/μL).[25] Meningitis is essentially ruled out in immunocompetent patients with a normal opening pressure, fewer than 5 white blood cells/μL, and a normal CSF protein concentration.[26] In critically ill immunocompromised patients whose inflammatory response is further compromised, a higher clinical suspicion for infection should be maintained, regardless of initial cell counts and chemistry results, until final cultures are available. CSF lactate measurements may be useful in neurosurgical patients to distinguish infection from postoperative aseptic meningitis.[27,28]

LABORATORY EVALUATION OF DIARRHEA

Diarrhea in critically ill patients is most commonly of noninfectious origin and due to high osmolar tube feedings, medications, microvillus atrophy, hypoalbuminemia, or due to nonspecific alterations of the bowel microflora secondary to antimicrobials.

However, diarrhea due to *Clostridium difficile* colitis is the most common infectious cause of nosocomial diarrhea and a serious entity which requires early diagnosis so specific treatment modalities can be administered. Nonspecific laboratory markers of *C. difficile* colitis include a leukemoid peripheral leukocyte count and evidence of enteric inflammation by the presence of fecal leukocytes on a Wright stain.[29] The gold standard for diagnosis is the tissue cytotoxin assay for the presence of toxin B, which has the highest sensitivity and specificity. This test requires a 24- to 48-hour period and has 90% sensitivity for one specimen and 95% to 100% sensitivity with a second specimen.[30,31] Many laboratories now employ the enzyme immunoassay (EIA), which detects toxins A and B and is more rapidly performed than the tissue cytotoxin assay, with a turnover time of hours, but has a sensitivity at least 5% to 15% lower than the tissue assay.[32] EIA tests that detect only toxin A are not recommended since 2% to 3% of *C. difficile* strains produce only toxin B.[33] Stool cultures for *C. difficile* are not indicated since nontoxigenic strains of *C. difficile* may exist.[34] The diagnostic yield of enteric (*Shigella, Salmonella, Campylobacter, Escherichia coli 0157, Yersinia, Entamoeba histolytica*) cultures or ova and parasite exams for new onset nosocomial diarrhea are extremely low and are recommended only if epidemiological circumstances warrant them. Expanded enteric cultures and stains for *Mycobacterium avium* complex, *Cryptosporidium, Microsporidium, Strongyloides stercoralis*, and other parasites should be considered in immunosuppressed patients.

NOVEL LABORATORY TESTS IN FEVER AND SEPSIS

Several biomarkers have been investigated for their utility in rapidly discriminating true infection from other inflammatory processes causing fever. Pro-inflammatory cytokines such as tumor necrosis factor-α and interleukin-6 have been shown to be predictive of survival outcome but are neither sensitive nor specific markers for the presence or etiology of infection in critically ill patients.[35,36]

The endogenous acute phase reactant C-reactive protein and procalcitonin are two of several markers studied in suspected infection and sepsis. Procalcitonin is a 116 amino-acid prohormone moiety elaborated by peripheral blood mononuclear cells.[37] A meta-analysis of 12 studies comparing procalcitonin to C-reactive protein for the diagnosis of bacterial infection (vs. nonbacterial causes of inflammation) showed procalcitonin to have superior sensitivity (88% vs 75%) and specificity (81% vs. 67%),[38] although only six studies selectively included adult ICU patients.

A more sensitive serum procalcitonin assay (BRAHMS, Berlin) is now approved for the early detection of bacterial infections and sepsis in patients during the first day of ICU admission. Procalcitonin level elevation higher than 0.5 ng/mL occurring within 2 to 3 hours of onset was observed along the continuum from systemic inflammatory response syndrome (0.6-2.0 ng/mL), to severe sepsis (2-10 ng/mL), to septic shock (>10 ng/mL). Most importantly, viral infections, recent surgery, and chronic inflammatory states are not associated with an increment in procalcitonin levels. Thus, procalcitonin levels may be a valuable and rapidly available diagnostic tool but, at present, only as an adjunct to conventional diagnostic procedures.

Key Points

1. To maximize the sensitivity and specificity of blood cultures, at least 20 to 30 mL of blood per culture set should be obtained and two to three sets of cultures sent.
2. Catheter cultures should be paired with peripheral blood cultures and should be requested only when there is reasonable suspicion of catheter infection.
3. Invasive (bronchoscopic) and quantitative culture methodologies for the diagnosis of ventilator-associated pneumonia may yield more precise information than noninvasive, semi-quantitative methods, but they have not been shown thus far to change outcome.
4. The tissue cytotoxin assay remains the most sensitive and specific test for *Clostridium difficile* colitis although a negative initial test should be repeated at least once.
5. An expanded spectrum of tests to detect less common opportunistic pathogens should be ordered in epidemiologically appropriate circumstances, particularly for respiratory, gastrointestinal, and central nervous system presentations.

Key References

1. O'Grady NP, Barie P, Bartlett JG, et al, for the Task Force of the Society of Critical Care Medicine and the Infectious Diseases Society of America: Practice guidelines for evaluating fever in critically ill adult patients. Clin Infect Dis 1998; 26(5):1042-1059.
3. Cockerill FR 3rd, Wilson JW, Vetter EA, et al: Optimal testing parameters for blood cultures. Clin Infect Dis 2004;38(12): 1724-1730.
7. Guidelines for the management of adults with hospital-acquired, ventilator-associated, and healthcare-associated pneumonia. Am J Respir Crit Care Med 2005;171(4):388-416.
12. Heyland D, Dodek P, Muscedere J, Day A: A randomized trial of diagnostic techniques for ventilator-associated pneumonia. N Engl J Med 2006;355(25):2619-2630.
30. Bartlett JG: Narrative review: The new epidemic of *Clostridium difficile*–associated enteric disease. Ann Intern Med 2006;145(10):758-764.

See the companion Expert Consult website for the complete reference list.

Clinical Syndromes

CHAPTER 159

The Sepsis Syndrome

Jean-Louis Vincent

OBJECTIVES

This chapter will:
1. Provide current definitions of sepsis syndrome.
2. Discuss the characteristics of sepsis syndrome according to the PIRO (predisposing factors, infection, response, and organ dysfunction) framework.
3. Define the epidemiology of sepsis syndrome in terms of incidence, causative organisms, and outcome.

The sepsis syndrome was defined by Roger Bone and colleagues[1] as the systemic response to infection expressed as tachycardia, fever or hypothermia, tachypnea, and evidence of inadequate organ perfusion or organ dysfunction. The sepsis syndrome is now generally termed severe sepsis; when accompanied by hypotension, severe sepsis becomes septic shock. Over the years much debate has focused on how best to define sepsis, and inconsistencies and lack of clear definitions has hampered research into the pathogenesis of sepsis and the development of potential new therapies. Each "septic" patient is an individual with a different background, underlying disease process, and onset and origin of infection, and the immune response will be different in different patients and at different times in the same patient. The challenge is, therefore, to find a means to better classify the immune response in critically ill patients, to define the clinical syndrome of the systemic inflammatory response to infection, so that potential therapies can be appropriately targeted and timed for those patients most likely to benefit. This chapter provides an overview of current definitions and epidemiology of sepsis and severe sepsis; septic shock is covered in Chapter 160.

DEFINITIONS—PAST AND PRESENT

In 1991, in a first attempt to standardize definitions of sepsis, a North American Consensus Conference introduced the term *systemic inflammatory response syndrome* (SIRS) as a new concept; any patient having two of four parameters (temperature higher than 38° C or lower than 36° C; heart rate greater than 90 beats per minute; respiratory rate of more than 20 breaths per minute or partial pressure carbon dioxide ($PaCO_2$) less than 32 mm Hg; white blood cell count more than $12 \times 10^9/L$ or less than $4.0 \times 10^9/L$) was said to fulfill the SIRS criteria.[2] Sepsis was then defined as the presence of SIRS plus infection, severe sepsis as sepsis plus evidence of organ dysfunction, and septic shock as severe sepsis associated with cardiovascular failure necessitating the administration of vasopressor agents. These definitions have been widely used and the SIRS concept was embraced by many; however, most patients in intensive care units (ICUs) fulfill the SIRS criteria at some time during their ICU stay,[3] making these criteria too sensitive and nonspecific to be of use in identifying patients with sepsis.

In December 2001, responding to continuing dissatisfaction with current sepsis definitions, a consensus conference of 29 experts in the field of sepsis from around the world was held in Washington, DC, under the auspices of the Society of Critical Care Medicine (SCCM), the European Society of Intensive Care Medicine (ESICM), American College of Chest Physicians (ACCP), American Thoracic Society (ATS), and Surgical Infection Society (SIS), in an attempt to "provide a conceptual and a practical framework to define the systemic inflammatory response to infection, which is a progressive injurious process that falls under the generalized term 'sepsis' and includes sepsis-associated organ dysfunction as well."[4] The conference participants concluded that the definitions of *sepsis*, *severe sepsis*, and *septic shock*, as defined in the 1991 North American Consensus Conference,[2] remain useful to clinicians and researchers, but that the diagnostic criteria for SIRS were overly sensitive and nonspecific. They suggested that an expanded list of signs and symptoms of sepsis might better reflect the clinical response to infection (Table 159-1). In addition, the participants commented that the definitions did not allow precise staging or prognostication of the host response to infection, and a new approach to staging, the PIRO (predisposing factors, infection, response, organ dysfunction) system, modeled to some degree on the tumor-nodes-metastasis (TNM) staging system for cancers, was proposed.[4]

PIRO (PREDISPOSING FACTORS, INFECTION, RESPONSE, ORGAN DYSFUNCTION) SYSTEM

Although the PIRO system needs further development to establish how it can best be used clinically, the four PIRO components are key elements of the sepsis response and

TABLE 159-1

Some Signs of Sepsis

Fever or hypothermia
Increased cardiac output or low systemic vascular resistance
Increased oxygen consumption
Unexplained tachycardia
Altered white blood cell count
Increased C-reactive protein
Increased procalcitonin
Increased neopterin, elastase
Increased cytokine levels (e.g., TNF-α, IL-6, IL-10)
Increased cytokine receptors (e.g., TNF-α receptors)
Unexplained lactic acidosis
Thrombocytopenia or disseminated intravascular coagulation
Unexplained hyperventilation or respiratory alkalosis
Unexplained disorientation or confusion
Unexplained alteration in liver function tests
Unexplained alteration in renal function

IL-6, interleukin-6; IL-10, interleukin-10; TNF-α, tumor necrosis factor-α.

provide a framework by which the characteristics of the sepsis syndrome can be discussed.

Predisposing Factors

There are many predisposing factors that influence whether or not an individual will develop sepsis, how severe sepsis will be if it does develop, and how patients will respond to treatment. Such factors include age, sex, presence of chronic diseases, and prolonged treatment with immuno-depressant medications. The influence of sex on the risk of developing sepsis and on the outcome of sepsis has been studied only relatively recently. The multiple confound-ing factors, including age, comorbidities, and genetic poly-morphisms, make it difficult to tease out the effects of sex, and complex statistical modeling is required. In a large study in the United States, men were more likely to have sepsis than women in every year of the 22-year study, with a mean annual risk of 1.28.[5] Other studies have also shown men to be at greater risk of developing infection and sepsis.[6,7] However, the effect of sex on the outcome from sepsis is less clear, and studies have yielded conflicting results.[7,8]

Genetic makeup is also increasingly being recognized as a key factor in determining who will develop sepsis and the severity and outcome of disease when it does develop. In an early, long-term follow-up study of 960 Danish fami-lies with children who were adopted at an early age, the death of either biological parent from a severe infection before age 50 was associated with an almost sixfold increase in the relative risk of death of the child from infection.[9] There was no significant association between the risk of death due to infection in adopted children and their adoptive parents. This study thus supported a strong predilection for severe infection and septic shock based on the genetic background of individuals. Since this early study, several genetic polymorphisms have been identified that are associated with an increased risk of infection and of mortality from sepsis. A polymorphism of the tumor necrosis factor-α (TNF-α) gene, the TNF-2 allele, is associ-ated with increased serum levels of TNF and a greater risk of mortality from septic shock.[10] A polymorphism within the intron 2 of the interleukin-1 receptor antagonist (IL-1ra) gene (IL-1RN*2) has been associated with reduced

IL-1ra production and increased mortality rates.[11] Poly-morphisms in the Toll-like receptor and interferon-γ (IFN-γ) genes have also been identified as influencing individual responsiveness to endotoxin or sepsis.[12-14] Advances in genetics technology and development of DNA microarrays will facilitate research into the genetic factors associated with a predisposition to sepsis.[15]

Infection

Sepsis is the host response to infection and may vary in severity, response to treatment, and outcome according to various infection-specific factors, for example, gram-negative versus gram-positive, antimicrobial resistant versus antimicrobial sensitive, urinary tract infection versus respiratory tract infection, and so on. It is widely understood that urinary tract infections are less likely to be associated with severe sepsis than are lower respiratory tract infections or meningitis, and that more virulent organisms, for example, *Pseudomonas* sp., are likely to be associated with a greater risk of death, but it is difficult to quantify these relative effects. In a systematic literature review of 510 articles describing the outcome of infections, Cohen and colleagues[16] recently generated specific risk codes for bacteremia, meningitis, pneumonia, skin and soft tissue infections, peritonitis, and urinary tract infec-tions. For each infection site and organism, a two-digit code was generated according to the mortality rate associ-ated with that infection (from 1, meaning less than or equal to 5%, to 4, meaning greater than 30%), and the level of evidence available to support the mortality risk (level A representing evidence from more than five studies with more than 100 patients, through to level E representing insufficient evidence from case reports). For example, *Pseudomonas aeruginosa* pneumonia had a code of 4A, representing a mortality risk of greater than 30% with A level evidence, while *Escherichia coli* urinary tract infec-tion was coded 1A, representing a mortality risk of less than or equal to 5%, supported by grade A evidence. Cohen and colleagues called the system the Grading System for Site and Severity of Infection (GSSSI). Although it needs to be validated, this system could be a useful means of better characterizing the different risks associ-ated with infections caused by different organisms in dif-ferent sites.

Response

The host response in sepsis is highly complex and varies among patients, making it difficult to put together a clear picture of how sepsis develops and evolves, and yet defin-ing the response in an individual is crucial in determining how best to treat individuals with sepsis. As discussed in the section "Predisposing Factors," many individual fea-tures influence a patient's response, including age, sex, underlying disease, and prior therapy. Some patients with sepsis may develop a state of relative hyperstimulation of the immune system while others, or the same patients at a different stage of their disease process, may have relative immune suppression. Clearly, therefore, not all patients will respond to the same immune-modulating therapies; some are more likely to require anti-inflammatory thera-pies, whereas others will likely respond better to immune stimulation. The challenge is how best to assess and monitor the degree of host response, which represents a continuum between the two extremes (immune hyper-

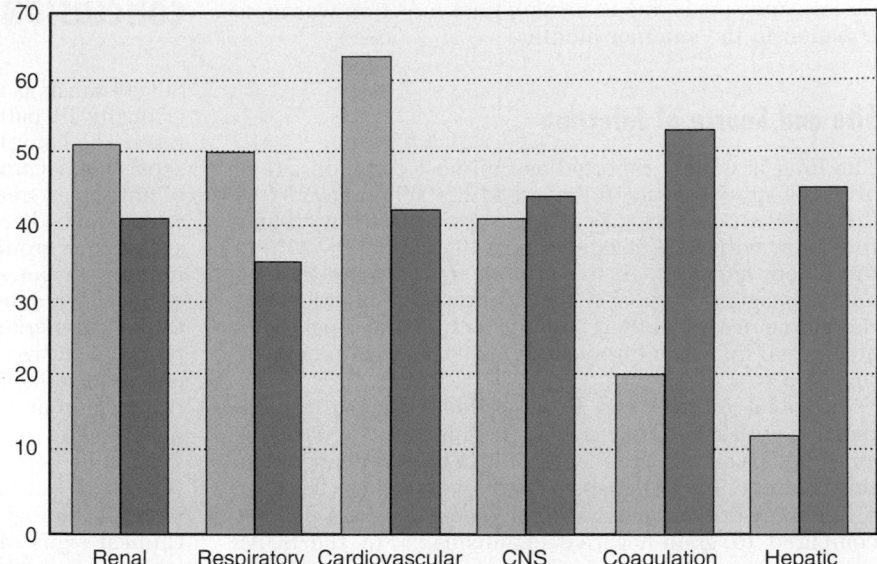

FIGURE 159-1. Incidence (light blue) of organ failure (alone or in combination) and associated intensive care unit (ICU) mortality (dark blue) in patients with severe sepsis in the Sepsis Occurrence in Acutely ill Patients (SOAP) study. CNS, central nervous system. (Data from Vincent JL, Sakr Y, Sprung CL, et al: Sepsis in European intensive care units: Results of the SOAP study. Crit Care Med 2006;34:344-353)

stimulation vs. immune suppression), such that treatments can be appropriately administered and adjusted as necessary. The sepsis response can be characterized by various markers of sepsis, including C-reactive protein (CRP) and procalcitonin. CRP is an acute-phase protein produced by the liver, and plasma levels rise with infection. CRP levels have been reported to be a useful indicator of the presence of sepsis,[17,18] and a fall in CRP levels suggests resolution of sepsis.[18] Procalcitonin has been introduced more recently and analysis of procalcitonin levels is not universally available in hospital laboratories. Procalcitonin levels have been shown to correlate with the severity of sepsis,[19-21] and a recent meta-analysis reported that procalcitonin was more sensitive and specific than CRP for diagnosing sepsis, severe sepsis, and septic shock.[22] In addition, procalcitonin is produced and cleared more rapidly than is CRP, making it potentially more useful for identifying infection early and for following disease progress. Procalcitonin-guided therapy has been shown to reduce total antibiotic exposure and antibiotic treatment duration in patients with community-acquired pneumonia,[23] but this approach needs to be validated in different patient populations. Improvements in rapid, functional genomics and proteomics will facilitate the classification of host response, with complex immune profiles being produced at the bedside from a single blood sample. Repeated sampling could assess changes in the profile over time, theoretically allowing treatments to be adapted accordingly.[24]

Organ Dysfunction

Sepsis-associated organ dysfunction represents the tissue response to sepsis and is critically associated with outcome.[5,25] The degree of organ involvement and changes in patterns of organ dysfunction over time can be assessed with various scoring systems such as the Sequential Organ Failure Assessment (SOFA) score.[26] The most common organ dysfunctions in patients with severe sepsis are cardiovascular, respiratory, and renal dysfunction (Fig. 159-1).[5,27,28] Importantly, the sequence and pattern of organ dysfunction in sepsis varies among patients and understanding why some patients develop acute respira-

tory failure and others acute renal failure or disseminated intravascular coagulation may provide some insight into the pathogenesis of sepsis.

EPIDEMIOLOGY OF SEVERE SEPSIS

In recent years, several large observational studies have provided important epidemiological data on the frequency, causative organisms, sites of infection, and outcomes of sepsis.[5,27,29-33]

Incidence

The occurrence of severe sepsis varies according to the population of patients studied and the precise definitions used, but reported values lie between 12% and 34% of ICU patients.[27,28,30,32-34] In the United Kingdom, Harrison and colleagues[34] reported an increase in the numbers of ICU patients admitted with severe sepsis, from 23.5% in 1996 to 28.7% in 2004. In the recent Sepsis Occurrence in Acutely ill Patients (SOAP) study, which studied 3147 patients in 198 ICUs across Europe, 30% of patients had severe sepsis at some time during their ICU stay[28]; the incidence varied from 10% in Switzerland to 63% in Portugal. A recent study also reported geographic variations in the incidence of severe sepsis, with lower rates of occurrence in the western United States than in the Northeast and South.[35] Perhaps not unexpectedly, the risk of severe sepsis varies according to season, being lower in the summer months than in the winter months.[27] In a retrospective cohort study using the National Hospital Discharge Survey, Danai and coworkers[35] reported that the seasonal rates for severe sepsis were lowest in the fall and highest in the winter, at 13.0 (95% confidence interval [CI], 12.6-13.3) and 15.3 (95% CI, 14.9-15.7) cases per 100,000 population, respectively, representing a 17.7% seasonal increase. This was due largely to the increased incidence of respiratory infections in the winter. There were no seasonal differences in the incidence of sepsis originating in the gastrointestinal system, skin, or soft tissues, and sepsis due to urinary tract infection was more common in the summer months.

Site and Source of Infection

The lung is widely reported as the most common site of origin of severe sepsis, followed by the abdomen.[28,32,33] In the SOAP study, 68% of cases of sepsis were due to lung infection, with 22% originating in the abdomen, 20% in the blood, and 14% in the urinary tract.[28] Brun-Buisson and colleagues[32] reported that pulmonary infection was the source in 49% of their patients with severe sepsis, with abdominal infection implicated in 24% and urinary infection in 5%.

Microbial culture can be a problem in critically ill patients with severe sepsis who are often already receiving antibiotics, and an organism is cultured in only about two thirds of patients with sepsis.[28,32,36] Overall there has been a trend toward increasing involvement of gram-positive compared to gram-negative organisms.[5,37] In the SOAP study, gram-positive organisms were isolated from 40% of patients, gram-negative from 38%, and fungi from 17%; 18% of infections were mixed.[28] *Pseudomonas* sp. (14%) and *Escherichia coli* (13%) were the most common gram-negative organisms, and methicillin-resistant *Staphylococcus aureus* (MRSA) was isolated from 14% of cultures. Brun-Buisson and associates.[32] reported that, in the 62% of their patients with severe sepsis in whom cultures were positive, gram-positive organisms were isolated in 44%, gram-negative organisms in 42%, and fungi in 8%.

Outcome

Severe sepsis was associated with an ICU mortality rate of 32% in the SOAP study[28]; rates varying from 27% to 35% have been reported in other studies.[27,33,34] Sepsis also increases the risk of death for up to 5 years after the septic episode even after comorbidities are accounted for.[38] Although hospital mortality rates seem to have decreased slightly in recent years, the incidence of sepsis, and hence the overall number of deaths, is increasing.[34]

Several studies have identified risk factors for mortality in patients with sepsis or severe sepsis. These include severity scores on admission,[28,32,39] age,[28,39,40] positive fluid balance,[28] presence of organ dysfunction,[28,32,39] bloodstream infection,[28] comorbidity including cirrhosis[28,32] and malignancy,[39] specific infecting organisms including *Pseudomonas* sp.,[28] and inadequate initial antimicrobial therapy.[39]

In addition to its effects on mortality, patients with severe sepsis have prolonged ICU stays and consume more ICU resources than patients without sepsis. Padkin and coworkers[27] reported that although admissions with severe sepsis accounted for 27.1% of all ICU admissions in their study, they consumed 44.9% of all ICU bed days and 33.3% of all hospital bed days. Survivors of sepsis may also have reduced health-related quality of life compared to other ICU survivors.[41]

CONCLUSION

Severe sepsis is an increasingly common disease entity in critically ill patients and associated with high mortality rates. The complexities of the immune response to severe sepsis are becoming increasingly apparent, and the failure of antisepsis treatments to have any impact on mortality rates may be because drugs have been tested in large heterogeneous groups of patients with likely widely differing immune responses. Clinical signs of sepsis are not specific or sensitive enough to categorize the immune response. Biological markers of sepsis may provide a greater indication, but further study is necessary to determine the best and most reliable means of defining the degree of immune response in any individual at any time. The PIRO system may provide a means of characterizing patients with sepsis syndrome. For the clinician, it is not new terminology that is needed, but rather a clearer understanding of the basic pathophysiology underlying the development of sepsis. Clinical signs of sepsis are not always reliable, and the immune response may vary between patients and with time in the same patient.

Key Points

1. Some 12% to 34% of patients will have severe sepsis at some point during their stay in the intensive care unit.
2. The most common source of severe sepsis is the lung.
3. Patients with severe sepsis have mortality rates of about 30%.
4. Better characterization of patients with severe sepsis will help improve understanding of the pathogenesis of sepsis and facilitate development and evaluation of new therapies.

Key References

4. Levy MM, Fink MP, Marshall JC, et al: 2001 SCCM/ESICM/ACCP/ATS/SIS International Sepsis Definitions Conference. Intensive Care Med 2003;29:530-538.
5. Martin GS, Mannino DM, Eaton S, Moss M: The epidemiology of sepsis in the United States from 1979 through 2000. N Engl J Med 2003;348:1546-1554.
22. Uzzan B, Cohen R, Nicolas P, et al: Procalcitonin as a diagnostic test for sepsis in critically ill adults and after surgery or trauma: A systematic review and meta-analysis. Crit Care Med 2006;34:1996-2003.
26. Vincent JL, de Mendonça A, Cantraine F, et al: Use of the SOFA score to assess the incidence of organ dysfunction/failure in intensive care units: Results of a multicentric, prospective study. Crit Care Med 1998;26:1793-1800.
28. Vincent JL, Sakr Y, Sprung CL, et al: Sepsis in European intensive care units: Results of the SOAP study. Crit Care Med 2006;34:344-353.

See the companion Expert Consult website for the complete reference list.

CHAPTER 160

Septic Shock

Asjad Khan and David T. Huang

OBJECTIVES

This chapter will:
1. Review the definition and epidemiology of septic shock.
2. Review the proposed PIRO (predisposing factors, infection, response, and organ dysfunction) staging template for sepsis.
3. Review the protean clinical features of septic shock.

Sepsis, severe sepsis, and *septic shock* are terms used to describe the body's systemic responses to infection. Consensus definitions were created in 1991[1] and again endorsed in a follow-up consensus conference in 2002.[2] Sepsis was defined as presence of infection plus one of the following conditions: body temperature higher than 38° C or lower than 36° C; heart rate greater than 90 beats per minute; respiratory rate of more than 20 breaths per minute or arterial partial pressure carbon dioxide ($PaCO_2$) less than 32 mm Hg; white blood cell count of more than 12,000 cells/mm^3 or fewer than 4000 cells/mm^3, or less than 10% immature (band) forms. *Severe sepsis* was defined as sepsis and organ dysfunction.[1]

Levy and colleagues[2] defined *septic shock* as a state of acute circulatory failure secondary to infection characterized by persistent arterial hypotension not attributable to other causes. Hypotension has been defined as a systolic arterial blood pressure less than 90 mm Hg, a mean arterial pressure of less than 60 mm Hg, or a reduction in systolic arterial blood pressure of greater than 40 mm Hg from baseline, which does not respond to adequate volume replacement.[2] However, early in the course of septic shock, patients frequently present with "cryptic shock," which is the presence of global tissue hypoperfusion with normal vital signs.[3]

EPIDEMIOLOGY

Most sepsis epidemiology work has focused on the broader syndrome of severe sepsis; hence, the data regarding septic shock per se are somewhat limited. A recent epidemiological study of sepsis did not mention any data specific to septic shock.[4] About a decade ago the annual incidence of severe sepsis in the United States was estimated to be 751,000, accounting for 2.1% to 4.3% of hospitalizations and 1% of all intensive care unit (ICU) admissions. Overall mortality was estimated to be 30%, or around 215,000 annual deaths.[5]

Sepsis is the second most common cause of death in the noncoronary ICUs,[6] and the 10th leading cause of death in the United States.[7] The incidence of sepsis is increasing at an annual rate of 9%, partly related to advances in medical care which allow patients to live longer and possibly from increased use of invasive procedures, immunosuppressive drugs, organ transplantation, and increased microbial drug resistance.[4]

A more recent epidemiological study focusing on septic shock found it accounted for 8.2% of all ICU admissions, with an average ICU length of stay of 15 days and a crude mortality of about 60%.[8]

DEMOGRAPHICS

Peak occurrence of sepsis and related syndromes was noted to be in the sixth decade.[4,8,9] There was also a greater predisposition of males developing septic shock than females.[4,10] It was also noted that patients of nonwhite ethnic origin had an increased risk.[4]

Certain patient populations, notably those with immunodeficiency states, malignancy, chronic renal failure, human immunodeficiency virus (HIV)–related disease, and chronic lung disease, have a greater incidence of septic shock as compared to healthy individuals.[4,11] In small heterogeneous populations, certain genetic polymorphisms have been associated with an increased susceptibility to, and mortality from, severe sepsis; no definite causal relationship has yet been established.[12]

MICROBIOLOGICAL AND ANATOMICAL FACTORS

In the majority of cases, the sites of infection are either lung, gastrointestinal tract, genitourinary system, or primary bloodstream infections.[4,8,11] The incidence of gram-negative bacteria as a cause of sepsis has been decreasing over the years (25%-30% in 2000) with a steady increase every year in the gram-positive bacteria (30%-50%) causing sepsis (Table 160-1).[4,8,13] In a recent epidemiological study in the United States, it was found that gram-positive organisms accounted for more than 50% of cases of sepsis, with gram-negative bacteria causing about 37% of the cases. This study also found that fungi caused about 5% of the cases of sepsis, an increase of about 200% in the past two decades.[4]

No obvious source of infection can be found in approximately one third of the cases with severe sepsis and septic shock.[8,14] The morbidity and mortality rates among the culture-negative and culture-positive groups have been similar.[14] Experts speculate that because of improvement in microbiological diagnostic techniques and increased use of antibiotics, the incidence of infection secondary to multiresistant bacteria, like *Pseudomonas* and methicillin-

TABLE 160-1

Pathogens in Septic Shock

PATHOGEN	ESTIMATED FREQUENCY (%)
Gram-Positive Bacteria	30-50
Methicillin-susceptible *Staphylococcus aureus*	14-24
Methicillin-resistant *S. aureus*	5-11
Other *Staphylococcus* sp.	1-3
Streptococcus pneumoniae	9-12
Other *Streptococcus* sp.	6-11
Enterococcus sp.	3-13
Anaerobes	1-2
Other gram-positive bacteria	1-5
Gram-Negative Bacteria	25-30
Escherichia coli	9-27
Pseudomonas aeruginosa	8-15
Klebsiella pneumoniae	2-7
Other *Enterobacter* sp.	6-16
Haemophilus influenzae	2-10
Anaerobes	3-7
Other gram-negative bacteria	3-12
Fungi	
Candida albicans	1-3
Other *Candida* sp.	1-2
Yeast	1
Parasites	1-3
Viruses	2-4

Adapted from Annane D, Bellissant E, Cavaillon JM: Septic shock. Lancet 2005;365(9453):63-78.

resistant *Staphylococcus aureus* and fungi, has increased significantly with time.[8]

PATHOGENESIS

The culmination of complex interactions between micro-organisms that cause infection and the hosts' immune, inflammatory, and coagulation responses results in the syndrome of septic shock.[15] The specific roles of innate immunity and inflammation, as well as the cellular and humoral responses to sepsis, are detailed in Chapters 148 through 153 and will not be discussed here. The immune response to sepsis involves leukocytes, cytokines, coagulation factors, and oxidative stress.

STRATIFICATION

At the International Sepsis Definitions Conference,[2] a template was proposed for staging sepsis in a manner analogous to the tumor-nodes-metastasis (TNM) staging system used in oncology. The model stratifies patients on the basis of predisposing factors, infectious insult, response, and organ dysfunction, generating the acronym PIRO.

Predisposing Factors

Premorbid patient characteristics can have a big impact on the incidence and outcome of sepsis and septic shock. A patient's age, gender, genetics, and past history (immunosuppression, alcoholism, tobacco abuse) can influence their susceptibility to, and the severity of, the disease.

Infection

This component of the PIRO model encompasses the characteristics of the infection. Source of infection (lung and intra-abdominal infections are associated with a greater risk of mortality than urinary tract), degree of extension (e.g., single lung pneumonia vs. bilateral pneumonia), type of microbe (bacteria vs. fungus, gram-positive vs. gram-negative infections), type of infection (health care related vs. community acquired) are all factors that may influence the patient's response to that infection, to treatment, or to both.

Response

The host immune response to the inflammation can be characterized by the presence or absence of the various clinical signs (temperature, respiratory rate, heart rate) and the measurement of various markers (white blood cell count, lactate, procalcitonin, saturated venous oxygen (SvO$_2$), C-reactive protein, interleukin-6).

Organ Dysfunction

Organ dysfunction is the final tissue sequela in response to severe sepsis and the ultimate determinant of survival. It has been amply demonstrated that septic hosts who have progressive multiple-organ failure are much more likely to succumb to severe sepsis than those who develop a single or no organ dysfunction in response to sepsis.[4,16,17]

Multiple-Organ Dysfunction (MOD)[16] and Sequential Organ Failure Assessment (SOFA)[18] are examples of scoring systems that try to objectively quantify organ dysfunction.

The PIRO model is a conceptual framework still in its infancy and needs to be directly tested in both the research laboratory and in clinical trial designs to determine its practical value and clinical relevance.

CLINICAL FEATURES

Prospective studies of the natural history of critical illness have shown that patients generally progress from sepsis to severe sepsis to septic shock, suggesting that these entities are a part of a continuum. One study found that more than two thirds of patients who developed septic shock had been previously classified as having severe sepsis, sepsis, or systemic inflammatory response syndrome (SIRS).[14,19] There are also instances when such a progression is not clear; some patients suddenly develop septic shock without any signs of sepsis in the preceding hours.[20]

GENERAL SIGNS AND SYMPTOMS

The constitutional symptoms of sepsis usually are nonspecific and include fever, chills, tachypnea, tachycardia, diaphoresis, and altered mental status (Table 160-2). Fever is defined as a temperature higher than 38.3° C. A core temperature should be obtained, especially in a hyperventilating patient.[21] Hypothermia (core temperature lower than 36° C) is seen in 20% of patients and is associated with

TABLE 160-2

Clinical Characteristics of Severe Sepsis

Infection, documented or suspected, and some of the following:

General Variables
Fever (core temperature >38.3° C)
Hypothermia (core temperature <36° C)
Heart rate >90 beats per minute or >2 SD above the normal value for age
Tachypnea
Altered mental status
Significant edema or positive fluid balance (>20 mL/kg over 24 hr)
Hyperglycemia (plasma glucose >120 mg/dL or 7.7 mmol/L) in the absence of diabetes

Inflammatory Variables
Leukocytosis (WBC count >12,000/μL)
Leukopenia (WBC count <4000/μL)
Normal WBC count with >10% immature forms
Plasma C-reactive protein >2 SD above the normal value

Hemodynamic Variables
Arterial hypertension[†] (SBP <90 mm Hg, MAP <70, or an SBP decrease >40 mm Hg in adults or <2 SD below normal for age)
$S\bar{v}O_2$ >70%[†]
Cardiac index >3.5 L/min/m²

Organ Dysfunction Variables
Arterial hypoxemia (PaO_2/FIO_2 <300)
Acute oliguria (urine output <0.5 mL/kg/hr or 45 mmol/L for at least 2 hr)
Creatinine increase >0.5 mg/dL
Coagulation abnormalities (INR >1.5 or aPTT >60 sec)
Ileus (absent bowel sounds)
Thrombocytopenia (platelet count <100,000/μL)
Hyperbilirubinemia (plasma total bilirubin >4 mg/dL or 70 mmol/L)

Tissue Perfusion Variables
Hyperlactatemia (>1 mmol/L)
Decreased capillary refill or mottling

aPTT, activated partial thromboplastin time; FIO_2, fraction of inspired oxygen; INR, international normalized ratio; MAP, mean arterial pressure; PaO_2, arterial partial pressure of oxygen; SBP, systolic blood pressure; SD, standard deviation; $S\bar{v}O_2$, mixed venous oxygen saturation; WBC, white blood cell.
From Levy MM, Fink MP, Marshall JC, et al: 2001 SCCM/ESICM/ACCP/ATS/SIS International Sepsis Definitions Conference. Crit Care Med 2003;31(4):1250-1256.

higher mortality rates.[22] Tachypnea and hyperventilation with respiratory alkalosis are also common findings, particularly in the early stages of sepsis. These findings are felt to be secondary to direct stimulation of the medullary respiratory center by inflammatory mediators or as compensation for metabolic (lactic) acidosis.

GENERAL HEMATOLOGICAL AND INFLAMMATORY REACTION

Leukocytosis (white blood cell count higher than 12,000/μL) is a common hematological finding. Infection by bacteria may also cause a left shift, which refers to a predominant neutrophilia in the white blood cell count differential or an increased number of immature forms,

bands causing a bandemia. Alternatively, leukopenia (white blood cell count lower than 4000/μL) can be seen as a result of sepsis-mediated marrow suppression. Patients in septic shock can have normal neutrophil counts, which is indicative of the nonspecificity of this hematological parameter; this is especially seen in the elderly population.[23] Thrombocytopenia is another common hematological manifestation of sepsis due to platelet aggregation or immune-mediated platelet destruction, or secondary to diffuse intravascular coagulation.[24,25]

Extensive work has been done on potential sepsis biomarkers such as endotoxin, procalcitonin, and triggering receptor expressed on myeloid cells-1 (TREM-1), but further research is needed to define their roles in routine clinical care.[26] Measurement of endotoxin levels as a marker for gram-negative infection lacks precision and accuracy and is not currently recommended for routine clinical use.[27] However, a recent study found that the presence of endotoxin may be a useful marker of illness severity and outcome.[28] Plasma procalcitonin concentrations can be elevated (more than 2 standard deviations above normal value) in sepsis, but debate exists regarding its clinical utility and ability to differentiate between inflammation and infection.[29] However, Uzzan and coworkers[59] performed a meta-analysis of procalcitonin and found it to be an accurate marker in the diagnosis of septic shock and related diseases.[30] Levels of another biomarker, soluble TREM-1, are increased in bacterial infections. Its plasma levels higher than 60 ng/mL can predict infectious process with septic shock, but the test is limited in its availability.[31]

HEMODYNAMIC ALTERATIONS

Tachycardia is an early response to maintaining cardiac output. Septic hemodynamic parameters are classically described as "hyperdynamic" and refer to an increased cardiac index and a decreased systemic vascular resistance (SVR). In view of the decreased SVR, the normal or the marginally raised cardiac output still indicates a diminished cardiac performance. The early septic shock hemodynamic changes can be considered as "hypodynamic," with the so-called "hyperdynamic" circulatory state developing only after fluid resuscitation.[32]

As the disease process progresses, the decrease in SVR can overwhelm the body's ability to compensate, leading to the development of hypotension. Although a high $S\bar{v}O_2$ (greater than 70%) is seen with the hemodynamic profile of septic shock, it can also be low (less than 65%).[33] A decreasing $S\bar{v}O_2$ may be indicative of myocardial dysfunction, which is characterized by ventricular dilatation, increased end-diastolic volume, decreased ejection fraction, and decreased response to fluid resuscitation. Certain circulating myocardial depressant factors (tumor necrosis factor-α and interleukin-1β) are thought to be the cause of this myocardial suppression, which is reversible in survivors.[34]

OTHER SIGNS OF ORGAN DYSFUNCTION

Pulmonary dysfunction is common in septic shock from diffuse alveolar epithelial injury leading to capillary leak.

The right-to-left shunt fraction is increased and compliance decreased, often necessitating mechanical ventilation. The clinical diagnosis of acute lung injury is made when there are new bilateral infiltrates on a chest radiograph, arterial partial pressure of oxygen (PaO_2) to fraction of inspired oxygen (FIO_2) ratio less than 300, and no evidence of left heart failure. A PaO_2/FIO_2 ratio of less than 200 is defined as acute respiratory distress syndrome.[35]

Encephalopathy is frequently seen and patients can be lethargic, somnolent, agitated, confused, or frankly obtunded. Patients with acute sepsis–related encephalopathy are associated with an increased mortality.[36,37]

Septic shock can lead to renal dysfunction, which can range from mild proteinuria to anuria and profound renal failure. Hypovolemia, renal vasoconstriction, hypotension, and nephrotoxic agents are the mechanisms by which acute kidney injury occurs. Renal failure in septic patients is associated with a mortality of 50%.[38]

The gastrointestinal tract can be affected, and patients may develop ileus, leading to malabsorption of medicines and intolerance to enteral feeding. The barrier function of the gut mucosa may be impaired, leading to translocation of bacteria into the lymph system and bloodstream. Liver dysfunction and cholestasis are common and cause an increase in direct bilirubin and alkaline phosphatase.[39]

The metabolic derangements seen in patients with septic shock include hypo- and hyperglycemia. Hypoglycemia occurs early and may cause mental status changes and seizures. Impaired gluconeogenesis by the liver and increased peripheral uptake are thought to be the cause of it. Being a stress state, septic shock leads to an increased activity of catecholamines, corticosteroids, and glucagons, leading to a hyperglycemic state. Although adrenal insufficiency is common in septic shock patients, its diagnosis is controversial.[40]

CONCLUSION

Septic shock remains a major cause of morbidity and mortality and is a burden on health care systems despite advancements in medicine. Although sepsis, severe sepsis, and septic shock can be considered as a continuum of syndromes, data representing septic shock are limited. There has been a shift in the microbiological causes of septic shock, with more cases being caused by gram-positive bacteria as well as increased incidence of sepsis due to fungi and multiple drug–resistant organisms. The lung is the most common source of infection in septic shock. Many complex mechanisms are involved in the pathogenesis of septic shock, including the inflammatory response, cytokine release, neutrophilic activation, coagulation cascade, tissue hypoxia, and oxidative stress. These pathways have extensive complementary and synergistic interactions, causing a significant delay from the start of the disease process to the presentation of the patient for medical care. For a better classification of the patient with septic shock, the PIRO system has been introduced. This system might help in more appropriate tailoring of therapeutic interventions to the individual patient. Identification of new biomarkers holds promise for early identification of septic shock.

Key Points

1. Septic shock is a major cause of morbidity and mortality and is likely to increase with the "graying" of the U.S. population.
2. Current consensus definitions of septic shock focus on blood pressure; however, hypoperfusion can be present, even with apparently normal vital signs.
3. The pathogenesis of septic shock is protean and not fully understood.
4. The clinical presentation of septic shock is protean and can affect every organ system. A high index of suspicion must be maintained for timely recognition.

Key References

2. Levy MM, Fink MP, Marshall JC, et al: 2001 SCCM/ESICM/ACCP/ATS/SIS International Sepsis Definitions Conference. Crit Care Med 2003;31(4):1250-1256.
5. Angus DC, Linde-Zwirble WT, Lidicker J, et al: Epidemiology of severe sepsis in the United States: Analysis of incidence, outcome, and associated costs of care. Crit Care Med 2001; 29(7):1303-1310.
8. Annane D, Aegerter P, Jars-Guincestre MC, et al: Current epidemiology of septic shock: The CUB-Rea Network. Am J Respir Crit Care Med 2003;168(2):165-172.
18. Vincent JL, Moreno R, Takala J, et al, for the Working Group on Sepsis-Related Problems of the European Society of Intensive Care Medicine: The SOFA (Sepsis-related Organ Failure Assessment) score to describe organ dysfunction/failure. Intensive Care Med 1996;22(7):707-710.

See the companion Expert Consult website for the complete reference list.

CHAPTER 161

The Kidney in Sepsis

Joseph McKenna and Jonathan Himmelfarb

OBJECTIVES

This chapter will:
1. Review the epidemiology and importance of sepsis as a cause of acute kidney injury.
2. Review the initiation, maintenance, and recovery phases of acute kidney injury.
3. Describe the pathophysiological mechanisms that cause acute kidney injury in sepsis.
4. Review promising targets for current and future therapy.

Infection is commonly associated with a decline in renal function. Although pathogens rarely invade the kidney directly, the sepsis syndrome is a precipitant for a wide spectrum of kidney diseases, including immune complex glomerulonephritis, vasculitis, interstitial nephritis, and transplant nephropathy. The most common renal manifestation of infection is acute kidney injury (AKI), related to abnormalities in effective circulating volume, coagulation proteins, inflammatory mediators, endothelial function, and increased oxidative stress. This chapter outlines the mechanisms responsible for AKI and the subsequent recovery of function in sepsis. One theory of kidney dysfunction in sepsis is organized around the concepts of initiation, maintenance of injury, and recovery of function. In the initiation phase, a susceptible kidney, often preconditioned by chronic injury, is damaged by a combination of factors: decreased renal blood flow (RBF), systemic inflammation, nephrotoxic drugs, and bacterial products, culminating in the histological picture of acute tubular necrosis. In the maintenance phase, RBF has often been restored, but inflammatory cytokines, coagulation disturbances favoring thrombosis, and oxidative stress create an injurious milieu that propagates and perpetuates injury. In the recovery phase, necrosis and apoptosis must be outweighed by dedifferentiation and cellular proliferation, restoring the renal architecture and reestablishing function.

EPIDEMIOLOGY

In the United States, sepsis accounts for approximately 750,000 hospital admissions annually, with an overall mortality rate of approximately 30%.[1] Half of these patients require intensive care unit (ICU) admission. In the United States, the incidence of sepsis-related hospital admissions appears to be rising at a rate of 1.5% to 8% per year (Fig. 161-1),[1,2] and international epidemiological studies suggest that sepsis now accounts for 17% of all medical ICU admissions.[3] Increasing in parallel to the incidence of sepsis is the incidence of AKI (Fig. 161-2).[4] Kidney injury among the elderly as a complication of sepsis is especially common; of the 6% of ICU patients who develop AKI, the median age is 67, with 30% of these patients having pre-existing renal dysfunction. The dominant risk factor for AKI among hospitalized patients is sepsis, occurring in about half of those with kidney failure in the ICU setting.[3]

Though recent advances in critical care management have improved overall ICU survival (Fig. 161-3), the same cannot be said for the critically ill with AKI.[2] Rangel-Frausto and colleagues[5] reported a stepwise increase in AKI as patients progressed from sepsis to septic shock. In this series, AKI occurred in 19% of patients with sepsis, 23% with severe sepsis, and 51% with septic shock when blood cultures were positive. Even in patients not requiring dialysis, AKI is shown to worsen prognosis in critical illness, and when dialysis is required, the ICU mortality rises to 45% to 80%.[6-8] While the development of AKI clearly is a marker of disease severity that portends a worse prognosis, the extent to which the development of AKI actually contributes to multiple-organ system failure remains an area of active inquiry.

While it is true that AKI worsens the prognosis of sepsis, the converse is also true in that sepsis worsens the outcomes for patients with AKI. Patients in whom AKI develops during sepsis have a worse prognosis than the critically ill with preexisting end-stage renal disease,[9] suggesting that the outcome is associated with systemic disease in addition to the renal dysfunction itself.[9,10]

PATHOPHYSIOLOGY

In the kidney, sepsis may be clinically manifested by a decline in glomerular filtration rate (GFR) or the development of oliguria. Historically, the resulting decline in GFR was felt to stem from ischemic injury and damage to the tubular epithelium. This injury initially occurs within the S3 segment and medullary thick ascending limb where, from medulla to cortex, a declining oxygen gradient is coupled with an increased cellular energy requirement. This ischemic injury leads to the loss of cellular polarity and destruction of the typical brush border, where the bulk of solute and water transport occurs. Subsequently there is redistribution of adhesion molecules (integrins) and separation of epithelial cells from the basement membrane. As injury progresses, the epithelium is sloughed into the tubular lumen, where adhesion with other cells, cellular debris, and Tamm-Horsfall proteins lead to obstruction and cast formation, further contributing to the decline in GFR.[11]

In recent years, the primacy of this hemodynamic mechanism has been called into question,[12] and more credence has been given to the respective roles of endothelial dysfunction, coagulation abnormalities, and systemic inflam-

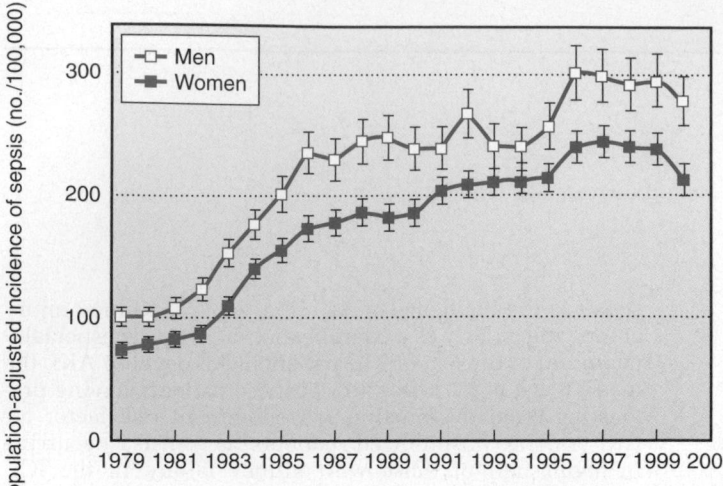

FIGURE 161-1. Increasing incidence of sepsis from 1979 to 2001. (Martin GS, Mannino DM, Eaton S, Moss M: The epidemiology of sepsis in the United States from 1979 through 2000. N Engl J Med 2003;348[16]:1546-1554.)

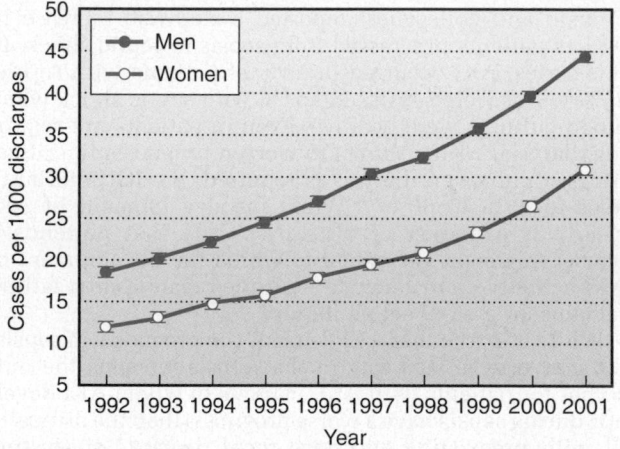

FIGURE 161-2. Increasing incidence of acute kidney injury (AKI) over the past decade. (Xue JL, Daniels F, Star RA, et al: Incidence and mortality of acute renal failure in Medicare beneficiaries, 1992 to 2001. J Am Soc Nephrol 2006;17[4]:1135-1142.)

mation, endothelial dysfunction, and oxidative stress. These mechanisms are discussed next.

Hemodynamics

The hemodynamic profile in sepsis is complex and dynamic, changing over the course of the disease. Initially sepsis is characterized by a hyperdynamic state with increased cardiac output. The systemic vascular resistance is low despite elevated levels of circulating catecholamines, vasopressin, and activation of the renin-angiotensin system.[13,14] An apparent decrease in effective circulating volume is mediated by nitric oxide–induced vasodilatation, impaired vascular reactivity, and a state of increased capillary permeability.[15] If the situation is not rapidly reversed, progressive development of cardiac dysfunction and relative vasopressor deficiency can contribute to circulatory compromise, hypotension, septic shock, and death.[16,17]

The effects of decreased relative effective circulating volume on RBF are unclear. Animal models of lipopoly-

saccharide-induced sepsis have suggested renal vasoconstriction and reduced total RBF[18,19]; however, a recent review of multiple animal models of RBF in sepsis demonstrated a marked heterogeneity of the hemodynamic responses to sepsis. Using renal vascular resistance as a surrogate for RBF, half of these studies reported an increase in renal vascular resistance and the remainder showed either a decrease in renal vascular resistance or no change.[20] In fact, animal size and cardiac output were the only independent determinants of renal vascular resistance. This variability may reflect either the inadequacy of existing animal models or heterogeneity of the sepsis syndrome itself.

Few human data are available regarding RBF in sepsis. Brenner and coworkers[21] measured both RBF and renal vascular resistance in eight septic patients using a percutaneous thermodilution catheter in the renal vein. In their series, AKI occurred in the majority of cases despite hemodynamic measurements, suggesting preserved RBF. However, GFR as measured by inulin clearance correlated closely with the fraction of cardiac output going to the kidneys, suggesting a state of *relative* renal vasoconstriction.[21] It should be remembered that GFR depends upon the intraglomerular pressure gradient generated by differences in afferent and efferent vascular tone, and even when RBF is relatively preserved, there may be microcirculatory redistribution of blood flow resulting in regional areas of ischemia and hypoperfusion.

Microcirculatory Dysfunction
Nitric Oxide

In addition to its constitutively expressed form, nitric oxide synthesis can be induced in renal tissues by endotoxin, tumor necrosis factor–α (TNF-α), interleukin-1 (IL-1), and thrombin.[22,23] Circulating nitric oxide is commonly elevated during sepsis and causes vasodilation via a pathway in which dephosphorylation of myosin light chains leads to vascular smooth muscle relaxation.[24] Additionally, nitric oxide may lead to activation of vascular adenosine triphosphate (ATP)–sensitive K channels (K_{ATP}), which hyperpolarize vascular smooth muscle and impair the vasoconstrictor response to both endogenous and exogenous pressors.[15,25] In the kidney, the primary function of nitric oxide appears to be the maintenance of

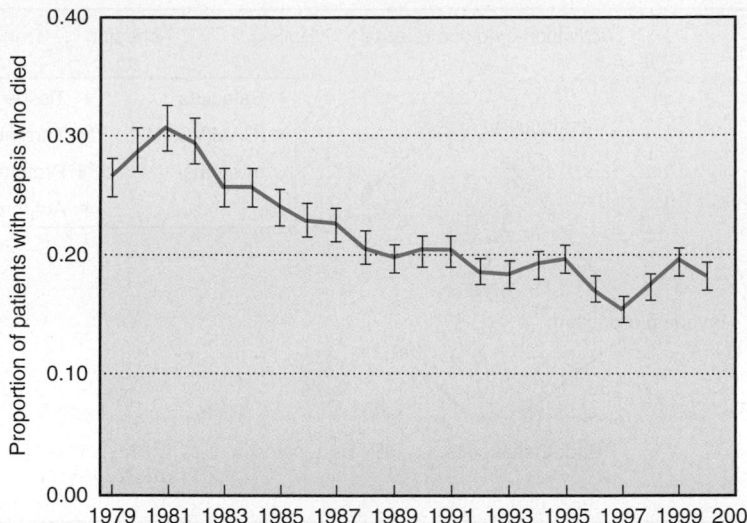

FIGURE 161-3. Overall in-hospital mortality rate among patients hospitalized for sepsis, 1979-2000. (Martin GS, Mannino DM, Eaton S, Moss M: The epidemiology of sepsis in the United States from 1979 through 2000. N Engl J Med 2003;348[16]:1546-1554.)

RBF through its effects on the afferent arteriole. Blockade of nitric oxide minimizes systemic vasodilation in sepsis, but in the kidney it decreases RBF and markedly impairs GFR.[26-28] At the microcirculatory level, this vasodilatory effect of nitric oxide may be confined to early sepsis, as animal models suggest impaired reactivity over time despite progressively increasing levels of nitric oxide.[29] Additionally, protracted exposure to nitric oxide appears to both increase oxidative stress and promote apoptosis, which may contribute to the extension phase of AKI.[30,31]

Other Local Mediators of Vascular Tone

Endothelin-1 is a potent endothelium-derived peptide upregulated in sepsis by angiotensin II, vasopressin, and IL-1. In the kidney, its actions are mediated via two endothelin receptors: ET_A and ET_B. ET_A is located primarily on the vascular endothelium (afferent, efferent, and tubular capillaries), and its activation induces potent vasoconstriction. Nonselective blockade of endothelin-1 or its receptor appears to mitigate the decline in RBF and urine output seen in dog and rat models of endotoxemia and sepsis.[32,33] Additionally, TNF-α, angiotensin II, thromboxane A2, leukotrienes, and enhanced sympathetic nerve activity are all augmented in sepsis and appear to promote the vasoconstrictive phenotype seen in the kidney.

Endothelial Activation

The vascular endothelium plays a crucial role in the regulation of hemostasis, inflammation, vasomotor tone, and angiogenesis. As the endothelium is commonly recognized as a major site of inflammatory and oxidative injury in sepsis, endothelial dysfunction has become one of the unifying themes in an evolving understanding of the pathogenesis of multiple-organ system failure (MOSF).[34] Initial alterations in endothelial function during sepsis are diverse and include enhanced cytokine production, immune cell recruitment, and triggering of a procoagulant state (Fig. 161-4).[35] As sepsis progresses and normal physiological responses fail, the transition from a physiological to pathological state occurs. Leukocytes adhere to the endothelium and infiltrate vessel walls. The endothelial barrier is broken, capillary leakage ensues, tissue factor is exposed to the circulation, and widespread imbalances in the coagulation cascade allow for microvascular thrombosis as the blood's viscosity rises and flow through capillary beds decreases.

Although the endothelial response to injury is tissue specific, certain recurrent pathological themes emerge.[36] In models of ischemia-reperfusion injury, upregulation of luminal adhesion molecules such as P-selectin, E-selectin, and intercellular adhesion molecule-1 (ICAM-1) occurs diffusely, and leukocytes are recruited. The resultant tissue infiltration is commonly implicated in the extension phase of renal injury.[37-39] In sepsis-induced MOSF, pathological examination of other vascular beds have demonstrated a remarkably similar pattern of adhesion molecule expression.[40] Adhesion molecules are also found in the circulation, where levels in sepsis correlate with disease severity.[41,42]

This early endothelium–leukocyte interaction appears pivotal in tissue injury, and in animal models pretreatment with soluble ligand or anti-ICAM-1 antibodies mitigate leukocyte infiltration and subsequent renal dysfunction.[38,43] Although the anti-ICAM-1 antibody enlimomab has not been studied in sepsis, it was used in a human trial for treatment of ischemic stroke; results showed increased mortality in the treatment arm.[44] A phase 2 trial of the same drug after renal transplantation showed no decrease in delayed graft function or acute rejection despite promising results in animal models.[45]

Coagulation Abnormalities

In addition to mononuclear cell infiltration, microvascular thrombosis has been widely implicated in the propagation of tissue injury. Widespread fibrin deposition in the intravascular space, including the glomerular capillaries, is a frequent finding in both animal models and human pathological specimens of sepsis.[46,47] In animal and human studies, it appears that abnormalities in the three primary endogenous anticoagulant pathways—heparin–antithrombin, tissue factor pathway inhibitor, and protein C—underlie most of the hemostatic disturbance in sepsis.[48]

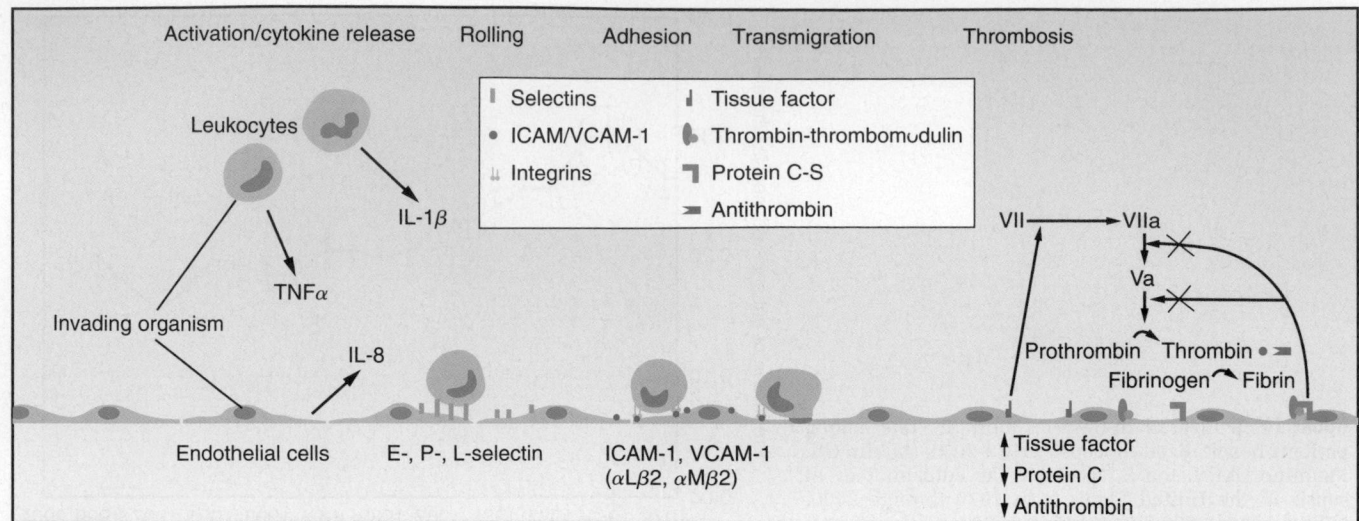

FIGURE 161-4. Mechanism of endothelial activation and coagulation abnormalities. ICAM-1, intercellular adhesion molecule-1; IL-1β, interleukin-1β; TNF-α, tumor necrosis factor-α; VCAM-1, vasocellular adhesion molecule-1. (Modified from Peters K, Unger RE, Brunner J, Kirkpatrick CJ: Molecular basis of endothelial dysfunction in sepsis. Cardiovasc Res 2003;60[1]):49-57.)

The antithrombin system interacts with heparin proteoglycans on the vascular endothelium to accelerate inactivation of thrombin. Animal models suggest that heparin proteoglycans are downregulated or functionally inactivated in sepsis.[48] Additionally, levels of antithrombin decline dramatically in septic shock. Unfortunately, a large multicenter trial of high-dose antithrombin replacement in severe sepsis found no effect on mortality or the incidence of renal dysfunction.[49]

Tissue factor expression is upregulated on both infiltrating monocytes and the exposed subendothelium following injury from diverse causes (ischemia-reperfusion, lipopolysaccharide, IL-1). Tissue factor pathway inhibitor expressed primarily on vascular endothelial cells serves to limit coagulation beyond the injured endothelium. While promising in animal models, a clear mortality or organ-specific benefit has not been observed in human trials.[50]

The protein C pathway is activated by a complex between thrombin and thrombomodulin on the endothelial membrane. Reduced levels are frequently found in sepsis and often precede the clinical manifestations of severe sepsis.[51] Infusion of recombinant activated protein C (rAPC) for severe sepsis has been a remarkable success, with an almost 20% relative risk reduction in mortality among the sickest subgroup of patients.[52] The direct effects of rAPC on renal function remain less clear. In animal models of renal ischemia-reperfusion injury, rAPC appears to inhibit leukocyte activation and reduce the associated tissue injury.[53] However, analysis of secondary endpoints from the Recombinant human protein C Worldwide Evaluation in Severe Sepsis (PROWESS) study found no statistical difference in renal outcomes in treated patients at 7 and 28 days.[54]

Inflammation and Apoptosis

When infection breaches local boundaries, elaboration of both inflammatory and anti-inflammatory cytokines modulate the systemic host response. Most human studies evaluating these inflammatory biomarkers have found that progressive increases in circulating cytokine titers predict both organ failure and mortality.[55] Two large therapeutic trials in sepsis have shown a correlation between a reduction in systemic cytokine levels and improvements in morbidity and mortality. The PROWESS study group investigators documented lower levels of IL-6 in those patients treated with APC.[52] Although not a primary endpoint, the Acute Respiratory Distress Syndrome Clinical Trials Network investigators showed that low tidal volume ventilation resulted in lower levels of IL-6, IL-8, and IL-10, which correlated with a reduction in nonpulmonary organ failure.[56]

The cytokine milieu of sepsis likely plays a role in promoting apoptosis. In a series of animal experiments, Imai and colleagues[57] found higher levels of IL-8 and increased rates of epithelial cell apoptosis in the kidneys of animals treated with a "lung-injurious" ventilation strategy. Likewise, apoptosis was increased in renal tubular epithelial cells incubated with plasma from these animals. This response was markedly attenuated by co-incubation with a blocking antibody to the fas ligand, a potent inducer of apoptosis. When plasma samples from patients ventilated with a lung protective strategy were compared with those of patients treated with "conventional" ventilation, increases in soluble fas ligand correlated with a rising creatinine.[57] Taken together, this suggests a role for fas ligand induced apoptosis in AKI.

RECOVERY

Little is known about the recovery phase from acute kidney injury. Historically, it was thought that when patients survived severe sepsis or MOSF, recovery of kidney function was the rule. But literature from the critical care population shows that more than 40% of patients who survive critical illness with AKI are discharged with newly impaired renal function, and up to 14% require renal replacement therapy at the time of discharge.[3,58] Currently few data are available regarding the long-term consequence of this renal injury, and further characterization has become a priority for future investigation.

Clinically, when renal recovery occurs, it is often heralded by a progressive increase in urinary output that precedes the correction of other metabolic derangements. Histologically, tubular repair after ischemic injury is characterized by a state of cellular dedifferentiation. During recovery, epithelial precursors display a phenotype remarkably similar to that seen in organogenesis (phylogeny recapitulating ontogeny) with cellular proliferation, migration, and ultimately differentiation which restores the denuded basement membrane. A detailed description of this process is beyond the scope of this chapter, and the reader is referred to a more comprehensive review.[59]

The correlate of recovery from AKI to organogenesis has prompted research into therapeutics that target repair mechanisms, such as insulin growth factor-1 and hepatocyte growth factor.[60,61] Initial animal studies suggest that both hormones may accelerate renal recovery, but in humans, a randomized multicenter trial of insulin growth factor-1 infusion to treat renal failure in the ICU did not show benefit in terms of renal recovery, and there was a trend toward slower return of urine output and GFR in the treated arm.[62] Thus far, no treatment has been better than standard supportive care to accelerate renal recovery once sepsis-related AKI has occurred.

CONCLUSION

Many factors contributing to kidney injury in sepsis have now been elucidated, but a comprehensive mechanistic understanding has not yet been achieved. Each phase of AKI in sepsis represents an opportunity for intervention that may improve patient outcomes. Early recognition of the initiation phase may allow for treatment that reverses the basic pathophysiology of injury before AKI is established. Therapy targeting the inflammatory, thrombotic, and oxidative environment of sepsis may shorten the maintenance phase, decrease the extent of injury, and make ultimate recovery of function more likely. Finally, identification and protection of the regenerative factors necessary for regrowth of the tubulointerstitium may optimize renal recovery and prevent long-term morbidity. The separation of sepsis-associated AKI into the induction, maintenance, and recovery phases will help clinicians and researchers target specific biochemical and hemodynamic abnormalities in the appropriate time frame to prevent or ameliorate kidney injury and thereby reduce mortality in these critically ill patients.

Key Points

1. Sepsis is an important cause of acute kidney injury (AKI).
2. AKI consists of three phases: Initiation, maintenance, and recovery.
3. Sepsis was initially thought to cause AKI via ischemic injury and damage to the tubular epithelium.
4. Recent research has placed more emphasis on the roles of endothelial dysfunction, coagulation abnormalities, systemic inflammation and oxidative stress in causing AKI.
5. Each phase of AKI in sepsis (initiation, maintenance, and recovery) represents an opportunity for intervention which may improve patient outcomes.

Key References

3. Uchino S, Kellum JA, Bellomo R, et al: Acute renal failure in critically ill patients: A multinational, multicenter study. JAMA 2005;294(7):813-818.
4. Xue JL, Daniels F, Star RA, et al: Incidence and mortality of acute renal failure in Medicare beneficiaries, 1992 to 2001. J Am Soc Nephrol 2006;17(4):1135-1142.
30. Wang W, Jittikanont S, Falk SA, et al: Interaction among nitric oxide, reactive oxygen species, and antioxidants during endotoxemia-related acute renal failure. Am J Physiol Renal Physiol 2003;284(3):F532-F537.
54. Vincent JL, Angus DC, Artigas A, et al: Effects of drotrecogin alfa (activated) on organ dysfunction in the PROWESS trial. Crit Care Med 2003;31(3):834-840.
55. Simmons EM, Himmelfarb J, Sezer MT, et al: Plasma cytokine levels predict mortality in patients with acute renal failure. Kidney Int 2004;65(4):1357-1365.

See the companion Expert Consult website for the complete reference list.

CHAPTER 162

Human Immunodeficiency Virus Infection and Acute Renal Failure

Scott D. Cohen, Lakhmir S. Chawla, and Paul L. Kimmel

OBJECTIVES

This chapter will:
1. Review the epidemiology of acute kidney injury in the setting of human immunodeficiency virus infection.
2. Evaluate the etiology and pathogenesis of acute kidney injury in the setting of human immunodeficiency virus infection.
3. Discuss the potential for highly active antiretroviral therapy nephrotoxicity.

The introduction of highly active antiretroviral therapy (HAART) has revolutionized outcomes in patients with human immunodeficiency virus (HIV) infection. However, HAART may also be a cause of the spectrum of renal disease associated with HIV infection. This chapter reviews the epidemiology and pathogenesis of acute renal failure (ARF) associated with HIV infection. HIV infection is associated with the same causes of ARF that are seen in the general population. HIV-infected patients have an increased risk of developing ARF as a result of numerous comorbid conditions. Prerenal azotemia, from volume depletion, remains the most common cause of acute kidney injury (AKI) in HIV-infected patients. Acute tubular necrosis (ATN) is the most common intrinsic cause of AKI. Postrenal obstructive uropathy and other intrinsic renal causes must be considered each time AKI occurs in the HIV-infected patient. There can also be rare cases of ARF in the setting of opportunistic infections and neoplasms associated with the immunosuppressed state, such as Kaposi's sarcoma, that create space-occupying lesions in the kidney.

EPIDEMIOLOGY

ARF is common in HIV-infected patients admitted to the hospital.[1-5] In a retrospective cohort of patients evaluated from Brooklyn, New York, sepsis-related hemodynamically mediated ARF was the cause of 52% of cases between 1984 to 1993; 23% of cases were attributable to nephrotoxic-induced ATN. The nephrotoxins included aminoglycosides, amphotericin B, pentamidine, intravenous acyclovir, and radiocontrast agents.[5] The remaining 25% of causes included acute interstitial nephritis in the setting of trimethoprim-sulfamethoxazole, allopurinol, phenytoin, or rifampin use. Other causes were use of nonsteroidal anti-inflammatory drugs (NSAIDs), rhabdomyolysis,

thrombotic microangiopathy, immune complex glomerulonephritis, and plasma cell dyscrasias causing interstitial nephritis.[5] Rao and Friedman[5] found a 60% mortality rate due to ARF in their patient population, highlighting the importance of this condition.

Franceschini and colleagues[6] studied a prospective cohort of 754 HIV-infected patients from the University of North Carolina Center for AIDS Research to determine the incidence rate and causes of ARF. ARF occurred with an incidence rate of 5.9 per 100 person years. Of the cases of ARF, 71% were acquired in the community, with prerenal azotemia the most common cause, comprising 38% of all cases. Intrinsic etiologies of ARF followed, with ischemia and drug-induced nephrotoxic ATN predominating. There were two cases of thrombotic microangiopathy in this cohort. Obstructive ARF occurred in the setting of crystal nephropathy from indinavir nephrotoxicity. This study found a higher incidence of ARF in males, patients coinfected with hepatitis C virus (HCV), patients with lower CD4 counts, higher HIV ribonucleic acid viral loads, and underlying infection. Similar to the results of Rao and Friedman, 52% of ARF cases occurred in the setting of acute infection such as meningitis, encephalitis, pneumonia, and bacteremias. Twenty percent of the cases of ARF in the setting of HIV-HCV coinfection occurred in the setting of cirrhosis.[6]

Wyatt and colleagues[7] performed a retrospective cohort study to evaluate the incidence of ARF in hospitalized HIV-infected patients in 1995 and in 2003 after the introduction of HAART therapy. ARF was found to be twice as common in 2003 compared to 1995; however, mortality was lower for hospitalized HIV-infected patients during the HAART era. Risk factors for ARF among HIV-infected patients included increased age, male gender, black race, diabetes, HIV-hepatitis coinfection, and a history of underlying chronic liver or kidney disease. ARF in HIV-infected patients was also associated with a 5.8 times greater mortality among hospitalized HIV patients.

Peraldi and coworkers[8] performed a single-center retrospective cohort study of 92 HIV-infected patients admitted to the hospital with ARF or "rapidly progressing renal failure" from June 1988 to January 1997. Patients were included in the study if they had an increase in serum creatinine to more than 180 µmol/L after 20 days, and if they had normal or increased kidney size on renal ultrasound. Renal biopsy data were available on 60 of the 92 HIV-infected patients. Hemolytic uremic syndrome was the most frequent cause of ARF in this cohort, found in 34.8% of cases. Biopsy confirmation of hemolytic uremic syndrome was documented in 26 of 32 cases. ATN occurred in 26.1% of cases. Six of the 24 cases were attributed to rhabdomyolysis, and 18 were thought to be due to ischemic or other nephrotoxic etiologies. Obstruction occurred in 17.4% of patients with ARF in this one hospital. There were two cases of biopsy-proven drug-induced acute interstitial nephritis, both in patients treated with trimethoprim-sulfamethoxazole. There were two cases of membranoproliferative glomerulonephritis. Both patients had active hepatitis. There were also two cases of lupus nephritis in this cohort. It is likely that this retrospective cohort study underestimates the true incidence of prerenal azotemia and ATN, since clear-cut ARF cases would not be evaluated by renal biopsies.

PRERENAL AZOTEMIA

It is important to assess the volume status of every patient that presents with ARF. Volume depletion from prerenal azotemia remains the most common cause of ARF in HIV-infected patients.[3,5]

HIV-infected patients are at increased risk for prerenal azotemia for a number of reasons. Gastrointestinal illnesses, with vomiting and diarrhea, are common whether from the HAART regimen, the HIV infection itself, or its associated opportunistic infections. The underlying HIV infection may also be associated with anorexia and decreased oral fluid intake, further predisposing to volume depletion. Volume depletion was the most common etiology of ARF, accounting for 38% of all cases in HIV-infected patients according to a retrospective analysis by Valeri and Neusy.[10]

States of decreased effective circulatory volume can also lead to prerenal azotemia. Unique factors that predispose HIV-infected patients to this condition include their increased risk for sepsis, which can cause prerenal azotemia through capillary leak, hypotension, endotoxin- or pressor-induced renal arteriolar vasoconstriction.[9] HIV infection has also been associated with hepatitis B or C virus co-infection and therefore an increased risk of developing cirrhosis. Cirrhosis is a known cause of prerenal azotemia, due to hypoalbuminemia and ascites formation with associated intravascular volume depletion. Finally, HIV infection can induce a cardiomyopathy which can also lead to prerenal azotemia in the setting of decompensated congestive heart failure.[9]

INTRINSIC RENAL FAILURE

Acute Tubular Necrosis

Nephrotoxic and ischemic ATN are common causes of ARF in HIV-infected patients. There are a number of nephrotoxic medications that are administered to treat opportunistic infections associated with HIV infection. These include amphotericin B, used to treat fungal infections; foscarnet, used to treat ganciclovir-resistant cytomegalovirus infection; pentamidine, used as second-line therapy for treating *Pneumocystis* infection; cidofovir, used to treat cytomegalovirus infection; and aminoglycosides to treat gram-negative bacteremias.[9] HIV-infected patients who are admitted to the hospital are frequently exposed to intravenous contrast to evaluate abdominal, pulmonary, and central nervous system pathology. This patient population is at increased risk for the development of contrast nephropathy, especially when presenting in volume-depleted states or with preexisting renal failure.[11,12] HIV-infected patients often report various myalgias and arthralgias requiring analgesics, including NSAIDs.[9]

NSAIDs have the potential to cause hemodynamically mediated ARF, especially in volume-depleted states when renal perfusion is dependent on the vasodilatory properties of renal prostaglandins.[9]

Ischemic ATN can occur in hypotensive HIV-infected patients who are admitted with sepsis, congestive heart failure, cirrhosis, or underlying endocrinopathies related to HIV infection, including adrenal insufficiency.[13]

Rhabdomyolysis

Myoglobinuric ARF from rhabdomyolysis is another common cause of ATN in the setting of HIV infection.[8,14,15] HIV-infected patients have a number of predisposing risk factors for rhabdomyolysis, including substance abuse, the direct myotoxic effects of the viral infection or its associated opportunistic infections, and medication side effects.[8,14-17] In a European study, rhabdomyolysis was the cause of approximately 10% of the cases of ARF that necessitated a renal biopsy at a single institution.[8]

Chariot and colleagues[14] evaluated 20 HIV-infected patients with rhabdomyolysis and ARF. Three of the 20 cases of rhabdomyolysis were felt to be secondary to direct effects of the HIV infection itself. There are data that polymyositis may be caused by cytopathic effects of the HIV infection on muscle tissue.[18,19] Data from an autopsy series of HIV-infected patients identified alterations in muscle histology in approximately two thirds of cases.[20] There have also been reports of rhabdomyolysis in the setting of acute HIV seroconversion syndrome when viral loads are often quite elevated, further supporting the role of a direct myotoxic effect of the virus.[21] Other opportunistic infections secondary to HIV infection may also cause direct muscle damage. *Pneumocystis*, *Toxoplasma gondii*, *Cryptococcus neoformans*, and *Staphylococcus aureus* infections all have been associated with potential links to rhabdomyolysis in the setting of HIV infection.[14]

Six of the 20 HIV-infected patients were felt to have rhabdomyolysis from antiretroviral medications, including nucleoside analogues such as zidovudine and didanosine.[14] Zidovudine inhibits mitochondrial DNA polymerase, leading to declines in mitochondrial DNA synthesis.[22,23] This could account for the mechanism by which zidovudine causes a myopathy. There is also evidence that zidovudine may promote deletional mutations in mitochondrial DNA.[24] Antiretroviral medications also have the potential to interact, via the cytochrome P450 (CP450) system, with a number of commonly prescribed medications.

HIV-infected patients treated with protease inhibitors often require statin therapy because of the atherogenic side effects of protease inhibitors.[25] There have been numerous reports of rhabdomyolysis in HIV-infected patients treated with statins.[25-32] Castro and Gutierrez[32] described a case of rhabdomyolysis and ARF in an HIV-infected patient taking delavirdine, lamivudine, stavudine, and atorvastatin. The authors attributed the rhabdomyolysis and ARF to the effects of delavirdine to decrease CYP3A4 enzyme activity, thereby decreasing the metabolism of atorvastatin. Myopathy is a major adverse reaction to statin therapy.[25-32] Any inhibition of metabolism of a statin may increase its potential myotoxicity. Therefore, caution must be used any time protease inhibitors and statins are concurrently prescribed. Lowering the dose of statin or use of pravastatin, which is not metabolized through CYP3A4 system, should be considered.

Joshi and Liu[15] evaluated the etiology of rhabdomyolysis in a case series of seven patients with HIV infection from the Presbyterian Medical Center in Philadelphia.[15] Three of the seven patients developed AKI. Acute infection was present in four of seven patients. Ongoing substance abuse including alcohol, heroin, barbiturates, or cocaine use occurred in six patients. Two of seven patients had recently had a history of seizures in the setting of concomitant substance abuse.

Cocaine can induce myonecrosis because of its vasoconstrictive properties.[15,33] There may also be a direct myotoxic effect of the drug.[15,34] Through stimulation of catecholamines, cocaine may promote the release of calcium from the sarcoplasmic reticulum and increase calcium entry into muscle cells, thereby leading to muscle injury.[15] Alcohol abuse is also a potential cause of rhabdomyolysis in HIV-infected patients.[15,35] Alcohol has been associated with myotoxicity through effects on the sarcolemma, increases in calcium and sodium transport into the muscle cells, and associated hypophosphatemia and hypokalemia, which all can precipitate muscle injury.[15,36-38]

Thrombotic Thrombocytopenic Purpura/ Hemolytic Uremic Syndromes

Thrombotic microangiopathy (TMA) consists of the following characteristics: microangiopathic hemolytic anemia, fever, renal dysfunction, neurological deficits, and thrombocytopenia.[39,40] Boccia and colleagues[41] reported the first case of hemolytic uremic syndrome in the setting of the acquired immunodeficiency syndrome in 1984. Since that time, further data have indicated an association between HIV infection and TMA.[42-45] Risk factors for thrombotic thrombocytopenic purpura in the setting of HIV infection include the medications used to treat the HIV, the direct cytopathic effects of the HIV infection, or its associated opportunistic infections.[44-47] The p24 antigen, specific for HIV, has been found in the endothelium of infected patients, supporting a direct role for HIV in causing thrombotic microangiopathies.[48] In addition, a decrease in ADAMTS 13 activity, the von Willebrand factor–cleaving protease, has been found in HIV-infected patients who have thrombotic thrombocytopenic purpura.[49]

The incidence and prevalence rates of TMA in HIV-infected patients vary depending on the patient population examined and whether or not HAART was available at the time of the study. Becker and colleagues[50] performed a prospective observational cohort study of 6022 HIV-infected patients between 1997 and 2003. They found a 0.3% incidence of TMA in their study, and a significantly higher incidence of TMA in HIV-infected patients who had lower CD4 counts and higher viral loads. The presence of *Mycobacterium avium* complex and HCV infection was also associated with significantly higher rates of developing TMA.[50] HIV-infected patients with TMA also had a higher mortality rate compared to HIV-infected patients without the underlying disease.[50] Moore[51] found a 7% incidence of TMA in a prospective cohort of 350 hospitalized HIV-infected patients. Gervasoni and colleagues[52] performed a retrospective cohort study of 1223 HIV-infected patients in the pre-HAART era from 1985 to 1996 and found a 1.4% incidence of TMA. This was then followed by a prospective cohort of 347 HIV patients treated with HAART from 1997 to 2000, in which there were no cases of TMA.[52]

It is still not clear if HAART therapy has a protective effect on the incidence of TMA because of decreased viral loads and burden of illness or whether the medications

themselves may precipitate the disease. Further studies in this area are needed to answer this question.

There are limited data on the treatment of TMA in the setting of HIV infection.[53] Similar to primary forms of TMA, plasmapheresis is the primary treatment option, but outcomes remain poor given the frequent association with advanced HIV infection.[53-55] It is unclear if additional immunosuppressive agents commonly employed in refractory thrombotic thrombocytopenic purpura, such as steroids or rituximab, may have a role in HIV-infected patients with preexisting altered immunity.[56,57] Careful attention to any secondary causes, such as drug-induced TMA, is always necessary.

Nephropathy Related to Use of Highly Active Antiretroviral Therapy

Indinavir has been commonly associated with crystal-induced nephropathy and is therefore not typically used in the common contemporary antiretroviral regimens for HIV infection.[58-60] Gagnon and coworkers[59] found a 67% prevalence of indinavir crystals at the beginning of therapy with this protease inhibitor. Kopp and colleagues[60,61] reported four major renal complications from indinavir use: crystalluria, nephrolithiasis, interstitial nephritis, and lower urinary tract inflammation. Kopp and colleagues[60] evaluated 240 patients initiated on indinavir to determine the incidence of complications. Seven of the 240 patients developed nephrolithiasis, and 19 of the patients developed "symptomatic urinary tract disease" defined as "nephrolithiasis with frank renal colic, flank pain or back pain without evidence of renal stones, and dysuria or urgency." Of the patients taking indinavir in this study, 20% had evidence of crystalluria without any symptoms.[60] Voigt and coworkers[62] found a 33% incidence of nephrolithiasis among 57 patients treated with indinavir over 48 weeks. Indinavir crystals can occur throughout the nephron down through the renal collecting system. Alkaline urine and volume depletion are the usual risk factors for indinavir crystal formation.[63,64] There is a 9% to 25% incidence rate of ARF in the setting of indinavir use.[58,64-66] Renal failure is usually reversible within 3 months after discontinuation of the drug.[58,66] Indinavir crystallization can lead to chronic tubulointerstitial nephritis if the drug is improperly continued despite early evidence of renal damage.[66] There are rare cases of permanent renal dysfunction despite indinavir withdrawal, highlighting the importance of using alternative protease inhibitors, especially in patients with known risk factors for obstructive uropathy and chronic tubulointerstitial disease.[58,66] The presence of sterile leukocyturia and renal failure in patients treated with indinavir should prompt concern for tubulointerstitial damage and discontinuation of the drug.[58] Because indinavir is metabolized mainly through the CYP3A 450 system, caution is advised when prescribing this drug along with other known CYP3A 450 inhibitors.[67] Administration of indinavir along with ketoconazole, clarithromycin, and itraconazole can raise the concentration of indinavir in blood.[67] Administration of indinavir along with rifampin may require use of a higher dose of indinavir, since rifampin is an inducer of the CYP 3A system.[67]

Ritonavir is another protease inhibitor that has been linked to AKI.[58,68-72] However, the data are limited and the kidney injury may be more likely to occur because of other drug interactions.[58,71,72] Additional studies are needed to determine if ritonavir is a distinct cause of ARF.

Tenofovir is a nucleotide reverse transcriptase inhibitor that, in contrast to indinavir, has become increasingly used in antiretroviral regimens because of a perceived lower incidence of adverse events. It belongs to the class of acyclic nucleoside phosphonates. Tenofovir nephrotoxicity is classically characterized by Fanconi's syndrome with or without ARF.[73-77] Initial randomized controlled trials suggested that the drug would have limited nephrotoxicity.[78,79] However, since the introduction of tenofovir, there have been numerous case reports of drug-related proximal tubular injury as well as diabetes insipidus.[74-77,80,81] Izzedine and colleagues[81] reported a case series of 19 patients with signs of proximal tubular damage attributed to initiation of tenofovir therapy. Nephrotoxicity was seen after a mean period of 20 weeks of tenofovir treatment. Fanconi syndrome resolved 4.7 ± 2.9 weeks after stopping the drug. Once signs of early proximal tubulopathy are evident, including hypophosphatemia, normoglycemic glycosuria, alkaline urine, and mild proteinuria, discontinuation of the drug should be strongly considered to avoid potential development of ATN. Close consultation with infectious disease specialists is needed to determine the optimal antiretroviral regimen with the least nephrotoxic potential. The mechanism of Fanconi's syndrome with tenofovir administration may be related to the uptake and secretion of the drug from the proximal tubular cell.[80,82] Tenofovir is reabsorbed from the blood into the proximal tubular cell by human organic anion transporters 1 and 3. The drug is secreted from the proximal tubule into the lumen by multidrug resistance protein 4.[80,82,83] Izzedine and colleagues and others[80,82,83] speculate that other antiretroviral drugs, such as ritonavir, which inhibit the activity of multidrug resistance protein channels, may interact to increase tenofovir concentrations inside the proximal tubular cell, thereby increasing its nephrotoxic potential. Further studies are needed to elucidate the exact mechanism of tenofovir nephrotoxicity and its potential interactions with other antiretroviral regimens.[83] Prevention of toxicity is currently directed at early detection of injury, avoiding the drug if there is underlying renal disease, and adequate volume repletion.[80]

Other drug classes of HAART, including the nucleoside reverse-transcriptase inhibitors, the non-nucleoside reverse-transcriptase inhibitors, and the fusion inhibitors, are only rarely associated with renal failure.[84] The evidence for nephrotoxicity with these drugs is mainly limited to isolated case reports.[84-88] Because of the multiple medications HIV-infected patients take, it is often difficult to determine causality between administration of specific medications and the development of AKI.

Acute Interstitial Nephritis

Acute interstitial nephritis (AIN) is another cause of ARF in the setting of HIV infection. HIV-infected patients often take numerous medications, all of which can potentially cause AIN. Sulfonamides, including trimethoprim-sulfamethoxazole, beta-lactam antibiotics, H2 receptor blockers, quinolones, allopurinol, phenytoin, rifampin, and NSAIDs, have all been linked to the development of AIN in the setting of HIV infection.[9] Valeri and Neusy[10] reported 9% of cases of ARF were caused by AIN from trimethoprim-sulfamethoxazole. Also, HIV is believed to have direct cytotoxic effects that can lead to AIN.[89] There is also the potential to develop opportunistic infections that can cause AIN, including tuberculosis, cytomegalovirus, candidiasis, and histoplasmosis.[89] Prompt recognition of this syndrome, classically characterized by fever, rash,

and eosinophilia, is essential to prevent ongoing renal injury which can lead to fibrosis if not detected early. Once AIN is suspected, discontinuation of the agent in question is indicated. Renal biopsy is needed to confirm the diagnosis of AIN.

Human Immunodeficiency Virus and Acute Glomerulonephritis

Glomerulonephritides, in the setting of coexisting HIV infection, are more often a cause of chronic kidney disease. However, rapidly progressive glomerulonephritis can also occur.[54] A number of acute glomerulonephritides, in the setting of HIV infection, are related to coexisting infectious diseases, which can cause proliferative glomerulonephritides presenting as either postinfectious glomerulonephritides or membranoproliferative glomerulonephritis.[54,90-92] Patients with HIV infection are frequently coinfected with either hepatitis B or C virus; both viruses have been associated with membranoproliferative glomerulonephritis, cryoglobulinemic vasculitis, and membranous nephropathy.[90-92] Glomerulonephritis is typically more common in Caucasian patients infected with HIV.[54,90,92] There has also been an association between HIV and immunoglobulin (Ig) A nephropathy. Kimmel and colleagues[93] showed nephritogenic IgA antibodies are directed against IgM or IgG antibodies produced in response to HIV glycoproteins p24 and gp120 in HIV-infected patients with IgA nephropathy. In addition, the response to HIV infection may culminate in circulating immune complexes which can result in the development of glomerulonephritis.[90]

Crystal Nephropathy

HIV-infected patients commonly take several medications that have been linked to the development of crystalluria and crystal nephropathy. These medications include sulfadiazine, acyclovir, and indinavir, which can all promote obstructive uropathy especially in volume-depleted states.[74,80] Indinavir nephrotoxicity has been discussed elsewhere in this chapter. Acyclovir most commonly causes ARF when given in the intravenous form as a rapid bolus, because this is more likely to lead to precipitation in the renal tubules. Volume depletion and inadequate adjustment of dose with renal insufficiency are the main factors predisposing to the development of drug-induced crystal nephropathies.[80] Ganciclovir has also been associated with intratubular precipitation of crystals, particularly in bone marrow transplant recipients who are administered prolonged intravenous courses for treatment of cytomegalovirus infection.[80] Sulfadiazine, used to treat toxoplasmosis, is another cause of crystal nephropathy in HIV-infected patients.[74] Almost 50% of HIV-infected patients taking sulfadiazine in one series developed ARF.[74] The drug tends to precipitate in acid urine; therefore alkalinization, in addition to volume repletion, is the optimal therapy for the prevention and treatment of sulfadiazine-induced crystal nephropathy.[74]

POSTRENAL FAILURE

HIV-infected patients have a number of risk factors predisposing them to developing obstructive uropathy. Nephrolithiasis can develop especially in the setting of administration of sulfadiazine, indinavir, or acyclovir. Moreover, there is an association between HIV infection and retroperitoneal lymphadenopathy, fibrosis and tumors, obstructing fungus balls, blood clots, and neuropathic and structural bladder abnormalities.[9,94,95] The typical clinical presentation is that of anuric or oliguric acute renal failure.[9] However, at times patients show signs of oliguria intermittently with polyuria in the setting of partial obstruction.[9] High-grade lymphomas with large tumor burden, including retroperitoneal lymphadenopathy, are associated more with advanced HIV infection.[95]

CONCLUSION

AKI is common in the setting of HIV infection. Prerenal failure from volume depletion remains the most common cause of ARF. Careful attention to potential intrinsic and postrenal causes, including nephrotoxic and ischemic ATN, drug-induced AIN, thrombotic microangiopathies, rapidly progressive glomerulonephritis, and obstructive uropathy, is critical when evaluating HIV-infected patients with ARF. HAART has also been linked to AKI. As HAART becomes more widely available in developing parts of the world, there may be an increase in the incidence of ARF from toxicity related to these medications. Further research is needed to determine the exact mechanisms underlying HAART-related nephropathy and how the various HIV-related medications interact to cause acute tubular injury.

Key Points

1. Acute renal failure is becoming increasingly common in human immunodeficiency virus–infected patients admitted to the hospital.

2. Prerenal azotemia from volume depletion remains the most common cause of acute kidney injury in this patient population.
3. Careful attention to other intrinsic and postrenal etiologies should be considered each time acute kidney injury occurs in the human immunodeficiency virus–infected patient.
4. There is an increase in reports of nephrotoxicity in the setting of highly active antiretroviral therapy.
5. Early detection and surveillance for tubular damage in the setting of highly active antiretroviral therapy is critical to avoiding the development of acute tubular necrosis and kidney failure.

Key References

6. Franceschini N, Napravik S, Eron JJ Jr, et al: Incidence and etiology of acute renal failure among ambulatory HIV-infected patients. Kidney Int 2005;67:1526-1531.
7. Wyatt CM, Arons RR, Klotman PE, Klotman ME: Acute renal failure in hospitalized patients with HIV: Risk factors and impact on in-hospital mortality. AIDS 2006;20:561-565.
83. Izzedine H, Launay-Vacher V, Deray G, et al: Renal tubular transporters and antiviral drugs: An update. AIDS 2005;19:455-462.
90. Kimmel PL, Phillips TM, Ferreira-Centeno A, et al: HIV-associated immune-mediated renal disease. Kidney Int 1993;44:1327-1340.
92. Kimmel PL, Barisoni L, Kopp JB: Pathogenesis and treatment of HIV-associated renal diseases: Lessons from clinical and animal studies, molecular pathologic correlations, and genetic investigations. Ann Intern Med 2003;139:214-226.

See the companion Expert Consult website for the complete reference list.

Specific Disorders

CHAPTER 163

Urinary Tract Infections in the Intensive Care Unit

François Marquis, Stéphane P. Ahern, and Martine Leblanc

OBJECTIVES

This chapter will:
1. Recognize urinary tract infection as an important cause of mortality and morbidity in the intensive care unit.
2. Identify risk factors for developing urinary tract infection.
3. Develop an appropriate approach to reduce morbidity and mortality related to urinary tract infection in the intensive care unit.
4. Distinguish community-acquired urinary tract infection from hospital-acquired urinary tract infection.
5. Describe specific urinary tract infections and their respective treatments.

Although not recognized as an important cause of mortality in the intensive care unit (ICU),[1] urinary tract infections (UTIs) are an important cause of morbidity, associated with prolonged hospitalizations, and the economic burden associated with their treatment is growing.[2-4] In a recent cohort study of emergency department visits, 13% of the patients in sepsis were found to have a UTI as the primary process.[5] UTIs represent more than 21% of nosocomial infections in the ICU and nearly 40% of all nosocomial infections in the United States.[6,7] The incidence of ICU-acquired UTIs was 7% (9.6 episodes per 1000 ICU days) in a recent prospective cohort study.[4] The incidence of catheter-associated UTI is usually between 2% and 16% for the first 10 days, and nearly universal at 30 days.[6] UTI remains an important topic for the ICU community and an opportunity to increase patient safety. However, few randomized clinical trials have been conducted, and recent reviews of the literature and meta-analyses have failed to show clear results or guidelines.

DEFINING URINARY TRACT INFECTION AND UROSEPSIS

Asymptomatic bacteriuria is a self-explaining term underlining the importance given to clinical manifestations in the evaluation of UTIs. Such manifestations are hardly appropriate in critically ill patients who are frequently delirious, sedated, or simply unable to communicate. Defining urosepsis remains a challenge in the catheterized ICU patient. Since many patients in the ICU remain asymptomatic, it is critical but difficult to differentiate between a microbial contaminant and a real infection. The International Sepsis Forum Consensus Conference on Definitions of Infection in the ICU suggested critical definitions regarding UTI and urosepsis.[6]

After a general description of pathogens and mechanisms of infection, catheter-related UTIs and bacteriuria—a critical opportunity for improved patient care and safety—are explored and specific treatments are discussed.

UROPATHOGENS

Most UTIs are caused by facultative anaerobes originating from the bowel reservoir. Greater prevalence of indwelling urinary catheters and antimicrobial-induced resistance of bowel and environmental flora contribute to the altered distribution of ICU uropathogens. Depending on the rate of cross-infection, ICUs are variably prone to epidemic infections caused by these antibiotic-resistant pathogens. In recent years, *Candida* species and gram-positive bacteria have been recognized as growing sources of UTIs in the ICU. *Candida* species now account for as many as one third, while gram-positive infections are responsible for 27.1%, of all ICU-acquired UTIs.[4,8]

In the ICU, monomicrobial UTIs are common, since only 5% to 12% of UTIs are polymicrobial. Rarely, true polymicrobial infection is found in association with an indwelling catheter, a stone, a neoplasia, or when a fistula exists between the bowel or the vagina and the urinary tract. Contamination of the urine specimen at the time of collection remains the most frequent cause of polymicrobial growth. Understanding the local epidemiology is critical because susceptibility to antibiotics may differ greatly between centers, according to differences in drug usage and types of patients.[7]

Escherichia coli seems to be consistently responsible for the majority of UTIs in the ICU, with an incidence of 26.0% in a recent analysis of data from the National Nosocomial Infection System from 1986 to 2006.[9] Other significant pathogens in this study were *Pseudomonas aeruginosa* (16.3%) and *Klebsiella pneumoniae* (9.8%). Approximately 20% of *K. pneumoniae* infections and 31% of *Enterobacter* species infections in ICUs in the United States now involve strains not susceptible to third-generation cephalosporins.[10] Laupland and colleagues[8] described 14% of antibiotic-resistant isolates. Resistance to two different classes was not rare (13 out of 53 isolates). *Corynebacterium* group D2, recognized as a nosocomial uropathogen, is highly resistant to most antimicrobials, with the exception of vancomycin. Group B streptococcal infections can be observed in diabetics, while elderly males with obstructive uropathy are prone to enterococcal infections. *Staphylococcus aureus* is an important pathogen, as its finding in a urine culture may signal a disseminated infection.[1]

These numbers contrast strongly with the fact that over 85% of community-acquired UTIs are caused by *E. coli*, whereas other enteric gram-negative bacteria such as *Proteus* and *Klebsiella* species are far less common.

MECHANISMS OF INFECTION

The presence of an indwelling urinary catheter is now recognized as the major risk factor for developing UTIs. While microorganisms from the meatus or distal urethra may be introduced directly into the bladder during catheterization, the safe use of intermittent catheterization showed that this is not a common source of infection.[11] Microorganisms will more likely invade the bladder by ascending the thin mucus film between the catheter and the urethra.[12] Another possible access is from the internal lumen, after the collection bag or the tube junction has been contaminated. The presence of a biofilm composed of proteins (Tamm-Horsfall protein), electrolytes, and organic molecules from the host's urine provides a suitable milieu in which they are protected from urine flow, host defenses, and antibiotics.[12,13] Biofilm formation does not only occur on synthetic materials; *E. coli* showed its capacity to create intracellular pod-like biofilms to protect itself from the host's defenses and induce recurrent UTIs.[14]

RISK FACTORS

Other than the presence of an indwelling urinary catheter, there are many recognized risk factors of developing UTIs in the ICU.[7,8] The mere fact of being in the ICU seems to be an independent risk factor, as showed by a recent study from Mnatzaganian and colleagues.[15] Length of stay in the ICU appears also as an independent risk factor.[7,8] Female sex is another well-recognized risk related to the shorter urethral length and contamination with nearby perineal flora.[8,13,15] Prolonged estrogen deficiency and a relative alkaline vaginal pH contribute to the enhanced UTI risk of postmenopausal and pregnant women, respectively.[16] Males are relatively protected by a longer urethra and antibacterial prostatic secretions.

Obstruction enhances susceptibility to UTIs; most congenital and acquired obstructive uropathies are associated with a higher incidence of infection, particularly of the upper urinary tract. Calculi predispose and perpetuate UTIs both by obstructing urine flow and serving as a nidus for bacteria.

Many other risk factors have been proposed, but their relative importance differs according to the population studied: previous and current antimicrobial agents, age, and catheter care.[7] Disease severity is accepted by many as an independent risk factor, but a recent study failed to show such an association.[4] The exact impact of comorbidities such as diabetes mellitus, immune suppression, structural urological and anatomical abnormalities, and urine flow are not completely understood.[7]

PREVENTION OF URINARY TRACT INFECTIONS

Unjustified prolonged urinary catheter use is frequent in critically ill patients.[3] Since the presence of an indwelling urinary catheter is the only modifiable risk factor, emphasis should be directed at discontinuing all catheters as soon as possible and refraining from installing one when not absolutely necessary.[3,11,17] Manipulations should be restricted to a minimum, and proper aseptic techniques should be used at all times.[3]

The use of a closed system with the drainage bag lower than the bladder to prevent any reflux or urine stagnation is still the single most efficient method to prevent infection, as it will reduce short-term catheterization infection rate from 100% (when open drainage is employed) to less than 25%.[11] Complex antireflux systems failed to show any advantage over the usual closed drainage and are not recommended for now.[18] Efforts should be directed at keeping the system closed and sterile.

Anti-infective urinary catheters have been studied for their capacity to reduce bacteriuria in patients hospitalized on regular wards rather than in ICU patients. Conflicting results have been published.[3] The benefit of such devices remains uncertain in the ICU, and more studies will be needed to assess their impact on ICU-acquired UTIs, cost-effectiveness, and infectious complications.

Antibiotics, antimicrobial bladder washes, antimicrobial drainage bags, and topical disinfectants will only reduce bacteriuria for a short time and will not prevent UTIs. Therefore, they are not recommended.[12] Biofilm-disrupting strategies are under investigation.[17]

ASYMPTOMATIC BACTERIURIA

Asymptomatic bacteriuria is defined by the presence of more than 10^5 cfu/mL of pathogenic microorganisms in the absence of related symptoms. Asymptomatic bacteriuria is common in the ICU. In asymptomatic men, 10^4 cfu/mL of voided specimen is likely to represent true bacteriuria.[19] The presence of a lesser count or of more than one organism suggests contamination.

Contrasting relevant UTI with asymptomatic bacteriuria requires the integration of clinical and laboratory information. Pyuria (defined as 5 to 10 leukocytes/high-power field of a clean-catch centrifuged urine specimen) is suggestive but nonspecific for the presence of asymptomatic or symptomatic UTI. Using a stricter criterion, more than 10 leukocytes/high-power field on microscopic examination is more accurate.[19] Rapid detection methods, such as the dipstick leukocyte esterase and nitrite tests, are useful adjuncts. Bacteria observed in uncentrifuged Gram-stained urine are indicative of a UTI.[20]

For women younger than 65 years, nondiabetic, nonpregnant, uncatheterized, and free of uropathy, asymptomatic bacteriuria can be left untreated. Asymptomatic bacteriuria is rare in middle-aged men, being usually encountered in patients over 50 years in association with a prostatic infectious process or uropathy. A concomitant prostatic infection, found in nearly 50% of cases, requires a prolonged treatment course and relapses frequently. Men with asymptomatic bacteriuria should be treated before urological surgery or procedures are performed.[12] The greater potential for complications in diabetics (such as ascending upper tract involvement, silent or associated with sepsis, altered glucose control, papillary necrosis, and further kidney compromise) justifies antimicrobial treatment.

In patients with valvular heart disease or prosthetic device, eradication of bacteriuria should be seriously considered before any urological manipulation. Asymptomatic bacteriuria should also be treated in immunosuppressed patients, with special considerations to renal transplant recipients.[21] In dialysis patients, UTIs, including asymptomatic bacteriuria, are not infrequent. Those with polycystic kidneys or stones need treatment.[22]

CATHETER-ASSOCIATED BACTERIURIA

In ICU patients with indwelling urinary catheter, silent bacteriuria is an important reservoir of potentially resistant microorganisms. Moreover, a count as low as 10^3 cfu/mL organisms is highly predictive of infection as it will progress rapidly to a 10^5 cfu/mL concentration when antibiotics are not given.[6]

It is preferable to remove the infected catheter, initiate antibiotic treatment, and reinsert a new catheter and drainage system only if necessary. Following catheter removal, bacteriuria will clear spontaneously in over 75% of young females but in less than 5% in older women.[23] Persistent bacteriuria 2 to 3 days after catheter removal should be treated in patients who are symptomatic, elderly, or at risk for complications.

Candida species are clearly associated with urinary infection, especially in catheterized patients and may be the only sign of a deep candidiasis. However, isolated candiduria (no evidence of *Candida* colonization or infection at other sites) is rarely treated. The literature suggests to treat counts of 10^4 cfu/mL or higher, as counts lower than 10^3 cfu/mL rarely progress and usually remain asymptomatic.[6]

The frequency of urinary tract infections is reduced but not eliminated with intermittent catheterization.[24] Although not free of infectious complications, a condom catheter can be a safer alternative to bladder catheterization in male patients. Suprapubic catheterization is associated with UTI rates similar or slightly lower than those associated with urethral catheterization.[24]

When indicated, the initial antibiotic regimen should be as that for complicated UTIs and subsequently modified depending on identified organisms and sensitivities. Parenteral antibiotics are reserved for signs of upper tract or systemic infection. A 7- to 10-day course will generally suffice, although the optimal management of catheter-acquired UTIs in ICU has not been evaluated.[13,21] Follow-up urine cultures should be performed 10 to 14 days after treatment completion to verify eradication.[21]

Funguria in catheterized patients at low risk for upper tract involvement or hematogenous dissemination can be managed by simply removing the catheter without further treatment. Amphotericin B bladder irrigations are now replaced by the use of fluconazole.[13,25] Not only is fluconazole safer, but studies show better survival.[25] Experience with other "azoles" is more limited because these agents achieve a limited concentration in the urinary tract. Caspofungin is probably an adequate treatment for parenchymal disease, but the drug only poorly penetrates the urinary tract. Intravenous amphotericin B has been proposed as alternative treatment, as well as flucytosine.[25]

LOWER URINARY TRACT INFECTIONS

Urethritis and cystitis are infections confined to the superficial mucosa of the urethra and bladder and are generally bacterial in origin. Related symptoms include dysuria with burning and discomfort on urination, urgency, frequency with small-volume micturition, nycturia, suprapubic discomfort, and sometimes incontinence. Over 80% of recurrent infections are due to reinfections, whereas relapses usually arise after insufficient treatment and may suggest a persistent renal focus of infection, an associated prostatic infection, an underlying calculus, or another urological abnormality.

All symptomatic infections should be treated with antimicrobial agents. The traditional regimen for lower UTIs consists of an oral antibiotic for 3 days, and cure rates usually exceed 90%. Single-dose therapy, particularly with oral beta-lactam agents, has been associated with more frequent relapses.[21]

If a lower UTI relapses after a first 3- or 7-day treatment, a 14-day course with an appropriate agent (based on repeated sensitivities since the bacteria may have developed resistance) is indicated. If another relapse occurs, a 6-week antibiotic course should be administered and urological investigation conducted.

Urological abnormalities are present in 25% to 75% of males with UTIs, and a urological investigation, including cystoscopy in patients over 50 years, is recommended after the first or second episode. If an acute prostatitis is associated, antibiotic treatment should be extended 4 to 6 weeks after an initial parenteral course. For chronic prostatitis, an oral course of 6 to 12 weeks is usually necessary. Trimethoprim, trimethoprim-sulfamethoxazole, and quinolones remain the preferred agents since they concentrate particularly well in prostatic tissues.

UPPER URINARY TRACT INFECTIONS

Acute Pyelonephritis

Acute pyelonephritis, a parenchymal bacterial infection of the kidney, is rarely an issue in the critical care unit. UTIs are usually detected and treated before evolving to overt pyelonephritis, and a patient presenting with a pyelonephritis will not be admitted in the ICU unless it progresses to a severe sepsis or septic shock. As for other UTIs, the clinical presentation may differ from classic unilateral flank pain, exquisite tenderness on percussion of the costovertebral angle, fever, chills, and prostration. Bacteriuria constitutes the expected mode of presentation. Approximately 50% of patients complain of lower urinary tract symptoms preceding the clinical picture by a few days. Gastrointestinal symptoms, such as nausea, vomiting, abdominal pain, or change in stool habits, result from an associated paralytic ileus. White cell casts and bacterial casts on urine microscopic examination suggest the diagnosis. Infection of the kidney by the hematogenous route is rare. *S. aureus, Salmonella, Mycobacterium tuberculosis,* and *Candida* are the most common species that can invade the kidney following bloodstream spread. An acute pyelonephritis developing in an ICU patient mandates parenteral treatment.

Lobar Nephritis

Acute bacterial nephritis or lobar nephritis, a severe form of acute pyelonephritis, is relatively uncommon and is believed to be the early stage of renal abscess formation. Lobar nephritis will usually present itself as a focal inflammatory mass which might have some resemblance to a malignant lesion.[26] The poorly marginated sonolucent and ovoid mass seen on imaging studies represents the focal inflammatory area with some tissue necrosis and can mimic an abscess, but there is no frank liquefaction. Computed tomography is now the preferred imaging modality.[27,28] The more severe multilobar grade has been found mainly in diabetics and immunocompromised patients and is associated with increased mortality.[29] These patients are septic, but their blood and urine cultures may be negative.[26] The most common pathogen causing lobar nephritis is *E. coli,* but *K. pneumoniae* and *P. aeruginosa* also can be found.[26,28]

No treatment guidelines have been clearly defined, especially for ICU patients. Medical treatment with parenteral antibiotics until fever abates is usually recommended.[27] Recent data suggest a total treatment of no less than 3 weeks. Surgery is rarely needed, except for patients with concomitant urological abnormalities.[28]

RENAL ABSCESS AND CARBUNCLE

A renal abscess may be consequent to an episode of acute pyelonephritis that was either unrecognized or insufficiently treated. The mortality rate, known to be 36% to 56% with surgical treatment, has been reduced to 12% with percutaneous drainage.[30] Diabetes mellitus and nephrolithiasis are the leading underlying diseases.[31] Generally, a gram-negative bacillus is the responsible organism (*E. coli, K. pneumoniae, Proteus mirabilis,* and *P. aeruginosa*).[32] Small abscesses (less than 3 cm) in immunocompetent patients may respond to medical treatment with antibiotic only, but larger ones are likely to need drainage.[33] A 4- to 6-week course of systemic antibacterial treatment is given in addition to percutaneous drainage.[32,34] Because percutaneous drainage is simple, rapid, and feasible at the bedside, and its efficacy is well documented, it is probably the procedure of choice for critically ill patients.[31,32]

A renal carbuncle is a cortical, circumscribed, multilocular abscess usually consequent to an infection with *S. aureus* or streptococci. The primary focus of the infection is extrarenal, with spread to the kidney by hematogenous dissemination. These lesions can be discovered quite late after a documented episode of bacteremia, with reported delays as long as 7 weeks.[34] Intravenous drug abusers, hemodialysis patients, and diabetics are populations at risk. Fever, sometimes of unknown origin, intermittent abdominal pain, and flank tenderness without lower urinary tract symptoms constitute the clinical picture. Urinalysis and culture will be negative unless the carbuncle communicates with the collecting system. Sonography and computed tomography are helpful diagnostic modalities. Parenteral anti-staphylococcal antibiotics are the treatment of choice and should be continued for at least 10 to 14 days, followed by an oral regimen of 2 to 4 weeks. Rarely, percutaneous aspiration or open incision and drainage will be required.

PERINEPHRIC ABSCESS

A perinephric abscess is a purulent collection localized between the kidney and Gerota's fascia that may extend to pararenal and subphrenic spaces, or into the psoas muscle or peritoneal cavity.[34] It is most often the result of a real parenchymal abscess rupture and is rarely secondary to hematogenous dissemination or extension of a retroperitoneal abscess. The clinical picture is insidious, although fever, chills, and flank pain are usually present, and fever is more likely to persist despite antibiotics, compared with renal abscesses or pyelonephritis.[32] There is typically a long delay before the diagnosis is made. Patients with uropathy and stone disease are most predisposed, and *Proteus* species are isolated almost as frequently as *E. coli.* Sonogram and computed tomography are more sensitive diagnostic tests. Early surgical or percutaneous drainage is mandatory, and antimicrobial therapy should be used as a therapeutic adjunct. Unfortunately, nephrectomy is frequently necessary, and mortality rates may be higher than 50% despite adequate treatment.[20,35]

INFECTED RENAL CYSTS

This entity occurs mainly in female patients with polycystic kidneys.[16] Usually, gram-negative organisms have invaded the upper tract by the ascending route or following urological instrumentation. The clinical presentation is similar as for renal abscess. Accurate diagnosis is not always straightforward because both ultrasound and computed tomography may be negative. However, presence of debris and material can be a valuable clue.[16] A gallium-67 scan will confirm the diagnosis in 50% of patients. As the response to antibiotic is inversely proportional to cyst size, a prolonged antibiotic course with a liposoluble agent is recommended. Surgical drainage is preferably avoided, and percutaneous drainage should be tried first.[16,34]

EMPHYSEMATOUS PYELONEPHRITIS

Emphysematous pyelonephritis, an acute pyelonephritis generally encountered in diabetics (80% to 96%) or patients with ureteral obstruction is caused by gas-forming uropathogens (*E. coli* and *Klebsiella, Proteus, Aerobacter, Citrobacter,* and *Pseudomonas* species).[36] Traditionally, urgent nephrectomy (within hours) has been the only treatment shown to decrease mortality rates from 75% to 25%. However, recent literature showed that percutaneous drainage with appropriate antimicrobial therapy is an acceptable therapy in selected patients.[21,37]

UROSEPSIS

As a primary disease, urosepsis is rarely asymptomatic, except in very debilitated or immunosuppressed patients. However, as a nosocomial infection in an already critically ill patient, urosepsis may be asymptomatic and the clinician must rely on the vitals (fever, tachycardia, low blood pressure), blood work, urine analysis, and cultures to reach an accurate diagnosis.[6]

General sepsis treatment guidelines apply for urosepsis as for any sepsis. Rapid liquid repletion with concomitant parenteral wide-spectrum antibiotics should be started immediately. The source (pyelonephritis, renal or perirenal abscess, but rarely simple UTIs) should be identified.[6] Indwelling urinary catheters should be removed and replaced only if necessary. When the source and the nature of the microorganism are known, targeted actions should be taken and antibiotic spectrum should be narrowed. The clinician should remember that even if the urinary tract is one of the most frequent sites of origin for gram-negative bacteremia, gram-positive bacteremia and fungus cannot be ignored, especially in a critically ill patient.

Complications such as adult respiratory distress syndrome and disseminated intravascular coagulation can be seen as a result of cytokine release and activation of several mediators involved in the pathophysiology of gram-negative sepsis.

FUNGAL URINARY TRACT INFECTIONS

Candida species account for most fungal UTIs. The vast majority are endogenous in origin, as many fungi are usual commensals of the gastrointestinal and female genital tracts and commonly of the skin. Based on autopsy evidence, the kidney is the organ most frequently involved following hematogenous *Candida* spread. Renal involvement is usually a clinically silent process and is manifested only by the presence of candiduria. The role of the ascending route with regard to fungal invasion of the kidney is unclear. The accumulation of fungal material in the renal pelvis may form bezoars (fungal ball). Imaging studies, such as sonography, computed tomography, and retrograde or anterograde urography, may be of value in demonstrating fungal invasion of the upper tract.

Patients with upper-tract urinary fungal infections need to be treated as for disseminated candidiasis with fluconazole for 2 to 4 weeks.[35] Fluconazole penetrates extremely well into the urinary tract and might be the preferred agent when *Candida albicans* is the infecting pathogen.

URINARY TRACT INFECTION AFTER RENAL TRANSPLANTATION

UTIs are a frequent problem following kidney transplantation, with prevalence rates as high as 40% within the first year.[38] The routine administration of trimethoprim-sulfamethoxazole for prophylaxis of *Pneumocystis jiroveci* has reduced the incidence of UTIs post transplantation.[39] Reported risk factors include prolonged bladder catheterization, recipient age, prior urological complications, as well as the degree of organ mismatch, probably reflecting the need for a higher degree of immunosuppression. Unless absolutely necessary, the urinary catheter should be kept for the shortest possible period and removed if bacteriuria occurs.

Aerobic gram-negative bacilli and enterococci are the predominant uropathogens. Early UTIs post transplantation are commonly associated with graft involvement and bacteremia (in over 90% and 10% of cases, respectively), while UTIs occurring after 6 months post transplantation are generally restricted to the lower urinary tract. Because of feared complications, early bacteriuria, with or without associated symptoms, should be treated early and aggressively with parenteral antibiotics; a total antibiotic course of 4 to 6 weeks is desirable. Tapering of immunosuppression is rarely indicated, except when secondary bacteremia and sepsis supervene. Follow-up urine cultures are indicated after the treatment and on a regular basis thereafter. Currently, graft or native nephrectomy is rarely justified unless the upper tract infection is severe, complicated by irreversible dysfunction, and unresponsive to conventional therapy. Infected fluid collections in the first few weeks after transplantation or a perinephric abscess may occur following repeated aspirations. An abscess may infect the arterial anastomosis, resulting in the formation of a mycotic aneurysm with the risk of acute hemorrhage and potential loss of the allograft.

Key Points

1. Urinary tract infections are a major source of nosocomial infections in the intensive care unit.
2. Urinary tract infections are a major source of morbidity in the intensive care unit.
3. The presence of an indwelling urinary catheter is the only modifiable risk factor for urinary tract infections.
4. Urinary catheter should be discontinued as soon as possible and avoided when not necessary.
5. Rapid diagnosis and treatment are essential in the management of complicated urinary tract infections and urinary sepsis.
6. Empirical antibiotic treatment should be tailored to local patterns of resistance.

Key References

1. Cohen J, Cristofaro P, Carlet J, Opal S: New method of classifying infections in critically ill patients. Crit Care Med 2004; 32(7):1510-1526.
3. Saint S, Savel RH, Matthay MA: Enhancing the safety of critically ill patients by reducing urinary and central venous catheter-related infections. Am J Respir Crit Care Med 2002; 165(11):1475-1479.
7. Bagshaw SM, Laupland KB: Epidemiology of intensive care unit-acquired urinary tract infections. Curr Opin Infect Dis 2006;19(1):67-71.
8. Laupland KB, Zygun DA, Davies HD, et al: Incidence and risk factors for acquiring nosocomial urinary tract infection in the critically ill. J Crit Care 2002;17(1):50-57.
19. Rubin RH, Shapiro ED, Andriole VT, et al, for the Infectious Diseases Society of America and the Food and Drug Administration: Evaluation of new anti-infective drugs for the treatment of urinary tract infection. Clin Infect Dis 1992;15(Suppl 1):S216-S227.

See the companion Expert Consult website for the complete reference list.

CHAPTER 164

Acute Kidney Injury in Malaria

Vivekanand Jha and Kirpal S. Chugh

OBJECTIVES

This chapter will:
1. Give an overview of the history, epidemiology, and distribution of malaria and the life cycle of the causative organism, the *Plasmodium*.
2. Describe the clinical features, pattern of organ involvement, and renal, electrolyte, and acid-base abnormalities encountered in acutely ill patients with malaria.
3. Elucidate the diagnostic tests and management principles of severe acute malaria.
4. Provide an insight into the pathogenesis of kidney injury in acute malaria.

HISTORY

Malaria, an ancient disease caused by the *Plasmodium* parasite, is described in cuneiform script, where it is attributed to Nergal, the Babylonian god of destruction and pestilence pictured as a double-winged, mosquito-like insect. The connection between malaria and swamps was known in antiquity, and the word *malaria* is derived from *malus* (bad) and *aeris* (air) that came from marshes. References to disease akin to malaria are found in Chinese, Sumerian, Egyptian, and Indian Vedic and Brahmanic writings. The *Athārva Veda* details the fact that fevers were common particularly after excessive rains or when there was a great deal of grass cover. The relationship between malaria and microorganisms was suspected in the 18th century, but the parasite was identified only in 1880 by Charles Laveran, a French physician working in Algeria and a student of Louis Pasteur. Camillo Golgi, an Italian neurophysiologist, recognized at least two forms of the disease, one with tertian periodicity (fever every other day) and one with quartan periodicity (fever every third day). In 1886, he observed differing numbers of segmentations on maturity in tertian and quartan forms, implying that the two diseases were caused by two distinct parasites. After years of painstaking research, Ronald Ross, a British scientist working in Indian Medical Service, proved mosquitoes to be disease carriers, and Italian physician Giovanni Battista Grassi identified the species as *Anopheles claviger* in 1898. Rapid strides have been made in understanding the biology of malaria in the last two decades, culminating in the publication of the complete *Plasmodium falciparum* genome sequence in 2002.

EPIDEMIOLOGY

With the exception of a few islands in the East Pacific, malaria is encountered throughout the tropics, affecting 300 to 500 million people annually and is responsible for 1 to 3 million deaths. About 90% of all deaths are in Africa, where children are the most affected.[1] Four *Plasmodium* species—*P. falciparum, P. vivax, P. malariae,* and *P. ovale*—cause human disease. *P. falciparum* predominates in sub-Saharan Africa, New Guinea, and Haiti, and *P. vivax* is more common in Central America and the Indian subcontinent. An increase in *P. falciparum* infections has been observed in India over the past decade. These two protozoal infections are equally prevalent in South America, eastern Asia, and Oceania. *P. malariae* and *P. ovale* infections are rare outside Africa. Generally, *P. falciparum* predominates in warmer regions closer to the equator and causes intense year-round transmission.

In addition to being a burden to the native communities, malaria is a danger to travelers to endemic areas. Even though transmission has been eliminated in North America and Western Europe, cases still occur, mostly in returning travelers or immigrants ("imported malaria"). Other mechanisms of transmission include "airport" malaria (malaria caused by infected mosquitoes that are transported rapidly by aircraft from a malaria-endemic country to a non-endemic country), locally transmitted mosquito-borne cases, congenital malaria, and through blood transfusions and organ transplants.

LIFE CYCLE

The sporozoite forms of *Plasmodium* are introduced into the bloodstream by female *Anopheles* mosquitoes during a blood meal. They are rapidly carried to the liver where they invade the hepatocytes and begin a cycle of asexual reproduction. After 6 to 16 days, the affected cells rupture to release motile merozoites into the bloodstream. In the cases of *P. vivax* and *P. ovale,* some sporozoites remain dormant in the liver and can give rise to relapsing infections months or years later. *P. falciparum* and *P. malariae* may persist as inapparent low-grade parasitemia and cause symptomatic recrudescences. Merozoites invade erythrocytes via specific receptors, become trophozoites, and multiply 10- to 20-fold every 2 to 3 days. Symptoms appear after the parasitemia exceeds $50/\mu L$. Some of the parasites develop into morphologically distinct gametocytes, which can be taken up by mosquitoes to undergo a sexual cycle in the midgut, producing sporozoites, which migrate to salivary glands and await inoculation into another human. The usual intervals between the mosquito bite and the appearance of parasitemia are 10 days for *P. falciparum,* 8 to 13 days for *P. vivax,* 9 to 14 days for *P. ovale,* and 15 to 16 days for *P. malariae.*

An important interspecies difference is the differential ability to invade human erythrocytes of different ages. *P. vivax* and *P. ovale* infect young red cells only; *P. malariae* infects only aging cells, but *P. falciparum* can invade cells of all ages and produces heavy parasitemia and severe disease.

GENETICS

A number of genetic traits confer resistance to malaria in humans. These include thalassanemias; hemoglobins S, E, and C; South East Asian ovalocytosis; glucose-6-phosphatase dehydrogenase deficiency; and polymorphisms in interferon-α and -γ receptors;[2] whereas certain polymorphisms in Toll-like receptor 4 and the promoter region of macrophage migration inhibitory factor gene predispose to more severe infection.[3,4]

CLINICAL FEATURES

Malaria is a common cause of fever in tropical countries. Initial symptoms include malaise, myalgia, headache, and chills; malaria also can cause confusion with a viral illness. In some patients, headache, chest pains, cough, abdominal pain, arthralgias, or diarrhea may be prominent. Soon, the characteristic high-grade fever and severe chills accompanied by tachycardia, nausea, orthostatic dizziness, and extreme weakness appear. The fever abates after several hours, and the patient becomes diaphoretic and exhausted. The paroxysms may occur at regular intervals corresponding to the length of the erythrocytic cycles, but they are often absent in malaria caused by *P. falciparum* or in persons who have received chemoprophylaxis. Absence of focal symptoms, lymphadenopathy, and rash (except herpes labialis) help distinguish malaria from other causes. Physical findings are nonspecific; splenomegaly may be present in advanced disease.

Rapid organ involvement leading to life-threatening complications can be encountered in untreated *P. falciparum* because of its ability to cause high parasitemia levels leading to sequestration and capillary sludging. Complications include cerebral malaria characterized by somnolence, coma, delirium, and seizures; respiratory failure due to noncardiogenic acute pulmonary edema; hematological abnormalities, including intravascular hemolysis, thrombocytopenia, and disseminated intravascular coagulation; jaundice as a result of hemolysis, malarial hepatitis, or both; acute renal failure (ARF) and severe metabolic abnormalities. Risk factors for complicated disease include extremes of age, immunocompromised state, pregnancy, asplenia, failure to take chemoprophylaxis, and delayed diagnosis.[5]

Clinically significant kidney disease is seen following infections with *P. falciparum* and *P. malariae*. *P. malariae* causes an immune-complex glomerulonephritis leading to nephrotic syndrome, whereas *P. falciparum* produces a wide range of structural and functional abnormalities (Table 164-1), including ARF, non-nephrotic proteinuria, microscopic hematuria, hemoglobinuria, or dyselectrolytemias. Proteinuria, both glomerular and tubular, has been documented in 85% to 100% of cases with falciparum malaria.

ARF is encountered following *P. falciparum* malaria. Some authors have described ARF in vivax malaria, but the cause-and-effect relationship between the two has not been proved and the possibility of dual infection has not been carefully investigated. The overall prevalence is less than 1% but may rise to 60% in patients with severe infection.[5] Populations in endemic areas acquire varying degrees of immunity to the infection, and the incidence among them is 2% to 5%. Nonimmune visitors to an endemic area and semi-immune children develop severe infection and

TABLE 164-1

Metabolic and Renal Abnormalities in Malaria Caused by *Plasmodium falciparum*

Extrarenal Manifestations
  Abnormalities in fluid balance
    Hypervolemia
    Normovolemia
    Hypovolemia
  Abnormalities in serum electrolytes
    Hyponatremia
    Hypokalemia
    Hypocalcemia
    Hypernatremia
    Hyperkalemia
    Hypophosphatemia
  Metabolic abnormalities
    Lactic acidosis
    Hypoglycemia
Renal Manifestations
  Hemoglobinuria
  Methemoglobinuria
  Myoglobinuria
  Mild glomerulonephritis (proteinuria with mild urinary sediment changes)
  Acute nephritis
  Nephrotic syndrome
  Acute renal failure

Adapted from Eiam-Ong S, Sitprija V: Falciparum malaria and the kidney: A model of inflammation. Am J Kidney Dis 1998;32:361-375.

are more likely to experience renal failure than the local residents; reported figures are 25% to 30%.[6,7] Recent studies have shown a high prevalence of decreased glomerular filtration rate, as indicated by elevated serum cystatin C levels in over 55% of uncomplicated falciparum malaria, and suggest that renal involvement may be more common than that realized so far.[8]

ARF is usually seen by the end of the first week and can be non-oliguric in about 50% of the cases.[9] It is usually hypercatabolic, and the blood urea and serum creatinine increase rapidly. Cholestatic jaundice, characterized by elevated alkaline phosphatase concentration out of proportion to the transaminases, is seen in over 75% of cases of malarial acute renal failure (MARF). Anemia and thrombocytopenia are encountered in more than two thirds of patients. Patients deficient in glucose-6-phosphate dehydrogenase may develop intravascular hemolysis.[5] A recent increase has been encountered in the poorly understood "blackwater fever" among non-immune European expatriates in the endemic areas.[10] The most commonly accepted explanations for this condition include hypersensitivity and oxidant-stress-induced intravascular hemolysis in patients deficient in glucose-6-phosphate dehydrogenase. Renal failure lasts from a few days to several weeks, with an average of 2 weeks.[5,9,11] Cerebral malaria and ARF usually are not seen in the same patient.

A host of metabolic abnormalities can be encountered.[12] Of the dyselectrolytemias, hyponatremia is the most common, seen in 55% to 60% of cases.[13] The postulated mechanisms are renal sodium loss in the initial phase and hemodilution in the later stages. Increased secretion of antidiuretic hormone and resetting of osmostat are the other possible mechanisms. It is mild and asymptomatic and usually does not require treatment. Hyperkalemia can be life-threatening in those with intravascular hemolysis and necessitates early dialysis. Hyperphosphatemia and hypocalcemia can be seen in severe infection. Hypoglycemia and lactic acidosis are common and portend a poor prognosis.[14] A combination of increased glucose consumption, failure of hepatic gluconeogenesis, and increased pancreatic insulin secretion by quinine and quinidine (the drugs used for treatment) lead to hypoglycemia.[15] Increased lactate production by the parasites and tissue hypoxia leading to anaerobic glycolysis and a failure of hepatic and renal lactate clearance contribute to lactic acidosis. Renal failure compounds the acidosis. The plasma concentrations of bicarbonate or lactate are the best biochemical prognosticators in severe malaria.

Patients with severe disease are at risk of developing superadded infections involving respiratory or urinary tracts. *Salmonella* bacteremia has been described specifically in association with *P. falciparum* infection.[11]

DIAGNOSIS

Most patients exhibit a normocytic normochromic anemia. Severe cases may be associated with leukocytosis, thrombocytopenia, and prolonged prothrombin and partial thromboplastin times, indicating consumptive coagulopathy. Hyponatremia and lactic acidosis are encountered commonly. In later stages, the clinical picture of severe falciparum malaria resembles other tropical infections including leptospirosis, scrub typhus, and hantavirus infection. A high index of suspicion is essential for making a timely diagnosis and prompt institution of therapy. The history should include details of recent travels to endemic areas, recent antimalarial therapy or prophylaxis, previous attacks of malaria, and diminishing urine output or alteration in urine color.

Diagnosis can be established by the demonstration of asexual forms of the parasite in thick and thin peripheral blood smears stained with Giemsa (pH 7.2), Wright, Field, or Leishman stains. Red blood cells in the tail of the thin blood smear are examined under oil immersion (×1000 magnification). *P. falciparum* is identified by the presence of small ring forms with double-chromatin knobs within the erythrocyte, multiply infected rings in individual red blood cells, presence of crescent-shaped (banana-shaped) gametocytes, and parasitemia exceeding 4%. Initial smear is positive in over 90% of cases, but parasitemia may be absent if the parasitized erythrocytes are sequestered from the bloodstream. If parasitemia is not seen in the stained thin smear, a thick smear that concentrates blood cells may provide the diagnosis. Mixed infection with *P. falciparum* should be suspected in any patient with severe malaria, but whose blood film shows only *P. vivax, P. ovale,* or *P. malariae.* In suspicious cases, the test should be repeated at least twice daily for 2 to 3 days to exclude malaria completely. Repeat smears should also be obtained to assess response to treatment. A microtube concentration method followed by staining with the fluorescent dye acridine orange is useful for processing a large number of samples, but it does not allow species identification. Recently, simple but specific antibody-based card tests that detect *P. falciparum*–specific, histidine-rich protein 2 or lactate dehydrogenase antigens in finger-prick blood samples have been introduced.[16] They allow differentiation of falciparum from non-falciparum malarias but have the disadvantage of remaining positive for several weeks after acute infection.

MANAGEMENT

Severe falciparum malaria is a medical emergency and requires intensive nursing care and careful medical management. Prompt assessment of volume status, blood glucose, and acid-base status are essential.[5,9,11] A central venous or pulmonary artery catheter is useful for fluid volume monitoring. Blood glucose levels should be measured every 4 to 6 hours in an unconscious patient, and hypoglycemia should be corrected with intravenous dextrose. Lumbar puncture may be required to exclude intracranial infection in those with altered sensoria. Antibiotics may be required in those with associated bacterial sepsis, and vitamin K administration is useful in those with coagulation abnormalities. Blood transfusions should be given to those with rapidly falling hemoglobin. Parenteral loop diuretics may be required to reduce the risk of fluid overload. Those with respiratory complications such as acute respiratory distress syndrome need ventilatory support.

All patients with severe *P. falciparum* infection should be presumed to have chloroquine-resistant infection.[5,9,11] Because of their activity against chloroquine-resistant strains, cinchona alkaloids (quinine or quinidine) are the mainstay of treatment.[17] Quinine is started intravenously at a dose of 7 mg of the salt per kg body weight, infused over 30 minutes, followed by 10 mg/kg body weight over 4 hours. Infusion is continued at the rate of 10 mg/kg every 8 hours until the patient can take oral quinine sulfate at a dose of 650 mg three times a day for a total of 7 days. Quinidine, more readily available outside the tropics, may be given as an infusion at a dose of 10 mg of the base per kg body weight over 1 to 2 hours, followed by 0.02 mg/kg/min, keeping blood concentrations at 3 to 7 mg/L until parasitemia decreases to less than 1% and the patient can take quinine orally. The dose should be decreased by 30% to 50% after the first 2 days if renal failure persists. Both these agents should be administered by slow intravenous infusion using a drip with a metered chamber or an infusion pump. Normal therapeutic doses can be used safely during pregnancy. Uterine activity and fetal heart rate should be assessed before starting treatment to avoid confusing the effects of malaria and high fever per se from those of the drug.

Cinchonism (giddiness, tinnitus, high-tone deafness, tremors, blurred vision, nausea, and vomiting) can develop at plasma concentrations in excess of 5 mg/L, and concentrations above 20 mg/L may cause blindness, deafness, hypotension, electrocardiogram abnormalities, and central nervous system depression. Quinine therapy often causes hyperinsulinemia, and hypoglycemia should be watched for. Many centers administer a continuous infusion of 5% to 10% dextrose to all patients treated with intravenous quinine or quinidine. Cardiovascular monitoring is required during quinidine infusion to detect cardiotoxicity (QT interval >5.5 seconds, arrhythmia, or saline-unresponsive hypotension).

Artesunate, artemether, and arteether are compounds derived from artemisinin, a sesquiterpene lactone isolated from *Artemisia annua,* a herb that has been used traditionally in China for the treatment of malaria. In large comparative studies, their use has been shown to reduce case fatality of severe falciparum malaria as effectively as quinine. They are particularly valuable in areas with quinine resistance and in patients with recurrent quinine-induced hypoglycemia.[18] Artesunate, a water-soluble hemisuccinate derivative of dihydroartemisinin, is reconstituted with 5% bicarbonate immediately before intravenous use and given at 4 mg/kg loading dose on the first day followed by 2 mg/kg once a day for 6 days. Artemether and arteether are oily suspensions and can be administered by intramuscular injection at 2.4 to 3.2 mg/kg as a loading dose on the first day, followed by 1.2 to 1.6 mg/kg daily for a minimum of 3 days or until the patient can take oral therapy to complete a 7-day course. The daily dose can be given as a single injection. Although neurological and fetal toxicities have been shown in animals treated with artemether and arteether, these effects have never been observed in tens of thousands of human patients who have received these drugs. In children, the use of a tuberculin syringe is advisable since the injection volume will be small.

All patients should receive gametocidal therapy (tetracycline 250 mg four times a day for 7 days, or pyrimethamine-sulfadoxine, three tablets in a single dose). Atovaquone, halofantrine, and lumefantrine have actions similar to quinine and are other possible alternatives for resistant falciparum malaria.

Medical therapy alone is unlikely to reduce the parasite burden when the count exceeds 10%, and exchange transfusions are recommended for bringing about a rapid reduction in the level of parasitemia.[19]

Treatment of renal failure is the same as that due to other causes. Fluid should be administered cautiously in the absence of signs of frank dehydration, as a delayed response to water load may precipitate pulmonary edema.[20] Patients with evidence of intravascular hemolysis should receive adequate hydration and parenteral sodium bicarbonate to alkalinize the urine (pH > 7.0). Some earlier studies found dopamine and frusemide to be beneficial in maintaining the renal blood flow and urine volume in patients with serum creatinine less than 440 µmol/L (5 mg/dL),[21] but more recent studies suggest that these drugs have no effect on renal function.[22] Since renal failure is usually hypercatabolic, frequent dialysis may be needed. Evidence of severe hyperkalemia should be watched for and adequately treated. The peritoneal microcirculation is impaired as a result of infected erythrocytes and vasoconstriction, reducing the efficacy of peritoneal dialysis. However, in practice, peritoneal dialysis is simple to perform and more readily available than hemodialysis. Continuous peritoneal dialysis has been shown to lower the blood urea and serum creatinine concentrations. In a recent comparative trial between state-of-the-art continuous venovenous hemofiltration and suboptimal peritoneal dialysis using a rigid catheter and an open drainage system, the former was associated with quicker resolution of acidosis and azotemia and with reduced risk of death and subsequent dialysis.[23]

PROGNOSIS

The mortality of MARF varies between 10% and 40%.[7,11,14,15,24-31] The outcome is good in patients who receive early medical attention and adequate dialysis. The mortality came down from 75% to 25% in one hospital in India after the setting up of a MARF task force. Late referral, high parasitemia, involvement of multiple organs, respiratory and liver failure, and infection in previously unimmunized subjects are associated with a poor prognosis. Younger age and absence of splenomegaly are risk factors for increased mortality among the pediatric population.[32] In a recent study, a high-serum interleukin-6/interleukin-10 (IL-6/IL-10) ratio was found to be predictive of mortality in patients with MARF.[33]

PATHOLOGY

Acute tubular necrosis is the most common histological lesion. Tubular changes may be subtle and not obvious on light microscopy in those with mild renal failure. Severe cases reveal cloudy swelling, degeneration, and necrosis of tubular cells involving predominantly distal tubules. Casts loaded with malarial pigment are often seen in the proximal tubules. The tubular cells contain hemosiderin granules. Hemoglobin casts may be seen in the lumina of the distal and collecting tubules in patients with intravascular hemolysis.[5] Tubules and vascular endothelia show enhanced expression of tumor necrosis factor-α (TNF-α), IL-1, IL-6, and granulocyte-macrophage colony-stimulating factor (GM-CSF).[34] Varying degrees of interstitial edema and mononuclear cell infiltrate are commonly encountered. In contrast to human infection, experimental animals exhibit marked interstitial inflammation.

Glomerular lesions are noted in around 20% of autopsies of falciparum malaria. The common changes are endocapillary proliferation, mild mesangial hyperplasia, and increased mesangial matrix. The glomerular basement membrane is usually normal. Peritubular capillaries may be packed with parasitized erythrocytes. Fibrin thrombi, malarial pigment-laden macrophages, lymphocytes, and plasma cells also may be seen. The larger blood vessels are unremarkable. Immunofluorescence may show finely granular deposition of IgM and C3 in the mesangial areas and along capillary walls.[35] Electron microscopy shows subendothelial and mesangial electron-dense deposits.

PATHOGENESIS

A number of hemodynamic, immunological, and metabolic perturbations in falciparum malaria contribute to acute kidney injury (Fig. 164-1). Out of these, the most important are the hemodynamic alterations, produced by unique properties of this parasite, which lead to renal ischemia. The growing parasite consumes and degrades erythrocyte proteins, mainly hemoglobin, and alters the transport properties of the red cell membrane, making it more spherical and less deformable. The parasite induces formation of membrane protuberances or "knobs" on the erythrocyte surface. These knobs are cup-shaped, electron-dense structures about 60 to 100 nm in diameter, overlying accretions of histidine-rich proteins, and extruding a strain-specific adhesive-variant protein of high molecular weight that mediates red cell attachment to receptors on venular and capillary endothelium, causing a phenomenon called cytoadherence. The major adhesive protein family is called Plasmodium falciparum erythrocyte membrane protein. The main member of this family, Plasmodium falciparum erythrocyte membrane protein-1, exhibits tremendous structural and antigenic variability between generations and is the main determinant of malarial morbidity.[36,37] Other families of histidine-rich proteins are rifins and rosettins.[38] These knobs are engaged by cell-surface receptors: CR-1 and glycosaminoglycans on the red blood cells, intercellular adhesion molecule-1 in the brain; chondroitin sulfate B in the placenta; and CD36, platelet-endothelial cell adhesion molecule-1 (PECAM-1)/CD31, thrombomodulin, E- and P-selectins, and vascular cellular adhesion molecule-1 elsewhere.[39] Some of these are constitutively expressed, whereas others are induced by inflammatory mediators released in severe disease. In

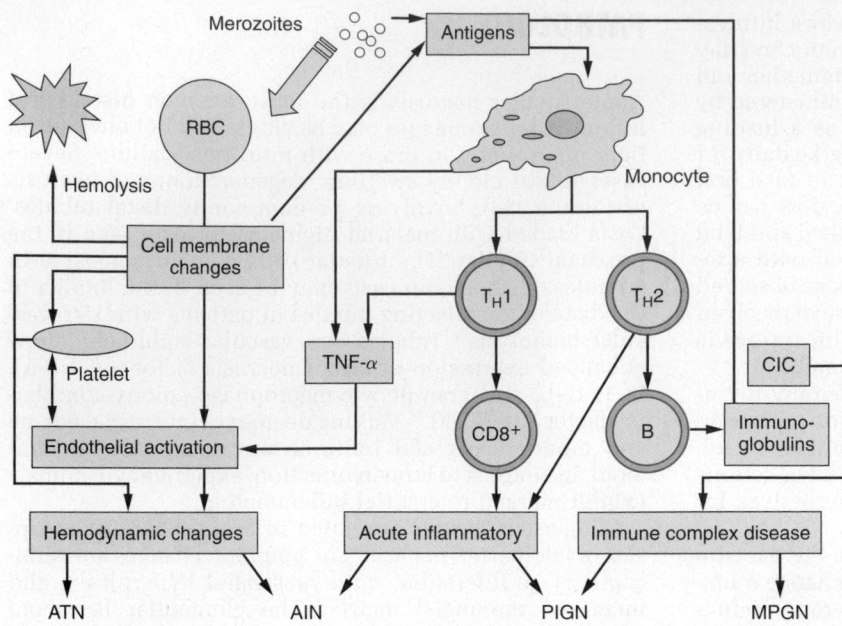

FIGURE 164-1. Pathogenetic mechanisms of development of acute kidney injury in falciparum malaria. AIN, acute inflammatory nephritis; ATN, acute tubular necrosis; CIC, circulating immune complexes; MPGN, membranoproliferative glomerulonephritis; PIGN, postinfectious glomerulonephritis; RBC, red blood cell; T_H1, type 1 helper T cell; T_H2, type 2 helper T cell; TNF-α, tumor necrosis factor-α. (From Barsoum RS: Malarial acute renal failure. J Am Soc Nephrol 2000;11:2147-2154.)

addition to the vascular endothelium, infected erythrocytes adhere to uninfected red cells platelets, monocytes, and lymphocytes. These aggregated and sequestered red cells interfere with microcirculatory flow. This phenomenon is unique to *P. falciparum* and has not been observed with other species.[11] Sequestration avoids the clearance of infected cells by liver or spleen.

The parasite induces the expression of several novel antigens on the surface of host cells by exposing the cryptic erythrocyte antigen and inserting antigens of parasitic origin. These include "var" gene products of the parasite, ring-infected erythrocyte surface antigen, Pf332 and heat-shock proteins.[40] These lead to activation of types 1 and 2 helper T cell (T_H1 and T_H2) arms of the immune response and to release of cytokines, for example, TNF-α, IL-6, interferon-γ, IL-4, IL-5, and IL-10.[41,42] Nonspecific B-lymphocyte proliferation leads to generation of anticardiolipin, antiphospholipid, and antineutrophil cytoplasmic antibodies. Anti-triosephosphate isomerase antibody has been associated with complement-dependent hemolytic anemia. Circulating IgE levels are elevated in severe falciparum malaria and lead to TNF-α generation from monocytes.[43] Glycosyl phosphatidylinositol moieties covalently linked to the surface antigens of malarial parasites are capable of acting as endotoxin and activating a monocyte receptor, CD14.[12] Soluble CD14 levels have been shown to be elevated and can be used as a marker for MARF.[44] Soluble CD14 causes release of TNF-α from monocytes and neutrophils and reactive oxygen species from neutrophils. Finally, *P. falciparum* activates the alternate complement pathway and intrinsic coagulation cascade.[45] The cumulative effect of these pathophysiological alterations is renal vasoconstriction. Human and experimental studies have shown a correlation between organ involvement in falciparum malaria and circulating IL-10, IL-6, IL-1, and TNF-α concentrations. Another study showed elevated IL-6 and soluble IL-6 receptor concentration in MARF. Successful treatment lowered the IL-6 levels but the soluble IL-6 receptor levels increased further, suggesting a role in clearing of the inflammatory state.[46]

As in sepsis, there is peripheral vasodilatation with increased cardiac output and decreased renal blood flow. Patients with severe infections often become hypovolemic

secondary to a cytokine-induced increase in capillary permeability, decreased fluid intake, and increased insensible fluid loss. A decreased response to water loading, attributed to excessive antidiuretic hormone action, is common in falciparum malaria. The blood volume depends on the stage and severity of infection, fluid administration, and systemic and renal hemodynamics.[20]

Increased catecholamine activity has been observed in both animal and human malaria.[47] Animal experiments showed reversible constriction of splanchnic blood vessels. Sitprija[48] showed restoration of renal hemodynamics with phenoxybenzamine in patients with malaria and decreased glomerular filtration rate. Levels of the potent vasoconstrictor, endothelin-1, are elevated and correlate with TNF-α levels in patients with MARF.[49]

An increase in plasma viscosity secondary to an increase in plasma fibrinogen and acute phase proteins has also been incriminated in the genesis of ARF in falciparum malaria. The decreased deformability of parasitized erythrocytes increases the whole blood viscosity.[50] Some authors have documented rhabdomyolysis in patients with severe falciparum malaria, which can contribute to ARF.[51]

CONCLUSIONS

Malaria caused by *P. falciparum* is a common protozoal infection encountered throughout the tropics. This propensity to infect erythrocytes of all ages leads to heavy parasitemia and alteration of red cell membrane characteristics, which causes microvascular sludging leading to tissue ischemia and dysfunction of various organs, including the kidneys. The metabolic demands of the parasite can lead to a variety of electrolyte and acid-base disorders. As the clinical picture is nonspecific, diagnosis requires a high index of suspicion and can be confirmed by demonstration of the parasite on blood smear or by modern molecular techniques. Management entails using parenteral quinine, quinidine, or artemisinin compounds. In view of the hypercatabolic state, patients with renal failure require intensive management including early and frequent hemodialysis or hemofiltration.

Key Points

1. Malaria is encountered throughout the tropical region. *Plasmodium falciparum* can cause severe life-threatening disease, especially in non-immune travelers to endemic areas.
2. Severe falciparum malaria presents with a multisystem illness in which renal, hepatic, and hematological systems show prominent involvement.
3. Diagnosis requires high index of suspicion and confirmation using simple laboratory techniques.
4. Organ involvement occurs as a result of hemorheological alterations produced by heavy parasitemia and capillary sludging leading to tissue ischemia.
5. In view of the high prevalence of chloroquine resistance, treatment must be with cinchona alkaloids (quinine or quinidine) or artemisinin derivatives.

6. Patients with acute renal failure require intensive management with hemodialysis or hemofiltration.

Key References

1. Breman J, Stekette R: Malaria. In Wallace RB (ed): Maxcy–Rosenau–Last Public Health and Preventive Medicine, 13th ed. Norwalk, CT, Appleton Lange, 1992, pp 240-253.
5. Chugh K, Sitprija V, Jha V: Acute renal failure in the tropical countries. In Davison A, Cameron J, Grunfeld J-P, et al (eds): Oxford Textbook of Nephrology. Oxford, Oxford University Press, 2005, pp 1614-1629.
7. Ehrich JH, Eke FU: Malaria-induced renal damage: Facts and myths. Pediatr Nephrol 2007;22:626-637.
11. Barsoum RS: Malarial acute renal failure. J Am Soc Nephrol 2000;11:2147-2154.
12. Eiam-Ong S, Sitprija V: Falciparum malaria and the kidney: A model of inflammation. Am J Kidney Dis 1998;32:361-375.
23. Phu NH, Hien TT, Mai NT, et al: Hemofiltration and peritoneal dialysis in infection-associated acute renal failure in Vietnam. N Engl J Med 2002;347:895-902.

See the companion Expert Consult website for the complete reference list.

CHAPTER 165

Poststreptococcal Glomerulonephritis

Peter Mount and Judy Savige

OBJECTIVES

This chapter will:
1. Describe the epidemiology, pathogenesis, diagnosis, and clinical course of poststreptococcal glomerulonephritis.
2. Discuss the general principles of management of poststreptococcal glomerulonephritis.
3. Emphasize the management of patients with poststreptococcal glomerulonephritis who require admission to the intensive care unit.

Poststreptococcal glomerulonephritis is characterized by the development of hematuria 1 to 3 weeks after a streptococcal throat or skin infection. The disease affects mainly children, and worldwide it is common in communities with crowded living conditions and poor standards of hygiene. Most affected individuals are asymptomatic, but some develop the nephritic syndrome with edema, hypertension, and an elevated serum creatinine. This usually resolves without specific treatment, and the prognosis is excellent. However, occasional patients with poststreptococcal glomerulonephritis require admission to the intensive care unit for management of acute renal failure due to crescentic glomerulonephritis or acute tubular necrosis; for fluid overload, especially in older patients with underlying cardiac disease; or for the encephalopathy that occasionally results from hypertension or infection. Furthermore, recent evidence suggests poststreptococcal glomerulonephritis in indigenous communities is a risk factor for the development of proteinuria and chronic renal disease in later life.[1]

EPIDEMIOLOGY

There are at least half a million cases of poststreptococcal glomerulonephritis worldwide annually.[2] Nearly 90% of these are children, mainly between the ages of 2 and 12 years, with boys affected twice as often as girls. Poststreptococcal glomerulonephritis is much less common in adults because of immunity from repeated streptococcal infections.

Poststreptococcal glomerulonephritis occurs four times as frequently per head of population in the developing world compared with Europe and the United States,[2] where its incidence is falling because of higher standards of living and widespread antibiotic use.[3] However, it remains a significant cause of renal disease in parts of Asia,[4] South America, and Africa,[5] as well as in Australian Aboriginal communities.[6]

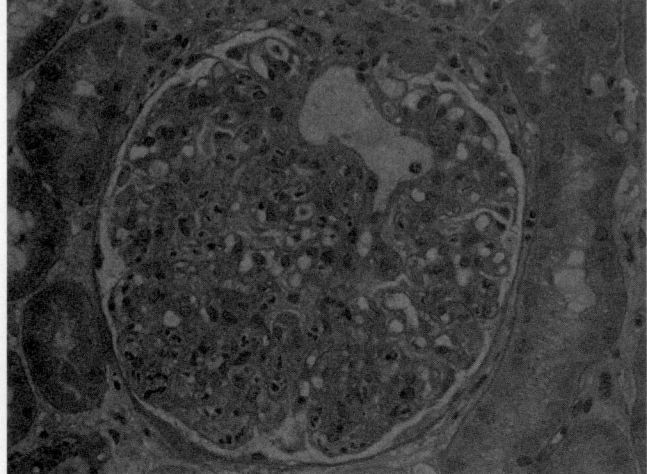

A

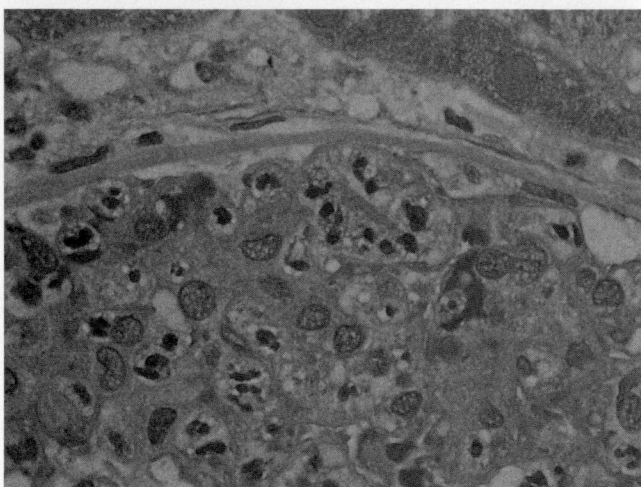

B

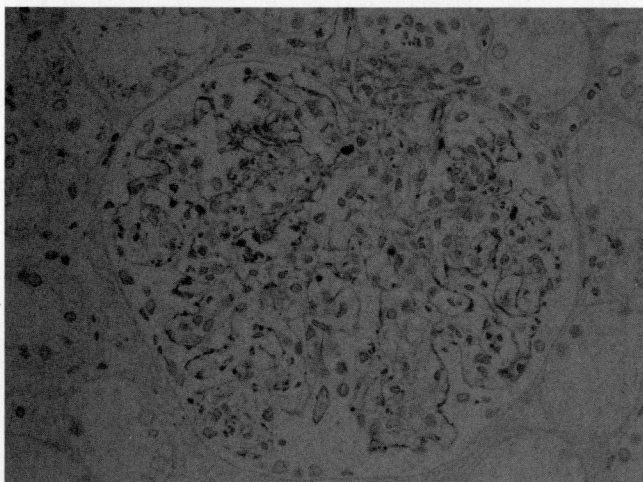

C

FIGURE 165-1. See also color plates. **A,** Diffuse endocapillary glo-merulonephritis with glomerular hypercellularity due to increased numbers of endothelial and mesangial cells and a neutrophil infiltrate (hematoxylin and eosin, ×400). **B,** Occasional small sub-epithelial humps (*stained red*) outline the slightly irregular glo-merular basement membrane and protrude into Bowman's space (Masson, ×1000). **C,** Granular staining of the capillaries for C3 (×400). (**A-C** courtesy of Dr. Moira Finlay, Department of Anatomi-cal Pathology, Melbourne Health, Parkville, Victoria, Australia.)

Poststreptococcal glomerulonephritis occurs after epi-demics of throat and skin infections with nephritogenic strains of group A β hemolytic *Streptococcus pyogenes.* Most cases of poststreptococcal glomerulonephritis occur after skin infections in the developing world. Sporadic cases occur with chronic scabies and other skin conditions in disadvantaged communities[6,7] and, in adults, often in alcoholics.[8]

PATHOGENESIS

In epidemics, 5% to 10% of patients with streptococcal throat infections and 25% of those with skin infections develop poststreptococcal glomerulonephritis. The major nephritogenic strains of *S. pyogenes* are types 12 and 49 in throat and skin infections, respectively, but the ability to cause nephritis is known now to be more widespread than previously thought.

Poststreptococcal glomerulonephritis results, at least in part, from antigen deposition in the glomerular capillary subendothelium and mesangium and subsequent antibody binding in situ to form immune complexes. However, circulating immune complexes also cross the damaged glomerular basement membrane and accumulate in the subepithelial space.

The evidence for nephritogenic antigens is best for the streptococcal plasmin receptor, which has glyceraldehyde phosphate dehydrogenase (GAPDH) activity, and for the cationic proteinase exotoxin B (SPE B) and its zymogen precursor.[9-11] These proteins induce a long-lasting anti-body response that means poststreptococcal glomerulone-phritis does not recur. Both streptococcal plasmin receptor and SPE B are deposited in affected glomeruli and bind plasmin, which activates complement, and induces neu-trophil chemotaxis and glomerular basement membrane degradation by matrix metalloproteinases.[12]

PATHOLOGY

Histologically there is a diffuse endocapillary glomerulo-nephritis with increased endothelial and mesangial cells, as well as a neutrophil infiltrate (Fig. 165-1A). The parietal and visceral epithelial cells occasionally proliferate to form crescents, and there may be a vasculitis of the intra-renal vessels. Special stains and ultrastructural examina-tion demonstrate subepithelial deposits, or "humps" (Fig. 165-2B). The glomerular capillary loops usually stain for IgM and C3 and less commonly stain for IgG (Fig. 165-2C). The "garland" pattern of immune deposits is particularly associated with heavy proteinuria.

CLINICAL FEATURES

Poststreptococcal glomerulonephritis occurs typically 1 to 2 weeks after the pharyngitis and 3 weeks after a skin infection. Streptococcal pharyngitis is characterized by fever, purulent tonsillar exudate, and tender cervical lymphadenopathy. Streptococcal impetigo comprises clusters of small vesicles that break to leave a thick crust (Fig. 165-2).

The clinical features of poststreptococcal glomerulone-phritis vary from asymptomatic hematuria in at least 80%

TABLE 165-1

Features of Different Forms of Glomerulonephritis Associated with Low Complement Levels*

GLOMERULONEPHRITIS	DISTINGUISHING CLINICAL FEATURES	CH50	C3	C4	OTHER INVESTIGATIONS	TREATMENT
Poststreptococcal glomerulonephritis	Preceding streptococcal throat or skin infection	↓	↓	N	ASOT, anti-DNase antibodies	Supportive care
Lupus nephritis	Arthralgia, rash	↓	↓	↓	Anti-dsDNA antibodies	Corticosteroids, cytotoxics
Infective endocarditis	Fever, new and regurgitant murmurs, embolic phenomena	↓	↓	↓	Positive blood cultures	Antibiotics
Membranoproliferative glomerulonephritis type I	No specific features	↓	↓	↓	For underlying cause, e.g., infections, malignancy, autoimmune	Treat underlying cause, (uncertain role) immunosuppression
Membranoproliferative glomerulonephritis type II	Partial lipodystrophy	↓	↓	N	C3 nephritic factor	(uncertain role) immunosuppression
Mixed cryoglobulinemia	Purpuric rash	↓	↓	↓	Cryoglobulins, rheumatoid factor, hepatitis C antibodies and RNA	Antiviral agents, (uncertain role) plasma exchange

*Complement levels may also be low after cardiopulmonary bypass and with cholesterol emboli, and where synthesis is reduced, for example, in severe sepsis and chronic liver disease.
ASOT, anti-streptolysin O titers; DNase, deoxyribonuclease; dsDNA, double-stranded DNA.

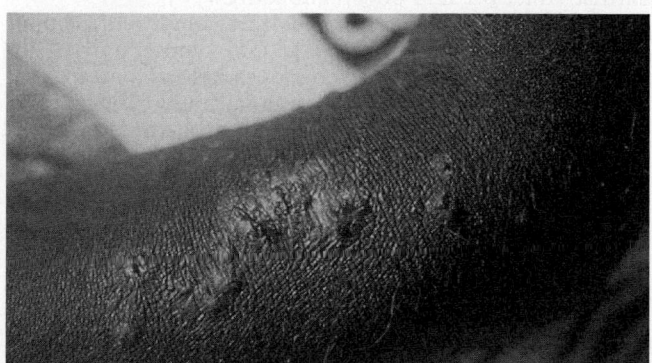

FIGURE 165-2. See also color plates. Streptococcal impetigo in an Australian Aboriginal child. (Courtesy of Dr. Bart Currie, Menzies School of Health Research, Darwin, Northern Territory, Australia.)

of children through to the nephritic syndrome with macroscopic hematuria, proteinuria, oliguria, generalized edema, and hypertension together with an elevated serum creatinine. Macroscopic hematuria and edema are the most common presenting complaints. Systemic features include lethargy, lumbar tenderness, and nausea. About 5% of patients develop the nephrotic syndrome, and 1% have acute renal failure usually due to a rapidly progressive glomerulonephritis with extensive crescentic change.[13,14] Other causes for acute renal failure include acute tubular necrosis from renal hypoperfusion, macroscopic hematuria,[15] or the nephrotic syndrome, and coincidental drug-induced interstitial nephritis.

Occasional patients develop encephalopathy from malignant hypertension or the effects of streptococcal toxins on the central nervous system.[16-18] Encephalopathy occurs more often in children than in adults and is characterized by headache, vomiting, confusion, drowsiness, and convulsions.

INVESTIGATIONS

All patients with poststreptococcal glomerulonephritis have microscopic hematuria. Phase contrast microscopy demonstrates the dysmorphic nature of the red blood cells (RBCs) and hence their glomerular origin, which is confirmed by the presence of RBC and hemoglobin casts, and proteinuria. Urinary RBC numbers are usually high, and counts greater than 500,000/mL correlate with crescentic change, but with rapid urinary bleeding, the RBC appearance may confusingly be isomorphic, incorrectly suggesting a nonglomerular lesion. Macroscopic hematuria corresponds to urinary RBC counts greater than 5,000,000/mL.

The diagnosis of poststreptococcal glomerulonephritis is usually made clinically but requires evidence of a preceding streptococcal infection. A throat or skin swab and culture is positive in fewer than 50% of cases because the infection has been treated or resolved prior to presentation; a positive throat swab may simply reflect the carrier state. However, the antistreptolysin O (ASO) titer is commonly elevated after a streptococcal pharyngitis, and antibodies against deoxyribonuclease (DNase) B antigen are often present after skin infections. A recent study has shown that testing for both ASO and anti-DNase B antibodies is the most sensitive (96%) and specific (89%) method for identifying recent streptococcal infections and hence an increased likelihood of poststreptococcal glomerulonephritis.[19] While testing for anti-GAPDH and anti-SPE B antibodies is even more accurate, these tests are rarely available.

Levels of total complement and C3 are reduced, but C4 levels are normal in 90% of patients with poststreptococcal glomerulonephritis. This pattern is consistent with activation of the alternative complement pathway (Table 165-1).

Rheumatoid factor is common in up to one third of patients. Cryoglobulins and low levels of anti-DNA antibodies are infrequent. Antineutrophil cytoplasmic antibodies (ANCA) are found occasionally, especially in patients with crescentic glomerulonephritis and acute renal failure.[20]

A renal biopsy is not usually necessary in poststreptococcal glomerulonephritis because the diagnosis can be made clinically, the prognosis is excellent, and there is no specific treatment. However, a biopsy is justified when the clinical features are atypical, for example, when there is a rapidly progressive glomerulonephritis, nephrotic syndrome, or normal complement levels and when other diagnoses cannot be excluded.

The presence of encephalopathy may be confirmed by the demonstration of a reversible posterior leukoencephalopathy on magnetic resonance imaging.[17,18]

DIFFERENTIAL DIAGNOSIS

The diagnosis of poststreptoccocal glomerulonephritis is usually made clinically but must be distinguished from other common causes of hematuria, namely IgA glomerulonephritis and thin basement membrane nephropathy. IgA glomerulonephritis is characterized by recurrent episodes of macroscopic hematuria occurring 3 to 5 days after the onset of pharyngitis, with persistent microscopic hematuria and often proteinuria at other times. Patients with thin basement membrane nephropathy typically have lifelong isolated microscopic hematuria, normal renal function, and a positive family history.[21]

Poststreptococcal glomerulonephritis must also be distinguished from other causes of infection-associated proliferative glomerulonephritis, such as bacterial endocarditis, malaria, hepatitis C, and typhoid fever, and from other forms of glomerulonephritis associated with hypocomplementemia, such as lupus nephritis, infective endocarditis, membranoproliferative glomerulonephritis types I and II, mixed cryoglobulinemia, and hemolytic uremic syndrome/thrombotic thrombocytopenic purpura. Poststreptococcal glomerulonephritis must occasionally be differentiated from other causes of rapidly progressive glomerulonephritis, nephrotic syndrome, and malignant hypertension, where the likely cause will depend in part on the age of the individual. The subepithelial "humps" seen on electron microscopy of the renal biopsy are not pathognomonic for poststreptococcal glomerulonephritis but also occur with endocarditis-associated glomerular disease, cryoglobulinemia, and lupus nephritis.

GENERAL PRINCIPLES OF TREATMENT

Most patients with poststreptococcal glomerulonephritis are asymptomatic and unrecognized. The disease is usually mild and resolves without specific treatment. However, patients are treated with antibiotics to prevent the spread of the nephritogenic bacteria,[22] and penicillin is the antibiotic of choice. No cases of penicillin resistance have been described with nephritogenic strains of S. pyogenes. Poststreptococcal glomerulonephritis does not recur, and long-term antibiotics are not necessary. Family members should be investigated for streptococcal throat or skin infections, and antibiotic treatment is justified in siblings of index cases and other at-risk individuals during epidemics.

Usually only supportive therapy is needed for the acute nephritis. Bed rest is frequently advocated but of no proven benefit. Fluid retention is the major reason for hospitalization. In mild cases, salt and fluid restriction is sufficient, but sometimes loop diuretics are needed for a maximum of 48 hours. Hypertension usually responds to removal of fluid and conventional antihypertensive agents.[23]

More severe cases with acute renal failure may require aggressive management of fluid retention, as well as treatment for hyperkalemia, acidosis, and hyperphosphatemia. There is no established role for corticosteroids or cytotoxics,[17] but anecdotal reports suggest pulse methylprednisolone may be beneficial in cases with acute renal failure due to crescentic glomerulonephritis.[24,25]

MANAGEMENT OF POSTSTREPTOCOCCAL GLOMERULONEPHRITIS IN THE INTENSIVE CARE UNIT

Patients with poststreptococcal glomerulonephritis rarely require admission to the intensive care unit, but the most common indications are for management of acute renal failure, fluid overload in the elderly patient with poor cardiac function, and encephalopathy.

In patients with acute renal failure, renal replacement therapies such as hemodialysis and hemofiltration are indicated for fluid overload that does not respond to loop diuretics and for progressive uremia, hyperkalemia, and acidosis.[26] Patients with acute renal failure due to crescentic poststreptococcal glomerulonephritis often require dialysis. The choice of treatment modality should be individualized according to the patient's clinical features and local expertise.

Elderly patients with poststreptococcal glomerulonephritis have a high risk of acute pulmonary edema caused by the rapid onset of circulatory volume overload. At-risk patients may benefit from early admission to an intensive care unit where pulmonary congestion, oxygenation, and cardiovascular hemodynamics can be monitored and treated more aggressively than in a general medical ward.

The mainstay of treatment of encephalopathy complicating poststreptococcal glomerulonephritis is control of blood pressure,[27] but in the event of convulsions, sedation and intubation are required.

CLINICAL COURSE

The prognosis of subclinical poststreptococcal glomerulonephritis is usually excellent. In most other patients the clinical features resolve spontaneously over 10 to 14 days. The macroscopic hematuria settles as the oliguria returns to normal within days of presentation, renal function normalizes within 2 weeks, and complement levels normalize within 2 months. However, microscopic hematuria commonly persists for a year or even more.

The long-term prognosis of poststreptococcal glomerulonephritis in children was formerly considered excellent, but there is now reason to be more guarded, at least in the developing world. In one study of 534 children followed for 12 to 17 years after presentation in Trinidad, the rates of hematuria, proteinuria, hypertension, and renal disease in the children were no different from those in the general population.[28] However, in the Australian Aboriginal community, 13% of patients with poststreptococcal glomerulonephritis had proteinuria at follow-up compared with only 4% of controls,[1] and a history of this disease in childhood correlated with a poor long-term renal prognosis.[1] This risk may be explained in part by the additional renal burdens of reduced nephron number, as well as the high prevalence of diabetes and arterial hypertension in this population. It remains unclear whether poststreptococcal glomerulonephritis has a similar long-term effect on renal prognosis in other disadvantaged groups.

The outcome for adults is less optimistic than in children,[29] especially if there is a history of alcoholism[24] or nephrotic-range proteinuria at presentation.[30] About 1% of patients with poststreptococcal glomerulonephritis develop irreversible end-stage renal failure. These are typically patients with diffuse crescentic lesions.

In general, older adults have an even worse prognosis, with a 20% mortality rate. This is determined largely by the severity of fluid retention and hypertension, the risk of cardiovascular complications, and the nature of medical comorbidities.[31]

CONCLUSION

Poststreptococcal glomerulonephritis is often subclinical, but some patients develop the nephritic syndrome with macroscopic hematuria, oliguria, edema, hypertension, and renal insufficiency. Although poststreptococcal glomerulonephritis has become less common in affluent societies, it remains an important cause of renal disease in the developing world and among indigenous populations. In children, it is usually a self-limiting illness, but occasionally in adults life-threatening complications such as acute renal failure, pulmonary edema, and encephalopathy ensue.

Key Points

1. Poststreptococcal glomerulonephritis is the prototypical cause of the nephritic syndrome and remains an important cause of renal disease in the developing world and among indigenous populations.
2. Poststreptococcal glomerulonephritis is usually a self-limiting disease, and supportive care is the mainstay of management.
3. Management in the intensive care unit is required for severe cases of poststreptococcal glomerulonephritis, with acute renal failure usually due to extensive crescentic disease or with fluid overload or encephalopathy.
4. Children with poststreptococcal glomerulonephritis have a good long-term renal prognosis, but the outcome is less favorable in adults and among indigenous populations.

Key References

9. Batsford SR, Mezzano S, Mihatsch M, et al: Is the nephritogenic antigen in poststreptococcal glomerulonephritis pyrogenic exotoxin B (SPE B) or GAPDH? Kidney Int 2005; 68:1120-1129.
11. Yoshizawa N, Yamakami K, Fujino M, et al: Nephritis-associated plasmin receptor and acute poststreptococcal glomerulonephritis: Characterization of the antigen and associated immune response. J Am Soc Nephrol 2004;15: 1785-1793.
14. Fairley C, Mathews DC, Becker GJ: Rapid development of diffuse crescents in post-streptococcal glomerulonephritis. Clin Nephrol 1987;28:256-260.
19. Blyth CC, Robertson PW: Anti-streptococcal antibodies in the diagnosis of acute and post-streptococcal disease: Streptokinase versus streptolysin O and deoxyribonuclease B. Pathology 2006;38:152-156.
25. Raff A, Hebert T, Pullman J, Coco M: Crescentic post-streptococcal glomerulonephritis with nephrotic syndrome in the adult: Is aggressive therapy warranted? Clin Nephrol 2005; 63:375-380.

See the companion Expert Consult website for the complete reference list.

CHAPTER 166

Spontaneous Bacterial Peritonitis and Hepatorenal Syndrome

Vicente Arroyo and Javier Fernández

OBJECTIVES

This chapter will:
1. Review the etiology, microbiology, and treatment of spontaneous bacterial peritonitis.
2. Discuss the interaction of spontaneous bacterial peritonitis and hepatorenal syndrome.
3. Describe the most applicable treatments of hepatorenal syndrome.

SPONTANEOUS BACTERIAL PERITONITIS

Spontaneous bacterial peritonitis (SBP) is the most characteristic infection in cirrhosis. It consists of the spontaneous infection of the ascitic fluid in the absence of any intra-abdominal source of infection. It is usually a monobacterial infection. *Escherichia coli, Klebsiella* species, and nonenterococcal streptococci are the most frequently causative organisms.[1,2] The concentration of bacteria is very low and the ascitic fluid culture is negative in approximately 50% of cases. Gram stain is positive in less than 10% of cases. Diagnosis of SBP, therefore, does not rely on these techniques. The inflammatory response in the peritoneum, however, is important. The concentration of polymorphonuclear leukocytes in ascitic fluid is always over 250, and often greater than 2000, cells per cubic millimeter. The concentration of cytokines (tumor necrosis factor-α and interleukin-6) is also very high.[3]

The pathogenesis of SBP is multifactorial.[1] The initial event is a translocation of bacteria from the intestinal lumen to the mesenteric lymph nodes and the systemic circulation. Intestinal bacterial overgrowth related to the sympathetic overactivity present in patients with decompensated cirrhosis, which causes intestinal hypomotility, and an increase in intestinal permeability due to structural abnormalities in the intestinal wall associated with portal hypertension are the most important mechanisms of bacterial translocation. Another important factor in the pathogenesis of SBP is an impaired Kupffer cell function, the most important cellular component of the reticuloendothelial system. In addition to a decrease in the number and functionality of these cells, a lack of contact of blood with Kupffer cells due to intrahepatic shunting (blood that circulates through the liver but not in contact with the hepatic cells because of interstitial fibrosis) and extrahepatic shunting (blood that bypasses the liver through the collateral circulation) is an important mechanism. The impairment in the phagocytic activity associated with this decrease in Kupffer cell function predisposes to the development of persistent bacteremia after bacterial translocation. An additional important factor is the concentration of proteins in the ascitic fluid, which decreases with the progression of portal hypertension. When the ascitic fluid protein concentration is below 10 to 15 g/L, the antibacterial activity of the ascitic fluid, which is related to proteins with opsonic capacity (fibronectin, complement), is low, and this favors the colonization of the ascitic fluid by the circulating bacteria.[1]

Diagnosis of SBP is based on the measurement of the concentration of polymorphonuclear leukocytes in the ascitic fluid, and treatment consists of the intravenous administration of third-generation cephalosporins.[2] In cases not responding to this treatment, antibiotics should be changed according to the results of the cultures (i.e., ampicillin). Resolution of the infection is obtained in almost 90% to 95% of cases in 3 to 5 days. Despite this rapid response, approximately 30% of patients die during hospitalization, mainly as a consequence of an acute deterioration of circulatory, renal, and hepatic function, a condition known as type-1 hepatorenal syndrome (HRS).[3,4]

The overall likelihood of a cirrhotic patient with ascites to develop an episode of SBP at one year is approximately 10%. Patients who recover from an episode of SBP have a 60% probability of developing SBP recurrence within one year after the resolution of the infection. A similar probability has been reported in patients without previous episodes of SBP having low protein ascites and advanced liver insufficiency (serum bilirubin >3-4 mg/dL). Patients with ascites and gastrointestinal hemorrhage are also predisposed to develop SBP (27%) within the first two weeks after the bleeding episode.[1,2] Long-term selective intestinal decontamination with oral norfloxacin is highly effective in the primary prophylaxis of SBP in patients with low protein ascites and advanced liver failure[5] and in the secondary prophylaxis of SBP in patients recovering from an episode of this infection.[6] It is also effective in preventing SBP in patients with gastrointestinal hemorrhage, although a recent trial indicates that intravenous ceftriaxone is more effective than oral norfloxacin in bleeding cirrhotic patients with severe liver failure.[7] Since patients with severe circulatory dysfunction, as indicated by abnormal serum creatinine (≥1.2 mg/dL) and/or dilutional hyponatremia (serum sodium ≤130 mEq/L) are predisposed to develop type-1 HRS after SBP, these patients should also be considered as potential candidates for primary prophylaxis.[5]

HEPATORENAL SYNDROME: CONCEPT, CLINICAL TYPES, AND DIAGNOSIS

HRS is a frequent complication in patients with cirrhosis, ascites, and advanced liver failure. The annual incidence in patients with ascites has been estimated as 8%.[8] HRS is a functional renal failure due to low renal perfusion.[8-11] Renal histology is normal or shows lesions that do not justify the decrease in the glomerular filtration rate (GFR). The traditional concept is that HRS is caused by deterioration in circulatory function secondary to an intense vasodilation in the splanchnic circulation (peripheral arterial vasodilation hypothesis). During the last few years, however, several features suggest a much more complex pathogenesis. In fact, two types of HRS with different clinical courses and prognostic implications have been identified. Moreover, effective therapies of HRS have been developed, and differences also exist in treatment response between type-1 and type-2 HRS. Type-1 and type-2 HRS are, therefore, not different expressions of a common disorder but probably two syndromes with distinct pathogeneses.

The first step in the diagnosis of HRS is the demonstration of a reduced GFR, and this is not easy in advanced cirrhosis. The muscle mass, and therefore the release of creatinine, is considerably reduced in these patients, and they may present normal serum creatinine concentration in the setting of a very low GFR. Similarly, urea is synthesized by the liver and may be reduced as a consequence of hepatic insufficiency. Therefore, false negative diagnosis of HRS is relatively common.[12,13] There is consensus to establish the diagnosis of HRS when serum creatinine has risen above 1.5 mg/dL or creatinine clearance has decreased to less than 40 mL/min.[14] The second step is the differentiation of HRS from other types of renal failure. The traditional parameters used to differentiate functional renal failure from acute tubular necrosis (oliguria, low urine sodium concentration, urine-to-plasma osmolality ratio greater than unity, normal fresh urine sediment and no proteinuria) are not useful in decompensated cirrhosis with ascites. Acute tubular necrosis in patients with cirrhosis and ascites usually courses with oliguria, low urine sodium concentration, and urine osmolality greater than plasma osmolality.[15] On the contrary, relatively high urinary sodium concentration has been observed in patients with HRS and high serum bilirubin.[16] Diagnosis of HRS is based on the exclusion of other disorders that can cause renal failure in cirrhosis (Table 166-1).[14]

Type-1 HRS is characterized by a severe and rapidly progressive renal failure, which has been defined as doubling of serum creatinine, reaching a level greater than 2.5 mg/dL in less than 2 weeks. Although type-1 HRS may

TABLE 166-1

International Ascites Club's Diagnostic Criteria of Hepatorenal Syndrome

Major Criteria
- Chronic or acute liver disease with advanced hepatic failure and portal hypertension
- Low glomerular filtration rate, as indicated by serum creatinine >1.5 mg/dL or 24-hr creatinine clearance <40 mL/min
- Absence of shock, ongoing bacterial infection, and current or recent treatment with nephrotoxic drugs. Absence of gastrointestinal fluid losses (repeated vomiting or intense diarrhea) or renal fluid losses (weight loss >500 g/day for several days in patients with ascites without peripheral edema or 1000 g/day in patients with peripheral edema)
- No sustained improvement in renal function (decrease in serum creatinine to ≤1.5 mg/dL or increase in creatinine clearance to ≥40 mL/min) following diuretic withdrawal and expansion of plasma volume with 1.5 L of isotonic saline
- Proteinuria <500 mg/day and no ultrasonographic evidence of obstructive uropathy or parenchymal renal disease

Additional Criteria
- Urine volume <500 mL/day
- Urine sodium <10 mEq/L
- Urine osmolality greater than plasma osmolality
- Urine red blood cells <50 per high-power field
- Serum sodium concentration <130 mEq/L

From Ginès P, Rodés J: Clinical disorders of renal function in cirrhosis with ascites. In Arrovo V, Ginès P, Rodés J, Schrier RW (eds): Ascites and renal dysfunction in liver disease: Pathogenesis, diagnosis, and treatment. Malden, MA, Blackwell, 1999, pp 36-62.

MEDIAN SURVIVAL

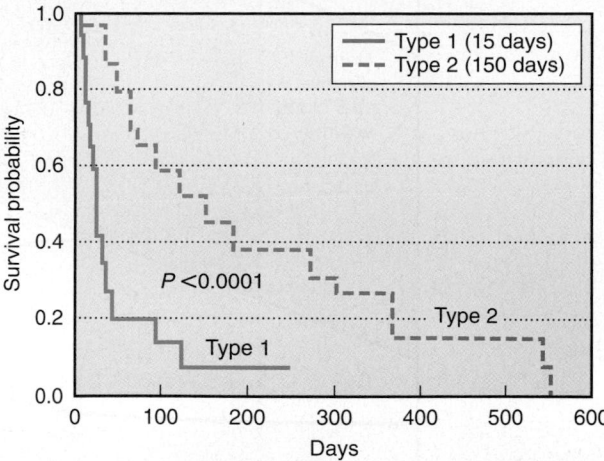

FIGURE 166-1. Survival of patients with cirrhosis after the diagnosis of type 1 or type 2 hepatorenal syndrome (HRS). (Ginès P, Guevara M, Arroyo V, Rodés J: Hepatorenal syndrome. Lancet 2003;362: 1819-1827.)

develop spontaneously, it frequently occurs in closed relationship with a precipitating factor, such as severe bacterial infection, mainly SBP, gastrointestinal hemorrhage, major surgical procedure, or acute hepatitis superimposed to cirrhosis. The association of HRS and SBP has been carefully investigated.[3,4,17] Type-1 HRS develops in approximately 25% of patients with SBP despite a rapid resolution of the infection with non-nephrotoxic antibiotics. Patients with severe circulatory dysfunction prior to infection (moderate increase in serum creatinine and high levels of plasma renin activity and norepinephrine concentration) or intense inflammatory response (high concentration of polymorphonuclear leukocytes in ascitic fluid and high cytokine levels in plasma and ascitic fluid) are prone to develop type-1 HRS after the infection. Besides renal failure, patients with type-1 HRS associated with SBP show signs and symptoms of a rapid and severe deterioration of liver function (jaundice, coagulopathy, and hepatic encephalopathy) and circulatory function (arterial hypotension, very high plasma levels of renin and norepinephrine).[3,4,17,18] In contrast to SBP, sepsis related to other types of infection in patients with cirrhosis induces type-1 HRS only when there is a lack of response to antibiotics.[19] In most patients with sepsis unrelated to SBP who respond to antibiotics, renal impairment, which is also a frequent event, is reversible. Without treatment, type-1 HRS is the complication of cirrhosis with the poorest prognosis, with a median survival time after the onset of renal failure of only 2 weeks (Fig. 166-1).[8]

Type-2 HRS is characterized by moderate (serum creatinine <2.5 mg/dL) and slowly progressive renal failure. Patients with type-2 HRS show signs of liver failure and arterial hypotension but to a lesser degree than patients

with type-1 HRS. The dominant clinical feature is severe ascites with poor or no response to diuretics (a condition known as refractory ascites). Patients with type-2 HRS are predisposed to develop type-1 HRS following SBP or other precipitating events.[3,4,17] The median survival of patients with type-2 HRS (6 months) is worse than that of patients with non-azotemic cirrhosis with ascites (see Fig. 166-1).[20]

Portal hypertension in cirrhosis is associated with arterial vasodilation in the splanchnic circulation due to the local release of nitric oxide and other vasodilatory substances.[21,22] The peripheral arterial vasodilation hypothesis proposes that renal dysfunction and type-2 HRS in cirrhosis is related to this feature (Fig. 166-2). Early in the course of the disease, when splanchnic arterial vasodilation is moderate, the decrease in systemic vascular resistance is compensated by the development of a hyperdynamic circulation (increased heart rate and cardiac output).[23] However, as the disease progresses and arterial vasodilation increases, the hyperdynamic circulation is insufficient to correct the changes in circulatory function.[24] Effective arterial hypovolemia develops, leading to arterial hypotension, activation of high-pressure baroreceptors, and reflex stimulation of the renin-angiotensin and sympathetic nervous systems and antidiuretic hormone. Arterial pressure increases to normal or near-normal levels but induces sodium and water retention and ascites formation. At this stage of the disease, arterial pressure is critically dependent on the vascular effect of the sympathetic nervous activity, angiotensin II, and antidiuretic hormone. Since the splanchnic circulation is resistant to the effect of angiotensin II, noradrenaline, and vasopressin due to the local release of nitric oxide and other vasodilators,[25] the maintenance of arterial pressure is due to vasoconstriction in extrasplanchnic vascular territories such as the kidneys, muscle, skin, and brain.[26,27] Type-2 HRS represents the extreme expression in the progression of splanchnic arterial vasodilation. The homeostatic stimulation of the renin-angiotensin system, the sympathetic nervous system, and antidiuretic hormone leads to intense renal vasoconstriction and a marked decrease in renal perfusion and GFR.

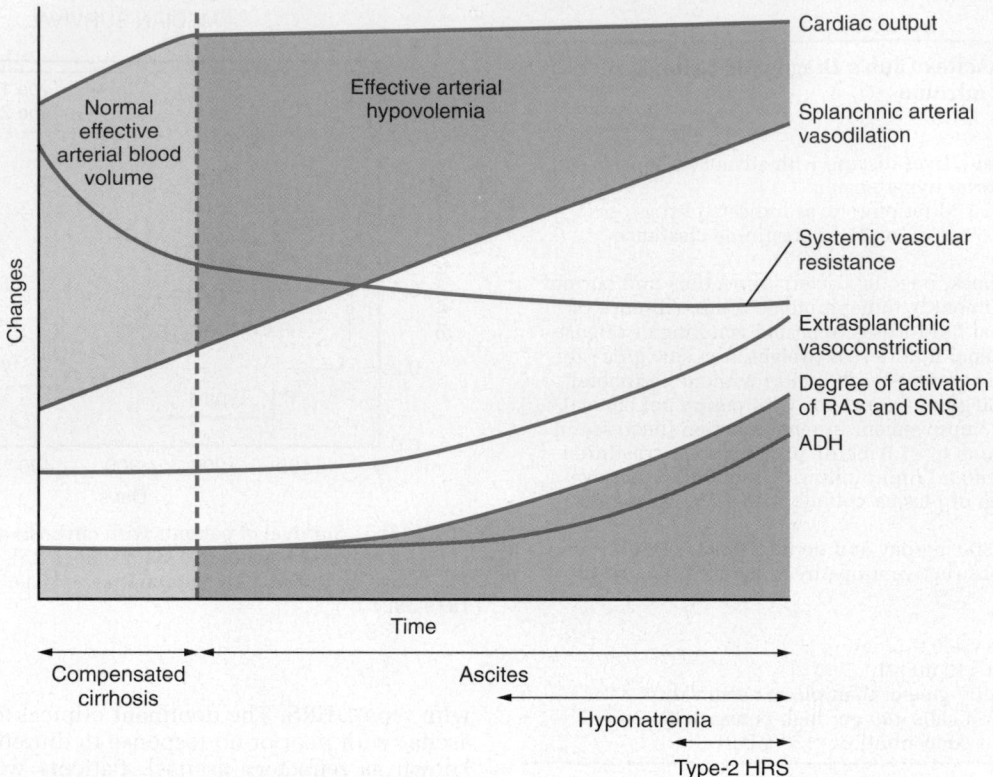

FIGURE 166-2. Peripheral arterial vasodilation hypothesis and renal dysfunction in cirrhosis. AHD, antidiuretic hormone; HRS, hepatorenal syndrome; RAS, renin-angiotensin system; SNS, sympathetic nervous system.

Most hemodynamic investigations in cirrhosis have been performed in nonazotemic patients with and without ascites, and the peripheral arterial vasodilation hypothesis was based on these studies. It assumed that type-2 HRS develops in the setting of a hyperdynamic circulation and increased cardiac output. However, there were two prior studies assessing cardiovascular function in patients with HRS or refractory ascites (most of them with type-2 HRS) showing that cardiac output was significantly reduced compared to patients without HRS.[28,29] In some cases cardiac output was even lower than in normal subjects, suggesting that circulatory dysfunction associated with HRS is due not only to arterial vasodilation but also to a decrease in cardiac function. A recent study by Ruiz-del-Arbol and colleagues[30] supports this feature. It consisted of a longitudinal investigation in 62 nonazotemic cirrhotic patients with ascites. Forty percent of them developed HRS during follow-up. These patients were studied at inclusion and following the development of HRS. In the initial study, those patients who went on to develop HRS had significantly lower mean arterial pressure and cardiac output and significantly higher plasma renin activity and norepinephrine concentration compared to those who did not develop HRS. Moreover, those who developed type-2 HRS had a further decrease in arterial pressure and cardiac output and an increase in renin and norepinephrine plasma levels without changes in peripheral vascular resistance (Table 166-2). These findings, therefore, support that progression of circulatory dysfunction in cirrhosis is

due to both an increase in arterial vasodilation and a decrease in cardiac function and that type-2 HRS occurs when there is a marked splanchnic vasodilation and a reduction in cardiac output (Fig. 166-3).

TYPE-1 HEPATORENAL SYNDROME ASSOCIATED WITH SPONTANEOUS BACTERIAL PERITONITIS: A SPECIAL FORM OF MULTIPLE-ORGAN FAILURE

Type-1 and type-2 HRS have two features in common: They occur in patients with cirrhosis and ascites, and renal failure is an important component of both syndromes. However, they show important differences. Type-2 HRS develops imperceptibly in patients with cirrhosis and ascites who are otherwise in stable clinical condition. These patients do not differ clinically from patients with cirrhosis and ascites without renal failure. They respond poorly to diuretics, but this also occurs in a significant number of patients with serum creatinine concentration below 1.5 mg/dL. Circulatory function, although severely deteriorated, remains steady or progresses slowly over several months as it occurs with the renal failure. Patients have advanced cirrhosis, but the degree of liver failure is also stable. Hepatic encephalopathy is infrequent. The

TABLE 166-2

Chronological Changes of Vasoactive Systems and Cardiovascular Function from Nonazotemic Cirrhosis with Ascites (NA) to Type-2 Hepatorenal Syndrome

	NA-1[†]	NA-2[‡]	AT DIAGNOSIS OF TYPE-2 HEPATORENAL SYNDROME
Mean arterial pressure (mm Hg)*	88 ± 9	86 ± 10	79 ± 7
Plasma renin activity (ng/mL/hr)*	3 ± 2	7.5 ± 3.7	11.9 ± 4.8
Norepinephrine (pg/mL/hr)*	221 ± 256	412 ± 155	628 ± 320
Systemic vascular resistance (dyn.s/cm^{-5})	962 ± 256	1058 ± 265	1014 ± 276
Cardiac output (L/min)*	7.2 ± 1.8	6.2 ± 1.4	5.8 ± 1.2
Heart rate (bpm)	87 ± 15	84 ± 12	80 ± 14
Hepatic blood flow (mL/min)*	1123 ± 328	1064 ± 223	824 ± 180
Portal pressure gradient (mm Hg)*	16.5 ± 3	19 ± 3	19.5 ± 2

*$P < 0.01$.
[†]NA-1: Baseline measurement in nonazotemic cirrhotic patients who did not develop hepatorenal syndrome in the follow-up.
[‡]NA-2: Baseline measurement in nonazotemic cirrhotic patients who developed type-2 hepatorenal syndrome in the follow-up.
From Ruiz-del-Arbol L, Monescillo A, Arocena C, et al: Circulatory function and hepatorenal syndrome in cirrhosis. Hepatology 2005;42:439-447.

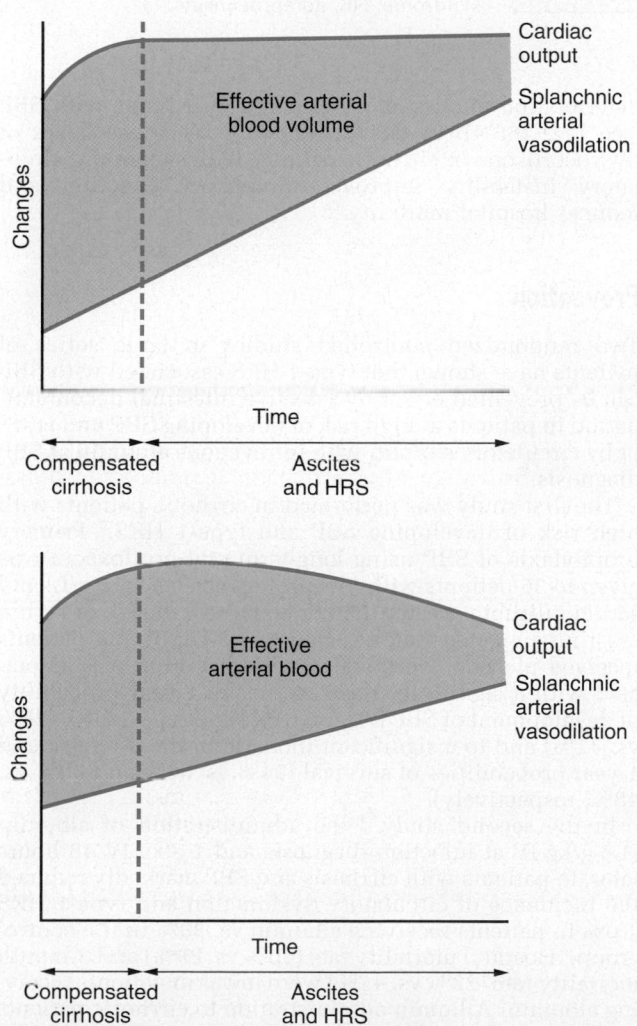

FIGURE 166-3. Peripheral vasodilation hypothesis (*top graph*) and modified peripheral vasodilation hypothesis (*bottom graph*). According to the latter hypothesis, impairment in arterial blood volume in cirrhosis could be the consequence of a progression of splanchnic arterial vasodilation and of a decrease in cardiac output. HRS, hepatorenal syndrome.

main clinical problem of patients with type-2 HRS is refractory ascites. In contrast, type-1 HRS is an extremely unstable condition. It frequently develops in the setting of an important clinical event that acts as a precipitating factor. On the other hand, there is a rapid deterioration of circulatory and renal function within days after the onset of the syndrome, leading to severe arterial hypotension and acute renal failure with intense oliguria. Finally, there is also a rapid deterioration of hepatic function, with increase in jaundice and encephalopathy.

Recent studies in patients with SBP have presented data indicating that type-1 HRS represents a special form of acute multiple-organ failure related to the rapid deterioration in circulatory function (Fig. 166-4). The syndrome develops in the setting of a significant decrease in arterial pressure and a marked stimulation of the renin-angiotensin and sympathetic nervous systems in the absence of changes in systemic vascular resistance, which is consistent with an increase in the arterial vasodilation obscured by the vascular effect of these vasoconstrictor systems. There is also an acute decrease in the cardiac output that contributes to the effective arterial hypovolemia.[18] The mechanism of this impairment in cardiac function is complex. There is a cirrhotic cardiomyopathy that weakens the cardiac response to stress conditions. On the other hand, in patients developing type-1 HRS associated with SBP, there is a decrease in cardiopulmonary pressures, suggesting a decrease in cardiac preload. Finally, despite the stimulation of the sympathetic nervous system, there is no increase in heart rate indicating an impaired cardiac chronotropic function.

In addition to renal vasoconstriction, patients with type-1 HRS associated with SBP develop vasoconstriction in the intrahepatic circulation, with a marked reduction in hepatic blood flow and an increase in portal pressure.[18] The acute deterioration of hepatic function and hepatic encephalopathy may be related to this feature. Cerebral vascular resistance is increased in patients with decompensated cirrhosis and correlates directly with the activity of the renin-angiotensin and sympathetic nervous systems and renal vasoconstriction (Fig. 166-5). Reduction in cerebral blood flow could, therefore, play a contributory role to hepatic encephalopathy.

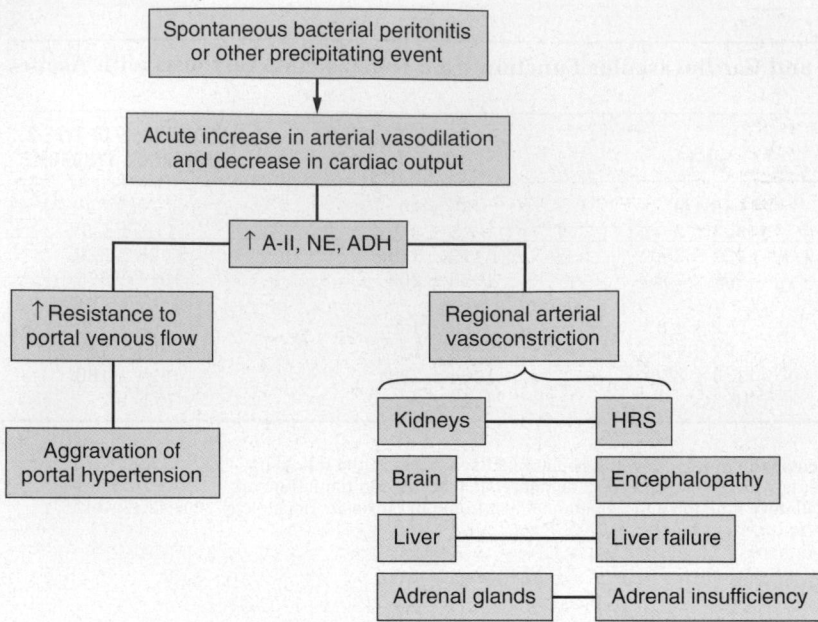

FIGURE 166-4. Hepatorenal syndrome as part of a multiple-organ failure. ADH, antidiuretic hormone; A-II, angiotensin II; HRS, hepatorenal syndrome; NE, norepinephrine.

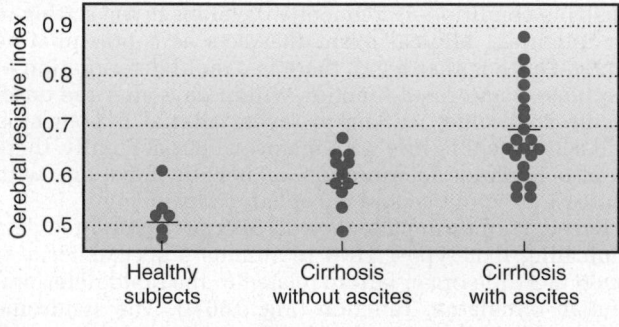

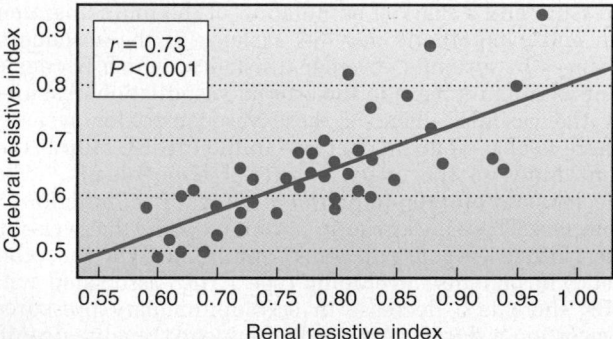

FIGURE 166-5. Resistive index in the middle cerebral artery in patients with compensated cirrhosis, patients with ascites, and healthy subjects (*upper graph*). Relationship between the renal resistive index and the resistive index in the middle cerebral artery in cirrhotic patients (*lower graph*). (Guevara M, Bru C, Ginès P, et al: Increased cerebrovascular resistance in cirrhotic patients with ascites. Hepatology 1998;28:39-44.)

Two studies in patients with cirrhosis and sepsis showed a surprisingly high incidence of relative adrenal insufficiency in patients with hemodynamic instability and renal failure.[31,32] Vasoconstriction of the suprarenal arteries is an attractive mechanism for the feature. Since cortisol is essential for the vascular effect of angiotensin II and noradrenaline, adrenal insufficiency may contribute to the deterioration of circulatory function in patients with SBP (see Fig. 166-4). In fact, treatment with stress doses of hydrocortisone in cirrhotic patients with sepsis and circulatory instability improves circulatory function and reduces hospital mortality.[32]

Prevention

Two randomized controlled studies in large series of patients have shown that type-1 HRS associated with SBP can be prevented either by selective intestinal decontamination in patients at high risk of developing SBP and HRS[5] or by circulatory support with intravenous albumin at SBP diagnosis.[33]

The first study was performed in cirrhotic patients with high risk of developing SBP and type-1 HRS.[5] Primary prophylaxis of SBP using long-term oral norfloxacin was given to 35 patients with low protein ascites (<15 g/L) and serum bilirubin greater than or equal to 3 mg/dL or serum creatinine greater than or equal to 1.2 mg/dL; 33 patients received placebo. Norfloxacin administration was associated with a significant decrease in the 1-year probability of development of SBP (7% vs. 61%) and type-1 HRS (28% vs. 41%) and to a significant increase in the 3-month and 1-year probabilities of survival (94% vs. 62% and 60% vs. 48%, respectively).

In the second study,[33] the administration of albumin (1.5 g/kg IV at infection diagnosis and 1 g/kg IV 48 hours later) to patients with cirrhosis and SBP markedly reduced the incidence of circulatory dysfunction and type-1 HRS (10% in patients receiving albumin vs. 33% in the control group). Hospital mortality rate (10% vs. 29%) and 3-month mortality rate (22% vs. 41%) were lower in patients receiving albumin. Albumin administration to cirrhotic patients with SBP induces not only an expansion of the plasma volume but also an increase in systemic vascular resistance. The efficacy of albumin in the prevention of type-1 HRS could, therefore, be related to both an increase in cardiac preload and cardiac output and a vasoconstrictor effect of albumin in the arterial circulation related to an attenuation of endothelial dysfunction.[34]

Treatment

Several therapeutic measures can be used in patients developing type-1 HRS associated with SBP. The most effective is liver transplantation. However, the applicability of this procedure is low. The most applicable treatment consists of the administration of plasma volume expansion with albumin and vasoconstrictors. The insertion of a transjugular intrahepatic portosystemic shunt (TIPS) is another possibility that can be used either alone or after reversal of HRS with vasoconstrictors plus albumin. Finally, extracorporeal albumin dialysis (molecular adsorbent recirculating system [MARS]) can be used in these patients. Each of these treatments should be considered after the infection resolution, as HRS may reverse following effective antibiotic treatment in a significant number of patients.

Liver Transplantation

Liver transplantation is the treatment of choice of patients with type-1 HRS.[35,36] Immediately after transplantation a further impairment in GFR may be observed, and many patients require hemodialysis (35% of patients with HRS as compared with 5% of patients without HRS).[35] After this initial impairment in renal function, GFR starts to improve and reaches an average of 30 to 40 mL/min by 1 to 2 months postoperatively. This moderate renal failure persists during follow-up, is more marked than that observed in transplant patients without HRS, and is probably due to a greater nephrotoxicity of cyclosporine or tacrolimus in patients with renal impairment prior to transplantation. The hemodynamic and neurohormonal abnormalities associated with HRS disappear within the first month after the operation, and patients regain a normal ability to excrete sodium and free water.

Patients with HRS who undergo liver transplantation have more complications, spend more days in the intensive care unit, and have a higher in-hospital mortality rate than do transplant patients without HRS. The long-term survival of patients with HRS who undergo liver transplantation is good, however, with a 3-year probability of survival of 60%. This survival rate is only slightly reduced compared to that observed after transplantation in patients without HRS (which ranges between 70% and 80%).[36]

The main problem of liver transplantation in type-1 HRS is its applicability, as most patients die before transplantation. The introduction of the Model for End-stage Liver-Disease (MELD) score, which includes serum creatinine, bilirubin, and the international normalized ratio for listing, has partially solved the problem, as patients with HRS are generally at the top of the waiting list for liver transplantation. Treatment of HRS with vasoconstrictors and albumin increases survival in a significant proportion of patients (thus increasing the number of patients eligible for liver transplantation), decreases early morbidity and mortality after transplantation, and prolongs long-term survival.

Vasoconstrictors and Albumin

The intravenous administration of vasoconstrictor agents (vasopressin, ornipressin, terlipressin, noradrenaline) or the combination of oral midodrine (an alpha-agonist agent) and intravenous or subcutaneous octreotide associated with intravenous albumin for 1 to 2 weeks is an effective treatment of type-1 HRS.[37-41] The rate of positive response, as defined by a decrease in serum creatinine below 1.5 mg/dL, reported in several pilot studies, is approximately 60%. An important observation of these studies is that type-1 HRS does not recur after the discontinuation of treatment in most patients. This finding contrasts sharply with that of other studies in patients with type-1 HRS not receiving specific treatment or treated with plasma volume expansion alone or associated with vasodilators (dopamine) or octreotide or with peritoneovenous shunting. Reversal of HRS was observed in less than 5% of the patients included in these studies. One- and 3-month probability of survival after treatment in the studies using vasoconstrictors and albumin were approximately 40% and 30%, respectively. The corresponding figures reported in the studies using other treatments were less than 5%.

Reversal of type-1 HRS when terlipressin is given alone (25%)[40] is lower than that observed in studies in which vasoconstrictors are associated with intravenous albumin, suggesting that albumin administration is an important component in the pharmacological treatment of type-1 HRS. As indicated earlier, studies[34] suggest that the beneficial effect of albumin on circulatory and renal function in patients with type-1 HRS is related not only to the expansion of the plasma volume but also to a direct vasoconstrictor effect on the peripheral arterial circulation.

Two randomized controlled trials comparing terlipressin plus albumin versus terlipressin alone have been reported.[42,43] Their results confirm that terlipressin plus albumin is an effective therapy in patients with type-1 HRS and that reversal of HRS improves survival. However, the effectiveness of the treatment reported by these trials (40% rate of reversal of HRS) is lower than those reported in the pilot studies.

Terlipressin is the most widely used vasoconstrictor in patients with type-1 HRS. Dosage should be progressive, starting with 0.5 mg every 4 hours. If serum creatinine does not decrease by more than 30% in 3 days, the dose should be doubled. The maximal dose of terlipressin has not been defined, although there is consensus that patients not responding to 12 mg/day will not respond to higher doses. Albumin should be given starting with a priming dose of 1 g/kg of body weight followed by 20 to 40 g/kg body weight per day. It is advisable to monitor central venous pressure. In patients responding to therapy, treatment should be kept until normalization of serum creatinine (<1.5 mg/dL).

Transjugular Intrahepatic Portosystemic Shunt

Three pilot studies have evaluated TIPS in type-1 HRS.[44-46] In the first study,[11] 14 patients with type-1 HRS (12 with alcoholic cirrhosis, 9 with active alcoholism) and 17 with refractory ascites (some of them with type-2 HRS) not suitable for liver transplantation were treated. Patients with bilirubin greater than 15 mg/dL, a Child-Pugh score greater than 12, or hepatic encephalopathy were excluded. Eleven of the 31 patients developed de novo hepatic encephalopathy or deterioration of previous hepatic encephalopathy. The 3-, 6- and 12-month survival rates in patients with type-1 HRS were 64%, 50%, and 20%, respectively. The second study[45] was performed in 7 patients (4 alcoholics) with type-1 HRS and a Child-Pugh score less than 12. Marked decrease in serum creatinine was observed in 6 patients and reversal of HRS in 4. Five patients developed episodes of hepatic encephalopathy after TIPS, but they responded satisfactorily to medical treatment. Five patients were alive 1 month after TIPS, but only 2 patients were alive after 3 months. The third study[46] was performed in 14 patients (13 with alcoholic cirrhosis) with type-1 HRS, treated initially with vasoconstrictors (midodrine and octreotide) plus albumin. Reversal of HRS was obtained in 10 patients. TIPS was subsequently inserted in 5 of these 10 patients who had bilirubin less than 5 mg/dL, international normalized ratio less than 2, and a Child-Pugh score less than 12. Normalization of GFR was obtained in all cases, and patients were alive from 6 to 30 months after TIPS. TIPS, therefore, is effective in normalizing serum creatinine in a significant proportion of patients with cirrhosis and severe azotemia and is an alternative treatment for type-1 HRS.

Extracorporeal Albumin Dialysis (MARS)

Three pilot studies including 29 patients (26 with type-1 HRS and 21 with alcoholic cirrhosis, severe acute alcoholic hepatitis, or both) aimed at assessing MARS in patients with type-1 HRS have been reported.[47-49] Since MARS incorporates a standard dialysis machine or a continuous venovenous hemofiltration monitor and GFR was not measured, it is not possible to know the effect of this treatment on renal function. The decrease in serum creatinine observed in most patients could be related to the dialysis process. However, clear beneficial effects on systemic hemodynamics and on hepatic encephalopathy were observed. The survival rate 1 and 3 months after treatment was 41% (12 patients) and 34% (10 patients), respectively. A recent randomized controlled trial in a large series of cirrhotic patients with hepatic encephalopathy,[50] many of them with HRS, demonstrated a clear beneficial effect of MARS on the rate and time of recovery of encephalopathy. Because the endpoint of this trial was encephalopathy, no conclusion could be drawn in relation to survival.

CONCLUSION

The main precipitating factor of HRS is SBP. Its pathophysiological hallmark is a vasoconstriction of the renal circulation. The syndrome develops in the setting of a significant decrease in arterial pressure and a marked stimulation of the renin-angiotensin and sympathetic nervous systems secondary to a marked vasodilation of the splanchnic vascular bed. There is also impairment in the cardiac function that contributes to the effective arterial hypovolemia. So, type-1 HRS represents a special form of acute multiple-organ failure related to a rapid deterioration in circulatory function. Several therapeutic measures can be used in patients developing type-1 HRS associated with SBP. The most applicable treatment consists of the administration of plasma volume expansion with albumin and vasoconstrictors. The insertion of a TIPS is another effective option. HRS associated with SBP can be prevented either by selective intestinal decontamination in patients at high risk of developing SBP and HRS or by circulatory support with intravenous albumin at SBP diagnosis.

Key Points

1. Spontaneous bacterial peritonitis is the main precipitating factor of hepatorenal syndrome.
2. Cardiac dysfunction is involved in the pathogenesis of hepatorenal syndrome in cirrhosis.
3. The most applicable treatment of type-1 hepatorenal syndrome is the administration of albumin and vasoconstrictors (terlipressin or noradrenaline). The insertion of a transjugular intrahepatic portosystemic shunt is another effective option.
4. Liver transplantation must be performed early after reversal of type-1 hepatorenal syndrome.
5. Selective intestinal decontamination in patients at high risk of developing spontaneous bacterial peritonitis and hepatorenal syndrome and circulatory support with intravenous albumin at spontaneous bacterial peritonitis diagnosis effectively prevent hepatorenal syndrome associated with spontaneous bacterial peritonitis.

Key References

4. Follo A, Llovet JM, Navasa M, et al: Renal impairment after spontaneous bacterial peritonitis in cirrhosis—incidence, clinical course, predictive factors and prognosis. Hepatology 1994;20:1495-1501.
14. Arroyo V, Ginès P, Gerbes AL: Definition and diagnostic criteria of refractory ascites and hepatorenal syndrome in cirrhosis. Hepatology 1996;23:164-176.
18. Ruiz-del-Arbol L, Urman J, Fernández J, et al: Systemic, renal, and hepatic hemodynamic derangement in cirrhotic patients with spontaneous bacterial peritonitis. Hepatology 2003;38:1210-1218.
30. Ruiz-del-Arbol L, Monescillo A, Arocena C, et al: Circulatory function and hepatorenal syndrome in cirrhosis. Hepatology 2005;42:439-447.
33. Sort P, Navasa M, Arroyo V, et al: Effect of intravenous albumin on renal impairment and mortality in patients with cirrhosis and spontaneous bacterial peritonitis. New Engl J Med 1999;341:403-409.

See the companion Expert Consult website for the complete reference list.

CHAPTER 167

Tropical Infections Causing Acute Kidney Injury

Rashad S. Barsoum

OBJECTIVES

This chapter will:
1. Describe the spectrum of tropical infections that may cause acute kidney injury.
2. Review the pathogenetic mechanisms involved in those conditions.
3. Provide an approach to the clinical diagnosis and differential diagnosis of kidney injury along the course of a severe tropical infection.
4. Outline a broad management strategy.

Infection remains the prime cause of morbidity and mortality in tropical and many subtropical countries. Several international agencies are concerned with this major health problem, including the World Health Organization (http://www.who.int/en/) and the Edna McConnell Clark Foundation (http://www.emcf.org/). Both define the term *tropical infections* as those which either occur uniquely in tropical and subtropical regions (which is rare) or, more commonly, are more widespread, or more difficult to prevent or control, in the tropics. This applies to a number of viral, bacterial, and parasitic infections (Table 167-1). Although many mycotic infections are highly prevalent in the tropics, they do not satisfy either of the definition criteria and hence are not considered as tropical infections.

It is generally believed that three major factors aggravate tropical infections: (1) widespread poverty leading to malnutrition and inadequate primary care; (2) poor sanitation leading to spread of droplet and waterborne infections; and (3) climatic influences which favor the spread of disease via a bioecological environment rich with animal reservoirs, vectors, and intermediate hosts.

Acute kidney injury (AKI) is a significant complication of tropical infections. However, since it is usually a confounding factor in a severe systemic illness, it may be overlooked by primary health care providers and underreported in respective primary health statistics. Accordingly, all relevant information originates from secondary care facilities, which confers an obvious bias on any statistical information. In addition, the majority of regional hospitals in endemic areas do not keep accurate registries, which further confines information on this topic to sporadic cohorts, published or presented in local, more often than international, periodicals or conferences. With all these factors in mind, it is generally believed that tropical infections contribute to more than two thirds of acute renal failure (ARF) cases in the tropics,[1] which may amount up to 800 per 1 million population according to certain calculations.[2]

SPECTRUM

Of the numerous tropical infections reported to cause AKI, only a few are characteristically incriminated in over half of reported AKIs (see Table 167-1). These include malaria, leptospirosis, cholera, shigellosis, dengue, and human immunodeficiency virus (HIV). These typically trigger multiple mechanisms of potential nephrotoxicity, which seems essential for clinically significant renal failure within the overall concert of a severe systemic infection.

Tropical infections can lead AKI in four major ways: (1) direct invasion of the renal parenchyma by microbial agents, (2) induction of an immune response that leads to renal inflammation, (3) induction of hemodynamic disturbances that lead to tubular necrosis, and (4) iatrogenic renal injury associated with treatment or prophylaxis against tropical infections.

Direct Parenchymal Invasion

Many bacterial agents may cause acute interstitial nephritis that may be diffuse or focal, the latter taking the form of microabscesses, as with septicemic melioidosis, or typical solitary abscesses, as with typhoid. Diffuse interstitial inflammation may be encountered in leptospirosis (Fig. 167-1), diphtheria, scrub typhus, tuberculosis, and leprosy.[1] It is unusual for these forms of renal invasion to cause ARF, although a transient oliguria and marginal retention of nonprotein nitrogen is not uncommon. However, ARF may occur if the infection is associated with significant hemodynamic effects, as with septicemia,[3] intravascular hemolysis,[4] rhabdomyolysis,[5] or disseminated intravascular coagulation.[3]

Viral interstitial nephropathies are more likely to cause ARF by direct invasion. Typical examples are dengue[6] and hanta viral[7] infections, which cause an acute hemorrhagic syndrome with reversible ARF. ARF with severe interstitial nephritis has been reported with tropical nonfulminant hepatitis A infection,[8] viral invasion being the proposed pathomechanism. Direct glomerular invasion by viral particles has been suggested to explain the glomerular lesions that appear with HIV, hepatitis C virus, and other infections.

Kala-azar is the prototype of parasitic infections that may cause acute interstitial nephritis leading to ARF, particularly in immunocompromised patients.[9] Leishmanial amastigotes tend to reside inside the interstitial monocytes

TABLE 167-1

Principal Tropical Infections

	A	B	C	AKI
Viral				
Bunya		*		
Chikungunya		*		
Dengue	*	*		+++
Ebola		*		
Hanta			*	++
Hepatitis A,B,C,E			*	++
HIV			*	+++
Lassa		*		
Marburg		*		
Yellow fever		*		+
Bacterial				
Cholera		*		++
Diphtheria			*	+
Leptospirosis		*		+++
Leprosy	*	*		+
Melioidosis			*	+
Salmonellosis			*	+
Scrub typhus			*	+
Scabies			*	++
Shigella dysentery			*	+
Tetanus			*	+
Tuberculosis	*		*	
Yaws		*		
Parasitic				
African trypanosomiasis	*	*		+
Chagas disease	*	*		
Filariasis	*	*		+
Leishmaniasis	*	*		+
Lymphatic filariasis	*	*		+
Malaria	*	*		+++
Schistosomiasis	*	*		

*, included in groups A-C; +, ++, +++, strength of association with AKI. **A,** Included in the Special Program for Research and Training in Tropical Diseases (TDR) of the World Health Organization; **B,** Occurring only or mostly in the tropics; **C,** Occurring elsewhere but more severe and difficult to control in the tropics; **AKI,** Reportedly associated with acute kidney injury.

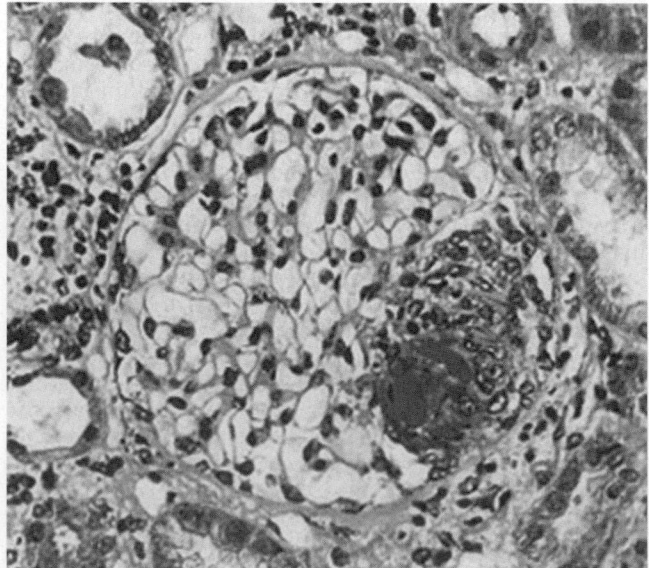

FIGURE 167-1. See also color plates. Leptospirosis. Note the interstitial infiltration, tubular necrosis, and blood casts.

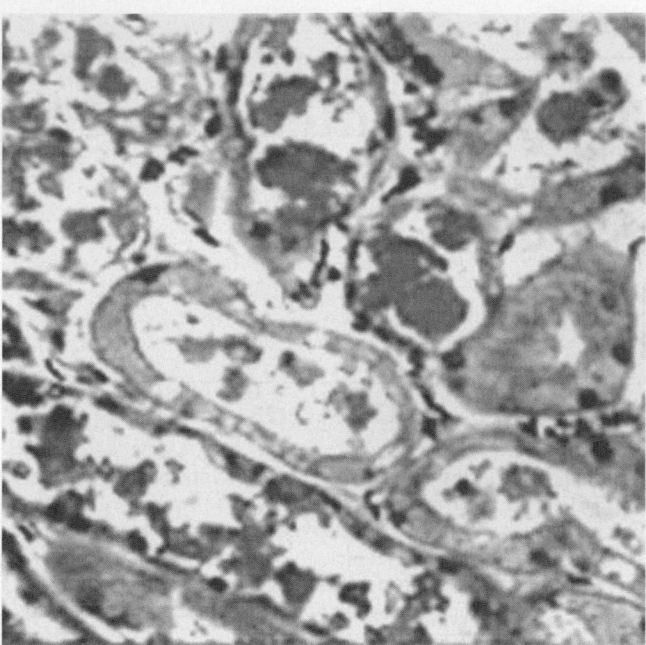

FIGURE 167-2. See also color plates. Hepatitis B; ANCA-negative vasculitis. Note the small cellular crescent adjacent to the focus of fibrinoid necrosis. ANCA, antineutrophil cytoplasmic antibody.

and evade their phagocytic function; yet they continue to release mediators that induce AKI.

Although mycotic infections are not categorized as tropical, it is worthwhile alluding to the recent reports, exclusively from the tropics, on ARF complicating renal mucormycosis in diabetics and immunocompromised individuals. In this condition, fungal hyphae are seen in abundance within the acute inflammatory reaction in the renal interstitium.[10]

Immune-Mediated Renal Lesions

Immune complex-mediated acute postinfectious glomerulonephritis, occasionally associated with transient, mild to moderate renal insufficiency, has been described with streptococcal infections of the skin in African children as opposed to the pharynx in the developed world. Typical tropical infections that may cause acute nephritis include typhoid, paratyphoid leptospirosis, and others.

A severe form of postinfectious glomerulonephritis, exudative glomerulonephritis, is often seen in tropical infections as typhoid, particularly when superimposed on hepatosplenic schistosomiasis,[11] filariasis,[12] and occasionally falciparum malaria.[13]

Crescentic glomerulonephritis is more often associated with acute or rapidly progressive renal failure. This has been described with HIV, hepatitis B virus, and hepatitis C virus nephropathies.[14] It may occur with secondary syphilis and lepromatous leprosy.[15] Many of these conditions may be associated with Type II or III mixed cryoglobulinemia.[14]

Tropical crescentic glomerulonephritis may also be pauci-immune, being associated with perinuclear antineutrophil cytoplasmic antibody (PANCA)–positive vasculitis in severe streptococcal infection and falciparum malaria. Similar lesions are occasionally seen in hepatitis B viral

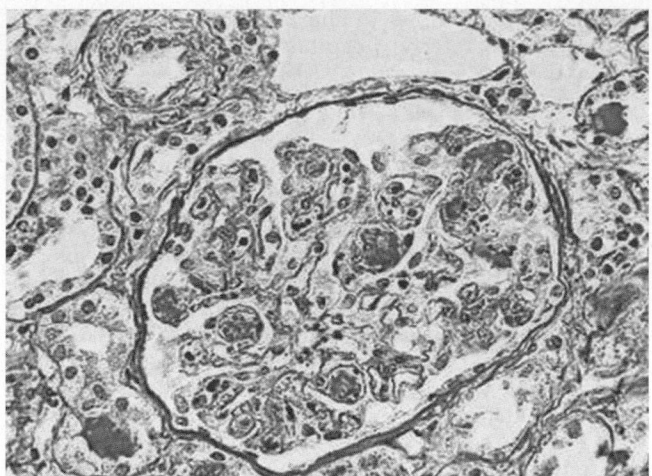

FIGURE 167-3. See also color plates. Shigella dysentery; glomerular capillary thrombi associated with the hemolytic uremic syndrome.

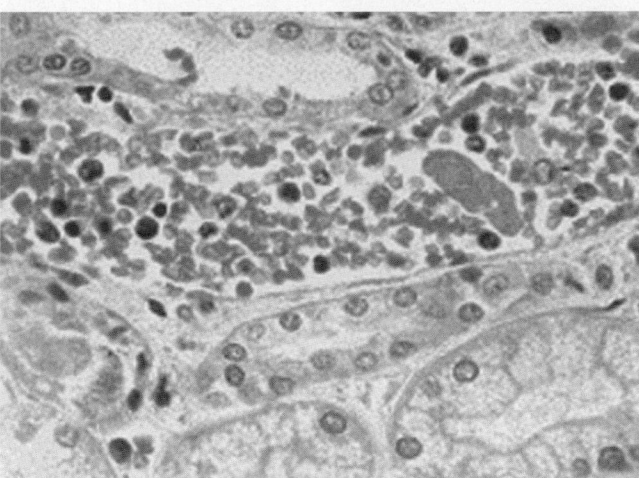

FIGURE 167-4. See also color plates. Malaria; sludging of red cells and platelets in a renal venule.

infection (Fig. 167-2), where antineutrophil cytoplasmic antibodies (ANCAs) are not detected.[14]

A distinct type of immune-mediated AKI is the hemolytic uremic syndrome, which is notoriously common in North India and Bangladesh.[16] Children in that region tend to develop the syndrome after an episode of bacterial dysentery. Shiga exotoxins directly attach to Gb3 receptors leading to the massive endothelial activation which underlies the development of microangiopathic hemolysis, capillary thrombosis (Fig. 167-3), and ARF.

Hemodynamically Mediated Acute Renal Failure

Pyrexial illness in the warm tropical climate leads to excessive fluid loss with perspiration and sweating. Many infections are associated with gastrointestinal fluid losses, which add to the dehydration. For obvious reasons, shrinkage of blood volume becomes particularly critical in children. Disseminated bacterial infection may lead to peripheral blood pooling, and extravascular colloid exudation may lead to decrease in the effective blood volume. Several mediators have been incriminated in such peripheral response including nitric oxide, tumor necrosis factor-α (TNF-α), dilatory prostaglandins, kinins, and free oxygen radicals.

Although renal failure in these cases is often prerenal and responds to adequate fluid therapy, associated endothelial activation in the glomerular and peritubular capillaries often leads to critical ischemia and structural damage. This may be the consequence of local or systemic release of endotoxins, cytokines, or free oxygen radicals as a part of the local or systemic inflammatory response. Certain infections may cause an outrageous release of catecholamines (e.g., tetanus),[17] thereby further amplifying the renal ischemia.

Sludging of red cells and platelets, due to the associated hemoconcentration, is often encountered in the renal microcirculation. This factor is considerably augmented in falciparum malaria (Fig. 167-4), owing to increased stickiness of the red cells and platelets, induced by certain de novo proteins, which form characteristic knobs at the red

cell membranes. These facilitate the adhesion of red cells to each other, to blood platelets, and to the capillary endothelium.[13] Furthermore, parasitized red cells tend to be less plastic and tend to clog the small capillaries. All the previously mentioned factors also lead to intravascular hemolysis, which adds to the pathogenesis of AKI by the classic well-known pathomechanisms. Apart from the notorious effects of malaria on the red cells, many other infections—such as viral hepatitis,[18] typhoid,[19] and typhus[20]—may lead to intravascular hemolysis in patients with glucose-6-phosphate dehydrogenase (G6PD) deficiency. The same and other infections may also lead to disseminated intravascular coagulation, which further compromises the renal circulation.

Although fluid loss through the skin becomes minimal with the development of hyperpyrexia in severe tropical infections such as malignant malaria, this may contribute to further renal injury by nonspecifically leading to muscle necrosis (rhabdomyolysis), thereby releasing free myoglobin, which has deleterious hemodynamic and tubulopathic effects,[21] in addition to its known tendency toward intratubular deposition.

A particularly notorious syndrome of rhabdomyolysis is "tropical pyomyositis."[22] This is a severe bacterial infection of skeletal muscles following trauma or intensive muscular exercise in 25% of patients. It may occur spontaneously in diabetic, alcoholic, undernourished, or immunosuppressed individuals, or those with autoimmune disorders or HIV infection. The usual causative organism is *Staphylococcus aureus*, but a variety of other organisms may be responsible. ARF may occur in advanced cases.

Tubular injury also may be induced by intrinsic pigments released in severe tropical infections as hemoglobin and bilirubin, as well as extrinsic microbial factors or medications. Tubular obstruction by hemoglobin, myoglobin casts, cell debris, and even detached viable tubule cells concludes this sad scenario.

Iatrogenic Renal Injury

Renal injury in acute tropical infections may be attributed to treatment rather than to the primary disease. Typical examples are different antibiotics, notoriously amphotericin B, aminoglycosides, cephalosporins, and vancomycin. Nephrotoxicity is considerably augmented when these agents are used in combination and when diuretics or nonsteroidal anti-inflammatory agents are added.

In the most underdeveloped countries, the iatrogenic component extends to traditional medicines that are often used by Sangomas and witch doctors for the treatment of fevers. Many of these are of unknown composition, yet their nephrotoxicity has been documented.[23]

Another interesting example of iatrogenic ARF is the vasculitic ARF occurring with interferon treatment for hepatitis C viral infection.[24] This complication is often encountered with the first few injections and is characterized by severe systemic effects, including pyrexia, hypotension, leukopenia, and thrombocytopenia. The renal lesion is dominated by interstitial edema, cellular infiltration, and variable degrees of tubular atrophy. Most patients respond to steroid treatment, which has led to the inclusion of these agents in several interferon-based protocols in viral hepatitis.

ARF also may occur as a result of vaccination. Anaphylactic and serum-sickness types of immune response leading to ARF have been described in association with the use of vaccines. A report from Brazil incriminates vaccination for transmitting yellow fever, resulting in fatal hemorrhagic ARF.[25]

CLINICAL FEATURES OF TROPICAL ARF

The clinical profile of ARF in the tropics is often modified by a number of factors. Most significant is the overlap between the manifestations of ARF and those of severe systemic infection or intoxication. In many cases, there is severe toxemia, shock, dehydration, disseminated intravascular coagulation, hepatocellular or pulmonary injury, or central nervous system involvement. These may impose difficulties for the selection of certain treatment modalities as hemodialysis in the presence of shock or severe thrombocytopenia.

The complexity of pathogenetic factors involved in tropical ARF often leads to aggravation of the uremic syndrome. Most patients reaching the hospital are already severely anemic, thrombocytopenic, severely acidotic, and critically hyperkalemic. Coma, convulsions, pericarditis, ascending paralysis, urea frost, and similar clinical signs, which are now seldom seen in the industrialized world, are an everyday experience in tropical ARF. Extremely high serum creatinine concentrations and serum potassium levels of 9 or 10 mEq/L associated with electrocardiographic signs may be seen when there is significant rhabdomyolysis. People living in the tropics also may have multiple chronic parasitic infestations and significant protein-calorie malnutrition. The added catabolic effects of the new infection or intoxication, and subsequently that of the uremic state, result in a considerable negative nitrogen balance that has a major impact on outcome.

Finally, there is the effect of delayed referral. Lack of adequate information in the primary care units, patients' reluctance to leave their own territories to be treated in central hospitals, and inefficient and unsafe transfer vehicles may contribute to a very high mortality from ARF,[26] which has been estimated in a consensus meeting to approach 80%. This is in sharp contrast to the reported mortality from referral hospitals, which ranges between 20% and 30%.

DIAGNOSIS

The diagnosis of ARF in the context of a severe systemic infection can be intriguing. Any severe infection may be associated with oliguria due to extrarenal fluid losses, azotemia and hyperkalemia due to the supervening catabolic state, and lactic acidosis due to tissue hypoxia. This may progress to renal shutdown with all its functional consequences but without significant structural damage. In those patients, urine is concentrated ($U_{osm} > 350$ mOs/kg), with a high urea ($U/P_{urea} > 3$), creatinine ($U/P_{creat} > 20$), and low sodium ($U_{Na} < 40$ mEq/L, FeNa $> 1\%$) content, and the adequate response to intravenous fluid challenge is diagnostic.

On the other hand, some patients develop a "high urine output" ARF, where the blood chemistry displays all the features of renal failure, yet shows preserved or increased urine volume. These patients are easier to manage and generally have a better prognosis.

The diagnosis of AKI in tropical infections is, therefore, based on the constellation clinical, laboratory, and therapeutic observations. Awareness of the infections that typically cause AKI should raise the index of suspicion and impose specific alertness to changes in urine volume and specific gravity and blood chemistry, particularly when the response to adequate hydration is poor.

Imaging is rarely necessary. Ultrasonography may show evidence of interstitial edema, cortical infarction, or calcifications in a few weeks following the occurrence of acute cortical necrosis, which is seen mostly in those who survive disseminated intravascular coagulation. Isotopic studies should confirm adequate preservation of renal perfusion (which is usually around 30% of the normal values), with persistence of the isotopic marker in the kidneys owing to the impaired tubular flow and interstitial leakage.

Renal biopsy is needed only in those with prolonged oliguria, to make the diagnosis of cortical necrosis, interstitial fibrosis, or a preexisting condition.

MANAGEMENT OF TROPICAL ARF

As with conventional ARF, the most effective intervention is prevention. Awareness of the potential renal complications of tropical infections and their treatment is the single most cost-effective measure. Unfortunately, very little attention is paid by different medical specialties to this important issue.

Timely intervention at the onset of ARF is usually rewarded by excellent results. Adequate attention to a primary infection, prompt control of pyrexia, correction of shock, adequate hydration, and avoidance of nephrotoxic drugs or drug combinations are simple and most effective. There is no evidence that induction of diuresis by osmotic or loop diuretics would change the outcome, nor would the use of dopamine, calcium channel blockers, or angiotensin-converting enzyme (ACE) inhibitors.

Adequate nutrition is of vital importance. Patients who are unable to eat or drink must be supported by enough fluids, electrolytes, calories, and amino acids parenterally.

This may be difficult with severe oliguria, when the total permissible fluid intake is restricted. Patients treated in the tropical climate may lose a lot of fluid in sweat and insensible routes, which provides more room for intravenous fluid administration.

Taking the multifactorial nature of ARF into consideration, dialysis is often needed as soon as the patient has reached the hospital. Fortunately, facilities for peritoneal dialysis, acute hemodialysis, and even continuous renal replacement therapy are now available in most tropical countries, though they are typically restricted to teaching or army hospitals.[27] In addition to logistic difficulties in transfer and acceptance of patients in these hospitals, there may be technical problems in implementing dialysis and other extracorporeal therapies due to vascular access problems, bleeding tendencies, circulatory instability, and so on. It is hoped that the use of peritoneal dialysis finds its way to smaller territorial hospitals where prompt renal replacement therapy can be implemented when needed.

The challenge facing the medical profession will continue for many decades. Patients will continue to die of ARF until the value of proper education of the primary care physician is appreciated and implemented. Unfortunately, this simple fact is lost within the jungle of politics, inappropriate diversion of funds, and inequity of health care.

Key Points

1. Tropical infections may be responsible for acute kidney injury in up to 800 million inhabitants in the tropics.
2. More than 20 tropical infections may be associated with acute kidney injury; the most widely known are malaria, leptospirosis, cholera, shigellosis, dengue, and human immunodeficiency virus.
3. Direct parenchymal invasion, hemodynamic disturbance, and immunological perturbation are the major mechanisms of kidney injury, in addition to the frequent nephrotoxicity of drugs and herbs used for treatment.
4. The clinical syndrome of acute kidney injury varies from mild to fatal interaction in between the original systemic illness and the confounding manifestations of acute renal failure.
5. Owing to the complexity of the resulting illness, and the relative lack of treatment facilities, the mortality from acute kidney injury complicating tropical infection may be up to 80%.

Key References

6. Tkachenko EA, Lee HW: Etiology and epidemiology of hemorrhagic fever with renal syndrome. Kidney Int Supp 1991;35: S54-S61.
9. Barsoum RS: Parasitic infections in transplant recipients. Nat Clin Pract Nephrol 2006;2:490-503.
13. Barsoum RS: Malarial acute renal failure. J Am Soc Nephrol 2000;11:2147-2154.
23. Kadiri S, Arije A, Salako BL: Traditional herbal preparations and acute renal failure in south west Nigeria. Trop Doct 1999;29:244-246.
25. Vasconcelos PF, Luna EJ, Galler R, et al: Serious adverse events associated with yellow fever 17DD vaccine in Brazil: A report of two cases. Lancet 2001;358:91-97.

See the companion Expert Consult website for the complete reference list.

General Treatment Concepts

CHAPTER 168

Principles of Antibiotic Prescription in Intensive Care Unit Patients and Patients with Acute Renal Failure

Penny L. Sappington

OBJECTIVES

This chapter will:
1. Describe how to select the appropriate antibiotic to treat critically ill patients in intensive care units.
2. Highlight the issues that pertain to prescribing antibiotics to patients with acute renal failure in intensive care units.
3. Discuss antibiotic resistance as a consequence of antibiotic choices.
4. Compare strategies that can minimize antibiotic resistance.

Prescribing appropriate antibiotics in the intensive care unit (ICU) remains an important task in the daily routines of physicians taking care of critically ill patients. Initial antibiotic therapy should be prompt, dosed correctly, and be broad-spectrum in coverage, since treatment delay and inappropriate antibiotic therapy are risk factors for mortality in ICU patients.[1] When making the choice of empirical antibiotic coverage, physicians must consider patient-specific factors, microbiological factors, and pharmacological factors. Patient-specific factors include the presumed source of infection, presence of comorbid conditions, and previous antibiotic administration history. Microbiological factors include the identification of the most likely pathogens and their unit-specific susceptibility patterns. Pharmacological factors include the potential toxicity and bioavailability of any particular antibiotic. As soon as possible, empirical antibiotic coverage should be de-escalated to what the patient's specific organisms are based on cultures and sensitivities. The chosen antibiotic should be the least toxic and the most cost-effective therapy available.

Risk factors for nosocomial infections in ICU patients include severity of the underlying disease, length of hospital stay, the presence of invasive devices (e.g., endotracheal tubes, intravascular catheters, urinary catheters); prior antibiotic exposure, and the high prevalence of mul-

tidrug-resistant organisms. Infections that require antibiotic use have become prevalent in the ICU. An average of 20% of the most critically ill ICU patients will develop a nosocomial infection while in the ICU.[2]

Prevalence studies have shown regularly in past decades that 40% of patients present in acute hospitals on a given day were treated with one or several antibiotics. This proportion rises to 70% or more in ICU patients, as confirmed in the European Prevalence of Infection in Intensive Care (EPIC) study.[2] In this large, multicenter, pan-European study with more than 10,000 patients, 71% of patients were treated with antibiotics on the very day of the survey. Combination therapy with two or more drugs represented 40% of antibiotic courses. Empirical treatments were frequent, representing 50% of those courses. In an EPIIC report the most frequently diagnosed ICU-acquired infections were pneumonia and infections of the lower respiratory tract (together 63%), followed by urinary tract infections (16%), sepsis (16%), and wound infections (11%). The most frequently cultured pathogens were gram-negative bacteria (92%), especially Enterobacteriaceae (34%) and *Pseudomonas aeruginosa* (30%), followed by *Staphylococcus* (37%), *Enterococcus* (20%), and, surprisingly, fungi (10%). The most-prescribed antibiotics were the cephalosporins (30%), followed by broad-spectrum penicillins (17%), metronidazole (17%), and aminoglycosides (13%).[3]

APPROPRIATE ANTIBIOTIC SELECTION

In selecting the appropriate antibiotic for therapy in the ICU patient, a number of factors have to be considered. A definitive diagnosis should be established before antibiotic therapy is initiated. This is accomplished by performing a comprehensive clinical evaluation, identifying the site of infection as well as the possible source; ordering the appropriate diagnostic tests and appropriate specimen for culture and susceptibility testing; and evaluating for noninfectious causes of fever. The selection of the antibiotic regimen should be broad-spectrum in coverage to ensure that the appropriate organisms are effectively covered. In determining what the appropriate antibiotic regimen should be, clinicians should consider the likely pathogens associated with the possible site of infection; any previous cultures as well as the associated susceptibility testing; ICU-wide antibiograms (resistance rates for even the same organism may differ between community-acquired and nosocomial sources); and host factors (which may affect the pharmacodynamics or pharmacokinetic properties of the agents used), such as history of adverse reactions to antibiotic agents, renal and hepatic function, pregnancy, genetic or metabolic abnormalities, and age. As the results of cultures and susceptibility tests become available, clinicians must reassess and make appropriate changes to empirical antibiotic regimens. The appropriate antibiotic regimen should provide suitable biological activity against the organism, while using the most cost-effective and narrowest regimen that has the most appropriate coverage. Many physicians continue empirical antibiotic coverage even when there are no clinical data suggesting that there is an infection. This practice often results in the excessive use of antibiotics for long durations, both of which are significant risk factors for resistance. Clinicians should change to the appropriate antibiotic coverage as soon as possible, narrow the coverage of the antibiotic regimen as soon as results of susceptibility testing are known, and limit the duration of the antibiotic regimen when possible. Short courses of antibiotics are desired over long courses to help prevent resistance and, in patients with no documented infection, antibiotic therapy should be assessed for possible discontinuation. Table 168-1 provides guidelines for selecting the appropriate antibiotic.

ANTIBIOTIC SELECTION IN PATIENTS WITH ACUTE RENAL FAILURE

Acute renal failure (ARF) is a common complication in patients admitted to the intensive care unit, and mortality rates are high. When selecting an antimicrobial dosing regimen for critically ill patients with severe renal failure, clinicians should consider the effects of renal failure itself, other acute and chronic disease states, and extracorporeal drug clearance by renal replacement therapies on drug pharmacokinetics. Most antibiotics are removed from the body largely unchanged in urine. Consequently oliguria potentially leads to drug accumulation. An increased volume distribution due to critical illness and fluid overload at the onset of oliguria, however, would dictate that the normal loading antibiotic doses should at least remain unchanged if not increased, while subsequent doses are given less frequently. Most patients are supported by renal replacement therapy, which will clear antibiotics in a similar manner to a native kidney with glomerular filtration rates approximating 35 mL/min. Whereas aminoglycoside and glycopeptide dosage intervals are greatly simplified by routine monitoring of concentrations, other antibiotics can not easily be measured, and toxic levels may be apparent only with the onset of a complication such as seizures. Guidance to doses and dosing intervals are well established in the literature on acute renal failure; however, with very severe infections such as endocarditis and meningococcal septicemia treated with penicillin, the narrow line between ensuring effectiveness and toxicity is best managed by introducing synergy with a second antibiotic.

TABLE 168-1

Guidelines in Antibiotic Selection in the Critically Ill and Acute Renal Failure Patient

Establishing a Diagnosis
Clinical examamination
Suspected site of infection
Diagnostic workup
  Blood cultures
  Chest radiograph
  Quantitative bronchoalveolar lavage
  Urinalysis and urine culture and sensitivity
  Computed tomography scan—sinuses, chest, abdomen
  Lumbar puncture
Antibiotic selection
  Broad-spectrum
  Prior cultures and susceptibility
  Antibiograms (unit specific)
Reevaluation of Patient and Clinical Data
Evaluate patient's clinical response at 72 hours
  Fever
  White blood cell count
  Organ function improvement
If clinical response:
  Narrow antibiotic according to culture data
  Monitor duration of appropriate therapy
If no clinical response, reevaluate for:
  Superinfection
  Induced resistance
  Another source or site of infection
  Complicated infection
  Noninfectious cause of fever
Antibiotic Selection for Patients with Acute Renal Failure (ARF)
Use the same principles for antibiotic selection in the critically ill patient, except
  Avoid nephrotoxic antibiotics if possible
  Adjust antibiotic dosages for calculated renal clearance
  Consider intermittent hemodialysis (HD)
  Establish dosing schedule (i.e., dose after HD)
  Consider continuous venoveno hemodiafiltration (CVVHD)

Typically penicillins, aminoglycosides, cephalosporins, carbapenems, glycopeptides, and fluconazole have prolonged half-lives ($t_{1/2}$) on renal replacement therapy and need increased dosage intervals, whereas chloramphenicol, ceftriaxone, clindamycin, erythromycin, metronidazole, itraconazole, amphotericin B, acyclovir, rifampicin, and, to a lesser extent, ciprofloxacin have substantial nonrenal clearances and $t_{1/2}$ during replacement therapy is only marginally increased. Antibiotics such as glycopeptides and aminoglycosides can additionally be monitored and provide an indication of what is likely to be happening to other concomitant antibiotics. As a general rule, severely infected patients with poor renal function and patients who are dialysis dependent should receive normal antibiotic doses given less frequently. Ideally postdialysis troughs and postadministration peaks are monitored to help prevent nonrenal antimicrobial toxicity in these patients. Table 168-2 summarizes the appropriate adjustments to antimicrobials in the treatment of patients with acute renal failure.[4-6]

ANTIBIOTIC RESISTANCE

Antibiotic resistance is becoming a worldwide problem. It has been estimated that 50% to 60% of all nosocomial

TABLE 168-2

Dosage and Interval Alterations of Antimicrobials in Patients with Acute Renal Failure

DRUG	CHANGE D OR I	Modified Dosage for Measured or Estimated C_{Cr} (mL/min)			COMMENTS
		≥50	10-50	≤10	
Penicillin					
Penicillin	D	ND	75% ND	50% ND	Dose after HD
Oxacillin	D	ND	ND	ND	
Piperacillin	I	ND q4-6h	ND q8h	ND q12h	Dose after HD
Nafcillin	—	ND	ND	ND	
Ampicillin	I	ND q4-6h	ND q8h	ND q12h	Dose after HD
Ampicillin/sulbactam	I	ND q6h	ND q8-12h	ND q24h	
Piperacillin/tazobactam	I	ND q6-8h	ND q8-12h	ND q12h	
Aztreonam	D	ND q8h	ND q8-12h	ND q24h	Dose after HD
Imipenem	D, I	0.5 g q6-8h	0.5 g q8-12h	0.5-0.25 g q12h	
Meropenem	D, I	1 g q8h	0.5-1 g q12h	0.5 g q24h	Dose after HD
Cephalosporin					
Cefazolin	D	ND q8h	ND	50% ND	Dose after HD
Cefotetan	I	ND q12h	ND q24	ND q24-48h	Dose after HD
Cefuroxime	I	ND q8h	ND q8-12h	ND q24h	Dose after HD
Cefotaxime	I	ND q8h	ND q12-24h	ND q24h	Dose after HD
Ceftriaxone	—	ND q24h	ND	ND	
Ceftazidime	I	ND q8h	ND q12-24h	ND q24-48h	Dose after HD
Cefepime	D, I	2 g q12h	1-2 g q24h	0.5g q24h	Dose after HD
*Aminoglycoside					
Amikacin	D, I	60%-90% ND q12h	30%-80% ND q12-18h	20%-30% ND q24-48h	Modify per serum levels; redose level <1 µg/mL
Gentamicin	D, I	Same	Same	Same	Same
Tobramycin	D, I	Same	Same	Same	Same
Quinolones					
Ciprofloxacin	D, I	ND	50%-75% ND	50% ND	Dose after HD
Levofloxacin	D, I	ND	50% ND	25% ND	Dose after HD
Moxifloxacin	—	ND	ND	ND	
Glycopeptides					
Vancomycin	I	20 mg/kg q12-24h	20 mg/kg q1-4d	20 mg/kg q4-7d	Modify per serum levels; redose level <20 µg/mL
Synercid	—	7.5 mg/kg q8h	ND	ND	
Daptomycin	I	3 mg/kg q12h	3 mg/kg q24h	3 mg/kg q48h	
Other Antibiotics					
Metronidazole	—	ND	ND	ND	
Clindamycin	—	ND	ND	ND	
Azithromycin	—	ND	ND	ND	
Linezolid	—	ND	ND	ND	
Bactrim	D, I	ND q18h	ND q24h	NR	
Antifungals					
Amphotericin B	I	ND	ND	ND q24-36h	
Fluconazole	D	ND	50% ND	50% q48h	
Voriconazole	—	ND	ND	ND	
Caspofungin	—	ND	ND	ND	
Antivirals					
Acyclovir	D, I	5-12 mg/kg q8h	5-12 mg/kg q12-24h	2.5-5 mg/kg q24-48h	Dose after HD
Ganciclovir	D, I	5 mg/kg q12h	5 mg/kg q24h	2.5 mg/kg q24h	Dose after HD

*Alternative dosing once-daily aminoglycosides 5-7 mg/kg, estimated C_{Cr} (mL/min): >60 dose every 24 hours; 40-60 dose every 36 hours; 20-40 dose every 48 hours; and <20 after the initial dose, follow through and redose for a level <1 mg/mL. Data from references 4-6.
D, dosage; I, intervals; ND, normal dosage; 50% ND, reduce dose to 50% of normal; NR, not recommended.
Modified from Mandell GL, Bennett JE, Dolin R, et al: Principles and Practices of Infectious Diseases. Dallas, TX, Antimicrobial Therapy, Inc., 1992, p 116; and Amsden GW: Tables of antimicrobial agent pharmacology. In Mandell GL, Bennett JE, Dolin R (eds): Mandell, Douglas, and Bennett's Principles and Practice of Infectious Diseases, 6th ed. Philadelphia, Churchill Livingstone, 2005, pp 635-700.

infections in the United States are caused by antibiotic resistance.[7] Multidrug-resistant gram-positive organisms, such as methicillin-resistant *Staphylococcus aureus*, vancomycin-resistant enterococci, and multidrug-resistant *Streptococcus pneumoniae*, are some of the pathogens found in critically ill patients. Resistance also is an increasing problem with gram-negative bacilli. Of particular concern is resistance mediated by extended-spectrum beta lactamases among organisms such as *Klebsiella pneu-*

moniae and *Escherichia coli*. Resistance of *Pseudomonas aeruginosa* to fluoroquinolones and imipenem also increased rapidly. Furthermore, an increasing cause of infection in critically ill patients is *Candida* species; in the United States 105 of isolates from bloodstream infections were found to be resistant.[8]

An appropriate broad-spectrum antibiotic regimen should take into account local resistance patterns, which, if not implemented as quickly as possible, could have a dramatic impact on mortality in the most critically ill patients.[9,10] Antibiotics are unique and powerful drugs, and antibiotic resistance has become one of the leading problems in modern medicine. For many years, physicians took a fairly lackadaisical attitude toward antibiotic resistance, because there was always a new antibiotic. However, over the past few decades, there have been few new antibiotics developed, especially antibiotics covering gram-negative organisms. Numerous factors are associated with high rates of antimicrobial resistance in the ICU. Heavy antibiotic use among critically ill patients is likely the most important cause. The use of antibiotics, as well as prior exposure, is associated with emergence of resistant therapy. Increased resistance is related to several variables associated with the higher severity of illness found among ICU patients. These variables include the presence of invasive devices, such as endotracheal tubes and intravascular and urinary catheters; prolonged length of hospital stay; immunosuppression; malnutrition; and cross-contamination by health care providers.[11,12] Antibiotics have a tendency to select out the most resistant microorganisms, leading to major issues of multidrug-resistant microorganisms worldwide. Therefore the level of resistance to many antibiotics of most bacteria (including those historically considered to be very susceptible), is becoming a serious problem worldwide.[13-15] Thus, given that ICUs represent epicenters for the development of resistance, medical staffs have the crucial responsibility of managing antibiotic therapies in severely infected patients.

STRATEGIES FOR PREVENTION OF RESISTANCE

In prescribing the appropriate antibiotic for ICU patients, clinicians must take into account the various strategies that will ultimately minimize resistance. The following section describes the most commonly employed antimicrobial modification strategies aimed at limiting antibiotic resistance.

Appropriate Pharmacokinetic and Pharmacodynamic Properties

Ineffective antibiotic dosing is a common yet often unrecognized factor associated with clinical treatment failure and the emergence of resistance. Antibiotic levels must be high enough to kill bacteria in both blood and infected tissues. Thus, it is of considerable importance to select appropriate dosages, especially at the beginning of treatment, because of the severity and high risk of morbidity and mortality associated with infections in critically ill patients. The concept of inhibitory quotient, which is the quotient between the antibiotic level in the considered area (in the blood and in the tissue) and the minimum inhibitory concentration (MIC) of the given strain for the given antibiotic, or the area under the curve over time, is becoming increasingly stressed in the literature. Drugs such as beta lactams, aztreonam, carbapenems, and vancomycin are characterized as concentration-independent antibiotics, and their efficacy is based on maintaining concentrations of the agent above the MIC of the organisms for prolonged periods.[16] The use of continuous antibiotic infusions has been endorsed for time-dependent drugs to optimize their pharmacodynamic properties and minimize the risk of resistance.[17,18] Concentration-dependent antibiotics, particularly aminoglycosides and fluoroquinolones, exert their maximal antibacterial activities when peak drug concentrations are well above the MIC of the organism.[16] More recently Forrest and colleagues[19] showed a relationship between the number of clinical and bacteriological failures and the area under the curve of the antibiotic in patients treated with quinolones for severe pneumonia. Newer strategies include the use of extended-interval dosing regimens for aminoglycosides and the use of high doses of fluoroquinolones to achieve high concentrations relative to the pathogen MICs.[20,21]

Studies have shown that dosing strategies that optimize the pharmacodynamic properties of antibiotics often result in improved bacterial eradication, decreased mortality, and decreased length of ICU and hospital stays. The application of pharmacodynamic principles to ICU patients is complicated by the potential for significantly altered drug pharmacodynamics in critically ill patients.[22] Larger volumes of distribution secondary to volume overload, decreased serum protein concentrations leading to decreased protein binding, decreased metabolism and clearance owing to organ dysfunction or hypoperfusion, and increased metabolism and clearance owing to hypermetabolic states have been described in ICU patients, and all may lead to clinically significant changes in antibiotic pharmacokinetics.[22] Antibiotic resistance can be reduced by optimizing antibiotic dosing based on better characterization of pharmacokinetic alteration in ICU patients, and the appropriate application of pharmacodynamic principles offers significant potential for improved outcomes.

Once the most appropriate drug has been determined, not only the route of administration but the dosages must be determined as well. Aggressive antibiotic dosing is the general recommendation in critically ill patients. Low doses of antibiotics may fail to eradicate the organism and predispose the organism to the development of resistance. High dosing strategies may potentially compensate for pharmacokinetic alterations, increasing the likelihood that patients are receiving adequate drug levels for eradication of the organism. Although drug dosing should be aggressive, it must be based on appropriate clinical considerations involving issues such as drug toxicities, presence of renal or hepatic dysfunction that may lead to drug accumulation, the presumed site of infection and the ability of the drug to achieve adequate concentrations in that site, susceptibilities of presumed or documented pathogens, and pharmacodynamic properties of the drugs in question.

Narrow Spectrum

Another proposed strategy to curtail the development of antimicrobial resistance, in addition to the judicious overall use of antibiotics, is to use drugs with a narrow antimicrobial spectrum. Similarly, the avoidance of broad-spectrum antibiotics (e.g., cephalosporins) and the reintroduction of narrow-spectrum agents (penicillin, trimethoprim, gentamicin) along with infection-control practices have been successful in reducing the occurrence of *Clostridium difficile* infections.[23] Unfortunately, ICU patients often have already received antimicrobial treatment, making it more probable that they will be infected with an antibiotic-resistant pathogen.[24] Initial empirical treatment with broad-spectrum agents is therefore often necessary in order to avoid inappropriate treatment until culture results become available.[1,25] The need for appropri-

TABLE 168-3

Indications for Antibiotic Combination Therapy

	BROAD-SPECTRUM COVERAGE	BACTERICIDAL EFFECT	SYNERGISTIC EFFECT	PREVENTION OF RESISTANCE
Endocarditis		+	+	
Septic shock	+	+	+	
Neutropenic patients	+	+	+	
Polymicrobial infections	+			
Late nosocomial infections	+			+

ate initial therapy must be carefully balanced against the risk of increased resistance as a consequence of unnecessary drug exposure. Empirical therapy should be adjusted promptly, based on clinical response of the patient and culture and susceptibility reports. Even when initial reports show an isolate is susceptible to the prescribed therapy, clinical failure indicates a change in antibiotic therapy, because resistance may be reducible, and expression of such treatment-emergent resistance may not be observed until after therapy has been initiated.

De-escalation involves switching to a narrower spectrum agent, reducing the number of antibiotics, stopping therapy altogether in patients not likely to have infection, and making efforts to reduce duration of therapy. Outcomes of the use of this strategy include improvements in the frequency of secondary infection, antimicrobial resistance, and mortality.[26]

Antibiotic Combination Therapy

The use of antimicrobial combination therapy has been proposed as a strategy to reduce the emergence of bacterial resistance, as has been employed for *Mycobacterium tuberculosis*.[27] Unfortunately, no convincing data exist to validate this hypothesis for nosocomial infections. Several recent meta-analyses recommend the use of monotherapy with a beta-lactam antibiotic for the definitive treatment of neutropenic fever and severe sepsis, once antimicrobial susceptibilities are known.[28] Additionally, there is no definitive evidence that the emergence of antibiotic resistance is reduced by the use of combination antimicrobial therapy. However, empirical combination therapy directed against high-risk pathogens such as *P. aeruginosa* should be encouraged until the results of antimicrobial susceptibility become available. Such an approach to empirical treatment can increase the likelihood of providing appropriate initial antimicrobial therapy with improved outcomes.[29,30] However, Table 168-3 shows some clinical settings where combination therapy may be advisable.

DURATION OF THERAPY

Optimal duration of antibiotic therapy has been poorly defined. Prolonged administration of antibiotics in ICU patients has been shown to be an important risk factor for the emergence of colonization and infection with antibiotic-resistant bacteria.[31,32] Recent attempts have therefore been made to reduce the duration of antibiotic treatment for specific bacterial infections. Several clinical trials have found that 7 to 8 days of antibiotic treatment is acceptable for most nonbacteremic patients with ventilator-associated pneumonia.[32-34] Similarly, shorter courses of antibiotic treatment have been employed successfully in patients at low risk for ventilator-associated pneumonia,[35] in patients with pyelonephritis,[36] and in patients with community-acquired pneumonia.[37]

CONCLUSION

Appropriate antibiotic selection in critically ill patients in the ICU, as well as those with ARF, is extremely important to the clinical care of these patients, and it remains a challenge. The basic principles for appropriate antibiotic selection and optimal dosing, especially for those patients with ARF, for both empirical and definitive therapy must be emphasized to not only improve outcome but also to reduce the possibility of resistance. Many controversies remain concerning the ideal antibiotic management of critically ill patients, including the role of selective digestive decontamination in the prevention of nosocomial pneumonia in ventilated patients, the role of antibiotic-coated catheters,[38] the use of quinolones in the ICU, the interest in combination therapy, the ideal length of therapy, the effectiveness of antibiotic policies (i.e., cycling), and the roles of guidelines and evidence-based medicine. The long-term effects of each of these strategies continue to be debated and each, by itself, is unlikely to be optimal in preventing antibiotic resistance. The combination of these strategies offers the greatest potential for preventing the spread of resistance and improving outcomes in critically ill ICU patients as well as those patients with ARF.

Key References

1. Kollef MH, Sherman G, Ward S, Fraser VJ: Inadequate antimicrobial treatment of infections: A risk factor for hospital mortality among critically ill patients. Chest 1999;115:462-474.
9. Ibrahim EH, Sherman G, Ward S, et al: The influence of inadequate antimicrobial treatment of bloodstream infections on patient outcomes in the ICU setting. Chest 2000;118:146-155.
12. Kollef MH, Fraser VJ: Antibiotic resistance in the intensive care unit. Ann Intern Med 2001;134:298-314.
26. Niederman MS: The importance of de-escalating antimicrobial therapy in patients with ventilator-associated pneumonia. Semin Respir Crit Care Med 2006;27:45-50.
38. Hanna HA, Raad II, Hackett B, et al: Antibiotic-impregnated catheters associated with significant decrease in nosocomial and multidrug-resistant bacteremias in critically ill patients. Chest 2003;124:1030-1038.

See the companion Expert Consult website for the complete reference list.

CHAPTER 169

Renal Replacement Therapy in Acute Renal Failure Secondary to Sepsis

Rinaldo Bellomo, John A. Kellum, Claudio Ronco, and Sean M. Bagshaw

---

OBJECTIVES

This chapter will:

1. Describe the unique aspects of sepsis-associated acute renal failure.
2. Examine some of the unique aspects of renal replacement therapy in severe sepsis and septic shock–associated acute renal failure.
3. Discuss the importance of timing of intervention with renal replacement therapy in patients with sepsis-associated acute renal failure.
4. Describe the potential effect of renal replacement therapy choice on renal recovery.
5. Explain the possible role of renal replacement therapy and new techniques of renal replacement therapy in the adjunctive treatment of the sepsis syndrome.

Septic shock, severe sepsis, and the multiple-organ dysfunction syndrome remain the most common causes of death in the intensive care unit (ICU), a source of prolonged ICU and hospital stay in survivors, and the trigger for a great deal of ICU expenditure.[1] In this context, acute renal failure (ARF) is common, and severe sepsis and septic shock are now the most common causes of ARF in critically ill patients.[2]

Although sepsis is the most common cause of ARF in critical illness, there is limited epidemiological information on sepsis-associated ARF. Among the 1753 patients studied as part of the Beginning and Ending Supportive Therapy for the Kidney (BEST Kidney) project,[2] sepsis was considered the cause in 833 (47.5%). The predominant sources of sepsis were chest and abdomen (54.3%). Sepsis-associated ARF appeared unique in that it was associated with greater aberrations in hemodynamics and laboratory parameters, greater severity of illness, and higher need for mechanical ventilation and vasoactive therapy. There was no difference in enrollment kidney function or in the proportion of patients receiving renal replacement therapy (RRT). Oliguria, however, was more common in sepsis-associated ARF (67% vs. 57%), and sepsis-associated ARF was associated with a higher in-hospital case-fatality rate compared with nonsepsis-associated ARF (70.2% vs. 51.8%). After adjustment for covariates, sepsis-associated ARF remained associated with higher odds of death (OR 1.48, 95% CI, 1.17-1.89). Patients with sepsis and acute kidney injury (AKI) had a longer duration of hospitalization. Yet, sepsis-associated AKI showed trends toward

greater renal recovery and independence from RRT at hospital discharge.

Thus, sepsis-associated ARF is clinically distinct (Table 169-1) and deserves special consideration, especially with regard to RRT.

Renal replacement therapy (and blood purification techniques in general) in the context of sepsis-associated ARF should logically aim to achieve several specific goals:

1. Replacement of lost renal function
2. Maintenance of physiological homeostasis
3. Facilitation of renal recovery
4. Additional beneficial effect on the humoral immune response that might participate in the pathogenesis of organ injury in this context

REPLACEMENT OF RENAL FUNCTION AND HOMEOSTASIS IN SEPSIS-ASSOCIATED ACUTE RENAL FAILURE

In patients with sepsis-associated ARF, all general aspects of artificial renal support apply. They include the need to substitute for several components of renal function.

Fluid status control is vital in all patients with ARF but particularly important in patients with multiple-organ failure and sepsis. In those patients with adult respiratory distress syndrome (ARDS), a recent multicenter randomized trial showed that the achievement of a daily negative fluid balance was an important determinant of earlier weaning from ventilation.[3] In this study close to 80% of ARDS patients had severe sepsis. Fluid control is particularly important also in patients with sepsis who are suffering bleeding complications or require the administration of plasma products. In such patients the ability to simultaneously remove fluid is important in preventing the development of pulmonary edema as a complication.

Uremic control is also important. This aims to prevent the clinical complications of uremia but also the less visible adverse molecular biological and immune effects of uremia.[4-6] In sepsis-associated ARF, where catabolism is pronounced and urea generation high, intensity of RRT is important to avoid such complications. Both adequate fluid status and uremic control are vital in allowing nutrition to proceed without restriction. The importance of adequate nutrition in the setting of multiple-organ failure, ARF, and sepsis is widely recognized.[7]

Acid-base control is also a renal function that requires substitution. In patients with sepsis, disorders of acid-base status are common, in particular metabolic acidosis with

TABLE 169-1

Baseline Characteristics between Septic and Nonseptic Acute Kidney Injury for Patients Receiving Renal Replacement Therapy

CHARACTERISTIC	TOTAL (N = 1250)	SEPTIC (N = 596)	NONSEPTIC (N = 654)	P-VALUE
Age (yr) [mean (SD)]	61.6 (15.4)	62.1 (15.4)	61.2 (16.6)	0.32
Male sex (%)	64.6	64.9	64.4	0.86
Weight (kg) [mean (SD)]	75.3 (18.2)	75.5 (18)	74.2 (18.3)	0.78
Surgical admission (%)	50.6	42.5	57.9	<0.001
SAPS II [mean (SD)]	50.2 (17.7)	53.8 (18.1)	46.9 (16.7)	<0.001
SOFA [mean (SD)]	10.9 (3.4)	11.9 (3.2)	9.9 (3.3)	<0.001
Mechanical ventilation (%)	80.2	89.2	71.7	<0.001
Vasoactive drugs (%)	73.9	82.5	66.2	<0.001

SAPS II, Simplified Acute Physiology Score; SD, standard deviation; SOFA, Sequential Organ Failure Assessment.
Data from Uchino S, Kellum JA, Bellomo R, et al, for the Beginning and Ending Supportive Therapy for the Kidney (BEST Kidney) Investigators: Acute renal failure in critically ill patients: A multinational, multicenter study. JAMA 2005;294:813-818.

acidemia. In this setting RRT should be able to both prevent and treat such acidemia.[8]

Electrolyte disorders are also common in severe sepsis and septic shock in the setting of ARF. These disorders include hyponatremia, hyperkalemia, hyperphosphatemia, and hypocalcemia.[9] Optimal RRT should prevent such disorders or reestablish electrolyte homeostasis.

Hemodynamic instability is the hallmark of severe sepsis and septic shock. In this setting, it is particularly important that RRT should be delivered without aggravating such instability.[10]

Several patients with sepsis and concomitant illness such as traumatic brain injury, fulminant liver failure, or both, are at particular risk of cerebral edema. In this setting RRT should deliver substitution of renal function without increasing the risk of cerebral edema.[11,12]

Most patients with severe sepsis and septic shock are febrile. While an elevated temperature of a moderate degree may be immunologically beneficial in terms of antiviral or antibacterial efficacy, a very high temperature significantly contributes to patient discomfort, delirium, and vasodilatory hypotension. In some extreme cases, it can induce rhabdomyolysis. In these patients, RRT can be used to control body temperature.[13]

All of the previously mentioned aspects must be taken into account when choosing the timing of initiation of RRT and the modality of RRT in sepsis-associated ARF.

TIMING OF RENAL REPLACEMENT THERAPY IN SEPSIS-ASSOCIATED ACUTE RENAL FAILURE

Data from the BEST Kidney study show that RRT started late, regardless of how timing was defined, was associated with a longer duration of RRT support. Also length of stay in hospital was considerably longer for those who had late initiation of RRT. Third, differences in hospital mortality rates were sensitive to how timing was defined. A temporal delay in starting RRT after ICU admission was associated with a greater than twofold increase in the odds of hospital death. Moreover, this temporal increase in mortality persisted in a sensitivity analysis restricted to only those patients with severe ARF at the time of ICU admission. Finally, RRT started late, when defined by serum urea or creatinine, was associated with reduced recovery

of kidney function and a higher rate of dialysis dependence at hospital discharge.

The decision to start RRT in critically ill patients with severe AKI can depend on numerous factors, and is, therefore, a complex process.[14] Accordingly, timing of RRT has been difficult to study and has shown considerable variations between clinicians and across institutions and remains controversial.[14] Theoretically, however, there is a rationale for considering that the timing of RRT might affect the outcome of critically ill patients with severe AKI. Specifically, the timing of RRT might affect the control of uremia, acidemia, electrolyte imbalances, extracellular volume expansion, attenuation of inflammation in sepsis-associated ARF, or all of these.[15-19] These physiological effects might then translate into a clinically important impact on patient outcomes. Gettings and colleagues[15] addressed this issue in a retrospective single-center study of trauma-related AKI where the absolute values of serum urea were used as criteria for start of RRT. These investigators found that "early" RRT (serum urea <21.4 mmol/L) was associated with a shorter stay in hospital and a lower hospital mortality.[18] Data from the BEST Kidney study also show important differences in additional clinically by relevant outcomes when timing was defined by either traditional serum biomarkers or temporally from date of ICU admission. Together, these potentially translate into significant increases in both patient morbidity and health resource utilization. Unfortunately, no sufficiently large randomized controlled trials exist to appropriately assess the issue of timing on outcome.

RENAL RECOVERY AND SEPSIS-ASSOCIATED ACUTE RENAL FAILURE

RRT might contribute to nonrecovery from dialysis dependence, possibly as a result of the occurrence of intratreatment hypotension or perhaps through other mechanisms related to differences in volume and solute control. In the BEST Kidney study, intratreatment hypotension was reported more than twice as often during intermittent hemodialysis (IHD) compared to continuous renal replacement therapy (CRRT) (24.0% vs. 11.1%, respectively).[20] Furthermore, patients who received CRRT were sicker and yet they recovered to dialysis independence more often compared to patients who received IHD. Indeed, logistic

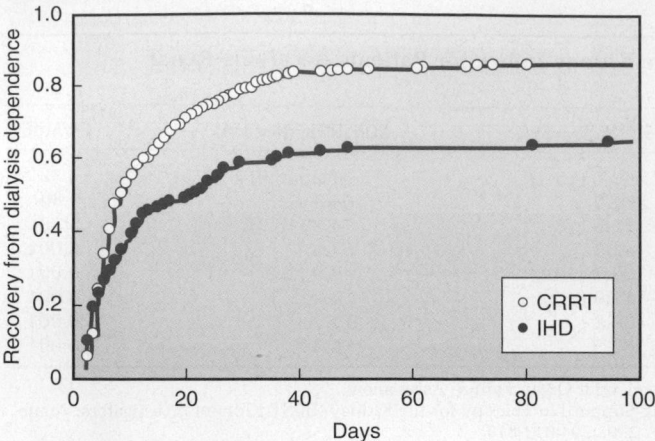

FIGURE 169-1. Inverted Kaplan-Meier graph showing recovery to dialysis independence after acute renal failure according to choice of renal replacement modality. Choice of continuous renal replacement therapy (CRRT) as the first modality of artificial renal support is associated with a greater chance of renal recovery than is intermittent hemodialysis (IHD).

regression analysis showed that CRRT was a significant predictor of recovery to dialysis independence among survivors, with the likelihood of recovery approximately 3 times greater than that seen with IHD (Fig. 169-1).[20] Although patients who received IHD had chronic renal dysfunction more frequently, the logistic regression model confirmed that it remained significant after adjustment of this confounding factor. Furthermore, to exclude the possibility that treatment modality was merely a marker of other center-specific process-of-care variables (i.e., that centers with better resources or more resources used CRRT), the analysis was repeated after excluding sites that performed only one type of therapy. Once again, CRRT remained a robust predictor of dialysis independence at hospital discharge ($p = 0.001$).

These findings are in keeping with previous clinical evidence. In a randomized controlled trial, Mehta and coworkers[21] reported that CRRT was associated with a significantly higher rate of complete renal recovery in the subgroup of surviving patients who received an adequate trial of therapy without crossover (CRRT: 92.3% vs. IHD: 59.4%). Therefore, animal studies, some observational studies, and a randomized study all suggest that IHD might delay or prevent renal recovery when compared to CRRT. This is likely to apply to sepsis-associated ARF as well.

CHOICE OF MODALITY

The issue of choice of modality is important in sepsis-associated ARF, as it is in other forms of ARF. Notwithstanding concerns about the effect of IHD on renal recovery, it is important to note that no randomized controlled trials of sufficient statistical power have addressed the issue of modality in sepsis-associated ARF. In the otherwise relatively small randomized controlled trials conducted so far, there has not been any specific consideration for subpopulations of patients with sepsis-associated ARF. Nonetheless, outside of less developed countries, peritoneal dialysis has been essentially abandoned in adult patients, leaving the debate to the issue of intermittent versus

continuous therapy. However, such therapies have also changed in a dynamic fashion. Recently, for example, intermittent therapy has been adjusted in intensity and duration into a technique broadly known as sustained low-efficiency daily dialysis (SLEDD). On the other hand, CRRT is evolving in dosage from the common 20 mL/kg/hr of urea clearance to the now widely recommended 35 mL/kg/hr. Two large multicenter randomized controlled trials are currently under way in the United States and Australia and New Zealand to address these important issues. The results are likely to be available in 2008 and 2009.

POTENTIAL IMMUNOLOGICAL EFFECTS OF RENAL REPLACEMENT THERAPY IN SEPSIS

Substantial progress has been made toward understanding the mechanisms whereby sepsis is associated with multiple-organ failure, including acute renal failure. Although hemodynamic factors might play a role in the pathogenesis of sepsis-associated ARF, other mechanisms are likely to be involved, which are immunological, toxic, or inflammatory in nature. Indeed, much clinical and molecular biology research suggests that cytokines and other septic mediators contribute to the pathogenesis of septic shock and multiple-organ failure, including ARF.[22]

The major initial immunological event in the pathogenesis of sepsis-associated ARF appears to be a generalized innate immunological system response to infection, which includes a large array of so-called soluble mediators (proteins, peptides, and lipid-derived products that circulate in blood and have pathophysiological properties). Under physiological conditions, the biological activity of these mediators is under control of specific inhibitors at different levels. In sepsis such immune homeostasis is altered with a large spillover of mediators into the circulation, where they exert autocrine and paracrine pro-inflammatory and immunosuppressive effects.[22-25]

Given the fact that many of these mediators are water soluble, present in plasma, and probably of pathophysiological significance, it has been suggested that their removal and a decrease in their concentration in blood may be beneficial.

In creating new concepts of blood purification therapy, clinicians have carefully considered the nature (targets, timing, and self-regulation) of the immune response to infection to achieve the restoration of near-normal hemodynamic and immunological homeostasis, perhaps by decreasing the peak concentration of several cytokines at different time intervals. This concept of cutting peaks of soluble mediators, for example, through continuous hemofiltration, has been called the *peak concentration theory* by Ronco and colleagues.[26]

The vast majority of cytokines are free, nonprotein-bound, water-soluble substances of middle molecular weight (8-51 kD), which are often eliminated by the kidney. These properties make them potentially removable by RRTs, such as hemofiltration.[27] Recently, these conventional tasks of RRT in sepsis-associated ARF have been extended to a new concept of blood purification which includes the aim of removing septic mediators.

In fact, hemofiltration can affect a wide array of inflammatory mediators, and virtually every known cytokine can be removed by it to some degree. However, hemofiltration would most likely only affect the circulating pool of septic mediators rather than significantly reducing local concentrations where their activity may be needed.

Second, this strategy has the capacity to autoregulate such that, as one compound of the response increases, so too does the effect on that compound by hemofiltration.

Third, as hemofiltration is provided in continuous mode, its effect might not depend on the identification of an ideal time point for intervention.

Fourth, sepsis does not fit a one-hit model but shows complex and multiple rises in mediator levels that change over time. Neither single-mediator directed nor one-time interventions therefore seem appropriate. This would also favor hemofiltration.

Fifth, as the ability of hemofiltration to remove substances of middle molecular weight is determined mostly by pore size–based exclusion, it is nonspecific in nature. Thus, one of the major criticisms attributed to continuous blood purification therapy in sepsis—its lack of specificity—could turn out to be a major strength.

Finally, since ARF is a frequent part of sepsis-associated multiple-organ failure, blood purification by RRT would be undertaken anyway. In addition to removing excess fluid and waste products, slightly modified hemofiltration may provide a simple adjunctive treatment option in patients with sepsis, preventing tissue and organ damage (see Chapter 170).

DOES PRACTICE REFLECT THEORY?

The issue of the true capability of hemofiltration to remove septic mediators has remained controversial. Numerous studies have shown that hemofiltration with commonly used synthetic high-flux membranes (nominal cutoff point 30-40 kD, estimated in vivo cutoff point 15-25 kD; cutoff point defined by convention as sieving coefficient of 0.1) can extract nearly every substance involved in the pathogenesis of sepsis to a certain degree.[28-31] Regarding plasma cytokines, however, decreases in concentration appear minor in extent. In fact, some studies could not show any influence of hemofiltration on circulating cytokines.[32] These observations have suggested the need to modify RRT technology in sepsis-associated ARF.

Approaches to achieve higher removal rates of septic mediators by hemofiltration are to increase ultrafiltration rate or increase the porosity of membranes.

Even using current technology, increasing ultrafiltration rates might add clinically important benefits, as suggested by Ronco and colleagues.[33] The degree of hemofiltration could be increased further (high-volume hemofiltration) to optimize blood purification in patients with sepsis. This approach has been tested in animal studies and pilot studies in humans, and promising results have been reported.[34-36] A phase II randomized controlled study is now under way.

EVOLVING TECHNOLOGY IN SEPSIS-ASSOCIATED ACUTE RENAL FAILURE

In spite of some encouraging results, useful convective removal of mediators from the human septic circulation has not been achieved to date, probably because many cytokines have a molecular weight above the true cutoff point of commercially available membranes when used in the clinical setting. Thus, the extent of achievable clinical benefit with conventional hemofiltration (conventional filters and flow rates) in sepsis has generally been disappointing.[32] Also, standard hemofiltration membranes, even when used in high-volume hemofiltration mode, demonstrate little removal by either convection or diffusion.[31] This is most likely attributable to the limited pore size of standard membranes. Several animal and human investigations have demonstrated that clinicians' ability to remove middle molecules (especially those >5 kD, such as cytokines and complement compounds) is limited when using current technology.

Higher removal of middle-molecular-weight substances could be achieved by increasing the porosity of membranes primarily by means of enlarging their pore size.

Such an increase in pore size would approximate the size of filtration pores of the glomerular basal membrane. This approach specifically aims to increase the clearance of larger septic mediators (approximately 15-51 kD). This additional task for RRT is most likely needed in those patients with sepsis-associated ARF who are not able to excrete septic mediators.

Recently, such high cutoff–point (HCO) membranes have been developed and tested with promising results. HCO membranes have an estimated industrial or nominal cutoff point of 100 to 150 kD and an estimated in vivo cutoff point of 60 kD, whereas conventional membranes appear to have an estimated nominal cutoff point of 25 to 40 kD and an estimated in vivo cutoff point of 15 to 20 kD.

Apart from an increased cutoff point, most HCO membranes use the same process of manufacture and chemical composition as conventional or commercially available membranes.

HCO membranes were found to have greater cytokine removal capacity compared to standard high-flux membranes in *ex vivo* experiments,[37] animal experiments,[38] and preliminary clinical studies.[39]

In a 100% lethal animal model, Lee and coworkers[38] found improved partial pressure of arterial oxygen (PaO_2), reduced platelet loss, and a smaller increase in liver enzymes but mainly a prolonged survival in HCO hemofiltration–treated animals compared to controls. In these animal models the authors speculated that their findings were most likely explained by removal of "cardiodepressant" or other septic mediators exclusively removed by HCO membranes.

To date, 84 patients have been enrolled in three trials comparing HCO membranes of identical type with standard high-flux membranes in patients with sepsis-induced ARF. In these studies, continuous venovenous hemofiltration was used as RRT.[39-41]

In all studies, blood flow was set at 150 mL/min and filtration flow ranged from 17 to 42 mL/min. Study duration was between 2 and 5 days. Maximum interleukin-6 (IL-6) clearance was 40 mL/min and maximum interleukin-1 receptor antagonist (IL-1ra) clearance was 42 mL/min. A significant reduction in levels of circulating IL-6 (AUC) was achieved with HCO membranes. Also, in a recent study, Morgera and colleagues[39] found a significant reduction of plasma IL-6 and IL-1ra levels for patients treated with HCO hemofiltration from baseline to end of treatment, whereas values remained unchanged within the control group treated with a standard high-flux membrane. HCO hemofiltration restored reduced peripheral blood mononuclear cell (PBMC) proliferation back into normal range, whereas standard hemofiltration did not. When HCO filtrate of patients with sepsis was incubated *ex vivo* with PBMC from healthy volunteers, PBMC proliferation was reduced, whereas neither standard filtrates of patients with sepsis nor HCO filtrates of healthy volunteers reduced such proliferation. In a similar fashion, a beneficial effect on the phagocytosis rate of polymorphonuclear leukocytes (PMNs) of patients with sepsis could be demonstrated.

Compared to standard hemofiltration, HCO hemofiltration was associated with a significant relative reduction in the requirement of norepinephrine infusion in patients with sepsis-associated ARF.

Data on replacement of albumin and coagulation factors is small, but HCO does not appear to be associated with increased need for substitution. However, there have been no studies of sufficient statistical power to detect differences in survival.

CONCLUSION

The application of RRT to sepsis-associated ARF poses unique challenges and has unique pathophysiological goals. Although particular choices of timing, modality, and membrane or filtration technology can be shown to affect biological events and pathophysiological states in vitro, in experimental animals, and in humans, no randomized controlled trials of sufficient quality and statistical power exist to guide clinicians in their choice of RRT, and changes in clinical outcome remain elusive. Accordingly, at this time, although the use of early intervention and continuous therapy appear physiologically and pathophysiologically more rational, they cannot be strongly recommended due to lack of convincing clinical data. Finally, new technologies such as high-volume hemofiltration and high cutoff hemofiltration remain experimental.

Key Points

1. The application of renal replacement therapy in sepsis-associated acute renal failure poses unique challenges.
2. Preservation of homeostasis over the entire period of treatment appears biologically important and physiologically desirable.

3. Early intervention aimed at preventing complications also appears desirable.
4. Choice of modality of renal replacement therapy may affect renal recovery.
5. There is insufficient evidence to recommend any particular modality of treatment in sepsis-associated acute renal failure.
6. Immunological modulation appears important but has not been achieved to a sufficient degree with commercially available technology.
7. New technologies such as high-volume hemofiltration and high cutoff hemofiltration are being studied as new approaches to renal replacement therapy in sepsis-associated acute renal failure.

Key References

8. Phu NH, Hien TT, Mai NT, et al: Hemofiltration and peritoneal dialysis in infection-associated acute renal failure in Vietnam. N Engl J Med 2002;347:895-902.
20. Uchino S, Bellomo R, Kellum JA, et al, for the Beginning and Ending Supportive Therapy for the Kidney (B.E.S.T. Kidney) Investigators Writing Committee: Patient and kidney survival by dialysis modality in critically ill patients with acute kidney injury. Int J Artif Organs 2007;30:281-292.
21. Mehta RL, McDonald B, Gabbai FB, et al, for the Collaborative Group for Treatment of ARF in the ICU: A randomized clinical trial of continuous versus intermittent dialysis for acute renal failure. Kidney Int 2001;60:1154-1163.
35. Honore PM, Jamez J, Wauthier M, et al: Prospective evaluation of short-term, high-volume isovolemic hemofiltration on the hemodynamic course and outcome in patients with intractable circulatory failure resulting from septic shock. Crit Care Med 2000;28:3581-3587.
39. Morgera S, Haase M, Kuss T, et al: Pilot study on the effects of high cut-off hemofiltration on the need for norepinephrine in septic patients with acute renal failure. Crit Care Med 2006;34:2099-2104.

See the companion Expert Consult website for the complete reference list.

CHAPTER 170

Blood Purification for Sepsis

Zhiyong Peng, John A. Kellum, Rinaldo Bellomo, and Claudio Ronco

OBJECTIVES
This chapter will:
1. Introduce the concept of blood purification.
2. Explain the mechanisms of blood purification in sepsis.
3. Evaluate the commonly used blood purification technologies.
4. Discuss the limitations and future directions of blood purification technologies.

Extracorporeal blood purification (EBP) is a treatment in which a patient's blood is passed through a device (e.g., membrane, sorbent) where solute (waste products, toxins) and possibly also water are removed. When fluid is removed, replacement fluid is added. EBP is used primarily in patients with renal failure (a procedure called *renal replacement therapy*). More than a decade ago, it was observed that renal replacement therapy could remove inflammatory mediators from the plasma of septic patients. Subsequently, clinical improvements (e.g., hemodynamics, gas exchange) with hemofiltration were reported in animal studies. A short time later, cytokine removal from the circulation of humans with sepsis was also demonstrated. Furthermore, a survival benefit associated with hemofiltration was reported. With these advances, blood purification as a treatment for human septic shock was born. Since that time many technological advances have occurred, along with substantial changes in medical professionals' basic understanding of sepsis and the inflammatory response. Modifications of existing technologies and new approaches have created a vast array of possible therapies to use or investigate.

MECHANISMS OF BLOOD PURIFICATION IN SEPSIS

Removal of Inflammatory Mediators

The pathophysiology of sepsis is complex and not completely understood. However, it is generally accepted that the circulating pro-inflammatory and anti-inflammatory mediators participate in the complex cascade of events that lead to cell and organ dysfunction and, in many cases, death. These soluble mediators include eicosanoids, leukotrienes, complement components, cytokines, chemokines, coagulation factors, and other potentially important small peptides and vasogenic substances. Multiple attempts have been made to block the inflammatory response. Early efforts to block specifically the pro-inflammatory mediators failed. However, recent successes in patients with severe sepsis have come from a broad spectrum of immunomodulatory effects, such as activated drotrecogin alpha and low-dose corticosteroids, rather than from specific blockers of inflammatory mediators. Moreover, growing evidence suggests that the anti-inflammatory response to sepsis induces immunoparalysis and may be just as, or even more, deleterious compared to the pro-inflammatory response. Thus, the goal of EBP is to restore homeostasis rather than to selectively inhibit pro- or anti-inflammatory mediators.

Most immune mediators are water soluble and fall into the middle-molecular-weight category (roughly 5-50 kD) and hence can theoretically be removed by EBP using standard equipment. EBP technologies can remove these inflammatory mediators via convection, diffusion, or adsorption. The effects are broad-spectrum, auto-regulating, and limited to the circulating pool of inflammatory mediators rather than influencing local tissue concentrations. These advantages provide a powerful rationale for blood purification used in sepsis.

Organ Support

Although the modulation of inflammatory mediators appears to be the major objective of blood purification in sepsis, this therapy also may offer additional physiological benefits, including temperature control, acid-base control, fluid balance control, cardiac support, protective lung support, brain protection, bone marrow protection, and blood detoxification and liver support. The extracorporeal circulation can be a potent modulator of body temperature and overall thermal balance. Negative thermal balance can be obtained depending on the length of blood lines,

room temperature, and the replacement fluid temperature. Cardiac support can be achieved by optimizing fluid balance, reducing organ edema, and restoring preload and afterload to desirable levels. Optimizing the patient's volume state and removing interstitial fluid through the use of extracorporeal therapy may provide additional support to the failing lung. Blood purification may improve the encephalopathy of sepsis by removing uremic toxins and amino acid derivatives and correcting acidemia. Through the removal of uremic toxins, blood purification also offers bone marrow support. Through the combination of membrane separation processes and adsorption mechanisms, the blood purification system is available for detoxification and potentially has some role in liver support.

PURIFICATION TECHNOLOGIES AND THEIR EVALUATION IN SEPSIS

Blood purification therapies designed to remove substances from the circulation now include hemodialysis (continuous high-flux), hemofiltration (high-flow or ultrafiltration), plasma therapy, hemadsorption, or some combination thereof (Table 170-1). Despite considerable advances in knowledge and technical capability in recent years, there still is no consensus over the optimal method and optimal conditions under which to use these therapies.

Continuous High-Flux Dialysis

Solutes are transported across a semi-permeable membrane generated by a concentration gradient. The extent of clearance is determined by the molecular weight of the solute; the concentration gradient across the membrane; temperature; and the membrane surface area, thickness, and pore size. Small solutes such as urea, creatinine, and electrolytes are cleared efficiently by diffusion. Therefore, conventional hemodialysis is suitable for renal replacement therapy in renal failure. During continuous renal replacement therapy, the addition of countercurrent dialysate flow accomplishes diffusive clearance by maximizing the concentration gradient between blood and dialysate through the length of membrane. Dialysis membranes are further classified based on their ultrafiltration coefficients into high-flux and low-flux membranes. For a given transmembrane pressure gradient, high-flux membranes have a higher filtration rate than do low-flux membranes.

This continuous high-flux dialysis technology uses a highly permeable dialyzer with blood and dialysate following in a countercurrent direction and in which ultrafiltrate production is controlled by a blood pump whereby there is a balance of filtration and backfiltration, with ultrafiltrate produced in the proximal portion of the fibers and reinfused by backfiltration in the distal portion of the fibers so that replacement fluid is not required. It was developed mainly to optimize the clearance of middle molecules without compromising the clearance of urea, and it is available for use in sepsis. Unfortunately, there are limited studies on the use of continuous high-flux dialysis as a mode of blood purification in human sepsis. Early studies have shown cytokine removal, however, and

TABLE 170-1

Comparison of Commonly Used Technologies in Sepsis

TECHNOLOGIES	PRINCIPLES	FLUID BALANCE	PARAMETERS	COMMENTS
CVVH	Convection	Ultrafiltrate replaced by replacement solution	Q_B: 50-200 mL/min Q_{UF}: 20-35 mL/min K: 12-36 L/24 hr	High Q_{UF} needed to achieve meaningful cytokine removal
CHFD	Diffusion and convection	Replacement not required	Q_B: 50-200 mL/min P_F: 2-8 mL/min Q_D: 50-200 mL/min K: 40-60 L/24 hr	Limited data in sepsis
CPFA	Plasma filtration (convection) and hemadsorption	Maintained	Q_B: 50-200 mL/min P_F: 20-30 mL/min	Requires plasma separation
TPE	Plasma filtration/exchange	Replaced with donor plasma	Q_B: 100-180 mL/min P_F: 39-82 mL/min	Sepsis with hematological and other plasma-borne humoral diseases

CHFD, continuous high-flux dialysis; CPFA, coupled plasma filtration adsorption; CVVH, continuous venovenous hemofiltration; K, clearance (urea); P_F, flow of plasma filtration; Q_B, blood flow; Q_D, flow of dialysate; Q_{UF}, flow of ultrafiltrate; TPE, therapeutic plasma exchange.

so the potential to exploit this therapy for sepsis certainly exists.[1]

High-Volume Hemofiltration

Hemofiltration is achieved by convective clearance, in which solutes are transported across a semi-permeable membrane, along with movement of solvent (ultrafiltration) that occurs in response to a positive transmembrane pressure gradient. Here, the clearance depends on the ultrafiltration rate and sieving characteristics of the membrane and solute and, to a lesser extent, on the molecular size of the solute. Studies comparing convective clearance and diffusive clearance have shown that middle-molecular-weight substances and large molecules are better removed by convection. Although most of the inflammatory mediator molecules fall in the middle-molecular-weight category and theoretically can be removed by hemofiltration, they have very high generation rates relative to uremic toxins. Thus, the intensity of blood purification and the beneficial effects have been relatively modest with the traditionally used effluent flow rates of 1 to 2 L/hr. It is generally agreed that conventional hemofiltration is not effective for treatment of sepsis. Subsequently, investigators seeking to achieve "adequate blood purification" in sepsis hypothesized that higher ultrafiltration rates would be necessary. Defined by an ultrafiltration flow rate in excess of 35 mL/kg/hr and often as high as 75 to 120 mL/kg/hr, high-volume hemofiltration (HVHF) may be necessary to achieve clinically meaningful convective removal of inflammatory mediators. To achieve HVHF, it is necessary to use a high permeability membrane with a large surface area and sieving coefficient close to 1 for a wide spectrum of molecules.

Numerous studies have shown that synthetic filters used in hemofiltration can extract a wide array of substances involved in sepsis—at least to a certain degree.[1] HVHF has been shown to improve hemodynamics and survival either in endotoxic animal models or in septic patients. However, these studies either involved small numbers of patients or were nonrandomized and uncontrolled. Despite these early promising studies, larger trials looking at HVHF as an adjunctive therapy in human sepsis are needed before such therapy can be routinely advocated. Furthermore, the application of HVHF routinely in humans still raises substantial organizational, technical, and financial difficulties.

Hemadsorption

Hemadsorption is a technique in which a sorbent is placed in direct contact with blood in an extracorporeal circuit. Nonspecific adsorbents, typically charcoal and resins, attract solutes through a variety of forces, including hydrophobic interactions, ionic (or electrostatic) attraction, hydrogen bonding, and van der Waals interactions. By manipulating the porous structure of solid-phase sorbents, it is possible to increase the selectivity of nonspecific adsorbents for particular solutes. In this case, solute molecules are separated according to their size and by their ability to penetrate the porous network of the sorbent materials. The adsorptive capacity for resins and charcoals is often quite high, in excess of 500 m^2 per gram of sorbent. Until recently, poor biocompatibility has been the major clinical limitation of these materials. Newer resin sorbents appear to have solved this issue with the addition of a biocompatible outer layer. In view of the high-molecular-weight adsorption characteristics of sorbents, it is possible to target larger molecules, exceeding the molecular weight cutoff of synthetic high-flux dialysis membranes. This makes sorbents potentially ideal for intervention in sepsis. Sorbents have been applied in combination with different treatment modalities, including being coupled with hemodialysis or coupled with plasma filtration.[2] The choice of modality is based on the properties of the sorbent and the technique used.[3-4]

Plasma Therapy

The term *plasma therapy* encompasses two therapies: plasmapheresis and plasma exchange.[4] Plasmapheresis is a two-step process in which blood is first separated into its components (cells and plasma) by means of a centrifugal pump or filter. Then the separated plasma is allowed to flow along column(s) containing different adsorbents, allowing the selective removal of components, and the processed plasma is reinfused in the patient. Hence, in plasmapheresis, no (or minimal) replacement fluids are necessary. However, plasma exchange is a single-step process in which blood is separated into plasma and cells similarly through the use of centrifugation pumps or a filter, and the cells are returned to the patient while the plasma is replaced with either donor plasma or albumin. Replacing volume lost with fresh frozen plasma is also done to replete any factor(s) (immunoglobulins) necessary to restore homeostasis and often to correct the underlying disorder for which the plasma therapy was prescribed. Simply put, plasma exchange is used to remove "bad" things and replace "good" things, whereas plasmapheresis simply removes harmful substances. It has been argued that plasma therapy is most likely to be effective in patients with sepsis-associated thrombotic microangiopathy.[5-6] *Plasma filtration* is an imprecise term because it can be used to perform either plasmapheresis (if the treated plasma is reinfused) or plasma exchange (if donor plasma is used). Plasma exchange using filtration has advantages over centrifugal plasma exchange in that it is less expensive and can be performed with the same machines used for continuous renal replacement therapy. Recent animal studies and clinical trials show plasma filtration and/or adsorption are promising blood purification technologies in sepsis.[7-14] To overcome the shortcomings of plasma filtration and improve the removal efficiency, a technology called *coupled plasma filtration adsorption* (CPFA) uses an activated charcoal sorbent cartridge placed in series with, but downstream of, the plasma filter.[2] CPFA improves the removal of nonspecific mediators. Another kind of sorbent cartridge is an immunosorbent column with mono- or polyclonal antibody-coated resin through which filtered plasma is pumped. This set-up, called *coupled plasma filtration immunoadsorption*, could improve the removal of specific mediators.

INDICATION AND INTERVENTION OUTCOMES

Even though available blood purification technology has no proven value in sepsis, patients with refractory septic shock often benefit from the blood purification intervention, at least in terms of improvement in blood pressure. Furthermore, some humoral immuonopathogenic diseases that can complicate sepsis, such as thrombotic thrombocytopenic purpura and thrombocytopenia-associated multiple-organ failure, respond to plasma therapy.

Possible physiological and biological outcomes for the blood purification therapy include improved organ dysfunction (cardiopulmonary and renal function), decreased need for vasopressor drugs, improved vital signs, improved acid-base homeostasis, and decreased cell toxicity of plasma and blood levels of mediators. Among these mediators, interleukin-6 and procalcitonin appear to show the tightest correlation with clinical outcome and might be particularly useful markers in sepsis. For thrombotic thrombocytopenic purpura and thrombocytopenia-associated multiple-organ failure, removal of ultralarge von Willebrand factors and possibly other mediators is essential.[8]

CONCLUSION

Although this wider approach to blood purification in sepsis seems logical and promising and opens new perspectives, many questions still remain unanswered, including the timing, duration, and frequency of these therapies in the clinical settings. Current technologies still remain inadequate for the removal of middle-molecular-weight substances and the current practice worldwide is extremely variable. Moreover, there is lack of large-scale randomized clinical trials.

To address these limitations, several approaches are worthy of further investigation. One of them would be to increase the porosity of membranes to improve middle molecular clearance. Such high-porosity hemofiltration has now been tested in animals with promising results. Increasing ultrafiltration rates (HVHF) to an optimized range would produce clinically important benefits in septic patients. Large multicenter trials evaluating the efficacy of these therapies to improve valid clinical outcomes (i.e., mortality or organ failure), rather than surrogate markers such as mediator clearance or transient improvement in physiological variables, are required to define the precise role of these therapies in the management of sepsis.

Key Points

1. There is currently a clear biological rationale for blood purification used in sepsis. Immunomodulation and organ support play important roles in the application of blood purification.
2. Conventional continuous venovenous hemofiltration and hemodialysis have been shown not to be effective in sepsis in the absence of concomitant acute renal failure.
3. Plasma therapies, high-volume hemofiltration, hemadsorption, or combinations of these therapies appear promising.
4. Multicenter randomized controlled trials are needed to test these promising blood purification technologies.

Key References

2. Bellomo R, Tetta C, Ronco C: Coupled plasma filtration adsorption. Intensive Care Med 2003;29:1222-1228.
4. Venkataraman R, Subramanian S, Kellum JA: Clinical review: Extracorporeal blood purification in severe sepsis. Critical Care 2003;7:139-145.
7. Kellum JA, Song M, Venkataraman R: Hemoadsorption removes tumor necrosis factor, interleukin-6, and interlekun-10, reduces nuclear factor-κB DNA binding, and improves short-term survival in lethal endotoxemia. Crit Care Med 2004;32:801-805.
8. Nguyen T, Stegmayr BG, Busund R, et al: Plasma therapies in thrombotic syndromes. Int J Artif Org 2005;28:459-465.

See the companion Expert Consult website for the complete reference list.

Acute Intoxication and Poisoning

Basic Physiology

CHAPTER 171

Characteristics, Pathophysiology, and Effects of Common Toxic Substances

Babak Mokhlesi and Ryan C. Kamp

OBJECTIVES

This chapter will:

1. Summarize current knowledge regarding the wide variety of toxins and the clinical presentations of poisoning.

2. Review the general signs and symptoms of common toxic ingestions—toxidromes.

3. Present an overview of the basic pathophysiology of the most commonly encountered toxins.

The diagnosis of acute intoxication challenges even the most talented clinicians; in many cases, therefore, a high index of suspicion is required to make the diagnosis (Table 171-1). The epidemiology of poisonings in the United States is recorded annually by poison control centers, and a summary of the most common causes of poisoning is presented in Table 171-2. The signs, symptoms, and laboratory aberrations that occur with intoxications are as varied as the toxins themselves, and the recognition of specific toxidromes can be extremely helpful in making the diagnosis. These toxidromes are presented in Table 171-3. The practice of routinely admitting poisoned patients to the intensive care unit (ICU) has been questioned.[1] Certain clinical risk factors can predict the need for critical care monitoring and intervention (Table 171-4).[2,3] Ultimately, the clinician's judgment may be superior to strict admission criteria.

This chapter examines the basic pathophysiology and clinical presentation of specific poisons. Diagnostic strategies and therapeutic interventions are described in greater detail in later chapters and are therefore mentioned only briefly here.

ACETAMINOPHEN

According to the 2005 American Association of Poison Control Centers annual report, acetaminophen (paracetamol) is the most common medicinal overdose reported to poison information centers. Acetaminophen, alone or in combination with other drugs, was involved in 138,000 overdoses in the United States in 2005. Over 77,000 of these cases were treated in health care facilities; 20,257 of the patients received *N*-acetylcysteine either in oral or intravenous forms, 333 of whom died.[4] Fatal hepatic injury is the most serious complication of acetaminophen toxicity. In a multicenter, prospective study by Larson and associates that included 662 patients with acute liver failure, 42% of the cases were due to acetaminophen ingestion.[5] Of these 275 patients, 178 (65%) survived, 74 (27%) died, and 23 (8%) underwent liver transplantation. Among patients with acute fulminant hepatic failure who do not receive liver transplantation, survival is highest among those with acetaminophen-induced fulminant hepatic failure.

After oral ingestion, acetaminophen is rapidly absorbed, achieving peak plasma levels in less than an hour. The liver is the primary site of metabolism, utilizing mainly glucoronidation as well as sulfation. Sulfation is an additional important pathway in young children. Extended-release acetaminophen preparations demonstrate a longer elimination half-life (up to 12 hours, compared with 2 to 4 hours for immediate-release preparations), owing to a longer absorption phase.

The toxicity of acetaminophen results from a metabolite, *N*-acetyl-*p*-benzoquinonimine (NAPQI), which is produced by the hepatic cytochrome P-450 mixed-function oxidase enzyme system and constitutes only 5% of acetaminophen metabolism.[6] At usual therapeutic doses, NAPQI is rapidly

TABLE 171-1

Most Lethal Human Toxin Exposures Reported to Poison Control Centers in 2005*

SUBSTANCE/TOXIN CATEGORY	TOTAL ADULT EXPOSURES (% OF ALL ADULT EXPOSURES)	TOTAL DEATHS PER CATEGORY INCLUDING CHILDREN AND ADULTS[‡]
Analgesics	126,901 (15%)	696
Sedatives/hypnotics/antipsychotics	101,853 (12%)	384
Antidepressants	65,573 (7.7%)	317
Stimulants and street drugs	23,238 (2.7%)	253
Cardiovascular drugs	49,096 (5.8%)	234
Alcohols (ethanol and nonethanol)	44,173 (5.2%)	131

*Data obtained from cases reported by 61 poison control centers during 2005. Not all poisonings and intoxications are reported to poison control centers.[4]
[‡]Number of deaths is based on an unlimited number of substances coded per exposure.

TABLE 171-2

Common Toxidromes

TOXIDROME	FEATURES	DRUG OR DRUG CLASS/TOXIN	DRUG TREATMENT
Anticholinergic	"Hot as a hare, dry as a bone, red as a beet, mad as a hatter" Mydriasis Blurred vision Fever Dry skin Flushing Ileus Urinary retention Tachycardia Hypertension Psychosis Coma Seizures Myoclonus	Antihistamines Atropine Baclofen Benztropine Tricyclic antidepressants Phenothiazines Propantheline Scopolamine Methylpyroline	Physostigmine (for life-threatening events, not to be used in cyclic antidepressant overdose because of potential for worsening conduction disturbances)
Cholinergic	"SLUDGE" *S*alivation *L*acrimation *U*rination *D*iarrhea *G*astrointestinal cramps *E*mesis Wheezing Diaphoresis Bronchorrhea Bradycardia Miosis	Carbamate Organophosphates Physostigmine Pilocarpine	Atropine Pralidoxime for organophosphates
β-Adrenergic	Tachycardia Hypotension Tremor	Albuterol Caffeine Terbutaline Theophylline	Beta blockade (caution in asthmatics) Potassium replacement
α-Adrenergic	Hypertension Bradycardia Mydriasis	Phenylephrine Phenylpropanolamine	Treat hypertension with phentolamine or nitroprusside; not with beta blockers alone
β-Adrenergic and α-adrenergic	Hypertension Tachycardia Mydriasis Diaphoresis Dry mucous membranes	Amphetamines Cocaine Ephedrine Phencyclidine Pseudoephedrine	Benzodiazepines
Sedative-hypnotic	Stupor and coma Confusion Slurred speech Apnea	Anticonvulsants Antipsychotics Barbiturates Benzodiazepines Ethanol Meprobamate Opiates	Naloxone Flumazenil Urinary alkalinization for phenobarbital

TABLE 171-2

Common Toxidromes—cont'd

TOXIDROME	FEATURES	DRUG OR DRUG CLASS/TOXIN	DRUG TREATMENT
Hallucinogenic	Hallucinations Psychosis Panic Fever Mydriasis Hyperthermia Synesthesia	Amphetamines Cannabinoids Cocaine LSD Phencyclidine (patient may present with miosis)	Benzodiazepines
Extrapyramidal	Rigidity/tremor Opisthotonos Trismus Hyperreflexia Choreoathetosis	Haloperidol Phenothiazines Risperidone Olanzapine	Diphenhydramine Benztropine
Narcotic	Altered mental status Slow shallow breaths Miosis Bradycardia Hypotension Hypothermia Decreased bowel sounds	Dextromethorphan Opiates Pentazocine Propoxyphene	Naloxone
Serotonin	Irritability Hyperreflexia Flushing Diarrhea Diaphoresis Fever Trismus Tremor Myoclonus	Fluoxetine Meperidine Paroxetine Sertraline Trazodone Clomipramine	Benzodiazepine Withdrawal of drug Cyproheptadine

Epileptogenic	Hyperthermia
	Hyperrreflexia
	Tremors
	May mimic stimulant pattern
		Strychnine
		Nicotine
		Lindane
		Lidocaine
		Cocaine
		Xanthines
		Isoniazid
		Chlorinated hydrocarbons
		Anticholinergics
		Camphor
		Phencyclidine
			Antiseizure medications
			Pyridoxine for isoniazid toxicity
			Extracorporeal removal of drug
			  (lindane, camphor xanthines)
			Physostigmine for anticholinergic
			  agents
			Avoid phenytoin for
			  theophylline-induced seizures

Solvent	Lethargy Confusion Headache Restlessness Incoordination Derealization Depersonalization	Hydrocarbons Acetone Toluene Naphthalene Trichloroethane Chlorinated hydrocarbons	Avoid catecholamines Withdrawal of toxin

Uncoupling of oxidative phosphorylation	Hyperthermia
	Tachycardia
	Metabolic acidosis
		Aluminum phosphide
		Salicylates
		2,4-Dichlorophenol
		Dinitrophenol
		Glyphosate
		Phosphorus
		Pentachlorophenol
		Zinc phosphide
			Sodium bicarbonate for metabolic
			  acidosis
			Patient cooling
			Avoid atropine and salicylates
			Hemodialysis in refractory
			  acidosis

LSD, lysergic acid diethylamide.

and irreversibly detoxified through conjugation with the sulfhydryl group of glutathione and then excreted by the kidneys as mercapturic acid and cysteine conjugates. In overdose, however, the supply of glutathione becomes depleted, and NAPQI cannot be detoxified. NAPQI then binds to macromolecules of hepatocytes, inducing centrilobular hepatic necrosis with periportal sparing.[7] The binding of NAPQI to cellular proteins, including mito-

chondrial proteins, may lead to dysfunction of mitochondrial respiration as well as ATP depletion, inducing further injury by oxidative stress.[8] The production of NAPQI occurs in the liver, making it the primary target of toxicity; but other organs can be affected. The toxic threshold with the potential to produce liver damage is 150 mg/kg or 7.5 to 10 g in healthy adults and 200 mg/kg in children (due to enhanced sulfation).[9-11] Ingestion of only 4 to 6 g of

TABLE 171-3

Clinical Features Mandating Consideration of Toxic Ingestion

Past history of drug overdose or substance abuse
Suicidal ideation or previous suicide attempt
History of other psychiatric illness
Agitation and hallucinations
Stupor or coma
Rotary nystagmus
Delirium or confusion
Seizures
Muscle rigidity
Dystonia
Cardiopulmonary arrest
Unexplained cardiac arrhythmia
Hypertension/hypotension
Ventilatory failure
Aspiration
Bronchospasm
Liver failure
Renal failure
Hyperthermia/hypothermia
Rhabdomyolysis
Osmolal gap
Anion gap acidosis
Hyperglycemia/hypoglycemia
Hypernatremia/hyponatremia
Hyperkalemia/hypokalemia
Polypharmacy

TABLE 171-4

Criteria for Admission of the Poisoned Patient to the Intensive Care Unit

Respiratory depression ($PaCO_2 > 45$ mm Hg)
Emergency intubation
Seizures
Cardiac arrhythmia (second- or third-degree atrioventricular block)
Systolic blood pressure <80 mm Hg
Unresponsiveness to verbal stimuli
Glasgow Coma Scale score <12
Need for emergency dialysis, hemoperfusion, or ECMO
Increasing metabolic acidosis
Pulmonary edema induced by toxins (including inhalation) or drugs
Hypothermia or hyperthermia including neuroleptic malignant syndrome
Tricyclic or phenothiazine overdose manifesting with anticholinergic signs, neurological abnormalities, QRS duration >0.12 second or QT duration >0.5 second
Exposure related to body packing/body stuffing
Emergency surgical intervention
Administration of pralidoxime in organophosphate toxicity
Need for continuous infusion of naloxone
Hypokalemia secondary to digitalis overdose (or need for digoxin-immune antibody Fab fragments)

ECMO, extracorporeal membrane oxygenation.

acetaminophen may be enough to cause toxicity in some higher-risk patients such as chronic alcohol users, patients with induced cytochrome P-450 enzymes, malnourished persons, and patients with depleted glutathione stores (for example, recent sublethal acetaminophen ingestion).[12,13] These patients either have decreased ability to detoxify the NAPQI (in alcoholics and the malnourished) or an increased rate of production of NAPQI (in those with induced cytochrome P-450 enzymes).

Acetaminophen toxicity is divided into four phases.[9] Most frequent signs and symptoms in phase I, usually occurring in the first 24 hours, are anorexia, malaise, pallor, diaphoresis, nausea, and vomiting. Phase II occurs during the 24 to 48 hours after untreated overdose. This phase is notable for right upper quadrant pain and abnormalities on liver function tests; these will occur even while signs and symptoms of phase I resolve. Patients progressing to phase III (48 to 96 hours) display symptoms of severe hepatotoxicity, including encephalopathy, coagulopathy, and hypoglycemia. Liver function abnormalities typically peak during this period, usually showing extreme elevations in alanine aminotransferase (ALT) and aspartate aminotransferase (AST) (10,000 IU/L or higher), and total bilirubin and prolongation of prothrombin time. The rise in transaminases tends to be disproportionate to the rise in total bilirubin, helping to differentiate acetaminophen-induced hepatotoxicity from viral hepatitis, biliary ob-struction, and cholestatic disease. Rarely, phase III of acetaminophen overdose may include hemorrhagic pancreatitis, myocardial necrosis, and acute renal failure. Acute renal failure results from acute tubular necrosis induced by the acetaminophen itself.[14] Rarely does it occur without the presence of fulminant hepatic failure.[15] Despite treatment with N-acetylcysteine, the renal failure may not be prevented.[16] Phase IV describes the period beyond 96 hours after ingestion. During this period, the patient may fully recover (without chronic liver disease) or may require emergency liver transplantation, or may expire. Hepatic enzyme levels that decline may signal recovery or continued massive hepatocellular necrosis. The latter is associated with rising prothrombin time and bilirubin and ammonia levels. If it occurs, recovery will be significant by 5 to 7 days after ingestion.

Investigators from King's College Hospital Liver Unit demonstrated that an Acute Physiology and Chronic Health Evaluation (APACHE) II score[17] of 15 or higher provided an accurate estimation of risk of in-hospital death and identified patients in need of transfer for possible transplantation in the setting of acetaminophen-induced acute liver failure. Because intensivists are more familiar with APACHE II than with specialist liver scores (e.g., King's criteria), this may expedite appropriate transfer to liver units.[18,19]

ALCOHOLS

The most commonly ingested nonethanol alcohols include ethylene glycol, methanol, and isopropanol. Ethylene glycol is odorless and tastes sweet. Products that contain ethylene glycol, such as antifreeze, deicers, and industrial solvents, usually contain an added blue or green fluorescent dye. The presence of the dye explains the occasional positive urinary fluorescence under Wood's lamp.[20] This method of detection is of limited clinical usefulness.[21,22] Methanol, also a colorless and odorless liquid, has a bitter taste and is highly volatile. Many paint removers, gas-line antifreeze, windshield washer fluid, and solid canned fuel contain methanol. Isopropanol, a similarly colorless and bitter-tasting alcohol, has an odor of acetone or alcohol. Products such as rubbing alcohol, skin lotions, hair tonics, aftershave, deicers, and glass cleaners may contain isopropanol. These alcohols are themselves weak toxins; however, their metabolic products can be quite toxic.

Intoxication by nonethanol alcohols manifests with signs and symptoms of inebriation in the setting of a low or absent ethanol level, making determination of an ingestion history very important. The cardinal features of ethylene glycol and methanol poisoning include a metabolic acidosis with an elevated anion gap and presence of an elevated osmolal gap.

Ethylene glycol is metabolized by the enzyme alcohol dehydrogenase to glycoaldehyde and glycolic acid; these are further metabolized to glyoxylic acid and oxalic acid. Precipitation of oxalic acid to calcium oxalate and its accumulation in the renal tubules lead to the production of calcium oxalate crystals, further contributing to the development of acute tubular necrosis. Additionally, hypocalcemia (due to precipitation by oxalate) and myocardial dysfunction are features of ethylene glycol poisoning. In an adult patient, ingestion of as little as 100 mL can be lethal. Serum levels greater than 50 mg/dL are associated with significant toxicity.

The clinical course of ethylene glycol poisoning contains three phases: Stage 1 (from 30 minutes to 12 hours after ingestion) includes signs and symptoms of inebriation, ataxia, and seizures, as well as variable levels of elevated anion gap metabolic acidosis with Kussmaul's breathing, elevated osmolal gap, crystalluria, and hypocalcemia. Development of cerebral edema may lead to coma or death. Complications in stage 2 (from 12 to 24 hours) include myocardial dysfunction with high- or low-pressure pulmonary edema. Death during this stage usually results from myocardial dysfunction or aspiration pneumonia. In stage 3 (from 2 to 3 days), acute renal failure usually develops as a result of acute tubular necrosis with an element of tubular obstruction from calcium oxalate precipitation.[23-25] In survivors of later stages (from 6 to 18 days), neurological sequelae also have been described.[26,27]

Methanol also is metabolized by alcohol dehydrogenase, leading to the formation of formaldehyde. Aldehyde dehydrogenase then further converts the formaldehyde to formic acid. Formic acid is the primary toxic metabolite responsible for the metabolic derangements and ocular disturbances observed in methanol poisoning. Intoxication may occur after oral ingestion, inhalation, or even dermal absorption. Again, a small amount, only 30 mL, may lead to significant morbidity. Approximately 150 to 240 mL of 40% solution may lead to death (lethal serum levels, 80 to 100 mg/dL). Methanol ingestion leads to an initial period of headache, inebriation, dizziness, ataxia, and confusion, followed by more pronounced visual symptoms and elevation of the anion gap as formic acid accumulates over 6 to 72 hours. Visual loss or optic nerve swelling on funduscopy also suggests methanol intoxication. Pancreatitis and acute renal failure also have been reported as additional features of methanol poisoning.[28-30] Concomitant ethanol ingestion may delay onset of manifestations of ethylene glycol and methanol ingestion. Alcohol dehydrogenase more rapidly metabolizes ethanol, delaying the production of the toxic metabolites of ethylene glycol and methanol.

The treatment of ethylene glycol intoxication and that of methanol poisoning are very similar.[31] The inhibition of the formation of toxic metabolites and urgent dialytic removal of these alcohols and their metabolites constitute the cornerstones of therapy. Inhibitors of alcohol dehydrogenase include fomepizole (4-methylpyrazole) and ethanol, and their use is described in later chapters.

Finally, isopropanol also is metabolized by alcohol dehydrogenase, leading to the formation of acetone, which is then excreted through the kidneys and by respiration.[32] Signs of ingestion of isopropanol include a combination of ketonemia (sweet-smelling breath, ketones in the urine, and absence of an elevated anion gap or metabolic acidosis), hemorrhagic gastritis, and an elevated osmolal gap. Detection of isopropanol in the serum confirms the diagnosis. Treatment of isopropanol ingestion usually is supportive and is discussed further later on.

AMPHETAMINES

In the United States and the United Kingdom, methamphetamine use has increased rapidly over the past decade, particularly in inner city areas.[33,34] Amphetamine and amphetamine-like prescription drugs such as methylphenidate, dextroamphetamine, and pemoline are used primarily for narcolepsy and hyperactivity-attention deficit disorder. In addition, various anorectic medications used for weight loss, including diethylpropion and phentermine, are derivatives of amphetamines. Illicit drugs include methamphetamine ("crank" or "ice") and 3,4-methylenedioxymethamphetamine (MDMA) (i.e., "ecstasy").[35]

The toxicity of amphetamines is exerted through stimulation of the central nervous system (CNS), peripheral release of catecholamines, inhibition of the reuptake of catecholamines, and inhibition of monoamine oxidase. Molecularly, these chemicals are very similar to the neurotransmitters epinephrine and dopamine. Their biological effects are most similar to those of these chemicals, in addition to serotonin.[36] MDMA, in particular, has significant serotoninergic effects. These compounds generally have a quite narrow therapeutic window. The pharmacokinetics of amphetamines vary with each drug type; however, in the case of MDMA, absorption is very rapid, within the first 2 hours of ingestion.[36]

Overdose of amphetamines usually causes confusion, tremor, anxiety, agitation, and irritability. Mydriasis, tachyarrhythmias, myocardial ischemia, hypertension, hyperreflexia, hyperthermia, rhabdomyolysis, renal failure, coagulopathy, and seizures also may frequently be encountered.[33,37] Additionally, severe hepatotoxicity requiring liver transplantation has been reported with ecstasy abuse.[38,39] Death usually results from complications of hyperthermia, arrhythmias, status epilepticus, intracranial hemorrhage, fulminant liver failure, or aspiration pneumonitis.[37]

BARBITURATES

Barbiturates exert their effect through enhancement of the inhibitory effects of the neurotransmitter γ-aminobutyric acid (GABA), as well as direct GABA receptor stimulation, both leading to antiepileptic effects as well as sedative effects. Phenobarbital is readily absorbed, with a bioavailability greater than 95% when taken orally, and reaches peak plasma levels within 0.5 to 4 hours. In addition, phenobarbital has a prolonged half-life of 3 to 5 days in adults.[40]

Barbiturate overdose, at mild to moderate levels, manifests with reduced level of consciousness, slurred speech, and ataxia. Higher doses cause hypothermia, hypotension, bradycardia, flaccidity, hyporeflexia, coma, and eventually apnea. Patients with severe overdose may appear to be dead, with absence of electroencephalographic activity.

Cardiovascular depression, due to a combination of decreased arterial tone and myocardial depression, leads to a high filling pressure, low cardiac output, and hypotensive state. Barbiturate overdose also leads to respiratory depression, with hypercapnia and hypoxemia being common findings. This impairment usually leads to a mixed respiratory and metabolic acidosis. Not surprisingly, patients who are unresponsive to painful stimuli tend to be significantly more acidemic and hypoxemic than those who show some response to pain, a finding that is not explained by differences in alveolar ventilation alone.[41] Hypoxemia may be aggravated by ventilation-perfusion mismatch or increased capillary permeability, with acute lung injury possibly related to aspiration pneumonitis.

Diagnosing barbiturate overdose usually can be made on clinical grounds and confirmed by urine toxicology screening. Blood levels do correlate with severity, but such findings rarely alter management.[42] Treatment of barbiturate overdose first involves general supportive measures, because no specific antidote is available.

BENZODIAZEPINES

Benzodiazepines are used for a variety of purposes—primarily as hypnotics, anxiolytics, muscle relaxants, and sedatives. The half-life of benzodiazepines can range from 2 hours to several days, depending on the specific drug. These drugs are frequently involved in drug overdoses, because of their widespread use, as either a single agent or in combination with other drugs. Routine urine toxicology screening leads to rapid confirmation of exposure.

Benzodiazepines display their biological effects by enhancing the inhibitory effects of the neurotransmitter GABA; this potentiation leads to generalized CNS depression. Symptoms and signs of overdose range from slurred speech and lethargy to respiratory arrest and coma, depending on the dose and compound ingested. In general, patients who are comatose as a result of benzodiazepine poisoning tend to be hyporeflexic, with small to midsized pupils that do not respond to naloxone administration. Patients will respond to the cautious administration of flumazenil.

BETA BLOCKERS

Beta blockers are competitive antagonists of β-adrenergic receptors. β_1-Adrenergic receptors are found in the heart; β_2-adrenergic receptors are found in the bronchial tree and blood vessels. Some beta blockers (e.g., acebutolol, betaxolol, pindolol, propranolol) have myocardial membrane–stabilizing activity that can cause QRS widening and lead to decreased myocardial contractility.

The mechanism of action of beta blockers, as well as calcium channel blockers, is through the decrease of intracellular calcium in the myocardial cells they affect. This leads to a variety of effects including the slowing of sinoatrial (SA) node automaticity, slower conduction through the atrioventricular (AV) node, and decreased myocardial contractility. Beta blockers constitute a very heterogeneous group of medications with a variety of pharmacokinetic properties and receptor affinities.[43]

Features of beta blocker overdose depend on the drug type, amount and timing of overdose, co-ingestions, and comorbid conditions. The diagnosis usually can be made on clinical grounds; blood levels are available but do not correlate closely with severity of overdose.[44] The risks of development of a cardiovascular morbidity with β-antagonist ingestion include co-ingestion of another cardioactive drug and a beta blocker with myocardial membrane–stabilizing activity (e.g., acebutolol, betaxolol, pindolol, propranolol).[45] In most of the patients (97%) in whom toxicity will develop, manifestations appear within 4 hours of ingestion. Patients who are asymptomatic and have a normal electrocardiogram (ECG) after 6 hours generally do not require ICU monitoring.[46]

Cardiovascular complications of beta blocker toxicity include hypotension, bradycardia, AV block of different degrees, and congestive heart failure, with or without pulmonary edema. Hypotension usually is due to decreased myocardial contractility rather than bradycardia. Other manifestations may include bronchospasm, hypoglycemia, hyperkalemia, lethargy, stupor, coma, and seizures. A risk of seizure is recognized, usually with propranolol, particularly when the QRS complex duration is longer than 100 ms.[47] In a large retrospective review of 52,156 cases of beta blocker overdose, 164 deaths were reported.[48] Propranolol was responsible for the greatest number of toxic exposures (44%) and was implicated as the primary cause of death in a disproportionately higher percentage of fatalities (71%). Cardiac arrest developed in 59% of patients after they reached the attention of health care personnel.

CALCIUM CHANNEL BLOCKERS

Calcium channel blockers function by selectively inhibiting the movement of calcium ions through the membrane of cardiac and vascular smooth muscle during the slow inward phase of excitation-contraction. These agents have cardiovascular effects of variable degree. For example, verapamil has a more negative inotropic effect, whereas nifedipine has more vasodilatory effects. Verapamil and diltiazem depress the sinus node, as well as slowing conduction through the AV node. Hypotension is the most common cardiovascular effect, generally occurring within 6 hours of calcium channel blocker overdose (except in overdose with sustained-release preparations, in which toxicity may not be evident for up to 12 hours). The hypotension usually follows a period of nausea and vomiting. In comparison with beta blocker toxicity, calcium channel blocker–induced hypotension is secondary to peripheral vasodilation, as opposed to myocardial depression. As stated previously, conduction abnormalities are worsened with concurrent beta blocker ingestion[49] and existing cardiovascular disease. In addition to the cardiovascular effects, lethargy, confusion, and coma also have been attributed to calcium channel blocker overdose, although seizures are not common. The influx of calcium also regulates the release of insulin from pancreatic islet cells, and calcium channel blocker overdose can inhibit this process, leading to hyperglycemia.

CYCLIC ANTIDEPRESSANTS

Antidepressants were third after analgesics and sedative-hypnotic-antipsychotic medications as a cause of overdose-related death, according to the most recent report from the American Association of Poison Control Centers. Nearly 50% of antidepressant fatalities were secondary to cyclic antidepressants.[4] Cyclic antidepressants (including the tricyclics, tetracyclics, bicyclics, and monocyclics) continue to be commonly encountered causes of self-poisoning. The tricyclic antidepressants include amitriptyline, desipramine, doxepin, imipramine, nortriptyline, protriptyline, and amoxapine. These drugs most often are used for depression, chronic pain syndromes, obsessive-compulsive disorder, panic and phobic disorders, eating disorders, migraines, insomnia, and peripheral neuropathies. With the development of newer and safer antidepressants, such as the selective serotonin reuptake inhibitors (SSRIs), a decline in the use of cyclic antidepressants is occurring. Tricyclic antidepressant overdoses are more likely to be associated with severe toxicity, admission to the intensive care unit, and death when compared with the newer SSRI antidepressants.[50,51] In overdose, the CNS and cardiovascular system are mainly affected. These drugs have significant anticholinergic effects and inhibit the neural reuptake of norepinephrine or serotonin, leading to the CNS toxicity seen in overdose. Cardiovascular manifestations also stem from anticholinergic effects and inhibition of neural uptake of norepinephrine or serotonin, as well as peripheral α-adrenergic blockade and membrane-depressant effects.

The clinical manifestations of toxicity may be divided into anticholinergic effects, cardiovascular effects, and seizures. Anticholinergic manifestations include mydriasis, blurred vision, fever, dry skin and mucous membranes, lethargy, delirium, coma, tachycardia, ileus, myoclonus, and urinary retention. The cardiovascular toxicity consists of sinus tachycardia as well as prolongation of the QRS, QTc, and PR intervals. Occasionally, sinus tachycardia with an extremely prolonged QRS may be difficult to distinguish from ventricular tachycardia, which also can occur in cyclic antidepressant overdose. Torsades de pointes, however, is relatively rare. Of importance, a limb-lead QRS interval longer than 0.10 second has been shown to predict seizures, and QRS duration over 0.16 second has been associated with ventricular arrhythmias.[52] The degree of interrater agreement in the measurement of QRS interval is adequate to make this measurement a useful part of the overall assessment of toxicity.[53] Although the electrocardiogram (ECG) can neither unequivocally confirm nor rule out impending toxicity, it has value as a bedside tool in combination with other clinical data gathered during patient assessment.[54] Comparatively, a maximal limb-lead QRS duration less than 0.1 second is rarely associated with seizures or ventricular arrhythmias. Various forms of AV block may accompany cyclic antidepressant overdose, most commonly right bundle branch block. Hypotension due to venodilation and a direct drug effect on myocardial contractility also may be features. Seizures may be short-lived and self-limited, or prolonged and refractory to treatment. Neurological deterioration may be abrupt and unpredictable. Metabolic acidosis from seizures or arrhythmias promotes unbinding of the drug from proteins, contributing to increased toxicity.[55]

The diagnosis of cyclic antidepressant overdose depends on a compatible history and clinical features, combined with a high index of suspicion. Cyclic antidepressant overdose should be considered in all patients with QRS prolongation. Confirmation of exposure is available by urine toxicology screening. Blood levels generally are not followed because of the reliability of the QRS duration to predict severity.

Cyclic antidepressant overdose causes death primarily by cardiac toxicity, and death tends to occur in the first 24 hours of arrival. In most cases, clinical manifestations develop within the first 6 hours after ingestion.[56] Patients with altered mental status, seizures, hypotension, metabolic acidosis, and cardiac arrhythmias require ICU monitoring. Patients should remain in the ICU up to 12 hours after discontinuation of all therapeutic interventions and should be asymptomatic and demonstrate a normal ECG and arterial pH before transfer to regular care.[57,58]

γ-HYDROXYBUTYRATE

γ-Hydroxybutyrate (GHB), or sodium oxybate, also known as "liquid ecstasy," "liquid G," the "date-rape drug," and "fantasy," has been used as a recreational drug in the younger population. When first developed, in the 1980s, the drug was promoted to bodybuilders as a growth hormone stimulator and muscle-bulking agent. It was claimed to cause euphoria without a hangover and to increase sensuality and disinhibition with recreational use. Because of this, GHB was banned outside of clinical trials approved by the U.S. Food and Drug Administration (FDA) in 1990. A precursor of GHB, γ-butyrolactone, continued to be available until a recent ban by the FDA.[59,60]

GHB, derived from γ-aminobutyric acid (GABA), is thought to function as an inhibitory transmitter through specific brain receptors for GHB and through GABA receptors.[61,62] Stage IV of non–rapid eye movement sleep (slow-wave deep sleep) has been shown to increase when normal human subjects are given GHB.[63] In narcolepsy, sodium oxybate has been shown in clinical trials to decrease cataplexy, sleep paralysis, hypnagogic hallucinations, and daytime sleep attacks.[64-66]

The clinical manifestations of GHB ingestion are dose-dependent. Tolerance and dependence has developed in patients with regular usage of GHB. Abrupt discontinuation can produce withdrawal delirium and psychosis.[67,68] In lower doses, GHB can induce a state of euphoria. In addition, emesis, hypothermia, symptomatic bradycardia, hypotension, and respiratory acidosis on arterial blood gas analysis all have been described.[69,70] Deep coma and death have been reported with larger overdoses; however, agitation also has been described with GHB toxicity without concomitant stimulant ingestion.[71] The last five years have seen a steady decline in the use of GHB in the United States.[72]

Laboratory diagnosis of GHB ingestion can be challenging. Normal toxicology screens do not include GHB. In cases of drug-facilitated sexual assault, however, it may be important to document GHB ingestion. Specialized laboratories can detect GHB in both urine and blood by gas chromatography–mass spectroscopy.[73,74] GHB also can be detected by hair analysis.[75]

LITHIUM

Lithium, a monovalent cation used for treatment of bipolar affective disorders, is rapidly absorbed through the gastrointestinal tract. Virtually no protein binding occurs, and the volume of distribution is small at 0.66 to 0.8 L/kg. Elimination of lithium is by glomerular filtration, with 80% of excreted lithium undergoing tubular reabsorption. The rate of reabsorption is even higher in states of dehydration. The 18-hour elimination half-life seen in healthy adults is prolonged in the elderly or in patients on long-term therapy.[76] Volume depletion, use of loop diuretics and angiotensin-converting enzyme (ACE) inhibitors, and renal insufficiency commonly precipitate lithium toxicity.[77] Deliberate acute lithium overdosage by ingestion with suicidal intent also is common.[78] Chronic use can result in nephrogenic diabetes insipidus, renal insufficiency, hypothyroidism, and leukocytosis.

The therapeutic index of lithium is quite low (target range, 0.5 to 1.25 mEq/L). Levels above 1.5 mEq/L are common with lithium intoxication and usually are due to unintentional overdose during chronic therapy. Clinical symptoms and intracellular levels of lithium correlate poorly with serum levels of lithium; however, with chronic use and in acute-on-chronic intoxication, the levels correlate more closely. Severe toxicity may occur at a lower serum level in chronic Li ingestion than in acute intoxication. Tremors, ataxia, nystagmus, choreoathetosis, photophobia, and lethargy are indicative of relatively mild intoxication (levels below 2.5 mEq/L). At higher levels of intoxication (2.5 to 3.5 mEq/L), agitation, fascicular twitching, confusion, nausea, vomiting, diarrhea, and signs of cerebellar dysfunction predominate. Worsening neurological dysfunction (seizures, coma), and cardiovascular instability (sinus bradycardia, hypotension) characterize severe toxicity (greater than 3.5 mEq/L). Decreased serum anion gap (less than 6 mEq/L) is an interesting consequence of severely elevated lithium levels and may be an important clue to the diagnosis.

The morbidity and mortality associated with lithium intoxication remain low with adequate therapy.[79] Treatment, including seizure control and use of vasopressors for hypotension refractory to fluids, tends to be supportive.

METHEMOGLOBINEMIA

Methemoglobin, formed by oxidation of circulating hemoglobin, is incapable of binding and transporting oxygen as compared to reduced hemoglobin. Small amounts of methemoglobin are formed by auto-oxidation even under normal circumstances. Reduced cytochrome $b5$ reacts with circulating methemoglobin to restore hemoglobin and oxidized cytochrome $b5$; the red blood cell enzyme NADH–cytochrome $b5$ reductase (methemoglobin reductase) regenerates reduced cytochrome $b5$ and thereby ensures insignificant concentrations of methemoglobin in circulating blood.[80]

Methemoglobinemia may be associated with a variety of etiologic factors including hereditary, dietary or drug-induced, and idiopathic.[81] Acquired methemoglobinemia, which can be severe and life-threatening, generally occurs in the setting of use of oxidant drugs or toxin exposure.

Hemoglobin concentration is cut in half in the presence of 50% methemoglobin concentration. Additionally, the oxyhemoglobin dissociation curve is shifted to the left in methemoglobinemia, thereby interfering with off-loading of oxygen in peripheral tissues. Despite evident cyanosis, patients tend to remain asymptomatic in mild methemoglobinemia (methemoglobin less than 15% of total hemoglobin). In patients with critical coronary artery disease, in whom angina or myocardial infarction may develop in the presence of mild functional anemia, mild methemoglobinemia may be more significant. Dyspnea, headache,

and weakness develop with more profound methemoglobinemia. Severe methemoglobinemia (methemoglobin greater than 60% of total hemoglobin) is associated with confusion, seizures, and death.

Detection of methemoglobinemia can at times be difficult. Arterial blood gas analysis with co-oximetry makes it possible to display the absorption of four or more different wavelengths, allowing the direct measurement of oxyhemoglobin, reduced hemoglobin, carboxyhemoglobin, and methemoglobin levels. By comparison, pulse oximetry estimates oxygen saturation by emitting a red light (wavelength of 660 nm), absorbed mainly by reduced hemoglobin, and an infrared light (wavelength of 940 nm), absorbed by oxyhemoglobin.[82] Methemoglobin absorbs equally at both wavelengths. At high methemoglobin levels (35%), oxygen saturation measured by pulse oximetry tends to regress toward 85% and plateaus at that level despite further increments in methemoglobin level. Thus, if the actual oxygen saturation by co-oximetry is above 85%, then the pulse oximeter will underestimate it; if it is less than 85% by co-oximetry, it will overestimate oxygen saturation.[83] Pulse oximetry may therefore be unreliable in this setting, registering falsely high readings in patients with severe methemoglobinemia and falsely low readings in those with mild methemoglobinemia. In addition, methylene blue also can cause false elevation in methemoglobin levels measured by co-oximetry and pulse oximetry.[84] "Chocolate-colored" venous blood that does not change color on exposure to air is another clue to the presence of methemoglobinemia.[85]

ORGANOPHOSPHATES AND CARBAMATE INSECTICIDES

Organophosphates and carbamates are the active ingredients in most insecticides used in the United States; additionally, they can be used as warfare nerve agents. They are rapidly degraded in the environment, which has led to their relative popularity. Both compounds exert their toxicity through inhibition of acetylcholinesterase (AChE). Organophosphates inhibit AChE irreversibly, whereas carbamate inhibition of AChE is reversible. Inhibition of AChE causes accumulation of acetylcholine at the synapses, giving rise to the cholinergic syndrome. Carbamates, which exhibit poor penetration of the CNS, do not produce CNS toxicity.

Absorption through the gastrointestinal tract accounts for most intoxications. Of note, however, the skin, conjunctiva, and respiratory tract are able to absorb most insecticides. Organophosphates typically are lipophilic and are rapidly absorbed.[86] Most exposures are accidental in the United States, but in some developing countries, organophosphates are commonly used for suicide.[87] In addition, poisoning from contamination of food has occurred.[88] Inadvertent contact with poisoned patients has been reported to have poisoned emergency department personnel.[89]

Clinical manifestations of acute toxicity occur within the first 12 to 24 hours after exposure.[90] Signs and symptoms can be nonspecific but commonly include weakness, blurred vision, nausea, vomiting, headache, abdominal pain, and dizziness. Other signs and symptoms include miosis (affecting 85% of patients), vomiting (58%), salivation (58%), respiratory distress (48%), depressed mental status (42%), and muscle fasciculations (40%).[91] In one large study, tachycardia occurred more often than brady-cardia.[92] Noncardiogenic pulmonary edema, arrhythmias, and conduction abnormalities comprise other cardiac manifestations of toxicity. Additionally, an odor of garlic in the breath or sweat may be noted.

Clinical features secondary to overstimulation of mus-carinic, nicotinic, and central receptors are the hallmark of organophosphate poisoning. Signs and symptoms of muscarinic overstimulation may be prolonged and can be characterized by the acronym SLUDGE (*s*alivation, *l*acri-mation, *u*rination, *d*iarrhea, *g*astrointestinal cramps, and *e*mesis), along with blurred vision, miosis, bradycardia, and wheezing. Nicotinic overstimulation, usually more transient, manifests with muscular weakness and fascicu-lations, progressing to paresis and paralysis, hypertension, and tachycardia. Organophosphates, as opposed to carba-mates, can overstimulate central receptors, inducing anxiety, confusion, seizures, psychosis, and ataxia owing to their ability to pass the blood-brain barrier.

Two principal cholinesterases, red blood cell (RBC) cho-linesterase (i.e., AChE), present in RBCs and nerve endings, and pseudocholinesterase (PChE), found primarily in liver and serum, aid the diagnosis of organophosphate poison-ing. Organophosphates and carbamates inhibit both cho-linesterases, and although clinical toxicity is due primarily to their action on AChE, PChE is more readily quantified. AChE is considered more specific when measured, however. In patients with liver disease, anemia, or malnu-trition, a falsely low PChE may be found. Low PChE also may represent a genetic variant (familial succinylcholine sensitivity). Normal levels of enzyme activity vary widely, therefore, not excluding poisoning. Confirmation of organophosphate exposure, in the absence of baseline plasma AChE levels, can be made with the use of sequen-tial postexposure plasma AChE levels.[93] Typically, levels less than 20% to 50% are seen with severe poisoning. The plasma AChE level, however, may not correlate with severity of intoxication.[94] Because of these limitations, the diagnosis of organophosphate and carbamate poisoning remains primarily a clinical one.

Organophosphate and carbamate poisoning lead to serious complications including respiratory failure, ven-tricular arrhythmias, CNS depression, and seizures. Most patients require 5 to 14 days of intensive care monitoring, on average. Recovery from carbamate poisoning is quicker than from organophosphates. Between 60% and 70% of patients require mechanical ventilation, and the mortality rate has been reported to range from 15% to 36%.[95,96]

PHENCYCLIDINE

Phencyclidine (PCP), also called "angel dust," has variable anticholinergic, opioid, dopaminergic, CNS stimulant, and α-adrenergic effects. It can be delivered by means of a variety of methods, including smoking, nasal inhalation, oral ingestion, and intravenous injection. Co-ingestants such as ethanol, marijuana, and lysergic acid diethylamide (LSD) are frequently encountered.

Behavioral and CNS effects also are quite varied. Akmal and colleagues[97] evaluated 1000 patients presenting with acute PCP intoxication. The incidence of violence was 35%; bizarre behavior was noted in 29% of cases, and agitation in 34% of cases. Only 46% of patients were alert and oriented; the others demonstrated alterations in mental status ranging from lethargy to coma. Nystagmus (which may be vertical or horizontal) and hypertension occurred

in only 57% of cases. Rare manifestations included grand mal seizures, muscle rigidity, dystonic reactions, and athetosis. Diaphoresis, hypersalivation, bronchospasm, and urinary retention occurred in less than 5% of cases. Twenty-eight of the patients (2.8%) were apneic, and 3 patients (0.3%) presented in cardiac arrest. Common findings include hypoglycemia and elevated serum cre-atine kinase (CK), uric acid, and AST and ALT. PCP intoxication complicated by rhabdomyolysis can cause acute renal failure.[97] Additionally, hypertensive crisis[98] and intracranial and subarachnoid hemorrhage have been reported.[99,100]

PCP intoxication should be considered in patients with fluctuating behavior, signs of sympathomimetic overstim-ulation, and vertical nystagmus. PCP toxicity may be sug-gested by the finding of pinpoint pupils. Confirmation of PCP intoxication is by qualitative urine toxicology screen-ing; serum drug levels do not correlate with the severity of clinical findings.[97]

SALICYLATES

Salicylates, most commonly acetylsalicylic acid (aspirin), continue to be frequent ingredients in a variety of prescrip-tion and nonprescription preparations, such as Soma Compound, Norgesic, Trilisate (choline magnesium tri-salicylate), Percodan, Darvon, and Pepto-Bismol (bismuth subsalicylate). Topical products containing salicylates, such as Ben-Gay, salicylic acid (keratolytic), and oil of wintergreen (methyl salicylate) (1 teaspoon contains 7000 mg of salicylate), can cause salicylate toxicity with ingestion.[101,102]

Reliance on alternative analgesics and the use of child-resistant containers have decreased the incidence of salic-ylate poisoning in the pediatric population. Additionally, improvements in packaging and pack size restrictions have reduced the likelihood of severe intentional poison-ings in adults.[103,104]

Acetylsalicylic acid (aspirin) is rapidly converted to salicylic acid, its active moiety, after being ingested. Absorption from the stomach and small bowel also is rapid. The liver metabolizes salicylic acid, and elimina-tion occurs in 2 to 3 hours with therapeutic doses. Serum levels of 10 to 30 mg/dL are considered therapeutic. The half-life increases to more than 20 hours with chronic usage.[105]

Serum levels above 40 mg/dL usually are associated with the development of clinical aspirin toxicity; in chronic intoxication, severe poisoning occurs at lower serum levels (particularly in elderly patients). At toxic levels, salicylates are metabolic poisons that affect a mul-titude of organ systems by uncoupling oxidative phos-phorylation and interfering with the Krebs cycle.[106]

Tinnitus, vertigo, nausea, vomiting, and diarrhea are features in mild cases of toxicity. Respiratory alkalosis or a mixed metabolic acidosis and respiratory alkalosis develop in adults with more significant ingestion.[107,108] Exceptions to this would include co-ingestion of a CNS depressant causing a respiratory acidosis. Respiratory alkalosis occurs through direct central stimulation, in addition, uncoupling of oxidative phosphorylation leads to accumulation of organic acids (including lactic acid and ketoacids) and a metabolic acidosis with elevation of the anion gap. Salicylic acid itself contributes minimally to the measured anion gap (3 mEq/L with a 50-mg/dL level).

Noncardiogenic pulmonary edema, mental status changes, seizures, coma, gastrointestinal bleeding, liver and renal failure, hypoglycemia (including low cerebrospinal fluid glucose), and death also develop with more significant poisoning.[109] Thisted and coworkers described the clinical findings in 177 consecutive admissions to an ICU with acute salicylate poisoning.[110] Neurological abnormalities occurred in 61% of patients, acid-base disturbances in 50%, pulmonary complications in 43%, coagulation disorders in 38%, fever in 20%, and circulatory disorders such as hypotension in 14%. In a two-year review of salicylate deaths in Ontario, 31% of the patients were dead on arrival at the treatment facility.[111] ICU mortality rates for severe salicylate poisoning continue to be high, having been reported to be nearly 15%.[110]

Approximately 10 to 30 g or 150 mg/kg (35 tablets or more) is a lethal dose in adults; however, serum levels correlate poorly with lethality of ingestion. A critical review of the commonly used Done nomogram[105] has revealed that it is of no value in the assessment of acute or chronic salicylism.[112] Its use may be misleading in cases with an incorrect time of ingestion, ingestion of more than a single dose, use of enteric-coated preparations,[113] or long-term use of salicylates. At particular risk for unintentional poisoning are elderly patients and a high index of suspicion is thus required to avoid delays in diagnosis that may contribute to higher mortality.[114] Patients with chronic intoxication commonly present with CNS injury,[115] noncardiogenic pulmonary edema,[116] or isolated elevation of the prothrombin time.

SELECTIVE SEROTONIN REUPTAKE INHIBITORS (SEROTONIN SYNDROME)

Psychiatrists, emergency room physicians, and intensivists should expect to see increasing numbers of patients with serotonin syndrome as a result of their more frequent and widespread usage.[117,118] The increased use of these medications reflects their relatively nontoxic drug profile compared with other antidepressants (such as the tricyclics and monoamine oxidase [MAO] inhibitors).[119] The list of SSRIs and noncyclic serotoninergic antidepressants has been growing rapidly in the past decade: sertraline (Zoloft), paroxetine (Paxil), fluoxetine (Prozac), fluvoxamine (Luvox), citalopram (Celexa), trazodone (Desyrel), nefazodone (Serzone), and venlafaxine (Effexor). Although these agents are relatively nontoxic when taken alone, combinations of MAO inhibitors or tryptophan and either SSRIs or tricyclic antidepressants with serotomimetic effects may result in serotonin syndrome and death.[120] For this reason, SSRI antidepressants should not be combined with MAO inhibitor antidepressants or other agents that have serotomimetic effects.[121,122] Other serotomimetic agents associated with this syndrome include 3,4-methylenedioxy-methamphetamine, dextromethorphan, and meperidine.[123] Serotonin syndrome also has been associated with linezolid and SSRI combination.[124] The presumed pathophysiological mechanism involves brainstem and spinal cord activation of the 1A form of the serotonin (5-hydroxytryptamine [5-HT]) receptor.

Toxic combination therapy may not be apparent for days to weeks owing to the long half-life of some of these medications. Association with a risk for clinically significant drug interactions, in part due to cytochrome P-450 inhibition, is more common with the newer SSRIs.[125,126]

Clinical manifestations can be mild, moderate, or severe.[127] The most frequent features are changes in mental status, restlessness, myoclonus, hyperreflexia, diaphoresis, shivering, tremor, flushing, fever, nausea, and diarrhea. Disseminated intravascular coagulation, convulsions, coma, muscle rigidity, myoclonus, autonomic instability, orthostatic hypotension, and rhabdomyolysis can occur in more severe cases.[121] Other findings include hyponatremia and syndrome of inappropriate antidiuretic hormone secretion (SIADH).[128,129] Fortunately, recovery within 1 day is usual, and death is rare.

The diagnosis, particularly with a history of depression and the use of serotoninergic drugs, should be considered in any patient with compatible clinical features. Additionally, consideration of serotonin syndrome in any agitated patient presenting to the emergency department also is important.[130] Unfortunately, blood and urine assays are currently not readily available and are not part of routine toxicology screening panels.

THEOPHYLLINE

Theophylline is a dimethylxanthine bronchodilator used in the management of patients with obstructive lung disease. It remains an important cause of intoxication with significant morbidity and mortality, despite the decline in its use.[131] A narrow and low therapeutic index, patient and physician dosing errors, and conditions that decrease drug clearance (i.e., drug interactions, smoking cessation, and congestive heart failure or hepatic dysfunction) are the primary reasons for its toxicity.[132] Mild toxicity can occur within the therapeutic range. Significant toxicity generally occurs with plasma levels above 25 mg/L. Acute ingestion or chronic use may lead to intoxication. Chronic intoxication causes more severe clinical sequelae as a result of larger total body stores of drug, compared with the same plasma levels in an acute ingestion.[131,133,134]

Clinical features of theophylline toxicity are divided into neurological, cardiovascular, and metabolic categories.[135] Seizures, less likely in acute intoxication unless levels exceed 80 to 100 mg/L, can occur in chronic intoxication at serum levels of 35 to 70 mg/L.[131,136] Uncontrolled seizures leading to hyperthermia and rhabdomyolysis can occur. Tachyarrhythmias (both supraventricular and ventricular) are associated with theophylline levels of 20 to 30 mg/L. At these serum levels, however, the need for antiarrhythmic therapy is uncommon.[137] With levels over 50 mg/L, cardiovascular collapse can also occur. Hypokalemia, hypomagnesemia, hyperglycemia, hypophosphatemia, hypercalcemia, and respiratory alkalosis are the commonly reported metabolic abnormalities.[138]

CONCLUSION

Intoxications manifest in many forms: known drug overdose or toxic exposure, illicit drug use, suicide attempt, or accidental exposure. A high index of suspicion in addition to familiarity with toxidromes can lead to a rational and systematic approach in critically ill poisoned patients. Early and appropriate admission to an ICU for monitoring and interventions can be lifesaving.

Key Points

1. The clinician must have a high degree of suspicion to identify patients with toxin exposure.
2. Recognition of specific signs and symptoms of individual toxins improves the clinician's ability to make a more rapid diagnosis.
3. The pathophysiology of each toxin is unique, and this knowledge can assist the clinician in making the diagnosis as well as initiating the correct treatment.
4. The clinical risk factors in an individual poisoned patient will predict the need for critical care monitoring and intervention.

Key References

1. Mokhlesi B, Corbridge T: Toxicology in the critically ill patient. Clin Chest Med 2003;24:689-711.
2. Mokhlesi B, Leiken JB, Murray P, et al: Adult toxicology in critical care: Part I: General approach to the intoxicated patient. Chest 2003;123:577-592.
3. Mokhlesi B, Leikin JB, Murray P, et al: Adult toxicology in critical care: Part II: Specific poisonings. Chest 2003;123:897-922.
4. Lai MW, Klein-Schwartz W, Rodgers GC, et al: 2005 Annual Report of the American Association of Poison Control Centers' national poisoning and exposure database. Clin Toxicol (Phila) 2006;44:803-932.
35. Mokhlesi B, Garimella PS, Joffe A, et al: Street drug abuse leading to critical illness. Intensive Care Med 2004;30:1526-1536.

See the companion Expert Consult website for the complete reference list.

Laboratory Tests and Diagnostic Methods

CHAPTER 172

Laboratory Testing in Toxicology

Stephen George

OBJECTIVES

This chapter will:
1. Provide a general overview of the recommended approach to support the clinical diagnosis and management of patients who are suspected of being poisoned.
2. Review the types and range of techniques that are commonly used to determine the presence of a toxicant in a patient, including simple and rapid screening techniques as well as more complex and specific techniques.
3. Summarize possible problems associated with the interpretation of analytical findings subsequent to specimen analysis, and highlight the importance of close liaison between the laboratory and the clinician.
4. Identify the commonly available compounds that may be specifically associated with critical illness and nephrotoxicity, including drugs, chemicals, and herbal remedies.

DECISION-MAKING PROCESS FOR CLINICAL INVESTIGATION OF SUSPECTED POISONING

More than 69,000 hospital admissions requiring 154,000 bed-days due to poisoning by medicine intake were reported in England for the period 2003 to 2004, costing an estimated £54 million (approximately $107 million).[1] These figures illustrate the scale of the problem, which may require toxicological investigations to be performed to aid in the effective diagnosis of poisoned patients. Appropriate laboratory support is recognized to reduce the average length of hospital stay for these patients, especially in complicated cases[2]; however, close clinician-laboratory liaison must be maintained throughout to permit the most effective application of laboratory resources and interpretation of analytical results.[3]

Three main areas must be addressed in the investigation of poisoning. First, it is important to collect as complete a patient history as possible, including identification of any drugs that may have been prescribed by general practitioners or after previous hospital visits; any drugs that may be available in the home or where the patient became unwell; any over-the-counter products that may have been taken; and any herbal or alternative remedies that may be part of the patient's health regimen. This information may be difficult to obtain, especially if the patient is unconscious, but all such information is useful to determine the approach and scope that the investigating laboratory may need to apply. Before the collection of any samples, the laboratory should be provided with details about any medication that may have been given to stabilize the patient's clinical condition, because such agents may then be excluded from any further investigations likely to be performed, or from influencing the interpretation of analytical findings.

Second, it is vital to obtain the required specimens as soon as possible after hospital admission of the patient to maximize the likelihood of detecting any drug or poison. Rapid procurement of specimens is especially important in the case of fast-acting, low-dose, high-potency drugs, such as those associated with drug-facilitated sexual assault.[4] Typically, a urine specimen (approximately 30 mL) collected into a plain sterile container without preservative will be adequate for screening for common drugs, metals, and chemical poisons. In addition, a sample of venous blood (approximately 5 to 10 mL) collected into a lithium heparin container (without gel separator) will allow measurement of the concentration of the toxicant to determine the need for antidotal treatment, if appropriate. It also may be useful to collect a sample into a fluoride oxalate tube for alcohol measurement, especially if the particulars of the case include medicolegal considerations such as involvement in a highway traffic accident. The use of fluoride oxalate as a preservative in a sample will prevent the loss or gain of alcohol that may potentially arise from the effect of microorganism contamination.

Third, provided that all possible information has been gathered regarding the potential exposure of the patient to drugs and poisons (including any medical interventions), and that the required specimens have been collected, the laboratory can start to select which techniques to apply to the case (see later on). In an unconscious patient, common sedative-hypnotic agents would be the primary agents to be considered responsible for the observed condition. Of note, however, patients who are postictal (have just had a seizure) or are exhausted after the binge use of stimulants also may present with this clinical picture—hence the need for a full and comprehensive screen to be performed for each case.

Without complete investigation of each of these three major issues, the nature and identity of the toxicant may never be discovered, and the treatment and management of the patient may rely solely on supportive measures, with the clinical manifestations of the true nature of the poison being observed sometime later.

COMMON TECHNIQUES USED TO DETERMINE POISONING

The laboratory can follow either of two general approaches to the investigation of poisoned patients; in both approaches, results depend primarily on the accuracy of the initial data collected on hospital admission. The first such approach is an *unknown drug screen* (UDS). The general concept of a UDS is to apply a broad range of analytical techniques to determine the presence or absence of drugs commonly taken in overdose. These include illicit drugs, therapeutic agents, and analgesics (Table 172-1). The UDS usually is performed on a urine specimen because this will contain both parent drug and metabolite(s) and chemical poisons in significant concentrations, thereby facilitating their identification. Whenever possible, screening processes are automated to facilitate rapid results generation with minimal sample volume requirements. More and more, this procedure is being performed using near patient testing devices, but these techniques are not without risk of misinterpretation.[5] In laboratories, such work is routinely performed using an automated platform (Fig. 172-1) with appropriate quality control and assessment.

These screening techniques may be followed by confirmatory analysis to identify specific substances that may be present in the specimen. For example, was an amphetamine-positive screening result due to an over-the-counter nasal decongestant containing pseudoephedrine or to "ecstasy," with the potential for rhabdomyolysis and subsequent renal failure? In addition to this qualitative (presence-or-absence) approach, quantitative measurements subsequently may be made using a plasma sample to test for compounds such as ethylene glycol, methanol, and acetaminophen, which would require treatment with an antidote to prevent the occurrence of life-threatening adverse reactions.

A second approach is known as *target analysis*, wherein very specific analytical methods are used to determine the presence or absence of individual toxicants. This approach may be slightly faster but runs the risk of missing other compounds that may have been taken by the patient.

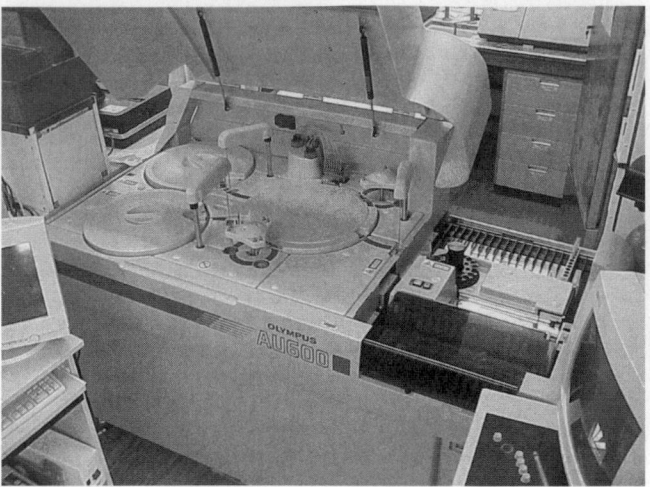

FIGURE 172-1. An example of a high-throughput automated screening platform. The Olympus AU600 System illustrated is capable of performing 800 photometric (drug) tests per hour.

Of note, no simple technique can identify or quantify all known drugs and chemicals that are likely to be ingested accidentally or nonaccidentally. Basic chemical "spot tests" can yield rapid results for certain compounds—for example, ferric chloride (Trinder's) reagent to detect salicylate intoxication or the sodium dithionite test to confirm paraquat ingestion. Similarly, immunoassay techniques can provide very rapid screening results for illicit drugs and alcohol using small sample volumes. This capability is particularly useful in pediatric cases, in which sample volumes tend to be limited.

Classic chromatographic techniques such as high-performance liquid chromatography (HPLC) or gas chromatography are performed to target the search for certain individual compounds or to confirm the presence or measure the concentration of specific drugs after screening. "Hyphenated" combination techniques such as HPLC–diode array detection or gas chromatography–mass spectroscopy (Fig. 172-2) can yield even more information and are currently assumed to be the gold standard in analytical techniques. In medicolegal cases, they should always be used to confirm potential unexpected findings.

Ultimately, the technique of choice will depend on the physical and chemical properties of the drug under inves-

TABLE 172-1

Hospital Admissions and Bed Days Required after Poisoning with Medicines*

CATEGORY	NUMBER OF ADMISSIONS	BED DAYS USED
Nonopioid analgesics (mainly acetaminophen)	40,711	62,712
Psychotropic drugs (e.g., antidepressants, tranquilizers)	18,174	25,400
Antiepileptic and antiparkinsonian drugs	14,684	24,550
Hallucinogens	7,670	13,560
Diuretics	7,325	11,013
Hematological drugs (e.g., anticoagulants such as antileukemic agents or warfarin)	2,043	4,218
Autonomic drugs (e.g., atropine, epinephrine)	1,886	2,975
Hormonal drugs (e.g., oral contraceptives)	1,632	3,814
Cardiovascular drugs (e.g., digoxin, beta blockers)	1,364	4,832
Antibiotics (e.g., penicillin)	776	1,225
Total	96,265	154,299

*Data reported from England during the period 2003 to 2004.

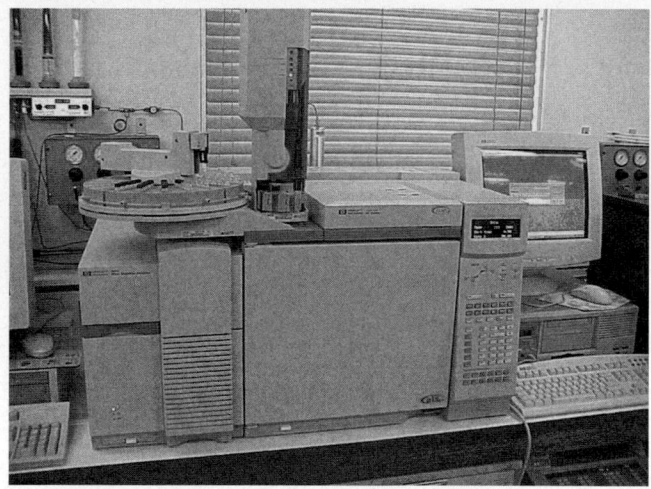

FIGURE 172-2. An example of a gas chromatography–mass spectrometry system used for the confirmation of screening tests, or defined target analysis. The Agilent system illustrated has been designed for rapid analysis to maximize analytical throughput.

tigation (e.g., molecular size and volatility), the urgency of the case, and potential future ramifications (e.g., medicolegal or nonaccidental injury cases) associated with the investigation. Nevertheless, it is only through the application of a combination of different techniques that the true identity of one or many toxicant(s) can be determined.

FACTORS THAT MAY CONFOUND ANALYTICAL INTERPRETATION

The number of issues surrounding the interpretation of analytical results increases with the degree of complexity of the system used to perform the analysis. Often several explanations are possible for the presence of a compound in the specimens analyzed, and the most obvious reasons may not always be the correct ones. Accordingly, the interpretation of analytical results needs to be performed by persons with a thorough working knowledge of the analytical systems to be used, including their limitations.[3]

Basic spot tests will, by their very nature, be subjective in their interpretation. Different compounds may yield very similar reactions, so various analytical system operators could arrive at numerous conclusions regarding the specific identity of the toxicant involved. Most laboratories, therefore, prefer to use well-characterized techniques yielding "hard" data that can be archived for future referral, rather than relying on results derived from the subjective interpretation of color reactions.

Apart from the subjective factors affecting analytical data interpretation, limitations such as sensitivity and specificity of techniques come into play.[6] The *sensitivity* of a technique relates to its ability to detect the compound of interest in a specimen. This ability is a direct function of the technique as well as the time elapsed between exposure to the toxicant and the collection of the specimen for analysis. Rapidly eliminated drugs may be completely cleared from the body before a sample can be taken for analysis, leading to obvious problems in identifying the "causative agent" associated with the patient's symptoms.

The *specificity* of the technique relates to its ability to identify a particular compound in a complex mixture of similar compounds or in a complex sample matrix. For example, the analysis of illicit drug use includes the differentiation of opiate drugs. Heroin, poppy seeds, and codeine all will be metabolized into morphine, but the dilemma facing the analyst in this case is the differentiation between an illicit drug, dietary foodstuffs, or an over-the-counter analgesic.[7]

BENEFITS OF LIAISON BETWEEN LABORATORY AND CLINICIAN

It can be seen from the preceding section that the analyst needs to be acutely aware of the limitations of the techniques at his or her disposal. It also is vital that the clinician be aware of these limitations to ensure correct understanding of the laboratory test results.[8] The response "not detected" may not be the same as "not exposed." Lack of detection may simply be a result of the sensitivity or specificity of the technique used, highlighting the importance of the correct information-gathering exercises as well as rapid specimen collection on admission of the patient.

Furthermore, it is important to inform the laboratory of any and all medications that may have been given to a patient before specimen collection. These details often may be overlooked on the grounds of expedience during the initial assessment and treatment of the patient, but such omissions may lead to analytical complications during subsequent laboratory investigations. There seems little point in the laboratory's having to spend valuable time and potentially use the available specimens simply to confirm what has been used in treatment, rather than concentrating on the detection of the initial toxicant.

TOXICANTS OF NOTE WITH REGARD TO CRITICAL ILLNESS AND NEPHROTOXICITY

Toxicological investigations or drug measurements may aid clinical diagnosis and management in patients exposed to three main groups of potential toxicants:

- Substances that lead to acute illness necessitating hospitalization
- Substances that primarily affect renal function
- Substances that necessitate close monitoring if renal function is compromised

The indicated investigations will depend on the clinical presentation of the patient and the toxicant potentially involved.

The most common agents associated with hospitalization for "intoxication" are the analgesics (e.g., acetaminophen), illicit drugs (e.g., opiates, cocaine), and therapeutic agents due to noncompliance or taken in overdose (e.g., antidepressants). In addition, there are less frequent admissions due to the intake of chemicals such as ethylene glycol and methanol (antifreeze), herbicides (e.g., paraquat), and herbal remedies that may contain heavy metals or be contaminated with toxic plant products. The medicines that were most frequently associated with hospital admission in England in 2003 to 2004 are shown in Table

TABLE 172-2

Frequency of Hospital Admissions Associated with Illicit Drug Use*

CATEGORY	NUMBER OF ADMISSIONS	BED DAYS USED
Opioid drugs	3,690	44,164
Multiple drug use	2,690	57,787
Cannabinoids	947	22,257
"Other" stimulants	447	7,577
Cocaine	328	3,745
Sedatives, hypnotics	206	3,848
Hallucinogens	128	2,005
Volatile solvents	44	493
Total	8,480	171,876

*Data reported from England during the period 2003 to 2004.

172-1, whereas the scale of the illicit drug problem for the same period is shown in Table 172-2.[1] It can be seen that more than 42% of hospital admissions due to poisoning with medicines are accounted for by the ingestion of analgesic agents, primarily acetaminophen. This finding probably reflects the ease of access to such medication. Similarly, more than 43% of admissions due to illicit drug use are associated with opioid drugs.

The kidney is exposed to relatively high concentrations of drugs or other compounds and their metabolites during excretion, and these may give rise to direct or indirect adverse reactions on an acute (e.g., acute tubular necrosis) or chronic (e.g., tubulointerstitial disease) exposure basis. The compounds that are particularly associated with renal impairment fall into four classes: certain prescribed therapeutic medicines, illicit drugs, chemicals, and metals.[9-11]

- Medicines—analgesics, nonsteroidal anti-inflammatory drugs, immunosuppressive agents
- Illicit drugs—cocaine, heroin
- Chemicals—solvents (methanol, ethylene glycol), herbicides, contrast agents
- Metals—arsenic, cadmium, chromium, gold, lead, mercury

Each of these classes of compounds will demonstrate various degrees of impact on renal function, and this effect may persist long after any trace of the compound may be detected in the system. In some cases, it may be necessary to investigate the potential for current or historic occupational exposure to harmful substances.

An important point is that one of the most important factors affecting toxicological investigations is renal function. Patients with normal renal function will excrete drugs, metabolites, and other toxicants fairly readily. In cases of reduced or declining renal clearance, the adverse effects of a drug will become more pronounced, and some active metabolites may accumulate, leading to even greater problems. This is especially true in elderly patients, in whom renal function is known to be reduced, and potential dose adjustments to prescribed medication need to be made.[12] Such considerations also are important in patients exhibiting renal impairment due to disease or injury. Accordingly, in renally compromised patients, particular care needs to be taken with the following categories of drugs:

- Drugs that are primarily renally excreted
- Drugs with a narrow therapeutic index (e.g., digoxin)
- Drugs that produce active metabolites (e.g., benzodiazepines, opiates)
- Drugs that may further reduce renal function (e.g., antidepressants, anti-inflammatory drugs)

Without appropriate surveillance in this group of patients, precipitation of further injury or more severe adverse reactions is likely, even with use of standard dosing regimens for the treatment and management of chronic illness.

CONCLUSION

Myriad compounds may potentially lead to critical illness. Paracelsus (1493-1541) is widely credited with the phrase "All things are poison and nothing (is) without poison; only the dose makes that a thing is no poison"—that is, it is merely the dose that makes a compound poisonous.[13] It would be impossible, however, to screen for every compound that could possibly be taken in overdose or give rise to adverse clinical reactions.

Some investigations are required to be performed in response to the acute onset of symptoms or signs, and other tests will be requested to support the diagnosis and management of patients exhibiting a progressive deterioration in clinical status. As described earlier, it is difficult for the laboratory to fully or appropriately investigate requests for evaluation in acute cases without prior full discussion of the case with the requesting physician. Occasionally, requests will arrive in a laboratory stating merely "drug overdose" or "unconscious—query cause," and without ascertainment of a more detailed clinical picture, time could be wasted investigating medications given in treatment, rather than the substances suspected of being implicated in the case. In general terms, the laboratory concentrates on looking for the presence of common sedative, hypnotic, and illicit drugs in unconscious patients, or in the absence of a full medical history, because these are the agents most likely to be responsible for the clinical presentation, and confirmation would support rapid, effective intervention.

Similarly, it is difficult to aid in the diagnosis of patients who are deteriorating in a setting of chronic exposure, because the tests likely to be routinely performed may not be appropriate. In such instances, a more thorough investigation may be required but should target compounds suggested by the signs and symptoms and history obtained, with the results used to guide management to minimize further injury or adverse postexposure sequelae. This clinical setting again highlights the importance of both clinical liaison and early collection of specimens for possible investigation, especially if a patient fails to respond to supportive treatment.

Key Points

1. The patient history should be as comprehensive as possible to identify all drugs prescribed, available, or given in treatment.
2. Both urine and blood samples should be collected into appropriate containers as soon as possible, and the details of the case should be communicated to the laboratory that will be involved in the investigations.
3. The analytical results generated should be discussed directly with the laboratory involved in the case to ensure complete and full understanding of the scope, limitations, and implications of the findings.
4. Further laboratory studies may be necessary because preliminary investigations may not be conclusive.
5. It is important for the clinician to be aware of the types of drugs and other substances that may give rise to renal insufficiency and the need to adjust doses in accordance with the individual patient's level of renal function.

Key References

2. Lee V, Kerr JF, Braitberg G, et al: Impact of a toxicology service on a metropolitan teaching hospital. Emerg Med (Fremantle) 2001;13:37-42.
3. Hammett-Stabler CA, Pesce AJ, Cannon DJ: Urine drug screening in the medical setting. Clin Chim Acta 2002;315: 125-135.
5. George S, Braithwaite RA: Use of on-site testing for drugs of abuse. Clin Chem 2002;48:1639-1646.
9. International Program on Chemical Safety: Principles and methods for the assessment of nephrotoxicity associated with exposure to chemicals. 1991. Available at http://www.inchem.org/documents/ehc/ehc/ehc119.htm (accessed May 2006).
11. Guo X, Nzerue C: How to prevent, recognize, and treat drug induced nephrotoxicity. Cleve Clin J Med 2002;69:289-312.

See the companion Expert Consult website for the complete reference list.

General Treatment Concepts

CHAPTER 173

Drugs and Antidotes in Acute Intoxication

George Braitberg

OBJECTIVES

This chapter will:
1. Provide an overview of drugs and antidotes in acute intoxication.
2. Highlight clinical pitfalls in the management of toxicity.
3. Identify the clinically significant toxidromes.
4. Describe the effects of sodium and potassium channel blockers.
5. Present a review of specific poisons and antidotes.
6. Review poisons that have significant effects on the kidney.

Deliberate self-poisoning, accidental poisoning, and recreational drug abuse and chemical exposure are increasing in frequency across the world. The Toxic Exposure Surveillance System (TESS) database of poison control centers of the United States gives a frequency of approximately 8.2 exposures per 1000 population since the year 2000.[1] Although children younger than 6 years of age were involved in a majority of poisoning reports, they incurred just 1.9% (24) of the recorded 1261 fatalities. Fifty-six percent of poisoning fatalities occurred in persons 20 to 49 years of age. Analgesics were thought to be responsible for most of the fatalities, with the next most common cause attributable to stimulants and "street drugs." Of all reported exposures, 83.8% were classified as unintentional; 12.6% were classified as intentional, a majority as a result of a suicidal act (8.13%). As might be expected, the frequency of unintentional ingestions demonstrates a peak in children younger than 6 years of age; the peak age for intentional ingestions was greater than 19 years of age.[1] Of note, therapeutic errors accounted for 9.9% of exposures. Overall, 22.8% of the patients required evaluation in a health care facility, of whom half (11.7%) underwent treatment and were released and 5.1% were admitted to an acute inpatient bed (3.3% in a critical care unit). Of all of the reported exposures, use of an antidote was reported in only 3%. The top 10 antidotes are listed in Figure 173-1.

Although poisoning should be suspected in any patient with multisystem involvement of unknown etiology until proven otherwise, the clinician also should be aware of common pitfalls in the workup of the patient with suspected or known poisoning. Common concerns are listed in Table 173-1.

TOXIDROMES

In many clinical circumstances, the poison is unknown, at least initially. In these circumstances, after appropriate life support measures have been instituted, the toxic treatment paradigm is to group signs and symptoms together into a toxidrome. *Toxidrome* describes clinical presentations common to a number of toxins.

The most common toxidromes are
- Anticholinergic (antimuscarinic)
- Cholinergic
- Adrenergic
- GABAergic
- Sodium and potassium channel blocker–related
- Serotoninergic
- Opiate-related

Anticholinergic Toxidrome

The most common toxidrome by far is due to anticholinergic toxicity. In 2003,[3] the TESS reported 3094 symptomatic anticholinergic drug presentations. Fifty-two percent were unintentional ingestions and 38% were intentional ingestions. Adverse reactions occurred in 7% of cases, with moderate morbidity (requiring specific treatment) reported in 20%, major morbidity (life-threatening reactions) in 3.7%, and death in 5 cases (0.16%).

Anticholinergic toxicity is more appropriately defined as antimuscarinic poisoning. It occurs when the acetylcholine postsynaptic muscarinic receptor is antagonized. This receptor is found on the parasympathetic postganglionic receptor.

Anticholinergic toxicity can be central, peripheral, or both. Peripheral toxicity may or may not be present before central toxicity develops, and vice versa.

Characteristics of *central* anticholinergic toxicity include the following:
- Biphasic effect of central nervous system (CNS) excitation followed by depression
- Distinctive mumbling or fragmentary speech pattern
- Atypical behavior, especially inappropriate undressing
- Repetitive "picking" movements. (e.g., tugging at the bedclothes or a catheter or grasping at space)
- Hallucinations, more commonly visual
- Movement disorders of an ataxic or clonic nature in some cases

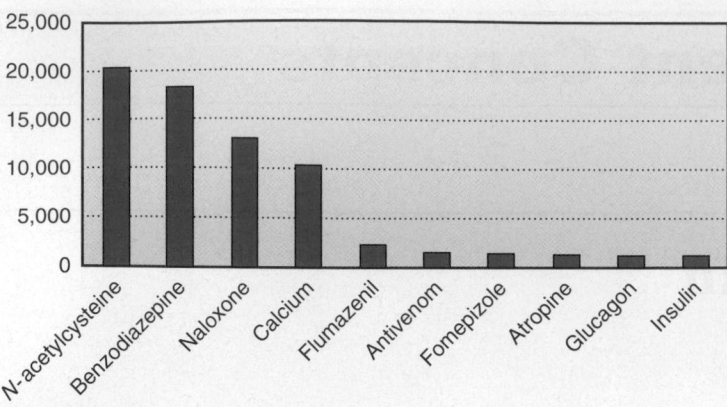

FIGURE 173-1. Top 10 antidotes by frequency of use. (Adapted from Lai MW, Klein-Schwartz W, Rodgers GC, et al: 2005 Annual Report of the American Association of Poison Control Centers' National Poisoning and Exposure Database. Clin Toxicol 2006;44:803-932.)

TABLE 173-1

Pitfalls in Clinical Management of Suspected Toxicity

- Not all patients with a presumed overdose have, in fact, overdosed. The young patient with altered state of consciousness may have suffered a primary neurological event, and a careful neurological examination looking for focal signs must always be part of the evaluation in such cases.
- A poisoned patient may have suffered a secondary event after the overdose or exposure (e.g., neurological and cardiac sequelae of cocaine intoxication are well documented).
- Polypharmacy is the rule. In one study, acetaminophen was the drug most commonly implicated in overdose (54%), but polypharmacy ingestions were the next most frequent (38%).[2] In multiple-ingestion overdoses, the poisoned patient will not follow a "predictable" path of recovery, because other substances may have different time courses for the development of toxicity (e.g., a patient who has overdosed on sustained-release verapamil may not display any signs of poisoning for up to 18 hours, at a time when toxicity from other substances co-ingested may be resolving).
- Recovery may be prolonged as a result of therapeutic intervention (e.g., development of aspiration pneumonia after gastrointestinal tract decontamination).
- Poisoning may occur from routes other than oral. Dermal absorption, as in the case of organophosphate poisoning, poses a particular risk for the rescuer or health care worker who attends the patient, without protective clothing, before decontamination. Inhalation absorption, as with exposures involving some noxious gases (e.g., products of combustion), puts both rescuer and victim at risk.
- Intravenous substance abuse has been associated with risk of infection, of which hepatitis and HIV infection are well known, but at present the leading cause of botulism in the United States is the use of contaminated needles.

HIV, human immunodeficiency virus.

Patients with severe central manifestations (e.g., hallucinations, psychoses, seizures, coma) have the highest morbidity rates.

Characteristics of *peripheral* anticholinergic syndrome, in order of onset, include the loss of ability to salivate, sweat, and lacrimate, followed by blurred vision (caused by decreased ability to accommodate and papillary mydriasis) and then an increase in heart rate and a decrease in bladder motility (leading to urinary retention). Finally, gut peristalsis is lost, leading to constipation.

An important *clinical clue* is that tachycardia with dry axillae distinguishes the anticholinergic toxidrome from the adrenergic toxidrome.

Anticholinergic syndrome can be summarized as follows:

Mad as a hatter*
Hot as a hare
Blind as a bat
Red as a beet
Dry as a bone

Many drugs and substances cause anticholinergic toxicity. Table 173-2 provides a list of common anticholinergic agents.

Antidote Considerations: Physostigmine

Little role exists for the routine use of physostigmine in the management of a patient displaying anticholinergic toxicity. Physostigmine is an acetylcholinesterase inhibitor and, unlike neostigmine, crosses the blood-brain barrier. Thus, it can increase both central and peripheral levels of acetylcholine.

Although physostigmine can dramatically reverse the anticholinergic toxidrome, its use is not without adverse effects, with seizure, bradycardia, and even asystole being reported when used in the management of overdose, especially in the setting of tricyclic antidepressant toxicity.[4] It is postulated that in this situation, the anticholinergic-induced tachycardia, which may be helpful in offsetting the negatively inotropic effect of sodium channel blockade, when antagonized acutely leads to cardiac or pump failure and dysrhythmia.

Physostigmine should be used only after consultation with a toxicologist, in a setting in which full resuscitation facilities are available. In one case report, its use was justified as a safer alternative to managing an agitated patient outside a critical care area with further administration of benzodiazepines.[5] A more desirable alternative, however, may be to transfer the patient to a critical care unit with appropriate airway protection.

The *dose* is 2.0 mg administered intravenously in 0.5-mg aliquots, given 5 to 10 minutes apart.

---

*Hat manufacturers applied mercury to the felt of their hats and as a result developed mercury poisoning. Thus, in reality, hatters were mad for reasons other than anticholinergic poisoning.

TABLE 173-2

Common Anticholinergic Agents

Antihistamines
  Chlorpheniramine
  Cyproheptadine
  Doxylamine
  Hydroxyzine
  Dimenhydrinate
  Diphenhydramine
  Meclizine
  Promethazine
Tricyclic antidepressants
  Amitriptyline
  Amoxapine
  Clomipramine
  Desipramine
  Doxepin
  Imipramine
  Nortriptyline
  Protriptyline
Mydriatics (easily systemically absorbed)
  Atropine
  Cyclopentolate
  Homatropine
  Tropicamide
Class 1 antiarrhythmics
  Disopyramide
Plants
  Atropa belladonna (deadly nightshade)
  Cestrum nocturnum (night-blooming jasmine)
  Datura suaveolens (angel's trumpet)
  Datura stramonium (jimson weed)
  Hyoscyamus niger (black henbane)
  Lantana camara (red sage)
  Solanum carolinensis (wild tomato)
  Solanum dulcamara (bittersweet)
Mushrooms (e.g., *Amanita muscaria*)
Antipsychotics
  Phenothiazines (e.g., chlorpromazine)
  Clozapine
  Mesoridazine
  Olanzapine
  Quetiapine
  Thioridazine
Antiparkinsonian drugs
  Benztropine (also used to control extrapyramidal effects
    from the major tranquilizers)
Motion sickness preparations
  Scopolamine patches
Muscle relaxants
  Orphenadrine (Norflex).
Others
  Carbamazepine

Cholinergic Toxidrome

The parasympathetic nervous system has acetylcholine as its neurotransmitter at both central and peripheral receptors. The central preganglionic receptor is a nicotinic receptor (Nn type). The sympathetic nervous system uses two neurotransmitters: Acetylcholine acts on Nn receptors in the preganglionic central chain, and norepinephrine acts on the peripheral alpha and beta receptors. The somatic nervous system has acetylcholine as its neurotransmitter, acting on the nicotinic Nm receptor subtype to innervate striped (skeletal) muscle.

The cholinergic toxidrome is manifested by signs of stimulation of both the muscarinic and the nicotinic receptors in both autonomic and somatic nervous systems.

Stimulation of the muscarinic receptors leads to the "classic" SLUDGE syndrome:
- Salivation
- Lacrimation
- Urination
- Diarrhea
- GI cramps
- Emesis

In addition, muscarinic cholinergic stimulation leads to bronchoconstriction and bronchorrhea.

Stimulation of central nicotinic receptors affects sympathetic and parasympathetic neurons. This causes a release of both norepinephrine and acetylcholine. An initial excitation phase, manifested by tachycardia and hypertension, may occur as a result of sympathetic nervous system stimulation. After the initial stimulation, however, prolonged ganglionic blockade and adrenal suppression occur (nicotinic receptors also are located in the adrenal medulla). At this point in the course, hypotension and bradycardia predominate. Nicotinic receptor stimulation in the brain leads to altered mental status, with confusion, agitation, restlessness, and vomiting. This may be followed by onset of seizure and neurological depression with coma.

Acetylcholinergic stimulation of Nm receptors on skeletal muscle causes initial excitation, with fasciculation and tonic clonic jerks, followed by blockade and muscle weakness. Hypotonia, decreased tendon reflexes, and motor paralysis sequentially occur.

Agents that cause a cholinergic toxidrome can be divided into two main groups according to their mechanism of action:
- Direct nicotinic receptor stimulation
  Plant alkaloids such as nicotine and coniine (found in poison hemlock)
  Nicotine-based insecticides
  Cigarette butts (at least three whole butts in a young child)
- Increased acetylcholine levels
  Organophosphates and carbamates

Organophosphates

Organophosphates are agricultural insecticides. These agents inhibit the enzyme acetylcholinesterase, which is responsible for the degradation of acetylcholine. The organophosphate binds to the enzyme, causing it to undergo a conformational change at its binding site to acetylcholine. If the organophosphate does not leave the acetylcholinesterase enzyme within 24 to 48 hours, it is irreversibly bound to the enzyme, which is permanently inactivated; this process is called "aging." Recovery from poisoning will occur only with resynthesis of new enzyme, a process that takes several weeks. The treatment of organophosphate poisoning is two-pronged:
1. Symptomatic treatment with atropine to overcome muscarinic stimulation by acetylcholine. The dose given is that sufficient to "atropinize" the patient—to abolish signs and symptoms (see later).
2. Reactivation of acetylcholinesterase with an oxime such as pralidoxime. Oximes cleave the organophosphate from acetylcholinesterase and bind circulating free organophosphate. In addition, pralidoxime displays antimuscarinic properties of its own. Because of the aging of the organophosphate-acetylcholinesterase complex, the earlier oximes are administered, the earlier acetylcholinesterase can be re-formed. Resolution of

symptoms and a rising acetylcholinesterase level indicate response to therapy.

In military or disaster scenarios, atropine and an oxime are combined in "autoinjectors." Pralidoxime is discussed here, but in other parts of the world, including the United States, other oximes are used, the most frequent being obidoxime. Oxime effectiveness and dosing have been the subject of much discussion because of the lack of randomized trials evaluating organophosphate treatment. A recently published article by Pawar and colleagues showed that higher-dose continuous infusion of pralidoxime iodide (1 g/hour of pralidoxime for 48 hours) was superior to intermittent dosing (a bolus of 1 g/hour every 4 hours).[6]

Antidote Considerations

ATROPINE. Atropine is a physiological antidote to the muscarinic features of organophosphate toxicity, acting to competitively inhibit acetylcholine at muscarinic receptors but with no effect at ganglionic or neuromuscular nicotinic receptors. It also may be useful in carbamate toxicity, which may be clinically indistinguishable from organophosphate toxicity.

The *dose* is 2 mg (0.05 mg/kg in children), repeated at 10- to 30-minute intervals until drying of excessive secretions occurs. There is no upper limit of dose in the treatment of a severe organophosphate poisoning. Severe toxicity may require extremely large doses to achieve atropinization (up to 1000 mg/24 hours has been used). An atropine infusion at 5 to 20 mg/hour may be required. Pupillary dilatation and tachycardia are not reliable therapeutic endpoints. Normalization of peripheral vascular resistance may be a better endpoint but is not normally measurable outside an ICU environment. Atropine may be useful in the treatment of hypotension without bradycardia. In the recently published randomized controlled trial, the atropine was administered as a 1.8- to 3.0-mg bolus on admission, followed by an infusion with intermittent boluses to achieve control of secretions from the tracheobronchial tree, return pupils to their normal size, and stabilize the pulse rate at between 80 and 100 beats per minute.[6]

Adverse reactions to atropine may include the following:
- Ventricular arrhythmias may occur if adequate tissue oxygenation is not achieved before the use of atropine.
- Atropine excess may cause anticholinergic symptoms: mydriasis, tachycardia, hyperpyrexia, ileus, delirium, facial flushing, urinary retention, drying of secretions.

PRALIDOXIME. The *dose* is 1 to 2 g (25 to 50 mg/kg in children) given over 30 minutes, followed by an infusion of 200 to 500 mg/hour. Infusions usually need to be continued for at least 48 hours in significant exposures. The dose should be reduced in the presence of renal failure.

Adverse reactions reported after pralidoxime iodide injection include dizziness, blurred vision, diplopia and impaired accommodation, headache, drowsiness, nausea, tachycardia, hyperventilation, and muscular weakness, but it is very difficult to differentiate the toxic effects produced by the organophosphate compounds from those of the drug. When atropine and pralidoxime iodide injection are used together, the signs of atropinization may occur earlier than might be expected when atropine is used alone, and less atropine may be required.[6] Excitement and manic behavior occurring immediately after recovery of

TABLE 173-3

Common Causes of the Adrenergic Toxidrome

Recreational drugs
- Cocaine
- Amphetamines and other "designer drugs"*—"ecstasy" (3,4-methylenedioxymethamphetamine [MDMA]); 3,4-methylenedioxyamphetamine (MDA); 3,4-methylenedioxyethylamphetamine (MDEA); paramethoxyamphetamine (PMA); methamphetamine

β_1-Adrenergic agents
- Salbutamol
- Theophylline

Inotropic agents
- Norepinephrine
- Epinephrine
- Isoproterenol

Over-the-counter cough and cold preparations and nasal decongestants
- Phenylpropanolamine
- Pseudoephedrine

Amphetamine-like agents prescribed for ADD or weight loss
- Methylphenidate
- Dextroamphetamine

Psychostimulants

*Up to 80% of ecstasy tablets sold in Australia are actually methamphetamine.
ADD, attention deficit disorder.

consciousness have been reported in several instances. However, similar behavior has been described in cases of organophosphate poisoning that were not treated with pralidoxime iodide injection.[7]

Adrenergic Toxidrome

Table 173-3 lists common causes of the adrenergic toxidrome. The adrenergic toxidrome is caused by sympathomimetic agents. Neurological manifestations include hyperthermia, agitation, seizures, and coma. Cardiovascular effects include tachycardia, hypertension, peripheral vasoconstriction, arrhythmias, and myocardial infarction. Metabolic disturbances from increased circulating catecholamines cause elevation of glucose levels and the white blood cell count. Hypokalemia in the absence of vomiting does not usually require correction because the cause is not a potassium deficit but rather an intracellular shift, which will settle as the toxidrome abates. Other signs and symptoms include bronchodilation, nausea, and vomiting; diaphoresis and rhabdomyolysis also may occur.

No specific antidotes are available. Management consists of lowering body temperature and blood pressure and achieving central sedation, usually with a benzodiazepine and other supportive measures. Hypertension requiring pharmacological intervention is treated with a specific alpha blocker or smooth muscle antihypertensive (e.g., hydralazine or sodium nitroprusside). Beta blockers have the potential to precipitate a vasoconstriction crisis by unopposed alpha stimulation.[8] If the patient exhibits psychosis in the setting of amphetamine or cocaine toxicity without significant cardiovascular toxicity, an agent such as haloperidol may improve the patient's mental status by means of dopamine antagonism. Phenothiazines such as chlorpromazine should be avoided because they lower the seizure threshold and may exacerbate hyperthermia due to anticholinergic activity. "Ecstasy" (i.e., 3,4-methylene-dioxymethamphetamine [MDMA]) poisoning may respond to antiserotoninergic medication such as cyproheptadine (see later).[9]

A Note about Recreational Drugs

In the 2004 national drug survey, more than 9% of Australians older than 14 years of age had tried amphetamine or methamphetamine, 7.5% had tried ecstasy, and nearly 5% had tried cocaine. From this survey, it is estimated that over half a million people used ecstasy at least once in 2004, and a similar number had used amphetamines. By contrast, only 1% had used cocaine in the previous year.[10]

Methamphetamines are produced by reduction of ephedrine or pseudoephedrine, found in decongestants and other household products, making them relatively simple drugs to produce.

Psychostimulants cause an overall increase in the amount of monoamine neurotransmitters—norepinephrine, dopamine, and serotonin—by increasing their release and blocking reuptake. Amphetamines, MDMA, and cocaine have the greatest effect on norepinephrine, serotonin, and dopamine, respectively.[11] Ecstasy primarily increases serotonergic activity, whereas methamphetamine primarily increases adrenergic activity. Cocaine also blocks fast sodium channels, causing local anesthetic and proarrhythmic effects.

A majority of ecstasy users do not experience adverse events that precipitate a hospital visit. Serious complications are rare and partly dependent on individual susceptibility and circumstances. The common adverse acute physiological and psychological effects that psychostimulants elicit constitute an exaggerated "fight or flight" response.

Extreme dehydration and water intoxication have been associated with MDMA toxicity. Dehydration is due to a lack of awareness of thirst in the setting of extreme physical activity. Water intoxication can be a consequence of increased antidiuretic hormone secretion and consumption of too much water (to prevent dehydration), leading to complications associated with hyponatremia. Cardiac ischemia can occur with any of these drugs but is particularly associated with cocaine. It is due to a combination of increased myocardial demand, coronary vasoconstriction, and increased thromboxane A_2 activity and thrombus formation.[12]

The most commonly repeated findings in studies of MDMA, methamphetamine, and cocaine use have been problems in the area of learning and memory. Both animal and human studies have yielded evidence of neurotoxicity, but whether this is permanent and irreversible after chronic use in humans is inconclusive. However, the evidence for neurotoxicity continues to accumulate.[13]

GABAergic Toxidrome

γ-Aminobutyric acid (GABA) is a naturally occurring inhibitory neurotransmitter located in the CNS. The other important inhibitory neurotransmitter, glycine, is situated both centrally and peripherally, where it is involved in inhibitory stimuli to tendon stretch reflexes. This peripheral action is demonstrated in strychnine poisoning, in which glycine receptors are inhibited by strychnine,

leading to abnormal muscle activity and painful spasms in affected patients, who retain a normal mental status.[14]

The GABAergic toxidrome refers to the effects of stimulation of the $GABA_A$ receptor. The $GABA_A$ receptor is a chloride ion receptor complex that causes chloride ions to enter the nerve cell, causing hyperpolarization on stimulation. This action produces inhibitory neurotransmission. Antagonism of the $GABA_A$ receptor causes excitation.[14]

Most CNS depressants work by enhancing $GABA_A$ neurotransmission. Benzodiazepines and barbiturates, anticonvulsants such as valproate, and to some degree, carbamazepine, general anesthetics, and ethanol are some examples. All of these agents must bind to GABA to produce their neuroinhibitory effect. In isoniazid overdose, in which GABA formation has been stopped, seizures are refractory to control with GABA-dependent anticonvulsants, such as barbiturates and benzodiazepines.[15]

Antagonists of the $GABA_A$ receptor include toxins such as chlordane, an organochlorine pesticide, and lindane, used in the treatment of lice. High-dose penicillin, used in animal models to induce seizures, antagonizes the receptor, as does the administration of ciprofloxacin. All of these agents may precipitate seizures.[14]

Antidote Considerations: Flumazenil

Flumazenil is a benzodiazepine antagonist that binds to the benzodiazepine receptor, displacing other benzodiazepine agonists, without neuroinhibitory effects.[16,17] Thus, it antagonizes the neuronal depression caused by GABA stimulation at the $GABA_A$ receptor. The routine use of flumazenil in the management of benzodiazepine overdose is not recommended, because withdrawal seizures may be precipitated in patients who are chronically dependent on benzodiazepines, or in those who are not, the abrupt reversal of benzodiazepines may unmask the effect of an excitatory drug taken as a co-ingestant (e.g., tricyclic antidepressants), also with the potential for causing seizures. A further consideration is the relatively high safety index (toxic-to-therapeutic dose ratio) of benzodiazepines.[14]

Sodium and Potassium Channel–Blocking Agents
Sodium Channel

In addition to the class I antiarrhythmic agents, numerous other drugs, including tricyclic antidepressants, amantadine, carbamazepine, antihistamines (e.g., diphenhydramine), beta blockers (propranolol, acebutolol, and oxprenolol), cocaine, and propoxyphene, have sodium channel–blocking properties. Many other drugs can cause sodium channel blockade when taken in overdose. Tricyclic antidepressants such as imipramine exert cardiovascular toxicity through their anticholinergic effects and ion channel–blocking effects in cardiac muscle.[18] Class Ic agents are the most potent sodium channel blockers but do not affect potassium channels; therefore, these agents cause QRS prolongation without QT prolongation on the electrocardiographic tracing.[19] Bicarbonate is considered by most toxicologists to be the treatment of choice for cardiac toxicity in the setting of sodium channel blocker poisoning. In Europe, hypertonic sodium lactate is used in place of bicarbonate. Both agents overcome sodium channel blockade by mass effect and by increasing serum pH, which inhibits binding of at least some sodium channel blockers to sodium channels. Serum alkalinization has been shown to be of benefit in reversing toxicity from tricyclic antidepressants, cocaine, quinidine, flecainide, procainamide, mexiletine, and bupivacaine.[18,20-25]

Potassium Channel

The QT interval is an electrocardiographic measure that includes both depolarization and repolarization. It begins with the onset of ventricular depolarization (Q wave) and ends with completion of repolarization (T wave). Because the QT interval shortens with increasing heart rates, it usually is corrected for heart rate (QTc). Depolarization of ventricular cells is the result of a rapid influx of sodium ions through selective sodium channels, and its duration is measured by the QRS interval. Repolarization involves calcium, sodium, and several potassium channels, but potassium channels play the pivotal role in drug-induced torsades de pointes (TdP). The potassium channel most often involved in drug-induced QT syndromes is the potassium rectifier (I_{Kr}) channel. Drugs blocking the I_{Kr} channel can induce torsades de pointes and sudden death in apparently healthy adults and after poisoning.[26,27] Although most drugs that block I_{Kr} result in QT prolongation, which is a requisite for TdP, QT prolongation alone is not sufficient to result in TdP. Indeed, amiodarone usually results in significant QT prolongation, but TdP from amiodarone is exceedingly rare. Heterogeneity of repolarization across cell types within ventricular myocardium is being increasingly recognized as one explanation for the lack of direct correlation between QT prolongation and proarrhythmia.[28]

Prolonged QTc interval has been associated with the risk of sudden death in epidemiological studies.[29,30] Many classes of agents produce this effect in both therapeutic and toxic doses, as listed in Table 173-4.[31-33]

In 1991, Mehtonen and associates[34] reviewed all medicolegal autopsies (coroners' cases) in Finland. Analyzing 24,158 cases, they found 49 sudden unexpected deaths among apparently healthy adults taking psychotropic medication. Forty-six of these 49 deaths involved a phenothiazine, primarily thioridazine (28 of the 46 cases). Although sudden unexpected death occurs almost twice as often (relative risk, 2.39; 95% confidence interval [CI], 1.77 to 3.22) in populations receiving antipsychotics as in normal populations, nevertheless only 10 to 15 such events occur in 10,000 person-years of observation.[35,36]

Treatment

Athough prolonged QTc after drug exposure may place the patient at greater risk of arrhythmia, it is important to realize that TdP can occur with a narrow QTc as well.[37] Although the evidence for treatment is based on case reports and in vivo experiments, the general consensus is to treat drug-induced TdP with magnesium sulfate given as a bolus (2 to 5 g over 60 seconds), to decrease the amplitude of early afterdepolarizations and suppress triggered rhythms. Treatment for patients with electrocardiographic evidence of prolonged QTc, particularly in the presence of any arrhythmia (e.g., bigeminy), has even less evidence base, but the current practice is to administer a slower infusion of magnesium.[38]

TABLE 173-4

Drugs or Conditions That Cause Prolonged QTc Interval

Antihistamines
    Diphenhydramine
    Astemizole
    Terfenadine
    Cetirizine
Antidepressants
    Citalopram
    Escitopram
    Fuoxetine
    Tricyclic antidepressants*
    Bupropion
    Lithium
    Moclobemide
Antipsychotic medications
    Olanzapine
    Respiradone
    Quetiapine†
    Thioridazine†
    Haloperidol
    Droperidol
    Ziprasadone
    Chlorpromazine
    Mesoridazine
    Amisulpride
Cardiac drugs
    Class 3 and class 1a antiarrhythmics
Antibiotics
    Erythromycin
    Clarithromycin
    Pentamidine
    Chloroquine
Metabolic disturbances
    Hypokalemia
    Hypomagnesemia
    Hypocalcemia
Other drugs and toxins
    Carbamazepine
    Cisapride
    Organophosphates
    Methadone
    Levomethadyl
    Arsenic
    Carbon monoxide
    Fluoride

*QT lengthening with tricyclic antidepressants is primarily the result of the QRS change and not primarily related to a delay in repolarization.
†Most pronounced QT prolongation; data from Hustey, 1999.[32]
Adapted from Proudfoot AT, Donovan JW: Diagnosis of poisoning. In Brent J, Wallace KL, Burkhart KK, et al (eds): Critical Care Toxicology. Diagnosis and Management of the Critically Poisoned Patient. Philadelphia, Mosby, 2005, pp 225-238.

Serotonin Syndrome

The diagnosis of serotonin toxicity is based on clinical findings. Although several diagnostic criteria have been developed, the decision rules described in Figure 173-2, originated by Boyer and Shannon,[39] are more sensitive (84% versus 75%) and specific (97% versus 96%) for diagnosing the syndrome. Clonus (inducible, spontaneous, and ocular) is a highly specific feature for establishing the diagnosis. Clinicians should always be aware that hyperthermia and hypertonicity occur in life-threatening cases, but muscle rigidity may mask the highly distinguishing findings of clonus and hyperreflexia, thereby clouding the diagnosis.

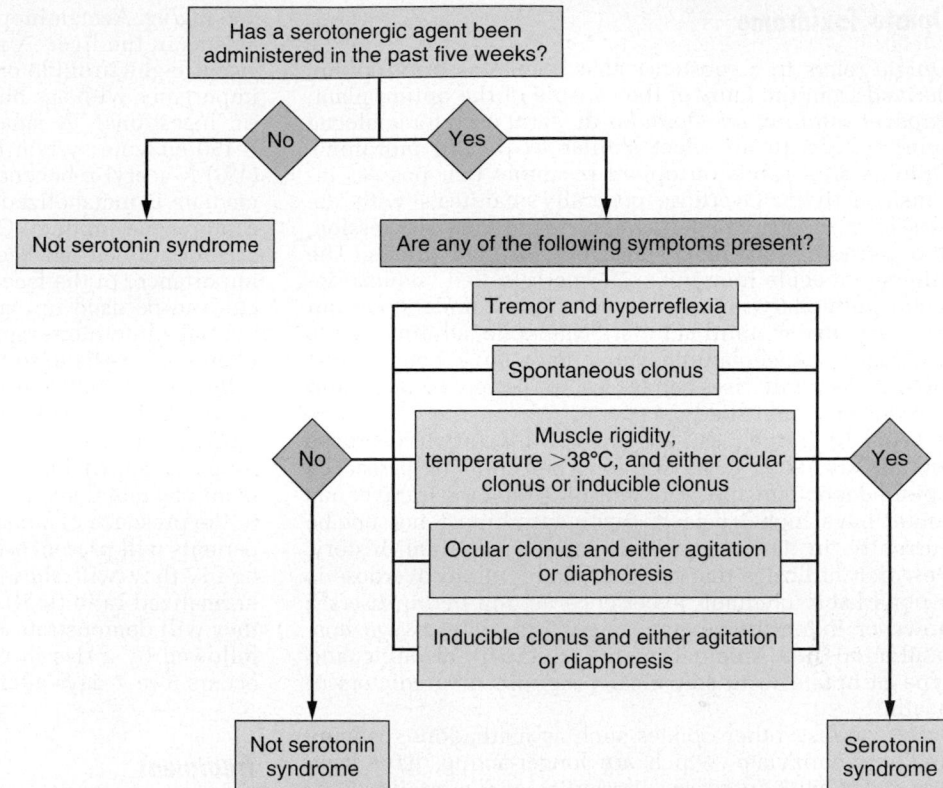

FIGURE 173-2. Algorithm for diagnosis of serotonin syndrome. (Redrawn from Boyer EW, Shannon M: The serotonin syndrome. N Engl J Med 2005;352:1112-1120.)

Treatment is essentially supportive, with intravenous hydration and close monitoring. Removal of the precipitating drug(s) and managing agitation, autonomic instability, and hyperthermia are essential. The administration of a 5-hydroxytryptamine type 2A ($HT_{[2A]}$)antagonist should be considered (see later).

The intensity of therapy depends on the severity of illness. Mild cases (e.g., with hyperreflexia and tremor but no fever) usually can be managed with supportive care and treatment with benzodiazepines. Moderately ill patients should have all cardiorespiratory and thermal abnormalities aggressively corrected and may benefit from the administration of 5-$HT_{(2A)}$ antagonists. Hyperthermic patients (with body temperature higher than 41.1° C) are severely ill and should receive the aforementioned therapies and also should undergo immediate sedation, neuromuscular paralysis, and orotracheal intubation.[40]

Control of agitation with benzodiazepines is essential in the management of the serotonin toxicity, regardless of its severity. Benzodiazepines such as diazepam improve survival in animal models and blunt the hyperadrenergic component of the syndrome.[40,41] Physical restraints are ill-advised in any drug-induced agitated state and may contribute to the risk of death by enforcing the isometric muscle contractions that are associated with severe lactic acidosis and hyperthermia.[42] If physical restraints are initially used, they must be rapidly replaced with chemical sedation.

Pharmacologically directed therapy involves the administration of a 5-$HT_{(2A)}$ antagonist. Cyproheptadine is currently recommended, although its efficacy has not been rigorously established. Treatment of the serotonin syndrome in adults may require 12 to 32 mg of the drug during a 24-hour period, a dose that binds 85%

to 95% of serotonin receptors.[43] In general, an initial dose of 8 to12 mg of cyproheptadine is recommended. Maintenance dosing involves the administration of 8 mg of cyproheptadine every 6 hours. Cyproheptadine is available only in oral form, but tablets may be crushed and administered by nasogastric tube.[39] Atypical antipsychotic agents with 5-$HT_{(2A)}$ antagonist activity may be beneficial in treating serotonin syndrome. The sublingual administration of 10 mg of olanzapine has been used successfully, but its efficacy has not been rigorously determined.[44] If a parenteral agent is needed, the intramuscular administration of 50 to 100 mg of chlorpromazine may be considered.[40] Care should be taken, however, with use of this drug in patients with hypotension, or those in whom the neuroleptic malignant syndrome is a possibility, because the drug may potentially exacerbate these conditions.[39]

Control of autonomic instability involves stabilization of fluctuating pulse and blood pressure. Hypotension arising from monoamine oxidase (MAO) inhibitor interactions should be treated with low doses of direct-acting sympathomimetic amines (e.g., norepinephrine, phenylephrine, epinephrine). Direct agonists do not require intracellular metabolism to generate a vasoactive amine, as distinct from indirect agents such as dopamine, which must be metabolized to epinephrine and norepinephrine by way of MAO. When inhibited, however, MAO cannot control the amount of epinephrine and norepinephrine produced, and an exaggerated hemodynamic response may ensue.

Other therapies for serotonin toxicity, including propranolol, bromocriptine, and dantrolene regimens, have not been shown to decrease morbidity and mortality rates.[39,45]

Opiate Toxidrome

Opiate refers to a substance that originates from opium, derived from the latex of the capsule of the opium plant, *Papaver somniferum*. *Opioid* is the term used for analogue substances with an effect similar to that of morphine. Opioids are ligands on opioid receptors that possess intrinsic activity. Overdose generally manifests with the classic triad of CNS depression, respiratory depression, and pinpoint (myopic), sluggishly reactive pupils. The etiology of acute lung injury, formerly called "noncardiogenic pulmonary edema," is not clearly understood but is likely to be multifactorial. Naloxone administration causing a catecholamine surge may be a contributing factor.[46] Troponin rises can be seen in patients with heroin overdose (unpublished data).

Typically in their late 20s or early 30s, heroin overdose victims are likely to have a long heroin-using career, be opioid dependent and regular users, prefer the intravenous route, have high levels of treatment contact but not be currently in treatment, and have a criminal history. Research indicates that nonfatal acute opioid overdose is a remarkably common experience among heroin users[47]; however, in multiple logistic regression analyses, age, hospital admission, suicidal intent, principal poisoning, and type of opiate were statistically significant predictors of death.[48]

By contrast, other opiates such as methadone, codeine and diphenoxylate, which are longer-acting, have been associated with increased morbidity and mortality. Care must be taken in patients at the extremes of age or those with renal or hepatic impairment.

Antidote Considerations: Naloxone

Two important early studies demonstrated the efficacy of naloxone in reversing opiate poisoning. Evans and coworkers[49] reported a study in which naloxone (0.4 to 1.2 mg given intravenously) resulted in recovery of consciousness within 1 to 2 minutes in nine patients with a history of opiate ingestion. This was associated with improvement in respiratory function in the six patients in whom this could be assessed by measurement of minute volume and respiratory rate. This rapid and clear benefit of therapy also was reported by Buchner and colleagues in 1972,[50] who studied the effects of naloxone (0.005 to 0.01 mg/kg) in 10 children with methadone poisoning.

The *recommended dose* of naloxone for a 70-kg adult is 0.2 to 0.4 mg given intravenously, for a maximum dose of 10 mg, and titrated to response. A high incidence (45%) of adverse events was reported during out-of-hospital naloxone administration. It is likely that the observed events mainly represented opioid withdrawal effects caused by naloxone. They also could be related to hypoxia and to the extensive use of heroin in combination with other agents. Most events were not serious.[51]

SPECIFIC POISONS AND ANTIDOTES

Acetaminophen

Acetaminophen (paracetamol) is one of the most common drugs taken in overdose. It is easily accessible and requires no prescription. Acetaminophen causes liver toxicity. Toxic levels are more likely to occur with ingestions over 150 mg/kg. Acetaminophen is metabolized by three mechanisms in the liver. A major portion of the drug is conjugated to glucuronide or sulfate (the latter is of decreasing importance with age but is extremely important in pediatric ingestions). A small amount is metabolized by the P-450 enzyme system to a potentially toxic intermediate (4%) N-acetyl-p-benzoquinoneimine (NAPQI). This intermediate is metabolized by glutathione to a nontoxic mercaptopurine product. Only when an excessive amount of acetaminophen has been ingested is this pathway of any importance. In the face of an overdose, however, glutathione can be used up, and when levels fall below 30% of normal, glutathione can no longer detoxify the acetaminophen intermediate, so toxicity develops.[52]

Because P-450 distribution is mostly confined to the centrilobular area of the liver, the characteristic histopathological change seen in acetaminophen-induced liver injury is centrilobular necrosis. Very rarely, renal impairment or mental status changes and acidosis may develop in the presence of a massive overdose. Without treatment, patients will present with nausea and vomiting. Within 24 hours, they will show an elevation in the international normalized ratio (INR). At 36 to 48 hours after ingestion, they will demonstrate an elevation in liver transaminases, followed by a rise in bilirubin levels. Frank liver failure occurs 5 to 7 days after the ingestion.

Treatment

The management of acetaminophen poisoning is determined by the drug level measured at least 4 hours after ingestion (after distribution has occurred). A nomogram plots the level against the probability of liver damage. A 4-hour level of 1000 mmol/L is an indication to begin treatment with N-acetylcysteine. If the level is above the line for the time after ingestion, antidotal therapy with N-acetylcysteine is indicated. If the level falls below the line, and the history of time of ingestion is accurate, then antidotal treatment is not required. The nomogram is adjusted down (by 30%) for patients with glutathione deficiency states. All patients who present within 1 hour of an acetaminophen overdose should be given activated charcoal if their airway is secure. If the patient can be given N-acetylcysteine within 8 hours after ingestion, then liver damage despite a high blood level is highly unlikely.

N-acetylcysteine acts by donating a sulfhydryl group to detoxify the P-450–formed intermediate. It also replenishes glutathione stores. People at risk for acetaminophen toxicity are those with lowered glutathione stores, including alcoholic persons and those on medication that increases P-450 activity, such as phenobarbital.

There is *no* time at which N-acetylcysteine *cannot* be given. Early reports, especially from the United Kingdom, suggested that N-acetylcysteine was of no benefit if given 16 hours after ingestion. This suggestion has proved to be false, and in more recent studies, even patients with fulminant hepatic failure from acetaminophen ingestion have benefited from the administration of N-acetylcysteine.[53] In fact, one school of thought advocates the use of N-acetylcysteine for any cause of liver failure, in accordance with the rationale that restored glutathione stores are helpful in combating oxidant stress on liver that has failed from any cause. Animal studies have shown that N-acetylcysteine may improve the survival of isolated perfused rat livers and may improve liver function in pigs.[54,55] The use of N-acetylcysteine in orthotopic liver transplantation had modest but not statistically significant hemodynamic effects in a study of 50 patients with chronic end-stage liver disease.[56]

In a recent study, Kerr and colleagues[57] showed no difference in anaphylactoid reaction rate when the initial bolus injection was given in 60 minutes rather than 15 minutes. (Of note, however, a trend toward decreased anaphylactoid reactions in the slower infusion group was demonstrated, with a 4% absolute risk reduction in the 60-minute group.) The lack of statistical difference has since been supported in a smaller retrospective study.[58] The rate of adverse reactions to intravenous *N*-acetylcysteine is variously quoted between 6% and 45%.[57-59] In their study, Merl and coworkers[58] found the most common adverse reaction to be flushing (noted in 14 patients [6%]), with urticaria (in 13 [5%]), bronchospasm (in 9 [4%]), and pruritus (in 3 [1.2%]) also reported. Patients were more likely to have an adverse reaction if they had not received *N*-acetylcysteine previously (10% versus 20%) and if the initial infusion was administered within 15 minutes (45% versus 28%), but neither factor reached statistical significance.

The anaphylactoid reaction seen in *N*-acetylcysteine administration is dose- and dose-rate–dependent. Because this reaction does not represent mast cell degranulation, if a rash or wheeze develops, the infusion should be stopped, antihistamines with or without steroids should be administered, and when the symptoms abate, the infusion should be cautiously restarted.

The *loading dose* of *N*-acetylcysteine is 150 mg/kg in 200 mL of 5% dextrose given over 15 minutes to 1 hour (note alteration from conventional recommendation of 15 minutes). Then 50 mg/kg in 500 mL of 5% dextrose is given over 4 hours, followed by 100 mg/kg in 1000 mL of 5% dextrose over 16 hours.

Ethylene Glycol

In the 2005 American Association of Poison Control Centers (AAPC) report,[1] fomepizole, the alcohol dehydrogenase antagonist used in the treatment of ethylene glycol poisoning was reported to be used 1206 times, representing 0.5% of all human exposures. The ingested amount of ethylene glycol required to produce toxicity in animals is approximately 1 to 1.5 mL/kg.[60] Glycoxylic and glycolic acid are the major toxins formed by the metabolism of ethylene glycol, but the parent compound is not readily measured, nor are these metabolites. Acid-base measurement and calculated osmolar gap often are used as indirect indicators of ethylene glycol toxicity, but the sensitivity and specificity of these measures is dependent on time from ingestion. Late presenters may have low or immeasurable concentrations of unchanged ethylene glycol and a consequently normal osmolar gap (less than 10 mOsm/kg).[61] In a survey of U.S. teaching hospitals, only 25% performed analysis of ethylene glycol on site, with a median turn-around time of 42 hours reported for off-site results.[62]

Clinical Manifestations

CNS depression is most severe within 6 to 12 hours after ingestion, when the acidic metabolites reach maximal concentration. Pneumonitis, pulmonary edema, and acute lung injury also have been reported.[63] Renal involvement becomes apparent 24 to 72 hours later as the metabolites of ethylene glycol, notably glycolic acid, accumulate.[64] If

TABLE 173-5

Recommended Biochemical Tests for Screening Patients with Suspected Toxicity in Small, Rural, or Remote Hospitals

- Arterial blood gases
- Electrolytes
- Anion gap
- Serum osmolality
- Urine oxalate crystals
- Lactate analysis
- Serum creatinine
- Ethylene glycol screening by enzymatic method or gas chromatography

In larger toxicology centers, testing should include all of the above and ethylene glycol confirmatory test and screening and quantification of glycolic acid on a 24-hour basis (<2-hour turn-around time).
Adapted from Fraser AD: Clinical toxicologic implications of ethylene glycol and glycolic acid poisoning. Ther Drug Monit 2002;24:232-238.

TABLE 173-6

AACT Criteria for Treatment of Ethylene Glycol Poisoning with an Antidote

Plasma ethylene glycol level >20 mg/dL (3 mmol/L)
or
Documented recent history of ingestion of ethylene glycol with an osmolar gap >10 mOsmol/kg
or
Strong suspicion of poisoning and at least 2 of the following:
- Arterial pH <7.3
- Serum bicarbonate <20 mEq/L (20 mmol/L)
- Osmolar gap >10 mOsmol/kg
- Urinary oxalate crystals present

AACT, American Academy of Clinical Toxicology.
Adapted from Barceloux DG, Krenzelok EP, Olsen K, et al: American Academy Practice Guidelines on the treatment of ethylene glycol poisoning. Ad Hoc Committee. J Toxicol Clin Toxicol 1999;37:537-560.

untreated, ethylene glycol toxicity may be fatal within 24 to 36 hours (Tables 173-5 and 173-6).

Treatment

FOMEPIZOLE. The loading dose is 15 mg/kg, with a maintenance dose 10 mg/kg every 12 hours for 4 doses followed by 15 mg/kg every 12 hours until ethylene glycol levels fall below 20 mg/dL (3 mmol/L). A separate treatment regime is used for the administration of fomepizole during hemodialysis.[65]

ETHANOL INFUSION. Intravenous ethanol (10% diluted in 5% dextrose) is given as a loading dose of 10 mL/kg over 30 minutes, followed by an infusion of 1.4 to 2.0 mL/kg per hour. Ethanol acts as an alternative substrate for alcohol dehydrogenase.

HEMODIALYSIS. American Academy of Clinical Toxicology (AACT) guidelines for hemodialysis in the setting of ethylene glycol poisoning include deteriorating vital signs despite intensive care support, significant metabolic acidosis (pH < 7.25), and renal failure or electrolyte imbalances unresponsive to conventional therapy.[60] Glycolic acid has a half-life of up to 18 hours, which is reduced by a factor of 6 with hemodialysis.[66]

OTHER AGENTS. Pyridoxine (50 to 100 mg every 6 hours) and thiamine (100 mg daily) both help promote the metabolism of intermediate byproducts to nontoxic metabolites.

Hypoglycemia Secondary to Sulfonylureas and Other Long-Acting Diabetic Medications

Sulfonylureas are responsible for 4000 poisoning exposures each year.[67] These medications can produce toxicity after a single tablet ingestion in children.[68] By binding to the sulfonylurea receptor on the beta cell of the pancreas, they promote the release of insulin. In nondiabetics, this excess insulin can lead to prolonged hypoglycemia.

Treatment

The mainstay of treatment is dextrose replacement, often at high infusion rates or concentrations. Octreotide is a long-acting synthetic octapeptide analogue of somatostatin and has been used to treat a variety of endocrine problems and esophageal variceal bleeding. In the hyperinsulinemic state after a sulfonylurea overdose, octreotide inhibits further insulin release from pancreatic beta cells. In human studies, octreotide decreases the number of hypoglycemic episodes and the required duration of dextrose therapy.[69,70] Octreotide is given by infusion at 50 µg/kg per dose, divided, every 6 to 8 hours.

Cyanide

Cyanide is a metabolic poison. Although the precise in vivo action of cyanide has yet to be determined, it is thought that its major effect is due to binding with the ferric ion (Fe^{3+}) in cytochrome oxidase, the last cytochrome in the respiratory chain causing inhibition of oxidative phosphorylation. As a result of this action, the clinical signs and symptoms of acute cyanide poisoning reflect gross metabolic disruption. As a consequence of inhibition of oxidative phosphorylation, there is a net accumulation of hydrogen ions and a change in the nicotinamide adenine dinucleotide (NAD)/NADH ratio, with greatly increased lactic acid production.[71]

Clinical Manifestations

CNS signs and symptoms, in order of increasing severity of cyanide exposure, include headache, anxiety, disorientation, lethargy, seizures, respiratory depression, CNS depression, and, finally, cerebral death.

Respiratory manifestations include initial tachypnea, which gives way to respiratory depression as CNS depression emerges.

Cardiovascular signs and symptoms include hypertension, usually followed by hypotension, tachycardia followed by bradycardia and the development of a variety of arrhythmias, including atrioventricular block. Systemic vascular resistance usually is decreased, and cardiac output usually is increased. The arteriovenous oxygen difference, a measure of oxygen extraction, is decreased. In the event of cardiovascular collapse, bright red skin or blood will not be a feature (with decreased oxygen consumption) in patients in whom significant myocardial, respiratory, or CNS depression has already occurred. In these situations, the patient will appear cyanotic. Cyanosis also may "appear" after treatment with amyl nitrite and induction of methemoglobinemia.[72,73]

Treatment

Cyanide poisoning is treated differently in different parts of the world. The treatment approach will differ according to whether cyanide is to be directly chelated with a cobalt-containing moiety (dicobalt edetate 300 mg and hydroxocobalamin 2.5 to 5 g as an initial dose) or whether the cyanide is provided with an alternative ferric ion source, thereby competitively removing it from the cytochrome, using a cyanide antidote kit containing amyl nitrite perles, sodium nitrite 10 mL (30 mg/mL), and sodium thiosulfate, 50 mL (250 mg/mL). The rationale for use of the cyanide antidote kit is that the nitrites produce methemoglobin (ferric hemoglobin) to which the cyanide combines to form cyanomethemoglobin, releasing the cyanide from the cytochrome. The addition of sodium thiosulfate converts the cyanide to thiocyanate, which is renally excreted, while the iron in the hemoglobin is restored to the ferrous state.

Currently the only labeled antidote available in Australia is dicobalt edetate, known as Kelocyanor. A major consideration is that administration of Kelocyanor is associated with a high rate of allergic reactions, particularly in the nonpoisoned patient. The cyanide antidote kit may be unsuitable for use in patients with carboxyhemoglobin poisoning. It has been shown that the mean peak amount of methemoglobin levels achieved after the administration of 300 mg of sodium nitrite is 10.5%.[74] This amount is below levels expected to affect significant exposure to carbon monoxide alone. Nevertheless, in the presence of coexisting carboxyhemoglobin poisoning and the reduced aerobic metabolism of cyanide toxicity, methemoglobin represents a potential (as yet undetermined) insult. Thus, the decision to use the kit presents a dilemma in the management of victims of potential smoke inhalation.

Hydroxocobalamin is a therapeutic agent with few side effects that can be safely given to nontoxic patients and is currently in use in Europe. A paucity of scientific data is available comparing the efficacy of hydroxocobalamin and dicobalt edetate, thereby precluding any definitive conclusion about which antidote is best. More is known about the fate of hydroxocobalamin in humans and its safety. In the emergency situation, hydroxocobalamin appears to offer a greater margin of safety. Hydroxocobalamin is recognized as an efficacious, safe, and easily administered cyanide antidote.[75,76]

Because of its extremely low adverse effect profile, hydroxocobalamin is ideal for out-of-hospital use in suspected cyanide intoxication. It has been recently recommended as the antidote of choice in the event of a cyanide chemical disaster to prevent needless morbidity and mortality.[77] The combination of hydroxocobalamin and thiosulfate has been reported to provide effective treatment for patients with extremely high levels of cyanide poisoning, and this combination is to be recommended.[78]

Heavy Metals

A variety of heavy metals have been taken (or given) as poison, both deliberately and accidentally. Common poisons include lead, arsenic, mercury, copper, and thallium. Although an exhaustive list of potential poisons is beyond the scope of this chapter, each of the available antidotes, dimercaprol (British antilewisite [BAL]), dimercaptosuccinic acid (DMSA) (i.e., succimer), 2,3-dimercaptopropane-1-sulfonic acid (DMPS), and calcium edetate (calcium disodium ethylenediaminetetra-acetic acid [EDTA]) is discussed next.

Treatment

DIMERCAPROL. Dimercaprol was developed during World War II as an antidote to the war gas lewisite. Based on observations that arsenoxide drugs acted on thiol groups, and that these reactions could be mitigated by sulfhydryl groups, BAL was found to be an effective treatment for the severe reactions associated with organoarsenical antibiotics used in the treatment of syphilis.[79] Subsequently, BAL was found to be effective in the treatment of mercury poisoning as well.[80] Dimercaprol is an oily, colorless solution that has a peanut odor associated with the peanut oil vesicant in which it is dissolved. It forms 1:1 or 1:2 complexes with several metals and then promotes urinary excretion of the metal.

FDA-labeled indications are as follows:
- Arsenic toxicity (mild)
- Arsenic toxicity (severe)
- Gold toxicity (mild)
- Gold toxicity (severe)
- Lead poisoning (mild)—when used concomitantly with edetate calcium disodium injection
- Lead poisoning (severe)—when used concomitantly with edetate calcium disodium injection
- Mercury toxicity—effective for acute poisoning by mercury salts if therapy starts within 1 to 2 hours after ingestion; not very effective for chronic mercury poisoning

The major concern with BAL is the required method of administration and the theoretical possibility of mobilization of metal with redistribution to the brain, seen in animal models.[81] BAL is given as deep intramuscular injections (by spinal needle), with dose and frequency dependent on the type of metal poisoning, as evident in Table 173-7.[82]

Adverse reactions are dose-dependent and include transient hypertension, tachycardia, gastrointestinal effects, salivation, and muscular aches and pains. CNS effects include headache, paresthesia, tremor, and seizures at high doses.[83] Dermatitis is common, and the formation of a sterile abscess at the injection site has been reported.[84]

Contraindications include the following:
- Acute renal insufficiency that develops during therapy (in such cases, use at a reduced dosage with extreme caution or discontinuation of therapy is recommended)
- Hepatic insufficiency except in postarsenical jaundice
- Iron, cadmium, or selenium poisoning (more toxic in complex with dimercaprol)[85,86]

Use in copper, silver, and tellurium intoxications is limited.

Calcium Edetate

In 1950, calcium edetate (calcium disodium EDTA) was used for the treatment of hypercalcemia and in 1952 was first reported to be used in the treatment of lead poisoning.[87] EDTA acts to reduce blood concentrations and depot

TABLE 173-7

Dosages for Dimercaprol

- **Arsenic toxicity—mild:** 2.5 mg/kg IM 4 times daily for 2 days, 2 times on day 3, then once daily for 10 days or until recovery
- **Arsenic toxicity—severe:** 3 mg/kg IM every 4 hr for 2 days, 4 times on day 3, then twice daily for 10 days or until recovery
- **Gold toxicity—mild:** 2.5 mg/kg IM 4 times daily for 2 days, 2 times on day 3, then once daily for 10 days or until recovery
- **Gold toxicity—severe:** 3 mg/kg IM every 4 hr for 2 days, 4 times on day 3, then twice daily for 10 days or until recovery
- **Lead poisoning—mild:** When used concomitantly with edetate calcium disodium injection: 4 mg/kg IM for initial dose, then 3 mg/kg every 4 hr for 2 to 7 days in combination with edetate calcium disodium injection at separate injection site
- **Lead poisoning—severe:** When used concomitantly with edetate calcium disodium injection: 4 mg/kg IM every 4 hr for 2 to 7 days in combination with edetate calcium disodium injection at separate injection site
- **Mercury toxicity:** Effective for acute poisoning by mercury salts if therapy starts within 1 to 2 hr after ingestion; not very effective for chronic mercury poisoning: 5 mg/kg IM for 1 day, followed by 2.5 mg/kg 1 or 2 times daily for 10 days

Micromedia Health Care Series, accessed through Clinicians Health Channel. Available at http://micromedexudc.hcn.net.au/hcs/librarian/ND_PR/Drugs/SBK/4/PFPUI/VW3ZKGJ1HfKwV0/ND_PG/PRIH/CS/A08525/ND_CPR/SearchByDatabase/ND_T/HCS/ND_P/Drugs/DUPLICATIONSHIELDSYNC/EDCB94/ND_B/HCS/PFActionId/hcs.common.RetrieveDocumentCommon/DocId/181240/ContentSetId/42/SearchOption/BeginWith (accessed January 21, 2007).

stores of lead. The calcium is replaced by divalent and trivalent metals, especially any available lead, to form stable, soluble complexes that are readily excreted. EDTA also will complex with zinc, and during therapy, serum zinc levels decline by 60% to 70%, returning to normal at the cessation of treatment.[88]

FDA-labeled indications are as follows:
- Lead poisoning, acute—to reduce blood levels and depot stores of lead
- Lead poisoning, chronic—to reduce blood levels and depot stores of lead
- Toxic encephalopathy due to lead—to reduce blood levels and depot stores of lead

Contraindications include the following:
- Anuria or active renal disease
- Hepatitis

Adverse effects with EDTA may include injection site pain, nausea, vomiting, myalgia, headache, and hypotension. Fever, thrombophlebitis, hypersensitivity reactions, and nephrotoxicity are said to occur relatively frequently.

The preferred *route of administration* is continuous intravenous infusion, rather than intermittent inramuscular injections. The *dose* for adults with severe lead poisoning is 2 to 4 g per 24 hours.

Succimer (DMSA)

Orally active succimer is a heavy metal–chelating agent that forms stable, water-soluble complexes with lead and consequently increases the urinary excretion of lead.

The *FDA-labeled indication* for this agent is lead poisoning, but succimer chelates other heavy metals such as arsenic and mercury. In a study of the relative effectiveness or therapeutic index of the various dimercapto compounds in protecting mice from the lethal effects of a 99% lethal dose (LD99) of sodium arsenite, Aposhian and coworkers[89] found that DMSA is more effective than DMPS, DMPA, and BAL, with relative efficacy of 42:14:4:1, respectively. In addition, unlike in BAL, DMPS, DMPA, and DMSA will not increase the arsenic content of the brain of rabbits injected with sodium arsenite.[89]

The *dose* is 30 mg/kg daily for 5 days, followed by 20 mg/kg daily for 14 days.

Hypersensitivity is a *contraindication* to use of succimer. Reported *adverse events* include rash (occurring in approximately 4% of exposed people), diarrhea, loss of appetite, nausea, vomiting, abnormalities on liver function tests, and neutropenia.[90]

Monitoring of the following is recommended with use of this agent:

- Blood lead levels at least once weekly after therapy until the patient is stable
- Complete blood count (including white cell count with differential and direct platelet counts), before and weekly during treatment
- Measurement of serum transaminases before and weekly during treatment

2,3-Dimercaptopropane-1-Sulfonic Acid (Unithiol)

Unithiol is a chelator structurally related to dimercaprol. It is water-soluble and reported to be less toxic than dimercaprol. Unithiol is used in the treatment of poisoning by heavy metals including arsenic, lead, and inorganic and organic mercury compounds. It also has been used in poisoning with chromium or cadmium, although its efficacy in such cases is not established.

Unithiol is administered orally in a *dose* of 100 mg given three or four times daily in chronic poisoning. It also may be given parenterally in patients with severe toxicity; a suggested intravenous dose is 3 to 5 mg/kg every 4 hours, reducing the frequency or changing to oral therapy after 1 to 2 days.[91]

ARSENIC POISONING. Complete recovery, without renal or neurological sequelae, has been reported after the use of unithiol in patients with potentially lethal acute arsenic poisoning.[92,93] Increased urinary arsenic excretion, with some reduction in clinical signs and symptoms, also has been reported with unithiol in chronic arsenic toxicity.[94,95]

LEAD POISONING. Unithiol may be used in lead poisoning, although other chelators generally are preferred. In a study of 12 children, unithiol reduced lead concentrations in blood but did not affect the concentrations of copper or zinc in plasma, although the urinary excretion of lead, copper, and zinc was increased during treatment.[96]

MERCURY POISONING. Unithiol is used in poisoning with mercury and mercury salts and has been administered by various routes. In seven patients with poisoning due to mercury vapor or mercuric oxide, unithiol 100 mg, given twice daily by mouth for up to 15 days, was found to enhance urinary elimination of mercury.[97] The urinary elimination of copper and zinc also was increased in most patients; skin rashes developed in two patients. A dose of 5 mg/kg given intramuscularly three times daily, reduced

to once daily by the third day of treatment, effectively reduced the half-life of mercury in the blood after poisoning with methylmercury.[98] Unithiol also has been used with hemofiltration in patients with inorganic mercury poisoning and acute renal failure.[99,100]

WILSON'S DISEASE. Unithiol 200 mg twice daily was used successfully to maintain cupriuresis in a 13-year-old boy with Wilson's disease after systemic lupus developed during treatment with penicillamine and trientine dihydrochloride. Unithiol was started in two similar patients, but both withdrew from treatment, one because of fever and a fall in leukocyte count after a test dose and the other because of intense nausea and taste impairment.[101]

ADVERSE EFFECTS. Rash and pruritus have been reported in patients receiving unithiol (200 to 300 mg/day).[97,102] Nausea has been reported after use of unithiol.[101-103] Elevated liver enzymes occurred in a patient receiving unithiol 400 mg/day. Leukopenia and fever have been reported in a patient after a test dose of unithiol.[98] An allergic reaction with bronchospasm occurred in a patient after intravenous administration of unithiol 2 mg/kg; however, treatment was not necessary.[104] Headache has been reported in patients receiving unithiol (300 to 400 mg/day).[102,103] Bronchospasm occurred in a patient after intravenous administration of unithiol 2 mg/kg; treatment was not necessary.[104]

Digoxin

For those toxins with a high volume of distribution (V_d), a potential for enhancing removal of absorbed drug is recognized. The best illustration of such therapy is for digoxin overdose. Digoxin has a high V_d and in toxic doses causes a multitude of cardiac dysrhythmias and is responsible for considerable morbidity and mortality.

Treatment: Digoxin-Fab₂ Fragments (Digibind)

If an ingested toxin can be seen as a foreign agent, like an invading microbe, then the use of immunotherapy to combat the "invasion" was a logical concept. Antidigoxin antibodies raised in sheep have been available for some years; administration of such antibodies is now the standard of care in the treatment of digoxin toxicity. The antibodies use only the Fab fragment of the antibody so they have a low likelihood of producing an anaphylactic reaction on administration but carry the important antibody-binding site.

Fab fragments should be administered to severely cardiac glycoside–intoxicated patients who fail to respond to immediately available conventional therapy. Severe cardiac toxicity includes ventricular arrhythmias (ventricular tachycardia, ventricular fibrillation), progressive bradyarrhythmias (severe sinus bradycardia), or second- or third-degree heart block not responsive to atropine. Use of Digibind should be *considered* in adults who have ingested more than 10 mL of digoxin or children who ingested more than 4 mL of digoxin, in patients with a postdistribution serum concentration greater than 10 ng/mL (6 to 8 hours after ingestion), or in those patients with progressive elevation of serum potassium concentration associated with an ingestion of digoxin.

The *dose* of Digibind varies according to the amount of digoxin to be neutralized. A 76-mg dose of digoxin–immune Fab will neutralize approximately 1 mg of digoxin or digitoxin. The following dosing calculations and principles are used:

1. Digibind dose (number of vials) = body load (mg)/0.5 (mg/vial), *or*

2. Dose calculated from serum level: Digibind dose (number of vials) = [serum digoxin concentration (ng/mL) × patient's weight (kg)]/100.

3. If the estimated amount ingested or digitalis serum concentration is not available, 20 vials (760 mg) can be administered.

4. Four to six vials (152 mg to 228 mg) will be adequate to treat 90% to 95% of cases of chronic digoxin toxicity.[105]

Digibind is administered intravenously over 30 minutes, infused through a 0.22-μg filter. Intraosseous administration is *not* recommended. Earliest-possible administration is recommended in life-threatening intoxication.[105] A bolus injection can be given if cardiac arrest is imminent.

After therapy, free digoxin levels rebound, peaking approximately 3 to 24 hours after Fab administration in patients with normal renal function; then a slow, steady decline in free digoxin occurs at a rate dependent on Fab and renal and nonrenal routes of elimination.[106]

Adverse reactions have been reported with use of Fab fragment therapy. Congestive heart failure and low cardiac output states may be exacerbated by withdrawal of the inotropic effects of digitalis. Reactivation of ATPase may lead to hypokalemia. Withdrawal of the effects of digitalis on the atrioventricular node may result in the development of a rapid ventricular response in patients with atrial fibrillation.[107] Digoxin–Fab fragments should be used with caution in patients with severe renal failure. The use of Fab therapy in a patient with renal disease is considered as effective as in patients with normal renal function, although the increased risk of rebound digoxin toxicity mandates a longer period of observation. In patients with kidney failure, neither digoxin nor Fab can be removed efficiently from the systemic circulation by hemodialysis or continuous arteriovenous hemofiltration.[108]

Other Immunotoxicological Therapies

No other antibodies (other than antivenoms) are available for clinical use in Australia at the present time. However, antibodies to the antimetabolite colchicine have been developed and used in a patient. Although colchicine poisoning is not especially common, it does appear to meet most of the requirements for a Fab antidote, because the usual ingested amount is small and colchicine is extremely toxic, with a high mortality rate from progressive hemodynamic collapse. The use of a Fab antidote for human colchicine poisoning was reported in a young woman who took a large overdose in a suicide attempt. Subsequently, progressive severe cardiopulmonary compromise resistant to fluid administration and inotrope infusion developed, but she improved rapidly with administration of goat-derived colchicine-specific Fab fragments.[109]

Fab therapy for cyclic antidepressant toxicity in experimental use has reduced lethality, but it is worth noting that such intoxications are not ideal for an immunological antidote because ingested amounts typically are large; thus, the required Fab dose for human poisoning is very large.[110-112] Experimental antibodies specific for other intoxicants including phencyclidine,[113] the herbicide paraquat,[114] amanitin,[115] and tetrodotoxin[116] also have been reported, but clinical experience is lacking for these agents.

SOME RENAL CONSIDERATIONS

Acute renal toxicity from poisoning or overdose can be due to organ specific injury or be part of a generalized multiorgan pattern. The unusual susceptibility of the kidney to toxic injury stems from its function of regulating the volume and composition of body fluids. The physiological role of the kidneys in filtration, concentration, excretion, and secretion directly affects how toxins and poisons are handled. Lithium, for example, almost exclusively eliminated in the urine (98%), can reach toxic levels in conditions that alter kidney function. Drug interactions, acute intercurrent medical illness, low-salt diet, dehydration and volume depletion, cardiac failure, thiazide diuretics, and concurrent use of nonsteroidal anti-inflammatory medication can predispose patients to develop acute or acute-on-chronic lithium poisoning, without having a direct tubulotoxic effect. By contrast, ethylene glycol causes renal toxicity by elaboration of a toxic metabolite glycolic acid, which in isolated rodent proximal tubule cells causes direct cellular damage.[64] The inherent toxicity of unmetabolized ethylene glycol is low compared with its many metabolites, and this knowledge has driven the treatment of toxicity, including the introduction of the antidote fomepizole, an alcohol dehydrogenase inhibitor that blocks the metabolism of ethynene glycol and slows the metabolism.

In salicylate toxicity, for example, the normal mechanisms for handling the poison are exceeded (zero-order kinetics), and renal excretion becomes time-dependent, renal absorption is pH-dependent, renal toxicity is both direct and indirect, and a major treatment modality involves manipulation of kidney processes.

Normally salicylate undergoes both glomerular filtration and tubular secretion. At therapeutic doses, the metabolic pathways for salicylates become saturated. Renal excretion is therefore very important in the elimination of salicylate at both therapeutic and toxic levels. Only the unbound fraction of salicylate is available for glomerular filtration, but in toxicity, this portion increases. Salicylate is reabsorbed at the proximal convoluted tubules (PCTs). This latter process depends on both urine flow rate and urine pH, and in an acid environment, salicylate is maximally nonionized, facilitating transfer across cell membranes and hence PCT reabsorption.

The mechanism by which aspirin exerts its toxicity is complex and not fully understood. Recognized effects, however, include direct respiratory center stimulation, uncoupling of oxidative phosphorylation, inhibition of the tricarboxylic acid cycle, inhibition of amino acid metabolism, stimulation of glyconeogenesis and lipid metabolism, and increased tissue glycolysis. In addition, interference with hemostatic mechanisms also is seen. Together, these features contribute to the total picture of aspirin poisoning.[117]

Renal toxicity may be explained either by a reduction in renal blood flow or as a result of direct nephrotoxicity. Typically it is thought salicylates acutely inhibit prostaglandin synthesis, resulting in vasoconstriction and reduced renal blood flow and glomerular filtration.[118] The resultant oliguria is exacerbated by the presence of dehydration. Preexisting renal disease may predispose affected patients to the development of renal impairment.[119] Other toxic manifestations include pulmonary edema and fluid retention from inappropriate antidiuretic hormone secretion, hypernatremia, and hypokalemia. The presence of a significant acidemia may result in a normal serum K$^+$ level but mask a true total body potassium deficiency.

Although acid-base disturbance is one of the most common manifestations of salicylate toxicity, toxicity itself is influenced by serum and urinary acid-base balance. Because biliary elimination of salicylate is minimal,[120] the renal handling of salicylate after poisoning is highly relevant to clinical management. In order to prevent CNS penetration and promote urinary excretion, the serum and urine of the patient should be alkalinized to shift the salicylate moiety to the ionic form. Chapman and Proudfoot[121] described patients in four categories of acid-base disturbance, with mixed respiratory alkalosis and metabolic acidosis or respiratory alkalosis alone predominating in 61% and 19% of patients, respectively. The arterial pH, rather than the class of acid-base disturbance, was of greater value in determining clinical severity and mortality. Reabsorption of salicylate by the kidney is pH dependent.

CONCLUSION

Paracelsus, the father of toxicology, wrote: "All things are poison and nothing is without poison, only the dose permits something not to be poisonous." The potential source matter for a chapter on drugs and antidotes is therefore as extensive as a pharmacopedia. Accordingly, many toxins, including plant and animal toxins and mushrooms to any great degree, have been omitted here, with the focus on the common and the challenging and with a renal perspective. The reader is encouraged to consult textbooks of toxicology for a broader review.

Key Points

1. Identification of toxidromes enables the clinician to identify the type of poisoning and initial treatment even if the identity of the substance is unknown.

2. The most common toxidrome is from anticholinergic poisoning.
3. Consideration of antidotal therapy is limited to specific toxins. Supportive care is the mainstay of treatment.
4. Antidotal therapy depends on the pharmacokinetic (toxicokinetic) properties of the poison.
5. Although poisoning is part of the differential diagnosis in all cases of poorly defined illness, consideration of nontoxic causes, such as head or environmental trauma, which may occur concomitantly, is vital to ensure that treatable conditions are not overlooked.

Key References

14. Wallace KW: Toxin-induced seizures. In Brent J, Wallace KL, Burkhart KK, et al (eds): Critical Care Toxicology. Diagnosis and Management of the Critically Poisoned Patient. Philadelphia, Mosby, 2005, pp 225-238.
31. Proudfoot AT, Donovan JW: Diagnosis of poisoning. In Brent J, Wallace KL, Burkhart KK, et al (eds): Critical Care Toxicology. Diagnosis and Management of the Critically Poisoned Patient. Philadelphia, Mosby, 2006, pp 13-28.
57. Kerr F, Dawson A, Whyte IM, et al: The Australian Clinical Toxicology Investigators Collaboration randomized trial of different loading infusion rates of N-acetylcysteine. Ann Emerg Med 2005;45:402-408.
89. Aposhian HV, Carter DE, Hoover TD, et al: DMSA, DMPS, and DMPA as arsenic antidotes. Toxicol Sci 1984;4:58-70.
98. Clarkson TW, Magos L, Cox C, et al: Tests of efficacy of antidotes for removal of methylmercury in human poisoning during the Iraq outbreak. J Pharmacol Exp Ther 1981;218: 74-83.

See the companion Expert Consult website for the complete reference list.

Hemodialysis, Hemofiltration, and Hemoperfusion in Acute Intoxication and Poisoning

Nikolas Harbord, Steven J. Gruber, Donald A. Feinfeld, and James Frank Winchester

OBJECTIVES

This chapter will:
1. Present the indications for extracorporeal therapies in the treatment of acute poisoning.
2. Review principles of drug removal and how they apply to selection of modality.
3. Describe the utility and complications of combining chelating agents to improve clearance of heavy metals.
4. Discuss clinical presentation and treatment (including extracorporeal therapy) with regard to specific intoxicants.

The treatment of acute intoxications involves application of nonspecific measures such as cardiopulmonary support and administration of activated charcoal and specific measures such as use of antidotes and modulation of urinary pH to enhance elimination. Extracorporeal therapies, including hemodialysis, hemofiltration, and hemoperfusion, are useful adjuncts in the treatment of acute poisoning.[1]

Criteria for initiating drug (or poison) removal by extracorporeal methods and for the selection of modality are reviewed next, followed by a discussion of the use of chelating agents to enhance removal of metals. Finally, detailed consideration is given to specific intoxicants where extracorporeal methods can play a major therapeutic role.

CRITERIA FOR CONSIDERATION OF EXTRACORPOREAL THERAPY

Discrete indications to recommend the use of dialysis exist for several types of intoxications, including agents with delayed toxicity such as mushrooms, paraquat, methanol, and ethylene glycol. Dialysis also should be considered when endogenous drug clearance is impaired or markedly slower (e.g., cardiac, renal, or hepatic failure) than can be achieved with available extracorporeal therapy.

In most cases, the decision to use dialysis for drug clearance during intoxication is clinical. Signs and symptoms to consider include abnormalities in vital signs suggesting hemodynamic instability, clinical deterioration despite adequate supportive treatment, and evidence of mental status deterioration, including confusion, lethargy, stupor, and coma. Further indications include pneumonia due to coma and midbrain dysfunction, as indicated by hypothermia, hypotension, and bradycardia.

In addition to removing the offending agent, dialysis may reverse electrolyte abnormalities and correct the metabolic acidosis that may accompany some types of poisoning. Dialytic therapies should be considered in the setting of concomitant metabolic disorders.

Hypotensive patients requiring hemodynamic support with an indication for dialysis should receive an infusion of adrenergic or vasopressin-agonist pressors distal to the dialysis or sorbent cartridge. Furthermore, careful monitoring of circulatory status is essential, because pressor clearance will be increased and requirements may change.

Hemodialysis

Hemodialysis is the most commonly used method of extracorporeal drug removal in this setting.[2] Factors governing the efficiency of drug removal with hemodialysis are both drug-related and dialysis-related.

Drug factors that increase removal are small molecular size (molecular weight less than 500), high water solubility, low degree of protein binding, small volume of distribution (less than 1 L/kg), and rapid equilibration of plasma and tissue to maintain a concentration gradient.[3] Limited drug clearance should be expected with drugs that are highly lipid soluble, tightly tissue bound, with large volumes of distribution, and slow plasma equilibration.

Dialysis factors include access type, blood and dialysate flow rates, and dialyzer properties (material, surface area, and pore size). The use of low blood flow rates may prevent hemodynamic instability but may necessitate longer or continuous treatments for adequate clearance. Although higher dialysate flow rates will increase diffusive clearance to some degree, no benefit is achieved with flow rates greater than 1.5 times that of blood.

With the use of membranes of larger pore size, larger-molecular-weight drugs can be cleared. For example, vancomycin is readily cleared with large-pore (high-flux) membranes despite a molecular weight of 1400.[4] As molecular weight increases, drug removal is less a function of diffusion than of convection (because of the creation of an ultrafiltrate).[5]

Efficient clearance of a large-molecular-weight intoxicant is best accomplished by ultrafiltration dialysis. This modality, *hemodiafiltration*, uses ultrafiltration across a high-flux dialysis membrane and countercurrent flow of dialysate for combined diffusive and convective clearance. The principle of hemofiltration, which relies on convective clearance alone, is considered further in the following discussion.

A list of readily dialyzable drugs is provided in Table 174-1.

Hemofiltration

Hemofiltration is employed in a continuous manner with several possible variations. In the simplest form, blood circulates under arterial pressure, as in continuous arteriovenous hemofiltration (CAVH), or is pumped out of the

TABLE 174-1

Drugs Removed with Hemodialysis*

Antimicrobials	*Other antimicrobials*	Nonbarbiturate hypnotics, sedatives,	Acetaminophen
Cephalosporins	Clavulanic acid	tranquilizers	Acetylsalicylic acid
Cefadroxil	PAS	Carbromal	Colchicine
Cefamandole	Moxalactam	Carbemazepine	(*d*-Propoxyphene)
Cefazolin	Metronidazole	Chloral hydrate	Acetophenetidin
Cephradine	Nitrofurantoin	Chlordiazepoxide	Methylsalicylate
Cefmenoxime	Sulfonamides	(Diazepam)	Salicylic acid
Cefmetazole	Tetracycline	(Diphenylhydantoin)	Antidepressants
(Cefonicid)	(Doxycycline)	(Diphenhydramine)	(Amitriptyline)
(Cefoperazone)	(Minocycline)	Ethiamate	Amphetamines
Ceforanide	Ethambutol	Ethchlorvinyl	(Imipramine)
(Cefotaxime)	Colistin	Ethosuximide	Isocarboxazid
Cefotetan	Trimethoprim	Gallamine	MAO inhibitors
Cefotiam	Aztreonam	Glutethamide	(Pargylline)
Cefoxitin	Cilastatin	(Heroin)	(Phenelzine)
Cefpirome	Imipenim	Meprobamate	Tranylcypromine
Cefroxadine	Chloramphenicol	(Methaqualone)	Tricyclics
Cefsulodin	Amphotericin	Methsuximide	Solvents/gases
Ceftazidime	Ciprofloxacin	Methprylon	Acetone
(Ceftriaxone)	(Norfloxacin)	Paraldehyde	Camphor
Cefuroxime	Ofloxacin	Primidone	Carbon monoxide
Cephacetrile	(Clindamycin)	Valproic acid	(Carbon tetrachloride)
Cephalexin	(Cycloserine)	Cardiovascular agents	(Eucalyptus oil)
Cephalothin	Isoniazid	Acebutolol	Thiols
(Cephapirin)	Vancomycin	(Amiodarone)	Toluene
Penicillins	Pyrizinamide	Atenolol	Trichloethylene
Penicillin	Pentamidine	Betaxolol	Sodium citrate
Amoxicillin	(Praziquantel)	(Bretyllium)	Plants/animals/herbicides/pesticides
Ampicillin	Rifampin	(Calcium channel blockers)	Alkyl phosphates
Carbenicillin	Chloroquine	Captopril	Amanitin
(Cloxacillin)	Quinine	Enalapril	Demetan sulfoxide
(Methicillin)	(Itraconazole)	Fosinopril	Dimethoate
(Nafcillin)	(Fluconazole)	Lisinopril	Diquat
Ticarcillin	(Ketoconazole)	Quinapril	Methylmercury complex
Temocillin	(Miconazole)	Ramipril	(Organophosphates)
Pipericillin	(Ribavarin)	(Diazoxide)	Paraquat
(Mezlocillin)	Acyclovir	(Digoxin)	Snake venom
Mecillinam	Amantadine	(Encainide)	Sodium chlorate
Floxicillin	Didanosine	(Flecainide)	Potassium chlorate
(Dicloxicillin)	Foscarnet	(Lidocaine)	Miscellaneous
Macrolides	Ganciclovir	Metoprolol	Acipimox
(Erythromycin)	Zidovudine	Methyldopa	Allopurinol
(Azithromycin)	Antineoplastics/cytotoxics	(Ouabain)	Aminophylline
(Clarithromycin)	5-Fluorocytosine	*N*-acetylprocainamide	Aniline
Aminoglycosides	Methotrexate	Nadolol	Borates
Amikacin	Azathioprine	Pindolol	Boric acid
Dibekacin	Cyclophosphamide	Practolol	(Chlorpropamide)
Fosfomycin	Vidarabine	(Quinidine)	Chromic acid
Gentamicin	Barbiturates	(Timolol)	(Cimetidine)
Kanamycin	Amobarbital	Sotalol	Dinitro-*o*-cresol
Neomycin	Aprobarbital	Tocainide	Folic acid
Netilimicin	Barbital	Alcohols	Mannitol
Sisomicin	Butabarbital	Ethanol	Methylprednisolone
Streptomycin	Phenobarbital	Ethylene glycol	Potassium dichromate
Tobramycin	Cyclobarbital	Isopropanol	Theophylline
(Enoxacin)	(secobarbital)	Methanol	Thiocyanate
Bacitracin	Pentobarbital	Analgesics/antirheumatics	Ranitidine
Fleroxacin	Quinalbital		

*Drugs in parentheses are not well removed with hemodialysis.
MAO, monoamine oxidase; PAS, *p*-aminosalicylic acid.
Modified from Winchester JF: Active methods for detoxification. In Haddad LM, Shannon MW, Winchester JF (eds): Clinical Management of Poisoning and Drug Overdose, 3rd ed. Philadelphia, WB Saunders, 1997.

venous circulation to return passively, as in continuous venovenous hemofiltration (CVVH). Blood in the circuit enters the filtration cartridge (consisting of hollow fibers with large pores), and an ultrafiltrate of plasma forms from pressure across the membrane. Solutes are cleared into the ultrafiltrate by solvent drag, while cells and solutes larger than the pore size remain in the blood and return to the circulation. Hemofiltration requires both anticoagulation of the blood circuit and continuous replacement of fluid and electrolytes lost into the ultrafiltrate.

Depending on pore size, hemofiltration can remove molecules with molecular weight up to 50,000. In addition to molecular weight, the principal determinant of clearance is degree of protein binding. As plasma proteins are filtered (or not ultrafilterable), convective clearance across the pore is greatest with unbound molecules. The ability of a molecule to pass convectively across the membrane is quantifiable, and called the sieving coefficient (SC). Clearance is equal to the sieving coefficient multiplied by the ultrafiltration rate, and for molecules that pass completely (an SC of 1), the plasma clearance is equal to the ultrafiltration rate. Increasing the ultrafiltration rate will thus increase clearance of any intoxicant with an SC over 0.

Drug and membrane interactions, such as binding of aminoglycosides (e.g., with tobramycin and Biospal AN69 membranes), may impair sieving.[6] Furthermore, in vitro measurements of SC obtained using saline rather than blood may not closely reflect clinical drug sieving and actual clearance.

Continuous hemofiltration, with fluid and electrolyte replacement, is likely to be useful for the removal of drugs for which diffusive modalities are inadequate (despite large dialyzer pores) and dialysate requirements would be excessive. Drugs with a large volume of distribution or slow equilibration (such as procainamide) are examples.

Data on drug removal from patients and treatment of poisoning by continuous hemofiltration are extremely limited. However, this modality has been used to remove large-molecule antibiotics such as aminoglycosides and vancomycin, as well as complexes of metals and chelators. (For more on chelators, see later on.)

Some investigators have reported clinical improvement (cardiac function, drug levels) in patients with digoxin overdose treated with hemofiltration. In animal studies, CAVH was ineffective in the removal of digoxin-Fab complexes. These complexes are molecules with molecular weights of 45,000 to 50,000, the size limit for passage through hemofiltration pores.[7]

Hemoperfusion

Although it has been available for several decades, *hemoperfusion* is used infrequently to treat acute intoxications. In practice, the apparatus consists of a blood circuit identical to that for hemodialysis, including blood pumps and pressure monitors, but with a cartridge containing a large-surface-area column of charcoal or resin. The column is first primed with saline, and then anticoagulated blood is pumped through the cartridge, wherein drugs with molecular weights between 100 and 40,000 are removed by adsorption. Activated charcoal has greater affinity for water-soluble molecules, whereas resins have greater affinity for lipid-soluble molecules.

The rate of removal of drugs adsorbed to charcoal may exceed that achieved with hemodialysis. For example, the extraction of theophylline is 99% with hemoperfusion, compared with 50% with hemodialysis. However, the sorbent column may become saturated, and extraction ratios may progressively decline throughout treatment.

High extraction ratios and clearance rates may not predict improved clinical outcomes. In fact, no controlled studies in poisoned patients have been performed to determine if hemoperfusion (or hemodialysis) reduces morbidity or mortality when compared with supportive measures. Evidence of effectiveness is based on pharmacokinetic data, animal studies, case reports, and retrospective studies. Adverse effects of hemoperfusion, including flushing, dyspnea, and thrombocytopenia, have largely been reduced with changes to preparatory methods and the coating of absorbents with polymers.

Clinical experience has shown that a "rebound" of drug concentration may occur after hemoperfusion as the drug redistributes from tissues into the plasma compartment. The use of short, intermittent hemoperfusion sessions provides several advantages: less "rebound" effect with possible clinical improvement, reduction in the hematological side effects, and, as devices saturate with longer treatments, overall improved drug clearance.

If a poison is eliminated equally well with hemodialysis, hemodialysis is preferred over hemoperfusion because it is less expensive and can address any superimposed metabolic disorder or hypothermia. For some poisonings, however, hemoperfusion is superior and is the preferred modality: lipid-soluble drugs, cardiac glycosides, barbiturates, and other types of hypnotics-sedatives-tranquilizers.

Table 174-2 lists some chemicals and drugs removed by hemoperfusion.

Use of Chelating Agents with Extracorporeal Modalities

Dialysis and hemoperfusion do not efficiently remove heavy metals or metalloids or their salts. The addition of chelating agents, before (and possibly after) treatment, will improve total clearance through dialysis, filtration, or adsorption of the metal-chelator complex.

In the past, when aluminum hydroxide was used as a phosphate binder, aluminum intoxication in patients maintained on dialysis was effectively treated with deferoxamine and either hemodialysis or hemoperfusion, with clinical improvement in those with osteomalacia, anemia, or encephalopathy.[8] The use of dialysis with high-flux polysulfone membranes probably results in clearance equivalent or superior to that achievable with charcoal hemoperfusion.[9] Furthermore, hemodialysis is less expensive and will not result in the thrombocytopenia and leukopenia due to hemoperfusion. Although not a common acute intoxicant, iron also can be effectively removed from the body with deferoxamine and hemodialysis or charcoal hemoperfusion.[8]

None of the available evidence supports the addition of dialytic therapies to standard chelation in arsenic, mercury, or thallium poisoning. In the future, chelating microspheres in specialized hemoperfusion columns may improve clearance of many metallic poisons.[10]

TABLE 174-2

Drugs and Chemicals Removed with Hemoperfusion*

Barbiturates	Doxorubicin
Amobarbital	Gentamicin
Butabarbital	Isoniazid
Hexabarbital	(Methotrexate)
Hentobarbital	Thiabendazole
Phenobarbital	(5-Fluorouracil)
Quinalbital	Antidepressants
Secobarbital	(Amitriptyline)
Thipental	(Imipramine)
Vinalbital	(Tricyclics)
Nonbarbiturate hypnotics, sedatives, tranquilizers	Metals
Carbromal	(Aluminum)†
Chloral hydrate	(Iron)†
Chlorpromal	Plants/animals/herbicides/pesticides
(Diazepam)	Amantin
Diphenhydramine	Chlordane
Ethchlorvinyl	Demetan sulfoxide
Glutethamide	Dimethoate
Meprobamate	Diquat
Methaqualone	Methyparathion
Methsuximide	Nitrostigmine
Methprylon	(Organophosphates)
Promazine	Phalloidin
Promethazine	Polychlorinated biphenyls
(Valproic acid)	Paraquat
Solvents/gases	Parathion
Carbon tetrachloride	Cardiovascular drugs
Ethylene oxide	Digoxin
Trichloroethane	Diltiazem
Xylene	(Disopyramide)
Analgesics/antirheumatics	Flecainide
Acetaminophen	Metoprolol
Acetylsalicylic acid	N-acetylprocainamide
Colchicine	Procainamide
d-Propoxyphene	Quinidine
Antimicrobials/anticancer agents	Miscellaneous
(Doxorubicin [Adriamycin])†	Aminophylline
Ampicillin	Cimetidine
Carmustine	(Fluoroacetamide)
Chloramphenicol	(Phencyclidine)
Chloroquine	Phenols
Clindamycin	(Podophyllin)
Dapsone	Theophylline

*Drugs in parentheses are not well removed by hemoperfusion; those in parentheses with † are removed with addition of a chelator; drugs with ↑ are well removed regionally.
Modified from Winchester JF: Active methods for detoxification. In Haddad LM, Shannon MW, Winchester JF (eds): Clinical Management of Poisoning and Drug Overdose, 3rd ed. Philadelphia, WB Saunders, 1997.

INTOXICATION WITH SPECIFIC AGENTS

Table 174-3 lists the optimal techniques for removing specific poisons.

Lithium

Lithium, with an atomic number of 3 and an atomic weight of 6.94, is the lightest of all metals. Carbonate and citrate salts of lithium are used in the treatment of bipolar affective disorder; and despite known toxicity, its substantial

TABLE 174-3

Suggested Optimal Techniques for Removing Poisons

HEMODIALYSIS	HEMOPERFUSION
Lithium	Lipid-soluble drugs
Bromide	Barbiturates
Ethanol	Nonbarbiturate hypnotics, sedatives, tranquilizers (e.g., carbamazepine, valproic acid)
Methanol	
Ethylene glycol	
Salicylates	Digitalis glycosides*
Theophylline	Procainamide

*Anecdotal evidence only.

clinical efficacy as a "mood stabilizer" explains its persistent widespread use. In addition to acute toxicity, chronic effects include a variety of neurologic sequelae, persistent nephrogenic diabetes insipidus, chronic cystic interstitial nephritis, and nephrotic glomerulopathies.[11]

In other than sustained-release preparations, lithium is rapidly (1 to 2 hours) and completely absorbed from the gastrointestinal tract. If administered shortly after ingestion, sodium polystyrene sulfonate resin modestly reduces the oral bioavailabilty of lithium.[12] The effective dose and schedule are uncertain, however, and potassium lowering may result. Once absorbed, lithium distributes freely in body water, where it competes with other cations (in order of effect, sodium, potassium, magnesium, and calcium), displacing them from bones and cells. Uptake by and release of lithium from the central nervous system (CNS) may be delayed by as much as 24 hours owing to slow passage across the blood-brain barrier. Lithium is eliminated by the kidneys, and clearance parallels creatinine clearance. In adults, the average half-life is 29 hours. Factors that decrease lithium clearance include any decrease in glomerular filtration rate and conditions that promote proximal tubular reabsorption of lithium along sodium pathways: hypovolemia, NSAID use, and distal tubule (thiazide) diuretics. Conversely, clearance can be increased with volume expansion, loop diuretics, and interruption of distal sodium (and lithium) reabsorption with amiloride or triamterene.

The clinical effects of acute lithium intoxication are primarily neurological and renal. Neurological signs and symptoms increase with blood concentrations and include progression from confusion and lethargy to stupor and coma, as well as motor signs such as fine motor tremor, spasticity and hyperreflexia, dystonia or choreiform movements, and cogwheel rigidity and cerebellar signs. The principal renal manifestation is nephrogenic diabetes insipidus, resulting in polyuria and polydipsia and possibly hypernatremia. Lithium impairs urinary concentrating ability through interruption of cyclic adenosine monophosphate (AMP) signaling and insertion of aquaporins into the luminal surface of collecting duct cells. Cardiovascular effects include hypotension, myocarditis, ST segment depression, lateral T wave inversions, heart block, and premature atrial beats. Finally, gastrointestional manifestations include vomiting, diarrhea, and gastroenteritis.

Acute overdosage is fatal in approximately 25% of cases; intoxication during maintenance therapy has a mortality rate of 9%.[13] Approximately 10% of patients with acute intoxication will have permanent neurological or renal damage.

No toxicity generally is apparent (except in very elderly patients) with blood levels of drug below 1.3 mEq/L; mild toxicity with levels of 1.5 to 2.5 mEq/L; moderate toxicity with levels of 2.6 to 3.5 mEq/L, and severe (life-threatening) toxicity with levels greater than 3.6 mEq/L.

For acute lithium intoxication, with levels less than 2.5 mEq/L, general measures such as gastric lavage, volume expansion with fluids, and use of diuretics (loop, amiloride, or triamterene) usually are sufficient. For levels higher than 2.5 mEq/L, or if three or more measurements at different intervals plotted on a log-linear scale suggest prediction levels above 0.6 mEq/L at 36 hours, then extracorporeal removal is indicated.

Hemodialysis and hemofiltration are both effective, since lithium extraction by hemodialysis is more than 90%. Plasma levels may rebound after treatment as a result of redistribution or continued gastrointestinal reabsorption and should be monitored carefully. Intermittent hemodialysis treatments are recommended until levels remain below 1 mEq/L. A single, 6-hour hemodialysis session with a high-efficiency membrane or 24 hours of hemofiltration also probably is sufficient for adequate clearance to achieve a low serum lithium level.

Methanol

Methanol is a widely available commercial and industrial solvent and a potentially fatal intoxicant. Although toxicity is possible after skin absorption or inhalation, ingestion is the major route of poisoning. Ingestion usually is isolated to cases involving alcoholic derelicts; however, outbreaks of "wood alcohol" poisoning traced to counterfeit liquor sources also have occurred. As little as 60 to 240 mL of methanol, or 15 to 30 mL of 40% solution, can be fatal.[14] Peak blood levels of methanol follow ingestion by 30 to 90 minutes, with a volume of distribution of 0.6 to 0.7 L/kg.[15] Elimination is by biotransformation in the liver and kidneys to formaldehyde and then formic acid, with only 5% of ingested methanol excreted unchanged into the urine. The metabolites of methanol are, in fact, principally responsible for toxicity.

Early signs of intoxication include inebriation and drowsiness. Delayed signs and symptoms may be ocular and may include blurred vision, dilated pupils, and retinal toxicity (optic disc hyperemia and possible blindness) secondary to local conversion to formaldehyde. Other delayed manifestations include vomiting, diarrhea, back pain, vertigo, cold and clammy extremities, bradycardia, delirium, agitation, and an odor of formaldehyde to the urine. Severe intoxications may result in Kussmaul respiration, coma, inspiratory apnea, and death with opisthotonos and convulsions. Pancreatitis also has been found at autopsy.

Laboratory findings include high serum osmolal gap (early in intoxication, from unmetabolized methanol), high anion gap (due to formate retention), metabolic acidosis with low bicarbonate, high hematocrit, high mean corpuscular volume, high glucose, and high serum amylase.

Patients with suspected methanol toxicity should first receive gastric lavage to remove residual gastric methanol. Because onset of signs and symptoms often is delayed, treatment then involves prevention of formation and, if necessary, removal of toxic metabolites. The enzymatic oxidation of methanol to formaldehyde requires alcohol dehydrogenase (ADH), an enzyme with greater affinity for ethanol and hence increased efficiency in handling this compound. Ethanol or another ADH inhibitor, 4-methyl pyrazole (4-MP), should be administered to patients to prevent conversion to formaldehyde. Folic and folinic acid also help to convert formate to water and carbon dioxide.[16] Most authorities recommend giving 4-MP as soon as the diagnosis is considered, if it is available from hospital pharmacies.[17,18]

Hemodialysis is an effective modality to remove methanol and metabolites and to correct the metabolic acidosis. It should be considered when patients have serum methanol levels above 50 mg/dL, serious symptoms, or refractory acidosis. Dialysis should continue until levels are below 20 mg/dL, with monitoring for rebound of plasma concentrations. If ethanol is administered, it may be placed into the dialysate or replaced after dialytic removal.[17]

Ethylene Glycol

Another intoxicant involved in ingestions among alcoholics, as suicide attempts, and occasionally by accident is ethylene glycol. This irritant alcohol is widely found in cosmetics and antifreeze (car radiator) fluid, is sweet to the taste, and may contain fluorescent dye added to aid in identification. Like methanol, ethylene glycol undergoes biotransformation into metabolites with fatal toxic potential.

Peak blood levels follow ingestion by 1 to 4 hours, and ethylene glycol is filtered and reabsorbed in the kidneys. The toxic metabolites of ethylene glycol are glycoaldehyde, glycolate, glyoxalate, lactate, and oxalate. Deposition of birefringent calcium oxalate crystals in the renal tubules causes renal failure with interstitial nephritis and hemorrhagic necrosis. Similar tissue destruction occurs in meningeal blood vessels, liver, and pericardium. A profound metabolic acidosis occurs from lactic acidosis and production of glyoxalate metabolites, which inhibit the citric acid cycle and produce further lactate. Furthermore, glycolate recondenses to form glycine and carbon dioxide with further consumption of bicarbonate.

Early signs of intoxication include inebriation with absent alcoholic breath. Focal seizures, nystagmus, paralysis of eye muscles, hyperreflexia, tetany, and coma may be evident. This initial CNS depression is due to glycoaldehyde and occurs approximately 30 minutes to 12 hours after ingestion. The second phase of intoxication begins 12 to 14 hours after ingestion and results from calcium oxalate deposition and tissue destruction. Signs include tachycardia, hypotension, pulmonary edema, and congestive heart failure. The final phase occurs 24 to 72 hours after ingestion and manifests with flank pain and tenderness with oliguric acute tubular necrosis. Kussmaul respiration may accompany acidosis.

Laboratory findings include high serum osmolal gap, azotemia, and high–anion gap metabolic acidosis. Hypocalcemia and hyperkalemia also may be present. Urinary abnormalities may include calcium oxalate crystalluria, hematuria, proteinuria, oliguria, and low specific gravity.

Most authorities recommend giving 4-MP as soon as the diagnosis is considered, if 4-MP is available from hospital pharmacies.[17,18] Hemodialysis removes ethylene glycol and metabolites and will correct the metabolic acidosis. It should be considered when metabolites are present and acidosis complicates the clinical picture. If ethanol is administered, it can be mixed with dialysate or given intravenously.

Patients also should receive gastric lavage to remove residual ethylene glycol. Ethanol or 4-MP should be administered to prevent conversion to metabolites. Intramuscular pyridoxine (500 mg four times daily), used to stimulate glyoxalate conversion to α- or β-ketoadipate, and thiamine (100 mg four times daily), used to convert glyoxalate to glycine, also are recommended.

Salicylates

Salicylates are a subclass of nonsteroidal anti-inflammatory drugs (NSAIDs) with well-described acute and chronic toxicity. The following discussion is limited to acute intoxication only.

Salicylates are absorbed in the jejunum of the small intestine. Delayed gastric emptying (e.g., presence of food in the stomach) and enteric coating of pills may prolong absorption time up to 12 hours. During first-pass metabolism, acetysalicylic acid is hydrolyzed into salicylic acid, which is then slowly cleared from the blood (half-life of 20 to 30 hours). Excretion occurs by conjugation with glycine and glucuronic acid to form salicyluric acid, salicylphenolic acid, and acylglucuronides.

Clinical features of acute intoxication invariably include tinnitus, deafness in varying degrees, bounding pulse, profuse sweating, and flushing with warm extremities. Nausea and vomiting may result from gastrointestinal irritation. Acid-base disorders with salicylate toxicity are common but variable in presentation according to patient age. These disturbances include a respiratory alkalosis, from central hyperventilation with increased rate and depth of breathing, and high–anion gap metabolic acidosis from accumulation of salicylates and bicarbonate consumption. In younger children, younger than 4 years of age, acidosis predominates. In older children and adults, respiratory alkalosis is more common. CNS signs are more common in children and include agitation and uncommunicative behavior followed by coma. CNS manifestations correlate with the degree of acidemia, which further facilitates entry of salicylates into the cerebrospinal fluid. Increased vascular permeability may result in pulmonary edema. Petechiae of the eyelids, face, and neck may be present.

Laboratory findings include mixed acid-base disorders with high anion gap metabolic acidosis and respiratory alkalosis or respiratory acidosis if respiratory failure develops. Hypocalcemia or hypercalcemia and hypokalemia also may be present. The clotting profile may show prolonged vitamin K–dependent coagulation.

Recommended gastrointestinal decontamination involves the use of single- and multiple-dose activated charcoal; ipecac is no longer recommended for gastric emptying in children. In patients with acidosis and organ dysfunction with levels greater than 60 mg/dL in adults or 35 mg/dL in children, forced alkaline diuresis is recommended to enhance elimination. Aggressive administration of bicarbonate to patients with alkalemia or pulmonary edema, however, is contraindicated.

Hemodialysis is effective for removal of salicylates. It is recommended for patients with levels greater than 80 to 100 mg/dL, acidosis, CNS dysfunction, and risk of pulmonary edema. Although hemoperfusion also will effectively remove salicylates, hemodialysis is preferred to correct acid-base disturbances.

Theophylline

Despite significant toxic potential and a narrow therapeutic index, theophylline is used in the treatment of chronic respiratory illnesses. Toxic ingestions may occur in suicide attempts or with maintenance therapy if drug clearance is reduced.

Theophylline is quickly absorbed, and blood levels peak within 2 hours of ingestion, although with sustained-release preparations, blood concentration may peak between 4 and 6 hours. Most of the drug is metabolized by the several enzymes within the P-450 system, with less than 10% excreted unchanged into the urine. A variety of drugs that inhibit these enzymes can increase theophylline concentrations to toxic levels.

Clinically evident toxicity occurs in 30% of patients with levels greater than 15 mg/dL and in 48% of those with levels greater than 25 mg/dL. Chronicity of toxicity, extremes of age, and smoking tend to worsen the signs of toxicity, and in patients with cirrhosis, neonates, and the elderly, protein binding of theophylline is decreased. Signs and symptoms such as nausea and vomiting may occur with levels greater than 20 mg/dL. Seizures may occur at levels of 40 mg/dL in chronic toxicity but only at levels of 80 to 100 mg/dL in acute ingestions. Arrhythmias may be supraventricular or ventricular tachycardia and fibrillation. Agitation, rhabdomyolysis, elevated cardiac creatine kinase type MB (CK-MB) concentration, and psychosis are further toxic signs.

Hypokalemia, hypomagnesemia, hypercalcemia, hypophosphatemia, and metabolic acidosis may be evident on laboratory analysis and should be corrected. Treatment also should include measures to reduce absorption, including gastric lavage and administration of activated charcoal, especially with ingestion of sustained-release theophylline. Propranolol may be the best choice to treat arrhythmias and will improve blood pressure.

Hemoperfusion using charcoal or a polystyrene resin is effective in the removal of theophylline during intoxication. Hemoperfusion should be considered when levels are 80 to 100 mg/dL and at lower levels (such as 40 mg/dL) in neonates, the elderly, or patients with underlying heart or liver failure.

Key Points

1. Indications for use of extracorporeal therapies in drug intoxication are primarily clinical.
2. Extracorporeal therapy should be considered for removal of agents with delayed toxicity, when endogenous clearance is impaired, or when evidence exists for clinical benefit.
3. Dialysis may reverse electrolyte abnormalities and correct the metabolic acidosis that may accompany some types of poisoning.
4. Dialysis efficiently removes drugs of small molecular size, high water solubility, low protein binding, and small volume of distribution.

5. Hemofiltration removes drugs of large molecular size and volume of distribution.
6. Hemoperfusion removes lipid-soluble drugs, cardiac glycosides, barbiturates, and other types of hypnotics-sedatives-tranquilizers but may be associated with thrombocytopenia.
7. Use of the chelator deferoxamine with hemodialysis or hemoperfusion improves clearance of aluminum and iron.
8. Hemodialysis effectively removes lithium, methanol, ethylene glycol, and salicylates.
9. Hemoperfusion is effective in the removal of theophylline during intoxication.

Key References

2. Watson WA, Litovitz TL, Rodgers GC Jr, et al: 2004 Annual Report of the American Association of Poison Control Centers Toxic Exposure Surveillance System. Am J Emerg Med 2005;23:589-666.
5. Depner T, Garred L: Solute transport mechanisms in dialysis. In Horl W, Koch KM, Lindsay RM, et al (eds): Replacement of Renal Function by Dialysis, 5th ed. Dordrecht, Kluwer Academic Publishers, 2004, pp 73-93.
8. Chang TMS, Barre P: Effect of desferrioxamine on removal of aluminium and iron by coated charcoal haemoperfusion and haemodialysis. Lancet 1983;2:1051.
11. Hansen HE, Hestbech J, Sorensen JC, et al: Chronic interstitial nephropathy in patients on long-term lithium therapy. Q J Med 1979;48:577.
18. Amathieu R, Merouani M, Borron SW, et al: Prehospital diagnosis of massive ethylene glycol poisoning and use of an early antidote. Resuscitation 2006;70:285-286.

See the companion Expert Consult website for the complete reference list.

CHAPTER 175

Plasmapheresis in Acute Intoxication and Poisoning

François Madore

OBJECTIVES

This chapter will:
1. Present an overview of the possible mechanisms of action of plasmapheresis in poisoning and drug overdose.
2. Review the pharmacokinetic factors that affect the elimination of poisons and drugs by plasmapheresis.
3. Summarize the limitations of published studies on the efficacy of plasmapheresis in poisoning and drug overdose.
4. Review published data on the efficacy of plasmapheresis for specific poisons and drugs.

Plasmapheresis is widely accepted as a therapeutic modality for a number of immunological, metabolic, and inherited diseases.[1] Plasmapheresis also is reported as a useful extracorporeal blood purification technique in the treatment of various intoxications and poisonings. The basic premise of plasmapheresis use in poisoning and drug overdose is that removal of circulating toxin or drug will reduce toxic-induced damage and minimize related complications.

MECHANISMS OF ACTION

The therapeutic benefit of plamaspheresis in acute poisoning and drug overdose is based on the rapid removal of drugs or toxins that cannot be eliminated adequately by usual therapeutic interventions. Plasmapheresis can remove rapidly toxins of all size, including protein- and lipid-bound toxins with a low volume of distribution.[2] The procedure removes toxins only from the blood compartment, however, so tissue stores remain unaffected except for re-equilibration with decreasing plasma concentration. Other possible benefits of plasmapheresis in the treatment of poisoning and drug overdose are its effects on toxin-induced complications such as hemolysis or thrombotic thrombocytopenic purpura.[2] For instance, in cases of drug-induced hemolysis, plasmapheresis has the potential for removing products of red blood cell destruction and hemoglobin.[3,4] In addition, infusion of normal plasma may itself have beneficial effects, independent of removal of toxic circulating compounds. For example, plasmapheresis with autologous plasma as replacement fluid provides a chance to give active cholinesterase in organophosphate poisonings.[5]

TECHNICAL OVERVIEW

Plasmapheresis involves withdrawal of venous blood, separation of plasma from blood cells, and reinfusion of cells plus autologous plasma or another replacement solution. Plasma and blood cells are separated by centrifugation or membrane filtration. Usually, the equivalent of 1 to 1.5 plasma volumes (or 2.5 to 4.0 L) is removed during a session. To maintain plasma volume, the removed plasma is replenished with an equal amount of replacement fluids. The typical replacement fluids are fresh frozen plasma, 5% albumin or other plasma derivatives (e.g., cryosupernatant), and crystalloids (e.g., 0.9% saline, Ringer's lactate). The choice of fluid has implications for the efficacy of the procedure, oncotic pressure, coagulation, and spectrum of side effects. Albumin usually is preferred to plasma because of the risk of hypersensitivity reactions and transmission of viral infections with the latter. Albumin (5%) generally is combined with 0.9% saline on a 50%:50% (volume-for-volume) basis. However, for some indications for which infusion of normal plasma may be beneficial (e.g., organophosphate poisoning), fresh frozen plasma is the preferred replacement solution.

COMPARISON WITH OTHER EXTRACORPOREAL DETOXIFICATION METHODS

Some advantages of plasmapheresis over other extracorporeal detoxification methods, such as hemodialysis and hemoperfusion, are recognized. For instance, toxin removal may be more rapidly accomplished with plasmapheresis than with hemodialysis and hemoperfusion.[2] In addition, the removal of toxins by plasmapheresis is not dependent on the size of the molecule, as is the case for hemodialysis.[2] Plasmapheresis can remove a number of substances that are not removed effectively by either hemodialysis or hemoperfusion (e.g., protein-bound compounds).[2] Plasmapheresis also can remove active metabolites as well as

TABLE 175-1

Poison/Drug Characteristics

Pharmacological
Volume of distribution
Binding to protein
Binding to peripheral tissues
Spontaneous metabolism and excretion
Half-life
Toxicity of unchanged poison/drug
Toxicity of metabolites
Clinical
Severity of symptoms and complications
Related complications (e.g., hemolysis)
Efficacy of standard therapy (e.g., forced diuresis)
Availability of specific antidote
Efficacy of other detoxification methods (e.g., hemodialysis, hemoperfusion)

unchanged drugs.[3] Nevertheless, although plasmapheresis is the best method for protein-bound toxins with low volume of distribution, other intoxications, such as with water-soluble substances (e.g., methanol, ethylene glycol), are best treated with hemodialysis. In addition, certain drugs that induce metabolic complications in poisoned patients are more appropriately treated with hemodialysis, which can correct the acid-base and electrolyte abnormalities associated with these poisons (e.g., aspirin).[3] Accordingly, the choice of the extracorporeal detoxification modality clearly depends on the characteristics of the drugs or toxins implicated. Table 175-1 shows the characteristics of poisons and drugs that need to be considered in the choice of detoxification method.

PHARMACOKINETIC CONSIDERATIONS

The elimination of drugs or toxins by plasmapheresis is governed by several factors. The extracorporeal elimination efficiency for a given substance depends on the volume of distribution, the protein binding, the intercompartment equilibration, and the plasma exchange volume.[6] The ideal drug for removal by plasmapheresis is one that is highly protein-bound and has a small volume of distribution. Some experts advocate that plasmapheresis is useful only when the plasma protein binding is greater than 80% and the volume of distribution is lower than 0.2 L/kg of body weight.[6] In addition, plasmapheresis should be considered only for drugs or toxins that have a prolonged half-life. For substances that are metabolized rapidly, plasmapheresis is unlikely to accelerate the removal rate significantly. Drug clearance due to plasmapheresis also must increase overall clearance by at least 30% to affect drug removal significantly. In addition, a clinical benefit may require that the level of a toxin be reduced to lower than the level that can be achieved using plasmapheresis.

LIMITATIONS OF PUBLISHED REPORTS

Several limitations complicate the interpretation of published reports that evaluated the efficacy of plasmapheresis in acute intoxication and poisoning. First, no

TABLE 175-2

Plasmapheresis and Poisoning

SPECIFIC POISON	POSSIBLE BENEFIT*	NO OR LITTLE BENEFIT	REFERENCE(S)
Amanita	X		7-11
Acetic acid	X		12
Dichromate/chromic acid		X	14
Heavy metals			
Aluminum		X	15
Gold		X	16
Mercury		X	17-19
Silver		X	20, 21
Thallium		X	22
Vanadium		X	23
Organophosphates			
Dimethoate	X		25
Parathion	X		12
Paraquat		X	26
Sodium chlorate	X		13

*Possible benefit in selected cases.

randomized controlled trial has been carried out to determine the range of indications, the potential benefits, and the cost-effectiveness of plasmapheresis in acute intoxication and poisoning. Most reports evaluating plasmapheresis efficacy were case reports or case series. Second, in most studies, patients were receiving concurrent treatment with hemodialysis or specific antidotes, rendering it difficult to evaluate the effect of plasmapheresis per se. Third, a majority of published studies failed to report important pharmacokinetic data to evaluate the efficacy of plasmapheresis in eliminating the drugs or toxins. For instance, most reports failed to quantify the total amount of the drug or toxin removed and to document the procedure's contribution to total drug clearance. Hence, treatment recommendations on the use of plasmapheresis in acute poisoning and drug overdose are of limited validity.

EFFICACY OF PLASMAPHERESIS IN SPECIFIC INTOXICATIONS

The treatment of poisoning with plasmapheresis has been reported for a number of agents (Table 175-2).

Amanita phalloides

Amanita phalloides, the death cap mushroom, contains the most deadly toxin (the amanita toxin) of all poisonous mushrooms. Reported mortality rates after ingestion of *Amanita phalloides* range from 25% to 50%.[7] The lethal dose of amanita toxin is 0.1 mg/kg of body weight, so severe poisoning can occur with as little as 5 to 7 mg of amanita toxin, an amount that can be present in a single mushroom.[7] The amanita toxin is eliminated by the kidneys and usually is undetectable in the plasma 48 hours after ingestion. Hence, rapid therapeutic intervention is required to avoid serious complications. More than 9 case series of the use of plasmapheresis in *Amanita phalloides* poisoning have been published over the last 25 years. Taken together, these case series (reviewed by Jander and

Bischoff[7]) reported improved survival when compared with historical survival rate. In a representative study of 17 patients, Jander and coworkers used plasmapheresis in addition to other ancillary treatments (charcoal, penicillin, thioctic acid) and reported an overall mortality rate of 4.8%.[8] By contrast, other studies have raised doubts about the efficacy of plasmapheresis in the treatment of *Amanita phalloides* poisoning. In a study of another 17 cases treated with forced diuresis and plasmapheresis, in which the amanita toxin concentrations were measured in the urine and plasma, Piqueras and associates found that forced diuresis eliminated between 20,000 and 350,000 ng of toxin, whereas plasmapheresis never eliminated more than 10,000 ng.[9] In addition, some studies using supportive measures without plasmapheresis found survival rates identical to those reported with use of plasmapheresis.[10,11] Thus, because of the uncontrolled nature of all of the studies published to date, it is impossible to determine if the improvement in patient survival reported in many studies is attributable to plasmapheresis or to other factors such as adjunctive therapies. If plasmapheresis is used, however, it probably should be instituted in the first 24 to 48 hours after ingestion because of the spontaneous elimination of the amanita toxin by the kidneys.

Acetic Acid and Sodium Chlorate

The successful use of plasmapheresis has been reported in poisoning with acetic acid and sodium chlorate.[12,13] The removal of these compounds by plasmapheresis is minimal, however, because neither is highly protein-bound. The beneficial effect of plasmapheresis is thought to be due to removal of red blood cell destruction products and hemoglobin, because these agents cause severe hemolysis. Therefore, plasmapheresis is not intended to clear the toxic compound, but it may be useful in removing free hemoglobin and blood cell debris from the circulation.[3]

Dichromate and Chromic Acid

Plasmapheresis has been used in the treatment of ammonium dichromate and chromic acid intoxications and

TABLE 175-3

Plasmapheresis and Drug Overdose

SPECIFIC DRUG*	POSSIBLE BENEFIT†	NO OR LITTLE BENEFIT	REFERENCE(S)
Acetaminophen (5%)		X	27-29
Anticonvulsants			
Phenobarbital (38%)		X	2
Phenytoin (11%)		X	30-32
Valproic acid (7%)		X	33
Benzodiazepines		X	4
Carbamazepine (6%)		X	50
Calcium channel blockers			
Diltiazem		X	47
Verapamil		X	45, 46
Chemotherapeutic agents			
Cisplatin	X		35
Vincristine	X		34
Cyclosporine (1%)		X	52
Digoxin (0.5%)		X	36, 37
L-Thyroxine (33%)	X		38-40
Prednisone (1%)		X	51
Propranolol (30%)		X	44
Quinine (1%)		X	48
Salicylates (10%)		X	41
Theophylline	X		25, 42, 43
Tobramycin (8.8%)		X	49
Tricyclic antidepressants	X		25

*Figures in parentheses are estimated % of total body toxin removed in one plasmapheresis session (data not available for all drugs).
‡Possible benefit in selected cases.

exposures.[14] Plasmapheresis has been reported to be ineffective in removing significant amounts of toxins or in causing sustained clinical improvement, however.[14]

Heavy Metals

Plasmapheresis has been attempted in cases of heavy metal intoxication. Removal of aluminum by plasmapheresis has been reported to be disappointing, with approximately 1% of total body aluminum removed.[15] Removal of other heavy metals by plasmapheresis has been attempted for gold,[16] mercury,[17-19] silver,[20,21] thallium,[22] and vanadium.[23] Although some heavy metal removal is possible with plasmapheresis, the evidence is anecdotal for the most part.

Organophosphates

Organophosphates are among the most commonly used insecticides in the world. The organophosphates cause a specific and irreversible inhibition of acetylcholinesterase. Treatment of organophosphate poisoning consists of specific antidotes including atropine and pralidoxime.[24] Plasmapheresis has been attempted in cases of organophosphate poisonings such as with parathion[12] and dimethoate.[25] Plasmapheresis with fresh frozen plasma as replacement fluid has been reported to be successful in a patient unresponsive to administration of atropine and pralidoxime whose cholinesterase levels were declining despite antidotal therapy.[5] Fresh frozen plasma contains active cholinesterase and may be used to augment plasma cholinesterase levels.[5] Accordingly, plasmapheresis with autologous plasma as replacement fluid may be beneficial by rapidly increasing cholinesterase levels.

Paraquat

Paraquat is a toxic herbicide that impairs renal function. This compound is not significantly protein-bound and has a short half-life. Its persistence in the circulation may be prolonged because elimination depends on renal function.[3] The total removal by plasmapheresis has been reported as nonsignificant in the context of endogenous metabolic clearance.[26]

EFFICACY OF PLASMAPHERESIS IN SPECIFIC DRUG OVERDOSE

The treatment of drug overdose with plasmapheresis has been reported for a number of agents (Table 175-3).

Acetaminophen

Plasmapheresis has been attempted in cases of severe acetaminophen intoxication with acute liver failure.[27,28] Although clinical benefit has been reported in some patients, the total amount of acetaminophen removed during a typical plasmapheresis session is less than 5%.[29] Thus, plasmapheresis provides no significant benefit in acetaminophen intoxication.

Anticonvulsants

Phenytoin often is considered an ideal drug for removal by plasmapheresis because of its high degree of protein binding (approximately 90%) and its small volume of distribution. During a typical plasmapheresis session, it is estimated that the total phenytoin clearance increases from 20.8 mL/minute to 42.5 mL/minute.[30] Plasma concentrations of the drug are not significantly altered by plasmapheresis after redistribution, however, because only a small percentage (less than 11%) of total body stores is removed during pheresis.[30-32] No advantage of plasmapheresis has been reported for poisoning with phenobarbital, which responds favorably to urinary alkalinization, forced diuresis, and dialysis.[2] Plasmapheresis makes only a minor contribution to valproic acid elimination, at approximately 7% of total body stores.[33]

Benzodiazepines

Plasmapheresis may appear useful in benzodiazepine intoxication because of the high degree of protein binding (up to 95%) characteristic of this group of drugs. Plasmapheresis has no significant role to play in this setting, however, because the extravascular compartment cannot be cleared effectively by extracorporeal detoxification methods.[4] In addition, an effective antidote for all benzodiazepines is available: flumazenil (Annexate).

Chemotherapeutic Agents

Plasmapheresis has been attempted in cases of vincristine and cisplatin overdose.[34,35] Treatment with plasmapheresis was associated with a significant reduction in the plasma concentrations of vincristine and platinum and with concomitant reduction in clinical symptoms. The use of plasmapheresis may be justified because of high protein binding of these agents and because of the absence of recognized therapy. Limited data are available, however, to appraise the contribution of plasmapheresis in the removal of these drugs.

Digitalis

Plasmapheresis is not effective for treatment of digitalis intoxication because of the extensive tissue binding and large volume of distribution for this drug.[36] In patients who receive treatment with digoxin–immune antigen–binding fragments (Digibind), plasmapheresis has been reported to increase the clearance of the digoxin-antidigoxin complexes.[37] Because these complexes are renally excreted, plasmapheresis may be useful only in patients with renal failure, who may experience renewed intoxication when the antigen-antibody combination dissociates in the absence of renal excretion.

L-Thyroxine

Reports of plasmapheresis for the removal of thyroid hormones have been encouraging.[38,39] At least 25% of total-body thyroxine (T_4) is present in plasma, readily removable by plasma exchange. A single-exchange procedure may not significantly decrease serum T_4 levels, owing to the rapid rebound of thyroid hormone from the tissues into the plasma.[3] Both plasmapheresis and charcoal hemoperfusion may be effective in decreasing the duration of thyroxine intoxication. Some investigators have reported that plasmapheresis is more effective than hemoperfusion in the extraction of thyroxine.[38,40]

Salicylates

The effects of plasmapheresis on the removal of salicylate have been studied by White and associates in a group of volunteers who were administered 3900 mg of salicylate per day.[41] The total amount of salicylate removed during a 6-hour plasmapheresis session was 191 mg (i.e., less than the amount found in one aspirin tablet). In addition, because as-pirin intoxications respond favorably to urinary alkalinization, forced diuresis, and dialysis, plasmapheresis has no indication for the treatment of salicylate intoxication.

Theophylline

The usual recommendations for the treatment of theophylline intoxication are that hemodialysis and hemoperfusion are the preferred detoxification methods because of their high levels of efficacy.[25] The use of plasmapheresis has been reported in several instances.[25,42,43] Because theophylline is 50% to 60% protein bound and its volume of distribution is low, plasmapheresis may be as effective as hemoperfusion in removing the drug and may have the advantage of not causing thrombocytopenia or hypoglycemia.[2] To date, no controlled study has compared the efficacy of plasmapheresis and that of hemoperfusion in theophylline intoxication.

Tricyclic Antidepressants

Although tricyclic antidepressants are highly bound to plasma proteins, plasmapheresis is relatively ineffective because of their large volume of distribution. Successful use of plasmapheresis has been reported in cases with severe cardiac and central nervous system toxicity.[25] In one such case, a 64% reduction in amitriptyline plasma levels has been reported with plasmapheresis associated with significant improvement in clinical condition.[25] Thus, plasmapheresis may be attempted in patients presenting with severe life-threatening complications.

Other Agents

The effects of plasmapheresis on propranolol elimination were reported in a nonoverdose situation.[44] The half-life of propranolol was reduced to one third of normal during plasmapheresis. These results, however, may not be an accurate reflection of the elimination of propranolol in an overdose situation.

Plasmapheresis also has been reported in cases of verapamil and diltiazem intoxication with possible clinical benefit.[45-47] Limited data are available to appraise the contribution of are in the removal of these drugs, however. Plasmapheresis also has been compared with hemodialysis and forced diuresis in cases of quinine intoxication.[48] In a report by Sabto and colleagues, forced diuresis accounted for removal of 1625 mg of quinine over 75 hours, hemodialysis recovered 30 mg over 6 hours, and 8.5 mg was eliminated with the use of plasmapheresis.[48] Similarly low percentages of total body toxin removal with plasmapheresis have been reported with tobramycin at 8%,[49] carbamazepine at 6%,[50] prednisone at 1%,[51] and cyclosporine at 1%.[52] Because of these minimal reductions, the use of plasmapheresis is not warranted for these agents, in view of the cost and the risks involved with the procedures.

COMPLICATIONS

The prevailing belief that "plasmapheresis is a benign procedure" undoubtedly has contributed to its use in poisoning and drug overdose despite the lack of evidence in favor of a clear benefit in the case of many toxins and drugs. Although plasmapheresis is relatively safe when performed by skilled clinicians, complications related to either vascular access or the composition of replacement fluids are frequent. The reported overall incidence of adverse reactions ranges from 1.6% to 25%, with severe reactions occurring in 0.5% to 3.1% of patients undergoing plasmapheresis.[53] Hematoma formation, pneumothorax, and catheter infections are the most frequent complications of vascular access. Complications related to the replacement fluids include anaphylactoid reactions to fresh frozen plasma, coagulopathies induced by inadequate replacement of clotting factors, and transmission of viral infections. Other complications include hypocalcemia resulting from citrate infusion and hypotension triggered by delayed or inadequate volume replacement, hypo-oncotic fluid replacement, or anaphylaxis. Plasmapheresis also may predispose patients to an increased incidence of infection; this effect is mostly observed with repeated plasmapheresis treatments. Other complications are related to the removal of therapeutically prescribed drugs during plasmapheresis and the requirement for supplementary doses of these drugs after plasmapheresis. Finally, several reports have described deaths directly attributable to plasmapheresis. Of note, however, because plasmapheresis often is undertaken as a last measure against inexorably fatal intoxications, it may be difficult to measure how the procedure itself contributes to the death of a patient.

CONCLUSION

Although plasmapheresis has been applied for the treatment of various intoxications and drug overdoses, clear evidence of benefit is lacking. Most reports evaluating treatment with plasmapheresis are case reports or case series in which many of the patients also received concurrent treatment with dialysis or specific antidotes. No randomized controlled trial has been conducted to compare plasmapheresis with other treatment modalities. Thus,

because of the uncontrolled nature of all of the studies reported to date, it is impossible to determine whether the improvement in patient survival reported in many studies is attributable to plasmapheresis or to other factors such as patient selection, earlier diagnosis, wide variability in presentation, or advances in general supportive measures or other adjunctive therapies. Therefore, recommendations for the treatment of poisonings and overdose are difficult to establish.

The use of plasmapheresis should be limited to research protocols or to exceptional cases in which the patient presents with life-threatening complications unresponsive to conventional therapy. If plasmapheresis is attempted, the total amount of drug or toxin removed should be documented to assess the contribution of the procedure to total clearance.

Key Points

1. Treatment recommendations for the use of plasmapheresis in acute poisoning and drug overdose are limited because of the lack of randomized controlled trials.
2. The ideal drug for removal by plasmapheresis is one that is highly protein-bound, has a small volume of distribution, and has a prolonged half-life.
3. The use of plasmapheresis should be limited to research protocols or to exceptional cases in which the patient presents with life-threatening complications unresponsive to conventional therapy.

Key References

1. Winters JL, Pineda AA, McLeod BC, Grima KM: Therapeutic apheresis in renal and metabolic diseases. J Clin Apher 2000;15:53-73.
2. Kale-Pradhan PB, Woo MH: A review of the effects of plasmapheresis on drug clearance. Pharmacotherapy 1997;17:684-695.
3. Jones JS, Dougherty J: Current status of plasmapheresis in toxicology. Ann Emerg Med 1986;15:474-482.
4. Seyffart G: Plasmapheresis in treatment of acute intoxications. Trans Am Soc Artif Organs 1982;28:673-676.
25. Nenov VD, Marinov P, Sabeva J, Nenov DS: Current applications of plasmapheresis in clinical toxicology. Nephrol Dial Transplant 2003;18(Suppl 5):v56-v8.

See the companion Expert Consult website for the complete reference list.

CHAPTER 176

Poisoning: Kinetics to Therapeutics

Dingwei Kuang, Claudio Ronco, and Nicholas A. Hoenich

> ### OBJECTIVES
> This chapter will:
> 1. Review the fundamentals of pharmacokinetics and toxicology.
> 2. Present an overview of therapeutic management of poisoning by conventional and extracorporeal circulatory methods.
> 3. Describe the role of supportive treatments.

Accidental or premeditated ingestion of poisons is a significant health problem worldwide and is a frequent cause of admission to emergency departments and intensive care units (ICUs). Serious clinical effects occur in less than 5% of acutely poisoned patients, and the overall in-hospital mortality rate is less than 0.5%.[1] The treatment of poisoning requires knowledge of the pathophysiology and toxicokinetics of the compound ingested, as well as the most appropriate method(s) of removal from the body. Reflecting the necessarily urgent nature of the clinical response to poisoning, randomized controlled trials evaluating the effectiveness of methods often are lacking, and evidence-based information on the management of poisoning is scarce.

After entering the body, a drug is eliminated by excretion and by metabolism. Although elimination can occur through a variety of different routes, most drugs are cleared by the kidney or by metabolism in the liver. The study of drug absorption, distribution, metabolism, and excretion requires the application of mathematical techniques, or modeling (pharmacokinetics or pharmacokinetic modeling). A variant of this approach is toxicokinetics, which relates to the absorption, distribution, and elimination processes of compounds that produce toxic effects in the body. Of note, however, almost all substances are toxic under the right conditions. As Paracelsus (1493-1541), the father of modern toxicology, said: *Sola dosis facit venenum* ("only dose determines the poison").[2]

THE EPIDEMIOLOGY OF POISON INGESTION

The incidence of accidental and intentional poisonings worldwide is unknown. In many countries, however, poisoning with organophosphorus pesticides is an important cause of morbidity and mortality.[3,4]

Within the United States, since 1983, the American Association of Poison Control Centers has compiled data covering 63 poison centers, which for 2004[5] reported a total of 2,438,644 cases. Children younger than 3 years were involved in 38.5% of these cases, and 51.3% occurred in children younger than 6 years. A male predominance is found among poison exposure victims younger than 13 years, but the sex distribution is reversed in teenagers and adults. In 5.3% of cases (130,056 cases), multiple patients were implicated in the poison exposure episode (e.g., siblings "shared" a household product, or multiple patients inhaled vapors at a hazardous material spill). Approximately 92.7% of exposures occurred at home, 2.0% at the workplace, 1.4% at school, 0.3% at health care facilities, and 0.4% at restaurants. A total of 1183 fatalities were reported, with analgesics, antidepressants, stimulants and street drugs, sedative-hypnotic-antipsychotic agents, and cardiovascular drugs being the most common agents responsible. Although involved in a majority of poisoning reports, children younger than 6 years incurred just 2.3% of the fatalities. Fifty-six percent of poisoning fatalities occurred in persons 20 to 49 years of age. 50.6% of fatal cases involved two or more drugs or products. The overwhelming majority of human exposures were acute (91.9%), compared with 55.9% of poison-related fatal exposures. The vast majority (84.1%) of poison exposures were unintentional; a suicidal intent was identified in 8.0% of cases. Therapeutic errors accounted for 9.1% of exposures (222,644 cases), with unintentional nonpharmaceutical product misuse accounting for another 3.9% of exposures.

PHARMACOKINETICS AND TOXICOKINETICS

The study of the time course of drug and metabolite concentrations in biological fluids, tissues, and excreta, with suitable models to interpret such data, is known as *pharmacokinetics*. The principles of this field of study were first described in 1937 by a Swedish physiologist and biophysicist, Torsten Teorell, who is regarded as the "father of pharmacokinetics" and was responsible for the introduction of compartmental modeling to analyze the behavior of drugs in physiological systems.[6,7]

The actual term "pharmacokinetics" was introduced into clinical and experimental research some years later and is attributed to a German pediatrician, F. H. Dost. Such research led to a rapidly increasing understanding of the mechanisms of drug disposition and of host factors determining drug concentration and drug effect within the organism. These advances in turn led to the evolution of what today is known as *clinical pharmacology*.[8] *Toxicokinetics* is a more recent branch of pharmacokinetics and extends the concepts to potentially toxic substances. It is essentially the same as pharmacokinetics, with the major difference being the dose, in that, as Paracelsus stated, "All substances are poisons, there is none which is not a poison. The right dose differentiates a poison from a remedy."[9]

Pharmacokinetic Modellng

Pharmacokinetic modeling provides a mathematical basis for the understanding of the pharmacological response. It is simply the study of the time course of drug and metabolite levels in different fluids, tissues, and excreta of the body, coupled to mathematical relationships to permit the interpretation of the data. A number of different approaches may be used; two well-known approaches are *compartment modeling*, in which the body is assumed to be made up of one or more compartments, which may be spatial or chemical in nature, and *physiological modeling*, based on blood flow rates through particular organs or tissues and experimentally determined blood tissue concentrations. The latter approach offers a substantial advantage over the compartmental model in that drug concentrations or movements can be predicted in specific organs, and changes in tissue concentrations arising from pathological conditions such as fever or congestive heart failure may be incorporated into the model.

Pharmacokinetics also may be established without the use of models (*model-independent pharmacokinetics*), and such an approach is sufficient to characterize plasma profiles in terms of maximum plasma concentrations, the time of the maximum concentration, the area under the plasma curve, and also the elimination half-life. These parameters generally can be obtained with reasonable accuracy using serial sampling. In addition to these approaches, a fourth approach known as *population pharmacokinetics* or *mixed effect modeling* may also be used. In such an approach, rather than using individual data profiles, the approach focuses on the data collected across a specific patient or subject population and on the interindividual variability of such data. Accordingly, intensive characterization of an individual patient is not critical. On the other hand, the limited sampling associated with population pharmacokinetics has been perceived as a major disadvantage of this approach.[10,11]

THERAPEUTIC MANAGEMENT OF POISONING

The management of poisoning is not uniform, because every toxin has different properties, as is evident in Table 176-1. A toxin injures the body in different places and compartments, ranging from the skin to internal organs. Once the toxin enters the blood compartment of the patient, the most important factor determining its removal is the distribution to other body compartments. Such distribution is determined by the route of ingestion, plasma and tissue protein binding, lipophilia, ionization (pK_a), blood flow rate to the organs, intercompartmental transfer,

and diffusion. Therapeutic management may thus be considered to be the removal or enhancement of the removal of the toxin from the body, coupled with supportive or general management.

The challenge for the clinician is to identify at an early stage those patients who are most at risk for the development of serious complications and who therefore may potentially benefit from specific measures in addition to general supportive care. As noted earlier, reflecting the urgent nature of the treatment, randomized controlled trials comparing methods of removal are lacking. The position statements prepared by the American Academy of Clinical Toxicology (AACT) and the European Association of Poison Centres and Clinical Toxicologists (EAPCCT) may be considered to constitute an evidence base for the use of different techniques in the treatment of poisonings. The position statements were formulated after a review of all relevant scientific literature by acknowledged experts using agreed-on criteria. Clinical and experimental studies were given precedence over anecdotal case reports, and abstracts usually were not considered. A draft of the position statement was initially produced and subjected to detailed peer review before being approved by the boards of the two societies. Position statements have been published for a range of commonly used therapeutic measures.[12-18]

Antidotes and Chelating Agents

An antidote is a special pharmacological or toxicological antagonist that can favorably alter the toxic effects of a poison. Some antidotes are toxic themselves and therefore should be used with caution.[19] Antidotes are available for only a limited number of drugs and poisons. With the exception of *N*-acetylcysteine (acetaminophen), naloxone (opioids), and flumazenil (benzodiazepines), very few antidotes are used on a consistent basis in the management of poisoning victims. Two relatively new antidotes are fomepizole (Antizol, orphan medical) for use in ethylene glycol poisoning or suspected ethylene glycol ingestion. Antivenin (Crotalidae) polyvalent immune Fab (Wyeth) may be used in the case of snake bites and is capable of neutralizing the toxic effects of venoms of crotalids (pit vipers) native to North, Central, and South America, including rattlesnakes (*Crotalus, Sistrurus*); copperhead and cottonmouth moccasins (*Agkistrodon*), including *A. halys* of Korea and Japan; the fer-de-lance and other species of *Bothrops*; the tropical rattler (*Crotalus durissus* and similar species); the Cantil (*A. bilineatus*); and bushmaster (*Lachesis mutus*) of South and Central America.[20]

Methods for the Removal or Enhancement of Removal of Toxins from the Body
Administration of Activated Charcoal

The vast majority of poisoning cases seen in emergency departments involve ingestion. In such cases, adsorption may be limited by the administration of activated charcoal either as a single dose or in multiple doses. Activated charcoal is a highly porous form of carbon with a surface area of 950 to 2000 m^2/g that is capable of adsorbing poisons with a molecular weight of 100 to 1000 Daltons. If a patient has ingested a potentially toxic amount of a poison that is known to be adsorbed to charcoal, single-dose activated charcoal in powder form may be considered up to 1 hour after ingestion. This approach remains widely used despite the fact that many overdose patients present at least 2 hours after taking a medication, when most of the toxin has been absorbed or has moved well into the intestine, limiting the usefulness of charcoal. Nevertheless, if absorption has been delayed or gastrointestinal motility is impaired, activated charcoal may reduce the final amount absorbed.

The use of gastric emptying in addition to activated charcoal has generated intense debate. Several large comparative studies have failed to demonstrate a benefit for gastric emptying before administration of activated charcoal. Because complications of such two-stage decontamination protocols include higher rates of intubation, aspiration, and ICU admission, gastric emptying in addition to use of activated charcoal cannot be considered a routine approach to management of these patients.[21] The *AACT-EAPCTC position statement* recommends that single-dose activated charcoal should not be administered routinely in the management of poisoned patients and may be considered only if a patient has ingested a potentially toxic amount of a poison (which is known to be adsorbed to activated charcoal) up to 1 hour previously.[22]

Multiple (two or more) doses of activated carbon also may be used to enhance the elimination of poisons already absorbed into the body. The removal of poisons with a small distribution volume, low pK_a, low plasma protein binding, and prolonged elimination half-life is enhanced by the administration of multiple doses of activated carbon. The *AACT-EAPCTC position statement* notes that although many studies in animals and volunteers have demonstrated that multiple doses of activated charcoal significantly increase drug elimination, this therapy has not yet been shown in a controlled study to reduce morbidity and mortality in poisoned patients. As indicated by experimental and clinical studies, multiple doses of activated charcoal should be considered only if a patient has ingested a life-threatening amount of carbamazepine, dapsone, phenobarbital, quinine, or theophylline.[13]

Enhancement of Gastric Emptying: Emesis

Enhancement of gastric emptying, or emesis, relies on the use of emetics, such as ipecac, prepared from the dried rhizome and roots of the *Cephalis acuminata* or *Cephalis ipecacuana* plant and administered in the form of a syrup. Ipecac may be administered to patients before referral to the emergency department in an attempt to start the gastric emptying process as early as possible; however, this approach is controversial.[23]

Ipecac syrup induces vomiting in a high percentage of patients to whom it is administered, and the resultant decrease in the gastrointestinal absorption of ingested substances will be time-dependent. Its effectiveness in preventing drug absorption has been documented for only a limited number of substances and is substantially reduced if it is given more than 30 to 90 minutes after ingestion of the toxic material.[24] Furthermore, potentially significant contraindications, adverse effects, and related problems may be associated with its use. The *AACT-EAPCTC position statement* states that syrup of ipecac should not be administered routinely in the management of poisoned patients, because no evidence is available from clinical studies to suggest that it would eliminate some portion of the poison and thereby reduce morbidity and mortality among poisoned patients[17]; a more recent review reiterates this opinion.[25]

Gastric Lavage

In cases of serious and potentially life-threatening intoxication, gastric lavage can be performed up to 1 hour after ingestion. It should not be considered as a routine treatment. Observational clinical studies suggest that most drugs are unlikely to be recoverable by gastric lavage in significant quantities more than 2 hours after ingestion. Even if a toxin is present in the stomach, gastric lavage may not recover a clinically significant amount. Experimental studies indicate that the amount of marker removed is highly variable and decreases with time. No convincing clinical evidence has demonstrated that the use of gastric lavage later than 1 hour after ingestion of a poison is of therapeutic value. Serious risks associated with its use include hypoxia, dysrhythmias, laryngospasm, electrolyte abnormalities, and aspiration pneumonitis.

The *AACT-EAPCTC position statement* recommends that gastric lavage should not be used routinely in the management of poisoned patients. It may be considered only in a patient who has ingested a potentially life-threatening amount of toxin within 60 minutes, or if the ingestant was an agent that delays gastric emptying (e.g., tricyclic antidepressants) or a drug not adsorbed by activated charcoal (e.g., ferrous sulfate, lithium).[16]

Laxatives and Cathartics

Cathartics (e.g., sorbitol, magnesium citrate) frequently are used to shorten gastrointestinal transit time, thereby shortening the period of absorption. Their use can lead to volume depletion and electrolyte disturbances, and the efficacy remains largely unproved. The doses used are mainly empirical. The *AACT-EAPCTC position statement* states that on the basis of available data, the routine use of cathartics and laxatives is not endorsed. Furthermore, if these agents are used, their application should be limited to a single dose, to minimize adverse effects.[15,20]

Whole-Bowel Irrigation

Whole-bowel lavage has some advantages over the use of cathartics or laxatives in that this approach washes the contents mechanically without drawing water into the bowel. A number of solutions are suitable for use, including mannitol, Ringer's lactate, and isotonic polyethylene glycol electrolytes. Whole-bowel irrigation is the least studied and the least used of the gastrointestinal decontamination modalities. Although some volunteer studies have shown substantial decreases in the bioavailability of ingested drugs, no controlled clinical trials have been performed, and conclusive evidence is lacking that such an approach improves outcomes for poisoned patients.

The *AACT-EAPCTC position statement* concluded that whole-bowel irrigation is not a recommended procedure to be used routinely in the management of the poisoned patient. Nevertheless, it remains a viable treatment option after the ingestion of drugs not adsorbed to activated charcoal (e.g., lithium, iron) or with large ingestions of enteric-coated or sustained-release tablets (e.g., calcium channel blockers). The use of whole-bowel irrigation for the removal of ingested packets of illicit drugs (in "body packers") also is a potential indication. Contraindications to use of this procedure include obstructed bowel, ileus, gastrointestinal hemorrhage, hemodynamic instability, or a compromised, unprotected airway.[14,27]

Text continued on p. 950

TABLE 176-1

Poison Index

DRUG OR POISON[*][†]	Pharmacokinetics						Toxicity	
	MW (Da)	PPB (%)	V_D (L)	SB	$T_{1/2}$ (hr)	EU	NEPHROTOXICITY	OTHER SYSTEMIC TOXICITY
Acebutolol[1,2]	336.4	11-25%	1.4-3	Lipophilic	8 hr	<10%	?	CV toxicity, CNS manifestations
Acarbose	643.6	?	?	Hydrophilic	2 hr	<2%	?	GI symptoms, flatulence, pharyngitis
Acetazolamide[3,4]	222.2	80-92%	0.2	Hydrophilic	4 hr	Mostly	Yes	GI disturbances, electrolyte imbalance
Acetic acid[5,6]	60	?	?	Hydrophilic	?	?	Yes	High level of causticity, acidosis, hemolysis, DIC, hepatotoxicity
Acetohexamide	324.4	90%	?	Hydrophilic	1.3 hr	?	?	Hypoglycemia, GI, dermatological, miscellaneous symptoms
Acetonitrile[7,8]	41.1	?	Large	Lipophilic	?	?	?	See Cyanide/hydrogen cyanide
Aconitine[9,10]	645.8	?	Large	Hydrophilic	?	Little	?	GI symptoms, neurotoxicity, cardiotoxicity
Acyclovir[11]	225.2	9-22%	0.8	Hydrophilic	2.5 hr	14%	Yes	Hepatotoxicity, hematotoxicity, neurotoxicity, skin rashes
Ajmaline[12]	326.4	61-76%	6.17	Hydrophilic	1.5 hr	4%	Yes	GI symptoms, cardiac and CNS toxicity, hepatotoxicity
Allobarbital	208.2	?	?	?	?	25-30%	?	CNS and respiratory depression, relaxation of skeletal smooth muscle and myocardium
Alprazolam[13]	308.8	70-80%	1	Lipophilic	6-12 hr	20%	?	CNS depression
Alprenolol	249.3	80-85%	3.3	Lipophilic	2-3 hr	Little	?	CV toxicity, respiratory and CNS symptoms
Aluminum	27	80-95%	Very large	?	Longer	Little	Yes	Multisystem toxicity
Amanita phalloides[14-16]		Very low	Very small	Hydrophilic	12 hr	90%	Yes	GI symptoms, fatal hepatic failure
Aminocaproic acid	131.7	Low	Large	Hydrophilic	1-3 hr	64%	Yes	GI symptoms, cardiotoxicity, acute muscle necrosis
Amiodarone[17]	681.8	95%	9-20	Lipophilic	5-7 hr	Little	?	Hepatotoxicity, cardiotoxicity, pulmonary toxicity
Amitriptyline[18,19]	277.4	95%	6-36	Lipophilic	12-24 hr	5%	?	Cardiotoxicity, coma, seizures, hyperthermia, urinary retention, ARDS
Amlodipine[20,21]	408.6	97%	2	Lipophilic	36 hr	5%	?	CV toxicity
Amobarbital	226.3	55-60%	0.9-1.4	Lipophilic	15-40 hr	10%	?	CNS depression, respiratory depression, relaxation of skeletal smooth muscle and myocardium
Amoxapine	313.8	High	Large	Lipophilic	8 hr	Little	?	Coma, repiratory depression, cardiotoxicity, seizures, hyperthermia
Amphetamines[22,23]		15-35%	3-33	Lipophilic	10 hr	5-50%	Indirect	CNS and CV symptoms, hyperthermia
Aniline[24]	93	?	?	Hydrophilic	?	?	?	Relaxation of smooth muscle, production of methemoglobin
Aprobarbital	210.2	35%	0.6-0.7	Lipophilic	14-34 hr	13-25%	?	CNS depression, respiratory depression, relaxation of skeletal smooth muscle and myocardium
Arsenic[25,26]	74.9	60%	Large	?	?	22.4-57.9%	Yes	Hepatotoxicity, cardiotoxicity, CNS toxicity, hematotoxicity
Arsine	77.9	?	Large	Lipophilic	7 hr	20%	Yes	Neurotoxicity, hemolytic anemia, cardiotoxicity, hepatotoxicity
Aspirin	180.2	99.5%	0.2-0.5	?	3-9 hr	Little	Yes	Tinnitus, abdominal pain, hypokalemia, hypoglycemia, pyrexia, CNS symptoms
Astemizole[27]	458.6	97%	Large	Lipophilic	24 hr	5-6%	?	CNS toxicity, dry mouth, GI symptoms, cardiotoxicity
Atenolol[28,29]	266.3	3%	0.7	Hydrophilic	6 hr	Mostly	?	CV toxicity, CNS manifestations
Atropine[30,31]	289.4	40-50%	2-4	Lipophilic	2-3 hr	33-50%	?	Symptoms of vagal stimulation, brainstem depression with respiratory and circulatory failure
Azalea		?	?	Hydrophilic	?	?	?	GI symptoms, neurotoxicity, cardiotoxicity, respiratory paralysis
Baclofen[32]	213.7	30%	0.8	Lipophilic	3.5 hr	80%	?	CNS inhibition, respiratory depression, cardiotoxicity, hypothermia

				Enhancement of Removal					
GD	IAC	FD	SA	HD	HP$_A$	HP$_R$	PD	PE	SUPPORTIVE TREATMENT
□□, <6 hr	□□	(+)	No	+	(+)	?	?	?	Intensive supportive care, management of arrhythmias and hypotension
(++)	?	0	No	(+)	?	?	0	?	Symptomatic treatment, close monitoring of blood glucose
?	?	?	No	+	(++)	?	0	?	Symptomatic treatment
+	?	+	No	□□	0	0	?	□	Analgesics, treatment of asphyxia and metabolic acidosis
(++)	?	?	No	(++)	?	?	(++)	?	Symptomatic treatment, close monitoring of blood glucose
?	?	?	No	(++)	□	?	?	?	
□□	□□	+	No	?	□	?	?	?	Immediate cardiac monitoring and oxygen administration
(++)	?	(+)	No	□□	(++)	?	+	0	
++	++	0	No	(+)	(++)	(+++)	?	?	Continuous ECG monitoring, control arrhythmias, sodium substitution
□□, <8 hr	□	0	No	(++)	(++)	(++)	0	?	Stabilization of circulatory and respiratory function, good nursing
□□, <3 hr	□	0	Yes	?	?	?	?	?	
□□, <3 hr	(++)	0	No	+	?	?	?	?	Intensive supportive care, management of arrhythmias and hypotension
(++)	?	0	Yes	+	+	?	?	?	DFO: 5 mg/kg IV once a week until serum aluminum increment <75 µg/L is attained
□□, <15 hr	□□	□□□	No	+	++	+++	?	□□	Fluid, electrolyte, and glucose supplementation; corticosteroids; liver protection or transplantation
(++)	?	?	No	(+)	?	?	?	?	Symptomatic treatment
□□	□□	0	No	0	(+)	(+)	?	?	
□□□	□□□	0	?	0	□□	+	0	□	Sodium bicarbonate infusion; monitoring of CV, CNS, and respiratory function
□□, <3 hr	□□	+	?	0	0	0	?	?	See *Verapamil*
□□, <8 hr	□	0	No	□□	□□□	□□□	0	?	Stabilization of circulatory and respiratory function, good nursing
□□□	□□□	0	?	0	(+)	(+)	0	?	Sodium bicarbonate infusion; monitoring of CV, CNS, and respiratory function
□□□	□	□	No	0	0	0	0	?	Cooling measures, benzodiazepines
□□	0	□	0	++	?	?	?	?	Monitoring blood gas, oxygen therapy
□□, <8 hr	□	0	No	□□	□□□	□□□	0	?	Stabilization of circulatory and respiratory function, good nursing
□□	□	++	Yes	+	□	?	0	?	Four chelating agents: BAL, D-penicillamine, DMSA, DMPS; exchange transfusion
0	?	□	?	+	?	?	+	?	Alkalinizing urine; monitoring of cardiac function, electrolyte, and blood gases
□, <8 hr	□	□□□	No	□□□	□□	□□	□	?	Correction of acidosis, electrolyte imbalance, dehydration, hypoprothrombinemia
□□	□□	0	No	0	0	0	?	?	ECG monitoring is mandatory
(+++)	(++)	++	No	++	++	?	?	?	Intensive supportive care, management of arrhythmias and hypotension
□□	□□	□□	Yes	0	?	?	?	?	Physostigmine is the antidote: 0.02-0.06 mg/kg IV over 5 min; treatment of hyperthermia
(++)	(++)	(+)	No	?	?	?	?	?	No experience; see *Aconitine*
□	□	□□	No	0	?	?	0	?	Early supportive measures; continuous monitoring of ECG, respiration, and temperature

TABLE 176-1

Poison Index—cont'd

DRUG OR POISON[+†]	Pharmacokinetics						Toxicity	
	MW (Da)	PPB (%)	V_D (L)	SB	$T_{1/2}$ (hr)	EU	NEPHROTOXICITY	OTHER SYSTEMIC TOXICITY
Barbital	184.2	<5%	0.4-0.6	Hydrophilic	48-65 hr	60-90%	?	CNS depression, respiratory depression, relaxation of skeletal smooth
Barium[33,34]	137.3	?	Large	Lipophilic	?	7%	?	Stimulation of cardiac, smooth, and skeletal muscle; hypokalemia; hypertension
Benzydamine[35]	309.4	15-20%	3	Lipophilic	8-13 hr	50%	?	Auditory and visual hallucination, GI symptoms
Bismuth[36]	209	?	?	Lipophilic	?	2.50%	Yes	CNS toxicity
Boric acid[37]	61.8	0%	Large	Hydrophilic	5-21 hr	90%	Yes	GI symptoms, skin signs, CNS symptoms
Bromates[38,39]		?	?	?	?	?	Yes	GI symptoms, deafness
Bromazepam[40]	316.2	70%	1.2	Lipophilic	15 hr	<1%	?	Intoxication is rare
Bromides	79.9	?	0.4	Lipophilic	12 days	Little	?	Neuropsychiatric, dermatological. and GI symptoms
Bromisoval	233.1	?	?	Lipophilic	?	Little	Yes	CNS toxicity, respiratory and cardiac toxicity, hepatotoxicity
Brotizolam	393.7	90-95%	0.6	Lipophilic	4-8 hr	1%	?	CNS depression
Buflomedil[41,42]	364.4	25-80%	0.5-1	?	2-3.5 hr	Little	?	CNS toxicity, cardiorespiratory arrest
Buprenorphine[43]	467.7	95-98%	Large	Lipophilic	1.2-7.2 hr	15%	?	Little information on its toxicity
Butabarbital	212.2	26-50%	?	Lipophilic	34-42 hr	10%	?	CNS depression, respiratory depression, relaxation of skeletal smooth muscle and myocardium
Butalbital	224.3	?	?	?	?	<10%	?	CNS depression, respiratory depression, relaxation of skeletal smooth muscle and myocardium
Cadmium	112.41	Low	?	?	10-30 yr	Little	Yes	Respiratory toxicity, CV toxicity, hepatotoxicity
Caffeine[44,45]	194.2	35-40%	1	Hydrophilic	3-6 hr	1%	?	CNS, CV, and GI signs and symptoms
Camphor[46]	152.2	61%	2-4	Lipophilic	167 min	Little	?	GI toxicity, CNS toxicity
Carbamates[47,48]		?	?	?	?	?	?	Cardiotoxicity, GI symptoms
Carbamazepine[49-53]	236.3	65%	0.8-1.8	Lipophilic	18 hr	1-2%	Indirect	Anticholinergic symptoms, hepatotoxicity, hyponatremia
Carbon monoxide	28	?	?	Lipophilic	?	?	Yes	Brain, heart, and almost every organ affected
Carbon tetrachloride	153.8	?	?	Lipophilic	?	?	Yes	CNS toxicity, hepatotoxicity
Carbromal	237.1	?	?	Lipophilic	?	Little	Yes	CNS toxicity, respiratory and cardiac toxicity, hepatotoxicity
Carisoprodol[54]	260.3	?	?	Lipophilic	?	Mostly	?	CNS depression
Carvedilol[55]	406.5	98%	115	Lipophilic	7-10 hr	42%	?	Asthenia, fatigue; CV, CNS, and GI symptoms
Chloral hydrate[56,57]	165.4	None	Large	Lipophilic	4-14 hr	Little	Yes	CNS depression, cardiotoxicity, hepatotoxicity
Chlorambucil	304.2	99%	?	?	1.5 hr	<1%	?	Corrosive action, neurotoxicity
Chloramphenicol	323.1	50%	0.9-1.4	?	4 hr	5-10%	?	Bone marrow toxicity, peripheral neuritis, GI symptoms
Chlorates[58]		?	?	Hydrophilic	?	95%	Yes	Hematotoxicity, GI symptoms
Chlordiazepoxide[59]	299.8	95%	<0.4	Hydrophilic	15 hr	1%	?	CNS depression
Chlorine and chloramine	70.9	?	?	Hydrophilic	?	?	?	Respiratory symptoms, headache, dizziness, nausea
Chlormezanone	273.1	None	?	?	20-24 hr	1-2%	?	CNS depression
Chlorophenoxy compounds		?	?	?	?	?	?	GI symptoms, respiratory symptoms, CNS toxicity
Chloroquine[60-63]	319.9	50-60%	93.6	Lipophilic	50 hr	40-70%	Indirect	CNS, CV, GI, and other systemic toxicity
Chlorpheniramine[64,65]	274.8	72%	?	?	21-27 hr	?	?	Convulsion, coma, tachycardia, fever, and fatigue
Chlorpromazine	318.9	91-99%	20	Lipophilic	18 hr	1-6%	?	CNS toxicity, cardiorespiratory toxicity, hypothermia
Chlorpropamide[66,67]	276.7	?	?	Lipophilic	36 hr	80-90%	?	Hypoglycemia; GI, dermatologic, hematologic, endocrine symptoms

				Enhancement of Removal					
GD	**IAC**	**FD**	**SA**	**HD**	**HP$_A$**	**HP$_R$**	**PD**	**PE**	*SUPPORTIVE TREATMENT*
□□, <8 hr	□	□	No	□□□	□□□	□□□	0	?	Stabilization of circulatory and respiratory function, good nursing
□□	?	□	No	□	?	?	?	?	Calcium administration, cardiac monitoring, control of respiration; magnesium sulfate?
□□, <1 hr	?	(+)	No	?	0	(+)	?	?	Treatment of convulsions: chlorpromazine and chlordiazepoxide
□□, <10 hr	□□	+++	Yes	++	?	?	□	?	Antidotes: BAL, DMSA, DMPS, D-penicillamine and its N-acetyl derivative
□□	0	□	No	□□□	0	0	□□□	?	Supportive and symptomatic treatment
□□	?	0	No	□□	?	?	□□	?	Intravenous administration of sodium thiosulfate
(+++)	(++)	0	Yes	?	□□	?	?	?	
□□	0	□	No	□□□	0	0	?	?	Supportive and symptomatic treatment
□□	□□	0	No	□□□	□□□	□□□	□□	?	Prevention of DIC, respiratory support, administration of digitalis and glycosides
□□, <3 hr	□	0	Yes	?	?	?	?	?	
□	□	(+)	No	0	?	?	?	?	Supportive and symptomatic treatment
?	?	(+)	No	0	?	?	?	?	See morphine
□□, <8 hr	□	0	No	□□	□□□	□□□	0	?	Stabilization of circulatory and respiratory function, good nursing
□□, <8 hr	□	0	No	(++)	(++)	(++)	0	?	Stabilization of circulatory and respiratory function, good nursing
□□, <3 hr	?	0	No	0	0	0	0	?	Supportive and symptomatic treatment
□□, <4 hr	□□	0	No	□	(++)	□□	?	?	See *Theophylline*
□□, <2 hr	0	0	No	0	0	0	?	?	Supportive and symptomatic treatment
++	++	0	Yes	++	++	++	?	?	Antidote: atropine; see *Organochlorines*
□□□, <10 hr	□□□	□	No	□□	□□	□□	□	□	Monitoring of respiratory and cardiac function
0	**0**	**0**	No	**0**	**0**	**0**	**0**	?	Hyperbaric oxygen therapy
□□	?	0	Yes	(+)	(++)	?	?	?	Administration of acetylcysteine, treatment of hypercoagulation, and hyperventilation
□□	□□	0	No	□□□	□□□	□□□	□□	?	Prevention of DIC, respiratory support, administration of digitalis and glycosides
(++)	(++)	(++)	No	?	?	?	?	?	See *Meprobamate*
(++)	?	0	No	+	?	?	(+)	?	Symptomatic treatment
□□	?	0	No	□□□	□□	(+++)	?	?	Supportive and symptomatic treatment
(+)	?	0	No	0	?	?	?	?	Supportive and symptomatic treatment
□□, <1 hr	□□	0	No	0	++	++	0	?	Supportive and symptomatic treatment
□□	?	0	?	□□□	?	?	□□□	?	Antidotes: sodium thiosulfate, methylene blue, ascorbic acid?
(++)	(++)	0	Yes	?	?	?	?	?	The antidote for an overdose of chlordiazepoxide (or any other benzodiazepine) is flumazenil (Anexate)
?	?	?	No	?	?	?	?	?	Supportive and symptomatic treatment
(++)	?	0	No	?	?	?	?	?	Supportive and symptomatic treatment
□□	□□	0	No	?	(+)	?	?	?	Supportive and symptomatic treatment
□□	□□	0	No	0	++	++	0	?	Diazepam and epinephrine combined with mechanical ventilation, symptomatic treatment
(++)	?	?	No	(++)	?	?	(++)	?	Symptomatic treatment
□□	□□	0	No	0	+	?	0	?	Treatment of respiratory depression and cardiac abnormalities, symptomatic treatment
(++)	?	(++)	No	(++)	□□	?	□□	?	Treatment of hypoglycemia

TABLE 176-1

Poison Index—cont'd

| DRUG OR POISON[*†] | Pharmacokinetics | | | | | | Toxicity | |
	MW (Da)	PPB (%)	V_D (L)	SB	$T_{1/2}$ (hr)	EU	NEPHROTOXICITY	OTHER SYSTEMIC TOXICITY
Chlorprothixene	315.9	99%	11-23	Lipophilic	8-12 hr	5%	Indirect	CV toxicity, CNS toxicity, hepatotoxicity
Cinoxacin	262.2	60-80%	?	?	1.5 hr	60%	?	GI and CNS signs and symptoms, hypersensitivity
Ciprofloxacin[68-71]	331.3	20-40%	?	?	4 hr	40-50%	Yes	GI and CNS signs and symptoms, hepatic injury, rash
Citalopram[72-74]	324.4	50%	12	Lipophilic	35 hr	10%	?	Asthenia, GI symptoms, dizziness, insomnia, somnolence, agitation
Clobazam	300.7	90%	1.4	Lipophilic	50 hr	1%	?	CNS depression
Clomipramine[75,76]	314.9	97%	12	Lipophilic	17-28 hr	3%	?	Drowsiness, ataxia, seizures, respiratory depression, cardiotoxicity and coma
Clonazepam	315.7	47-82%	3.3	Lipophilic	23-36 hr	1%	?	Intoxication is rare
Clonidine[77-80]	230.1	30-40%	3-5.5	Lipophilic	5-13 hr	50%	?	Respiratory depression, CNS depression, hypotension, bradycardia, hypothermia
Clorazepate	332.7	?	?	Hydrophilic	36-100 hr	?	?	See *Oxazepam*
Clotiazepam	318.8	?	2-3	Lipophilic	?	Little	?	CNS depression
Cocaine[81-83]	303.4	?	1.2-1.9	Lipophilic	1 hr	5-10%	Indirect	CNS stimulation, sympathomimetic effects, "body packer" syndrome
Codeine	299.4	7-25%	3.5	?	3-4 hr	Little	?	Respiratory depression; CV, dermatological, and GI signs and symptoms
Colchicine[84-87]	399.4	0-50%	1.4-3.0	Lipophilic	20 min	20%	Yes	GI symptoms, multiorgan failure, hypothermia
Cresol	108	High	Large	Lipophilic	?	?	Indirect	Corrosive effects, CNS depression, hemolysis, Heinz bodies
Cyanide/hydrogen cyanide[88-92]	27.04	?	Large	Lipophilic	1 hr	Little	?	Respiratory, CV, CNS symptoms
Cyclobarbital	236.3	25%	?	Lipophilic	8-17 hr	7%	?	CNS depression, respiratory depression, relaxation of skeletal smooth muscle and myocardium
Cyclobenzaprine[93]	275.4	93%	?	?	1-3 days	<1%	?	Symptoms of central and peripheral cholinergic blockade
Cyclopentobarbital		?	?	?	?	?	?	CNS depression, respiratory depression, relaxation of skeletal smooth muscle and myocardium
Cycloserine	102.1	<2%	0.6	Hydrophilic	10 hr	60%	?	Extremely rare; headache, dizziness, abnormal behavior, ataxia, pyramidal signs
Dapsone[94,95]	248.3	80%	1-2	Lipophilic	20-40 hr	15%	?	Methemoglobinemia, hemolysis, damage in various organs due to hypoxia
Desipramine	266.4	70-95%	40	Lipophilic	25 hr	5%	?	Intoxication is rare
Dextromoramide	392.5	?	?	?	?	Mostly	?	?
Diacetylmorphine	369.5	20-39%	Large	Lipophilic	<1 hr	Little	Yes	CNS and CV toxicity, GI symptoms, infections, immune dysfunction, leukoencephalopathy, heroin lung, rhabdomyolysis, "body packer" syndrome
Diazepam[96]	284.8	98%	1.1	Lipophilic	30-45 hr	<1%	?	Tiredness, sleep, stupor, respiratory depression, CV symptoms
Diazoxide[97]	230.7	90%	0.2	?	28 hr	50%	?	Tachycardia, headache, vomiting, nausea, hyperglycemia, hypotension
Dibenzepin[98]	295.5	96%	Large	Lipophilic	4 hr	Little	?	Cramps and areflexia, severe tachycardia, cardiac insufficiency, brochospasm
Dichloroethane[99,100]	98.96	?	?	Hydrophilic	?	?	Yes	See *Carbon tetrachloride*
Dicyclomine	310.5	?	?	?	?	?	?	Drowsiness, irritability, respiratory symptoms
Dieffenbachia[101]		?	?	?	?	?	?	Pain, inflammation, swelling of lips, dysphagia, edema, contact dermatitis, respiratory arrest
Diethylene glycol[102,103]	106.1	?	?	Hydrophilic	?	?	?	Metabolic acidosis, edema, GI and pulmonary bleeding

				Enhancement of Removal					
GD	IAC	FD	SA	HD	HPₐ	HP_R	PD	PE	SUPPORTIVE TREATMENT
□□	□□	0	No	0	++	?	0	?	Treatment of dysrhythmias
(++)	?	(++)	No	(++)	?	?	(++)	?	Symptomatic treatment
(++)	□□	(+)	No	(+)	?	?	(+)	?	Symptomatic treatment
(++)	?	0	No	(++)	?	?	(+)	?	Symptomatic treatment
□□, <3 hr	□	0	Yes	?	?	?	?	?	
(++)	0	0	?	0	(+)	(+)	0	?	See *Amitriptyline*
(+++)	(++)	?	Yes	?	?	?	?	?	
□□	□□	0	Yes	+	□	?	?	?	Antidotes: naloxone and tolazoline; supportive and symptomatic treatment
(+++)	(++)	?	Yes	?	?	?	?	?	
□□, <3 hr	□	0	Yes	?	?	?	?	?	
0	0	0	No	+	+	?	?	?	Supportive and symptomatic treatment
□□	□□	□□	Yes	0	(+)	?	?	?	Antidote: naloxone; establish adequacy of respiratory function and circulation
□□□, <12 hr	□□□	0	No	0	0	0	0	?	All intensive care measures required, supportive and symptomatic treatment
□□		□□	No	+++	?	?	?	?	See *Phenol and derivatives*
□□	□□	0	Yes	++	□	?	?	?	Antidotes: thiosulfate, sodium nitrite, amyl nitrate, aminophenols, hydroxocobalamin, dicobalt-EDTA
□□, <8 hr	□	0	No	□□□	(+++)	(++)	0	?	Stabilization of circulatory and respiratory function, good nursing
(++)	?	0	?	0	(+)	?	?	?	See *Amitriptyline*
□□, <8 hr	□	0	No	(++)	(++)	(++)	0	?	Stabilization of circulatory and respiratory function, good nursing
□□	?	(++)	No	□□	?	?	□□	?	
□□, <6 hr	□□	++	Yes	0	++	?	?	?	Antidote: methylene blue; supportive and symptomatic treatment
(++)	?	0	?	0	(+)	(+)	?	?	See *Amitriptyline*
(++)	?	(++)	?	?	?	?	?	?	See *Morphine*
□□	□□	0	Yes	0	+	?	?	?	Antidote: naloxone; establish adequacy of respiratory function and circulation, withdrawal and dependence
□□, <3 hr	□□	0	Yes	0	0	0	0	?	Antidotes: flumazenil and physostigmine
(+)	?	(++)	No	+	?	?	+	?	Treatment of hyperglycemia, hypotension; prolonged surveillance more than 7 days
(++)	(++)	(++)	?	0	(+)	(+)	0	?	See *Amitriptyline*
(++)	(++)	0	Yes	?	□	?	?	?	See *Carbon tetrachloride*
?	?	?	No	?	?	?	?	?	Supportive and symptomatic treatment, physostigmine may be tried
?	?	?	?	?	?	?	?	?	Supportive and symptomatic treatment
□□	□□	□	Yes	□□	?	?	?	?	Antidote: fomepizole; see *Ethylene glycol*; symptomatic treatment

TABLE 176-1

Poison Index—cont'd

DRUG OR POISON[*†]	Pharmacokinetics						Toxicity	
	MW (Da)	PPB (%)	V$_D$ (L)	SB	T$_{1/2}$ (hr)	EU	NEPHROTOXICITY	OTHER SYSTEMIC TOXICITY
Digitalis[104-107]	764.9	90-97%	0.6-0.8	Lipophilic	180-220 hr	60%	?	GI and neurological signs and symptoms, visual disturbances, cardiac manifestations, electrolyte abnormalities
Digoxin[108,109]	780.9	20-30%	512	Lipophilic	30-50 hr	70%	?	GI and neurological symptoms, visual disturbances, cardiac manifestations, electrolyte abnormalities
Dihydrocodeine[110,111]	301.4	?	1	?	20 min	13-22%	?	Respiratory depression, miosis, hypothermia, CV depression
Diltiazem[112,113]	414.5	80%	5	Lipophilic	2 hr	0.2-4%	?	CV toxicity
Dimenhydrinate[114]	470	98%	Very high	?	4-7 hr	Little	?	CNS depression, anticholinergic stimulation, sedation
Dinitrophenol	184.11	High	Large	Lipophilic	?	?	Indirect	Corrosive effects, hemolysis, CNS depression, respiratory and CV signs and symptoms
Dinitro-o-cresol	198.13	High	Large	Lipophilic	?	?	Indirect	Corrosive effects, hemolysis, CNS depression, respiratory and CV signs and symptoms
Diphenhydramine	255.4	90-98%	3-7	?	4-10 hr	2-4%	?	Peripheral and central anticholinergic symptoms, rhabdomyolysis
Disopyramide[115]	339.5	<5%	0.5-1.2	?	5-9 hr	42-62%	Indirect	Anticholinergic effects, cardiac toxicity, hypokalemia, metabolic acidosis, hypotension
Dothiepin[116,117]	331.9	80-90%	10	?	20 hr	<0.5%	?	Intoxication is rare; see *Amitriptyline*
Doxepin[118]	279.4	75%	20	?	16 hr	Little	?	See *Amitriptyline*
Doxorubicin	543.5	74-76%	20-30	?	0.6 hr	4-5%	?	Cardiac toxicity
Doxylamine[119]	270.4	?	2.6-3.2	?	10 hr	60-85%	?	Dry mouth, headache, tachycardia, dizziness, GI symptoms, rhabdomyolysis
Encainide	352.5	70%	Large	Lipophilic	4 hr	Mostly	?	Seizures, hypotension, marked QRS widening on ECG
Enoxacin	320.3	40%	?	Hydrophilic	3-6 hr	>40%	?	GI and CNS signs and symptoms, hepatic injury, rash
Ergotamines[120]		?	2	?	2 hr	<5%	Indirect	Hemorrhagic vesiculation, pruritus, nausea, vomiting, peripheral nervous system symptoms
Erythromycin	733.9	90%	?	Lipophilic	1.5 hr	<5%	?	Abdominal pain, diarrhea, nausea, vomiting
Escitalopram[121]	324.4	56%	12	Lipophilic	27-32 hr	8%	?	Somnolence, tremor, dizziness, ejaculation failure, dry mouth, GI symptoms
Esmolol	331.8	55%	?	Hydrophilic	9 min	Little	?	CV toxicity, CNS manifestations
Ethchlorvynol	144.6	35-50%	4	Lipophilic	10-25 hr	10%	Yes	Respiratory depression, hypothermia, cardiac toxicity, GI symptoms, hemolysis
Ethinamate	167.2	?	?	?	2.3 hr	2%	No	CNS depression, respiratory depression, nausea, hyperthermia
Ethyl alcohol	46	?	?	Hydrophilic	?	2-10%	?	Neurological symptoms, abdominal pain, hypoglycemia, metabolic acidosis, hypothermia
Ethylene glycol[122,123]	62.4	None	0.7-0.8	Hydrophilic	3 hr	25%	Yes	Severe metabolic acidosis, neurological, cardiopulmonary manifestations
Fenfluramine[124]	231.3	30%	8-10	Lipophilic	8 hr	10~30%	?	CNS toxicity, cardiac toxicity, hepatotoxicity
Fentanyl[125,126]	336.5	80-85%	1-5	Lipophilic	1.5-6 hr	6-10%	?	Respiratory depression, CNS and CV toxicity, dermatitis, hypothermia
Flecainide[127-129]	414.4	48%	9-10	Lipophilic	7-23 hr	27%	?	CV toxicity, vertigo, blurred vision, headache, nausea
Flunitrazepam[130]	313.3	80%	3-4	Lipophilic	15 hr	1%	?	CNS depression
Fluorine and fluorides[131]		None	?	Hydrophilic	2-9 hr	50%	Yes	Respiratory and cardiac toxicity, neurological disturbances
Fluoxetine[132,133]	309.3	94%	20-45	?	2 days	11%	?	Nausea, agitation, vomiting, hypomania, insomnia, tremor
Fluoxetine[134]	349	94.5%	?	Hydrophilic	2-4 days	80%	?	Nausea, headache, nervous, sedation, insomnia, dry mouth
Flurazepam[135]	387.9	15%	22	Lipophilic	2-3 hr	1%	?	CNS depression

				Enhancement of Removal					
GD	*IAC*	*FD*	*SA*	*HD*	*HP$_A$*	*HP$_R$*	*PD*	*PE*	*SUPPORTIVE TREATMENT*
□□, <2 hr	□□	0	Yes	0	+	+	?	□	Antidote: Fab fragments; supportive and symptomatic treatment
□□, <3 hr	□□	0	Yes	0	0	0	0	□	Antidote: Fab fragments; supportive and symptomatic treatment
(++)	(++)	(+)	Yes	?	?	?	?	?	See *Codeine*
□□, <3 hr	0	0	?	0	0	0	?	□	See *Verapamil*
□□	□□	0	No	?	?	?	?	?	Symptomatic treatment; see *Diphenhydramine*
□□	□□	□□	No	++	?	?	?	?	See *Phenol and derivatives*
□□	□□	□□	No	+++	?	?	?	?	See *Phenol and derivatives*
□□	?	0	Yes	0	+++	+++	?	?	Antidote: physostigmine?; symptomatic treatment
□□	□□	□	No	++	□□	□□□	?	0	Arterial cardiac monitoring, evaluation of respiratory function, treatment of arrhythmias
□	□□	(+)	?	0	(+)	(+)	0	?	See *Amitriptyline*
(++)	(+)	0	?	□	(+)	□□	0	?	See *Amitriptyline*
?	?	0	?	0	0	0	0	?	Symptomatic treatment
(+)	?	(++)	?	?	?	?	?	?	Supportive treatment
(++)	?	(++)	?	+	?	?	?	?	Sodium substitution; see *Flecainide* and *Quinidine*
(++)	?	(+)	No	(+)	?	?	(+)	?	Symptomatic treatment
□□	□□	0	?	?	?	?	?	?	Intravenous administration of vasodilators; supportive treatment
(++)	?	0	No	(+)	?	?	(+)	?	Symptomatic treatment
(++)	?	0	No	(++)	?	?	(+)	?	Symptomatic treatment
?	?	(+++)	No	(++)	?	?	?	?	Intensive supportive care, management of arrhythmias and hypotension
□□□	□□□	0	No	++	□□	□□□	+	?	Physical assessment, treatment of severe respiratory depression
(++)	(++)	0	No	□□	?	?	?	?	See *Pentobarbital*
□□, <90 min	?	0	Yes	□□□	□	0	□□□	?	Antidotes: naloxone and physostigmine; supportive treatment
□□, <12 hr	□□	□	Yes	□□□	(+)	?	□□	□	Antidote: 4-methylpyrazole; treatment of respiratory insufficiency, acidosis; ethanol administration
□	□	?	No	0	?	?	0	?	Careful cardiac monitoring, symptomatic treatment
?	?	□	Yes	0	?	?	?	?	Antidote: naloxone; management of respiratory depression
□□	□□	□	?	+	++	?	?	?	Sodium substitution, symptomatic treatment
□□, <3 hr	□	0	Yes	?	?	?	?	?	
□□, <45 min	0	0	Yes	++	?	?	?	?	Antidote: calcium; supportive treatment
□□, <8 hr	□□	0	No	0	0	0	0	?	
(++)	?	□□	No	(++)	?	?	(+)	?	Symptomatic treatment
□□, <3 hr	□	0	Yes	?	?	?	?	?	

TABLE 176-1

Poison Index—cont'd

| DRUG OR POISON[*][1] | Pharmacokinetics | | | | | | Toxicity | |
	MW (Da)	PPB (%)	V_D (L)	SB	T_{1/2} (hr)	EU	NEPHROTOXICITY	OTHER SYSTEMIC TOXICITY
Fluvoxamine	318.3	77-80%	25	Lipophilic	15.6 hr	2%	?	Diarrhea, fatigue, anxiety, sexual dysfunction, anorexia
Formic acid	58	?	?	Hydrophilic	45 min	?	Yes	High causticity, cytotoxicity
Gemifloxicin	389.4	60-70%	4.18	Hydrophilic	5-9 hr	36%	?	Rash, diarrhea, urticaria, vomiting, headache, dizziness
Germanium[136,137]	72.6	?	?	?	?	Mostly	Yes	Hepatotoxicity, muscle and CNS toxicity
Gliclazide[138]	323.4	?	?	?	11 hr	?	Yes	Hypoglycemia; respiratory, GI, and musculosketetal signs and symptoms
Glimepiride	490.6	>99.5%	8.8	Lipophilic	5 hr	60%	?	Hypoglycemia, dizziness, asthenia, headache, nausea
Glipizide	444.5	98-99%	11	?	2-5 hr	<10%	?	Hypoglycemia; GI, dermatological, and miscellaneous symptoms
Glutethimide	217.3	50%	Large	Lipophilic	40 hr	0-2%	?	Profound and prolonged coma, respiratory and CV toxicity
Grepafloxacin	359.4	50%	4-6	Hydrophilic	12-18 hr	<10%	?	GI and CNS symptoms, hypersensitivity
Halazepam	352.7	95%		Lipophilic	35 hr	Little	?	CNS depression
Haloperidol	375.9	90%	20-30	Lipophilic	20 hr	1%	?	Severe extrapyramidal reactions, hypotension, sedation, cardiotoxicity
Heptabarbital	250.3	?	?	?	10 hr	Little	?	CNS depression, respiratory depression, relaxation of skeletal smooth muscle and myocardium
Hexachlorophene	407	92%	Large	Lipophilic	24 hr	?	Indirect	Neurotoxicity, GI disturbances
Hexobarbital	236.3	20%	1.0-1.2	Lipophilic	2-7 hr	<10%	?	CNS depression, respiratory depression, relaxation of skeletal smooth muscle and myocardium
Hydralazine	160.2	87%	7-8	Hydrophilic	3-4 hr	3-14%	?	Cardiovascular toxicity, headache, skin flushing
Hydrochloric acid	36.5	?	?	Lipophilic	?	?	Yes	High causticity, cytotoxicity
Hydrocodone	299.4	?	?	?	4-8 hr	?	?	?
Hydromorphone	285.3	?	1.2	?	2-5 hr	<10%	?	Respiratory depression, somnolence, progressing stupor or coma, hypotension, bradycardia
Imipramine[139-141]	280.4	76-95%	20-40	?	9-20 hr	1-3%	?	See Amitriptyline
Iron[142-146]	55.8	?	?	?	?	Little	Indirect	GI and cellular toxicity. Impaired liver, function, impairment of the hematological system necrosis, gastric scarring
Isocarboxazid[147]	231.3	?	?	?	?	Little	Indirect	CNS, CV, hepatic toxicity
Isoniazid[148-150]	137.2	30%	0.6	Hydrophilic	2-3 hr	4-20%	?	Recurrent seizures, metabolic acidosis, hepatic dysfunction
Isoprenaline	?	?	?	?	?	?	?	Headache, cardiotoxicity
Isopropyl alcohol[151,152]	60	None	0.6-0.8	Lipophilic	7.6-26 hr	10-30%	Yes	GI signs and hemorrhage, CNS effects, cardiac depression and hypotension
Lactic acid	90.1	?	?	?	?	?	Yes	High causticity, acidosis, hemolysis, DIC, hepatotoxicity
Lead[153-156]	207.2	?	?	?	?	?	Indirect	Gastrointestianl symptoms, hematological effects, CNS and neuromuscular effects
Levofloxacin	741.8	24-39%	?		6-8 hr	Mostly	?	Transient decreased vision, fever, headache, ocular pain, pharyngitis
Lidocaine[157,158]	234.3	40-80%	1.5	?	6-15 min	5-10%	?	CNS, CV, GI tract toxicity
Lithium[159-163]	6.94	None	0.6-0.9	?	24 hr	95%	Yes	CNS, GI, CV, hematopoietic system toxicity
Lofepramine	419	32-96%	Large	Lipophilic	44-76 hr	Little	?	See Amitriptyline
Lomefloxacin	351.3	10%	?	Hydrophilic	8 hr	65%	?	Headache, GI symptoms, photosensitivity, dizziness
Lorazepam	312.2	80%	?	Lipophilic	<10 hr	3%	?	CNS depression
Lorcainide[164]	370.9	75-85%	8-10	?	7.7 hr	2%	?	CNS, cardiac toxicity, GI symptoms
Lormetazepam	335.2	85%	4.6	Lipophilic	9-15 hr	<1%	?	CNS depression

				Enhancement of Removal					
GD	IAC	FD	SA	HD	HP_A	HP_R	PD	PE	SUPPORTIVE TREATMENT
(++)	?	0	No	(++)	?	?	(+)	?	Symptomatic treatment
+	?	?	No	□□□	0	0	?	?	Analyosics, treatment of asphyxia and metabolic
(++)	?	(+)	No	(++)	?	?	(+)	?	Symptomatic treatment
?	?	?	?	?	?	?	?	?	
(++)	?	?	No	(+)	?	?	(+)	?	Symptomatic treatment, close monitoring of blood glucose
(++)	□□	(++)	No	(++)	?	?	(++)	?	Symptomatic treatment, close monitoring of blood glucose
(++)	?	0	No	(++)	?	?	(++)	?	IV dextrose, use of octreotide as an antidote, restoring acid-base balance
□□	□□	0	No	(+)	□□□	□□□	(+)	?	Treatment of respiratory depression and cerebral edema
(++)	?	0	No	(++)	?	?	(+)	?	Symptomatic treatment
□□, <3 hr	□	0	Yes	?	?	?	?	?	
□□, <8 hr	□□	0	No	0	□	□	?	?	Treatment of respiratory depression, hypertension, and arrhythmias
□□, <8 hr	□	0	No	(++)	(++)	(++)	0	?	Stabilization of circulatory and respiratory function, good nursing
□□	□□	□□	No	0	(+)	?	0	?	See *Phenol and derivatives*
□□, <8 hr	□	0	No	(++)	(+)	(+)	0	?	Stabilization of circulatory and respiratory function, good nursing
□□, <1 hr	□□	0	No	?	?	?	?	?	Support to relieve CV symptoms
+	?	?	No	?	?	?	?	?	Analgesics, treatment of asphyxia and metabolic acidosis
?	?	?	Yes	?	?	?	?	?	Antidote; levallorphan; see *Morphine*
?	?	0	Yes	?	?	?	?	?	Antidote: naloxone; see *Morphine*
?	?	?	?	?	?	?	?	?	See *Amitriptyline*
□	0	?	Yes	0	+	?	?	?	Chelator: DFO
□□	□□	0	?	?	?	?	?	?	Close monitoring for at least 24 hours, symptomatic treatment
□□, <2 hr	□□	□□□	Yes	+++	(+)	?	++	?	Antidote: pyridoxine (vitamin B_6)
(+)	?	?	No	?	?	?	?	?	Supportive and symptomatic treatment
□□, <30 min	0	0	No	□□□	□	0	□□	?	Supportive and symptomatic treatment for hypotension, respiration, and hypothermia
+	?	?	No	□□□	0	0	□□	?	Analgesics, treatment of asphyxia and metabolic acidosis
□□	□□	□□	Yes	0	0	0	0	?	Chelator: calcium-sodium-EDTA, BAL, D-penicillamine, DMSA
(++)	?	(++)	No	(+)	?	?	0	?	Symptomatic treatment
□□	□□	□□	No	?	?	□□	?	?	Symptomatic treatment
□, <8 hr	0	□	No	□□□	0	?	□	?	Symptomatic treatment
(++)	?	?	?	0	(+)	(+)	?	?	See *Amitriptyline*
(++)	?	(++)	No	(+)	?	?	(+)	?	Symptomatic treatment
□□, <3 hr	□	0	Yes	?	?	?	?	?	
(++)	?	0	No	?	?	?	?	?	Symptomatic treatment; see *Flecainide* and *Quinidine*
□□, <6 hr	□	0	Yes	?	?	?	?	?	

TABLE 176-1

Poison Index—cont'd

DRUG OR POISON*†	Pharmacokinetics						Toxicity	
	MW (Da)	PPB (%)	V_D (L)	SB	T_1/2 (hr)	EU	NEPHROTOXICITY	OTHER SYSTEMIC TOXICITY
Mannitol	182.2	7%	0.18	?	1.5-3 hr	Mostly	Yes	Severe fluid overload, CNS disturbance, hyponatremia, hyperosmolality
Maprotiline	277.4	88%	23	Lipophilic	30 hr	Little	?	CV, psychiatric, neurological, hematological toxicity; GI disorders; anticholinergic activity
Medazepam	270.8	100%	?	Lipophilic	2 hr	<1%	?	Intoxication is rare
Mephobarbital	246.3	40-60%	2.6	Hydrophilic	48-52 hr	?	?	CNS and respiratory depression, relaxation of skeletal smooth muscle and myocardium
Meprobamate	218.3	15-0%	0.7	?	8-12 hr	10%	?	CNS, CV toxicity
Mercury[165-168]	200.6	>90%	20	?	40 day	Mostly	Yes	Neurological and GI symptoms; cardiac, hepatic, endocrine, immune system toxicity; metabolic changes
Metformin[169-174]	129.2	None	296-1012	Hydrophilic	6.2 hr	Mostly	Yes	Hypoglycemia, diarrhea, nausea
Methadone[175-177]	309.5	8-44%	4-7	Lipophilic	2-3 hr	Little	Yes	Respiratory depression, hypotension, hypothermia, miosis, bradycardia, vomiting, euphoria
Methaqualone	250.3	70-90%	2.5-6	Lipophilic	2-6 hr	1-3%	Indirect	CNS depression, pulmonary edema, increased muscle tone and motor activity
Methohexital	262.3	73%	1.1	Lipophilic	1-2 hr	1%	?	CNS depression, respiratory depression, relaxation of skeletal smooth muscle and myocardium
Methotrexate[178-185]	454.4	35%	1	Hydrophilic	2hr	90%	Yes	GI and bone marrow toxicity
Methotrimeprazine	328.5	50-60%	20-40	Lipophilic	16-31 hr	1%	?	Intoxication is extremely rare
Methsuximide	203.2	None	?	?	2.6-4 hr	1%	?	Delayed onset of stupor and coma
Methyl alcohol[186]	32.04	None	0.6-0.7	Hydrophilic	?	2-5%	?	Systemic acidosis, CNS depression, neurotoxicity, blindness
Methyldopa	211.2	0-20%	0.5	?	0.2-0.5 hr	50%	?	Hepatotoxicity, CNS depression
Methylphenobarbital	246.3	20-45%	?	Hydrophilic	?	Little	?	CNS and respiratory depression, relaxation of skeletal smooth muscle and myocardium
Methyprylon	183.2	60%	Large	?	3-6 hr	<3%	?	CNS depression; pulmonary, GI tract, CV manifestations
Metoprolol[187,188]	267.4	12%	5.6	Hydrophilic	3-4 hr	5%	?	CV toxicity, CNS manifestations, acute shoulder syndrome
Mexiletine[189,190]	179.3	60-75%	5.5-12	?	5-15 hr	10%	?	Prolongation of ventricular depolarization, motor seizures
Mianserin	264.4	90%	40-50	Lipophilic	17 hr	4-7%	?	Cardiac arrhythmias
Midazolam[191]	325	95%	1.7	Lipophilic	2 hr	<1%	?	CNS depression
Minoxidil[192,193]	209.3	None	3-5	?	4 hr	90%	?	Skin rashes, polymenorrhea, headache, hypertrichosis
Monochloroacetic acid[194,195]	94.5	?	?	Hydrophilic	?	?	Indirect	Malaise, vomiting; CNS, CV, hepatic toxicity; metabolic acidosis; hypokalemia
Morphine	303.4	35%	3-4	?	3.5 hr	10%	?	Coma, respiratory depression, miosis
Moxifloxacin[196]	401.4	50%	?	?	11.5-15.6 hr	?	?	CNS and GI symptoms, conjunctivitis, dry eyes, keratitis, ocular hyperemia
Nadolol	309.4	20-30%	2.5	Lipophilic	14-2 hr	70%	?	CV toxicity, respiratory and CNS signs and symptoms
Nalidixic acid	232.2	93%	?	?	1.1-2.5 hr	85%	?	CNS, GI, allergic symptoms
Nateglinide[197]	317.4	98%	10	Lipophilic	1.5 hr	16%	?	Upper respiratory tract infection, headache, back pain, sinusitis, diarrhea
Nifedipine[198,199]	346.3	99%	0.6-1.2	?	4 hr	<1%	?	CV toxicity, flushing
Nitrazepam	281.3	87%	1.9-2.4	Lipophilic	20-50 hr	1%	?	CNS depression
Nitric acid	63	?	?	Hydrophilic	?	?	Yes	High causticity, acidosis, hemolysis, DIC, hepatotoxicity
Nitrites and nitrates	191.1	<4%	?	?	5 hr	Little	?	Methemoglobinemia; CV, respiratory, and CNS toxicity
Norfloxacin[200]	319.3	10-15%	?	Lipophilic	3-4 hr	26-32%	?	Dizziness, GI symptoms, headache, asthenia
Nortriptyline	263.4	High	Large	?	36 hr	?	?	See *Amtriptyline*

				Enhancement of Removal					
GD	IAC	FD	SA	HD	HP_A	HP_R	PD	PE	SUPPORTIVE TREATMENT
0	0	0	No	□□	?	?	□	?	Supportive treatment
□□	□□	0	No	0	+	+	0	?	Supportive treatment
(+++)	(++)	?	Yes	?	?	?	?	?	
□□, <8 hr	□	□	No	(++)	(++)	(++)	0	?	Stabilization of circulatory and respiratory function, good nursing
□□, <4 hr	□□	++	No	□□	□□□	□□□	++	?	Treatment of hypotension, respiratory failure, convulsion
□	□	++	Yes	+	□	?	+	□	Antidotes: BAL, DMSA, DMPS, D-penicillamine and its N-acetyl derivative
(++)	?	□□	No	□□□	?	?	(+++)	?	Symptomatic treatment, close monitoring of blood glucose
□	□	0	Yes	0	0	0	0	?	Antidote: naloxone; stabilization of vital function
□□, <4 hr	□□	0	No	+	+++	+++	+	?	Supportive treatment
□□, <8 hr	□	0	No	(++)	(++)	(++)	0	?	Stabilization of circulatory and respiratory function, good nursing
□	□	□	Yes	□	□□	□□	0	□□□	Antidote: folinic acid
(+++)	?	0	No	0	?	?	0	?	
(+)	?	0	No	+	++	?	+	?	
□□□, <8 hr	□□	0	Yes	□□□	□	0	□	?	Antidote: pyrazole and 4-methylpyrazole; ethanol substitution, adequate ventilation
□□	□□	(++)	No	+++	?	?	++	?	Symptomatic treatment
□□, <8 hr	□	□	No	(++)	(++)	(++)	0	?	Stabilization of circulatory and respiratory function, good nursing
□□, <4 hr	□□	0	No	+	+	?	+	?	Supportive treatment
□□, <3 hr	□□	++	No	+	?	?	?	?	Intensive supportive care, management of arrhythmias and hypotension
(++)	□□	?	No	?	?	?	?	?	See *Lidocaine*
□□, <2 hr	?	0	No	0	(+)	(+)	?	?	Symptomatic treatment
□□, <3 hr	□	0	Yes	+++	?	?	?	?	
?	?	?	?	?	?	?	?	?	
0	0	?	?	?	?	?	?	?	Symptomatic treatment
□□	□□	0	Yes	0	+	?	0	?	Antidote: naloxone; establish adequacy of respiratory function and circulation
(++)	□□	?	No	(++)	?	?	(+)	?	Symptomatic treatment
□□, <8 hr	□□	0	No	+	?	?	?	?	Intensive supportive care, management of arrhythmias and hypotension
(++)	?	(++)	No	(++)	?	?	(++)	?	Symptomatic treatment
(++)	?	0	No	(++)	?	?	(++)	?	Symptomatic treatment, close monitoring of blood glucose
□□, <3 hr	□	0	?	0	□	?	?	?	See *Verapamil*
□□, <6 hr	□	0	Yes	?	?	?	?	?	
I	?	?	No	?	0	0	?	?	Analgesics, treatment of asphyxia and metabolic acidosis
□□	0	□	Yes	?	?	?	?	?	Antidote: methylene blue; supportive treatment
(++)	?	(+)	No	0	?	?	0	?	Symptomatic treatment
□□□	□□□	0	?	0	(+)	(+)	0	?	See *Amitriptyline*

TABLE 176-1

Poison Index—cont'd

DRUG OR POISON*[†]	Pharmacokinetics						Toxicity	
	MW (Da)	PPB (%)	V_D (L)	SB	T_{1/2} (hr)	EU	NEPHROTOXICITY	OTHER SYSTEMIC TOXICITY
NSAIDs		90-99%	0.1-0.17	?	?	Little	Yes	GI, CNS, CV, hepatic, neuromuscular activity symptoms
Ofloxacin	361.4	32%	?	?	9 hr	65-80%	?	Nausea, insomnia, headache, dizziness, diarrhea, rash, pruritus
Oleander/oleandrin[201-206]	576.7	?	Large	?	?	?	?	Irritation of mucosa, GI symptoms, CV symptoms
Orciprenaline	?	?	?	?	?	?	?	Headache, cardiotoxicity
Organochlorines		?	?	Lipophilic	?	?	?	Tremor, seizures, CNS and GI symptoms, arrhythmias, metabolic acidosis
Organophosphates[207,208]		?	15-27	?	?	?	?	Stimulation of autonomic nervous system muscarinic receptors, nicotinic receptors, cholinergic receptors in CNS
Orphenadrine[209]	269.1	20%	?	Hydrophilic	10 hr	8%	?	CNS, CV, hepatic toxicity
Oxaflozane[210]	273.3	?	?	?	2 hr	?	?	Seizures, mydriasis, tachycardia, coma
Oxalic acid	90	None	33	Hydrophilic		Mostly	Yes	Corrosive effects, hypocalcemia, hematemesis, petechial bleeding, diarrhea, CNS symptoms
Oxazepam	286.7	97%	1	Lipophilic	12 hr	<1%	?	Intoxication is extremely rare
Oxprenolol	265.3	70-80%	1.3	Lipophilic	2 hr	<5%	?	CV toxicity, respiratory and CNS symptoms, hypokalemia
Oxycodone	315.4	?	?	?	2-3 hr	?	?	See Codeine
Paracetamol[211-213]	151.2	15-20%	0.9-1	Lipophilic	8 hr	1-4%	Yes	Hepatotoxicity, CNS and cardiac toxicity, respiratory symptoms
Paraphenylenediamine[214,215]	108.1	?	?	?	?	?	Yes	Dermatitis, asthma, anemia, cardiac and CNS toxicity, hepatitis, vasculitis
Paraquat[216-218]	257.16	None	1.2-1.6	Hydrophilic	5-84 hr	7-8%	Yes	Hepatocellular necrosis, cerebral and adrenal hemorrhage, myocardial necrosis, pulmonary fibrosis
Pargyline	152.9	?	?	?	?	<1%	Indirect	CNS, CV, and hepatic toxicity
Paroxetine	329.4	95%	Large	Hydrophilic	24 hr	2%	?	CNS and GI symptoms, asthenia, ejaculation failure
Pefloxacin[219]	333.4	20-30%	?	Hydrophilic	8.6 hr	?	?	Peripheral neuropathy, nervousness, agitation, anxiety, phototoxic events
Pentachlorophenol[220,221]	266.4	?	Large	Lipophilic	10-35 hr	80%	Yes	Central, peripheral, and vegetative system effects, bone marrow injury, hepatomegaly
Pentobarbital[222]	226.3	65%	0.8-1.0	Lipophilic	20-30 hr	1%	?	CNS and respiratory depression, relaxation of skeletal smooth muscle and myocardium
Phencyclidine	243.4	65%	6	Lipophilic	21-24 hr	<10%	Yes	CNS, respiratory, and CV symptoms; hyperthermia
Phenelzine	136.2	?	?	Hydrophilic	1.2 hr	<2%	Indirect	CNS, CV, and hepatic toxicity
Phenobarbital	232.2	15-45%	0.5-0.6	Hydrophilic	48-144 hr	25%	?	CNS and respiratory depression, relaxation of skeletal smooth muscle and myocardium
Phenol and derivatives[223]		High	Large	Lipophilic	?	?	Indirect	Corrosive effects, hemolysis, CNS depression, respiratory and CV symptoms
Phenylbutazone[224]	308.4	88-98%	0.17	?	70 hr	1%	Yes	Toxic hepatitis, gastric ulceration, acidosis
Phenytoin[225-227]	252.3	90-95%	5-6	Lipophilic	24-230 hr	5%	?	Respiratory depression, CV and CNS symptoms, hepatotoxicity, hyperglycemia
Philodendron	?	?	?	?	?	?	?	Pain, inflammation, swelling of lips, dysphagia, edema, contact dermatitis, respiratory arrest
Phosphoric acid	98	?	?	Hydrophilic	5-11 hr	?	Yes	High causticity, acidosis, hemolysis, DIC, hepatotoxicity
Phosphorus	31	?	Large	?	?	?	Yes	GI and CNS symptoms, hepatotoxicity
Pindolol	248.3	60%	2	Lipophilic	3-4 hr	40%	?	CV toxicity, respiratory and CNS symptoms

Enhancement of Removal									
GD	IAC	FD	SA	HD	HP_A	HP_R	PD	PE	SUPPORTIVE TREATMENT
□	□	0	No	0	□□	□□	0	?	Supportive treatment
(++)	?	(++)	No	(+)	?	?	(+)	?	Symptomatic treatment
□□, <2 hr	□□	0	Yes	0	+	+	?	?	See *Digitalis*
(+)	?	?	No	?	?	?	?	?	Supportive and symptomatic treatment
□□	□□	0	No	?	++	++	?	?	Respiratory support, treatment of seizures and arrhythmias
□□	□□	□	Yes	+	□□	□□	?	□	Antidote: atropine; treatment of respiratory problems, blood gas, and cardiac monitoring
□, <1 hr	?	0	Yes	+++	?	?	?	?	Antidote: physostigmine; symptomatic treatment
?	?	?	?	?	?	?	?	?	
□	?	□	No	□□□	0	0	□□□	?	Prevention of hypocalcemia, tetany
(+++)	(++)	?	Yes	?	?	?	?	?	
□□, <3 hr	□□	0	No	+	?	?	?	?	Intensive supportive care, management of arrhythmias and hypotension
(++)	(++)	0	?	?	?	?	?	?	See *Morphine*
0	□□	0	No	□□	?	?	□	+++	Intensive supportive treatment
?	?	?	No	?	?	?	?	?	Symptomatic treatment
□□	□	0	No	□	□□	+	0	++	Oxygenation, anti-inflammatory drugs, prevention of lung fibrosis
□□	□□	0	?	?	?	?	?	?	Close monitoring for at least 25 hours; symptomatic treatment
(++)	?	0	No	(++)	?	?	(+)	?	Symptomatic treatment
(++)	?	?	No	(+)	?	?	□	?	Symptomatic treatment
□□	□□	(++)	No	?	?	?	?	□	Symptomatic treatment
□□, <8 hr	□	0	No	□□	□□□	□□□	0	?	Stabilization of circulatory and respiratory function, good nursing
□□	□□	□	No	0	?	?	0	?	Symptomatic treatment
□□	□□	0	?	?	?	?	?	?	Closely monitoring for at least 26 hours; symptomatic treatment
□□, <8 hr	□	□	No	□□	□□□	□□□	0	?	Stabilization of circulatory and respiratory function, good nursing
□□	□□	□□	No	0	□□	?	0	?	Symptomatic treatment
□	□	0	No	+	□□	□□	?	□	Supportive treatment
□	□	0	No	0	□□	+	0	0	Symptomatic treatment
?	?	?	?	?	?	?	?	?	Supportive and symptomatic treatment
+	?	?	No	□□□	(+)	(+)	?	?	Analgesics, treatment of asphyxia and metabolic acidosis
□□	□□	0	No	0	0	0	0	?	Symptomatic treatment
□□, <3 hr	□□	(++)	No	?	?	?	?	?	Intensive supportive care, management of arrhythmias and hypotension

TABLE 176-1

Poison Index—cont'd

DRUG OR POISON[*†]	Pharmacokinetics						Toxicity	
	MW (Da)	PPB (%)	V_D (L)	SB	$T_{1/2}$ (hr)	EU	NEPHROTOXICITY	OTHER SYSTEMIC TOXICITY
Pioglitazone	356.4	>99%	0.22-1.04	Lipophilic	3-7 hr	Little	?	Upper respiratory tract infection, headache, back pain, sinusitis, diarrhea
Platinum[228]	195.1	?	?	?	?	?	?	Gastroenteritis, hypovolemia, fever, muscle cramps
Potassium permanganate[229,230]	158	?	?	Hydrophilic	?	?	?	Corrosion, dyspnea, stridor, hepatotoxicity
Prajmaline	518.6	60%	?	?	5-7 hr	10%	Yes	CV, respiratory tract, and CNS toxicity
Prazepam	324.8	97%	?	Lipophilic	1-2 hr	Little	?	CNS depression
Prazosin	382.4	90%	0.5	?	2.5 hr	3.50%	?	Orthostatic hypotension, syncope
Primidone	218.3	<20%	0.64-0.86	Hydrophilic	12-22 hr	15-25%	?	CNS and respiratory depression, relaxation of skeletal smooth muscle and myocardium
Procainamide[231]	235.3	15%	1.7-2.2	Hydrophilic	3 hr	50-60%	?	Lethargy, confusion, hypotension, ventricular arrhythmias, SLE-like syndrome
Propafenone[232-234]	341.5	95%	2.5-4	?	4 hr	<1%	?	CV, neurological, and GI symptoms
Propoxyphene	339.5	73-80%	10-20	Lipophilic	4 hr	<10%	Indirect	CNS depression, respiratory depression
Propranolol	259.3	93%	3.5	Lipophilic	2-3 hr	Mostly	?	CV toxicity, respiratory and CNS symptoms
Protriptyline	263.4	92%	Large	Lipophilic	55-92 hr	2%	?	Cardiotoxicity, coma, seizures, hyperthermia, urinary retention, ARDS
Pyrethrum	?	?	?	Lipophilic	?	?	?	Contact dermatitis, anaphylactic reactions, GI symptoms, CNS excitation
Pyrithyldione	167.2	?	?	Hydrophilic	10-20 hr	3%	?	Drowsiness, mydriasis, GI disturbances, hepatic injury, respiratory depression
Quinidine	360.5	60-95%	2-3.5	?	6-8 hr	15-40%	Indirect	Tinnitus, dizziness, GI disturbances, CV and CNS effects, hypotension
Quinine[235,236]	324.4	69-92%	1.8-2.2	Lipophilic	9-15 hr	25%	?	Hypersensitivity, gastric distress, hemolysis, cinchonism, amblyopia
Repaglinide	452.6	>98%	31	Lipophilic	1 hr	0.10%	?	Hypoglycemia; respiratory, GI, musculoskeletal symptoms
Reserpine	608.7	40-95%	Very large	Lipophilic	4-5 hr	8%	?	CNS and CV toxicity
Rosiglitazone	357.4	99.8%	17.6	Lipophilic	3-4 hr	0	?	Upper respiratory tract infection, headache, back pain, sinusitis, diarrhea
Salbutamol[237,238]	239.3	?	?	?	2.7-5 hr	?	?	Fine tremor of skeletal muscle, hypotension, tachycardia
Salicylates[239-242]	180.15	50-80%	0.2-0.5	Lipophilic	2-30 hr	3-30%	Yes	Respiratory and acid-base disturbances; GI, hepatic, and CNS toxicity; hyperthermia
Secobarbital	238.3	30-70%	1.6-1.9	Lipophilic	22-30 hr	5%	?	CNS and respiratory depression, relaxation of skeletal smooth muscle and myocardium
Sertraline[243,244]	306.2	98%	?	Lipophilic	26 hr	Little	?	Somnolence, tremor, dizziness, ejaculation failure, dry mouth, GI symptoms
Sodium azide[245,246]	66	?	?	Hydrophilic	2.5 hr	?	?	CV, pulmonary, hematological and neurological effects, electrolyte disturbances
Sodium chloride[247]	58.5	None	0.6	Hydrophilic	?	?	Yes	CNS and GI toxicity, hyperthermia, metabolic acidosis
Sodium nitroprusside	298	?	?	?	3-11 min	20-50%	?	Vasodilatation, hypotension, circulatory collapse
Sotalol	272.4	None	1.6-2.4	Hydrophilic	15-17 hr	>80%	?	CV toxicity, respiratory and CNS symptoms
Sparfloxacin	392.4	45%	3.1-4.7	Lipophilic	20 hr	50%	?	Photosensitivity, GI symptoms, insomnia, QT interval prolongation
Strychnine[248-251]	334.2	Low	13	Lipophilic	10-16 hr	5-20%	Indirect	Muscle spasms, respiratory and cardiac failure, hyperthermia, lactic acidosis
Sulfuric acid	98	?	?	Hydrophilic	?	?	Yes	High causticity, acidosis, hemolysis, DIC, hepatotoxicity
Temazepam	300.7	97%	1	Lipophilic	6-16 hr	2%	?	CNS depression
Terbutaline[252,253]	225.3	?	?	?	3-4 hr	?	?	Fine tremor of skeletal muscle, headache, tachycardia

				Enhancement of Removal					
GD	*IAC*	*FD*	*SA*	*HD*	*HP$_A$*	*HP$_R$*	*PD*	*PE*	*SUPPORTIVE TREATMENT*
(++)	?	0	No	(++)	?	?	(++)	?	Symptomatic treatment, close monitoring of blood glucose
(++)	(++)	?	No	0	?	?	?	?	Symptomatic treatment
(+)	?	0	No	++	0	0	?	?	Symptomatic treatment
?	?	□□	No	?	?	□□	?	?	
□□, <6 hr	□	0	Yes	?	?	?	?	?	
?	?	?	?	?	?	?	?	?	
□□, <8 hr	□	□	No	++	□□□	□□□	0	?	Stabilization of circulatory and respiratory function, good nursing
□□, <4 hr	□□	□□	No	□	□	+++	0	?	Treatment of dysrhythmias
?	?	0	No	+	?	++	?	?	See *Quinidine*
□□, <5 hr	□□	0	Yes	0	0	0	0	?	Antidote: naloxone; supportive treatment
□□, <3 hr	□□	(++)	No	+	+	+	?	?	Intensive supportive care, management of arrhythmias and hypotension
□□□	□□□	0	?	0	(+)	(+)	0	?	See *Amitriptyline*
?	?	?	No	?	?	?	?	?	Supportive treatment
□□, <4 hr	□□	0	No	+	+	?	+	?	See *Methyprylon*
□□, <5 hr	□□	□	No	+	+	(+)	+	?	Symptomatic treatment
□□, <6 hr	□	0	No	+	+	?	+	?	Symptomatic treatment
(++)	?	0	No	(++)	?	?	(++)	?	Symptomatic treatment, close monitoring of blood glucose
□	□	(+)	No	0	0	0	0	?	Maintenance of blood pressure
(++)	?	0	No	(++)	?	?	(++)	?	Symptomatic treatment, close monitoring of blood glucose
□	□	?	No	?	?	?	?	?	Supportive and symptomatic treatment
□□, <8 hr	□□	□□	No	□□	□□	□□	□	?	Urine alkalinization; correction of acidosis, electrolyte imbalance, and dehydration
□□, <8 hr	□	0	No	□□	□□□	?	0	?	Stabilization of circulatory and respiratory function, good nursing
(++)	?	0	No	(++)	?	?	(+)	?	Symptomatic treatment
□□	?	?	No	?	?	?	?	?	Symptomatic treatment
□□	0	□□	No	□□□	0	0	□□□	?	Dilution therapy; symptomatic treatment
□□	□□	0	Yes	++	?	?	?	?	See *Cyanide/hydrogen cyanide*
□□, <6 hr	□□	□□	No	++	?	?	?	?	Intensive supportive care, management of arrhythmias and hypotension
(++)	?	(++)	No	(++)	?	?	(+)	?	Symptomatic treatment
□, <2 hr	□	0	No	0	0	0	0	?	Support of respiration, prevention of convulsions, treatment of hyperthermia
+	?	?	No	?	?	?	?	?	Analgesics, treatment of asphyxia and metabolic acidosis
□□, <6 hr	□	0	Yes	?	?	?	?	?	
(+)	?	?	No	?	?	?	?	?	Supportive and symptomatic treatment

TABLE 176-1

Poison Index—cont'd

DRUG OR POISON[*†]	Pharmacokinetics						Toxicity	
	MW (Da)	PPB (%)	V_D (L)	SB	T_{1/2} (hr)	EU	NEPHROTOXICITY	OTHER SYSTEMIC TOXICITY
Tetrachloroethylene[254]	165.9	?	8.1	Lipophilic	6-8 day	>80%	Yes	CNS, GI, and CV symptoms; coagulopathy, hepatotoxicity
Tetrazepam	288.8	30-70%	3.3	Lipophilic	10-20 hr	Little	?	CNS depression
Thallium[255-258]	205.4	?	11	Hydrophilic	10-30 day	3%	?	GI, neurological, and CV symptoms; hair loss, frank alopecia; Mees lines
Theophylline[259-263]	180.2	40%	0.5	Hydrophilic	7-9 hr	10%	?	CNS, GI, and CV symptoms; metabolic and acid-base disturbance
Thiamylal	276.3	>70%	Large	Lipophilic	?	?	?	CNS and respiratory depression, relaxation of skeletal smooth muscle and myocardium
Thiopental	241.3	72-86%	1.4-1.7	Lipophilic	5-17 hr	Little	?	CNS and respiratory depression, relaxation of skeletal smooth muscle and myocardium
Tocainide	192.3	50%	1.5-3.2	?	7-15 hr	40%	?	CNS, CV, and GI toxicity
Tolazamide	311.4	?	?	?	7 hr	85%	?	Hypoglycemia, GI and dermatologic symptoms
Tolbutamide[264]	270.3	96%	?	?	4.5-6.5 hr	?	?	Hypoglycemia, dizziness, asthenia, headache, nausea
Toluene[265]	92.1	?	?	Lipophilic	21 hr	?	?	Eyes, lungs, skin, and GI mucosa effects
Tranylcypromine	133.2	?	?	Hydrophilic	1.9-3.5 hr	2%	Indirect	CNS, CV, and hepatic toxicity
Trazodone[266,267]	371.9	90%	0.8-1.3	?	1 hr	Little	?	Drowsiness, vomiting, priapism, respiratory arrest, seizure
Triazolam	343.2	80-90%	1.0-1.5	Lipophilic	3 hr	2%	?	CNS depression
Trichloroacetic acid[268]	147.4	?	?	Hydrophilic	Longer	?	Yes	See *Chloral hydrate*
Trichloroethylene[269-272]	131.4	High	10	Lipophilic	0.5 hr	Little	?	CNS, cardiac, respiratory, GI, and hepatic toxicity
Troglitazone	441.5	>99%	10.5-26.5	Lipophilic	16-34 hr	<3%	?	Hepatic injury, GI symptoms, asthenia, back pain, dizziness
Trovafloxacin	416.4	76%	Large	?	9.1-12.2 hr	6%	?	Convulsions, decreased activity, diarrhea, sleepiness, tremor
Valproic acid[273-277]	144.2	90%	0.1-0.5	Lipophilic	1 hr	2-3%	Indirect	GI, hepatic, CNS, hematological, and CV toxicity
Vancomycin[278-281]	1449.2	55%	0.5-1	?	5.5 hr	Mostly	Yes	Hypotension, cyanosis, ototoxicity, neurotoxicity, hematological toxicity
Verapamil[282-285]	454.6	90%	4-6	Lipophilic	2-7 hr	Little	?	CV and CNS toxicity
Viloxazine	237.3	80-90%	?	?	3 hr	Little	?	GI and CNS symptoms
Vincristine[286,287]	824.9	75%	Large	?	7 min	15%	?	CNS toxicity
Vinyl chloride[288]	62.5	?	?	Lipophilic	?	?	?	CNS, cardiac, and respiratory toxicity

*Data from Seyffart G: Poison Index: The Treatment of Acute Intoxication. Lengerich, North Rhine–Westphalia, Germany, Pabst Science Publishers, 1997.

†See the companion Expert Consult website for the references for this table.

ARDS, acute respiratory distress syndrome; BAL, British anti-lewisite (dimercaprol); CNS, central nervous system; CV, cardiovascular; DFO, deferoxamine; DIC, disseminated intravascular coagulation; DMSA, dimercaptosuccinic acid; DMPS, 2,3-mercapto-1-propanesulfonic acid; ECG, electrocardiogram; EDTA, ethylenediaminetetra-acetic acid; EU, excreted in urine as the parent drug; FD, forced diuresis; GD, gastrointestinal decontamination; GI, gastrointestinal; HD, hemodialysis; HP_A, hemoperfusion using activated charcoal; HP_R, hemoperfusion using resin (Amberlite XAD-4); IAC, instillation of activated charcoal; MW, molecular weight; NSAIDs, nonsteroidal anti-inflammatory drugs; PD, peritoneal dialysis; PE, plasma exchange; PPB, plasma protein binding; SA, special antidote; SB, solubility; SLE, systemic lupus erythematosus; T_{1/2}, plasma half-life; V_D, apparent volume of distribution (L/kg). **0**, not recommended, or removal negligible for various reasons; □, □□, □□□, good and effective removal, method indicated; +, ++, +++, removal appreciable but clinical effect minimal, not uniform or controversial; (+), (++), (+++), no experience, but appreciable removal can theoretically be expected; ?, no published experience.

Urine Alkalinization

Urine alkalinization is a treatment regimen that increases poison elimination by the administration of intravenous sodium bicarbonate to produce urine with a pH of 7.5. Forced alkaline diuresis (alkaline diuresis) was introduced into clinical practice at a time when toxicokinetic principles were unknown or in their infancy. Because the ionized poison is not reabsorbed from the renal tubular lumen back into the blood and because the ionization of a weak acid is increased in an alkaline environment, manipulation of the urine pH potentially can enhance renal excretion. Because the dissociation constant (pK_a) is a logarithmic function, then, theoretically, a small change in urine pH could have a disproportionately larger effect on clearance. Each change in urine pH of one unit theoretically is accompanied by a 10-fold change in renal clearance, whereas at best, the renal clearance of a reabsorbed drug varies directly

					Enhancement of Removal					
GD	IAC	FD	SA	HD	HP_A	HP_R	PD	PE		SUPPORTIVE TREATMENT
□	?	0	No	0	?	?	0	?		Carbon dioxide–induced hyperventilation, avoid catecholamines
□□, <3 hr	□	0	Yes	?	?	?	?	?		
□	□	□	Yes	□□□	□□	□□	0	□		Chelator: Prussian blue
□	□□	0	No	++	□□	□□	0	□		Monitoring of vital functions, symptomatic treatment
□□, <8 hr	□	0	No	(++)	(++)	(++)	0	?		Stabilization of circulatory and respiratory function, good nursing
□□, <8 hr	□	0	No	(++)	(++)	(++)	0	?		Stabilization of circulatory and respiratory function, good nursing
□□	□□	□□	No	(+)	?	?	?	?		See *Lidocaine*
(++)	?	(++)	No	(++)	?	?	(+)	?		Symptomatic treatment, close monitoring of blood glucose
(++)	□□	?	No	(++)	?	?	(++)	?		Symptomatic treatment, close monitoring of blood glucose
□	?	□	No	□	?	?	?	?		Removal from the area of exposure, irrigate eyes, avoid catecholamines
□□	□□	0	?	++	?	?	?	?		Close monitoring for at least 27 hours; symptomatic treatment
?	?	?	No	?	?	?	?	?		Symptomatic and supportive treatment
□□, <3 hr	□	0	Yes	?	?	?	?	?		
+	?	□	No	□□□	?	?	?	?		Analgesics, treatment of asphyxia and metabolic acidosis
++, <2 hr	0	0	No	0	0	0	0	?		Artificial ventilation, avoid catecholamines
(++)	?	0	No	(++)	?	?	(++)	?		Symptomatic treatment, close monitoring of blood glucose
(++)	?	0	No	(++)	?	?	(+)	?		Symptomatic treatment
□	□	0	No	□□□	□□	□□	?	?		Symptomatic treatment
□	□	0	No	□	□	(+)	0	□		
□□, <3 hr	□	+	?	0	□	0	?	□		Antidotes: calcium, 4-aminopyridine, glucagon?; supportive and symptomatic treatment
□□□	□□□	0	?	0	+	+	0	?		See *Amitriptyline*
?	?	0	No	?	?	?	?	□		Monitoring of vital functions, symptomatic treatment
+	?	□	No	?	?	?	?	?		Removal from the area of exposure, irrigate eyes, avoid catecholamines

with the urine flow rate. Clinical evidence demonstrating that forced alkaline diuresis is superior to urine alkalinization alone is lacking, however. The effectiveness of urine alkalinization depends on the relative contribution of renal clearance to the total body clearance of active drug. Urine alkalinization increases the urinary elimination of chlorpropamide, 2,4-dichlorophenoxyacetic acid, diflunisal, fluoride, mecoprop, methotrexate, phenobarbital, and salicylate. Urine alkalinization should be considered a first-line treatment in patients with moderately severe salicylate poisoning who do not meet the criteria for hemodialysis.

The AACT-EAPCTC–endorsed *position paper* adopts the term *urine alkalization* to emphasize that urine pH manipulation, rather than a diuresis, is the prime objective of treatment. It recommends that the terms "forced alkaline diuresis" and "alkaline diuresis" be abandoned.[12]

Enhancement of Elimination by Extracorporeal Methods

Schreiner in 1958 provided the basis for the use of such an approach and laid down the criteria for the use of hemodialysis in the treatment of poisonings.[28] Subsequently, new methods of enhancing removal have become available, and the indications for the use of such treatments have been summarized in the literature.[29,30]

Today, extracorporeal methods have a key position in the enhancement of removal of a variety of poisons and drugs, and all rely on the use of either diffusion, convection, or adsorption to enhance removal from the blood. Although such methods are widely applied, randomized controlled trials relating to their efficacy and to resulting modulation of mortality and morbidity are lacking. Furthermore, their use frequently superimposes additional complications and difficulties on those invoked by the poison, such as vascular instability arising from fluid removal and the need to maintain adequate levels of anticoagulation, as well as to provide access to the patient's circulation.

Hemodialysis

Hemodialysis relies on the use of diffusion to remove the compound from the bloodstream. For hemodialysis to be effective, a poison must be of low molecular weight (less than 500 Daltons), be relatively water soluble, and have a relatively low plasma protein binding fraction, a small distribution volume (less than 1 L/kg of body weight), a long half-life, and low endogenous clearance (less than 4 mL/kg per minute). Hemodialysis has the additional benefit of correcting concomitant electrolyte or acid-base disturbance in anuric patients. The use of this modality may be considered in life-threatening toxicity from lithium, salicylates, theophylline, methanol, boric acid, and ethylene glycol and also for heavy metal chelation in patients with renal failure. Efficiency of removal is governed not only by physicochemical characteristics but also by procedural factors such as the blood flow rate, dialysate flow rate, dialyzer surface area, and pore structure of the chosen membrane.

Treatment is not time-limited, because the permeability of the membrane is not usually affected and the dialysis solution is prepared continuously. Sustained or extended dialysis also may be used; although such an approach is less efficient, it offers advantages in terms of maintaining the patient's vascular stability.

Hemoperfusion

Hemoperfusion is an extracorporeal treatment in which blood comes into direct contact with an adsorbent material such as activated carbon or anion exchange resin. This contact results in adsoption and removal of compounds from the blood stream. With early devices, this procedure carried the risk of thrombocytopenia, hypocalcemia, hypoglycemia, hypothermia, access complications, charcoal embolization, and cartridge saturation[31,32]; these problems have been overcome by coating the particles with a polymer solution, without loss of adsorptive capacity.[33] Historically, charcoal was used, but today nonionic (i.e., electrostatically neutral) resins such as Amberlite XAD-2 or XAD-4 also are available.[30] Resin-based hemoperfusion is effective for removal of lipid-soluble drugs. Water- and lipid-soluble substances with molecular weights ranging from 113 to 40,000 Daltons are well adsorbed. Efficiency for higher-molecular-weight adsorption drops when hemocompatible coatings, such as cellulose or albumin, are used.[30] Hemoperfusion has been effectively used to enhance elimination of theophylline, phenobarbital, phenytoin, carbamazepine, paraquat, and glutethimide.[30,34]

Hemofiltration

Hemofiltration is a method whereby the removal of a compound occurs primarily by convective solute transport, rather than diffusion. It is performed using highly permeable membranes, with replenishment of the fluid or plasma water removed during treatment. Hemofiltration is potentially useful for removal of substances with a low plasma protein binding fraction, a small volume of distribution (less than 1 L/kg), or a fast rate of equilibrium from peripheral tissue to bloodstream,[29] as well as for the removal of high-molecular-weight solutes or complexes, such as combined digoxin–Fab fragment complexes or deferoxamine complexes with iron or with aluminum.[34] It also may be of benefit in iron and lithium overdose.[35]

Clinical application of this modality to date has been confined to case reports, rather than being studied in randomized controlled trials.[36-38]

Peritoneal Dialysis

Peritoneal dialysis allows the diffusion of poison or its metabolite from the mesenteric capillaries across the peritoneal membrane into the dialysis solution within the peritoneal cavity. It has only a limited role in poison removal and should not be used if facilities for hemodialysis are available.[39]

Plasmapheresis

Plasmapheresis involves removal of the patient's plasma with substitution by crystalloid solution or fresh frozen plasma. Plasmapheresis is the best option available to remove drugs or poisons that are highly protein bound and therefore will not be effectively removed by hemodialysis or hemofiltration.[40-44] Its rationale for use must be confirmed in each type of intoxication by evidence of effective clearance.[42,45]

Continuous Renal Replacement Therapies

Continuous venovenous hemofiltration (CVVH), continuous venovenous hemodialysis (CVVHD), and continuous arteriovenous hemodialysis (CAVHD) all are forms of *continuous renal replacement therapy* (CRRT). In general, because of slower flow rates, clearance rates for dialyzable substances are lower with CRRT than with conventional hemodialysis. The application of continuous therapies is indicated in the treatment of poisonings in which removal of the offending compound from the plasma is associated with a redistribution from tissues, such as lithium, valproic acid, or theophylline. Both CAVHDF and CVVHDF provide gradual but good clearance of lithium after overdose without an apparent post-treatment rebound, as has been described in cases treated by hemodialysis.[46]

Combination Therapies

Combination therapies combine one or more of the aforementioned extracorporeal techniques. The first such approach was described by de Broe and coworkers, who combined hemoperfusion with hemodialysis.[47] It combines diffusion and absorption, thereby increasing the overall clearance of the compound, and is particularly useful in the treatment of poisonings by compounds with a small volume of distribution.[48-50]

A recent variant of combination therapy is the Molecular Adsorbents Recirculating System (MARS), which has the potential to remove substantial quantities of albumin-bound toxin.[51,52] Several animal and clinical studies have shown that MARS can remove both albumin and other protein-bound drugs such as phenytoin,[53] midazolam, and fentanyl.[54] However, its use can be associated with complications.[55]

GENERAL SUPPORTIVE TREATMENT

The aim of supportive treatment is to preserve vital organ functions until detoxification is accomplished and the patient regains normal physiological homeostasis, using the specific measures outlined next.

Respiratory Complications

Respiratory depression, hypoventilation, hypoxia, and pulmonary edema are common, because drugs that induce depressed consciousness also impair respiration. Supportive measures should be directed at maintaining a patent airway and providing respiratory support, with immediate access to suction equipment, oxygen, or mechanical ventilation if it is necessary. Agitation may require sedation.

Cardiovascular Complications

Patients may present with hypotension, hypertension, myocardial depression, systemic vasodilation, bradyarrhythmias, or tachyarrhythmias, depending on the toxin involved, and electrocardiographic monitoring is advisable. Treatment should be individualized, but an initial strategy of rapid infusion of normal saline solution is indicated in most instances. Management of refractory hypotension may require the use of vasopressors.

Neurological Complications

The ingestion of toxins may induce depression of consciousness, seizures, cerebral edema, and peripheral nerve injuries. If the toxicity is associated with acid-base and electrolyte disturbances, treatment requires correction of these abnormalities. A reduction in intracranial pressure, hyperventilation, elevation of the head, and fluid restriction also may be required. Seizures may occur as a result of metabolic disturbances or cerebral hypoxia or from a direct toxic effect. To minimize neural damage, correction of metabolic defects and termination of the seizures should be rapid. Seizures that do not respond to first-line benzodiazepines (lorazepam or diazepam) or to second-line antiepileptic drugs (phenytoin or fosphenytoin, phenobarbital, or valproate) usually are considered refractory, requiring more aggressive treatment. The optimal treatment has not been defined, but patients should be managed in an ICU because artificial ventilation and hemodynamic support are required. Invasive hemodynamic monitoring is often necessary, and electroencephalographic monitoring is essential. Once seizures have been controlled for 12 to 24 hours, continuous intravenous therapy should be gradually tapered off if the drug being administered is midazolam or propofol. Gradual tapering probably is not necessary with pentobarbital or thiopental sodium. Continuous electroencephalographic monitoring is required during high-dose treatment and while therapy is being gradually withdrawn. During withdrawal of anesthetic therapy, intravenous phenytoin or fosphenytoin or valproate should be continued to ensure an adequate baseline of antiepileptic medication, to prevent the recurrence of status epilepticus. If additional medication is needed, the most appropriate antiepileptic drugs are gabapentin for focal seizures and levetiracetam and topiramate for all seizure types, because these drugs can be started at high doses with a low risk of idiosyncratic reactions. Even with current best practice, the mortality rate among patients who experience seizures is approximately 50%, and only a minority return to their premorbid functional baseline.[56]

Hypoglycemia

Significant hypoglycemia should be treated initially with an intravenous bolus of 50 mL of 50% dextrose in water.[57] In treating hypoglycemia induced by sulfonylurea or meglitinide after initial euglycemia is achieved, it should be followed by the administration of oral carbohydrates. Continued hypoglycemia may be treated using octreotide (initial dose of 50 µg, repeated two to three times per day), which decreases intravenous dextrose requirements, thereby minimizing the risk of glucose-stimulated insulin release.[1,58]

Hypothermia and Hyperthermia

Central nervous system impairment may cause hypothermia (body temperature below 35° C) or hyperthermia (higher than 39° C). Appropriate management for hypothermia includes passive rewarming, intravenous fluid warming, and warm water humidification in artificial ventilation. Hyperthermia may be treated with cool intravenous fluids and active cooling measures. For patients in whom hyperthermia is secondary to excessive sympathetic stimulation, such as that associated with cocaine and amphetamines, treatment may include intravenous benzodiazepines. Patients with resistant hyperthermia may benefit from peripherally acting muscle relaxants (dantrolene), centrally acting serotonin antagonists (cyproheptadine), or general sedation.[1]

Metabolic Complications

Indices of hepatic and renal function, electrolytes, blood glucose, and arterial blood gas and urine samples should be checked routinely. Renal failure may be due to tubular necrosis arising from hypotension hypoxia or a direct effect of poison on tubular cells. Hemoglobinuria or myoglobinuria may further precipitate renal failure. The patient should be catheterized, and urine output should be maintained at 0.5 mL/kg per hour. Metabolic acidosis is frequently encountered, and sodium bicarbonate may be needed if pH falls below 7.1.

CONCLUSION

Enhancement of removal of the ingested toxin, supplemented by general supportive management, remains the cornerstone of management of poisoning. According to the limited evidence-based data available, many of the traditional management interventions do not improve clinical outcome and may subject the patient to a certain degree of risk. In consequence, whether it is better to use a treatment that may be of some benefit but also may be associated with risk, or not to use a treatment that carries any risk unless it has a proven benefit, remains unresolved and controversial.

Key Points

1. Enhancement of removal of the ingested toxin, supplemented by general supportive measures, constitutes the cornerstone of management of poisoning.
2. Randomized controlled trials comparing methods of removal are lacking. The position statements prepared by the American Academy of Clinical Toxicology and the European Association of Poison Centres and Clinical Toxicologists may be considered to constitute an evidence base for the use of conventional treatments in the management of poisonings.
3. Methods commonly used in an outpatient setting, such as gastrointestinal decontamination, have little or no impact on patient outcome and should be abandoned.
4. The use of extracorporeal circulatory procedures is well established in the treatment of poisoning, allowing fast elimination of the intoxicating agent and effective restoration of homeostasis.
5. Reflecting the necessarily urgent nature of the clinical response to poisoning, treatment often is based on clinical experience; well-designed, evidence-based studies are needed.

Key References

1. Greene SL, Dargan PI, Jones AL: Acute poisoning: Understanding 90% of cases in a nutshell. Postgrad Med J 2005; 81:204-216.
2. Guzelian PS, Victoroff MS, Halmes NC, et al: Evidence-based toxicology: A comprehensive framework for causation. Hum Exp Toxicol 2005;24:161-201.
10. Beal SL, Sheiner LB: Estimating population kinetics. Crit Rev Biomed Eng 1982;8:195-222.
19. Mokhlesi B, Leiken JB, Murray P, Corbridge TC: Adult toxicology in critical care: Part I: General approach to the intoxicated patient. Chest 2003;123:577-592.
31. Borkan SC: Extracorporeal therapies for acute intoxications. Crit Care Clin 2002;18:393-420, vii.

See the companion Expert Consult website for the complete reference list.

Part II

Organ Interaction

The Heart and the Kidney

CHAPTER 177

Hypertensive Emergencies

Frank M. van der Sande, A. A. Kroon, Jeroen P. Kooman, and Karel M. Leunissen

---

OBJECTIVES

This chapter will:
1. Describe the epidemiology, pathogenesis, diagnosis, and clinical course of hypertensive emergencies.
2. Review the general principles of management of hypertensive emergencies.
3. Summarize the management of patients with a hypertensive emergency and renal failure and discuss treatment under other specific conditions.

Hypertension is an exceedingly common disorder in Western societies. In particular, hypertensive emergencies and hypertensive urgencies are commonly encountered in hospitals.[1,2] Hypertensive emergencies were defined by the 7th Joint National Committee (JNC) on Detection, Evaluation and Treatment of High Blood Pressure as those conditions in which a severe increase in blood pressure coincided with acute or ongoing end-organ damage (of note, in this definition, no absolute blood pressure level is needed for the diagnosis).[3] A number of different terms have been applied to acute and severe elevations in blood pressure. *Hypertensive crisis* or *emergency* is defined as a sudden increase in systolic and diastolic blood pressures associated with acute end-organ damage, such as to the cardiovascular, renal, or central nervous system, and requires immediate management. Hypertensive emergencies may arise as a result of malignant or accelerated hypertension, hypertensive encephalopathy, eclampsia, or an adrenergic crisis associated with pheochromocytoma. It has been shown that the subdivision between malignant and accelerated hypertension on the basis of the severity of retinal encephalopathy is not useful anymore because the prognoses for grade III and that for grade IV retinopathy are identical.[4] Conditions in which an increase in blood pressure leads to an aggravation of an underlying disorder, such as cerebrovascular accident (stroke), cardiac failure, myocardial infarction, or dissecting aortic aneurysm, are considered to be hypertensive emergencies.

A severe elevation of blood pressure without signs of acute end-organ damage constitutes a *hypertensive urgency*.[5,6] A point worthy of emphasis is that the clinical distinction between hypertensive emergency or crisis and hypertensive urgency depends on the presence of acute target organ damage, rather than the absolute level of blood pressure.

The term "malignant hypertension" has been used to describe a syndrome characterized by elevated blood pressure accompanied by encephalopathy or acute nephropathy[7,8]; however, this term has been removed from national and international blood pressure control guidelines.[3,7] Because it consists of both hypertensive emergency and hypertensive urgency, the condition is best referred to as a *hypertensive crisis*. This term is therefore used instead of "malignant hypertension" throughout the chapter.

Hypertensive crisis and urgency are quite common. Approximately 1% of all patients with hypertension will experience a hypertensive crisis at some point during their lives.[9] In a recent report, the contribution of hypertensive crisis and urgencies in relation to all emergencies was 6.4% and 20.8%, respectively.[10] A majority of the patients in the reported series, however, suffered from acute myocardial infarction and pulmonary edema.

The prevalence of hypertensive crisis is declining. In a more recent study in the United States, severe hypertension (systolic blood pressure higher than 220 mm Hg and diastolic blood pressure higher than 120 mm Hg) was the reason for referral in 4.9% of patients referred to a hospital.[11] In a study from Brazil, university-affiliated hospital hypertensive crisis accounted for 0.5% of all clinical emergency cases studied and for 1.7% of all clinical emergencies, hypertensive urgency being more common than hypertensive emergency.[12]

This chapter gives special attention to the etiology, pathophysiology, and treatment of hypertensive crisis in relation to acute renal failure. Hypertensive encephalopathy and hypertension in acute renal failure without signs of hypertensive crisis also are discussed. The treatment of adrenergic crises and hypertension in combination with cerebrovascular accident and postresuscitation hypertension also is reviewed, whereas the treatment of hypertension in combination with myocardial infarction, cardiac failure, or a dissecting aortic aneurysm, which generally is in the hands of the cardiologist, is covered only briefly in the following pages. Eclampsia is covered in another chapter.

ACCELERATED HYPERTENSION OR HYPERTENSIVE CRISIS

Hypertensive crisis is defined as a condition manifesting with severe hypertension, grade IV retinopathy with papilledema, and, often, impaired renal function.[13] In the past, *accelerated hypertension* was distinguished from hypertensive crisis by the presence of retinal hemorrhages and soft exudates without papilledema.[14] It is questionable, however, whether this distinction is of clinical importance, because in more recent series, no difference in outcome was seen between patients with grade III and those with grade IV retinopathy.[15,16] In the study by Ahmed and colleagues, some difference in survival was seen between patients with grade IIIa (incomplete retinal features) and grade IV (papilledema) retinopathy.[15] Furthermore, the diagnosis of early-stage papilledema is difficult and prone to interobserver variability,[16] and the pathogenesis and treatment of accelerated hypertension and of hypertensive crisis do not differ.[6] Therefore, in the following discussion, no distinction is made between accelerated hypertension and hypertensive crisis.

Although most patients have a diastolic blood pressure above 120 to 130 mm Hg, no absolute blood pressure level distinguishes hypertensive crisis from benign hypertension. By contrast, blood pressure values can even be higher in some patients with uncomplicated essential hypertension than in patients in hypertensive crisis.[17] The absolute level of blood pressure may not be as important as the *rate* of increase.

Incidence, Etiology, and Prognosis for Hypertensive Crisis

The true incidence of hypertensive crisis is not well known. In earlier studies, the incidence of hypertensive crisis in the hypertensive population ranged between 1% and 7%.[17-19] In a recent study, the incidence was found to be 1 to 3 cases per 100,000 per year in the general population.[20]

Several investigators have noted a declining incidence of hypertensive crisis,[21,22] probably owing to improvements in detection and therapy of patients with essential hypertension. This impression was not corroborated in a recent single study by Lip and coworkers, in which no decline in the incidence of hypertensive crisis was found—an observation that the investigators hypothesized to be due partly to racial factors.[23]

Indeed, for poorly understood reasons, the incidence of hypertensive crisis is higher in blacks than in whites.[24] Perhaps the relative resistance of black patients to some classes of antihypertensive therapy plays a role in this aspect.[25] Patients with hypertensive crisis are more commonly male, as is also the case in essential hypertension. By contrast, the peak incidence of hypertensive emergencies is at age 40 to 50 years and differs from the incidence of uncomplicated essential hypertension, which increases with age.[13] Smokers appear to have a higher risk for the development of hypertensive crisis.[26]

The factors that lead to severe and rapid elevation of blood pressure in patients with hypertensive crisis are poorly understood. Many patients who experience hypertensive emergencies had preexisting essential hypertension.[20,23,27] In this respect, temporary discontinuation of prescribed antihypertensive drugs is a frequent cause of a

TABLE 177-1

Causes of Hypertensive Crisis

Essential hypertension
Renal parenchymal disease
   Acute glomerulonephritis
   Vasculitis
   Hemolytic uremic syndrome
   Thrombotic thrombocytopenic purpura
Renovascular hypertension
   Renal artery stenosis
Pregnancy
   (Pre)eclampsia
Endocrine diseases
   Pheochromocytoma
   Cushing's disease
   Renin-producing tumor
   Mineralocorticoid-induced hypertension
Systemic diseases and vasculitis
   Scleroderma
Medication and intoxication
   Cocaine, amphetamine, erythropoietin, cyclosporine, sympathomimetics, tricyclic antidepressants
   Withdrawal of central-acting medication (e.g., clonidine)
   Interaction with monoamine oxidase blockers (e.g., tyramine)
   Lead intoxication
Autonomic hyperreactivity
   Guillain-Barré syndrome
   Acute intermittent porphyria
Cerebral diseases
   Trauma capitis
   Cerebral stroke or hemorrhage
   Brain tumors

hypertensive crisis.[28] In some series, however, the incidence of underlying renal disease was found to be even higher than 50%, as discussed in detail later on. Other causes of hypertensive crisis, such as pheochromocytoma,[23,29] oral contraceptives[30,31] and several other drugs,[13] primary hyperaldosteronism,[32] renal carcinoma,[33] and cholesterol embolism,[34] are less common. With the appearance of the drug called "ecstasy," a new cause of hypertensive crisis has been introduced.[35] Table 177-1 presents an overview of causes of hypertensive crisis.

In earlier days, the prognosis for patients in hypertensive crisis was grim: Almost all patients died within 5 years, with less than a 20% 1-year survival rate.[11] Most of these patients died from complications of uremia.[14,17] The introduction of antihypertensive agents and dialysis has greatly improved prognosis: Nowadays, the 5-year survival rate is approximately 75%.[21,36] Renal function at presentation still appears to be an important prognostic factor, however.[21,36,37] Also, differences in underlying factors may be related to survival: Kawazoe and associates observed a better long-term prognosis in patients with underlying renal disease than in those with essential hypertension,[38] although this observation is not consistent with earlier findings.[36]

Renal Disease in the Etiology of Hypertensive Crisis

The prevalence of preexisting renal disease in patients presenting with hypertensive crisis ranges from 40%[23] to as high as 80%[22] in several surveys. The incidence of underlying renal disease appears to be lower in the black population.[39] Renal parenchymal disease accounts for up to 80% of all secondary causes, with chronic pyelonephritis and glomerulonephritis, and especially immunoglobulin A (IgA) nephropathy, as the most common causes of hypertensive crisis in patients with underlying renal disease.[22,40]

Patients with renal vasculitis and lupus glomerulonephritis can present with hypertensive crisis, whereas the presence of lupus anticoagulant alone without systemic features also is associated with hypertensive crisis.[41] An interesting observation is that in scleroderma, renal crisis, which is characterized by highly elevated renin levels, the renal abnormalities precede the development of hypertensive crisis.[42,43] Although a less frequent cause of hypertensive crisis compared with chronic glomerulonephritis, a significant percentage of patients with renal disease presenting with hypertensive crisis also have tubulointerstitial disease.[44] The incidence of renovascular disease as a cause of hypertensive crisis ranges between 3% and 43% in various series.[23,39]

Pathophysiology of Hypertensive Crisis

Although the pathogenesis of hypertensive crisis is still not fully understood, a critical level of blood pressure elevation is mandatory in its development, so the role of mechanical stress on the vessel wall appears to be critical in its pathogenesis. The blood pressure level probably is not the only explanatory factor because, as mentioned earlier, the increased blood pressure levels in patients in hypertensive crisis can vary widely.[45] The chance for the development of a hypertensive crisis is higher at high levels of blood pressure (systolic blood pressure greater than 220 mm Hg; diastolic blood pressure greater than 120 to 130 mm Hg); however, acute elevations of blood pressure, as can be found in acute glomerulonephritis or preeclampsia, may induce a crisis at relatively low blood pressure levels.[46] The release of humoral vasoconstrictor substances from the stressed vessel wall certainly plays a role, because elevated levels of renin, angiotensin II, and aldosterone usually are found in patients with hypertensive crisis.[6,47] Also, increased levels of vasopressin have been observed.[48] Furthermore, enhanced sympathetic activity, assessed by microneurography, was reported in patients in hypertensive crisis,[49] possibly related to the activated renin-angiotensin system.

The precise role of the increased vasoactive hormones is not entirely clear. In any case, an initial, rapid increase in vascular resistance due to elevated blood pressure must be one of the first predisposing factors, resulting in an imbalance between vasodilating (nitric oxide [NO] and prostacyclin, i.e., prostaglandin I_2 [PGI_2]) and vasoconstrictive substances (endothelin-1 [ET-1] and thromboxane A_2 [TXA_2]).[50] In experimental animals, infusion of vasoactive hormones was followed by the development of hypertensive crisis.[51] Locally acting factors, such as cytokines, NO, endothelin, and platelet-derived growth factor, may be implicated in the pathogenesis of hypertensive crisis. In a recent report, extremely high plasma ET-1 levels were found in patients in hypertensive crisis.[52] Whether endothelin plays a pathogenetic role or is just a marker of vascular damage[53] needs to be addressed in future studies. In this respect, worthy of note is the observation that hypertensive subjects with the DD-genotype of the I/D polymorphism, who have higher levels of the angiotensin-converting enzyme (ACE), have a threefold higher risk for the development of a hypertensive crisis compared with other hypertensive subjects without this genotype.[54] Increased levels of vasoactive substances will not be the only pathogenetic factor, however, because hypertensive crisis also occurs in patients with normal or reduced levels of renin.[27,38] Most probably, a vicious circle is triggered in which the increased blood pressure in combination with hormonal changes leads to vascular damage, tissue ischemia, or a further increase in the levels of vasoconstrictor substances. Kincaid-Smith proposed that an increased level of vasoactive hormones together with increased vascular reactivity leads to pressure natriuresis and hypovolemia, which in turn triggers a further activation of vasoactive hormones, (such as angiotensin II) and an increase in sympathetic nervous system activity.[55]

Increased blood pressure and endothelial dysfunction lead to alternating constriction and dilatation ("sausage string") of arterioles, creating intravascular turbulence, followed by platelet activation and ongoing endothelial damage, in microangiopathic hemolytic anemia and intravascular coagulation. In addition, mitogenic factors (such as angiotensin II) may lead to myointimal proliferation. This change, in combination with thrombus formation, will lead to narrowing of the vascular lumen, followed by end-organ ischemia. In the kidney, narrowing of the lumen will again trigger the activation of vasoconstrictor substances, thereby completing the vicious circle. Several experimental and clinical findings are in agreement with this hypothesis.[50,53,56] In the late stage of a hypertensive crisis, disintegration of the endothelin may occur, with vasodilation and increase in the permeability of the endothelin. Such changes result in hyperperfusion of the end organs, arteriolar fibrinoid necrosis, and perivascular edema.

Clinical Findings in Hypertensive Crisis

The clinical manifestations of hypertensive crisis are those associated with end-organ dysfunction, and vary from patient to patient (Table 177-2). Patients with hypertensive crisis present most often (in greater than 75% of cases) with headache, which often is located in the occipital region and may have been present for several months, depending on preexisting blood pressure.[13,45]

Visual disturbances, due to retinopathy, commonly are present (in more than 60% of cases).[6,13,45] Funduscopic changes constitute the hallmark of malignant hypertension. In Grade III retinopathy, retinal hemorrhages or soft exudates are present. Soft exudates result from ischemic infarction of nerve fibers, whereas hard exudates result from exudation of plasma components. Flame-shaped

TABLE 177-2

Clinical Findings in Hypertensive Crisis

- Diastolic blood pressure greater than 130 mm Hg (sometimes a crisis can occur at lower pressure, especially in cases of sudden increase in blood pressure, such as in acute glomerulonephritis and preeclampsia).
- Confusion, sometimes insult or transient pareses; consciousness and coma
- Retinopathy grade III or IV (exudates, hemorrhage, papilledema)
- Cardiomegaly, sometimes signs of cardiac decompensation
- Gastrointestinal signs and symptoms: nausea, vomiting
- Reduced glomerular filtration

hemorrhages are caused by loss of endothelial integrity.[45,57] Grade IV retinopathy is characterized by papilledema, which is caused by intracranial hypertension but is not necessarily related to cerebrospinal fluid pressure.[17] With adequate treatment, the ophthalmologic findings resolve within 2 to 12 weeks.[45] In patients with hypertensive crisis, more severe neurological signs and symptoms also can occur, such as focal cerebral ischemia or cerebral hemorrhage.[58] They have to be distinguished from the syndrome of hypertensive encephalopathy, discussed later on.

In other patients, the cardiovascular manifestations of hypertensive crisis may predominate, with angina, acute myocardial infarction, or acute left ventricular failure.[10,49] Less specific symptoms, such as malaise, nausea, and weight loss, the last probably due to pressure natriuresis, commonly are observed. Rarely, the vascular lesions may lead to acute pancreatitis and bowel ischemia.[48,59] A small proportion of patients may remain asymptomatic.[23] In a Nigerian study, more than 75% of patients with hypertensive crisis presented without clinical signs or symptoms, although this finding does not appear to be representative for the white population.[60] The renal signs and symptoms of hypertensive crisis are covered later on.

Laboratory findings in patients with hypertensive crisis often include an elevated erythrocyte sedimentation rate.[17] Coombs-negative hemolytic anemia with fragmented red cells and a low platelet count may be present, especially in patients with renal failure.[61] The fragmented red cells may lead to difficulties in the differential diagnosis with thrombotic thrombocytopenic purpura and the hemolytic uremic syndrome.[61,62]

As a result of increased activity of the renin-angiotensin-aldosterone system, hypokalemic metabolic alkalosis may ensue.[45] Changes on the electrocardiogram (ECG) typical of left ventricular hypertrophy will be seen in a majority of patients; however, the ECG tracing may be normal.[23]

Renal Failure Due to Hypertensive Crisis

Hypertensive crisis very often manifests with elevated serum creatinine levels, which may progress to overt acute renal failure, although some patients may present with normal creatinine levels.[17] Microscopic hematuria with granular casts and proteinuria, with a protein level that may exceed 2 g/L, commonly is seen, although the range of the latter may vary widely.[6,19,63] In a recent report, 63% of patients presenting with hypertensive crisis had significant proteinuria and 21% had hematuria, these abnormalities being more pronounced in patients with higher serum creatinine levels.[23] Rarely, red cell casts are seen.[6] Most patients present with increased creatinine levels, although renal function may be normal at presentation.[17] Four different types of renal impairment have been described[64]: (1) progressive subacute deterioration of kidney function over several weeks, especially in patients with initial mild impairment of kidney function that has been inadequately treated; (2) transient deterioration of renal function after initiation of antihypertensive treatment, which is due to a decrease in renal perfusion; (3) established renal failure, in which, as discussed later on, the differential diagnosis between primary renal disease and renal failure due to hypertensive crisis is clinically difficult; and (4) acute oliguric renal failure with active urinary sediment, an entity that is less commonly observed. Impairment of renal function has prognostic implications: In earlier days, uremia was the most common cause of death in this population.[14,17] Initial serum creatinine level is still related to survival,[65] possibly through its association with end-organ damage. Hemodialysis and adequate antihypertensive therapy, however, have greatly improved the outlook for survival, turning death from uremia into a very rare event. Although the prognosis for renal function has greatly improved since the availability of adequate antihypertensive therapy, it is still poor for patients with preexisting renal failure.[63,66] In the overall group, the 1-year survival rate is approximately 30%; the 5-year renal survival rate lies between 37% and 65%.[36,44,66]

Although renal function often deteriorates after initial antihypertensive therapy, renal function may recover after blood pressure control,[64] whereas partial recovery may occur even after several months.[67-69] Once the patient presents with renal insufficiency as one of the initial manifestations of a hypertensive crisis, however, complete recovery of renal function is unlikely.[70] Of interest, the efficacy of antihypertensive treatment is not influenced by the degree of underlying renal insufficiency.[71] Recently, it was stated that the combined renal length (length of both kidneys) may be a marker for recovery.[72,73] In one study, all patients with a combined renal length less than 18 cm remained dependent on dialysis.[73]

Histological Findings in Renal Failure Due to Hypertensive Crisis

The role of renal biopsy in patients with renal failure and hypertensive crisis is controversial.[64] Renal biopsy in patients with small kidneys seen on echography usually will not alter treatment and is therefore not indicated. In patients with normal kidneys and significant proteinuria and hematuria, a renal biopsy is desirable to exclude glomerulonephritis and vasculitis. Because lupus nephritis and vasculitis may be underlying causes of hypertensive crisis, serological studies (e.g., atrial natriuretic factor [ANF], anti–double-stranded DNA [anti-dsDNA], cytoplasmic anti–neutrophil cytoplasmic antibody [c-ANCA]) may be performed if the diagnosis is suspected on clinical grounds. Inadequately controlled hypertension and significant coagulation abnormalities constitute relative contraindications to renal biopsy.

Characteristic findings on renal biopsy in patients with hypertensive crisis are fibrinoid necrosis and proliferative endarteritis. The latter probably is due to long-standing pressure overload. It manifests as intimal thickening, with cellular proliferation and concentric deposition of extracellular matrix, with a characteristic "onion skin" appearance in the interlobular arteries.[6,13,45,53] Proliferative endarteritis also may be seen in sustained essential hypertension[74] and is not rapidly reversible with treatment.[75]

Although fibrinoid necrosis is a characteristic finding in hypertensive crisis and was long assumed to be diagnostic, this lesion also can be observed in patients with other disorders, such as scleroderma renal crisis, hemolytic uremic syndrome, and postpartum renal failure.[62,76,77] Fibrinoid necrosis is characterized by deposition of eosinophilic material consisting of fibrin, extracellular debris, and necrotic muscle cells in the arteriolar wall. It probably results from leakage of fibrin and other plasma components through the damaged endothelium. Fibrinoid necrosis is present in the afferent arterioles and may extend into the glomerular capillaries. Because its distribution may be patchy, it may be missed on renal biopsy.[17] In contrast with proliferative endarteritis, effective treatment leads to rapid disappearance of fibrinoid necrosis.[78]

Another histological finding may be acute tubular necrosis, especially in patients presenting with acute renal failure.[69] Even after renal biopsy, the differential diagnosis with hemolytic uremic syndrome and thrombotic thrombocytopenic purpura can still be difficult.[77] In the latter two entities, renal biopsy also often is not possible, owing to the severe coagulation abnormalities, and the diagnosis must rely on clinical parameters.

The relation between renal impairment and histological findings is still unclear. It has been hypothesized that fibrinoid necrosis is largely responsible for renal impairment in patents with hypertensive crisis, and the improvement of renal function after successful treatment is due to its resolution.[13] This opinion is challenged by some authorities, who state that renal impairment is due to irreversible renal ischemia and that the improvement of renal function after successful treatment of hypertensive crisis results from hypertrophy of the remaining nephrons.[79] Recently, it was hypothesized that reversal of acute renal failure may be due to a decrease in the intense renal vasoconstriction after successful treatment of hypertensive crisis.[80]

Further Diagnostic Approach

After the patient has been stabilized and normal blood pressure values have been obtained, the next step is to search for the underlying cause of the hypertensive crisis. It is especially important to look for a renal artery stenosis, because this is a potentially treatable cause of hypertension.[81] Radionuclide tests are not always reliable in this respect,[82] so angiography is the diagnostic test of choice,[83] although special attention must be given to the patient with increased serum creatinine levels, because contrast nephropathy can exacerbate renal failure. Magnetic resonance imaging (MRI) may be a helpful tool, when contrast medium is contraindicated, although recently several cases of gadolinium-induced nephrogenic systemic fibrosis have been published.[84] Moreover, MRI can miss renal artery stenosis. A rare cause of hypertensive crisis, pheochromocytoma, also should be excluded, preferably by assay of plasma catecholamine samples obtained during the hypertensive crisis.[85]

HYPERTENSIVE ENCEPHALOPATHY

Hypertensive encephalopathy is defined as decreased alertness, impaired cognitive function, delirium, and in some cases, generalized seizures or cortical blindness, unexplained by other disease and reversible with blood pressure lowering.[58] The diagnosis should be questioned when the neurological symptoms do not abate with antihypertensive treatment. Patients with hypertensive encephalopathy often present with headache, visual disturbances, convulsions, and sometimes even overt coma, preceded by an abrupt increase in blood pressure. Hypertensive encephalopathy may occur in the absence of retinal changes[86] and does not always coincide with the other clinical features of malignant hypertension.[45,64] Possible etiological factors include eclampsia, pheochromocytoma, acute withdrawal of antihypertensive therapy, and renovascular disease.[13] Recently, the use of erythropoietin has been implicated in its pathogenesis.[87] Primary cerebral stroke, which also may be followed by severe increases in blood pressure,[88] can be difficult to distinguish clinically

from hypertensive encephalopathy. An important point, however, is that primary cerebral stroke is common and hypertensive encephalopathy is uncommon.

Hypertensive encephalopathy probably results from loss of cerebral autoregulation secondary to a severe rise in blood pressure ("breakthrough theory"), leading to cerebral hyperperfusion and focal cerebral edema.[89] An intense vasoconstriction in response to an acute blood pressure rise also has been proposed as a pathogenetic mechanism ("overregulation theory").[13,64] Especially patients with previously normal blood pressure levels, such as occurs in eclampsia or acute renal failure, are at risk for the development of this intense vasoconstriction condition.[86,90] In these patients, hypertensive encephalopathy may occur at relatively low blood pressure levels (as low as 100 mm Hg diastolic).[91] In patients with hypertensive encephalopathy, the computed tomography (CT) scan may appear completely normal or display only signs of cerebral edema. Parallel to the clinical presentation of hypertensive encephalopathy, posterior leukoencephalopathy can be seen on a MRI scan. The latter are mostly bilateral abnormalities of the parieto-occipital white matter regions of cerebrum, cerebellum, or cerebral cord.[92] These abnormalities probably are caused by perivascular edema of areas with an intensive sympathetic innervation of the vessels.[93] These abnormalities, which are reversible when appropriately treated, constitute the well-characterized posterior leukoencephalopathy syndrome (PLS).[94] The treatment of hypertensive encephalopathy is covered later on.

SEVERE HYPERTENSION WITHOUT END-ORGAN DAMAGE

Much more commonly observed than patients with hypertensive crisis or hypertensive emergencies are patients presenting with severe hypertension (diastolic blood pressure greater than 115 to 120 mm Hg) without signs of end-organ damage. These patients often have essential hypertension that has not yet been diagnosed or inadequately controlled. The elevation in blood pressure often is discovered during routine blood pressure checks. Patients with severe uncomplicated hypertension often are asymptomatic or have only nonspecific symptoms such as dizziness or headache. Although these patients are at severe risk for long-term complications if their hypertension is not adequately controlled, they usually are not in immediate danger. Therefore, as discussed later on, the risks associated with immediate and vigorous blood pressure control probably are greater than those associated with more gradual blood pressure control in these hypertensive emergencies.

Severe Hypertension in Acute Renal Failure

Nearly all forms of acute renal failure can manifest with severe hypertension, which can be due to activation of vasoactive substances and renal pressor reflexes, decreased renal production of vasodilating factors, and fluid overload. In the case of severe blood pressure elevation, the differential diagnosis with hypertensive crisis may be difficult, because the renal failure itself is a predisposing factor for the development of hypertensive crisis[62]; if possible, a renal biopsy is needed. When microangiopathic hemolytic anemia is present, the distinction among hypertensive crisis, hemolytic uremic syndrome, and thrombotic thrombocytopenic purpura can be hard to make, because also the findings on renal biopsy may be more or less identical (see earlier). In most cases, however, blood pressure will be lower and retinal changes less pronounced in the latter syndromes, although occasionally, severe hypertension may ensue.[77]

Scleroderma renal crisis may manifest as hypertensive crisis and is characterized by the preexistent signs and symptoms of systemic sclerosis, although it may be seen in patients without prior skin or other organ involvement.[43,95]

Many patients with hypertension and acute renal failure not due to hypertensive crisis present with volume overload, in contrast with patients with hypertensive crisis, who generally are fluid depleted.[17] This has important consequences for therapy: Whereas patients with hypertensive crisis generally should not receive diuretics, fluid removal (by diuretics or ultrafiltration) is mandatory for patients with volume overload and constitutes the first step of treatment (see "Treatment" section). Therefore, a careful assessment of fluid status is necessary, and invasive pressure monitoring will sometimes have to be used. Apart from diuretic therapy, however, drug therapy of hypertension in acute renal failure generally is the same in patients with and those without signs of hypertensive crisis, as detailed later on. ACE inhibitors and beta blockers should be used with caution, because they may decrease glomerular filtration rate and induce hyperkalemia.

Severe Hypertension in Patients with Renal Transplantation

Severe hypertension is relatively common after renal transplantation and may lead to hypertensive encephalopathy if inadequately controlled. In the postoperative period, hypertension can be due to overhydration, thrombosis of the transplanted kidney, or pressor effects of the residual kidneys. Hypertension occurring later after transplantation may also be due to hypertensive effects of the remnant kidneys. Moreover, acute or chronic rejection or renal artery stenosis in the transplanted kidney are common causes of post-transplantation hypertension. In patients who receive treatment for acute rejection, high-dose steroid therapy or the use of antilymphocyte antibodies may lead to a severe increase in blood pressure.[96,97] Therapy for patients with severe post-transplantation hypertension is not essentially different from that for hypertensive crises in other patients and depends on the clinical picture. ACE inhibitors should be used only with extreme caution, however, because they may induce renal insufficiency in patients with renal artery stenosis of the transplanted kidney, or severe hyperkalemia, especially when used in combination with cyclosporine. Also, beta blockers are not desirable for monotherapy because they may decrease renal blood flow and induce hyperkalemia.[13]

TREATMENT

A targeted medical history and physical examination supported by appropriate laboratory evaluation are essential in patients with a possible hypertensive emergency or crisis. Previous hypertensive history and blood pressure

TABLE 177-3

Approach to Hypertensive Emergency or Crisis

General Measures
- Maintain patient on bed rest in a quiet environment.
- Insert a peripheral intravenous line.
- Perform a quick laboratory evaluation (electrolytes, renal function, parameters of coagulation, urinary evaluation, electrocardiography).
- Monitor blood pressure (preferably with an intra-arterial line).
- Prevent a too-rapid decrease in blood pressure. Generally, blood pressure should not be lowered below diastolic levels of 110 mm Hg during the first several hours.
- Patients with hypertensive crisis may be hypovolemic; intravenous fluid supplementation may be necessary.
- After the critical phase, start oral medication (avoid nifedipine in case of myocardial ischemia or encephalopathy) and taper intravenous medication (do not immediately stop intravenous medication after the start of oral medication!).
- Search for the cause of the hypertensive crisis.

Specific Therapy
- Start intravenous therapy: Give labetalol in a bolus of 10-20 mg, followed by continuous infusion of 5-20 mg/hour; adjust according to blood pressure response.
- When labetalol has no effect, change to nitroprusside (which also may be used as a first-line agent). Starting dose is 0.3-3 µg/kg per minute.

control should be ascertained, as should any history of renal and cardiac disease. Likewise, the use of prescribed or nonprescribed medications should be documented. Blood pressure in both arms should be measured with use of appropriately sized cuffs. Physical examination must include palpation of pulses in all extremities, auscultation for renal bruits, a focused neurological examination, and finally a funduscopic examination.

General Guidelines in Hypertensive Emergencies

Adequate treatment of severe hypertension is a challenge (Table 177-3). It will be essential to balance between a too-rapid lowering of blood pressure, which may lead to a symptomatic decrease in end-organ perfusion, and exposing the patient to severe hypertension for too long a period, which may exacerbate vascular damage.[4] Most patients with hypertensive crisis are chronically hypertensive and will have a rightward shift of the pressure-flow (cerebral, renal, and coronary) autoregulation curve.[98] Rapid reduction in blood pressure below the cerebral, renal, or coronary autoregulatory range will result in a marked reduction in organ blood flow, leading to ischemia and infarction.[99]

By means of autoregulation, blood flow to the brain, heart, and kidneys is maintained constant within a wide range of blood pressure levels in healthy persons and in patients with chronic hypertension. In normotensive subjects, blood flow to the brain is controlled by autoregulation at a mean arterial pressure between 60 and 120 mm Hg,[13] whereas in untreated patients with chronic hypertension, these limits may be much higher (between 120 and 160 mm Hg mean arterial pressure).[96,100,101] This differential in autoregulatory limits explains why cerebral ischemia may occur during uncontrolled lowering of blood pressure,

TABLE 177-4

Specific Drug Therapy: Intravenous Agents

MEDICATION	DOSAGE	FIRST EFFECT	DURATION OF EFFECT	SIDE EFFECT(S)
Diazoxide	10-30 mg/minute in 15-30 minutes	1-5 minutes	4-12 hours	Myocardial ischemia, orthostatic hypotension, hyperglycemia, salt retention
Enalapril	1.25-5.0 mg as bolus	15 minutes	4-6 hours	Hypotension, renal insufficiency
Esmolol	0.5-1 mg/kg in 1-4 minutes, followed by 50-300 mg/kg/minute	1-2 minutes	10-20 minutes	Dizziness, nausea, pruritus, AV block
Fenoldopam	0.1-1.6 µg/kg/minute	5-10 minutes	10-15 minutes	Hypotension, reflex tachycardia, headache, intraocular increase in pressure, tolerance (after 48 hours of infusion)
Fentolamine	1-5 mg as bolus; 0.5-1.0 mg/hour continuously	1-2 minutes	3-5 minutes	Reflex tachycardia
Hydralazine	10-20 mg as bolus	2-6 hours	2-6 hours	Reflex tachycardia
Labetalol	10-20 mg as bolus; 5-20 mg/hour continuously	2-4 hours	2-4 hours	Nausea, vomiting, pruritus, AV block
Nicardipine	2-10 mg/hour	5-10 minutes	2-4 hours	Reflex tachycardia, flushing
Nitroglycerin	0.5-10 mg/hour	2-5 minutes	3-5 minutes	Headache, dizziness, nausea, vomiting, tolerance
Nitroprusside	0.3-10 µg/kg/minute	Direct	1-2 minutes	Hypotension, nausea, vomiting, reflex tachycardia, (thio)cyanate intoxication

AV, atrioventricular.

especially in patients with chronic untreated hypertension.[102] Because of preexisting atherosclerosis, elderly patients appear to be at greater risk for ischemia when blood pressure is acutely lowered to normal values.[98]

Therefore, a gradual decline in blood pressure is desirable, except for special cases, such as a dissecting aortic aneurysm or overt cardiac failure, in which blood pressure has to be lowered very quickly to normal levels.[103] In hypertensive encephalopathy, blood pressure probably should be reduced more quickly over several hours to systolic values of approximately 160 to 170 mm Hg and diastolic values of approximately 100 to 110 mm Hg.[45,86] During the first hour of treatment, blood pressure probably should not be reduced below more than 20% of the initial blood pressure, or below values of 150 to 160 mm Hg systolic or 100 to 110 mm Hg diastolic, whatever occurs first.[6,45] Too-rapid lowering may worsen cerebral ischemia in this disorder.[101] In other instances, a recommended approach is to decrease mean arterial blood pressure not below 120 mm Hg, or not below 170/110 to 160/100, whatever occurs first, during the first 24 hours, and then to establish complete normalization using oral antihypertensive medication during the next week.[6,13]

Bed rest in a quiet environment is mandatory. Fluid status, renal function, and serum electrolytes should be monitored carefully, especially in patients with severely elevated creatinine levels; further deterioration of renal function may be expected, and hemodialysis may be needed.[44] Use of this procedure is not a contraindication to further antihypertensive therapy, however, because it will protect from further damage to other organs, whereas renal impairment can be reversible (see earlier). In our opinion, all patients with hypertensive emergencies should be transferred to an intensive care unit, and intra-arterial pressure measurements should be performed continuously when intravenous antihypertensive therapy is used.

At presentation, a choice between oral and intravenous drugs has to be made. Some investigators have proposed the use of oral antihypertensive agents in hypertensive "emergencies,"[104] but the decrease in blood pressure with

the use of oral antihypertensive agents is not always entirely predictable and cannot be regulated very precisely. It is therefore our opinion that in case of a direct threat to life or organ function, such as hypertensive encephalopathy, rapidly progressive renal failure, adrenergic crisis, or acute intracerebral hemorrhage (discussed later on), intravenous antihypertensive therapy is mandatory; this recommendation also applies for management of acute pulmonary edema, dissecting aortic aneurysm, and myocardial infarction. When blood pressure is controlled by parenteral therapy and the patient is stabilized, oral agents can be started. Intravenous therapy should not be stopped immediately after initiation of oral therapy, however, because this may lead to severe rebound hypertension before oral therapy has had time to work.[64] In less severely affected patients, oral therapy can be used as primary therapy. This also is appropriate management for scleroderma renal crises, which respond very well to treatment with ACE inhibitors.[76]

General Guidelines in Hypertensive Urgencies

In hypertensive "urgencies"—severe elevations in blood pressure without direct threat to organ function—immediate blood lowering is not justified, because overzealous treatment can put the patient at greater risk for cerebral or cardiac ischemia (see Table 177-3).[105,106] It is reasonable to first observe the effects of rest on blood pressure levels. When blood pressure remains severely elevated, it can be lowered using oral agents gradually over 24 to 48 hours.[1]

Specific Drug Therapy
Intravenous Agents

Specific drug therapy with intravenous agents is summarized in Table 177-4.

Intravenous labetalol, an agent that combines alpha- and beta-blocking properties, has proved to be the most useful agent in the treatment of hypertensive crisis.[107-109] The theoretical advantage is that the reflex tachycardia usually associated with vasodilatation due to the alpha blockade is diminished because of its beta-blocking properties.[110] The onset of action after intravenous bolus administration is rapid and occurs within 5 minutes.[99] With constant intravenous infusion, an effect generally is seen within 5 to 10 minutes.[111] Its antihypertensive effect may last for several hours.[6,45] With the use of labetalol, systemic vascular resistance declines while cardiac output remains stable or slightly decreases.[13,112] Renal hemodynamics is little affected. Cerebral blood flow is minimally affected during the use of labetalol.[113]

Because of its beta-blocking properties, labetalol should not be used in patients with heart block or obstructive pulmonary disease.[110] Because it is cleared mainly by hepatic metabolism, it can be used safely in patients with renal insufficiency. Excessive hypotension can occur when large intravenous boluses are given.[114] With the use of continuous infusion (starting at a rate of 5 to 10 mg/hour), which may be preceded by a small initial bolus (10 to 20 mg given over 1 minute), the risk of hypotension is smaller.[99] After adequate blood pressure levels have been reached, labetalol can be given orally (starting dose, 100 to 200 mg twice daily; maximum daily dose, 1200 to 2400 mg).[110] Because of the risk of hypotension, we recommend that intra-arterial monitoring be used when intravenous labetalol is prescribed.

Sodium nitroprusside is a very effective and easily titratable hypertensive drug with a nearly immediate onset of effect.[115] It usually is given as a continuous intravenous infusion at 0.3 to 10 μg/kg per minute; the dose can be titrated until the desired blood pressure level is reached. Doses larger than 3 μg/kg per minute are rarely needed.[45] The duration of action of sodium nitroprusside is approximately 1 to 2 minutes. Sodium nitroprusside acts as both a venous and an arteriolar dilator. Therefore, reflex tachycardia is almost absent.[115] Cardiac output remains fairly constant during its use, whereas renal blood flow and glomerular filtration rate increase.[13] Although it is a weak cerebral vasodilator, conflicting data exist regarding its effect on cerebral blood flow, which may be dose-dependent—increasing at low doses and decreasing at high doses.[100,116] Generally, however, it is considered a useful drug for the treatment of hypertensive encephalopathy, because of its quick reversibility and easy titration.[1,6,13] Because of its very rapid action and the risk of hypotension, however, intra-arterial blood pressure monitoring is mandatory. The drug is photosensitive, and the infusion solution and lines should be protected from light. When sodium nitroprusside is given for more than 72 hours, or at rates exceeding 3 μg/kg per minute, thiocyanate intoxication can develop, especially in patients with renal insufficiency.[117] With use of lower doses used over shorter periods, however, this complication is rare.

Nitroglycerin can be useful in the treatment of hypertensive crisis, especially when cardiac failure or myocardial ischemia is present. However, because it is less effective than nitroprusside as a blood pressure–lowering agent,[118] sodium nitroprusside should be the drug of choice in the case of hypertensive crisis and myocardial ischemia. Recently, newer agents such as nicardipine[109] (a calcium antagonist), dilevalol (a beta blocker with β₂-adrenergic– stimulating properties),[119] and enalaprilat (ACE inhibitor)[120] also were found to be effective as intravenous agents in the treatment of severe hypertension. However, their effectiveness has not yet been directly compared with that of more established agents.

Fenoldopam is a selective peripheral dopamine receptor agonist. The antihypertensive action is based on a combination of systemic and renal vasodilation and stimulation of natriuresis.[121] In Western countries, it typically has been used when a short duration of decline in blood pressure is of importance.[121]

In most patients with hypertensive crisis, plasma volume is decreased, so diuretics generally should be avoided. Of interest, sodium infusion was followed by a decrease in blood pressure levels in one clinical study.[122] In patients with acute renal failure, however, overhydration can be present, and treatment with loop diuretics may be necessary to normalize fluid status.[45] In these cases, high doses of loop diuretics are needed: Up to 500 to 1000 mg/day can be given as a continuous infusion.[123] These high doses should never be given as a bolus because ototoxicity may result. In combination with furosemide, thiazide diuretics may further increase the diuretic response. Especially with this combination, sodium and potassium levels should be monitored closely.[124] When diuretic therapy does not succeed, ultrafiltration will be needed.

Beta blockade is not recommended as a single first-line treatment because of the potential for decrease in cardiac function and increase in systemic vascular resistance, especially in agents without intrinsic sympathetic activity (ISA),[13] which may lead to a reduction in glomerular filtration rate in patients with impaired renal function[1] and can exacerbate hyperkalemia. In combination with vasodilating agents, however, beta blockers may be a valuable adjunct because they reduce reflex tachycardia. General contraindications to the use of beta blockers include cardiac failure, heart block, obstructive pulmonary disease, and severe peripheral vascular disease.

Intravenous diazoxide and hydralazine have been regularly used in the treatment of hypertensive crisis and hypertensive encephalopathy. They have major shortcomings, however, and may cause cerebral edema as a result of predominant arteriolar vasodilatation, when blood pressure is not lowered intensively.[6,13,125,126] We also do not use intravenous therapy with clonidine, because of the possibility of an initial pressor effect and its relatively slow onset of action and sedative properties.[13]

Oral Agents

Labetalol also has been used for oral treatment for severe hypertension,[110,127] although in some cases, it may be ineffective.[128] Blood pressure is lowered within 1 to 3 hours after oral administration.[129] Because hypotension may be observed after higher doses, a starting dose of 100 to 200 mg twice daily is recommended.

ACE inhibitors are effective in the treatment of severe hypertension. Captopril starts to work within 5 minutes when administered sublingually[130] and within 15 to 30 minutes when administered orally.[131] The maximal fall in blood pressure after sublingual administration is reached within 1 hour, and within 1 to 2 hours after oral administration. The antihypertensive effect lasts for 2 to 6 hours.[13,130] A recommended starting dose is 6.25 to 12.5 mg, although no hypotensive periods were observed in a study when a starting dose of 25 mg was used.[130] In patients with renal failure, however, intravascular volume depletion and renal artery stenosis are especially sensitive to the effect of ACE inhibitors.[132] Therefore, we advise a more cautious approach. Administration of captopril may lead to a slight increase in cardiac output.[133] Captopril may increase cerebral perfusion without inhomogeneous flow distribution. Favorable effects on the cerebral autoregulatory curve have been observed in animals.[134] Enalapril can be used in the case of severe hypertension. Its onset of action is somewhat slower, but the effect is longer acting.[1] Both captopril and enalapril are very useful in the treatment of scleroderma renal crises.[42,135] They should, however, be used with caution with renal insufficiency, because they can induce hyperkalemia. In patients with bilateral renal artery stenosis or in post-transplant hypertension due to stenosis of the vascular anastomosis, the use of ACE inhibitors may lead to a severe decrease in glomerular filtration rate, owing to preferential dilation of efferent glomerular arterioles.[136]

In the past, clonidine, a central alpha receptor agonist, frequently was applied in the treatment of severe blood pressure elevation. Today, however, the risk of rebound hypertension after discontinuation,[105] the potential for drowsiness as a side effect,[64] and the relatively slow onset of action[13] have resulted in declining popularity of clonidine,[137] especially now that equally effective agents with fewer side effects are available.

Nifedipine, the calcium antagonist that is most widely used for the treatment of hypertensive emergencies, is effective and fast-acting. The recommended starting dose is 5 to 10 mg, administered orally or sublingually. The maximal effect of 10 mg nifedipine is reached within 1 hour,[13,130] but a blood pressure–lowering effect may already be seen 3 minutes after sublingual and 15 to 20 minutes after oral administration.[13] The difference in onset of action between the oral route and the sublingual route does not seem to be due to oral absorption, because this is poor, but rather to quicker gastric absorption. When nifedipine is bitten and swallowed, the same onset of action is observed as for the sublingual route.[138] The effect of nifedipine lasts for 3 to 4 hours after oral or sublingual administration.[139] This agent usually will not suffice for monotherapy for the treatment of severe hypertension.[140] Nifedipine generally is well tolerated, although some patients complain of headache, dizziness, flushing, and palpitations.[130] When it is given in larger doses or as an additional dose during too short a period (especially within 1 hour), hypotension with cerebral and myocardial ischemia may occur.[141] In addition, although cardiac output, heart rate, renal blood flow, and glomerular filtration rate increase with nifedipine,[13,142] its cerebral vasodilating properties may exacerbate cerebral edema, leading to an increase in inhomogeneous brain perfusion in patients with hypertensive encephalopathy.[64] Therefore, some experts strongly discourage especially the use of sublingual nifedipine because of its unpredictable effects.[143] We strongly encourage this view that when immediate blood pressure control is needed, parenteral drugs are the therapeutic agents of choice, because they can be better titrated. Accordingly, the use of nifedipine is "relatively" contraindicated in hypertensive crisis.

If a hypertensive urgency is refractory to treatment with the oral agents discussed previously, minoxidil, a direct vasodilator, often will be effective, especially in combination with a beta blocker and a diuretic.[144] These drugs are necessary to blunt the reflex tachycardia and to deal with salt and water retention. Other side effects include headache, nausea, and hypertrichosis. The usual starting dose is 2.5 to 5 mg, three to four times a day, continued until the blood pressure is controlled. The usual maintenance dose is 5 to 10 mg twice daily. The onset of the effect of minoxidil is within 1 to 2 hours, peak action is achieved

TABLE 177-5

Treatment Considerations in Specific Clinical Situations

- **Dissecting aneurysm:** Immediate blood pressure lowering to low-normal values is necessary; use β-adrenergic blockers with sodium nitroprusside.
- **Myocardial infarction:** Use β-adrenergic blockers with nitroglycerin (*alternative*: nitroprusside).
- **Cardiac asthma:** Give nitroglycerin (or sodium nitroprusside) with furosemide.
- **Intracerebral bleeding/infarction:** Use labetalol; in general, treat only if diastolic blood pressure is greater than 130 mm Hg.
- **Postoperative hypertension:** Use labetalol.
- **Pheochromocytoma:** Use phentolamine.
- **Severe hypertension without signs of end-organ damage:** Maintain patient on bed rest; when blood pressure remains elevated, give captopril or nifedipine orally (avoid nifedipine with signs of myocardial ischemia or cerebral dysfunction) (*alternative*: labetalol orally).

in 4 to 8 hours, and the duration of action is approximately 12 hours.[13]

SPECIFIC CLINICAL PROBLEMS

Treatment considerations in the management of selected clinical problems are summarized in Table 177-5.

Adrenergic Crisis

Adrenergic crises occur primarily in the presence of a pheochromocytoma. However, they can also occur after acute withdrawal of clonidine (or possibly methyldopa).[145] In the past, adrenergic crises also were seen after the ingestion of monoamine oxidase inhibitors in combination with tyrosine-rich food.[6]

Hypertension is due to an abrupt increase in sympathetic activity with elevated plasma catecholamine levels. Also, patients with spinal cord lesions (especially above the midthoracic level) may experience severe hypertensive episodes as a result of release of catecholamines from the denervated spinal cord, especially in response to stimulation of hollow organs, such as bladder and bowel.[146]

Clinical features of an adrenergic crisis include palpitations, intense diaphoresis, headache, abdominal discomfort, and pallor of the extremities. In these circumstances, drugs with alpha-blocking activity are particularly useful. Both intravenous phentolamine and labetalol have been successfully used,[51,147] although with the latter agent, the β-antagonistic effect is (theoretically, at least) undesirable.[6] Also, sodium nitroprusside lowers the blood pressure effectively.[148] The recommended starting dose of phentolamine in an adrenergic crisis is 1 to 5 mg administered as bolus, followed by a continuous infusion of 5 mg/minute.[6]

For further information regarding pathogenesis, diagnosis, and treatment of pheochromocytoma, the reader is referred to recent reviews.[149]

Cerebrovascular Accidents

A markedly elevated blood pressure also may be found in patients who have suffered an ischemic stroke, cerebral hemorrhage, or subarachnoid hemorrhage.[88,150] Controversy exists regarding whether hypertension should be treated in these circumstances.[151-154] Often, the blood pressure decreases spontaneously during the first few days.[155]

To limit edema formation, treatment seems desirable, whereas for the maintenance of perfusion to the brain, observation may be more appropriate.[152] Indeed, in patients with thrombotic stroke, cerebral autoregulation may be impaired,[156] and quick blood pressure lowering may compromise cerebral blood flow, potentially leading to a further increase in the cerebral infarction.[157,158] A study that assessed the possible neuroprotective role of the calcium antagonist nimodipine was stopped prematurely because of a dose-dependent decline in neurological status in patients in the treatment group.[159] Therefore, patients with a mild blood pressure elevation should not be given antihypertensive agents; this injunction is supported by a recent randomized controlled trial.[160] Although no consensus on this subject has been reached,[152,154] most authorities recommend antihypertensive treatment only in patients with severe blood pressure elevation (to greater than 130 mm Hg diastolic), with reduction in blood pressure to be achieved gradually (over approximately 24 hours) to diastolic levels not lower than 100 to 110 mm Hg.[100,107,151,153,161]

When treatment is started, an easily titratable drug such as intravenous labetalol or nitroprusside probably constitutes the best choice, despite concern regarding the cerebral vasodilating effect of nitroprusside.[152] Calcium antagonists probably are best avoided because they also may increase intracerebral pressure.[162] ACE inhibitors appear to have no effect on cerebral blood flow[152] but may induce a quick drop in blood pressure when given in too large a dose, especially in patients with volume depletion. Even in patients with intracerebral hemorrhage, the value of immediate antihypertensive treatment is unclear. Lowering of blood pressure may reduce the chance of rebleeding and cerebral edema[6,13,151] but also may compromise cerebral perfusion as a result of the loss of cerebral autoregulation.

So, in patients with a cerebrovascular accident, immediate treatment of mild hypertension is not indicated. In patients with severe hypertension, the value of treatment is not clear. If treatment seems desirable, a gradual decrease in blood pressure (not below 20% of the initial value[64]), using short-acting parenteral agents, probably is justified. The value of blood pressure lowering in patients with subarachnoid hemorrhage also is unclear. One investigator advocates an aggressive approach, to decrease the chance of rebleeding.[163] Cerebral vasospasm, resulting in cerebral infarction, is a feared complication after subarachnoid hemorrhage,[164] however, and quick blood pressure control may potentially further exacerbate cerebral ischemia. In one study of the use of nimodipine (a dihydropyridine calcium blocker), a cerebral vasodilator at doses that do not affect mean arterial pressure was found to be useful in preventing cerebral infarction.[165] Further studies are needed to confirm these results.

Myocardial Infarction

Hypertension in patients with myocardial ischemia or infarction increases the burden and therefore the oxygen demand of the heart. Moreover, postinfarction hypertension may put the patient at greater risk for myocardial rupture.[64] Reduction of blood pressure reduces the oxygen demand of the heart and may limit the size of the infarct.

The aim of treatment should be to reduce the blood pressure to low-normal levels. Intravenous nitroglycerin is the agent of choice because it can be easily titrated, decreases myocardial oxygen consumption, and usually does not induce significant reflex tachycardia.[6] The adjunctive use of (oral or intravenous) beta blockade is very advantageous because this reduces further myocardial oxygen demand by a decrease in heart rate and cardiac contractility.[64] Contraindications to the use of beta blockers include heart block, obstructive pulmonary disease, and severe peripheral vascular disease. Oral calcium antagonists are less desirable because they induce an uncontrollable reduction in blood pressure and may precipitate reflex tachycardia and heart failure. Moreover, it was recently reported that the use of nifedipine after myocardial infarction may increase mortality.[166]

In patients with severe hypertension that is uncontrollable by nitroglycerin and beta blockade, sodium nitroprusside may be administered. This agent has less desirable actions than nitroglycerin, in that it may induce a "steal" effect by means of the arterial vasodilation,[167] leading to reflex tachycardia if no beta blocker is administered.

Cardiac Failure

Patients with cardiac failure may present with severe hypertension as a result of an increase in peripheral vascular resistance induced by activation of vasopressor systems.[6,168]

Severe hypertension is seen particularly in patients with diastolic dysfunction of the left ventricle, in whom the systolic function of the heart often is maintained. In these patients, pulmonary edema develops owing to an increased stiffness of the left ventricle, which may hamper diastolic filling. Such patients may benefit most from beta blockade. In patients with left ventricular failure accompanied by hypertension, lowering of the blood pressure by nitroglycerin or nitroprusside often is very effective.[1,6,64]

Dissecting Aortic Aneurysm

Dissection of the aorta is initiated by a tear in the intima, which often is caused by degeneration of the aortic media. Preexisting hypertension is an important risk factor. Patients with acute aortic dissection most often present with severe chest pain of acute onset that may migrate to other areas as the dissection advances. Also, neurological complications may be present. Most patients with acute aortic dissection have elevated blood pressure at presentation.[169,170]

Proximal aortic dissections should always necessitate surgical treatment, whereas operation in the case of distal dissections is more controversial. Nevertheless, in all cases of acute aortic dissection, immediate blood pressure lowering to the lowest level compatible with adequate perfusion to other organs is mandatory. Blood pressure lowering should be achieved by intravenous administration of sodium nitroprusside. The concurrent administration of intravenous beta-blocking agents (for propranolol, the recommended dose is 0.05 to 0.15 mg/kg/body weight every 4 to 6 hours; for esmolol, the dose is 80 mg infused over 15 to 30 minutes, followed by 50 mg/kg per minute, for a maximum of 300 mg/kg per minute) is imperative, because administration of sodium nitroprusside alone may increase cardiac output, which is highly undesirable in this setting. In the case of an absolute contraindication to beta blockade, verapamil (5 to 10 mg given every 6 to 8 hours) can be used in combination with sodium nitroprusside. Intravenous trimetaphan (a ganglionic blocker) also can be used as the sole agent (at a dosage of 1 to 2 mg/minute). With the latter agent, side effects due to parasympathetic inhibition (e.g., obstipation, urinary retention) are rather common.[13]

Postresuscitation Hypertension

In patients with hypovolemic shock, severe hypertension may develop after aggressive resuscitation, especially with the use of colloid solutions. This form of hypertension most often is due to acute hypervolemia and also may lead to respiratory failure secondary to pulmonary edema. In the case of fluid overload, loop diuretics should be given to improve sodium and water excretion. Also, the use of a vasodilating agent, such as intravenous nitroglycerin, may be useful to reduce the volume burden on the heart.[171]

Perioperative Hypertension

Perioperative hypertension may occur after any operation, although the incidence is especially high for coronary bypass procedures, carotid endarterectomy, abdominal aortic aneurysm procedures, and peripheral vascular operations. Especially large increases in blood pressure are especially likely to occur during intubation and after recovery from anesthesia. Severe increases in blood pressure may lead to complications such as myocardial ischemia or cardiac failure and neurological problems, and to leakage of vascular sutures and bleeding episodes.[64,172] Perioperative hypertension occurs especially in patients with insufficiently controlled blood pressure before surgery (especially in patients with systolic blood pressure levels higher than 200 mm Hg and diastolic blood pressure levels lower than 110 mm Hg). Perioperative hypertension is, in the absence of fluid overload, generally characterized by an increase in vascular resistance due to an increase in vascular tone.[173] Short-acting and easily titratable agents such as labetalol and nitroprusside should be used for treatment, to avoid hypotensive periods, which may lead to myocardial or cerebral ischemia.[172] An alternative to the latter two drugs may be ketanserine administered intravenously (a bolus of 5 to 10 mg given over 10 minutes, followed by a continuous infusion of 2 to 6 mg/hour),[174] especially after peripheral artery surgery.

In patients with hypertension after coronary bypass surgery, nitroglycerin is the agent of choice, because it reduces myocardial oxygen consumption. The treatment for post–carotid endarterectomy hyperperfusion syndrome has recently been reviewed.[175] In such cases, labetalol treatment is advocated. In other circumstances, sodium nitroprusside is preferable because it is very effective and easily titratable.[176]

Key Points

1. Renal disease is an important underlying cause and consequence of a hypertensive emergency.
2. In contrast with hypertensive urgencies, managing hypertensive emergencies necessitates immediate intravenous therapy in an intensive care unit setting.
3. During a hypertensive emergency, it is essential to balance the immediate need for lowering of blood pressure against the lower risk of complications associated with temporary maintenance of a higher blood pressure level.
4. With hypertensive emergencies, partial or complete recovery of renal function may occur after several months when optimal blood pressure control is initiated.

Key References

3. Chobanian AV, Bakris GL, Black HR, et al: The seventh report of the Joint National Committee on Prevention, Detection, Evaluation, and Treatment of High Blood Pressure. The JNC 7 Report. JAMA 2003;289:2560-2572.
20. van den Born BJ, Koopmans RP, Groeneveld JO, van Montfrans GA: Ethnic disparities in the incidence, presentation and complications of malignant hypertension. J Hypertension 2006;24:2299-2304.
36. Guerin C, Berthoux F: Prognostic factors in malignant hypertension selected by multivariate analysis. Nephrol Dial Transplant 1990;5:563-568.
50. Vaughan GJ, Delanty N: Hypertensive emergencies. Lancet 2000;356:411-417.
54. Stefansson B, Ricksten A, Rymo L, et al: Angiotensin-converting enzyme gene I/D polymorphism in malignant hypertension. Blood Press 2000;9:104-109.

See the companion Expert Consult website for the complete reference list.

CHAPTER 178

Cardiac Surgery and the Kidney

Andrew Shaw, Dipen Parikh, and Mark Stafford-Smith

OBJECTIVES

This chapter will:
1. Describe the effects of cardiac surgery on the kidney.
2. Present an overview of risk stratification and the link between acute kidney injury and outcome.
3. Review measures used to assess for acute kidney injury after cardiopulmonary bypass and cardiac surgery.
4. Outline an approach to prevention of acute kidney injury during cardiac surgery.

Acute kidney injury (AKI) is a major medical problem that is of particular concern after heart surgery.[1] The renal failure following cardiac surgery is addressed in detail in Chapter 197; this chapter focuses on the effects of cardiac surgery, medications used during these procedures, and cardiopulmonary bypass on the kidney.

Perioperative AKI is independently highly predictive of short-term morbidity, increased costs of treatment, and poor long-term outcome.[2] This is especially the case when acute deterioration is superimposed on chronic kidney disease.[3] Although diverse mechanisms contribute to the renal insult sustained during cardiac surgery, ischemia-reperfusion, inflammation, and atheroembolism are common etiological factors. In addition, the oxygen diffusion shunt characteristics of the renal microcirculation, along with the high metabolic demands of tubular reabsorption, make the kidney uniquely vulnerable to ischemic injury.

INCIDENCE AND SIGNIFICANCE OF ACUTE KIDNEY INJURY

The type of cardiac surgical procedure is important in characterizing the incidence and severity of postoperative AKI, because each operation has its own characteristic pattern of dysfunction.[4] As shown in Figure 178-1, the average peak serum creatinine rise after primary elective aortocoronary bypass graft (CABG) surgery is approximately 29%, the peak occurring most often on the second day and declining to levels at or lower than baseline by the fourth or fifth day.[5] Of importance, timing varies among patients such that the highest creatinine value for each individual patient (postoperative peak), averaged for a cohort, will always considerably exceed the greatest daily average value (see Fig. 178-1). The average peak creatinine rise is most valuable to describe AKI in a group of patients (rather than the highest daily average value), because this value reflects the most significant renal impairment and is highly correlated with adverse outcome.[6] When assessed by peak creatinine rise, approximately 8% of coronary bypass patients sustain moderate AKI (greater than 1.0 mg/dL peak rise), and 1% to 3% will require dialysis.[6] Reflect-

ing a lack of effective preventive therapies, the incidence of renal dysfunction after cardiac procedures and the associated mortality risk in numerous case series has changed very little over the last four decades.[6-9] In-hospital mortality rate after CABG surgery increases from less than 1% to 20% in the presence of moderate AKI and exceeds 60% when dialysis is required.[6] In survivors, escalating resource utilization is strongly associated with greater degrees of acute renal injury, including duration of intensive care and hospital stay and need for extended care after hospital discharge.[9] Excess morbidity and mortality can be demonstrated even when creatinine rise never exceeds the normal range. Up to 20% of bypass surgery candidates have evidence of renal dysfunction preoperatively, and for these patients, AKI predicts a particularly high risk of adverse outcomes including accelerated long-term renal decline.[10] Although the relation between acute renal injury and risk of adverse outcome is best characterized for coronary bypass surgery, similar associations exist for all types of cardiac surgery wherever it has been studied.

Care for patients with postoperative renal impairment figures centrally in the overall costs of cardiac surgery, with estimated in-hospital costs for CABG surgery ranging from $32,680 for uncomplicated cases to $100,593 if dialysis is required.[11] The cost per quality-adjusted life-year saved for patients needing dialysis after cardiac surgery is estimated at $274,100. Given that more than 800,000 cardiac surgical procedures occur annually worldwide,[12] and that CABG surgery consumes more medical resources in the United States than any other medical treatment, any effective renoprotective intervention would have significant potential to influence total health care costs.

PATHOPHYSIOLOGY OF ACUTE KIDNEY INJURY

During cardiopulmonary bypass, renal artery blood flow is pressure-dependent.[13] This resembles the normal change in renal blood flow in this blood pressure range and probably does not represent a pathological condition (i.e., loss of renal blood flow autoregulation), because the renal artery myogenic response serves primarily to protect the kidney from pressure overload (lower threshold approximately 80 mm Hg).[14] By contrast, the effect of bypass on autoregulatory tubuloglomerular feedback control of solute delivery, and on blood flow regulation through the microvasculature of the renal medulla, is largely unknown.[14]

AKI following cardiac surgery is the net result of several perioperative insults, some or all of which may occur in any given patient. These consist primarily of tissue ischemia-reperfusion with reactive oxygen species (ROS) elaboration, inflammation, and atheroembolism. The consequence of these insults is a cascade of reflex changes within the kidney leading to a common presentation of AKI manifesting as impairment of renal function, persis-

PATTERNS OF RENAL DYSFUNCTION AFTER CARDIAC SURGICAL PROCEDURES

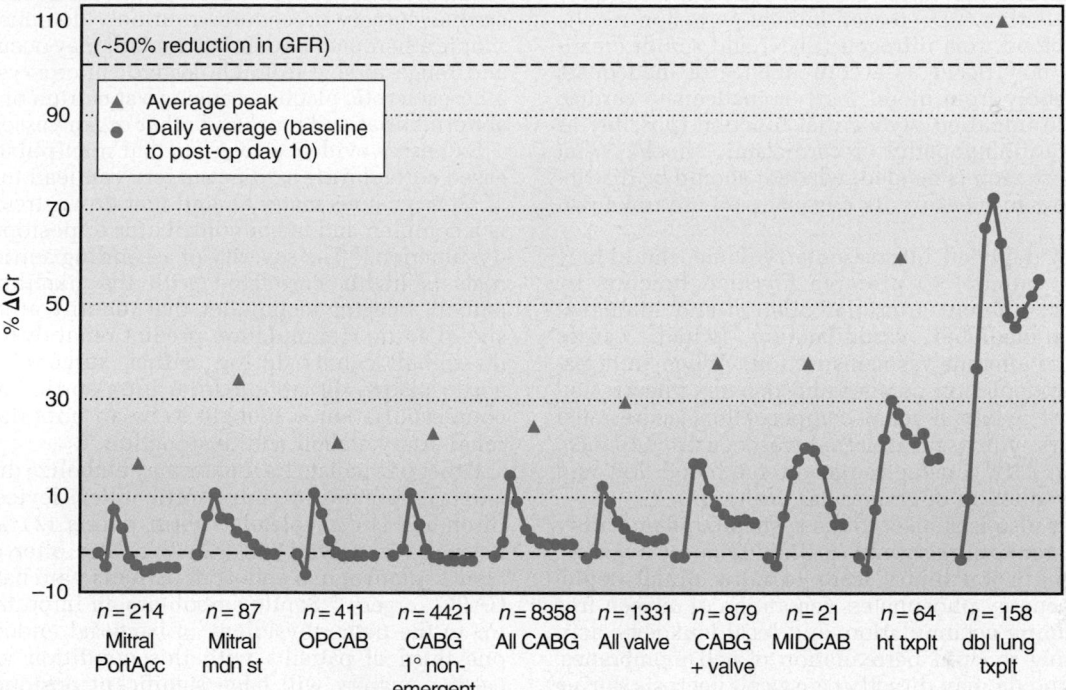

FIGURE 178-1. Average peak *(triangles)* and average daily *(circles)* serum creatinine values, relative to preoperative, for the first 10 days after several different cardiac surgery procedures. Note that each procedure has its own "signature" pattern of renal impairment. Wide variation in the timing of creatinine rise among patients undergoing the same procedure explains why the average peak value always considerably exceeds the highest average daily value. CABG, coronary artery bypass grafting; % ΔCr, peak fractional serum creatinine rise; dbl lung txplt, double lung transplant; ht txplt, heart transplant; mdn st, median sternotomy mitral valve surgery; MIDCAB, minimally invasive coronary artery bypass surgery; OPCAB, off-pump coronary artery bypass surgery; PortAcc, port access mitral valve surgery; 1°, primary.

tent renal vasoconstriction, an exaggerated response to exogenous vasoconstrictors, and vascular endothelial and tubular epithelial cell death due to necrosis and apoptosis.

Although renal artery blood flow delivers oxygen in excess of the kidneys' metabolic need, marked differences in regional perfusion make the medulla paradoxically vulnerable to ischemic injury. The term *medullary hypoxia* refers to the relatively low PO_2 values normally observed in the renal medulla (10 to 20 mm Hg). This relative hypoxia is attributable primarily to the sluggish perfusion and high metabolic activity of the medullary tubules, a phenomenon that is exaggerated by the hairpin loop vascular anatomy of capillaries accompanying the loop of Henle that allow "O_2 escape" from entrance to exit vessels. Stress such as hypoperfusion causes medullary PO_2 to further decline as glomerular filtration is preserved. In fact, during experimental cardiopulmonary bypass, oxygen levels in the medulla are unmeasurable.[15] Post-bypass urine PO_2 measurements are known to correlate with medullary PO_2 and can be used to predict postoperative acute renal dysfunction.[15,16]

The few studies addressing the genetically attributable risk of post–cardiac surgery acute renal dysfunction have identified factors that independently may explain the greater than twofold risk in this setting compared with known clinical risk factors.[17] Some gene variants associated with changes in the acute inflammatory response and modulation of vasoconstriction demonstrate strong associations with postoperative renal impairment.[17,18] Co-possession of the IL-6 572C and angiotensinogen (AGT) 842C polymorphisms in whites predicts a 121% peak creatinine rise after coronary artery bypass surgery. Similarly, the combination of IL-6 572C and tumor necrosis factor (TNF)-α 308A polymorphisms predicts a doubling of postoperative serum creatinine. Endothelial nitric oxide synthase (eNOS) and renin-angiotensin-aldosterone (RAA) system signaling pathways are known to affect systemic and intrarenal paracrine regulation of vascular tone. In African Americans, co-possession of the eNOS 894T and the angiotensin-converting enzyme (ACE) deletion polymorphisms predicts a 162.5% creatinine rise. Possession of the eNOS 894T allele also is associated with exaggerated responsiveness to intravenous phenylephrine during cardiopulmonary bypass and predicts post–cardiac surgery renal dysfunction when combined with other RAA system variants such as the angiotensin receptor 1 (i.e., angiotensin II type 1 receptor [AGTR1]) polymorphism 1166C. Although the mechanism underlying apolipoprotein E (apoE)-related renal dysfunction remains obscure, the e2 and e3 alleles of the *ApoE* gene predict increased risk, and the e4 allele predicts decreased risk for numerous renal disorders, including post–cardiac surgery renal dysfunction.[19]

Ischemia-Reperfusion and Inflammation

Ischemia-reperfusion and inflammation are major causes of AKI in critically ill and cardiac surgical patients.[20]

Ischemia-reperfusion within the kidney triggers local inflammation, and mediators are released from the kidney into the circulation.[21] Decreased kidney perfusion results in elevated blood urea nitrogen (BUN) and serum creatinine, which may occur as a consequence of inadequate volume (possibly from blood loss) or inadequate cardiac output due to impaired myocardial function (possibly as a result of cardiomyopathy or cardiogenic shock). What amount of perfusion is needed, where it should be distributed, and how to measure its adequacy all are unknown factors.

In cases of depleted intravascular volume, the kidney initially will attempt to preserve filtration function by autoregulatory afferent arteriolar dilation and intrarenal prostaglandin-mediated vasodilatation (which causes attenuation of afferent vasoconstriction). When intravascular volume depletion persists and remains uncorrected in the face of maximal renal compensation, acute renal failure occurs. Intense intrarenal vasoconstriction also may result in AKI, causing reduced renal blood flow and subsequent reduction of glomerular perfusion.

The kidney also is subject to the systemic inflammatory response related to surgery and cardiopulmonary bypass.[22] Ischemia-reperfusion injury leads to intracellular depletion of high-energy phosphates, generation of oxygen free radicals, calcium accumulation, and local leukocyte activation, leading to lipid peroxidation of cell membranes. Although hypoxia may directly cause cell necrosis during renal ischemia-reperfusion, programmed cell death (apoptosis) also is important. Apoptosis involves an intracellular biochemical cascade that leads to activation of various executioner enzymes (caspases). Apoptotic cell bodies may themselves instigate further renal inflammation and injury.[23] Of interest, caspase inhibition is effective in blocking apoptotic cell death in animal models of renal ischemia-reperfusion.[23]

Inflammation within the kidney is a direct consequence of ischemia-reperfusion injury. Intracellular ATP depletion and accumulation of ionized calcium trigger the activation of nuclear factor-κB (NF-κB).[24] In turn, NF-κB–mediated activation of pro-inflammatory genes contributes to the pathophysiology of renal ischemia-reperfusion injury.[24] Finally, direct inhibition of NF-κB ameliorates ischemia-reperfusion injury in animals.

Atheroembolism

Cholesterol atheroemboli constitute a common vascular cause of intrinsic renal failure. Embolic phenomena, including formation of atheroemboli, thromboemboli, other particulate emboli, fat droplets, and air bubbles, are common during mechanical disruption of plaque during angiographic or surgical procedures; rarely, embolization occurs spontaneously. A review of data for 221 patients with cholesterol atheroembolism as the cause of nephrotoxicity revealed that only 5% of the patients were younger than 50 years of age. Associated conditions included hypertension, coronary artery disease, aortic aneurysm, cerebrovascular disease, congestive heart failure, and diabetes mellitus. Detection tools demonstrate high embolic rates, particularly during aortic manipulation such as cross-clamping and unclamping. Embolic renal vascular obstruction is poorly tolerated, and infarcts manifest in a wedge-shaped distribution involving both cortex and medulla.

Renal atheroembolism can be confused with angiography-related radiocontrast agent–induced nephropathy and is occasionally a dominant cause of post–cardiac surgery renal dysfunction. Intra-aortic filter devices used during cardiac surgery procedures routinely demonstrate macroscopic atheromatous debris.[25] Emboli may occur in showers and range in size from cholesterol microcrystals to large atherosclerotic plaques, causing a spectrum of biochemical abnormalities and renal and other organ vessel occlusion.

Extensive evidence suggests that manipulation of a diseased aorta during cardiac surgery can lead to detachment of atheromatous material, and that downstream embolism is a common and major contributor to postoperative renal dysfunction.[26] The severity of ascending aortic atherosclerosis is highly correlated with the likelihood of renal emboli. Imaging techniques that identify atheroma at the site of aortic manipulation predict renal dysfunction,[27] as do emboli counts during cardiac surgery.[28] Descending aortic plaque disruption from intra-aortic balloon pump counterpulsation is thought to be an important source of renal artery emboli and dysfunction.[29]

Other particulate fragments may embolize during cardiac surgery. A study of intra-aortic filter devices identified thrombus (14%), platelet fibrin debris (21%), and even normal vessel wall (3%) in the filter after aortic cross-clamp removal in a cohort of patients who had undergone CABG surgery.[25] Septic emboli are an important contributor to the pathophysiology of bacterial endocarditis, and one third of patients with this condition who undergo cardiac surgery will have significant postoperative renal dysfunction.

Small lipid droplets from sternal bone marrow that enter the circulation in scavenged blood also are a significant source of microemboli. These droplets probably cause "small capillary arteriolar dilatations" (SCADs), observed by funduscopy in patients who have undergone cardiac surgery. Although lipid droplets can significantly affect renal cortical blood flow, their relevance as contributors to renal insult is unclear. Nonetheless, strategies to reduce or eliminate return of lipid droplets to the circulation seem prudent, and differences exist between scavenging strategies and perfusion technologies in the clearance of these particles.

The severity of cholesterol atheroembolism is highly variable, and the degree of renal failure depends on the extent of renal involvement. The diagnosis of atheroembolism involves an initial high index of suspicion. Laboratory data may show eosinophilia, eosinophiluria, and hypocomplementemia. Typically, the onset of renal failure is delayed, but the renal failure gradually worsens during subsequent months. Although many strategies aimed at reducing atheroemboli are being incorporated into routine practice, including intraoperative epiaortic scanning and use of aortic filters and saphenous vein connector devices, very few of these innovations have been demonstrated to improve outcome. A randomized trial evaluating an intra-aortic filtration system in 1289 patients found no difference in ischemic events; however, a post hoc analysis in high-risk patients noted reduced renal complications (14% versus 24%; $P = .04$).[30]

Aprotinin

A meta-analysis of aprotinin studies in cardiac surgery populations performed between 1991 and 2005, including 27 double-blind randomized clinical trials, confirms an increase in the incidence of renal dysfunction with use of aprotinin compared with placebo (115 of 889 versus 75 of 889; $P = .006$), but not for renal failure requiring dialysis

(35 of 2349 versus 31 of 2332; $P = .71$).[31] Aprotinin is effective in reducing other insults related to cardiac surgery (e.g., anemia and transfusion) relative to placebo and even other antifibrinolytic therapies (e.g., lysine analogues).[32] Consideration of the renal risks and benefits of aprotinin must be part of any decision to use this agent. The renal risk from lysine analogue antifibrinolytic agents has not been studied in prospective outcome studies, but a single retrospective analysis of ε-aminocaproic acid (EACA) in 1502 patients did not demonstrate a change in the incidence of renal dysfunction or dialysis associated with use of EACA from that observed with no antifibrinolytic agent.[33]

RENAL RISK STRATIFICATION

A plethora of risk factors have been identified over the 45 years since the first report of acute renal failure after cardiac surgery.[34] More recent studies evaluating intermediate renal injuries in large cohorts of patients undergoing cardiac surgery with the full range of baseline renal functions have helped identify more subtle effects. Even though a wide variety of patient and procedural factors predict renal impairment, and although preoperative risk stratification algorithms have been developed, unfortunately these have little use as clinical tools in the setting of cardiac surgery. For patients with normal renal function, the current paradigm relies heavily on patient characteristics and poorly identifies those at risk.

Known risk factors for postoperative renal impairment (e.g., advanced age, African-American ethnicity, increased body weight, hypertension, carotid or peripheral atherosclerotic vascular disease, diabetes and elevated preoperative serum glucose, reduced left ventricular function and obstructive pulmonary disease, procedure-related factors [such as emergency and "redo" operations, aortic valve procedures, and operations requiring a period of circulatory arrest or extended cardiopulmonary bypass]) fail to account for much of the variation in postoperative creatinine levels relative to baseline. Knowledge of baseline renal function (serum creatinine) explains approximately 30% of creatinine rise, but this is simply due to the nonlinear response of creatinine rise with different starting creatinine values—baseline renal dysfunction is not a definitive predictor of risk of renal injury. Owing to their proximity to the dialysis threshold, however, patients with preexisting renal dysfunction are at greater risk for dialysis; nevertheless, they are *not* at greater risk for renal impairment relative to baseline.[35]

ANIMAL MODELS OF ACUTE KIDNEY INJURY IN CARDIOVASCULAR SURGERY

Animal studies play a key role in many aspects of investigation into human disease, including as tools to investigate pathophysiology and identify therapeutic strategies worthy of testing in humans. Although numerous animal models exist involving reproducible renal insults and injury that have been invaluable in elucidating the pathomechanisms of this disorder, the same cannot be said for their value as a tool to identify candidates for human renoprotective therapies.[20] For example, agents with reno-

protective properties in animal studies, such as low-dose dopamine, fenoldopam, dopexamine, furosemide, mannitol, atrial natriuretic peptide, and calcium channel blockers, all have failed when used subsequently for renoprotective interventions in randomized double-blind clinical trials involving cardiac surgery in humans.

It has been suggested that a re-evaluation of the optimal animal model to identify renoprotective agents for study in humans is due.[20] Existing acute renal injury models differ from cardiac surgery in that they usually involve a single insult, typically either renal artery clamping or exposure to a nephrotoxic agent, or rarely a combination of two renal insults.[20] Alternate models that more closely resemble cardiac surgery conditions may facilitate the search for useful renoprotective interventions. Animal models of cardiac surgery now exist,[15] including technical innovations that permit rodents to undergo cardiopulmonary bypass[35] (Fig. 178-2) and even deep hypothermic circulatory arrest. These animal models demonstrate reproducible renal impairment, including creatinine rise and histological evidence of injury, and may be useful for evaluation of candidate renoprotective therapies.[36] It remains to be seen, however, whether these models will be more reliable simulations of human post–cardiac surgery acute renal injury.

RENAL PREVENTION OUTCOME STUDIES

Interventions aimed toward improving renal outcome after cardiac surgery can be categorized in accordance with their timing relative to the occurrence of renal insult or impairment of kidney function.[37] Although rationales for strategies aimed at prophylaxis and prevention are distinctly different from those aimed at limiting extension of renal injury or hastening recovery, the term *renoprotection* has come to include them all. In the following discussion, all data regarding a specific intervention are reviewed together.

Procedure Planning and Other Nonpharmacological Modifiable Clinical Factors

Several nonpharmacological strategies aimed at reducing postoperative renal injury have been adopted in cardiac surgery. Some of these strategies have achieved limited success, whereas others have been disappointing. Nonpharmacological interventions are summarized in Table 178-1.

Preoperative decisions regarding chronic medication may influence perioperative renal risk. Despite the fact that ACE inhibitors and angiotensin I receptor blockers may precipitate acute renal failure in special circumstances, such as renal artery stenosis, these agents have not been associated with postoperative renal impairment or mortality. In fact, renal artery stenosis does not appear to significantly affect renal risk during cardiac surgery. By contrast, one retrospective study found that chronic diuretic therapy was associated with increased postoperative complications in CABG surgery.

Adequate preoperative fluid rehydration during the preoperative period may be beneficial in preventing

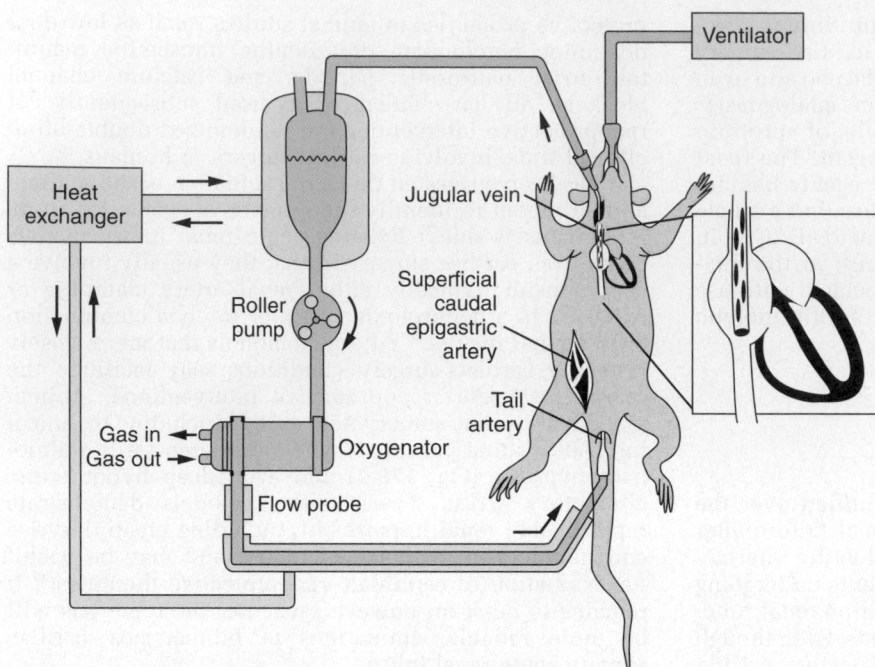

FIGURE 178-2. Schematic diagram of a rat model of cardiopulmonary bypass and deep hypothermic circulatory arrest.

postoperative renal dysfunction.[38] The use of hydroxy-ethyl starch (HES) for volume expansion is associated with renal dysfunction in surgical and critically ill patients in several retrospective reports. A randomized study of 129 critically ill septic patients found higher peak serum creatinine values and frequency of acute renal failure in patients receiving 6% HES compared with 3% gelatin.[39]

Because the duration of cardiopulmonary bypass independently predicts post–cardiac surgery renal impairment, a widely embraced renoprotective strategy is the avoidance of bypass techniques. Although small prospective studies have shown reductions in occult renal injury, until a recent paper from the Cleveland Clinic reported a lower incidence of AKI in off-pump cases than in on-pump cases,[40] the literature generally had not shown off-pump techniques to confer significant renal benefit over conventional CABG surgery. Studies of devices that reduce atheroma detachment and embolic showers during aortic manipulation have been similarly inconclusive regarding renal protection.[41] Catheter-based minimally invasive surgery, on the other hand, has been consistently associated with improved renal outcome, particularly in mitral valve surgery. Of note, however, randomized clinical trials have not focused on renal outcomes. Endovascular repair of aortic pathology may be beneficial with regard to postoperative renal dysfunction in comparison with open procedures. This benefit has been shown principally in the treatment of abdominal aortic aneurysms. More extensive studies involving thoracic aortic pathology are awaited.

Strategies aimed at modifying cardiopulmonary bypass management have been investigated for their renal effects. Hemodilution, common during cardiopulmonary bypass, is associated with postoperative renal dysfunction. Ironically, one alternative to tolerating extreme bypass hemodilution—transfusion—also has been implicated as a renal risk factor. Although extreme hemodilution (to less than 20%) has been associated with worse renal outcome in several retrospective studies, maintenance of high hemat-

ocrit also has been associated with renal dysfunction. A single prospective report evaluated three cardiopulmonary bypass hematocrit strategies but did not establish a safe "middle ground" or target hematocrit. Hypothermia during bypass, once thought to confer universal organ protection, does not provide intraoperative protection for the kidneys. Although use of higher perfusion pressures during cardiopulmonary bypass is widely practiced, this strategy does not protect against postoperative renal dysfunction. Flow during cardiopulmonary bypass, rather than pressure, may be the important determinant of renal function. Selection of one vasoactive agent over another has been suggested as a chance for renoprotection: Although vasopressin may be preferable to conventional catecholamines as a treatment for vasodilatory shock, comparison studies of the renal effects of these agents in cardiac surgery patients have not been performed.

Pharmacological Interventions

Although numerous agents showing promising renoprotection in animal models have been extensively investigated in cardiac surgical populations, very few pharmacological options are available to prevent or treat post–cardiac surgery acute renal dysfunction (Table 178-2). These various options are discussed in specific chapters and are not repeated here.

Insulin

Insulin is perhaps the one pharmacological option that is more relevant to cardiac surgery. Beyond maintenance of adequate hydration and renal perfusion, meticulous perioperative glucose management probably is the most important renal preservation strategy currently available. Return of filtered glucose by the kidney to the circulation is an active oxygen-consuming process that occurs in the proximal tubule by the phlorizin-sensitive sodium-glucose

TABLE 178-1

Nonpharmacological Interventions Assessed as Renoprotective Therapies, with Evidence-Based Assessment of Usefulness in Patients Undergoing Cardiac Surgery

PROCEDURE MODIFICATION	Evidence LEVEL*	CLASS†	NO. OF RCTS	SUMMARY COMMENT(S)
Transfusion avoidance	B	I	1	High Hct, as well as "older" blood, associated with renal dysfunction
Intravenous fluid therapy	B	IIa	1	Preoperative hydration found to be beneficial in single trial in patients with baseline renal impairment
Port access approach	B	IIa	0	Mechanism of benefit unclear
Hypothermic CPB	A	IIb	3	No benefit of hypothermia
OPCAB	B	IIb	6	Inconsistent findings in published studies
Aortic manipulation avoidance	B	IIb	1	Device use may increase manipulation and embolic showers
Endovascular aortic aneurysm repair	C	IIb	0	Benefit may be from less inflammation
CPB perfusion pressure	B	IIb	2	No benefit from higher pressures; pump flow more important than perfusion pressure
Hemodilution	B	III	1	Extreme hemodilution (Hct < 20%) worse than "mild" (Hct 24%) Ideal CPB Hct undetermined
"Fast track" management	B	III	0	Retrospective evidence of more renal failure

*A: Consistent finding across more than one RCT. B: Limited evidence. C: Very scant evidence.
†Class I: Intervention should be used; benefit >> risk. Class IIa: Reasonable to use intervention; benefit > risk. Class IIb: Intervention may be considered; benefit may outweigh risk in some circumstances. Class III: Intervention is not helpful and may be harmful; risk > benefit.
CPB, cardiopulmonary bypass; Hct, hematocrit; OPCAB, off-pump coronary artery bypass graft surgery; RCT, randomized controlled trial.

TABLE 178-2

Agents Assessed for Renoprotective Therapy, with Evidence-Based Assessment of Usefulness in Patients Undergoing Cardiac Surgery

DRUG	Evidence LEVEL*	CLASS†	NO. OF RCTS	SUMMARY COMMENT(S)
Insulin	B	I	2	Benefit is from glycemic control
α_2-Adrenergic agonists	B	IIa	23	Survival and MI benefit
Fenoldopam	B	IIb	8	May be useful in certain groups
Dopexamine	B	IIb	21	Not available in United States
Anaritide	B	IIb	2	Hypotensive effect may offset renal effect
Urodilantin	B	IIb	4	High control group dialysis rates
N-acetylcysteine	B	IIb	3	No benefit, no harm
Calcium channel blockers	B	IIb	5	No clear overall benefit
Nesiritide	C	IIb	1	Positive trial in abstract form only
Prostaglandins	B	IIb	2	Increased CrCl in treatment group
Erythropoietin	C	IIb	0	Works in animals
Growth factors	C	IIb	2	No evidence of benefit in humans
Omapatrilat	C	IIb	0	Not evaluated in humans
Pentoxifylline	C	IIb	1	Possible benefit but study small
Dopamine	A	III	>60	Should no longer be used
Loop diuretics	A	III	3	May protect mTAL at expense of DCT
Mannitol	B	III	3	Used in forced diuresis
Steroids	B	III	1	Small numbers in trial
NSAIDs	B	III	8	RCTs suggest possible harm
Adenosine antagonists	B	III	2	Underpowered studies
Endothelin antagonists	C	III	1	May be harmful
ACEIs and ARBs	C	III	0	Role largely unexplored

*A: Consistent finding across more than one RCT. B: Limited evidence. C: Very scant evidence.
†Class I: Intervention should be used; benefit >> risk. Class IIa: Reasonable to use intervention; benefit > risk. Class IIb: Intervention may be considered; benefit may outweigh risk in some circumstances. Class III: Intervention is not helpful and may be harmful; risk > benefit.
ACEIs, angiotensin-converting enzyme inhibitors; ARBs, angiotensin receptor blockers; CrCl, creatinine clearance; MI, myocardial infarction; mTAL, medullary thick ascending limb; NSAIDs, nonsteroidal anti-inflammatory drugs; RCT, randomized controlled trial.

cotransporter. Renal oxygen demand is significantly increased with hyperglycemia. Although no trials in humans have assessed intraoperative renoprotection with insulin, the Leuven study[42] enrolled 1548 critically ill patients (greater than 75% of whom were post–major surgery) randomized to intensive or conventional insulin therapy; this study found that improved glucose management resulted in better renal outcome and improved survival. Compared with conventional therapy (target glucose, 180 to 200 mg/dL), intensive insulin therapy (target in

ICU, 80 to 110 mg/dL; post-ICU target, 180 to 200 mg/dL) was associated with lower peak serum creatinine values, a 41% reduction in the need for dialysis ($P = .007$), and a 34% lower in-hospital mortality rate ($P = .01$). Analysis indicated that better metabolic control, rather than insulin dose per se, explained the beneficial effects. Of note, beyond glucose control, effects such as improved immune function, suppression of inflammation, better macrophage function, and normalization of dyslipidemia are cited as clinically relevant benefits of intensive insulin therapy on renal dysfunction, renal failure, and death.

CONCLUSION

Despite intense research efforts, renal dysfunction continues to be a major complication of cardiac surgery. Nevertheless, significant advances have occurred in characterization of this disorder, including its pathophysiology, risk factors, and relationship with outcome. In addition, advances also have been achieved in elucidation of the mechanisms of renoprotection: Although many currently used interventions aimed at renoprotection probably should be abandoned and others with promise remain incompletely investigated, several practice points remain to guide the cardiac anesthesiologist, surgeon, and intensivist. Foremost among these practice points are that (1) meticulous attention to maintenance of perioperative normoglycemia is essential and (2) transfusion can contribute to renal dysfunction and, particularly during cardiopulmonary bypass, should be considered only after all sources of hemodilution have been minimized. In addition to continuing the search for renoprotective interventions, the future of this area of concern lies in advancing animal models that more closely represent the condition and defining the role of genetic markers and other potential renal risk stratification tools (such as proteomics, metabolomics, and progenitor or stem cell reserve). Moreover, better understanding of the role of acute uremic toxins and the pathophysiological links between postoperative renal impairment and adverse outcome may allow identification of new opportunities to improve the care of patients undergoing cardiac surgery.

Key Points

1. Acute kidney injury is common after heart surgery, and the type of surgical procedure is important in determining its incidence and severity.
2. The etiology of acute kidney injury includes both clinical and genetic risk factors.
3. Few effective strategies for the prevention of acute kidney injury have been described to date.

Key References

3. Cooper WA, et al: Impact of renal dysfunction on outcomes of coronary artery bypass surgery: Results from the Society of Thoracic Surgeons National Adult Cardiac Database. Circulation 2006;113:1063-1070.
17. Stafford-Smith M, et al: Association of genetic polymorphisms with risk of renal injury after coronary artery bypass graft surgery. Am J Kidney Dis 2005;45:519-530.
40. Hix JK, et al: Effect of off-pump coronary artery bypass graft surgery on postoperative acute kidney injury and mortality. Crit Care Med 2006;34:2979-2983.

See the companion Expert Consult website for the complete reference list.

CHAPTER 179

Renal Function in Congestive Heart Failure

Mark Crandall and Sunil Mankad

OBJECTIVES

This chapter will:
1. Present an overview of the epidemiology of and proposed definitions for aggravated renal dysfunction in congestive heart failure.
2. Identify clinical predictors of renal failure in the setting of congestive heart failure.
3. Review the pathophysiology of the cardiorenal syndrome and identify renal adaptations to congestive heart failure.

Decreased renal function often is seen in congestive heart failure.[1] Furthermore, the specific treatments for acute decompensated heart failure, including the use of diuretics and vasodilators, can further exacerbate renal dysfunction.[2] *Cardiorenal syndrome* is the name used to describe the downward spiral of worsening heart failure and kidney failure that leads to further volume overload, low renal plasma flow, and diuretic resistance. A common alternative name for this syndrome in the literature is *aggravated renal dysfunction* (ARD).

The complex pathophysiology behind the cardiac and renal interactions in the cardiorenal syndrome remains unclear, but emerging data suggest that the decline in cardiac function is synergistic with the decline in renal function, and that the cardiorenal syndrome has distinct properties not occurring in conditions that affect either organ alone.[3] The definition of the cardiorenal syndrome is somewhat arbitrary, however. Several studies in patients hospitalized for management of heart failure have used a threshold of a 0.3-mg/dL (26.5-mmol/L) rise in serum creatinine to define the cardiorenal syndrome.[4-6] Changes of this magnitude occur in 25% to 45% of patients hospitalized for heart failure treatment.[7] Other studies have defined the cardiorenal syndrome as a 25% or greater increase in serum creatinine.[8]

Because of the lack of a uniform definition, the true prevalence of the cardiorenal syndrome has been difficult to ascertain. It is estimated that renal insufficiency develops in one third to one half of patients with heart failure,[9] defined by the National Kidney Foundation as a glomerular filtration rate (GFR) of less than 60 mL/minute per 1.73 m^2 of body surface.[10,11] In the Evaluation of Losartan in the Elderly (ELITE) heart failure trial, in which the effects of captopril (an ACE inhibitor) were compared with those of losartan (an angiotensin receptor blocker), 29.7% of the patients in the captopril group and 26.1% of those in the losartan group experienced worsening renal function.[12] Similarly, Forman and colleagues found that renal function deteriorated in 27% of patients hospitalized for heart failure treatment.[4] Weinfeld and colleagues reported that ARD developed in 21% of patients hospitalized for management of heart failure, occurring more often in older patients with lower baseline creatinine clearance.[8]

CLINICAL PREDICTORS AND OUTCOMES IN PATIENTS WITH CARDIORENAL DYSFUNCTION

Patients with the cardiorenal syndrome have high rates of mortality and morbidity. Butler and colleagues demonstrated that an increase in creatinine of 0.3 mg/dL or greater predicted in-hospital mortality with 65% sensitivity and 81% specificity.[13] In addition, this degree of renal dysfunction in hospitalized heart failure patients is associated with longer length of stay, increased risk of death at 6 months after discharge, and higher rates of readmission.[14] Weinfeld and colleagues confirmed that ARD was not only common in patients admitted for treatment of advanced heart failure but also associated with worse survival at 1 year[8] (Fig. 179-1).

Several studies have identified risk factors for worsening renal function in patients with advanced heart failure. Patients in whom ARD develops generally are older and have a higher prevalence of diabetes, hypertension, and prior heart failure and a greater degree of renal dysfunction.[4,5] Low ejection fraction was associated with the development of renal insufficiency in the Studies of Left Ventricular Dysfunction (SOLVD) trial.[15] By contrast, however, other studies have suggested that patients with heart failure in whom ARD develops are not more likely to have systolic dysfunction and that ejection fraction does not correlate with the development of the cardiorenal syndrome.[4,5,13] Of interest, worsening renal function does not always appear to be characterized by a "low-output state," as indicated by the fact that a greater proportion of these patients actually have higher blood pressures and less fatigue compared with patients who do not go on to

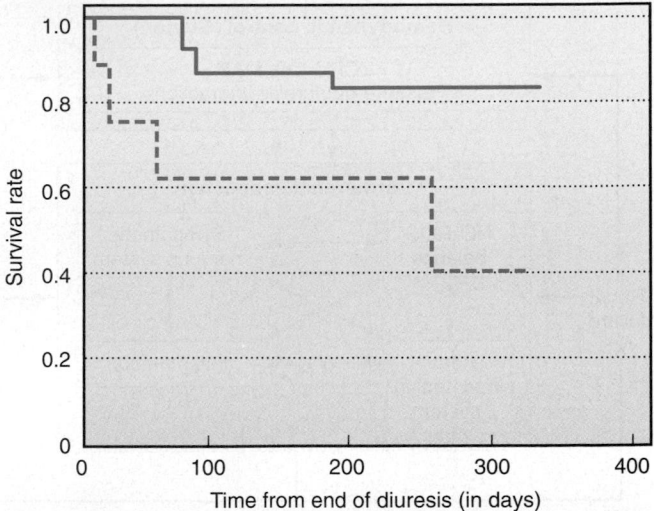

FIGURE 179-1. Kaplan-Meier plot of survival rate versus time from end of diuresis in days for 10 patients with *(dashed line)* and 38 patients without *(solid line)* aggravated renal dysfunction (ARD), demonstrating worse survival with ARD (*P* = .002). (From Weinfeld MS, Chertow GM, Stevenson L: Aggravated renal dysfunction during intensive therapy for advanced chronic heart failure. Am Heart J 1999;138:285-290.)

TABLE 179-1

Clinical Predictors of Renal Failure in Patients with Heart Failure

- Old age
- Low ejection fraction
- Low systolic blood pressure
- Elevated baseline serum creatinine level
- Diabetes mellitus
- Hypertension
- Use of antiplatelet therapy, diuretics, or beta blockers

develop renal failure.[13] It now appears that vascular mediators such as nitric oxide, prostaglandins, natriuretic peptides, and endothelin affect renal perfusion independently of cardiac hemodynamics.[4] Although higher doses of diuretics in patients hospitalized for heart failure have been independently associated with increased risk of death,[13] the degree of diuresis and weight loss does not appear to predict the development of the cardiorenal syndrome.[13] Another interesting and unexpected finding in the study by Weinfeld and colleagues was an association between atrial fibrillation and the development of ARD.[8] Table 179-1 lists factors that correlated with worsening renal function in the Studies of Left Ventricular Dysfunction (SOLVD) trial although not all of these factors were reproduced in all studies evaluating risk factors for development of the cardiorenal syndrome.[12,15]

THE CARDIORENAL SYNDROME

The interactions and feedback mechanisms involved in heart and kidney failure are much more complex than was previously thought. The classic understanding of kidney

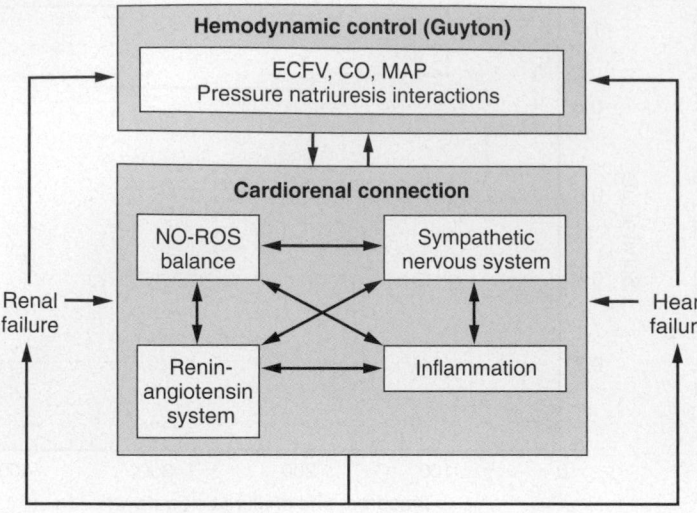

FIGURE 179-2. Pathophysiological basis of the severe cardiorenal syndrome. The model of Guyton explains heart-kidney interaction with respect to blood pressure and extracellular fluid volume (ECFV). When one of the organs fails, a vicious circle develops in which the renin-angiotensin system, nitric oxide (NO)–reactive oxygen species (ROS) balance, the sympathetic nervous system, and inflammation interact and synergize. CO, cardiac output; MAP, mean arterial pressure. (Redrawn from Bongartz LG, Cramer MJ, Braam B: The cardiorenal connection [letter]. Hypertension 2004;43:14.)

dysfunction in heart failure was that low renal plasma flow signaled the kidneys to retain sodium and water to bolster circulatory pressure and improve perfusion to vital organs.[14] It is now thought that both hemodynamic adaptations of the kidney and mechanisms that are independent of cardiac hemodynamics are involved (Fig. 179-2). The renal hemodynamic response to chronic heart failure is characterized by low renal plasma flow with relative preservation of GFR. This relative preservation of GFR results in an increased filtration fraction. Filtration fraction is preserved until cardiac function is severely impaired. The major mechanism for this preservation of GFR and filtration fraction is through a striking increase in efferent arteriolar resistance and glomerular capillary hydrostatic pressure. Because of this degree of constant efferent arteriolar vasoconstriction, further compensation is not possible in case of decreases in renal perfusion pressure, so hypotension can lead to a major decrease in GFR.[16] In addition to these changes in GFR control, enhanced sodium reabsorption in the loop of Henle also appears to play a significant role in the cardiorenal syndrome.[17]

Multiple neurohormonal factors are responsible for most of the alterations associated with the cardiorenal syndrome. Most important are the sympathetic system and the renin-angiotensin system. This neurohumoral activation occurs together with increased arginine vasopressin release and endothelin release, resulting in systemic vasoconstriction, preservation of GFR, and antidiuresis.[18] This initially compensatory response attempts to preserve or optimize cardiac output, arterial blood pressure, and GFR. GFR preservation is further supported by the release of prostaglandins, which induce afferent arteriolar vasodilation, although low baseline resistance to renal blood flow also may be maintained through nitric oxide release.[19] In heart failure, however, the final result of this neurohormonal response may be the development of a congestive state with peripheral edema. Inappropriate activation of the renin-angiotensin system also leads to activation of nicotinamide adenine dinucleotide phosphate (reduced) (NADPH) oxidase by angiotensin II, leading to the formation of reactive oxygen species.[3,20] The critical role that the renin-angiotensin system plays in the cardiorenal syndrome suggests the possibility of a treatment paradox: ACE inhibitor therapy in patients with heart failure plus renal insufficiency is clearly associated with significant long-term benefits but hypothetically may acutely exacerbate

the cardiorenal syndrome. In fact, however, this does not appear to occur, because ACE inhibitors are not associated with worsening renal function in patients hospitalized for management of heart failure.[13] Clinical decisions will need to be individualized, but in most patients with heart failure who are already on an ACE inhibitor, slight worsening of renal function as a result of the cardiorenal syndrome does not constitute an indication to stop ACE inhibitor therapy.

Nitric oxide is involved in vasodilation, natriuresis, and desensitization of tubuloglomerular feedback.[21] It also inhibits several components of atherogenesis, inhibits smooth muscle cell proliferation,[22] and increases angiogenesis by ensuring delivery of vascular endothelial growth factor.[23] Nitric oxide also inhibits platelet aggregation, endothelial adhesion molecule expression, and leukocyte–endothelial cell interactions.[24] In renal failure, the balance between nitric oxide and reactive oxygen species is shifted. A relative deficiency of nitric oxide results from the reaction of nitric oxide and free radicals. The aforementioned mechanisms offer a plausible explanation for how decreased nitric oxide and increased oxidative stress in patients with renal failure lead to increased risk for cardiac events.

Atherosclerosis is now understood to be essentially an inflammatory process,[25] and several markers of inflammation are increased in both congestive heart failure and chronic renal insufficiency.[3] C-reactive protein has numerous pro-inflammatory and proatherogenic effects and is thought to have a role in the pathogenesis of atherosclerosis.[26] It is elevated in end-stage renal failure and probably has a synergistic role in the progression of both renal and cardiovascular disease.[27] In one study, elevated C-reactive protein combined with renal insufficiency had more than an additive effect on the incidence of myocardial infarction and death.[28]

The sympathetic nervous system stimulates the release of renin by means of sympathetic neurons. Catecholamines produce hemodynamic changes in the glomerulus similar to those of angiotensin II (elevated systemic vascular resistance and sodium retention).[14] Peripheral sympathetic nerve activity increases in end-stage renal disease but corrects when the diseased kidneys are removed.[29] The complex interactions involved in ARD eventually lead to a compensatory response that involves several natriuretic factors, such as atrial natriuretic factor, brain natriuretic factor, and urodilatin.[30] The clinician must therefore appreciate that a deceptively normal GFR in patients with CHF often represents a fragile level of pathophysiological compensation. Alteration of any of its components may result in a clinically important degree of decompensation. Also of importance, despite the compensatory role that brain natriuretic factor plays in heart failure, nesiritide does not appear to improve renal function in patients with decompensated heart failure, mild chronic renal insufficiency, and renal function that had worsened from baseline.[32]

CONCLUSION

Worsening renal function in the setting of congestive heart failure has been termed the cardiorenal syndrome. Patients with this clinical syndrome are at greater risk for mortality and morbidity than would be predicted by either disease entity alone. Renal and heart failure are synergistic, and the pathophysiology involves complex mechanisms beyond hemodynamic interactions. The exact interplay among the renin-angiotensin system, the sympathetic nervous system, nitric oxide, reactive oxygen species, and inflammation remains poorly understood.

Key Points

1. Cardiorenal syndrome is the term used to characterize the downward spiral of worsening renal function that leads to further volume overload, low renal plasma flow, and diuretic resistance often seen in patients with heart failure.

2. The cardiorenal syndrome is not always associated with a low cardiac output state, but clinical predictors such as older age and poor baseline renal function are well recognized.

3. Although the pathophysiology of the cardiorenal syndrome remains incompletely understood, it appears to be characterized by abnormalities in the renin-angiotensin system, the sympathetic nervous system, nitric oxide, reactive oxygen species, and inflammation.

4. The initial compensatory mechanisms eventually fail, and the changes associated with the cardiorenal syndrome become pathological, with increased morbidity and mortality.

Key References

4. Forman DE, Butler J, Wang Y, et al: Incidence, predictors at admission, and impact of worsening renal function among patients hospitalized with heart failure. J Am Coll Cardiol 2004;43:61-67.
6. Hillege HL, Girbes AR, deKam PJ, et al: Renal function, neurohormonal activation, and survival in patients with chronic heart failure. Circulation 2000;102:203-210.
7. Shlipak MG, Massie BM: The clinical challenge of cardiorenal syndrome. Circulation 2004;110;1514-1517.
8. Weinfeld MS, Chertow GM, Stevenson L: Aggravated renal dysfunction during intensive therapy for advanced chronic heart failure. Am Heart J 1999;138:285-290.
13. Butler J, Forman DE, Abraham WT, et al: Relationship between heart failure treatment and development of worsening renal function among hospitalized patients. Am Heart J 2004;147:331-338.

See the companion Expert Consult website for the complete reference list.

CHAPTER 180

Acute Renal Failure after Cardiac Surgery

Charuhas V. Thakar and Emil P. Paganini

OBJECTIVES
This chapter will:
1. Examine the incidence of acute renal failure after cardiac surgery.
2. Evaluate the evidence regarding risk factors for postoperative acute renal failure.
3. Summarize the effects of acute renal failure on morbidity and mortality after cardiac surgery.
4. Review the present evidence regarding early diagnosis and treatment of postoperative acute renal failure.

Acute renal failure (ARF) after cardiac surgery is one of the most serious postoperative complications. The incidence of postoperative ARF is relatively low, but the mortality rate in ARF is strikingly high, usually exceeding 50% in patients in whom ARF requiring dialysis develops. Although attempts to prevent or treat ARF have yielded limited success, the clinical setting of cardiac surgery offers an exciting opportunity to improve patient outcomes in kidney injury—a setting in which, optimally, renal insult could be anticipated, preoperative risk factors could be identified, and ARF of variable degree could be correlated with morbidity and mortality during the postoperative period. These efforts have an inherent benefit of risk stratification to optimize clinical management, as well as maximizing awareness of postoperative outcomes, including health care utilization both during hospitalization and beyond.

This chapter discusses the incidence of and risk factors for the development of ARF after cardiac surgery, summarizes the effects of ARF on postoperative outcomes, and reviews modalities of therapy that have been used to prevent or treat kidney injury. A point worthy of emphasis is that the available clinical evidence related to this topic derives almost entirely from observational studies, with the exception of a few small interventional studies. Thus, the risk of renal failure or prediction of associated hospital outcome has to be interpreted after the clinical decision for cardiac surgery was made. Thus, strictly from a study design point of view, in absence of randomized data with feasible alternative therapies, the risk of poor postoperative outcome is hardly a contraindication to the performance of cardiac surgery. Rather, it can be viewed as an opportunity to improve patient outcomes in ARF.

INCIDENCE OF AND RISK FACTORS FOR ACUTE RENAL FAILURE

Incidence of ARF after cardiac surgery depends on its definition. When ARF is defined in its most severe form as requiring dialysis, the incidence of ARF usually is low, at less than 5%.[1,2] With milder degrees of renal dysfunction, the incidence shows a wide variation in the reported literature. When ARF is defined as a 50% drop in estimated GFR (or an analogous rise in serum creatinine), the frequency of ARF ranges between 5% and 10%.[3,4] Although a clinically relevant threshold of renal dysfunction in the setting of cardiac surgery remains undetermined, recent evidence strongly suggests that even a 25% to 30% increase in serum creatinine level in the immediate postoperative period is an independent predictor of increased morbidity and mortality.[4,5]

Several studies have identified risk factors for ARF after cardiac surgery.[3,6-9] The risk of ARF is influenced by preoperative comorbid diseases, intraoperative events and factors including type of surgical procedure, and postoperative complications. As shown in Table 180-1, demographic characteristics such as female gender and older age have been identified as predictors of ARF in large cohort studies. Insulin-requiring diabetes, peripheral vascular disease, and functional classification of congestive heart failure are some of the important risk factors for ARF, also consistently shown to be associated with ARF in several studies. Additionally, greater than 70% blockage of the left main coronary artery, prior open heart surgery, need for emergency surgery, and preoperative use of intra-aortic balloon pump (IABP) all predict increased risk for ARF and may serve as surrogates for the severity of ischemic heart disease.

Although multiple intraoperative events are recognized to facilitate ischemic renal injury, few have been studied rigorously. Duration of cardiopulmonary bypass probably is the most important surrogate to the intraoperative events. Additionally, exposure to the bypass circuit is known to activate inflammatory cascades, but a direct causal effect on renal injury remains unclear in clinical settings. Epidemiological data suggest that median bypass time greater than 100 minutes is associated with a signifi-

TABLE 180-1

Risk Factors for Development of Acute Renal Failure after Cardiac Surgery

Preoperative Risk Factors	Intraoperative Risk Factors
Age	Duration of cardiopulmonary bypass
Female gender	Valvular surgery
Insulin-requiring diabetes mellitus	Combined CABG and valve procedure
Chronic obstructive pulmonary disease	Increased requirement for transfusion
Congestive heart failure	On-pump versus off-pump surgery
Left ventricular fraction <40%	Aortic cross-clamp time
Use of intra-aortic balloon pump	**Postoperative Risk Factors**
Prior cardiac surgery	Cardiovascular complications
Emergency surgery	Sepsis syndrome, septic shock
Left main coronary artery occlusion >70%	
Peripheral vascular disease	
Preoperative chronic kidney disease	

CABG, coronary artery bypass grafting.

cant increase in the risk of development of ARF. The type of cardiac surgical procedure also influences the risk of postoperative ARF, independent of bypass time. Patients undergoing valvular surgery, with or without coronary artery bypass grafting (CABG), are at a greater risk for the development of ARF, compared with those undergoing CABG alone.

Chertow and colleagues were among the first to develop a preoperative renal risk stratification algorithm based on the VA Coronary Artery Surgery Study experience.[6] Patients, predominantly males, were stratified on the basis of dichotomous variables of comorbid disease burden in order to calculate the estimated probability (area under the curve [AUC] = 0.72) of postoperative ARF requiring dialysis. To improve the clinical utility of risk assessment, a more recent study incorporated graded severity of comorbid disease burden in a cohort consisting of 70% males and 30% females. Thakar and colleagues examined the Cleveland Clinic Cardiothoracic Registry to create an ARF scoring model (Fig. 180-1) with an improved predictive accuracy (AUC = 0.85) that incorporated the simultaneous effects of multiple risk factors on the risk of ARF.[10] Predicting postoperative ARF risk can be viewed as either a clinical or a clinical research tool. It is important to increase the overall awareness of risk of ARF, because despite its low incidence, ARF portends a poor hospital outcome. In programs with a high volume of cardiac surgical procedures performed, predictive algorithms also could be used as policy-making tools, in terms of anticipating the burden of resource utilization. Additionally, identification of high-risk patients provides an opportunity to modify and optimize preoperative care. As a research tool, preoperative risk stratification provides an "epidemiological platform" from which to plan translational studies related to early diagnosis or intervention in ARF.

Most of the risk factors considered thus far include the effect of preoperative or intraoperative status on the risk of ARF. The interrelationship between nonrenal postoperative complications and development of ARF after cardiac surgery is less well understood. In a recent

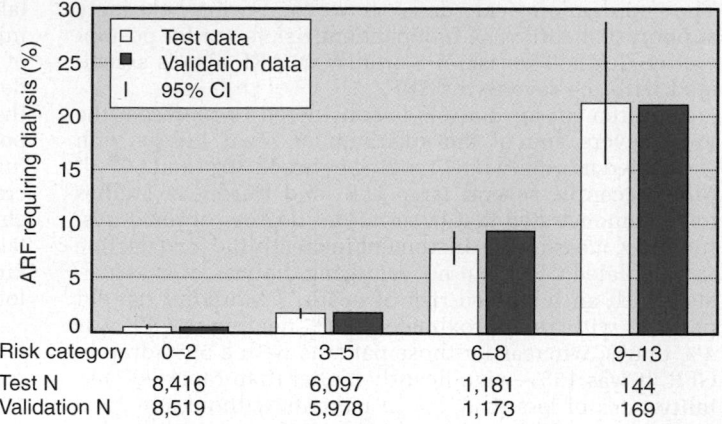

Risk category	0–2	3–5	6–8	9–13
Test N	8,416	6,097	1,181	144
Validation N	8,519	5,978	1,173	169

FIGURE 180-1. Score to predict acute renal failure requiring dialysis. ARF, acute renal failure; CABG, coronary artery bypass grafting; CHF, congestive heart failure; COPD, chronic obstructive pulmonary disease; IABP, intra-aortic balloon pump; IDDM, insulin-dependent diabetes mellitus; LVEF, left ventricular ejection fraction. (Data from Thakar CV, Arrigain S, Worley S, et al: A clinical score to predict acute renal failure after cardiac surgery. J Am Soc Nephrol 2005;16:162-168.)

Risk factor	Score points
Female	1
CHF	1
LVEF<35%	1
Pre-op IABP	2
COPD	1
IDDM	1
Prior surgery	1
Emergency surgery	2
Surgery type:	
Valve only	1
CABG + valve	2
Other	2
Pre-op creatinine:	
1.2 to < 2.1 mg/dL	2
2.1 mg/dL or greater	5

study of patients undergoing cardiac transplantation, researchers examined the temporal association between severe ARF and other serious, nonrenal complications developing in the intensive care unit (ICU).[11] Of interest, a majority of patients who required postoperative dialysis had sustained cardiovascular or serious infection complications before the initiation of dialysis. Sepsis syndrome or septic shock developed in relatively few patients after initiation of dialysis for ARF. Similar observations have been confirmed by demonstrating an association between postoperative cardiogenic shock and postoperative ARF.[12] These data suggest that, more often than not, postoperative multiorgan system failure usually precedes severe ARF.

Of note, much of the current understanding regarding risk stratification or interrelationship between renal and nonrenal postoperative complications involves patients in whom severe ARF requiring dialysis develops. Very few studies have examined the renal risk assessment to predict milder yet clinically relevant degrees of ARF. As the definition of ARF becomes more "liberal," the accuracy of prediction, based on clinical and comorbid factors, becomes poorer. It is increasingly recognized that milder degrees of renal dysfunction independently influence patient outcomes, and that a graded association exists between degree of renal injury and magnitude of association with death. It is possible that patients with ARF requiring dialysis form a more "homogeneous" group of patients wherein this definition of ARF is a rather accurate measure of the degree of severity of injury. By contrast, in the group of patients with milder degrees of ARF, a proportion of those with prerenal azotemia may suffer transient reversible reductions in glomerular filtration rate (GFR), as reflected by mildly elevated creatinine levels. Targeting those patients who are at a higher risk of poor hospital outcome remains a challenging task, in absence of a consensus on clinically relevant threshold of renal dysfunction in non–dialysis-requiring patients.

ACUTE RENAL FAILURE AND MORBIDITY AND MORTALITY AFTER CARDIAC SURGERY

From early studies in the 1970s, it was correctly observed that ARF after cardiac surgery carries a "bad prognosis" during the postoperative period.[13] Although the overall mortality rates after cardiac surgery are low (2% to 5%), the mortality rate among patients in whom ARF subsequently develops usually exceeds 50%. A prevalent notion had been that ARF is a proxy to the severity of other medical illnesses, and its causal association is still debated.

The epidemiological data, however, overwhelmingly support that ARF is an independent risk factor for postoperative death. The risk of mortality in ARF also is associated with the severity of ARF.

Requirement for dialysis is considered to represent the most severe end of the spectrum of renal injury, with associated mortality rates ranging between 30% and 60%.[14] More recently, several large U.S. and European studies have demonstrated that even milder degrees of renal dysfunction, measured as increment in creatinine (or a decline in calculated GFR), but not requiring dialysis, was associated with an increased risk of death.[4,5] Mortality rate for patients with an approximately 30% decline in GFR was 4% to 6%, whereas for those patients with a 50% drop in GFR, it was 15%—significantly higher than reported mortality rates of less than 1% in patients without any renal dysfunction. These data raise an important question regarding the clinically relevant threshold for ARF. For example, a 10% to 20% drop in GFR (or an equivalent increase in serum creatinine) independently predicts a bad hospital outcome, but whether it truly represents kidney tissue damage or reversibility remains unclear. One possible explanation is that a very mild increment in serum creatinine may not necessarily represent a significant ischemic injury; however, it does serve as a marker for poor prognosis. Thus, changes in creatinine may not be necessarily viewed as an accurate measure of GFR but rather may be regarded as a marker for poor hospital outcome. Unless tissue-specific biomarkers that can accurately assess kidney damage (à la renal troponin) are identified, such considerations will remain a matter of debate. Regardless of certain gaps in current understanding, the evidence leads to the consensus that the risk of death in ARF is proportional to the degree of severity of acute kidney injury, measured according to the prevalent standards of care. Undoubtedly, attempts to prevent or treat ARF are key to improving patient outcomes.

Level of baseline renal function is an important predictor of postoperative ARF—higher the preoperative creatinine, greater the risk of postoperative ARF. Additionally, it also influences the risk of mortality independent of ARF. Thus, the interaction between preoperative renal function and postoperative ARF for its effect on mortality is of important clinical relevance. For example, an absolute change in creatinine (or estimated GFR) may not portend similar mortality risk for a different baseline renal function. The data indicate that as the baseline kidney disease advances, it becomes an increasingly important contributor to postoperative mortality, even with very subtle acute changes in GFR.[4] Such observations are especially important in evaluating the occurrence of postoperative ARF in patients with underlying chronic kidney disease, because the episode of ARF will affect the short-term hospital outcome and may have an influence on renal recovery.

Although ARF after cardiac surgery predicts poor prognosis during hospitalization, the rates of recovery of renal function among those patients who survive are encouraging. Of those patients who sustain severe ARF requiring dialysis and who survive the hospitalization, a majority (more than 90%) recover sufficient renal function to allow discontinuation of dialysis. In the same study, Loef and colleagues observed that of those patients who experience a milder increment in serum creatinine during the postoperative period, approximately 70% exhibit a return to baseline levels at the time of discharge.[12] The effect of episodes of ARF on chronic progression of kidney disease remains unclear in the clinical setting. Ample experimen-

tal evidence, however, indicates that ischemia-reperfusion injury leads to kidney tissue damage with progressive loss of structure and function.[15,16] It is possible that the current definitions of "recovery" of renal function are limited in that they are based on rather short-term follow-up endpoints, such as discharge from the hospital. Additionally, functional recovery of glomerular filtration rate (i.e., serum creatinine) may not necessarily represent irreversible changes in kidney parenchyma that may become important in influencing either the underlying natural history of kidney disease progression or other organ systems in the long term.

ARF after cardiac surgery is associated with poor long-term survival. Patients in whom ARF develops during the postoperative period have twice as much risk of dying at 100 months as that in patients in whom ARF did not develop.[14] Of note, the observed long-term mortality rates were similar in ARF patients whether or not they had recovered their renal function at the time of hospital discharge. It raises the question regarding the ability of serum creatinine determination to accurately quantify "kidney function," in that it does not describe how other organ systems are affected. An important limitation to these findings is that such evidence relies on long-term outcomes reported on surveys or questionnaires. These are valid tools in acquiring information on mortality, but their value is limited in examining the influence of other risk factors that may have changed over the duration of follow-up. Thus, the association of long-term mortality with an event such as ARF during index hospitalization needs to be interpreted with caution in the absence of detailed longitudinal data.

The interrelationship between ARF and other major postoperative complications is complex. It has been long recognized that ARF after cardiac surgery was associated with bleeding complications, including gastrointestinal bleeding, in critically ill patients. Patients with ARF are at increased risk for the development of nonrenal complications such as infections in the ICU, including sepsis syndrome and septic shock[17] (Fig. 180-2). This risk seems to be strikingly accentuated in patients in whom severe ARF requiring dialysis develops but also is high in milder degrees of ARF, compared with patients without ARF. Thus, the epidemiological findings suggest that intervention in ARF may offer benefit in reducing nonrenal serious postoperative complications.

ACUTE RENAL FAILURE AFTER CARDIAC TRANSPLANTATION

Cardiac transplantation represents a relatively unique setting among patients undergoing cardiac surgery. By historical comparison, the incidence of severe ARF requiring dialysis is greater after transplantation (6%) than after nontransplantation cardiac surgery (less than 2%).[18,19] The reasons behind this difference may have to do with different patient characteristics and exposure to nephrotoxic agents during the postoperative period. In a recent large single-center study, preoperative serum creatinine, serum albumin, insulin-requiring diabetes status, and duration on cardiopulmonary bypass were identified as independent predictors of severe ARF.[11] Such risk-stratifying tools may assist in deciding postoperative protocols to determine the exposure to nephrotoxic immunosuppressive agents.

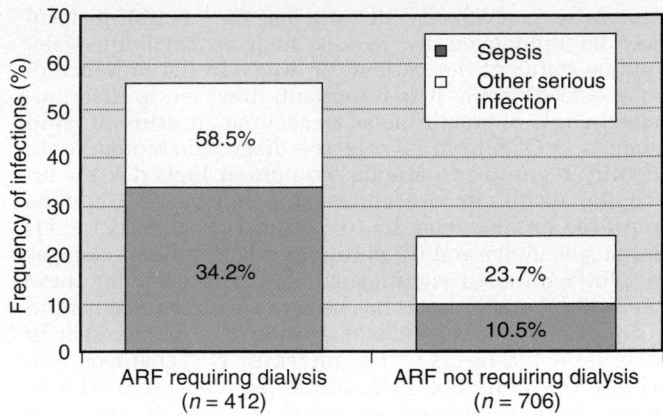

FIGURE 180-2. Risk of infections and sepsis in acute renal failure after cardiac surgery. ARF, acute renal failure. (Data from Thakar CV, Yared JP, Worley S, et al: Renal dysfunction and serious infections after open-heart surgery. Kidney Int 2003;64:239-246.)

(Chi-square test of dependence: Serious infection: $P < .001$; sepsis: $P < .001$)

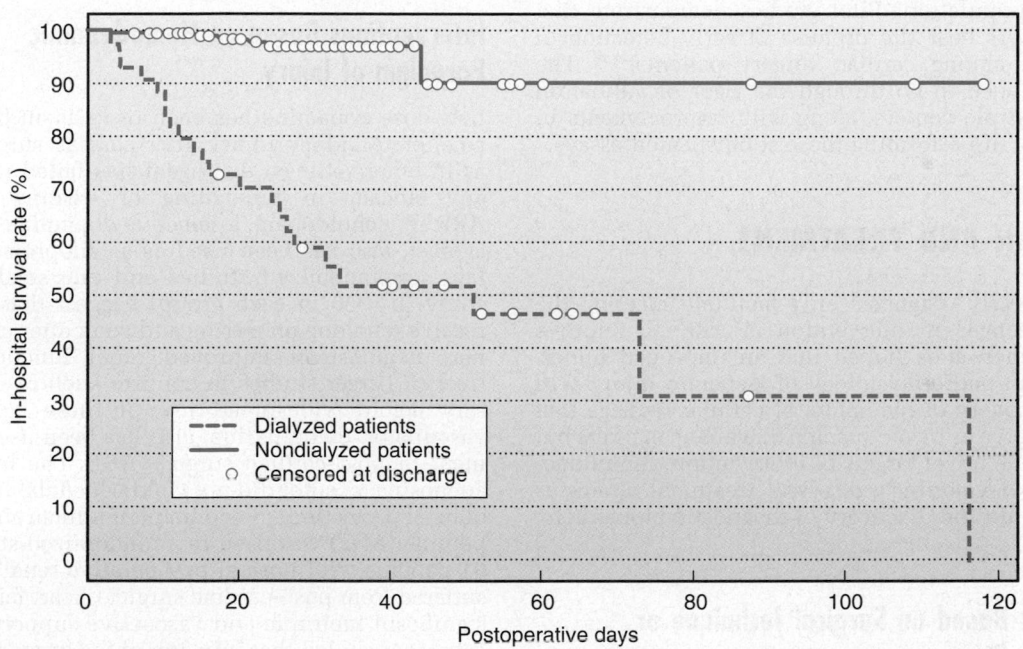

FIGURE 180-3. Survival in acute renal failure after cardiac transplantation. (Data from Boyle JM, Moualla S, Arrigain S, et al: Risks and outcomes of acute kidney injury requiring dialysis after cardiac transplantation. Am J Kidney Dis 2006;48:787-796.)

The outcomes in ARF after cardiac transplantation are similar to those for nontransplantation cardiac surgery and may represent a much more serious impact in view of the shortage of replacement organs. Among patients with severe ARF requiring dialysis, the mortality rate during hospitalization is 50%[11] (Fig. 180-3). A majority of the patients who survived were able to recover sufficient renal function to allow discontinuation of dialysis before hospital discharge. Availability of longitudinal follow-up, by way of institutional or national transplant registries, allows the transplantation setting to evaluate long-term outcomes in ARF in a much more useful manner than is available for nontransplantation cardiac surgery. A large cohort study that examined the United Network for Organ Sharing (UNOS) experience found that an episode of ARF during the immediate post-transplantation period was an independent risk factor for progression to end-stage renal disease in cardiac and other nonrenal solid organ trans-

plant recipients.[20] In the "clinical model" of renal disease in solid organ transplantation, however, the natural history of progression is dominated by exposure to long-term calcineurin use; thus, these findings are difficult to generalize to other clinical settings.

EARLY DIAGNOSIS

The topic of early diagnosis in ARF is discussed in much greater detail in other sections. The following discussion is limited to the present evidence related to cardiac surgery patients. An ideal diagnostic biomarker still evades the morbidity of ARF. As a component of standard care, determination of serum creatinine remains the widely used measure of changes in GFR. The use of serum creatinine as a surrogate for rapid changes in GFR has its limitations:

Especially in critically ill patients, the creatinine level may be influenced by factors such as catabolic state, volume status of the patient, or drugs, in the presence of a non–steady state. It is important, however, to discriminate the role of creatinine as an accurate measure of rapid changes in GFR from its role as a diagnostic biomarker to identify a group of patients who are at high risk for in-hospital death. Its usefulness as a biomarker could be improved on, however, by two critical characteristics: (1) tissue specificity and (2) ability to reflect sudden changes in GFR without a significant delay. The need for these latter two characteristics has been the driving force behind a rapidly advancing field of discovery of biomarkers in early ischemic injury.[21] It is increasingly recognized that within the complex pathophysiology of acute kidney injury, several biomarkers represent various stages of kidney injury. Interleukin-18 and neutrophil gelatinase-associated lipocalin (NGAL) are two proteins involved in inflammatory cascade of ischemic injury that have been tested in the clinical setting of cardiac surgery in a pediatric patient population. Pilot studies demonstrate that these biomarkers bear the promise of early detection of kidney injury among cardiac surgery patients.[22,23] The markers now need to go through the rigor of validation studies at multiple centers, along with improvements in the technology of performing these sophisticated assays.

PREVENTION AND TREATMENT

Advances in early diagnosis only facilitate meeting the next immense task of intervention in ARF: to improve patient outcomes. It is hoped that an improved understanding of the pathophysiology of ischemic injury will allow the discovery of mediators of cellular damage that not only can serve as tissue specific diagnostic markers but also can provide novel targets of intervention. Simultaneous efforts at developing successful treatment strategies are needed to aid the discovery of diagnostic biomarkers.

Interventions Based on Surgical Technique or Dialysis Modality

Probably the most compelling evidence, albeit retrospective, of any intervention that is associated with a reduced risk of ARF after cardiac surgery is the role of off-pump coronary artery surgery. Off-pump bypass is increasingly offered as an alternative technique in suitable patients that is comparable to on-pump surgery in terms of short-term and long-term cardiovascular outcomes. Although the randomized controlled studies focused on cardiovascular outcomes, they did not report any benefit in terms of ARF risk reduction. Owing to very low event rates of ARF requiring dialysis, however, the studies were underpowered to test renal outcomes. Ascione and coworkers reported changes in creatinine clearance during the intraoperative and immediate postoperative periods in 50 patients randomized to undergo on- or off-pump surgery. The study indicated a significant decline in creatinine clearance within the first two postoperative days in the on-pump group compared with the off-pump group.[24] Hix and associates examined the effect of off-pump surgery in a propensity-matched cohort of more than 1000 patients.[25] The odds of developing ARF (defined in two ways as AKI requiring dialysis or 50% decline in GFR but not requiring dialysis)

were twofold higher with exposure to the bypass circuit. Additionally, the study demonstrated a link between reduced risk of ARF and improved survival after off-pump cardiac surgery. These reports have been confirmed in different centers in separate cohorts of cardiac surgery patients, which increase their validity.[26] Taken together, the data suggest that in suitable patients, off-pump procedures may be preferable.

Modalities of dialysis support (or dose) in severe ARF have not been well studied in the cardiac surgery setting. Thus, the prevalent standards of dialysis support in critically ill patients still apply to this patient population. Certain intraoperative techniques, such as modified ultrafiltration during cardiopulmonary bypass, have been studied to examine its effect on postoperative outcomes, but randomized studies did not yield any beneficial results in terms of mortality or health resource utilization.[27]

Interventions Based on Hemodynamic Paradigm of Injury

Low-dose dopamine has been used as an intervention to ameliorate kidney injury after cardiac surgery; however, as in other settings, this agent has failed to demonstrate any efficacy in preventing or treating postoperative ARF.[28,29] Fenoldopam, a selective dopamine DA-1 receptor agonist, also has been used as a renoprotective agent. A few nonrandomized studies and one small randomized study ($n = 80$ in each group) suggest that patients who receive fenoldopam during and soon after cardiac surgery may demonstrate improved renal function postoperatively.[30] Larger studies to confirm such results are necessary before widespread use of these agents. Another vasodilator, theophylline, also has been used in the treatment of post–cardiac surgery ARF. The blockade of A_1 adenosine receptor did not yield beneficial results in terms of renal protection.[31] Recombinant human atrial natriuretic peptide (ANP) was used in a randomized study involving 61 patients with normal preoperative renal function who suffered from post–cardiac surgical heart failure requiring significant inotropic and vasoactive support. The investigators concluded that infusion of the drug (at 50 ng/kg per minute) enhanced renal excretory function, decreased the probability for dialysis, and improved dialysis-free survival in early, ischemic acute renal dysfunction after complicated cardiac surgery.[32]

Diuretic use, based on the rationale that such agents may reduce oxygen consumption and limit tubular obstruction, has always been a matter of controversy in ARF treatment. In the setting of cardiac surgery, a double-blind, randomized controlled trial involving 126 patients demonstrated that use of furosemide was associated with a higher rate of renal impairment, defined as increase in serum creatinine of 0.5 mg/dL over baseline.[33] Similar results were confirmed by other studies, suggesting that diuretic use, as a measure to treat ARF, should be avoided.[34] Studies involving mannitol have been less unequivocal to show a detrimental effect. In pediatric cardiac surgery, mannitol, added in increasing doses to the bypass priming solution, allowed maintenance of better urine output during the postoperative period; however, these findings remain unconfirmed.[35] By contrast, another small study showed increased excretion of β_2-microglobulin in patients receiving mannitol, which is a nonspecific marker of proximal tubular injury.[36]

Interventions Based on Cell Fate or Inflammation Paradigm of Injury

Pro-inflammatory cytokines have been extensively studied as mediators or markers of acute ischemia-reperfusion injury in experimental models of ARF. Their role in patients undergoing cardiac surgery is of particular interest because of the potential stimulation of inflammatory mediators on exposure to the extracorporeal circuit. Use of therapeutic agents to interfere with these mediators, however, has been less than promising in terms of reducing risk of ARF in the clinical setting of cardiac surgery. Steroids, such as dexamethasone, have been used to treat ARF during the perioperative period but failed to demonstrate any beneficial renoprotective effect.[37] The use of *N*-acetylcysteine to prevent radiocontrast agent–induced nephropathy has yielded conflicting results. Most clinicians would agree, however, that the absence of known adverse effects and the finding of some potential benefit have allowed its widespread use before contrast administration in high-risk patients. Available data on *N*-acetylcysteine use in the cardiac surgery setting are scarce; several large randomized controlled studies did not show any benefit of administering this agent to provide renal protection during the perioperative period.[38-40]

Taken together, as in other clinical settings, pharmacological interventions to prevent or treat ARF after cardiac surgery have resulted in equivocal results with limited success. Some of the key impediments to successful strategies in performing clinical trials in ARF include (1) improper preoperative risk stratification; (2) the multifaceted nature of the paradigm of injury in clinical setting, as opposed to the expected mechanism of action of particular agents; (3) inconsistency in defining ARF, either to start an intervention or to measure an outcome; and (4) lack of early diagnosis leading to delay in proposed intervention. It is encouraging, however, that attempts to unify the definition of ARF, based on its association with hard clinical endpoints, and data regarding diagnostic markers of early kidney injury have demonstrated some promise. It is hoped that the existing epidemiological data will allow planning of clinical trials of ARF using cardiac surgery as a "clinical model" in executing translational research concepts.

Key Points

1. The incidence of postoperative acute renal failure varies according to its definition; it ranges from 2% to 10%, depending on the degree of severity of kidney injury.
2. Various preoperative and intraoperative risk factors can predict the occurrence of severe acute renal failure requiring dialysis during the postoperative period. The risk factors for milder degrees of renal failure remain less well established.
3. Regardless of its severity, postoperative acute renal failure is associated with a strikingly high risk of serious morbidity and mortality during the postoperative period. The effect of acute renal failure on patient survival lasts well beyond the duration of hospitalization.
4. Although recent advances have been achieved in identifying tissue-specific biomarkers, the clinical application of such strategies to effectively ameliorate renal injury, and to improve patient survival, remains a challenging task.

Key References

2. Mangano CM, Diamondstone LS, Ramsay JG, et al: Renal dysfunction after myocardial revascularization: Risk factors, adverse outcomes, and hospital resource utilization. The Multicenter Study of Perioperative Ischemia Research Group. Ann Intern Med 1998;128:194-203.
5. Lassnigg A, Schmidlin D, Mouhieddine M, et al: Minimal changes of serum creatinine predict prognosis in patients after cardiothoracic surgery: A prospective cohort study. J Am Soc Nephrol 2004;15:1597-1605.
6. Chertow GM, Lazarus JM, Christiansen CL, et al: Preoperative renal risk stratification. Circulation 1997,95:878-884.
10. Thakar CV, Arrigain S, Worley S, et al: A clinical score to predict acute renal failure after cardiac surgery. J Am Soc Nephrol 2005;16:162-168.
23. Parikh CR, Mishra J, Thiessen-Philbrook H, et al: Urinary IL-18 is an early predictive biomarker of acute kidney injury after cardiac surgery. Kidney Int 2006;70:199-203.

See the companion Expert Consult website for the complete reference list.

CHAPTER 181

Renal Function and Acute Renal Failure in the Setting of Heart and Heart-Lung Transplantation

R. John Crew and David J. Cohen

OBJECTIVES

This chapter will:
1. Discuss the pretransplantation prevalence of renal insufficiency in wait-listed heart and heart-lung transplant candidates.
2. Describe the incidence, causes, and impact of acute renal failure in the perioperative period in heart and heart-lung transplant recipients.
3. Review the prevalence, severity, and impact of chronic renal insufficiency after heart and heart-lung transplantation.
4. Identify the options and limitations for modifying immunosuppression after transplantation in the face of chronic renal insufficiency.

Renal insufficiency is common in candidates awaiting heart transplantation, because many risk factors for renal disease and ischemic heart disease overlap, and reduced glomerular filtration is a frequent consequence of severely reduced cardiac output. In patients with end-stage heart failure, differentiating abnormal renal function due to renal parenchymal disease from that due to hypoperfusion can be exceedingly difficult. Nevertheless, proper perioperative management as well as deciding between combined heart-kidney transplantation versus heart transplantation alone requires making this clinical judgment. This assessment must attempt to balance an anticipated improvement in glomerular filtration rate (GFR) resulting from increased renal perfusion with the negative impact of immunosuppression with calcineurin inhibitors (CNIs) on future renal function. Acute renal failure is common in the perioperative period, frequently necessitating renal replacement therapy and alterations in medication and immunosuppression management. After heart transplantation, mild degrees of renal dysfunction are virtually universal, with more severe disease present in 10.9% of patients after heart transplantation and in 6.9% after heart-lung transplantation.[1] This chapter provides an overview of current practice in the assessment and management of renal disease at each stage in heart transplantation.

EPIDEMIOLOGY

Heart transplantation is the third most common solid organ transplant procedure performed in the United States, behind kidney and liver. Annually, between 2000 and 2200 heart-alone transplant procedures are done, with an additional 30 to 40 combined heart-lung transplant procedures. Approximately 2800 patients are on the waiting list for heart transplants and 140 for heart-lung transplants. Based on Organ Procurement and Transplantation Network (OPTN) data from December 2006, the most common causes of heart failure in currently wait-listed patients include ischemic cardiomyopathy (seen in 32.6%), idiopathic dilated cardiomyopathy (in 31.2%), congenital heart disease (in 6.5%), and valvular heart disease (in 2.4%).

Many of these patients have underlying conditions that are common risk factors for both ischemic heart disease or cardiomyopathy and chronic kidney disease (CKD). Most notably, these include hypertension and diabetes mellitus. These are the two leading causes of renal disease in the United States and are present in approximately 18% and 6.5%, respectively, of patients awaiting cardiac transplantation.[1,2] Other risk factors in common include smoking and hyperlipidemia, although available data on their prevalence in wait-listed patients are limited. In addition, GFR is highly dependent on renal blood flow. Thus, many patients with cardiac dysfunction severe enough to be judged suitable candidates for transplantation will have compromised renal function based on hemodynamic factors, rather than, or in addition to, structural abnormalities. It is not surprising, therefore, that preexisting renal insufficiency at the time of transplantation is a common finding.

In a study of renal dysfunction after nonrenal transplantation, Ojo and associates reviewed the United Network for Organ Sharing (UNOS) database for evidence of baseline renal insufficiency in patients receiving heart transplants between 1990 and 2000.[1] These investigators reported that 2.5% of patients who underwent transplantation had a GFR of 29 mL/minute or less, including 1% receiving hemodialysis. An additional 22.4% had a calculated GFR between 30 and 59 mL/minute (stage 3—moderate CKD). In more recent analyses of the national UNOS data, covering heart transplant recipients between 1995 and 2005, Russo and coworkers found that 4.8% of wait-listed patients had an estimated GFR less than 30 mL/minute (stage 4 CKD—severe), with a serum creatinine greater than 2.5 mg/dL in 6% of wait-listed patients (7.7% for those with diabetes and 5.6% for those without).[2,3] In a review of a large, single-center experience covering 1994 to 2001, the prevalence of GFR less than 40 mL/minute was noted to be 15%.[4] Renal insufficiency in patients awaiting heart transplantation remains a widespread and persistent problem whose prevalence may in fact be increasing.

For wait-listed heart-lung transplant candidates, the most frequent primary diagnoses are Eisenmenger's syndrome (in 31%), primary pulmonary hypertension (in 11%), congenital heart defects (in 28%), and sarcoidosis (in 7%) (www.optn.org). Compared with heart-alone transplant candidates, somewhat fewer heart-lung transplant candidates experience serious renal dysfunction, with 1.2% having an estimated GFR of 29 mL/minute or less, and 10.8%, between 30 and 59 mL/minute.[1]

EVALUATION OF RENAL DYSFUNCTION IN POTENTIAL HEART TRANSPLANT RECIPIENTS

The two most important aspects of assessing patients with renal dysfunction before heart transplantation are (1) distinguishing renal hypoperfusion from intrinsic renal disease and (2) deciding if combined heart-kidney transplantation is indicated. These two considerations are related in that patients without intrinsic renal disease are likely to recover renal function once they undergo transplantation, whereas patients with any significant degree of intrinsic disease are likely to experience progressive renal failure once started on CNIs.

The past medical history and prior laboratory results are invaluable in determining the likelihood of intrinsic disease, particularly in patients with acute cardiac decompensation. Recently, normal serum creatinine levels suggest that renal function will recover once renal blood flow is improved following transplantation, whereas prolonged prior elevations in serum creatinine suggest but do not prove irreversibility. Many patients with heart failure are managed with increasing doses of diuretics and angiotensin-converting enzyme (ACE) inhibitors or angiotensin receptor blockers (ARBs), resulting in chronic, progressive elevations in serum creatinine level in the absence of structural renal damage.

Unfortunately, the determination of renal function may itself be problematic. Serum creatinine levels that are normal or only mildly elevated may be misleading. At low levels, serum creatinine is an insensitive marker for renal dysfunction, particularly in patients with severe congestive heart failure, many of whom are malnourished and have experienced significant muscle wasting. Measurement of creatinine clearance by 24-hour creatinine collection may be instructive. Formulas that estimate renal function have been tested for accuracy against isotopically measured GFR in patients with heart failure.[5] In this study, the Cockcroft-Gault and MDRD equations, as well as 24-hour urine creatinine clearance, overestimated renal function at low GFR and underestimated renal function at high GFR. All measurements performed better in patients with stage 3 or 4 heart failure.

In the evaluation of patients with acute renal failure who are awaiting cardiac transplantation, the prerenal state due to poor cardiac output is by far the most frequently encountered scenario. Other potentially causative disorders and conditions should be excluded, however, particularly acute tubular necrosis from episodes of hypotension, drug toxicity from antibiotics or nonsteroidal anti-inflammatory drug (NSAID) use, the hemodynamic effects of ACE inhibitors or ARBs, exposure to intravenous radiocontrast agents, rhabdomyolysis from 3-hydroxy-3-methylglutaryl–coenzyme A (HMG-CoA) reductase inhibitor use, and obstructive nephropathy. As in other forms of renal disease, the presence of proteinuria or persistent microscopic hematuria can indicate underlying acute or chronic glomerular disease. Renal imaging can be helpful: Small or severely echogenic kidneys indicate chronic disease, although normal-appearing kidneys do not necessarily exclude significant pathology.

Screening for renal artery stenosis would seem reasonable in patients with ischemic heart disease and a history of hypertension, because studies using screening abdominal aortography at time of coronary angiography detect 50% or greater stenoses in approximately 20% of patients.[6] The frequency of renal artery stenosis is likely to be lower among patients preselected for heart transplantation. In a study of screening aortography in heart transplant recipients within 1 year of surgery, only 0.9% had a significant renal artery lesion.[7] Urine sodium or the fractional excretion of sodium (FE_{Na}) frequently is used to distinguish prerenal azotemia from intrinsic renal disease, but both are difficult to interpret in patients with heart failure because diuretics increase urine sodium excretion. The fractional excretion of urea (FE_{urea}) may be a helpful alternative. In one study, the FE_{Na} was less than 1% in only 48% of patients with prerenal azotemia on diuretics, but the FE_{urea} was less than 35% in 89% of patients with prerenal azotemia, including those on diuretics.[8]

Despite noninvasive testing, the etiology of renal dysfunction and the degree of reversibility will be unclear in some patients. In this group, a renal biopsy may help in identifying patients who have significant underlying renal pathology and would be better served by combined heart-kidney transplantation.[9] In a single-center report, 11 patients with either an estimated GFR less than 40 mL/minute or proteinuria (urinary protein excretion rate more than 500 mg/24 hours) underwent renal biopsy before heart transplantation. On the basis of the renal biopsy findings, 4 patients were able to undergo heart transplantation alone, 3 underwent combined heart-kidney transplantation, and 4 were not listed for transplantation (i.e., were not considered for combined organ transplantation). In 4 of the 11 patients, a form of ischemic nephropathy was found, with dramatic expansion of the juxtaglomerular apparatus, presumably from chronic expression and release of angiotensin, as well as significant tubular atrophy or interstitial fibrosis (Fig. 181-1). This histopathological finding confirms that chronic hypoperfusion alone can lead to progressive structural lesions over time. This type of abnormality would not be expected to regress with heart transplantation alone. The remaining 7 biopsy specimens showed amyloidosis in 2 patients and 1 case each of diabetic nephropathy, membranous nephropathy, obesity-related focal segmental glomerulosclerosis, fibrillary glomerulonephritis, and myeloma cast nephropathy.

No consensus has been reached on the level of renal dysfunction that precludes transplantation, although in two thirds of U.S. transplantation centers, a serum creatinine level greater than 3 mg/dL is considered a contraindication to transplantation.[10] With improved surgical techniques and medical management, dual organ transplantation is an increasingly acceptable option. Currently, no nationally accepted criteria are available to identify patients for combined heart-kidney transplantation. In an era with a severe shortage of donor organs, kidney transplants should not be wasted on those who will not need them, nor should cardiac transplantation alone be performed in patients whose outcomes will be compromised by poor renal function. Renal dysfunction before heart transplantation is a risk factor for the later development of stage 4 or 5 CKD and end-stage renal disease requiring dialysis, which in turn is associated with a fourfold

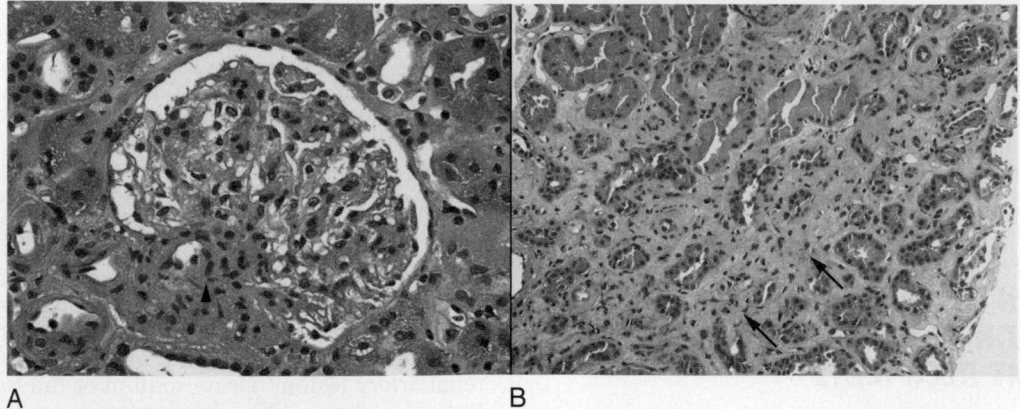

FIGURE 181-1. See also color plates. Pathological features of ischemic nephropathy in heart failure. **A,** The *arrowhead* marks the hypertrophied juxtaglomerular apparatus. **B,** *Arrows* identify the severe tubular atrophy and interstitial fibrosis present in a different high-power field.

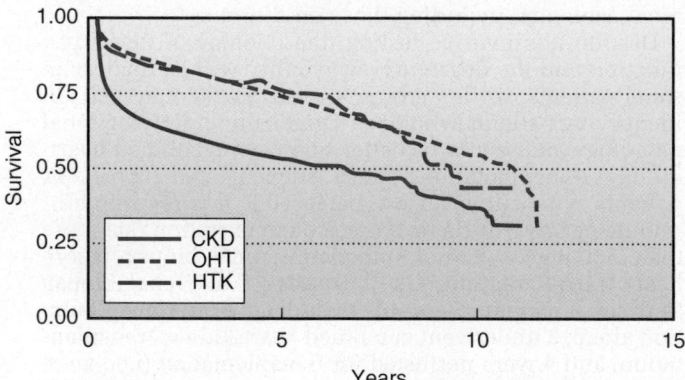

FIGURE 181-2. Survival in combined heart-kidney (HTK) and isolated heart transplant with (CKD) and without (OHT) chronic kidney disease. OHT, orthotopic heart transplantation. (From Russo M, Chen JM, Stewart AS, et al: Long-term survival following combined heart-kidney transplant compared with isolated heart transplant: An analysis of the UNOS database [abstract]. Am J Transplant 2006;6:382, with permission.)

increased risk of death.[1] In addition, preoperative renal dysfunction (estimated GFR less than 40 mL/minute) has been associated with a twofold increased early mortality after transplantation.[4] A recent analysis of the UNOS database found improved recipient survival with combined organ transplantation, compared with heart-alone transplantation, when the estimated GFR at the time of listing was less than 30 mL/minute (Fig. 181-2).[2]

The addition of renal transplantation to heart transplantation can make the organ selection process more complicated. Renal transplantation requires a crossmatch (a test for preformed anti-donor antibodies in the serum of the potential recipient) before surgery. The additional time needed to complete the crossmatch limits the acceptable geographical area from which the donor organs can be retrieved. Also, patients may be too unstable after cardiac surgery to permit renal transplantation to be safely performed, although this procedure usually can be delayed for hours if necessary. Hypotension and the subsequent

requirement of pressor and inotrope support, frequently administered after heart transplantation, may increase the risk of delayed graft function in a transplanted kidney. Over the past several years, between 25 and 50 combined heart-kidney transplant procedures have been performed annually in the United States.[11]

If no other cause of renal dysfunction is found, treatment relies on maximizing renal perfusion. Successful management requires close monitoring of fluid status, avoiding electrolyte disorders with appropriate diet restrictions, appropriate dosing of antibiotic and other medications for level of renal function, avoiding nephrotoxins, and inotrope support. In many patients with end-stage heart failure, fluid balance cannot be maintained despite maximum inotrope and other medication support; continued fluid retention and worsened pulmonary edema lead to upregulation of the renal-angiotensin-aldosterone axis and sympathetic nervous system, causing progressive sodium and water retention.[12] In these cases, fluid balance can be maintained by slow continuous ultrafiltration (SCUF) or continuous venovenous hemodiafiltration (CVVHDF). Brief fluid removal with SCUF may lead to improvement in cardiac function and response to diuretics.[13] We also have successfully used peritoneal dialysis in selected cases.

Despite maximal medical therapy, a smaller subset of patients will require mechanical support as a bridge to transplantation. The 2006 report of the International Society for Heart and Lung Transplantation (ISHLT) comments on the need for pretransplantation mechanical support. Between January 1, 2003, and June 30, 2005, 22.7% of patients awaiting heart transplants had received left ventricular assist devices (LVADs), 5.1% were on intra-aortic balloon pumps (IABPs), 0.6% had received right ventricular assist devices (RVADs), and 0.2% had received an artificial heart.[14] Many patients with elevated serum creatinine before LVAD placement have improvements in renal function after surgery.[15] Unfortunately, renal failure requiring renal replacement therapy is also common after LVAD insertion, ranging from 24% to 34% in two recent series.[16,17] Acute renal failure after LVAD insertion carries a terrible prognosis, with mortality rates ranging from 50% to 93% at 6 months. In addition, patients with acute renal failure after LVAD insertion are less likely to successfully undergo transplantation (52% versus

83%).[17] Finally, LVAD use at the time of transplantation is associated with a 28% increased relative risk for death at 1 year after transplantation.[14] Although no randomized trials have been conducted on the subject, CVVHDF is the initial renal replacement therapy of choice in these patients, providing closer control of fluid balance, avoiding fluctuations in filling pressures compared with hemodialysis, and allowing the administration of intravenous medications and blood products as needed.

ACUTE RENAL FAILURE IN THE IMMEDIATE POSTOPERATIVE PERIOD

In patients not on dialysis before cardiac transplantation, renal failure requiring dialysis occurs postoperatively in 5% to 15% of patients.[4,18-20] Renal function before transplantation was a risk factor for the need for dialysis in some but not all studies. In the immediate postoperative period, the most frequent causes of acute renal failure are acute tubular necrosis from ischemia, prerenal azotemia from hypoperfusion, and the hemodynamic effects of CNIs. Other causes of acute renal failure include rhabdomyolysis, thrombotic microangiopathy due to CNIs, renal failure due to starch-containing oncotic fluids used during resuscitation, obstruction due to a malfunctioning Foley catheter in the bladder, and other drug toxicities. Causes of hypoperfusion immediately after transplantation include left ventricular failure due to donor organ dysfunction, cardiac tamponade, right ventricular failure due to elevated central venous pressures or to elevated pulmonary vascular resistance, hypovolemia due to bleeding, and vasodilatory shock from temporary vasopressin deficiency after cardiopulmonary bypass, sepsis, or drug reaction in the case of some induction therapies (particularly antithymocyte sera or OKT3 use).

Because cardiac instability is common and the potential causes of hypoperfusion are diverse, measurement of intracardiac pressures and cardiac output with a Swan-Ganz catheter is essential. Particular attention needs to be paid to the possibility of right ventricular failure, because this accounts for 50% of cardiac complications and is a frequent cause of early death.[21] The most important preoperative risk factor for right-sided heart failure is abnormal pulmonary hemodynamics, manifested as an elevated pulmonary vascular resistance, transpulmonary pressure gradient, or measured pulmonary arterial pressure.[22] The donor heart's right ventricle is not prepared to generate the pressures needed to contract against elevated filling pressure and elevated outflow resistance. Fortunately, in most patients with reversible pulmonary hypertension before transplantation, the pulmonary vascular resistance decreases within the first week after surgery. Pharmacological measures used to decrease pulmonary vascular resistance and improve right-sided heart function include inhaled nitric oxide, inhaled prostacyclin (Iloprost), intravenous prostaglandins, and milrinone, among others.[23]

Because these patients are hypotensive, hypoperfused, and receiving multiple medications or blood products, oliguric renal failure or at least loss of ability to maintain negative fluid balance frequently ensues. Managing fluid balance frequently requires initiation of CVVHDF. Despite hypotension and cool extremities, it is imperative to maintain the central venous pressure at a level suitable to the new right ventricle, which may mean fluid removal despite the hypotension. The pharmacological reduction in pul-

monary vascular resistance and improved contractility in the setting of reduced central venous pressures act to restore renal (and whole-body) perfusion.

As in the management of acute renal failure in the setting of severe heart failure, the major goals of therapy are to improve renal perfusion, limit nephrotoxins, and prevent metabolic complications from impairing renal clearance. Improving renal perfusion requires coordinating inotrope use, vasopressor use, and fluid balance with the heart transplant team. Limiting nephrotoxins may be a challenge, because complicated cases may dictate the need for imaging studies with intravenous contrast, or the use of nephrotoxic antibiotics in the setting of increasingly resistant hospital-acquired infections. Finding alternative imaging strategies and using careful antibiotic dosing with close monitoring of blood levels become paramount. Modification of the immunosuppressive regimen also should be considered. Minimizing use of the nephrotoxic CNIs cyclosporine and tacrolimus in the setting of acute renal failure can be accomplished by starting immunosuppression with antibody induction therapy. Protocols exist using either antithymocyte sera (horse ATG/ATGAM or rabbit ATG/Thymoglobulin) or muromonab OKT3. All of these agents lead to effective depletion of T lymphocytes, allowing adequate immunosuppression while awaiting renal recovery before institution of CNI immunosuppression. However, a cytokine release syndrome resulting in reduced renal blood flow due to renal vasoconstriction may be seen with any of these agents, an effect that usually is mildest with equine ATG. Additional toxicity results if prolonged courses are given, particularly infections, leukopenia, thrombocytopenia, and long-term risk of lymphoproliferative disorders. The interleukin-2 receptor antagonists basiliximab (Simulect) and daclizumab (Zenapax) are better tolerated than the polyclonal antithymocyte sera and also have been used to delay CNI introduction. It is uncertain whether they provide adequate immunosuppression without concomitant CNI administration.[24] Although it would seem intuitive that CNIs, known nephrotoxins, should be minimized or avoided in the setting of acute renal failure, data from randomized trials in kidney transplantation suggest that CNIs cause little delay in renal recovery.[25,26] In patients with prolonged acute tubular necrosis, the added infectious risk and hematological complications of antithymocyte sera must be balanced against the potential for prolonging the duration of acute tubular necrosis with early initiation of CNI therapy.

A newer, oral immunosuppressant, sirolimus (Rapamune), does not share the same nephrotoxic effect of CNIs. It has been used successfully in heart transplant recipients with chronic renal insufficiency as a replacement to CNIs (see later on) and has been tried for primary immunosuppression immediately after heart transplantation.[27] It remains unknown, however, if a CNI-free regimen with sirolimus provides adequate immunosuppression early after cardiac transplantation. Moreover, experience from kidney transplantation suggests that sirolimus, because of its potent antiproliferative effect, may prolong recovery from ATN and also may impair wound healing.[28]

CVVHDF is the preferred method of renal replacement therapy for renal failure immediately after transplantation. Patients frequently can be switched to intermittent hemodialysis once hemodynamic stability has returned and fluid balance can be adequately maintained with intermittent dialysis treatments. Most studies show a significant increase in early mortality in patients requiring renal replacement therapy immediately after heart transplantation.[4,18,19,29] The increased mortality appears to be mostly from increased risk of infections.[22] This risk may be related to the need for central venous catheters for dialysis access, as well as the added immunosuppressive effect of uremia on an immune system that is already undergoing intense immunosuppression. Despite the increased risk of early death, those patients who required dialysis perioperatively and survived the first month enjoy 5-year survival rates similar to those for patients without perioperative renal failure.[22]

CHRONIC RENAL FAILURE AFTER HEART TRANSPLANTATION

Incidence

Before the introduction of cyclosporine, 1-year success rates after cardiac transplantation were so low that little opportunity arose for concern regarding long-term complications. The introduction of cyclosporine in the early 1980s dramatically improved short- and long-term survival rates. Renal insufficiency was immediately recognized as a common complication. By 1984, Myers and coworkers noted a mean GFR of 51 mL/minute at 12 months after transplantation in patients receiving cyclosporine, compared with 93 mL/minute in those receiving azathioprine, despite similar cardiac allograft function.[30] Histologically, interstitial fibrosis with focal segmental glomerular sclerosis was seen. The same group of investigators found renal function to remain depressed at the 2-year follow-up evaluation.[31] Despite constancy of GFR, however, histological evidence of progressive parenchymal injury was observed. By 1991, 3% of heart or heart-lung recipients on long-term cyclosporine therapy (9 years) were noted to have progressed to end-stage renal failure.[32] Another early report found that virtually no patients had completely normal renal function by 3 years after cardiac transplantation.[33] With the considerably lower doses of cyclosporine used today compared with those used in the 1980s and early 1990s, however, it appears that the incidence of advanced renal insufficiency may currently be less.[34]

Reviewing more recent results, Ojo and associates observed that 11% of heart transplant recipients have an estimated GFR less than 30 mL/minute at 5 years[1] (Fig. 181-3). Similarly, the ISHLT Heart Recipient Registry shows that more than 14% of patients have a serum creatinine level greater than 2.5 mg/dL at 8 years.[14] Longer follow-up, from the ISHLT Registry 2006 Report, found that 42% had abnormal renal function at 10 years after transplantation.[14] The annual risk of end-stage renal disease was estimated to be 0.37% in the first year after transplantation, increasing to 4.49% by the sixth post-transplantation year.[35] Our own experience demonstrated that at long-term follow-up, end-stage renal disease eventually developed in 6.5% of heart transplant recipients who received cyclosporine[36]—a rate similar to that noted by other investigators[34,37] but somewhat less than the 20% cumulative incidence noted at 10 years by Rubel and colleagues.[38]

The 2006 ISHLT Lung and Heart-Lung Registry indicates that 27.7% of heart-lung recipients have abnormal renal function at the 5-year follow-up evaluation, with only 1% reported as requiring dialysis.[39] In a study combining lung and heart-lung recipients, 55% of those surviving more than 6 months doubled their serum creatinine concentration, with 7.3% progressing to ESRD.[40] Other single-center studies found a long-term ESRD incidence ranging from 4.5% in heart-lung recipients to 16.5% in a combined lung and heart-lung transplant cohort.[41,42] Ojo and associates found a steadily increasing incidence of chronic renal failure (GFR less than 30 mL/minute) after heart-lung transplantation, reaching 6.9% at 60 months, from 1.7% at 12 months and 4.2% at 36 months.[1]

Pathology

No systematic reviews of renal pathology in long-term surviving heart or heart-lung transplant recipients have been performed. Although the pathological findings in the vast majority of cases are undocumented, the clinical course and histopathological changes (when available) are identical to those seen in liver and lung transplant recipients, all of whom have in common long-term use of cyclosporine or tacrolimus, leaving little doubt about the main culprit. Our own unpublished data, as well as the early experience of Myers and colleagues[31] and, more recently, Silva and associates,[43] all confirm that CNI toxicity is the primary lesion. As would be expected in a population as large as heart transplant recipients, a number of cases of other primary and secondary renal diseases have been documented.[44] Proteinuria usually is minimal, because the principal CNI toxicity is tubulointerstitial; with advanced toxicity, however, nephrotic-range proteinuria can occur, with lesions of focal segmental glomerular sclerosis.[45]

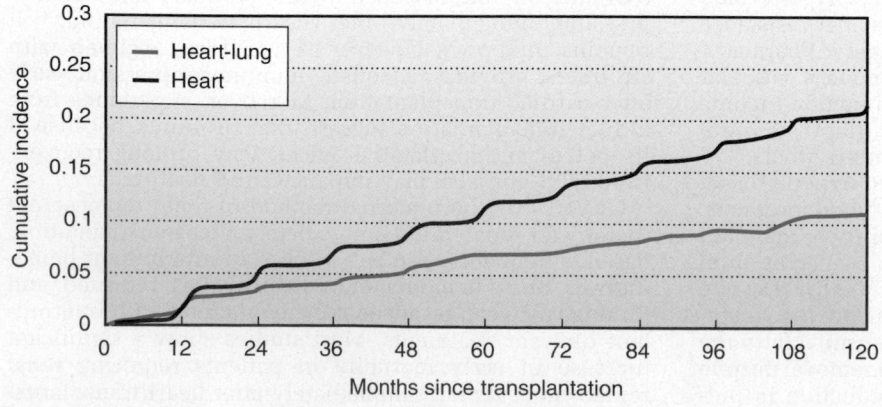

FIGURE 181-3. Incidence of chronic renal insufficiency, defined as estimated glomerular filtration rate of 29 mL/minute or less or the onset of end-stage renal disease, among heart and heart-lung transplant recipients in the United States between 1990 and 2000. (Courtesy of A. Ojo. Adapted from Ojo A, Held PJ, Port FK, et al: Chronic renal failure after transplantation of a nonrenal organ. N Engl J Med 2003;349:931-940.)

Clinical Course

The clinical course typically consists of three phases. An *initial improvement* in renal function soon after surgery is common, as a result of improved renal blood flow. This is followed by a *significant decline* in renal function (due to the hemodynamic effect of the CNI); function then stabilizes for a variable period of time, most commonly years.[46-48] Serum creatinine slowly *increases*—again, over a period of years—in those patients in whom progressive renal insufficiency develops. With advanced disease, nephrotic syndrome can occur, as noted earlier.

Impact on Outcome

Several groups of investigators have documented the adverse impact of renal insufficiency on outcomes after cardiac transplantation. Elevated serum creatinine and, in particular, the need for dialysis are associated with increased mortality, early as well as long-term, more than double that for patients with well-preserved renal function in many studies. This includes pretransplantation renal dysfunction, as well as the development of abnormal renal function after transplantation.[4,44,49-52] With the annual cost of dialysis over $60,000 in the United States, this elevated rate of renal failure contributes significantly to post-transplantation costs. One study calculated that the added cost of end-stage renal disease after cardiac transplantation increases the average per-patient cost of transplantation by more than $10,000.[35]

Risk Factors for Chronic Kidney Disease and Progression to End-Stage Renal Disease after Transplantation

In light of the frequency and impact of renal insufficiency after cardiac transplantation, identification of patients at particular risk and investigation of preventive measures have been undertaken by many investigators. Those factors predictive of compromised renal function after transplantation include preoperative renal insufficiency, older recipient age, elevated creatinine at 1 month after transplantation, male gender, and the development of hypertension.[41,47,48] Much effort is being put forth to find markers that identify patients at higher risk for the development of progressive CNI toxicity. In one study, elevated levels of urinary retinol-binding protein, a marker of proximal tubule dysfunction, identified a subgroup of heart transplant recipients at higher risk for chronic renal insufficiency before any change in renal function was observed.[53] No definite relationship between renal function and CNI doses or levels has been established. This lack of association probably is due to two factors: (1) All patients are by protocol dosed similarly, and (2) dose reductions are common in the face of increased serum creatinine levels. The most commonly identified potentially treatable risk factors for the development of renal insufficiency are pre-operative renal insufficiency itself and postoperative acute renal failure.

In a study combining lung and heart-lung transplant recipients, older age at transplantation, lower GFR at 1 month, and cyclosporine use versus tacrolimus use were identified as predictors for the development of chronic kidney disease.[40]

MANAGEMENT OF RENAL FAILURE AFTER CARDIAC TRANSPLANTATION

Immunosuppressive Strategies

Because CNI nephrotoxicity is the most common cause of renal insufficiency in heart transplant recipients, many attempts have been directed at finding less nephrotoxic, yet equally effective, immunosuppressive regimens. These studies have focused on either dose reduction or complete elimination of CNIs, along with modification of concomitant immunosuppressives. Virtually all have been single-center, nonrandomized observational studies in small numbers of patients. Conversion from cyclosporine to either azathioprine, tacrolimus, or sirolimus has been reported. All studies demonstrated short-term improvement in renal function in a majority of patients. An early attempt at substitution of azathioprine for cyclosporine resulted in a very high incidence of rejection.[54] One report found that conversion from cyclosporine to tacrolimus was beneficial in selected patients.[55]

More recently, several groups of investigators have noted significantly improved renal function after conversion from CNI-based immunosuppression to mycophenolate and sirolimus, with CNI discontinuation.[56-60] The frequency of rejection episodes appeared to be acceptably low. Other reports, however, suggested that a sirolimus-mycophenolate regimen had unacceptable side effects or was not associated with any improvement in renal function.[61,62]

An alternative to CNI discontinuation has been 50% CNI dose reduction, accompanied by substitution of mycophenolate mofetil for azathioprine.[63,64] With this protocol, renal function improved, and rejection episodes were infrequent. These findings were confirmed in a multi-center, prospectively controlled study evaluating renal functional response to adjustments in immunosuppression.[65] In a single-center randomized, prospectively controlled study, sirolimus substitution for cyclosporine resulted in further improvement in renal function compared with cyclosporine dose reduction.[66] Table 181-1 summarizes the design and results of several recent studies aimed at improving renal function through altering immunosuppression. At present, no single, agreed-upon approach is recognized, although a reduction in CNI exposure appears prudent, and most centers report favorable results with sirolimus substitution for cyclosporine. Further randomized, prospective, controlled long-term studies are clearly needed.

Other Management

Other approaches have been suggested to reverse or stabilize declining renal function. These include the addition of omega-3 fatty acids,[67] use of calcium channel blockers or ACE inhibitors or ARBs for blood pressure control, and aggressive lipid lowering. Inhibition of angiotensin may have the added benefit of muting TGF-β–driven interstitial fibrosis.

END-STAGE RENAL DISEASE

In those unfortunate patients in whom progressive renal disease develops, hemodialysis, peritoneal dialysis, and

TABLE 181-1

Protocols to Reduce CNI Exposure as Treatment for Renal Insufficiency after Orthotopic Heart Transplantation

STUDY	DESIGN	OUTCOME(S)
Gleissner et al., 2006[66]	39 pts already on low-dose Cy (target <80 ng/mL) + MMF, with SCr 1.7-3.5 > 6 months after transplantation, were randomized to receive continued therapy vs. converting to sirolimus + MMF.	SCr 2.1 ± 0.4 mg/dL reduced to 1.6 ± 0.4 mg/dL in sirolimus group, compared with no change in control arm.* No rejection episodes of ISHLT grade 2 or higher.
Bestetti et al., 2006[56]	10 pts on CNI/MMF with SCr > 1.5 mg/dL despite CNI reduction underwent conversion to sirolimus (target 10-14 ng/mL). Compared with 28 contemporaneous patients without CRF.	SCr 3.8 ± 1.8 mg/dL reduced to 1.3 ± 0.4 mg/dL at 180 days after conversion.
Hunt et al., 2005[60]	80 pts on CNI/Pred ± MMF underwent conversion to sirolimus/MMF/Ster; 60 of these pts had SCr > 2.0 mg/dL. No comparison group.	SCr 2.04 ± 0.57 mg/dL reduced to 1.64 ± 0.48 mg/dL in CRF group. 5 episodes of ISHLT grade 3A rejection overall.
Groetzner et al., 2004[58]	30 pts on CNI/MMF with SCr > 1.9 mg/dL and >30% increase in SCr over >3 months underwent conversion to sirolimus/MMF. Compared with historical controls.	SCr decreased from 3.1 ± 0.81 mg/dL to 2.2 ± 0.6 mg/dL. No rejection episodes.
Angermann et al., 2004[65]	Multicenter study of 161 pts >6 months after transplantation with SCr > 1.7 mg/dL on Cy ± Aza ± Ster; 109 pts received MMF with Cy reduced to target 50 ng/mL. Control group: 52 contemporaneous pts without medication change, followed at a single center.	7.6 mL/min increase in GFR in MMF arm vs. no change in control arm; 3% rejection rate in MMF arm.

*$P < .001$ for within-group and between-group comparisons with control.
Aza, azathioprine; CNI, calcineurin inhibitor; CRF, chronic renal failure; Cy, cyclosporine; ISHLT, International Society for Heart and Lung Transplantation; MMF, mycophenolate mofetil; Pred, prednisone; pts, patients; SCr, serum creatinine; Ster, steroids.

kidney transplantation all are viable options. Heart transplant recipients on peritoneal dialysis may have more episodes of peritonitis, increased risk of peritoneal dialysis failure due to infections, and shorter survival times after institution of peritoneal dialysis.[68] ESRD is associated with a three- to fourfold increase in mortality over that observed in heart transplant recipients without renal dysfunction, but this rate was similar to that observed in other patients with ESRD in one study.[69] Kidney transplantation from live or deceased donors is the preferred option for patients with adequate cardiac allograft function. Most single-center reports are limited to fewer than 10 patients but suggest good results.[69-71] Analysis of UNOS data suggests that kidney transplantation is highly successful for appropriate patients, with a mortality rate approximately half of that expected without transplantation.[1] Because these patients are already on immunosuppressant drugs, the long-term cost of kidney transplantation also is likely to be much less than that of continued dialysis.

CONCLUSION

Renal insufficiency constitutes a major clinical challenge in the care of heart (and, to a lesser extent, heart-lung) transplant candidates and recipients. Reduced cardiac output associated with end-stage heart failure frequently leads to renal insufficiency as a result of poor renal perfusion. Although the injury generally is reversible, if the impaired perfusion is severe enough or prolonged enough, irreversible renal injury may result. Those patients with fixed GFR less than 40 mL/minute may benefit from combined heart-kidney transplantation. The hemodynamic alterations of the transplant operation followed by the widespread long-term use of nephrotoxic immunosuppressive medications have created a population of post-transplantation patients among whom moderate to severe chronic kidney disease is common. As long-term survival rates continue to improve, increasing numbers of these patients are likely to reach end-stage renal failure requiring either dialysis or kidney transplantation. Increased understanding of those factors leading to irreversible renal damage in those on the waiting list, coupled with careful management of blood pressure and lipid levels and the continued development of non-nephrotoxic immunosuppressive regimens, is essential in the management of these patients and potentially should minimize the number of patients experiencing progressive renal insufficiency.

Key Points

1. Renal insufficiency occurs in 20% to 25% of heart transplant candidates and may be due to reversible hemodynamic factors or irreversible renal parenchymal damage.
2. Selected patients with advanced renal insufficiency are likely to derive benefit from combined heart-kidney transplantation, rather than from heart-alone transplantation.
3. After transplantation, the vast majority of heart (and a somewhat smaller number of heart-lung) recipients experience a significant reduction in renal function as a result of the long-term widespread use of calcineurin inhibitor–based immunosuppression.
4. Reduced dosing or discontinuation of calcineurin Inhibitors in those patients experiencing progressive renal failure may improve renal function while maintaining adequate immunosuppression.

5. For selected patients who reach end-stage renal failure, renal transplantation is an appropriate therapy, with excellent success rates.

Key References

1. Ojo AO, Held PJ, Port FK, et al: Chronic renal failure after transplantation of a nonrenal organ. N Engl J Med 2003; 349:931-940.
4. Odim J, Wheat J, Laks H, et al: Peri-operative renal function and outcome after orthotopic heart transplantation. J Heart Lung Transplant 2006;25:162-166.

35. Hornberger J, Best J, Geppert J, McClellan M: Risks and costs of end-stage renal disease after heart transplantation. Transplantation 1998;66:1763-1770.
40. Canales M, Youssef P, Spong R, et al: Predictors of chronic kidney disease in long-term survivors of lung and heart-lung transplantation. Am J Transplant 2006;6:2157-2163.
56. Bestetti R, Theodoropoulos TA, Burdmann EA, et al: Switch from calcineurin inhibitors to sirolimus-induced renal recovery in heart transplant recipients in the midterm follow-up. Transplantation 2006;81:692-696.

See the companion Expert Consult website for the complete reference list.

CHAPTER 182

The Kidney in Acute Heart Failure Syndromes and Cardiogenic Shock

Adrian Salmon, Vijay Karajala-Subramanyam, and John A. Kellum

OBJECTIVES

This chapter will:
1. Review the definitions of heart failure, acute heart failure syndromes, and cardiogenic shock.
2. Outline pathophysiological mechanisms of kidney response in acute heart failure syndrome.
3. Describe the mechanism of kidney injury in cardiogenic shock.
4. Discuss clinical aspects in the management of cardiogenic shock.

Heart failure is a complex clinical syndrome that can result from any structural or functional cardiac disorder that impairs the ability of the ventricle to fill with or eject blood.[1] States of high-output heart failure, such as with arteriovenous fistula, hyperthyroidism, and beriberi, also may be seen.[2,3] An *acute heart failure syndrome* (AHFS) may be defined as heart failure with a relatively rapid onset of signs and symptoms, resulting in hospitalization or unplanned office or emergency room visits. As the term indicates, AHFSs can result from a variety of different pathophysiological conditions. Most AHFS events (70%) are the result of worsening chronic heart failure. Other causes of AHFS include new-onset heart failure caused by an acute coronary event, such as a myocardial infarction (MI), and end-stage or refractory heart failure that is not responsive to therapy. Clinical presentation may vary, encompassing worsening congestion, worsening chronic heart failure, pulmonary edema, hypertensive crisis, or cardiogenic shock.[4]

In all forms of heart failure, the kidney responds in a similar manner, retaining sodium and water despite expansion of the extracellular fluid volume (ECFV). AHFS can manifest as cardiogenic shock, characterized by impaired tissue perfusion. The cardial signs of cardiogenic shock are tachycardia, cold extremities, and oliguria.[5,6] Renal dysfunction has significant importance in the clinical manifestations of AHFS. An increase in plasma creatinine concentration has been identified as a strong predictor of mortality in patients with heart failure.[7] This chapter discusses AHFS and cardiogenic shock; a review of chronic heart failure and the cardiorenal syndrome can be found in Chapter 196.

In AHFS, two main pathophysiological mechanisms are operative, beginning with an abnormal perception of inadequate volume by sensors within the afferent limb, followed by a disturbance in the response by neurohormonal mechanisms (the efferent limb) that alters the balance of sodium and water retention by the kidney.

KIDNEY RESPONSE IN ACUTE HEART FAILURE SYNDROME

Decrease in cardiac output is perceived by the kidney as a hypovolemic state that triggers the response of neurohormones (such as angiotensin II and aldosterone from the renin-angiotensin-aldosterone system). Angiotensin II induces secretion of vasopressin by the anterior pituitary gland and endothelin-1 by endothelial cells. Neurohormonal activation and, particularly, increased vasopressin levels result in fluid retention, sodium retention, vasoconstriction, and high venous pressure, which increase myocardial wall stress and decrease cardiac performance. In addition, increased venous pressure may contribute to renal dysfunction. Vasoconstriction also decreases glomerular filtration, thereby impairing renal function and increasing sodium and water retention. This establishes a deleterious positive feedback loop, resulting in the chronic elevation of neurohormones and the worsening of heart

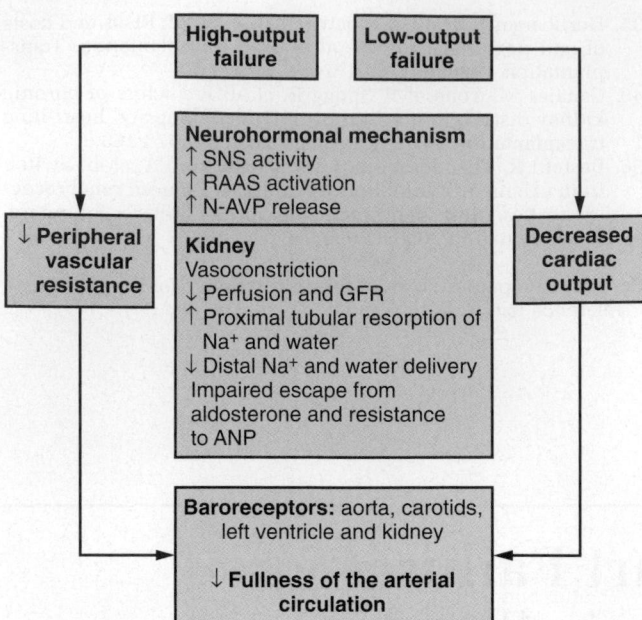

FIGURE 182-1. Summary of pathophysiology: Neurohormonal mechanisms and kidney response in heart failure and cardiogenic shock. ANP, atrial natriuretic peptide; GFR, glomerular filtration rate; N-AVP, nonosmotic arginine vasopressin (vasopressin); RAAS, renin-angiotensin-aldosterone system; SNS, sympathetic nervous system; ↓, decreased; ↑, increased. (Redrawn with permission from Gorfinkel HJ, Szidon JP, Hirsch LJ, Fishman AP: Renal performance in experimental cardiogenic shock. Am J Physiol 1972;222(5):1260-1268.)

failure[3] (Fig. 182-1). See Chapter 196 for detailed discussion.

ACUTE KIDNEY INJURY IN CARDIOGENIC SHOCK

Although the kidneys receive approximately 20% of the cardiac output, blood flow distribution within the kidney is very heterogeneous. The cortex receives more than 85% of the blood flow, even though the medulla is highly active metabolically. Tissue PO_2 is approximately 50 to 100 mm Hg in the cortex, whereas it is as low as 10 to 15 mm Hg in the medullary thick ascending limb. This progressive fall in tissue PO_2 from the cortex to the medulla is secondary to countercurrent oxygen exchange. Energy is required for the various active transport mechanisms, especially in the metabolically active thick ascending limb of the loop of Henle. Accordingly, the medulla is thought to be more prone to ischemic injury. During periods of ischemia, sympathoadrenal activation redistributes blood preferentially to the medulla to attenuate medullary ischemia.[8]

Under normal circumstances, renal blood flow and glomerular filtration rate are maintained by autoregulation (i.e., at a constant rate over a wide range of renal perfusion pressures).[9] The afferent arterioles dilate and the efferent arterioles constrict in response to a decrease in perfusion pressure, to maintain the transglomerular pressure. Only when the mean arterial pressure (MAP) drops below 70 mm Hg do the transglomerular pressure and glomerular filtration rate (GFR) decrease as well. It is thought that

afferent arterioles contain myogenic stretch receptors that cause vasoconstriction in response to stretch secondary to an increase in perfusion pressure. However, the exact mechanism of renal autoregulation is not completely understood. Tubuloglomerular feedback is a negative feedback loop that induces preglomerular arteriolar constriction in response to increased solute delivery to the distal nephron, thereby reducing GFR and solute resorptive demands. Adenosine, which is a systemic vasodilator, acts as a vasoconstrictor in the kidney and is thought to mediate tubuloglomerular feedback.[10] These mechanisms that redistribute blood flow from cortex to medulla also are important in maintaining oxygen balance by decreasing oxygen utilization. The extent to which autoregulation can increase renal medullary blood flow is limited, however.

Literature on human renal circulation in cardiogenic shock is sparse. Using animal models, Gorfinkel and coworkers, in 1971,[11] studied the renal response in cardiogenic shock and conducted a parallel study in hemorrhagic shock. These investigators showed that renal blood flow behaved differently in both shock states, decreasing drastically during hemorrhagic shock and moderately in cardiogenic shock. Urine production decreased moderately and concentrating capability was preserved in cardiogenic shock, whereas they deteriorated rapidly and markedly in hemorrhagic shock.

The intrarenal distribution of blood flow remains normal in cardiogenic shock, whereas hemorrhagic shock is associated with large areas of cortical ischemia. The investigators concluded that renal vasoconstriction occurs only preterminally in experimental cardiogenic shock. They also raised the possibility that the occurrence of oliguria in human cardiogenic shock may represent a particularly advanced phase of the clinical syndrome.

CLINICAL ASPECTS OF THE MANAGEMENT OF ACUTE HEART FAILURE SYNDROME AND CARDIOGENIC SHOCK

AHFS can have different clinical presentations. One important presentation is that of severe hypertension resulting in pulmonary congestion; typically, the patient is older, with relatively preserved left ventricular function but with diastolic dysfunction, who presents with acute pulmonary edema caused by an abrupt increase in pulmonary capillary wedge pressure (PCWP). Another relatively common presentation is one of less severe pulmonary congestion and peripheral edema but worsening symptoms due to a gradual increase in PCWP. The patient does not have hypertension and maintains a relatively preserved cardiac output. A third clinical presentation is one of cardiogenic shock with possibly severe systolic dysfunction. The patient presents with end-stage or advanced heart failure refractory to conventional medical therapy.

Standard medical therapy for heart failure, such as diuretics, beta blockers, angiotensin-converting enzyme (ACE) inhibitors, or angiotensin receptor blockers, should be started or maximized in patients in the setting of AHFS when they present with pulmonary congestion but with adequate systemic perfusion pressures. The role of B-type natriuretic peptide (nesiritide) in AHFS management

TABLE 182-1

Causes of Cardiogenic Shock

Systolic dysfunction
Diastolic dysfunction
Valvular dysfunction
Cardiac arrhythmias
Coronary artery disease/myocardial infarction
Mechanical complications:
  • Ventricular septal defect
  • Acute valve dysfunction
  • Free wall rupture
  • Pericardial tamponade
Others:
  • Sepsis
  • Prolonged cardiopulmonary bypass

remains controversial. Nesiritide may have a role in the management of moderate to severe heart failure in absence of hypotension. Large prospective, randomized clinical trials are needed, however, to further clarify the safety of this agent and to determine the place it will occupy in acute heart failure management. Two studies have questioned the safety of the drug. The first meta-analysis showed increased risk of worsening renal failure at any time after exposure to the drug. A second analysis showed increased mortality at day 30 after treatment with nesiritide.[12,13] Subsequent analysis of pooled data showed that in-hospital mortality rates were similar for nesiritide and for nitroglycerin.[14]

Management of patients with cardiogenic shock can be challenging because of the limited effectiveness of pharmacological therapy and the severity of illness in the setting of systemic organ hypoperfusion. Cardiogenic shock in patients with chronic renal disease is associated with an increased risk of recurrent hospitalization, subsequent coronary artery bypass graft (CABG) surgery, and death. This increased risk of death is independent and additive to the risk associated with diabetes.[15] Among patients requiring emergency CABG surgery as a lifesaving strategy in the setting of ischemic cardiogenic shock, the in-hospital mortality rate is as high as 20%, with a high incidence of stroke (8%), renal failure requiring dialysis (8.3%), and bleeding (63.3%).[16] The most important goal in the management of cardiogenic shock is rapid restoration of cardiopulmonary stability and assessment of the underlying disease process. Intravascular volume guided by invasive monitoring is an important tool and remains critical to achieve therapeutic goals in tissue oxygenation and organ function. It is very important to make a rapid assessment of the etiology of cardiogenic shock and to get an immediate echocardiogram if a mechanical cause that may necessitate invasive intervention is suspected on clinical grounds (Table 182-1).

Inotropic support remains the central therapy for a depressed myocardium, and correction of the underlying cause such as ischemia will improve outcomes and produce less kidney injury. An important point is that when pharmacological therapy fails to produce adequate organ perfusion to maintain renal function, multiple organ failure will rapidly ensue.[17,18] In this clinical situation mechanical circulatory support such as with intra-aortic balloon pump (IABP) counterpulsation or placement of a ventricular

assistance device needs to be considered to serve as a bridge therapy to percutaneous or surgical revascularization or other cardiac surgical interventions.

MECHANICAL CIRCULATORY SUPPORT IN CARDIOGENIC SHOCK AND ITS EFFECTS ON RENAL FUNCTION

IABP support is indicated for medically refractory cardiogenic shock during acute myocardial infarction or after cardiac surgery and for refractory angina.[19-21] It also can be used for other causes of cardiogenic shock and treatment-refractory malignant ventricular arrhythmias.[22]

The physiological effects of IABP support include increasing coronary perfusion pressure by increasing diastolic pressure and increasing cardiac output, primarily by a reduction in left ventricular afterload that occurs after balloon deflation just before systole. The net effect is to greatly improve the balance between myocardial oxygen supply and demand while creating a modest improvement in systemic perfusion and blood pressure.[23,24]

Indications for ventricular assist device (VAD) placement include stabilization of patients in postcardiotomy shock, bridging patients with refractory heart failure to heart transplantation, and, to a limited extent, cardiac support in patients with myocardial infarction with cardiogenic shock.[26,27] The development and progression of renal dysfunction help to identify patients in acutely deteriorating condition that would benefit most from stabilization with early institution of mechanical circulatory support. Contemporary use of ventricular assist devices has been shown to lead to resolution of severe renal dysfunction in most patients with cardiogenic shock, with long-term outcomes comparable to those in patients without renal dysfunction.[28] The improvements in renal function probably are explained by not only improved cardiac function but also subsequent correction of the abnormal neurohormonal balance found in cardiogenic shock.[29] Extracorporeal membrane oxygenation (ECMO) constitutes the last option for circulatory or pulmonary support for treatment-refractory postoperative cardiopulmonary failure. A venoarterial (ECMO)-based approach can be used for temporary, complete circulatory support until myocardial recovery occurs or during assessment for suitability for heart transplantation. Mortality rates are comparable to those for other cardiac assist devices, with approximately 30% of patients able to be discharged from the hospital.[30]

ROLE OF CONTINUOUS RENAL REPLACEMENT THERAPY IN CARDIOGENIC SHOCK

Currently, continuous renal replacement therapy (CRRT) is the best way to support patients with advanced AKI and cardiogenic shock. It allows controlling volume and correction of electrolyte and acid-base disorders with less hemodynamic impact. In recent years, other forms of extracorporeal fluid removal have been developed (e.g., aquaphoresis), but existing data provide no evidence of advantage relative to CRRT, and the absence of solute clearance is a significant disadvantage.

CONCLUSION

Renal impairment confers a clinically significant risk for excess mortality in patients with AHFS or cardiogenic shock, and the magnitude of the increased mortality is comparable to that associated with traditional prognostic indicators in AHFS, such as ejection fraction.

Worsening renal function leads to fluid retention and further cardiac descompensation. The role of pharmacological therapy is controversial. Inotropes are useful acutely, whereas diuretics and natriuretics can be effective for treating volume overload but can worsen shock. Fluid also can be removed with extracorporeal therapy.

Key Points

1. In acute heart failure syndromes, two main pathophysiological mechanisms operate to maintain extracelluluar fluid volume homeostasis: first, an abnormal perception of inadequate volume by sensors within the circulation and second, a disturbance in the response by neurohormoral mechanisms that will alter the balance of sodium and water retention by the kidney.
2. The faster the perfusion is restored, the better the recovery from acute kidney injury.
3. When pharmacological therapy fails to produce adequate organ perfusion to maintain renal function, multiple organ failure will rapidly ensue.

4. Nesitiride can be considered in moderate to severe cases of acute heart failure syndrome in the absence of hypotension.
5. Renal failure in shock is associated with higher mortality. Early recognition and treatment are essential.

Key References

2. Ho KK, Pinsky JL, Kannel WB, Levy D: The epidemiology of heart failure: The Framingham Study. J Am Coll Cardiol 1993;22(4 Suppl A):6A-13A.
3. Hunt SA, Abraham WT, Chin MH. et al: ACC/AHA 2005 Guideline Update for the Diagnosis and Management of Chronic Heart Failure in the Adult: A report of the American College of Cardiology/American Heart Association Task Force on Practice Guidelines (Writing Committee to Update the 2001 Guidelines for the Evaluation and Management of Heart Failure): Developed in collaboration with the American College of Chest Physicians and the International Society for Heart and Lung Transplantation: Endorsed by the Heart Rhythm Society. Circulation 2005;112:e154-e235.
6. Hollenberg SM, Kavinsky CJ, Parrillo JE: Cardiogenic shock. Ann Intern Med 1999;131:47-59.
7. Hillege HL, Girbes AR, de Kam PJ, et al: Renal function, neurohormonal activation, and survival in patients with chronic heart failure. Circulation 2000;102:203-210.
25. Boehmer JP, Popjes E: Cardiac failure: Mechanical support strategies. Crit Care Med 2006;34(9 Suppl):S268-S277.

See the companion Expert Consult website for the complete reference list.

CHAPTER 183

Renal Function during Cardiac Mechanical Support and the Artificial Heart

Charuhas V. Thakar

OBJECTIVES

This chapter will:
1. Review the available types of mechanical cardiac support.
2. Evaluate the clinical evidence regarding the impact of mechanical cardiac devices on renal function in patients with severe congestive heart failure.
3. Summarize renal and patient outcomes in recipients of mechanical heart devices.

Congestive heart failure (CHF) remains one of the leading causes of hospitalization and is associated with significant morbidity and mortality. It is estimated that approximately 5 million Americans suffer from heart failure, with more than 500,000 new cases diagnosed each year. The aggregate 5-year survival rate for patients with heart failure is approximately 50%; for those with advanced heart failure, the 1-year mortality rate can be as high as 50%.[1] Cardiac transplantation, as a successful treatment for end-stage CHF, was first performed in 1967. According to the United Network for Organ Sharing (UNOS), 2000 heart transplantation procedures were carried out in the United States in 2004 (www.unos.org). Thus, the epidemiological impact of transplantation as a potential treatment for advanced heart failure remains very limited.

Various short-term and long-term circulatory support devices have been used to treat intractable heart failure since the inception of the artificial heart program at the National Institutes of Health (NIH) in 1964. Several different types of mechanical devices have since been approved, either for short-term use, as a bridge to transplantation, or as destination therapy for heart failure.

INDICATIONS FOR AND TYPES OF MECHANICAL CARDIAC SUPPORTS

Severe cardiogenic shock that is not responsive to medical therapy is a well-recognized indication for considering mechanical cardiac support. Depending on the etiology of cardiac failure and whether the expected duration of support is short-term or long-term, various modalities can be used. Intra-aortic balloon pump (IABP) counterpulsation is a temporary form of inotropic support. IABP support commonly is used in cardiogenic shock due to acute myocardial infarction, in association with cardiopulmonary bypass surgery, or with high-risk coronary angioplasty. Influence of IABP support on renal function can be divided into two major categories:

Procedure-related complications such as renal artery occlusion, dissection, or atheroembolic and thromboembolic complications. These anatomical and embolic events may lead to a spectrum of abnormalities ranging from mild temporary renal dysfunction to a more catastrophic event such as renal infarction and cortical necrosis.[2]

Postoperative acute renal failure (ARF). Preoperative IABP support has been consistently demonstrated to be an independent risk factor for severe postoperative ARF.[3,4] Whether the effect is causal, via direct interference with renal blood flow or embolic phenomena, or whether the need for IABP support is a surrogate for the severity of hemodynamic state during the preoperative period remains unclear. Yet it can be used as one of the key predictors to identify patients who are at higher risk for the development of postoperative kidney injury.

The past few decades have seen tremendous advances in another type of mechanical cardiac support—ventricular assist devices (VADs). The following sections focus on types of devices, selection of patients, and renal and related patient outcomes in VAD recipients.

VADs are "blood pumps" and can be classified in multiple ways. One approach to classification of these devices is presented in Table 183-1. In terms of expected response, candidates for VAD placement can be broadly categorized as the following groups: (1) bridge to recovery, in which the disease is expected to be of short-term duration, such as postcardiotomy shock or myocarditis; (2) bridge-to-bridge support, in which a center has the ability to insert a VAD but usually requires that the patient be transferred to an institution that is geared to provide long-term support including transplantation; (3) bridge to transplantation, in which the patient either is already a wait-listed transplantation candidate or is considered suitable for possible transplantation; and (4) destination therapy, in which the patient is deemed unsuitable for transplantation but may benefit from long-term mechanical support.

Indications for VADs include postcardiotomy shock, cardiogenic shock occurring as a consequence of myocardial ischemia, decompensated heart failure regardless of transplantation eligibility, myocarditis, and ventricular arrhythmias refractory to treatment.

PATHOPHYSIOLOGICAL CONSIDERATIONS

The intricate interrelationship of kidney and cardiac function is well recognized. Worthy of emphasis here, however, is that normal renal blood flow averages approximately 1.2 L/minute (normal cardiac output = 6 L/minute) such that it receives 20% of the total cardiac output in the physiological state. This translates to a blood flow of approximately 400 mL/minute per 100 g of kidney tissue, whereby it has the highest oxygen delivery of all major vital organs (84 mL/minute per 100 g). Additionally, the renal outer medulla has the highest ratio of oxygen consumption to oxygen delivery (79%).[5] With progressive heart failure, various compensatory changes in the sympathetic activity, renin-angiotensin system, and vasopressin axis can have a spectrum of effects on renal circulation and renal function. Regional blood flow, especially to the kidney, can be affected independent of central venous pressures in the setting of CHF. The vascular resistance of regional vascular beds, such as renal or hepatic blood flow, is better correlated with systemic vascular resistance than with the recorded mean arterial pressure.[6]

Mechanical support devices may influence renal blood flow, depending on the type of devices, as indicated by experimental models. It has been suggested that intrarenal distribution of renal blood flow can be influenced by pulsatile versus nonpulsatile blood flow; pulsatile-assisted devices may have a better intrarenal vascular redistribution.[7,8] Additionally, early institution of right ventricular support with its associated changes in filling pressures also has been implicated in preservation of renal function.[9]

TABLE 183-1

Summary of Types of Ventricular Assist Devices (VADs)

TYPE OF DEVICE	MECHANISM(S)	EXAMPLE(S)*
Pulsatile VAD	Pneumatic	ABIOMED BVS 5000 Thoratec VAD
	Electric	Thoratec-HeartMate Novacor
Nonpulsatile VAD	Axial flow	MicroMed DeBakey HeartMate II Jarvik 2000
	Centrifugal flow	HeartMate III
Total artificial heart (TAH)	Biventricular, orthotopic, pneumatic, pulsatile blood pump	CardioWest
	Biventricular, orthotopic, nonpulsatile, centrifugal flow pump	AbioCor

*The devices named here are meant to be representative examples in each category; the listing may not include all available devices currently in use.

Whether data from experimental models translate to the clinical setting of heart failure remains less clear. It is no surprise, however, that in disorders of progressive cardiac failure (or institution of cardiac support), kidney function remains a direct downstream target. Epidemiological data increasingly support the striking impact of abnormal kidney function on morbidity and mortality associated with cardiac failure.[10] Worsening kidney function, to the point of end-organ failure, carries a poor prognosis in severe heart failure, and more important, it influences the decisions regarding medical treatment, mechanical support strategies, and cardiac transplantation. Of course, this chapter presents a very introductory and simplistic view of the interrelationship between the heart and the kidney, and the pathophysiology of these interactions is discussed in much greater detail in other chapters of this book. The following sections focus on the clinical aspects of renal function in patients receiving mechanical cardiac support for severe CHF.

PREOPERATIVE ASSESSMENT

With increased understanding of the important issues, significant expansion of the pool of patients considered to be eligible for VAD placement has occurred. Before insertion of a VAD, several aspects unrelated to patient characteristics play a role in patient or device selection. These include institutional expertise, availability of sophisticated postoperative care, and a functioning transplant program. Both the devices and techniques continue to improve over time, and the selection criteria will concurrently change with it. Insertion of a VAD is absolutely contraindicated in patients with active infections or sepsis. Additionally, irreversible neurological injury is widely accepted as a contraindication to provide mechanical support. Other end-organ failure, particularly renal failure, has been associated with poor postoperative outcomes. With early initiation of renal replacement therapy and improved strategies of ultrafiltration, however, the presence of renal failure as a contraindication to mechanical support needs to be evaluated on a case-by-case basis. The present evidence limits the possibility of robust predictive assessments, in terms of patient outcomes, after instituting support.

Hemodynamic criteria considered for eligibility have been those traditionally representative of cardiogenic shock, including cardiac index less than 2.0 L/minute per m^2 of body surface, systolic blood pressure less than 90 mm Hg, left or right atrial pressures greater than 20 mm Hg, and systemic vascular resistance greater than 2100 dyne-sec/cm^{-5}.[11,12] Additional criteria to screen patients for VAD use are based primarily on the estimate of postoperative success. Oz and colleagues published a single-center experience that proposed a scoring system to predict immediate postoperative mortality after VAD insertion.[13] Urine output less than 30 mL/hour (3 points), central venous pressure greater than 16 mm Hg (2 points), mechanical ventilation (2 points), prothrombin time greater than 16 (2 points), and prior surgery (1 point) were selected as independent predictors of death. At a score higher than 5, the operative mortality rate was 38%, compared with 13% in patients with a score of 5 or lower, with a receiver operating characteristic (ROC) value of 0.73. Of note, urine output during the immediate preoperative period, and not serum creatinine level, was a better predic-

tor of postoperative survival. This scoring system was validated a decade later in a separate cohort of patients, albeit at the same institution, when neither creatinine nor urine output predicted postoperative survival.[14] It was postulated that patients may have received aggressive therapy aimed at improving urine output, or volume status in general, which may have been related to the change in the association between urine output and post–VAD insertion survival.

In another study from the European Cardiothoracic Registry, Friedel and colleagues evaluated organ recovery during mechanical assistance for respiratory, hepatic, and renal dysfunction parameters in patients who underwent bridge-to-transplantation procedures.[15] The study found that preimplantation data such as serum creatinine, liver enzymes, and pulmonary gas exchange did not provide predictive indicators of irreversible organ damage. More than 85% of patients experienced functional recovery from preexisting respiratory, hepatic, and renal dysfunction after VAD insertion. Subsequent transplantation, however, was affected by the number of failing organs before institution of mechanical support. Of 17 patients with isolated organ failure before assist, 14 (82%) underwent transplantation. By contrast, only 9 (75%) out of 12 with combined failure of two organs and only 6 (54%) out of 11 patients with three failing organ systems received transplants. In all patients who underwent successful transplantation, however, rapid functional organ recovery occurred within 10 to 15 days after the initiation of mechanical (VAD) assistance.

Although these observational data provide some guidelines for physicians in screening patients, the studies include relatively small numbers of patients and the predictive accuracy of the scoring models approaches ROC values of 0.75. Larger prospective validation studies across multiple centers, including a comparison of the devices used, are necessary before such criteria can be widely accepted as a standard of care.

PREIMPLANTATION RENAL FUNCTION

The relationship between preimplantation renal function and patient outcomes after VAD insertion has been reported in observational studies. A majority of such studies emanate from registries of clinical trials, in which subsequent nested analyses were performed. In one such study involving placement of a Novacor (Worldheart, Oakland, CA) left ventricular assist device (LVAD), 220 patients who underwent surgeries between 1996 and 2003 were examined.[16] Overall, 38% patients died while on LVAD support. Preoperative creatinine clearance significantly influenced post-LVAD survival. Patients with creatinine clearance greater than 95 mL/minute had 30-, 180-, and 365-day survival rates of 90%, 78%, and 66%, respectively, compared with 74%, 41%, and 26% in patients with preoperative creatinine clearance less than 45 mL/minute. The relationship between level of baseline renal function and survival after LVAD placement was directly proportional.

The association between preoperative renal function and post–LVAD insertion survival was independent of transplantation status. A similar relationship existed when patients who received a transplant were assessed separately for survival to transplantation or 30 days after transplantation. Additionally, the investigators examined the effect of change in renal function after LVAD support as a predictor of survival. Patients were stratified at a preoperative creatinine clearance level of 50 mL/minute and followed postoperatively to study the changes in renal function. For those patients whose creatinine clearance started out at lower than 50 mL/minute but increased to greater than 50 mL/minute after LVAD insertion, the 30-day survival rate was 84%, compared with 66% in those whose renal function did not improve after LVAD placement. The difference in survival was not statistically significant.

In another observational study that specifically addressed the impact of preoperative renal dysfunction, 18 patients with pre–VAD insertion creatinine level greater than 3.0 mg/dL were observed for postoperative outcome.[17] Seven patients required post–LVAD insertion hemodialysis for further worsening of renal function. Another 7 patients died before transplantation; 3 were on hemodialysis at the time of death, and the remaining 4 had demonstrated improvement in renal function and died of other causes. Overall, 11 patients were successfully bridged to transplantation, including 4 patients who had required postoperative dialysis. None of the 11 patients were on dialysis at the time of transplantation, and the mean creatinine level had significantly improved compared with that at the time of LVAD placement (1.6 mg/dL versus 4.1 mg/dL, respectively).

These findings could be interpreted to suggest that the level of preoperative renal function affects both short-term and long-term survival (30 days to 1 year) after VAD placement. As expected, the key to long-term survival is the successful replacement of cardiac function by transplantation. Once the bridge to transplantation has been accomplished, the pretransplantation renal function does not seem to influence long-term survival after transplantation. The analyses do not establish an independent relationship between preoperative renal dysfunction and postoperative survival. The data suggest, however, that VAD insertion leads to improvement in renal function. Thus, level of renal function should not preclude patients from receiving mechanical support, especially if they are considered suitable transplantation candidates. Additionally, current ability to accurately predict reversibility of renal function after VAD insertion remains limited.

POSTIMPLANTATION RENAL AND PATIENT OUTCOMES

Patient outcomes and renal outcomes after VAD insertion need to be assessed in the context of whether the indication for VAD use was bridge to transplantation or destination therapy. Most of the data regarding renal outcomes are derived from clinical trials conducted with various devices in these two categories of patient population. Of note, both of these groups can be distinctly different with respect to certain comorbid conditions that determine eligibility for transplantation.

In patients in whom VAD placement has been used as a destination therapy, a randomized controlled trial— Randomized Evaluation of Mechanical Assistance for Treatment of Congestive Heart Failure (REMATCH)— enrolled 129 patients who were not candidates for transplantation. Patients were randomized to receive either medical therapy or VAD insertion as a destination therapy.[18] Sixty-eight patients underwent VAD placement.

The study found a 48% risk reduction for death from any cause in the VAD group, as compared with the medical management group, over a 2-year period. Reported 1-year survival estimates were 52% in the device group and 25% in the medical management group; at 2 years, the survival estimate in the device group was 23%, as opposed to 8% in medically managed patients. Median survival was 408 days in device-placed patients, whereas it was 150 days in the other group. The study also reported quality of life, as assessed by physical function, emotional well-being, and the Minnesota Living with Heart Failure questionnaire score, which were significantly better in the device group at 1- and 2-year follow-up evaluations.

Patients with device placement were at a greater risk for adverse events. Within 3 months after implantation, the likelihood of infection of VAD was 28%, including fatal sepsis. The frequency of bleeding as an adverse event was 42% within 6 months of implantation. No device failure occurred within 1 year of follow-up, but the probability of failure of device was 35% at 24 months. Based on the survival advantage in this randomized controlled trial, it is estimated that for every 1000 patients with end-stage heart failure, 270 deaths could be prevented, as indicated by a 27% absolute risk reduction in mortality. Although these estimates are far superior to improved survival due to advances in drug treatment, the results need to be considered in the context of both the complexity and the costs of care involved in treating patients with VAD. Nevertheless, little doubt exists that in suitable patients, the option of VAD can contribute to meaningful improvement in survival and quality of life in otherwise fatal end-organ failure.

A true comparison of improved survival weighed against costs and complexity of care is difficult because the technology of artificial cardiac support continues to evolve over time. Additionally, ethical considerations as well as dynamics of the health care system and health care delivery need to be accounted for before generalizing the protocols for use of these therapies. The randomized controlled trials of device placement tend to select patients who may be destined to have some short-term success, and the therapies are naturally not instituted with severely ill patients with a high predicted mortality. As is evident from the data, the mean baseline serum creatinine level of patients randomized to undergo VAD insertion was approximately 1.7 mg/dL. Thus, on the basis of existing observational evidence of perioperative renal function, these patients were in the lower risk category in terms of the influence of renal function on postoperative outcomes. None of the reported adverse events in the 2-year period included severe ARF.

The data regarding renal outcomes associated with VAD placement, when used as bridge to transplantation, point to slightly different findings. In a prospective multicenter trial conducted at 24 centers in the United States, 280 transplantation candidates were implanted with a Thoratec-HeartMate (vented electrical left ventricular system) (Thoratec Corp., Pleasanton, OH).[19] Post–VAD insertion renal dysfunction was defined as a serum creatinine greater than 2.2 mg/dL or a blood urea nitrogen greater than 50 mg/dL. Mean baseline serum creatinine in the 280 patients was 1.72 mg/dL. In this cohort, 158 patients (56%) experienced postoperative renal dysfunction. The renal function had significantly improved, however, at the time of transplantation or death, relative to baseline. Median waiting time from VAD placement to transplantation was 105 days. Of the 280 patients, 67%

($n = 188$) were successfully bridged to transplantation, 4% elected to remove the device, and 29% ($n = 82$) died before transplantation. Four major risk factors associated with poor survival included level of baseline creatinine, age, prior cardiac surgery, and elevated total bilirubin level. Probability of survival to transplantation was approximately 60% at 1 year; once the patients received a transplant, the 1-year survival rate was 84%.

Quiani and associates examined the VAD experience from the European registry between 1986 and 1993, during which 258 patients underwent surgeries for VAD placement.[20] In 69% of patients, the placement was intended as a bridge to transplantation, whereas in the remaining patients, various other indications included cardiogenic shock, postcardiotomy, and graft failure or rejection. Of the total number of patients, 56% received pneumatic devices, 30% received a total artificial heart, and 14% received nonpulsatile devices. Postoperative ARF occurred in 25% of cases. When ARF was defined as a need for dialysis, the incidence of ARF was 13%. The overall mortality rate during support was 38%, whereas 62% received an organ transplant. Risk factors for death during support included renal failure, infection, and neurological complications. One hundred sixty patients underwent transplantation, of whom 105 patients were discharged from the hospital (40% of the VAD recipients). The study also analyzed predictors of mortality in all VAD recipients who were not able to be discharged from the hospital, including transplant recipients. Graft failure and renal failure were the two most important determinants of mortality in this subgroup.

Another single-center experience from the United States examined the experience with different devices with respect to VAD outcomes.[21] In 243 patients, the Thoratec-HeartMate was placed as a bridge to transplantation between 1990 and the end of 2003. The study included 174 (72%) patients with single-lead vented electrical devices (SLVEDs), 17 (7%) patients with dual-lead vented electrical devices (DLVEDs), and the remaining 21% with pneumatic VADs. Overall, 70% of 243 patients received a transplant, and the rate of transplantation was the highest in the SLVED group (72%). Survival rates at 1, 3, 5, and 10 years after transplantation were not influenced by pretransplantation placement of VAD. Overall actuarial survival rates after transplantation were 90% at 1 year and 40% at 10 years.

Although several studies report the incidence of postoperative renal dysfunction, detailed analyses of predictors of postoperative ARF remain unclear. In one study, 201 patients undergoing VAD placement between 1996 and 2004 were examined.[22] Postoperative continuous renal replacement therapy (CRRT) was required in 65 patients (32%). Advanced age, preoperative use of IABP, lower albumin, and higher LVAD score were associated with postoperative CRRT in an unadjusted analysis, but only LVAD score was the independent predictor of postoperative CRRT. Baseline creatinine levels at the time of VAD implantation were similar in both ARF and no-ARF groups. Although long-term postoperative survival was lower in those patients who require CRRT, a majority of deaths in the CRRT group occurred either during the hospitalization or within the first few months after surgery. When survival was examined based on transplant status, for those who received a cardiac transplant, the long-term survival was not influenced by postoperative requirement for CRRT. These findings could be interpreted to suggest that postoperative ARF necessitating CRRT is a marker of overall poor clinical outcome during the postoperative period, as predicted by the LVAD score. It is not clear whether postoperative ARF adds discriminatory function to the existing LVAD score used to predict postoperative mortality. If the patients were successfully bridged to transplantation, however, their long-term outcomes were not influenced by pretransplantation need for CRRT.

In contrast with the U.S. data, data from the German group indicated much poorer outcomes associated with postoperative ARF. Kaltenmaier and colleagues examined 227 LVAD recipients (Berlin Heart System [Worldheart, Oakland, CA], Novacor, or HeartMate 2000) between 1988 and 1995.[23] The VAD was used as a bridge to transplantation in 72% of the patients. Postoperative ARF requiring dialysis developed in 55 patients (24%). Survival rate at 30 days was 61% in the non-ARF group, compared with 38% in the ARF group. At 6 months, the survival rate in the non-ARF group was 40%, as opposed to a meager 7% in the ARF group. The investigators conclude that post-LVAD ARF portends an extremely poor short-term or long-term outcome regardless of the indication for VAD placement, particularly including patients with bridge to transplant status.

Clearly, similar to the observations related to preoperative renal function, the data on postoperative ARF do not establish an independent association with death in this group of patients. It may be prudent to suggest at this time that on the basis of existing evidence, if the patient is deemed a suitable candidate for transplantation, then aggressive support with renal replacement therapy along with VAD insertion will improve the outcome with bridge to transplantation.

COMPLICATIONS

The complications associated with VAD placement are related to the device itself or the surgical procedure involved. The rate of device failure has continued to decline as the technology advances. In recent randomized studies, the reported rates of failure are less than 5% at 1 year but increase to above 30% at 24 months. Depending on the device surface, anticoagulation can be necessary to prevent thrombosis and embolic complications. Improvements in the biocompatibility of the materials used to construct these devices have reduced the risk of thromboembolic or inflammatory complications. Use of short-term or long-term anticoagulation is associated with perioperative bleeding, one of the most frequent complications associated with VAD insertion. For various reasons, the need for blood transfusions, including platelet transfusions due to consumptive coagulopathy, is increased in these patients. The high frequency of transfusions can sensitize these patients, further complicating their transplant recipient status. No clinical studies have examined this risk factor in an analytical way, however.

Infection and sepsis after VAD insertion are associated with poor patient outcome. Infection of the pocket or the parts of the device itself can be difficult to treat and may result in explantation. Sepsis leading to multiorgan system failure is the most frequently reported cause of death. Insertion of LVAD can lead to increased load on the right ventricle and to right ventricular failure. Central venous pressure monitoring, both before and soon after LVAD insertion, may allow determination of early indications for a right ventricular assist device (RVAD). A list of commonly occurring complications after VAD insertion is shown in Table 183-2.

TABLE 183-2

Complications Associated with Use of Ventricular Assist Devices

- Bleeding
- Infection/sepsis
- Device failure
- Multiorgan system failure
- Right ventricular failure
- Thromboembolic events
- Immune sensitization

TOTAL ARTIFICIAL HEARTS

The use of the total artificial heart is still very limited. At present, two approved devices are available in the United States: the CardioWest (SynCardia, Tucson, AZ) total artificial heart, used for bridge to transplantation, and the AbioCor (ABIOMED, Danvers, MA), used for destination therapy. The Jarvik-7 total artificial heart was first implanted in 1982 and was previously used in the United States and France as a bridge-to-transplantation support.[24] A slightly modified version, now available in the United States as the CardioWest total artificial heart, has been approved for use by the U.S. Food and Drug Administration (FDA) as a bridge to transplantation. Between 1993 and 2002, 62 consecutive recipients of these devices were studied.[25] Twenty-three percent of the patients died before receiving a cardiac transplant. A total of 48 patients (77%) received a transplant, of whom 42 survived to be discharged from the hospital. Average preimplantation creatinine was 1.7 mg/dL (range, 0.4 to 5.2 mg/dL). Postimplantation renal dysfunction was defined as an increase in serum creatinine greater than 0.5 mg/dL or new requirement for dialysis. ARF developed after implantation in 12 patients, 5 of whom subsequently showed improvement in renal function. In the 7 remaining patients, ARF was associated with death.

Another device, the AbioCor (ABIOMED) total artificial heart, has been placed as a destination therapy in a small group of patients. The device was recently approved for use by the FDA. In the initial published experience, seven patients, with an expected 30-day mortality rate greater than 70%, received this device; one of these died intraoperatively, and four patients died between postoperative days 51 and 151.[26] Two patients were able to be discharged from the hospital.

Based on the numbers of patients, the available evidence is inadequate to allow meaningful commentary on the impact of renal function on patient outcomes; however, descriptive data suggest that acute renal dysfunction continues to represent a marker of poor outcomes. Whether it will be a modifiable risk factor remains to be answered. In view of the very high mortality with end-stage organ failure, these supportive therapies represent a significant advance in medical technology and techniques to prolong survival. As these therapies become more prevalent, an assessment of costs of care and benefits in terms of survival or quality of life will need to be addressed further.

In a field that continues to evolve and has seen rapid advances, it is difficult to examine past evidence and be confident about practice guidelines in the future. Outcomes in VAD recipients represent a perfect example of such a scenario. Preoperative care has seen changes in duration of use of IABP support, early selection of patients for VAD insertion, different approaches to optimize fluid status, and broad-spectrum antibiotic prophylaxis. In addition to the development of newer generations of devices and techniques, certain intraoperative practices such as use of inotropes, vasodilators, or antibiotics also have changed over many years. Improvements in postoperative ICU care, timing of institution of CRRT, and aggressive use of RVADs to prevent pulmonary hypertension and right-sided heart failure are some of the postoperative practices that have changed over time. These factors are important in examining epidemiological data related to outcomes in critically ill patients. Some evidence suggests that trends in incidence of survival change over time independent of the characteristics of the patient population. It is extremely difficult, however, to quantify these changes in order to examine them as study variables.

Key Points

1. Level of preoperative renal function influences short-term and long-term outcomes after placement of ventricular assist devices. Yet a majority of the patients do demonstrate improvement in glomerular filtration rate after ventricular assist device insertion. At present, level of preoperative renal function does not seem to be a contraindication for instituting mechanical cardiac support.
2. Postoperative acute renal failure also portends a poor short-term prognosis and is a predictor of mortality after left ventricular assist device insertion. The studies are limited in identifying specific predictors of kidney injury in the postoperative period.
3. Once bridged to successful transplantation, pre–ventricular assist device renal function or post–ventricular assist device renal failure does not influence post-transplantation outcomes. Thus, if deemed suitable for transplantation, the degree of renal insufficiency may not preclude patients from receiving ventricular assist device support. Available data comparing the effects of different devices on renal function are insufficient for adequate assessment.

Key References

2. Boehmer JP, Popjes E: Cardiac failure: Mechanical support strategies. Crit Care Med 2006;34(9 Suppl):S268-S277.
14. Rao V, Oz MC, Flannery MA, et al: Revised screening scale to predict survival after insertion of a left ventricular assist device. J Thorac Cardiovasc Surg 2003;125:855-862.
18. Rose EA, Gelijns AC, Moskowitz AJ, et al: Long-term mechanical left ventricular assistance for end-stage heart failure. N Engl J Med 2001;345:1435-1443.
25. Copeland JG, Smith RG, Arabia FA, et al: Total artificial heart bridge to transplantation: A 9-year experience with 62 patients. J Heart Lung Transplant 2004;23:823-831.
26. Dowling RD, Gray LA Jr, Etoch SW, et al: Initial experience with the AbioCor implantable replacement heart system. J Thorac Cardiovasc Surg 2004;127:131-141.

See the companion Expert Consult website for the complete reference list.

CHAPTER 184

The Role of Extracorporeal Blood Purification Therapies in the Prevention of Radiocontrast Agent–Induced Nephropathy

Dinna N. Cruz, Mark A. Perazella, and Claudio Ronco

OBJECTIVES

This chapter will:
1. Provide a brief overview of the epidemiology and impact of radiocontrast agent–induced nephropathy after cardiology procedures.
2. Summarize studies on removal of radiocontrast by extracorporeal blood purification therapies.
3. Review the available data on intermittent hemodialysis for the prevention of radiocontrast agent–induced nephropathy.
4. Discuss the studies on continuous renal replacement therapies for the prevention of radiocontrast agent–induced nephropathy.

EPIDEMIOLOGY OF RADIOCONTRAST AGENT–INDUCED NEPHROPATHY

Radiocontrast agent–induced nephropathy (RCIN) is the third leading cause of hospital-acquired acute kidney injury (AKI) worldwide, accounting for 11% of cases, and is associated with significant morbidity.[1] The most common definition of RCIN today is an increase in serum creatinine of 25% or more, or an absolute increase of 0.5 mg/dL or more, from the baseline value, within 48 to 72 hours after radiocontrast exposure. Using these definitions, the reported incidence of RCIN ranges from 3.3% to 23%.[2] It is, however, significantly higher in certain patient subsets, particularly in the elderly, patients with advanced chronic kidney disease (CKD) including renal transplant recipients, patients with diabetes, and those undergoing percutaneous coronary interventions (PCIs).[3,4] Certain patients are at particularly high risk for the development of RCIN related to hemodynamic instability—for example, patients with myocardial infarction or those requiring use of an intra-aortic balloon pump or high dye loads.[3]

The clinical significance of seemingly minor changes in serum creatinine values is not negligible but unfortunately often is ignored. Such changes not only are associated with higher in-hospital mortality (odds ratio, 6.56 to 13.8 with respect to patients who did not develop RCIN)[4,5] but also increases long-term mortality (odds ratio, 2.37 to 7.4).[5,6] This increased risk is more pronounced among patients with preexisting CKD[6] and in patients with AKI severe enough to require dialysis (odds ratio, 13.54).[4] Risk for nonrenal complications also is increased in the setting of RCIN: A greater incidence of periprocedural cardiac com-

plications, including acute myocardial infarction, cardiac arrest, and the need for emergency coronary bypass grafting, has been described.[3] Vascular and systemic procedural complications, such as femoral and gastrointestinal bleeding, also occur with greater frequency in patients with RCIN.[3] A significantly greater cumulative 1-year incidence of major cardiac adverse events, regardless of the presence of CKD at baseline, also complicates RCIN.[6]

In addition to adverse patient-related outcomes, RCIN imparts a significant economic burden. This dramatic increase stems from more widespread exposure of patients to iodinated contrast media, particularly in the field of cardiology. Over the past 10 to 15 years, the number of cardiac catheterizations has increased by 390% in the United States, and the number of PCIs increased by 324%.[7] These diagnostic and therapeutic procedures are performed in an older population, with half of the patients being at least 65 years of age. Europe is following a similar trend: The number of cardiac catheterizations has more than doubled, and the rate of PCI has tripled.[8]

The resulting RCIN after PCI is associated with increased medical resource utilization such as increased length of stay in the intensive care unit (ICU) and in the hospital.[6,9,10] Despite its infrequent occurrence, RCIN requiring either acute or chronic dialysis adds substantially to health care costs. An economic analysis of a CKD database showed a cost of $128,000 per quality-adjusted life-year for patients requiring post-discharge hemodialysis after PCI and a cost of $51,000 per year for chronic maintenance hemodialysis.[10]

PATHOPHYSIOLOGY OF RADIOCONTRAST AGENT–INDUCED NEPHROPATHY

The pathogenesis of RCIN is complex and not fully understood, but iodinated contrast agents induce intense and prolonged vasoconstriction at the corticomedullary junction of the kidney.[11] Moreover, high-osmolar dyes directly impair the autoregulatory capacity of the kidney through a reduction in nitric oxide synthesis. These effects, coupled with direct tubular toxicity of iodinated radiocontrast, lead to overt acute tubular necrosis and the syndrome of RCIN. Pathophysiological effects of hyperosmolar radiocontrast, perturbations of glomerular blood flow, increased oxidative stress, and disturbed endothelin, adenosine, and prostaglandin metabolism have been implicated (Table 184-1). It is beyond the scope of this chapter to discuss

TABLE 184-1

Pathogenesis of Radiocontrast Agent–Induced Nephropathy

Ischemic acute tubular necrosis
- Adenosine
- Endothelin
- Nitric oxide
- Tubuloglomerular feedback (osmotic effects)
- Direct endothelial damage
- Smooth muscle injury

Direct tubular toxicity
- Tubular cell dysfunction and swelling due to hyperosmolarity
- Reduced tubular cell ATP
- Increased intracellular calcium concentration

Oxidative stress and lipid peroxidation
- Generation of reactive oxygen species

Apoptosis of tubular cells
- Tubular cell injury from osmotic stress
- Hypoxia of tubular cells

TABLE 184-2

The Choyke Questionnaire

Six questions for patients:
- Have you ever been told you have renal problems?
- Have you ever been told you have protein in your urine?
- Do you have high blood pressure?
- Do you have diabetes?
- Do you have gout?
- Have you ever had kidney surgery?

Adapted from Choyke PL, Cady J, DePollar SL, Austin H: Determination of serum creatinine prior to iodinated contrast media: Is it necessary in all patients? Tech Urol 1998;4:65-69.

these mechanisms in detail, and the reader is referred to excellent reviews on this topic.[11]

Despite observational data showing strong associations between RCIN and mortality rate, it remains unclear whether the development of AKI in this setting is a marker of multisystem failure in critically ill patients or directly contributes to mortality, or both. Observed associations of AKI with recent myocardial infarction, shock, and a history of congestive heart failure suggest that hemodynamic deterioration plays a central role in the pathogenesis of RCIN that parallels the poor prognosis of patients in whom RCIN develops.[3]

PREVENTION OF RADIOCONTRAST AGENT–INDUCED NEPHROPATHY

The first step in reducing the likelihood of RCIN is to identify patients at risk. Nonmodifiable risk factors include advanced age, diabetes mellitus, preexisting CKD, congestive heart failure, acute myocardial infarction, and cardiogenic shock.[2,3,12] Modifiable risk factors include hypotension, intravascular volume depletion, use of certain drugs (e.g., nonsteroidal anti-inflammatory drugs [NSAIDs], diuretics), and the volume and type of contrast media administered. The Contrast-Induced Nephropathy (CIN) Consensus Working Panel recommended that a simple yet rational approach to risk prediction should focus on kidney dysfunction and diabetes mellitus as the most important risk markers. Patients with a GFR of 60 mL/minute per 1.73 m² or less (CKD stage 3 and higher) are at increased risk for RCIN.[12] The GFR is easily estimated using the abbreviated Modification of Diet in Renal Disease (MDRD) formula (which is easily downloadable for portable personal computer devices)[13]:

$$GFR \ (mL/min/1.73 \ m^2)$$
$$= 186 \times serum \ creatinine^{-1.154} \ (\mu mol/L) \times age^{-0.203}$$
$$(\times 0.742 \ if \ the \ patient \ is \ a \ woman)$$
$$(\times 1.21 \ if \ the \ patient \ is \ black)$$

In the absence of a GFR calculation, the Working Panel agreed that serum creatinine levels of 1.3 mg/dL or greater (114.9 µmol/L or greater) in men and 1.0 mg/dL or greater (88.4 µmol/L or greater) in women were indicative of higher risk.[12]

A serum creatinine value measured up to 6 months before performance of the radiological procedure was deemed acceptable. A serum creatinine measurement is considered highly desirable, although the Working Panel acknowledged that this may be impractical in certain circumstances.[12] In these situations, the Panel supports the use of a simple questionnaire, such as that developed by Choyke and associates (Table 184-2),[14] or dipstick testing for urine protein[15] as a rapid screen. A negative answer to all six questions on the questionnaire or the absence of proteinuria identifies many patients who can undergo radiocontrast studies without serum creatinine measurement.

In an attempt to favorably influence prognosis, a number of prophylactic measures are used to prevent RCIN. Among these are periprocedural hydration, reduced contrast volume, low or iso-osmolar contrast agent administration, and withdrawal of agents that induce a prerenal state (diuretics and NSAIDs) or possess nephrotoxic potential.[16,17] Although proven to be effective in reducing the incidence of RCIN, adequate intravenous hydration may be difficult to achieve in patients at highest risk—that is, those with advanced CKD or congestive heart failure—or when not enough time is available for administration of fluids before the contrast is given, as in patients with acute myocardial infarction. Currently, it is not clear that isotonic sodium bicarbonate is more effective than isotonic or hypotonic saline prophylaxis.[18-20] N-acetylcysteine has been extensively studied, with trials showing either benefit or no effect, but no harm. Thus, N-acetylcysteine is a reasonable and safe agent for prophylaxis. Although controversial, the prophylactic use of theophylline, ascorbic acid, and prostaglandin E₁ may offer some nephroprotection.[21,22] Discussion of these pharmacological approaches to the prevention of RCIN is beyond the scope of this chapter, and the reader is referred to several excellent reviews on these topics.[16,17,23,24] This chapter focuses on the use of extracorporeal blood purification (EBP) therapies to prevent RCIN.

CLEARANCE OF CONTRAST WITH EXTRACORPOREAL BLOOD PURIFICATION THERAPIES

Radiocontrast media are excreted almost exclusively by the kidneys, and elimination of these agents is delayed in patients with underlying kidney disease. The rationale for

TABLE 184-3

In Vivo Studies on Radiocontrast Clearance by Extracorporeal Therapies

STUDY	RADIOCONTRAST AGENT	DIALYSIS TIME	CONTRAST ELIMINATION AND/OR CLEARANCE
Baars et al., 1984[25]	Diatrizoate	>10 hr	80.7 ± 4.7%
Kierdorf et al., 1989[26]	Iopromide	3 hr	65% 80 mL/min
Donnelly et al., 1993[27]	Iopamidol	4 hr	55.7%
Moon et al., 1995[28]	Iohexol	6 hr	77% 70.4 ± 24.6 mL/min
Ueda et al., 1996a[29]	Iopremol	4 hr	4.6% 131-133 mL/min
Ueda et al., 1996b[30]	Ioversol	4 hr	82.5 ± 5.1% 114-129 mL/min
Furukawa et al., 1996[31]	Iohexol	4 hr	78.4 ± 6.5%
	Ioxaglate	4 hr	72.4 ± 6.0%
Lehnert et al., 1998[32]	Iopentol	3 hr	32%
Matzkies et al., 1999[33]	Iopromide	3 hr	62% (low-flux) 110 ± 1.4 mL/min
		3 hr	58% (high-flux) 108 ± 1.9 mL/min
Matzkies et al., 2000a[34]	Iopromide	NS	87-121 mL/min (cuprophane)
		NS	147-162 mL/min (polysulfone)
Matzkies et al., 2000b[35]	Iopromide	2 hr	59% (cuprophane) 102 ± 7 mL/min
		2 hr	66% (polysulfone) 153 ± 4 mL/min
Sterner et al., 2000[36]	Iohexol, iodixanol, ioxaglat	4 hr	79%
Lorusso et al., 2001[37]	Iomeprol	4 hr	40% 80.6 mL/min
Berger et al., 2001[38]	Iopromide	2-3 hr	83% after 24 hr
Schindler et al., 2001[39]	Iopromide, iomeprol	NS	64 ± 1% (low-flux) 82 ± 2.3 mL/min
		NS	74 ± 3% (high-flux) 100 ± 2.2 mL/min
		NS	82 ± 1% (HDF) 114 ± 4 mL/min
		NS	62 ± 3% (HF) 86 ± 5 mL/min
Frank et al., 2003[40]	Iomeprol	4 hr	54 ± 15 mL/min
Gabutti et al., 2003[41]	Ioversol	10 hr	30.9% (CVVHDF)

CVVHDF, continuous venovenous hemodiafiltration; HDF, hemodiafiltration; HF, hemofiltration; NS, not stated.

use of EBP therapies in the prevention of RCIN is based on the concept of enhanced clearance of nephrotoxic radiocontrast in patients with kidney dysfunction. EBP therapy may reduce contrast exposure and theoretically prevent the development of RCIN in this high-risk group of patients.

Several studies have evaluated the removal of radiocontrast media by hemodialysis. Contrast elimination ranges from 32% to 83% in various studies (Table 184-3).[25-41] Clearance is affected by various factors, including blood flow, duration of dialysis, type of dialyzer, and use of diffusive, convective, or combined modalities. As little as one third of the contrast dose was removed in a study that performed 3-hour hemodialysis at low blood flows.[32] Conflicting reports on the ability of different dialyzers to remove contrast media have been published. In vitro studies have demonstrated that with increasing transmembrane pressure, a high-flux polyacrylonitrile dialyzer has a higher sieving coefficient than a low-flux cuprophane dialyzer.[42] These findings are congruent with those in an in vivo randomized study of patients on chronic dialysis as well as "predialysis" patients.[39] By contrast, Matzkies and colleagues demonstrated no difference in iopromide clearance between high-flux and low-flux dialyzers among their patients.[33] These same investigators reported that

iopromide elimination with polysulfone membranes was more effective than with cuprophane membranes.[34,35] The effect of residual renal function and endogenous radiocontrast removal was not considered in any of these studies, however. Similar uncertainty exists in terms of data on the convective modalities, such as hemodiafiltration and hemofiltration. An in vitro study using a bovine tank model reported that hemodiafiltration could remove contrast media more effectively than hemofiltration.[43] This finding is not unexpected in view of the molecular weight of radiocontrast studied (iomeprol has a molecular weight of 723). With regard to in vivo studies, a higher extraction ratio for contrast media was noted with hemodiafiltration than with both hemofiltration and low-flux hemodialysis.[39] By contrast, another study demonstrated comparable iopromide elimination with hemofiltration and with hemodialysis.[34]

Clearance of ioversol with continuous venovenous hemodiafiltration (CVVHDF) was evaluated in 12 patients. CVVHDF performed for 10 hours with a blood flow of 100 to 150 mL/minute and dialysis and replacement fluid rate of 2000 mL/hour provided a fractional removal of contrast media of 30.9% ± 20.7%.[41] Ioversol elimination was considered to be modest and approximately equal to the intrinsic renal removal of radiocontrast (mean ioversol

TABLE 184-4

Studies on Extracorporeal Blood Purification (EBP) for the Prevention of Radiocontrast Agent–Induced Nephropathy

| STUDY | RADIOCONTRAST AGENT | EBP Group | | | | Standard Medical Therapy Group | | RANDOMIZATION |
		N	BASELINE SCr (mg/dL)	EBP MODALITY/FILTER	N	BASELINE SCr (mg/dL)	
Moon et al., 1995[28]	NS	13	4.6	HD/cuprophane	0	N/A	No comparison group
Huber et al., 2002[49]	Iomeprol	31	4.01	HD/Fresenius F60	0	N/A	No comparison group*
Lehnert et al., 1998[32†]	Iopentol	15	2.58	HD/Fresenius F50	15	2.26	Yes
Sterner et al., 2000[36†]	Iohexol, iodixanol, ioxaglat	15	3.36-3.86†	HD/low-flux cellulose acetate or diacetate	17	2.62-3.43‡	Yes
Vogt et al., 2001[45†]	Low-osmolality	55	3.58	HD/Fresenius F50, F60	58	3.48	Yes
Berger et al., 2001[38†]	Iopromid	7	2.9	HD/Fresenius F6	8	2.5	Yes
Frank et al., 2003[40†]	Iomeprol	7	3.9	HD/Fresenius F60	10	4.2	Yes
Marenzi et al., 2003[46†]	Iopentol	58	3.0	CVVH/Renaflow HF700	56	3.1	Yes
Marenzi et al., 2006[47§]	Iopentol	31 (pre-post) 31 (post)	3.7 (pre-post) 3.6 (post)	Pre-post CVVH/post CVVH/Renaflow HF700	30	3.6	Yes
Hsieh et al., 2005[48†]	Iopromid	20	3.9	HD/AM-Bio HX90	20	3.3	No
Gabutti et al., 2003[41†]	Ioversol	26	2.6	CVVHDF/Prisma M100	25	>2.0 mg/dL¶	No

To convert creatinine values from mg/dL to mmol/L, multiply by 88.4.
*Described their results in the context of previous studies.
†Included in systematic review by Cruz et al.[44]
‡Different inclusion criteria for serum creatinine for diabetics and nondiabetics; the median is given for each subgroup.
§This study evaluated CVVH performed 6 hours before, plus 18 to 24 hours after contrast ("pre-post") and CVVH performed only after contrast ("post").
¶Mean value not stated in paper.
CVVH, continuous venovenous hemodialysis; CVVHDF, continuous venovenous hemodiafiltration; HD, hemodialysis; NS, not stated; SCr, serum creatinine.

urinary-CVVHDF extraction rate of 1.00 ± 0.46). Because only one CVVHDF treatment was examined, it is not clear whether higher ultrafiltration rates would have enhanced ioversol clearance.

EXTRACORPOREAL BLOOD PURIFICATION THERAPIES FOR THE PREVENTION OF RADIOCONTRAST AGENT–INDUCED NEPHROPATHY

EBP therapies have been studied in the prevention of RCIN (Table 184-4). A recent systematic review identified six randomized controlled trials and two nonrandomized trials comparing EBP with standard therapy (n = 412).[44] Of these, six evaluated intermittent hemodialysis,[32,36,38,40,45,48] one CVVHDF,[41] and one continuous venovenous hemofiltration (CVVH),[46] immediately before, during, or within 2 hours of administration of radiocontrast. Most studies included patients undergoing diagnostic or interventional cardiac procedures. RCIN incidence, defined as an increase in serum creatinine concentration of at least 0.5 mg/dL (44 μmol/L), was 35.2% with standard medical therapy (e.g., saline, calcium channel blockers, aminophylline), and 27.8% with extracorporeal therapies.[44] RCIN incidence was not significantly reduced with EBP compared

with standard therapy (Fig. 184-1) (relative risk [RR], 0.97; 95% confidence interval [CI], 0.44 to 2.14), but the results of the trials were heterogeneous.

Hemodialysis

Separate analysis of the 6 intermittent hemodialysis trials demonstrated a nonsignificant trend favoring standard therapies over periprocedural hemodialysis (RR, 1.35; 95% CI, 0.93 to 1.94). One study[45] found a trend for more complications in the hemodialysis group. EBP, whether intermittent or continuous, also did not markedly affect the need for temporary acute renal replacement therapy (RRT) (Fig. 184-2) (RR, 0.92; 95% CI, 0.09 to 9.30), or the combined incidence of death and the need for permanent RRT.

These observations are consistent with previous animal studies demonstrating the rapid effect of radiocontrast on renal blood flow and imply that kidney injury occurs very rapidly. Injury develops even after only a brief delay in the initiation of hemodialysis. It was likewise disappointing that even simultaneous hemodialysis[40] or CVVHDF[41] does not reduce the incidence of RCIN. Although hemodialysis is not useful for reducing the risk for RCIN, the CIN Consensus Working Panel agreed that for patients with severe renal impairment (estimated GFR less than 20 mL/minute) who require radiocontrast administration, procedure preparation should include planning for hemodialy-

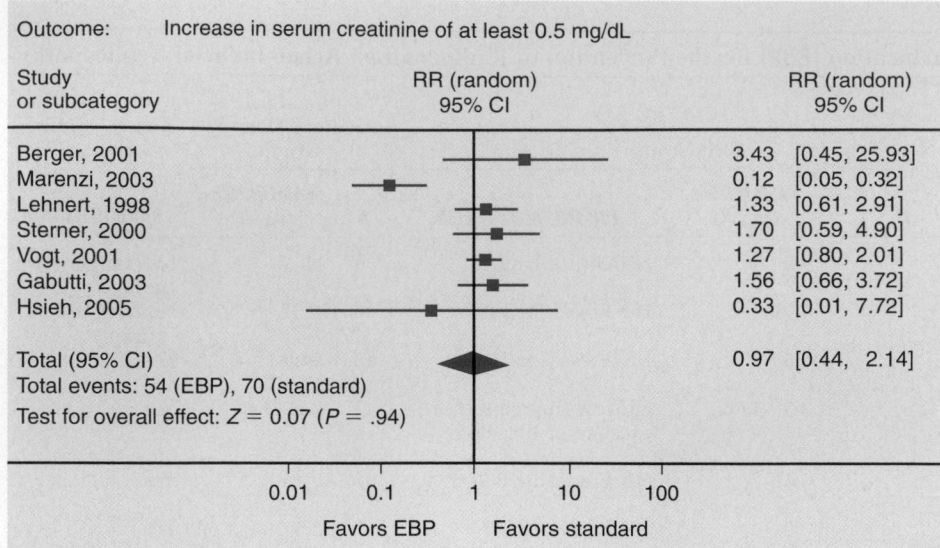

FIGURE 184-1. Relative risk (RR) for radiocontrast agent–induced nephropathy. CI, confidence interval; EBP, extracorporeal blood purification.

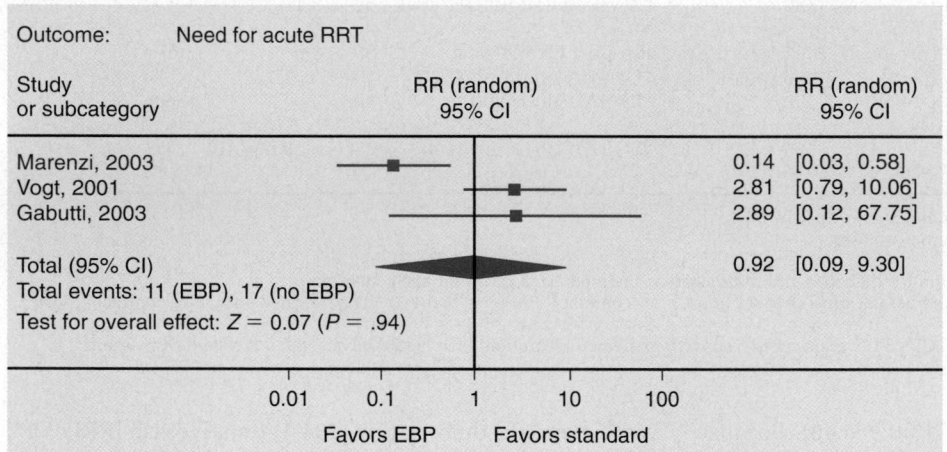

FIGURE 184-2. Relative risk (RR) for need for acute temporary renal replacement therapy (RRT). CI, confidence interval; EBP, extracorporeal blood purification.

sis in the event that severe RCIN occurs despite prophylaxis.[50]

Continuous Renal Replacement Therapies

Continuous renal replacement therapies (CRRTs) have been studied in the prevention of radiocontrast nephropathy.[41,46,47] The results of three separate studies are divergent, perhaps because of differences in the study population, the amount of radiocontrast given, the CRRT technique itself, or ancillary care.

Gabutti and colleagues studied 26 patients with various degrees of kidney disease (mean creatinine, 2.6 ± 0.9 mg/dL) who underwent CVVHDF.[41] Treatment was initiated immediately before the contrast procedure, and continued during and after the procedure for 10 hours. The incidence of RCIN in the CVVHDF group, defined as an increase in serum creatinine of at least 0.5 mg/dL above baseline within 3 days of contrast, was 37%, compared with 24% in a historical control group of 25 patients (*P* = not significant). One patient in the CVVHDF group subsequently required temporary dialysis, and although not specifically mentioned, it is implied that none of the historical group did. All cases of RCIN in the CVVHDF group occurred in

patients who underwent aortofemoral angiography or angioplasty, who received more radiocontrast than their counterparts who underwent coronary procedures. Unfortunately, it is not simple to draw conclusions from these results. The characteristics of the CVVHDF group are described in a table; those of the control group are nonexistent except for minimum baseline creatinine (higher than 2 mg/dL) and type of contrast procedure.

The historical control group received treatment with prophylactic saline infusion or withdrawal of potentially nephrotoxic medications, whereas only 16 patients in the CVVHDF group received saline prophylaxis. Moreover, 8 of the treatment group patients had either absolute or relative hypovolemia; of these, 2 had frank cardiogenic shock. This subgroup would be expected to have a poor outcome in terms of RCIN and also would likely suffer from further renal ischemia from any extracorporeal therapy, especially if fluid is performed. With respect to the prescribed CRRT, the dialysis and replacement fluid flow rates were 2000 mL/hour. On the basis of the mean weight of study patients and an assumption of no net fluid removal, the mean ultrafiltration rate can be estimated at 27.8 mL/kg per hour. This is lower than the dose recommended by Ronco and colleagues for the treatment of AKI in critically ill patients.[51] It is not clear whether these recommendations are applicable for prevention of RCIN. CVVHDF was successfully performed during the contrast procedure, hemodynamic tolerance was described as excellent (except in one patient), and complications were minimal. The investigators concluded that although it is feasible to perform CVVHDF simultaneously during contrast procedures, radiocontrast clearance was modest and did not affect the occurrence of RCIN.[41]

Marenzi and colleagues performed two randomized trials comparing CVVH with isotonic saline volume expansion.[46,47] In the first study, 114 patients undergoing PCI (mean creatinine level, 3.0 ± 1.0 mg/dL) were randomized to undergo periprocedural CVVH ($n = 58$) or to receive intravenous saline ($n = 56$).[46] Exclusion criteria included cardiogenic shock and overt congestive heart failure—one of the differences from the CVVHDF study previously described. RCIN was defined as a greater than 25% increase in baseline serum creatinine concentration. CVVH was initiated 4 to 6 hours before PCI and continued for 18 to 24 hours. Replacement fluid rate was set at 1000 mL/hour, lower than in the CVVHDF study (2000 mL/hour). Other than a decreased likelihood of RCIN (5% versus 50%; $P < .001$), a reduction in the requirement for acute temporary RRT (3% versus 25%; $P < .001$) and in in-house mortality (2% versus 14%; $P = .02$) and 1-year mortality (10% versus 30%; $P = .01$) rates was noted.[46]

This study has been criticized for the inequality of treatment between the CVVH and the control group, as the former were monitored in the intensive care unit while the latter were observed in the step down unit.[52] It is possible that the survival and renal benefit attributed to CVVH is instead related to the higher level of care given to the CVVH patients. The location of the patients in the CVVHDF study was not stated,[41] and it is not possible to make any comparisons with the CVVH study. It is certainly plausible that a difference in location or staffing ratio also obtained in this study. It is likewise possible that intermittent hemodialysis for RCIN prophylaxis may show a positive result if performed in an ICU.

Heparin administration in the CVVH (not given in the control group) has been suggested to explain the difference in RCIN reduction.[52] This speculation is based on the effect of heparin to inhibit acute inflammation, attenuate ischemia-reperfusion injury, and reduce oxidant stress.[53] However, patients in CVVHDF study and at least one of the intermittent hemodialysis studies also received heparin, making this explanation less tenable. Despite its limitations, the Marenzi group study should be credited for the use of computer randomization, description of the randomization process and sample size calculations, and for monitoring renal function with both serum creatinine concentration (creatinine clearance) and urine output. It is the only study to report the course of diuresis in these patients. In the patients who received CVVH, urine output remained stable, whereas a transient decrease was observed in patients in the control group, suggesting at least that the CVVH procedure did not adversely affect renal hemodynamics.

This same group of investigators subsequently published a second randomized study with three arms: CVVH performed before and after the contrast procedure ("pre- plus post-contrast"), CVVH performed after contrast administration only, and isotonic saline prophylaxis without CVVH.[47] The hemofiltration and saline prophylaxis protocols were identical to those in the first study, except that the post-contrast hemofiltration group started CVVH after the contrast procedure and continued it for 18 to 24 hours. A beneficial effect of pre- plus post-contrast hemofiltration on the incidence of RCIN (3% versus 26% versus 40% in the pre- plus post-contrast hemofiltration, post-contrast hemofiltration, and control groups, respectively; $P = .001$), need for acute temporary RRT (zero versus 10% versus 30%; $P = .002$), and in-hospital mortality (zero versus 10% versus 20%; $P = .03$) was described.[47] The effect of post-contrast CVVH was less marked, but this protocol still reduced the need for acute temporary RRT and in-hospital mortality. The investigators suggest that controlled high-volume hydration, rather than contrast removal, underlies the beneficial effect. They hypothesize that vigorous bicarbonate infusion given to the pre- plus post-hemofiltration group may counterbalance the osmotic diuretic effect of contrast agents, increase circulating volume and glomerular filtration, decrease renal vasoconstriction, enhance contrast elimination, and decrease residence time of contrast within the tubules.[47] The explanation is not that straightforward, however, because bicarbonate-based solutions were used in the CVVHDF study that did not show a benefit.[41] The mechanisms underlying the observed clinical benefits of pre- plus post-contrast CVVH in these two studies remain unclear. At present, with the level of currently available evidence, the high cost and need for ICU admission will limit the usefulness of this prophylactic approach.[50]

Adverse Events

Reported adverse events associated with EBP were few. They included clotting of blood lines ($n = 1$), catheter dysfunction ($n = 1$), arteriovenous fistula formation at the site of the access ($n = 1$), bleeding at the site of vascular access ($n = 3$), and need for blood transfusion ($n = 1$).[41,45,46] In one study, 7 patients had palpable groin hematomas, but because this also was the site of the arterial catheter for the coronary angiogram, the actual cause of the local bleeding could not be determined.[41]

Limitations of Present Knowledge

One aspect to consider in use of both intermittent and continuous EBP therapies is the use of serum creatinine concentration to define the presence or absence of RCIN. The extracorporeal therapies themselves lower the serum creatinine concentration through solute removal, making these markers imprecise and susceptible to error. Because the most commonly used definition of RCIN indeed relies on the measurement of changes in serum creatinine concentration, this study flaw cannot be completely avoided. Also, the cosmetic effect of dialysis on serum creatinine concentration persists only for a day after the treatment. Thus, measurements at 48 to 72 hours after the procedure would not be unreasonable if the slopes of the changes in serum creatinine concentration were evaluated in the two groups. Moreover, any definition of RCIN based on creatinine concentrations would be unable to distinguish between AKI due to radiocontrast itself and that due to renal atheroemboli. Prospective studies using markers and endpoints unaffected by the experimental intervention itself, such as AKI markers including kidney injury molecule-1 (KIM-1), Cyr 61, and NGAL,[54-56] or "hard" clinical endpoints such as need for acute RRT or death, will clarify these issues. To make such studies applicable to current clinical practice, standard and novel protective therapies such as bicarbonate-based prophylaxis or N-acetylcysteine should be used in the standard medical therapy arm.

CONCLUSION

RCIN is a common complication associated with significant morbidity. It also is associated with increased in-hospital, 1-year, and 5-year mortality rates. Currently available prophylactic measures remain only modestly effective in preventing RCIN in high-risk patients. Extracorporeal blood purification, including hemodialysis and the various forms of CRRT, also appears to be ineffective in the prevention of this complication. Until adequately powered studies demonstrate efficacy and safety of EBP in the prevention of RCIN, it cannot be recommended at this time.

Key Points

1. Radiocontrast-induced nephropathy is a common and potentially serious complication occurring after diagnostic and therapeutic cardiology procedures using radiocontrast media.
2. The first and most important step in reducing the likelihood of radiocontrast-induced nephropathy is to identify patients at risk by medical history and measurement of serum creatinine concentration to allow calculation of estimated glomerular filtration rate.
3. Extracorporeal blood purification effectively removes radiocontrast agents from the circulation.
4. Periprocedural extracorporeal blood purification (hemodialysis or continuous renal replacement

therapy) does not reduce the incidence of radiocontrast agent–induced nephropathy compared with standard medical therapy and cannot be recommended at this time.
5. The potential benefit of continuous venovenous hemofiltration, reported by a single center, should be confirmed with further studies before this modality can be recommended or disregarded, and higher doses of continuous renal replacement therapy also may merit further investigation.

Key References

17. McCullough PA, Soman SS: Contrast-induced nephropathy. Crit Care Clin 2005;21:261-280.
44. Cruz D, Perazella M, Bellomo R, et al: Extracorporeal blood purification therapies for prevention of radiocontrast-induced nephropathy: A systematic review. Am J Kidney Dis 2006; 48:361-371.
45. Vogt B, Ferrari P, Schonholzer C, et al: Prophylactic hemodialysis after radiocontrast media in patients with renal insufficiency is potentially harmful. Am J Med 2001;111:692-698.
47. Marenzi G, Lauri G, Campodonico J, et al: Comparison of two hemofiltration protocols for prevention of contrast-induced nephropathy in high-risk patients. Am J Med 2006;119: 155-162.
50. Stacul F, Adam A, Becker CR, et al for the CIN Consensus Working Panel: Strategies to reduce the risk of contrast-induced nephropathy. Am J Cardiol 2006;98(suppl): 59K-77K.

See the companion Expert Consult website for the complete reference list.

The Lung and the Kidney

CHAPTER 185

Lung Function in Uremia

Özgür Karacan and Emre Tutal

OBJECTIVES

This chapter will:
1. Review pulmonary function tests commonly used in clinical practice.
2. Summarize the current literature on pulmonary function abnormalities in uremic patients.
3. Outline the effects of different renal replacement treatment modalities, including hemodialysis, continuous ambulatory peritoneal dialysis, and renal transplantation, on pulmonary function abnormalities.

As well known by the reader, uremia is a clinical syndrome developing secondary to loss of metabolic, hormonal, and excretory functions of the kidneys, in acute or chronic background and characterized mainly by accumulation of nitrogenous catabolism end products and water and electrolyte imbalances. Similar to every other organ system, the lungs also are under the adverse influence of renal failure and are highly affected by uremia of any cause. Patients with renal failure of any stage (acute, chronic, end-stage) are at risk for a group of clinically significant pulmonary complications including, most commonly, pulmonary edema, pulmonary fibrosis, pulmonary calcification, pulmonary hypertension, hemosiderosis, and pleural fibrosis.[1-6] These patients also may have some degree of pulmonary dysfunction that may not be clinically significant and detectable only by a series of noninvasive evaluations called pulmonary function tests. Pulmonary dysfunction may be the direct result of circulating uremic toxins or may result indirectly from volume overload, anemia, immune suppression, extraosseous calcification, malnutrition, electrolyte disorders, or acid-base imbalances. Also, available renal replacement therapy (RRT) modalities for renal failure—hemodialysis, continuous ambulatory peritoneal dialysis (CAPD), and renal transplantation—may cause some specific pulmonary side effects. This chapter provides comprehensive and in-depth information, derived from the most recent medical literature, about lung function in uremia that may not be found in traditional medical textbooks.

Physiological tests of lung function can be separated into those that evaluate the lung as a mechanical object (volumes, flows, compliance, resistance, maximal respiratory pressures, work of breathing) and those that focus on the gas exchange function of the lung (pressures of arterial oxygen and carbon dioxide, diffusing capacity, alveolar-arterial oxygen pressure difference). Accordingly, pulmonary function tests can be categorized as follows[7]:

Airway function tests
- Basic spirometry—basic lung volumes and capacities (e.g., vital capacity, expiratory reserve volume)
- Forced vital capacity maneuver—forced vital capacity (FVC), forced expiratory volume in first second (FEV_1)
- Maximum voluntary ventilation
- Maximum inspiratory and expiratory pressures
- Airway resistance and compliance

Lung volumes and ventilation
- Diffusion capacity
- Arterial blood gases and gas exchange tests
- Cardiopulmonary exercise testing

Using these tests, the clinician can assess the general efficacy of the ventilatory apparatus, such as the operative condition of central respiratory units, neural pathways, and neuromuscular junctions; differentiate obstructive from restrictive-type pulmonary disorders; and evaluate respiratory muscle strength and gas exchange functions. Cardiopulmonary exercise testing also allows assessment of the patient's exercise capacity and effects on the respiratory, cardiovascular, skeletal, hematological, and psychoneurological systems. In uremia and related conditions, pulmonologists commonly use airway function tests such as basic spirometry and the FVC maneuver as initial tests to evaluate expiratory flow rates and lung volumes. Such testing in patients with chronic renal disease may reveal a wide variety of disorders, ranging from those in which normal pulmonary function is normal, to those with minimal reduction in parameters of small airway function, to disorders with profoundly reduced lung volumes, as in the case of overt pulmonary edema.

This chapter summarizes the current literature on pulmonary function test abnormalities in patients with renal failure, and on the effects of different RRT modalities on these findings.

DIFFUSION CAPACITY AND LUNG VOLUME CHANGES IN UREMIC PATIENTS

As already mentioned, the most common pathological condition of lungs in patients with renal failure is pulmonary edema, usually resulting from a combination of fluid overload and abnormal permeability of pulmonary microcirculation secondary to uremic toxins.[1-3] Although many pulmonary function abnormalities may be attributed to this pathological condition, Wallin and coworkers, using an indocyanide green indicator dilution technique, reported that decrease in lung fluid volume may be independent of weight loss during a hemodialysis session.[8] Similarly, Morrison and colleagues reported that changes in diffusion capacity for carbon monoxide (DLCO) and pulmonary capillary blood flow were occurring independently of pulmonary volume changes during hemodialysis sessions.[9] As suggested by these reports and clinical experiences, a patient who achieves a planned posthemodialysis dry weight may nevertheless still have subclinical pulmonary dysfunction that may be hard to identify in routine clinical practice. So it is important to ensure that the patient with renal failure is not in a hypervolemic state before interpretation of pulmonary function test findings.

The earliest relevant studies reported that the most common abnormalities of lung functions in uremic patients were reduced DLCO and small airway disease.[1] In 1965 Daum and associates reported a 55% reduction in DLCO in 15 patients with acute and 2 with chronic renal failure.[10] Similarly, in 1973 Zidulka and coworkers studied 6 fluidoverloaded patients just before and after hemodialysis; they reported that all 6 patients had reduced lung volume and DLCO before hemodialysis, whereas after hemodialysis, closing capacity decreased (an important marker of improvement in small airway function) and basal ventilation and perfusion increased significantly in 5 patients.[11] On the basis of these findings, these investigators suggested that these changes were due to dialyzable pulmonary edema and irreversible uremic lung fibrosis. Similarly, Crosbie and Parsons, Wolf and associates, and Forman and coworkers reported decreased DLCO as the most common lung function abnormality in uremic patients in 1974, 1979, and 1981, respectively.[12-14] In the study by Wolf and associates, which included 43 uremic patients (serum creatinine between 1.5 and 14.0 mg/100 mL), DLCO values were found to be correlated with patients' hemoglobin instead of serum creatinine levels; accordingly, the investigators concluded that reduction in DLCO was due to renal anemia, rather than to uremic damage of interstitial lung disease.[14]

The first published study (1991) comparing effects of different RRT modalities on pulmonary function tests was that of Bush and Gabriel,[15] who reported pulmonary function analysis results for 80 patients without any significant lung disease history, who were distributed equally into four management groups: no RRT, CAPD, hemodialysis, and renal transplantation. Only 9 of the 80 patients were found to have normal lung function. DLCO was decreased in all patient groups including transplant recipients; patients on CAPD had significantly lower DLCO values than those measured in patients on other RRT modalities. The investigators concluded that the likeliest explanation of decreased DLCO that does not respond to renal transplantation, unlike many other complications of uremic syndrome, was subclinical pulmonary edema that progressed to pulmonary fibrosis before a succesful renal transplantation could be performed.

Subsequent studies that also reported decreased DLCO in patients on hemodialysis usually presented similar conclusions, emphasizing that this situation may be mainly secondary to subclinical pulmonary edema, pulmonary fibrosis, or dialysis membrane reactions (complement activation, leukocyte sequestration[16-19]). Duration of dialysis also was speculated to be an important factor for development of DLCO abnormalities in patients on hemodialysis. In 2002, Herrero and coworkers studied 43 patients maintained on hemodialysis and reported that those receiving regular hemodialysis for more than 5 years showed significantly lower values of DLCO and carbon monoxide transfer coefficient compared with patients before dialysis and patients receiving regular hemodialysis for less than 12 months.[16] Seventy-five percent of patients on long-term hemodialysis had markedly reduced DLCO or KCO, compared with 17% of patients before dialysis and 10% of patients dialyzed for less than 12 months. On the basis of these findings, they concluded that patients undergoing long-term regular hemodialysis with bioincompatible membrane are prone to experience selective loss of DLCO, possibly owing to chronic pulmonary fibrosis.

Studies of patients on peritoneal dialysis have yielded conflicting results. Beasley and colleagues reported that instillation of 2 L of dialysis fluid in patients on CAPD does not result in a clinically significant deterioration in pulmonary functions, after measuring lung volumes and DLCO in 20 patients with and without dialysis solution in the abdominal cavity.[20] Contradictory findings also were reported recently by Mydlik and coworkers and Tang and associates.[21,22] Mydlik's group found significantly decreased DLCO values for 15 patients on CAPD and concluded that this reduction was due mainly to low hemoglobin levels and minimal interstitial pulmonary edema.[21] Tang and associates measured DLCO in 50 uremic patients just before and again after initiation of CAPD and found that these patients had low DLCO values that did not improve but also deteriorated after initiation of CAPD, whereas indices of pulmonary ventilation (FVC, maximum breathing capacity, FEV$_1$, peak expiratory flow rate, maximum midexpiratory flow rate) improved significantly with initiation of dialysis.[22]

We also could not demonstrate any decrease in DLCO in two different studies that included 27 patients on hemodialysis and 22 on CAPD, respectively.[23,24] An interesting finding was that DLCO was not only preserved but also increased in the patients on hemodialysis, which potentially may be secondary to use of biocompatible membranes in the hemodialysis unit, or to minimal pulmonary congestion, which could cause vascular changes and increase DLCO.[23] Similar findings indicating an increase in DLCO were reported by Chan and colleagues, who studied pulmonary function in a group of patients on hemodialysis who underwent renal transplantation.[25] The patients' DLCO and residual volume (RV) were in the high range of predicted values (115.7% and 157.8%, respectively) before transplantation, but the values dropped steadily after transplantation and normalized at 6 months after surgery. The investigators attributed the high pretransplantation DLCO and RV values to chronic vascular congestion. Their results were similar to the DLCO and RV values we recorded in our own studies.[23,24]

Contradicting our speculations,[23] some studies reported that dialyzer membranes do not have any important effect on lung functions. Recently, Lang and colleagues reported data for 14 patients on hemodialysis in whom a cellulose dialyzer membrane and a synthetic high-flux dialyzer membrane were used at different times.[26] A spirometric evaluation (VCmax, FEV$_1$, FEF$_{25-75}$, PEF) was performed in each patient for each membrane just before and after a hemodialysis session. The investigators found no signifi-

TABLE 185-1

Diffusion Capacity and Lung Volume Changes in Uremic Patients

STUDY	STUDY POPULATION	FINDING(S)
Daum et al.[10]	15 acute renal failure patients, 2 chronic renal failure patients	$DL_{CO} \downarrow$
Zidulka et al.[11]	6 HD patients	$DL_{CO} \downarrow$
Crosbie and Parsons[12]	6 chronic renal failure patients with volume overload	$DL_{CO} \downarrow$
Forman et al.[13]	18 HD patients	$DL_{CO} \downarrow$
Wolf et al.[14]	43 uremic patients (serum creatinine between 1.5 and 14.0 mg/100 mL)	$DL_{CO} \downarrow$ (highly correlated with low hemoglobin levels)
Bush and Gabriel[15]	80 uremic patients distributed equally into four groups (no RRT, CAPD, HD, renal transplantation)	$DL_{CO} \downarrow$ in all patient groups CAPD group had lowest DL_{CO} DL_{CO} reduction does not resolve after transplantation
Herrero et al.[16]	17 uremic patients (no dialysis) 10 HD patients (duration <12 months) 16 HD patients (duration >5 years)	75% of long-term HD, 17% of predialysis, 10% of short-term HD patients had $DL_{CO} \downarrow$
Beasley et al.[20]	20 CAPD patients	Normal DL_{CO}
Mydlik et al.[21]	15 CAPD patients	$DL_{CO} \downarrow$
Tang et al.[22]	50 uremic patients (before and after initiation of CAPD)	$DL_{CO} \downarrow$ (does not resolve after initiation of CAPD) FVC, MBC, FEV_1, PEF, MMEF $\downarrow$ (all improve after initiation of CAPD)
Karacan et al.[23]	20 HD patients	DL_{CO}, RV $\uparrow$ PI_{max}, PE_{max} $\downarrow$
Karacan et al.[24]	27 HD, 22 CAPD, 24 renal transplantation patients	RV, TLC $\uparrow$, $FEF_{25-75} \downarrow$ in HD and CAPD groups $DL_{CO} \uparrow$ in HD patients PI_{max}, $PE_{max} \downarrow$ in all groups (CAPD significantly lowest)
Chan et al.[25]	10 HD patients (before and after transplantation)	$DL_{CO} \uparrow$ before transplantation but normalized at 6 months after surgery
Tkacova et al.[28]	20 patients with ESRD (GFR <0.2 mL/sec), 29 with chronic renal failure (GFR >0.2 mL/sec)	Small airway disease in both groups, but FEV_1 and FEF_{25-75} significantly lower in ESRD patients GFR significantly correlated with FEV_1 and FEF_{25-75}
Ewert et al.[38]	79 renal transplantation patients	$DL_{CO} \downarrow$ in a majority of patients
Kalender et al.[39]	20 predialysis and 20 renal transplantation patients	Significantly better spirometric and diffusion capacity results in renal transplant recipients

CAPD, continuous ambulatory peritoneal dialysis; DL_{CO}, lung diffusion capacity for carbon monoxide; ESRD, end-stage renal disease; FEV_1, forced expiratory volume in 1 minute; FEF_{25-75}, forced midexpiratory flow rate during the middle half of the FVC; FVC, forced vital capacity; GFR, glomerular filtration rate; HD, hemodialysis; MBC, maximal breathing capacity; MMEF, mean midexpiratory flow; PE_{max}, static maximal expiratory pressure; PEF, peak expiratory flow; PI_{max}, static maximal inspiratory pressure; RRT, renal replacement therapy; RV, residual volume; TLC, total lung capacity;

cant difference between biocompatible and bioincompatible membranes in means of pulmonary function tests. In an older study, however, Davenport and Williams reported that dialyzer reuse causes an improvement in pulmonary functions, possibly by altering its biocompatibility characteristics in a positive manner.[27]

As indicated by the foregoing review of findings in relevant studies, much of the evidence regarding changes in DLCO capacity in uremic patients and effects of RRT modalities and dialyzer membranes is contradictory. Although consensus is lacking on the underlying mechanisms for pulmonary dysfunction, pulmonary edema was suggested as the main underlying pathological condition in nearly all of the studies. Effects of transplantation on DLCO are discussed in the following sections. A summary of the aforementioned studies is presented in Table 185-1.

Another common lung function abnormality is flow limitation in small airways in patients with end-stage renal disease in whom clinical signs of cardiopulmonary disease are absent. Improvement in small airway dysfunction and in ventilation-perfusion relationships was found after initiation of dialysis in uremic patients, and again,

pulmonary edema was suggested as the underlying pathological mechanism for these abnormalities, as with DLCO abnormalities.[22] Other possible causative disorders and lesions underlying small airway disease are extraosseous calcifications, vasculitis, and infections.[1] Because pulmonary edema seems to play a significant and central role in all pulmonary function abnormalities in uremic patients, findings in patients with chronic renal failure in the predialysis period whose urinary output remains adequate gain importance for differentiating between effects of uremic toxins and those of fluid overload. In a similar study, Tkacova and colleagues evaluated 49 patients with reduced renal function who never received RRT and who exhibited stable volume status, without any evidence of fluid overload. These investigators reported that most common spirometric abnormalities were reflective of small airway dysfunction (characterized by decreased FEV_1 and FEF_{25-75}), and that these parameters were closely correlated with glomerular filtration rate.[28] On the basis of these findings, they concluded that small airway dysfunction should be expected not only in patients with end-stage renal disease receiving dialysis but also in those with moderate reductions in glomerular filtration rate.

CARDIOPULMONARY EXERCISE TESTING AND RESPIRATORY MUSCLE STRENGTH IN UREMIC PATIENTS

Patients with end-stage renal disease maintained on either hemodialysis or CAPD frequently have impaired endurance exercise capacity and often have diminished muscle strength. Significant atrophy and increased noncontractile tissue are present in the muscle of patients on hemodialysis.[29] Other potential causes of impaired exercise capacity in chronic renal failure patients are shown in Table 185-2.[30] In clinical practice, symptom- or maximal heart rate–limited cardiopulmonary exercise testing is used to assess exercise capacity and related parameters, such as work rate (WR), peak oxygen uptake ($\dot{V}O_2$), carbon dioxide output ($\dot{V}CO_2$), maximal minute ventilation (MVE), breathing reserve (BR), anaerobic threshold (AT), oxygen pulse, and respiratory quotient (RQ). The most widely used protocol, the incremental exercise test, consists of a 3-minute baseline rest period followed by a 3-minute warm-up period; the periodic work rate increased by 10 to 15 watts for each minute. Cardiopulmonary exercise test findings in uremic patients in selected published studies are summarized in Table 185-3.[31-34]

In summary, studies to date have shown impaired exercise capacity in uremic patients, with reduction in exercise duration, peak $\dot{V}O_2$, and WR on cardiopulmonary exercise testing. The exact mechanism underlying this impairment is not clear. Possible explanations are deconditioning, uremic toxins, malnutrition, sedentary lifestyle, electrolyte imbalances, and structural and functional alterations in skeletal muscles (see Table 185-2).

Using spirometry, overall respiratory muscle strength in uremic patients also can be assessed. A widely used method for measuring static inspiratory and expiratory pressures (PI_{max} and PE_{max}, respectively) was defined by Black and Hyatt.[35] Two recent studies reported reduced PI_{max} and PE_{max} scores in patients on hemodialysis and in those on CAPD.[23,24] Impairment of static pressures also has been noted.[36] As with cardiopulmonary exercise testing, the mechanism(s) responsible for this impairment is still unknown.

TABLE 185-2

Potential Causes of Impaired Physical Exercise Capacity in Patients with Advanced Chronic Renal Failure

Anemia
Comorbid diseases
Associated with impaired blood flow or oxygen delivery to muscle
  Impaired cardiac output
  Reduced pulmonary function
  Peripheral vascular insufficiency
Other disease states
  Infection
  Diabetes mellitus with or without neuropathy
  Other neurological diseases
  Liver disease
  Non–infection-related inflammatory states
Malnutrition
  Protein-energy
  Vitamin
  Mineral (e.g., potassium, magnesium)
Consequences of renal failure per se
  Abnormal muscle ultrastructure
  Mitochondrial dysfunction
  Fluid and electrolyte disorders
  Deficiency of 1,25-dihydroxycholecalciferol and its analogues
  Uremic neuropathy
  Resistance to endogenous anabolic compounds: insulin, growth hormone, insulin-like growth factor-1
  Elevated levels of the antianabolic hormones: glucagons, parathyroid hormone
  Inflammation?
  Oxidative stress?
  Carbonyl stress?
  Other uremic toxins
Physical deconditioning

RENAL TRANSPLANTATION AND PULMONARY FUNCTIONS

Renal transplantation is the preferred treatment for renal failure in clinically available patients and is an ultimate solution for many problems associated with renal failure or dialysis-related complications. Many studies also have investigated the effects of transplantation on uremia-related pulmonary function abnormalities. As already mentioned, Bush and Gabriel's study in 1991 was the first to report reduced DLCO in uremic patients that fails to normalize after renal transplantation. The investigators speculated that the irreversibility of the deficit was due to pulmonary fibrosis that developed secondary to chronic pulmonary edema.

Pulmonary fibrosis is a common pathological finding both in patients maintained on hemodialysis and in transplant recipients, as reported by Fairsther and coworkers in two different studies.[4,37] Similarly, Ewert and associates studied 79 renal transplant recipients with pulmonary

TABLE 185-3

Cardiopulmonary Exercise Testing Findings in Various Cohorts of Patients with End-Stage Renal Disease

STUDY	STUDY POPULATION	TEST FINDING(S)
Ulubay et al.[31]	22 CAPD patients	Exercise duration ↓, peak $\dot{V}O_2$ ↓, maximum WR ↓
Pattaragarn et al.[32]	Hemodialysis (pediatric): 24 patients, 8 healthy controls	Treadmill time ↓, $\dot{V}O_2$ ↓, $\dot{V}O_2$AT ↓
Beasley et al.[33]	18 CAPD patients	$\dot{V}O_2$ max ↓
Painter et al.[34]	12 CAPD, 20 renal transplantation patients	$\dot{V}O_2$ max ↓, maximal HR ↓

CAPD, continuous ambulatory peritoneal dialysis; HR, heart rate; $\dot{V}O_2$, peak oxygen uptake; $\dot{V}O_2$AT, peak oxygen uptake anaerobic threshold; WR, work rate.

function testing and pulmonary computed tomography (CT) and reported that DLCO was less than 80% of predicted in 57% of the patients.[38] Of note, however, they were unable to demonstrate any relationship between interstitial CT features and pulmonary function abnormalities. They concluded that reduced DLCO in transplant recipients may be a result of pulmonary microvascular injury in combination with long-term decrease in pulmonary perfusion. Contradicting these previous results, we reported data for 24 renal transplant recipients with normal DLCO (96.2% of predicted value) but with low PI_{max} and PE_{max} values.[24] Chan and colleagues also reported that DLCO is increased in patients on hemodialysis and normalizes to lower levels at 6 months after surgery.[25] Comparing data for 20 patients with predialysis chronic renal failure and for 20 patients who underwent successful transplantation, Kalender and associates reported that mean spirometry and diffusion capacity values for the transplant recipients were in the normal range and significantly better than those for the predialysis patients.[39]

The different findings may reflect differences in lung histology between patients in each study. Pulmonary fibrosis is a well-known cause of decreased DLCO, which may develop on a background of chronic pulmonary volume overload with long-term dialysis treatment and has been reported as a common pathological finding in uremic patients and transplant recipients.[4,37] Evidently, no study has yet evaluated lung fibrosis demonstrated by pathological examination and pulmonary function abnormalities in transplant recipients versus that in patients maintained on dialysis. Additional studies directed at elucidating this issue would be very useful to clarify whether the presence and extent of pulmonary fibrosis are significant, or to determine the underlying cause of documented pulmonary function abnormalities in both groups of patients.

CONCLUSION

Pulmonary function abnormalities are common in renal failure of any cause. The most commonly reported ones are small airway disease and DLCO abnormalities. The most commonly reported DLCO abnormality is reduction in diffusion capacity; however, a few authors, including Chan and colleagues[25] and Karacan and associates,[23,24] also have reported increased DLCO values. Nevertheless, the general consensus is that uremic patients have decreased

cardiopulmonary exercise capacity and pulmonary muscle strength. Still unresolved is whether a successful transplantation is effective in correcting uremia-related pulmonary dysfunction or ineffective in resolving those abnormalities that occur on a background of chronic pathological changes such as pulmonary fibrosis.

Key Points

1. Pulmonary function test results usually are abnormal in patients with renal failure of any etiology.
2. Small airway disease (obstructive dysfunction) is a common finding and develops because of pulmonary volume overload.
3. Both reduction and increase in carbon monoxide diffusing capacity are seen in dialysis patients, and the reasons are not well documented.
4. Decreased cardiopulmonary exercise capacity and respiratory muscle strength (PI_{max} and PE_{max}) are nearly universal findings in dialysis patients.
5. Although transplantation is the ultimate treatment choice in chronic dialysis patients, its effects on already established pulmonary dysfunction are not well documented.

Key References

1. Bush A, Gabriel R: The lungs in uraemia: A review. J R Soc Med 1985;78:849-855.
15. Bush A, Gabriel R: Pulmonary function in chronic renal failure: Effects of dialysis and transplantation. Thorax 1991; 46:424-428.
16. Herrero JA, Alvarez-Sala JL, Coronel F, et al: Pulmonary diffusing capacity in chronic dialysis patients. Respir Med 2002;90.487-492.
24. Karacan O, Tutal E, Colak T, et al: Pulmonary function in renal transplant recipients and end-stage renal disease patients undergoing maintenance dialysis. Transplant Proc 2006;38: 396-400.
38. Ewert R, Opitz C, Wensel R, et al: Abnormalities of pulmonary diffusion capacity in long-term survivors after kidney transplantation. Chest 2002;122:639-644.

See the companion Expert Consult website for the complete reference list.

CHAPTER 186

The Kidney during Mechanical Ventilation

Jan Willem Kuiper, A. B. Johan Groeneveld, and Frans B. Plötz

---

OBJECTIVES

This chapter will:
1. Describe the epidemiological relationship between mechanical ventilation and acute renal failure and address the indications for mechanical ventilation.
2. Review the adverse effects of mechanical ventilation on the lung and distant organs.
3. Outline the effects of mechanical ventilation on systemic hemodynamics and local renal blood flow and on the kidney.
4. Discuss the possible effects of hypercapnia and hypoxemia on kidney function.
5. Introduce the concept of biotrauma and describe its effects on the kidney.

Mechanical ventilation has been of great value in improving the survival of many patients suffering from respiratory failure. A common cause of respiratory failure is acute lung injury (ALI), of which the most severe form is the acute respiratory distress syndrome (ARDS), with an associated mortality rate of 38.5%.[1] Although the most obvious clinical abnormalities in ALI and ARDS are referable to the lung, the most common cause of death is multiple organ dysfunction including acute renal failure (ARF).[2] Respiratory failure is a risk factor for developing ARF, and mechanical ventilation is very common in patients with ARF; more than 75% of patients in the intensive care unit (ICU) with ARF receive mechanical ventilation.[3] Mechanical ventilation has been shown to be an independent risk factor for in-hospital death in critically ill patients with ARF, more than doubling the risk of dying.[3] This chapter describes possible mechanisms through which mechanical ventilation affects the kidney in patients requiring ICU management and how these may contribute to the development of ARF.

MECHANICAL VENTILATION VERSUS SPONTANEOUS BREATHING

During spontaneous breathing, respiratory muscles establish negative intrathoracic and intrapulmonary pressures and, by downward movement of the diaphragm, a positive intra-abdominal pressure. The resulting intrathoracic pressure–to–ambient pressure gradient allows air to flow into the lungs. The physiological mechanism of spontaneous breathing facilitates venous return, thereby supporting hemodynamics. In contrast with spontaneous breathing, mechanical ventilation uses positive pressure to inflate the lungs.

In most patients with ALI or ARDS, either volume-controlled or pressure-controlled ventilation is used. In the volume control mode, a volume is preset on the ventilator, resulting in a variable airway pressure, whereas in the pressure control mode, the inspiratory pressure is preset, resulting in a certain tidal volume. Thus, the airway pressure results from the applied tidal volume or preset inspiratory pressure and on the preset basic end-expiratory volume and depends on lung compliance, airway resistance, and air flow.

During mechanical ventilation, pressure gradients are altered considerably compared with pressure gradients in spontaneously breathing subjects. Intrathoracic, intrapulmonary, and intra-abdominal pressures increase during inspiration and remain positive during the breathing cycle. Only at the end of expiration do they equalize with ambient pressure, when no positive end-expiratory pressure (PEEP) is applied. PEEP usually is applied to prevent the alveoli from collapsing at end expiration. Consequently, mechanical ventilation exerts systemic hemodynamic effects through a complex interaction among intrathoracic pressure, intravascular volume, and cardiac performance. Mechanical ventilation decreases cardiac output by decreasing preload, affecting both left ventricular geometry and pulmonary vascular volume and resistance, and, in addition, increasing right ventricular afterload. Evidence for these proposed mechanisms has been known for decades, based on studies in animal models and human subjects during spontaneous ventilation or controlled mandatory ventilation in combination with PEEP.[4,5]

INDICATIONS FOR MECHANICAL VENTILATION

The most common and obvious indication for mechanical ventilation in patients under ICU care is ALI (or ARDS). This condition can be defined qualitatively as any respiratory pathological process associated with failure of arterial oxygenation and inadequate alveolar ventilation, with a subsequent decrease in PaO_2 or rise in $PaCO_2$, or both. Although in most mechanically ventilated patients, normal gas exchange is targeted, in many patients with ALI or ARDS managed in the ICU, the maintenance of normal gas exchange is impossible. In such cases, in order to avoid ventilator-induced lung injury (VILI), a low PaO_2 or a high $PaCO_2$ is accepted.[6] The former occurs despite measures to improve oxygenation and despite avoidance of high, potentially toxic inspired oxygen concentrations. The latter may be associated with a strategy of small tidal volume ventilation with adequate mean airway pressure to achieve satisfactory oxygenation, thereby avoiding toxic inspired oxygen concentrations and allowing $PaCO_2$ to increase if necessary. These strategies are called *permissive hypoxemia* and *permissive hypercapnia*, respectively. In this regard, it is important to recognize that patients in the ICU may be subjected to acute changes in PaO_2 and $PaCO_2$, or to mild chronic hypoxemia or hypercapnia, as a result of the applied ventilatory strategy or their underlying condition.

VENTILATOR-INDUCED LUNG INJURY

Besides the adverse effects mechanical ventilation has on systemic hemodynamics, it also can cause direct damage to the lungs.[7] Initial experimental research on the induction and course of VILI focused primarily on the contribution of mechanical factors such as pressure and volume.[8] Based on these studies, innovative and lung-protective strategies have been proposed to avoid VILI by limiting tidal volume and plateau pressure and by maintaining recruitment of alveolar regions with sufficient PEEP. Clinical trials subsequently made clear that ventilator management can alter mortality in patients with ARDS.[6,9] In 2000 the ARDS Network clinical trial revealed that mortality rate was significantly lower for the group of patients managed with lower tidal volumes than for those patients managed with traditional tidal volumes (31.0% versus 39.8%). The mean tidal volumes on days 1 to 3 were 6.2 ± 0.8 and 11.8 ± 0.8 mL/kg of predicted body weight ($P < .001$), respectively, and the mean plateau pressures were 25 ± 6 and 33 ± 8 cm of water ($P < .001$), respectively.[9]

Recent research has focused on how mechanical stresses caused by mechanical ventilation can affect cellular and molecular processes in the lung, a mechanism that has been called *biotrauma*.[10] Two independent pathways of the biotrauma hypothesis have been distinguished: (1) Ventilation may cause release of mediators, and (2) these mediators have biological activity. Most research has focused on the first part of this hypothesis. It has become clear that ventilation strategies using "large" tidal volumes and zero PEEP in already injured lungs can promote the release of inflammatory mediators in the lungs. This potentiation of the inflammatory response is supported by evidence from experimental models ranging from mechanically stressed cell systems to isolated lungs and intact animals and humans. The possible pivotal role for biotrauma in the development of multisystem organ failure was based on the suggestion that this inflammatory reaction may not be limited to the lungs but, by way of spillover of mediators in the circulation, also may initiate and propagate a systemic inflammatory response.[11] Indirect evidence from experimental models ranging from an isolated perfused and ventilated mouse lung, intact animals with preinjured lungs, and humans with ALI or ARDS supports this hypothesis. Whether the same phenomena occur in noninjured lungs remains unclear. In contrast with the first part of the biotrauma hypothesis, the second pathway of the biotrauma hypothesis—whether these mediators have biological activity—has only recently begun to be addressed.

In addition, other mechanisms by which mechanical ventilation may affect distant organs include suppression of peripheral immune response and translocation of bacteria and endotoxin from both lung and intestine to the systemic circulation.[12]

MECHANICAL VENTILATION AND THE KIDNEY

Acute tubular necrosis most often is ischemic or toxic in origin. Prerenal failure and ischemic tubular necrosis represent points along a continuum, with the former leading to the latter when blood flow is sufficiently compromised.[13] Many clinical conditions can lead to kidney ischemia as a result of either extrarenal or intrarenal factors that compromise renal blood flow.[14] After ischemia, toxins account for the largest number of cases of acute intrinsic renal failure by directly damaging tubular cells or by various other mechanisms.[14]

Mechanical ventilation may contribute to the development of ARF by three different mechanisms (Fig. 186-1): First, the effect of mechanical ventilation on systemic hemodynamics can alter renal blood flow; second, changes in $PaCO_2$ and PaO_2 can affect renal hemodynamics; and third, the systemic release of inflammatory mediators may have biological activity that affects the kidney.[15]

Effects of Mechanical Ventilation on Renal Blood Flow

Based largely on renal ischemia-reperfusion studies, it is well known that a compromised renal blood flow contributes to renal vascular endothelial and tubular damage and influences long-term renal function. The mechanisms by which mechanical ventilation alters renal perfusion include a reduction in cardiac output and stimulation of hormonal and sympathetic pathways.[15,16]

First, a decreased cardiac output during mechanical ventilation in patients with respiratory failure may lead to decreased renal perfusion and is associated with reduced renal function as reflected in sodium handling, glomerular filtration rate (GFR), urinary output, and urea and creatinine clearance. Hemodynamic studies demonstrated an immediate decline in urinary output after start of mechanical ventilation—an effect that appears to be exacerbated by PEEP.[15,16] The reported effects of mechanical ventilation on GFR and renal blood flow are variable and may reflect differences in hydration status, patient acuity, possible underlying pulmonary dysfunction, and anesthetics used. Dispute exists, however, regarding the relative contribution of effects of cardiac output and the stimulation of water- and sodium-retaining hormonal systems.

Second, various regulatory hormonal mechanisms that affect renal function during mechanical ventilation have been proposed. Thus far, no definite correlation between antidiuretic hormone (ADH), prostaglandin, catecholamine, atrial natriuretic factor (ANP), or vasoactive peptide levels and renal function during mechanical ventilation has been established.[17-21]

Third, mechanical ventilation with PEEP increases sympathetic tone, resulting in increased plasma renin activity and thereby decreasing GFR by reducing blood flow.[22] Mechanical ventilation also has a transient effect on aortic blood pressure, which reflexively activates the sympathetic nervous system through aortic and (sino)carotid baroreceptors and, more slowly, affects intravascular volume by changing renal function.[23] Whether the effect of atrial stretch receptors on renal vascular tone also alters renal function during mechanical ventilation remains to be evaluated.[24] In conclusion, the effects of a reduced cardiac output on kidney function during mechanical

TABLE 186-1

Inflammatory, Vasoactive, and Pro-apoptotic Mediators That Potentially Mediate the Effects of Mechanical Ventilation on the Kidney

INFLAMMATORY MEDIATORS	VASOACTIVE MEDIATORS	PRO-APOPTOTIC MEDIATORS
IL-1β	Nitric oxide	Soluble Fas ligand
IL-6	Vasopressin (ADH)	MCP-1
IL-8	Catecholamines	
IL-10	RAAS	
TNF-α	Prostaglandins	
Soluble IL-1RA	ANF	
Soluble TNF receptors	Endothelin	

ADH, antidiuretic hormone; ANF, atrial natriuretic factor; IL, interleukin; MCP-1, monocyte chemotactic protein-1; RA, receptor antagonist; RAAS, renin-angiotensin-aldosterone system; TNF, tumor necrosis factor.

ventilation have been documented extensively. By contrast, the relative role of neurohumoral regulatory systems remains to be investigated.

$PaCO_2$, PaO_2, and the Kidney

Hypercapnia

The effect of hypercapnia on renal blood flow has been well documented in normal persons and in patients in respiratory failure or with chronic obstructive pulmonary disease. $PaCO_2$ levels have been found to correlate inversely with renal blood flow.[25] Hypercapnia can reduce renal blood flow by direct and indirect mechanisms. Hypercapnia directly causes renal vasoconstriction and stimulates norepinephrine release, acting on the sympathetic nervous system.[26] Increased sympathetic activity can reduce renal blood flow and, to a lesser extent, GFR and may contribute to nonosmotic release of vasopressin.[27] Indirectly, hypercapnia causes systemic vasodilation that decreases systemic vascular resistance, "inactivating" the baroreceptors with a subsequent release of norepinephrine and stimulation of the renin-angiotensin-aldosterone system, leading to a fall in renal blood flow.[25]

Human, post–renal transplantation, and animal studies suggest that local neurogenic mechanisms play a role in the response of renal blood flow to hypercapnia.[28] In addition, other factors such as circulating catecholamines and neuropeptides also affect the renovascular response to hypercapnia, in addition to effects on renal innervation (Table 186-1). Of importance clinically, the rapid and marked decrease in renal blood flow in response to hypercapnia also occurs in the presence of normal or increased PaO_2. This finding suggests that changes in $PaCO_2$, independent from PaO_2, play a pivotal role in determining the renovascular response to changes in arterial blood gas pressures.

Hypoxemia

Severe hypoxemia (PaO_2 less than 40 mm Hg) generally is thought to reduce renal blood flow and can lead to functional renal insufficiency.[29] Reports on the renal effects of moderate hypoxemia are conflicting, however. Several studies suggest that mild hypoxemia without concomitant hypercapnia exerts no significant effect on renal hemodynamics. Other studies have demonstrated that acute normocapnic hypoxemia increases renal vascular resis-

tance, leading to renal hypoperfusion and decreased GFR. The underlying mechanisms whereby changes in oxygenation induce vasomotor nephropathy are not fully understood. Possible mechanisms include (in)activation of vasoactive factors such as nitric oxide (NO), angiotensin II, endothelin, and bradykinin and a chemoreceptor-mediated sympathetic reflex (see Table 186-1).[15]

BIOTRAUMA AND THE KIDNEY

A number of mediators have been reported to increase in the systemic circulation during mechanical ventilation and may potentially contribution to ARF (see Table 186-1). The simultaneous detection of both proinflammatory and anti-inflammatory mediators may reflect altered regulation of the inflammatory response. A persistent activation of the inflammatory response is associated with organ failure.[30] Inflammatory mediators may affect renal function through several mechanisms, some of which may be synergistic. Suggested mechanisms include (1) a direct effect on renal blood flow through the release of several vasoactive mediators or through (2) induction of a local renal inflammatory response by proinflammatory mediators from pulmonary origin. (3) A third mechanism involves the direct induction of apoptosis by pro-apoptotic factors. Soluble Fas ligand is known to induce apoptosis of glomerular cells, and interleukin (IL)-1β, IL-6, and tumor necrosis factor (TNF)-α may facilitate this process by activating platelet-activating factor and inducing an inflammatory reaction, both contributing to the apoptotic effects of soluble Fas ligand. A combination of the aforementioned processes may also be involved. By compromising renal blood flow, a critical threshold may be reached and inflammatory mediators may exert a direct effect on renal endothelial and epithelial cells, thereby inducing or contributing to ARF (see Fig. 186-1).

Only a few studies have addressed the role of biotrauma in association with the kidney. In a clinical study, Ranieri and associates observed that a conventional mechanical ventilation strategy was associated with a local and systemic cytokine response that was sustained over 36 hours in patients with ARDS, whereas in a second group of patients, the inflammatory response was attenuated by a lung-protective strategy. Patients in the latter group had significantly lower concentrations of a number of cytokines (TNF-α, IL-1β, IL-6, IL-8, soluble TNF receptors, IL-1 receptor antagonist) in plasma and bronchoalveolar lavage

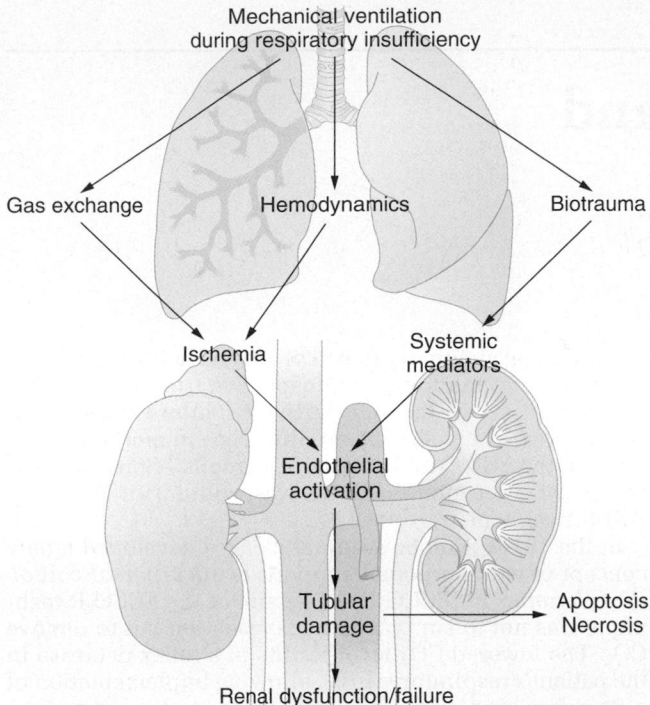

Mechanical ventilation
during respiratory insufficiency

Gas exchange   Hemodynamics   Biotrauma

Ischemia   Systemic mediators

Endothelial activation

Tubular damage   Apoptosis Necrosis

Renal dysfunction/failure

FIGURE 186-1. Mechanical ventilation affects the kidney through three distinct mechanisms: (1) through direct effects on gas exchange that can activate vasoactive mechanisms and decrease renal blood flow; (2) through depressing effects on systemic hemodynamics, thereby decreasing renal blood flow; and (3) secondary to biotrauma from mechanical ventilation, with the subsequent systemic release of inflammatory and pro-apoptic mediators that may affect the kidney. These effects may be more pronounced in patients with severe acute respiratory distress syndrome or with circulatory compromise.

fluid at 36 hours.[31] A post hoc analysis revealed that an increase in IL-6 plasma concentrations correlated with the development of acute renal failure.[32] Recently, other studies found significant correlations between increased pro- and anti-inflammatory cytokine levels, including IL-1β, IL-6, IL-8, IL-10 and TNF-α, and mortality in patients with ARF compared with healthy controls and patients with end-stage renal disease.

In the aforementioned studies, specific issues need to be evaluated. First, the source of the mediators remains uncertain. Lung-borne mediators may spill over into the systemic circulation and exert their effect on distant organs.[33] However, these mediators also may be produced locally in the kidneys as a result of a compromised renal blood flow and exert their effect directly in the organs where they are produced. Second, it is important to prove a cause-and-effect relationship between mediators and renal dysfunction, rather than simply recognizing an association.[34]

CONCLUSION

Mechanical ventilation plays an important role in the care of patients in the ICU and is critical to survival in many cases. Despite the emergence of new modes of ventilation and new ventilator strategies, the effects of mechanical

ventilation remain complex and extend to organ systems other than the lung. In the ICU, patients usually suffer from ALI or ARDS, both of which significantly alter lung mechanics, thereby aggravating the adverse effects of mechanical ventilation—further depression of hemodynamics and exacerbation of the pulmonary inflammatory processes. In addition, the harmful effects of mechanical ventilation on the kidney become more significant when comorbid conditions are present. In the presence of ALI, it is more difficult to maintain normal gas exchange, and moderate arterial hypoxemia and hypercapnia often are accepted, which potentially decrease renal blood flow. Renal blood flow is further compromised because of a decreased cardiac output secondary to high intrathoracic pressures. Furthermore, the impact of biotrauma is not limited to the lungs but may lead to a systemic inflammatory reaction. These effects on renal function can be aggravated during sepsis, when prerenal blood flow is further compromised. This series of events may reflect a multifactorial process that eventually may result in the development of ARF. Despite difficulties in differentiating between the effects of mechanical ventilation per se and the underlying disease on renal function, it is likely that mechanical ventilation itself greatly affects the kidney.

Key Points

1. Mechanical ventilation has been shown to be an independent risk factor for in-hospital death in critically ill patients with acute renal failure, more than doubling the risk of dying.
2. Through various mechanisms, mechanical ventilation exerts effects on both the lungs and extrapulmonary organ systems, including the kidney.
3. Mechanical ventilation exerts effects on systemic hemodynamics and local renal blood flow that may in turn influence renal function.
4. Mechanical ventilation strategies of permissive hypercapnia and hypoxemia may compromise renal blood flow, thereby affecting renal function.
5. Biotrauma, the propagation of a pulmonary inflammatory reaction and spillover of inflammatory mediators into the systemic circulation, also may affect renal function.

Key References

1. Rubenfeld GD, Caldwell E, Peabody E, et al: Incidence and outcomes of acute lung injury. N Engl J Med 2005;353: 1685-1693.
7. Pinhu L, Whitehead T, Evans T, Griffiths M: Ventilator-associated lung injury. Lancet 2003;361:332-340.
9. Ventilation with lower tidal volumes as compared with traditional tidal volumes for acute lung injury and the acute respiratory distress syndrome. The Acute Respiratory Distress Syndrome Network. N Engl J Med 2000;342:1301-1308.
12. Plotz FB, Slutsky AS, van Vught AJ, Heijnen CJ: Ventilator-induced lung injury and multiple system organ failure: A critical review of facts and hypotheses. Intensive Care Med 2004;30:1865-1872.
15. Kuiper JW, Groeneveld AB, Slutsky AS, Plotz FB: Mechanical ventilation and acute renal failure. Crit Care Med 2005;33: 1408-1415.

See the companion Expert Consult website for the complete reference list.

CHAPTER 187

Extracorporeal Support and Renal Function

Chiara Sala, Nicolò Patroniti, and Roberto Fumagalli

OBJECTIVES

This chapter will:
1. Define the different types of extracorporeal support devices.
2. Review their functions and their clinical applications.
3. Describe their components, management, and complications.
4. Discuss the influence of extracorporeal support on renal function.

Extracorporeal support had been used to support both circulation and gas exchange. This chapter focuses mainly on extracorporeal support for respiratory failure.

Despite the many technical improvements over the years in the management of severe acute respiratory distress syndrome (ARDS), the primary treatment for refractory hypoxemic ARDS is still extracorporeal support. Whereas the ventilator can substitute for respiratory muscle function alone, the extracorporeal support system can provide the entire range of lung functions, including gas exchange.

Extracorporeal support is accomplished by means of an external system that bypasses heart and lungs and substitutes for their functions: Venous blood is drawn from the patient through vascular tubing and driven from a pump to an artificial lung, which oxygenates the blood and removes CO_2; then arterial blood is circulated back to the patient.

EXTRACORPOREAL MEMBRANE OXYGENATION AND EXTRACORPOREAL CARBON DIOXIDE REMOVAL

Extracorporeal oxygenation was first used in cardiovascular surgery to substitute heart and lung function during an open heart procedure in 1953.[1] In those years, oxygenators involved direct contact between oxygen and blood: Oxygenation was achieved by bubbling oxygen through the blood (bubble oxygenators). This technique caused several complications that limited the use of these devices to a few hours.[2] Subsequently, Clowes and coworkers developed a new oxygenator in which oxygen was separated from blood by a membrane, and the technique of *extracorporeal membrane oxygenation* (ECMO) was born.[3] The first application of ECMO for the treatment of ARDS dates back to 1972, when Hill reported the survival of a young multitrauma victim with ARDS treated with ECMO.[4] In 1973, the first randomized prospective trial of ECMO for patients in severe acute respiratory failure began. The study revealed not significant difference in mortality rates for both the ECMO and the control groups.[5] Consequently, in almost all centers, ECMO was withdrawn for adult ARDS treatment.

In the 1970s, Kolobow and associates developed a new concept of extracorporeal support: *extracorporeal carbon dioxide removal* (ECCO₂R).[6] The aim of the ECCO₂R technique was not to support lung oxygenation but to remove CO_2. The lowered CO_2 level results in a reflex decrease in the patient's respiratory drive, allowing implementation of a stressless kind of mechanical ventilation known as low-frequency positive-pressure ventilation, characterized by few ventilator breaths with use of low tidal volumes and peak inspiratory pressures.[7] In 1986, Gattinoni and colleagues reported a survival rate of 50% in patients with severe ARDS treated with ECCO₂R.[8] This result was not supported by the randomized controlled trial performed in 1994 by Morris and coworkers, however. Even if the survival rate was improved from the previous studies, outcomes were not significantly different between the two groups.[9]

Although no randomized controlled trial has demonstrated an evidence-based rationale for application of extracorporeal support in the treatment of severe ARDS, several centers around the world continue to perform ECMO and ECCO₂R in life-threatening and treatment-refractory acute respiratory failure. Several case studies report successful results with extracorporeal support in patients in whom all other treatment options have failed.

PHYSIOLOGY OF EXTRACORPOREAL SUPPORT AND CLINICAL APPLICATION

ECMO techniques generally are understood to incorporate a high-flow venoarterial bypass system like that used in the original ECMO trial. The main goal of this system is blood oxygenation, which is accomplished by means of an artificial membrane lung, with high blood flow. By contrast, ECCO₂R is characterized by a low-flow venovenous bypass system, the goal of which is CO_2 removal.

Blood oxygenation and CO_2 removal take place by means of different physiological mechanisms. Oxygenation is a diffusion-limited process that requires high blood flow through the lung but delivery of a small amount of oxygen; by contrast, CO_2 removal is a ventilation-limited process that requires high ventilation but can be achieved at low blood flow. During extracorporeal support, therefore, oxygenation is enhanced by setting high blood flow for the membrane lung, whereas CO_2 removal is enhanced by setting low blood flow and high gas flow.

Several experimental studies[10] show that when CO_2 is removed by an artificial lung, the natural lung decreases spontaneous ventilation, with reduction in both respiratory frequency and tidal volume. Consequently, removal of the total amount of CO_2 produced by the body allows a use of a ventilatory mode characterized by low volumes and low peak inspiratory pressures. This is one of the most important advantages of extracorporeal support. In the late 1970s and 1980s, in fact, the deleterious effects of mechanical ventilation were elucidated, and ventilator-induced lung injury began to be a subject of clinical study.[11] The evidence that mechanical ventilation itself can augment or cause pulmonary damage led to a new approach in the treatment of ARDS: *lung-protective ventilation.*[12]

Today the conventional treatment of ARDS is based on low tidal volumes, low plateau pressure, and a clinically set positive end-expiratory pressure (PEEP). In severe hypoxemic ARDS, several adjunctive therapies have been proposed: recruitment maneuvers, steroid, prone position and inhaled nitric oxide. Nevertheless, in refractory hypoxemic ARDS, it often is impossible to effect adequate gas exchange with a safe mode of mechanical ventilation. In such instances, extracorporeal support offers many advantages: It performs gas exchange, allowing a reduction of ventilation; moreover, it keeps the lung at rest, allowing its recovery. Accordingly, extracorporeal support should be included in the context of a lung-protective strategy.

EXTRACORPOREAL SYSTEM COMPONENTS

Basically, an ECMO or $ECCO_2R$ system consists of vascular access (cannulas), tubing, a driving force (pump), and a gas exchange unit (oxygenator or membrane lung). As noted previously, whereas the ECMO system generally involves venoarterial bypass, $ECCO_2R$ is a venovenous system.

Venous drainage usually is achieved by cannulation of the right atrium through the right internal jugular vein or, alternatively, through the right or left femoral vein. In venovenous bypass, arterialized blood is returned through cannulation of the right or left femoral vein; in venoarterial bypass, instead, blood is returned through cannulation of the right common carotid artery or the right or left femoral artery.[13] Cannulas used during extracorporeal support generally are heparin-coated and spiral-armed, have a multiholed tip, and are percutaneously inserted. All internal surfaces of the extracorporeal system are coated with covalently bound heparin to minimize the need for systemic anticoagulation.[14]

Mostly roller or centrifugal pumps are used to drive blood from the patient to the artificial lung. In both kinds of pumps, the mechanical stress sustained by red blood cells and the blood deposition on the pump itself lead to hemolysis, which requires periodic changing of the pump for a new one.[15]

Heparin-coated silicone membrane oxygenators and hollow-fiber oxygenators are in use for extracorporeal support. Because of their smaller priming volumes, their higher gas transfer rates, and their lower resistance, hollow-fiber oxygenators are preferred over silicone membrane lungs. In the past, a serious complication associated with use of hollow-fiber artificial lungs was plasma leakage, but nowadays, the use of newly developed fibers has solved this problem.[16] A continuous gas flow runs through the membrane lung to guarantee oxygen delivery to the blood and the washout of CO_2. The flow rate is set to the required arterial CO_2 tension levels.

CLINICAL MANAGEMENT AND COMPLICATIONS

Anticoagulation is achieved by continuous heparin infusion throughout the period of bypass. The anticoagulation level is monitored through determination of activated clotting time (ACT), which is kept at a value of 150 to 200 seconds. In the case of heparin-induced thrombocytopenia, alternative anticoagulant drugs can be used. A laboratory screen is performed daily, to include prothrombin time, partial thromboplastin time, fibrinogen level, platelet count, and assays for fibrinogen degradation products and antithrombin. Because use of heparinized surfaces requires normal levels of antithrombin, a continuous infusion of antithrombin III is often necessary.[17] At the beginning of treatment, the patient is kept sedated and paralyzed, but as soon as possible, reestablishment of spontaneous breathing should be attempted to prevent a further reduction in functional residual capacity and to conserve the functionality of the patient's respiratory muscles. In patients with acute renal failure, a continuous hemofiltration device can be connected directly to the extracorporeal system.

Weaning from extracorporeal support can be easily accomplished when the natural lung recovers its normal functions. Extracorporeal blood flow is gradually lowered, and FIO_2 settings on the ventilator and the membrane lung are decreased to reduce CO_2 removal.[17]

The possible complications of extracorporeal support can be classified into mechanical and medical complications.[18] Mechanical complications are much less frequent than resultant medical problems and include tubing disruption, pump malfunction, cannula displacement, and membrane lung failure. Of the possible medical complications, the most frequent is bleeding, which in some cases may be life-threatening. Several improvements have been introduced during the years to reduce bleeding, such as the use of percutaneous cannulation and of heparinized surfaces into the circuit and the creation of new materials that are more biocompatible.

RECENT DEVELOPMENTS

In recent years, a pumpless arteriovenous system for extracorporeal support has been introduced in clinical practice—pumpless extracorporeal lung assist (ECLA).[19] This new device exploits cardiac output to drive arterial blood from the patient to the membrane lung and then back to the patient. This technique is made possible by a new kind of membrane lung with a very low blood flow resistance. The pumpless extracorporeal device has numerous advantages: It is small and easily handled, with short tubing, and it causes fewer hemolysis problems and requires lower levels of anticoagulation than the traditional system. The principal disadvantages are as follows: Pumpless ECLA does not allow a direct blood flow control, so its efficiency depends on cardiac output. For this reason, its use is contraindicated in hemodynamically unstable patients.

Moreover, it requires arterial cannulation, and it does not provide efficient blood oxygenation.[15,16]

EXTRACORPOREAL SUPPORT AND RENAL FUNCTION

Patients with respiratory distress can present with several abnormalities of renal function. Some of these abnormalities are consequences of the primary disease (e.g., cardiogenic pulmonary edema due to heart failure), some are consequences of treatment (e.g., mechanical ventilation, diuretic therapy, nephrotoxic drugs such as aminoglycosides), and some are physiological consequences of the primary disease (e.g., low oxygen tension, cytokines, and local effects).

The interactions of extracorporeal support with the aforementioned factors have been addressed only in some animal experimental studies, so the available clinical data are scarce. In the following discussion, the effects of extracorporeal respiratory support on renal function are considered in three categories:

• Hemodynamic effects
• Respiratory effects
• Metabolic effects

Hemodynamic Effects

Systemic hemodynamics can be directly influenced by the type of extracorporeal support and by the magnitude of extracorporeal blood flow. Venoarterial bypass is able to increase systemic blood pressure and, theoretically, renal blood flow; venovenous bypass has only marginal effects on pressure. Despite these considerations, some studies found no significant differences in renal blood flow and perfusion pressure during prolonged venovenous and venoarterial bypass in ARDS.[20] Different considerations hold for use of arteriovenous bypass: In animal studies, organ blood flow was evaluated during arteriovenous CO_2 removal. When measured, arteriovenous shunt was found to be between 5% and 25% of cardiac output, and renal blood flow was maintained within 80% of the baseline level.[21]

Several studies explored the effect of the pulsatility of blood flow on renal perfusion and concluded that renal blood flow was significantly greater in pulsatile flow than in nonpulsatile flow.[22,23] These observations have not been confirmed by other reports, however.[24]

Another effect due to hemodynamic manipulation during ECMO has been observed in neonates[25]: Despite no differences in mean blood pressure, protein intake, serum albumin, or use of diuretics, neonates managed with ECMO had higher positive fluid balance, lower urine flow rates, and higher blood urea nitrogen and creatinine levels than neonates managed without ECMO. A possible explanation for these findings is the alteration in the balance of circulating vasoactive mediators observed in patients undergoing ECMO; these substances may affect renal blood flow and, consequently, renal function.

Respiratory Effects

During extracorporeal circulation lung management is usually modified. Different approaches have the same target: decrease barotrauma. This goal can be achieved reducing alveolar pressure (PEEP and plateau pressure) and respiratory rate in order to decrease the stretching force applied per time. The ability of the artificial lung to remove CO_2 allows the application of this lung-protective ventilation mode.

Metabolic Effects

The effects of acute hypoxemia on kidney are debated. A review of the published data shows that opposite findings are possible: Glomerular filtration can be decreased,[26] unaffected,[27] or increased.[28]

By contrast, the effect of hypoxemia on Na^+ reabsorption is widely accepted: Tubular Na^+ transport is the major component of renal oxygen consumption and can be impaired in conditions of reduced blood oxygen concentration.[29] Diuretic response to hypoxemia seems to be independent of prostaglandin release or respiratory alkalosis but it is evidently mediated by cardiovascular response to hypoxia.[28]

Renal perfusion is unaffected by mild respiratory acidosis but is decreased by severe acidosis. Extracorporeal support allows manipulation of blood gases and pH, and its effect will reflect the extent of such manipulation.

ECMO treatment can cause several different types of electrolyte disturbance by various mechanisms. The ECMO circuit usually is primed with blood. This blood has a low pH, with hyperkalemia of variable degree, depending on storage time; moreover, it contains citrate, which is a calcium-chelating agent and can precipitate hypocalcemia. Prolonged treatment with ECMO can also produce oncotic dysequilibrium, which requires frequent albumin administration.

During extracorporeal circulation, blood is continuously exposed to the nonbiological, synthetic surfaces of the ECMO circuit. This exposure leads to activation of the systemic inflammatory response, cytokine release, and coagulation activation.[30] This phenomenon has been widely studied in cardiopulmonary bypass, but data on prolonged ECMO for severe ARDS are scarce.

Key Points

1. Extracorporeal support is used in severe refractory hypoxemic respiratory failure to substitute for lung function and to perform gas exchange in order to allow protective lung ventilation and to keep the natural lung at rest.
2. *Extracorporeal membrane oxygenation* generally refers to a high-flow venoarterial bypass with the principal aim of blood oxygenation. *Extracorporeal carbon dioxide removal* refers to a low-flow venovenous bypass with the aim of blood carbon dioxide removal.
3. Anticoagulation is indispensable to perform extracorporeal circulation, but it is also responsible for the most severe complications of extracorporeal membrane oxygenation.
4. Extracorporeal support can affect renal function because of its interactions with systemic hemodynamics, blood gases and pH, electrolytes, and the inflammatory system.

Key References

17. Pesenti A, Gattinoni L, Bombino M: Extracorporeal carbon dioxide removal. In Tobin MJ (ed): Principles and Practice of Mechanical Ventilation, 2nd ed. New York, McGraw-Hill, 2006.
19. Reng M, Philipp A, Kaiser M: Pumpless extracorporeal lung assist and adult respiratory distress syndrome. Lancet 2000; 27:1340-1351.
21. Brunston RL Jr, Tao W, Bidani A, et al: Organ blood flow during arteriovenous carbon dioxide removal. ASAIO J 1997; 43:M821-M824.

25. Roy BJ, Cornish JD, Clark RH: Venovenous extracorporeal oxygenation affects renal function. Pediatrics 1995;95:573-578.
30. Butler J, Rocker GM, Westaby S: Inflammatory response to cardiopulmonary bypass. Ann Thorac Surg 1993;55:552-559.

See the companion Expert Consult website for the complete reference list.

CHAPTER 188

Acute Respiratory Distress Syndrome and the Kidney: Lung and Kidney Crosstalk

Mallar Bhattacharya, Michael A. Matthay, and Hamid Rabb

OBJECTIVES

This chapter will:
1. Review the pathophysiology of acute lung injury.
2. Summarize the emerging understanding of lung-kidney crosstalk in critical illness.
3. Identify the mechanisms by which acute kidney injury may potentiate acute lung injury.
4. Outline the significance of acute lung injury during acute kidney injury.

Patients admitted to the intensive care unit (ICU) for management of acute respiratory failure who require renal replacement therapy for acute kidney injury face short-term mortality rates of up to 80%.[1]

PULMONARY PHYSIOLOGY IN CRITICAL CARE

Structure and Function

The structure of the lung facilitates its major function—specifically, to absorb oxygen and to excrete carbon dioxide. The alveoli and the respiratory bronchioles lie in direct apposition to the lung interstitium, through which course the pulmonary capillaries (Fig. 188-1). The capillaries are derived from both bronchial and pulmonary arteries. The bronchial circulation delivers oxygenated blood to interstitial tissue lacking close apposition to the airspaces, and the pulmonary circulation carries blood that is hypoxic and hypercarbic before equilibration with alveolar air.

Major Mechanisms for Abnormal Gas Exchange

Gas exchange can be impaired by several mechanisms. Insufficient carbon dioxide (CO_2) excretion leads to arterial hypercapnia, which can result from alveolar hypoventilation due to decreased respiratory frequency, as in drug-induced coma, diaphragmatic dysfunction, muscle weakness, and acute or chronic obstructive lung disease. Hypercapnia may be worsened in the critically ill, in whom oxygen consumption and carbon dioxide production are increased, as in patients with fever and sepsis. Arterial hypoxemia usually results from (1) alveolar hypoventilation ($PaCO_2$ greater than 40 mm Hg), which reduces alveolar oxygen tension because of the associated increase in alveolar carbon dioxide concentrations; (2) ventilation-perfusion mismatch from perfused capillaries with poorly ventilated alveoli; or (3) right-to-left shunting at the cardiac or intrapulmonary level. Ventilation-perfusion mismatch and intrapulmonary shunting in the critical care setting result from alveolar filling processes, such as pulmonary edema, alveolar hemorrhage, inflammation, infection, and atelectasis.

ACUTE LUNG INJURY

Epidemiology and Pathophysiology

Acute lung injury (ALI) and its severest manifestation, the acute respiratory distress syndrome (ARDS), are major causes of morbidity and mortality in critically ill patients. Since its initial description in 1967,[2] ALI-ARDS has been a major clinical cause of acute respiratory failure in critically ill patients. ALI-ARDS is a type of noncardiogenic pulmonary edema that results primarily from an increase

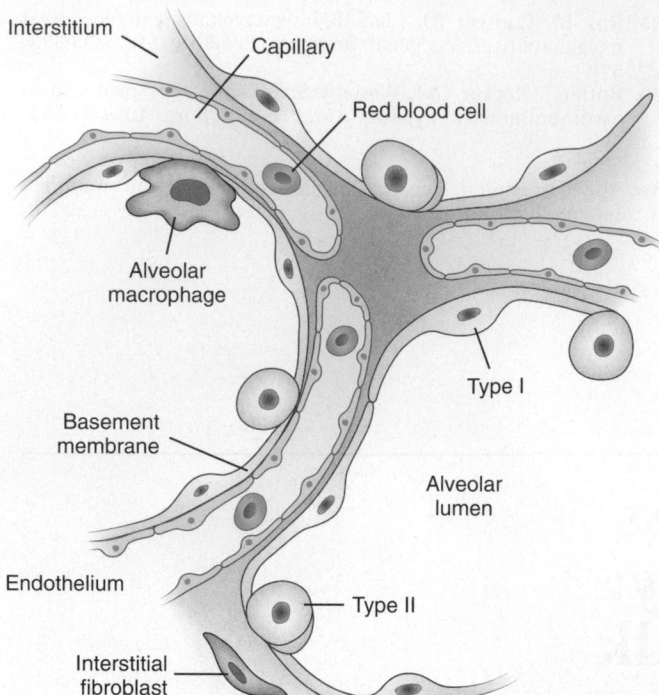

FIGURE 188-1. Alveolar structure. (Redrawn from Sabourin PJ: Pulmonary toxicology. In Hodgson E, Levi PE [eds]: Introduction to Biochemical Toxicology, 2nd ed. Norwalk, CT, Appleton & Lange, 1994, pp 491-517.)

in lung endothelial and epithelial permeability. A recent prospective population-based study established that approximately 200,000 cases of ALI occur annually in the United States alone.[3] The most common clinical disorders associated with the development of ALI are pneumonia, sepsis, aspiration of gastric contents, and major trauma with shock, as well as severe pancreatitis, severe burn injury, and anaphylaxis.[4] The extent of ALI is classified according to the requirement of fractional inspired oxygen. If cardiac filling pressures are not elevated, a ratio of the arterial oxygen tension to the fractional inspired oxygen concentration (PaO_2/FIO_2) less than 300 meets diagnostic criteria for ALI, and a value less than 200 is defined as the full-blown syndrome (i.e., ARDS).

Conceptually, ALI requires increased lung water (pulmonary edema) in the absence of elevated pulmonary capillary pressures. It is useful to review the determinants of fluid flux across the lung microvascular barrier, as determined by the Starling equation:

$$\text{Transcapillary fluid flux} = K_f[(P_{mv} - Pi) - \sigma(\pi mv - \pi i)]$$

where K_f = filtration coefficient (a function of surface area of filtration and hydraulic conductivity)
Pc = capillary hydrostatic pressure
Pi = interstitial hydrostatic pressure
πc = capillary protein osmotic pressure
πi = interstitial protein osmotic pressure
σ = osmotic reflection coefficient

The Starling equation describes the determinants of transvascular fluid filtration in the lung. Once the filtered fluid has collected in the interstitium, fluid is drained by pulmonary lymphatics. The tight alveolar-epithelial

barrier is important in preventing alveolar flooding by interstitial edema fluid. Thus, alveolar flooding varies with the capacity for lymphatic drainage of interstitial fluid and with the integrity of the alveolar-epithelial cell-cell junctions. Although the primary determinant of ALI is an increase in lung endothelial permeability, several experimental and clinical studies have established that elevated lung intravascular pressures often compound the degree of lung edema. For example, the recent multicenter ARDS Clinical Trials Network report noted that 29% of patients with ALI had coexistent pulmonary arterial wedge pressures greater than 18 mm Hg.[5] Only a small fraction of these patients had a decreased cardiac output, so the higher intravascular pressures probably were the result of fluid administered for resuscitation in conditions associated with the development of ALI, such as major trauma and sepsis.

Alveolar edema fluid is removed from the distal airspaces by active sodium and chloride transport across the alveolar epithelium.[6-8] Both type I and type II pneumocytes express apical sodium channels (ENaC) and basolateral sodium-potassium ATPases that actively pump sodium into the interstitium, with osmotically driven movement of water across the alveolar epithelium, potentially facilitated by aquaporin 5 water channels. Alveolar fluid clearance can be upregulated by cAMP agonists that require functional ENaC and CFTR.[6] The potential value of treating patients with β_2-adrenergic agonists to accelerate the resolution of pulmonary edema in ALI are being tested in a large multicenter, phase III ARDS Network clinical trial.

In summary, the accumulation of pulmonary edema fluid is a function of (1) lung endothelial and epithelial permeability, (2) lung capillary hydrostatic pressure, (3) lung lymphatic clearance, and (4) the efficiency of vectorial salt and water transport across the alveolar epithelium. The primary molecular and cellular determinants of ALI, on the other hand, are incompletely understood and are likely to be heterogeneous, including cytokines, leukocytes, and vascular thombi[9]; the end result is endothelial and epithelial injury, with increased capillary and epithelial permeability. Increased permeability leads in turn to flux of protein solutes that increase oncotic pressure, favoring alveolar flooding. Furthermore, as explained earlier, lung edema fluid accumulation is exacerbated by an increase in capillary hydrostatic pressure, as in coexistent heart failure or volume overload, conditions that often develop in the setting of renal failure. Impaired alveolar edema fluid clearance can be mediated by several mechanisms, including apoptosis and necrosis of the alveolar epithelium or injury to the apical or basolateral transporters by cytokines, oxygen radicals, and severe hypoxia or from microbial products.[6]

Clinical Strategies in the Care of Patients with Acute Lung Injury

Lung-protective mechanical ventilation, with the use of a low tidal volume (6 mL/kg of ideal body weight) and a plateau pressure limit (less than 30 cm of water), has been shown to protect lung parenchyma from mechanical trauma, which enhances lung endothelial and epithelial injury. High levels of positive end-expiratory pressure, although not proved to have a mortality benefit, often are necessary to maintain minimum arterial oxygen tensions because of alveolar flooding and collapse in ALI. Corticosteroids do not reduce morbidity or mortality in patients with ALI whether they are given early or late in the clinical course.[10] Finally, a recent trial showed that a conservative fluid strategy designed to achieve a net even daily fluid balance driven by reducing central venous or pulmonary artery wedge pressure, as opposed to net positive fluid delivery, significantly reduced the length of mechanical ventilation without higher rates of organ dysfunction, including renal failure.[5] All of these parameters—fluid management, mechanical ventilation strategies, and lung injury itself—are potentially relevant to kidney function in critical illness, as described subsequently.

COMBINED ACUTE LUNG INJURY AND ACUTE KIDNEY INJURY

The profound increase in mortality attributable to combined lung and kidney failure reflects in large part the severity of underlying illness in patients with multiorgan dysfunction. One recent analysis of clinical data from ARDS Network trials demonstrated that in patients with ALI, the development of acute kidney injury (defined as a rise in serum creatinine greater than 50% from baseline over the first four study days) resulted in an increase in the mortality rate of 58%, compared with a mortality rate of 28% in those patients with ALI in whom acute kidney injury did not develop.[11] New data focused on the interactive effects of lung and kidney dysfunction have emerged in recent years in several experimental studies (Fig. 188-2). These experiments are heterogeneous and multidisciplinary, pointing to the complex nature of crosstalk between whole organs; however, two major domains of inquiry have emerged: the *biomechanical* and the *inflammatory*.

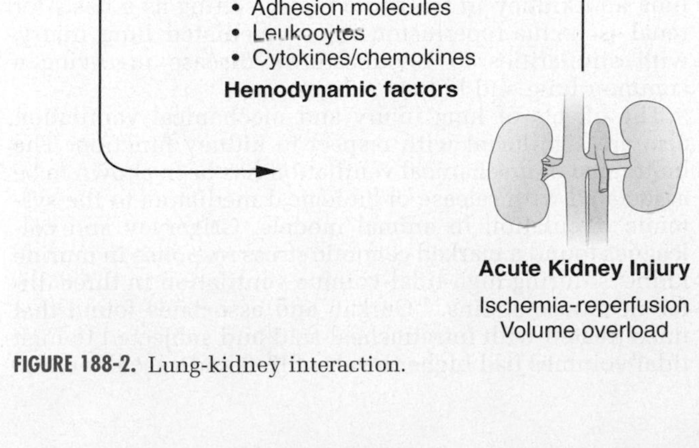

Acute Lung Injury

Ventilator-induced injury

Inflammation pathways
- Adhesion molecules
- Leukocytes
- Cytokines/chemokines

Hemodynamic factors

Acute Kidney Injury

Ischemia-reperfusion
Volume overload

FIGURE 188-2. Lung-kidney interaction.

Biomechanical Interaction between Lung and Kidney

The chief biomechanical effect of acute kidney injury is to increase intravascular volume and pressures. The resulting increased hydrostatic pressure in the pulmonary venules and capillaries leads to flooding of the interstitium and alveoli, particularly with conditions of increased capillary permeability and impaired alveolar epithelial clearance that are typical of ALI. Furthermore, markedly increased pressures themselves may damage and further increase the permeability of the pulmonary microvasculature; animal studies have demonstrated a phenomenon of capillary and extra-alveolar vascular "stress injury" that worsens pulmonary edema at moderately elevated vascular pressures.[12,13]

Conversely, the biomechanical effects of ALI and mechanical ventilation also can compromise renal function. Positive end-expiratory pressure (PEEP), used in ALI to maintain acceptable levels of systemic oxygenation, has been shown in animal studies to exacerbate hemodynamic instability in certain settings. Because pulmonary pressures are directly transmitted to the pericardium, right atrial collapsing pressures may be achieved in the setting of low central venous pressure and high mean airway pressures, as in volume depletion combined with high PEEP. Animal and clinical studies have borne out the importance of volume resuscitation in maintaining venous return, cardiac output, and renal blood flow in this context.[14,15]

Hypercapnia, tolerated to a variable extent in mechanically ventilated patients, also compromises renal blood flow. Studies in animals, normal subjects, and patients with hypercarbic respiratory failure have demonstrated an inverse relationship between $PaCO_2$ and renal blood flow, independent of PaO_2.[16] The mechanism is both direct and indirect: Hypercapnia causes renal vasoconstriction and also stimulates sympathetic activity. Furthermore, hypercapnia results in vasodilatation of other vascular beds, indirectly leading to activation of the sympathetic and renin-angiotensin-aldosterone axes and diminution of renal blood flow.

Pro-inflammatory Interaction between Lung and Kidney

Given that it is well established that inflammation and apoptosis are important mechanisms underlying ALI, how can renal injury contribute to the pro-inflammatory state leading to ALI? Early data showed upregulation of pulmonary vascular adhesion molecules after murine renal ischemia-reperfusion injury.[17] Next, studies using Evans blue dye extravasation demonstrated increased pulmonary capillary permeability and leukocyte and erythrocyte microvascular sludging after kidney ischemia-reperfusion injury in rats in a vascular clamp model (Fig. 188-3).[18] The molecular correlates of these physiological data were provided by ischemia-reperfusion injury studies in mice showing upregulation in lung tissue of inflammatory signaling pathways, such as by stress-regulated protein kinase phosphorylation, within 30 minutes of renal reperfusion after ischemia.[19] Acute kidney injury in mice results in genomic inflammatory changes in lung, and a pulmonary apoptotic response has been reported.[20] A potential mediator of acute kidney injury–induced

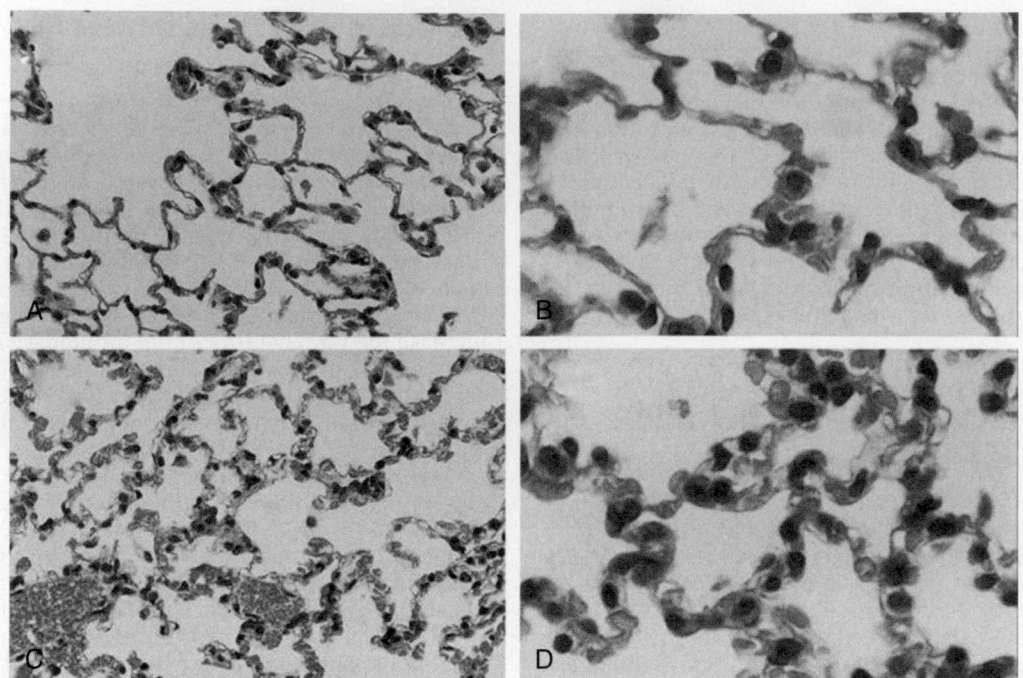

FIGURE 188-3. See also color plates. Increased interstitial edema in lung in response to renal ischemia-reperfusion. Preparations from sham-operated rats display clear alveolar spaces and minimal fluid or blood cells in the interstitial spaces at low (20×) and at high (40×) power (**A** and **B**). By contrast, preparations from rats with ischemic acute kidney injury exhibit lung interstitial edema, leukocyte sludging, and erythrocyte rouleaux formation, with occasional areas of alveolar hemorrhage (**C** and **D**). (From Kramer AA, Postler G, Salhab KF, et al: Renal ischemia/reperfusion leads to macrophage-mediated increase in pulmonary vascular permeability. Kidney Int 1999;55:2362.)

pulmonary capillary permeability is interleukin (IL)-10, with IL-10 antagonism attenuating distant effects of acute kidney injury.[21]

The pulmonary effects of renal injury are not limited to the endothelium: Renal failure can adversely affect pulmonary epithelial function. Rats subjected to either nephrectomy or renal ischemia-reperfusion injury were examined for histological changes in aquaporin 5, ENaC, and sodium-potassium ATPase.[22] Both nephrectomized and renal ischemia-reperfusion injury animals showed downregulation of ENaC, sodium-potassium ATPase, and aquaporin 5 compared with controls, independent of volume status. Of interest, the effect was observed in both the ischemia-reperfusion–injured and nephrectomized rats, suggesting that uremia itself, not reperfusion products, may play the greater role in the observed effect.

Further work has explored the potential effectors of these remote and rapid effects of renal injury. In one study, rats subjected to ischemia-reperfusion injury by vascular clamping were treated with CNI-1493, a macrophage pacifant that has been shown to inhibit pro-inflammatory signaling selectively in macrophages.[23-25] Rats treated with CNI-1493 before and after induction of renal ischemia-reperfusion injury displayed protection against the increase in pulmonary vascular permeability seen in control animals. No effect on the course of renal failure assessed by serum creatinine levels was observed, suggesting that the increase in permeability was independent of renal dysfunction and that macrophages or macrophage products activated by ischemia reperfusion injury were responsible for the lung injury.[18]

Recent data from the acute kidney injury literature suggest that the inflammatory cascade set in motion by ischemia-reperfusion or uremia is mediated in part by lymphocytes. Whereas clear evidence points to an innate immune response to ischemia-reperfusion injury, an immune mechanism of injury was unexpected, with considerable impact on both elucidation of mechanisms and development of therapies. Burne and coworkers demonstrated the importance of T cells in renal ischemia-reperfusion injury in finding that CD4-deficient mice were protected from renal injury, an effect that was both IFN-γ– and CD28-dependent.[26] Subsequent data provided evidence that this T cell response to ischemia-reperfusion injury is major histocompatibility complex (MHC)-dependent: Mice lacking the αβ T cell receptor were protected from renal ischemia-reperfusion injury and had a blunted cytokine response.[27] Whether the classic antigen-dependent pathway is activated by endogenous "alloantigens" liberated in ischemia-reperfusion injury, or by some antigen-independent pathway, remains to be studied. Moreover, further studies must address the relevance of the T cell dependence of acute kidney injury to ALI; it is tempting to speculate a potential antigenic link between lung and kidney in the acute injury setting as a basis for renal ischemia-reperfusion injury–mediated lung injury, with similarities to Goodpasture's disease involving a common lung and kidney antigen.

The effects of lung injury and mechanical ventilation also are significant with respect to kidney function. The biotrauma of mechanical ventilation has been shown to be associated with release of biological mediators to the systemic circulation in animal models. Grigoryev and colleagues found a marked genomic stress response in murine kidneys during high-tidal-volume ventilation in three different mouse strains.[28] Gurkan and associates found that mice treated with intratracheal acid and subjected to high tidal volumes had higher levels of IL-6 and vascular endothelial growth factor (VEGF) receptor-2 in kidney than the low-tidal-volume protocol group.[29]

In a randomized controlled clinical study, higher levels of pro-inflammatory cytokines in bronchoalveolar lavage fluid and plasma were detected in patients ventilated at higher lung volumes compared with controls.[30] A post hoc analysis showed that patients in the higher-tidal-volume protocol group had higher rates of renal failure at 72 hours, and that the degree of multiorgan failure was correlated with IL-6 levels. Additional evidence for acute kidney injury is available in a recently published mouse model of transfusion-associated lung injury.[31]

The interaction between lung and kidney in the setting of acute injury is complex, and recent work has raised the possibility that organ failure even may have distant protective effects. Acute kidney injury leads to reduced capacity for tissue injury in both systemic and kidney leukocytes.[32,33] Consistent with this finding are recent data showing that murine renal injury leads to decreased hypoxia after high tidal volume and lung acid injury, with the intriguing speculative conclusion that acute kidney injury may protect from ventilator-induced injury.[34] Clearly, further study is needed to expand the understanding of the effects, and effectors, of the inflammatory cascade triggered by concomitant lung injury, mechanical ventilation, and renal failure.

PULMONARY EFFECTS OF RENAL REPLACEMENT THERAPY

Management of kidney failure often requires renal replacement therapy. The impact of nonbiological polymers and plastics found in the dialysis circuit has long been known, and the pro-inflammatory effects have been found to extend even to the biocompatible membranes in use today. A growing literature has described the platelet- and leukocyte-activating effects of dialysis membranes.[33-37] The clinically relevant consequences of dialysis membrane reactions, as well as differences in effect between intermittent dialysis and continuous dialysis on ALI, remain to be explored. However, it is likely that continuous dialysis provides more physiological support for the critically ill patient with renal dysfunction and thus is more likely to be useful in multiorgan failure.

Key Points

1. The biomechanical and pro-inflammatory pathways that characterize acute lung injury and acute kidney injury suggest some common pathomechanisms for organ injury.
2. Because acute lung injury and renal dysfunction frequently coexist in the critical care setting, the effects of failure of one organ system are particularly relevant to the function of the other.
3. Recent experimental evidence provides new support for the existence of important pulmonary-renal interactions, some mediated by mechanical ventilation–associated lung injury.
4. Lung-kidney crosstalk has clinical relevance and may suggest novel mechanisms of multiorgan dysfunction, conceivably leading to new therapeutic strategies.

Acknowledgments

The work on which this chapter was based was supported by NHLBI P0HL073994 and NIDDK R01 DK054770 (for H.R.) and NHLBI RO1 HL 51854, R01 HL 51856, and P50 HL74005 (for M.M.).

Key References

4. Ware LB, Matthay MA: The acute respiratory distress syndrome. N Engl J Med 2000;342:1334.
9. Matthay MA, Zimmerman GA, Esmon C, et al: Future research directions in acute lung injury: Summary of a National Heart, Lung, and Blood Institute working group. Am J Respir Crit Care Med 2003;167:1027.
18. Kramer AA, Postler G, Salhab KF, et al: Renal ischemia/reperfusion leads to macrophage-mediated increase in pulmonary vascular permeability. Kidney Int 1999;55:2362.
23. Rabb H, Wang Z, Nemoto T, et al: Acute renal failure leads to dysregulation of lung salt and water channels. Kidney Int 2003;63:600.
34. Zarbock A, Schmolke M, Spieker T, et al: Acute uremia but not renal inflammation attenuates aseptic acute lung injury: A critical role for uremic neutrophils. J Am Soc Nephrol 2006;17:3124.

See the companion Expert Consult website for the complete reference list.

CHAPTER 189

Early High-Volume Hemofiltration to Prevent Invasive Ventilation in Critically Ill Patients

Pasquale Piccinni and Nereo Zamperetti

OBJECTIVES

This chapter will:
1. Review the pathophysiological rationale for the use of early high-volume hemofiltration to prevent the need for invasive ventilation in critically ill patients.
2. Summarize recent data on the use of hemofiltration during cardiopulmonary bypass, which has specific effects that collectively can be considered to represent a technically induced and replicable form of the systemic inflammatory response syndrome.
3. Present experimental data on the use of hemofiltration in critical patients in sepsis or septic shock.
4. Discuss the possible clinical implications of such data.

The multiple organ dysfunction syndrome (MODS)[1] is the most frequent cause of death in patients admitted to the intensive care unit (ICU) with severe sepsis. The mortality rate for these patients remains very high, exceeding 50% in spite of intensive care and full organ support.[2-5]

The lungs and the kidneys are the two organs most commonly affected by MODS.[6] Both organs may develop injury and dysfunction because of the systemic effects of numerous and diverse immunomodulating substances (humoral mediators) released into the circulation during severe infection.[7,8] Consequently, it is possible to hypothesize that treatment with techniques and modalities that can nonselectively affect a wide range of such modulators may potentially prove beneficial if applied early and at an appropriate level of intensity. One such modality is high-volume hemofiltration (HVHF).

Recent experimental studies on animal models have provided support for this conceptual framework. Published studies in humans focused on the effects of hemofiltration either on patients undergoing cardiopulmonary bypass, which is a well-known and replicable source of the systemic inflammatory response syndrome (SIRS), or on critically ill patients in sepsis or septic shock.

HEMOFILTRATION IN EXPERIMENTAL STUDIES IN ANIMALS

Back in 1991, Stein and colleagues demonstrated that continuous hemofiltration can modify endotoxin-induced lung injury in a porcine endotoxic shock model.[9] These workers hypothesized that such an effect probably was caused by the convective transport of mediator substances.

In 1994, Grootendorst and colleagues, studying the influence of high-volume continuous hemofiltration on the hemodynamics of pigs subjected to bowel ischemia and subsequent reperfusion, demonstrated that animals treated with HVHF had better hemodynamics and survival.[10]

In 2000, Bellomo and colleagues assessed the effect of intensive plasma water exchange by hemofiltration on hemodynamics and soluble mediators in canine endotoxemia.[11] They showed that intensive continuous venovenous hemofiltration (CVVH) can attenuate the early component of endotoxin-induced hypotension and reduce serum concentrations of endothelin-1. In this study, the hemodynamic effect of CVVH is not explained by convective clearance of the mediators. Unfortunately, in these two last studies, the possible impact of the therapy on respiratory function was not addressed.

HEMOFILTRATION AND CARDIOPULMONARY BYPASS

Cardiopulmonary bypass has been shown to induce complement activation, activation of leukocytes, expression of adhesion molecules, and release of endotoxins and of many inflammatory mediators including oxygen free radicals, arachidonic acid metabolites, cytokines, platelet-activating factor, nitric oxide, and endothelins.[12] In this sense, cardiopulmonary bypass creates a clinical condition that can be considered a replicable form of SIRS.

Journois and colleagues[13] studied the effects of hemofiltration performed during the rewarming phase of cardiopulmonary bypass in children undergoing surgical correction of tetralogy of Fallot. Hemofiltration was found to improve hemodynamics and early postoperative oxygenation and to reduce postoperative blood loss and duration of mechanical ventilation. Hemofiltration also proved capable of removing some major mediators of the inflammatory response.

Subsequently, the same group of investigators[14] assessed clinical effects and inflammatory mediator removal for high-volume, zero-fluid-balance ultrafiltration, also during rewarming after cardiopulmonary bypass in children. The results suggested that hemofiltration can exert some beneficial clinical effects. Of interest, both time to extubation and postoperative alveolar-arterial oxygen gradient significantly improved, among other variables. In the investigator's opinion, such effects are due neither to water removal nor to a direct removal of cytokines but probably are secondary to early removal of factors triggering the inflammatory response.

Recently, Oliver and colleagues compared perioperative corticosteroids with hemofiltration during cardiopulmonary bypass, in terms of attenuation of inflammation, to assess which approach could best reduce duration of mechanical ventilation after cardiac surgery.[15] These investigators demonstrated that even if both hemofiltration and steroids attenuated the inflammatory response, only hemofiltration was able to reduce time to tracheal extubation in adults after cardiopulmonary bypass.

HEMOFILTRATION IN CRITICALLY ILL PATIENTS

Some less recent data from studies using low-dose intervention (such as CVVH at 2 L/hour of ultrafiltration)[16] or low-grade continuous plasma filtration[17] have failed to show a benefit of blood purification in sepsis. In these studies, however, different results could have been obtained using early HVHF.

Honore and coworkers[18] studied prospectively 20 patients with severe septic shock, which had failed to respond to conventional therapy, to evaluate the effects of short-term (4-hour) HVHF (35 L of ultrafiltrate was removed, and neutral fluid balance was maintained). They reported that early initiation of therapy and adequate dose may improve hemodynamic and metabolic responses and 28-day survival. Unfortunately, this study failed to include a control group.

Oudemans-van Straaten and associates studied intermittent HVHF (mean ultrafiltration rate, 63 mL/minute; SD 20) in a cohort of patients in an ICU setting acquired over a period of 30 months.[19] Observed mortality was significantly lower than predicted. As suggested by this study, treatment with HVHF appears to be safe and feasible. Unfortunately, these researchers also failed to include a control group and to pay specific attention to possible changes in respiratory function.

In a controlled, randomized cross-over clinical trial, Cole and associates[20] assigned patients to either 8 hours of HVHF (at 6 L/hour) or 8 hours of standard CVVH (at 1 L/hour) in random order. They demonstrated changes in hemodynamic variables, dose of norepinephrine required to maintain a mean arterial pressure greater than 70 mm Hg, and plasma concentrations of complement anaphylatoxins and several cytokines. An 8-hour period of HVHF was associated with a greater reduction in norepinephrine requirements than that obtained with a similar period of CVVH. Both therapies were associated with a temporary reduction in plasma concentration of C3a, C5a, and interleukin 10 within 2 hours of initiation, but HVHF was associated with a greater reduction in the area under the curve for C3a and C5a. The investigators concluded that compared with standard CVVH, HVHF decreases vasopressor requirements in human septic shock and affects anaphylatoxin levels differently.

In a prospective randomized study of the impact of different ultrafiltration doses in continuous renal replacement therapy on survival, Ronco and colleagues[21] randomly assigned patients to different ultrafiltration protocols (20, 35, and 45 mL/hour per kg of body weight, respectively). Overall mortality was high, but increase in the rate of ultrafiltration improved survival significantly. The investigators recommend that ultrafiltration be prescribed according to the patient's body weight and should reach at least 35 mL/hour per kg ($n = 140$).

Joannes-Boyau and colleagues studied the effect of high-volume continuous venovenous hemofiltration (HVCVVH) on hemodynamics and outcome in patients with septic shock.[22] These workers showed that the hemodynamic parameters increased consistently during treatment by HVCVVH and suggested a beneficial effect of HVCVVH on 28-day mortality rates (46% versus 70%).

In view of some concerns expressed about the feasibility and costs of continuous HVHF, in 2005 Ratanarat and colleagues evaluated the efficacy of "pulse HVHF" (on a 24-hour schedule: HVHF at 85 mL/kg per hour for 6 to 8 hours, followed by CVVHF at 35 mL/kg per hour for 16 to 18 hours).[23] These workers demonstrated that pulse HVHF is a feasible modality that improves hemodynamics both during and after therapy. Consequently, it may be a beneficial adjuvant treatment for severe sepsis or septic shock in terms of patient survival, and it represents a compromise between traditional CVVH and HVHF.

Unfortunately, none of these studies focused on the respiratory effects of the technique. On the contrary, Piccinni and colleagues performed the first study to compare the clinical effects of HVHF in septic patients with ALI, in the absence of fully established acute renal failure, and in a control group.[24] These investigators studied the effect of a change in protocol that included early isovolemic HF (EIHF) in patients with septic shock, ALI, and oliguric acute renal injury. According to the new protocol, patients received EIHF at 45 mL/kg per hour of plasma water exchange over 6 hours with neutral fluid balance, followed by conventional CVVH. Benefits of this protocol included improved recovery of gas exchange and urine production (Table 189-1), earlier weaning from mechanical ventilation, shortened duration of ICU stay, and increased survival (Table 189-2).

The change in the survival curves became significant at day 13 (Fig. 189-1). This finding is particularly interesting, because in most published studies on HVHF, the so-called nonresponders or nonsurvivors appear to die within 24 hours from refractory shock[18] or within 72 hours from early multiple organ failure.[22] Perhaps this is due to the fact that EIHF works not only by removing pro-inflammatory mediators (thereby explaining the hemodynamic changes) but also by removing anti-inflammatory mediators, with restoration of immune competence.[25] This fact may explain the "late" difference in mortality between groups and is in line with the peak concentration hypothesis[26] and the possible effect of prolonging the initial EIHF effect with standard CVVH throughout the day. In fact, the high volume exchange of plasma water may be beneficial in removing substantial amounts of mediators; at the same time, the continuous application of the extracorporeal therapy may be important to cut the peaks of both pro-inflammatory and anti-inflammatory mediators in the circulation, and to reset the immune system to a more physiological level of function.

CONCLUSION

All of the foregoing data suggest a true biological effect of early HVHF in patients with sepsis requiring ICU care. They also are consistent with the paradigm of the humoral theory of sepsis that provides a rationale for blood purification therapies in sepsis.[27-31] Even if they are not conclusive, such data nevertheless suggest the feasibility of a moderately large, multicenter, phase IIb randomized con-

TABLE 189-1

Physiological Changes from Baseline to 48 Hours after Treatment with Standard Care and with Early Isovolemic Hemofiltration (EIHF)*†

PHYSIOLOGICAL PARAMETER	Baseline Values		Values After 48 Hours	
	GROUP A	GROUP B	GROUP A	GROUP B
Heart rate (beats/minute)	135 ± 9	140 ± 10	130 ± 10	120 ± 12‡
Mean arterial pressure (mm Hg)	60 ± 12	50 ± 10	65 ± 10	95 ± 10‡
Central venous pressure (mm Hg)	7 ± 2	5 ± 3	14 ± 2	10 ± 2
Pulmonary artery pressure (mm Hg)				
Systolic	25 ± 2	27 ± 3	24 ± 3	22 ± 2
Diastolic	10 ± 2	12 ± 2	18 ± 2	12 ± 3
Mean	16 ± 2	17 ± 2	22 ± 2	18 ± 2
Pulmonary artery wedge pressure (mm Hg)	8 ± 2	9 ± 3	12 ± 2	13 ± 2
Cardiac index (L/minute/m²)	3.0 ± 0.8	3.0 ± 0.7	3.3 ± 0.9	4 ± 0.5
Systemic vascular resistance (dynes-sec/cm⁵)	600 ± 260	800 ± 200	900 ± 350	1100 ± 200‡
Pulmonary vascular resistance (dynes-sec/cm⁵)	270 ± 30	402 ± 38	390 ± 40	310 ± 31
Urine output (mL/day)	550 ± 170	600 ± 200	650 ± 180	1200 ± 250‡
BUN (mg/dL)	110 ± 38	120 ± 30	98 ± 48	88 ± 40
Creatinine (mg/dL)	1.7 ± 2	1.8 ± 2	1.9 ± 2	1.6 ± 2
Norepinephrine dose (µg/kg/minute)	0.20 ± 2	0.20 ± 2	0.20 ± 0.2	0.02 ± 0.2‡
PaO₂/FIO₂	125 ± 55	117 ± 59	160 ± 50	240 ± 50‡

*Note in particular the significant increase in PaO₂/FIO₂ in patients managed with early isovolemic hemofiltration compared with their baseline values and with values for patients receiving standard care.
†Patients in Group A received standard care treatment; patients in Group B received EIHF.
‡P < .05 compared with baseline and between groups. The reported values are means ± SD.
BUN, blood urea nitrogen; PaO₂/FIO₂, ratio of arterial oxygen tension to fractional inspired oxygen concentration.
From Piccinni P, Dan M, Barbacini S, et al: Early isovolaemic haemofiltration in oliguric patients with septic shock. Intensive Care Med 2006;32:80-86.

TABLE 189-2

Comparison of Clinical Outcomes in Patients Receiving Standard Care Treatment and Those Managed with Early Isovolemic Hemofiltration (EIHF)*

OUTCOME	EIHF (N = 40)	CONTROL (N = 40)	P
Successful weaning	28 (70%)	15 (37%)	<.001
Duration of MV (days)	11 ± 3	20 ± 5	<.001
Independence from vasopressor support	30 (75%)	10 (25%)	<.001
ICU stay (days)	12 ± 5	16 ± 4	.002
Hospital stay (days)	19 ± 5	34 ± 4	<.001
ICU survival (predicted survival based on	28 (70%)	16 (40%)	.003
individual risk of death)	41 ± 12	40 ± 10	(NS)
28-day survival rate (predicted survival based on	22 (55%)	11 (27.5%)	.005
individual risk of death)	41 ± 12	40 ± 10	(NS)

*Note in particular the significant difference in rate of successful weaning (70% versus 37%) and in duration of mechanical ventilation (11 ± 3 versus 20 ± 5 days) in patients managed with EIHF compared with patients on standard care.
ICU, intensive care unit; MV, mechanical ventilation; NS, not significant. Values expressed as means with standard deviation or as numbers with percentage.
From Piccinni P, Dan M, Barbacini S, et al: Early isovolaemic haemofiltration in oliguric patients with septic shock. Intensive Care Med 2006;32:80-86.

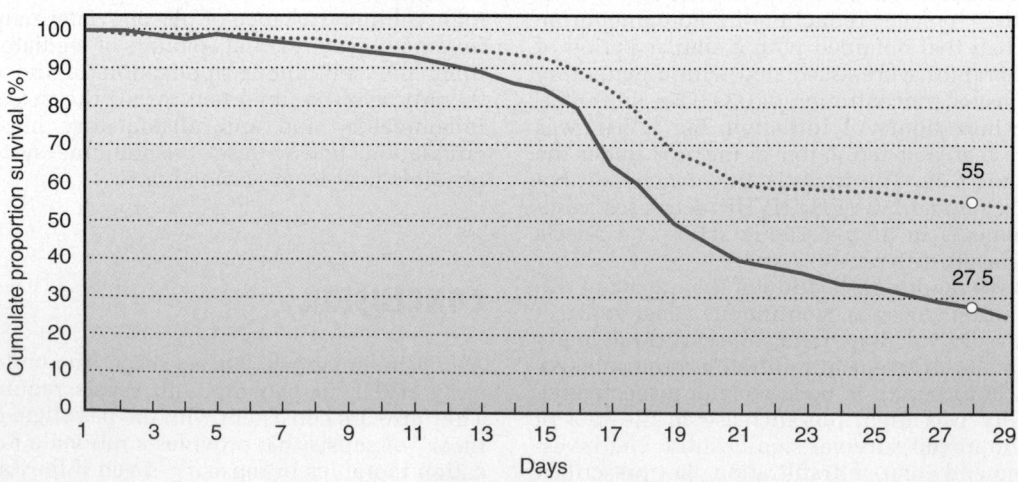

FIGURE 189-1. Kaplan-Meier estimate of survival rates in patients receiving standard care treatment (solid line) compared with patients receiving early isovolemic hemofiltration (dotted line). (From Piccinni P, Dan M, Barbacini S, et al: Early isovolaemic haemofiltration in oliguric patients with septic shock. Intensive Care Med 2006;32:80-86.)

trolled trial of early HVHF in critically ill patients with sepsis. Such a trial is the necessary step to justify a larger phase III study, in view of the cost of therapy and the associated technical demands.

Key Points

1. Published experimental and clinical data support the hypothesis that early high-volume hemofiltration can exert positive effects on the respiratory function of critically ill patients with sepsis and may limit the need for invasive ventilation.
2. Because the findings are not conclusive, it seems necessary to perform a moderately large, multicenter, phase IIb randomized controlled trial of early high-volume hemofiltration in such patients.

Key References

1. Brivet FG, Kleinknecht DJ, Loirat P, Landais PJ: Acute renal failure in intensive care units—causes, outcome, and prognostic factors of hospital mortality; a prospective, multicenter study. French Study Group on Acute Renal Failure. Crit Care Med 1996;24:192-198.
5. Tonelli M, Manns B, Feller-Kopman D: Acute renal failure in the intensive care unit: A systematic review of the impact of dialytic modality on mortality and renal recovery. Am J Kidney Dis 2002;40:875-885.
18. Honore PM, Jamez J, Wauthier M, et al: Prospective evaluation of short-term, high-volume isovolemic hemofiltration on the hemodynamic course and outcome in patients with intractable circulatory failure resulting from septic shock. Crit Care Med 2000;28:3581-3587.
19. Oudemans-van Straaten HM, Bosman RJ, van der Spoe JI, Zandstra DF: Outcome of critically ill patients treated with intermittent high-volume haemofiltration: A prospective cohort analysis. Intensive Care Med 1999;25:814-821.

See the companion Expert Consult website for the complete reference list.

CHAPTER 190

Pulmonary Renal Syndromes

Richard K. S. Phoon, A. Richard Kitching, and Stephen R. Holdsworth

OBJECTIVES

This chapter will:
1. Define the spectrum of conditions causing immune alveolar and glomerular injury inducing acute pulmonary and renal impairment, often with lung hemorrhage.
2. Explain the immunopathogenesis and the major clinical features of Goodpasture's syndrome.
3. Outline the diagnostic pathways.
4. Discuss the recent advances in treatment based on multicenter prospective trials.

Acute renal failure and respiratory failure both are common problems in the intensive care unit (ICU) and frequently occur together. This chapter deals with the syndrome of immune-mediated systemic disease that simultaneously targets both lung and kidney: *Goodpasture's syndrome* (GPS). A useful working definition of GPS is acute pulmonary parenchymal immune inflammation (with or without pulmonary hemorrhage) occurring together with acute proliferative glomerulonephritis. This is a syndrome, not a disease, and can result from several different diseases and immune processes. It is now recognized that a majority of the cases are autoimmune diseases and fall into one of three groups: small-vessel vasculitis associated with anti-neutrophil cytoplasmic antibodies (ANCAs), immune complex diseases (including systemic lupus erythematosus [SLE]), and anti–glomerular basement membrane (anti-GBM) disease (Table 190-1). It should be noted that the term *Goodpasture's disease* is widely used to refer to pulmonary hemorrhage and crescentic glomerulonephritis associated with circulating anti-GBM antibodies.

IMMUNOPATHOGENESIS

Accumulating evidence suggests that most of the diseases causing GPS are autoimmune in nature. Many of the disease-initiating autoantigens have been defined, and useful serological diagnostic assays have become available. The tissue lesions result from small-vessel inflammation triggered by either deposition of autoantibody or local recognition of autoantigens as peptides by autoimmune effector T cells. These humoral and cellular effectors induce complement activation and recruitment of injurious leukocytes (neutrophils and macrophages). Infiltrating leukocytes release soluble mediators, including enzymes, reactive oxygen species, arachidonic acid–derived products, cytokines, and chemokines, that induce local inflammation, tissue injury, and increased capillary permeability. Exudation of plasma proteins and red cells results. Vessel injury may be of a severity that allows hemorrhage in the lung and macroscopic hematuria in the kidney. The resulting tissue injury and disruption of physiological processes (i.e., gas transfer in the lung and glomerular filtration in the kidney) can induce loss of function of both organs, resulting in acute respiratory failure and rapidly progressive glomerulonephritis. In severe cases, fatal pulmonary hemorrhage and acute oligoanuric renal failure are seen. GPS is commonly acute (days) and constitutes a medical emergency. Almost all of the diseases inducing GPS are

TABLE 190-1

Diseases Causing Goodpasture's Syndrome (GPS): Renal Biopsy Diagnosis

CLASSIFICATION	ANTIBODY PATTERN	CAUSATIVE DISORDER(S)
Anti-GBM GN	Linear	Anti-GBM GN (Goodpasture's disease)
Immune complex	Granular	SLE
		SBE
		Infection-associated GN, hepatitis C
		Idiopathic GN—mesangiocapillary, IgA, HSP
Immune-negative	Pauci-immune	Small-vessel vasculitis
		Wegener's granulomatosis
		Microscopic polyangiitis

Anti-GBM, anti–glomerular basement membrane; GN, glomerulonephritis; HSP, Henoch-Schönlein purpura; IgA, immunoglobulin A; SBE, subacute bacterial endocarditis; SLE, systemic lupus erythematosus.

treatable and potentially reversible if recognized and treated aggressively early in the course.

Vasculitis

GPS may be induced by a subgroup of vasculitides. These forms of vasculitis have in common the targeting of small blood vessels, arterioles, capillaries, and venules, explaining the effects on gas transfer and renal filtration. They are strongly associated with ANCAs. It is likely that ANCAs are pathogenic and result from autoimmunity to leukocyte lysosomal enzymes. Several of the target autoantigens have been identified; the two major targets are myeloperoxidase (MPO)[1] and proteinase 3 (PR3).[2,3] Paradoxically, the affected tissues are frequently injured without the local deposition of ANCAs, although T cells and the delayed-type hypersensitivity (DTH) effectors they recruit—macrophages, fibrin, and neutrophils—are almost always present.[4,5] The presence of such effectors suggests that this nephritogenic immune response is driven by T_H1[6] or T_H17[7] CD4+ subsets. It is likely that ANCAs bind their target autoantigens when a trigger such as sepsis induces translocation of PR3 or MPO to the cell membrane.[8] ANCA-bound neutrophils become localized in the glomerular microcirculation[9] (and probably the pulmonary microcirculation), where MPO and PR3 become deposited, acting as local targets for autoimmune effector T cells that recruit local DTH effectors. Because the target autoantigens circulate (in neutrophils), many different organs also can be targeted, and multisystem involvement is a feature of ANCA-associated small-vessel vasculitis.

Several subgroups of small-vessel vasculitis have been defined and are collectively known as *ANCA-associated systemic vasculitis* (AASV). In the kidney, the inflammation includes acute proliferative focal and segmental necrotizing crescentic glomerulonephritis with little antibody deposition–hence the term *pauci-immune crescentic glomerulonephritis*. This designation is somewhat erroneous because "pauci-immunity" refers only to the humoral immunity; cellular immune effectors are prominent in almost all cases.[4,5] In the lung, interstitial infiltrates and hemorrhage are the major features. The inflammation can include granulomata, and if it does, the condition is termed *Wegener's granulomatosis*. This syndrome is associated predominantly, but not exclusively, with autoimmunity to PR3. The combination of lung infiltrates and glomerulonephritis (and other organ involvement) without granulomata is termed *microscopic polyangiitis* and is predominantly, but not exclusively, associated with autoimmunity to MPO.[10]

Anti–Glomerular Basement Membrane Disease

Anti-GBM disease is an autoimmune disease in which the target autoantigen is the noncollagenous domain of the α3 chain of type IV collagen.[11] This antigen is expressed in basement membranes of glomerular and alveolar capillaries. It is a cryptic epitope, and case studies suggest that hydrocarbons, infections, cigarette smoking, and lithotripsy[12] may be associated with the onset of disease, perhaps by revealing the epitope to the systemic autoimmune process. The antibody is directly pathogenic and can induce nephritis in primates.[13] The presence of T cells and macrophages in glomerular lesions suggests that cellular immunity also is involved. Strong linear deposition of immunoglobulin G (IgG) is seen in renal biopsy specimens and also is observed in biopsied lung tissue. A strong association with the human leukocyte antigen HLADR2 has been recognized.[14] Genotyping shows that the HLADRB1*1501 and *1502 alleles confer increased susceptibility, whereas DRB1*07 and *01 confer protection.[15] In the presence of circulating antibody, kidney allografts rapidly develop recurrent disease.[16]

Immune Complex Goodpasture Syndrome
Autoimmune Disease

The best-described autoimmune immune complex cause of GPS is SLE. Pulmonary involvement is uncommon but clearly can occur and can manifest with pulmonary hemorrhage. The target antigens are multiple, but those most clearly associated include nuclear antigens (antinuclear antibody [ANA]) and double-stranded DNA (dsDNA). The renal and lung lesions show granular deposition of immunoglobulins of several different subclasses, a characteristic pattern of injury resulting from SLE-induced immune complex deposition. Lupus nephritis is subclassified on the basis of histological pattern; type IV proliferative crescentic glomerulonephritis is most frequently associated with GPS.

Other Immune Complex Diseases

A number of different diseases can cause acute, rapidly progressive glomerulonephritis and occasionally also simultaneously involve the lung. These diseases include subacute bacterial endocarditis (SBE), in which host immunity to persistent intravascular microbial antigens causes immune complex–induced vasculitis,[17] occasion-

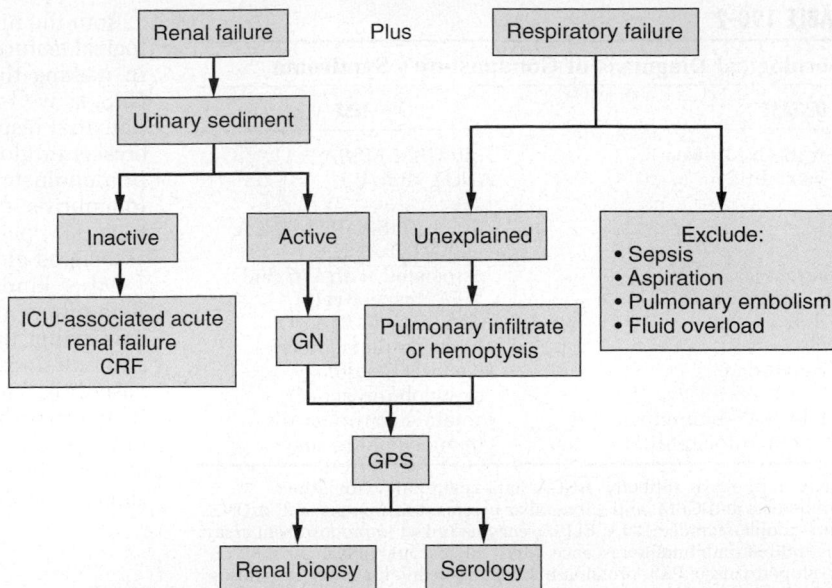

FIGURE 190-1. Diagnosis of Goodpasture's syndrome (GPS). CRF, chronic renal failure; GN, glomerulonephritis; ICU, intensive care unit.

ally postinfectious glomerulonephritis, and other infections[18] such as hepatitis C–induced cryoglobulinemia.[19] Other crescentic forms of glomerulonephritis of uncertain (but likely autoimmune) etiology can occasionally cause this syndrome: mesangiocapillary glomerulonephritis, immunoglobulin A (IgA) disease, Henoch-Schönlein purpura,[20] idiopathic cryoglobulinemia,[21] and fibrillary and immunotactoid glomerulonephritis.[22,23]

CLINICAL FEATURES AND DIAGNOSTIC APPROACHES

GPS requires the presence of acute renal impairment due to glomerulonephritis. Urine analysis is a simple and essential prerequisite to making the diagnosis (Fig. 190-1). Nephritis in GPS is associated with an active urinary sediment and proteinuria with abnormal hematuria, with urinary red cells exhibiting a "glomerular" dysmorphic appearance under phase contrast microscopy. Red cell casts also may be present, suggestive of heavy glomerular bleeding.

The respiratory features of GPS are nonspecific. Alveolar bleeding manifests as overt hemoptysis in a minority of affected persons. A history of breathlessness and presence of cough are more common features. The chest x-ray appearance is one of diffuse alveolar shadowing and is not specific for bleeding. A computed tomography (CT) scan is a more sensitive study for showing multilobular involvement, a common pattern of bleeding in GPS. Sputum microscopy may reveal red cells or hemosiderin-laden macrophages, or bronchoscopy may show diffuse bleeding.

Most patients with anti-GBM disease have an acute illness with few, if any, symptoms beyond those due to pulmonary and renal involvement. A bimodal age distribution is recognized. Vasculitis-associated GPS typically occurs in the elderly (although all ages can be affected), with an inflammatory prodrome of weeks to months (weight loss, anorexia, sweats). Evidence of vasculitis in multiple organ systems beyond the kidney and lungs,

especially the skin on the lower limbs, is common but not essential to the diagnosis in this multisystem disease. Lupus occurs mainly in young women, with multisystem features such as skin rash, serositis, dermal vasculitis, central nervous sytem (CNS) involvement, and the other typical features of SLE.

Nonimmune Causes of Pulmonary Disease in Patients with Renal Disease

Fluid overload, especially compounded by increased capillary permeability due to proteinuria-induced hypoalbuminemia, commonly occurs with acute renal failure. Chronic renal failure is associated with pericardial and pleural effusions. Pneumonia, aspiration, and pulmonary embolism are not uncommon in patients with renal failure in the ICU setting. It is important to exclude these conditions and rigorously review the urinary sediment to exclude glomerulonephritis. Unexplained pulmonary infiltrates, in association with nephritis, should strongly raise the suspicion of GPS. The corrected carbon monoxide transfer factor (K_{CO})[24] is a sensitive test for pulmonary hemorrhage (it is increased with pulmonary hemorrhage) and also can be used for monitoring treatment response and disease relapse. If nephritis and unexplained pulmonary infiltrates are present, two main diagnostic options are available: serological diagnosis and renal biopsy.

Serological Diagnosis of Goodpasture's Syndrome

The serological diagnosis of GPS is summarized in Table 190-2. ANCAs are strongly associated with vasculitis. Recommended assays include enzyme-linked immunosorbent assay (ELISA)-based assays for antibodies to MPO and PR3 and neutrophil immunostaining "slide testing" using alcohol-fixed neutrophils, which give characteristic patterns of cytoplasmic staining. Perinuclear staining ("p"-pattern ANCA) is associated with anti-MPO reactivity, whereas diffuse cytoplasmic staining ("c"-pattern

Serological Diagnosis of Goodpasture's Syndrome

DISEASE	TEST
Anti-GBM disease	Anti-GBM ELISA
Vasculitis	ANCA slide IIF
	plus
	ANCA ELISA (PR3-ANCA and MPO-ANCA associated with WG and MPA, respectively)
SLE	ANA, anti-dsDNA, hypocomplementemia
Hepatitis C	Hepatitis C serology, cryoglobulin screen
Fibrillary/immunotactoid glomerulonephritis	Protein electrophoresis (monoclonal bands)

ANA, antinuclear antibody; ANCA, anti–neutrophil cytoplasmic antibodies; anti-GBM, anti–glomerular basement membrane; anti-dsDNA, anti–double-stranded DNA; ELISA, enzyme-linked immunosorbent assay; IIF, indirect immunofluorescence; MPA, microscopic polyangiitis; MPO, myeloperoxidase; PR3, proteinase 3; SLE, systemic lupus erythematosus; WG, Wegener's granulomatosis.

ANCA) correlates with anti-PR3 activity. This combination of assays, especially in patients selected for a high pretest probability of GPS (by the presence of red cells, white cells, and cellular, particularly red cell, casts in the urinary sediment), has a high sensitivity (approximately 98%) and specificity (approximately 70%).[25,26]

Assays for anti-GBM antibodies are widely available. ELISAs using purified GBM generally are more reliable than indirect immunofluorescence testing using kidney sections. These tests have not been subject to the rigorous standardization of ANCA, but they have found general acceptance. Case reports of serum anti-GBM–negative but positive linear antibody–staining renal biopsy specimens[27] and the realization that many normal sera have low-level GBM reactivity[28] are sources of concern. Reports show that sera from up to 30% of patients who are anti-GBM–positive are also positive for ANCA, whereas sera from up to 5% of patients who are ANCA-positive are also positive for anti-GBM antibodies.[29]

Screening for SLE is well accepted, and negative results on ANA and anti-dsDNA assays militate strongly against this diagnosis. Some ANA-positive sera also contain genuine ANCAs, but ANA testing can give a false-positive p-ANCA result. This can be checked using non–alcohol-fixed neutrophil slides, in which MPO does not move to a perinuclear location (as occurs with alcohol fixation). Other useful screening tests for less common GPS-inducing disease include serum complement levels, hepatitis serology, serum protein immunoelectrophoresis, and cryoglobulin quantitation.

Renal Biopsy

The presence of urinary evidence of nephritis plus renal impairment in a patient with unexplained pulmonary infiltrates or hemoptysis is a strong indication for urgent renal biopsy. The argument could be made that a positive result on an ANCA assay in this setting is sufficient to initiate treatment, but in view of the potential toxicity of current therapies, a biopsy would generally still be recommended.

Both the histological appearance and the immunohistological features of the renal biopsy specimen are important in making the diagnosis of the specific disease causing GPS, as well as in giving important information regarding potential responses to therapy. In fact, the classification of crescentic glomerulonephritis rests heavily on renal biopsy immunohistological findings (type 1: anti-GBM glomerulonephritis; type 2: immune complex glomerulonephritis; type 3: pauci-immune or immune-negative ANCA-associated glomerulonephritis) (see Table 190-1).

Other kinds of tissue sampling should be considered. Skin biopsy rarely is performed but is a simple method of confirming the presence of a leukocytoclastic vasculitis, and immunostaining usually helps distinguish lupus from vasculitis. Lung biopsy is sometimes helpful, particularly if the renal biopsy specimen shows evidence of disease not typically associated with GPS. Other involved organs also may be sampled for diagnostic tissue in some circumstances, particularly in multisystem diseases.

APPROACH TO TREATMENT OF GOODPASTURE'S SYNDROME

Most patients have aggressive autoimmune vascular inflammation, which potentially will respond to immunosuppressive or anti-inflammatory drug therapy. The diseases for which the best evidence base has been established are small-vessel vasculitis, anti-GBM disease, and lupus nephritis. Many of the other, less common diseases that occasionally cause GPS also are immune or inflammatory diseases. Although their infrequency has made the evidence base for therapeutic decision making much less robust, their probably similar immunopathology gives some justification for adopting therapeutic protocols successful in vasculitis and anti-GBM disease.

PRINCIPAL DISEASES CAUSING IMMUNE ALVEOLITIS AND NEPHRITIS

Anti–Glomerular Basement Membrane Disease
Clinical Features

Anti-GBM disease is a rare disorder, with an incidence of approximately 1 case per 1 million population per year. It typically manifests as acute, rapidly progressive glomerulonephritis with lung hemorrhage.[30] In approximately 40% of cases, however, the glomerulonephritis occurs as an isolated entity. The disease is more common in whites, and males are more commonly affected than females. A bimodal age distribution that peaks in the third and sixth decades is recognized.[12] In most cases, acute nephritic syndrome with significant renal impairment or oligoanuric acute renal failure constitutes the major renal manifestations. Pulmonary involvement can be dramatic, with overt hemoptysis. Less specific signs and symptoms including breathlessness and cough are more common with pulmonary infiltrates detected radiologically.

Although the disease is rare, it is overrepresented in the group of patients presenting with rapidly progressive glomerulonephritis and hemoptysis, constituting around 20% of the cases. Pulmonary hemorrhage is more common and severe in smokers.[24] In most patients, clinical manifestations are limited to the lung and kidney; however, a minority experience a systemic nonspecific prodrome of malaise and weight loss and suffer from fatigue. The cause of these symptoms may be anemia, or such cases may represent the 20% of patients with anti-GBM disease who also have circulating ANCA.[29] Untreated, the disease carries a very poor prognosis with a high mortality rate.

Treatment

The largest and best-documented experience in anti-GBM disease comes from the Hammersmith group in England.[12,30,31] This disease is the most aggressive form of GPS, with the worst renal prognosis. The use of oral cyclophosphamide and prednisolone (based on the National Institutes of Health [NIH] Wegener's granulomatosis protocol) is the best-evaluated protocol: oral prednisolone beginning at 1 mg/kg tapered over 6 months, combined with cyclophosphamide 2 to 3 mg/kg (1 to 2 mg/kg in patients older than 55 years of age). Based on the presence of circulating antibody of proven pathological capacity, plasma exchange aiming to radically reduce the circulating level has been widely used. One small randomized trial has been undertaken,[32] although in only 17 patients. The addition of plasma exchange to cyclophosphamide and prednisolone was associated with 75% retention of renal function (33% without plasma exchange). The Hammersmith protocol includes daily exchange at 60 mL/kg, with albumin or with fresh frozen plasma if bleeding is a risk, for 14 days or until anti-GBM antibody testing results become negative.

This group of investigators reported a 12-month survival rate of 85%, with dialysis-independent renal function in approximately 50% of the patients. The renal prognosis for patients who are dialysis-dependent at presentation (who generally show histological evidence of very extensive crescent formation, interstitial damage, and evidence of sclerosis—all poor prognostic markers) is 7%, compared with 90% for patients with serum creatinine less than 500 µmol/L,[33] so less aggressive therapy is recommended for these patients because of the high risk-to-benefit ratio. Pulmonary hemorrhage generally responds to active treatment with cyclophosphamide, prednisolone, and plasma exchange. Some clinicians use pulse steroids in this situation, although trial evidence showing additional benefit is lacking. Once recovery has occurred and anti-GBM antibody levels are unmeasurable, therapy can be tapered. Recurrences of this disease are distinctly uncommon. Transplantation should not be undertaken until antibody levels are unrecordable.

Anti-Neutrophil Cytoplasmic Antibody–Associated Systemic Vasculitis and Goodpasture's Syndrome
Clinical Features

Systemic vasculitis is the predominant cause of GPS.[34] Although most forms of primary vasculitis have been reported to manifest with GPS, lung and kidney involvement is most characteristic of the small-vessel vasculitides, which include Wegener's granulomatosis, microscopic polyangiitis, and Churg-Strauss syndrome. Most cases of small-vessel vasculitis are associated with the presence of

ANCA (Wegener's granulomatosis and microscopic polyangiitis are strongly associated with PR3-ANCA and MPO-ANCA, respectively, whereas ANCA predominantly of MPO reactivity is found in approximately 40% of patients with Churg-Strauss syndrome), and case series report the incidence of ANCA in GPS as between 55% and 86%.[35-37] Pulmonary hemorrhage portends a particularly poor prognosis in small-vessel vasculitis and occurs in up to 42%, 29%, and 3% of patients with Wegener's granulomatosis, microscopic polyangiitis, and Churg-Strauss syndrome, respectively.[38,39]

Constitutional signs and symptoms such as fever, malaise, weight loss, myalgias, and arthralgias commonly accompany GPS secondary to ANCA-associated systemic vasculitis (AASV). Involvement of small vessels in the skin (e.g., leukocytoclastic vasculitis), nerves (e.g., mononeuritis multiplex), and gastrointestinal tract (e.g., ischemic ulceration of the gut) also may be a feature. Wegener's granulomatosis is differentiated clinically from other diagnostic possibilities by its predilection for upper respiratory tract disease (manifested as sinusitis, subglottic stenosis, otitis media, or nasal septal disease, present in up to 90% of patients[26]) and, histologically, by the presence of necrotizing granulomatous inflammation of small vessels. By contrast, microscopic polyangiitis is defined by the presence of necrotizing inflammation of small vessels, almost invariably associated with so-called pauci-immune glomerulonephritis, in the absence of granuloma formation.[10] Several classification systems for the diagnosis of Churg-Strauss syndrome have been proposed,[10,40,41] reflecting the variable clinical presentation of patients with this rare disorder, although the triad of small-vessel vasculitis, asthma, and peripheral eosinophilia usually is present. Among the vasculitides, Churg-Strauss syndrome is an uncommon cause of GPS (accounting for 3% or less of the cases).

The severity of pulmonary hemorrhage secondary to AASV varies, ranging from mild hemoptysis to severe pulmonary hemorrhage. Occult hemorrhage in the presence of a normal appearance of the chest radiograph also may be suggested by an elevated K_{CO} to greater than 30% above the predicted value.[42] Non–immune-mediated causes of hemoptysis also should be considered, as indicated by the recent Wegener's Clinical Occurrence of Thrombosis (WeCLOT) study, which demonstrated an increased incidence of venous thromboembolic events in patients with Wegener's granulomatosis.[43]

Treatment

Pulmonary hemorrhage in AASV is an ominous sign and generally is agreed to warrant early and aggressive intervention. Although incompletely supported by controlled studies, initial (induction) treatment typically consists of combination therapy, as follows:

1. High-dose corticosteroids (oral prednisolone, 1 mg/kg per day, up to a daily maximum of 80 mg, which initially may be preceded by 3 days of intravenous methylprednisolone, 500 to 1000 mg per day)
2. Cyclophosphamide (either orally, 2 mg/kg per day, or as intravenous pulses of 15 mg/kg every 2 to 4 weeks)
3. Plasma exchange (60 mL/kg for seven exchanges over 2 weeks).

The introduction in the 1970s of combination therapy using corticosteroids and cyclophosphamide[44] dramatically improved the outcome of patients with AASV. Complete remission can now be expected in 75% to 85% of patients, whereas corticosteroid monotherapy is reported to yield lower remission and higher relapse rates than can be achieved in combination with cyclophosphamide.[26,45,46] Relapse, however, occurs in approximately half of those patients who achieve complete remission, and cyclophosphamide therapy is limited by significant potential toxicity (including opportunistic infections secondary to cyclophosphamide-induced leukopenia, hemorrhagic cystitis, bladder cancer, and amenorrhea). Additionally, resistant vasculitis occurs in approximately 10% of patients.[31]

As a minimum standard of care, appropriate prophylaxis should be provided to patients receiving cyclophosphamide, including maintenance of adequate hydration, administration of mercaptoethane sulfonate (mesna) to prevent cystitis, and the use of trimethoprim-sulfamethoxazole for *Pneumocystis jiroveci* (formerly *carinii*) pneumonia (PCP) prophylaxis. Some evidence suggests that this antimicrobial regimen also may be beneficial in patients with Wegener's granulomatosis by reducing chronic nasal carriage of *Staphylococcus aureus*, a known risk factor for relapse.[47] Strategies have been proposed to minimize exposure to cyclophosphamide, including (1) the use of intravenous versus oral cyclophosphamide, (2) the use of alternative induction agents, and (3) timely conversion to non–cyclophosphamide-based maintenance therapy.

Pulse intravenous cyclophosphamide may be less toxic than daily oral cyclophosphamide. Despite early reservations regarding inferior relapse rates with the use of intravenous cyclophosphamide,[48] the preliminary reports of the CYCLOPS (*Cyclo*phosphamide Daily *O*ral versus *Pulsed*) trial demonstrated equivalent survival, remission, and relapse rates with intravenous and oral cyclophosphamide regimens using an approximately 50% reduced cumulative cyclophosphamide dose.[49] This trial, however, excluded patients with life-threatening disease. Various studies have investigated the usefulness of adjunctive induction therapy. Use of methotrexate, in the NORAM (*N*on-*R*enal Wegener's Granulomatosis Treated *A*lternatively with *M*ethotrexate) trial,[50] and etanercept, in the Wegener's Granulomatosis Etanercept Trial (WGET),[51] yielded disappointing results: Neither treatment provided additional benefit. Relapse rates also were higher in the NORAM trial methotrexate treatment group, whereas the incidence of solid cancers was increased in the WGET etanercept treatment group. In addition, most patients with GPS have moderate to severe renal impairment, excluding the use of methotrexate. By contrast, initial results from small, uncontrolled series (predominantly in refractory or relapsing AASV) evaluating the efficacy of rituximab, a chimeric monoclonal antibody directed at the B cell surface antigen, CD20, have been more promising.[52-54] Two larger studies, Rituximab for ANCA-Associated Vasculitis (RAVE) and RITUXVAS, are in progress to further investigate its efficacy in induction of remission.

Most experts would recommend plasma exchange for patients with AASV presenting with pulmonary hemorrhage, dialysis-dependent renal failure on presentation,[55] or the presence of concurrent anti-GBM antibodies. Klemmer and colleagues[56] performed a retrospective, single-center analysis of data for 20 patients with diffuse alveolar hemorrhage secondary to AASV treated with plasma exchange and standard induction therapy. Subsequently, hemorrhage resolved in all patients, and half of the patients who had initial azotemia had improved renal function on discharge. The recent MEPEX (*Me*thyl *P*rednisolone versus *Plasma Ex*change as Additional Therapy for Severe ANCA-Associated Glomerulonephritis) study

was a randomized trial conducted in 137 patients with severe glomerulonephritis (serum creatinine greater than 500 μmol/L) secondary to AASV who were randomized to receive treatment with either plasma exchange or methylprednisolone.[57,58] Patients treated with plasma exchange were more likely to be alive and dialysis-independent at 3 months (69% versus 49%; $P < 0.02$) and there was a 24% reduction in the risk for progression to end-stage kidney disease. The greatest benefit was found in those patients who were dialysis-dependent at presentation, and no differences in adverse events were observed between groups.

Rarely, AASV is resistant to standard induction therapy with cyclophosphamide. Data recommending specific therapy are scarce; however, some medications that have been evaluated with variable success include antithymocyte globulin,[59] intravenous immunoglobulin,[60] rituximab,[52-54] mycophenolate,[61] and 15-deoxyspergualin (gusperimus).[62] Once remission has been achieved (usually within 3 to 6 months), patients should be switched to non–cyclophosphamide-based maintenance therapy with azathioprine (2 mg/kg daily) or methotrexate if normal or near-normal renal function remains (up to 20 to 25 mg/week) for 12 to 18 months. The CYCAZAREM (*Cy*clophosphamide versus *Aza*thioprine during *Rem*ission for Generalised Vasculitis) study evaluated outcomes in 155 patients who were randomized to receive maintenance therapy with either azathioprine or cyclophosphamide and found no differences in rate of relapse.[63]

GPS secondary to AASV carries a high mortality rate (approximately 80% within 1 year) if left untreated. However, the advent of effective cyclophosphamide-based induction therapy has led to 5-year survival rates on the order of 65% to 75% (lower if irreversible dialysis-dependent renal failure is present).[31] Clinical relapses are not uncommon, and risk factors include presence of PR3-ANCA and lung or upper respiratory tract involvement.[45] End-stage kidney disease occurs in approximately 20% to 25% of patients, the major predictors of which include impaired renal function on presentation and histological appearance of the kidney. Many patients with AASV eventually require renal replacement therapy.

Lupus Nephritis with Lung Hemorrhage

A number of case studies have reported on outcomes with pulmonary hemorrhage in SLE.[64-67] These studies described the outcomes in 88 patients. Most of these patients had both pulmonary hemorrhage and active glomerulonephritis (in more than 90%) and thus qualify as having GPS. Hemorrhage was overt in a minority and revealed by bilateral diffuse infiltrates in a majority and was commonly associated with a significant fall in hemoglobin concentration. DLCO was increased in 90% of the patients. Immunohistological studies revealed pulmonary capillary inflammation in 70%. The overall mortality rate was significant at 38%. All patients received pulse steroids and cyclophosphamide therapy. Plasma exchange was frequently used, but without obvious benefit (no controlled studies have been performed).

Key Points

1. Three main groups of disorders cause so-called Goodpasture's syndrome: small-vessel vasculitis associated with anti–neutrophil cytoplasmic anti-

bodies, immune complex diseases (including systemic lupus erythematosus), and anti–glomerular basement membrane disease.

2. It is likely that anti–neutrophil cytoplasmic antibodies are pathogenic and result from autoimmunity to leukocyte lysosomal enzymes.

3. Anti–neutrophil cytoplasmic antibody–bound neutrophils probably become localized in the glomerular and pulmonary microcirculation) acting as local targets for autoimmune effector T cells.

4. Anti–glomerular basement membrane disease is an autoimmune disease, with the target autoantigen being the noncollagenous domain of the α3 chain of type IV collagen.

5. Combined plasma exchange with prednisolone and cyclophosphamide is recommended for the treatment of anti–glomerular basement membrane disease and anti–neutrophil cytoplasmic antibody–associated systemic vasculitis.

6. Rituximab, a chimeric monoclonal antibody directed toward the B cell surface antigen, CD20, has shown initial promising results in treatment of anti–neutrophil cytoplasmic antibody–associated systemic vasculitis.

Key References

8. Morgan MD, Harper L, Williams J, et al: Anti-neutrophil cytoplasm–associated glomerulonephritis. J Am Soc Nephrol 2006;17:1224-1234.
12. Pusey CD: Anti-glomerular basement membrane disease. Kidney Int 2003;64:1535-1550.
31. Little MA, Pusey CD: Rapidly progressive glomerulonephritis: Current and evolving treatment strategies. J Nephrol 2004; 17(Suppl 8):S10-S19.
58. Jayne DR, Gaskin G, Rasmussen N, et al for the European Vasculitis Study Group: Randomized trial of plasma exchange or high-dosage methylprednisolone as adjunctive therapy for severe renal vasculitis. J Am Soc Nephrol 2007;18:2180-2188.

See the companion Expert Consult website for the complete reference list.

The Liver and the Kidney

CHAPTER 191

Liver-Kidney Interaction

Edmund Bourke

OBJECTIVES

This chapter will:
1. Give the reader an understanding of liver as an acid-base organ.
2. Provide an appreciation of the complexities of liver-kidney interaction at the molecular level.
3. Describe the limitations of the traditional view and the advantages of recent conceptual developments.

The concept of acid-base balance and its application to mammalian pH homeostasis have undergone a number of paradigm shifts in the last century.[1] Recent texts and reviews have centered on two concepts: the so-called "traditional" view,[2-5] which sees a single regulatory organ, the kidney, and a more recent conceptual view, which points to the liver as a major pH homeostatic organ and emphasizes the coordinated actions of the liver and kidney in the overall regulatory response to metabolic acid-base disturbances.[6-10] The latter concept is emphasized in this chapter. (See also Chapters 117, 118, and 121 for an expanded discussion and reference to physical and chemical acid-base analysis.)

THE TRADITIONAL VIEW

The traditional view, first proposed by Pitts,[11] remains predominant among renal physiologists. It envisages NH_3, derived in most part from the amino acid glutamine in renal tubular cells, as combining with hydrogen ions in acid urine to form NH_4^+. This is excreted, with resultant removal of hydrogen ions from the body. These hydrogen ions from the body are also derived from renal tubular cells, from the dissociation of H_2CO_3 through the action of carbonic anhydrase. Their secretion and trapping in the urine leaves behind an HCO_3^- ion. The return of this HCO_3^- to the circulation replenishes the depleted bicarbonate stores which induced the adaptation in the first place. The challenge of metabolic acidosis stimulates renal ammonia-genesis with enhanced urinary trapping and elimination of H^+ as NH_4^+; this, in a nutshell, is the traditional view.

A major inadequacy of the traditional view is its incompatibility with physical chemistry. The misapprehension centers on the practice of representing glutamine in the un-ionized form (Fig. 191-1A), as it frequently is in biochemistry textbooks. Such a representation can be theoretically envisaged as giving rise to two NH_3 molecules after glutamine deamidation and deamination, respectively. However, glutamine is ionized in vivo (see Fig. 191-1B). Like other amino acids, it is a dipolar ion containing an anionic carboxylate group (-COO^-) and a cationic substituted ammonium (-NH_3^+) group. Conversion of the α-NH_3^+ group of glutamine to NH_4^+ and its movement into the urine do not result in any uptake or release of hydrogen ions from the body's stores. The nitrogen was protonated from the beginning. Although the amide nitrogen of glutamine is not protonated, hydrolysis of an amide yields NH_4^+ and a carboxylate anion, with no uptake of protons. Glutamine, therefore, does not generate the NH_3 that could mop up H^+ derived from the dissociation of H_2CO_3, so an alternative explanation of the observed facts is required.

THE ROLE OF α-KETOGLUTARATE

After the removal of two NH_4^+ groups from glutamine, the remaining carbon skeleton, α-ketoglutarate, has two negatively charged carboxylate groups. Most of this α-ketoglutarate is metabolized within the kidney to glucose or CO_2. Whatever its metabolic fate, conservation of charge demands that two HCO_3^- ions be produced from each molecule of α-ketoglutarate:

$$OOC-CH_2-CH_2-\overset{\overset{\displaystyle O}{\|}}{C}-COO^- + 4O_2$$
$$\rightarrow 3CO_2 + 2HCO_3^- + H_2O$$

$$^-OOC-CH_2-CH_2-\overset{\overset{\displaystyle O}{\|}}{C}-COO^- + O_2 + 2H_2O$$
$$\rightarrow 1/2C_6H_{12}O_6 + 2HCO_3^-$$

An early modification of the traditional view postulated an acidosis-induced increase in renal α-ketoglutarate–derived bicarbonate.[12] This interpretation, however, is an

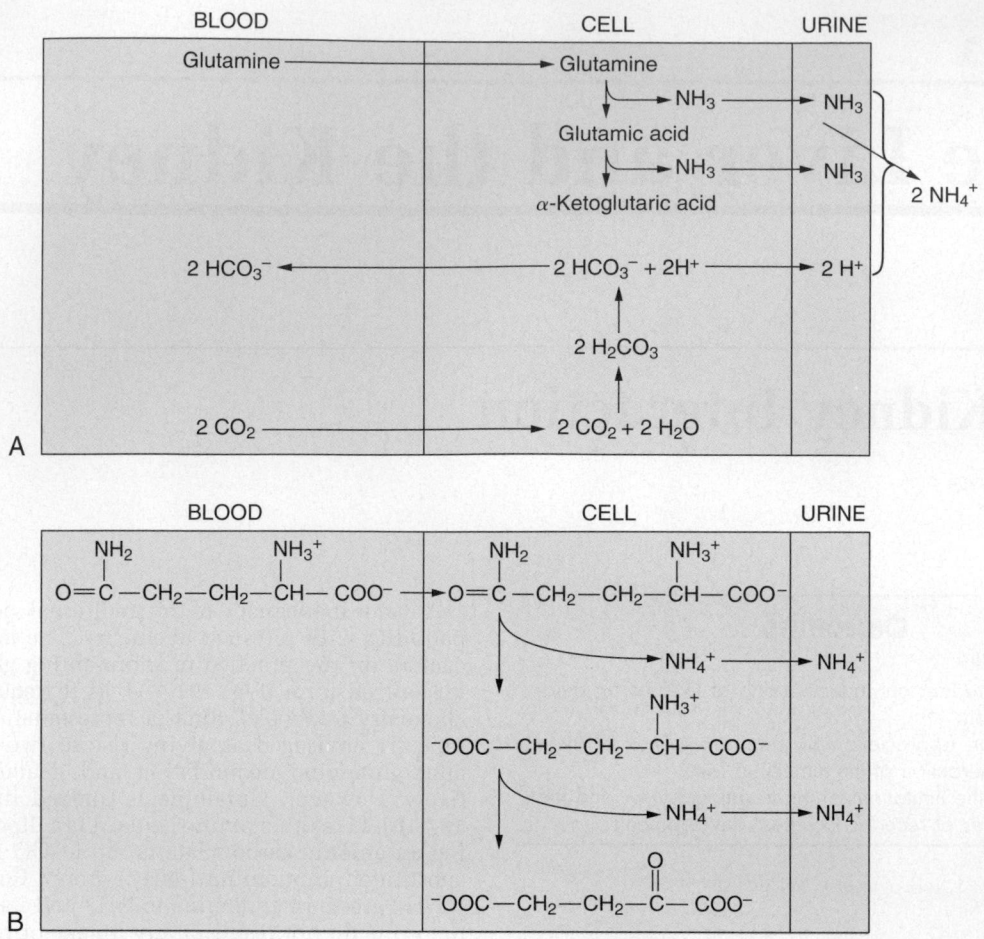

FIGURE 191-1. Deamidation and deamination of glutamine in the kidney. **A,** The conventional Pitts formulation. NH_3, derived from glutamine, moves into the lumen and combines with H^+ that was obtained from the body buffer, with generation of an equimolar amount of HCO_3^- which moves into the blood. **B,** The chemically valid formulation, taking ionization into account. NH_4^+, rather than NH_3, is the product of deamidation and deamination of glutamine, and excretion of NH_4^+ has no effect on the body buffer.

oversimplification. Renal metabolism of other carboxylate-containing bicarbonate precursors, such as lactate, is reciprocally decreased in acidosis. There is a change in the renal utilization of metabolic fuels—a shift in the utilization of bicarbonate precursors, as it were—but total renal energy production (and, hence, bicarbonate generation) is the same in acidosis and alkalosis.[13,14] The conclusion that the sequestration into the urine of ammonium from the amino acid glutamine in metabolic acidosis leads to a stoichiometric addition of new, renally generated bicarbonate to the body, which is the essence of the traditional view, is not substantiated by experimental data. More importantly, even were such an increase in renal bicarbonate production to occur, it would not affect systemic acid-base balance. Glutamine that is not used in the kidney will be metabolized elsewhere (Fig. 191-2).[15] Metabolic acidosis, in addition to increasing renal glutamine utilization, deceases hepatic glutamine utilization. But whether it is used in the liver or transported to the kidney and used there, two bicarbonate ions are generated from each molecule of glutamine, and the alkalinizing effect on the blood is the same in both cases. Therefore, this modification of the traditional view fails to explain the observed facts, and a revised interpretation is still required.

PROTEIN CATABOLISM AS A BICARBONATE-GENERATING PROCESS

A prerequisite to a revised interpretation of these facts requires a broader look at amino acid metabolism, which necessarily leads to as many bicarbonate ions as the number of carboxylate groups on the amino acid, and an approximately equal number of ammonium ions:

$$\overset{\overset{\displaystyle NH_3^+}{\|}}{CH_3-CH-COO^-} + 3O_2$$
$$\rightarrow 2CO_2 + HCO_3^- + NH_4^+ + H_2O$$

$$2\,\overset{\overset{\displaystyle NH_3^+}{\|}}{CH_3-CH-COO^-} + 4H_2O + 2CO_2$$
$$\rightarrow 2C_6H_{12}O_6 + 2NH_4^+ + 2HCO_3^-$$

It is self-evident and readily demonstrable that ammonium bicarbonate is alkalinizing. Indeed, ammonium bicarbonate is almost equivalent, in its direct effect on acid-base status, to the addition of an equimolar amount

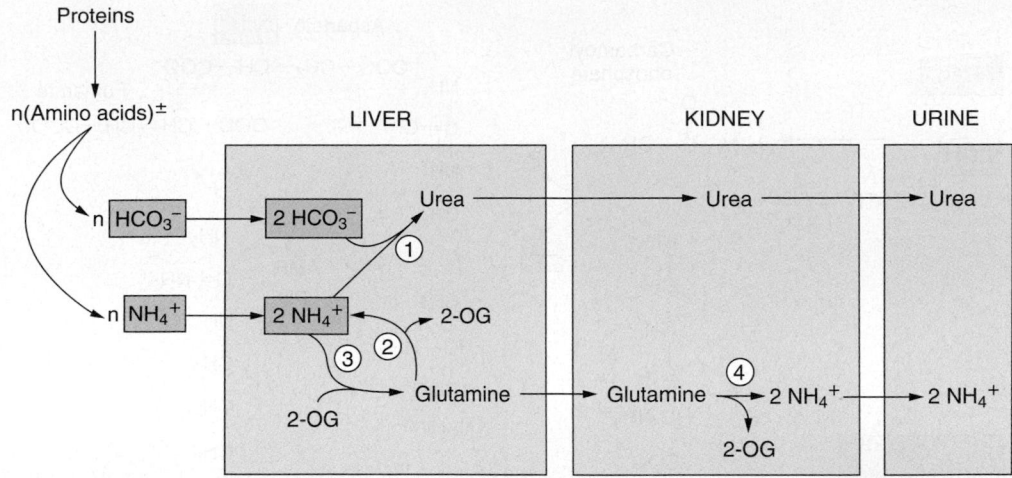

FIGURE 191-2. Ammonium metabolism and bicarbonate homeostasis. NH_4^+ and HCO_3^- generation are ultimately linked in a 1:1 stoichiometry during protein catabolism because of the irreversible elimination of both compounds via hepatic urea synthesis. Flux through the urea cycle is sensitively controlled by the extracellular acid-base status. The mechanisms involved adjust bicarbonate-consuming urea synthesis to the requirements of acid-base homeostasis. When urea synthesis decreases relative to the rate of protein catabolism in acidosis, bicarbonate is spared and NH_4^+ is excreted as such in the urine; there is no net production or consumption of α-ketoglutarate (2-oxoglutarate, or 2-OG) in the organism. Numbers in circles refer to major points of flux controlled by the acid-base status. In metabolic acidosis, flux through the area cycle (reaction 1) and hepatic glutaminase (reaction 2) are decreased, whereas flux through hepatic glutamine synthesis (reaction 3) and renal glutaminase (reaction 4) are increased. This interorgan "team effort" between the liver and the kidney results in NH_4^+ disposal without concomitant removal of HCO_3^- from the organism. (From Haussinger D, Gerok W, Sies H: The effect of urea synthesis on extracellular pH in isolated perfused rat liver. Biochem J 1986;236:261-265.)

of sodium bicarbonate.[10] Herein lies the first key insight to understanding the conceptual change in acid-base homeostasis: Protein catabolism overall is an alkalinizing process.[16] It is also true that some acid is liberated in the metabolism of sulfur-containing amino acids, but the amount is small. Some 1000 to 1500 moles of NH_4HCO_3 is derived from a typical daily protein intake of a male adult in the United States. It needs to be disposed of. Our marine ancestors disposed of this load of bicarbonate (and ammonium) through the gills. The alligator, when aquatic, excretes bicarbonate and ammonium via a prodigious flow of urine. An alternative evolutionary development for bicarbonate disposal was required for air-breathing land animals to emerge. The disposal mechanism in mammals such as humans is ureagenesis in the liver.

UREAGENESIS AS A BICARBONATE-CONSUMING PROCESS

The second key insight underlying the conceptual change in acid-base homeostasis is the realization that ureagenesis is a bicarbonate-consuming process (Fig. 191-3).[6,7,9] The role of hepatic urea synthesis in acid-base physiology was overlooked in the past, because attention focused mainly on ammonium detoxification. In hepatocytes, NH_4^+, derived partly from the portal blood and partly from the action of pH-dependent glutaminase, reacts with bicarbonate from carbamoyl phosphate, with the self-evident consumption of bicarbonate. In the subsequent formation of citrulline in the urea cycle, a proton is released; it, in turn, converts HCO_3^- to CO_2 and H_2O. Thus, two bicarbonates are consumed with each revolution of the urea cycle. This can be represented in summary fashion as follows:

$$2NH_4^+ + 2HCO_3^- \rightarrow NH_2{-}CO{-}NH_2 + CO_2 + 3H_2O$$

Because NH_4^+ (pK = 9.3) is a very weak proton donor at physiological pH levels, it would be thermodynamically impossible to titrate HCO_3^- (pK = 6.1) directly (as indicated earlier, NH_4HCO_3 is similar in physiological solutions to $NaHCO_3$). The only means by which protons of NH_4^+ can be obtained for titration of HCO_3^- is through incorporation of the nitrogen into an uncharged group of an organic molecule with liberation of protons. Metabolic energy is required, and the process is made energetically feasible by being coupled to the conversion of four molecules of adenosine triphosphate (ATP) to adenosine diphosphate (ADP); this forces the titration of HCO_3^- by a proton donor that is much too weak to effect the titration directly. This generation of protons appears to be a major metabolic function of ureagenesis. The relevance of this energy-consuming biosynthesis becomes evident from numerous studies showing that hepatic ureagenesis is responsive to the needs of systemic pH regulation[7]; indeed, the increase in urinary ammonium long known to accompany hydrochloric acidosis in humans has been shown to be accompanied by an equimolar decrease in urea execration.[16] By decreasing urea production, the liver decreases the consumption of bicarbonate stores, which is what induced the adaptation in the first place.

THE COORDINATED ACTIONS OF THE LIVER AND KIDNEYS

To summarize the conceptual change in our understanding of pH homeostasis thus far, the catabolism of proteins is a bicarbonate-generating process. In mammals, there is a liver-specific pathway for irreversible removal of metabolically generated bicarbonate—namely, urea synthesis. In acidosis, a decrease in urea synthesis relative to the rate of protein catabolism results in sparing of bicarbonate as

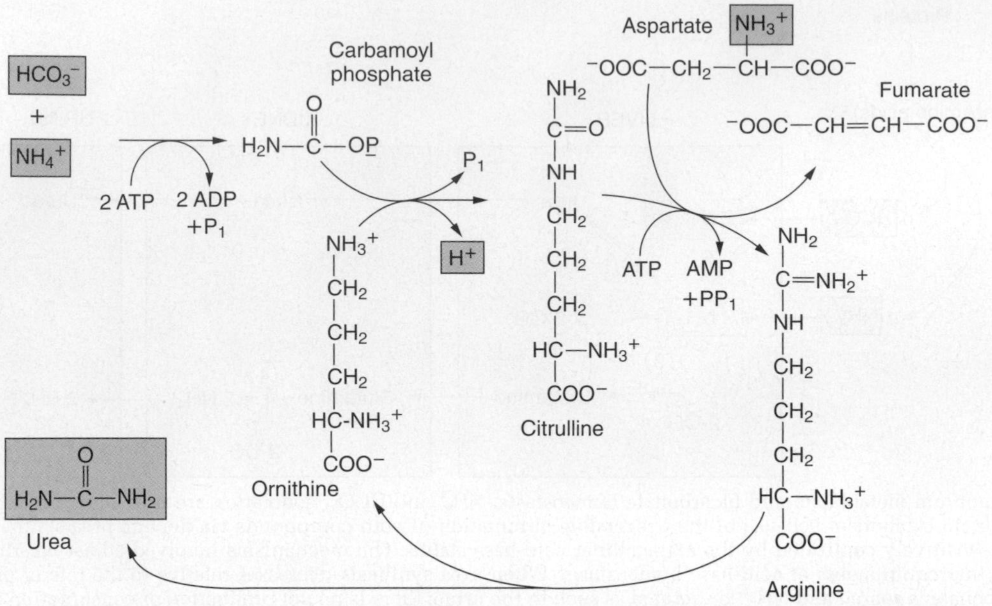

Aspartate NH_3^+

HCO_3^-

NH_4^+

Carbamoyl phosphate

$^-OOC-CH_2-CH-COO^-$

Fumarate

$^-OOC-CH=CH-COO^-$

$2\ ATP$ $2\ ADP +P_1$

$H_2N-C-OP$ P_1

H^+

ATP $AMP +PP_1$

Citrulline

Ornithine

Urea $H_2N-C-NH_2$

Arginine

FIGURE 191-3. The pathway of urea synthesis. Compounds and ions that are consumed or produced are enclosed in boxes. In each turn of the cycle, two bicarbonate ions (one of which is retained in the product, urea) are titrated with protons derived from two ammonium ions. This titration, which would be thermodynamically impossible as a direct reaction, is made energetically favorable by being coupled to the conversion of four molecules of adenosine triphosphate (ATP) to adenosine diphosphate (ADP). (From Atkinson DE, Boorke E: pH Homeostasis in terrestrial vertebrates: Ammonium ion as a proton source. In Heisler N [ed]: Mechanisms of Systemic Regulation: Acid-Base Regulation, Ion Transfer and Metabolism, no. 22 [Advances in Comparative and Environmental Physiology]. Berlin, Springer, 1995, pp 1-26.)

a pH homeostatic response by the liver. This places a major component of metabolic acid-base regulation in the liver. What, then, is the relevance of the acid-base–induced adaptation in renal glutamine and ammoniagenesis, which is the hallmark of the traditional view? The answer becomes clearer when the increased utilization of glutamine by the kidney in metabolic acidosis is seen in the context of overall glutamine metabolism by the body as a whole, and particularly by the liver (see Fig. 191-2). Several studies have shown an increased net release, or a decreased utilization of glutamine, or both, by the liver in acidosis,[6,7,9] The data are compatible with the following interpretation: In metabolic acidosis, a considerable amount of the substituted ammonium of amino acids that is ordinarily incorporated into urea with prorogation of bicarbonate is diverted via glutamine to be extracted into the urine as NH_4^+ by a mechanism that does not utilize bicarbonate yet simultaneously maintains nitrogen homeostasis. The overall effect is mitigation of the challenge of acidosis, but a concomitant hyperammonemia is also prevented. This, in a nutshell, is the new conceptual change. It establishes the liver as a major pH homeostatic organ, but it also emphasizes the coordinated actions of liver and kidney in the overall regulatory response to metabolic acid-base disturbances.

The paradigm shift from a single regulatory organ to a two-organ system incorporates all of the experimental facts on which the traditional view is based, without making interpretations that are incongruent with physical chemistry and without the need for the kidney to add new bicarbonate to the body's stores (see Fig. 191-3). Because the metabolism of protein produces a large bicarbonate overload, all that is necessary is to curtail its consumption. This is what the liver does in metabolic acidosis. Teleologically, it would not make sense to add new bicarbonate while its consumption continued unabated. Instead, what happens in response to an acid challenge is that the liver consumes less bicarbonate, leaving more behind to replenish the body's stores.

Ureagenesis occurs to the extent needed for the disposal of bicarbonate, with the leftover NH_4^+ being incorporated into glutamine for transport to and release by the kidney. In this way, the coordination of both processes, hepatic ureagenesis and urinary ammonium excretion, contributes to overall regulation of homeostasis. Hepatic and renal nitrogen metabolism are linked by an interorgan glutamine flux, which couples both renal ammoniagenesis and hepatic ureagenesis to systemic acid-base regulation. Furthermore, this interorgan "team effort" facilitates a structural-functional arrangement within the liver, outlined in the next paragraph, whereby the urea cycle flux in response to metabolically generated bicarbonate can be uncoupled from the need to maintain ammonium homeostasis.

THE REGULATORY ROLE OF HEPATOCYTE HETEROGENEITY

The revised interpretation of the traditional view is strongly supported by the sequential distribution of enzymes within the functional units of the liver. The acini, which give precedence to the regulation of ureagenesis over glutamine synthesis, enable the rate of ureagenesis to respond to pH change while leftover NH_4^+ is packaged into glutamine for export. The arrangement that facilitates this regulated sequence can be summarized as follows (Fig. 191-4): Each acinus extends from a terminal portal venule along a sinusoid to a terminal hepatic venule. The hepatocytes near the sinusoidal inflow are termed *periportal* and those near the sinusoidal outflow are termed *perive-*

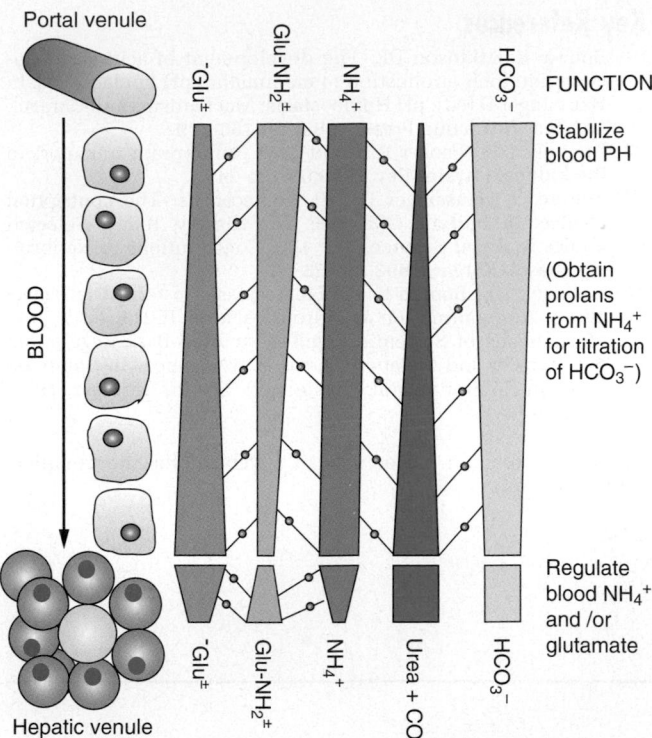

Portal venule

BLOOD

Hepatic venule

⁻Glu⁺

Glu-NH₂⁺

NH₄⁺

HCO₃⁻

FUNCTION

Stabilize blood PH

(Obtain prolans from NH₄⁺ for titration of HCO₃⁻)

Regulate blood NH₄⁺ and /or glutamate

⁻Glu⁺

Glu-NH₂⁺

NH₄⁺

Urea + CO₂

HCO₃⁻

FIGURE 191-4. Schematic representation of nitrogen metabolism in the liver. As blood flows from the portal venule through the sinusoid, it first passes cells that contain glutaminase and the enzymes of the urea cycle. Glutamine is hydrolyzed to a greater or lesser extent. NH_4^+ is generated from the hydrolysis and from the metabolism of amino acids (not shown); incorporation of NH_4^+ into urea generates protons that serve to titrate HCO_3^-, half of which is incorporated into urea, with the other half converted to CO_2. The last rank of cells around the hepatic venule takes up glutamate and NH_4^+ and synthesizes glutamine. Changes in widths of the bars represent changes in concentrations of the corresponding substances. Glu, glutamate; Glu-NH₂⁺, glutamine. (From Atkinson DE, Boorke E: pH Homeostasis in terrestrial vertebrates: Ammonium ion as a proton source. In Heisler N [ed]: Mechanisms of Systemic Regulation: Acid-Base Regulation, Ion Transfer and Metabolism, no. 22 [Advances in Comparative and Environmental Physiology]. Berlin, Springer, 1995, pp 1-26.)

nous hepatocytes. A remarkable functional hepatocyte heterogeneity with respect to nitrogen metabolism occurs; it involves metabolic zonation of ureagenesis and glutamine synthesis, respectively, which is attributable to a special separation of the key enzymes between the periportal (urea cycle enzymes, glutaminase) and the perivenous (glutamine synthetase) hepatocytes of the hepatic acinus. Accordingly, along the sinusoid, the pathways of urea and glutamine synthesis are arranged in sequence. This organization prevents competition for the available ammonium between the two processes. Instead, there exists an established priority for ureagenesis. From the periportal venule, throughout a substantial length of the hepatic acinus, the enzyme glutaminase that contributes to the supply of ammonium for ureagenesis and also the enzymes of the urea cycle itself share, as it were, a common hepatic compartment, giving prevalence to ureagenesis. Downstream, separately compartmentalized in the last rung of cells of the perihepatic venule, is the enzyme glutamine synthetase, which acts as a high-affinity scavenger

for ammonium that has not been used in the periportal synthesis of urea. As the blood moves downstream through the sinusoid from the portal toward the hepatic venule, there is, initially, the formation of urea from the consumption of bicarbonate, which is derived from the metabolism of carboxylate groups of keto acids, and of ammonium, which is derived in part from the portal blood but is kept in adequate supply by the action of glutaminase. Acidosis reduces this bicarbonate-utilizing process. As a consequence, there is ammonium left over which is not used for ureagenesis. This leftover ammonium is taken up by the last rung of cells of the acinus, where glutamine synthetase incorporates it into glutamine, thereby controlling the blood ammonium concentration and serving as a transport mechanism for ammonium to the kidney.

ACID-BASE BALANCE IN HEPATIC FUNCTIONAL IMPAIRMENT

Reports as to the consequences of functional liver impairment for acid-base status vary. A failure of experimental partial hepatectomy (85%) to influence acid-base homeostasis, despite decreased urinary urea, led to the conclusion that a major role for the liver in acid-base regulation was unlikely.[17] Other interpretations of this study are possible, however. The net rate of protein and amino-acid catabolism may have been decreased in the hepatectomized animals, requiring a lower than normal rate of ureagenesis for the maintenance of normal blood pH, and the reported results may merely indicate that residual liver tissue was sufficient to meet the reduced needs. In chronic liver disease in humans, a different picture emerges.[18-20] In a series of patients with histologically stratified liver disease, the in vivo plasma bicarbonate increased, with progressive loss of in vivo urea cycle capacity; in these patients, other causes of metabolic alkalosis, such as diuretics, antacids, vomiting, hyperaldosteronism, and renal dysfunction, were rigorously excluded.

Because alkalosis in turn is a potent stimulus for the ammonia amplifier, glutaminase,[18] a feedback circuit between urea synthesis, bicarbonate accumulation, and amplification of hepatic ammoniagenesis via glutaminase has been proposed, as follows[18-20]: A decrease of urea cycle capacity leads to hyperbicarbonatemia and alkalosis, which, in turn, activates hepatic glutaminase. Glutaminase activation augments urea synthesis and restores a normal urea flux, despite diminished capacity to synthesize urea.[6] Because the net consequence of this metabolic shift is stimulation of hepatic bicarbonate consumption, metabolic alkalosis may have a self-limiting effect in the stable cirrhotic patient, which would predictably increase to a new steady state with progressive loss of hepatic functional reserve.

Interestingly, the progressive loss of urea cycle capacity in cirrhosis is paralleled by an increase in renal ammonium excretion, despite coexisting metabolic alkalosis, indicating that the kidney undertakes the task of eliminating ammonium when urea synthesis fails.[18-20] This increase is not attributable to the small rise in plasma NH_4^+ concentration (which remains within normal range) but requires de novo renal generation. This opens up a new facet in the regulation of renal ammoniagenesis. It appears that renal ammonium production is activated when ureagenesis decreases; this occurs not only in metabolic acidosis, when urea synthesis is inhibited due to homeostatic regulation, but also during alkalosis, when urea synthesis fails due to liver disease.

Key Points

1. Contrary to the traditional view, glutamine does not generate NH_3 and therefore cannot remove H^+.
2. Ureagenesis is an acidifying process, whereas glutaminogenesis is alkalinizing.
3. The kidney's role in acid-base regulation requires cooperation with the liver.
4. Renal ammonium production is activated when ureagenesis decreases; this occurs not only in metabolic acidosis, when urea synthesis is inhibited due to homeostatic regulation, but also during alkalosis, when urea synthesis fails due to liver disease.

Key References

1. Bourke E, Atkinson DE: The development of acid-base concepts and their application to mammalian pH homeostasis. In Haussinger D (ed): pH Homeostasis: Mechanisms and Control. London, Academic Press, 1988, pp 163-179.
2. Knepper MA, Packer R, Good DW: Ammonium transport in the kidney. Physiol Rev 1989;69:179-249.
7. Bourke H, Haussinger D: pH Homeostasis: The conceptual change. In Berlyne GM (ed): The Kidney Today. Selected Topics in Renal Science, vol. 100. Contributions to Nephrology. Basel, Karger, 1992, pp 58-88.
10. Atkinson DE, Boorke E: pH Homeostasis in terrestrial vertebrates: Ammonium ion as a proton source. In Heisler N (ed): Mechanisms of Systemic Regulation: Acid-Base Regulation, Ion Transfer and Metabolism, no. 22 (Advances in Comparative and Environmental Physiology). Berlin, Springer, 1995, pp 1-26.

See the companion Expert Consult website for the complete reference list.

CHAPTER 192

Pathophysiology of the Hepatorenal Syndrome

Elena Mancini and Antonio Santoro

OBJECTIVES

This chapter will:
1. Describe the clinical aspects of hepatorenal syndrome, a dramatic complication of cirrhosis and portal hypertension.
2. Discuss the pathological mechanisms of this disorder—including circulatory, renal, and cardiac dysfunction; the hepatorenal reflex; the compartment syndrome; and other mechanisms of renal damage.
3. Present the therapeutic approach, which is based on the pathogenetic aspects of hepatorenal syndrome.

The onset of renal damage during liver disease strongly affects prognosis, as does liver deficit during renal insufficiency. In 1994, an Indian group led by Amarapurkar[1] published an interesting work in the *Indian Journal of Gastroenterology* concerning the prognostic importance of renal function in patients with uncompensated cirrhosis. Sixty-eight patients who were monitored for 6 months had differential survival based on creatinine clearance. Patients with a creatinine clearance greater than 80 mL/min had a mortality rate of just 9%, whereas patients with clearance of less than 50 mL/min had a mortality rate of 36%. Intermediate results were obtained for those with a clearance between 50 and 80 mL/min. Moreover, patients with cirrhosis were predisposed to the onset of acute renal insufficiency owing to a series of factors such as portal hypertension, ease of bleeding, and the administration of nephrotoxic drugs (e.g., aminoglycosides).

Hepatorenal syndrome (HRS) primarily develops in patients with advanced liver disease, and there is an association between the degree of liver dysfunction and the development of renal dysfunction. The pathophysiological situation of HRS is the development of a picture of severe renal insufficiency in a patient with a severe hepatic deficit (acute or chronic) in the absence of other identifiable causes of renal pathology. Renal function normalization after liver transplantation is a strong indicator that the liver is directly involved in renal dysfunction.[2] In 1996, the International Ascites Club[3] defined the diagnostic criteria of HRS (Table 192-1), which was differentiated into two types. Type 1 is an acute form with rapid progression and unfavorable prognosis (<2 weeks) that appears in a patient with a serious hepatic pathology. This form is characterized by a rapid deterioration in renal function with a doubling of the serum creatinine concentration to more than 2.5 mg/dL or with a creatinine clearance rate lower than 20 mL/min.[3] Type 2 is more subtle in its onset, appearing in patients with ascites resistant to diuretics, and the renal deficit can even take months to set in.

It is hard to evaluate the real incidence of HRS type 1, because many of the studies are old and did not use the diagnostic criteria later established.[4] In a prospective study involving 229 patients with chronic liver disease and who had no signs of compromised renal function, HRS developed during the first year in 18% of those patients with cirrhosis, and within 5 years in 39%.[4] HRS developed

TABLE 192-1

Diagnostic Criteria for HRS as Defined by the International Ascites Club*

Major Criteria

Chronic or acute liver disease with advanced hepatic failure and portal hypertension

Low GFR (serum creatinine >1.5 mg/dL or 133 μmol/L) or 24-hr clearance <40 mL/min

Exclusion of shock, ongoing bacterial infection, use of nephrotoxic drugs, volume depletion

No sustained improvement in renal function after stopping diuretics and volume repletion with 1.5 L of saline

Proteinuria <500 mg/dL with no ultrasonographic evidence of obstructive uropathy or parenchymal renal disease

Minor Criteria

Urine volume <500 mL/day

Urinary sodium <10 mEq/L

Urine osmolality >plasma osmolality

Urine red blood cells <50 per high-power field

Serum sodium concentration <130 mEq/L

GFR, glomerular filtration rate; HRS, hepatorenal syndrome.
*All major criteria must be present for the diagnosis of HRS; minor criteria support but are not necessary for the diagnosis.

much more easily in patients with hyponatremia and high plasma renin and in those with spontaneous bacterial peritonitis. The patients with primitive biliary cirrhosis seemed to be better protected as a result of the chronic retention of biliary salts, which gave them a greater natriuresis and an intrarenal vasodilatation.

DIAGNOSIS, CLINICAL PRESENTATION, AND RENAL MORPHOLOGY

The diagnosis of type 1 HRS is largely based on exclusion criteria: a rapid rise in creatinine, often accompanied by oliguria and by concentrations of urinary sodium lower than 10 mEq/L, in the absence of other renal pathologies, with no response to intravascular volume expansion.[5] Serum creatinine is not actually an ideal marker for renal function in liver patients, because of a reduced endogenous production related to reduced muscle mass coexisting with an increased tubular secretion. Cystatin C, an accurate marker of glomerular filtration, has been proven to have a diagnostic accuracy greater than that of creatinine in identifying a reduced glomerular filtration rate (GFR) in patients with liver disease,[6] but it is not yet available in all settings.

Precipitating factors of HRS are gastrointestinal bleeding, excessive administration of diuretics, large-volume paracentesis, and infections, particularly peritoneal infections. However, at least 24% of patients with type 1 HRS develop renal failure with no obvious precipitating factor.[7] Instead, acute tubular necrosis (ATN) may occur due to the administration of aminoglycosides or contrast media or during sepsis, persistent hyperbilirubinemia, or protracted bleeding. At the laboratory level, it is hard to distinguish between an ATN and HRS, because several factors overlap. In ATN during cirrhosis, it is not absolutely certain that the sodium excretion fraction will exceed 2% (a typical diagnostic element in classic ATN), because the chronic renal ischemia induces continuous sodium reten-

tion also with important tubular damage. Furthermore, the frequent concomitant presence of hyperbilirubinemia during both HRS and ATN may alter the urinary sediment and make cellular and epithelial cylinders appear in either of the two diseases, although they are generally typical of ATN.

Hyponatremia is an almost universal hallmark of HRS; it results when antidiuretic hormone (ADH) induces retention of solute-free water disproportionate to the amount of retained sodium (dilutional hyponatremia). If the plasma sodium concentration is normal, the diagnosis of HRS is highly unlikely, and the patient should be investigated for another cause of renal insufficiency.[4]

In type 2 HRS, the increase in serum creatinine and urea nitrogen has a slight tendency to progress, at least in the short term, and a sudden progression of renal failure may eventually develop after a long period of stability.

From the structural standpoint, the kidney in HRS is perfectly normal, with its glomerular and tubular functions intact.[3] The proof lies in its rapid functional recovery when it is transplanted into a person with renal insufficiency but normal liver function. Naturally, in the later phases, typical structural alterations appear because of the acute tubular damage along with glomerular ischemia.

PATHOPHYSIOLOGY

Hemodynamic Derangements: Circulatory and Renal Dysfunction

The underlying mechanisms leading to HRS onset are complex and include interactions between increased portal pressure, changes in the systemic arterial circulation, activation of vasoconstrictive pathways and factors, and suppression of vasodilator factors acting on the renal circulation.[8]

The regulation of renal circulation in cirrhosis depends on the interaction between vasoconstrictor and vasodilator substances acting on the renal vasculature (Table 192-2).

In the early stages of cirrhosis, in the pre-ascitic phase, renal blood flow may be kept within normal limits due to the effects of local vasodilators that antagonize the action of the systemic vasoconstrictors on the renal vasculature. When there is a stimulation of the endogenous vasoconstriction (e.g., modest hypotension), renal vasodilators (prostaglandin, nitric oxide, natriuretic peptides) also become activated, to maintain renal perfusion and the GFR. Actually, even in these very early stages of the disease, despite near-normal systemic hemodynamics, there is increased tubular sodium reabsorption in the kidney, the sodium excretion after a saline load is reduced, and the excretion of free water is reduced.[9]

With the progression of liver disease, and above all with the formation of ascites, the renal function progressively worsens[10] due to intrarenal vasoconstriction, which is no longer efficiently counterbalanced by the vasodilator substances.

The pathophysiological hallmark of HRS is severe vasoconstriction of the renal circulation, but the initial pathogenetic factor responsible for the chain of events leading to HRS lies inside the liver itself. It is the *sinusoidal portal hypertension*, which develops with the chronic liver disease, inducing the opening of portosystemic shunts. Splanchnic and systemic vasodilatation are the result, with consequent *arterial underfilling*, according to the

TABLE 192-2

Vasodilator and Vasoconstrictor Factors That Affect the Regulation of Renal Circulation during Cirrhosis and Are Involved in the Pathogenesis of Hepatorenal Syndrome

VASODILATORS	VASOCONSTRICTORS
Nitric oxide, endotoxins	Angiotensin II
Prostacyclin	Norepinephrine
Prostaglandin E_2	Endothelin-1
Atrial natriuretic peptide	Isoprostane F_2
Kallikrein-kinin system	Thromboxane
Glucagon	Cysteinyl leukotrienes
	Adenosines
	Neuropeptide Y

peripheral arterial vasodilatation hypothesis.[11] There is a compensatory increase in the cardiac load *(hyperdynamic circulation)*, but it is unable to maintain an effective blood volume,[4,10,12] and arterial hypotension, which is the clinical epiphenomenon of the arterial underfilling, arises.

The reduction in central effective arterial blood volume stimulates the baroreceptors and induces an increase in the sympathetic tone, due to the activation of the sympathetic nervous system (SNS), with intrarenal *preglomerular* vasoconstriction, which plays the major role in the decrease of the GFR (Fig. 192-1).[3]

Secondary hyperaldosteronism is also established, due to activation of the renin-angiotensin system (RAS), with a consequent increase in distal tubular sodium reabsorp-

tion. At the same time, the increase in sympathetic tone and angiotensin II further stimulate sodium reabsorption at the levels of the proximal tubule and loop of Henle.[13]

Massive sodium-water retention is the result,[11] on the one hand, of the reduction in GFR, secondary to extreme intrarenal vasoconstriction, and, on the other hand, of the reduction in natriuresis due to both decreased filtration and increased reabsorption, as well as the reduction in excretion of free water.[10] Hyponatremia appears, despite an extreme sodium reabsorption tendency, because of the very low free water excretion *(dilutional hyponatremia)*, with consequent water overload. Moreover, because of the high proximal reabsorption of sodium, its delivery to the distal nephron is limited, accounting for the poor effect of both diuretics that act on the loop of Henle (furosemide) and those that act on the distal tubule (spironolactone).

The derangements of *renal circulatory autoregulation* play a pivotal role. In noncirrhotic, healthy subjects, autoregulation protects the kidney from hypoperfusion in the event of a reduction in arterial pressure. When the mean arterial pressure is lower than 70 mm Hg, this mechanism is lost, and the renal blood flow is directly correlated to the renal perfusion pressure (arterial blood pressure – renal venous pressure). In patients with SNS hyperactivity (e.g., patients with cirrhosis), the autoregulation curve is shifted rightward,[14] and even a minor reduction in blood pressure may precipitate hypoperfusion, maximally reducing the filtration capacities and resulting in a marked contraction in urinary output. The importance of arterial hypotension in cirrhosis has been stressed by various authors, who have reported a relationship between the degree of arterial hypotension and the severity of liver dysfunction, signs of decompensation, and even survival.[15,16]

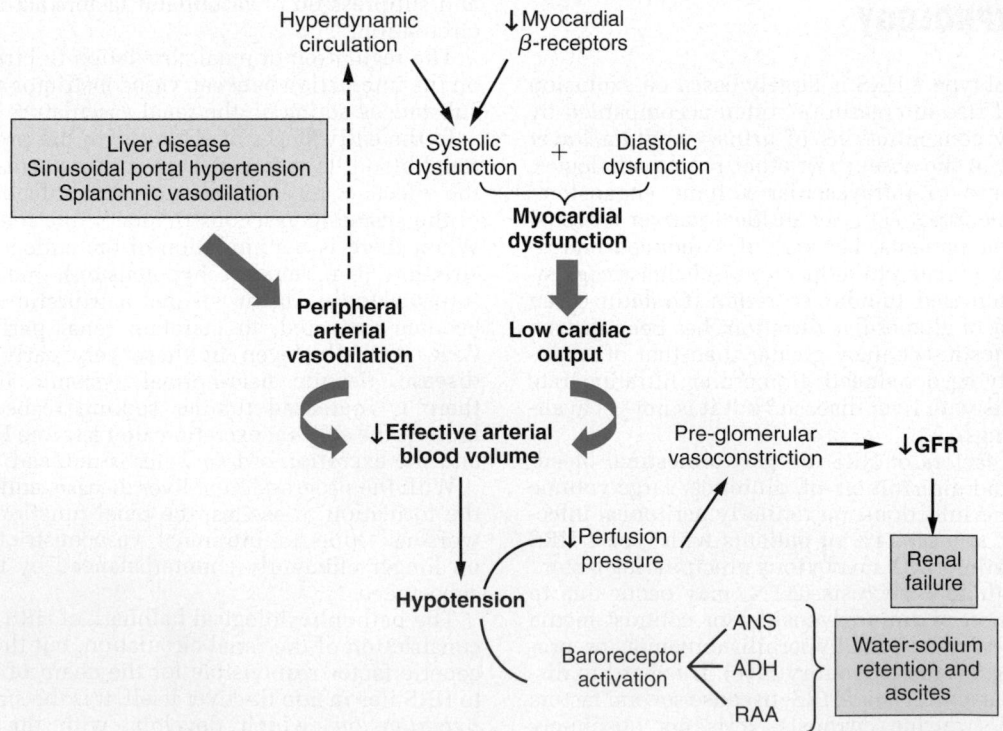

FIGURE 192-1. Schematic representation of the pathogenetic mechanisms leading to the appearance of the hepatorenal syndrome as a complication of chronic liver disease. ADH, antidiuretic hormone; ANS, autonomic nervous system; GFR, glomerular filtration rate; RAA, renin-angiotensin-aldosterone.

However, Platt and colleagues[17] showed, in a longitudinal study in 180 cirrhotic patients with a normal renal function, that 55% of those with a resistance index (RI) greater than 0.7 on renal echo-Doppler ultrasound developed HRS, whereas only 6% of those with an RI lower than 0.7 did so.

Therefore, renal hypoperfusion and vasoconstriction seem to represent an extreme expression of arterial underfilling secondary to marked vasodilatation of the splanchnic vascular bed.[4] Once vasoconstriction develops, intrarenal mechanisms perpetuate HRS due to the development of intrarenal vicious circles, in which vasoconstrictive mechanisms and factors prevail over the vasodilating ones.

Hemodynamic Derangements: Cardiac Dysfunction

The pathophysiological model of HRS, deriving the drop in GFR from arterial underfilling consequent to portal hypertension, is probably not complete. A cardiac dysfunction may also be involved in the pathogenesis of renal failure. *Cirrhosis-related cardiomyopathy* is the term identifying this condition[18] of progressive involvement of the heart in the course of cirrhosis.

Both systolic and diastolic functions may be affected. The increased blood volume of the hyperdynamic circulation, with the constant increase in preload, may, in the long run, overload the heart itself, progressively affecting the *contractile capacity*.[18-20] Diminished myocardial β-adrenergic receptor signal transduction function has also been reported.[18] Neurohumoral hyperactivity induces a thickening of the walls of the left ventricle, progressively leading to fibrosis and resulting in a *diastolic dysfunction*, which is known to be more pronounced in the presence of severe ascites.[21,22]

The work by Ruiz-del-Arbol and colleagues opened the possibility that HRS may be caused by mechanisms other than splanchnic vasodilation and arterial underfilling alone.[23] In decompensated patients with spontaneous bacterial peritonitis who developed the HRS, they found significant reductions in both cardiopulmonary pressures (right atrial and pulmonary capillary wedge pressure) and stroke volume. The authors hypothesized that heart rate does not adequately change in response to the reduction in stroke volume, so a low cardiac output ensues. In this perspective, the arterial underfilling could derive from a low cardiac output condition during systemic vasodilatation, with secondary activation of intrinsic renal mechanisms for vasoconstriction.

A concomitant myocardial contractile deficit may be a further mechanism compromising the stroke volume (see Fig. 192-1).[19]

Once the cardiac output is reduced, arterial pressure homeostasis is solely dependent on the activity of the RAS, the SNS, and ADH, which together impair circulation not only in the kidneys but also in other organs and tissues.[23] The cutaneous, muscular, and cerebral vascular blood flow are reduced in patients with HRS.[3] Ruiz-del-Arbol and coworkers demonstrated that even the liver is underperfused, due to an intense reduction in the hepatic blood flow. Vasoconstriction affects several organs, thus inducing something akin to multiorgan failure; it affects vital organs such as the kidneys, the brain, and the liver and appears to be the most likely explanation for the organ failure (renal and hepatic function) and perhaps even for encephalopathy.[22-24]

Endotoxins, Endocannabinoids, and Nitric Oxide

Gastrointestinal mucosal damage, which is very frequent in alcoholic cirrhosis, and portosystemic shunting facilitate the passage of gut-derived bacterial endotoxins into the systemic circulation, without detoxification by the liver.[25] Endocannabinoids and nitric oxide are gut-derived humoral factors implicated as possible mediators of the peripheral vasodilation in cirrhosis and portal hypertension.

Endogenous endocannabinoids are lipid-like substances with a vasodilator effect.[26] The anandamide receptor, an endogenous endocannabinoid, has been found to be upregulated in the vascular endothelium of patients with cirrhosis,[26] thus increasing end-organ sensitivity to the vasodilating effect.

Endotoxins also overstimulate the production of *nitric oxide* (NO). In effect, although the expression of the endothelial-constitutive NO synthase (eNOS) decreased in the liver microcirculation in a cirrhotic rat model,[27] *systemic* NO production is increased in cirrhotic patients and in animal models and promotes systemic vasodilation.[28] Indeed, some studies have demonstrated that the vasoconstriction capacities are reestablished by NO synthesis inhibitors in both animals and humans.[28,29]

These results strongly support the hypothesis that increased NO production is a major factor in the peripheral arterial vasodilation in cirrhosis.

Other factors stimulating NO production include cytokines such as tumor necrosis factor-α (TNF-α), interleukin-1 (IL-1), IL-6, and interferon-γ (IFN-γ). Moreover, the endotoxins bond to the cellular and serum-soluble CD14 receptors, through activation of the nuclear factor-κB (NF-κB), fostering the expression of TNF-α, IL-6, and IL-8, with a subsequent vasodilator effect that can be blocked by anti-TNF-α antibodies.[30] A decrease in cardiac index and portal pressure, together with an increase in mean arterial pressure and systemic vascular resistance, was also demonstrated by Lopez-Talavera and associates by means of anti-TNF-α antibodies.[31]

Prostaglandins

In patients who have decompensated cirrhosis without renal failure, the renal production of prostaglandin E_2 and prostacyclin (prostaglandin I_2) is often increased[32]; if HRS is present, however, the urinary excretion of these prostaglandins has been found to be decreased, compared with levels in patients who have ascites without HRS. This is due partly to a fall in the GFR and partly to decreased production.[33] The administration of nonsteroidal anti-inflammatory drugs (NSAIDs), which are cyclooxygenase inhibitors, may favor the onset of intrarenal vasoconstriction.[34]

Glucagon

Glucagon, which is increased in cirrhotic patients, is another substance that desensitizes the mesenteric vascular wall to the vasoconstrictor stimuli favoring vasodilation.[35] It also stimulates the production of cellular cyclic adenosine monophosphate (cAMP), which, as for the endotoxins, favors NO production.

Intrarenal Vasoconstriction: The Hepatorenal Reflex

The increase in intrarenal vascular tone is initially a reflex response to adrenergic stimulation, with activation of the RAS occurring consequent to the arterial underfilling and hypotension. A global renal vascular dysfunction with glomerular ischemia and a reduction in glomerular filtration arises. Moreover, the overproduction of vasoconstrictor substances (endothelin, isoprostane F_2, thromboxane, and leukotrienes) prevails over the intrarenal vasodilatation potential, enhancing arteriolar constriction but also inducing mesangial cell contraction and thereby reducing the glomerular filtration surface.[4,10,36]

Endothelins are powerful vasoconstrictors, and increased circulating levels and hepatic release of endothelins have been found in patients with ascites and HRS.[37] Endothelin-1 (ET-1) has a wide variety of biological effects, among which are the constriction of cortical and medullary vessels and mesangial cell contraction.[29,38] ET-1 is involved in renal disorders characterized by increased renal vasculature resistance, such as ischemic acute renal failure, calcineurin inhibitor toxicity, endotoxemia, and HRS. It is elevated in HRS as a result of both intrarenal ischemia and oxidative stress (lipid peroxidation with synthesis of isoprostane F_2, which is a powerful stimulator of endothelin synthesis). Levels of ET-1 and renal ET_A correlate with excretory liver function assessed by bilirubin.[39] Its increase is also correlated with GFR reduction.[40] Moreover, ET-1 levels decrease rapidly after orthotopic liver transplantation,[41] together with the improvement in liver failure and before recovery of renal function, further supporting the possibility of a strong endothelin involvement in the intrarenal vasoconstriction of HRS.

The activation of the SNS is also the result of a *hepatorenal reflex*. Under experimental conditions, Kostreva and colleagues[42] showed that the increase in intrahepatic pressure generates an increase in intrarenal adrenergic activity, probably mediated by hepatocyte swelling and activation of the sympathetic hepatorenal reflex, with decreased renal blood flow and decreased GFR. In human cirrhosis, the reduction in renal blood flow after an increase in portal pressure with a concomitant increase in renal release of ET-1 supports the presence of a hepatorenal reflex. Moreover, recent experimental data indicate that the retention of sodium and water that results from a decrease in portal venous blood flow may be abolished by hepatic denervation or by administration of an adenosine receptor antagonist, suggesting a role for adenosine receptors in the hepatorenal reflex.[43]

The hepatorenal reflex works as a counter-regulatory system, aimed at maintaining an efficient filtration fraction through vasoconstriction of the efferent arteriole in spite of the low renal perfusion pressure. In this situation, the administration of angiotensin-converting enzyme (ACE) inhibitors or angiotensin-II receptor blockers or V_1 vasopressin antagonists may be responsible for arterial hypotension, further decreases in renal blood flow, vasodilation of postglomerular arterioles, and then prerenal failure and oliguria.[44,45]

Compartment Syndrome

When tense ascites is present, a true compartment syndrome secondary to *intra-abdominal hypertension* may arise, worsening renal perfusion both on the arterial side of the circulation and on the venous side.[46] Renal perfusion pressure results from the difference between mean arterial pressure and abdominal pressure, which can be easily evaluated by measuring the intravesical pressure.[46] Intra-abdominal pressure has been recognized as an independent factor for acute renal failure.[47]

Another important consequence is that intra-abdominal hypertension may induce a release of proinflammatory cytokines, with an increase in intestinal permeability that favors bacterial translocation to intestinal mesenteric lymph nodes and the liver.[46]

Because the pathophysiological implications of intra-abdominal hypertension are varied (neurological, cardiovascular, respiratory, renal, and gastrointestinal), the risk of the progression to multiple organ system failure should always be taken into consideration.

Other Renal Damage Mechanisms

Apart from intrarenal vasoconstriction, the accumulation of toxic substances consequent to advanced hepatic deficit can also contribute to kidney dysfunction. The same applies to biliary acids, endotoxins, and the inflammatory mediators. *Biliary acids* are capable of damaging the structure of cellular membranes. Experimentally, the biliary acids induce an increase in oxidative stress and damage to the cellular and mitochondrial membranes, with alterations in the processes of oxidative phosphorylation. In those patients with persistent hyperbilirubinemia, alterations in the tubular renal cells, decreased GFR, and reduced excretion of sodium and water occur.[40] Bilirubin removal with plasmapheresis or recirculation dialysis with albumin can improve renal function in patients with persistent jaundice and HRS.[48]

Endotoxins, as mentioned previously, accumulate in patients with cirrhosis, inducing an overproduction of NO but also the activation of an *inflammatory cascade*. The endotoxins are capable of activating neutrophils, as well as causing ischemia. The activated neutrophils adhere to the endothelium of the renal capillaries and pass through it; once they are in the endothelial space, they release enzymes and cytokines, causing direct local damage and the recall of the other flogosis cells, such as monocytes and macrophages. Blocking of TNF-α[49] or of the adhesion molecules such as intercellular adhesion molecule 1 (ICAM-1) and P-selectin is experimentally capable of preventing the damage induced by the activated neutrophils. Renal ischemia in ICAM-1 knockout rats does not cause a renal deficit.[50]

Furthermore, complement alterations and circulating immune complexes can worsen inflammatory damage. Cirrhosis is accompanied by low levels of C3, C4, and total complement, because of both reduced production and increased consumption (classical and alternative pathway activation, secondary to the presence of endotoxin and various circulating immunocomplexes).

In short, damage of an exclusively vasofunctional nature in HRS is complicated by toxic damage and an inflammatory substratum, which in turn aggravates the damage to the microcirculation and tissue ischemia.

PATHOPHYSIOLOGY-BASED THERAPEUTIC APPROACH

The prognosis of type 1 HRS is fatal, with a mortality rate of 80% at 2 weeks without treatment.[3,6] Occasionally, kidney recovery occurs after hepatic functional improve-

TABLE 192-3

Preventive Strategies to Preserve Renal Function

Avoid the following:
Aminoglycosides
ACE inhibitors
Angiotensin-II receptor antagonists
NSAIDs
High-dose diuretics
Contrast media
Large-volume paracentesis
Prevent the following:
Intrarenal vasoconstriction
Systemic vasodilatation
Intravascular volume depletion and hypotension
SBP (antibiotic regimen prophylaxis)
Portal hypertension (TIPS, when indicated)
Gastrointestinal bleeding

ACE, angiotensin-converting enzyme; NSAIDs, nonsteroidal anti-inflammatory drugs; SBP, spontaneous bacterial peritonitis; TIPS, transjugular intrahepatic portosystemic shunt.

ment, and this is more frequent in the case of acute liver disease or the alcoholic forms. Much less severe is the type 2 HRS, which can take months to set in and is more easily controlled with a meticulous therapeutic regimen.

Given the severity of the HRS and its poor outcome, prevention is particularly important, aimed at reduction in the incidence of HRS in chronic disease. If HRS is already ongoing, it is necessary to start a series of therapeutic procedures ranging from the administration of vasoactive drugs to the use of replacement therapies and, lastly, orthotopic liver transplantation (OLT).

Prevention

The preventive measures that allow the incidence of HRS to be reduced are reported in Table 192-3. Spontaneous bacterial peritonitis (SBP) is one of the factors precipitating HRS through a vaso-mediated mechanism in which some inflammatory cytokines, such as the TNF-α, aggravate a state of systemic vasodilatation which, in the presence of a relative hypovolemia, generates acute renal ischemia. A recently published randomized trial demonstrated that *selective intestinal decontamination* with norfloxacin is of paramount importance and partially reverses the hyperdynamic circulatory state in cirrhotic patients, thus confirming a possible role for the endotoxin-NO pathway.[51]

Because bacterial peritonitis and acute alcoholic hepatitis are high-risk conditions for HRS occurrence, some studies are particularly relevant. In 1999, Sort and coworkers reported an interventional protocol with the combined administration of albumin (1.5 g/kg IV at infection diagnosis and 1 g/kg IV 48 hr later) and specific antibiotics (cefotaxime) in patients with cirrhosis and SBP, which proved capable of preventing the circulatory dysfunction and occurrence of type 1 HRS, compared to cefotaxime alone.[52]

More recently, Fernandez and associates compared the effect of albumin and the synthetic plasma expander, hydroxyethyl starch, on the systemic hemodynamics of patients with SBP. Treatment with albumin, but not with the artificial plasma expander, was associated with an increase in arterial pressure and a suppression of the renin

activity. Moreover, serum nitrates and nitrites increased in patients treated with the starch but not in those treated with albumin, suggesting an inhibitory effect of albumin on endothelial cell functions.[53]

The administration of pentoxifylline, an inhibitor of TNF (400 mg three times daily), to patients with severe acute alcoholic hepatitis reduced the occurrence of HRS, compared with placebo (8% versus 35%, respectively) in a study by Akriviadis and colleagues.[49]

Contrast media can, under situations of chronic hypovolemia such as that of many cirrhotic states, generate renal damage through a mechanism of vasoconstriction and direct tubular damage. Therefore, investigations with contrast should be limited to situations of absolute need and should be substituted whenever possible with magnetic resonance or with radionuclide investigations using radiopharmaceuticals. Should the need for use of contrast media arise, it is necessary to maintain a good hydration level and to effect a prophylaxis with antioxidant drugs such as acetylcysteine.[54]

Also critical may be the administration of drugs that interfere with the RAS, such as ACE inhibitors or the angiotensin II-receptor blockers.[55] The same can be said for the NSAIDs that cancel out the intrarenal vasodilatation. The type of antibiotic, doses, and administration intervals often become crucial in the appearance or worsening of a renal deficit. Aminoglycosides, in particular, are often responsible for a worsening of renal function.

Paracentesis

If tense ascites is present, paracentesis may improve renal perfusion by reducing the venous pressure.[56] A vicious circle may, however, take place, because abdominal decompression may be responsible for a *postparacentesis circulatory dysfunction (PCD)*, involving hyponatremia, functional renal failure, and rapid ascites reaccumulation. After a large tap, in fact, there is an early hemodynamic effect, secondary to the decompression of the vena cava and improvement in cardiac output with suppression of vasoconstrictors and antinatriuretic factors. It has been demonstrated that simultaneous intravenous administration of albumin (6 to 8 g per liter of fluid removed) may minimize the activation of the vasoactive systems, suggesting that hypovolemia may be responsible for the PCD.[57,58]

However, several studies have failed to demonstrate a significant reduction in intravascular volume after paracentesis. Recent studies suggest that the sudden abdominal decompression, per se, could play a role in PCD, aggravating the already present vasodilation of the splanchnic vascular bed. The initial beneficial effects deriving from vena cava decompression may be followed by the negative effects of the abdominal decompression, with consequent further aggravation of renal perfusion and function.[59] In this perspective, a controlled decrease of intra-abdominal pressure that avoids abrupt changes in systemic hemodynamics could help prevent the development of acute PCD.

Pharmacological Approach

Given that there are no pharmacological means capable of resolving HRS completely, numerous drugs have been used for its treatment, with varying effect. Drugs with the best pathophysiological rationale are vasoconstrictors—vasopressin analogues and α-adrenoreceptor agonists—

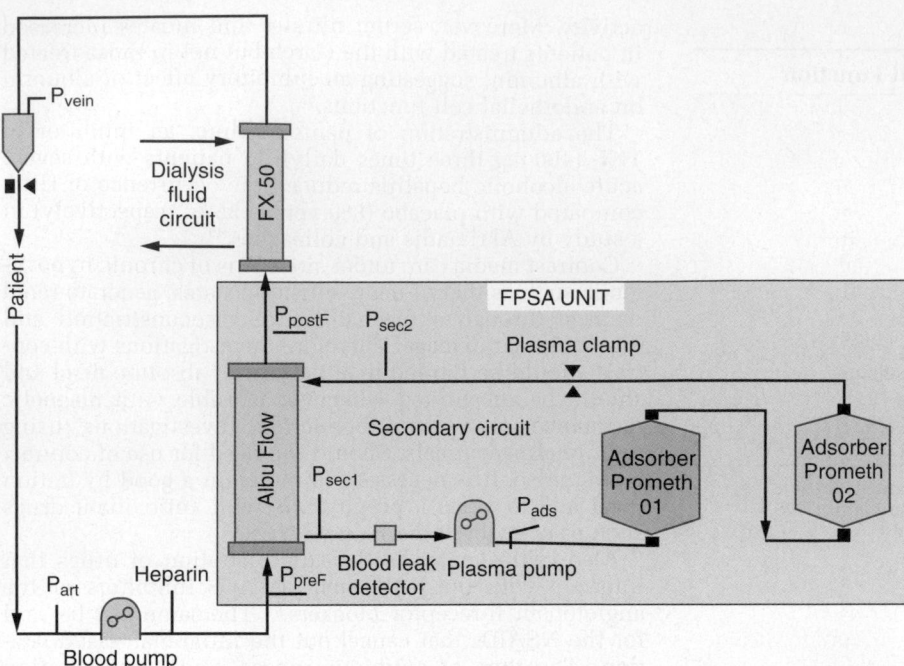

FIGURE 192-2. Schematic representation of the Prometheus extracorporeal circuit. After separation through an albumin-permeable membrane (Albuflow), the patient's plasma flows through a secondary circuit where protein-bound toxic substances are removed by two adsorbers (Prometh 01 and 02). Plasma is then returned to the venous blood line, where a high-flux hemodialyzer removes water-soluble substances. FPSA, fractionated plasma separation adsorption; P_{ads}, adsorption pressure; P_{art}, arterial (negative) pressure; P_{postF}, postfilter pressure; P_{preF}, prefilter pressure; P_{sec1}, preplasma pump pressure; P_{sec2}, postadsorption pressure; P_{vein}, venous pressure.

which act, respectively, on V_1 vasopressin receptors and α_1-adrenergic receptors present in vascular smooth muscle cells. These drugs, in fact, have collected the most data in their favor in clinical practice.

Terlipressin in particular has vasoconstrictive properties akin to those of vasopressin, but with a much lower incidence of ischemic complications. Its use, combined with albumin, seems to get the best results, with improvement in renal function and an increased survival.[60,61]

In a recent meta-analysis evaluating 10 clinical trials in 154 unique patients (only two studies were randomized controlled trials), the rate of reversal of HRS after terlipressin therapy was 52%, and the odds ratio for mortality among patients who did not respond to terlipressin was 5.746.[62]

Terlipressin may therefore be a valid "bridge" therapy to OLT, because the appearance of renal failure has a great impact on the course before and after transplantation.

Drugs that are able to induce a renal vasodilation (misoprostol and *N*-acetylcysteine), endothelin blockers, and adenosine antagonists have now mainly a speculative interest.

The prevention of portal hypertension is the most effective element in preventing HRS,[29] but also reduction of the pressure regime in the portal territory can have some beneficial effects. This is the rationale for use of the *transjugular intrahepatic portosystemic shunt* (TIPS). This consists of the intrahepatic placing of a shunt between the portal and the suprahepatic region. The portal decompression and direct transfer of a certain amount of blood from the portal to the systemic circulation has the dual advantage of reducing the pressure regimes in the portal territory and increasing the intravascular volume and, therefore, the effective volemia and cardiac output.[63] Suppression of the RAS is observed within the first week after TIPS insertion, whereas suppression of ADH requires a greater length of time. Increases in serum sodium and GFR are also observed, indicating an improvement in renal perfusion and free water clearance, in 1 to 3 months.[9]

Extracorporeal Support

New extracorporeal support systems, specific for liver insufficiency, are now available,[64] with the aim of removing liver toxins such as bilirubin, biliary salts, and ammonia, as well as aromatic amino acids, mercaptans, endogenous benzodiazepines, and cytokines. Selective plasmapheresis, the Molecular Adsorbents Recirculating System (MARS) method (see Chapter 196), and the new plasmafiltration Prometheus system are now available.[65] We believe that systems based on plasmapheresis and adsorption are best for this pathology.

The Prometheus system is a new plasmafiltration technique that couples plasma adsorption and hemodialysis, with the aim of blood purification in liver failure. After separation through an albumin-permeable membrane, plasma enters a secondary circuit wherein protein-bound toxic substances are removed by two adsorbers: Prometh 01, a neutral resin, and Prometh 02, an anion exchanger. Plasma is then returned to the venous blood line, where a high-flux hemodialyzer removes water-soluble substances (Fig. 192-2).[66] We started using this technique in 2004 and have performed almost 90 treatments, with excellent results in terms of protein-bound solutes (bilirubin, biliary salts) as well as water-soluble substances (ammonia). An international, multicenter, randomized clinical trial is now ongoing to compare standard medical therapy with and without Prometheus in patients with acute-on-chronic liver failure, using hard end points such as survival and time to transplantation or liver function recovery.

ORTHOTOPIC LIVER TRANSPLANTATION

OLT is the treatment of choice; it allows for the recovery of renal function, albeit incomplete compared with that of patients without HRS at transplantation.[66] The use of the

Model of End-stage Liver Disease (MELD) score (bilirubin, creatinine, and international normalized ratio) for organ allocation attaches paramount importance to the renal function.[4] Everything should be attempted to improve renal function, because patients with HRS who undergo liver transplantation have higher morbidity and in-hospital mortality than those without HRS[66,67]; in particular, there is a greater need for hemodialysis. Patients treated with vasopressin analogues and albumin before transplantation have a good outcome, similar to that of non-HRS patients, and the 3-year survival likelihood after OLT is very good (60% to 100%). In some experiences, survival has been slightly lower than for patients transplanted without HRS,[66] and in others slightly better.[68]

Combined liver and kidney transplantation for patients with HRS does not improve the overall results obtained with liver transplantation alone and should not be used.[69]

filtration rate are the consequences. Renal failure with increased sodium and water reabsorption is the final picture. An impairment in cardiac function, generating a reduction in cardiac output, is probably associated.

4. Type 1 HRS has a dramatic course with a very poor prognosis. New pharmacological options (vasoconstrictors and albumin) seem, however, to have a positive impact on the clinical course of the syndrome. Type 2 HRS is a chronic form, with a slow deterioration of renal function developing over weeks.

5. Liver transplantation is the best treatment. Extracorporeal systems to support liver function are now available to offer a bridge to transplantation.

Key Points

1. Hepatorenal syndrome is a functional renal failure without significant morphological changes in the kidney. The pathogenetic mechanisms leading to the hepatorenal syndrome are mainly of a hemodynamic nature, in the setting of a circulatory dysfunction with arterial hypotension.
2. Central hypovolemia consequent to splanchnic arterial vasodilation activates various compensatory mechanisms, including the sympathetic nervous system, the renin-angiotensin-aldosterone system, arginine-vasopressin release, and renal endothelin production.
3. Preglomerular vasoconstriction with reduced renal hypoperfusion and a decreased glomerular

Key References

4. Ginès P, Guevara M, Arroyo V, Rodés J: Hepatorenal syndrome. Lancet 2003;362:1819-1827.
23. Ruiz-del-Arbol L, Monescillo A, Arocena C, et al: Circulatory function and hepato-renal syndrome in cirrhosis. Hepatology 2005;42:439-447.
29. Wong F, Blendis L: New challenge of hepatorenal syndrome: Prevention and treatment. Hepatology 2001;34:1242-1251.
63. Moreau R, Lebrec D: The use of vasoconstrictors in patients with cirrhosis: Type 1 HRS and beyond. Hepatology 2006;43:385-394.
64. Santoro A, Mancini E, Buttiglieri S, et al: Extracorporeal support of liver function: Part II. Int J Artif Organs 2004;27: 176-185.

See the companion Expert Consult website for the complete reference list.

CHAPTER 193

The Liver in Kidney Disease

Naem Raza and John A. Kellum

OBJECTIVES

This chapter will:
1. Discuss the role of hepatic replacement therapies.
2. Explore the clinical impact of uremia on liver metabolism.
3. Review systemic diseases affecting both liver and kidney.
4. Discuss current understanding of drugs and toxins leading to liver and kidney dysfunction.
5. Review congenital diseases involving the kidney and liver.

The liver and kidneys are vitally important for maintenance of physiological homeostasis. Although a person can survive without normal renal function due to advances in dialysis therapy, one cannot survive very long with poor hepatic function. Indeed, death is virtually certain within 48 hours in the anhepatic state. There is currently no form of hepatic replacement therapy except for liver transplantation. Various extracorporeal liver assist devices have been used in animal studies and, rarely, in patients with fulminant hepatic failure, but generalized use outside isolated research centers has not yet occurred, and support is partial at best. The liver and kidneys are often affected by the same systemic diseases, toxins, infections, and physiological perturbations, albeit to varying degrees. Isolated disease of one organ often affects the function of the other. This chapter reviews this inter-relationship in various disease states and the physiological response of the liver to disease of the kidney; renal dysfunction secondary to liver disease is discussed in Chapters 192 and 195 of this section.

EFFECT OF UREMIA ON LIVER FUNCTION

Uremia is a clinical syndrome associated with fluid, electrolyte, and hormone imbalances and metabolic abnormalities that develop in parallel with deterioration of renal function. The term *uremia* literally means urine in the blood; it used to describe the clinical condition associated with renal failure. Uremia more commonly develops with later stages of chronic kidney disease marked with creatinine clearance of less than 10 mL/min, but it also may occur with acute renal failure (ARF) in cases of rapid loss of renal function. As yet, no single uremic toxin has been identified that accounts for all of the clinical manifestations of uremia, but β_2-microglobulin, polyamines, advanced glycosylation end products, and other molecules are thought to contribute to the clinical syndrome. The effect of uremia on the liver is also part of the multiorgan system involvement of renal failure. A decreases in serum albumin has been shown to be an independent marker of prognosis in patients with chronic renal failure. Uremia can also lead to many endocrine dysfunctions, including decreased insulin clearance, which causes a decrease in gluconeogenesis and ureagenesis by approximately 20% to 45%.[1] Clinically, there is improvement in glucose control in patients with diabetes, but it may be an ominous sign of worsening renal function and uremia. Plasma concentrations of urea, creatinine, fibrinogen, and glutathione are increased significantly in rats after nephrectomy.[2] In addition, the hepatic excretion of urea, creatinine, phospholipids, cholesterol, and aldosterone are significantly increased.[3] The ability of the liver to clear certain toxins in the presence of uremia may be altered.

Patients with chronic renal failure have decreased dietary intake, leading to reduced expression of insulin-like growth factor 1 (IGF-1) receptor on the hepatocyte membrane.[4-6] The reduced expression leads to reduced IGF-1 binding in the liver and a subsequent increase in plasma levels. These findings may be partially responsible for the growth failure seen in chronic renal failure. Moreover, the ratio of adenosine triphosphate (ATP) to the monophosphate (ADP) in hepatocyte mitochondria is decreased in uremia, suggesting impaired bioenergetics.[1] In normal persons, the liver can readily form tyrosine from phenylalanine, but in patients with ARF or chronic renal failure, phenylalanine infusion does not raise the tyrosine concentration, indicating impairment in conversion.[7]

In a recent study, a high-sucrose diet given to uremic rats led to worsened anorexia and stunted growth compared with controls. Both weight gain and liver weight were lower, and the levels of glycogen, fructose 1,6-diphosphate, and several other intermediates of glucose and phosphate metabolism were markedly reduced.[8] In addition, liver lactate and pyruvate levels were increased.

Amino acid uptake and elimination by the liver is also disturbed in the presence of renal failure. There are significant alterations in lipid metabolism in patients with ARF; increases in triglycerides and very-low-density lipoproteins (VLDL) and decreases in high-density lipoproteins (HDL) have been observed secondary to impairment in hepatic lipase.[8]

Several hormonal aberrations related to the liver have been identified in renal failure. As noted there is reduced expression of IGF-1–binding protein on the hepatocyte. Similarly, there is marked reduction in iodide production from thyroxine by the rat hepatocyte, and this reduction is not due to inhibition of deiodinase activity.[9] Instead, the deiodination of reverse triiodothyronine (rT_3) is affected, leading to the euthyroid sick syndrome frequently seen in uremia and other chronic illnesses. Moreover, the inhibition of deiodination is partially reversed with dialysis, suggesting the existence of circulating inhibitors. Surprisingly, no qualitative differences in hepatic aldosterone metabolism have been shown in uremic animals compared with controls.[2,3] In patients with cirrhosis and sepsis, renal failure is considered as an important and common outcome and is associated with significant morbidity and mortality. Sepsis, spontaneous bacterial peritonitis, renal vasoconstriction, and hepatorenal syndrome are considered common associated pathways leading to renal failure in patients with cirrhosis (see Chapter 192).

SYSTEMIC DISEASE AFFECTING THE LIVER AND KIDNEY

Cardiac Disease

Any disease process that prevents the heart from providing an adequate cardiac output and perfusion pressure will lead to multisystem organ dysfunction. The severity of heart failure and the acuteness of the process affect various organs differently. ARF secondary to acute tubular necrosis is well recognized as a consequence of hypotension and decreased tissue perfusion.[10] Acute myocardial infarction, valvular insufficiency, or arrhythmia can lead to passive congestion of liver presenting as a shock liver or ischemic hepatopathy. In some case reports, arterial hypoxia secondary to respiratory failure or obstructive sleep apnea has led to ischemic hepatitis, severe coagulopathy, ARF, and encephalopathy.[11] Acute elevation of serum aminotransferase levels is a hallmark of this clinical picture. Coagulation abnormalities with elevation of prothrombin time, high bilirubin levels. and encephalopathy can also occur. Ascites is associated with a high albumin gradient (>1:1).

Most of the drugs needed for treatment of heart failure require elimination through liver or kidney metabolism, and reduced elimination can lead to toxicity of these medicines, resulting in arrhythmias and other side effects.[12] Moreover, long-standing heart failure leads to an increase in B-atrial natriuretic factor, with a concurrent increase in antidiuretic hormone production leading to hypo-osmolar hyponatremia.[13,14] The presence of hyponatremia in heart failure has been correlated with poor survival. The hypo-osmolar state causes an increase in hepatic protein and glycogen synthesis, amino acid uptake, and several other metabolic effects on the liver. These metabolic changes may have a profound impact on the patient's health by altering protein metabolism and the ability to withstand oxidative stress and resist viral infection. In patients with severe hyponatremia, there is also increased association of renal dysfunction; this usually develops in the acute-on-chronic pattern and also is associated with both heart failure and liver failure.[15]

Vascular Disease

Vascular diseases affecting either the arterial or the venous system can have marked effects on both the hepatic and the renal vasculature. Acquired platelet dysfunction is at least partially corrected by hemodialysis, suggesting that accumulation of uremic toxins in the blood may contribute to the observed effects.[16] Hypercoagulable states secondary to deficiencies of protein C, protein S, and antithrombin III may predispose an individual to venous thrombosis of the renal and hepatic or portal veins. Likewise, thromboembolism may lead to pulmonary hypertension and subsequent hepatic and renal insufficiency by passive congestion. Budd-Chiari syndrome, or hepatic vein thrombosis, has been associated with abdominal trauma,[17] use of oral contraceptives,[18] paroxysmal nocturnal hemoglobinuria,[19] and leiomyosarcomas.[20] Hypercoagulable states associated with pregnancy, such as lupus anticoagulant and other circulating antiphospholipid antibodies and antifactor antibodies, can lead to development of multiple venous thrombosis, including the renal and portohepatic veins.[21] Multiple venous thrombosis (Trousseau's sign) is a well-recognized complication of solid tumors, notably pancreatic cancer.[22] Bone marrow transplantation is also associated with a significant incidence of veno-occlusive disease. This veno-occlusive disease is related to renal failure and cardiopulmonary and liver damage. Insult to the liver is a common complication of cytoreductive therapy, and the most common site is the terminal hepatic venule. This clinical syndrome is most commonly called veno-occlusive disease of the liver.[23]

Several arterial diseases are worth mentioning, because they have profound effects on multiple organ systems, including the liver and kidneys. Arteritides (discussed later) resulting from various autoimmune processes can lead to hepatic artery and renal vascular disease. Hypertensive emergencies lead to marked end-organ dysfunction, particularly of the kidneys, central nervous system, and heart, but they may also affect liver function. Acute fatty liver of pregnancy, preeclampsia, eclampsia, and the HELLP syndrome (*h*emolysis, *e*levated *l*iver enzymes, and *l*ow blood *p*latelet count) have all been demonstrated as important causes of severe hepatic failure in pregnancy and are associated with significant maternal and perinatal mortality. Failure to control the hypertension by medical therapy or emergency delivery can result in irreversible damage to many organs.[24] Preeclampsia affects 5% to 7% of all women during the second and third trimesters of pregnancy, and a subset of these patients also develop HELLP syndrome. Renal insufficiency frequently occurs; initially, there is a decrease in the clearance of uric acid, followed by proteinuria leading to hypoalbuminemia. Liver function tests reveal a significant increase in alkaline phosphatase. These pathological processes may lead to further complications, including veno-occlusive disease, hepatic rupture, renal failure, and neurological complications such as seizures and are associated with significant mortality.[24] Hepatorenal syndrome (HRS) is discussed in Chapters 192 and 195.

Infectious Diseases

Both acute and chronic renal disease have been linked to a number of infectious agents, of which several may also cause significant liver abnormalities. The most widely recognized agents are hepatitis B virus (HBV) and hepatitis C virus (HCV), which may lead to fulminant hepatic failure and chronic hepatitis but have also been associated with membranous glomerulopathy[25,26] and with mixed essential cryoglobulinemia.[27] There is a strong association between chronic HCV infection and glomerular disease, particularly three types: mixed (immunoglobulin G [IgG]/IgM) cryoglobulinemia, membranoproliferative glomerulonephritis, and membranous nephropathy. In patients with mixed cryoglobulinemia, HCV-containing immune complexes are strongly associated with disease, and there are reports of detection of HCV antigens in glomerular capillary wall and mesangium in patients with HCV-positive mixed cryoglobulinemia.[28] Membranous glomerulopathy is the most common cause of nephritic syndrome in adults and is idiopathic in most cases. However, a small percentage is secondary to antecedent HBV infection. Mixed essential cryoglobulinemia is a disease of middle-aged women characterized by recurrent bouts of fever, palpable purpura, hepatosplenomegaly, hypocomplementemia (C4, C1q, and total hemolytic complement [CH_{50}]), Raynaud's phenomenon, arthralgias, and muscle weakness. The kidney exhibits a diffuse proliferative glomerulonephritis with intraluminal hyaline thrombi, and the serum immunoelectrophoresis is characteristic for IgG-IgM complexes that precipitate at 4° C.[25] Treatment with interferon has resulted in improvement in renal disease and reduces flare-ups, but relapses are common.[29]

Nonstreptococcal postinfectious ARF has been linked to malaria,[30] schistosomiasis,[31] syphilis (*Treponema pallidum*),[32] and Leptospirosis (*Leptospira interrogans*).[32,33] Malaria[34] is widely prevalent throughout southeast Asia, Africa, and Latin America. Malaria sporozoites mature into schizonts after being cleared by hepatocytes from circulation. Two species, *Plasmodium vivax* and *Plasmodium ovale,* produce dormant forms in the liver that may mature into infectious schizonts up to 1 year after initial infection, resulting in febrile illness. The resulting acute or relapsing febrile illness may be associated with marked hemolysis and ARF due to hemoglobinuria (black water fever). The clinical presentation and prognosis of the disease are worse when anemia, hepatosplenomegaly, and cerebral and renal involvement occur as complications of disease. *Plasmodium falciparum* and *Plasmodium malariae* usually cause renal involvement in malaria. *P. vivax* has also been reported in recent cases. In general, *P. falciparum* is linked with ARF and *P. malariae* with chronic progressive glomerulopathy. The hepatic dysfunction associated with malaria is caused by intravascular hemolysis, disseminated intravascular coagulation, and, in some cases, malaria hepatitis.

Schistosomiasis (caused by the *Schistosoma* species *mansoni, japonicum, haematobium, intercalatum,* and *mekongi*) can lead to a marked immune response to the presence of ova in the portal vein and a resulting fibrotic process that ultimately results in hepatosplenomegaly, portal hypertension, and granuloma formation.[35] *S. haematobium* often inhabits the venous plexus around the lower end of the ureters and urinary bladder, leading to an obstructive uropathy.[36] In zoonoses such as Rocky Mountain spotted fever (RMSF), leptospirosis, and ehrlichiosis, renal failure, hepatic injury, and aseptic meningitis can be major manifestations. One of the differential aspects in these three infections is the white blood cell count, which is usually elevated in RMSF and leptospirosis, whereas the presence of leukopenia is more suggestive of ehrlichiosis.[37]

Leptospirosis (Weil's disease) is a spirochetal disease characterized by widespread vasculitis caused by pathogenic leptospira whose main reservoirs are wild and domestic animals (rodents, foxes, livestock, dogs, and frogs). Transmission to humans is usually through infected urine or other tissue of infected animals. Weil's disease is characterized by widespread hemorrhage, jaundice, hepatic and renal dysfunction, and bile staining.[38-40] The kidneys may also show acellular tubular injury or interstitial nephritis and focal areas of hemorrhage with elevation of urinary protein, hematuria, pyuria, and hyperkalemia.[32,33] Interstitial involvement of the kidney is the basic lesion. Renal failure is observed in about 44% to 67% of leptospirosis cases and is mostly secondary to tubular necrosis and interstitial nephritis.[41] Jaundice results as vascular damage in hepatic capillaries, and liver biopsy demonstrates nonspecific inflammatory changes, cholestasis, and hemorrhage.[41] Oliguria and high levels of bilirubin are considered to be independent factors associated with death.

Hemolytic uremic syndrome (HUS) is a multisystem disorder characterized by a clinical triad of microangiopathic hemolytic anemia, thrombocytopenia, and ARF. In North America, the most common cause of HUS is *Escherichia coli* O157:H7. Fibrin deposition and thrombosis of the submucosal and intramural vessels occur in kidneys, pancreas, liver, and other organs. Complications of acute HUS include stroke, seizure, hemorrhagic colitis, cholelithiasis, and hyperbilirubinemia. Hyperbilirubinemia seen in HUS is usually unconjugated and is most likely a manifestation of hemolysis and increased bilirubin load. Also reported is a more severe form of hepatocellular injury associated with HUS in which the histology shows fibrin deposition in the hepatic sinusoids.[42]

Neoplastic Disease

Malignant neoplasms may affect organ function by several different mechanisms, whereas benign tumors principally affect local organs by disruption of anatomic architecture. Malignant neoplasms may distort local anatomy by compression or invasion or both, but they may also affect distant organs by metastatic disease or alteration of function via paraneoplastic syndromes. Moreover, a pelvic malignancy, such as ovarian carcinoma, may progress to involve multiple abdominal organs, including the liver, while leading to an obstructive uropathy. The only significant primary malignancy that has direct effects on both organs is renal cell carcinoma (hypernephroma). Paraneoplastic syndrome and bizarre metastatic sites are not uncommon. Clinical manifestations may include fever, hypertension, erythrocytosis, hypercalcemia, and anemia.[43] Stauffer's syndrome is a well-characterized hepatic disorder associated with renal cell carcinoma that features elevated alkaline phosphate and α-globulin, prolonged prothrombin time, hypercholesterolemia, and low albumin.[44] These abnormalities may occur even without metastasis to the liver. Hepatic dysfunction is usually associated with poor prognosis and may be the result of cytokines such as granulocyte-macrophage colony-stimulating factor (GM-CSF) and possibly interleukin-6.[45,46] In patients with renal cell carcinoma, paraneoplastic elevation of serum alkaline phosphatase is associated with poor prognosis, and persistent elevation after radical nephrec-

TABLE 193-1

Drugs and Toxins Affecting Renal and Liver Function

Nephrotoxins	Hepatotoxins
Antibiotics	Antibiotics
Amoxicillin-clavulanate	Oxacillin
Gentamicin	Isoniazid
Tobramycin	Tetracycline
Streptomycin	Nitrofurantoin
Amikacin	Acetaminophen
Amphotericin B	Aspirin
NSAIDs	Steroids
Metals	Anabolic steroids
Lead	Corticosteroids
Cadmium	Chemotherapeutic agents
Mercury	Allopurinol
Iron	Methotrexate
Arsenic	6-Thioguanine
Solvents	Vinyl chloride
Tetrachloroethylene	Other drugs
Iodinated contrast media	Ethanol
Carbon tetrachloride	Halothane
Chemotherapeutic agents	Chlorpromazine
Cisplatin	Phenylbutazone
	α-Methyldopa

NSAIDs, nonsteroidal anti-inflammatory drugs.

tomy suggests distant metastasis or residual tumor.[47] Hepatocellular cancer associated with polymyositis, presenting as fulminant rhabdomyolysis and ARF, was also mentioned in one case report.[48]

Drugs and Toxins

The list of drugs and toxins that may lead to both renal and liver dysfunction is long, and a discussion of each is beyond the scope of this chapter. A brief list of the more commonly encountered drugs is given in Table 193-1. Acetaminophen (paracetamol, Tylenol), the most commonly reported toxic pharmaceutical ingestion in the United States, is particularly worth mentioning in detail.[49] On average, 500 deaths and more than 56,000 emergency room visits in each year in the United States are related to acetaminophen toxicity.[50] Almost half of the cases result from unintentional overdose due to the presence of acetaminophen in multiple preparations.[51] According to the prescribing label, the maximum recommended dose is 65 mg/kg and 4 g/24 hr in an adult.[52] There are many case reports in which patients with alcohol abuse suffered from combined hepatocellular and renal injury secondary to therapeutic acetaminophen use.[53] The exact toxic dose varies depending on factors such as underlying liver injury and glutathione levels. If a toxic amount is ingested (140 mg/kg in children, or about 7.5 g in an adult), the capacity of the liver to metabolize it to nontoxic glucuronide and sulfate conjugates is overwhelmed. This leads to formation of excessive amounts of N-acetyl-para-benzoquinoneimine, a highly reactive and toxic intermediate.[54-56] This leads to acute hepatocellular and renal toxicity, and the extent of toxicity is directly related to the quantity of drug ingested, the serum level obtained, and the time before therapy with N-acetylcysteine, although wide individual variation may still occur. Recently, measurement of acetaminophen-protein adducts have been evaluated in diagnosing acetaminophen-induced hepatotoxicity especially if no clear history is available and acetaminophen levels are undetectable.[50] Renal function abnormalities are common in patients with documented hepatotoxicity, and ARF requiring dialysis may develop.

There are reported incidences of ARF and hepatic failure after ingestion of raw carp gallbladder. This syndrome is more prevalent in Asian populations of Taiwan, Hong Kong, Japan, and South Korea, but some cases were also reported in the United States. In some cases, hepatic manifestations proceed renal failure, but the two may be concomitant.[57,58]

Congenital Abnormalities

The most common hereditary disease in the United States is autosomal dominant polycystic kidney disease (ADPKD), with approximately 500,000 people affected.[59] The disease is transmitted as an autosomal dominant gene, with one form localized to chromosome 16 and the other to chromosome 4.[60] ADPKD is a disease in adults, with symptomatic presentation rarely before age 25 years. Flank pain and hematuria are the most common clinical presentations, with most patients developing hypertension, nocturia, and frequent urinary tract infections. Prevalence of liver disease is the most common extrarenal manifestation, and up to two thirds of patients have multiple, asymptomatic hepatic cysts as well. The number and size of hepatic cysts increase such that approximately 20% of the liver volume is affected, 20% in the third decade to approximately 75% after the sixth decade.[61] Rarely, these cysts cause functional impairment of the liver. However, the disease often progresses to end-stage renal failure by late adulthood.

Unlike ADPKD, autosomal recessive polycystic kidney disease (ARPKD) is a disease of infants and children and is a significant cause of renal- and liver-associated morbidity and mortality. This is a rare disease, with an incidence of about 1 in 20,000 live births. It manifests with abdominal masses, failure to thrive, hypertension, and urinary tract infections.[60] Children usually progress to end-stage renal failure before adolescence, but neonates may develop renal failure within a few weeks of diagnosis. Despite improvement in intensive care, neonatal mortality is still as high as 25% to 35%. In contrast to ADPKD, many children with ARPKD also have hepatic fibrosis and portal hypertension as part of their disease. The characteristic findings associated with ARPKD liver disease are biliary dysgenesis secondary to primary ductal plate malformation with associated periportal fibrosis leading to congenital hepatic fibrosis and dilatation of intrahepatic bile ducts (Caroli's disease).[61]

A number of inborn errors of metabolism have both renal and hepatic manifestations. Hypertyrosinemia type 1 results from a defect in the enzyme, fumarylacetoacetate hydrolase, which leads to an accumulation of the amino acid, tyrosine.[62] Hepatic cirrhosis and renal tubular failure develop, with death usually occurring unless tyrosine is restricted from the diet. Wilson's disease (hepatocellular degeneration) is an inherited disorder characterized by the accumulation of copper in many tissues of the body, particularly the liver, brain, kidneys, skin, and eyes.[63] Fanconi's syndrome and renal calculi are not uncommon, but the most devastating manifestations are secondary to accumulation of copper in the basal ganglia and liver, leading to severe neurological impairment and cirrhosis. Massive hemolysis may also occur, leading to ARF.

Collagen Vascular Disease

Systemic lupus erythematosus (SLE) is a disease of unknown etiology characterized by inflammation of many different organ systems. Most patients with SLE exhibit some degree of renal impairment, but few develop severe disease that threatens organ survival. In SLE, renal failure may develop in the form of rapidly progressive glomerulonephritis or membranous disease associated with liver dysfunction. Rarely, chronic hepatitis occurs. Elevation of liver enzymes is common but usually is not of clinical significance.[64]

Polyarteritis nodosa is a rare systemic necrotizing vasculitis involving small and medium-sized arteries with a peak onset of disease in the fifth and sixth decades of life. Typically, patients present with chronic symptoms of fever, abdominal pain, weight loss, and arthralgia. But it can be catastrophic, with acute complications such as intestinal ischemia, infarction of a kidney or other major organ, and sudden loss of multiple nerves (mononeuritis multiplex). The widespread nature of this disease leads to diverse clinical presentations, but renal involvement is very common. Renal disease occurs as renal arteritis, infarction of kidneys, or glomerulonephritis and is the leading cause of death in two thirds of patients with polyarteritis nodosa.[65,66] Involvement of the liver is shown frequently at autopsy, and in other situations it can manifest as hepatomegaly with or without jaundice, or as extensive hepatic necrosis.[66,67]

Key Points

1. There is currently no form of hepatic replacement therapy except for liver transplantation.
2. The ability of the liver to clear toxins is significantly altered by uremia.
3. Fulminant hepatic failure, chronic hepatitis, and membranous glomerulopathy are serious complications of hepatitis B virus and hepatitis C virus infections.
4. Acetaminophen (paracetamol) is the most commonly reported toxic pharmaceutical ingestion in the United States, and almost half of the cases are related to unintentional overdose.
5. *N*-acetyl-para-benzoquinoneimine is a highly reactive and toxic intermediate of paracetamol that leads to acute hepatocellular and renal toxicity.

Key References

5. Fleck C: Biliary amino acid excretion in rats before and after bilateral nephrectomy. Physiol Res 1992;41:273-278.
6. Tonshoff B, Eden S, Weiser E, et al: Reduced hepatic growth hormone (GH) receptor gene expression and increased plasma GH binding protein in experimental uremia. Kidney Int 1994;45:1085-1092.
25. Lai KN, Li PK, Lui SF, et al: Membranous nephropathy related to hepatitis B virus in adults. N Engl J Med 1991;324:1457-1463.
27. Han MK, Hyzy R: Advances in critical care management of hepatic failure and insufficiency. Crit Care Med 2006;34(9 Suppl):S225-S231.
42. Riley MR, Lee KK: Escherichia coli O157:H7–associated hemolytic uremic syndrome and acute hepatocellular cholestasis: A case report. J Pediatr Gastroenterol Nutr 2004;38:352-354.
53. Kaysen GA, Pond SM, Roper MH, et al: Combined hepatic and renal injury in alcoholics during therapeutic use of acetaminophen. Arch Intern Med 1985;145:2019-2023.

See the companion Expert Consult website for the complete reference list.

CHAPTER 194

Kidney Dysfunction after Liver Transplantation

Phuong-Thu Pham, Phuong-Chi Pham, and Alan H. Wilkinson

OBJECTIVES

This chapter will:
1. Present the risk factors for early postoperative acute renal failure after orthotopic liver transplantation (OLT), including pre-OLT factors, intraoperative factors, and post-OLT factors.
2. Present the factors affecting renal dysfunction in long-term survivors after OLT.
3. Suggested strategies to reduce risk factors.

Acute renal failure (ARF) is common immediately after orthotopic liver transplantation (OLT), whereas chronic kidney disease (CKD) and end-stage renal disease (ESRD) increase in incidence with time. Identifying the risk factors for renal dysfunction after OLT and developing strategies to either minimize the risks for de novo renal dysfunction or retard the progression of preexisting renal dysfunction should be an integral part in the management of OLT. An overview of the literature on the risk factors for early postoperative ARF and on the factors affecting renal dysfunction in long-term survivors is presented. Suggested therapeutic approaches to prevent, halt, or ameliorate renal dysfunction are also discussed.

RISK FACTORS FOR EARLY POSTOPERATIVE ACUTE RENAL FAILURE AFTER ORTHOTOPIC LIVER TRANSPLANTATION

ARF after OLT has been reported to occur at incidences ranging from 17% to 95%.[1] This broad range may be partly due to the wide disparity in the criteria used to define "acute renal failure." Nonetheless, severe ARF requiring renal replacement therapy has been documented in 5% to 35% of patients after OLT.[2] Although the risk factors for ARF are often multifactorial and difficult to establish, they can be linked to three distinct time frames in relation to the OLT: the pre-OLT, intraoperative, and post-OLT periods (Table 194-1).

Pretransplantation Risk Factors

Pretransplantation renal dysfunction and preexisting hepatorenal syndrome (HRS) are well-established risk factors for post-transplantation ARF, and higher serum bilirubin levels, hypoproteinemia, hypoalbuminemia, and Acute Physiology and Chronic Health Evaluation (APACHE) II scores have been reported to be associated with a greater incidence of postoperative ARF.

In a retrospective study consisting of more than 600 recipients of liver-only transplants, Sanchez and colleagues showed that a preoperative serum creatinine concentration (SCr) greater than 1.9 mg/dL, preoperative blood urea nitrogen (BUN) greater than 27 mg/dL, intensive care unit stay longer than 3 days, and a Model for End-Stage Liver Disease (MELD) score greater than 21 were significant predictive indicators of the need for renal replacement therapy after OLT.[3] Similarly, Contreras and associates showed that elevated pretransplantation BUN and SCr and low urine output are associated with the need for renal replacement therapy during the first week after OLT.[2] With regard to low urine output, volume overload may dictate the need for renal replacement therapy irrespective of electrolyte abnormalities.

Although the association between high serum bilirubin level and postoperative renal failure has been long recognized, its pathogenic mechanism remains incompletely understood. Nonetheless, it has been speculated that jaundice-related nephropathy is a tubulopathy. Both normal renal architecture and extensive renal tubule necrosis have been observed in renal biopsies of patients with jaundice and renal insufficiency.[4]

The mechanisms whereby low serum albumin increases the risk of postoperative ARF remain speculative. Although controversial, it has been suggested that hypoalbuminemia modifies Starling's forces in the systemic capillaries and results in the reduction of glomerular filtration.[5] Hypoalbuminemia has also been suggested to alter the pharmacokinetics of potentially nephrotoxic drugs, thereby increasing the risk of ARF. In a prospective study consisting of 104 patients treated with intravenous amikacin for at least 36 hours, Contreras and coworkers showed that low serum albumin is associated with amikacin accumulation in the plasma and an increased risk of nephrotoxicity.[6]

More recently, the presence of hyponatremia, defined as a serum sodium concentration of less than 130 mEq/L at the time of transplantation, has also been suggested to be associated with a high rate of complications after OLT, including neurological disorders, infectious complications, and renal failure during the first month after transplantation.[7] It is well established that the presence of hyponatremia identifies a group of patients with cirrhosis who have severe impairment in circulatory function.[7] It is speculated that this acts in concert with the intraoperative and perioperative hemodynamic changes to increase the risk of postoperative ARF.

Strategies to Reduce Risk Factors

Every effort should be made to prevent or minimize the risk of developing pretransplantation renal dysfunction or HRS. The potential benefits of diuretics, lactulose, contrast dye exposure, nephrotoxic medications, nonsteroidal anti-inflammatory drugs (NSAIDS) and selective cyclooxygen-

TABLE 194-1

Risk Factors for Early Postoperative Acute Renal Failure

Pretransplantation Factors
Pretransplantation renal dysfunction
Hepatorenal syndrome
High bilirubin levels
Hypoproteinemia, hypoalbuminemia
APACHE II scores
Hyponatremia
Intraoperative Factors
Hemodynamic instability during anesthesia induction and anhepatic phase
Intraoperative bleeding and volume of transfused blood products
Standard surgical technique (with or without VVB) vs piggyback technique*
Conventional risk factors*
Postoperative Factors
Acute tubular necrosis secondary to ischemic or toxic insults
Delayed liver graft function or primary nonfunction
Postreperfusion syndrome
Contrast nephropathy
Drug-induced interstitial nephritis
Prolonged use of dopamine or vasopressors
Bacterial infection
Repeat laparotomy
Perioperative volume of transfused blood products
Calcineurin inhibitor immunosuppressive therapy

APACHE II, Acute Physiology and Chronic Health Evaluation II; VVB, venovenous bypass.
*See text for details.

ase-2 (COX-2) inhibitors must be carefully balanced against the risk of precipitating HRS. Large-volume paracentesis in patients with severe hypoalbuminemia or ascites without peripheral edema is thought to increase risk for the development of acute volume depletion and potential HRS. In such cases, the use of plasma expanders has been advocated. In general, albumin is believed to be more effective than artificial plasma expanders in the prevention of circulatory dysfunction.[8] Nevertheless, not all investigators agree that plasma expanders are necessary during large-volume paracentesis or that paracentesis can precipitate HRS. However, the use of albumin infusion in cirrhotic patients with spontaneous bacterial peritonitis has been suggested to reduce the risk of renal failure and mortality, especially among those with renal insufficiency and hyperbilirubinemia at presentation.[9]

Intraoperative Risk Factors

Cross-clamping of the portal vein and inferior vena cava during the anhepatic phase (phase II) interrupts the venous return from the lower extremities and splanchnic bed and may result in decreased cardiac output and blood pressure, increased systemic vascular resistance, and reduced perfusion to vital organs. The latter may lead to renal hypoperfusion and potential ischemic renal injury. Although veno-venous bypass (VVB) has been shown to improve or restore normal hemodynamic physiology during the anhepatic phase, the use of VVB has not been consistently shown to decrease the incidence of perioperative or early postoperative renal failure.[1] In a retrospective study of 87 recipients of OLT, Shaw and coworkers showed that the use of VVB was associated with a lower SCr level at postoperative day 3 and a decreased requirement for postoperative dialysis.[10] In contrast, in a more recent pro-

spective controlled trial involving 77 recipients of OLT randomized to receive either VVB support or no VVB support, the degree of renal dysfunction (assessed by inulin clearance) measured at various perioperative periods (anesthesia induction, hepatectomy, anhepatic phase, biliary anastomosis, and 24 hours after surgery) was not significantly different between the two groups at any time point, with the exception of the anhepatic phase, in which a more marked renal function impairment occurred in patients without VVB support. Nevertheless, renal function on the seventh postoperative day and need for hemodialysis/hemofiltration during the first week were similar in both groups. Deterioration of renal function occurred in both groups, and renal impairment persisted in a subset of patients during the early postoperative period. A multivariate analysis revealed that low mean arterial pressure at anesthesia induction was an independent risk factor for early postoperative severe renal failure (inulin clearance <10 mL/min/1.73 m^2 at the 24th postoperative hour).[11]

Although large, prospective clinical trials are lacking, it is conceivable that intraoperative risk factors for the development of perioperative and early postoperative ARF in OLT are similar to those in other surgical settings. These may include an anesthesia-induced decrease in effective blood volume, preexisting cardiovascular disease or severe cardiomyopathy, a prolonged episode of hemodynamic instability or hypotension, severe intravascular volume depletion, use of drugs that can adversely affect intrarenal hemodynamics, older age, preexisting renal insufficiency, and diabetes mellitus. In this respect, hemodynamic instability associated with a prolonged anhepatic phase and major bleeding during hepatectomy can potentially predispose patients undergoing OLT to postoperative ARF. Cabezuelo and colleagues showed that, compared with the standard surgical technique (with or without VVB), the piggyback technique significantly reduces the probability of ARF after liver transplantation. It is speculated that this is partly due to the reduction in retroperitoneal blood loss, because the piggyback technique does not require retrocaval dissection. In addition, it permits venous return to the heart during the anhepatic phase and avoids hemodynamic variation during inferior vena cava clamping.[12]

Strategies to Reduce Intraoperative Risk Factors

Control of bleeding during surgery, careful attention to management of fluid and electrolytes, and avoidance of hypotensive episodes are imperative in the perioperative period. Whether use of the piggyback technique, as opposed to the standard surgical technique (with or without VVB), significantly reduces the probability of ARF after liver transplantation remains to be determined.

Postoperative Risk Factors

Factors that have been shown to cause or predispose OLT recipients to postoperative ARF, particularly acute tubular necrosis (ATN), include ischemic or toxic insult to the kidneys, prolonged hypotension, sepsis, sustained prerenal renal failure, the use of nephrotoxic drugs, delayed liver graft function or primary graft nonfunction, postreperfusion syndrome, and contrast nephropathy. Other suggested predictive factors include prolonged treatment with dopamine or vasopressors, repeat laparotomy, and perioperative volume of transfused blood products.[5,13] The use of

TABLE 194-2

Induction Therapy after Orthotopic Liver Transplantation*

N	INTERVENTION	OUTCOME	FOLLOW-UP	REF. NO.
298	Thymoglobulin/delayed CNI	Early AR prevented without compromising patient and graft survival	1 yr	14
45	Basiliximab/delayed tacrolimus vs control (tacrolimus on day 1, no basiliximab)	Early renal dysfunction prevented without ↑ risk of graft rejection and infection compared with control	22 mo (median)	15
148	Daclizumab/delayed low-dose tacrolimus vs "standard" tacrolimus induction/maintenance dosing	Early renal function preserved compared with "standard" therapy without ↑ AR; patient survival and AR episodes were comparable between the two treatment groups	12 mo	16

AR, acute rejection; CNI, calcineurin inhibitor.
*See text for details.

cyclosporine or tacrolimus in the post-transplantation period may further exacerbate renal dysfunction. Finally, polypharmacy, and specifically the use of multiple antibiotics, may contribute to postoperative renal failure due to drug-induced interstitial nephritis.

Strategies to Reduce Postoperative Risk Factors

Bleeding and infectious complications in the perioperative period should be sought and treated aggressively. The use of contrast studies or nephrotoxic drugs should be minimized or avoided. Therapeutic approaches in the postoperative period should be modified in patients with preexisting HRS or pretransplantation renal dysfunction. The use of calcineurin inhibitor (CNI) minimization or avoidance protocols to reduce postoperative ARF and chronic renal failure has met with variable results. The following section provides an overview of the literature on the various strategies that have been used to prevent or retard the progression of renal dysfunction in recipients of OLT (summarized in Tables 194-2 through 194-6).

REDUCTION OF CALCINEURIN INHIBITOR NEPHROTOXICITY

In a retrospective analysis consisting of 298 recipients of OLT, Tchervenkov and coworkers showed that induction therapy with Thymoglobulin may allow a delay in the initiation of CNI without compromising patient and graft survival, while preventing early rejection even among patients with baseline renal dysfunction (defined as a baseline SCr > 1.5 mg/dL).[14]

With the advent of the monoclonal antibodies, anti-IL2 receptor antibodies (basiliximab and daclizumab), mycophenolate mofetil (MMF), and sirolimus, independent investigators have developed various immunosuppressive protocols that avoid the nephrotoxic effects associated with CNI therapy while providing adequate immunosuppression.

Table 194-2 summarizes the studies in this and the following section.

Early Experiences with the Anti-IL2R Antibodies Basiliximab and Daclizumab as Renal-Sparing Agents

In a small prospective, open-label, nonrandomized study consisting of 45 recipients of adult living donor liver transplants, Lin and colleagues showed that, compared with a control group (tacrolimus on postoperative day 1 without basiliximab), basiliximab induction could prevent early renal dysfunction by delaying the initiation of tacrolimus and reducing its dose requirement without increasing the risk of graft rejection and infection, despite worse preoperative conditions and higher MELD scores in the basiliximab treatment group (basiliximab on days 0 and 4, delay in tacrolimus administration [median, 36 hours; range, 24 to 108 hours]). In addition, at 3 months' follow-up, creatinine clearance (CrCl) was higher (72 versus 57 mL/min; $P = .04$) and the incidence of renal insufficiency was lower (26% versus 67%; $P < .01$) in the basiliximab induction group compared with the control group.[15]

In a multicenter, randomized clinical trial consisting of 148 OLT recipients, Yoshida and associates showed that daclizumab induction and delayed low-dose tacrolimus (target trough, 4 to 8 mg/dL, starting on day 4 to 6) preserved early renal function, compared with "standard" tacrolimus induction/maintenance dosing (target trough, 10 to 15 mg/dL for the first 30 days) without the risk of increased acute rejection. The estimated glomerular filtration rate (GFR) assessed by the Cockcroft-Gault formula for the daclizumab versus the standard group was 110.7 versus 89.6 mL/min ($P = .019$) at the end of the first week; no significant differences were noted thereafter. The GFR derived from the Modification of Diet in Renal Disease (MDRD) study equation, however, revealed significant improvement in renal function in the daclizumab versus the standard group at 1 month (86.8 versus 70.1 mL/min; $P < .001$) and at 6 months (75.4 versus 69.5 mL/min; $P = .038$) after transplantation. There was no statistical difference between the two treatment groups at post-transplantation months 2, 3, and 12. Patient survival and acute rejection episodes were comparable between the two groups.[16]

Early Experiences with Mycophenolate Mofetil as a Renal-Sparing Agent

The studies described in this section are summarized in Table 194-3.

In a small series consisting of 19 adults, long-term (>1 year) OLT recipients with renal dysfunction (defined as a CrCl decreased by more than 25% compared with the first month after transplantation), Cantarovich and colleagues showed that the introduction of mycophenolate mofetil (MMF) followed by tapering of cyclosporine (CsA)

TABLE 194-3

Mycophenolate Mofetil as a Renal-Sparing Agent (in Patients with Renal Dysfunction)*

N	RENAL FUNCTION	INTERVENTION	OUTCOME	FOLLOW-UP	REF. NO.
19	>25% decrease in CrCl compared with first month after OLT	Institution of MMF; CsA tapered to 25 mg bid	Significant improvement in renal function; AR in 29%	1 yr	17
27	>20% decrease in renal function since OLT or SCr = 1.8-4.0 mg/dL or CrCl = 20-60 mL/min	Institution of MMF; 50% ↓ in CsA or Tac dose or discontinuation	Significant improvement in renal function; AR in 14% with MMF/↓Tac or MMF/no Tac; AR in 9% with MMF/↓CsA but 38% with MMF/no CsA	52 wk	18
45	SCr > 1.36 mg/dL or CrCl < 50 mL/min	2 g MMF monotherapy† or 2 g MMF + low-dose CNI	Improvement in SCr at long-term follow-up	32.5-34 mo (median)	19
12	SCr > 1.8 mg/dL	Introduction of MMF + 30-50% ↓ in Tac dose	Improvement in renal function in 7, deterioration in 4, no change in 1	6 yr	20
9	SCr > 2.2 mg/dL (biopsy-proven CNI toxicity)	Institution of MMF or AZA; CsA/Tac withdrawal	No significant improvement in renal function	9 mo	21
5	SCr > 1.7 mg/dL	MMF monotherapy (CNI ↓ and ultimately discontinued)	Severe AR requiring retransplantation in 2, severe steroid-responsive AR in 1	Trial halted	22

*See text for details.
†All other immunosuppressants withdrawn at 1 month.
AR, acute rejection; AZA, azathioprine; CNI, calcineurin inhibitor; CrCl, creatinine clearance; CsA, cyclosporin A (cyclosporine); MMF, mycophenolate mofetil; SCr, serum creatinine concentration; Tac, tacrolimus.

to a very low dose (25 mg twice a day) resulted in a significant improvement in renal function. At 1-year follow-up, the SCr had decreased from 141 ± 24 to 105 ± 22 μmol/L (*P* = .002), and the GFR had increased from 40 ± 13 to 64 ± 18 mL/min (*P* = .002). However, acute rejection occurred in 29% of the subjects studied, suggesting that this strategy may be associated with a risk of acute rejection.[17]

In a recent prospective, randomized, multicenter pilot study, Reich and coworkers demonstrated that in OLT recipients with renal dysfunction (defined as >20% reduction in renal function since OLT, an SCr of 1.8 to 4.0 mg/dL, or a CrCl of 20 to 60 mL/min), institution of MMF along with 50% dose reduction or discontinuation of cyclosporine or tacrolimus resulted in significant improvement in renal function at 52 weeks' follow-up. Five of six patients in the group receiving MMF and no CsA demonstrated greater than 15% improvement in renal function, and the remaining patient had no change in renal function. In the MMF/CsA reduction group, four of nine patients had greater than 15% improvement, three had no change in renal function, and two experienced deterioration in renal function. In the MMF/no tacrolimus group, two of five patients had greater than 15% improvement in renal function, and the remaining three had no change. In the MMF/tacrolimus dose reduction group, four of seven patients had greater than 15% improvement in renal function, and the remaining three had no change. The incidence of biopsy-proven acute rejection (BPR) was 14% for both groups in the tacrolimus trials; in the CsA trials, the rate of BPR was 9% for the CsA reduction groups and 38% for the CsA withdrawal groups. All BPRs were of mild to moderate intensity, and all were successfully treated with steroids, CNI increase or resumption, or both. Further analysis revealed that a prior history of rejection and high CsA levels before CsA withdrawal were risk factors for BPR after CNI withdrawal.[18]

In a series consisting of 45 patients with SCr levels greater than 120 μmol/L or CrCl rates of less than 50 mL/min, 2 g MMF, administered either as monotherapy (with all other immunosuppressants—CNI, azathioprine, and steroids—withdrawn in 1 month) or in combination with low-dose CNI, resulted in considerable improvement in SCr values at long-term follow-up.[19] In the MMF monotherapy group, death occurred in 3 of 11 patients at 7 to 18 months after beginning MMF monotherapy, but none of these deaths was the result of rejection. Of the remaining 8 patients, 5 had normal SCr and one required dialysis at a median follow-up of 35 months. Improvement in SCr was also seen in the MMF/low-dose CNI groups with a median follow-up of 32.5 to 34 months. Frequent rejection was seen only in those with previous repeated episodes of rejection and did not result in graft loss.

In a small series consisting of 12 patients with SCr greater than 1.8 mg/dL, the introduction of MMF along with 30% to 50% tacrolimus dose reduction resulted in improvement in renal function in seven patients, deterioration in four, and no change in one patient.[20] Overall mean SCr declined from 2.5 to 1.9 mg/dL at 6 months but increased to 2.2 mg/dL at 18 to 24 months. Thereafter, renal function remained stable for 72 months in all seven patients. Iothalamate clearance showed 18.5% improvement at 1 year. Suggested poor prognostic indicators included a starting SCr greater than 4.0 mg/dL and combined size of native kidney less than 20 cm. Elevated hepatic enzymes were noted in three patients during the first year. However, increasing baseline immunosuppression resulted in normalization of hepatic enzymes in all three patients.[20]

In contrast, Neau-Cransac and colleagues failed to demonstrate any significant improvement in renal function in OLT recipients (*N* = 9) with severe renal failure (defined as SCr ≥ 200 μmol/L or ≥2.2 mg/dL) and biopsy-proven chronic CNI nephrotoxicity despite cyclosporine or tacrolimus withdrawal and institution of either MMF or azathioprine. On the other hand, there was no increase in the incidence of graft rejection at a median follow-up of 9 months after CNI withdrawal. Of note, baseline biopsies revealed 60% glomerulosclerosis in 1 of the 9 patients (11%), 50% glomerulosclerosis in 2 (22%), 30% sclerosis in 2 (22%), 20% sclerosis in 1 (11%), and 10% sclerosis in 1 (11%). Glomerulosclerosis was not seen in 2 patients (22%). Interstitial fibrosis was seen in all 9 cases and tubular atrophy in 8.[21]

TABLE 194-4

Studies with Sirolimus as a Renal-Sparing Agent*

N	IMMUNOSUPPRESSION	OUTCOME	FOLLOW-UP	REF. NO.
185	Sirolimus monotherapy vs sirolimus + CNI vs CNI alone	Comparable patient and graft survival and AR rates in all 3 groups; in patients with baseline renal insufficiency, greatest improvement was seen with sirolimus monotherapy	12 mo	23
64	De novo sirolimus (29 patients) vs CNI to sirolimus conversion due to CNI nephrotoxicity or rejection (35 patients)	Higher rate of AR in the de novo compared with conversion group[†]	2 yr	24

AR, acute rejection; CNI, calcineurin inhibitor.
*See text for details.
[†]Note: patients with hepatocellular carcinoma or autoimmune disorders were selected to receive de novo sirolimus therapy per center protocols. See text for discussion.

Whereas most series studied to date have reported a low or acceptable rate of acute rejection when MMF was used as a renal-sparing agent, severe acute rejection episodes after manipulation of CNI therapy have also been reported. In a randomized, controlled trial of MMF monotherapy in long-term liver transplant patients (>1 year after OLT) who developed renal failure (SCr > 150 μmol/L or >1.7 mg/dL) associated with CNI therapy, two of five patients receiving MMF monotherapy developed severe rejection requiring retransplantation after 2 and 3 months, respectively, of MMF monotherapy. Of the remaining three patients, one developed steroid-responsive severe acute rejection after 3 weeks of monotherapy, and two patients had normal liver function tests after 2 weeks and 2 months of monotherapy, respectively. Although renal failure improved when the CNI dose was reduced and ultimately discontinued, the trial was halted due to the prohibitive risk of rejection.[22]

Early Experiences with Sirolimus as a Renal-Sparing Agent
De novo Sirolimus Immunosuppressive Therapy after Orthotopic Liver Transplantation

The studies described in this section are summarized in Table 194-4.

Sirolimus is a potent immunosuppressant with a mechanism of action and a side effect profile distinct from that of calcineurin inhibitors. When used as base therapy without a CNI, sirolimus has been shown to be devoid of nephrotoxicity. In a retrospective analysis consisting of 185 patients who underwent OLT, Zaghla and colleagues showed that sirolimus alone or in conjunction with CNI is safe and effective as an initial immunosuppressive agent in OLT.[23] One-year patient and graft survival and the rate of acute cellular rejection at 12 months were comparable among those who received sirolimus monotherapy ($n = 28$), sirolimus in combination therapy with CNI ($n = 56$), or CNI alone for immunosuppression ($n = 101$). The overall incidence of acute cellular rejection during the 12-month follow-up period for the sirolimus alone, sirolimus plus CNI, and CNI alone groups was 20%, 35%, and 31%, respectively ($P = .42$). In all patients, steroids were tapered off by the sixth month based on toxicity and rejection episodes, and the proportion of patients receiving MMF was comparable among the three treatment groups. Among patients with baseline renal insufficiency, the greatest improvement was seen in those receiving sirolimus without CNI therapy.

In a small series consisting of 29 recipients of OLT who were started on sirolimus immediately after transplantation (de novo group) and 35 OLT recipients who were converted from CNI to sirolimus due to nephrotoxicity or rejection, Sanchez and associates found a higher rate of acute cellular rejection in the de novo compared with the conversion groups: 17.2% (40% of which were steroid resistant) versus 2.8%, respectively, during a 2-year follow-up period. The investigators suggested that the use of sirolimus is not indicated in the immediate period after liver transplantation.[24] However, these data should be interpreted with caution. In their studies, patients with hepatocellular carcinoma or autoimmune disorders were selected to receive de novo sirolimus therapy according to center study and hepatocellular protocols, and recipients with autoimmune liver disease are at higher risk for both acute and chronic rejection.[25]

Sirolimus Conversion Therapy in Patients with Presumed or Biopsy-Proven Calcineurin Inhibitor Nephrotoxicity

The studies described in this section are summarized in Table 194-5.

In a retrospective study consisting of 16 long-term (>3 years) OLT recipients with renal insufficiency ranging from mild (CrCl > 70 mL/min) to severe (CrCl 20 to 40 mL/min), conversion from cyclosporine or tacrolimus to sirolimus-based immunosuppression resulted in variable improvement in renal function and no rejections at 6 months' follow-up.[26]

Similarly Sanchez and colleagues recently showed that sirolimus conversion after liver transplantation resulted in improvement in the GFR (assessed by iodine 125–labeled sodium iothalamate) at 2 years after conversion.[24] In their prospective study consisting of 2005 OLT recipients, 64 patients were administered sirolimus for various indications. In 32 patients, therapy was converted to sirolimus—in 27 because of nephrotoxicity (GFR ≤ 30 to 40 mL/min) and in 5 because of acute cellular rejection refractory to CNI optimization and steroid recycle therapy. Although a small number of patients in the postconversion group showed progressive decline in GFR, most regained GFR to match with case-control subjects at 1 and 2 years after conversion. (17 patients [56.7%] at 1 year and 8 [44.4%] at 2 years showed stable or continued improvement in GFR; progressive decline in GFR was

TABLE 194-5

Sirolimus Conversion Therapy (Cyclosporine or Tacrolimus to Sirolimus)

N	COMMENTS	RENAL FUNCTION AT CONVERSION	OUTCOME	FOLLOW-UP	REF. NO.
16	Time at conversion >3 yr post-OLT	CrCl range: >70 to 20-40 mL/min; no rejection	Variable improvement in renal function	6 mo	26
32	Conversion due to nephrotoxicity (27 patients) or refractory rejection (5 patients)	—	A small number of postconversion patients showed progressive ↓ in GFR, but most regained GFR to match case-control subjects at 1 and 2 yr after conversion; AR occurred in 2.8% of those converted due to CNI nephrotoxicity	—	24

AR, acute rejection; CNI, calcineurin inhibitor; CrCl, creatinine clearance; GFR, glomerular filtration rate; OLT, orthotopic liver transplantation.

seen in 8 patients [26.7%] at 1 year and in 5 patients [27.8%] at 2 years.) Conversion to sirolimus due to CNI nephrotoxicity resulted in one episode of acute cellular rejection (2.8%) and no episodes of steroid-resistant rejection.[24]

Our own opinion on the use of induction therapy and maintenance immunosuppression with sirolimus or MMF (or both) in CNI-sparing protocols is as follows. Due to the lack of large, prospective, controlled trials and the mixed results obtained from small series of patients, manipulation of immunosuppressive therapy to avoid nephrotoxicity should be tailored to each patient. In patients with HRS, MMF in conjunction with low-dose tacrolimus and standard steroid therapy appears to be safe and effective (unpublished observation). Although the use of interleukin-2 (IL-2) receptor blocker induction therapy in a CNI-sparing protocol has been reported to result in improvement in renal function without an increased risk of rejection, there have been anecdotal reports suggesting that the use of IL-2 receptor blockers in combination with MMF or sirolimus increases the risk of viral reactivation and/or the development of more severe hepatitis C recurrence after liver transplantation.[27,28] An increased incidence of hepatitis C virus (HCV) reactivation associated with IL-2 receptor blockers has also been observed at our center, reemphasizing that modification of immunosuppressive therapy should be individualized. Although early studies suggested that MMF may have a ribavirin-like antiviral effect and may provide synergism when used with interferon-alfa, its use in the post-transplantation period has not been consistently shown to be either beneficial or deleterious.

Studies on the association between an increased incidence and/or severity of HCV recurrence and the use of polyclonal antilymphocyte preparations and/or anti-OKT3 monoclonal antibody have also resulted in contradictory results.[1] In our opinion, these agents should be reserved for patients with delayed recovery of HRS or pretransplantation renal dysfunction, and for the treatment of acute rejection. Their routine use in a CNI-sparing protocol as prophylactic therapy is not recommended. In a subset of patients with renal dysfunction attributed to CNI nephrotoxicity, CNI to MMF or sirolimus conversion therapy can improve renal function without an increased risk of acute rejection. Withdrawal or minimization of CNI therapy appears to be safe and effective in patients with no prior rejection episodes and in those with minimal CNI requirement before withdrawal. Manipulation of immunosuppressive therapy in the face of severe renal failure (defined as SCr > 3.5 to 4 mg/dL) may be futile, and the added risks of acute rejection should be carefully weighed against the benefits.

Although they are invasive, renal biopsies may help direct therapy. When more than 25% to 40% of glomeruli were sclerosed or when greater than 20% to 30% interstitial fibrosis was present, progressive renal function deterioration has been observed in both primary renal disease and after renal transplantation.[29] However, it should also be noted that there is currently no proven cutoff value for the degree of glomerulosclerosis or interstitial fibrosis that accurately predicts the inexorable development of ESRD regardless of intervention. In patients with chronic renal insufficiency who have unrelenting renal failure despite drastic CNI dose reduction or withdrawal, the options available to prevent further decline in renal function remain contentious. Although angiotensin-converting enzyme inhibitors and/or angiotensin receptor blockers have been suggested to retard the progression of interstitial fibrosis, the role of these agents in halting or alleviating the progression of chronic CNI nephrotoxicity remains to be determined.

FACTORS AFFECTING RENAL DYSFUNCTION IN LONG-TERM SURVIVORS AFTER ORTHOTOPIC LIVER TRANSPLANTATION

Commonly suggested causes or risk factors for the development of progressive CKD or ESRD in long-term survivors of OLT include CNI nephrotoxicity (discussed in the previous section), pre-OLT HRS, preexisting renal insufficiency, development of hypertension, diabetes mellitus (before or after transplantation), and the use of nephrotoxic drugs. Postoperative ARF, dialysis requirement before and/or after transplantation, HCV infection, and older age have also been variably shown to be associated with an increased risk for development of CKD.[30-33] In patients undergoing transplantation for chronic hepatitis C, disease recurrence has been reported to accompany the development of HCV-associated cryoglobulinemia, leading to irreversible renal failure.[34] More recently, Campbell and colleagues suggested that the duration, but not the cause, of renal dysfunction in the pretransplantation period predicts renal outcome in OLT recipients.[35] Regardless of the etiological factors causing CKD, it is likely that the incidence of ESRD increases with time after transplantation.

TABLE 194-6

Factors Affecting Renal Dysfunction in Long-Term Survivors

Chronic CNI nephrotoxicity
Pre-OLT HRS
Preexisting renal insufficiency
Hypertension
Diabetes mellitus (preexisting or posttransplant diabetes mellitus)
Use of nephrotoxic drugs
Postoperative renal failure
Renal replacement therapy requirement in the pre- or post-transplant period
Hepatitis C infection
Duration of renal dysfunction prior to OLT
Older age

CNI, calcineurin inhibitor; HRS, hepatorenal syndrome; OLT, orthotopic liver transplantation.

Strategies to Reduce Risk Factors in Long-Term Survivors

In those patients with established CKD secondary to chronic CNI nephrotoxicity and no or minimal prior rejection episodes, the administration of MMF or sirolimus in conjunction with CNI dose reduction or withdrawal can be safe and effective. In addition, blood pressure control and aggressive management of comorbid conditions such as diabetes mellitus and dyslipidemia are recommended. Statins have been shown to be safe and effective in treating hypercholesterolemia after liver transplantation. Nonetheless, close monitoring of liver function tests following statin therapy is mandatory. Table 194-6 summarizes factors affecting renal dysfunction in long-term survivors after OLT.

CONCLUSION

In summary, ARF is common after OLT, whereas CKD and ESRD increase in incidence in long-term survivors who often have excellent function of their allograft. Identifying the risk factors for renal dysfunction and developing strategies to prevent, halt, or ameliorate renal function should be an integral part of management for candidates or recipients of liver transplants. Bleeding and infectious complications in the perioperative period should be sought and treated aggressively. Careful attention to management of fluid and electrolytes and avoidance of hypotensive episodes are imperative. Whether the use of the piggyback technique compared with the standard surgical technique (with or without VVB) significantly reduces the probability of ARF after liver transplantation remains to be defined. Therapeutic approaches in the postoperative period should be modified in patients with preexisting HRS or pretransplantation renal dysfunction. The use of IL-2 receptor blocker or antilymphocyte preparations may allow for the delayed introduction of CNI and preserve early renal function. Sirolimus-based immunosuppression without CNI may improve renal function in patients with baseline renal dysfunction. Delayed wound healing and development of severe thrombocytopenia may limit its use in the immediate postoperative period, particularly in recipients of liver transplantation. Whether de novo sirolimus immunosuppressive therapy increases the risk of acute rejection compared with conventional CNI therapy is unknown, and studies are awaited. The use of contrast studies or neph-

rotoxic drugs should be minimized or avoided. Although early transplantation of patients with baseline renal dysfunction may improve renal outcome after transplantation, the duration of renal failure in the pretransplantation period continues to be prolonged despite adoption of the MELD score for allocation of OLT,[29] which was designed to prioritize patients with renal insufficiency. Hence, careful selection of candidates for combined kidney-liver transplantation avoids added renal-related complications after liver transplantation.

Key Points

1. Pretransplant renal dysfunction and preexisting hepatorenal syndrome are well-established risk factors for post-transplant acute renal failure. The potential benefits of diuretics, lactulose, contrast dye exposure, or nephrotoxic medications must be carefully balanced against the risk of precipitating acute renal failure or hepatorenal syndrome.
2. Although large, prospective clinical trials are lacking, it is conceivable that intraoperative risk factors for the development of perioperative acute renal failure are similar to those in nontransplant surgical settings. Aggressive control of intraoperative bleeding, management of fluid and electrolyte abnormalities, and avoidance of hypotensive episodes are imperative in the perioperative period.
3. Post-transplant acute renal failure is likely multifactorial and may include ischemic or toxic insult to the kidneys, prolonged hypotension, sepsis, sustained prerenal renal failure, and the use of calcineurin inhibitors or other nephrotoxic drugs. Bleeding and infectious complications should be treated promptly and aggressively. The use of calcineurin inhibitor sparing protocols in patients with preexisting hepatorenal syndrome or pretransplant renal dysfunction should be individually tailored.
4. Manipulation of immunosuppressive therapy such as calcineurin inhibitor minimization or withdrawal in the face of severe renal failure may be futile. The added risks of acute rejection should be carefully weighed against the benefits.

Key References

1. Pham PT, Pham PC, Wilkinson AH: Renal failure in adult liver transplant recipients. In Busuttil RW, Klintmalm GB (eds): Transplantation of the Liver, 2nd ed. Philadelphia, Elsevier Saunders, 2005, pp 891-914.
3. Sanchez EQ, Gonwa TA, Levy MF: Preoperative and perioperative predictors of the need for renal replacement therapy after orthotopic liver transplantation. Transplantation 2004; 78:1048-1054.
5. Cabezuelo JB, Ramirez P, Rios A, et al: Risk factors of acute renal failure after liver transplantation. Kidney Int 2006;69: 1073-1080.
8. Pham PT, Pham PC, Rastogi A, Wilkinson AH: Current management of renal dysfunction in the cirrhotic patient [review article]. Aliment Pharmacol Ther 2005;21:949-961.
35. Campbell MS, Kotlyar DS, Bresinger CM, et al: Renal function after orthotopic liver transplantation is predicted by duration of pretransplantation creatinine elevation. Liver Transpl 2005;11:1048-1055.

See the companion Expert Consult website for the complete reference list.

CHAPTER 195

Pharmacological Treatment for Hepatorenal Syndrome

Emilios Andrikos and Olga Balafa

OBJECTIVES

This chapter will:
1. Report on the drugs used in clinical trials for patients with hepatorenal syndrome.
2. Describe their mechanisms of action.
3. Comment on their effectiveness, side effects, and clinical use.

Renal failure commonly complicates the clinical course of patients with cirrhosis. There are several factors contributing to renal function deterioration in cirrhosis (e.g., volume depletion, hemorrhagic shock, nephrotoxic drugs), but renal failure in these patients is most commonly characterized as hepatorenal syndrome (HRS). HRS is a unique form of functional and reversible renal failure in which the kidneys are histologically normal in the early stages. Two types are observed: HRS-1, which is characterized by rapidly progressive renal failure (serum creatinine >2.5 mg/dL or glomerular filtration rate [GFR] <20 mL/min) and a bad prognosis, and HRS-2, a chronic form that is characterized by moderate renal failure (serum creatinine >1.5 mg/dL or GRF < 40 mL/min) and a better prognosis.[1,2]

Liver cirrhosis is characterized by circulatory dysfunction due to splanchnic arterial vasodilation secondary to portal hypertension, which leads to a fall in systemic vascular resistance, hyperdynamic circulation, and sodium and water retention. The pathophysiological hallmark of HRS is severe vasoconstriction of the renal circulation. The underlying mechanisms are complex and not totally clarified. The most explanatory theory suggests that renal hypoperfusion and vasoconstriction represent an expression of arterial underfilling secondary to a marked vasodilation of the splanchnic vascular bed. Arterial underfilling leads to activation of the renin-angiotensin system (RAS) and the sympathetic nervous system (SNS), resulting in vasoconstriction. In the early stages, renal vasodilators maintain renal perfusion. However, with progression of the disease, the balance breaks and HRS occurs.[2,3]

GENERAL ASPECTS

Untreated HRS carries a high mortality rate. Spontaneous recovery occurs in only 3.5% of patients.[4] Liver transplantation is the only available treatment for HRS-1. However, not all patients with HRS-1 are suitable candidates for transplantation. Moreover, an organ is often not available in a timely manner for those who are candidates for transplantation, and patients with HRS have a lower probability of postoperative survival than patients without HRS.[5] Therefore, pharmacological treatment for all of these patients is essential.

The ideal treatment of HRS-1 must fulfill at least the following aims: (1) reduction of serum creatinine to less than 1.5 mg/dL; (2) prolongation of survival, which may increase the chance of receiving a liver transplant; and (3) avoidance of serious adverse events.[6]

The most important goal in HRS treatment is improving renal perfusion and GFR. The best results have been obtained with systemic vasoconstrictors that reduce the splanchnic vasodilation, increase the arterial pressure, and suppress the vasodilators activated in HRS. These drugs include vasopressin analogues and α-adrenergic agonists. Their use in combination with plasma volume expanders (e.g., albumin) seems to be effective in reversing some of the clinical features of HRS-1 and may even postpone renal failure (Table 195-1).[7]

Patients with HRS-2 are less sick, and their refractory ascites can be managed with large-volume paracentesis accompanied by albumin infusion and/or transjugular intrahepatic portosystemic shunt (TIPS). Limited data support the efficacy of vasoconstrictors in the treatment of HRS-2.

Vasopressin Analogues

Ornipressin and terlipressin (a synthetic derivative of vasopressin) act on V_1 receptors present on vascular smooth muscle cells in the mesentery and skin. These agents reverse the overactivity of the SNS and RAS and stimulate release of atrial natriuretic protein (ANP). Both drugs are nonselective splanchnic vasoconstrictors that reduce blood flow to splanchnic organs, diminishing portal pressure. Vasopressin analogues are not universally available (e.g., in the United States).

Acute intravenous administration of ornipressin induces splanchnic vasoconstriction, increases mean arterial pressure and pulmonary capillary wedge pressure, and increases plasma renal flow and GFR.[8] In clinical studies, it seems to be effective in reversing HRS, but the high frequency of ischemic side effects limits its use.[9-11]

The most studied agent effective in managing HRS is the vasopressin analogue, terlipressin. The administration of terlipressin (0.5 to 2 mg IV every 4 to 6 hours) is associated with an improvement in renal function in 42% to 92% of patients treated in various studies, with an average of 63%.[12-27] In a small study, Therapondos and colleagues demonstrated that a bolus injection of terlipressin produced an increase in median arterial pressure and systemic vascular resistance, along with a reduction in cardiac output without a reduction in renal blood flow.[12] However, most of the reported studies have been retrospective, nonrandomized, and performed in small numbers of patients

TABLE 195-1

Recommendations for Using Vasoconstrictor Agents in Patients with Hepatorenal Syndrome Type 1

1. Goal of treatment: reduction of the serum creatinine concentration to <1.5 mg/dL
2. Recommended drugs and doses
   A. Terlipressin, 0.5 mg IV q4h-q6h. The dose can be increased every 2-3 days up to 1 mg/4 hr. The maximum dose should not exceed 2 mg/4 hr
   B. Midodrine, 2.5-7.5 mg PO tid (maximum, 12.5 mg tid) *plus* octreotide, 100 µg SC tid (maximum, 200 µg tid)
   C. Noradrenaline, 0.5-3 mg/hr IV
3. Concomitant infusion of albumin solution
4. Terlipressin should be avoided in patients with a history of coronary heart disease, cerebrovascular disease, hypertension, or asthma

including both HRS-1 and HRS-2. To date, the only prospective controlled trial was performed by Solanki and colleagues and evaluated treatment of HRS-1 with terlipressin versus placebo.[13] At 2 weeks after initiation of treatment, none of the patients in the placebo group but 5 (of 12) patients in the terlipressin group were still alive. All survivors had improved renal function and increased arterial pressure. Improvement of renal function has been associated with increased survival in retrospective studies.[14,15] The predictive factors for survival were the absence of a precipitating factor for HRS, terlipressin-induced improvement in renal function, and a Child-Pugh score of 11 or less at inclusion.

The optimal dose and duration of the therapy are not well defined, although in most studies dosages of 4 to 6 mg/day (divided into two to three doses) are used. The recommended dose is 0.5 mg IV every 4 hours; it can be increased in a stepwise fashion (every 2 to 3 days) to 1 mg/4 hr and then up to 2 mg/4 hr in refractory cases.[7] It seems that the higher the Child-Pugh score, the greater the dose required.[7] Most patients respond in the first days, and the treatment is continued until HRS resolves. The duration of therapy ranges from 7 to 15 days. Many patients relapse after treatment is discontinued (50%). Retreatment of recurrence may be effective.[21,22]

The explanation for the lack of improvement in some patients is unknown. Probably vasoconstriction/vasoactivation is not the only mechanism of HRS in cirrhotic patients. The terlipressin may also elicit a cardiac output reduction by inducing coronary vasoconstriction.[28] Moreover, the drug may be ineffective due to arterial hyporeactivity in cirrhotic patients in response to exogenous vasoconstriction.[29]

The drug is often administered with human albumin solution. This combination is effective, but whether the albumin has a role other than for volume expansion is controversial.[16,18] Certain patients treated with albumin seem to become "good hemodynamic responders" to terlipressin and thus become renal responders to the drug. However, hemodynamic monitoring studies investigating this theory are absent.

Ischemic side effects with terlipressin are uncommon (15%). The drug acts as a vasodilator in cerebral arteries, and it seems that its use in patients with severe acute liver failure may cause deleterious consequences on cerebral hemodynamics.[30] In general, its use should be avoided in older patients with a history of coronary heart disease, cerebrovascular disease, hypertension, or asthma.[7]

Although its use is controversial, the drug may have a role in the prevention of renal failure in patients with advanced liver disease who develop bacterial peritonitis. This effect may be due to prevention of postparacentesis circulatory instability.[31,32]

α-Adrenergic Agonists
Midodrine

Midodrine is an oral α-adrenergic agonist. Combination therapy with octreotide (a somatostatin analogue) may be effective and safe. In small studies, treatment with midodrine and octreotide appeared to be associated with a significant reduction of creatinine and reduction in mortality.[33-36] The relative contribution of octreotide or midodrine to the successful treatment is unknown, and a synergistic effect seems to exist. Midodrine acts as a systemic vasoconstrictor, whereas octreotide is an inhibitor of the release of endogenous vasodilators (glucagons and vasoactive intestinal peptide).

Octreotide alone does not appear to be effective.[33] One study compared octreotide and a combination of midodrine and octreotide. Midodrine significantly decreased cardiac index and heart rate and increased mean arterial pressure and systemic vascular resistance. Octreotide caused a decrease in renal vascular resistance and increased renal blood flow but significantly reduced GFR. The addition of midodrine to octreotide did not modify renal hemodynamics and function, compared with baseline, but caused an almost insignificant minor increase in renal vascular resistance and a significant minor decrease in renal blood flow, compared with octreotide alone.[34]

In one study of 13 patients with HRS-1, 5 were given midodrine (7.5 to 12.5 mg three times daily) and octreotide (100 to 200 µg three times daily), and 8 were given dopamine. Both groups also received albumin daily. All of the patients receiving the combination therapy had improved renal function (higher GFR, lower serum creatinine, and increased urine volume), and four of them successfully underwent transplantation. On the other hand, seven of the patients receiving dopamine alone died during the first 12 days, although their renal function was stabilized or improved.[35]

Norepinephrine

Norepinephrine has been evaluated in the treatment of HRS. Duvoux and colleagues treated 12 patients with norepinephrine (0.5 to 3 mg/hr IV to obtain an increase in mean arterial pressure of at least 10 mm Hg), albumin and furosemide. Ten responded completely and three underwent successful transplantation. However, when the short-term effect of norepinephrine on GFR or renal plasma flow was evaluated, no effect was measured. One patient sustained an episode of myocardial hypokinesia.[37]

Other Drugs
Misoprostol

Oral ingestion of high doses of the prostaglandin analogue misoprostol (0.4 mg four times daily) with albumin infusion was used in one study to improve renal hemodynamics. However, the data are preliminary and conflicting, so its use in HRS is not recommended.[38-40]

N-Acetylcysteine

It is known that N-acetylcysteine improves serum creatinine in an experimental animal model of acute cholestasis and renal failure.[41] Infusion of N-acetylcysteine was evaluated in a pilot study in patients with HRS. It appears to improve creatinine clearance, urine output, and sodium excretion. It is well tolerated and probably minimizes splanchnic vasodilation and NO production.[42] However, NAC also decreases serum creatinine without changes in GFR in healthy humans, suggesting that other mechanisms, including decreased creatinine production and tubular secretion, may be responsible for the apparent beneficial effect.[43]

Endothelin Antagonist

Endothelin-1 is a potent vasoconstrictor, and recent studies have sustained its probable role in HRS.[44] The endothelin receptor antagonist BQ123 was associated with an increase in GFR in four patients with HRS, but all died.[45]

CONCLUSION

Vasoconstrictor drugs seem to be effective for treatment of HRS-1. However, large randomized, controlled studies are needed to evaluate the best treatment option in HRS. Furthermore, no study has compared terlipressin to α_1-agonists. Future studies should also evaluate the use of these drugs in the treatment of HRS-2.

Key Points

1. Vasoconstrictor drugs (vasopressin analogues and α-adrenergic agonists) seem to be effective for treatment of hepatorenal syndrome type 1.
2. Their action is based on the reduction of splanchnic vasodilation and increased arterial pressure to suppress the vasoconstrictors activated in hepatorenal syndrome.
3. Among them, the most effective agents appear to be terlipressin and the combination of midodrine and octreotide.

Key References

2. Arroyo V, Colmenero J: Ascites and hepatorenal syndrome in cirrhosis: Pathophysiological basis of therapy and current management. J Hepatol 2003;38:S69-S89.
7. Moreau R, Lebrec D: The use of vasocontrictors in patients with cirrhosis: Type 1 HRS and beyond. Hepatology 2006;43:385-394.
13. Solanki P, Chawla A, Garg R, et al: Beneficial effects of terlipressin in hepatorenal syndrome: A prospective, randomized placebo-controlled clinical trial. J Gastroenterol Hepatol 2003;18:152-156.
15. Moreau R, Durand F, Poynard T, et al: Terlipressin in patients with cirrhosis and type 1 hepatorenal syndrome: A retrospective multicenter study. Gastroenterology 2002;122:923-930.
33. Pomier-Layragues G, Paquin SC, Hassoun Z, et al: Octreotide in hepatorenal syndrome: A randomized, double-blind, placebo-controlled, crossover study. Hepatology 2003;38:238-243.

See the companion Expert Consult website for the complete reference list.

CHAPTER 196

Extracorporeal Liver Support and the Kidney

Ashita Tolwani and Keith Wille

OBJECTIVES

This chapter will:
1. Discuss the indications for liver support systems.
2. Describe the design of the nonbiological and biological liver support systems.
3. Review the current literature on the application of liver support devices in the care of the patient with liver failure.

PURPOSE OF LIVER EXTRACORPOREAL DEVICES

The objective of liver support systems is to bridge patients with liver failure to either transplantation or recovery through detoxification, biosynthesis of products, and regulation of inflammation (Table 196-1). Liver support systems can be divided into two broad categories: nonbiological systems and biological systems (Table 196-2). Nonbiologi-

TABLE 196-1

Goals of Therapy with Liver Support Devices

Primary Goal
In acute liver failure: recovery to normal health
In acute-on-chronic liver failure: recovery to the state before
  decompensation
Alternative Goals
Bridge to liver transplantation
Prevention of progression to liver failure
Improvement of end-organ function in established
  multiorgan failure

TABLE 196-2

Extracorporeal Liver Support Systems

Nonbiological Systems
Hemofiltration
Hemoperfusion techniques
Plasma exchange
Albumin dialysis
Biological Systems
Extracorporeal whole liver perfusion
Cross-circulation
Hybrid bioartificial liver support systems

cal systems do not incorporate tissue and provide only detoxification functions using membranes and adsorbents. Biological systems aim to provide the excretory, synthetic, and metabolic functions of the liver through the use of living liver cells. This chapter focuses on the evolution and adaptation of kidney dialysis concepts to liver support systems.

NONBIOLOGICAL SYSTEMS

The success of hemodialysis in removing toxins in cases of renal failure led to the rationale for using extracorporeal therapy to remove circulating toxins resulting from liver failure by means of filtration or adsorption techniques.

Hemodialysis

Hemodialysis was introduced in the 1950s as a successful technique for treating renal failure by removing uremic toxins with a molecular weight of less than 5 kDa through diffusion. This approach was applied to patients with liver failure as an attempt to remove dialyzable, small-molecular-weight toxins, such as ammonia, that were thought to cause hepatic encephalopathy. Hemodialysis was first tried by Kiley and coworkers in 1958, who noted improved neurological function in four of five patients but no improvement in survival.[1] Uncontrolled small trials throughout the 1970s and 1980s failed to show a survival benefit with conventional dialysis in acute-on-chronic liver failure (ACLF) or fulminant hepatic failure (FHF) with low-permeability membranes; this led to the conclusion that the protein-bound toxins in liver failure could not be removed by the traditional dialysis membrane.

Hemofiltration

In 1976, the development of the polyacrylonitrile (PAN) membrane permitted the removal of molecules up to a molecular weight of 15 kDa using filtration techniques, and there was renewed interest in applying this therapy to patients with liver failure.[2] However, uncontrolled trials again demonstrated no survival benefit for either high-permeability dialysis or hemofiltration, and investigators began combining hemofiltration with other techniques. Continuous hemofiltration has been used in liver failure to avoid the increase in intracranial pressure caused by rapid changes in plasma osmolality during intermittent hemodialysis.[3]

Hemoperfusion

Because hemodialysis and hemofiltration remove only water-soluble toxins, hemoperfusion was introduced in the 1960s to increase the efficacy of dialysis by circulating blood over a sorbent material for the purpose of removing protein-bound toxins. These sorbents included charcoal, synthetic resins, and ion exchange resins. Charcoal removes water-soluble and protein-bound molecules in the range of 0.5 to 5 kDa but requires coating with albumin or encapsulation in hydrophilic gels to prevent complement activation and the removal of platelets and leukocytes. Synthetic resins remove lipid-soluble and protein-bound molecules, whereas ion exchange resins remove both ionic and organic compounds. Although initial studies and clinical reports with charcoal demonstrated improved neurological status, a randomized controlled trial by O'Grady and colleagues demonstrated no survival benefit.[4]

Plasmapheresis

Plasmapheresis, or plasma exchange, has been used in patients with liver failure since the 1970s. Plasma is separated from the cellular blood components with the use of a centrifuge or a membrane. The separated plasma is discarded and replaced with an equivalent volume of fresh plasma. This technique removes circulating liver toxins such as mercaptans, γ-aminobutyric acid, phenols, and aromatic amino acids and supplies proteins normally synthesized by the liver. Although numerous small, uncontrolled trials have been performed with various forms of plasmapheresis, including standard plasma exchange, high-volume plasma exchange with hemofiltration, continuous-flow membrane plasmapheresis, and high-volume plasmapheresis, none has shown a definite survival benefit despite improvements in neurological function and coagulation indices. Furthermore, the usefulness of this approach is limited by the large amount of plasma needed, ineffective removal of intracellular protein- and tissue-bound toxins, and complications of pulmonary edema, infection, and hypocalcemia from citrate intoxication.

Hemodiabsorption

Hemodiabsorption is a cross between hemodialysis and hemoperfusion; blood is passed through a hemodialyzer that contains a suspension of sorbents on the dialysate side. The smaller particle size and larger surface area of the charcoal in the sorbent suspension allow for a greater capacity of adsorption than with hemoperfusion columns. The BioLogic-DT sorption-suspension dialyzer made by HemoCleanse, Inc. (West Lafayette, Indiana), was the first device available for clinical use. The patient's blood is circulated, via a venous catheter, through a cellulose plate dialyzer, a sodium-loaded cation exchange resin suspension, and a charcoal suspension, permitting clearance of positively charged molecules and liver toxins up to 5 kDa. The largest prospective randomized trial enrolled 56 patients and demonstrated improved neurological status and blood pressure in patients treated with the device.[5] In 1996, the HemoCleanse BioLogic-DT was approved for use in the United States by the Federal Drug Administration (FDA) for the treatment of hepatic encephalopathy and serious drug overdose.

Albumin Dialysis

Albumin is an abundant plasma protein that binds to many non–water-soluble toxins that accumulate in liver failure, including bilirubin, bile acids, nitric oxide, fatty acids, mercaptans, thiols, and copper endogenous benzodiazepines. Various detoxification methods allowing for the removal of albumin-bound toxins have been investigated. Whereas whole blood exchange and plasma exchange techniques discard the patient's albumin and do not regenerate it, the albumin dialysis systems aim to remove the albumin-bound toxic ligands without removal of the patient's albumin.

Molecular Adsorbents Recirculating System

The Molecular Adsorbents Recirculating System (MARS; Teraklin, Rostock, Germany) is the best studied liver support device worldwide and to date has been used in approximately 4500 patients in more than 100 hospitals. MARS is commercially available and removes both water-soluble and albumin-bound toxic metabolites by utilizing a standard hemodialysis machine, a specialized high-flux dialyzer, and an albumin-enriched dialysate. The indications and contraindications of MARS are listed in Table 196-3.

The MARS uses a hollow-fiber membrane with albumin-related binding sites of 50 to 60 kDa and dialyzes the patient's blood while maintaining a constant flow of albumin-enriched dialysate in the extracapillary compartment (Fig. 196-1). The 50- to 60-kDa size limit prevents endogenous albumin, hormones, and carrier proteins from

passing through the membrane. After the toxins are transported across the MARS membrane, they attach to the albumin in the dialysate. The dialysate containing the albumin-bound toxins is then itself dialyzed against a bicarbonate-based dialysate, allowing for removal of water-soluble toxins such as urea and creatinine. Next, it passes through two adsorber columns containing activated charcoal and an anion exchange resin. These columns extract albumin-bound toxins, thereby regenerating the albumin dialysate for recirculation and additional toxin removal.

Although there are few randomized controlled trials comparing MARS with standard medical therapy, most studies have demonstrated that MARS improves both patient survival and clinical markers of disease severity in ACLF. The latest randomized, controlled trial included 24 patients with ACLF and hyperbilirubinemia who were randomized to either MARS ($n = 12$) or standard medical therapy ($n = 12$).[6] Patients receiving MARS had a greater reduction in bilirubin, bile acid, and creatinine levels, with improvement in mean arterial pressure and encephalopathy grade, compared to controls. Patients treated with MARS also had a significant improvement in 30-day survival (11/12 patients, versus 6/11 in the control group). However, a recent meta-analysis based on four, small randomized trials concluded that MARS offered no significant survival benefit over standard medical care for patients with liver failure.[7] Larger. multicenter, randomized trials examining MARS therapy in ACLF are currently being conducted.

MARS is also being used in some instances for the treatment of acute liver failure (ALF). Experience from a single center in Helsinki suggests a potential benefit in sustaining patients until either liver transplantation can be performed

TABLE 196-3

Indications and Contraindications of MARS Therapy

Indications
Acute-on-chronic liver failure
Severe alcoholic hepatitis
Severe pruritus due to cholestasis
Intoxication from protein-bound substances
Relative Contraindications
Progressive coagulopathy indicative of DIC
Uncontrolled sepsis
Uncontrolled bleeding

DIC, disseminated intravascular coagulation; MARS, Molecular Adsorbents Recirculating System.

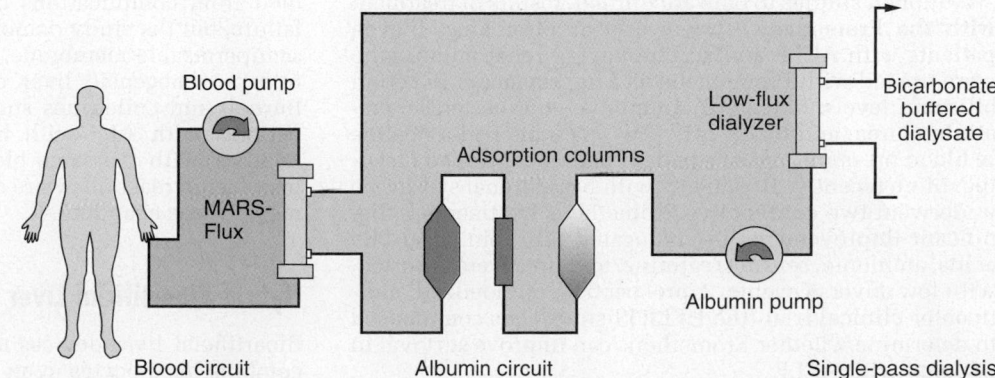

FIGURE 196-1. Schematic representation of the Molecular Adsorbent Recirculating System (MARS) circuit. (Reproduced with permission from Teraklin, Rostock, Germany).

or recovery occurs. Controlled clinical trials will be necessary before any firm recommendations for the use of this system in ALF can be made.

Other potential applications of MARS include primary biliary cirrhosis, Wilson's disease, benign recurrent intrahepatic cholestasis, drug-induced liver injury, liver failure after paracetamol intoxication, primary nonfunction after liver transplantation, cytotoxic mushroom poisoning, and acute chromium-copper intoxication. MARS therapy has been variably successful in these clinical situations.[8-14]

In general, MARS treatment is well tolerated, and the only consistently reported adverse effect is thrombocytopenia. The thrombocytopenia associated with MARS is usually asymptomatic and rarely requires discontinuation of therapy. However, there is consensus that MARS should be contraindicated in patients with disseminated intravascular coagulopathy (DIC). Unlike some liver assist devices, MARS is not associated with the loss of clotting factors, hormone-binding proteins, or acute phase reactants.[15] Yet, MARS may lower the concentration of albumin-bound drugs, and therefore appropriate drug level monitoring with MARS is typically warranted.

Single-Pass Albumin Dialysis

Single-pass albumin dialysis (SPAD) is a modification of MARS in which the albumin solution is passed only once through the dialysate compartment of the dialyzer and then discarded. One study found that SPAD was as effective as MARS in removing albumin-bound toxins and even more efficient than MARS in removing ammonia.[16]

Prometheus

The Prometheus liver support system (Fresenius, Bad Homburg, Germany) is a variant of albumin dialysis that combines fractionated plasma separation and adsorption (FPSA) with high-flux hemodialysis using a 250-kDa semipermeable membrane. The Prometheus device uses a special filter that separates blood cells and larger proteins from plasma, albumin, and smaller protein molecules. The albumin-containing plasma-like solution then passes through two adsorbers that detach and bind toxins associated with albumin. After adsorption, the patient's plasma and purified albumin are recombined with blood cells, and dialysis is performed to remove water-soluble toxins. Because the entire process requires no exogenous albumin, the method is more cost-effective than MARS or SPAD. Prometheus, in sum, blends adsorption for the removal of albumin-bound toxins with diffusion for the management of water-soluble substances.

Although studies to date are limited, results of treatment with the Prometheus system appear promising. Eleven patients with ACLF and accompanying renal failure who were treated with Prometheus had improvement in serum bilirubin levels, bile acids, ammonia, cholinesterase, creatinine, urea, and blood pH.[17] Two patients had a decline in blood pressure, and one patient had uncontrolled bleeding. More recently, 10 patients with hepatorenal syndrome underwent two consecutive Prometheus treatments.[18] Significant improvements in conjugated bilirubin, total bile acids, ammonia, serum creatinine, and urea were reported, with few adverse events. A prospective, randomized, multicenter clinical trial (the HELIOS study) has commenced to determine whether Prometheus can improve survival in patients with ACLF.

BIOLOGICAL SYSTEMS

The inability of nonbiological filtration techniques to perform the multiple functions of the liver provided a rationale for the development of biological liver support systems in which living liver tissue is used to perform hepatic functions.

Extracorporeal Whole Liver Perfusion

The need for hepatic tissue for the effective treatment of liver failure led to the concept of using the whole liver in an extracorporeal perfusion system. Through a circuit configuration, the patient's arterial blood is pumped to the portal vein of an isolated xenogeneic or allogeneic whole liver and from the inferior vena cava of the liver back to the patient's venous circulation. Eiseman performed the first clinical study in 1965, using extracorporeal pig liver perfusion for the treatment of severe hepatic encephalopathy.[19] There was some improvement in encephalopathy but no improvement in survival. Multiple small studies utilizing mainly porcine livers have demonstrated improvement in neurological outcome. However, most of these studies have been reports of single cases and cannot be used to make a definitive conclusion about the efficacy of this treatment. Furthermore, the immunological implications of perfusion of human blood through a xenogeneic liver and the potential for transmission of disease are unknown. Extracorporeal perfusion using human or baboon livers may provide additional benefits, but these techniques are limited by the supply of suitable donors.

Liver-tissue hemoperfusion using fresh or frozen liver slices rather than whole organs has also been studied; however, obtaining tissue pieces and maintaining adequate nutrient and oxygen supplies have been problematic. Direct implantation of hepatocytes in the peritoneal cavity and spleen is another technique that has been used to treat liver failure, but there is no agreement on the method, site of implantation, or volume of cells needed.

Cross-Circulation

Cross-circulation involves connecting the circulation of the patient with liver failure to that of another person to allow blood from the patient to be treated by the liver of the healthy person. In 1959, Kimoto first studied cross-dialysis using a cation exchange filter between a human patient and a dog.[20] The nitrogenous waste products were dramatically reduced in the human blood, and no anti-canine antibodies were detected. The patient eventually died from complications of volume overload and heart failure, but the study demonstrated that, with the use of a semipermeable membrane, detectable immune activation from a xenogeneic liver could be prevented. In 1967, Burnell and colleagues successfully treated one of three patients with ALF with human cross-circulation using relatives with the same blood groups.[21] However, severe transfusion reactions were observed in all donors, and this method was abandoned.

Hybrid Bioartificial Liver Support Systems

Bioartificial liver devices are extracorporeal devices that combine hepatocytes in an extracorporeal circuit, through which the patient's blood or plasma is perfused. The "biological" portion is designed to provide the synthetic functions of the liver, while the "artificial" portion provides detoxification through methods used in dialysis. The basic components of a bioartificial liver consist of hepatocytes within a reactor, membranes for cell retention and mass transfer, oxygenation to maintain cell function and viability, and heat exchangers to maintain cells at physiological temperatures. Charcoal columns are incorporated in some systems to allow removal of certain organic substances prior to cell contact. Some systems use whole blood, and others use plasma. Use of the patient's whole blood allows for a simpler configuration of the device but is associated with thrombocytopenia and hemolysis and requires anticoagulation with heparin. Use of plasma complicates the design of the system but decreases the need for anticoagulation and provides an additional separation between the hepatocytes and blood.

The most popular design uses capillary hollow-fiber membranes, made of small-diameter cellulose acetate tubes enclosed within a rigid polycarbonate housing. This system provides for a large surface area and minimizes the mass transfer distance between the intraluminal compartment within the fibers and the extraluminal compartment outside the fibers. Communication between the two compartments occurs through pores in the fiber walls. Hepatocytes, in conjunction with microcarriers, attach to the extraluminal compartment of the hollow-fiber membranes or are entrapped within a gel biomatrix within the intraluminal compartment. Nutrient medium is circulated through the compartments, and the hollow-fiber membranes are perfused with the patient's blood or plasma.

Difficulties in the Design of Bioartificial Liver Support Systems

Difficulties in designing an effective bioartificial liver support system include issues related to the source and storage of hepatocytes, cell mass, and membrane type.

SOURCE AND STORAGE OF HEPATOCYTES. Human and porcine hepatocytes are the most predominant sources of hepatocytes used in bioartificial livers. Primary human hepatocytes are the preferred cellular components but are short in supply. In addition, they have limited viability in culture, because they replicate only for a finite time and lose function rapidly. Human cell lines provide an endless supply of cells but lack important metabolic activities because they are not fully differentiated as normal hepatocytes. The C3A/HepG2 cell line, developed by Sussman and colleagues,[22] is derived from human hepatoblastoma cells and can express many normal liver-specific metabolic pathways; however, concern exists regarding its tumorigenic potential. HHY41, another immortalized human hepatocyte cell line that retains many liver-specific functions and is particularly resistant to acetaminophen, is currently under investigation.[23] The advantage to using primary porcine hepatocytes is easy availability; disadvantages include immunological risks related to porcine protein exposure and the potential for transmission of infectious agents, such as the porcine endogenous retrovirus (PERV), across species.

The bioartificial livers can be seeded with fresh cells or with thawed hepatocytes after cryopreservation. Cryopreservation results in a 10% to 25% loss of viability.[24] Culture of the cells in the reactor before treatment increases their functionality due to cell-cell interactions, but the cells must be maintained with circulating medium for a

TABLE 196-4

Bioartificial Liver Support Device Designs

HepatAssist 2000
ELAD (Extracorporeal Liver Assist Device)
BLSS (Bioartificial Liver Support System)
MELS (Modular Extracorporeal Liver System)
LIVERX2000 System
AMC-BAL (Academic Medical Centre Bioartificial Liver)

specific amount of time before they can be used for treatment. Factors that influence the viability and function of cultured hepatocytes include the presence of an extracellular matrix, growth factor availability, and preservation of three-dimensional hepatocyte orientation.

CELL MASS. The minimal quantity of cells needed to provide adequate liver function in a bioartificial liver is unknown. Based on hepatic resection studies in humans, approximately 10% to 30% of liver parenchyma is required for effective support. This corresponds to approximately 150 to 450 g of hepatocytes to support an adult patient.[16]

MEMBRANE TYPE. Bioartificial livers utilize membranes to retain the hepatocytes, prevent hepatocyte–blood cell contact, and maximize mass transfer of toxins, oxygen, and nutrients to the hepatocytes and synthetic products to the patient's blood. As a result, membranes require a pore size that is large enough (typically a molecular weight cutoff of 100 kDa) to allow for the influx of albumin-bound liver toxins but small enough to prevent exposure of hepatocytes to immunoglobulins, complement, and immunocompetent cells. Pore sizes of about 200 nm allow passage of immunological mediators. However, viral particles range from 30 to 200 nm in size and can pass through membranes with a molecular weight cutoff of 100 kDa, increasing the risk of xenozoonosis during treatment with porcine hepatocytes.[25] Hepatoma cells have also been found to pass through membranes with a 100-kDa cutoff.

Bioartificial Liver Support Device Designs

The various bioartificial liver support devices are listed in Table 196-4.

HEPATASSIST SYSTEM. The HepatAssist System (Circe Biomedical, Lexington, MA) is an extracorporeal, porcine-based liver assist device. With this technique, patients first undergo plasmapheresis, and the separated plasma passes through an activated charcoal adsorption column, where small-molecular-weight toxins are removed. Second, a heat exchanger and membrane oxygenator are used to warm the plasma and provide oxygen for the hepatocytes. Third, the plasma passes through a microporous hollow-fiber cartridge lined with viable porcine hepatocytes (5 to 7 × 10⁹ cells). This cartridge contains a matrix that provides surface area for hepatocyte attachment and promotes cell-cell matrix interaction. The porcine hepatocytes are cryopreserved but can be thawed and available in as little as 3 hours for treatment. After detoxification by the hepatocytes, plasma and blood components are returned together to the patient.

The largest controlled trial to date examining the HepatAssist System was published in 2004.[26] In this multi-center trial, Demetriou and colleagues randomly assigned 171 patients (147 with FHF and 24 with primary graft nonfunction) to the HepatAssist System or standard medical care. There was no difference in 30-day survival between groups for the entire study population (71% for HepatAssist versus 62% for standard treatment; $P = .26$); however, for patients with FHF, HepatAssist appeared to offer a survival benefit (73%, versus 59% for standard treatment; $P = .12$). This finding was not observed for patients with primary graft nonfunction. The results of this study were notably confounded by the impact of liver transplantation, which was ultimately performed in 54% of participants. After controlling for transplantation as well as other factors (e.g., etiology, encephalopathy grade) that might have influenced survival, HepatAssist was found to reduce mortality by 47% in patients with FHF. Despite these findings, the FDA has requested a phase III trial. A second-generation HepatAssist device is also under evaluation.

EXTRACORPOREAL LIVER ASSIST DEVICE. The Extracorporeal Liver Assist Device (ELAD; Vital Therapies, San Diego, CA) is similar to the HepatAssist System, except that it incorporates human hepatocytes from the hepatoblastoma-derived C3A/HepG2A cell line. This system comprises four hollow-fiber cartridges that each contain approximately 200 g of hepatocytes. The patient's plasma is separated and then circulated through the ELAD System, where detoxification occurs. The C3A human hepatocyte cell line can be produced in unlimited quantities and easily stored for delivery.

A pilot controlled trial (24 patients, of whom 17 were considered to have recoverable causes of liver failure) showed that ELAD, compared with standard medical care, led to marginal improvements in ammonia levels and encephalopathy in patients with ALF.[27] Survival did not differ between treatment and control groups, although the trial was not sufficiently powered for this end point. In a more recent phase I randomized trial in patients with FHF listed for liver transplantation, 11 (92%) of 12 ELAD patients underwent transplantation, compared with 3 (43%) of 7 controls ($P < .05$).[28] Ten of 12 ELAD patients survived to 30 days, compared with 3 of 7 controls ($P = .12$). Given the potential benefit of ELAD for patients awaiting and receiving liver transplantation, additional randomized trials are underway.

BIOARTIFICIAL LIVER SUPPORT SYSTEM. The Bioartificial Liver Support System (BLSS; Excorp Medical, Oakdale, MN) also uses primary porcine hepatocytes (cell mass, 70 to 100 g) embedded in a collagen medium and a hollow-fiber design. In contrast to other systems, whole blood is perfused through the BLSS system, and heparin is used as an anticoagulant. In a phase I pilot safety study, four patients with ALF or ACLF were evaluated.[29] Treatments lasted 12 hours and were well tolerated. Some improvement in serum ammonia, but not bilirubin, was observed. Although three patients died several days after treatment, one underwent successful transplantation 16 days after BLSS. The results of additional clinical trials are anticipated.

MODULAR EXTRACORPOREAL LIVER SYSTEM. The Modular Extracorporeal Liver System (MELS; Charite Virchow Clinic, Berlin) is a hollow-fiber system that utilizes human hepatocytes from livers considered to be unsuitable for transplantation. The MELS device consists of several components, including hepatocytes within a bioreactor, albumin-based dialysis, and continuous venovenous hemofiltration, which together detoxify plasma. The hepatocyte aggregates (cell mass, 400 to 600 g) are incubated for about 3 weeks after inoculation of the bioreactor and form a three-dimensional framework resembling sinusoids. Cells may survive within this system for

as long as 8 weeks. Studies to date have shown that MELS is well tolerated and can serve as a successful bridge to transplantation. However, continued investigation of MELS may be limited by the availability of human hepatocytes.

LIVERX2000 SYSTEM. The LiverX2000 system (Algenix/University of Minnesota, MN) uses a hollow-fiber design with porcine hepatocytes suspended within a colloid solution. Two cartridges containing hepatocytes (cell mass, 40 g each) connect in series, and the patient's whole blood is circulated around the hollow fibers. The small pore diameter of the hollow-fiber membrane permits diffusion of toxins but not larger molecules or blood cells. Like some of the other hepatocyte-based devices, the LiverX2000 utilizes a nutrient-rich medium to maintain cell viability. Early clinical trials are underway.

ACADEMIC MEDICAL CENTRE BIOARTIFICIAL LIVER. The Academic Medical Centre Bioartificial Liver (AMC-BAL; Amsterdam) uses approximately 200 g of primary porcine hepatocyte aggregates, contained within a hollow-fiber cartridge, to detoxify patient plasma. The rate of immunological problems is reduced by the presence of two plasma filters. The results of a phase I clinical trial, in which seven patients with ALF and advanced encephalopathy were treated, have been reported.[30] All patients had neurological improvement, and bilirubin and ammonia levels improved. One patient improved and did not require transplantation; the remaining six underwent liver transplantation.

CONCLUSION

Extracorporeal liver support devices fall into two major categories, nonbiological and biological systems, and use dialysis concepts for removal of toxins. A summary of selected nonbiological and biological liver support devices is provided in Table 196-5. The nonbiological systems provide detoxification but do not replace other important liver functions. Data on the efficacy of the nonbiological systems are limited. Biological systems use liver cells in an attempt to replace the functions of the liver beyond detoxification. Bioartificial liver devices vary in regard to the source, volume, and maintenance of hepatocytes. Although studies demonstrate that these systems may improve neurological status and physiological parameters, a definite survival benefit has not been demonstrated. Properly conducted controlled trials are needed to determine the appropriate utility of these systems in liver failure.

Key Points

1. Liver support systems use basic dialysis concepts and can be divided into nonbiological or biological systems.
2. Nonbiological systems provide only the detoxification function of the liver.
3. Biological systems use cells in an attempt to provide all the functions of the liver.
4. Most liver support systems have been shown to be safe in phase I studies, but no studies have clearly demonstrated long-term survival benefits.

TABLE 196-5

Comparison of Selected Biological and Nonbiological Liver Support Systems

CHARACTERISTIC	MARS	PROMETHEUS	HEPATASSIST	ELAD	BLSS	MELS	LIVERX2000	AMC-BAL
Manufacturer (location)	Teraklin AG (Germany)	Fresenius Medical Care AG (Germany)	Circe Biomedical (KY)	Vital Therapies (CA)	Excorp Medical (MN)	Charite Virchow Clinic (Germany)	Algenix (MN)	Academic Medical Centre (Amsterdam)
Cell type	Acellular	Acellular	Porcine	Human, tumor derived	Porcine	Human	Porcine	Porcine
Cell source	—	—	Cryopreserved	Cultured C3A hepatoma	Freshly isolated	Freshly isolated	Freshly isolated	Freshly isolated
Cell amount	—	—	$5\text{-}7 \times 10^9$	200-400 g	70-120 g	Up to 600 g	Up to 80 g	10×10^9
Bioreactor	Hemodialyzer with hollow-fiber membrane	Hemodialyzer with AlbuFlow filter and fractionated plasma separation and adsorption	Hollow-fiber cartridge with collagen-coated dextran beads and sorbent compartments	Ultrafiltrate generator with fiber semipermeable membrane	Hollow-fiber cartridge	Hollow-fiber, albumin dialyzation	Hollow-fiber cartridge	Polypropylene hollow-fiber membrane
Plasma/blood perfusion	Blood	Plasma	Plasma	Blood	Blood	Plasma	Blood	Plasma
Treatment time	6-8 hr	4-6 hr	6 hr	Up to 168 hr	12 hr	7-74 hr	8 hr	Up to 24 hr
Anticoagulation	Heparin	Heparin/citrate	Citrate	Heparin	Heparin	Heparin	Heparin	Heparin

AMC-BAL, Academic Medical Centre Bioartificial Liver; BLSS, Bioartificial Liver Support System; ELAD, Extracorporeal Liver Assist Device; MARS, Molecular Adsorbents Recirculating System; MELS, Modular Extracorporeal Liver Support.

5. Larger randomized, controlled trials of liver support systems with subjects of similar disease and severity, with well-defined end points, are needed.

Key References

5. Ash SR: Extracorporeal blood detoxification by sorbents in treatment of hepatic encephalopathy. Adv Renal Replace Ther 2002;9:3-18.
7. Khuroo MS, Khuroo MS, Farahat KL: Molecular adsorbent recirculating system for acute and acute-on-chronic liver failure: A meta-analysis. Liver Transpl 2004;10:1099-1106.
23. Jalan R, Sen S, Williams R: Prospects for extracorporeal liver support. Gut 2004;53:890-898.
24. Tsiaoussis J, Newsome PN, Nelson LJ, et al: Which hepatocyte will it be? Hepatocyte choice for bioartificial liver support systems. Liver Transpl 2001;7:2-10.
26. Demetriou AA, Brown RS, Busuttil RW, et al: Prospective, randomized, multicenter, controlled trial of a bioartificial liver in treating acute liver failure. Ann Surg 2004;239:660.

See the companion Expert Consult website for the complete reference list.

The Brain and the Kidney

CHAPTER 197

Treatment of Combined Acute Renal Failure and Cerebral Edema

Andrew Davenport

OBJECTIVES

This chapter will:
1. Present the basic pathophysiology of cerebral edema.
2. Give the characteristics of patients at risk of cerebral edema.
3. Describe the standard supportive management of cerebral edema.
4. Discuss the issues to consider when prescribing renal support for the patient with cerebral edema.

BASIC PATHOPHYSIOLOGY OF CEREBRAL EDEMA

In the normal, healthy adult, the skull acts as a rigid box, containing the brain (approximately 80% of the intracranial volume), with its vasculature (10%), and the cerebrospinal fluid (CSF) (10%). Because the skull is not compressible, the Monro-Kellie doctrine states that any increase in the volume of its contents will result in an increase in intracranial pressure (ICP), unless there is a compensatory reduction or displacement in the volume of the other components.

Intracranial volume can increase as a result of cerebral edema. Typically, cerebral edema is divided into cytotoxic and vasogenic edema.[1,2] Cytotoxic edema develops as a consequence of both neuronal and astrocyte cell swelling with maintenance of the integrity of the blood-brain barrier. Because glial cells outnumber neurons by 20:1, edema is mainly due to astrocyte swelling. Cytotoxic edema is usually caused by increased sodium (Na^+) and potassium (K^+) permeability of the cell membrane, energy depletion followed by failure of the energy-dependent ion pumps, the sustained uptake of osmotically active solutes, or some combination of these. In vasogenic edema, on the other hand, the integrity of the blood-brain barrier, comprising the endothelium and adjoining astrocytes, is disrupted, resulting in a protein-rich exudate with increased interstitial edema. Other causes of cerebral edema include interstitial edema that occurs in cases of severe hydrocephalus, wherein the CSF penetrates into adjacent brain due to the high CSF pressure, and osmotic cerebral edema, which is typified by the syndrome of inappropriate secretion of antidiuretic hormone, with an osmotic imbalance between the cerebral tissue and plasma.

ICP can also increase in association with increased cerebral blood volume, which can be caused by prolonged epileptiform neuronal activity, loss of vasoregulation due to disease, or physiological stimuli such as hypercarbia or pharmacological cerebral vasodilators. Similarly, hydrocephalus and space-occupying lesions can result in raised ICP.

Initially, the increasing intracranial volume is compensated by the combination of compression of the ventricles, displacement of CSF from the cerebral to the spinal subarachnoid space, increased CSF reabsorption by the arachnoid villi, and compression of the cerebral vasculature. CSF is produced in the choroid plexuses, mainly by the hydrostatic pressure gradient, so the CSF production rate falls as a result of the reduced arterial inflow and increased cerebral tissue pressure.

Because of these compensatory mechanisms, there is only a relatively small increase in ICP with increasing cerebral edema. However, eventually the buffering systems fail to compensate for further volume expansion, and then the ICP increases rapidly. This is shown in Figure 197-1. The ICP tracing shows not only a higher mean value but also the increasing pulse wave amplitude as the swollen brain becomes less compliant during systolic arterial inflow.

The rate of change of ICP with increasing intracranial volume depends on the cause of the cerebral edema. Slowly expanding mass lesions can be better compensated than rapidly evolving edema. Even so, the development of hypoxia and/or hypercarbia can lead to a sudden increase in ICP in a patient with a slowly expanding mass. Similarly, acute falls in mean arterial pressure (MAP), which lead to a reduction in cerebral perfusion, can trigger reflex vasodilatation with increased vascular flow and a secondary increase in ICP (Fig. 197-2).

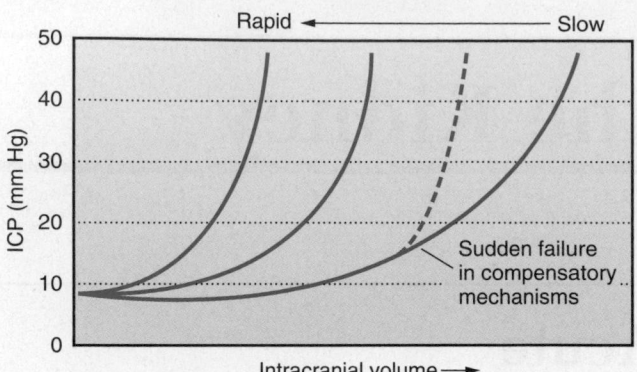

CHANGE IN INTRACRANIAL VOLUME

FIGURE 197-1. Relationship between intracranial pressure (ICP) and increasing intracranial volume. The change in ICP depends on the rapidity of the increase in intracranial volume. If the process is slow, then the compensatory mechanisms can potentially buffer changes more effectively than when there is a sudden increase in intracranial volume.

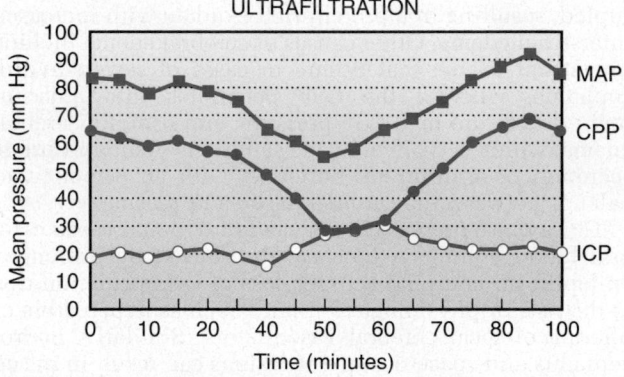

ULTRAFILTRATION

FIGURE 197-2. Changes in intracranial pressure (ICP), mean arterial pressure (MAP), and cerebral perfusion pressure (CPP). In this case, ultrafiltration initially led to a reduction in ICP and MAP, which was then followed by a rebound increase in ICP due to cerebral hypoperfusion.

PATIENTS AT RISK OF CEREBRAL EDEMA

In addition to patients with known space-occupying lesions (including tumors and abscesses), traumatic head injury, extradural or subdural hemorrhage, or acute intracranial or subarachnoid hemorrhage and those who have undergone neurosurgery, many medical patients are at risk of cerebral edema. These include patients with endothelial damage resulting from vasculitis, such as the primary small vessel vasculitides, including systemic lupus erythematosus, microscopic polyangiitis, and secondary forms of vasculitis associated with infections such as leptospirosis. Cerebral ischemia ranges from small-vessel occlusion associated with cerebral malaria; to thrombosis seen with thrombotic thrombocytopenic purpura, hemolytic uremic syndrome, or antiphospholipid syndrome; to larger-vessel ischemia including acute embolic and/or ischemic stroke. Infections, particularly those causing generalized enceph-

alitis or severe bacterial meningitis, may be complicated by severe cerebral edema. Prolonged epileptic seizures also lead to cerebral edema.

Metabolic causes of cerebral edema in adults are generally restricted to acute and acute-on-chronic liver failure, although, rarely, cerebral edema has been reported in chronic liver disease. Occasionally, runners develop cerebral edema on a hot day due to substantial retention of ingested water and renal failure caused by rhabdomyolysis and heat exhaustion. Patients can develop cerebral ischemia and edema after solid organ transplantation associated with abrupt changes in plasma sodium concentration and also related to immunophilin toxicity. Other drugs that can cause cerebral edema include the monoclonal antilymphocyte agent OKT3, and valproate (encephalopathy due to hyperammonemia).

In children, inborn errors of metabolism, including those affecting the urea cycle, may predispose to cerebral edema during times of stress and supplemental feeding. Similarly, cerebral edema may occur during the treatment of diabetic ketoacidosis, particularly in young children, which is associated with a rapid fall in plasma glucose.[3]

SUPPORTIVE MANAGEMENT OF PATIENTS WITH CEREBRAL EDEMA

General Standard Care

Brain perfusion, or the cerebral perfusion pressure (CPP), depends on the difference between the MAP, traditionally measured at the level of the carotid artery siphon, and the ICP. Under normal circumstances, brain perfusion is autoregulated, and cerebral blood flow is maintained above a lower limit of 50 mm Hg. Below that limit, further reduction in CPP may lead to reflex vasodilatation (see Fig. 197-2), with increased cerebral blood volume and consequent increased ICP, which results in a further fall in CPP. Increased ICP within the limits of the cranial cavity can then result in brain herniation and death. It has been suggested that a higher CPP, greater than 60 mm Hg, is required in patients with traumatic brain injury or hepatic encephalopathy to prevent further cerebral ischemia, although there are case reports of patients surviving with lower CPPs.

The key basic management strategy for a patient with cerebral edema is to maintain normal physiology (Table 197-1). Because both hypoxia and hypercarbia exacerbate ICP, patients should maintain a PaO_2 of greater than 11 kPa (82.5 mm Hg), with a $PaCO_2$ of between 4.5 and 5 kPa (49.5 to 55 mm Hg). To achieve these levels, patients may require elective intubation and ventilation. In those with raised ICP on the steep part of the ICP/intracranial volume curve (see Fig. 197-1), a modest reduction in $PaCO_2$ can lead to a significant fall in ICP. However, overventilation, by reducing the PaO_2 too far, can result in further reduction in cerebral blood flow with resultant cerebral ischemia and further increase in ICP.[4] Nevertheless, in an acute emergency when there are signs of herniation or a severe sustained surge in ICP, a short period of hyperventilation ($PaCO_2 < 3.33$ kPa or 25 mm Hg) can be used. Some centers have used jugular venous oxygen monitoring to determine optimal hyperventilation, aiming for a venous saturation greater than 65%, but this technique can be affected by the relative amount of extracerebral blood flow, light intensity, and movement artefacts.[5]

TABLE 197-1

Standard Support for Patients Who Have or Are at Risk of Intracranial Hypertension

Standard Support	
Normoxia	PaO$_2$ >11 kPa (83 mm Hg)
Normocapnia	PaCO$_2$ 4.5-5 kPa (34-38 mm Hg)
Maintain CPP	≥60 mm Hg
Moderate hypothermia	32-35°C
Actively Treat	
Precipitating factors	Seizures/pyrexia
	Hyperglycemia
	Electrolyte imbalances
	Hypo/hyperosmolality
With Sustained ↑ ICP	
Hypertonic saline	Plasma Na 145-155 mmol/L (mEq/L)
Mannitol	200 mL 20% over 15-30 min
Anesthetic agents	Propofol/thiopentone
Hyperventilation	PaCO$_2$ 4.0 kPa (28 mm Hg)
	Surgical decompression

CPP, cerebral perfusion pressure; ICP, intracranial pressure.

Similarly, patients should be fluid loaded and given vasoactive agents to maintain a CPP higher than 60 mm Hg,[6] or a MAP at 75 to 90 mm Hg if the ICP is not monitored. Traditionally, patients are nursed with 30 degrees head-upright tilt, because this helps to reduce the incidence of nosocomial pneumonia and causes a modest reduction in ICP. However, in those patients on the steep part of the ICP/intracranial volume curve, the associated reduction in MAP caused by sudden tilting of the patient may result in an acute reduction in CPP,[7] and a lower tilt of 15 to 20 degrees is more appropriate in patients who require pressors.

Potential exacerbating factors, such as epileptic seizures, pyrexia, sepsis, blood glucose abnormalities, and electrolyte (particularly hyponatremia) and osmolality abnormalities should be sought and treated appropriately.

Specific Medical Treatments for Intracranial Hypertension/Cerebral Edema

Steroids, which are effective in reducing peritumoral edema by regulating astrocyte aquaporin 4 channel expression, have no role in traumatic cerebral injury or metabolic edema. However, early steroid administration has been shown to improve the outcome in childhood acute bacterial meningitis, although meta-analysis failed to show any advantage in cerebral malaria.[7a]

Mannitol superseded urea therapy for the treatment of raised ICP in the 1950s. Initially, mannitol expands the intravascular compartment, by drawing water out of the tissues, and similarly reduces red cell volume. In hypovolemic patients, this can result in hypotension. The initial effect of mannitol on blood rheology causes reduced cerebrovascular resistance with increased cerebral blood flow and consequent autoregulatory deceased cerebral blood volume and ICP. After 30 minutes, the osmotic gradient that develops between the plasma and the brain may then lead to a further reduction in brain volume and ICP. Traditionally, mannitol is infused at a dose of 0.5 to 1.5 g/kg

over 15 to 30 minutes,[5] and this is repeated provided that the plasma osmolality remains at 325 mOsm/L or lower. Mannitol therapy may subsequently cause an increase in ICP. The reason for this is not well established but may be related to mannitol accumulation within brain tissue, with a resultant oncotic pressure gradient moving water back into the brain. In patients with acute renal failure, the baseline plasma osmolality is increased because of the raised urea concentration. The plasma osmolality should be carefully monitored before repeated boluses, because accumulating plasma mannitol may predispose to cerebral accumulation.

More recently, there has been increased use of osmotherapy with hypertonic saline for treating cerebral edema associated with head trauma and acute liver failure. Typically, 30% hypertonic saline is infused to maintain plasma sodium concentrations between 145 and 155 mmol/L (mEq/L), or it is given as a 20-mL bolus.[8] Other centers have used a 75-mL bolus of 10% hypertonic saline. Hypertonic saline is thought to work in a similar fashion to mannitol, with initial plasma volume expansion and increased cardiac output, caused by either increased preload or a possible additional inotropic effect, followed by a subsequent osmotic effect. Hypertonic therapy has been reported to be successful in patients with acute renal failure.[8] As with mannitol, later complications have included subsequent increased or "rebound" intracranial hypertension. In addition, many patients with cerebral edema have a degree of hyponatremia, and too rapid an increase in plasma sodium has been observed to cause seizures and central pontine myelinosis. The sodium and chloride load may also result in congestive heart failure or chloremic acidosis, so volume replacement has to be carefully monitored in the patient with acute renal impairment.

To reduce the risk of fluid overload, newer solutions containing a mixture of 7.5% saline in combination with 6% dextran have been developed; in early trials, these have been reported to be more effective than equimolar mannitol in reducing ICP.[9]

Physiotherapy and patient movement can result in increased ICP. Patients should therefore be nursed in a quiet environment if possible. Thiopentone is used to control status epilepticus and was therefore tried to control ICP, on the basis of reducing neuronal metabolism and cerebral blood volume. Initial studies showed promise in controlling ICP,[10] but thiopentone boluses were often complicated by hypotension. Similarly, propofol was also used as both continuous infusion and bolus to control ICP, but, as with thiopentone, boluses could also reduce MAP. What has not been established is whether patients treated with thiopentone and/or propofol infusion are more susceptible to hypotension resulting from the administration of other drugs, such as alfentanil, or hypotension during renal replacement therapy.

More rarely, children treated by propofol infusion developed a severe metabolic acidosis. The majority of units in the United Kingdom currently use benzodiazepine sedatives such as midazolam and opiate analgesics such as fentanyl, both of which accumulate in renal failure.

Moderate controlled hypothermia in patients with acute liver failure has been reported to result in an increase in MAP and CPP, associated with a reduction in arterial ammonia, brain metabolism, cerebral blood flow, brain cytokine production, and markers of oxidative stress.[11] However, randomized, multicenter, controlled trials in neurosurgical trauma have not shown an overall survival benefit of cooling patients to 33°C,[5] possibly because of the time taken to cool patients and the increased complications in the hypothermic group (e.g., pneumonia). In subsequent trials, hypothermia proved superior to barbiturate coma in treating patients with raised ICP, and cooling to 35°C resulted in better indices of cerebral metabolism with least side effects of hypothermia.[12]

CHOOSING RENAL SUPPORT FOR THE PATIENT WITH CEREBRAL EDEMA

The key issue when deciding on the choice of renal support for the patient with cerebral edema is the CPP and the cardiovascular stability of the patient. The ideal treatment would have no adverse effect on the CPP or cerebral blood flow (Table 197-2). Secondly, too rapid a fall in plasma osmolality could lead to a further increase in ICP (see Chapter 199).

Several studies have reported that middle cerebral arterial flow velocity is reduced after standard intermittent hemodialysis[13] in stable, healthy, chronic dialysis patients without neurological disease. Similarly, changes in cerebral blood flow in response to carbon dioxide were observed to be maintained, although this response has been shown to be reduced in anemic patients undergoing chronic dialysis.[14] However, intermittent hemodialysis was noted to reduce both stroke volume and cardiac output by 20%, even though there was no significant change in blood pressure.[15] In critically ill patients, intradialytic hypotension is more common, with a corresponding decrease in CPP. This typically accounts for the initial increase in ICP observed during intermittent hemodialysis and/or hemofiltration.[16] Until the advent of continuous hemofiltration and/or dialysis, peritoneal dialysis was the main alternative to intermittent hemodialysis for renal replacement, and it caused much fewer adverse changes in ICP and CPP. However, peritoneal dialysis can result in increased ICP and reduced CPP in compromised patients[17] because of changes in cardiac output and blood pressure associated with standard 2-L exchanges using higher glucose solutions.[18] Therefore, continuous renal replacement modalities have become the standard therapy for treatment of cerebral edema.[19]

PRESCRIBING RENAL SUPPORT FOR PATIENTS WITH CEREBRAL EDEMA

Modality

If intermittent hemodialysis is to be performed, then it should preferably be daily, and therapy time should be prolonged to minimize cardiovascular instability by reducing the ultrafiltration rate. Dialysis machines with relative blood volume monitoring and ultrafiltration feedback control are preferred. A high dialysate sodium concentration is required to both improve cardiovascular stability and maintain plasma osmolality. Dialysate temperature should be cooled to 35°C or set to isothermic, again to improve cardiovascular stability during treatment. By opting for daily treatment with extended time, dialysate flow rates can be slowed down to reduce the rate of fall in plasma osmolality; similarly, bicarbonate concentration can be reduced to 28 to 30 mmol/L (mEq/L) to prevent too rapid a correction of plasma bicarbonate.[20] Compared with standard routine intermittent hemodialysis, dialyzers with larger surface area and fast blood pump speeds are not required, and smaller dialyzers with lower blood flow rates should be chosen. Potential hypotensive reactions at the initiation of treatment caused by bradykinin production may be reduced by choice of membrane composition and by priming with isotonic sodium bicarbonate rather than normal saline.

These precautions for intermittent hemodialysis also apply to hybrid techniques of extended daily dialysis. For continuous renal replacement modalities, hyponatremic replacement solutions and dialysates should be avoided, and warming should be minimized to deliberately cool the patient. Sodium balance is better maintained with hemofiltration than with dialysis mode, because the sodium sieving coefficient is less than 1.0.

If peritoneal dialysis is chosen, a cycling machine should be used, with a tidal regime to avoid large and relatively abrupt changes in intraperitoneal volume. Peritoneal dialysis fluids are relatively hyponatremic, and patients may well require additional hypertonic sodium infusions to maintain a high plasma sodium concentration.

TABLE 197-2

Advantages and Disadvantages of Currently Used Renal Replacement Modalities

TECHNIQUE	ADVANTAGE	DISADVANTAGE
CRRT	Minimizes changes in intravascular volume Slow rate of change in plasma osmolality Cooling	Risk of hemorrhage if systemic anticoagulants are used with ICP monitors
Peritoneal dialysis	Slow rate of change in plasma osmolality Cooling No anticoagulation	Hyponatremic dialysates Hypertonic exchanges may result in reduction in CPP
Intermittent hemodialysis	No anticoagulation	Risk of reduction in CPP with rise in ICP Risk of dialysis dysequilibrium
Slow extended daily dialysis (hybrid dialysis)	Potentially anticoagulant free Possible reduced chance of nosocomial infection Cooling	Depending on duration of therapy, may not be as cardiovascularly stable as CRRT

CPP, cerebral perfusion pressure; CRRT, continuous renal replacement therapy; ICP, intracranial pressure.

Anticoagulation

It must be remembered that there is an increased risk of local bleeding around the site of ICP monitoring devices (risk greatest for intraventricular drain > subdural catheter > extradural monitor).[21] Therefore, patients should preferably receive no anticoagulation, or only a regional anticoagulant such as citrate, nafamostat, or prostanoids. The potent vasodilatory agent, prostacyclin, may provoke an increase in ICP by causing hypotension.[22]

CONCLUSION

Patients who develop acute renal failure with cerebral edema should receive standard supportive medical care designed to augment cerebral perfusion and maintain CPP. These patients require adequate fluid resuscitation, and pressors are necessary to support MAP. Sepsis should be actively sought and treated appropriately, as should electrolyte imbalances, and patients should be rendered euglycemic. Cerebral perfusion can be improved by the use of hypertonic saline and by maintaining an increased plasma sodium concentration. In addition, boluses of mannitol may have an additive effect. Cerebral volume can be reduced by controlled hyperventilation, although excessive hyperventilation may result in a reduction in cerebral blood flow. Mild hypothermia may also help to reduce ICP and cerebral metabolic demand. Sedative anesthetic agents reduce ICP, but thiopentone and propofol also cause vasodilatation and may result in hypotension, limiting their effectiveness.

Preferably, renal replacement therapy should have a minimal impact on cerebral perfusion and CPP, because a reduction in either can result in a further increase in ICP. Therefore, continuous modalities are preferred, because they allow the least changes in intravascular volume and have slower rates of change in plasma osmolality. If intermittent techniques are to be used, then treatment times should be extended, with reduced blood and dialysate flows, similar to slow extended daily dialysis/hemofiltration.

Key Points

1. The astrocyte is designed to maintain cerebral homeostasis and initially responds to osmotic stresses by changing intracellular electrolyte and water content.
2. Transcellular water transport through aquaporin channels is faster than urea transport through urea transporters.
3. Cerebral ischemia results in cerebral edema with a corresponding increase in intracranial pressure.
4. During renal replacement therapy, cerebral edema can occur because of osmotic changes—too rapid a reduction in urea and other plasma osmolytes—and also secondary to intradialytic hypotension.
5. Renal replacement therapy in patients at risk of cerebral edema/ischemia should be designed to minimize hypotensive episodes by utilizing cooled high-sodium dialysates coupled with slower blood and dialysate flows.

Key References

1. Unterberg AW, Stover J, Kress B, Kiening KL: Edema and brain trauma. Neuroscience 2004;129:1021-1029.
4. Soustiel JF, Mahamid E, Christyakov A, et al: Comparison of moderate hyperventilation and mannitol for control of intracranial pressure control in patients with severe traumatic brain injury: A study of cerebral blood flow and metabolism. Acta Neurochir 2006;148:845-851, discussion 51.
5. Adamides AA, Winter CD, Lewis PM, et al: Current controversies in the management of patients with severe traumatic brain injury. A N Z J Surg 2006;76:163-174.
6. The Brain Trauma Foundation, The American Association of Neurological Surgeons, The Joint Section on Neurotrauma and Critical Care: Guidelines for the management of severe traumatic brain injury. 3rd ed., 2007. Available at http://www.braintrauma.org/site/PageServer?pagename= Guidelines.
20. Davenport A: Renal replacement therapy in the patient with acute brain injury. Am J Kidney Dis 2001;37:457-466.

See the companion Expert Consult website for the complete reference list.

CHAPTER 198

Renal Protection in the Organ Donor

Helen Opdam

OBJECTIVES

This chapter will:
1. Describe the physiological sequelae of brain death, the effect on organ function, and protective strategies that may prevent damage to transplantable organs.
2. Review the evidence surrounding pituitary dysfunction in brain death and the efficacy of hormonal resuscitation in the supportive treatment of potential organ donors.
3. Provide an overview of the clinical management of the potential organ donor that will facilitate successful organ procurement, minimize organ damage, and optimize outcome for the kidney transplant recipient.

Kidney transplantation for the treatment of chronic renal failure results in improved health and longevity.[1] A kidney may be donated by a living person or a deceased person (cadaveric donation). In the United States and Australia, 60% of transplanted kidneys are from deceased donors, whereas in Europe this figure is 80%.[2-4]

Cadaveric donation is of two types: (1) donation from persons declared deceased using neurological criteria—that is, donation after brain death (DBD); and (2) donation after irreversible cessation of the circulation, otherwise known as donation after cardiac death (DCD) or "non–heart-beating organ donation."

Because of the universal shortage of organs for transplantation, there has been renewed interest in DCD. Although there is potential to expand this pool of donors, such donors currently provide only 5% of transplanted kidneys from cadaveric donors in Europe, Australia, and the United States.[4-6] Recipients who receive kidneys from DCD and DBD donors have the same outcome in terms of long-term allograft and patient survival, although there is a higher incidence of delayed graft function in kidneys from DCD donors.[7] This chapter focuses on the more common form of cadaveric donation, DBD.

MEDICAL SUITABILITY

Because of the shortage of donated organs and advances in transplantation medicine, the criteria for donor suitability are constantly broadening.

Absolute contraindications to donation are few and include infection with the human immunodeficiency virus (HIV), active malignant disease, and a history of malignancy that poses a high risk for transmission (e.g., melanoma, breast cancer). Patients with a history of malignancy and a long cancer-free interval represent a small risk of transmission and should be considered as potential donors.[8] Patients with treated bacterial infection, including meningococcal infection, may also be suitable donors. Organs from potential donors infected with hepatitis B or hepatitis C virus may be transplanted into recipients infected with the same virus or considered for noninfected individuals who are in need of a life-saving transplant. Patients with a history of intravenous drug use or other risk factors for HIV and viral hepatitis should be referred to the donor agency for careful exploration of the risk to potential recipients.

Acute organ dysfunction, in particular acute renal failure in a potential donor with prior normal renal function, is not a contraindication to donation. Older persons and those with a history of hypertension and diabetes mellitus are also often suitable donors of kidneys and other organs. Although many transplant units uncommonly transplant kidneys from persons older than 75 years of age, in Spain individuals as old as 90 years have provided kidneys that have resulted in successful transplantation.[9]

BRAIN DEATH AND PHYSIOLOGICAL SEQUELAE

Brain death is associated with progressive physiological instability that can ultimately affect kidney graft function after transplantation (Fig. 198-1). Timely confirmation of brain death, referral to the organ donor agency, and procurement of organs minimizes the loss of donors and maximizes the number of organs suitable for transplantation. Reported loss of potential donors through failed physiological support ranges from 5% to 25%.[10,11] Those who medically manage the potential donor and oversee the logistics of organ donation should work to minimize this loss through ensuring timely procurement and provision of excellent supportive treatment.

Brain death may develop as a result of progressive brain swelling in the hours or days after a severe brain injury (e.g., trauma, cerebral hemorrhage, cerebral infarction). Because the brain is contained within a rigid skull that limits its expansion, progressive edema and/or hemorrhage results in rising intracranial pressure and inadequate cerebral perfusion pressure. A cycle of cerebral infarction, edema, and further increase in intracranial pressure occurs with eventual loss of blood flow to the entire brain. This rise in intracranial pressure also results in downward dis-

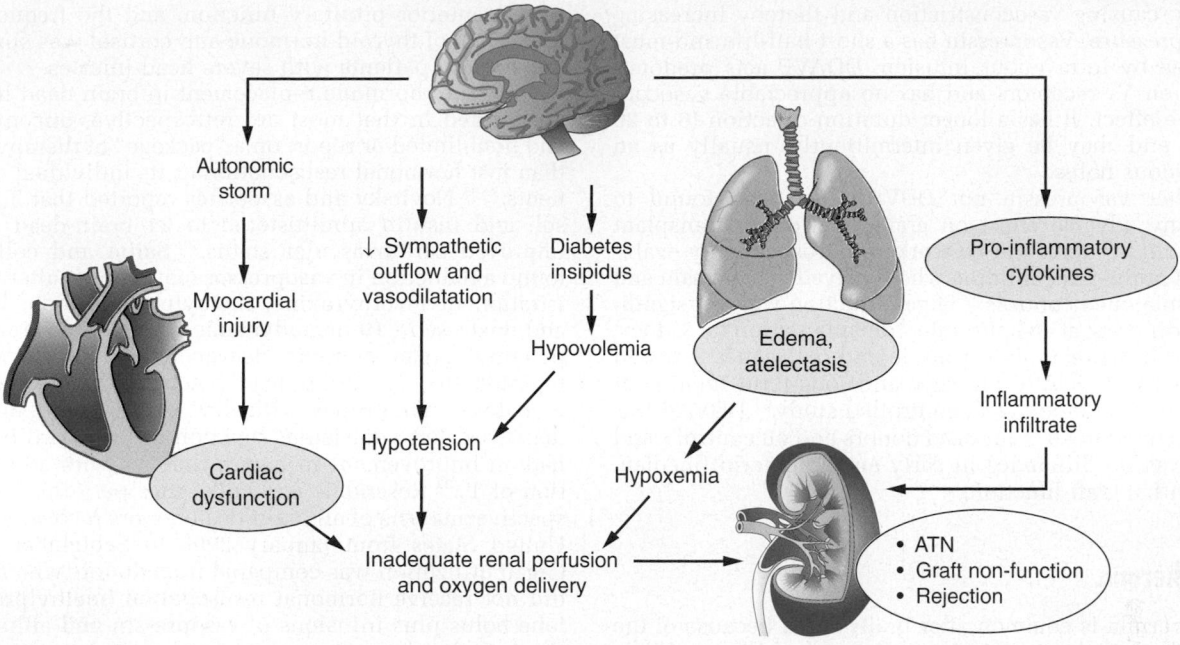

FIGURE 198-1. Brain death and effect on kidney function. ATN, acute tubular necrosis.

placement of the brain (herniation) with compression of the brainstem and loss of brainstem reflexes.

Cardiovascular

This process of brainstem compression may result in an intense sympathetic surge with marked hypertension, tachycardia (or reflex bradycardia [Cushing's reflex]) and/or arrhythmias, known as the "autonomic storm." This is usually short-lived but may result in cardiac ischemia and myocyte necrosis, electrocardiographic changes, and cardiac dysfunction.[12,13] Animal studies indicate that blunting of the sympathetic activity that occurs with brainstem compression reduces myocardial injury.[12] Any drugs administered in an attempt to minimize myocardial injury should have a very short duration of action, because longer-acting agents will exacerbate the hypotension that usually follows this period.

Subsequent to the autonomic storm, there is usually loss of sympathetic outflow, resulting in vasodilation and hypotension. This may be exacerbated by preexisting hypovolemia, polyuria from diabetes insipidus (DI), and cardiac dysfunction. Cardiac dysfunction may be chronic or secondary to myocardial injury associated with brain death.

Adequate support of blood pressure and cardiac output is necessary to optimize organ perfusion and, hence, the outcome of kidney transplantation. Pressor agents and/or inotropic drugs are required for persisting hemodynamic disturbance after correction of volume depletion. More than 90% of brain-dead potential donors require administration of pressor agents to maintain adequate blood pressure.[5] There is a paucity of research to guide the choice of agent in terms of optimizing organ perfusion and recipient outcome. In Australia and New Zealand, norepinephrine is used in 75% of patients.[5] Some protocols recommend dopamine or dobutamine.[14,15] Vasopressin has also been recommended as first-line therapy, especially if DI is present.[11]

Deficiency in vasopressin (antidiuretic hormone, or ADH) is thought to occur in the majority of brain-dead potential donors due to posterior pituitary dysfunction. Administration of low-dose arginine vasopressin in hemodynamically unstable brain-dead patients frequently results in a reduction or discontinuation of catecholamine pressor agents.[16,17] It is possible to sustain brain-dead patients for a longer period of time with the addition of vasopressin than with epinephrine alone.[18] At high doses (>2.4 U/hr), vasopressin causes vasoconstriction of coronary, renal, and splanchnic vasculature and may result in regional ischemia.[19] Because vasopressin is likely to be deficient in brain death, its use seems rational. However, it is not known whether the addition of vasopressin is preferable to using catecholamine agents alone in terms of organ perfusion and kidney recipient outcome.

Diabetes Insipidus

DI occurs in approximately 80% to 90% of brain-dead potential donors and is caused by the loss of posterior pituitary function, which results in deficiency of ADH.[11] This results in polyuria, hypernatremia, and hypovolemia. Prior treatments for raised intracranial pressure, such as hypertonic saline and mannitol, may also contribute to hypernatremia and hypovolemia.

Polyuria can be marked if untreated, often exceeding 1 L of urine output per hour. Attempts to correct the free water loss through the administration of large volumes of fluid may result in further derangements, such as hyperglycemia and hypothermia. Hypernatremia in the donor has been associated with a higher rate of post-transplantation acute tubular necrosis and primary kidney nonfunction.[20]

Therefore, it is important to diagnose DI early and to replace deficient ADH using either arginine vasopressin or desmopressin (1-desamino-8-D-arginine vasopressin, or DDAVP). The antidiuretic effect of vasopressin and DDAVP is mediated via V_2 receptors in the renal collecting ducts. Vasopressin also acts on V_1 receptors located within blood vessels, causing vasoconstriction and thereby increasing blood pressure. Vasopressin has a short half-life and must be given by intravenous infusion. DDAVP acts predominantly on V_2 receptors and has no appreciable vasoconstrictive effect. It has a longer duration of action (6 to 20 hours) and may be given intermittently, usually as an intravenous bolus.

Neither vasopressin nor DDVAP has been found to have any adverse effect on graft function in transplant recipients.[17,21] Katz and co-workers retrospectively evaluated 34 brain-dead children who received vasopressin and 28 age-matched controls.[17] Organ function was not significantly different at 48 hours after transplantation for kidney, liver, or heart recipients. Guesde and colleagues assessed the effects of DDAVP on early and long-term renal graft function in a randomized, controlled study.[21] DDVAP was administered to 49 brain-dead donors and 48 controls, and there was no difference in early and long-term (median, 45 months) graft function.

Hypothermia

Hypothermia is common after brain death because of the loss of hypothalamic thermoregulation, inability to shiver, and loss of vasoconstriction. Hypothermia may be exacerbated by the administration of large volumes of relatively cool fluids in the treatment of DI. Adverse effects include cardiac dysfunction, arrhythmias, coagulopathy, and a leftward shift of the oxyhemoglobin dissociation curve with reduced oxygen delivery to tissues. Temperatures lower than 35°C preclude or delay the declaration of death via clinical brain death testing.

Hyperglycemia

Administration of large volumes of dextrose-containing fluids in the treatment of DI may cause hyperglycemia. Hyperglycemia may also be caused by preexisting diabetes mellitus or by increases in the levels of counter-regulatory hormones and peripheral resistance to insulin.[22] It may result in an osmotic diuresis and electrolyte abnormalities.

Anterior Pituitary Dysfunction

Conflicting evidence exists as to the occurrence and clinical significance of hypothalamic-pituitary-adrenal/thyroid dysfunction in brain death. Animal models demonstrate that a deficiency of thyroid hormone, cortisol, and adrenocorticotropic hormone (ACTH) occurs with brain death[23] and that exogenous hormone administration may improve hemodynamics and myocardial contractility.[24,25]

It is unclear whether clinically significant thyroid hormone or cortisol deficiency occurs in humans after brain death. Most studies suggest that anterior pituitary function is partially preserved, with normal levels of cortisol and thyroid hormone, or with low thyroid hormone in the setting of normal or increased levels of thyroid stimulating hormone (TSH) consistent with the sick euthyroid syndrome.[26-28] In these studies, no correlation was found between low levels of cortisol or thyroid hormone and blood pressure or vasopressor requirement. In a further study of 32 patients, serial measurements up to 80 hours after brain death failed to show a progressive decline in the level of free triiodothyronine (T_3) or cortisol.[29] ACTH remained constant and TSH increased, suggesting pre-

served anterior pituitary function, and the frequency of low levels of thyroid hormone and cortisol was similar to that seen in patients with severe head injuries.

Studies of hormone replacement in brain-dead humans are limited in that most are retrospective, uncontrolled, and nonblinded or report on a "package" of therapy rather than just hormonal resuscitation or its individual components.[30-33] Novitsky and associates reported that T_3, cortisol, and insulin administered to 21 brain-dead donors improved cardiovascular status.[30] Salim and colleagues found a reduction in vasopressor requirement after administration of levothyroxine, methylprednisolone, insulin, and dextrose in 19 hemodynamically unstable brain-dead potential organ donors.[31] Jeevanandam and co-workers reported that six brain-dead potential donors receiving high doses of inotropes, with elevated filling pressures and depressed left ventricular function on echocardiography, had an improvement in hemodynamics with administration of T_3.[32] Rosendale and colleagues performed a retrospective analysis of all brain-dead donors recovered in the United States from January 2000 to September 2001.[33] Organ utilization was compared from donors who did and did not receive hormonal resuscitation (methylprednisolone bolus plus infusions of vasopressin and either T_3 or thyroxine). A greater number of organs were obtained and transplanted if the donor received hormonal resuscitation.

However, two randomized, controlled studies of thyroid hormone use failed to show a benefit on hemodynamics in brain-dead patients. Randell and Hockerstedt reported a lack of effect on hemodynamics in 12 patients who received T_3 intraoperatively during organ procurement, compared with 13 control patients in a nonblinded study.[34] In a blinded randomized, placebo-controlled study, T_3 administered as a bolus to 19 subjects, compared with 18 controls, resulted in no improvement in hemodynamic or echocardiographic parameters.[35]

A number of studies have looked at steroids independently of other components of hormonal resuscitation (vasopressin and thyroid hormone). A placebo-controlled study of pigs with induced brain death found that methylprednisolone, administered either before or after brain death, was associated with preserved left ventricular function.[36] Zaroff and co-workers published a retrospective review of 16 potential donors who underwent serial echocardiography during donor management that included corticosteroids in 75% of the donors and dopamine in 15 donors.[37] Thirteen subjects had an initial ejection fraction of less than 50%; the ejection fraction improved in 12 subjects after intensive donor management.

The uncontrolled and unblinded nature of most of these studies raises the possibility that factors apart from hormonal resuscitation, such as other aspects of physiological management, may have contributed to the observed differences. A number of reports indicate increased organ utilization from donors after implementation of donor management protocols and transformation of "unacceptable" to "acceptable" donors by resuscitation implemented with the arrival of organ procurement teams.[38,39] Rosendale and associates examined donors from 88 critical care units after the introduction of a donor management algorithm.[38] The total number of organs transplanted per 100 donors was significantly greater after implementation of the pathway, compared with retrospective data collected in the same institutions. Salim and co-workers found a similar increase in the number of organs recovered and a reduced loss of donors due to hemodynamic instability after introduction of aggressive donor management.[39] This approach included donor management by dedicated physicians, pulmonary artery catheterization, aggressive fluid resuscitation, early use of vasopressors, and use of thyroid hormone in hemodynamically unstable donors.

Such experience is the basis for including pulmonary artery catheterization in algorithms such as that arising from the consensus conference, Maximizing Use of Organs Recovered from the Cadaver Donor: Cardiac Recommendations, held in 2001.[15] Hormonal resuscitation was also included in this algorithm and has been incorporated into the United Network for Organ Sharing (UNOS) critical pathway for heart donor management and other reviews.[11,14,40] Whether such interventions improve organ utilization and recipient outcome beyond that attained with careful physiological management of potential donors by critical care physicians remains untested.

Inflammatory and Immunological Changes

Significant changes in the cytokine profiles, including elevation of pro-inflammatory cytokines such as interleukin 6 (IL-6), are observed in humans after brain death.[41] High-dose steroids may block inflammatory cytokines, stabilize membranes and prevent lysosomal enzyme release, and reduce cell-mediated cellular injury, thus minimizing injury to transplanted organs. Pratschke and colleagues demonstrated, in a rat model of brain death and kidney donation, that administration of steroids after induction of brain death resulted in less inflammatory infiltrate in transplanted kidney grafts.[42] They suggested that organs transplanted from steroid-treated donors may be more inert and may not trigger host immunity, thus attenuating rejection in the recipient.

A retrospective review of lung donors found steroid administration to be associated with increased donor lung oxygenation and utilization.[43] The authors hypothesized that steroids may reduce pro-inflammatory cytokines or prevent lysosomal membrane disruption, reducing development of the adult respiratory distress syndrome.

The nutritional state of the brain-dead organ donor may also influence the function of transplanted organs.[44] Provision of nutrition up until organ procurement may restore energy reserves, reduce cytokine generation, and protect against ischemia and reperfusion injury.

Respiratory and Hematological Changes

Other contributors to failed physiological support of the potential organ donor, or loss of otherwise suitable organs for transplantation, relate to respiratory and hematological sequelae of brain death. Hypoxia from atelectasis and pulmonary edema may contribute to deterioration in cardiopulmonary status, leading to cardiac arrest before organ procurement. Anemia may be dilutional, resulting from bleeding due to trauma and exacerbated by coagulopathy. Coagulopathy may occur as an effect of substances released from necrotic brain that induce fibrinolysis (especially in traumatic brain injury), or as a result of dilution from bleeding and fluid administration, and it may be worsened by hypothermia.[45]

MANAGEMENT OF THE POTENTIAL ORGAN DONOR

The approach to management for the potential organ donor is similar to that for other critically ill patients in the intensive care unit. The aim is to maintain normal physiology, and the usual spectrum of monitoring and interventions should be employed. An awareness of the specific perturbations that may occur in brain death and timely institution of appropriate supportive treatment is essential.

Autonomic Storm

This is usually self-limited, and no treatment is required. If antihypertensive agents are used, they should be short-acting (e.g., esmolol, sodium nitroprusside). Antihypertensives with a longer duration of action are best avoided, because they will exacerbate the hypotension that usually follows this period.

Arrhythmias

Arrhythmias may be prevented by minimizing the time between brain death and organ procurement and maintaining normal serum electrolyte concentrations, blood pressure, volume state, and temperature. Standard therapy may be administered for atrial and ventricular arrhythmias (e.g., amiodarone, cardioversion). In the event of cardiac arrest, cardiopulmonary resuscitation may result in recovery of cardiac function and successful organ transplantation.[20] Bradycardia is usually resistant to atropine, but adrenaline, isoprenaline, or pacing may be effective.[46]

Hypovolemia

The volume state should be optimized by administration of intravenous fluids. Competing requirements for optimization of organ function may produce conflicting strategies for fluid replacement. Higher rates of lung procurement are associated with a minimally positive fluid balance,[47] whereas liberal fluid administration favors kidney function. Early determination of the suitability for transplantation of specific organs facilitates the development of focused medical management strategies (e.g., more aggressive fluid therapy if lung donation is contraindicated).

Hypotension and Low Cardiac Output

An adequate perfusion pressure should be targeted (e.g., mean arterial pressure approximately 60 to 70 mm Hg) by optimizing the volume state and by use of pressor/inotropic agents (e.g., norepinephrine, epinephrine, dopamine, or dobutamine). Vasopressin may also be used, and most protocols recommend between 0.5 and 4 U/hr,[14,15,40] although it has been suggested that doses greater than 2.4 U/hr may cause regional ischemia.[19]

Use of a pulmonary artery catheter may assist with the optimization of hemodynamics.[15,38,48] High inotrope requirements do not preclude successful donation, and recent series have suggested a limited or no relationship between inotrope dose in the donor and recipient outcome.[20,49] Nonetheless, doses of inotropes should be minimized if possible, and most donors can be managed successfully with fluid resuscitation and low-dose vasopressors.

Hormonal therapy should be considered, especially if there is persistent hemodynamic instability.[15] Suggested hormonal resuscitation regimens include the following[14,15,40]:

Triiodothyronine (T_3): 4 µg IV bolus, then 3 µg/hr by IV infusion

Methylprednisolone: 15 mg/kg IV single bolus

Arginine vasopressin (AVP): 0.5 to 4.0 U/hr

Diabetes Insipidus

Urinary volume loss should be replaced with intravenous 5% dextrose or, if there is resistant hyperglycemia, with sterile water administered via a central venous catheter.

DDAVP or arginine vasopressin should be administered. DDAVP may be given intravenously, intramuscularly, subcutaneously, or intranasally at a dose between 1 and 4 µg every 2 to 6 hours, or as required if urine output exceeds a particular volume (e.g., 300 mL/hr). Vasopressin is given as an intravenous infusion at a dose of 0.5 to 4.0 U/hr (see earlier discussion).

Early administration of antidiuretic agents in suspected DI (polyuria and rising serum sodium in a patient with likely or confirmed brain death), rather than awaiting confirmation from serum or urinary osmolalities, may avoid physiological instability caused by hypovolemia and hypothermia from large-volume intravenous replacement fluids.

Metabolic Derangement

Serum electrolytes (sodium and potassium) should be monitored in the potential donor every 2 to 4 hours to guide fluid replacement and electrolyte supplementation. Insulin may be given by infusion to maintain blood glucose within the normal range.

Hypothermia

Hypothermia is easier to prevent than to reverse, and it may be avoided by using warming blankets and ensuring that inhaled gases are warmed and humidified. Fluids should be warmed if large-volume intravenous fluid replacement is required.

Respiratory Changes

Careful respiratory management, including frequent suctioning, repositioning and turning, ventilatory techniques that reduce atelectasis (e.g., positive end-expiratory pressure, recruitment maneuvers), and appropriate management of volume state, help maintain adequate oxygenation and oxygen delivery to organs.

Anemia and Coagulopathy

Blood transfusion may be required, as may the administration of coagulation factors and/or platelets in the setting of coagulopathy. Procurement should be expedited if there is worsening coagulopathy.

Nutritional State

Continued enteral feeding in the potential donor up until the time of organ procurement may have beneficial effects on post-transplantation kidney graft function.[44]

CONCLUSION

With attentive provision of supportive treatment, most potential organ donors should be able to be supported until the time of organ procurement. Optimal medical management is required to maximize the number of organs suitable for transplantation in each donor and to produce the best outcomes in renal transplant recipients.

Key Points

1. Brain death results in progressive physiological instability. Timely confirmation of brain death and procurement of organs minimizes loss of donors resulting from progressive physiological instability and maximizes the number of organs suitable for transplantation.
2. An understanding of the mechanism of brain death and the ensuing physiological derangements is important in being able to institute appropriate supportive treatment in a timely manner.
3. The most common sequelae of brain death include hypotension, diabetes insipidus, and hypothermia. Conflicting evidence exists as to whether clinically significant anterior pituitary–adrenal/thyroid dysfunction occurs.
4. Clinical management by staff skilled in critical care practice is essential in ensuring successful support of potential donors for organ procurement and optimal post-transplantation kidney function.
5. Careful physiological monitoring should be employed, with the aim of maintaining normal electrolyte levels and temperature, identifying and treating diabetes insipidus, and ensuring adequate organ perfusion through optimizing the volume state and use of pressor and/or inotropic agents. Respiratory care and blood product support may be required.
6. Hormonal resuscitation (vasopressin, thyroid hormone, and steroids) should be considered in the setting of hemodynamic instability.

Key References

14. Phongsamran PV: Critical care pharmacy in donor management. [Erratum appears in Prog Transplant 2004 Sep;14(3):264]. Progress in Transplantation 2004;14:105-111.
15. Zaroff JG, Rosengard BR, Armstrong WF, et al: Consensus conference report. Maximizing use of organs recovered from the cadaver donor: Cardiac recommendations, March 28-29, 2001, Crystal City, Virginia. Circulation 2002;106:836-841.
29. Gramm HJ, Meinhold H, Bickel U, et al: Acute endocrine failure after brain death? Transplantation 1992;54:851-857.
35. Goarin JP, Cohen S, Riou B, et al: The effects of triiodothyronine on hemodynamic status and cardiac function in potential heart donors. Anesth Analg 1996;83:41-47.
40. Wood KE, Becker BN, McCartney JG, et al: Care of the potential organ donor. N Engl J Med 2004;351:2730-2739.

See the companion Expert Consult website for the complete reference list.

CHAPTER 199

Dialysis Dysequilibrium Syndrome

Sean M. Bagshaw, Natalia Polanco, Catalina Ocampo, Rinaldo Bellomo, and Andrew Davenport

---

OBJECTIVES

This chapter will:
1. Describe the clinical presentation of dialysis dysequilibrium syndrome (DDS).
2. Describe the pathophysiology of DDS.
3. Present strategies for the prevention of DDS.

Dialysis dysequilibrium syndrome (DDS) is the clinical phenomenon of acute central nervous system dysfunction attributed to cerebral edema that occurs during or after renal replacement therapy (RRT). DDS has not traditionally been described in the setting of critical illness, yet critically ill patients may represent a unique cohort at particular risk for the development of this complication of RRT. Epidemiological studies of critically ill patients have shown that acute renal failure (ARF) is a common and serious clinical problem that is independently associated with both morbidity and mortality.[1-5] Moreover, the majority of these patients go on to need, at least provisionally, some form of RRT.[2,4,5] Yet, there are virtually no data available on the epidemiology of DDS in critically ill patients with ARF treated with RRT. This chapter focuses on the clinical presentation, risk factors, pathophysiology, and prevention of DDS with an emphasis on the critically ill patient.

CLINICAL PRESENTATION

DDS occurs most often during or after initiation of the first hemodialysis sessions and was originally described by Kennedy and associates in 1962.[6] In those days, severely symptomatic and uremic patients were dialyzed on consecutive days, leading to abrupt falls in serum urea, after which hemodialysis treatment was withdrawn and restarted again only when they became symptomatic. This pattern of hemodialysis commonly predisposed patients to or precipitated many of the symptoms attributed to DDS. Following the introduction of thrice-weekly hemodialysis for patients with chronic renal failure, the frequency of DDS symptoms was markedly reduced. However, even in modern clinical practice, DDS can still occur. The precise epidemiology of DDS is poorly described, and it is probably under-reported, particularly in the critically ill population. This is most likely a result of the wide spectrum of clinical manifestations that can occur and the numerous potential confounding factors present in critically ill patients.

DDS has classically been described in patients receiving conventional intermittent hemodialysis. However, it has occasionally been observed with peritoneal dialysis. Specifically, DDS has been reported to occur during acute intermittent peritoneal dialysis when hyperosmolar dialysate solutions are used.[7] In addition, evolving strategies for delivery of continuous RRT (e.g., high-volume hemofiltration) in critically ill patients with ARF, whereby high rates of urea clearance are targeted, may predispose to the development of DDS.[8-12] Thus far, however, no clinical studies have assessed for or observed DDS in critically ill patients undergoing continuous RRT. Yet, there are anecdotally documented episodes of acute nervous system dysfunction consistent with DDS in critically ill patients receiving continuous hemodiafiltration at 40 mL/kg/hr for ARF.

The symptoms of DDS can vary in spectrum and severity. Mild symptoms such as headache, nausea, vomiting, blurred vision, muscle cramps, tremors, disorientation, anorexia, restlessness, hypertension, and dizziness are still commonly described during or following hemodialysis and attributed to DDS (Table 199-1).[13,14] A more serious form of DDS can be characterized by greater central nervous system dysfunction, manifested by delirium and myoclonus. In some instances, these symptoms have been reported to persist for several days.[15] In the most severe instances, patients can develop generalized tonic-clonic seizures, papilledema, raised intraocular pressure, cardiac arrhythmias, central pontine myelinolysis, and coma.[16-19] Death is an extremely rare occurrence, with most fatalities having occurred before 1970, although cases have been reported in modern clinical practice.[19,20]

In general, the clinical course and temporal profile of DDS have not been well described. However, symptoms can develop acutely during hemodialysis or can be delayed for 24 hours or longer after the session.

DDS has been shown to cause acute focal electroencephalographic (EEG) alterations in patients undergoing rapid hemodialysis.[15] Concomitant cerebral angiography has shown evidence of normal blood flow and no ischemia. These asymmetrical EEG findings corresponded to acute central nervous system dysfunction and slow but reversible neuropsychiatric disturbances.[15] In a small series of critically ill neurosurgical patients, intermittent hemodialysis was associated with significant increases in intracranial pressure.[21]

Several studies have shown significant global densitometric changes of brain tissue after rapid intermittent hemodialysis that suggest a gain in cerebral water content.[7,22,23] In addition, focal abnormalities have also been detected.[18,19] Focal hypodense lesions in pontine and extrapontine locations on computed tomography (CT) scans of the brain have been associated with severe DDS after peritoneal dialysis.[19] In another report, imaging showed focal white matter changes in the posterior parietal and occipital lobes consistent with changes seen in reversible posterior leukoencephalopathy syndrome after initiation of hemodialysis.[18] Similarly, in a small study of chronic hemodialysis patients, volumetric T1-weighted

TABLE 199-1

Spectrum of Clinical Features Reportedly Associated with Dialysis Dysequilibrium Syndrome

Headache
Nausea/vomiting
Blurred vision
Anorexia
Tremors/restlessness
Muscle cramps
Hypertension
Disorientation
Dizziness
Myoclonus
Seizures
Central pontine myelinolysis
Altered level of consciousness/coma

TABLE 199-2

Potential Risk Factors for Dialysis Dysequilibrium Syndrome

Pediatric patient
Severe/symptomatic uremia
Acute renal failure or acute on chronic renal failure
Efficient intermittent hemodialysis
Acute or chronic brain injury
Severe sepsis

magnetic resonance imaging (MRI) scans were performed immediately before and after a standard hemodialysis session.[24] Although no patients developed significant neurological dysfunction, MRI studies showed an average 3% (32.8 mL) increase in brain volume consistent with cerebral edema. However, findings of acute EEG or densitometric changes on brain CT scan have not always been replicated in patients with stable end-stage renal disease (ESRD) and chronic uremia.[25]

RISK FACTORS FOR DIALYSIS DYSEQUILIBRIUM SYNDROME

DDS is most common in patients with severe symptomatic uremia or ARF; in patients receiving rapid, efficient and intermittent hemodialysis for generally longer than 4 hours; and in pediatric patients (Table 199-2). In addition, patients with preexisting or acute neurological disease, such as head trauma, stroke, or malignant hypertension, may be at greater risk for development of DDS.[21,26] For example, in brain-injured patients, cerebral blood flow autoregulation may be impaired and subtle changes to the $PaCO_2$ can have dramatic effects on perfusion.[27] In these circumstances, the rapid correction of serum osmolality or acid-base disturbance due to ARF, by an efficient strategy of RRT, may not only worsen brain injury but also precipitate DDS. Similarly, ARF is common in the setting of severe sepsis and/or multiorgan failure where there is widespread immune activation that can act to alter the permeability of the blood-brain barrier.[28,29] As a result, the threshold for development of DDS in this population may

be lower compared with the initiation of RRT for stable ESRD. Moreover, discriminating the clinical symptoms of DDS in septic patients with ARF from those of septic encephalopathy may be challenging. Despite no evidence from experimental or clinical studies, these theoretical risks warrant consideration and may have particular relevance for clinicians prescribing RRT for critically ill septic patients.

BASIC PATHOPHYSIOLOGY OF THE BRAIN IN RENAL FAILURE

In renal failure, not only urea but also a whole series of nitrogenous metabolites accumulate. These include guanidino compounds, uric acid, hippuric acid, various amino acids, polypeptides, polyamines, phenols, phenolic and indolic acids, acetone, glucuronic acid, carnitine, myoinositol, sulfates, phosphates, and so-called middle molecules.[30] The guanidino compounds, in particular, have excitatory effects on the central nervous system, through activation of excitatory N-methyl-D-aspartate receptors and concomitant inhibition of inhibitory γ-aminobutyric acid (GABA)-ergic neurotransmission.[31] Retention of these guanidino compounds (i.e., creatinine, guanidine, guanidinosuccinic acid, methylguanidine) in either acute or chronic renal failure can cause a corresponding significant increase in their concentrations in serum, cerebrospinal fluid, and brain. The increased levels in the central nervous system, in turn, lead to an overall increase in cerebral osmolality.

Glial cells within the brain, which considerably outnumber the neurons, are pivotal for maintaining homeostasis of the extracellular milieu. Astrocytes, the most abundant glial cell type and a building block of the blood-brain barrier, play a central role in regulating the chemical environment and preserving the intracellular volume of neurons. Astrocytes respond to changes in extracellular fluid osmolality by regulating sodium/potassium exchange and by generating and accumulating intracellular osmoles. These intracellular osmoles (e.g., urea, glycerol, sorbitol) help safeguard cerebral extracellular volume. This adaptation, the accumulation of intracellular osmoles, occurs in response to the increased serum osmolality seen in renal failure.

Despite the significant cerebral chemical adaptations to uremia, the regulation of cerebral blood flow appears to be preserved. Studies in healthy, nonanemic, chronic hemodialysis patients have shown that cerebral blood flow, as assessed by transcranial Doppler measurements of the middle cerebral artery, is normal and, similarly, cerebral blood flow responds appropriately to changes in arterial carbon dioxide tension.[32]

PATHOPHYSIOLOGY OF DIALYSIS DYSEQUILIBRIUM SYNDROME

Although it is generally accepted that DDS is associated with cerebral edema, the pathophysiology remains debated and incompletely understood.[33-35] However, two central hypotheses have been proposed: (1) the "reverse urea effect" and (2) the "idiogenic osmolyte" hypothesis (Table 199-3).

TABLE 199-3

Pathophysiology of Dialysis Dysequilibrium Syndrome

DDS HYPOTHESIS	DURING HEMODIALYSIS	CEREBRAL EDEMA
Reverse urea effect	Serum [urea] << [brain]	Water movement → brain
Idiogenic osmolytes	Osmolality serum << brain	Water movement → brain
	Hypotension	
	↑↑ Serum bicarbonate	

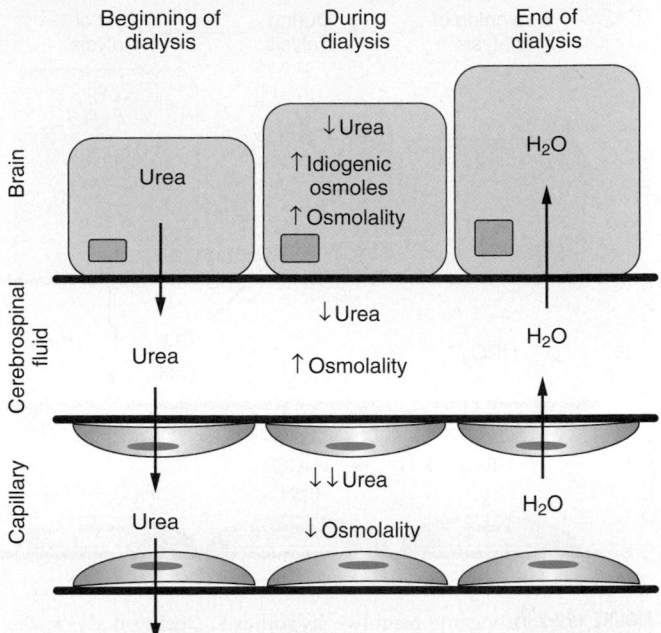

FIGURE 199-1. Reverse urea effect hypothesis. Pathogenesis of dialysis dysequilibrium syndrome caused by increased removal of plasma urea; with slower removal from cerebrospinal fluid and brain tissue; water moves into brain cells, leading to edema.

Numerous investigations of brain tissue density in patients with chronic kidney disease treated by intermittent hemodialysis have shown significant and measurable changes to brain density after hemodialysis, consistent with water influx into the brain.[7,22,23] Although these brain density changes may in some instances represent restoration of normal intracellular hydration in a brain that appeared dehydrated before the hemodialysis session, this remains speculative. The theory is supported by findings that the mild increases in brain water content that occur after routine outpatient hemodialysis are asymptomatic.[24,25] However, additional diagnostic imaging studies in similar patient populations have also shown abnormal changes consistent with the formation of pathological cerebral edema.[15,18,24,36] These pathological changes to brain tissue density are generally seen only in association with rapid or intermittent hemodialysis, whereas these findings were avoided with the greater physiological stability offered by continuous therapies.[36]

DDS was originally attributed to the slower removal of urea from the brain, compared with the serum, during acute hemodialysis; this differential creates an osmotic gradient, and results in the reverse inflow of water into the brain, causing cerebral edema.[26] This hypothesis has been referred to as the "reverse urea effect" (Fig. 199-1). In support of this theory, experimental evidence has shown that, after acute hemodialysis in a rat model, a substantial brain-to-serum urea concentration difference develops and is associated with an increase in brain water content.[13,33] Similarly, in vivo studies have documented that the brain urea concentration remains lower than that in the serum for several hours after the serum urea is acutely raised.[37] In addition, the transfer of urea across the blood-brain barrier has been shown to be one-twentieth that of water.[38] On the assumption that the brain and the serum are in osmotic equilibrium, then the urea concentration gradient after hemodialysis would be sufficient to explain the amount of water influx into the brain.[33,39] Finally, brain water content does not increase after experimental hemodialysis if rapid removal of serum urea is prevented by the addition of urea to the dialysate.[39,40]

Recently, further insights into the pathophysiology of DDS have been made with the discovery and characterization of membrane transporters for both urea and water.[41,42] These membrane transporters are constitutively expressed on all cerebral astrocytes, the key cell that maintains the integrity of the blood-brain barrier and protects the brain from significant changes in osmolality. In a rat model of chronic renal failure, the expression of urea transporters (UT-B1) in the brain was decreased by 30% to 50% at 1 week after nephrectomy, whereas expression of the aqua-

porin (AQ) transporters AQ4 and AQ9 was increased by 50% and 65%, respectively.[41,42] The downregulation of UT-B most likely causes urea exit from astrocytes to be delayed during rapid removal of plasma urea through hemodialysis. This physiological adaptation, coupled with the dramatic upregulation of AQ4 and AQ9 in the setting of rapid and efficient hemodialysis, increased the risk for dysequilibrium. The serum urea was rapidly reduced, yet the brain intracellular urea was slower to clear, providing the stimulus for water movement into the brain.

The reverse urea effect theory was challenged by a series of experimental studies by Arieff and colleagues, mostly conducted in the 1970s.[13,35,43,44] These studies, while confirming that urea was retained in the cerebrospinal fluid immediately after hemodialysis, showed that it was rapidly cleared from cortical gray matter.[35] In addition, they suggested that the gradient in urea concentration across the brain after hemodialysis was insufficient by itself to completely account for the resulting cerebral edema.[35] Direct measurements of brain osmolality after hemodialysis showed that this value was considerably higher than serum osmolality and that the gradient could not be explained by the measured concentrations of brain urea and simple electrolytes. Therefore, it was hypothesized that adaptations occurred in the brain that resulted in the formation and accumulation of new osmolytes.[34,35] This hypothesis has been referred to as the "idiogenic osmolyte" hypothesis (Fig. 199-2).

Experimental studies have shown that the brain adapts to the increases in serum osmolality seen in renal failure by accumulation of intracellular brain osmolyte content.[34] The rapid correction of a high plasma osmolality with hemodialysis can generate a significant osmotic gradient across the blood-brain barrier. This gradient, in turn, promotes an influx of water into the brain. Additional studies

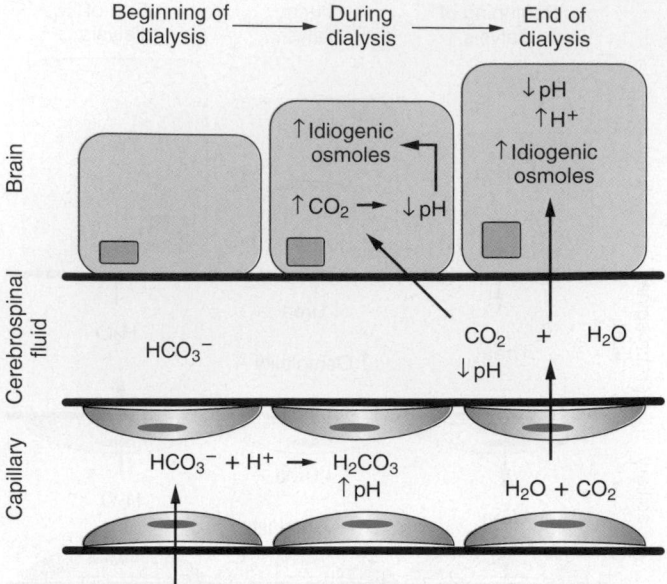

Beginning of dialysis → During dialysis → End of dialysis

FIGURE 199-2. Idiogenic osmolyte hypothesis. During dialysis, the plasma bicarbonate level rapidly increases, but bicarbonate cannot pass across the blood-brain barrier. However, carbon dioxide diffuses rapidly and increases its level into the cerebrospinal fluid, leading to a reduction in pH; intracellular acidosis results in the breakdown of intracellular proteins to create idiogenic osmoles. These osmoles create an osmotic gradient for water movement into the brain.

have shown significant decreases in intracellular pH in the brain after hemodialysis that contributed to decreases in cerebrospinal fluid pH and bicarbonate concentrations.[44] It was suggested that the fall in pH occurs through the acute formation of organic acids and that these osmolytes caused an increase in brain osmolality. In addition, plasma metabolic acidosis is generally rapidly corrected during hemodialysis by diffusion of bicarbonate from the dialysate and, in part, by loss of volatile carbon dioxide into the dialysate. Because bicarbonate is a charged molecule, it can not readily cross into cells, whereas carbon dioxide is freely diffusible. This differential has been speculated to lead to an initial paradoxical intracellular acidosis, which exacerbates cerebral idiogenic osmolyte generation and further contributes to brain water influx and cerebral edema.

Overall, mechanisms involved in both hypotheses probably contribute to a final common pathological increase in brain water content seen with rapid and efficient hemodialysis and lead to the spectrum of symptoms that characterize the DDS.

PREVENTION OF DIALYSIS DYSEQUILIBRIUM SYNDROME

Prevention of DDS is the mainstay of therapy, particularly during initiation of hemodialysis in new patients (Table 199-4). Once it was apparent that DDS was more likely to occur when severely uremic patients were rapidly dialyzed for extended durations, clinicians invoked widespread changes to practice. Despite the absence of

TABLE 199-4

Strategies for Prevention of Dialysis Dysequilibrium Syndrome

Reduce reduction in serum osmolality	Shorter hemodialysis session
	Small surface area hemofilter
	Low blood flow rate
	Low dialysate flow rate (CRRT)
	High dialysate sodium
	Avoid supraphysiological dialysate [bicarbonate]
	Apply CRRT (low-dose hemofiltration or hemodiafiltration)
Improve cardiovascular stability	Cooled dialysate
	High dialysate sodium
	Volumetric machine
	Blood volume control

CRRT, continuous renal replacement therapy.

evidence-based guidelines, the conventional aim has been to prescribe a slower and more gradual initial clearance of urea. This can be achieved by several strategies, including (1) limiting the duration of the first hemodialysis session to 1 hour or less, (2) using a small surface area or less efficient dialyzer, and (3) targeting lower blood flow rates of 150 to 200 mL/min to limit the rate of change in serum urea and osmolality. In addition, attention should be given to preserving hemodynamic stability. Improvements in hemodialysis practice designed to improve cardiovascular stability have included cooling of the dialysate and use of higher sodium content in the dialysate. These measures can further aid in reducing the frequency of DDS.[14] Moreover, the higher dialysate sodium concentrations can prevent significant reductions to serum osmolality and thus avoid large brain-to-serum osmotic gradients.[45] The use of a lower bicarbonate dialysate in severely acidotic patients with long-standing ESRD can reduce the risk of significant intracellular acidosis.

In the critically ill population at risk for DDS, additional strategies may include use of alternative modalities for RRT, such as sustained low-efficiency dialysis (SLED) or continuous renal replacement therapy (CRRT), to ensure a more gradual and stable clearance of urea.[13,46,47] Clinical studies have shown that CRRT, when compared with intermittent hemodialysis, may be superior for prevention of DDS because of the more gradual decreases of intravascular volume, slower changes in serum osmolality, improved compensation of metabolic acidosis, more stable $PaCO_2$ levels throughout RRT, less paradoxical acidosis in cerebrospinal fluid, and a lower urea concentration gradient between cerebrospinal fluid and plasma.[46] These differences in acute physiology have practical relevance for the prescription of RRT in both critically ill patients and those who may be at risk for DDS.

The prophylactic administration of bolus mannitol or benzodiazepines during the first hemodialysis sessions has been proposed to reduce mild symptoms of DDS, yet there exist no data from randomized, controlled trials showing that these measures can altogether prevent or reduce the severity of symptomatic DDS.[16,48] Although case studies have reported use of urea-containing and high-glucose-concentration dialysates for prevention of DDS, these measures remain unproven and cannot be recommended.[17,49]

CONCLUSION

In summary, the precise epidemiology and pathophysiology of DDS remain unclear. In the pioneering days of hemodialysis, DDS was more common and was a potentially life-threatening condition, with acute encephalopathy, seizures, and even death attributed to cerebral edema. In modern clinical practice, the occurrence of DDS in ESRD patients undergoing regular hemodialysis is rare. Whether this is due to a combination of greater clinical awareness of the risks for DDS, improvements in strategies for the application of hemodialysis (e.g., earlier initiation of RRT in patients with ARF, shorter initial but more frequent treatment sessions, higher-sodium and cooler dialysates) or to improvements in hemodialysis technology (e.g., introduction of volumetrically controlled dialysis machines) remains to be answered. In the critically ill population, the occurrence and risks for DDS are poorly characterized. However, selected critically ill patients may represent a unique population in which coexisting illnesses such as sepsis, brain injury, multiorgan dysfunction, and need for continuous sedation can be confounding and present obstacles in the diagnosis of DDS. In general, as outlined in this chapter, identification of those patients at risk for DDS and appropriate tailoring of RRT measures (i.e., low-dose CRRT) are fundamental measures for prevention. Future research may further describe the epidemiology and risk factors in critically ill patients and advance understanding of the pathophysiology of DDS.

Key Points
---

1. The epidemiology of dialysis dysequilibrium syndrome is poorly described.

2. The pathophysiology is likely a combination of the "reverse urea effect" and "idiogenic osmolyte" hypotheses.
3. Critically ill patients with sepsis, multiorgan failure, or brain injury may be at higher risk for dialysis dysequilibrium syndrome when initiating renal replacement therapy.
4. Dialysis dysequilibrium syndrome can be prevented by appropriate identification of those at risk and adjustment of initial renal replacement therapy prescription.

Key References

13. Arieff AI: Dialysis dysequilibrium syndrome: Current concepts on pathogenesis and prevention. Kidney Int 1994;45: 629-635.
34. Trachtman H, Futterweit S, Tonidandel W, Gullans SR: The role of organic osmolytes in the cerebral cell volume regulatory response to acute and chronic renal failure. J Am Soc Nephrol 1993;3:1913-1919.
35. Arieff AI, Massry SG, Barrientos A, Kleeman CR: Brain water and electrolyte metabolism in uremia: Effects of slow and rapid hemodialysis. Kidney Int 1973;4:177-187.
36. Ronco C, Bellomo R, Brendolan A, et al: Brain density changes during renal replacement in critically ill patients with acute renal failure: Continuous hemofiltration versus intermittent hemodialysis. J Nephrol 1999;12:173-178.
42. Trinh-Trang-Tan MM, Cartron JP, Bankir L: Molecular basis for the dialysis dysequilibrium syndrome: Altered aquaporin and urea transporter expression in the brain. Nephrol Dial Transplant 2005;20:1984-1988.

See the companion Expert Consult website for the complete reference list.

CHAPTER 200

Effect of Renal Replacement Therapy on the Brain

Natalia Polanco, Catalina Ocampo, Claudio Ronco, and Andrew Davenport

---
OBJECTIVES
This chapter will:
1. Describe the effect of chronic uremia on the brain and on the peripheral nervous system.
2. Describe changes in brain function with chronic renal replacement therapies.
3. Describe the short-term impact of renal replacement therapies on cerebral function.
4. Describe anticoagulation for patients with cerebral disorders.

End-stage renal disease (ESRD), irrespective of the primary cause of renal disease, occurs when chronic renal failure progresses to the point at which the kidneys are functioning at less than 10% of their normal capacity. This is frequently associated with other organ dysfunction, and cardiovascular and neurological disorders remain an important cause of morbidity and mortality in the ESRD population.[1,2]

EFFECT OF CHRONIC UREMIA ON THE BRAIN

Uremic Encephalopathy

Encephalopathy, in patients with renal failure, is a common problem that may be caused by uremia, but other causes such as thiamine deficiency, dialysis treatment, transplant rejection, hypertension, fluid and electrolyte disturbances, or drug toxicity may also play a role.[3]

Uremic encephalopathy is an organic brain syndrome that occurs in patients with untreated renal failure. It was very common before the introduction of routine chronic dialysis treatment. Typically, uremic encephalopathy is more severe and progresses more rapidly when renal failure is acute.

The clinical course is characterized by variability from day to day, and early symptoms may be subtle, including fatigue, apathy, clumsiness, and impaired concentration. As the encephalopathy worsens, the patient becomes emotionally labile and more lethargic, makes perceptual errors, and develops sleep inversion. Impaired abstract thinking and behavioral changes are the manifestations of frontal lobe damage. There can be motor symptoms at this time, including paratonia, grasp problems, and palmomental reflexes. In the later stages of uremic encephalopathy, the patient may become delirious, with visual hallucinations, disorientation, and agitation, and may progress to stupor, preterminal coma, and convulsions, which are usually generalized tonic-clonic seizures, although focal motor seizures may occur. Typically, these symptoms and signs improve or disappear after one or more dialysis treatments.[4]

Although the clinical symptoms of uremic encephalopathy are well described, its pathophysiology remains uncertain and is probably multifactorial. Postmortem studies on the brains of patients dying with chronic renal impairment often show mild, nonspecific changes related more to concomitant illness than to the renal failure.[1] In renal impairment, uremic toxins accumulate (urea, guanidino compounds, uric acid, hippuric acid, various amino acids, polypeptides, polyamines, phenols, phenolic and indolic acids, acetone, glucuronic acid, carnitine, myoinositol, sulfates, phosphates and "middle molecules"); they may possibly act as uremic neurotoxins, but no single metabolite has been identified as the only cause of uremia.[5] Removal of these uremic toxins by dialytic treatments and/or renal transplantation is associated with an improvement in uremic encephalopathy, supporting a pathophysiological role. Guanidine compounds are markedly increased in serum, cerebrospinal fluid, and the brain of uremic patients, and it has been postulated that these compounds have excitatory effects on the central nervous system, by activation of the excitatory N-methyl-D-aspartate receptors and concomitant inhibition of inhibitory γ-aminobutyric acid (GABA)-ergic neurotransmission.[6] In uremic animal and in vitro studies, intermediary metabolism is affected, with increased levels of creatine phosphate, adenosine triphosphate, and glucose and decreased levels of monophosphate, adenosine diphosphate, and lactate. These biochemical changes are associated with reduced metabolic rate of the brain and a decrease in cerebral oxygen consumption.[1] In addition, hormonal disturbances have been suggested to play a role in the pathogenesis of uremic encephalopathy. For example, the calcium content of the cerebral cortex is almost twice that of normal brain. This increase is probably caused by secondary hyperparathyroidism, because both electroencephalographic (EEG) abnormalities and brain calcium accumulation were prevented by parathyroidectomy in dog models of acute and chronic renal failure.[7]

It is difficult to establish a diagnosis of uremic encephalopathy with certainty, because the level of azotemia correlates poorly with the degree of neurological dysfunction. Laboratory blood tests only confirm the existence of chronic kidney disease (CKD) but cannot exclude other causes for the encephalopathy. EEG has been widely used to evaluate metabolic encephalopathy, since as long ago as 1937, when Berger first observed slow brain activity induced by hypoglycemia.[8] EEG findings in uremic patients are usually most abnormal in the acute encephalopathic state. There is a generalized slowing of the EEG, with an excess of delta and theta waves, with suppression of normal alpha and beta wave activity, and occasionally bilateral spikes and wave complexes occurring in absence of evident clinical seizure activity (Fig. 200-1). As the uremic state progresses and the serum creatinine concentration increases, the EEG wave activity becomes slower.[1,8,9] Cerebral imaging with CT or MRI does not provide additional diagnostic information, although it is useful to exclude other causes of encephalopathy, such as subdural hematoma or hydrocephalus. Reversible signal changes in the basal ganglia, periventricular white matter, and internal capsule have been described on MRI in chronic uremic encephalopathy and disappear after dialysis. The pathophysiological mechanisms and the relevance of these changes are as yet unclear.[1,10]

Initiation of renal replacement therapy or renal transplantation usually improves the symptoms of uremic encephalopathy, although many patients fail to fully respond to these therapies.

Dementia

Dementia is more common in patients with renal failure than in the general population. Cerebral atrophy is common in patients with CKD, even in those without evident cognitive, affective, or behavioral changes. On psychometric testing, there is often evidence of intellectual deficits in these patients. The atrophy might be caused by endogenous uremic toxins, arterial hypertension, or cerebral hypoperfusion due to atherosclerosis.[11] Increasing the dose of dialysis, by switching patients from standard thrice weekly to daily nocturnal dialysis, improves psychomotor performance and memory.[11]

Dementia should be differentiated from delirium and depression, which are also common in CKD.

Cerebrovascular Disease

Patients with CKD are prone to the development of arteriosclerosis, atherosclerosis, and ischemic stroke, and these are important causes of morbidity and mortality.

Ischemic stroke in renal failure mainly results from atherosclerosis, thromboembolic disease, intradialytic hypotension, or some combination of these.

Atherosclerosis in patients with chronic renal failure is generally more diffuse and distally located than in the general population, probably because of a combination of traditional atherogenic risk factors such as male gender, age, diabetes mellitus, hypertension, dyslipidemia, and smoking, together with factors more specifically related to renal failure and its treatment,[12] including accumulation

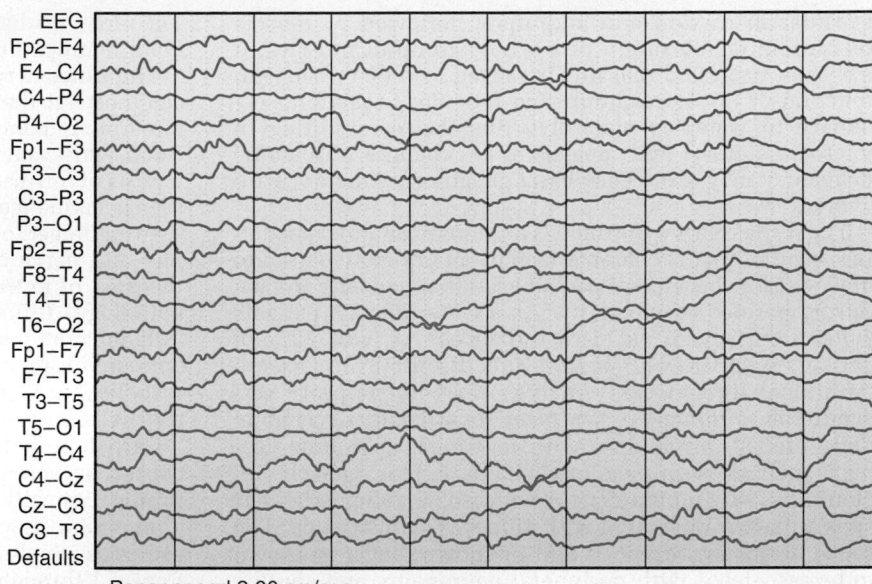

EEG
Fp2–F4
F4–C4
C4–P4
P4–O2
Fp1–F3
F3–C3
C3–P3
P3–O1
Fp2–F8
F8–T4
T4–T6
T6–O2
Fp1–F7
F7–T3
T3–T5
T5–O1
T4–C4
C4–Cz
Cz–C3
C3–T3
Defaults

Paper speed 3.00 cm/sec
Sensitivity 100 μV/cm
Time constant 0.30 sec
Filter 70 Hz

FIGURE 200-1. Electroencephalogram from a patient with end-stage renal failure showing a marked reduction in normal beta and alpha wave activity with increased slow-wave theta and delta wave activity.

of guanidine compounds, oxidative and carbonyl stress, hyperhomocysteinemia, and disturbances of the calcium-phosphate metabolism.[13-15]

Accumulation of endogenous guanidino compounds may be an important factor in endothelial dysfunction. One of these guanidine compounds can competitively inhibit the synthesis of nitric oxide, reducing the vasodilatory effects of endothelium-derived relaxing factor, and consequently affects vasomotor tone in several vascular beds, including the cerebral circulation.[13,14,16] Other guanidine compounds might potentiate the deleterious effects of cerebral hypoxia under uremic conditions.[17]

Oxidative and carbonyl stress in CKD are associated with the inflammatory milieu that plays a central role in the pathogenesis of atheroma. Besides an accumulation of oxidized low-density lipoproteins, advanced glycation end products (AGEs) also increase in these patients. This could be due to impaired renal clearance of AGEs in combination with increased endogenous formation and dietary intake. AGE formation can be inhibited by angiotensin-converting enzyme inhibitors, angiotensin receptor blockers, or aminoguanidine.[18,19]

Large observational studies have established that hyperhomocysteinemia is an independent risk factor for atherosclerosis, and this condition is prevalent in 85% to 100% of patients with CKD.[20]

Soft tissue calcification, with an increased risk of medial vascular calcification, arterial stiffness, and worsening of arteriosclerosis, can also occur due to disturbances in calcium metabolism. Soft tissue and vascular calcification is increased in patients with ongoing inflammation, often accompanied by malnutrition and hypoalbuminemia. In addition, both patients with low bone turnover and those with secondary hyperparathyroidism due to reduced active vitamin D production by the kidneys and phosphate retention (which can lead to tertiary hyperparathyroidism)[21] are at increased risk of soft tissue calcification.

During routine hemodialysis, intradialytic hypotension is often encountered, and repetitive hypotensive episodes may lead to cerebral hypoperfusion and small vessel isch-

emia with lacunar infracts. It has also been shown that particulate matter is generated during hemodialysis treatments, and these microemboli could potentially cause small-vessel cerebral ischemia in patients with a patent foramen ovale or other right-to-left shunt.[21a]

Because renal anemia has been shown to be an independent risk factor for stroke and cardiovascular events in chronic renal failure, treatment with recombinant human erythropoietin would appear to be an important preventive measure.[22]

Hemorrhagic stroke may include intracerebral, subarachnoid, or subdural hemorrhage. The uremic state per se causes platelet dysfunction and altered platelet-vessel wall interaction, resulting in a bleeding tendency that is partially corrected by effective dialysis. However, hemodialysis itself is associated with higher incidence of intracerebral hemorrhage (8.7 to 10.3 per 1000 patient-years; relative risk [RR], 10.7 compared to normal) and subarachnoidal hemorrhage (0.8 per 1000 patient years; RR, 4.0). The prognosis of hemorrhagic stroke in patients with chronic renal failure is poor, having a morbidity and mortality as high as 60%.[23,24] Recent studies have confirmed that patients in renal failure are at increased risk of spontaneous hemorrhage when prescribed warfarin and other coumarin anticoagulants.[24a]

Movement Disorders and Restless Legs Syndrome

Movement alterations in patients with CKD can be the result of encephalopathy, medication, or structural lesions.

In metabolic encephalopathy, several types of involuntary movements may occur. Asterixis or "flapping tremor" can be caused by sudden loss of tone originating from cortical dysfunction; it clinically comprises multifocal, action-induced jerks that can mimic drop attacks in severe cases. Myoclonus can also occur as sudden contractions, irregular in rhythm and amplitude, followed by muscle relaxation, or relaxation of a whole group of muscles. It has been suggested that this is caused by a disturbance in function of the lower brainstem reticular formation, secondary to water or electrolyte imbalances resulting in microcirculatory and degenerative changes. Thiamine deficiency may also cause basal ganglia dysfunction with chorea.[25-27]

The restless legs syndrome is a common and incapacitating disorder that is characterized by an imperative need to move the legs because of paresthesias that typically worsen during periods of inactivity. As a consequence, patients suffer from severe sleep disturbances. At least 20% of patients with CKD suffer from this disorder.[28] In general, traditional thrice-weekly dialysis does not improve this syndrome, although it has been reported to respond to daily dialysis. Treatment with levodopa, dopamine agonists such as pramipexole, benzodiazepines, gabapentin, clonidine, or opioids can provide some relief. There is substantial improvement with kidney transplantation. The cause of this syndrome is still unknown, but it is known to be associated with peripheral neuropathy and chronic renal failure.[29]

Opportunistic Infections

Uremia can be associated with defective polymorphonuclear white blood cell phagocytosis, leading to an acquired immunodeficiency–like state, especially against bacterial infections. Immunosuppressed patients can present with ambiguous signs and symptoms and infections with uncommon and atypical microorganisms. Neurological infections in patients with renal failure mainly present as acute, subacute, or chronic meningitis, encephalitis, myelitis, or brain abscess.[30,31]

Opportunistic bacterial infections include pathogens such as *Nocardia asteroides*, *Mycobacterium tuberculosis*, and *Listeria monocytogenes*.[32] The most common fungal infections are caused by *Cryptococcus neoformans*, *Aspergillus fumigatus*, and *Candida*, *Histoplasma*, *Mucor*, and *Paracoccidioides* species.[33] Latent viral infections that can be reactivated include herpes simplex, cytomegalovirus, and JC polyomavirus.[34]

Lumbar puncture is often needed for diagnosis, but it should be performed only after exclusion of intracranial space-occupying lesions by neuroimaging. If a definitive diagnosis cannot be made, then, depending on the clinical condition, a trial of empirical therapy may be required.[1]

Neoplasms

The immunosuppressive state of patients with CKD is associated with an increased incidence of de novo neoplasia, but neurological tumors are rare. Malignant meningioma and primary central nervous system lymphoma have been reported.[35,36]

PERIPHERAL NERVOUS SYSTEM COMPLICATIONS IN UREMIA

Mononeuropathy

Patients with uremia have an increased susceptibility to compression and local ischemia of the peripheral nerves.

The ulnar, median, and femoral nerves are prone to entrapment neuropathies.

The ulnar nerve can be damaged by uremic soft tissue calcinosis at the wrist and in Guyon´s canal in the midforearm. Depending on the site of compression in the canal, this may cause purely motor dysfunction with paresis of intrinsic hand muscles; sensory loss of the hypothenar eminence, the small finger, and the lateral part of the ring finger; or mixed symptomatology. Electromyography and nerve conduction studies are useful to confirm the area of entrapment and document the extent of the pathology. Initially, conservative treatment with anti-inflammatory medication, tricyclic antidepressants, and anticonvulsants can be used. If the patient shows no response, or if motor deficits develop, then surgical neurolysis is indicated.

Carpal tunnel syndrome is far more common and is caused by entrapment of the median nerve in the carpal tunnel, typically due the deposition of dialysis-associated β_2-amyloidosis.[37] Symptoms include burning pain and paresthesias involving the ventral surface of the hands and fingers I through III and the medial surface of finger IV. Thenar muscle atrophy may occur. Renal transplantation may relieve the symptoms but does not reverse β_2-amyloidosis.[38]

Acute femoral neuropathy may occur as a complication of renal transplantation as a result of perioperative compression of the nerve by retractors or nerve ischemia. Patients develop weakness of the thigh and suffer pain or sensory deficit on the thigh and inner calf.[39]

Polyneuropathy

Uremic polyneuropathy occurs in approximately 60% of patients with CKD and can affect motor, sensory, autonomic, and cranial nerves.[40,41] There is an unexplained male predominance, and patients typically present with symmetrical distal sensory loss for all modalities, more pronounced in the lower extremities. These effects are minimal at glomerular filtration rates (GFR) greater than 12 mL/min; but as the GFR falls, nerve conduction studies become abnormal, and patients begin to demonstrate clinical signs of peripheral nerve dysfunction when the GFR is lower than 6 mL/min. Early findings include increased vibratory threshold and impaired temperature sensation. Paradoxical heat sensation, paresthesias, and pain are common. Later in the course, ascending hyperesthesia to pinprick or to touch, areflexia, restless legs, muscle weakness, cramps, and atrophy may be found.[40] The neuropathy usually evolves over several months, but rarely an acute or subacute course is seen. Pruritus is often present in renal failure, especially during dialysis. Autonomic neuropathy can play a role in the pathogenesis of intradialytic and orthostatic hypotension, incontinence, diarrhea, constipation, esophageal dysfunction, hyperhidrosis, and impotence.[40] Besides parasympathetic vagal dysfunction, neuropathy of other cranial nerves—especially optic, trigeminal, facial, and vestibulocochlear neuropathy—have been described anecdotally. Electrophysiological studies typically demonstrate axonal loss with secondary demyelination. This is thought to be caused by the retention of guanidino compounds that interfere with the assembly of tubulin proteins in the myelin sheath. The most sensitive parameters in the diagnosis of uremic neuropathy are F-wave measurements from the lower limbs, vibration detection thresholds in the foot, and sural nerve sensory action potential amplitudes with decreased nerve conduction velocity.[41]

CHANGES IN BRAIN FUNCTION WITH CHRONIC RENAL REPLACEMENT THERAPIES

Since the introduction of dialysis, the spectrum of neurological complications has changed, and different neurological alterations have emerged. Dialysis dysequilibrium syndrome (see Chapter 199), dialysis dementia, hypertensive encephalopathy, and cerebrovascular accident can occur as a direct consequence of dialysis. Furthermore, dialysis is associated with accelerated arteriosclerosis and may contribute to the development of hemorrhagic stroke, subdural hematoma, Wernicke's encephalopathy, osmotic myelinosis, and intracranial hypertension.[3]

Dialysis Dementia

Dialysis dementia, also known as dialysis encephalopathy or progressive myoclonic dialysis encephalopathy, is a slowly progressive but fatal neurological condition. It was first clearly documented by Alfrey and colleagues in 1972,[42] but it was some 4 years later that the link was made between increased aluminum levels in the brain gray matter, bone, and other tissues of patients with dialysis dementia and the use of aluminum-containing phosphate binders.[43] However, only a small minority of dialysis patients suffered dialysis dementia, even though, at that time, the majority were prescribed aluminum-based phosphate binders. In the late 1970s, the prevalence of dialysis dementia in Europe was 600 per 100,000 dialysis patients, with marked variation among centers.[44] In 1982, Prior showed a strong association between the aluminum content in dialysate water, dialysis dementia, and severe dialysis osteodystrophy. From this observation, the importance of trace element contamination of the dialysate was realized, and reverse osmosis was introduced to the preparation of dialysates.

Even though water treated with reverse osmosis was used for dialysate, dialysis dementia still occurred in hemodialysis patients with high serum aluminum.[45] Aluminum absorption is now known to be increased in iron deficiency, by citrate, and from cooking in aluminum pans when bicarbonate or acids are added. On the other hand, residual renal function protects against aluminum overload.

How aluminum interferes with neuronal function to cause dementia is still unknown. Potential mechanisms include complexing with high-energy phosphates, impaired enzymatic function, deoxyribonucleic acid binding, impaired hydrolysis of phosphoinositides, impaired microtubular function, reduced calmodulin activity via binding, and reduced neurotransmitter uptake.[1]

After 35 years, many questions about dialysis dementia remain unsolved. The use of purified water, new phosphate binders, and attention to dialysis adequacy and nutritional status have reduced but not eliminated dialysis dementia.

Dialysis dementia is a subacute, progressive, and invariably fatal disorder unless treated. This syndrome may be part of a multisystem disorder that includes vitamin D–resistant osteomalacia, proximal myopathy, and a non–iron-deficient, microcytic, hypochromic anemia. When Dr. Allen Alfrey reported the first series of patients in 1972, he referred to this clinical entity as "a syndrome of dyspraxia and multifocal seizures associated with chronic hemodialysis."[42] The first clinical features of dialysis dementia include dysarthria, dysphasia, and dysgraphia; a mixture of these three symptoms has been reported as one of the earliest signs of dialysis dementia in up to 95% of cases. The patient may initially have a stuttering speech that occurs only during and immediately after dialysis. As the disorder progresses, language function becomes more severely and more persistently affected. Patients may also suffer from personality changes and psychosis with hallucinations and paranoid delusions that become prominent in the later stages. Myoclonus occurs in up to 80% of cases, and patients may become both ataxic and dyspraxic. Seizures develop in up to 60% as patients progress to frank dementia. Death usually follows 6 to 9 months after the onset of symptoms in most untreated cases.[1,3,46]

To establish the diagnosis of dialysis dementia, the concentrations of aluminum in cerebrospinal fluid or serum are of only limited assistance. Dialysis dementia has been reported in patients with serum concentrations ranging from 15 to more than 1000 µg/l. Although dementia is uncommon with serum concentrations of 50 µg/L or lower, such concentrations by no means exclude the diagnosis.[1] The European guidelines (1986) suggested that the aluminum content of dialysis fluid should not exceed 10 µg/L and that plasma monitoring of aluminum should be carried out at least quarterly. However, with the improvement of water quality and decreased use of aluminum phosphate binders, the regular routine monitoring of plasma aluminum in patients not treated with aluminum phosphate binders may no longer be necessary. Plasma aluminum measurements are also required in other groups of patients at risk from aluminum toxicity, including those receiving total parenteral nutrition with renal disease, aluminum-containing infant formulas or plasma exchange, and people at risk from industrial exposure, such as aluminum smelter workers.[47]

Because aluminum is mainly stored intracellularly, serum and plasma estimations may underestimate the total body burden. The desferrioxamine chelation test has been used as an additional diagnostic test for aluminum overload. In the standard test protocol, 40 mg/kg of desferrioxamine is infused over the last 30 minutes of a dialysis session, and the change in serum aluminum concentration is determined between the baseline value (before administration of desferrioxamine), and the value 48 hours later (before the next dialysis session). Increments of 100 and 200 µg/L have been suggested to be associated with an increased aluminum body burden requiring active chelation therapy.

Abnormalities in the EEG, with intermittent bursts of high-voltage slowing and spike and wave activity, particularly in the frontal leads, may precede clinically overt symptoms by up to 6 months and are therefore useful to help establish the diagnosis. The EEG may show an initial deterioration after treatment with desferrioxamine has commenced.[1,48] Neuroimaging studies are useful to help exclude other diagnoses if the clinical picture is atypical.

The use of aluminum-free dialysate may arrest or even improve the established case, but, because aluminum is so avidly bound to plasma protein, very little is actually removed at subsequent dialysis. Although several approaches have been tested, no satisfactory treatment exists. The mainstay of treatment of dialysis dementia is desferrioxamine infusions. Desferrioxamine is a chelating agent which binds aluminum with greater affinity than that of the plasma proteins to which the metal is usually bound. The resulting complex has a molecular weight of 600 and therefore is removed by dialysis. The clinical improvement is slow, and therapy may need to be given once weekly for over a year.[1,49-53] It has been reported that some patients initially deteriorate with desferrioxamine treatment even with low doses.[54] These adverse effects are unusual if desferrioxamine is administrated 4 to 5 hours before the beginning of dialysis, but long-term use of desferrioxamine may result in ocular toxicity. The only other treatment that has been successful in removing aluminum is kidney transplantation.[55]

CEREBROVASCULAR DISEASE

Cerebrovascular disease (CVD) in chronic dialysis patients is associated with significant morbidity and mortality. In 2002, researchers in the Dialysis Outcomes and Practice Patterns Study (DOPPS) reported that approximately 18% and 13.7% of patients undergoing dialysis in the United States and Europe, respectively, had a history of CVD (defined as stroke, transient ischemic attack, or carotid endarterectomy).[56] More recently, a secondary analysis of data from the Hemodialysis (HEMO) Study found a similar prevalence of CVD (19.5%).[57] Seliger and colleagues, analyzing U.S. Renal Data System and national Hospital Discharge Survey data, determined that incident dialysis patients are at 5 to 10 times the risk of either an ischemic or a hemorrhagic stroke requiring hospitalization, compared to patients without renal failure.[58] Furthermore, in the dialysis population, the 2-year mortality rate after a stroke is 64%, an outcome almost as poor as that after acute myocardial infarction.[57]

Comorbid conditions such as hypertension, diabetes, and hyperlipidemia, which are known risk factors of CVD in the general population, are common in chronic dialysis patients. However, in uremic patients, the pathogenesis of vascular disease may be somewhat different from that in the general population because of the high prevalence of nontraditional risk factors, such as disturbances in the calcium-phosphate product, inflammation, hyperhomocysteinemia, and oxidative stress.[59] In the dialysis population, a greater risk for stroke was found with lower serum albumin levels, older age, greater mean blood pressure,

and diabetes mellitus. With the exception of blood pressure, those baseline risk factors also were associated with CVD death.[57,60] In the same way, despite the technological improvements in hemodialysis treatment, there are diverse cardiovascular risk factors directly associated with dialysis therapy (Table 200-1). To date, no randomized trial has been undertaken to analyze whether one modality of dialysis is better to decrease the incidence of stroke-related death in patients with end-stage renal disease. In the analysis of data from the HEMO study, neither the flux nor dose had an effect on the rate of CVD death, but in subgroups without baseline evidence of CVD or with duration of hemodialysis therapy longer than 3.7 years, high flux was associated with decreased risk for CVD death.[57]

Hemorrhagic Complications

The incidence of cerebral hemorrhage seems to be higher than that of cerebral infarction in patients undergoing chronic hemodialysis in Japan,[23] although these results may not be generalizable to the European and North American dialysis populations.

Hypertension and anticoagulant therapy are the two main nontraumatic causes of intracranial hemorrhage. Many hemodialysis patients have a long history of hypertension in the predialytic phase, and hypertension often persists during the period of dialysis. Patients with polycystic kidney disease may have underlying cerebral aneurysms, which are at increased risk of bleeding if blood pressure is not adequately controlled. In addition, the uremic state, with platelet dysfunction and altered platelet–vessel wall interaction, results in a bleeding propensity,[24,61] and this may account for the increased risk of bleeding in patients prescribed coumarin anticoagulants. The platelet defects are partially corrected by effective dialysis, but on the other hand the routine use of heparin and antiplatelet agents in dialysis patients is an additional factor in the high potential risk of cerebral hemorrhage in this population.[1,60,62]

Subdural hematoma has been reported in 1% to 3.3% of patients undergoing hemodialysis in all age ranges, and it is not an exceptional cause of death in this population. Although subdural hematoma is well recognized as a complication in hemodialysis patients, it may be overlooked because of clinical similarity to encephalopathy and dementia. The clinical features may have a sudden onset, followed by a gradual or rapid evolution phase. Early symptoms such as headache, nausea and vomiting are not uncommon, and a high index of suspicion is necessary,

TABLE 200-1

Cardiovascular Risk Factors in the Dialysis Population

CLASSIC RISK FACTORS	UREMIA-ASSOCIATED RISK FACTORS	DIALYSIS-ASSOCIATED RISK FACTORS
Older age	Anemia	Dialysate
Male gender	Calcium-phosphorus alterations	Bioincompatibility
Hypertension	Hyperhomocysteinemia	Inadequate dialysis
Diabetes	Chronic inflammation	Episodes of hypotension
Hyperlipidemia	Oxidative stress	Volume overload
Previous CV disease	Low level of albumin	Arteriovenous access
Current smoker	Sleep alterations	
LVH		
Sedentary		

CV, cardiovascular; LVH, left ventricular hypertrophy.

but if these symptoms are followed by signs of increased intracranial pressure (ICP), such as loss of consciousness and coma, a diagnosis of cerebral bleeding should be excluded. Subacute and chronic subdural hematoma may cause pseudodementia, drowsiness, confusion with marked day-to-day fluctuations, or focal signs such as hemiparesis. The diagnosis can be confirmed by CT scan or by MRI.[1,48,62]

Subarachnoid hemorrhage can be considered as an important cause of death in hemodialysis patients. Hypertension, polycystic kidney disease (with an increased risk for development of cerebral vascular malformations), and the use of anticoagulation and/or antiplatelet agents are the most important risk factors. A CT scan may help in the diagnosis by showing hemorrhages 1.5 cm or greater in width.

The prognosis of hemorrhagic stroke in patients with CKD is poor, with high morbidity and mortality of up to 60% to 70%.[23,63] Large hematoma size,[62,64] reduced Glasgow Coma Scale score on admission, age greater than 65 years, and diabetes mellitus[23,60,64] are all reported to be adverse prognostic factors.

Wernicke's Encephalopathy

Wernicke's encephalopathy (WE) is caused by thiamine deficiency. Although WE is most closely linked to alcoholism, its development is a rare but probably underdiagnosed occurrence outside the usual context of alcoholism.[1,62] A growing number of reports have referred to this diagnosis in the setting of other conditions affecting thiamine uptake and metabolism, including dialysis.[65,66]

This syndrome is characterized by the triad of ataxia, changes in ocular motility (nystagmus, abducens palsy), and disturbance of consciousness. In nonalcoholic patients, this triad is rarely present, which is one reason why this disorder often remains unrecognized. Moreover, dialysis patients not infrequently suffer from a large variety of neurological disorders, including uremic encephalopathy, dysequilibrium syndrome, dialysis dementia, hypertensive encephalopathy, and cerebral vascular diseases.

Thiamine is a water-soluble vitamin that is not removed by dialysis to any greater degree than that with normal excretion in urine. It was reported that no significant differences were observed in plasma thiamine levels between chronic dialysis patients and controls.[67] However, in some patients, plasma thiamine concentrations fluctuate widely during dialysis, probably because of concomitant comor-

bidities (malabsorption, undernutrition, inflammation, malignancy, genetic predisposition) and/or an acute precipitating event (sepsis, acute cardiovascular episode).[65,66]

WE has a fatal prognosis if unrecognized, but a good outcome can be obtained if the diagnosis is suspected and thiamine is administered immediately.[65,66] This condition should be differentiated from the various other neurological disorders associated with dialysis and should be suspected in all dialysis patients who present with at least one of the clinical triad of symptoms of WE.

Short-Term Impact of Renal Replacement Therapies on Cerebral Function

The management of dialysis after acute cerebral hemorrhage or infarction is problematical because dialysis itself may cause specific problems, including increased ICP and cerebral edema with cerebral hypoxia.[68] Although intermittent dialysis treatments can result in cerebral edema due to the dialysis dysequilibrium syndrome (DDS; see Chapter 199), ICP can also increase within the first hour of treatment due to hypotension resulting in cerebral hypoperfusion and a rebound increase in ICP (Fig. 200-2). It is therefore very important when managing dialysis in patients with acute brain injury that cardiovascular stability be maintained (Table 200-2). During routine hemodi-

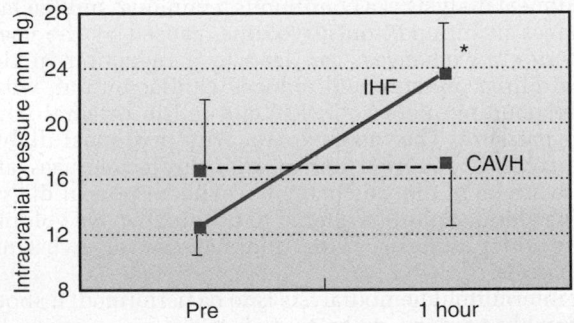

FIGURE 200-2. Maximum recorded sustained intracranial pressure (ICP) during the first hour of treatment with continuous arteriovenous hemofiltration (CAVH) and intermittent hemofiltration (IHF)—16 L exchange in 3.5 hours. Mean values are shown; bars represent the standard error of the mean (SEM). Pre, pretreatment. *, $P < .05$ versus pretreatment ICP.

TABLE 200-2

Hemodialysis in the Brain-Injured Patient

RISK FACTOR	CLINICAL STRATEGY TARGET	CLINICAL MANAGEMENT
Cerebral edema	Serum urea <15 mmol/L	Daily treatment
	Serum sodium >145 mmol/L	High-sodium dialysate
	Reduce fall in plasma osmolality	Slower blood pump speed
		Smaller surface area dialyzer
		May need hypertonic saline bolus
	Prevent hypotension	Prolong treatment time
		Minimize ultrafiltration rate
		Cool dialysate
		Blood volume monitoring
	Avoid sudden alkalosis	Reduce dialysate bicarbonate
Cerebral hemorrhage	Avoid systemic anticoagulation	No anticoagulation
		Regional anticoagulant

TABLE 200-3

Effects of Chronic Dialysis on the Nervous System

NEUROLOGICAL DISORDER	ETIOLOGY	RISK FACTOR
Encephalopathy	Uremia	Unexpected presentation
Dementia	Aluminum	Contaminated dialysate/drugs
	Cerebrovascular disease	Hypertension
Stroke	Acute ischemia	Hypertension
	Hemorrhage	Hypotension
	Aneurysm	Hypertension
		Polycystic kidney
Wernicke's encephalopathy	Thiamine deficiency	Poor nutrition
Peripheral neuropathy	Axonal/demyelination	High-flux dialysis
	β_2 amyloid deposition	Uremia
		Entrapment neuropathy
Myoclonus/restless legs	Neuropathy	Uremia

alysis in stable patients, cerebral blood flow falls during treatment, in association with a reduction in plasma volume due to ultrafiltration.[69] Although blood flow velocity decreases, reactivity to carbon dioxide remains intact, provided that patients are not anemic.[70]

In the head-injured patient, or in the patient with pre-existing cerebral edema, the fall in mean arterial blood pressure resulting from ultrafiltration can provoke a surge in ICP.[71] Because cardiovascular stability tends to be greater for continuous rather than intermittent renal replacement modes, the former are preferred.[72,73] Although peritoneal dialysis is a continuous technique, sudden large changes in intraperitoneal volume, caused by the use of hypertonic exchanges, can lead to a reduction in right atrial filling pressure and reduced cardiac output, with a corresponding increase in ICP and fall in cerebral perfusion pressure. This may explain why peritoneal dialysis was recently reported not to offer any advantages after acute stroke in dialysis patients.[63] The peritoneal dialysis prescription should be altered to use small cycle volumes, as in tidal dialysis, with minimal use of hypertonic exchanges.

If intermittent hemodialysis is to be performed, it should preferably be done daily, to maintain a serum urea concentration of less than 15 mmol/L (preferably <12 mmol/L), to minimize the osmotic effects of dialysis-induced fluxes of urea on cerebral volume. In addition, dialysis therapy time should be prolonged to minimize cardiovascular instability by reducing the absolute ultrafiltration rate. Daily dialysis allows the use of reduced blood flow rates and smaller surface area dialyzers to reduce the rate of fall in plasma osmolality. Dialysis machines with relative blood volume monitoring and ultrafiltration feedback control are preferred. A high dialysate sodium concentration is required to both improve cardiovascular stability and maintain plasma osmolality. In this respect, patients undergoing peritoneal dialysis with a dialysate sodium concentration of 132 mmol/L may benefit from additional hypertonic saline, as may patients treated by CRRT with a serum sodium concentration of less than 145 mmol/L. Sodium balance is better maintained with hemofiltration than with dialysis mode, because the sodium sieving coefficient is less than 1.0.

Dialysate temperature should be cooled to 35°C or set to isothermic, again to improve cardiovascular stability during treatment. Daily treatment with extended time allows dialysate flow rates to be slowed down, to reduce the rate of fall in plasma osmolality; similarly, the bicar-

bonate concentration can be reduced to 28 to 30 mmol/L (mEq/L) to prevent too rapid a correction of plasma bicarbonate.[20] Compared with standard routine intermittent hemodialysis, larger surface area dialyzers and fast blood pump speeds are not required, and smaller dialyzers with lower blood flow rates should be chosen. Potential hypotensive reactions at the initiation of treatment, which are caused by bradykinin production, may be reduced by choice of membrane composition and by priming the equipment with isotonic sodium bicarbonate rather than normal saline.

These precautions for intermittent hemodialysis also apply to hybrid techniques of extended daily dialysis.

Anticoagulation

It must be remembered that there is an increased risk of local bleeding around the site of ICP monitoring devices (the risk is greatest for intraventricular drains > subdural catheter > extradural monitor).[74] Therefore, patients with ICP devices; those with intracranial, subarachnoid, or subdural hemorrhage; and those treated immediately after ischemic stroke should preferably receive no anticoagulation, or only regional anticoagulation, such as citrate, nafamostat, or prostanoids.

Citrate has an advantage in that trisodium citrate leads to a positive sodium load, but, because each citrate is indirectly metabolized to three bicarbonates, patients may become alkalemic. For this reason, careful monitoring is required for patients who may be hyperventilated to a $PaCO_2$ of 4.5 kPa (33.5 mm Hg). Prostacyclin and epoprostenol are potent vasodilators and may provoke an increase in ICP by causing hypotension.[75] Therefore, these agents must be used cautiously and, if necessary, covered by increased inotropic support to maintain the cerebral perfusion pressure. Nafamostat is a very effective regional anticoagulant but is readily available only in Japan.

CONCLUSION

Chronic uremia, if left untreated, can result in peripheral neuropathy, movement disorders, and encephalopathy, which generally respond to initiation of dialysis. The effects of chronic dialysis on the nervous system are summarized in Table 200-3.

Patients undergoing dialysis can develop dementia due to contamination of the dialysate water supply, concomitant drug therapy, or CVD. Ischemic CVD can be exacerbated by hypertension but also by repetitive hypotensive events during hemodialysis, and possibly by microemboli produced during dialysis. Long-term dialysis patients can develop entrapment neuropathies, both entrapment of peripheral nerves (e.g., carpal tunnel compression) and spinal cord involvement due to β_2-microglobulin deposition, with secondary vertebral destruction and collapse. Similarly, poor nutrition coupled with high-flux dialysis and hemodiafiltration can lead to vitamin deficiencies.

Standard routine outpatient hemodialysis causes an increase in cerebral water content, which in most patients is asymptomatic. In addition, ultrafiltration is associated with a reduction in middle cerebral artery flow. This combination of effects leads to increased risk of cerebral ischemia during episodes of intradialytic hypotension. In the patient with acute or preexisting brain injury, these effects are exacerbated, and treatment must be altered to minimize shifts of urea and other osmolytes and maintain cardiovascular, and thereby intracranial, stability.

Key Points

1. Both acute and chronic renal failure can adversely affect cerebral function.
2. Patients with renal failure are more susceptible to cerebral side effects of drug toxicity, and drug dosages should be adjusted accordingly.
3. Cerebral edema commonly occurs after a routine outpatient hemodialysis session.

4. Renal replacement therapies should be adjusted to minimize the change in plasma osmolality by reducing blood and dialysate flows and using high-sodium dialysates and/or replacement solutions to minimize cerebral edema.
5. Similarly, renal replacement therapies should be adjusted to minimize falls in systemic blood pressure and to prevent falls in cerebral perfusion pressure.

Key References

11. Savazzi GM: Pathogenesis of cerebral atrophy in uremia: State of the art. Nephron 1988;49:94-103.
68. Davenport A: Renal replacement therapy in the patient with acute brain injury. Am J Kidney Dis 2001;37:457-466.
70. Skinner H, Mackaness C, Bedford N, Mahajan R: Cerebral haemodynamics in patients with chronic renal failure: Effects of haemodialysis. Br J Anaesth 2005;94:203-205.
71. Davenport A, Will EJ, Losowsky MS: Rebound surges of intracranial pressure as a consequence of forced ultrafiltration used to control intracranial pressure in patients with severe hepatorenal failure. Am J Kidney Dis 1989;14:516-519.
72. Gondo G, Fujitsu K, Kuwabara T, et al: Comparison of five modes of dialysis in neurosurgical patients with renal failure. Neurol Med Chir 1989;29:1125-1131.
73. Yorioka N, Oda H, Ogawa T, et al: Continuous ambulatory peritoneal dialysis is superior to hemodialysis in chronic dialysis patients with cerebral hemorrhage. Nephron 1994;67:365-366.

See the companion Expert Consult website for the complete reference list.

Uremic Toxins

CHAPTER 201

Metabolic Waste Products in Acute Uremia

Griet Glorieux, Eva Schepers, Wim Van Biesen, Norbert Lameire, and Raymond Vanholder

---

OBJECTIVES

This chapter will:
1. Discuss the possible factors responsible for the uremic syndrome in acute kidney injury (AKI).
2. Underline the contribution of the retention and accumulation of uremic solutes, especially the low-molecular-weight toxins.
3. Stress the importance of optimal toxin removal in the treatment of AKI.

The uremic syndrome is characterized by a progressive deterioration of biochemical and physiological functions, and a quantitative and qualitative deterioration of performance, in parallel with the progression of renal failure. This is largely attributed to the retention of a myriad of compounds that under normal conditions are excreted by the healthy kidneys. The clinical characteristics are aspecific, in a way mimicking the picture of poisoning by drug overdosage. The most pronounced changes are found in the cardiovascular, neurological, hematological, and immunological systems (Table 201-1).

The basic pathophysiological mechanisms are related to the dysfunction of several hormonal, homeostatic, and metabolic systems. Although extensive knowledge is available about the basic functional disturbances in uremia, most studies regarding this issue have focused on chronic kidney disease (CKD); one of the reasons for this preference may be the relatively stable clinical condition of CKD patients, which allows the planning of clinical, biochemical, and functional investigations. The patient with acute kidney injury (AKI) is in an unstable condition, and, in addition, many interfering factors (sepsis, pulmonary dysfunction, hemodynamic instability) can obscure the picture. Therefore, most of the accumulated experience on the pathophysiology of uremic toxicity has been obtained in CKD patients. It is, however, conceivable that much can be extrapolated to AKI, in as far as both conditions emanate in uremic toxin accumulation and/or changes in the specific metabolic conditions induced by renal failure.

INTERFERING FACTORS RELATED TO RENAL REPLACEMENT THERAPY

Renal replacement therapy, in spite of its beneficial effect on uremic retention, may cause a number of side effects or trade-off effects that mimic uremic toxicity.

Dialysis with dialyzers containing complement- and leukocyte-activating membranes may affect the immunological, metabolic, and hematological status, irrespective of general toxicity.[1] The insertion of central vein catheters for acute hemodialysis, as well as the use of peritoneal dialysis catheters, may enhance the risk of infection. Both fresh and spent peritoneal dialysis fluid affects leukocyte functional capacity, but in spent dialysate part of the functional depression may be a consequence of the presence of toxic solutes in the fluid.

Hemodialysis fluid may also have pro-inflammatory activity, if it contains microbiological contaminants.[2,3] Although the problem of water purity has been solved in many chronic maintenance dialysis units, appropriate water purification systems are more frequently missing in intensive care units (ICUs). Batch hemodialysis with the Genius system (Fresenius Medical Care, Bad Homburg, Germany), which makes ultrapure dialysis water available at the bedside, may solve this problem.[4]

Arteriovenous fistulas may cause cardiac decompensation. The use of immunosuppressive agents after renal transplantation and in autoimmune diseases enhances the risk of infection and cancer. All of these factors may cause problems that at first glance could be related to uremia, in CKD as well as in AKI.

BIOCHEMICAL ALTERATIONS

The uremic syndrome is characterized by a virtually ubiquitous disturbance of biochemical functions. They are at the basis of the clinical epiphenomena. In as far as toxin accumulation is similar in AKI and CKD, these functional

TABLE 201-1

Organ Systems Affected by Uremia

AFFECTED SYSTEM	EFFECT
Cardiovascular	Severe inflammation, with the potential to modify the vascular status
	Cardiac hypertrophy and dilated cardiomyopathy due to fluid overload and hypoproteinemia
Neurological	Functional and morphological nervous damage leading to neuropathy (e.g., complex reflex pathways such as F-waves and H-reflexes)
Hematological	Repeated blood losses or samplings, overt inflammation, and malnutrition might aggravate anemia
Coagulation	Presence of inflammation should result in a procoagulatory effect
Immunological	Extra morbidity and mortality due to an enhanced susceptibility to infection
	The presence of a number of uremic retention solutes (guanidines, AGEs, p-cresylsulfate, cytokines) has the potential to modify the immune response
Endocrinological	
Carbohydrate metabolism	Inadequate response to insulin results in inadequate cellular uptake of glucose and inadequate calorie utilization
Thyroid hormone	TSH release in response to TRH is suppressed
Growth hormone	Administration of growth hormone to ICU patients was shown to have a negative impact on outcome; nevertheless, it appeared to have a positive metabolic effect on critically ill patients with acute renal failure

AGEs, advanced glycosylation end products; ICU, intensive care unit; TRH, thyroid-releasing hormone; TSH, thyroid-stimulating hormone.

disturbances can, by extrapolation, be expected to be similar.

Enzymatic Processes

In the course of renal failure and uremic retention, a host of enzymatic and metabolic functions are depressed,[5] including gluconeogenesis, lactate dehydrogenase. mitochondrial storage of calcium, mitochondrial oxygen consumption, alkaline phosphatase isoenzyme activity, and insulin degradation. Also, the activity of glutathione peroxidase and reduced glutathione levels in erythrocytes are decreased in CKD,[6,7] resulting in higher glutathione plasma levels.[6]

Due to a host of enzymatic and functional disturbances, resting cellular and cytosolic concentrations of calcium (Ca^{2+}) are enhanced, which results in the impairment of various metabolic processes (e.g., pancreatic glucose-dependent insulin secretion).[8] Increased intracellular or cytosolic Ca^{2+} has been related to increased peripheral vascular resistance and, hence, to hypertension,[9] as well as to a blunted phagocytic response.[10] According to Gafter

and colleagues, uremic high red blood cell calcium can at least in part be attributed to deficient extrusion after deactivation of Ca^{2+}-ATPase.[11] Lindner and colleagues demonstrated the presence of a circulating inhibitor of the red blood cell membrane calcium pump in uremic plasma ultrafiltrate.[12] The responsible factor was partially identified and characterized as being of low molecular weight, dialyzable, and heat stable.

Both production and metabolic clearance of calcitriol were demonstrated to be disturbed in AKI as well as in CKD.[13-15] In further studies, it was demonstrated that uremic ultrafiltrate contained factors inhibiting both production and metabolism of calcitriol.[16] Some of these factors showed an elution pattern on high-performance liquid chromatography consistent with purines such as uric acid or xanthine. Administration of purines induced alterations similar to uremic ultrafiltrate.[17] Infusion of uremic ultrafiltrate to normal rats further reduced the intestinal calcitriol receptor concentration as well as the receptor interaction with DNA in vitro, pointing to a reduction of the biological action of calcitriol in renal failure.

From these data, it becomes clear that a host of biological processes are depressed or altered in uremia, and that the causative factors are variable and remain to a large part unidentified.

Drug Protein Binding

As reviewed elsewhere,[18,19] two binding defects are possible: in one group of essentially acidic drugs binding is decreased, which means an increase of the free, active fraction. Because, for most drugs, it is the total (bound plus unbound) concentration that is monitored, lower than normal total concentrations should be aimed at in this situation. At "normal" levels, toxic side effects are to be expected. Current examples are theophylline, phenytoin, methotrexate, diazepam, digoxin, and salicylate.[20,21] Basic drugs, such as propranolol, cimetidine, clonidine, and imipramine, show increased protein binding. This causes a decrease in the available free concentration, diminishing the therapeutic effect. For these drugs, higher total concentrations should be pursued.

Attempts to identify the ligands responsible for decreased protein binding have been scant. Several studies suggested that hippuric acid is one of the main contributing compounds,[21-23] but its relative importance remains undefined. Other potential competitors are indoxyl sulfate,[23] derivates of furanpropanoic acid[24,25] and other furancarboxylic acids,[26] β-(m-hydroxyphenyl)-hydracrylate and p-hydroxyphenylacetate.[22] The rise in binding site number for basic drugs is related to a rise in the concentration of α_1-acid glycoprotein,[27] caused by its decreased removal by the kidneys.

The altering relations between bound and unbound drug fractions emphasize the importance of monitoring free rather than total drug concentrations in uremic patients. It should be stressed that changes in drug protein binding are not the only side effect of uremia related to pharmacology. Decreased renal clearance and/or metabolism and changes in distribution volume may also enhance drug toxicity. Increments in active concentration may be compensated by alternative pathways of metabolism (e.g., hepatic, intestinal). In addition, accumulation of active drug metabolites may add to the toxicity of the accumulation of the genuine drug per se, as is the case for theophylline.[28]

Protein binding is not the only effect that is related to the efficacy and toxicity of drugs. In addition, uremic solute protein binding also may alter toxicity, because, conceivably, only the free, non-bound compounds may exert toxicity. Many potential toxins are protein bound (e.g., indoxyl sulfate, the hippuric and propionic acids, phenols and indoles). Guanidino compounds provoke structural alterations of albumin, decreasing its binding capacity for homocysteine and thus generating more free homocysteine with the potential to enhance the toxic impact of this compound.[29] Peritoneal dialysis may induce a more efficient removal of protein-bound compounds than hemodialysis.[30] Also, albumin-leaking hemodialysis membranes have the capacity to enhance removal of protein-bound molecules.[31]

Changes in protein binding of drugs may be an extra source of pathophysiology in AKI because of the multiplicity of drugs that are often administered to these patients. In addition, patients with AKI often have low plasma protein levels due to inflammation, malnutrition, and protein losses through capillary leaks. All of these conditions, together with uremic toxin accumulation, tend to liberate drugs from their binding sites, thus increasing potential toxicity.

FACTORS RESPONSIBLE FOR THE UREMIC SYNDROME

Knowledge about the factors responsible for the uremic syndrome remains inconsistent and incomplete. The concept that one single uremic toxin is responsible for the uremic syndrome is very likely incorrect. In a review, approximately 90 uremic retention solutes were identified as having been reported in the literature.[32] It is likely, however, that a much larger number of solutes with a toxic potential remain unidentified.[33] Also the extrapolation of in vitro data to the clinical situation has sometimes resulted in incorrect hypotheses, whereas trivial factors that can potentially bias the results, such as use of incorrect concentrations[32] or determination errors due to analytical mistakes,[34] have been overlooked too often.

The uremic syndrome results from the retention of compounds that are cleared by the healthy kidneys; the intake of precursors, mainly via nutrition, also plays a role. This concept is underscored by the success of dialysis in end-stage renal failure and the symptomatic improvement after decreases in dietary protein intake. However, the uremic syndrome is the result not only of retention of compounds but also of deranged hormonal and enzymatic homeostasis. Several secondary factors contribute to the uremic syndrome, such as the speed of progression of renal failure and fluctuations in toxin concentration. In analogy to drugs, peak levels may be more important than trough levels.

Historically, uremic toxicity was at first attributed to low-molecular-weight compounds (molecular weight <500 Da). However, this theory could not explain the favorable results with continuous ambulatory peritoneal dialysis, and, as a consequence, the concept of "middle molecules" was developed. Middle molecules are hypothetical uremic toxins with a molecular weight roughly between 500 and 12,000 Da.[35] At the time when the middle molecule hypothesis was formulated no compounds with their characteristics and a definite biological impact were known, so attention was focused again in the direction of low-molecular-weight solutes. Urea was identified as a

useful marker for the biochemical follow-up of dialysis patients; urea kinetics during and between dialyses were applied for the calculation of parameters related to dialysis adequacy (Kt/V, where K = dialyzer clearance of urea, t = dialysis time, and V = patient's total body water) and nutritional and metabolic status (protein catabolic rate, or PCR). One drawback of urea is that reports on its toxic capacity remain scanty. For that reason, the most recent research has focused on the characterization of other responsible toxins that might follow a kinetic behavior different from that of urea.

With improved analytical techniques, it became evident that presumed middle molecular fractions are in fact heterogeneous mixtures containing many lower-molecular-weight compounds.[36] The reason may be that molecular weight is only one factor influencing solute behavior in uremia. Factors that play additional roles include electrostatic charge, hydrophobicity, steric configuration, protein binding, compartmental behavior, and resistance of cell membranes toward gradient-dependent solute transfer. Each of these factors may slow intradialytic solute movement, either from the plasma to the dialysate compartment or from the intracellular compartment to the plasma. Thus, the definition of middle molecules may be extended to much smaller molecules with protein binding and/or multicompartmental distribution.

MAJOR LOW-MOLECULAR-WEIGHT UREMIC RETENTION PRODUCTS

The definition of uremic retention in acute renal failure, compared with chronic renal failure, might be a matter of debate. Most studies on uremic toxicity have been undertaken in patients with CKD, which can be considered the more stable condition. Nevertheless, in both conditions glomerular filtration decreases substantially, so it is conceivable that similar compounds would be retained to a fairly similar extent. However, enhanced tissue breakdown, deficient nutritional status, and/or altered bacterial production in the gut may provoke substantial differences in generation despite similar disturbances of excretion. Whether this might result in differences in retention pattern remains largely unknown. The currently determined low-molecular-weight retention solutes, such as urea, creatinine, phosphorus, potassium, and uric acid, are retained to a similar extent in AKI and in CKD.

In this section, the current knowledge about low-molecular-weight uremic toxins is reviewed; conceivably, some of those toxins show a middle molecular behavior. In Chapter 202, toxins with a higher molecular weight are discussed. Many data have been obtained in CKD. Most of the collected knowledge may probably be extrapolated in a fairly reliable way to AKI.

Advanced Glycosylation End Products

AGEs are generated and retained at increasing concentrations during the aging process but also during diabetes mellitus and uremia.[37] They intrinsically result from nonenzymatic glycosylation, and their presence in diabetes is related to cumulative glucose concentrations resulting in the production of ligands that are linked in a progressive way to other compounds, mainly proteins.[38] In uremia, AGEs are rather generated by oxidative processes. The production process takes a substantial period of time (several weeks). At the end of this period, the resulting modified proteins have changed, not only structurally but also functionally. The molecules at the basis of these modifications have a low molecular weight[38]; because of the linkage to amino acids that are part of (poly)peptides, the end products are larger, often in the middle molecular range. Because the development of these compounds takes several weeks, their pathophysiological importance in AKI, with its relatively short course, may be less prominent, although less stable precursors, such as Schiff's bases and Amadori products, develop in the range of hours to days and may also exert toxicity.

There is not much debate that AGEs are retained in uremia[39] and that they interfere with biological function. Among those, a pro-inflammatory effect has been found consistently.[40] However, most data in that direction have been obtained with artificially prepared AGEs, which do not necessarily conform to the structures retained in uremia. A more recent study showed similar immune-stimulating effects for AGEs definitely retained in uremic patients but not for all compounds submitted to evaluation.[41] Dialytic removal of AGEs is difficult, and only highly efficient strategies, applying very open membranes and convection, seem to positively affect removal of AGEs.[42]

Creatinine

The rise in serum creatinine during kidney failure is not linearly related to the decrease in glomerular filtration rate (GFR), which may decrease by 50% or more without marked changes in serum creatinine. Changes become more prominent in the lower range of filtration. There are virtually no convincing arguments in favor of a toxic effect of creatinine, although it may be a precursor of the toxic compound methylguanidine.[43]

Serum creatinine concentration is affected not only by kidney failure but also by the muscular status. In AKI, creatinine levels may be at the origin of an overestimation of GFR and a false feeling of safety in the case of patients with muscular wasting, which is common after a prolonged stay at the ICU in an inflammatory status.[44] It has been suggested that serum creatinine may be more elevated than can be expected from renal function in the presence of acute massive muscle necrosis in rhabdomyolysis, but this supposition could not be corroborated clinically.

Dimethylarginine

Asymmetric dimethylarginine (NG, NG-dimethylarginine, ADMA) is an endogenous structural analogue of L-arginine, the latter compound being a precursor of nitric oxide (NO) synthesis. NO synthesis, which contributes to endothelial protection, is blocked by excess ADMA accumulation in the blood, as is the case in renal failure.[45] In CKD, ADMA concentrations are related to indices of vascular damage,[46] although concentrations in many studies are below the level at which NO synthase blockade is induced. Convective strategies enhance ADMA removal in AKI.[47]

Guanidines

Several guanidines have been related to neurotoxic effects.[48,49] Recently, it was demonstrated that guanidines interfered with immune function, in either an immune-inhibiting or an immune-enhancing way[50]; guanidino compounds were shown to suppress the natural killer cell response to interleukin-2.[51]

Although guanidino compounds are small and water soluble, most of them distribute over a much larger volume than urea, resulting in a substantial postdialytic rebound.[52] Therefore, it can be supposed that long, slow dialysis strategies, as often applied in AKI, may benefit their removal.

Hippuric Acid

Indirect data reported by Gulyassy[22] and by MacNamara[23] and their colleagues, as well as more direct studies on ultrafiltrate collected in dialyzed patients,[21] demonstrated that hippuric acid interferes with the protein binding of drugs such as phenytoin and theophylline. It also interferes with tubular transport of organic acids. Hippuric acid (molecular weight, 179 Da) behaves like larger molecules because of its protein binding, which even tends to increase during dialysis.[53]

The role of hippuric acid in AKI might be substantial as a result of its interference with drug protein binding and tubular organic acid excretion. Because most patients with AKI receive many drugs, hippuric acid retention results in the liberation of protein-bound drugs from their binding sites and in an enhanced risk for drug toxicity, which is often difficult to quantify. Most drug concentrations are actually monitored as total, and in that case pursuing a maximal "acceptable" total drug concentration will lead to too high a concentration of free, active drug. To our knowledge, the problem of drug protein binding in AKI has not been subjected to in-depth evaluation.

Homocysteine

Homocysteine concentration increases in inverse relation to the evolution of renal function.[54] Hyperhomocysteinemia has been limited to premature arterial occlusion in the general population, but it has been more difficult to demonstrate such a relationship in CKD.[55] One might wonder whether exposure to homocysteine in AKI is sufficiently long to induce vascular damage. Dialytic removal of homocysteine is difficult, but it is more efficacious with larger pore sizes.[31]

Indoxyl Sulfate

Indoxyl sulfate, an indole derivative, is found at high concentrations in uremic serum. It is to a large extent bound to protein. Indoxyl sulfate has been associated with decreases in drug protein binding[23] and with defects of cellular organic acid transport.[56]

Because of its substantial protein binding (about 100% in normal subjects and 90% in uremic patients), indoxyl sulfate has an intradialytic behavior that is not typical of other low-molecular-weight compounds such as creatinine.

Phosphate

Phosphate levels are related to itching and stimulate parathyroid activity, resulting in hyperparathyroidism.

Phosphate has been linked to vascular damage through deposition of calcium-phosphorus complexes in vessel walls.[57] Because phosphate also accumulates in AKI, and because calcium-phosphorus complexes are generated readily once the product exceeds a certain threshold, phosphate retention might be deleterious in AKI as well, but this is not necessarily taken into account clinically. Intradialytic kinetics are not straightforward and are not comparable to those of urea, creatinine, or uric acid.[58] Dialytic phosphate removal is followed by a marked rebound,[59] suggesting multicompartmental behavior, and does not correlate with urea elimination. Standard dialysis as applied in CKD (alternate days, 4 hours) might be insufficient for phosphate removal in AKI.

Purines

Several purine analogues are retained in uremia, including uric acid, xanthine, and hypoxanthine. It has been demonstrated that purines are involved in disturbances of calcitriol production and metabolism. Uric acid, xanthine, and hypoxanthine also inhibit the monocytic response to the cytokine effect of calcitriol.[60]

Urea

It is accepted that, in general, urea may be toxic only at higher concentrations than those currently encountered in uremia. In AKI, urea has been used as a marker for making the decision whether to start dialysis; in this case, the molecule is considered as an indicator of both protein catabolism and uremic retention.

CONCLUSION

The uremic syndrome is related to a complex set of biochemical and pathophysiological alterations that result in a state of malaise and generalized dysfunction. The basic process at the origin of this malfunction is the retention of toxic solutes, which should be corrected by the removal of these toxins. In AKI, functional disturbances attributable to toxins may be induced to an equal extent as in CKD but may be paralleled or even overwhelmed by other pathophysiological events, such as sepsis, fluid overload, inflammation, blood losses, malnutrition, and vitamin deficiency. For that reason, it is not always possible to induce functional improvement by specifically removing uremic solutes alone; this aim can rather be reached by applying a whole set of therapies. Optimal toxin removal should, however, be one of the primary aims.

Key Points

1. In acute kidney injury, the specific metabolic conditions induced by renal failure are obscured by many interfering factors (e.g., sepsis, pulmonary dysfunction, hemodynamic instability).
2. Many low-molecular-weight uremic retention solutes contribute to the uremic syndrome.
3. Optimal toxin removal should be one of the primary aims in the treatment of acute kidney injury.

Key References

32. Vanholder R, de Smet R, Glorieux G, et al: Review on uremic toxins: Classification, concentration, and interindividual variability. Kidney Int 2003;63:1934-1943.
33. Weissinger EM, Kaiser T, Meert N, et al: Proteomics: A novel tool to unravel the pathophysiology of uraemia. Nephrol Dial Transplant 2004;19:3068-3077.
46. Zoccali C, Benedetto FA, Maas R, et al: Asymmetric dimethylarginine, C-reactive protein, and carotid intima-media thickness in end-stage renal disease. J Am Soc Nephrol 2002; 13:490-496.
47. Kielstein JT, Boger RH, Bode-Boger SM, et al: Low dialysance of asymmetric dimethylarginine (ADMA): In vivo and in vitro evidence of significant protein binding. Clin Nephrol 2004; 62:295-300.
55. Suliman ME, Qureshi AR, Barany P, et al: Hyperhomocysteinemia, nutritional status, and cardiovascular disease in hemodialysis patients. Kidney Int 2000;57:1727-1735.

See the companion Expert Consult website for the complete reference list.

CHAPTER 202

Granulocyte-Inhibitory Proteins and Other Proteinaceous Molecules in Acute Kidney Injury

Griet Glorieux, Eva Schepers, Wim Van Biesen, Norbert Lameire, and Raymond Vanholder

OBJECTIVES

This chapter will:
1. Describe the biological action of identified middle molecules.
2. Discuss the problems related to middle molecule removal.
3. Suggest strategies to improve removal of middle molecules.

MIDDLE MOLECULES

A substantial number of uremic retention solutes with a molecular weight in excess of 500 Da (so-called middle molecules) have been identified (Table 202-1).[1-32] Most of them exert biological action and interfere especially with immune function and cardiovascular response.

Among those middle molecules, the *peptides* constitute a heterogeneous group of molecules. Granulocyte-inhibiting protein 1 (GIP 1, 28 kDa), recovered from uremic sera or ultrafiltrate, suppresses the killing of invading bacteria by polymorphonuclear cells.[19] The compound has structural analogy with the variable part of κ light chains. Another peptide with granulocyte inhibitory effect, GIP 2 (9.5 kDa), is partially homologous with β2-microglobulin and inhibits granulocyte glucose uptake and respiratory burst activity.[13] A degranulation-inhibiting protein (DIP, 24 kDa), identical to angiogenin, was isolated from plasma ultrafiltrate of uremic patients.[31] The structure responsible for the inhibition of degranulation is different from the sites that are responsible for the angiogenic activity of angiogenin. A structural variant of ubiquitin inhibits polymorphonuclear chemotaxis (chemotaxis-inhibiting protein or CIP, 8.5 kDa).[4] The presence of these granulocyte-inhibitory proteins might hamper immune defenses, which might be deleterious in patients with acute kidney injury (AKI), who suffer often from infection. Also κ and λ light chains have a negative impact on immune activity.[3]

Leptin is a 16-kDa compound which, in addition, is protein bound and thus difficult to remove by dialysis. Its pathophysiological role has been linked to malnutrition, again a frequent problem in AKI.[33]

Parathyroid hormone is secreted in a compensatory reaction to hypocalcemia, hyperphosphatemia, and a shortage of active vitamin D analogues, all of which are induced by kidney failure.[34] Also, parathyroid levels start to rise soon after the development of AKI.[35] The toxic role of parathyroid hormone is essentially linked to its capacity to enhance calcium uptake into the cell, with a modification of several essential functions as a consequence.[36]

β2-Microglobulin is a 11.8-kDa molecule that has been connected most essentially to renal failure and dialysis-related amyloidosis.[37] The latter is a complication that develops slowly over many years of dialysis in pro-inflammatory conditions; the course of AKI is probably too short in most cases to induce this disease. The further role of β2-microglobulin is related to its frequent use as a marker of large molecule removal by dialysis.

Perhaps the middle molecules with the greatest pathophysiological relevance in AKI are the *cytokines*, which are retained in renal failure and generated in infection. Because many patients with AKI are septic, they often develop overwhelmingly high cytokine concentrations in the blood. These cytokines are essential for the immune response but may become toxic by themselves through induction of inflammatory damage (multiorgan failure).

FACTORS INFLUENCING THE PLASMA CONCENTRATION OF UREMIC SOLUTES

It is difficult to define in an individual patient which concentration of a middle molecule is useful and which one is deleterious, and this weighs on the decision of whether or not to remove these molecules. Standard dialysis removes none, or almost none, of the middle molecules. Removal becomes possible only by increasing the pore size, adding convection, and/or increasing dialysis length and frequency.[38,39] In a setting of continuous renal replacement therapy (CRRT), blood and dialysate flow rates are generally low, so that removal is restricted, unless extreme quantities of ultrafiltration and substitution fluid are imposed.[40] Alternatively, intermittent dialysis may be applied with larger-pore, high-flux membranes. In general, however, intermittent dialysis for AKI is conducted with low-flux membranes, essentially because the guarantees about water purity are insufficient in intensive care units. In this setting, middle molecule removal is nil. For that reason, dialysis strategies with large-pore membranes and ultrapure water, possibly prolonged, performed daily and at intermediate blood and dialysate flow rates, should be preferred.

It has been claimed that membranes for CRRT provoke substantial removal by adsorption of middle molecules, especially cytokines. However, careful kinetic studies have shown that adsorptive and global removal by these

TABLE 202-1

Thirty-two Identified Middle Molecules

MIDDLE MOLECULE	MOLECULAR WEIGHT (kDa)	REF. NO.
Adiponectin	30.0	29
Adrenomedullin	5.7	20
Atrial natriuretic peptide	3.1	8
β_2-Microglobulin	11.8	21, 28
β-Endorphin	3.5	14
Basic fibroblast growth factor (bFGF)	18-24.0	30
Calcitonin gene-related peptide (CGRP)	3.8	24
Chemotaxis-inhibiting protein	8.5	4
Cholecystokinin	3.9	1
Clara cell protein	15.8	21
Complement factor D	23.7	25
Cystatin C	13.3	21
Degranulation-inhibiting protein	14.1	27
Delta sleep–inducing peptide	0.8	16
Endothelin	4.3	8
Guanylin	1.5	23
Granulocyte-inhibiting protein (GIP 1, GIP 2)	28; 9.5	13, 19, 31
Hyaluronic acid	25.0	7
Interleukin-1β	32.0	26
Interleukin-6	24.5	22
Interleukin-18	20.0	12
κ-Immunoglobulin light chain	25.0	3, 5
λ-Immunoglobulin light chain	25.0	3, 5
Leptin	16.0	6, 18
Methionine-enkephalin	0.5	14
Motilin	2.7	17
Neuropeptide Y	4.3	1
Parathyroid hormone	9.2	32
Retinol-binding protein	21.2	21
Substance P	1.3	15
Tumor necrosis factor-α	26.0	9, 22
Uroguanylin	1.7	11
Vasoactive intestinal peptide (VIP)	3.3	10
Vasopressin	1.1	2

devices is relatively small and is rapidly overwhelmed by massive generation; even more importantly, removal of both pro-inflammatory and anti-inflammatory cytokines is similar, resulting in a neutral net effect on the immune system.[41]

CONCLUSION

The decrease of glomerular filtration rate, whether due to chronic kidney disease or AKI, is characterized by the retention of several compounds that are difficult to remove by standard dialysis strategies, such as protein-bound and larger "middle" molecules. It has been demonstrated that several of these compounds exert biological and biochemical actions and therefore may induce complications and affect clinical conditions. Solute retention and removal are estimated by studying the behavior of small, water-soluble compounds such as urea and creatinine, which, however, are biochemically inert.

In analogy with chronic kidney disease, it might be reasonable also in AKI to enhance removal of the difficult-to-remove molecules by increasing membrane pore size, convection, dialysis frequency, and dialysis length. One drawback in this setting might be the relative impurity of

dialysis water in intensive care units. Therefore, dialysis water purity should be another aim to be pursued.

Key Points

1. Middle molecules are an important group of biologically active uremic retention solutes.
2. Removal by standard dialysis strategies is limited.
3. Increasing pore size, adding convection, and increasing dialysis length and frequency improve removal.

Key References

22. Kimmel PL, Phillips TM, Simmens SJ, et al: Immunologic function and survival in hemodialysis patients. Kidney Int 1998;54:236-244.
26. Pereira BJ, Shapiro L, King AJ, et al: Plasma levels of IL-1 beta, TNF alpha and their specific inhibitors in undialyzed chronic renal failure, CAPD and hemodialysis patients. Kidney Int 1994;45:890-896.
33. Stenvinkel P, Pecoits R, Lindholm B: Leptin, ghrelin, and proinflammatory cytokines: Compounds with nutritional

impact in chronic kidney disease? Adv Renal Replace Ther 2003;10:332-345.

40. Ronco C, Bellomo R, Homel P, et al: Effects of different doses in continuous veno-venous haemofiltration on outcomes of acute renal failure: A prospective randomised trial. Lancet 2000;356:26-30.

41. De Vriese AS, Colardyn FA, Philippe JJ, et al: Cytokine removal during continuous hemofiltration in septic patients. J Am Soc Nephrol 1999;10:846-853.

See the companion Expert Consult website for the complete reference list.

CHAPTER 203

Uric Acid as a Toxin

Martino Marangella and Claudio Ronco

OBJECTIVES

This chapter will:
1. Describe the molecular characteristics of uric acid and its metabolism.
2. Characterize the mechanisms involved in renal toxicity by uric acid.
3. Report the most common syndromes in which uric acid is involved as a toxin.

Uric acid (UA) is an end product of purine metabolism handled by both the kidney and the intestine. The genetic silencing of uricase, which promotes oxidation of UA to allantoin in other species, and a complex four-phase renal handling, which results in only 10% fractional clearance, produce relatively high plasma UA levels in humans.[1] The potential evolutionary advantage of the loss of uricase has been the subject of much discussion, substantially based on a hypothetical capability of UA to act as a scavenger of free radicals.[2,3] Conversely, the frequent association of hyperuricemia (HUA) with a number of cardiovascular and renal diseases has focused attention on the possible harmful actions of UA against vessels, heart, and kidney.[4] All of these actions would occur through a common mechanism involving endothelial dysfunction.

PATHOPHYSIOLOGY

The more common clinical consequences of UA are related to its poor solubility in body fluids. The solubility product in serum is low (7.0 mg/dL) and is very close to reference values in the general population.[5] In urine, UA solubility is critically related to pH; at pH 5, saturation is reached at a concentration of 1 mmol/L (168 mg/L).[6] Gouty arthritis and gouty nephropathy are the consequences of oversaturated media in serum, and UA nephrolithiasis is the result of oversaturated urine. However, in none of these clinical settings is the harmful action of UA toxin-like, because the injury is substantially caused by crystal formation, aggregation, and precipitation in either synovial or renal structures.

A toxic role of UA has been hypothesized from the frequent association of elevated plasma UA levels with a number of pathological conditions (Table 203-1).[4] The essential core of the UA theory is that, at higher concentrations, UA could cause endothelial dysfunction, which is the hallmark of most of the diseases associated with UA.[7]

URIC ACID AND ENDOTHELIAL DYSFUNCTION

Earlier studies showed that UA could be harmful via crystal-mediated mechanisms. In human platelets, UA crystals induced activation and release of serotonin.[8] Later on, UA, whose local production can increase fivefold in response to vasoconstriction or under ischemic conditions, was shown to increase the expression of a platelet factor capable of stimulating vascular smooth muscle cell proliferation.[9] A crystal-independent role of UA in endothelial dysfunction was also confirmed in experiments conducted on human vascular smooth muscle cells, in which UA at 6 to 12 mg/dL increased expression of C-reactive protein, reduced nitric oxide (NO) release, and promoted cell proliferation and migration (Fig. 203-1).[10] UA was also found to decrease serum NO and to inhibit both basal and vascular endothelial growth factor–induced production in bovine aortic endothelial cells.[11] In humans with essential hypertension, endothelial function, studied by means of hemodynamic response to acetylcholine in the forearm, was found to be influenced by UA levels: a 1 mg/dL increase in UA induced a 41% decrease in relaxation.[12] Aortic smooth muscle cells were shown to express the urate transporter, UAT1,[13] thereby facilitating the influx of UA into these cells. Furthermore, activation of xanthine oxidase contributed to endothelial injury through the increased production of reactive oxygen species (ROS). Allopurinol induced beneficial effects on endothelial function, and this was closely associated with decreases in UA levels.[14]

Overall, the harmful effect of UA on endothelial function would seem to be caused by its ability to worsen oxidative stress, inflammation, NO production, and platelet activation.

URIC ACID AND THE METABOLIC SYNDROME

The main features that define the metabolic syndrome are well known and include dyslipidemia, abdominal obesity, hypertension, fasting hyperglycemia, and insulin resistance.[15] Metabolic syndrome, which affects as many as 27% of the United States population,[16] is mainly characterized by insulin resistance and high insulin levels. Insulin has been shown to reduce UA fractional clearance in both normal and hypertensive subjects, thereby favoring HUA.[17]

An interesting contribution to the understanding of a possible link between UA and metabolic syndrome came from studies of Nakagawa and colleagues.[18] They suggested that the increasingly high intake of fructose may be the common underlying cause of both HUA and metabolic syndrome. In experimental studies, feeding rats with fructose, but not glucose, induced features of the metabolic syndrome as well as endothelial dysfunction, glomerular hypertension, and microvascular damage.[18,19] These changes were prevented by drugs able to reduce UA, leading the authors to speculate that UA could be the mediator of fructose-induced metabolic syndrome.

Finally, both metabolic syndrome and elevated UA are frequently and associatedly found in patients with cardiovascular and renal diseases. Both are probably involved in the increasing incidence of these diseases seen in Western countries.[20]

TABLE 203-1

Pathological Conditions Often Associated with Hyperuricemia

Metabolic syndrome
Hypertension
Cardiovascular diseases
Gouty nephropathy
Renal insufficiency
Cyclosporin A nephropathy
Eclampsia

URIC ACID AND HYPERTENSION

The relationship between UA and hypertension is well established, in that HUA occurs in about 25% of hypertensives, in 50% of those treated with thiazides, and in more than 70% of those with malignant hypertension or associated renal insufficiency. The mechanisms invoked to explain hypertension-induced HUA include microvascular injury, renal ischemia, tubulointerstitial damage, local activation of xanthine-oxidase, lactic acidosis, and consequent reduction of tubular secretion.[21]

Much concern was recently focused on a direct effect of UA in causing hypertension. This hypothesis was tested on rats with oxonic acid–induced HUA. The animals developed a salt-sensitive form of hypertension that was preventable with allopurinol or benziodarone.[7] The mechanisms whereby UA could directly induce hypertension include activation of the renin-angiotensin-aldosterone system and inhibition of endothelial NO synthase, in addition to the effects mentioned earlier. These could finally result in vascular smooth muscle cell proliferation and renal microvascular damage.[4,18,19]

In humans, some, but not all, epidemiological studies have reported the association between UA and hypertension. UA was shown to be an independent predictor of both hypertension and progression of blood pressure in 3329 normotensive participants of the Framingham Study over a 4-year prospective follow-up.[22] Similarly, in the Normative Aging Study, the development of hypertension over 21.5 years of follow-up was predicted by serum UA, and the association held, at a low significance level, after correction for calculated renal function.[23] Conversely, no independent association between UA level and risk for incident hypertension was found among older men in an 8-year follow-up study.[24]

URIC ACID AND RENAL INJURY

In the oxonic acid–induced HUA rat model, a primary arteriolar vasculopathy and glomerular hypertension were seen.[25] In the remnant rat kidney, HUA increased protein-

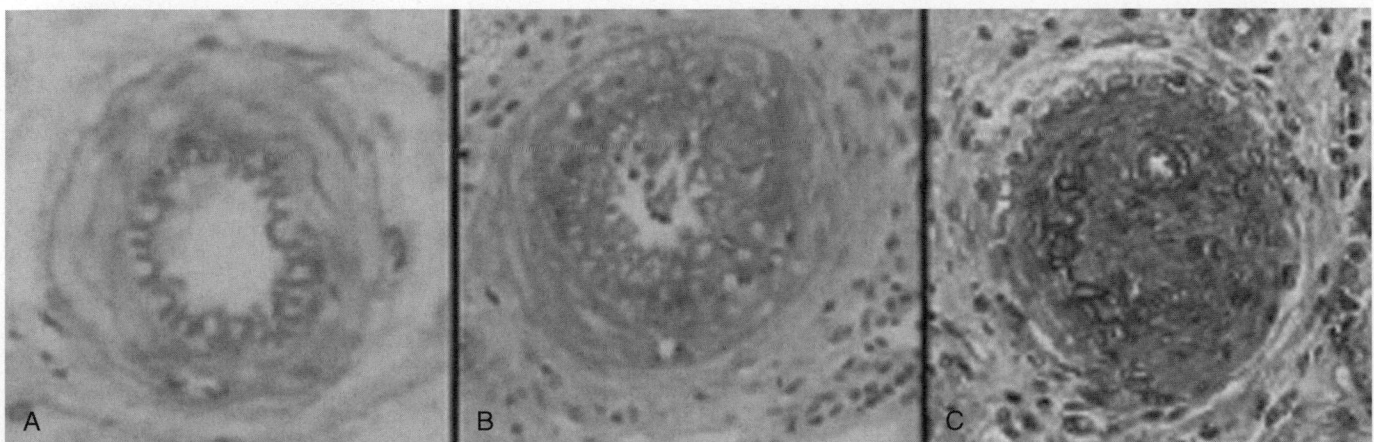

FIGURE 203-1. Preglomerular vessels in remnant kidney rats **(A)** and in remnant kidney rats rendered hyperuricemic with oxonic acid **(B** and **C),** Note thickening of the arterial wall and smooth muscle cell proliferation in oxonic acid–treated rats. (From Kang DH, Park SK, Lee IK, Johnson RJ: Uric acid-induced C-reactive protein expression: Implication on cell proliferation and nitric oxide production of human vascular cells. J Am Soc Nephrol 2005;16:3553.)

uria and worsened glomerulosclerosis and tubulointer-stitial fibrosis, and both effects were preventable by angiotensin-converting enzyme (ACE) inhibitors but not by thiazides.[26] Rats with fructose-induced HUA developed glomerular hypertension and renal microvascular damage.[19] These negative effects on kidney morphology and function occurred via mechanisms involving endothelial dysfunction. The fact that ACE inhibitors but not thiazides prevented renal damage suggests that UA action may be pressure independent.[27]

UA was independently associated with microalbuminuria in patients defined as prehypertensives but not in normotensive patients.[28] Over a 2-year follow-up period, patients with HUA had a significantly higher prevalence of serum creatinine greater than 1.2 mg/dL in females or 1.4 mg/dL in males.[29] In association with high triglycerides, UA represented a risk factor for the progression of immunoglobulin A nephropathy.[30] From a clinical viewpoint, HUA was reported to exacerbate chronic cyclosporine nephropathy.[31]

URIC ACID AS AN ANTIOXIDANT

As mentioned earlier, the hypothetical advantages of the genetic silencing of uricase are based on evidence supporting antioxidant properties of UA. Ames and associates showed that UA is as effective as ascorbic acid as an antioxidant in serum; because its concentration in humans is much higher than that of ascorbate, UA would stand as a major natural scavenger of oxygen radicals.[2] In a prospective case-control study using samples that had been stored for 13 to 15 years before measurement of carotid wall thickness, UA and serum antioxidant capacity were found to be higher in samples from patients who eventually developed atherosclerosis, compared with those who did not. This behavior of UA was understood as a reaction to greater oxidative potential among patients who were to develop atherosclerosis.[32] Inactivation of extracellular superoxide dismutase (SOD) by oxidative stress was attenuated by physiological levels of UA in mice.[33] In experiments, UA in the presence of SOD and H_2O_2 was transformed into hydroxyl radicals and these, in the presence of ascorbate, were easily reconstituted to UA. In this way, UA maintained the activity of SOD, despite the addition of H_2O_2, resulting in a decrease of free radical production.

A natural scavenging activity of UA against peroxynitrite was described in the course of allergic encephalomyelitis and multiple sclerosis.[3]

In summary, from this incomplete review, UA emerges as an important component of the natural antioxidant potential in humans, hypothetically involved in the defense against free radical–caused aging, cancer, and other diseases, perhaps including atherosclerosis.

The positive and negative effects of UA are summarized in Table 203-2.

CONCLUSION

The ultimate evidence of a crystal-independent, toxic action of UA is as yet lacking. Studies in humans are epidemiological or association studies, by which it is very

TABLE 203-2

The Uric Acid Paradox

Uric Acid as a Toxin
Endothelial dysfunction
Hypertension
Link to fructose-induced metabolic syndrome
Uric Acid as an Antioxidant
Scavenger activity against free radicals
Hyperuricemia as a compensatory response to oxidative stress

difficult to state whether UA is causally or casually linked to a given pathology. On the other hand, all of the experimental studies showing that UA exerts harmful actions have been conducted in animals with conserved uricase activity. In these animals, normal levels of UA are lower by far than in those in which UA is experimentally induced to look at a given effect.

Therefore, we are still waiting for prospective studies in humans designed to investigate whether early correction of HUA can prevent or modify endothelial dysfunction and its consequences in human pathology.

Key Points

1. The frequent association of hyperuricemia with a number of cardiovascular and renal diseases has driven attention to a potential harmful action of uric acid against vessels, heart, and kidney.
2. Organ and tissue damage seems to occur through a common mechanism involving endothelial dysfunction.
3. The harmful effect of uric acid on endothelial function appears to depend on its ability to worsen oxidative stress, inflammation, production of nitric oxide, and platelet activation.
4. The negative effects of uric acid on kidney morphology and function are likely to be mediated by the effects on endothelial dysfunction.

Key References

6. Marangella M: Uric acid elimination in the urine: Pathophysiological implications. Contrib Nephrol 2005;147:132-148.
7. Johnson RJ, Kang DH, Feig D, et al: Is there a pathogenetic role for uric acid in hypertension and cardiovascular and renal disease? Hypertension 2003;41:1183-1190.
10. Kang DH, Park SK, Lee IK, Johnson RJ: Uric acid-induced C-reactive protein expression: Implication on cell proliferation and nitric oxide production of human vascular cells. J Am Soc Nephrol 2005;16:3553-3562.
11. Khosla UM, Zharikov S, Finch JL, et al: Hyperuricemia induces endothelial dysfunction. Kidney Int 2005;67:1739-1742.
21. Hayden MR, Tyagi SC: Uric acid: A new look at an old risk marker for cardiovascular disease, metabolic syndrome, and type 2 diabetes mellitus—The urate redox shuttle. Nutr Metab 2004;1:10.

See the companion Expert Consult website for the complete reference list.

CHAPTER 204

Myoglobin as a Toxin

Carlo Crepaldi, Catalina Ocampo, and Claudio Ronco

OBJECTIVES

This chapter will:
1. Describe myoglobin as a nephrotoxic agent that develops its toxicity on the kidney with various mechanisms and pathways.
2. Promote an early and efficient conservative management of rhabdomyolysis that may prevent the development of acute renal failure.
3. Describe the extracorporeal renal replacement therapies in patients with severe acute renal failure that, together with adequate medical and surgical support, are effective to maintain survival until renal function recovers. These continuous renal therapies contribute to maintain fluid and solute homeostasis in patients with severe myoglobin-induced acute renal failure.

Literally, rhabdomyolysis means "dissolution of striated muscle." In practice, this term refers to traumatic or nontraumatic damage to the striated muscle cells which results in the release into the systemic circulation of intracellular elements that trigger many clinical and laboratory systemic abnormalities.[1] Rhabdomyolysis ranges from an asymptomatic illness with elevation in the creatine kinase to a life-threatening condition associated with extreme elevation in creatine kinase, electrolyte imbalances, acute renal failure (ARF), and disseminated intravascular coagulation (DIC).

Muscular trauma with crush syndrome is one of the major causes of rhabdomyolysis. Less common causes include muscle enzyme deficiency, electrolyte abnormalities, infectious causes, drugs, toxins, and endocrinopathies. Rhabdomyolysis is commonly associated with myoglobinuria, and, if it is sufficiently severe, it can result in ARF. Weakness, myalgia, and tea-colored urine are the main clinical manifestations.

Rhabdomyolysis was observed in ancient times.[2] The Old Testament refers to a plague suffered by the Israelites during their exodus from Egypt after abundant consumption of quail (Numbers 11:31-35). Myolysis after the consumption of quail is well known in the Mediterranean region. It is the result of intoxication by hemlock herbs, which are consumed by quail during spring migration.[3] There is indirect evidence that the biblical episode occurred during springtime. In more recent times, the first cases of crush syndrome and ARF were reported during the Sicilian earthquake in Messina in 1908 and in the German medical literature during the First World War,[4] referring to soldiers who were buried in trenches.

The first modern description of rhabdomyolysis dates back to 1941. Bywaters and Beall described four patients with crush injury sustained during the bombing of London in the Battle of Britain. All of them developed ARF and died within 1 week. Pigmented casts were found in the renal tubules at autopsy, although the relationship between muscle injury and renal failure was unclear.[4] During the next 30 years, numerous case reports of rhabdomyolysis with and without ARF were published, and the spectrum of etiological factors expanded to include surgical trauma, toxins, extreme exertion, and drug overdoses.

In 1959, the causes of rhabdomyolysis were divided into exertional and nonexertional types. For the former group, a tendency to have recurrent attacks was described, with onset in young adulthood, often with a positive family history of recurrent myoglobinuria. This group most commonly included patients with inherited enzyme deficiencies. For the nonexertional group, infection was recognized as the most important cause of rhabdomyolysis.[5] Additional nontraumatic causes of rhabdomyolysis were recognized and identified as potential causes of ARF in the 1960s and 1970s.[6,7]

MECHANISMS OF TISSUE DAMAGE BY MYOGLOBIN

Rhabdomyolysis develops as the result of an imbalance between energy production and energy consumption in the muscles. Factors causing an insufficient supply of the substrates and/or oxygen required for energy production (e.g., crush injury, ischemia), impaired cellular energy production (e.g., hereditary enzymatic defects), or increased calcium influx into the cell (e.g., malignant hyperthermia) are predisposing factors for rhabdomyolysis. On the other hand, if the cell consumes an excessive amount of energy (e.g., increased muscle metabolism caused by strenuous exercise in a hot and humid environment) and this energy cannot be replaced in a parallel manner, again rhabdomyolysis can develop. Sometimes a definite factor cannot be determined, and, in most cases, multiple factors play a role in the etiology.

In normal muscle cells, as in other cells, sodium enters by passive diffusion and is actively extruded by a process that requires metabolic energy. This process is coupled to an exchange for potassium ions from the outside of the cell and is dependent on the sodium/potassium adenosine triphosphatase (Na^+-K^+-ATPase) pump, which extrudes sodium at a greater rate than that of potassium entry. The pump is responsible not only for the generation of a high gradient of sodium across the cell wall, which in turn facilitates calcium removal by a sodium-calcium exchange carrier in the sarcolemmal membrane, but also for the generation of a negative electrical force in the cell. Active sodium efflux from cells produces an electrical and chemical gradient, both of which drive sodium back into the cell, where it can be exchanged for potassium and calcium.[8,9]

Under normal circumstances, muscular contraction is initiated by the release of calcium from the sarcoplasmic reticulum; for its relaxation, calcium should go back into the intracellular stores, which also requires ATP-based energy production. If calcium cannot return to its stores and high levels are sustained in the cytosol, continuous muscle contraction ensues, which causes energy depletion and then cellular damage.

If the function of the sarcolemmal Na^+-K^+-ATPase is impaired, as occurs in damaged muscles, there is a reduced extrusion of sodium from the sarcoplasm, which indirectly lowers the efflux of calcium from the cell; the sodium/potassium pumps are then activated, and sodium ions are pumped out of the cell while calcium ions are taken in.[9] Therefore, free calcium increases and activates a series of cytolytic enzymes, such as proteases, nucleases, glycogen-phosphorylases, and many others,[10] that lead to proteolysis, impair the integrity of the cell membrane, and result in more calcium influx into the cell. These enzymes interfere with mitochondrial functions and ATP production as well, so that intracellular ATP stores progressively decrease, and extrusion of calcium ceases. Mitochondrial dysfunction caused by increased cytosolic calcium levels results in an excessive production of superoxide and subsequent cellular injury.

It is also important to note that ischemia (i.e., physical causes) produces damage and necrosis in the muscle that is not very evident at the onset of the ischemia but rather develops at a later stage, when tissue perfusion is restored. This phenomenon, known as ischemia-reperfusion injury, can be explained as follows. When blood flow to the traumatized muscle is impaired, muscles are partially protected from systemic pathophysiological events; when the flow is restored (reperfusion), many important mediators of ischemia-reperfusion become effective and expose the body to their adverse effects.

With ischemia, vascular occlusion prevents blood from reaching the compromised tissue, and, as a result, calcium influx to the cytosol is relatively insignificant; as reperfusion begins, increased cytosolic calcium triggers rhabdomyolysis. There is also an increased production of mitochondrial oxygen free radicals that promotes intracellular and extracellular damage to molecules such as hyaluronic acid and deoxyribonucleic acid; activated or damaged macrophages additionally lead to lipid peroxidation. These oxygen free radicals that are formed during reperfusion readily attack the unsaturated bonds of free fatty acids in the phospholipid bilayer of the cell membrane. This reaction is propagated through the cell membrane and can result in fragmentation and severe structural and functional alterations in the membrane, leading to cell swelling, interstitial edema, and, ultimately, cell death and tissue necrosis. When this damage impairs the integrity and permeability of the sarcolemma, it results in an influx of sodium, calcium, and water into the cell, thus contributing to cell lysis.

There is also an alteration in local pH (intracellular and extracellular) that results from tissue ischemia. Acidosis has a protective effect on tissue injury, and it improves with reperfusion, so that cell damage becomes more prominent.

Therefore, in the pathogenesis of physically induced rhabdomyolysis, compression of the muscles (baromyopathy) is the key event. In this case, stretching of the sarcolemma results in an increase in its leakiness to substances abundant in the muscle cells (e.g., potassium, myoglobin, phosphate, creatine) and efflux of these substances to the extracellular environment. On the other hand, sodium, chloride, water, and calcium in the extracellular milieu diffuse into the cell below their electrochemical gradients. This phenomenon results in cellular swelling. Compartment syndrome, the typical finding in many patients with crush syndrome, results from this edema. An important consequence of increased sarcolemmal permeability is an elevation in enzymes, which causes lysis of the muscle fibers, leading to rhabdomyolysis. Increased cytosolic calcium also results in mitochondrial calcification as well as the release of reactive oxygen metabolites, which altogether contribute to the pathogenesis of rhabdomyolysis.

ACUTE KIDNEY INJURY AND ACUTE RENAL FAILURE

Impaired renal perfusion from any cause results in loss of tubular cell membrane polarity and destruction of cellular interactions, as well as several other subsequent reactions (e.g., impairment of sodium transport, activation of phospholipases, depletion of purines, acidosis and destruction of cytoskeleton integrity), all of which play a role in the pathogenesis of ischemic ARF.

Various factors contribute to this impaired perfusion of the kidneys during rhabdomyolysis, including hypovolemia, hypotension, and cardiovascular depression. At early stages, almost all patients with rhabdomyolysis are hypovolemic, mainly due to fluid accumulation in the compartment, fluid losses, bleeding, and vasodilation mediated by nitric oxide (NO), which causes deviation of blood into the muscles and release of systemic vasoconstrictors that intensify renal hypoperfusion. There is also a decrease in cardiac output, primarily in patients with crush syndrome, because of the effects of hyperkalemia and hypocalcemia.

If impaired renal perfusion cannot be restored at an early stage, ischemic (and toxic) tubular necrosis develops. Similar to the pathogenesis of rhabdomyolysis, the key event in ischemic tubular necrosis is depletion in renal ATP stores. Renal ischemia as well as leakage of ATP precursors (e.g., adenosine, inosine, hypoxanthine) from the damaged tubular epithelium plays a role in this depletion. Derangement in ATP metabolism impairs the function of ionic pumps, and the subsequent increase in cytosolic calcium triggers tubular necrosis.

Myoglobin exerts its toxic effect at the level of the nephron by various mechanisms:

1. *Renal vasoconstriction* is probably the result of the NO scavenging characteristics of myoglobin, and it is more accentuated in the presence of hypovolemia and hypotension. There is an important release of endotoxins and cytokines that can increment vasoconstriction.
2. Formation of *intratubular casts* with obstruction caused by plugs of myoglobin is part of the pathogenesis of ARF. The casts are the result of a combination of multiple factors: (1) As tubular flow rate slows down because of a decrease in the glomerular filtration rate (GFR), more sodium and water are reabsorbed, and the intraluminal myoglobin concentration increases; high urine osmolality in dehydrated patients further increases the myoglobin concentration in the tubules. (2) Metabolic acidosis and aciduria lead to tubular obstruction by myoglobinuria, and acidic pH of the urine stimulates the interaction between myoglobin and Tamm-Horsfall proteins. (Precipitation of myoglobin in aqueous solutions and formation of casts is possible only in the presence of Tamm-Horsfall proteins.)

TABLE 204-1

Causes of Rhabdomyolysis

NONPHYSICAL CAUSES	PHYSICAL CAUSES
Electrolyte Abnormalities	**Trauma and/or Compression of the Muscles**
Hypokalemia, hypocalcemia, hypophosphatemia, hyponatremia, hypernatremia	Natural and manmade disasters
Alcohol, Drugs, and Toxins	Traffic or working accidents
Legal and illegal drugs	Torture, beating
Toxins	Long-term confinement in the same position
Snake and insect venoms	**Occlusion or Hypoperfusion of the Muscular Vessels**
Fish toxins	Thrombosis
Infections and Infestations	Embolism
Infections localized to muscles (pyomyositis)	Vessel clamping
Metastatic infections (sepsis)	Shock
Systemic effects: toxic shock syndrome, *Legionella, Streptococcus,*	**Straining Exercise of Muscles**
Staphylococcus, Clostridium perfringens, Francisella tularensis, Salmonella,	Strenuous exercising
Plasmodium falciparum, human immunodeficiency virus, herpesvirus, and	Epilepsy
coxsackievirus infections	Delirium tremens
Endocrine Disorders	Tetanus
Hypothyroidism, diabetic coma and resulting electrolyte imbalances	Status asthmaticus
Disseminated Intravascular Coagulation (DIC)	**Electrical Current**
Polymyositis, dermatomyositis	High-voltage electrical injury
	Cardioversion
	Hyperthermia
	High ambient temperatures
	Neuroleptic malignant syndrome
	Malignant hyperthermia
	Sepsis
	Exercise

3. *Direct tubular toxicity* of myoglobin is a controversial theory. Some argue that the toxic effect on tubular epithelial cells is due to myoglobin ferrihemate, which is formed when the urinary pH drops to less than 5.5, in addition to dehydration and acidemia. It has also been suggested that other toxic substances released from damaged muscles contribute to tubular necrosis. The toxic effects of myoglobin are effective by several mechanisms: (1) Reabsorption of the heme proteins into the tubular cells predisposes them to ischemia and stimulates the formation of cytokines and free radicals. (2) Moreover, the porphyrin ring of myoglobin is metabolized in the tubular cell, which results in release of free iron; it is normally rapidly converted into ferritin, but in rhabdomyolysis, as large quantities of iron are presented, the capacity to convert iron to ferritin is overwhelmed. (3) As free iron levels increase, it readily accepts or donates electrons and has the capacity to generate oxygen and non-oxygen free radicals, leading to oxidant stress and injury to renal cells.

Reperfusion injury, which takes place when blood flow is reestablished, is important also in the pathogenesis of ARF. At this time, leukocytes migrate from the circulation into the injured tissues, contributing to their damage. Also, when oxygen is supplied, free radicals are produced, resulting in direct and indirect renal damage through the initiation of lipid peroxidation.

Almost every organ is compromised in the ischemia process, and many complications can occur, including gastritis, mesenteric ischemia, ischemic colitis, pancreatitis, acalculous cholecystitis, and ischemic hepatitis. Endotoxins absorbed from the gastrointestinal tract cause inflammatory reactions and increase hemodynamic instability and can lead to multiple organ dysfunction syndrome.

Together with myoglobin, considerable amounts of uric acid and phosphate are released from the damaged muscles into the systemic circulation. Hyperphosphatemia can cause calcium phosphate precipitation in the renal tissue that can lead to local tissue damage. Hyperuricemia and subsequent hyperuricosuria can form uric acid plugs, leading to tubular obstruction, although this mechanism is not completely accepted by all authors.

Thromboplastin released from injured muscles can induce DIC, which in turn causes the formation of microthrombi in the glomerular capillaries and contributes to the development of ARF.

Rhabdomyolysis can result in other systemic complications. Infections (especially sepsis) originating from infected traumatic or fasciotomy wounds can directly or indirectly lead to ARF. Various agents used in the treatment of other complications (e.g., nonsteroidal antiinflammatory drugs, anesthetics, blood and blood products) may also contribute to renal damage.

Table 204-1 shows the main causes of rhabdomyolysis from an etiological point of view. According to this classification, rhabdomyolysis may be caused not only by direct muscle injury but also by nontraumatic events such as those associated with increased muscle oxygen consumption (e.g., severe exercise, delirium tremens, seizure, heat stroke, hyperthermia, malignant neuroleptic syndrome), decreased muscle energy production (hypokalemia, hypophosphatemia, hypothermia, genetic enzymatic deficiencies), decreased muscle oxygenation, infections, and direct toxins. Multiple factors, capable of damaging muscles by different mechanisms, may be present in the same category. In conclusion, any process that interferes with delivery, storage, or utilization of oxygen by the muscle cells can predispose them to injury or necrosis.

CLINICAL FEATURES

There is a wide variation in the clinical presentation of rhabdomyolysis. The typical clinical features of a patient with rhabdomyolysis are muscle pain, stiffness, weakness, tenderness, and swelling. A "classic triad" of symptoms has been described: muscle pain, weakness, and dark urine.[11] The clinical manifestations can be subdivided into musculoskeletal signs, general manifestations, and complications.

Musculoskeletal Signs

Musculoskeletal signs vary in a wide range of possibilities. The muscle pain, weakness, tenderness, and contracture may involve specific groups of muscles or may be generalized.[12] The calves and the lower back are the muscle groups most frequently compromised. They can be tender and swollen, and there can be skin changes indicating pressure necrosis. Fewer than 10% of all patients present with the "classic triad."

It has been demonstrated that a large quantity of fluids, appearing as edema, may be sequestered in damaged muscles within hours or days, and muscle swelling due to sequestration of fluids may appear only after intravenous therapy. Therefore, limb swelling after parenteral therapy used for resuscitation may be an important clue to recent rhabdomyolysis.[13-15]

Some patients present with excruciating pain, which may lead the clinician to rule out other possibilities: the calf pain may result in a workup for deep venous thrombosis, and the back pain may mimic a renal colic. If there is involvement of the chest musculature, the patient may present with anginal-type chest pain. More than 50% of patients do not complain of muscle pain or weakness.[15]

General Manifestations

The initial clinical sign of rhabdomyolysis may be the appearance of discolored urine, which can change from pink-tinged, to cola-colored, to dark black.[16]

The general manifestations include malaise, fever, tachycardia, nausea, and vomiting.

In the crush syndrome, clinical features can be classified as follows:

1. *Local findings:* At admission, the typical local sign is the compartment syndrome. It is more frequent in the lower extremities, plays a central role in the initial hypovolemia of crush casualties, and may progress to a shock state. Usually, skin and subcutaneous tissues over the traumatized muscles are intact. Myalgia, muscular weakness, and rigidity are prominent, and pain is more severe than expected for the local findings.
2. *Systemic findings:* These can vary according to the compromised organs and systems affected by the primary event. The most common findings are hypotension, shock, and ARF, but cardiac and respiratory failure may be present in some patients. ARF is more complicated in patients with crush syndrome than in those with ARF generated by other etiologies.

Complications

The complications can be classified as early or late. The former include hyperkalemia, which occurs because of massive muscle breakdown; hypocalcemia; elevated liver enzymes in 25% of patients; cardiac dysrhythmias; and cardiac arrest. The latter include ARF and DIC; these complications usually develop 12 to 72 hours after the acute insult.[17]

Medical and surgical complications lead to an increase in morbidity and mortality. The most common complications in patients with the crush syndrome are hyperkalemia and infections. Hypertension is usually difficult to control, and psychiatric problems are observed in the majority. The leading causes of mortality in these victims are infections, hyperkalemia-induced arrhythmias, and other cardiovascular complications, which are augmented in those who also present with DIC and acute respiratory distress syndrome, making it mandatory to treat such patients in an intensive care unit.

In exertional rhabdomyolysis, patients appear pale, confused, and sometimes unconscious and unresponsive, with important hypotension, tachycardia, fever, and hyperventilation. Infusion of fluids causes rapid improvement; deterioration appears 12 to 24 hours later, manifesting as ARF, hypocalcemia, or signs of DIC.[18]

In cases related to overdoses of ethanol, heroin, or other depressant drugs, patients are comatose or lethargic, often dehydrated, and show painful swelling, without pitting edema, of one or more parts of the body, due to prolonged immobilization.[13]

The "second wave phenomenon" is sometimes present in patients with massive muscle necrosis affecting the legs. After an initial decrease in heat, pain, and swelling, patients may show a severe worsening of these signs on the second or third day, followed by ischemic necrosis if rhabdomyolysis has occurred in the tight fascial compartment. As mentioned previously, this is caused by accumulation of fluids in the injured muscle, resembling thrombophlebitis, and can lead to an erroneous diagnosis of vascular thrombosis.

In spite of this wide spectrum of possibilities, some patients have minimal symptoms or are asymptomatic. In these cases, anamnesis usually helps; age, gender (women are rarely affected by exertional rhabdomyolysis[19]), and a family history of chronic weakness or muscle cramps associated with minimal exercise are important clues.

DIAGNOSIS

Although the history and physical examination may provide clues, the diagnosis of rhabdomyolysis is confirmed by laboratory studies.[20]

Urinalysis

The most common, typical, and important finding observed in urinalysis of crush syndrome victims is a visible, dirty-brown discoloration of the urine, which results from myoglobinuria.

In a normal subject, myoglobin has a half-life of 1 to 3 hours and completely disappears from circulation in approximately 6 hours. Normal plasma concentration varies between 0 and 0.003 mg/dL, and 50% to 85% is bound weakly to plasma globulins. In healthy people, a very small amount passes to the urine (5 ng/mL). It and its metabolite, bilirubin, have a rapid renal clearance (the threshold value is 15,000 mg/L for myoglobin), so serum levels may be normal at admission to the hospital. A plasma concentration of about 100 mg/dL is necessary to cause visible staining in plasma, but this level would represent enormous muscle destruction. The concentration of myoglobin in the muscle is 4 mg/g, and its volume of distribution is approximately 28.5 L; the staining of this volume would require elaboration of 28,500 mg of myoglobin derived from the destruction of 7.1 kg of muscle. This quantity of muscle contains a huge amount of potassium, and its release would cause sudden death even before the plasma myoglobin concentration reached a visible level. This possibility, together with the high myoglobin renal clearance rate, could explain why, in rhabdomyolysis, unless there is a markedly depressed GFR or myonecrosis is very severe, the plasma is usually clear, whereas the urine stains red, red-brown, or brown according to its pH.[18,21]

Myoglobinuria is detected by the dipstick test. A positive test without any erythrocytes in the urinary sediment can indicate myoglobinuria, but it is not very helpful in the differential diagnosis. In crush syndrome, other urinary findings in the later course are proteinuria, isosthenuria, and necrotic tubular epithelial cells, all suggestive of acute tubular necrosis.

Blood Chemistry

The most sensitive and often diagnostic marker for muscle injury is the elevation of serum creatine phosphokinase (CPK), and particularly its isoenzyme middle molecule. Various reports suggest that serum CPK levels need to be higher than 500, 1000, or even 3000 IU/L for a definite diagnosis. However, values of this enzyme can be greater than 100,000 IU/L and reach a peak level within 12 to 24 hours. Without further muscle injury, CPK should decline by 50% in each 48-hour period. A second rise may accompany the second wave phenomenon.[18,19] A direct correlation between the serum CPK concentration and injured muscle mass is an expected finding.[22] Contradictory opinions exist on the prognostic value of serum CPK. Some authors have pointed out that increased levels of CPK may lead to an increased risk for ARF,[22,23] but others have not found this relationship.[15]

A significant correlation was found between the duration of dialysis support and serum CPK levels[24] in victims of the Kobe earthquake; in this same disaster, serum CPK levels were related to the extent of muscle damage, and higher levels led to higher risk of mortality.[45]

Other enzymatic increases involve transaminases (aspartate transaminase [AST] increases more than alanine aminotransferase [ALT]), aldolase, and lactic dehydrogenase (LDH$_4$ and particularly LDH$_5$).[25]

The most common abnormalities in the blood count are anemia, leukocytosis, and thrombocytopenia. Anemia may point to traumatic hemorrhage or hemodilution, whereas leukocytosis may be the result of rhabdomyolysis per se and/or infection. Thrombocytopenia may suggest DIC.

Hyperkalemia, which can sometimes be life-threatening, is often present during muscular destruction. Muscle cell potassium content is about 100 mmol/kg[18]; necrosis of about 150 g of muscle releases more than 15 mmol, sufficient to elevate the plasma and extracellular concentrations by 1 mmol/L.[15] Hyperkalemia associated with acidosis can cause severe cardiac arrhythmias. Renal function is the most important determinant of potassium levels in rhabdomyolysis.

The phosphorus content of skeletal muscle is about 2.25 g/kg. Massive muscle disruption causes an important elevation of serum phosphorus levels, sometimes up to 20 mg/dL. The highest values have been reported in rhabdomyolysis caused by crush syndrome or exhaustive exercise; less elevated levels are reported with impaired muscular energy production, toxins, and infectious diseases.[18]

Hypocalcemia is present frequently and early in the course of rhabdomyolysis. It varies directly with hyperphosphatemia and has been attributed to the precipitation of calcium phosphate salts in injured muscles.[26,27] Low plasma levels of 1,25-dihydroxycholecalciferol (1,25-(OH)$_2$), depressed by hyperphosphatemia, could also be responsible for the hypocalcemia of rhabdomyolysis. Hyperphosphatemia also stimulates the production of parathyroid hormone (PTH), but, despite high levels of PTH, the hypocalcemia is not corrected, suggesting bone resistance to the calcemic action of the hormone.[28] During the recovery phase of rhabdomyolysis-induced ARF, initially hypocalcemic patients may become hypercalcemic. This could be a result of healing of the injured muscles and a fall in the phosphorus levels, which would allow remobilization of calcium previously deposited in damaged muscles.

Severe hyperuricemia, often greater than 20 mg/dL, resulting from release of purines from injured muscles and their conversion to uric acid in the liver, is frequently seen in rhabdomyolysis, particularly in those patients with exertional rhabdomyolysis. In these patients, a disproportionate elevation of uric acid compared to blood urea nitrogen (BUN) has been reported.[18]

The serum anion gap in patients with metabolic acidosis and rhabdomyolysis-related ARF was significantly higher than in patients with non-rhabdomyolysis–related ARF. The mean anion gap was also significantly higher in patients with rhabdomyolysis without renal failure than in other patients randomly selected on a single day from the wards of the hospital, suggesting that unidentified organic acids are of some importance in rhabdomyolysis.[15]

The most frequent major complication of rhabdomyolysis is ARF, which may develop, as described by Gabow and colleagues, in about one third of the patients.[15] Many researchers have devoted their attention to what factors may be predictive of renal dysfunction. In a retrospective study, Ward noted that renal failure could be predicted by higher degrees of serum CPK, potassium, and phosphorus.[29]

Gabow's group introduced the following formula to help predict the risk of developing ARF:

$$R = 0.7([K]) + 1.1([Creat]) + 0.6([Alb]) - 6.6$$

where [K] is the serum potassium concentration in micromoles per liter (mmol/L), [Creat] is the serum creatinine concentration in milligrams per deciliter (mg/dL), and [Alb] is the serum albumin concentration in grams per deciliter (g/dL). R values equal to or higher than 0.1 and R values lower than 0.1 represent high- and low-risk conditions for ARF, respectively.[15]

PROPHYLAXIS AND THERAPY

The management of rhabdomyolysis involves identifying the cause and, if possible, its specific treatment; implementing measures to prevent ARF, or its treatment if it is established; and, finally, institution of renal replacement therapy if conservative measures have been inadequate to control hyperkalemia or volume overload or if clinical features of uremia have developed.

Conservative Management

ARF is a major cause of morbidity and mortality in patients with rhabdomyolysis; therefore, its prevention is of vital importance for decreasing the death toll. A variety of interventions have been tested for their ability to prevent or attenuate the injury or hasten the recovery of acute tubular necrosis (ATN) caused by rhabdomyolysis. Some of these interventions are effective in altering the course of experimental models of ATN. However, only a few have consistently been shown to be of benefit in clinical ATN.

Fluid replacement has been suggested as the most useful therapy in the prophylaxis of this disorder, even while the cause of the rhabdomyolysis is sought. The timing of fluid resuscitation is vitally important in the prevention of ARF. Clinical observations in injured people as well as in animal models with extensive muscle injury suggest that volumes equal to the entire extracellular fluid volume may diffuse into injured muscles ("third spacing") within hours to days after injury. Because the hypovolemia is the most important factor in the pathogenesis of rhabdomyolysis in hypovolemic patients, early and vigorous plasma volume expansion with intravenous isotonic saline should be given as soon as possible. The administration of fluids is important even in patients who are not hypovolemic, to increase urine flow in an attempt to protect kidney tubules from myoglobinuric damage. Patients with rhabdomyolysis may require massive amounts of fluid to maintain a vigorous diuresis because of fluid sequestration in the areas of injury.

Several reports have focused on determining the amount of fluid needed for prophylaxis of ARF caused by rhabdomyolysis. In patients with sufficient urine production, it has been suggested that isotonic saline could be initiated at a rate of 1 to 1.5 L/hr, with a total of 6 to 14 L/day. Even as much as 24 L of fluids per day was administered to some of the earthquake victims. However, one must be very cautious when administering such large volumes to elderly patients, who are prone to develop cardiovascular complications as a result of volume overload. To observe a more modest and gentle volume replacement protocol in these patients, it has been suggested that a central venous catheter be placed as soon as possible for monitoring volume status. Urinary output should be monitored closely in all the patients with rhabdomyolysis, and subsequent volume of fluids should be individualized.

Treatment after initial fluid resuscitation consists of a forced saline-mannitol or alkaline-mannitol diuresis. The usual requirement for bicarbonate is 200 to 300 mEq for the first day. The objective is to keep the urinary pH higher than 6.5. In those patients who pass adequate volumes of urine, 50 mL of 20% mannitol can also be added to each liter of isotonic or bicarbonate solution. The target is to maintain normal perfusion of the kidneys and to alkalinize the urine, thus preventing intratubular obstruction by myoglobin casts or urate crystals, because hyperuricemia and hyperuricosuria are common complications of crush myopathy and other causes of rhabdomyolysis. Also, in the crush syndrome, the mannitol component of this regimen can decompress and protect swollen muscles, reducing the leak of nephrotoxic myoglobin and urate from the muscle.

Nevertheless, there is no clear clinical evidence that an alkaline diuresis is more effective than saline diuresis, and there is a potential risk of alkalinization, because the precipitation of calcium phosphate can be promoted and hypocalcemia induced or exacerbated. Therefore, patients who are being treated by vigorous alkaline-mannitol diure-

TABLE 204-2

Effects of Mannitol Administration

Extrarenal Effects
Expansion of extracellular volume with subsequent increase in cardiac output and stabilization of mean blood pressure
Increase of cardiac contractility
Stimulation of release of atrial natriuretic factors
Decrease in intracompartmental pressure and improvement in compartment syndrome; reduction in efflux of myoglobin, purine, and phosphate from the injured muscles; protection of kidneys from toxic effects of these substances
Restoration of normal tonus of the dilated blood vessels in crushed muscles

Renal Effects
Increase in glomerular filtration rate through decreased blood viscosity and oncotic pressure
Dilation of glomerular capillaries and stimulation of release of prostaglandins E and I
Increase in proximal intratubular urine flow and prevention of obstruction
Prevention of tubular cell edema and damage
Increase in clearances of myoglobin, urate, and phosphate
Scavenging of oxygen free radicals

sis are potential candidates for hypokalemia, and they should be monitored closely for cardiac arrhythmia.

There are some theoretical arguments for the use of mannitol in either prevention or treatment of ATN caused by rhabdomyolysis. Mannitol can induce diuresis, potentially washing out obstructing cellular debris and casts. In addition, many other renal and extrarenal beneficial effects of mannitol have been described (Table 204-2).

In a systematic review of the literature, Karajala and colleagues have observed that there is no benefit with the use of mannitol as an osmotic diuretic over hydration in rhabdomyolysis,[47] so the use of mannitol in rhabdomyolysis is still controversial.

Extracorporeal Therapies

Once ARF has been established, or severe hyperkalemia and acidosis are present, the patient requires dialysis. Fluid overload is a rare indication to start dialysis, because patients tend to be dehydrated due to massive fluid accumulation in the damaged muscle; hyperkalemia, acidosis, and ARF are the factors that trigger the initiation of renal replacement therapy. Hemodialysis has several advantages in these severely catabolic patients. It provides:
1. Efficient removal of solutes, including potassium, phosphate, and protons
2. The possibility of dialysis without anticoagulants in severely traumatized patients
3. The opportunity to treat several patients per day on the same dialysis station

Continuous hemodialysis or hemofiltration strategies allow for the gradual removal of solutes and slow correction of fluid overload. The need for continuous anticoagulation is a disadvantage, especially in traumatized patients. Locoregional anticoagulation with sodium citrate, neutralized by administration of equivalent quantities of calcium salts, is dependent on the availability of staff familiar with this procedure.

Peritoneal dialysis is difficult to administer in patients with abdominal trauma and often is inefficient for the removal of potassium and other catabolic metabolites. It might offer temporary help, however, especially if mechanically driven dialytic options are not readily available in a disaster situation.

Removal of myoglobin by plasma exchange has no demonstrated benefit and also is debatable, because the metabolic turnover of myoglobin is fast.

Plasma exchange and charcoal hemoperfusion have been used. The former was associated with only a 10% clearance of serum myoglobin in a porcine model.[30]

Plasma adsorption perfusion might be a good technique to remove myoglobin, but a specific cartridge for myoglobin is not yet available.

The definitive approach to extracorporeal therapy for rhabdomyolysis has not been established but almost all of the possibilities have been tried.[31]

Although myoglobin may be more amenable to removal by convection than by diffusion because of its molecular weight, the timing and application of either hemofiltration or hemodialysis in this situation remain investigational.[31]

Both continuous veno-venous hemofiltration (CVVH) and continuous arteriovenous hemofiltration have been successfully applied to patients with rhabdomyolysis and ARF for the removal of serum myoglobin.[32-36]

One study found that the mean clearance of myoglobin was 22 mL/min (mean ultrafiltration rate, 2153 ± 148 mL/hr), but the clearance rate later decreased to 14 mL/min. The sieving coefficient (the percentage of the concentration of a plasma solute that appears in the ultrafiltrate) for myoglobin was reduced from 0.6 during the first 9 hours of therapy with an acrylonitrile membrane (AN69, 0.9 m² surface area) to 0.4 during the subsequent 7 hours. In contrast, sieving coefficients for urea, creatinine, and phosphorus remained stable at 1.0 during the first 16 hours of CVVH treatment. Similarly, other authors found that CVVH provided a constant fraction of free myoglobin removal and that a steady state was reached after 14 days of therapy, possibly because of binding of myoglobin to plasma proteins.[36] Others[37] have reported removal of serum myoglobin in CVVH with the use of a high-flux F80 polysulfone membrane and an ultrafiltration rate of 1 L/hr. Other investigators have either employed continuous hemodiafiltration[38,39] or detected rapid decreases in serum myoglobin levels independent of changes in renal function or extracorporeal blood purification method.[24,40,41]

Recently, Bellomo's group[39] tested the ability of a novel super high-flux (SHF) membrane with a larger pore size to clear myoglobin from serum. SHF hemofiltration achieved a much greater clearance of myoglobin than conventional hemofiltration, and it may provide a potential modality for the treatment of myoglobinuric ARF.

Because myoglobin has a minimal nephrotoxic capability in the absence of aggravating factors such as volume depletion, acidosis, and aciduria,[43-45] prophylactic renal replacement therapies based on the presence of an elevated CPK level alone cannot be recommended.

Moreover, not all rhabdomyolysis leads to ARF, and the prognosis of rhabdomyolysis-induced ARF is benign,[46] because recovery of renal function is usually expected within 3 months after the initial insult, if the patient survives.[22]

CONCLUSION

Rhabdomyolysis ranges from an asymptomatic illness with elevation in the creatine kinase level to a life-threatening condition associated with extreme elevations in creatine kinase, electrolyte imbalances, ARF, and DIC. Rhabdomyolysis may occur sporadically or as an "epidemic" after an earthquake. The management of this syndrome is quite different according to its severity and the situation in which it developed.

The main goal of intensivists and nephrologists has to be early and effective conservative treatments to prevent the development of ARF. Once ARF has developed, the use of extracorporeal substitutive renal techniques may maintain an adequate homeostasis of fluids and solutes, improving the prognosis of this severe clinical condition.

Key Points

1. Rhabdomyolysis with release of myoglobin from the muscle is one of the most frequent causes of development of acute renal insufficiency in intensive care units.
2. Myoglobin induces renal impairment via many different mechanisms and pathways.
3. Some simple conservative procedures are very important to prevent acute renal insufficiency and to reduce the myoglobin-related renal damage.
4. Continuous renal replacement therapies are very efficient in restoring the homeostatic equilibrium of patients who have developed rhabdomyolysis.
5. There is no clear evidence of early efficacy of continuous renal replacement therapies to prevent or reduce the myoglobin-related renal impairment.

Key References

1. Sever MS: The Crush Syndrome (and Lessons from the Marmara Earthquake). Basel, Karger, 2005.
10. Better OS, Abbasi Z, Rubinstein I, et al: The mechanism of muscle injury in the crush syndrome: Ischemic versus pressure stretch myopathy. Miner Elect Matab 1990;16:181-184.
39. Bellomo R, Daskalakis M, Parkin G, Boyce N: Myoglobin clearance during acute continuous hemodiafiltration. Intensive Care Med 1991;17:509.
40. Schetz M: Non-renal indications for continuous renal replacement therapy. Kidney Int Suppl 2002;56:S88-S94.
43. Zager RA: Rhabdomyolysis and myohemoglobinuric acute renal failure. Kidney Int 2002;46:314-376.

See the companion Expert Consult website for the complete reference list.

CHAPTER 205

Nanoparticles: Potential Toxins for the Organism and the Kidney?

Antonietta M. Gatti, Marco Ballestri, and Gianni Cappelli

OBJECTIVES

This chapter will:

1. Present the state of the art regarding the possible toxicity of nanoparticles.
2. Introduce a new diagnostics tool that verifies the presence of tiny foreign bodies inside the pathological tissue.
3. Show examples of the presence of some microparticles and nanoparticles in renal tissues.

All substances are poisons. There is none which is not a poison. The right dose distinguishes a poison from a remedy.

Paracelsus

The toxic effects of a chemical on an organism are related to the amount of exposure to the chemical. The toxicity is an inherent quality of the chemical that cannot be changed without changing the chemical to another form.

For many decades, some chemicals, including drugs, have been known to be toxic to the kidneys, and other substances, which have a primarily renal elimination from the body, have been recognized as potential local or systemic toxins if their excretion is compromised by a damaged kidney function. Excluding drugs, Table 205-1 summarizes most of the known renal toxic substances and describes their related clinical effects.

Renal toxicity is usually described in terms of pure chemical composition (e.g., ion, salt, metal), without taking into account any other important parameter such as physiochemical properties (e.g., size, charge, surface).[1] Modern developments in the technology of nanoparticles have allowed the separation of microparticles and nanoparticles from chemical toxins—that is, the particulates from the bulk form. Nanoparticles are generally in the range of 1 to 100 nm, and their properties are very different from those of their respective bulk material, because 40% to 50% of the atoms are on the surface, resulting in greater reactivity. Biological activity, in fact, is inversely related to particle size: smaller particles occupy less volume, resulting in a higher number of particles and greater surface area per unit mass, with potentially higher biological activity.[2] Some nanomaterials occur naturally or represent byproducts of natural, chemical, or combustive processes, whereas others are engineered or manufactured. Each of these types offers wide differences in properties and, most important, in biological interferences.[3] Nanotoxicology is growing as a separate field to investigate possible harmful effects from exposure to nanoparticles.[4] Nanoparticles may enter the body through oral ingestion, inhalation, skin dermal passage, or direct intravenous injection.

In relation to experimental pathology, various studies have been performed, ranging from in vitro cell cultures to in vivo animal studies (Fig. 205-1). Earlier papers dealt with environmental pollution and particulate inhalation, reporting respiratory tract toxicity due to increased oxidative stress, inflammatory cytokine production, and apoptosis.[5] Some particles preferentially localize in mitochondria, where they induce damage and activate oxidative stress.[6] When the particle structure consists of fibrous and tubular nanoparticles, the result is an inflammation process with fibrotic tendency and increased risk of carcinogenesis.[7]

UPTAKE AND DISTRIBUTION OF NANOPARTICLES IN THE BODY

Uptake of nanoparticles has been demonstrated to occur not only from epithelial and endothelial cells but also from the kidneys, where glomerular mesangial cells are more active in comparison to tubular epithelial cells.[8] Kidney cells in culture exhibit reduced adhesive ability and cell proliferation, as well as increased apoptosis, when in contact with single-walled carbon nanotubes, a manufactured nanoparticle with great potential for biomedical applications.[9] Fullerenes, carbon-based nanoparticles, have also been demonstrated to be toxic; for example, a polyalkylsulfonated C60, given intraperitoneally or intravenously at high doses to rats, induced a phagolysosomal nephropathy with phagolysosomal and/or lysosomal inclusions in the cytoplasm of the renal tubular epithelium.[10] A dose- and size-dependent toxicity of nano-copper particles was demonstrated in rats and resulted in glomerulonephritis and proximal tubular cell damage.[11] Also, nanoscale zinc powder, after oral ingestion in mice, induced renal histologic damage even when the biochemical data did not evidence a significant alteration in kidney function.[12]

Once they have entered the body, nanoparticles have the ability to translocate and to be distributed to other organs. This has been demonstrated for silver and carbon in rat liver, brain, and kidney.[13] As within other organs or cells, renal parenchymal toxicity is mediated by induction of an inflammatory process activated through several primary mechanisms[14]:

1. Direct nanoparticle-membrane interaction and/or particle intracellular phagocytosis activating oxidative stress with increased intracellular Ca^{2+}
2. Release of transition metals carried by nanoparticles at the membrane surface inducing pro-inflammatory intra-

TABLE 205-1

Most Known Renal Toxic Compounds

CHEMICAL	SITE OF ACTION	REFERENCE
Lead	Proximal tubule and interstitium lesions	Cramer K, Goyer RA, Jagenburg R, Wilson MH: Renal ultrastructure, renal function, and parameters of lead toxicity in workers with different periods of lead exposure. Br Ind Med 1974;31:113-127.
Cadmium	Proximal tubule and interstitium lesions	Nordberg OF, Herber RFM (eds): Cadmium in the Human Environment: Toxicity and Carcinogenicity. Lyon, France, IARC, 1992.
Mercury	Proximal tubule lesions and necrosis	Gerstner HB, Huff JE: Selected case histories and epidemiologic examples and human mercury poisoning. Clin Toxicol 1977;11:131.
Uranium	Acute tubular necrosis	Leggett RW: The behavior and chemical toxicity of uranium in the kidney: A reassessment. Health Phys 1989;57:365-383.
Arsenic	Proximal and distal tubule lesions	Fowler BA, Weissberg JB: Arsine poisoning. N Engl Med 1972;291:1171.
Chromium	Proximal tubule damage; unusual	Kaufman DB, Di Nickola W, McIntosh R: Acute potassium dichromate poisoning. Am J Dis Child 1970;119:374.
Copper, thallium, nickel, antimony, silver	Tubular and/or vascular lesions; very unusual	Lilis R, Valciukas JA, Weber JP, et al: Epidemiologic study of renal function in copper smelter workers. Environ Health Perspect 1984;54:181-192.
Gold	Glomerulopathy and/or tubulointerstitial nephritis	Francis KL, Jenis EH, Hensen GE, et al: Gold-associated nephropathy. Arch Pathol Lab Med 1984;108:204.
Platinum	Tubulointerstitial injury	Hardaker WT, Stone RA, McCoy R: Platinum nephrotoxicity. Cancer 1974;34:1030-1034.
Hydrocarbons	Acute tubular necrosis, chronic interstitial nephritis, and glomerulonephritis	Yaquoob M, Bell GM, Stevenson A, et al: Renal impairment with chronic hydrocarbon exposure. Q J Med 1993;86:165-174.
Silica and silica compounds	Proliferative glomerulonephritis, vasculitis	Tervaert KW, Stegeman CA, Kallenberg CG: Silicon exposure and vasculitis. Curr Opin Rheumatol 1998;10:12-17.

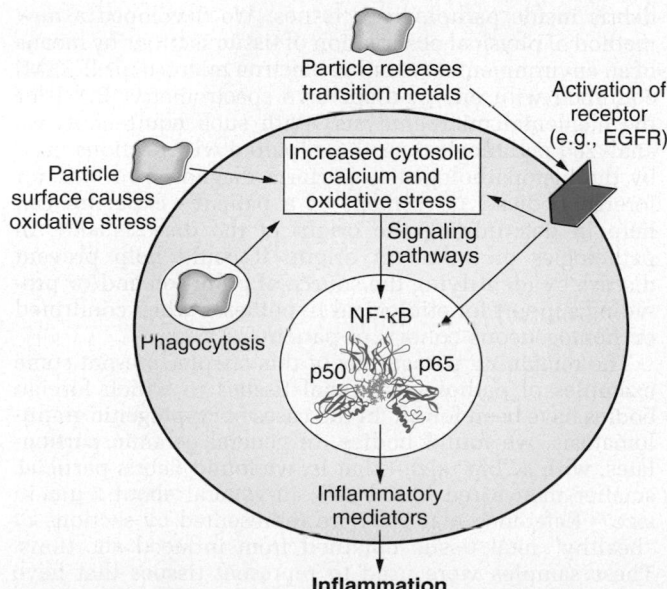

FIGURE 205-1. Mechanisms of the interactions of nanoparticles with the cell. Nanoparticles can induce oxidative stress, cytokine production, and apoptosis. EGFR, epidermal growth factor receptor; NF-κB, nuclear factor κB.

cellular signal induction, either directly or mediated through activation of membrane receptors (e.g., epidermal growth factor receptor [EGFR])

3. As a result of the previous two mechanisms, nuclear gene activation (NF-κB) with consequent induction and release of pro-inflammatory mediators resulting in local and systemic inflammation

PATHOPHYSIOLOGY

In a clinical experimental study carried out by the Leuven School,[15] researchers verified in five volunteers the dissemination of 100-nm technetium radiolabeled carbon nanoparticles after inhalation. After 60 seconds, the nanoparticles passed through the lung barrier and were inside the blood circulation; after 60 minutes, they reached the liver. The experiment showed that the physiological barrier is ineffective for these nanoparticles. The digestive barrier likewise cannot stop their free distribution inside the body; when nanoparticles are in the blood circulation they have the possibility of reaching every organ, including kidneys, brain, and gonads.[16-19]

Notwithstanding these documented pathophysiological processes, rare clinical reports of human toxicology from

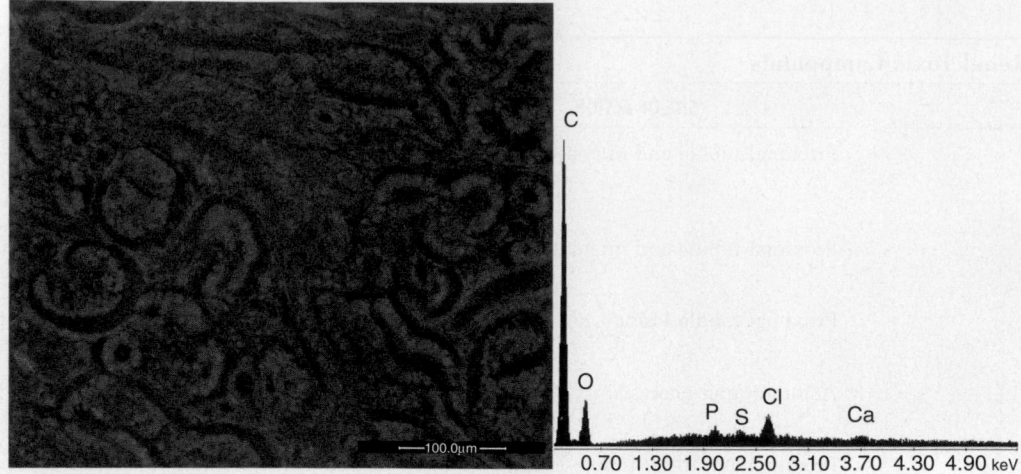

FIGURE 205-2. Environmental scanning electron microscope (ESEM) image of a section of a fetal liver with its energy-dispersive spectrometry (EDS) spectrum. The liver of a fetus never exposed to environmental pollution is free of any inorganic contamination. The tissue contains only carbon, oxygen, and small quantities of phosphorus, sulfur, chlorine, and calcium.

nanoparticles are found in the literature. Most data are linked to pulmonary disorders (from acute phlogosis to chronic asthma) related to occupational or environmental exposures.

The kidneys represent a main excretory route for nanoparticles, and, like laboratory animals, humans could be damaged by these new toxins. In theory, the kidney could be affected by particles reaching the bloodstream after oral ingestion or inhalation, so environmental pollutants as well as oral ingestions of contaminated nutrients or medical prosthetic devices represent a potential source of kidney damage. Very recent awareness of the problem and difficulties in microscopy techniques are probably the reasons for the poor clinical documentation of these effects. In most cases, because of the size of the particles and analysis of nonvital cells, mostly a cellular reaction with granuloma formation has been demonstrated, resembling a granuloma response to a foreign body.

A kidney and liver cryptogenic granulomatosis was described as a reaction to feldspar (nonfibrous silicate from dental porcelain prostheses), and debris with varying chemical composition and dimensions from 100 μm to 50 nm was found in 18 colon tissue samples from cancer patients.[20,21] Some particles with variable chemical composition have also been reported at the blood-thrombus surface from removed temporary vena cava filters.[22,23]

FUTURE RESEARCH

In the future, an increasing confidence with nanoparticle toxicology and amelioration in the manufacture of these substances could result in the possibility of drug targeting by nanoparticles to renal cells involved in inflammatory processes, especially mesangial cells and macrophages. Nanoparticles could also be used not only to induce experimental kidney damage in laboratory animals[24] but also to decrease drug concentration in tubular cells or to reduce any other tubular toxicity.[25]

To detect the impact of nanoparticles on the human body will probably require some years, because the duration of possible exposure to nanopollution among workers in nanotechnological industries is still too short. In the case of "nanoparticles" of asbestos, the interval from the beginning of exposure to evidence of symptoms was long, 20 to 27 years. The Nobel Prize winner, Prof. Richard E. Smalley, who discovered the fullerenes ("bucky balls"), died in October 2005 with simultaneous lung cancer and leukemia. There has been no evidence of a correlation between these diseases and inhalation of the nanoparticles he synthesized over more than 8 years, but nobody has looked for a possible correlation as yet.

STUDIES OF NANOPARTICLES IN PATHOLOGICAL TISSUES

During our studies in the European Community Project "Nanopathology" (QOL-2002-147), it became evident that microparticles and nanoparticles were already present as debris inside pathological tissues. We developed a new method of physical observation of tissue sections by means of an environmental scanning electron microscope (ESEM) equipped with energy-dispersive spectrometry (EDS) for the elemental microanalysis. With such equipment, we analyzed pathological sections (paired with sections used by the histopathologist to perform diagnosis) to look for foreign bodies. Assessment of a patient's exposure can help in determining the origin of the disease, and, in pathologies of unknown origin, it could help prevent disease by identifying the source of pollution and/or providing support for etiological hypotheses when confirmed on homogeneous cohorts of patients.

The remaining paragraphs of this chapter present some examples of pathological renal tissues in which foreign bodies have been found. In the cases of cryptogenic granulomatosis, we found bodies, in general ceramic particulates, with a "big" size—that is, we found debris particles smaller than a red blood cell, in general about 5 μm in size.[26] Reference materials are represented by sections of "healthy" fetal tissue obtained from induced abortions. These samples were used to represent tissues that have never been exposed to environmental pollution and are free from any inorganic contamination.

Figure 205-2 shows a microimage taken with an ESEM (Quanta 200, Fei Company, The Netherlands) of the kidney section of a healthy fetus used as reference material with

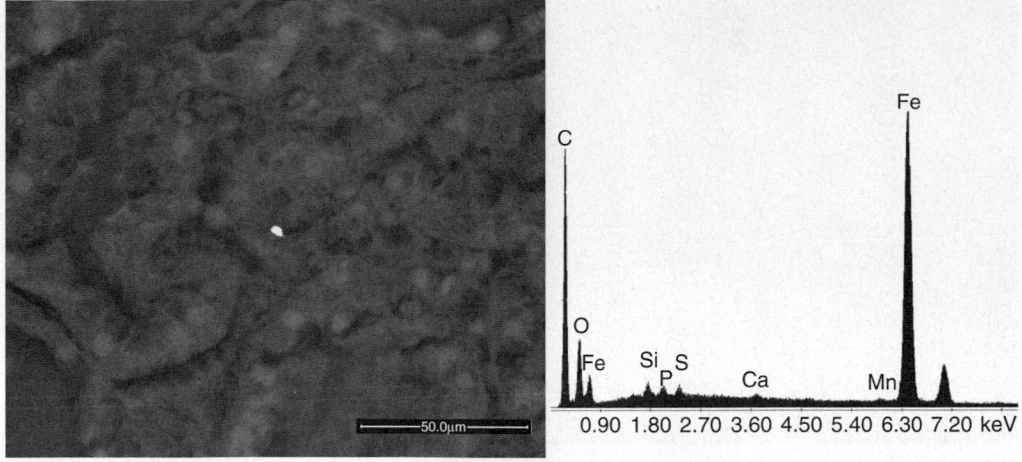

FIGURE 205-3. ESEM image of an iron-manganese-silicon-calcium particle found in a patient with acute renal failure due to septic shock.

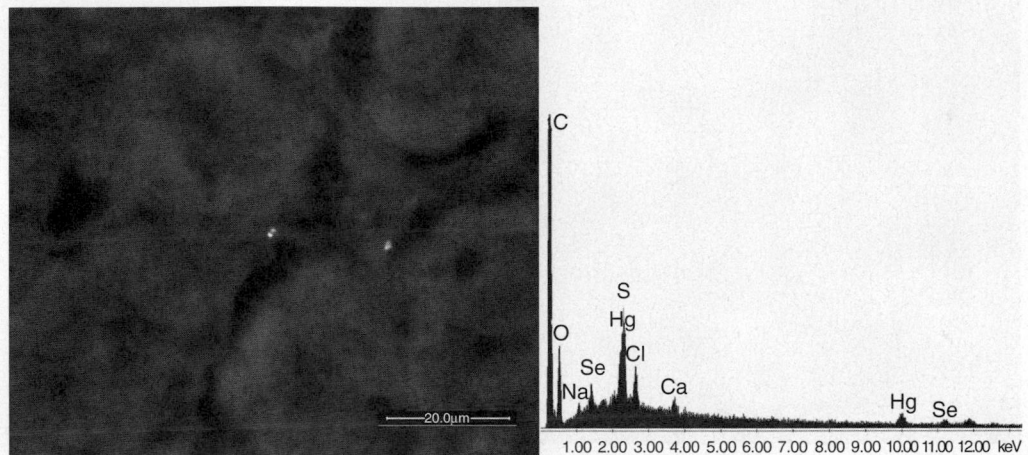

FIGURE 205-4. ESEM image of a section of a kidney from a soldier with Gulf War syndrome, showing nanoparticles of metallic materials. The particles are composed of mercury-selenium, sulfur, and calcium. This is a toxic compound that was found disseminated in the patient's entire body.

its chemical composition after fixation in formalin. The biological tissue contains carbon, oxygen, and small quantities of phosphorus, sulfur, chlorine, and calcium. This can be considered as the basic composition of renal tissue, and therefore the following reports list only the findings of other, additional elements.

In a tissue section of a patient with oligoanuric acute renal failure due to septic shock with disseminated intravascular coagulation, we found small particles of iron, manganese, cadmium, and silicon (Fig. 205-3). These particles are not biodegradable, and, because of their size, they could result in vascular glomerular occlusion. In order to link these data with clinical pictures, a systemic evaluation for the presence of these foreign bodies would have to be confirmed and interpreted for causative effect.

In other cases, really nanoscaled particles were found, and the patients were mainly soldiers or civilians exposed to a new type of environmental pollution created by the explosions of high-technology bombs during the First Gulf War and the Balkans War in the 1990s. The high temperature developed during explosions of depleted uranium and tungsten weapons (>3000°C) sublimates everything in the volume affected by the explosion (e.g., tanks, armor-

ies, factories). Immediately after the explosion, aerosols are formed and dispersed in the environment. Because of its reduced size, this particulate matter, if inhaled or digested (by ingestion of food contaminated by fallout of this nanopollution), can enter through the blood circulation to the body and all organs. A biological reaction of the tissues and organs can be triggered by presence of these foreign bodies, whose composition sometimes includes chemical toxins. Submicronic particles are created also in some workplaces where specific high-temperature processes are developed, as in laser and plasma melting or soldering facilities.

Figure 205-4 shows the case of a Canadian soldier who developed chronic fatigue syndrome and other systemic symptoms after 2 months of service in Iraq. Over a period of 8 years, he developed also some neurological pathologies resembling Parkinson's and Alzheimer's diseases. Nanoparticles of mercury-selenium were detected as singlet particles dispersed in the kidneys. We analyzed other autoptic samples from this soldier and found nanoparticles in most organs. The chemical composition included some chemically toxic metals potentially leachable as ions, with related toxicity apart from specific organ

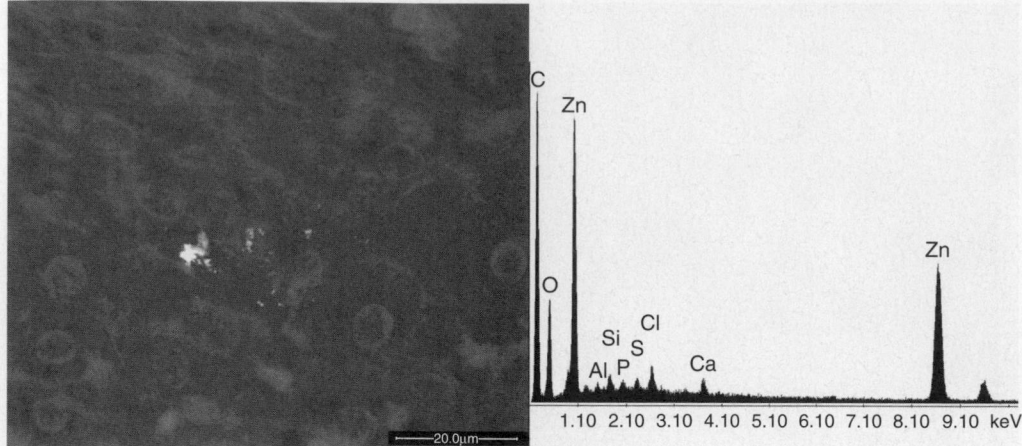

FIGURE 205-5. ESEM image of a section of kidney from a fetus delivered prematurely and dead. The section shows the presence of nanoparticles of zinc-chlorine-silicon-aluminum-calcium which were disseminated throughout the organ. Note: The EDS spectrum shows the primary peaks of the elements and secondary peak of zinc.

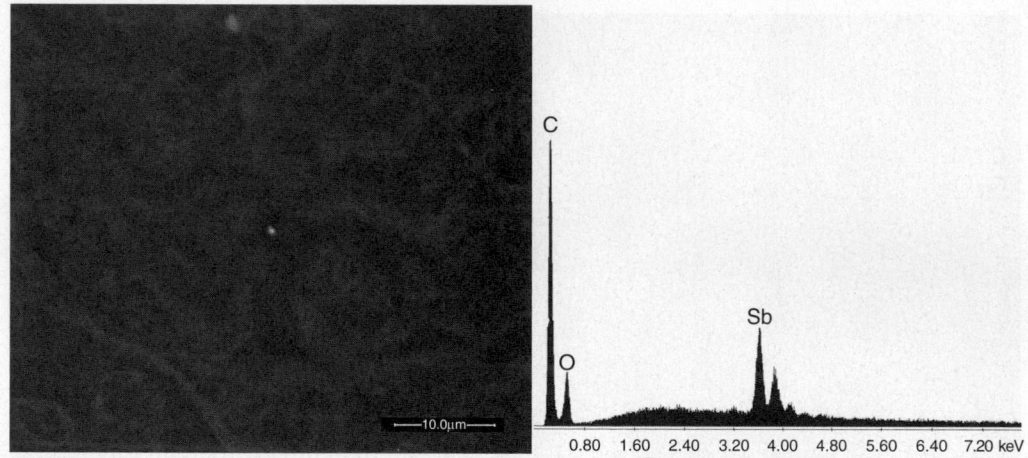

FIGURE 205-6. ESEM image of a section of kidney from a malformed fetus affected with Neu-Laxova syndrome. Nanoparticles of antimony were found disseminated in all internal organs.

reaction to foreign bodies. The dissemination of these particles was peculiar in that they did not aggregate to form the usual clusters but remained as singlet particles. This situation is atypical and very difficult to reproduce in laboratory animals.

Figure 205-5 shows the presence of nanoparticles composed of zinc-silicon-aluminum from the kidney of a fetus delivered prematurely and dead. The mother was exposed to this pollution and transmitted the contamination to the embryo through the fetal circulation.

Figure 205-6 presents other findings in a fetus affected by the rare Neu-Laxova syndrome, in which particles of antimony were found. In another patient with a cancer of the kidney, we found a wide dissemination of precipitates of iron-phosphorus and sodium. The difference between a "bulk" particle and a precipitate can be understood by looking at the images. The particle is compact, more brilliant, and white. The precipitates show a non-compact structure; they are grayish because their atomic density is poor (less than a similar particle of iron), so they appear less white, with a color similar to that of the tissue. However, these particles are not biodegradable, so they represent foreign bodies even if they are composed of elements present in the human body. A similar situation was verified in the liver of a patient with siderosis.

Figure 205-7 shows a singular case of calcium-phosphate crystals precipitated within renal tubules (at both apical and distal sites). The patient had consumed repeated enormous doses of a cathartic agent composed of a sodium-phosphate. In blood, the absorbed phosphorus ions coprecipitated with calcium, inducing a serum hypocalcemia. At kidney level, needle-shaped crystals formed in the tubule segment, where the absorption of water occurs with increased relative ion concentration.

Figure 205-8 shows another image in which there is an area rich in balls of different sizes, composed of calcium, phosphorus, sodium, and magnesium. The small granuloma is a concentrate of microsized and nanosized balls almost impossible to better define. The more credited hypothesis is that they are bacteria at various stages of proliferation that have calcified.

CONCLUSION

In conclusion, every foreign body that is not biodegradable and not biocompatible and is free in the blood circulation can reach the kidney; it is only a matter of size. Also, some diagnostic injectable compounds or dialytic fluids could

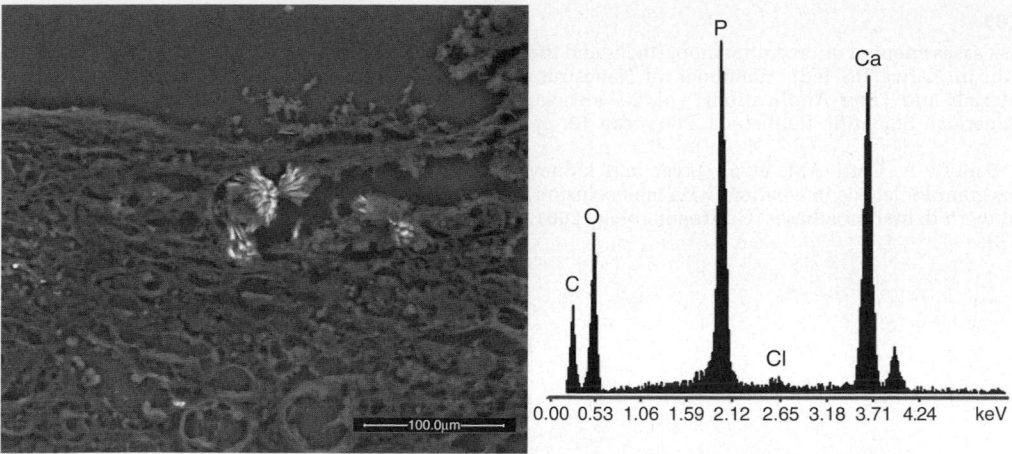

FIGURE 205-7. ESEM image of crystals of calcium-phosphate found in a renal tubule (white needles). This local formation was correlated to repeated enormous doses of a cathartic agent composed of a sodium-phosphate.

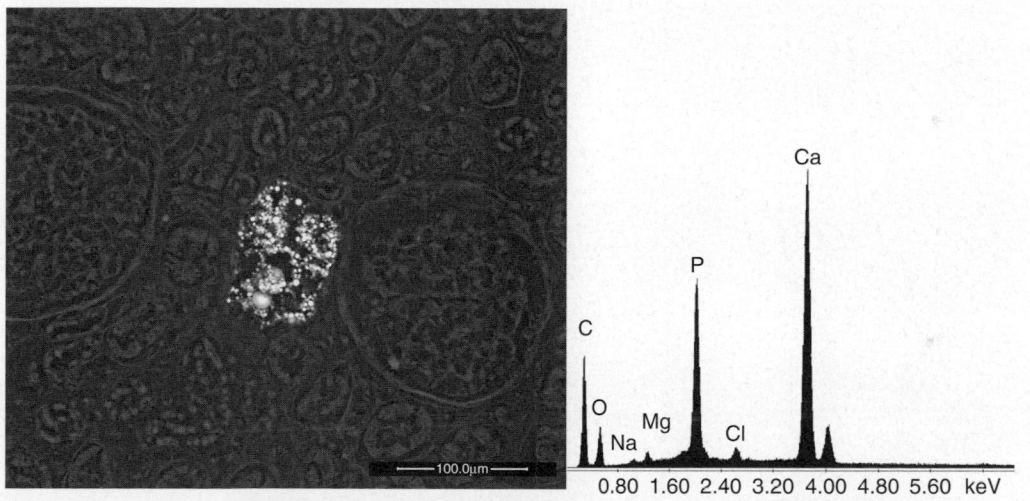

FIGURE 205-8. ESEM image of a small granuloma containing small, spherical particles of calcium-phosphorus-magnesium-sodium. It is hypothesized to be the result of a calcification of unknown organic bodies.

contain nanoparticles and could cause problems similar to those analyzed here with chronic administration. When this contamination occurs, actual drug therapy is ineffective.

In the case of renal contamination by particles, two different reactions are possible:

1. The "large" particles (>5 μm) could be stopped in the glomerulus at a vascular level, causing capillary occlusion. When entrapped, if degradable, they could release toxic ions with related symptoms.
2. Very tiny particles circulate in the bloodstream and cause local and systemic reactions. They enter the renal parenchyma (tubular and mesangial cells), and their internalization has been already verified. In these cases, we do not know exactly what they cause: effects could be different from those of normal toxicity. We have already found cells in a replicating phase with nanoparticles inside. This does not represent a safety assurance, and the possibility of genomic alterations cannot be excluded.

The European Project DIPNA (Development of an Integrated Platform for Nanoparticle Analysis to verify their possible toxicity and eco-toxicity) is investigating these questions and could within 3 years begin providing specific results about the interactions between nanoparticles and cells.

Key Points

1. A new diagnostic tool is available for the detection of microparticles and nanosized foreign bodies.
2. Nanosized environmental pollution, if inhaled or digested, can reach the blood circulation and can then be entrapped in filter organs and trigger diseases.
3. Foreign bodies can be identified in pathological samples of the kidneys.
4. The origin of the nanopollution can be investigated and found.
5. Dialytic processes can introduce contamination that is easily detectable and identifiable.

Key References

19. Gatti AM: Risk assessment of micro and nanoparticles and the human health. In Nalwa HS (ed): Handbook of Nanostructured Biomaterials and Their Applications, vol. 2. Valencia, California, American Scientific Publishers, 2005, cap 12, pp 347-369.
20. Ballestri M, Baraldi A, Gatti AM, et al: Liver and kidney foreign bodies granulomatosis in a patient with malocclusion, bruxism, and worn dental prostheses. Gastroenterology 2001; 121:1234-1238.

21. Gatti AM: Biocompatibility of micro- and nano-particles in the colon. Part II: Biomaterials. 2004;25:385-392.
23. Gatti AM, Montanari S: Retrieval analysis of clinical explanted vena cava filters. J Biomed Mater Res B Appl Biomater 2006;77:307-314.
26. Gatti AM, Ballestri M, Bagni A: Granulomatosis associated to porcelain wear debris. Am J Dent 2002;15:369-372.

See the companion Expert Consult website for the complete reference list.

Part III

Renal Replacement Therapy

General Principles of Acute Renal Replacement Therapy

CHAPTER 206

History and Development of Acute Dialysis Therapy

Orly F. Kohn, Carl M. Kjellstrand, and Todd S. Ing

OBJECTIVES

This chapter will:
1. Recognize the major contributors to the development of dialysis.
2. Identify the key obstacles that had to be overcome to make renal replacement therapy practical.
3. Explain the historical context in which dialysis evolved.

Just over 60 years ago, the diagnosis of oliguric acute renal failure (ARF) lasting more than a few days carried a grave prognosis. The high fatality rate extended even to young patients with no comorbidities. Patients with ARF succumbed to hyperkalemia, acidosis, volume overload, and uremic coma. The evolution of all aspects of dialysis therapy, from dialyzer to access, has been extraordinary and life-saving. Today, with the availability of a variety of renal replacement options, safely and reliably delivered, almost no patient is expected to die of ARF unless also affected by multiorgan failure or serious comorbidities. The progress in this area of medicine started evolving in the 1850s and gained momentum with the parallel improvement in understanding of membranes and their production, anticoagulation, devices that allow safe repeated access to the circulation or peritoneal cavity, machines with adequate safety features, and improved monitoring of blood chemistries. The therapy for acute kidney failure benefited also from the interest in application of renal replacement therapy to patients with chronic kidney failure and from industry research.

DIALYSIS: EARLY EXPERIMENTS

In the mid-19th century, a chemist from Scotland, Thomas Graham (1805-1869), made the trailblazing declaration that: "It may perhaps be allowed me to apply the conve-nient term *dialysis* to the method of separating by diffusion through a system of gelatinous matter."[1] Thus the word *dialysis* was born (Table 206-1). According to the dictionary definition, *dia-* means "through" or "across," *-lysis* means "loosening" or "dissolution," and *dialysis* means "the separation of substances in solution by means of semipermeable membranes through which the smaller molecules and ions diffuse readily whereas the larger molecules and colloidal particles diffuse very slowly or not at all."[2]

In spite of Graham's brilliant discovery, the world had to wait for half a century, until November 10, 1912, before Abel, Rowntree, and Turner, of the Johns Hopkins University in Baltimore, succeeded in performing hemodialysis on a rabbit for 2 hours. In their 41-page classic paper published in 1914, they noted that, in kidney failure, numerous substances accumulate in the body "whose presence in excessive amount is detrimental to life processes. In the hope of providing a substitute in such emergencies, which might tide over a dangerous crisis . . . we have devised a method by which the blood of a living animal may be submitted to dialysis outside the body and again returned to the natural circulation. . . . The process may be appropriately referred to as vivi-diffusion."[3] They went on to state, "the apparatus constitutes what has been called an artificial kidney."[3] By the time they described their discovery in a printed format, they had already toured Europe and made presentations to the Association of American Physicians in Washington. Their semipermeable membrane was made of collodion, a product of nitrated cellulose. After cellulose dinitrate was dissolved in alcohol and ether, the mixture was poured into glass tubes, coating the inside evenly. Once the ether evaporated, a delicate film remained that retained its tubular shape when carefully retrieved. A series of such fragile collodion tubes were tied to glass manifolds of great intricacy. The manifolds directed the flow of blood from the vascular access through the collodion tubes, which were bathing in a dialysis solution. Hirudin, extracted from hundreds of leech heads, was given to the animals to prevent clotting. The hirudin used was not pure, and its potency was variable and dependent on many factors, including the leeches' nutritional status.

TABLE 206-1

Some of the Milestones in Acute Dialytic Therapy

DATE	EVENT
1861	Graham coins the word "dialysis" and studied solute movement across semipermeable membranes.
1912	Abel, Rowntree, and Turner dialyze a rabbit for a couple of hours using collodion membranes and hirudin anticoagulation.
1916	Maclean discovers heparin.
1923	Ganter carries out the first human peritoneal dialysis.
1924	Haas performs the first human hemodialysis using collodion membrane and hirudin anticoagulation.
1937	Thalhimer hemodialyzes dogs using cellophane membrane and heparin anticoagulation.
1938	Wear successfully treats, with peritoneal dialysis, a uremic patient suffering from a urinary obstruction—an historic first.
1943	Kolff hemodialyzes a patient with the rotating drum kidney, using cellophane membrane and heparin anticoagulation.
1945	Kolff saves the life of a patient with intrinsic acute renal failure with hemodialysis—an historic first.
1945	Fine, Frank, and Seligman, using peritoneal dialysis, save the life of a patient with intrinsic acute renal failure.
1946	Murray, Delrome, and Thomas perform the first successful human dialysis in North America.
1946	Alwall dialyzes the first patient with the Alwall kidney; he also advances the concept of controlled ultrafiltration.
1953	Teschan champions the concept of early, prophylactic dialysis.
1960	Quinton, Dillard, and Scribner place their first arteriovenous shunt into a patient.
1961	Shaldon introduces percutaneous catheterization of vessels for dialysis access using the Seldinger technique.

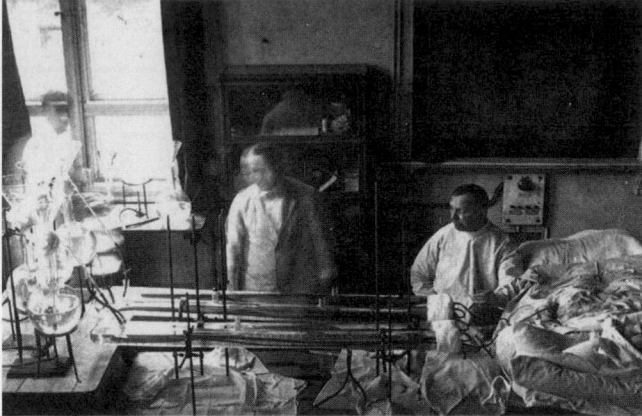

FIGURE 206-1. George Haas, seated at the right, dialyzing one of his patients, ca. 1925.

The supply of leeches was unreliable and the cost high. Based on the solute transport studies, Abel and associates showed that the efficiency of the apparatus could be augmented by increasing the number of collodion tubes and, hence, the dialyzing surface area. Abel's research ground to a halt with the outbreak of World War I, possibly due to difficulty in obtaining leeches from Europe or perhaps due to separation of the original research team.

The Clinical Pioneers

The first human dialysis was performed in October of 1924 in Giessen, Germany, by Georg Haas (1886-1971). Haas experimented with various membranes for hemodialysis and ultimately constructed a variant of Abel's artificial kidney using long collodion tubes connected in series and providing a surface area of about 0.4 m². The first few dialysis sessions lasted less than 1 hour and did not bring about clinical improvement. The hirudin used caused excessive bleeding and some febrile reactions. The efficacy of dialysis was assessed by using iodine as a tracer and measuring total dialysate urea nitrogen content. In 1928, Haas dialyzed two patients using heparin anticoagulation and observed a temporary clinical improvement (Fig. 206-1). His experiments were summarized in several articles that appeared between 1926 and 1928[4,5] and in

"Die Methodik der Blutauswaschung" (Methods of Dialysis in Vivo), an entry in the *Handbuch der Biologischen Arbeitsmethoden.*[6] Haas gave up further development of dialysis because of the difficulties with collodion tubes. He wrote that their production was "complicated, time consuming and, above all, . . . so brittle, that blood-washing with these membranes, in order to be performed without problems, needed both specific precautions to be taken and well-experienced coworkers!"[7] Like many of the other pioneers, Haas encountered active resistance from an entrenched, conservative academic medical establishment. However, he lived long enough to witness the realization of his lifelong dream—namely, dialysis as a life-saving therapy.

Heparin

The discovery of heparin was crucial to the development of dialysis as a viable therapeutic option, and its intriguing story is inseparable from the history of dialysis. Jay Maclean, a medical student from California working in the laboratory of William Henry Howell at the Johns Hopkins Hospital in Baltimore, discovered the anticoagulant in liver extract rather serendipitously, while pursuing thromboplastic substances: "The hepatophosphatid on the other hand . . . had no thromboplastic effect, and in fact shows a marked power to inhibit coagulation."[8] He published this discovery in a paper he authored alone. Howell and Holt subsequently named the substance *heparin,* characterized it as a glycosaminoglycan,[9] and quickly gained recognition for its discovery, while Maclean's contribution remained obscure during his lifetime. In about 1923, crude, low-potency heparin became available for experimental use. The team of Charles Best in Toronto further purified and standardized the drug.

Cellophane

A critical development came in the late 1930s with the introduction of cellophane to dialysis by William Thalhimer. Cellophane was synthesized from cellulose almost 50 years earlier and became widely used for food packing in the 1920s. Its advantages over collodion were clear: easy sterilizability, resistance to breaks, and commercial availability. Thalhimer, a Johns Hopkins graduate, obtained cellophane from the Visking sausage casing manufacturer of Chicago, and used it in an Abel-type artificial kidney to dialyze dogs using heparin anticoagulation in the late 1930s.[10] His experiments were successful, demonstrating the removal of 200 to 700 mg of urea during a 3- to 5-hour dialysis. He did not proceed to human studies, but the stage was then set.

EARLY MACHINES FOR DIALYSIS

In the mid-1940s, two nephrology giants, Willem ("Pim") Johan Kolff and Nils Alwall, established hemodialysis as a method to treat uremia. Each contributed to the concepts that are the foundation of dialysis as it is practiced today. Kolff was born on February 14, 1911, in Leiden, the Netherlands. He graduated from the Leiden Medical School in 1938. In 1940, he was experimenting with cellophane tubing at the Groningen University in an effort to determine the length of tubing needed for a certain amount of urea removal. After Hitler's army invaded the Netherlands that year and a Nazi was appointed to the chair of medicine at Groningen, Kolff moved to Kampen, a small city in eastern Netherlands.[11] There, with the assistance of Hendrik Berk of Berk Enamel Works, he constructed the rotating drum dialyzer. It had a cylindrical drum, around which a 20- to 30-meter long cellophane tubing was wound, providing a relatively large surface area. When the drum was rotated in an open tub of dialysis solution, blood was propelled through the tubing by the 2000-year-old method of Archimedes' screw. A pump kneading the rubber tube on the venous side prevented sudden swelling of the cellophane tubing, averting a prompt fall in the patient's blood volume. This artificial kidney was first used to dialyze a 29-year-old woman with end-stage uremia and malignant hypertension on March 17, 1943. Clear clinical benefit was noted with repeated treatments, but access sites to the circulation became exhausted after 10 treatments, foreshadowing the emergence of access as a major problem in dialysis for years to come. Kolff's 1944 paper[12] is a remarkable document describing the construction of his dialysis machine and the treatment of his first patient.

Kolff and his team labored under tremendous difficulties, with occupation-related shortages severely affecting their dialysis operation. Rubber, for example, was extremely scarce, so rubber tubing had to be reused multiple times; with time, such tubing became so scarce that long segments had to be replaced by glass ones. The enamel factory, under close German scrutiny, could no longer make the drums and frames; these essential items then had to be made of wood. All of the first 16 patients treated with the artificial kidney died. However, Kolff's 17th patient, who was unconscious with a blood urea concentration of 67 mmol/L (400 mg/dL) and severely hyperkalemic (14 mmol/L or 55 mg/dL) as a result of ARF in the presence of cholecystitis, was dialyzed for 11 hours in September 1945, regained consciousness, and ultimately recovered—the first person to survive intrinsic ARF after being saved by hemodialysis. One major drawback of the rotating drum was the difficulty in achieving ultrafiltration. Since the compliant tubing was not contained, it expanded in the face of a positive pressure on the blood side. Glucose had to be added to the dialysis solution in large quantities to promote osmotic ultrafiltration.

Kolff's experiences were summarized in two extraordinary books: *The Artificial Kidney*,[13] which described the

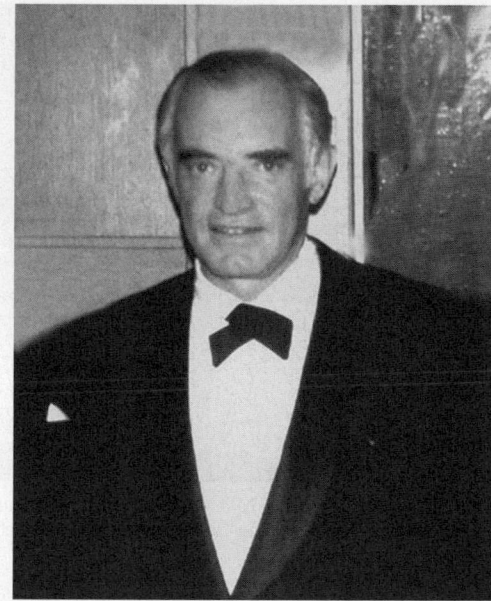

FIGURE 206-2. John P. Merrill, MD, in a 1960 photograph taken when he received an award from the New York Academy of Medicine. (Courtesy of Dr. Eli Friedman.)

construction of his machine and clinical experiences with his first 16 patients, and *New Ways of Treating Uremia: The Artificial Kidney, Peritoneal Lavage, Intestinal Lavage*,[14] which reviewed other potential treatment methods and concluded that "vividiffusion" was the most efficient method. Kolff also described another survivor of ARF treated by an alternative form of dialysis: A man with sepsis-related ARF regained renal function after two treatments with peritoneal dialysis during 10 days of oligoanuria.

After the war, Kolff donated many of his machines to institutions in Europe and North America. The most successful modification of the rotating drum dialyzer was the Kolff-Brigham machine developed from blueprints at the Peter Bent Brigham Hospital in Boston. At that institution, John P. Merrill (Fig. 206-2) treated more than 100 ARF patients over 3 years and trained many physicians on dialysis and the overall care of patients with renal failure.[15] The Kolff-Brigham machine and the knowledge gained were applied to save lives among U.S. casualties during the Korean War in 1952.[16]

Paul Teschan (Fig. 206-3) established the principle of "prophylactic dialysis," which is dialysis started earlier to prevent the complications of advanced uremia. Before this time, dialysis was initiated only when death was imminent, because conservative medical authorities unduly overemphasized the dangers of dialysis. Teschan rightly stressed that it was unreasonable to let patients, particularly those who were hypercatabolic from trauma and infection, to suffer unnecessarily severe disturbances in their internal milieu.[17]

Kolff moved to the United States in 1950 and was the head of the Department of Artificial Organs at the Cleveland Clinic in Cleveland, Ohio. Along with Watschinger, he developed the first mass-fabricated disposable dialysis filter, the twin coil dialyzer, in 1955. The dialyzer was manufactured by the Travenol Laboratories (the predecessor of Baxter Healthcare Corporation) and gained popularity in the 1960s because of its ease of operation and disposability.[18]

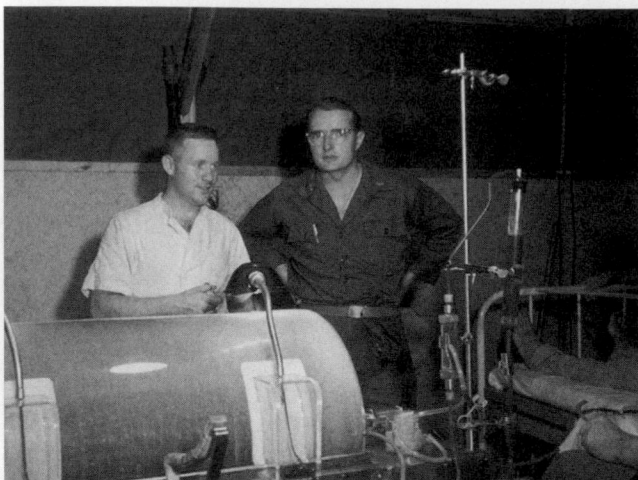

FIGURE 206-3. Paul E. Teschan, MD *(right),* operating the Kolff-Brigham dialysis machine during the Korean War. (Courtesy Dr. Eli Friedman.)

Unaware of Kolff's rotating drum artificial kidney, Gordon Murray, Edmund Delorme, and Newell Thomas at the Toronto General Hospital constructed a dialysis machine which also had a coil design built on a steel frame. In December 1946, they successfully dialyzed a young anuric, uremic, and volume-overloaded woman who recovered after three treatments. Thus, Murray and colleagues performed the first successful human dialysis in North America less than 4 years after Kolff's first human dialysis.[19,20] Murray accessed the circulation in a unique manner, by inserting two catheters into the inferior vena cava via a saphenous vein and the contralateral femoral vein. Murray's interest in dialysis was peripheral to his greater interest in heparin use, and it was the application of heparin in an extracorporeal circuit that drew him to dialysis.

Nils Alwall was born on October 7, 1904, in Kiaby, southern Sweden. He came to the University of Lund in 1923 and received his MD in 1932 and his PhD in 1935. Alwall began his studies in dialysis in the mid-1940s. Originally unaware of Kolff's work, he later determined to build a better dialysis machine. The Alwall dialyzer, used with some technical changes till the early 1960s, had three major improvements over the rotating drum. First and foremost, the cellophane tubing was sandwiched between two perforated cylinders that restricted its expansion, so the ultrafiltration rate could be controlled by changes in the transmembrane pressure. Second, the dialyzer was stationary while the dialysate circulated over it with the use of a propeller, avoiding the complicated rotating fittings of the rotating drum. Third, blood was pushed into the cellophane compartment with a finger pump massaging a rubber segment, thus allowing easy control of the flow and, hence, the speed of urea removal. Controlled ultrafiltration was achieved by the use of a tight-fitting cover over the dialysis solution reservoir. This approach made the generation of a negative pressure on the dialysis solution side possible, either by using a water Venturi pump or by simply letting a long hose hang out through a window in the dialysis room. Finally, instead of creating a negative pressure, a positive pressure could be generated by tightening a small screw-clamp on the venous blood-line. Alwall was able to remove several kilograms of fluid

from a patient with cardiac failure, hypertension, and nephrosclerosis in 1947.[21]

Alwall's knowledge of physiology and ability to control fluid balance with his device allowed him to elegantly solve an important clinical controversy. Many patients with acute uremia died of pulmonary problems. A large number of prestigious physicians thought at the time that this problem was the result of a specific "uremic pneumonitis." Alwall argued that it was caused by volume overload brought on by the popular but totally misdirected "fluid shot" therapy, the practice of giving huge amounts of fluids to anuric patients in the false hope of "flushing open the kidneys." To prove his point Alwall showed that 15% of overhydrated rabbits (with normal renal function) developed pulmonary edema. Nephrectomized rabbits with the same degree of overhydration also had pulmonary edema, which was cured with ultrafiltration alone (no dialysis at all), proving that fluid excess, not uremia, was the culprit. A focus on the importance of maintaining homeostasis is evident throughout the body of Alwall's work. A series of 30 articles, each beginning with "On the artificial kidney" in the title, was published in *Acta Medica Scandinavica* (Vols. 128 through 152) between 1947 and 1955. His writings cover a wide range of nephrology topics, including chemical analysis of blood and dialysis solution, percutaneous renal biopsy (1945), arteriovenous shunt for repeated blood access (which failed because of the materials used), ultrafiltration guided by serial chest radiograms and the use of a bed scale during dialysis, recovery from acute tubular necrosis, treatment of severe barbiturate intoxication by dialysis (1953), and radiocontrast-induced renal failure (1955). In 1963, Alwall summarized his experience of treating 1075 patients in *Therapeutic and Diagnostic Problems in Severe Renal Failure.*[22] Alwall's dedication and inspiration gave Lund two world firsts: a dedicated dialysis unit and an independent nephrology department. Alwall worked at the University of Lund till his death in February 1986.

HEMODIALYSIS ACCESS

It was recognized early that long-term vascular access is critical for multiple hemodialyses. The initial usual approach was to perform a cut-down on a vessel and insert a glass cannula; once the cannula clotted, a new site had to be found, and, before long, usable vessels were no longer available. Even Alwall's approach with arteriovenous shunts in rabbits in 1948 usually lasted less than 1 week because the materials used for construction were thrombogenic.[23]

A breakthrough came in 1960 with the creation of a Teflon (trademark for preparations of polytetrafluoroethylene, PTFE) arteriovenous shunt by Wayne Quinton, David Dillard, and Belding Scribner.[24] Thin-walled Teflon cannulas were inserted into vessels through subcutaneous tunnels while the other ends of those cannulas were allowed to emerge from the skin through tight-fitting puncture wounds. Between dialyses, a Teflon connecting segment was placed between the protruding ends of the cannulas without the use of anticoagulants. Clyde Shields, a 39-year-old Boeing machinist, was the first end-stage kidney disease patient to have this type of arteriovenous shunt created in his arm in March of 1960. He survived on dialysis until 1971. The initial report by Quinton and colleagues included four ARF patients who presented a substantial challenge due to the frequent occurrence of thrombosis in their arm veins; this necessitated the cannulation of more distant intact veins, with the resultant lengthening of the distance between the cannulas and the development of more clotting. The durability of arteriovenous shunts was improved greatly by the advent of silicone rubber.

In 1961, Stanley Shaldon and associates performed percutaneous femoral vessel catheterization using the Seldinger technique,[25,26] gaining immediate access to the circulation for dialysis. Initially, a time-consuming task was self-fashioning of the required catheters, which were not commercially available. The use of this method to obtain femoral vein access for short-term dialysis is still popular today.

Another preferred route for urgent and shorter-term hemodialysis in ARF at present is via the right internal jugular vein using a dual-lumen catheter.

DIALYSIS SOLUTION

Originally, hemodialysis solutions were made in batches just before use, with bicarbonate as the alkalinizing base. Carbon dioxide was bubbled through the bath to lower the pH to less than 7.6, in order to ensure the solubility of calcium and magnesium salts.[27] Bacterial growth in bicarbonate-containing dialysis solutions mandated their prompt use after preparation. Because of these issues, sodium acetate was chosen to replace sodium bicarbonate as the alkalinizing base in the 1960s.[28] A final acetate-based dialysis solution could then be prepared from product water and a liquid concentrate containing sodium acetate and the other necessary constituents. Acetate-based dialysis was poorly tolerated by some patients because of the occurrence of vasodilatation and cardiac depression. Therefore, when the dual-concentrate, bicarbonate-containing dialysis solution delivery system became available, bicarbonate-based dialysis promptly returned. The avoidance of acetate-based dialysis is particularly important in patients in intensive care units because of the adverse effects of acetate on the cardiovascular system.

At the beginning, it was common to use a dialysis solution with a sodium level slightly less than that of serum (approximately 130 mmol/L), in an attempt to facilitate removal of sodium from the body. However, a dialysis solution with such a low sodium value can foster the occurrence of the dialysis dysequilibrium syndrome and of hypotension. In the past few decades, owing to the shortening of dialysis sessions, it has become customary to use a higher sodium level in the dialysis solution, such as 135 to 140 mmol/L, in an attempt to maintain an adequate blood volume and, hence, a proper blood pressure during dialysis.

HISTORY OF PERITONEAL DIALYSIS IN ACUTE RENAL FAILURE

In the late 1800s, physiologists including Wegner (Berlin), Starling, Tubby, and Leathes (London), and Orlow (St. Petersburg) made important observations on peritoneal transport. They found that peritoneal fluid volume rose after instillation of hypertonic solutions and fell with hypotonic solutions and that the peritoneal membrane displayed bidirectional permeability to larger molecules. In 1923, Putnam described "the living peritoneum as a dialyzing membrane,"[29] having demonstrated the changes in the values of urea, chloride, trypan, and fluid volume over time after introduction of a variety of solutions into the abdominal cavity of animals. Heinrich Necheles, a contemporary of Haas and Putnam, used animal peritoneum ex vivo as the dialyzing membrane in his flat-plate hemodialyzer.[30] When one considers the difficulty of constructing an artificial kidney, it is not surprising that the idea of in situ utilization of the peritoneal membrane for dialysis readily came to mind.

The first human peritoneal dialysis is attributed to Georg Ganter (1884-1940), a German physician who experimented with repeated peritoneal lavage in uremic animals. He performed a single 1.5-L exchange on a woman with obstructive ARF as a result of uterine carcinoma in 1923. Under the Nazi regime, Ganter's exemplary ethical conduct sadly led to his untimely demise after he had been banned for refusing to deny treatment to Jewish patients.[31] Stephen Rosenak, "the father of the peritoneal catheter,"[32] was the first to use a special cannula with multiple distal holes to instill and retrieve fluid from the peritoneal cavity. In 1934, Rosenak and Balázs dialyzed two women with ARF secondary to mercurial poisoning, employing much larger volumes of dialysis solutions than previously reported, along with hypertonic dextrose to foster ultrafiltration. Despite reductions in urea and mercury levels, both patients died.[32]

In 1938, John Wear performed the first peritoneal dialysis treatment in the United States; one of his five patients survived and recovered after removal of a urinary tract obstruction.[33] This was the first patient who was saved by peritoneal dialysis. Wear used a physiological solution containing 28 mmol/L of bicarbonate. In 1946, less than a year after Kolff's first surviving intrinsic ARF patient, the group of Howard Frank, Arnold Seligman, and Jacob Fine at the Beth Israel Hospital in Boston successfully dialyzed an anuric, uremic patient with continuous peritoneal dialysis for a period of 4 days, achieving a prompt recovery from sulfonamide-induced ARF. These investigators inserted into the peritoneal cavity two catheters through which dialysis solution flowed continuously. The number of connections was minimized by using large volumes of dialysis solution housed in 20-L carboys.[34] Kop and Kolff dialyzed five ARF patients with peritoneal dialysis in the middle to late 1940s, with three survivors. The group of Dérot and Legrain in Paris treated 38 ARF patients in the late 1940s with peritoneal dialysis; 26 of those patients recovered, an astounding percentage.[35]

Originally, peritoneal dialysis solutions were bicarbonate based and were prepared in batches just prior to use.[36] In addition, peritoneal dialysis catheters were introduced either percutaneously, using conventional, large-bore trocars and cannulas, or via peritoneotomy. These cumbersome approaches involving solution and catheter use impeded the growth of peritoneal dialysis for ARF therapy. The barriers for peritoneal dialysis application were later overcome with simplification of the technique as a result of the following advances. Baxter Healthcare Corporation began producing a lactate-based dialysis solution (Dianeal) with disposable Y-tubing sets as designed by Maxwell of California.[37] Weston and Roberts designed a peritoneal dialysis catheter with a sharp stylet within for easy introduction into the peritoneal cavity while at the same time minimizing pericatheter leaks. The catheter was commercialized by Baxter as Trocath.[38] In the 1960s, peritoneal dialysis was used extensively for the treatment of ARF because of its relative simplicity, avoiding the need for complicated machines, anticoagulation, and vascular access. The decline in utilization of peritoneal dialysis in ARF over the last couple of decades in all groups but the very young is due to competition from better hemodialysis technology and the advent of hemofiltration and hemodiafiltration.

PERSPECTIVE

All the clinical trailblazers of dialysis encountered seemingly insurmountable difficulties. World War I and World War II, which took place when dialysis was in its infancy, led to tremendous human suffering and affected these pioneers to varying degrees, only a glimpse of which has been exposed in this chapter. In addition, many pioneers were confronted by hostile, suspicious medical conservatives who made every effort to marginalize and ridicule the science of dialysis. These obstructionists could not envision the tremendous impact that dialysis was soon to have on medical practice, while the life-saving promise of the new horizon catalyzed and spurred the innovators and their courageous patients. As the phenomenal accomplishments of these visionaries slowly sink back into history and fade from memory, perhaps not many nephrologists realize the tremendous debt that they owe the early dialysis researchers who created the intellectual and knowledge structure that make renal replacement therapy possible. What appears most obvious today is only so because we follow their footprints on the sands of time.

Finally:

> It is difficult to say what is impossible,
> for the dream of yesterday is the hope
> of to-day and the reality of to-morrow.
>
> *Robert H. Goddard*

Key Points

1. Dialysis as a means of treating kidney failure was first conceived by J. Abel, L. Rowntree, and B. Turner, who performed hemodialysis in rabbits in 1912 using a dialyzer made of intricate glass conduits and tubes of collodion membrane and hirudin for anticoagulation.
2. Major developments in hemodialysis occurred in the 1940s with the first successful application in patients with acute intrinsic renal failure using cellophane membrane and heparin anticoagulation by W. Kolff, N. Alwalls, and G. Murray
3. The first successful peritoneal dialysis in a patient with acute intrinsic renal failure was also performed in the 1940s by H. Frank, A. Seligman, and J. Fine.
4. The concept of "prophylactic dialysis" for acute renal failure evolved during the Korean War.
5. Vascular access breakthrough occurred in the 1960s with the development of the Scribner shunt.

Key References

3. Abel JJ, Rowntree LG, Turner BB: On the removal of diffusible substances from the circulating blood of living animals by dialysis. J Pharmacol Exp Ther 1913-1914;5:275-316.
11. Kolff WJ: First clinical experience with the artificial kidney. Ann Intern Med 1965;62:608-619.
21. Alwall N, Norvitt L, Steins AM: On the artificial kidney. VII: Clinical experiences of dialytic treatment of uremia. Acta Med Scand 1949;132:587.
24. Quinton WE, Dillard DH, Scribner BH: Cannulation of blood vessels for prolonged hemodialysis. Trans Am Soc Artif Intern Organs 1960;6:104-113.
31. Cameron JS: History of the Treatment of Renal Failure by Dialysis. Oxford, Oxford University Press, 2002.

See the companion Expert Consult website for the complete reference list.

CHAPTER 207

Renal Replacement Therapy in the Intensive Care Unit

Allen Nissenson and Anjay Rastogi

> ### OBJECTIVES
>
> This chapter will:
> 1. Present the incidence and prevalence of acute renal failure (ARF) in the critical care setting.
> 2. Discuss the etiopathogenesis of ARF with special emphasis on sepsis.
> 3. Describe the management of ARF in the critical care setting with emphasis on renal replacement therapy (RRT).
> 4. Review the indications for RRT in the critical care setting.
> 5. Evaluate the timing, modality, dose, and complications of RRT in the critical care setting.
> 6. Describe new modalities of RRT on the horizon.

ACUTE RENAL FAILURE

Acute renal failure (ARF) is a common occurrence in the critical care setting and its incidence has been estimated at up to 10% of the intensive care unit (ICU) admissions. As many as 50% of ICU patients who develop ARF currently require some form of renal replacement therapy (RRT), which may be temporary or permanent. Despite recent advances in critical care and nephrology, mortality from ARF remains unacceptably high[14] and has shown only a modest improvement, at best, over the last 3 decades. Although it is true that an increase in the severity of comorbid conditions present might account significantly for this dismal outcome, the assertion that, after the advent of dialysis, patients died *with* renal failure rather than *from* it might not be entirely true, based on more recent data.[1-2,15] Among patients who do survive, however, the renal prognosis in general is good, with the majority regaining independent renal function.[25]

ARF causes a myriad of problems related to solute and toxin clearance, fluid and electrolyte balance, and acid-base homeostasis. These include, but are not limited to, azotemia and uremia, fluid overload, acidosis/acidemia, hyponatremia, hyperkalemia, hyperphosphatemia, and hypocalcemia. Uremic symptoms, including anorexia, nausea, vomiting, weakness, lethargy, altered mentation, and pruritus, may develop. Other associated findings include gastrointestinal ulcerations, bleeding from platelet dysfunction, increased predisposition to infections due to abnormal leukocyte function, impaired wound healing, and malnutrition from the hypercatabolic state.

Causes of Acute Renal Failure in the Intensive Care Unit Setting

ARF in the ICU setting is usually multifactorial. ARF has traditionally been classified as prerenal, renal, and postrenal based on etiology. Prerenal ARF is caused by hypoperfusion of the kidneys due to hypovolemia, decreased effective arterial volume, or poor cardiac function. Postrenal failure is caused by obstruction from stones, strictures, tumor, and other factors. Renal causes should be considered in terms of the major site affected: glomerulus, blood vessels, tubules, and interstitium. In the hospital setting, prerenal ARF and acute tubular necrosis (ATN) are the predominant causes of acute decline in renal function, the latter being caused both by ischemia and by nephrotoxic agents.[26] Acute kidney injury resulting from either of these conditions is potentially reversible, provided the insulting agent is removed.

Patterns of ARF are changing with time as the patient population ages, because of the development of substantial risk factors including cardiovascular disease and diabetes, exposure to complex surgical procedures, and multiple medications with increased nephrotoxicity potential. There are also substantial geographical differences in the causes of ARF. In tropical countries, ATN from diarrhea is a common cause of ARF, especially in children. Obstetrical causes of ARF are also more common in third world countries. There are also regional differences in the causes of ARF based on the local use of potential nephrotoxins, such as certain herbs in African countries. Severe hemolysis-induced ARF is seen in places where malaria is endemic, such as certain regions of Asia and Africa.

Sepsis and Acute Renal Failure

ARF is a common complication of sepsis and carries a grave prognosis.[21] Mortality in patients with septic ARF was reported to be higher than in those with other causes of ARF. Although other comorbid conditions and multiorgan failure definitely contribute to this trend of higher mortality in septic patients, ARF has been shown to increase morbidity and mortality independently as well.

The etiology of ARF in patients with sepsis is multifactorial.[19-21] A generalized inflammatory response and activation of the coagulation and fibrinolytic pathways result in endothelial injury. There is an outpouring of humoral mediators into the systemic circulation in the septic state. These humoral mediators include multiple cytokines (interleukins, tumor necrosis factor [TNF]), lipid mediators (platelet-activating factors, arachidonic acid metabolites), endothelins, and components of the complement system. Inflammatory infiltrates cause local damage by release of reactive oxygen species and proteolytic enzymes. Endothelial injury and abnormalities of the coagulation and fibrinolytic pathways lead to intraglomerular thrombosis. Reduced renal blood flow also contributes to the decline in renal function seen in septic states. Both systemic hypotension and local intrarenal vasoconstriction contribute to this reduced state of renal blood flow. Imbalance between vasodilatory and vasoconstrictor substances accounts for the intrarenal vasoconstriction. The abnormality in renal blood flow predominantly affects the outer medulla, which is predisposed to ischemic insult. Tubular damage leads to detachment of cells, back-leakage of glomerular filtrate, and tubular obstruction.

Management of Acute Renal Failure

Optimal therapy for ARF requires proper identification of the etiology and pathogenesis of the disease state and intervention to address these directly, if possible. Prerenal causes are best treated with optimization of renal perfusion. This can be done by increasing intravascular volume through repletion or treating the cause of reduced effective intravascular volume (e.g., heart failure, liver failure, sepsis). Intrarenal causes of ARF are best treated by treating the cause. Postrenal causes of ARF require rapid identification of the obstructive process and intervention to reveal the obstruction. However, a significant proportion of these patients will need some form of RRT to tide them over the acute insult. The dose, timing, and modality of RRT that will lead to the best outcomes in patients with acute kidney injury are not known, and this is an area of intense research.[16]

RENAL REPLACEMENT THERAPY IN THE INTENSIVE CARE UNIT SETTING

ARF in the ICU setting, compared to ARF occurring elsewhere in the hospital or in the outpatient setting, is associated with higher morbidity and mortality. There are several characteristics that distinguish critically ill patients and explain the poorer clinical outcomes.[3] ICU patients usually suffer from multiorgan failure that may occur before, after, or concomitantly with ARF. Patients in the ICU setting are also more likely to be septic, acidemic, and overloaded with fluid. They also are more likely to be hemodynamically unstable, requiring blood pressure support, and to be receiving mechanical ventilation for respiratory support. They also tend to have higher catabolic rates.[17-18] It should be noted that the principle of "steady-state" kinetics does not apply to patients with ARF, because they are in a dynamic state of catabolism and rarely, if ever, are truly in the steady state. Critically ill patients also often require massive amounts of fluids in the form of blood and various blood products (freshfrozen plasma, platelets), nutritional support, and intravenous therapeutic agents. All of these features and many others differentiate these patients from other, less ill inpatients with ARF and need to be taken into consideration when deciding on therapy.

TABLE 207-1

Life-Threatening Complications That Arise from Renal Failure

Acidemia—life-threatening and causing hemodynamic instability
Hyperkalemia—life-threatening
Intoxications
Volume overload unresponsive to diuretics
Uremia including pericarditis and encephalopathy

Indications

The indications and decision to start RRT in ICU patients have historically been based on the presence of lifethreatening complications that arise from renal failure and are refractory to conservative management (Table 207-1). However, as knowledge about the pathophysiology of ARF in critically ill patients expands, so will the management and indications for RRT in this setting.

Mehta separated the indications to start dialysis in the ICU setting into two broad categories: renal replacement and renal support. The indications for renal replacement are the classic ones and are listed in Table 207-1.

Renal support, as defined by Mehta,[13] focuses on minimizing and ameliorating the effects of complications arising from the failure of organs other than the kidneys in the setting of multiorgan failure, as opposed to treatment for complications arising from renal insufficiency itself. An example of renal support is fluid management in the setting of volume overload without oliguria/anuria: adequate fluid removal can allow for proper nutrition and better fluid management in the setting of multiorgan failure and congestive heart failure. There is also some evidence for the notion that continuous renal replacement therapy (CRRT) is more beneficial in the setting of sepsis and inflammation because of removal of cytokines and other biological agents.[22] The thought is that the nonspecific elimination of inflammatory humoral mediators with CRRT could be an adjunctive treatment in the septic patient. This is based on two assumptions for which there is some, although not convincing, support[23]: (1) cytokines and other mediators can be effectively removed during CRRT, and (2) the nonspecific removal of mediators, including the removal of some potentially beneficial mediators, is beneficial for the patient. Even though several studies have shown removal of inflammatory mediators with CRRT, the effect was not significant or sustained. The cytokines were shown to be removed mainly by adsorption, which was limited by rapid saturation of the dialyzer membrane.[22] RRT has also been used in refractory heart failure, hepatic failure, tumor lysis syndrome, prevention of radiocontrast-induced renal failure, and several other conditions.[27] The goal of renal support therapy in general is to increase survival time, so as to allow for recovery of other organs, including kidneys.

Timing

The decision to initiate RRT in the ICU setting is a complex and multifaceted one. Historically, practitioners have waited for life-threatening indications before initiating dialysis. More recently, however, there is evidence that early intervention might be more beneficial, especially when the need for and value of renal support and the high mortality rate in this patient population are considered.

Modality

RRT can be provided in various forms depending on the availability of resources, the needs of the patient, and the expertise of the staff. These may include the use of an extracorporeal circuit containing an artificial membrane (hemodialysis) or use of the abdominal cavity and the patient's own peritoneal membrane (peritoneal dialysis). Even though peritoneal dialysis is rarely used for management of ARF in the United States, the intensivist and the nephrologist should familiarize themselves with the technique; in certain situations, it might be the only modality available.

The two major types of RRT currently used are CRRT and intermittent hemodialysis (IHD). The actual technique might be predominantly based on convection (hemofiltration), diffusion (hemodialysis), or a combination of the two (hemodiafiltration). With so many techniques available, it is no wonder that there is controversy about the best technique for a particular patient. Often, the modality chosen will depend on the experience and skill of the physicians and staff overseeing the treatment.

IHD is usually done daily or every other day for 3 to 4 hours per session in the setting of ARF. CRRT offers several theoretical advantages over IHD but also has some limitations and disadvantages. The advantages of CRRT include hemodynamic stability; more gentle fluid and solute shifts, which is specially advantageous in the setting of cerebral edema; better solute clearance and correction of acid-base and electrolyte abnormalities; and the capability to remove a greater amount of fluids without causing a hemodynamic compromise. CRRT has also been used in sepsis and in some other conditions, as mentioned earlier.

There are several disadvantages of CRRT, including limited availability, need for continuous anticoagulation, patient immobilization, and heavy resource requirement, including the need for ICU monitoring and advanced nursing care. CRRT is also potentially more expensive than IHD.

Slow, low-efficiency dialysis (SLED) is another variation of RRT used in ICU patients. Treatments are prescribed at low blood and dialysate flow rates over extended periods of time, and conventional hemodialysis machines and dialyzers are used. The advantages of SLED compared to CRRT include increased patient mobility, decreased requirements for anticoagulation, and decreased need for ICU monitoring and staffing, while volume and hemodynamic control are maintained. Slow continuous ultrafiltration (SCUF) is another variant of RRT. SCUF is performed using a CRRT machine in which the dialysate flow rate is set at zero and no replacement fluids are given, with resultant pure ultrafiltration. SCUF is used for patients who have volume overload but do not have other indications for RRT (e.g., heart failure, cirrhosis with ascites).

Dose

The appropriate and optimal dosage of RRT, whether it be intermittent or continuous, has not been as well defined in ARF as in end-stage renal disease (ESRD) and is currently an area of great interest and research. Available data indicate that the prescribed RRT dose in ARF does not even meet the minimum accepted recommended RRT

dosage for ESRD patients. In addition, the delivered dose often fails to meet the prescribed dose for multiple reasons, including catheter malfunction and early termination of treatment. Furthermore, while deciding the RRT dosage in critically ill patients, the physician must keep in mind both renal replacement and renal support indications. In a recent landmark trial, Ronco and colleagues showed that survival at 15 days after the last treatment was improved when the dose of CRRT was increased from 20 to 35 mL/kg/hr.[4] A retrospective study at the Cleveland Clinic showed that patients receiving a higher dose of dialysis had better survival. Schiffl and colleagues, in a randomized, controlled trial, showed daily dialysis to be better than every-other-day dialysis.[5] Continuous hemofiltration was associated with better survival when compared to peritoneal dialysis.[6] High intensity of CRRT treatment has also resulted in better clinical outcomes.[7] Another study recently showed increased survival with higher doses of CRRT. ATN and RENAL are two ongoing multicenter prospective randomized parallel group studies that should shed more light on whether higher doses of RRT improve outcomes and justify a change in practice if results are positive. In summary, at this point, it would be prudent to wait for the results from these high-quality, appropriately powered, multicenter trials before deciding on the most appropriate dose and modality of RRT in patients with ARF.

Vascular Access

The National Kidney Foundation's Kidney Disease Outcomes Quality Initiative (NKF-K/DOQI) practice guidelines recommend that acute hemodialysis access should initially be obtained by percutaneous placement of a double-lumen catheter in the femoral, internal jugular, or subclavian vein. If the dialysis is expected to extend beyond several days, consideration should be given to early placement of a tunneled catheter in the internal jugular vein, provided the patient is not bacteremic. The femoral vein is technically easiest to cannulate, and thoracic catheters have the advantage of less recirculation. However, it should be kept in mind that subclavian vein cannulation is associated with higher rates of both immediate (pneumothorax and hemorrhage) and delayed (stenosis) complications and should be placed only if all the other options have been exhausted. Use of portable ultrasound machines has improved the success rate of cannulation and decreased rates of complications and they should be routinely used if available. Temporary catheters have been shown to increase the rate of septicemia. Adequate precautions should be taken to minimize the risks of infection. If there is an access-related infection, appropriate antibiotic coverage should be provided, and consideration should be given to removal of the catheter, if needed.

Membrane

The effect of type of membrane on outcomes in patients with ARF in the ICU setting was reviewed recently by Modi and coworkers.[24] The bio-incompatibility of the dialyzer membrane can potentially worsen outcomes by activating the inflammatory cascade. Clinical studies to date, however, have not established unequivocally the benefits of using synthetic membranes over unsubstituted cellulose membranes. With synthetic membranes being used more routinely, this should be a lesser issue when selecting membranes for the dialyzer. Newer membranes that mimic glomerular permselectivity while retaining high rates of hydraulic permeability are being designed using novel engineering techniques including nanofabrication and microfluidics.

Complications

The major complications seen during RRT are related to rapid shifts in plasma volume and solutes, vascular access, anticoagulation, and dialysis membrane compatibility. Intradialytic hypotension is common during acute IHD; it adversely affects solute clearance and dialysis efficiency and can further compromise renal perfusion and exacerbate tubular necrosis. Intradialytic hypotension is usually triggered by excessive fluid removal during ultrafiltration. This might happen if the fluid removed is not matched with the flux of fluid into the intravascular space from the interstitial and intracellular compartments; that is, if the fluid removed is excessive or the patient has impaired neurocardiovascular responses and reflexes. Careful attention needs to be paid to volume status, dialysis prescription, and clinical observation of the patient.

The dialysis dysequilibrium syndrome is caused by rapid movement of water into brain cells due to a rapid, transient drop in plasma osmolality as solutes are rapidly cleared from the blood during dialysis. It is usually self-limited and is characterized by nausea, vomiting, headache, altered consciousness, stupor, and, rarely, coma and seizures. It can be avoided by a less aggressive dialysis prescription initially.

The blood in the extracorporeal circuit is prone to clotting, which often leads to blood loss, decreased dialysis efficiency, and increased costs stemming from the need to replace the system. In ARF, the situation is compounded by the increased propensity to bleed in these patients, which precludes the use of systemic anticoagulation. Several alternatives to conventional systemic heparinization, including regional anticoagulation (heparin and citrate), are available. Several factors guide the choice of modality, including staff experience, resources available, and patient considerations.

NEW MODALITIES ON THE HORIZON

The renal tubule cell assist device (RAD) is an innovative step in dialysis.[8,9] Adult kidney tubule cells are isolated and expanded in culture and then grown along the inner surface of the fibers in a standard hemofiltration cartridge. This device is placed in series with a conventional filter. The goal of this approach is to mimic and replace the metabolic, endocrine, and active transport properties of the renal tubule as much as possible. Promising preclinical data from studies in dogs and pigs led the U.S. Food and Drug Administration to approve phase I/II studies on 10 critically ill patients with ARF and multiorgan failure receiving CRRT. Phase I studies confirmed the safety of the device, and phase II studies are underway.

Key Points

1. Acute renal failure is a common occurrence in the critical care setting and is associated with high morbidity and mortality.
2. Sepsis is a major cause of acute renal failure in the critical care setting.
3. Renal replacement therapy is the major means of managing acute renal failure in critically ill patients.
4. Indications for dialysis for acute renal failure in critical care are much wider than those in outpatient or routine hospital wards.
5. Special attention needs to be paid to the indications, timing, modality, and dose of dialysis in critically ill patients.
6. There are several new modalities of renal replacement therapy on the horizon, including the bioartificial kidney.

Key References

See the companion Expert Consult website for the complete reference list.

CHAPTER 208

Indications for Renal Replacement Therapy in the Critically Ill

Michael Joannidis

OBJECTIVES

This chapter will:
1. Review the renal indications for renal replacement therapy (RRT).
2. Review the nonrenal indications for RRT.
3. Discuss the timing of RRT in the intensive care unit.

The primary goal of renal replacement therapy (RRT) is to compensate for the abrupt loss of renal function that characterizes acute renal failure (ARF). Disturbances associated with ARF are volume overload, accumulation of nitrogenous waste products and uremic toxins, hyperkalemia, and metabolic acidosis. In patients admitted to the intensive care unit (ICU), acute kidney injury (AKI) is often encountered at a very early stage, so symptoms may

TABLE 208-1

Indications for Renal Replacement Therapy in the Intensive Care Unit

RENAL INDICATIONS	NONRENAL INDICATIONS
Uremic signs and symptoms	Thermoregulation (hyperthermia)
Progressive azotemia	Intoxication/drug overdose
Volume overload/oliguria	Sepsis
Electrolyte disturbances	Crush injury/rhabdomyolysis
Metabolic acidosis	

not be as prominent as in community-acquired ARF. Consequently, the decision to start RRT in critically ill patients is frequently based on very early signs of AKI, such as prolonged oliguria. In general, renal and nonrenal indications can be discriminated (Table 208-1).

RENAL INDICATIONS

Uremia and Progressive Azotemia

Although the development of overt uremic symptoms (pericarditis, neuropathy, coma) represents an obvious indication for initiation of RRT, the start of RRT in ICU patients is rarely delayed until the full-blown uremia develops. On the other hand, early signs such as anorexia, nausea, vomiting, and changes in mental state are usually nonspecific and may be difficult to discriminate from symptoms of other diseases present in critically ill patients. Consequently, progressive azotemia is frequently used as an indication to start RRT for critically ill patients developing AKI. However, there is no generally accepted threshold for when to start RRT.

The concept of prophylactic hemodialysis in ARF was established by Teschan and coworkers more than 50 years ago.[1] Based on several retrospective case series between 1950 and 1970 and two prospective trials in the 1970s and 1980s, the recommended threshold of blood urea nitrogen (BUN) for initiation of hemodialysis decreased from between 165 and 200 mg/dL or higher to levels ranging from 60 to 100 mg/dL.[2-7] In a retrospective trial investigating timing in continuous veno-venous hemodialysis (CVVH) and using a BUN of 60 mg/dL for defining "early" versus "late" initiation of RRT, Gettings and colleagues[8] found significantly improved survival in the "early" group (average BUN, 43 mg/dL) compared to the "late" group (average BUN, 94 mg/dL). Another retrospective analysis on 243 ICU patients with ARF from the Program to Improve Care in Acute Renal Disease (PICARD) study used the median BUN value of 76 mg/dL for defining early versus late initiation of dialysis. The authors found that a higher degree of azotemia (>76 mg/dL; mean BUN, 114.8 mg/dL) at initiation of dialysis was associated with an increased relative risk of 1.85 for death.[9] Considering all randomized, controlled trials on RRT in ARF performed in ICUs, comprising at least 100 patients and defining mortality as the endpoint, it becomes obvious that RRT is usually initiated at a BUN level between 50 and 110 mg/dL or at a serum creatinine level between 3.5 and 5 mg/dL.[10-14]

Volume Overload and Oliguria

Volume overload due to salt and water retention is a frequent complication in ARF; it occurs in 30% to 70% of those patients in the ICU.[15] Although diuretics are frequently tried for antagonizing oliguria,[16,17] their benefit has not been proven in this situation.[18] Patients with volume overload exhibit greater risk for increased morbidity and mortality. Patients who are responsive to diuretics show improved outcome, and restrictive fluid management has proved to be beneficial both in surgical patients[19] and in those with acute respiratory distress syndrome (ARDS).[20] Consequently, in the presence of severe volume overload that does not respond to diuretic therapy, initiation of RRT appears indicated. In fact, in the ICU setting, initiation of RRT is more frequently guided by oliguria expected to result in volume overload than by increases in creatinine or BUN.[21,22]

A few retrospective studies investigating early initiation of RRT compared oliguria to conventional criteria (BUN or creatinine) for starting RRT. In two studies investigating patients who underwent cardiac surgery,[23,24] continuous RRT was started when urine output was less than 100 mL over 8 hours; a third study,[25] in patients with septic shock, used oliguria present for longer than 12 hours as the criterion. All three studies showed significantly reduced hospital or 30-day mortality in patients for whom RRT was started in the presence of oliguria instead of waiting for an increase in BUN or serum creatinine. The only prospective study investigating dose and initiation found no difference between "early" and "late" initiation[14]; however, the mortality rate was low in this study, and the sample size was very small. Translating to the classification system of RIFLE or AKIN, this would suggest using the presence of RIFLE Injury or AKI Stage II as an indication to start RRT in critically ill patients.

Electrolyte Disturbances

Hyperkalemia is a common finding in ARF, because potassium homeostasis relies mainly on renal excretion. Consequently, potassium accumulation does occur frequently in ARF. Additional factors contributing to hypokalemia are shifts from intracellular space due to acidosis and insulin resistance in critical illness. Sometimes rhabdomyolysis, hemolysis, and adverse effects of certain drugs (angiotensin-converting enzyme inhibitors, calcineurin inhibitors, cotrimoxazole, beta blockers) contribute to hyperkalemia. If not treated, hyperkalemia may lead to intractable ventricular arrhythmias or heart failure and can be rapidly fatal. Most medical therapies for hyperkalemia provide transitory improvement by shifting potassium into the intracellular space. The only effective measures to decrease the whole-body potassium load are diuretic therapy, enteric potassium-binding resins, and RRT.

Hemodialysis is the most effective way to remove potassium in renal failure, because it provides substantially higher potassium clearance (removal of 50 to 80 mmol of potassium in a 4-hour session[26]) than continuous forms of RRT. Alternatively, continuous veno-venous hemodiafiltration (CVVHDF) should be applicable if it provides sufficient total solute effluent rates. Long-term control of potassium can be more satisfactorily provided by continuous RRT.

A specific threshold for initiation of RRT in hyperkalemia cannot be generally recommended, because the decision depends on the acuteness of the serum potassium changes and their effect on cardiac rhythm and the patient's overall condition. Usually, RRT is not established at serum potassium values lower than 6.5 mmol/L.[27]

Both hypernatremia and hyponatremia occur in ARF, depending on the patient's volume status and remaining water clearance by the kidneys. However, as long as there is residual renal function, it rarely appears necessary to start RRT based on such a diagnosis.

Severe hypercalcemia may occur in the setting of hyperparathyroidism or malignancy and can lead to crystal nephropathy, tubular obstruction, and renal failure. In addition to pharmacological treatment such as bisphosphonates, RRT may be considered as a last-resort treatment for acute derangements of serum calcium and ARF or heart failure.[28]

Metabolic Acidosis

The kidney is a major player in acid-base regulation. Renal failure results in a continuous increase in organic acids and other unmeasured anions[29] due to continuous acid production of approximately 50 to 100 mEq H^+ per day. Furthermore, severe acidosis occurring as a consequence of intoxication with alcohols is an indication for acute hemodialysis. These high anion gap acidoses are usually associated with an increased osmolar gap (i.e., the difference between measured and calculated osmolality; normally $\leq$10 mOsm/L). The role of RRT in other settings of metabolic acidosis, especially lactic acidosis, is not yet answered by clinical studies. However, both hemodiafiltration and extended hemodialysis have been reported to control acidosis in these situations.[30] Although no clear studies exist to define the exact threshold, an intractable acidosis is usually considered as an indication to start RRT.

NONRENAL INDICATIONS

Sepsis

Severe sepsis and septic shock are associated with AKI in up to 50% of patients.[31] However, septic patients in the ICU often do not show prominent azotemia when developing AKI. Consequently, other criteria, such as prolonged oliguria or severe metabolic acidosis, may provide sufficient indication to start RRT.[25] "Prophylactic" RRT has been discussed in association with the hypothesis that it can possibly influence mediators released during sepsis. The only prospective, randomized study investigating this indication did not find any beneficial effect of RRT in severe sepsis without AKI.[32] Therefore, on basis of the current evidence, such a procedure cannot be recommended routinely.

Thermoregulation (Hyperthermia, Therapeutic Hypothermia)

The use of an extracorporeal circuit is associated with significant cooling of the blood. Although this is considered an unwanted side effect during regular RRT, this property may be used in case of intractable hyperthermia, such as occurs in malignant neuroleptic syndrome, malignant hyperthermia, and heat stroke. Case reports of cooling with the use of an extracorporeal circuit exist for all forms of intractable hyperthermia.[33]

A randomized, prospective study reported favorable outcomes after cardiopulmonary resuscitation with either high-volume hemofiltration (HVH) at 37° C or HVH with cooling.[34] In the meantime, several devices have reached the market that allow cooling either externally or by special central venous catheters using a cooled water circuit. Because these devices are easy to use and do not require anticoagulation, RRT for thermoregulation appears to have become obsolete.

Drug Overdose and Intoxications

Overdose of drugs or toxins that can be dialyzed is another important indication for RRT in the ICU. Drugs and toxins that can be effectively removed by dialysis are characterized by water solubility, low protein binding, low molecular weight (<500 Da), and small distribution volume. RRT may be considered in cases of overdosing or intoxication with certain alcohols (e.g., methanol, ethylene glycol), salicylates, lithium, theophylline, or methotrexate.[35] Extended dialysis has also been described as successful in paraquat intoxication, although hemoperfusion appears to be more effective.[36]

Rhabdomyolysis

Rhabdomyolysis occurs in the setting of myocyte necrosis secondary to either traumatic injury (crush injury, excessive exercise) or nontraumatic injury (ethanol, inherited defects in cellular metabolisms, toxins). This results in release of myoglobin (molecular weight, 17 kDa), which may cause ARF by the mechanisms of vasoconstriction, tubular cell damage via oxidant injury, and tubular obstruction by myoglobin casts. Rhabdomyolysis and myoglobinuria are responsible for about 5% of the cases of ARF in the United States.[37] RRT is typically initiated after failure of conservative measures (alkaline-fluid hydration, mannitol, diuretics) to prevent ARF. However, early initiation of RRT for removal of myoglobin in case of excessive rhabdomyolysis accompanied by acidosis and volume depletion, a setting in which ARF must be expected, is recommended by some authors.[38] Because conventional membranes provide insufficient sieving coefficients for myoglobin (0.4 to 0.6), usage of super-high-flux membranes for continuous RRT has been described to effectively clear myoglobin.[39]

Radiocontrast-Induced Nephropathy

Radiocontrast-induced nephropathy remains a prominent cause of hospital-acquired ARF and is associated with significant mortality.[40] A prospective, randomized trial investigating the effect of CVVH started before administration of radiocontrast media reported a significantly reduced incidence of contrast nephropathy.[41] However, the invasive nature of this procedure and unresolved questions about the pathophysiological concept of this intervention raise concerns about the utility of this approach in daily practice.

CONCLUSION

Based on current evidence, there is no evidence-based nonrenal indication for RRT with the exception of drug overdose or intoxication.

Key Points

1. Established indications for RRT are uremic signs or symptoms, progressive azotemia, volume overload/oliguria, electrolyte disturbances (mainly hyperkalemia), and metabolic acidosis.
2. Blood urea nitrogen levels between 50 and 100 mg/dL are usually considered an indication for application of renal replacement therapy (RRT) in the intensive care unit (ICU).
3. Oliguria lasting longer than 12 hours may be considered an indication for RRT in ICU patients with sepsis.
4. With the possible exception of contrast nephropathy, there is no evidence supporting the use of prophylactic RRT in ICU patients.

Key References

2. Vinsonneau C, Camus C, Combes A, et al: Continuous venovenous haemodiafiltration versus intermittent haemodialysis for acute renal failure in patients with multiple-organ dysfunction syndrome: A multicentre randomised trial. Lancet 2006;368:379-385.
9. Liu KD, Himmelfarb J, Paganini E, et al: Timing of initiation of dialysis in critically ill patients with acute kidney injury. Clin J Am Soc Nephrol 2006;1:915-919.
14. Bouman CS, Oudemans-van Straaten HM, Tijssen JG, et al: Effects of early high-volume continuous venovenous hemofiltration on survival and recovery of renal function in intensive care patients with acute renal failure: A prospective, randomized trial. Crit Care Med 2002;30:2205-2211.
25. Piccinni P, Dan M, Barbacini S, et al: Early isovolemic haemofiltration in oliguric patients with septic shock. Intensive Care Med 2006;32:80-86.
32. Cole L, Bellomo R, Hart G, et al: A phase II randomized, controlled trial of continuous hemofiltration in sepsis. Crit Care Med 2002;30:100-106.

See the companion Expert Consult website for the complete reference list.

CHAPTER 209

The Bases of Mass Separation Processes

Edward F. Leonard

OBJECTIVES

This chapter will:
1. Recognize diffusion and reaction as the bases of mass separation.
2. Distinguish convection and diffusion and describe their complementary roles in mass separation.
3. Explain the difference between ordinary and forced diffusion.
4. Recognize the importance of dimensional scale in all separation processes.

This chapter first enumerates the basic possibilities for separating biological molecules, without distinguishing between those that occur naturally and those that are used in therapeutic systems. Then those mechanisms that appear in nature and those that are deployed in manmade systems are described, and an attempt is made to identify the principal reasons for the differences between. Finally, the foreseeable developments that might mitigate the shortcomings of current artificial separation processes are indicated.

The separation of selected molecules from a mixture may occur based on the intrinsic state of the molecules, or it may be the result of a sophisticated process that is driven by and dependent on external forces. For example, water may evaporate spontaneously on the absorption of heat, leaving precipitated solutes behind. In contrast, very sophisticated regulatory processes are needed to produce a urine that precisely meets the volumetric and compositional requirements of a complex organism. Although the degree of regulation and the complexity of the operation may vary between these extreme cases, the basic means available for selective molecular separations are the same.

TRANSPORT-BASED SEPARATION

Molecules can do only two things: move and react. Both movement and reaction can effect separation, but only to the degree that either is selective with respect to the molecular species that are present. Molecular movement is also termed "transport." Transport can be accomplished either by convection or by diffusion.

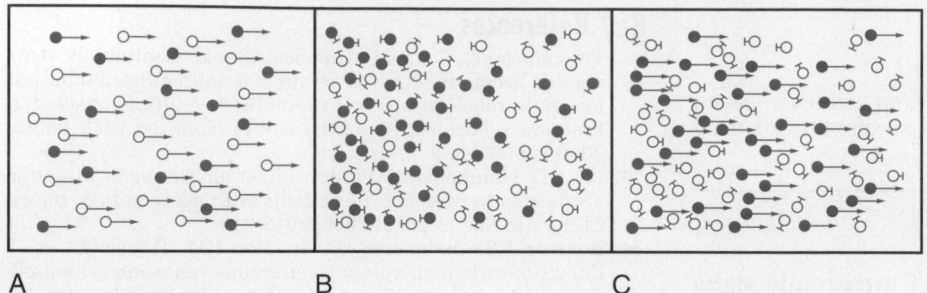

A   B   C

FIGURE 209-1. Diffusion is the result of microscopic molecular movements. **A,** Convection without diffusion moves all molecules equally and does not result in separation. **B,** Unhindered ordinary diffusion causes initially separated molecules to move together. **C,** Forced diffusion, provided by an external force, separates molecules when the force acts differently on different molecular types.

Convection

Convection is, by definition, the movement of a species with the medium in which it is imbedded.[9] Each component moves with the same speed (Fig. 209-1A). Thus, convection is of little value in separating molecular species because it requires all species to move together—the antithesis of separation. However, convection provides the essential function of delivering and removing streams of molecules to and from a boundary at which they may be separated, and thus it is an essential concomitant of all practical separation processes. Convection is sometimes claimed to effect separation itself when it delivers a mixture to a boundary, as in hemodiafiltration,[6] but it is the boundary that does the work, and the backward diffusion of what is not passed controls the process.

Diffusion

Diffusion is a highly variegated phenomenon. Ordinary or Fickian diffusion is defined as the molecular movement of a species that is induced by microscopic random movements coupled to the non-uniform distribution in space of the species.[5] (This phenomenon is illustrated in Figure 209-1B, where the larger proportion of blue molecules at the left will, because of many random movements, lead ultimately to their uniform distribution in the mixture.) In mathematical terms, the diffusive flux of a substance is related to its concentration variation, or gradient. (The flux is the number of molecules or moles of a species that passes through a unit area in unit time.) The flux of a typical molecular species, A, is designated as J_A, and it is proportional to the gradient of the concentration of the diffusing substance:

$$N_A = -D_A \nabla c_A$$

In this equation, the general expression for the gradient, ∇c, is used. When diffusion takes place in a prescribed direction, the gradient can be replaced by the spatial derivative (e.g., dc/dx). This equation is known as *Fick's law,* and D is termed the *Fickian diffusivity.* The negative sign in the equation declares that movement is always such that the distribution becomes more uniform with time: concentrated pockets of material move into less concentrated surroundings. Ordinary diffusion is contrasted with forced diffusion (discussed later), in which an external force acts selectively on some molecules, causing them to move relative to other molecules in the system (see Fig. 209-1C).

Ordinary Diffusion

Ordinary diffusion assists convection in delivering molecules to a boundary and is, in fact, the essential final step in the delivery of molecules from a fluid to a boundary. However, because ordinary diffusion dissipates molecular concentration, it, like convection, is not of itself useful in molecular separations. Although diffusion in solutions depends on the properties of the solution and the sizes of the different molecular species, this dependence is not strong. Most small molecules, such as glucose, urea, and ionized salts, have D values near 10^{-5} cm^2/sec in physiological solutions at ambient and physiological temperatures. For molecules that are large relative to those comprising the medium, D varies with the cube root of the molecular weight, as described by the Stokes-Einstein equation

$$D = \frac{k_B T}{6 \pi \mu R}$$

with the usual assumption that most molecules are globular, with their effective radius for diffusion, R, proportional to their molecular weight (or molecular mass), M. In this equation, k_B is the Boltzmann constant, T is the absolute temperature, and μ is the viscosity of the medium.[4,5] Thus, the diffusion coefficient of albumin is only about 15 times smaller than that of urea, even though its molecular weight is about 1000 times larger.

However, if a third molecule is introduced that affects the two molecules to be separated in radically different manners, large differences in effective diffusion coefficients and rates can be observed. The third molecule typically hinders the passage of some molecules. Hindered ordinary diffusion is the basis of many separations accomplished in nature and in artificial systems. It may be accomplished by *membranes,* which are thin, almost two-dimensional arrays, or by three-dimensional *gel structures,* exemplified by extravascular tissue and synthetic gels. Table 209-1, taken from a much more extensive compendium,[10] shows both how diffusion coefficients change with molecular weight and how they are affected by the presence of a polymer matrix, either natural or artificial. The polymer matrix of typical dialysis membranes changes the diffusivity ratio of albumin versus a typical small molecule from a value in the neighborhood of 0.1 to a value that may be 0.001 or lower.

Figure 209-2 shows a membrane with a molecular structure (lines in the figure) that permits passage of small, but not larger, molecules. The flow is from right to left. The rejected molecules accumulate on the membrane surface. If they are not to clog it, they must either diffuse away, against the impinging stream of molecules, or be carried away sidewards (upward or downward in the figure) by a "crossflow." With respect to rejection by the membrane, size is only one principle, albeit an important one, that sets its selectivity.

True pores are not seen in gels and homogeneous polymeric membranes. Such polymer membranes and gels are

TABLE 209-1

Diffusivities in Free and Hindered Diffusion

SOLUTE	MW (Da)	D (FREE) cm²/sec × 10⁵	D (MATRIX) cm²/sec × 10⁵	TISSUE OR GEL
Glucose	180	0.96	0.48	Cartilage
Sodium chloride	58.5	1.22	0.76	Cartilage
Lactalbumin	14,200	1.01	0.63	3.9% Agarose
Lactalbumin	14,200	1.01	0.32	7.5% Agarose
Ovalbumin	45,000	0.72	0.40	7.5% Agarose
Serum albumin	68,000	0.60	0.16	7.5% Agarose

D, Fickian diffusivity; MW, molecular weight.

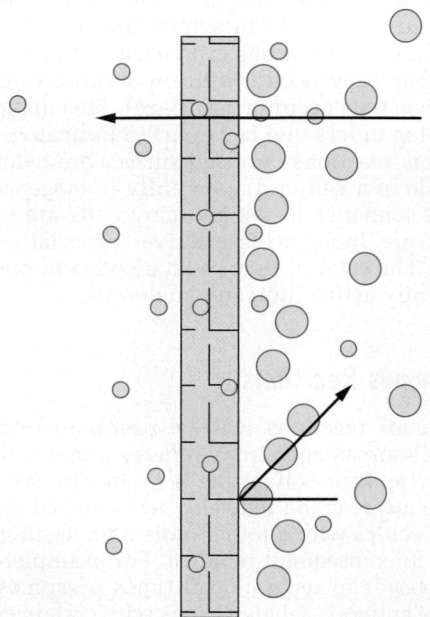

FIGURE 209-2. Hindered ordinary diffusion, typically provided by a membrane or a gel structure, separates molecules. The hindering structure must act differently on the different types of molecules to be separated.

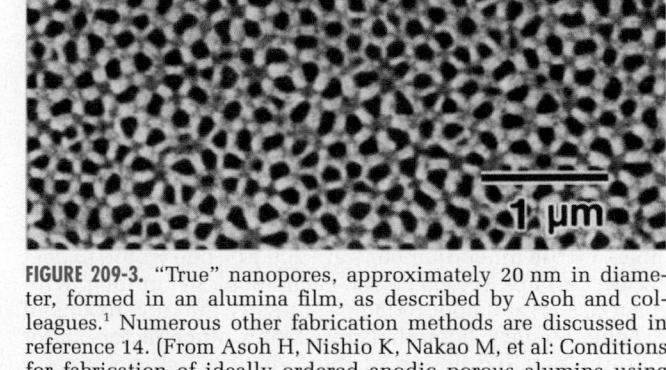

FIGURE 209-3. "True" nanopores, approximately 20 nm in diameter, formed in an alumina film, as described by Asoh and colleagues.[1] Numerous other fabrication methods are discussed in reference 14. (From Asoh H, Nishio K, Nakao M, et al: Conditions for fabrication of ideally ordered anodic porous alumina using pretextured Al. J Electrochem Soc 2001;148:B152-B156.)

characterized by a network of fixed, even if somewhat "wiggly," molecular chains that act like a structure perforated by pores with a more or less narrow distribution of diameters. Microporous and nanoporous membranes possess actual pores with walls that do not wiggle. These membranes can have a very narrow distribution of pore diameters. They provide a new means for separating molecular species, at present primarily on the basis of molecular size (Fig. 209-3).

There is a great advantage in making any membrane thin, but this goal is limited by the need for any membrane to be supported over relatively large surface areas. Although the thickness of a biological membrane is on the order of a nanometer, it is usually called upon to span areas only on the order of a cell diameter. Artificial membranes are much thicker, indeed seldom thinner than about 100 µm. Recent efforts to improve artificial membranes have taken different forms in polymers and gels,[8] as opposed to recently realized structures that include "true" pores.[14] In both instances, these efforts have been directed toward achieving a thin discriminating layer or "skin" on a thicker substrate that provides strength but offers less resistance to molecular movement.

Some membranes discriminate among molecular species based on a combination of solubility and diffusive mobility within the membrane structure. For example, elastomeric, notably silicone, membranes[13] have been used to transport respiratory and anesthetic gases between blood and a gas stream while blocking almost completely the movement of solute molecules. Transport through these structures is considered to be proportional to the product of a "mobility" and a solubility.

All ordinary diffusion is limited by the available concentration gradient, which, in turn, is limited by the concentration of the solute to be separated (one often wishes it could be higher) and by the distance to be traveled in order to achieve separation (one often wishes it could be shorter). The work of Collander, summarized in reference 3 and reproduced in Figure 209-4, shows clearly the roles of both mobility, as represented by molecular size, and solubility, expressed as an oil-water partition coefficient.

Diffusive processes can be graded in terms of their speed: by a "characteristic time," τ, equal to D/l^2, where l is a diffusion length.[4] When this length is chosen appropriately (e.g., the radius of a hollow fiber or the thickness of a membrane), the diffusion time can be roughly estimated. For example, if the average path required for a urea

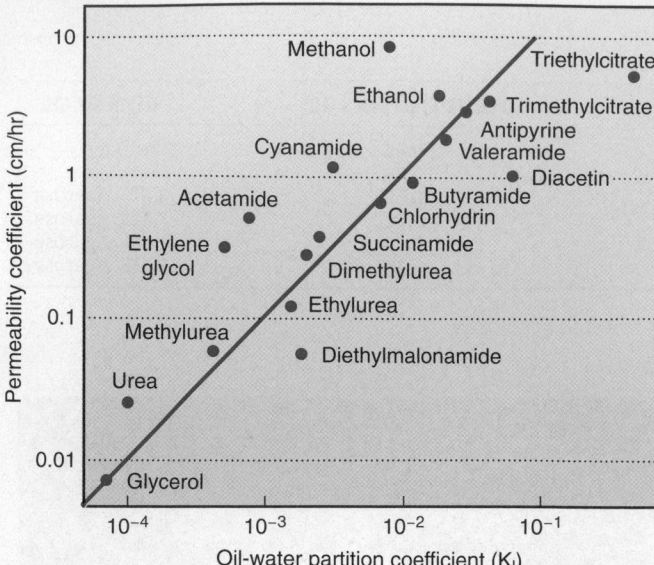

FIGURE 209-4. The diffusivity of molecules depends on both the size and the solubility of the molecule in the diffusion medium. The size of the circles on the figure are proportional to the diameters of the designated molecules. (Adapted from Byrne JH, Schultz SG: An Introduction to Membrane Transport and Bioelectricity. New York, Raven Press, 1988.)

molecule to leave a hollow fiber is 150 μm, the time needed within the fiber for this molecule to be extracted would be about 23 seconds. At a blood flow of 300 mL/min, the blood volume within the fibers would be 115 mL. For fibers whose inner diameters are 200 μm, one would expect to use perhaps 10,000 fibers, each about 30 cm long, with a surface area of about 1.8 m^2—roughly the dimensions of a contemporary hemodialyzer. Many other factors enter into the detailed design of these devices, but none more importantly than the diffusion time and the factors that determine it.

Forced Diffusion

Forced diffusion (see Fig. 209-1C) induces relative molecular motion by the application of an external force that acts differently on the different molecular species present in a mixture. If the force does not act differently, it has the effect of moving the entire mixture; this is convection, the inutility of which was discussed earlier. The force field can be electrical, magnetic, gravitational, or centrifugal.[2] Even a fluid shear field can be an effective separator if the species to be moved is a deformable cell.[7,15] The separation of cells can be effected by any of the forced diffusion modalities. Cells may be separated from their suspending fluid, typically plasma, or from each other. Centrifugal separations are commonplace. Magnetic separations of one cell type from another can be achieved either by exploiting intrinsic differences in the magnetic properties of different cell types or by labeling a target population with magnetic beads. Electrical separations are achieved in certain cell-sorting devices and in electrophoretic gels. The transport of charged molecules across membranes is a combination of ordinary and forced diffusion that has been treated in great detail.[11]

TABLE 209-2

Separation Principles

Transport	Convection
	Diffusion—free
	Diffusion—forced
Reaction	Homogeneous
	Heterogeneous

REACTION-BASED SEPARATION

Direct interaction with another molecule (i.e., reaction) is the remaining principle by which molecular separations can be achieved. Reactions can be categorized as homogeneous (when they occur within a solution) or heterogeneous (when they occur on a surface). This distinction can be confusing unless one is careful to indicate the *scale* of observation: reactions on a cell surface are heterogeneous at the scale of a cell and apparently homogeneous at the scale of a container in which many cells are suspended. Reactions are inherently selective, especially catalyzed reactions. The catalyst may be an enzyme or one of a host of chemically active inorganic materials.

Homogeneous Reactions

Homogeneous reactions may be useful in either of two ways. A dissolved agent may remove a molecular species by destroying it or converting it to an inactive molecule. Homogeneous reaction may also allow the combination of target molecules with another molecule, tagging the target molecule for subsequent removal. For example, the use of magnetic beads to separate cell types presumes the prior reaction of antibody-labeled beads with certain cells which are then selectively removed in a magnetic field. Photoreaction is essentially a homogeneous reaction that is conducted in a light field. It may depend on the intrinsic photosusceptibility of target molecules or on pretreatment of the solution to make certain components more photoreactive.

Heterogeneous Reactions

Most sorbents achieve separations by reacting chemically with a molecule that diffuses to, and perhaps into, the sorbent. The sorbent is usually a solid but can be a liquid. Some sorbents contain an immobilized enzyme. One example is the Redy cartridge, which contains immobilized urease. Other important sorbents include ion exchange resins, which function in a fairly specific manner to substitute one ion for another, and activated carbon, which functions in a largely nonspecific manner, preferentially binding large molecules.

The possible separation principles, discussed to this point, are summarized in Table 209-2.

WATER REMOVAL

Water removal from biological fluids is a special separation process, because the amount of water to be removed is usually so much greater (in either molar or gravimetric terms) than that of any other species. It is often stated that water is removed only by convection, but such is not the case. It seems as if ultrafiltration is convection dominated; however, the whole medium is not moved, but rather only the preponderant component (water). Further, the process is not limited by what is removed, but rather by what is done with what is not removed, namely the cells and molecules that are held back on the high-pressure side of an ultrafiltration membrane. Water removal is accomplished in most systems by forced, hindered diffusion. (The diffusion is forced by pressure fields in hemodialysis and hemodiafiltration or by an osmotic gradient in peritoneal dialysis.) Because of its relatively high vapor pressure, it is possible to remove water as vapor from the surface of an artificial membrane—a mimicry of the insensible water movement that occurs across biological surfaces exposed to air. The artificial process is known in industry as pervaporation.[12]

NATURAL VERSUS ARTIFICIAL SYSTEMS

In the world of artificial separation processes, there is one natural process that has gone largely unduplicated: the membrane permease. A permease that does not require high-energy compounds to facilitate transport might seem to be almost as easy to introduce into an artificial system as its close relative, the enzyme. Such a view begs an important difference between biological membranes and artificial interfaces: membrane thickness. A permease in a biological system need only translate a molecule over a distance measured in angstroms, whereas, as noted earlier, most artificial barriers are much thicker.

Therefore, the crucial difference between transport and separation in natural as opposed to artificial systems is scale, particularly as measured along the diffusion path. As was shown earlier, diffusion affects (usually limits) all molecular separation processes. The time required for a small molecule to transit a cell membrane is on the order of 1 μsec, whereas the time required to traverse a typical polymer membrane in a hollow-fiber dialyzer is on the order of 10 sec. This correct calculation has sometimes been incorrectly interpreted. A membrane as thin as a cell membrane, if realized and given structural integrity in an artificial system, would be limited not by its own thickness or pore area but by the thickness of the fluid layer that it would be servicing. Natural systems couple thin membranes with two requisites: support for the membrane, and very thin fluid layers juxtaposed to these membranes, achieved by the branching, thinning structure of the vascular system that occurs in all large-scale plant and animal organisms. The analysis of natural systems for molecular separation, and the synthesis of artificial ones, requires an appreciation of scale. The point was first made quantitatively in the detailed work of August Krogh,[16] but it is just as cogent in relation to contemporary tissue engineering.

FUTURE DEVELOPMENTS

As delineated in this chapter, one must assess the bases of transport with two criteria in mind. The first is *selectivity*. Separation is inexorably tied to selection. As one must exclude convection as a principle of separation, so must one look askance at separation processes that are not adequately selective. The second criterion is *speed*, whose determinants are process time, volume, and the characteristic dimension. Artificial processes are slow because their characteristic dimensions are large compared with those of cells and capillaries. Any improvement must address the largest of the relevant dimensions, because making the smallest dimensions smaller or the fastest parts of the overall process faster will not help appreciably.

CONCLUSION

Diffusion and chemical reaction are the sole bases for the separation of mass. Convection assists these bases in all macroscopic processes, both natural and artificial. Ordinary diffusion is ubiquitous and can be augmented by forced diffusion. The crucial difference between diffusion in living and manmade systems is the length of the path that molecules must traverse to be separated. Manmade mass separation processes have never been closer to the paradigm presented by nature, but they still have a long way to go. In fact, however, these processes must be conducted at a steadily smaller scale, so our task might better be stated as how to find a very short way to go.

Key References

2. Bird RB, Steward WE, Lightfoot EN: Transport Phenomena. New York, J. Wiley, 2002.
3. Byrne JH, Schultz SG: An Introduction to Membrane Transport and Bioelectricity. New York, Raven Press, 1988.
9. Lightfoot EN: Transport Phenomena and Living Systems: Biomedical Aspects of Momentum and Mass Transport. New York, Wiley, 1974.
11. Schultz SG: Basic Principles of Membrane Transport. Cambridge, Cambridge University Press, 1981.
13. Stern SA: Polymers for gas separations: The next decade. J Membr Sci 1994;94:1-65.

See the companion Expert Consult website for the complete reference list.

CHAPTER 210

Renal Replacement Techniques: Descriptions, Mechanisms, Choices, and Controversies

Zaccaria Ricci, Rinaldo Bellomo, and Claudio Ronco

OBJECTIVES

This chapter will:
1. Describe the implications of the principal mechanisms of water and solute transport as the basis of renal replacement therapies.
2. Describe the application of these mechanisms to clinical practice and to various renal replacement modalities.
3. Describe the potential advantages and disadvantages of various renal replacement modalities.

The term *dialysis* literally means to "pass across." The mechanisms involved in renal replacement therapies (RRT) are based on the principle of water and solute transport whereby the composition of a solution is exposed to a second solution through a semipermeable membrane.[1-8] Water and low-molecular-weight molecules can pass through the membrane pores, but larger molecules are not "sieved," depending on the membrane pore size cutoff. There is a wide range of artificial membranes and techniques available for RRT, and treatments today can be tailored to individual patient needs. The general principles of the various techniques are summarized in Figure 210-1.

Membranes can be divided into cellulose-based or synthetic (noncellulose) types. The cellulosic-hydrophilic membranes include cuprophan, hemophan, and cellulose acetate, and the synthetic-hydrophobic membranes include polysulfone, polyamide, polyacrylonitrile, and AN69S. Cellulose-based membranes are generally considered to be low-flux membranes, meaning that their permeability coefficient to water, Km, is less than 10 mL/hr × mm Hg/m². They are extremely thin (wall thickness, 5 to 15 µm) and have a symmetrical structure with uniform porosity. They are essentially hydrophilic. Synthetic membranes are high-flux membranes with a Km greater than 30 mL/hr × mm Hg/m². Wall thickness ranges between 40 and 100 µm, and the structure is asymmetrical, with an inner skin layer and a surrounding sponge layer. Synthetic membranes have larger pores and are hydrophobic. They have high sieving coefficients for solutes of a wide range of molecular weights and therefore are more suitable for convective treatments. Because of these properties, high filtration rates are achieved with these membranes mainly by a method of convection.

In peritoneal dialysis, the peritoneal mesothelium is utilized as a living membrane to separate the dialysis solution infused into the peritoneal cavity from the blood of the peritoneal microcirculation.

MECHANISMS OF SOLUTE AND WATER TRANSPORT ACROSS SEMIPERMEABLE MEMBRANES

Solutes that can pass through membrane pores are transported by two different mechanisms, diffusion and ultrafiltration (convection).

Diffusion

The term *diffusion* defines the movement of a solute with a statistical tendency to reach the same concentration in the available distribution space on each side of the membrane. The practical result is a passage of molecules from the more concentrated compartment into the less concentrated one. Solute transport is governed by the following formula:

$$Jd = DTA \, (\delta c / \delta x)$$

where J is the solute flux, D is the diffusion coefficient, T is the temperature of the solution, A is the surface area of the membrane, δc is the concentration gradient between the two compartments, and δx is the thickness of the membrane.

In dialysis, blood and dialysate are separated by a membrane. Bidirectional diffusive transport of molecules occurs in response to a concentration gradient. Clearances (K) can be calculated in dialysis from the following formulas:

$$K = [(Qbi \times Cbi) - (Qbo \times Cbo)]/Cbi$$

or

$$K = (Qdo \times Cdo)/Cbi$$

where Qbi and Qbo are the inlet and outlet blood flows, respectively; Cbi and Cbo are the inlet and outlet blood concentrations, respectively; Qdo is the dialysate effluent flow; and Cdo is the solute concentration in the effluent dialysate (i.e., that leaving the dialyzer or the peritoneal cavity).

Convection (Ultrafiltration)

Convection occurs when water is driven by either a hydrostatic or an osmotic force across a semipermeable membrane carrying solutes that can pass through the membrane pores. This is also referred to as "solvent drag." The water pushed through the membrane is accompanied by solutes at concentrations similar to those in the original solution.

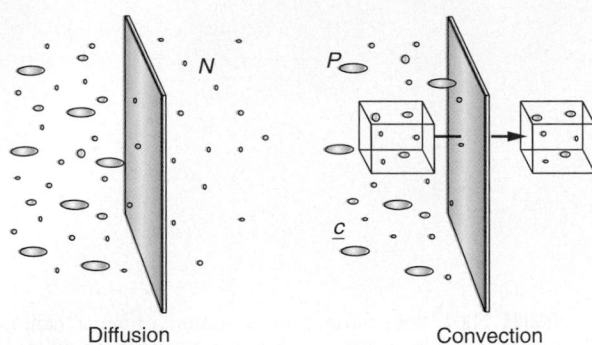

Diffusion   Convection

FIGURE 210-1. Diffusion and convection are schematically represented. During diffusion, the solute flux (Jx) is a function of the solute concentration gradient (dc) between the two sides of the semipermeable membrane, the temperature (T), the diffusivity coefficient (D), the membrane thickness (dx), and the surface area (A), according to the following equation:

$$Jx = DTA\ (dc/dx)$$

Convective flux of solute (Jf) requires instead a pressure gradient between the two sides of the membrane (transmembrane pressure, or TMP), which moves a fluid (plasma water) with its crystalloid content in a process called ultrafiltration (which is also dependent on the membrane permeability coefficient, or Kf). Colloids and cells will not cross the semipermeable membrane, depending on the pores' size.

$$Jf = Kf \times TMP$$

and

$$TMP = Pb - Pd - \pi$$

where Pb is the blood hydrostatic pressure, Pd is the hydrostatic pressure on the ultrafiltrate side of the membrane, and π is the oncotic pressure.

Larger molecules are held back. Filtration occurs in response to a transmembrane pressure gradient according to the following formula:

$$Qf = Km \times TMP = Km\ (Pb - Puf - \pi)$$

where Km is the coefficient of permeability of the membrane, TMP is the transmembrane pressure, Pb is the hydrostatic pressure of blood, Puf is the hydrostatic pressure in the ultrafiltrate compartment, and π is the oncotic pressure of blood.

Once ultrafiltration occurs, solutes are carried to the other side of the membrane at various rates according to their membrane rejection coefficient (σ), with σ being near 1 for albumin and near 0 for small solutes such as urea. The sieving coefficient for a solute (S) is inversely correlated with the membrane rejection coefficient, assuming a relation of $S = 1 - \sigma$. In clinical practice, S is measured from the ratio between the concentration of solute in the ultrafiltrate and its concentration in plasma water. In convective treatments, therefore, the transport (Jc) of solute x is governed by the formula,

$$Jc = UF \times [X]_{UF}$$

where UF is the volume of ultrafiltrate and $[x]_{UF}$ is the concentration in the ultrafiltrate of the solute, x. From this, we may derive the formula for clearance (K) in convective treatments:

$$K = Qf[x]_{UF}/[x]_{Pw}$$

where Qf is the ultrafiltration rate and $[x]_{UF}/[x]_{Pw}$ is the ratio of the solute concentrations in the ultrafiltrate and

plasma water (i.e., the sieving coefficient, S). From this formula, we may observe that when the sieving is 1, the clearance is equal to the ultrafiltration rate.

Despite these distinctions, diffusion and convection often act simultaneously, and it is almost impossible to physically divide these transport mechanisms.

Osmosis

Osmosis is especially utilized in peritoneal dialysis. Glucose is utilized as an osmotic agent in the peritoneal dialysis solution. The low rate of glucose absorption from the peritoneal cavity enables the dialysis solution to have the osmotic property of permitting water transport. In this particular modality, water movement proportional to the osmotic power of the solution is achieved, and patient hydration can be controlled. However, the net fluid removal also takes into account other processes such as transcapillary ultrafiltration and lymphatic reabsorption.

CONTINUOUS RENAL REPLACEMENT THERAPIES

The goals of any RRT in the critically ill patient should be mimicking the functions and physiology of the native organ, ensuring qualitative and quantitative blood purification, restoring and maintaining homeostasis, avoiding complications, achieving good clinical tolerance, and facilitating organ recovery. Continuous renal replacement therapy (CRRT) might achieve such goals. It has practical and theoretical advantages over intermittent therapies in hemodynamically unstable or severely catabolic patients with acute renal failure (ARF).

Use of CRRT for the management of ARF has grown to the point that, according to a recent survey, 80% of the intensive care units worldwide routinely choose this strategy.[9] This therapy is not new. Starting from previous innovations by Henderson[4] and Silverstein,[10] who used ultrafiltration as a treatment for fluid overload and azotemia, Peter Kramer developed this technique in 1977 by accidentally accessing the femoral artery instead of the vein, creating an arteriovenous circuit, which gave birth to a very primitive but innovative approach.[11] Problems with low-circuit flow and coagulation left this idea dormant until Lauer and colleagues (1983) described the unique operational characteristics of the system and the enormous potential for the treatment of ARF in intensive care departments.[12] After the application of blood pumps and the substitution from arteriovenous to veno-venous circuitry, finally CRRT practice as we currently know it was born: since then, the concept has remained unchanged, but the technology has improved enormously.

Continuous arteriovenous treatments are no longer used because of multiple technical problems, including low flow rates, poor efficiency, prolonged arterial cannulation, and the requirement of a satisfactory mean arterial pressure to drive the circuit. Arterial access itself can have grave complications such as hemorrhage, distal ischemia, arterial thrombosis, traumatic fistula formation, and pseudoaneurysms. With the advent of compact and efficient peristaltic blood pumps, venous circuitry is the method of choice, and arterial driven circuits have been superseded.

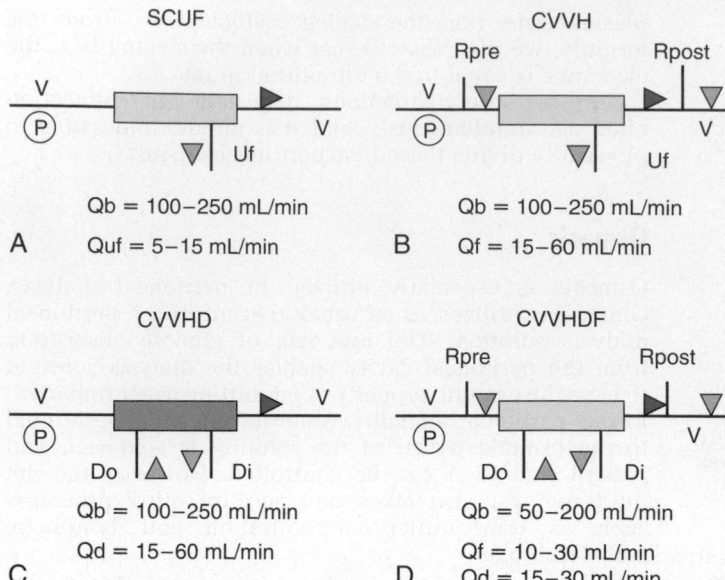

FIGURE 210-2. Schematic representation of most common continuous RRT setups. **A,** Slow continuous ultrafiltration (SCUF). **B,** Continuous veno-venous hemofiltration (CVVH). **C,** Continuous veno-venous hemodialysis (CVVHD). **D,** Continuous veno-venous hemodiafiltration (CVVHDF). See text for specifications. Dark triangles represent blood flow direction; light triangles indicate the flow of dialysate/ replacement solutions. Di, dialysate in; Do, dialysate out; P, pump; Qb, blood flow; Qd, dialysate solution flow; Qf, replacement solution flow; Quf, ultrafiltration flow; Rpre, replacement solution prefilter; Rpost, replacement solution postfilter; Uf, ultrafiltration; V, vein.

INTERMITTENT AND HYBRID RENAL REPLACEMENT THERAPIES

Intermittent and hybrid techniques require an adequate vascular access and specifically trained nurses to carry out the dialysis session. Efficient and suitable equipment able to achieve the prescription intended is important. A specific water-softening setup that can de-ionize water is required to achieve pure water for dialysate preparation. In some cases, despite the use of reverse osmosis as a water treatment system, on-line ultrafilters are needed to achieve bacterial- and pyrogen-free dialysate. The dialysis machine must respond to the standards of reliability and safety and must have an adequate blood module, as well as a precise dialysate preparation module with adequate warming and deaeration systems, and all parts must have active alarms to avoid any possible accident. Until recently, this resource could be facilitated and carried out only by nephrology units, but modern intensive care units are becoming autonomous, initiating treatment without the need of nephrological liaison.

Hybrid techniques have been given a variety of names but have the common purpose of optimizing the advantages offered by continuous and intermittent modalities, including efficient solute removal with minimum solute dysequilibrium, reduced ultrafiltration rate with hemodynamic stability, optimized delivery to the prescribed ratio, low anticoagulant needs, diminished cost of therapy, efficiency of resource use, and improved patient mobility. These hybrid techniques have been defined as sustained low-efficiency dialysis (SLED), slow low-efficiency extended daily dialysis (SLEDD), prolonged intermittent daily renal replacement therapy (PIDRRT), extended daily dialysis (EDD), extended daily dialysis with filtration (EDDf), or simply extended dialysis (ED),[13-18] depending on variations in schedule and type of solute removal (convective or diffusive). The benefit of this form of treatment is that it provides a high dialysis dose, which can be applied even in unstable patients with the advantage of allowing unrestricted access to patients for daytime procedures.

RENAL REPLACEMENT TECHNIQUES AND MODALITIES

Several techniques and modalities are today available for RRT. Techniques may differ in terms of vascular access and extracorporeal circuit design, as well as frequency and intensity of treatment (continuous, extended, intermittent); they differ essentially in regard to mechanism of transport and type of membrane utilized (dialysis, hemofiltration, hemodiafiltration, plasmafiltration, perfusion). The following paragraphs briefly describe the types of equipment utilized, the operational parameters normally employed, and the target efficiencies as far as solute and fluid control are concerned. Typically, *intermittent hemodialysis* (IHD) is carried out in a session of 3 to 5 hours with a blood flow of 250 to 500 mL/min. A low-permeability membrane such as cuprophan or hemophan may be used, with an average surface area of 1 to 1.5 m². Dialysate flow is 500 mL/min, and the rate of ultrafiltration can be set as clinically indicated.

Sustained low-efficiency extended dialysis (SLED) is a recently developed hybrid technique of RRT that applies a conventional hemodialysis machine but with reduced blood flow (100 to 200 mL/min) and dialysate flow rates (100 to 200 mL/min); it is usually performed nocturnally for an extended time (10 to 12 hours). Different prescriptions, variable amounts of ultrafiltrate, and other "variations on the theme" have been described.

Slow continuous ultrafiltration (SCUF) is a treatment typically employed for 24 hr/day or for only some hours during a day with a venovenous access (with pump) (Fig. 210-2A). The treatment is carried out with high-flux membranes, and the objective is to achieve volume control in patients with fluid overload. The operational parameters are generally those described in the figure. Because low filtration rates are required, filters with small surface area are employed. An ultrafiltration control system should be applied to prevent excessive fluid loss and hypovolemia. Because of the low filtration rates, the treatment is not suitable to achieve blood purification but only volume control.

Continuous veno-venous hemofiltration (CVVH) is normally applied for an extended period, up to several weeks. The treatment is performed in veno-venous mode (see Fig. 210-2B). The technique utilizes high-flux membranes, and the prevalent mechanism of solute transport is convection. The operational conditions are described in the figure. An ultrafiltrate is produced and is partially or totally replaced by fresh substitution fluid. In CVVH, the flow is regulated by a pump, and the rate of ultrafiltration can significantly increase. In the presence of high filtration rates, systems for ultrafiltration and reinfusion control are used. Different machines use either volumetric control systems or volumetric pumps regulated by one or more scales. Heparin is typically infused in the arterial line to prevent clotting of the circuit. The replacement solution can be infused either before the filter (predilution) or after the filter (postdilution). In the first case, ultrafiltration must be relatively increased to maintain the same efficiency observed in postdilution mode. Because the ultrafiltrate is replaced by the substitution fluid which is toxin free, the treatment is used for blood purification and volume control. Once the blood flow is set, the average ultrafiltrate (filtration fraction) ideally should not exceed 20% of the overall blood flow rate.

Continuous veno-venous hemodialysis (CVVHD) is a treatment carried out over an extended period using a circuit driven by either an arteriovenous access or a veno-venous pump. The treatment as originally described used a low-flux membrane such as cuprophan and a countercurrent flow of dialysate at 15 to 20 mL/min. Because of the nature of the membrane and the gradient provided by the dialysate, the prevalent mechanism of solute transport in this technique is diffusion (see Fig. 210-2C). An ultrafiltrate volume is obtained exactly in the range of values adequate to maintain the patient's fluid control without the requirement of fluid reinfusion. With the availability of blood pumps, blood flows and dialysate flow rates can be increased, and dialyzers with higher surface areas and modified cellulosic membranes such as triacetate can be effectively used. When dialysate is run at low flow rates, fluid saturation is almost complete. When dialysate flow is increased, despite a progressive desaturation of the spent dialysate, there is an increase in clearance of small-molecular-weight solutes. In most cases, designated machines must be used to control inlet and outlet dialysate flows and to achieve the desired volume of ultrafiltrate.

A further modification of these techniques is called continuous venovenous hemodiafiltration (CVVHDF).[19] In this technique, high-flux dialyzers are used in a continuous hemodialysis circuit with continuous ultrafiltrate volume control. Because the spontaneous filtration occurring in the hollow-fiber dialyzer would be much greater than the desired fluid loss, in this condition a positive pressure is automatically applied to the dialysate compartment and the transmembrane pressure gradient is reduced significantly. This, in turn, results in a very special pressure profile inside the dialyzer. Large amounts of filtration and consequently of convective transport are maintained in the proximal part of the hemodialyzer despite a moderate net filtration. The net fluid balance is obtained because of a significant amount of backfiltration of fresh dialysate in the distal portion of the dialyzer. With this technique, diffusion and convection are conveniently combined. The system can be run in either single-pass or recirculation mode, and clearance of middle- to high-molecular-weight solutes can reach values as high as 60% of those observed for small molecules such as urea.

Continuous veno-venous hemodiafiltration (CVVHDF) (see Fig. 210-2D) is a treatment that requires a high-flux hemodiafilter and operates combining the principles of hemodialysis and hemofiltration. Dialysate is circulated in countercurrent mode to blood, and at the same time ultrafiltrate is obtained in excess of the desired fluid loss from the patient. This is totally or partially replaced with substitution fluid, in either predilution or postdilution mode. Recent modifications allow a combination of predilution and postdilution substitution, aiming at combining the advantages of both modalities. Because this therapy is supposed to combine the best aspects of diffusion and convection, optimal clearances are expected for both small- and large-molecular-weight solutes.

High-volume hemofiltration (HVHF) is a pure convective therapy that can be performed with two basic schedules: continuous HVHF or "pulsed" HVHF (PHVHF).[20,21] In the first case, the therapy is performed for 24 hours with a fluid exchange rate greater than 3 L/hr. Clearances in the range of 80 L/day can be obtained. Technical requirements for this modality especially address the increased blood flow rates and the availability of large volumes of substitution fluid. PHVHF can be performed for some hours (3 to 6) during the day, exchanging 6 to 8 L/hr, while the patient continues with standard CVVH for the rest of the day. These therapies have been shown to produce a beneficial effect on patient hemodynamics, with a significant reduction in the requirement for vasopressor drugs. The technology involved is, in most cases, borrowed from the chronic hemodialysis setting. The large volumes of fluid exchanged may render the treatment impractical. Newer methods for on-line production of substitution fluid may contribute in the future to reduce the costs and the problems of fluid supply.

Continuous plasmapheresis (CPF) and continuous plasma exchange (Pex) are techniques that are basically derived from the classic plasma therapies with the same names but are performed with lower flow rates and for extended periods of time. The rationale for these therapies is based on the attempt to remove plasma proteins and immune complexes that are considered the pathophysiological cause of the patient's disease. Because plasma is filtered across highly porous membranes, large quantities of plasma substitutes, such as fresh-frozen plasma, are required for these procedures. Single or repeated sessions can be performed in isolation or in conjunction with other blood purification techniques.[22]

Continuous plasmafiltration coupled with adsorption (CPFA) is a special technique that was recently introduced in an attempt to combine the advantages of CRRT and CPF without requiring large amounts of plasma substitutes.[23] The technique consists in two steps: (1) blood is circulated through a plasmafilter, and a pump then drives the plasmafiltrate through a cartridge containing a mixture of hydrophobic resin and uncoated charcoal; (2) the regenerated plasma is returned to the main circuit, where blood is reconstituted and eventually dialyzed. Because the patient's own plasma is used for reinfusion, there is no need for substitution fluids, and unwanted protein losses are avoided. The technique has been effective in reducing circulating levels of various cytokines and at the same time has allowed a significant reduction in vasopressor requirements in the early stages of the septic syndrome.

Continuous hemoperfusion-hemodialysis is another combination therapy which was mostly used in the past for acute intoxications.[24] The technique is based on the placement of a sorbent cartridge in series with the dialyzer, in an attempt to remove those toxins that are not removed by classic blood purification techniques. One of the major limitations imposed by this technique in the past was the poor biocompatibility of the sorbent, but newer sorbent materials are coated with biocompatible surfaces that prevent platelet trapping and clotting activation. Among the sorbent techniques, the attempt to remove circulating endotoxin with polymyxin B coated fibers should be mentioned. The cartridge contains fibers that are coated with an antibiotic (polymyxin B) with high affinity for lipopolysaccharide. The critical factor in making this therapy effective seems to be its early application, when high levels of circulating endotoxin can be detected in plasma and the systemic effects of the humoral response to lipopolysaccharide have not yet fully developed.

TECHNICAL ASPECTS

The evolution of CRRT has been accompanied by a parallel evolution in the related technology. Several machines have incorporated the heparin pump or other systems for regional heparinization and citrate anticoagulation. The most common anticoagulant remains heparin, although high blood flows and predilution techniques allow for a smooth conduction of CRRT without any anticoagulant in patients at risk. Regional heparinization and the use of citrate are mostly reserved for special situations, as is the case for low-molecular-weight heparin and prostacyclin. In recent years, catheters, blood circuit lines, and filters with heparin bound on the inner surface have been developed. However, their use is still experimental and requires further evaluation.

Dialyzers with different membranes have been created, making it possible to choose among a variety of membrane materials. Membranes with different porosity and ultrafiltration coefficients are available. There is a tendency to increase the filter surface area, because the pumped circulation can operate at higher blood flows compared to arteriovenous circuits. A series of on-line monitoring techniques are today under evaluation, including blood volume monitoring and blood temperature monitoring. Finally, a great deal of development has taken place in the operator interface of the CRRT machines. Most of these machines are equipped with large color screens and step-by-step guidelines for priming the circuit and running the treatment smoothly and effectively.

Integrated system accuracy and safety features are today a priority in CRRT equipment, to the point that a so-called third-generation machine has been released into clinical practice. Technical complications related to CRRT, potentially challenged by increased safety standards and higher dialytic dose prescriptions, are seldom observed in clinical practice, and the recent technological developments deliver the highest protection ever for patients and operators. Nonetheless, there is no solution to the unwise utilization of a near-perfect system.[25,26]

THE CONTROVERSIES

The scientific community has not yet established whether an ideal RRT strategy exists.[27,28] Studies comparing inter-mittent and continuous therapies can be misleading and, at the moment, have not delivered a definitive answer. Continuous therapies are certainly achieving extensive uptake all over the world,[9] because of their ease of use and the possibility of tailoring the management of ARF to the needs of critically ill patients. This is similar to what happens for all modern intensive care treatments (such as ventilation, antibiotic regimens, infusions of inotropes and vasopressors) that require dynamic and continuously modifiable prescriptions (i.e., ultrafiltration rates in CRRT). Hence, the presence of a wide range of therapeutic options, from totally continuous to hybrid to highly intermittent therapies, should be seen in the light of flexible prescriptions, with the possibility of changing machine settings in response to the patient's clinical progress. This opportunity is enhanced by a vast assortment of modern machines that allow great technical versatility. For example, several monitors currently used for intermittent therapies are now adapted to hybrid or semicontinuous therapies. Conversely, machines specifically dedicated to CRRT can reach elevated blood and dialytic flow rates with extreme accuracy for prolonged periods.

Finally, no consensus exists about which modality should be prescribed for critically ill patients: diffusive, convective, or other combined or more complex therapies. Again, scientific evidence is unlikely to reach adequate levels of evidence to suggest a specific standard. The key point is still a deep knowledge of blood purification mechanisms and their adaptation to clinical needs. For the same reason, a dynamically changing RRT modality during the course of the intensive care unit admission seems desirable. As a practical suggestion, CVVHDF seems to be an adequate compromise technique, with the advantages of diffusion and convection, which might maximize the combined clearance of small and larger molecules. CVVHDF appears to be an optimal technical approach also, because of the ease of operation by nursing staff even at high exchange volumes.[29]

CONCLUSION

The era of having only a few treatment modalities available for ARF (i.e., peritoneal dialysis and intermittent therapies) has well and truly passed. The development of continuous therapies has deeply modified ARF management. Nephrologists and intensive care clinicians now have technically advanced machines with multiple functions, which can tailor treatment on an individual basis. They provide simple, reliable, and efficient treatment options for a variety of different methods, such as pure diffusive or convective mode or combination modes. They can be utilized in most clinical scenarios, including cardiovascular instability in critically ill subjects, without serious limitations. Membrane technology has opened new horizons for more efficient and broader purification. Uremic toxins of variable molecular weight can now be removed. Newer modalities such as hemoperfusion technology, still under investigation, may help achieve even higher levels of blood purification. The future of RRTs looks positive. Ultimately, the ideal machine will simulate normal kidney function, and the available technology is rapidly approaching this point. An improved expertise on correct selection between intermittent and continuous therapies will certainly represent a step forward in the treatment of ARF in coming years.

Key Points

1. The mechanisms involved in renal replacement therapy are based on the principle of water and solute transport according to two fundamental principles: diffusion and convection.
2. These mechanisms can be applied in clinical practice as different techniques (intermittent, extended, or continuous renal replacement therapy) and different modalities (hemofiltration, hemodialysis, hemodiafiltration, plasmafiltration, hemoperfusion, and coupled plasmafiltration and adsorption).
3. A precise understanding of the technical and clinical implications of such therapies seems important in delivering a correct renal replacement therapy prescription.

4. No consensus exists yet on which technique or which modality should be administered to critically ill patients with acute renal failure.

Key References

4. Henderson LW: Blood purification by ultrafiltration and fluid replacement (diafiltration). ASAIO Trans 1967;17:216-221.
9. Uchino S, Kellum JA, Bellomo R, et al: for the Beginning and Ending Supportive Therapy for the Kidney (BEST Kidney) Investigators: Acute renal failure in critically ill patients: A multinational, multicenter study. JAMA 2005;294:813-818.
19. Clark WR, Ronco C: Renal replacement therapy in acute renal failure: Solute removal mechanism and dose quantification. Kidney Int 1998;53(Suppl 66):S133-S137.
23. Ronco C, Brendolan A, Lonnemann G, et al: A pilot study of coupled plasma filtration with adsorption in septic shock. Crit Care Med 2002;30:1250-1255.

See the companion Expert Consult website for the complete reference list.

CHAPTER 211

Principles of Extracorporeal Circulation

Richard A. Ward

OBJECTIVES

This chapter will:
1. Define the functions of the extracorporeal circuit.
2. Describe the components of the extracorporeal circuit that perform these functions.
3. Describe the protective systems of the extracorporeal circuit.

THERAPEUTIC FUNCTIONS OF THE EXTRACORPOREAL CIRCUIT

The extracorporeal circuit is designed to remove blood from the patient's circulation, deliver that blood to some form of blood purification device, and then return the purified blood to the patient. These tasks must be performed without damaging blood components, without losing blood to the environment, and without exposing the patient to potentially harmful contaminants from the extracorporeal circuit or the environment.

COMPONENTS OF THE EXTRACORPOREAL CIRCUIT

A typical extracorporeal circuit is shown in Figure 211-1. The three basic blood-contacting elements of the circuit are a means of accessing the circulation, a blood tubing set, and a blood purification device.

Blood Access

Most patients receiving renal replacement therapy (RRT) in an acute setting do not have an established blood access route. In these patients, access to the circulation is usually provided by a catheter placed in an appropriate blood vessel. A single catheter with two lumens may be used for both withdrawal and return of the blood. Less commonly, two single-lumen catheters may be used. If the patient does have an established blood access, such as a fistula or synthetic graft, 15- to 16-gauge needles may be used for blood access. More details on blood access are given in Chapter 253.

Blood Tubing

Blood is conveyed to and from the blood purification device by a disposable blood tubing set. The blood tubing set consists of two segments: an arterial segment that connects the outflow from the blood access to the inlet port of the blood purification device, and a venous segment that connects the outlet port of the blood purification device to the return blood access. Blood tubing sets are usually manufactured from plasticized polyvinylchloride and may be sterilized with ethylene oxide or gamma irradiation. Conventional hemodialysis machines typically use generic blood tubing sets, whereas some systems specifically designed for continuous RRT applications combine the blood tubing set and the blood purification device in a system-specific integrated unit. Blood tubing sets typically include side arms for the administration of fluids and anticoagulants, as well as chambers for capturing any air

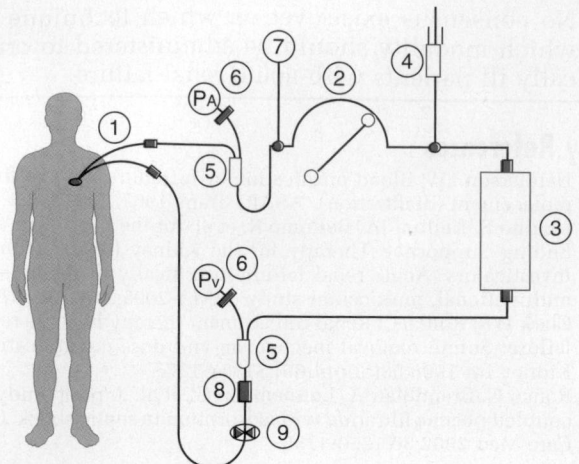

FIGURE 211-1. Typical extracorporeal circuit for hemodialysis. Convective therapies, such as hemodiafiltration and hemofiltration, use a similar circuit with the addition of lines for the infusion of replacement solution before or after the hemodialyzer or hemofilter. The major components of the extracorporeal circuit are as follows: 1, a blood access device (shown as a central venous catheter); 2, a blood pump; 3, a blood purification device (hemodialyzer, hemofilter, or sorbent cartridge); 4, an anticoagulant infusion pump; 5, air-capture chambers; 6, pressure-monitoring systems (shown as a pressure transducer isolated from the blood path by a pressure-transmitting sterile barrier); 7, a side line for priming the extracorporeal circuit with saline; 8, an ultrasonic air and foam detector; and 9, a line clamp.

that may inadvertently enter the blood circuit and for pressure monitoring.

Blood Pump

The pressure at the inlet to the catheter or needle used to withdraw blood from the patient into the extracorporeal circuit is usually insufficient to provide the desired flow rate of blood through the extracorporeal circuit. Therefore, almost all extracorporeal circuits for RRT use a blood pump to provide a controlled flow of blood to the blood purification device. These blood pumps are usually peristaltic pumps, also known as roller pumps, although one recently introduced system uses a diaphragm pump. A typical peristaltic pump uses a rotating arm fitted with diametrically opposed spring-loaded rollers that occlude the blood tubing as it enters the pump and force the blood in the section of tubing before the point of occlusion to the outlet of the pump as the arm rotates. The blood flow rate displayed by the machine is calculated from the geometry of the pump, the inner diameter of the blood tubing, and the rotational speed of the pump.

Blood Purification Device

Most blood purification devices used in critical care nephrology are hollow-fiber membrane devices that allow exchange of solutes using diffusion and/or convection and removal of water by ultrafiltration. The relative importance of diffusion versus convection depends on the therapy selected. Standard hemodialysis relies mostly on diffusive solute removal, particularly for small waste metabolites, electrolytes, and non-protein-bound drugs, whereas hemofiltration achieves the same goals through convection. Still other therapies, such as hemodiafiltra-

tion, rely on a combination of diffusion and convection. More details on these processes are given in other chapters. Other blood purification devices incorporate, or consist entirely of, a cartridge containing various types of adsorption resin (see Section 20).

Ancillary Components

Extracorporeal circuits include various other components, depending, in part, on the nature of the therapy being performed. All extracorporeal circuits activate coagulation pathways through contact of blood components with foreign surfaces and any air within the circuit, together with the generation of shear stresses. For this reason, allowance is usually made for infusion of an anticoagulant into the extracorporeal circuit, whether or not an anticoagulant is actually infused during the treatment. Common anticoagulants used for extracorporeal circulation in critical care RRT are heparin and citrate (see Chapters 244 and 277). Heparin may be administered by intermittent bolus or by continuous infusion into the arterial segment of the extracorporeal circuit, using a syringe pump that is a standard feature of most machines used for RRT. Two infusion pumps may be necessary for citrate anticoagulation, depending on the protocol followed; one pump is used to infuse citrate into the arterial segment of the extracorporeal circuit, and a second pump is used to infuse calcium into the venous segment of the circuit. The extracorporeal circuit may also allow for infusion of the sterile replacement solutions required for therapies involving controlled convective transport, such as hemofiltration and hemodiafiltration. In critical care applications, these replacement solutions are usually provided in prepackaged plastic bags and are infused into the arterial segment (predilution) or into the venous segment (postdilution) of the extracorporeal circuit, using a peristaltic pump.

PRESSURE PROFILES IN THE EXTRACORPOREAL CIRCUIT AND THEIR EFFECTS ON PERFORMANCE

Because the pressure at the inlet to the catheter or needle used to withdraw blood from the patient is usually only 10 to 40 mm Hg and may vary during the course of a treatment, a blood pump is needed to generate the pressure required to achieve the desired flow of blood through the extracorporeal circuit. The extracorporeal blood circuit can be envisioned as a series of resistances to flow; the blood pump creates a pressure profile along the length of the extracorporeal circuit that is dependent on the flow rate, the geometry of the circuit, and the properties of the blood.[1] A typical pressure profile is shown schematically in Figure 211-2. The change in pressure along each segment of the extracorporeal circuit is governed by the laws of fluid mechanics, including the Hagen-Poiseuille law and the Bernoulli equation.[1] These laws relate change in pressure to the dimensions of the flow path, the blood flow rate, and physical properties of the blood, such as viscosity and density. In general, the change in pressure along a segment of the extracorporeal circuit increases as the flow rate and viscosity increase and as the diameter of the flow path decreases. Viscosity increases exponentially with hematocrit over the range of values encountered in extracorporeal circulation for RRT[2] and, therefore, may change markedly along the length of the extracorporeal circuit and

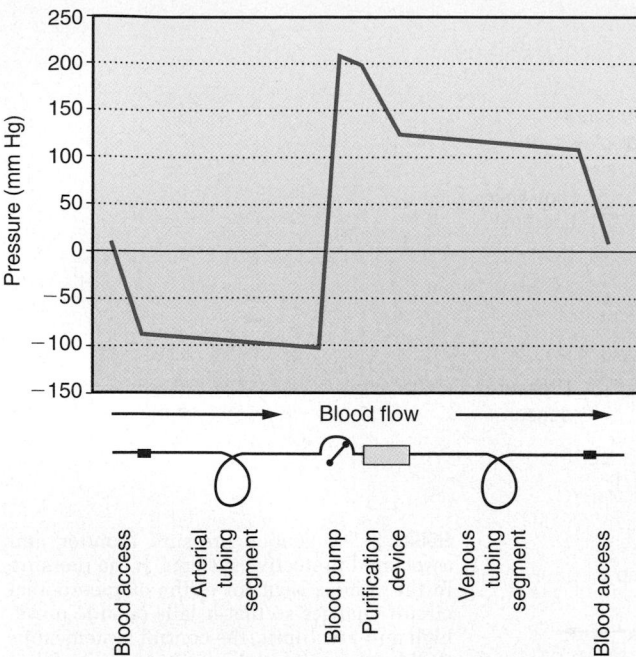

FIGURE 211-2. Typical pressure profile along the extracorporeal circuit. For a given treatment, actual pressures will depend on the nature of the circuit used and the operational parameters. In particular, pressures are affected by the blood flow rate, the patient's hematocrit, and the type and internal diameter of the blood access devices.

with time of treatment, depending on ultrafiltration and fluid infusion.

Although the prescribed operating parameters, such as blood flow rate and ultrafiltration rate, establish the pressures in the extracorporeal circuit, these pressures may, in turn, affect the operating parameters. For example, as the pressure in the tubing at the inlet to the blood pump decreases, the ability of the tubing to expand back to a circular cross-section at the end of each stroke of the pump decreases. This failure to undergo complete elastic recoil decreases the cross-sectional area of the tubing, resulting in a lower stroke volume and a consequent decrease in actual blood flow rate.[3] This phenomenon is dependent on the elasticity of the blood pump segment of the tubing[4] and is usually most evident at high blood flow rates and with the use of catheters for blood access.[5] However, even when a graft or fistula is used for blood access, low pressures may be generated at the inlet to the blood pump with relatively low blood flow rates if small-diameter needles are used in combination with a high hematocrit. Some machines measure the pressure at the inlet to the blood pump and use an algorithm to calculate and display a corrected blood flow rate.

SAFETY FEATURES OF THE EXTRACORPOREAL CIRCUIT, PROTECTIVE SYSTEMS, AND THEIR LIMITATIONS

Extracorporeal circuits should be designed to minimize the risk of adverse events during extracorporeal circulation. The incorporation of active protective systems should

form part of this design process. In general, a protective system independently monitors some operational parameter of a device and causes the device to assume a safe state if the operational parameter enters a hazardous range. The major hazards associated with the extracorporeal circuit are loss of blood to the environment after a break in the integrity of the extracorporeal circuit, loss of blood and therapeutic efficacy resulting from clotting in the extracorporeal circuit, and air embolism.

System Integrity

To avoid accidental separations, the extracorporeal circuit should be designed so that all connections between the blood access, the tubing set, the blood purification device, and any other ancillary tubing are made with locking connectors. Although the use of locking connectors reduces the likelihood of inadvertent line separation, this protection is not absolute. Locking connectors of the Luer-Lok type have been observed to separate via dissipation of torsional energy stored in the lines when a connection is made with one of the lines immobilized close to the point of connection (e.g., a catheter immobilized against the skin with an adhesive dressing) or when the surfaces of the connector are inadvertently lubricated. For this reason, connections in the extracorporeal circuit should remain visible throughout a treatment, and consideration should be given to external stabilization of the connection, particularly for long-duration therapies, during which staff surveillance may be intermittent. The use of extracorporeal circuits in which the blood tubing and blood purification device are integrated in a single unit may improve safety by eliminating unnecessary tubing and reducing the number of connections between components.

Pressure Monitoring

In conventional hemodialysis systems, pressure is usually monitored at two points in the extracorporeal circuit: in the arterial segment between the blood access and the inlet to the blood pump, and in the venous segment between the blood purification device and the blood access. Systems that are used for convective therapies also monitor pressure between the blood pump and the blood purification device. Pressure in the blood tubing is measured via an air-capture chamber connected to a pressure transducer or by use of a load cell that senses expansion or contraction of the walls of a pressure pillow in the blood tubing. When pressure is sensed with an air-capture chamber, a pressure-transmitting sterile barrier is used to isolate the blood pathway from the pressure transducer in the machine, to prevent contamination of the transducer and inadvertent transmission of infectious agents from patient to patient.[6]

Monitoring of pressure in the extracorporeal circuit serves as the basis for protective systems to guard against blood line separation or occlusion. High and low alarm limits are set about the monitored pressure. The alarm limits are usually set automatically by the machine at some predetermined amount above and below the measured operating pressure at the start of the treatment; however, some machines allow the operator to adjust the magnitude of these preset high and low alarm offsets. The difference between the low- and high-pressure limits and the operating pressure should be small enough to detect a hazardous condition but not so small as to cause frequent nuisance alarms when small excursions in operating pressure occur (e.g., when the patient moves).

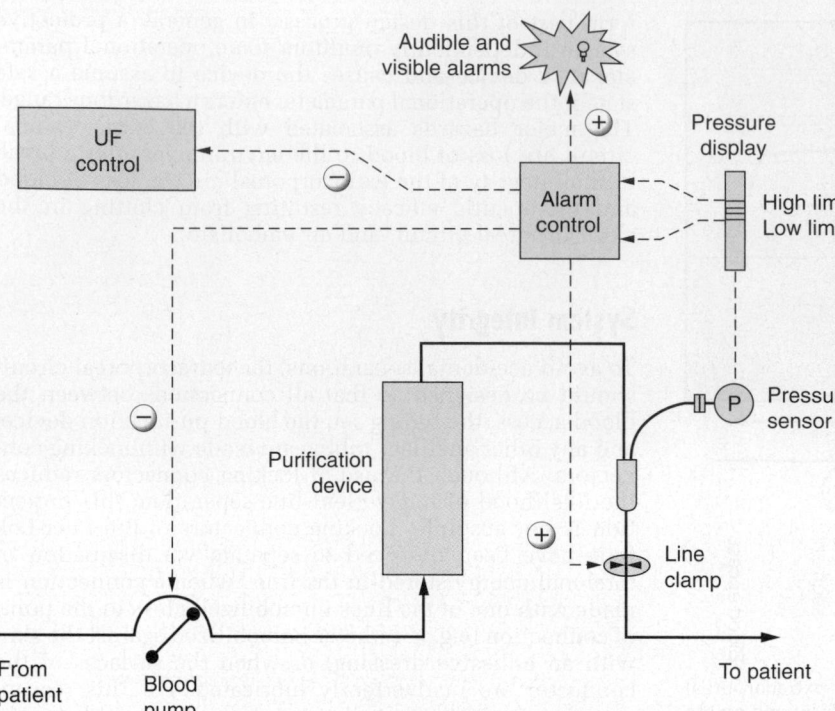

FIGURE 211-3. Venous pressure monitor and associated protective systems. If the pressure in the venous segment of the extracorporeal circuit changes so that it falls outside preset high and low limits, the control system stops the blood pump (−), minimizes net ultrafiltration (−), closes the line clamp (+), and activates audible and visible alarms (+).

Venous Pressure Monitors

The components of a protective system based on monitoring pressure in the venous segment of the blood tubing are shown schematically in Figure 211-3. If the pressure decreases below the lower alarm limit (e.g., line separation) or increases above the upper limit (e.g., line occlusion), audible and visible alarms are activated, the blood pump is stopped, the line clamp is activated, and the fluid balancing system is set to a neutral condition so that there is neither volume expansion nor volume contraction in the extracorporeal circuit.

Arterial Pressure Monitors

Because the pressure in the arterial blood tubing proximal to the blood pump is almost always less than atmospheric pressure, air can be drawn into the blood tubing if any connection in this segment of the tubing does not form a tight seal or if the arterial needle slips out of the access. Any air drawn into the system has the potential to promote clotting in the blood purification device or to result in an air embolus if the air and foam detector fail simultaneously. Monitoring of the pressure in the arterial segment of the blood tubing proximal to the blood pump serves as the basis for a protective system to guard against these hazards. Because the pressure in this segment of the blood tubing is less than atmospheric, a break in system integrity will lead to an increase in pressure, so that the upper alarm limit is exceeded. The same protective system also guards against occlusion of the blood tubing proximal to the pressure monitor, which can occur if the blood tubing becomes kinked or there is a problem with the blood access. In this instance, the pressure will decrease and breach the lower alarm limit. If either alarm limit is breached, the protective system alerts the operator and places the machine in a safe mode, as described previously for the venous pressure monitor.

Monitoring of pressure between the blood pump and the inlet to the blood purification device can alert the user to clotting or mechanical occlusion downstream of the pressure monitor. An increase in the post-pump arterial pressure, together with an increase in the difference between the post-pump arterial pressure and the pressure in the venous segment of the blood tubing, usually signifies clotting in the blood purification device. An increase in the post-pump arterial pressure with little or no change in the difference between the post-pump arterial pressure and the pressure in the venous segment of the blood tubing usually signifies clotting of the blood access device or occlusion of the tubing beyond the venous pressure monitor. Post-pump arterial pressure may also be used as one input to a system monitoring the transmembrane pressure, particularly in convective therapies such as hemofiltration and hemodiafiltration.

Limitations of Pressure Monitors

Pressure-based protective systems are not perfect. Depending on the pressures in the extracorporeal circuit, disconnection of the blood tubing from the blood access device or dislodgment of a blood access needle may not result in a pressure change sufficient to activate the protective system. This situation is most likely to occur at low blood flow rates when the pressure drop across the blood access device is small, as described earlier, or when the alarm limits are spread widely apart. For this reason, connections to the blood access device, as well as to the access site itself, should always be kept visible, and the low pressure alarm limit should be set as close to the operating pressure as possible. Protective systems based on monitoring of the pressure in the venous segment of the blood tubing also may not detect occlusion of the tubing between the blood pump and the blood purification device. Partial occlusion of this line has been reported to cause significant hemolysis because of the high shear rates generated by narrowing of the tubing lumen at the point of partial occlusion.[7] Integrated tubing sets help avoid this hazard. If an integrated tubing set is not used, the tubing should be positioned carefully using the line clips on the face of the machine.

Prevention of Air Embolism

Separation of the venous segment of the tubing set from the blood access device will lead to blood loss, but separation of the arterial segment from the blood access device will cause air to be drawn into the extracorporeal circuit and pumped into the patient. The protective system against this hazard is based on use of an ultrasonic sensor to detect air or foam in the venous segment of the blood tubing. In conventional hemodialysis machines and in some machines designed for continuous RRT, the air and foam detector is located at the air-capture chamber that is used to measure the pressure in the venous segment of the tubing set. In other machines, the air and foam detector is independent of the air-gap chamber. If air or foam is detected, audible and visible alarms are activated, the blood pump is stopped, the fluid balancing system is set to a neutral condition so that there is neither volume expansion nor volume contraction in the extracorporeal circuit, and the blood tubing is clamped downstream of the air and foam detector. Some blood tubing sets incorporate a sample port downstream of the air and foam detector. In addition to sample withdrawal, that port can be used for administration of medications. However, that port should not be used for pumped infusion of fluids, because any air inadvertently administered through the port will not be detected by the air and foam detector.

Key References

1. Polaschegg HD: Pressure and flow in the extracorporeal circuit. Clin Nephrol 2000;53(Suppl 1):S50-S55.
3. Depner TA, Rizwan S, Stasi TA: Pressure effects on roller pump blood flow during hemodialysis. ASAIO Trans 1990;31:M456-M459.
4. Ahmed J, Besarab A, Lubkowski T, Frinak S: Effect of differing blood lines on delivered blood flow during hemodialysis. Am J Kidney Dis 2004;44:498-508.
6. Delarocque-Astagneau E, Baffoy N, Thiers V, et al: Outbreak of hepatitis C virus infection in a hemodialysis unit: Potential transmission by the hemodialysis machine? Infect Control Hosp Epidemiol 2002;23:328-334.
7. Sweet SJ, McCarthy S, Steingart R, Callahan T: Hemolytic reactions mechanically induced by kinked hemodialysis lines. Am J Kidney Dis 1996;27:262-266.

See the companion Expert Consult website for the complete reference list.

CHAPTER 212

Membranes and Filters for Use in Acute Renal Failure

Nicholas A. Hoenich and Claudio Ronco

OBJECTIVES

This chapter will:
1. Describe the fundamentals of solute and fluid transport in therapies used for the treatment of acute renal failure.
2. Review the factors influencing solute and fluid transport in clinical practice.

Support for acute renal insufficiency relies on the use of various dialysis methods whose origin may be traced to methods used in the treatment of chronic renal disease or to the seminal work of Kramer.[1] Methods of treatment may be intermittent or continuous and may include the use of a membrane separation device or filter to facilitate solute and fluid removal from the patient by diffusion, convection, or a combination of both. In this chapter, the physical properties and functional performance of devices and membranes are discussed.

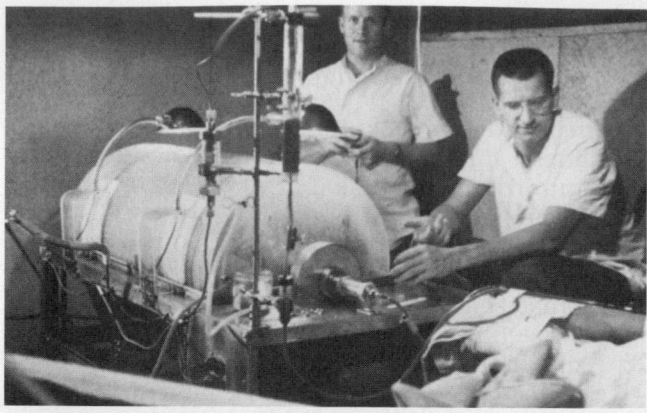

FIGURE 212-1. Early (c. 1950) treatment of acute renal failure using the Kolff-Brigham dialysis system.

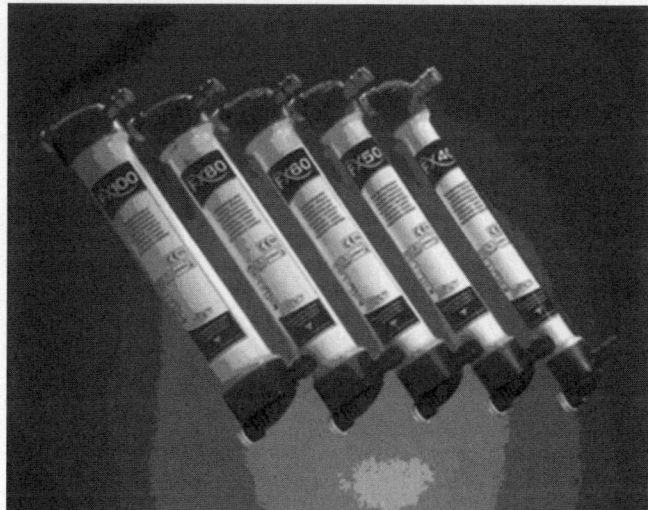

FIGURE 212-2. A series of modern hollow-fiber hemodialyzers of differing surface area suitable for use in the treatment of both chronic and acute renal failure. The devices shown utilize fibers with a three-dimensional microwave structure incorporated into a specifically designed housing to provide optimized flow distributions in both the blood pathway and the dialysate pathway. (Photograph courtesy of Fresenius Medical Care, Bad Homburg, Germany.)

DEVICES AND MEMBRANES

Devices

The early treatments of acute renal failure (ARF) relied on the use of hemodialysis systems; initially, devices in which the membrane in the form of a tube was made from unmodified cellulose wound around a rotating drum were used (Fig. 212-1). Today, treatment is undertaken with specially designed equipment used in conjunction with either a hollow-fiber device or, less commonly, a parallel-plate device (Figs. 212-2 and 212-3). In both types, the blood flows on one side of the membrane (blood pathway). In diffusive and combination techniques, dialysis fluid flows on the outer side of the membrane, and the composition of this fluid can be varied to achieve specific clinical goals, such as correction of electrolyte imbalances or correction of acidemia. When devices are used without a fluid

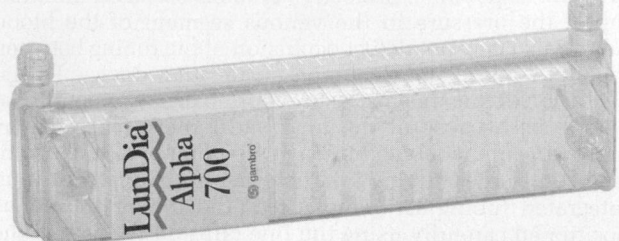

FIGURE 212-3. A modern, multiple-pathway, flat-plate hemodialyzer. (Photograph courtesy of Gambro, Lund, Sweden.)

in the dialysate pathway, they are generally referred to as hemofilters.

Membrane Materials

A variety of membranes are available for clinical use (Fig. 212-4). Membranes may be classified according to their chemical structure, with further subclassifications based on hydraulic permeability or ultrafiltration characteristics. In terms of chemical structure, one type of membrane comprises unmodified cellulose membranes (e.g., cuprophan) and modified cellulose membranes in which the bioreactive hydroxyl (-OH) groups have been reduced, either by substitution (e.g., cellulose acetate) or by the bonding of synthetic materials to the cellulose (e.g., polyethylene glycol). The most common membrane type used today, however, is the family of membranes manufactured entirely from synthetic materials. On their own, the base materials used are hydrophobic; to permit their clinical use, they are blended with a hydrophilic agent such as polyvinylpyrrolidone (PVP). The amount of blending, together with subsequent phase inversion used to manufacture the membrane, are commercially sensitive determinants of the membrane structure. In general, synthetic membranes, in contrast to those manufactured from cellulose, have an asymmetrical structure. A typical structure (Fig. 212-5) is characterized by a skin on the blood-contacting surface supported by a thicker spongy region, with interstices that cover a wide size range and with a structure ranging from open- to closed-cell foam, as determined by the manufacturing process and the polymer composition.

Within the synthetic group of membranes, the most widely available variant is that based on polysulfone. Although there is a tendency to refer to this material as a single group, chemical differences exist between polysulfone membranes.[2] A more appropriate grouping based on their chemistry has been suggested. With this approach, membranes containing isopropyliden groups are classed as polysulfone, whereas materials that do not contain isopropyliden are classed as polyarylethersulfones or polyethersulfones.[3]

DEVICE PERFORMANCE

Manufacturers characterize device performance using methodology detailed in international standards (European Committee for Standardization [CEN] EN 1283, haemodialyser, haemodiafilters, haemofilters, haemoconcentrators, and their extracorporeal circuits, or International Standard Organization [ISO] 8637: 2004 ardiovascular implants and artificial organs—haemodialysors, haemodiafilters,

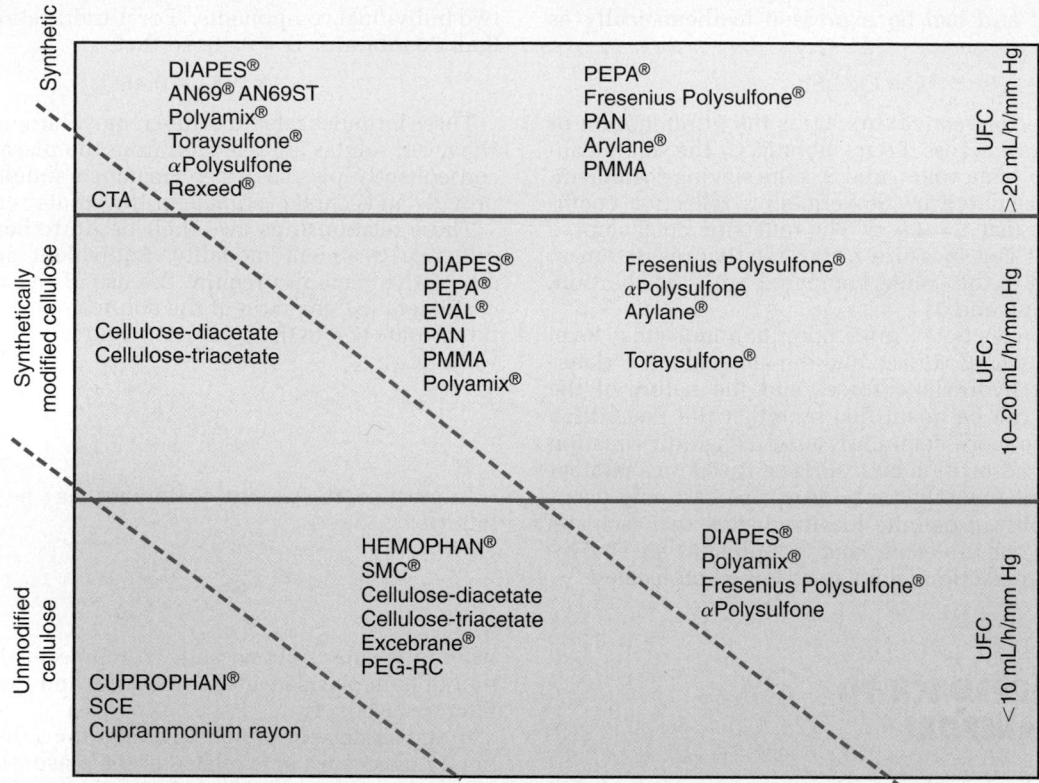

FIGURE 212-4. The clinically used range of membranes. The horizontal lines subdivide the membranes according to their ultrafiltration coefficients (UFC), and the diagonal lines subdivide them according to chemical composition.

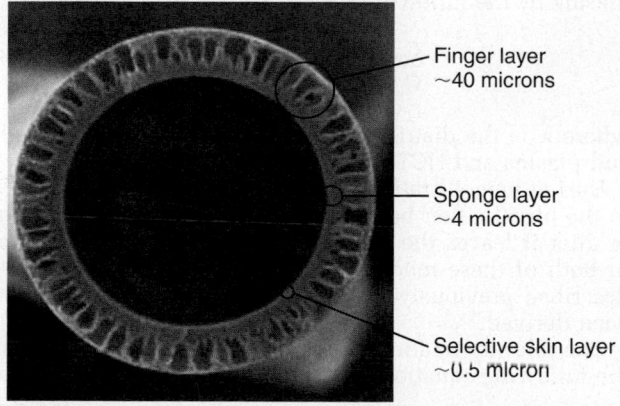

FIGURE 212-5. Synthetic membrane structure.

haemofilters, and haemoconcentrators), and this forms the basis of the product insert for the device. Such methods characterize the performance of the device in the laboratory and focus on the solute transport and fluid removal characteristics of the device, parameters of importance in the clinical setting. In addition, data relating to the pressure losses in the blood and dialysate pathways are also provided. It is not the intention to catalog performance but to provide the user with an appropriate background to understand the product specification sheet and enable measurements to be made during the clinical use of the device.

MECHANISMS OF SOLUTE TRANSPORT

Solute transport across membranes occurs by two different mechanisms: diffusion and convection. In addition, there is also an interaction between the solutes and the membrane surface, leading to their adsorption to the membrane surface.

The relative contributions to total solute transport from diffusion and from convection are determined by the treatment modality. For example, in hemodialysis the dominant mode of solute transport is diffusive, whereas in convective techniques such as ultrafiltration and hemofiltration the dominant solute mechanism is convective. Adsorption occurs with all treatment modalities and can be considered either as a negative attribute (membrane fouling leading to a reduction in transmembrane transport) or a positive attribute (adherence of endotoxins to the membrane).[4]

Mathematically, diffusive solute transport across the membrane is governed by Fick's law and can be expressed as follows:

$$J_D = -DA\frac{dC}{dx}$$

where J_D is the diffusive flux, D is the solute diffusion coefficient, A is the area available for transport, and dC/dx is the concentration gradient.

Convective solute transport is movement of solute across the membrane that results from the bulk movement of the solvent and can be expressed mathematically as follows:

$$J_C = Q_F C_B S$$

where J_C is the convective flux, Q_F is the ultrafiltration or fluid transfer rate across the membrane, C_B the solute concentration in plasma water, and S is the sieving coefficient, a parameter regulated by Stavermann's reflection coefficient (σ), such that $S = 1 - \sigma$. The reflection coefficient, a parameter that is a measure of the relative restriction of the membrane to the solute compared with the solution, varies between 0 and 1.

Adsorption reflects the interaction at a molecular level between the material surface and the molecule; it is determined by the hydrostatic forces and the nature of the compound. It can be quantified by either the Freundlich equation or the more commonly used Langmuir equation for monolayer adsorption on a surface, based on a number of assumptions—namely, that adsorption can only occur at a fixed number of definite localized sites, that each site can hold only one molecule, and that all sites are equivalent with no interaction between adsorbed molecules.

CLINICAL APPROACH TO SOLUTE TRANSPORT

The expressions described in the previous section define the physical phenomena governing solute transport across the membrane and, as such, are of limited interest or use in the clinical setting. Solute transport in the clinical setting is frequently defined as clearance (K), a term analogous to the clearance concept of the human kidney. It focuses on solute removal by the device and can be defined as "the amount of solute removed from the blood per unit of time, divided by incoming blood concentration (i.e., the volumetric rate of removal by the device)," expressed mathematically as follows:

$$K = Q \frac{(C_i - C_o)}{C_i}$$

where Q is the volumetric flow rate, C the concentration, and the subscripts i and o represent inlet and outlet, respectively.

Because the blood flow entering and that leaving the device are not identical (due to fluid removal during its passage through the device), it is necessary to modify this relationship, so that it becomes

$$K = Q_{Bin} \frac{(C_i - C_o)}{C_i} + Q_F \frac{C_o}{C_i} \quad \text{because } Q_{Bin} - Q_{Bout} = Q_F$$

It should be noted that this correction does not provide a quantification of solute transport via convection but merely corrects the diffusion equation for differences in the flow rates entering and leaving the device. For the quantification of clearance in the presence of convection it is possible to present clearance as

$$K = K_0 + Tr Q_F$$

where K_0 is a pure diffusive clearance (no ultrafiltration, equivalent to $Q_{Bin} = Q_{Bout}$), Q_F is the ultrafiltration flow rate, and Tr is the transmittance coefficient.

Experimental studies have indicated, however, that overall solute removal is generally less than the sum of the two individual components.[5] For ultrafiltration rates lower than 70 mL/min, Tr = 0.46, so that

$$K = K_0 + 0.46 Q_F$$

These formulas refer to solute removal from whole blood. However, solutes are removed from the plasma water, and consequently plasma water clearance should be used to provide an accurate estimate of the solute removal.

These relationships owe their origin to hemodialysis, a diffusive treatment modality. Equivalent approaches to convective therapies require the use of the solute sieving coefficient (S), the ratio of the solute concentration in the ultrafiltrate (C_F) to the solute concentration of bulk plasma water (C_w):

$$S = \frac{C_F}{C_W}$$

In practice, the sieving coefficient may be calculated as follows:

$$S = \frac{2 C_F}{C_{wi} + C_{wo}}$$

where the subscripts wi and wo represent the concentration of bulk plasma water at the inlet and the outlet of the filter, respectively.

In the absence of protein binding, the solute concentration in plasma water is related to the plasma concentration as follows:

$$\frac{C_P}{C_w} = 1 - \phi$$

where ϕ is the volume fraction of hydrated proteins and is 0.0107 of the concentration in plasma (C_P).

The concentration in the blood is related to that in plasma by the following formula:

$$\frac{C_P}{C_w} = 1 - HCT + \lambda HCT$$

where λ is the distribution coefficient between red cells and plasma and HCT is the hematocrit.

During hemofiltration, the diluting fluid may be added to the blood either before it enters the filter (predilution) or after it leaves the filter (postdilution). Solute removal in both of these modalities is more complex than those described previously, but mathematical expressions have been derived.[6]

The relevant relationships for predilution are shown by the following equation:

$$K = Q_B \left(\frac{1 - HCT}{1 - HCT + HCT\,\lambda} \right)$$
$$\left[1 - \left\{ \frac{(1-\phi)(1-HCT) + \dfrac{Q_B}{Q_D}\left(1 - \dfrac{Q_F}{Q_D}\right)}{(1-\phi)(1-HCT) + \dfrac{Q_D}{Q_B}} \right\}^S \right]$$

and those for postdilution as follows:

$$K = Q_B \left(\frac{1 - HCT}{1 - HCT + HCT\,\lambda} \right) \left[1 - \left\{ \frac{(1-\phi)(1-HCT) + \dfrac{Q_F}{Q_D}}{(1-\phi)(1-HCT)} \right\}^S \right]$$

where Q_F is the filtrate addition rate and S is the solute sieving coefficient.

In continuous therapies involving substitution, the whole blood clearance is equivalent to the plasma clearance, such that:

$$K = \frac{Q_F C_F}{C_{Bin}}$$

When the effects of the exclusion volume of the hydrated proteins are neglected, this relationship simplifies to

$$K_B = Q_F S$$

In conventional hemodialysis (i.e., in treatments using a blood flow rate >200 mL/min and a dialysis fluid flow rate ≥500 mL/min), clearance increases with increasing blood and/or dialysis fluid flow rate and with a parameter, koA, which characterizes the mass transfer across the membrane. This parameter is the product of the area (A) and the overall mass transfer coefficient (ko). The inverse of the overall mass transfer resistance (R_T) represents the sum of three resistances to transport—in the blood pathway (R_B), in the membrane (R_M), and in the dialysis fluid pathway (R_D):

$$R_T = R_B + R_M + R_D$$

This expression can be thought of as the barrier to solute transport in the fluid film layers adjacent to the membrane surface in each compartment and the membrane. The fluid dynamic conditions within the blood and dialysis fluid pathways determine R_B and R_D, whereas R_M is a function of membrane thickness and solute diffusive permeability.

Mathematically, it is possible to relate the mass transfer coefficient of a dialyzer (koA) to the clearance (K) by the following relationship:

$$K = Q_B \left\{ \frac{\exp\left[\frac{koA}{Q_B}\left(1 - \frac{Q_B}{Q_D}\right)\right] - 1}{\exp\left[\frac{koA}{Q_B}\left(1 - \frac{Q_B}{Q_D}\right)\right] - \frac{Q_B}{Q_D}} \right\}$$

where Q_B and Q_D represent the blood and dialysis fluid flow rates.

A number of caveats to the use of this approach apply: it does not take into consideration the convective mass transport, and it assumes that the value of koA is constant throughout varying operating conditions. A number of experimental studies have indicated that this assumption may not be true, because increasing the dialysate flow rate results in an alteration of the koA characteristics resulting from better flow distribution within the fiber bundle for hollow-fiber dialyzers.[7,8]

Combined convective and diffusive therapies used in the treatment of ARF generally use lower dialysate flow rates than those used in the treatment of chronic kidney disease, and the dependence of dialyzer clearances and mass transfer-area coefficients for small solutes at low flow rates has not received extensive study. In a recent publication by Leypoldt and associates, however, the in vitro dialyzer clearances for urea and creatinine at dialysate flow rates of 40, 80, 120, 160, and 200 mL/min and ultrafiltration flow rates of 0, 1, and 2 L/hr, were analyzed. The results indicated that mass transfer-area coefficients at low dialysate flow rates for all dialyzers tested were substantially lower than those reported under conventional conditions.[9]

CLINICAL FACTORS INFLUENCING SOLUTE TRANSPORT PERFORMANCE

Flow Rates

Solute transport during extracorporeal treatments is a function of the blood flow and dialysate flow rates (Fig. 212-6). In contrast to conventional hemodialysis, the blood flow rates are in the lower range of those used for the treatment of chronic renal failure (approximately 200 mL/min), but the dialysate fluid flows are substantially reduced and range between 10 and 40 mL/min. This means that the dialysis fluid leaving filter will be 100% saturated with easily diffusible solutes, and the clearance will be equal to the dialysate flow rate.

Treatment Duration

Treatment duration for ARF is longer than that used for the treatment of chronic renal disease. During such extended use, membrane fouling and thrombus generation can substantially reduce solute transport. Interruptions during treatment can additionally cause clinically significant therapy downtime, leading to a discrepancy between prescription and delivery.[10,11]

FLUID REMOVAL

Fluid removal across the membrane during treatment is governed by the presence of a pressure gradient and the plasma oncotic pressure. Mathematically, this can be expressed in terms of the membrane permeability, the membrane area, and the pressure gradient:

$$Q_F = L_h A [P]$$
$$Q_F = L_h A \left[\frac{P_{Bin} + P_{Bout}}{2} + \frac{P_{Din} + P_{Dout}}{2} - P_{osm} \right]$$

where the product of hydraulic permeability (L_h) and area (A) is the ultrafiltration coefficient. With clinical use of a device, particularly over an extended period of time, this relationship will be nonlinear due to protein and fibrin deposition on the membrane surface (Fig. 212-7).

The dependence of ultrafiltration on the fluid dynamic conditions within devices is complex and has not been studied extensively. Its role is particularly important in hemofilters, where the filtration flux is dependent on the shear rate or the velocity gradient at the blood membrane interface, which in turn are influenced by the concentration of red blood cells.

PRESSURE DROPS AND FLOW RESISTANCES

The relationship between flow and pressure in a tube is governed by the Hagen-Poiseuille law, which, in the context of a hollow-fiber blood pathway, can be expressed as follows:

$$\Delta P = \frac{128 \mu L}{\pi N d_i^4} Q_B$$

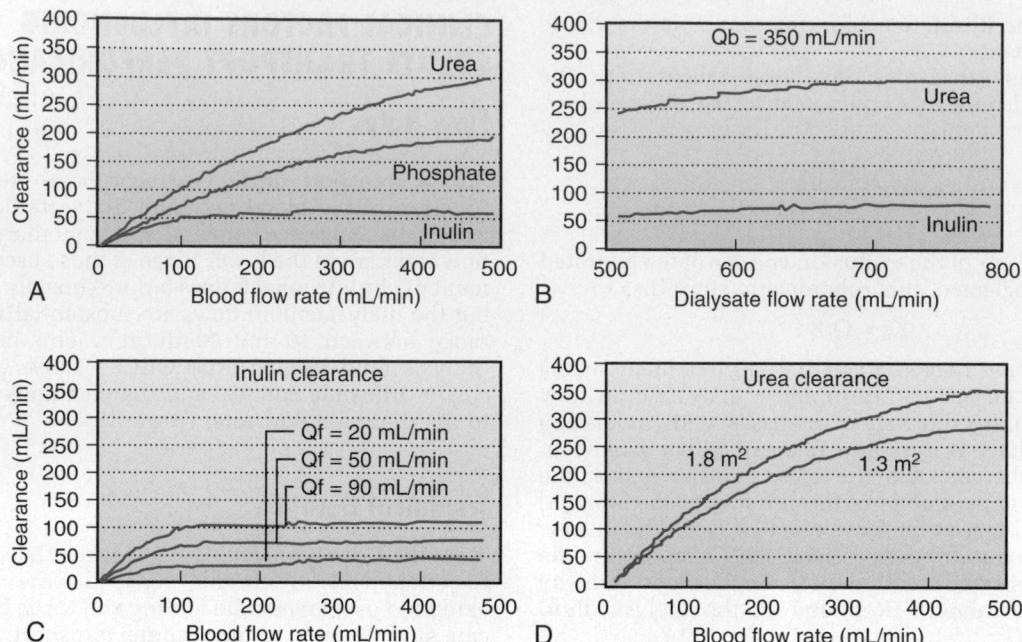

FIGURE 212-6. The influence of operating parameters on clearance characteristics. **A,** Influence of blood flow rate (Qb) at a constant dialysate flow rate on the clearance of small and large molecules. **B,** Influence of varying the dialysis fluid flow rate on the clearance of small and large molecules. Qf, ultrafiltration flow rate. **C,** Influence of flux on the clearance of large molecules. **D,** Influence of surface area on the clearance of small molecules.

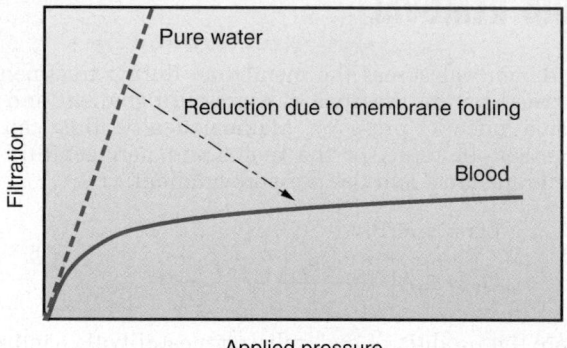

FIGURE 212-7. The influence of fluid composition on filtration.

and for a parallel-plate design device in which the ratio of blood pathway height to width is large, flow resistance is shown by

$$\Delta P = \frac{12\mu L}{Wh_B^3 N} Q_B$$

where μ is the blood viscosity, N is the number of fibers or layers for plate devices, L is the length, W is the width of the layers in plate devices, d_i is the internal diameter of the fibers, and h_B is the blood film thickness.

Early variants of continuous therapies relied on the patient's heart to provide the driving force for the flow in the extracorporeal circuit. To minimize the pressure drop in the filter, such devices were much shorter than those used today.

These relationships are critically dependent on the blood pathway dimensions. For example, in the case of a hollow fiber, the pressure is dependent on the fourth power of the fiber diameter. In practical terms, this means that a 10% variation in fiber diameter will result in a 46% variation in flow through the fibers.

These relationships assume that the blood viscosity is constant, but blood is a non-Newtonian fluid in which the viscosity is dependent on the shear rate. Shear rate is dependent on flow through the device as well as the ultrafiltration rate, and, for accuracy, more complex mathematical relationships, determined by the nonparabolic flow profile for non-Newtonian fluids, should be used.

The equations governing dialysate pathway resistance and flow rate are comparable to those shown for the blood pathway and for hollow-fiber devices; the flow resistance will be governed not only by the pathway dimensions but also by the fiber packing density.

OPTIMIZATION OF PERFORMANCE

Filtration

As blood flows into the fibers, water is removed by ultrafiltration. As a consequence, the protein concentration increases and so does the oncotic pressure, resulting in an axial variation of both hydraulic and oncotic pressures. At low blood flow rates, the local transmembrane pressure approaches the value of the plasma oncotic pressure, so that the net driving force for fluid removal approaches zero. This means that, under these conditions referred to as filtration pressure equilibrium, fluid removal or ultrafiltration is limited to the inlet end of the filter.[12] This phenomenon can be reduced or avoided by increasing the blood flow and reducing the filtration rates. Alternately, modification of the fiber geometry by adjustment of either the length of the fibers or their internal diameter may be used.[13]

Solute Transport

The primary determinants of solute transport are the flow rates in the blood and the dialysate pathways of the device. The manipulation of operating conditions involving the dialysate inflow rate, the ultrafiltration rate, and the substitution fluid replacement rate are used to achieve desired clearances. For the diffusion-based therapies, dialysate saturation (i.e., the concentration in the dialysis fluid) exiting the system approximates the inflowing plasma water urea nitrogen, simplifying such manipulations.

Solute clearance is also influenced by the presence of an uneven flow or maldistribution of flow in the blood pathway. Such maldistribution can occur for a variety of reasons, such as variability in the internal diameter of the fibers or alteration in the internal diameter secondary to wetting of the fibers during priming of the device. A number of experimental studies have investigated the flow distribution in the blood pathways of hollow-fiber devices. Early experiments of this type used simple Newtonian solutions, whereas more recent approaches have used not only sophisticated imaging techniques (e.g., helical computed tomography scanning) but also blood containing a range of red cell concentrations comparable to those that would be seen in a clinical setting. These latter studies demonstrated a more apparent maldistribution at higher red cell concentrations.[8,14]

Flow maldistribution in the blood pathway may also be influenced by the pressure profile within the header or device inlet manifold, and novel approaches to minimize these effects have been developed.[15]

The role of packing density on flow distribution optimization has similarly been demonstrated for the dialysis fluid pathway.[16] In devices used for the treatment of End Stage Renal Disease (ESRD), this has led to the use of spacers or moiré patterned fibers to improve the flow distribution.[17,18]

Studies on optimizing solute transport have focused primarily on flow rates used during the treatment of chronic renal disease, and, with the exception of the recent study by Leypoldt and colleagues,[9] results at low dialysis fluid flow rates are at present lacking.

THE SELECTION OF FILTERS AND MEMBRANES

The selection of filters and membranes is linked, not only to the delivery of treatment dose and the role that the membrane may play in outcomes, but also to the treatment regimen used. Although the maintenance of fluid balance and improved vascular stability favor the use of continuous treatment modalities, circuit patency and fluid removal rates tend to decrease with elapsed treatment time and may necessitate the application of strategies to prolong performance and patency.[19] As during hemofiltration, the rate of small molecular solute removal is equivalent to the rate of fluid removal. Such rates may not be sufficient in the treatment of catabolic patients. The treatment of such patients may necessitate the use of alternate strategies such as hemodiafiltration.

Dialysis adequacy in patients with chronic renal disease involves the use of urea kinetic modeling, a reflection of both dietary protein intake and efficiency of small solute clearance. In recent years, there has been a growing effort to measure dialysis adequacy in patients with ARF using urea kinetic modeling.[20,21] In contrast to patients with chronic renal disease, there is no definition of "adequate" dialysis in those with ARF. Since the publication of results from a large prospective, randomized trial on the effects of treatment dose on outcome of patients with ARF,[22] it appears that a degree of consensus has been achieved

that 35 mL/kg/hr of clearance is adequate in continuous therapies.[23]

Membranes as well as the treatment regimen play an important role in the removal of solutes. In critically ill patients, it is important to remove not only small molecular compounds but also inflammatory mediators. The removal of inflammatory mediators is favored by the use of high-permeability membranes, a combination of convective and diffusive mass transport, and membranes in which there is significant removal by adsorption.[24]

Experimental and clinical studies have suggested that dialysis membrane biocompatibility may influence the morbidity and mortality of patients with ARF, and complement activation by dialysis membranes may also prolong the recovery from ARF. As discussed elsewhere, meta-analyses relating biocompatibility to treatment outcomes have not found an unequivocal benefit for synthetic membranes over unsubstituted cellulose membranes.[25]

FUTURE DEVELOPMENTS

Current membranes are nonselective, and future focus will be on enhancing selectivity such that it replicates glomerular selectivity.[26]

Many patients with ARF are subject to sepsis, and in such patients, current techniques of treatment offer only a limited removal of cytokines and some improvement in outcome.[27,28] They remain insufficient to reverse the complicated biological dysregulation resulting from sepsis-associated ARF. The development of a bioartificial kidney consisting of a conventional hemofiltration device in series with a renal tubule assist device containing renal proximal tubule cells represents a new therapeutic approach that currently is under investigation and has been shown to improve survival in ARF.[29]

Key Points

1. A variety of membranes are used in devices intended for the treatment of ARF. Meta-analyses have not demonstrated an unequivocal benefit for membranes manufactured from synthetic polymers compared to those manufactured from cellulose.
2. Primary determinants of solute transport are the blood and the dialysate flow rates, while fluid removal is influenced primarily by the pressure gradient across the membrane and the membrane's hydraulic permeability.
3. All devices demonstrate a decline in performance with time, necessitating the application of strategies to prolong performance and circuit life.
4. When treating hypercatabolic patients, conventional hemofiltration in which convective mass transport dominates may be inadequate and consideration should be given to the use of treatments involving both diffusive and connective mass transport.

Key References

5. Jaffrin MY, Ding LH, Laurent JM: Related simultaneous convective and diffusive mass transfers in a hemodialyser. J Biomech Eng 1990;112:212-219.

13. Ronco C, Brendolan A, Crepaldi C, et al: Importance of hollow-fiber geometry in continuous arteriovenous hemofiltration. Contrib Nephrol 1991;93:175-178.
15. Ronco C, Ghezzi PM, Metry G, et al: Effects of hematocrit and blood flow distribution on solute clearance in hollow-fiber hemodialyzers. Nephron 2001;89:243-250.
25. Alonso A, Lau J, Jaber BL: Biocompatible hemodialysis membranes for acute renal failure. Cochrane Database of Systemic

Reviews 2008;1. Article CD005283. DOI 10.1002/14651858. CD005283.pub2.
26. Humes HD, Fissell WH, Tiranathanagul K: The future of hemodialysis membranes. Kidney Int 2006;69:1115-1119.

See the companion Expert Consult website for the complete reference list.

CHAPTER 213

Evolution of Machines for Acute Renal Replacement Therapy

Claudio Ronco and Hans Dietrich Polaschegg

OBJECTIVES

This chapter will:
1. Summarize the history of hemodialysis in acute renal failure.
2. Describe the history of continuous renal replacement therapy (CRRT) devices.
3. Describe the basic aspects of CRRT devices.
4. Analyze current and alternative devices for CRRT.

HISTORICAL DEVELOPMENT

The history of renal replacement therapy begins with "acute" treatments. During the quest for an effective and safe treatment, many ideas were tried. Some of those ideas were reinvented decades later, when new technology became available. An example is continuous arteriovenous hemofiltration (CAVH), which was described by a U.S. patent 10 years before Kramer[1] used it in Göettingen[2] (see Fig. 213-3). A more recent example is the invention of dialysate containing citrate by Ahmad,[3] which was described 50 years earlier by Alwall.[4]

HEMODIALYSIS

Kolff, who performed the first successful hemodialysis treatment, was not only a medical pioneer but also became a successful promoter of the artificial kidney and other artificial organs. Immediately after the Second World War, he sent replicas of his machine to four places. One came to the United States and was rebuilt by a company; this machine was later used by U.S. researchers and clinicians.

The successful use of the Kolff-Brigham machine during the Korean War[5,6] (Fig. 213-1) may have helped to promote the development of the artificial kidney in the United States. The rotating drum machine provided no support for the tubular membrane through which blood was trans-

ported and was therefore operated without added pressure. It required a pump for pumping blood back to the patient. The Kolff-Brigham machine used a pneumatically driven pump with ball valves for this purpose.

When maintenance dialysis became possible with the Quinton-Scribner shunt and, later, the Cimino-Brescia fistula, the need for small, safe machines that could also be used in patients' homes became urgent. This led to the development of single-patient machines and water treatment systems used today in dialysis clinics and homes. A decade later, the basic features of today's dialysis machines, with the exception of controlled ultrafiltration, were well described.[7-10] Volumetric control of ultrafiltration was developed in the 1970s and became widely available in the 1980s. These machines were operated in the well-organized environment of dialysis units or in the patient's home. Inside hospitals, patients had to be moved to the dialysis ward for treatment, because dialysis machines and water treatment systems were too bulky to be taken to the intensive care unit (ICU).

HEMOFILTRATION

Ultrafiltration of blood was described at the end of the 19th century and was used for analyzing blood water solutes. Hemofiltration with replacement of fluid was described by Malinow and Korzon.[11] They employed self-made cellophane filters with 400 cm² surface area; up to 20 of these were arranged in parallel to increase the filtration capacity. Ringer-Krebs solution was used for replacement. In animal tests, up to 7 L of fluid was exchanged. The authors concluded that the method was not as efficient as the Kolff kidney, because the amount of ultrafiltrate that could be achieved was too low. Nevertheless, theirs was the first paper describing in vivo hemofiltration with positive and negative pressure-driven ultrafiltration. The situation changed 20 years later, when Michaels at Amicon[12] developed a method to cast asymmetrical high-flux (then called high-flow) membranes with approximately 50-fold higher permeability, which were used by Henderson and colleagues[13] for in vitro testing. The authors concluded that 0.65 m² of this membrane would be sufficient for human

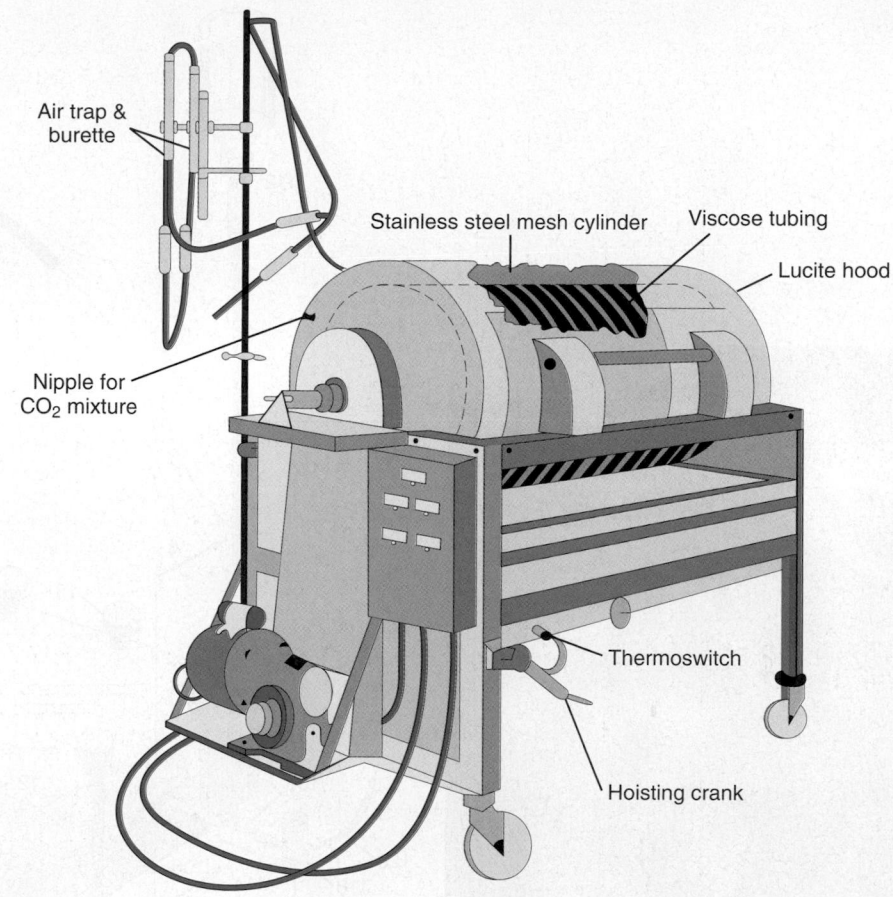

FIGURE 213-1. Kolff-Brigham machine.

treatment. By the end of the 1960s, hemofiltration became feasible with the progression of membrane technology and the availability of a suitable capillary hemofilter made from polysulfone.[14] In spite of this pioneering work, hemofiltration or hemodiafiltration never gained acceptance in the United States outside the ICU.

Also at the end of the 1960s, the company Rhone Poulenc in France developed a high-flux membrane based on acrylonitrile,[15] which was used in the parallel-plate high-flux dialyzer, RP6. In Germany, Quellhorst and coworkers[16] used the RP6 high-flux dialyzer for the first clinical trials with postdilution hemofiltration. The cooperation of the Quellhorst group with the German company Sartorius (Göttingen, Germany) led to the development of the Hemoprocessor (Fig. 213-2), a microprocessor-controlled machine comprising three pumps and two balances for fluid balancing and weight loss control. The German company Dialysetechnik (now Baxter Dialysetechnik, Ettlingen, Germany) developed a hemofiltration machine employing a single weight cell for fluid balancing and a volumetric ultrafiltration pump for weight loss.[17] These machines were used in the ICU and in chronic dialysis wards.

THE BEGINNING OF CONTINUOUS RENAL REPLACEMENT THERAPY

In 1974, Silverstein and associates[18] presented results of a clinical trial on 100 hemodialysis patients with fluid

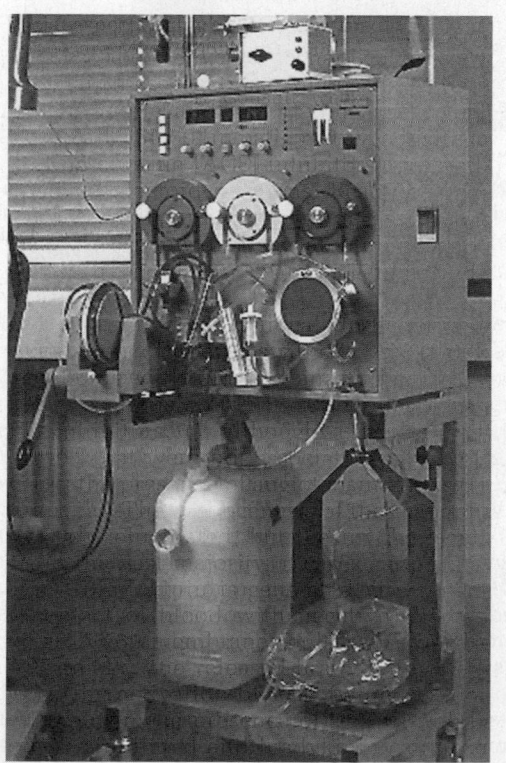

FIGURE 213-2. Hemoprocessor (Sartorius). A machine used for hemofiltration c. 1980.

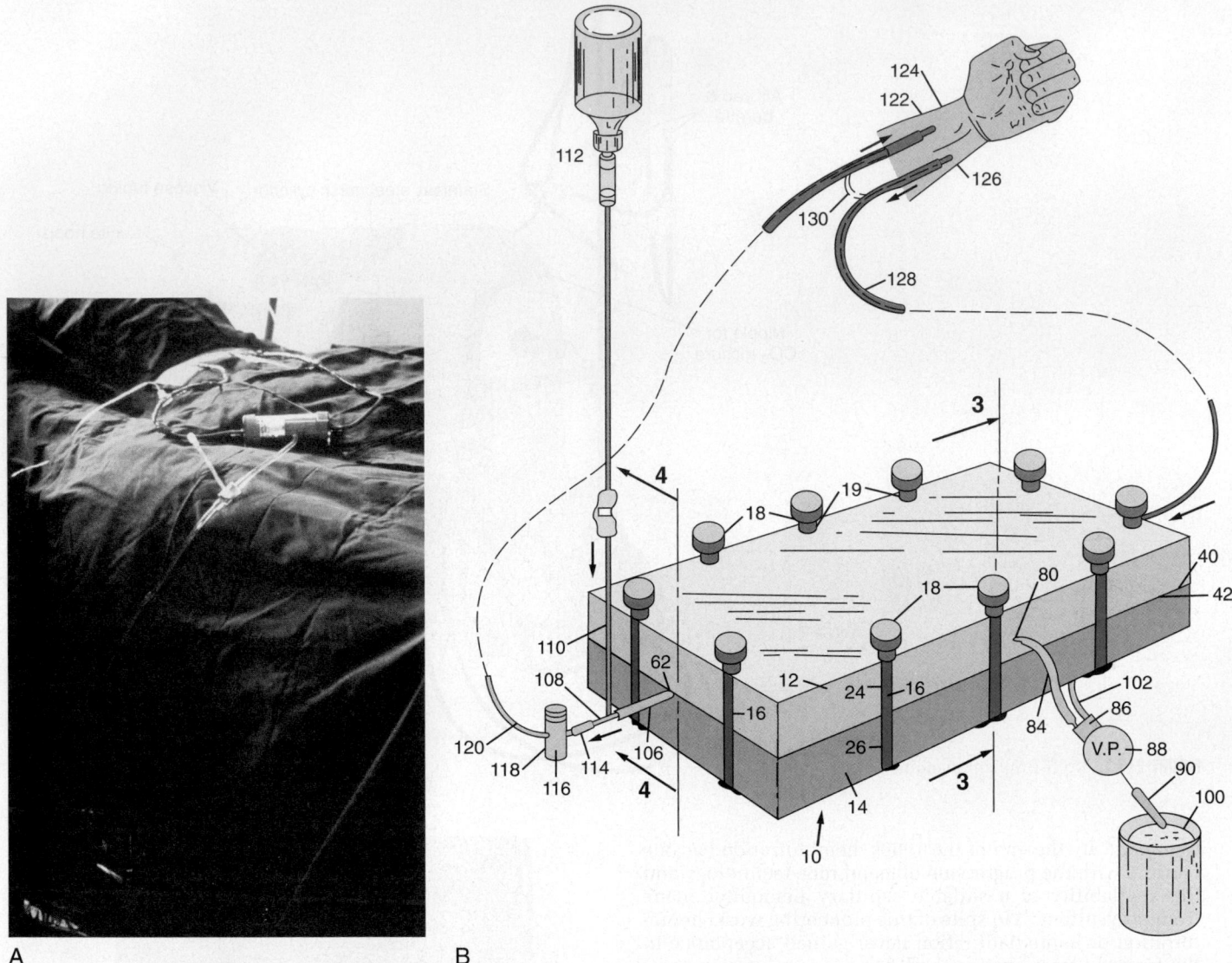

FIGURE 213-3. A, Continuous arteriovenous hemofiltration (CAVH). **B,** Typical circuit for CAVH described in U.S. patent 3483867 by Markovitz 10 years before Kramer's work. Blood from peripheral blood vessels is driven through a flat membrane filter by the arterial-venous pressure difference. Ultrafiltrate collected in vessel 100 is replaced by substitution fluid from vessel 112.

overload. A new ultrafiltration device with a small poly-sulfone capillary filter of 0.2 m² surface area, made by the U.S. company Amicon (Beverly, MA) was used. The filter was inserted into a conventional extracorporeal circuit with a blood pump and standard monitoring. This small but highly permeable capillary filter soon became available in Europe and was used as described by Silverstein and colleagues.

This Amicon filter was also used in 1977 by Kramer and colleagues,[1] who perceived "arteriovenous hemofiltration" (Fig. 213-3), later called CAVH, as a simple, machine-free method for the treatment of overhydrated patients resistant to diuretics. The simple setup consisted of arterial and venous catheters connected to a capillary hemofilter by tubing. Filtrate pressure was produced by the difference between blood pressure and environmental pressure. The only mechanical device used was a syringe pump for heparin. The authors emphasized the simplicity of this method as compared to any pump-assisted method.

In 1984, Eisenhauer[19] gave some information on how CAVH was conceived: In preparation for a treatment with a hemofiltration machine, a catheter was inadvertently placed into the femoral artery. It was Peter Kramer's idea to put the filter between the arterial and the venous bloodline, observing that ultrafiltrate was produced.

This method was rapidly accepted worldwide. Researchers, clinicians, and technicians used it as a starting point for technical improvements. The conference proceedings from the International Conference on CAVH, held in Aachen in 1984, provide an overview of the state of the art at that time, including the addition of fluid-balancing devices[20,21] and additional ultrafiltration pumps.[22,23] Already known from commercially available hemofiltration machines, fluid-balancing devices typically consisted of one or two weight cells. Ultrafiltrate was collected in an ultrafiltrate bag, and gravity infusion of substitution fluid was controlled so that the total weight of ultrafiltrate and substitution fluid remained constant or increased according to a prescribed rate.

A commercial machine for CVVH was presented that allowed single-needle access. Better control of the ultrafiltration rate and better safety measures were emphasized.

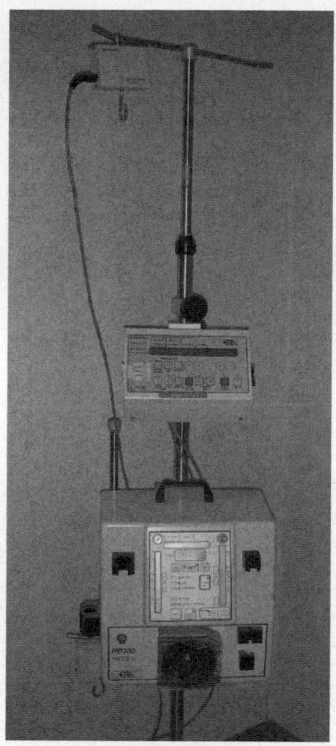

FIGURE 213-4. EQUAline fluid balancing device plus Equapump blood module HP300 (by Medica).

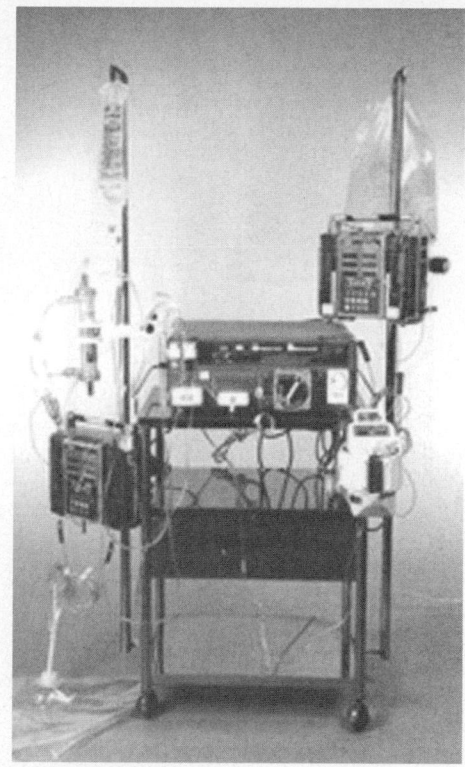

FIGURE 213-5. Gambro AK10 hemodialysis machine equipped for continuous veno-venous hemofiltration.

Stiller and Mann[24] modeled continuous slow hemodialysis (SLED). Clinical results with this method had been reported in the same year by Geronemus and Schneider.[25] To improve the efficacy of the original, machine-free procedure, Ronco[26] introduced continuous arteriovenous hemodiafiltration (CAVHDF).

A commercial device combining fluid balancing with gravity infusion was the EQUAline fluid control system from Medica (Fig. 213-4).

FIRST-GENERATION DEDICATED CRRT MACHINES

The first-generation CRRT machines were simple devices derived from components of standard hemodialysis equipment used for maintenance dialysis. An example was the Hospal BSM32 IC, which was originally derived from the blood module of the Monitral system (Hospal, Lyon, France) for maintenance hemodialysis. The system consisted of two roller pumps: the blood pump (30 to 700 mL/min) and the fluid pump (100 to 2000 mL/hr). A heparin pump allowed for continuous infusion or infusion of boluses. Standard monitoring of the extracorporeal circuit included three pressure sensors (prepump arterial, postpump prefilter, and venous) and an air/foam detector. There was also a colorimetric blood leak detector on the filtrate/spent dialysate line and an "empty bag" detector for fluid replacement. The device did not include fluid balancing, which had to be performed manually by the operator.

The blood module of the AK10 hemodialysis machine (Gambro, Stockholm, Sweden) was used as well. Fluid balancing was performed with infusion pumps (Fig. 213-5).

An example of a device with separate modules for blood pumping and for fluid balancing that could be combined or operated independently was the HP300 system by Medica (Medolla, Italy). It consisted of the HP300 pump (see Fig. 213-4), which comprised a peristaltic roller pump and standard monitoring for the extracorporeal circuit, and the EQUAline fluid-balancing system (see Fig. 213-4), to allow for automatically controlled CVVH.

Another modular machine was the B. Braun (B. Braun, Melsungen, Germany) trio, which consisted of three interfaced modules that were derived from the infusion pump technology of the company. Fluid balancing in this system was done volumetrically with rigid, disposable measuring chambers. This concept was soon abandoned, however.

Also abandoned soon was the modular system ADM08/ABM made by Fresenius Medical Care (Bad Homburg, Germany) which used small weight cells for gravimetric fluid balancing in quasicontinuous mode.

Other machines of this period came from the companies Sorin (Salugia, Italy), Carex (Mirandola, Italy), and RenalSystems (division of Minntech, Minneapolis, MN); Miren (Mirandola, Italy) made a device for Amicon.

An integrated machine of this generation was the Baxter BM25, which consisted of the modules BM11 + BM14 (Fig. 213-6). This device is still available from Edwards Life Sciences (Irvine, CA). Originally developed by the German company Dialysetechnik, which was acquired by Baxter, it is now produced by MeSys (Hannover, Germany). The system comprises a blood pump and standard monitoring of the extracorporeal circuit. Fluid balancing is controlled with two pumps and two scales.

Monitoring and user interfaces with these machines were derived from machines used for chronic dialysis:

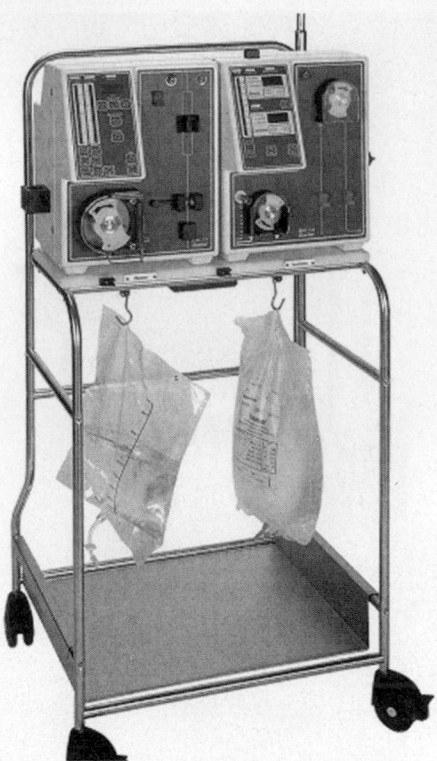

FIGURE 213-6. Baxter BM25 machine. The blood pump module is on the left, and the fluid balancing module is on the right.

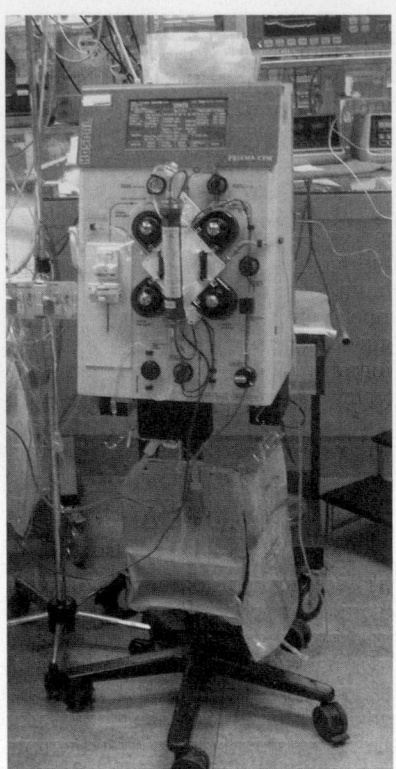

FIGURE 213-7. The PRISMA machine by Gambro.

Indicators and buttons were distributed over the modules. Priming was at best semiautomatic, and, because flat panel displays were not affordable, user guidance was rudimentary.

SECOND-GENERATION CRRT MACHINES

A major step was made when the company Cobe (later acquired by Gambro) introduced the PRISMA machine (Fig. 213-7).[27] This device was specifically developed for continuous treatment in the ICU, allowing hemodialysis, hemofiltration, and hemodiafiltration using pharmaceutical replacement fluid and/or dialysate. In addition to four pumps for blood, dialysate, substitution fluid, and waste, this machine had three scales for dialysate, substitution fluid, and waste. The specific progress made with this machine was the air-free, optimized disposable cassette system with integrated dialyzer. Both the extracorporeal blood circuit and the dialysate/replacement fluid circuit used color-coded tubing with 3-mm inner diameter throughout. The tubing system was operated air free, without drip chambers or clot filters, to improve hemocompatibility. Pressure is transmitted through flexible but tight membranes (pressure pots). This machine included the usual safety monitors and a state-of-the-art user interface guiding the user through the various steps required for setting up the machine and rectifying problems. Optimized for slow continuous treatment, blood flow in this machine was limited to 180 mL/min. The balances could handle approximately 5 L of fluid.

The PRISMA machine triggered the development of integrated, specialized CRRT machines all over the world (described in another chapter of this book). These newer machines included three to five pumps and three to four balances able to handle 12 to 20 L of replacement fluid or dialysate and capable of producing blood flows up to 400 to 600 mL/min. Some machines used conventional blood tubing systems that differed little from extracorporeal circuits used for standard dialysis machines; others used cassette systems for the tubing but without integration of the dialyzer/hemofilter. A newer version of the PRISMA, the Prismaflex, still comes with an integrated but more sophisticated cassette system that allows for automatic loading and priming and free choice of treatment modality using a single disposable cassette system.

The general trend was toward a fully automatic, universal machine that would allow all treatment modes. In addition, competition drove development toward larger fluid-handling capacity and higher flows of blood, dialysate, and substitution fluid.

SPECIAL MACHINES AND MODIFIED HEMODIALYSIS MACHINES

Within less than 30 years, CRRT equipment had become even more complicated than the dialysis machines CAVH was designed to replace. The original purpose of CAVH was fluid removal. This treatment can still be performed with the latest CRRT machines, but at comparably high cost. With some machines, cassette systems containing all tubes necessary for the most complicated treatment (pre-

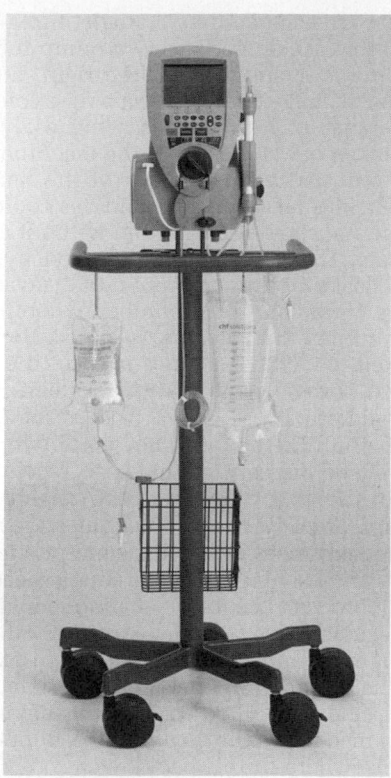

FIGURE 213-8. Aquadex FlexFlow (CHF Solutions) used for slow continuous ultrafiltration.

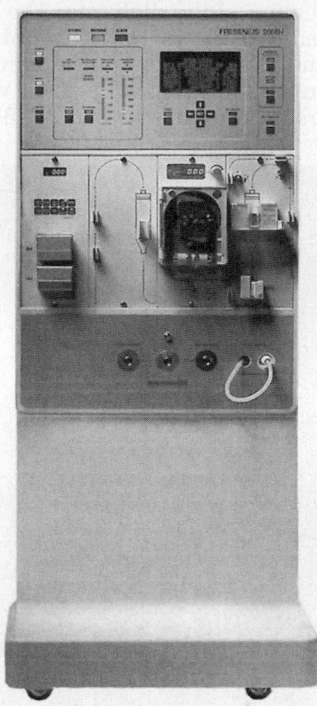

FIGURE 213-9. The 2008H by Fresenius, a machine used for sustained low-efficiency dialysis (SLED).

post continuous veno-venous hemodiafiltration [CVVHDF]) are used.

As an alternative to the "universal" machine, a simple device for fluid removal, hemofiltration, and hemodialysis at moderate flows was developed in the 1990s: the Acumen (Fresenius).[28] This device consisted of a pneumatic blood pump and a volumetric balancing chamber integrated together with the filter in a disposable cassette system for easy loading from the front. Fluid removal was restricted by the volume ratio of the balancing chamber to the blood pump chamber (1 : 5). The blood pump generated tidal flow, producing higher shear rates in the filter in order to reduce concentration polarization and increase filtration performance. It has been shown that tidal flow is as efficient as continuous flow for hemodialysis if the tidal volume is smaller than the filling volume of the dialyzer.[29] This machine has since been abandoned, however.

A small machine capable of controlled ultrafiltration became available recently in the United States. The Aquadex FlexFlow (CHF Solutions, Brooklyn Park, MN) (Fig. 213-8) weighs less than 10 kg (as opposed to up to 80 kg for standard CRRT machines) and uses a smooth, air-free extracorporeal circuit with three integrated pressure sensors. It was designed for low blood flows and can be used with peripheral vein blood access. The disposable part consists of two cassettes, one containing the blood pump tubing and the prepump pressure sensor, and the other one containing the filter, the filtration pump tubing, the return, and the filtrate pressure sensors. Filtrate is additionally weighed by a balance. The air-free circuit permits safe temporary flow reversal of the blood pump if the withdrawal cannula sucks to the vessel wall. Because of its small size and weight, the machine can easily be

transported and operates up to 30 minutes on battery power.

The high capital and operating costs of CRRT machines have motivated the development of adapted treatment modalities for standard hemodialysis machines. The treatment called sustained low-efficiency dialysis (SLED) is, in fact, highly efficient when compared to standard CRRT treatment but operates at lower dialysate flow rates than intermittent treatment does. In order to operate the dialysis machine at low clearance, the dialysate flow is reduced to 100 mL/min, which allows operation for 12 hours with a single set of concentrate containers. Fresenius Medical Care North America has adapted the 2008 H and 2008 K (Fig. 213-9) machines to allow operation at low dialysate flows of 100 mL/min. Standard dialysis machines usually are unable to operate at this low flow. Standard hemodialysis machines are designed for dialysate flows between 300 and 800 to 1000 mL/min. The typical dialysate pumps (gear pumps) capable of producing this flow are not stable when run at very low flows. Low flow is achieved by running the dialysate pump at 300 mL/min, but in intermittent flow mode with a duty cycle of 1 : 2. This intermittent flow is generated by delayed switching of the balancing chambers used for fluid balancing. As mentioned earlier, tidal flow is as efficient as continuous flow of blood if the tidal volume is smaller than the filling volume of the dialyzer. The same applies for the dialysate side. With balancing chamber volumes of 30 mL, this condition is satisfied even for small filters.

The GENIUS machine (Fresenius) (Fig. 213-10), designed by the late Dr. Bernd Tersteegen,[30] is used for SLED as well. This machine is unique because it uses a tank system containing 90 L of fresh dialysate, which is circulated through the dialyzer back to the bottom of the same tank without mixing. Thanks to the design of the system, the dialysate is "ultrapure," a state that is achieved by ultraviolet irradiation of the dialysate. The thermally isolated tank is filled with dialysate at a central filling station, and the machine is wheeled to the point of use. The machine is operated with low voltage (24 V) and can run for several hours on the built-in battery. Blood flow and dialysate flow are generated by a single, three-roller peristaltic pump that accommodates two pump tubes. Precise fluid balancing is guaranteed by the rigid, air-free tank. Mixing of fresh and spent dialysate is avoided by the density difference of fresh versus spent dialysate. Fresh dialysate is taken out at the top of the machine, and spent dialysate is returned at the bottom of the tank. Because spent dialysate has taken up urea and has cooled down, it is more dense and stays at the bottom without mixing with fresh dialysate. Ultrafiltration is achieved by a separate roller pump; leaks are the only potential cause of ultrafiltration errors. With a minimal number of components and limited monitoring, this machine has recently been favorably compared to CRRT machines used in the ICU.[31]

The Allient Sorbent hemodialysis system (Renal Solutions, Warrendale, PA) (Fig. 213-11),[32] is a complete redesign of the REDY machine employing dialysate regeneration. The concept of dialysate regeneration was developed in the 1970s and has been slightly improved over the years. Some of the old machines are still in use. The machine comprises a two-ventricle pneumatic blood pump that can also be used for single-needle access. Single-needle access has been abandoned almost completely in regular dialysis because of low efficiency, but the efficiency is acceptable for SLED. Single-lumen access overcomes the most severe safety problem related to extracorporeal circulation: blood loss to the environment in case of disconnection of the blood tubing from the catheter (discussed elsewhere in this book).

Peristaltic roller pumps circulate dialysate through a sorbent column that removes uremic substances but also electrolytes. For this reason Ca, Mg, and K are added to the reconstituted dialysate by an additional pump. Ultrafiltration control is achieved with the help of a scale which also accommodates a heater. The electrical power require-

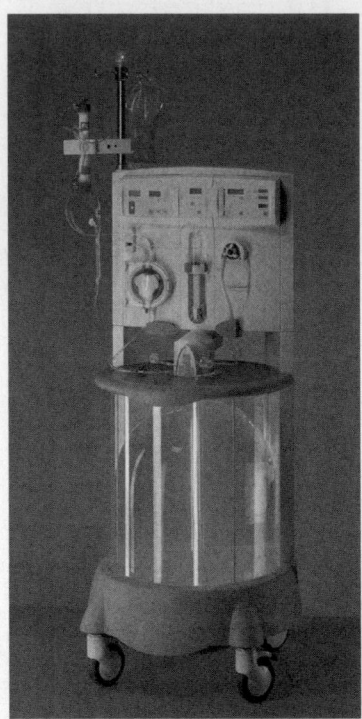

FIGURE 213-10. The GENIUS machine (Fresenius) used for sustained low-efficiency dialysis (SLED).

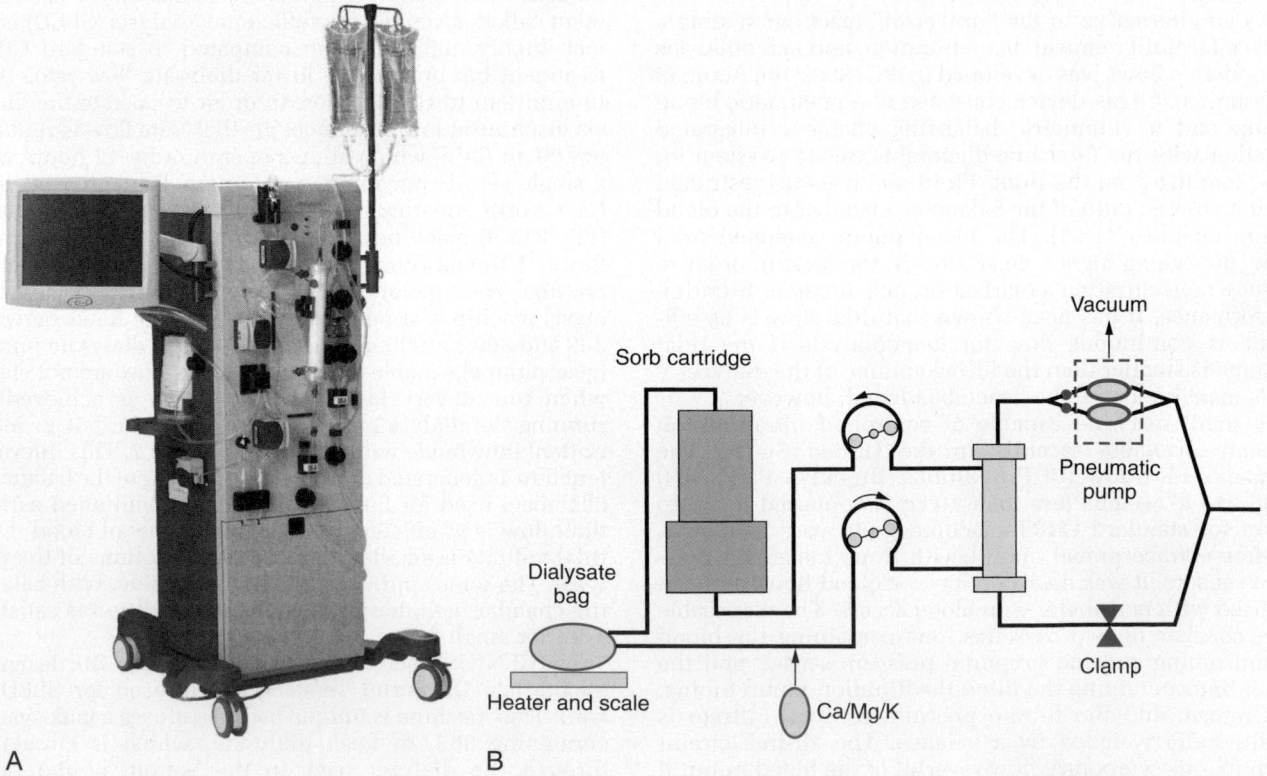

FIGURE 213-11. **A,** Allient Sorbent hemodialysis system (Renal Solutions) used for sustained low-efficiency dialysis (SLED). **B,** Simplified flow schematic of the Allient machine.

ment of this machine is low, because the heater must only replace heat lost to the environment when dialysate is recirculated. Like standard CRRT machines, it does not require connections to water and drain and uses disposable components for the dialysate circuit.

The sorbent cartridge of the Allient machine contains layers of activated charcoal that adsorb most organic substances but not urea, which is converted by urease to ammonium carbonate. Ammonium but also K, Ca, and Mg ions are exchanged against Na and H ions in an ion-exchange layer consisting of zirconium phosphate. Anions such as phosphate or fluoride are captured in the final layer. Because of the ion-exchange mechanism, treatment of electrolyte disturbances with this system may require a different approach than that with standard CRRT machines.

All CRRT machines working with pharmaceutical fluid use weight scales for fluid balancing. The disadvantage of these systems are their limitations when handling large fluid volumes. Because fresh and spent dialysate fluid must be positioned on the machine, even large and heavy machines can handle only four 5-L bags simultaneously. Bags must be changed frequently for a highly efficient treatment. Although the change of bags is guided by the machines, thanks to modern electronics, the process is still prone to human error. In addition, weight scales are sensitive to vibration and movements. These limitations can be overcome by the use of volumetric fluid balancing, which is used by most conventional hemodialysis machines. This principle is employed by the NxStage System One (NxStage Medical, Lawrence, MA) (Fig. 213-12).[33] It is a compact hemodialysis/hemofiltration machine utilizing pharmaceutical dialysate and/or replacement fluid. The flat, disposable cassette system contains tubes and chambers for pumping, monitoring, and volumetric fluid balancing. Balancing chambers are employed for fluid balancing that are functionally equivalent to the balancing chambers in standard hemodialysis machines. Like other advanced CRRT machines, the System One cassette system loads automatically and only needs to be connected to fluid and waste bags for priming. The outstanding feature is the lack of weight cells for fluid balancing. The volumetric balancing system works continuously and handles large fluid volumes. Effluent need not be collected but can be dumped to drain during the treatment. The blood path is air free.

DIALYSERS AND FILTERS FOR ACUTE THERAPIES

CRRT started with CAVH. Because this method does not use a blood pump, blood flow through the filter is a function of the arterial-venous pressure difference and the flow resistance of the extracorporeal system. The latter is the sum of the flow resistances of the catheter, the blood tubing, and the filter. Because capillary dialyzers were already predominantly in use when CAVH was introduced, short filters with larger than usual diameters (240 μm instead of 200 μm) of the capillaries were used for CAVH filters, to reduce the flow resistance.

With pump-driven blood flow and pump-controlled ultrafiltration, the ultrafiltration rate is no longer limited by the blood flow rate resulting from the arterial-venous pressure difference and the flow resistance. The maximum ultrafiltration rate that can be achieved for a given blood flow depends on the filter design and the operating parameters. These operating parameters have been studied by

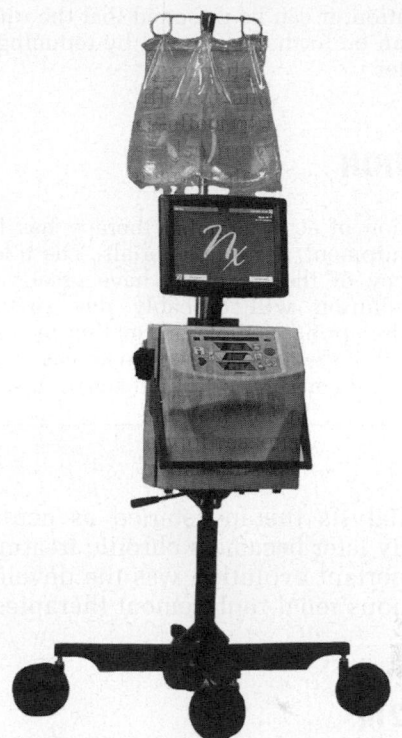

FIGURE 213-12. NxStage System One (NxStage Medical) hemodialysis machine.

Okazaki and Yoshida.[34] Their results can be summarized as follows: When plasma or colloid solutions are filtered, a gel layer forms at the surface which limits the solvent flux. The gel layer thickness is controlled by the filtrate flux and the diffusion of the gel molecules back into the fluid stream. This relation is modified by the wall shear rate. Ultrafiltrate flow becomes independent of transmembrane pressure above a certain limit and after that is a function only of the wall shear rate. Red blood cells cause local turbulence but also hinder backdiffusion of protein molecules. Low hematocrits enhance filtration, and high hematocrits hinder it. At high hematocrits, the ultrafiltration flux is much reduced compared to plasma at low shear rates, but it approaches the same value at wall shear rates greater than 1000 L/sec. Higher shear rates would further increase ultrafiltration but would also increase the risk of mechanical hemolysis.

The practical consequences are as follows: With the surface area kept constant, long, thin filters allow higher ultrafiltration rates than short, thick filters. Smaller inner-diameter capillaries result in higher shear rates, reducing concentration polarization.

Düngen and colleagues[35] were surprised about the result when they tested short and long filters of equal surface area in the clinic under controlled conditions. The explanation presented by the authors for the fact that long filters were better is not plausible; the Fahraeus-Lindquist effect is dependent on the capillary diameter, which had been kept constant (220 μm). They also mentioned the viscosity of blood, which depends on the shear rate. However, an estimate of the mean shear rate showed that it was larger than 400 L/sec, and the viscosity change in this range is negligible. Using the correction factor of Okazaki and Yoshida, the observed difference in ultrafiltration flow rate between long and short filters can be reproduced. From this calculation, it can be reasoned that the ultrafiltration flow rate can be further improved by reducing the capillary diameter.

CONCLUSION

The evolution of acute dialysis therapy has led to new devices, equipment, and biomaterials. The tolerance and the efficiency of the treatment have greatly improved. Further evolution will probably deal with software advances, the application of information technology, and improvement of the user interface, with easier application of multiple and complex treatment schedules.

Key Points

1. Hemodialysis therapy started as acute therapy and only later became a chronic treatment.
2. An important evolution was the development of continuous renal replacement therapies.

3. Specific devices and equipment have been developed over the years to accomplish a series of multiple and complex tasks.

Key References

1. Kramer P, Wigger W, Rieger J, et al: Arteriovenous haemofiltration: A new and simple method for treatment of overhydrated patients resistant to diuretics. Klin Wochenschrift 1977;55:1121-1122.
7. Grimsrud L, Cole JJ, Eschbach JW, et al: Safety aspects of haemodialysis. Trans Am Soc Artif Intern Organs 1967; 13:1-4.
29. Polaschegg HD, Wojke R: Constant blood flow during single-needle dialysis is unnecessary. Int J Artif Organs 1993;16: 505-509.
34. Okazaki M, Yoshida F: Ultrafiltration of blood: Effect of hematocrit on ultrafiltration rate. Ann Biomed Eng 1976;4: 138-150.
35. Dungen HD, von Heymann C, Ronco C, et al: Renal replacement therapy: Physical properties of hollow fibers influence efficiency. Int J Artif Organs 2001;24:357-366.

See the companion Expert Consult website for the complete reference list.

CHAPTER 214

Principles of Anticoagulation in Extracorporeal Circuits

Donald F. Cronin and Ravindra L. Mehta

OBJECTIVES

This chapter will:
1. Review the basic mechanisms involved in the coagulation cascade and clotting, with emphasis on how they pertain to patients with kidney dysfunction.
2. Discuss how the various components of extracorporeal circuits, the dialysis procedure in general, and critical illness can alter the normal balance between coagulation and anticoagulation.
3. Discuss the various techniques and maneuvers available to promote circuit patency while not increasing the risk of hemorrhage to the patient.

There is a fine balance between hemostasis and hemorrhage in the human body, managed by a complex system of plasma, cellular, and endothelial factors.[1] *Coagulation* is the normal process occurring when vascular injury results in formation of a fibrin clot; *thrombosis* refers to the pathological formation of clot in response to injury, stasis, and hypercoagulability.[1] Intermittent and continuous dialysis therapies depend on adequate anticoagulation occurring in the extracorporeal circuit (ECC), so as to maximize circuit and filter longevity, which increases clearance and lessens costs and nurse time requirements. Insufficient anticoagulation results in decreased filter performance, clotting, and blood loss; excessive anticoagulation leads to bleeding complications, reported to occur in 5% to 26% of treatments. Patients with end-stage renal disease are known to be hypercoagulable, and this imbalance probably extends to critically ill patients with acute kidney injury as well. They are at risk for both hemorrhagic and thrombotic complications. Bleeding can be caused by uremic platelet dysfunction or by the anticoagulants used for dialysis. The activation of coagulation during dialysis can lead to blood loss, estimated to be 300 to 750 mL/yr in patients undergoing chronic hemodialysis.[2] This chapter deals with the principles of anticoagulation in the ECC, the disturbances that occur in critically ill patients with renal insufficiency, and the importance of the intrinsic pathway, platelet activation, and the fibrinolytic system in affecting ECC patency. Circuit design, contributions of membrane/blood interaction, and how these factors might be modified are also addressed. Specific anticoagulation strategies are covered in Chapter 216.

COAGULATION IN CRITICALLY ILL PATIENTS

Prevention of blood coagulation depends on a complex interaction of endothelial cells, blood cells, and plasma

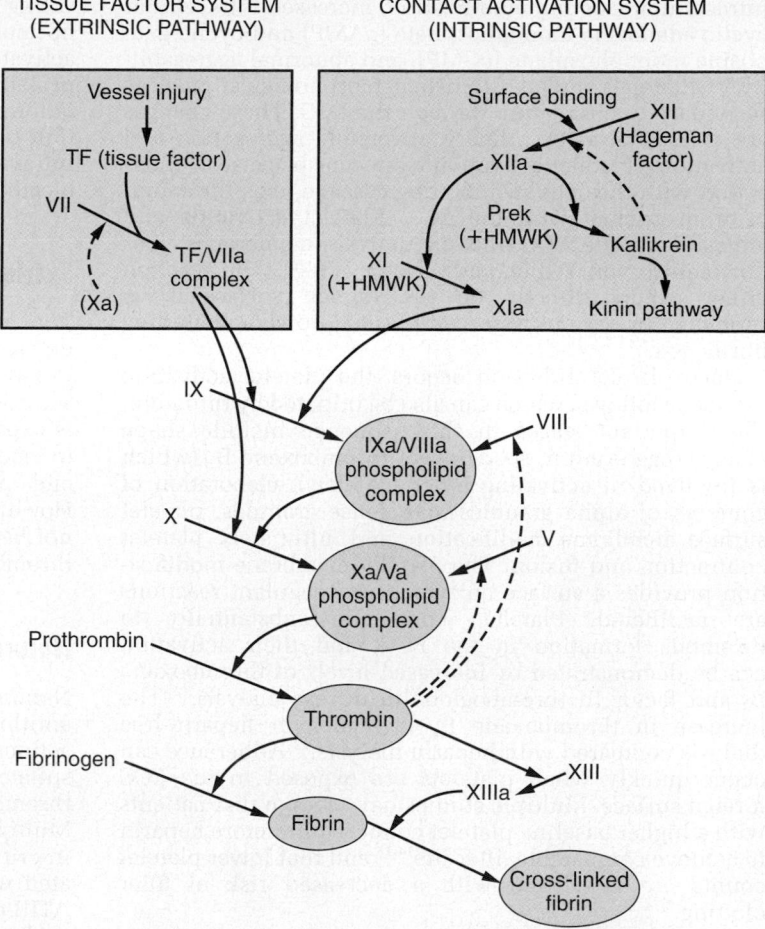

TISSUE FACTOR SYSTEM
(EXTRINSIC PATHWAY)

CONTACT ACTIVATION SYSTEM
(INTRINSIC PATHWAY)

FIGURE 214-1. The anticoagulation cascade. *Straight arrows* indicate conversion of a coagulation protein from an inactive to an activated form. *Curved arrows* show a catalytic effect or the enzymatic action of an activated factor or complex on the next factor in the cascade. *Dashed arrows* show positive feedback loops. The intrinsic pathway is activated by foreign surfaces such as dialysis membranes. Heparin binds to and activates antithrombin III, which is a natural inhibitor of factor IXa, factor Xa, and thrombin. Low-molecular-weight (LMW) is more active in inhibiting factor Xa and less potent against thrombin than is unfractionated heparin. Citrate is an anticoagulant because it chelates calcium ions, which are needed for the formation of all complexes shown in the figure, for the enzymatic activity of factor XIa, and for the conversion of XIII to XIIIa by thrombin. HMWK, high molecular weight kininogen; PreK, prekallikrein. (From Ward D: Anticoagulation in patients on hemodialysis. In Nissenson AR, Fine RN [eds]: Clinical Dialysis, 4th ed. New York, McGraw-Hill, 2005.)

factors.[3] This balance between procoagulant and anticoagulant activity is a delicate one, and it is disturbed when blood is forced through an ECC, because the endothelial component is temporarily removed from the mix. As a result, the balance is shifted toward coagulation. There are numerous routes through which activation can occur, with the end result being platelet aggregation and formation of a clot. Shifting back the balance requires addition of an anticoagulant to the ECC, which can then lead to an imbalance in the other direction in the systemic circulation, favoring bleeding. In critically ill patients with sepsis and multiorgan failure, the imbalance in the normal clotting mechanisms can be extreme, with activation of multiple inflammatory pathways and downregulation of anticoagulant pathways.[3,4] Activated monocytes and polymorphonuclear cells add to the coagulation cascade via increased expression of tissue factor and production of reactive oxygen species. Despite heparinization, clotting can occur in the ECC in these patients, as well as concomitant systemic bleeding.

The processes of hemostasis and coagulation are well reviewed elsewhere[5]; they involve many functional areas, including platelet function, coagulation enzyme cascades, contact activation, natural anticoagulants, the endothelium, and fibrinolysis.[3] When blood is exposed to the foreign surface of an ECC, two principal mechanisms of thrombus formation have traditionally been thought to be important: the intrinsic pathway of blood coagulation and platelet adhesion and activation. The traditional theory postulates that the intrinsic pathway in ECC can begin with the "contact activation factors," such as factor XII, high-molecular-weight kallikrein, and prekallikrein, which occur more readily on a negatively charged surface. However, a recent study looking at blood parameters in continuous veno-venous hemodialysis (CVVH) circuits without heparin did not demonstrate any change in plasma levels of factor XIIa-C1 inhibitor complex or the kallikrein-C1 inhibitor complex,[6] findings that would argue against significant involvement of contact activation of the intrinsic pathway in clotting in CVVH. These results were in keeping with those of a previous study, which did not find an increase in contact activation factors in a system using polyacrylonitrile membranes and systemic heparinization.[7] The generation of thrombin can also start with the activation of factor X, either on the surface of activated platelets or by the integrin receptor membrane attack complex 1 (MAC-1) on leukocytes.[8] However it is initiated, it then proceeds through an amplifying series of enzyme reactions, is moderated by multiple negative and positive feedback loops, and culminates in the production of thrombin and the formation of a stable, cross-linked fibrin clot (Fig. 214-1).

Platelet Dysfunction

Many abnormalities have been described in uremic platelets, including decreased thromboxane A_2, abnormal intracellular calcium mobilization, increased intracellular cyclic adenosine monophosphate (cAMP) and cyclic guanosine monophosphate (cGMP), and abnormal aggregability.[9,10] Platelets undergo transient morphological changes secondary to circulating through the ECC. These changes are consistent with primary, reversible aggregation and activation.[3] Platelet activation can occur because of interaction with the activated clotting cascade (e.g., thrombin) or from contact with the ECC. Platelet activation and adhesion in the ECC and on dialysis membranes does not require von Willebrand's factor (vWF). The reaction either occurs directly on the foreign surface or is promoted by various adsorbed plasma proteins, including fibrinogen.[5,11]

Once platelet adhesion occurs, the platelet activation sequence follows, which can also be initiated by thrombin. The important stages in this sequence include shape change, aggregation, secretion of thromboxane B_2 (which is involved in activating other platelets), elaboration of contents of alpha granules and dense granules, platelet surface membrane modification, and, ultimately, platelet contraction and fusion. The platelet membrane modification provides a surface on which procoagulant reactions are facilitated. Platelets contribute substantially to thrombus formation in the ECC, and their activation can be demonstrated by increased levels of thromboxane B_2 and factor III thromboglobulin during dialysis.[12] The increase in thromboxane B_2 is higher in heparin-free dialysis compared with heparin dialysis.[13] Adherence can occur quickly when platelets are exposed to the ECC foreign surface. Multiple studies have shown that patients with a higher baseline platelet count require more heparin to achieve comparable filter life[14-16] and that lower platelet counts are associated with a decreased risk of filter clotting.[6,14]

Fibrinolytic System

The fibrinolytic system has as its main enzyme plasmin, an active fibrin protease that is produced from plasminogen. There is an increase in fibrinolytic activity during dialysis, secondary to an increase in the endothelial release of tissue plasminogen activator (t-PA). It is believed that the blood contact with the dialysis membrane provides the stimulus for this reaction. There is no evidence that this response limits clotting in the ECC.[5] However, in the study by Bouman, already mentioned, baseline levels of factor XIIa-C1 inhibitors and kallikrein-C1 inhibitor complexes were lower in the subgroup of patients with early increased thrombin generation, which would be consistent with decreased fibrinolysis. Confusing these results was the presence of a trend toward increased levels of plasmin-antiplasmin complex (normally associated with increased fibrinolysis) in the patients with early clotting. The authors hypothesized that these levels of plasmin-antiplasmin complexes may have been more a marker of coagulation than of fibrinolytic activity. Alternatively, it was speculated that these same elevated complex levels may have reflected a higher baseline thrombin generation, which could then have activated endogenous anticoagulant protein C and resulted in less coagulation in the CVVH circuit.[6] Factor XIIa and kallikrein are believed to be important in the activation of fibrinolysis. Factor XII can activate fibrinolysis both by activating prekallikrein (and with subsequent urokinase-type plasminogen activator), causing the prekallikrein-driven generation of kallikrein (leading to increased t-PA), and by directly activating plasminogen. Activated protein C also promotes fibrinolysis because of its inhibitory effect on plasminogen activator inhibitor. Thus, decreased levels of activated protein C with sepsis may tip the balance toward coagulation; however, this effect may be offset by the consumption of coagulation factors associated with disseminated intravascular coagulation (DIC), which would favor bleeding.[3]

Extrinsic Pathway

The extrinsic pathway begins with factor VII, which depends on the release of the tissue factor thromboplastin to have an effect on its natural targets, factors IX and X. Thromboplastin is released from injured vessel walls and is expressed by activated monocytes, usually in response to endotoxins, cytokines, hypoxia, advanced glycation end products, growth factors, and oxidative stress.[17] However, the extrinsic pathway and its mechanisms have not been found to be important in the formation of ECC thrombi.[5]

Natural Anticoagulants

Natural anticoagulant systems are in place and include antithrombin III (ATIII), a serine protease inhibitor. Its actions, which are potentiated by heparin and heparin sulfate (located in vessel walls), include inhibition of thrombin; factors Xa, IXa, XIa, and XIIa; and kallikrein. Multiple studies have shown subnormal levels of ATIII in critically ill patients, and low levels have been associated with filter failure.[18] A retrospective study of septic, ATIII-deficient patients undergoing continuous renal replacement therapy (CRRT) showed reduced filter clotting when heparin anticoagulation was supplemented with ATIII.[19] Protein C, in reactions catalyzed by protein S, inactivates factors Va and VIIIa, thus limiting thrombin generation. Protein C is activated by the binding of thrombin to vascular endothelial-associated thrombomodulin.[3] Decreased levels of activated protein C with sepsis may tip the balance toward coagulation (however, as mentioned previously, this coexists with DIC-associated consumption of coagulation factors, which favors bleeding). In a study of patients with severe sepsis undergoing CVVH, treatment with continuous intravenous recombinant human activated protein C removed the need for additional anticoagulation. Filter life compared favorably with that observed with the use of unfractionated heparin.[20]

Hypercoagulable State

A hypercoagulable state exists to some extent secondary to uremia itself. Patients with end-stage renal disease and those who are critically ill with acute kidney injury/uremia have intrinsic clotting system activation. They have increased levels of procoagulant factors VII and VIII, decreased levels of coagulation inhibitors such as ATIII and proteins C and S, and impaired fibrinolysis.[5] Dialysis can be associated with the release from endothelial cells of other procoagulant substances such as vWF, 6-keto-prostaglandin $F_{1\alpha}$, and t-PA.[5,12] There is also a large dialysis-associated increase in the levels of prothrombin and thrombin-antithrombin complexes (TAT), even more so when anticoagulation is suboptimal or withheld.[21]

CONTRIBUTIONS TO CLOTTING

Catheter

The length and internal diameter of dialysis catheters, as well as any kinks, can affect blood flow, promoting clotting. Position-related changes in blood flow rates can lead to clotting. Femoral lines have been shown in some studies to increase chances of clotting.[19] Large-bore, small-length catheters are preferable for arteriovenous, nonpumped systems, to allow a high blood flow rate. In pumped systems, the size of the catheter depends on the site of insertion (internal jugular, femoral, or subclavian).[22]

Circuit, Tubing, and Membrane

Improving the laminar flow configuration, minimizing stagnant areas in dialyzer headers, keeping tubing lengths short, avoiding dependent loops, minimizing reservoir volumes, and decreasing air-blood interface in traps can all help prevent clotting.[3] The air-blood interface in the bubble trap can be the initial site for clotting. However, direct heparin injection into the air trap was not found to improve circuit life, although the dose used may have been insufficient.[23] Recently, an experimental model was developed to test biochemical markers of coagulation activation at various times and sites in a dialysis circuit. The authors measured TAT and found that the blood lines alone, without a dialyzer attached, did not significantly activate coagulation during the first 20 minutes of circulation; in contrast, when a dialyzer was included in the system, only 5 minutes of circulation was needed to activate coagulation.[24]

Pumped ECC systems have the advantage of ensuring more consistent blood flows, regardless of the patient's blood pressure, which can contribute to circuit life. In nonpumped systems such as continuous arteriovenous hemofiltration (CAVH), membrane geometry may be important, because parallel-plate dialyzers result in greater urea clearance than hollow-fiber configurations do in this setting. Parallel plates have less flow resistance, which may result in less unstirred layers at the membrane-blood interface and potentially less clotting. However, in pumped systems such as CVVH, flat-plate dialyzers were not shown to have an advantage over hollow-fiber designs in terms of prolonging circuit longevity, and there was a nonsignificant trend favoring the latter.[23]

The membrane represents approximately 95% of the blood contact area in the circuit.[5] The perfect nonthrombogenic membrane material remains elusive. Membrane failure occurs secondary to red blood cell, platelet, and protein coating of the membrane. The filter can represent the point in the ECC where the flow is the slowest, creating an environment favorable to red blood cell aggregation, especially if macromolecules such as fibrinogen and artificial plasma substitutes are present and facilitate the creation of molecular bridges.[3,25] However, when experiments using membranes with larger surface areas were carried out,[23] the thought being that the larger the membrane, the longer the period of time before saturation and failure, no difference was observed in circuit life between membranes of 0.75 versus 1.3 m².

The degree of biocompatibility may affect the thrombotic potential of a membrane. Both cellulosic and synthetic polymer membranes activate the complement system, but synthetic membranes adsorb the activated products more readily, leading to less overall stimulation of the system.[26] It has been difficult to determine whether thrombogenicity differs between cellulose and synthetic membranes; the results have been contradictory, possibly because of the variety of anticoagulation methods chosen. Polyacrylonitrile (PAN) membranes have been found to be associated with a higher clotting frequency than polyamide membranes in a number of studies.[15,27] This may have to do with the high negative charge of a PAN membrane, which has been shown to correlate with the degree of activation of Hageman's factor, kallikrein, and bradykinin. In keeping with this hypothesis, a study comparing polyamide and PAN membranes showed that the latter was associated with a greater effect on the levels of TAT.[28] Membranes with higher porosity may lead to removal of the anticoagulant (e.g., r-hirudin), whereas an unmodified cellulosic membrane may result in its accumulation.

Some membranes can be precoated with heparin (e.g., AN69-ST [Hospal, Lyon, France], Hemophan [Akzo, Wuppertal, Germany]), which allows circuits to remain patent longer with either no anticoagulant or with reduced anticoagulant.[5,29] Grafting of polyethyleneimine onto an AN69 PAN membrane decreases surface electronegativity, and the surface then repels cationic plasma molecules, including high-molecular-weight kininogen. Conversely, strongly anionic heparin is tightly bound to the modified membrane and is included in the blood-derived membrane coating the synthetic polymer.[29] Multiple studies have looked at the increased biocompatibility of heparin-coated surfaces and have found a decreased adsorption of fibrinogen, diminished platelet activation and aggregation, decreased complement activation, and less formation of platelet-leukocyte aggregates.[30-32] The advantages of such a heparin-bonded circuit would theoretically benefit patients most if low ATIII levels were first supplemented.

Low-molecular-weight heparin (LMWH)-coated circuits also were shown to be effective, without additional anticoagulation, in intermittent hemodialysis patients with normal coagulation parameters.[32] This study confirmed the increased biocompatibility of heparin-coated surfaces, although TAT levels rose after the fourth hour of dialysis if no additional dalteparin was given. There remains some controversy as to the relative importance, in regard to hemocompatibility, of the interaction of surface-bound heparin with ATIII (and subsequent inactivation of key coagulation factors), compared with the adsorption and cleavage of plasma proteins with these coated membranes.[30] Studies have shown that, to produce valid results, in vitro experiments evaluating the thrombogenic potential of membranes using platelet adhesion and protein adsorption measurements should always use non-anticoagulated blood.[31]

The optimal life requirement of a filter used for CRRT remains controversial. Some studies show that high-flux membranes become maximally coated with pro-inflammatory molecules by 24 hours, and if attempts are made to extend the life beyond that point, these molecules are released back into the circulation.[33] A low dialysate pH can contribute to dialyzer clotting, although data are scarce since the initial mention of this problem in 1977.[34]

Blood Flow

In pumped systems, the pump speed setting does not necessarily reflect actual delivered blood flow. A recent study utilizing a customized miniature Doppler flow probe (mounted on the tubing before the filter) coupled to a computer allowed for flow wave analysis during CRRT.[35] The results showed a high frequency of flow reductions in the medium range (34% to 67% reduction) in the diastolic phase (the trough period after the forward stroke of the roller cam) which were not detected by the machine's alarms. The authors found a strong inverse correlation between the frequencies of these medium-level flow reductions and filter life. The correlation was even stronger than the correlation with standard anticoagulation variables. The reductions in flow were associated with backward flow of blood and stasis, which, in the setting of continued ultrafiltration, would result in further hemoconcentration across the filter, contributing to clotting. Additionally, shear stress could be increased, and stasis could increase the duration of the interaction between blood and membrane, leading to prolonged exposure to the activated coagulation cascade. The authors speculated that possible triggers to these flow reductions might include catheter kinking or dysfunction and changes in patient position, such as sitting up with subsequent underfilling of neck veins. Any degree of catheter dysfunction would contribute to these low blood flows.

Effects of Ultrafiltration

Low blood flow rates and excessive ultrafiltration can lead to detrimental increases in filtration fraction, resulting in local increases in the hematocrit at the level of the dialyzer membrane, which leads to increased clotting. This results not only from the alterations in flow characteristics (rheological effects) but also from the effect of convective mass transfer. In an experiment using polysulfone dialyzers, this variable was higher with hemofiltration/hemodiafiltration than with high-flux hemodialysis, because of the greater total ultrafiltration volume, and resulted in increased procoagulatory activity, as measured by TAT (associated with intravascular thrombin formation) and D-dimer levels.[36] Although this finding was not associated with increased filter clotting risk, the increased procoagulatory profile was believed to be secondary to the fluid shear stress generated by the filtration of large amounts of fluid from the blood, with the platelets at the periphery being more affected, and subsequent activation of the coagulation system.[37] Maintenance of filtration fractions of 20% or less is optimal. This can be accomplished through the use of prefilter dilution and adjustments in blood flow rates.[38]

Predilution versus Postdilution

Predilution reduces the viscosity of the blood, which can help prevent buildup of cellular sludge at the level of the membrane. Several studies have demonstrated increased circuit life with predilution versus postdilution.[39] One such study showed a median circuit life of 18 versus 13 hours,[40] and another, more recent, study achieved durations of 45.7 versus 16.1 hours with predilution versus postdilution, respectively.[41] A recent crossover study did not demonstrate such a difference, but it was limited by small sample size.[10] However, the study did demonstrate that postdilution resulted in a higher number of filters clotting within the first hour—two to seven, as opposed to none when predilution was used.

Use of Erythropoietin

Erythropoietin has been found to decrease bleeding time, to increase the levels of vWF and fibrinogen, and to reduce the levels of ATIII and protein C.[5,42-45] It has been blamed for contributing to increased thrombosis. A direct effect on platelets, in terms of increased adhesion and aggregability, has also been demonstrated in hemodialysis patients after 20 weeks of therapy.[46] It is possible that the effect is dosage related, because higher doses were found to be associated with lower prothrombin fragment concentrations.[21]

Hematocrit

Hematocrit is the most important determinant of viscosity, and a higher hematocrit can increase the chances of thrombosis. Exogenous erythropoietin can add to this risk, apart from its effects on platelets. Blood transfusion into the circuit proximal to the filter can lead to clotting and should be avoided, especially if no anticoagulant is being used. The advantages of the better flow that mild anemia might provide need to be balanced against the risks of decreased oxygen delivery to the tissues.

Side Effects of Anticoagulants

Heparin binds to platelet factor IV and forms an epitope; it is this site that can trigger the formation of antibodies in 20% to 30% of patients, with 1% to 3% of patients developing clinical thrombocytopenia and heparin-induced thrombocytopenia.[47] Two-thirds of these patients will go on to develop thromboembolic manifestations. Heparin does block thrombin generation, resulting in decreased fibrin formation; however, it does not prevent the interactions of platelets, leukocytes, and factor XII with foreign surfaces; indeed, it can facilitate these interactions.[3] Heparin can also lead to consumption of ATIII. The LMWH enoxaparin does not cause endothelial cell activation and release of cell adhesion molecules.[36,48] It is believed to reduce monocyte adhesion to vascular endothelial cells by inhibiting lipopolysaccharide-induced E-selectin expression as well as intercellular adhesion molecule 1 (ICAM-1) expression induced by tumor necrosis factor.[48]

Citrate anticoagulation has been associated with greater increases in ATIII over time. In a scanning electron microscopy study, citrate anticoagulation resulted in a lower dialyzer clotting score than unfractionated heparin or LMWH, potentially contributing to improvement in biocompatibility.[49] The use of citrate has also been shown to decrease lactoferrin release from neutrophils in hemodialysis; this is secondary to citrate's effects on ionized calcium, which is believed to be an important mediator of neutrophil degranulation.[50]

The Endothelium

Normally, the vascular endothelium performs both anticoagulant and antithrombotic functions. Endothelial cells produce heparin sulfate, which binds ATIII and potentiates its protease inhibitor activity. This results in excellent local control of thrombin generation. The various factors produced by or associated with the endothelium are numerous. Those with procoagulant activity include plasminogen activator inhibitor, tissue factor, and vWF. The endothelium contributes anticoagulant activity through ATIII, glucose aminoglycans, nitric oxide, prostacyclin, protein S, thrombomodulin, tissue factor pathway inhibitor, and t-PA.[3] Disruption of normal endothelial cell function, such as occurs in sepsis and inflammatory disorders, can decrease the anticoagulant and fibrinolytic activity and shift the balance toward clotting.[3]

CONCLUSION

Patients with renal dysfunction are at risk for thrombosis secondary to being in a hypercoagulable state. If they require dialysis, the risk is increased because of blood and circuit interactions. On the other hand, they are at risk for hemorrhage secondary to the effects of uremia on platelet function, as well as the effects of any anticoagulant used during their treatments. Whether and when circuit clotting ultimately occurs depends on a balance among these factors and other contributing factors from the patient's clinical situation, such as the presence of sepsis or DIC. The goal of the nephrologist remains prolongation of ECC life, in the safest manner possible for the patient. Precoating of membranes with unfractionated heparin or LMWH seems to render them more biocompatible. The use of these membranes, as well as the smart use of activated protein C in certain situations, may allow for less clotting with reduced doses of systemic heparin. More experience is accumulating with the use of citrate, which in experienced centers is safe. Studies of citrate show less activation of neutrophils and less dialyzer clotting compared with heparin. Use of replacement fluids in prefilter mode and avoidance of excessive ultrafiltration and blood flow reductions can also lead to improved circuit patency.

Key Points

1. There exists a fine balance between clotting and bleeding, which is affected by various plasma, cellular, and endothelial factors.

2. This balance is upset in patients with severe kidney disease, with most of these patients being hypercoagulable.

3. The extracorporeal circuit adds an additional element of complexity, because it removes the endothelial component from the mix.

4. Favorable extracorporeal circuit design, catheter characteristics, membrane biocompatibility, avoidance of excessive ultrafiltration and variations in blood flow rate, and the use of prefilter fluid replacement all figure importantly in maintaining circuit patency.

5. Knowledge of these elements, as well as the judicious use of proper anticoagulants, can help the clinician to safely balance the need for circuit longevity with the need to avoid unwanted bleeding.

Key References

3. Webb AR, Mythen MG, Jacobson D, Mackie IJ: Maintaining blood flow in the extracorporeal circuit: Haemostasis and anticoagulation. Intensive Care Med 1995;21:84-93.
5. Ward DM: Anticoagulation in patients on hemodialysis. In Nissenson AR, Fine RN (eds): Clinical Dialysis, 4th ed. New York, McGraw-Hill, 2005.
21. Ambuhl PM, Wuthrich RP, Korte W, et al: Plasma hypercoagulability in haemodialysis patients: Impact of dialysis and anticoagulation. Nephrol Dial Transplant 1997;12:2355-2364.
23. Baldwin I, Tan HK, Bridge N, Bellomo R: Possible strategies to prolong circuit life during hemofiltration: Three controlled studies. Ren Fail 2002;24:839-848.
35. Baldwin I, Bellomo R, Koch B: Blood flow reductions during continuous renal replacement therapy and circuit life. Intensive Care Med 2004;30:2074-2079.

See the companion Expert Consult website for the complete reference list.

CHAPTER 215

Principles of Fluid Manufacturing and Sterilization for Renal Replacement Therapy in the Intensive Care Unit

Ingrid Ledebo and Anders Wieslander

OBJECTIVES

This chapter will:
1. Define the role of the fluids used for various forms of renal replacement therapy (RRT).
2. Discuss specific fluid requirements and their impact on manufacturing and sterilization.
3. Describe commercial manufacturing of sterile solutions and discuss the use of these fluids for RRT in the intensive care unit (ICU).
4. Discuss the preparation of sterile solutions in hospital pharmacies.
5. Describe the preparation of sterile solutions as an integrated part of the RRT treatment system (i.e., on-line preparation) and discuss the use of these fluids in the ICU.

THE FLUID ROUTE DETERMINES THE MODE OF THERAPY

In all forms of renal replacement therapy (RRT), fluid of special composition is the vehicle for the blood purification, and a membrane is the means of separation and selection. The relation between fluid and blood determines the mode of treatment (Fig. 215-1). In hemodialysis, fluid and blood are separated by the membrane, forming a concentration gradient that drives diffusive transport. The fluid is referred to as *dialysis fluid* (Europe) or *dialysate* (United States) in this application, and because it is separated from blood, there is no requirement for it to be sterile. In hemofiltration, the fluid is infused into the blood, and solute removal is achieved via convective transport as a consequence of ultrafiltration. In this case, the fluid is referred to as the *substitution* or *replacement solution*, and it must be sterile and nonpyrogenic. Hemodiafiltration is a combination of both therapies; it requires both dialysis fluid for diffusive transport and substitution solution for convective transport. These modes of dialysis and their requirements for fluids of different quality are valid for all forms of RRT, whether acute or chronic, continuous or intermittent.[1] Substitution solution can be administered either before the filter (predilution) or after the filter (postdilution). In predilution mode, the fluid should more correctly be referred to as *diluting solution*; in postdilution mode, the term *substitution solution* is appropriate because the fluid substitutes for excess ultrafiltration.

GENERAL FLUID REQUIREMENTS

The composition of the purifying fluid, whether it is used as dialysis fluid or for dilution or substitution, should in principle mirror the composition of normal plasma water, because normalization of body fluids is the goal. A slight concentration gradient should be created in favor of the desired direction of transport. The gradient could be somewhat larger for dialysis fluid than for substitution solution, because the former must cross an initial barrier, the membrane, before it can be effective. The gradient could also be larger for intermittent treatments of short duration compared with longer, more frequent or continuous treatments, because long treatment intervals require a certain overcorrection of the blood composition. To achieve more rapid exchange of a solute, the concentration gradient for that specific solute should be increased. This applies in both directions, and it means that solutes not present in the fluid will be lost from blood. However, large concentration gradients and rapid solute exchange should be avoided, because such conditions may lead to disequilibrium symptoms.

The amount of fluid required for a specific therapy depends on the flow rates and the duration of treatment. The trend today favors increasing fluid volumes for all forms of acute RRT, because there is evidence that this might improve the outcome.[2,3] A state-of-the-art prescription for continuous veno-venous hemofiltration (CVVH) requires approximately 60 L of substitution solution, and a continuous veno-venous hemodiafiltration (CVVHDF) treatment would need additionally 25 to 35 L of dialysis fluid, both applied in postdilution to an average-size patient over a period of 24 hours. For similar therapies and modes, the total amount of fluid is an overall indicator of the degree of blood purification. When quantifying therapies with predilution, compensation should be made for the degree of dilution, which affects the ultrafiltrate to the same extent as the blood.[4]

SPECIFIC FLUID REQUIREMENTS

Buffer

The buffer component of fluids for dialysis needs special attention. Acid-base disturbances are common in patients with acute kidney injury, and correction of the acid-base balance is one of the main objectives of the RRT. From a

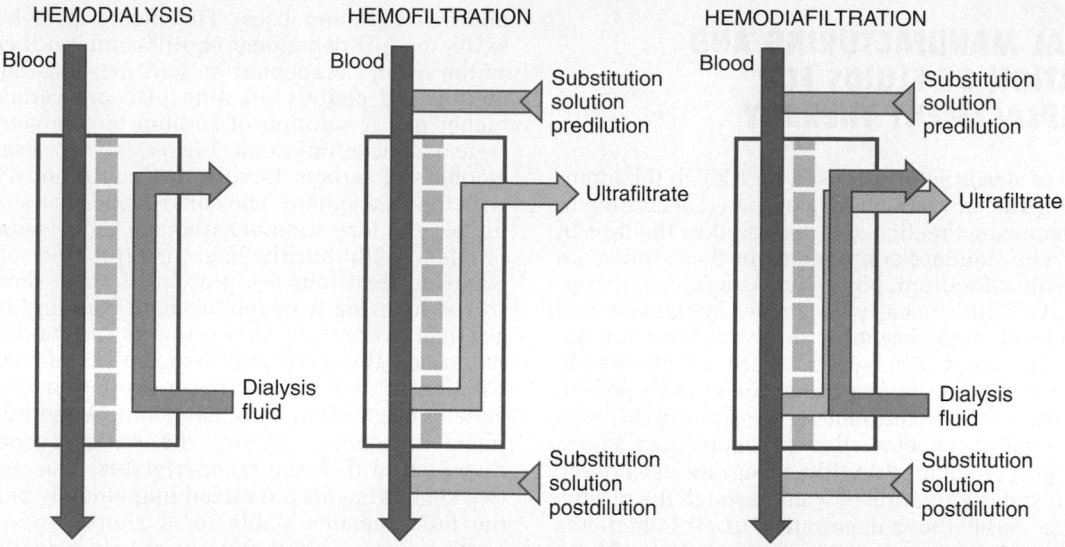

FIGURE 215-1. The relationship between fluid and blood determines the type of renal replacement therapy. In hemodialysis, the dialysis fluid is separated from blood by the membrane in the filter. In hemofiltration, the sterile and nonpyrogenic substitution solution is mixed with blood, either before the filter (predilution) or after it (postdilution). Hemodiafiltration is a combination of hemodialysis and hemofiltration.

physiological point of view, bicarbonate is the ideal buffer, but practical and economical issues limit the use of bicarbonate-containing fluids, and many patients with acute conditions are still treated with lactate-based fluids. Lactate and other possible buffer sources (e.g., acetate, citrate) need to be metabolized before buffer equivalents are generated. If this metabolism is disturbed or delayed, bicarbonate will be lost from blood, and the acidosis will be aggravated. At the same time, lactate accumulates, and this may be associated with hemodynamic instability. However, in patients without severe metabolic problems, it appears that lactate can be safely used as a buffer source, although there is widespread preference for the physiological buffer, bicarbonate.[5,6] The practical problems with bicarbonate-containing fluids are mainly of chemical nature. A physiological solution containing ions of calcium, magnesium, and bicarbonate is supersaturated, and in vitro precipitation will proceed with time. Although a lower pH would keep the bicarbonate ions in solution, it would also lead to an unstable situation, with formation and evaporation of carbon dioxide. All of this can be avoided by keeping bicarbonate separated from the divalent ions and the acid during storage.

Microbiology

All fluids for infusion must be sterile and nonpyrogenic. Although this statement is obvious, the practical interpretation may not be so, and we need to refer to the *European Pharmacopoeia* for a definition. *Sterility* means absence of all viable microorganisms with a degree of assurance of 1 in 1 million.[7] To appreciate this criterion, we need to remember that bacteria grow logarithmically, and reduction of the number of cells in a solution to an acceptable level does not mean that the number will remain as such. This is the reason for the safety margin of 6 magnitudes. Pyrogens, or more specifically endotoxins, are parts of dead bacteria that originate mainly from the cell wall and

have a strong immunogenic effect, leading to cell activation and cytokine release. All sterile solutions used for CRRT should be regarded as infusion solutions, whether they are used as substitution solution or dialysis fluid, and whether they are classified as drug or device, respectively. According to the *Pharmacopoeia*, these solutions may contain up to 0.25 endotoxin unit per milliliter (EU/mL), a level that appears to be based on infusion of limited quantities of fluid.[7] However, considering that a safe dose in healthy humans should not exceed 5 EU per kilogram of body weight and per hour, fluid quality in RRT with large volumes of infusion solution becomes a critical issue.

As already stated, dialysis fluid need not be sterile because it is separated from blood by a membrane that is impermeable to intact bacterial cells. However, some dialysis membranes are permeable to bacterial products in the fluid, as evidenced by monocyte activation across membranes under in vitro conditions.[8] When patients are dialyzed with purified fluid, clinically relevant differences in terms of reduced levels of the major inflammatory markers, C-reactive protein and interleukin-6, have been observed.[9,10] Based on such evidence, ultrapure dialysis fluid ($<10^{-1}$ colony-forming units [CFU]/mL and <0.03 EU/mL) is now recommended by some clinical guidelines.[11] When using high-flux membranes in sustained low-efficiency dialysis (SLED) applications, there may be concern that contaminants from the nonsterile dialysis fluid are backfiltered into blood. However, as long as ultrapure fluid is used and the dialyzer membrane can adsorb small quantities of endotoxin, backfiltration can be considered safe.[12] Most modern dialysis machines for chronic treatment are equipped with an ultrafilter in the flow path to provide ultrapure dialysis fluid, and this is as strongly recommended for acute as for chronic applications. CRRT machines that are specially designed for acute treatments do not have fluid preparation capability and operate with prepackaged fluid, which therefore must be sterile.

INDUSTRIAL MANUFACTURING AND STERILIZATION OF FLUIDS FOR RENAL REPLACEMENT THERAPY

The majority of sterile solutions used for RRT in the intensive care unit (ICU) are industrially prepared according to Good Manufacturing Practice and delivered to the unit in plastic bags. The standard components in these fluids are the chloride salts of sodium, potassium, calcium, and magnesium; a buffer that is usually lactate or bicarbonate; and glucose. The label on the bag must show the exact composition of the fluid, and concentrations are not allowed to deviate more than ±5% during the entire storage period, usually 2 years. The requirement on sodium is even stricter, and pharmacopoeias allow no more than ±2.5% deviation. If polyvinylchloride (PVC) bags are used, there may be significant evaporation of water through the plastic; this slowly increases the concentration of all ingredients and thus determines the maximum storage time. These fluids are prepared by dissolving the chemicals in water that has been treated in several steps to remove particles, ions, and microbiological contaminants. The quality should correspond to "water for injection" (i.e., <0.25 EU/mL). Large tanks which typically contain thousands of liters are used, and the composition of the fluid is verified by analysis of samples. When the solution fulfils the specification, it is filtered and packaged in 5 L plastic bags. Each bag is covered with an overwrap, placed on a large trolley, and brought to terminal heat sterilization. To avoid excessive microbiological growth, the entire process, from dissolving of the chemicals in the tank until terminal sterilization, should take no more than 24 hours.

The required sterility assurance level (SAL) of 10^{-6} is achieved by exposure to superheated water in autoclaves loaded with up to 1000 bags. The unit used to quantify the sterilization effect, F_0, is the exposure time in minutes at 121°C. F_0 relates to temperature exponentially and to time linearly; the total sterilizing effect is calculated as the sum of all effective time-temperature combinations throughout the autoclaving process. To guarantee sterility of all products in a batch, it is important that each and every bag reach a minimum F_0 value of 8; that is, the sterilizing effect should correspond to 8 minutes at 121°C. This is valid for products with a bioburden (number of microorganisms in the fluid before sterilization) of less than 100 CFU/L. In well-controlled production facilities, the bioburden is normally close to 0 CFU/L. In reality, most manufacturers apply a concept of "overkill" and aim at an F_0 of 15 or greater to secure sterility of all products. It should be noted that each sterilization cycle takes hours, rather than minutes, because of the time needed to heat and cool several tons of fluid. The obtained F_0 value for individual bags may vary considerably, depending on product design and position in the autoclave.

Buffer-Related Problems Connected with Sterilization and Storage

The common electrolytes do not normally give rise to any stability problems during sterilization or storage, but the choice of buffer can complicate the issue. Lactate, acetate, and citrate are stable buffer sources that can be mixed with the other electrolytes in single-compartment bags without problems. Bicarbonate, however, is unstable and requires multicompartment bags. The bicarbonate buffer system exists in a pH-dependent equilibrium, with carbonic acid as the major component at acid pH, bicarbonate ions at neutral and slightly alkaline pH, and carbonate ions at higher pH. A solution of sodium bicarbonate, in physiological concentration or higher, always contains small amounts of carbon dioxide that continuously equilibrate with the atmosphere. The consequence is a slowly increasing pH and formation of carbonate. This leads to the other problem with bicarbonate: precipitation of carbonates when divalent ions are present. Both of these issues are solved by using two-compartment bags and multilayered, gas-tight overwraps. This prevents carbon dioxide evaporation and therefore stabilizes the pH of the bicarbonate solution. It also avoids the precipitation of calcium carbonate, magnesium carbonate, and, when relevant, phosphate carbonate, because the critical components are dissolved in different compartments. The contents of the two compartments are mixed immediately before use, and the fluid remains stable for a short period of time. In certain cases, a small amount of acid, usually acetic acid or lactic acid, is needed to create the necessary pH and keep the bicarbonate ions in solution. The anion is later metabolized to generate buffer equivalents. Any evidence of precipitation in bicarbonate solutions immediately after mixing indicates composition errors, and the solution might be unsafe to use.[13]

Glucose-Related Problems Connected with Sterilization and Storage

Historically, fluids designed for peritoneal dialysis were utilized as dialysis fluid or replacement fluid in CRRT treatments because of lack of alternatives. Because these fluids contain at least 1.5% glucose, there is a risk of hyperglycemia. Today, many RRT fluids contain physiological concentrations of glucose to avoid loss of energy. Whenever glucose solutions are exposed to light or elevated temperatures, glucose degradation products (GDPs) are generated. Research with peritoneal dialysis fluids has shown that GDPs are strongly cytotoxic and promote decline in the residual renal function.[14-16] They have also been associated with reduced long-term survival in patients undergoing peritoneal dialysis.[17] To avoid GDP formation, glucose should always be sterilized at pH 2 to 3.5, preferably in a concentrated solution.[18] This necessitates dilution and mixing with a slightly alkaline solution before use, which is facilitated by multicompartment bags. In analyzing some of the commercially available, single-compartment, glucose-containing solutions used for RRT, we have identified elevated levels of the following toxic components: formaldehyde (approximately 5 μmol/L), acetaldehyde (100 μmol/L), 3-deoxyglucosone (25 μmol/L), and 3,4-dideoxyglucosone (2 μmol/L) (unpublished data). Although these concentrations are only 10% to 20% of those found in peritoneal dialysis fluids, the total exposure may be considerable, because the volumes are large and the solutions are often mixed directly with blood. Another source of GDPs may be the glucose solutions given as intravenous nutrition supplements to patients in ICUs. These fluids are heat sterilized and contain up to 800 μmol/L of 3-deoxyglucosone, a highly toxic GDP. Exposure to GDPs might well have contributed to the recently observed association between the amount of infused glucose and mortality in an ICU populaton.[19] Although the clinical relevance of GDPs has not been

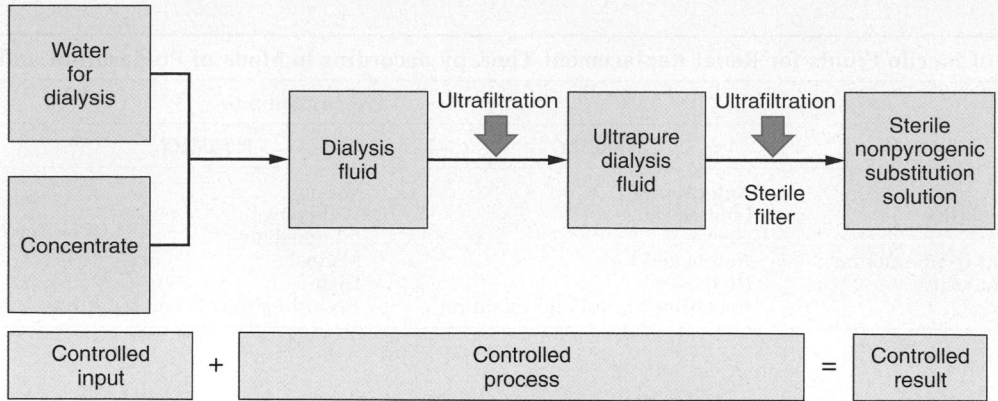

FIGURE 215-2. Process control for on-line preparation of sterile, nonpyrogenic substitution solution for convective renal replacement therapy. To achieve the required quality levels, the entire process must be operated with validated components and appropriate hygiene.

investigated for critically ill patients, one should probably avoid exposing these patients to fluids containing reactive carbonyls such as GDPs.

Preparation of Sterile Solutions for Renal Replacement Therapy on Prescription

Today, several fluid compositions are available as commercially prepared sterile solutions for renal intensive care. However, the introduction of new fluids is delayed by regulatory procedures, and bicarbonate-containing substitution solutions have only recently become available in North America. There may also be a need for specialized fluids to treat certain disorders. To satisfy these requirements, and motivated by economic incentives, it is not uncommon for hospital pharmacies to deliver solutions on prescription. Fluid preparation in local pharmacies may range from full production, consisting of weighing and mixing raw chemicals with water and sterilizing the solution, to simply spiking bags of sterile water or saline with the desired electrolytes.[20] Although the flexibility of in-house–produced, tailor-made fluids is valuable, manual preparation can never reach the same level of quality control as that applied industrially. Risks are associated with microbiological contamination and with compounding errors, either of which could lead to significant adverse clinical outcome. A recent analysis from several pediatric critical care programs demonstrated that most of the reported medication errors in CRRT were due to incorrect composition of the dialysis fluid.[21] All compounding errors were reported from programs using manually prepared fluids. One example of a severe mistake during preparation of CRRT fluids was a mix-up of potassium and sodium that led to death from hyperkalemia in at least one patient.[22]

GENERAL PRINCIPLES FOR ON-LINE PREPARATION OF STERILE FLUID

Patients undergoing chronic treatment with convective therapies may use 20 to 100 L of sterile substitution solution per session, depending on the mode of therapy. Today, this fluid is most commonly prepared by the dialysis equipment itself, as an integrated part of the treatment. The absolute characteristics of on-line prepared fluid are that it is continuously prepared and immediately used, without intermediate packaging or storage. This way of preparing sterile fluids involves mixing water and dialysis concentrates, both of well-defined microbiological quality, in a hygienically maintained flow path and subjecting the fluid to stepwise ultrafiltration using validated filters with known retention properties (Fig. 215-2).[23] The chain of strict quality control must not be broken by sampling or packaging, which would introduce a risk of external contamination followed by bacterial growth. Because the fluid cannot be tested before use, strict quality control of input components and process parameters is necessary to safeguard the quality of the final fluid.

On-Line Preparation, Regulations, and Safety

On-line preparation involving sterile filtration and immediate use is not listed among the sterilization methods in the *Pharmacopoeia*, and it has therefore been important to demonstrate that such fluid can meet the regulatory requirements for sterility.[7] The *Pharmacopoeia* recognizes that sterility cannot be proven by testing and that it must be assured by validation of the production process. The entire on-line process has been validated by in vitro studies in which the fluid was tested at critical sampling points along the flow path, using sensitive microbiological methods.[23] The final fluid quality is achieved by application of sterile ultrafilters with a guaranteed reduction of 7 logarithms to fluid that is at least ultrapure ($<10^{-1}$ CFU/mL). This combination more than fulfills the SAL of 10^{-6} required by the *Pharmacopoeia*. Satisfactory fluid quality has also been shown in practice by the absence of viable bacteria in volumes of fluid corresponding to those typically used for a treatment. In vivo testing of the fluid has shown that there is no sign of cell activation or cytokine production when large volumes of on-line prepared fluid are used in convective treatments, and judging from these results, on-line prepared fluids may even be of superior quality compared to bag-sterilized fluid.[24,25]

TABLE 215-1

Characteristics of Sterile Fluids for Renal Replacement Therapy according to Mode of Preparation and Sterilization

	Preparation Site		
CHARACTERISTIC	INDUSTRY	PHARMACY	DIALYSIS UNIT
Sterilization	Autoclaving	Various	Filtration
Composition flexibility	Limited range	Wide range	Wide range
Cost	High	Intermediate	Low
Labor component in production	Automated	Manual	Automated
Labor component at use	High	High	Low
Volume limitation	According to cost and handling	According to cost and handling	No

On-Line Prepared Fluid for Renal Replacement Therapy in the Intensive Care Unit

Considering the present demands for increasing fluid volumes for RRT in the ICU, on-line fluid preparation fulfills an important requirement, because practically unlimited volumes of high-quality fluids—ultrapure dialysis fluid as well as sterile substitution solution—of individualized composition can be prepared at the bedside as part of the RRT. Still, dialysis equipment with on-line capability is not widely used in the ICU setting, because of a combination of regulatory obstacles, lack of proper water treatment, and staff issues. On-line dialysis machines for convective therapies, although widely used in Europe and Asia, are not approved in the United States. The water required for all forms of dialysis must comply with current standards for "water for dialysis" (<100 CFU/mL and <0.25 EU/mL). All chronic dialysis units have special water treatment equipment consisting of appropriate pretreatment with particle filters, carbon filters, and softeners, followed by single or double reverse osmosis. Intensive care units may not have access to water of this quality, and, although compact water treatment equipment could be installed, it still presents a drawback. Finally, ICU staff are not trained to operate chronic dialysis equipment and often do not see it as their task.

Realizing the advantages of on-line prepared solutions, it may be tempting for staff in the pharmacy or the dialysis unit to set up a minifactory for fluid manufacturing and fill bags with on-line prepared fluid. However, even if they take all possible precautions (e.g., disinfected connections, sterile bags, aseptic filling technique), this process is associated with a great risk of contamination. To allow time for microbiological testing, the fluids would need to be stored for at least a couple of days, but no tests are sensitive enough to prove sterility, and storage of the solutions would increase the potential bioburden. This procedure is neither approved nor recommended. However, in hospitals without access to commercially prepared or pharmacy-prepared sterile solutions, it may be the only possibility to treat patients with CRRT in the ICU.

CONCLUSION

Blood purification in RRT requires physiological fluids of high quality. In convective therapies, fluids are used to dilute blood or to substitute for ultrafiltered volume. These fluids must be sterile and nonpyrogenic, because they are mixed with blood. When diffusive transport is applied, the fluid is not in direct contact with blood and can therefore be ultrapure. In chronic dialysis units, these different fluids are prepared by the dialysis machines. However, in ICUs, the infrastructure required for such fluid preparation (i.e., water treatment, dialysis equipment, and trained staff) may not be available, and prepacked, sterile solutions are used (Table 215-1). These solutions should be prepared and stored in multicompartment bags to avoid chemical problems with bicarbonate and glucose. As long as the volume requirement is reasonable and fluid of appropriate composition is available, it is most convenient to work with prepackaged solutions. Patient safety and clinical efficiency favor commercially produced fluids, whereas flexibility and price may support local pharmacy production. Still, the risks associated with any preparation involving manual steps should not be underestimated. Today, a wide range of commercially prepared, sterile solutions with physiological composition is available in most countries for all forms of RRT in the ICU.

Key Points

1. The role of fluids in all forms of renal replacement therapy is to drive the blood purification.
2. The composition of these fluids should be physiological, mirroring the composition of plasma water.
3. When mixed with blood for convective transport, the fluids must be sterile and nonpyrogenic; when separated from blood by a semipermeable membrane and used for diffusion, the fluids can be ultrapure.
4. Industrially prepared fluids, prepared according to Good Manufacturing Practices, carry less risk than hospital-prepared fluids. Multicompartment bags should be used for fluids containing bicarbonate or glucose.
5. Sterile fluids can also be prepared as an integrated part of the treatment using validated on-line equipment, provided that the required infrastructure is available in the intensive care unit. This approach is labor-saving and cost-effective, especially for the large volumes increasingly required for continuous renal replacement therapy.

Key References

9. Ward RA: Ultrapure dialysate. Semin Dial 2004;17:489-497.
18. Erixon M, Wieslander A, Lindén T, et al: How to avoid glucose degradation productions in peritoneal dialysis fluids. Perit Dial Int 2006;26:490-497.
20. Palevsky PM: Continuous renal replacement therapy component selection: Replacement fluid and dialysis solutions. Semin Dial 1996;9:107-111.

23. Ledebo I: On-line preparation of solutions for dialysis: Practical aspects versus safety and regulations. J Am Soc Nephrol 2002;13:S78-S83.

See the companion Expert Consult website for the complete reference list.

CHAPTER 216

Starting and Stopping Renal Replacement Therapy in the Critically Ill

John T. Bestoso, Roy Mathew, and Ravindra L. Mehta

OBJECTIVES

This chapter will:
1. Evaluate the factors that determine need for dialytic intervention in critically ill patients and describe the current status of initiation of renal replacement therapy in the intensive care unit (ICU).
2. Define and contrast approaches for renal replacement and renal support in the ICU.
3. Discuss the practical aspects of initiating and withdrawing dialysis in critically ill patients.

Most cases of acute kidney injury (AKI) in critical care settings are caused by acute tubular necrosis, effective volume depletion, or their variants, including sepsis syndrome and toxic nephropathy. Although these generally are reversible processes, a significant number of patients require renal replacement therapy (RRT). When renal replacement or renal support is required, there is a far worse prognosis than with lesser degrees of renal injury.[1-3] Several dialysis techniques are now available for RRT to manage AKI. Acute intermittent hemodialysis, peritoneal dialysis, and continuous techniques are the main treatment modalities. Considerable debates have ensued over the choice of modality in the acute setting, especially for the critically ill, and are discussed in Chapter 218.

An important consideration in the dialytic management of AKI is defining the goals of therapy. Several issues must be considered, including the timing of the intervention, the amount and frequency of dialysis, and the duration of therapy. In practice, these issues are based on individual preferences and experience, and no set criteria are followed. There is a paucity of information on the criteria for initiating and stopping RRT. Dialytic intervention in AKI is usually considered when there is clinical evidence of uremic symptoms or biochemical evidence of solute and fluid imbalance. Most nephrologists will intervene with dialysis if the patient has a blood urea nitrogen (BUN) value greater than 100 mg/dL, hyperkalemia, or marked acidosis, or if there is evidence of fluid overload unresponsive to diuretics, central nervous system manifestations, a pericardial rub, or gastrointestinal hemorrhage attributed to uremia. Unfortunately, there is no consensus on the timing of intervention for AKI. In patients with end-stage renal disease, dialysis is usually not initiated until creatinine clearances are less than 5 mL/min (range, 5 to 10 mL/min) or the patient is symptomatic. Extrapolation of these criteria to AKI is common but is problematic, because the strategy in treating AKI is to minimize and avoid uremic complications, whereas in end-stage renal disease the aim is to keep the patient off dialysis as long as possible. Therefore, it is not necessary to wait for progressive uremia to initiate dialytic support. It is apparent that there needs to be a reappraisal of current practices in this area. This chapter addresses the pertinent issues that should be considered for initiating and stopping RRT in the critically ill patient.

TRADITIONAL INDICATIONS FOR RENAL REPLACEMENT THERAPY

There is little consensus among nephrologists and intensivists regarding indications for starting RRT in a specific patient. In a survey by Ricci and associates,[4] 560 attendees of a critical care nephrology conference listed 90 combinations of indications for initiating treatment. Oliguria/anuria was the most frequent choice, at only 27%. This is less surprising when one considers that AKI has multiple causes and clinical manifestations. The unique combination of factors in a particular case should dictate the timing and type of therapy offered. Although the balance between risks and benefits of invasive procedures must be considered carefully in the individual patient, evidence in favor of early intervention has grown steadily. In 1998, Bellomo and Ronco proposed 12 indications for initiating dialysis in critically ill patients.[5] In their schema, combinations of two or more indications make initiation of RRT "urgent

TABLE 216-1

Some Criteria for Initiation of Renal Replacement Therapy (RRT) in Adult Critically Ill Patients*

Commonly Encountered Indications
Volume overload with severe respiratory or cardiac manifestations
Oliguria or anuria
Output <400 mL/day
Output less than obligatory input
Hyperkalemia with $[K^+] > 6.5$
Acidemia with pH < 7.1-7.2
Azotemia with BUN > 76-100[†]
Creatinine clearance <10 mL/min[†]
AKI after cardiac surgery
Less Commonly Encountered Indications
Poisoning or drug overdose with dialyzable toxin
Uremic encephalopathy and neuropathy
Uremic platelet dysfunction

AKI, acute kidney injury; BUN, blood urea nitrogen.
*The presence of any one of these indications may be sufficient to initiate RRT. The presence of two or more makes RRT urgent. Combined derangements should lead to initiation of therapy before the suggested limits have been reached.
[†]When prolonged for 1-2 days without evidence of renal recovery.
Adapted from Bellomo R, Ronco CS: Indications and criteria for initiating renal replacement therapy in the intensive care unit. Kidney Int 1998;66(Suppl):S106-S109.

and mandatory." Their original indications are presented in Table 216-1.

Hyperkalemia, severe hyperphosphatemia, severe hyperuricemia, severe acidemia, and uremia-related complications (coma, pericarditis, seizures) are all accepted indications for starting dialysis. However, there is wide variability regarding the timing of initiation of dialysis, even when these indications are present. Aside from situations in which there are severe derangements, most nephrologists have a tendency to avoid dialysis for as long as possible. Two major factors contribute to the decision to delay dialysis. First, the dialysis procedure itself is not without risk. Hypotension, arrhythmias, and complications of vascular access placement are not uncommon.[6] Second is the concern that dialysis may delay recovery of renal function.[7,8] Therefore, in general, dialysis in current practice is initiated when clinical features of significant volume overload and solute imbalance dictate a need for intervention. Common parameters used to define the indication and timing of dialysis in patients with AKI include the levels of BUN and creatinine, presence of oliguria, evidence of heart failure and pulmonary edema, and an estimate of the catabolic state.[9,10]

Blood Urea Nitrogen

BUN is generally considered to be nontoxic, except for its impact on platelet function and, rarely, when initiating dialysis in the face of elevated intracranial pressures. However, many observational and retrospective studies have shown improved survival for patients who start dialysis at lower levels of BUN. In a multicenter study of 243 patients with AKI, Liu and colleagues[11] found that mortality was significantly greater when dialysis was started with BUN levels greater than 76 mg/dL, despite an apparently lower burden of comorbidities than those

patients with lower BUN. In contrast, a randomized, control trial conducted in oliguric critically ill patients in the Netherlands revealed no significant difference in hospital mortality with early (mean BUN, 46 mg/dL) versus late (105 mg/dL) initiation of hemofiltration.[12] These findings, and those of earlier studies, have been disputed because they did not account for nonrenal processes that influence BUN. Volume depletion, hyperalimentation, gastrointestinal bleeding, and exogenous glucocorticoids all raise BUN, and all are commonly seen in AKI patients in critical care settings. Further, the low-BUN groups may have included many patients who would have improved without dialysis.[13] Nonetheless, until appropriate prospective studies have been conducted, it is prudent to consider the level of BUN carefully in the decision to initiate dialysis.

Creatinine and Creatinine Clearance

Many studies have demonstrated that serum creatinine alone is an insensitive indicator of AKI. Use of creatinine as a marker is confounded by the finding that AKI survivors tend to have higher creatinine levels than nonsurvivors.[11,14] Rhabdomyolysis may be an exception, because serum creatinine appears to correlate with both AKI and the eventual need for RRT in these patients.[15] In actual practice, one is often confronted with a patient whose AKI is manifested only by increases of BUN and creatinine. The creatinine clearance may be calculated from a timed urine collection over 6 to 24 hours, with the longer interval preferred. The average of serum creatinine values obtained at the beginning and at the end of the collection should be used in the clearance calculations to account for the dynamic nature of AKI. Clearances that are sustained for several days below 10 mL/min should prompt initiation of RRT in the absence of other signs of renal recovery. Some providers calculate urea clearance on the same collection and average the value with the creatinine clearance. Although there are few data to support this practice, it permits consideration of the apparently increased mortality in high-BUN states. At the present time, there is no compelling outcome-based evidence for substituting exogenous markers such as inulin for creatinine or urea.

Urine Output

Oliguria and its associated complications is a serious contributor to morbidity in AKI. Daily urine output of less than 400 mL that does not improve with diuretics in a patient who is volume replete is typically cited as an indication for RRT. Higher thresholds should be considered for the patient with significant obligate inputs, such as blood products, antibiotics, and nutritional support. Trends in output should be respected, regardless of the current hourly flow. Decreasing output in the face of evolving sepsis is poorly tolerated and is unlikely to respond to diuretics. Anuria is indicative of a severe kidney injury. It rarely improves quickly enough to forestall need for dialysis in the absence of volume depletion. The use of diuretics to support urine flow has been debated in the literature with no clear indication that it either hurts or helps in oliguria.[16-19] Diuretics generally are ineffective without at least some preexisting urine flow. It sometimes is important to remind other providers that anuria is consistent with a glomerular flow rate of zero.

Given the added comfort of volume control, maintenance of urine volume with or without diuretics may unnecessarily delay the onset of dialysis in select individuals. Liangos and colleagues examined the relationship of urine volume to timing of initiation of dialysis and overall mortality. Nonsurvivors had significantly higher urine volumes and severity of illness than survivors (1.5 versus 0.7 L/day). Nonsurvivors also had lower BUN values at the start of the nephrology consultation (42 versus 76 mg/dL; $P = .01$). What this study demonstrated was the increasing complexity of the natural history of AKI. Seemingly mild clinical deterioration (as evidenced by a lower Acute Physiology and Chronic Health Evaluation [APACHE II] score at consultation) resulted in delayed initiation of therapy and, ultimately, poor outcomes.

Fluid Balance

Volume overload is often the immediate indication for starting RRT. Several pieces of evidence point to the importance of fluid overload in determining outcomes from AKI. We showed in a randomized, controlled trial comparing intermittent therapies to continuous therapies that patients dialyzed for solute control had a better outcome than those dialyzed for volume control.[20] Moreover, patients dialyzed for both solute and volume control had the worst outcome. Mukau and Latimer showed that 95% of their patients with postoperative acute renal failure had fluid excesses of more than 10 L at initiation of dialysis.[21] Recent studies suggested that achieving a negative fluid balance within the first 3 days after admission for septic shock was a predictor of better survival.[22] Foland and colleagues showed that pediatric patients receiving continuous veno-venous hemodialysis (CVVH) who have greater than 10% fluid overload before initiation of CVVH have a poor prognosis.[23] Consequently, fluid regulation seems to be an important consideration when deciding to initiate dialysis in the intensive care unit (ICU) patient with acute renal failure. Moreover, such renal support provides volume "space," which permits the administration of nutritional support without limitations.[24] Generally, RRT is considered preferable to intubation and mechanical ventilation. Conservative strategies involve minimizing inputs, increasing oxygen delivery, maximizing diuretics, controlling the heart rate, and employing vasodilators.[25] When those options fail to maintain the oxygen saturation at 90% or higher, extracorporeal volume removal becomes necessary. If placement of a temporary dialysis catheter is delayed until oxygen saturation reaches this threshold, the patient may not tolerate lying supine for the procedure. Therefore, the clinician should consider the patient's ability to lie flat long enough for catheter placement in determining when to start RRT.

Hyperkalemia

There is no universally accepted serum potassium level for initiation of RRT. However, a value greater than 6.5 mEq/L should prompt consideration of dialysis. In many cases, hyperkalemia can be treated conservatively.[25-27] RRT becomes more urgent under the following conditions:

1. The potassium concentration is too high to be lowered rapidly into a safe range by shifting it into the intracellular space. Administration of insulin and glucose or high-dose β-adrenergic therapy can each lower potassium by up to 1 mEq/L. The effects of bicarbonate therapy are less predictable.
2. The electrocardiogram (ECG) demonstrates changes typical of serious hyperkalemia. The absence of ECG changes should not be the sole criterion for delaying dialysis, however, because the changes can evolve quite rapidly to asystole.
3. There is ongoing addition of potassium to the extracellular fluid. Typical cases would involve massive cell lysis, as can be observed in hepatic necrosis, rhabdomyolysis, and some myeloproliferative disorders.
4. There is a concomitant acidosis or beta blockade. Both can inhibit the passage of potassium into the intercellular fluid, minimizing the ability to compensate for a potassium load.
5. There is a loss of ability to remove potassium from the body with potassium-exchange resins. These are active in the colon. It is important to determine whether the colon has been removed or whether the patient has intestinal obstruction or ileus before using this method.

Acidosis

Acidosis is variably associated with ICU mortality, depending on the underlying disease process and available compensatory mechanisms. Severe acidemia contributes to hypotension (by multiple mechanisms), hyperkalemia, hyperventilation, and respiratory fatigue. A pH of 7.20 is a reasonable therapeutic target for avoiding these and other complications.[28] Inability to achieve pH 7.20 with conservative measures such as exogenous bicarbonate replacement and hyperventilation should prompt initiation of RRT. Respiratory acidosis appears to be better tolerated than a metabolic acid load, although there is evidence that uncompensated acidosis is a risk factor for mortality in chronic obstructive pulmonary disease[29] and status asthmaticus.[30]

Platelet Dysfunction

Uremic patients have a bleeding tendency due to multifactorial platelet dysfunction that correlates with the bleeding time. Although there is considerable debate about the clinical utility of bleeding time in the individual patient, the bleeding tendency has been well documented, starting at relatively modest degrees of kidney failure. For instance, Anderson and colleagues demonstrated a significant increase in bleeding complications and the need for blood product transfusions in cardiac surgery patients with creatinine concentrations higher than 1.5 mg/dL.[31] Using the same cutoff points, O'Brien and coworkers similarly found excess bleeding risk in general surgery patients.[32] In the ICU, this is clinically important when dealing with gastrointestinal and intracranial hemorrhage or when contemplating invasive procedures. The initial step in management should be to increase the hematocrit to 30%, to improve red cell rheology. The specific platelet defects can be addressed by administering desmopressin (DDAVP) to increase levels of preformed von Willebrand's factor, transfusing cryoprecipitate, and, if sufficient time is available, administering conjugated estrogens. Should these be ineffective, dialysis may substantially improve the bleeding time, although there are few available outcome data to support the institution of RRT.[33,34]

Uremic Encephalopathy and Neuropathy

Acute uremia can contribute to alterations of mental status or clouding of consciousness in critically ill patients.[35,36] Uremic encephalopathy is rarely clinically significant in the absence of a separate central nervous system process, such as posterior reversible encephalopathy, stroke, hypercalcemia, or hepatic failure. Similarly, acute uremic peripheral neuropathy usually is an exacerbation of a pre-existing process such as diabetic neuropathy. Patients with these conditions may improve with institution of dialysis, sometimes dramatically. However, in most cases, institution of dialysis will not provide a substantial benefit unless the underlying processes are also addressed.

The nephrologist may be asked to provide RRT to an encephalopathic patient near death, either to ascertain the patient's wishes or to permit a family to say farewell. Dialytic intervention in such hopeless cases should probably be considered futile therapy.

RENAL SUPPORT VERSUS RENAL REPLACEMENT

In spite of the absence of standards for initiation of dialysis in the ICU, several important factors need to be considered when making the decision to provide RRT. An important distinction in the ICU patient is the recognition that acute renal failure does not occur in isolation from other organ system dysfunction. Consequently, providing dialysis can be viewed as a form of *renal support* rather than mere replacement.[37] For example, in the presence of oliguric renal failure, administration of large volumes of fluid to patients with multiple organ failure may lead to impaired oxygenation. In such a setting, early intervention with extracorporeal therapies for management of fluid balance may significantly affect the function of other organs irrespective of more traditional indices of renal failure, such as BUN. This terminology serves to distinguish between the strategy of replacing individual organ function and one of providing support for all organs. Continuous RRTs are particularly suited to provide renal support in the ICU patient. The freedom to provide continuous fluid management permits the application of unlimited nutrition, adjustments in hemodynamic parameters, and achievement of steady-state solute control which is difficult with intermittent therapies. It is thus possible to widen the indications for renal intervention and provide a customized approach for the management of each patient.

PROPHYLACTIC DIALYSIS

There are a few specific clinical situations in which early dialysis can be recommended to improve survival. The use of early dialysis to remove poisons such as lithium and ethylene glycol is unchallenged. There is increasing evidence that early intervention reduces mortality after cardiac surgery.[38,39] Likewise, several studies have demonstrated improved survival if intermittent or continuous dialysis is offered early to trauma patients with AKI.[40] There is a suggestion that early use of dialysis to maintain euvolemia may have a positive impact on survival in AKI after pediatric bone marrow transplantation[41] or in the treatment of complex congenital heart defects.[42] There was

hope that AKI due to massive rhabdomyolysis could be forestalled or moderated with early hemofiltration to remove myoglobin; however, it appears that myoglobin elimination is not substantially improved with continuous veno-venous hemodiafiltration (CVVHDF) compared with noninvasive measures.[43] Super high-flux membranes with larger pore sizes offer significantly greater myoglobin removal, but they are not readily available.[44] Early intervention has also been explored in sepsis and contrast nephropathy.

Sepsis

Early conventional dialysis has not been shown to improve outcomes in sepsis-associated AKI.[45,46] This may reflect the dose of dialysis delivered. Ronco and colleagues found a trend toward improved survival with higher doses of CRRT.[47] Piccini and colleagues[48] demonstrated a 50% improvement in 28-day survival in patients with sepsis and oliguric AKI who were treated with RRT within 12 hours after ICU admission. Their protocol included 6 hours of isovolemic, high-flux hemofiltration at high blood flow rates, followed by 18 hours of conventional CVVH daily. The improved survival was tentatively attributed to cytokine removal. The authors noted in their discussion that the retrospective nature of the study and the use of historical controls could make generalization of the results problematic for some. In addition, the demand on resources with this approach is quite high.[49] Nonetheless, the remarkable results achieved in this study should spur further investigations of hemofiltration in sepsis.

Contrast Nephropathy

There does not appear to be a role for RRT in the prevention of contrast nephropathy. Intermittent dialysis is ineffective at best.[50] A 2003 study by Marenzi and associates demonstrated that hemofiltration can provide some renal protection, but the protocol is far too cumbersome to be recommended except in extraordinary circumstances.[51] A recent economic analysis raised substantial questions regarding cost-effectiveness of the technique when compared with other strategies.[52]

PREDICTORS FOR DIALYSIS REQUIREMENT

Neither laboratory nor clinical data alone seem to predict when dialysis should be initiated. The combination provides the basis for the decision-making process in initiating therapy with dialysis. A key issue is the timing of involvement of the nephrologist in the care of individuals with AKI. Late consultation with a nephrologist was associated with lower BUN (mean, 47 versus 77 mg/dL with late versus early consultation, respectively) and higher urine output (mean, 1180 versus 608 mL, respectively) in a prospective observation trial conducted among ICU patients requiring nephrology consultation.[53] Late nephrology consultation was also associated with higher in-hospital mortality and lower recovery of renal function in survivors (adjusted odds ratio, 1.5), although the difference was not statistically significant. AKI involves a complex physiological milieu that requires early aggressive collaborative management to provide appropriate therapy in a timely manner. Careful clinical assessment of the patient, review of laboratory parameters for trends, and knowledge of anticipated events are key to the appropriate management of these ICU patients. The following parameters should be considered.

Urine Studies and Biomarkers

Examination of urine sediment and calculation of fractional excretion of sodium have long been used to estimate the reversibility of AKI and, by extension, the need for RRT. The literature supporting this practice is weak and contradictory, particularly in patients with septic pathophysiology.[54,55] The utility of biomarkers such as cystatin C and interleukin 18 in the diagnosis of AKI is still being evaluated. Outside research protocols, they do not yet have an established role in deciding whether to start RRT.

Scoring Systems

The utility of disparate scoring systems such as APACHE II; the Risk, Injury, Failure, Loss of kidney function, and End-stage kidney disease (RIFLE) system; and the Simplified Acute Physiology Score (SAPS II) in the timing of dialysis remains unclear. Although these systems have been studied largely in the prediction of mortality, it is logical to assume that RRT might be started sooner if a patient is known to have a higher risk of death. The members of the Project to Improve Care in Acute Renal Disease (PICARD) study group, in a multicenter observational study, found that models had poor predictive power as of the day of AKI diagnosis.[56] The reproducibility and general applicability of these models in the patient with AKI have been questioned.[57] Large prospective studies and further refinement are needed before they can be used with confidence to predict the need for RRT. Although there are currently no trials exploring the timing of intervention for acute dialysis, the availability of the Acute Kidney Injury Network (AKIN) staging system should permit an improved characterization of AKI. Ongoing analyses are being performed on the utility of RIFLE as a predictor of mortality as well as an indicator for therapy initiation.[2,58-60]

DISCONTINUING RENAL REPLACEMENT THERAPY

There is very little literature to guide the decision to discontinue RRT in patients recovering from AKI. The underlying insult must have resolved, the patient must have enough urine output to avoid volume overload, creatinine clearance should be greater than 10 to 12 mL/min, and metabolic homeostasis must be assured.[61] In addition, the patient must be able to receive sufficient nutrition. Ideally, a patient undergoing CRRT would continue to receive that therapy until sufficient function is regained. However, competing clinical requirements and the need to mobilize the patient often compel transition to intermittent hemodialysis. Care should be taken to avoid further injury to the recovering kidney. The treatments should be spaced closely enough to avoid possible deleterious hemodynamic consequences of excessive ultrafiltration.[62] The

intervals can be extended, as urine output and laboratory indices permit, until it is clear that the patient will not need further therapy.

SOCIAL ISSUES

Although this chapter emphasizes the medical aspects of starting dialysis, social issues sometimes supervene. It is not uncommon for the nephrologist or intensivist to be faced with decisions regarding the use of dialysis as a life-sustaining therapy. Several factors may influence the decision to offer dialysis support for critically ill patients and also influence the duration of therapy. It is also not uncommon for there to be a lack of agreement among caregivers and family members on the best course of action. For some patients and family members, dialysis remains an extraordinary therapy that can be declined or delayed for personal or financial reasons. It is not unusual for a patient or family to stipulate that dialysis should not be initiated under any circumstances, or not unless the patient's life is directly and immediately threatened by kidney failure. It is prudent to communicate early and regularly with the patient and family members to ascertain their desires, to gauge their level of understanding, and to provide focused education to assist their decision making.

In some circumstances, RRT needs to be withdrawn because further therapy is futile. Although this is a difficult decision, a collaborative approach with discussion among the intensivist, nephrologist, family members, and other caregivers is a prerequisite for defining the endpoints for therapy. An appropriate management strategy can be developed based on general ethical principles and an understanding of the process of care in the ICU setting. For instance, patients who have severe underlying chronic organ failure (e.g., decompensated cirrhosis, cardiomyopathy) can be offered a "trial of therapy" with predefined end points to establish improvement or deterioration over a set duration. This approach permits a standardized method to provide renal support.

Key Points

1. Most patients with acute kidney injury (AKI) in critical care settings will ultimately require dialysis.
2. There have been very few rigorous, prospective trials of sufficient power to guide decision making when faced with AKI in critical care settings. As a result, clinicians use more than 90 combinations of indicators to decide when to start renal replacement therapy.
3. Traditional blood and urinary indicators of AKI, such as urinary sediment and fractional excretion of sodium, should be interpreted with caution, because they have not been studied carefully in the critical care setting. Scoring systems and biomarkers are being studied more systematically, but this method is not yet mature enough to guide initiation of renal replacement therapy.
4. Early dialysis improves survival in AKI after cardiac surgery and probably after trauma. Early conventional dialysis, including continuous renal replacement therapy, has not been shown to

improve survival in sepsis-associated AKI. However, there may be a role for early and aggressive hemofiltration in oliguric, septic patients.

5. Approaches to discontinuation of renal replacement therapy are entirely empirical at this point.

6. Dialysis decisions for critically ill patients should be collaborative and should involve discussions with family members and the caregiver team. A "trial of therapy" concept should be considered for patients with potentially irreversible organ dysfunction.

Key References

See the companion Expert Consult website for the complete reference list.

CHAPTER 217

The Concept of Renal Replacement Therapy Dose and Efficiency

Zaccaria Ricci, Rinaldo Bellomo, John A. Kellum, and Claudio Ronco

OBJECTIVES

This chapter will:
1. Describe the main components of renal replacement therapy (RRT) dose: efficiency, intensity, and clinical efficacy.
2. Describe the most important studies addressing the impact of RRT dose on the survival of critically ill patients.
3. Describe some practical concepts guiding the clinician to RRT prescription.

The conventional view of renal replacement therapy (RRT) dose is that it is a measure of the quantity of blood purification achieved by means of extracorporeal techniques. However, this broad concept is too difficult to measure and quantify. The *operational* view of RRT dose is that it is a measure of the quantity of a representative marker solute which is removed from a patient. This marker solute is considered to be reasonably representative of similar solutes that require removal for blood purification to be considered adequate. This premise has several major flaws: The marker solute cannot and does not represent all the solutes that accumulate in renal failure. Its kinetics and volume of distribution are also different from those of the solutes of interest. Finally, its removal during RRT is not representative of the removal of other solutes. This is true both for end-stage renal disease (ESRD) and acute renal failure (ARF).

However, a significant body of data in the ESRD literature[1-6] suggests that, despite these major limitations, single solute marker assessment of dialysis dose appears to have a clinically meaningful relationship to patient outcome and, therefore, to clinical utility. Nevertheless, the Hemodialysis (HEMO) Study, which examined the effect of intermittent hemodialysis (IHD) doses, enforced the concept that "less dialysis is worse" but failed to confirm the intuition that "more dialysis is better."[6] Therefore, this premise seems useful in ESRD and is accepted to be potentially useful in ARF for operational purposes.

Hence, the amount (measure) of delivered dose of RRT can be described by various terms: efficiency, intensity, and clinical efficacy. Each of these is discussed in the following sections.

EFFICIENCY, INTENSITY, EFFICACY: Kt/V

Efficiency of RRT is represented by the concept of clearance (K)—the volume of blood cleared of a given solute over a given time. K does not reflect the overall solute removal rate (mass transfer); rather, its value is normalized by the serum concentration. Even when K remains stable over time, the removal rate will vary if the blood levels of the reference molecule change. K depends on solute molecular size, transport modality (diffusion or convection), and circuit operational characteristics such as blood flow rate (Qb), dialysate flow rate (Qd), ultrafiltration rate (Qf), and hemodialyzer type and size. K can be used to compare the treatment dose during each dialysis session, but it cannot be employed as an absolute dose measure to compare treatments with different time schedules. For example, K is typically higher in IHD than in continuous renal replacement therapy CRRT or sustained low-efficiency daily dialysis (SLEDD). This is not surprising, because K represents only the instantaneous efficiency of the system. However, mass removal may be greater during SLEDD or CRRT. For this reason, information about the time span during which K is delivered is fundamental to describe the effective dose of dialysis.

Intensity of RRT can be defined by the product "clearance × time" (Kt). Kt is more useful than K for comparing different RRTs. A further step in assessing dose must include the frequency of the Kt application over a particular period (e.g., 1 week). This additional dimension is given by the product of intensity × frequency (Kt × treatment days/week, or Kt · d/w). Kt · d/w is superior to Kt, because it offers information beyond a single treatment, and patients with ARF typically require more than one treatment. This concept of Kt · d/w offers the possibility of comparing disparate treatment schedules (e.g., intermittent, alternate-day, daily, continuous). However, it does not take into account the size of the pool of solute that needs to be cleared. This requires the dimension of efficacy.

Efficacy of RRT represents the effective solute removal outcome resulting from the administration of a given treatment to a given patient. It can be described by the fractional clearance of a given solute (Kt/V), where V is the volume of distribution of the marker molecule in the body. Kt/V is an established marker of adequacy of dialysis for small solutes correlating with medium-term (several years) survival in patients undergoing chronic hemodialysis.[6] Urea is typically used as a marker molecule in ESRD to guide treatment dose, and a Kt/V_{UREA} of at least 1.2 is currently recommended.

As an example, we can consider the case of a 70-kg patient who is treated for 20 hr/day with a postfilter hemofiltration of 2.8 L/hr at a zero balance. His K_{UREA} will be 47 mL/min (2.8 L/hr = 2800 mL/60 min), because we know that during postfilter hemofiltration the ultrafiltered plasma water will drag all urea across the membrane, making its clearance identical to the ultrafiltration flow. His treatment time (t) will be 1200 minutes (60 minutes for 20 hours). His urea volume of distribution will be approximately 42,000 mL (60% of 70 kg), roughly equal to total body water. Simplifying this patient's Kt/V_{UREA}, we will have 47*1200/42000 = 1.34.

However, Kt/V_{UREA} application in patients with ARF has not been rigorously validated. In fact, although the application of Kt/V to the assessment of dose in ARF is theoretically intriguing, many concerns have been raised, because problems intrinsic to ARF can hinder the accuracy and meaning of such dose measurement. These problems include lack of a metabolic steady state, uncertainty about the volume of distribution of urea (V_{UREA}), a high protein catabolic rate, labile fluid volumes, and possible residual renal function, which changes dynamically during the course of treatment. To evaluate V_{UREA} in patients with ARF, Himmelfarb and colleagues[7] undertook a systematic study in a cohort of 28 patients with ARF. They determined V_{UREA} by various approaches to anthropometrical measurements (Watson, 42.5 ± 7.0 L; Hume-Weyer, 43.6 ± 7.1 L; Chertow, 46.8 ± 8.1 L) and found that they yielded significantly lower measures than V_{UREA} determined by physiological formulas or by bioimpedance (51.1 ± 11.6 L and 51.1 ± 13.3 L, respectively). Finally, all measures of V_{UREA} by blood-based kinetics exceeded measurements by any other method (7% to 50% difference). The investigators inevitably concluded that estimates of V_{UREA} cannot be reliably used in patients with ARF.[7]

Furthermore, delivery of prescribed dose in ARF can be limited by technical problems (access recirculation, poor blood flows with temporary venous catheters, membrane clotting, and machine malfunction) and by clinical issues (hypotension and vasopressor requirements that can be responsible for solute dysequilibrium within tissues and organs). These aspects are particularly evident during IHD, less so during SLEDD, and even less so during CRRT. This difference occurs because, after some days of CRRT, patients' urea levels approach a real steady state: Because the therapy is applied continuously, the effect of compartmentalization of solutes is minimized; from a theoretical point of view, purification of total body water can be considered uniform in all organs, and single-pool kinetics can be applied (spKt/V).

Despite all the uncertainty surrounding its meaning and the gross shortcomings related to its accuracy in patients with ARF, the idea that there might be an optimal dose of solute removal continues to have a powerful hold in the literature. This is likely due to evidence from ESRD, where a minimum Kt/V of 1.2 thrice weekly is indicated as standard.[6] However, the benefits of greater Kt/V accrue over years of therapy, whereas, in ARF, any difference in dose would apply for days to weeks, and the view that it would still be sufficient to alter clinical outcomes remains somewhat optimistic. Nonetheless, the hypothesis that higher doses of dialysis may be beneficial in critically ill patients with ARF must be considered by analogy and investigated. Several reports exist in the literature dealing with this issue. Furthermore, the concept of predefined dose is a powerful tool to help clinicians to a correct prescription and to at least avoid undertreatment.

Brause and coworkers,[8] using continuous veno-venous hemofiltration (CVVH), found that higher Kt/V values (0.8 versus 0.53) were correlated with improved uremic control and acid-base balance. This would be expected. No clinically important outcome was affected. Investigators from the Cleveland Clinic[9] retrospectively evaluated 844 patients with ARF requiring CRRT or IHD over a 7-year period. They found that, when patients were stratified for disease severity, dialysis dose did not affect outcome in patients with very high or very low scores, but it did correlate with survival in patients with intermediate degrees of illness. A mean Kt/V greater than 1.0 was associated with increased survival. This study was retrospective, with a clear post hoc selection bias. The validity of these observations remains highly questionable.

Daily IHD, compared with alternate-day dialysis, also seemed to be associated with improved outcome in a 2002 trial.[10] Daily hemodialysis resulted in significantly improved survival (72% versus 54%; $P = .01$), better control of uremia, fewer hypotensive episodes, and more rapid resolution of ARF. However, several limitations affected this study. First, sicker, hemodynamically unstable patients were excluded and underwent CRRT instead. Furthermore, according to reported mean time–averaged concentration of urea (TAC_{UREA}), it appears that patients receiving conventional IHD were underdialyzed. In addition, this was a single-center study with all the inherent limitations with regard to external validity. Furthermore, alternate-day dialysis was associated with significant differences in fluid removal and dialysis-associated hypotension, suggesting that other aspects of "dose" beyond solute control (e.g., inadequate and episodic volume control) might have explained the findings. These observations suggest that further studies should be undertaken to assess the effect of dose of IHD on outcome.

In a randomized, controlled trial of CRRT dose, postdilution CVVH at 35 or 45 mL/kg/hr was associated with improved survival, compared to 20 mL/kg/hr, in 425 critically ill patients with ARF.[11] Applying Kt/V dose assessment methodology to CVVH at a dose of 35 mL/kg/hr in a 70-kg patient treated for 24 hours, a treatment day would be equivalent to a Kt/V of 1.4 also applied daily. Despite uncertainty regarding the calculation of V_{UREA}, CVVH at 35 mL/kg/hr would still provide an effective *daily* delivery of 1.2, even if V_{UREA} were underestimated by 20%. Many technical and/or clinical problems, however, can make it difficult, in routine practice, to apply such strict protocols by pure postdilution hemofiltration. They include filter clotting; high filtration fraction in the presence of access

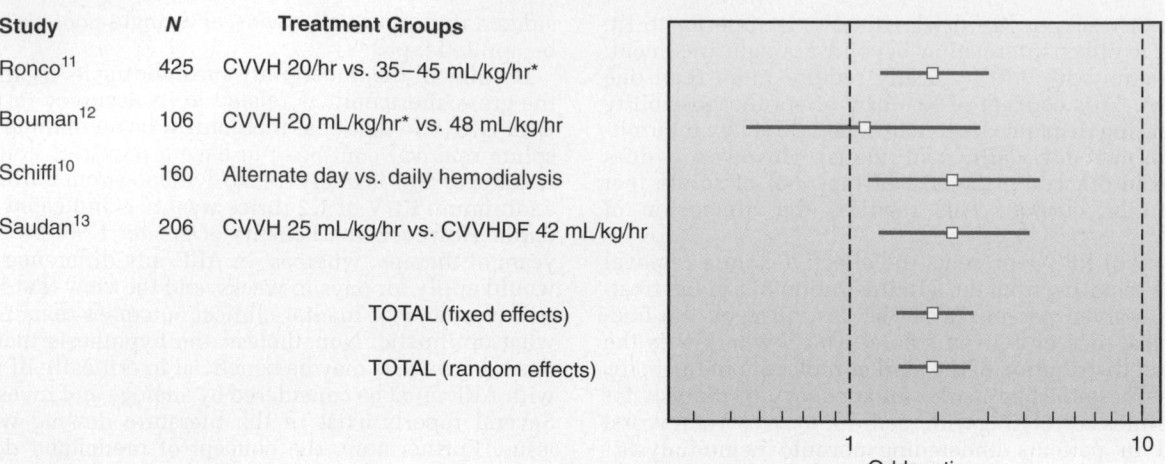

Study	N	Treatment Groups
Ronco[11]	425	CVVH 20/hr vs. 35–45 mL/kg/hr*
Bouman[12]	106	CVVH 20 mL/kg/hr* vs. 48 mL/kg/hr
Schiffl[10]	160	Alternate day vs. daily hemodialysis
Saudan[13]	206	CVVH 25 mL/kg/hr vs. CVVHDF 42 mL/kg/hr
TOTAL (fixed effects)		
TOTAL (random effects)		

FIGURE 217-1. Pooled results from four main studies on dose (references 10 through 13) indicate a very large effect on survival in favor of augmented renal replacement therapy dosing. *For purposes of analysis, the two high-dose arms in Ronco were combined, as were the two low-dose arms in Bouman. If these groups are removed, the odds ratio is unchanged (1.94; $P < .001$). (From Kellum JA: Renal replacement therapy in critically ill patients with acute renal failure: Does a greater dose improve survival? Nat Clin Pract Nephrol 2007;3:128-129.)

dysfunction and fluctuations in blood flow; and circuit down-time during surgery, radiological procedures, and filter changes. Equally important are the observations that this study was conducted over 6 years in a single center, that uremic control was not reported, that the incidence of sepsis was low compared with that in the typical populations reported to develop ARF in the world, and that its final outcome was not the accepted 28-day or 90-day mortality typically used in ICU trials. Therefore, the external validity of this study remains untested.

Another prospective, randomized trial, conducted by Bouman and associates,[12] assigned patients to three intensity groups: early high-volume hemofiltration (72 to 96 L/24 hours), early low-volume hemofiltration (24 to 36 L/24 hours), and late low-volume hemofiltration (24 to 36 L/24 hours). No difference was found in terms of renal recovery or 28-day mortality. Unfortunately, prescribed doses were not standardized by weight, making the potential variability in RRT dose large. Furthermore, the number of patients was small, making the study insufficiently powered, and, again, the incidence of sepsis was low compared with that in the typical populations reported to develop ARF in the world. A recent randomized trial from a Swiss group[13] enrolled 371 patients with ARF, assigning 102 to CVVH and 104 to continuous veno-venous hemodiafiltration (CVVHDF), and prescribed 25 mL/kg/hr ultrafiltration in the CVVH group and 24 mL/kg/hr in the CVVHDF group; patients receiving CVVHDF were prescribed an adjunctive mean dialysis dose of 18 mL/kg/hr. The CVVHDF patients had significantly higher mean urea and creatinine reduction ratios 48 hours after the initiation of continuous RRT than did the CVVH patients (50% versus 40%, $P < .009$, and 46% versus 38%, $P < .014$, respectively). Survival rates at 28 days and 90 days were higher with CVVHDF than with CVVH. Like previous trials, this study was underpowered; furthermore, it confounded the effects of dose and technique by adding dialysis to filtration.

Nevertheless, pooled results from all four of the studies described here (Schiffl,[10] Ronco,[11] Bouman,[12] Saudan[13] indicate a very large effect on survival in favor of augmented dosing, with an odds ratio of 1.95 (Fig. 217-1).[14] Although these data may still not be definitive, the best evidence to date supports the use of at least 35 mL/kg/hr for CVVH, CVVHDF, or daily IHD. The exact method with which to achieve an augmented dose, and indeed what the correct dose should be, remain matters of clinical judgment.

During the third International Course on Critical Care Nephrology held in Vicenza, Italy, a survey on various aspects of ARF, including treatment prescription, was conducted among about 550 participants (equally distributed between nephrologists and intensivists) from about 500 different centers.[15] More than one third of responders declared that they did not prescribe any specific RRT dose for ARF patients, and 75% did not monitor RRT delivered dose. In fact, although a clear understanding of the adequate dose of RRT has not yet been achieved, it is also true that, as for antibiotic blood levels during severe infections, adequate prescription should be followed by adequate administration. Recently, two multicenter trials were devised, one in the United States and the other in Australia. These efforts ultimately became the Acute Renal Failure Trial Network (ATN) study[16] and the Randomised Evaluation of Normal versus Augmented Level of RRT (RENAL) study,[17] respectively, both of which are currently underway. Pretrial surveys of prospective study sites in both trials indicated that a specific dose of RRT had not been adopted in clinical practice.[17]

These observations underline the recommendation that RRT prescriptions for ARF patients in the ICU should be monitored closely if one wishes to ensure adequate delivery of prescribed dose. The use of a software called Adequacy Calculator for ARF was recently tested. This is a Microsoft Excel-based program[18] that calculates urea clearance and estimates fractional clearance and Kt/V_{UREA} for all RRT modalities. The software allowed us to strictly monitor our treatments during the study period, and an average 10.7% ($P < .05$) reduction of therapy delivery was found, compared with the prescribed dose.[19] This delivery reduction was sometimes due to calculator overestimation and, more often, to an operative treatment time that was shorter than prescribed (because CRRT is not administered during bag substitution, troubleshooting of alarms, and filter changes). Of note, in the CVVH dose trial,[11] only patients who achieved more than 85% of the prescribed dose were included: In order to obtain this goal, compensation for interruptions in treatment due to ICU procedures was made by increasing effluent flow rates in the subsequent hours.

FROM BENCH TO BEDSIDE: THE CLINICAL MEANING OF DOSE

These observations described in this chapter indicate that, unlike in the field of chronic hemodialysis, only major changes in the application of dose (e.g., changing from alternate-day to daily dialysis) can be reasonably believed to truly deliver a "different" dose in the setting of ARF. More subtle adjustments, such as prescribing a calculated Kt/V of 1 versus 1.2, can easily be criticized as being within the calculation error associated with each prescription and not necessarily representing a reliable change in dose delivery.

The major shortcoming of the traditional solute marker–based approach to dialysis dose in ARF lies well beyond any methodological critique of single-solute kinetics–based prescriptions. In patients with ARF, the majority of whom are in intensive care, a restrictive (solute-based only) concept of dialysis dose seems grossly inappropriate. In these patients, the therapeutic needs that can be or need to be affected by the "dose" of RRT are more than the simple control of small solutes as represented by urea. They include control of acid-base, tonicity, potassium, magnesium, calcium, phosphate, intravascular volume, extravascular volume, and temperature and avoidance of unwanted side effects associated with the delivery of solute control.

In the critically ill patient, it is much more important (e.g., in the setting of coagulopathic bleeding after cardiac surgery) for 10 units of fresh-frozen plasma, 10 units of cryoprecipitate, and 10 units of platelets to be administered rapidly without inducing fluid overload (because 1 to 1.5 L of ultrafiltrate is removed in 1 hour) than for the Kt/V to be of any particular value at all. Dose of RRT is about prophylactic volume control. In a patient with right ventricular failure, ARF, and acute respiratory distress syndrome who is receiving lung-protective ventilation with permissive hypercapnia and who has acidemia inducing a further life-threatening deterioration in pulmonary vascular resistance, the "dose" component of RRT that matters immediately is acid-base control and normalization of pH 24 hours/day. The Kt/V (or any other solute-centric concept of dose) is almost just a byproduct of such dose delivery. In a young man with trauma, rhabdomyolysis, and rapidly rising serum potassium already at 7 mmol/L, dialysis dose, to begin with, is all about controlling kalemia. In a patient with fulminant liver failure, ARF, sepsis, and cerebral edema who is awaiting urgent liver transplantation and whose cerebral edema is worsening because of fever, RRT dose is all about lowering the temperature without any tonicity shifts that might increase intracranial pressure. Finally, in a patient with pulmonary edema after an ischemic ventricular septal defect requiring emergency surgery, ARF, ischemic hepatitis, and the need for inotropic and intra-aortic balloon counterpulsation support, RRT dose is all about removing fluid gently and safely so that the extravascular volume falls while the intravascular volume remains optimal. Solute removal is just a byproduct of fluid control.

These aspects of dose must explicitly be considered when discussing the dose of RRT in ARF, for it is likely that patients die more often from incorrect "dose" delivery of this kind than from incorrect dose delivery of the Kt/V

kind. Although each and every aspect of this broader understanding of dose is difficult to measure, clinically relevant assessment of dose in critically ill patients with ARF should include all dimensions of dosing, not just one dimension picked because of a similarity with ESRD: There is no evidence in the acute field that such solute control data are more relevant to clinical outcomes than volume control or acid-base control or tonicity control.

FROM BENCH TO BEDSIDE: THE PRESCRIPTION

During RRT, clearance depends on circuit blood flow (Qb), ultrafiltration rate (Qf) or dialysate flow rate (Qd), the molecular weights of the solutes, and hemodialyzer type and size. Qb, as a variable in delivering RRT dose, is mainly dependent on vascular access and operational characteristics of machines used in the clinical setting. Qf is strictly linked to Qb, during convective techniques, by filtration fraction. Filtration fraction does not limit Qd, but when the Qd/Qb ratio exceeds 0.3 it can be estimated that dialysate will not be completely saturated by blood-diffusing solutes. The search for specific toxins to be cleared has not been successful despite years of research, and urea and creatinine are generally used as reference solutes to measure renal replacement clearance for renal failure. Although the available evidence does not allow direct correlation of the degree of uremia with outcome in chronic renal disease, in the absence of a specific solute, clearances of urea and creatinine blood levels are used to guide treatment dose.

During ultrafiltration, the driving pressure jams solutes, such as urea and creatinine, against the membrane and into the pores, depending on the membrane sieving coefficient (SC) for that molecule. SC expresses a dimensionless value and is estimated by the ratio of the concentration of the solutes in the filtrate divided by that in the plasma water or blood. An SC of 1.0, as is the case for urea and creatinine, demonstrates complete permeability, and a value of 0 reflects complete rejection. Molecular size larger than approximately 12 kDa and filter porosity are the major determinants of SC.

The K during convection is measured by the product of Qf × SC. Therefore, in contrast to diffusion, there is a linear relationship between K and Qf, the SC being the changing variable for different solutes. During diffusion, the linear relationship is lost when Qd exceeds about one-third of the Qb. As a rough estimate, we can consider that, during continuous slow-efficiency treatments, the RRT dose is a direct expression of Qf – Qd, independently of which solute must be removed from the blood. Continuous treatment is now suggested to deliver a urea clearance of at least 2 L/hr, with the clinical evidence that 35 mL/kg/hr might be the best prescription (i.e., about 2.8 L/hr in a 70-kg patient). Other authors have suggested a prescription based on patient requirements, according to the urea generation rate and the catabolic state of the individual patient. However, it has been shown that, during continuous therapy, a clearance rate of less than 2 L/hr will almost definitely be insufficient in an adult critically ill patient. For more exact estimations, simple computations have been shown to adequately estimate clearance.[19,20]

Tables 217-1 and 217-2 show an algorithm and an example that could be followed each time an RRT prescription is indicated.

TABLE 217-1

Algorithm for Prescription of Renal Replacement Therapy

CLINICAL VARIABLES	OPERATIONAL VARIABLES	SETTING
Fluid balance	Net ultrafiltration	Continuous management of negative balance (100-300 mL/hr) is preferred in hemodynamically unstable patients. Complete monitoring (CVC, S-G, arterial line, ECG, pulse oximeter) is recommended.
Adequacy and dose	Clearance/modality	Prescribe 2000-3000 mL/hr K (or 35 mL/kg/hr) for CRRT; consider first CVVHDF. If IHD is selected, a daily 4-hr prescription is recommended. Prescribe a Kt/V > 1.2.
Acid-base balance	Solution buffer	Bicarbonate-buffered solutions are preferable to lactate-buffered solutions in cases of lactic acidosis and/or hepatic failure.
Electrolyte balance	Dialysate/replacement fluid	Consider solutions without K^+ in cases of severe hyperkalemia. Manage accurately $MgPO_4$.
Timing	Schedule	Early and intense RRT is suggested.
Protocol	Staff/machine	Well-trained staff should routinely utilize RRT monitors according to predefined institutional protocols.

CRRT, continuous renal replacement therapy; CVC, central venous catheter; CVVHDF, continuous veno-venous hemodiafiltration; ECG, electrocardiogram; IHD, intermittent hemodialysis; S-G, Swan-Ganz catheter.

TABLE 217-2

Schematic Example of a Possible Prescription for Continuous Treatment*

TREATMENT MODALITY	ESTIMATED UREA CLEARANCE	NOTES	VALUE OF Q REQUIRED TO OBTAIN 35 mL/kg/hr	VALUE OF Q REQUIRED TO OBTAIN A Kt/V OF 1
CVVH Postdilution	$K_{CALC} = Qrep$	Always keep filtration fraction <20% (Qb must be 5 × Qrep)	Qrep = 41 mL/min (2450 mL/hr)	Qrep = 29 mL/min (1750 mL/hr)
CVVH Predilution	$K_{CALC} = Quf/[1 + (Qrep/Qb)]$	Filtration fraction computation changes (keep <20%)	For a Qb of 200 mL/min, Qrep = 53 mL/min (3200 mL/hr)	For a Qb of 200 mL/min, Qrep = 35 mL/min (2100 mL/hr)
CVVHD	$K_{CALC} = Qdo$	Keep Qb at least 3 × Qd	Qdo = 41 mL/min (2450 mL/hr)	Qdo = 29 mL/min (1750 mL/hr)
CVVHDF Postdilution (50% convective and diffusive clearance)	$K_{CALC} = Qrep + Qdo$	Consider all of the above notes	Qrep = 20 mL/min + Qdo = 21 mL/min	Qrep = 14 mL/min replacement solution + Qdo = 15 mL/min

BW, body weight; CVVH, continuous veno-venous hemofiltration; CVVHD, continuous veno-venous hemodialysis; CVVHDF, continuous veno-venous hemodiafiltration; K_{CALC}, estimated urea clearance (mL/min); Kt/V_{CALC}, estimated fractional clearance; t, prescribed treatment time (min); Qb, blood flow rate; Qdo, dialysate solution flow rate; Qnet, patient's net fluid loss; Qrep, replacement solution flow rate; Quf, ultrafiltration flow rate (Quf = Qrep + Qnet); V_{UREA}, urea volume of distribution (mL).
*Assuming a 70-kg patient ($V_{UREA} = 42$ L) during an ideal session of 24 hours (t = 1440 minutes), with net ultrafiltration (patient fluid loss) considered to be zero in K_{CALC} for simplicity. V = BW × 0.6. $Kt/V_{CALC} = K_{CALC} × t$. A clearance rate of 35 mL/kg/hr roughly corresponds to a Kt/V of 1.4; a Kt/V of 1 approximately corresponds to 25 mL/kg/hr. Postdilution filtration fraction = Qrep/Qb × 100; Predilution filtration fraction = Qrep/(Qb + Qrep) × 100.

Key Points

1. The best evidence to date supports a renal replacement therapy dose of at least 35 mL/kg/hr, with a single-pool fractional clearance (spKt/V) of 1.4, for continuous veno-venous hemofiltration or hemodiafiltration or daily intermittent hemodialysis.
2. The exact method with which to achieve an augmented dose is still a matter of clinical judgment.
3. A specific dose of renal replacement therapy has not been adopted in clinical practice; a standard dose prescription and strict control of delivered dose should be automated if one wishes to ensure adequate delivery of the prescribed dose.

Key References

9. Paganini EP, Tapolyai M, Goormastic M, et al: Establishing a dialysis therapy/patient outcome link in intensive care unit acute dialysis for patients with acute renal failure. Am J Kidney Dis 1996;28(Suppl 3):S81-S89.
10. Schiffl H, Lang SM, Fischer R: Daily hemodialysis and the outcome of acute renal failure. N Engl J Med 2002;346:305-310.
11. Ronco C, Bellomo R, Homel P, et al: Effects of different doses in continuous veno-venous haemofiltration on outcomes of acute renal failure: A prospective randomised trial. Lancet 2000;356:26-30.
12. Bouman C, Oudemans-van Straaten H, Tijssen J, et al: Effects of early high-volume continuous veno-venous hemofiltration on survival and recovery of renal function in intensive care patients with acute renal failure: A prospective randomized trial. Crit Care Med 2002;30:2205-2211.
13. Saudan P, Niederberger M, De Seigneux S, et al: Adding a dialysis dose to continuous hemofiltration increases survival in patients with acute renal failure. Kidney Int 2006;70:1312-1317.
14. Kellum JA: Renal replacement therapy in critically ill patients with acute renal failure: Does a greater dose improve survival? Nat Clin Pract Nephrol 2007;3:128-129.

See the companion Expert Consult website for the complete reference list.

CHAPTER 218

Quantification of Acute Renal Replacement Therapy

Mark R. Marshall and Francesco G. Casino

OBJECTIVES

This chapter will:
1. Provide a clinical context for acute renal replacement therapy (RRT) dosing.
2. Discuss the role and limitations of urea kinetic modeling for the quantification of dose.
3. Discuss the concepts and demonstrate the use of practical tools for the quantification of dose that are specific to either intermittent or continuous RRT.
4. Discuss the concept and demonstrate the use of equivalent renal urea clearance as a unified expression of dose for all acute RRT modalities.

In critically ill patients treated with acute renal replacement therapy (ARRT), the fraction of mortality that is attributable to acute kidney injury (AKI) is estimated to be between 25% and 50%.[1] The prevailing view among opinion leaders is that adequate replacement of failing renal function will minimize this attributable risk and optimize patient outcomes. This chapter presents and clinically contextualizes tools for dose quantification of ARRT.

Uremic toxicity in critically ill patients with AKI is uncommon, insofar as it is not in the familiar form seen in end-stage renal disease (ESRD). Deaths in this setting occur in the context of nonspecific physiological derangement, such as nonresolving infection, hemorrhage, or nonresolving shock despite optimal care. These conditions may therefore constitute an acute uremic syndrome specific to AKI. It follows that mediators and markers of this acute uremic injury may also be unique. There is promising research evaluating dose-response relationships for various ARRT modalities in terms of their capacity for immunomodulation.[2] In time, it is possible (and even probable) that data from such studies may fundamentally change practice patterns, although definitive studies are lacking at present. To date, dose-response relationships have been defined only in terms of solute clearance, using either empirical means or urea kinetic modeling (UKM).

Studies of ARRT dose have used different expressions for solute clearance for different modalities. These expressions can be unified on a small-solute therapy map, although there is not as much experience in assessing larger-solute clearance. Because of these difficulties, true dose equivalence across the full range of purported uremic toxins has not been established for intermittent hemodialysis (IHD) compared with continuous renal replacement therapy (CRRT), or among continuous veno-venous hemo-

filtration (CVVH) hemodialysis (CVVHD) and hemodiafiltration (CVVHDF).

CLINICAL DOSING TARGETS FOR ACUTE INTERMITTENT HEMODIALYSIS

A number of studies have suggested a relationship between small-solute control or clearance and patient outcomes during acute IHD. In the 1950s and 1960s, it was conclusively demonstrated during the Korean and Vietnam wars that IHD saved lives,[3,4] although subsequent underpowered and clinically outdated studies arising from that experience fell short of proving the case for "early" IHD (initiated when the blood urea nitrogen [BUN] level was <100 to 150 mg/dL) or for "intensive" IHD (maintaining BUN <60 mg/dL and serum creatinine <5 mg/dL).[5]

Since then, no clinical trials have evaluated the effect of small-solute clearance as an intervention on outcomes in the critically ill AKI population, although there are studies in progress that are likely to be informative.[6] The most compelling observational data were from Schiffl and colleagues,[7] who used IHD to provide an average single-pool fractional clearance (spKt/V) of 0.92 on 6.2 occasions per week (resulting in a time-averaged BUN concentration [TAC$_{BUN}$] of 60 mg/dL), which was associated with a lower mortality rate and a shorter duration to resolution of AKI than was IHD providing an average spKt/V of 0.94 on 3.2 occasions per week (TAC$_{BUN}$ = 104 mg/dL).[7] The internal validity of this study is questionable; overtly inadequate uremic solute control in the low-dose group most likely exaggerated the results in the high-dose group. Notwithstanding this criticism, the findings were clinically plausible and are supportive of a relationship between dose and outcome for acute IHD.

Further support is found in observational data from Paganini and associates: IHD providing an average spKt/V greater than 1.0 per treatment was associated with better survival than that providing less than 1.0 fractional clearance per treatment, after adjustment for illness severity.[8] A major deficiency of these data is that they do not account for treatment frequency, which limits their utility in establishing clinical dosing targets.

There are no data supporting a relationship between larger-solute clearance and outcomes for acute IHD. Intermittent hemodiafiltration (IHDF) and high-flux IHD for critically ill AKI patients have demonstrated no clinical or laboratory advantage over low-flux IHD. This is likely due to the low clearances of larger solutes afforded by these modalities. Whereas low-flux IHD clears approximately

3 mL/min of β_2-microglobulin from blood water during the course of treatment, high-flux IHD clears only about 35 mL/min, and even IHDF clears only 50 to 150 mL/min, depending on the substitution fluid rate.[9] Given the short duration over which these modalities are applied, a meaningful clinical effect seems unlikely. The effect of IHD on solute control is therefore, for the most part, restricted to small solutes.

In summary, data suggest that patient outcomes can be improved by achieving spKt/V of 0.92 on no less than 6.2 occasions per week. There are no published data relating clearance of larger solutes to outcome for acute IHD.

CLINICAL DOSING TARGETS FOR CONTINUOUS RENAL REPLACEMENT THERAPY

The first study to link solute clearance to outcomes for CRRT was performed almost 20 years ago. However, it is only recently that clinical dosing targets have been refined. In a prospective, randomized clinical trial from Ronco and colleagues, mortality was lowest for patients receiving postdilution CVVH with an ultrafiltration rate (UFR) of 35 mL/kg/hr or greater (indexed to patient premorbid weight), provided it was applied more than 85% of the time.[10] The external validity of this study is perhaps questionable, because the participants were relatively small (average weight, 68 kg) and had a low incidence of sepsis (12%). However, the results are strongly supportive of a standard for solute clearance during CRRT. Although a subsequent trial failed to confirm these findings, it was underpowered and also was performed in patients who had undergone cardiosurgical procedures, for whom factors other than solute control were likely to be relatively more important as determinants of outcomes.[11]

It is uncertain from the study of Ronco and colleagues whether the superior survival with higher UFR was related to clearance of small or larger solutes. Small-solute clearance would be equal to the UFR, but clearance of larger solutes was not reported. This issue was addressed in a later study from Saudan and associates, which showed that the addition of approximately 18 mL/kg/hr of diffusive clearance using CVVHD to a basal amount of approximately 24 mL/kg/hr of convective clearance using CVVH resulted in superior patient survival.[12] This finding demonstrated that at least some of the benefit of a higher dose of CRRT in Ronco's study was the result of increased small solute clearance.

Even higher doses of CRRT may benefit those with septic shock and a high predicted mortality risk. In Ronco's study, there was a trend to lower mortality for septic patients receiving a UFR of 45 mL/kg/hr or greater. These findings were supported by observational data from Honore and colleagues, who found that the dose of high-volume CVVH was greater (average UFR, 132.5 mL/kg/hr) in those patients whose hemodynamic parameters improved during treatment than in those whose parameters did not improve (average UFR, 107.5 mL/kg/hr).[13] These studies are suggestive but not definitive.

In summary, data suggest that patient outcomes can be improved by achieving an indexed small-solute clearance of 35 mL/kg/hr or greater, provided the therapy is applied for more than 85% of the time. There are no published data relating specifically to larger-solute clearance to outcomes during CRRT.

CALCULATION OF FRACTIONAL CLEARANCE FOR INTERMITTENT HEMODIALYSIS

To calculate Kt/V, UKM must be applied. UKM is based on the mass balance principle that "urea accumulation equals urea input minus urea output." Practically, this principle is embodied in a model that estimates urea concentration based on three patient-dependent parameters—urea distribution volume (V), urea generation rate (G), and renal urea clearance (Kr)—and three treatment-dependent parameters—dialyzer urea clearance (K_D), session length (T), and treatment schedule. A differential equation can be developed from this model, whose solution provides the general equations for UKM that are presented later.

Urea kinetics can be assessed through either blood measurements or direct dialysate quantification. The former option is logistically more feasible, although the role of partial dialysate collection or on-line urea and ionic dialysate monitors warrants further study in this setting. For the moment, however, the standard approach is to use blood measurements. The BUN and available estimates of UKM parameters are entered into the general equations for UKM. These equations are iteratively solved to impute UKM parameters that are not provided to the model (usually G and V) from those that are (usually K_D). This allows the calculation of Kt/V.

Studies of urea kinetics show four major differences between the critically ill AKI population and the ESRD population.[14] First, critically ill patients often have markedly increased values for G, attributable to a more catabolic state. Second, they often have markedly increased V at 65% to 70% of their body weight, compared with ESRD patients at 55% to 60% of body weight. Some of this increase is attributable to Na^+ and H_2O loading (and concurrent loss of lean body mass) in critical illness, although most of the increase is attributable to the dissociation of V from its usual anatomical correlate of total body water (TBW): V is between 10% and 30% higher than TBW in critically ill AKI patients.[15] This discrepancy is not just a byproduct of UKM but a literal one demonstrable with the use of radiolabeled (^{13}C) urea and deuterium oxide.[16] Of note, this discrepancy is not satisfactorily explained by intercompartmental urea dysequilibrium (i.e., delayed entrance of urea into the blood from body pools that have high resistance to solute transfer due to a low ratio of tissue perfusion to water, such as muscle or skin), which is, in fact, surprisingly similar to that seen in patients with ESRD.[14]

Third, critically ill patients often have values for K_D that are lower than expected, and specifically lower than those calculated by usual means (e.g., Michael's formula).[17] Veno-venous angioaccess leads to high recirculation rates, especially in short femoral catheters, where it can approach 25%, and this is exacerbated by the frequent need for line reversal in 25% to 50% of treatments. Fiber-bundle clotting also reduces K_D, especially in the absence of anticoagulation.

Finally, critical illness is associated with marked variation in all of these UKM parameters over time.[14] The assumption of urea steady state underlies many of the UKM calculations in the maintenance IHD population and affords convenience (e.g., model fitting using two BUN points rather than three). However, urea steady state cannot be assumed for critically ill AKI patients or for the modeling of IHD dose in this setting.

TABLE 218-1

Useful Equations for Calculating Single-Pool Kt/V (spKt/V) during Intermittent Hemodialysis (IHD)

Formal Iterative Urea Kinetic Modeling (UKM) Equations Derived from the Variable-Volume, Single-Pool (VVSP) Model by Sargent and Gotch

$$V = \frac{(BW_{PRE} - BW_{POST})}{\left[\dfrac{BUN_{PRE} \times (K_D - (BW_{PRE} - BW_{POST})/T + K_R) - G}{BUN_{POST} \times (K_D - (BW_{PRE} - BW_{POST})/T + K_R) - G}\right]^{\frac{((BW_{PRE}-BW_{POST})/T)}{(K_D-(BW_{PRE}-BW_{POST})/T+K_R)}} - 1}$$

$$G = ((BW_\Phi - BW_{POST})/\Phi + K_R) \times \left[\frac{BUN_\Phi \times \left[\dfrac{V + (BW_\Phi - BW_{POST})}{V}\right]^{\frac{(BW_\Phi-BW_{POST})/\Phi+K_R}{(BW_\Phi-BW_{POST})/\Phi}} - BUN_{POST}}{\left[\dfrac{V + (BW_\Phi - BW_{POST})}{V}\right]^{\frac{(BW_\Phi-BW_{POST})/\Phi+K_R}{(BW_\Phi-BW_{POST})/\Phi}} - 1}\right]$$

BUN refers to blood urea nitrogen (mg/mL). *T*, Φ, and *BW* refer to intradialytic time (min), interdialytic time (min), and body weight (g), respectively, and the subscripts of *PRE*, *POST*, and Φ refer, respectively, to predialysis values, immediate postdialysis values, and values measured before the following dialysis. K_D and K_R refer, respectively, to effective intradialytic patient urea clearance (which can be estimated by in vivo hemodialyzer urea clearance) and residual renal urea clearance (mL/min). K_D is provided to the equations, which are then solved for stable values of urea distribution volume (*V*) and generation rate (*G*), with *V* used in the final calculation of the fractional clearance (*Kt/V*). (See Table 218-2.)

Simplified UKM Equations of Daugirdas and Garred

$$Kt/V = -\ln(R - 0.008 \times T) + (4 - 3.5 \times R) \times UF/W = \frac{-\ln(R) + 3 \times UF/W}{1 - 0.01786 \times T}$$

R refers to the ratio of postdialysis to predialysis BUN. *T*, *UF*, and *W* refer to intradialytic time (hr), ultrafiltrate volume (L), and postdialysis weight (kg), respectively.

Calculations using UKM equations provide a critical and extremely important benefit when dealing with the uncertainties and sources for error mentioned previously, in that they allow for the mathematical phenomenon whereby erroneous UKM parameters are offset. In this manner, any error in the calculation of, for instance, K_D leads to proportional overestimates (or underestimates) of both V and G and little or no error in the final value of Kt/V or normalized protein catabolic rate (nPCR). Such offsetting of error does not occur if UKM techniques are not used. Occasionally, we see Kt/V directly calculated from values of K_D and V that have been measured by other means (e.g., K_D from Michael's equation, V from bioimpedance analysis). We do not recommend this. As shown previously, values for K_D and V are unpredictable in critically ill AKI patients, and any error in their assessment will result in a proportional error in Kt/V during direct substitution. We therefore recommend that such measurements be used as input UKM parameters.

The most common UKM equations for formal iterative calculation of Kt/V are those derived from the variable-volume single-pool (VVSP) model developed by Sargent and Gotch.[18] Alternatively, simplified (noniterative) calculation of Kt/V is possible using equations such as those of Daugirdas and Garred (Tables 218-1 and 218-2).[19,20] Formal UKM calculation is preferable for accuracy, although some data suggest that the simplified equations may provide reasonable estimates of dose.[21] All of these approaches calculate spKt/V. To obtain the equilibrated Kt/V (eKt/V), the Daugirdas rate equation (eKt/V = [spKt/V − 0.47] × (K/V) + 0.02) has been shown to be as accurate as complicated double-pool variable-volume modeling in this setting.[19,22]

The eKt/V undoubtedly provides a more realistic reflection of acute IHD dose; however, spKt/V defines dosing targets from the literature and should be preferentially used in clinical practice.

In summary, spKt/V can be calculated most accurately using formal three-point UKM, or less accurately by simplified formulas. The eKt/V can be calculated using the Daugirdas rate equation but is correspondingly harder to relate to clinical dosing targets. It should be remembered that Kt/V by itself is an inadequate assessment of IHD dose; concurrent consideration of the frequency of treatments is essential.

CALCULATION OF INDEXED SOLUTE CLEARANCE FOR CONTINUOUS RENAL REPLACEMENT THERAPY

To calculate CRRT dose, one considers the effluent (dialysate and/or filtrate) flow rate of the particular CRRT and the saturation of the effluent with the solute in question. After indexing of solute clearance to body weight, the units of CRRT dose are therefore milligrams per kilogram per hour. Unlike IHD and its variants, effect of CRRT on solute control applies to both small and larger solutes. For the moment, however, we will consider small-solute clearance only.

Theoretically, the effluent during CRRT should be completely saturated with small solutes. During CVVHD, dialysate flow rates are sufficiently low for complete

TABLE 218-2

Formal Iterative Urea Kinetic Modeling (UKM) for the Calculation of Single-Pool Kt/V (spKt/V) Using Microsoft Excel (Microsoft Corporation, Seattle, WA)

Worked Example	SYMBOLS	CYCLE 1
Clinical Data (Units)		
Predialysis body weight (g)	BW_{pre}	90000
Postdialysis body weight (g)	BW_{post}	89000
Next predialysis body weight (g)	BW_Φ	91000
Predialysis blood urea nitrogen (BUN) (mg/mL)	BUN_{PRE}	0.952
Postdialysis BUN (mg/mL)	BUN_{POST}	0.392
Next predialysis BUN (mg/mL)	BUN_Φ	0.756
Residual renal urea clearance (mL/min)	K_R	0
Intradialytic patient urea clearance (mL/min)	K_D	190.1
Treatment duration (min)	T	240
Interdialytic duration (min)	Φ	1440
Equations		
Seeded G	$G^\#$	12.10
$BW_{PRE} - BW_{POST}$	wl	1000
$BW_\Phi - BW_{POST}$	wg	2000
wl/T	dwl	4.17
wg/Φ	dwg	1.39
$BUN_{PRE} * (K_D - dwl + K_R)$	$Z1$	177.01
$BUN_{POST} * (K_D - dwl + K_R)$	$Z2$	72.89
$(K_R + dwg)/dwg$	$Z3$	1.00
$dwl/(K_D - dwl + K_R)$	$Z4$	0.02
$[(Z1 - G^\#)/(Z2 - G^\#)]^{Z4}$	$Z5$	1.02
$wl/(Z5 - 1)$	V	44212.12
$((V + wg)/V)^{Z3}$	$Z6$	1.05
$(K_R + dwg) * (BUN_\Phi * Z6 - BUN_{POST})/(Z6 - 1)$	G	12.23
$(G - G^\#)/G^\# * 100$	Convergence of G and $G^\#$	1.00
$(G + G^\#)/2$	Suggested New $G^\#$	12.16
$Kd * T/V$	Kt/V	1.03

Practice Tips
Step 1. Create a spreadsheet with the equations entered as shown.
Step 2. Enter clinical data including an estimated value for K_D, and an arbitrary seeding value for $G^\#$ between 10 and 20.
Step 3 (Manual). Manually input new values for G by overwriting the "$G^\#$" cell with values suggested in the "Suggested New $G^\#$" cell. Usually four to five iterations will be needed to bring the value in the "convergence" cell to 1 (i.e., to bring modeling accuracy to within 1%).
Step 3 (Automated). Use the Microsoft Excel Solver add-in function, specifying the "convergence" cell as the target cell to equal 1 (i.e., modeling accuracy to within 1%) and the "$G^\#$" cell as that which Solver is to change.

equilibration of small solutes between dialysate and blood water by diffusion across the membrane. During CVVH, solutes are dragged across the membrane in association with ultrafiltered water, unless they are above a certain weight, at which point sieving occurs. For small solutes, the sieving coefficient (proportionality constant between the rate of solute movement and fluid movement across the membrane) approximates 1. The ultrafiltrate will therefore have the same concentration of small solutes as the blood water, and the CRRT dose will equal the effluent flow rate (Table 218-3).[14]

Practically, however, there are common situations in which complete saturation of effluent does not occur. The first of these occurs when the filter is performing poorly. Filters typically develop progressive fiber-bundle clotting over time, and they may also develop concentration polarization, a condition in which protein fouling of the membrane leads to diffusive transport of especially larger solutes back into the blood from a concentrated layer immediately adjacent to the membrane. In both of these situations, the concentration of all solutes is lower in effluent than in blood water.

The second situation is during predilution, a modality that involves infusion of substitution fluid before the filter in the extracorporeal circuit. The concentration of all solutes again is lower in effluent than in blood water.

Predilution reduces clearance of small solutes by approximately 15% for low-dose prescriptions (UFR <2 L/hr), and by about 40% for high-dose prescriptions (UFR ≈ 4.5 L/hr).[23,24] The impact of the predilution modality on small-solute clearance can be estimated by a number of formulas (see Table 218-3).

The final situation in which complete saturation of effluent does not occur is when the blood flow rate (Qb) is very low or the dialysate flow rate (Qd) is very high. In this case, the mismatch of flow results in incomplete equilibration of small solutes between dialysate and blood water. This can also occur if the dialyzer is large in relation to Qb and Qd as a result of incomplete fiber-bundle penetration.

Because of these uncertainties, opinion leaders recommend regular monitoring of the ratio between effluent urea nitrogen (EUN) and BUN (the EUN/BUN ratio) (see Table 218-3).[25] In addition to providing a measure of small solute clearance, it also provides a measure of filter performance: A decrease of 20% has been suggested as a threshold for action and replacement of the extracorporeal circuit. The measurement of simultaneous effluent and blood concentrations is also the only way to determine the clearance of larger solutes, which have a sieving coefficient of less than 1 and therefore saturate the effluent to a lower degree than the blood water.

TABLE 218-3

Useful Equations for Calculating Small Solute Clearance (K) during Continuous Renal Replacement Therapy

Continuous Veno-Venous Hemofiltration (CVVH), Hemodialysis (CVVHD), and Hemodiafiltration (CVVHDF), Respectively, Assuming Complete Saturation of Effluent

$$K = UFR = QD = UFR + QD$$

where UFR is the ultrafiltration rate and QD is the dialysate flow rate.

Predilution CVVH and CVVHDF, Respectively, Assuming Complete Saturation of Effluent Other than for the Predilution Modality

$$K = UFR \times [QB_{H_2O}/(QB_{H_2O} + UFR)] = (UFR + QD) \times [QB_{H_2O}/(QB_{H_2O} + UFR)]$$

where QB_{H_2O} is the blood water flow rate, equal to the product of blood flow rate and (1 – hematocrit). The influence of plasma water fraction and red cell water fraction can be ignored with acceptable error at the bedside.

CVVH, CVVHD, CVVHDF, Respectively, Using the Ratio of Effluent Urea Nitrogen (EUN) to Blood Urea Nitrogen (BUN)

$$K = UFR \times \frac{EUN}{BUN} = QD \times \frac{EUN}{BUN} = (UFR + QD) \times \frac{EUN}{BUN}$$

UFR (mL/kg/hr) Needed in Predilution CVVH to Provide 35 mL/kg/hr of Small Solute Clearance, Assuming Complete Saturation of Effluent Other than for the Predilution Modality

$$UFR = \frac{QB_{H_2O} \times 35 \times (BW/60)}{(QB_{H_2O} - 35 \times (BW/60))} \times 60/BW$$

where BW is body weight. For example, for an 80-kg person, QB is 267 mL/min and hematocrit is 0.25; therefore QB_{H_2O} is 200 mL/min at the blood pump. The UFR required to achieve a small solute clearance of 35 mL/kg/hr is 45.65 mL/kg/hr.

UFR (mL/hr/kg) and QD (mL/hr/kg) Needed in Predilution CVVHDF to Provide a Combination of Small Solute Clearance by Filtration ($K_{CONV-TARG}$) and Dialysis ($K_{DIFF-TARG}$), Assuming Complete Saturation of Effluent Other than for the Pre-Dilution Modality

$$UFR = \frac{QB_{H_2O} \times K_{CONV-TARG} \times (BW/60)}{(QB_{H_2O} - K_{CONV-TARG} \times (BW/60))} \times BW/60; \quad \text{UFR is then substituted in}$$

$$QD = K_{DIFF-TARG} \times \frac{QB_{H_2O} + UFR \times (BW/60)}{QB_{H_2O}}$$

For example, for an 80-kg person when a total small solute clearance of 35 mL/kg/hr is desirable through a combination of $K_{CONV-TARG}$ equal to 20 mL/kg/hr plus $K_{DIFF-TARG}$ equal to 15 mL/kg/hr, assuming again that QB_{H_2O} is 200 mL/min, the UFR required to achieve this $K_{CONV-TARG}$ is 23.1 mL/kg/hr, and the QD to achieve this $K_{DIFF-TARG}$ is 17.3 mL/kg/hr.

In summary, small-solute clearance during CRRT can be estimated empirically as the effluent flow rate, although the practitioner should be alert to situations in which complete saturation of the effluent cannot be assumed. We recommend regular measurement of the EUN/BUN ratio for more accurate quantification of CRRT dose and quality assurance of therapy delivery.

UNIFIED EXPRESSIONS OF DOSE FOR ACUTE RENAL REPLACEMENT THERAPY

The ideal expression for ARRT dose should be numerically comparable across all modalities and treatment schedules. The expression should also be simple to calculate without sacrificing accuracy. This does not mean necessarily that the mathematics need be simple, because the most complex of calculations are easily made on modern computers. Instead, this means that the UKM input parameters should be simple and, in particular, readily available to the practitioner. An expression of ARRT dose, no matter how elegant, is clinically unworkable if the input variables are wholly unknown to the practitioner. Furthermore, the ideal expression of dose should be intuitively meaningful,

guiding the practitioner in optimizing the process of solute removal.

As described previously, CRRT dose is expressed as mL/kg/hr. This unit is attractive, because it is numerically comparable with glomerular filtration rate (GFR) and has clear meaning to the practitioner. Moreover, one of the major controversies in ARRT is the timing of therapy initiation in relation to residual renal function, and future studies are likely to utilize GFR as at least one criterion for therapy initiation. Such studies may result in a single clinical target for solute clearance to optimize patient outcomes, which could be met by any combination of residual renal function and ARRT. Occasionally, we see attempts to express CRRT dose as a daily Kt/V. We do not recommend this. The calculations require potentially unreasonable assumptions about V, and they result in an expression for dose that is generally less meaningful than mL/kg/hr.

As also described earlier, IHD dose is expressed as Kt/V. There are difficulties with the use of unit of dose in critically ill AKI patients. The main issue is that there is dissociation between Kt/V and solute mass removal over the course of an IHD treatment: Clearance stays the same, but the mass removal rate goes down as solute concentrations decrease in the body (Fig. 218-1). This dissociation does not affect comparisons of Kt/V within a given dosing schedule (e.g., daily, three times a week). It does mean, however, than cumulative Kt/V does not change propor-

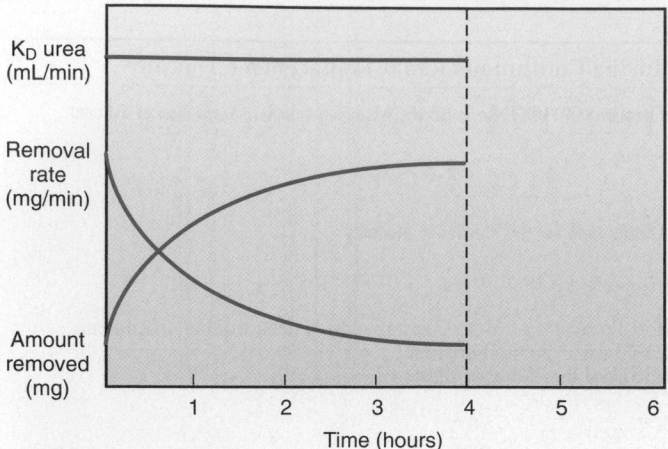

FIGURE 218-1. A representation of solute transport during single-pass intermittent hemodialysis. The curves demonstrate the relationship between the clearance rate of urea (K_D) and urea removal with time.

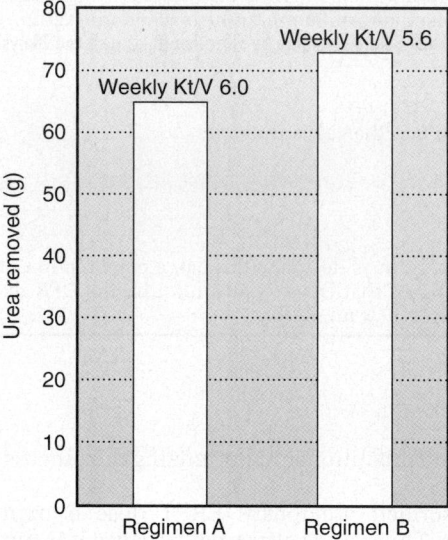

FIGURE 218-2. A comparison of urea nitrogen removed per week during two dialysis regimens, where residual renal function is absent, normalized protein catabolic rate (nPCR) is 0.8 g/kg/day, and starting blood urea nitrogen concentration (BUN) for the week is 93 mg/dL. In regimen A, three hemodialysis (HD) treatments are given per week, with a duration of treatment of 240 minutes, a volume (V) of 40 L, and a clearance rate (K_D) of 333 mL/min. In regimen B, seven HD treatments are given per week, with a duration of 120 minutes, V of 40 L, and K_D of 267 mL/min).

tionally with cumulative solute mass removal for IHD regimens that vary in terms of frequency. It is therefore invalid to quantify cumulative IHD over a given time period by simple addition of Kt/V. It is also invalid to compare the sum of Kt/V per week, for instance, unless the number of treatments within the period of observation is the same. As an example, Figure 218-2 illustrates the increased removal of urea, despite a lower cumulative weekly Kt/V, that occurs as a result of more frequent treatments.

The most reasonable approach to a unified expression for ARRT dose is to model small-solute clearance using UKM. The dose of all ARRT modalities can be expressed in this manner, at least in terms of small-solute clearance. We do acknowledge that uremic toxicity in the setting of AKI is far from well characterized, but we believe that the evidence associating clearance of larger solutes with outcomes is too preliminary to be incorporated into dosing paradigms at the present time.

There are several competing UKM equations that provide unified expressions of dose across different modalities. Gotch derived the "standard Kt/V" (stdKt/V)[26] and Keshaviah and Star derived the "solute removal index" (SRI) in the 1990s.[27] Both expressions are based on the peak urea concentration hypothesis; kinetically equivalent therapy prescriptions are those that produce the same urea mass removal rate at the same predialysis BUN. There are two difficulties with this paradigm in critically ill AKI patients. First, BUN concentrations can be very asymmetrical and variable as a result of urea non–steady state or irregular IHD schedules, and arbitrary definitions of peak BUN concentration are likely to have less validity. Second, the peak urea concentration hypothesis is legitimized in the ESRD setting by the clinical equivalence of IHD and continuous ambulatory peritoneal dialysis (CAPD) and the coincidence that adequate doses of IHD and CAPD are characterized by numerically equal values for stdKt/V and SRI. However, these arguments cannot be extrapolated to critically ill AKI patients. A comparison of IHD and CAPD by Phu and colleagues showed disparate clinical outcomes, despite adequate doses of dialysis by ESRD standards and therefore similar values for stdKt/V and SRI.[28] This finding undermines the validity of the peak urea concentration hypothesis in this setting, as well as the use of stdKt/V and SRI as unified expressions of dose.

In our opinion, the most suitable expression of ARRT dose is the equivalent renal urea clearance (EKR), which has the unit of milliliters per minute.[29] When applied to intermittent ARRT, EKR expresses dose as the continuous urea clearance that will result in the same TAC_{BUN} for a given amount of urea mass removal over the period of observation. When applied to CRRT, EKR is simply the time-averaged continuous urea clearance over the period of observation. EKR is modeled using time-averaged as opposed to peak urea concentration, which is easier to define and likely to be more valid for critically ill AKI patients. EKR is corrected in a manner analogous to GFR to account for different body sizes (EKRc). The correction factor is still based on the archetypal 70-kg male, and his ideal V of 40,000 mL (rather than body surface area) is used as the correction factor (EKRc = EKR/V × 40,000). This correction is critical, because it allows for the previously mentioned mathematical phenomenon that offsets error in the input UKM variables so that there is little or no error in the final value of EKRc. Such offsetting of error does not occur if EKR is corrected to actual body weight or body surface area, which are parameters that are less tightly bound to the kinetic parameter V.

EKRc has also been used in research settings to determine kinetic equivalence between ARRTs for the clearance of larger solutes.[30] There are fewer studies validating this approach, and a workable tool that might be applied in the clinical setting has not yet been presented. Our own preliminary work suggests that the methodology described in the next section could be developed into a unified expression of β_2-microglobulin clearance as well, although the tool is still under development.

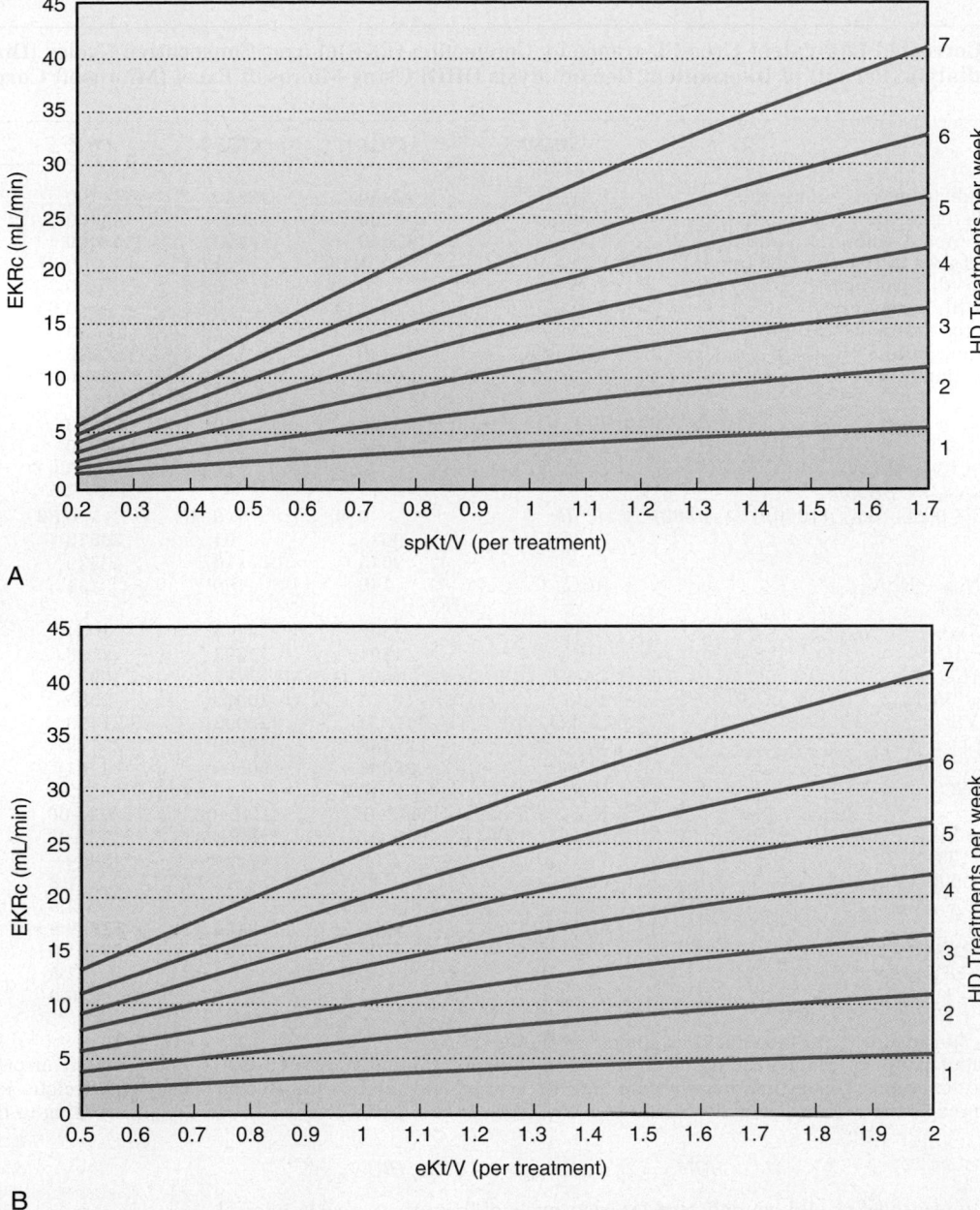

A

B

FIGURE 218-3. A, Relationship between corrected equivalent renal urea clearance (EKRc) and single-pool fractional clearance (spKt/V) per treatment for a frequency of one to seven treatments per week. **B,** Relation between EKRc and equilibrated Kt/V (eKt/V) per treatment for a frequency of one to seven treatments per week.

PRACTICAL QUANTIFICATION OF ACUTE RENAL REPLACEMENT DOSE USING CORRECTED EQUIVALENT RENAL UREA CLEARANCE

Approximate EKRc values can be calculated for acute IHD from the Kt/V per treatment and the treatments per week, using nomograms based on either single-pool or double-pool modeling (Fig. 218-3).[29,31] However, these nomograms are based on the traditional formula for calculating for EKR (G/TAC$_{BUN}$). This formula is valid only during the urea steady state, because it underestimates when the TAC$_{BUN}$

is falling and overestimates when it is rising. The urea non–steady state can render error as high as 30% to 40%.[9]

More accurate values can be calculated by discarding the assumption that the urea mass removal rate for solute J (Jm) is equal to the urea generation rate (G) and modeling instead using the core equation EKRj = Jm/TAC$_{BUN}$. We have previously presented simple algebraic formulas that derive the necessary input data for the calculation of EKRj and corrected EKRj (EKRjc) from BUN time-concentration profiles over the weekly interval (Table 218-4).[32] These formulas can be used in any commercial spreadsheet program, with input of sequential pre-IHD and post-IHD BUN and paired estimations of pre-IHD and post-IHD V.

TABLE 218-4

Calculation of Corrected Equivalent Urea Clearance by Convection (EKRjc) over Consecutive Cycles (Dialysis and following Interdialytic Period) of Intermittent Hemodialysis (IHD) Using Microsoft Excel (Microsoft Corporation, Seattle, WA)

Worked Example	SYMBOLS	CYCLE 1	CYCLE 2	CYCLE 3	CYCLE 4 ... N
Clinical Data (Units)					
Predialysis urea distribution volume (mL)	$V_{PRE(n)}$	43440	42640	44190	45090
Postdialysis urea distribution volume (mL)	$V_{POST(n)}$	42700	42000	44100	44000
Next predialysis urea distribution volume (mL)	$V_{\Phi(n)}$	42640	44190	45090	46590
Predialysis blood urea nitrogen (BUN) (mg/mL)	$BUN_{PRE(n)}$	1.43	1.04	0.77	0.68
(Equilibrated) postdialysis BUN (mg/mL)	$BUN_{POST(n)}$	0.93	0.66	0.39	0.36
Next predialysis BUN (mg/mL)	$BUN_{\Phi(n)}$	1.04	0.77	0.68	0.66
Residual renal urea clearance (mL/min)	K_R	3.2	2.8	3	2.6
Treatment duration (min)	$T_{(n)}$	120	180	240	240
Interdialytic duration (min)	$\Phi_{(n)}$	1380	3000	3720	2880
Equations					
$TT = T + \Phi$	TT	1500	3180	3960	3120
Sum TT	ΣTT	1500	4680	8640	11760
$G = (V_{\Phi} * BUN_{\Phi} - V_{POST} * BUN_{POST})/$ $\quad \Phi + K_R * (BUN_{POST} + BUN_{\Phi})/2$	G	6.4	4.1	5.3	6.5
$nPCR = (9.35 * G + 0.294 * V_{POST}/1000)/(V_{POST}/580)$	$nPCR$	0.98	0.70	0.82	0.98
$A_{CY} = G * TT$	A_{CY}	9615	13101	20813	20420
Sum $A_{CY} = \Sigma A_{CY}$	ΣA_{CY}	9615	22716	43529	63949
$AUC_D = T * (BUN_{PRE} - BUN_{POST})/$ $\ln(BUN_{PRE}/BUN_{POST})$	AUC_D	140	150	134	120
$AUC_I = \Phi * (BUN_{POST} + BUN_{PRE})/2$	AUC_I	1362	2143	1984	1464
$AUC_T = AUC_D + AUC_I$	AUC_T	1501	2293	2118	1585
Sum $AUC_T = \Sigma AUC_T$	ΣAUC_T	1501	3795	5913	7498
$V_{\Phi} * BUN_{\Phi} - V_{PRE} * BUN_{PRE}$	ΔVC	−17774	−10319	−3365	88
Sum $\Delta VC = \Sigma\Delta VC$	$\Sigma\Delta VC$	−17774	−28093	−31458	−31370
$M_{CY} = A_{CY} - \Delta VC$	M_{CY}	27388	23420	24178	20332
Sum $M_{CY} = \Sigma M_{CY}$	ΣM_{CY}	27388	50809	74987	95318
$EKRj = \Sigma M_{CY}/\Sigma AUC_T$	$EKRj$	18.2	13.4	12.7	12.7
$V_{POST} * TT$	$V_{POST} * TT$	6.4E+07	1.34E+08	1.75E+08	1.37E+08
Sum $V_{POST} * TT = \Sigma V_{POST} * TT$	$\Sigma V_{POST(M)} * TT$	6.4E+07	1.98E+08	3.72E+08	5.1E+08
$V_{POST(M)} = \Sigma V_{POST} * TT/\Sigma TT$	$V_{POST(M)}$	42700	42224	43084	43327
$EKRjc = EKRj * 40000/V_{POST(M)}$	$EKRjc$	17.1	12.7	11.8	11.7
$K_{RC}^{\#} = K_R * 40000/V_{POST(M)}$	$K_{RC}^{\#}$	3.0	2.7	2.8	2.4
$K_{RC}^{\#} * TT$	$K_{RC}^{\#} * TT$	4496.5	8434.9	11029.6	7489.1
Sum $K_{RC}^{\#} * TT = \Sigma K_{RC}^{\#} * TT$	$\Sigma K_{RC}^{\#} * TT$	4496.5	12931.4	23961.0	31450.1
$K_{RC} = \Sigma K_{RC}^{\#} * TT/\Sigma TT$	K_{RC}	3.0	2.8	2.8	2.7
$dEKRjc = EKRjc - K_{RC}$	$dEKRjc$	14.1	9.9	9.0	9.1

Practice Tips

Step 1. Create a spreadsheet with the equations entered as shown.

Step 2. Enter data for input variables including an estimated value for volume of distribution (V). Because any error is offset in the subsequent calculations, this estimation does not need to be exact and can be estimated as 0.65 × body weight. Postdialysis BUN can be entered as immediate postdialysis values (BUN_{POST}) or as equilibrated values ($BUN_{POST(EQ)}$) according to the equation from Tattersall:

$$BUN_{POST(EQ)} = BUN_{PRE} \times (BUN_{POST}/BUN_{PRE})^{T/T+35}$$

Columns in the spreadsheet should be replicated for every cycle of IHD over a weekly interval.

These estimations of V need not be exact, because the accuracy of the calculated value for EKRjc by this method is not compromised until the estimation error of V is greater than 25% to 50% in either direction. Our own practice is to estimate V by using a value of 0.65 times body weight. The calculated value for EKRjc using this spreadsheet method is not compromised by the urea non–steady-state or by variations in G. In addition, EKRjc can be calculated in a manner that accounts for compartment effects by adjusting the post-IHD BUN for urea dysequilibrium using the formula from Tattersall.[33]

For CRRT, the approximate EKRjc values can be calculated from small-solute clearance. The only difference between EKRjc (mL/min) and CRRT dose (mL/kg/hr) is that the former is corrected to a V of 40 L and the latter is indexed to body weight. To calculate EKRjc (mL/min), one can assume V to be 0.65 × body weight and divide the indexed small-solute clearance by 0.975.[9]

More accurate values for EKRjc for CRRT can be calculated in a similar manner as for IHD, but using a different set of algebraic formulas from those used for IHD, based on a differently modeled BUN time-concentration profile over the weekly interval.[32]

It should be emphasized that EKRc is not simply time-averaged hemodialyzer urea clearance. By way of an example, EKRc would not triple if hemodialyzer clearance were to be tripled for a given IHD regimen. EKRc is a true mass balance parameter that accounts for the inefficiency of intermittent therapies.

In summary, it is our opinion that EKRjc is the best expression to unify dose of ARRT between different modalities and schedules. We believe that acute IHD dose should be preferentially expressed as EKRjc, to provide an expression that accounts for the frequency of treatments and also allows some comparison with CRRT in terms of small solute clearance. Furthermore, we believe that CRRT dose can be legitimately expressed as EKRjc, which can certainly be used in the research setting to quantify dose across a range of solutes and clarify the relative impact of small versus larger solute clearance on patient outcomes.

CONCLUSION

The prescription and quantification of ARRT according to dosing standards is an increasingly popular and widespread practice pattern and will become ubiquitous in the future if various studies that are currently underway provide definitive results proving a causal relationship between ARRT dose and clinical outcomes.

We have presented an overview of methods to calculate small-solute clearance during ARRT that are comparable between modalities and schedules. This does not mean that we believe large-solute clearance to be unimportant, merely that small-solute clearance is currently the best correlate of outcomes for patients treated with ARRT. We believe that there are as yet insufficient data to support the inclusion of large-solute clearance in clinical dosing targets for ARRT.

Two major uncertainties arise when using solute clearance to define ARRT dose. First, it is unknown whether solute control per se (i.e., levels of uremic toxins or markers) is more important than solute clearance per se. Second, it is increasingly apparent that mass transfer across membranes may play a relatively minor role in the removal of certain potential uremic toxins, such as pro-inflammatory cytokines. Their sieving coefficient is frequently much less than 1, and their removal has been shown to be due to an adsorptive mechanism resulting in up to a 10-fold higher removal of such mediators in comparison to mass transfer alone.[34] Adsorption is critically dependent on membrane composition and structure, and it may become necessary to stratify or adjust expressions for ARRT dose for membrane type, if studies in the future show adsorption to be clinically important.

Key Points

1. In critically ill patients with acute renal injury treated with acute renal replacement therapy (ARRT), the relationship between solute clearance and clinical outcomes is best defined for small solutes, although there are preliminary data supporting a similar relationship for larger solutes.
2. The "best" expression for ARRT dose is determined by whatever expression has been correlated with clinical outcomes in the literature: that is, single-pool fractional clearance (spKt/V) for intermittent hemodialysis and ultrafiltration rate for continuous renal replacement therapy (CRRT).
3. Urea kinetics are different in critically ill patients with AKI; and spKt/V is most accurately calculated using formal iterative three-point urea kinetic modeling, and less accurately using simplified formulas.
4. The ultrafiltration rate is known directly in post-dilution conventional CRRT. In other situations, it can be estimated by a variety of formulas depending on the exact modality, or, alternatively, by the ratio of the urea concentration in the effluent to that in the blood (EUN/BUN ratio).
5. The corrected equivalent renal urea clearance (EKRjc) is the most accurate unified expression for ARRT dose, and it is easy to calculate using commercial spreadsheet programs.

Key References

6. Palevsky P, O'Conner T, Zhang J, et al: Design of the VA/NIH Acute Renal Failure Trial Network (ATN) Study: Intensive versus conventional renal support in acute renal failure. Clin Trials 2005;2:423-435.
7. Schiffl H, Lang S, Fischer R: Daily hemodialysis and the outcomes of acute renal failure. N Eng J Med 2002;346:305-310.
8. Paganini EP, Tapolyai M, Goormastic M, et al: Establishing a dialysis therapy/patient outcome link in intensive care unit acute dialysis for patients with acute renal failure. Am J Kidney Dis 1996;28(Suppl):S81-S89.
25. Sigler M: Critical care nephrology. Transport characteristics of the slow therapies: Implications for achieving adequacy of dialysis in acute renal failure. Adv Renal Replace Ther 1997;4:68-80.
32. Casino F, Marshall M: Simple and accurate quantification of dialysis in acute renal failure patients during either the urea non-steady state or treatment with irregular or continuous schedules. Nephrol Dial Transplant 2004;19:1454-1466.

See the companion Expert Consult website for the complete reference list.

CHAPTER 219

Principles of Pharmacodynamics and Pharmacokinetics of Drugs Used in Extracorporeal Therapies

Federico Pea and Mario Furlanut

OBJECTIVES

This chapter will:
1. Identify the major factors affecting drug removal during renal replacement therapy (RRT).
2. Define the principles for appropriate dosage adjustments during RRT.
3. Describe the potential relevance of RRT in modifying the pharmacodynamic behavior of antimicrobial agents during RRT.

When a drug is administered for therapeutic purposes, its pharmacodynamic effect is the result of the achievement and maintenance of adequate therapeutic free concentrations at the site of action. This result depends on several complex pharmacokinetic processes occurring in the body after the administration according to the drug's peculiar physicochemical properties. As a consequence, each individual drug may present different plasma protein binding, distribution with tissue accumulation, metabolism (mainly by the liver), and/or elimination (mainly by the kidney), and, in order to guarantee the therapeutic effect, appropriate dosing regimens must be defined.

When starting a drug therapy, the loading dose (i.e., the initial dose) is administered with the intent of rapidly achieving therapeutically effective concentrations, and its amount is essentially dependent on volume of distribution (Vd).[1] The subsequent doses (i.e., the maintenance doses) are administered with the intent of maintaining these effective levels over time by replacing the amount eliminated from the body during the dosing interval, so their amount depends mainly on drug clearance (K).

In the presence of acute renal failure, the application of renal replacement therapies (RRTs) may consistently alter the clearance of drugs, especially of those compounds that are normally cleared by the kidney.[2] Consistently, the maintenance dose, but not the loading dose, of a given drug might require significant modification during the application of RRT, to avoid both toxicity risks related to overexposure and therapeutic failure related to underexposure, especially when drugs with a low therapeutic index are used.

The amount of drug removal may greatly vary according to several factors related to the functioning processes of RRT, the peculiar physicochemical and pharmacokinetic properties of the drug, and the properties of the device.

FACTORS AFFECTING DRUG CLEARANCE DURING RENAL REPLACEMENT THERAPY

Principles of Drug Removal

RRT may employ two different physicochemical processes, diffusion and convection, to replace renal function in the elimination of several solutes from blood through semipermeable membranes, and these processes may greatly influence drug removal by RRT (Table 219-1).[3]

Diffusion represents the typical working principle of hemodialysis; it occurs passively through a semipermeable membrane, according to the concentration gradient and in countercurrent respect to blood flow, and generally needs time to reach equilibrium. Diffusive clearance is inversely correlated to the molecular weight (MW) of the solutes, being especially efficient for small drug molecules (MW < 500 Da).[4]

Conversely, convection represents the typical working principle of hemofiltration; it is an active process similar to glomerular filtration and occurs rapidly and efficiently thanks to a pump-driven pressure gradient. Drug removal is independent of the MW, considering that almost all drug molecules are smaller than the very high hemofilter cutoffs, which are expressly targeted to allow the filtration of large solutes (e.g., inflammatory cytokines).[5] Similarly to the glomerular filtration process in the kidney, hemofiltration produces an ultrafiltrate, so a replacement fluid must be administered in order to preserve adequate circulatory volume.

The most frequently applied RRTs in patients with acute renal failure are intermittent hemodialysis (IHD), continuous veno-venous hemofiltration (CVVH), and continuous veno-venous hemodiafiltration (CVVHDF). Whereas IHD is essentially a diffusive technique, CVVH is a convective technique, and CVVHDF is a combination of both.

Drug Properties

The drug characteristics that affect clearance during RRT are shown in Table 219-2.

Molecular Weight

Drug removal is expected to be dependent on MW only if the filter membrane cutoff is lower than the size of the considered drug. This aspect is completely irrelevant for

TABLE 219-1

Comparison of Characteristics of Drug Removal during Renal Replacement Therapy

DIFFUSION	CONVECTION
Typical of dialysis	Typical of hemofiltration
Passive process	Active process
Movement results from concentration gradient and is countercurrent to blood flow	Movement results from pump-driven pressure gradient
Dependent on drug molecular weight	Independent of drug molecular weight
Long time to equilibrium	Rapid equilibrium
No need for replacement fluid	Need for replacement fluid to reconstitute blood volume (predilution or postdilution mode)

TABLE 219-2

Factors Potentially Affecting Drug Clearance during Renal Replacement Therapy

DRUG PROPERTIES	DEVICE PROPERTIES
Molecular weight	Composition
Plasma protein binding	Surface area
Volume of distribution	Pore size
Proportion of renal clearance	Adsorption

hemofiltration techniques such as CVVH or CVVHDF, because almost all therapeutic drugs have MW less than 2000 Da—a value significantly lower than the hemofilter cutoffs, which are optimized to be impermeable to plasma proteins (about 30,000 to 50,000 Da). On the other hand, MW becomes relevant in IHD because the filters are optimized for small solutes, often with a cutoff value of less than 800 to 1000 Da. Accordingly, almost all drugs are expected to be at least partially removed by CVVH and CVVHDF, whereas most, but not all drugs, will be removed by IHD.[4] For example, the glycopeptide antibiotics vancomycin and teicoplanin are not removed during classic IHD because they have an MW higher than 1500 Da.[6]

Plasma Protein Binding

The second relevant factor conditioning drug clearance during RRT is the amount of plasma protein binding. Only the unbound moiety of a drug is available for elimination by RRT, so that higher plasma protein binding means lower drug clearance.

Volume of Distribution

The Vd reflects where a given drug is compartmentalized in the body, and it can vary greatly according to the drug's physicochemical properties, namely hydrophilicity or lipophilicity. Hydrophilic compounds, because of their inability to passively cross the plasmatic membrane of the eukaryotic cell, present a distribution limited to the plasma and to the extracellular space; therefore, they are promptly and efficiently removed by RRT. This is typically the case with most antibacterials belonging to β-lactam, glycopep-

tide, and aminoglycoside classes, for which supplemental dosing (in comparison with the regimen used in patients with complete renal failure) is often mandatory during RRT.[7] On the other hand, most of the available therapeutic drugs are lipophilic compounds, which, thanks to their ability to freely cross the plasmatic membrane of the eukaryotic cells according to the concentration gradient, may significantly accumulate in the intracellular compartment. The larger the Vd, the less likely it is that the drug will be removed by RRT. For most lipophilic drugs with wide Vd, only a small fraction of the total drug amount present in the body can be removed, even with 100% extraction across the RRT filter, so supplemental dosing during RRT is unnecessary.[7]

Proportion of Renal Clearance

Drug clearance from the body is the result of elimination by renal excretion and by extrarenal pathways (nonrenal clearance), usually hepatic metabolism. Because RRT replaces renal function, it is clear that drug clearance during RRT is clinically relevant only with those drugs for which renal clearance is normally dominant (i.e., ≥30% of the total body clearance). This is usually the case with most hydrophilic antibiotics, for which supplemental doses (beyond the regimen used in patients with complete renal failure) are usually needed during RRT. Conversely, drugs exhibiting mainly nonrenal clearance are expected to be only minimally cleared by RRT, so no major dosing modification (compared with the full dosing regimen in patients with normal renal function) is needed.

Estimation of Drug Clearance During Hemofiltration

Although estimation of drug removal may be difficult for IHD, it is more easily calculated for continuous treatments.[4]

The sieving coefficient (S) identifies the drug fraction cleared during continuous hemofiltration and may be defined by the following equation:

$$S = C_{UF}/C_P$$

where C_{UF} is the drug concentration in the ultrafiltrate, and C_P is the drug concentration in plasma.

The efficiency of drug clearance during CVVH depends on the administration mode of the replacement fluid. If the replacement fluid used to reconstitute blood volume is added in the postdilution mode (i.e., hemofiltration), drug clearance by the hemofilter (K_{HF}) is equal to the ultrafiltration rate (Q_{UF}) so that:

$$\text{Postdilution } K_{HF} = Q_{UF} \times S$$

Conversely, in the predilution mode, drug clearance will be lower, because plasma entering the filter is diluted by the substitution fluid, so that a dilution factor (DF) must be taken into account:

$$DF = Q_{BF}/(Q_{BF} + Q_{RF})$$

where Q_{BF} is the blood flow rate and Q_{RF} is the replacement flow rate. Drug clearance in these circumstances is defined by the following formula:

$$\text{Predilution } K_{HF} = Q_{UF} \times S \times Q_{BF}/(Q_{BF} + Q_{RF})$$

Accordingly, it may be postulated that during CVVH drug removal will increase in a manner directly propor-

TABLE 219-3

Factors Potentially Increasing Drug Clearance during Renal Replacement Therapy (RRT)

RRT OPERATING CONDITIONS	PATIENT'S PATHOPHYSIOLOGY
Hemodiafiltration	Hypoalbuminemia
High-volume ultrafiltration	Residual renal function

tional to the applied ultrafiltration rate and will generally be higher in the postdilution mode.[3,8]

Considering that the hemofilter cutoffs are typically greater than the MW of almost all drugs, S in most cases should be equal to the unbound moiety of the drug, and, theoretically, K_{HF} should be easily estimated. However, several authors have demonstrated that predicted and observed S frequently do not correspond.[2] If drug removal is higher than expected, the explanation might lie in the influence of several factors related to the properties and operating conditions of the device and to the patient's pathophysiological status.

Device Properties

Devices present different characteristics in terms of composition, surface area, and ultrafiltration coefficient (see Table 219-2), and these factors may be directly correlated to both diffusive and convective transport.[9] Additionally, drug removal may be increased because of drug adsorption to the hemofilter.[10,11] This adsorption rate may vary significantly over time, because it is expected to be maximal immediately after starting RRT and then to progressively decrease until filter exhaustion.

Operating Conditions

The efficiency of drug removal for a specific compound is expected to be greater for continuous than for intermittent RRT, and, generally speaking, the order is CVVHDF > CVVH > IHD. However, the total removed amount can vary greatly, even according to the ultrafiltration flow rate (Table 219-3). The application of high-volume ultrafiltration rates (>35 mL/kg/hr), as recently suggested to improve survival in acute renal failure,[12] may significantly increase the extracorporeal clearance of hydrophilic antimicrobials with low Vd and low protein binding, so that more aggressive dosing regimens must be advocated under these circumstances.[13]

Patient's Pathophysiology

In severely critically ill patients, there are often some peculiar pathophysiological conditions that may concur in altering drug clearance during CRRT (see Table 219-3). First of all, the unbound fraction of a drug that is usually moderately to highly bound may vary in critically ill patients who present with hypoalbuminemia; in some cases, drug clearance may be expected to increase under this circumstance.[2,14] It was recently shown that this effect may be clinically relevant for some highly protein-bound antimicrobial agents, namely ceftriaxone[15] and teicoplanin.[16]

Additionally, the presence of residual renal function must eventually be taken into account, considering that it may significantly increase the total clearance of drugs that are highly removable by RRT, such as most hydrophilic antibiotics.[9,17]

Finally, for drugs with limited extracellular distribution, the presence of an extra volume in the interstitial compartment of critically ill patients may greatly enlarge their Vd. For example, this may occur because of capillary leakage due to sepsis or polytrauma.[18,19] In these situations, when starting therapy with hydrophilic antimicrobials, an increased loading dose should be administered, with the intent of promptly achieving therapeutic concentrations.

PRINCIPLES FOR DOSAGE ADJUSTMENTS DURING CONTINUOUS RENAL REPLACEMENT THERAPY

In critically ill patients with acute renal failure, different approaches for drug dosage adjustments should be pursued according to the relative importance of the extracorporeal clearance (K_{CRRT}) compared with the total body clearance (K_T).

One of the most investigated field concerns the use of antibacterial agents. The clinical relevance of CRRT during antimicrobial treatment is mainly related to the need to prevent underdosing by administering substitutional or increased doses, with the double intent of avoiding the risk of therapeutic failure and containing the spread of breakthrough bacterial resistance.

As a general rule, four different situations may be encountered (Table 219-4). First, when using drugs with low Vd and normally high renal clearance, for which K_{CRRT} represents a significant percentage of K_T, additional doses (in comparison with those used for anephric patients) are usually required. It is clear that the relative importance of CRRT in drug removal is maximal for hydrophilic compounds with low plasma protein binding (Table 219-5), this being the typical profile of several hydrophilic antimicrobial agents, such as most β-lactams and aminoglycosides.

Second, when using drugs with moderately high Vd but normally high renal clearance, for which K_{CRRT} represents a significant percentage of K_T (e.g., levofloxacin), additional doses in comparison with anephric patients are frequently required.

Third, when using drugs with high Vd for which renal clearance normally varies because of the presence of other compensatory mechanisms, for which K_{CRRT} may represent a moderate and variable percentage of K_T (e.g., ciprofloxacin), doses similar to those used in patients with moderately impaired or even normal renal function may be required.

Fourth, when using drugs with normally low renal clearance, for which K_{CRRT} is expected to represent a poor percentage of K_T, doses similar to those used in patients with normal renal function are frequently required.

From all of the above considerations, it appears that, when hydrophilic antibacterial agents highly cleared by extracorporeal therapies are used during CVVH or CVVHDF in critically ill patients with acute renal failure, significant dosage increases (versus anephric patients) may sometimes be necessary, especially in the presence of high-volume ultrafiltration rates.[7,13]

TABLE 219-4

Handling of Some Antimicrobial Agents during CRRT (CVVH and/or CVVHDF)*

CHARACTERISTICS OF ANTIMICROBIAL AGENT	DOSAGE ADJUSTMENT	EXAMPLE DRUGS
1. Low Vd + normally high renal clearance: K_{CRRT} is a significant part of K_T	Require additional doses, compared with anephric patients	**Aminoglycosides:** Amikacin Gentamicin Netilmicin Tobramycin **Penicillin:** Amoxicillin or amoxicillin-clavulanate Ampicillin or ampicillin-sulbactam Piperacillin or piperacillin-tazobactam **Cephalosporins:** Cefepime Cefotaxime Ceftazidime **Carbapenems:** Imipenem-cilastatin Meropenem **Monobactams:** Aztreonam **Glycopeptides:** Vancomycin Teicoplanin[†]
2. High Vd + normally high renal clearance: K_{CRRT} is a significant part of K_T	Require additional doses, compared with anephric patients	**Fluoroquinolones:** Levofloxacin
3. High Vd + normally variable renal clearance: K_{CRRT} is a variable part of K_T	May require doses similar to those for patients with moderately impaired renal function	**Fluoroquinolones:** Ciprofloxacin
4. Normally low renal clearance: K_{CRRT} is a poor part of K_T	Require doses same as those for patients with normal renal function	**β-Lactams:** Ceftriaxone[†] Oxacillin **Fluoroquinolones:** Moxifloxacin **Others:** Clindamycin Linezolid Quinupristin/dalfopristin

CVVH, continuous veno-venous hemofiltration; CVVHDF, continuous veno-venous hemodiafiltration; K_{CCRT}, extracorporeal clearance; K_T, total body clearance; Vd, volume of distribution.
*For theoretical dosages, see Trotman et al.[7] and at Scheetz et al.[13]
[†]Higher doses may be necessary in the presence of hypoalbuminemia.

TABLE 219-5

Drug Properties Conditioning the Highest Potential Clearance during Renal Replacement Therapy

Low molecular weight*
Low plasma protein binding
Low volume of distribution
High renal clearance

*Relevant only for intermittent hemodialysis.

PHARMACODYNAMICS AND DOSAGE ADJUSTMENTS OF ANTIMICROBIAL AGENTS DURING RENAL REPLACEMENT THERAPY

Considering that dosage increase may be performed in two different ways, by enlarging the amount of each single dose or by shortening the dosing interval, the approach chosen should be based on the pharmacodynamic behavior of the specific drug.

Anti-infective agents may exhibit time-dependent or concentration-dependent antimicrobial activity. For time-dependent antimicrobial agents, namely β-lactams, macrolides, glycopeptides, oxazolidinones, and azole antifungals, the time (t) during which concentrations are maintained above the minimum inhibitory concentration (MIC) of the etiological agent (t > MIC) is considered the most relevant pharmacodynamic parameter.[20] For these agents, exposure may be optimized by maintaining trough plasma levels (C_{min}) greater than the MIC (C_{min} > MIC).[18] Accordingly, for those time-dependent agents significantly removed by CRRT, the most suitable approach for dosage increment to preserve efficacy would be to increase the frequency of drug administration by shortening the dosing interval.

For concentration-dependent antimicrobials, namely aminoglycosides and fluoroquinolones, the most important pharmacodynamic parameter, both to ensure efficacy and to prevent the spread of bacterial resistance, is the ratio between the peak plasma level (C_{max}) and the MIC (C_{max}/MIC), which must be at least 10.[21] Additionally, the total daily drug exposure, in terms of the area under the curve of plasma concentration versus time (AUC), must be many times higher than the MIC, the thresholds for optimal pharmacodynamic exposure being AUC/MIC = 125 for gram-negative microorganisms[22] and AUC/MIC = 40 for gram-positive microorganisms.[23] Accordingly, to improve efficacy during extracorporeal therapy with those concentration-dependent agents that are highly removable by CRRT, it may be more useful to increase the amount of each single dose while extending the dosing interval.

CONCLUSION

Drug removal during RRT is a complex process that may vary greatly even in a brief period as a consequence of frequent variations in CRRT characteristics and operating conditions or in the patients' pathophysiological status.

Several authors have suggested different approaches with the intent of estimating drug clearance during CVVH or CVVHDF in order to calculate the appropriate dose,[2,4,8,9,24] and useful dosage recommendations during CRRT, specifically for antimicrobial agents, have recently been published.[7,13] Although these might be helpful in starting therapy, several pharmacokinetic studies carried out in critically ill patients during extracorporeal therapies have documented very large interindividual and intraindividual pharmacokinetic variability. Of note, higher than currently recommended dosages may be especially needed for some hydrophilic compounds during the application of high-volume ultrafiltration rates[25] or in the presence of residual renal function.

Tailored therapy with hydrophilic antimicrobials by means of therapeutic drug monitoring should be considered in critically ill patients undergoing CRRT, because this is probably the only way to optimize exposure in each individual patient.[26] Moreover, it was recently demonstrated that discrepancies between predicted and observed CVVH removal of antimicrobial agents in critically ill patients may be especially relevant for drugs having both a narrow therapeutic index and a predominantly renal clearance (e.g., vancomycin).[27]

Key Points

1. The drugs most completely removable by renal replacement therapy are those with a low volume of distribution, low protein binding, and high renal clearance; this is true for most hydrophilic antibiotics belonging to the β-lactam and aminoglycoside classes.
2. Continuous veno-venous hemodiafiltration (CVVHDF) is generally the most efficient technique in drug removal.
3. High-volume ultrafiltration rates may significantly increase drug removal.
4. The presence of hypoalbuminemia and/or sepsis may cause underdosing.
5. Therapeutic drug monitoring of plasma concentrations should be applied to optimize drug exposure, especially with hydrophilic antimicrobials and with drugs that have a low therapeutic index.

Key References

3. Bugge JF: Influence of renal replacement therapy on pharmacokinetics in critically ill patients. Best Pract Res Clin Anaesthesiol 2004;18:175-187.
4. Bohler J, Donauer J, Keller F: Pharmacokinetic principles during continuous renal replacement therapy: Drugs and dosage. Kidney Int Suppl 1999;72:S24-S28.
7. Trotman RL, Williamson JC, Shoemaker DM, et al: Antibiotic dosing in critically ill adult patients receiving continuous renal replacement therapy. Clin Infect Dis 2005;41:1159-1166.
14. Golper TA: Update on drug sieving coefficients and dosing adjustments during continuous renal replacement therapies. Contrib Nephrol 2001;(132):349-353.
19. Pea F, Viale P, Furlanut M: Antimicrobial therapy in critically ill patients: A review of pathophysiological conditions responsible for altered disposition and pharmacokinetic variability. Clin Pharmacokinet 2005;44:1009-1034.

See the companion Expert Consult website for the complete reference list.

CHAPTER 220

Ethical Considerations in Acute Renal Replacement Therapy

Nereo Zamperetti, Maurizio Dan, and Pasquale Piccinni

OBJECTIVES

This chapter will:
1. Present the main bioethical problems associated with the management of continuous renal replacement therapy (CRRT) in critically ill patients.
2. Discuss the use of moral principles to guide difficult decisions.
3. Present a protocol to guide a practical possible approach to difficult decisions in critically ill patients.
4. Present and discuss some of the problems associated with clinical research in CRRT in critically ill patients.
5. Present some biosocial issues related to CRRT.

Renal replacement therapy (RRT) has always had a strict connection with bioethics. Information and consent for a life-saving therapy (dialysis), clinical research, management of vital support procedures, procurement of vital organs for transplantation, and maintenance of waiting lists for expensive and scarce devices are only a few examples of how the history of RRT has strongly marked the development of bioethics. For this reason, a specific chapter dealing with some ethical considerations can find its proper place in this manual.

The goals of this chapter are to ensure that the moral principles for delivery of care and their practical applications are understood, to promote a bioethical culture for the best management of RRT for care and for research, and to ensure that readers can make responsible choices in the management of RRT, even for terminally ill patients.

The chapter is divided in three parts. The first part deals with some bioethical considerations when caring for critically ill patients in need of RRT. Because renal failure in such patients is significantly associated with poor prognosis, the problem of forgoing restorative care and optimizing palliative care is particularly examined. The second part of the chapter deals with clinical research in RRT. Finally, some biosocial issues related to RRT are discussed.

RENAL REPLACEMENT THERAPY IN THE CARE OF THE CRITICALLY ILL PATIENT

Is Renal Replacement Theory Moral?

The ethical management of intensive care support procedures can be very difficult. A basic question refers to the question of whether RRT is moral. If it is, where does its

morality stand? The answers can only come from our view of health and health care. Health could be considered just a physical accident (such as beauty, height, or the color of the eyes) and health care a commercial commodity reserved to those who can pay for it. If this happens, perhaps RRT (and, indeed, any other medical activity) is only a technical act, one that must be managed with attention, commitment, and honesty but does not have any relevant intrinsic moral content.

On the contrary, we believe that health is a fundamental good of every human being and that health care is a basic human right.[1] Consequently, RRT is more than a mere technical act. Attending to a suffering person and doing the most possible to help that person recover *is* a moral action. Obviously, its morality is not absolute. It must be related to the patient's willingness of being cured, acceptance of the reasonable results, view of life, and moral and religious beliefs. Nevertheless, a clinically sound and compassionately administered medical action should be considered a good and adequate approach until proven otherwise. The best proof is the patient's valid refusal of therapy.

Three factors—clinical indication, informed consent, and compassionate administration—are the basis of the ethical foundation of RRT.

Information and Consent for Renal Replacement Therapy

People with chronic renal failure necessitating long-term ambulatory RRT (dialysis) are usually able to be informed and to give valid consent or refusal. In fact, the refusal or discontinuation of dialysis is the cause of approximately 25% of deaths of patients in irreversible renal failure.[2,3]

Such valid consent or refusal is not usually possible for the critically ill patient in an intensive care unit (ICU) who requires RRT as part of intensive support. The competence of these patients is typically inadequate at the time when important therapeutic decisions are made.[4-6] Consequently, such patients might receive care they would not have chosen and whose aim is inconsistent with their wishes.[7-10]

Yet, at least some patients are competent at the time of hospitalization. Whenever possible, their involvement in the decision-making process is mandatory. Every piece of information regarding a patient's health status is a private property of that individual patient. Health care workers (HCWs) have the right and duty to manage such data only in order to make sense of them and to give them back to the patient so that she or he can make the best choice. Once the patient has been adequately informed, it is possible to agree with her or him on the course of care that is most fitting. Obviously, the competent patient can change her or his position in time; in this sense, informed consent is a continuous process and not a punctual event.

The process of advance care planning, in which the patient is informed and agrees with the HCWs on a course of therapy, can take different forms. Advance directives can include a "living will" (an instruction directive wherein the patient specifies the level of acceptable therapy) and/or a proxy directive ("durable power of attorney for health care," wherein the patient indicates the person who can make sound decisions in her or his place, should she or he become incompetent).

Unfortunately, information to the patient is often inadequate, and both advance care planning and advance directives are rare in everyday clinical practice.[11] Even worse, these directives have not proved to be able to affect significantly the course of care of critically ill patients, because they are often ignored by HCWs.[7,12,13]

The HCWs and the Relatives of the Incompetent Patient

HCWs alone are not likely to be the best decision makers for their incompetent patients, especially when end-of-life decisions have to be made.[14-19] An extreme variability among doctors in defining a patient's prognosis and in decision making about forgoing life-sustaining therapies (including continuous RRT) has been shown.[4,14-16,20]

If the patient's competence is inadequate and her or his wishes are not known, the patient's relatives should be included in the decision-making process.[21] This does not mean that the relatives should decide the course of therapy, which is always a medical decision. Nonetheless, the family may be a precious source of information about the patient's wishes, especially when future quality of life is considered. Relatives should be able to clarify what the patient would consider as her or his own best interest. On the other hand, what the relatives say could be conditioned by their own experience, moral and religious beliefs, or external interests, as well as anxiety and depression.[22] Relatives' and surrogates' decisions do not always accurately reflect the patient's wishes and preferences.[23-27]

For these reasons, the family of an incompetent patient and the HCWs should work together to determine the patient's desires and expectations and the level of cure the patient would have chosen for herself or himself in that situation.[25] This requires a great amount of attention, time, and sensitivity. Successful and effective communication is extremely important, and its lack is the main cause of family dissatisfaction.[28-30]

Guidelines and Moral Principles

Guidelines are very useful because they provide the clinical, moral, and legal background for decision making. Yet, they are not always sufficient. No guideline would be able to determine the best decision for every patient. Each situation is unique, because patients, families, and relatives are always different, and so are the HCWs.

So, having adequate references from official guidelines, the solution to every individual situation is best found within that situation. For this task, shared ethical principles are indispensable: *autonomy, beneficence, nonmalefi-*

cence, and *justice* are the ones currently accepted in the Western world. They can guide reasoning and decision making according to the needs of the case.

The aim of decision making is promoting patients' dignity; the principles are the means to reach such a goal. In case of conflict among principles, the one that best promotes the patient's dignity in the specific situation must be privileged. Therefore, the moral principles are not absolute and admit exceptions. Obviously, such exceptions must always be dealt with in the most careful way.[31] Any exception to any moral principle must be accepted only exceptionally and only if it is indispensable to best promote the patient's dignity, which is the goal of care. In such decisions, those who decide which principle should be sacrificed must assume the burden of proof. In conclusion, moral principles are clear and valid in general terms, but their specification, application, and weighing depend on circumstances.

Again, an optimal decision can be obtained only with continuous, overt, and honest circular communication among everyone involved in the care of the patient, in order to determine clear goals of treatment, verify which therapies actually satisfy those goals, and define subsequent adequate strategies.

In Table 220-1, part A, a protocol is proposed to guide the decisional process for the terminally ill incompetent patient.

Managing the Refusal of Renal Replacement Treatment

Involving patients/relatives and searching for consent means accepting that a potentially life-saving treatment (e.g., RRT) can be refused. Such refusal may be expressed by the sufficiently competent patient (directly or through advance care planning) or mediated by the relatives. This situation can be difficult to manage if the HCWs do not subscribe to the patient's decision.

Great care should be used in evaluating whether the refusal concerns the proposed therapy or the reasonably expected outcome. The therapy is just a means; the goal is the outcome. If the informed patient refuses the proposed therapy but accepts the possible outcome of therapy, then a duty exists to make effective therapy as agreeable as possible. On the contrary, if the patient reliably refuses the outcome, there is no reason to administer any therapy save for the compassionate ones.

A reliable therapeutic refusal must be honored. Consequently, the duty of the HCW is to assess the trustworthiness of the patient's refusal. This should not lead to mistaking competence for rationality. What should be assessed is not whether the family or the HCW agrees with the patient's decision but whether the patient's decision is coherent with his or her view of life and moral and religious beliefs (as witnessed by the patient's relatives and friends).

In this sense, a few words on the difference between "facts" and "values" must be sketched out. HCWs may be expert on the facts, but they are not always experts on the underlying values. Furthermore, many HCWs believe that questions such as forgoing of life supports can be based on purely factual grounds (e.g., by claiming that treatments are "not medically indicated"), when in fact these questions have many value dimensions that need to be taken into consideration. In other words, making end-of-life

TABLE 220-1

A Protocol for the Management of Care for Incompetent, Terminally Ill Patients in Intensive Care Units

Part A—The Decisional Phase

1. Every patient, considered in her or his particular clinical condition, should receive the best possible treatment to fulfill her or his interests. The adequate level of intensivity and palliation should be officially defined. In the absence of such definition, the patient must be considered in full treatment until officially stated otherwise.
2. In emergency conditions, such a decision can be made by the clinician and the nurse in charge, after a reasonable clarification of the diagnosis and prognosis of the patient and, whenever possible, an adequate discussion with the patient's relatives (to whom the final decision must be communicated).
3. In nonemergency conditions, the patient's course of care may be discussed on the request of the patient, with the patient's relative or an HCW (MD or RN). Such a request should activate a meeting (even informal), as soon as possible. Every HCW involved in the patient's care should be allowed to attend; among them, the clinician in charge of the ICU, the clinicians and nurses who best know the patient's case, and, if necessary, an external consultant (e.g., surgeon, nephrologist, cardiologist). If the request comes from the patient's relatives, they can be allowed to attend the meeting. The discussion will deal with the following:
    a. The clinic—Which are the relevant clinical data? Are they sufficient to define diagnosis and prognosis with reasonable certainty? Are particular data necessary and achievable for a more certain diagnosis/prognosis?
    b. The involved subjects—Are the patient's wishes and preferences known? Is it possible to meet them? Which subjects can or must be involved in the discussion? Are diagnosis and prognosis sufficiently clear for all of them? For each subject, what needs must be respected in the final decision?
    c. A possible solution—Taking into account points 3a. and 3b., which solution most respects the rights and needs of all those involved (above all, those of the patient): (1) full treatment without limitation, (2) full treatment with re-evaluation within a specific time interval *(time limit)* or in case of a specific event *(event limit)*, or (3) treatment with a diagnostic or therapeutic limit *(specifying what is limited)*? Are there predictable obstacles to the implementation of such a decision? Are there internal interventions (among the involved subjects) or external interventions (e.g., specialist consultant, psychologist, Ethics Committee) that could help increase the agreement on such a decision?
4. The final decision—taken in the patient's interest after adequate involvement of the patient's relatives—becomes operative after it has been communicated, understood, and shared by all of the subjects involved in the decision (the patient whenever possible, the patient's relatives, and all of the HCWs).
5. Such a decision must be reported and explained in the patient's chart.

Part B—The Operational Phase

6. The decision (see points 2 and 3) should be communicated to the relatives by the clinician and nurse who are in charge of care for that patient.
7. Whenever possible, the decision to limit intensive support will be implemented by trying to wean the patient and transfer him or her to a normal ward, where the presence of relatives and friends can be assured more easily.
8. If discharge from the ICU appears to be impossible because of the patient's strict dependence on intensive life support, every drug, instrumentation, and monitoring device that is not indispensable for the patient's comfort will be forgone, according to the previous decision (point 3c.). The management of the endotracheal tube will be decided in each case, according to the patient's conditions and wishes and the relatives' understanding of the situation. However, there are no contraindications to the extubation of a terminal patient.
9. Whenever indicated, adequate analgesia and sedation will be provided. There are neither clinical, moral, nor legal reasons why a patient should die with pain or discomfort.
10. The patient's relatives should be constantly and adequately informed of what is being done.
11. Except for exceptional situations, the relatives' access to the patient's bed will be more unrestrained. In particular, it is recommended to call relatives in time, to relax restrictions on visitation, and to remove every obstacle to physical contact (e.g., lowering bed rails and other restraints and obstacles to hand-holding).
12. The relatives' needs should be taken into consideration. Some of the most important of these are the need to be with the dying person, to feel helpful to the dying person, to the informed of the dying person's changing condition, to understand what is being done to the patient and why, to be assured of the patient's comfort, to be comforted and to express emotions, to be assured that the final decision was right, to find meaning in the dying of their loved one, to be involved in the caring activities (e.g., mouth care), and to be fed, hydrated, and rested.
13. Times and modalities of the relatives' presence at the patient's bedside will be managed by the nurse in charge of the patient, in relation to his or her global caring engagements and obligations.
14. The relatives should always be offered the possibility of being present at the moment of the patient's death, together with the clinician and nurse who are in charge of care for that patient.
15. Opportunity for debriefing should always be considered.

HCW, health care worker; ICU, intensive care unit.

decisions often involves many assumptions about values that must be taken into careful consideration.

As a practical approach, the consequence of refusal of an effective therapy should be weighed against the patient's acceptability of the predictable outcome. If the consequence of the refusal is clearly in contrast with the patient's view of life and moral and religious beliefs, so much so that the decision can be considered unreliable, every effort should be undertaken to make the therapy acceptable. Adequate sedation—if clinically indicated—can be a final but acceptable resource in the patient's best interest. Actually, cases of patients who were happy to have received successful treatment despite their previous rejection of it have been reported.[32,33]

On the contrary, if the patient does refuse the outcome, and such a decision can be considered reliable, then this position should be respected until the end. The same should be done even if the outcome is desirable but is obtainable only through means that the patient refuses because of religious or well-grounded personal beliefs (Fig. 220-1).

Ethical consultation can be useful. Legal advice is also recommended, such as for adequate application of domestic laws.

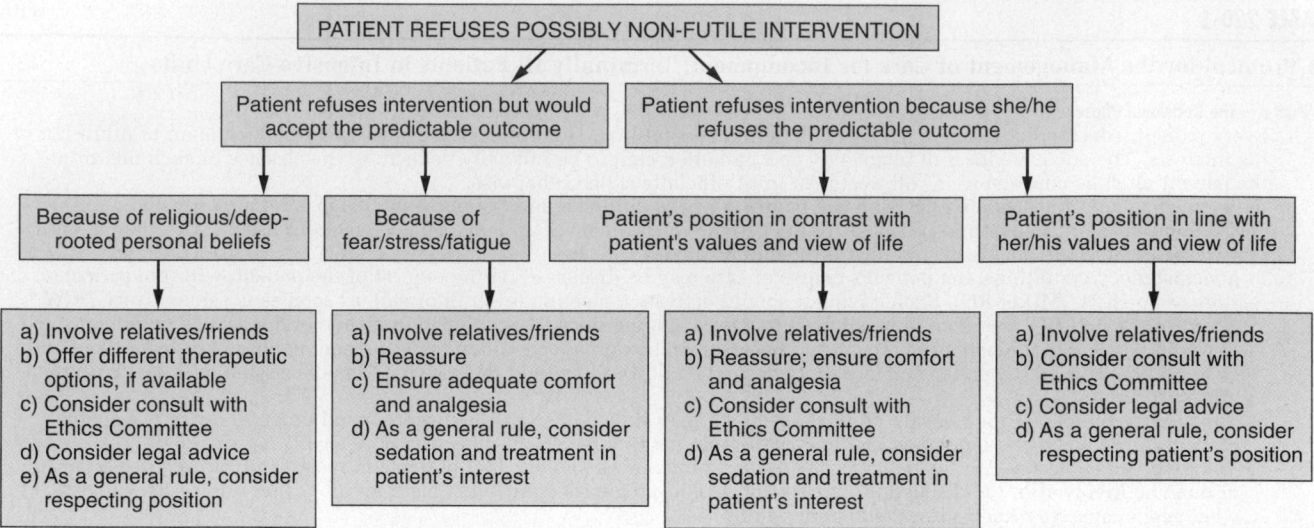

FIGURE 220-1. Suggested management of the patient's refusal of possibly nonfutile intervention (see text for discussion).

The Right to Die without Renal Replacement Therapy

Honoring the patient's refusal of a possibly life-saving RRT means acknowledging a right to die without RRT. Such right can have at least three different meanings, applying to different categories of patients.

In terminally ill patients, for whom an intensive approach could only unduly prolong the process of dying, RRT could be defined as incorrect per se, because it infringes the principles of *beneficence, nonmaleficence,* and *distributive justice.*[34,35] Futile treatments should not be offered.[36] In such situations, even the term *life-saving* supports can be misleading when supports turn out to be just *agony-prolonging.* The term *intensive* supports may be preferable, and it is the one used in this chapter. As for patients in these conditions, dying without RRT means that the way and the time of dying should be respected and dignified. A corresponding clinicians' duty to fulfill the patient's wish can be affirmed. Every communicative effort should be made to reduce the request for futile treatment from relatives of the patient who has become incompetent.[25] Yet, when patients or surrogates claim what the HCW believes is a futile treatment, the HCWs should not limit treatment on the basis of their personal view of futility; rather, they should rely on institutional and professional policies.[37]

The second category is those patients who have poor life expectancy, even if it is not unequivocally definable. These are, for instance, patients with severe chronic obstructive pulmonary disease in fleeting compensation, patients with critical inoperable cardiac disease, and cancer patients who have multimetastatic disease but are still nonmoribund. In these situations, an acute crisis (e.g., a septic episode) can be cured and overcome with intensive care, but without a substantial improvement in prognosis. For this group, the right to not prolong an untreatable and terminal disease or condition against the will of the sufferer should be acknowledged. Again, a corresponding HCW duty should be affirmed.

The third category covers those patients who have a fair prognosis for survival, usually thanks to chronic care, but at the expense of a quality of life that they judge unacceptable. Quadriplegic patients and patients in a vegetative state with previously ascertained refusal of invasive therapies are typical representatives of this group, for which a right of not being kept alive by artificial means is admissible. Such a right can pose particular bioethical and legal problems. Each situation should be resolved in light of the individual circumstances.

Justifying Forgoing of Renal Replacement Therapy

Justifying forgoing of intensive supportive measures such as RRT is rarely painless. Actually, such supports tend to be self-justifying for the mere reason that they are at least temporarily life-saving. They tend also to expand from the acute to the chronic phase of the illness and from single to the multiorgan support. Decisions to limit supportive therapy are often hindered by prognostic uncertainty, because the available prognostic indexes cannot predict the outcome of the individual patient with sufficient accuracy to justify end-of-life decisions.[38,39] Finally, such decisions are made even more difficult by the usual temporal correlation with the death of the patient.

Nevertheless, a fundamental concept is that the aim of intensive supportive care is not to cure diseases. If this were the case, it would be impossible to recognize any diagnostic or therapeutic limit. Even worse, the patient would become an accident of the illness, the mere biological substrate necessary for the disease to occur and by which the disease can be fought. In reality, the object (or, better, the subject) of the curing/caring process is the patient. If this is true (and we believe it is), intensive support procedures should be used as long as they are useful to the patient, according to the patient's wishes and project of life. Beyond that point, they should be limited.[40]

The Practice of Forgoing Renal Replacement Therapy

Recognizing the patient's right to die without RRT can have little meaning if it does not lead to adequate actions. In particular, the rights of the patient and the needs of all the involved subjects must be recognized.

The patient's needs and rights are usually well known, and adequate care is usually best aimed at the relief of physical, psychological, and emotional suffering. Whenever necessary, an adequate sedation is recommended, as long as the true intention of the HCW is to alleviate pain and distress even if a shortening of the terminal process of dying may result. However, adequate palliation must be kept distinct from active shortening of the dying process.[41] The principle of the *double effect* regulates this aspect of care.[42]

Great regard must be paid to the family's needs. Many little considerations are necessary to gratify these needs,[43] which cannot be included in any guideline but which can come only from the careful presence of the health care team. The commitment of the HCW should not be to give a corpse back to the family, but to help the patient's relatives to accompany their loved one in the dying process and to participate in it. This can be done only with a "caring for the family while caring for the patient" approach. In this regard, nurses, as the HCWs who spend the most time at the bedside, play a pivotal role in communication.[44] Unfortunately, disagreement between clinicians and nurses in end-of-life decisions has been described,[45-48] and it, together with dissatisfaction because of inadequate involvement in the decision-making process,[49,50] can lead to frustration on the part of nurses. The needs of the clinical team must also be recognized and satisfied; these include cooperation among team members, competence in the care of patients and relatives, administrative support, and opportunity for debriefing. A protocol is proposed in Table 220-1, part B, wherein the operative phase (how to implement what has been decided) is considered.

Limiting Treatments, Not Care

Finally, three concepts must be emphasized. The first one is that the patient's decision to give up cures that she or he considers disproportionate should never lead to abandonment. Caring opportunities exist even after the attainment of a therapeutic limit. "No RRT" should never come to mean "No care." Yet, it is also fundamental to remember that palliation is not a separate option to be reserved for the terminal phase. There is not one time for invasive restorative care and a separate time (and perhaps separate HCW) for palliation. In every moment of care, HCWs should always act as intensivists and palliativists at the same time. The prevalence of intensivity and palliativity should vary according to the patient's conditions. Restorative care is justified as long as it is useful to the patient. Palliation should always be present. At the end, when there is no more meaning for intensivity, palliation alone remains as the most adequate form of caring.

The second aspect is that a decision to limit supportive procedures is made with the intention of avoiding futile therapies, not in order to lead a patient to death. Actually, limiting support does not imply the immediate death of the patient[4] and is consequently well compatible with maintaining other therapies, if indicated. A decision to forgo futile continuous RRT, for instance, does not conflict with the use of diuretics to stimulate a residual diuresis (if present) or with careful treatment of distressing symptoms of fluid overload.

Finally, clinicians should always be ready to re-evaluate the patient's situation. The decision to forgo an intensive care procedure is adequate as much as it is based on clinical facts and on the wishes of the patient; if clinical facts change, the decision should be revised. Indeed, survival of patients following revision of end-of-life decisions has been described.[51]

CLINICAL RESEARCH IN RENAL REPLACEMENT THERAPY

RRT cannot exist without good research, which includes the patients' informed consent. Unfortunately, patients' incompetence is common in clinical research in the intensive setting, which leads to inadequate provision of information to the patient. A recent European Directive on clinical trials could interfere with emergency research in intensive care because of this issue.[52] Furthermore, introduction of a waiver of consent in clinical trials has been shown to increase patients' recruitment[53] and to reduce the time needed to achieve satisfactory research endpoints.[54]

The problem is complex also because clinical research regarding critical conditions treatable with RRT cannot be performed on healthy volunteers: Inducing renal failure or sepsis in healthy people for mere research purposes would be simply inconceivable.

Perhaps going back to the core question can help: Why is patients' consent so important?

A first answer is that informed consent is a way of honoring the principle of *autonomy*. If the patient is not adequately competent, the only acceptable decision should be the one that corresponds to what the patient would have decided. Unfortunately, the reliability of HCWs and relatives[55] to predict patients' wishes is still unclear.

A second point is that informed consent is usually considered a form of patient self-protection.[56,57] Yet, studies of cancer patients demonstrate unacceptably low comprehension by patients of the protocols they consented to enter.[58,59] The competence of critically ill patients in need of RRT is much less adequate. Therefore, it is not clear how informed consent could protect them.

Nevertheless, patients must be protected.[60] Relatives are not always an adequate protection and could be unavailable for emergency research.[59] Researchers can have both nonfinancial and financial conflicts of interest.[61-63] Randomized controlled trials (RCTs) have proved to be possibly subject to bias and potentially dangerous to patients in many ways. Inadequate or ineffective control treatment,[64] useless RCTs,[65] overemphasized statistical significance of clinically meaningless results,[66] use of composite outcomes where good minor results rarely affect major ones,[67] publication bias,[68] and influence of pharmaceutical industries[69-71] have been described.

For all these reasons and in spite of all obvious difficulties, informed consent should not be abandoned, because it clarifies that clinical research is for the patients (and not the other way around) and promotes respect for critically ill patients and their rights.[59]

TABLE 220-2

Ethical Requirements for Clinical Research

1. Social value: The research must improve health or advance knowledge.
2. Scientific validity: The research must be scientifically rigorous and provide reliable results.
3. Fair participant selection: The research must expose the vulnerable and the privileged to the same risks and benefits.
4. Favorable risk/benefit ratio: The research must minimize risk and maximize benefit to participants whenever possible.
5. Independent review: The research must be reviewed, approved, amended, or terminated by unaffiliated observers.
6. Informed consent: The research participants or their surrogates must be informed about the research, must understand it, and must agree to it voluntarily and without coercion.
7. Respect for enrolled participants: The research participants' privacy must be respected, their withdrawal permitted, and their safety monitored.

From Luce JM, Cook DJ, Martin TR, et al; American Thoracic Society: The ethical conduct of clinical research involving critically ill patients in the United States and Canada: Principles and recommendations. Am J Respir Crit Care Med 2004;170:1375-1384.

TABLE 220-3

An Ethical Checklist for Clinical Research

Research Design
1. Will the study results provide social or scientific value?
2. Is the study design scientifically valid?
3. Is the intended participant selection fair and suitable for the research question?
4. Is there a favorable risk/benefit ratio?
5. Has the design undergone, or will it undergo, independent review before the study is started?
6. Are adequate procedures in place to ensure informed consent, and have they been reviewed?
7. Are adequate procedures in place to ensure respect for potential and enrolled participants?
8. Are data and safety monitoring in place?
9. Have conflicts of interest been identified and minimized?

Research Implementation and Monitoring
1. Do new data or hypotheses undermine the social or scientific value of the ongoing study?
2. Do new results from this or other studies unfavorably alter the risk/benefit ratio?
3. Is the participant selection process working as intended and designed?
4. Are investigators carrying out the study as intended and designed?
5. Are the data and safety monitoring procedures, including the detection and reporting of adverse events, working as intended and designed?

From Luce JM, Cook DJ, Martin TR, et al; American Thoracic Society: The ethical conduct of clinical research involving critically ill patients in the United States and Canada: Principles and recommendations. Am J Respir Crit Care Med 2004;170:1375-1384.

On the other hand, it is evident that informed consent is not enough. Also, the quality of research should be improved as much as possible. Less-than-optimal therapy for the control group of patients should be carefully avoided. The number of research protocols in RRT (and in general in critical care) could be reduced and their quality increased. A few large, multicenter trials are more desirable than many statistically underpowered studies. Great care is needed in designing, conducting, and evaluating protocols of clinical studies. Also, other methodological options (e.g., using different treatments separately at different times or in different centers and then comparing them[72]) have been suggested.

Ethics Committees and Institutional Review Boards must ensure careful evaluation of research protocols; however, the effectiveness of these institutions has also been questioned.[73] Thorough discussion and evaluation of protocol from all the staff involved in the research is also recommended.

Finally, the introduction of a registry of protocols[74,75] is a extremely positive step.

As for local situations, readers are invited to refer to specific papers. One is the result of a conference on the ethical conduct of clinical research involving critically ill patients in the United States and Canada.[76] Ethical requirements for clinical research were specified (Table 220-2), and an ethical checklist for clinical research design, implementation, and monitoring was proposed (Table 220-3). Other reports take into account also the European situation.[77,78]

BIOSOCIAL ASPECTS OF RENAL REPLACEMENT THERAPY

RRT is a fundamental component of modern high-technology medicine. High-technology medicine can be extremely effective in individual cases, but it also poses important biosocial problems. One of them relates to the possibility of manipulating virtually every aspect of the process of dying and prolonging low-quality lives. HCWs should be aware that all they actually manage is not life or death but clinical data, drugs, and devices in order to reach the best possible quality of life for their patients. Because death is a inevitable event, the quality of each death and of the relationships involved in each death is a major indicator of quality of care.

Another problem is related to the extraordinary amount of resources necessary for high-technology medicine.[79-82] For this reason, it is likely that HTM will be increasingly available only to those patients who can have access to it. We proposed the word *presentism* to describe the fact that a huge amount of money is spent to cure a limited number of patients (those who are "present" to receive it), whereas much less is offered to all those who are "absent."[83]

As a consequence, high-technology medicine can work only in highly developed countries. As a mere example, 90% of the 100,000 patients who develop end-stage renal disease each year in India die without seeing a nephrologist, and only 4% of those who begin hemodialysis are still being treated after 1 year, often with unacceptable standards of treatment.[84]

In the other hand, in the United States, total spending on health care is increasing and already accounts for 16% of the gross domestic product.[85] Critical care alone consumes more than 1% of the gross domestic product.[86] Yet, in spite of its enormous costs, this system has negligible positive impact on global health and life expectancy of the U.S. population.[83] The risk is that, for many patients, high-technology medicine could reduce to an extremely expensive way to manage unavoidable death: by now, one out of five Americans already dies in an ICU,[87] often in relation to the refusal or limitation of supportive care.[4,5]

Obviously, the solution cannot be abolishing high-technology medicine (and consequently RRT). We must avoid "throwing the baby away with the dirty bathwater." Yet, even if causes and remedies are above all political and societal, it is important that every HCW be aware of these biosocial issues.

Key Points

1. A clinically sound and compassionately administered medical approach should be considered good and adequate unless refused by the patient. Clinical indication, informed consent, and compassionate administration are the bases of the ethical foundation of renal replacement therapy.

2. Decisions regarding the course of therapy for an incompetent patient are always a medical task; the relatives or surrogate and health care workers should work together to determine the patient's desires and expectations. The aim of the decisions is promoting patients' dignity; guidelines and principles are the means to reach such a goal. They are not absolute, and exceptions can be admitted; guidelines can be ignored and principles can be sacrificed, if this is necessary to best promote patient dignity in a specific situation.

3. The aim of intensive life support is to care for patients, not to cure diseases; consequently, such procedures should be used only so long as they are useful to the patient. A right to die without renal replacement therapy exists, and a reliable request should be honored. In carrying out a decision to limit intensive supports, the rights of the patient and the needs of all the involved subjects must be recognized and satisfied.

4. Informed consent clarifies the fact that clinical research is for the patients and promotes respect for critically ill patients and their rights. However, it cannot solve all the problems related to research in continuous renal replacement therapy. Also, the maximum possible quality of research should be ensured.

5. Health care workers should be aware that renal replacement therapy (like all the other components of modern high-technology medicine) poses important biosocial problems; the most important ones relate to the possibility of manipulating the process of dying and to the amount of resources necessary.

Key References

40. Carlet J, Thijs LG, Antonelli M, et al: Challenges in end-of-life care in the ICU. Statement of the Fifth International Consensus Conference in Critical Care, Brussels, Belgium, April 2003. Intensive Care Med 2004;30:770-784.

43. Truog RD, Cist AF, Brackett SE, et al: Recommendations for end-of-life care in the intensive care unit: The Ethics Committee of the Society of Critical Care Medicine. Crit Care Med 2001;29:2332-2348.

59. Luce JM: Is the concept of informed consent applicable to clinical research involving critically ill patients? Crit Care Med 2003;31(3 Suppl):S153-S160.

76. Luce JM, Cook DJ, Martin TR, et al; American Thoracic Society: The ethical conduct of clinical research involving critically ill patients in the United States and Canada: Principles and recommendations. Am J Respir Crit Care Med 2004;170:1375-1384.

83. Zamperetti N, Bellomo R, Dan M, Ronco C: Ethical, political, and social aspects of high-technology medicine: Eos and care. Intensive Care Med 2006;32:830-835.

See the companion Expert Consult website for the complete reference list.

Intermittent Hemodialysis and Sustained Low-Efficiency Daily Dialysis in the Intensive Care Unit

Basic Principles

CHAPTER 221

Intermittent Techniques for Acute Dialysis

John K. Leypoldt

OBJECTIVES

This chapter will:

1. Discuss the basic principles of prescribing intermittent hemodialysis for patients with acute renal failure.
2. Review the evidence regarding the effect, on outcome for the patient with acute renal failure, of the type of dialysis membrane and the dialysis dose.
3. Compare treatments using conventional intermittent hemodialysis with those using sustained, low-efficiency intermittent hemodialysis.

BACKGROUND

Intermittent hemodialysis (IHD) remains a common form of renal replacement therapy for treating critically ill patients with acute renal failure (ARF, also called acute kidney injury). Although continuous renal replacement therapies (CRRTs) have certain theoretical advantages, IHD achieves comparable, and perhaps even superior, overall patient outcomes.[1-4] The reasons for these findings are debatable; nonetheless, IHD will likely remain a therapy of choice for many patients with ARF. The extent to which IHD is used in this setting varies widely in different geographical regions[5-9] and is related largely to practical considerations, such as familiarity with alternative technologies, access of physicians to them, and the cost of these technologies.

There are two fundamentally different types of IHD therapies. The first and most common type of IHD closely resembles that performed in dialysis centers in patients with end-stage renal disease (ESRD) or chronic renal failure. The second type of IHD therapy consists of several variations of long, low-efficiency hemodialysis techniques. Both therapies are described in this chapter; further details of various aspects of these IHD therapies are described in other chapters of this monograph.

INTERMITTENT, CONVENTIONAL HEMODIALYSIS

Intermittent hemodialysis in the intensive care unit (ICU) is performed with the use of equipment and medical reasoning comparable to those in the long-term dialysis center. For example, the machines used for IHD in the ICU are usually the same as those used in the affiliated long-term dialysis center. Ideally, these machines should provide volumetrically controlled ultrafiltration and should use bicarbonate-containing dialysis solutions. Such equipment is important in this setting because it provides optimal control of patient volume status; however, such machines are often too complex to be used independently by ICU staff and therefore require operation (or oversight) by a dialysis nurse.

The dialysis prescription for patients with ARF is largely empirical; a blood flow rate of 350 mL/min and a dialysate flow rate of 500 mL/min have been recommended for a standard 70-kg patient.[10] Lower blood flow rates are also commonly used in regions where they are standard practice. Because temporary catheters are most commonly employed as vascular access in patients with ARF, there is likely significant access recirculation in these applications, decreasing the efficiency of the dialysis procedure, especially at relatively high blood flow rates. The amount of recirculation is variable and depends on the site of catheter placement and the type of catheter. Standard therapy for IHD is a treatment length of 3 to 4 hours, with treatments three or four times per week.

The composition of the dialysis solution employed is similar to that used during routine hemodialysis for patients with ESRD, although certain small, but significant, variations in dialysate composition are clinically relevant.[10] Thus, the standard dialysis solution used for patients with ESRD who are hyperphosphatemic, hyperkalemic, and acidotic is not always optimal for use in patients with ARF. In this case, the composition of the dialysis solution must be altered to normalize patient blood chemistry, especially with respect to electrolyte and acid-base concentrations. These latter concerns are patient specific.

Technically advanced hemodialysis machines have a number of new features, such as ultrafiltration profiling, sodium profiling, blood volume monitoring, and blood temperature monitoring. These technologies have theoretical benefit in the ICU because their application may optimize patient hemodynamic and volume status and may help avoid further renal insults. Direct evidence that these new technologies are beneficial in IHD for patients with ARF is sparse, however. Combined ultrafiltration and sodium profiling was found to improve patient hemodynamic stability in a crossover trial of 10 critically ill patients[11]; in a prospective observational study of 20 patients with ARF, however, blood volume monitoring had no benefit.[12] Additional studies using these novel technologies are needed to demonstrate their utility during IHD in the ICU.

Dialysis Membrane

Two properties of dialysis membranes may affect patient outcomes, their biocompatibility and their porosity.

The type of polymers used in the manufacture of dialysis membranes largely determines the extent to which blood cells and proteins are activated when they initially come into contact with the membrane in the extracorporeal circuit. Dialysis membranes are often divided into three categories on the basis of base polymer materials: unsubstituted cellulosic, substituted cellulosic, and synthetic. These basic categories are used because complement proteins are activated differently by these membranes. In general, unsubstituted cellulosic membranes activate complement proteins to a high degree and are considered bioincompatible, whereas synthetic membranes activate complement proteins to a low degree and are considered biocompatible. Substituted cellulosic membranes are of intermediate biocompatibility. These concepts of membrane biocompatibility are derived from studies in patients with ESRD undergoing long-term hemodialysis; few biocompatibility studies have been performed in patients with ARF.[13]

The importance of the type of dialysis membrane and, by implication, its biocompatibility, to outcomes in patients with ARF remains unclear. Early studies suggested that outcomes (overall patient survival and recovery of renal function) were better for patients in whom synthetic or biocompatible membranes were used.[14,15] Other, later studies reported the opposite—that patient outcomes were not influenced by the type of dialysis membrane used.[16-18] Most of these later studies were small and too underpowered to support robust conclusions. Interestingly, two meta-analyses using combined literature data also reported disparate conclusions—one reporting that biocompatible membranes improved patient survival,[19] and the other concluding that the type of membrane made no difference.[20] In summary, there is no conclusive evidence to suggest that dialysis membrane material influences outcome of patients with ARF undergoing IHD.

The porosity of dialysis membranes may also affect patient outcomes by increasing the removal of low-molecular-weight proteins, which may be biologically active and detrimental to patient recovery. Although adsorption of proteins to membranes may be the main removal mechanism, enhanced membrane porosity can also improve protein adsorption.[21,22] Clinical studies to address the importance of dialysis membrane porosity during IHD in the ICU are few. In one small study, no clinical advantages could be demonstrated for the use of more porous (high-flux) dialysis membranes in this setting.[23] Another study found no evidence of better patient outcomes with the use of high-flux membranes for intermittent hemodiafiltration.[24] If removal of low-molecular-weight proteins is shown to be beneficial in future studies using intermittent therapies, comparisons between IHD and CRRT using high-flux (and super-high-flux) membranes must be performed, because CRRT has been shown to achieve better clearance of such solutes in kinetic modeling studies.[25]

Dialysis Dose

Historically, the dose of dialysis prescribed during IHD has been largely based on the clinical or biochemical state of the patient, without a general quantitative basis. Hemodialysis prescription for patients with ARF typically used practices extrapolated from those in patients with ESRD. The extent of such prescription practices on the delivered dose of dialysis in patients with ARF has been examined in several studies.

The use of urea kinetic modeling to prescribe dialysis dose during IHD in patients with ARF has often been criticized, because the assumptions for these models, for example, a constant urea generation rate, are not strictly valid. The relevant assumptions are probably applicable, but only over the period of a single hemodialysis treatment and its interdialytic interval; thus, dialysis dose has been examined with the use of urea kinetic models in several studies. Evanson and colleagues[26] determined dialysis dose as urea clearance (K) multiplied by treatment time (t) normalized to urea distribution volume (V), or urea Kt/V, in 40 patients with ARF who underwent 136 IHD treatments. These investigators reported that approximately half the dialysis prescriptions were for urea Kt/V values less than 1.2, a marginal dose as defined by National Kidney Foundation Kidney Disease Outcomes Quality Initiative (KDOQI) Guidelines for patients with ESRD.[27] Moreover, the delivered urea Kt/V in this study was low, 1.04 ± 0.49 (mean $\pm$ SD). Further analysis of these data showed that delivered urea Kt/V was inversely related to patient body size and was lower for both low achieved blood flow rates and treatments without the use of anticoagulants. These findings suggest that dialysis dose was

TABLE 221-1

Studies of Delivered Dialysis Dose per Treatment during Intermittent Hemodialysis in Patients with Acute Renal Failure

STUDY (YEAR)	Urea Volume of Distribution (Kt/V)*	
	Kt/V or spKt/V	Urea eKt/V
Paganani et al (1996)[32]	0.90 ± 0.04 (survivors)	ND
	0.76 ± 0.05 (nonsurvivors)	ND
Evanson et al (1998)[26]	1.04 ± 0.49	ND
Schiffl et al (2002)[33]	0.94 ± 0.11	ND
	0.92 ± 0.16	ND
Kanagasundaram et al (2003)[40]	1.02 ± 0.27	0.91 ± 0.26
Klouche et al (2007)[41]	1.2 ± 0.3	ND

eKt/V, equilibrated (or double-pool) volume of distribution; spKt/V, single-pool volume of distribution.
*Values given are mean ± standard deviation.

prescribed largely without consideration of patient body size.

Additional studies using more detailed calculations confirmed and extended these findings. Himmelfarb and associates[28] calculated urea Kt/V using both single-pool and double-pool urea kinetic models and showed that the reason for low delivered values of urea Kt/V is that urea distribution volume in patients with ARF is significantly larger than anthropometric and bioelectric impedance–derived estimates of total body water. Thus, these investigators concluded that the use of total body water to prescribe dialysis dose in patients with ARF leads to significant underestimates of prescribed and delivered urea Kt/V. A subsequent study by Ikizler and coworkers[29] using isotopic tracer solutes confirmed that the urea distribution volume is significantly larger than the total body water volume in patients with ARF. It is interesting to note that this relationship, of urea distribution volume with total body water volume, is opposite to that observed in patients with ESRD.[30,31] A summary of studies evaluating dialysis dose as assessed by urea Kt/V during IHD is shown in Table 221-1. In general, the delivered dialysis dose during IHD for patients with ARF is less than that recommended for patients with ESRD.

The association between dialysis dose during IHD and patient survival has been addressed in only two studies. Paganini and colleagues[32] retrospectively examined the relationship between patient survival and dialysis dose in patients with ARF treated with both IHD and CRRT. For patients treated with IHD, the delivered doses were significantly higher in surviving patients than in nonsurvivors (see Table 221-1); however, these differences were only marginal and were not statistically significant when illness severity and other variables (i.e., hemodynamic status, Acute Physiology and Chronic Health Evaluation II [APACHE II] score, comorbidities) were taken into account. When all patients treated by either IHD or CRRT were considered together, a preliminary analysis suggested that higher dialysis dose improved patient survival only in patients with moderate illness severity (i.e., neither very ill nor only modestly ill).

Additional evidence indicating better patient outcome with higher dialysis dose was reported by Schiffl and associates,[33] who performed a prospective clinical trial of 160 patients treated with IHD performed either daily or every other day. Patients with ARF who underwent daily dialysis had better control of uremia and fewer hypotensive

episodes, and the weekly total delivered urea Kt/V was 5.8 ± 0.4 in patients treated daily, compared with 3.0 ± 0.6 in patients treated every other day. In this study, patient mortality (14 days after the last hemodialysis treatment session) was 28% for daily dialysis compared with 46% when treatments were performed every other day. After adjustment for illness severity (APACHE II score) and other patient variables, the odds ratio for death was almost four times higher (estimate, 3.92; 95% confidence interval [CI], 1.68-9.18) for patients treated by every-other-day dialysis than in those treated daily. Other clinical parameters that were favorably altered during daily dialysis were faster recovery of renal function, fewer intradialysis hypotensive episodes, and lower rates of development of oliguria, sepsis, respiratory failure, and gastrointestinal bleeding. These studies are supportive of a significant role of dialysis dose during IHD in patients with ARF, similar to that reported by Ronco and colleagues[34] during the use of CRRT.

It should be noted that the effect of dialysis dose during IHD on survival in patients with ARF is not widely accepted because of several limitations in the generalizability of the findings from the study by Schiffl and associates.[35] Furthermore, whether better clinical outcomes for daily dialysis in that study were due to the higher dialysis dose or the greater treatment frequency is unknown. It is anticipated that more robust conclusions about the influence of dialysis dose and frequency on clinical outcome of patients with ARF will be reported by the ongoing VA/NIH Acute Renal Failure Trial Network (ATN) Study.[36,37]

SUSTAINED LOW-EFFICIENCY DIALYSIS

A later application of IHD in the ICU has been to perform hemodialysis treatments with prolonged treatment times but under conditions in which the dialyzer operates at low efficiency. Such therapies have been called by various names, but it is convenient to lump them together into a single entity, sustained low-efficiency dialysis (SLED). The essential characteristic of these therapies is the prolonged treatment time; such conditions permit slow removal of fluids and better hemodynamic stability during treatment. The longer treatment time also permits the

TABLE 221-2

Studies of Prescription Parameters during Sustained Low-Efficiency Dialysis for Patients with Acute Renal Failure

STUDY (YEAR)	BLOOD FLOW RATE (mL/min)	DIALYSATE FLOW RATE (mL/min)	TREATMENT TIME (Hours)
Kumar et al (2000)[42]	200	300	6-8
Lonnemann et al (2000)[43]	70	70	18
Marshall et al (2001 & 2002)[39,44]	200	100	12
Kielstein et al (2004)[45]	200	100	12

achievement of an adequate dialysis dose (for small solutes) even with the dialyzer operating at low blood and dialysate flow rates. Such treatments also probably increase removal of middle molecules and putative inflammatory mediators. Thus, in many respects, SLED is an IHD therapy with several of the advantages of CRRT; as such, these therapies are commonly referred to as hybrid therapies.

SLED therapies are covered in more detail in other chapters of this book; however, it is worth briefly noting their similarities and advantages when compared with conventional IHD.

The Technology

The equipment used during SLED is often identical to that used during conventional IHD with only minor modifications. For example, conventional hemodialysis machines do not often permit the use of the low dialysate flow rates that are employed during SLED; however, newer versions of the machine do have an option for SLED. Thus, an advantage of SLED over CRRT is that it is simpler from a technical perspective.

Other aspects of SLED therapies are very similar to those of conventional IHD. Although low-flux dialysis membranes have been used in certain SLED therapies, high-flux dialysis membranes are often preferred. Dialysis solutions can either be prepared on-line from concentrated solutions or prepared in batches for use.[38] Various dialysis prescription parameter combinations have been previously used in SLED therapies, some of which are listed in Table 221-2. Only one study performed detailed analysis of the delivered dose of dialysis,[39] demonstrating that this version of SLED achieved a delivered urea Kt/V between 1.2 and 1.4, depending on how it was measured. These data suggest that the dialysis dose per treatment achieved with SLED is at least as large as that with conventional IHD. Indeed, Liao and associates[25] have calculated theoretically that daily treatments using SLED achieve therapy adequacy equivalent to that with predilution continuous venovenous hemofiltration, at least with respect to clearances of small solutes such as urea.

Additional concerns with SLED therapies require additional study, such as the potential loss of certain solutes and pharmacological agents. Thus, routine monitoring of serum phosphorus and antibiotic plasma concentrations should be performed in patients receiving SLED therapy.

Key Points

1. Intermittent hemodialysis performed three or four times per week is a common modality for treating patients with acute renal failure.
2. The delivered dose of dialysis, as assessed by urea Kt/V, for patients with acute renal failure is often less than recommended by guidelines for treatment of patients with chronic renal failure.
3. Evidence to support the use of synthetic or biocompatible dialysis membranes or higher doses of dialysis to improve patient outcomes remains limited.
4. Intermittent hemodialysis can be used to treat hemodynamically unstable patients with acute renal failure if applied as sustained, low-efficiency dialysis (SLED).

Key References

14. Himmelfarb J, Tolkoff Rubin N, Chandran P, et al: A multicenter comparison of dialysis membranes in the treatment of acute renal failure requiring dialysis. J Am Soc Nephrol 1998;9:257-266.
18. Jorres A, Gahl GM, Dobis C, et al: Haemodialysis-membrane biocompatibility and mortality of patients with dialysis-dependent acute renal failure: A prospective randomised multicentre trial. International Multicentre Study Group. Lancet 1999;354:1337-1341.
26. Evanson JA, Himmelfarb J, Wingard R, et al: Prescribed versus delivered dialysis in acute renal failure patients. Am J Kidney Dis 1998;32:731-738.
33. Schiffl H, Lang SM, Fischer R: Daily hemodialysis and the outcome of acute renal failure. N Engl J Med 2002;346:305-310.
43. Lonnemann G, Floege J, Kliem V, et al: Extended daily venovenous high-flux haemodialysis in patients with acute renal failure and multiple organ dysfunction syndrome using a single path batch dialysis system. Nephrol Dial Transplant 2000;15:1189-1193.

See the companion Expert Consult website for the complete reference list.

CHAPTER 222

Vascular Access for Intermittent Renal Replacement Therapy

Bernard Canaud

OBJECTIVES

This chapter will:
1. Review central venous catheter as the vascular access standard reference for intermittent renal replacement therapy in acute renal failure.
2. Describe the two main categories of central venous catheters: short-term, made of semi-rigid polymer (polyurethane, carbothane) and bearing usually two lumens, and long-term tunneled, made of soft polymer (silicone, polyurethane) and bearing two lumens.
3. Discuss the insertion of central venous catheters by percutaneous route under local anesthesia in various sites based on the Seldinger method. Short-term catheters are inserted in a vein using a metallic guidewire, whereas long-term catheters require in addition the use of a vein dilator with desilet introducer and a tunneler.
4. Describe the need for central venous catheter insertion to be secured by preliminary ultrasound vein location and confirmed expertise of the operator.
5. Discuss the importance of adequate monitoring of central venous catheter performances and of hygienic sterile care and management from the nursing team to prevent complications.

Vascular access is the basic tool required to launch all forms of extracorporeal renal replacement therapy (RRT). Central venous catheters (CVCs) are the preferred form of vascular access in the acute renal failure setting. Catheters provide rapid and easy blood access for starting hemodialysis in critically ill patients.[1] Despite significant technical advances in catheter design and great progress in care management, CVCs remain a major cause of morbidity in intensive care units that can be minimized by respecting best practice guidelines.[2,3] CVCs are used in patients with acute renal failure to provide renal replacement support during the wait for renal recovery, which takes 4 to 0 weeks.

RRT in the intensive care unit relies on two options based on weekly frequency and blood flow regimen. In brief, RRT may be indicated in either an intermittent high-flow modality or a continuous low-flow modality. The choice of modality relies on the clinical condition of the patient with acute renal failure, in whom hemodynamic instability and number of failing organs (sepsis being regarded as a failing organ) are predominant factors in the decision.[4,5] Dialysis catheters are not similar in design and performance.[6] This chapter addresses the following issues related to catheters used in intermittent RRT: catheter material and geometry, indications, insertion procedure, catheter care management, catheter performance, and outcomes.

CATHETER CHARACTERISTICS: MATERIAL, GEOMETRY, AND DESIGN

CVCs are classified in two main categories according to their intended duration of use. Short-term CVCs are used less than 2 weeks, whereas long-term (or permanent) CVCs may be used for extended periods, up to several months or years. The difference between these two types of device relies on the fact that long-term CVCs could be tunneled. Cannulas are made of synthetic polymers (e.g., polyvinyl chloride, polytetrafluoroethylene, polyethylene, polyurethane, silicone elastomer, thermoplastic polyurethane elastomer [Tecoflex]), which give them their specific characteristics (resistance, softness, hemocompatibility). Several models of large-bore hemodialysis catheters are currently available but not are necessarily equivalent in performance.[7] Both design and cannula engineering (inner lumen diameter, length, tip design, central and/or side holes) affect the performance of the catheter (maximum blood flow, flow resistance, recirculation). Different models of catheters are shown in Figures 222-1 to 222-4. When choosing the catheter material, the physician should know these characteristics and should be aware of CVC-related hazards.[8]

Catheter stiffness depends on polymer nature, plasticizer content, and extrusion mode. Polyurethane and silicone rubber are the materials most widely used for CVCs. Catheter stiffness dictates the procedure for insertion. Rigid and semirigid CVCs are easily introduced percutaneously by means of the Seldinger method, over a soft metallic guidewire (see Fig. 222-1).

Soft and flexible CVCs (e.g., silicone) require a two-step technique, which uses first an introducer and then a sheath vein dilator (peelable or nonpeelable) to introduce the catheter. Soft CVCs have the following major advantages over rigid ones: (1) they are less traumatic to the host vein and more biocompatible with the blood, (2) they are subcutaneously tunneled, and (3) they have a subcutaneous anchoring system (Dacron cuff, pursestring suture).[9]

Single-lumen or double-lumen cannulas may be used for hemodialysis. Single-lumen catheters have a single port used alternatively for both inflow and outflow. In the past, two single-lumen catheters (inflow and outflow) inserted in the same central vein were used to optimize flow performances (Figures 222-5 to 222-8). Double-lumen catheters, which have one arterial flow port and one venous flow port, are now more widely indicated and may be used in clinical practice instead of short-term CVCs (Figures 222-6 to 222-8).[10] Designs of the lumen and distal tips vary considerably among catheters. Schematically, one can consider two main types of catheter: one with port sites arranged in a double-barreled gun fashion (coaxial, double-D, double-O) (see Fig. 222-2) and the other with independent or separated port sites (dual catheter or split catheter) (see Figs. 222-3 and 222-4).

From a flow perspective, it has been proved that independent catheter lines offer more consistently adequate and high flow than the attached lines.[11,12] Improved functionality is due to the catheter design, which reduces risk of catheter occlusion by arterial wall suction or sidewall contact.

INDICATIONS FOR CENTRAL VENOUS CATHETERS

Methods of catheter insertion have been improved over the last decade, contributing to reductions in the morbidity associated with CVCs. Ultrasonography- or fluoroscopy-based methods to locate and to guide the vein cannulation has reduced the incidence of failure, the time spent in catheterization, and the incidence of traumatic complications.[13,14] Catheter-assisted methods have been shown to be particularly beneficial for inexperienced physicians and in case of abnormal vein location (20% to 30% of cases).

The choice of central venous site depends on the clinical context, the state of the patient's health, and the physician's experience.[15] The femoral approach is preferred in critically ill patients with respiratory distress (pulmonary edema, respiratory failure), hemodynamically unstable patients, and comatose or ventilation-supported patients. Internal jugular vein access is preferable in the absence of life-threatening conditions; it uses an easily accessible vein that gives access for transjugular renal biopsy at the same time.[16] Subclavian vein access should be considered as a third option and last resort when no other possibility exists, because it is associated with high risk of late stenosis.[17] In all cases, the percutaneous vein cannulation option must be performed after skin preparation, with local anesthesia, and in very strict aseptic conditions.

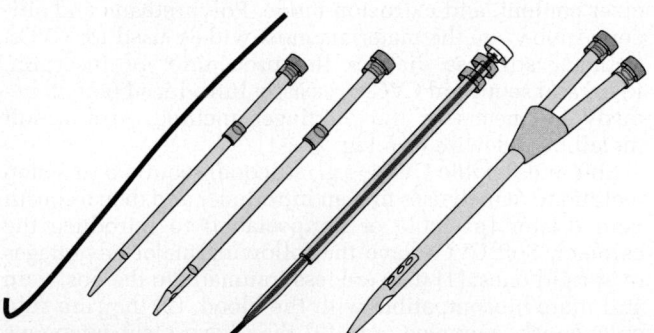

FIGURE 222-1. Different models of short-term central venous catheters.

Short-term CVCs are usually indicated for blood access in cases of urgently required RRT. In these cases, a nontunneled double-lumen polyurethane catheter inserted in the femoral vein with local anesthesia is usually the best option (Figs. 222-9 and 222-10). On the other hand, long-term CVCs are indicated in cases of nonurgent and planned RRT or when the expected duration of use exceeds 2 weeks. In these cases, a tunneled soft polyurethane or silicone rubber double-lumen catheter or duo-catheter inserted in the internal jugular vein is considered the best option.[18]

Femoral vein access represents a primary option in emergency conditions and a secondary option in patients who are bedridden with severe neurological disorders, are receiving ventilatory assistance (tracheotomy), or have multiple-organ failure (Fig. 222-11). A double-lumen semirigid polyurethane catheter is the best catheter for starting the dialysis. The right and left femoral veins offer the same facility for insertion. The length of a femoral catheter for optimal flow performance is 25 to 35 cm. The insertion site is located approximately 1 to 2 cm below the crural arcade and 1 cm medial to the femoral artery. For safety reasons, it is reasonable to use these catheters for less than 2 weeks. Two single-lumen polyurethane catheters inserted in the same femoral vein may be an alternative to achieve adequate blood flow. Tunneled soft silicone catheters have been also successfully used in acute conditions.[19,20] Such angioaccess is a quite interesting and innovative option that should be promoted.[21]

Internal jugular cannulation has gained popularity over the last two decades and should be considered when the expected duration of treatment exceeds 2 weeks. The incidence of deep venous thrombosis and stenosis is reduced with use of the internal jugular vein, in comparison to that of femoral and subclavian catheter use. Straight or kinked double-lumen catheters exiting near the ear are clearly more exposed to infections and should not be used anymore. Tunneled soft polyurethane and silicone rubber catheters (double-lumen catheter, use of two catheters, split catheter) inserted into the internal jugular vein are clearly preferable to reduce the infectious risk (Figs. 222-12 and 222-13). Percutaneous catheter insertion into the internal jugular vein in a low position is suitable to prevent catheter kinking. The right internal jugular vein is the best location. The left internal jugular approach should be used only when the right vein is not possible. The percutaneous insertion and tunneling procedure (upward or downward) depends on the type of catheter. A subcutaneous anchoring system (Dacron cuff, pursestring suture) should be used to secure and protect the catheter.

Subclavian vein cannulation for hemodialysis should no longer be used or should be regarded as the last resort. Subclavian placement of a catheter entails a major risk of

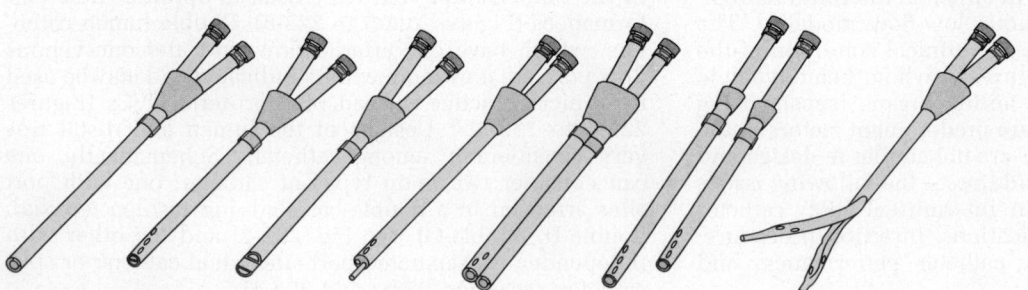

FIGURE 222-2. Several models of double-lumen long-term central venous catheters.

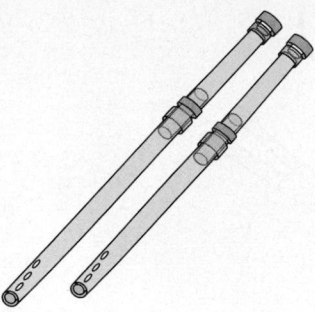

FIGURE 222-3. Double-lumen silicone long-term central venous catheter.

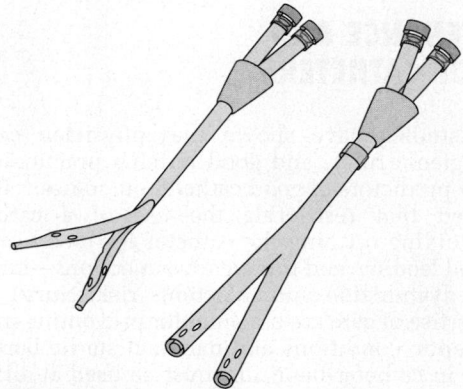

FIGURE 222-4. Double-lumen silicone long-term central venous catheter.

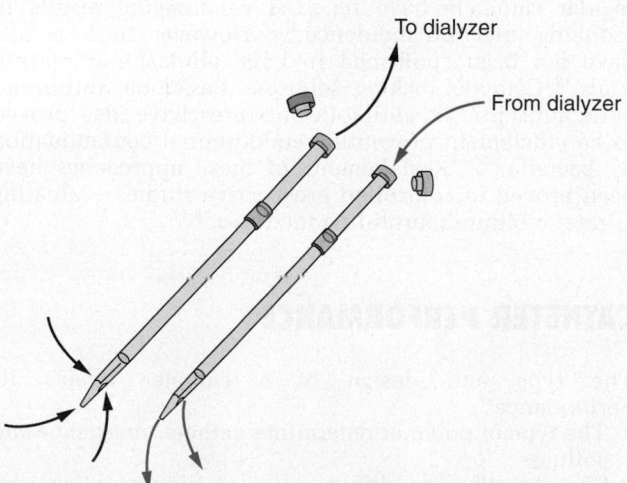

To dialyzer

From dialyzer

FIGURE 222-5. A double-lumen polyurethane central venous catheter for short-term use.

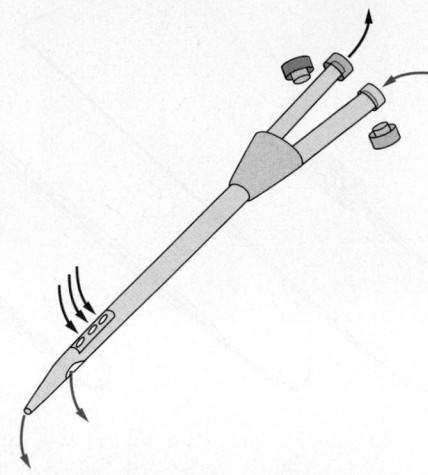

FIGURE 222-6. A double-lumen polyurethane central venous catheter for short-term use.

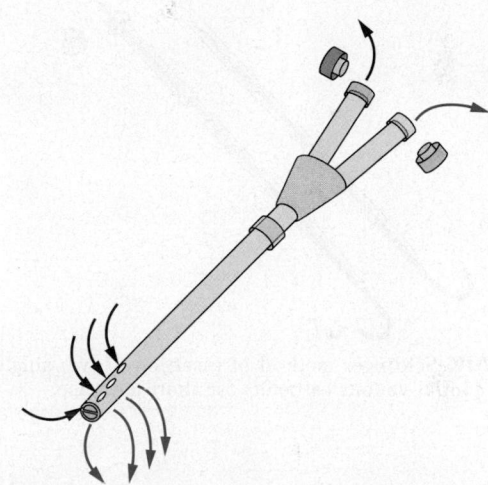

FIGURE 222-7. Double-lumen silicone (2D) central venous catheter for long-term use in action.

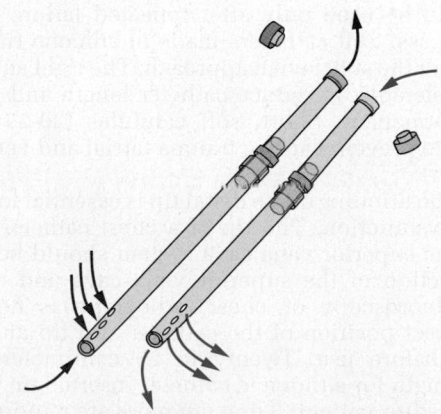

FIGURE 222-8. Silicone dual central venous catheter for long-term use in action.

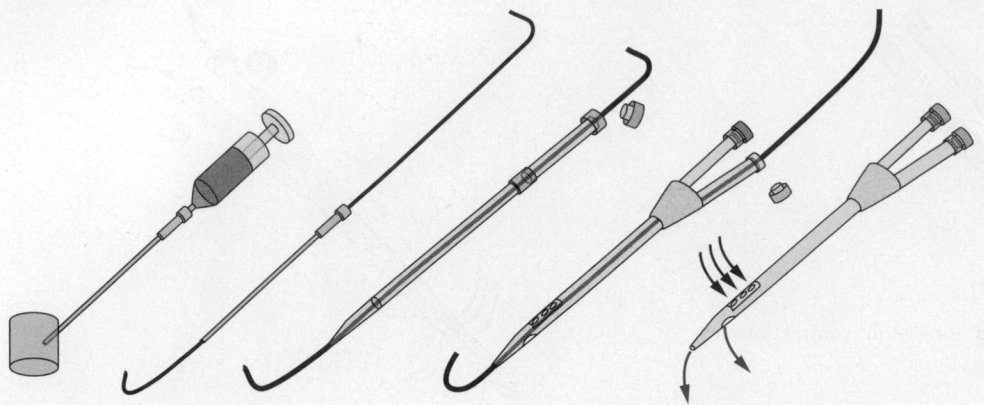

FIGURE 222-9. Seldinger method of insertion of a double-lumen polyurethane central venous catheter for short-term use.

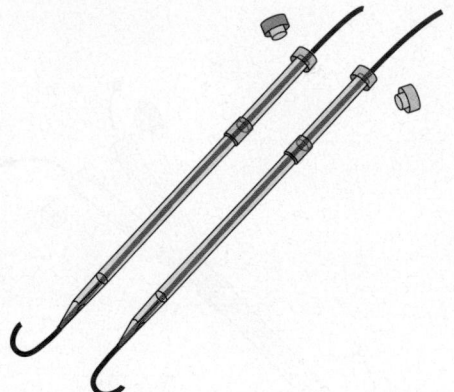

FIGURE 222-10. Seldinger method of insertion of two single polyurethane central venous catheters for short-term use.

stenosis or thrombosis of the host vein, compromising the chance of creating a fistula.[22] Indeed, subclavian cannulation should be used only after repeated failure of other venous access. Soft catheters made of silicone rubber are preferred for the subclavian approach. The right subclavian vein is preferable, to reduce catheter length and improve flow performances. Short, soft cannulas (20-25 cm) are indicated to prevent cardiac trauma (atrial and ventricular perforation).

Correct positioning of the distal tip is essential to prevent catheter dysfunction. The tip of a chest catheter passing through the superior vena cava system should be located at the junction of the superior vena cava and the right atrium. Fluoroscopy or chest radiograph is needed to check correct position of the catheter and tip after insertion and before use. Twenty to 25 centimeters is the optimal length for a thoracic catheter inserted on the right side in an adult patient; 3 or 4 cm more are required when a catheter is inserted on the left side.

The tip of a femoral catheter accessing the inferior vena cava system should be positioned in the central lumen of the inferior vena cava. Thirty to 35 centimeters is the length needed for a femoral catheter to reach the inferior vena cava in an adult.

MAINTENANCE AND CARE OF CATHETERS

Several studies have shown that physician expertise, strict hygienic rules, and good nursing practices are the strongest predictors of good catheter outcomes.[23] It is well recognized that restricting the use of a catheter to RRT—avoiding opening the catheter for blood sampling, parenteral feeding, and intravenous injections—minimizes catheter dysfunction and infectious risk. Nurse training and expertise of care are essential for preventing infection. Strict aseptic conditions and maximal sterile barrier precautions in catheter handling must be used at all times.[24] The use of antiseptic ointment or a protective box on catheter hubs significantly reduces the incidence of bacteremia in patients undergoing hemodialysis.[25] A catheter dressing is recommended to protect the emergence site of a catheter; indeed, tight occlusive dressings promote moisture and proliferation of cutaneous bacteria. Preliminary studies comparing surface-treated catheters or bioactive material (silver- or antibiotic-impregnated material) with regular catheters have reported encouraging results in reducing infection incidence.[26,27] However, these results have not been confirmed in large clinical randomized trials.[28] Catheter locking solutions based on antithrombotic/antiseptic or antibiotic mixtures have also proved to be efficient in preventing endoluminal contamination by bacteria.[29-32] Real benefits of these approaches have been proved in controlled prospective studies evaluating citrate or citrate/taurolidine mixtures.[33-36]

CATHETER PERFORMANCE

The type and design of a catheter affects its performance[37]:
- The type of polymer determines catheter resistance and softness
- The length and inner catheter diameter governs maximum flow rate and resistance
- The presence or lack of distal holes affects blood flow stability.

Intermittent RRT modalities require usually high blood flows (300-400 mL/min) with low resistance (venous and arterial pressures <200 mm Hg). An internal lumen diam-

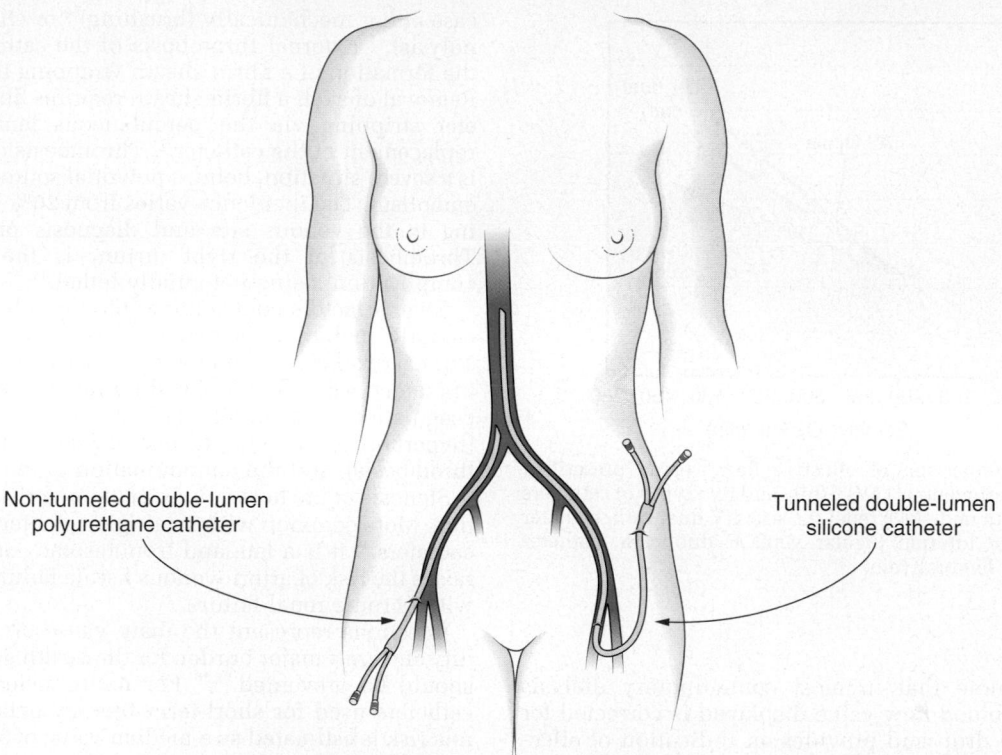

Non-tunneled double-lumen
polyurethane catheter

Tunneled double-lumen
silicone catheter

FIGURE 222-11. Double-lumen central venous catheter for either short-term or long-term catheter inserted in the femoral veins.

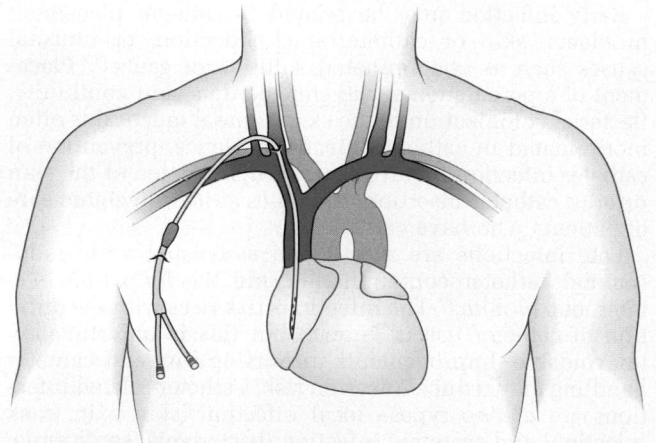

FIGURE 222-12. Double-lumen silicone central venous catheter for long term use inserted in the right internal jugular vein.

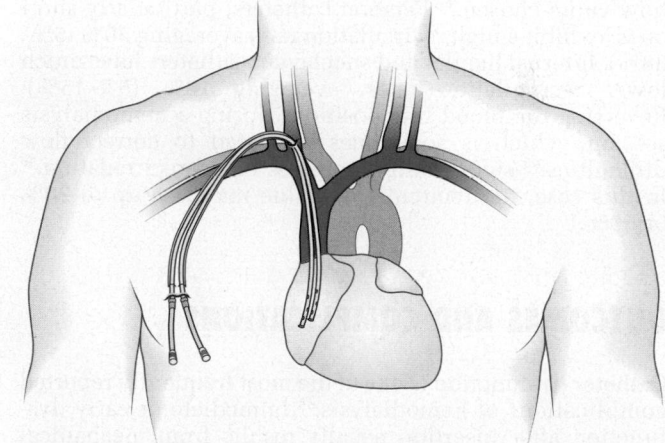

FIGURE 222-13. Double-lumen silicone central venous catheter for long term use inserted in the right internal jugular vein with subcutaneous anchoring.

eter between 2.0 and 2.2 mm (10F) is necessary in these cases to provide an optimal flow-resistance regimen. One must recognize that the effective blood flow with a CVC is usually 10% to 20% lower than the prescribed blood flow (Fig. 222-14). Two independent catheters (or a split catheter) bearing circular distal holes are essential to reduce the probability of catheter dysfunction (parietal suction, partial lumen obstruction, fibrin sleeve formation).[38] Permeability of the internal lumen and stability of the cannula in the venous bulk flow are key factors in the proper operation of a catheter.[39] In all cases, the objective

is to deliver an adequate dialysis dose to the patient with acute renal failure,[40] meaning that effective blood flow should be achieved regularly and recirculation should be minimized.[41,42]

Extracorporeal blood pressures (arterial and venous) recorded by the dialysis machine provide indirect evidence of the catheter's permeability. The negative pressure recorded on the inflow side and the positive pressure recorded on the outflow side reflect blood resistance in the extracorporeal circuit. These values may be used as indirect bedside indicators of partial catheter obstruction. It is

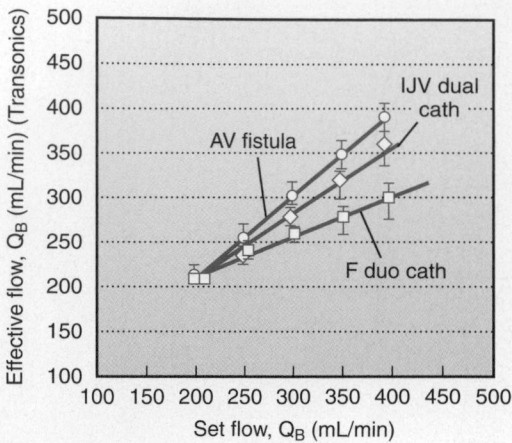

FIGURE 222-14. Comparison of effective flow versus prescribed blood flow in arteriovenous (AV) fistula and two types of catheters in 10 patients with end-stage renal disease. IJV dual cath, catheter inserted into the internal jugular vein; F duo cath, catheter inserted into the femoral vein.

important to note that in most contemporary dialysis machines, the blood flow value displayed is corrected for blood pressure drop and provides an indication of effective blood flow. The use of two catheters provides better effective flow rate than a double-lumen catheter.[43]

Recirculation, a common feature of catheters, reduces dialysis efficacy. The recirculation value depends on type of catheter, catheter tip positioning, vein used, and blood flow value chosen.[44] Femoral catheters, particularly short ones, exhibit a high recirculation rate, averaging 20% (5%-38%). Internal jugular and subclavian catheters have much lower recirculation rates, averaging 10% (5%-15%). Reversing the blood line positions during a hemodialysis session, which is sometimes indicated to correct flow difficulties,[45] significantly increases blood recirculation.[46] In this case, the recirculation value may rise up to 20% or 30%.[47]

OUTCOMES AND COMPLICATIONS

Catheter dysfunction is one of the most frequently reported complications of hemodialysis.[48] Immediate or early dysfunction after insertion usually results from mechanical problems, including malpositioning of catheter tips, kinking of catheter, and constriction due to ligatures or aponeurosis. On the other hand, late dysfunction (>2 weeks after insertion) is often caused by thrombotic problems, such as partial or total obstruction of the catheter lumen, thrombosis or stenosis of the host vein, external sheath formation on the distal end of the catheter (external fibrin sleeve), and internal coating of the catheter (endoluminal fibrin sleeve). Partial or total occlusion of the lumen and distal and/or lateral perforations of CVCs greatly increase the extracorporeal resistances and accordingly reduce the effective blood flow. Short-term catheters are more prone to dysfunction than long-term CVCs.[49]

Thrombosis is a common complication that is indicated usually by intermittent or permanent dysfunction, or, less frequently, by unexplained fever or edema of the ipsilateral arm. Endoluminal thrombosis of the catheter is the most common form. The catheter may be reopened in this case either mechanically (brushing)[50] or chemically (fibrinolysis).[51] External thrombosis of the catheter represents the formation of a fibrin sheath wrapping the catheter tip. Removal of such a fibrin sheath requires fibrinolysis, catheter stripping via the percutaneous femoral route, or replacement of the catheter.[52] Thrombosis of the host vein is a severe situation, being a potential source of pulmonary embolism. The incidence varies from 20% to 70% according to the venous site and diagnosis procedure used. Thrombosis of the right atrium is the most serious complication, being potentially lethal.[53]

Several factors contribute to the thrombogenicity of the cannula, including the material (type of polymer, softness, surface regularity), the mode of insertion, the type of vein (diameter, vein flow), the duration of cannulation, the coagulation and inflammation profiles of the patient (hyperfibrinemia, hyperthrombocytemia, previous venous thrombosis), and the contamination of the catheter.[30]

Stenosis of the host vein is a common risk of catheterization. More common with semirigid catheters than with soft catheters,[54] it is a late and troublesome complication that raises the risk of arteriovenous fistula failure in the patient with chronic renal failure.

Infections represent the main cause of catheter morbidity and are a major burden for the health system, and they should be prevented.[55,56] For nontunneled polyurethane catheters used for short-term therapy entail, the bacteremia risk is estimated as a median value of 5.9 episodes per 1000 patient-days in intensive care units. The incidence of bacteremia varies greatly according to specific practices.[57] Nontunneled internal jugular access has a higher risk of infections, particularly if located in the femoral groin area.[58]

Early infection may be related to catheter placement problems, skin or catheter track infection, or unusual causes such as contaminated solution or gauze.[59] Placement of a percutaneous catheter disrupts skin continuity. Bacterial colonization of the skin or nasal mucosal is often incriminated in catheter infections. Hence, prevention of catheter infection requires careful disinfection of the skin prior to catheter insertion as well as strictly hygienic care of patients who have catheters.[60]

Late infections are most often associated with endoluminal catheter contamination and the formation of a microbial biofilm.[61] The infectious risk rises with the duration of catheter use is known, but this is unfortunately unavoidable. Improvements in nursing care and catheter handling may reduce infection risk. Catheter-related infections are of two types—local infection (skin exit, track infection) and systemic infection (bacteremia, septicemia, infected thrombosis).

Skin exit and bacteremia, the most common forms of infection, may be treated with local and systemic antibiotic therapy with the catheter kept in situ and use of an antiseptic locking solution.[62-64] Catheter track infection, septicemia, and infected venous thrombosis are the most severe forms of infection, requiring both catheter withdrawal and systemic antibiotic therapy. Endoluminal contamination from catheter hubs may be the source of microbial biofilm. In this case, bacteria enter the lumen, adhere to the catheter surface, grow, produce glycocalyx (slime), and become resistant to antibiotics. Occasionally, bacteria may be released from this biofilm as a result of the high shear stress of the blood pump during hemodialysis session; the result is an acute bacteremia with a sudden shivering episode.

When an unexplained septic condition is observed in a patient with a catheter, it is reasonable to assume that the catheter is the primary source of infection. Some authorities have proposed replacing the catheter over a guidewire in this situation.[65] Other researchers regard this action as an unsafe approach that bears the risk of disseminating bacteria from the subcutaneous track into the bloodstream.[66] Another approach to infection is to remove the catheter, maintain the systemic antibiotic therapy, and insert a new catheter several days later in another vein. Whether this catheter exchange is pertinent or not remains highly debatable.[66-68] In all cases, it is essential to culture the withdrawn catheter.

The insertion of a soft-tunneled catheter with an anchoring system appears highly preferable to prevent catheter infection hazards. Strict aseptic rules, including the use of gloves, mask, drapes, and antiseptic solution, must be observed whenever a catheter is handled or is being connected to dialysis machine bloodlines, to prevent the endoluminal passage of bacteria present on the catheter's hub. The prophylactic use of antiseptic or antimicrobial locking solutions is a new and quite appealing option to preventing bacteremia.[69-72]

PERSPECTIVES

Despite related hazards, dialysis catheters represent the only means of blood access in patients requiring extracorporeal RRT. Biomaterials research may yield solutions to improve the safety of catheters in the near future.

Surface treatment of catheters that render them softer and smoother reduces hemoreactivity and prevents activation of the coagulation cascade, reducing the risk of thrombosis.[73] Fixation of bioactive materials on the polymer surface (silver impregnation, anticoagulant, antibiotic/antiseptic adsorption) is intended to prevent platelet adhesion, to avoid clotting, and to protect against bacterial adhesion. Studies comparing the incidences of infection with impregnated-antibiotic catheters and with regular catheters have confirmed the protective role of bioactive material.[74] However, this beneficial protective effect must be proven over a longer period.

Catheter locking solutions, using antithrombotic and antiseptic mixture, appear more appealing in this context to prevent infection.[75] Such locking solutions prevent biofilm formation and eradicate microbial catheter contamination.[76,77] All such solutions need to be evaluated in term of cost-effectiveness before they can be recommended for routine clinical practice.

CONCLUSION

Nowadays, CVCs represent the vascular access common to venovenous RRT modalities. A semirigid double-lumen polyurethane catheter inserted in the femoral vein is the emergency access of choice and must be restricted to short-term use (<2 weeks). Insertion of a soft silicone or polyurethane double-lumen catheter or two single-lumen catheters seems better indicated for medium- and long-term use. The internal jugular vein (right side) yields a properly functioning catheter and has a lower risk of stenosis. Subclavian access should be avoided or restricted

to a last resort; if it must be used, a silicone catheter is indicated for risks of stenosis and/or thrombosis. Catheter-related morbidity may be significantly reduced by better catheter care and regular use of an antithrombotic/antiseptic locking solution. Bioactive materials will probably make catheters safer in the near future.

Key Points

1. Short-term central venous catheters are intended to be used less than 14 days, while long-term tunneled central venous catheters are intended to be used up to 90 days or even longer.
2. A soft-tunneled dual lumen catheter (or dual catheter) is indicated in a patient with acute renal failure when renal replacement therapy is expected to exceed two weeks, in order to prevent complications.
3. Catheter insertion in the internal jugular vein and femoral vein are clearly recommended to prevent vein stenosis or thrombosis.
4. Catheter-related morbidity (dysfunction, thrombosis, infection) is in part due to the type of catheter (chronic tunneled catheter is better than acute catheter) but is mainly driven by nursing and medical practices implicated in catheter care.
5. Catheter performances (blood flow, resistance, recirculation) governing directly the efficacy of the renal replacement therapy should be regularly monitored.
6. Catheter-locking solutions (antithrombotic and/or antiseptic solution) are clearly a step forward in preventing catheter-related complications.

Key References

3. Canaud B, Desmeules S, Klouche K, et al: Vascular access for dialysis in the intensive care unit. Best Pract Res Clin Anaesthesiol 2004;18:159-174.
12. Trerotola SO, Kraus M, Shah H, et al: Randomized comparison of split tip versus step tip high-flow hemodialysis catheters. Kidney Int 2002;62:282-289.
18. Weijmer MC, Vervloet MG, ter Wee PM: Compared to tunnelled cuffed haemodialysis catheters, temporary untunnelled catheters are associated with more complications already within 2 weeks of use. Nephrol Dial Transplant 2004;19:670-677.
21. Klouche K, Amigues L, Deleuze S, et al: Complications, effects on dialysis dose, and survival of tunneled femoral dialysis catheters in acute renal failure. Am J Kidney Dis 2007;49:99-108.
29. Weijmer MC, Debets-Ossenkopp YJ, Van De Vondervoort FJ, ter Wee PM: Superior antimicrobial activity of trisodium citrate over heparin for catheter locking. Nephrol Dial Transplant 2002;17:2189-2195.
35. Betjes MG, van Agteren M: Prevention of dialysis catheter-related sepsis with a citrate-taurolidine-containing lock solution. Nephrol Dial Transplant 2004;19:1546-1551.

See the companion Expert Consult website for the complete reference list.

CHAPTER 223

Solute and Water Transport across Artificial Membranes in Conventional Hemodialysis

Zhongping Huang, Jeffrey J. Letteri, Claudio Ronco, Dayong Gao, and William R. Clark

---

OBJECTIVES

This chapter will:
1. Explain the basic differences between cellulosic and synthetic membranes and how these differences influence their solute and fluid removal properties.
2. Explore how membrane pore size effects influence both the diffusive solute and water permeability of dialysis membranes.
3. Describe the fundamental difference between solute clearance and mass removal rate.
4. Discuss the ways in which solute clearance can be expressed.
5. Present the major determinants of blood-side and dialysate resistance in a dialyzer.

Conventional hemodialysis remains an important renal replacement modality for critically ill patients with acute kidney injury. Because prescription of hemodialysis requires goals to be set with regard to the rate and extent of both solute removal and fluid removal, a thorough understanding of the mechanisms by which solute and fluid are removed during hemodialysis is necessary. This chapter provides an overview of solute and water transfer during hemodialysis. First, the major characteristics of hollow fiber membranes influencing solute and water removal are discussed. Within this section, the chemical composition and physical characteristics of commonly used dialysis membranes and the features determining their solute and water permeability properties are reviewed. The remainder of the chapter emphasizes the major determinants of dialyzer performance.

HOLLOW-FIBER MEMBRANES: CLASSIFICATION BY MATERIAL

Cellulosic Membranes

The relatively long duration of popularity of cellulosic membranes can be explained largely by their particular suitability for a diffusion-based procedure like hemodialysis.[1] The underlying hydrogel structure of these membranes and their tensile strength allow the combination of thinner walls (see later) and high porosity to be achieved in the fiber spinning process.[2] These characteristics allow the attainment of high rates of diffusive membrane transport and efficient removal of small, water-soluble uremic solutes, such as urea and creatinine. Another characteristic feature of these membranes is symmetry with respect to composition, implying an essentially uniform resistance to mass transfer over the entire wall thickness.

The most commonly used cellulosic dialyzers contain cellulose acetate (rigorously, cellulose diacetate) membranes,[3] in which approximately 75% of the hydroxyl groups on the cellulosic backbone are replaced with an acetate group. As opposed to a hydroxyl group, an acetate group does not bind avidly to a C3 molecule to initiate activation of the complement cascade. Consequently, in dialysis using cellulose acetate membranes, complement activation is attenuated, as is the leukopenic response, in comparison with dialysis using unmodified cellulosic membranes. Because production of cellulose triacetate membranes involves complete hydroxyl group substitution with acetate groups, further attenuation of complement activation and leukopenia is achieved.[4]

Synthetic Membranes

Synthetic membranes were developed essentially in response to concerns about the narrow scope of solute removal and the pronounced complement activation associated with unmodified cellulosic dialyzers. The AN69 membrane, a copolymer of acrylonitrile and an anionic sulfonate group, was first employed in flat sheet form in a closed-loop dialysate system in the early 1970s.[5] Since that time, a number of other synthetic membranes have been developed, including polysulfone,[6] polyamide,[7] polymethyl methacrylate (PMMA),[8] polyethersulfone,[9] and polyarylethersulfone/polyamide.[10] Largely in relation to the interest in hemofiltration as a therapy for end-stage renal disease in the late 1970s and early 1980s, along with the inability to use low-flux unmodified cellulosic dialyzers for this therapy, these membranes were initially formulated with high water permeability.[11] The large mean pore size and thick wall structure of these membranes allowed the high ultrafiltration rates necessary in hemofiltration to be achieved at relatively low transmembrane pressures. However, with the waning of interest in hemofiltration as a long-term dialysis therapy in the mid-1980s, dialyzers with these highly permeable membranes were used subsequently in the diffusive mode as high-flux dialyzers. This latter mode continues to be the most common application of these membranes, although they are increasingly being employed for long-term hemodiafiltration now.[12]

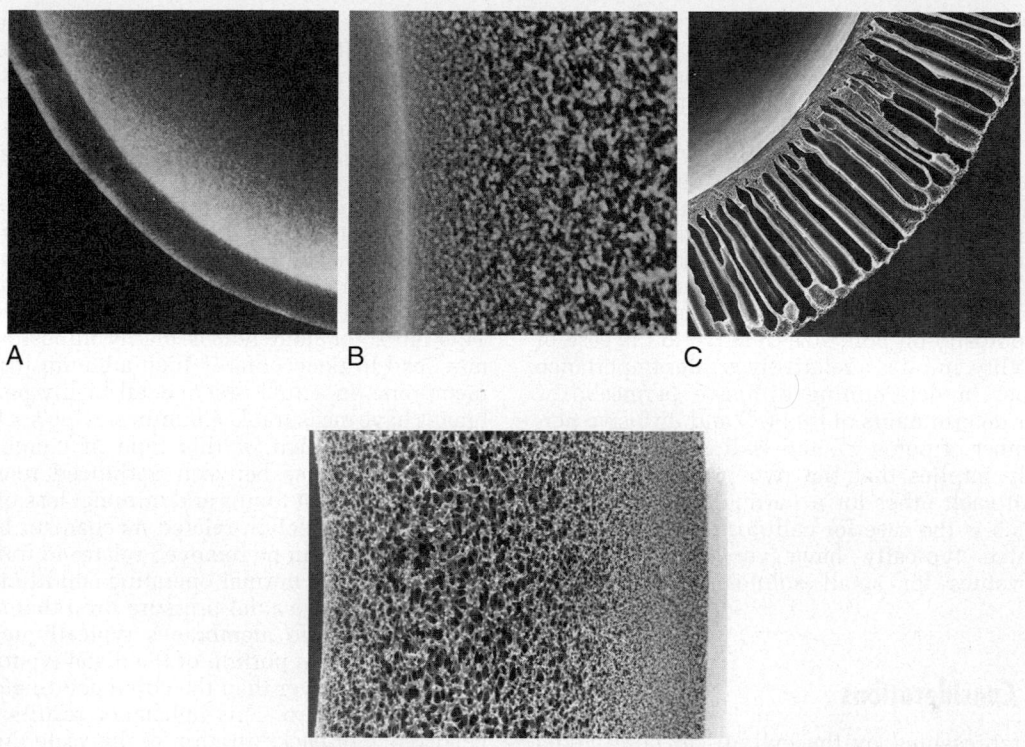

FIGURE 223-1. Structure of different membranes used for clinical hemodialyzers. **A,** Cellulose-based membrane with no visible porosity. **B,** Foamlike synthetic membrane. **C,** Macroreticular anisotropic synthetic membrane. **D,** Three-layer foamlike synthetic membrane.

An obvious difference between synthetic and cellulosic membranes is chemical composition. Unlike naturally occurring cellulose membranes, synthetic membranes are manufactured polymers that are classified as thermoplastics. In fact, the hemodialysis market represents only a small fraction of the industrial utilization of most synthetic membranes. As noted previously, another feature differentiating cellulosic and synthetic membranes is wall thickness (Fig. 223-1). Synthetic membranes have wall thickness values of at least 20 μm and may be structurally symmetrical (e.g., AN69, pPMMA) or asymmetrical (e.g., polysulfone, polyamide, polyethersulfone, polyarylethersulfone/polyamide). For asymmetrical structures, a very thin "skin" (approximately 1 μm) contacting the blood compartment lumen acts primarily as the membrane's separating element with regard to solute removal. The structure of the remaining wall thickness ("stroma"), which determines a synthetic membrane's thermal, chemical, and mechanical properties, varies considerably among the various synthetic membranes.[13] For example, the stroma has a relatively homogeneous, spongelike consistency in the Fresenius polysulfone membrane (Fresenius Medical Care AG & Co. KGaA, Bad Homburg, Germany). On the other hand, the Polyflux membrane (Gambro AB, Stockholm), which is actually a blend of polyamide and polyarylethersulfone, has three distinct layers; as in the Fresenius polysulfone membrane, one layer of the Polyflux membrane is a thin blood-contacting inner lumen, composed of polyarylethersulfone enriched with polyvinylpyrrolidone (PVP), and the outer surface is composed of relatively PVP-free polyamide. Interspersed between these two layers is a polyarylethersulfone stroma.[10,13] Finally, the DIAPES polyethersulfone membrane (Membrana GmbH, Wuppertal, Germany) contains both inner

and outer skin layers surrounding a spongelike stroma.[9] For this membrane, the average pore radii of the inner and outer skin layers are approximately 5 and 10 nm, respectively. Takeyama and Sakai[14] have suggested that an effective mean pore radius between 5 and 8 nm achieves the appropriate balance between β_2-microglobulin removal and albumin loss.

PROPERTIES OF HEMODIALYZER MEMBRANES THAT INFLUENCE DIALYZER PERFORMANCE

Water Permeability

A hollow-fiber dialyzer membrane can be modeled as having straight cylindrical pores, all of the same radius (r) and all with a directionality perpendicular to the flow of blood and dialysate.[2] (As discussed later, this model does not exactly replicate a clinical dialyzer but is nevertheless useful from a quantitative perspective.) The major determinants of plasma ultrafiltrate flow rate through the pores are the number of pores (i.e., number per unit area of membrane surface area), transmembrane pressure, and pore size. Just as the Hagen-Poiseuille equation[15] can be used to model axial (i.e., lengthwise) blood flow through an individual hollow fiber, it can also be employed to assess ultrafiltrate flow through an individual pore. Thus, the rate of ultrafiltrate flow actually depends on the fourth power of the pore radius (i.e., r^4). As such, the membrane characteristic that most directly influences water permeability is mean pore size.

Diffusive Permeability

Membrane wall thickness is one important determinant of diffusive transport.[16] The relatively thin-walled structure of cellulosic membranes (usually 6-15 μm) is largely responsible for their particular suitability in the setting of diffusive hemodialysis. The other major determinant of dialyzer membrane diffusive transport is porosity, also known as pore density. On the basis of the cylindrical pore model described previously, membrane porosity is directly proportional to both the number of pores and the square of the pore radius (r^2). Therefore, the smaller dependence of membrane porosity on pore size, relative to the ease of water permeability, implies a relatively greater importance of pore number in determining diffusive permeability. That the major determinants of flux (r^4) and diffusive permeability (number of pores, r^2, and wall thickness) differ so significantly implies that the two properties can be independent of each other for a particular hemodialysis membrane. Such is the case for cellulosic high-efficiency dialyzers, which typically have very high diffusive permeability values for small solutes but low water permeability.

Nondiffusive Considerations

A membrane represented by the cylindrical pore model previously described deviates from an actual membrane used for clinical hemodialysis, in that the latter actually has a distribution of pore sizes. Ronco and colleagues[17] have discussed the manner in which pore size distribution may differ among hemodialysis membranes and the manner in which this distribution influences a membrane's sieving properties (see Chapter 277 for a detailed discussion of sieving coefficient). In Figure 223-2, which has been reproduced from their study, the membrane represented by curve A on the left diagram has a large number of relatively small pores, whereas the membrane represented by curve B has a large number of relatively large pores. On the basis of the relatively narrow pore size distributions, the solute sieving coefficient versus molecular weight profiles for both membranes (left diagram) have the desirable sharp cutoff, similar to that of the native kidney. However, the molecular weight cutoff for membrane A (approximately 10 kDa) is consistent with a high-efficiency membrane

whereas that of membrane B (approximately 60 kDa) is consistent with a high-flux membrane. In addition, primarily due to the large number of pores, both membranes would be expected to demonstrate favorable diffusive transport properties. On the other hand, the membrane represented by curve C exhibits a pore size distribution that is unfavorable from both a diffusive transport and sieving perspective. The relatively small number of pores accounts for the poor diffusive properties. In addition, the broad distribution of pores explains not only the "early" drop-off in sieving coefficient at relatively low molecular weight but also the "tail" effect at high molecular weight. This latter phenomenon is highly undesirable because it may lead to unacceptably high albumin losses across the membrane. In actual practice, all highly permeable membranes have measurable albumin sieving coefficient values, so that the design of this type of membrane involves striking a balance between optimized removal of high-molecular-weight toxins and minimal loss of albumin.

Another convection-related mechanism by which large uremic toxins can be removed relates to fluid flow within the filter. Under normal operating conditions of high-flux dialysis, the large axial pressure drop that occurs in such highly permeable membranes typically results in pressures in a certain portion of the distal (venous) end of the fiber that are lower than the corresponding dialysate compartment pressure. This imbalance results in the routine occurrence of back-filtration of dialysate during high-flux hemodialysis.[18] Although the combination of significant back-filtration and contaminated dialysate raises concerns related to "back-transfer," this internal filtration mechanism ("Starling's flow") can significantly augment removal of larger molecules. In fact, under normal operating conditions of high-flux hemodialysis, this mechanism typically is the predominant mechanism by which large solute removal occurs. Attempts to accentuate this internal filtration mechanism, through either a decrease in hollow-fiber inner diameter or manipulations in dialysate compartment pressure, have been described.[19]

Adsorption (membrane binding) is another mechanism by which hydrophobic compounds like peptides and proteins may be removed during hemodialysis. Although adsorption during hemodialysis is a relatively poorly understood phenomenon, certain membrane characteristics play an important role. First, adsorption occurs primarily within the pore structure of the membrane rather than at the nominal surface contacting the blood only.[20] Therefore, the open pore structure of high-flux membranes affords more adsorptive potential than the pores of low-flux membranes. Second, synthetic membranes, many of which are fundamentally hydrophobic, generally are much more adsorptive than hydrophilic cellulosic membranes.[21]

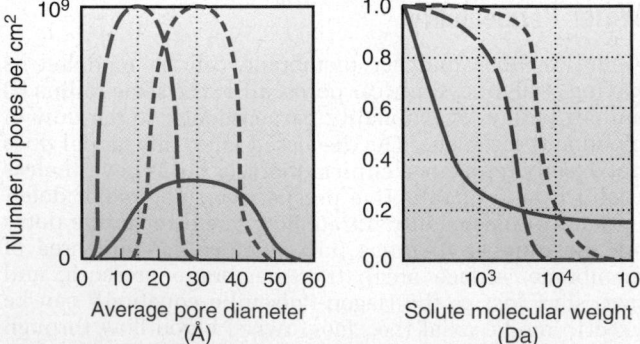

FIGURE 223-2. Pore size distribution and sieving coefficient profiles for three hypothetical membranes. *Left,* The relationship between number of pores and pore size. *Right,* Sieving coefficient as a function of solute molecular weight. (From Ronco C, Ballestri M, Gappelli G: Dialysis membranes in convective treatments. Nephrol Dial Transplant 2000;15[Suppl 2]:31-36.)

CHARACTERIZATION OF DIALYZER PERFORMANCE: CLEARANCE AND ULTRAFILTRATION COEFFICIENT

Clearance

Whole Blood Clearance

By definition, solute clearance (K) is the ratio of mass removal rate (N) to blood solute concentration (C_B) as follows[22]:

$$K = \frac{N}{C_B} \qquad [1]$$

For a hemodialyzer, the mass removal rate is simply the difference between the rate of solute mass (i.e., product of flow rate and concentration) presented to the dialyzer in the arterial blood line and the rate of solute mass leaving the dialyzer in the venous blood line. This mass balance applied to the dialyzer results in the following classic (i.e., arteriovenous) whole-blood dialyzer clearance equation[23]:

$$K_B = \frac{(Q_{Bi} \times C_{Bi}) - (Q_{Bo} \times C_{Bo})}{C_{Bi} + Q_F \times (C_{Bo}/C_{Bi})} \qquad [2]$$

where K_B is whole blood clearance, Q_B is blood flow rate, C_B is whole blood solute concentration, and Q_F is net ultrafiltration rate; the subscripts i and o refer to the inlet (arterial) and outlet (venous) blood lines.

It is important to note that diffusive removal, convective removal, and, possibly, adsorptive removal of solutes occur simultaneously in hemodialysis. For a nonadsorbing solute like urea, diffusion and convection interact in such a manner that total solute removal is significantly less than what would be expected if the individual components were simply added together. This phenomenon is explained in the following way: Diffusive removal results in a decrease in solute concentration in the blood compartment along the axial length (i.e., from blood inlet to blood outlet) of the hemodialyzer. Because convective solute removal is directly proportional to the blood compartment concentration, convective solute removal decreases as a function of this axial concentration gradient. On the other hand, hemoconcentration resulting from ultrafiltration of plasma water causes a progressive increase in plasma protein concentration and hematocrit along the axial length of the dialyzer. This hemoconcentration and resultant hyperviscosity cause an increase in diffusive mass transfer resistance and a decrease in solute transport via this mechanism. The effect of this interaction on overall solute removal has been analyzed rigorously by numerous investigators. The most useful quantification has been developed by Jaffrin,[24] as follows:

$$K_T = K_D + Q_F \times Tr \qquad [3]$$

where K_T is total solute clearance, K_D is diffusive clearance under conditions of no net ultrafiltration, and the final term, $Q_F \times Tr$, is the convective component of clearance, being a function of the ultrafiltration rate (Q_F) and an experimentally derived transmittance coefficient (Tr), as follows:

$$Tr = S\left(1 - \frac{K_D}{Q_B}\right) \qquad [4]$$

where S is the solute sieving coefficient. Thus, Tr for a particular solute depends on the efficiency of diffusive removal. At very low values of K_D/Q_B, diffusion has a very small effect on blood compartment concentrations, and the convective component of clearance closely approximates the quantity $S \times Q_F$. However, increasing efficiency of diffusive removal (i.e., increasing K_D/Q_B) significantly influences blood compartment concentrations. The result is a decrease in Tr and, consequently, in the convective contribution to total clearance.

BLOOD WATER AND PLASMA CLEARANCE. An implicit assumption in the determination of whole blood clearance is that the volume from which the solute is cleared is the actual volume of blood transiting through the dialyzer at a certain time. This assumption is incorrect for two reasons. First, in both the erythron and plasma components of blood, a certain volume is composed of solids (proteins or lipids) rather than water. Second, for solutes like creatinine and phosphate, which are distributed in both the erythron and plasma water, slow mass transfer from the intracellular space to the plasma space (relative to mass transfer across the dialyzer) results in relative sequestration (compartmentalization) in the former compartment.[25] This reduces the *effective* volume of distribution from which these solutes can be cleared *in the dialyzer*. As such, derivation of whole blood dialyzer clearances from plasma water concentrations in conjunction with blood flow rates—a common practice in dialyzer evaluations—results in a significant overestimation of actual solute removal. The more appropriate approach is to employ blood water clearances, which account for the previously described hematocrit-dependent effects on effective intradialytic solute distribution volume, as follows[26]:

$$Q_{BW} = 0.93 \times Q_B \left[1 - Hct + K(1 - e^{-\alpha t})Hct\right] \qquad [5]$$

where Q_{BW} is blood water flow rate. In this equation, for a given solute, K is the red blood cell (RBC) water–plasma water partition coefficient for a given solute, α is the transcellular rate constant (units: time^{-1}), and t is the characteristic dialyzer residence time. Estimates for these parameters have been provided by numerous prior studies and have been summarized by Shinaberger and colleagues.[27] (The factor 0.93 in Equation 5 corrects for the volume of plasma occupied by plasma proteins and lipids). Finally, K_{BW} can be calculated by substituting Q_{BW} for Q_B in Equation 2.

Although the distribution volume of many uremic solutes approximates that of total body water, it is much more limited for other toxins, particularly those of larger molecular weight. For example, the distribution space of β_2-microglobulin and many other low-molecular weight proteins is the plasma volume. Consequently, when Equation 2 is used to determine β_2-microglobulin clearance, plasma flow rates (inlet and outlet) should replace blood flow rates in the first term of the right side of the equation.

The distinction between whole blood, blood water, and dialysate-side clearances is very important in the interpretation of clinical data. However, clearances provided by dialyzer manufacturers are typically in vitro data generated from experiments in which the blood compartment fluid is an aqueous solution. Although these data provide useful information to the clinician, they overestimate the actual dialyzer performance that can be achieved clinically (under the same conditions). This overestimation is related to the inability of aqueous solution–based experiments to capture the effects of RBCs (as discussed previously) and plasma proteins (see later) on solute mass transfer.

Dialysate-Side Clearance

As indicated in Equation 1, solute clearance is the ratio of mass removal rate to blood concentration. Although blood-side measurements are typically used to determine solute mass removal rate, clearance can also be estimated from dialysate-side measurements, as follows:

$$K_D = \frac{Q_{Do} \times C_{Do}}{C_{Bi}} \qquad [6]$$

where Q_{Do} is venous dialysate flow and C_{Do} is dialysate solute concentration. In this equation, dialysate-side solute clearance (K_D) is determined by measurement of the rate of mass appearance in the effluent dialysate stream ($Q_{Do} \times C_{Do}$). Dialysate-side measurements provide more accurate mass transfer information than blood-side determinations and are generally considered the gold standard for evaluating dialyzer performance. Relative to dialysate-side values, whole blood clearances substantially overestimate true dialyzer performance. Blood water clearances also moderately overestimate dialyzer performance, although the agreement between these values and simultaneously determined dialysate-side values (for non-adsorbing solutes) are usually within 5% of each other under rigorous test conditions. The major disadvantage of dialysate-based clearance techniques is the need to assay solute concentrations at very low concentrations. For some solutes (e.g., phosphate), these dilute concentrations may be difficult to assay with standard automated chemistry devices.

Clearance versus Mass Removal Rate

It is important to recognize that clearance is *not* a measure of actual mass removal of a particular solute by dialysis. As Equation 1 indicates, clearance is the ratio of mass removal rate to blood concentration for a given solute. In hemodialysis, the mass removal rate of small solutes like urea is very high during the early stage of an intermittent hemodialysis treatment owing to a favorable transmembrane concentration gradient for diffusion at this time. As the treatment proceeds, proportional decreases in blood urea nitrogen value and urea mass removal rate, which is determined by the instantaneous blood urea nitrogen value, occurs.[22] Equation 2 predicts that a proportional decrease in these parameters results in a constant dialyzer clearance during the treatment (provided that dialyzer function is preserved) (Fig. 223-3). Despite not being a measure of actual dialytic solute removal, clearance

remains a very reasonable parameter to assess dialyzer function. The discordance between solute clearance and mass removal rate described above is a much more relevant consideration when a whole body (rather than dialyzer) clearance approach is used (see below).

Whole-Body Clearance versus Dialyzer Clearance

The discussion to this point has focused on clearance of a solute by the dialyzer and has included the implications of solute compartmentalization within the dialyzer for solutes such as creatinine and phosphate. Compartmentalization may also occur during hemodialysis within the patient's body. During hemodialysis, direct removal of a particular solute can occur only from that portion of its volume of distribution that actually perfuses the dialyzer, and sequestration of solute occurs in the remaining volume of distribution. Solute compartmentalization involves interplay between dialyzer solute clearance and patient/solute parameters, such as compartment volumes and intercompartmental mass transfer resistances. Even if solute removal by the dialyzer is relatively efficient, overall (effective) solute removal may be limited by slow intercompartmental mass transfer.

To account for these effects of "intracorporeal" solute compartmentalization on overall solute removal, many clinicians prefer to use whole-body rather than dialyzer clearance, believing that the former is a better measure of overall treatment efficacy.[28] Whole-body clearance methodologies employ blood samples obtained before and after the hemodialysis treatment. An example of a widely used whole-body clearance approach is the second-generation Daugirdas equation. In this approach, a logarithmic relationship between delivered urea Kt/V and the extent of the intradialytic reduction in blood urea nitrogen is assumed. Two issues complicate the use of these methodologies. One is the assumed distribution volume of the solute for which the clearance is being estimated and whether or not this volume is multicompartmental. The second important consideration, incorporation of the effects of post-hemodialysis rebound, is closely tied to multicompartment kinetics.

Relationship of Dialyzer Clearance and Treatment "Efficiency"

Although not precisely defined, hemodialysis treatment efficiency is very closely related to a dialyzer's small solute removal capabilities. The term "high-efficiency," currently in wide use, actually had its origin as a therapy first described by Keshaviah and associates,[29] rather than a specific type of dialyzer. These investigators employed large–surface area cellulose acetate dialyzers and relatively high blood flow rates to achieve sufficiently high urea clearances to allow reductions in treatment time. The use of large–surface area dialyzers capable of achieving these high urea clearances has increased to the point that a separate, albeit somewhat indistinct, class of high-efficiency dialyzers now exists.

Ultrafiltration Coefficient

There is considerable confusion about the precise meaning of *dialyzer flux*. By definition, *flux* is the transmembrane

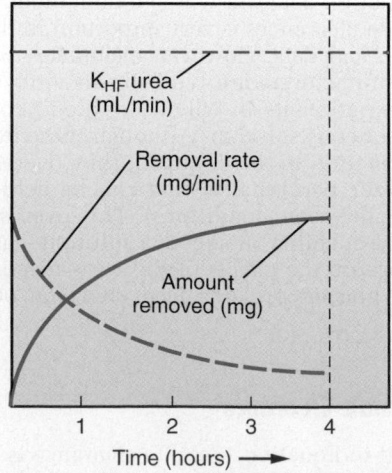

FIGURE 223-3. Relationship among solute clearance, mass removal rate, and cumulative removal during a 4-hour hemodialysis treatment. Even with constant dialyzer clearance, mass removal rate falls during the treatment because of a reduced concentration gradient. (From Clark WR, Henderson LW: Renal vs continuous vs intermittent therapies for removal of uremic toxins. Kidney Int 2001;59[Suppl 78]:S298-S303.)

rate of transfer of a substance, normalized to membrane surface area. Thus, one may define a diffusive or convective flux for a membrane-based process with respect to solute removal as the mass removal rate normalized to membrane surface area. Likewise, the hydraulic flux of membrane is the volumetric rate (normalized to surface area) at which ultrafiltration of water occurs. Although numerous classification schemes have been proposed,[30] hemodialysis membranes are traditionally classified according to *water flux*, a term synonymous with *water permeability*. The clinical parameter used to characterize the water permeability of a dialyzer is the ultrafiltration coefficient (K_{UF}, in mL/hr/mm Hg). The water permeability of a dialyzer is usually derived from in vitro experiments in which bovine blood is ultrafiltered at varying transmembrane pressure (TMP). The relationship between plasma ultrafiltration rate and TMP is linear at relatively low TMP values for all membranes, whereas a plateau in ultrafiltration rate occurs at relatively high TMP values.[31] Dialyzer K_{UF} is defined by the slope of the linear portion of this ultrafiltration rate plotted against the TMP curve. The membrane characteristic with the largest effect on water permeability is pore size, such that ultrafiltrate flux is roughly proportional to the fourth power of the mean membrane pore radius.[2] Therefore, small changes in pore size have a very large effect on water permeability.

DETERMINANTS OF DIFFUSIVE SOLUTE CLEARANCE

Diffusion is the dominant mass transfer mechanism mediating small solute removal in hemodialysis. Diffusive solute removal involves sequential mass transfer from the dialyzer blood compartment, through the membrane, and into the dialysate compartment. To quantify a dialyzer's diffusive capabilities, the concept of mass transfer resistance is frequently employed, as shown in the following equation[32]:

$$R_O = R_B + R_M + R_D \qquad [7]$$

where R_O is the overall resistance to diffusive mass transfer of a particular solute by a dialyzer, R_B is blood compartment resistance, R_M is resistance due to the membrane itself, and R_D is dialysate compartment resistance. In turn, R_O is the inverse of the overall mass transfer coefficient (K_O), which is a component of the overall mass transfer–area coefficient (K_OA) discussed later.

Blood Compartment

A fundamental relationship exists between diffusive clearance and blood flow rate for all solutes. For a given solute, a graph of clearance versus blood flow rate (Q_B) has two domains.[33] In the relatively low Q_B regimen, an effectively linear relationship exists between these two parameters. For all solutes, the line defined by this relationship falls below the line of identity, thus indicating that dialyzer clearance can never exceed the blood flow rate. For a given dialyzer, the slope of the line defining this flow-limited regimen is inversely related to solute size. Beyond a certain Q_B, the curve defining the clearance versus Q_B relationship for a given solute-dialyzer combination demonstrates a plateau. This plateau defines the K_OA-limited region. For a given solute-dialyzer combination, the K_OA parameter

can be regarded as the maximal clearance attainable under a given set of flow conditions. Both the Q_B at which the transition from the blood flow–limited to the K_OA-limited region and the plateau clearance value are specific for a given solute-dialyzer combination.[33] For a given solute, an increase in either membrane diffusivity (K_O) or area (A) has the effect of increasing both the transition Q_B and the plateau clearance value.

Minimizing the mass transfer resistance in the blood compartment is achieved primarily through the use of relatively high flow rates (i.e., shear rates), which minimize effects related to boundary (unstirred) layers. A *boundary layer* can be conceptualized as a stagnant film of fluid residing on the membrane surface. However, another important factor influencing blood compartment resistance is hematocrit. Blood is a complex fluid in which RBCs are suspended in plasma. Plasma is an aqueous solution but it does have a solid component (approximately 7% by volume) consisting of proteins and lipids. The erythron is also primarily aqueous, with water constituting approximately 70% of the total erythron and the remaining solid component primarily comprising cellular membranes. Although many uremic solutes are distributed in the aqueous phase of both the RBC and plasma fractions of blood, solute removal during hemodialysis (hemodialysis) can occur only from plasma water.

Before actual dialytic removal of solutes with this type of distribution can be achieved, mass transfer from the RBC water to the plasma water must occur. In turn, the rate at which this latter process occurs is solute-specific. Prior data indicate that urea movement across the RBC membrane is relatively fast.[34] Therefore, during hemodialysis, urea in the plasma water leaving the dialyzer is in equilibrium with urea in the RBC water, with the ratio of these concentrations (approximately 0.76) being determined by the ratio of the water fractions of the aqueous and RBC compartments. On the other hand, the transcellular rate of movement for other uremic solutes, such as creatinine and phosphate, is small (or negligible) relative to the rate of dialytic removal.[35] For a given unit volume of whole blood, a rise in hematocrit causes a relative increase in the distribution of solute in the RBC water, resulting in a relative sequestration of solutes with low RBC membrane diffusivity.

The application of rheological principles to the flow of blood in a dialyzer also raises concerns that blood compartment mass transfer may be impaired by increasing hematocrit. For a given solute, diffusive mass transfer resistance in the blood compartment of a dialyzer is the ratio of effective diffusive path length (x) to effective solute diffusivity (D), both of which may be influenced by hematocrit.[36] Because the volume of RBC mass per unit volume of blood increases with rising hematocrit, solutes diffusing to the membrane surface are relatively more likely to encounter a RBC, causing an effective lengthening of the diffusion distance. In addition, solute diffusivity may decrease as a function of rising hematocrit because of the latter's effect on viscosity, which is itself a determinant of mass transfer resistance.

Lim and coworkers[26] studied five patients in whom the pre-hemodialysis hematocrit was raised from a mean of 22.9% to 37.8% with the use of erythropoietin. Whole blood (K_B) and dialysate-side (K_D) clearances of urea, creatinine, and phosphate were measured under the following (prescribed) conditions: Q_B, 400 mL/min; dialysate flow rate (Q_D), 500 mL/min; and treatment time, 180 min. Dialysate-side clearance was used as the truer (gold standard) estimate of mass removal. The ratio K_D/K_B, an

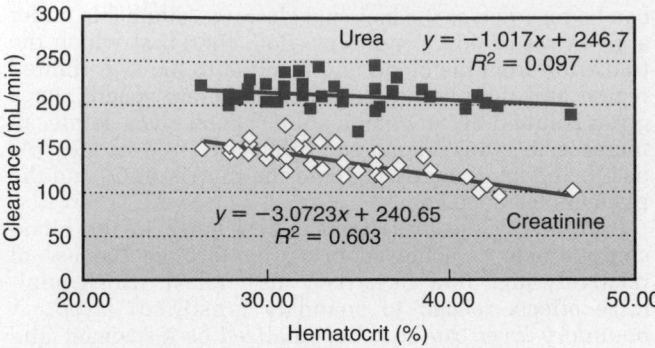

FIGURE 223-4. Small solute clearance as a function of hematocrit in hemodialysis. (From Ronco C, Brendolan A, Crepaldi C, et al: Blood and dialysate flow distributions in hollow fiber hemodialyzers analyzed by computerized helical scanning technique. J Am Soc Nephrol 2002;13[Suppl 1]:S53-S61.)

estimate of the extent to which whole blood clearance overestimates mass removal, was observed to diminish significantly for both creatinine and phosphate but not for urea. In urea kinetic analyses (based on the direct dialysate quantification method), both Kt/V (1.21 vs. 1.17) and percentage of urea reduction (64.2% vs. 61.6%) decreased, but not significantly. Interestingly, in a separate group of seven patients in whom hematocrit was raised from 19.1% to 29.5% with RBC transfusions, both Kt/V (1.32 vs. 1.19) and percentage reduction (66.4% vs 62.7%) decreased significantly.

Data from Ronco and colleagues[35] suggest that the hematocrit value may also influence flow distribution within the blood compartment of a dialyzer. These investigators employed a computed tomography–based technique to measure fiber bundle perfusion of blood with varying hematocrit values (25%-40%). A centralized distribution of flow was observed. Moreover, the extent of this maldistribution was proportional to hematocrit. In fact, at a hematocrit value of 40%, the flow velocity and wall shear rate were twofold to threefold higher in the central region of the bundle than in the peripheral region. For clinical correlation, these investigators also measured dialyzer urea and creatinine clearances as functions of hematocrit. As shown in Figure 223-4, this study corroborated the differential effect of increasing hematocrit on urea and creatinine clearance reported by Lim and coworkers.[26]

Dialysate Compartment

Higher efficiency of both blood compartment and transmembrane small solute mass transfer has been attained through the use of high blood flow rates and improved membrane designs, respectively. Consequently, efforts have now focused on dialysate-side mass transfer. On the basis of the K_OA concept already described, both the dialysate-side mass transfer coefficient and membrane surface area may influence mass transfer. The dialysate-side mass transfer coefficient is determined largely by boundary layer phenomena, as in the blood compartment. As discussed later, effective mass transfer area (A) is not necessarily equal to the manufacturer-reported (nominal) value.

Dialyzer characteristics that influence dialysate-side mass transfer include packing density, fiber undulation

(also known as crimping), and the presence or absence of spacer yarns. *Packing density* is defined as the ratio of the area composed of hollow fibers to the area of the dialyzer housing, based on a cross-sectional cut through the dialyzer. Recent magnetic resonance imaging and computed tomography studies suggest that nonoptimized packing density may be the cause of channeling of dialysate at standard flow rates.[35,36] These investigations demonstrated that a large proportion of the dialysate stream may flow peripheral to the fiber bundle in dialyzers that are not optimally configured. From a physical perspective, the interior of a fiber bundle packed too tightly represents a path of relatively large resistance, and the peripheral pathway is the path of least resistance. Obviously, an inwardly situated hollow fiber cannot participate in diffusive mass exchange if it is not perfused with dialysate. Packing density values beyond the optimum may account for the finding that large–surface area dialyzers (i.e., greater than 1.7 m^2) are generally associated with less efficient mass transfer of dialysate small solutes, relative to dialyzers of smaller surface area.[37]

Another dialyzer characteristic that influences hollow fiber perfusion with dialysate is fiber bundle spacing. Dialysate may not be able to perfuse the area between adjacent fibers that are too close to one another. As is the case for non-optimized packing density, this situation reduces the effective membrane surface area available for mass exchange. Two approaches have been developed to address this fiber spacing problem. First, *spacer yarns* are multiple-filament, linear structures interspersed longitudinally in a specific spatial distribution within the fiber bundle.[35] Second, all hollow fibers are manufactured with a relatively specific periodicity (amplitude and frequency); however, as discussed later, evidence now suggests that *specific fiber undulation patterns* improve dialysate flow distribution and small solute mass transfer.

In a clinical evaluation already cited, Ronco and colleagues[35] measured the effect of microcrimping and spacer yarns on both small solute removal and dialysate flow distribution. The microcrimped polysulfone fibers contained in the dialyzers used in this study have a relatively low amplitude and high frequency. In comparison with conventional dialyzers (i.e., that have fibers with standard undulation and no spacer yarns), urea clearances were found to be significantly higher for dialyzers with both microcrimped fibers and spacer yarns. Using a computed tomography–based technique, these investigators also found that dialysate flow distribution was most homogeneous in dialyzers with microcrimped fibers, least homogeneous in conventional dialyzers, and intermediate in dialyzers with spacer yarn technology (see Fig. 224-6 in Chapter 224). These data suggest that both of these newer approaches improve dialysate flow distribution and, thus, increase effective membrane surface area.

In addition to this influence on effective surface area, microcrimping may also reduce dialysate-side mass transfer resistance, essentially by disrupting ("agitating") the boundary layer. Another way in which boundary layer effects may be attenuated is through creation of a turbulent flow regimen with a relatively high Q_D. At a relatively common combination using Q_B 300 mL and Q_D 500 mL/min, it is possible that dialysate-side mass transfer is rate-limiting under certain conditions. For several high-efficiency and high-flux dialyzers, Leypoldt and associates[37] reported a mean increase of 14% in in vitro urea K_OA when Q_D was increased from 500 to 800 mL/min at a constant Q_B of 450 mL/min. These laboratory data have been corroborated clinically.[38,39]

Two important points about Q_D-related effects on small solute mass transfer require comment. First, for Q_D to have a significant effect on K_OA, a minimal Q_B value must be achieved. Specifically, if the blood flow rate is much less than 50% of the dialysate flow rate at baseline, an increase in the latter cannot be expected to confer much benefit.[40] Second, it is important to note that the beneficial effect of increasing Q_D on small solute mass transfer may also be due to a reduction in channeling with improved perfusion of the inner fiber bundle. Thus, the mass transfer benefit of both microcrimping and increased dialysate flow mechanisms may be due to dissipation of boundary layer effects, an increase in effective membrane surface area, or both.

CONCLUSION

The major characteristics of hollow-fiber membranes that influence solute and water removal have been discussed, along with the features determining their solute and water permeability properties. The major dialyzer properties that affect solute and fluid transfer, including those of the blood and dialysate compartments, have also been discussed. It is hoped this overview will provide clinicians with a rational approach to prescription of hemodialysis in acute kidney injury.

Key Points

1. Cellulosic and synthetic dialysis membranes have chemical and structural differences that influence dialyzer performance.
2. Both mean pore size and the distribution of pore sizes affect the diffusive properties, sieving profiles, and water permeability of dialysis membranes.
3. Solute clearance is defined as the ratio of mass removal rate to solute blood concentration.
4. Solute clearance can be expressed in the following ways: whole blood, blood water, plasma, dialysate-side, and whole body.
5. Data indicate that dialysate flow distribution is an important determinant of solute clearance.

Key References

See the companion Expert Consult website for the complete reference list.

CHAPTER 224

Flow Distribution and Cross-Filtration in Hollow-Fiber Hemodialyzers

Claudio Ronco

OBJECTIVES

This chapter will:
1. Describe the structure and design of membranes and dialyzers utilized for extracorporeal therapies.
2. Explore the nature of the mechanisms involved in membrane separation processes inside hemodialyzers.
3. Characterize the fluid mechanics inside hollow-fiber hemodialyzers in respect to blood and dialysate flow distribution and cross-filtration.

Since the beginning of dialytic therapy, diffusion and convection have been combined in an attempt to replace renal function.[1] The knowledge of diffusion came from industrial chemistry, and dialyzers were designed to be ideal countercurrent exchangers. Only later was convection used in clinical practice, showing its potential advantages. Although ultrafiltration was employed first to treat over-hydrated patients, convective solute removal was subsequently used to enhance solute removal. Blood flow greatly affects the clearance of small solutes like urea, whereas ultrafiltration rate primarily affects the removal of larger solutes like inulin. Rises in dialysate flow rate become important only with large–surface area dialyzers and mostly affect the clearance of small solutes. In addition to all of these aspects of dialysate, type of membrane utilized and the hydraulic conditions within the hemodialyzer must also be considered.

DIFFUSION AND CONVECTION

Diffusion is a process in which molecules randomly move in all directions. Statistically this movement results in a passage of solutes from a more concentrated area to a less concentrated one. In addition to the concentration gradient (dc), the solute diffusive flux (Jd) through a semipermeable membrane depends on the temperature (T), the surface area (A), and the diffusivity (D) of the solute and is inversely proportional to the membrane thickness (dx), as shown by the following equation:

$$Jd = D \times A \times T \left(\frac{dc}{dx}\right)^{1}$$

The convective process requires a fluid movement caused by a transmembrane pressure gradient. Therefore, the convective flux of a solute (Jc) will depend on the ultrafiltration rate (Q_F), the solute concentration in plasma water (C_B), and the solute sieving coefficient (S), as shown in the following equation:

$$Jc = Q_F \times C_B \times S^2$$

in ideal conditions, that is, $S = 1 - \sigma$, where σ is the reflection coefficient of the membrane. These definitions present convection and diffusion as two separate phenomena. However, it is impossible to precisely define the contribution of the individual process in the removal of solutes because of their continuous interactions.

MEMBRANE STRUCTURE AND INTERACTION WITH SOLUTES

Membranes used in dialysis are of natural or synthetic origin. A simple but comprehensive summary of existing membranes is shown in Table 224-1. Different membranes have been generated from numerous basic materials and have subsequently utilized in extracorporeal therapy over the years. Membranes can be characterized on the basis of several aspects, as shown in Table 224-2.

Membranes derived from natural polymers such as cellulose are considerably hydrophilic, with wall thicknesses ranging from 5 to 15 μm (Fig. 224-1). These membranes offer remarkable diffusive performances with limited

solute sieving properties. When wet, such a membrane becomes a hydrogel and often increases in thickness by 20% or more. Original synthetic high-flux membranes had an internal skin layer surrounded by a microporous structure with a total thickness up to 100 μm. The polymer was hydrophobic, and its efficiency in diffusion was poor. Mixed hydrophilic-hydrophobic synthetic membranes with reduced wall thickness and high sieving capacity have been developed, permitting the combination of diffusion and convection, as in high-flux dialysis or hemodiafiltration.

As solute molecular weight increases, the diffusivity coefficient tends to decrease. Thus, the characteristics of the solute are extremely important, and diffusion of solutes in the range of 5000 to 20000 Da may be poor even in the presence of a very permeable membrane. In this case, transport is limited mainly by the low diffusivity of the molecule rather than the sieving characteristics of the membrane. In addition to the hydrophobic nature of the membrane, the membrane wall thickness and a considerable amount of unstirred fluid inside the support structure slow down solute transport remarkably. The structure of the newer synthetic high-flux membranes partially avoids the problems just described, combining a

TABLE 224-1

Membranes for Renal Replacement Therapy

CHEMICAL COMPOSITION	NATURAL	SYNTHETIC
Structure	Homogeneous	Asymmetrical
Porosity	Hydrogel	Microporous
Interaction with water	Hydrophilic	Hydrophobic
Thickness	Small	Large
Biocompatibility	Low	High
Electrical charges	Mixed	Negative
Hydraulic permeability	Low-flux	High-flux

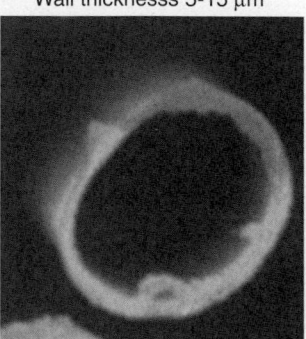
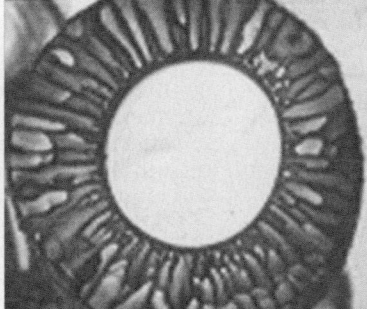
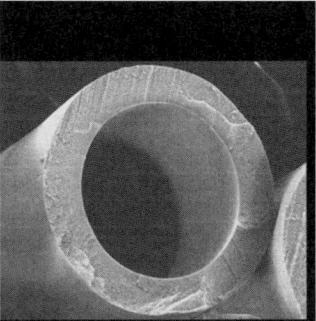

Wall thicknesss 5-15 μm

Wall thicknesss 75-100 μm

Wall thicknesss 30 μm

Natural polymer
Hydrophilic (hydrogel)
Low hydraulic permeability
Dm/Dw = 0.3
Prevalent use in diffusion

Synthetic polymer (asymmetrical)
Hydrophobic
High hydraulic permeability
Dm/Dw = 0.6
Exclusive use in convection

Synthetic copolymer (micropore)
Hydrophobic-hydrophilic
High hydraulic permeability
Dm/Dw = 0.6
Combined use diffusion-convection

FIGURE 224-1. Dialysis membranes can be characterized according to different parameters. Among them are composition (natural or synthetic) and permeability (high-flux and low-flux). The ratio between diffusivity in membrane and diffusivity in water (Dm/Dw) also describes the capacity of the membrane to perform in diffusive treatments. The last parameter is the thickness of the membrane, which may interfere with the process of diffusion. Low-flux membranes are mostly utilized in hemodialysis, in which the prevalent solute transport mechanism is diffusion. High-flux membranes are utilized in hemofiltration, in which the mechanism is convection, and hemodiafiltration, in which the mechanism is mixed diffusion and convection.

TABLE 224-2

Membranes for Renal Replacement Therapy

Cellulosic Membranes	
Classic	Cuprophan (AKZO NV, Arnhem, The Netherlands)
	RC (Asahi Kasei Medical, Tokyo)
	RC (Teijin, Tokyo, Japan)
	RC (Terumo Corp., Japan)
	SCE (Teijin; Althin Medical AB, Ronneby, Sweden)
Modified	Diaphan CA 2.5 (AKZO)
	CA (Toyobo Co., Ltd, Osaka, Japan; Althin)
	CTA (Toyobo; Althin)
Synthetically modified	Hemophan (AKZO)
	SMC (AKZO)
	Polyethylene glycol (Asahi)
	PAN-RC (Asahi)
	Excebrane (Terumo)
Synthetic Membranes	
Hydrophilic (native)	EVAL C (Kuraray Co., Ltd, Tokyo)
	EVAL D (Kuraray)
Hydrophilic (modified mixture)	PA (Gambro AB, Stockholm)
	PSF (Toray Industries, Inc., New York)
	PSF (Minntech Corporation, Minneapolis, MN)
	Polyester polymer alloy (PEPA) (Nikkiso Company, Ltd., Tokyo)
	DIAPES (Membrana GmbH, Wuppertal, Germany)
Hydrophilic/hydrophobic	PC (Gambro)
	Helixone (PSF) (Fresenius Medical Care AG & Co. KGaA, Bad Homburg, Germany)
	PUREMA (Membrana)
	PAN-DX (Asahi)
	PAN (AN69) (Hospal Zaventem, Belgium)
	PMMA (Toray)

AN69, polyacrylonitrile–sodium methallylsulfonate; PAN, polyacrylonitryl; PC, polycarbonate; PMMA, polymethyl methacrylate; PSF, polysulfone; RC, regenerated cellulose; SCE, saponificaton of cellulose acetate; SMC, synthetically modified cellulose.

relatively less hydrophobic nature with a thinner wall and a more homogeneous structure.

Solute diffusivity also plays an important role in blood and dialysate. The resistance (R) generated by blood (R_B), dialysis fluid (R_D), and membrane (R_M) can be reported as percentages of the overall resistance (R_O) to solute transport, as follows:

$$R_O = R_B + R_M + R_D$$

At the cutoff value, the resistance of the membrane represents 100% of the total resistance. This resistance progressively decreases for smaller solutes, and the resistances in the blood and dialysate compartments become increasingly important.

The resistance to the transport of larger solutes, which is due to their poor diffusion coefficients, can be overcome by the use of convection. The convective flux is influenced by the permeability of the membrane, which is characterized by the observed sieving coefficient curve. The *sieving coefficient* is the ratio between the solute concentration in the filtrate and the solute concentration in plasma water, in the absence of a gradient for diffusion. However, solute distribution in the blood compartment is not homogeneous, because it is influenced by polarization and other phenomena. As ultrafiltration increases, part of the solute tends to accumulate at the blood-membrane interface, thus creating gradients for diffusion both toward the bulk region inside the hollow fiber and toward the dialysate compartment across the membrane. As a consequence, diffusion is continuously interfering with convection, and the sieving coefficient can be overestimated. In fact, the concentration in the bulk region (which is the value measured empirically) is generally lower than that at the blood-membrane

interface. Therefore, the difference between the observed sieving coefficient (S_O) and the true sieving coefficient (S_T) can be significantly affected by the amount of convection used. With low ultrafiltration values, S_O and S_T tend to be equal, but large differences can be observed at high ultrafiltration rates.[2]

HEMODIALYZER DESIGN

Hemodialyzers have been designed over the years to be ideal solute exchangers and excellent hydraulic units for filtration. In fact, the process of diffusion is optimized by a countercurrent configuration of blood and dialysate flow that ensures the maximal gradient for diffusion in any single point along the length of the filter. Since the beginning of dialysis, dialyzer design has featured a three-compartment structure consisting of a blood compartment, a semipermeable membrane, and a dialysate compartment. Blood brought to the dialyzer through a tube (blood line) is distributed inside the blood compartment by a blood port. Blood ports with conic or spiral distributors have been designed to obtain an even distribution of the flow in all available spaces of the blood compartment. Both plate and hollow-fiber devices have been developed in an attempt to obtain the best configuration for ideal countercurrent solute exchange (Fig. 224-2). Plate devices had lower resistance, but the volume of the blood compartment varied according to the pressures applied and was often too high. Hollow-fiber dialyzers overcome many of the limitations imposed by plate devices and offer the best compromise between blood volume and surface area

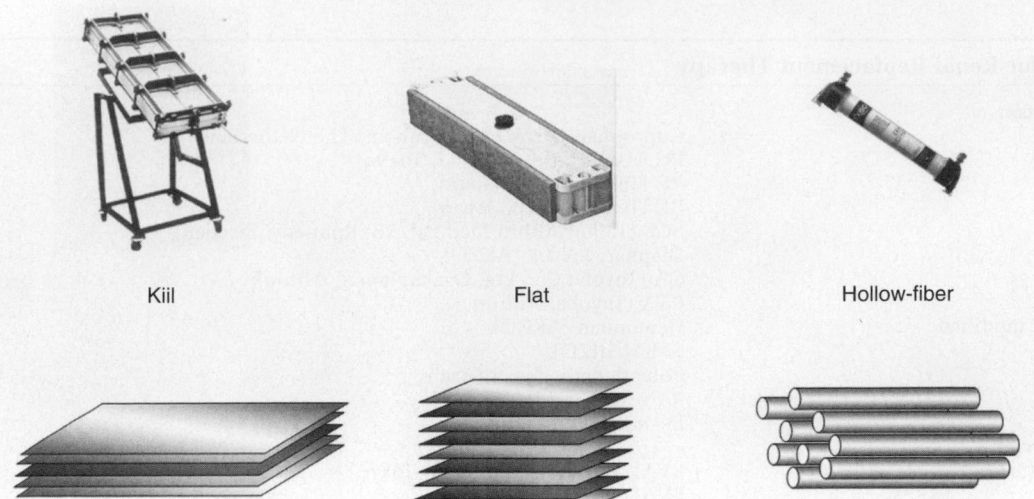

FIGURE 224-2. The evolution of hemodialyzers. Hemodialyzers can have a plate configuration or hollow-fiber configuration. In either case, the unit consists of three main components: the blood compartment, the membrane, and the dialysate compartment.

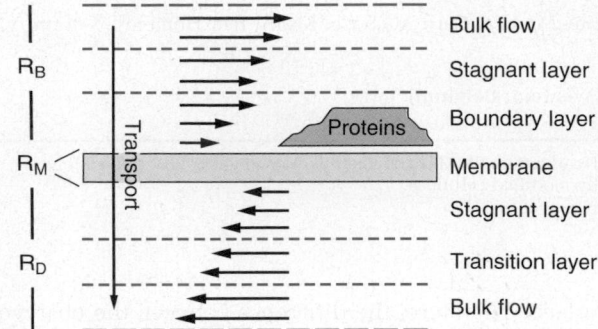

FIGURE 224-3. The resistance to transport consists of the blood compartment with blood stagnation layers and concentrated proteins at the blood membrane interface, the membrane, and the dialysate compartment with unstirred layers and bulk flow.

exposed for exchanges. One deficiency of the hollow-fiber design however is that the resistance is higher than in plate devices, and the mechanics of fluid inside the filter becomes more complex. Finally, the dialysate compartment is generally designed to provide an easy flow of dialysate with minimal trapping of bubbles and reduced stagnation or channeling of dialysis fluid. To obtain these results, specific dialysate inlet ports have been created; furthermore, to uniformly distribute the flow among the fibers, spacer yarns and fiber waving have been developed in an attempt to optimize the countercurrent configuration.

The Blood Compartment of the Hemodialyzer

With all dialyzer membranes to some extent, but particularly with synthetic membranes, a protein layer is deposited on the internal surface of the fiber. This layer slightly reduces the membrane sieving coefficient with a rather constant trend. However, in case of high ultrafiltration rates or high filtration fractions, a thick protein deposit on the membrane is induced by the additional phenomenon of polarization (Fig. 224-3). This factor progressively

reduces the membrane permeability, and S_O becomes proportional to a new reflection coefficient ($\sigma 1$) of the membrane. This layer is a function of several variables, above all the value of "shear rate" at the wall. As the blood enters the hollow fiber, the shear stress generates different layers of blood from the bulk phase to the membrane interface, all of which flow at different velocities. The ratio between the differential velocity of the fluid threads in the fiber and the differential distances from the center of the fiber (shear rate, expressed in sec^{-1}) is a function of blood viscosity and shear stress. The shear rate is also proportional to the blood flow per single fiber. The thickness of the protein layer at the blood-membrane interface depends on the wall shear rate value and is extremely important for membrane performance. The shear rate value correlates linearly with the shear stress in case of newtonian fluids, and the velocity profile is regularly parabolic. Blood approaches newtonian behavior only at shear rates higher than 200 sec^{-1}.[3] Thus, blood flow distributors are used at the filter entrance (conic or spiral ports) to prevent uneven distribution of blood flow. Nevertheless, velocity of blood flow is often lower in the peripheral regions of the bundle (Fig. 224-4).

Ultrafiltration and solute sieving coefficients are considerably influenced by the wall shear rate because it contributes to keeping the polarization layer very thin. This is particularly important for solutes in the middle to high range. Diffusion is also affected by the value of shear rate, because high shear rates help keep the diffusion distance from blood to dialysate at a minimum. The reason is that concentration polarization and the secondary layer of proteins lead to the formation of a pseudo-membrane, the thickness of which is added to that of the original membrane. In clinical practice, high wall shear rates are obtained with high blood flows and appropriate device geometry, with relative preservation of ultrafiltration rates and solute clearances. In studies carried out with dye injection in the blood compartment of different hollow-fiber dialyzers, Ronco and associates[4] could demonstrate that in peripheral fibers, blood flows and shear rates are much lower than those observed in the central fibers of the bundle. This difference is even more evident when hematocrit rises above 35%. On the basis of all the issues just discussed, one could speculate that blood flows higher

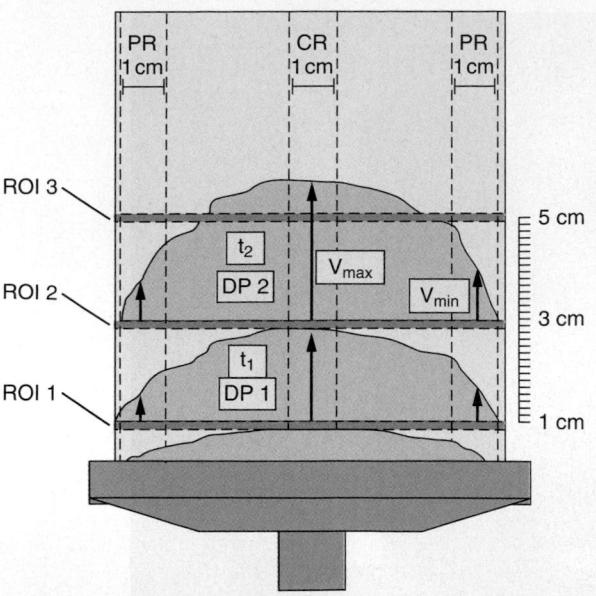

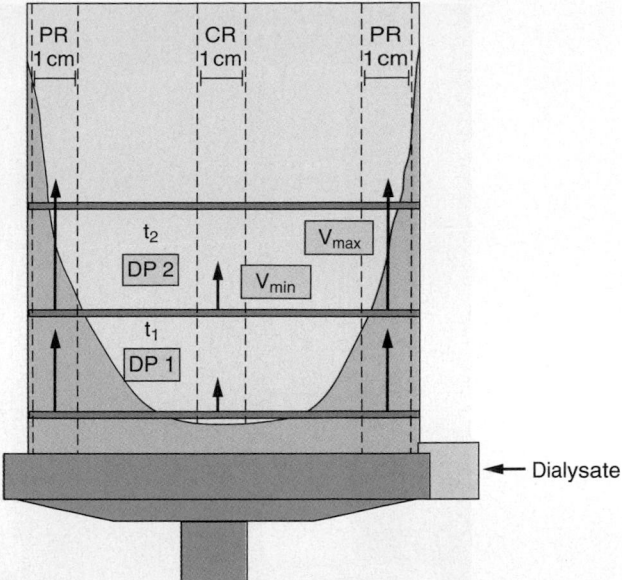

FIGURE 224-4. When blood enters the hemodialyzer, its velocity (V_{max}) in the central region of the fiber bundle (CR) may be higher than that (V_{min}) in the peripheral region (PR). This uneven velocity distribution may result in dialyzer malfunction and inadequate performance. The internal diameter of the case for this dialyzer is 33 mm. DP, density profile; ROI, region of interest; t_1, t_2, subsequent times of analysis. The average flow velocity (V) can be calculated as follows:

$$V = \frac{4Q_B}{(\pi d^2 n)}$$

where Q_B is blood flow, d is inner fiber diameter, and n is number of fibers. Wall shear (wSh) can be calculated as follows:

$$wSh = \frac{4Q_B}{\pi r^2} = \frac{4V\pi r^2}{\pi r^3} = \frac{4V}{\pi r}$$

where V is flow velocity in the fiber and r is inner radius of the fiber.

than 350 to 400 mL/min must always be utilized in the presence of a 1.8 to 2.0 m^2 dialyzer in order for the performance of all the fibers to be optimal. On the other hand, new blood port designs and new bundle configurations have shown an excellent flow distribution in the blood compartment at various blood flow and hematocrit values.[5]

The Dialysate Compartment of the Hemodialyzer

Several attempts have been made to optimize the blood compartment, by creating adequate blood ports and flow distributors at the inlet of the dialyzer, but very little attention has been paid to the dialysate compartment. The dialysate distribution may, in fact, be asymmetrical inside the dialyzer, presenting nonhomogeneous distribution within the fiber's bundle and the consequent phenomenon of channeling. This process may prevent optimal performance of the dialyzer and may affect the efficacy of treatment (Fig. 224-5).

Some investigators have attempted to avoid dialysate channeling through new filter design. For example, longer

FIGURE 224-5. As with blood (see Fig. 224-4), when dialysate enters the hemodialyzer, its velocity (V_{min}) in the central fibers (CR) may be lower than that (V_{max}) in the peripheral fibers (PR). This uneven velocity distribution may result in dialyzer malfunction and inadequate performance. DP, density profile; t_1, t_2, subsequent times of analysis.

fibers reduce contact because of their uneven configuration or surface. An external irregular surface avoids perfect contact of adjacent fibers. Different systems of nonparallel orientation of the fibers or the use of tissue structures within the bundle may further ensure adequate distances between adjacent fibers. The latest approach is the use of spacing filaments ("spacer yarns") between the fibers or the creation of uneven fiber surface (moiré structure). Ronco and colleagues[5] carried out a complex evaluation of the newer fibers using helical computed tomography to achieve detailed imaging of the dialysate distribution pattern after dye injection. The modified dialysate compartments with the spacing filaments (spacer yarns) between the fibers and the moiré structure displayed more homogeneous distributions of the dye than standard dialyzers, in which a typical channeling effect was displayed in the peripheral regions (Fig. 224-6).[5]

Interference between Diffusion and Convection

Although convection and diffusion are described as two separate phenomena, their single contributions cannot be distinguished in practice. Moreover, especially in treatments that involve the combined utilization of diffusion and convection, there is a continuous interference between the two transport mechanisms.[9] In such circumstances, enhancement of one type of transport can produce effects on the other, which may be beneficial or detrimental.

In hemodiafiltration, solutes are carried across the membrane at the same concentration as in plasma water because of high ultrafiltration rate. This phenomenon takes place principally in the proximal side of the filter and reduces the driving force for diffusion. In this case, convection negatively affects diffusion, a fact that becomes more

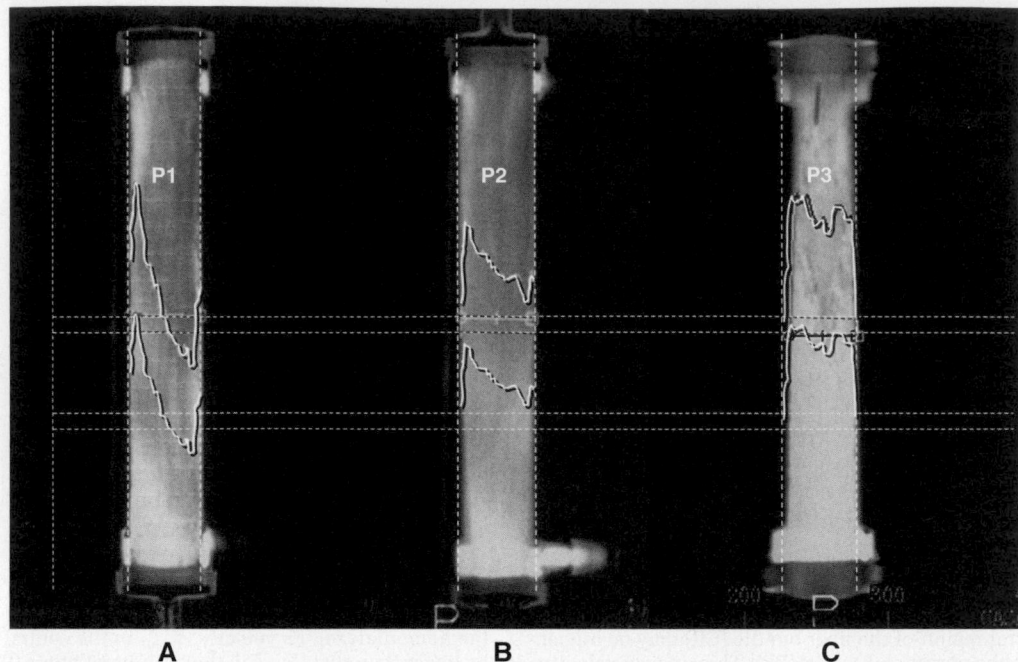

FIGURE 224-6. Distribution of dialysate in three different hemodialyzer configurations: **A,** standard fibers; **B,** fibers with spacer yarns; **C,** hollow fibers with moiré structure, which corresponds to microcrimping. It is evident that the most homogeneous distribution is obtained with the micro-undulation design of the hollow fibers (**C**).

important on the distal side of the filter, where the ultrafiltration rate approaches zero. This effect emphasizes the importance of the surface area for diffusive performance in hemodiafiltration. However, the back-diffusion of substances such as buffers from dialysate into the blood may also be negatively affected, at least in the proximal side of the filter, where ultrafiltration is higher. In high-flux dialysis, a typical filtration-backfiltration profile occurs.[6] The minimal interference between convection and diffusion is achieved in the central part of the dialyzer, at which the water flux in both directions is near zero. In the region near the blood ports, convection may interfere with diffusion in both the filtration and backfiltration modes.

Internal Filtration and Backfiltration

Hemodiafiltration enhances middle molecule clearances, but the need to replace the ultrafiltrate with sterile solutions makes this modality complex and costly. Volumetrically controlled hemodialysis with high-flux membranes (high-flux dialysis) also achieves better middle molecule clearances than standard hemodialysis, and without the need for substitution fluid. In this latter modality, however, the convective removal of middle molecules is limited by the rate of internal filtration.

Internal filtration is governed by the hydraulic and oncotic forces acting along the length of the dialyzer on each side of the membrane. As each point of the dialyzer, the local pressure differential is termed *transmembrane pressure* (TMP). When the TMP is positive, the water flux is from the blood compartment to the dialysate compartment. When the TMP is negative, backfiltration occurs (Fig. 224-7). Thus, removal of middle molecules can be enhanced by raising the positive-pressure differential in the proximal part of the dialyzer, thus increasing internal filtration. Adequate net filtration is maintained by the

ultrafiltration control system through a parallel increase in the negative-pressure differential in the distal part of the dialyzer. This results in greater proximal filtration and distal backfiltration without affecting the "net" filtration rate.

When high rates of backfiltration are utilized, high-quality dialysate is needed to prevent side effects related to pyrogen transfer into the patient's circulation. For this treatment, use of the latest-generation hemodialysis machines is strongly suggested. New machines are equipped with a built-in pyrogen filter to prepare ultrapure dialysate. The re-infusion via backfiltration provides extra safety because the fluid is filtered again across the hemodialysis membrane before it reaches the blood compartment.

Several possible ways to increase the rate of internal filtration have been investigated, including modifications of the geometry of the dialyzer and the application of an O-ring in the middle portion of the hemodialyzer.[7,8] The most practical modification has been shown to be a reduction of the inner diameter of the hollow fiber. This is an interesting way to increase the positive-pressure differential across the membrane in the proximal and distal regions of the hemodialyzer without introducing major changes in dialyzer design. One study has found this approach to result in a definite increase of internal filtration.[9]

The difference in pressure drop between the two filters is significant, as it is predicted by the Hagen-Poiseuille equation, as follows:

$$\Delta P = Q_B \times \frac{8\eta L}{\pi r^4}$$

where ΔP is the end-to-end pressure drop, Q_B is blood flow, η is blood viscosity, L is the length of the fiber, and r is the internal radius of the fiber. Since the pressure drop in a fiber correlates with r^4, it seems logical to attempt solu-

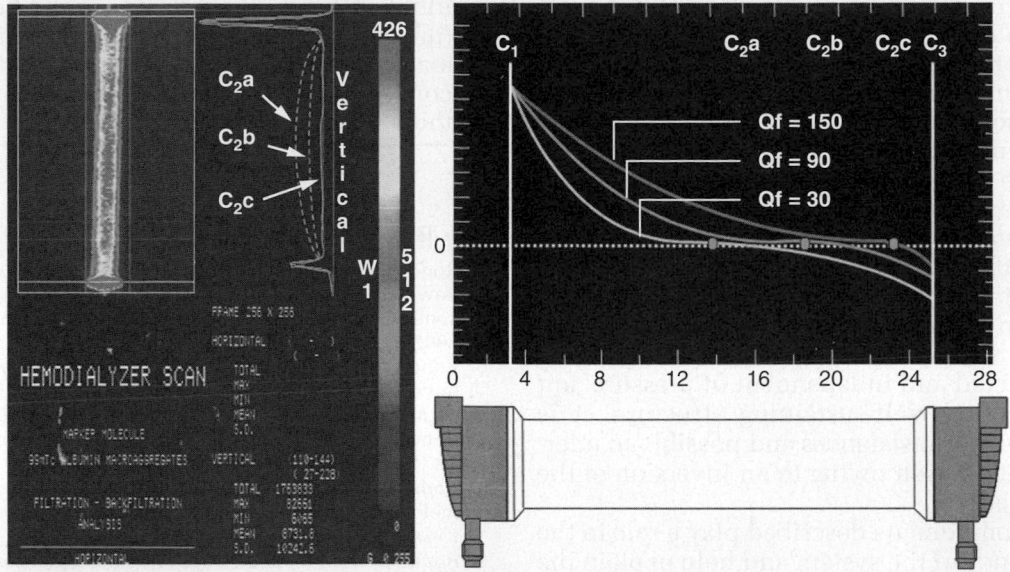

FIGURE 224-7. See also color plates. *Left,* Images of a dialyzer filter analyzed with the gamma camera after injection of a specific marker molecule in blood. The increased concentration of the labeled nondiffusible marker molecule in the central portion of the hemodialyzer can be visually captured from the change in color. The curve of the radioactive count is displayed on the right side of the filter image. The peak changes in concentration C_2a, C_2b, C_2c differ according to the net filtration rates. The lower the filtration rate is, the higher the peak concentration change and the higher the internal filtration-backfiltration (*right*). The different lines describe the local cross-filtration along the length of the fiber bundle. In the proximal portion (*left*), the cross-filtration is positive, and in the distal portion (*right*) the cross-filtration is negative (backfiltration).

tions that involve modifications of the fiber geometry. In this case, even small changes in the inner diameter of the fiber may cause dramatic changes in its performance. With net filtration rates near zero, the increases in filtration and backfiltration can be doubled with specific dialyzer and fiber designs.

One may speculate that reduction of the inner diameter of the hollow fiber will also result in an increase in the average blood flow velocity per fiber and a consequent rise in wall shear rates. This additional factor may in fact result in a "cleaning" effect at the blood-membrane interface. In fact, higher shear rates lead to a reduction in the thickness of the protein boundary layer and improve membrane permeability, counterbalancing the concentration polarization phenomenon. So reducing the inner diameter will certainly help obtain not only better performance of the membrane in terms of filtration rates at a given local transmembrane pressure gradient but also optimal utilization of the sieving capacities of the membrane.

In vivo analysis of middle molecule removal has demonstrated the benefits of increased internal filtration resulting from the change in hollow fiber geometry. Although urea, creatinine, and phosphorus clearances were not changed as expected from their high diffusion coefficients (poorly affected by changes in convection), clearances of vitamin B_{12} and inulin were improved by more than 30% by use of the modified dialyzers.

Therefore, modifications in the design of hollow fibers may lead to new and interesting improvements in hemodialyzer performances. Newly conceived dialyzers may therefore appear in the future with enhanced convective transport, leading to simplified hemodiafiltration techniques that do not require replacement solutions, but simply utilize internal filtration as a major way to improve convective transport.

CONCLUSION

Hemodialyzers are designed to optimize both diffusion and convection processes. The blood and dialysate compartments are optimized to maintain the best concentration gradient for diffusion, whereas convection and internal filtration depend mostly on operational conditons. Once these aspects are well known, the optimal unit can be chosen to achieve the desired results with the treatment.

Key Points

1. Dialysis membranes can be characterized according to different parameters. Among them are composition (natural or synthetic) and permeability (high flux and low flux). The ratio of diffusivity in membrane to diffusivity in water (Dm/Dw) also describes the capacity of the membrane to perform in diffusive treatments. The last parameter is the thickness of the membrane that may interfere with the process of diffusion.
2. Low-flux membranes are mostly utilized in hemodialysis, in which the prevalent solute transport mechanism is diffusion. High-flux membranes are utilized in hemofiltration (prevalent mechanism, convection) and hemodiafiltration (prevalent mechanism, mixed diffusion and convection).
3. Hemodialyzers can have a plate or hollow-fiber configuration. In either case, the unit consists of three main components, the blood compartment, the membrane, and the dialysate compartment.

4. Blood flow is of paramount importance in providing fresh blood for diffusion and convection in the dialyzer. Special blood ports are created to achieve a uniform distribution of the flow inside the blood compartment and to obtain full utilization of the membrane surface.
5. The surface of the membrane is important but it can achieve maximal efficiency only when blood and dialysate flows are adequate. In the flat hemodialyzers, the blood compartment is subject to lower resistance but its thickness may increase in response to high positive transmembrane pressures. In hollow-fiber dialyzers, the priming volume is fixed and independent of pressure, but because of such self-sustaining structure, it is subject to higher resistances and possibly to internal reverse filtration owing to an inversion of the pressure gradient.
6. All of the components described play a role in the final efficiency of the system and help explain the mechanisms operating in different techniques, such as hemodialysis (prevalently diffusion-based with low-flux membranes), high-flux dialysis (mixed diffusion and convection with internal filtration and backfiltration), hemodiafiltration (mixed diffusion and convection with reinfusion external to the filter), and hemofiltration (pure convective therapy with re-infusion external to the filter).

Key References

5. Ronco C, Brendolan A, Crepaldi C, et al: Blood and dialysate flow distributions in hollow-fiber hemodialyzers analyzed by computerized helical scanning technique. J Am Soc Nephrol 2002;13:S53-S61.
6. Ronco C, Brendolan A, Crepaldi C, et al: Dialysate flow distribution in hollow fiber hemodialyzers with different dialysate pathway configuration. Int J Artif Organs 2000;9:601-609.
7. Ronco C: Backfiltration: A controversial issue in modern dialysis. Int J Artif Organs 1988;11:69-74.
8. Ronco C, Brendolan A, Feriani M, et al: A new scintigraphic method to characterize ultrafiltration in hollow fiber dialyzers. Kidney Int 1992;41:1383-1393.
9. Ronco C, Brendolan A, Lupi A, et al: Enhancement of convective transport by internal filtration in a modified experimental hemodialyzer. Kidney Int 1998;54:979-985.

See the companion Expert Consult website for the complete reference list.

CHAPTER 225

Biocompatibility of the Dialysis System

Nicholas A. Hoenich

OBJECTIVES

This chapter will:
1. Present the fundamentals of biocompatibility of membranes used along with other factors contributing to the biocompatibility of dialysis.
2. Discuss the findings of meta-analyses concerned with the effect of biocompatibility on treatment outcomes.

The treatment of acute renal failure (ARF) encompasses a variety of different treatment modalities, including intermittent hemodialysis, continuous therapies relying on convective removal of fluid and solutes, and hybrid therapies involving both convective and diffusive solute transport. All such treatments use a membrane separation device. The passage of blood through this device as well as through the extracorporeal circuit exposes the patient's blood to nonphysiological surfaces, the largest of which is the membrane.

For years, the dialysis membrane was considered inert; however, this assumption is no longer appropriate, owing to the recognition that blood-membrane contact activates a variety of pathways with clinical sequelae (Fig. 225-1).

A *biocompatible membrane* may be defined as one in which there is minimal interaction between material and blood. This definition is subject to shortcomings, however, because there is no standard technique available for the measurement of biocompatibility. Furthermore, because of a membrane's chemical composition and surface, universal biocompatibility is not feasible; the absence of response in one pathway (e.g., complement activation) does not translate into the absence of response in other pathways. In extracorporeal treatments, biocompatibility is governed not only by the membrane—which as the largest contact surface has received extensive study—but also by other elements, such as the tubing sets and fluids used. This chapter discusses the concepts of biocompatibility as applied to the dialysis system together with its relevance in treatment and in outcome of ARF.

MEMBRANES

The membranes used for solute transport in devices forming part of the extracorporeal circuit may be classified according to their chemical structure, with further subclassifications based on hydraulic permeability or ultrafiltra-

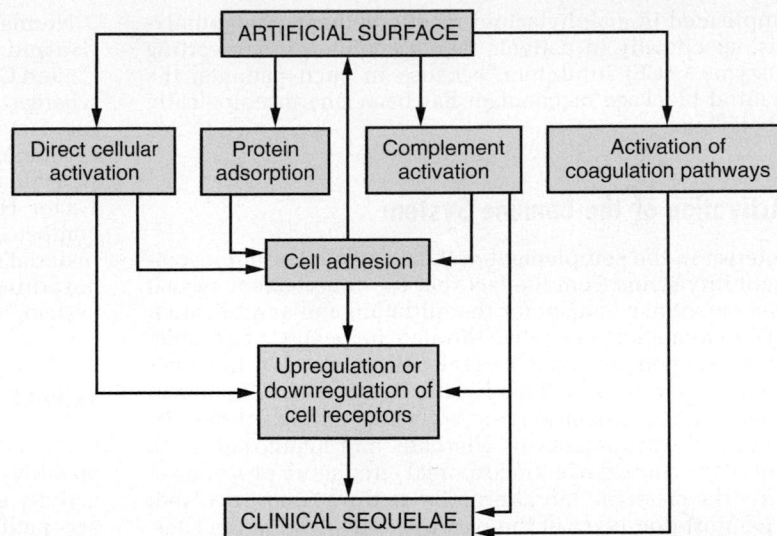

FIGURE 225-1. The activation of multiple physiological pathways within blood after contact with a foreign material such as a dialysis membrane.

tion characteristics. Broadly, on the basis of chemical structure, three categories of membrane are currently produced: those based on unmodified cellulose, those based on cellulose in which the chemical structure or composition has been altered, and those based on synthetic polymers (see Fig. 212-4 in Chapter 212). All currently used membranes exhibit reactivity when blood comes into contact with them. Despite considerable uncertainty about the effect of such reactivity on treatment outcomes, there has been a considerable shift toward use of the more biocompatible synthetic membranes in the treatment of end-stage renal disease.[1]

Basic Mechanisms of Blood Membrane Interactions
Protein Adsorption

Contact of blood with a foreign surface leads to the rapid adsorption of proteins onto the surface. The sequence of protein adsorption is governed by the physical interaction between the protein and the material surface, with flow rate, the surface character of the protein, material surface roughness, and chemical composition of the material playing key roles.[2] Adsorption is hierarchical and called the *Vroman effect*.[3] Sequentially albumin, immunoglobulins, fibrinogen, fibronectin, high-molecular-weight kininogen, and factor XII are involved. Once the proteins are adsorbed onto the surface, they undergo conformational changes owing to their relatively low structural stability and their tendency to unfold, permitting further bond formation. The adsorbed protein layer can confer a degree of bioreactivity to the material surface but may also modulate solute and fluid transport across the membrane.

The presence of proteins on the surfaces of materials induces platelet adhesion, followed by the movement of glycoproteins (β-thromboglobulin, serotonin, platelet factor-4, adenosine diphosphate [ADP], thromboxane B_2, and thrombospondin) from internal storage to the surface as well as an increase in the number of platelet surface markers. There is an interaction between the platelets on the material surface and the intrinsic coagulation pathway, arising from procoagulants liberated from platelets and

from factor XII activation stimulated by ADP release; this interaction leads to the formation of thrombin, the production of fibrin on the surface further promoting platelet aggregation and adhesion.[4,5]

Coagulation System

The human coagulation system consists of two pathways, intrinsic and extrinsic. The pathways differ from each other with respect to the initiating stimulus and the subsequent chain of events that occur until the activation of factor X, which activates prothrombin. Thereafter, the two pathways follow the same course (the common pathway), which culminates in the formation of thrombus.

Thrombus formation after contact of blood with material involves platelet activation, fibrin formation, and the activation of the extrinsic and intrinsic coagulation systems. The extrinsic coagulation pathway is considered the major initiator of the coagulation cascade when blood comes in contact with biomaterial surfaces—more specifically, with surfaces that are negatively charged. Activation of the extrinsic pathway occurs contact phase activation (through factor XII). This activation is governed by the material's surface, and surface-related factors, in particular a negative surface charge that induces a conformational change in factor XII or Hageman factor.

Heparin does not block thrombin formation, but merely blunts activation of the coagulation cascade. Furthermore, the amount of thrombin produced is influenced by both patient-related, such as age and comorbid disease, and material-related factors, including surface area, duration of exposure to the surface, turbulence, stagnation, and, to a lesser extent, temperature.

As discussed previously, negatively charged surfaces adsorb positively charged factor XII onto the surface. The adsorbed factor XII undergoes a conformational change, resulting in self-activation to factor XIIa, which in turn transforms pre-kallikrein into kallikrein on the surfaces of biomaterials. The major function of kallikrein is to amplify the activation of coagulation and the fibrinolytic systems. It also cleaves high-molecular-weight kinin to produce bradykinin, a potent inflammatory mediator that causes vasodilation. Such bradykinin production has been implicated in anaphylactoid reactions during hemodialysis, specifically in patients taking angiotensin-converting enzyme (ACE) inhibitors, because in such patients, the natural blockage mechanism has been pharmacologically abolished.[6]

Activation of the Immune System

Interest in the complement system as a marker of biocompatibility stems from the fact that the complement system is a potent mechanism for the initiation and amplification of inflammation mediated through fragments of complement components capable of releasing histamine and other mediators from cells (anaphylatoxin activity). The human complement system may be activated through three distinct pathways (classical, alternate, and mannose-lectin), but in the context of extracorporeal circulatory procedures, only the classical and alternative pathways are involved. The most dominant of the pathways involved is the alternative pathway, although contact between heparinized blood and the synthetic surfaces of the extracorporeal circuit also results in the activation of contact plasma proteins and, thus, the classical complement pathway.

Complement activation is rapid and peaks within the first 15 to 30 minutes of treatment. Thereafter it gradually returns to pretreatment levels owing to adsorption of complement fractions by cellular receptors as well as their deposition onto the membrane surface.

Within the classical pathway, activation of C1, possibly by activated factor XIIa, sequentially activates C2 and C4 to form C4b2a (classical C3 convertase), which cleaves C3 to form C3a and C3b. The generation of C3b activates the alternative pathway, involving factors B and D in the formation of C3bBb, the alternative pathway C3 convertase that cleaves C3 to form C3a and C3b. Although the classical pathway proceeds in sequential steps, the alternative pathway contains a feedback loop that greatly amplifies cleavage of C3 by membrane-bound C3 convertase to membrane-bound C3b and C3a. This activation is a consequence of the fact that artificial membranes do not have the protective proteins on their surfaces that normally control complement activation. The two C3 convertases effectively merge and are involved in the production of C3b, which cleaves C5 to C5a and C5b. C3a and C5a are potent vasoactive anaphylatoxins contributing to greater pulmonary vascular resistance, edema, neutrophil sequestration, and an increase in extravascular water associated with extracorporeal circulatory procedures. Of the two anaphylatoxins, C3a is the principal circulating compound, as C5a binds to neutrophils and is difficult to detect in plasma. C3b acts as an opsonin, which binds target cell hydroxyl groups and renders them susceptible to phagocytic cells expressing specific receptors for C3b. The production of C5b secondary to the cleavage of C5 ultimately leads to formation of the membrane attack complex (MAC, or C5b-9), which causes cellular death by intracellular swelling after loss of the intracellular-interstitial osmotic gradient.

Together, C5a and C5b-9 play major roles in promoting neutrophil-endothelial cell interactions through upregulation of specific adhesion molecules. Importantly, C5b-9 may also activate platelets and promote platelet-monocyte aggregates.

These complement proteins also contribute to neutrophil loss from the circulation through adhesion to surface-bound platelets and, more importantly, to endothelial cells and have been implicated in causing organ damage after cardiopulmonary bypass procedures.[7,8]

Normally, regulatory proteins modulate the actions of C5a and C5b-9 by inactivating convertases, which cleave C3 and C5. Two such proteins, factors H and I, are soluble, whereas complement receptor 1 (CD35), decay-accelerating factor, and membrane cofactor protein (CD46) are membrane bound. Factor I cleaves C3 into inactive iC3b, which cannot form C3 convertase but can be an opsonin. Factor H, the dominant complement regulatory protein, competes with factor B in binding to C3. Adsorption to the material's surface by these control proteins is pivotal in governing the material's ability to activate the complement system.[9]

Cellular Effects of Complement Activation

Cells have complement receptors on their surfaces, enabling the complement system to influence their activity either directly or indirectly.[10] The cells involved are neutrophils, monocytes, platelets, and endothelial cells.

Neutrophils are strongly activated after exposure to chemoattractants, but their activation varies considerably among individuals. The presence of diabetes, oxidative stress, and, perhaps genetic factors, influences neutrophil activation. The principal agonists are kallikrein and C5a. One of the recognized effects of such upregulation is the increased adhesion and margination of neutrophils in the lung vasculature, which leads to neutropenia during the initial phase of treatment. This neutropenia, which is rapid, occurring within the first few minutes of dialysis and reaching its nadir by 15 minutes, leads to clinically measurable hypoxemia during dialysis. After the initial neutrophil activation, there is a gradual return to predialysis levels, although the downregulation of L-selectin and CD43 may result in levels exceeding those seen at the commencement of dialysis.

The mechanism by which monocytes are activated is not fully elucidated, with C5a, thrombin, platelet factor-4), and bradykinin—four potent agonists generated from blood contact with material surfaces—likely to be involved. C3a and C5a can affect monocytes directly, leading to production of interleukin-1 and priming the monocytes for production of tumor necrosis factor (TNF).

C5b-9, also known as the membrane attack complex (MAC), is a potent platelet activator contributing to both local prothrombotic events and transient bleeding due to the circulation of activated platelets. Endothelial cells are activated by C5a during extracorporeal circulatory procedures.

Membrane-Related Factors Modulating Biocompatibility

Materials used in a clinical setting undergo biocompatibility testing as part of the development process. The nature of the testing is determined by the intended body contact and the duration of that contact and is governed by U.S. Food and Drug Administration (FDA) guidance and International Organization for Standardization (ISO) 10993 standards. The characterization of membranes in terms of biocompatibility can be made on the basis of a number of different parameters. Historically, complement activation (and the associated neutropenia due to the activation of complement receptors on the cells) was widely used. Current emphasis focuses on the elucidation of the molecular mechanisms involved, with a view to minimizing reactivity.

Although the membrane within a device used for the solute transport and fluid removal is the largest contact surface within the extracorporeal circuit, it forms an integral part of the device, and there is interaction between the two. For example, the device design determines the blood flow dynamics (flow rates and potential turbulence) and the duration of blood contact, and the membrane governs the surface area for contact.

The responses elicited are governed by a variety of factors, including chemical composition and surface character. Synthetic membranes generally outperform those based on cellulose, although the distinction between modified cellulose and synthetic materials is less distinct. Both cellulose-based and synthetic membranes tend to be treated as generic groups. However, despite a similarity in the base material, membranes can behave in different ways when in contact with blood. A clear understanding of the reasons for differences between membranes manufactured from similar blends of materials such as polysulfone is lacking, but some studies suggest that the differences may be a result of variation in the extent of cross-linkage between the polymers used.[11]

Two membrane-related factors are important in determining the material's biocompatibility profile. The first is the membrane's surface, in terms of chemistry and roughness. The second is the membrane's pore size distribution, which determines the range of complement fractions that can be removed from the blood or adsorbed into the material matrix.[12-15]

Controlled chemical modification can lead to the development of predictable biocompatibility profiles, and considerable activity has been extended into understanding of the material-related factors. For example, hydrophilic domains on the material surface have a stimulatory effect on the complement activation potential of the material, but play little effect in determining the material's ability to activate platelets. On the other hand, hydrophobic domains show a reduced influence on the activation of the complement system, but stimulate platelet adhesion.[16]

THE EXTRACORPOREAL CIRCUIT

The tubing sets used in extracorporeal circuits are generally manufactured from polyvinylchloride (PVC), which affords easy construction and sterilization and contains a plasticizer to permit malleability. The most widely used plasticizer is diethylhexyl phthalate (DEHP). One of a class of agents called hypolipidemic hepatocarcinogens, DEHP migrates in small quantities into blood from the tubing; exposure to DEHP has been linked to damage to the reproductive system and to higher risks for asthma and cancer. Furthermore, the repeated action of the blood pump rolls on the tubing segment results in luminal damage and particulate release.[17,18]

In consideration of these issues, a number of regulatory agencies have evaluated the safety of this compound. An FDA Safety Assessment undertaken in 2001 reported that DEHP may not be safe for infants, children, and adults receiving certain medical treatments that involve PVC medical devices.[19] A Health Canada Expert Advisory Panel in 2002 recommended that health care providers not use DEHP-containing devices in the treatment of pregnant women, breastfeeding mothers, infants, males before puberty, or patients undergoing cardiac bypass, hemodi-

alysis, or heart transplant surgery. This report also named certain patient groups and medical procedures that require urgent action, as follows: "Alternate measures are immediately justifiable and should be introduced as quickly as possible to protect those sub-populations at greatest risk, namely, the fetus, newborns, infants and young children receiving transfusions, ECMO [extracorporeal membrane oxygenation], cardiopulmonary by-pass, exchange transfusion, hemodialysis, TPN [total parenteral nutrition] and lipophilic drug formulations."[20]

Potential approaches that have been explored to minimize such leaching or release of particles include coating the inner lumen of the tubing to improve the migration resistance and the use of an alternative plasticizer.[21-23] It is of note, however, that only certain types of coating can diminish release of DEHP into the blood,[22] and luminal coating fails to influence the complement activation (C3a) associated with exposure of blood to tubing material.[24]

Polyolefins represent a suitable alternative to the widely used PVC. They have a similar flexibility, which is achieved by the use of three dimensional molecular configurations based on hydrogen and carbon molecules. Polyolefins employed in medical devices include polyethylene, polypropylene, and their co-polymers. Of these, low-density polyethylene is used in rigid and opaque containers and tubings.

DIALYSIS FLUID

Continuous therapies tend to use sterile reinfusion fluids, but because of the volumes used in dialysis and their cost, some centers favor the use of "on-line" therapies in which the fluid for infusion is derived from the dialysis fluid. Such an approach requires that rigorous attention be paid to the microbiological quality of the fluid, because it is generally accepted that although membranes in current clinical use do not allow bacteria to pass through, endotoxins and bacterial fragments have the potential to cross such membranes.[25] Furthermore, in conventional dialysis, the quality of the dialysis fluid may be suboptimal owing to the contamination of the water distribution system and the hydraulic circuit of the dialysis machine by biofilm.[26,27]

DOES BIOCOMPATIBILITY PLAY A ROLE IN THE OUTCOMES OF ACUTE RENAL FAILURE?

The biological consequences of blood-dialyzer interactions in the setting of ARF are the subject of considerable controversy. Membranes with poor biocompatibility have the potential to worsen the catabolic state, aggravate the proinflammatory state, and predispose patients to bacterial infections.[28-30]

Deposition of leukocytes in the pulmonary vasculature may aggravate pulmonary injury, and animal studies have suggested that the use of unsubstituted cellulose membranes delays the recovery of ARF through leukocyte activation and infiltration of renal parenchyma, especially after ischemia-reperfusion injury.[31]

Several meta-analyses have reviewed the effects of biocompatibility on outcomes of ARF.[32-34] Jaber and colleagues,[32] analyzing seven studies involving a total of 722 patients, concluded that available evidence does not permit a recommendation for or against the use of biocompatible membranes in patients with ARF. Subgroup analyses, however, indicated that modified cellulose membranes (cellulose acetate) may offer a survival advantage over synthetic membranes, which in turn may be more beneficial than unmodified cellulose membranes. Subramanian and associates[33] analyzed the results of ten studies, of which eight (867 patients) provided survival data and six (641 patients) provided data on recovery of renal function. These researchers concluded that synthetic membranes appear to confer a significant survival advantage over cellulose-based membranes; however, the analysis did not demonstrate a benefit for synthetic membranes in respect to recovery of renal function. Furthermore, the researchers suggested that the survival disadvantage for cellulose-based membranes may be limited to unsubstituted cellulose membranes. A later analysis by Alonso and coworkers[34] was based on nine studies involving a total of 1062 patients; the conclusions of this group concurred with those of the Jaber group.[32]

Thus, the importance of membrane biocompatibility in ARF remains unresolved. It is possible that the attainment of a clear answer may never be possible because the underlying severity of illness remains the overwhelming determinant of the outcome, especially in the setting of multiple-organ failure.

CONCLUSION

The treatment of acute renal failure by extracorporeal circulatory procedures activates a number of physiological pathways, and efforts to minimize activation of pathways has focused principally on minimizing the activation of complement. The blood activated after its passage through the extracorporeal circuit eventually comes into contact with wounds and the intravascular compartment. Although such contact has the potential to cause harm, there is no conclusive evidence to suggest that the biocompatibility of the extracorporeal circuit plays a significant role in determining treatment-related outcomes.

Key Points

1. In extracorporeal treatments, elements other than a membrane's chemical composition contribute to its biocompatibility.
2. The biological consequences of biocompatibility in the setting of acute renal failure remain the subject of considerable uncertainty.

Key References

22. Hildenbrand SL, Lehmann HD, Wodarz R, et al: PVC-plasticizer DEHP in medical products: Do thin coatings really reduce DEHP leaching into blood? Perfusion 2005;20:351-357.
27. Tapia G, Yee J: Biofilm: Its relevance in kidney disease. Adv Chronic Kidney Dis 2006;13:215-224.
34. Alonso A, Lau J, Jaber BL: Biocompatible hemodialysis membranes for acute renal failure. Cochrane Database Syst Rev 2005;(2):CD005283.

See the companion Expert Consult website for the complete reference list.

CHAPTER 226

Composition of Hemodialysis Fluid

Anton Verbine and Claudio Ronco

OBJECTIVES
This chapter will:
1. Describe the main electrolyte components of modern dialysate.
2. Characterize clinical effects of changes in concentration of major dialysate constituents.
3. Outline the requirements for purity of dialysis water.

In a general sense, hemodialysis fluid can be considered a temporary "extension" of the patient's extracellular fluid.[1] As a result of a blood-dialysate contact via pores in extracorporeal semipermeable membranes, bidirectional diffusion takes place. Solutes tend to reach similar concentrations on the two sides of a dialysis membrane; uremic toxins from blood diffuse into toxin-free dialysate, and buffers from dialysate are back-transported to blood. Some other solutes also cross the membrane via concentration gradient and via convection, with water movement in both directions. Therefore, the chemical, physical, and microbiological characteristics of dialysate are crucial for safe and effective dialysis.

The complexity of modern dialysate composition has increased significantly since 1914, when 0.9% sodium chloride with some potassium was used by Abel, Rowntree, and Turner at Johns Hopkins University for dialysis in experimental animals (history of dialysis is reviewed by Ronco and colleagues[2]). The problem of precipitation of calcium in the presence of bicarbonate buffer was approached in the Kolff-Brigham kidney in 1948 by bubbling carbon dioxide through low-calcium dialysate, with intravenous calcium supplementation. In those coil-type devices, the dialyzer was completely immersed in a tank with premade dialysate, which was changed every 2 hours.

In the 1960s, the first central-delivery machines became available, which distributed ready-to-use dialysate to dialysis stations. The typical cation composition of premade dialysate was as follows:
• Na 140 mmol/L
• K 1.5 mmol/L

- Ca 1.87 mmol/L
- Mg 0.5 mmol/L

Because the use of calcium bicarbonate as a dialysate buffer was linked to the risk of calcium precipitation and bacterial growth, more stable acetate has been used since 1964. The dextrose content was progressively reduced and in some cases eliminated.

After 1974, modern-type machines with bedside proportioning systems became available, which continuously improved reliability and precision of dialysate composition. Extemporaneous preparation of dialysate from treated water and concentrated solution or dry salts at the patient's bedside has made it possible to return to bicarbonate-buffered dialysis. Since that time, individualizing dialysate content for particular patient needs and maintaining water purity have been major fields of interest in dialysis practice.

With the modern dialysis machines, composition of dialysis fluid can be significantly modified to individualize the treatment. The concentration of almost any dialysate component can be changed independently and maintained to the desired level during any given period. Meanwhile, certain "standard" dialysate prescriptions are offered in most centers and serve as the starting point for adjustments to meet patients' needs.

Certainly, any change in dialysis fluid formulas will in turn change the patient's electrolyte homeostasis, with both desired and undesired physiological effects.

DIALYSATE COMPONENTS

Sodium

Sodium is the major determinant of volume and tonicity of extracellular fluids. Because sodium freely crosses dialysis membrane, its concentration in dialysis fluid (Na_D) plays a role in cardiovascular stability during extracorporeal therapy. Acute changes in plasma sodium concentrations are known risks for brain cell damage. Long-term changes in sodium balance can affect patient morbidity via dialysis prescription noncompliance worsening of edema, and hypertension control.

Because plasma is an aqueous solution of crystalloids and proteins, and plasma proteins (on average 70 g/L) occupy a certain volume, the volume of plasma water is somewhat less than that of whole plasma. Therefore, the concentration of sodium in plasma water, Na_{PW}, is always greater than that measured in total plasma and can be estimated through the use of certain formulas.[3]

However, the concentration of sodium in the ultrafiltrate, Na_{UF}, is lower than that in plasma water because of the Donnan effect—some cations cannot cross the membrane because they are kept in the blood vessels by negatively charged proteins. In calculations of the concentration of sodium available for diffusion, Na_{PW} (calculated or measured) must be corrected for the Donnan effect.[4,5]

Dialysate with both "high" and "low" Na_D values has been tried, with different clinical effects. Hyponatric dialysate (130 mmol/L) is reported to result in less thirst and interdialytic weight gain.[6] However, not all of the patients treated with hyponatric dialysate in one study showed improvement in hypertension control, presumably because of a stimulated renin secretion.[7] In another study, dialytic dehydration in hyponatremic patients was obtained predominantly from extracellular volume, with

a high incidence of dialysis dysequilibrium, cramps, and hypotension.[8]

Raising Na_D from 130 to 136 mmol/L resulted in a decrease in rate of muscle cramps,[9] and in another study, raising the Na_D from 132.5 through 135 mmol/L to 142 through 145 mmol/L led to lower rates of headache, nausea, and vomiting.[10,11] Moreover, some patients achieved better immediate hypertension control with higher dialysate sodium concentration, probably as a result of better achievement of "dry weight." On the other hand, when excretion of sodium is limited in anuric patients undergoing long-term dialysis, sodium balance at the end of dialysis sessions can contribute to thirst, greater interdialytic weight gain, and "volume-dependent" arterial hypertension over the long term.[12]

There are different approaches to "normalizing" Na_D concentration. One is to adjust it to Na_{PW}, to prevent a drop in plasma osmolarity secondary to diffusive losses.[10,13] Then, the only sodium removed is by convection. Another approach is to aim for normal sodium balance at the end of treatment. Because daily sodium and water intakes are about 100 mmol and 1 L, respectively, adequate Na_D should permit sodium and water removal in this proportion, resulting in an Na_D of approximately 145 mmol/L.[14]

With modern dialysis machines it is possible to change Na_D during the treatment continuously, performing so-called sodium profiling. Usually, Na_D is hypertonic at the beginning of treatment, counteracting urea flux from cells to extracellular space while urea removal is at its peak.[15] Then Na_D is progressively reduced, approaching normal at the end of dialysis. Increased Na_D at the time of peak ultrafiltration rate can increase refilling of extracellular compartment with improved venous refill.[16,17] The limitations of using sodium profiling to limit intradialytic symptoms are the risk of positive sodium balance at the end of dialysis, difficulties in modeling complex interactions among Na_{PW}, serum protein concentration, total body water, and plasma refilling rate,[18,19] and variations in the temporal relationship between decreased circulating blood volume and hypotension.[20] In the future, improved sodium kinetic modeling may help create a software biofeedback loop based on online signals from the patient-machine complex.[21]

Potassium

In patients undergoing long-term dialysis and consuming a liberal diet, daily potassium intake varies between 60 and 80 mmol. With that fact taken into account, thrice-weekly dialysis with a potassium bath of 1.5 to 2.0 mmol/L seems to produce an acceptable potassium balance in most patients.[22] However, relative hypoinsulinemia and metabolic acidosis can shift potassium from the intracellular space to the extracellular space. Clinical scenarios of cytolysis (ischemia, hemolysis, trauma, internal bleeding), renal tubular acidosis type 4 or fasting in diabetics, administration of various medicines (angiotensin-converting enzyme inhibitors, angiotensin receptor blockers, nonsteroidal anti-inflammatory drugs, trimethoprim, and nonselective beta-blockers) can also contribute to hyperkalemia. Rapid correction of hyperkalemia in metabolic acidosis theoretically can hyperpolarize the cells, with persistence of intracellular acidosis.[23] All of these factors, together with dietary variations, dictate personalization of dialysate potassium content. For life-threatening hyperkalemia, a zero-potassium bath is feasible. The contribution of dialysis with a low-potassium bath to the risks of dangerous ventricular ectopy and cardiac arrest is unclear.[24] For patients with poor potassium intake or increased losses through diarrhea, dialysis fluid containing 4 mmol/L of potassium can be advised.[22]

Calcium

The content of calcium in dialysate is an important component in the total management of calcium balance, and both high and low serum calcium levels may in turn contribute to bone disease, cardiovascular morbidity, and mortality in patients undergoing hemodialysis.[25,27]

The National Kidney Foundation's Kidney Disease Outcomes Quality Initiative (KDOQI) opinion, based on level III and IV evidence, recommends that in a patient with stage 5 kidney disease, the predialysis albumin-corrected serum calcium level should be kept within the normal laboratory reference range, preferably toward the lower end (2.1-2.4 mmol/L), provided that keeping serum calcium at this level does not worsen hyperparathyroidism.[28]

With the modern water treatment, the calcium content of final dialysate depends completely on composition of the liquid concentrate and, therefore, on dialysis prescription. To reach and maintain the goal serum calcium level, calcium concentration in dialysate may have to be individualized. The diffusible fraction of calcium, available for dialysis exchange, has been reported to be higher in uremic patients (57.6%-64.3% of total plasma calcium).[29] That amount corresponds to an average concentration of 1.6 mmol/L (6.5 mg/dL). Therefore, dialysate with a calcium concentration of 1.25 to 1.75 mmol/L[30,31] will likely provide a net calcium balance close to zero, depending on the patient's calcium intake and calcium losses by convective means with ultrafiltrate. Increasing the dialysate calcium concentration to 1.75 to 2.0 mmol/L may help control hyperparathyroidism and metabolic bone disease but is linked to a risk of post-dialysis hypercalcemia, arrhythmias, and hypertension[32,33] as well as decreased bone turnover.[28] On the other hand, for some patients taking calcium-containing phosphate binders and vitamin D analogues, a calcium bath containing 1.05 to 1.35 mmol/L can normalize serum ionized calcium and control osteodystrophy.[34] Generally, however, calcium dialysate levels below 1.5 mmol/L tend to promote hyperparathyroidism.[35,36]

For a subgroup of patients with cardiopathy who were undergoing hemodialysis, particularly those with left ventricular dysfunction, a dialysate calcium concentration less than 1.75 mmol/L was associated with a significant decrease in both myocardial contractility[37] and intradialytic blood pressure.[38,39]

Calcium-free dialysate can be used for the treatment of hypercalcemia (mean decrease in serum calcium 1.71 ± 0.54 mmol/L per session), but should be reserved for patients with hypercalcemic crisis or renal impairment because of the significant risk of adverse cardiovascular effects.[40]

Magnesium

Major guidelines do not comment on dialysate magnesium concentration, and trials of this topic with morbidity and/or mortality end points are lacking.

Magnesium is distributed predominantly intracellularly and in the bone tissue. Therefore, serum magnesium levels (0.70-1.05 mmol/L) only partially reflect changes in total body magnesium content. The kidney is a major regulator of serum magnesium concentration, and renal insufficiency,[41] as well as consumption of magnesium-based drugs, can increase the serum magnesium concentration. However, the magnesium content of food and its absorption from food in patients undergoing dialysis can also be reduced, so both high and low magnesium concentrations can occur.

Although only about 70% of serum magnesium is diffusible across dialysis membranes, the magnesium concentration in dialysate strongly affects total balance at the start of dialysis.[42,44] Intracellular (muscle and blood cell) magnesium content in dialysis populations seems to be normal and not to be influenced by magnesium in the dialysate, while both extracellular fluid and bone magnesium levels change in parallel with the dialysate magnesium.[42] Most commercial dialysates contain 0.25 to 0.75 mmol/L of magnesium. In bicarbonate hemofiltration and hemodiafiltration, the replacement solution is generally magnesium-free to prevent precipitation, unless bags with the option of mixing bicarbonate- and magnesium-containing components immediately before dialysis are available.

The relationship between serum magnesium levels, parathyroid hormone, and bone disease in dialysis populations is rather complex. Chronic hypermagnesemia seems to inhibit parathyroid hormone secretion, but to a lesser extent than was previously thought.[41,42,45] In several studies, however, decreasing dialysate magnesium concentrations for some, particularly hypermagnesemic patients from 0.5 to 0.25 mmol/L reduced the rate of osteomalacia without a change in bone resorption.[43,45] Also, chronic magnesium depletion can stimulate parathyroid hormone secretion. In one study, 10 of 12 studies of patients undergoing hemodialysis showed a significant inverse relationship between levels of serum magnesium and serum intact parathyroid hormone,[46] even though the serum calcium concentration was kept at a normal value. Four of the studies on magnesium concentration and dialysis also suggest an inverse relationship between serum magnesium concentration and vascular calcification in patients undergoing hemodialysis.

Buffer

Correction of chronic metabolic acidosis is one of the tasks of renal replacement therapies. Hemodialysis cannot remove significant amounts of free hydrogen ions (H^+) because of their low concentration and rapid buffering in blood. Therefore, acidosis is decreased mainly through providing alkaline equivalents (in the form of bicarbonate or acetate) that are diffusing from dialysate via concentration gradient to be consumed in blood for buffering H^+.

Acetate

Sodium salts of organic acids (NaOA) can bind H^+ according to the following formula:

$$NaOA + H_2CO_3 \rightarrow HOA + NaHCO_3$$

To deplete H^+, organic compounds should be metabolized to CO_2 and H_2O. Of all potential substrates, only acetate is widely used.

Sodium acetate has a molecular weight of 136 Da and is almost completely dissociated in body fluids because of low pK.[47] Acetate is mostly metabolized in peripheral tissues (and to a lesser extent in the liver), capturing one H^+ and forming acetyl–coenzyme A as an intermediate product. Acetyl–coenzyme A may enter via several metabolic pathways (Krebs cycle, ketone body formation, fatty acid synthesis, gluconeogenesis), and buffering is delayed until it is fully decarboxylated. Oxidation of 1 mol of acetate consumes 2 mol of O_2 and produces net 1 mol of CO_2 (1 mol of CO_2 is consumed with H^+ to form acetic acid from acetate).

About 54% of infused acetate is immediately oxidized, and the rest enters alternative pathways.[47] Consequently, if glucose-free acetate dialysate is used, increases in ketone bodies and free fatty acids[48] and a decrease in insulin level are noted. If ketone bodies persist in body fluids, they often dissociate, with a disappearance of their buffering effect.

The lower rate of oxidation can be explained by the fact that acetate is not commonly a major metabolic fuel. The maximal rate of acetate metabolism in normal subjects is estimated to be 5 mmol/min and seems to be lower in patients undergoing dialysis (3-4 mmol/min). When blood acetate levels exceed 7 mmol/L, blood concentrations of maleate and citrate increase,[49] imposing a higher risk that metabolic acidosis will persist.

In the past, during acetate dialysis with no bicarbonate in the dialysate, acetate concentrations ranged from 35 to 40 mmol/L. Taking into account the concurrent blood bicarbonate loss, the total amount of buffer gain at the end of a 4-hour session was 120 to 360 mmol.[2] This may not be enough to compensate for metabolic acid production during the interdialytic period, so low pre-dialysis levels of blood bicarbonate (16-20 mmol/L) were usually seen. Moreover, the higher the urea clearance, the more bicarbonate is lost in dialysate. Raising the acetate content of the dialysate is not a valid option because of the risk of exceeding metabolic capacity, with resulting symptomatic metabolic acidosis and vasodilatation due to high plasma acetate levels during and after dialysis.[50,51] The major role of acetate in modern dialysis solutions is stabilization of ready-to-use bicarbonate and calcium-containing mixes, and the majority of the base load is provided by bicarbonate.

Bicarbonate

Bicarbonate is a physiologic buffer in the body fluids. It is a part of a complex system that includes carbonic acid, carbonate, and carbon dioxide, which can be described as follows:

$$CO_2 + H_2O \leftrightarrow H^+ + HCO_3 \leftrightarrow 2H^+ + CO_3^-$$

When dissolved CO_2 leaves the system or acid is added, the reaction equilibrium shifts to the left. Carbonic anhydrase, which shifts the reaction to the right, is ubiquitous, so the carbonic acid concentration in body fluids is proportional to the dissolved CO_2 concentration. The second dissociation of carbonic acid, $HCO_3 \leftrightarrow H^+ + CO_3^-$, has a pK of 9.8; usually it is not important for body fluids but can be seen in bone or in dialysis solution. In both settings, divalent cations of Mg and Ca are present, with the possibility of carbonate precipitation.

$$Ca(HCO_3)_2 \leftrightarrow CaCO_3\downarrow + H_2O + CO_2$$

Slow precipitation can start at pH higher than 7, and is inhibited by high CO_2 content. Historically the main problems with using high-bicarbonate dialysis solutions were instability and risk of bacterial contamination. The modern

solution to those problems is the use of dry bicarbonate in a container (e.g., BiCart BiBag), in which saturated solution is prepared on the spot and automatically proportioned as needed.

The usual concentration of bicarbonate in dialysate, 30 to 35 mmol/L, is enough to provide a dialysate-blood gradient and repletion of buffer stores[52] in most patients.

Evidence from some small randomized trials suggests that increasing the dialysate bicarbonate concentration from 30 or 35 mmol/L to 40 mmol/L—which raised the serum bicarbonate concentration from a predialysis value less than 19 mmol/L to 23 to 24 mmol/L—might improve bone metabolism[52] and nutrition.[53] On the other hand, alkalosis may cause both acute symptoms and chronic calcium deposition in vessels and other tissues. The bicarbonate profiling feature of new dialysis machines might help smooth the pH correction, but specific indications for this technique are yet to be determined.

Chloride

The chloride concentration in most dialysis fluids varies from 98 to 112 mmol/L. Because chloride and buffer are the only anions in the solution, the chloride concentration is determined by the differences between the sum of total prescribed concentrations of cations (Na, K, Ca, Mg) and anions (acetate and bicarbonate) to maintain neutral ionic charge.

Glucose

The osmotic pressure of glucose, which was utilized for fluid removal during the early years of dialysis, is not important with the pressure-driven ultrafiltration of modern hemodialysis machines. Therefore contemporary dialysis fluids may contain from 0 to 200 mg/dL of glucose. Glucose losses of 30 ± 9 g per session have been reported with the use of dextrose-free dialysate, whereas a positive glucose balance of 15.8 ± 12 g per session was observed after the use of high-glucose dialysate (200 mg/dL). Meanwhile, the clinical significance of either positive or negative glucose parameter after dialysis is unclear, and both hypertriglyceridemia and hypercholesterolemia seem to develop independently of dialysate glucose in this population.[54]

However, in critically ill patients, in children, and in some other patient groups, a physiologic concentration of glucose in dialysis fluid may help avoid hypoglycemia,[55] particularly with continuous techniques. In selected cases, the presence of glucose in the dialysate can also help counteract osmotic dysequilibrium.[56] However, glucose in a solution can be a substrate for bacteria if contamination occurs.[57]

DIALYSATE QUALITY

Treated water is the most abundant component consumed during dialysis sessions. Dialysis patients undergoing dialysis can be exposed to 300 to 600 liters of water per week. Water purification to remove both inorganic and organic compounds, the choice of "pure" concentrate, disinfection of dialysis machines, and control of the chemical and microbiological purity of the final dialysate solution are of paramount importance in achieving quality dialysis.

TABLE 226-1

Comparison of Maximum Water Contaminant Levels Recommended by the Association for the Advancement of Medical Instrumentation (AAMI) and European Pharmacopoeia

CONTAMINANT	CHEMICAL SYMBOL	Maximum Concentration (mg/L)	
		AAMI	*European Pharmacopoeia*
Aluminum	Al	0.0100	0.0100
Antimony	Sb	0.0060	0.0060
Arsenic	As	0.0050	0.0050
Barium	Ba	0.1000	0.1000
Beryllium	Be	0.0004	0.0004
Cadmium	Cd	0.0010	0.0010
Calcium	Ca	2 (0.05 mmol/L)	2 (0.05 mmol/L)
Chloramines	NH_2Cl, $NHCl_2$, NCl_3	0.1000	0.1000
Chromium	Cr	0.0140	0.0140
Copper	Cu	0.1000	0.1000
Cyanide	CN	0.0200	0.0200
Fluoride	F	0.2000	0.2000
Free chlorine	Cl	0.5000	0.5000
Lead	Pb	0.0050	0.0050
Magnesium	Mg	4 (0.16 mmol/L)	2 (0.08 mmol/L)
Mercury	Hg	0.0002	0.0010
Nitrate	NO_3	2.0000	2.0000
Potassium	K	8 (0.2 mmol/L)	2 (0.08 mmol/L)
Selenium	Se	0.0900	0.0900
Silver	Ag	0.0050	0.0050
Sodium	Na	70 (3.0 mmol/L)	50 (2.2 mmol/L)
Sulfate	SO_4	100	100
Thallium	Tl	0.0020	0.0020
Zinc	Zn	0.1000	0.1000

Adapted from European Best Practice Guidelines for Hemodialysis: SECTION IV: Dialysis fluid purity. Available at http://www.ndt-educational.org/images/Hemodialysis%201%20Section%20IV.pdf/ and European Best Practice Guidelines: Section IV: Dialysis fluid purity. Nephrol Dial Transplant 2002;17(Suppl 7):45-62.

TABLE 226-2

Comparison of Maximum Microbial Contaminant Levels in Water with Different Purity Grades

MAXIMUM CONTAMINANT LEVEL	AAMI WATER	European Pharmacopoeia		
		Regular Water	*Ultrapure Water*	*Sterile Water*
Microbial contamination (CFU/mL)	200	100	0.1	0.000001
Bacterial endotoxins (IU/mL)	2	0.25	0.03	0.03

From European Best Practice Guidelines for Hemodialysis: SECTION IV: Dialysis fluid purity. http://www.ndt-educational.org/images/Hemodialysis%20 1%20Section%20IV.pdf/ and or European Best Practice Guidelines: Section IV: Dialysis fluid purity. Nephrol Dial Transplant 2002;17(Suppl 7):45-62.

Different substances are removed by specific modalities applied sequentially. Combining different methods meets the standards of water purity.[58,61] First, particles (dust, sand, rust fragments) are removed by sediment or media filters. Then organic compounds (chloramine, endotoxin, various agricultural contaminants) are removed by absorbent carbon filters. Inorganic substances, such as trace elements, sodium, calcium, and fluoride, can be effectively removed by softeners, de-ionizers, and reverse osmosis equipment.

The most important substances with established toxicity for patients undergoing hemodialysis are aluminum, chlorine compounds (including trihalomethanes such as chloramine), copper, zinc, nitrates, and sulfates. Their effects include dementia, hemolytic anemia, osteomalacia, and acidosis.[58,59,62,67] Other monitored substances may also cause injury if present in excess amounts.[68,69]

Standards for water used in hemodialysis have been established in guidelines issued by the Association for the Advancement of Medical Instrumentation (AAMI) and European Best Practice; they are outlined in Table 226-1.

The water cleaning system itself, as well as storage tanks and piping materials, can be the sources of contamination of dialysate. Most notable is bacterial contamination from water treatment system exhaustion, water stagnation, inaccurate disinfection of dialysis machines, and the use of infected concentrate.[70,73] Guidelines specify allowable levels of both live bacteria (measured in colony-forming units [CFU]) and membrane components of dead gram-negative microorganisms (endotoxins of which are detected by the *Limulus* amebocyte lysate test) in dialysate water (Table 226-2). Large synthetic membranes can be placed in the dialysate line before the dialyzer to further reduce bacterial contamination and endotoxin content.[2] The resulting "ultrapure" dialysate, defined as containing less than 0.1 CFU/mL and less than 0.03 endotoxin unit per mL (EU/mL),[74,75] can improve chronic inflammation, anemia, and nutrition parameters (reviewed by

Masakane[76]).[77] The European Best Practice Guidelines for Haemodialysis now recommend the use of ultrapure dialysis fluid as a goal for all patients and all modalities,[60] and ongoing debates by some other authorities about its use appear to have an economic rather than a clinical basis.[76]

CONCLUSION

Modern dialysis machines, which use pretreated water and precisely calculate dosage of dialysate concentrate components, can prepare dialysate of virtually any composition needed. To individualize dialysis prescription, it is essential to understand both short-term and long-term physiologic effects of changes in dialysate composition. Given the frequency of dialysis treatments and their profound effects on patients' body fluid composition, dialysate can be viewed as one of the most important "medicines" prescribed for the uremic patient.

Key Points

1. Raising dialysate osmolarity by increasing the sodium concentration (Na_D up to 145 mmol/L) generally reduces morbidity during a dialysis session but poses the long-term risk of positive sodium balance.
2. Changes in dialysate calcium may have both short-term effects on the cardiovascular system and long-term effects on hyperparathyroidism and total calcium balance.
3. The relationship between dialysate magnesium concentration and bone disorders in patients undergoing hemodialysis is complex and needs further study for clarification.
4. The main role of acetate in modern dialysate solutions is stabilization, not provision of buffer ions.
5. Bicarbonate load during dialysis provides patients with buffer stores for interdialytic periods. The long-term risks and benefits of post-dialytic alkalosis versus interdialytic acidosis needs further study.
6. Most problems of water contamination by chemicals are successfully managed by sequential purification in modern dialysis water treatment systems. Treated dialysate water is never sterile, but less contaminated, "ultrapure" water is increasingly being used.

Key References

2. Ronco C, Fabris A, Feriani M: Hemodialysis fluid composition. In Jacobs C, Kjellstrand CM, Koch KM, et al (eds): Replacement of Renal Function by Dialysis, 4th ed. Dordrecht, The Netherlands, Kluwer, 1996, p 256.
16. van Kuijk WH, Wirtz JJ, Grave W, et al: Vascular reactivity during combined ultrafiltration-haemodialysis: Influence of dialysate sodium. Nephrol Dial Transplant 1996;11:323.
58. Association for the Advancement of Medical Instrumentation: Dialysate for Hemodialysis. Standard ANSI/AAMI RD 52:2004. Arlington, Virginia, Association for the Advancement of Medical Instrumentation, 2004.
60. European Best Practice Guidelines: Section IV: Dialysis fluid purity. Nephrol Dial Transplant 2002;17(Suppl 7):45.
74. Ledebo I: Ultrapure dialysis fluid—how pure is it and do we need it? Nephrol Dial Transplant 2007;22:20.

See the companion Expert Consult website for the complete reference list.

Clinical Aspects

Indications for and Contraindications to Intermittent Hemodialysis in Critically Ill Patients

Christophe Vinsonneau, Christophe Ridel, and Jean-François Dhainaut

---

OBJECTIVES

This chapter will:

1. Describe the major technical differences between intermittent hemodialysis and continuous renal replacement therapies to treat acute renal failure in acutely ill patients.
2. Discuss the advantages and limitations of intermittent hemodialysis in this setting.
3. Describe some technical aspects of both methods to help physicians in the choice of the best method for the clinical situation.

Until the early 1980s, intermittent hemodialysis (IHD) was the only available method to treat patients with acute renal failure (ARF) in intensive care units (ICUs). IHD was first developed for patients with chronic renal failure and was implemented by nephrologists. This is why nephrologists became the specialists who administered IHD to patients in ICUs who had ARF. However, the implementation of IHD as derived from nephrology practices raised some concerns, especially about hemodynamic tolerance. The description of a new mode of renal replacement therapy (RRT), known as continuous arteriovenous hemofiltration, by Kramer and associates[1] in 1977 offered a new way to treat ARF. Given the arteriovenous access, the treatment was directly controlled by the arterial pressure, which led to better hemodynamic tolerance. In the absence of well-conducted comparative studies, venovenous hemofiltration or hemofiltration (corresponding to the evolution of continuous arteriovenous hemofiltration) gained wide acceptance in ICUs[2] for the treatment of ARF because of its supposedly better hemodynamic tolerance and its ease of use at the bedside.[3] Meanwhile, IHD improved, in particular for the treatment of ARF. Results of clinical studies led to IHD standards for patients in ICUs that were quite different from those for patients with chronic renal failure. Hemodynamic tolerance and therefore efficiency was improved by the use of synthetic membranes, bicarbonate-based buffers, and specific settings.[4]

An abundant literature has compared IHD with hemofiltration in critically ill patients, but no significant differences in terms of mortality or renal recovery have ever been shown,[5-12] even in the latest prospective randomized studies.[7-12] Therefore, it appears that both methods can be used in critically ill patients and that almost all patients can be treated with IHD.[12] The two methods appear complementary and can be used for specific indications according to their advantages and limitations.

OPERATIONAL CHARACTERISTICS OF INTERMITTENT HEMODIALYSIS AND HEMOFILTRATION

In IHD, molecule removal is driven by a concentration gradient between the vascular compartment and the dialysate side. This method favors removal of small molecules because their high diffusibility across the membrane provides a high efficiency (clearance around 200 mL/min). This high clearance is responsible for a rapid decrease in the concentration gradient, which in turn leads to a drop in the removal rate, thus limiting the amount of solute removed (Fig. 227-1). These characteristics explain why IHD is used discontinuously, usually for 4 to 6 hours every day or every other day. Taking into account the high urea volume distribution and the high efficiency of the treatment, the refilling of urea from the interstitium to the vascular compartment is limited during the IHD session but occurs soon after the end of treatment. This explains the increase in serum urea after each session, called *urea rebound*. This phenomenon limits IHD efficiency.

Because of the rapid exchange of solute, high and fast osmolality variations may occur during treatment. These variations involve the vascular compartment and may induce or worsen cellular edema, leading to cerebral edema. In addition, along with the high ultrafiltration rate of IHD needed by the shortness of the session, these osmolality variations precipitate hemodynamic impairment. However, the short duration of IHD sessions offers some advantages (Table 227-1). The nurse's workload is diminished, the patient's mobility is preserved, and bleeding risk is decreased because of low exposure to anticoagulants. Moreover, treatment can be performed without anticoagulation, with good efficiency given the short duration and the high blood flow.[13] In addition, from a practical point of view, one machine can treat several patients a day, whereas continuous therapies require one monitor for each patient-day. Yet IHD presents some technical limitations (see Table 227-1): It demands a specific water production, more complex training of care providers and, in many countries, the intervention of a nephrology team.

Hemofiltration refers to all extrarenal therapies that use convection as the mechanism of solute or water removal. Therefore, solute and water removal is driven by a pressure gradient between the blood and ultrafiltrate sides of the membrane. The solute concentration in the ultrafiltrate side is then similar to the blood concentration, and small molecule clearance rate exactly correlates with the ultrafiltration rate (around 35 mL/min). This low clearance rate explains the necessity to use hemofiltration continuously. Two other RRT methods use continuous patterns, either based on diffusion (continuous venovenous hemodialysis [CVVHD]) or combining diffusion and convection (continuous venovenous hemodialfiltration). All of these continuous therapies are collectively called continuous renal replacement therapy (CRRT). The specific characteristics of hemofiltration account for many advantages: no abrupt variation of osmolality, the management of net ultrafiltration over 24 hours, and an increase in the amount of urea removed, considering the interstitium's potential to refill the plasma compartment. This explains the better hemo-

dynamic tolerance and efficiency usually reported with the use of hemofiltration. In addition, the convection mechanism allows a higher efficiency of removal of middle-molecular-weight substances, with a potential effect on inflammatory mediators. In contrast, the continuous aspect of this method entails some limitations (see Table 227-1): high dose of anticoagulation, lack of patient mobility, higher nurse's workload, and frequent unplanned interruptions of treatment.

INTERMITTENT HEMODIALYSIS AND CONTINUOUS RENAL REPLACEMENT THERAPY: IS ONE BETTER THAN THE OTHER?

The debate between the proponents of IHD and CRRT is ongoing, with valuable arguments on both sides. Several studies have compared the two methods, but most of them were nonrandomized, retrospective trials.[14-23] Many methodological biases preclude conclusions to be drawn from the results of these studies: The membranes were not standardized (biocompatible in CRRT, cuprophane in IHD), different therapies were pooled in CRRT (arteriovenous and venovenous methods) or in IHD (peritoneal dialysis and IHD), and some studies compared two groups enrolled at different times (historical IHD group). Probably the most important limitation is the lack of standardization for efficiency (i.e., dialysis dose) and hemodynamic tolerance in IHD. Indeed, nowadays, we know that hemodynamic tolerance can be significantly improved with the use of specific settings in IHD for critically ill patients[4] and that dialysis dose is a powerful prognostic factor.[24,25] Nevertheless, these studies reported conflicting results, some showing a significantly higher mortality with CRRT,[19-21,23] some a lack of significant difference between the two methods,[14,15,17] and some a lower mortality with CRRT.[16,18]

To date, six prospective randomized studies have been published.[7-12] The study by Mehta and colleagues[7] found a significantly higher mortality in the CRRT group, whereas the five other studies found no significant difference between the methods in terms of mortality.[8-12] In the Mehta study,[7] however, despite randomization, the IHD and

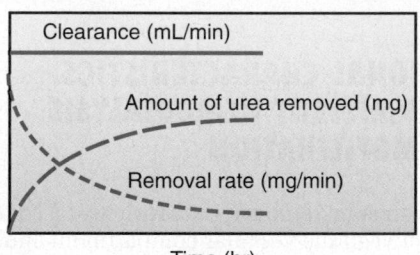

FIGURE 227-1. Representation of urea removal rate and amount of urea removed during intermittent hemodialysis.

TABLE 227-1

Advantages and Limitations of Intermittent Hemodialysis and Hemofiltraion

	ADVANTAGES	LIMITATIONS
Intermittent hemodialysis	High clearance for small molecules Patient's mobility Several patients treated per day with one machine Low or no anticoagulation, low bleeding risk Lower cost	Hemodynamic tolerance Abrupt osmolality variations Fluid management over short period Dialysis dose not predictable Microbiological dialysate safety Nurse training
Hemofiltration	Good hemodynamic tolerance Continuously adaptable metabolic control Low osmolality variations Better fluid management Removal of medium-molecular-weight substances Sterile fluid bags	Anticoagulation and bleeding risk Low patient mobility Frequent unplanned interruptions (coagulation +++) One monitor needed per day for each patient Fluid storage Nurse workload Higher cost

CRRT patient groups were not comparable for several covariates (number of organ failures and severity score), but the multivariate analysis showed no relation between the mode of RRT and mortality. It is important to note that most of those studies involved small numbers of patients (from 30 to 166 patients). Also, various studies had major weaknesses, such as randomization failure,[7] modifications of therapeutic protocol during the study period,[9] combination of different types of CRRT,[7] and small number of heterogeneous groups of patients enrolled.[8-11] However, the Hemodiafe study, conducted by Vinsonneau and coworkers,[12] enrolled 360 patients and found no significant difference in survival between the two groups (60-day survival, 32% for IHD vs. 33% for CRRT). In that study, both techniques were standardized for membrane polymers and dialysis buffers, factors known to affect the ability of patients to tolerate renal replacement therapies. In addition, guidelines based on results of the study by Schortgen and colleagues[4] were provided to improve hemodynamic tolerance of IHD.

Regarding renal recovery, no convincing data exist to support the ability of CRRT to decrease duration of RRT or patients' dialysis dependency at discharge from the ICU or hospital. Except for a few studies that report a significant benefit for CRRT[17-23] or a trend toward a benefit,[7,19] published studies found no effect. In addition, the latest prospective randomized studies found no significant difference between CRRT and IHD in terms of RRT duration or rate of dialysis dependency.[10-12]

One can conclude, therefore, that the two methods seem to provide similar outcomes in critically ill patients as long as they are performed by experienced teams with strict adherence to guidelines to improve hemodynamic tolerance. This conclusion agrees with that of the latest consensus conference.[26] The fourth international Acute Dialysis Quality Initiative[27] conference also concluded, "When analyzed on the basis of combined outcome of mortality or non recovery of renal function, the data does not favor either modality (grade A)."

Therefore, the operational characteristics of each method with its advantages and limitations (see Table 227-1) permit one to propose some good indications for IHD and some debatable ones. In fact, there is no a priori contraindication to IHD, given that prospective studies report similar survival rates for patients with ARF,[8,11] even with multiple-organ dysfunction syndrome, who undergo the treatment.[12] Moreover, the literature provides an insight into the feasibility of and interest in IHD in clinical practice. In the study by Mehta and colleagues,[7] which included patients who had multiple-organ dysfunction syndrome without hemodynamic instability, the rate of crossover was 19.3% and was well-balanced between the two treatment groups. In the study by Vinsonneau and coworkers,[12] the crossovers were controlled by predefined criteria. The overall rate of crossover was quite low (6%); the rate was 3% in the IHD patients (mainly for hemodynamic instability) and 10% in the continuous venovenous hemodiafiltration patients (for bleeding or contraindication to anticoagulant, technical problems, or insufficient metabolic control). Nevertheless, in some cases, hemofiltration may appear more suitable, as for example, in patients with severe hemodynamic instability, especially when high ultrafiltration rates are needed. Finally, the advantages of one method compensate for the limitations of the other—situations in which one should probably not be used are ideal for use of the other. Therefore, it is possible to propose more specific indications for IHD, even though either method can provide adequate treatment for ARF in

the ICU. This is all the more true when new developments are implemented such as high-volume hemofiltration to enhance efficiency in hemofiltration or sustained low-efficiency dialysis to enhance the tolerance of IHD.

The choice should be determined in light of the two main objectives of RRT, adequate delivered dialysis dose and good hemodynamic tolerance to avoid ischemic events. Therefore, the better method is the one that permits these objectives to be achieved for each patient.

SITUATIONS IN WHICH INTERMITTENT HEMODIALYSIS SHOULD BE PREFERRED

IHD is indicated to treat the metabolic syndrome of acute ARF and to manage fluid balance.[28] The best indications are acute metabolic or toxic situations in acutely ill patients without uncontrolled hemodynamic instability. The need to treat a patient without using anticoagulation and the preference to permit patient mobility are other good indications. Inefficient hemofiltration for repeated filter clotting despite adequate anticoagulation and insufficient metabolic control can be good indications as well. Given the low efficiency of diffusion in removing middle-molecular-weight substances, IHD cannot be considered for standard modulation of inflammatory processes. The use of a very-high-permeability membrane could perhaps have interesting effects in inflammatory states,[29] but this issue is not discussed further here.

Complications of Acute Renal Failure

IHD is certainly the most powerful method to easily and quickly control life-threatening situations associated with ARF. This is the case for severe hyperkalemia, for severe metabolic acidosis, and also for pulmonary edema with fluid overload in oliguric patients without severe hemodynamic impairment. These situations require rapid control of the disorder and are usually associated with an uncompromised hemodynamic situation.

Hyperkalemia

The advantage of IHD for removal of small molecules is more evident in transient disorders (hyperkalemia complicating the acute phase of ARF), but could be questionable in case of persistent abnormalities such as tumor lysis syndrome and severe hyperphosphatemia.[30] These situations can justify a combination of IHD early in the course of treatment followed by the use of a continuous modality once sufficient initial control is achieved.[31] This strategy enables good metabolic control without iterative peaks of concentration.

Metabolic Acidosis

Severe uncontrolled metabolic acidosis in shock remains a classic indication for RRT despite the lack of consensus.[26] Lactic acidosis related to tissue hypoperfusion accounts for the major etiology, and bicarbonate infusion is usually insufficient. Using hemofiltration in a standard way may achieve insufficient control, especially when liver dysfunction is present. Indeed, Levraut and associates[32] demonstrated that standard hemofiltration clearance accounted only for 3% of blood clearance in patients with normal lactate levels and stable hemodynamic status.[32] IHD offers a higher clearance of lactate and a greater bicarbonate exchange. IHD must be used repeatedly during the acute phase, and hemofiltration can be used thereafter but without a lactate buffer.

Other situations of life-threatening lactic acidosis in which IHD is useful are metformin intoxication and complications of nucleoside analogue treatment in patients with human immunodeficiency virus.[33] Hemofiltration and IHD have been successfully used in such situations, according to various case reports. It appears, however, that low-volume hemofiltration is unable to control the situation, so high-volume hemofiltration is mandatory.[34] In contrast, hemodialysis providing high clearance can lead to significantly better lactate removal during the emergency phase.[35]

Azotemia

For azotemia control, IHD is a good method, although its efficiency can be limited by urea rebound. In addition, time-averaged urea concentration is reported to be higher with IHD than that obtained with hemofiltration.[7,16] IHD can, however, be improved to obtain similar time-averaged urea values.[11,12] As reported by Clark and associates,[36] who used a computer-based model designed to permit individualized RRT prescription, IHD and CRRT can achieve similar efficiency in azotemia if IHD is performed every day. Nowadays, since the study reported by Schiffl and coworkers,[25] daily IHD has become the gold standard for improving both tolerance and prognosis. Moreover, in some hypercatabolic patients, IHD is probably the best method to control azotemia, given the inability of hemofiltration to deliver target dialysis doses in some patients. In fact, the mean duration of hemofiltration reported in clinical studies is between 16 and 20 hours,[11,37] leading to a decrease in efficiency with no steady-state situation.[37] This approach can be supported by the crossover rate from hemofiltration to IHD in the Hemodiafe study, in which the catabolism in three patients was uncontrolled with hemofiltration.[12]

Poisoning

Many toxic substances can be removed from the blood by extrarenal therapies. Some poisonings require rapid removal because they are life-threatening. How efficient the extrarenal therapy is in removing the toxic substance is determined by the latter's characteristics. The toxin must be of low molecular weight (<500 Da), with high water solubility, low protein-bound fraction, and low volume of distribution (<1.5 L/kg). In addition, the clearance offered by the extrarenal technique is of paramount importance, because one of the main prognostic factors is the rapidity of toxic elimination. IHD is the best method in these situations because it can remove toxic substances from the blood more rapidly than hemofiltration. In fact, hemofiltration could be considered in poisoning with a substance that has a high volume of distribution and low refilling rate, such as prolonged-release lithium intoxication, but it must be performed with high performance[38] and only after initial management with IHD to rapidly improve the symptoms.

Risk of Hemorrhage and Contraindication to Anticoagulants

Filter patency and line patency are major determinants of filter life span and therefore of delivered dialysis dose. IHD can be performed with the use of a low dose of or no anticoagulant, representing a major advantage in patients who are at high risk for bleeding or have any contraindication to anticoagulation. In addition, it seems easier to use IHD to treat patients with heparin-induced thrombopenia and as an alternative treatment to heparin (danaparoid), given the pharmacological properties of these molecules and the difficult management of these treatments in continuous methods.[39] IHD's advantages are related mainly to the short duration of each session (4-6 hours) and to a higher blood flow than that of hemofiltration. With shorter hemodialysis, the coagulation activation induced by extracorporeal circuit should be less.[40] Heparin-free hemodialysis has been reported in ICU patients to be safe and efficient, delivering dialysis doses equivalent to those of hemodialysis using heparin.[13] Continuous therapies using saline flush and predilution hemofiltration without anticoagulant have been reported.[41] However, this method may be time-consuming for nurses, and predilution clearly reduces the delivered dialysis dose. In the near future, when automated machines are available, citrates will allow the use of continuous therapy without major bleeding risk.[42]

Other Indications

After primary care in patients treated with hemofiltration, when the hemodynamic situation improves, switching to IHD improves both ICU care and patient comfort. Moreover, patients' greater mobility makes transport of the patient outside the ICU for diagnostic evaluations such as computed tomography and magnetic resonance imaging easier, aids in the prevention of bedrest-related complications (decubitus ulcer, venous thrombosis, atelectasis), and helps start rehabilitation. Indeed, IHD can be an alternative for some patients for whom hemofiltration is not suitable because of iterative surgical procedures and frequent treatment interruptions that would lead to low delivered dialysis doses.

SITUATIONS IN WHICH INTERMITTENT HEMODIALYSIS SHOULD BE AVOIDED

Given the operational characteristics of IHD, this method is probably not the best one in severely hemodynamically unstable patients or in patients at risk of cerebral edema. Also, fluid balance management in patients with fluid overload seems to be easier with continuous methods of dialysis.

Severe Hemodynamic Instability

Several studies performed with small sample sizes have reported better hemodynamic tolerance with CRRT than with IHD.[8,10] The two latest prospective studies comparing IHD and hemofiltration, however, did not find significant differences, in terms of mean arterial pressure, in the two treatment groups.[11,12] IHD tolerance can be significantly improved in acutely ill patients, as reported by Schortgen and colleagues,[4] although in the Hemodiafe study, three patients were switched from IHD to continuous venovenous hemodialfiltration because of hemodynamic instability. Thus, even with strict guidelines, IHD may not be well tolerated. Use of IHD in patients with severe hemodynamic instability can be a real problem for a clinician with little experience with the method. Schiffl and associates[25] reported that alternate-day IHD for 3.5 hours with a mean net ultrafiltration around 1 L/hr leads to a hypotension rate of 25 ± 5% and worsening of organ dysfunction. Thus, given the deleterious effects of hypotension and ischemic events in kidney function, continuous methods appear better suited to patients with severe hemodynamic instability. This conclusion is in agreement with the guidelines of the Surviving Sepsis Campaign.[26]

Fluid Overload

Basically, it seems obvious that managing net fluid loss for 24 hours is easier and better tolerated than doing so over 4 or 6 hours. To demonstrate this beneficial effect of continuous treatment, Augustine and coworkers[10] performed a study comparing continuous venovenous hemodialysis with IHD in critically ill patients with optimized setting for hemodynamic tolerance. These investigators found better hemodynamic stability with continuous therapy despite a significant increase in net fluid loss during 3 days (cumulative median value), −4 liters versus +1.5 liters ($P < .001$). Mehta and colleagues[7] reported in their prospective randomized study that target net fluid loss was not achieved in 28% of the IHD group compared with 9% in the continuous therapy group.[7] A particular situation is the patient with congestive heart failure and major fluid overload that is refractory to diuretics. Slow continuous ultrafiltration is probably the best method for such a patient and can be given along with hemofiltration in patients with ARF. Two other studies report a decrease in fluid overload and neurohormonal activation and no safety problems with the use of continuous hemofiltration or slow continuous ultrafiltration.[43,44]

Risk of Cerebral Edema

Rapid osmolality variations with IHD may induce cerebral edema in patients at risk—for instance, those with brain injury or trauma or who have undergone neurosurgery. Very few studies have addressed these issues, but in small or case report studies, continuous methods of hemodialysis seem to be superior to IHD as far as keeping the risk of intracranial hypertension or cerebral edema low.[45]

Davenport and associates[46,47] performed two studies to compare IHD and hemofiltration in patients with severe hepatic failure associated with acute renal failure. Both studies report better results for hemofiltration in terms of mean arterial pressure, cardiac index, intracranial pressure, and cerebral edema. However, the beneficial effect of continuous methods must be evaluated against the bleeding risk induced by anticoagulation. In fact, IHD using

increased sodium concentration in the dialysate can be performed with caution by trained physicians in patients at risk for cerebral edema.

CONCLUSION

IHD is still helpful in the management of life-threatening situations if performed by physicians and nurses well trained and experienced in its use. However, the advantages and limitations of IHD and continuous methods appear complementary. Technological advances to improve the efficiency and the tolerance of either method (high-volume hemofiltration, sustained low-efficiency dialysis) will allow their routine use for any clinical situation in the near future. In addition, progress in anticoagulation, such as the use of citrate in continuous therapy, will enable easier management. Consequently, the choice of method will rest mainly on availability and the best experience of the ICU team.

Key Points

1. Intermittent hemodialysis is suitable for patients with transient life-threatening conditions and without hemodynamic instability.
2. In some specific settings, use of intermittent hemodialysis leads to better hemodynamic tolerance than continuous methods of dialysis.
3. Intermittent hemodialysis and hemofiltration are two complementary methods for the treatment of acute renal failure and can be used at different times in the same patient according to the evolution of the disease.
4. Intermittent hemodialysis still has a place in the range of renal replacement methods used in the intensive care unit.

Key References

10. Augustine JJ, Sandy D, Seifert TH, Paganini EP: A randomized controlled trial comparing intermittent with continuous dialysis in patients with ARF. Am J Kidney Dis 2004;44: 1000-1007.
12. Vinsonneau C, Camus C, Combes A, et al: Continuous venovenous haemodiafiltration versus intermittent haemodialysis for acute renal failure in patients with multiple-organ dysfunction syndrome: A multicentre randomised trial. Lancet 2006;368:379-385.
24. Ronco C, Bellomo R, Homal P, et al: Effects of different dose In continuous veno-venous haemofiltration on outcomes of acute renal failure: A prospective randomised trial. Lancet 2000;356:26-30.
25. Schiffl H, Lang SM, Fischer R: Daily hemodialysis and the outcome of acute renal failure. N Engl J Med 2002;346: 305-310.
42. Monchi M, Berghmans D, Ledoux D, et al: Citrate vs. heparin for anticoagulation in continuous venovenous hemofiltration: A prospective randomized study. Intensive Care Med 2004; 30:260-265.

See the companion Expert Consult website for the complete reference list.

CHAPTER 228

Technical and Clinical Complications of Intermittent Hemodialysis in the Intensive Care Unit

Alexandra I. Voinescu and Madhukar Misra

OBJECTIVES

This chapter will:
1. Discuss the technical and clinical complications of hemodialysis in the intensive care unit.
2. Explain how to recognize and treat clinical and technical complications of this treatment.

Acute renal failure (ARF) requiring renal replacement therapy (RRT) in the intensive care unit (ICU) is a serious condition with a reported mortality rate as high as 50% to 80%.[1,2] The choice of RRT depends on logistics and the patient's clinical condition. Although intermittent hemodialysis (IHD) may be used to manage ARF in the ICU, sustained low-efficiency dialysis (SLED) has become an increasingly popular therapy for critically ill patients. This latter modality has evolved as a conceptual and technical hybrid of continuous and intermittent therapies, with therapeutic aims that combine the desirable properties of each of these component modalities, as follows[3]:

- A lower rate of ultrafiltration for optimized hemodynamic stability
- Low-efficiency removal of solutes to minimize solute dysequilibrium
- Intermittent treatments allowing patients to leave the unit for diagnostic and therapeutic procedures during scheduled down-time

This chapter reviews the various hazards complicating the course of IHD/SLED in patients with ARF receiving treatment in the ICU. Complications may generally be classified into two broad categories, clinical and technical. The clinical complications are vascular access problems, air embolism, hemolysis, and electrolyte and acid-base disorders. The clinical complications are bleeding, thrombosis, hypoxemia, hypotension, biocompatibility and allergic reactions, arrhythmias, febrile reactions, and dialysis dysequilibrium syndrome. The chapter also discusses other, miscellaneous issues related to dialysis in ARF, including recovery of renal function, nutrition, and dialysis dosing.

TECHNICAL COMPLICATIONS

Vascular Access Problems

Table 228-1 lists the vascular access problems associated with hemodialysis performed to treat ARF in patients receiving intensive care.

At present, double-lumen, noncuffed dialysis catheters are the preferred means of obtaining acute dialysis vascular access. If it is anticipated that a catheter will be needed for more than a week, a tunneled cuffed catheter should be inserted to take advantage of the lower infection rates and higher blood flow rates associated with such catheters. Noncuffed, double-lumen catheters are inserted percutaneously, by means of the Seldinger insertion method, at any of three different deep venous sites: femoral, internal jugular, or subclavian. The anatomical venous site is usually chosen according to the clinical context and the physician's experience. Ideally, such dialysis catheters should be placed in the internal jugular or femoral position, the right internal jugular usually preferred. Insertion into the right jugular vein is associated with the lower probability of major complications because there is an almost straight venous path from the insertion site to the right atrium.[5,6] The subclavian route should be avoided whenever possible, because insertion of subclavian catheters is associated with an unacceptable rate of central venous thrombosis and stenosis, leading to loss of potential sites for future arteriovenous fistulas and grafts. This issue is of particular importance, because it is frequently difficult to determine which patients with ARF will need continuous renal replacement therapy either at the time of discharge or in the future. The stenosis that forms in association with a subclavian catheter may be silent until an arteriovenous fistula or graft is created on the ipsilateral arm; the most common clinical presentation in this situation is ipsilateral arm swelling with subclavian vein stenosis.

The causes of dialysis catheter malfunction depend on the time of introduction. In general, immediate catheter malfunctions are related to catheter position, whereas late malfunctions (more than 2 weeks after insertion) are more often related to thrombus or fibrin sheath formation.[7]

Thrombosed, noncuffed catheters can be exchanged over a guidewire or treated with thrombolytics as long as the exit site and tunnel are not infected. Exit site, tunnel tract, or systemic infections should prompt the removal of noncuffed catheters.[8] The thrombolytic agent used to treat thrombosis of a catheter varies with local practice. In the United States for example, tissue plasminogen activator (t-PA) is commonly used for catheter thrombolysis. This agent may be effective even in low doses of 1 mg per lumen.[9] Thrombosis of cannulated veins is another complication of indwelling catheters. The incidence of venous thrombosis ranges from 20% to 70%, depending on the site and diagnostic modalities used.[7,10] Deep vein thrombosis develops after activation of the coagulation cascade by an inflammatory process, which is itself triggered by

TABLE 228-1

Types of Vascular Access for Hemodialysis in the Intensive Care Unit

	FEMORAL CATHETER	INTERNAL JUGULAR CATHETER	SUBCLAVIAN CATHETER
Complications of insertion	Puncture of the femoral artery Groin hematoma Retroperitoneal hematoma Increased risk of infection	Puncture of the carotid artery Local hematoma Risk of pneumothorax, hemothorax Rupture of the superior vena cava Pericardial tamponade	Puncture of subclavian artery Risk of pneumothorax, hemothorax Rupture of the superior vena cava Pericardial tamponade Lesions of the brachial plexus
Advantages	Technically easy procedure; used by inexperienced operators Used when the cardiovascular condition of patient (pulmonary edema) does not allow thoracic catheterization	Low recirculation rate Low venous stenosis rate Ambulation possible	Low recirculation rate Low infection rate Ambulation possible
Disadvantages	Highest infection rate Highest recirculation rate (longer catheters [>19 cm] required) Used only in bed-bound patients Should not be left in place longer than 5 days	Technically difficult More prone to infectious complications, particularly in patient with tracheotomy Trendelenburg position required for placement	Technically difficult High rate of central venous stenosis Trendelenburg position required for placement

the presence of the intraluminal foreign body and venous endothelial lesions. The patient presents with edema of the ipsilateral limb, which may be tender and painful. The presence of vein thrombosis is confirmed by ultrasonography. Treatment consists of catheter removal and anticoagulation.[11]

Infection is a common complication in dialysis-dependent patients in whom a catheter is used. Bacteremia usually results either from migration of microorganisms from the skin through the exit site and down the catheter into the bloodstream or from contamination of the catheter lumen.[12] The cuff represents a significant barrier for periluminal bacterial penetration, and infection rates with cuffed catheters are markedly lower than those with uncuffed catheters. Reported bacteremia rates vary from 3.8 to 6.5 per 1000 catheter-days[13,14] for uncuffed catheters and 1.6 to 5.5 for tunneled cuffed catheters.[15,16] The infection rates for nontunneled femoral and internal jugular catheters are higher than for subclavian vein catheters. In one study, the risk of bacteremia was higher after 1 week at the femoral site and after 3 weeks at the internal jugular site, and increased threefold with the use of the femoral rather than the internal jugular site.[13] In another study, this risk was increased sixfold by the use of the internal jugular rather than the subclavian site (no femoral catheters were used in this study).[14] A third study that compared the outcomes of uncuffed and cuffed catheters found an infection rate of 2.9 per 1000 catheter-days for tunneled cuffed catheters, 15.6 for uncuffed jugular catheters, and 20.2 for uncuffed femoral catheters.[17]

Prevention of infection requires strict aseptic care at the time of catheter insertion as well as optimal exit site care with regular review of the exit site and aseptic dressing change. The use of either povidone-iodine ointment or mupirocin ointment has been shown in randomized controlled trials to significantly reduce the risk of bacteremia from tunneled cuffed catheters. For temporary catheters, both povidone-iodine and mupirocin ointments with dry gauze exit site dressings are reported to be similarly useful.[18-22] There is also growing interest in the use of

antimicrobial solution to lock catheters between treatments, but this approach is yet to be studied for temporary catheters.

Access recirculation has not been as well defined for temporary cuffed catheters as for tunneled cuffed catheters. Access recirculation depends on the design and site of the catheter. Access recirculation is higher in femoral catheters than in those located elsewhere, especially if the catheter is shorter than 20 cm. Recirculation rates of 4%, 5%, and 10% (depending on whether the site was internal jugular, subclavian, or femoral) have been reported with temporary venous catheters and a fixed blood flow of 250 mL/min.[23] Interestingly, these recirculation rates did not significantly change at higher blood flow rates (up to 400 mL/min). On the other hand, short femoral catheters (15 cm) exhibit higher recirculation rates, which further rise with higher blood flow rates.[23] Finally, it is worth remembering that in up to half of the treatments, catheters will have to be used with inflow and outflow lines in reversed configuration—using the arterial line for venous return and the venous line for blood aspiration. In this context, recirculation rates of about 20% to 30% have been measured.[18] The impact of access recirculation on dialysis dose has been shown by the study of Leblanc and colleagues,[24] who reported that the urea reduction ratio (URR) was significantly higher with subclavian catheters (62.5%) than with femoral catheters (54.5%) despite identical IHD operating parameters for both sites.

Air Embolism

With the development of modern hemodialysis machines, the incidence of life-threatening air embolism has diminished. Modern machines contain air bubble detectors, which can stop perfusion when air is detected in the system. The two types of air embolism—venous and arterial—are distinguished by the mechanism of air entry and the site where the embolism ultimately lodges.

The three possible areas for air entry through the hemodialysis circuit are as follows:

- The arterial line, into which air can be sucked because of subatmospheric pressure between the arterial access and the blood pump. Leaks in this segment, which may occur from a loose connector or a crack in the polymeric silicone (Silastic) tubing of the blood pump, may result in air embolism.
- Air in the dialysate fluid may diffuse across the dialysis membrane into the blood, forming bubbles in the venous air trap.
- Central venous catheters.

Most causes of air embolism are reported during catheter insertion, incorrect catheter removal, or disconnection of central venous catheters.[25] During dialysis, the emboli are typically venous. The clinical severity depends on the quantity of the injected air, the rate of air entry, and the site of entry. The patient's body position at the time of embolization determines the clinical manifestations. With the patient in the sitting position, the air may first migrate to the cerebral blood vessels, causing neurological decompensation and unconsciousness. With the patient in the recumbent position, air reaches the right atrium and right ventricle; foam develops in those chambers and flows into the pulmonary vasculature, which becomes occluded, causing pulmonary hypertension. Symptoms of this complication are dyspnea, chest pain, and cough followed by cardiovascular collapse.[26,27] In rare cases, air that has entered venous circulation can reach the left heart and then the systemic arterial circulation, where it may provoke coronary and cerebral embolization. Embolization can happen through "paradoxical embolism" via a patent foramen ovale, through passage through physiologic pulmonary arteriovenous shunts, or from incomplete filtering of a large air embolus by the pulmonary capillaries.

Because the majority of affected patients present with nonspecific symptoms, air embolism may be difficult to diagnose in the absence of a high level of suspicion for such a possibility. Air embolism should be suspected in dialysis-dependent patients after insertion, manipulation, or removal of a central venous catheter in whom sudden onset of cardiopulmonary or neurological decompensation develops. Transesophageal echocardiography is a definitive method for detecting intracardiac air. If an air embolism occurs, the venous blood line should be clamped immediately to prevent further entry of air. Management is supportive, with the patient being placed in flat, supine position. This position is now recommended for both venous and arterial air embolism, rather than the traditionally advocated left lateral and Trendelenburg positions. The recommendation is based on the echocardiographic observation that with the body in the lateral position, air persists longer in the right ventricle, thus worsening and prolonging right ventricular dilatation. Adequate oxygenation is often possible only with an increase in the oxygen concentration of the inspired gas up to 100%. If the patient does not show response within minutes, mechanical ventilation and inotropic support may be needed. If significant foaming has occurred in the right ventricle, causing cardiac arrest, cardiac puncture and aspiration should be performed to remove the foam. Hyperbaric oxygen therapy is an additional aid in treating air embolism.[28,29]

Hemolysis

Clinically significant hemolysis can occur during the dialysis procedure. There are numerous reported causes of acute hemolysis, including oxidant damage (from chloramines, zinc, copper, or nitrate contamination of the dialysate), reduction injury (from formaldehyde used to disinfect reprocessed dialyzers or water treatment system), osmolar injury (from hypotonic or hypertonic dialysate), thermal injury (from overheated dialysate), and mechanical injury (e.g., kinking of blood lines, narrowed aperture of the blood tubing set, pump malocclusion, and the presence of a blood clot at the tip of a subclavian catheter). Clinical manifestations include headache, abdominal pain, nausea, vomiting, chest or back pain, malaise, shortness of breath, and severe hyperkalemia due to red blood cell destruction. Immediately after acute hemolysis is suspected or diagnosed, the blood pump should be stopped, the venous blood lines clamped, and the blood discarded. Dialysis should be restarted as soon as the patient is stable, owing to potential fatal hyperkalemia if it is not.[28,30]

Electrolyte and Acid-Base Disorders

Hyponatremia or hypernatremia can occur if there is an error with the preparation of electrolyte solution and the conductivity monitors fail or the alarms are not set properly. Acute hyponatremia causes water intoxication, cerebral edema, and hemolysis. Its clinical manifestations include neurological symptoms, abdominal pain, leg cramps, hypertension, and hyperkalemia. Treatment consists of stopping the dialysis session and starting another dialysis using a dialysate sodium concentration level of 120 to 130 mEq/L or, if hyponatremia is life-threatening, a hypertonic saline infusion to raise the plasma sodium concentration to 120 to 125 mEq/L. Complete normalization of plasma sodium concentration should be avoided in order to reduce the level of cerebral edema.[26]

Hypernatremia causes intracellular (including cerebral) volume depletion as water shifts into the extracellular space. Its symptoms include thirst, headache, nausea and vomiting, seizures, hot flushes, weakness, and even coma and death. If severe hypernatremia occurs, the dialysis treatment should be stopped. Oral water or an infusion of 5% glucose should be given, and dialysis restarted with an appropriate sodium concentration in the dialysate. To prevent cerebral edema, plasma sodium levels should not be allowed to fall below 145 mEq/L.[26]

Hypokalemia can occur when patients, especially those with acidemia, undergo dialysis with a low-potassium dialysate, because the correction of acidosis results in a rapid shift of potassium from the extracellular space to the intracellular space. Hypokalemia is associated with muscle weakness, fatigue, cardiac arrhythmias, and cardiac arrest. Dialysis-induced hypokalemia can be prevented by raising the dialysate potassium concentration. Intravenous potassium can be administered during dialysis when needed. The serum potassium level should be determined frequently to minimize the risk of hyperkalemia.[28] Dialysis-induced *hyperkalemia* is rare. Theoretically, the use of high-potassium dialysate or inadvertent potassium supplementation could lead to hyperkalemia during dialysis. The most common cause of hyperkalemia is hemolysis. Hyperkalemia should be suspected in any patient undergoing dialysis who has weakness, dysrhythmia, or hypotension. Treatment consists of dialysis with a low-potassium dialysate.[28]

Hypophosphatemia can become a significant problem in patients undergoing daily IHD or SLED in the ICU setting. Phosphorus is removed during dialysis, and hypophosphatemic patients require phosphorus supplementation during dialysis to prevent muscle weakness and cardiac arrhythmias.[30] Because phosphate is distributed predominantly intracellularly, its removal is enhanced by more frequent and longer dialysis, which may require monitoring and replacement.

Hypercalcemia can occur because of faults in the ICU water supply. In absence of proper safeguards and/or faults in the deionized/water softener systems, dialysate calcium or magnesium concentration may rise inappropriately, leading to what some call hard water syndrome. Symptoms of this condition consist of nausea, vomiting, increased warmth, headache, tachycardia, and hypotension. The dialysate concentration should be immediately checked for any patient exhibiting such symptoms, and corrected if necessary.

Metabolic acidosis due to dialysis is not a common complication. It occurs as a consequence either of defective conductivity or defective pH sensors in the dialysis equipment or of incorrect buffer concentration. Metabolic acidosis causes nonspecific symptoms, including malaise, nausea, headache, and hypotension. It also predisposes to ventricular arrhythmias. Treatment consists of administration of sodium bicarbonate and the use of dialysis fluid with the correct concentration of buffer.[26]

CLINICAL COMPLICATIONS

Bleeding and Thrombosis

Anticoagulation is an essential component of all extracorporeal therapies. The passage of blood through an extracorporeal circuit causes platelet activation and induces a variety of inflammatory and prothrombotic mediators, resulting in fibrin deposition on filter membranes. The extracorporeal circuit is prone to clotting during acute treatments unless some form of anticoagulation is employed. Clotting of the system leads to loss of blood, decreased delivery of therapy and/or reduced clearance, and higher costs of therapy. On the other hand, excessive anticoagulation may result in bleeding complications. Patients with ARF can have many comorbidities that further raise hemorrhagic risk, such as disseminated intravascular coagulation, sepsis, and hepatic failure. Uremia per se is thought to cause bleeding diathesis by impairing platelet aggregation and platelet–vessel wall interaction.[31] Studies over the last 30 years suggest that gastrointestinal bleeding is the most common bleeding complication of ARF, observed in 10% to 36% of cases.[32] Other, less common manifestations are intracranial bleeding, hemorrhage of surgical wounds, retroperitoneal hematoma, hemorrhagic pleural effusion, subcapsular hepatic hematoma, and hemopericardium.

Systemic anticoagulation with heparin is commonly used for anticoagulation in patients undergoing dialysis in the ICU. However, the major drawback of systemic heparin therapy is the risk of life-threatening bleeding episodes, which ranges from 25% to 30%.[33,34] Alternative methods for anticoagulation have been proposed, such as regional heparinization with protamine, low-molecular-weight heparin, regional citrate anticoagulation, prostacyclin, and saline flushes with no anticoagulant. Combination regimens using heparin and prostacyclin are more popular in Europe and are reported to be fairly efficacious.[35,36] Regional citrate anticoagulation has been found to be an effective alternative to heparin anticoagulation in patients

at high risk for bleeding.[34,37,38] Regional citrate anticoagulation may be complicated by metabolic alkalosis, particularly if high doses of citrate are required; therefore, frequent monitoring of the acid-base status is mandatory with its use.[39] Dialysis with citrate may induce a rise in total calcium concentration during and after dialysis.[40]

Compared with continuous CRRT, SLED has some important advantages with regard to anticoagulation and bleeding risk. One study found that patients treated with SLED required significantly less heparin than those treated with CRRT; 31.9% of the subjects receiving SLED could be dialyzed without anticoagulation, compared with 2.7% of those undergoing CRRT.[41] SLED using saline flushes can also be safely and efficiently performed without anticoagulation.[42,43]

Treatment of patients with bleeding who are undergoing dialysis is similar to that in patients without dialysis. It consists of volume and blood replacement, identification of the bleeding sites, and appropriate definitive therapy, which depends on the severity and site of bleeding. The administration of desmopressin acetate (DDAVP), cryoprecipitate, and conjugated estrogens may be beneficial.[28,44]

Repetitive thrombosis of the extracorporeal circuit and hemofilter is a common consequence of inadequate anticoagulation. The hemofilter's life span is directly correlated to the activated partial thromboplastin time (APTT): The likelihood of hemofilter plugging decreases by 25% with every 10 second increase in APTT.[11,45] It appears that polyamide membranes are less thrombogenic than acrylonitrile membranes.[46]

Hypoxemia

During dialysis treatment, arterial partial pressure of oxygen (PaO_2) falls by about 10 to 20 mm Hg. The clinical implication of the dialysis-induced hypoxemia is of immediate importance to the patient whose cardiopulmonary function is already compromised. Hypoxemia is multifactorial in etiology but it is principally related to the use of acetate dialysate (rarely used) and bioincompatible membranes. Acetate causes hypoxemia by at least two mechanisms, increased oxygen consumption due to acetate metabolism and hypoventilation secondary to carbon dioxide loss across the dialyzer membrane.[47,48] Hypoxemia is observed particularly with use of unmodified cellulose membranes. The interaction between blood and cellulosic membranes activates the alternate complement pathway, leading to intrapulmonary leukostasis, which in turn causes ventilation-perfusion mismatch and hypoxemia. This phenomenon is significantly decreased if biocompatible noncellulosic membranes such as polyacrylonitrile and polysulfone are used.[49-52]

In critically ill patients, who may already have some predialysis hypoxia, it is necessary to increase the ventilated volume and/or the fraction of inspired oxygen (FiO_2) during dialysis. The use of bioincompatible membranes and acetate dialysis should be avoided.[28]

Hypotension

Although hypotension is very common with hemodialysis, it becomes all the more significant in the ICU setting owing to a much sicker patient population with multiple comorbidities. Hypotension is common in patients receiving intensive care. It may be a special problem in kidneys with acute tubular necrosis, which appear to be particularly

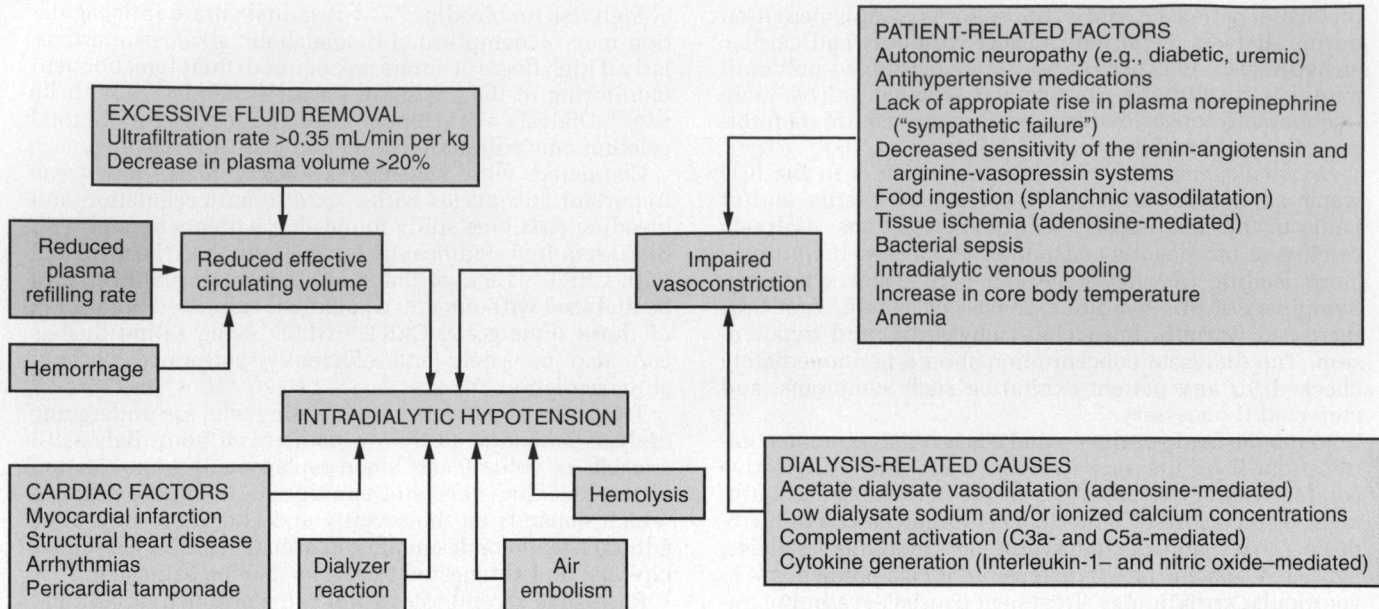

FIGURE 228-1. Causes of intradialytic hypotension.

sensitive to diminished perfusion. Normal kidneys vasodilate in the presence of ischemia as part of the autoregulatory response to keep renal blood flow and glomerular filtration rate near baseline levels. Autoregulation is impaired in acute tubular necrosis, perhaps because ischemic endothelial injury reduces the release of vasodilating substances such as prostacyclin and nitric oxide.[53,54] Hemodynamic instability experienced by patients with such problems can be further enhanced by initiation of RRT. The mechanisms of dialysis-related hypotension are complex (Fig. 228-1). In addition, hypovolemia secondary to blood loss or third spacing of fluids may contribute to hypotension in this patient group.

The most important factors causing hemodynamic instability seem to be aggressive reduction of circulating blood volume owing to ultrafiltration, rapid decrease in extracellular osmolality associated with sodium removal, and coexisting imbalance between ultrafiltration and plasma refilling.[55] The rate-limiting step for removal of fluid from the body is the transport rate between the extravascular and the intravascular compartments. In many patients in the ICU, the fluid transport between the intravascular and extravascular fluid compartments is altered by changes in the permeability of the capillaries due to inflammation and by alterations in plasma colloid or crystalloid osmolarity due to hypoalbuminemia and/or electrolyte disturbances. The fluid removal rate is thus often limited because of inadequate "refilling" of the vascular bed.[56] If ultrafiltration takes place at a rate exceeding the capacity of the interstitial fluid to migrate into the intravascular compartment, a rapid fall in plasma volume with consequent hypotension will result.[57] The usual response to a reduction in circulating plasma volume consists of increases in cardiac output, peripheral vascular resistance, and venoconstriction. Hypotension can occur when one or more compensatory responses are defective. Several factors, including autonomic dysfunction, acetate in the dialysate, dialysate temperature, membrane biocompatibility, splanchnic fluid sequestration, and tissue ischemia, could impair the normal compensatory response of patients to intravascular volume depletion.

The situation may be compounded by a reduction in venous capacitance reactivity, which is in part related to the cardiopulmonary redistribution of blood flow that may occur if patients undergo dialysis through an arteriovenous fistula or arteriovenous graft. The combined effect is a further reduction in cardiac filling pressures. Initially the reduction is compensated by increased sympathetic nervous and neuroendocrine activity. However, in some patients, these compensatory mechanisms fail for a variety of causes (autonomic dysfunction, acetate in the dialysate, dialysate temperature, membrane biocompatibility, splanchnic fluid sequestration, and tissue ischemia). This failure may lead to the Bezold-Jarisch reflex, a cardiodepressant reflex typified by a relative bradycardia and hypotension. Clinically, patients experience muscle cramps due to reduced muscle blood flow, abdominal pain due to mesenteric angina and/or ischemic pancreatitis, cardiac angina, transient ischemic brain damage, and, in severe cases, unconsciousness and even a full-blown stroke or myocardial infarction. Repetitive hypotension may result in numerous small cerebral infarcts.

The composition of the dialysate may also influence blood pressure in several ways. Sodium and calcium concentrations, the nature of the buffer (i.e., bicarbonate or acetate), and the temperature of the dialysis fluid are among the factors that influence the frequency of hypotension during dialysis. Acetate, a peripheral vasodilator, may also predispose to hypotension by reducing myocardial contractility. Hypoxemia during dialysis is exacerbated by acetate-buffered dialysate and contributes to hypotension. Patients undergoing dialysis are often receiving antihypertensive agents or other medications that can interfere with the normal hemodynamic response to ultrafiltration. Beta-blockers reduce myocardial contractility and also exert a negative chronotropic effect. Such agents, by preventing a compensatory increase in the heart rate, interfere with a major defense supporting blood pressure during dialysis. Verapamil can be expected to exert a similar effect. Vasodilators can prevent the vasoconstriction response to ultrafiltration.[58]

There is concern that hypotensive episodes during RRT may impede renal recovery.[59] Conversely, reduction of hypotensive episodes should have a positive effect on the recovery of renal function. On the basis of the premise that SLED is hemodynamically "gentler" and thus less prone to cause hypotension, it also has been studied in this regard.[60-63] The first randomized, prospective, controlled trial, performed by Kielstein and associates,[61] compared cardiovascular tolerability of extended dialysis with that of continuous venovenous hemofiltration in severely ill patients with ARF in the ICU. The results of the study showed no difference in mean arterial blood pressure or use of catecholamines between the treatment groups.[61] Some other studies have also shown cardiovascular tolerability associated with SLED to be similar to that associated with continuous RRT, even in severely ill patients.[62,63] SLED is an increasingly utilized mode of RRT that may have a favorable hemodynamic profile, even in critically ill patients with ARF in the ICU.[64]

Preventive measures to avoid hypotension consist of using cool dialysate (35° C) and use of selective alpha-agonists like midodrine. Treatment of intradialytic hypotension depends on its mechanism. Hypovolemia-induced hypotension (low cardiac output, low preload) should be managed with either isolated or sequential ultrafiltration or SLED. Patients with cardiogenic shock (low cardiac output, high filling pressures) requiring RRT may benefit from inotropic support, reduction of afterload, and a higher dialysate calcium concentration. Finally, if vasodilatory shock is present (high cardiac output, low systemic vascular resistance), the use of vasopressors (norepinephrine, phenylnorepinephrine, vasopressin) and/or corticosteroids may be required. Dosage of vasopressors may have to be increased at the start of RRT for patients already receiving vasopressors. In general, measures such as reducing or stopping ultrafiltration and performing volume replacement with normal saline, hypertonic saline solution, mannitol, dextran 70, hydroxyethyl starch (higher-molecular-weight preparations sometimes precipitate out in the small dermal capillaries, resulting in an intensely irritating skin rash) are commonly used. Salt-poor albumin has not been shown to be more effective than normal saline in this setting.[65-67]

Biocompatibility

Several studies in experimental animals with ARF have shown that complement activation during the blood-dialyzer interaction with cuprophane membranes (but not with more compatible membranes) can lead to neutrophilic infiltration into the kidney (and other tissues) and prolonged ARF. Animal studies have shown the adverse effects of infiltrating leukocytes on recovery of renal function[60] and on whole-kidney glomerular filtration rate when activated neutrophils are infused into a mildly ischemic kidney.[69] In studies of rats with ARF, dialysis using a membrane that activated complement and neutrophils was found to lead to a slower resolution of renal failure and to be associated with a threefold rise in the number of neutrophils per glomerulus in histological sections in comparison with dialysis using a membrane that did not activate complement.[70,71]

These findings may be applicable to humans, because some prospective randomized trials have shown that survival rate and rate of recovery from ARF in critically ill patients were significantly higher and that the recovery occurred earlier when dialysis was performed with bio-compatible rather than bioincompatible cuprophane membranes.[72-74] Other studies, however, have not detected a difference in survival with use of these different membranes.[75-77] Several meta-analyses have been performed, with inconsistent results.[78-80] In the 2005 meta-analysis of the Cochrane database, nine studies involving a total of 1062 patients reviewed. The values for relative risk of death and rate of recovery of renal function were similar for biocompatible and bioincompatible membranes.[81]

Another issue of some importance in this context is the choice of membranes for dialysis of patients with concomitant hepatic failure. Because these patients may be particularly prone to harmful effects of elevated intracranial pressure, owing to their tendency for development of cerebral edema, the choice of membranes becomes important. In this regard, polyacrylonitrile and polyamide membranes are preferable to cuprophane membranes. The former, being more biocompatible (polyacrylonitrile more than polyamide), has a lesser tendency to affect intracranial pressure.[82]

Hypersensitivity Reactions

Hypersensitivity reactions are observed occasionally during dialysis therapy for ARF. There are two types of first-use reactions, a hypersensitivity type (type A) and a nonspecific type (type B).

Type A reactions usually occur in the first few minutes of dialysis, immediately after the return of blood from the dialysis circuit to the patient; however, the onset may be delayed up to 30 minutes into treatment. The symptoms may be mild to moderate, consisting of itching, urticaria, flushing, rhinorrhea or lacrimation, cough, sneezing, wheezing, abdominal cramping, diarrhea, and dyspnea. However, severe reactions—bronchospasm, bradycardia, hypotension, cardiac and/or respiratory arrest, and death—have been described. Several mechanisms have been suggested to explain these reactions. Among these, pretreatment with ethylene oxide and use of polyacrylonitrile membranes, especially AN69 (in patients treated with angiotensin-converting enzyme [ACE] inhibitors) are well-defined causes of anaphylactoid reactions. Reactions to ethylene oxide are uncommon with improved degassing techniques, thorough rinsing of new dialyzers and tubing, and replacement of ethylene oxide by steam or gamma radiation to sterilize dialyzers.[83,84]

Since 1990, a number of clinical studies have shown a strong correlation of use of synthetic AN69 polyacrylonitrile membrane with induced anaphylactoid reactions. Most of the reactions were observed in patients treated with ACE inhibitors,[85-88] although a few episodes have been reported that were not associated with ACE inhibition,[86,89] or in the presence of angiotensin II receptor antagonist therapy.[90,91] The pathogenesis of these anaphylactoid reactions is not elucidated, but the involvement of ACE inhibitors in the vast majority of cases suggests a role for bradykinin.[89] Bradykinin is generated via contact activation, so, contact of blood with negative charges on the surface of an AN69 membrane could cause release of bradykinin. Normally, the released bradykinin is effectively degraded by the activation of ACD (which is identical to kininase II), but in the presence of an ACE inhibitor, the degradation is inhibited and bradykinin can accumulate, allowing the full development of the clinical picture.[89,92] If the reaction occurs, dialysis should be stopped immediately and the tubing should be clamped. The dialyzer and tubing, along with the blood contained therein, should be discarded. The patient should be treated, depending on the severity of the symptoms, with antihistamines, corticosteroids, epinephrine, bronchodilators, and/or vasopressors.[93]

Type B reactions are less severe than type A reactions. The most common symptoms are chest and back pain, dyspnea, cramps, nausea, vomiting, and hypotension. Symptoms of type B first-use reactions are usually observed during the first hour of dialysis and disappear or lessen dramatically during subsequent hours.[93] The pathogenesis of type B reactions is not clear. It is thought that they might be related to complement activation. Treatment with oxygen and analgesics is sufficient.

Cardiac Arrhythmias

Arrhythmias are one of the major cardiovascular complications of dialysis, because their occurrence might result in severe cardiovascular collapse and sudden death. Both patient- and treatment-related factors are involved in their occurrence. Patient-related factors include age, heart and/or lung failure, rapid reduction of extracellular fluid volume, electrolyte and acid-base derangements, cardiac and major vascular surgery, digoxin therapy, and sympathetic dysfunction. Treatment-related factors include changes in serum potassium or calcium concentrations as well as in acid-base balance produced by dialysis.[28] Hypokalemia increases the vulnerability of the heart to arrhythmias because of a higher ratio between intracellular and extracellular potassium concentrations, which results in a negative membrane potential. Dialysis leads to rapid changes in serum potassium level, especially when a low-potassium bath is used. The concomitant use of digoxin increases the sensitivity of the heart to rapid changes in serum potassium and may augment the risk for arrhythmias in patients undergoing dialysis.[26,94,95] Acetate in the dialysate has also been implicated in the pathogenesis of arrhythmias during dialysis, and a reduction in the incidence has been demonstrated with a switch to bicarbonate-buffered dialysis fluid[96,97]; however, these findings have not been universal.[98]

Dialysate calcium level can also influence the incidence of arrhythmias. Use of a dialysate with high calcium concentration raises the serum calcium concentration and may induce life-threatening arrhythmias during dialysis through an increase in reentry or triggered activity.[99] If arrhythmia develops in a patient undergoing dialysis, blood samples should be drawn immediately for measurement of sodium, potassium, calcium, magnesium, bicarbonate, and glucose levels. An electrocardiogram should be obtained and evaluated for supraventricular or ventricular arrhythmias. Treatment is based on the same principles as for arrhythmias in patients not receiving dialysis.

Febrile Reactions

Febrile reactions can be observed after bacterial contamination of the circuit or the contamination of water or bicarbonate dialysate. These exposures result in bloodstream infections, which are related to exposure of the patient's blood to bacterial endotoxins or lipopolysaccharides. Another important cause of febrile reactions during dialysis is vascular access infection. Such an infection is usually caused by *Staphylococcus aureus*, and treatment requires removal of the infected catheter.

Dialysis Dysequilibrium Syndrome

Dialysis dysequilibrium syndrome is a neurological disorder that occurs in patients starting on IHD, especially if they have a high predialysis blood urea nitrogen (BUN) value. Early clinical manifestations include nausea, vomiting, and headache. In more severe cases, hypertension, confusion, disorientation, seizures, coma, and sometimes death are observed. The cause of this syndrome is controversial. Most authorities believe it to be related to an acute rise in brain water content. When the plasma solute level is rapidly lowered during dialysis, the plasma becomes hypotonic with respect to the brain cells, and water shifts from the plasma into brain tissue. Other researchers incriminate acute changes in the pH of the cerebrospinal fluid during dialysis.[100] Dialysis dysequilibrium syndrome is generally a self-limited condition. For severe cases, dialysis should be discontinued. Seizures can be treated with intravenous diazepam. In several studies, the syndrome has been treated with the addition of osmotically active solutes (mannitol, glucose, fructose, glycerol, sodium chloride) to the dialysate. Because dialysate sodium levels can be changed easily in modern dialysis machines, the use of high-sodium dialysate may be the most convenient approach.[28]

MISCELLANEOUS COMPLICATIONS

Nutritional and Metabolic Problems

It is important to note that dialysis (SLED or IHD) may affect nutrition and metabolism in a multitude of ways in a patient with ARF. Besides substrate losses affecting protein and amino acid metabolism, the treatment may also inhibit protein synthesis. Dialysis may also result in loss of low-molecular-weight nutrients (vitamins and amino acids) with small volume of distribution and sieving coefficients less than 1. Amino acid losses may amount to 5 to 10 g/day. Although there is an obligatory loss of amino acids with dialysis, nutritional amino acid infusions (1 to 1.5 g/kg/day) do not increase this elimination (or plasma concentrations) substantially, because the endogenous clearance of amino acids is several-fold higher. The other possible ways in which dialysis could remove clinically relevant molecules are convection (peptides/hormones) and adsorption (hormones, interleukins, complement factors, etc). However, the clinical relevance of such removal is minimal.

Prolongation of Renal Recovery

There are several putative mechanisms by which recovery of renal function may be adversely affected by hemodialysis (Table 228-2). Of these, hemodynamic compromise and inflammatory burden–induced injury (secondary predominantly to microbiological infections) are the most important.

The kidney in acute kidney injury is vulnerable to further insult owing to impairment in renal autoregulation.[55] Thus, repeated episodes of hypotension with hemodialysis may prolong or worsen renal ischemic injury and delay recovery.[101] Whether "gentler" therapies like continuous venovenous hemodialysis, which conventionally utilize lower blood flow rates over a longer period, may be less injurious in this respect is yet to be proven.[102] Similar evidence in favor of SLED is also lacking. Whenever blood

TABLE 228-2

Mechanisms by which Recovery of Renal Function May Be Adversely Affected by Hemodialysis

| FREQUENCY | IMPACT ON RENAL FUNCTION | | |
	HIGH	UNCERTAIN	LOW
High	Hemodynamic compromise Catheter-associated infection		Access malfunction Anticoagulation-associated complications Membrane bioincompatibilty
Unknown	Human error	Vitamin and micronutrient depletion Hormone depletion Amino acid depletion Hyperglycemia Impaired thermal balance	Electrolyte complications
Low	Catheter-associated hemorrhage Catheter-associated vascular/visceral organ injury Membrane-associated bradykinin activation	Microbiological contamination Acid-base disturbances	Catheter-associated thrombosis Mechanical dysfunction Chemical contamination

is exposed to an extracorporeal circuit, blood-membrane interaction results in activation of several important biological pathways. Blood-membrane interactions are important in humans with biocompatible membranes because they lead to a higher rate of renal recovery and patient survival.[73,74] Although this issue is still not completely settled,[81] the use of bioincompatible membranes in patients with ARF is generally not recommended.

Dialysis Dosing and Recovery of Renal Function in Acute Renal Failure

There is some evidence that time to recovery of renal function is shorter in patients receiving IHD than in those receiving daily dialysis. Thus, daily dialysis may mitigate ongoing renal injury by decreasing the ultrafiltration requirements per treatment in addition to causing fewer hypotensive episodes.[103] Lastly, the decrease in the amount of urine produced over a 24-hour period usually falls with the institution of dialysis. Both ultrafiltration (convective) and urea (diffusive) removal may contribute to this effect. However, whether the decrease in urine output affects the overall renal recovery from ARF has never been proven.

Issues with the Dose of Dialysis in the Intensive Care Unit

ICU patients requiring dialysis are usually hypercatabolic. Consequently, the dosing parameters derived for maintenance hemodialysis may not be applicable in this circumstance and may even pose a risk of under-dialysis. Computer models show that for a 50-kg man in ARF, 4.4 dialyses per week will maintain a steady-state BUN of 60 mg/dL; however, even daily 4-hour hemodialysis may be insufficient to maintain the same steady-state BUN for a 90-kg man.[104] Although solute removal is only one of the goals of RRT in ARF, data do support aiming for higher clearances with RRT to improve patient survival, at least in patients with ARF of intermediate severity.[105] Efforts to achieve a steady-state BUN of 60 to 70 mg/dL or an equilibrated efficacy value (eKt/V) of 1.0 (single-pooled Kt/V 1.2), as an index of providing intensive hemodialysis in ARF, may be hampered by the fact that the prescribed dose may not match the delivered dose.[106,107]

Poor blood flow, hypercatabolic state, difficulties with anticoagulation leading to frequent filter clotting and increase in down time, and increased body water (higher V) are some factors that may be responsible for failure to achieve dosing targets in ARF. Dialysis dosing in ARF is a controversial issue, and a recent trial has shown no benefit of a more intensive dialysis regimen.[108]

Key Points

1. Both sustained low-efficiency dialysis and intermittent hemodialysis are successful in managing acute renal failure in the intensive care unit.
2. Both therapies can have technical as well as clinical complications.
3. Poorly functioning vascular access is often a cause of treatment down time.
4. Bleeding/thrombosis and hypotension are major clinical problems that require prompt recognition and management.
5. Intermittent hemodialysis and sustained low-efficiency dialysis provide viable alternatives to continuous therapies in managing acute renal failure in the intensive care unit.

Key References

9. Haymond J, Shalansky K, Jastrzebski J: Efficacy of low dose alteplase for treatment of hemodialysis catheter occlusions. J Vasc Access 2005;6:76-82.
13. Oliver MJ, Callery SM, Thorpe KE, et al: Risk of bacteremia from temporary hemodialysis catheters by site of insertion and duration of use: A prospective study. Kidney Int 2000;58:2543-2545.
56. Sulowicz W, Radziszewski A: Pathogenesis and treatment of dialysis hypotension. Kidney Int Suppl 2006;104:S36-S39.
86. Tielemans C, Madhoun P, Lenaers M, et al: Anaphylactoid reactions during hemodialysis on AN69 membranes in patients receiving ACE inhibitors. Kidney Int 1990;38:982-984.
108. The VA/NIH Acute Renal Failure Trial Network, Palevsky PM, Zhang JH, O'Connor TZ, Intensity of renal support in critically ill patients with acute kidney injury. N Engl J Med 2008;359:7-20.

See the companion Expert Consult website for the complete reference list.

CHAPTER 229

Correction of Water, Electrolyte, and Acid-Base Derangements by Hemodialysis and Derived Techniques

Ryan Brown and Patrick Murray

OBJECTIVES

This chapter will:
1. Discuss the clinical implications of using different dialysate sodium concentrations when performing intermittent hemodialysis.
2. Describe how to safely manage patients with different degrees of hyponatremia and hypernatremia using intermittent hemodialysis.
3. Review the factors that influence potassium removal during intermittent hemodialysis.
4. Explain the effects of different dialysate calcium concentrations on patients' electrolyte abnormalities and hemodynamics.
5. Show how to adjust dialysate bicarbonate concentration to manage acid-base abnormalities and to understand its effects on serum calcium and potassium concentrations.

Acute kidney injury (AKI) frequently develops in the most critically ill patients in the intensive care unit (ICU), often as a component of multiple-organ system failure. The constellations of electrolyte and acid-base abnormalities seen in these patients vary according to the clinical situation but are often highly complex. The introduction of hemodialysis can have profound effects on these metabolic perturbations, and the clinician must understand these mechanisms in order to optimize clinical outcomes of dialytic intervention and avoid further complications.

This chapter explores the use of intermittent hemodialysis (IHD) to correct electrolyte and acid-base abnormalities. A great deal of the literature concerning this topic comes from the end-stage renal disease (ESRD) population and must be extrapolated with caution; patients with ESRD have chronically developed compensatory physiological responses to the uremic milieu, generally have better vascular access than patients with AKI, and are as a rule more hemodynamically stable than patients in the ICU. However, the data collected from studies on ESRD do provide valuable insight into the utility of IHD to correct acid-base and electrolyte abnormalities in patients with renal failure in the ICU. Finally, it should also be noted that patients with ESRD who are undergoing maintenance hemodialysis are frequently cared for in the ICU, and the presence of existing arteriovenous access (fistula or graft) is a major incentive to optimize and continue the use of intermittent dialysis in such patients whenever possible, as opposed to placement of temporary dialysis access to switch to continuous renal replacement therapy (RRT).

SODIUM ABNORMALITIES

Abnormalities of sodium concentration are commonly seen in critically ill patients. Sodium is the principal determinant of both plasma and dialysate osmolality, and the use of IHD can dramatically affect a patient's osmotic homeostasis. As water flows from an area of lower osmolality to one of higher osmolality, the associated fluid shifts can adversely affect hemodynamic stability (when water moves from intravascular to tissue compartments), cerebral fluid and osmolyte homeostasis (when fluid shifts in either direction), or both. Much of the data regarding the effect of hemodialysis on plasma sodium concentration comes from the ESRD population but may be extrapolated cautiously to determine the correct approach to dialyze patients with acute renal failure (ARF).

Sodium crosses hemodialysis membranes by means of diffusion or convection. Diffusion depends on the concentration gradient and the molecular weight of the solute, but not all ionized sodium is diffusible. The presence of negatively charged plasma proteins results in some cation retention to maintain electrical neutrality (the Donnan effect). The ionized sodium in the dialysate, however, is completely available for diffusion, because there are no anionic proteins there. Because of this discrepancy, one can achieve a diffusive gradient of zero only by choosing an ionized sodium concentration in the dialysate of about 5 to 10 mEq/L less than the ionized sodium concentration in plasma water.[1-3] Other factors that might change the amount of sodium available for diffusion are dialysate temperature and pH, and the addition of other ions, such as carbonate, bicarbonate, and phosphate. In contrast, convective transport (ultrafiltration) of sodium occurs when plasma water is driven across the membrane by either a hydrostatic or an osmotic force.

The choice of dialysate sodium concentration depends on the goals to be achieved and has historically changed over the years. In the past, a lower dialysate sodium concentration, typically less than 135 mEq/L, was used to limit interdialytic hypertension and thirst. This approach, however, can be complicated by headaches, muscle cramps, nausea, and vomiting,[3] and may play a role in the dialysis dysequilibrium syndrome.[4] The use of a dialysate sodium concentration below the serum sodium concentration results in fluid shifts from the extracellular compartment to the intracellular compartment, as diffusion lowers serum sodium and plasma osmolality. Ultimately, the total water loss from the extracellular space exceeds the total water loss from the body. In contrast, the use of a dialysate with a higher sodium concentration than the serum sodium concentration causes water removal from both intracellular and extracellular compartments and minimizes the effect of plasma volume loss.[5]

The mechanism by which higher dialysate sodium concentration maintains a greater proportion of plasma volume while accomplishing ultrafiltration is especially important in the context of ARF. Many patients with ARF are hypervolemic but are also hypotensive from cardiogenic or septic shock, and the ability to produce significant ultrafiltration while minimizing hemodynamic impact is an important tool in such cases. The side effects of increased thirst and polydipsia, which can defeat the purpose of these techniques in the outpatient setting, are often less relevant in the critically ill patient. For this reason, the use of a dialysate sodium concentration of 140 to 145 mEq/L is often advised for acute dialysis,[6] and the same principle underlies the use of sodium modeling to prevent or manage intradialytic hypotension.

Hemodialysis of a patient with an abnormally low or elevated serum sodium concentration deserves special consideration. Dialysis is not typically used to treat these conditions but is often necessary in patients with ARF in whom dysnatremias have developed or in critically ill patients with ESRD. The correct approach to acute dialysis of a patient with significant hyponatremia or hypernatremia depends on both the severity and chronicity of the dysnatremia, and dialysis should never be initiated in such a patient without consideration of both factors. Hyponatremia, a common complication in the critically ill patient, is usually asymptomatic but can cause central nervous system manifestations, generally at serum sodium concentrations below 125 mEq/L. The correction of hyponatremia can be complicated by osmotic demyelination if the serum sodium concentration is raised rapidly in the setting of chronic hyponatremia (with associated cerebral accommodation to hypotonicity). Even in the symptomatically hyponatremic patient, it is generally believed that a targeted extent of correction should not exceed 8 mmol/L on any day of treatment. Similarly, in patients with severe, symptomatic hyponatremia, the initial rate of correction may be 1 to 2 mmol/L/hr for the first several hours, until clinical improvement is seen, and is then slowed to less than 0.5 mmol/L/hr. In the setting of asymptomatic hyponatremia, there is no indication for acute correction, and the targeted rate of correction should not exceed 10 to 12 mmol/L/day.[7] During a typical average-efficiency, 4-hour hemodialysis session, the expected postdialysis serum sodium concentration is typically at the midpoint between the predialysis serum sodium concentration and the dialysate sodium concentration. Because the change in serum sodium generated with this method may be too rapid, it may become necessary to use a lower dialysate sodium concentration, shorter dialysis time, or a slower blood flow rate to dialyze the patient safely. Accordingly, more frequent dialysis may be necessary to achieve adequate clearance for azotemia control while safely correcting hyponatremia.

A similar approach is necessary in the hypernatremic patient undergoing dialysis. In patients with elevated serum sodium levels that have developed suddenly (over the course of hours), rapid correction (1 mmol/L/hr) is recommended and is associated with minimal side effects. However, in the patient with hypernatremia of prolonged or unknown duration, an accumulation of organic solutes in the brain cells requires several days to dissipate. The maximal rate of correction in chronic hypernatremia should not exceed 0.5 mmol/L/hr, with a targeted drop in serum sodium concentration of up to 10 mmol/L/day.[8] As described previously, the use of a dialysate sodium concentration below the serum sodium concentration can be complicated by hemodynamic instability as fluid shifts from the extracellular to the intracellular compartment and the plasma volume contracts. Therefore, use of a dialysate sodium concentration similar to that found in the serum and slow correction of the hypernatremia with hypotonic intravenous fluids are generally recommended.

There are, however, several published case reports describing the treatment of hypernatremia with hemodialysis. In one report, three patients with severe hypernatremia and volume overload were treated with low dialysate sodium concentrations (110 mEq/L), causing reductions in serum sodium of 19 to 34 mEq/L over the course of 3.5 to 4 hours.[9] Other reports have described the use of IHD, one with a dialysate sodium of 138 mEq/L in a hypovolemic hypernatremic patient who required daily 2-hour treatments,[10] and the other in burn patients with hypernatremic ARF.[11] Despite the lack of neurological complications seen in these selected patients, large changes in serum sodium concentrations are best avoided over the time span of IHD. Correction of severe hypernatremia with RRT is probably more safely achieved with less efficient, more titratable techniques, such as sustained low-efficiency daily dialysis (SLEDD) or continuous RRT.

POTASSIUM ABNORMALITIES

Hyperkalemia is a common and potentially fatal complication in critically ill patients with AKI. The causes of hyperkalemia are myriad and include some disorders resulting in tissue breakdown and release of intracellular potassium (rhabdomyolysis, tumor lysis syndrome, visceral ischemia), which may make metabolic control difficult even with dialysis. These etiologies include some acutely reversible and correctable causes, such as compartment syndromes. Regardless of the etiology of the hyperkalemia, hemodialysis is generally recognized as the most rapid means of lowering the serum potassium concentration.[6,12] This is particularly important because the patient with AKI has not developed some of the protective measures of the patient with ESRD, such as chronically upregulated colonic potassium secretion, and is often subjected to conditions causing decreased cellular uptake of potassium, such as metabolic acidosis and catecholamines. The role of catecholamines is particularly complicated, because α-adrenergic receptor stimulation is known to cause potassium efflux from cells, whereas β-adrenergic receptor stimulation mediates cellular uptake of potassium.[13]

The rate of potassium removal with hemodialysis and the associated changes of serum potassium concentration have been the subjects of many studies. The principal factors affecting these issues in the ESRD population include the initial serum potassium concentration, the surface area of the dialyzer, the blood flow rate, the duration of treatment, and the dialysate potassium concentration.[13] An additional factor to consider in the less stable patient is the level of potassium generation, because intracellular potassium is released into the serum. A variety of studies have demonstrated similar patterns of potassium removal during a typical hemodialysis session (Fig. 229-1).[14-17] Mass removal of potassium is greatest in the first 60 minutes, a period that correlates with the time of the greatest decrease in serum potassium

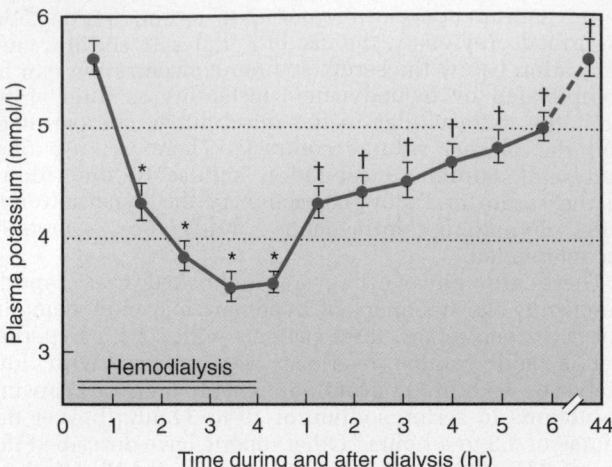

FIGURE 229-1. Changes in plasma potassium (mmol/L) during and up to 6 hours after hemodialysis. *, Significantly lower than pre-dialysis value ($P < .001$); †, significantly higher than end-dialysis value ($P < .001$). (From Blumberg A, Roser HW, Zehnder C, Müller-Brand J: Plasma potassium in patients with terminal renal failure during and after haemodialysis: Relationship with dialytic potassium removal and total body potassium. Nephrol Dial Transplant 1997;12:1629-1634.)

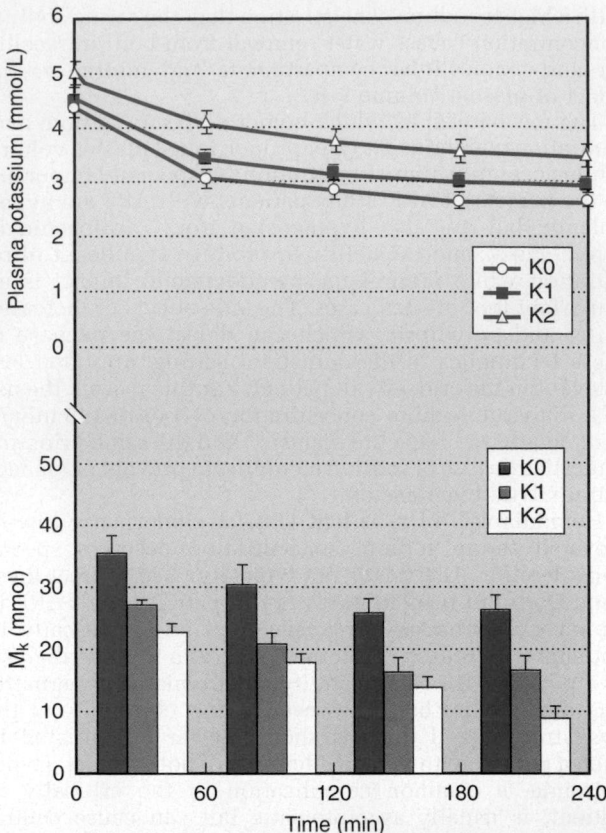

FIGURE 229-2. Plasma potassium concentrations (*top*) and potassium mass removed (M_K) (*bottom*) during standardized high-flux hemodialysis with potassium-free (K0), potassium 1 mmol/L (K1), and potassium 2 mmol/L (K2) dialysates. Potassium concentrations and M_K values were measured at 60-minute intervals. (From Zehnder C, Gutzwiller J-P, Huber A, et al: Low-potassium and glucose-free dialysis maintains urea but enhances potassium removal. Nephrol Dial Transplant 2001;16:78-84.)

concentration. The extent of potassium removal and the drop in its serum concentration are generally less impressive over the next 2 hours, creating a plateau in serum potassium decline after 3 hours. This tapering in the rate of potassium removal is to be expected because the potassium concentration gradient between the serum and dialysate diminishes throughout the treatment.

Potassium does not freely diffuse between the intracellular and extracellular compartments, and the amount removed from each compartment during hemodialysis depends on a number of factors. Several studies have shown that potassium elimination in dialysate occurs with little change in serum potassium during the fourth and subsequent hours of conventional hemodialysis (Fig. 229-2).[14-18] One study of nine patients undergoing dialysis for 5 hours with a dialysate potassium concentration of 1.5 mmol/L demonstrated that two thirds of the potassium removed during the first hour of dialysis was from the extracellular compartment and that only 15% of the potassium removed in the last 2 hours came from the same compartment.[15] It has been estimated that 28% to 47% of the potassium dialyzed in a standard 4-hour treatment comes from the extracellular compartment.[13,19] These findings demonstrate the inequality in the rates of potassium transport across the dialyzer membrane and the cell membrane and also the difficulty in predicting the kinetics of potassium removal, which cannot be adequately described with a "single-pool" model.

There is another consequence to these findings with more serious clinical implications, the routinely significant rebound of serum potassium in the hours following dialysis. The rise in serum potassium after a short-lived nadir achieved at the end of hemodialysis has been well described in the past. An average of 35% of the serum potassium concentration reduction achieved during dialysis is reversed within the first hour after dialysis, and 47% to 68% of the reduction is degraded within 5 to 6 hours.[14,16] Although the extent of rebound is not entirely predictable, a close correlation between the predialysis and 6-hour

postdialysis serum potassium concentrations has been described. This finding should be considered in the patient who presents with severe hyperkalemia; a greater rebound should be expected after the treatment. Unlike the patient with ESRD, the patient with AKI treated with conventional hemodialysis may require repeated courses of dialysis more often than thrice weekly to control refractory hyperkalemia.

The amount of potassium removed by a single hemodialysis session varies considerably, depending on the dialysate potassium concentration. Most studies have used dialysate baths with potassium concentrations ranging from 0 to 3 mmol/L.[14,16-20] Zehnder and colleagues[17] measured potassium removal in 12 patients with ESRD who underwent high-flux hemodialysis with a polysulfone filter using a blood flow rate of 300 mL/min and a dialysate flow rate of 500 mL/min over a 4-hour session.[17] In these patients, potassium removal was 117.1 ± 10.3 mmol with the zero-potassium bath and 63.3 ± 5.2 mmol with the 2 mmol/L dialysate. The greater potassium removal with low-potassium dialysate is tempered by the concern for intradialytic or early postdialytic hypokalemia and its complications. Although there is conflicting evidence in the ESRD population regarding the association between lower dialysate potassium levels and increased ventricular arrhythmias,[20-22] there are no data on patients with AKI.

Particular caution should be taken in choosing the dialysate potassium concentration for patients with preexisting or acute heart disease, especially if they are receiving digitalis therapy.

Another factor that must be considered is the blood flow rate, which is typically lower with the use of temporary catheters in the setting of AKI. In a cross-over prospective study reported by Gutzwiller and associates, 13 patients with ESRD underwent dialysis using blood flow rates of 200, 250, and 300 mL/min. Potassium removal was significantly higher with the use of higher blood flow rates and correlated with higher dialysis efficacy (Kt/V) values.[23] This finding provides further evidence that methods that improve solute clearance, such as higher blood flow rates and limiting of recirculation, should be expected to improve the efficacy of potassium removal. Furthermore, observations of SLEDD have shown significant declines in potassium levels over longer periods,[24] but these findings require further study and comparison with results in IHD.

Furthermore, several clinical situations can affect the transport of potassium between the intracellular and extracellular compartments and the extent of potassium removal. A higher dialysate sodium concentration results in a higher serum sodium concentration, which causes a significant rise in serum potassium. Twelve patients were enrolled in a crossover trial to receive hemodialysis using a dialysate sodium concentration of 143 mmol/L or 138 mmol/L; the treatments using the higher sodium bath were associated with a greater rebound, which was statistically significant at 1 hour after dialysis.[18] The underlying mechanism is thought to be a solvent drag caused by the increased tonicity of the extracellular fluid, which inhibits the transfer of potassium into cells.

The presence of glucose in dialysate also influences potassium removal. Studies comparing dialysate glucose concentrations of zero and 200 mg/dL have shown that the higher glucose bath is associated with less potassium removal but a similar decline in serum potassium concentration.[19] The higher dialysate glucose concentration results in higher serum glucose and insulin levels, which in turn cause the transport of potassium into the cells, lowering the serum potassium concentration. However, the corresponding decrease in serum potassium concentration results in a diminished potassium gradient between the serum and dialysate, impairing diffusive dialytic potassium clearance. Similarly, some of the methods used to lower serum potassium acutely in the patient with AKI act by shifting potassium into cells, decreasing the efficacy of dialytic potassium removal, and causing greater rebound levels in the following hours. For example, a study examining the effects of nebulized albuterol on potassium removal in seven patients with ESRD showed that the albuterol caused a substantial decrease in the magnitude of potassium removal by dialysis.[25]

Theoretically, intracellular potassium shifts induced by insulin or glucose therapy and, perhaps, sodium bicarbonate could similarly degrade the efficacy of dialytic potassium removal. In fact, acute administration of sodium bicarbonate has mixed effects on serum potassium levels; the associated acute increase in osmolality actually shifts potassium out of tissue and raises serum potassium transiently, but ultimately, alkalinization results in intracellular potassium shift, and this in turn may impair dialytic potassium removal. One study that examined the effects of different dialysis bicarbonate concentrations, ranging from 27 to 39 mmol/L, during the hemodialysis of eight patients with ESRD found that the serum potassium diminished significantly more with the higher bicarbonate bath, with a difference seen in the first 15 minutes of treatment. However, the cumulative potassium removal was not significantly different among the different treatments, suggesting a large effect of intracellular potassium shift.[26] These findings also reinforce the practice of using lower dialysate bicarbonate concentrations, such as 25 mmol/L, along with higher potassium concentrations in patients with hypokalemia who are undergoing hemodialysis.

ABNORMALITIES OF DIVALENT IONS

Calcium abnormalities are very common in the critically ill population for a variety of reasons. Hypocalcemia, the most common finding, is associated with ARF because of phosphate retention, impaired formation of 1,25-dihydroxycholecalciferol, and parathyroid hormone resistance. Hypocalcemia can also be seen in the critically ill patient regardless of renal function and is frequently associated with sepsis and burn injury.[27,28] Together with the importance of serum calcium concentration in determining myocardial contractility and the stability of excitable membranes, careful consideration of the impact of dialytic therapy on calcium homeostasis is critically important in the ICU.

The diffusion of calcium during hemodialysis depends on the gradient between serum and dialysate calcium concentrations. Ultrafiltration is a critical component as well, especially in modalities using larger volumes, such as hemofiltration and hemodiafiltration, because the calcium losses by convective transport can exceed the gain of calcium by diffusion. Calcium mass balance studies have shown that in the normocalcemic patient undergoing long-term dialysis, a dialysate calcium concentration of 2.5 mEq/L is associated with a negative calcium balance during treatment and a concentration of 3.5 mEq/L is associated with a gain.[29] Given these findings, the standard dialysate calcium concentration for chronic hemodialysis in many institutions has been reduced to 2.5 mEq/L to decrease the potential long-term impact of dialysate-derived calcium on vascular calcification in atherosclerotic patients and to avoid hypercalcemic suppression of parathyroid hormone as a potential contributor to adynamic bone disease.

However, that approach is not recommended in the setting of AKI, particularly in the hemodynamically compromised patient. Serum ionized calcium concentration during dialysis has been shown to correlate directly with myocardial contractility and vascular reactivity.[30] Similarly, small studies comparing dialysate calcium concentrations of 2.5 mEq/L and 3.5 mEq/L have found significantly lower blood pressures in patients dialyzed with the lower calcium concentration, with more clinically relevant differences in patients who have a greater degree of heart dysfunction (Fig. 229-3).[31,32] Dialysate calcium concentrations of 2.5 mEq/L have also been associated with an increased QT dispersion, which may predispose patients with cardiac disease to ventricular arrhythmias.[33] On the basis of these studies, a dialysate calcium concentration of 3.0 mEq/L or greater is generally recommended for the patient with AKI. This is especially true in the patient with combined hypocalcemia and metabolic acidosis; the alkalinizing effect of acute dialysis initiation in such a patient may precipitate tetany by lowering serum ionized calcium concentration. Accordingly, the

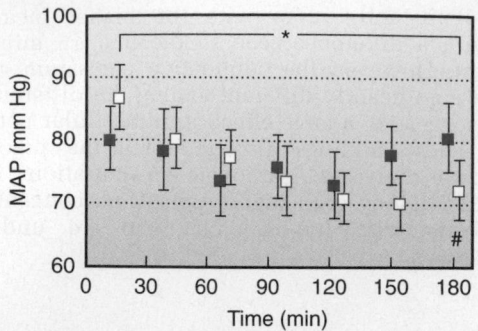

FIGURE 229-3. Mean arterial pressure (MAP) with 1.25 mmol/L dialysate calcium concentration (*open squares*) and 1.75 mmol/L dialysate calcium (*closed squares*) during 3 hours of hemodialysis. Measurements are given every 30 minutes. (From Van der Sande FM, Cheriex EC, van Kuijk WHM, Leunissen KML: Effect of dialysate calcium concentrations on intradialytic blood pressure course in cardiac-compromised patients. Am J Kidney Dis 1998;32:125-131.)

use of a lower-bicarbonate bath (25 mEq/L) is recommended for initial dialytic therapy of severely hypocalcemic patients with AKI, even if they have concomitant metabolic acidosis, to decrease the potential for precipitating this complication of dialysis initiation. Challenges in treating these patients persist despite such modifications. A retrospective study examining 44 patients who received IHD with a dialysate calcium concentration of 3.5 mEq/L found that there was no change in the proportion of patients with calcium abnormalities, which remained near 50% of the sample, although hypercalcemia made up 36.1% of these abnormalities after treatment.[34]

Hypercalcemia is encountered less commonly in the ICU but can occur in a patient with ARF, especially in the setting of a malignancy. Hemodialysis is indicated when the presence of renal or cardiac failure prevents the administration of large volumes of intravenous fluids to lower calcium levels. In these cases, a lower calcium concentration can be used with hemodialysis, and case series of patients treated with dialysate calcium concentrations of 0 to 1 mEq/L have reported minimal complications.[35,36] Generally, to minimize the possibility of an overly rapid decrease in the serum ionized calcium level, the use of concentrations lower than 2.0 mEq/L is not recommended.

AKI requiring dialysis is often associated with hyperphosphatemia. When tissue breakdown results in AKI and severe hyperphosphatemia, such as in tumor lysis syndrome or rhabdomyolysis, hypocalcemia may be life-threatening, and acute dialysis (intermittent or continuous) is required to safely raise serum calcium concentration while lowering serum phosphate concentration. As for potassium, a rebound effect is seen after phosphate removal with hemodialysis because the bones act as a reservoir, returning phosphate to the serum towards the end or shortly after the cessation of treatment. When serum phosphate levels were drawn from six patients with ESRD every 30 minutes during their treatments, a nadir was reached at 30 to 150 minutes and the levels 4 hours after dialysis did not significantly differ from the predialysis levels.[37,38]

In patients with chronic kidney disease, who generally are able to achieve higher blood flow rates with superior hemodialysis access, only approximately 900 mg of phos-

phorus is removed with each treatment[39]; such patients require a low-phosphorus diet and phosphate binders to minimize intake. Improved clearance has been demonstrated with 8-hour nocturnal hemodialysis, suggesting that longer periods of treatment with higher solute clearance may be useful in patients with greatly elevated phosphate concentrations.[40] A similar improvement was noted in a series of SLEDD therapies performed over 12 hours nocturnally. In this study of 145 treatments, there was a drop in average serum phosphate concentration from 5.9 ± 2.1 mg/dL before treatment to 3.4 ± 1.0 mg/dL 1 hour after treatment was completed.[24] Continuous RRT also effectively lowers serum phosphorus levels, typically requiring supplementation within 1 to 2 days of initiation. This modality may be preferred for control of severe hyperphosphatemia in patients with tumor lysis syndrome or other tissue breakdown and may be combined with an initial hemodialysis therapy to rapidly lower the serum potassium concentration if severe hyperkalemia is also present.

ARF in malnourished patients can be accompanied by hypophosphatemia as well. In these cases, it is especially important to provide oral or intravenous supplementation prior to initializing hemodialysis in order to prevent worsening of the hypophosphatemia with resultant multiple-organ dysfunction. Methods of using phosphate-enriched hemodialysate for patients with normal phosphate levels who present with acute overdose of dialyzable intoxicants requiring prolonged dialysis (e.g., lithium, ethylene glycol, methanol) have also been described; the dialysate can be prepared by adding sodium phosphate salts to liquid concentrates of a bicarbonate-based dialysate generating system.[41]

Magnesium has been shown to have significant hemodynamic and excitable membrane effects, which may play a role in the treatment of the critically ill patient. Although hypomagnesemia has been a factor in cardiac arrhythmias, higher levels of magnesium may be detrimental because the substance acts as a vasodilator and can contribute to hypotension in the unstable patient. The kidneys are the dominant site of magnesium excretion, which typically measures 100 mg a day, so AKI is often accompanied by hypermagnesemia. Different dialysate magnesium concentrations have been examined to see what effect they have on patients' clinical outcomes and laboratory measurements. A study of 78 patients randomly assigned to dialysis with dialysate magnesium concentrations of either 0.75 mEq/L or 1.5 mEq/L found that the group receiving the higher magnesium concentration had lower mean arterial pressures and more episodes of intradialytic hypotension.[42] Dialysates with lower magnesium concentrations are available, but the use of zero-magnesium dialysate is often complicated by severe muscle cramps. Interestingly, one study showed that when a dialysate solution contains low magnesium (0.5 mEq/L) and a calcium concentration of 2.5 mEq/L, hypocalcemia and hypomagnesemia can be induced, causing a greater degree of intradialytic hypotension.[43] The changes in both calcium and magnesium can be more dramatic when convective clearance becomes dominant, such as with the higher ultrafiltration volumes used in hemofiltration and hemodiafiltration.

ACID-BASE ABNORMALITIES

Hemodialysis plays an important role in management of acid-base abnormalities associated with AKI. Normally a decrease in renal function causes an accumulation of acids with a corresponding decline in serum bicarbonate levels, resulting in metabolic acidosis. In the critically ill patient, however, the acid-base abnormalities can be highly complex and less predictable. In the context of metabolic acidosis, dialysis provides a buffer source that moves by diffusion into the blood to replace the bicarbonate titrated by the excess acid. Historically, this buffer source has been bicarbonate or acetate, but acetate is no longer routinely used as an alkali source in patients with AKI. Although sodium acetate undergoes oxidation to become bicarbonate in the blood, the delivery of acetate has been shown to exceed the body's capacity to metabolize it. Acetate acts as a direct peripheral vasodilator and myocardial depressant, and its accumulation can have severe clinical ramifications in the critical care setting. Several factors play a role in contributing to this complication, including those related to the influx of acetate from the dialysate to the patient, such as shorter treatment time, higher efficiency dialyzers, and higher blood flow rates, and those related to the acetate metabolism, such as a reduction in muscle mass, malnutrition, elderly patients, hepatic dysfunction, and female gender.[44,45]

Bicarbonate solutions are prepared separately from the remainder of the dialysate because of the low solubility of sodium bicarbonate and its incompatibility in combined solution with calcium. The two components (bicarbonate and calcium-containing) are then combined in a given proportion by the dialysis machine, offering a wide range of final bicarbonate concentrations depending on the clinical situation. In the majority of patients with kidney failure, the dialysate bicarbonate concentration is kept at 32 to 37 mmol/L to maintain a more physiologic pH.[46] The correction of acid-base disturbances with IHD occurs through the mechanism of diffusion, which is well suited for clearing the small solutes that factor into the calculation of pH and the strong ion difference (SID). The performance of hemodialysis is one of many factors in the patient's serum bicarbonate concentration and depends on the dialysate composition, the duration of the treatment, the membrane used, blood and dialysate flow rates, and the extent of ultrafiltration. The mechanism of convection plays a larger role with other forms of intermittent RRT, such as hemofiltration and hemodiafiltration. The same solutes that determine pH and SID easily cross the membrane with the ultrafiltration. As a result, maintenance of the serum bicarbonate concentration depends on the contents of the replacement fluid.[46] Acetate-free biofiltration has been described as an alternative hemodiafiltration method to the on-line addition of bicarbonate by the dialysis machine. In this model, bicarbonate is administered in the replacement solution in the outflow blood line and can be adjusted on an hourly basis to reach a specific serum bicarbonate concentration.[47]

The administration of bicarbonate through hemodialysis is part of a larger discussion regarding the role of bicarbonate in the treatment of metabolic and respiratory acidoses. It has been argued that alkali therapy can be used to maintain a more physiologic pH in the patient with severe acidosis in order to prevent or reverse the detrimental consequences of severe acidemia.[48,49] However, it has also been shown that intravenous administration of bicarbonate may raise the partial pressure of arterial carbon dioxide and, paradoxically, lower intracellular pH, because carbon dioxide, unlike bicarbonate, freely crosses cell membranes.[50] Much of this debate centers on the treatment of lactic acidosis, because the supplementation of bicarbonate in bicarbonate-losing metabolic acidoses, such as those seen with diarrhea or renal tubular acidosis, is widely accepted.

Another clinical situation in which intravenous bicarbonate use is controversial involves acute respiratory distress syndrome (ARDS), a common entity in the ICU. The role of protective lung ventilation in ARDS generally leads to an elevation in carbon dioxide tension, resulting in what has been termed "permissive hypercapnia."[51-53] The buffering of the acidosis that often results from this strategy is a common technique and has been advocated in review articles[51] and used in one of the seminal studies showing a mortality benefit with the use of lower tidal volumes.[52] Hemodialysis is often necessary in patients with severe acidemia who have a respiratory acidosis that cannot be metabolically compensated by the injured kidneys. In these cases, the use of a higher bicarbonate concentration on hemodialysis is recommended to maintain a more physiologic pH and provide more comprehensive RRT.

The advent of hybrid therapies, such as SLEDD and sustained low-efficiency daily diafiltration (SLEDDF), has changed the management of critically ill patients in many centers. Specific information related to handling of the acid-base balance using these therapies is still being acquired, but previous studies have shown a general increase in serum bicarbonate after treatment. In a study of 37 patients who underwent SLEDD using a dialysate flow rate of 100 mL/min, a blood flow rate of 200 mL/min, and a dialysate bicarbonate concentration of 35 mmol/L over 12 hours, the average serum bicarbonate level after treatment was 24.4 ± 3.2 mmol/L.[24] A study of 56 treatments using sustained low-efficiency daily diafiltration in 24 critically ill patients with similar flow rates over a span of 8 hours using a dialysate bicarbonate concentration of 26 mmol/L resulted in an average serum bicarbonate level of 23.3 ± 2.7 mmol/L after treatment.[54]

CONCLUSION

IHD continues to play an important role in the management of critically ill patients with renal failure. Many of the electrolyte and acid-base disturbances present in these individuals can be corrected with proper management and an understanding of the capabilities and limitations of hemodialysis and other renal replacement techniques. Some critical electrolyte abnormalities are best corrected rapidly with acute hemodialysis, particularly severe hyperkalemia. Other abnormalities, however, such as symptomatic hyponatremia with severe renal failure, are probably better managed with slower, more titratable techniques such as CRRT. A combination approach using IHD followed by CRRT to prevent rebound elevation of serum potassium and phosphorus with recurrent acidosis is probably optimal for patients with tissue necrosis or some intoxications, such as with lithium. Despite the growing range of renal replacement modality options, IHD remains an essential option for RRT in the ICU setting.

Key Points

1. A higher dialysate sodium concentration, 140 to 145 mEq/L, is typically used in the setting of acute renal failure in order to improve hemodynamic stability.

2. A primary goal of intermittent hemodialysis should be to limit dramatic changes in the serum sodium concentration, especially in the setting of chronic hyponatremia.
3. Potassium removal by hemodialysis and its subsequent rebound are subject to several factors, including the sodium and glucose content of the dialysate.
4. The bicarbonate concentration of dialysate can be manipulated at the time of hemodialysis to control the delivery of alkali to the patient with acid-base abnormalities.
5. The choice of calcium and magnesium concentrations used in dialysate can have clinical implications for the hemodynamically unstable patient.

See the companion Expert Consult website for the complete reference list.

CHAPTER 230

Urea Kinetics, Efficiency, and Adequacy of Hemodialysis and Other Intermittent Treatments

Thomas A. Depner and Jane Y. Yeun

OBJECTIVES

This chapter will:
1. Examine methods for measuring intermittent renal replacement therapy in critically ill patients.
2. Review data documenting the response to different modes of intermittent renal replacement therapy.
3. Examine the effect of variables that affect the efficiency of solute removal.
4. Recommend methods to assess and improve the adequacy of renal replacement therapy in the intensive care unit.

Hemodialysis was first used during the 1940s to sustain life in patients with acute renal failure. After a series of initial failures, it became clear that life could be prolonged and death from uremia prevented while the native kidneys recovered.[1] The early pioneers in hemodialysis were likely impressed with its eventual success but were limited by rudimentary equipment, arterial access, and adverse reactions, so little attention was given to optimizing its adequacy. In the 1960s, soon after hemodialysis began to be used in patients with chronic renal failure, attempts were made to shorten the duration of treatment as a means of cost reduction and to satisfy patients who naturally prefer short versus long treatment sessions. Symptoms such as muscle cramps and malaise often occur toward the end of treatment, and patients mistakenly believe these symptoms will be reduced or eliminated by shortening the treatment. Despite less need to shorten treatment time in hospitalized patients, dialysis in the ICU setting was also shortened to an average of 3 hours three times weekly, usually without measuring the dose. When the urea clearances achieved with this approach are compared with those achieved in the outpatient setting, it is clear that the average ICU patient treated three times weekly receives less hemodialysis than the average outpatient despite the theoretical need for at least as much dialysis (Fig. 230-1).[2] In fact, an argument can be made for more treatment in the ICU because of the high rates of catabolism often found in critically ill patients.

The enormous experience with hemodialysis in outpatients has generated excellent tools for measuring adequacy that can also be applied to patients in the ICU. The intermittence of treatments both in the outpatient setting and in the ICU facilitates measurement of small solute clearance and also provides the clinician with an opportunity to measure the patient's protein catabolic rate and water volume simply by sampling the blood at the beginning and end of the treatment.[3] As discussed later, these opportunities are not as readily available in patients treated continuously or in patients with native kidney function. This chapter focuses on hemodialysis—more specifically, on the dose of dialysis and its adequacy in critically ill patients requiring intensive care. Although the techniques are similar to measurements used in stable outpatients, the scene is very different and the stakes are much higher in terms of risks from the underlying disease as well as the procedure itself.[4] The good news is that recovery is possible and that near-normal kidney function after recovery is a strong possibility.

GOALS OF DIALYSIS

The primary goal of hemodialysis replacement therapy is to reduce the concentrations of small toxic solutes in the patient. The proven success of dialysis confirms that small solutes account for uremic toxicity, especially considering that earlier membranes effectively removed solutes of molecular weight only up to about 2000 Da.[5] Ideally, the adequacy of this effort could be assessed by measuring concentrations of toxic solutes in the patient's blood, but experience has proven otherwise. Urea, the most abundant small organic solute to accumulate in patients with kidney failure, is a poor indicator of dialysis effectiveness, primarily because its concentration in the blood depends as much on its generation from protein catabolism as on its

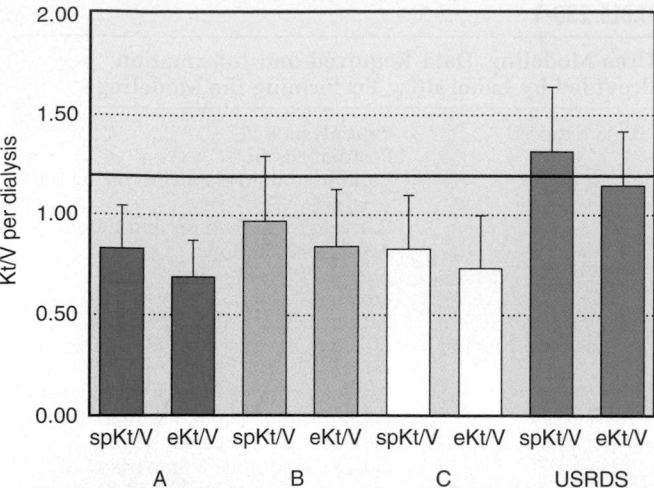

FIGURE 230-1. Hemodialysis adequacy in the intensive care unit. The average delivered dose of dialysis, expressed as single-pool Kt/V (spKt/V), in three studies (A, B, C) published from 1997 to 2002 was lower than the accepted minimum target spKt/V established for outpatient hemodialysis (*horizontal line*). Equilibrated Kt/V values (eKt/V) and actual delivered spKt/V values in the United States, obtained from the United States Renal Data System [USRDS] during 1997, are shown for comparison. Data from Teehan GS, Liangos O, Jaber BL: Update on dialytic management of acute renal failure. J Intensive Care Med 2003;18:130-138.

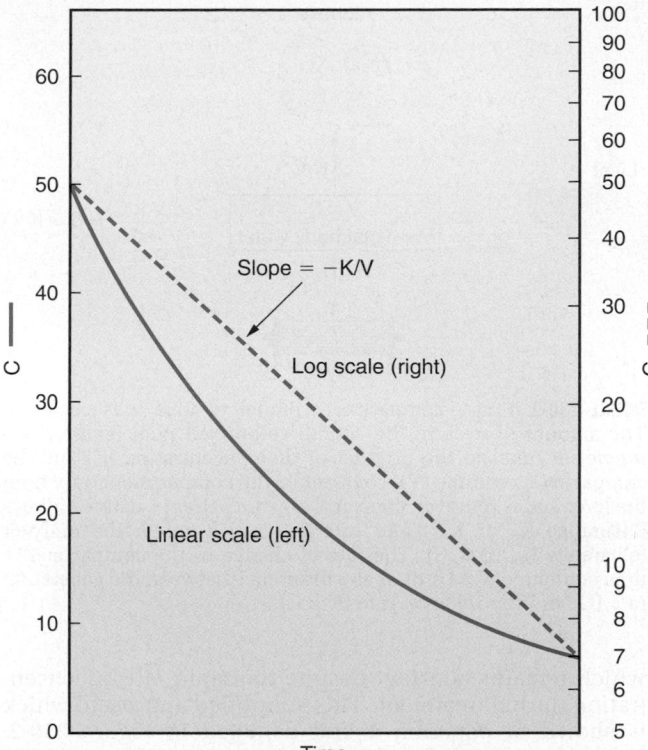

FIGURE 230-2. Origin of Kt/V. If the generation rate and changes in compartment volume are ignored, the solution to the single-compartment model is simplified. The linear decline in log BUN (blood urea nitrogen) during a single idealized dialysis session has a constant slope of –K/V (*dashed line*), where K is the total clearance and is equal to $K_d + K_r$, where K_d is the dialyzer clearance and K_r is the native kidney residual clearance. The slope is the difference between the log of the initial C and the log of the final C (which is also the log ratio of predialysis to post-dialysis C) divided by time t.

removal by dialysis. In stable patients, both high urea generation rates and high urea removal rates are associated with better outcome.[6] The source of uremic toxins is unknown, but the generation rates likely vary from solute to solute and from time to time, forcing the clinician to measure all of them if the goal is to reliably assess adequacy at any point in time. An alternative approach is to pick a representative solute and measure the rate at which the dialyzer removes it. Because both diffusion and convection of solute across the dialyzer membrane are first-order processes (removal is proportional to the concentration), removal can be expressed as a clearance, which is the constant ratio of the removal rate to the concentration, as follows:

$$\text{Clearance} = \frac{\text{Solute removal rate}}{\text{Solute concentration}} \quad [1]$$

This well-known expression is especially valuable during intermittent hemodialysis or intermittent hemofiltration, when concentrations of easily dialyzed solutes fall rapidly. If expressed as a clearance, the dialysis dose is constant, independent of absolute solute concentrations, and is freed from the errors caused by differences in solute generation rates.

Removing or clearing small solutes from the blood is the major accomplishment of dialysis and is clearly vital to survival of the patient with kidney failure. Other techniques can be used to control fluid balance, hormone deficiencies or excesses, electrolyte balance, or larger solutes, but if small solute removal is inadequate, patient outcome is poor.[6] Therefore, providing an adequate clearance of small solutes must be the primary focus of any attempt to measure dialysis adequacy.

HOW TO MEASURE THE DOSE

As previously noted, the net flux (removal rate) of a diffusible solute across the dialyzer membrane is proportional to the solute concentration (C):

$$dC/dt = -kC \quad [2]$$

where *k* is the elimination constant (fractional removal rate), which can also be expressed as K/V, where *K* is the clearance and *V* is the volume of solute distribution. Integration of equation 2 from the beginning to the end of dialysis yields a simple expression:

$$C = C_0 e - Kt/V \quad [3]$$

where C_0 is the initial predialysis concentration and *C* is the concentration at time *t*, usually at the end of dialysis. Taking logarithms of both sides of equation 3 yields the following simple expression:

$$Kt/V = \ln\left(\frac{C_0}{C}\right) \quad [4]$$

Kt/V is determined primarily from the ratio of predialysis to postdialysis solute concentrations and is a measure of the dialysis dose expressed as an integrated or average dialyzer clearance (*K*) throughout the entire dialysis time (*t*), and factored for the patient's size. Size is represented by the volume of urea distribution, which is equated to total body water (*V*). Kt/V is essentially a clearance per dialysis and is therefore a measure of dialyzer function independent of absolute solute concentrations or removal rates.

Figure 230-2 shows that the slope of the line connecting log urea concentrations during dialysis is the ratio K/V,

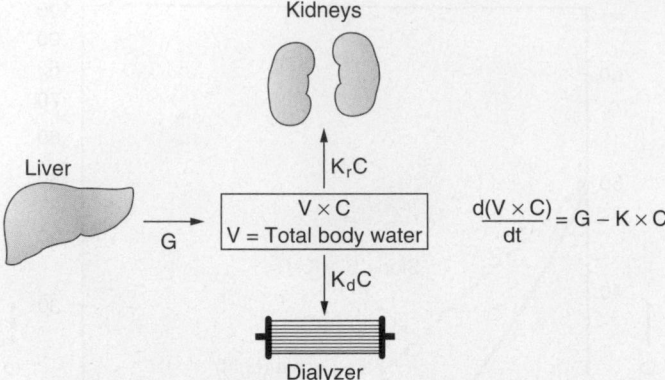

FIGURE 230-3. Single-compartment model of urea mass balance. The amount of urea in the single well-mixed pool (*central rectangle*) is equal to the product of the concentration (C) and the compartment volume (V). Urea enters the compartment only from the liver and is removed constantly by the patient's native kidneys (clearance K_r, or K_rC) and intermittently through the dialyzer (clearance K_d, or K_dC). The rate of change in the compartment's urea content, $d(V \times C)/dt$, is the difference between the generation rate (G) and the removal rate ($K \times C$).

which remains constant despite the rapid fall in concentration during treatment. This simplified approach, which is shown in equation 4 and depicted in Figure 230-2, although helpful for demonstration purposes, is more complicated than shown here because several other modifying variables must be included. A more complete mass balance diagram is shown in Figure 230-3, which also contains a slightly more complex but more accurate equation describing the rate of change in concentration (dC/dt) as a function of C but modulated to a lesser extent by changes in V, urea generation, and native kidney clearance during dialysis. An explicit solution to this equation, although more complicated and therefore more accurate, has the same basic form as equation 3 (exponential function of C_0), as follows[7]:

$$C = C_0 \left(\frac{V + Bt}{V} \right)^{-\frac{k+B}{B}} + \left(\frac{G}{K+B} \right) \left(1 - \frac{V + Bt}{V} \right)^{-\frac{k+B}{B}} \quad [5]$$

where V_0 is the volume of urea distribution before dialysis, K is the sum of dialyzer clearance and native kidney clearance during dialysis and native kidney clearance alone between dialyses, and B is the rate of fluid gain between or during dialyses (negative during).

To measure the dose of dialysis, one would apply equation 5 in reverse. Predialysis and postdialysis serum urea concentrations are measured, and the parameters K/V and G are solved by iterative computer techniques, a process called "urea modeling."

UREA MODELING

Urea modeling is performed by laboratories that service outpatient dialysis clinics. The clinic provides the blood samples together with the input data listed in Table 230-1, and a report is issued by the laboratory that comprises the outcome data shown in Table 230-1. If the laboratory has access to routinely collected data in the dialysis clinic, the process is further simplified. Urea modeling is not automated in the ICU so is rarely done. The patient's status and dialysis parameters often change from day to day, so

TABLE 230-1

Urea Modeling: Data Required and Information Provided by Laboratory Performing the Modeling

Data required	Predialysis BUN
	Postdialysis BUN
	Volume of fluid removed during the dialysis
	Dialyzer manufacturer and model
	Average blood flow
	Average dialysate flow
	Treatment time
	Patient height and weight
Information provided	Effective dialyzer urea clearance
	Delivered Kt/V
	Patient's volume of urea distribution
	Patient's urea generation rate
	Patient's protein catabolic rate
	Quality assurance (comparison of prescribed with delivered Kt/V)

BUN, blood urea nitrogen; Kt/V, clearance per dialysis.

a steady state of urea balance is rarely reached. This situation does not affect the calculation of dose but confounds the interpretation of urea generation and its derivative, protein catabolism.

MODELING PROTEIN CATABOLISM

The urea generation rate provided by formal urea modeling can be used to calculate the patient's net protein catabolic rate by means of a simple conversion equation.[8] As applied in the outpatient setting, a week-to-week steady state with respect to protein intake and output is assumed. Unfortunately in the ICU setting, this assumption is most often inappropriate. To avoid this error, modeling can be done with three BUN measurements, the third being performed at the beginning of the next dialysis treatment. In an oversimplified state in which there is no residual clearance and no weight change, the normalized protein catabolic rate (nPCR; the patient's protein catabolic rate normalized to an ideal body weight based on V [g/kg body wt/day]) is a simple function of the rate of rise in urea concentration between treatments, as follows[9]:

$$nPCR = 5420 \left(\frac{C'_0 - C}{t_i} \right) + 0.17 \quad [6]$$

where C'_0 is the second predialysis BUN (mg/mL), C is the postdialysis BUN (mg/mL), and t_i is the time interval between dialyses (minutes). Measuring the third BUN also eliminates the mathematical coupling between Kt/V and nPCR found in two-BUN measurements.[10] The generation rate and nPCR derived from equation 6 and more formal urea modeling apply only to the interval between the two dialysis treatments, but they can be useful, especially in febrile, injured, or corticosteroid-treated patients, in whom rates of net protein catabolism are expected to be high, or in patients receiving parenteral nutrition.[11]

ON-LINE METHODS

The dose is usually calculated in retrospect, often several days after the treatment, when the laboratory finishes mea-

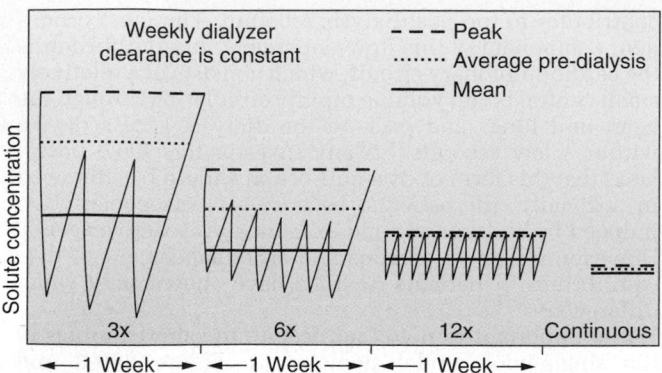

FIGURE 230-4. Effect of more frequent dialysis on solute levels. Despite no change in the weekly dialysis clearance, fragmenting the dose among more treatments (3×, 6×, 12×) results in a significant decline in peak, average pre-dialysis, and mean solute concentrations. The most efficient treatment is the continuous mode (*right*).

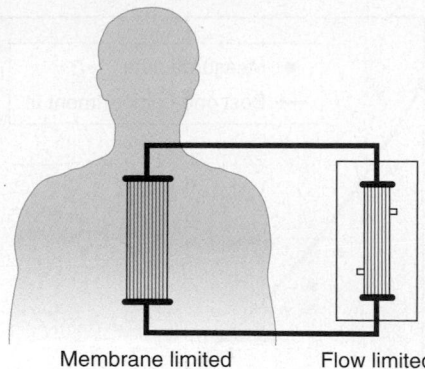

FIGURE 230-5. Two membranes, two barriers to diffusion. Therapeutic hemodialysis requires two sites of solute exchange, one at the dialyzer-blood interface and the other at the patient-blood interface. For highly diffusible solutes, removal by the dialyzer tends to be limited by blood flow, whereas transport across cell membranes in the patient tends to be limited by membrane resistance.

suring predialysis and postdialysis BUN values and returns the data. Because the essence of dose measurement as previously described is the dialyzer clearance of small solutes, methods have been developed to provide clearances in real time, during the treatment, by measuring individual or collective small solute levels.[12-16] Both blood-side and dialysate-side approaches have been studied; urea is used as the marker for clearance on both sides of the membrane, and conductivity has been used on the dialysate side. The latter is essentially a measure of sodium movement across the membrane and closely approximates urea clearance because the two molecules are both highly diffusible.[14,15]

DIALYSIS EFFICIENCY

The rapid fall and subsequent rise in solute concentration caused by intermittent scheduling of treatments provides a ripe opportunity for measurement that is not available in people with native kidney function, in patients managed with continuous peritoneal dialysis, or in patients undergoing continuous renal replacement in the ICU. However, this advantage is offset by the reduction in dialysis efficiency when treatments occur infrequently.

The most efficient form of renal excretory replacement is the continuous process of solute removal provided by the native kidney. *Efficiency* can be defined as a ratio of effective output to energy input. In the case of dialysis, energy input is represented by the dialyzer clearance, and output is measured as a controlled reduction in solute concentrations. Uremic toxicity is probably best represented by the predialysis or average concentration of solute in the patient rather than the postdialysis concentration, but regardless of the output measure selected, the effectiveness of intermittent solute removal, whether by diffusion (dialysis) or by convection (filtration), depends on the frequency of treatments, as shown in Figure 230-4. The reason for this dependence is threefold:

1. Rapid removal causes solute concentrations to fall precipitously in the patient. This decline reduces and eventually extinguishes the solute gradient across the membrane, the driving force for dialysis.
2. Unfettered generation of a solute between dialysis treatments raises its concentration independent of the vigor

of dialysis. This accumulation of solute between treatments limits the capacity of the dialysis to control solute concentrations in the patient.
3. For most solutes, high-intensity (high-clearance) dialysis causes a gradient to develop within the patient, further limiting delivery of solute to the dialyzer membranes.

SOLUTE DYSEQUILIBRIUM: AN IMPEDIMENT TO DELIVERING AN ADEQUATE DOSE

Removal of solute widely distributed in the body, via the blood compartment, depends on movement of solute from other compartments into the blood. The movement into the blood is caused by concentration gradients that result from the dialysis-induced reduction in blood concentrations. Although solute movement across the dialyzer membrane can be easily calculated on the basis of blood concentrations and dialyzer permeability, movement of solute within the body is less predictable. Figure 230-5 highlights two diffusion processes, one a compilation of multiple pathways in the patient, and the other across the dialyzer. Movement in each sphere depends on characteristics of the solute and of the diffusive pathways. Acting together, these two processes of diffusion cause a rapid decrease in solute concentration during dialysis and a rebound in concentration afterwards (Fig. 230-6), neither of which is predicted by the mass balance model shown in Figure 230-3.

The location of the most significant change in solute concentration during dialysis is within the dialyzer itself. The red cell component of blood flowing through the dialyzer represents the second pathway of diffusion that, for urea, is nearly instantaneous, owing to facilitated diffusion pathways (Fig. 230-7). Urea is a uniquely diffusible molecule for which transport pathways exist in erythrocyte and other cell membranes to facilitate its movement.[17] Nearly all other solutes diffuse less rapidly than urea within the body, a finding that probably explains much of the improvements in patient outcome that have been reported when dialysis frequency and treatment time are

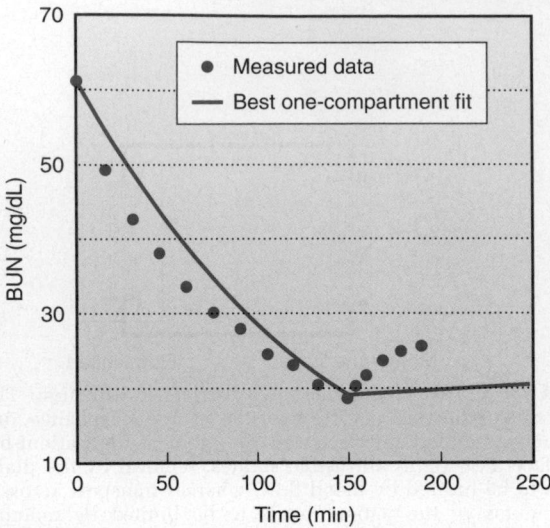

FIGURE 230-6. Potential problems with the single-compartment model. Blood urea nitrogen (BUN) levels measured every 15 minutes during and every 10 minutes after a single dialysis are lower during and higher after the treatment than predicted by the model.

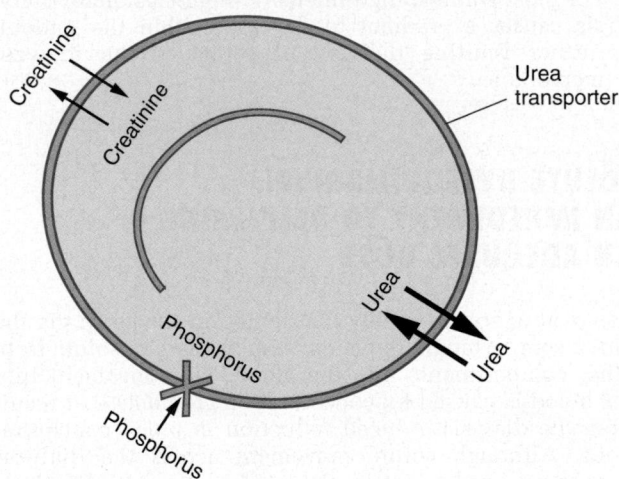

FIGURE 230-7. Erythrocyte diffusion barriers within the dialyzer. Robust transporters allow urea to move freely across the red blood cell membrane. Lacking such transporters, creatinine diffuses at a slower pace and equilibrates incompletely during passage through the dialyzer. The membrane is impermeable to phosphorus. See text for further discussion. (Data from Lim VS, Flanigan MJ, Fangman J: Effect of hematocrit on solute removal during high efficiency hemodialysis. Kidney Int 1990;37:1557-1562; and Gotch FA, Panlilio F, Sergeyeva O, et al: Effective diffusion volume flow rates [Qe] for urea, creatinine, and inorganic phosphorous [Qeu, Qecr, QeiP] during hemodialysis. Semin Dial 2003;16:474-476.)

increased.[18,19] The pattern of divergence from single-compartment predictions shown for urea in Figure 230-6 is greater for nearly all other solutes. For example, creatinine diffuses only partially, and phosphate does not move at all across the erythrocyte membrane (see Fig. 230-7).[20,21]

Another form of dysequilibrium, dictated by differences in blood flow among body compartments, further impedes solute removal.[22,23] Independent of solute concentration gradients, this form of dysequilibrium causes similar rapid reductions in solute concentrations during dialysis and

contributes to the postdialysis rebound. The most prominent component of this flow-dependent dysequilibrium is the cardiopulmonary circuit, which consists of a relatively small central blood volume rapidly circulating through the heart and lungs and back to the dialysis access device within a few seconds.[23] Many investigators have postulated that this form of dysequilibrium should be enhanced in critically ill patients because of vasoconstriction induced by endogenous and exogenous vasoactive agents. However, efforts to demonstrate an enhancement of dysequilibrium in patients in ICUs have shown only small differences.[24,25]

It is important to note that despite the shortcomings of the single-pool model depicted in Figure 230-3 and described by equation 5, the dialyzer clearances are reasonably accurate when dialysis is delivered three times weekly. The reason for this accuracy is the combined canceling effects of overestimating urea concentrations during dialysis and underestimating concentrations during the rebound phase (see Fig. 230-6).[3] Therefore, for accurate determination of dialyzer clearance (expressed as single-pool or spKt/V) with the single-pool model, the method for drawing the postdialysis blood sample must be consistent and timed to avoid errors due to access recirculation and cardiopulmonary recirculation.[26] The method recommended by the National Kidney Foundation's Kidney Disease Outcomes Quality Initiative (KDOQI) is to slow the blood pump to 100 mL/min for 10 seconds, then stop the pump and draw the sample.[27]

To partially account for the effect of rebound, single-pool Kt/V has been modified to use the equilibrated postdialysis BUN value instead of the immediate postdialysis BUN.[28-30] The resulting equilibrated Kt/V (eKt/V) is proposed as a more accurate measure of the effect of dialysis in the patient (patient clearance). Further modifications have sought to develop an expression of intermittent dialysis that would describe its effect as if it were given continuously, a continuous equivalent clearance, or continuous equivalent Kt/V.[31-33] A widely used version, called standard Kt/V (stdKt/V), expresses Kt/V as a weekly clearance that would produce average predialysis urea concentrations identical to the constant concentration produced by a continuous clearance of the same magnitude.[33] When expressed as a continuous equivalent clearance, the dose is theoretically independent of the frequency or duration of dialysis, thus facilitating the comparison of outcomes in patients dialyzed more versus less frequently or undergoing short versus long treatment times.

MINIMUM DOSE, FREQUENCY, AND TREATMENT TIME

In the setting of chronic renal failure, hemodialysis is an extremely effective therapy that has an impressive potential for preserving life almost indefinitely despite total loss of a vital organ. Extensive outcome studies have established a dose ceiling below which patient outcome is coupled with the dose, and above which no additional improvement in measurable parameters of outcome, including hospitalization and mortality rates, can be discerned in population studies.[6,34] In the setting of acute renal failure, in which patients are often anuric, it is logical to expect that the same minimal doses should apply.[4] However, compromises due to patient intolerance of dialysis, interruptions by the need to perform other procedures, clotting in the dialyzer from withholding heparin, and dysequilibrium in the patient have resulted in doses in the ICU that are often lower than doses considered adequate for outpatient therapy (see Fig. 230-1).[2,24] It is clear that the standard "3/3" approach—3 hours three times weekly—is inadequate for most patients in the ICU.[35] For patients dialyzed more frequently or continuously, several outcome studies suggest that a higher weekly dose improves survival (see Chapter 264). In addition, extrapolations based on small solute kinetics at lower frequencies suggest that more frequent dialysis provides better solute control, lower levels in the patient, and an expected improvement in outcome.[27,33,36,37] These analyses also suggest that once dialysis frequency is increased, the ceiling of responsiveness rises, and extending the treatment time provides further benefit that is not evident when the frequency is limited to three treatments per week.[36,38]

PATIENT SIZE AND UREA VOLUME: IMPEDIMENTS TO DIALYSIS?

Total body water is a mathematically convenient denominator but it may not be appropriate, especially because body surface area is more widely recognized as the appropriate denominator to normalize native kidney function and other physiological functions.[39,40] The concentration of uremic toxins in body fluids is thought to modulate toxicity and, therefore, the need for dialysis, but for first-order processes, the concentration is a function of generation and removal and does not depend on the space of distribution. For a patient whose clearance (K) is constant, and whose toxin generation rate (G) is equal to the removal rate, changes in the volume of distribution (V) have no effect on concentration in the steady state, or:

$$C = \frac{G}{K}$$

For example, an increase in V from edema formation or a decline in V from muscle loss would not affect toxin concentrations after equilibrium is reached if all else remains constant. Larger animals and larger people logically require larger kidneys and more dialysis, not because of larger V but because of higher G. In general, patients receiving intensive care have expanded extracellular volumes.[41,42] But accumulation of edema fluid or expansion of the urea space[43] is unlikely to affect G, so patients in the ICU with expanded extracellular volumes should not require more dialysis for purposes of solute removal.

HEMODIALYSIS VERSUS HEMOFILTRATION

Convective clearance by hemofiltration is discussed in more detail in Chapters 283 and 286. For purposes of adequacy testing, however, if hemofiltration is applied intermittently with either prefilter or postfilter dilution, the method of measuring adequacy is similar to that for hemodialysis. Measurements of BUN before and after treatment provide the input for urea modeling to assess the adequacy of small solute removal. In addition to urea and other small solutes, attention is often directed to larger solutes that hemofiltration has the potential to remove more efficiently than hemodialysis. However, one must recall that diffusive clearance remains the major transport mechanism within the patient regardless of the method of removing solute in the extracorporeal circuit (see Fig. 230-5). Consequently, increasing the intensity of removal by using a larger dialyzer, a larger filter, a more permeable filter or higher flow rates can have significant limitations.[36] Ward and colleagues[44] showed that a sevenfold increase in extracorporeal clearance had only a modest effect on β_2-microglobulin removal and solute levels in patients when treatment was administered three times weekly.[44] However, levels fell significantly when the same dose was administered more frequently. To make more effective use of devices that clear larger, poorly diffusible substances, the frequency of treatments must increase, followed by an increase in treatment time; the former must precede the latter.

ACCOUNTING FOR RESIDUAL CLEARANCE

Logically, if the patient's native kidneys clear small solutes, their clearance (K_r) should be added to the dialyzer clearance (K_d) during treatment. No objections to this addition have been raised, but methods differ for assessing the continuous clearance afforded by the native kidneys between treatments. Because a continuous clearance removes solute more efficiently than an intermittent clearance (see preceding discussion), simple addition of $K_d \times t_d$ to $K_r \times t_i$ underestimates the effect of the native kidney (t_d being the time of treatment and t_i the interdialysis time).

Two methods for resolving this inequity have been proposed. The first and original method is an inflation of the native kidney clearance prior to adding $K_r \times t_i$.[45] The result is a dialyzer equivalent clearance that, if provided by the dialyzer alone, would result in approximately the same solute concentrations. More recently, the continuous equivalent of intermittent clearance (see standard Kt/V, discussed previously) has been used as a measure of dialysis. Because stdKt/V can be treated as a continuous clearance, residual kidney clearance can be added to it directly. For example, if stdKt/V is 2.0/week, and K_r(urea) is 3 mL/min in a 35-liter patient, the combined stdKt/V is calculated as follows:

$$2.0/\text{week} + (3 \text{ mL/min}) \times \frac{10,080 \text{ min/week}}{35,000 \text{ mL}} = 2.9/\text{week}$$

DRUG DOSING DURING AND BETWEEN TREATMENTS

Intermittent treatments are often intense, achieving high clearance rates for urea and other small solutes, especially when the frequency is limited to three treatments per week. Because drugs given intravenously may achieve high initial plasma concentrations, infusions are usually restricted to the interval between dialysis treatments or are given near the end of the treatment to avoid losses through the dialyzer.[46] If plasma protein binding is not limiting, removal during dialysis can be accelerated, requiring a supplemental dose after or during the treatment.[47,48] Documents supplied by the pharmaceutical company usually indicate when such supplements are required. Significant rebound in plasma concentrations can be expected for most drugs, so blood samples taken immediately after dialysis may give falsely low trough concentrations (e.g., gentamicin).[49] Waiting a variable time, usually 30 to 60 minutes, after dialysis results in higher, more representative drug concentrations. Drugs that depend on renal function for elimination can be expected to have prolonged half-lives between treatments similar to those in patients with advanced renal failure that does not yet require dialysis (stage 4 chronic kidney disease).

SIMPLIFIED METHODS

To circumvent the need for complex mathematical programs and equipment and to provide tools for quick bedside estimates, simplified approaches to urea modeling have been developed to calculate Kt/V, eKt/V, and nPCR.[28,50,51] The most commonly used is the Daugirdas formula for calculating Kt/V, as follows[28]:

$$Kt/V = -\ln(R - 0.03) + (4 - 3.5R)UF/W \qquad [7]$$

where R is the ratio of postdialysis/predialysis BUN, UF is the total ultrafiltrate volume in liters/dialysis, and W is the patient's weight in kilograms. The equilibrated Kt/V (see eKt/V discussed previously) can be calculated from spKt/V by means of one of several formulas, each of which gives a result that is only slightly different from the others.[28-30] The first formula of this type was developed and validated during the recent National Institutes of Health–sponsored HEMO Study. Called the "rate equation" because it is based on the rate or intensity of dialysis (K/V), this formula is as follows[28]:

$$eKt/V = spKt/V - 0.6\ K/V + 0.03 \qquad [8]$$

These two equations (7 and 8) were developed for treatments given three times weekly and should not be applied to treatments given more frequently. For more frequent dialysis, the following simplified approach to calculating standard Kt/V (see stdKt/V discussed previously), using spKt/V, eKt/V, frequency (N per week), and treatment time (t), has been proposed[30,33]:

$$stdKt/V = \frac{10{,}080\dfrac{1 - e^{-eKt/V}}{t}}{\dfrac{1 - e^{-eKt/V}}{spKt/V} + \dfrac{10{,}080}{Nt} - 1} \qquad [9]$$

This formula assumes a symmetrical week (i.e., that the time intervals between each dialysis treatment are equal). The formula has not been thoroughly tested but at present is the simplest available.

OTHER BENCHMARKS OF ADEQUACY

Replacement of kidney function entails more than renal excretory function. Physiologists have taught us for several decades that the kidney's responsibility is to maintain the integrity of the internal milieu. Although excretion is a major part of that job, control of electrolyte concentrations, acid-base balance, and calcium-phosphate-magnesium balance must be included. Replacement of renal hormones cannot be ignored, and control of water volume is critical, especially in patients with multiple-organ dysfunction, as

discussed in Chapter 263. Experience in the outpatient clinic has shown, with respect to small solute control, that renal replacement therapy should be considered only barely adequate. It prevents immediate death from uremia but leaves the patient susceptible to cardiovascular disease, infection, and other complications that are reflected in the high yearly mortality rates. Rates of mortality in patients undergoing dialysis in the ICU are even higher than in outpatients and than in patients in the ICU who do not have kidney failure, suggesting that renal replacement therapy is incomplete. Experience with more frequent and continuous replacement techniques is encouraging, and renal hormone replacement has markedly improved the tolerance of dialysis and has reduced mortality. Additional efforts are needed to search for other renal factors that require replacement and to examine the role of poorly dialyzed larger solutes (e.g., polypeptides) and protein-bound solutes.

CONCLUSION

While considering all the known and unknown risks affecting survival in critically ill patients, the nephrologist must remember that for patients requiring renal replacement therapy in the ICU, his or her primary responsibility is to maintain low concentrations of uremic toxins in patients by ensuring adequate removal of small solutes. Other issues must also be addressed, but the primary focus must be on solute removal. Each patient is different, so the clinician must tailor renal replacement therapy to the individual patient's needs, making adjustments in the timing, frequency, duration, flow rates, and other parameters to fit, keeping in mind the dictum to first do no harm, and remembering that the prescribed dose of dialysis is often lower than the dose ultimately delivered to the patient.[2,24]

Key Points

1. Solute removal is the major goal of renal replacement therapy.
2. Rapid changes in solute concentrations caused by intermittent renal replacement therapy provide an opportunity to easily measure the replacement dose as well as the patient's solute generation rate and volume of distribution.
3. Dysequilibrium within the patient limits the efficiency of intermittent renal replacement therapy.
4. Increasing the frequency of renal replacement therapy theoretically raises its ceiling of effectiveness and increases the benefits from extending treatment time.
5. The primary responsibility of clinicians managing the patient who has lost kidney function is to maintain low levels of toxic solutes in the patient.

See the companion Expert Consult website for the complete reference list.

CHAPTER 231

Assessment of Fluid Status and Body Composition and Control of Fluid Balance with Intermittent Hemodialysis in the Critically Ill Patient

Peter Kotanko

OBJECTIVES

This chapter will:
1. Discuss body composition in health and disease.
2. Describe the evaluation of body composition and fluid status.
3. Consider intermittent hemodialysis in the critically ill patient for control of fluid balance and prevention of intradialytic hypotension.

BODY COMPOSITION IN HEALTH AND DISEASE

Body composition can be viewed from five perspectives—atomic, molecular, cellular, tissue, and whole body levels.[1] At the atomic level, six elements form 98% of the body mass: 61% oxygen, 23% carbon, 10% hydrogen, 2.6% nitrogen, and 1.4% calcium; 2% of the mass consists of 44 other elements.

More than 100,000 distinct molecules constitute the molecular composition, ranging from simple molecules such as water to highly complex ones such as lipids and proteins. Water, which accounts for about 60% of a 70-kg "reference male" and about 50% of a "reference female," is thus the major chemical component of the body and essential for the interior milieu. The total body water (TBW) is distributed between two major compartments, the intracellular volume (ICV) and the extracellular volume (ECV); the latter can be divided into the interstitial compartment, which constitutes the extracellular environment of the cells, and the vascular space. Body fat depends heavily on nutrition and training status, ranging from less than 10% to more than 50%. Protein and minerals account for 15% and 5% of body composition, respectively. The 10^{18} cells forming the cellular body composition domain can be divided into connective tissue cells (fat cells, blood cells, bone cells), epithelial cells, neural cells, and muscle cells. In terms of tissue composition, bone, adipose tissue, and muscle make up 75% of body weight. The *lean body mass* is the mass of the body minus the fat mass (storage lipid).

In healthy adults, body composition is maintained over the short term within narrow limits. Gender, age, race,

nutrition, physical activity, and hormonal status are the main determinants of body composition. Illness may have a significant effect on body composition with malnutrition being a major complication. Malnutrition, which develops when nutritional intake falls short of nutritional requirements, leads to organ dysfunction, reduced body cell mass, abnormal blood chemistry, and worsened clinical outcomes.[2] Critically ill patients in particular are prone to malnutrition and consecutive unfavorable alterations in body composition. Malnutrition is frequently observed in patients regardless of type of illness.[3] In critically ill patients, hypermetabolism is caused by an activation of the sympathetic nervous system and the pituitary-adrenal axis, resulting in high plasma levels of catecholamines, adrenocorticotropic hormone, growth hormone, and cortisol. These metabolic adaptations contribute to protein-calorie malnutrition (defined as a negative balance of 100 g nitrogen and 10,000 kcal within a few days). Assessment of nutritional status and body composition in the critically ill patient is of major importance and guides adequate and aggressive nutritional support.

EVALUATION OF FLUID STATUS AND BODY COMPOSITION

The assessment of fluid status, body composition, and nutritional status is in most instances performed in a subjective manner by experienced health care workers. The fluid status can be clinically judged (with well-known pitfalls) from the presence or absence of edema, the skin turgor, jugular venous pressure, predialysis blood pressure, and changes in blood pressure and heart rate during dialysis. Imaging techniques such as chest radiography, ultrasonography to delineate the diameter of the inferior vena cava (IVC), and echocardiography may yield additional important information. Bioimpedance techniques are capable of providing an integrative view of body composition.

Anthropometric models have been developed to estimate body composition (see Tables 231-1 and 231-2 for a summary of anthropometric algorithms; see www.medal.org). The anthropometric models are straightforward to apply but are not well validated in the dialysis population.

TABLE 231-1

Anthropometric Algorithms

DOMAIN	MODEL
TBW (males > 16 years) in L [Hume and Weyers]	$(0.194786 \times [\text{height in cm}]) + (0.296785 \times [\text{weight in kg}]) - 14.012934$
TBW (females > 16 years) in L [Hume and Weyers]	$(0.344547 \times [\text{height in cm}]) + (0.183809 \times [\text{weight in kg}]) - 35.270121$
TBW (males) in L [Watson]	$(-0.09516 \times [\text{age in years}]) + (0.1074 \times [\text{height in cm}]) + (0.3362 \times [\text{weight in kg}]) + 2.447$
TBW (females) in L [Watson]	$(0.1069 \times [\text{height in cm}]) + (0.2466 \times [\text{weight in kg}]) - 2.097$
LBM (males > 16 years) in kg [Hume and Weyers]	$(0.32810 \times [\text{body weight in kg}]) + (0.33929 \times [\text{height in cm}]) - 29.5336$
LBM (adult males) in kg [Boer]	$(0.407 \times [\text{body weight in kg}]) + (26.7 \times [\text{height in m}]) - 19.2$
LBM (females > 30 years) in kg [Hume and Weyers]	$(0.29569 \times [\text{body weight in kg}]) + (0.41813 \times [\text{height in cm}]) - 43.2933$
LBM (adult females) in kg [Boer]	$(0.252 \times [\text{body weight in kg}]) + (47.3 \times [\text{height in m}]) - 48.3$
LBM (males) in kg [James]	$(1.10 \times [\text{body weight in kg}]) - (128 \times ([\text{body weight in kg}]^2)/(\text{body height in cm}^2)$
LBM (females) in kg [James]	$(1.07 \times [\text{body weight in kg}]) - \left(148 \times \dfrac{[\text{body weight in kg}]^2}{[\text{body height in cm}]^2} \right)$
Corrected arm muscle area in cm² [Heymsfield]	$\left(\dfrac{(\text{Midarm circumference in cm}) - (\pi \times [\text{triceps skinfold thickness in cm}])^2}{4 \times \pi} \right)$ $- (\text{gender factor for bone area})$ Gender factor = 10 in males and 6.5 in females
Total body muscle mass in kg [Heymsfield]	$(\text{height in cm}) \times (0.0264 + [0.0029 \times (\text{CAMA})])$

CAMA, corrected arm muscle area.
Data from medal.org. Available at www.medal.org. Accessed September 30, 2008.

TABLE 231-2

Anthropometric Models to Estimate Extracellular Volume and Intracellular Volume

GENDER	PARAMETER*	EXTRACELLULAR VOLUME (L)	INTRACELLULAR VOLUME (L)
Male	Height in m	$9.78 \times \text{height}$	$7.92 \times \text{height}$
	Weight in kg	$0.245 \times \text{weight}$	$0.198 \times \text{weight}$
	BSA in m²	$9.22 \times \text{BSA}$	$7.45 \times \text{BSA}$
	LBM in kg	$0.303 \times \text{LBM}$	$0.244 \times \text{LBM}$
Female	Height in m	$8.44 \times \text{height}$	$7.04 \times \text{height}$
	Weight in kg	$0.220 \times \text{weight}$	$0.186 \times \text{weight}$
	BSA in m²	$8.18 \times \text{BSA}$	$6.84 \times \text{BSA}$
	LBM in kg	$0.302 \times \text{LBM}$	$0.248 \times \text{LBM}$
Both	LBM in kg	$0.3027 \times \text{LBM}$	$0.2456 \times \text{LBM}$

BSA, body surface area; LBM, lean body mass.
*LBM is computed with Boer's equation (see Table 231-1).
Data from medal.org. Available at www.medal.org. Accessed September 30, 2008.

Ultrasonography is frequently used as a bedside tool to assess fluid status, and several indices related to IVC measures have been proposed (Table 231-3). The indexed vena cava diameter (VCDi) is calculated as follows:

$$\text{VCDi} = \frac{\text{maximal IVC diameter (IVCmax)}}{\text{body surface area (in m}^2)}$$

The IVC collapsibility index (IVCCI) is computed as follows:

$$\text{IVCCI}(\%) = \left[\frac{\text{IVCmax} - \text{IVCmin}}{\text{IVCmax}} \right] \times 100$$

These indices can be easily determined[4] and are a feasible option for rapid assessment of intravascular volume status in an outpatient dialysis setting by operators with limited formal training in ultrasonography, but there is a poor relationship between dry weight goals and IVC collapsibility. Echocardiography is useful in determining volume status measures in addition to cardiac indices.

Biochemical markers, most prominently natriuretic peptides, have been advocated as noninvasive means to determine hydration status, but the levels of brain natriuretic peptide (BNP) correlate poorly with volume status.[5]

Bioimpedance analysis (BIA) is increasingly used in patients undergoing dialysis and in critically ill patients[6] to determine TBW, ECV, ICV, and other aspects of body composition. Body composition analysis by means of BIA has been compared to magnetic resonance imaging (MRI) analyses, and appropriate regression models have been developed to enable estimation of fat and muscle content.[7,8] Basically, impedance (Z) expresses the opposition to current flow that a system offers to injected alternating electric current; Z has two components (both expressed in ohms), resistance (R) and reactance (Xc). Resistance and

TABLE 231-3

Cutoffs for Indexed Vena Cava Diameter (VCDi) and Inferior Vena Cava Collapsibility Index (IVCCI)

VOLUME STATUS	VCDi CUTOFF (mm/m²)	IVCCI CUTOFF (%)
Hypovolemia	<8	>75
Euvolemia	≥8 and ≤11.5	≥40 and ≤75
Hypervolemia	>11.5	<40

reactance change with alternating current frequency, and an increase in frequency results in a decrease in impedance. According to current concepts, the fluid volume component is largely reflected in the resistance, and reactance represents the cell membrane, which is related to nutrition. In biological systems, lower-frequency currents travel preferentially in the extracellular space, whereas currents with higher frequencies pass through both extracellular and intracellular compartments.

With injection of multiple-frequency currents (standard range 5 kHz to 1000 kHz), ECV and ICV can be estimated, in a procedure called multifrequency bioimpedance spectroscopy (MFBIS). Single-frequency bioimpedance analysis (SFBIA) with an injection current frequency of 50 kHz has been used for many years.[9] SFBIA is simpler and easier to use than MFBIS. However, the inability to make accurate distinction between ECV and ICV is its major limitation. Different BIA approaches, such as wrist-to-ankle ("whole body") and segmental methods,[2,4,10-15] have been used to measure ECV, ICV, and TBW in patients undergoing dialysis. These studies aimed to measure hydration status and estimate dry weight by employing ratios of ECV to ICV, ECV to TBW, and ECV to body weight.[16-20]

Nutritional status relates strongly to morbidity and mortality in patients undergoing dialysis. BIA-based measurement of muscle mass and of subcutaneous and total adipose tissues can be routinely made. Body cell mass estimated by BIA is correlated with body cell mass determined by dual energy x-ray absorptiometry (DEXA), as is TBW estimated by BIA and determined by D₂O dilution.[20] Some researchers have proposed analyzing the impedance vector in the R–Xc plane to assess body composition and nutritional state according to tolerance ellipses defined in healthy subjects.[21-23] However, because patients undergoing hemodialysis have abnormal distribution of body fluid content, thus affecting resistance, the error of estimation may be significant with this approach. Therefore, segmental BIA of the arm or leg has been suggested as an alternative approach.[7,24] Kaysen and associates[7] developed a model to estimate total body muscle mass on the basis of BIA-derived ICV (Table 231-4), which was as precise as methods based on total (40)K counting, a measure of body cell mass.

INTERMITTENT HEMODIALYSIS IN THE CRITICALLY ILL PATIENT: CONTROL OF FLUID BALANCE AND PREVENTION OF INTRADIALYTIC HYPOTENSION

Removal of uremic toxins and excessive fluid are the main goals of renal replacement therapy. In contrast to continuous techniques such as continuous venovenous hemofil-

TABLE 231-4

Body Composition Analysis Based on Bioimpedance

TISSUE	MODEL
Fat-free mass in kg [Deurenberg]	$(0.671 \times (10^4) \times \dfrac{(\text{height in m})^2}{\text{resistance in ohms}} + (3.1 \times (\text{gender value})) + 3.9$
	Gender value = 0 if female, 1 if male
Total body water (hemodialysis patients) in kg [Chertow]	$(-0.07493713 \times (\text{age})) - (1.01767992 \times (\text{points for gender})) + (0.12703384 \times (\text{height})) - (0.04012056 \times (\text{weight})) + (0.57894981 \times (\text{points for diabetes})) - (0.00067247 \times (\text{weight}) \times (\text{weight})) - (0.03486146 \times (\text{age}) \times (\text{points for gender})) + (0.11262857 \times (\text{points for gender}) \times (\text{weight})) + (0.00104135 \times (\text{age}) \times (\text{weight})) + (0.00186104 \times (\text{height}) \times (\text{weight}))$
	Height in cm; weight in kg; age in years
	Gender point = 0 if female, 1 if male
	Diabetes point = 1 if diabetic, 0 if not
Total body muscle mass in kg [Kaysen]	$9.52 + 0.331 \times$ ICV (by BIS; in mL) $+ 2.77$ (male; 0 if female) $+ 0.180 \times$ weight (kg) $- 0.133 \times$ age (in years)
Fat-free mass (in kg) [Chumlea]:	
Males	$-10.68 + \dfrac{0.65 \times \text{height (in cm)}^2}{\text{resistance (in ohm)}} + 0.26 \times$ weight (in kg) $+ 0.02 \times$ resistance (in ohm)
Females	$-9.53 + \dfrac{0.69 \times \text{height (in cm)}^2}{\text{resistance (in ohm)}} + 0.17 \times$ weight (in kg) $+ 0.02 \times$ resistance (in ohm)

BIS, bioimpedance spectroscopy; ICV, intracellular volume
Data from medal.org. Available at www.medal.org. Accessed September 30, 2008.

tration, removal of fluid with intermittent hemodialysis is frequently limited by hemodynamic instability, which manifests in most circumstances as intradialytic hypotension (IDH). IDH and orthostatic hypotension after hemodialysis are independent predictors of mortality in patients undergoing hemodialysis.[25]

IDH is the most common intradialytic problem, with an incidence of 5% to 40% of treatments depending on the definition of this complication, which varies from an asymptomatic percentage fall in systolic blood pressure to symptomatic hypotension requiring active treatment. Females, elderly patients with isolated systolic hypertension, diabetic patients, and patients with autonomic neuropathy are at increased risk. In healthy subjects, blood pressure is maintained after removal of as much as 30% of the blood volume. In the dialysis population, however, the combination of autonomic dysfunction, ventricular dysfunction and decreased venous return, and increased body temperature impairs the body's ability to cope with the hemodynamic stress caused by ultrafiltration.

Major factors determining the hemodynamic response are the ultrafiltration rate, the plasma refilling rate, and their instantaneous difference. The *plasma refilling rate* is the unit per time difference between filtration and absorption of plasma water in the capillary bed plus the lymphatic flow. Fluid dynamics in the capillary are governed by Starling forces, with the plasma oncotic pressure as a main absorptive factor.

The threat of IDH can be reduced by reduction of the ultrafiltration rate (through reduction of the interdialytic weight gain and, thus, the ultrafiltration volume and/or prolongation of ultrafiltration time) and by support of the body's ability to deal with the hemodynamic challenges caused by ultrafiltration—through improving vasoconstriction, treating congestive heart failure, or raising the serum albumin concentration.

Diastolic dysfunction results from impaired myocardial relaxation and reduced distensibility of the left ventricle. Systolic dysfunction is in most cases due to myocardial ischemia from coronary artery disease. Autonomic neuropathy is common in diabetic patients. Therapy with drugs that interfere with vasoconstriction and other hemodynamic responses to ultrafiltration should be avoided immediately before or during hemodialysis.

Raising the dialysate sodium concentration to 150 mmol/L at the beginning of treatment is effective in reducing the chance of episodes of hypotension and maintaining blood pressure, but the price paid consists of increases in interdialytic weight gain and blood pressure as well as aggravation of the problems of overhydration.

Reduction of interdialytic weight gain with a low-salt diet (3 g/day) is an important preventive measure for IDH. Iatrogenic salt loading results from high dialysate sodium concentration or from application of intravenous saline solutions during dialysis.

Monitoring of relative changes in blood volume with a blood volume monitor helps estimate plasma refilling rate in relationship to ultrafiltration rate. A drop in blood volume greater than 15% during a hemodialysis session sharply raises the risk of IDH. On the other hand, IDH is unusual with a drop in blood volume smaller than 5%. An unchanged blood volume despite ongoing ultrafiltration suggests overhydration.

Maggiore and colleagues[21] first reported the beneficial effects of cooling dialysate on systematic hypotensive episodes during dialysis. A systematic review of the current literature on this issue concluded that reducing dialysate fluid temperature reduces IDH frequency by a factor of 7.1 and that postdialysis mean arterial pressure was 11.3 mm Hg higher with cool-temperature dialysis.[26] There may be an advantage in maintaining or reducing the core temperature with an automated feedback device (BTM, Fresenius Medical Care, Homburg, Germany) rather than making arbitrary reductions of dialysate temperature. Investigators in major randomized European trials concluded that active control of body temperature with an automated feedback device can significantly improve intradialytic tolerance in hypotension-prone patients, reporting a 50% reduction in rate of hypotensive episodes[27]

Midodrine, an α_1-adrenergic receptor agonist, administered 30 minutes (5 mg orally) before the dialysis session improves intradialytic blood pressure. This agent should be used cautiously in patients who have congestive heart failure or who are taking beta-blockers, digoxin, or a non-dihydropyridine calcium channel blocker.

Symptomatic IDH should be treated promptly through reduction of ultrafiltration rate and changing the patient to the Trendelenburg position; resistant IDH should be treated with 200 to 500 mL saline. If severe IDH persists, an extended investigation including physical examination, electrocardiogram, emergency echocardiography, and laboratory studies is warranted. Arrhythmia, myocardial infarction, pericardial tamponade, hemorrhage, hemolysis, pulmonary embolism, and air embolism should be considered in the differential diagnosis. K/DOQI guidelines on the evaluation and treatment of IDH are available.[28]

Key Points

1. Knowledge of body composition is of paramount importance in the care of critically ill patients.
2. Fluid status and nutritional condition can be delineated by clinical, anthropometric, biochemical, imaging, and bioimpedance means.
3. Body composition can reliably be assessed by bioimpedance techniques.
4. Reducing interdialytic weight gain is the cornerstone in the prevention of intradialytic hypotension (IDH). Cool dialysate is of proven benefit in IDH prone patients.

Key References

1. Wang ZM, Pierson RN Jr, Heymsfield SB: The five-level model: A new approach to organizing body-composition research. Am J Clin Nutr 1992;56:19-28.
2. Cerra FB, Benitez MR, Blackburn GL, et al: Applied nutrition in ICU patients: A consensus statement of the American College of Chest Physicians. Chest 1997;111:769-778.
3. Weinsier RL, Hunker EM, Krumdieck CL, Butterworth CE Jr: Hospital malnutrition: A prospective evaluation of general medical patients during the course of hospitalization. Am J Clin Nutr 1979;32:418-426.
11. Zaluska WT, Schneditz D, Kaufman AM, et al: Relative underestimation of fluid removal during hemodialysis hypotension measured by whole body bioimpedance. ASAIO J 1998;44:823-827.
14. Donadio C, Consani C, Ardini M, et al: Estimate of body water compartments and of body composition in maintenance hemodialysis patients: Comparison of single and multifrequency bioimpedance analysis. J Ren Nutr 2005;15:332-344.
26. Selby NM, McIntyre CW: A systematic review of the clinical effects of reducing dialysate fluid temperature. Nephrol Dial Transplant 2006;21:1883-1898.

See the companion Expert Consult website for the complete reference list.

CHAPTER 232

Outcome of Intermittent Dialysis in Critically Ill Patients with Acute Renal Failure

Norbert Lameire, Wim Van Biesen, Eric A. J. Hoste, and Raymond Vanholder

---

OBJECTIVES

This chapter will:
1. Summarize the comparative studies of intermittent hemodialysis and continuous renal replacement therapy and their effects on survival of patients with acute renal failure.
2. Compare the effects of intermittent hemodialysis and continuous renal replacement therapy on renal outcome.
3. Discuss some particular problems associated with intermittent hemodialysis (membrane biocompatibility, anticoagulation, vascular access).

In the absence of a universally accepted definition for *acute renal failure* (ARF), and with the recognition that ARF actually comprises a spectrum of clinical conditions, from subclinical injury to complete failure of the organ, the Acute Kidney Injury Network (AKIN) group has recommended using the term *acute kidney injury* to reflect the entire spectrum of the syndrome.[1] The term acute kidney injury (AKI) is thus proposed to apply in all patients with an acute injury to the kidney, irrespective of a concomitant decrease in glomerular filtration rate (GFR), whereas the term acute renal failure (ARF) should be reserved for dialysis-requiring AKI. Consequently, this chapter continues to use the term ARF.

Administrative databases indicate that the overall incidence rate of ARF is rising by approximately 11% per year.[2] The disease certainly has a negative impact on overall hospital mortality; in a study of discharge documents for Medicare beneficiaries from 1992 to 2001, Xue and colleagues[2] found the overall in-hospital death rate to be 4.6% in patients without ARF, 15.2% in those for whom ARF was the principal diagnosis, and 32.6% in those for whom ARF was a secondary diagnosis. In-hospital death rates were 32.9% in patients with ARF that required dialysis and 27.5% in those with ARF that did not require dialysis. These data show ARF to be a major contributor to morbidity and mortality in hospitalized patients.

ARF is a common complication in the critically ill patient admitted to the intensive care unit (ICU), in whom it is also associated with greater morbidity, greater mortality, and higher health care costs.[3] Although a portion of the death rate is directly related to the seriousness of the patients' underlying illnesses, multiple studies have demonstrated that ARF in the ICU poses an independent risk for death.[3]

Data on the mortality of critically ill ARF patients is conflicting. Some studies report unchanged mortality for ARF patients treated in ICUs over the last several decades,[4] but another study reports that the overall mortality for these patients, whether or not they undergo dialysis, is declining.[5] The last study is based on administrative coding on hospital discharge documents and was not limited to patients receiving intensive care.

Several dialysis modalities have been applied and have been mutually compared as treatment of critically ill patients with ARF.[6-9] This chapter summarizes the different outcome trials comparing intermittent hemodialysis (IHD) and continuous renal replacement therapies (CRRTs) in the critically ill patient with ARF.

For sake of clarity, the intermittent character of hemodialysis is considered only if the dialysis session is not longer than the "classic" 4 to 5 hours; the sustained low-efficiency daily dialysis (SLEDD) techniques, a hybrid form of CRRT and intermittent dialysis, is not included in this analysis. This modality is discussed in other chapters and has been summarized in other studies.[7,10]

CONTINUOUS RENAL REPLACEMENT THERAPY VERSUS INTERMITTENT HEMODIALYSIS

Although the most obvious difference between the two modalities is the time span over which they are applied (4-5 hours versus, theoretically, 24 hours), some other technical differences may be more relevant. IHD is performed as a highly efficient technique, relying mainly on diffusion and thus necessitating high dialysate flow rates to maintain high concentration gradients. CRRT is mostly performed as a low-efficiency technique, relies mainly on convection, and implies the need for sterile substitution fluids. Consequently, a water treatment system and a dialysis monitor are mandatory for IHD, whereas CRRT can in principle be performed with simpler hardware. These technical peculiarities imply also that an IHD machine can be programmed to perform continuous therapy but that a CRRT machine cannot be used to perform intermittent treatment, because the low-efficiency nature of the setup necessitates prolonged treatment duration to achieve adequacy goals. To enhance efficiency, CRRT has evolved from continuous arteriovenous hemofiltration, without a blood pump, to high-volume continuous venovenous hemofiltration (CVVH) or continuous venovenous hemodiafiltration (CVVHDF), involving the application of sophisticated blood pumps and fluid balance systems equilibrating hemofiltered and substituted fluids. The initial technical simplicity that was the major advantage of CRRT is lost with this evolution.

In addition, intermittent modalities require a shorter duration of anticoagulation or even no anticoagulation, whereas continuous forms need longer exposure to anticoagulating agents. Hence, the evolution to hybrid therapies, whereby IHD machines are used to perform extended treatments, is a logical next step.

TIMING OF INITIATION OF RENAL REPLACEMENT THERAPY

A 2006 review by Palevsky[8] concluded that there are at present inadequate data to enable definitive recommendations to be made as to the optimal time to initiate RRT in the patient with ARF. The predominantly retrospective data from the first three decades of clinical dialysis strongly support the prophylactic initiation of dialysis before the onset of advanced uremia—in other words, treatment should be initiated by the time the blood urea nitrogen value reaches 80 to 100 mg/dL.

Evaluation of this issue with an appropriately powered, randomized controlled trial is obviously needed. One study compared the relationship between urine volume at the time of initiation of IHD and mortality in patients with ARF.[11] Although oliguria is well established as a predictor of mortality in ARF, this study found that hospital mortality was independently associated with a higher urine volume at the time of initiation of IHD. Higher urine volume was also independently associated with increased time to initiation of dialysis. The investigators of the study speculate that physician bias toward later initiation of dialysis in nonoliguric ARF may have contributed to the reversal of the usual mortality benefit associated with nonoliguric state. Interpretation of these data must take into account the highly selected population involved in the study, which excluded patients who did not survive at least 7 days after initiation of dialysis, did not receive at least three dialysis sessions in the first week of treatment, or underwent treatment modalities other than IHD.

DOSE OF DIALYSIS

An analysis of the effects of dose of dialysis on outcome of ARF patients has summarized the numerous difficulties related to this problem.[12] The dose requirement in ARF depends on the catabolic state, patient size, desired level of metabolic control, and volume status. It is well known that in critically ill patients suffering from ARF, classic measures of dialysis dose such as the clearance for urea (Kt/V_{urea}) are not as suitable as in patients undergoing long-term dialysis. In addition, "prescribed dose" is sometimes substantially different from "delivered dose."[13] Dialysis dose can be increased in several ways: lengthening treatment time (e.g., extended daily dialysis), increasing treatment frequency (e.g., daily dialysis), or using CRRT (e.g., CVVH or CVVHDF).

In a small group of patients, Gillum and colleagues[14] found no survival advantage to intensive dialysis (BUN < 60 mg/dL, serum creatinine < 5 mg/dL, usually daily 5-6 hours of IHD) over nonintensive dialysis (BUN < 100 mg/dL, serum creatinine < 9 mg/dL, 5 hours of IHD every third day). This study did not stratify patients according to disease severity but did match them for cause of ARF.

In contrast, Paganini and associates[15] retrospectively evaluated 844 patients with ARF requiring CRRT or IHD who were treated in their institution over a 7-year period. When patients were classified according to disease severity, dialysis dose did not affect outcome in patients with very high or very low scores but did correlate with survival in patients with intermediate degrees of illness. A mean Kt/V_{urea} greater than 1.0 with IHD or time-averaged concentration of urea (TAC_{urea}) less than 45 mg/dL with CRRT was associated with longer survival.

Schiffl and coworkers[16] found that daily IHD was associated with fewer dialysis-related complications, a shorter time to renal recovery, and a significantly lower mortality than alternate-day IHD (28% vs. 46%, respectively). A criticism of this article, however, highlights the fact that patients in the conventional group may have received inadequate dialysis.[17]

OUTCOME STUDIES COMPARING INTERMITTENT HEMODIALYSIS AND CONTINUOUS RENAL REPLACEMENT THERAPIES IN ACUTE RENAL FAILURE

The majority of studies comparing IHD and CRRT have been nonrandomized or retrospective case series in which analysis is confounded by variations in disease severity between study groups. Many of these studies have been reviewed earlier.[18] In an attempt to mitigate this confounding, Swartz and colleagues[19] used multivariate regression analysis to adjust for severity of illness in 349 patients. Although univariate analysis demonstrated an odds ratio for death associated with CRRT more than double that associated with IHD, the odds ratio yielded by multivariate risk analysis was 1.09 for CRRT compared with IHD.

The same study group[20] attempted to perform a better comparative study of survival with CRRT and IHD. They performed multivariable Cox proportional hazards regression to analyze the impact of dialysis modality choice (CRRT vs. IHD) on in-hospital and 100-day mortality rates among patients with ARF receiving RRT during 2000 and 2001; these researchers used an "intent-to-treat" analysis adjusted for multiple comorbidity and severity factors. The overall in-hospital mortality before adjustment was 52%. Assignment by triage to CRRT was associated with higher severity and unadjusted relative risk (RR) of in-hospital death of 1.62. Adjustment for comorbidity and severity of illness reduced the RR of death for patients triaged to CRRT and suggested a possible survival advantage (RR = 0.81). Analysis restricted to patients in the ICU for more than 5 days and receiving at least 48 hours of total RRT showed the RR of in-hospital mortality with CRRT to be nearly 45% lower than that for patients receiving IHD (RR = 0.56), a difference that indicates a strong trend for lower in-hospital mortality for CRRT. Analysis of the 100-day mortality also suggested a potential survival advantage for CRRT in all cohorts, particularly among patients who were treated in the ICU for more than 5 days and who received at least 48 hours of RRT.

A prospective multicenter observational study reported an unadjusted mortality of 79% in patients treated with CRRT, compared with 59% in patients treated with IHD. After adjustments were made for other clinical factors, however, the modality of dialysis was not independently associated with survival.[21]

A retrospective study from South Korea compared outcomes in critically ill patients with ARF managed with either IHD or CVVHDF.[22] Overall survival was 46% with IHD and 21% with CVVHDF. However, as in many other studies, CVVHDF was utilized in more severely ill patients with a higher number of failed organs and higher initial Acute Physiology and Chronic Health Evaluation (APACHE) III scores. The investigators concluded that CVVHDF may give a chance of survival to patients with APACHE III scores higher than 103 and may be more useful than IHD in patients with failure of three or fewer organs, but that the trend toward better survival was not statistically significant.

Few prospective randomized studies comparing IHD and CRRT have been published in peer-reviewed journals. Mehta and associates[23] randomly assigned 166 patients with ARF at four academic medical centers in Southern California to undergo either IHD or CRRT. In the primary intention-to-treat analysis, 28-day all-cause mortality was 60% for CRRT compared with 42% for IHD ($P < .02$). However, randomization was unbalanced, with the result that patients with significantly higher APACHE III scores and a higher prevalence of liver failure were in the CRRT group, and both of these features were independently related to mortality in the ICU setting. Adjustment for this imbalance yielded an adjusted odds ratio for death associated with CRRT of 1.58. Similarly, a time-to-event analysis using a Cox proportional hazards model demonstrated an adjusted hazard ratio associated with CRRT of 1.35.

A single-center, randomized controlled study[24] did not show differences in survival or incidence of episodes of hemodynamic instability between 52 patients receiving daily IHD and 52 patients treated with CRRT; in the latter group, 31 received a dose of 18 mL/kg/hr ultrafiltration, and 21 received a dose of 35 mL/kg/hr. Nonetheless, the dose of CRRT did not have an effect on the outcome. These patients all suffered from ARF associated with multiple-organ failure. This study, however, was not adequately powered to detect small differences between modalities.

In another single-center trial involving 80 patients randomly assigned to CVVHD or IHD, the investigators observed no difference between modalities in all-cause hospital mortality (CVVHD 68%, IHD 70%; $P > .05$) or recovery of renal function.[25] These equal outcomes were observed despite greater hemodynamic stability and more effective fluid removal in the patients treated with CVVHD. There was a significant decrease in mean arterial blood pressure in patients undergoing IHD therapy that was not seen in those undergoing CVVHD therapy. However, the study, too, was not adequately powered for survival as an endpoint.

Uehlinger and colleagues[26] randomly assigned 125 patients to treatment with either CVVHDF or IHD from a total of 191 patients with ARF in a tertiary-care university hospital ICU. Over 30 months, 66 patients were omitted from randomization for nonmedical reasons, but no patient was omitted for medical reasons. Of the 125 randomized patients, 70 were treated with CVVHDF and 55 with IHD. The two groups were comparable at the start of RRT with respect to age, gender, number of failed organ systems, Simplified Acute Physiology Score, septicemia, shock, and surgery. Mortality rates in the hospital (47% for

CVVHDF vs. 51% for IHD) or in the ICU (34% for CVVHDF vs. 38% for IHD) were independent of the technique of RRT applied. Hospital length of stay in the survivors was comparable in the two groups. The duration of RRT required was the same in the two groups. Although no evidence for a survival benefit of either modality was provided, it should be noted that this study was also inadequately powered for finding a difference. In addition, other factors—the technique of CRRT, the use of different membranes, and the absence of standardization of dialysis protocols—preclude correct interpretation of these results.

It is clear that up till 2006, many of the published prospective studies were underpowered, and the largest one, performed by Mehta and associates,[23] was flawed by unbalanced randomization. Resolution of this issue required a prospective trial designed with sufficient power to detect clinically important differences in outcomes, with a randomization strategy to ensure the absence of bias between the treatment groups. In addition, the study design needed to address the common practice of switching patients between IHD and CRRT in response to changes in hemodynamic status.

Such a study has been published by Vinsonneau and coworkers.[27] These investigators performed a prospective, randomized, multicenter study between October 1, 1999, and March 3, 2003, in 21 medical or multidisciplinary ICUs from university or community hospitals in France. Guidelines were provided to achieve optimum hemodynamic tolerance and effectiveness of solute removal in both groups. IHD was compared with CVVHDF in predilution mode and with the use of bicarbonate-based substitution solution. IHD was performed with the machine available in the center. All treatments had to be given with the same membrane polymer as in CVVHDF with a high surface area (2 m²) and bicarbonate-based dialysate. After randomization, every patient was treated with the allocated technique. Patients in the CVVHDF group could be switched to IHD (planned switch) either once multiple-organ dysfunction syndrome had resolved (defined as a logistic organ dysfunction score <5 for 3 days) or after 3 weeks of CVVHDF to allow easier management after the acute period. A change from one treatment to the other for any other reason was not allowed according to the protocol.

A total of 360 patients were involved in the study, and the primary endpoint was 60-day survival based on an intention-to-treat analysis. The survival rates (32% for IHD vs. 33% for CRRT) at 60 days and at any other time did not differ between the groups. These data suggest that, provided strict guidelines to improve tolerance and metabolic control are used, almost all patients who have ARF as part of multiple-organ dysfunction syndrome can be treated with IHD.

An editorial accompanying the publication of this study pointed out two difficulties in it; one was the perhaps hidden bias toward IHD in the study, and the second was related to the dose of dialysis applied in the IHD group.[28] A previous study by Schiffl and coworkers[16] had demonstrated that daily dialysis was associated with better outcome than alternate-day dialysis as was applied in the study by the Vinsonneau group. Vinsonneau and coworkers counteracted the editorial's argument, however, by showing that the time-averaged urea concentration in the IHD group (15.7 mmol/L) was lower than that achieved in the best group in the study reported by Schiffl and colleagues (21.7 mmol/L).

In 2006, Cho and associates[29] published their analysis of the data from the Program to Improve Care in Acute Renal

Disease (PICARD), a multicenter observational study of AKI. Among 398 patients who required dialysis, the risk for death within 60 days was examined according to assigned initial dialysis modality (CRRT vs. IHD) using standard Kaplan-Meier product limit estimates, proportional hazards (Cox) regression methods, and a propensity score approach to account for selection effects. Crude survival rates were lower for patients treated with CRRT than for those treated with IHD (survival at 30 days 45% vs. 58%, respectively; $P = .006$). After adjustments for age, hepatic failure, sepsis, thrombocytopenia, and blood urea nitrogen and serum creatinine levels and stratification by site of hemodialysis catheter insertion, the relative risk for death associated with CRRT was 1.82 (95% confidence interval [CI], 1.26 to 2.62). Further adjustment for the propensity score did not materially alter the association (RR 1.92; 95% CI, 1.28 to 2.89). Although the results could reflect residual confounding by severity of illness, these latest data provide no evidence for a survival benefit from CRRT.

Two meta-analyses have been published comparing CRRT and IHD. An analysis by Kellum and colleagues[30] reviewed 13 studies encompassing 1400 patients. Only 3 of the 13 studies were prospective, randomized studies, including the study by Mehta and associates[23] discussed previously. Overall, there was no difference in mortality (RR 0.93; 95% CI, 0.79-1.09; $P = .29$); however, the study quality was poor, and only 6 of the studies compared groups with equal baseline severity of illness. Adjusting for study quality and severity of illness, Kellum and colleagues[30] calculated a relative risk of death in patients treated with CRRT of 0.72 (95% CI, 0.60 to 0.87). In the 6 studies with a similar baseline severity of illness, the unadjusted relative risk of death with CRRT was 0.48 (95% CI, 0.34 to 0.69). These researchers concluded that, given the weakness in study quality, the evidence was insufficient to draw strong conclusions about the mode of renal support; at least, however, this analysis suggested a potential benefit of continuous over intermittent therapy.

In contrast, Tonelli and associates[31] limited their meta-analysis to six randomized controlled studies, including data from the articles by Mehta and associates[23] and Augustine and colleagues,[25] as well as data from three additional studies that had not been published in peer-reviewed journals. These researchers concluded that no survival benefit was associated with a given modality of RRT.

After publication of these studies, has the question that has been debated for so many years—which modality, intermittent or continuous RRT, is best in ARF—now been put to rest definitely? We agree with Kellum and Palevsky[28] that at least the Vinsonneau study and the data from PICARD indicate that virtually all critically ill patients with ARF can be treated with IHD and that, for the time being, no survival benefit has been demonstrated for any of the modalities.

Schortgen and colleagues[32] showed previously that adherence to specific guidelines to improve hemodynamic tolerance of IHD progressively improved the tolerance also in critically ill patients. Table 232-1 summarizes these guidelines. After implementation of these guidelines, these researchers observed fewer systolic blood pressure drops at initiation and during the IHD sessions. Although the ICU mortality rates before and after implementation of the guidelines were similar, death rate and length of ICU stay after the implementation were significantly less than predicted from SAPS II scores. Whether this approach is

TABLE 232-1

Practice Guidelines for Intermittent Hemodialysis in the Intensive Care Unit

Recommendation for systematic use	Use only modified cellulosic membranes rather than cuprophane
	Connect the two lines of the circuit, which have been filled with 0.9% saline, to the catheter simultaneously
	Set dialysate sodium concentration to ≥145 mmol/L
	Limit the maximal blood flow to 150 mL/min with a minimal session duration of 4 hrs
	Set dialysate temperature to ≤37° C
Advice for use in the most hemodynamically unstable patients	Start session with dialysis and continue with ultrafiltration alone
	Cool dialysate to 35° C
Additional recommendations	Stop vasodilator therapy
	Start dialysis session without ultrafiltration, then adapt hourly ultrafiltration rate according to hemodynamic response
	Set ultrafiltration rate strictly according to patient's volemic status and weight loss requirements

Modified from Schortgen F, Soubrier N, Delclaux C, et al: Hemodynamic tolerance of intermittent hemodialysis in critically ill patients: Usefulness of practice guidelines. Am J Respir Crit Care Med 2000;162:197-202.

as good as or even better than treating all patients with CRRT cannot be answered by the Vinsonneau study, given its limited statistical power.

Other important practical questions, such as whether a patient will do better with continuous therapy or IHD and when it is most appropriate to switch from one method to the other, remain unanswered.

IMPACT OF DIALYSIS MODALITY ON RECOVERY OF RENAL FUNCTION

Although RRT is the mainstay of supportive care in patients with severe ARF, performance of this life-sustaining treatment can have untoward effects that may contribute to the prolongation of renal failure or impede the ultimate recovery of renal function. Palevsky and colleagues[33] have elegantly summarized all these untoward effects and their potential effects. Both dialysis-associated hypotension and the activation of cellular and humoral mediators by exposure to the extracorporeal circuit have been proposed as mechanisms of ongoing parenchymal injury.[34]

Although several retrospective studies have reported a lower rate of hypotension with CVVHDF than with IHD, three prospective randomized studies provided inconsistent results.[25,35,36] Also, in the latest randomized trial comparing IHD and CVVHDF, no significant differences in arterial hypotension were observed.[27] Access catheter–associated complications, metabolic and electrolyte disturbances related to the performance of RRT, and the use

TABLE 232-2

Impact of Complications of Renal Replacement Therapy on Prolongation of Renal Injury

FREQUENCY	COMPLICATIONS WITH HIGH IMPACT	COMPLICATIONS WITH UNCERTAIN IMPACT	COMPLICATIONS WITH LOW IMPACT
High	Hemodynamic compromise Catheter-associated infection		Access malfunction Anticoagulation-associated complications Membrane bioincompatibility
Unknown	Human error	Vitamin and micronutrient depletion Hormone depletion Amino acid depletion Hyperglycemia Impaired thermal balance Peritonitis	Electrolyte complications
Low	Catheter-associated hemorrhage Catheter-associated vascular/visceral organ injury Membrane-associated bradykinin activation	Microbiological contamination Acid-base disturbances	Catheter-associated thrombosis Mechanical dysfunction Chemical contamination

Adapted from Palevsky PM, Baldwin I, Davenport A, et al: Renal replacement therapy and the kidney: Minimizing the impact of renal replacement therapy on recovery of acute renal failure. Curr Opin Crit Care 2005;11:548-554.

of impure dialysate may also affect outcomes in patients with ARF.

Which Adverse Effects Has the Greatest Effect on Prolongation of Renal Failure or Impedance of Renal Recovery?

Rigorous data on these potential adverse effects of renal replacement therapy on renal function are not available. Table 232-2, adapted from the review by Palevsky and colleagues,[33] categorizes these adverse events as occurring with high, low, or unknown frequency and as being associated with high, low, or unknown effect.

Hemodynamic compromise and catheter-associated infections occur with the highest frequency and are likely to be associated with the greatest effect. Catheter-associated infections are included in this category with the caveat that although they are thought to be strongly associated with morbidity and mortality in critically ill patients, specific data regarding their effect on renal recovery are not available.[33]

Access malfunction and anticoagulation-associated complications also occur with high frequency but are likely to have a relatively low effect on recovery of renal function; however, additional data are required to define this effect better.

Is There a Relation Between Modality of Therapy and Risk for Ongoing Renal Injury?

Recovery of renal function has been evaluated as a secondary outcome in several trials comparing IHD with CRRT. CRRT is thought to afford greater hemodynamic stability than IHD, particularly in critically ill patients with underlying hemodynamic compromise.[30] This benefit was demonstrated in a prospective randomized trial of 80 patients in which continuous venovenous hemodialysis (CVVHD) was associated with a small rise in mean arterial blood pressure, and IHD with a drop in mean arterial blood pressure despite greater net fluid removal during CRRT.[25] Despite the greater hemodynamic stability in the CRRT-treated patients, this study did not detect any difference in survival or recovery of renal function between groups.

Several other studies have suggested that CRRT is associated with improved recovery of renal function in surviving patients, although the researchers were unable to demonstrate a survival benefit.

Mehta and associates[23] reported a significantly higher rate of complete renal recovery in surviving patients treated with CRRT who received an "adequate" exposure to therapy and did not cross over from one modality to the other modality than in those treated with IHD (92% vs. 59%, respectively; $P < .01$).

In a retrospective analysis of 261 patients from two tertiary ICUs, Manns and colleagues[37] also observed a higher rate of recovery of renal function in surviving patients who had been treated with CRRT than in those treated with IHD (80% vs. 62%; $P = .06$). Jacka and coworkers[38] reported similar findings in a retrospective analysis of 93 patients and observed recovery of renal function in 87% of surviving patients treated with CRRT, compared with 36% of surviving patients treated with IHD. Pooling of the data from all three studies shows that recovery of renal function was observed in 80% of surviving patients treated with CRRT and in 58% of patients treated with IHD ($P < .001$). However, limiting the analysis of recovery of renal function to surviving patients does not take into account the competing risk of mortality. When the composite endpoint of death or nonrecovery of renal function is used, 75% of patients receiving CRRT in these three studies reached the endpoint, compared with 69% of patients treated with IHD ($P = .17$). Thus, although there does appear to be a higher rate of recovery of renal function in surviving patients treated with CRRT, no benefit can be ascribed when the competing risk of mortality is taken into account.[8] In addition, the meta-analysis reported by Tonelli and associates[31] could not find a difference in renal outcome between patients treated with IHD and CRRT. Finally, in the trial reported by Vinsonneau and coworkers,[27] the rate and time to recovery of renal function did not differ significantly between the two treatment groups. After discharge from the ICU, 6 of 61 (10%) patients remained dialysis dependent in the IHD group compared with 4 of 61 (7%) patients in the CVVHDF group ($P = 0.5$). After hospital discharge, only 1 patient (from the CVVHDF group) remained dependent on dialysis.

Relatively few studies have analyzed the long-term prognosis of patients surviving ARF and their quality of life after several years of follow-up. Noble and associates[39] analyzed outcome data from 126 patients with ARF and acute respiratory failure who required treatment with RRT and mechanical ventilation. This study described a cohort of patients treated in 1984 with either continuous hemodialysis with ultrafiltration (CHDF) using biocompatible membranes and prostacyclin and heparin anticoagulation or IHD using cuprophane membranes and heparin anticoagulation; in the long-term survivors, the health-related quality of life was assessed with the Medical Outcomes Study SF-36 (short-form) questionnaire. No difference in ICU mortality (73.5% for IHD vs. 71.8% for CHDF) or hospital mortality (83% IHD vs. 76.5% CHDF) between the two treatment groups was observed. By 1999, there were 16 surviving patients; only 12 of these survivors completed SF-36 forms (10 CHDF vs. 2 IHD). The overall physical health summary score and scores for seven of the health domains were significantly reduced. The mental health summary score and the domain mental health score did not differ from those in the general population. The researchers concluded that the method of RRT used in patients with ARF who were receiving intensive care had no influence on survival and that the long-term survivors of multiple-organ failure have poor physical health.

BIOCOMPATIBILITY OF DIALYSIS MEMBRANES

There is considerable controversy about whether the use of biocompatible dialysis membranes in patients with ARF can positively influence patient survival and recovery of renal function compared with bioincompatible membranes. The *biocompatibility* in this discussion is limited to the property of some dialyzer membranes, such as cuprophane, to activate leukocytes and complement. Different trials yielded contradictory results. The discussion is hampered by the divergence of definitions of biocompatibility. Some studies compared cellulosic with synthetic membranes, in which cellulosic is considered bioincompatible.

However, modified cellulosic membranes (e.g., hemophan) have a lower complement-activating capacity than cuprophane and should hence be considered biocompatible. It has also been argued that differences in flux are responsible for the observed differences, whereby one must understand that the nonmodified cellulosic membranes are always low flux, whereas biocompatible (either synthetic or modified cellulose) membranes may be either low or high flux. Increasing flux improves the removal of middle- and high-molecular-weight uremic retention products, which might be important in patients in the ICU, who are often catabolic.[40] Whether the removal of cytokines by RRT is possible and/or beneficial remains controversial.[41-44]

In a meta-analysis of data from a total of 867 patients, Subramanian and colleagues[45] observed a 1.37 relative risk of mortality for the use of cellulosic membranes (CI,

1.02 to 1.83). A separate subanalysis of studies in which only unmodified cellulose membranes served as the controls versus studies in which both unmodified and modified cellulose membranes served as controls showed that the observed survival benefit for synthetic membranes was largely due to the difference from unmodified cellulose. When only correctly randomized trials were involved in the meta-analysis, the statistical significance of the survival advantage of biocompatible membranes was lost. Jaber and coworkers[46] performed another meta-analysis comparing use of unmodified cellulose (bioincompatible) membranes with use of synthetic and modified cellulose membranes (biocompatible) in a total of 722 patients. The survival advantage for the biocompatible membranes did not reach statistical significance. In neither of these two meta-analyses was an attempt made to dissect the impact of biocompatibility from that of flux.

ANTICOAGULATION IN INTERMITTENT HEMODIALYSIS

A detailed review of this issue has been performed by Davenport.[47]

One of the major advantages of IHD is the lower need for anticoagulation compared to CVVH, in which a continuous struggle is fought between filter coagulation and patient hemorrhage.[48] In most patients, a 2-hour dialysis session can be performed without anticoagulation, but even longer sessions can be completed without the occurrence of clotting in patients with thrombocytopenia or coagulation disorders. Saline flushes can be administered into the afferent blood lines to maintain the patency of the circuit. Prerinsing of the circuit with heparinized saline has largely been abandoned nowadays. Traditionally, standard heparin has been used for IHD in ARF. Several alternative anticoagulation strategies have been described that can be applied in both RRT modalities: minimal heparinization, regional heparinization combined with neutralization with protamine, regional citrate anticoagulation, and the use of low-molecular-weight heparins, heparinoids, hirudin, prostacyclin, or nafamostat.[49]

Regional anticoagulation with citrate is based on its binding with calcium. The citrate solution is infused into the afferent blood line, and from the infusion site on, the blood is anticoagulated. The level of anticoagulation is related to the citrate concentration in the extracorporeal circuit. We favor concentrations between 3.5 and 4.3 mmol/L. The infusion rate of citrate can be calculated from the target citrate concentration, the citrate concentration in the infusion solution, and the blood flow. The higher the blood flow, the higher the amount of citrate needed. The calcium concentration in the infusion solution should be based on frequent monitoring of blood ionized calcium levels.

The rate of removal of citrate by dialysis is also related to the dialysate flow. Dialysis with low dialysate flows and high blood flows can result in citrate retention, a potential cause of hypocalcemia and metabolic alkalosis. Therefore, on theoretical grounds, citrate anticoagulation is safer in IHD than in CVVHD and especially CVVH, in which less citrate is removed. With citrate anticoagulation, different dialysate calcium concentrations have been applied.

When the blood passes through the artificial kidney, citrate completed with calcium is removed by dialysis. If, however, calcium-free dialysate is used, the blood is not repleted with calcium and anticoagulation persists in the outlet blood line. In contrast, if a calcium-containing dialysate is used, calcium diffuses toward the blood and the coagulation cascade is no longer inhibited, so clotting can occur, especially in the venous chamber. Short dialysis sessions (up to 3 hours) can be completed with regional citrate anticoagulation using a calcium-containing dialysate. In contrast, extended dialysis frequently results in clotting of the venous chamber unless a dialysate without calcium is used. The use of calcium-containing dialysate avoids $CaCl_2$ infusions and makes the procedure easier and safer.

Conversely, a major drawback of IHD is the need for a catheter lock to prevent clotting of the catheter once the session is finished. The standard solution applied in this context contains 5000 IU of heparin per mL. Because leakage of heparin from the catheter results in systemic anticoagulation, it is recommended to decrease the heparin concentration in patients with a bleeding risk. A specific device (CLAVE Connector, ICU Medical, San Clemente, CA) makes it possible to prevent clotting of the catheter without using heparin, through the creation of a positive-pressure fluid displacement by a flushing device in the scaling cap; to date there are no published data on the use of this device.

Vascular Access

More detailed discussions of this issue have been published.[50,51] Angioaccess for IHD is usually via single- or double-lumen polyurethane or silicone temporary catheters in the internal jugular, subclavian, or femoral veins. Tunneled cuffed catheters, usually present in patients with end-stage renal disease, may also be used; they probably perform better than temporary catheters but are more difficult to insert and exchange and are therefore rarely used in short-term RRT in the ICU.

Subclavian catheters are associated with a higher incidence of procedural complications as well as of stenosis and thrombosis in the vein; they are therefore not recommended.

Catheter performance is more important for IHD than for CRRT.[50] Higher blood flows are necessary during IHD to provide sufficient overall solute clearance, whereas lower blood flows are sufficient to achieve adequate clearance by CRRT owing to its continuous nature. In general, blood flow rate can be safely increased during IHD until the venous and arterial pressures are ±350 mm Hg, respectively, after which hemolysis can occur. Left-sided internal jugular and subclavian catheters tend to provide unreliable blood flow, at a rate that is typically up to 100 mL/min lower than at other insertion sites, because their tips abut the walls of the superior vena cava and innominate vein, respectively. Femoral vein and right-sided internal jugular or subclavian vein catheters provide the best blood flows.[52] There are significant differences between blood flows achieved with different catheter brands, and larger-bore lines are preferred.

Access recirculation has not been as well defined for temporary as it is for tunneled cuffed catheters. Measurements with ultrasonographic saline dilution showed that access recirculation for all sites is approximately 10% at blood flow rates 250 to 350 mL/min and may rise to as much as 35% at blood flow rates greater than 500 mL/min.[52] Access recirculation depends on the design and site of the catheter. Up to half of treatments require catheters

to be utilized with inflow and outflow lines in reversed configuration, so that the original venous line is used for blood inflow (relative to dialyzer), and the original arterial line for outflow. In this situation, access recirculation is ap-proximately doubled, in the order of 20% at blood flow rates of 250 to 350 mL/min.[53] This phenomenon has an impact on the delivered dose of dialysis.

Infection of temporary catheters sometimes resulting in sepsis is also common, occurring at rates several times those for tunneled cuffed catheters.

CONTRAINDICATIONS TO INTERMITTENT HEMODIALYSIS

In specific conditions, for instance, in patients with cerebral edema[54] or liver failure, CRRT is an absolute preference.[55] Alternatively, IHD may be preferable in patients with increased bleeding risk.

Ronco and colleagues[54] studied patients who were treated for 2 subsequent days in random sequence with IHD (one 4-hour session; Kt/V ≥ 1) and CVVH (one 24-hour session; Kt/V ≥ 1). Brain computed tomography scans were obtained before and after the IHD and CVVH sessions in each patient. Under baseline conditions, the only macroscopic morphological alteration was a slight brain edema in some patients. Significant changes in the density of white matter and gray matter were observed after IHD in all patients, whereas no changes were observed after CVVH. The investigators concluded that in contrast to CVVH, IHD may lead to higher water content in the brain after each session, leading to a postdialytic brain edematogenic state. No other study has been performed in this area.

Davenport and colleagues[55] investigated the effect of various modes of RRT in 30 consecutive patients referred with both fulminant hepatic failure and ARF. Cardiac output decreased during the first hour of 30 intermittent machine hemofiltration treatments, as did tissue oxygen delivery and tissue oxygen uptake. In contrast, there was no significant change during 30 continuous hemofiltration and/or dialysis treatments. Intracranial pressure remained stable during the continuous modes but increased during intermittent machine hemofiltration, with the greatest increase, 55% ± 9%, within the first hour. Mean arterial blood pressure was stable during treatment with the continuous modes, but decreased during the first hour of intermittent machine hemofiltration, resulting in a maximum reduction in cerebral perfusion pressure of 35%. In this group of critically ill patients suffering from combined liver and renal failure, continuous modes of RRT seem to result in better cardiac and intracranial stability than standard intermittent modes of treatment.

Key Points

1. Although considerable advances have been made in the dialytic treatment of intensive care unit–related acute renal failure, several important issues still remain a matter of debate.
2. It has repeatedly been suggested that continuous renal replacement therapy was linked to better outcomes than intermittent hemodialysis, but

convincing evidence is lacking. Even for secondary endpoints such as hemodynamic stability and removal of water and solutes, data on the superiority of continuous methods are missing or at least contradictory.

3. Currently, there are thus no unequivocal data demonstrating the superiority of any modality of renal replacement therapy for critically ill patients with acute renal failure.

4. We recommend a pragmatic and individualized approach to renal replacement therapy.

5. In patients requiring renal replacement therapy in the intensive care unit, the skills and experience of the dialysis staff providing the therapy probably influence outcomes at least as much as the type of therapy per se.[18]

Key References

3. Lameire N, Van Biesen W, Vanholder R: Acute renal failure. Lancet 2005;365:417-430.
8. Palevsky PM: Dialysis modality and dosing strategy in acute renal failure. Semin Dial 2006;19:165-170.
12. Luyckx VA, Bonventre JV: Dose of dialysis in acute renal failure. Semin Dial 2004;17:30-36.
27. Vinsonneau C, Camus C, Combes A, et al: Continuous venovenous haemodiafiltration versus intermittent haemodialysis for acute renal failure in patients with multiple-organ dysfunction syndrome: A multicentre randomised trial. Lancet 2006;368:379-385.
33. Palevsky PM, Baldwin I, Davenport A, et al: Renal replacement therapy and the kidney: Minimizing the impact of renal replacement therapy on recovery of acute renal failure. Curr Opin Crit Care 2005;11:548-554.

See the companion Expert Consult website for the complete reference list.

CHAPTER 233

Intermittent Hemofiltration for Management of Fluid Overload and Administration of Contrast Media

Giancarlo Marenzi, Gianfranco Lauri, and Emilio Assanelli

OBJECTIVES

This chapter will:
1. Discuss the clinical relevance of renal dysfunction in congestive heart failure.
2. Explore the problem of radiocontrast agent–induced nephropathy in high-risk patients.
3. Describe hemofiltration for management of fluid overload in congestive heart failure.
4. Consider application of hemofiltration for prevention and treatment of radiocontrast-induced acute renal failure.

There is growing awareness that renal dysfunction represents an important epidemiological, clinical, and prognostic problem in both acute and chronic cardiovascular conditions, in particular in the settings of coronary artery disease and congestive heart failure (CHF). Evolution in the quality of care of these two conditions and consequent improvement in long-term survival of patients with cardiac disease have led physicians to treat progressively older patients who have more severe cardiac diseases, and associated comorbidities. Because the prevalence of coronary artery disease and CHF is dramatically growing, hospitalization for acute destabilization of patients with chronic disease has markedly increased. Considerable efforts are continuously being made to improve the health-related quality of life and the clinical outcome for patients with cardiac disease as well as to reduce hospitalizations and demands on health service resources.

Diagnosis and treatment of coronary artery disease relies heavily on cardiovascular imaging. Contrast-enhanced imaging studies and interventions are a relevant part of modern medical practice. An increasing number of patients, estimated at 30 million per year in the United States, receive contrast agents during diagnostic or interventional procedures.[1] Iodinated contrast media occupy a strategic place in this expanding field, and although they are essential for contrast enhancement and diagnostic precision, they are also toxic to the kidney. Indeed, one of the most troublesome complications of the administration of contrast agents is kidney toxicity, and radiocontrast agent–induced nephropathy (RCIN) represents one of the leading causes of renal impairment and the third cause of in-hospital acquired renal failure.

Renal replacement therapies (RRTs), as supportive care in patients with coexisting cardiovascular and renal disorders, are clearly emerging as useful therapeutic strategies and have received extensive investigation. Their use continues to grow in both elective and emergency situations, and the European Society of Cardiology has recently included the hemofiltration device in its recommended technical equipment for modern intensive cardiac care units.[2] Nevertheless, surprisingly, no official guidelines for the use of RRT in patients with cardiac disease have been defined. Information about clinical indications, therapeutic protocols, and impact of these adjunctive treatments on hard clinical endpoints is still lacking. The possible reasons are the limited number of randomized, controlled studies conducted in selected cardiovascular populations and the exclusion of patients with renal disease from the majority of cardiovascular disease trials.[3] Thus, most of the existing knowledge on the use of RRTs has been indirectly acquired from noncardiological clinical backgrounds, such as nephrology and intensive care settings.

In this chapter, the potential applications of hemofiltration in cardiovascular medicine are discussed on the basis of clinical and investigational experience, with special emphasis on fluid overload withdrawal in severe CHF and the prevention and treatment of acute renal failure due to RCIN in patients undergoing percutaneous cardiovascular interventions (PCIs). A brief updated overview on the objective impact of these two conditions is provided to better define the clinical scenario in which hemofiltration therapy may have its positive effects.

THE CLINICAL IMPACT OF CONGESTIVE HEART FAILURE AND ASSOCIATED RENAL DYSFUNCTION

Current estimates of the prevalence of CHF vary widely, but it is reported to be 5% or higher in the general population older than 65 years. Patients with advanced CHF have a very high 1-year mortality rate, which reaches about 50% for patients with New York Heart Association class IV disease. In addition to cardiac mortality, all-cause mortality has been shown to be threefold higher in patients with CHF than in the general population. Renal dysfunction has been clearly recognized as the most important independent predictor of mortality in both chronic and acute CHF.[4,5] Even small rises in serum creatinine concentration (>0.3 mg/dL) during hospitalization for CHF, occurring in almost 30% of cases, have been shown to have prognostic relevance, including a sevenfold greater in-hospital mortality rate.[6] Data on hospitalizations in patients with CHF are even more impressive, occurring, on the average, about four times per patient per year. Although patients with severe (New York Heart Association class IV) CHF represent only 13% of the whole CHF patient population, their care accounts for almost 50% of the cost of CHF hospitalizations, mainly owing to their more frequent need for hospital admissions, in both intensive and nonintensive care units.[7]

The precise triggers of acute destabilization and congestion in CHF are not known. However, excess salt intake, renal dysfunction, neurohormonal and cytokine activation, and medications may contribute to fluid retention.

HEMOFILTRATION FOR MANAGEMENT OF FLUID OVERLOAD IN CONGESTIVE HEART FAILURE

The primary therapeutic goals for acute exacerbation of CHF include removal of fluid overload, reduction of ventricular filling pressures, increase in cardiac output, myocardial protection, neurohormonal modulation, and renal preservation. Although intensive intravenous treatment with loop diuretics may initially facilitate fluid loss, reduce left ventricular pressure, and improve symptoms, their use is associated with strengthening of neurohormonal activation, intravascular volume depletion, and renal function decline. Moreover, a worse outcome has been associated with diuretics, and a dose-dependent inverse relationship between loop diuretics use and survival has been demonstrated in advanced CHF.[8,9]

Because fluid overload heavily affects quality and expectancy of life for patients with CHF, alternative therapeutic strategies are needed to counteract the development of refractoriness, particularly in cases in which progressively increasing doses of diuretics are required.

Hemofiltration was first utilized for the treatment of fluid overload in CHF more than 50 years ago; in the last 25 years, several studies have confirmed its clinical efficacy as well as its safety profile.[10-13] When applied to CHF patients, hemofiltration in the short term stops the vicious circle responsible for the progression of the disease—in which cardiac output reduction, neurohormonal activation, and renal dysfunction negatively affect one another.[14] The peculiar feature of hemofiltration is its capacity for removing excessive fluid from the extravascular space without affecting circulating volume; most of the observed clinical, hemodynamic, and respiratory effects are the result of this feature.[11-14]

Reduction of extravascular lung water via hemofiltration allows the rapid improvement in respiratory symptoms (dyspnea and orthopnea), pulmonary gas exchange, and radiological signs of pulmonary vascular congestion and alveolar and interstitial edema (Fig. 233-1). Removal of systemic extravascular water allows resolution of peripheral edema and, when present, ascites and pleural and pericardial effusions.[12] The removal of extravascular pulmonary water, by reducing the intrathoracic pressure and, thus, the diastolic burden on the heart, exerts a positive influence on cardiac dynamics. The hemodynamic improvement after hemofiltration is the result of both the reduction of the extracardiac constraint and the optimization of circulating volume. Even withdrawal of several liters of fluid, over a period of a few hours, can be safely performed without detrimental hemodynamic consequences, and clinical improvement is usually maintained for a long time after a single session.[12,13] During hemofiltration, circulating volume—the true cardiac preload—is preserved, or even optimized, by fluid refilling from the extravascular space. The decrease in the ventricular filling pressures reflects the reduction of intrathoracic pressure and of pulmonary stiffness due to absorption of the excessive extravascular lung water that burdens the heart (Fig. 233-2). Recovery in pulmonary mechanics favorably affects the heart, with a reduction in its size and in Doppler imaging–derived ventricular restrictivity as well as an improvement in circulatory hemodynamics.[15-17]

In addition to edema removal, hemofiltration allows for effects that are particularly useful in patients with advanced CHF: correction of hyponatremia, restoration of urine output and diuretic responsiveness, reduction of circulating levels of neurohormones, and, possibly, removal of other cardiac-depressant mediators.[12,14,18,19] The mechanism by which hemofiltration induces renal improvement is still unclear, but it can be possibly explained by the interaction of multiple factors, such as resolution of kidney congestion, recovery of an effective transrenal arteriovenous pressure gradient that increases glomerular filtration rate, and reduction of the activity of several neurohumoral factors with vasoconstrictive and water- and salt-retaining properties.

Recovery of diuretic responsiveness is a major clinical effect, because it allows for maintenance, and even improvement in the following days and months, of the clinical benefits achieved at the end of a single session of hemofiltration. Moreover, it permits the use of lower dosages of diuretics, with consequent minor exposure to side effects.

It should be pointed out that the favorable effects of hemofiltration are not reproducible when equivalent fluid

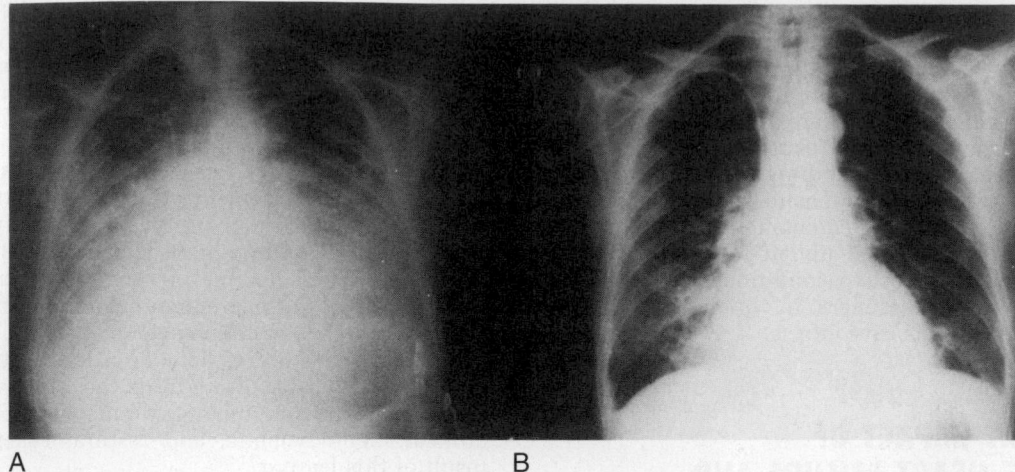

FIGURE 233-1. Chest radiograph findings (**A**); improvement after hemofiltration in a patient with acute pulmonary edema (**B**).

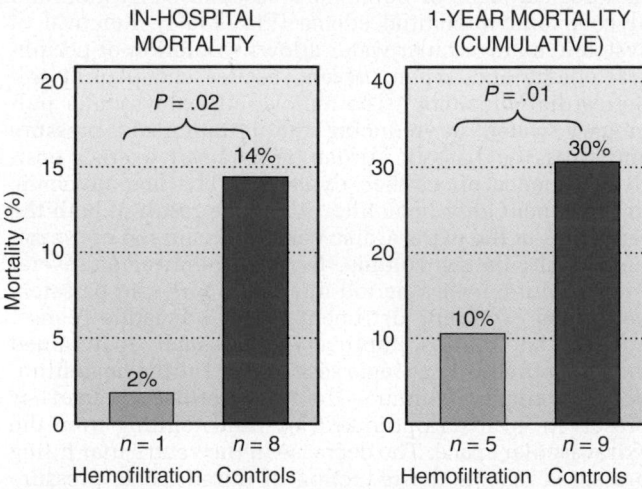

FIGURE 233-2. In-hospital and 1-year mortality rates in patients with chronic renal failure treated with hemofiltration for prevention of radiocontrast agent–induced nephropathy and in control subjects. (Data from Marenzi G, Marana I, Lauri G, et al: The prevention of radio-contrast-agent-induced nephropathy by hemofiltration. N Engl J Med 2003;349:1331-1338.)

volume is removed by high doses of diuretic infusion.[20] When the two strategies for fluid withdrawal—mechanical and pharmacological—are compared, divergent effects on sodium removal capacity, intravascular volume, and renin-angiotensin system activity are usually achieved. Indeed, the fluids removed with the two treatments have a different tonicity, isotonic with hemofiltration, and hypotonic with furosemide; intravascular volume is preserved with hemofiltration and reduced with furosemide. These differences in the amount of sodium removed and the intravascular volume, in spite of a similar fluid volume withdrawn, are assumed to be responsible for the diverse neurohormonal reaction, with consequent achievement of a more favorable water and salt balance after hemofiltration (less input of water without recovery in body weight), and rapid gain of the baseline condition after furosemide. This hypothesis emphasizes the clinical relevance of a more "physiologic" dehydration in CHF.

Hyponatremia, hypokalemia, and renin-angiotensin system activation associated with long-term diuretic treatment are recognized to be negative prognostic indicators

in CHF. Presumably, long-term treatment with periodic sessions of hemofiltration, which typically does not affect sodium and potassium serum concentrations and does not activate the renin-angiotensin axis, could have a positive impact on the progression of the disease, edema formation, and, finally, mortality.

To date, the ability of hemofiltration to prolong survival in patients with CHF has not been established. The first randomized trials designed to evaluate the long-term effectiveness of ultrafiltration and hemofiltration in acute and chronic CHF are ongoing. The results of these studies should definitely establish their clinical impact in CHF in terms of morbidity (rate and duration of hospitalizations), mortality, and overall cost of care. The first studies have been published in 2007. In particular, the UNLOAD trial[20a] has demonstrated that early treatment with ultrafiltration in patients with acute heart failure safely produces greater weight and fluid loss than intravenous diuretics and is associated with a 44% reduction of rehospitalizations for heart failure in the following three months. Because CHF imposes a heavy burden on individuals, in terms of low tolerance of physical exertion, lengthy hospital admissions, and short life expectancy, any improvement in quality of life and any reduction in number and duration of hospitalizations via hemofiltration are clearly attractive.

Future randomized studies are needed to compare the efficacy of different RRT modalities in CHF, with particular emphasis on their possible diverse capacities for sodium removal. One more point of investigative interest is the possible advantage of combining techniques in different phases of the clinical course of patients with CHF, that is. hemofiltration for removal of fluid overload and rapid clinical stabilization and long-term treatment with peritoneal dialysis for prevention of water and salt retention and of hospitalization.[21]

THE CLINICAL IMPACT OF RADIOCONTRAST AGENT–INDUCED NEPHROPATHY

Radiocontrast agent–induced nephropathy implies acute transient impairment in renal function after intravascular

TABLE 233-1

Risk Factors for Radiocontrast-Induced Nephropathy

Patient-related factors	Chronic kidney disease (stage III or greater)
	Diabetes mellitus (type 1 or type 2)
	Volume depletion
	Age
	Congestive heart failure (or left ventricular ejection fraction <40%)
	Hypertension
	Anemia
	Hypoalbuminemia
	Nephrotoxic drug use (nonsteroidal anti-inflammatory drugs, cyclosporine, aminoglycosides)
	Hypotension or preprocedural hemodynamic instability
	Urgent procedure (acute myocardial infarction)
	Intra-aortic balloon pump use
Non–patient-related factors	Contrast agent properties: High osmolarity Ionic state Viscosity
	Contrast agent volume
	Intra-arterial administration of contrast agent

administration of contrast medium. It is usually defined as an absolute (>0.5 mg/dL) or a relative (>25%) increase in serum creatinine concentration within 48 to 72 hours after contrast agent exposure. In patients with normal renal function, the frequency of RCIN is low, less than 3%, but it may be as high as 50% in high-risk patients.

Development of RCIN is linked to a higher risk of cardiovascular complications, prolonged hospitalization, and higher rate of in-hospital and long-term mortality. Several risk factors, including chronic renal failure, diabetes mellitus, intravascular volume depletion, and use of a high volume of contrast agent, confer an increased risk for RCIN (Table 233-1). In most cases RCIN is predictable, so that the only effective therapeutic approach is the employment of preventive strategies. Accordingly, several studies have focused on strategies to prevent RCIN, primarily by pharmacological means. However, none of the drugs tested (furosemide, mannitol, dopamine, calcium channel blockers, endothelin receptor antagonists, theophylline, fenoldopam, N-acetylcysteine, and prostaglandin) has been conclusively shown to be efficacious, particularly in patients with severe chronic renal insufficiency. To date, the probability of RCIN in high-risk patients undergoing PCI still approximates 50%, with a 30% associated rate of cardiovascular death within 1 year.[22]

Although spontaneous recovery of renal function ensues within 1 to 2 weeks in patients in whom RCIN develops, severe nephropathy requiring in-hospital dialysis may occur, which is associated with a very poor clinical outcome. Hence, more effective prophylactic strategies are needed to attenuate the particularly high risk associated with PCI in patients with severe renal insufficiency.

INTERMITTENT HEMOFILTRATION FOR MANAGEMENT OF CONTRAST MEDIA ADMINISTRATION

The potential preventive effects and therapeutic advantage of hemodialysis, hemodiafiltration, and hemofiltration have been a matter of intense investigative interest. Contrast media are excreted mainly by glomerular filtration, and effective removal of contrast media by the artificial membranes, through a process mimicking spontaneous glomerular filtration, has been demonstrated in patients with renal failure.[23] Hemodialysis was first proposed for the prevention of RCIN after radiographic procedures in patients with chronic renal insufficiency, but no clear benefit of this approach over hydration, or even of potential harm, was demonstrated.[24-27]

The incongruence between the effective removal of contrast media by hemodialysis and the lack of a preventive effect against RCIN has been postulated to be either the result of hemodialysis-related nephrotoxicity (activation of inflammatory reactions, acute hypotension, etc.), or of the delay between exposure to and elimination of the contrast agents—given the rapid onset of renal injury after dye administration. However, two studies in which hemodialysis and hemodiafiltration were started immediately before contrast agent administration and continued for some hours did not demonstrate appreciable protection against RCIN.[28,29] In contrast to these results, Marenzi and colleagues[22] found evidence that hemofiltration offers protection against RCIN in high-risk patients. Hemofiltration, with fluid replacement of 1000 mL/hr without weight loss, was started 6 hours before contrast exposure in patients with advanced renal failure undergoing PCI, and was then continued for 18 to 24 hours after the procedure. RCIN occurred in only 5% of patients in the hemofiltration group and in 50% of patients in the control group ($P <$ .001). Overall mortality in the hemofiltration group was significantly lower than in the control group (see Fig. 233-2).

However, the hypothesis that the positive effects of hemofiltration derive from removal of contrast agent from the circulation is strongly contradicted by the results of a randomized clinical study in which two different hemofiltration protocols for the prevention of RCIN, in patients with severe renal insufficiency (creatinine clearance <30 mL/min) scheduled for elective PCI, were compared.[30] In one group, intravenous hydration was performed for 12 hours before administration of contrast medium, and hemofiltration was given for 18 to 24 hours after the angiographic procedure (post-hemofiltration group); in another group, hemofiltration was performed for 6 hours before and then for 18 to 24 hours after contrast administration (pre/post-hemofiltration group). RCIN occurred in 26% of patients in the post-hemofiltration group, compared with only 3% of patients in the pre/post-hemofiltration group ($P =$ .0013). Rates of in-hospital clinical complications and mortality (10% and 0%, respectively) paralleled the incidence of RCIN in the two groups. This study confirmed that prophylactic hemofiltration is particularly effective in preventing RCIN in high-risk patients but also demonstrated that a preprocedural session is required to obtain a full clinical benefit. These findings represent a limitation in the use of hemofiltration, because its indications remain restricted to patients treated with elective procedures, and patients undergoing emergency PCI cannot benefit from this prophylactic strategy. The results of this study also

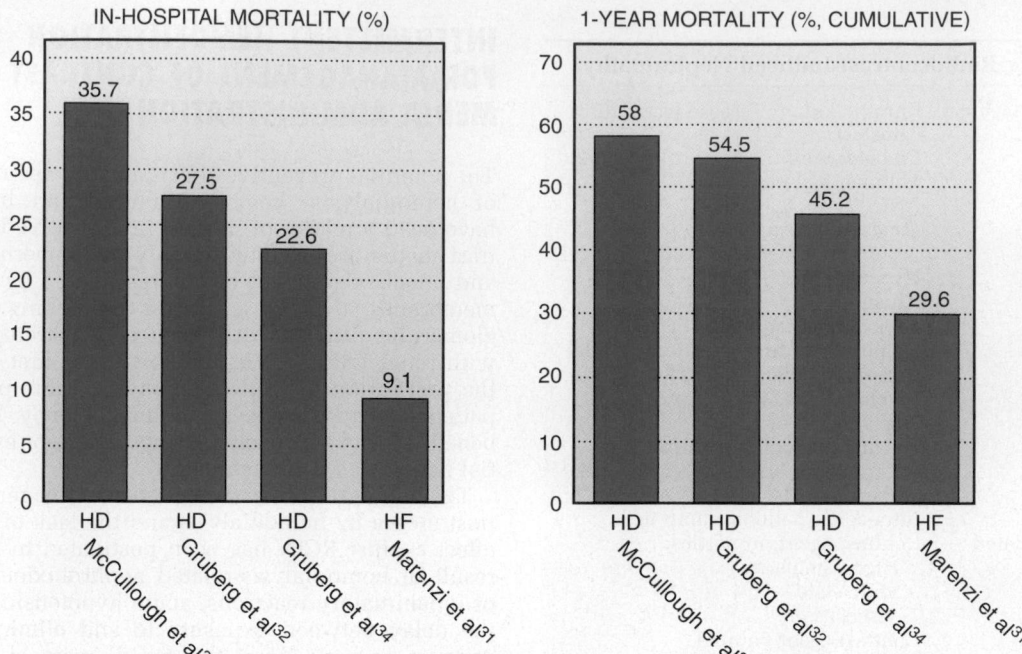

FIGURE 233-3. In-hospital and 1-year mortality rates in patients treated with hemodialysis (HD), reported by three studies, and with hemofiltration (HF), reported by one study, for acute renal failure due to radiocontrast agent-induced nephropathy.

suggest that other mechanisms may be involved in its prophylactic effect, such as high-volume controlled and safe hydration, removal of mediators of contrast-induced toxicity by convective filtration and adsorption to the filter membrane, and alkalinization by bicarbonate-based solutions.

When acute renal failure due to severe RCIN occurs, and RRT is required, intermittent hemodialysis continues to be the preferred form of treatment. However, no clear evidence of its superiority over other kinds of RRT has ever been demonstrated. In particular, hemofiltration could be superior to hemodialysis because it allows more effective fluid volume control and grants better cardiovascular stability, a clear advantage in critically ill patients with cardiac insufficiency. Moreover, hemofiltration does not require specifically trained dialysis personnel.

As reported by Marenzi and colleagues,[31] treatment with hemofiltration in patients in whom acute renal failure and oligoanuria developed after PCI, with or without concomitant overt CHF, was associated with a recovery of spontaneous diuresis, improvement of renal function parameters, and correction of fluid and electrolyte imbalance in most cases. In this population, in-hospital mortality rate was 9%, and the cumulative 1-year mortality was 27%—significantly lower than that reported in previous studies in which patients were treated with intermittent hemodialysis (Fig. 233-3). Gruberg and associates[32] reported in-hospital and 1-year mortality rates of 27% and 54%, respectively, in 51 patients requiring hemodialytic treatment after PCI. An in-hospital mortality rate of 35% and a 2-year survival of 19% were reported by McCullough and coworkers.[33] In another study by Gruberg and associates,[34] in-hospital mortality in patients requiring hemodialysis was 23%, whereas the cumulative 1-year mortality was 45%. In this setting, the remarkably lower in-hospital and 1-year mortality rates in hemofiltration-treated patients suggests a potential clinical advantage of this technique over hemodialysis.

CONCLUSION

The application of hemofiltration for the treatment and prevention of renal failure associated with cardiovascular diseases is continuously evolving. In patients with CHF, hemofiltration allows for improvement of clinical and hemodynamic conditions without interfering with cardiac performance, reestablishes neurohormonal imbalances, and restores diuresis and diuretic responsiveness. Furthermore, hemofiltration represents an important advance for prevention of RCIN, because it expands the group of patients with advanced chronic renal insufficiency who can undergo invasive cardiovascular procedures safely. The interest in using RRT for the prevention of RCIN in high-risk patients has not vanished but has progressively shifted from a post-procedural to a pre-procedural application (Fig. 233-4), and has focused on a safe and hemodynamically tolerated high-volume hydration rather than a mechanical removal of contrast agents.

Further investigation is needed to confirm the positive clinical effect of hemofiltration in such cardiovascular conditions, to better define protocols and compare different RRT modalities, to identify patients and clinical settings in which the greatest benefit can be obtained, and, finally, to definitively establish the effect of its use on hard clinical endpoints.

Key Points

1. Hemofiltration has gained a decisive role in the management of various forms of cardiovascular disease, namely congestive heart failure and radiocontrast agent–induced nephropathy.
2. In patients with severe congestive heart failure, withdrawal of fluid overload by hemofiltration allows for (a) resolution of pulmonary edema

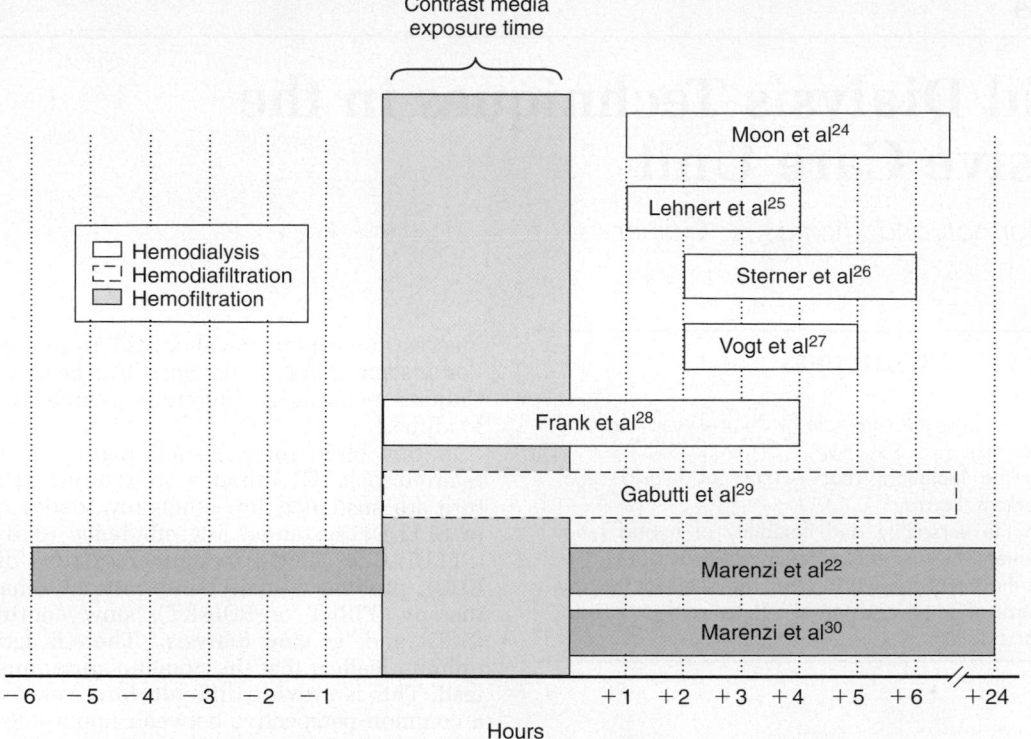

FIGURE 233-4. Comparison of duration and time of treatment of different renal replacement therapies in relation to duration and time of exposure to contrast media.

with improvement in respiratory symptoms (dyspnea, orthopnea), respiratory gas exchanges, radiographic signs of vascular congestion and alveolar and interstitial edema, (b) resolution of peripheral edema, ascites, pleural and pericardial effusions, (c) hemodynamic stability, (d) correction of hyponatremia, (e) restoration of urine output and diuretic responsiveness, (f) reduction of circulating levels of neurohormones, and (g) reduction of number of hospitalizations as well as duration of stay in intensive care units and hospitals.

3. In patients with severe renal insufficiency undergoing interventional cardiovascular procedures requiring contrast media exposure, hemofiltration allows for marked reduction in the incidence of radiocontrast agent–induced nephropathy as well as associated short-term and long-term mortality rates.

Key References

2. Hasin Y, Danchin N, Filippatos GS, et al; Working Group on Acute Cardiac Care of the European Society of Cardiology: Recommendations for the structure, organization, and operation of intensive cardiac care units. Eur Heart J 2005;16: 1676-1682.

3. Coca SG, Krumholz HM, Garg AX, Parikh CR: Underrepresentation of renal disease in randomized controlled trials of cardiovascular disease. JAMA 2006;296:1377-1384.

15. Agostoni PG, Marenzi G, Pepi M, et al: Isolated ultrafiltration in moderate congestive heart failure. J Am Coll Cardiol 1993;21:424-431.

22. Marenzi G, Marana I, Lauri G, et al: The prevention of radiocontrast-agent–induced nephropathy by hemofiltration. N Engl J Med 2003;349:1331-1338.

30. Marenzi G, Lauri G, Campodonico J, et al: Comparison of two hemofiltration protocols for prevention of contrast-induced nephropathy in high-risk patients. Am J Med 2006;119: 155-162.

See the companion Expert Consult website for the complete reference list.

CHAPTER 234

Hybrid Dialysis Techniques in the Intensive Care Unit

Mark R. Marshall and Thomas A. Golper

OBJECTIVES

This chapter will:
1. Define and give the rationale for hybrid renal replacement therapy.
2. Discuss the technical requirements of hybrid renal replacement therapy.
3. Explain the versatility and flexibility of hybrid renal replacement therapy prescription and provision.
4. Discuss the effects of hybrid renal replacement therapy on control of small and larger solutes and on cardiovascular stability.

Hybrid renal replacement therapy (HT) is a newly described modality of acute renal replacement therapy (ARRT) with the following features:

- Outpatient nephrology intermittent hemodialysis (IHD) machinery is used to deliver treatments, as opposed to dedicated intensive care unit (ICU) continuous renal replacement therapy (CRRT) machinery.
- Treatment sessions may be deliberately intermittent rather than necessarily being continuous.
- Treatment sessions are of longer duration than outpatient nephrology IHD treatments.
- The rate of solute and fluid removal is slower than with outpatient nephrology IHD treatments but faster than with conventional CRRT.

The technical elements of HT are not novel. In the extreme, it can be argued that Kolff actually performed the first HT treatments more than 50 years ago.[1] The clinical context of HT is novel, however, as a conceptual and logistic compromise between the modern applications of IHD and CRRT. With this rationale, HT was first presented 10 to 15 years ago as a way of combining the advantageous features of IHD and CRRT while minimizing their respective disadvantages.[2-5] The major advantages of IHD are that it is inexpensive and has the convenience of scheduled downtime that allows the patient to be available for out-of-unit radiological and surgical procedures. The major advantages of CRRT are that it allows fluid removal with minimal hemodynamic instability and provides consistent solute control. In general, HT has lived up to this rationale, and reported experience to date has shown this modality to be effective among a wide range of patients, popular with nurses, and inexpensive.[6]

HT is increasingly utilized. For example, 7% of patients in the Acute Renal Failure Trial Network (ATN) Study receive HT as primary treatment, and 25% of practitioners participating in this study routinely prescribe this modality.[7] These proportions are reported to be similar in Europe on the basis of data from around the same time.[8] It is important to note that there is a lot of unpublished or inaccessible experience about HT in the world literature. For instance, important work has been reported in the Chinese nephrology literature, which is not listed by Medline.[9]

In this topic review, such regimens are collectively referred to as HT, although other terms used in the literature are sustained low-efficiency (daily) dialysis (SLED or SLEDD), sustained low efficiency (daily) diafiltration (SLEDD-f or SLED-f), extended (daily) dialysis (ED or EDD), prolonged (daily) intermittent renal replacement therapy (PIRRT or PDIRRT), slow continuous dialysis (SCD), and "go slow dialysis." There is agreement among opinion leaders that the nomenclature must be standardized. This is proving difficult, however, owing to lack of a common perspective between nephrologists and intensivists: Hybrid therapy is "low efficiency" and "prolonged" to nephrologists, but "high efficiency" and "foreshortened" to intensivists. In the authors' opinion, nomenclature is likely to remain a local affair and to depend on which of the disciplines has responsibility for the therapy in an institution. It would seem that the only two terms that would be acceptable to both disciplines are hybrid therapy and prolonged (daily) intermittent renal replacement therapy.

TECHNICAL ISSUES

An overall summary of HT programs from published literature is shown in Table 234-1.[9-19] A few key technical issues are discussed here; issues related more to prescription are discussed in Chapter 235.

Machinery

A fundamental feature of HT is the use of outpatient nephrology IHD machinery. Maintenance IHD programs are very common throughout the world, and hospitals that have such programs are in possession of all the technical elements necessary to an HT program. In some hospitals, there has been a clear mandate to adapt and share existing machinery between maintenance IHD and HT programs, thereby reducing the cost of program implementation and maintenance. In fact, one of the main motivating factors for nocturnal HT was the need to use the machinery in outpatient IHD facilities during the day.[16] In other hospitals (particularly where ICU provides ARRT), machinery for HT is owned and maintained by the ICU as a separate going concern, although it remains the same as (or technically very similar to) that used by nephrology services.[17,18]

Almost any IHD machine *can* be used for HT. However, blood and dialysate flow rates (Q_B and Q_D, respectively)

TABLE 234-1

Hybrid Dialysis Therapy Programs Reported in Published Literature

	Study									
	SCHLAEPER ET AL[19]	FINKEL AND FORINGER[12]	LONNEMANN ET AL[15]	MARSHALL ET AL[16]	MARSHALL ET AL[17]	NAKA ET AL[18]	KUMAR ET AL[13,14]	FIACCADORI ET AL[11]	LI ET AL[9]	BERBECE ET AL[10]
Hemodialysis machine	Fresenius 2008H	Fresenius 2008H	Fresenius GENIUS	Fresenius 2008H	Fresenius 4008S ARrT-Plus	Fresenius 4008S ARrT-Plus	Fresenius 2008H	Gambro AK200S Ultra	Fresenius 4008S or Toray TR123	Gambro Integra
Hemodialyzer	Fresenius F40	Fresenius F7	Fresenius F60S	Fresenius F8	Fresenius AV600S	Fresenius AV600S	Toray 1.0	Fresenius F7HPS	Fresenius AV600S	Bellco Diapes 140G
Membrane composition	Polysulfone	Polysulfone	Polysulfone	Polysulfone	Polysulfone	Polysulfone	Polymethyl methacrylate	Polysulfone	Polysulfone	Polysulfone
Area (m²)	0.7	1.6	1.25	1.8	1.4	1.4	1.0	1.6	1.4	1.4
Flux	High	Low	High	Low	High	High	High	Low	High	High
Duration (hours)	Continuous	Continuous	8-18	12	8-10	8-10	8	8-9	10	8
Time of day	Continuous	Continuous	Nocturnal	Nocturnal	Nocturnal/ Diurnal	Diurnal	Diurnal	Diurnal	Nocturnal/ Diurnal	Diurnal
Frequency	Continuous	Continuous	Daily	Daily/5-6 days per week	Daily/5-6 days per week	Daily/5-6 days per week	Daily/6 days per week	Daily/6 days per week	Daily/ alternate days	6 days per week
Blood flow rate (QB) (mL/min)	150-200	150	70	200	200-350	100	150-200	200	150-200	200
Dialysate flow rate (QD) (mL/min)	100	100	70	100	200	200	300	100	300	350
Filtration rate (QF) (mL/min)	0	0	0	0	100	25	0	0	0	17
Dialysate	Bicarbonate	Bicarbonate	Bicarbonate	Bicarbonate	Bicarbonate	Bicarbonate	Bicarbonate	Bicarbonate	Bicarbonate	Bicarbonate

TABLE 234-2

Machines from Major Vendors Used for Hybrid Dialysis Therapy

MACHINE	LOWER LIMIT OF BLOOD FLOW (mL/min)	UPPER LIMIT OF TREATMENT TIME	EASY TRANSITION TO HT MODE?
Fresenius 2008H	300*	Nil	N/A
Fresenius 2008H + P/N 190178	100	Nil	Yes
Fresenius 2008K	100	Nil	Yes
Fresenius 4008S	300	10[†]	N/A
Fresenius 4008S ARrT Plus	200	10[†]	Yes
Fresenius 5008S	100	Nil	Yes
Gambro AK95/100/200	300	10	N/A
Gambro Integra	350	10	N/A
Toray TR-123	300	10	N/A

HT, hybrid dialysis therapy; N/A, specific HT mode not available.

*Can set QD 100mL/min by manually recalibrating dialysate temperature sensors, a procedure that takes ~45 minutes (details in Ref 45)

[†]Treatments can be restarted at the end of 10 hrs by re-entering new treatment parameters, to effectively carry the treatment on beyond his time limit without having to disinfect or drain the machine and setting up again with new lines.

and treatment session duration are typically different from that of conventional IHD (see Table 234-1), and machines must be capable of being changed to any of these variations in a convenient fashion. The ideal HT machine, therefore, is versatile over a wide range of operating conditions and easy to use. Specifically, the following features should be considered in the choice of a machine for HT:

- Flexibility of Q_D from as low as 100 mL/min up to the dialysis flow rates used for conventional IHD.
- Flexibility of treatment session length from as short as those used for conventional IHD up to continuous duration.
- Clear interface between machine and staff conducting treatment.
- Easy transition between IHD and HT modes.

In the first descriptions of HT, dialysate for treatments was produced in batches and used in now-outdated batch dialysis machinery.[2,3] In the modern practice of HT, only one such batch machine remains in common use, the GENIUS therapy system (Fresenius Medical Care, Bad Homburg, Germany).[15,20,21] This machine is only sold in Europe at present. For this machine, dialysate is generated in the outpatient nephrology dialysis unit through the use of a separate machine called a "preparator" and stored in a 75- or 90-L tank within the machine. A single roller pump is used to move both dialysate and blood (max Q_B 300 mL/min) through the extracorporeal circuit at a ratio of 1:1 to 1:2. This ratio is determined by the staff conducting treatment, who choose between lines that have different lumen widths for the segments in the roller pump that provide Q_B and Q_D. Fresh dialysate is pumped from the top of the dialysate storage tank, and spent dialysate is returned to the bottom. Despite the lack of a physical barrier between these fluids, there is little mixing within the tank. Separation is maintained by small but important differences in fluid density and temperature between fresh and spent dialysate. One HT session using the GENIUS machine can last up 15 hrs with a Q_D of 100 mL/min.

The GENIUS machine has several advantages over single-pass machines. Treatments can be performed in the ICU without the need for a water supply. It is very easy to set operating parameters via independent and simple controls, allowing unlimited combinations of Q_B, Q_D, and session duration. An argument has been made that dialysate sterility in this machine is superior to that in single-pass machines, although this contention has not been proven and is not likely. Disadvantages of the GENIUS machine are its weight (approx 165 kg) and its fixed clearance, which is due to the fixed aliquot of dialysate per treatment. Nevertheless, this machine is regarded by some opinion leaders as the best HT machine on the market.[22]

Generally around the world, HT is performed using single-pass machines, whereby solutions for blood purification in HT are generated on-line from purified tap water and dialysate concentrate. Few of these machines are ideally suited for HT (Table 234-2), and most have some limitations around the lowest Q_D and the longest HT session length that can be provided. With regard to Q_D, these limits do not impose any critical clinical limitation. A Q_D of 300 mL/min is perfectly satisfactory in most clinical circumstances, and there are often means to reduce effective Q_D without drastically modifying machine hardware. For instance, one group of researchers has used the Gambro AK200S Ultra machine (Gambro AB, Stockholm, Sweden) in hemofiltration mode; the replacement fluid is used as countercurrent dialysate within the dialyzer at 100 mL/min, the operational QD on the machine interface set to zero (E. Fiaccadori, personal communication, 7 September, 2005; P. Van Malderen, personal communication, 9 September 2005). Another group has developed a simple shunt to be used with the Fresenius 4008H machine (Fresenius Medical Care), which allows a proportion of the dialysate to bypass the hemodialyzer.[23,24] There are probably easier and simpler ways to reduce the effective Q_D from 300 mL/min to the equivalent of 100 mL/min, such as reducing hemodialyzer size and using co-current dialysate flow.

With regard to treatment session length, many machines in North America can perform treatments for 24 hours or even continuously (e.g., Fresenius 2008K, Fresenius Medical Care North America, Lexington, MA), but most in Europe and the Asia Pacific region can perform treatments for only 10 hours (e.g., Fresenius 4008S, Fresenius Medical Care). This difference is due to different regulatory environments between the continents. This trend is changing, and some of the newer European machines from major vendors have an option for 24-hour or continuous treatment (e.g., Fresenius 5008S, Fresenius Medical Care).

Many vendors are selling or developing machines that switch easily and instantaneously between IHD and HT modes (so-called universal platforms). Fresenius Medical Care has undoubtedly taken the lead in this regard, having developed the two or three leading machines in terms of ease of operation—the Fresenius 2008K (US), 4008S ARrT Plus (Asia Pacific), and 5008S (Europe). All of these machines allow selection of CRRT or HT from their startup screens and enable easy changes of operating parameters.

Water Quality

Fluids for blood purification in HT are usually generated on-line from purified tap water and dialysate concentrate. In contrast are those used in CRRT, which are pharmacy-made or commercially purchased and delivered to the point of service, for both batch and single-pass machinery. A growing concern is the possibility of exposure to bacterial contaminants—and specifically endotoxin—from these fluids. Such exposure might arise during direct infusion of on-line replacement fluid and also from backfiltration via dialysate into the patient. It is therefore generally accepted that water quality for on-line fluids should conform to the same standards that are used in the outpatient nephrology IHD setting.

The critical question, however, is whether water purity for ARRT should actually be higher than this standard. In the absence of any definitive clinical trial data, many opinion leaders opt for dialysate sterilization using ultrafilters in the dialysate pathway, especially if high-flux membranes are being used. These ultrafilters remove bacteria and endotoxin by virtue of a pore size of about 0.22 μm and specific adsorptive properties.[25] It must be stressed that this decision is based on observational evidence or surrogate endpoints. A counterargument has been made that bacterial contaminants are removed sufficiently by the dialyzer during backfiltration by most common membranes and that dialysate sterilization is unnecessary.[26,27] Clearly, a definitive trial is urgently needed to determine optimal clinical practice.

There is less debate about water quality for on-line replacement fluid for hemodiafiltration. This fluid is a fraction of dialysate that is infused directly into the extracorporeal circuit either before or after the diafilter. The ionic composition of replacement fluid does not differ from that of dialysate. Such fluid should be sterile (no growth, endotoxin concentration <0.03 endotoxin units). This is achieved by passing water and/or dialysate through two (Fresenius) or three (Gambro) ultrafilters before being infused. This process has been shown to yield a fluid that is at least as sterile as commercially available fluids.[28,29] The U.S. Food and Drug Administration has not approved such a process, and a similar situation exists in some European countries. In these countries, on-line replacement fluid preparation is not used in patients, and hemodiafiltration during HT is performed using pharmacy-made or commercially purchased fluids or, more commonly, normal saline.[10]

Hemodialyzers

Hemodialyzers used for HT can be the same as those used for conventional IHD and intermittent hemodiafiltration (IHDF). Hemodialyzer membranes can be low-flux or high-flux. High-flux membranes contain large pores that theoretically allow for greater permeability of larger putative uremic toxins. There are no comparisons of low-flux and high-flux membranes in HT; the only available data pertain

to comparisons involving conventional IHDF or high-flux IHD versus low-flux IHD. In studies of ARRT in the ICU population, the more permeable membranes demonstrate no clinical or laboratory advantages over the less porous ones.[30-32] This negative result may be biased by residual confounding in these studies from unrecognized back-transport of potentially harmful waterborne molecules (see previous discussion). Alternatively, the negative results may be true, resulting from the low mass removal of larger solutes (in absolute terms) afforded by these modalities. For instance, low-flux IHD clears about 3 mL/min of β_2-microglobulin from blood water during the course of treatment, high-flux IHD only clears about 35 mL/min, and even IHDF clears only about 50 to 150 mL/min, depending on the hemofiltration (Q_F) rate.[33] Given the short duration over which these modalities are applied, a meaningful clinical effect seems unlikely. In contrast, the longer duration for HT makes a clinical effect seem more plausible, although it remains to be proven.

The effect of membrane biocompatibility on outcomes (when present) is consistently beneficial, although the data overall are conflicting.[34,35] Notwithstanding, such membranes can now be obtained cheaply, and because cost has been eliminated as a deciding factor, it is recommended that all patients be treated with these membranes.

On-line hemodiafiltration is being increasingly used during HT.[10,17,18] The rationale for this technique is predicated on a survival benefit conferred by combined convection and diffusion that is not conferred by diffusion alone. This assumption has some support in the literature but is not proven. Hemofiltration rates reported during convective HT vary from 17 to 100 mL/min. Higher convection leads to increased clearance of middle-sized and larger uremic solutes, which can amount to more than 50% of the small solute clearance. Moreover, other features of on-line hemodiafiltration, such as thermal energy transfer, may also affect clinical outcomes. Several groups of investigators have demonstrated the logistic feasibility of convective HT.[10,17,18,24] Further studies are still needed, however, to compare outcomes of this modality and diffusive HT. These studies should explore not only the relationship between removal of middle-sized and larger uremic solutes and clinical outcomes but also the role of thermal energy transfer and other features of convective ARRT in general.

Hemodialyzer size is probably not critical. Two groups have reported experience with moving from a larger to smaller hemodialyzers for HT, for the purposes of reducing extracorporeal circuit clotting.[14,19] Neither group has reported any deterioration in solute control or clearance. It should be noted that the relationship between hemodialyzer urea mass-transfer area coefficient (K_0A), Q_D, and Q_B is not predictable during HT because of a mismatch between dialysate and blood flows due to incomplete fiber bundle penetration at low flows that creates a shunt within the dialyzer.[36] Further studies on this important area are needed before a recommendation can be made.

CLINICAL OUTCOMES

The major surrogate endpoint in ARRT is optimal control of solute and fluid balance, but the true clinical endpoints are patient mortality and recovery of renal function. As with all ARRT, outcomes studies in HT have mostly related practice patterns to the former rather than the latter outcomes. All reports of HT have consistently shown that

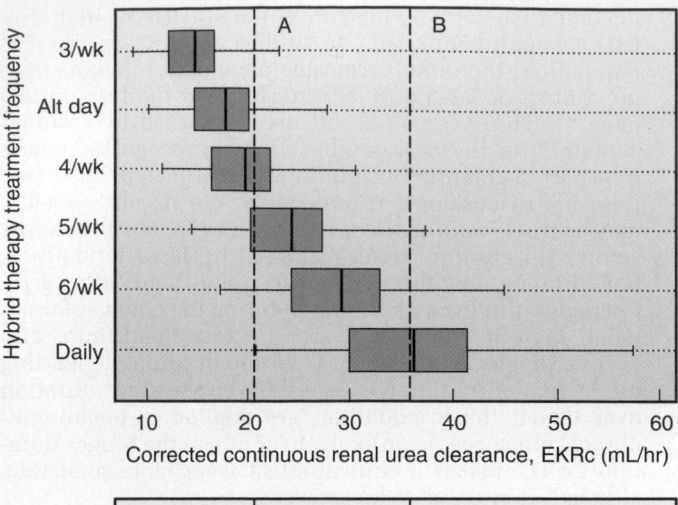

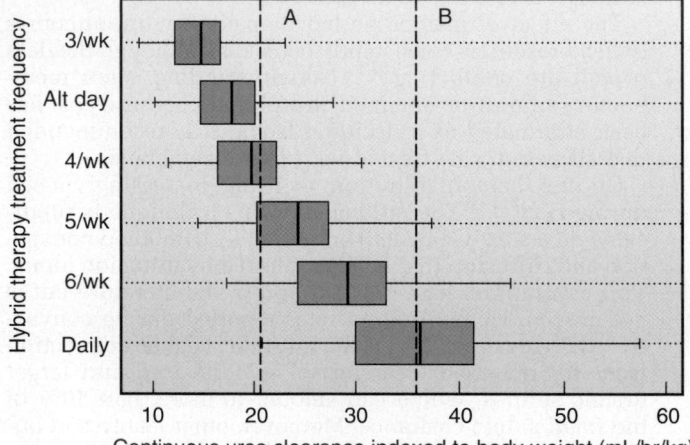

FIGURE 234-1. Small solute clearance achieved in the first 100 patients in the hybrid therapy program at Middlemore Hospital, New Zealand.

electrolyte concentrations can be maintained within normal limits.

There are no agreed standards for solute control in ARRT. In terms of small solutes, however, strong suggestions have been made in various reports that clinical outcomes are optimized during CRRT with a urea clearance of 35 mL/kg/hour or more and during IHD with Kt/V of 0.92 at a frequency of 6.2 per week.[37,38] Although not experimentally verified, these different expressions for small solute clearance can be unified using the corrected equivalent renal urea clearance (EKRc), which reexpresses the preceding doses as a continuous clearance that provides the same time-averaged concentration of BUN for the same mass of urea removed, corrected for a urea redistribution volume of 40 L.[39,40] Expressed in this way, the values for EKRc that correspond to the two suggestions above are 35.9 mL/min for CRRT and 20.7 mL/min for IHD (assuming V = 0.65 × body weight).[41] Readers are referred to the chapters in this book on ARRT quantification for a more detailed explanation of these concepts and calculations.

The small solute clearance achieved in the first 100 patients in the HT program at Middlemore Hospital, New Zealand, is illustrated in Figure 234-1. Small solute kinetics from other published HT experiences are shown in Table 234-3.[9-19,39,40,42] In general, metabolic control in most case series is comparable to that observed during CRRT, with one quasi-randomized controlled trial also reporting similar conclusions.[14]

It should be noted that multicompartmental effects due to urea dysequilibrium do not occur to a significant degree during HT, as indicated by the parity between whole body and hemodialyzer urea clearances, minimal post-dialysis BUN rebound, conformity between observed intradialytic time-concentration BUN profiles and those predicted from a standard single-pool urea kinetic model, and monexponential dialysate urea nitrogen time-concentration profile (Fig. 234-2). These findings all indicate minimal urea dysequilibrium.[36,43]

It should also be noted that small solute clearance is actually reduced by hemodialyzer clotting. In fact, the on-line clearance or ratio of dialysate/filtrate (effluent) urea nitrogen to BUN (i.e., EUN/BUN) has been used to permit an elective change of a failing filter before it clots. This strategy is based on the observation that there is a decline in EUN/BUN over the treatment course, probably due to a combination of concentration repolarization and diafilter clotting. Although this issue has not been prospectively validated, it is the firm recommendation from opinion leaders that a EUN/BUN less than 60% mandates diafilter replacement (R. Mehta, personal communication, 15 July 1999).

There are fewer data on larger solute clearance during HT. As discussed previously, interest in these particular solutes arises from the potential for removal of middle-molecule inflammatory mediators. Notwithstanding, the greatest removal of such molecules can be achieved with hemodiafiltration, although some removal also occurs

TABLE 234-3

Reported Rates of Small Solute Clearance Delivered By Hybrid Dialysis Therapy

	Study									
	SCHLAEPER ET AL[19]	FINKEL AND FORINGER[12]	LONNEMANN ET AL[15]	MARSHALL ET AL[16]	MARSHALL ET AL[17]	NAKA ET AL[18]	KUMAR ET AL[13,14]	FIACCADORI ET AL[11]	LI ET AL[9]	BERBECE ET AL[10]
BUN (mg/dL):										
Before treatment	21*	17*	82	71.6	54.9	53.8	24	75	69.5	26.6
After treatment	N/A	N/A	38	31	20.4	37.0	N/R	37	12.5	10.4
Serum creatinine (mg/dL):										
Before treatment	1.7*	1.5*	3.93	3.4	3.85	3.1	2.5	N/R	8.74	1.07*
After treatment	N/A	N/A	1.96	1.6	1.81	2.43	N/R	N/R	1.87	N/R
spKt/V per treatment	2.4 (daily)	24 (daily)	1.25[†]	1.45	1.43	0.56[†]	1.14	1.17[†]	1.60[‡]	1.39
EKRc per treatment (mL/min)	54[§]	N/R	31.68[ǁ]	31.9[§]	35.7	15.5[ǁ]	25.1[¶]	28.9[ǁ]	39.6[ǁ]	29[§]
Urea nitrogen removed (g/day)	N/R	N/R	33.1	28.6	N/R	N/R	N/R	N/R	N/R	N/R

BUN, blood urea nitrogen; EKRc, corrected equivalent renal urea clearance; N/A, not applicable; N/R, not reported; spKt/V, single-pool Kt/V.
*Steady state solute concentrations.
[†]spKt/V calculated using reported data either (a) from direct dialysate quantification using reported pre- and post-treatment BUN and urea nitrogen mass removal, or (b) iteratively by formal single pool urea kinetic modeling using reported pre- and post-treatment BUN combined with hemodialyzer clearance calculated using manufacturer reported KoA.
[‡]spKt/V calculated using reported data from pre- and post-treatment BUN by method of Basile et al.[42]
[§]EKRc calculated from reported continuous urea clearances or EKR by correcting for V = 40L with correction for urea non-steady state by method of Casino and Marshall.[40]
[ǁ]EKRc calculated from Kt/V values using nomogram method of Casino and Lopez assuming daily treatments.[39]
[¶]EKR as originally reported unable to be corrected to V = 40L.

Hours	0	2	4	6	8	10	12	13
○ Modeled BUN	76.9	64.5	54.5	46.4	39.9	34.7	30.4	32.6
□ Observed BUN	76.9	62.1	52.2	44.4	38.6	33.7	30.2	33.9

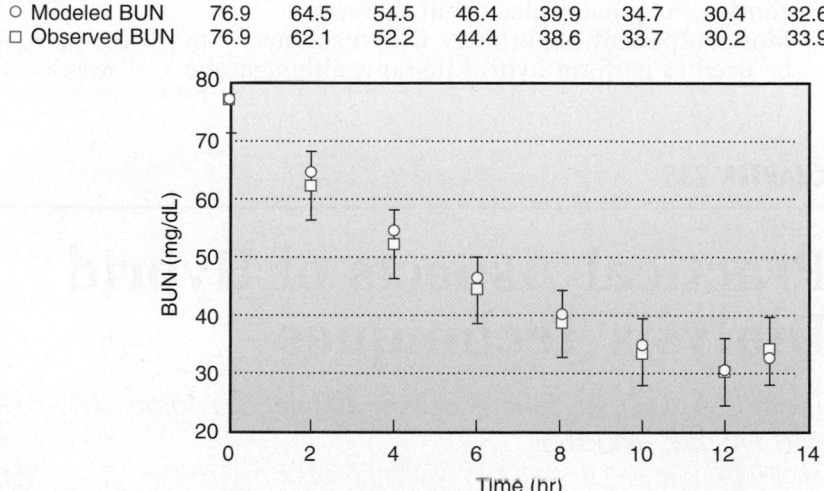

FIGURE 234-2. Graphic description of BUN profiles during hybrid renal replacement therapy under the condition of single pool urea kinetics, with *hollow squares* representing observed BUN profile and *hollow circles* representing the modeled BUN profile. Points of data are presented in graph as mean +/− standard error and in tabulated form as mean (n = 9; correlation coefficient = 0.99).

with HT based on high-flux dialysis without filtration. The literature as a whole suggests that clearance of larger solutes is between 50% and 66% of that of small solutes using high-flux HT or hemodiafiltration, and very low with low-flux HT.[17,21,44,45] Support for beneficial immunomodulation by HT can be found in one study reporting restoration of function for stimulated but exhausted circulating monocytes,[46] and in two studies showing improvement in the ratio of anti-inflammatory to pro-inflammatory mediators.[9,47]

All reports of HT have shown ultrafiltration to be well tolerated and not to be associated with undue cardiovascular instability. In some series, a minor temporary increase in inotrope dose has been noted during treatments, especially in patients with more severe illness and greater cardiovascular instability.[16,17] In the literature as a whole, between zero and 7% of patients were reported to have discontinued HT treatment because of intractable hypotension. Many of these patients also could not be supported by CRRT. A quasi-randomized controlled trial reported similar conclusions.[14]

The most rigorous assessment of cardiovascular stability during hybrid treatments comes from a randomized controlled trial of HT versus CRRT. Thirty-nine critically ill patients were randomly assigned to either arm, achieving total ultrafiltration of 3.0 L over 12 hours and 3.3 L over 24 hours during the hybrid treatment and CRRT, respectively. There was no significant difference in inotrope dose or number between the groups. There was an insignificant trend to slightly lower blood pressure and cardiac output in the HT group, and a slightly higher peripheral vascular resistance. This trend was not reflected in outcomes, and any associated cardiovascular instability that might exist is likely to be of little clinical significance.[21]

No modality of ARRT in the critically ill patient with acute renal failure has been shown to confer a survival benefit.[48,49] All of the reported experiences with HT suggest that patients' outcomes are no different from those predicted by the patients' illness severity scores. A single-center observational study found no change in patient mortality rates over time with a facility-level change from CRRT to HT.[50]

CONCLUSION

HT is effective, safe, and cheap. It is likely that HT will become the dominant ARRT in the next 10 years. Appropriate machinery is now emerging from major vendors that will facilitate the growth of this modality.

Key Points

1. Hybrid renal replacement therapy is a conceptual and logistic compromise between the modern applications of intermittent hemodialysis and continuous renal replacement therapy.
2. Most outpatient nephrology IHD machinery can be used to perform hybrid therapy, although one should be aware of the limitations of the machines in terms of the lowest dialysis flow rate and the longest hybrid therapy session length that can be provided.
3. The prescription and provision of hybrid therapy is very flexible and can be varied when desired to suit the requirements of the institution and patient.
4. Hybrid renal replacement therapy provides high small solute clearance and significant larger solute clearance.
5. This modality allows ultrafiltration with a minimum of cardiovascular instability and is well tolerated by patients with severe illness.

Key References

10. Berbece AN, Richardson RM: Sustained low-efficiency dialysis in the ICU: Cost, anticoagulation, and solute removal. Kidney Int 2006;70:963-968.
15. Lonnemann G, Floege J, Kliem V, et al: Extended daily venovenous high flux haemodialysis in patients with acute renal failure and multiple organ dysfunction syndrome using a single path batch dialysis system. Nephrol Dial Transplant 2000;15:1189-1193.
16. Marshall M, Golper T, Shaver M, et al: Sustained low-efficiency dialysis for critically ill patients requiring renal replacement therapy: Clinical experience. Kidney Int 2001; 60:777-785.
18. Naka T, Baldwin I, Bellomo R, et al: Prolonged daily intermittent renal replacement therapy in ICU patients by ICU nurses and ICU physicians. Int J Artif Organs 2004;27:380-387.
43. Marshall M, Golper T: Sustained low-efficiency or extended daily dialysis. UpToDate Available at www.uptodate.com/ [search using keyword SLED].

See the companion Expert Consult website for the complete reference list.

CHAPTER 235

Practical Aspects of Hybrid Dialysis Techniques

Thomas A. Golper, John A. Clark, Daniel S. Majors, Maureen Craig, and Mark R. Marshall

OBJECTIVES

This chapter will:
1. Describe the technical requirements and delivery aspects of hybrid renal replacement therapies.
2. Discuss the differences among intermittent, hybrid, and continuous renal replacement therapies and explain how these differences can become the strengths and/or weaknesses of the therapies.
5. Explain how to modify hybrid therapies to suit a specific hospital's or patient's needs.
6. Review the cost differences among these therapies.
7. Identify future research needs regarding hybrid therapies.

WHY HYBRID THERAPIES?

Hybrid renal replacement therapies combine the most useful components of intermittent treatments with those of continuous therapies. These therapies have compelling advantages, such as improved ease of operation, versatility, reduced costs, and widespread availability.

Ease of Operation

Operational characteristics of hybrid therapies are detailed later. The fact that virtually every hospital facility caring for patients with end-stage kidney failure provides some form of hemodialysis already implies an existing skill set and infrastructure. The modifications of traditional intermittent hemodialysis (IHD) that characterize hybrid therapies are simple extensions or expansions of the existing skill set that are easily translated to the critical care setting within any institution.

Versatility

Hybrid therapies can be applied to virtually any clinical situation that requires renal replacement therapy (RRT). The major functions of RRTs span the spectrum from pure solute removal to pure fluid removal and can be achieved with either continuous or intermittent delivery. Hybrid RRTs have the capacity to deliver any combination of functions along the entire RRT spectrum, for any duration, with the simple adjustment of machine controls. No new solutions are required from the pharmacy or supply depot, and no new connections are made. Essentially all the tools needed are already in place mechanically and conceptually. Thus, the versatility of hybrid RRTs is beyond comparison.

Cost

Clearly, the manner in which the treatment is performed will influence costs. However, the variations of operational characteristics in hybrid therapies have a much smaller impact on costs than do the variations of operational characteristics for continuous renal replacement therapies (CRRTs).

Hybrid therapies are most cost-effective if treatments are nocturnal, thereby allowing machines to be used for IHD treatments during the day. At Vanderbilt University Medical Center, University of California, Davis, and Middlemore Hospital, all of the chapter authors perform hybrid therapies during the day.[1,2] Even under these circumstances, hybrid therapies appear to be sixfold less expensive than continuous therapies on a daily basis.[3] The calculations and assumptions that apply in the derivation of the sixfold figure are detailed in Tables 235-1 and 235-2. If regular dialysate is used, the difference is even greater than if citrate-containing dialysate (Citrasate) is used. With regional citrate anticoagulation, the regimens used for hybrid therapies versus CRRTs are similar, such that the costs attributed to anticoagulation are similar if the hybrid therapy runs continuously. If hybrid therapy runs for less than continuous periods, the cost of the regional citrate anticoagulation is less than that with CRRT. The cost of citrate is a function of both duration of therapy and blood flow rate (Q_B) (because it determines citrate infusion rate). This issue is discussed later (see "Anticoagulation"). Under all circumstances, the costs of hybrid therapies are considerably less than the costs of CRRTs, as corroborated by others.[4]

Availability

Hybrid therapy programs are often limited by the availability of suitably trained nursing staff. The programs are less limited by the availability of medical staff, because any nephrologist or intensivist who understands the principles and techniques of IHD can prescribe and manage hybrid therapies. Nursing staff assignments (dialysis staff vs. intensive care unit staff) are discussed later. Whether dialysis or ICU nurses, the personnel providing RRT for patients with ARF have, in general, embraced hybrid therapies as being easier than and preferable to CRRTs.[1]

HYBRID THERAPY SETUP

Equipment

Essentially *any hemodialysis machine* can be utilized for hybrid therapy. However, the more modern machines are more suitable because they have built-in components that make operational changes easier (see later discussion of operational characteristics). Furthermore, because hybrid therapy running times are extended and/or dialysate flow rates are increased, patients are exposed to larger volumes of dialysate, and the processing of dialysate water requires modern methods for purification from bacterial byproducts. Dialysate and blood flow variations for hybrid therapy are typically different from those in standard IHD, and the machines must be able to vary these flows in the least labor-intensive manner. Many vendors already have machine platforms that switch easily and instantly between hybrid therapies and standard IHD. Thus, the equipment serves multiple purposes for a dialysis facility. This approach is typified by the scheduling of nocturnal sustained low-efficiency dialysis (SLED) and two or three diurnal IHD treatments per machine in a 24-hour period.

Portable reverse osmosis machines are needed when central on-line water delivery systems are unavailable. This requirement exists whether IHD or hybrid therapies are performed and is the alternative to using pharmacy-made or commercially purchased dialysate or replacement solutions in CRRT.

Dialyzers used for hybrid therapies can be the same as those used for IHD, depending on the operating conditions (see later), and may actually be smaller and cheaper. In any case, they are considerably cheaper than those used in most CRRTs (see Table 235-1).

The modality determines whether one uses *dialysate* or *replacement fluids*. When the modality involves hemodialysis, dialysate is generated by a proportioning system for which there is either a central or local water source. Central sources may utilize a processing system in one locale, then a delivery system throughout the hospital. Most hospital dialysis units are fed water locally (in the ICU or the patient's room) that is subsequently processed by a portable system (reverse osmosis machine plus dialysis machine). When the modality involves additional hemofiltration, on-line replacement fluids can be generated from purified dialysate; this technique is not yet approved in the United States, however. The generation of the cleansing solutions in hybrid therapies is in clear contradistinction to those in CRRT, in which pharmacies or commercial vendors bag solutions that are delivered in bulk to the point of service. This difference creates much of the cost differential between hybrid therapies and CRRTs (see Table 235-1).

The proportioning systems in hemodialysis machines require containers of dialysate concentrate. Depending on the operating conditions elected (see later), the concentrate container may last for 12 to 18 hours. This arrangement reduces labor costs, in that nurses spend time on direct patient care instead of changing out the solution bags as required in CRRTs. Essentially, the nurse can devote more attention to patient care, whether for the patient undergoing hybrid therapy or for another patient.

TABLE 235-1

Cost Comparisons for Sustained Low-Efficiency Dialysis (SLED) using a Fresenius K Machine and Continuous Renal Replacement Therapy (CRRT) using a Gambro PRISMA Machine

SUSTAINED LOW-EFFICIENCY DIALYSIS		CONTINUOUS RENAL REPLACEMENT THERAPY	
MACHINES AND SUPPLIES	*COST**	*MACHINES AND SUPPLIES*	*COST**
Fresenius K (Fresenius Medical Care, Homburg, Germany)	20,000	PRISMA (Gambro AB, Stockholm)	25,000
Portable reverse osmosis machine (RO)	5,000		
F50 dialyzer (each)	17	PRISMA circuit includes dialyzer	170
Bloodlines	2.90		
Liquid bicarbonate (4 gal)	12.32	Baxter Pre-mixed dialysate ($27/5 L) @ 2 L/hr use over 24 hours	324
		or	
		Gambro Prismasate with bicarbonate ($35/5 L) @ 2 L/hr use over 24 hours	420
Citrasate, 4 gal	27		
or			
8 gal	54		
Normal saline prime (2 L)	1.26	Saline prime (4 L)	2.52
—		Heparin (per day)	15
Diasafe ultrafilter for Fresenius K, $50.00/ filter; replacement every 7 weeks $1485.72 per year + Biomed labor for installation	$4/day over whole year	—	
Monthly AAMI standard culture and endotoxin for each Fresenius K and each RO plus biannual AAMI standard chemical analysis per RO $2144.00 per year + follow-up samples as needed	$6/day over whole year	—	
Supply cost 1 SLED setup and projected run 14 hours (8 gallons of Citrasate)†	97.48	Supply cost 1 CRRT setup bicarbonate premixed dialysate and average 24-hour run per circuit	511.52 (Baxter) or 607.52 (Gambro)

AAMI, American Association for Medical Instrumentation
*Costs given in 2004 U.S. dollars.
†Assuming Citrasate is used; cost will be lower if standard dialysate is used.
Modified from Golper TA: Hybrid renal replacement therapies for critically ill patients. Contrib Nephrol 2004;144:278-283.

Dialysate for RRT in the critically ill patient should probably be ultrapure, especially when porous membranes are used for dialysis. Dialysate is usually purified by passing it through an ultrafilter, which removes bacteria and endotoxins by virtue of a pore size of about 0.22 μm and specific adsorptive properties. Thus, the water in dialysate is purified by passage through a reverse osmosis membrane, one ultrafilter, and, finally, the dialyzer membrane before it enters the patient's circulation during backfiltration.

Fluid preparation differs for replacement fluid that is directly administered intravenously during on-line hemodiafiltration. Replacement fluid for direct intravenous administration is generated from a fraction of dialysate that is redirected prior to entering the dialyzer. This frac-

tion is sterilized by being passed through at least two ultrafilters before being infused directly into the blood lines. The U.S. Food and Drug Administration has not approved such a process. A similar situation exists in some European countries; and as a result of such restrictions in these countries, replacement fluid preparation and on-line hemodiafiltration are not available to patients.

STAFFING

Across the world there are many different models of care for the provision of IHD. In general, IHD requires a nephrology/dialysis nurse who has been fully trained in the use

TABLE 235-2

Comparisons of Labor Requirements for Sustained Low-Efficiency Dialysis (SLED) and Continuous Renal Replacement Therapy (CRRT)

PERSONNEL	SLED	CRRT
Dialysis Registered Nurse (RN)	• Set up and monitor over first hour • Then check at least three times/day Provide 24/7 coverage for troubleshooting and new setups when needed	• Set up and monitor over first hour • Then check at least three times/day Provide 24/7 coverage for troubleshooting and new setups when needed because of clotting
Intensive care unit RN	• Monitor and calculate ultrafiltration each hour • Perform basic troubleshooting for alarms and termination if needed Notify dialysis staff of anything unusual	• Monitor and calculate ultrafiltration each hour • Change dialysate bags every 2.5 hours and empty effluent bag every 2.5 hours • Perform basic troubleshooting for alarms and termination if needed Notify dialysis staff of anything unusual

of both the water system and the dialysis delivery system, including setup and dismantling of the dialysis machine and circuit. Where legally applicable, suitably credentialed patient care dialysis technicians may also perform the technical aspects of the dialysis. In the United States, the ICU nurse generally has no responsibility for this form of RRT, other than for collaborating with the dialysis nurse in demarcated of areas of responsibility, such as intravenous fluid loading and vasopressor administration for hypotension.

Models of care for hybrid therapies are as versatile as the modalities themselves. There are two broad fundamental types of care, those pertaining to "open" ICUs such as those at Vanderbilt University Medical Center and the University of California, Davis, and those pertaining to "closed" ICUs such as those at Middlemore Hospital. In "open" ICUs, hybrid therapies are performed through collaboration between nephrology and ICU nursing personnel. At Vanderbilt University Medical Center and the University of California, Davis, the nephrology nurse, who has been fully trained in the use of both the water system and the dialysis delivery system, including setup and dismantling of the dialysis machine/circuit, is responsible for the following tasks:

1. Setting up the water system: Initial testing and verification of water quality as well as ensuring that the water pressure is adequate to keep the water system running continuously. Location of the water system and the safe and unobtrusive placement of water lines are also a concern.
2. Setting up the dialysis delivery system: Setting up the dialysis machine, testing the alarms, verifying that the conductivity of the dialyzing fluid is acceptable, and priming the dialyzer and tubing.
3. Assessing the patient's blood access, especially the determination that blood flow will be adequate for the prescribed treatment.
4. Assessing the patient's volume, solute, and electrolyte status.
5. Initiating SLED or other hybrid treatment, and verifying that the parameters of the treatment match the physician's orders.
6. Ending the treatment and disassembling and disinfecting the equipment.
7. Developing and implementing a training and educational process for the ICU nurses that includes both theoretical and practical approaches.
8. Training the ICU nurses in basic troubleshooting (as well as determining the difference between basic trou-

bleshooting and advanced troubleshooting) for the dialysis access, the water treatment system, and the dialysis machine.
9. Acting as a resource for the ICU nurse and being available to assist in basic troubleshooting.
10. Collaborating with the nephrologist in the entire process from giving end-user/expert opinions during the equipment acquisition process and program setup to the end of the treatment and evaluation of the whole operation.
11. Acting as a patient advocate and liaison, coordinating patient care from multiple services.

The ICU nurse is responsible for the following:
1. Monitoring the equipment during the intradialytic period:
    • Troubleshooting the system and alarms. At the two institutions mentioned, flows are intentionally set to minimize alarms. For example, in the setting of a tenuous access, the blood flow rate may be turned down so the ICU nurse is not dealing with access pressure alarms.
    • Adjusting ultrafiltration rate.
    • Being familiar with the machines (location of knobs, dials, touch screens, etc.) and how they work.
    • Securing lines and monitoring for integrity of connections.
    • Assessing the dialysis catheter for integrity and function.
2. Assessing and documenting the patient's response to treatment.
3. Collaborating with the nephrology nurse and nephrologists.
4. Acting as a patient advocate and liaison, coordinating patient care from multiple services.
5. When required, knowing how to terminate the treatment and to preserve the dialysis catheter.
6. Drawing and monitoring laboratory specimens (eventually).
7. Titrating flow rates according to specific algorithms in the physician's orders—citrate/calcium, heparin, and ultrafiltration rate.

As is the norm in most aspects of modern medicine, standing orders and protocols simplify issues, allow reproducible methods and troubleshooting techniques (quality controls), and thus prevent many problems. A sample standing order set for extended daily dialysis from the dialysis program at the University of California, Davis, is presented in Figure 235-1.

Slow EDD or Continuous HD Orders with Regional Citrate Anticoagulation

Date/Time: _____   *For Date/Time:* _____

Directions: Check and complete those orders to be implemented (order renewal daily).

For assistance, Monday-Friday 0700-1930, call x48730; other hours, call operator for on-call nurse.

1. ☐ EKG monitoring required.

2. ☐ Patient weight: _____.

3. ☐ Priority: ☐ 1 ☐ 2   Vascular access: _____.

4. ☐ Dialysis type: ☐ SLEDD (8 hrs) ☐ CHD (24 hrs/day).

5. ☐ Dialyze _____ hours.

6. ☐ UF volume: _____liters (SLEDD)   UF Rate = Total patient input ± _____mL/hr (CHD).

7. ☐ Dialyzer: _____.

8. ☐ Blood flow rate _____ (100-200) mL/min. Dialysate flow rate_____ (SLEDD 300 or CHD 200) mL/min.

9. ☐ Dialysate: K^+_____(mEq/L) Na^+ _____ (135 mEq/L)
Phos_____(2.5 mg/dL)
Ca^{2+}_____(0 mEq/L) HCO_3^-_____(25-30 mEq/L).

10. ☐ Support SBP < _____ mm Hg with 0.9% NaCl or _____PRN. (SLEDD)

11. ☐ Call Nephrology if fluid bolus > 250 mL/shift is ordered for BP support or if MAP < 60 mm Hg. (CHD)

12. ☐ (Optional) Replacement fluid: Normal saline_____(1000-2000 mL/hr).

13. ☐ (Optional) Replace patient output (urine, stool, drains) mL for mL with replacement fluid.

Medications

14. ☐ ACD-A through arterial line _____ (150-250 mL/hr).

15. ☐ Adjust ACD-A to maintain **system** (venous port) ionized calcium 0.35-0.50 mMol/L:

*If **system** (venous port) ionized calcium is:*	*Adjust ACD-A as follows:*
<0.35	Decrease by 25 mL/hr
0.35-0.50	No change
>0.50	Increase by 25 mL/hr

16. ☐ Calcium gluconate 40 mg/mL (20 g in 500 mL NS) @ _____(60-180 mL/hr) in separate line or at venous return. (Avoid blood line reversal. Liver failure or increased ACD-A rates will require more calcium.)

17. ☐ Adjust calcium gluconate to maintain **arterial line or port** ionized calcium of 1.11-1.31 mMol/L:

*If **arterial line/port** (patient) ionized calcium is:*	*Adjust calcium gluconate as follows:*
<1.01	Increase by 20 mL/hr, see order #19, and call Nephrologist
1.01-1.10	Increase by 20 mL/hr

FIGURE 235-1. Sample of orders for slow extended daily dialysis or continuous hemodialysis with regional citrate anticoagulation, from Maureen Craig, University of California, Davis. ACD-A, 2.2% trisodium citrate plus 7% citric acid; BFR, blood flow rate; CBC, complete blood count; CHD, continuous hemodialysis; Chem-20, serum test for 20 chemicals; DFR, dialysate flow rate; EKG, electrocardiogram; ICU, intensive care unit; MAP, mean arterial pressure; NS, normal saline; Post-BUN, blood urea nitrogen concentration after dialysis; Pre-BUN, blood urea nitrogen concentration before dialysis; SLEDD, sustained low-efficiency daily dialysis; SPB, system blood pressure; UF, ultrafiltration.

| 1.11-1.31 | No change |
| >1.31 | Decrease by 20 mL/hr |

18. ☐ Give calcium gluconate 1 g in 50 mL NS @ 200 mL/hr for symptoms of hypocalcemia and/or for patient ionized calcium < 1.01 mMol/L.

Laboratory

19.   ☐ Draw pretreatment specimen for patient ionized calcium.

     ☐ Draw ionized calcium specimens from both system and patient 60 minutes after start and 60 minutes after prescribed BFR, DFR, ACD-A, or calcium gluconate infusion rate change, then every 2-3 hours for SLEDD or every 4-6 hours for CHD when rates are stable.

     ☐ Draw ionized calcium specimens if patient is symptomatic of hypocalcemia or hypercalcemia.

     ☐ Draw patient ionized calcium specimen 20 minutes after discontinuing treatment.

20   ☐ Chem-20   ☐ CBC   ☐ Pre-BUN   ☐ Post-BUN   ☐ Hepatitis screen

Ordering Nephrologist

_____

 P.I.#_____   Beeper # _____   Signature/Print Name
 Noted by

_____ R.N.

 (Nephrology Nurse)   Signature/Print Name
 Noted by

_____ R.N.

 (ICU Nurse)   Signature/Print Name

FIGURE 235-1, cont'd

At Middlemore Hospital, as for the vast majority of ICUs in Australia and New Zealand, which are "closed," the nephrology nurse has no responsibility for the performance of hybrid therapy.[5,6] All the responsibilities itemized in the preceding lists lie with ICU nursing personnel, including those pertaining to machine maintenance such as disinfection, and water testing and troubleshooting. In this arrangement, ICU nurses have the same training in the technical elements of dialysis as nephrology nurses, and arguably have a better appreciation of the patient's overall treatment goals in the ICU and, therefore, a better appreciation of the optimal hemodynamic and fluid status and response to therapeutic measures.

OPERATIONAL CHARACTERISTICS

Table 235-3 summarizes the operational characteristics of RRT and the factors that determine them. For any particular patient, operating conditions of RRT are determined in a logical and sequential manner from clinical conditions (Fig. 235-2). Understanding the interactions among operating characteristics is critical to the skillful prescription of hybrid therapies.

Hemodynamic stability is the prime determinant of RRT modality choice and prescription. For patients who are stable, ultrafiltration and solute removal goals can be achieved over a short time, and IHD is a suitable modality. For patients who are unstable, the fluid status becomes the next determinant of other operating conditions. Low ultrafiltration rates are needed to accommodate the hemodynamic instability. Time becomes the savior in this setting, and the ultrafiltration rate needed to achieve fluid removal goals determines the *duration of therapy* as well as the need for prolonged or even continuous therapies that attempt to utilize all minutes of the day.

The duration of therapy determines the solute removal rate. If the hemodynamics are so unstable that continuous therapy is needed, per-minute clearance goals can be less as time compensates for lower per-minute clearances. On the other hand, if hemodynamics allow-fluid balance to occur in 8 to 12 hours, the per-minute solute clearance must be higher. Blood flow rate and/or dialysate flow rate (Q_D) is increased to achieve higher per-minute clearances.

In continuous therapies, solute clearance is limited by the rate of ultrafiltration and fluid replacement in convective treatments, or by dialysate flow rates in diffusive treatments. Generally, the *blood flow* is not a factor for solute clearance if a blood pump is utilized. This issue became clear as CRRTs evolved from arteriovenous circuits to pump-driven venovenous circuits. So even if Q_B is as low as 100 mL/min or as high as 400 mL/min, solute clearance generally depends on Q_D (Fig. 235-3).

When hybrid therapies were designed in the late 1990s, it was assumed that hemodynamic instability would mandate daily application. Because solute clearance in hybrid therapies depends on Q_D and because duration of hybrid therapy depends on the patient's tolerance of ultra-

TABLE 235-3

Determinants of Operating Characteristics for Renal Replacement Therapy

OPERATING CHARACTERISTIC	DETERMINANT(S)
Ultrafiltration rate (UFR)	Initial volume status
	Hemodynamic instability
	Tolerance of fluid removal
Frequency	Volume status
	UFR tolerance
	Solute load
Duration	Volume status
	UFR tolerance
Blood flow rate (Q_B)	Set as high as can be without triggering flow alarms
Dialysate flow rate (Q_D)	Duration
	Frequency
Dialyzer size	Probably not important unless extracorporeal blood commitment is a concern
Dialyzer membrane	High-flux membrane preferred for removal of higher-molecular-weight electrolytes
Dialysate composition	Blood levels
	Form of anticoagulation

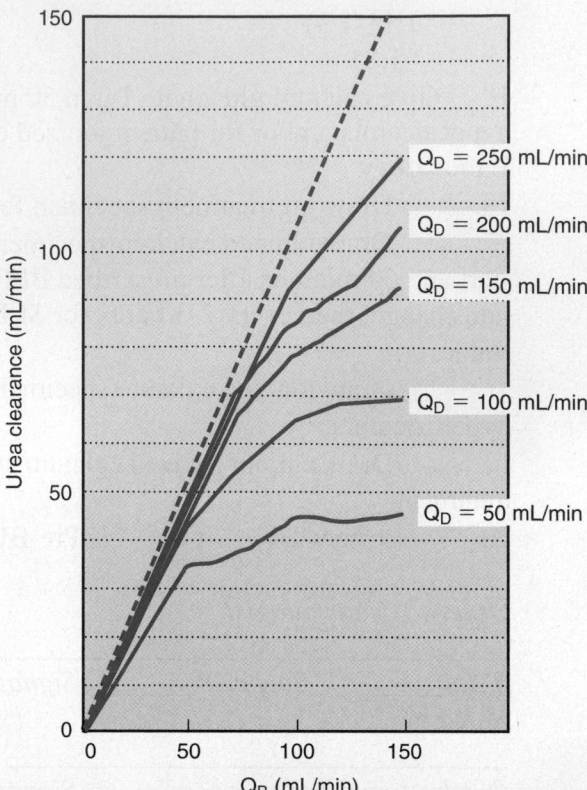

FIGURE 235-3. Determinants of urea clearance during hybrid hemodialysis treatments. This example is for sustained low-efficiency dialysis, showing the relationships among urea clearance, blood flow rate (Q_B), and dialysate flow rate (Q_D). The flattening of the urea clearance curves describe the conditions in which further rises in Q_B do not enhance clearance. (From Rose BD [ed]: UpToDate. Waltham, MA, UpToDate, 2006. Available at www.uptodate.com; with data from Kudoh Y, Iimura O: Slow continuous hemodialysis—new therapy for acute renal failure in critically ill patients—Part 1: Theoretical consideration and new technique. Jpn Circ J 52:1171-1182, 1988.)

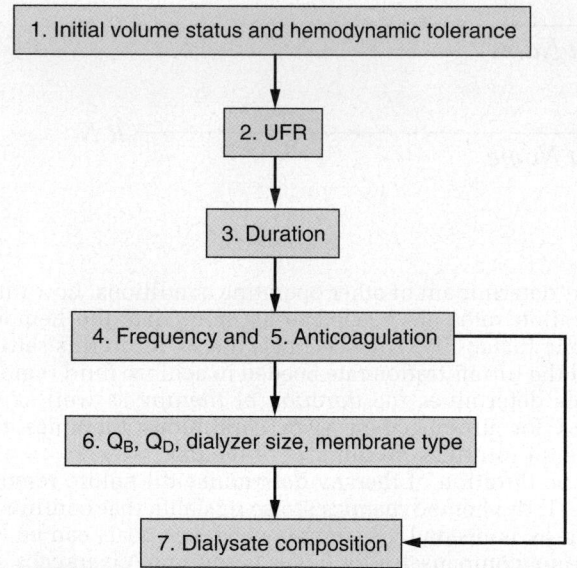

FIGURE 235-2. The sequence of decisions in determining the operating characteristics for a hybrid hemodialysis treatment. Duration determines both the frequency and the anticoagulation regimen, and the anticoagulation regimen influences dialysate composition—as do Q_B (blood flow rate), Q_D (dialysate flow rate), dialyzer size, and membrane type. UFR, ultrafiltration rate.

filtration rate, it becomes clear that operational conditions follow a logical sequence, as depicted in Figure 235-3. For purposes of simplicity, let us consider three durations of hybrid dialysis: 8 hours, 12 hours, and 24 hours. Adequate solute removal must now occur over this 8, 12, or 24 hours of therapy. A Q_D of 100 mL/min will deliver a urea clearance rate of about 65 mL/min and will provide a urea clearance (Kt/V_{urea}) of 1.2 to 1.6 over 10 to 12 hours.[7] On a daily basis, this is substantial clearance of small solutes. For higher-molecular-weight solutes, this arrangement

still provides substantial clearance, as depicted in Figure 235-4. For an 8-hour treatment, it is probably more prudent to utilize a Q_D of 300 mL/min to enhance per minute clearances. A simple approach is to set Q_D at 300 mL/min for treatments of 8 to 10 hours treatment and a Q_D of 100 mL/min for treatments of 10 to 24 hours. More study can precisely determine the best Q_D for a given expected duration of treatment time (see later discussion of research). High-Q_D hybrid treatments require considerably more calcium replacement during regional citrate anticoagulation because of the high clearance of the calcium-citrate complex (see discussion of anticoagulation).

Dialyzer size is probably not important but has not been studied. Larger devices require a larger extracorporeal blood commitment, which certainly is clinically significant in children. Small devices adequately ultrafilter and clear solute but may require longer duration of therapy or more frequent treatments. It should be noted that it is difficult to predict treatment clearance during low-Q_D and low-Q_B hybrid treatments from dialyzer mass transfer coefficients derived at higher blood and dialysate flows, because mismatch of these low flows within the hemodialyzer creates a shunt in which no solute transfer occurs. In a previous study of 9 patients undergoing SLED, Q_B

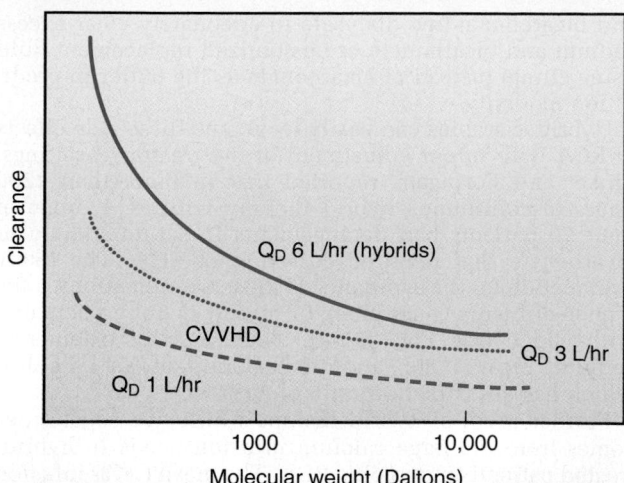

FIGURE 235-4. The relationship between clearance and molecular weight for different continuous/hybrid renal replacement therapies. The *dotted line* represents a dialysate flow rate (Q_D) of 3 L/hr, which is similar to the clearance recommended by Ronco et al[39] for the dose of renal replacement in acute renal failure. CVVHD, continuous venovenous hemodialysis.

200 mL/min and Q_D 100 mL/min were used with a 1.8-m^2 polysulfone low-flux hemodialyzer. Measured urea clearance by direct dialysis quantification averaged 78 mL/min, as opposed to the theoretical values of about 100 mL/min predicted from urea kinetic models.[7] The authors generally use high-flux dialyzers measuring 1 to 2 m^2 and often let cost and availability dictate practice.

Dialyzer membrane is preferentially a high-flux synthetic for both clearance and adsorptive characteristics. Backfiltration occurs under the usual operating conditions, explaining the concern about the quality of dialysate water.

Dialysate composition is determined by assessing the patient's metabolic and electrolyte status. Na^+, K^+, Ca^{2+}, HCO_3^-, and PO_4^{-3} are the main electrolytes that should be monitored and adjusted according to patient laboratory assessment and the patient's response to prior treatments.

Approximately 1.5 g of phosphorus are removed during a 12-hour hybrid treatment with Q_B 200 mL/min, Q_D 100 mL/min, and a low-flux 1.8-m^2 dialyzer.[1] Intravenous phosphorus supplementation is therefore required in patients having daily treatments, 0.1 to 0.2 mmol/kg or through the addition of 45 mL of Fleet Phospho-Soda to 9.5 L of bicarbonate concentrate to give a final concentration of 0.81 mmol/L.[8]

Changes in dialysate composition are often necessary during regional citrate anticoagulation (RCA; see later). For example, if hypernatremia occurs, perhaps secondary to trisodium citrate, the dialysate Na^+ concentration can be reduced to compensate and correct the problem. Alkalosis from citrate can be rectified by a reduction in the bath HCO_3^- concentration. A citrate gap can be corrected by an increase in Q_D. RCA requires a reduction or elimination of Ca^{2+} in the dialysate.

On-line hemodiafiltration is being used increasingly during hybrid therapies. The rationale for this technique is predicated on an added survival benefit with combined convection and diffusion compared with diffusion alone. This assumption has some support but is not yet proven. The ionic composition of replacement fluid does not differ from that of dialysate. The hemofiltration rate during hybrid treatments varies from 21 to 100 mL/min. Clearance of middle-sized and larger uremic solutes increases with rising hemofiltration rate, such that it can achieve 50% of the small solute clearance rate. Logistic feasibility of the technique has been demonstrated, although the clinical benefit is yet to be proven.

It is also important to remember the effect of RRT on amino acid levels. As with other RRTs, significant losses of amino acids occur during hybrid therapy, reportedly between 6.2 and 15.7 g per treatment. This loss mandates supplementation of protein prescriptions by 0.2 g/kg/day.[9,10]

ANTICOAGULATION

All of the anticoagulation strategies used in hybrid therapies have been used in clinical practice with CRRT and IHD for more than 30 years. The lower blood flow rates in CRRT predispose to clotting in the extracorporeal circuit. This effect is probably delayed by saline flushes and greatly reduced by systemic or regional (in the circuit only) anticoagulation.[4] Patients who might benefit from hybrid therapies are often at high risk for clotting or bleeding, and the added anticoagulation may further promote bleeding. The major anticoagulation strategy has traditionally been systemic administration of unfractionated heparin. Later strategies using regional anticoagulation free the patient from complications of systemic anticoagulation.

The lower Q_B used in hybrid therapies provides a reasonable dialysis dose achieved over a longer duration. Some authorities recommend that Q_B be maximized to the tolerance of the catheter to improve the patency of the circuit, and others recommend the use of smaller (and particularly shorter) dialyzers.[8,11] All of these interventions affect the other operating conditions (see Fig. 235-1).

Heparin

A polymucosaccharide composed of equal amounts of D-glucosamine and uronic acid, heparin has a molecular weight ranging from 3000 to 30,000 Da. It prolongs clotting time via potentiation of antithrombin III, which inhibits a number of clotting factors. Heparin is the most commonly used anticoagulant in all RRTs. Regimens include initial priming of the circuit by flushing with 5000 to 20,000 U heparin. Before initiation of CRRT, a heparin bolus of 2000 to 5000 U is administered, followed by a continuous infusion of 400 to 1000 U/hr.[12-15] Heparin anticoagulation is predictable. Heparin regimens in hybrid therapies typically consist of a 1000- to 2000-U bolus, followed by an infusion of 500 to 1000 U/hr to keep the activated partial thromboplastin time 10 to 20 seconds above or 1.5 times the control value.[1,5,6,16,17] In some protocols, hourly heparin infusion rates are 1080 U/hr for CRRT versus 643 U/hr for hybrid therapy, a 40% lower exposure to heparin.[18]

Saline Flushes

The use of saline flushes is a heparin-free approach in IHD treatments that is widely accepted and applied to hybrid therapies if nursing time can be devoted to such an intervention.[1,2,4] In one study in which 68% of patients received

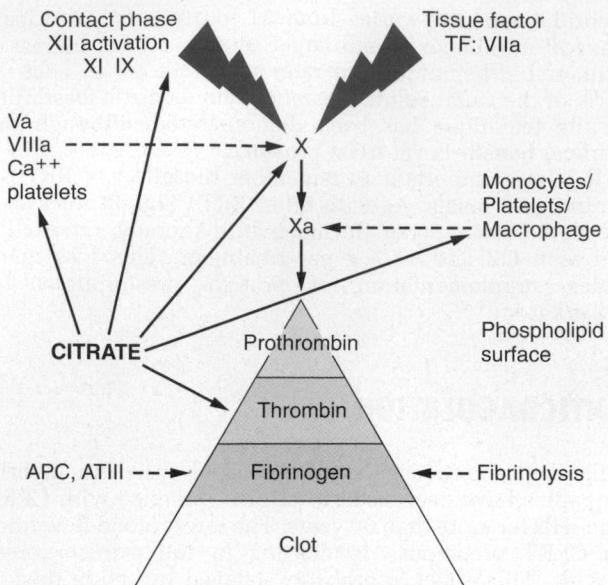

FIGURE 235-5. The role of citrate in the clotting cascade. APC, activated protein C; ATIII, antithrombin III.

heparin, filter clotting occurred in 17% of heparin treatments and 27% of heparin-free treatments.[2] In another description of hybrid therapies, 28% of treatments were performed without heparin and filter clotting occurred in 26% of all the treatments; the researchers concluded that there was no observed difference in clotting rate between treatments with and without heparin.[1] In a study reported from Toronto, heparin was used in 35% of SLED treatments (18% filter clot rate) and saline flushes in the remainder (29% filter clot rate).[4] Hybrid therapies are readily performed without systemic anticoagulation under certain circumstances, however, with the acknowledgment of the nuisance and expense that clotting poses in routine day-to-day practice.

Regional Citrate Anticoagulation

Calcium ions have pivotal roles in the coagulation cascade (Fig. 235-5). Usually added in the form of trisodium citrate, citrate ions bind (chelate) ionized (free) calcium in the blood. This decalcified blood does not clot. RCA, which was first introduced in 1983,[19] has expanded to and been modified for each dialysis modality. To date, the main application of RCA has been in CRRT, but it is being adapted to hybrid therapies.

There are two recognized citrate solutions in the United States. The first is trisodium citrate (TSC 4% sodium citrate) and the second is anticoagulant citrate dextrose (ACD), which is available in two formulations; ACD-A consists of 2.2% TSC plus 7% citric acid, and ACD-B of 1.32% TSC plus 0.48% citric acid. The most commonly used ACD solution in anticoagulation circuits is the ACD-A formulation. Citrate is metabolized to bicarbonate in skeletal muscle and liver tissue, generating about 2.8 mmol of sodium bicarbonate from 1 mmol of trisodium citrate. The final metabolism of these citrate solutions therefore produces several hundred mmols of sodium bicarbonate per dialysis, potentially resulting in metabolic alkalosis and hypernatremia. These results have been observed in CRRT and usually require either the use of hyponatremic

and bicarbonate-free dialysate to adequately clear excess sodium and bicarbonate or customized replacement fluid using citrate instead of bicarbonate as the buffer in predilution modality.

Hybrid therapies can easily overcome these side effects of RCA with minor adjustment of the treatment settings. Finkel and Foringer[20] reported that in more than 2200 hours of continuous hybrid therapy with RCA, none of their 20 patients had derangements in serum sodium or bicarbonate that required cessation of RCA. The likely explanation for the avoidance of those complications is the higher diffusive capabilities of hybrid therapy compared with CRRT (see Fig. 235-4). This capacity extends to sodium, bicarbonate, and the calcium-citrate complex, which has an extraction ratio of 70%.[21]

Further proof of hybrid therapy's diffusive capabilities comes from the large calcium infusion needs in hybrid-treated patients undergoing RCA. The mean $CaCl_2$ infusion rate with continuous venovenous hemodialysis is approximately 8 mmol/hour when the Q_D is 33 mL/min. During hybrid therapy sessions, Q_D can vary from 100 to 300 mL/min. Under these varying operating conditions, the required mean $CaCl_2$ infusion rate rises to approximately 14 to 40 mmol/hour of elemental Ca^{2+} to maintain a normal serum ionized calcium level. As in other institutions, the protocol for RCA in hybrid therapy used at Vanderbilt University Medical Center has achieved safe and reliable citrate anticoagulation (Table 235-4). Other, less widely utilized regimens have also been published that use RCA with low calcium dialysate concentrations and no post-dialyzer calcium replacement.[18,20]

Citrisate

An alternative to heparin therapy and RCA is Citrisate, a commercially available dialysate that uses citric instead of acetic acid as buffer. Back-diffusion of citrate from the dialysate to the blood in the fibers of the dialyzer essentially decalcifies the blood at the membrane luminal surface, hence postponing coagulation at that site. The use of Citrisate during IHD has been reported to have rates of extracorporeal circuit clotting that were 60% to 70% less than rates for heparin-free dialysis.[22] However, the citrate content of the dialysate is only 2.4 mEq/L in the final diluted concentration within the dialyzer, which is well below the 7 to 15 mEq/L threshold required for true anticoagulation.[23] Calcium levels in the patient remain within the normal range when citrate dialysate is used, and no supplemental calcium replacement measures are needed. There is preliminary evidence supporting the use of Citrasate dialysate in hybrid therapy.[24] Madison and colleagues[24] reported a 26% clotting rate with hourly saline flushes alone versus 14% with Citrasate plus saline flushes, and 2% with ACD-A. Replication of this study is indicated before definitive recommendations can be made, but these findings are promising.

Other Regimens

There are many other anticoagulants, but they have all been used in either CRRT or IHD and only rarely with hybrid therapies. They are mainly used as alternatives to heparin for contraindications like heparin-induced thrombocytopenia (HIT) and active bleeding.

Low molecular weight heparins (LMWHs) are products of depolymerization of unfractionated heparin and have

TABLE 235-4

Regional Citrate Anticoagulation for Sustained Low-Efficiency Dialysis as Performed at Vanderbilt University Medical Center

Machine, flow rates, duration	• Fresenius 2008K machine • Blood flow rate (Q_B) 250 mL/min • Dialysate flow rate (Q_D) 300 mL/min • 8- to 10-hour treatment duration daily
Fluids and infusion rates: Dialysate	0 calcium 3-4 mmol/L K^+ Standard bicarbonate concentration
Calcium chloride ($CaCl_2$) solution	160 mL of 10% $CaCl_2$ in 250 mL 0.9% NaCl Pharmacy to prepare and deliver ×1 premix (39 mg/mL) $CaCl_2$ solution or 1 mmol Ca^{2+}/mL
Citrate solution	4% sodium citrate solution in 250 mL (40 gm/L = 144 mmol/L) Pharmacy to provide 10 × 250 mL premix bags of 4% sodium citrate
Run sodium citrate infusion PRE-FILTER @ 231 mL/hr Start $CaCl_2$ infusion POST-FILTER @ 41 mL/hr Titration protocol:	9.24 gm/hr = 33 mmol/hr of Na citrate 1.6 g/hr = 14.5 mmol/hr of $CaCl_2$ = 40 mmol/hr of Ca^{2+} Caution on use of units; use the units as the laboratory reports ionized calcium [iCa^{2+}] values

Conversions:
  To convert mmol/L of ionized calcium to mg/dL
  To convert mmol/L of ionized calcium to mEq/L
  To convert mmol/L of sodium citrate to mg/dL
	
	Multiply by 2
	Multiply by 4
	Multiply by 27.6

Rate adjustment protocol: If circuit iCa^{2+} < 0.8 mg/dL If circuit iCa^{2+} is 0.8-1.6 mg/dL	 Decrease citrate rate by 5 mL/hr Do not change the citrate rate; this is the optimal laboratory value range
If circuit iCa^{2+} is 1.6-2.0 mg/dL If circuit iCa^{2+} > 2.0 mg/dL If patient iCa^{2+} > 5.8 mg/dL If patient iCa^{2+} is 4.8-5.8 mg/dL If patient iCa^{2+} is 4.0-4.8 mg/dL If patient iCa^{2+} is 3.6-4.0 mg/dL If patient iCa^{2+} < 3.6 mg/dL Notify Nephrology fellow if	Increase citrate rate by 5 mL/hr Increase citrate rate by 10 mL/hr Decrease $CaCl_2$ rate by 10 mL/hr Decrease $CaCl_2$ rate by 5 mL/hr Do not change $CaCl_2$ rate; this is optimal laboratory value range Increase $CaCl_2$ rate by 5 mL/hr Give bolus $CaCl_2$, 10 mg/kg, and increase $CaCl_2$ rate by 10 mL/hr Patient's serum HCO_3^- rises >10 mEq/L Patient's serum Na rises by >10 mEq/L or is >155 mEq/L*

*Serum HCO_3^- and serum Na should be measured prior to initiation of the procedure, at 4 hours, and at 6 hours.

molecular weights of around 5000 Da. Like unfractionated heparin, LMWHs bind to antithrombin III and potentiate its protease activity on the coagulation factors Xa, IXa, XIa, XIIa, and thrombin. Their activity can be monitored by measuring anti-Xa activity.[25] The use of LMWHs has not been studied in hybrid therapies.

There is a single report of *prostacyclin* (PGI₂) as anticoagulation during hybrid therapy.[26] It was infused at 6 ng/kg per min before the hemodialyzer. Although there was no control arm in this study, PGI₂ was associated with clotting in 11% of treatments, and no undue cardiovascular instability was observed.

The direct thrombin inhibitor *argatroban* can be used as a substitute for heparin. At Vanderbilt University Medical Center, a bolus of 100 to 250 μg/kg followed by a 2 μg/kg/min infusion throughout the treatment has been used in patients without liver failure.

Hirudin, a direct inhibitor of thrombin, has no cross-reactivity with heparin or LMWH. It has been used successfully in IHD as a substitute for heparin and has been shown to have the same protection against thrombosis at a lower activated partial thromboplastin time.[27,28] Although it has yet to be studied during hybrid therapies, hirudin may have a role in the patient with heparin-induced thrombocytopenia.

Nafamostat mesylate is a synthetic protease inhibitor with a very short half-life. It has been used in both intermittent and continuous renal replacement therapy, but not in hybrid treatments.[29,30] This agent shows considerable promise because its action on thrombin may prevent clotting, and its short half-life limits systemic anticoagulation. Experience with its use is still limited to countries outside the United States.

Anticoagulation Summary

Because the duration of exposure carries the greatest risk, the longer the therapy, the more important and the more complex becomes any form of anticoagulation. Therefore, it is generally easier and safer to anticoagulate for shorter therapies than for CRRTs. So even systemic anticoagulation, such as with heparin, will probably carry less risk in hybrid treatments than it would in the same patient undergoing CRRT. When RCA is used in the aggressive solute-removing, short-duration hybrid treatments (extended daily dialysis or 8-hour SLED), there is significant dialytic clearance of the calcium-citrate complex, so that much more calcium may be needed to recalcify the blood. Also, with the use of RCA, the higher the Q_B, the more citrate is needed,[31] but with the use of heparin, the opposite may be the case. Other than using RCA or Citrasate, all anticoagulation strategies lead to some level of systemic anticoagulation that increases the risk of bleeding. Although labor intensive, saline flushes remain a valid alternative to anticoagulation in hybrid therapies owing to shorter duration and higher Q_B than in CRRT. The operational characteristics of each hybrid therapy prescription determine the type and need for safe and reliable anticoagulation (see Fig. 235-1). The area of anticoagulation in hybrid therapy is evolving and needs continued investigation.

NEEDED RESEARCH IN HYBRID THERAPIES

Convective therapies remove higher-molecular-weight solutes more effectively than do diffusive therapies. Hybrid therapies generally emphasize diffusion, but in some countries where large quantities of on-line sterile water are allowed, hemodiafiltration is performed.[5] It follows then that comparisons between convective and diffusive hybrids will be made, and rightly so, as we need to see whether removing larger-molecular-weight species leads to better outcomes. Figure 235-4 summarizes the relationships between clearance and molecular weight in the different CRRTs.

Operational characteristics must be optimized to achieve cost-effective care, to minimize nursing time committed to the therapy, and to achieve the best possible outcomes. There are few data comparing the effect of different dialyzer sizes and membranes on RRT dose. Given that solute clearance is a potentially important determinant of outcomes, this area may be critical in the future. The role of on-line clearance measurements must be clarified. These measurements in themselves cannot produce a unified expression of dialysis dose that would be numerically comparable to expression of RRT dose for continuous therapies.[32] However, they are very likely to be useful as an input to other calculations that can produce such unified expressions. In the era of in-line plasma volume monitoring, one could predict ultrafiltration tolerance. Then, as noted in Figure 235-1, one could calculate the other operational characteristics and reassess results on a daily basis. Feedback control systems will be developed. This is based on observations in the setting of chronic dialysis treatments, in which blood pressure–plasma volume relationships are reasonably understood. This relationship is more variable in acute renal failure, however.

Short-duration hybrid treatments using heparin for 8 to 12 hours carry a bleeding complication risk that certainly is less than a 24-hour therapy but is still clinically significant. The operational characteristics to minimize anticoagulation requirements should be determined (e.g., very high Q_B). Regional citrate anticoagulation can be complicated by citrate accumulation, metabolic alkalosis, and hypernatremia. All three of these metabolic complications are readily correctable through adjustments in operating characteristics. Predicting the problem and estimating the necessary adjustment will take experience and clinical research. As for clearance, feedback control systems will be developed for anticoagulation status.

CONCLUSION

Because CRRT has not been shown to be superior in outcomes to IHD, CRRT will not be superior to hybrid therapy.[33-38] Hybrid renal replacement therapies will supplant CRRTs in the management of critically ill patients in the very near future. Their ease of operation, versatility, adaptability, simplicity, broad availability, and reduced costs will be persuasive arguments for their application in patients otherwise too unstable for IHD.

Key Points

1. Hybrid therapies are much easier and cheaper to perform and potentially more readily available than continuous renal replacement therapies.
2. The operational characteristics of hybrid therapies follow a logical sequence based on a patient's clinical needs.
3. The versatility of hybrid therapies allows any form of anticoagulation needed.
4. Complications and side effects of hybrid therapies are essentially self-correcting.
5. Hybrid therapies will replace the currently used, expensive continuous therapies within the next few years.

Acknowledgments

We are grateful to our physician colleagues, the inpatient dialysis nursing staff, the intensive care unit nursing staff, and our pharmacy staff for their continuous efforts to make our RRT programs improve. Without their efforts, no progress would be made.

Key References

1. Marshall M, Golper TA, Shaver MJ, et al: Sustained low efficiency dialysis for critically ill patients requiring renal replacement therapy: Clinical experience. Kidney Int 2001; 60:777-785.
2. Kumar V, Craig M, Depner T, Yeun J: Extended daily dialysis: A new approach to renal replacement therapy for acute renal failure in the intensive care unit. Am J Kidney Dis 2000;36: 294-300.
3. Golper TA: Hybrid renal replacement therapies for critically ill patients. Contrib Nephrol 2004;144:278-283.
8. Kumar VA, Yeun JY, Depner TA, Don BR: Extended daily dialysis vs. continuous hemodialysis for ICU patients with acute renal failure: A two year single center report. Int J Artif Organs, 2004;27:371-379.
17. Kielstein JT, Kretschmer U, Ernst T, et al: Efficacy and cardiovascular tolerability of extended dialysis in critically ill patients: A randomized controlled study. Am J Kidney Dis 2004;43:342-349.
18. Morgera S, Scholle C, Melzer C, et al: A simple, safe and effective citrate anticoagulation protocol for the Genius dialysis system in acute renal failure. Nephron Clin Pract 2004;98: c3514.

See the companion Expert Consult website for the complete reference list.

CHAPTER 236

Acute Dialysis with the GENIUS System

Detlef Kindgen-Milles, Thomas Roy, and Ciro Tetta

> ### OBJECTIVES
> This chapter will:
> 1. Describe the technical and operational features of the GENIUS therapy system.
> 2. Discuss the advantages of this system in the intensive care unit.
> 3. Review the clinical application of the GENIUS therapy system in the treatment of acute renal failure and multiple organ failure.
> 4. Report on single-center experience with this system.

Slow-extended daily dialysis (SLEDD) and so-called hybrid renal replacement therapy (RRT) have received more and more attention. A 2001 survey showed that resource availability, convenience, and practical limitations as well as the increased pressure on costs are bound to be more decisive in the choice of a given RRT modality than the conviction that one is superior over another.[1] It is not therefore surprising that the GENIUS therapy system (Fresenius Medical Care, Bad Homburg, Germany) is now being revaluated in the context of hybrid RRT in the intensive care unit (ICU).

This chapter is limited to the technical description of the GENIUS system and illustration of its clinical use in the ICU. The interested reader is referred to other sections of this chapter and to excellent reviews on SLEDD and other hybrid RRTs.[2-4]

THE GENIUS SYSTEM

Rationale and Technical Details

For more than 10 years, the GENIUS therapy system has been successfully used in Europe and Latin America for the dialysis of patients with chronic kidney disease. Originally developed by the late B. Tersteegen (1939-1995) in Düsseldorf, this system is used in more than 150 dialysis centers. For many years the GENIUS system was used for long-term hemodialysis. Later, however, several advantages derived from its use have made it a concrete and feasible alternative treatment for acute renal failure (ARF) in the context of multiple-organ failure.

The first hemodialysis systems were all based on the principle of the so-called tank or batch system: Batches of dialysate required for the dialysis session were prepared prior to the treatment in a tank, using water and the necessary electrolytes. The heater for the dialysate was integrated in the tank. A dialysate pump was employed to circulate the dialysate through the entire system. This technique implied that fresh and spent dialysate were mixed, which meant a gradual decrease of treatment efficiency related to the gradual increase of solute loading of the dialysate flowing through the hemodialyzer. The inadequate hygienic properties of these systems led to extreme microbiological contamination of the dialysate within a relatively short time. These two major deficiencies led to the replacement of the batch systems by so-called single-pass systems, in which the fresh dialysate is discarded after passing through the hemodialyzer.

The development of the GENIUS system was intended primarily to overcome the obvious deficiencies of classic batch systems while retaining their obvious advantages, such as technical simplicity and flexibility with regard to dialysate composition. The Rhodial 75 (Rhone Poulenc, Paris, France) was the first system to employ volumetrically controlled ultrafiltration (Fig. 236-1). All volumetric balancing single-pass systems that followed were built on more or less the same principle, with considerable technical effort and complexity.

Theory of Operation
Design Principle

The objective—retention of the advantages of a batch system while overcoming the known deficiencies—could be achieved by a suitable design. The technical features of the GENIUS therapy system offer important advantages for use in the ICU setting. The machine is supplied with electrical power from the 230V main circuit via a safety isolation transformer internally powered by 24V. An accumulator ensures continued operation also in the case of main power failure. Depending on its charge, it is possible to carry out dialysis for up to 8 hours without need for an external power supply. These features, together with the excellent mobility of the dialysis machine, which is mounted on four large castors (Fig. 236-2), facilitate a highly efficient treatment at any location without requiring the usual energy, water, and drainage installations.

The dialysis fluid is contained in a completely filled and thus air-free glass tank with a maximal capacity of 90 L (see Fig. 236-2). The thermal insulation of the transparent container prevents an excessive cooling of the prewarmed dialysis fluid, so there is no need for a separate heater. The distribution rod made from quartz glass is positioned along the central axis of the dialysis fluid container. The ultraviolet radiator, located in the center of the tube, facilitates operation with an ultrapure dialysis fluid.

During dialysis treatment, fresh dialysis fluid is aspirated from the upper part of the tank via the distribution rod and a peristaltic pump. After passage through the hemodialyzer, the fluid is returned to the lower part of the tank.

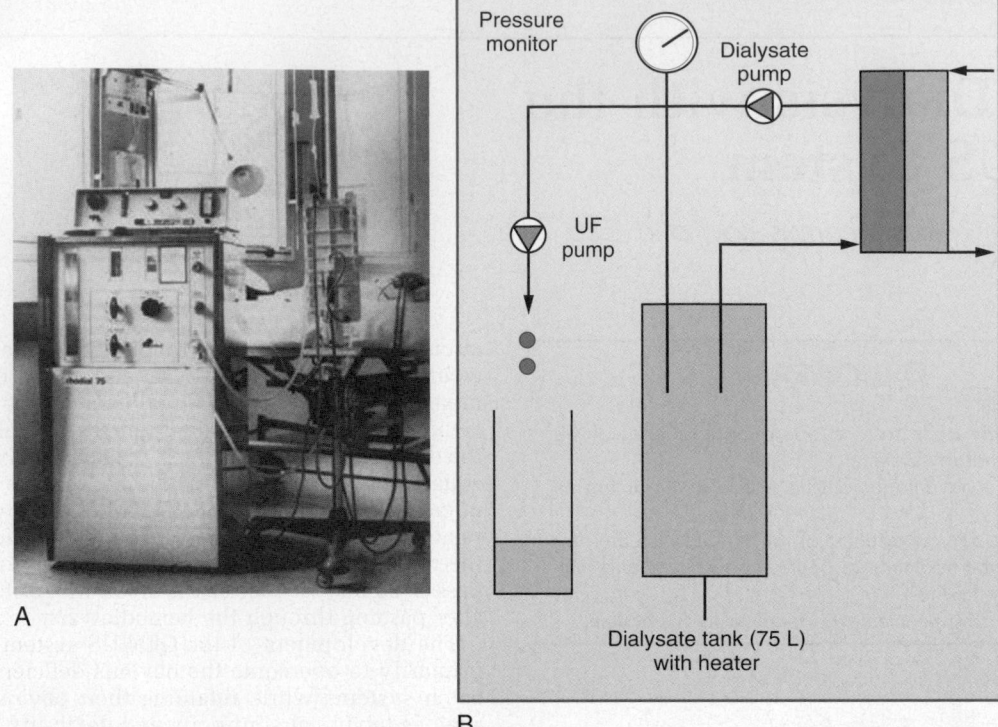

FIGURE 236-1. **A,** Illustration of the historical batch-system Rhodial 75 dialysis machine. **B,** Schematic drawing depicting the concept of the batch system and the control of ultrafiltration.

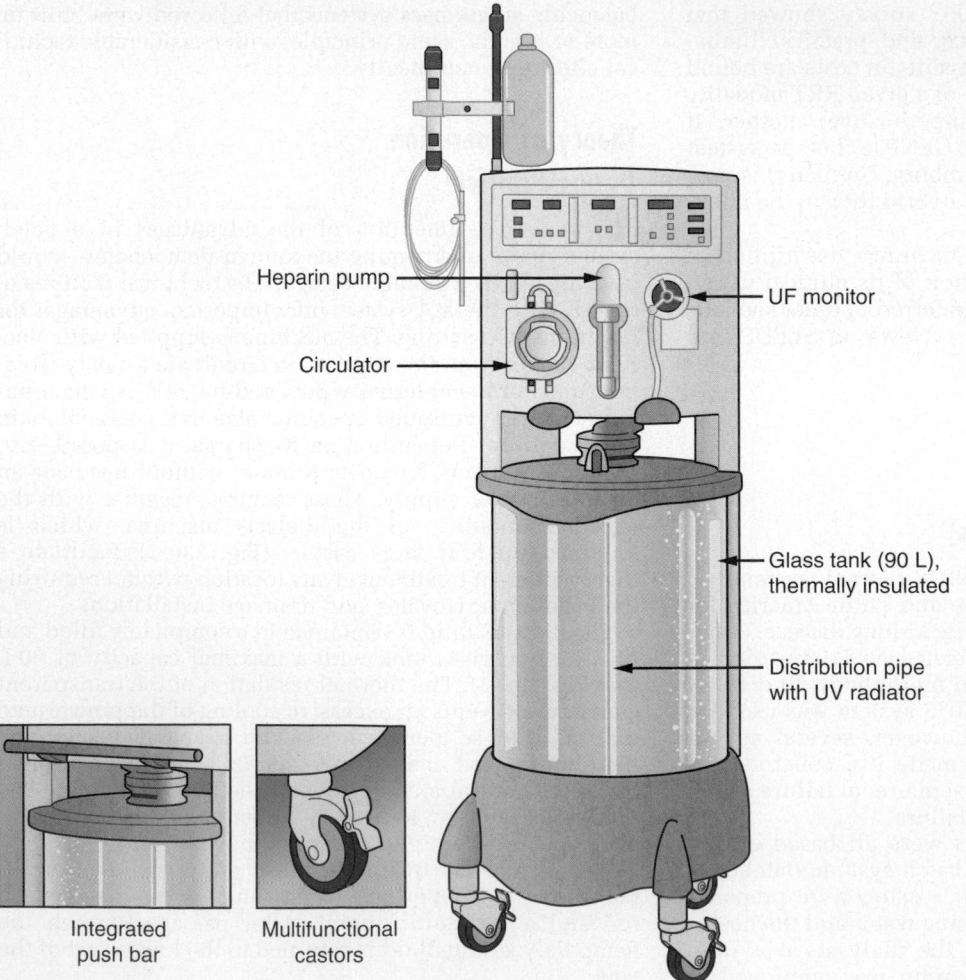

FIGURE 236-2. Today's GENIUS therapy machine and its main features.

The physical separation of used and fresh dialysis fluid in the reservoir makes the practical operation of GENIUS as a single-pass system possible, providing 90 L of fresh dialysis fluid for a single treatment. Figure 236-3 shows that the separating layer is clearly visible. This clear separation between fresh and used dialysis fluids can also be chemically demonstrated for other substances, such as electrolytes, urea, creatinine, and drugs.

The double-sided peristaltic pump transports both the patient's blood and the dialysis fluid in such a way that they pass the hemodialyzer in countercurrent flow direction (Fig. 236-4). Blood flow and dialysis fluid flow are coupled in a set ratio, 1:1 or 2:1, at a maximal flow rate of 350 mL/min. Because of the single pump it is always necessary to place a double-lumen catheter or the patient must have a well-functioning dialysis shunt that can be punctured at two sites, because a so-called single-needle dialysis is not possible.

The extremely simple tubing system consists of the following five parts:

• Arterial line
• Venous line
• Line from the tank to the hemodialyzer
• Line from the hemodialyzer to the tank
• Line from the tank to the ultrafiltration-controlling pump

The entire closed system is completely filled with fluid (i.e., air-free) and does not need the usual air-filled chambers ("air traps"). This arrangement allows the placement of the air detector between the (blood) pump and the hemodialyzer (see Fig. 236-4). It protects the patient against air infusion and also safely prevents a loss of filter effectiveness due to the entry of air into the hemodialyzer. Furthermore, the air-free system is clearly less thrombogenic and coagulation-activating, favorably influencing heparin consumption. Because of both the tight coupling of the hydraulic pressures in the blood and dialysis fluid compartments of the hemodialyzer and the minimal compliance of the totally fluid filled hydraulic system, any pressure change in the blood compartment is transferred to the dialysis fluid compartment and is reflected by a change of the system pressure which is measured (noninvasively) at the dialysis fluid compartment.

The completely closed system permits an easy and reliable volumetric ultrafiltration control from 50 to 1000 mL/hr by means of a pump. The fluid volume removed from the system is directly balanced by an equivalent volume from the patient's circulation.

The GENIUS system does not require the invasive measurement of venous return pressure usually required in conventional dialysis systems as a safeguard against blood loss into the environment. Because the entire system is completely filled with fluid, any change in pressure on the blood side affects the system pressure measured noninvasively on the dialysate side, where the change will be detected. The completely closed system allows volumetric ultrafiltration control in its most simple and reliable form: Any fluid volume which leaves the system is controlled

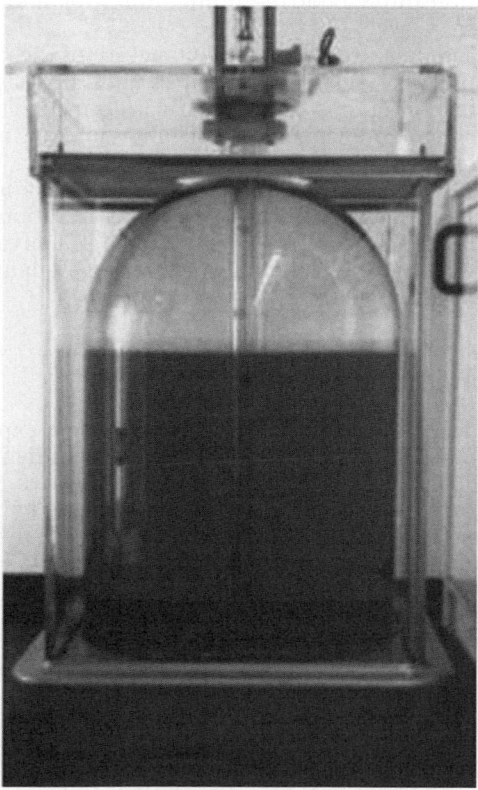

FIGURE 236-3. Spent dialysate sediment stays in the lower part of the tank because of the difference in density between it and fresh dialysis fluid. The picture is taken from in vitro experiments using vitamin B_{12}.

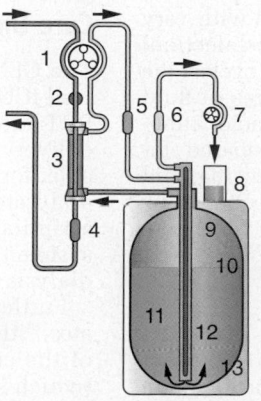

FIGURE 236-4. Schematic representation of the countercurrent GENIUS therapy system circuit.

1 Double-sided roller pump (blood, dialysate)
2 Air detector
3 Dialyser
4 Venous flow chamber (no air gap)
5 Blood leak detector
6 System pressure monitor
7 UF controller
8 UF volume
9 Preheated fresh dialysate
10 Boundary layer between fresh and used dialysate
11 Used dialysate
12 Distribution pipe with UV radiator
13 Glass vessel (90 L), thermally insulated

by the ultrafiltration monitor and represents the fluid removed from the patient.

Preparation of Dialysis Fluid, Drainage, and Cleaning

In the first step, a dry concentrate, consisting of the prescribed amounts of sodium bicarbonate and glucose as well as the majority of the prescribed amount of sodium chloride, is placed in a mixing vessel, dissolved with warmed ultrapure water, and flushed into the dialysis fluid tank. In the second step, a liquid concentrate containing the prescribed amounts of the chloride salts of potassium, magnesium, and calcium as well as a small portion of the prescribed sodium chloride is added. Supplemental concentrates or any water-soluble additives may also be added to the dialysis fluid (for example, water-soluble vitamins). The wide choice of various concentrates allows the physician to individualize the composition of the dialysis fluid. Furthermore, the small volume of the concentrates takes up little storage space. During the entire filling process, the ultraviolet radiator is operating to kill any possible microorganisms that might have entered.

For the production of ultrapure dialysis fluid, a reverse osmosis system is required. Tap water is processed therein, and the resulting reverse osmosis water is stored in a large tank called an aquator. The preparator is used for automated production of dialysis fluid and filling of the dialysis machine. The composition of the dialysis fluid, which is tailored to the needs of the patient, is prescribed by the treating physician.

At the end of the filling process, the dialysis fluid is checked for temperature and conductivity, and the data are recorded in a printed report. After the filling process, which takes about 5 to 10 minutes, the GENIUS system is ready for operation and can be moved to the location dedicated for the treatment.

Bicarbonate is used exclusively as buffer substance in the dialysis fluid. The entire system is completely closed and under constant positive pressure, preventing the loss of CO_2 from the solution and maintaining stability of the dissolved bicarbonate.

After completion of the treatment, the dialysis machine is returned to the preparator and disinfected. The dialysis fluid left in the container is drained with the help of air that has been sterile-filtered and washed over peracetic acid. Thereafter, the system is subjected to three rinsing and emptying phases. The rinsing volume amounts to only 3 to 5 L; a spraying head located in the tank directs the rinsing fluid onto the inner walls of the container. The ultraviolet radiator is operating during the entire procedure to support and enhance the effect of the peracetic acid. This outstanding disinfection is achieved with very low consumption of disinfectant (0.4 mL per disinfection) and a short operation time. At the end of these cycles, the dialysis fluid container is almost completely free of fluid and filled only with an enriched peracetic acid atmosphere. The machine can now be either prepared for another treatment or put away. Drainage, cleansing, and disinfection are performed as an automated sequence by the preparator.

Hygiene

The hygienic properties of the GENIUS system are essential design features that help to consistently avoid common errors. On the basis of the fact that hygiene is never the result of a single measure, the following multiple factors contribute to ensuring the exceptional hygiene of the machine:

- The machine is supplied with ultrapure water, because the quality of the product water has a decisive influence on the properties of the dialysate.
- The use of dry concentrate ingredients reduces the risk of contamination.
- GENIUS uses connectors other than Hansen couplings, one of the most critical components in dialysis as far as hygiene is concerned.
- Microorganisms that may have entered the system are destroyed by the ultraviolet radiator, which is in operation throughout the filling, draining, and rinsing process.
- The materials used for the manufacture of the GENIUS system (mainly glass) and their structural design with smooth, continuous, straight surfaces impede colonization by microorganisms while allowing for effective cleaning and sterilization.

The combination of all these features results in a hygienic standard unequaled in dialysis without filtration of the dialysate—which is sometimes employed in conventional systems—and without the need to use large quantities of chemical disinfectants.

Long-Term Experience

Several articles have described the long-term experience with the GENIUS therapy system in long-term hemodialysis. Kleophas and colleagues,[5] in a retrospective analysis of data from 399 patients, showed survival rates in between those for Tassin and those for European Dialysis and Transplant Association (EDTA) and the United States. Sixty-five percent of the patients in the Kleophas study were free of antihypertensive medication, versus 97% in the Tassin study,[6] 18% in EDTA statistics,[7] and 18.4% in U.S.[8] statistics. These researchers also could show high albumin plasma levels and a very low incidence of carpal tunnel syndrome, underlining the importance of water and dialysate quality. Later, Fassbinder[9] and Kleophas and Backus[10] independently reviewed the clinical experience emphasizing the simplicity and flexibility of the GENIUS therapy system. Various aspects of the experience with this system, such as the microbiological safety and the high quality of the dialysate, have also been dealt with in several independent publications.[11-13]

Use of the System in the Intensive Care Unit

The GENIUS therapy system is best located in a centralized ICU where a consistent number of patients in need of RRT are treated. The use of the preparator ensures the delivery of ultrapure dialysate. This piece is easily placeable, for instance, in the technical room of any ICU. The dialysate prepared according to an individualized prescription is then pumped into the container. The GENIUS system therefore has several advantages over conventional dialysis machines that require a central delivery system.

Furthermore, as elegantly shown by Dhondt and associates,[14] the fresh dialysate (which is pumped from the top of the container) seldom mixes with the spent dialysate (which is pumped back into the tank at the bottom), owing to physiochemical differences. In a prospective randomized study, these investigators treated 39 critically ill patients who were undergoing mechanical ventilation and had oliguric ARF in one of two ways, as follows:

- Continuous venovenous hemofiltration (CVVH) and a substitution fluid rate of at least 30 mL/kg/hr for 24 hours; 19 patients with Acute Physiology and Chronic Health Evaluation II (APACHE II) scores 32.3 ± 1.2 and a 79% sepsis rate
- GENIUS therapy for 12 hours; 20 patients with APACHE II scores 33.6+1.0 and an 85% sepsis rate.

Dhondt and associates[14] reported no significant differences in average mean arterial blood pressure, heart rate, cardiac output, systemic vascular resistance, or epinephrine dose between the treatment groups. Urea reduction rates were similar for extended dialysis (53% ± 2%) and CVVH (52% ± 3%; P not significant) despite an average rate of substitution fluid with the latter of 3.2 ± 0.1 L/hr.[15]

The adoption of SLEDD using the GENIUS therapy system is facilitated by several of the system's features: the easy-to-handle equipment and user-friendly interface, flexibility of the therapy, and personalization of the treatment for the patient's needs. Furthermore, use of regional citrate anticoagulation with this system in a simple and effective protocol has been also reported.[16] In a crossover study design, 27 patients with ARF were allocated to either citrate-anticoagulated or heparin-anticoagulated dialysis sessions (4-6 hrs). For citrate anticoagulation, a 4% sodium citrate solution was infused into the arterial line of the extracorporeal circuit. A low calcium dialysate concentration (1 mmol/L) was used for all dialysis sessions. Citrate dosing was adjusted according to the postfilter ionized calcium concentration (targeted values 0.5-0.7 mmol/L). There was no routine calcium substitution. Heparin anticoagulation was started with a heparin loading dose followed by an individual, patient-adjusted continuous heparin infusion. Electrolyte disarrangements, namely hypernatremia, hypocalcemia, and hypercalcemia, did not occur in either group. Although the highest bicarbonate levels were achieved during citrate anticoagulation, the acid-base values remained equilibrated in both groups. Filter longevity was excellent, and the targeted dialysis time was achieved in all but 1 patient. Citrate anticoagulation was well tolerated with respect to cardiovascular hemodynamics.

A SINGLE-CENTER EXPERIENCE

The University Hospital Düsseldorf is a major tertiary referral hospital with 1300 beds and an interdisciplinary surgical ICU containing 40 beds. There are about 3500 admissions per year to the ICU, which provides care to all surgical departments except neurosurgery. The majority of patients are admitted after elective surgical procedures, including cardiac, vascular, general, and trauma surgery.

The ICU provides all forms of extracorporeal life support, including continuous and intermittent RRT, liver support (with the Prometheus system, Fresenius Medical Care), ventricular assist devices, and extracorporeal membrane oxygenation. The ICU is organized as a "closed ICU," with a full-time ICU director, three consultants specialized in intensive care, and 24 physicians from the anesthesiology and surgical departments. Because the delivery of care is organized in the closed form, the majority of RRTs are prescribed and performed by the ICU staff. Nephrological consulting is available around the clock.

Until 2003, nearly all patients with ARF—most of them in the complex setting of multiple-organ impairment (≈80% of patients undergoing mechanical ventilation, ≈70% receiving catecholamine therapy, ≈50% with severe sepsis)—were treated with continuous venovenous hemodiafiltration (CVVHDF) as the first-line RRT. Patients with single-organ or with stable hemodynamics and those in the later course of ARF were treated with intermittent hemodialysis.

The ICU has a policy of initiating RRT early in the course of a patient's illness and of delivering a higher dialysis dose because both interventions have been shown to improve survival.[17,18] Therefore, during continuous RRT (CRRT), to achieve a target of about 35 mL per kg body weight per hour of ultrafiltration or combined ultrafiltration/dialysis, the initial dose of CVVHDF is at least 40 mL per kg body weight per hour. Intermittent hemodialysis is performed daily.

Over the last ten years, the number and severity of comorbidities of admitted patients and the mean age have increased significantly. More patients are admitted after high-risk surgical procedures and severe trauma. Thus, in 2003, almost 10,000 hours of CRRT were applied per year and in 2004, in line with implementation of new surgical procedures, almost 15,000 hours were applied. The workload imposed on the ICU staff exceeded the tolerable amount and treatment costs exploded, particularly because of the use of large amounts of sterile hemofiltration fluids.

As a consequence, alternative procedures to maintain the high quality of RRT despite limited resources were sought. A switch to more frequent use of conventional hemodialysis did not seem to be the right choice because the majority of patients suffered from impaired hemodynamics. In this setting, prolonged treatments offer better cardiovascular stability, allowing continuous removal of excess fluid and greater clearance rates. In addition to these medical considerations, intermittent hemodialysis is technically demanding and requires the availability of trained dialysis staff during the whole treatment period.

Fortunately, at that time, promising data on the use of extended daily dialysis were reported by Kielstein and associates.[15] In 2004, the decision was made to install a GENIUS therapy system exclusively for use in the ICU. The complete system was set up in a separate room of the ICU, and initially three, and later five GENIUS machines, each with a 90-L tank, were purchased. The following discussion summarizes this experience.

Hemodynamic Stability

The GENIUS system is used regularly in patients with multiple-organ failure who are undergoing vasopressor therapy. The duration of a treatment session in such patients is extended to at least 8 hours per day; in the majority, a dialysis session lasts 10 to 12 hours. The initial blood and dialysate flow rates are set to 100 mL/min (using the system with a 1:1 tubing) and then is increased to a maximum of 150 mL/min. In patients with severe hemodynamic instability, dialysate flow rate is not increased but left at 100 mL/min until all dialysate has been used. In patients with fluid overload, the treatment is prolonged to allow gentle removal of excess fluid. Compared with use of CRRT, no greater hemodynamic instability or higher demand for vasopressors has been associated with use of extended dialysis. Also, in patients with septic shock, treatments are well tolerated, and as with CRRT, effective temperature control is achieved in hyperthermic patients.

Dialysis Dose and Anticoagulation

The goal of dialysis in normal adults with body weights higher than 70 kg is to use the whole 90 L of dialysate during one dialysis session. The standard anticoagulant is unfractionated heparin, which is infused into the extracorporeal circuit. The typical dose is 500 to 1000 IU/hr during RRT, unless higher doses are required by the underlying disease of the patient. With this approach, premature clotting is absent in more than 80% of all treatments, and the prescribed dialysis dose is delivered to the patient. A major advantage of the GENIUS system is that the amount of blood that has circulated through the system is depicted on a monitor. Thus, with a 1:1 tubing arrangement, this figure is equivalent to the amount of dialysis fluid used, and the control of delivered dialysis dose is available at first glance.

In patients with higher risk of bleeding or other contraindications against the use of heparin, regional anticoagulation with citrate is used. In the ICU of the University Hospital Düsseldorf, a modification of the Berlin algorithm published by Morgera and colleagues[19] is used. The calcium dialysate concentration is 1.0 mmol/L, and a 4% citrate solution is infused via a three-way stopcock into the arterial line of the extracorporeal circuit at the connection site to the dialysis catheter. With citrate flows of 100 to 150 mL/hr, the prefilter concentration of the ionized calcium is 0.5 to 0.7 mmol/L, which is sufficient for effective anticoagulation. With this technique, the serum ionized calcium concentration exceeds 1.1 mmol/L in the majority of patients without an additional infusion of calcium. If this parameter falls below 1.1 mmol/L, an infusion of calcium chloride is started. Filter longevity is excellent, and the prescribed dialysis duration is achieved in more than 90% of all patients. The ionized calcium levels in both the serum and the extracorporeal circuit are monitored 10 to 15 minutes after the start of therapy and thereafter every 1 to 4 hours. It must be kept in mind that the ultrafiltration rate must be increased to remove the additional fluid infused with the citrate. Because regional citrate anticoagulation is required only for short periods in most patients, this approach, which does not require an additional infusion pump for calcium, is very convenient. Significant hypocalcemia does not occur. However, if citrate anticoagulation is required for longer periods (defined in the Düsseldorf ICU as the need for more than seven treatments), substitution of calcium is mandatory to avoid a negative calcium balance with its potential adverse effects.

Staff

The physicians in the ICU prescribe the dialysis therapy. The GENIUS circuit is set up by dialysis technicians and connected to the patient in the presence of an intensive care physician, who stays in the patient's room for the first few minutes, especially for patients undergoing catecholamine therapy. The ICU staff performs the further management of the system, including anticoagulation and eventual adjustments of ultrafiltration rate.

The acceptance of the system by the ICU staff is high. New members of the team acquaint themselves very quickly with the system because it is quite easy to use. At present, a large number of nurses prefer extended dialysis with the GENIUS system to classic CRRT, particularly because of its significantly lower workload. With CRRT, at least 72 or even more liters of hemofiltration fluids must be moved into a patient's room. The 5-kg bags have to be lifted onto the machine, and the same amount of fluid plus the ultrafiltrate must be moved out of the room. With the GENIUS system, this workload is completely abolished, and the nurses gain time that can be dedicated to patient care.

Compared with other machines, a reduced number of alarms occur with the GENIUS system, because of the simplicity of the pressure monitoring and a reduced number of clotting events. Thus, the operational features of the machine reduce the noise level in the patient's room, another factor in its greater acceptance by the staff, and also by the patient if he or she is awake.

Treatment Costs and Reimbursement

Prolonged GENIUS therapies are equivalent to CRRT with regard to reimbursement by health insurance providers, although different reimbursing systems in different countries render comparisons difficult. Nevertheless, the running costs are significantly lower mainly because the use of hemofiltration fluids is avoided and clotting is rarely observed. On the other hand, the initial investment is higher than that for a CRRT system, making the GENIUS system economically attractive only for large ICUs.

In the Düsseldorf experience, however, the avoidance of costs for additional dialysis staff is more important. For uncomplicated cases, as in many other institutions, RRT is performed with intermittent hemodialysis. Because the GENIUS system can also be used to deliver a short (3-5 hours) hemodialysis session, the following approach is used to reduce costs for staff. In the morning, the GENIUS machines are used for intermittent hemodialysis in stable patients. Thereafter, the systems are drained, sterilized, and prepared by the dialysis nurses. Each machine is then connected to another patient for extended therapy, either as a SLEDD or for an overnight therapy of more than 10 to 12 hours. After all dialysate is spent, the machine is disconnected from the patient by the staff of the ICU. Draining and sterilization are performed in the morning by the dialysis nurses. Thus, one single shift of dialysis nurses is sufficient to treat two patients per day with one machine. The major reduction in costs associated with RRT in this ICU is therefore achieved through the avoidance of staffing a late shift of dialysis nurses.

CONCLUSION

Taken together, the introduction of extended daily dialysis using a single-batch system has proved safe and effective in the clinical setting of large ICUs such as that of the University Hospital Düsseldorf. Thus, the data published in controlled and randomized studies on efficacy, hemodynamic tolerance, and cost effectiveness have been confirmed by daily experience. In this 40-bed ICU, broadening the spectrum of available RRTs with the GENIUS system has certainly improved quality of care and significantly reduced the RRT costs.

Key Points

1. Originally conceived and used in the treatment of patients with chronic kidney disease, the GENIUS therapy system has become a concrete and feasible alternative for treatment of acute renal failure in the context of multiple-organ failure.
2. This system is a batch (90-L) system that provides ultrapure dialysis fluid. During dialysis treatment, fresh dialysis fluid is aspirated from the upper part of the tank via the distribution rod using a peristaltic pump. After passage through the hemodialyzer, it is returned into the lower part of the tank. The physical separation of used and fresh dialysis fluid in the reservoir makes possible the practical operation of GENIUS as a single-pass system, providing 90 L of fresh dialysis fluid for a single treatment.
3. Consolidated experience now exists showing that the GENIUS therapy system is an efficient therapy applicable to patients with multiple-organ failure.
4. Broadening the spectrum of available renal replacement techniques with the GENIUS system

has certainly improved quality of care and significantly reduced the costs of renal replacement therapy.

Acknowledgment

The authors thank Dr R. Pohlmeier and Mr. A. Heinz for critically reviewing the manuscript.

Key References

2. Van Biesen W, Lameire N: SLEDD and hybrid renal replacement therapies for acute renal failure in the ICU. In Vincent JL (ed): Yearbook of Intensive Care and Emergency Medicine 2003. New York, Springer, 2003, pp 663-678.
13. Dhondt A, Eloot S, Wachter DD, et al: Dialysate partitioning in the Genius® batch hemodialysis system: Effect of temperature and solute concentration. Kidney Int 2005;67: 2470-2476.
14. Kielstein JT, Kretschmer U, Ernst T, et al: Efficacy and cardiovascular tolerability of extended dialysis in critically ill patients: A randomized controlled study. Am J Kidney Dis 2004;43:342-349.

See the companion Expert Consult website for the complete reference list.

CHAPTER 237

Daily Dialysis in the Intensive Care Unit: Nursing Perspectives

Ian Baldwin

OBJECTIVES

This chapter will:
1. Describe what daily dialysis is through a review of nomenclature used and discussion of some of the implications for nursing in the ICU setting.
2. Highlight the importance of planning and scheduling for the use of a limited-time treatment.
3. Discuss important differences among continuous therapies in terms of anticoagulation requirements, fluid balance, electrolyte prescription, drug administration, and access catheter care.
4. Introduce some of the technical and practical considerations for the use of a dialysis machine and reverse-osmosis–treated water.
5. Propose a suitable education program for teaching daily dialysis to nurses.

Despite reports of clinical use of daily dialysis for more than 10 years, nursing literature for the application of daily dialysis in the intensive care unit (ICU) is very sparse. This chapter provides information and discussion relevant to nurses with the aim of developing the protocols and procedures required. This limited-time treatment, often performed "daily," has many advantages for nursing—treatment fluids and waste disposal are easier to manage; a "treatment-free" period can be better for the patient and creates efficiency for nursing care. Before the key nursing issues are presented, a review, of how daily dialysis evolved and what it is, provides a useful background to improve the understanding of how nursing protocols and care for patients may best be provided. Daily dialysis required many modifications of the protocols developed for use of continuous renal replacement therapy (CRRT) in the ICU. As discussed further, there are several different acronyms to describe a daily dialysis technique

TABLE 237-1

Common Settings for Renal Replacement Therapy

TREATMENT MODE	BLOOD FLOW (mL/min)	Replacement Fluid		Dialysate Fluid		Filtrate Loss	
		mL/min	L/hr	mL/min	L/hr	mL/min	L/hr
Continuous venovenous hemofiltration	150-200	33	2.0	—	—	33*	2.0*
Continuous venovenous hemodiafiltration	150-200	17	1.0	17	1.02	33*	2.0*
Sustained low-efficiency extended (daily) dialysis	100-150	—	—	150-200	9.0-12.0	150*-200*	9.0*-12.0*
Sustained low-efficiency dialysis with filtration/extended daily dialysis with filtration	100-150	21	1.26	100-200	6.0-9.0	121*-221*	7.26*-13.26*
Intermittent hemodialysis	300-350	—	—	500	30.0	500+	30.0+

*Indicates an additional loss per hour for negative fluid balance.

for critically ill patients; however, for convenience, the term *sustained low-efficiency dialysis* (SLED) is used for all variants unless a specific technique is being discussed.

NOMENCLATURE

Several acronyms are used to describe the application of daily, limited-time renal replacement therapy. Although the acronym SLED is used to generally describe sustained low-efficiency dialysis therapy as used in the ICU setting, some important variations of the technique are worthwhile understanding, because they are not all the same. A 1994 report by Kihara and associates[1] used the term slow hemodialysis (slow HD), which was applied for 10 hours in the daytime for critically ill patients, by means of a modified dialysis machine operated by nurses in the ICU. In 1999, Schlaeper and colleagues[2] reported their use of slow continuous dialysis (SCD) with a modified dialysis machine that reduced the dialysate flow rate to 100 mL/min. This was also used in the ICU for critically ill patients, in collaboration with nephrology nurses; however, treatment times were continuous rather than fixed. In 2000, Kumar and coworkers[3] applied the term *extended daily dialysis* (EDD) to describe a slow–flow rate dialysis using a conventional dialysis machine over an extended period (6-8 hours) during the day, also through a collaborative relationship between nephrology and ICU nurses.[3] In the same year, Lonnemann and associates[4] reported experience with a technique they called *extended daily high-flux hemodialysis* (HFD), which used a dialysis machine with a pre-prepared tank of water that had been treated with reverse osmosis and received additions of electrolytes and bicarbonate, as a treatment "batch" via the GENIUS therapy machine (Fresenius Medical Care, Bad Homburg, Germany).[5] In 2001, Marshall and colleagues[6] used the term *sustained low-efficiency dialysis* (SLED) to describe the application of a 12-hour treatment using a dialysis machine at low flow rates (by selecting a "slow dialysis" option), as a shared ICU and nephrology nursing activity. These treatments were also performed overnight, and were referred to as nocturnal SLED. A further and similar technique was described using the acronym SLEDD, for slow low-efficiency daily dialysis.[7]

Up to this time, all reported techniques consisted of dialysis with diffusion as the key solute removal mechanism. In 2004, Marshall and colleagues[8] used the acronym SLEDD-f to describe a diafiltration circuit that added convective solute clearance to the largely diffusive technique in SLED variants. This use of predilution fluids, which requires an additional treatment process for production of ultrapure fluid production, is also referred to as extended daily diafiltration[9] or prolonged intermittent renal replacement therapy (PIRRT).[10]

These reports together highlight an important difference from standard intermittent hemodialysis (IHD), in which much higher blood and dialysate flow rates are used for a shorter time. The machine settings in SLED and its variants are lower than those used in IHD but higher than those used in CRRT. The SLED treatment uses water that has been treated with reverse osmosis and electrolyte and bicarbonate additives. This machine-manufactured fluid is necessary to provide higher flow rates not feasible with the commercial fluid bags used in CRRT. However, unlike with conventional dialysis, treatment time is longer but not continuous. Table 237-1 lists the common settings used for renal replacement techniques, enabling a comparison and identification of how the techniques differ in respect to blood and fluid flow rates.

The common denominators of these terms and acronyms are as follows:
- A daily treatment of limited duration, but not necessarily performed during the day
- A mostly diffusive technique commonly using a machine built for dialysis
- Often provided as a collaborative effort between ICU and nephrology nurses

Van Biesen and colleagues[11] summarized the advantages of SLED and its variants, suggesting that they are likely to be used more frequently because they combine the technical efficiency and fluid economy advantages of IHD with the smooth metabolic control of CRRT. This combination is achieved with reduced anticoagulation, a smaller workload, and more time for medical and nursing interventions during the treatment-free period each day.

From a nursing perspective, SLED variants mean a treatment for a fixed time, using a dialysis machine, usually over one nursing shift. This treatment must suffice for solute, acid-base, and fluid balance control for the "day." Therefore, it must be successful and must be completed

TABLE 237-2

Protocol Items List for Use of Daily Dialysis in the ICU Setting

PROTOCOL ITEM	RECOMMENDATION	EXAMPLE
Scheduling treatments	Scheduling and preferences for treatment start and stop times Evening or night treatments can provide many advantages and be better for both patient and nursing staff	8-hr treatment between 1200 and 2000 hrs
Anticoagulation	Anticoagulation and dosing decided on and set as a standard approach for all patients Heparin at lower dose, such as 5.0-7.5 IU/kg/hr, or no anticoagulation for patients with coagulopathy or at risk for bleeding	For 70-kg patient, use 350 IU/hr Bolus dose of 2500 units given at start
Machine, circuit preparation	Setup of machine and circuit; membrane priming For machine used, use a checklist Preparation of the machine away from the bed area is helpful in most settings	Use manufacturer checklist routine, or make one Keep copies with machine

Fluid balance	Fluid balance and management:
	    Consider all fluid intake; use plan that may set goals over 2 or 3 days
	    Loss of 350 mL/hr is a reasonable prescription
		Fluid loss:
		    Day 1: 2.5 L
		    Day 2: 2.0 L
		    Day 3: 1.5 L

Electrolyte, potassium control	Potassium and prescription for these solutes should be part of daily dialysis orders Consider potential for serum potassium rise during time without treatment Calcium, phosphate, and magnesium may also require replacement during or after treatment	Use K$^+$ bath of 2.0 mmol/L on day 1 Modify for days 2 and 3 Check daily results for all electrolytes
Drugs administered during SLED	Rescheduling some drug administration until after the daily treatment, in discussion with the prescribing physician, should be part of the daily dialysis orders Other drugs, such as antibiotics, may require blood level monitoring before and after treatment, with changes to dose according to results	Consult physician and/or pharmacy for drug clearance (e.g., vancomycin, meropenem)

Access catheter use and care	Access catheter management:
	    Secure with adhesive dressing and redress whenever this becomes loose
	    Label "for dialysis only"
	    Inspect each nursing shift even when not in use
	    Flush and instill anticoagulant into lumens after each treatment
		Use polyurethane dressings in "sandwich" technique
		Use heparin, 1000 IU, as concentrate to instill into lumens when not in use

Time period without treatment (off or down time)	Planning activities for the time without treatment should be part of a daily dialysis nursing care plan Wait for some period after treatment before beginning activities, when fluid "shifts" and effect of anticoagulation are reduced	Discuss and make a list of activities to be done during treatment-free period
Machine use	Planning the treatment for additional patients is efficient use of a machine in the ICU This goal requires planning and negotiation each day	Consider other patients, and integrate care Provide an evening treatment in one patient followed by a night treatment in a second patient
Teaching others; education for SLED	Use the protocol and policy documents as a training and educational tool Provide this tool as reading material for all nurses managing SLED treatments	Make protocol copies available Conduct a SLED education program annually

ICU, intensive care unit; SLED, sustained low-efficiency dialysis.

without interruption or failure. These issues are discussed further in a nursing context. For each point presented and discussed, a summary protocol recommendation is presented at the end of each section and listed in Table 237-2.

PLANNING THE TREATMENT; TIMING AND DURATION OF THE TREATMENT

Daily treatments in the ICU require planning and scheduling, with consideration given to the nursing expertise

necessary, machine availability, patient care needs, and, importantly, patient solute and solvent clearance requirements.

Some centers apply daily dialysis only during the day, when more highly skilled ICU nurses or nephrology nurses are available, particularly when a center is starting a new program for SLED.[6,10] It may be also necessary to start and complete a treatment within a nursing shift if there will be no skilled nurse on the next shift or to limit the use of overtime payments. Different nursing models for the management of RRT in the ICU also influence the scheduling of treatments. For example, in centers where ICU nurses manage the treatment alone or independent of nephrology nurses, RRT may be performed in the evening

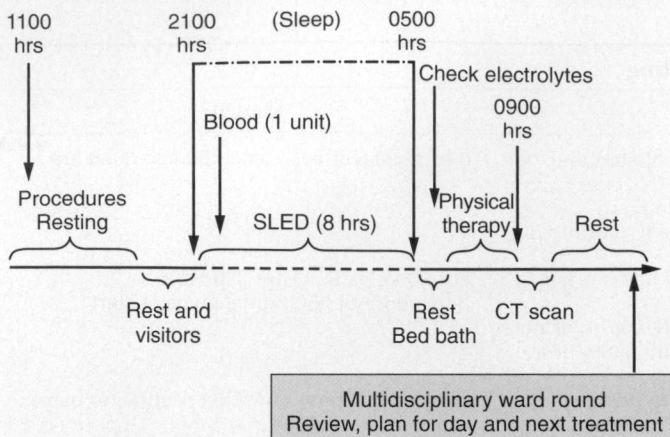

FIGURE 237-1. Example of a care plan and schedule for the use of nocturnal sustained low-efficiency dialysis (SLED) in the intensive care unit.

or during the night and given the name "nocturnal SLED"[6]; one center reported that almost 50% of treatments were done at night.[12] Evening or night treatments have some advantages, allowing patient mobilization as well as performance of physiotherapy procedures during the day before treatment begins.

Such scheduling also allows for patient care goals to be determined in association with the multidisciplinary team. This issue is important in regard to forecasting fluid balance requirements and making predictions about acid-base and electrolyte control. It is better to know before a treatment is started whether a patient will be administered blood products, will require computed tomography, or is undergoing a change in antibiotic therapy, so that these interventions can be considered in the prescription of the SLED treatment "recipe." This goal is usually best achieved through a focused discussion between the nurse (ICU and/ or nephrology) managing the patient and the prescribing physician. A written and verbal plan must be completed. Documenting the plans in the patient medical file or suitable "orders" sheet makes them clear and useful for next shift staffing to refer to. An example of such a treatment schedule using nocturnal SLED is provided in Figure 237-1.

A further advantage of SLED is the potential to use the same machine for two or three patients in a single 24-hour period.[12] Therefore day, evening, and night treatments are feasible, with each treatment lasting between 6 and 7 hours to allow for changeover. This arrangement is not possible with CRRT, in which one machine is used continuously for one patient. However, depending on patient requirements, treatments may be of varying times. For example, a patient in recovery from acute renal failure with oliguria may need only 4 to 5 hours of RRT, mostly for small solute clearance, and another in an acute admission situation may require a 10-hour treatment because of anuria, high serum small solute levels (e.g., urea, creatinine, potassium), and severe acid-base derangement.

The ability to manipulate blood and dialysate flow rates and, therefore, clearance intensity in association with treatment duration means that therapy can be truly "tailor made" for each patient each day.[13]

Protocol recommendation: A preference within the ICU for treatment start and stop times should be included in the protocol. Evening or night treatments can provide many advantages and can be better for both patient and nursing.

ANTICOAGULATION NEEDS AND DIFFERENCES

Use of daily dialysis places a much greater emphasis on the need for the treatment to be successful and completed. Many patient activities may be scheduled around the treatment period, or a treatment may have to be completed during one nursing shift. In this respect, premature clotting is of greatest concern; many patients in the ICU can be treated without anticoagulation,[14] particularly when the treatment time is limited to 6 or 8 hours, but others require anticoagulation. The anticoagulation method used must be sufficient for the prescribed treatment period without clotting, and therefore, a lower dose or a less aggressive approach is possible. Published reports comparing SLED with CRRT indicate use of either lower doses of heparin in SLED[3,14,15] or no anticoagulation in up to 65% of patients treated with SLED.[16] Heparin is most commonly used, but the use of citrate has been reported for prolonged SLED treatments—up to and for more than 12 hours.[17] It is also important to remember that a short and fixed-time treatment may require a fluid (ultrafiltration [UF]) loss rate of 300 to 400 mL/hr, which poses a greater potential for clotting in the dialysis membrane, where the filtration fraction will be high.[18] Therefore, membranes with larger surface area (1.4 to 1.6 m^2) are suggested for SLED treatments in 70- to 80-kg adults, for high blood flow rates (>200 mL/ min), and/or for the use of predilution (>20 mL/min) in diafiltration treatments.

Protocol recommendation: Anticoagulation method and dosing are chosen by prescribing physicians and used for all patients. Heparin is administered at lower doses, such as 5.0 to 7.5 IU/kg/hour. No anticoagulation is used in patients with coagulopathy or at risk for bleeding.

THE MACHINE FOR SUSTAINED LOW-EFFICIENCY DIALYSIS

The faster solute clearance necessary in shorter daily dialysis treatments requires a machine capable of generating high dialysate fluid flow rates—usually meaning dialysate fluid flows equal to or exceeding blood flow rates and maximizing diffusion. For example, the reported use of dialysate and blood flow rates of 70 mL/min[4] is "slow" in comparison with conventional dialysis and most SLED treatments. In CRRT, dialysate flow rates rarely exceed 34 mL/min despite blood flow rates of 150 to 200 mL/min.[19]

For SLED treatments, therefore, a machine incorporating the use of reverse osmosis (RO) and electrolyte-added water is required. This process may occur in a "master" RO unit with outlets to individual bed areas or via a small single RO unit for each dialysis machine.[13] In both systems, electrolyte and bicarbonate additives are required and are commercially prepared in a bottle or bag with machine programming to control specific electrolytes or bicarbonate concentration in the dialysate. In addition to the priming and flushing routine for the circuit and membrane, the machine must undergo a "self-testing" and water preparation phase before use. Most dialysis machines use this RO water mixture for the priming phase before use of the fluid during treatment. This approach differs significantly from that in CRRT, which involves use of commercial fluids in treatment and saline solution for priming. Preparation and priming are simple with the SLED machine despite being more "manual" than the automated CRRT machines that use cartridge-style circuits.

Some tubing sections in a SLED machine have end caps that must be removed for air displacement, and the removal of air from the membrane requires inverting (outflow port uppermost or to the top) the membrane while dialysate flow is drawing air and fluid out of the membrane. After priming is complete, the membrane, with the blood and dialysis lines connected to create a blood flow in one direction and a dialysate flow in the opposite direction, can be left in any position. Some nurses position the membrane vertically with the blood passing downward from top to bottom and the dialysate flow entering the bottom port flowing from bottom to top. With this arrangement, any bubbles in the dialysate flow come out into the waste pathway because they rise to the top along with the dialysate countercurrent flow. However, with sealed tubing hoses, such bubbles are minimal, and any position of the membrane in the machine clamp is satisfactory. However, countercurrent flow of blood and dialysate fluid are considered important to maximizing solute clearance.[20,21] Machines are sensitive to sequence during the preparation phase, and if the sequence is not followed, the self-test or priming phase will fail.

When space is limited around a patient bed, when dialysis must be delayed until other nursing activities are complete, or when family members are present, it can be more efficient to prepare the machine elsewhere, in an open space and without interruptions. Machines that can be powered down after priming and powered up after being moved to the patient's bedside and/or that can access a temporary battery-power mode during such a move are very useful.

Protocol recommendation: The setup of the machine, circuit, and membrane in accordance with manufacturer directions must be established as a procedure with an accompanying checklist. Preparation of the machine away from the bed area is helpful in most settings.

FLUID BALANCE APPROACH

One limiting factor in daily dialysis for critically ill patients, particularly those with anuria, is the need to provide continuous, hourly negative fluid balance. This requirement may prohibit the use of a daily treatment in some groups, such as those with neurotrauma or acute liver failure with brain edema and raised intracranial pressure.[22] In other patients in whom a daily negative fluid balance is required, 2 or 3 L per treatment may be necessary with ultrafiltration rates of 250 to 500 mL/hr. The rate per hour is relative to the total treatment time. This higher ultrafiltration rate may be possible for the first few hours of a treatment, but in some vasopressor-dependent patients, an increase in vasopressor dose may be necessary to achieve the fluid loss target. It is possible with some machines to "profile" or taper the fluid loss so that hourly loss rates diminish over time, in an attempt to minimize dialysis-induced hypovolemia.[23]

High negative fluid loss requirements may be related to excessive fluid inputs, suggesting that patients in the ICU who are treated with daily dialysis may need some fluid restriction. Fluid restriction is often now not considered in critically ill patients treated with CRRT, because continuous fluid removal is performed without concern for limiting fluid intake with concentrated drug preparations, lower volume nasogastric feeds, or minimizing any small fluid infusions for bolus medications. This view is supported in a report by Kumar and associates,[14] who reported on a 2-year experience using a continuous dialysis treatment or EDD in 54 ICU patients; they found that the average input in the continuous treatment group was 5.8 L/day and that in the EDD group was 3.3 L/day. The need for blood product administration can add further to negative fluid balance targets.

Daily dialysis requires some careful planning and consideration for both fluid input each day and the amount of fluid that should be removed during a treatment. In some cases, it is safer to plan this requirement over 2 or 3 days rather than attempting a large fluid loss prescription in one day or one treatment. In addition, the first SLED treatment may have to be extended to more than 12 hours to achieve the fluid loss requirements on the first day. Subsequent treatments can then be shorter with a focus on small solute clearance. There is a limit as to how much can safely be achieved in one treatment. The hypotension and cardiac arrhythmias associated with 4-hour IHD treatments in the past[24] are likely to occur if high negative fluid loss targets are attempted with short SLED treatments. A fluid loss rate of less than 350 mL/hr has been proposed[11] and seems reasonable in most cases. A review of five reports using variants of SLED in the ICU[3,6,8,15,25] in which fluid loss per hour was reported or could be calculated from the treatment times and total fluid loss volumes, concurs with this suggestion.[11] This calculation reveals that an average negative fluid loss of 2.8 L over 9.4 hours, or 355 mL/hour, can be achieved without instability or difficulty.

Nurses should discuss these issues and these limitations of daily dialysis with prescribing physicians and plan accordingly, generating treatment plans for day 1, day 2, day 3, and so on, as needed. If a patient can be accurately and reliably weighed each day, body weight is useful data for determining fluid balance and removes some of the guesswork, because fluid charts may not always describe the true fluid balance despite being quite comprehensive in ICU care.[26]

Protocol recommendation: Fluid balance and management of all patient fluids input must be considered, with a plan that may set goals over 2 or 3 days. A fluid loss of 350 mL/hour is a reasonable and safe prescription.

ELECTROLYTES AND DAILY DIALYSIS

All electrolyte concentrations must be monitored during RRT, potassium being monitored and manipulated the most. Concentrations of other electrolytes, such as phosphate, calcium, and magnesium, may also be abnormal and require management.[27,28]

Potassium is the electrolyte of greatest importance because both hypokalemia and hyperkalemia can give rise to life-threatening arrhythmias,[29] and despite acute renal failure, ICU patients may be hypokalemic during the first 24 hours after admission. Uchino and colleagues,[28] who retrospectively analyzed data from 47 patients treated with IHD and 49 patients treated with continuous venovenous hemodiafiltration (CVVHDF) in the ICU, reported a 45.8% incidence of hypokalemia in both groups.

For CRRT, potassium replacement is achieved through addition of potassium to bags of commercial fluid, which contain either 1 mmol/L or no potassium.[30] After the first 12 to 24 hours of any treatment, potassium supplementation is often required. One advantage to using commercial fluids is the ability to change the potassium dose in each new bag as indicated by serum concentrations, which are often obtained from arterial blood gas samples collected during treatment that also measure other key electrolytes. During a dialysis treatment, in contrast, the potassium concentration is established before treatment by additives to a concentrate bottle and can be changed only by changing the entire bottle during treatment; though possible, this approach is wasteful. It is much preferable to set the right potassium bath concentration at the start of treatment start, through discussion with the prescribing physician, and to use it for the entire treatment.

To prevent hyperkalemia due to the rise in a patient's potassium concentration between dialysis treatments, however, a lower dosing of dialysate potassium may be required. Nurses using CRRT would suggest that a preparation of 4.0 mmol/L is best, because it is aimed at achieving "normal" serum levels. However, to allow for the "off time" without RRT in a patient being treated with daily dialysis, a lower potassium concentration, such as 2.0 to 3.0 mmol/L, is often better. A patient may finish a treatment with a serum potassium level lower than would be commonplace in the ICU (3.0 to 3.5 mmol/L), but allowing a possible rise in the serum before the next treatment while minimizing the likelihood of hyperkalemia and the need to manage it with additional dialysis.[31] For longer treatment times, such as SLED over 12 hours, a dialysate potassium concentration of 4.0 mmol/L may be more appropriate. Some patients may also make some urine when off treatment, losing further potassium. Administration of potassium and/or blood products between dialysis treatments should be avoided. Blood products are best given during treatment so that additional potassium is removed in addition to the fluid loss needed to facilitate this blood product volume. A serum potassium check is advisable via either a blood gas sample (usually by local ICU machine) or a venous sample collected several hours after a daily treatment is complete, when some stabilization has occurred.

Protocol recommendation: Potassium and the prescription for it should be part of daily dialysis orders. The potential for a serum potassium rise between treatments should be considered. A dialysate potassium level of 2.0 to 3.0 mmol/L is appropriate for 6- to 8-hour treatments. Calcium, phosphate, and magnesium may also need to be replaced during or after treatment. Serum electrolyte levels should be checked 1 to 2 hours after the treatment finishes.

DRUG ADMINISTRATION IN THE PATIENT RECEIVING DAILY DIALYSIS TREATMENT

Because daily dialysis is a high-intensity, diffusive technique, delaying the administration of some drugs until after the treatment is complete may provide more therapeutic levels. However, antibiotics such as meropenem and vancomycin, commonly used in the ICU for life-threatening infections, may need close monitoring and dose adjustment, depending on the SLED treatment used, to avoid underdosing due to high clearance of the drug.[32,33] This is another issue that must be included in the nurse's planning of the daily treatment in association with the treating physician and should also be included in a daily dialysis nursing protocol along with prescriptions for drug dosing in relation to each treatment.

Protocol recommendation: Rescheduling administration of some drugs until after daily dialysis should be part of the daily dialysis orders after discussions between the nurse and the prescribing physician. Other drugs, such as antibiotics, may require blood level monitoring before and after treatment, so that changes to dosage may be made if required to maintain therapeutic drug levels.

ACCESS CATHETER MANAGEMENT AND CARE

During daily dialysis, the access catheter may be handled more frequently than during CRRT—twice per day, one connection and one disconnection. However, this frequency may be less than in some patients in whom frequent clotting is a problem with CRRT. Between SLED treatments, when the catheter is not in use, the access catheter must be flushed with saline and the dead space of the lumens must be filled with anticoagulant; this procedure is more important for SLED than for CRRT, which involves only short periods during which the access catheter is not in use. For circuit changeover or replacement with CRRT in a short time (60-90 minutes), saline flushing without anticoagulants is sufficient.

Some patients treated with daily dialysis may be mobilized with more enthusiasm than those tethered to a circuit and machine during CRRT, so the access catheter dressing must be well secured and dressed with a firm technique using either the polyurethane film "sandwich" technique[34] or a firm adhesive tape and gauze pad (single dressing). While the catheter is not in use, regular inspection of both catheter and the skin site is important and should be part of the nursing assessment each shift. It may also be necessary to label this catheter ("Dialysis only") in between treatments to prevent use of the lumens for other drug and/or fluid infusion—which would raise the risk for infection and also make the start of dialysis treatment more complicated because of the need to relocate infusions first. The need for multiple venous access points is a common problem in the ICU, where multiple drug infusions are used.

Protocol recommendation: Access catheter management: Secure adhesive dressing and redress whenever it becomes loose; label for "Dialysis only"; inspect catheter and skin site each nursing shift even when not in use; flush and instill anticoagulant into lumens after each treatment.

NURSING: TAKING ADVANTAGE OF THE DOWNTIME

The time between dialysis treatments must be used to full advantage because some activities may have been delayed or rescheduled because of treatment. Examples are physiotherapy, patient movement out of bed, standing, or walking, procedures, and diagnostics. Overnight treatment, termed *nocturnal SLED*,[35] has been proposed to allow for best use of day hours and related services. If nursing expertise permits night-time treatment, this approach has the potential to fully utilize the daylight hours for patient care without treatment. Some nurses may believe that the time without dialysis treatment is for patient rest. Rest may be needed for the time immediately after completion of treatment, when body fluids stabilize. Such a period would not be the best time for a patient to walk or sit out of bed. However, when day treatments are done, the patient could sit in a suitable chair (with reclining and footrest options) either before treatment is started or even during treatment. Provided that adequate care is taken, a slide board or slip sheet is used for the transfer, and the patient is generally stable, allowing the patient to sit in a chair during dialysis is safe (Fig. 237-2).

In addition, procedures that involve minor surgery may be best delayed until any anticoagulation used for dialysis, such as heparin administration, has become less effective. However, to take advantage of daily dialysis over CRRT, the off-treatment time must be effectively utilized. After a rest time of 1 or 2 hours, scheduled nursing activities and/or procedures can begin.

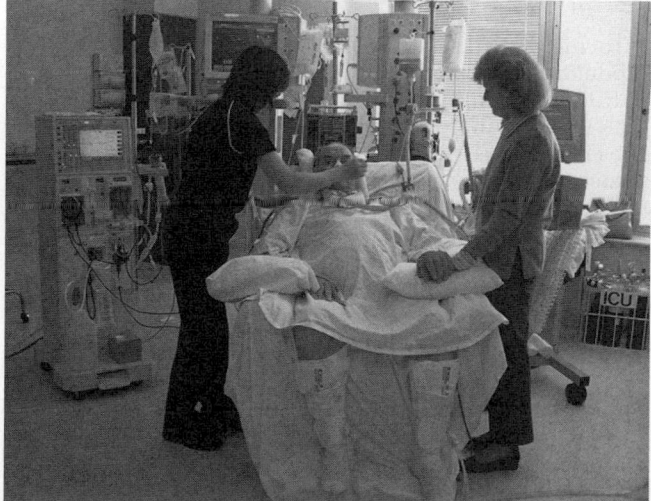

FIGURE 237-2. A patient in the intensive care unit is out of bed and sitting in a chair during a sustained low-efficiency dialysis treatment using a Fresenius 4008S ARrT plus machine (Fresenius Medical Care, Bad Homburg, Germany).

Protocol recommendation: Planning activities for the time without treatment should be part of a daily dialysis nursing care plan. Wait for some time after treatment (1-2 hours), after fluid shifts and effect of anticoagulation have subsided, to begin such activities.

BEST USE OF THE MACHINE: MORE THAN ONE PATIENT PER 24 HOURS

With daily dialysis treatment times of 6 to 7 hours, up to three patients could be treated with one machine in the ICU. A changeover of the machine to the next patient has to be well planned, but this practice is possible. With CRRT, each patient requires one machine all the time. This concept also suggests that night treatments would be required. However it is important to remember that the costs of some service and maintenance schedules are independent of the number of treatments. Given a purchase price similar to that for a CRRT machine, a dialysis-SLED machine can be worked harder and to the benefit of more patients. Having such a machine not in use is similar to an aircraft remaining on the ground, not taking any passengers.

Protocol recommendation: Planning the treatment for additional patients is efficient use of a machine in the ICU and would require planning and negotiation each day.

EDUCATION

Teaching and training nurses for daily dialysis requires new knowledge in addition to that necessary for CRRT. The machine, RO water connection, preparation, and priming sequence are very different and are performed manually, unlike the automatic priming cartridge circuits used in CRRT systems such as the PrismaFlex (Gambro Hospal, Lyon, France) and Aquarius (Edwards Life Sciences, Irvine, CA) machines. It may be more difficult for experienced CRRT nurses to learn a "manual" dialysis machine because they have to unlearn what they know about using an automated CRRT machine.

A lecture/theory program is useful for teaching a group, with "handout" reading materials and lecture notes. The reading material is often best made for a local setting with simple Microsoft Power Point slides. Pictures on slides and simple text descriptors are useful. Journal papers reviewing the use of daily dialysis for how, why, and when are a helpful adjunct. This material can all be prepared and bound into a booklet for each nurse. A 1-day program with a physician and nurse teachers and clinician presentations is useful. Table 237-3 summarizes a suitable study day or seminar for SLED training. This day must also include some machine demonstration with setup and priming. However, each nurse will then require one-to-one teaching during a live patient treatment, perhaps for three to four treatments before being able to work independently. Providing a nursing policy responding to the key headings of this chapter is also part of the reading material for the education process and a helpful reference during treatments. This policy or protocol also helps reinforce the important aspects of treatment with respect to the importance of planning activities for the off time, potassium and fluid balance management, anticoagulation, and the access catheter care.

TABLE 237-3

Sustained Low-Efficiency Dialysis: Education and Training Program for Nurses

TOPIC	TIME UNIT*	SUPPLEMENTARY MATERIALS AND SUITABLE SPEAKERS
Introduction: overview of day	0.25	List of day schedule/program
Introduction to and background for extended daily dialysis in ICU: What is it? How and why used?	1.0	ICU/Nephrology physician Handout of lecture slides Journal references from literature
Difference in application of SLED and CRRT	1.0	ICU/Nephrology nurse Handout of lecture slides Nursing policy or protocol document handout
Break		
The machine for SLED	1.0	Company/supplier display and/or demonstration Handout of machine specifications and/or brief operating guide
Reverse osmosis water and technical aspects of dialysis water	1.0	Dialysis technician or similar Handout of lecture slides Journal references from literature
Lunch break		Provided by medical suppliers/sponsored
Circuit components—"show and tell" review of priming procedure	1.0	ICU/Nephrology nurse Handout of lecture slides on sequence of routine for priming/preparation
Machine use and mock patient connection	1.0	ICU/Nephrology nurse Use simulation with resuscitation manikin or similar model at vacant bed in ICU ward
Conclusion and panel discussion	0.5	Lecture room with panel discussion
Questions and answers		Refreshments

CRRT, continuous renal replacement therapy; ICU, intensive care unit; SLED, sustained low-efficiency dialysis.
*1.0 unit = 60 minutes.

Protocol recommendation: Use the protocol and policy documents as a training and educational tool. Provide them as reading material for all nurses managing SLED treatments.

TECHNICAL ISSUES—DIALYSIS AND REPLACEMENT FLUIDS

Dialytic techniques for daily dialysis require high-volume fluid production. This is more easily achieved through use of a dialysis machine designed for it. Fluid production is routinely achieved in dialysis clinics through connection of each dialysis machine to a reverse osmosis (RO) water plant. The machine adds to this fluid, electrolytes, and bicarbonate to make a suitable dialysate and/or substitution fluid. In some ICU areas, this water is provided to each bedside, being linked as a "satellite" to the system of an adjacent dialysis unit. However, if the dialysis plant is too far away or the necessary piping is not in the ICU, a small portable RO water machine can be used for each machine, either connected to the bedside cold water tap or via purpose-built water connections at the bedside. In either case, the water is untreated for dialysis use and is usually a tap linked into the hand basin at the bedside. In addition, drains for both the patient waste fluid and "reject" water from the portable RO unit are necessary. When such a portable system is used, it may be necessary for the ICU nursing staff and/or technical staff in an ICU to understand how to monitor the quality of such water. Monitoring may also be done in association with an industry supplier of the RO units and dialysis machine or the hospital dialysis technical staff, conforming to industry standards.[36,37]

Simply, and in brief, the water used must undergo mineral, chemical, microbiological, chlorine/chloramine, and endotoxin assessment on a regular schedule.[10,38] Upon initial use of this technology, testing may be done frequently to establish a true baseline. After this initial process with satisfactory results, assessment of water quality follows a less frequent schedule and constitutes a routine quality assurance activity year round. The schedule is also set in coordination with the dialysis machine and RO unit services, which includes water filter and water purifying membrane changes. Records of machine services, filter and membrane changes, and other water quality testing must be made and maintained by an individual or group with this responsibility.

If water quality assessment is not a service provided by dialysis technicians or by a medical supplier of the machine, who will usually know these requirements well, it is an added knowledge and expertise area for staff in the ICU.

To highlight the difference in fluid management and production between CRRT, which uses fluid bags and SLED, Figure 237-3 shows the inside of a SLED-suitable dialysis machine during technical service. This machine is used for SLED with diafiltration, and the figure demonstrates the complex internal fluid tubing and valves needed for fluid management, including an internal balance system for measurement of fluids.

CONCLUSION

Nursing management for SLED in the ICU requires careful planning to ensure that the treatment is performed safely and achieves adequate solute and solvent removal. Completion of a successful treatment means that a treatment-free period can be used for other procedures, nursing care, and therapies not as easily done when CRRT is used. The machine uses dialysis technology with on-line fluids production necessary for a higher-clearance, mostly diffusive technique. When SLED is used in ICU, one machine

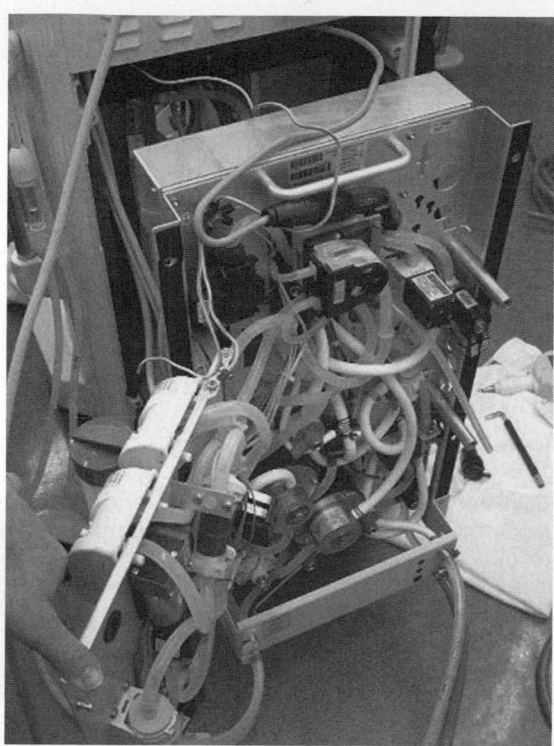

FIGURE 237-3. The internal fluid tubing and valves necessary to manufacture fluids and manage the fluid balance in the Fresenius 4008S ARrT plus machine (Fresenius Medical Care, Bad Homburg, Germany), a dialysis machine suitable for sustained low-efficiency dialysis with filtration.

can treat several patients each day. Administration of antibiotics and electrolyte supplements may need to be modified to ensure stable and therapeutic serum levels. In some ICUs where CRRT has been used for many years, a training and education program for SLED is useful, because there are many differences between the two techniques, and performing SLED requires new nursing knowledge.

Key Points

1. SLED (sustained low-efficiency dialysis) applies to several versions of dialysis.

2. Daily scheduling and prescription used for each treatment can vary and should be carefully considered because of the many nursing implications.

3. SLED requires a dialysis-designed machine incorporating the preparation of dialysis and/or intravenous replacement fluids.

4. Anticoagulation requirements for SLED are generally less than those needed for continuous renal replacement therapy. Lower-dose heparin is simple and is commonly used.

5. Fluid balance and electrolyte prescription require careful consideration, because these goals must be achieved over a limited time and must provide for the time without treatment.

6. Nursing education and training programs for the use of SLED help achieve success and ensure safety.

7. A policy document or protocol describing specific procedures, such as circuit preparation, access catheter care, and liaison between ICU and Nephrology nursing, is needed.

Key References

7. Vanholder R, VanBiesen W, Lamiere N: What is the renal replacement therapy of choice for intensive care? J Am Soc Nephrol 2001;12(Suppl 17):S40-S43.
8. Marshal M, Ma T, Galler D, et al: Sustained low-efficiency daily diafiltration (SLEDD-f) for critically ill patients requiring renal replacement therapy: Towards an adequate therapy. Nephrol Dial Transplant 2004;19:877-884.
9. Baldwin I, Naka T, Fealy N, et al: A pilot randomised controlled comparison of continuous veno-venous haemofiltration and extended daily dialysis with filtration: Effect on small solutes and acid-base balance. Intensive Care Med 2007;33:830-835.
10. Bellomo R, Baldwin I, Fealy N: Prolonged intermittent renal replacement therapy in the intensive care unit. Crit Care Resusc 2002;4:281-290.
21. O'Reilly P, Tolwani A: Renal replacement therapy III: IHD, CRRT, SLED. Crit Care Clin 2005;21:367-378.
38. Baldwin I, Bellomo R: Sustained low efficiency dialysis in the ICU. Int J Intensive Care 2002;Winter:177-187.

See the companion Expert Consult website for the complete reference list.

CHAPTER 238

Information Technology in Renal Replacement Therapy

James Tattersall

OBJECTIVES

This chapter will:
1. Describe the information needs of renal replacement therapy in critical care.
2. Discuss the principles underlying the information technology appropriate for critical care.

The provision of renal replacement therapy (RRT) in critical care is a complex logistical exercise that depends on accurate information for planning, implementation, and troubleshooting. The decision to start RRT is based on several criteria, some of which are scores that are themselves calculated from several other clinical or laboratory observations.[1] The provision of RRT requires the appropriate equipment, trained staff, fluids, and disposables at the bedside. The renal replacement process must be monitored and managed appropriately for safety and optimal outcome. This management consists of calculation of the appropriate dose of dialysis, measurement of dose, monitoring of machine settings, guarantee of an adequate supply of fluid and disposables, and application of the appropriate protocols.

Some of these data are acquired at the bedside, and others are supplied by laboratory reports, the Internet, or elsewhere. Staff involved in the support and planning of RRT may work outside the clinical area yet still require access to the information.

The entire process and all supporting information must be documented and saved for several years for legal reasons and to guide future treatment. The data are the property of the patient and are subject to human rights and privacy legislation.

Much of the information generated and required in RRT is specialized and not of interest to other departments of the health care system. Therefore, generalized information systems in use in a hospital are unlikely to provide the functions required for RRT. Conversely, some of the information generated and required in RRT forms part of the patient record and is used by other departments for medical care and administration.

This situation requires an information system that is secure, is accessible from various locations, provides the required functions, integrates with laboratory and other hospital systems, and is practical to use at the bedside.

INITIATING RENAL REPLACEMENT THERAPY

The decision to start RRT is based on a number of clinical and laboratory criteria (Table 238-1). Not only the absolute values but also the trends of these values over time are taken into account. It may be necessary to predict likely future need for RRT in an individual patient to allow adequate time for planning and preparation.

PRESCRIBING RENAL REPLACEMENT THERAPY

The prescription of RRT depends on a number of patient and other factors. In particular, the dose of dialysis,[2] choice of anticoagulant, and type of buffer are determined by patient factors and have been shown to affect outcome (Table 238-2).

Mathematical models have been developed that predict the effect of RRT on the patient. These models can be incorporated into the information system to guide prescription. Ideally, the information system should suggest a prescription appropriate to the patient and other input data. In future, the prescription modeling software would use published outcome data to predict the effect of any prescription on outcome.

If RRT is to be provided intermittently, advanced modeling methods may be required to determine the optimum timing and dose of each session.[3]

MONITORING RENAL REPLACEMENT THERAPY

RRT is typically monitored by the dialysis equipment. Analysis of the arterial and venous pressure provides information on the condition of the vascular access and can help detect disconnection or occlusion. The treatment time and the blood, dialysate, and/or filtrate flow rates may vary from the prescription and are used to estimate dialysis dose, which has been shown to affect outcome.

If RRT is provided intermittently with on-line dialysate/filtrate preparation, the equipment may also monitor dialysate/filtrate temperature, conductivity, and pH.

Some of the information collected by the equipment is valuable only during the treatment run (e.g., arterial and venous pressure); other data may usefully be retained as part of the patient record.

TABLE 238-1

Data Used to Plan Initiation of Renal Replacement Therapy

CRITERIA	SOURCE
Estimated glomerular filtration rate	Laboratory Demographics
APACHE II (Acute Physiology and Chronic Health Evaluation II) score*	Laboratory Bedside clinical findings Vital signs monitor Demographics
RIFLE (Risk of renal dysfunction, injury to the kidney, failure of kidney function, loss of kidney, end-stage renal disease) score	Laboratory
Urine output	Bedside clinical findings
Blood pressure trends	Vital signs monitor
Serum creatinine, electrolytes, bicarbonate.	Laboratory
Clinical assessment	Bedside clinical findings Medical record
Department protocols	Protocol database

*Bagshaw SM, Mortis G, Doig CJ, et al: One-year mortality in critically ill patients by severity of kidney dysfunction: A population-based assessment. Am J Kidney Dis 2006;48:402-409.

TABLE 238-2

Components of the Renal Replacement Therapy Prescription

COMPONENT	INFORMED BY
Dialysate/filtrate flow rate	Weight Height Blood urea Renal function
Blood flow rate	Type of access Blood urea level Electrolyte concentrations
Dialysate potassium concentration	Blood potassium concentration
Dialysate buffer content	Blood bicarbonate concentration Liver function
Dialysate additives	Blood calcium, magnesium, and phosphate concentrations
Dialyzer/filter type	Body weight
Anticoagulant type/dose	Clinical information
Modality (pre/post dilution, filtration/dialysis, continuous/intermittent)	Clinical information Availability of equipment and staff Logistical considerations Departmental protocol

OUTPUT FROM THE INFORMATION SYSTEM

Data stored in the information system are used to plan further care, for troubleshooting, and for administrative purposes (Table 238-3). An information system can alert users to the need for specific interventions such as RRT[4] or nutritional support.[5] Inappropriate treatment can be detected.[6] Reports on the disposables and equipment used

TABLE 238-3

Use of Output from Hospital Information Systems

REPORT	USED FOR OR BY
Patients likely to require renal replacement therapy	Clinical care Technical staff Stock control Staff management
Equipment in use	Technical staff
Disposables and fluids used	Stock control Accounting
Treatments and interventions	Staff management Accounting Clinical audit
Indications for renal replacement	Clinical audit Registry
Adverse events	Clinical audit Legal activities
Renal replacement prescriptions	Clinical audit Registry
Renal replacement, prescribed vs. delivered dose	Clinical audit Clinical care Registry
Outcome, predicted vs. actual	Clinical audit Registry
Nutritional status	Dietitian Clinical care Clinical audit

by the RRT can be used for stock control. For example, equipment for RRT may be prepared in advance by technical staff working in a hospital location relatively remote from the critical care areas. Technical staff are guided by the information system, which would list all current and predicted use of equipment, disposables used, and location of use.

These information reports are used remotely from the critical care areas. Some of the reports describe the current situation and are valid for only a short time. For these reasons, the reports should be accessible online in administrative and technical areas as well as the critical care area.

BEDSIDE DATA COLLECTION

Some of the data required by the information systems is clinical information that must be entered by hand. Good medical practice principles dictate that it is entered (1) by the clinical staff observing or acquiring the information and (2) as soon as it is observed or acquired. Staff should not be required to enter the same data twice (as this is wasteful of their time), and the data should not be transcribed by clerical staff (as this introduces error and delay).

The requirement for clinical staff to enter clinical details at a personal computer on the nursing station may adversely affect quality of care because that activity takes them away from the patient.[7] Data entry on shared workstations may be time-consuming because the staff has to log in and select the patient before entering any data. Ideally, data on each patient should be entered at the bedside by staff using a nearby or portable terminal allocated to the specific patient. Such an arrangement almost completely eliminates the need to log in and select the

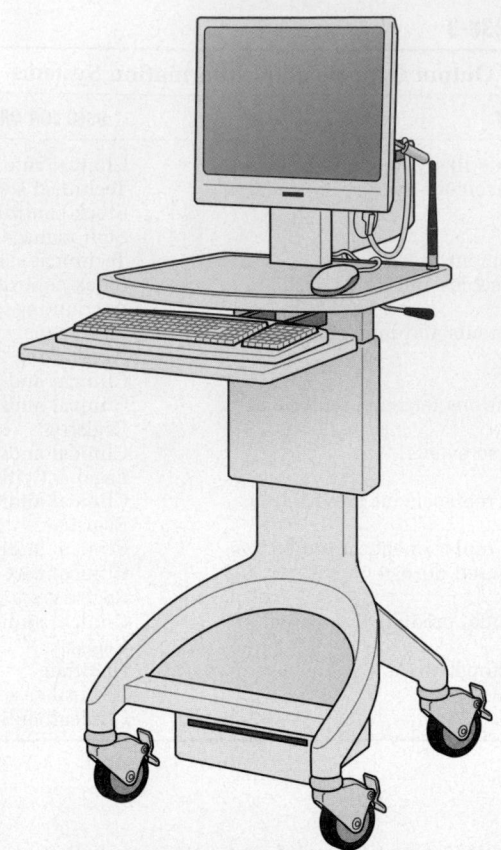

FIGURE 238-1. A typical mobile bedside computer workstation.

patient repeatedly. The use of touch screens, barcode scanners, and handwriting recognition can improve speed of data entry. The requirement for staff to type at the keyboard, the most time-consuming aspect of data entry, should be reduced to a minimum.

Various mobile computer workstation terminals are available that are suitable for bedside data access (Fig. 238-1). They can be connected to wired or, ideally, wireless networks. A bedside computer workstation occupies less space than the paper charts it replaces and can be used for multiple other tasks.

INTERFACE TO MONITORING EQUIPMENT

The monitoring equipment used in critical care provides information that may inform RRT or be part of its documentation. Ideally, the information system should capture this information automatically.

Most vital signs monitoring equipment in use in critical care areas can be supplied as a complete system, including a dedicated information management system and interfaces to transfer data. These proprietary monitoring information systems are unlikely to have the functions required to handle all aspects of RRT and other specific departmental needs.

Monitoring equipment can potentially be connected to any computerized information system. International Organization for Standardization (ISO) standard 11073 defines how medical devices communicate with computer systems. In theory, any ISO 11073–compliant monitoring equipment would be able to transfer data into information management software that implements the standard. Critical care departments may consider requiring all suppliers to comply with ISO 11073 or to provide interfaces to other computer systems where appropriate.

In the past, monitoring equipment has been connected to a computer system with a serial cable. This arrangement is not really practical when many devices are connected, as each requires its own cable and a dedicated port on a central computer. Modern monitoring equipment is likely to implement embedded computer processing, which is capable of communicating by means of standard network protocols.

Ideally, medical devices should communicate wirelessly using the well-established Institute of Electrical and Electronics Engineers (IEEE 803.11) standards. This form of wireless communication does not interfere with medical devices.[8] Separate standards mandate that all medical devices be immune to electromagnetic interference of a specified power and frequency, which includes IEEE 803.11 communication. Wireless networks are much cheaper to install and manage than wired networks and have been shown to be reliable. A growing number of measuring and monitoring devices are designed to communicate wirelessly using the IEEE 803.11 standard.[9] A further advantage of the IEEE 803.11 standard is that it is a network protocol compatible with hospital data networks and the Internet. Some existing mobile phones, many personal data assistants, and most notebook computers and tablet personal computers are designed to communicate in this way.

If the critical care area is covered by an IEEE 803.11-standard network, staff would also be able to access hospital, departmental, and Internet information systems and communicate wirelessly using inexpensive portable devices.

INTERFACE TO HEMODIALYSIS OR HEMOFILTRATION MACHINES

The typical modern hemodialysis or hemofiltration machine contains an onboard computer that accepts the prescription, controls the equipment, monitors the treatment, and displays information to the user. The machine is, therefore, in possession of much of the data that would be useful as part of the medical record. Ideally, the data should be automatically transferred into the main information system by means of the technology previously described for monitoring equipment.

Because hemodialysis or hemofiltration machines are heavy and mobile, wired data connections are particularly subject to mechanical stress when the machines are moved. The connections are also subject to exposure to saline and dialysis fluid. For these reasons, wireless data communication, using a transmitter located in the sealed electronics area of the machine, are particularly appropriate.

INTERFACE TO HOSPITAL SYSTEMS

The planning and management of RRT depend on laboratory results and other clinical information that are probably held in the main hospital information system. RRT in critical care has additional specialized information requirements that are unlikely to be met by the main hospital system. Therefore, the critical care area needs its own departmental information management system that complements existing hospital systems. Because some of the data are common to the two systems, the departmental system should be integrated with or at least communicate with the hospital systems. The departmental systems should implement the Health Level 7 (HL7) standard for clinical data exchange and interface with a single central hospital computer to keep the cost of developing and administering these interfaces as low as possible.

To reduce the cost and management burden, these departmental systems should be as simple as possible. They should be used only for those functions that are inadequately provided for by central systems. To avoid wasteful duplication, delay, and error, any data used by the departmental system and stored elsewhere on the main hospital system should be automatically downloaded into the departmental system. This downloaded data includes the patient identifying codes, demographic data, laboratory results, and any relevant clinical information. Data should be entered directly into the departmental systems only when it is not available elsewhere.

SECURITY

Medical information is the property of the patient and is subject to privacy and human rights laws. In general, the data can be stored and used only with the patient's permission and for a specific purpose. The data can be accessed by persons or organizations only with the patient's consent.

In practice, it is assumed that the patient gives permission to store any data required for direct clinical care. Staff involved with the patient's clinical care and its administration are assumed to have permission to access the data for this purpose. Information systems must be secure against unauthorized access and must ensure that the data are accurate, up to date, and complete.

New information systems should have the following features, at a minimum, to improve security:
- No data can be accessed without a valid log-in.
- A valid log-in consists of a user ID and password. Ideally, the ID should be supported by a card or biometric data (fingerprint or iris image).
- The log-in is specific to an individual user who is authorized to access the data.
- The user is a professional accountable to the organization (i.e., subject to disciplinary action).
- The log-in allows access only to specific data required for the user's professional role within the organization.

The administration of security is a significant management task.

BACKUP

Computer data are vulnerable to loss because of equipment failure. Data are normally copied to various secure locations periodically so that they can be recovered in case of equipment failure. Normally, a data file cannot be copied while it is in use, because it is frequently being

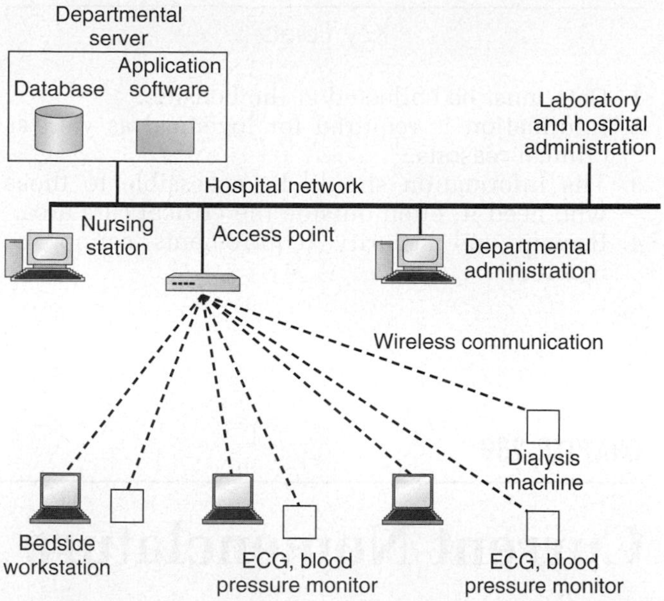

FIGURE 238-2. Diagram of an information system in the critical care area. ECG, electrocardiogram.

updated by users. The process of updating data commonly requires multiple steps. The data are unreadable or corrupted if the data file was copied midway through the update, when some of the steps had not been completed.

For secure backup, the data must be held in a central database that is designed for the task. Backups must be managed centrally, and the backup data stored securely.

SYSTEM DESIGN

Medical data are normally held in a central database located on a server in a secure area (Fig. 238-2). The data are accessed through client workstations, which may be standard desktop personal computers, laptop computers, or tablet computers. If specifically supported, the system may be accessed by personal digital assistants.

The client workstations are connected to the server over a network that could consist of wireless segments. To reduce cost and management complexity, most of the software required for processing data can be located on the server. This arrangement allows the client computer to be relatively simple, ideally requiring only an Internet browser to access the system. So-called thin client computers can be located at the bedside for convenient and economical access to the data.

CONCLUSION

Existing, well-developed, and standards-driven information technology can assist in the application of new medical knowledge to the management of RRT, improving safety and quality of care. The vast quantity of information required and generated by critical care demands a carefully planned and integrated approach to information management.

Key Points

1. Data must be collected at the bedside.
2. Information is required for logistical as well as clinical reasons.
3. The information should be accessible to those who need it, often outside the critical care area.
4. Backup and security requirements cannot be ignored.

5. The information systems used in critical care must be integrated with hospital systems and must implement recognized standards for communication.

See the companion Expert Consult website for the complete reference list.

CHAPTER 239

Current Nomenclature

Zaccaria Ricci, Rinaldo Bellomo, John A. Kellum, and Claudio Ronco

OBJECTIVES

This chapter will:
1. Review the current nomenclature for different renal replacement therapies (RRTs).
2. Make short recommendations for future proposals to modify renal replacement therapies.

The issue of nomenclature in the field of renal replacement therapy (RRT) was addressed for the very first time during an international conference more than 10 years ago.[1] The definitions were subsequently modified and were endorsed in 2000 by the Acute Dialysis Quality Initiative.[2] The consensus set of definitions, abbreviations, and nomenclature for RRT was produced with the following two indispensable premises:
1. The definitions were to be based on the operating characteristics of each method with emphasis on the primary forces for solutes and fluid removal.
2. The description of circuit components was not considered in the definition.
Since then, authors of scientific papers on the field of RRT substantially accepted this set of recommendations. Hundreds of papers referred to this initial framework and sometimes proposed new modifications and new terms for advanced or innovative therapies.

The aim of the present chapter is to provide a reasonably updated version of current RRT nomenclature, including mechanisms of solute transport, techniques, and modalities. The list of definitions is presented in the form of a glossary for a quick and rapid explanation. In-depth details on single terms can be found in specific chapters. Arteriovenous circuits are no longer used worldwide[3] and are systematically excluded from the present chapter.

Figures 239-1 and 239-2 schematically represent most common renal replacement techniques and modalities.

NOMENCLATURE FOR MECHANISMS OF WATER AND SOLUTE TRANSPORT AND RENAL REPLACEMENT THERAPY CIRCUIT SPECIFICATIONS

DIFFUSION. The movement of a solute (in this case across a semipermeable membrane) with a statistical tendency to reach the same concentration in the available distribution space on each side of the membrane. Diffusion is directly proportional to concentration gradient, temperature, surface area, and solute diffusivity across that membrane, and inversely proportional to the distance for diffusion (thickness of the membrane). The practical result is a passage of molecules from the more concentrated compartment into the less concentrated one.

CONVECTION. A process by which solutes are transported across the semipermeable membrane together with the solvent by means of a filtration mechanism (solvent drag), which occurs in response to a transmembrane pressure gradient. Convective transport depends on the filtration rate and the permeability of the membrane in the presence of a certain concentration of the solute in plasma water.

ULTRAFILTRATION. The transport of water across a semipermeable membrane (ultrafiltrate in biology is a fluid with the same concentration of crystalloids of plasma, but without cell or colloids). Also, a process by which plasma water and ultrafilterable solutes are separated from whole blood across a semipermeable membrane in response to transmembrane pressure. This term is utilized as a mechanism of (water) transport, as a treatment modality and, sometimes incorrectly, as a synonym for fluid balance or of hemofiltration. See longer discussion under "Modalities."

BACKFILTRATION. Also known as reverse filtration or back-ultrafiltration; a flux of water from the dialysis fluid compartment of a hollow fiber dialyzer into the blood caused by a local negative transmembrane pressure gradient. This process typically occurs in presence of ultrafiltration control systems during dialysis conducted

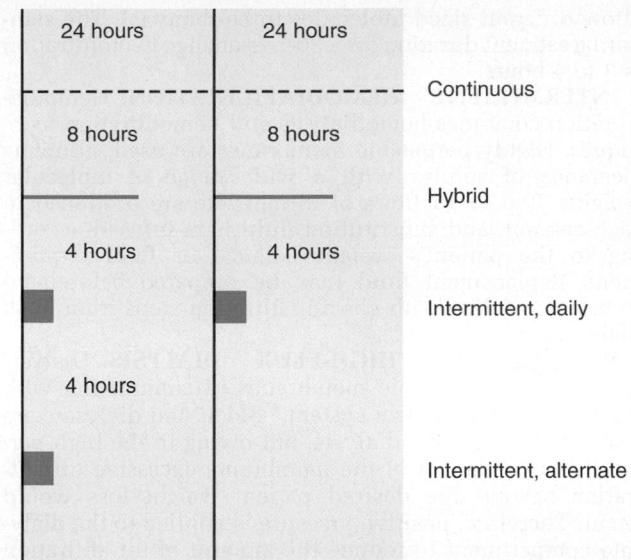

FIGURE 239-1. Schematic representation of different renal replacement techniques.

MODALITIES

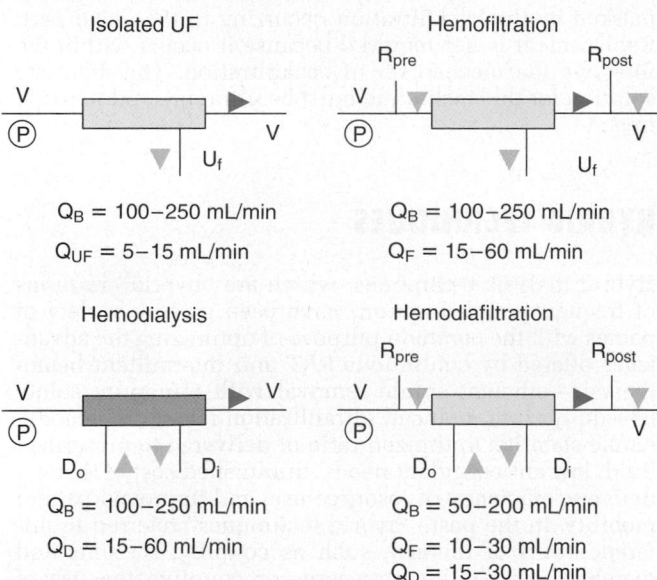

FIGURE 239-2. Schematic representation of different renal replacement modalities. Reported flows represent typical prescriptions of continuous renal replacement therapies. P, roller pump; Q_B, blood flow rate, Q_D, dialysis flow rate; Q_F, reinfusion flow rate; Q_{UF}, ultrafiltration flow rate; R_{post}, post-dilution reinfusion. R_{pre}, predilution reinfusion; UF, ultrafiltration; V, venous access.

with hollow-fiber dialyzers equipped with high-flux membranes.

TRANSMEMBRANE PRESSURE (TMP). In hollow fiber dialyzers, the gradient of pressure across the membrane. The components are the same as in human capillaries—the Starling forces. TMP represents the pressure gradient between blood and ultrafiltrate/dialysate and is derived from the difference between the hydrostatic and oncotic gradients.

VENOVENOUS (VV) CIRCUIT. The venous vascular access and associated tubing that carry blood into and out

of the hemofilter and back into the circulation. It is performed generally, but not necessarily, by means of one double-lumen catheter. Arteriovenous vascular access has been abandoned because of the uselessness of arteriovenous pressure gradient in pumped systems and the high morbidity linked to arterial puncture.

PREDILUTION. The administration of replacement fluid into the patient's blood before its entry into the hemofilter (prefilter delivery).

POSTDILUTION. Postdilution is the administration of replacement fluid into the patient's blood after its exit from the hemofilter (postfilter delivery).

MODALITIES

HEMODIALYSIS. A prevalently diffusive treatment in which blood and dialysate are circulated in countercurrent mode. If a low-permeability cellulose-based membrane is employed, solutes are removed exclusively by diffusion. With a high-flux synthetic membrane, diffusion and convection may variably participate in blood purification. Weight loss results from a low ultrafiltration rate, which derives from the difference between the dialysis fluid infused into the dialysate compartment and the effluent fluid that is produced from the dialysis compartment.

HEMOFILTRATION. An exclusively convective treatment performed with highly permeable membranes. The ultrafiltrate produced is replaced completely or in part by a sterile solution (re-infusion). Weight loss results from the difference between ultrafiltration and re-infusion rates (no dialysis fluid is used).

HEMODIAFILTRATION. A treatment in which diffusion and convection are combined and a highly permeable membrane is used. Blood and dialysate are circulated as in hemodialysis, but typically, an ultrafiltration in excess of the scheduled weight loss is produced. To achieve fluid balance, sterile solution is re-infused to the patient at an adequate rate.

ULTRAFILTRATION. A modality in which fluid removal is the main target of the therapy. Highly permeable filters are utilized and fluid is removed from the body without replacement. Ultrafiltration can be performed intermittently or daily with variable ultrafiltration rates applied, depending on the hemodynamic stability of the patients. In clinical practice, ultrafiltration has also been used in sequence with hemodialysis to improve cardiovascular tolerance or at very low filtration rates (1-2 mL/min) specific to remove only water.

This term is utilized as a mechanism of (water) transport, as a treatment modality, and, sometimes incorrectly, as a synonym for fluid balance or hemofiltration. The following is a definitive list of the correct uses of the term ultrafiltration and related concepts:

- *Total ultrafiltration*: Amount of ultrafiltration removed from the filter in a given time (typically, 24 hours).
- *Ultrafiltration rate:* Amount of ultrafiltration produced by the filter per minute (or per hour).
- Total re-infusion: Amount of fluid re-infused in the circuit in a given time (typically, 24 hours).
- *Re-infusion rate:* Amount of fluid re-infused in the circuit per minute (or per hour).
- *Net ultrafiltration:* Overall amount of fluid extracted from the patient in a given time (typically 24 hours).
- *Net ultrafiltration rate*: The amount of fluid extracted from the patient per minute (or per hour).

PLASMAPHERESIS. With use of a particular membrane with a molecular weight cutoff much higher than that of a plasma filter, whole plasma is filtered and blood is reconstituted by the infusion of plasma derivatives, fresh frozen plasma, albumin, or other fluids. The treatment is indicated for removal of proteins or protein-bound solutes that cannot be removed by simple hemofiltration.

HEMOPERFUSION. A form of treatment in which blood is circulated through a cartridge coated with activated charcoal or carbon to remove solutes by adsorption. The technique is specifically indicated in toxic acute renal failure, poisoning, or intoxication. Unlike hemodialysis, hemoperfusion has the ability to clear protein-bound substances because charcoal can compete with plasma proteins for drugs. It is also more effective than hemodialysis in the removal of lipid-soluble substances.

INTERMITTENT TECHNIQUES

Intermittent dialysis techniques require an adequate vascular access and specifically trained nurses to carry out the dialysis session. Efficient equipment capable of achieving the intended prescription is important. A specific water-softening setup that can de-ionize water is required in order to produce pure water for dialysate preparation. In some cases, despite the use of reverse osmosis as a water treatment system, on-line ultrafilters are needed to achieve a bacteria- and pyrogen-free dialysate. The dialysis machine must respond to the standards of reliability and safety with an adequate blood module, a precise dialysate-preparing module with adequate warming and de-aeration systems, and all parts must have active alarms to avoid possible accident. Until recently, this resource could be facilitated and carried out only by nephrology units, but modern intensive care units are becoming autonomous, initiating such treatment without the assistance of Nephrology staff. The prescribed schedule can vary according to single-center protocols or clinical needs: Treatments can be applied three times a week, on alternate days, or daily, or even used in a daily prolonged modality.

INTERMITTENT HEMODIALYSIS. A technique is carried out in a session of 3 to 5 hours with a blood flow of 250 to 500 mL/min. A low-permeability membrane such as cuprophane or Hemophan with an average surface area of 1 to 1.5 m^2 is used. Dialysate flow is 500 mL/min, and the rate of ultrafiltration can be set as clinically indicated. The technique relies on mainly diffusive mechanisms and low-molecular-weight solutes are removed faster than larger molecules. If a highly permeable membrane is utilized, the treatment is called "intermittent high-flux hemodialysis" (see later).

INTERMITTENT HEMOFILTRATION. Hemofiltration in which treatment time depends on the rate of ultrafiltration and the total amount of fluid to be exchanged. Blood flow must exceed 300 mL/min, and no dialysate is present. A highly permeable membrane is utilized, and solutes are removed by convection. Synthetic membranes like polysulfone have a sieving capacity of approximately 1 for a wide spectrum of molecular weights. Sieving coefficients in cellulosic membranes significantly decrease even for moderately larger molecules. For this reason, synthetic membranes are used in hemofiltration. Ultrafiltration is totally or partially replaced with sterile substitution fluid, and solute concentrations in plasma are essentially normalized. Net fluid balance is the difference between ultrafiltration and re-infusion. High-permeability membranes allow different sized molecules to be removed. The standard treatment duration for a 30-L exchange hemofiltration is 3 to 4 hours.

INTERMITTENT HEMODIAFILTRATION. Hemodiafiltration combines hemodialysis and hemofiltration techniques. Highly permeable membranes are used, allowing clearance of solutes with a wide range of molecular weights. Ten to 15 liters of ultrafiltrate are produced in each session, and substitution fluid is re-infused according to the patient's weight balance or fluid requirement. Replacement fluid may be prepared beforehand in bags or on-line with specific filtration steps from fresh dialysate.

INTERMITTENT HIGH-FLUX DIALYSIS. Dialysis using highly permeable membranes in conjunction with an ultrafiltration control system.[4] Blood and dialysate are circulated as in hemodialysis, but owing to the high permeability coefficient of the membrane, excessive ultrafiltration beyond the desired patient weight loss would occur. Therefore, positive pressure is applied to the dialysate compartment to reduce the amount of ultrafiltration and to avoid the need for replacement solution. Because of the peculiar structure of hollow-fiber dialyzers, filtration takes place in the proximal part of the filter, and backfiltration occurs in the distal part. Diffusion and convection therefore are still combined because the high filtration rate occurring in the proximal part of the dialyzer is masked by the backfiltration occurring in the distal part. Replacement is not required because it occurs within the filter via the mechanism of backfiltration. The dialysate solution for this technique must be ultrapure and pyrogen free.

HYBRID TECHNIQUES

Hybrid dialysis techniques, which are "hybrid" in terms of frequency and duration, have been given a variety of names with the common purpose of optimizing the advantages offered by continuous RRT and intermittent hemodialysis—efficient solute removal with minimum solute dysequilibrium, reduced ultrafiltration rate with hemodynamic stability, optimized ratio of delivered to prescribed fluid, low anticoagulant needs, diminished cost of therapy delivery, efficiency of resource use, and improved patient mobility. In the past, "hybrid techniques" referred to different forms of therapy, such as coupling sorbents and membrane separation processes or coupling the use of artificial membranes with living cells.

SUSTAINED LOW-EFFICIENCY DIALYSIS. Sustained low-efficiency dialysis is only one of many definitions that hybrid techniques have been given; others are slow low-efficiency extended daily dialysis (SLEDD), prolonged intermittent daily RRT (PDIRRT), extended daily dialysis (EDD), EDD with filtration (EDDf) or, simply, extended dialysis (ED),[5] depending on variations in schedule and type of solute removal (convective or diffusive). SLED is a recently developed hybrid technique of RRT that uses a conventional hemodialysis machine with reduced blood flow (100-200 mL/min) and dialysate flow rates (100-200 mL/min); it is usually performed nocturnally for an extended period (10-12 hours). The benefit of this form of treatment is that it provides a high dialysis dose, which can also be applied in unstable patients with the advantage of allowing unrestricted access to patients for daytime procedures. Different prescriptions, variable amounts of ultrafiltrate, and other "variations on the theme" have led to the description of this approach as a "genius" recirculation system.

CONTINUOUS TECHNIQUES

Continuous renal replacement therapy (CRRT) is delivered 24 hours a day. In terms of treatment efficiency, hemodynamic stability, and versatility of prescription, this treatment fits the needs of critically ill patients better than intermittent RRT. Nonetheless, the prolonged effort that a continuous treatment requires—the need for a specialized expertise and specific equipment, the necessity of continuous anticoagulation, the unremitting nurse workload, and the continuous alarm surveillance—make this therapy far from perfect. Most of these pitfalls are currently managed in modern intensive care units, and the use of CRRT for the management of acute renal failure has today grown to the point that, according to a 2005 survey, 80% of the intensive care units worldwide routinely choose this strategy.[3]

SLOW CONTINUOUS ULTRAFILTRATION. A treatment that may be employed for 24 hours a day or for only some hours each day through a venovenous access (with pump). It is carried out with high-flux membranes, and the objective to achieve volume control in patients with fluid overload. The operational parameters are generally those described in the figure. Because low filtration rates are required, filters with small surface area are generally employed. An ultrafiltration control system should be applied in order to prevent excessive fluid loss and hypovolemia. Because of the low filtration rates, the treatment is suitable to achieve only volume control, not blood purification.

CONTINUOUS VENOVENOUS HEMOFILTRATION. A technique performed in venovenous mode utilizing high-flux membranes in which the prevalent mechanism of solute transport is convection. It is normally applied for an extended period, up to several weeks. Ultrafiltrate is produced and it is partially or totally replaced by fresh substitution fluid. In this modality, the flow is regulated by a pump, and the rate of ultrafiltration can significantly increase. In the presence of high filtration rates, systems for ultrafiltration and re-infusion control are generally utilized. Different machines use either volumetric control systems or volumetric pumps regulated by one or multiple scales. Heparin is infused in the arterial line to prevent clotting of the circuit. The replacement solution can be infused either before the filter (predilution) or after the filter (postdilution). With predilution, ultrafiltration must be relatively increased to maintain the same efficiency observed in postdilution mode. Because the ultrafiltrate is replaced by the substitution fluid that is toxin free, the treatment is used for blood purification and volume control. Once blood flow is set, average ultrafiltration should not exceed 20% of the overall blood flow rate (filtration fraction).

CONTINUOUS VENOVENOUS HEMODIALYSIS. A treatment carried out over an extended period using either an arteriovenous access or a venovenous pump–driven circuit. The treatment was originally described as utilizing a low-flux membrane such as cuprophane and a countercurrent flow of dialysate of 15 to 20 mL/min. Because of the nature of the membrane and the gradient provided by the dialysate, the prevalent mechanism of solute transport in this technique is diffusion. Ultrafiltration is obtained precisely within the range of values adequate to maintain

the patient's fluid control without requirement of fluid re-infusion. The development of blood pumps to increase blood flows was then applied to dialysate flows. For this reason, dialyzers with higher surface area and modified cellulosic membranes such as triacetate could be effectively used. When dialysate is run at low flow rates, the fluid saturation is almost complete. When dialysate flow is increased in spite of a progressive desaturation of the spent dialysate, there is an increase in clearance of low-molecular-weight solutes. In most cases, designated machines must be used to control inlet and outlet dialysate flows and to achieve the desired volume of ultrafiltration. The system can be run either in single-pass or recirculation mode, and clearance of middle- to high-molecular-weight solutes can reach values as high as 60% of those observed for smaller molecules like urea. When this treatment is performed with a highly permeable membrane, the technique is more precisely called "continuous high-flux dialysis."

CONTINUOUS VENOVENOUS HEMODIAFILTRATION. A treatment that requires a high-flux hemodiafilter and combines the principles of hemodialysis and hemofiltration. Dialysate is circulated in countercurrent mode to the blood, and at the same time, ultrafiltration is obtained in excess of the desired fluid loss from the patient. This loss is totally or partially replaced with substitution fluid, either in predilution or postdilution mode. Newer machines allow a combination of predilution and postdilution modes, aimed at combining the advantages of both modalities. Because this therapy is supposed to combine diffusion and convection, optimal clearances are expected for both low- and high-molecular-weight solutes.

SPECIAL THERAPIES

HIGH-VOLUME HEMOFILTRATION. A purely convective therapy that can be performed with two basic schedules: continuous or pulsed.[6,7] With a continuous schedule, the therapy is performed for 24 hours with a fluid exchange rate higher than 3 L/hr, and clearances in the range of 80 liters/day can be obtained. Technical requirements for this technique consist especially on the increased blood flow rates and the availability of large volumes of substitution fluid. The pulsed schedule can be used for a short time (3-6 hrs) during the day, with a fluid exchange rate of 6 to 8 L/hr, and the standard continuous schedule and exchange rate used for the rest of the day. These therapies have been shown to have a beneficial effect on patient hemodynamics, with a significant reduction of vasopressor drug requirement. The technology involved is in most cases borrowed from the chronic hemodialysis setting. The large volumes of fluid exchanged may render the treatment impractical. Newer methods for on-line production of substitution fluid may in the near future, however, reduce the costs and the problems of fluid supply.

CONTINUOUS PLASMAPHERESIS–PLASMA EXCHANGE. Techniques that are basically derived from the classic plasma therapies with the same name, but performed with lower flow rates and for extended periods. The rationale for these therapies is to remove plasma proteins and immunological complexes that are believed to be the pathophysiological sources of the patient's disease. Because plasma is filtered across highly porous membranes, large quantities of plasma substitutes, such as fresh-frozen plasma, are required for these procedures. Single or repeated sessions can be performed in isolation or in conjunction with other blood purification techniques.[8]

HIGH-POROSITY HEMOFILTRATION. Also known as high-cutoff hemofiltration; a technique using a high-flux hemofilter with an in vivo cutoff point of approximately 60 kDa.[9] This technique can be regarded as a compromise between standard hemofiltration and plasmapheresis. In a pilot study comparing this technique with standard hemofiltration, high-porosity hemofiltration seemed to decrease adjusted norepinephrine dose over time.[9] Clearance rates for interleukins IL-6 and IL-1ra were significantly higher in the high-cutoff hemofiltration group, with a corresponding decline in such cytokine plasma levels. Because the rationale for this technique is the same as that for other special RRTs, the greater technical complexity of high-porosity appears to limit its usefulness. Compared with high-volume hemofiltration, the technique requires smaller quantities of replacement solution, lower blood flow rates, and lower anticoagulant dosages. High-porosity hemofiltration could be performed in selected patients as a standard treatment with this special membrane, with a particular attention to the protein and albumin losses that can occur over time. This technique has also been called "super-high-flux hemofiltration."

COUPLED PLASMAFILTRATION-ADSORPTION. A special technique that combines the advantages of CRRT and CPF without requiring large amounts of plasma substitutes.[10] The technique has two steps: (1) blood is circulated through a plasma filter, and plasma filtrate is pushed by a pump through a cartridge containing a mixture of hydrophobic resin and uncoated charcoal; (2) the regenerated plasma is returned to the main circuit, where blood is reconstituted and eventually dialyzed. Because the patient's own plasma is used for re-infusion, there is no need for substitution fluids, and unwanted protein losses are avoided. The technique has been effective in reducing circulating levels of various cytokines and at the same time has allowed significant reduction in the pharmacological requirement to maintain hemodynamic stability in patients in the early stages of sepsis syndrome.

CONTINUOUS HEMOPERFUSION-HEMODIALYSIS. A combination therapy that has been mostly used in the past for acute intoxications.[11] The technique is based on the placement of a sorbent cartridge in series with the dialyzer in an attempt to remove toxins that are not removed by classic blood purification techniques. One of the major limitations imposed by this technique was the poor biocompatibility of the sorbent. Newer sorbent materials, however, are coated with biocompatible surfaces that prevent platelet trapping and clotting activation. Among the sorbent techniques, the attempt to remove circulating endotoxin with polymyxin B–coated fibers should be mentioned. The cartridge contains fibers that are coated with an antibiotic with a high affinity for lipopolysaccharides (polymyxin B). The critical factor in making this therapy effective seems to be its early application, when high levels of circulating endotoxin can be detected in plasma and the systemic effects of the humoral response to lipopolysaccharides have not yet occurred.

Key Points

1. Definitions are important to avoid describing different treatment modalities with the same name.
2. Nomenclature is quintessential to the ability to compare reports of studies using the various modalities.
3. The mechanisms involved in renal replacement therapies should be known and used appropriately by investigators in order to describe the nature of the performed therapy accurately.

See the companion Expert Consult website for the complete reference list.

Continuous Renal Replacement Therapies

Basic Principles

CHAPTER 240

History and Development of Continuous Renal Replacement Therapy

Claudio Ronco and Hans Dietrich Polaschegg

OBJECTIVES

This chapter will:
1. Describe the birth of continuous arteriovenous hemofiltration.
2. Describe the evolution from arteriovenous to venovenous treatments.
3. Present the evolution of technology for continuous renal replacement therapy.
4. Present the evolution of the approach to the therapy of acute renal failure.

In the past decade, the change in the epidemiology of acute renal failure has made critical care nephrology an emerging subspecialty of intensive care medicine. Dedicated literature and a series of physicians and nurses have made an effort to bridge the knowledge and experience from nephrology and critical care medicine in response to an increased incidence of acute kidney injury in patients in intensive care units.[1]

THE BIRTH OF CONTINUOUS ARTERIOVENOUS HEMOFILTRATION

The origin of the new era of extracorporeal treatment of acute renal failure can be found in the mid-1970s, when continuous arteriovenous hemofiltration (CAVH) appeared on the scene (Fig. 240-1). Until that point, acute renal failure was treated with conservative measures, peritoneal dialysis, or intermittent hemodialysis. All techniques presented the limitations of low clearances, poor fluid management control, and many complications. CAVH was discovered by Peter Kramer in 1977, and it immediately became an important alternative treatment for acute renal failure in those patients where peritoneal dialysis or hemodialysis was clinically or technically precluded.[2] This opened the doors of intensive care units to a dedicated dialysis technology that experienced a flourishing evolution in subsequent years. In the mid-1980s, the technology of CAVH was extended to infants and children, and newly designed hemofilters permitted the application of the technique even to newborns (Fig. 240-2). CAVH presented important advantages over intermittent hemodialysis. These were particularly apparent in the areas of hemodynamic stability, control of circulating volume, and nutritional support. However, CAVH also had serious shortcomings, which included the need for arterial cannulation (or construction of a Scribner arteriovenous shunt) and the limited solute clearance that could be achieved even under optimal operating circumstances (10 ± 12 mL/min for small solutes such as urea). Initial technical modifications, such as predilution (i.e., the infusion of the replacement solution before the filter instead of after it), improved creatinine clearance, and the next major technical advance was the creation of an additional side port to the hemofilter. Through this port, countercurrent dialysate could be infused at slow flow rates (i.e., 1 L/hr) to achieve additional diffusive solute clearance. This modified technique was named continuous arteriovenous hemodiafiltration or hemodialysis (CAVHDF or CAVHD). With the arrival of CAVHDF, intermittent hemodialysis was utilized less often, as uremic control could be achieved in all patients, irrespective of their weight or

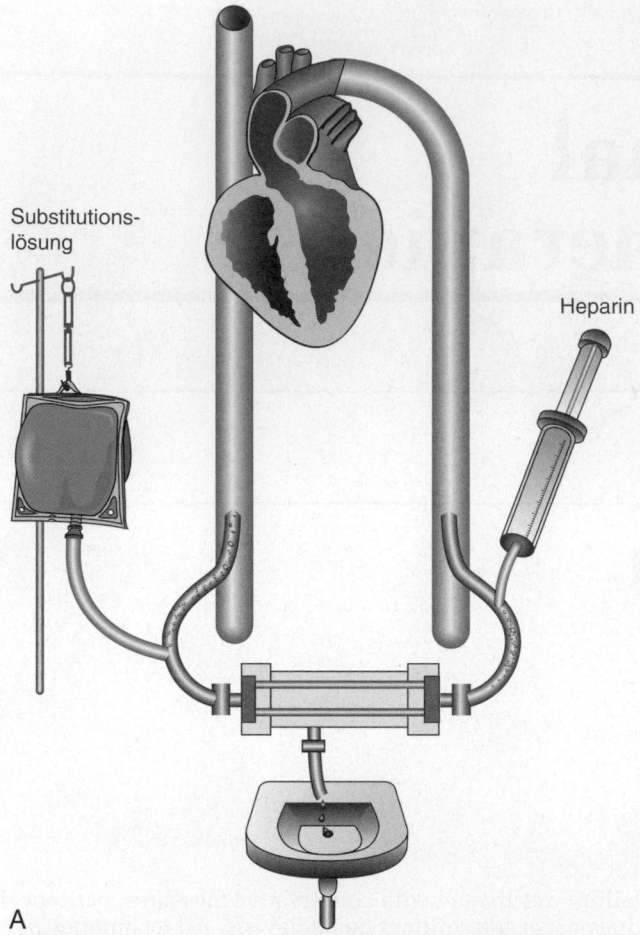

Substitutions-
lösung

Heparin

A

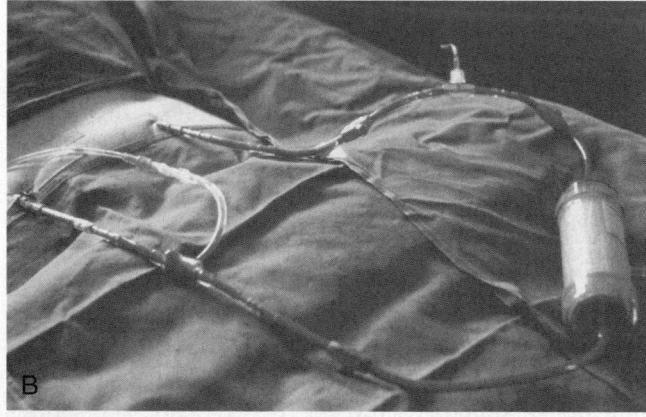

B

FIGURE 240-1. A, The original drawing of continuous arteriovenous hemofiltration (CAVH) by Peter Kramer. **B,** The first patient treated in Vicenza, Italy, with CAVH.

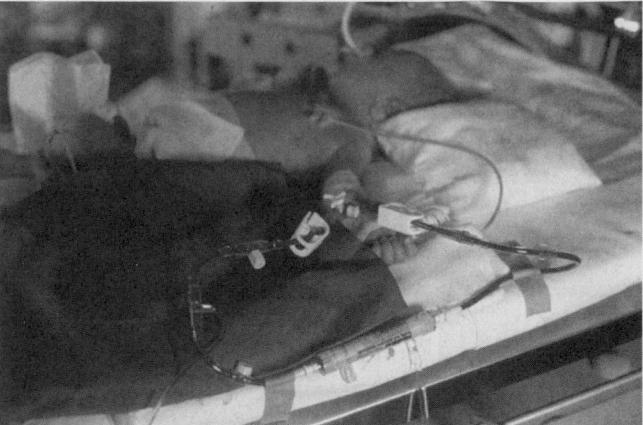

FIGURE 240-2. Application of the Amicon Minifilter to a newborn with acute renal failure (Vicenza 1985).

central venous catheter for vascular access were considered preferable and safer. Thus, within a few years, continuous venovenous hemofiltration (CVVH) replaced continuous arteriovenous hemofiltration because of its improved performance and safety. The advance was made possible by the use of blood pumps, calibrated ultrafiltration control systems, and double-lumen venous catheters (Fig. 240-3). In this setting, improved safety and reliability were then offered by CVVH or continuous venovenous hemodiafiltration or hemodialysis (CVVHDF or CVVHD). These treatments started to be widely utilized at the end of the 1980s, showing excellent uremic control employing high blood flows (150 mL/min or more) and large membrane surface areas (0.8 m^2 or more). To facilitate nursing care, ultrafiltration was soon controlled by devices with reasonable precision. Thus, for clinical purposes ultrafiltration and reinfusion could be fully regulated to achieve the desired therapeutic goals. In the late 1980s, specific machines for continuous renal replacement therapies (CRRTs) were designed (Fig. 240-4), and a new era of renal replacement in the critically ill patient began.[3] The therapy started to be standardized and clear indications began to be defined. The evolution of technology did not stop, however, and the recent demand for higher efficiency and exchange volumes has spurred new interest in a further generation of machines with better performance, integrated information technology, and easy-to-use operator interfaces.

RECENT ADVANCES IN CONTINUOUS RENAL REPLACEMENT THERAPY

The most recent generation of machines available on the market today and representing the evolution of the past decade of research and development are shown in Figure 240-5. Machines have been designed specifically to permit safe and reliable performance of the therapy. These new devices are equipped with a user-friendly interface that allows for easy performance and monitoring. The apparent complexity of the circuit is made simple by a self-loading circuit or a cartridge, which includes the filter and the blood and dialysate lines. Priming is performed automatically by the machine, and predilution or postdilution (reinfusion of substitution fluid before or after the filter)

catabolic state, simply by increasing countercurrent dialysate flow rates to 1.5 or 2 liters per hour as necessary.

EVOLUTION TOWARD VENOVENOUS PUMPED TECHNIQUES

Arteriovenous therapies were simple because they did not require a peristaltic blood pump, but the morbidity associated with arterial cannulation was substantial. For this reason, venovenous techniques utilizing a double-lumen

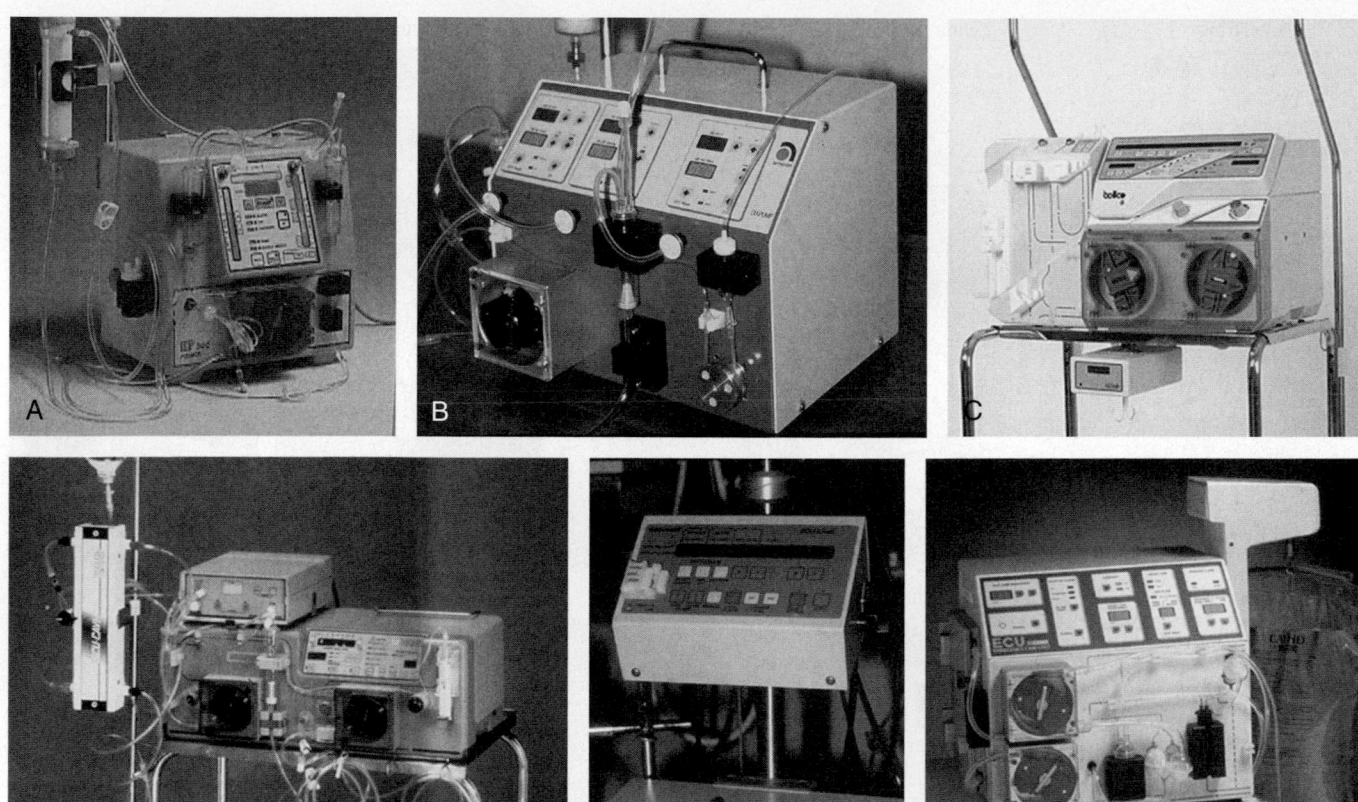

FIGURE 240-3. Pumps and ultrafiltration control systems for continuous venovenous hemofiltration (CVVH). **A,** Medica Pump. **B,** Amico dia-pump. **C,** Bellco Multimat B (Bellco-Sorin, Mirandola, Italy). **D,** Hospal BM 32. **E,** Equaline (Medica, Medolla, Italy). **F,** Carex ACU.

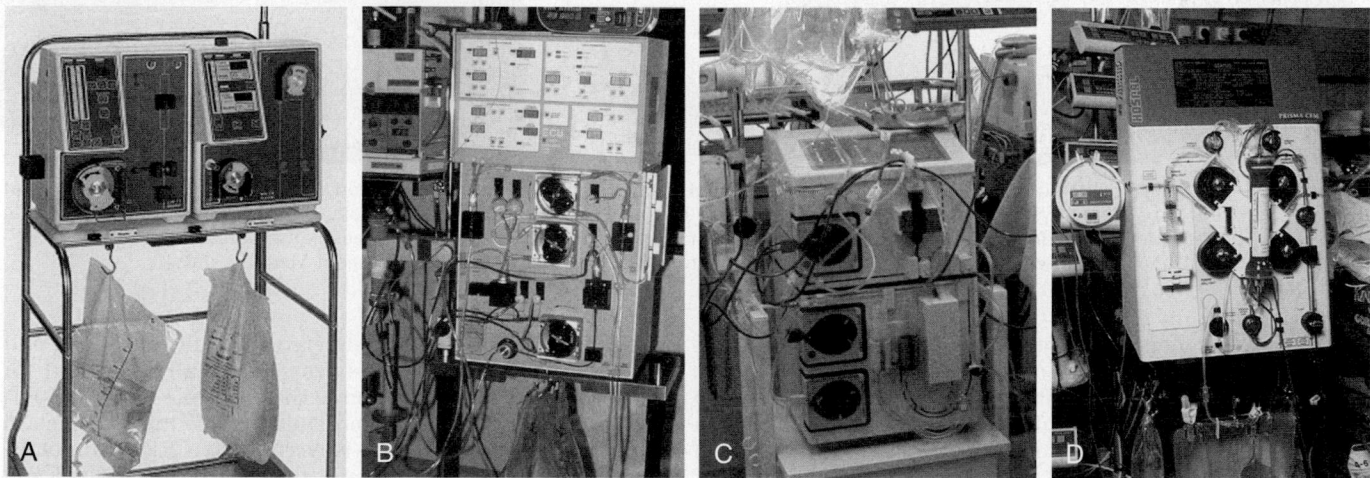

FIGURE 240-4. First generation of machines for continuous renal replacement therapy (CRRT). **A,** Baxter BM 25. **B,** Carex ECU. **C,** Fresenius ADM. **D,** Gambro-Hospal Prisma.

can be performed easily by changing the position of the reinfusion line. These new machines permit all CRRTs to be performed by programming the flows and the total amounts of fluid to be exchanged or circulated as a countercurrent dialysate at the beginning of the session.

A schematic drawing of different techniques available today for the therapy of the critically ill patient with renal and other organ dysfunction is given in Figure 240-6. Two interesting aspects of the evolution of renal replacement therapy in the intensive care unit over the past decade are

represented by the definition of an "adequate" dose of dialysis in acute kidney injury and the potential of high-dose therapies for the treatment of sepsis.[4] The first of these has identified 35 mL/kg/hr as a dose of dialysis capable of improving survival, whereas higher doses do not seem to give additional benefits in the general population.[4] The second concept introduces the rationale for high-volume hemofiltration (HVHF) in patients with acute renal failure and sepsis.[5] In this setting, the most important advance of the past decade has been the use of either

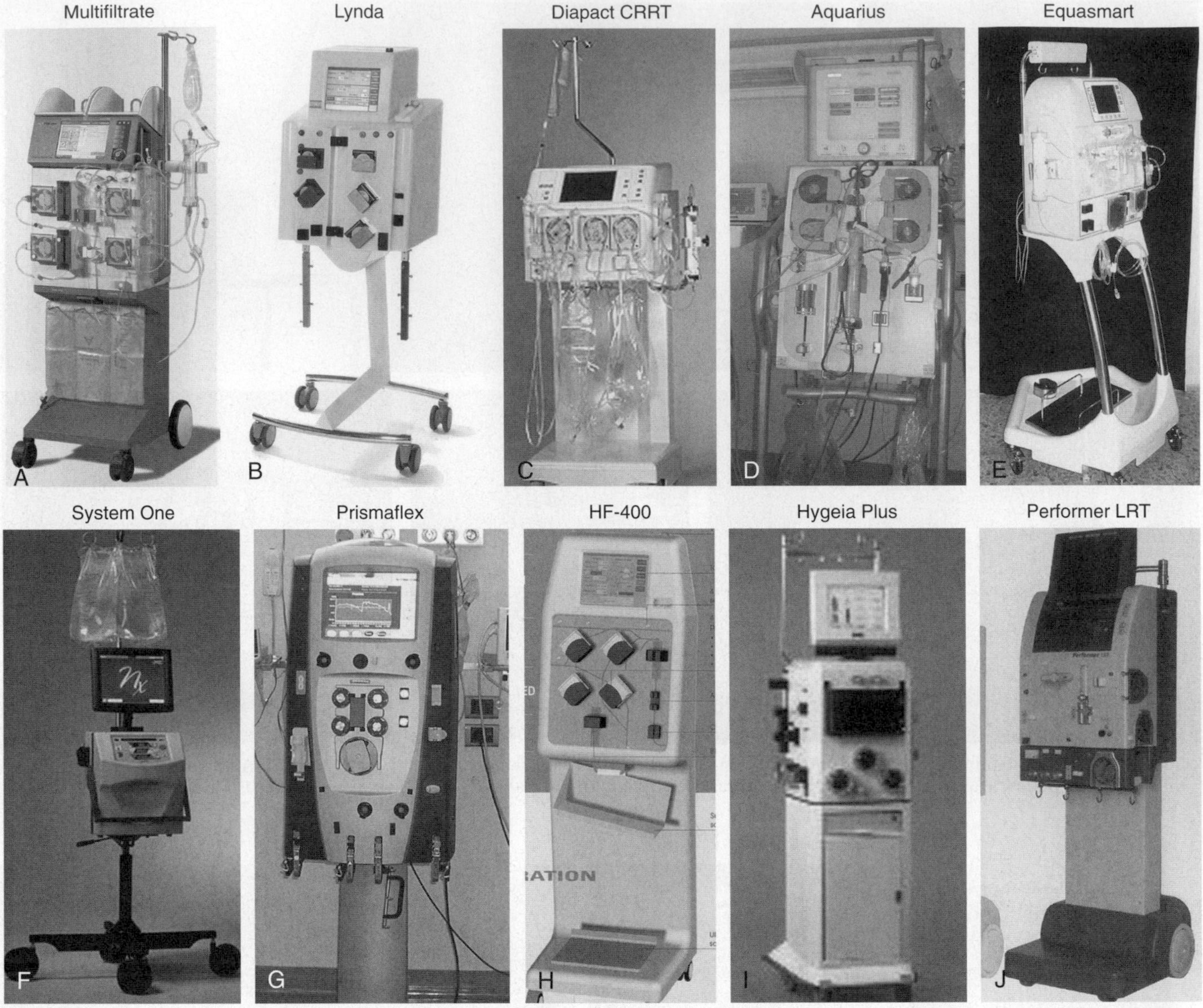

FIGURE 240-5. The last generation of continuous renal replacement therapy (CRRT) machines. **Top row:** Multifiltrate (Fresenius Medical Care, Bad Homburg, Germany); Lynda (Bellco, Mirandola, Italy); Diapact CRRT (B. Braun, Bethlehem, PA); Aquarius (Edwards, Irvine, CA); Equasmart (Medica, Medolla, Italy). **Bottom row:** System One (NxStage, Lawrence, MA); Prismaflex (Gambro, Lakewood, CO); HF-400 (Infomed, Geneva, Switzerland); Hygeia Plus (Kimal, London, UK); Performer LRT (RanD Biotech, Medolla, Italy).

increased exchange volumes in hemofiltration or the combined use of adsorbent techniques in systems where the needed to confirm the preliminary results on the positive effect of HVHF and coupled plasmafiltration-adsorption (CPFA) on outcome. Except for the beneficial effect of dialysis dose, the effect of HVHF on clinical outcome has been suggested for the group of patients suffering from severe sepsis and septic shock. The effect of different modalities of CRRT on length of stay and recovery of renal function in the general population is still under evaluation since the case mix is changing in every study and the population treated is not homogeneous. In this field further research is needed. Adequate technical support becomes mandatory, therefore, to fulfill all these expectations. The evolution of understanding of the previously mentioned concepts has led to the improvement of technology and the generation of new machines and devices compatible with the demand for increased efficiency, accuracy, safety, performance, and cost/benefit ratio. At present, almost all

CRRT therapies can be delivered in a safe, adequate, and flexible way, thanks to devices specifically designed for critically ill patients to a point that multiple-organ support therapy is envisaged as a possible therapeutic approach in the critical care setting.[6] Nevertheless, CRRT cannot be considered a simple therapy that can be prescribed and administered by everybody. Careful education and training are quintessential for the personnel dealing with these techniques. Specific nurses and knowledgeable specialists are required to carry out a therapy with optimal features of safety and efficacy.

HVHF or CPFA can be seen as a powerful immunomodulatory treatment for sepsis. Since sepsis and systemic inflammatory response syndrome are characterized by a cytokine network that is synergistic, redundant, autocatalytic, and self-augmenting, the control of such a nonlinear system cannot be approached by simple blockade or elimination of some specific mediators. Therefore, nonspecific removal of a broad range of inflammatory mediators by

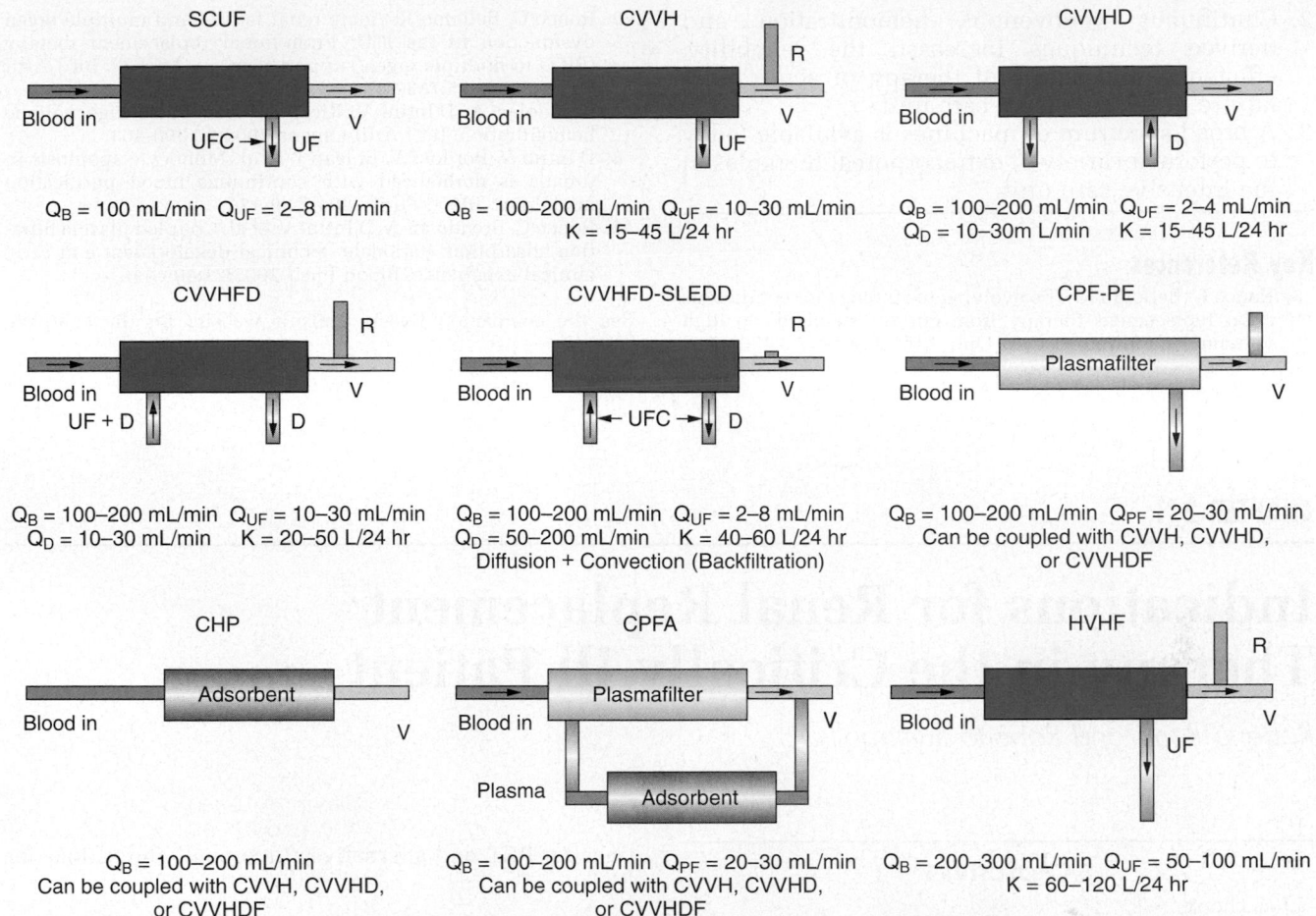

FIGURE 240-6. Techniques available today for renal replacement in the intensive care unit. CHP, continuous hemoperfusion; CPFA, coupled plasmafiltration-adsorption; CPF-PE, continuous plasmafiltration–plasma exchange; CVVH, continuous venovenous hemofiltration; CVVHD, continuous venovenous hemodialysis; CVVHDF, continuous venovenous hemodiafiltration; CVVHFD, continuous venovenous high-flux dialysis; D, dialysate; HVHF, high-volume hemofiltration; K, clearance; Q_{PF}, plasmafiltrate flow; Q_B, blood flow; Q_D, dialysate flow; Q_{UF}, ultrafiltrate flow; R, replacement; SCUF, slow continuous ultrafiltration; SLEDD, sustained low-efficiency daily dialysis; UF, ultrafiltration; UFC, ultrafiltration control system.

HVHF and CPFA may be beneficial, as recently suggested on the basis of the peak concentration hypothesis.[7] The high dose that characterizes HVHF can be delivered using a constantly high exchange rate or by delivering a "pulse" for 6 to 8 hours of very-high-volume hemofiltration (85-100 mL/kg/hr) followed by standard doses.[8] In both cases, cytokine half-lives and concentrations are affected, the first by the continuous modality and the second by the nonspecific decapitation of peaks. Therefore, rather than a detailed analysis of each molecule involved, what would be more interesting and useful is a teleological analysis of the impact of HVHF on more integrated events such as monocyte cell responsiveness, including apoptosis, neutrophil-priming activity, and oxidative burst.[9,10] More studies are needed to define the role of HVHF in hyperdynamic septic shock, with or without acute renal failure. A last comment should be dedicated to the use of sorbents, especially those cartridges dedicated to the adsorption of endotoxin and related material. A great deal of evolution has occurred in this area, but it seems that this is only the beginning of a long and possibly fruitful journey.[10]

CONCLUSIONS

A significant number of advances have taken place since CRRT was first introduced. Progress has been made in both the technology and the understanding of the pathophysiology of acute renal failure. New biomaterials and new devices are available today, and new options are on the horizon. Although improvements have been made, much remains to be done. The progress of technology in critical care nephrology has been enormous and more will come in the near future, with improvement in morbidity and mortality of the most severely ill patients.

Key Points

1. Continuous arteriovenous hemofiltration was the first treatment that permitted management of acute renal failure in critically ill patients and was an alternative to hemodialysis or peritoneal dialysis.

2. Continuous venovenous hemofiltration and derived techniques increased the reliability, efficiency, and safety of therapy of acute renal failure in the intensive care unit.

3. A broad spectrum of machines is available today to perform a variety of extracorporeal therapies in the intensive care unit.

Key References

3. Ronco C, Bellomo R: The evolving technology for continuous renal replacement therapy from current standards to high volume hemofiltration. Curr Opin Crit Care 1997;3:426-433.

6. Ronco C, Bellomo R: Acute renal failure and multiple organ dysfunction in the ICU: From renal replacement therapy (RRT) to multiple organ support therapy (MOST). Int J Artif Organs 2002;25:733-747.
7. Brendolan A, D'Intini V, Ricci Z, et al: Pulse high volume hemofiltration. Int J Artif Organs 2004;27:398-403.
8. D'Intini V, Bordoni V, Bolgan I, et al: Monocyte apoptosis in uremia is normalized with continuous blood purification modalities. Blood Purif 2004;22:9-12.
11. Ronco C, Brendolan A, D'Intini V, et al: Coupled plasma filtration adsorption: Rationale, technical development and early clinical experience. Blood Purif 2003;21:409-416.

See the companion Expert Consult website for the complete reference list.

CHAPTER 241

Indications for Renal Replacement Therapy in the Critically Ill Patient

Roberto Rona and Roberto Fumagalli

OBJECTIVES

This chapter will:
1. Explain and briefly describe the main clinical indications for extracorporeal blood purification in critically ill patients.
2. Promote a timely application of renal replacement therapy in the setting of acute renal failure in the intensive care unit.
3. Consider renal and nonrenal indications for starting renal replacement treatment.
4. Provide theoretical support for the early application of renal replacement therapy to control fluid overload, remove solute, and improve patient survival.
5. Illustrate nonrenal indications for the use of renal replacement therapy, because of renal replacement therapy's convective clearance of medium- and high-molecular-weight toxins.

Renal replacement therapy (RRT) is a key component of the clinical practice of critical care. Intensivists, in cooperation with nephrologists, often use artificial renal support to manage and resolve clinical problems in critically ill patients. The use of RRT is progressively increasing.

Few randomized clinical trials have been done on when to begin extracorporeal blood purification, and many clinicians believe that artificial renal support should start early in the course of patient management, especially in the setting of an acute renal failure (ARF).[1]

This chapter illustrates the main clinical indications for RRT in critically ill patients. The chapter describes the classification of RRT modalities, classic "renal" indications for RRT, and alternative, "nonrenal" indications for RRT.

CLASSIFICATION OF RENAL REPLACEMENT THERAPY

An ideal RRT should accomplish the following[2]:
• Ensure blood purification.
• Restore homeostasis, balance electrolytes, and provide adequate fluid volume.
• Support native kidney function recovery.

There are three main modalities of artificial renal support in the ICU setting: intermittent hemodialysis (IHD), continuous renal replacement therapy (CRRT), and peritoneal dialysis.

The indications for peritoneal dialysis have been progressively limited in developed countries, most likely because of several peritoneal dialysis limitations: poor solute clearance and fluid removal, high risk of glycemic disturbance, recurrent peritonitis, abdominal compartment syndrome, and respiratory failure.

Therefore, most of the recent controversy is related to the indications for, and preferential use of, CRRT versus IHD.[1] The differences between CRRT and IHD are debated elsewhere and are not discussed in this chapter.

CLASSIC RENAL INDICATIONS FOR RENAL REPLACEMENT THERAPY

Almost all the indications for RRT illustrated in this section are related to critically ill patients with ARF, a

TABLE 241-1

Main Worldwide Accepted Indications for Starting Continuous Renal Replacement Therapy in the Intensive Care Unit

- Nonobstructive oliguria (urine output <200 mL/12 hr) or anuria)
- Severe acidemia (pH < 7.1) due to metabolic acidosis
- Azotemia ([urea] >30 mmol/L)
- Hyperkalemia ([K$^+$] > 6.5 mmol/L or rapidly rising [K$^+$])*
- Suspected uremic organ involvement (pericarditis, encephalopathy, neuropathy, or myopathy)
- Progressive severe dysnatremia ([Na$^+$] >160 or <115 mmol/L
- Hyperthermia (core temperature >39.5° C)
- Clinically significant organ edema (especially lung)
- Drug overdose with dialyzable toxin
- Coagulopathy requiring large amounts of blood products in patients with, or at risk of, pulmonary edema or ARDS†

*Intermittent hemodialysis (IHD) removes potassium more efficiently than does continuous renal replacement therapy (CRRT).
†For example, patients with fulminant liver failure, adult respiratory distress syndrome (ARDS), international normalized ratio greater than 3, or spontaneous epistaxis. Unless volume is rapidly removed, as fresh frozen plasma is rapidly given, these patients are very likely to develop pulmonary edema.
From Bellomo R, Ronco C: An introduction to continuous renal replacement therapy. In Bellomo R, Baldwin I, Ronco C, Golper G (eds): Atlas of Hemofiltration. London, Bailliere Tindall, 2001, pp 1-9.

clinical condition associated with high rates of morbidity, mortality, and use of health care resources.

In a recent, multinational, multicenter, prospective epidemiological survey of ARF in ICU, Uchino and colleagues[3] found that out of 29,629 critically ill patients, renal failure occurred in 1768 patients (5.7%). The authors documented that almost two thirds of the patients affected by renal failure were managed by RRT (1260 out of 1768) and that CRRT was the most common modality used (80%), followed by IHD (16.9%) and peritoneal dialysis (3.1%). The mortality of ARF was 52% during ICU care and 8% after ICU discharge. Based on these data, the worldwide prevalence of ARF in ICUs is approximately 6%, and the use of acute RRT is approximately 4%.[3]

In another Canadian population-based study, Bagshaw and colleagues[4] estimated annual incidences of severe acute renal failure, long-term survival, and renal recovery outcomes. The collected results confirmed an average incidence of 4.2% of critically ill patients receiving RRT. The annual incidence of ARF in Canadian experience (11 per 100,000 population) was similar to that revealed by previous studies from Australia and Europe. Critically ill patients with ARF presented an increased risk of death (case fatality at 1 year was 64%), a longer duration of hospital length, and a poor quality of life after hospital discharge.[4]

The worldwide accepted indications for artificial renal support in critically ill patients are summarized in Table 241-1.

Fluid Overload in Nonobstructive Oliguria

Fluid overload may occur as a complication of acute renal failure or as a complication of other critical clinical syndromes, like acute myocardial dysfunction, congestive heart failure, iatrogenic fluid overload in shock, acute endothelial dysfunction, and acute respiratory distress syndrome.

A rational therapeutic approach consists of early identification of etiology and treatment, an accurate monitoring of volumic status, and finally the reduction of fluid overload.

Overhydration must be managed with fluid intake restriction, high-dose diuretics, and pharmacological interventions such as vasodilating drugs or inotropic agents. When this approach fails, extracorporeal removal is recommended, especially if urinary volume is lower than 400 mL over 24 hours.[5]

A recent consensus statement[6] about hemofiltration in cardiac surgery and heart failure recommends (1) isolated hemofiltration, which can improve patient survival and reduce hospital length of stay (Grade D recommendation), and (2) larger randomized clinical trials to identify precise clinical indications for RRT.

Solute Removal—Hyperazotemia

The uremic syndrome is characterized by multiple-organ deterioration. In the setting of critically ill patients, the most serious derangements are found in the cardiovascular, neurological, hematological, and immunological statuses.[7]

Patients with ARF in ICU differ greatly from patients affected by end-stage renal disease in that patients with ARF present an increased protein catabolic rate with negative nitrogen balance and a variable total body water urea distribution. An early and aggressive approach to hyperazotemia is an important therapeutic goal because the reduction of the level of urea plasma could reduce the rate of complications of ARF and improve survival in critically ill patients.[8]

Early artificial renal support for post-traumatic ARF can improve patient survival, especially if renal failure arises in the setting of multiple-organ failure.[9]

The principal recommendations for RRT in ARF are the following[10]:

- Patients affected by ARF should be managed by acute RRT (Grade D).
- RRT must continue as long as clinical criteria of severe ARF are present (Grade E).

Acid Removal

When a medical approach to acidosis (diuretics and bicarbonate administration) fails, RRT must be started to avoid myocardial electrical conduction and contractility alterations.

Hilton and colleagues[11] published a study in which 200 patients with ARF and lactic acidosis were managed with CRRT and bicarbonate-based replacement fluid. They demonstrated acidosis correction in 89 patients (45%), without inducing hypernatremia or extracellular volume expansion, and a survival rate of 25%.

Control of Electrolyte Derangements

Electrolyte derangements are common and serious complications in critically ill patients affected by ARF or metabolic acidosis. An extracorporeal management should be considered if the standard medical approach fails to correct

TABLE 241-2

Alternative, Nonrenal Indications for Continuous Renal Replacement Therapy in the Intensive Care Unit

Sepsis
Rhabdomyolysis
Thermoregulation
Refractory congestive heart failure and cardiopulmonary
 bypass
Hepatic failure
Tumor lysis syndrome
Adult respiratory distress syndrome
Radiocontrast-induced nephropathy
Osmoregulation
Lactic acidosis
Schizophrenia
Acute pancreatitis
Psoriasis

From Briglia AE: The current state of nonuremic applications for extracorporeal blood purification. Semin Dial 2005;18:380-390.

hyperkalemia (K$^+$ > 6.5 mmol/L with normal pH) and severe dysnatremia (Na$^+$ > 160 mmol/L or <115 mmol/L).[1] RRT should be used to prevent and manage electrocardiographic alterations in hyperkalemia and neurological impairment due to the rapid rise of dysnatremia.

The management of hyperkalemia and metabolic acidosis with RRT is now a consolidated clinical practice in the ICU setting. A retrospective report published in 1994 confirmed that continuous venovenous hemodialysis (CVVHD) provides excellent control of electrolytes without further hemodynamic alterations and with a mortality rate lower than predicted.[12] Intraoperative continuous venovenous hemofiltration (CVVH) also can be used during surgical treatment of complicated aortoiliac occlusion to prevent the development of severe ischemia-reperfusion injury, characterized by electrolyte and acid-base alterations.

In the setting of dysnatremia the therapeutic target is a slow correction at a rate of 0.5 mEq per hour, because both electrolyte derangements and their rapid improvement can cause clinical problems. CRRT can be utilized successfully to treat hypernatremia in order to progressively reduce the plasmatic imbalance and to avoid neurological disorders.

NONRENAL INDICATIONS FOR RENAL REPLACEMENT THERAPY

Studies conducted in the past decade have tried to define new RRT applications in "nonuremic" waste product removal.

The CRRT convective clearance of medium- and high-molecular-weight toxins (PM: 500-20,000 Da) is probably the most important mechanism contributing to this alternative effect. Therefore, these so-called nonrenal indications are related to CRRT, whereas IHD is limited to ARF or end-stage renal disease management.[13]

Table 241-2 lists the principal and worldwide accepted nonrenal indications for CRRT. This section describes the most common, nonrenal critical conditions that indicate a necessity for RRT.

Sepsis/Systemic Inflammatory Response Syndrome

Sepsis is probably exacerbated by a profound imbalance between pro- and anti-inflammatory substances. Theoretically, extracorporeal removal of the inflammatory mediators could improve patient outcome.

Ronco and Bellomo[14] described two opposite components of immune dysregulation in sepsis: an excessive pro-inflammatory status causing SIRS versus an anti-inflammatory condition of denominated compensated anti-inflammatory response syndrome (CARS). In sepsis, SIRS and CARS can coexist in different districts or systems and can induce severe organ failure. The new, so-called peak concentration hypothesis theorizes that a nonselective control of the pro- and anti-inflammatory cytokines can reduce immune imbalances and improve patient outcome.

In spite of these theoretical statements and promising preliminary results, no human randomized clinical trials have demonstrated a real increase in survival or in organ performance. Thus, the usefulness of CRRT in the setting of sepsis without acute renal failure is still strongly debated.[13-15]

In 2004 the Surviving Sepsis Campaign published international guidelines for management of sepsis and septic shock. The recommendations about renal replacement therapy are the following[16]:

- In the setting of ARF, CVVH and IHD are equivalent treatments (Grade B).
- Current evidence does not support the use of CVVH in sepsis in lack of renal replacement need.

Crush Syndrome and Rhabdomyolysis

A relevant muscular necrosis, caused by a traumatic or nontraumatic event, and the consequent increase of myoglobin plasmatic levels can be very dangerous to renal function.

In this context the mechanisms of renal toxicity are several: tubular obstruction by myoglobin casts, tubular damage by oxidant injuries, or renal vasoconstriction. Renal disorders develop in 15% to 30% of patients with creatine kinase levels greater than 5000 ui/L.[13]

Investigators found a rapid decrement of pigment plasmatic levels, regardless of renal performance and artificial blood purification, suggesting extrarenal removal mechanism.[13]

Based on these data, major "messages" about this concern are the following[13-17]:

- Adequate, early and aggressive fluid resuscitation combined with urinary and plasmatic alkalinization are the medical therapeutic goals in the setting of crush syndrome.
- Obtaining an elevated urine volume (>2-3 mL/kg/hr) is the best prophylactic measure to prevent renal damage.
- Prophylactic CRRT based only on creatine kinase–elevated plasmatic levels, without clinical manifestation of ARF, is not recommended.

Tumor Lysis Syndrome

This clinical condition, which is a real oncological emergency, occurs usually after chemotherapy. Tumor lysis syndrome is caused by a rapid and massive tumor lysis, with great amounts of uric acid, potassium, and phosphate plasmatic release. Tumor lysis syndrome develops usually in patients with lymphoproliferative malignancies, but also in those with solid tumors.

In this setting, kidneys could be damaged by renal tubular accumulation of uric acid and calcium phosphate crystals. Kidney impairment is often exacerbated by concomitant hypovolemia and urine volume contraction.[18,19]

Radiocontrast-Induced Nephropathy

Radiocontrast-induced nephropathy is an increasing clinical problem in critically ill patients because of the increasing use of intravenous or intra-arterial contrast for diagnostic or interventional radiological procedures. Contrast nephropathy is rare in patients with normal renal function but can develop in 5% to 15% of high-risk patients, especially in the setting of diabetic nephropathy or heart failure.[20]

Pathophysiological mechanisms of contrast nephropathy are intrarenal vasoconstriction and medullar ischemia, oxygen-derived free radical damage, sublethal cellular damage and apoptosis, and renal atheroembolism.

New recommendations and guidelines for contrast nephropathy prevention and management have been published. The main recommendation is the use of prophylactic hemofiltration in patients with severe cardiac and renal dysfunction (Grade B), whereas prophylactic hemodialysis is not recommended (Grade B).[20,21]

Renal Failure

Renal failure occurs frequently in the setting of ARF or end-stage liver disease. Pathophysiological mechanisms of the renal impairment[22] include intravascular depletion in acute upper gastrointestinal hemorrhage or vomiting and diarrhea; severe sepsis due to spontaneous bacterial peritonitis; hepatorenal syndrome developing in 25% of patients with severe acute alcoholic hepatitis; and nephrotoxic effects of drugs like nonsteroid antiinflammatory drug (NSAID), aminoglycoside antibiotic, and angiotensin-converting enzyme inhibitors.

Specific recommendations for the use of RRT in the setting of renal failure are the following[23]:

- CRRT is probably more adaptable than IHD to unstable hemodynamic patients suffering from ARF or end-stage liver failure.
- CRRT can remove protein-bound or neurotoxins and numerous proinflammatory cytokines that may be involved in liver disease and brain edema.
- High-volume hemofiltration may enhance membrane adsorption and convective exchange and dramatically improve neurological status in some children with ARF.
- The usefulness of CRRT in the setting of liver failure without ARF remains to be established by future investigations.

CONCLUSION

Artificial renal support is an important component of critical care medicine. A recent study of nearly 30,000 patients

from 23 countries reveals that 4% to 5% of critically ill patients are managed with RRT.[3]

This considerable use of RRT most likely is due to two main factors: (1) advances in technological devices, and (2) the recent demonstration that early aggressive extracorporeal blood purification can prevent serious classic ARF complications, improving patient survival rate.

There is a worldwide consensus by now, that CRRT or IHD can be a good therapeutic option when severe ARF is developing. There is a consensus, too, that extracorporeal treatment should be started early.

There are discussions and poor grade recommendations regarding nonrenal indications to RRT, especially in the setting of SIRS or sepsis. The usefulness of extracorporeal blood purification in patients with sepsis but no renal impairment is no longer recommended, in spite of the promising biological rationale of convective removal of sepsis mediators.

An unresolved but crucial issue is the efficacy and usefulness of the new blood purification modality. Objectives of future multicenter randomized clinical trials will be, therefore, clinical research about very-high-flux convective treatment in sepsis (pulse high-volume hemofiltration)[24] or coupled plasmafiltration-adsorption.[25]

Future perspectives will consider ARF as part of the multiple-organ dysfunction syndrome and RRT as a part of multiple-organ support therapy.[16] In the future multiple-organ support therapy could be a clinical and technological evolution of RRT, supporting physiological performances of all organs involved in critical illness.

Key Points

1. Acute renal failure in critically ill patients is a serious clinical condition with 60% mortality.
2. Early artificial renal support is recommended when acute renal failure develops in the intensive care unit. The rationale is to avoid the classic complications of renal failure and to improve patient survival.
3. Whereas peritoneal dialysis has several limitations, continuous renal replacement therapy and intermittent hemodialysis are accepted worldwide.
4. Despite interesting biological rationale, continuous renal replacement therapy treatment in systemic inflammatory response syndrome or sepsis without acute renal failure is no longer recommended.
5. In the setting of acute renal failure in association with systemic inflammatory response syndrome or sepsis, the minimum effective convective clearance during continuous renal replacement therapy is 35 milliliters per kilogram body weight per hour. Standard treatment with an ultrafiltration rate of less than 2 liters per minute is inadequate.

Key References

2. D'Intini V, Ronco C, Bonello M, Bellomo R: Renal replacement therapy in acute renal failure. Best Pract Res Clin Anesthesiol 2004;18:145-157.

3. Uchino S, Kellum J, Bellomo R, et al: Acute renal failure in ICU. A multinational, multicentre study. JAMA 2005;294:813-818.
4. Bagshaw SM, Laupland KB, Doig CJ, et al: Prognosis for long-term survival and renal recovery in critically ill patients with severe acute renal failure: A population based study. Crit Care 2005;9:700-709.

14. Schetz M: Non renal indications for continuous renal replacement therapy. Kidney Int Suppl 1999;56:S88-S94.
20. Barret BJ, Parfrey PS: Preventing nephropathy induced by contrast medium. N Engl J Med 2006;354:379-386.

See the companion Expert Consult website for the complete reference list.

CHAPTER 242

Beginning and Ending Continuous Therapies in the Intensive Care Unit

Shigehiko Uchino

OBJECTIVES

This chapter will:
1. Review current practice for beginning and ending continuous renal replacement therapy.
2. Recommend when to begin and end continuous renal replacement therapy, in view of limited evidence.

Compared to 30 years ago, hospital mortality for patients with severe acute renal failure (ARF) has hardly changed, staying at approximately 60%,[1] although patient acuity and treatment modality are quite different.[2] One of the improvements in the management of patients with severe ARF is the development and widespread use of continuous renal replacement therapy (CRRT) in the intensive care unit (ICU). Although CRRT is gaining in popularity and becoming more frequently used in the ICU, very few high-quality studies have been conducted to direct physicians how to prescribe CRRT. This situation is quite different from that of mechanical ventilation, for which many randomized controlled trials have been conducted and consensus recommendations published.[3-5] Therefore, there are no guidelines and few data to rely on in deciding which patients should be treated with CRRT or when to begin and end CRRT.

The BEST Kidney (Beginning and Ending Supportive Therapy for the Kidney) study is a multicenter, multinational, prospective, epidemiological study with the aim of elucidating the multiple aspects of ARF at an international level.[6-8] This study included more than 1700 patients from 54 centers in 23 countries. Among 1260 that were treated with renal replacement therapy (RRT), approximately 80% of patients received CRRT.[6] Therefore, the BEST Kidney study can provide current information about how clinicians worldwide begin and end CRRT.

This chapter presents current practice for indications and timing of beginning and ending CRRT, based on data from the BEST Kidney study. Some opinions for these issues are discussed, despite limited evidence. As nonrenal indications for use of CRRT are discussed in another chapter (see Chapter 241), this chapter specifically addresses the use of CRRT in patients with ARF.

INDICATIONS AND TIMING FOR BEGINNING CONTINUOUS RENAL REPLACEMENT THERAPY

Whether a patient with ARF should receive RRT or can be managed medically is a difficult issue, and very little information on this issue is available. Because of the lack of data in this area, current practice in the world for beginning CRRT is quite varied. In the BEST Kidney study (Fig. 242-1), the most common reason to begin CRRT was oliguria or anuria (70.2%), followed by high urea/creatinine levels (53.0%), metabolic acidosis (43.6%), and fluid overload (36.7%). This means that close to half of patients did not have high urea/creatinine and almost two thirds of them did not have fluid overload when CRRT was begun. These results are different from traditional indications for the application of RRT in patients with ARF. For example, the most common textbook of internal medicine states that the indications for use of RRT in ARF are "symptoms or signs of the uremic syndrome, management of refractory hypervolemia, hyperkalemia or acidosis" or a "BUN [blood urea nitrogen] level of greater than 100 mg/dL."[9]

Table 242-1 shows regional variations of renal variables at beginning CRRT in the BEST Kidney study. Australian and European centers seem to initiate CRRT earlier than the other regions (lower creatinine/urea and higher urine output). The ranges of these values were wide: from 282 to 399 µmol/L in creatinine, from 19 to 30 mmol/L in urea, and from 60 to 140 mL per 6 hours in urine output. Importantly, however, even in South America, where CRRT seemed to be begun the latest among the five regions, median urea when CRRT was begun was 30 mmol/L (BUN of 84 mg/dL), clearly below the 100 mg/dL of BUN described in textbooks. Put another way, essentially no one in this study of 54 units in 23 countries practices medicine as suggested in textbooks, which obviously appear outdated.

Several reviews for indications of CRRT have been published in the literature.[10-12] Among these, Bellomo and Ronco[10] proposed criteria for the initiation of RRT in critically ill patients. The criteria consisted of oliguria (<200 mL/12 hours), azotemia (urea >30 mmol/L), hyperkalemia (>6.5 mmol/L), acidemia (pH < 7.1) and other uremic symptoms. These criteria are more similar to current practice (see Table 242-1) than criteria described in textbooks.

However, it is unknown whether earlier start (e.g., before developing severe azotemia) is related to better outcome in patients with ARF. If CRRT is started too early, some patients who may not require CRRT may receive it, and

CRRT is not a treatment without complications, for example, bleeding tendency due to anticoagulation, immobilization, blood loss in clotted filters, thrombocytopenia, activation of white blood cells, and more. On the other hand, delayed initiation of CRRT also can cause problems, for example, fluid overload, electrolyte and acid-base abnormalities, immunosuppression due to uremia, and so on. Several studies have examined this issue.[13-16] For example, Gettings and colleagues[13] retrospectively reviewed 100 adult trauma patients treated with CRRT.[13] Patients were characterized as "early" or "late," based on whether BUN was less than or greater than 60 mg/dL at the beginning of CRRT. Although there was no difference in demographics or laboratory values between the two groups, the "early" group had a significantly higher survival rate than the "late" group (39.0% vs. 20%, $P = 0.041$). Kresse and colleagues[14] compared two periods (Period 1: from 1991 to 1993, 128 patients; Period 2: from 1994 to 1995, 142 patients). In Period 2, RRT was started earlier compared to Period 1 (creatinine 520 vs. 250 µmol/L, urine volume 500 vs. 900 mL/day). Although there was no significant difference in demographics or etiology of ARF, mortality was lower in Period 2 compared to Period 1 (59.6% vs. 78.9%, $P < 0.001$). However, all of these studies are single-center observational studies, and no randomized controlled trial has been conducted for this issue.[13-16]

The Acute Dialysis Quality Initiative (ADQI) recently reviewed the available evidence and published consensus recommendations for CRRT.[17,18] About selection of patients for CRRT, they stated, "No recommendations on the timing of initiation of renal replacement therapy are possible beyond those defined by the conventional criteria that apply to chronic renal failure patients."[17]

Although there is no high-quality evidence (i.e., multi-center randomized controlled trials), some epidemiological studies and physiological reasoning suggest that early initiation of RRT might achieve better outcomes for ARF patients; no evidence exists against such thinking. With current technology (biocompatible membranes and CRRT), early initiation is feasible and physiologically sound and should be the approach of choice until one or more randomized controlled trials are conducted to provide clinicians with better quality evidence to guide their practice.

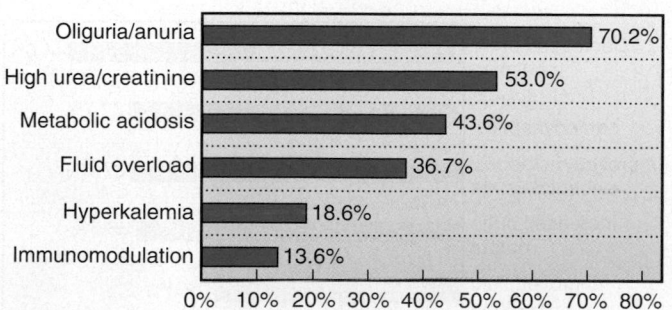

FIGURE 242-1. Reasons why continuous renal replacement therapy was begun in the Beginning and Ending Supportive Therapy for the Kidney (BEST Kidney) study.

TABLE 242-1

Variables at Beginning Continuous Renal Replacement Therapy in the Beginning and Ending Supportive Therapy for the Kidney (BEST Kidney) Study

	ASIA	AUSTRALIA	EUROPE	NORTH AMERICA	SOUTH AMERICA
Number of centers	9	6	26	8	5
Number of patients	151	195	478	120	62
ICU to start* (days)	0.7 (0.1-1.7)	0.6 (0.2-1.5)	1.8 (0.6-5.1)	2.5 (0.9-7.0)	3.1 (1.0-9.2)
Creatinine (µmol/L)	347 (175-571)	282 (187-402)	288 (193-399)	343 (236-454)	399 (286-533)
Urea (mmol/L)	19 (12-32)	21 (14-31)	25 (17-36)	25 (17-36)	30 (19-40)
Potassium (mmol/L)	4.6 (3.8-5.6)	4.6 (4.1-5.4)	4.5 (4.1-5.1)	4.5 (3.9-5.2)	4.9 (4.4-6.0)
pH	7.31 (7.2-7.42)	7.28 (7.16-7.37)	7.35 (7.28-7.41)	7.33 (7.23-7.39)	7.30 (7.24-7.36)
Urine output (mL/6 hr)	60 (15-195)	90 (20-290)	140 (40-353)	75 (20-212)	60 (28-200)

*Duration between intensive care unit (ICU) admission and starting continuous renal replacement therapy (CRRT).

EARLY COMPLICATIONS AT THE BEGINNING OF CONTINUOUS RENAL REPLACEMENT THERAPY

In the BEST Kidney study, hypotension related to CRRT occurred in 18.8% of patients and arrhythmias were observed in 4.3%. Critical arrhythmias (cardiac arrest, ventricular tachycardia, or fibrillation) considered related to CRRT occurred in eight patients and were fatal in three. When CRRT is started, a patient typically loses the equivalent of a circulating blood volume of approximately 150 to 200 mL. This acute change in circulating blood volume may induce hypotension in some unstable critically ill patients. In the BEST Kidney study, among patients that developed hypotension at the beginning of CRRT, most of them (15.6%) required an increase in vasopressor dose. In the severest cases, three patients suffered from cardiac arrest and could not be resuscitated. All of these three patients were on a high dose of vasopressors and had a very high serum lactate concentration (>10 mmol/L). These findings highlight the need to pay the highest level of attention to hemodynamics at the start of CRRT and to consider prophylactic steps (fluid loading before and during initiation, increasing vasopressor therapy, or both), especially when patients are on a high dose of vasopressors and have a high serum lactate concentration.

INDICATIONS FOR AND TIMING OF ENDING CONTINUOUS RENAL REPLACEMENT THERAPY

Since weaning from mechanical ventilation is a crucial aspect of mechanical pulmonary support, it has been extensively investigated, and several randomized controlled trials have been conducted.[19-21] However, there is a complete absence of evidence in the literature, including an absence of observational studies, on weaning patients from mechanical renal support.

Because of the lack of evidence, current practice for ending CRRT is quite varied in the world. Figure 242-2 shows reasons why CRRT was ended for patients who were treated with CRRT and survived in the BEST Kidney study. Decreased urea/creatinine was the most common

reason for ending CRRT (44.6%), followed by stable hemodynamics (37.7%), improved metabolic/electrolyte state (37.4%), and increased urine output (36.8%). No reason had more than 50% incidence, suggesting that there is no common practice for ending CRRT worldwide. Indeed, significant regional variations can be found in the BEST Kidney database (Table 242-2). In South America, patients with ARF were treated with CRRT for only 1.9 days in median, when urine output was only 25 mL in 6 hours. On the other hand, patients in Europe were treated with CRRT for a much longer period (5.1 days in median), when patients had very low creatinine (154 μmol/L) and high urine output (370 mL in 6 hours).

Several patterns of terminating CRRT exist. CRRT might be ended because a physician expects that a patient will improve renal function enough not to require RRT anymore. CRRT might be ended and switched to intermittent RRT (IRRT) because a patient has stable enough hemodynamics to tolerate IRRT or needs to be discharged from the ICU. Also, CRRT might be withdrawn because of futility. In the BEST Kidney study, approximately one third of patients (32.9%) died on CRRT. A similar number of patients (29.8%) recovered renal function after a median of 5 days of treatment and were discharged from ICU without need for RRT. After initial cessation of CRRT, 22.8% either switched to IRRT or needed to go back to CRRT. Renal replacement therapy was withdrawn in 13.4% of patients after a median of 5 days of CRRT.

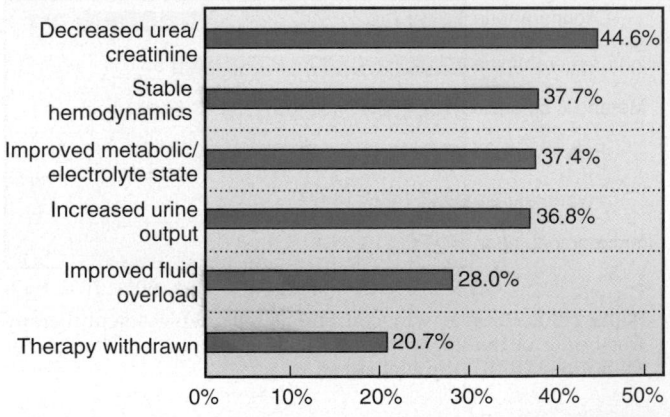

FIGURE 242-2. Reasons why continuous renal replacement therapy was ended for survivors in the Beginning and Ending Supportive Therapy for the Kidney (BEST Kidney) study.

TABLE 242-2

Variables among Survivors at Ending Continuous Renal Replacement Therapy in the Beginning and Ending Supportive Therapy for the Kidney (BEST Kidney) Study

	ASIA	AUSTRALIA	EUROPE	NORTH AMERICA	SOUTH AMERICA
Number of centers	9	6	26	8	5
Number of patients	75	122	248	61	23
CRRT days	4.0 (2.1-8.9)	3.8 (2.4-8.4)	5.1 (2.5-13.2)	5.3 (2.6-10.3)	1.9 (1-3.3)
Creatinine (μmol/L)	220 (107-341)	165 (123-234)	154 (108-229)	185 (122-246)	314 (212-383)
Urea (mmol/L)	13 (9-20)	12 (9-17)	15 (10-20)	15 (11-19)	18 (14-27)
Potassium (mmol/L)	3.9 (3.6-4.4)	4.0 (3.8-4.4)	4.1 (3.8-4.5)	3.9 (3.7-4.2)	4.0 (3.9-4.3)
pH	7.40 (7.36-7.45)	7.46 (7.41-7.48)	7.43 (7.39-7.48)	7.41 (7.36-7.47)	7.33 (7.3.0-7.37)
Urine output (mL/6 hr)	160 (13-645)	177 (64-431)	370 (80-680)	129 (10-413)	25 (0-120)

CRRT, continuous renal replacement therapy.

When a patient has stable hemodynamics, whether CRRT can be switched to IRRT or not is one of unresolved issues for conducting CRRT. Mehta and colleagues[22] conducted a randomized controlled trial comparing CRRT and IRRT and showed that patients who received CRRT with no crossover to IRRT had a 92.3% rate of renal recovery and that patients who crossed over from CRRT to IRRT had a 44.7% rate of complete renal recovery. These two groups are not easily compared because such crossover was not conducted randomly, and crossover groups might have had more severe renal injury and required longer duration of RRT. Nonetheless, IRRT might cause intravascular fluid depletion and hypotension and delay renal recovery.[23] Therefore, it might be beneficial for patients to continue CRRT until a patient recovers dialysis-independent renal function.

The difference between withdrawing CRRT and withdrawing other organ support technology (mechanical ventilation and vasopressors) is that patients usually do not die rapidly when CRRT alone is withdrawn. Zamperetti and colleagues[24] conducted a questionnaire of participants in the First International Course of Critical Care Nephrology. Their aim was to examine the ethical approach of intensivists and nephrologists to the initiation or withdrawal of CRRT. Only 43% of responders thought that CRRT and other organ supports are equivalent and that every support should be withdrawn when futile. The responders were asked to give a score to determine the difficulty of terminating different vital supports. The highest score was for mechanical ventilation as the most difficult support to terminate. It was followed by CRRT, artificial feeding or hydration, vasoactive drugs, antibiotics, and blood transfusion.

After reviewing the literature, ADQI stated, "CRRT should continue as long as the criteria defining severe ARF are present. No further recommendation can be made."[18] The ADQI workgroup recommended conducting observational studies of the clinical decision-making process and of physiological status at time of cessation in relation to ending CRRT.[18]

In my opinion, CRRT should be continued until a patient recovers dialysis-independent renal function. After ending CRRT, if a patient is found not to have adequate enough renal function to be free from dialysis, clinicians should have a low threshold for recommencing CRRT to avoid the development of fluid overload or uremic complications.

Switching from CRRT to IRRT might cause delay of renal recovery and, in some patients, impede it altogether.

Key Points

1. Very little information is available on which to base clinical decisions for when to begin and end continuous renal replacement therapy in patients with severe acute renal failure.
2. This lack of information causes a huge variability in current practice worldwide.
3. Research is urgently needed to improve this situation.
4. Until such evidence becomes available, it seems reasonable to begin continuous renal replacement therapy early and end it late.
5. The highest level of attention to hemodynamics needs to be paid at the start of continuous renal replacement therapy, especially when patients are on a high dose of vasopressors and have a high serum lactate concentration.

Key References

6. Uchino S, Kellum JA, Bellomo R, et al: Beginning and Ending Supportive Therapy for the Kidney (BEST Kidney) Investigators. Acute renal failure in critically ill patients: A multinational, multicenter study. JAMA 2005;294:813-818.
10. Bellomo R, Ronco C: Indications and criteria for initiating renal replacement therapy in the intensive care unit. Kidney Int 1998;66:S106-S109.
13. Gettings LG, Reynolds HN, Scalea T: Outcome in post-traumatic acute renal failure when continuous renal replacement therapy is applied early vs. late. Intensive Care Med 1999;25:805-813.
17. Kellum JA, Mehta RL, Angus DC, et al, for the Acute Dialysis Quality Initiative Workgroup: The first international consensus conference on continuous renal replacement therapy. Kidney Int 2002;62:1855-1863.
24. Zamperetti N, Ronco C, Brendolan A. et al: Bioethical issues related to continuous renal replacement therapy in intensive care patients. Intensive Care Med 2000;26:407-415.

See the companion Expert Consult website for the complete reference list.

CHAPTER 243

Vascular Access for Continuous Renal Replacement Therapy

Bernard Canaud

OBJECTIVES

This chapter will:
1. Discuss why the central venous catheter has become the vascular access standard reference for continuous renal replacement therapy in acute renal failure.
2. Describe the two main categories of central venous catheters: the acute catheter (for short-term use) and the chronic tunneled catheter (for long-term use).
3. Review central venous catheter insertion methods.
4. Highlight the importance of catheter design and nursing and maintenance care for successful catheter performance.

The central venous catheter (CVC) represents the only means for blood access in critically ill patients who require urgent renal replacement therapy (RRT). CVCs are used in patients with acute renal failure (ARF) to provide renal support and to permit care of multiple-organ failure.[1]

Renal replacement therapy in the intensive care unit (ICU) relies on two main schedules based on weekly frequency of treatment sessions. In brief, RRT may be indicated either as an intermittent high-flow modality or as a continuous low-flow modality. Intermittent renal replacement therapy (IRRT) modalities rely on sessions of various duration (3 to 12 hours) that vary from once every other day (4 sessions per week) to once a day (7 sessions per week). The choice between continuous renal replacement therapy (CRRT) and IRRT relies on the clinical condition of the ARF patient where hemodynamic instability and sepsis prevail and a number of organs may have failed.[2-4] Frequency and duration of RRT do not preclude the potential beneficial role of convective modalities (hemodiafiltration, hemofiltration) versus diffusive modalities (hemodialysis).[5]

Dialysis CVCs that are used to ensure CRRT in the ICU environment are different from those of IRRT in both design and performance. Renal support in patients with ARF may vary from a few days to several weeks. Basic objectives for CVC use are to ensure adequate and regular flow, with low morbidity, to deliver an optimal treatment dose.

This chapter addresses criteria for choosing the best catheter option for CRRT: catheter material and geometry, indications and insertion procedure, catheter care management, catheter performances and outcomes.

CATHETER CHARACTERISTICS: MATERIAL, GEOMETRY, AND DESIGN

The performance of CVCs is dependent on a patient's blood characteristics and the manufacturer's catheter design.[6,7] Users must know these intrinsic limitations since they negatively affect the dialysis dose delivered in RRT.[8]

On the patient side, CVC performance is impeded by two factors: One is the low pressure regime of the venous system; the other one is the blood viscosity. Venous pressure varies considerably according to the patient's volemic state, and it is well known that hypovolemia reduces the blood flow delivery in the extracorporeal blood circuit. In other words, the effective flow is usually 10% to 20% lower in the extracorporeal circuit than the blood flow set on the dialysis monitor. Moreover, this blood flow may change significantly over time. Blood viscosity is another factor that affects catheter performance. Note that at body temperature, blood viscosity is relatively constant but inversely proportional to the hematocrit and protocrit.

On the catheter side, CVC performance is obviously dependent on the manufacturer and the cannula engineering design.[9] Catheter manufacturers have competed to propose optimized and high-performance angioaccess devices. Improvements have been made in cannula design and in polymer material resistance and surface properties.[10] Clinicians can judge CVC performance based on three criteria: blood flow delivery, flow resistance, and recirculation.

Blood flow is a critical factor that directly affects the solute removal capacity and, consequently, the efficacy of the RRT modality. However, the role of blood flow is not unique. First, the mean effective flow over time (total amount of blood cleared per session) is more important that the instantaneous maximum flow achieved during a session. Second, the solute clearance is not proportional to blood flow above a threshold value of 200 to 300 milliliters per minute (mL/min). Third, the clearance value is membrane-dependent for middle and large solutes. In other words, the duration of session and the average blood flow are essential to delivering an adequate body clearance, and membrane permeability is crucial to the removal of large solutes.

Flow resistance (R) is proportional to the pressure (ΔP) generated by the blood pump and inversely proportional to the blood flow (Q_B); this translates into the following equation where $R = \Delta P/Q_B$. The blood pump is designed to generate pressure and move blood forward against resistance within the catheter and the extracorporeal blood circuit. Because the blood pump speed is limited and a high pressure regime is deleterious for red cells, the major objective of manufacturers has been to design catheters with a low resistance profile. In laminar flow conditions, the resistance to flow R can be obtained by rearranging the Poiseuille equation as follows:

$$R = \Delta P/Q_B = 8\,\mu L/\pi r^4$$

where μ is the viscosity, L the length of catheter, r the radius, a surrogate, of the inner lumen diameter. From this equation, it is easy to show that the resistance through a catheter is proportional to its length and is inversely proportional to the fourth power of its internal lumen diameter. Schematically, shortening the catheter by 50% reduces the resistance by half, whereas doubling the diameter of the catheter increases the flow 16-fold. In summary, to reduce the resistance to flow, it is more advantageous to increase the diameter of the inner lumen of the catheter rather than reduce its length.

Recirculation is a constant and unavoidable phenomenon with CVCs. Recirculation is 10% on average but varies from 5% to 30% according to the catheter design (double-lumen or double catheter, catheter tips, presence of side holes), the vein location, and the blood flow prescribed. Recirculation is more important with femoral vein than with subclavian and jugular veins.[11] It increased with high blood flow of more than 300 mL/min.[12] Physicians must be aware of this phenomenon since it reduces, by the same proportion, the dialysis dose delivered to the patient with ARF.

To summarize, catheter performance affects the dialysis efficacy in the CRRT options (low flow, extended duration of treatment) less than in the IRRT modalities (high flow, limited duration of treatment), since the overall solute clearance relies more on time duration rather than on instantaneous clearance.

CVCs are classified in two main categories according to their intended use and duration. Acute (or short-term) CVCs are used less than 2 weeks; chronic (or long-term) CVCs may be used for an extended period of time up to several weeks. The difference between these two types of catheters is that chronic CVCs can be tunneled. In both cases, the cannulas are made of synthetic polymers (e.g., polyvinyl chloride, polytetrafluoroethylene, polyethylene, polyurethane, silicone elastomer, Tecoflex [Lubrizol Advanced Materials, Cleveland, OH]), each with its own characteristics (resistance, softness, hemocompatibility). Several models of hemodialysis catheters currently available are presented in Figures 243-1, 243-2, and 243-3. Both design and cannula engineering (inner lumen diameter, length, tip design, central and side holes) affect the performance (blood flow, flow resistance, recirculation) of the catheter. When choosing a CVC, the physician should be aware of these differences.

Catheter stiffness depends on polymer nature, plasticizer content, and extrusion mode. Polyurethane and silicone rubber are the most widely used materials for manufacturing CVCs. Catheter stiffness dictates the procedure for insertion. Rigid and semi-rigid CVCs are easily introduced percutaneously using the Seldinger method over a soft metallic guidewire. Soft and flexible CVCs (e.g., silicone) require a two-step insertion technique, first using an introducer and then a sheath vein dilator (pealable or nonpealable). Soft CVCs have major advantages over rigid ones: They are less traumatic for the host vein and more biocompatible for the blood, they are subcutaneously tunneled, and they benefit from a subcutaneous anchoring system.

Single- and double-lumen cannulas may be used for hemodialysis. Single-lumen catheters have a single port used alternatively for both inflow and outflow. Two single-lumen catheters (inflow and outflow) need to be inserted in the same vein to optimize flow performance. Double-lumen catheters (one arterial port and one venous port) are now more widely used because they provide a more convenient and simple way to access blood. Layout of the lumen and distal tips varies considerably among catheters. Schematically, there are two main types of catheter: one with port sites attached in a double-barreled gun fashion (coaxial, double-D, double-O), the other one with independent or separated port sites (dual catheter, split catheter). Independent catheter lines offer a more consistently adequate and high flow compared with the attached catheter lines. Improved functionality is due to the catheter design, which reduces the risk of catheter occlusion by arterial wall suction or sidewall contact.

Acute nontunneled double-lumen CVCs are made of polyurethane. They are easy to insert into the femoral vein or the internal jugular vein and can be used within minutes to start RRT (Fig. 243-4). Chronic tunneled CVCs are gaining popularity in the ICU field (Fig. 243-5), since they provide better performance (blood flow, stability, longev-

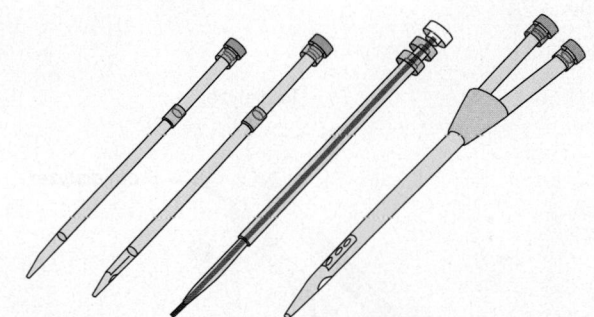

FIGURE 243-1. Acute central venous catheters (CVCs): different models.

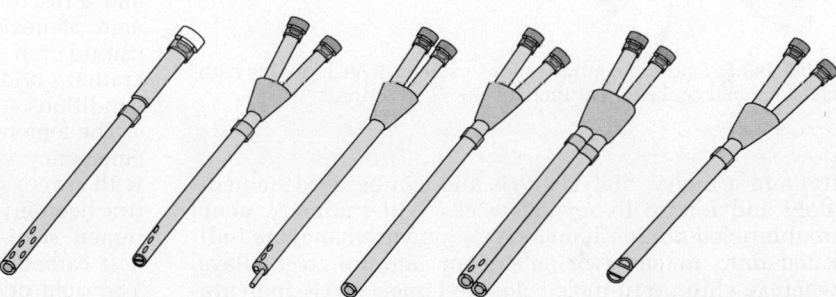

FIGURE 243-2. Chronic central venous catheters (CVCs): several types of single- and double-lumen silicone catheters for renal replacement therapy (RRT).

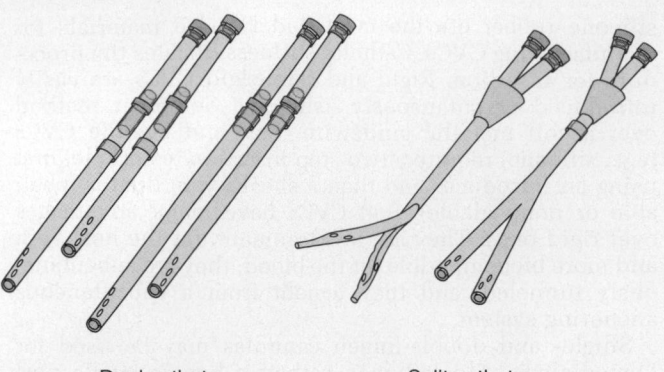

FIGURE 243-3. Chronic central venous catheters (CVCs): several types of double catheters for renal replacement therapy (RRT).

Dual catheter   Split catheter

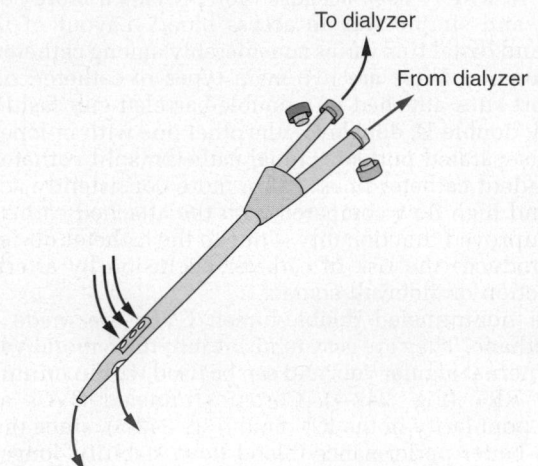

To dialyzer

From dialyzer

FIGURE 243-4. Acute central venous catheter (CVC): double-lumen polyurethane catheter for renal replacement therapy (RRT) in action.

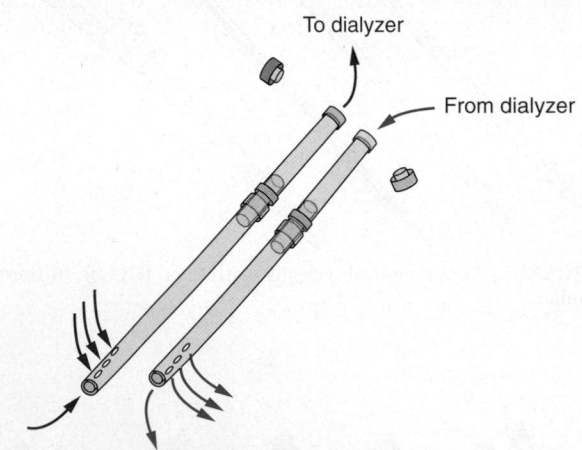

To dialyzer

From dialyzer

FIGURE 243-5. Chronic central venous catheter (CVC): double catheter for renal replacement therapy (RRT) in action.

ity) and a higher dialysis dose and can be used immediately and for up to several weeks.[13] In summary, acute nontunneled double-lumen CVCs (polyurethane) are indicated only in cases of emergency and up to 14 days, whereas chronic tunneled double-lumen CVCs (polyure-

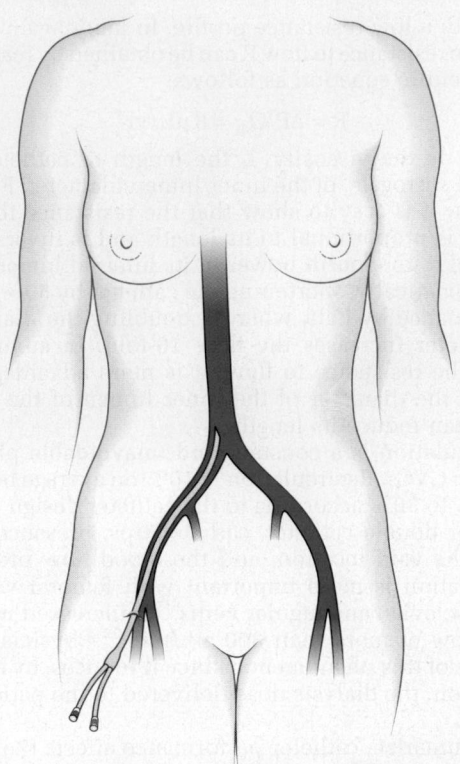

FIGURE 243-6. Acute central venous catheter (CVC): nontunneled double-lumen polyurethane catheter inserted in the right femoral vein.

thane, silicone rubber) are indicated after life-threatening conditions have resolved and may be used up to several weeks.

INDICATIONS FOR AND INSERTION OF CENTRAL VENOUS CATHETERS

Methods of catheter insertion have improved over the past decade, contributing to the reduction of morbidity associated with CVCs. Ultrasound- or fluoroscopy-based methods to locate the vein and to guide the vein cannulation have reduced the incidence of failure, the time spent for catheterization, and the incidence of traumatic complications.[14-16]

Choosing the venous site depends on the clinical context, the patient's state, and the physician's experience. The femoral approach is preferred in critically ill patients. Alternatively, the internal jugular approach is more appealing in the absence of a life-threatening situation. Subclavian access should be considered as the last resort and a rescue option because of the late and high risk of vein stenosis.[17,18] In all cases, the percutaneous vein cannulation option must be performed after skin preparation, under local anesthesia, and in strict aseptic conditions.

The femoral vein is the preferred cannulation site in an emergency condition and when patients are bedridden with severe neurological disorders, ventilatory assistance (tracheotomy), or multiple-organ failure. Acute double-lumen semi-rigid polyurethane catheters represent the best catheter option in these circumstances (Fig. 243-6). The right or left femoral vein offers the same facility for

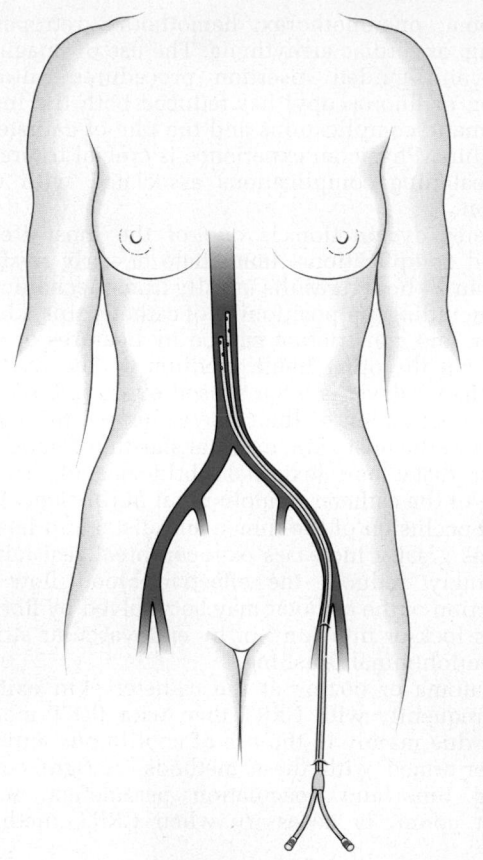

FIGURE 243-7. Chronic central venous catheter (CVC): tunneled dual catheter inserted in the left femoral vein.

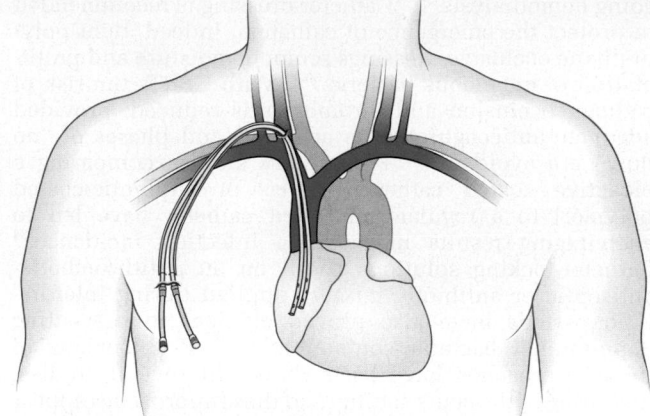

FIGURE 243-8. Chronic central venous catheter (CVC): dual catheter inserted in the right internal jugular vein.

insertion. The length of femoral catheters that provides optimal flow is between 30 and 35 cm. The insertion site is located approximately 1 to 2 cm below the crural arcade and 1 cm medially apart from the femoral artery. For safety reasons, these catheters should be used no more than 2 weeks. Chronic tunneled silicone CVCs have been successfully evaluated in the ICU setting (Fig. 243-7). A recent randomized comparison in ARF patients with acute versus chronic CVCs showed that tunneled CVCs provided a higher blood and dialysis dose delivered on a regular basis with less morbidity and longer permeability expectancy.[19] Long-term tunneled CVCs represent an interesting and innovative angioaccess that tends to be recognized as superior to the acute CVC in patients with ARF.[20,21]

Internal jugular cannulation has gained popularity over the past 2 decades.[22] Straight or kinked acute double-lumen CVCs exiting near the ear are clearly more exposed to infections and should be abandoned except to resolve an acute life-threatening condition. Chronic tunneled soft (polyurethane and silicone rubber) CVCs (double-lumen catheter, double catheter, split catheter) inserted into the internal jugular vein are preferable, to reduce the risk of infection (Fig. 243-8). Percutaneous insertion in the internal jugular vein in a low position is suitable to prevent catheter kinking. The right internal jugular vein is the best location. The left internal jugular approach is indicated only when the right is not possible. The percutaneous insertion and tunneling procedure (upward or downward) depends on the type of catheter. A subcutaneous anchoring system (Dacron cuff, purse-string suture) is

important, as it is a means of securing and protecting the catheter.

Subclavian vein cannulation for hemodialysis should be abandoned because it entails a major risk of stenosis or thrombosis, jeopardizing the further creation of a native arteriovenous fistula.[23,24] Indeed, subclavian cannulation should be considered as the ultimate rescue option in the setting of repeated venous access failure. Soft chronic CVCs are preferred when this approach is indicated. The right subclavian vein is preferable to reduce catheter length and improve flow performance. Short cannulas (20-25 cm) prevent cardiac trauma (atrium and ventricle perforation).

Correct positioning of the distal tip is essential to prevent catheter dysfunction. Chest catheters passing through the superior vena cava system have their tips located at the junction of the superior vena cava and the right atrium. Extemporaneous fluoroscopy, chest x-ray, or electrocardiogram should be used to check the correct position of the catheter and of its tip before catheter use.[25] The optimal length of a thoracic catheter to be inserted on the right side in adults is 20 to 25 cm, and 3 to 4 additional cm are required when catheters are inserted on the left side.

Femoral catheters accessing the inferior vena cava system should have their tips positioned in the central lumen of the inferior vena cava. For a femoral catheter to reach the inferior vena cava in adults, it must be 30 to 35 cm in length.

CATHETER MAINTENANCE AND CARE

Several recent studies have shown that strict hygienic rules and good nursing practices are the strongest predictors of good catheter outcomes. It is well recognized that restricting the use of catheters to RRT and avoiding catheter opening for blood sampling, parenteral feeding, and intravenous injection will minimize catheter dysfunction and infectious risk. Nurse training and care expertise are essential elements for preventing infection and maintaining catheter flow performance.[26] Strict aseptic conditions in catheter handling and maximum sterile precaution barriers must be in place at all times.[27] The use of antiseptic ointment or a protective box on catheter hubs reduces significantly the incidence of bacteremia in patients undergoing hemodialysis.[28,29] Catheter dressing is recommended to protect the emergence of catheters. Indeed, tight polyurethane occlusive dressings promote moisture and proliferation of cutaneous bacteria.[30,31] With CRRTs the risk of catheter occlusion and thrombosis is reduced, provided adequate anticoagulation is achieved and phases of "no flow" are avoided.[32,33] Preliminary studies comparing a bioactive coated catheter (silver- or antibiotic-coated polymer) to a regular noncoated catheter have led to encouraging results in reducing infection incidence.[34] Catheter-locking solutions based on an antithrombotic-antiseptic or antibiotic mixture applied during interdialytic periods have also proved efficient in preventing endoluminal bacteria contamination.[35] Real benefits of these approaches have been shown in several studies, including in the acute setting, and these approaches appear to be the most efficient preemptive actions.[36]

CATHETER PERFORMANCE

Catheter type and design affect catheter performance. The type of polymer the catheter is made of determines the catheter resistance and softness; length and inner catheter diameter govern maximum flow rate and resistance; presence or lack of distal holes affects blood flow stability. CRRT modalities usually require blood flows (200-300 mL/min) at low resistance (venous and arterial pressure less than 100 mm Hg). Internal lumen diameter between 2.0 and 2.2 millimeters is necessary in these cases to provide optimal flow and resistance. Two independent catheters (or a split catheter) bearing circular distal holes are essential to reduce probability of catheter dysfunction (parietal suction, partial lumen obstruction, fibrin sleeve formation).[37,38]

Extracorporeal blood pressure (arterial and venous sides) recorded by the dialysis machine provides indirect evidence for resistance to flow within the catheter. The pressure displayed may be used by nursing staff as an indicator of partial catheter obstruction. In most contemporary dialysis machines, blood flow is corrected for flow resistance and displayed as an effective blood flow.[39]

Recirculation is a common feature of catheters.[40] This phenomenon reduces the dialysis efficacy. Recirculation value depends on the type of catheter, the catheter tip positioning, the type of vein, and the blood flow used. Femoral catheters, particularly short ones, exhibit a high recirculation rate, averaging 20% (5%-38%). Internal jugular and subclavian catheters have a much lower recirculation rate, averaging 10% (5%-15%). Note that the inversion of the bloodlines during hemodialysis session, which is sometimes indicated to correct flow difficulties,[41] significantly increases blood recirculation rates. In this case the recirculation rate may rise to 20% or 30%.

CATHETER OUTCOMES AND COMPLICATIONS

Traumatic-related complications of catheter use are less frequent nowadays as a result of better expertise among operators. Catheter morbidity is still frequent, and medical personnel must be aware of potential catheter complications.[42] Depending on the venous site, complications of CVC insertion include arterial puncture, local bleeding, hematoma, pneumothorax, hemothorax, retroperitoneal bleeding, or cardiac arrhythmia. The use of imaging techniques and guided insertion procedures (ultrasound, Doppler, or fluoroscopy) has reduced both the incidence of traumatic complications and the rate of catheter insertion failure. Physician experience is crucial to preventing life-threatening complications associated with catheter insertion.

Catheter dysfunction is one of the most frequently reported complications. Immediate or early dysfunction (less than 24 hours) results usually from mechanical problems, including malpositioning of catheter tips, kinking of catheter, and constriction caused by ligatures or aponeurosis.[43] On the other hand, medium or late dysfunction (more than 2 days) is often caused by thrombosis: partial or total obstruction of the catheter lumen, thrombosis or stenosis of the host vein, external sheath formation on the catheter distal end (external fibrin sleeve), or internal coating of the catheter (endoluminal fibrin sleeve). Partial or total occlusion of the lumen and distal and lateral perforations greatly increases extracorporeal resistance and, accordingly, reduces the effective blood flow. Partial obstruction of the catheter may be resolved by fibrinolysis used as lock or infusion[44] or by endovascular stripping[45] or by endoluminal brushing.[46]

Hematoma or oozing at the catheter skin exit occurs more frequently with CRRT than with IRRT modalities. This is due mainly to the use of continuous anticoagulation performed with these methods. A tight control of clotting time and coagulation parameters, including platelet count, is necessary when CRRT methods are used.

Thromboses are frequent complications revealed usually by intermittent or permanent dysfunction of the CVC. Endoluminal thrombosis of the catheter is less common with CRRT when there is adequate anticoagulation but still may occur. In this case the catheter may be reopened either by mechanical (brushing) or chemical cleaning action (fibrinolysis).[47] External thrombosis of the catheter results from the formation of a fibrin sheath wrapping the catheter tip. This is a delayed complication (over 7 to 10 days) and happens less frequently in CRRT-treated patients because of the permanent flow maintained within the catheter. Several factors contribute to the thrombogenicity of the cannula, including material, mode of insertion, type of vein, duration of cannulation, coagulation, and inflammation profile (hyperfibrinemia, hyperthrombocytemia, previous venous thrombosis), and silent infection.

Stenosis of the host vein is a common risk related to use of all types of catheters. It happens more frequently with acute than with chronic soft catheters. It is a late and troublesome complication that jeopardizes the creation of arteriovenous fistula in patients with chronic renal failure.

Infections represent the main cause of catheter morbidity.[48,49] Nontunneled polyurethane catheters used as a short-term therapy entail a bacteremia risk estimated to occur at a median value of 5.9 episodes per 1000 patient-days in ICUs. However, the incidence of bacteremia varies greatly according to the units.[50] Nontunneled internal jugular access bears a higher risk of infection than does tunneled internal jugular access, notably in patients with a tracheotomy.

Early infection is due to catheter placement problems or skin and catheter track infection. Placement of a percutaneous catheter disrupts the skin continuity. Bacterial colonization of the skin or nasal mucosa is often incriminated in catheter-related infection. Hence, to prevent catheter infection there is a need for developing strict hygienic and aseptic rules for inserting and handling catheters.

Late infections are often associated with endoluminal catheter contamination. The infectious risk increases with the duration of catheter use. Improving nursing care and catheter handling alleviates the risk of infection. Catheter-related infections are of two types: local infection (skin exit, track infection) and systemic infection (bacteremia, septicemia, infected thrombosis). Skin exit and bacteremia are the most frequent forms of infection, which may be treated by local and systemic antibiotic therapy while keeping the catheter in situ with a dual antibiotic-antithrombotic lock solution.[51] Catheter track infection, septicemia, and infected venous thrombosis are the most severe forms of infection and require catheter withdrawal and systemic antibiotic therapy. In the context of infectious risk, the insertion of a chronic tunneled catheter with an anchoring system appears highly preferable to prevent infection hazards. Strict aseptic rules including the use of gloves, mask, drapes, and antiseptic solution must be applied at any time when handling catheters or hooking them to dialysis machine bloodlines to prevent the endoluminal passage of bacteria present on the catheter's hub.

Biomaterial research points to potential improvements in the safety of catheters. Surface treatment of catheters, rendering them softer and smoother, reduces hemoreactivity and prevents coagulation cascade activation which in turn reduces the risk of thrombosis.[52] Fixation of bioactive material on polymer surface (silver impregnation, anticoagulant, antibiotic-antiseptic adsorption) is intended to prevent platelet adhesion, avoid clotting, and protect bacterial adhesion.[53,54] Recent studies comparing the incidence of infection using impregnated-antibiotic catheters to regular catheters have confirmed the protective role of bioactive material.

CONCLUSION

The acute double-lumen polyurethane CVC represents the best short-term option for patients with ARF requiring urgent hemodialysis. The chronic silicone rubber central venous double catheter (or double-lumen catheter) is alternatively the most suitable option for medium- and long-term use, including in patients treated with CRRT. The femoral approach is particularly well indicated in multiple-organ failure or bedridden patients. Chronic tunneled CVCs have been shown to improve comfort, safety, and dialysis efficacy in all forms of RRT. The internal jugular vein warrants proper functioning of CVCs and reduces complication hazards. The subclavian approach should be avoided or restricted to multiple angioaccess failure and considered as a last resort, for example, in a rescue situation.

Key Points

1. Acute central venous catheters are intended to be used less than 14 days, while chronic tunneled central venous catheters are intended to be used up to 90 days or more.

2. Soft-tunneled dual-lumen catheters (or dual catheters) should be indicated in patients with acute renal failure when renal replacement therapy is planned for more than 2 weeks.

3. Femoral and internal jugular routes are recommended in immobilized patients with acute renal failure. The subclavian route should be avoided to prevent stenosis and thrombosis of the host vein.

4. Catheter-related morbidity (dysfunction, thrombosis, infection) is in part due to the type of catheter (the chronic tunneled catheter is less harmful than the acute catheter) but is mainly due to nursing and medical practices associated with catheter care.

5. Catheter performance (blood flow, resistance, recirculation) governing the efficacy of the renal replacement therapy should be monitored regularly. Because of the continuous mode of treatment, the overall dialysis efficacy is somewhat less sensitive to catheter performance.

6. Use of catheters for dialysis only is strongly recommended to prevent catheter dysfunction, thrombosis, or both.

7. To help prevent catheter-related complications, catheters should be locked with antithrombotic solution, antiseptic solution, or both, when not used for renal replacement therapy.

Key References

9. Depner TA: Catheter performance. Semin Dial 2001;14(6): 425-431.

12. Leblanc M, Bosc JY, Vaussenat F, et al: Effective blood flow and recirculation rates in internal jugular vein twin catheters: Measurement by ultrasound velocity dilution. Am J Kidney Dis 1998;31(1):87-92.

23. Barrett N, Spencer S, McIvor J, Brown EA: Subclavian stenosis: A major complication of subclavian dialysis catheters. Nephrol Dial Transplant 1988;3(4):423-425.

27. Raad II, Gilbreath J: Prevention of central venous catheter-related infections by using maximal sterile barrier precautions during insertion. Infect Control Hosp Epidemiol 1994;15: 231-236.

34. Chatzinikolaou I, Finkel K, Hanna H, et al: Antibiotic-coated hemodialysis catheters for the prevention of vascular catheter-related infections: A prospective, randomized study. Am J Med 2003;115(5):352-357.

51. Krishnasami Z, Carlton D, Bimbo L, et al: Management of hemodialysis catheter-related bacteremia with an adjunctive antibiotic lock solution. Kidney Int 2002;61(3):1136-1142.

See the companion Expert Consult website for the complete reference list.

CHAPTER 244

Anticoagulation Strategies for Continuous Renal Replacement Therapies

Roy Mathew and Ravindra L. Mehta

OBJECTIVES

This chapter will:
1. Identify the ideal anticoagulant for continuous renal replacement therapy.
2. Describe the technical aspects of continuous renal replacement therapy delivery that impacts on circuit patency.
3. Compare the advantages and disadvantages of available anticoagulation strategies.
4. Discuss the application of the available anticoagulation strategies in various continuous renal replacement therapy modalities.
5. Provide basic recommendations for the use of these anticoagulants for continuous renal replacement therapy depending on the clinical situation.

Maintaining circuit patency during continuous renal replacement therapy (CRRT) is important for adequate volume and solute clearance. Anticoagulation is necessary despite the increased risk in critically ill patients. The goals of ideal anticoagulation are the following:
1. Anticoagulation with high antithrombotic potential with low hemorrhagic risk
2. Brief anticoagulation action, limited to the CRRT circuit
3. Anticoagulation monitoring that is easy and suited for bedside use
4. Long-term use of anticoagulation that is not associated with severe systemic side effects
5. An antidote available in case of overdose

TECHNICAL ASPECTS: NON-ANTICOAGULANT CONSIDERATIONS

Access and Circuit

The traditional arteriovenous circuit is no longer commonly used and thus will not be discussed in this chapter. Venovenous circuits have several sites for potential thrombosis: access, dialysis tubing, blood pump, and venous air trap.[1] Catheter malfunction leads to sluggish blood flow rates and increased risk of circuit failure. Temporary cath-

eters for acute hemodialysis are made largely of polyurethane or silicone; both are hemocompatible. Polyurethane is a stiffer material and catheters utilized for this purpose are for acute use only (<3 weeks).[2] Silicone is less stressful on the vessel wall and more suitable for long-term use. Mechanisms for optimizing catheter function involve utilizing proper location and length. Femoral dual-lumen catheters are preferably 20 to 24 cm and possibly 30 cm in adults,[2] whereas internal jugular (preferably in the right internal jugular vein) catheters are 13.5 to 16 cm in length (in general, subclavian intravenous catheters are discouraged given the potential for subclavian stenosis and difficulties with future arteriovenous fistulas).[3,4] During treatment interruption, appropriate measures should be taken to maintain access patency. Catheter lock solutions should be selected to maintain catheter patency when the circuit is not being used. There is mounting evidence that citrate, as a catheter lock solution, offers better protection against bacteremia and adequate line patency as compared to heparin.[5,6]

Blood flow pumps, which have allowed the use of the venous circulation alone for blood access, contribute to thrombosis. Multiple pumps result in the requirement of each pump to spin faster, resulting in more hemolysis. At slower blood flows (50-100 mL/min), there is ample time for the tubing to recoil to full diameter and therefore fully fill with blood. With blood flow rates above 100 mL/min, tubing recoil is less, and if there is any impediment to the delivery of blood to the compressed segment, that is, access failure, then blood flow will slowly fall below the prescribed amount. These factors have not been studied extensively in the CRRT setting, and most of the current data are derived from the cardiopulmonary bypass literature.[1]

While different membranes are available for CRRT in hollow fiber configuration, few data are available regarding anticoagulant-coated fibers and tubing. Studies of patients receiving chronic dialysis have demonstrated the ability to carry out dialysis with these coated tubes (heparin and low-molecular-weight heparin) and no systemic anticoagulation.[7,8] Further studies are required in the critical care setting.

Air traps allow for a relatively slow-moving column of blood to have constant contact with air, potentiating the formation of clots. Baldwin and colleagues[9] examined if providing heparin into both a prefilter line and air trap could prolong filter life. As compared to single-site administration, the dual-site administration had a filter life of 18.1 ± 3.1 hours versus 17 ± 3.2 hours. Gretz and coresearchers[10] achieved slightly longer circuit life by raising the blood level in the air trap higher than the blood inlet port. By doing so, they diminished the amount of contact that the circulating blood had with air.

Predilution versus Postdilution

A key issue in maintaining circuit patency is to minimize concentrating the blood as ultrafiltrate is removed across the filter. Evidence has amassed that providing a dilutional fluid, either in the form of replacement fluid in continuous venovenous hemofiltration (CVVH) or as a continuous low-volume infusion of saline prefilter, prolongs filter life as compared to providing all replacement fluid postfilter. Uchino and colleagues[11] reported a median life span of 18 hours in predilution mode and 13 hours in post-dilution mode. De Pont and coworkers[12] reported a non-significant trend toward longer filter life in predilution mode (median filter life 28 hours in predilution and 15 hours in postdilution).[12] In a similar study design, van der Voort and colleagues[13] observed a filter life of 45.7 hours in predilution mode and 16.1 hours in postdilution mode. A related issue for filter fouling is the process of progressive protein adsorption, termed *concentration repolarization*. This leads to a progressive decline in the filtering surface and efficacy. Few studies have specifically examined this subject[14] and have observed no statistical difference in filter life between hemofiltration, hemodiafiltration, and hemodialysis.[15,16] To maximize filter life and filtration efficacy during ultrafiltration modalities, it is recommended that the ratio of ultrafiltrate to plasma flow (filtration fraction) be kept below 20%.[17]

AVAILABLE ANTICOAGULATION STRATEGIES

General Factors

Preventing thrombosis or coagulation along the tubing of the CRRT circuit requires adequate anticoagulation of the blood, optimal localization of anticoagulation administration, and optimal anticoagulation delivery method. Adequate anticoagulation will be discussed in more detail under each anticoagulant section. The location of administration has not been extensively studied. The practice in our institution involves administration of anticoagulant at the connection between access and tubing via a 3-way tap. A more dilute anticoagulation solution would allow greater mixing with the blood per dose delivered. However, a randomized crossover trial demonstrated no difference between dilute heparin (10 iu/mL) positioned proximally in the circuit versus standard heparin (100 iu/mL) posi-

tioned more distally (through prefilter); mean circuit life was 21.4 hours (standard deviation [SD] 19.2) and 20.1 (SD 14.6), respectively.[18]

No Anticoagulation

Several trials have looked at the use of no anticoagulation versus conventional anticoagulation. Median filter life has been reported to vary from 19 to 53 hours, the prime variable leading to longest life being low platelet count (<60,000/mL).[11,16,19-21] Current data suggest no anticoagulation be used when patients are actively bleeding or are at very high risk for bleeding complications (<48 hr postoperative; platelet count <60,000/mL; activated partial thromboplastin time [aPTT] >45 sec).[11,16,19-21]

Systemic Anticoagulation
Heparin

Heparin continues to be the most commonly used anticoagulant for CRRT. Unfractionated heparin is a mixture of glycosaminoglycans of varying molecular weight.[22] It is now known that the higher molecular-weight component reversibly binds to antithrombin-III (ATIII) and the lower molecular-weight heparins predominantly inhibit factor Xa. The molecular weight range is from 3000 to 30,000 daltons with a mean of around 15,000. The anti-Xa activity occurs predominantly around the 3000 range. Approximately one third of the intravascular heparin binds to ATIII. The remaining two thirds is nonspecifically bound to various plasma proteins and cell surfaces. The binding to ATIII gives the majority of its anticoagulant property; by binding to ATIII, heparin enhances thrombin binding and hence enhances its anticoagulant activity. The non-ATIII binding is the source of heparin's adverse effects and limitations.[22]

Conventional strategies include priming with heparinized saline (5-10 iu/mL). A bolus of 2000 to 5000 iu is injected into the circuit at commencement of the CRRT procedure. Continuous infusion is started at the arterial side at 3 to 15 international units per kilogram body weight per hour (iu/kg/hr) to maintain an aPTT 1.5 to 2 times the upper limit of normal.[15,19,23] In patients with preexisting coagulopathy, often the bolus is omitted and the lower end of the goal is the aim (Fig. 244-1).

Low-dose strategies also have been attempted in order to prolong filter life beyond the time achieved through use

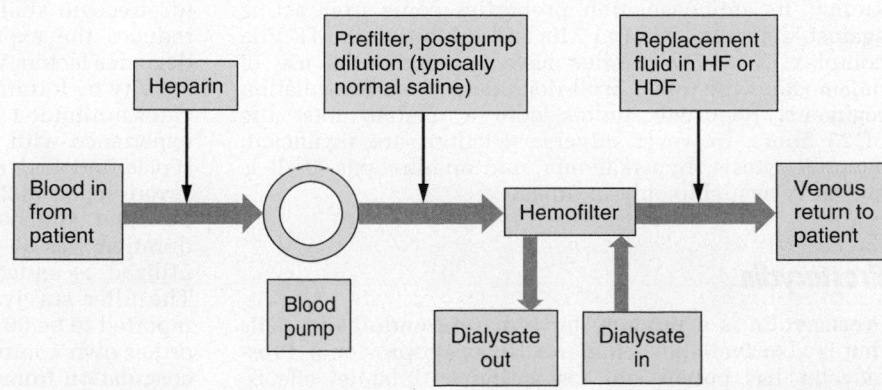

FIGURE 244-1. Schematic of heparin anticoagulation for continuous venovenous hemodiafiltration (CVVHDF). HDF, hemodiafiltration; HF, hemofiltration. (From Schetz M: Anticoagulation for continuous renal replacement therapy. Curr Opin Anaesthesiol 2001;14(2):143-149.)

of the no-anticoagulation strategy but avoid the potential hemorrhagic complications resulting from systemic heparin therapy. No bolus is administered. Heparin is infused at the rate of between 5 and 10 iu/kg/hr. Studies examining the efficacy of a low-dose heparin strategy are not promising by any means. Filter survival is less than, or no better than, regimens that use no anticoagulation.[20,21]

Current data comparing heparin to alternate forms of anticoagulation reveal that the risk-benefit ratio of heparin in critically ill patients is unfavorable. Prolonged heparin use is associated with significant hemorrhagic complications, thrombocytopenia (heparin-induced thrombocytopenia [HIT]) and subsequent thrombotic complications. In one observational study, 48 hemorrhagic episodes occurred, of which 3 resulted in death and 10 required cessation of CRRT.[15] A clear inverse relationship between filter-clotting episodes and hemorrhagic events based on aPTT was demonstrated in this study; no mention of HIT was made.

Low-Molecular-Weight Heparin

Low-molecular-weight heparin (LMWH) exerts its effects by inhibiting clotting factor Xa. The pharmacokinetic profile is more predictable than that of unfractionated heparin given that there is far less protein and cell binding. Monitoring is not typically done in persons with normal renal function. However, LMWH is eliminated via the kidneys, so it must be avoided in persons with renal dysfunction or, if used, monitored by anti-factor Xa activity (goal 0.25-0.35 iu/mL).[24,25] Protamine does not directly inhibit the action of LMWH but can be tried if significant bleeding occurs and there is only partial removal of LMWH by CRRT.[22,24] Dosing strategies depend on the brand used, as various polymerization strategies affect the pharmacokinetics.[26] In one study, dalteparin was given as a bolus dose of 25 u/kg and then maintenance infusion of 10 u/kg/hr.[23] Complications included HIT (1 patient) and bleeding (2 episodes). The filter life was not significantly different from that of unfractionated heparin. The cost of using LMWH was significantly higher than the cost of using unfractionated heparin. No monitoring of anti-Xa activity was performed during this study.

Nafamostat

Nafamostat (Torii Pharmaceutical, Tokyo) is a synthetic serine protease inhibitor that was originally intended for use in the treatment of acute pancreatitis, as it has activity against pancreatic enzymes such as trypsin and kallikrein.[27] Its anticoagulation properties come from acting against factors IIa, Xa, and XIIa and inhibiting the TF-VIIa complex. Very few studies have compared the use of nafamostat with other well-documented anticoagulation regimens. Reported studies note a median filter life of 23 hours. However, adverse reactions are significant: agranulocytosis, hyperkalemia, and anaphylaxis.[26,27] It is currently available only in Japan.

Prostacyclin

Prostacyclin is a product derived from endothelial cells that is also available commercially as epoprostenol. Prostacyclin has potent and fast-acting antiplatelet effects.

Current data on the use of prostacyclin as a sole anticoagulation agent reveals that, in the case of pump-driven venovenous modes of CRRT, there is insufficient filter longevity (12-48 hr).[28-30] Disadvantages of prostacyclin use are risk of clinically significant hypotension and difficulty in monitoring. Monitoring is via thromboelastography or bleeding time measurement.

Hirudin

Hirudin is a polypeptide produced by leeches that directly inhibits bound and unbound thrombin. Given in its natural form, it can produce marked hypersensitivity; recombinant formulations have been derived that do not elicit such a response. The system is primed with a hirudin saline solution of 33 micrograms per liter (μg/L) saline. Dosing strategies include prepump administration with a bolus of 0.08-0.15 milligrams per kilogram body weight (mg/kg) and then infusion rate at 10 μg/kg/hr. Hirudin is adjusted in increments of 2 μg/kg/hr based on a target ecarin clotting time of 80 to 100 seconds.[31] The main disadvantage of hirudin is its complete dependence on renal function for elimination. Furthermore, hemofiltration incompletely removes hirudin from the circulation.[32] Ecarin clotting time is not a readily available monitoring tool, and aPTT does not accurately reflect hirudin activity.

Argatroban

Argatroban is a direct thrombin inhibitor that is cleared predominantly by the liver. It is derived from arginine and it inhibits thrombin by reversibly binding to its catalytic site without the aid of a cofactor.[33] As an anticoagulant for CRRT, there are limited data and no controlled trials. Tang and colleagues[33] describe the pharmacokinetics and use of argatroban in one patient on CVVH who developed HIT (liver function was not reported in the study). aPTT was kept at "around 70 seconds" and activated clotting time "around 200 seconds"; CRRT clearance of argatroban was minor compared to systemic clearance. No complications were reported and no efficacy for the CVVH was mentioned. Dosing for argatroban ranged from 0.5 to 2 μg/kg/min.

Activated Protein C

Activated protein C (APC) is a naturally occurring anticoagulant that when given as the recombinant form (Xigris [drotrecogin alfa], Eli Lilly, Indianapolis, IN) inhibits and reduces the expression of tissue factor; proteolytically degrades factors V and VIII; and potentiates the fibrinolytic activity by forming tight junctions with plasminogen activator inhibitor-1.[34] de Pont and coworkers[34] describe their experience with three patients who had suffered severe sepsis and had required CVVH. They received APC for severe sepsis at 24 μg/kg/hr for 96 hours. During this time no other anticoagulation was provided. Reported filter duration was 55 ± 13 hours. Unfractionated heparin was utilized as anticoagulation once APC was discontinued. The filter survival time for unfractionated heparin was reported to be 66 ± 19 hours. Each patient was used as his or her own control, so it is likely there was residual anticoagulation from APC.

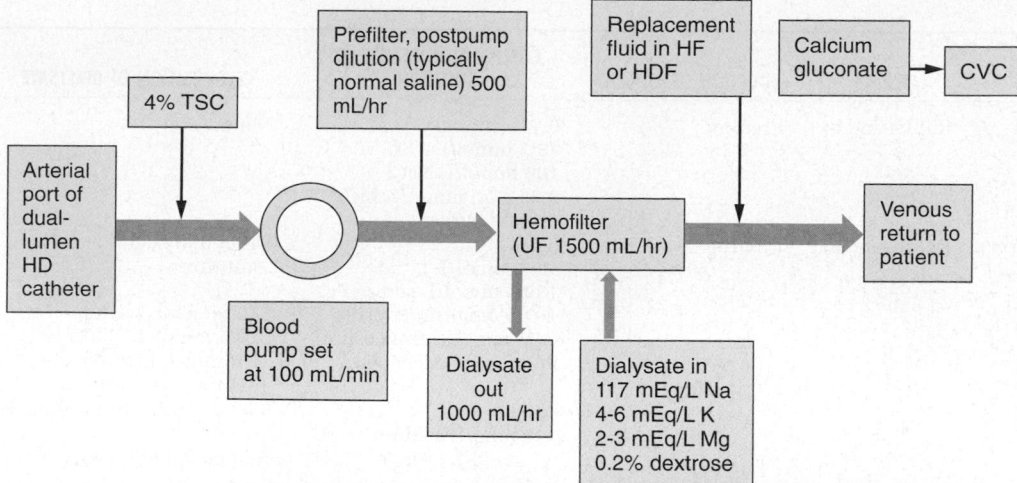

FIGURE 244-2. Schematic of UCSD citrate anticoagulation for continuous venovenous hemodiafiltration (CVVHDF). CVC, central venous catheter; HD, hemodialysis; HDF, hemodiafiltration; HF, hemofiltration; K, potassium; Mg, magnesium; Na, sodium; TSC, trisodium citrate; UF, ultrafiltration. (From Mehta RL: Anticoagulation during continuous renal replacement therapy. ASAIO J 1994;40(4):931-935.)

Regional Anticoagulation

Citrate

Citrate has been used as an effective anticoagulation for continuous dialysis circuits since the 1990s.[35-37] The mechanism of action involves chelation of unbound calcium, a requisite ion for coagulation. Citrate is provided at the entry port of the circuit. On return to the patient, the total body calcium, plus other divalent cations, inundates the circulating citrate, thereby normalizing the serum calcium. This is further supplemented by calcium administration at a non-CRRT-related venous line in the patient (typically a separate central venous catheter). Citrate has the added benefit in that, in those with adequate hepatic function, it is a source of bicarbonate. Means of citrate administration are as follows:

1. Standard protocol: Citrate solution (trisodium citrate or anticoagulation D) is administered at the site of blood entry into the CRRT circuit; the rate is adjusted to goal postfilter ionized calcium of 0.2 to 0.3. Calcium is supplemented by a separate central venous catheter (Fig. 244-2). Typically, the dialysate used for continuous venovenous hemodiafiltration (CVVHDF) is calcium free to avoid premature access and hemofilter coagulation. However, Gupta and colleagues[38] have described a protocol using a low-calcium peritoneal dialysate with anticoagulant citrate dextrose formula A solution as the anticoagulant for CVVHDF. Mean filter duration was 63 hours, and 49% of the filters were patent at 72 hours.[38]

2. Alternate protocols: In both CVVH and CVVHDF, methods have been proposed for the administration of citrate along with the replacement fluid.[39,40] A list of solutions is presented in Table 244-1.

Potential complications are hypernatremia, hypo- or hypercalcemia, hypomagnesemia, alkalosis, and citrate toxicity leading to metabolic acidosis.[41] Hypocalcemia has not been attributed to significant cardiac dysrhythmias or hypotension.[16,36,39,41,42] Citrate accumulation (>28.8 mg/dL [1.5 mmol/L], though not routinely measured) may lead to worsening metabolic acidosis and hypocalcemia and hypomagnesemia. Current data support the use of a total calcium to ionized calcium ratio greater than 2:1 or ionized calcium less than 0.8 mmol/L as markers of citrate toxic-

ity.[43,44] Citrate delivery needs to be reduced until the ratio reduces. Hetzel and coworkers[43] recommend discontinuation of citrate-CVVH to allow time for elimination of excess citrate. Bleeding due to over-anticoagulation with citrate occurs very rarely, in contrast to heparin anticoagulation.[16,36,39,42]

The major disadvantage of utilizing citrate is the lack of standardized solutions for dialysate administration. Specialized citrate or dialysate solutions require dedicated pharmacy support and nursing familiarity with the solutions.

Unfractionated Heparin-Protamine

Regional heparin anticoagulation involves providing heparin prefilter at the point of blood entry into the dialysis circuit and giving protamine at a ratio of 100:1 (units of heparin to milligrams of protamine) post filter prior to return of blood to the patient (see Fig. 244-2). This strategy has not consistently proved to provide adequate protection against hemorrhagic complications in the patient.[11,19,21] This is primarily due to the phenomenon of rebound anticoagulation. Protamine has a half-life that is shorter than that of heparin and therefore allows for a bolus of heparin once the protamine is turned off. The titration of protamine to heparin for proper antidote takes time, and the average patient aPTT tends to be slightly higher than the upper limit of normal, allowing for potential hemorrhagic possibilities. Protamine also carries the risk of significant hypotension and anaphylaxis-type reactions.[21,22]

MONITORING

Several parameters should be monitored for effective delivery of anticoagulants during CRRT. The goal is to maximize circuit efficiency and minimize complications.

1. Dialysis adequacy
   a. Decreasing CRRT efficacy, that is, the sieving coefficient of urea (UF urea/blood urea) less than 0.6, may precede overt clotting. Monitors of CRRT efficacy have been discussed elsewhere.[35]

TABLE 244-1

CRRT MODALITY	CITRATE	LOCATION OF CITRATE	COMPOSITION OF CITRATE SOLUTION	COMPOSITION OF DIALYSATE	CHAPTER REFERENCES
Hemofiltration	Replacement	Prefilter	0.4% citrate: 13.3 mmol/L TSC 100 mmol/L NaCl 0.75-1.75 mmol/L MgCl 0.1% dextrose	None	40, 51
Hemodiafiltration	Replacement	Prefilter	0.4%[53]: 13.3 mmol/L citrate 139.9 mmol/L sodium 101.5 mmol/L chloride 0.75 mmol/L magnesium Potassium as needed 0.5%[39]: 140 mEq/L sodium 18 mmol/L citrate 0.67%[39]: 140 mEq/L sodium 23 mmol/L citrate Hemocitrasol-20[52] 145 mmol/L sodium 100 mmol/L chloride 20 mmol/L citrate 10 mmol/L glucose 0-4 mmol/L potassium 0-1 mmol/L phosphorous	Same dialysate for 0.4% solution[53] 140 mmol/L sodium 118.5 mmol/L chloride 25 mmol/L bicarbonate 4 mmol/L potassium 0.58 mmol/L magnesium[39] As needed 0.9% saline[52]	39, 52, 53
Hemodiafiltration	Alone	3-way stopcock at arterial entry into circuit	ACD-A: 112.9 mmol/L citrate (3.22%) 123.6 mmol/L glucose 224.4 mmol/L sodium 114.2 mmol/L hydrogen ion	Variable: Hemosol B0+ (Gambro, Lund, Sweden) Hemosol B0 5.88% NaHCO₃ in varying amounts depending on patient's acid-base status. Baxter dialysate for hemodiafiltration (Baxter, Deerfield, IL) NORMOCARB HF (Dialysis Solutions, Whitby, ON, Canada)	16, 54
Hemodiafiltration	Alone	3-way stopcock at arterial entry into circuit	4% TSC: 136 mmol/L citrate 420 mmol/L sodium 0.4% TSC: 90 mL 4% TSC in 910 mL 5% dextrose solution	Custom dialysate: 117 mmol/L sodium 0-40 mmol/L bicarbonate 1.5-3 mEq/L magnesium 0.1-0.2% dextrose 0-6 mmol/L potassium 75-124 mmol/L chloride when using 4% TSC *or* 110 mmol/L sodium 110 mmol/L chloride 0.75 mmol/L magnesium when using 0.4% TSC	36, 41, 47

ACD-A, anticoagulant citrate dextrose-A; CRRT, continuous renal replacement therapy; MgCl, magnesium chloride; NaCl, sodium chloride; NaHCO₃, sodium bicarbonate; TSC, trisodium citrate.

TABLE 244-2

Anticoagulation for Continuous Renal Replacement Therapy

PATIENT CHARACTERISTICS	RECOMMENDATION
Low-bleeding risk*	Citrate, heparin, LMWH
High-bleeding risk†	Citrate, no anticoagulation
Active bleeding	No anticoagulation
Heparin-induced thrombocytopenia	Citrate, argatroban

*Platelet count > 60,000/mm³; aPTT < 45 sec; PT < 1.5 sec.
†Platelet count < 60,000/mm³; aPTT > 45 sec; PT > 1.5 sec.
aPTT, activated partial thromboplastin time; LMWH, low-molecular-weight heparin; PT, prothrombin time.

TABLE 244-3

METHOD	FILTER PRIMING	INITIAL DOSE	MAINTENANCE DOSE	MONITORING	MEAN FILTER LIFE (HOURS) (AS REPORTED IN LITERATURE)[26]	PRO	CON	OVER ANTICOAGULATION
No anticoagulation	None or with heparinized saline (5-8 iu/mL)	n/a	n/a	Filter thrombosis, filter pressure	3-70	No monitoring or risks associated with other anticoagulation regimens; adequate filter patency especially in high-risk patients with decreased platelets	Inadequate filter patency in all other patients	n/a
Heparin	Heparinized saline (5-8 iu/mL)	2000-5000 iu prefilter	3-15 iu/kg/hr prefilter	aPTT/ACT 1.5-2 times the upper limit of normal	15-50	Familiarity, effective anticoagulation, ease of monitoring in catheterized patient	Increased risk of hemorrhagic complications, HIT, adrenal insufficiency	Protamine administered 10 mg:100 u heparin (dose should be sum of prior 2-3 hours of heparin administration)
Low-dose heparin	None or heparinized saline (5-8 iu/mL)	None	500 iu/hr or 5 or 10 iu/kg/hr	Maintain normal or baseline range of systemic aPTT	19-32	Familiarity, defensive monitoring of AC rather than chasing the aPTT	Continued risk of bleeding, ineffective filter patency	As above
LMWH (dalteparin)	Heparinized saline or 1.5-2.5 u/mL of dalteparin	Bolus of 20 u/kg	Prefilter administration at 10 u/kg/hr	Recommendations are to monitor anti-Xa activity of 0.25-0.35 iu/mL	15.4-46.8	Similar patency rates as with heparin	More costly and pitfalls of heparin persist.	Protamine may be tried as above. Blood products may be required.
LMWH (enoxaparin)		750 u	0.05 mg/kg/hr	Anti-Xa activity 0.25-0.35 iu/mL	18-30 [range 0.75-72]	Similar patency rates as with heparin	More costly and pitfalls of heparin persist.	Same as above
Argatroban		250 µg/kg	0.5-2 µg/kg/min	aPTT aiming for 1 to 1.4 times the upper limit of normal	No significant data	Safe in renal failure. Established as treatment for HIT	No antidote for bleeding; aPTT may not absolutely correlate with anticoagulation	No antidote available. Blood products may be required.

TABLE 244-3—cont'd

METHOD	FILTER PRIMING	INITIAL DOSE	MAINTENANCE DOSE	MONITORING	MEAN FILTER LIFE (HOURS) (AS REPORTED IN LITERATURE)[26]	PRO	CON	OVER ANTICOAGULATION
Citrate (TSC or ACD-A administered alone prefilter)	None *or* with heparinized saline if no HIT present	140-160 mL/hr of 4% TSC given prefilter (3%-8% of the blood flow rates) or ACD-A citrate solution at 250 mL/hr	Vary rate of citrate in 5-10 mL/hr increments to maintain desired postfilter ionized calcium rates.	Maintain postfilter ionized calcium at 0.2-0.3 mmol/L. Use systemically administered calcium to maintain systemic ionized calcium within the normal range of the laboratory (1.0-1.2 mmol/L).	24-124	Ease of administration, ease of monitoring, low incidence of adverse events, ease of discontinuation if complications arise There may be improved biocompatibility with citrate.[49,50]	Difficulty in obtaining appropriate dialysate and citrate solution (depends on pharmacy availability); potential for metabolic alkalosis, hypernatremia, hyper- or hypocalcemia, or citrate toxicity	Rarely if ever occurs. If total calcium to ionized calcium ratio > 2:1 then lower citrate rate or turn off citrate anticoagulation.
Citrate (administered in replacement fluid prefilter)	None *or* with heparinized saline if no HIT present	Citrate can be given as a 0.4%, 0.5%, or 0.67% solution.	Varies depending on prescribed effluent dose (i.e., 35 mL/ kg/hr) or desired hourly fluid balance	Postfilter ionized calcium ranging 0.2-0.5 mmol/L. Systemic ionized calcium in normal range for laboratory.	48 to >72	Simpler than separate citrate administration; ability to utilize standardized dialysate or replacement fluids; similar filter longevity and metabolic stability as with citrate alone administration	Combining the goal of filter anticoagulation and dialysis dose leads to complexities in altering the rates of various fluids. The metabolic complications mentioned above are still a concern.	As above

AC, anticoagulation; ACD-A, anticoagulant citrate dextrose-A; ACT, activated coagulation time; aPTT, activated partial thromboplastin time; HIT, heparin-induced thrombocytopenia; LMWH, low-molecular-weight heparin; TSC, trisodium citrate.

2. Circuit functioning
   a. Positioning: Patient positioning may cause catheter kinking, especially with regard to femoral cannulation. Motorized hospital beds that change the bed-bound patient's position increase the potential for catheter kinking. Nursing care to avoid significant leg bending or avoidance of femoral catheters in these patients would be ideal.
   b. Access function: Venous and arterial pressure readings on the CRRT machine can give indirect evidence of access function and impending access failure. Peak venous pressures should remain less than 50% blood flow rate.[2] Increased pressure should lead to investigations of catheter positioning and patency.
   c. Visible clot formation: The hemofilter venous air trap should be periodically monitored for clot formation to indicate circuit failure.
3. Systemic effects: See Table 244-2.

RECOMMENDATIONS

Table 244-2 lists the recommendations for anticoagulation during CRRT. Table 244-3 lists anticoagulation dosing regimens and potential complications. These recommendations are made based on the available data regarding anticoagulation. (At our institution we use citrate for most situations, given the local support staff and the general success in providing sufficient CRRT support to most critically ill patients.) Less common agents such as prostacyclin, nafamostat, and APC are not included because the data on the safety and efficacy of their use are sparse. There is mounting evidence from prospective randomized and prospective cohort trials that citrate offers far better filter patency and a more favorable safety profile than heparin.[16,45-48] The local support staff, clinician expertise, and patient needs will ultimately guide anticoagulation choices. An established protocol for CRRT administration and system monitoring for clot formation should be established in each institution. Anticoagulation with citrate, heparin, or LMWH are well established in most health care centers, and efficacy and risk profile in appropriately selected patients are acceptable using any of these anticoagulants.

Key Points

1. Anticoagulation is necessary in the majority of cases requiring continuous renal replacement therapy to maintain filter life and efficacy; several options are available.
2. General measures such as circuit design (placement of anticoagulation at most proximal point; using dilute solutions; and, in the future, anticoagulation-coated filters or tubing) and operating characteristics (filtration fraction less than 20% to 30%; predilution) can set up to optimize filter life.
3. Citrate and heparin are the most extensively studied available anticoagulants for continuous renal replacement therapy. Data supporting the safety and efficacy of citrate over heparin are mounting. Continuous renal replacement therapy may be run without anticoagulation in selected individuals only (thrombocytopenia less than 60,000/µL being the key factor).
4. Systematic monitoring of appropriate clinical parameters will optimize efficacy and minimize systemic complications of anticoagulation (activated partial thromboplastin time for heparin; total ionized calcium ratio plus postfilter ionized calcium for citrate).
5. Choice and selection of appropriate anticoagulation are dependent on pathophysiological considerations of disease process, as well as available support systems for appropriate delivery of care.

Key References

6. Weijmer MC, van den Dorpel MA, Van de Ven PJG, et al: Randomized, clinical trial comparison of trisodium citrate 30% and heparin as catheter-locking solution in hemodialysis patients. J Am Soc Nephrol 2005;16(9):2769-2777.
16. Brophy PD, Somers MJ, Baum MA, et al: Multi-centre evaluation of anticoagulation in patients receiving continuous renal replacement therapy (CRRT). Nephrol Dial Transplant 2005;20(7):1416-1421.
26. Oudemans-van Straaten HM, Wester JP, de Pont AC, Schetz MR: Anticoagulation strategies in continuous renal replacement therapy: Can the choice be evidence based? Intensive Care Med 2006;32(2):188-202.
35. Mehta RL: Anticoagulation during continuous renal replacement therapy. ASAIO J 1994;40(4):931-935.
39. Tolwani AJ, Prendergast MB, Speer RR, et al: A practical citrate anticoagulation continuous venovenous hemodiafiltration protocol for metabolic control and high solute clearance. Clin J Am Soc Nephrol 2006;1:79-87.

See the companion Expert Consult website for the complete reference list.

CHAPTER 245

Strategies to Prevent Coagulation of the Extracorporeal Circuit

Ian Baldwin

OBJECTIVES

This chapter will:
1. Highlight that clotting in the continuous renal replacement therapy circuit is complex and affected by many factors in the critically ill patient.
2. Anticoagulant agents can prevent or delay clotting but are not the only preventive strategy necessary.
3. Indicate that clotting occurs either in the membrane or the venous air trap chamber and proposes how this clot may form.
4. Discuss the need to prevent clotting by ensuring the extracorporeal circuit is not mechanically obstructed and blood flow is maintained.
5. Describe the influence of the access catheter and site, membrane and venous chamber, predilution fluid administration, blood flow setting, and nursing competence on circuit clotting.

The mechanism for blood coagulation in the renal replacement therapy (RRT) extracorporeal circuit (EC) supporting a critically ill patient is complex. Acute renal failure, inflammation with critical illness, and other factors influence the normal roles of key mediators such as thrombin, tissue factor, platelets, and endothelium. A precise explanation of how clotting occurs, or why it does not occur, when blood is being pumped outside the body via plastic tubes is not easily explained.[1,2,3] This may also explain why a wide variation in response to anticoagulation strategies to prevent clotting in the EC can be observed, with time before clotting ranging from only hours to several days with and without anticoagulation, and despite improvements in RRT technology and clinician expertise over the past 10 years.[2,4] However, clotting in the EC is inevitable because this nonbiological environment places blood under stress, with coagulation occurring at places of high resistance, stasis, and positive or negative pressures with shearing forces. In this respect, the blood is behaving normally. During flow through the EC, cells and plasma separate, cellular aggregation occurs, proteins deposit or build up, and an inflammatory response occurs. This may explain why thrombin generation is increased during continuous hemofiltration by activation of the tissue factor pathway,[5] with this being only one of the many responses causing coagulation. Although anticoagulants can be successful in delaying clot formation and make a RRT procedure functional for long periods of time without clotting, there are components of the EC and other influences on the EC that are important as adjuncts to the use of anticoagulants and are very important when anticoagulation is not used.

CLOTTING: WHERE AND HOW?

The two components of the EC where clotting occurs are the hemofilter (membrane) and the venous bubble trap chamber.[1,6] Coagulation is not common along the circuit tubing or in the blood pump tubing segment. Additional chambers in the EC for fluid addition, or where smaller tubing enters the main blood path at a T junction, may also be sites of clot formation. However, clot development in these components is not a cause of circuit failure unless the clot formed at these junctions breaks off and embolizes into the main circuit path, obstructing flow into the membrane. This type of EC embolus clotting can obstruct blood flow at the entry of blood to the membrane or the exit of the venous chamber, causing an abrupt cessation to treatment by total blood flow obstruction, with an inability to return the EC blood to the patient. Figure 245-1 shows a clot obstructing blood flow into a membrane. The picture depicts a membrane autopsy: Immediately after clotting, the membrane is cut in half to reveal the site of the clot obstructing the membrane at blood entry rather than by clotting along the fibers of the membrane, which is a slower progressive process. Figure 245-2 shows a venous chamber with a large clot formed in the chamber, which can break off from the top section of the chamber and move down to the outlet, thereby causing an acute obstruction.

It is assumed that circuit life data reflect the time before membrane fiber clotting; however, the membrane entry port or the venous chamber may clot before, and independent of, the membrane fibers. Not only do these events constitute a failure of the circuit but also, in the case of the venous chamber, unless the venous tubing segment can be changed quickly, blood flow cannot continue and the circuit volume of blood may not be returned (discarded) to the patient despite the membrane(s) itself being unaffected.[7,8]

Therefore, strategies to prevent clot formation in the EC are essentially aimed at these two components: the membrane and the venous bubble trap. For a more complete understanding of this problem when using continuous RRT (CRRT), the discussion needs to include all of the EC components and their contribution to circuit clotting at these two sites.

ANTICOAGULANTS

Anticoagulant drugs prevent or delay the formation of clot in the EC, and many methods are used with variability in

Membrane autopsy: cross-section cut after clotting

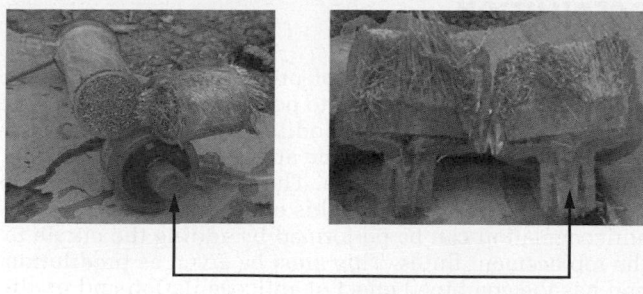

Clot formation at blood entry to membrane

FIGURE 245-1. A membrane autopsy revealing clot at the entrance to the membrane where resistance to flow occurs. A common site for clot formation independent of the membrane fibers.

Top: at blood level   Bottom: at chamber filter

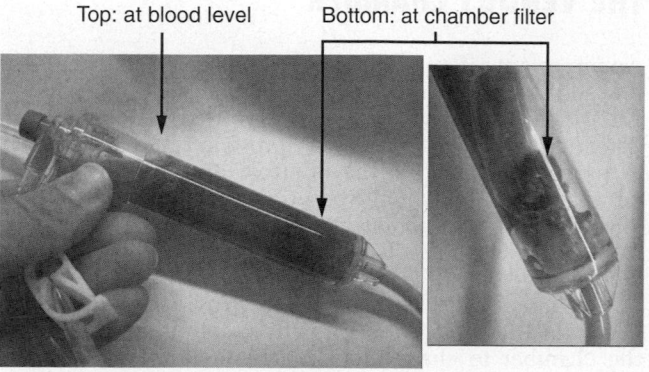

Clot formation in venous air trap chamber

FIGURE 245-2. The venous air trap chamber showing clot formation commonly occurring at the top of the chamber and at the bottom around the outlet filter.

the quality of evidence supporting their success and safety.[9] However, the effectiveness of any anticoagulant, or the dose used, may be limited by the component and mechanical design of the EC. This suggests that in addition to an effective anticoagulant drug, or more importantly when no anticoagulation is used in patients at risk of bleeding, other strategies to prevent clot formation in the EC are useful to implement at all times, in every patient treatment (see Chapter 244 for more on anticoagulants and anticoagulation strategies).

When clotting does occur in the EC, differentiating between component failure (mechanical obstruction) and anticoagulant failure (dose too low) is very important so that the correct remedy is used.[9-11] For example, prescribing an increase in heparin dose may not be appropriate when the cause is mechanical obstruction in the EC.

THE ACCESS CATHETER AND SITE

The double-lumen venovenous access catheter commonly used for CRRT is not a common place for clot formation.

However, the access catheter is implicated in the formation of clot. The essential task of the catheter is to allow blood to be drawn from the patient vein into the EC and to be returned to the vein from the EC. The catheter must be patent in order to allow both functions and, in addition, must not offer too much resistance to this flow. As blood pump speed increases, a greater demand is placed on the catheter (increasing negative arterial pressure) such that if the lumen size is inadequate, or the lumens are obstructed, the pump sucking blood from the catheter will fail and not deliver its prescribed output. This can then cause slowing of blood flow to the membrane and clotting, as ultrafiltration continues irrespective of blood-flow indicator speed.[12] Although not often an immediately identifiable event, covert access catheter failure leading to unrecognized reduced blood flow may be a causative factor in membrane clotting. Furthermore, if obstruction to the venous or return limb of the double-lumen catheter occurs (high venous pressure), this creates stasis and slowing of blood flow in the venous bubble trap chamber, also promoting clotting in this chamber.

The site (e.g., femoral, subclavian, internal jugular) of the venous access catheter may be related to more or less potential for obstruction. However, there is no published study for reference, despite many useful reviews of the topic.[13] Nurses' anecdotal experience can generate many opinions on this topic as they observe a strong relationship between patient positioning and access function. For example, when a patient is supine and not sitting up, the femoral vein site may function well; however, if this patient is sitting toward 90 degrees, the catheter may fail. This may also apply to the subclavian or internal jugular site, with no obstruction when the patient is lying flat due to higher venous pressure. Side lying can also create obstruction, particularly at the subclavian site, with shoulder flexion and kinking of the catheter. Nursing care and physical therapy must be managed with caution and with attention to changes in arterial and venous circuit pressures indicating catheter obstruction. In some situations it may be better to pause the fluid exchange process, slow the blood pump to 50% of set treatment speed, and then move the patient. After the move is complete, the blood pump can be slowly returned to treatment speed, the arterial and venous pressures should be monitored, and subtle maneuvers can be made to the patient position to preserve stability before restarting the fluid exchange. This strategy is highly recommended when moving a patient connected to CRRT out of bed to a suitable recliner chair in the intensive care unit (ICU).

THE BLOOD PUMP–FLOW SPEED

Blood flow controlled by the blood pump setting may have some influence on the development of EC clot formation.[11,14] In theory, a faster blood flow rate means less clot formation. A blood flow rate of 200 mL/min is commonly applied and is adequate to maintain flow across the length of the circuit, with minimal stasis, but not too fast to increase resistance and create turbulence and cell damage with shearing forces at resistance points, such as where blood is entering the membrane or exiting the venous chamber. When convective clearance is the sole mechanism for solute removal and replacement fluids are administered after the hemofilter (postdilution), blood flow must be adequate for the ultrafiltration rate setting to minimize concentration of blood in the hemofilter. For example, with an ultrafiltration rate of 2 L/hr or 33 mL/min, a blood flow rate of 200 mL/min is suitable as the plasma water removal is less than 15% of the blood flow.

When using diffusive clearance techniques, hemoconcentration such as this is less important, but blood flow up to 200 mL/min is used to maintain flow and prevent blood stasis. This suggests a relationship may exist between clearance mode or technique and potential for clotting in the EC. While there is currently no prospective study published, some clinicians suggest that convection clearance (continuous venovenous hemofiltration [CVVH]) may have a higher potential for clotting in comparison to diffusive clearance (continuous venovenous hemodiafiltration [CVVHDF]),[15,16] with data from a small study presented as an abstract indicating a significant difference in circuit life favoring CVVHDF.[17] This was a randomized crossover design study treating 45 patients with CVVH (50 circuits—mean life 8 hr 39 min) and CVVHDF (43 circuits—mean life 18 hr 6 min), $P < 0.001$.

MEMBRANES: TYPE, SIZE, HEPARIN COATING

Membranes used for CRRT vary in fiber composition and surface area. It is also common to add heparin into a circuit during or after priming to heparin-coat the membrane.[2,7,8,18] There is no good evidence to suggest this has any effect on all membranes; however, plastic and membrane surfaces do uptake heparin, particularly after treating to neutralize negative charge,[19,20] and thromboresistance with reduced clotting has been reported in bovine experiments[21] with a surface-coated membrane. Therefore, unless contraindicated, heparin can be added to a circuit after priming and before connection to the patient and circulated within the EC at a slow blood pump speed to promote distribution and the coating effect. Depending on dose used and the specific patient requirements, this heparin may be flushed out before it is connected to the patient, or a bolus dose prior to use of heparin during treatment can be considered—for example, 5000 international units of heparin into a circuit priming bag of 100 mL saline. Then set the blood pump machine at 50 mL/min for 10 to 20 minutes with both limbs of the circuit into the priming bag for continuous recirculation.

Different fiber types may also influence clotting.[22-24] Although synthetic membranes are considered biocompatible, one patient may have premature clotting when exposed to an acrylonitrile membrane as opposed to a polysulfone membrane, or vice versa. There may also be some differences in racial and genetic disposition to clotting for different membrane compositions.[25] If one type of membrane clots frequently despite anticoagulation and when no anticoagulation is used, trying a different membrane composition can be useful. Finally, larger surface area membranes may take longer to clot, possibly because of resistance to blood flow[26] or simply the surface area itself. This can be useful in the context of adults with frequent occurrence of membrane clotting. Increasing the membrane size from 1.4 m^2 to 1.42 or a 40% increase may create an increase in time before clotting and failure.

FLUID ADMINISTRATION— PREDILUTION

There is evidence that use of predilution reduces membrane clotting in comparison to postdilution in convection clearance CVVH.[27] The hemodilution of blood prior to passage through the membrane appears to reduce clot formation by hematocrit change. The amount of predilution volume required to achieve this effect is not clear. Citrate anticoagulation can be performed by adding the citrate to the replacement fluids. This must be given as predilution and has the combined effect of anticoagulation and predilution.[28] Predilution fluids must enter the CRRT circuit after the blood pump so that they increase the blood flow. If the fluids are administered before the blood pump, they become a percentage of the blood flow and reduce blood delivery to the membrane.

THE VENOUS CHAMBER

An important safety feature of any EC is an air trap chamber placed in the EC prior to the blood returning to the patient. An ultrasound wave is passed through the chamber to detect air. A mesh filter is also provided in this chamber to prevent a clot from the EC from entering the patient circulation. There should be no further line connections after the venous bubble trap bypassing these safety features. However, this EC component is often a site for clotting.[1,2,7,11,29]

A chamber must be included to provide a wider open space for these features. This allows blood after entering the chamber to change its flow characteristics, with the chamber level rising and falling consistent with the pulsatile flow of the blood pump, and the varying resistance at the return limb of the access catheter. It is necessary to permit a pocket of gas (air or CO_2) above the blood level to act as a conduit for pressure readings when connected to a pressure sensor and transducer. This is effective and adequate for a pressure display in millimeters of mercury (mm Hg), despite being damped in comparison to fluid-filled pressure-monitoring systems with high resonance. The blood level in this chamber fluctuates up and down with an amplitude and frequency directly proportional to the main blood pump speed and venous return pressure(s). This causes a constant blood smearing and cell deposition on the inside of the chamber and eventually creates a ring around the chamber that gradually builds to form a clot (Fig. 245-3). The process appears to be hastened by the coagulability of the blood, amount of gas allowed in the chamber, and the chamber profile-shape. To prevent this clot formation, readjustment of the blood level in this chamber to below the clot formation may reduce clot formation when frequent chamber clotting occurs. Therefore, starting treatment with a full chamber is desirable.

Attempts have been made to prevent this clotting by adding heparin into the chamber before and during use,[30] adding fluids into the chamber (postdilution), and using a design with incoming blood entering under the blood level. This last approach can create a cell-plasma separation with a small layer of plasma separating to the top of the chamber providing a blanket protecting the cells from exposure to the gas and reducing cell smearing with adhesion. None of these clot prevention methods is supported by data to suggest they are effective.

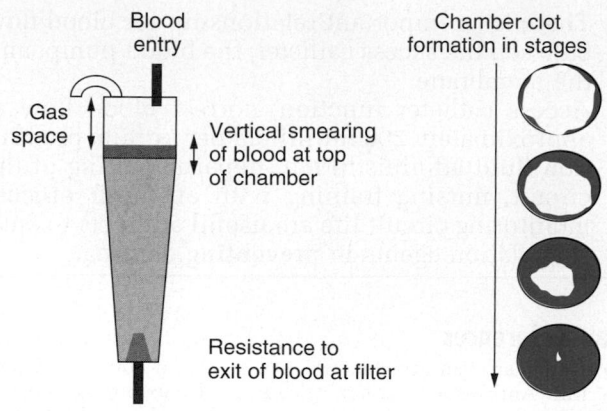

FIGURE 245-3. A schematic of the venous chamber showing the mechanism by which a clot forms. Smearing of blood at the top of the chamber with a fluctuating blood level is consistent with the blood pump rotations and access catheter resistance. This causes cell adhesion and clot formation with eventual obstruction.

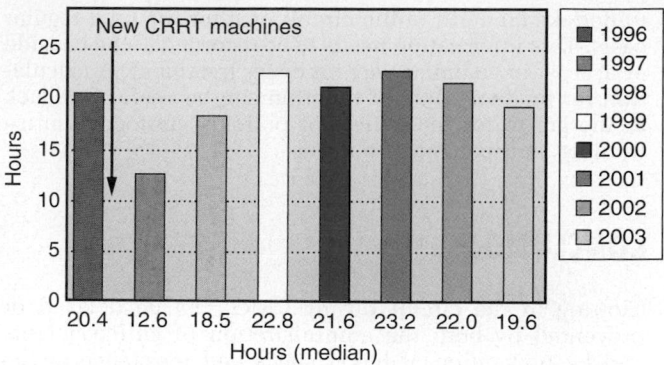

FIGURE 245-4. Filter life data indicated as the median. A reduction in median filter life can reflect loss of skills and poor troubleshooting ability among medical personnel, for example, after new continuous renal replacement therapy (CRRT) machines are introduced to an intensive care unit.

However, despite a lack of supporting evidence, it is common practice and may be useful to (1) keep the venous chamber full of blood, thereby minimizing the gas pocket, (2) adjust the level down when a ring of clot begins to form, (3) add postdilution fluids directly into this chamber when used, and (4) add heparin into the chamber during the priming procedure of heparin coating.

Manufacturers are attempting to modify and/or eliminate the venous chamber from the CRRT EC, but because the safety feature must be retained, this is difficult. Gambro did this with the Prisma machine (Gambro, Lyon, France), but it has reintroduced a de-aeration chamber with the latest Prismaflex machine.

CRRT AND MULTIDISCIPLINARY TEAM

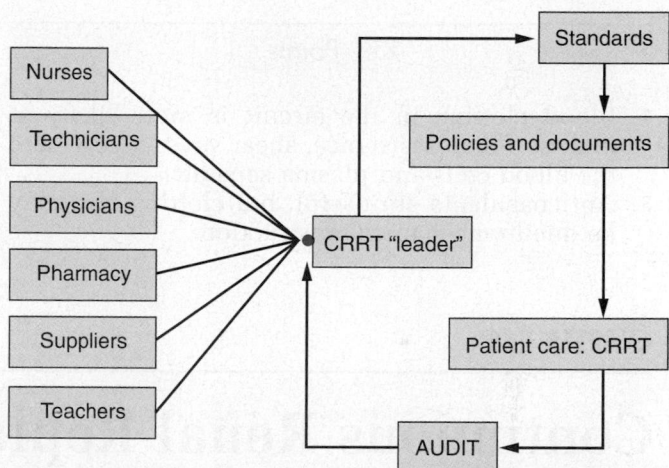

FIGURE 245-5. The team and audit concept for successful use of continuous renal replacement therapy (CRRT) as an important strategy to prevent excessive clotting.

TRAINING, EDUCATION, AND THE MULTIDISCIPLINARY TEAM

Safe and skilled use of CRRT machines requires nursing education and training activities. In addition, without a suitable education process providing both theoretical and practical information, patient safety and successful, effective therapy will be compromised. It is more likely that premature clotting of the EC will occur if nurses managing the treatment do not understand the strategies discussed in this chapter and have poor troubleshooting skills for maintaining blood flow. For example, in the event of blood pump stoppage for an alarm event such as arterial or negative access pressure, if the pump is stopped for a prolonged period, blood stasis and clot development are likely. Where nursing skills are poor in an ICU and nephrology nurses are required to attend the ICU for such troubleshooting, the time delay involved can cause a simple alarm event to be unrecoverable due to clotting without blood pump operation. Current machines have troubleshooting prompts on screen displays and unlatched alarms that reset the alarm and restart the treatment if the error corrects itself. However, other alarms, such as air in the line, are latched and will not reset, and the blood pump will stop until a reset function is selected and the air is removed. Although this event may be easily rectified by a skilled nurse, untrained nurses may take a prolonged time or fail to fix the alarm, thus prolonging a period of no blood flow.

There are many strategies to train nurses for these events, using simulation setup of the machine and EC, interactive video activities of these alarms, and simple tutorial activities on a drawing whiteboard.[7,31] Bedside records indicating circuit life are useful and, when audited, can reflect variations in nursing expertise. A reduction in median circuit life may be associated with a reduction in nursing expertise. Figure 245-4 indicates circuit life audits over many years in a large ICU setting and reflects the reduction in circuit life after the introduction of new CRRT machines, with a recovery of expertise following.

A multidisciplinary team is also important to success and without a leader or similar person(s) to champion the cause, poor outcomes of CRRT use, including frequent circuit clotting, may occur. This team must include senior medical, nursing, nursing teacher, pharmacy, technical, allied health, and industry or suppliers. A final and further strategy to prevent clotting in the EC is to develop and nurture such a team with suitable leaders and specialist clinicians (Fig. 245-5). The team must meet regularly and undertake an audit of the circuit or filter life on a regular basis. This information needs to be recorded at the bedside or at least in a similar way for every treatment. A calculation for median hours of function can be useful feedback to the group for the review of policies, protocols, nurse training, and patient care needs.

CONCLUSION

Clotting in the circuit during CRRT can be delayed or prevented by both the administration of anticoagulants and by prevention of blood stasis and resistance in the circuit. Clot formation is a complex hematological process in the critically ill patient, but clotting in the circuit membrane and venous chamber can be prevented by attention to blood flow mechanics, particularly when no anticoagulation is necessary. Nursing training and close monitoring of circuit life provide important feedback to a medical team focused on CRRT and preventive clotting strategies.

Key Points

1. Blood clotting in the circuit is more likely at places of high resistance, shear stress, and where the blood cells and plasma separate.
2. Anticoagulants are useful, but clotting also may be due to mechanical obstruction.

3. There is an important relationship for blood flow between the access catheter, the blood pump, and the membrane.
4. Access catheter function, correct blood flow at approximately 200 milliliters per minute predilution fluid administration, heparin coating of the circuit, nursing training with an audit process monitoring circuit life are useful adjuncts to anticoagulation agents in preventing clotting.

Key References

9. Oudemans-van Straaten HM, Wester JP, de Pont AC, Schetz MR: Anticoagulation strategies in continuous renal replacement therapy: can the choice be evidence based ? Intensive Care Med 2006;32:188-202.
10. Baldwin I, Bellomo R, Koch W: Blood flow reductions during continuous renal replacement therapy and circuit life. Intensive Care Med 2004;30:2074-2079.
11. Webb AR, Mythen, MG, Jacobsen D, Mackie IJ: Maintaining blood flow in the extracorporeal circuit: Haemostasis and anticoagulation. Intensive Care Med 1995;21:84-93.
12. Baldwin I, Bellomo R: The relationship between blood flow, access catheter and circuit failure during CRRT: A practical review. Contrib Nephrol 2004;144:203-213.
27. Uchino S, Fealy N, Baldwin I, Morimatsu H, Bellomo R: Predilution vs. post-dilution during continuous veno-venous hemofiltration: Impact on filter life and azotemic control. Nephron Clin Pract 2003;94:94-98.

See the companion Expert Consult website for the complete reference list.

CHAPTER 246

Continuous Renal Replacement Therapy: Hemofiltration, Hemodiafiltration, or Hemodialysis?

Rinaldo Bellomo and Claudio Ronco

OBJECTIVES

This chapter will:
1. Review the principles of continuous renal replacement therapy.
2. Discuss the practical application of continuous renal replacement therapy and the consequences of such application.
3. Examine the consequences of technical modifications to continuous renal replacement therapy.
4. Provide information pertaining to choices and prescription of continuous renal replacement therapy.

Endogenous toxins accumulate in blood as a result of many biochemical processes.[1] If their concentration exceeds certain levels, they cause illness. Some toxins are volatile (CO_2, ketones) and can be excreted by the lungs

through ventilation, others are lipophilic (bile acids, bilirubin) and can be excreted by the liver via the biliary system, and others are water soluble and nonvolatile and are excreted by the kidneys (Table 246-1).[1] When the kidneys fail acutely, removal of such water-soluble toxins requires acute artificial renal replacement therapy (RRT).[2]

Water-soluble toxins exist in blood at various concentrations. Blood is a complex fluid containing cells and plasma. Plasma is a complex solution, and it is the plasma compartment of blood that is available for purification by RRT. Plasma contains myriad solutes (electrolytes, proteins, lipids, carbohydrates, vitamins, amino acids), which are dissolved in plasma water (the solvent). Only those solutes that are water soluble and not protein bound (free solutes) are available for removal by classic RRT. This is because the conventional biosynthetic membranes used for RRT have an in vivo cutoff point of about 15 to 20 kilodaltons (kD), which does not allow the passage of

TABLE 246-1

Route of Blood Purification for Various Toxins

TOXIN	ROUTE
CO_2	Lung
Other volatile toxins	Lung
Ketones	Lung and kidney
Bilirubin	Liver and kidney
Biliary acids	Liver
Fat-soluble toxins	Liver and (after conjugation) kidney
Urea	Kidney
Water-soluble toxins	Kidney

anything beyond small proteins (such as β_2-microglobulin).[3] Accordingly, the following discussion of blood purification principles and techniques relates to free solutes of relatively small to small-medium molecular weight (<15 kD). The chapter does not discuss peritoneal dialysis where the dialyzing membrane is the peritoneum and where some larger proteins are removed during the blood purification process. Also not discussed in this chapter are different forms of plasma therapies where protein-bound solutes can be removed through high-porosity membranes.

Extracorporeal techniques are broadly named *renal replacement therapy* (RRT) and include continuous or intermittent hemofiltration, hemodialysis, or hemodiafiltration, each with its own technical variations. All of these techniques rely on the principle of removing unwanted solutes and water through a membrane separation process.

PRINCIPLES OF SOLUTE REMOVAL

The principles of RRT have been extensively studied and described.[2,4,5] This section provides a summary of some technical aspects of RRT, which are particularly relevant for the critical care physician.

Water Removal

The removal of excess solvent (water) is therapeutically at least as important as the removal of unwanted solutes (acid, uremic toxins, potassium, and the like). During RRT, water is removed through a process called *ultrafiltration*. This process is essentially the same as that performed by the glomerulus. It requires a pressure gradient (generated by blood flow and circuit resistance) to move water across a semipermeable membrane. This is because plasma water would normally be kept within the circulation due to oncotic pressure. This ultrafiltration is achieved by generating a positive hydrostatic pressure (as in hemofiltration or during intermittent hemodialysis) which is greater than oncotic pressure. The final result is a positive transmembrane pressure that drives fluid through the membrane at a rate dependent on the hydraulic permeability coefficient and the surface of the membrane.

Solute Removal

The removal of retention solutes can be achieved by creating a transmembrane pressure–driven "solvent drag," where solute moves together with solvent (convection) across a porous membrane. Solvent with unwanted solutes is discarded as effluent and then replaced with toxin-free fluid containing electrolytes (hemofiltration). The rate of transport of the solute depends on the relationship between solute radius (or molecular weight) and the radius of membrane pores. Solutes smaller than the pores will pass freely through the membrane and will not be "rejected" (rejection coefficient = 0), whereas solutes larger than the pores will be fully rejected (rejection coefficient = 1). Since it is difficult to establish a priori the rejection coefficient, in practice the physician can observe and measure the sieving coefficient, which is exactly the opposite of the rejection coefficient corrected for empirical factors. Solute clearance will be determined by the product of ultrafiltration rate by the value of measured sieving. Sieving is measured easily by the ratio between the concentration in the filtrate and that in plasma water.

Unwanted solutes also can be removed by creating a chemical gradient across the membrane using a "flow past" system with toxin-free dialysate (diffusion) as in hemodialysis.

The rate of diffusion of a given solute depends on (1) its molecular weight (diffusivity coefficient), (2) the porosity of the membrane, (3) its surface and its thickness, (4) the blood flow rate and the dialysate flow rate (which generates the concentration gradient and prevents equilibration due to blood and dialysate stagnation), (5) its concentration gradient across the membrane, (6) its binding to proteins, (7) its electrical charge, and (8) finally the temperature at which the process takes place. If standard, low-flux, cellulose-based membranes are used, middle molecules greater than 500 daltons (D) molecular weight can hardly be removed. If synthetic high-flux membranes are used (cutoff at 15 to 20 kD in molecular weight), larger molecules can be removed to a certain extent. However, with these membranes, convection is superior to diffusion in achieving the clearance of middle molecules.

CONTINUOUS RENAL REPLACEMENT THERAPY

First described in 1977, continuous renal replacement therapy (CRRT) has undergone several technical modifications. Initially, it was performed as an arteriovenous therapy (continuous arteriovenous hemofiltration [CAVH]), where blood flow through the hemofilter is driven by the patient's blood pressure. However, clearances were low because blood flow was low (often <80 mL/min) and ultrafiltration was low. Thus, countercurrent dialysate flow was soon added to double or triple solute clearances (continuous arteriovenous hemodialysis or hemodiafiltration [CAVHD or CAVHDF, respectively]), with or without spontaneous ultrafiltration. The need to cannulate an artery, however, is associated with 15% to 20% morbidity. Accordingly, double-lumen catheters and peristaltic blood pumps have come into use (continuous venovenous hemofiltration [CVVH]) with control of ultrafiltration rate. Because blood flow (often set at 200 mL/min) is no longer a limiting factor, venovenous technology has made hemofiltration easily able to deliver the necessary clearances

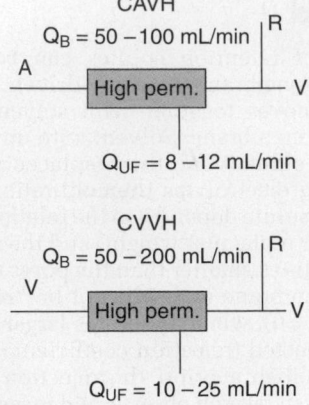

FIGURE 246-1. Diagrams illustrating an arteriovenous and a venovenous circuit for continuous hemofiltration. The top circuit represents continuous arteriovenous hemofiltration (CAVH) with spontaneous generation of ultrafiltrate (UF) and postfilter administration of replacement fluid (R). The bottom circuit represents continuous venovenous hemofiltration (CVVH). The letters A (arterial) and V (venous) refer to the source of blood. Ranges of possible values for blood flow (Q_B) and ultrafiltrate flow (Q_{UF}) are provided.

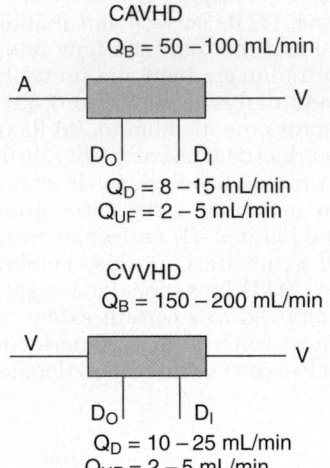

FIGURE 246-2. Diagrams illustrating an arteriovenous and a venovenous circuit for continuous hemodialysis. The top circuit represents continuous arteriovenous hemodialysis (CAVHD) with countercurrent dialysate flow. The bottom circuit represents continuous venovenous hemodialysis (CVVHD) with countercurrent dialysate flow. The letters A (arterial) and V (venous) refer to the source of blood. D_I and D_O represent the dialysate inflow and outflow ports. Ranges of possible values for blood flow (Q_B) and dialysate flow (Q_D) are provided.

again (Fig. 246-1). In the developed world, essentially all CRRT is now carried out in venovenous mode.[3]

In a venovenous system, dialysate can also be delivered countercurrent to blood flow (continuous venovenous hemodialysis [CVVHD]) to achieve almost purely diffusive clearance (Fig. 246-2). Purely diffusive clearance is, however, never possible as ultrafiltration is always necessary to remove some solvent. Accordingly, a degree of ultrafiltration with convective clearance must always occur, over a 24-hour cycle, even with CVVHD.

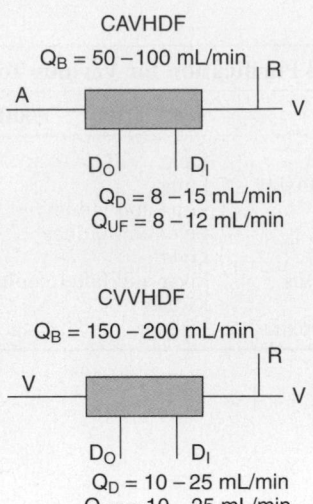

FIGURE 246-3. Diagrams illustrating an arteriovenous and a venovenous circuit for continuous hemodiafiltration. The top circuit represents continuous arteriovenous hemodiafiltration with countercurrent dialysate flow (CAVHDF) and postfilter replacement fluid (R). The bottom circuit represents continuous venovenous hemodiafiltration with countercurrent dialysate flow (CVVHDF) and postfilter replacement fluid. The letters A (arterial) and V (venous) refer to the source of blood. Q_B represents blood flow, Q_D, dialysate flow, and Q_{UF}, ultrafiltrate flow. D_I and D_O represent the dialysate inflow and outflow ports. Ranges of possible values for Q_B and Q_D are provided.

Furthermore, even without ultrafiltration, within the filter there are differences in hydraulic pressure and colloid oncotic pressure relationship such that the hydraulic pressure is greater than the colloid oncotic pressure, and transmembrane pressure is positive. Thus, there is a degree of convection within the membrane microenvironment in all patients. Also, depending on the type of membrane and the blood flow rate or dialysate flow rate and their relationship, other events such as backfiltration typically occur. Nonetheless, the feature that separates hemodialysis from hemodiafiltration is the fact that, in hemodialysis, no replacement fluid is given.

Finally, diffusion and convection can be coupled, as in continuous venovenous hemodiafiltration (CVVHDF) (Fig. 246-3).[6] In this mode, there might be, for example, ultrafiltration at 1 L/hr and dialysate flow at 1 L/hr resulting in an effluent of 2 L/hr and the need for 1 L/hr of replacement fluid, if no fluid loss is planned. This approach would combine convection and diffusion in almost equal proportions.

These concepts, as discussed for continuous therapies, also apply to intermittent therapies. The only differences will, of course, relate to blood flow, dialysate flow, or ultrafiltration rate and replacement fluid rate. The possible combinations of blood flow rate, dialysate flow rate, ultrafiltration rate, and replacement fluid rate are almost infinite.

No matter what technique is used, the clinician needs to understand the solute clearance implications of using one versus the other and the solute clearance implications of using so-called predilution (the replacement fluid is administered before the filter) or postdilution (the replacement fluid is administered after the filter).

Hemofiltration, Hemodialysis, and Hemodiafiltration

If replacement fluid is given after the filter (postdilution) and 2 L of effluent (the fluid that is discarded) is generated each hour, urea and creatinine clearance is essentially the same whether hemofiltration is performed with 2 L of replacement fluid per hour, hemodialysis with 2 L of dialysate fluid per hour, or hemodiafiltration with 1 L of dialysate fluid plus 1 L of replacement fluid per hour.

That is because, for all three techniques, the effluent-to-plasma concentration ratio for urea or creatinine will be essentially 1.

Thus, for small solutes, the choice of technique does not matter.

However, if replacement fluid is given postfilter, the hematocrit will rise within the filter as plasma water is removed (Fig. 246-4). For example, if blood flow is 150 mL/min and the hematocrit is 30% (50 mL), plasma flow will be 100 mL/min. If ultrafiltration is 2 L/hr, 33 mL/min of plasma water will then be removed. Thus, at the return end of the filter, the amount of plasma water will be 67 mL, which, added to 50 mL of cells, will deliver an intrafilter hematocrit of 42.7%. This is a significant increase, which will also be associated with a similar percentage increase in intrafilter platelet count and protein concentration. This

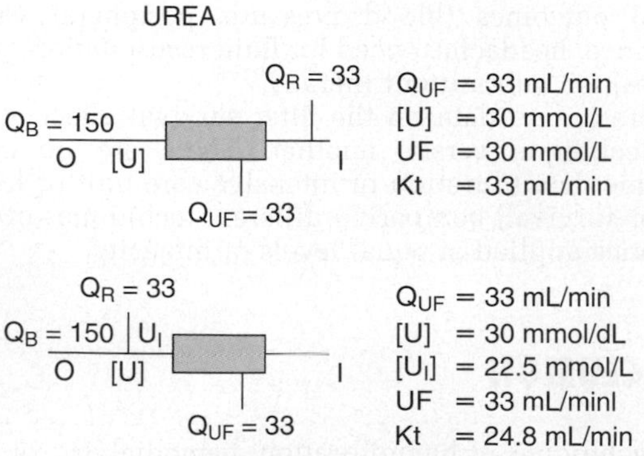

FIGURE 246-4. Diagrams illustrating the differences between continuous venovenous hemofiltration (CVVH) in postdilution and CVVH in predilution. The letters U and U_I refer to the concentration of urea in the patient's blood entering the circuit (U) and the same blood after dilution with prefilter replacement fluid (U_I) at the inlet of the filter. I, inflow port of the catheter; Kt, clearance; O, outflow port of the double-lumen catheter; Q_B, blood flow; Q_R, replacement fluid rate; Q_{UF}, ultrafiltration rate; UF, ultrafiltrate.

concentrating effect on red cells, platelets, and proteins will, of course, be attenuated by any increase in blood flow. However, even with a blood flow of 200 mL/min, the statistical probability of filter clotting will rise and filter life will shorten (see Fig. 246-4).[7]

In addition, if the filtration fraction (effluent flow rate/plasma flow rate) is high (>30%), some loss of clearance (especially for middle molecules) will occur as proteins and cells are pushed against the membrane by transmembrane pressure and form a proteinaceous layer (so-called concentration polarization) on top of it, which decreases functional pore size and number. These observations have clear implications if a clinician moves to perform so-called high-volume hemofiltration (need to increase blood flow, need to maintain acceptable filtration fraction).[8,9]

Finally, these observations not only apply to CVVH but also to the convective component of CVVHDF and to any intermittent therapy that employs substantial convective clearance. They do not apply to CVVHD or conventional intermittent hemodialysis or diffusive sustained low-efficiency dialysis.[10]

Faced with the problem of hemoconcentration if postdilution is used, the clinician could reasonably turn to so-called predilution. This approach to fluid replacement essentially eliminates hemoconcentration and can be expected to increase filter life.

However, predilution will also dilute the very solutes that one wishes to clear. The proportional dilution will be equal to the replacement fluid flow rate/plasma flow rate ratio (see Fig. 246-4). If replacement fluid is delivered pre–blood pump, dilution will also be greater than if it is delivered post–blood pump. For example, if blood flow is 150 mL/min and the hematocrit is 30%, plasma flow will be 100 mL. If predilution fluid is administered at 33 mL/min (2 L/hr) after the blood pump but before the filter, urea dilution will occur. If the rate was 30 mmol/L in the patient's plasma, it will then become 22.5 mmol/L when it enters the filter. As the clearance is equal to ultrafiltration rate × (urea) in the ultrafiltrate, urea clearance will be significantly decreased with predilution as compared with postdilution (see Fig. 246-4). However, other events happen, which tend to attenuate this decrease in clearance. They include diminished concentration polarization due to protein dilution, increased wall shear rate (i.e., an increased velocity gradient at the blood membrane interface, which keeps the inner membrane clean), minimized filtration fraction, and the movement of urea from red cells into plasma following dilution. Clearly, no such dilution would occur with CVVHD and only half the dilution would occur with CVVHDF, if half the effluent was replaced prefilter (Table 246-2).

TABLE 246-2

Estimated Clearances of Small Solutes with Various Techniques of Continuous Renal Replacement Therapy at Zero Fluid Balance*

TECHNIQUE	PLASMA FLOW (mL/min)	PREFILTER RF FLOW (mL/min)	EFFLUENT FLOW (mL/min)	DIAYSATE FLOW (mL/min)	CLEARANCE (mL/min)
CVVH	100	33.3	33.3	0	25
CVVH	100	0	33.3	0	33.3
CVVHD	100	0	33.3	33.3	33.3
CVVHDF	100	16.6	33.3	16.6	29.1
CVVHDF	100	0	33.3	16.6	33.3

*Effluent = the replacement fluid rate, the dialysate flow rate, or both. When the prefilter replacement fluid (RF) flow = 0, then the RF is given postfilter for CVVH and CVVHDF. If it is 16.6 mL/min, the other 16.6 mL/min is given postfilter.
CVVH, continuous venovenous hemofiltration; CVVHD, continuous venovenous hemodialysis; CVVHDF, continuous venovenous hemodiafiltration.

The final outcome of these processes has been measured in vivo by Brunet and colleagues.[11] These investigators compared urea and creatinine clearance with predilution CVVH, CVVHD, or CVVHDF (50% in predilution), all with an equal 2 L/hr of effluent generation and a blood flow of 150 mL/min. They found that, with CVVH, urea clearance was 28.5 mL/min compared to 33.1 mL/min with CVVHD and 29.8 mL/min with CVVHDF. For creatinine the values were 26.3, 30.1, and 28 mL/min, respectively.[11]

Given that dilution is dependent on blood flow, these differences would be further reduced if blood flow were 200 or 250 mL/min. Nonetheless, at 150 mL/min of blood flow, it would appear that CVVHD should be the therapy of choice, given that the costs of replacing the effluent would be the same for all three approaches and that small solute clearance is about 20% better than with CVVH and close to 10% better than with CVVHDF.

However, this assessment only tells part of the story. The picture is different with larger molecules. For example, one can use urate as a marker for somewhat larger small molecules because urate has a molecular weight of 168 daltons compared to 113 daltons for creatinine and 60 daltons for urea. As might be expected, the clearances for urate found by Brunet and colleagues were 26.2 versus 27.4 versus 27.1 mL/min for CVVH, CVVHD, and CVVHDF, respectively. Using β_2-microglobulin (11.2 kD in molecular weight) as a marker for middle molecules and the same operative settings, CVVH delivered a clearance of 17.4 mL/min compared to 8.3 mL/min with CVVHD and 10.7 mL/min with CVVHDF.[11]

Thus, for a 20% loss of small solute (molecular weight <150) clearance, CVVH appears to lose little at any molecular weight greater than 150, while achieving a 100% increase in middle-molecular clearance. This observation is important. A recent review of free, water-soluble uremic toxins identified 45 low-molecular-weight toxins.[1] Only 17 of these had a molecular weight below 150 daltons. The same review also identified 22 middle-molecular-weight toxins. Thus, even with predilution, CVVH (convective clearance) can be reasonably expected to double the clearance of 22 toxins compared to CVVHD, while having essentially equal clearance for another 28 and a 20% decrease in clearance for another 17. Given that the individual toxicity of each uremic toxin is unknown, one could allocate a score of 1 for its expected clearance with pure diffusion (CVVHD). With this approach, CVVHD would have a "uremic burden clearance" score of 67 (1 multiplied for all uremic toxins removed). Compared to this, predilution CVVH would score 0.8 for 17 molecules (loss of 20% clearance), 1 for 28, and 2 for 22 (doubled clearance compared to CVVHD). Thus, its uremic burden clearance score would be 85.6. This analysis does not take into account the fact that, in critically ill patients, a whole array of potentially pathological middle molecules accumulate (cytokines, myocardial depressant factors, chemokines, complement anaphylatoxins) which are all of middle molecular weight and can be expected to show a clearance pattern similar to that of β_2-microglobulin.[12,13] Accordingly, on the basis of the clearance measurements and given the knowledge available at this time, from a blood purification point of view, postdilution CVVH offers more "bang for the buck" at the same cost compared to CVVHD or CVVHDF. The limitations of CVVH are dependent only on the amount of ultrafiltrate one can achieve in a given time. Due to a sieving of 1 for several solutes, clearance equals ultrafiltration rate in postdilution mode. When ultrafiltration rate equals the effluent rate in CVVHD or CVVHDF, CVVH is always superior. There is no need

to go with CVVHD or CVVHDF if CVVH offers the ultrafiltration rate requested. The problem may arise when filtration fraction increases too much. At this point, either blood flow can be increased or diffusion can be used additionally. But once again, diffusion must consider the degree of effluent saturation. This is why CVVH was used in a recent CRRT dose randomized controlled trial.[8]

Accordingly, we have long been using and continue to use CVVH as the technique of choice.[14]

These observations apply to intermittent therapy as well, because the principles of convection and diffusion and solute clearance are the same. However, one must consider that, due to the high efficiency of these intermittent therapies, the blood compartment is often cleared faster than it can be replenished from tissues. Slower therapies, which are of intermediate efficiency and are applied for longer periods of time, offer greater potential for mass removal and may represent an ideal compromise.[15]

Impact on Outcomes

The final pertinent question is whether the differences in solute clearance discussed earlier in this chapter generate differences in outcomes. There is evidence that they generate differences in biochemical outcomes when compared in vivo.[16] Such differences favor hemofiltration when one focuses on middle-molecular-weight solutes such as cytokines.[16]

There are limited comparative data in terms of physiological outcomes (blood pressure, peripheral vascular resistance, headaches, need for fluid resuscitation, muscle cramps) for intermittent therapy.[17,18]

There are no data on the filter survival effect of using one technique versus another. There are no clinical outcome data (duration of intensive care unit or hospital stay or survival) comparing different techniques of solute clearance applied at equal levels of intensity.

CONCLUSION

The techniques of hemofiltration, hemodialysis, or hemodiafiltration, either continuously or intermittently, achieve excellent small-solute clearances. If postdilution is used, such small-solute clearances are essentially identical. If predilution is used, hemofiltration will be less efficient for small-solute removal than hemodialysis. However, such limited efficiency loss will come with a major gain in middle-molecular solute clearance. There are no differences in cost or ease of use among these techniques. Given the minimal differences in small-solute clearance, the same cost and the major gain in middle-molecular solute clearance, continuous hemofiltration appears the most logical technical approach to CRRT at this time. For intermittent therapies, due to the high blood flow requirements needed, hemofiltration is technically more demanding and may best be coupled with a degree of diffusive clearance (intermittent hemodiafiltration).

Key Points

1. Hemofiltration is equivalent in efficacy to hemodialysis for small-solute clearance.
2. Hemofiltration leads to better middle-molecular-weight solute clearance than hemodialysis.

3. Hemofiltration with prefilter replacement fluid administration leads to some loss of solute clearance due to dilution.
4. Hemodiafiltration with predilution is not as efficient as hemodiafiltration with postdilution.
5. Although postdilution increases solute clearance, it also leads to hemoconcentration.
6. Hemoconcentration increases the statistical probability of filter clotting.

7. Filter clotting is greater with postdilution compared to predilution.
8. Because of filter clotting, predilution delivers equivalent clearances over a 24-hour cycle with fewer episodes of filter clotting.

Key References

See the companion Expert Consult website for the complete reference list.

CHAPTER 247

Slow Continuous Ultrafiltration

Gabriella Salvatori

OBJECTIVES

This chapter will:
1. Discuss slow continuous ultrafiltration management and monitoring.
2. Present clinical indications and applications for slow continuous ultrafiltration.
3. Describe internal ultrafiltration and plasmafiltration devices.

Slow continuous ultrafiltration (SCUF) is a type of continuous renal replacement therapy (CRRT) used to achieve safe and effective management of severe fluid overload even in absence of acute renal failure.

In particular, this type of extracorporeal ultrafiltration has been assessed as an adjunctive therapy for patients with refractory congestive heart failure (CHF). These patients can be treated safely, achieving the normalization or the improvement of cardiac filling pressures, without dangerous reductions in circulating blood volume.[1]

This chapter briefly describes the treatment characteristics of SCUF, its principal physiological effects, and clinical indications for its use. Future technical developments and alternative therapeutic potential of this therapy also are considered.

TECHNICAL FEATURES

SCUF is the least complex treatment from among all CRRTs. It is employed usually for 24 hours per day in an intensive care setting, but it also may be applied for some hours per day with an arteriovenous or a venovenous access circuit (Fig. 247-1). The arteriovenous modality is rarely used any more because of frequent complications from arterial cannulation.[2] The venovenous modality is a pump-driven system that uses an ultrafiltration control system to maintain the ultrafiltration rate at the desired

levels. Access can be either an arteriovenous fistula or graft or a double-lumen venous catheter. Recently venous catheters for long-term use and subcutaneous prosthetic devices have been produced as efficient access to the extracorporeal circulation, contributing to a simplification of the procedures.[3] These devices represent potential resources to perform CRRTs at home with minimal training, significantly reducing the need of hospitalization.

Generally SCUF can be performed with low blood flow rates, between 50 and 200 mL/min in venovenous modality, and ultrafiltration rate is usually between 100 and 300 mL/hr according to fluid balance needs. Because of the low ultrafiltration and blood flow rates required, relatively small surface area filters can be employed with reduced heparin doses to maintain circuit patency.[4] Convective clearance of solutes is not significant and blood purification is ineffective. The main purpose of treatment is to achieve volume control; therefore, no fluids are administered either as dialysate or replacement fluids.[5,6] Synthetic high-flux membranes of polysulfone, polyamide, polymethylmethacrylate, or polyacrylonitrile are generally employed because of their excellent permeability and biocompatibility characteristics.[7,8]

TREATMENT MONITORING

Volume overload is a common occurrence in critically ill patients. The main clinical matter is deciding if these patients have an effective increase in circulating blood volume and therefore would benefit from specific fluid-removal therapies. To identify parameters adequate to monitor intravascular volume is, therefore, essential.

Conventional indicators of hydration status and tissue perfusion are systemic blood pressure, heart rate, body weight, jugular-venous pulsation, and peripheral edema. In critically ill patients, however, these indicators become defective measures of volume status because of the presence of positive pressure ventilation, especially positive end-expiratory pressure, or because numerous physiological and treatment variables affect them. Central venous pressure (CVP) and pulmonary capillary occlusion

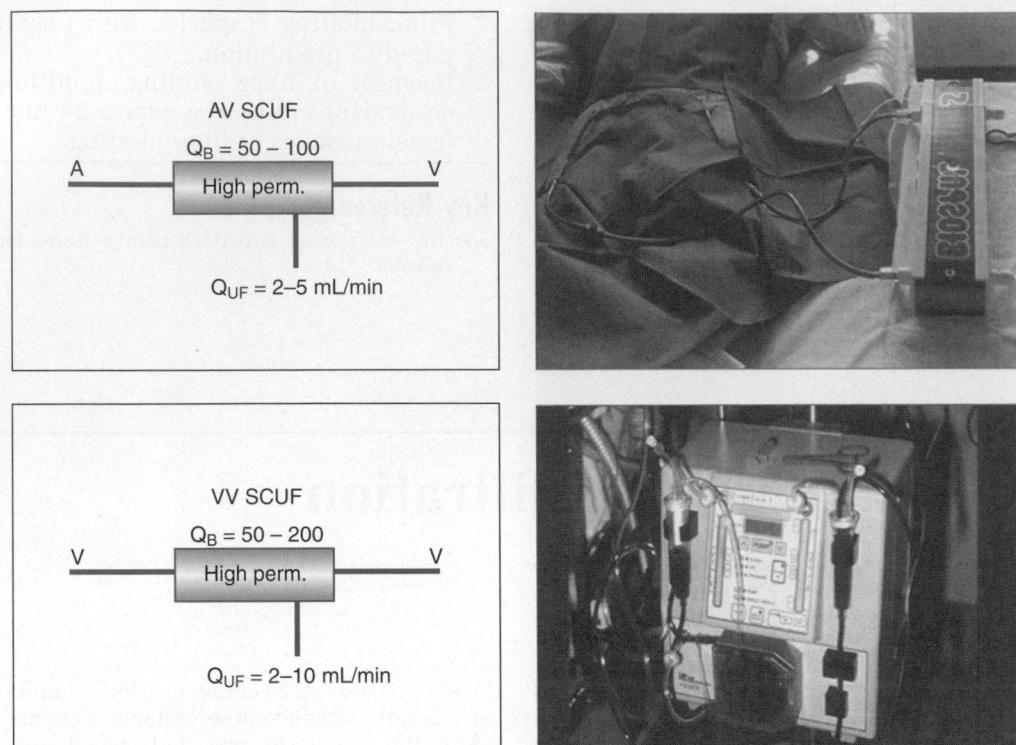

FIGURE 247-1. Arteriovenous (AV) and venovenous (VV) slow continuous ultrafiltration (SCUF): Scheme of the treatment circuit and its clinical application for each modality. Q_B, blood flow; Q_{UF}, ultrafiltrate flow. (Modified from Ronco C, Ricci Z, Brendolan A, et al: Ultrafiltration in patients with hypervolemia and congestive heart failure. Blood Purif 2004;22:150-163.)

pressure (PCOP) assess preload accurately, but they can guide therapy only when pressure values are low (<10 mm Hg). An increased CVP or PCOP does not ensure adequate filling pressures or hypervolemia. Total end-diastolic volume index and intrathoracic blood volume index may be more useful indicators of volume status than pressure variables, but they lack widespread clinical availability.[9] Response to single or multiple fluid challenges may not detect hypovolemia, depending on its degree. The mixed venous oxygen saturation can serve as a surrogate for cardiac output but does not define optimal filling. In patients who are on mechanical ventilation, the absence of arterial pulse-pressure variation provides a robust indicator of fluid loading and represents a better predictor of fluid responsiveness.[10] In other cases, echocardiography may provide the only reliable evidence of fluid optimization and may consent to adjust therapy.[11] Chest radiography may reveal an enlarged heart, pulmonary interstitial edema (Kerley B lines), pulmonary vascular engorgement, mediastinal silhouette of the great vessels, and an increased vascular pedicle width.[12] As far as laboratory parameters are considered, albumin levels and sodium concentration should be monitored in fluid overloaded states.

Such a difficult monitoring assessment of intravascular volume can be simplified during extracorporeal ultrafiltration by a new device recently implemented in the extracorporeal circuit. It is an online monitor (Crit-Line; Hema Metrics, Salt Lake City, UT) that allows a continuous monitoring of blood volume: When significant blood volume reduction occurs, ultrafiltration rate can be reduced or arrested until a complete refilling from the interstitial compartment has taken place.[13]

PAST ACKNOWLEDGMENTS AND FUTURE DEVICES

The clinical application of ultrafiltration for fluid removal dates from the advent of dialysis therapy. Ultrafiltration was first described in peritoneal dialysis utilizing hyperosmotic solutions to remove fluid from patients. In the early dialysis techniques, a negative pressure was applied to the external compartment of hemodialyzers to increase transmembrane pressure and to increase plasma water removal. In 1974 ultrafiltration was proposed in addition to the standard hemodialysis apparatus.[5] A blood purification technique based on the principle of convective transport was subsequently refined by Henderson and colleagues.[14] In the early 1980s CRRT was proposed as a new form of artificial renal support that allowed management of fluid overload together with hemodynamic stability in critically ill patients. Moreover, the development of pumps and double-lumen catheters enabled clinicians to perform extracorporeal ultrafiltration for fluid removal in a variety of modalities and techniques in almost all clinical settings.[15]

The future of this field is represented by an innovative simple experimental approach which uses a modified indwelling catheter that directly extracts plasma (SCIP catheter, Transvivo, Napa, CA).[16] It is formed by a new filtration membrane and fluid control system for selective exclusion of cells in vivo and the extraction and processing of plasma in an external ultrafiltration cartridge (Fig. 247-2).[17] These fibers are 3 times larger in diameter than "standard" ultrafiltration fibers, the mean pore size distribution is increased, and the filtration surface is inverted

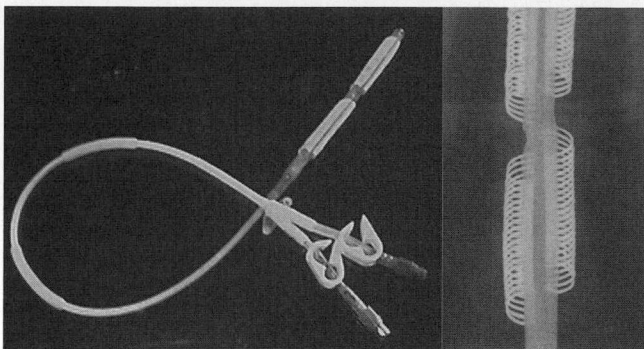

FIGURE 247-2. Prototype of a plasma separation catheter. (From Ronco C, Ricci Z, Bellomo R, et al: A novel approach to the treatment of chronic fluid overload with a new plasma separation device. Cardiology 2001;96:202-208.)

as it moves to the outer surface. Inversion of the filtration surface also diminishes clogging by eliminating static flow around the fiber. Venous blood flow rates approach 3 L/min in healthy adults, maximizing the shear rate over the membrane surface in contrast to near-static (<100 mL/min) blood flow within the central lumen of an individual fiber in a "standard" ultrafiltration cartridge. The exclusion of cells from the external circuit prevents platelet activation and aggregation within the removal circuit.

Another system replaces centrifuge-based plasmapheresis with a slow continuous intracorporeal plasmapheresis (SCIP; Transvivo, Napa, CA).[18] The SCIP system consists of four major components: a unique intravenous plasmapheresis (filtration) catheter, an extracorporeal tubing set, an extracorporeal fluid control module, and a standard hemofiltration cartridge. SCIP is envisioned as a platform technology for a variety of in vivo filtration applications, including ultrafiltration, dialysis, therapeutic apheresis, and in situ autologous cell culture or tissue engineering. The catheter is maintained by an external, self-monitoring control module. The module promotes the longevity of the plasmapheresis catheter by limiting the transmembrane access pressure and providing an intermittent reversal of flow, or "backflush," with heparinized saline (2.5 mL in 5 seconds every 5 minutes). The heparin dose is sufficient to provide localized anticoagulation without systemic effects. These characteristics increase the longevity of the system and allow fluid filtration to continue for more than 72 hours without interruption. The SCIP system is capable of removing up to 5 liters of plasma per day for plasma exchange, purification, or other purpose depending upon catheter size and design.[16] The combination of mechanical backflush, localized heparinization, biocompatible materials, and the high shear rates across the membrane result in a plasmapheresis fiber and catheter with exceptional longevity in vivo, minimal protein or clot deposition on the surface, and a continuous volume removal. The SCIP system of extracorporeal plasma SCUF has been shown to remove clinically significant amounts of fluid from pigs while maintaining stable blood chemistry over several days without requiring elevated systemic coagulation times.[19]

Data suggest that the therapeutic benefits of SCUF for acute care of fluid-overloaded patients may be extended to plasma SCUF with the SCIP system[20] to additionally reduce hospital staff and management resources and costs. This device may allow the development of longer term plasmapheresis implants and self-contained mobile fluid-maintenance systems.

TABLE 247-1

Main Clinical Conditions That Present Fluid Disorders in Critically Ill Patients

Excess Water Intake
Solute Depletion
Renal solute loss
  Diuretic therapy
  Hyperglycemia
  Mannitol
  Salt-wasting nephropathy
  Mineral corticoid deficiency
Nonrenal solute loss
  Gastrointestinal
  Cutaneous
  Blood
Solute Dilution
Increased proximal nephron reabsorption
  Cirrhosis
  Congestive heart failure (CHF)
  Nephritic syndrome
  Hypothyroidism
Impaired distal nephron dilution
  SIADH
  Glucocorticoid deficiency

SIADH, syndrome of inappropriate antidiuretic hormone.

CLINICAL INDICATIONS

Pathophysiological Understanding: Overhydrated Syndromes

Disorders of body fluids are among the most common problems encountered in the critical care setting.[21] Many of the different clinical conditions that present such disorders in critically ill patients are summarized in Table 247-1.

In fact, through different physiological mechanisms, all of these clinical conditions result in a common clinical syndrome: overhydration. They present an expansion of total body water with generalized or localized edema in the presence of increased, normal, or even reduced circulating blood volume.[22] The most important physiological mechanisms involved are a reduced capacity of excretion or an increased retention of salt and water in the presence of decreased effective circulating blood volume, loss of plasma oncotic power, generalized or local endothelial lesions and consequent loss of membrane selectivity and protein-retention capacity, iatrogenic disorders, and reduced renal perfusion due to impaired cardiac function. The final common pathway is an expansion of the extracellular fluid volume, which can be associated with oliguria or anuria.[23]

Any change in circulating blood volume activates different feedback systems[24-28] which become overcompensatory and self-maintaining: the activation of the sympathetic nervous system, the renin-angiotensin-aldosterone axis and the release or suppression of natriuretic peptides, atrial natriuretic factor, brain natriuretic factor, and urodilatin.[29-31] Indigenous substances, such as caspase and cathepsin, convert angiotensin-I to angiotensin-II by an alternate pathway when the primary pathway is blocked by the use of angiotensin-converting enzyme (ACE) inhibitors, thereby leading to increased levels of angiotensin-II and aldosterone, with consequent vasodilatation.[32-35] All of these factors vary in their relative significance in gener-

TABLE 247-2

Principal Causes of Myocardial Dysfunction and Organ Failure in Critically Ill Patients

Hemodynamic Instability
　　Trauma
　　Surgical interventions
　　Sepsis, septic shock
Bacteremia, Endotoxemia
　　Sepsis, septic shock
Acute Dysproteinemic Conditions
　　Liver failure
　　Nephritic syndrome
　　Rhabdomyolysis
Iatrogenic Fluid Overload
　　Shock
　　Acute respiratory distress syndrome (ARDS)
Acute Endothelial Dysfunction
　　Sepsis, septic shock
　　Trauma
　　Burns

ating water retention in different patients, but untreated patients have elevation of total blood volume, interstitial fluid volume, and body sodium. Such a congestive state with peripheral edema and cardiac dilatation has significant adverse consequences in the long run, particularly affecting kidney and heart function.

Treating extracellular fluid excess in absence of intravascular hypervolemia is not justifiable, but an optimization of fluid balance—through the reduction of organ edema and the restoration of desirable levels of preload and afterload—is essential to support cardiac function.[36] Myocardial dysfunction, in fact, almost always comes with the disruption of fluid homeostasis due to many syndromes frequently associated in critically ill patients (Table 247-2).[37-43]

Congestive Heart Failure

Currently, almost 12 million people in the United States and Europe suffer from CHF.[44] Its incidence and prevalence has increased markedly during the past 10 years as a direct consequence of the ever-increasing aging of the population[45] and the progressive reduction in mortality in patients with coronary artery disease.[35] CHF varies over a spectrum from chronic subclinical disease up to acute cardiogenic shock.[35,45] It represents one of the principal causes of mortality and morbidity in developed countries and has a significant impact on society and health care systems.[46-50]

In the United States, 90% of the hospitalizations for heart failure are due to symptoms of fluid overload.[51,52] Hypervolemia, a necessary physiological compensatory mechanism to maintain cardiac output through an elevated blood volume, contributes to CHF progression and mortality.[53-55]

The main purposes of CHF therapy are to prevent disease progression, decrease the incidences of mortality and morbidity, and optimize patients' quality of life by decreasing the rate of hospitalization.[56] Treatment guidelines recommend that therapy of CHF patients be aimed at achieving euvolemia.[57]

Standard treatments include early application of drug therapy combined with hygiene and dietary measures, in particular digitalo-diuretic treatment and ACE inhibitors (ACE-I).[55,56]

There is no documented benefit of co-administration of albumin with loop diuretics in extracellular fluid–overloaded patients who are hypoalbuminemic. Other medications have recently been shown to be beneficial in CHF, including carvedilol,[58] losartan,[59] and ibopamine.[60]

Traditional diuretic therapy for congestion in acute decompensated heart failure (ADHF) is often ineffective and expensive. Diuretics can precipitate renal dysfunction through intravascular volume depletion[61]; elevated plasma creatinine levels and drug resistance are the eventual result of continuous, long-term diuretic treatment,[62] especially in New York Heart Association class IV patients, and are related to a very poor prognosis.[45]

First findings on the improvement of cardiac functional performance through extracorporeal therapies go back to 15 years ago, suggesting that even in patients with moderate CHF and a deceptively normal glomerular filtration rate, ultrafiltration ameliorates diastolic function, which is of great importance in ischemic and idiopathic dilated cardiomyopathy.[63,64] Such beneficial effects are associated, in most patients, with a significant increase in diuresis and lead to a sustained beneficial clinical effect that can last for several weeks. Several reports have shown that myocardial elastance can improve with restoration of adequate fluid balance.[65]

The Acute Decompensated Heart Failure National Registry (ADHERE) recently showed that most ADHF hospitalizations are due to congestion in patients refractory to oral diuretics.[66] Unresolved congestion may contribute to high readmission rates. Approximately 25% to 30% of patients develop diuretic resistances, defined as reduced diuresis and natriuresis. Therapies for diuretic resistance have limited success,[67] and renal insufficiency and diuretic resistance are associated with prolonged hospitalization.[68,69] Such a refractoriness to treatment with increasing edema and diuretic-resistant oliguria can benefit from ultrafiltration.[52-54,70-72] Ultrafiltration has been shown to reduce right atrial and pulmonary artery wedge pressures and interstitial lung water with increased cardiac output, diuresis, and natriuresis without changes in heart rate, systolic blood pressure, renal function, electrolytes, or intravascular volume.[73] Circulating neurohormones drop below control values, explaining why its benefits last for a long period of time.[74]

Today, it is no longer justifiable to wait until severe symptoms are present, and an earlier intervention should be scheduled, as SCUF has been shown to be better tolerated and safe.[75] Early ultrafiltration safely and effectively reduces congestion in ADHF with diuretic resistance. It decreases length of stay and rehospitalizations in high-risk CHF patients. Moreover, clinical benefits last for more than 3 months.[76] SCUF has proved to be physiologically superior to diuretics in preventing rebound of interstitial fluid into the vascular space and allowing organ recovery.[77,78]

Possible increase in outcome and quick volume optimization are the main reasons to start such a therapy; risk due to anticoagulation and the high cost of the procedure remain frequent sources of skepticism and criticism.[74]

Studies have confirmed that ultrafiltration safely improves hemodynamics in patients with CHF.[79-82] The trial[83] showed that in hypervolemic RAPID-CHF patients, ultrafiltration produced greater weight and fluid loss and reduced the rate and the length of rehospitalization and unscheduled medical visits compared with intravenous diuretic therapy, whereas the two therapies produced similar improvement in dyspnea, quality of life, functional status, and biomarkers. This could be explained by the fact that for similar volumes of fluid removed, ultrafiltration removes more total body sodium.[84]

Extracorporeal ultrafiltration is another important advance in the management of fluid overload in newborns and children.[85] Small infants can be treated with specifically designed devices, and accurate fluid control can be achieved within a few hours.

In cases of a severe underlying myocardiopathy, extracorporeal ultrafiltration cannot be expected to be a cure for the underlying disease but only a supportive therapy or a bridge to heart transplantation. However, SCUF and derived therapies can be applied when the pharmacological support is temporarily failing or even beforehand, possibly on a preventive basis from time to time. The frequency could be twice monthly or even less frequent, with a remarkable improvement in the response to diuretics and an improved quality of life. Under these circumstances, it would be of interest to explore any possibility of a simplified therapy that could be carried out at home or self-administered by the patient. Devices and simple machines described in this chapter could be employed without complex training or equipment in such situations.

CONCLUSION

A multidisciplinary management of CHF or other clinical conditions characterized by refractory severe fluid overload is the best type of management considering the complex pathophysiological and biochemical mechanisms involved in their generation and progression. In fact, while diuretic-based therapy remains a first-level therapy, these drugs stimulate adaptive responses that may be counterproductive.

At present, the developments in the clinical application of different ultrafiltration therapies, from both the technical and the scientific point of view, together with their wider diffusion and accessibility, have made the use of SCUF one of the safest and most effective approaches for fluid overload in patients refractory to pharmacological treatment. It should be the first intervention because it achieves a safe and effective management of fluid overload in the simplest way.

Indications for these treatments have grown in number, although a curative effect cannot be expected.

The effects of these therapies in improving quality of life and reducing hospitalization, at least the need for intensive care hospitalization, may represent a remarkable outcome and should be explored on a large prospective scale.

The potential for a home-based application represents a further stimulating concept to be investigated. It should be explored in the coming years and considered as a simple effective answer to the enormous demand for treatment of fluid overload.

Key Points

1. Description of slow continuous ultrafiltration treatment.
2. Clinical benefits of ultrafiltration in overhydrated syndromes.
3. Slow continuous ultrafiltration as a model of heart and kidney support in congestive heart failure.
4. Novel device: the slow continuous intracorporeal plasmafiltration system.
5. Future approaches include multi-organ support therapy, peripheral ultrafiltration, and wearable devices.

Key References

17. Handley HH, Ronco F, Gorsuch R, et al: Artificial in vivo biofiltration: Slow continuous intravenous plasmafiltration (SCIP) and artificial organ support. Int J Artif Organs 2004; 27:186-194.
52. Clark WR, Paganini E, Weinstein D, et al: Extracorporeal ultrafiltration for acute exacerbation of chronic heart failure: Report from the acute dialysis quality initiative (Review). Int J Artif Organs 2005;28:466-476.
57. Hunt SA, Abraham WT, Chin MH, et al: ACC/AHA 2005 guideline update for the diagnosis and management of chronic heart failure in the adult. Circulation 2005;112:1825-1852.
73. Domanski M, Norman J, Pitt B, et al: Diuretic use, progressive heart failure, and death in patients in the Studies Of Left Ventricular Dysfunction (SOLVD). J Am Coll Cardiol 2003;42:705-708.
83. Bart BA, Boyle A, Bank AJ, et al: Ultrafiltration versus usual care for hospitalized patients with heart failure: The Relief for Acutely Fluid-Overloaded Patients with Decompensated Congestive Heart Failure (RAPID-CHF) trial. J Am Coll Cardiol 2005;46:2043-2046.

See the companion Expert Consult website for the complete reference list.

CHAPTER 248

Continuous Venovenous Hemofiltration

Heleen M. Oudemans–van Straaten

> ### OBJECTIVES
> This chapter will:
> 1. Describe the method and mechanisms of continuous venovenous hemofiltration.
> 2. Provide practical recommendations for continuous venovenous hemofiltration regarding indication, timing, dose, and replacement fluids using the Grading of Recommendations, Assessment, Development, and Evaluation (GRADE) system for gradation.[1]
> 3. Draw attention to the metabolic consequences of continuous venovenous hemofiltration.

PRINCIPLES

Continuous venovenous hemofiltration (CVVH) is a technique of continuous blood purification basically comparable to glomerular filtration. Blood is conducted along a semipermeable membrane. Ultrafiltration (the passage of water and solutes) is driven by hydrostatic pressure, a process called convection. Removal by convection depends on interplay of characteristics of the solute, the membrane, and the CVVH modality (Table 248-1). Apart from convection, adsorption to the membrane may, to a lesser degree, contribute to removal. To compensate for losses with ultrafiltration, water and electrolytes are replaced. Net solute removal by CVVH depends on the removal by ultrafiltration, adsorption, and the site and composition of the replacement. For adequate renal replacement therapy, 50 to 70 liters are exchanged per day, necessitating the use of a reliable device with an accurate balance, a sufficient heating capacity, five to six pumps, and sophisticated software enabling fine tuning of the process (Fig. 248-1). It should further be noted that hemofiltration is far from selective. Apart from uremic substances, beneficial substances are removed as well. CVVH therefore needs metabolic monitoring and knowledge of the process to adjust the potential derangements.

Convective Removal

Convective removal is determined by sieving coefficient (SC) and ultrafiltrate (UF) rate. The SC of a solute describes the ratio of its concentration in UF to its mean concentration in the plasma water along the filter. If a solute passes the membrane without restriction, its UF concentration equals plasma concentration and the SC equals 1. As larger molecules are partially or fully retained, their SC is less than 1 or falls to 0. However, even for smaller solutes, the process of sieving is more complex. Driven by the negative charge of the protein layer on the membrane, the SCs of negatively charged substances are greater than 1 and those of positive ions smaller than 1.[2] Observed SCs slightly greater than 1 can also be caused by convective forces acting on a concentration polarization layer and by the rapid mobilization from the intracellular to the plasma compartment, as may occur for urea. Furthermore, the SC is not constant for any given solute-membrane combination, but depends on UF flow, blood flow, filtration fraction (the ratio of UF to blood flow), and the site of replacement.[3] This process is complex. For example, the SC of middle molecules decreases as filtration fraction increases.

Adsorption

During the course of hemofiltration, plasma proteins adhere to the membrane and form a secondary membrane, the so-called *gel layer* or *protein cake*. This adsorbed layer gradually reduces the solute and hydraulic permeability of the membrane (clogging), especially affecting the middle-molecular and larger molecular clearance. Some membranes have a high adsorptive capacity. When these membranes are used, adsorption may contribute to the removal of proteins such as cytokines. It should be noted, however, that adsorption is subjected to saturation over time and secondary release from the membrane. As a result, the absolute effect of absorption on total body clearance is small.[4,5]

Concentration Polarization

Distinct from this secondary membrane formation, hemofiltration is associated with concentration polarization, a process describing the accumulation of rejected solutes at the membrane surface. The thickness of the polarized layer depends on an interplay of blood flow, UF rate, hematocrit, plasma (lipo)protein content, and site of replacement. Due to polarization, convection acts on the high concentration of proteins at the submembranous site, promoting the removal of low-molecular-weight proteins. Polarization explains the higher removal of low-molecular-weight proteins during convective, as compared to diffusive, removal.[6]

Replacement

Water, electrolytes, and buffer are replaced to compensate their loss by filtration and correct metabolic acidosis. The composition of the various commercial replacement solutions differs with respect to electrolyte and glucose concentrations, and type and content of buffer (Table 248-2). Electrolyte balances depend on the relation between the

TABLE 248-1

Factors Influencing Solute Removal in Continuous Venovenous Hemofiltration

Solute-Related Factors
Free plasma concentration
Size, charge, and geometry
Volume of distribution
Speed of intra- to extracellular mobilization
Membrane polarization
Membrane-Related Factors
Hydraulic permeability
Pore size
Adsorptive characteristics
Modality-Related Factors
Ultrafiltrate flow
Blood flow
Filtration fraction
Pre- or postdilution replacement

TABLE 248-2

Composition of Commercial Replacement Fluids

Na$^+$	138-142 mmol/L
K$^+$	0-4 mmol/L
Ca^{++}	1.00-2.00 mmol/L
Mg^{++}	0.50-1.0 mmol/L
Cl$^-$	100-120 mmol/L
Glucose	5.6-14.4 mmol/L
Bicarbonate	0 or 32-40 mmol/L
Lactate	3 or 30-46 mmol/L

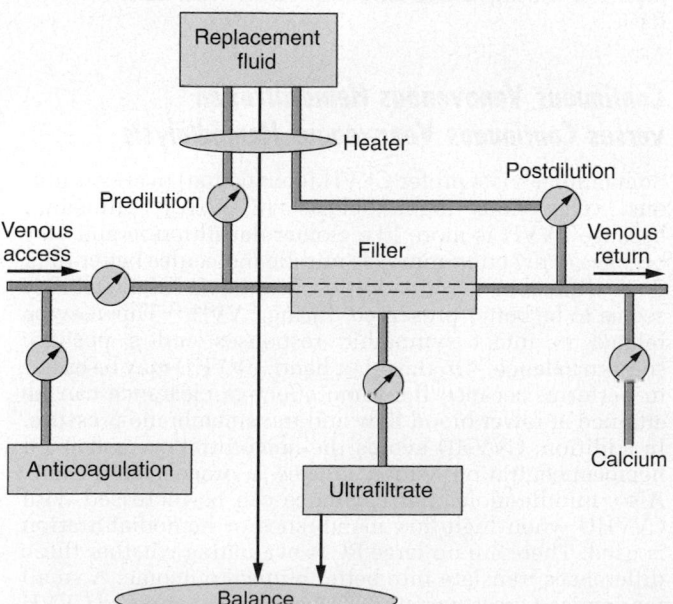

FIGURE 248-1. Schematic presentation of the continuous venovenous hemofiltration (CVVH) circuit. The circuit has a heater, a balance, and six pumps: a blood pump, an ultrafiltrate pump, two pumps for replacement (predilution and postdilution), an anticoagulation pump, and a calcium pump, to be used for citrate anticoagulation.

electrolyte concentration in the plasma and the replacement fluid in use, the UF rate, and the site of substitution.[2,7] Lactate, bicarbonate, acetate, and citrate are the available buffers. Acetate is generally not used anymore because of its lower buffer capacity, vasodilator, and negative inotropic effects.[8] Citrate is used in the setting of regional anticoagulation (see Chapter 277). The choice in daily practice is either lactate or bicarbonate.

Filtration Fraction

One of the problems with hemofiltration is the hemoconcentration occurring as a consequence of ultrafiltration. Within the filter, hematocrit and protein content of the blood increase, enhancing the tendency toward coagulation. Hemoconcentration explains why hemofiltration is associated with a shorter circuit life than is hemodialysis.[9] To minimize the procoagulant effects of hemoconcentration, it is recommended to keep filtration fraction below 25%. If larger volumes are exchanged, an increase in blood flow is often limited by vascular access and higher filtration fractions are accepted (up to 30%). Another option to reduce filtration fraction is to administer (part of) the replacement fluid before the filter (i.e., predilution).

Predilution and Postdilution

To reduce hemoconcentration, clinicians often administer replacement fluids before the filter (predilution), in contrast to the conventional method of replacement after the filter (postdilution) (see Fig. 248-1). By diluting the blood, hematocrit, platelet count, and the concentration of coagulation factors decrease at the filter inlet. Rheological conditions in the filter improve. Small studies have shown that predilution is associated with longer circuit survival time and reduced anticoagulant use.[10,11]

Predilution has several other effects. First, as a result of plasma dilution, convective clearance is reduced as compared to postdilution. To obtain a similar small-solute clearance, UF rate should be increased with the percentage dilution at the prefilter site. Predilution, however, has more complex effects on solute removal. It has been suggested that with predilution, membrane performance is better maintained by reducing protein adsorption. On the other hand, others have shown a greater protein adsorption and fouling with predilution.[3] This may be explained by the higher UF rate in predilution, opening a greater number of channels, thus increasing the actual surface and the amount of protein adsorbed. In addition, for equivalent UF rates, predilution is less effective than postdilution in the removal of low-molecular-weight proteins, because predilution decreases polarization of macromolecules.[6]

In the absence of large randomized controlled trials (RCTs) with clinical endpoints, the clinician has to weigh the pros and cons of predilution and postdilution. A combination can be considered. For more discussion on predilution and postdilution, see Chapter 249.

CLINICAL ISSUES

Before starting CVVH in a patient, the clinician must consider the following issues. The RIFLE (*r*isk, *i*njury, *f*ailure, *l*oss of kidney function, and *e*nd-stage kidney disease)

TABLE 248-3

Indications for Continuous Venovenous Hemofiltration (Grade 2C)

Acute renal injury without perspective of early recovery due to persistent shock or vasopressor need
Persistent oliguric acute renal failure with fluid overload
Acute renal failure with
  • A progressive rise of uremic toxins without a tendency of a decreasing slope
  • Metabolic derangement, e.g., acidosis or hyperkalemia
Cardiac failure with refractory fluid retention and progressive renal dysfunction

scoring system is used to define the severity of acute renal dysfunction (see Chapter 11).

Indications

General indications for CVVH are the removal of (uremic) toxins and fluid, and metabolic control. The primary setting is acute renal injury (ARI) or acute renal failure (ARF) in the critically ill. There is broad clinical consensus that patients with established ARF need renal replacement therapy. There are, however, no large RCTs to support this notion, and they likely will not appear. Practical indications for CVVH are formulated in Table 248-3.

Initiation

One RCT in critically ill patients with ARF, two controlled, and several retrospective controlled trials address this issue. In 106 ventilated patients with circulatory failure developing oliguric ARF, survival and recovery of renal function were not different in the patients randomized to early CVVH (i.e., 12 hours after the onset of oliguria) as compared to late (urea >40 mmol/L, severe pulmonary edema, or both).[12] However, early was not very early and late not very late, because a creatinine clearance below 20 mL/min (RIFLE-ARF) was required before the early group could start, and in nearly half of the patients in the late group, CVVH was initiated for pulmonary reasons before serum urea reached 40 mmol/L. In a retrospective controlled trial, clinical outcomes of 40 patients with septic shock with acute lung injury and ARI receiving early CVVH (45 milliliters per kilogram body weight per hour [mL/kg/hr] over 6 hours followed by CVVH 20 mL/kg/hr) were significantly better than outcomes of 40 patients receiving standard care including low-volume CVVH on late indications in the period before change of the unit protocol.[13] Three other retrospective studies showed a better survival when continuous renal replacement therapy (CRRT) was initiated early compared to late.[14]

In the aforementioned studies there is a trend, although not consistent, toward a better outcome with earlier timing of CRRT. In the absence of large RCTs comparing early to late initiation of CRRT, no firm overall recommendations for timing of renal replacement therapy can be made. However, when considering initiation of CRRT, it is important to realize that the consequences of uremic toxicity, metabolic acidosis, fluid overload, or all three, likely are more severe in the critically ill patient. Moreover, renal function is unlikely to recover soon if severe failure of other organs persists. Furthermore, various inflammatory mediators are cleared by the kidney. As a result, ARF enhances their toxic effects and CVVH can eliminate some of them (see Section 15).

Although evidence is weak, it is recommended to base the decision when to start CVVH not only on the severity of acute renal dysfunction but also on the severity of other organ failure. Early initiation is to be considered in ventilated patients with acute lung injury or shock at oliguric ARI or ARF (RIFLE) and/or a steep rise in serum creatinine despite adequate fluid resuscitation (Grade 2C). For more discussion on initiating CRRT, see Chapter 238.

Continuous Venovenous Hemofiltration or Other Modes of Renal Replacement Therapy
Continuous versus Intermittent

Although outcome of patients on CVVH may be beneficial,[15] none of the RCTs comparing CRRT to intermittent hemodialysis (IHD) showed a survival advantage for either therapy.[14] Some issues are worth mentioning, however. First, in many of the studies, patients with shock were excluded. Second, it is more difficult to attain an adequate dialysis dose with IHD, because treatment time is limited and solute dysequilibrium may occur as a result of delayed solute transfer between body compartments.[16] Third, although delivered replacement dose was not reported in many of the studies, none seems to have achieved the higher dose associated with a better survival in randomized CRRT studies.[17,18] Fourth, one of the RCTs suggests that CRRT is associated with an increased complete renal recovery.[19] Fifth, physicians prefer CRRT for patients in shock. Beneficial effects on cardiovascular stability, cerebral edema, and intestinal acidosis have been reported during CRRT in comparison with conventional IHD.[14]

Continuous Venovenous Hemofiltration versus Continuous Venovenous Hemodialysis

Some intensivists prefer CVVH (convection) over continuous venovenous hemodialysis ([CVVHD] diffusion), because CVVH is more like glomerular filtration and also because convection removes middle molecules better than does diffusion.[20,21] In addition, cardiovascular stability seems to be better preserved during CVVH.[22] This may be related to intact sympathic responses and a positive sodium balance.[2] On the other hand, CVVHD may be easier to perform, because the same effective clearance can be attained at lower blood flow and transmembrane pressure. In addition, CVVHD avoids the hemofiltration-associated hemoconcentration which creates a procoagulant state. Also, middle-molecular clearance can be increased with CVVHD when high-flux membranes or hemodiafiltration is used. There are no large RCTs evaluating whether these differences translate into better clinical outcome. A small randomized crossover study (15 patients) compared CVVH (mixed predilution and postdilution to keep filtration fraction below 20%) to equally dosed CVVHD.[9] CVVHD was associated with longer circuit survival. Small-molecular clearances were not different, but there was a trend toward a better middle-molecular clearance (β_2-microglobulin) with CVVH (16.3 vs. 6.3 mL/min, $P = 0.055$). This benefit should be weighed to the longer filter down-time in CVVH.

Based on the previously mentioned restrictions, it may be concluded that in patients with stable hemodynamics, continuous and intermittent treatments are equivalent regarding survival. However, despite the low to moderate level of evidence, CRRT is recommended over IHD for patients with ARF who are in shock, need liberal fluid management, or are at risk for cerebral edema. With CRRT, dose requirements are more easily attained. Despite many physiological differences, neither CVVH nor CVVHD can be recommended as superior in terms of a better clinical outcome. For more discussion, see Chapters 242 and 270.

Dose

Although physicians are generally satisfied when the CVVH machine is running, it is crucial to quantify actual performance of treatment and to prescribe a target for the individual patient. Targets are related to solute removal (clearance), fluid removal, and control of electrolyte and acid-base balance. Clearance by CVVH is generally expressed as UF volume time. This corresponds to the clearance of a solute with a SC of about 1, typically representing urea. When dose is prescribed, several issues have to be accounted for. First, if clearance of body water is the target of treatment, dose has to be adjusted to body weight. Second, two single-center large RCTs in critically ill patients show that survival was significantly better when CRRT was delivered at a rate of 35 to 45 mL/kg/hr than at 20 mL/kg/hr.[16,17] A smaller RCT, including 105 patients with at least three failing organs, could not support this finding.[12] Apparently factors other than dose contribute to outcome.[23] Third, for several reasons, CVVH does not run for 24 hours a day, causing delivered dose to be smaller than prescribed. Prescribed dose has to correct for "filter downtime." The issue of high-volume hemofiltration in septic shock is discussed in Chapters 279 and 280.

Up to now, evidence indicates that for treatment of ARI or ARF, an UF flow of 35 mL/kg/hr in postdilution should be delivered (Grade 1B). Prescribed dose needs adjustment for predilution, using the dilution factor, and for filter downtime. For more discussion, see Chapter 239.

Lactate or Bicarbonate Replacement

Achieving acid-base balance depends on the patient's metabolic acid production, pulmonary compensation, UF rate, the type and concentration of buffer in the replacement fluids (see Table 248-2), and predilution or postdilution replacement. Buffer balances should be calculated for each setting and each specific fluid. A septic patient with a high metabolic rate and a severe acidosis needs higher buffer replacement rates (and acid removal) than a stable patient with a normal base excess. In the latter, buffer balance may become increasingly positive and metabolic alkalosis may occur, especially at higher buffer replacement concentrations and higher UF flows.

Lactate acts as a buffer after conversion to pyruvate and subsequent oxidation in the Krebs cycle. Each mole of lactate consumes three moles of oxygen. For several reasons, lactate solutions must be used with caution. First, in a RCT in 117 patients comparing lactate to bicarbonate buffered replacement in low-volume CVVH (1 L/hr),

lactate replacement was associated with more metabolic acidosis, hypotensive periods and cardiovascular events, and a trend toward a higher mortality in patients with cardiac failure.[24] With lactate replacement in CVVH at 2 L/hr, mild hyperlactatemia occurs and is associated with a slightly acidifying effect.[7,25] Base excess is compensated in most patients due to a decrease in chloride and phosphate and an effective removal of strong anions, whereas lactate contributes to acidosis only by decreasing the strong ion difference. However, if liver function and tissue perfusion fail, lactate conversion is limited and, as a result, lactate is not the suitable buffer. With the use of high-volume hemofiltration and a replacement fluid containing 46 mmol lactate/L, plasma lactate increased from about 0.4-3.8 to 6.5-12 mmol/L.[24] The hyperlactatemia occurring during CVVH is due to a positive lactate balance. If, for example, 4 L/hr are exchanged in postdilution, lactate balance becomes positive for up to 168 mmol/hr (360 g/day), while metabolic capacity is about 60 mmol/hr in stable patients with multiple-organ failure.[26]

The use of lactate as a buffer has other metabolic effects as well. During CVVH (20 mL/kg/hr), lactate replacement was associated with higher glucose turnover and plasma glucose, despite higher insulin levels.[26] Normally, gluconeogenesis accounts for 20% of the lactate conversion; however, with high exogenous supply surpassing the capacity of the Krebs cycle, up to 70% of the lactate is used as substrate for gluconeogenesis. Thus, lactate buffering may increase glucose intolerance and contribute to caloric intake.

Bicarbonate-buffered solutions have the advantage that the buffer is available without prior metabolic conversion. Since the buffer has no caloric value, switching from lactate to bicarbonate replacement decreases caloric intake and may induce hypoglycemia if insulin dose is not timely adjusted. Bicarbonate solutions, however, are more expensive and have limited preservability after mixing the calcium and the bicarbonate compartments. The formation of air bubbles during use requires continuous venting.

Lactate-buffered replacement fluids should not be used in patients with liver failure, marginal tissue perfusion, poor myocardial function, glucose intolerance, or if higher volumes are exchanged. In these conditions, bicarbonate-buffered solutions are recommended (Grade 1B-C).

Other Metabolic Consequences

The clinician should take account of the electrolyte content of fluids. The composition of commercial replacement fluids varies widely, and the concentration of many of the solutes is far from physiological (Table 248-4) Potassium is low and phosphate absent. Both have to be replaced separately. The magnesium content in some solutions is too low and the calcium content too high. Despite equal concentrations of sodium in blood and replacement fluid, net sodium balance is positive, due to a SC below 1 for positive ions.[2] For more discussion on this topic, see Chapter 277.

Glucose Control

During CVVH, glucose is lost by filtration (SC about 1.1)[2] and subsequently replaced. Glucose balance depends on plasma concentration, UF rate, glucose content of the replacement fluids, and prefilter or postfilter replacement. Glucose concentration of the replacement fluids ranges

TABLE 248-4

Metabolic Consequences of Continuous Venovenous Hemofiltration

Electrolyte Imbalance
Hypokalemia
Hypophosphatemia
Metabolic acidosis
Metabolic alkalosis
Hypomagnesemia
Hypercalcemia
Hyperlactatemia
Loss and Gain of Macronutrients
Glucose
Amino acids
Loss of Micronutrients
Water-soluble vitamins
Trace elements such as selenium
Loss of Heat
Hypothermia
Modulation of the Inflammatory Response
Decrease of hyperthermia
Decrease of metabolic rate

TABLE 248-5

Monitoring of the Patient and the Continuous Venovenous Hemofiltration (CVVH) Treatment and Process

Patient
Hemodynamics
Fluid balance
Blood biochemistry
  Sodium, potassium
  Acid-base balance
  Calcium, magnesium
  Phosphate
  Glucose
  Anticoagulation
Body temperature
Venous access
Treatment
Actual ultrafiltrate flow
Actual replacement flow
Net CVVH balance
Filtration downtime
Process
Blood circuit
  Access pressure
  Prefilter pressure
  Venous pressure
Membrane
  Transmembrane pressure
Filtrate pressure
Temperature of the replacement fluid
Circuit life

from 5.6 and 14.6 mmol/L (1-2.6 g/L). As a result, glucose balance may vary from 0 to about 50 g/day with 2 L in predilution to about 150 g/day with 4 L in postdilution. While tight glucose control decreases glucose loss with ultrafiltration, replacement with high-glucose fluids implies a substantial net positive glucose balance, especially if high volumes are exchanged. This net glucose infusion may increase insulin needs. On the other hand, hyperglycemia increases glucose loss and causes a negative energy balance. Furthermore, lactate replacement increases gluconeogenesis.

Loss of Beneficial Substances

CVVH is associated with considerable losses of amino acids, water-soluble vitamins, and micronutrients, because filters do not allow reabsorption as the native tubules do. In low-volume CVVH (1.5 to 2 L/hr), daily losses of vitamin C, thiamine, copper, and selenium are considerably more than the recommended daily intake.[27,28] Other nutrients are lost as well, and losses are multiple if higher volumes are exchanged.

Loss of amino acids is especially relevant for glutamine, since this is the amino acid with the highest plasma concentration. Glutamine losses were measured in 17 patients on CVVH at a rate of 4 L/hr. Median total glutamine loss was 9.6 g (SC 1.1), but increased to 60 g in a patient needing prolonged CVVH. To compensate for nitrogen loss, nutrition should contain sufficient amounts of protein. Since RCTs are not available, recommended protein intake remains a matter for expert opinion but may be at least 1.2 g/kg/day.

Temperature

Since 50 to 70 liters of fluids are exchanged per day, loss of heat is a key issue. Hypothermia decreases metabolic rate and oxygen consumption, causes vasoconstriction, and increases arterial blood pressure. Mild hypothermia is applied in patients during chronic IHD to facilitate fluid removal. Although short-term hypothermia (2 hr) during

CVVH was not associated with a change in mixed venous oxygen saturation or splanchnic acidosis,[30] hypothermia sustained for days may have pronounced effects. Loss of heat implies loss of energy and discomfort to the conscious patient. Shivering increases oxygen needs tremendously. Hypothermia decreases tissue perfusion and cellular functions, increases the risk of infections, increases myocardial work, and impairs coagulation. In an ovine septic shock hemofiltration model, prevention of hypothermia by warming the blood improved hemodynamics and outcome.[31]

Although modern equipment pretends to provide adequate heating of replacement fluids, it is our experience that heating is inadequate when higher volumes were exchanged.

To prevent a drop in core temperature, monitoring of body temperature and timely external heating is recommended.

MONITORING

The aim of monitoring is to improve the safety and the quality of treatment. Monitoring of CVVH includes monitoring of the patient, the hemofiltration treatment, and the hemofiltration process (Table 248-5). CVVH balance has to be adjusted over the day in relation to the patient's needs. When circulation improves, a more negative CVVH balance can be achieved while zero-balanced CVVH is the option in patients with shock. Prescribed CVVH dose should be adjusted daily if delivered dose is less than target.[31] Temperature of the replacement fluid is monitored to detect whether the CRRT device provides insufficient heating. A relative decrease in peripheral to core temperature may indicate impending hypovolemia, a signal to reduce fluid removal with CVVH.

Hyperlactatemia, in addition to metabolic acidosis, warrants bicarbonate replacement, a higher CVVH dose, or both. Glucose monitoring should be intensified if net glucose infusion changes after transition to a replacement fluid with different glucose content.

Monitoring of the hemofiltration process includes monitoring of blood circuit pressures. Repeated access pressure alarms warrant inspection of the vascular access and correction of kinking or position and, if necessary, introduction of a new catheter. Prefilter pressures are monitored to detect impending clotting of the filter or the venous chamber and allow timely reinfusion of the blood before the circuit clots. An increase in transmembrane pressure indicates membrane fouling and a decreased effectiveness of larger molecular clearance. Circuit life is monitored to indicate timely disconnection of the circuit, because the integrity of the silicone segments is not guaranteed beyond 72 hours.

Most ideally, monitoring of the CVVH process is integrated in the patient data management system.

PRESCRIPTION

Before CVVH is prescribed, the clinician should consider the indications, the timing, and the alternatives for renal replacement therapy. When the indication is set, a prescription is made including CVVH dose, type of anticoagulation (Chapter 268), type and site of replacement fluid, target of net CVVH, and total fluid balance (adjusted to targets of circulation and fluid status), for additional supplementation and monitoring.

Key Points

1. The advantages of continuous venovenous hemofiltration include hemodynamic stability, liberal fluid management, and optimal clearance of uremic toxins, including middle molecules. The disadvantages are the requirement of a higher blood flow and the shorter circuit life as compared to continuous venovenous hemodialysis.
2. The decision when to start continuous venovenous hemofiltration should be based not only on the severity of acute renal failure but also on the severity of other organ failure. Early initiation should be considered in ventilated patients with acute lung injury or shock at oliguric acute renal

injury or acute renal failure (RIFLE criteria) and/or a steep rise in serum creatinine despite adequate fluid resuscitation (Grade 2C).
3. It is recommended to achieve a delivered ultrafiltrate flow of 35 milliliters per kilogram body weight per hour in postdilution for treatment of acute renal injury or acute renal failure (Grade 1B). Prescribed dose needs adjustment for predilution, using the dilution factor, and for filter downtime.
4. Full account must be taken of the composition of the replacement fluid and of the glucose balance.
5. Lactate-based replacement fluids should not be used in patients with liver failure, marginal tissue perfusion, poor myocardial function, glucose intolerance, or if higher volumes are exchanged. In these conditions, bicarbonate-buffered solutions are recommended (Grade 1B-C).
6. Continuous venovenous hemofiltration prescriptions should be individualized for dose, fluid balance, type of anticoagulation and site of replacement, additional supplementation, and monitoring.
7. The monitoring of the continuous venovenous hemofiltration process must be integrated into the patient data management system.

Key References

6. Clark WR, Gao D: Determinants of uraemic toxin removal. Nephrol Dial Transplant 2002;17(Suppl 3):30-34.
14. Bouman C, Oudemans-van Straaten HM: Guidelines for timing, dose, and mode of continuous renal replacement therapy for acute renal failure in the critically ill. Neth J Crit Care 2006;10:561-568.
17. Ronco C, Bellomo R, Homel P, et al: Effects of different doses in continuous veno-venous haemofiltration on outcomes of acute renal failure: A prospective randomised trial. Lancet 2000;356:26-30.
18. Saudan P, Niederberger M, De Seigneux S, et al: Adding a dialysis dose to continuous hemofiltration increases survival in patients with acute renal failure. Kidney Int 2006;70:1312-1317.
26. Bollmann MD, Revelly JP, Tappy L, et al: Effect of bicarbonate and lactate buffer on glucose and lactate metabolism during hemodiafiltration in patients with multiple organ failure. Intensive Care Med 2004;30:1103-1110.

See the companion Expert Consult website for the complete reference list.

CHAPTER 249

Predilution and Postdilution Reinfusion Techniques

Zhongping Huang, Jeffrey J. Letteri, Claudio Ronco, Dayong Gao, and William R. Clark

---

OBJECTIVES

This chapter will:
1. Explain the relationship between continuous renal replacement therapy dose and patient outcome.
2. Present the benefits and drawbacks of predilution and postdilution reinfusion approaches.
3. Elucidate the potential effect of location of reinfusion fluid delivery on continuous renal replacement therapy dose delivery.
4. Describe the manner in which blood flow rate is a limiting factor in dose delivery in both predilution and postdilution continuous venovenous hemofiltration.
5. Discuss the potential benefits of simultaneous predilution and postdilution reinfusion in continuous venovenous hemofiltration.

A reassessment of the dialytic management of critically ill patients with acute kidney injury (AKI) has occurred recently. In a landmark study, Ronco and colleagues[1] reported a direct relationship between daily ultrafiltrate volume and survival in critically ill patients with ARF who were treated with postdilution continuous venovenous hemofiltration (CVVH). A normalized ultrafiltration rate of 35 milliliters per kilogram body weight per hour (mL/kg/hr) or more (on average) was associated with a 30-day mortality of approximately 45%, while a more standard ultrafiltrate rate (mean, 20 mL/kg/hr) was associated with a 30-day mortality of approximately 65%. Likewise, Saudan and coworkers[2] reported significantly better outcomes in patients with ARF who received a mean normalized effluent rate of 42 versus 25 mL/kg/hr in predilution continuous venovenous hemodiafiltration ([CVVHDF] 30-day survival, 70% vs. 50%, respectively). Moreover, results of several recent studies[3-5] indicate that relatively early application of convection-based continuous renal replacement therapy (CRRT) also improves survival in critically ill patients with ARF, septic shock, or both.

These recent findings suggest the utilization of convective therapies in AKI will become more common in the future. An integral aspect of these therapies is the provision of reinfusion (replacement) fluids to achieve net solute removal and preserve fluid balance. Therefore, rational use of convective therapies requires a basic understanding of different reinfusion techniques. This chapter provides an overview of different reinfusion approaches, with the focus on the manner in which they influence solute clearance.

REINFUSION MODES IN CONVECTIVE RENAL REPLACEMENT THERAPIES

Postdilution Hemofiltration

Hemofiltration involves the simultaneous removal of plasma water by ultrafiltration and replacement with a buffered electrolyte solution (replacement or reinfusion fluid).[6] This exchange process achieves blood purification (i.e., reduction in blood concentration of toxins). The location of reinfusion fluid delivery in the extracorporeal circuit during hemofiltration has a significant impact on solute removal and therapy requirements. Reinfusion fluid can be delivered to the arterial blood line prior to the hemofilter (predilution mode) or to the venous line after the hemofilter (postdilution mode)[7] (Table 249-1). In postdilution hemofiltration, the relationship between solute clearance and ultrafiltration rate is relatively straightforward. In this situation, solute clearance is determined primarily by, and related directly to, the solute's sieving coefficient (i.e., the ratio of the solute concentration in the filtrate to the simultaneous plasma concentration) and the ultrafiltration rate.[8] For a given solute, the extent to which it partitions from the plasma water into the red blood cell mass and the rate at which it is transported across red blood cell membranes also influences clearance.[9] For example, the volume of distribution of both urea and creatinine includes the red blood cell water. However, while urea movement across red blood cell membranes is very fast, the movement of creatinine is significantly less rapid. Furthermore, red blood cell membranes are completely impermeable to many uremic toxins. A prominent example of this is the low-molecular-weight protein toxin class, for which the volume of distribution is the extracellular fluid.[10] These observations lead to the obvious conclusion that hematocrit also influences solute clearance in hemofiltration.

For a given volume of replacement fluid over a wide molecular-weight spectrum of uremic toxins, postdilution hemofiltration provides higher solute clearance than does predilution hemofiltration. As discussed later in this chapter, the relative inefficiency of the latter mode is related to the dilution-related reduction in solute concentrations, which decreases the driving force for convective mass transfer.[11] Despite its superior efficiency with respect to replacement fluid utilization, postdilution hemofiltration is limited inherently by the attainable blood flow rate. More specifically, the ratio of the ultrafiltration rate to the plasma flow rate delivered to the filter, termed the *filtration fraction*, is the limiting factor. In general, a maximal filtration fraction of approximately 25% usually guides prescription in postdilution hemofiltration in the acute renal replacement realm. At filtration fractions beyond

TABLE 249-1

Reinfusion Fluid Administration in Continuous Renal Replacement Therapy (CRRT)

Postdilution
- Reinfusion into venous line (postfilter)
- Disadvantage: ultrafiltration rate limited to certain percentage of blood flow rate due to hemoconcentration
- Advantages: relatively low volume of replacement fluids; clearance directly related to ultrafiltration rate

Predilution
- Reinfusion into arterial line (prefilter)
- Disadvantages: reduction of solute concentrations (lowered clearances); higher replacement fluid requirements
- Advantages: no ultrafiltration rate limitation; prolonged circuit life?

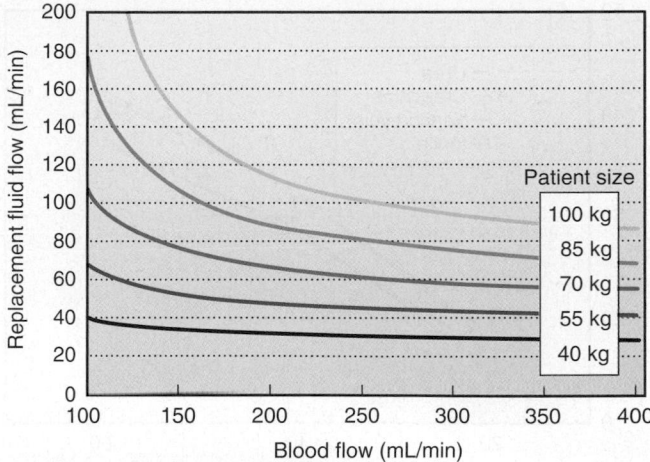

FIGURE 249-1. Reinfusion fluid requirements as a function of blood flow rate in predilution continuous venovenous hemofiltration (CVVH). (Reprinted with permission from Clark WR, Turk JE, Kraus MA, Gao D: Dose determinants in continuous renal replacement therapy. Artif Organs 2003;27:815-820.)

these values, concentration polarization and secondary membrane effects become prominent and may impair hemofilter performance (see Chapter 277).[12]

For acute hemofiltration (usually delivered continuously as CVVH), the blood flow limitations imposed by the use of temporary catheters accentuates the filtration fraction–related constraints on maximally attainable ultrafiltration rate in the postdilution mode. Therefore, the ultrafiltrate volumes shown by Ronco and colleagues[1] to improve survival can frequently be achieved only in the predilution mode. Efficient utilization of replacement fluid in acute predilution hemofiltration is an important consideration.

Predilution Hemofiltration

The use of predilution reinfusion has several advantages over postdilution with respect to solute removal. However, these mass transfer benefits must be weighed against the predictable dilution-induced reduction in plasma solute concentrations, one of the driving forces for convective solute removal. The extent to which this reduction occurs is determined mainly by the ratio of the replacement fluid rate to the blood flow rate.[11,12] In fact, a frequently overlooked consideration is the important influence of blood flow rate on solute clearance, particularly in acute hemofiltration. For small solutes, which are distributed in the blood water (BW) component within the blood passing through the hemofilter, the operative clearance equation in predilution hemofiltration is[13]

$$K = Q_{UF} \times S \times [Q_{BW}/(Q_{BW} + Q_R)]$$

where K is solute clearance, Q_{UF} is ultrafiltration rate, S is sieving coefficient, Q_{BW} is blood water flow rate, and Q_R is the reinfusion (replacement) fluid rate. At a given Q_{UF} value, predilution CVVH is always less efficient than postdilution CVVH with respect to fluid utilization. A sieving coefficient of 1.0 implies equivalence of blood water and ultrafiltrate concentrations, resulting in small-solute clearances that are effectively equal to Q_{UF} in postdilution CVVH. As the preceding equation indicates, the larger Q_R is relative to Q_{BW}, the smaller is the entire fraction represented by the third term on the right-hand side. In turn, the smaller this term is, the greater is the loss of efficiency (relative to postdilution) due to dilution. Since employing

a relatively low Q_R is not an option in high-dose CVVH, due to the direct relationship that exists between Q_{UF} and Q_R, attention needs to be focused on achieving blood flow rates that are significantly higher than what have been used traditionally in CRRT (i.e., 150 mL/min or less). In fact, widespread attainment of doses consistent with the intermediate- and high-dose arms in the study performed by Ronco and colleagues (35-45 mL/hr/kg) cannot occur unless blood flow rates of approximately 250 mL/min or more become routine in predilution CVVH.

Evidence supporting the critical importance of blood flow (Q_B) in predilution CVVH appears in Figure 249-1.[11] For this single-pool modeling analysis, a dose equivalent to 35 mL/hr/kg in postdilution is targeted. In addition, a filter operation of 20 hours per day is assumed to account for differences in prescribed versus delivered therapy time.[14] For patients of varying body weight, the reinfusion fluid requirements to attain the dose previously mentioned are shown as a function of Q_B. For low blood flow rates (<150 mL/min), these data suggest reinfusion fluid rates required to achieve this dose are impractically high in the majority of patients (>70 kg) due to a "chasing the tail" phenomenon. To achieve the dose target, a high ultrafiltration rate is required. However, the concomitant requirement of a similarly high reinfusion fluid rate has a relatively substantial dilutive effect on solute concentrations at low Q_B. On the other hand, for Q_B values greater than 250 mL/min, the dilutive effect of the reinfusion fluid is attenuated significantly and with the resultant improvement in fluid efficiency, the target dose can be delivered practically to a broad range of patients.

At least until recently, the ultrafiltration rate (Q_{UF}) in CVVH has typically been in the range of 1 to 2 L/hr. However, in response to recent dose and outcome data,[1,2] prescription of significantly higher Q_{UF} values is occurring. Although the relationship between ultrafiltration rate and clearance is relatively clear in postdilution, the same relationship may not be as predictable in predilution. Consequently, the claim that Q_{UF} is a dose surrogate in predilution hemofiltration needs to be demonstrated. To this end, Huang and colleagues[20] have investigated the effect of Q_{UF} on solute-removal parameters in predilution CVVH. For a

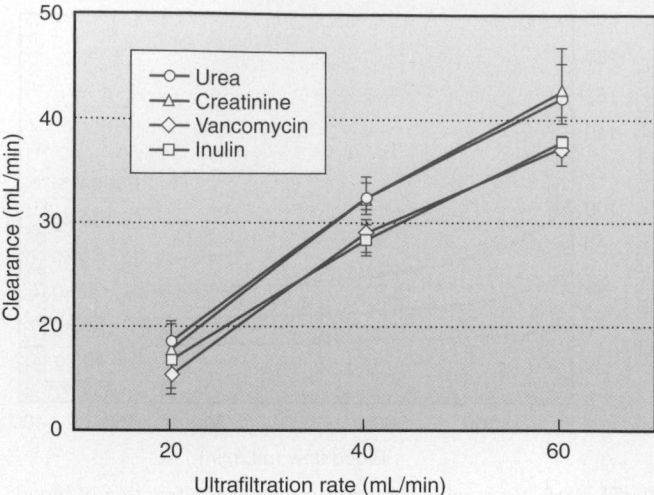

FIGURE 249-2. Solute clearance (mL/min) as a function of ultrafiltration rate (mL/min) in predilution continuous venovenous hemofiltration (CVVH). (Reprinted with permission from Huang ZP, Letteri JJ, Clark WR, et al: Ultrafiltration rate as a dose surrogate in pre-dilution hemofiltration. Int J Artif Organs 2007;30: 124-132.)

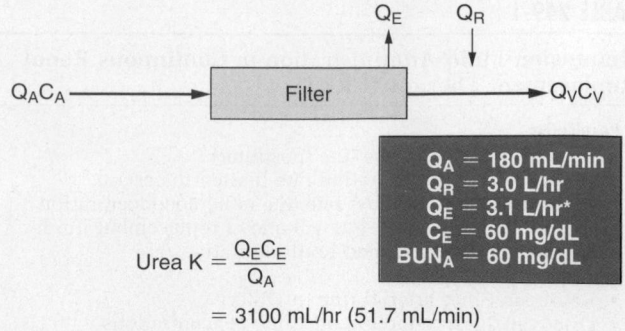

$$\text{Urea K} = \frac{Q_E C_E}{Q_A}$$

$$= 3100 \text{ mL/hr} \ (51.7 \text{ mL/min})$$

*Filtration fraction = 41%

FIGURE 249-3. Determinants of solute clearance in postdilution continuous venovenous hemofiltration (CVVH). C_E, concentration of effluent; K, clearance; Q_E, flow rate of effluent; Q_R, flow rate of reinfusion.

blood flow rate of 200 mL/min, removal parameters at Q_{UF} values of 20, 40, and 60 mL/min, corresponding to 17, 34, and 51 mL/hr/kg for a 70-kg patient were measured for solutes of varying molecular weight. The relationship between solute clearance and Q_{UF} for urea, creatinine, vancomycin, and inulin appears in Figure 249-2. Overall, these data are consistent with a convective therapy for two reasons. First, for each solute, the Q_{UF}-clearance relationship is linear, confirming a direct relationship between these two parameters. Second, for a given Q_{UF} over the solute molecular-weight range investigated, clearance is not strongly dependent on molecular weight, at least in comparison to hemodialysis. Specifically, very little difference in clearance is observed between the two small solutes and between the two middle-molecule surrogates as a function of Q_{UF}. On the other hand, reflecting its diffusive basis, hemodialysis is associated with much larger differences in clearance over the same molecular-weight range. The authors concluded that, because an orderly relationship exists between Q_{UF} and solute clearance, Q_{UF} is a reasonable dose surrogate in predilution CVVH, as has been suggested for postdilution CVVH[1] and for CVVHDF.[2] Overall, these data seem to validate the use of effluent-based dosing, which is being employed in two ongoing international trials evaluating the relationship between CRRT dose and outcome.

Hemodiafiltration

In 1978, Leber and coworkers[15] described a system employing simultaneous hemofiltration and hemodialysis for the treatment of end-stage renal disease. This hemodiafiltration approach was developed to overcome a major limitation of chronic hemofiltration. Because this time period preceded the development of online fluid generation systems,[17] reinfusion volumes were relatively small (20-25 L) and, based on these volumes, small-solute clearances were relatively low. Chronic hemodiafiltration has continued to be a popular modality even after the development of online fluid generation systems.

Hemodiafiltration is also widely used as a CRRT modality for patients with AKI.[2,18-20] One explanation for its widespread use is as an alternative to hemofiltration and the associated limitations associated with blood flow rate when high solute clearances are desired. In addition, with respect to the availability of commercially manufactured fluids in the United States, several dialysates have been cleared by the Food and Drug Administration (FDA) and used over the past several years. However, the FDA has only very recently approved the first commercially manufactured replacement fluids, and this is another explanation for the relative popularity to date of hemodiafiltration for AKI, specifically in the United States. The use of CVVH is expected to increase after the recent FDA decisions.

EFFECT OF REINFUSION LOCATION AND MODALITY ON SOLUTE CLEARANCE IN CONTINUOUS RENAL REPLACEMENT THERAPY: PRACTICAL CONSIDERATIONS

To demonstrate the effect of reinfusion location and modality on CRRT dose and solute clearance, a hypothetical patient having the following clinical and treatment characteristics is considered: (1) weight = 80 kg; (2) blood urea nitrogen (BUN) = 60 mg/dL; (3) Q_B = 180 mL/min; (4) total fluid (replacement fluid, dialysate, or both) (Q_R) administration rate = 3 L/hr; and (5) net fluid removal rate = 100 mL/hr. A schematic representation of treatment of this patient with postdilution CVVH appears in Figure 249-3. By definition, clearance is mass removal rate (mg of solute removed per minute) divided by the blood concentration of that solute entering the filter.[21] In CRRT, the mass removal rate is estimated by measuring the actual amount of solute appearing in the effluent, and mass removal rate is the product of the effluent flow rate (Q_E) and the effluent concentration of the solute (C_E). Based on the assumption of ideal operating conditions for the hemofilter in this situation, the sieving coefficient of urea is 1.0. If this is indeed the case, clearance is equal to the total effluent rate. This also implies the concentration of urea nitrogen in the effluent is the same as the concentration in the arterial blood. However, it is important to note this is really a theoretical clearance only because, as Figure 249-3 indicates, a filtration fraction of 41% would be required. This is much higher than the generally accepted maximum value of 25% and would most likely prevent the attainment of a urea sieving coefficient of 1.0. The other modalities considered are predilution CVVH, CVVHD, and predilution CVVHDF. For CVVHD, saturation of the effluent dialysate with respect to urea is assumed whereas an equal volume of replacement fluid and dialysate is assumed for CVVHDF.

Based on these considerations, the effluent-based CRRT dose and estimated urea clearance for the different modalities are shown in Table 249-2. Because the total effluent rate is the same for all scenarios, the effluent-based dose does not vary. However, as Table 249-2 shows, actual solute clearance differs significantly among the modalities. For predilution CVVH, the prefilter dilution of blood reduces solute concentrations and the filter is presented with less solute per unit time, as discussed previously. Compared to postdilution CVVH, this means less solute can be removed in the effluent for a given effluent volume. This translates into a lower effluent concentration (C_E), which leads to a lower clearance value. Based on the assumption of dialysate saturation in CVVHD, the clearance is simply equal to the effluent rate, as is the case in postdilution CVVH. Finally, for the case of predilution CVVHDF, urea clearance is intermediate between the value obtained for postdilution CVVH and CVVHD at the high end and predilution CVVH on the low end. The explanation for this is that the dialysate is achieving 1 mL/min of clearance for each 1 mL/min of fluid (due to dialysate saturation), while the predilution replacement fluid does not yield 1 mL/min of urea clearance for every 1 mL/min of fluid, as discussed previously.

SIMULTANEOUS PREDILUTION AND POSTDILUTION: A NEW REINFUSION TECHNIQUE IN CONTINUOUS RENAL REPLACEMENT THERAPY

One of the clinical aims of chronic hemodiafiltration or any filtration-based therapy is to provide convective solute removal. However, unless a blood flow rate of at least 400 mL/min can be achieved, filtration fraction constraints may become significant, likely resulting in high transmembrane pressures and potentially impaired filter performance. The possibility of this occurrence is especially high in patients who have end-stage renal disease and relatively high hematocrits. For this and other clinical scenarios, online hemodiafiltration systems with the capability to deliver simultaneous prefilter and postfilter replacement fluids[22,23] have been developed.

TABLE 249-2

Continuous Renal Replacement Therapy Dose: Urea-Based versus Effluent-Based*

	POST-CVVH	PRE-CVVH	CVVHD	CVVHDF
Urea dose[†]	38.8	29.5	38.8	34.1
Effluent dose	38.8	38.8	38.8	38.8

*Q_B = 180 mL/min; Q_E = 3.1 L/hr; patient weight loss = 100 mL/hr.
[†]Results expressed as mL/kg/hr, based on 80-kg body weight.
CVVH, continuous venovenous hemofiltration; CVVHD, continuous venovenous hemodialysis; CVVHDF, continuous venovenous hemodiafiltration; Q_B, blood flow rate; Q_E, effluent flow rate.

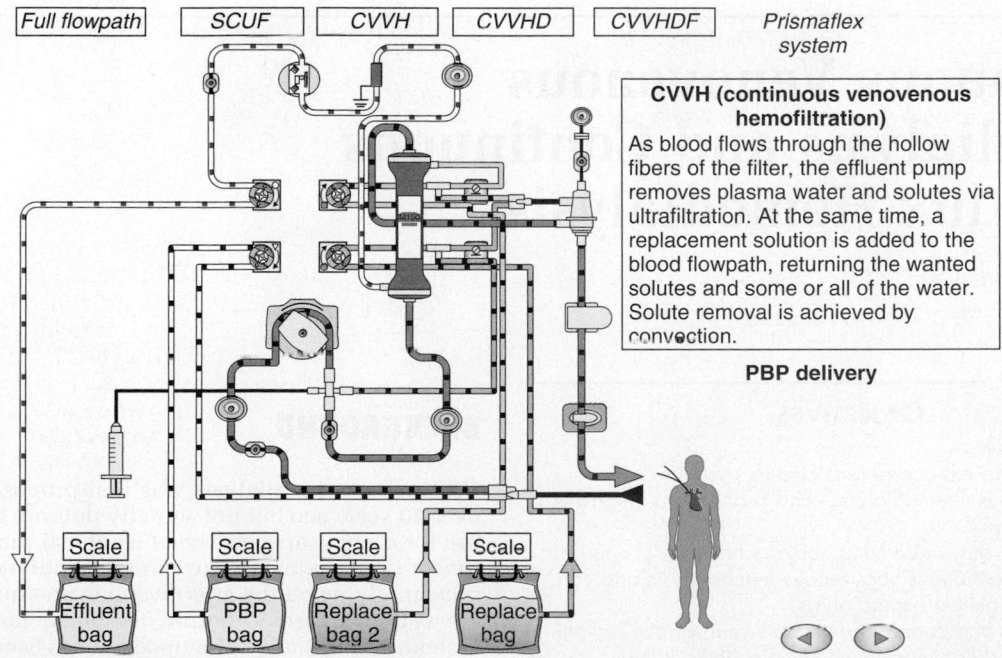

FIGURE 249-4. Diagram of Prismaflex (Gambro-Dasco, Lakewood, CO) extracorporeal circuit, showing different reinfusion capabilities. CVVH, continuous venovenous hemofiltration; CVVHD, continuous venovenous hemodialysis; CVVHDF, continuous venovenous hemodiafiltration; SCUF, slow continuous ultrafiltration.

As described previously, blood flow rate limitations are also an important consideration in convective CRRT modalities, from both a dose delivery and operational perspective. Therefore, in a manner analogous to the situation of chronic online convective modalities, systems with simultaneous predilution and postdilution reinfusion capabilities have been developed. One of these systems is the Prismaflex (Gambro-Dasco, Lakewood, CO) device.[24,25] With this type of machine, the clinician can take advantage of the benefits of both postdilution (e.g., low replacement fluid requirements for a given clearance target) and predilution (e.g., no filtration fraction constraints) while avoiding the drawbacks of each mode when used in a "pure" manner. A diagram of the system, with the different reinfusion points in the extracorporeal circuit, appears in Figure 249-4. When operated in the CVVH mode, in addition to simultaneous predilution and postdilution reinfusion, the capability to deliver fluid to a "pre–blood pump" location exists. As such, prefilter fluid reinfusion can occur at both the "traditional" (i.e., post–blood pump) and pre–blood pump locations, providing the clinician with greater flexibility in fluid delivery to the extracorporeal circuit.

CONCLUSION

Based on recent clinical data, convection-based CRRT provided at the appropriate dose can favorably influence AKI patient outcome. For these modalities, the location of reinfusion fluid within the extracorporeal circuit has a significant impact on solute clearance, dose delivery, and fluid utilization. This chapter has emphasized these issues, along with the important influence of blood flow rate on dose delivery in CVVH.

Key Points

1. Continuous renal replacement therapy dose is associated with patient outcome.
2. Reinfusion fluids can be delivered to the extracorporeal circuit before the filter (predilution) or after the filter (postdilution).
3. The location of reinfusion fluid delivery may have a significant impact on continuous renal replacement therapy dose delivery.
4. Blood flow rate is an important determinant of reinfusion fluid requirements for the attainment of a specific dose.
5. Newer generation continuous renal replacement therapy systems have the capability to deliver simultaneous prefilter and postfilter reinfusion fluids.

See the companion Expert Consult website for the complete reference list.

CHAPTER 250

Continuous Venovenous Hemodialysis and Continuous High-Flux Hemodialysis

R. T. Noel Gibney

OBJECTIVES

This chapter will:
1. Outline the extracorporeal circuits used in continuous venovenous hemodialysis and continuous high-flux hemodialysis.
2. Describe the underlying physiochemical properties used in continuous venovenous hemodialysis and continuous high-flux hemodialysis.
3. Compare and contrast continuous venovenous hemofiltration and continuous venovenous hemodialysis.
4. Discuss the clinical indications for and drug clearance with continuous venovenous hemodialysis.

BACKGROUND

Continuous hemodialysis was first proposed by Scribner over 40 years ago but not actually put into general clinical use for some years because of technical limitations at that time.[1,2] Continuous arteriovenous hemodialysis, a pumpless system relying on the arteriovenous pressure gradient and the patient's cardiac output for blood flow through the system, was initially developed but has been largely superseded by continuous venovenous hemodialysis (CVVHD), which uses a blood pump and provides more reliable operation and solute clearance.[2-4]

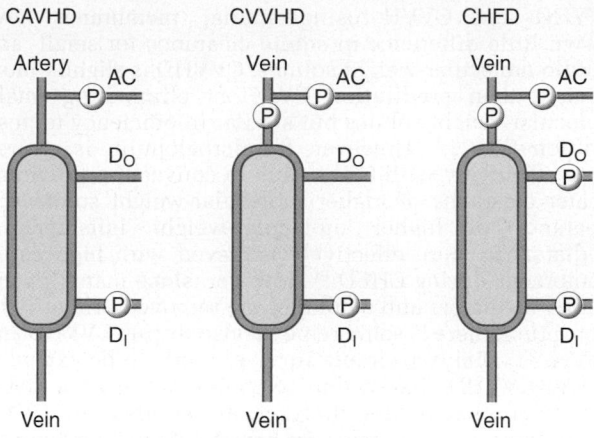

FIGURE 250-1. Schematic representation of continuous hemodialysis and continuous high-flux hemodialysis and the usual operational parameters used for these renal replacement therapies. AC, anticoagulation; CAVHD, continuous arteriovenous hemodialysis; CHFD, continuous high-flux dialysis; CVVHD, continuous venovenous hemodialysis; D_I, dialysate inflow; D_O, dialysate outflow; P, pump; Q_B, blood flow; Q_D, dialysate flow; Q_{UF}, ultrafiltration rate.

PHYSIOCHEMICAL PROPERTIES UNDERLYING CONTINUOUS VENOVENOUS HEMODIALYSIS

CVVHD is characterized by slow countercurrent dialysate flow into the ultrafiltrate/dialysate compartment of the dialyzer (Fig. 250-1). Ultrapure dialysate may be produced using online proportioning systems, or bags containing sterile dialysate may be used. Blood is pump driven through an extracorporeal circuit beginning and ending in a central vein and flowing through the blood compartment of a dialyzer countercurrent to the dialysate flow. Fluid replacement is not typically provided; consequently, solute clearance is primarily by diffusion with a small degree of backfiltration. Ultrafiltration may be used as required to maintain the desired patient fluid balance.[3-5]

At low flow rates, the dialysate is almost completely saturated with solute by the end of its course through the dialyzer. At higher dialysate flows small- and medium-molecular-weight solute clearance increases as solute concentration gradients across the membrane are maintained at higher levels. However, with some synthetic high-flux membranes, in addition to diffusive solute clearance there is also a major element of ultrafiltration and convective solute clearance. The rate of ultrafiltration is controlled by an ultrafiltration/dialysate volume control system and obviates replacement fluid. In this therapy, positive pressure in the dialysate compartment causes ultrafiltration in the proximal part of the dialyzer and backfiltration more distally. During backfiltration there is a flow of dialysate from the dialysate compartment across the membrane into the blood compartment. This form of renal replacement therapy is called continuous high-flux dialysis (CHFD).[3-5] CHFD, however, is not widely available as a modality on many continuous renal replacement therapy (CRRT) machines and has not gained wide usage.

HYBRID THERAPIES

CVVHD is a simple CRRT technique, suitable for intensive care unit staff with no trained dialysis nurses, which facili-

TABLE 250-1

Hybrid Forms of Continuous Venovenous Hemodialysis (CVVHD)

Continuous venovenous hemodiafiltration (CVVHDF)
Sustained low-efficiency daily dialysis (SLEDD)
Continuous sustained low-efficiency daily dialysis (C-SLEDD)
Albumin-enhanced CVVHD or single-pass albumin dialysis (SPAD)

tates an adequate control of uremia, fluid removal, acid-base homeostasis, and parenteral nutrition.[6-9] CVVHD and continuous venovenous hemofiltration (CVVH) have been combined as continuous venovenous hemodiafiltration to provide greater solute in some CRRT machines with limited blood and dialysate flows. In addition, the features of CVVHD and intermittent hemodialysis have been combined into the hybrid therapy of sustained low-efficiency daily dialysis (SLEDD), which uses dialysis over an extended time period (see Chapters 234 and 235) and recently came full circle with the development of continuous SLEDD (C-SLEDD), which effectively provides CVVHD using standard intermittent hemodialysis machines.[10-13] This form of CVVHD, which produces online ultrapure dialysate, is likely one of the most cost-effective CRRT modalities. Table 250-1 lists hybrid forms of CVVHD.

COMPARISON OF SOLUTE CLEARANCE BETWEEN CONTINUOUS VENOVENOUS HEMODIALYSIS AND CONTINUOUS VENOVENOUS HEMOFILTRATION

Membrane characteristics greatly influence solute clearance and, in this respect, some polyamide membranes are not designed for diffusive clearance.[14] Comparisons of

CVVHD and CVVH using similar membranes have shown little difference in solute clearance for small- and middle-molecular-weight solutes. CVVHD is slightly more efficient than predilution CVVH at eliminating small-molecular-weight solutes but similar in efficiency to post-dilution CVVH.[15] However, β_2-microglobulin is cleared more effectively with CVVH due to convection providing greater clearance of higher molecular-weight solutes.[16,17] Clearance of higher molecular-weight inflammatory mediators is more effectively achieved with high cutoff membranes during CHFD.[18] However, since many inflammatory mediators and cytokines are removed primarily by adsorption, there is some removal also during CVVHD and CVVH.[19-21] Dialyzer circuit survival tends to be extended during CVVHD, likely due to maintenance of a stable hematocrit across the dialyzer, in contrast to CVVH where there is an increase in hematocrit toward the end of the hemofilters due to plasma water loss from ultrafiltration.[17]

ANTICOAGULATION FOR CONTINUOUS VENOVENOUS HEMODIALYSIS

Anticoagulation for CVVHD is most commonly achieved using unfractionated heparin or low-molecular-weight heparin (see Chapter 269).[22] If the patient is at high risk of bleeding, it is reasonable to run the circuit without anticoagulation, although circuit life is usually only 12 to 18 hours unless the patient has significant coagulopathy.[22] Regional citrate anticoagulation during CRRT using either trisodium citrate or acid citrate dextrose is becoming increasingly popular. This provides regional anticoagulation within the extracorporeal circuit by chelating ionized calcium, which is then unavailable to participate at numerous points in the coagulation cascade. In addition, since citrate is a small-molecular-weight compound, it is also cleared diffusively during CVVHD. Regional citrate anticoagulation provides the longest dialyzer survival and minimizes interruptions of therapy caused by clotting.[23,24] Direct thrombin inhibitors such as danaparoid, lepirudin, and argatroban also have been used to provide anticoagulation, usually in the setting of heparin-induced thrombocytopenia.[25,26]

CONTINUOUS VENOVENOUS HEMODIALYSIS OUTCOMES

CRRT has been compared to intermittent hemodialysis in terms of outcomes. No study has shown survival benefit.[27-29] Some studies have suggested there may be less hypotension and lower vasopressor requirements during CRRT, although this did not appear to translate into a survival benefit.[30] In addition, some studies have suggested improved recovery of renal function with CRRT.[31-33] Factors that may affect current practice include local availability of equipment, commercial availability of dialysis fluids, and the lack of commercially available replacement fluid. Relative costs may play a significant role in local practice.

CVVHD has been used primarily to provide renal replacement therapy in critically ill, hemodynamically unstable adult patients with acute renal failure. It has also been used to treat infants and children with inborn errors of metabolism.[34,35] CVVHD also has been advocated as a means to effectively cool patients with hyperthermia or to improve hemodynamic stability in hypotensive patients, and it has been used to treat hypothermia using warmed dialysate.[36,37]

DRUG CLEARANCE AND DOSING DURING CONTINUOUS VENOVENOUS HEMODIALYSIS

Solute removal is particularly relevant to antimicrobial therapy, as sepsis is common in critically ill patients who require effective antimicrobial therapy, usually with a combination of a number of antibiotics. The pharmacokinetics of drug removal in critically ill patients receiving CRRT is complex, with many variables affecting clearance (see Chapter 291).[38] Protein-bound drugs have a higher molecular weight and lower clearance, whereas antimicrobials with lower protein binding are more readily cleared. Pharmacokinetic studies of a number of agents, mainly antibiotics, have been performed. Antimicrobials with good tissue penetration and tissue binding typically have lower clearance during CVVHD. Membrane pore size also significantly influences drug clearance. One of the potential challenges of antibiotic clearance during CVVHD (or any form of CRRT) is that combination agents such as piperacillin-tazobactam or imipenem-cilastatin have differential rates of removal of each of the combination drugs, potentially leading to accumulation of tazobactam or cilastatin, respectively. Whereas tazobactam is not toxic in higher doses, cilastatin accumulation during CRRT can cause hepatic toxicity, suggesting that meropenem, which does not require a dehydropeptidase inhibitor, may be a better choice in patients receiving CVVHD.[38,39]

ALBUMIN-ENHANCED CONTINUOUS VENOVENOUS HEMODIALYSIS

Albumin-enhanced CVVHD, also called single-pass albumin dialysis, has been used to treat drug intoxications with protein-bound substances and also to manage patients with fulminant hepatic failure or acute or chronic liver failure. This technique uses an albumin-containing dialysate to facilitate diffusive removal of protein-bound toxins or drugs across a concentration gradient.[40-43]

CONCLUSION

CVVHD is an effective and safe CRRT technique for critically ill patients with acute renal failure. Solute clearance during CVVHD is primarily diffusive; consequently, this technique is less effective than CVVH in removing inflammatory mediators. The C-SLEDD version of CVVHD with online ultrapure dialysate production is likely one of the most cost-effective CRRT modalities.

Key Points

1. Continuous venovenous hemodialysis provides effective diffusive clearance of lower molecular-weight solutes.
2. Continuous venovenous hemodialysis does not provide effective clearance of larger molecular-weight solutes such as inflammatory mediators.
3. Continuous venovenous hemodialysis has longer dialyzer survival as compared to continuous venovenous hemofiltration.
4. Continuous venovenous hemodialysis is associated with less hemodynamic compromise as compared to intermittent hemodialysis.
5. Continuous venovenous hemodialysis hybrids, such as sustained low-efficiency daily dialysis and continuous sustained low-efficiency daily dialysis, provide cost-effective solute clearance by using online production of ultrapure dialysate.

Key References

2. Geronemus R, Schneider N: Continuous arteriovenous hemodialysis: A new modality for treatment of acute renal failure. Trans ASAIO 1984;30:610-613.
4. Ronco C, Bellomo R: Continuous renal replacement therapy: Evolution in technology and current nomenclature. Kidney Int 1998;53(Suppl 66):S160-S164.
8. Sigler MH, Teehan BP: Solute transport in continuous hemodialysis: A new treatment for acute renal failure. Kidney Int 1987;32:562-571.
15. Parakininkas D, Greenbaum LA: Comparison of solute clearance in three modes of continuous renal replacement therapy. Pediatr Crit Care Med 2004;5(3):269-274.
17. Ricci Z, Ronco C, Bachetoni A, et al: Solute removal during continuous renal replacement therapy in critically ill patients: Convection versus diffusion. Crit Care 2006;10(2):R67.

See the companion Expert Consult website for the complete reference list.

CHAPTER 251

Solute and Water Kinetics in Continuous Therapies

Jeffrey J. Letteri, Zhongping Huang, Claudio Ronco, Dayong Gao, and William R. Clark

---

OBJECTIVES

This chapter will:
1. Outline the quantitative basis for the concept of solute clearance.
2. Describe the three basic mechanisms of solute removal (diffusion, convection, and adsorption) and the factors influencing these processes in continuous renal replacement therapy.
3. Present the factors influencing the effective water permeability of a continuous renal replacement therapy filter.
4. Describe the manner in which the basic principles of solute and water removal apply in the clinical application of the different continuous renal replacement therapy modalities.
5. Discuss the comparative solute-removal capabilities of various acute kidney injury modalities.

Renal replacement therapy is required in a significant percentage of patients developing acute kidney injury (AKI) in an intensive care unit (ICU) setting.[1] One of the foremost objectives of continuous renal replacement therapy (CRRT) is the removal of excess fluid and blood solutes that are retained as a consequence of decreased or absent glomerular filtration. Because prescription of CRRT requires goals to be set with regard to the rate and extent of both solute and fluid removal, a thorough understanding of the mechanisms by which solute and fluid removal occurs during CRRT is necessary. This chapter provides an overview of solute and water transfer during CRRT.

CHARACTERIZATION OF FILTER PERFORMANCE IN CONTINUOUS RENAL REPLACEMENT THERAPY

Clearance

Quantification of dialytic solute removal is complicated by the confusion relating to the relationship between clearance and mass removal for different therapies. By definition,[2] solute clearance (K) is the ratio of mass removal rate (N) to blood solute concentration (C_B):

$$K = N/C_B \qquad [1]$$

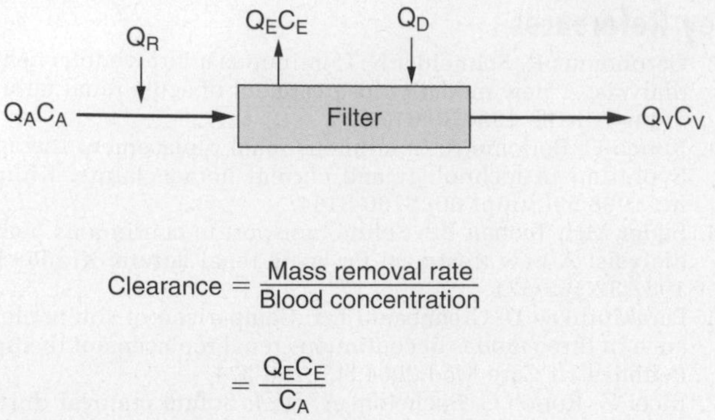

$$\text{Clearance} = \frac{\text{Mass removal rate}}{\text{Blood concentration}}$$

$$= \frac{Q_E C_E}{C_A}$$

FIGURE 251-1. Relevant flow considerations for the determination of solute clearance in continuous renal replacement therapy (CRRT). The modality represented is continuous venovenous hemodiafiltration (CVVHDF).

TABLE 251-1

Solute Clearance in Continuous Renal Replacement Therapy (CRRT)

CVVHD, CVHDF

$$K = E \times Q_D$$

$$\left(E = \frac{\text{concentration in effluent dialysate or diafiltrate}}{\text{concentration in blood}} \right)$$

Postdilution CVVH

$$K = S \times Q_{UF} \left(S = \frac{\text{concentration in filtrate}}{\text{concentration in blood}} \right)$$

Predilution CVVH

$$K = S \times Q_{UF} \times \left(\frac{Q_{BW}}{Q_{BW} + Q_R} \right)$$

CVVH, continuous venovenous hemofiltration; K, clearance; Q_{BW}, blood water flow rate; Q_D, dialysate flow; Q_R, replacement rate; Q_{UF}, ultrafiltration rate; S, sieving coefficient.

From a kinetic perspective, Figure 251-1 depicts the relevant flows for determining CRRT clearances and Table 251-1 provides the solute clearance expressions, which differ from those used in conventional hemodialysis. In the latter therapy, the mass removal rate (i.e., the rate at which the dialyzer extracts solute from blood into the dialysate) is estimated by measuring the difference in solute concentration between the arterial and venous lines. In other words, a "blood-side" clearance approach is used. On the other hand, in CRRT, the mass removal rate is estimated by measuring the actual amount of solute appearing in the effluent. The mass removal rate is the product of the effluent flow rate (Q_E) and the effluent concentration of the solute (C_E).

In continuous venovenous hemodialysis (CVVHD) and continuous venovenous hemodiafiltration (CVVHDF), the effluent is dialysate and diafiltrate, respectively. For these therapies, the extent of solute extraction from the blood is estimated by the equilibration ratio (E), also known as the degree of effluent saturation. The benchmark for efficiency in these therapies is the volume of fluid (dialysate, replacement fluid, or both) required to achieve a particular solute clearance target.

Clearance in postdilution continuous venovenous hemofiltration (CVVH) is the product of the sieving coefficient and the ultrafiltration rate (Q_{UF}).[3] For small solutes like urea and creatinine, the sieving coefficient is essentially 1

(under normal filter operation). Therefore, small-solute clearance in postdilution CVVH essentially is equal to the Q_{UF}. On the other hand, estimation of clearance in predilution CVVH has to account for the fact the blood solute concentrations are reduced by dilution of the blood before it enters the filter.[4] Thus, the clearance has a "dilution factor," which is represented by the third term on the right-hand side of equation 2. This term essentially is the ratio of the blood flow rate (Q_B) to the sum of Q_B and the replacement fluid rate (Q_{RF}) (the actual blood flow parameter, Q_{BW}, is blood water flow rate). In essence, the dilution factor can be viewed as a measure of the extent to which predilution differs from postdilution for a specific combination of Q_B and Q_{UF}.

These clearance equations are ultrafiltrate-side measurements. Thus, they are quite satisfactory for small solutes but are not always appropriate for larger molecules, which may have an adsorptive clearance component. As an example, for the AN69 membrane, sieving coefficient interpretations for larger molecules may be difficult due to its adsorptive nature.[5] Specifically, during the first two hours of use of an AN69 filter, adsorptive removal of large compounds like β_2-microglobin may predominate over transmembrane removal. If a β_2-microglobin sieving coefficient determination is made during this early period, the value may be very low (or zero), and the untrained observer may conclude that the membrane is not clearing any β_2-microglobin. However, significant clearance is occurring by adsorption—to appreciate this, a total clearance (i.e., blood side) measurement needs to be made. After the first two hours of treatment, the membrane may reach adsorptive saturation, and β_2-microglobin "breakthrough" into the filtrate may occur and a measurable sieving coefficient obtained. Thus, the timing of AN69 clearance determinations for larger molecules is important for correct interpretation.

Sieving Coefficient

When a dialyzer is operated as an ultrafilter (i.e., ultrafiltration with no dialysate flow), solute mass transfer occurs almost exclusively by convection. Convective solute removal is primarily determined by membrane pore size and treatment ultrafiltration rate.[6] Mean pore size is the major determinant of a dialyzer's ability to prevent or allow the transport of a specific solute. The sieving coefficient (S) represents the degree to which a particular membrane permits the passage of a specific solute:

$$S = C_{UF}/C_P \qquad [2]$$

In this equation, C_{UF} and C_P are the solute concentrations in the ultrafiltrate and the plasma (water), respectively. (As discussed later in this chapter, a sieving coefficient measurement is influenced by the flow operating conditions under which the determination is made). Irrespective of membrane type, all filters in the virgin state have small-solute sieving coefficient values of 1, and these values are typically not reported by dialyzer manufacturers. Sieving coefficient values for solutes of larger molecular weight are more applicable, and manufacturers frequently provide data for one or more middle-molecule surrogates, such as vitamin B_{12}, inulin, cytochrome C, and myoglobin. As is the case for solute clearance, the relationship between S and solute molecular weight is highly dependent on membrane mean pore size (i.e., flux).[7]

Sieving coefficient data provided by manufacturers are usually derived from in vitro experimental systems in which (non-protein-containing) aqueous solutions are

Diffusion is solute transport across a semipermeable membrane—molecules move from an area of higher to an area of lower concentration.

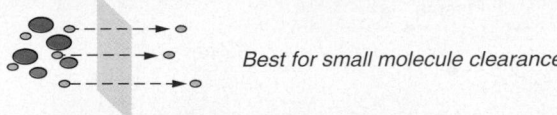

Best for small molecule clearance

Convection is a process where solutes pass across the semi-permeable membrane along with the solvent ("solvent drag") in response to a positive transmembrane pressure.

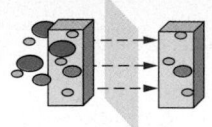

Effectiveness less dependent on molecular size

FIGURE 251-2. Mechanisms of diffusion and convection.

used as the blood compartment fluid. In actual clinical practice, nonspecific adsorption of plasma proteins to a dialyzer membrane effectively reduces the permeability of the membrane.[8] Consequently, in vivo sieving coefficient values are typically less than those derived from aqueous experiments, sometimes by a considerable amount.

MECHANISMS OF SOLUTE REMOVAL

Diffusion

Diffusion is the process of transport in which molecules that are present in a solvent and can freely move across a semipermeable membrane tend to move from the region of higher concentration into the region of lower concentration. In reality, molecules present a random movement. However, since they tend to reach the same concentration in the available space occupied by the solvent, the number of particles crossing the membrane toward the region of lower concentration is statistically higher. Therefore, this transport mechanism occurs in the presence of a concentration gradient for solutes that are not restricted in diffusion by the porosity of the membrane (see Chapter 246 for further details about membrane structure).[9] In addition to the concentration gradient (dc), the diffusive flux (J_X) is influenced by membrane characteristics, namely surface area (A) and thickness (dx), solution temperature (T), and the diffusion coefficient of the solute (D). Fick's law of diffusion then provides the diffusive flux, defined as the solute mass removal rate due to diffusion normalized to membrane surface area[10]:

$$J_X = DTA \, (dc/dx) \qquad [3]$$

Based on the earlier discussion, the clearance of a given solute can be predicted with reasonable certainty under a given set of operating conditions. However, several factors may lead to a divergence between theoretical and empirically derived values. As an example, protein binding or electrical charges in the solute may negatively impact the final clearance value. Conversely, convection or adsorption may result in a measured clearance value that is significantly greater than the value based on a "pure" diffusion assumption. Diffusion is an efficient transport mechanism for the removal of relatively small solutes, but as solute molecular weight increases, diffusion becomes limited and the relative importance of convection increases. Figure 251-2 describes the mechanisms of diffusion and convection.

Convection

Convection is the mass transfer mechanism associated with ultrafiltration of plasma water.[11] If a solute is small enough to pass through the pore structure of the membrane, it is driven ("dragged") across the membrane in association with the ultrafiltrated plasma water. This movement of plasma water is a consequence of a transmembrane pressure (TMP) gradient. Quantitatively, the ultrafiltration flux (J_F), defined as the ultrafiltration rate normalized to membrane surface area, can be described this way:

$$J_F = K_F \times TMP. \qquad [4]$$

In this equation, K_F is the membrane-specific hydraulic permeability (units: mL/hr/mm Hg/m^2) and TMP is a function of both the hydrostatic and oncotic pressure gradients.

Under theoretical conditions, the convective flux of a given solute (J_X), defined as the solute mass removal rate due to convection normalized to membrane surface area, is a function of J_F, solute concentration in the plasma water (C_B), and the sieving coefficient of the membrane (S):

$$J_X = J_F C_B (1 - \sigma) = J_F C_B S \qquad [5]$$

Under theoretical conditions, S is regulated by the reflection coefficient of the membrane (σ) according to

$$S = 1 - \sigma. \qquad [6]$$

In clinical practice, however, because plasma proteins and other factors modify the original reflection coefficient of the membrane, the final observed sieving coefficient is smaller than that expected from a simple theoretical calculation. As noted earlier, nonspecific adsorption of plasma proteins occurs instantaneously to an extracorporeal membrane after exposure to blood. This changes the effective permeability of the membrane, from the perspective of both water and solute permeability. This is explained by the action of proteins to essentially "plug" or block a certain percentage of membrane pores.

In Figure 251-3, percent rejection, which is essentially equal to 1 (sieving coefficient), is plotted against solute molecular weight. Results for both a protein-containing fluid (plasma) and a protein-free fluid (saline) are shown. For a test solute with a molecular weight of 5000, the percent rejection in saline is 0% (i.e., the sieving coefficient is 1). On the other hand, for that same solute, the percent rejection in plasma is approximately 60% (sieving coefficient of 0.4). This difference demonstrates the significant effect of secondary membrane formation on mem-

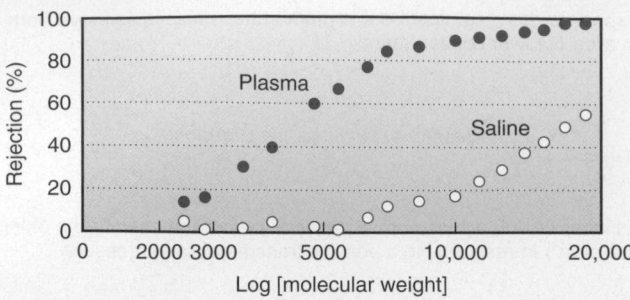

FIGURE 251-3. Effect of secondary membrane formation on membrane sieving properties.

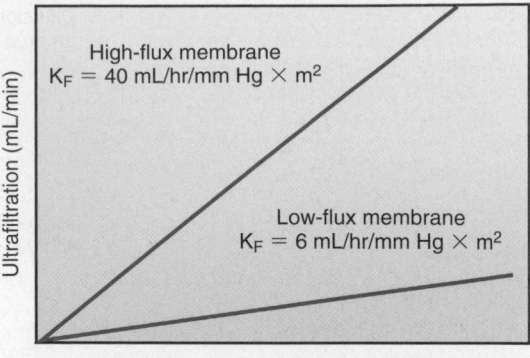

brane function. Postdilution tends to accentuate secondary membrane effects because protein concentrations are increased within the membrane fibers (due to hemoconcentration). On the other hand, higher blood flow rates work to attenuate this process because the shear effect created by the blood attenuates the binding of proteins to the membrane surface.

Adsorption

For certain membranes, adsorption (binding) may be the dominant or sole mechanism by which some hydrophobic compounds (i.e., peptides and proteins) are removed.[12] The adsorptive surface area of a membrane resides primarily in the pore structure rather than the nominal surface area. As such, the adsorption of a low-molecular-weight protein is highly dependent on access of the protein to a membrane's internal pore structure. Consequently, adsorption of peptides and low-molecular-weight proteins, such as β_2-microglobin, to low-flux membranes is not expected to be clinically significant, at least in comparison to that which occurs to high-flux membranes. The adsorption affinity of certain high-flux synthetic membranes for proteins and peptides is particularly high, attributable to the relative hydrophobicity of these membranes.

WATER PERMEABILITY (FLUX) OF CONTINUOUS RENAL REPLACEMENT THERAPY FILTERS

Extracorporeal membranes used for dialysis are classified according to their ultrafiltration coefficient as high flux or low flux (Fig. 251-4). In clinical practice, membranes are incorporated into specific devices designed to optimize the performance of the membrane itself. These devices may either be designed as dialyzers, working prevalently in diffusion with a countercurrent flux of blood and dialysate, or as hemofilters, working prevalently in convection. Improvements in membrane design have allowed diffusive and convective mass transport to be combined, leading to therapies (high-flux dialysis and hemodiafiltration) in which the advantages of both mechanisms are significantly enhanced.

Considerable confusion regarding the exact meaning of *flux* currently exists. As discussed earlier, the hydraulic flux of membrane is the volumetric rate (normalized to surface area) at which ultrafiltration of water occurs. The

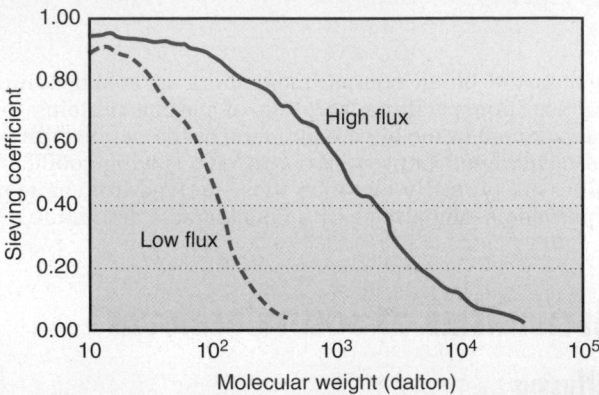

FIGURE 251-4. Differentiation between low-flux and high-flux properties.

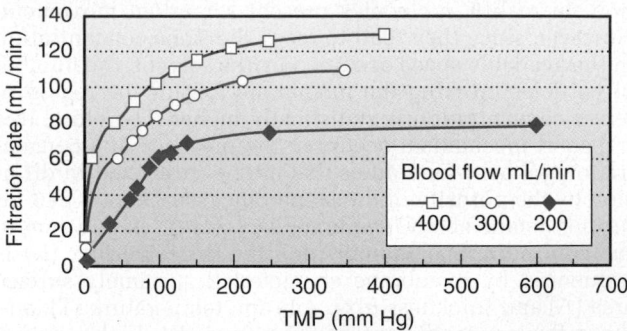

FIGURE 251-5. Relationship between ultrafiltration rate and transmembrane pressure during ultrafiltration. TMP, transmembrane pressure. (Reprinted from Kim S: Characteristics of protein removal in hemodiafiltration. Contr Nephrol 1994;108:23-37.)

clinical parameter used to characterize the water permeability of a specific dialyzer is the ultrafiltration coefficient (K_{UF}: mL/hr/mm Hg).[13] The K_{UF} of a filter is usually derived from in vitro experiments in which bovine blood is ultrafiltered at varying TMPs. The membrane characteristic having the largest impact on water permeability is pore size, such that ultrafiltrate flux is roughly proportional to the fourth power of the mean membrane pore radius. As such, small changes in pore size have a very large effect on water permeability.

As shown in Figure 251-5, a defined relationship exists between Q_{UF} (on the *y*-axis) and TMP (on the *x*-axis). (Although Fig. 251-5 is more relevant for chronic hemofiltration, it still has applicability to CVVH.) For each curve, at relatively low TMP values, there is a linear region; the slope of the line in this region is essentially the K_{UF} of the filter. As TMP increases, each curve eventually plateaus at a certain maximum Q_{UF}.[14] As mentioned previously, filter K_{UF} is a value that is specific to a certain set of flow operating conditions, including Q_B. In terms of clinical operation of a filter, the plateau portion of the curve is to be avoided because, in this region, an increase in TMP yields no additional increase in Q_{UF}.

Blood flow rate influences the nature of these curves in two ways. First, as Q_B increases, the slope of the curve in the linear (low TMP) region increases. Effectively, this means to achieve a certain Q_{UF}, a lower TMP is required. As an example, to achieve a Q_{UF} of 60 mL/min, a TMP of only about 10 mm Hg is required at a Q_B of 400 mL/min whereas TMPs of about 50 and 100 mm Hg are required at Q_B values of 300 and 200 mL/min, respectively. The second way in which Q_B influences the nature of these curves is its effect on the maximum achievable (plateau) Q_{UF}. This value is approximately 120 mL/min for a Q_B of 400 mL/min whereas it is only 100 mL/min for a Q_B of 300 mL/min and only 65 mL/min for a Q_B of 200 mL/min. The explanation for the behavior of these curves is related to the effect of higher Q_B in preserving filter membrane function. Specifically, as Q_B increases, a greater shear force is applied to the proteins comprising the secondary membrane. In this way, the secondary membrane is disrupted and its negative impact on membrane function is blunted.

KINETIC CONSIDERATIONS FOR VARIOUS CONTINUOUS RENAL REPLACEMENT THERAPY TECHNIQUES

Several techniques are today available in the spectrum of CRRT. Techniques may differ in terms of vascular access and extracorporeal circuit design, frequency and intensity of treatment, predominant mechanism of transport utilized, and type of membrane. The following descriptions are based primarily on the operational parameters normally employed and the target efficiency with respect to solute and fluid control.

Slow Continuous Ultrafiltration

In the intensive care unit, slow continuous ultrafiltration (SCUF) is typically employed for 24 hours a day but may also be applied during some portion of the day. The treatment is carried out with high-flux membranes, and the objective is to achieve volume control in patients with severe, diuretic-resistant volume overload. Relative to hemofiltration, low filtration rates (typically 2-8 mL/min) are required. As such, filters of relatively small surface area and low blood flow rates can be employed. Machines used for this therapy require an ultrafiltration control system to prevent excessive ultrafiltration. Although very effective for volume reduction, the low filtration rates and lack of substitution fluids render this therapy ineffective as a blood purification modality.

Extracorporeal ultrafiltration is increasingly being used as an adjunctive therapy for patients with refractory heart failure.[15,16] In this context, an important consideration is the type of vascular access type required. When conventional hemodialysis and venovenous CRRT systems are used in the acute dialysis setting, a central venous catheter is nearly always chosen as the vascular access. The achievable blood flow rate of such an access has a significant effect on solute clearances in the therapies delivered by these systems. In general, the desired solute clearances for these therapies can be achieved only with relatively high blood flow rates (>150 mL/min), the attainment of which requires a large-bore catheter in a central vein. However, isolated ultrafiltration is not a blood-cleansing modality, and solute clearance is not a relevant consideration. This suggests the possibility of using a smaller bore catheter in a peripheral vein for vascular access. From one perspective, the minimum blood flow rate is that required to avoid excessive hemoconcentration. To quantify this phenomenon, the filtration fraction (ratio of the ultrafiltration rate to the plasma flow rate delivered to the filter) has been employed traditionally. In general, a maximal filtration fraction of 25% usually guides prescription in acute postdilution hemofiltration, which is the relevant comparison in this instance. At filtration fractions beyond this value, hemoconcentration is associated with an environment that promotes interactions between both formed elements and proteins in the blood and the filter membrane, leading to a high risk of filter clotting. However, the ultrafiltration rates typically employed in isolated ultrafiltration (<10 mL/min) are significantly less than those in hemofiltration, which may be 40 mL/min or higher. Therefore, although the minimum blood flow rate may be 200 mL/min or higher in the setting of postdilution hemofiltration, a blood flow rate of 50 mL/min may be adequate to maintain the filtration fraction less than 25% in isolated ultrafiltration. For example, based on a blood flow rate of 50 mL/min prescribed to a patient with a hematocrit of 35%, isolated ultrafiltration at a rate of 8 mL/min (480 mL/hr) results in a filtration fraction of 25% *at the onset of therapy.*

Although the preceding analysis suggests that a blood flow rate as low as 50 mL/min may be used in isolated ultrafiltration, two caveats must be discussed. First, the filtration fraction calculation mentioned is based on a hematocrit of 35% at the start of therapy. However, as ultrafiltration proceeds and net volume removal occurs, hematocrit increases. Therefore, for a given volume of blood flowing through the filter, an increasing percentage of that volume is composed of red blood cells and a decreasing percentage is composed of plasma water during ongoing ultrafiltration therapy. At a fixed blood flow rate and ultrafiltration rate, this implies an increasing filtration fraction, since plasma water flow rate is the denominator in the filtration fraction equation. Thus, from the relatively narrow perspective of filtration fraction, a seemingly adequate blood flow rate at the onset of ultrafiltration may be inadequate after several hours of therapy. A second important consideration related to blood flow rate involves its effect on blood rheology at the membrane surface. The velocity that blood achieves while passing through an individual hollow fiber membrane is directly proportional to its blood flow rate.[51] In turn, the velocity (or more rigorously, the velocity gradient) of blood at the membrane surface is directly proportional to its shear rate at that membrane-blood interface. When continuous arteriovenous therapies were popular in the early years of CRRT, filters were designed specifically to overcome some of the drawbacks of the characteristically low blood flow rates achieved with these therapies. However, the design characteristics of contemporary filters are based on the higher blood flow rates achieved with continuous venovenous therapies. Thus, whether or not contemporary filters can achieve adequate ultrafiltration rates at blood flow rates delivered from a peripheral venous access (i.e., approximately 50 mL/min) will need to be assessed carefully.

Continuous Venovenous Hemofiltration

CVVH is normally applied for an extended period up to several weeks. The technique utilizes high-flux membranes, and the prevalent mechanism of solute transport is convection. Ultrafiltration rates in excess of the amount required for volume control are prescribed, requiring partial or total replacement of ultrafiltrate losses with reinfusion (replacement) fluid. Blood flow is regulated by a pump, and systems for ultrafiltration and reinfusion control are generally utilized. Different machines use either volumetric control systems or volumetric pumps regulated by one or multiple scales. As described in greater detail in Chapter 275, replacement fluid can either be infused before the filter (predilution) or after the filter (postdilution). Postdilution hemofiltration is inherently limited by the attainable blood flow rate and the associated filtration fraction constraint.

On the other hand, from a mass transfer perspective, the use of predilution has several potential advantages over postdilution.[17] First, both hematocrit and blood total protein concentration are reduced significantly prior to the entry of blood into the hemofilter. This effective reduction in the red cell and protein content of the blood attenuates the secondary membrane and concentration polarization phenomena described earlier, resulting in improved mass transfer. Predilution also favorably impacts mass transfer due to augmented flow in the blood compartment, because prefilter mixing of blood and replacement fluid occurs. This achieves a relatively high membrane shear rate, which also reduces solute-membrane interactions. Finally, predilution may also enhance mass transfer for some compounds by creating concentration gradients that induce solute movement out of red blood cells.

However, the major drawback of predilution hemofiltration is its relatively low efficiency, resulting in relatively high replacement fluid requirements to achieve a given solute clearance.[18] In a group of patients treated with a traditional blood flow rate for CRRT, Troyanov and colleagues[19] recently quantified the efficiency loss associated with predilution. This study demonstrated the significant negative effect on efficiency when a relatively low Q_B (<150 mL/min) is used with a relatively high Q_{UF} and Q_{RF} in predilution CVVH. This specific combination of Q_B = 125-150 mL/min and Q_{UF} = 4.5 L/hr (75 mL/min) is associated with a loss of efficiency of 30% to 40% relative to postdilution for several different solutes. In other words, to achieve the same solute clearance, 30% to 40% more replacement fluid is required in predilution under these conditions, relative to postdilution under the same conditions. However, it should be noted the likelihood of achieving such an ultrafiltration rate in postdilution is very remote at such a low blood flow rate, as this would require a filtration fraction in excess of 50%. This condition is likely to lead to very short-term filter patency.

Continuous Venovenous Hemodialysis

CVVHD is a treatment carried out over an extended period of time with a pump-driven circuit. Because of the nature of the membrane and the gradient provided by the dialysate, the prevalent mechanism of solute transport in this

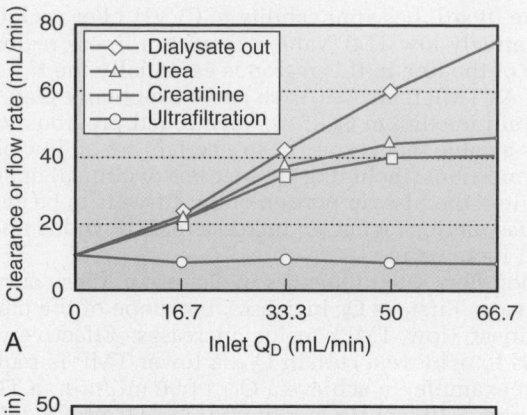

A

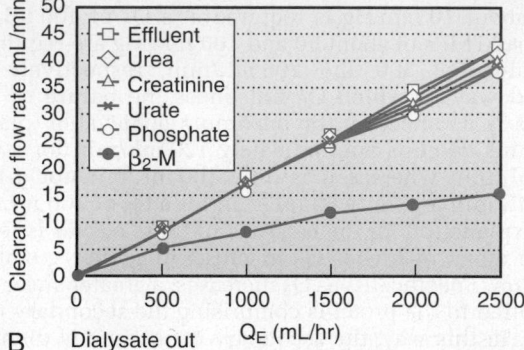

B   Dialysate out Q_E (mL/hr)

FIGURE 251-6. Relationship between solute clearance and dialysate flow rate for a 0.4 m² filter (**A**) and a 0.9 m² filter (**B**). β₂-M, β₂-microglobulin; Q_D, dialysate flow; Q_E, effluent flow. (**A**, Reprinted from Bonnardeaux A, Pichette V, Ouimet D, et al: Solute clearances with high dialysate flow rates and glucose absorption from the dialysate in continuous arteriovenous hemodialysis. Am J Kidney Dis 1992;19:31-38; **B**, reprinted from Brunet S, Leblanc M, Geadah D, et al: Diffusive and convective solute clearances during continuous renal replacement therapy at various dialysate and ultrafiltration flow rates. Am J Kidney Dis 1999;34:486-492.)

technique is diffusion. As such, either a low-flux or high-flux filter can be used, although the latter is typically prescribed. Ultrafiltration is obtained exactly in the range of values adequate to maintain patient's fluid control without requirement of fluid reinfusion. In most cases, designated machines must be used to control inlet and outlet dialysate flows and to achieve the desired rate and volume of ultrafiltration.

When CVVHD is performed with a relatively small surface area filter (<0.5 m²), saturation of the dialysate is only achieved at relatively low dialysate flow rates. For a 0.4 m² filter, Bonnardeaux and colleagues[20] showed saturation of the effluent dialysate for urea and creatinine is preserved only up to a dialysate flow rate of approximately 16.7 mL/min (1 L/hr) (Fig. 251-6A). For dialysate flow (Q_D) values in the 2-3 L/hr range (33.3-50 mL/min), an increase in Q_D results in an increase in clearance. However, the divergence between the urea/creatinine clearance curves and the effluent dialysate curve indicates the degree to which the dialysate is "nonsaturated." Of course, the greater the degree of nonsaturation, the more inefficient is the procedure. Beyond a Q_D value of approximately 3 L/hr, the urea/creatinine clearance curves plateau—beyond this Q_D value, further increases in Q_D no longer result in an increase in clearance.

A more contemporary study involving a larger surface area filter (0.9 m²) demonstrates clearly the important effect of surface area on preserving dialysate saturation

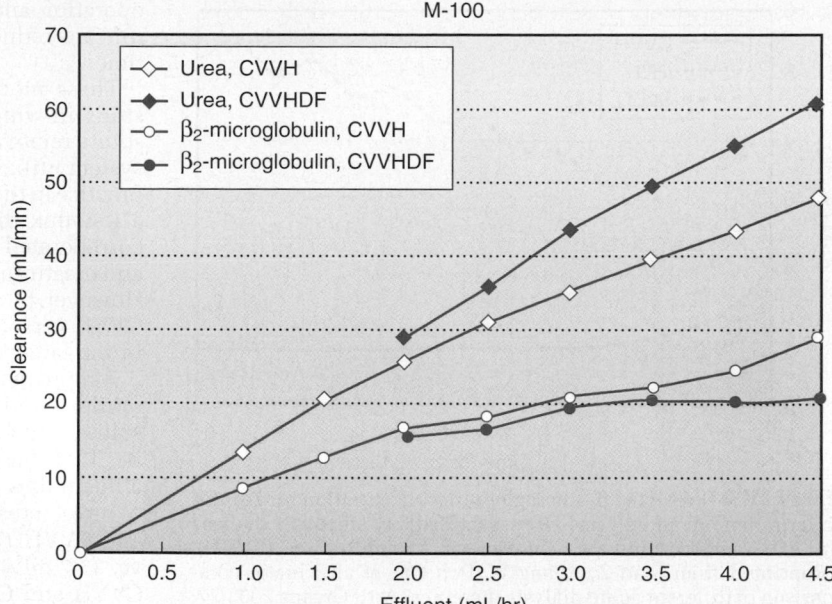

FIGURE 251-7. Comparison of solute clearance in predilution continuous venovenous hemofiltration (CVVH) and continuous venovenous hemodiafiltration (CVVHDF). (Reprinted from Troyanov S, Cardinal J, Geadah D, et al: Solute clearances during continuous venovenous haemofiltration at various ultrafiltration flow rates using Multiflow-100 and HF1000 filters. Nephrol Dial Transplant 2003;18:961-966.)

(Fig. 251-6B).[21] For this larger filter, preservation of effluent dialysate saturation was achieved essentially over the entire Q_D range, the only exception being β_2-microglobulin. The high molecular weight of this compound (approximately 200 times that of urea) severely limits its diffusive capabilities and, therefore, its ability to saturate the dialysate.

Continuous Venovenous Hemodiafiltration

CVVHDF requires a high-flux hemodiafilter and operates combining the principles of hemodialysis and hemofiltration. As such, this therapy may allow for an optimal combination of diffusion and convection to provide clearances over a very broad range of solutes. Dialysate is circulated in countercurrent mode to blood and, at the same time, ultrafiltration is obtained in excess of the desired fluid loss from the patient. The ultrafiltrate is partially or totally replaced with reinfusion fluid, either in predilution or postdilution mode. Later generation CRRT machines allow a combination of predilution and postdilution with the aim of combining the advantages of both reinfusion techniques (see Chapter 275 for further information). Information from the chronic hemodiafiltration literature suggests a combination of predilution and postdilution may be optimal in terms of clearance and operational parameters.[22] This may also be the case for CVVHDF in AKI although this possibility has not been assessed carefully. The optimal balance is most likely dictated by the specific set of CVVHDF operating conditions, namely blood flow rate, dialysate flow rate, ultrafiltration rate, and filter type.

The specific manner in which diffusion and convection interact in CVVHDF differs significantly from the situation when this treatment is applied in the end-stage renal disease setting. In the latter situation, diffusion and convection interact in such a manner that total solute removal is significantly less than what is expected if the individual components are simply added together.[23] This phenomenon is explained in the following way. Diffusive solute removal results in a decrease in solute concentration in the blood compartment of the filter along the axial length

(i.e., from blood inlet to blood outlet) of the hemodiafilter. As convective solute removal is directly proportional to the blood compartment concentration, convective solute removal decreases as a function of this axial concentration gradient. At the same time, hemoconcentration resulting from ultrafiltration of plasma water causes a progressive increase in plasma protein concentration and hematocrit along the axial length of the filter. This hemoconcentration and resultant hyperviscosity causes an increase in diffusive mass transfer resistance and a decrease in solute transport by this mechanism.

Due to the markedly lower flow rates used and clearances obtained in CVVHDF, the effect of simultaneous diffusion and convection on overall solute removal is quite different. Therefore, the small-solute concentration gradient along the axial length of the filter (i.e., extraction) is minimal compared to that which is seen in chronic hemodiafiltration, in which extraction ratios of 50% or more are the norm. Thus, the minimal diffusion-related change in small-solute concentrations along the filter length allows any additional clearance related to convection to be simply additive to the diffusive component. This has been demonstrated clearly in both continuous hemodialysis[24] and continuous hemodiafiltration.[21]

Troyanov and colleagues[19] performed a direct clinical comparison of CVVHDF and predilution CVVH with respect to urea and β_2-microglobin clearance at a traditional blood flow rate of 125 mL/min. The study compared clearances at the same effluent rate over an effluent range of up to 4.5 L/hr. As Figure 251-7 indicates, urea clearance was higher in CVVHDF than in predilution CVVH and, in fact, the difference between the two therapies increased as effluent rate increased. These results are consistent with the "penalizing" effect of predilution, which is especially pronounced at low blood flow rates. For β_2-microglobin, the results are contrary to the conventional wisdom, which would suggest a purely convective therapy like CVVH should inherently be superior to a partly convective therapy like CVVHDF for clearance of a molecule this size. However, once again, the penalty of predilution in CVVH is apparent, as the β_2-microglobin clearances for the two modalities are equivalent except at very high effluent rates (>3.5 L/hr). Until the impact of

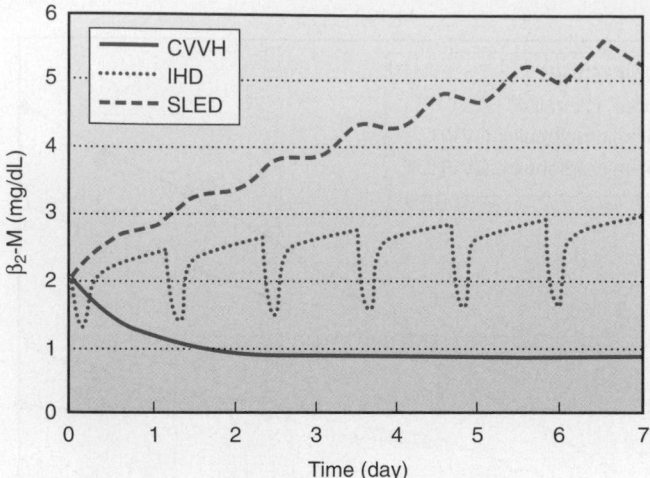

FIGURE 251-8. Predicted β_2-microglobulin concentration profiles for intermittent hemodialysis (IHD), sustained low-efficiency dialysis (SLED), and continuous venovenous hemofiltration (CVVH). (Reprinted from Liao Z, Zhang W, Poh CK, et al: Kinetic comparison of different acute dialysis therapies. Artif Organs 2003;27: 802-807.)

higher blood flow rates on solute clearances in CRRT can be assessed, these and other data suggest CVVHDF is a logical modality choice to achieve the broadest spectrum of solute molecular-weight range in the most efficient way.

COMPARISON OF DIFFUSIVE AND CONVECTIVE SOLUTE REMOVAL IN DIFFERENT ACUTE MODALITIES

The relationship between solute clearance and flow rate in diffusive therapies differs significantly from that in convective therapies. Based on mass transfer considerations, the expected clearance of small solutes during CVVHD and postdilution CVVH is the same. However, as solute molecular weight increases, the relevance of diffusion diminishes and the benefits of convection become increasingly apparent. For acute dialysis modalities, these principles have been substantiated in both modeling and clinical studies. Liao and colleagues[25] performed a kinetic comparison of intermittent hemodialysis (daily 4-hour treatments), sustained low-efficiency dialysis (SLED) (daily 12-hour treatments),[27,28] and predilution CVVH (ultrafiltration rate, 35 mL/kg/hr).[29] These investigators employed the equivalent renal clearance concept[30] to compare effective solute removal for these modalities. Their analyses indicated similar effective urea clearances for CVVH and SLED of 33 and 31 mL/min, respectively, both of which were substantially higher than that delivered by daily intermittent hemodialysis (21 mL/min). On the other hand, the estimated β_2-microglobulin clearances for CVVH and SLED were 18 and 4 mL/min, respectively. Daily intermittent hemodialysis with a high-flux dialyzer was estimated to provide an intermediate β_2-microglobulin clearance of 7 mL/min. The predicted β_2-microglobulin concentration profiles appear in Figure 251-8. The profile specifically predicted for SLED is the result of ongoing solute generation in the face of no removal by a low-flux filter. On the other hand, the combination of continuous

operation and convection permit CVVH to achieve a significant reduction in β_2-microglobulin concentration over time.

These modeled data are extended by a recent clinical study in which effluent collections were used to quantify solute removal in predilution CVVH (2.5 L/hr) and a SLED system utilizing a high-flux filter. (Consistent with clinical practice in the United States, this modeling study employed a low-flux dialyzer.[31]) Indeed, Kielstein and colleagues[31] corroborated Liao's findings by demonstrating that urea and creatinine removal during CVVH and SLED are similar. However, β_2-microglobulin removal was twofold greater in CVVH versus SLED, even with the use of a high-flux filter in the latter therapy.

A more recent study performed by Ricci and colleagues[32] reinforces the importance of convection in achieving solute clearance over a broad molecular-weight spectrum in CRRT. Based on a common prescription of 35 mL/kg/hr effluent flow rate,[29] these investigators measured clearance of urea, creatinine, and β_2-microglobulin during CVVH and CVVHD in a crossover study. The median urea (31.6 vs. 35.7 mL/min) and creatinine (38.1 vs. 35.6 mL/min) in CVVH and CVVHD, respectively, were similar. However, median β_2-microglobulin clearance in CVVH was higher than that in CVVHD (16.3 vs. 6.3 mL/min, respectively; P = 0.055). This borderline statistically significant difference was observed despite the fact this trial was markedly underpowered.

CONCLUSION

Rational prescription of CRRT to critically ill patients with AKI is predicated upon an understanding of the basic principles of solute and water removal. In this chapter, the major ways in which filter function is characterized clinically were reviewed. In addition, the fundamental mechanisms for solute and fluid transport were discussed. Finally, these principles have been applied in a therapeutic context to the various CRRT modalities used by clinicians managing AKI patients.

Key Points

1. Solute clearance in continuous renal replacement therapy is the ratio of mass removal rate to solute blood concentration.
2. In continuous venovenous hemodialysis, sufficient membrane surface area is a critical factor in attaining dialysate saturation of small solutes.
3. Secondary membrane effects play an important role in continuous venovenous hemofiltration, especially in postdilution.
4. For the flow rates used typically in continuous venovenous hemodiafiltration, diffusive and convective clearances are additive.
5. Of all dialysis modalities to treat acute kidney injury, continuous therapies have the greatest solute-removal capabilities over the broadest molecular-weight range.

See the companion Expert Consult website for the complete reference list.

Clinical and Technical Aspects

CHAPTER 252

Hemodynamic and Biological Response to Continuous Renal Replacement Therapies

Ciro Tetta and Didier Payen de La Garanderie

OBJECTIVES

This chapter will:
1. Describe the elimination of endotoxins and cytokines with continuous renal replacement therapy.
2. Analyze the modulation of the immune response seen with continuous renal replacement therapy.
3. Outline the major features of the systemic and regional circulatory responses to continuous renal replacement therapy.
4. Evaluate the evidence on the relevance of cooling in hemodynamic stability.

New insights into the pathogenesis of acute renal failure (ARF) have shown the inflammatory nature of the systemic[1] and renal tissue[2] response, as well as the possibility of "crosstalk" with other organs as the cause of acute lung injury (ALI).[3] The large study by Metnitz and colleagues[4] has convincingly shown that the occurrence of ARF increases the risk to die *of* ARF, thereby disproving the old perception that patients die *with* ARF.

Continuous renal replacement therapies (CRRTs) are commonly used for the treatment of ARF in critically ill patients but also are used in so-called extrarenal conditions such as the need for fluid control, congestive heart failure, acute respiratory distress syndrome (ARDS), and sepsis.[5,6] The main evidence on the hemodynamic and biological response to CRRT is reviewed next.

ELIMINATION OF ENDOTOXINS AND CYTOKINES BY CONTINUOUS RENAL REPLACEMENT THERAPY

Over the past decade, several studies have dealt with the ability of high-permeability membranes to filter and adsorb endotoxins and cytokines, pointing to a role for CRRT in reducing plasma concentrations of these substances. Several papers have presented evidence that continuous venovenous hemofiltration (CVVH) removes pro-inflammatory mediators such as cytokines[7-9] and that by removing these substances, this therapy may improve hemodynamics and clinical outcomes. Several studies have evaluated whether plasma cytokine concentrations decrease with CVVH as a consequence of transmembrane flux (i.e., convection) or of adsorption.[10-13]

Reduction of plasma concentrations occurring in either in vitro or animal studies turned out to be of little or no relevance in the clinical setting (reviewed by Tetta and colleagues[14]). In fact, the presence or absence of detectable levels of cytokines within a biological fluid (e.g., plasma or ultrafiltrate) reflects a complex balance between enhancing and inhibitory signals acting on producer cells, production and catabolism, cytokine binding to target cells, and their modulation.[15] Although these studies failed to demonstrate remarkable and steady reduction in plasma concentrations of different cytokines, other work has nonetheless implicated effects of CRRT on biological activities such as oxidative and carbonyl stress,[16,17] superoxide production,[18] removal of activated complement components,[19] reduction in serum priming activity of stimulated polymorphonuclear neutrophil chemiluminescence,[20] and septic plasma–induced pro-apoptogenic effects.[21,22] Although most of these studies are provocative from a biological point of view, they are not informative about whether the effects induced by the membrane transport affect these activities at the tissue level or may be ultimately relevant at the clinical level.

Clinically, CRRTs have been preferred for their effects on the hemodynamic and biological response in the critically ill patient.[23] Current thinking on the pathogenesis of ARF, as well as on the targets for any therapy including extracorporeal treatments, has evolved extensively over the past decade (reviewed by Vincent and Abraham[24]). Concepts such as immunoparalysis, immunomodulation, endotoxin tolerance (reviewed by Cavaillon and Adib-Conquy[25]), and organ crosstalk[26] and the emerging role of apoptosis and its regulation, as well as the regulatory mechanisms of defense and damage at the organ level, have made the overall picture increasingly much more complicated than was originally conceived (Fig. 252-1). Initially, CRRT was rather simplistically considered to work by eliminating biologically active substances produced in excess (by means of convection or adsorption); nowadays, CRRT is recognized to have a remarkable hemodynamic and biological impact through a more complex mode of action.

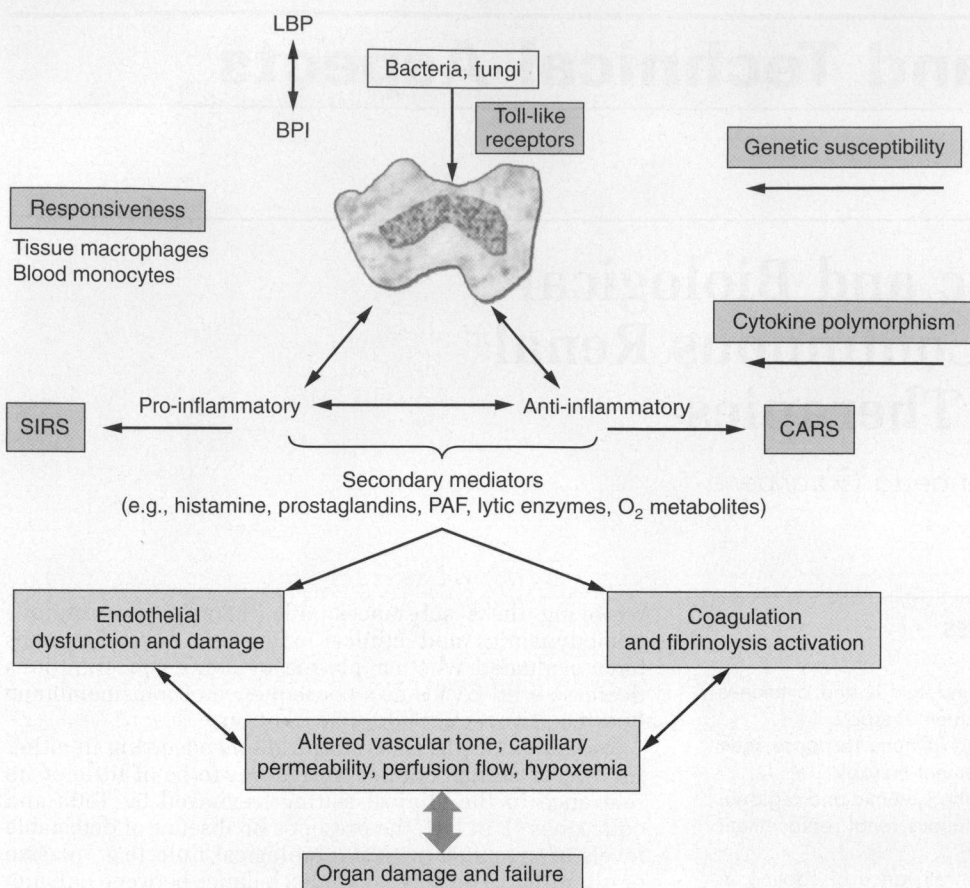

FIGURE 252-1. Schematic drawing of the cascade of events following the activation of innate immunity by bacterial and fungal constituents. In the case of bacterial endotoxin (LPS), at least two concurrent pathways with opposite biological effects are recognized: LPS may be bound by lipopolysaccharide-binding protein, which strongly enhances on a molar basis the effect of LPS. On the contrary, LPS may be bound to bacterial permeability-inducing protein (BPI) that allows the body clearance. The interaction with Toll-like receptors is instrumental to the monocyte-macrophage activation leading to the production and release of pro-inflammatory and anti-inflammatory mediators. Important secondary mediators later come into play that are responsible for endothelial dysfunction and damage, as well as the activation of fluid systems such as the coagulation and the fibrinolytic pathways. CARS, compensatory anti-inflammatory response syndrome; LBP, lipopolysaccharide-binding protein; PAF, platelet-activating factor; SIRS, systemic inflammatory response syndrome.

Three main hypotheses recently have been put forward, all of which help to provide a useful platform for understanding the mechanisms by which CRRT may have a hemodynamic and biological impact: the *peak concentration hypothesis*,[27] the *threshold hypothesis*,[28] and the *mediator delivery hypothesis*.[29] The first two deal with a "critical" level of cytokines in plasma or in tissues, respectively, whereas the mediator delivery hypothesis suggests that CRRT may in fact have an effect not only through removal (by convection or adsorption) but also through a washout effect at the level of the extracellular compartment. This possibility provides support not only for the use of high volumes but for a more adequate composition of the infusion fluid.

CONTINUOUS RENAL REPLACEMENT THERAPY AND ITS HEMODYNAMIC EFFECTS IN EXPERIMENTAL AND HUMAN SEPSIS

The pioneering studies by Grootendorst and associates showed the beneficial effect of high-volume hemofiltration (HVHF) on the hemodynamics of pigs in endotoxic shock.[30,31] The ultrafiltrate from endotoxin (LPS)-infused pigs caused a 50% decrease in mean arterial pressure (MAP), an eight-fold increase in mean pulmonary arterial pressure (PAP), and a threefold decrease in cardiac output

(CO). Later, interleukin (IL)-6 was implicated as the major cardiodepressant in sepsis caused by meningococci.[32]

Rogiers and coworkers[33,34] applied HVHF only after 6 to 12 hours, thereby allowing enough time for the animals to become hemodynamically unstable and to show early signs of multiple organ failure. In their studies, it also became evident that the early application of HVHF showed the most beneficial and the most impressive results. In an interesting compilation of the last 12 studies in the past 10 years based on animal models, the "middle dose" used in those experiments was approximately 100 mL/kg per hour, whereas in the human studies (the last 13 human studies), only 40 mL/kg per hour was given.[35] Therefore, it is quite clear that despite the remarkable hemodynamic impact in most experimental studies on hemofiltration, findings may be not be applicable to the clinical setting, because the model of endotoxin (LPS) infusion differs considerably from human sepsis, in which the release of endotoxin may occur continuously or intermittently.

In a clinical study of burn-injured patients and in a parallel set of experiments using a cecal ligation and puncture rodent model of sepsis, Kelly and associates[36] questioned the idea that circulating endotoxin (LPS) is the trigger for increased pro-inflammatory cytokine production, systemic inflammatory response syndrome (SIRS), and septic complications in injured patients and in the experimental model. More recently, however, the issue of whether removal of endotoxin from plasma may be instrumental in reducing the hemodynamic derangements associated with experimental models of septic shock has again been highlighted.[37-39] Many studies have indeed explored

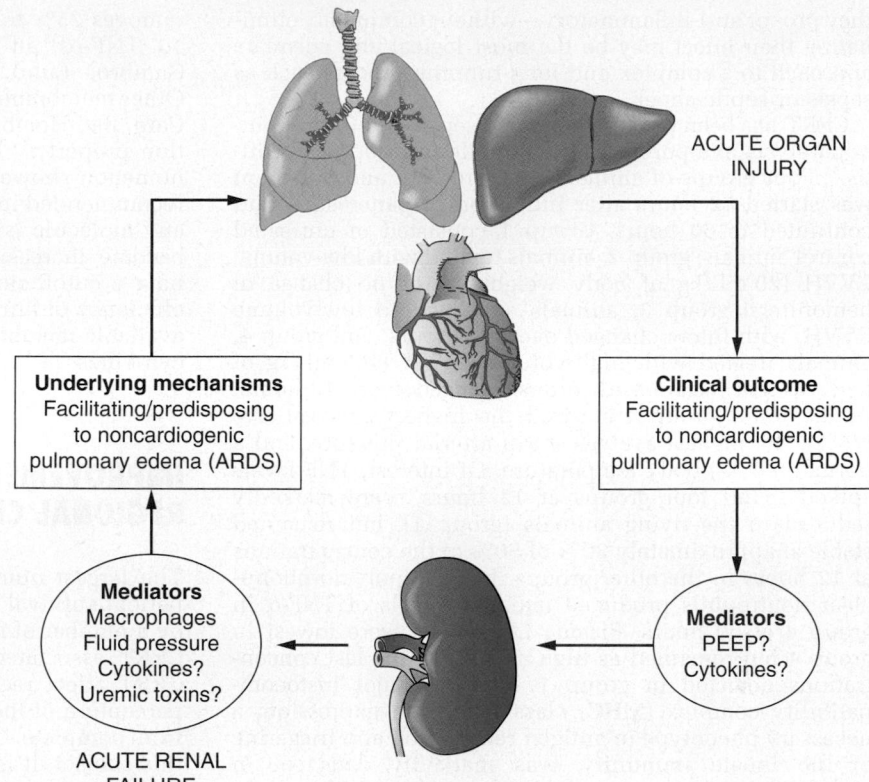

FIGURE 252-2. Schematic drawing of the hypothesized crosstalk between kidney and lung. ARDS, acute respiratory distress syndrome; PEEP, positive end-expiratory pressure. (Modified from Molls RR, Rabb H: Limiting deleterious cross-talk between failing organs. Crit Care Med 2004;32: 2358-2359.)

the possibility of removing clinically significant amounts of bacterial endotoxin (LPS) from plasma using chemically modified polymers (reviewed by Tetta and colleagues[40]). However, their effects in human studies are for an all-or-none response.[41] Although the removal of LPS theoretically constitutes a logical approach to blood purification in sepsis, it is essential to take into account the very short half-life of all microbe-based molecules, which have molecular patterns recognized by specific pattern recognition receptors that promptly induce cytokine expression (Fig. 252-2). Furthermore, these microbial patterns act synergistically with one another, with host mediators, and with hypoxia (reviewed by Annane and coauthors[42]). After intravenous injection of LPS, a lag phase occurs and is followed after 1 hour by a steep increase in tumor necrosis factor-α (TNF-α), reaching a peak at 1.5 hours. TNF-α plasma concentrations are sharply reduced at 3 hours, when both IL-6 and IL-8 sharply increase. LPS is no longer detectable in plasma after 1 minute from injection.

The concept of sepsis as a simply pro-inflammatory event has been challenged, as described next.[43]

IMMUNE MODULATION OF INFLAMMATORY CELL RESPONSIVENESS

Critically ill patients requiring intensive care are in a SIRS or, most often, a compensatory anti-inflammatory response syndrome (CARS) state. Hyporesponsiveness occurs not only in peripheral mononuclear cells but in whole blood.[44] Hyporesponsiveness is associated with increased plasma levels of IL-10 and prostaglandin E_2, which are potent

inhibitors of the production of pro-inflammatory cytokines.[45] Adib-Conquy and colleagues[46] demonstrated that on LPS activation, peripheral mononuclear cells from patients with SIRS show patterns of nuclear factor (NF)-κB expression that resemble patterns reported during LPS tolerance: global downregulation of NF-κB in survivors of sepsis and trauma patients and the presence of large amounts of the inactive homodimer in the nonsurvivors of sepsis.

In intensive care medicine, blocking one mediator has not led to measurable outcome improvement in patients with sepsis.[47] Possibly, more rigidly defined subgroups would benefit from TNF-α–antagonizing treatments.[48] On the other hand, antagonizing a cytokine may have deleterious consequences, leading to substantially higher mortality.[49] A low-level TNF-α response is necessary for mounting the host defense against infection,[50] high levels being modulated by an anti-inflammatory feedback mechanism. In sepsis, however, impaired regulation may cause an excessive anti-inflammatory response that generates monocyte "immunoparalysis," exposing the host to further infection. Both processes—inflammation and "anti-inflammation"—are designed to act in response to specific stimuli in a well-balanced fashion defined as immune homeostasis.

The time point of therapeutic intervention in sepsis seems to be crucial.[51] Because the network acts like a cascade, early intervention is intuitively optimal. Sepsis does not fit a one-hit model, however, but shows complex and multiple rises in mediator levels that change over time. Neither single mediator–directed nor one-time interventions, therefore, seem appropriate. One of the major criticisms of continuous blood purification treatment in sepsis—its lack of specificity—may turn out to be a major strength. Unspecific removal of soluble mediators—be they pro- or anti-inflammatory—without completely eliminating their effect may be the most logical and adequate approach to a complex and long-running process such as sepsis or septic shock.

CRRT has been proved to reverse sepsis-induced immunoparalysis in a porcine model of bile-induced pancreatitis.[52] Four groups of animals were studied, and treatment was started 12 hours after induction of pancreatitis and continued to 60 hours. Group 1 consisted of untreated control animals; group 2, animals treated with low-volume CVVH (20 mL/kg of body weight), with no change of hemofilters; group 3, animals subjected to low-volume CVVH, with filters changed every 12 hours; and group 4, animals treated with high-volume CVVH (100 mL/kg of body weight), again with filters changed every 12 hours. At 60 hours, group 4 showed the highest survival rate (75%), the highest average mean arterial pressure, and a normal (37° C) body temperature. Of interest, TNF levels spiked in all four groups at 12 hours, were markedly reduced in the dying animals (group 1), but remained stable at approximately 30% of 50% of the concentrations at 12 hours in the other groups. In vitro polymorphonuclear neutrophils produced maximal levels of TNF-α in group 4 at 60 hours. Plasma LPS levels were lowest in group 4 but remained as high as 40% of the last concentrations detected in group 1. Finally, major histocompatibility complex (MHC) class II antigen expression, a necessary phenotype in antigen recognition and triggering of the innate immunity, was markedly defective in group 1 but, of note, was reversed in group 4. This study was remarkable in that it introduced a pancreatitis model sharing many parallels with severe human pancreatitis—for example, the nonbacterial onset of the disease preceding nonbacterial translocation and endotoxemia, a hyperdynamic circulatory response, and characteristic laboratory and immunological features found frequently in the human clinical setting (e.g., high plasma C-reactive protein, reduced expression of MHC class II antigen expression, polymorphonuclear neutrophil–associated oxidative stress). The authors of this pioneering study suggested that convection and adsorption may be instrumental in the removal of various factors involved in the complex pathophysiology of pancreatitis. CVVH reversed or prevented neutrophil hyporesponsiveness to endotoxin. Also observed was a modulatory effect on anti-inflammatory cytokines such as IL-10, limiting the initial exorbitant response seen in control animals and avoiding a drop in both IL-10 and transforming growth factor-β (TGF-β).

Several questions are still to be answered: Is convection the only driving force for the mass transfer of cytokines and other biologically active substances involved in sepsis? For convection, differences are more pronounced for middle-size and large solute categories, and the equivalent renal urea clearance in CVVH is approximately two- and fourfold greater, respectively, than the corresponding values with daily hemodialysis and slow extended daily dialysis (SLEDD). The superiority of middle-size and large solute removal in CVVH stems from the powerful combination of convection and continuous operation. In CVVH, a decrease in the initial blood urea nitrogen (BUN) from 150 to 50 mg/dL is predicted to decrease the time-averaged concentration (TAC) (and therefore to increase equivalent renal urea clearance by approximately 35%).[53] Adsorption to the membrane itself is the initial mechanism for removal of proteins from the circulation. Molecules may be trapped within the supporting external sponge layer, rather than simply being adhered to the inner surface.[54] Adsorption

removes 25% to 43% of the cytokine load (IL-6, IL-8, IL-10, TNF-α)[55] in the first hour using an AN-69R (Hospal-Gambro, Lund, Sweden) polyacrylonitrile membrane. Other membranes, such as polysulfone (Fresenius Medical Care, Bad Homburg, Germany), show a negligible adsorption property.[56] Membrane adsorption is a transient phenomenon, however, and frequent filter changes are not recommended in daily practice. The convective transfer of any molecule is indicated by its filtration fraction. It has become increasingly clear that although all membranes have a cutoff sieving size of approximately 30,000 D, the efficiency of filtration declines over time. Accordingly, all available membranes can remove only small quantities of cytokines.

IMPROVEMENT IN SYSTEMIC AND REGIONAL CIRCULATION

The largest number of studies on CRRT are focused on patient survival and recovery of renal function (reviewed by a number of investigative teams[57-60]). Why, therefore, is CRRT associated with a hemodynamic response? Does CRRT affect regional circulation and how? The current perception of the hemodynamic alteration in sepsis is far from complete. Owing to the scarcity of clinical studies on this subject, it is necessary to evaluate experimental data in this context, with reservations concerning their extrapolation to human beings. Septic shock, a distributive shock, results from a homogeneous decline in vascular tone and therefore of regional blood flow. Nitric oxide and prostaglandins as well as cytokines produce direct or indirect vasodilatation with hypocontractility. In hyperkinetic shock in animals, dilatation of the mesenteric and coronary arteries occurs, with reduction in pancreatic, skin, and muscle flow rates. The hepatic, pancreatic, and mesenteric circulations are particularly threatened, their flow being reduced by 50% as a result of vaconstriction. In the kidney, the alteration in flow rate is biphasic: high first, then low. Restoration of normovolemia or treatment with vasopressors does not seem to improve kidney function, or to correct disorders in cardiac output distribution (reviewed by Payen[61]; see also the reports of Losser[62] and Bateman[63] and their coworkers).

Table 252-1 summarizes only the studies concerned with the hemodynamic alterations observed in different patient populations treated with various continuous therapy modalities. The effect of CRRT on hemodynamics is relative to the amount of volume exchanged and to the timing of initiation of the therapy. HVHF attenuates altered hemodynamics in the first 4 to 6 hours of treatment and represents a useful therapeutic approach to maintain stable circulatory conditions. Pulse or short high-volume therapies are being considered because of the very promising results in highly variable, critically ill populations studied in different centers, to the intensive workload and to the unequivocally higher costs of HVHF (see Table 252-1). A note of caution, however, is in order: Until now, no randomized control trials have been performed testing the impact of hemofiltration versus conventional therapy on the systemic or regional circulation. As a consequence, only experimental studies and a few clinical studies can be used to analyze such aspects of CVVH.

As mentioned earlier, hemofiltration is an integrated, unselective technique, which in itself may become an advantage for plasma content modification. Depending on

TABLE 252-1

Summary of Studies Describing Hemodynamic Effects during Continuous Renal Replacement Therapy (CRRT)

STUDY*	DESIGN	ENDPOINT(S)	TREATMENT	NO. OF PATIENTS	INCLUSION CRITERIA	TIMING	HEMODYNAMIC OUTCOME
Journois et al., 1996	Randomized, blinded, controlled	Respiratory and mediator response	4972 mL/m²	20 children	Cardiopulmonary bypass	During rewarming	Reduced postop. alveolar-arterial oxygen gradient at 3 hr
Honoré et al., 2000	Prospective, interventional	Hemodynamic and metabolic status, 28-day survival in patients with refractory septic shock	1. 35 L effluent at zero fluid balance, *followed by* 2. CVVH for at least 4 days	20 with circulatory failure	Early "fresh" septic shock + intractable CF; BUN <15 mmol/L	1. 4 hr 2. 4 days	Responders: 11 of 20 had hemodynamic improvement; 28-d mortality: 82%; no difference at 60 and 90 d
Cole et al., 2001	Randomized, crossover	Effect on hemodynamics and serum cytokine and complement concentrations	1. 6 L/hr 2. 2 L/hr (both isovolemic)	11 patients with septic shock and multiorgan failure	Septic shock	Late (mean 71 hr) after onset of septic shock	Hemodynamic response (reduced norepinephrine dose), but no difference in
Joannes-Boyau et al., 2004	Prospective case series	28-d mortality. Hemodynamics	40–60 mL/kg/hr	24	(Post-abdominal surgery) Sepsis + two-organ failure	From 6 hr to 4 days after onset of sepsis	Mortality 46% vs. predicted 70%; $P > .05$ for SAP, CI, SVRI (from 36 to 96 hr)
Cornejo et al., 2006	Protocol-guided, goal-directed earlier use of pulse HVHF	Reversal of progressive refractory hypotension, hypoperfusion in patients with severe hyperdynamic septic shock	Pulse HVHF at 100 mL/kg/hr for 12 hr	20	Hyperdynamic catecholamine-resistant septic shock (CI > 3.0 L/min/m²)	Immediate	11 of 20 patients showed decreased NE requirements and lactate levels (responders); 9 patients did not fulfill these criteria (nonresponders); NE dose, lactate levels, and heart rates decreased and arterial pH increased significantly in responders
Vinsonneau et al., 2006	Prospective, randomized multicenter	60-d survival/28-d, 90-day, LOS, time on dialysis, time to recover	1. CVVHDF (1 L/hr) 2. IHD (5 hr)	Total: 360 1. 184 2. 176	ARF (BUN > 36 mmol/L, Cr 310 µmol/L; need for dialysis; MOF	Not defined	No difference in hypotension
Piccinni et al., 2006	Retrospective study (8 years)	28-d survival, PaO₂/FiO₂ at 48 hr after CRRT initiation	1. 20 mL/kg/hr 2. 45 mL/kg/hr for 6 hr	Total: 80 1. 40 2. 40	Hyperdynamic sepsis with ARF and ALI	12 hr	Improved survival; higher dose increased ($P < .001$) PaO₂/FiO₂

*Data sources (in alphabetical order): Cole L, Bellomo R, Journois D, et al: High-volume haemofiltration in human septic shock. Intensive Care Med 2001;27:978-986; Cornejo R, Downey P, Castro R, et al: High-volume hemofiltration as salvage therapy in severe hyperdynamic septic shock. Intensive Care Med 2006;32:713-722; Honore PM, Jamez J, Wauthier M, et al: Prospective evaluation of short-term, high-volume isovolemic hemofiltration on the hemodynamic course and outcome in patients with intractable circulatory failure resulting from septic shock. Crit Care Med 2000;28:3581-3587; Joannes-Boyau O, Rapaport S, Bazin R, et al: Impact of high volume hemofiltration on hemodynamic disturbance and outcome during septic shock. ASAIO J 2004;50:102-109; Journois D, Israel-Biet D, Pouard P, et al: High-volume, zero-balanced hemofiltration to reduce delayed inflammatory response to cardiopulmonary bypass in children. Anesthesiology 1996;85:965-976; Piccinni P, Dan M, Barbacini S, Carraro R, et al: Early isovolaemic haemofiltration in oliguric patients with septic shock. Intensive Care Med 2006;32:80-86; Vinsonneau C, Camus C, Combes A, et al: Continuous venovenous haemodiafiltration versus intermittent haemodialysis for acute renal failure in patients with multiple-organ dysfunction syndrome: a multicentre randomised trial. Lancet 2006;29:379-385.

ALI, acute lung injury; ARF, acute renal failure; BUN, blood urea nitrogen; CF, cardiac failure; CI, cardiac index; Cr, serum creatinine; CVVH, continuous venovenous hemofiltration; CVVHDF, continuous venovenous hemodiafiltration; HVHF, high-volume hemofiltration; IHD, intermittent hemodialysis; LOS, length of (hospital) stay; MOF, multiple organ failure; PaO₂/FiO₂, ratio of arterial oxygen tension to fractional inspired oxygen concentration; SAP, systolic arterial pressure; SVRI, systemic vascular resistance index.

the hemofiltration mode used, such as the "classic" or high-volume technique, the resultant hemodynamic alterations may differ considerably. In theory, removing all substances released in sepsis may improve cell function, reducing mediator levels and altering the metabolic environment. In accordance with such a theory, a reasonable expectation is a better hemodynamic situation, with improved cardiac function and vascular function, decreased oxygen demand, and better organ perfusion during or after hemofiltration, especially if it is efficient enough to "purify" the plasma. In addition, CRRT seems to have advantages over intermittent techniques: It allows more gradual blood purification, avoiding large and rapid shifts in circulatory volume and blood pressure and limiting the ischemia-reperfusion insult.[27] This feature may be of great importance, because ventilatory support may in itself induce renal damage, through activation of circulating cells by the artificial circuit, potential imbalance between pro- and anti-inflammatory mediators such as nitric oxide–endothelin[64] or cytokine–anticytokine-soluble receptor,[15] and, finally, its hemodynamic consequences—hypotension or blood pressure instability, modification of renal blood flow in relation with cardiac output, and so on.[65]

In this respect, it is difficult to predict the impact of hemodynamic variation on the perfusion of different organs, some being strongly autoregulated and others only modestly so. In addition, little is known about the modifications induced by systemic inflammation on organ perfusion physiology. As an example, brain blood flow, which normally is independent from systemic blood flow, may become dependent on systemic blood flow.[66] Similarly, the normally autoregulated renal blood flow seems to be dependent on cardiac output during sepsis.[55] In general, the techniques used for supportive therapy also may have an impact on organ perfusion, because the increase in intrathoracic pressure always induces an antidiuresis with an antinatriuresis.[67] Pressors are supposed to improve the perfusion pressure and then the flow, when the organ blood flow is pressure-dependent.

Using animal models, it has been shown that hemofiltration may change the cardiovascular status such as the systemic parameters or the regional perfusion. Staubach and associates used an experimental model based on continuous perfusion of *Salmonella abortus-ovis*, with use of hemofiltration in one of the treatment groups.[68] Whole-body oxygen consumption, CO_2 production, oxygen delivery, ventilatory mechanics, cardiac output, and arterial blood pressure were less altered in the hemofiltration treatment than in the conventional treatment group. Nevertheless, no difference in outcome between the two groups was observed. Gomez and colleagues infused *E. coli* into dogs and then measured left ventricular function before and after hemofiltration.[69] Left ventricular pressure-volume curves had a better shape for the hemofiltration treatment group than for the control animal group. In addition, incubation of rat papillary muscles with concentrated plasma from these dogs demonstrated better isometric contraction in the hemofiltration group plasma.

In a dog model, hemofiltration was shown to reduce the pulmonary hypertension induced by LPS injection.[70] More convincingly, it was shown that hemofiltration used after LPS injection improved cardiac function. The landmark paper from Grootendorst and associates using high hemofiltration rate in pigs demonstrated a remarkable beneficial effect on the hemodynamics, with improvements on cardiac output, stroke volume, and right ventricular stroke work index.[30]

Only a few clinical studies have supported the beneficial impact of classic hemofiltration on systemic hemodynamic and regional blood flow or microcirculation. The most impressive and convincing study on HVHF came from Honoré and colleagues.[71] These investigators reported findings from an open study performed in patients with extremely severe and treatment-resistant septic shock who were receiving HVHF. Although the technique used cannot be recommended for routine application (40 to 60 mL/kg), it proved the effectiveness of blood purification, because responders improved their cardiac output by approximately 50%, with an arterial pH greater than 7.3 with a concomitant reduction in catecholamine infusion. Of more importance, such improvement was not merely cosmetic, because mortality was reduced in comparison with the patients who did not respond to the technique. Other reports using HVHF suggest such hemodynamic benefit, even if no randomized controlled trial has confirmed it. Cole and associates[72] have compared the impact of hemofiltration at 6 L/hour and at 1 L/hour on cardiovascular failure in patients with septic shock. These workers observed a reduction in catecholamine dose in the HVHF group. No information on outcome benefit could be derived from this study.

In conclusion, although HVHF may be beneficial to systemic hemodynamics, allowing reduction in pressor requirement, the impact on outcome remains to be demonstrated. Well-designed studies are needed to better characterize the effect of hemofiltration on regional circulation and the microcirculation, because new tools are now available for clinical research.

Effect on Core Temperature and Hemodynamic Stability

With use of HVHF, the rate of cooling is much faster. As a matter of fact, the cooling effect in hemofiltration on hemodynamics has long been recognized. Beneficial effects of hypothermia on hemodynamic tolerance due to extracorporeal therapy have been studied mainly during chronic intermittent hemodialysis. The decrease in the number of hypotension episodes in patients undergoing intermittent hemodialysis related to cooling of dialysis fluid was reported for the first time by Maggiore and coworkers in the 1980s.[73] The presumed effect of hypothermia induced by cooling the dialysate is counteracted by an increase in venous tone and systemic arterial resistance.[74,75] A systematic review of the studies performed in patients maintained with intermittent hemodialysis confirmed a beneficial effect of reduction in dialysate temperature on hemodynamic tolerance.[76] A recent publication has underlined the effect of cooling on left ventricular diameter and function.[77] The optimal temperature of the dialysate has not yet been identified.

Only a few studies hve analyzed the temperature variations in patients on CRRT. During intermittent hemodialysis, the mechanisms responsible for thermal losses are different from those involved during intermittent hemodialysis. Heat losses are due mainly to negative energy transfer along the extracorporeal circuit. The consequences of heat loss on body temperature seem to be more important during CVVH than with use of intermittent hemodialysis. In the absence of a fluid rewarmer within the circuit, the amount of fluid infused during CVVH may influence the decrease in body temperature.[78] Consequently, during CVVH, the potential risk of induced significant hypothermia is theoretically possible. Thus frequently, a rewarmer device is set in the venous return line of the circuit with the aim of limiting heat loss. Of note, however, such rewarming may alter vascular reactivity and induce hypotension during CVVH.[79]

Matamis and colleagues did not demonstrate any deleterious hemodynamic effect of hypothermia in 10 patients undergoing CVVHF.[80] Similarly, Yagi and associates did not show any significant hemodynamic consequence of hypothermia in patients receiving CVVHF. This study, however, featured great individual variation in the clinical data. Furthermore, comparisons were done using data obtained with various CVVH regimens.[81] More recently, Rokyta and coworkers[82] demonstrated that cooling was associated with significant decrease in heart rate, cardiac output, systemic oxygen delivery and consumption, and increase in MAP during CVVHF, without significant alteration in energy balance, in 9 septic patients. In this latter study, cooling was induced only during a 2-hour period. The feasibility of monitoring extracorporeal energy balance has been shown in vitro.[83]

Thus, further investigations in the field are of importance to determine the optimal recommended temperature to be achieved in ICU patients treated with CVVH.

Key Points

1. The effect on the cytokine network by continuous renal replacement therapy is more complex than in the simpler model conceived earlier. Removal and adsorption are not the only mechanisms. In fact, apart from eliminating the peak or threshold

---

concentrations of cytokines and other multiple sepsis-associated mediators, a washout effect linked to the infusion of fluids may be an additional mechanism in the extravascular or vascular compartment.

2. The hemodynamic effect of continuous renal replacement therapy is associated with the amount of volume exchanged and with timing of initiation of the therapy.

3. Animal and human studies support a beneficial effect of high-volume hemofiltration on hemodynamics, but randomized controlled studies are still lacking to confirm pioneering work on an outcome benefit.

4. Hyothermia may help to ensure improved hemodynamic stability.

Key References

27. Ronco C, Tetta C, Mariano F, et al: Interpreting the mechanisms of continuous renal replacement therapy in sepsis: The peak concentration hypothesis. Artif Organs 2003;27:792-801.
29. Di Carlo JV, Alexander SR: Hemofiltration for cytokine-driven illnesses. The mediator delivery hypothesis. Int J Artif Organs 2005;28:777-786.
32. Pathan N, Hemingway CA, Alizadeh AA, et al: Role of interleukin 6 in myocardial dysfunction of meningococcal septic shock. Lancet 2004;363:203-209.

See the companion Expert Consult website for the complete reference list.

CHAPTER 253

High-Volume Hemofiltration in the Intensive Care Unit

Olivier Joannes-Boyau, Patrick M. Honoré, and Gérard Janvier

OBJECTIVES

This chapter will:
1. Provide a current definition of high-volume hemofiltration.
2. Outline the rationale for using high-volume hemofiltration.
3. Review practical considerations for safe and optimal use of high-volume hemofiltration.
4. Summarize the clinical results with high-volume hemofiltration.
5.. Present an overview of the future of high-volume hemofiltration, including indications, insights for research, and interim reports on studies in progress.

High-volume hemofiltration (HVHF) currently is used in the intensive care unit (ICU) in the treatment of various pathological conditions, especially sepsis. Although the

definition and practice of and rationale for HVHF have changed in recent years with an increase in the volumes prescribed, consensus is lacking on the specifics of this technique. This chapter provides insights and recommendations regarding optimal use of this modality.

DEFINITION OF HIGH-VOLUME HEMOFILTRATION

In the past decade, standard hemofiltration often was provided at 1 or 2 L/hour of ultrafiltration and usually only in predilution mode. Practice began to change in 2001, however, when Ronco and colleagues reported a beneficial effect on outcome from increasing the ultrafiltration rate to 35 mL/kg per hour in patients with acute renal failure (ARF).[1] At that time, the old definition of HVHF was becoming the standard; since the year 2000, new concepts,

TABLE 253-1

Summary of Hemofiltration Doses, Definitions, and Correspondences

UF VOLUME INDEXED TO BODY SIZE	CATEGORY	EQUIVALENCE FOR 75-kg HUMAN
0 ↓ 35 mL/kg/hr	Very-low-volume hemofiltration (inadequate ICU dose)	0 ↓ 2.6 L/hr
35 ↓ 50 mL/kg/hr	Low-volume hemofiltration (renal ICU dose)	2.6 L/hr ↓ 3.75 L/hr
50 ↓ 100 mL/kg/hr	High-volume hemofiltration (sepsis ICU dose)	3.75 L/hr ↓ 7.5 L/hr
100 ↓ 120 mL/kg/hr	Very-high-volume hemofiltration (sepsis/ cardiodepression ICU dose)	7.5 L/hr ↓ 9 L/hr
150 ↓ 215 mL/kg/hr	Very-high-volume hemofiltration (?)	11.25 L/hr ↓ 16.125 L/hr

ICU, intensive care unit; UF, ultrafiltrate.

summarized in Table 253-1, have emerged.[2-4] Furthermore, two different HVHF methods have become common: (1) continuous high-volume treatment providing 50 to 70 mL/kg per hour 24 hours a day; and (2) intermittent hemofiltration with brief, very-high-volume regimens of 100 to 120 mL/kg per hour for 4 to 8 hours—sometimes called pulse HVHF. The principles involved and results for these two forms of HVHF are somewhat different, as described later on.

RATIONALE FOR USE OF HIGH-VOLUME HEMOFILTRATION

The first idea to justify the use of hemofiltration was for the treatment of ARF, which is an independent risk factor for severity and poor outcome. However, previous studies had shown that the mortality rate for patients requiring renal replacement therapy (RRT) for ARF in an ICU setting was nearly twice as high as that for patients without ARF (62.8% versus 38.5%).[5,6] This finding suggests that ARF is independently responsible for increased mortality, even if any form of RRT is used. In fact, although standard RRT significantly reduced mortality in patients with ARF in comparison with that observed before the introduction of dialysis, the mortality rate achieved was still not as low as in patients without ARF. Shortly thereafter arrived the new concept of "blood purification challenge," developed in an attempt to decrease mortality.

Systemic inflammatory response syndrome (SIRS), sepsis, and septic shock and severe acute pancreatitis (SAP) are the leading causes of ARF in the ICU, and they are known to create an immunological disturbance with a cytokine "storm." Sepsis and inflammatory conditions disrupt homeostasis with a cellular and humoral response, generating secretion of cytokines such as interleukins and tumor necrosis factor-α (TNF-α). In the past, many attempts were made to block some part of the inflammatory cascade or to destroy a specific component; results obtained in animal models did not translate to any clinical benefit.[7] In fact, it has been claimed that a large and unspecific cytokine reduction in the blood compartment could in theory reduce mortality more than by simply concentrating on one specific element.[2,8,9] However, this approach is com-

plicated by the fact that neither the pharmacodynamics nor the pharmacokinetics of cytokines and immune components is known in any detail, nor even their exact function.

Three main theories have been provided by investigators in the field of hemofiltration. First, the *peak concentration hypothesis* of Ronco and Bellomo postulates that by removing the peak cytokine concentration from the blood circulation during the early phase of sepsis could stop the inflammatory cascade and the accumulation of free cytokines, which are the leading cause of remote organ damage and homeostasis disruption.[10]

The second concept is called the *threshold immunomodulation hypothesis*, developed by the research group of Honoré.[2,11] In this concept, the removal of cytokines does not only affect the cytokine concentration in the blood stream but also their level in tissues. Indeed, when the cytokine concentration is reduced in blood, both concentrations may be equilibrated to extract the immune components trapped in the organs. This could explain why no crucial reduction in cytokine concentration is observed in the blood stream during hemofiltration, because cytokines from the organs permanently compensate their loss in the blood.

The third theory, advanced by Di Carlo and Alexander, sheds new light on the *mediator delivery hypothesis*, in which the use of hemofiltration with a high volume of crystalloid fluids (3 to 5 L/hour) is able to increase the lymphatic flow 20- to 40-fold.[12] Indeed, this increase is correlated with the infusion of a high dose of fluids. Because the cytokines and other immune components are transported by the lymphatic stream, this could explain their removal even though high quantities of cytokines were not found in ultrafiltration fluid.[13,14] Thus, the use of high volumes of exchange fluid may be the principal driver of cytokine removal.

To gain a wider view of these theories, a review of the new paradigm of chaos and complex, nonlinear systems in sepsis and SIRS is needed.[15] The principal goal underlying these theories is not only the removal of cytokines but also immunomodulation and control of the inflammatory response, which becomes deleterious when it becomes excessive. Indeed, the immune response of the host against septic aggression can be compared to a complex, nonlinear system that is defined by an infinity of solutions in response

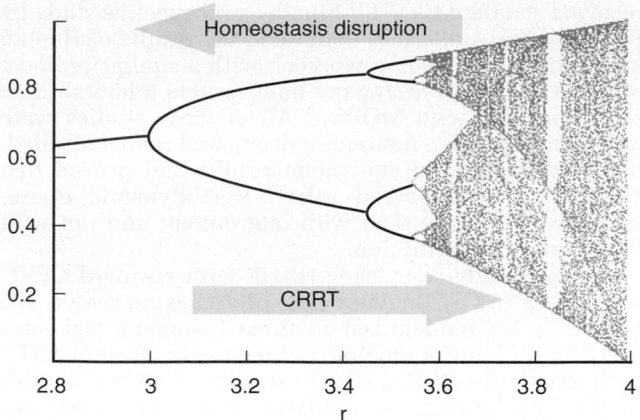

FIGURE 253-1. The change of system status, from complex nonlinear system to linear system during sepsis, and back to complex nonlinear system with continuous renal replacment therapy (CRRT). *r* = resource of system, representing the level of possibility; the higher the value of *r*, the more possibilities exist.

to a lone stimulus. In a complex, nonlinear system —exemplified by the chaos whereby a flight of butterflies in China can change the weather in Boston three days later—a bacterial attack or cytokine secretion will have repercussions throughout the whole body. This explains why homeostasis is not a state of stability per se but rather the capability to maintain stability while the status is continually changing. Yet this incredible adaptability is halted when the system is overwhelmed by an excess of information and when the "endocrine effects" of cytokines and other immune messengers are lost in the storm.[16,17] The resources of the body system become depleted, and the complex, nonlinear system becomes a linear system, with only one course of action. This change heralds the onset of multiple organ dysfunction syndrome (MODS). It may be that hemofiltration plays a role at this point by decreasing the cytokine storm through different modes and by allowing recovery of efficacy of the immune messenger system. Thus, the resources of the system increase, allowing restoration of the complex, nonlinear system and return of homeostasis (Fig. 253-1).

PRACTICAL CONSIDERATIONS WITH USE OF HIGH-VOLUME HEMOFILTRATION

New treatment volumes will require changes in hemofiltration practice aimed at ensuring the efficacy and safety of the technique. Indeed, to reach a treatment volume of 60 or 100 mL/kg per hour, important principles need to be respected. First, a high blood flow is necessary to maintain a filtration fraction below 25%, a level above which "protein cake" (clogging) in the membrane becomes a major concern. To attain such a blood flow, however, excellent vascular access is required, with use of a large catheter (13.5 or 14 Fr), appropriate location (the right jugular is the best, followed by the femoral vein approach; the subclavian route is not to be used), and good structure (permitting full-bore arterial intake). Second, the optimal restitution fluid probably is buffered bicarbonate, which should be administered one third in predilution and two

thirds in postdilution, to achieve the best compromise between loss of treatment efficacy and optimization of blood flow.[18] The choice of the membrane also is critical, and a highly biocompatible synthetic filter with a large exchange surface is recommended (1.7 to 2.1 m²). Temperature control is not important with low fluid exchange volumes but becomes essential when the volume increases dramatically. Two approaches are possible: heating the fluid before restitution or heating the blood directly. Empirically heating the replacement fluid seems preferable to heating the blood, owing to possible deleterious effects of high heat on blood. To date, however, no problems have been recorded, and both systems have demonstrated adequate safety as well as efficacy.

The new machines specially dedicated to high volumes have extremely sensitive and precise pressure control and volume balance functions. Furthermore, maintenance of a normal pressure range is essential for optimal use of hemofiltration. Indeed, an arterial pressure that stays below −120 mm Hg is indicative of a catheter problem and likely early machine failure. The same is true with a venous line: High pressure indicates catheter or bubble trap clotting. The transmembrane pressure reflects the presence or absence of clogging in the filter, whereas a high pressure indicates that many fibers are clogged. To alleviate the pressure problem, stopping the treatment is recommended during nursing interventions or repositioning, especially with use of high volumes. HVHF also requires adequate management and control of fluid exchange and small solutes. In fact, the small molecules are mainly removed during hemofiltration, and strict monitoring of sodium, glucose, and acid-base balance is mandatory.[19]

CLINICAL RESULTS WITH HIGH-VOLUME HEMOFILTRATION

Animal models have shown benefit in terms of survival when "early" and "strong" hemofiltration doses were applied in septic animals. Early use of hemofiltration has been thoroughly investigated in animal models.[20,21] Most of the initial studies used hemofiltration before or just after the injection of bolus or even infusion of endotoxin. It was only in the late 1990s that investigators started to wait approximately 6 to 12 hours before initiating HVHF, thereby allowing the animals to become extremely ill and hemodynamically unstable and to develop early MODS.[22] Thus, these animal models reproduced some aspects of the clinical setting. Only animal models in which HVHF was applied early proved to be very beneficial (some spectacularly so), mainly because of the fact that in addition to early application, the investigators administered a much stronger dose of HVHF. However, the differences between human and animal models did not allow these results to be extrapolated to humans.

One of the greatest remaining problems with human studies (and especially those addressing technical aspects of this modality) is the fact that the number of patients is very limited because HVHF technology is very expensive. Moreover, filtration exchange rates used in the clinical studies were much less than the mean rate of 100 mL/kg per hour used in animal models, being limited to only 40 mL/kg per hour. As a consequence, many anticipated effects seen in animal models can never be reproduced in the clinical setting, owing to the use of inadequate doses of HVHF. On the other hand, extreme variability is observed between clinical trials in range of doses applied, ranging from the basic dose to 15-fold in recent studies.[2,8]

The principles of the high-volume technique were established by Ronco and associates, who showed that in their subgroup of patients with sepsis, increasing the volume of treatment from 35 mL/kg hour to 45 mL/kg per hour improved outcome.[1] Their study effectively demonstrated that hemofiltration could be considered as a viable management approach in the ICU. The volume of treatment must be adapted not only to body weight but also to the patient's severity of illness. If nonseptic ARF is being treated, then a lower dose may be optimal. With septic ARF, however, a higher dose, close to 50 or 70 mL/kg per hour or greater, may be necessary, with different regimens for catecholamine-resistant septic shock (or refractory hypodynamic septic shock) or severe acute pancreatitis.

At the end of the 1990s, Journois and colleagues applied HVHF in 20 children during cardiac surgery (100 mL/kg per hour) and found a reduction in postoperative blood loss, earlier extubation time, and reduced cytokine plasma levels.[23] The first large study using pulse HVHF, by Honoré and colleagues, was conducted in 20 septic patients with refractory hypodynamic shock, with the ultrafiltration pump running at approximately 100 mL/kg per hour for 4 consecutive hours (and then back at 20 mL/kg per hour) as an important adjunctive treatment. This therapy dramatically increased survival in these severely ill patients as compared with conventional treatment.[24] The observed mortality rate (55%) was significantly lower than the predicted one (79%) established by severity score. However, some patients were hemodynamic nonresponders (9 of 20), with disastrous mortality. At the same time, in a single-center study by Oudemans-van Straaten and associates with a prospective cohort design and including mainly cardiac surgery patients with oliguria (306 patients), the observed mortality rate was statistically lower in the group undergoing intermittent HVHF with a mean volume of 3.8 L/hour (nearly 50 mL/kg per hour for a 70-kg patient) than the predicted mortality rate evaluated by three validated severity scores.[25] This treatment was shown to be most effective in the septic subgroup.

Thereafter, some studies in the early 21st century focused on hemodynamic response and cytokine removal, such as that by Cole and coworkers, who showed notable hemodynamic improvement in septic patients treated by HVHF.[26] A team of investigators from Chili headed by Cornejo recently completed a study similar to the one by Honoré's group and obtained comparable results. They created an algorithm based on the international recommendations for sepsis treatment and incorporated it at the end of an intermittent HVHF protocol (100 mL/kg per hour for a single 12-hour period) given as salvage therapy for patients in treatment-refractory septic shock.[27] Like the Honoré study, although the observed mortality rate (40%) was lower than predicted (60%), this study also included a responder and a nonresponder group.

By comparison, Joannes-Boyau and coworkers studied the effect of HVHF at 50 mL/kg per hour maintained for 96 hours in patients with septic shock and MODS.[28] Results in terms of mortality rate were comparable to those in previous studies (45% observed versus 70% predicted by three severity scores), but all of the patients were hemodynamic responders. A retrospective study by Piccinni and associates recently found similar results with continuous HVHF at 45 mL/kg per hour in 40 septic patients, in comparison with a historical group of patients who received standard CVVH.[29] Finally, a prospective study by Ratanarat and colleagues confirmed the results of Honoré and Cornejo and their coworkers, with a similar protocol of pulse HVHF (85 mL/kg per hour for 6 to 8 hours) in 15 septic patients with MODS.[30] All of these studies were only single-center, nonrandomized, and noncontrolled, but they all showed equivalent results and proved that HVHF can be delivered safely. Hemodynamic nonresponders were only seen with intermittent and not with continuous hemofiltration.

A single study comparing HVHF with standard CVVH was conducted by Bouman and colleagues, in which 106 patients were randomized to three treatment regimens: early HVHF (within the first 12 hours after onset of ARF), early standard CVVH, and late standard CVVH.[31] No difference was found in mortality at 28 days or in recovery of renal function, but no statistical conclusions could be drawn owing to the lack of power, with only 35 patients included in each group. In this study, the specific patient population, mostly cardiac surgery patients, explains the low mortality rate, so the possibility of finding any statistical difference between the groups was even more remote.

Several studies, in particular a few from Asia, also have explored the effects of HVHF on severe acute pancreatitis: Wang and associates in animal models[32] and human patients[33] and Jiang and coworkers in humans[34] proved its clinical benefit. They studied the effects of HVHF alone and in comparison with standard CVVH on mortality and organ function recovery and showed a clear benefit of using high volumes with early initiation.

Although all of these studies were promising, the findings did not allow clear-cut conclusions to be drawn. Accordingly, it is time for larger studies and randomized controlled trials.

FUTURE DIRECTIONS WITH HIGH-VOLUME HEMOFILTRATION

Regarding recommendations for clinical practice, patients with ARF should receive a renal replacement dose of at least 35 mL/kg per hour (level II evidence and grade C recommendation)[1] and probably a higher dose if sepsis is present. Catecholamine-resistant septic shock, either hypodynamic or hyperdynamic, may be an indication (level V evidence and grade E recommendation) for experienced clinicians in the field of HVHF.[2,8,9] Nevertheless, HVHF should be integrated into a treatment algorithm and used as a salvage therapy in many ICUs, because no other treatment has proved its efficacy in these patients with a very high risk of death. HVHF is reserved for patients with ARF, and although the benefit of early treatment has been shown, initiating RRT before renal injury has occurred is not recommended. In fact, the best time to begin hemofiltration may be at onset of renal injury (defined as a creatinine level of twice the baseline value or oliguria with urine production of less than 0.5 mL/kg in 12 hours), which may constitute the best compromise between early initiation and renal impairment.[35]

To evaluate HVHF, more numerous and larger prospective randomized studies are needed, and certain conditions should be respected:

- First, the safest technique must be used; this requirement is the easiest to meet, because the newer hemofiltration machines are much safer and more efficient.

- Second, it is essential to define the time to start hemofiltration from the beginning of sepsis and ARF. The best policy is to use a common classification for ARF such as RIFLE (*r*isk of ARF, presence of renal *i*njury, kidney *f*ailure, *l*oss of kidney function, *e*nd-stage renal disease) and start hemofiltration within the first 24 hours after onset of sepsis.
- Third, the volume of treatment (mL/kg per hour) must be determined according to body size.
- Finally, it is essential to develop a greater understanding of the mechanisms of sepsis and SIRS in order to identify appropriate targets for HVHF.

In future trials, it would be interesting to detect potential interferences or possible synergy between HVHF and activated protein C. The best design for the use of hemofiltration still remains to be defined, and the optimal sequences and duration of high-volume "pulses" need to be established. Prolonged HVHF seems better able to stop the initial inflammatory storm and late immunoparalysis; nevertheless, the efficiency and practicability of pulsed high volumes should be explored. Although several large randomized trials are currently in progress investigating hemofiltration doses in ARF patients, only one is designed to compare HVHF with standard CVVH[36]: The IVOIRE (h*I*gh *V*olume in *I*ntensive ca*RE*) study will try to apply the findings of the initial study by Ronco and colleagues to septic patients. Indeed, the study will accrue 480 patients in intensive care for management of septic shock plus acute renal injury, as defined by the RIFLE classification. After computerized randomization, patients will receive either 35 mL/kg per hour or 70 mL/kg per hour. This study aims to demonstrate that a higher dose (such as 70 mL/kg per hour) will incrementally improve the survival rate of patients with septic ARF in the ICU, respectively at 28, 60, and 90 days.

CONCLUSION

The use of hemofiltration treatment has steadily increased in the past decade, from the simple treatment of ARF to adjunctive therapy for sepsis or other acute episodes of pancreatitis. The story continues to unfold, and the development of technology and elucidation of pathology, hemofiltration doses, and true efficacy of the machines can be expected. For the moment, 35 mL/kg per hour remains the standard hemofiltration dose in ICUs for all patients, although in some situations such as sepsis, the dose should be increased to provide salvage therapy, in view of the disastrous mortality rate in this patient subgroup. More trials are needed, however, to allow confident recommendations for and further development of optimal HVHF protocols for use as routine treatment in ICUs, and to establish a consensus regarding this modality.

Key Points

1. The standard hemofiltration dose is 35 mL/kg per hour.
2. With high-volume hemofiltration, the dose begins at 50 mL/kg per hour and above.
3. Continuous high-volume hemofiltration and pulse high-volume hemofiltration are two available techniques but require additonal clinical evaluation.
4. Strict observance of practical recommendations is necessary for maximum safety and efficacy.
5. High-volume hemofiltration should be integrated into an algorithm and used as a salvage therapy.
6. High-volume hemofiltration should not be used only in patients who have acute renal failure.
7. Randomized controlled trials are needed. The ongoing IVOIRE study should bring additional answers, either positive or negative.

Key References

1. Ronco C, Bellomo R, Homel P, et al: Effects of different doses in continuous veno-venous haemofiltration on outcomes of acute renal failure: A prospective randomised trial. Lancet 2000;356:26-30.
24. Honoré PM, Jamez J, Wauthier M, et al: Prospective evaluation of short-term, high-volume isovolemic hemofiltration on the hemodynamic course and outcome in patients with intractable circulatory failure resulting from septic shock. Crit Care Med 2000;28:3581-3587.
27. Cornejo R, Downey P, Castro R, et al: High-volume hemofiltration as salvage therapy in severe hyperdynamic septic shock. Intensive Care Med 2006;32:713-722.
28. Joannes-Boyau O, Rapaport S, Bazin R, et al: Impact of high volume hemofiltration on hemodynamic disturbance and outcome during septic shock. ASAIO J 2004;50:102-109.
31. Bouman CS, Oudemans-van Straaten HM, Tijssen JG, et al: Effects of early high-volume continuous venovenous hemofiltration on survival and recovery of renal function in intensive care patients with acute renal failure: A prospective, randomized trial. Crit Care Med 2002;30:2205-2211.

See the companion Expert Consult website for the complete reference list.

CHAPTER 254

Pulse High-Volume Hemofiltration in Management of Critically Ill Patients with Severe Sepsis or Septic Shock

Eric Roessler, Ranistha Ratanarat, Alessandra Brendolan, and Claudio Ronco

---

OBJECTIVES

This chapter will:
1. Assess the safety, feasibility, and technical considerations with use of pulse high-volume hemofiltration as an adjuvant therapy for critically ill patients with sepsis or septic shock.
2. Review the rationale for the use of pulse high-volume hemofiltration in this clinical setting.
3. Evaluate the current clinical and experimental evidence supporting the use of pulse high-volume hemofiltration as an adjuvant therapy for critically ill patients with severe sepsis or septic shock.
4. Highlight possible future lines of investigation for applications of pulse high-volume hemofiltration.

Sepsis is the leading cause of morbidity and mortality among critically ill patients worldwide. Despite current advances in the understanding of the pathophysiology of this complex syndrome, mortality rates associated with sepsis remain between 30% and 50%, which seems unacceptably high.[1,2]

The sepsis syndrome is associated with an overwhelming systemic overflow of pro-inflammatory and anti-inflammatory mediators, leading to generalized endothelial damage, multiple organ failure, and altered cellular immunological responsiveness, inducing in turn a state of immunoparalysis or monocyte hyporesponsiveness.[3]

The last several years have seen a growing interest in the role of blood purification techniques with high ultrafiltration volumes in an attempt to enhance unselective clearance of water-soluble pro-inflammatory and anti-inflammatory cytokines produced during septic states, theoretically restoring humoral homeostasis and avoiding both excessive inflammation and "anti-inflammation." In a study by Ronco and colleagues that included 425 patients, continuous venovenous hemofiltration (CVVH) was used at three different ultrafiltration rates: 20 mL/kg per hour (group 1), 35 mL/kg per hour (group 2), and 45 mL/kg per hour (group 3). Survival rates were significantly lower in group 1 than in groups 2 and 3. The survival rates among patients from groups 2 and 3 were not significantly different from one another except for the subgroup of septic patients in which the survival increased with higher ultrafiltration volumes (18% in group 2 versus 47% in group 3), suggesting that this group may benefit from higher doses of blood replacement.[4]

High-volume hemofiltration (HVHF) is a variant of CVVH that uses ultrafiltration rates of 35 to 80 mL/kg per minute. In sepsis and multiple organ failure syndrome (MODS), HVHF is applied with the aim of nonselective removal of pro- and anti-inflammatory mediators by enhancing convective clearance and adsorption of these molecules by the filtering membrane.[5]

Multiple in vitro studies have demonstrated the ability of HVHF to remove cytokines involved in sepsis.[6] Animal studies have shown beneficial hemodynamic effects and improved survival with the use of HVHF in endotoxemic models, and human studies have shown trends toward improved survival.[7-12] Unfortunately, performing HVHF is problematic because of the associated need for high blood flows, tight ultrafiltration control, and large amounts of sterile fluids, which are expensive. The technical requirements of HVHF have generated some concern about its feasibility and cost for use as a continuous-treatment modality.[13]

DEFINITION AND RATIONALE

Recently, Ronco and colleagues proposed pulse high-volume hemofiltration (PHVHF) as a modality that reduces practical and technical difficulties associated with HVHF.

PHVHF is application of HVHF for short periods providing intensive plasma water exchange, followed by conventional CVVH. It consists of a daily schedule of HVHF (at 85 mL/kg per hour) for 6 to 8 hours, followed or preceded by CVVH (at 35 mL/kg per hour) for the remaining time, leading to a cumulative dose of approximately 48 mL/kg per hour (Fig. 254-1). The schedule can be modified according to the patient's response and needs, and as required by organizational considerations, in an attempt to maximize cost-effectiveness and practical application of HVHF.[13,14]

Previous studies, by Honoré[9] and Piccinni[15] and their coworkers, have evaluated the clinical outcomes for patients receiving pulses of high ultrafiltration volumes followed by conventional CVVH: In a retrospective study by Piccinni and associates, 80 oliguric septic patients underwent renal replacement therapy. Forty patients received conventional CVVH with ultrafiltration volume

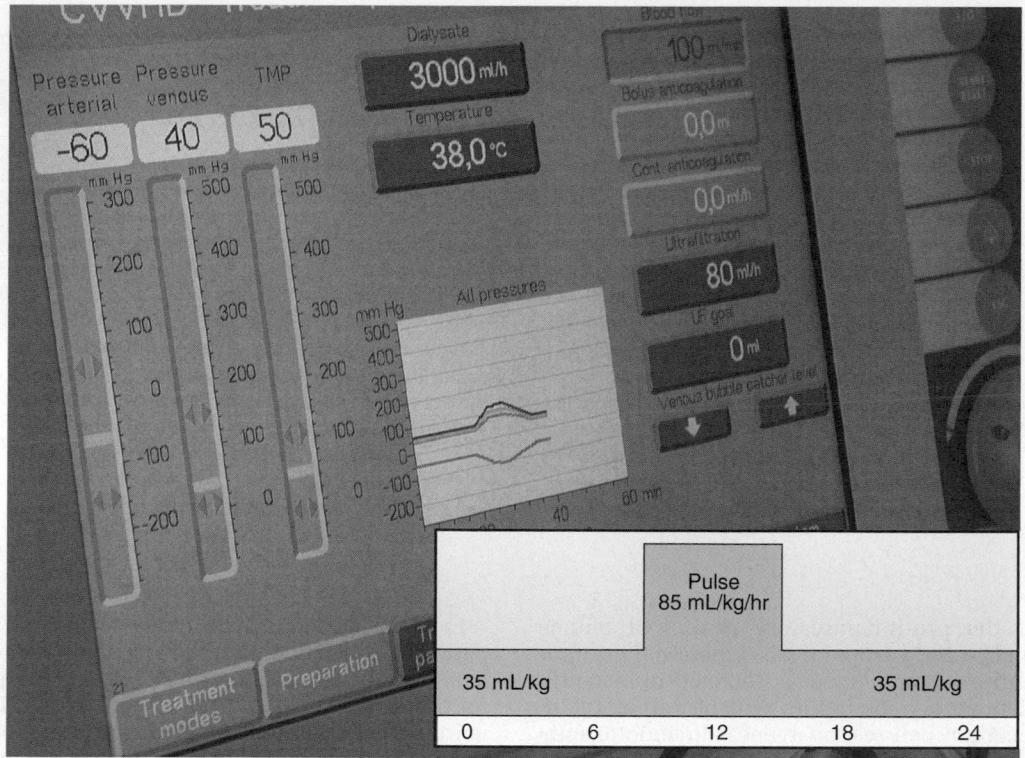

FIGURE 254-1. Pulse high-volume hemofiltration can be performed by modern continuous renal replacement therapy machines like the Multifiltrate (Fresenius Medical Care, Bad Homburg, Germany), pictured here. The rationale for use of this modality is as follows:
• Very high volumes are difficult to maintain over 24 hours.
• Solute kinetics may render high volume useless after a few hours.
• Standard continuous venovenous hemofiltration (CVVH) may contribute to maintain the effect of pulse.
• Sudden changes are achievable without post-treatment rebound.

20 mL/kg per hour only for conventional indications (control group), and the other 40 patients were selected to receive, within 12 hours of admission, 6 hours of HVHF (45 mL/kg per hour), followed by conventional CVVH (intervention group). The intervention group showed a significant decrease in norepinephrine dose and improvement in gas exchange, cardiac index, mean arterial pressure, systemic vascular resistance, and urine output compared with the control subjects. Although mortality rates predicted by Acute Physiology and Chronic Health Evaluation II (APACHE II) and Sequential Organ Failure Assessment (SOFA) severity scores were similar in both groups (41 ± 12% in intervention group patients versus 40 ± 10% in control subjects), the 28-day survival rate was significantly better in the intervention group (55%) than in the control group (11%).[15]

In a prospective trial by Honoré and colleagues, 20 patients with intractable cardiocirculatory failure complicating septic shock underwent 4 hours of HVHF with removal of 35 L of ultrafiltrate, followed by conventional CVVH exchanging 24 L per day for at least 4 days. Among the 11 patients considered responders (evidenced by a greater than 50% increase in cardiac index, greater than 25% increase in mixed venous saturation, increase in pH to above 7.3, and a greater than 50% reduction in epinephrine dose), the 28-day mortality rate was significantly lower in the responders group. After the 35-L exchange volume was indexed to individual patient body weight,

ultrafiltrate dose was found to be significantly higher in responders (0.53 ± 0.07 L/kg) than in nonresponders (0.43 ± 0.07 L/kg; $P < .003$).[9]

The pathogenic role of apoptosis in organ injury during sepsis is increasingly recognized. Apoptosis is accelerated in monocytes during sepsis, a fact that may contribute to "monocyte hyporesponsiveness" and impaired host defense capacity. D'Intini and coworkers recently studied the effect of PHVHF on monocyte apoptotic activity: Septic plasma induced pronounced apoptotic effects on U937 human monocytic cells compared with those observed in controls. PHVHF but not CVVH significantly reduced the apoptotic plasma activity by the first hour of therapy; this effect was maintained at 5 hours of treatment and at 5 hours after the end of the pulse therapy. These results highlight potential biological effects of PHVHF on sepsis beyond hemodynamic improvement.[16]

The rationale for use of PHVHF scheduling rests on practical and biological considerations. Practical advantages are related to easier management of large fluid exchanges for a short period of time as compared with continuous handling of large volume exchanges of expensive substitution fluids in HVHF. The biological rationale relies on the fact that pulse HVHF can remove a large amount of mediators, and the continuity of therapy with conventional CVVH may curtail the peak of proinflammatory and anti-inflammatory mediators such as IL-10. According to the peak concentration hypothesis, the

Table 254-1

Effects of Pulse High-Volume Hemofiltration on Hemodynamic Variables

VARIABLE	PRE-PHVHF	MID-PHVHF	END-PHVHF	6 hr AFTER PHVHF	12 hr AFTER PHVHF	P
Norepinephrine (μg/min)	48 (0-114)	40 (0-97)*	40 (0-93)	40 (0-69)†	33 (0-67)†	.001
SBP (mm Hg)	124.32 ± 25.63	126.64 ± 22.10	133.00 ± 24.55	133.06 ± 23.88	133.16 ± 25.15	.04
MAP (mm Hg)	82.16 ± 18.31	85.02 ± 18.82	86.88 ± 17.56	87.76 ± 20.65	87.26 ± 22.05	NS
CI (L/min/m²)	3.4 ± 1.1	3.4 ± 1.2	3.5 ± 1.0	3.5 ± 1.1	3.5 ± 1.3	NS
HR (beats/min)	97.28 ± 25.53	99.62 ± 22.94	100.06 ± 21.79	99.94 ± 20.71	95.62 ± 20.66	.04
Temperature (° C)	36.7 ± 1.0	36.8 ± 0.8	36.8 ± 0.8	36.9 ± 0.8	36.7 ± 0.9	NS
PaO₂/FIO₂	230.9 ± 109.1	232.8 ± 104.4	243.0 ± 105.6	230.2 ± 109.9	234.6 ± 106.4	NS

*$P < .005$.
†$P < .001$ versus baseline.
CI, cardiac index; HR, heart rate; MAP, mean arterial pressure; NS, not significant; PaO₂/FIO₂, ratio of arterial oxygen tension to fractional inspired oxygen; SBP, systolic blood pressure. Normally distributed variables are reported as mean ± standard deviation, and normally distributed variables are reported as median (between the 25th and 75th percentiles).
Adapted from Ratanarat R, Brendolan A, Ricci Z, et al: Pulse high volume hemofiltration in critically ill patients: A new approach for patients with septic shock. Semin Dial 2006;19:69-74.

amputation of the pro-inflammatory peak will reduce endothelial damage and vasoparalysis, whereas the amputation of the anti-inflammatory peak secreted in response to the pro-inflammatory mediators will be important in maintaining a certain cell responsiveness to endotoxemia and bacteremia, with preservation of the immunological response. The continuous nature of the technique and the double-pool kinetics for different mediators allow long-term maintenance of lowered levels.[6,13]

TECHNICAL CONSIDERATIONS

In order to achieve ultrafiltration rates of 85 mL/kg per hour, vascular access ensuring a constant blood flow rate (Q_b) of at least 300 mL/minute is required. This goal can be obtained with use of a 14 Fr catheter. If the catheter or the cannulated vessel is too small, the resistance of the arterial lumen of the catheter will create a negative pressure before the pump that can reach –300 mm Hg, with an adverse effect on dialyzer life.

With high rates of net ultrafiltration (i.e., volume of fluid removed from the patient—volume of substitution fluid infused), venous line pressure can rise because of hemoconcentration. Accordingly, pulse therapy net ultrafiltration must be kept as low as possible.

When high blood flow rates are used, the time of contact between blood and the artificial surface is reduced; in this setting, anticoagulation becomes less important. In cases of higher filtration fraction of more than 25% to 30%, however, the increased blood viscosity and hematocrit make it necessary to achieve adequate anticoagulation in order to avoid filter clotting.

PHVHF requires use of hemofilters with high surface area (81.8 to 2.0 m² in a 70-kg patient) in order to achieve high ultrafiltration rates. Highly biocompatible synthetic membranes with high ultrafiltration coefficients (between 30 and 40 mL/hour per mm Hg) are recommended. Such membranes have sieving coefficients close to 1 to remove a wide spectrum of molecular sizes.

Bicarbonate-buffered hemofiltration solutions (35 mmol/L) should be administered, combining predilution (33% to 50%) and postdilution (50% to 66%) with a temperature of approximately 38.5° to 39.5° C.

Even though compelling evidence that PHVHF improves patient survival is lacking, a reasonable approach is to start hemofiltration as early as possible as an adjuvant therapy for hypotensive patients with sepsis or MODS resistant to volume resuscitation and pressors, based on the recently proven benefits of early goal-directed therapy.[13,14]

CLINICAL EXPERIENCE

The efficacy of PHVHF was evaluated in a recently published prospective interventional trial by Ronco and colleagues, in which 15 critically ill patients with severe sepsis or septic shock underwent daily PHVHF with a 24-hour schedule that consisted of HVHF at 85 mL/kg per hour for 6 to 8 hours, followed by CVVH at 35 mL/kg per hour for the remaining 16 to 18 hours. The mean number of treatments per patient was 3.4.

By setting the temperature of the replacement fluid at 38.5° to 39° C, body temperature was maintained constant during the pulse treatment.

The mean APACHE II score was 31.2, the mean Simplified Acute Physiology Score II (SAPS II) 62, and the mean SOFA score 14.2.

Hemodynamic variables and norepinephrine dose to maintain mean arterial pressure (MAP) above 70 mm Hg were measured immediately before PHVHF, at mid-PHVHF, immediately after PHVHF, and at 6 and 12 hours after PHVHF completion (Table 254-1). Systolic blood pressure increased significantly over time, and the dose of norepinephrine required for maintenance of target MAP decreased significantly by the midpoint of the HVHF regimen; the effect was maintained at 6 and 12 hours after treatment. The observed patient 28-day all-cause hospital mortality was 46.7%, compared with a rate of 72% predicted by APACHE II and 69% predicted by SAPS II severity scores. Of interest, the mean number of PHVHF treatments per patient was significantly higher among the survivors (4.8 ± 2.7) than among nonsurvivors (1.9 ± 0.7; $P = .02$).

PHVHF was well tolerated in this group of critically ill patients and appeared to offer many of the benefits of continuous HVHF while avoiding its disadvantages. A regimen of 6 to 8 hours of daytime PHVHF was widely accepted by the ICU nursing staff because it reduced the labor-intensive requirements of the treatment protocol during the night.

The investigators were not able to demonstrate any differences in body temperature, arterial pH, or daily fluid balance before and after the PHVHF treatment. Accordingly, it is very unlikely that mediator-independent factors played a significant role in hemodynamic improvement; by contrast, the reduction in vasopressor requirements seems to be related to continuous removal of soluble vasodilatory mediators or molecules known to be present in sepsis by either convection or adsorption.

Although this preliminary clinical experience shows a trend toward reduction in mortality predicted by severity scores, prospective randomized controlled trials on a larger scale are needed to assess the exact role of this technique in altering mortality rates among septic patients. Undoubtedly, however, PHVHF is feasible and, as a treatment for severe sepsis or septic shock, has been shown to positively influence physiological endpoints.[16]

CONCLUSION

Sepsis is the leading cause of death among critically ill patients, with an associated mortality rate of 30% to 50%. Abundant clinical and experimental evidence suggests that unselective removal of cytokines by HVHF has a beneficial hemodynamic impact in severe sepsis or septic shock and may favorably influence mortality. The feasibility of HVHF has been questioned because of technical difficulties and considerable costs. PHVHF is presented as a feasible and well-tolerated alternative to HVHF as adjuvant therapy for severe sepsis or septic shock because it provides the benefits of continuous HVHF while avoiding its technical and economic problems. The benefits achieved during a short phase of very highly convective transport seem to be maintained over time and are stabilized by use of standard-dose CRRT until the next pulse phase.

Preliminary clinical evidence suggests hemodynamic improvement with the use of PHVHF in severe sepsis or septic shock, but its exact role in reducing mortality associated with this condition needs to be addressed by prospective randomized trials.

Key Points

1. Pulse high-volume hemofiltration represents a feasible modality of blood purification in critically ill patients that provides a compromise between continuous renal replacement therapy and high-volume hemofiltration.
2. Pulse high-volume hemofiltration is well tolerated in critically ill patients and appears to offer many of the benefits of continuous high-volume hemofiltration while avoiding its technical difficulties.
3. When applied to patients with severe sepsis or septic shock, pulse high-volume hemofiltration can achieve hemodynamic benefit with reduction in vasopressor requirements.
4. Hemodynamic improvement associated with pulse high-volume hemofiltration is maintained at 6 and 12 hours after pulse treatment.
5. Further prospective randomized trials are needed to assess the impact of this adjuvant therapy on mortality among critically ill patients with severe sepsis or septic shock.

Key References

6. Ronco C, Ricci Z, Bellomo R: Importance of increased ultrafiltration volume and impact on mortality: Sepsis and cytokine story and the role of continuous veno-venous haemofiltration. Curr Opin Nephrol Hypertens 2001;10: 755-761.
13. Ratanarat R, Brendolan A, Ricci Z, et al: Pulse high volume hemofiltration in critically ill patients: A new approach for patients with septic shock. Semin Dial 2006;19:69-74.
14. Brendolan A, D'Intini V, Ricci Z, et al: Pulse high volume hemofiltration. Int J Artif Organs 2004;27:398-403.
15. Piccinni P, Dan M, Barbacini S, et al: Early isovolemic haemofiltration in oliguric patients with septic shock. Intensive Care Med 2006;32:80-86.
17. Ratanarat R, Brendolan A, Piccinni P, et al: Pulse high volume hemofiltration for treatment of severe sepsis: Effects on hemodynamics and survival. Crit Care 2005;9:R294-R302.

See the companion Expert Consult website for the complete reference list.

CHAPTER 255

Removal of Mediators of Inflammation by Continuous Renal Replacement Therapy: An Open Debate of Pros and Cons

Patrick M. Honoré, Olivier Joannes-Boyau, and Willem Boer

OBJECTIVES

This chapter will:
1. Present an overview of the proven and theoretical benefits, contrasted with potential drawbacks and possible inefficacy, of inflammatory mediator removal during continuous renal replacement therapy.
2. Outline the evolution of theories concerning mediator removal in the past decade, highlighting the importance of mediator removal in sepsis and the systemic inflammatory response syndrome during continuous renal replacement therapy and emphasizing the importance of removal at the tissue level.
3. Summarize the latest concepts concerning mediator displacement, transport, and removal within and from body tissues in the context of continuous renal replacement therapy in sepsis and the systemic inflammatory response syndrome.
4. Review the "pleiotropic" properties of continuous renal replacement therapy, including its wide variety of effects, and compare this modality with other therapies for sepsis and the systemic inflammatory response syndrome.
5. Discuss the importance of volume exchange not only for mediator removal but mainly for mediator displacement between different body compartments.

In this chapter, the data on inflammatory mediator removal during continuous renal replacment therapy are presented in a "pros versus cons" format to help the clinician reach a balanced view on this important topic.

THE CASE *FOR* REMOVAL OF MEDIATORS OF INFLAMMATION BY CONTINUOUS RENAL REPLACEMENT THERAPY

Evolving Theories of Mediator Removal during Continuous Renal Replacement Therapy

It has been postulated since the early 1990s[1,2] that the reduction in cytokine levels in the blood compartment may potentially lead to a reduction in mortality. Although current understanding of the highly complex pharmacodynamics and pharmacokinetics of cytokines throughout the body remains limited, a number of concepts have been put forward concerning mediator removal during CRRT.

In the concept developed by Ronco and colleagues, the *peak concentration hypothesis*[3-5] (Fig. 255-1), removal of mediators and cytokines from the blood compartment during the pro-inflammatory phase of sepsis is the central feature. Reducing the amount of free cytokines in this compartment is expected to result in a dramatic decrease in remote organ (associated) damage, thereby decreasing the overall associated death rate. Effects on cytokines at interstitial and tissue levels are not taken into account in this hypothesis, although it stands to reason that such changes play an important part in organ damage.

In this setting, techniques enabling rapid and substantial removal of cytokines or mediators from the blood compartment are privileged. Among these highly specialized techniques, high-volume hemofiltration (HVHF) and very-high-volume hemofiltration feature prominently, as do a number of hybrid therapies encompassing high-permeability hemofiltration (HPHF),[6] super-high-flux hemofiltration (SHFHF),[7] hemoadsorption,[8] and coupled plasma filtration and adsorption (CPFA),[9] and any adsorptive techniques using physical or chemical forces rather than driving forces normally implemented in hemofiltration-derived techniques.

An important point worthy of emphasis here is that strictly speaking, *adsorption* is not the right term in this setting, because blood is not passing through a semipermeable membrane, and it is not the combined effect of convective plus oncotic forces that results in the passage of mediators through this kind of device. Rather, the term *absorption* is more appropriate, because chemical and physical forces are the drivers.[10]

The second concept is called the *threshold immunomodulation hypothesis* (Fig. 255-2) and sometimes is referred to as the "Honoré concept"[11,12] in the English-language literature. In this concept, the view of the system is much more dynamic. Experimental evidence demonstrates changes at interstitial (and at tissue) level when removal is taking place from the blood compartment side, whereby not only mediators but also "pro" mediators are removed, effectively shutting down certain pathways. At this "threshold point," the cascade is blocked, and no further harm can be done to the tissue of the organism. In clinical practice, however, it is difficult to know when this point is reached during extracorporeal removal. The fact that improvement in both hemodynamics and survival in the

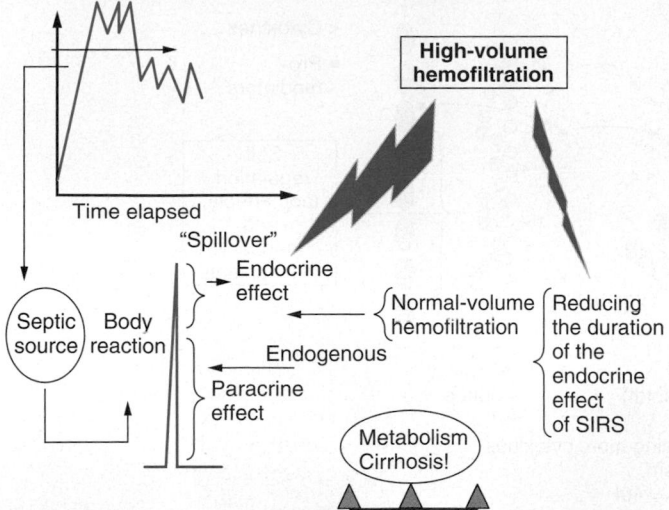

ECR: Rationale
"Peak concentration" hypothesis

Concept = Vascular removal and remote organ damage

FIGURE 255-1. Mediator removal by extracorporeal techniques—evolving theories of rationale: The peak concentration hypothesis. ECR, extracorporeal removal; SIRS, systemic inflammatory response syndrome. (Data from Brivet FG, Emilie D, Galanaud P: Pro- and anti-inflammatory cytokines during acute severe pancreatitis: An early and sustained response although unpredictable of death. Parisian Study Group on Acute Pancreatitis. Crit Care Med 1999;27:749-755; Honoré PM, Zydney AL, Matson JR: High volume and high permeability haemofiltration in sepsis: The evidence and the key issues. Care Criti Ill 2003;3:69-76; Ronco C, Tetta C, Mariano F, et al: Interpreting the mechanism of continuous renal replacement therapy in sepsis. The peak concentration hypothesis. Artif Organs 2003;27:792-801.)

clinical setting has been demonstrated by various studies using HVHF, without any significant drop in mediator levels in the blood compartment itself,[13-15] points to an effect outside this compartment. Although this benefit is obtained by a drop in cytokine or mediator concentrations at the tissue level (where they do harm), without any dramatic fall in plasma cytokine levels, this hypothesis does not explain how the increased mediator and cytokine flow between interstitium and the blood compartment, necessary for increased clearance by extracorporeal removal, is brought about.

The so-called *mediator delivery hypothesis* (Fig. 255-3),[16] otherwise known as the "Alexander concept," addresses this dilemma. In this theory, the use of HVHF, especially using high fluid delivery rates (3 to 5 L/hour), increases lymphatic flow 20- to 40-fold, thereby increasing mediator and cytokine flux through lymphatic drag. This phenomenon has been described in several papers[17-19] and points to a pivotal role for the use of larger volumes of exchange fluid (apart from extraction from the blood compartment) in order to increase the flow of lymphatic transport between the interstitial tissue and blood compartments.

Role of Volume in Displacement and Removal

It is therefore reasonable to assume that some forms of extracorporeal removal, such as high-flow hemofiltration, are able to dramatically increase lymphatic transport of mediators and cytokines from tissue and interstitial space to the blood compartment for potential removal later on. Accordingly, other forms of extracorporeal removal, such

ECR: Rationale
"Threshold modulation" hypothesis

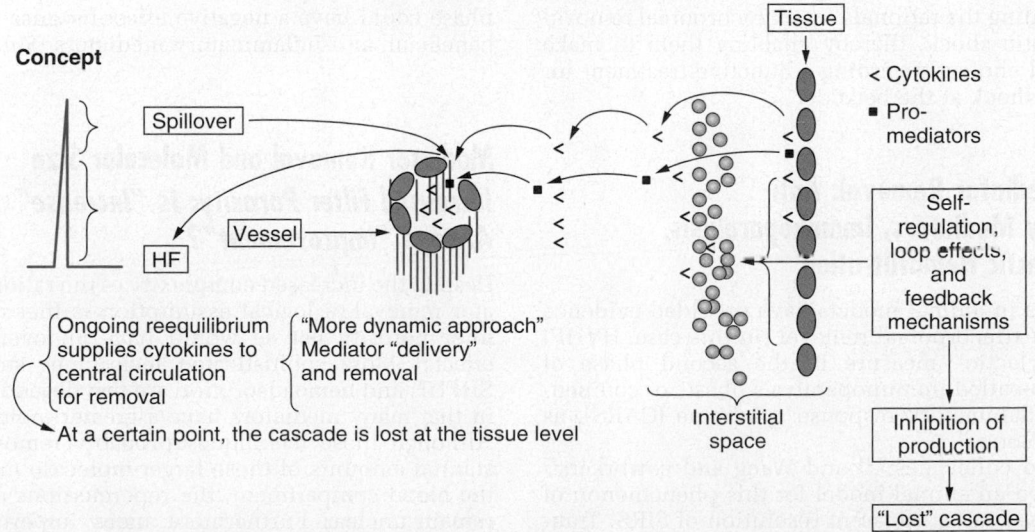

FIGURE 255-2. Mediator removal by extracorporeal techniques—evolving theories of rationale: The threshold modulation hypothesis. ECR, extracorporeal removal; HF, hemofiltration. (Data from Honoré PM, Joannes-Boyau O: High volume hemofiltration (HVHF) in sepsis: A comprehensive review of rationale, clinical applicability, potential indications and recommendations for future research. Int J Artif Organs 2004;27:1077-1082; Honoré PM, Matson JR: Extracorporeal removal for sepsis: Acting at the tissue level—the beginning of a new era for this treatment modality in septic shock. Crit Care Med 2004;32:896-897.)

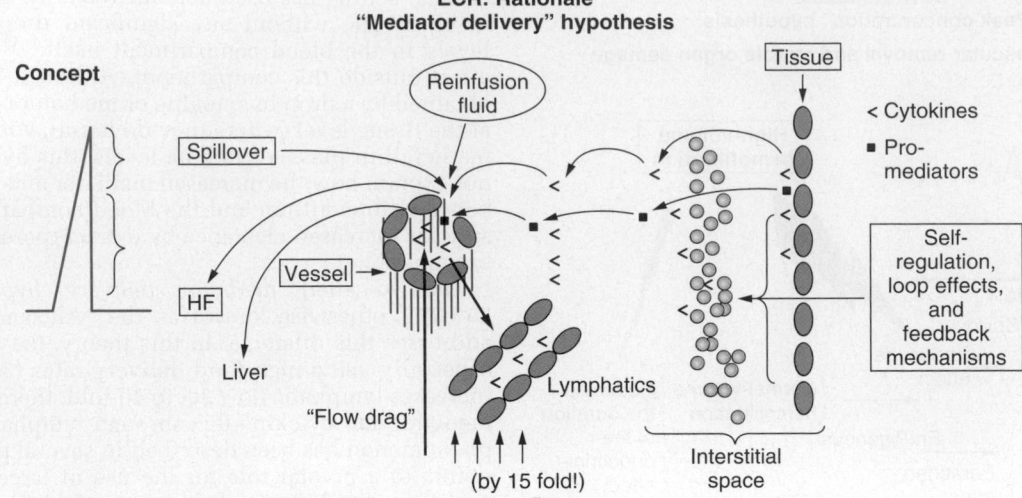

ECR: Rationale
"Mediator delivery" hypothesis

This scheme represents an "Interstitial protein washout"
"More dynamic approach" → Lymphatic flow → Bringing more cytokines
into the blood for hemofiltration, other organs' metabolism...
Lymph/serum ratio of albumin = 0.48/IL-8 = 9.8 but IL-6 = 40!

FIGURE 255-3. Mediator removal by extracorporeal techniques—evolving theories of rationale: The mediator delivery hypothesis. ECR, extracorporeal removal; HF, hemofiltration. (Data from Olszewski WL: The lymphatic system in body homeostasis: Physiological conditions. Lymphat Res Biol 2003;1:11-21; discussion 21-24).

as HPHF or CPFA with the capacity for the removal of larger amounts of mediators and cytokines from the blood compartment are, in their present form, unable to increase lymphatic flow and consequently are unable to mobilize crucial cytokines and mediators at interstitial and tissue levels (where they do harm).

This finding can go some way to explaining why, despite high hopes, some recent studies (e.g., a recent paper presented by Rogiers)[20] using these forms of extracorporeal removal (HPHF and other forms of highly permeable systems) have been shown to be ineffective in improving hemodynamics and survival in animal models for acute sepsis.

In conclusion, clinicians should be aware of these new insights regarding the rationale for extracorporeal removal in severe septic shock, thereby enabling them to make well-informed choices regarding adjunctive treatment for severe septic shock at the bedside.

Timing of Mediator Removal: Anti-inflammatory Mediators, Immunoparalysis, and Prophylactic Hemofiltration

Recent studies in animal models have provided evidence for a role for extracorporeal removal (in this case, HVHF) as a "prophylactic" measure in the second phase of sepsis—the so-called immunoparalysis phase, or compensatory anti-inflammatory response syndrome (CARS), as described by Bone.[21]

Yekebas and colleagues[22-24] and Wang and coworkers[25] both developed an animal model for this phenomenon of immunoparalysis after apparent resolution of SIRS. Traumatic pancreatitis was induced in healthy pigs, and hemofiltration was initiated 12 hours after trauma but before the onset of sepsis and shock. After 12 hours, fulminant peritonitis and intravascular sepsis due to bacterial translocation occurred, inducing a shock state in these pigs.

By comparing different hemofiltration regimens, especially low-dose (20 mL/kg per hour) hemofiltration plus adsorption and HVHF at a rate of 100 mL/kg per hour, the investigators were able to demonstrate that the early, prophylactic use of HVHF (100 mL/kg per hour) resulted in reduction in the severity of immunoparalysis and in subsequent risk of secondary infection and, ultimately, the death rate. For the first time, albeit in an animal model, HVHF was shown to have a beneficial effect not only in the pro-inflammatory phase but also, as a prophylactic measure, on the secondary immunoparalysis phenomenon itself.

This finding seems to dispel the fear that removal of mediators in a phase other than the pro-inflammatory phase could have a negative effect because of removal of beneficial, anti-inflammatory mediators (Fig. 255-4).

Mediator Removal and Molecular Size
Increased Filter Porosity: Is "Increase" Always "Improvement"?

Despite the increased complexity of the rationale for mediator removal, a logical assumption is that increasing the filter porosity per se would have an overall beneficial effect.[26] More sophisticated techniques such as HPHF, SHFHF, and hemoadsorption are privileged in this context in that many mediators have a greater molecular weight. Although these techniques probably remove more substantial amounts of these larger-molecule mediators from the blood compartment, the repercussions at tissue level remain unclear. Furthermore, many important nutrients, hormones, and drugs, particularly antibiotics, as well as many unknown metabolites, also may be lost.

For this reason, investigators have chosen to implement hybrid techniques, using the advantages of different techniques while avoiding some obvious drawbacks. Indeed,

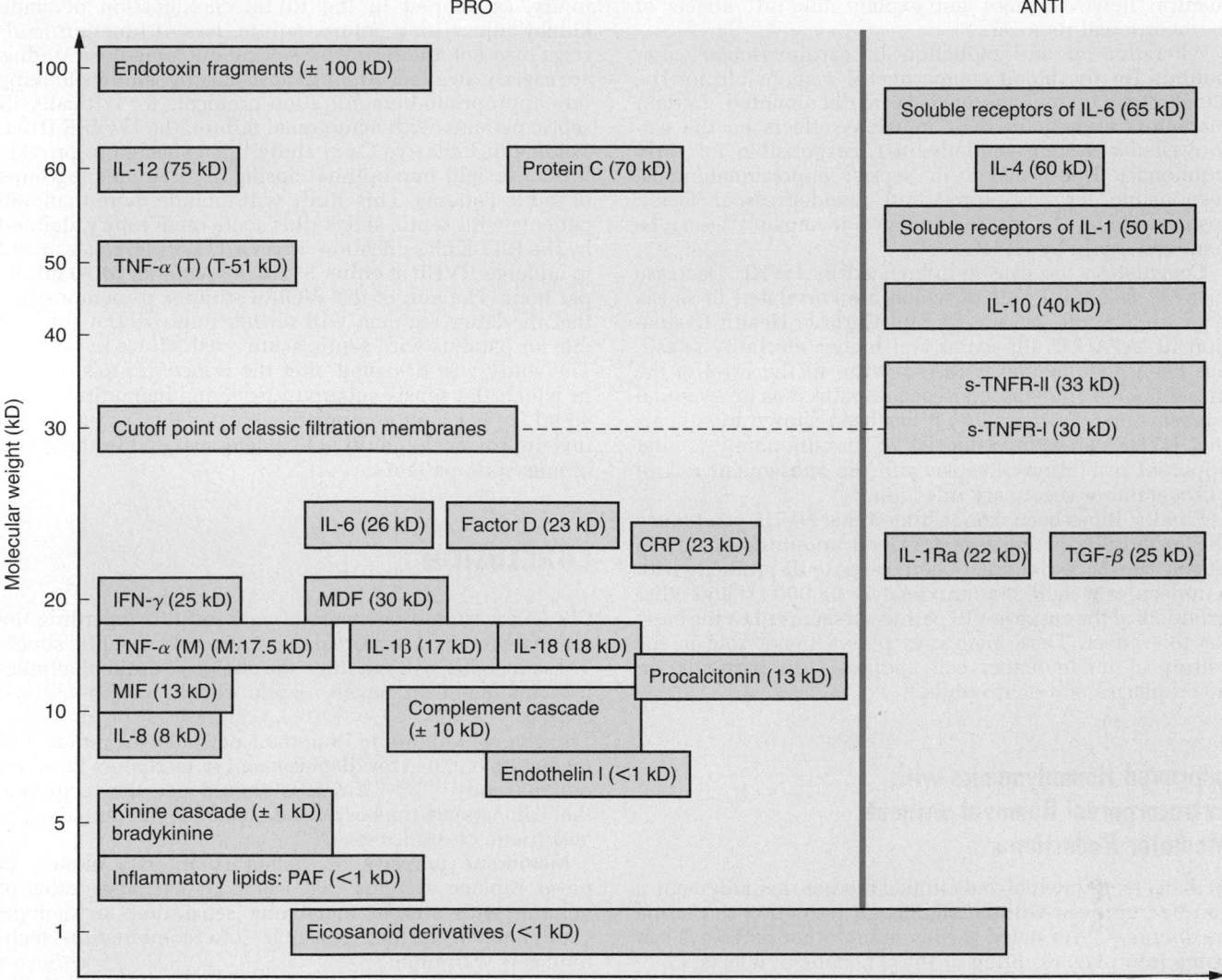

PRO   ANTI

FIGURE 255-4. Summary of pro-inflammatory and anti-inflammatory mediators in relation to the cut-off point of classic filtration membranes. CRP, C-reactive protein; IL, interleukin; MDF, myodepressant factor; MIF, macrophage inhibiting factor; PAF, platelet-activating factor; sTNFR-I, sTNFR-II, tumor necrosis factor receptors I and II; TGF, transforming growth factor; TNF, tumor necrosis factor.

because techniques such as CPFA and cascade hemofiltration (CCHF)[27] return a large portion of the treated blood to the patient, large amounts and large molecules can be retrieved without risking the loss of important nutrients. In theory, further development of hybrid techniques such as CCHF and CPFA will one day offer the possibility of optimal and precise targeting of molecules, with negligible loss of beneficial molecules.

The Neglected Domain in the Filter Porosity Spectrum: Midsize Molecules

At present, most activity in hemofiltration is concentrated at either end of the molecular spectrum. At the lower end, HVHF and HVHF-derived techniques seek to modify concentrations of molecules less than 45 kD in size, whereas at the higher end, in plasma filtration, molecules of approximately 900 kD are targeted. The domain in between begs attention from both clinicians and investigators and

remains largely neglected at present. A study using high-cutoff hemofiltration (filter cutoff at 60 kD), demonstrating better filter clearance of some mediators, is a small first step in the right direction.[28,29]

THE CASE *AGAINST* REMOVAL OF MEDIATORS OF INFLAMMATION BY CONTINUOUS RENAL REPLACEMENT THERAPY

Role of Multiple Pathways in Mediating Effects of Continuous Therapy

Extracorporeal removal can influence the pro-inflammatory phase and inhibit its expression by potentially reducing unbound cytokine levels and reducing the corresponding remote organ damage.[30,31] This simple mantra, however, does not explain the full effects of extracorporeal removal.

Alteration of and reduction in cardiovascular compounds (in the blood compartment) responsible for the shock state in humans have been documented. Certain mediators known for their injurious effects on the cardiovascular system—endothelin-1, responsible for early pulmonary hypertension in sepsis; endocannabinoids, responsible for vasoplegia; and myodepressant factor, responsible for the cardiodepression in sepsis[32-34]—can be removed easily by HVHF.

Coagulation too can be influenced by HVHF. Decrease in pPAI factor I, levels of which are correlated in sepsis with high Acute Physiology and Chronic Health Evaluation III (APACHE III) scores and higher mortality rates,[35] has been documented with reduction in the level of the disseminated intravascular coagulopathy[36] as an eventual consequence. Furthermore, it has been shown in animals that HVHF can reduce the risk of immunoparalysis after apparent resolution of sepsis and the subsequent risk of nosocomial or secondary infection.[22-25]

Finally, it has been demonstrated that HVHF can reduce the magnitude of inflammatory cell apoptosis occurring during sepsis. Extraction of both caspase III products with a molecular weight of approximately 35,000 Da and other products of the caspase VIII pathways seems to be the basis for this effect. These pathways play a major role in the setting of inflammatory cell apoptosis, in particular in macrophages and neutrophils.[37]

Improved Hemodynamics with Extracorporeal Removal without Mediator Reduction

In many experimental and clinical models, hemodynamics can be improved without significant reduction in plasma mediators.[15,38] As stated earlier, many other pathways can come into play, resulting in these beneficial effects. Catecholamine-resistant septic shock is an exception, however, because improvement in hemodynamics has been proved to be associated with a significant decrease in plasma mediator concentration (Table 255-1).[39]

CLINICAL IMPLICATIONS

The use of extracorporeal removal as an adjunctive therapy in sepsis has clinical implications for the bedside intensivist. Application of fluid substitution in hemofiltration at 35 mL/kg per hour continues to evade widespread use. Despite the evidence, recent unpublished surveys have shown that less than 20% of clinical centers (at least in continental Europe) are applying this regimen. A recent position paper published by an Acute Dialysis Quality Initiative (ADQI) group has emphasized that HVHF could be used by clinicians in catecholamine-resistant septic shock (level V evidence and grade E recommendation).[11-14,40] In the same paper, the ADQI group promoted extended use of fluid substitution at 35 mL/kg per hour, citing level II evidence and a grade C recommendation.[40] Indeed, adequate dosing is supported by the "pro" arguments put forward earlier, in order to displace and remove mediators at the tissue level.

In classic hyperdynamic septic shock, particularly in the setting of acute septic renal failure or acute septic renal injury, as defined in the RIFLE classification of acute kidney injury (*r*isk, *i*njury, *f*ailure, *l*oss of function, *e*nd-stage disease), the results of several outcome-dose studies are eagerly awaited. Among those ongoing studies looking into appropriate hemofiltration protocols for critically ill septic patients with acute renal failure, the IVOIRE (*H*igh *Vo*lume in *I*ntensive *Ca*re) study[41] is expected to provide further insight into optimal dosing in different subgroups of septic patients. This study will include more than 480 patients with septic shock plus acute renal injury, defined by the RIFLE classification, in an ICU setting, randomized to undergo HVHF at either 35 mL/kg per hour or 70 mL/kg per hour. The aim of the IVOIRE study is to demonstrate that the latter regimen will further improve the survival rate for patients with septic acute renal failure in the ICU. The study was designed after the Ronco group's study,[42] in which the sepsis subgroup receiving hemofiltration at 45 mL/kg per hour demonstrated better survival, although this improvement could not be demonstrated in the group of nonseptic patients.

CONCLUSION

Clinicians should be aware of new insights regarding the rationale for extracorporeal therapy in severe septic shock. These insights will facilitate the choice of optimal adjunctive treatment in severe septic shock in the clinical setting.

Exchange volume is important not only for removal of mediators but also for displacement of mediators throughout the body.[17-19,43] Clinicians should use the technique that can achieve the best blood clearance rate but also the best tissue clearance rate.[43-45]

Membrane porosity or system complexity alone can never replace systems that use high exchange rates of volume with simple membrane separation technology. Undoubtedly, further research into combination techniques is warranted.

The field of hemofiltration and associated hybrid therapies is still evolving rapidly. Both investigator and clinician should be aware of recent advances, because several ongoing dose-outcome studies may profoundly change daily practice. At the same time, critical evaluation and balanced views on published studies in this area are eagerly needed now more than ever.[46]

Key Points

1. Volume exchange is needed not only for mediator removal but mainly for mediator transport and displacement into the body, facilitating removal.
2. Reducing blood mediator levels is of limited value, because mediators exert their injurious effects at tissue level.
3. Recent theories demonstrate that mediator removal is not a linear process but the result of complex cascades. This complexity is addressed in a number of hypotheses for mediator removal.
4. Pleiotropism of continuous renal replacement therapy illustrates the complexity of numerous mediators working on many different pathways and denies the validity of the removal of a single mediator as a magic bullet.

TABLE 255-1

Summary of Recent Clinical Studies of Mediator Clearance by Continuous Extracorporeal Removal Techniques

STUDY*	N	DIAGNOSIS	DESIGN	VOLUME	TECHNIQUE: Mb + S	UF RATE (mL/hr)	EXTRACTED MEDIATOR(S)	CLINICAL EFFECT(S)	TIMING	WEIGHT	UF RATE INDEXED TO BW
Tonnesen et al., 1993	9	Sepsis	P, NC	TBV	CAVH, PS/S: NA	750	TNF-α, IL-1β	NA	NA	NA = 75 kg	10 mL/kg/hr (E)
Guegniaud et al., 1994	6	Brûlés graves, ARF	RS, NC	TBV	CVVH, CA-SMS: NA	NA	IL-6	↑ MAP	NA	NA	NA
Wakabayashi et al., 1996	6	SIRS	P, NC	TBV	CVVH, Mb + S: NA	NA	IL-6, IL-8	↑ MAP ↑ SVR	NA	NA = 75 kg (E)	NA
Hoffman et al., 1996	16	Sepsis	P, NC	TBV	LV-CVVH, PA/S: NA	2000	C3A, C5A	↑ MAP ↑ SVR	NA	NA = 75 kg (E)	26 mL/kg/hr (E)
Heering et al., 1997	33	Sepsis	P, C	TBV	LV-CVVH, PS/S: 1.35 m²	1000	TNF-α, IL-6, IL-8	→MAP CI	NA	NA = 75 kg (E)	13 mL/kg/hr (E)
Sander et al., 1997	26	SIRS	R, C	TBV	LV-CVVH 13 pts: CVVH 13 pts: IHD CA-SMS: 0.6 m²	1000	IL-6	↔ MAP ↔ CI	NA	NA = 75 kg (E)	13 mL/kg/hr (E)
Kellum et al., 1998	13	SIRS + ARF	R, Cros	TBV	LV-CVVH + CVVHD, PAN/S: 0.6 m²	2000	TNF-α	NA	NA	NA = 75 kg (E)	26 mL/kg/hr (E)
De Vriese et al., 1999	15	Sepsis	P, NC	TBV BV	MV-CVVH, CA-SMS: 1 m²	1500 2700	TNF-α, IL-6, IL-10, IL-1Ra, sTNFR-I, sTNFR-II	↑ SVR	NA	NA = 75 kg (E)	20 mL/kg/hr (E) 36 mL/kg/hr (E)
Hommel et al., 1999	5	Sepsis	P, NC	TBV	LV-CVVH, CA-SMS: 0.4 m²	1080	TNF-α, IL-6, TNF-α	NA	NA	NA = 75 kg (E)	14.4 mL/kg/hr (E)
Cole et al., 2001	11	Sepsis	R, Cros	THV	HV-CVVH, CA-SMA: 1.6 m²	6000	C3A, C5A	↓ vasopressors	NA	NA = 75 kg (E)	80 mL/kg/hr

*Data sources (in alphabetical order): Cole, et al.: Intensive Care Med 2001;27:978-986; De Vriese A, et al: J Am Soc Nephrol 1999;10:846-853; Guegniaud PY, et al: Crit Care Med 1994;22:717; Heering P, et al: Intensive Care Med 1997;23:288-296; Hoffman, et al: Intensive Care Med 1996;22:1360-1367; Hommel, et al: Rean-Urg 1999;8:209-213; Kellum J, et al: Crit Care Med 1998;26:1995-2000; Sander, et al: Intensive Care Med 1997;23:878-884; Tonnesen E, et al: Anaesth Intensive Care 1993;21:752-758; Wakabayashi, et al: Br J Surg 1996;83:393-394.

ARF, acute renal failure; BV, blood volume; BW, body weight; C, controlled; CA-SMA, copolymer acrylate–sodium metholyl acrylate; CA-SMS, copolymer acrylate–sodium methlyl sulfate; CAVH, continuous arteriovenous hemofiltration; CI, cardiac index; Cros, crossover study; C3A, conferent fraction 3A; C5A, conferent fraction 5A; CVVHD, continuous venovenous hemodialysis; CVVH, continuous venovenous hemofiltration; E, estimated; HV-CVVH, high-volume continuous venovenous hemofiltration; IHD, intermittent hemodialysis; IL, interleukin; LV-CVVH, low-volume continuous venovenous hemofiltration; MAP, mean arterial pressure; Mb, membrane; MV-CVVH, mid-volume continuous venovenous hemofiltration; NA, not available; NC, not controlled; P, prospective; PAN/S, polyacrylamide/surface; PA/S, polyamide/surface; PS/S, polysulfate/surface; R, randomized; RS, retrospective; S, study; SIRS, systemic inflammatory response syndrome; sTNFR-I, sTNFR-II, tumor necrosis factor receptors I and II; SVR, systemic vascular resistance; TBV, total blood volume; THV, total hemofiltrate volume; TNF, tumor necrosis factor; UC, uncontrolled; UF, ultrafiltration.

5. Removal of mediators during the second phase of sepsis can be beneficial in reducing secondary immunoparalysis and subsequent infection.

6. Type and timing of techniques are very important because evidence suggests that early, prophylactic treatment can be effective in the pro-inflammatory phase, whereas longstanding moderate techniques can be beneficial in the late phase of sepsis.

7. The technique that can remove the greatest amount of mediator from the bloodstream is not necessarily the best, because removal at the tissue level is accomplished by displacement to the blood compartment.

8. Improvements in clinical management can be expected if these new insights are integrated into the rationale of mediator removal by continuous renal replacement therapy–derived techniques.

Key References

8. Honoré PM, Matson JR: Hemofiltration, adsorption, sieving and the challenge of sepsis therapy design. Crit Care 2002;6:394-396.
10. Bellomo R, Honoré PM, Matson JR, et al: Extracorporeal blood treatment (EBT) methods in SIRS/sepsis. Consensus statement. ADQI III Conference. Int J Artif Organs 2005;28: 450-458.
16. Di Carlo JV, Alexander SR: Hemofiltration for cytokine-driven illness: The mediator delivery hypothesis. Int J Artif Organs 2005;28:777-786.
28. Matson JR, Zydney RL, Honoré PM: Blood filtration: New opportunities and the implications on system biology. Crit Care Resusc 2004;6:209-218.
43. Joannes-Boyau O, Honoré PM, Boer W: Hemofiltration: The case for removal of sepsis mediators from where they do harm. Crit Care Med 2006;34:2244-2246.

See the companion Expert Consult website for the complete reference list.

CHAPTER 256

Nonrenal Applications of Extracorporeal Treatments: Heart Failure and Liver Failure

Eduardo Rocha, William R. Clark, and Claudio Ronco

OBJECTIVES

This chapter will:
1. Review the clinical scope of the problem of heart failure on a global basis and the potential role of ultrafiltration in its management.
2. Identify the key factors determining the hemodynamic effects of extracorporeal ultrafiltration.
3. Summarize the major clinical trials evaluating the potential clinical benefits of ultrafiltration in heart failure.
4. Outline the fundamental differences between non–cell-based and cell-based liver support systems.
5. Summarize the major clinical trials performed to investigate ultrafiltration for liver support.

When conservative measures fail, critically ill patients with acute kidney injury (AKI) require dialytic renal replacement for the correction of metabolic disturbances and volume overload. For such patients, extracorporeal dialytic techniques constitute the predominant management approach. Specifically, conventional hemodialysis and continuous renal replacement therapy (CRRT) are the mainstays of treatment for AKI in the intensive care unit (ICU).

In recent years, interest in the use of extracorporeal techniques for the management of clinical conditions other than AKI has been growing. Examples of nonrenal applications of extracorporeal therapies are heart failure, liver failure, and sepsis. This chapter discusses the first two of these applications; sepsis is covered in another chapter.

EXTRACORPOREAL ULTRAFILTRATION FOR HEART FAILURE

Chronic Heart Failure
Scope of the Problem

Approximately 5 million people in the United States currently have the diagnosis of chronic heart failure, which has a prevalence of 10 events per 1000 in the elderly population (persons older than 65 years of age). This disorder is responsible for nearly 1 million hospitalizations and 300,000 deaths per year.[1] In contrast with many other cardiovascular disorders, the incidence of heart failure is increasing, and in excess of 500,000 new cases are now diagnosed annually. The total annual cost of caring for patients with chronic heart failure in the United States may be as high as $40 billion, most of which is incurred in the hospital setting. These figures are staggering, especially in light of the recent advances that have been made in elucidation of heart failure pathophysiology.

Pathophysiology and Clinical Aspects

Despite the benefits of the various agents used to treat heart failure, its therapy is not without adverse effects, especially in patients in New York Heart Association (NYHA) classes III and IV. In many of these patients, hypotension often precludes use of fully therapeutic doses of angiotensin-converting enzyme (ACE) inhibitors and beta blockers. Moreover, for a patient with advanced heart failure, blood pressure is quite variable because it is influenced directly by cardiac output, which in turn is modulated by filling pressures in accordance with Starling's curve. Another problem that commonly develops is diuretic resistance.[2] Many patients with advanced heart failure have "functional" renal insufficiency in which reduced cardiac output leads to decreased glomerular filtration but intact renal tubular function. Because the efficacy of most diuretics is dependent on entry into the renal tubular lumen by means of glomerular filtration, their function is impaired in advanced heart failure. Although larger diuretic doses may achieve the desired effect, the well-described adverse effects of diuretics, especially those related to electrolyte and acid-base disturbances, are much more likely to occur at such doses. These disturbances, especially hypokalemia, hypomagnesemia, and metabolic alkalosis, are particularly worrisome in this patient population characterized by a high incidence of cardiac arrhythmias. In addition, diuretics may induce effective intravascular volume depletion, potentially exacerbating both hypotension and hyponatremia and resulting in worsened renal function.

Isolated Ultrafiltration for Acute Exacerbations of Chronic Heart Failure: Overview

Owing to the underlying pathophysiology of heart failure, the therapeutic range for standard-of-care pharmacological agents is small, and titration in this narrow range is difficult. Indeed, it is not uncommon for this titration process to take several days in the hospital. Moreover, a significant proportion of this process may occur in an ICU setting. Clearly, conventional medical therapy has limitations, and an additional therapeutic alternative that addresses these limitations is desirable. A potential alternative to this is extracorporeal ultrafiltration.

Isolated ultrafiltration as a therapy for volume overload was first described formally by Silverstein and colleagues in 1974.[3] Using a blood flow rate of 200 mL/minute and a 1.0 m^2 filter, these investigators reported that ultrafiltration rates of up to 800 mL/hour could be tolerated, as determined by degree of volume overload and hemodynamic status in the individual patient. Subsequent studies[4-19] have characterized this modality's specific clinical benefits, which include decreases in cardiac filling pressures and improvements in diuretic responsiveness, hyponatremia, edema, renal function, and dyspnea. A common element of many of these studies has been the

capability of ultrafiltration to "reset" the neurohormonal axis, as evidenced by decreases in plasma norepinephrine, aldosterone, and renin activity. A relatively common prescription in these studies has been an ultrafiltration rate of 300 to 600 mL/hour, administered over a several-hour treatment period for consecutive days.

Physiological and Clinical Considerations in the Use of Ultrafiltration for Heart Failure

In ultrafiltration, removal of plasma water is achieved by application of a pressure gradient across an extracorporeal membrane. This pressure gradient can be generated by creation of a positive pressure in the blood compartment or a negative pressure in the ultrafiltrate compartment of the filter. Modern devices control transmembrane pressure automatically to achieve the desired rate and volume of ultrafiltrate production. Extracorporeal ultrafiltration is a dynamic process in which the rate of volume removal by the extracorporeal filter has to be viewed in the context of the manner in which it modifies Starling's forces governing fluid flow across the capillary wall. First, removal of plasma ultrafiltrate from the intravascular space decreases hydrostatic pressure in that compartment. This results in a hydrostatic pressure gradient across the capillary wall that favors entry of fluid from the extravascular (interstitial) space, which has a relatively high hydrostatic pressure as a result of tissue edema. Because the ultrafiltrate generated is relatively protein-free, another ultrafiltration-induced Starling force change promoting capillary refill is an increase in oncotic pressure in the intravascular compartment.

A fundamental concern relating to the use of ultrafiltration is the rate at which volume can be removed while maintaining hemodynamic stability, an important determinant of which is blood volume. Provided that the rate of removal from the intravascular compartment does not exceed the capillary refill rate, maintenance of blood volume is possible. Marenzi and colleagues[17] estimated capillary refill to be at least 800 mL/hour at the initiation of an ultrafiltration treatment, falling to 400 mL/hour at the conclusion of a treatment session achieving approximately 4 L of volume removal (Fig. 256-1). This finding is

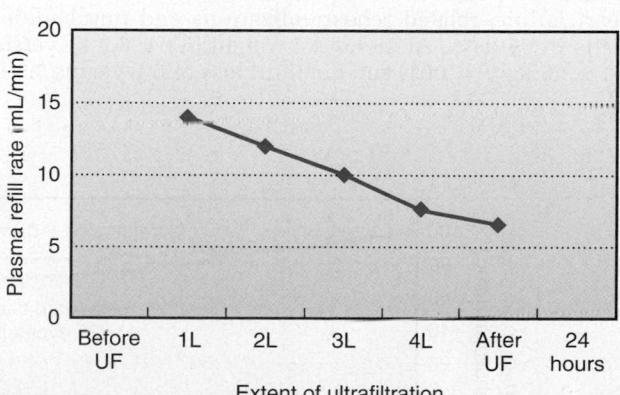

FIGURE 256-1. Plasma refilling rate as a function of extent of ultrafiltration in patients with chronic heart failure. (From Marenzi G, Lauri G, Grazi M, et al: Circulatory response to fluid overload removal by extracorporeal ultrafiltration in refractory congestive heart failure. J Am Coll Cardiol 2001;38:963-968.)

consistent with ultrafiltration rates reported in other published studies demonstrating clinical benefits of ultrafiltration therapy.

One of the aforementioned studies provides insight into the potential mechanisms explaining the benefits of ultrafiltration in patients with heart failure: Agostoni and coworkers measured neurohormonal and clinical parameters in NYHA class II and class III patients who received either high-dose intravenous furosemide or a single extracorporeal ultrafiltration treatment.[11] Ultrafiltration was performed at a rate of 500 mL/hour and achieved a cumulative volume removal of 1.7 L, which was similar to the urine volume in the diuretic treatment group during the study period. In the ultrafiltration treatment group, a significant decrease in plasma aldosterone, norepinephrine, and renin activity was observed within 48 hours, along with a reduction in degree of hyponatremia. Moreover, a significant improvement in functional capacity that persisted for 3 months occurred. On the other hand, these changes were not observed in the diuretic treatment group, in which elevated filling pressures and pulmonary congestion instead recurred within days. The clinical benefits reported in this study may relate to the difference in the composition of the volume removed by ultrafiltration versus diuretics. In ultrafiltration, the fluid removed is an ultrafiltrate of plasma and, as such, has electrolyte concentrations that are isotonic with respect to plasma water. By contrast, urine is inherently hypotonic with respect to plasma water. Therefore, sodium removal is significantly greater in ultrafiltrate relative to the same volume of urine. Moreover, owing to the isotonicity of the ultrafiltrate, ultrafiltration induces no acute changes in electrolyte concentrations.

A new approach to ultrafiltration for decompensated heart failure has recently been introduced in the United States. The Aquadex device (CHF Solutions, Brooklyn Park, MN) is a dedicated ultrafiltration system designed to be used with either central or peripheral venous access.[20-22] Several clinical evaluations with this system have been reported in the literature, most recently the UNLOAD (Ultrafiltration versus Intravenous Diuretics for Patients Hospitalized for Acute Decompensated Heart Failure) trial.[22] In this study, 200 patients hospitalized for heart failure with clinical signs of hypervolemia were randomized to receive ultrafiltration treatment or intravenous diuretics. The primary endpoints were weight loss and dyspnea assessment at 48 hours after randomization; secondary endpoints included net fluid loss at 48 hours and heart failure–related rehospitalizations and unscheduled visits in 90 days. At 48 hours, weight (5.0 ± 3.1 kg versus 3.1 ± 3.5 kg; $P = .001$) and net fluid loss (4.6 L versus 3.3 L;

$P = .001$) were greater in the ultrafiltration group; dyspnea scores were similar. At 90 days, the ultrafiltration group had fewer patients rehospitalized for heart failure (16 of 89, or 18%, versus 28 of 87, or 32%; $P = .037$); fewer heart failure–related rehospitalizations (0.22 ± 0.54 versus 0.46 ± 0.76; $P = .022$) and rehospitalization days (1.4 ± 4.2 versus 3.8 ± 8.5; $P = .022$) per patient; and fewer unscheduled visits (14 of 65, or 21%, versus 29 of 66, or 44%; $P = .009$) (Fig. 256-2). No significant serum creatinine differences between groups were noted, although the serum creatinine trended higher and early in the ultrafiltration group. Relative to the baseline value, for which the mean was 1.5 mg/dL in both groups, the mean serum creatinine increase was 0.2 to 0.3 mg/dL and 0.1 mg/dL in the ultrafiltration and control groups, respectively, during the first 10 days of the study.

Future Issues with Use of Ultrafiltration for Heart Failure

Although the available clinical data suggest a role for ultrafiltration in the management of patients with heart failure, a number of issues need to be addressed before ultrafiltration becomes a mainstream therapy in this population (Table 256-1). One critical issue relates to the technical requirements for an extracorporeal system used specifically in heart failure. Although the basic mechanism by which volume removal occurs (i.e., creation of a pressure gradient across a filter membrane) is similar to that in other extracorporeal therapies, devices used for patients with heart failure may require additional features. Device size and portability represent two such features. Standard

TABLE 256-1

Ultrafiltration for Heart Failure: Considerations in Clinical Application

- Device portability and ease of use
- Venous access: central or modified PICC line
- Modality: continuous versus intermittent daily ultrafiltration
- Cost-effectiveness (shorter hospital stays, decreased readmission rate)
- Close collaboration between nephrologist and cardiologist
- Clinical data requirements for therapy adoption

PICC, peripherally inserted central catheter.

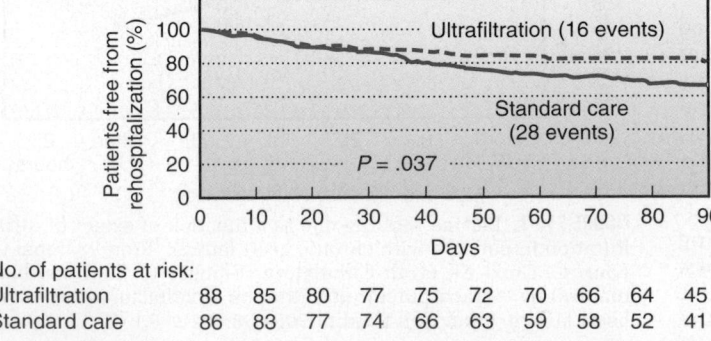

No. of patients at risk:

	0	10	20	30	40	50	60	70	80	90
Ultrafiltration	88	85	80	77	75	72	70	66	64	45
Standard care	86	83	77	74	66	63	59	58	52	41

FIGURE 256-2. Rehospitalization in control and ultrafiltration arms of the UNLOAD trial. (From Costanzo MR, Guglin MR, Saltzberg MT, et al: Ultrafiltration versus intravenous diuretics for patients hospitalized for acute decompensated heart failure. J Am Coll Cardiol 2007; 49:675-683.)

machines used for conventional hemodialysis and, in most cases, CRRT were developed largely for applications other than simple volume removal and are therefore more complex than is necessary for isolated ultrafiltration in the heart failure population. Moreover, these traditional devices tend to be relatively large and bulky, making portability difficult. Ease of use by nondialysis personnel and easy portability between cardiac units, ICUs, and even outpatient clinics are highly desirable features for a specialized ultrafiltration device.

One of the most important aspects of future clinical investigations of isolated ultrafiltration for heart failure is defining clinical and resource utilization endpoints. Potential clinical endpoints include those based on predetermined hemodynamic targets, such as pulmonary capillary wedge pressure or cardiac index; volume removal, such as the time required to meet a defined volume target; and changes in neurohormonal parameters. Other clinical endpoint considerations include the effect of ultrafiltration on required doses of diuretic and vasoactive medication and treatment-related adverse effects, such as arrthythmias, electrolyte disturbances, renal dysfunction, and myocardial ischemia. Of importance, cost-effectiveness parameters, including ICU and hospital length of stay and readmission rates, need to be evaluated, along with the effect of ultrafiltration therapy on quality of life. Finally, it is anticipated that these studies will involve a spectrum of ultrafiltration protocols with respect to flow rates and both frequency and duration of treatment.

Conclusion

Significant room for improvement exists in the management of patients with exacerbations of chronic heart failure. Finding a practical, economical treatment alternative for these patients is essential in view of the economic implications of providing in-hospital treatment for the rapidly growing heart failure population. Published literature suggests that isolated ultrafiltration has the potential to significantly influence morbidity, quality of life, hospital length of stay, and hospital readmissions for patients with heart failure. Broader adoption of this therapy would benefit from well-conducted clinical studies to characterize further the extent of ultrafiltration's benefits.

EXTRACORPOREAL THERAPY FOR LIVER FAILURE

General Considerations

For both acute liver failure (ALF) and acute-on-chronic liver failure (AOCLF), orthotopic liver transplantation is clearly the definitive therapy. Limited organ availability is a major problem, however, in both clinical scenarios. Moreover, as the incidence of decompensated cirrhosis and AOCLF due to hepatitis C continues to increase over the next 10 to 20 years, the demand for organs will increase significantly; at the same time, organ availability is projected to remain relatively constant. These projections lead to an inescapable conclusion: that alternative therapeutic modalities for liver failure are needed desperately. One potentially promising alternative is extracorporeal liver support, which not only may serve as a bridge to transplantation in patients with decompensated cirrhosis but also can provide a lifesaving option for patients with ful-

TABLE 256-2

Toxin Accumulation in Liver Failure: A Vicious Circle

- Because of failure of the detoxification function of the liver, byproducts of protein metabolism and other substances normally processed by the liver accumulate in the blood.
- These toxins propagate further damage to the liver or at least prevent liver regeneration.
- These toxins also may contribute to the multiorgan dysfunction that commonly accompanies liver failure.
- Ammonia is one such toxin, but many others exist.

minant hepatic failure at high risk of death due to inadequate hepatic regeneration.

In the past, a number of different extracorporeal approaches to the management of liver failure have been used, including standard hemodialysis, hemofiltration, cross-circulation and exchange transfusion, apheresis techniques, hemoperfusion, and extracorporeal liver cell perfusion. For a variety of reasons, these approaches did not meet the clinical needs of patients with liver failure. A critique of these older approaches is beyond the scope of this discussion—the reader is referred to a number of recent reviews for this purpose.[23,24] Instead, this chapter describes more contemporary techniques, especially those that have recently undergone clinical evaluation. By way of background, an overview of the two major types of artificial liver support is presented first.

Cell-Based versus Non–Cell-Based Therapies
Non–Cell-Based Therapies

One approach to liver support is focused almost exclusively on the detoxification aspect of liver function. It is well known that liver failure frequently is associated with dysfunction of many other organs, especially the kidney, heart, and brain. Proponents of non–cell-based approaches suggest that the accumulation of byproducts of protein metabolism and other substances normally processed by the liver is responsible for this multiorgan dysfunction.[25] Moreover, these same toxins also are viewed as propagating further damage to the liver itself, or at least preventing liver regeneration. A vicious circle feedback loop in which liver injury leads to toxin accumulation, which in turn results in further liver injury, is conceptualized (Table 256-2). Although ammonia, a small-molecule water-soluble compound, is one of the protein metabolites that accumulates in liver failure, most of the putative toxins are thought to be protein-bound.

In the view of many experts, the major drawback of this approach is its inability to fully replicate native hepatic function, especially with respect to synthetic function. The countering argument to this point, however, is that the clinically important products of hepatic synthesis, especially clotting factors, albumin, and glucose, can be provided with infusions of fresh frozen plasma and other intravenous solutions. Although the Molecular Adsorbents Recirculating System (Gambro)[26] is the prototypical device in this category, additional devices have been described.[27,28] These systems all involve the use of membrane-based cartridges and incorporate features designed to promote the removal of albumin-bound toxins.

Cell-Based Therapies

Proponents of cell-based therapies contend that a liver replacement therapy should mimic native hepatic function comprehensively and should not only provide detoxification but also have synthetic and excretory capabilities. The generic name most frequently given to a cell-based device is *bioartificial liver* (BAL), which is the term used in this chapter.[29-32]

At a minimum, all BAL devices contain both cellular and blood or plasma compartments separated by a membrane. The devices discussed here all use hollow-fiber membranes similar to (or the same as) those used for hemodialysis,[29-31] although other configurations have been described.[32]

The presence of hepatic cells in BAL systems renders them considerably more complex than non–cell-based therapies, and an obvious requirement for creation of a BAL is the ability to isolate and culture a sufficient number of cells. Although the ability to culture liver cells was demonstrated many years ago, the effects of an extracorporeal environment on hepatocyte function and the associated implications for optimal BAL design are still not understood entirely. Specifically, an understanding of what components in addition to the cells themselves are required for maintenance of hepatocellular function is required. In this regard, the extracellular matrix is a very important consideration. As is the case for many other types of cells, such as in the kidney and intestine, a liver cell requires attachment either to other liver cells or to an extracellular support material (matrix) to function properly. Both biological substances (e.g., collagen) and nonbiological materials have served as extracellular matrix platforms in BAL devices. Another issue is whether the liver cells are cultured *ex situ* (i.e., outside the environment of the BAL device) or cultured after delivery to the device. Finally, an abundance of data suggests that the manner in which hepatocytes aggregate in the extracorporeal environment also is important in retaining cell functionality. Specialized techniques are used to promote the development of specific three-dimensional cellular structures in this aggregation process.

A fundamental consideration is whether the liver cells used are from a human or animal source. Because of the critical shortage of human livers, procurement of primary cells from this source is not feasible. Sussman and Kelly,[30] however, have used a cloned (immortalized) human cell line (C3A cells) derived from patients with a specific type of liver tumor (hepatoblastoma) for their bioartificial liver, the *extracorporeal liver assist device* (ELAD). Although this approach provides essentially an unlimited supply of hepatocytes, a number of concerns have been voiced. The most serious of these relates to the possibility of transmembrane passage of either tumor cells or tumor-inducing proteins into the plasma or blood compartment of a BAL device. Approaches are being developed to ensure the safety of using immortalized cells in human applications, but it is not clear how they will apply specifically to the BAL. Consequently, most BAL devices currently undergoing clinical or preclinical evaluations use primary hepatocytes from an animal source. Although availability is not a limitation of this approach, the use of nonhuman (xenogeneic) cells has raised concerns about the induction of zoonoses (animal-related infections) in humans. In this regard, a specific virus, pig endogenous retrovirus (PERV), has been identified.[33] The possibility of PERV transfer across extracorporeal membranes and the associated implications for use of BAL devices are a matter of debate, because studies have reported conflicting results. Consequently, from a regulatory perspective, this remains an unsettled issue.

Extracorporeal Liver Therapies: Design Considerations

Non–Cell-Based Therapies

As suggested previously, the major aim of systems in this category is the removal of protein-bound toxins that accumulate in hepatic failure. A recent review by Patzer and Bane[34] notes that one of albumin's main physiological functions is to transport insoluble compounds. Hepatic failure involves the accumulation of such insoluble compounds (toxins), which not only maintains the presence of these toxins in the blood but also prevents albumin from performing its other physiological functions. Moreover, because water solubility is essentially a prerequisite for a solute to be removed by conventional dialysis techniques, protein-bound toxins are removed ineffectively by these therapies. Therefore, the removal of such toxins requires adaptation of standard dialysis techniques. For a system based on a dialyzer-type device containing a standard (albumin-impermeable) membrane, two fundamental principles apply. First, the system must promote the dissociation ("unbinding") of a protein-bound toxin in the blood compartment, thereby creating a relatively high *free* toxin concentration. Second, to maximize the transmembrane concentration gradient for removal, the *free* toxin concentration in the dialysate compartment must be maintained as close to zero as possible.

In the original development of the molecular adsorbent recycling system (MARS) by Stange and colleagues,[35] these principles were put into practice. In the original description, the system had three key features: (1) a high-flux dialyzer containing an asymmetrical, albumin-impermeable membrane in which the macroporous support layer is impregnated with albumin; (2) a closed-loop dialysate compartment containing an albumin-based solution serving as a toxin "sink"; and (3) a regenerating adsorbent system designed to remove bound toxins from albumin in the dialysate. The asymmetrical structure of a polysulfone membrane, in which the inner, blood-contacting layer is less than 1 μm thick, enabled albumin impregnated in the macroporous layer to be in close proximity to albumin-bound toxin in the blood compartment (Fig. 256-3). This proximity promoted the initial dissociation of bound toxins in the blood compartment. A toxin removed in this manner could subsequently be adsorbed to the membrane itself or be "shuttled" through the membrane by successive binding to and release from albumin molecules impregnated in the membrane.

A recent kinetic analysis of albumin dialysis[34] indicates that four parameters influence transport of a given protein-bound toxin:

- The strength of interaction between the toxin- and albumin-binding sites
- The ratio of the dialyzer mass transfer coefficient–area product (KA) to the blood flow rate
- The dialysate-blood flow rate ratio
- The ratio of total albumin concentration in the dialysate to that in the blood

As shown in this investigation, when albumin is present at even low concentration in the dialysate (1 g/L versus 100 g/L for the MARS), the dialyzer's mass transfer coefficient is the most important of these four parameters in

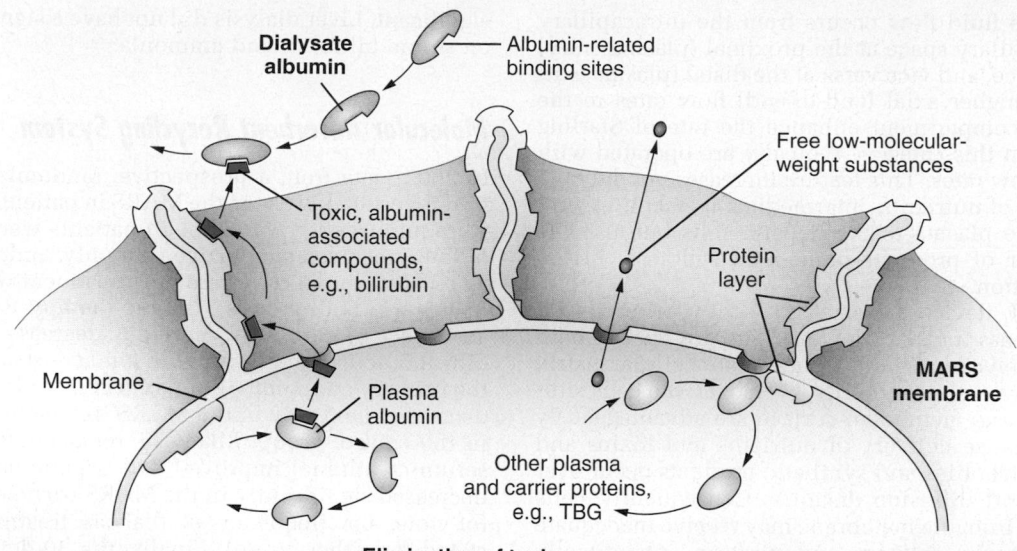

FIGURE 256-3. Schematic diagram of membrane mass transfer for the molecular adsorbent recycling system (MARS) device. *Note*: MARS is not approved by the U.S. Food and Drug Administration for use in liver failure.

influencing toxin removal. The data predict that until albumin saturation of the macroporous pore structure occurs, toxin removal occurs by diffusion or convection in the fluid phase of the pores. Once albumin saturation occurs, however, the rate of solute removal actually increases because the adsorbed albumin molecules provide a facilitated transport pathway for toxin molecules, as suggested previously.

Another system that uses an albumin-impermeable membrane is the Liver Dialysis System (formerly the Bio-Logic-DT) (Hemocleanse), in which a flat-plate dialyzer containing a low-permeability cellulosic membrane separates blood from a charcoal suspension.[36] The relatively thin-walled membrane (approximately 6 μm thick) allows reasonably close proximity between the blood and the adsorbing charcoal.

By contrast, two recently described systems incorporate protein-permeable membranes. In one system, designated as fractionated plasma separation and adsorption (FPSA),[37] plasma is ultrafiltered through a 250-kD cutoff polysulfone filter having albumin and fibrinogen sieving coefficients of 0.89 and 0.17, respectively. As in the MARS, the albumin in the ultrafiltrate is de-ligandized by passage through a dialyzer, charcoal column, and anion exchanger before reinfusion into the albumin-permeable filter. An adaptation of FPSA is the Prometheus system (Fresenius Medical Care, Bad Homburg, Germany),[28] for which an additional feature is an albumin-impermeable high-flux polysulfone dialyzer situated in series with the albumin-permeable filter.

Cell-Based Therapies

Although other configurations have been described, the following discussion focuses on hollow fiber–based BAL devices in which the blood-plasma and cellular compartments are the intracapillary and extracapillary regions, respectively. One of the most important design considerations for such a device is the manner in which oxygen and other nutrients, along with toxins, are delivered to the

extracapillary compartment from the intracapillary space. Adequate oxygen delivery is important not only to support hepatocellular function but also to promote cell attachment in this compartment. Yet exposure to excessively high oxygen concentrations also may adversely influence liver cell function. Striking the appropriate balance in oxygen delivery is complicated by its relatively low solubility in aqueous solutions. In addition to oxygen, the hepatocyte compartment of a BAL device requires nutrient (e.g., glucose) delivery from the intracapillary compartment. Finally, detoxification of blood-borne toxins requires efficient delivery of these compounds to the hepatocytes in the extracapillary space. On the other hand, the metabolic and synthetic products generated during BAL operation must be delivered from the extracapillary space to the blood compartment. Thus, the design of BAL devices requires consideration of this bidirectional solute transfer. It is important to note that export of clinically relevant amounts of high-molecular-weight synthetic products (e.g., albumin) from the cells and the delivery of protein-bound toxins to the cells require use of more permeable membranes than those used in standard dialysis therapies.

For transmembrane solute mass transfer and that occurring in the blood compartment, analytical techniques similar to those used for standard hemodialysis can be used for hollow-fiber BAL devices. However, the presence of cells in the extracapillary compartment renders a mass transfer analysis considerably more complex for a BAL device, relative to a standard dialyzer. Moreover, for the variety of BAL devices that are discussed next, the predominant mechanism of mass transfer (diffusion versus convection) differs widely. In some BAL devices, an ultrafiltrate of plasma is the fluid that perfuses the cells in the extracapillary space. Therefore, although some mass transfer may occur by diffusion, the predominant mechanism for these devices is convection. Of note, however, because the extracapillary compartment ports are sealed in these devices, their operation differs significantly from that of a conventional hemofilter. Instead, they are operated as Starling flow devices, in which transmembrane fluid flow occurs from the intracapillary to the extracapillary space at the proximal (plasma entry) end of the device, and vice versa at the distal (plasma exit) end. Because higher axial (end-to-end) flow rates in the intracapillary compartment enhance the rate of Starling flow, devices in this category typically are operated with high plasma flow rates. This feature increases not only the rate of transfer of nutrients, intermediate metabolites, and toxins from the plasma to the hepatic cells but also the rate of transfer of products of hepatic synthesis in the opposite direction.

Another BAL device approach is to rely primarily on diffusion for mass transfer. However, the presence of both the cells themselves and the associated extracellular matrix reduces diffusive solute mobility. Moreover, the cells situated closest to the membrane surface are advantageously positioned because delivery of nutrients and toxins and removal of metabolites and synthetic products occur over a relatively short diffusion distance. Consequently, cells located farther from the membrane may receive inadequate nutrient and toxin delivery and perform suboptimally with respect to synthetic functions.

Major Clinical Studies Evaluating Extracorporeal Liver Support Systems
Cedars-Sinai Bioartificial Liver

The phase II/III trial of the Cedars-Sinai BAL, the Circe device,[38] included 147 patients with acute liver failure and advanced-stage encephalopathy. The trial was performed at 20 centers in the United States and Europe, with a primary endpoint of 30-day survival. Each BAL treatment session lasted 6 hours; treatment could be performed as many as 14 times according to the protocol. Based on the primary data analysis, the survival rate in the BAL group (71%) was not significantly different from that in the control group (62%). Thus, on the basis of the primary endpoint, the study findings were negative. As indicated by a post hoc analysis adjusting for the effect of transplantation on survival, however, a significant 44% reduction in the risk of death was observed for the BAL treatment group.

Liver Dialysis System

Ash has summarized multiple randomized trials performed with the Liver Dialysis System (formerly BioLogic-DT) over the past several years.[39] A total of 31 patients (21 with an acute exacerbation of chronic liver failure and 10 with fulminant hepatic failure) comprised the treatment arm, and 25 patients comprised the control arm. The primary endpoints were recovery of liver function (or sufficient improvement in liver function to allow transplant eligibility), neurological improvement, and hemodynamic improvement. In the chronic liver failure group, liver dialysis resulted in improvement of liver function in a significantly higher percentage of patients relative to the control group. On the other hand, liver dialysis had no effect on this outcome in patients with fulminant hepatic failure. For both the neurological and hemodynamic outcome parameters, both patients with fulminant hepatic failure and those with chronic liver disease treated with liver dialysis experienced greater improvement than that noted for control patients. The small number of patients in the study, however, prevented these differences from being

significant. Liver dialysis did not have a significant impact on serum bilirubin and ammonia.

Molecular Adsorbent Recycling System

In 2002, data from a prospective, randomized controlled trial investigating use of the MARS in patients with AOCLF were published.[40] A total of 24 patients were enrolled; 12 of these received supportive care only, and the remaining 12 received supportive care plus treatment with the MARS device. (In both groups, dialytic therapy was considered an aspect of supportive care.) A decrease in the serum bilirubin to less than 15 mg/dL for 3 consecutive days was the primary endpoint. Serum bilirubin and bile acid levels decreased modestly in the MARS treatment group but not in the control group. Likewise, renal function (based on serum creatinine) improved and hepatic encephalopathy decreased significantly in the MARS treatment group only (of note, the frequency of dialysis treatments was not stated for either group). Finally, the 30-day survival rate was significantly higher in the MARS treatment group (93%) than in the control group (50%).

A more recent randomized, controlled, multicenter trial was conducted to investigate the clinical effects of the MARS device on grades 3 and 4 hepatic encephalopathy in patients with AOCLF. Patients were randomized to receive MARS therapy plus standard medical therapy (SMT) or SMT alone. Albumin dialysis was done daily for 6 hours for 5 days or until a patient experienced a two-grade improvement in hepatic encephalopathy grade. The primary endpoint of the study was the improvement proportion with respect to hepatic encephalopathy, and a total of 70 patients were enrolled. Precipitating events for hepatic encephalopathy were most commonly infection and bleeding. Based on an intent-to-treat analysis, improvement proportion for hepatic encephalopathy was significantly higher in the MARS therapy group (median, 30) than in the SMT-only group (median, 0) ($P = .044$) (Fig. 256-4). In addition, the MARS therapy group reached the first two-grade improvement in hepatic encephalopathy grade significantly more quickly and more frequently than the SMT group ($P = .045$). The investigators concluded that MARS therapy was significantly more efficacious than SMT in reversing severe grades of hepatic encephalopathy in patients with end-stage liver disease and acute decompensation. (*Note*: the MARS device has not been cleared by the U.S. Food and Drug Administration for use in patients with hepatic encephalopathy.)

Conclusion

The treatment of both fulminant hepatic failure and end-stage liver failure continues to be problematic owing to the critical shortage of organs for transplantation. Moreover, the severity of this problem is projected to increase over the next 2 decades as the epidemic of hepatitis C unfolds. Extracorporeal liver support is a potential solution to this problem. A number of systems have been developed over the past decade, many of which have undergone clinical evaluations. Of these systems, largely because of a less constrained regulatory pathway, the MARS device has been involved in the largest number of clinical trials. By contrast, because the cell-based systems are considered to be biologicals, rather than devices, by regulatory authorities in both Europe and the United States, their regulatory pathway is more stringent. Future clinical trials with these

IMPROVEMENT PROPORTION

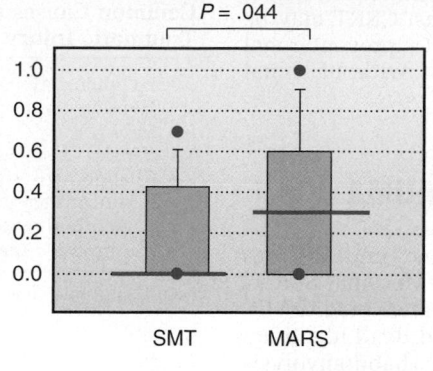

TIME TO IMPROVEMENT

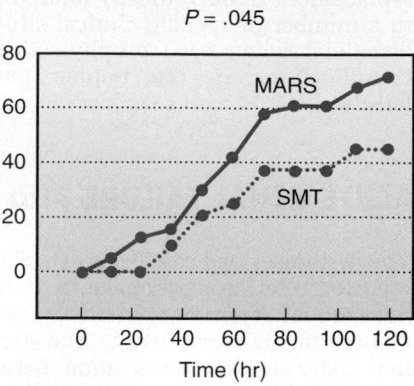

FIGURE 256-4. Mean cumulative number of improvements per person with molecular adsorbent recycling system (MARS) therapy versus standard medical therapy (SMT) by intent-to-treat analysis. *Note*: MARS is not approved by the U.S. Food and Drug Administration for use in liver failure. (From Hassanein TI, Tofteng F, Brown RS, et al: A prospective, controlled study of the clinical efficacy of extracorporeal albumin dialysis using the molecular adsorbent recirculating system [MARS] for the treatment of patients with hepatic encephalopathy. Hepatology 2007;46:1853-1862.)

systems will help establish their respective roles in the management of patients with liver failure.

Key Points

1. A worldwide epidemic of heart failure exists, and standard medical management for this problem has serious shortcomings.
2. Preservation of hemodynamic stability during ultrafiltration involves a dynamic balance between intravascular volume removal and refill.
3. Significant clinical outcome benefits for ultrafiltration in heart failure have been demonstrated in a randomized controlled trial.
4. A recent randomized controlled trial has demonstrated a significant clinical benefit (reduction in

hepatic encephalopathy) for the molecular adsorbent recycling system device in patients with acute-on-chronic liver failure.

Key References

1. American College of Cardiology/American Heart Association Task Force: Guidelines for the evaluation and management of chronic heart failure in the adult: Executive summary. Circulation 2001;104:2996-3007.
9. Marenzi G, Grazi S, Giraldi F, et al: Interrelation of humoral factors, hemodynamics, and fluid and salt metabolism in congestive heart failure: Effect of extracorporeal ultrafiltration. Am J Med 1993;94:49-56.
23. Sen S, Williams R: New liver support devices in acute liver failure: A critical evaluation. Semin Liver Dis 2003;23:283-294.

See the companion Expert Consult website for the complete reference list.

CHAPTER 257

Continuous Renal Replacement Therapy in Trauma

Deborah M. Stein and Maureen McCunn

OBJECTIVES

This chapter will:

1. Identify the causes of and risk factors for acute renal failure in the injured patient.
2. Describe the main benefits of continuous renal replacement therapy over intermittent hemodialysis in the setting of trauma.
3. List indications for continuous renal replacement therapy in trauma.
4. Review the special considerations with use of continuous renal replacement therapy in the trauma patient.
5. Outline potential uses of continuous renal replacement therapy in the injured patient at risk for renal dysfunction.

Trauma is a leading cause of death and disability worldwide. Early deaths following injury are most commonly the result of hemorrhage and traumatic brain injury (TBI); however, late deaths often are the result of sepsis and multiple organ dysfunction syndrome (MODS). Acute renal failure (ARF) is a common sequela of severe injury and can occur early or late after traumatic injury. Many of the underlying causes of ARF after trauma are relatively unique to the injured patient; some are the result of the common pathway of sepsis and MODS. The primary focus of intensive care after injury is to prevent the organ system dysfunction, but when organ systems fail, specific therapies are instituted. In the event of ARF, renal replacement therapy often is used. In clinical scenarios involving hemodynamic instability, concomitant TBI, or risk of ongoing hemorrhage, continuous renal replacement therapy (CRRT) often is the preferred modality of renal replacement in the critically injured patient. Additionally, in a number of specific clinical situations, CRRT may be beneficial when used prophylactically to prevent renal complications in the trauma patient without renal failure.

ACUTE RENAL FAILURE AND TRAUMA

The first-described case of "crush syndrome" and ARF was reported after an earthquake in 1909 in Messina, Sicily.[1] Subsequent reports appeared in the German medical literature during World War I.[2] Bywaters and Beall identified the first causative association between rhabdomyolysis and ARF after observing victims of the bombing of London during the Battle of Britain in 1940.[3] Since that time, renal failure secondary to traumatic injury has been repeatedly described throughout military conflicts and in civilian trauma situations.[4-7]

During World War II, the incidence of post-traumatic renal failure was approximately 42%, with a mortality rate of 96%.[8] After the introduction of dialysis for renal failure during the Korean War, the mortality rate decreased to 53%, and reports of civilian trauma in the 1950s and 1960s indicated that the mortality rate for ARF was approximately 60%.[9,10] During the Vietnam War, however, the mortality rate for ARF appears to have increased to 77%. This increase was attributed to delayed onset of sepsis in survivors of field combat.[11] The overall incidence of ARF requiring some form of renal replacement in modern-day trauma care systems ranges from less than 0.1% to 3.7% of injured patients.[5] In injured patients admitted to an intensive care unit (ICU), the rate has been reported to be as high as 31%.[7] Mortality in patients with post-injury renal failure remains high, however, with reported mortality rates in excess of 50%.[5,12,13] Death in patients with post-injury ARF may be related more directly to underlying injury and disease states and the etiology of the renal failure than to the presence of the renal failure itself.[14,15]

ETIOLOGY

Any of a number of disorders and conditions may be the cause of renal failure and renal insufficiency in the injured patient. Some of these are common in critically ill patients in general, and some are more unique to trauma patients. Typically, the etiology of renal dysfunction is multifactorial in patients who have sustained traumatic injury. Table 257-1 lists the common causes of ARF in trauma patients.

Decreased renal perfusion is an increasingly recognized cause of ARF.[5,12] In the injured patient, ongoing hemorrhage secondary to torso injury and long bone and pelvic fractures frequently cause shock, with the potential for renal hypoperfusion as a result of hypovolemia. Almost half of the injured patients in whom ARF developed in one study had significant hypotension.[5]

Sepsis is a well-recognized late complication of trauma and a leading cause of delayed death in trauma patients. Sepsis is a frequent precedent to renal failure in the ICU after severe trauma.[16,17] An important point is that even in the setting of single-organ injury, traumatic injury itself initiates a systemic inflammatory response that may actu-

TABLE 257-1

Common Causes of Acute Renal Failure after Traumatic Injury

- Hypotension
- Hypovolemia
- MODS
- Sepsis
- Rhabdomyolysis
- Radiocontrast administration
- Abdominal compartment syndrome
- Nephrotoxic medications

MODS, multiple organ dysfunction syndrome.

ally worsen with therapeutic or iatrogenic insults such as fracture stabilization.[18,19] Accordingly, severely injured patients may be at higher risk for organ system dysfunction and ARF than that typical of other critically ill patients.[20]

Rhabdomyolysis is a well-recognized cause of renal failure.[21-26] The incidence of acute renal insufficiency in the setting of rhabdomyolysis is 17% to 33%.[27] Rhabdomyolysis results from muscle breakdown and necrosis and frequently is seen in injured patients. Breakdown of muscle may occur as the result of significant soft tissue injury, long bone fractures, compartment syndrome, crush injury, or vascular injury with resultant ischemia-reperfusion. Typically, serum creatine kinase (CK) is measured in at-risk trauma patients and trended over time. The level of CK that is associated with an increased risk of renal failure is unclear, ranging between 500 IU/L and 75,000 IU/L in different studies.[28-32] The incidence of ARF clearly increases at higher serum CK levels. Serum myoglobin may be a more specific marker, and levels of this protein can similarly be measured and tracked over time.

Other toxic agents contribute significantly to acute renal insufficiency and ARF in injured patients. Severely injured patients are often subjected to administration of large and repeated doses of intravenous radiocontrast material during diagnostic or therapeutic studies. This intravenous radiocontrast material is well known to be nephrotoxic and can cause renal failure, particularly in the setting of hypoperfusion or hypovolemia, both of which are common in trauma patients.[33] Additionally, medications frequently used in brain-injured patients to treat elevated intracranial pressure, such as mannitol and propofol, have been reported to cause renal failure as well when excessive doses are used.[34-37] Intra-abdominal hypertension is a well-recognized complication of trauma and may be primary, as a result of intra-abdominal injury, or secondary, caused by ongoing resuscitation.[38] Elevated intra-abdominal pressure can lead to the clinical syndrome of abdominal compartment syndrome, with a constellation of clinical findings including renal insufficiency due to decreased renal perfusion. Other causative agents and presentations that may be associated with the development of renal failure in injured patients include high-dose vasoconstrictor agents, aminoglycosides, severe burns, spinal cord injury, severe beatings, torture, and recently, exercise in men taking performance-enhancing compounds that include creatine, amino acids, and ephedrine.[12,39-45]

Although not specifically causative of renal failure, risk factors for the development of renal dysfunction are seen in critically injured patients as well. The need for mechan-

TABLE 257-2

Risk Factors for the Development of Acute Renal Failure after Traumatic Injury

Shock on admission
Advanced age
Injury severity score (ISS) >17
Presence of hemoperitoneum
Presence of fractures
Serum creatine kinase >10,000 IU/L
Need for mechanical ventilation
Glasgow Coma Scale (GCS) score <10
Body mass index (BMI) >30 kg/m²
Male gender

TABLE 257-3

Advantages of Continuous Renal Replacement Therapy in Trauma

- Tolerance with hemodynamic instability
- Continuous removal of volume
- Prevention of hypovolemia
- Intracranial pressure stability
- Efficient urea clearance
- Clearance of myoglobin
- Route for provision of full nutritional support

ical ventilation in the treatment of acute lung injury (ALI) also has been found to increase the risk of renal failure in critically injured patients. This effect may be due to the fact that the high mean airway pressure needed to maintain adequate gas exchange reduces renal perfusion.[46] Other identified risk factors for renal failure after injury have been identified and include advanced age, injury severity score (ISS) greater than 17, presence of hemoperitoneum, presence of shock on admission, presence of fractures, CK level greater than 10,000 IU/L, Glasgow Coma Scale (GCS) score less than 10, body mass index (BMI) greater than 30 kg/m², and male gender.[7,47] Table 257-2 outlines the risk factors that have been found to be associated with the development of renal failure in injured patients.

POTENTIAL BENEFITS OF CONTINUOUS RENAL REPLACEMENT THERAPY IN TRAUMA PATIENTS

The use of continuous renal replacement modalities for patients who have sustained traumatic injuries is becoming more common, and this therapy has had a measurable impact on long-term recovery of renal function and mortality.[15] CRRT brings a number of theoretical—but unproven—advantages to the treatment of renal failure in trauma patients (Table 257-3). In the setting of hemodynamic instability, a common occurrence in trauma patients, CRRT is better tolerated than are intermittent forms of renal replacement.[48] CRRT allows for large-volume blood product administration without fluid overload, because the additional volume can be readily and continuously removed. Volume depletion and dehydration are avoided with CRRT,[49] and certain discrete disadvantages of inter-

mittent hemodialysis can be sidestepped in patients at risk for the development of elevated intracranial pressure.[50]

Despite the theoretical advantages of CRRT in treating ARF in critically ill patients, no studies have prospectively examined the use of CRRT exclusively in injured patients in the setting of ARF. Results from studies looking at mixed populations of critically ill patients with ARF have been conflicting. Although retrospective studies have mostly demonstrated benefit of CRRT, prospective studies have failed to show consistent advantage.[48] One prospective controlled study showed no improvement in patient survival with CRRT compared with intermittent hemodialysis, although the patients randomized to the CRRT arm of the investigation were more critically ill than those in the intermittent hemodialysis arm.[51] Similarly, a retrospective study by Swartz and coworkers compared continuous venovenous hemofiltration (CVVH) with intermittent hemodialysis for management of patients in the ICU and concluded that mortality was attributable more specifically to the patient's clinical status than to the modality of renal replacement itself.[52] Work by Kierdorf and Sieberth, on the other hand, demonstrated a survival advantage with CRRT over intermittent hemodialysis.[53] A meta-analysis of hemodialysis compared with CRRT in ARF has not yet shown an advantage for either mode of therapy.[54] The only study done looking at therapeutic CRRT in trauma patients was a retrospective review of early versus late use of CRRT in injured patients with ARF. This study, performed at the R Adams Cowley Shock Trauma Center in Baltimore, Maryland, indicated that earlier initiation of CRRT was beneficial in terms of survival and of recovery of native renal function.[15]

In the setting of ARF secondary to rhabdomyolysis, some clear advantages of CRRT over intermittent hemodialysis are recognized. In injured patients, rhabdomyolysis is the causative agent of ARF in 28% of cases.[5] The size of the myoglobin molecule (17,000 D) may be greater than the sieving limit of standard hemodialysis membranes. This size is well below the limit of hemofilters and is therefore amenable to removal by continuous hemofiltration.[55,56] The sieving coefficient of myoglobin is reported to be between 0.2 and 0.6, so myoglobin can be readily cleared by means of convection.[57,58] A second advantage of using CRRT in rhabdomyolysis is in the ability to control metabolic complications, such as hyperkalemia, metabolic acidosis, and severe hypocalcemia.[59]

SPECIAL CONSIDERATIONS IN THE TRAUMA PATIENT

Nutritional Considerations

Trauma leads to a profoundly hypercatabolic state.[60] In severely injured trauma patients, caloric requirements may be as high as 30 kcal/kg per day during the acute phase of the clinical course.[61] Additionally, daily protein requirements may exceed 2 g in such patients.[61] This combination of hypercatabolism and the need for large amounts of protein alimentation generates large urea nitrogen loads. In the setting of renal insufficiency or failure, the initial response may be to restrict protein intake to decrease this urea burden. In the critically injured patient, however, this strategy fails to provide the necessary nutritional requirements for wound healing and prevention of infection and results in a negative nitrogen balance.[62] CRRT has been demonstrated to provide uremic control superior to that possible with intermittent hemodialysis and allows for high-protein alimentation, resulting in improved nitrogen balance.[63-65] At the R Adams Cowley Shock Trauma Center, a study was conducted to compare urea nitrogen removal by continuous hemodiafiltration versus functional native kidneys in critically ill, septic patients with a protein intake of more than 2 g/kg daily.[66] The investigators concluded that urea nitrogen removal during CRRT is a function of effluent volume and can therefore be readily adjusted as needed. This finding led to the recommendation that amino acid intake need not be restricted in ill and injured patients with ARF. Additionally, studies have demonstrated improved survival in patients with ARF who are given full nutritional support.[67] The use of CRRT in the setting of renal dysfunction allows for the delivery of full protein and caloric support without restriction for critically ill patients after traumatic injury.

Anticoagulation

Trauma patients are unique in that they are almost uniformly at risk for hemorrhage. Forty percent of trauma deaths are related to failure of hemorrhage control, and coagulopathy is the leading cause of death from perioperative bleeding in injured patients.[68,69] Patients with TBI and spinal cord injury are at significantly increased risk of morbidity in the setting of ongoing hemorrhage and coagulopathy. In these patients, anticoagulation is specifically contraindicated. Anticoagulation also may be contraindicated in patients with significant fractures and visceral injury. Some patients, however, will require renal replacement therapy despite being at risk for bleeding.

CRRT typically requires some form of anticoagulation. Heparin most typically is applied but may be contraindicated in many trauma patients. Therefore, regional anticoagulation with trisodium citrate often is used.[70-72] Studies have demonstrated benefit compared with standard unfractionated heparin in terms of hemofilter life.[73] Use of trisodium citrate usually is a suitable alternative in patients in whom anticoagulation with heparin is contraindicated and does not carry the risk of heparin-induced thrombocytopenia. Trisodium citrate is administered in the prefilter portion of the circuit to bind calcium in the hemofiltration system. Administration of citrate to produce a post-filter hemofilter ionic calcium of 0.25 to 0.35 mmol/L is thought to be sufficient to inhibit coagulation in the circuit.[74,75] Owing to the potential for binding with calcium, care should be taken not to infuse a substitution fluid or dialysate with calcium.

Owing to the high content of trisodium citrate in these alternative anticoagulation regimens, hypocalcemia, hypernatremia, and metabolic alkalosis often are seen. Simultaneous with trisodium citrate administration, calcium chloride infusions should be initiated and titrated to a normal serum ionized calcium level. Metabolic alkalosis and hypernatremia is caused by the release of sodium and bicarbonate ions when the citrate is metabolized by the liver.[76] Hypernatremia may be offset by the use of a hyponatremic dialysis or replacement solution. Although an elevated sodium level may be advantageous in some trauma patients, such as patients with TBI, the compensatory CO_2 retention that occurs in response to the metabolic alkalosis may be deleterious. Individualization of management to each patient is therefore necessary.

Traumatic Brain Injury

Approximately one third of the 150,000 deaths following traumatic injury in the United States each year are due to TBI. Although 1 million patients with TBI survive each year, nearly 25% require extended inpatient care. The most severely brain-injured have the longest mean length of stay and highest mean hospital costs of all injured patients. Regardless of initial severity of injury, patients with TBI are at high risk for incurring disabilities, and patients who survive after their injury are more impaired than other trauma cohorts.[77] Most therapies for the treatment of TBI are aimed at attenuating or eliminating the secondary insults that occur in the injured brain. Edema, ischemia, and inflammation all compound the primary insult, leading to increased morbidity and mortality. It is therefore imperative to prevent secondary brain injury by eliminating risks that may lead to further damage, such as ongoing or recurrent intracranial hemorrhage. In addition, a single episode of hypotension is associated with an increase in morbidity and a doubling of mortality after severe TBI.[78] When renal failure occurs and renal replacement therapy is required, intermittent hemodialysis may be contraindicated in the setting of TBI because of the potential for episodes of hypotension during therapy.

Some evidence suggests that standard intermittent hemodialysis in patients with acute and chronic renal failure results in an increase in brain water content, which may be detrimental to patients with TBI.[79,80] When patients with cerebral edema or after acute brain injury are subjected to traditional hemodialysis, intracranial pressure has been shown to increase significantly during treatment.[81,82] CRRT results in greater intracranial stability than is obtained with standard intermittent hemodialysis or filtration.[80,83] Although studies comparing continuous and intermittent modalities have yet to show a treatment advantage in this patient population, CRRT may be the modality of choice for patients with brain injury who require renal support.[50,84]

POTENTIAL "INDICATIONS" FOR CONTINUOUS RENAL REPLACEMENT THERAPY IN TRAUMA

A number of clinical situations that arise in the injured patient with normal renal function may be amenable to management with CRRT. Although these applications are largely unstudied and therefore cannot be unconditionally recommended, they represent extended uses of this therapy and should be subjects of future clinical trials.

Clearance of Myoglobin

Muscle breakdown is extremely common in the injured patient. As discussed earlier, acute renal insufficiency may occur in one third of patients with rhabdomyolysis.[27] It is difficult to predict, however, which patients will develop renal dysfunction and which patients will be able to clear myoglobin using conventional means alone. The pathophysiological basis for the development of renal dysfunction in the setting of rhabdomyolysis is thought to have three components: decrease in renal perfusion, tubular obstruction from cast formation, and direct toxic effect of myoglobin of the kidney.[85] Typically, treatment of rhabdomyolysis is accomplished with early and aggressive hydration with isotonic fluids. Additional therapies include mannitol diuresis and alkalinization of the urine.[85,86] Some of these therapies may be detrimental in some patients and may not be well tolerated. In patients with volume overload, aggressive fluid administration may precipitate respiratory insufficiency, whereas in patients with TBI, alkalinization of urine may lead to CO_2 retention and worsening of intracranial pressure. In injured patients, other concomitant nephrotoxic agents may be administered that may increase the risks of renal insufficiency. Because CRRT is an effective way of rapidly and predictably clearing myoglobin,[55-57] its use in patients with rhabdomyolysis before the onset of renal dysfunction should be investigated.

Prevention of Intravenous Radiocontrast Agent–Induced Nephropathy

Intravenous radiocontrast is well known to be nephrotoxic. In volume-depleted injured patients, administration of intravenous radiocontrast material can precipitate renal failure.[33] Injured patients often are subjected to administration of multiple doses of contrast material for repeated CT scans and angiography and interventions with angiographic embolization. Conventional therapy aimed at the prevention of radiocontrast agent–induced renal dysfunction includes hydration with isotonic fluids, administration of bicarbonate solutions, and use of N-acetylcysteine.[33,87-89]

In a recent prospective randomized trial of nondialyzed patients with chronic renal failure undergoing coronary angiography, the periprocedural prophylactic use of CVVH was associated with a significant decrease in the percentage of patients with a greater than 25% increase in serum creatinine over baseline, in the need for renal replacement therapy, and in both in-hospital and 30-day mortality rates.[90] Although this study was conducted in a group of patients at high risk for worsening renal function, these conclusions may be extrapolated to other patient populations as well. Certainly, a number of injured patients will have baseline renal dysfunction even before their injury; in still other patients, renal insufficiency will develop during the clinical course. Both of these groups of patients may benefit from this prophylactic use of CRRT before additional intravenous radiocontrast administration. Clearly, this is an area worthy of additional study.

Inflammatory Mediator Clearance

Because trauma patients are at significant risk for ARF as a result of activation of the inflammatory cascade at the time of injury and then repeated activation of cytokines with additional interventions,[18,19] it could logically be speculated that instituting a therapy to remove inflammatory mediators may decrease the incidence of ARF or organ failure.[91] A number of cytokines and inflammatory mediators have been found to be elevated in injured patients, most prominently, IL-1α, IL-6, IL-8, and TNF-α.[92,93]

Studies that have examined the use of CRRT for cytokine removal have yielded mixed results. One study of 30 patients with trauma and multiple organ dysfunction found that despite removal of substantial amounts of cytokines with CVVH, serum concentrations remained similar in these patients and in control subjects.[94] Another study of postsurgical and injured patients demonstrated a decrease in IL-6 and IL-8 levels with CVVH that correlated with clinical improvement.[95] A prospective study of prophylactic use of CVVH in injured patients demonstrated a blunted cardiovascular response and increased oxygen extraction but noted a potentially significant risk of thrombocytopenia in the CVVH group.[96] A study conducted in burned septic patients demonstrated effective clearance of cytokines in the CVVH treatment group as measured by decreased serum levels when compared with the control group.[97] To better clarify the role of prophylactic CRRT for cytokine clearance in injured patients, significant additional investigation is warranted.

SPECIFIC CLINICAL EXPERIENCE WITH USE OF CONTINUOUS RENAL REPLACEMENT THERAPY

Our institution, the R Adams Cowley Shock Trauma Center in Baltimore, Maryland, admits more than 7000 trauma patients each year. A CRRT program was first established in the early 1980s, with the CRRT administered by the intensivists and intensive care nurses in the Multi-trauma and Neuro-trauma Intensive Care Units. Initially, the program was limited to continuous arteriovenous ultrafiltration (CAVH). The implementation of continuous venovenous hemodialysis (CVVHD) and continuous venovenous hemodiafiltration (CVVHDF) occurred from 1987 through the early 2000s. The primary aim of the intensivist-run CRRT program was to improve the timeliness of service and to guarantee continuous observation while decreasing mortality. The secondary aim of the CRRT program was threefold: to provide constant electrolyte control, to ease the management of volume status with less hemodynamic impact, and to improve the ability to administer unlimited fluids, blood products, and nutritional support, all vitally important in injured patients. The mortality rate among patients requiring CRRT at the Shock Trauma Center decreased 13.5% (from 67.4% to 58.3%) in the year after the institution of a multidisciplinary process improvement program.[98] Utilization and mortality data gathered for the fiscal year before implementation of the program and at the end of the first year thereafter demonstrated a 26% reduction in total CRRT patient-days, with a 31% reduction in average CRRT days per patient. No change in the annual number of patients receiving treatment was noted in this time period.

Despite the fact that studies are lacking that demonstrate a survival advantage or improvement in renal recovery with the use of CRRT in trauma patients, at our institution, CRRT is used routinely in all critically ill patients with renal failure and frequently in those patients considered to be at risk for renal failure. CVVH typically is used, but CVVHD also is used, depending on clinical indications. We also use CVVHDF as indicated. Typical blood flow rates range from 150 to 300 mL/minute, depending on the patient's hemodynamics and desired ultrafiltration rates. Substitution flow generally is targeted toward a minimum of 35 mL/kg per hour, because these rates have been shown to improve survival in the setting of ARF and sepsis.[99] Ultrafiltration rate is varied in accordance with the fluid balance desired. Trisodium citrate typically is selected as an anticoagulant, in view of the large percentage of patients who experience specific contraindications to systemic

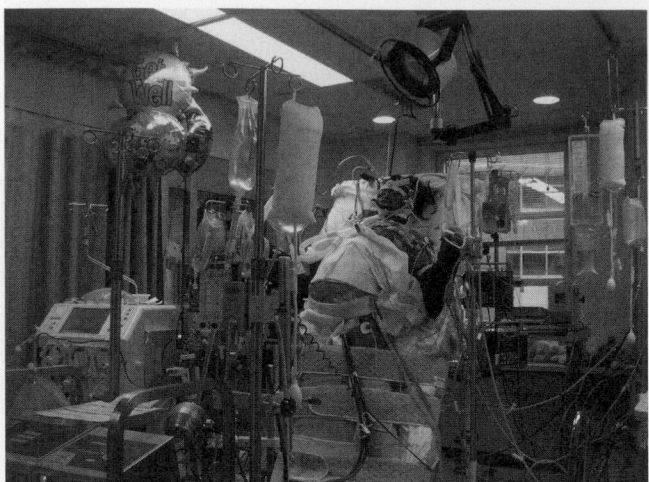

FIGURE 257-1. This patient at the R Adams Cowley Shock Trauma Center in Baltimore was a 16-year-old girl who sustained severe multisystem injuries after being struck by a motor vehicle while she was walking home from school. She suffered a severe traumatic brain injury and was in renal and respiratory failure. She has already undergone a decompressive laparotomy for abdominal compartment syndrome and has been placed on venovenous bypass and continuous venovenous hemodiafiltration. She is secured on a tilt table in an effort to maintain a low intracranial pressure, while positional respiratory support is being provided.

anticoagulation with heparin. Should the patient not recover renal function, the nephrology service is consulted for conversion to intermittent hemodialysis once the patient's clinical status permits. Figure 257-1 shows a patient from the center who was on CRRT and venovenous bypass after severe multisystem trauma.

CONCLUSION

Trauma is a common cause of morbidity and mortality. Late deaths typically are the result of MODS and sepsis developing after severe injury. ARF is a common cause of morbidity secondary to trauma. A number of clinical situations subject the injured patient to the risk of renal dysfunction. Hypovolemia, hemorrhage, and hypotension are common and may lead to ARF. Other causes of renal insufficiency subsequent to trauma include sepsis, rhabdomyolysis, and administration of nephrotoxic substances. The use of CRRT in injured patients with renal failure is becoming more commonplace owing to a number of discrete advantages over intermittent hemodialysis. These include tolerance of therapy in the setting of hemodynamic insta-

bility and the ease and efficient removal of volume and solutes. Continuous renal replacement is preferred in patients at risk for increased intracranial pressure due to TBI and allows for clearance of myoglobin. Additionally, CRRT allows for full calorie and protein administration, which is vitally important for healing after severe injury. In injured patients at risk for renal dysfunction, a role for "prophylactic" CRRT has been suggested. Some of these as-yet-unproven "indications" are in patients at risk for rhabdomyolysis and in those who receive large and repeated doses of intravenous contrast material for imaging studies. Additionally, the role of CVVH for removal of inflammatory mediators in the setting of severe injury is another potentially important use of CRRT after trauma. These areas warrant further investigation.

Key Points

1. Renal dysfunction is a common problem in patients with traumatic injury.
2. Many of the causes of and risk factors for development of acute renal failure after trauma are relatively unique to the severely injured patient.
3. Continuous renal replacement therapy has a number of discrete advantages over intermittent hemodialysis after trauma, especially in the presence of traumatic brain injury.
4. In many trauma patients, systemic anticoagulation is contraindicated, so alternative regional anticoagulation often is applied.
5. Injured patients at risk for renal dysfunction may benefit from continuous renal replacement therapy. More research is needed to elucidate the role of this modality in this setting.

Key References

5. Morris JA, Mucha P, Ross SE, et al: Acute post-traumatic renal failure: A multi-center perspective. J Trauma 1991;31:1584-1590.
84. Davenport A: Renal replacement therapy in the patient with acute brain injury. Am J Kidney Dis 2001;37:457-466.
94. Sanchez-Izquierdo JA, Perez Vela JL, Lozano Quintana MJ, et al: Cytokines clearance during venovenous hemofiltration in the trauma patient. Am J Kidney Dis 1997;30:483-488.
96. Bauer M, Marzi I, Ziegenfuss T, Riegel W: Prophylactic hemofiltration in severely traumatized patients: Effects on post-traumatic organ dysfunction syndrome. Intensive Care Med 2001;27:376-383.
98. McCunn M, McCourt T, McQuillan K, et al: Implementation of a multi-disciplinary continuous renal replacement therapy service: Process and progress. Crit Care Med 2002;30:A151.

See the companion Expert Consult website for the complete reference list.

Clinical Effects of Continuous Renal Replacement Therapies

Zaccaria Ricci and Claudio Ronco

OBJECTIVES

This chapter will:
1. Describe different renal replacement strategies and their clinical effects on critically ill patients.
2. Review the benefits and side effects of continuous renal replacement therapies.
3. Compare the clinical effects of continuous therapies with those of intermittent and hybrid techniques.

Different renal replacement therapy (RRT) modalities and the specific protocols as prescribed will result in various clinical effects in individual critically ill patients. These effects can be acknowledged either as desirable clinical outcomes of the dialytic treatment or as undesirable side effects that should be avoided. With extracorporeal RRT, an obvious antagonism between (s)low-efficiency continuous therapies and high-efficiency intermittent treatments has been growing since Kramer and colleagues first introduced the idea of continuous hemofiltration some 20 years ago.[1] As explored later in the chapter, consideration of the entire spectrum of possible applications may potentially lead to optimal treatment for all patients by means of hybrid techniques.

The kidneys remove water, various solutes, and nonvolatile acids, thereby maintaining homeostasis; they also metabolize inflammatory mediators and excrete administered drugs or their metabolites. The first point to be addressed, then, in examining clinical effects of RRT and their impact on the altered homeostasis of critically ill patients is to evaluate whether the optimal treatment should closely mimic the functions of the kidneys or if renal support can be safely managed on an intermittent basis, as with other therapies such as antibiotics or antiarrhythmics.

FLUID REMOVAL

Continuous RRT (CRRT) slowly and continuously removes fluid, approximating ongoing urinary output, whereas intermittent hemodialysis must extract up to 2 days' worth of administered fluid plus excess body water, which may be present in the anuric patient as a result of a pathological process, in one relatively brief session. The intravascular volume depletion associated with intermittent hemodialysis is due to both the high rate of fluid removal required and the transcellular and interstitial fluid shifts caused by the rapid dialytic loss of solute.[2] The major consequence of rapid fluid removal is hemodynamic instability. Critically ill patients need continuous volume infusions: blood and fresh frozen plasma, vasopressors and other continuous infusions, and parenteral and enteral nutrition, which must be delivered without restriction or interruption even in hypercatabolic patients. In the clinical setting of anuria, providing such infusions carries a constant risk for fluid overload and high daily ultrafiltration requirements. Examples of patients in whom sudden intravascular volume shifts may be catastrophic are the patient with acute respiratory distress syndrome (ARDS), the septic patient who is becoming refractory to vasopressors, and the patient with cerebral edema. Furthermore, all critically ill patients tolerate hypotension poorly, with a definite risk of cardiac arrest, particularly if they are already inotrope dependent. Indeed, the damaged kidneys, which have temporarily lost pressure-flow autoregulation, also may be threatened with fresh ischemic lesions occurring with each hemodialysis session,[3] leading to a delay in renal recovery.

Of interest, recent reports have suggested a benefit for CRRT with respect to recovery of renal function.[4-6] First, chronic renal insufficiency at either death or hospital discharge was diagnosed in 17% of patients whose initial therapy was conventional hemodialysis, versus only 4% of patients whose initial therapy was CRRT ($P = .01$). Second, for patients receiving a minimum exposure of 25 hours of CRRT and two treatments of 3 hours or more each of conventional hemodialysis, 92% of the patients undergoing CRRT had complete recovery of renal function, versus 59% of those receiving conventional hemodialysis ($P < .01$). Finally, a significantly higher percentage of patients crossing over from conventional hemodialysis to CRRT had complete recovery of renal function compared with those crossing over in the opposite direction (45% versus 7%; $P < .01$).

The importance of fluid balance management is enhanced in the specific category of patients with decompensated heart failure. In fact, it is just these patients who may well respond positively to continuous ultrafiltration with a rise in cardiac index, while avoiding a fall in arterial pressure, owing to a beneficial change in preload optimizing myocardial contractility on the Starling curve.[2] In many instances, congestive heart failure not responding to conventional therapy can now be successfully treated in this way.[7]

In critically ill children, the correction of water overload is considered a priority: It has been shown that restoring adequate water content in small children is the main independent variable for outcome prediction.[8,9] This concept is much more important in critically ill neonates, in whom a relatively larger volume of fluid must be administered to deliver an adequate amount of drug infusion, parenteral or enteral nutrition, and blood derivatives.

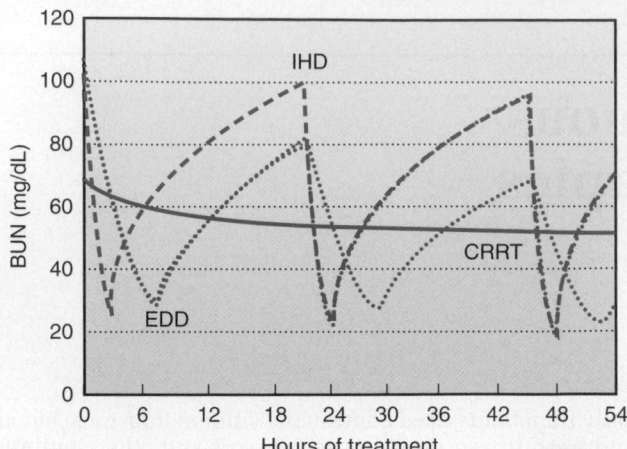

FIGURE 258-1. Example of changes in mean blood urea nitrogen (BUN) concentration during continuous renal replacement therapy (CRRT), intermittent hemodialysis (IHD), and extended daily dialysis (EDD) during 2 days of therapy.

SOLUTE REMOVAL, ACID-BASE CONTROL, AND ELECTROLYTE BALANCE

An attribute of intermittent hemodialysis often quoted by proponents is that it is highly efficient at clearing solutes such as urea. In fact, this is both a false argument and a disadvantage. The primary rationale for using continuous therapy is to maintain a more physiological, constant removal of fluid and solute, among other things. In the process, the cumulative clearance of urea and creatinine by a continuous method is significantly superior to that achieved by intermittent hemodialysis applied up to 4 times per week, even in septic patients. Indeed, intermittent hemodialysis sessions 6 times per week would be required to achieve the same uremic control[10] (Fig. 258-1).

The details of the physiological impact of better control have not been fully elucidated. Nevertheless, several facts have been established in patients with end-stage renal failure. In the National Cooperative Dialysis Study, rates for indices of morbidity, including cardiovascular events and hospitalization rate, were higher in the group of patients whose target average urea was 100 mg/dL (36 mmol/L) than in the patients whose target urea was 50 mg/dL (18 mmol/L).[11] An effect of uremia relevant to intensive care is immunosuppression, with impaired phagocytosis and defective lymphocyte and monocyte function. Uncertainty regarding the relative contributions of uremia, malnutrition, and bio-incompatible membranes is evident from previous studies.[12] Work needs to be done specifically in patients with ARF. A landmark study by Ronco and coworkers is at the moment the only randomized trial that showed how a high (adequate) dialytic dose (metabolic control) improved survival: In this study, continuous venovenous post-dilution hemofiltration at either 35 mL/kg per hour or 45 mL/kg per hour was associated with improved survival when compared with a hemofiltration rate of 20 mL/kg per hour in 425 critically ill patients with ARF.[13]

Nonvolatile acids, normally excreted by the glomerulus and renal tubules, cross hemofilters by diffusion and con-

vection. Once again, the main concern with intermittent hemodialysis is the physiological effects of rapid clearance, particularly in critically ill, catabolic patients with accelerated acid production. Acid accumulation may interfere with normal myocardial electrical conduction and contractility. Rapid delivery of bicarbonate during dialysis may exacerbate intracellular acidosis, although this point is still controversial. Bicarbonate is the standard buffer used with intermittent hemodialysis; a number of buffers have been used with CRRT—most commonly, lactate. Acetate, of course, should not be used because of its vasodilating, hypoxia-inducing, and cytokine- and complement-activating properties.[14,15] Some clinicians use citrate for its additional anticoagulant effects. No clinical difference has been observed in the relative merits of lactate versus bicarbonate buffering, apart from the need to avoid lactate buffering in patients with fulminant hepatic failure.[16,17] The essential point is that both can be delivered with continuous therapy.

One specific comment is in order regarding the difference between continuous venovenous hemofiltration (CVVH) and all other techniques, including dialysis and the use of diuretics. In all pharmacological and dialytic techniques, the removal of sodium and water cannot be dissociated, and the mechanisms are strictly correlated. In particular, the diuretic effect is based on a remarkable natriuresis, whereas ultrafiltration during dialysis may result in hypo- or hypertonia, depending on the interference with diffusion and removal of other molecules such as urea and other electrolytes. In such circumstances, water removal is linked to other solutes in proportions that are dependent on the technique used. In CVVH, the mechanism of ultrafiltration produces a fluid that is very similar to plasma water except for a minimal interference due to Donnan effects. In such a technique, ultrafiltration is basically iso-osmotic and isonatriemic, and water and sodium removal cannot be dissociated, with sodium elimination linked to the sodium plasma water concentration. In CVVH and hemofiltration in general, the ultrafiltrate composition is definitely similar to plasma water, but the sodium balance can be significantly affected by the sodium concentration in the replacement solution. Sodium removal can be dissociated from water removal in CVVH, thereby allowing definitive manipulation of the sodium pool in the body. This effect cannot be achieved with any other technique. The advantage is that not only plasma concentrations but also the electrolyte content in the extracellular and possibly intracellular volume can be normalized.[18]

One of the most active areas of research in intensive care in recent years involves the modulation of the septic response with the aim of reducing the persistently high mortality in this group of patients. One avenue has been to investigate the potential benefit of CRRT in the sepsis syndrome. Although skepticism counters the idea that any improvement is due to nonspecific changes such as fluid removal or lowering the core temperature in febrile patients, some evidence suggests that cytokines and complement, among other mediators, are cleared from the blood by convection or adsorption, or both, onto high-flux synthetic hemofilter membranes. Whether this removal translates to significant reversal of end-organ damage by inflammatory mediators and results in a reproducible reduction in mortality or morbidity is still being elucidated. There is little doubt, however, that use of biocompatible membranes is important, and that mediator removal, to be beneficial, needs to be continuous and convective, not intermittent and diffusive.[19]

SIDE EFFECTS OF CONTINUOUS RENAL REPLACEMENT THERAPY

Although considerable attention has focused on the perceived benefits of CRRT, less emphasis has been placed on the possibility that this modality may carry increased risk. As a continuous extracorporeal therapy, CRRT often requires continuous anticoagulation, which can increase bleeding risk. Conversely, clotting of the extracorporeal circuit also occurs frequently with CRRT, which may potentially contribute to blood loss, thereby exacerbating anemia in critically ill patients. The increased solute transfer associated with the use of CRRT may enhance removal of amino acids, vitamins, catecholamines, and other solutes with a beneficial function in critically ill patients.

Continuous therapies must be continuous to work: How many treatments really last more than 18 to 20 hours per day? Downtime due to filter-circuit-catheter clotting, circuit change, frequent replacement or substitution of solution bags, and patient mobility (surgery, diagnostics) should be carefully monitored; any of these factors may have significant impact on dialysis dose.[20] Also of concern are recent reports that technical problems with the delivery of CRRT, including machine malfunction, medication errors, and compounding errors, may contribute to increased patient morbidity and mortality. Detection of safety problems and adverse events is particularly difficult when the rates of expected morbidity and mortality are already high in the population undergoing a procedure, as is the case with CRRT in critically ill patients with AKI.

Currently, few available studies in the nephrology literature provide substantive information on the safety or adverse effects of CRRT or intermittent hemodialysis in the critically ill population. After the introduction of new technology and devices into medical practice, a natural tendency is to assume that the novel therapeutic approach is providing benefit. This is especially the case when a therapy is applied to a critically ill patient 24 hours a day and becomes part of the typical equipment of an ICU bed. The level of attention from ICU caregivers probably is superior when a dedicated dialysis nurse administers conventional hemodialysis for few hours during a day shift. Nonetheless, a new generation of dedicated CRRT machines has been recently released with strict safety features and the possibility of a broad range of prescriptions. In any case, the ideal therapy still does not exist, and specific ICU staff training is mandatory before the routine use of such modern monitors: There will never be a solution to the unwise use of a perfect system.[21]

TRIALS ON THE FINAL CLINICAL EFFECT: MORTALITY

Four recently published randomized clinical trials and one multicenter observational study have claimed that outcomes with CRRT are superior to those with intermittent hemodialysis.[22-26] None of these studies showed a superior outcome for CRRT compared with intermittent hemodialysis. The results often are surprising, and in some cases, the studies can be strongly criticized for methodology and group randomization.[27] Nevertheless, they certainly do not support the belief that CRRT provides better outcomes than those obtained with intermittent hemodialysis.

Of interest, a common key point that can be derived from these recent trials is that intermittent hemodialysis has become safer and more efficacious with contemporary dialytic techniques. Furthermore, liberal and extended use of CRRT may be less safe or efficacious than was previously considered or expected. The presumed ability of CRRT to provide more hemodynamic stability, more effective volume homeostasis, and better blood pressure support than intermittent hemodialysis has been the basis for the assumption that CRRT is a superior therapy. Over the past 2 decades, however, technical advances in the delivery of conventional hemodialysis have dramatically decreased the propensity of intermittent hemodialysis to cause intradialytic hypotension. These advances include the introduction of volume-controlled dialysis machines, the routine use of biocompatible synthetic dialysis membranes, the use of bicarbonate-based dialysate, and the delivery of higher doses of dialysis.

In an important study, Schortgen demonstrated a lower rate of hemodynamic instability and better outcomes after implementation of a clinical practice algorithm designed to improve hemodynamic tolerance to intermittent hemodialysis.[28] Recommendations included priming the dialysis circuit with isotonic saline, setting dialysate sodium concentration at above 145 mmol/L, discontinuing vasodilator therapy, and setting dialysate temperature to below 37° C. Thus, the original rationale for the widely held assumption that CRRT is a superior therapy may have dissipated over time. Analysis of the results of recently published observational studies and randomized trials reveals no convincing evidence to support superiority of CRRT over intermittent hemodialysis in the management of most critically ill patients with AKI.[29]

A POTENTIAL COMPROMISE: HYBRID TECHNIQUES

Hybrid techniques have been given a variety of names, such as slow-efficiency daily dialysis (SLEDD), prolonged intermittent daily RRT, extended daily dialysis (EDD), or simply extended dialysis,[30-33] depending on variations in schedule and type of solute removal (convective or diffusive). Theoretically, the purpose of such therapies would be consolidation of the advantages offered by either CRRT or intermittent hemodialysis, including efficient solute removal with minimum solute dysequilibrium, reduced ultrafiltration rate with hemodynamic stability, optimized delivered-to-prescribed ratio, low anticoagulant needs, diminished cost of therapy delivery, efficiency of resource use, and improved patient mobility. Initial case series have shown the feasibility and high clearance rates that potentially are associated with such approaches. A single short-term, single-center trial comparing hybrid therapies with CRRT has shown satisfying results in terms of dose delivery and hemodynamic stability. The arrival of technology that can be used by nurses in the ICU to deliver SLEDD with convective components offers further options from a therapeutic point of view. It is now possible, using user-friendly ICU technology, to generate ultrapure replacement fluid and administer it as in CRRT but at lower cost, in greater amounts, and for shorter periods of time, or to combine such hemofiltration with diffusion, or to use pure diffusion at any chosen clearance for a period that can encompass a given nursing shift, the "9 to 5" maximum staff availability period, or the nighttime period.

A recent randomized trial comparing CVVH and EDD with filtration (EDDf) found that both techniques achieved correction of several electrolyte abnormalities present before intervention.[34] Potential risk of hypophosphatemia in patients undergoing CVVH suggests the need for vigilance and frequent serum phosphate monitoring. Of importance, in all patients, hypo- or hyperkalemia and magnesemia were avoided with the prescriptions used. Although the serum sodium was maintained within the normal range and levels were similar in both groups, significant differences in the chloride concentration were noted. The relative hyperchloremia in the EDDf patients was almost certainly due to the greater concentration of chloride in the fluids used for EDDf (111.8 mmol/L) than in the fluids used for CVVH (100.75 mmol/L). The investigators found that the two therapies affected metabolic acid-base variables differently. First, the concentration of lactate was lower with EDDf throughout the study period. This difference probably was explained by the use of lactate as buffer during CVVH, versus bicarbonate during EDDf. Second, despite the increase in lactate with CVVH, median pH, bicarbonate, and base excess values were all less acidotic with continuous treatment. These findings are consistent with both the lower amount of buffer in EDDf fluids (26 mEq/L) than in CVVH fluids (45 mEq/L) and the relative hyperchloremia of these fluids. The effect of hyperchloremia also is likely to explain the difference in mean apparent strong ion difference (SID) between the two groups. A decrease in CO_2 in response to this metabolic acidosis accounted for the lower effective SID values observed during EDDf. Conversely, the strong ion gap was similar for both treatments, in keeping with probably equivalent clearance of unmeasured acids. Although the clinical significance of these differences is uncertain, a higher bicarbonate concentration in EDDf fluids may be desirable.

CONCLUSION

Comparing intermittent and continuous therapies can be misleading. Besides the difficulty of conducting a well-designed, adequately powered, randomized trial (requiring at least 1200 patients), continuous and intermittent therapies represent a continuum in the management of AKI. Sicker patients, for example, may potentially derive greater benefit from CRRT, whereas less severely ill patients may do well with daily extended or intermittent treatments.

The choices today are almost limitless: Should the therapy be 3 or 4 hours of intermittent hemodialysis with standard settings? Or should it be CRRT at 35 mL/kg per hour effluent flow rate? Or should it be SLEDD at blood and dialysate flow rates of 150 mL/minute for 8 hours

during the day? Or should SLEDD be applied for 12 hours overnight? Or should a convective component be added to SLEDD to make it SLEDDf? Or should CRRT and SLEDD be combined for the first 2 or 3 days when the patient is in the hyperacute phase, with SLEDD alone thereafter as recovery takes place? Indeed, from the point of view of the intensivist, the modes of RRT are beginning to resemble the modes of mechanical ventilation, with ventilator settings seamlessly being changed to fit the therapeutic goals and patient needs and phases of illness. Just as stereotypical approaches to ventilation are anachronistic, often resulting in an attempt to fit the patient into an inappropriate, fixed therapy, rather than tailoring the therapy to the patient, so should RRT be adjusted to fill the needs of the individual patient and his or her illness. Also, just as the possibility of showing that one mode of ventilation is better than another is apparently a lost cause, the same seems to hold true for RRT.

To summarize how to choose the most appropriate RRT modality at the start of treatment, *the optimal RRT is the safest, the simplest, and the most efficient.* Usually, this ideal treatment is the one the clinician knows best.

Key Points

1. Different renal replacement therapy prescriptions, modalities, and schedules can be administered to critically ill patients with acute kidney injury.
2. Clinical effects in critically ill patients depend on the selected renal replacement therapy protocol and on the severity and complexity of the clinical picture.
3. Modern, versatile machines and flexible prescriptions allow the clinician to choose from among various renal replacement therapies ranging from highly intermittent high-efficiency therapies to slow continuous hemofiltration, depending on the patient's hemodynamic stability, fluid balance needs, and acid-base and electrolyte status.

Key References

6. Clark WR, Letteri JJ, Uchino S, et al: Recent clinical advances in the management of critically ill patients with acute renal failure. Blood Purif 2006;24:487-498.
7. Costanzo MR, Guglin ME, Saltzberg MT, et al for the UNLOAD Trial Investigators: Ultrafiltration versus intravenous diuretics for patients hospitalized for acute decompensated heart failure. J Am Coll Cardiol 2007;49:675-683.
18. Ronco C, Ricci Z, Bellomo R, Bedogni F: Extracorporeal ultrafiltration for the treatment of overhydration and congestive heart failure. Cardiology 2001;96:155-168.

See the companion Expert Consult website for the complete reference list.

CHAPTER 259

Immunomodulation and Biological Effects of Continuous Renal Replacement Therapy

Achim Jörres and Claudio Ronco

OBJECTIVES

This chapter will:
1. Discuss the complexity of the mediator cascades during sepsis.
2. Review the main hypotheses that attempt to provide a rationale for the use of extracorporeal blood purification techniques in sepsis.
3. Present examples of the influence of continuous renal replacement therapy on more global aspects of immunomodulation.

Despite recent advances in critical care medicine, sepsis and septic shock remain the leading causes of acute renal failure, multiple organ system dysfunction, and death in the intensive care unit. A key element in the development of sepsis is the activation of monocytes and macrophages, which respond to stimulation by bacterial products with the release of a large array of immune mediators, such as the cytokines tumor necrosis factor-α (TNF-α), interleukin (IL)-1, IL-6, and interferon-γ (IFN-γ). Upon their binding to target receptors, the activation of the different signal transduction pathways will then initiate the various downstream cascades of cell activation, leading to the excess generation of cytokines, chemokines, products of the cyclooxygenase and lipoxygenase pathways, nitric oxide, and platelet-activating factor (PAF). At the plasma level, activation of the complement cascade and coagulation pathways may further trigger and sustain cell activation. Moreover, a multitude of other compounds such as endorphins, endocannabinoids, kinins, and myocardial depressant factors are generated, all of which contribute to the pathophysiology of systemic inflammation that ultimately leads to cell damage, enhanced apoptosis, and end-organ failure.[1]

In the 1980s, a wide variety of animal models of sepsis provided evidence that the deleterious course of systemic inflammation may potentially be ameliorated or even prevented by the inhibition of a single key mediator early on in the pro-inflammatory cascade. Since then, more than 50 prospective randomized clinical trials have been undertaken that evaluated such approaches as the neutralization of endotoxin or the blockage of pro-inflammatory mediators such as TNF-α, IL-1, nitric oxide, prostaglandins, or PAF. Other attempts were targeted at enhancing host defense with interferon-γ or granulocyte colony-stimulating factor (G-CSF); ultimately, however, these approaches were found to be unsuccessful in the clinical setting of sepsis and septic shock.[2]

On account of these experiences and in view of the enormous complexity of the inflammatory response during sepsis, it seems increasingly unlikely that the modulation of a single agent or pathway will achieve a significant outcome benefit in patients with sepsis or septic shock. On the other hand, because the clinical course in patients with sepsis also includes an anti-inflammatory phase, the *compensatory anti-inflammatory response syndrome* (CARS),[3] which may not strictly follow the pro-inflammatory or *systemic inflammatory response syndrome* (SIRS) phase but rather occur in parallel, as the *mixed antagonistic response syndrome*, an intervention at the wrong time may even increase mortality.

Under physiological conditions, the biological activity of the various mediators controlling inflammatory responses is under the tight control of specific inhibitors. In the sepsis syndrome, this homeostatic balance appears to be disturbed, leading to profound changes in the relative production of pro-inflammatory and anti-inflammatory mediators that may, however, not be reflected by corresponding changes in circulating mediator levels.[4,5] Thus, a more generalized approach to correct the disturbed immunohomeostasis by eliminating both excessive anti-inflammatory and pro-inflammatory mediators could prove more beneficial in sepsis than a "magic bullet" approach.[6]

It is precisely in this area in which continuous renal replacement therapy (CRRT) may eventually prove to be of value beyond its established role as kidney replacement therapy. Although the capability of hemofiltration to effectively lower the circulating levels of specific cytokines remains controversial, numerous studies have demonstrated that standard hemofiltration systems may extract a multitude of mediators, at least to some degree.[7] Of interest, some clinical studies have reported significant clinical benefit in terms of hemodynamic improvement even in the absence of a measurable reduction in circulating cytokine levels.[8] Conversely, the ultrafiltrate of septic patients was shown to contain compounds with significant immunomodulatory qualities,[9,10] as well as substances that induced significant cardiotoxic effects in rat cardiomyocytes,[11] suggesting that the elimination of mediators during CRRT through convection or diffusion may indeed be biologically significant. Nevertheless, clinical data available to date indicate that the greater part of cytokine elimination from septic patients' blood occurs through adsorption to the hemofiltration membrane, which is, however, quickly saturated.[12]

How, then, can the clinical benefits of CRRT that were observed in a number of clinical studies be explained? Three main hypotheses have been developed to explain its mechanism of action in the setting of sepsis (Fig. 259-1).

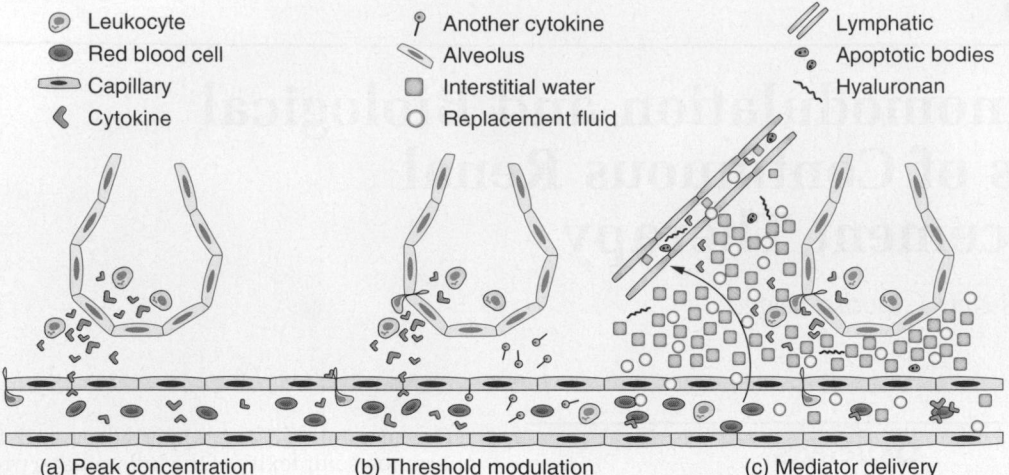

FIGURE 259-1. Theories of mediator clearance through hemofiltration. The peak concentration hypothesis (a) posits the attenuation of the inflammatory response by filtration of excess cytokine that has spilled into the central circulation. In the threshold modulation hypothesis (b), ongoing reequilibration supplies cytokine to the central circulation for removal at the hemofilter. The mediator delivery hypothesis (c) posits that interstitial and lymphatic flux is stimulated by the large-volume crystalloid replacement fluid infusion. This would result in the tissue clearance of multiple entities, including middle-molecular-weight molecules, filtered plasma proteins, extravasated blood cells, cellular byproducts and wastes, excessive ground matrix substances, apoptotic cells, and free DNA. Some of these entities would be delivered to various organs for scavenging or metabolism; some would be cleared at the hemofilter. (Redrawn from Di Carlo JV, Alexander SR: Hemofiltration for cytokine-driven illnesses: The mediator delivery hypothesis. Int J Artif Organs 2005;28:781.)

The *peak concentration hypothesis*, proposed by Ronco and coworkers,[6] suggests that an excess production of mediators that are primarily intended to exert autocrine or paracrine effects may lead to a spillover into the circulation during peak production. This spillover may then generate systemic effects such as endothelial damage, vasoparalysis, and coagulation abnormalities. In this scenario, the attenuation of the peak concentrations by CRRT may be enough to result in significant clinical improvement.[6] On the other hand, it is not clear how the attenuation of peak concentrations would affect local mediator production or mediator levels in the interstitial space. Quite clearly, a successful intervention aimed at effectively cutting off critical peak concentrations will require highly efficient removal procedures, a condition that probably is not met by "renal dose" CRRT. Consequently, extracorporeal therapies with a higher cytokine clearance capacity, such as high-volume hemofiltration protocols,[13-15] use of highly permeable membranes,[16-18] or hybrid approaches such as coupled plasma filtration and adsorption (CPFA),[19,20] may be required to achieve maximal clinical impact.

The *threshold immunomodulation hypothesis*, proposed by Honoré and colleagues, focuses on the complexicity and nonlinear characteristics of the inflammatory cascade.[13] The redundancy of pro-inflammatory mediator systems results in a network that is still functioning even if one or several particular components are blocked.[21] The nonspecific removal of various mediators by hemofiltration may potentially interrupt the cascade, and the depletion of a particular compound in the plasma could result in its redistribution from tissue into the circulation, thereby making more mediator material available for extracorporeal removal. This process continues to a point at which some pathways are shut down and cascades are blocked. This is the "threshold point" at which further tissue and organ injury is stopped. Although in this model, mediator reduction occurs at the level of tissue and interstitium, no concomitant decrease in mediator levels in the circulation is observed. It is therefore difficult to determine when the threshold point has been reached. Moreover, the mechanism by which hemofiltration facilitates mediator flow from the interstitium to the blood compartment remains unexplained by this hypothesis. On the other hand, this theory may help to explain why, for example, high-volume hemofiltration protocols sometimes exert substantial biological effects in the absence of significant changes in mediator concentrations in the blood compartment.[13]

Whereas both the peak concentration hypothesis and the threshold immunomodulation concept focus on elimination of circulating cytokines and mediators, the *mediator delivery hypothesis*, brought forward by Di Carlo and Alexander,[22] proposes that the kinetics of cytokine reduction by hemofiltration depends on cytokine washout at the interstitium. In this model, the infusion of large volumes of replacement fluid drives a dynamic interstitial circulation that delivers mediators and middle-molecular-weight toxins from the intercellular space by means of the lymphatics to the bloodstream and, subsequently, to various points of elimination, such as liver, kidney, the red blood cells, and the extracorporeal system. Indeed, it has been demonstrated previously that with large volumes of fluid infusion (3 to 5 L/hour), lymphatic flow can increase 20- to 40-fold.[23] Thus, the mediator delivery hypothesis suggests that hemofiltration may exert its effect at a more fundamental level than by direct immunomodulation. The invigoration of lymphatic flow and function may in itself be an effective adjunct in the therapy of sepsis because it may help to clear away filtered plasma proteins, extravasated blood cells, wastes of cellular metabolism, excessive ground matrix substances, apoptotic cells, and free DNA.[22]

At present, the available data do not allow determination of which of the foregoing concepts best reflects the observed clinical impact of hemofiltration on septic patients. It seems reasonable, however, to conclude that the ideal immunomodulating strategy would be one that restores immunological stability, rather than blindly inhibiting or stimulating one or another component of the complex network interacting in sepsis.[24] Accordingly, the focus of research has shifted toward nonspecific methods of influencing the entire inflammatory response without suppressing it.

The third Acute Dialysis Quality Initiative (ADQI) consensus conference[25] stated that a biological rationale exists for extracorporeal blood treatment (EBT) in SIRS and sepsis. However, EBT may work not only through SIRS modulation but by a "pleiotropic" effect that includes potential reduction in the degree of immunosuppression in the later phase of sepsis. Indeed, hemofiltration was demonstrated to reverse sepsis-induced immunoparalysis in a porcine model of bile acid–induced pancreatitis. CVVH ameliorated the initial serum TNF-α response and prevented sepsis-induced endotoxin hyporesponsiveness. At the same time, the downregulation of major histocompatibility complex (MHC) class II and CD14 expression on monocytes was significantly improved, and the oxidative burst and phagocytosis capacity in polymorphonuclear leukocytes was augmented.[26]

More recently, using a special high-permeability hemofilter for CVVH, it was demonstrated in an *ex vivo* study that HPHF, but not conventional CVVH, restores peripheral blood mononuclear cell (PBMC) proliferation in septic patients.[16] The underlying mechanism appeared to be the elimination of immunomodulatory mediators, because ultrafiltrates from patients with sepsis demonstrated a significant suppressive effect on anti-CD3–stimulated PBMC proliferation only when obtained with HPHF but not with conventional hemofilters. In a similar study, intermittent HPHF attenuated polymorphonuclear neutrophil phagocytosis.[17] Incubation of high-permeability filtrates with blood from healthy donors resulted in a significant induction of phagocytosis, whereas conventional filtrates had no phagocytosis-stimulating effects, lending further support to the hypothesis that the elimination of mediators by HPHF may exert immunomodulatory effects that are biologically significant.[17]

Another, more global aspect of immunomodulation is the modification of apoptosis. Apoptosis plays a fundamental role in the function of the "normal" immune response: It is critical to the normal control of leukocytes, which are continuously being generated at a basal rate; this control must be upregulated in response to infection and subsequently downregulated once the infectious stimulus has been eliminated.[27] In sepsis and SIRS, neutrophil apoptosis is delayed,[28,29] whereas lymphocyte apoptosis is increased.[30,31] Moreover, pro-apoptotic molecules that are generated during sepsis also may be responsible for alterations in organ function. In particular, apoptosis may be a critical factor in end organ damage such as septic acute kidney failure.[32] In turn, kidney failure and the subsequent accumulation of uremic toxins such as advanced-oxidation protein products (AOPPs) and carbonyls may influence apoptotic pathways.

A recently published small clinical study in dialysis patients reported a significant correlation between the extent of plasma-induced pro-apoptotic activity of monocytes and both plasma carbonyl and AOPP levels.[33] In vitro data indicate that pro-apoptotic factors induced by lipopolysaccharides can be effectively eliminated from blood by high-flux membranes.[34] Although clinical data on the potential impact of CRRT on apoptosis in septic patients

are lacking at present, it is tempting to speculate that extracorporeal blood purification techniques will favorably influence the underlying mechanisms, both through the removal of uremic toxins and by means of their immunomodulatory capacity.

CONCLUSION

In patients with SIRS or sepsis, the homeostatic balance between pro-inflammatory and anti-inflammatory mechanisms is profoundly disturbed. CRRT, particularly with high volume regimens or with high-permeability membranes, may result in significant clinical benefits even in the absence of changes in circulating mediator concentrations. These beneficial effects are most likely related not only to SIRS modulation but to a "pleiotropic effect" that includes vasoactive compounds, uremic toxins, the coagulation system, and cardiodepressant factors. Future studies of the immunomodulating effect of CRRT should therefore focus on more global aspects, such as apoptosis or monocyte functional properties, rather than concentrating on single mediators.

Key Points

1. In sepsis, the homeostatic balance between pro-inflammatory and anti-inflammatory mechanisms is profoundly disturbed.
2. Continuous renal replacement therapy may result in significant clinical benefits despite a lack of change in circulating mediator concentrations.
3. The beneficial effects of continuous renal replacement therapy are most likely not only related to systemic inflammatory response syndrome modulation but to a "pleiotropic effect" that includes vasoactive compounds, uremic toxins, the coagulation system, and cardiodepressant factors.
4. Future studies of the immunomodulating effect of continuous renal replacement therapy should focus on more global aspects such as apoptosis or monocyte functional properties rather than concentrating on single mediators.

Key References

1. Marshall JC: The pathogenesis and molecular biology of sepsis. Crit Care Resusc 2006;8:227-229.
22. Di Carlo JV, Alexander SR: Hemofiltration for cytokine-driven illnesses: The mediator delivery hypothesis. Int J Artif Organs 2005;28:777-786.
24. Venkataraman R, Subramanian S, Kellum JA: Clinical review: Extracorporeal blood purification in severe sepsis. Crit Care 2003;7:139-145.
25. Bellomo R, Honoré PM, Matson J, et al: Extracorporeal blood treatment (EBT) methods in SIRS/sepsis. Int J Artif Organs 2005;28:450-458.
32. Wan L, Bellomo R, Di Giantomasso D, Ronco C: The pathogenesis of septic acute renal failure. Curr Opin Crit Care 2003;9:496-502.

See the companion Expert Consult website for the complete reference list.

CHAPTER 260

Continuous Ultrafiltration and Dialysis with a Wearable Artificial Kidney

Victor Gura and Claudio Ronco

OBJECTIVES

This chapter will:
1. Examine the inadequacy of current dialysis schedules as the main reason for the dismal morbidity and mortality rates in the chronic dialysis population and emphasize the need for significant technological breakthroughs to provide feasible and practical solutions.
2. Review the challenges to be overcome in building a wearable artificial kidney.
3. Describe the use of the wearable artificial kidney as a continuous hemofiltration device for the treatment of fluid overload in patients with congestive heart failure.
4. Outline the advantages of a double-pulsation mechanism for blood and dialysate in opposite cycles as a method of achieving hemodiafiltration.

Renal replacement therapies have come a long way since the epic event of Willem Kolff's first successful dialysis in Kampen, Holland.[1] To this day, however, outcomes for patients with end-stage renal disease (ESRD) still leave a lot to be desired. Quality of life is poor, and mortality remains disappointingly high.[2,3] During the last few years, a growing body of literature indicates that prolonged and more frequent dialysis treatments are associated with strikingly improved outcomes in patients with ESRD.[4-6] As patients were shifted from a typical regimen of three dialysis treatments per week to one of daily dialysis, significant improvement in quality of life was reported (e.g., liberalization of the diet, removal of fluid restrictions), alongside substantial reductions in medication consumption, complications, psychological symptoms, and hospitalizations. In a healthy subject, the blood is filtered by two native kidneys, 24 hours a day, 7 days a week, for a total of 168 weekly hours of blood purification. Obviously, treatment for ESRD consisting of 9 to 12 hours of dialysis per week (typically prescribed in the United States) is both non-physiological and completely inadequate. This inadequacy may well explain, to a great extent, the poor quality of life and unacceptably high mortality among the ESRD population.

Unfortunately, logistical and economical obstacles have made the successful implementation of daily dialysis difficult, impractical, and financially unfeasible.[7,8] Accordingly, an innovative and practical approach to this challenge to make the benefits of daily dialysis available to patients with ESRD, without imposing further financial burden on health budgets and without increasing the demand for nursing support, is urgently needed. The solu-

tion to this dilemma may be a wearable artificial kidney (WAK), which could bring the many advantages of continuous renal replacement therapy (CRRT) to this patient population.

Attempts to build a WAK date back to the 1970s, when Kolff's group described a WAK consisting of a combined blood and dialysate pump (weighing 1.2 kg), rechargeable batteries, tubing, a dialyzer, and a charcoal regeneration module, with a total weight of 3.5 kg.[9] In the mid-1980s, further attempts were made by Murisasco and colleagues[10] to build a WAK with continuous hemofiltration and ultrafiltrate reinfusion into the bloodstream after purification with a sterile sorbent system. An additional attempt was made by Landis and associates and Roberts,[11,12] who designed a peritoneal dialysis WAK in which dialysate also was regenerated with a similar sorbent system. None of these systems was ever implemented in practice, owing to several challenges that had to be solved to achieve true wearability.

These challenges were as follows:
- *Weight*: The WAK must not impede the patient's ability to carry out activities of daily living. The design must incorporate very light and energy-efficient parts, to avoid the need for heavy batteries, and efficient use of smaller amounts of sorbents.
- *Ergonomics*: The WAK must adapt to body contours, to permit maximum mobility and comfort. The ergonomic adaptation most likely to permit carrying the device without undue effort is a belt.
- *Lightweight but powerful battery design*: Independence from an electrical outlet hookup requires batteries powerful enough to make the WAK work without adding excessive weight and capable of supplying power for a reasonable period to avoid frequent interruption of activities for recharging or replacement of batteries.
- *Safety*: The WAK must have adequate safety features to manage not only the same risks posed by conventional dialysis machines but also those risks generated when the treatment is not carried out in a clinic or hospital and nurses or physicians are absent.
- *Concerns with clotting and toxicity*: The WAK must mitigate or eliminate the risks of clotting and infection and provide toxin-free dialysate.

As the pressing need for a better solution to provide more dialysis hours became more acute, we decided it was time to renew the efforts of our predecessors in this regard. We therefore developed an experimental prototype WAK that provided reasonable solutions to all of these challenges.[13] The initial WAK version (Fig. 260-1) consisted of a Hemophan 0.2 m² dialyzer, a sorbent-based dialysate regeneration system, and a main pump with two channels, one for blood and another one for dialysate, whereby both

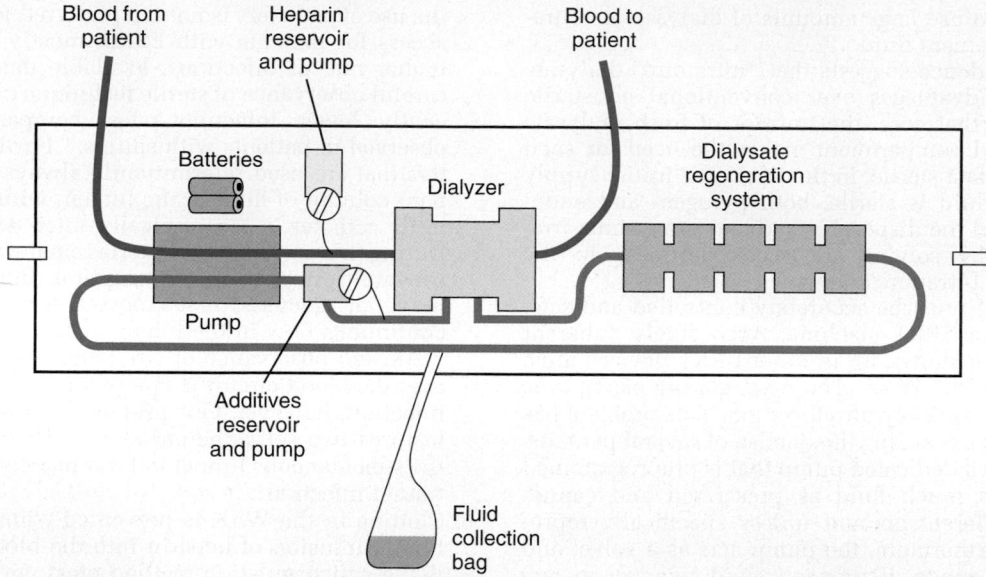

FIGURE 260-1. Schematic draft of the V1.0 wearable artificial kidney belt device. (Adapted from Gura V, Beizai M, Ezon C, Polaschegg HD: Continuous renal replacement therapy for end-stage renal disease: The wearable artificial kidney (WAK). In Ronco C, Brendolan A, Levin NW [eds]: Cardiovascular Disorders in Hemodialysis. Basel, Karger. Contrib Nephrol 2005;149:325-333.)

FIGURE 260-2. Flow behavior of both blood and dialysate in the wearable artificial kidney pump. Q_b, blood flow rate; Q_d, dialysate flow rate. Average Q_b = 95 mL/minute; average Q_d = 90 mL/minute. (Adapted from Gura V, Beizai M, Ezon C, Polaschegg HD: Pulsatile blood and dialysate counter phase flows, increased sorbent capacity and a high flux membrane explain the high efficiency of the wearable artificial kidney (WAK). J Am Soc Nephrol 2005;16:38A-39A.)

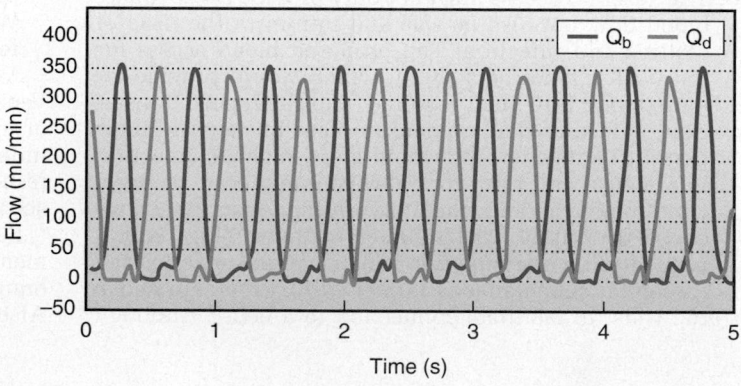

fluids are propelled in a pulsating fashion but on opposing cycles, so that pressures peak in one compartment when the other compartment pressures are at trough pressures, and vice versa (Fig. 260-2). The device also features reservoirs with heparin to be infused into the blood circuit as well as magnesium and calcium to be infused into the dialysate. These infusions are accomplished by auxiliary small pumps at prescribed rates. An additional auxiliary pump, volumetrically controlled, removes ultrafiltrate. The governing principles of this design are reflected in six specific considerations:

1. The optimal design would incorporate light, small, and energy-efficient parts requiring minimal amounts of energy from commonly available batteries but delivering efficient mass transfer across a dialyzer membrane to satisfy the highest dialysis adequacy. To meet this objective, hemodiafiltration was the most suitable modality. The double-pulsation mechanism for both blood and dialysate, oscillating at half-cycle differences, generates intermittent pressure changes across the dialyzer membrane, providing flow characteristics completely different from those of conventional dialysis machines. The transmembrane pressure (TMP) gradient

changes direction with each pulsation at different magnitudes along the hollow fiber: High increased convection forces higher mass transfer from the blood to the dialysate compartment in the proximal aspect of the fiber, while at certain parts of the pulsating cycle, fresh sterile fluid is propelled from the dialysate into the blood compartment, generating "post dilution," thus accomplishing hemodiafiltration.

2. The amount of dialysate necessary for a conventional dialysis treatment usually exceeds 100 L. With such a burdensome load, designing a wearable device would be impossible. The only way to overcome this problem is to use a sorbent regeneration system that constantly removes undesirable substances and excess electrolytes from the fluid so that a constant supply of fresh dialysate is provided. The WAK uses only 375 mL of fluid that is recirculated through several canisters containing urease, zirconium, and activated charcoal. These sorbents have been used successfully for several decades in the regeneration of dialysate with the REDY system,[14,15] and more recently a new conventional dialysis machine has been brought to market using this time-honored system. This solves the weight burden problem created

by the need to use large amounts of dialysate or ultrafiltrate replacement fluid.

3. Mounting evidence suggests that "ultrapure" dialysate has several advantages over conventional nonsterile dialysate. Furthermore, the transfer of fresh dialysate into the blood compartment makes the need for such fluid to be in fact sterile. In the WAK, the initial supply of dialysate fluid is sterile, both pyrogen- and endotoxin-free, and the disposable sorbents are gamma-irradiated, thereby solving all issues pertinent to the provision of "ultrapure" water.

4. Fluid removal must be accurately controlled and safe. The WAK is a CRRT machine. Accordingly, inherent risks that have shown up in other CRRT devices must be avoided in the WAK. The most glaring example is uncontrolled, runaway ultrafiltration. This problem has been reported as causing the demise of several patients. The WAK has a dedicated pump that is preprogrammed to remove as much fluid as prescribed and cannot remove a different amount unless specifically reprogrammed. Furthermore, the pump acts as a valve, and in its failure mode, it prevents fluid removal in any amount. Also, the WAK always can generate enough replacement fluid for any amount convectively removed, and it does not depend on scales monitoring the weight of fluid removed to determine the amount to be replaced.

5. The vascular access must not only provide for adequate blood flow but also be safe and minimize the risks of clotting and infection. The proposed blood access for the WAK cannot be a shunt, which would provide far more blood flow than required, and the repeated insertion of needles that are held in place by several flimsy pieces of adhesive tape would make such a connection impractical and risky for a device intended to be worn continuously in an ambulatory setting. Accordingly, we chose a central double-lumen catheter (Fig. 260-3) implanted in the superior vena cava and exteriorized through a subcutaneous tunnel exiting the skin above the waist to facilitate connection to a belt.[13] Although

the use of catheters is not the preferred form of vascular access for patients with ESRD, mostly because of the higher rate of infections, available data indicate that careful observance of sterile technique can yield significantly lower infection rates, comparable to those observed in patients with shunts.[16] Furthermore, catheters that are used intermittently always contain a stagnant column of fluid in the lumen, with no circulation until catheter reuse, typically after 48 to 72 hours. During this period, any bacteria remaining in the lumen can multiply with no interruption, impervious to the potential defenses of leukocytes and antibodies. The continuous flow in the lumen of the catheter using the WAK and observance of strict sterile technique whenever the blood circuit is open will minimize the risk of infection, however. Our proposed catheter design also features two self-adherent closure (Velcro) cuffs along the subcutaneous tunnel to form mechanical barriers to tunnel infection.

6. Clotting in the WAK is prevented primarily by a continued infusion of heparin into the blood circuit. This is the anticoagulation method most widely used today in patients undergoing dialysis. The use of alternatives such as argatroban, hirudin, and low-molecular-weight heparin has not been studied extensively in these patients. Although citrate has been used effectively in CRRT in an intensive care unit (ICU) setting, we cannot speculate at this point on the use of this agent in the WAK, although this would be at least theoretically feasible.

A summary of the initial animal studies with the WAK Version 1.0 (V1.0) is presented in Table 260-1. The amounts of urea and creatinine removed in 8 hours of treatment indicated that the continuous use of the device would result in adequate dialysis that meets or exceeds that achieved with a daily regimen.[13]

Further development of the WAK brought the replacement of the Hemophan dialyzer with a high-flux membrane dialyzer and a larger membrane surface (Fig. 260-4). Also, the dialysate pH was increased to 7.4 with the addi-

BLOOD ACCESS VIA OUTPATIENT CATHETER PLACEMENT

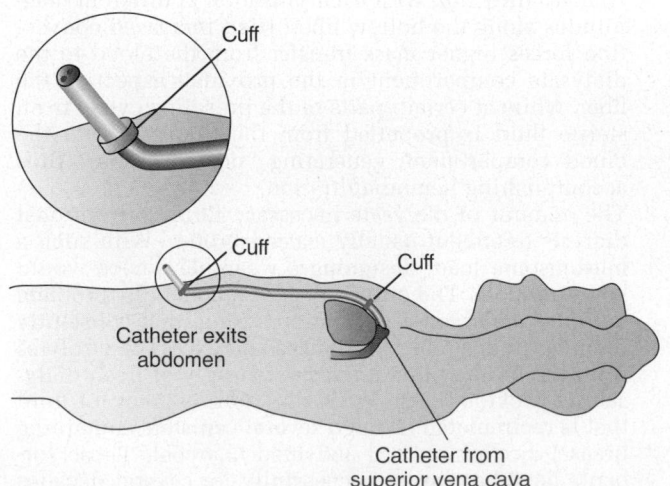

FIGURE 260-3. Schematic design of the wearable artificial kidney double-cuff catheter. (Adapted from Gura V, Beizai M, Ezon C: CRRT for CHF: The wearable continuous ultrafiltration system. ASAIO J 2006;52:59-61.)

TABLE 260-1

Summary of Findings in Initial Animal Studies of Wearable Artificial Kidney V1.0*

	Finding	
BIOCHEMICAL INDEX	*GROUP I*	*GROUP II*
Effective urea clearance (mL/min)	24.3 ± 1.4	23.9 ± 3.5
Effective creatinine clearance (mL/min)	25.5 ± 1.4	24.7 ± 3.2
Total urea removal (g)	12.7 ± 2.8	12.0 ± 2.9
Total creatinine removal (g)	0.9 ± 0.2	1.0 ± 0.1
Total phosphorus removal (g)	0.8 ± 0.2	0.84 ± 0.4
Total potassium removal (mmol)	71.9 ± 13.3	89.1 ± 25.7
Extrapolated standard Kt/V (urea)	5.4 ± 2.4	8.4 ± 1.5

*In uremic pigs. In Group I, a blood flow rate of 44 mL/minute was used; in Group II, blood flow rate was 75 mL/minute. Values are means ± SD. Data from Gura V, Beizai M, Ezon C, Polaschegg HD: Continuous renal replacement therapy for end-stage renal disease: The wearable artificial kidney (WAK). In Ronco C, Brendolan A, Levin NW (eds): Cardiovascular Disorders in Hemodialysis. Basel, Karger, Contrib Nephrol 2005;149:325-333.

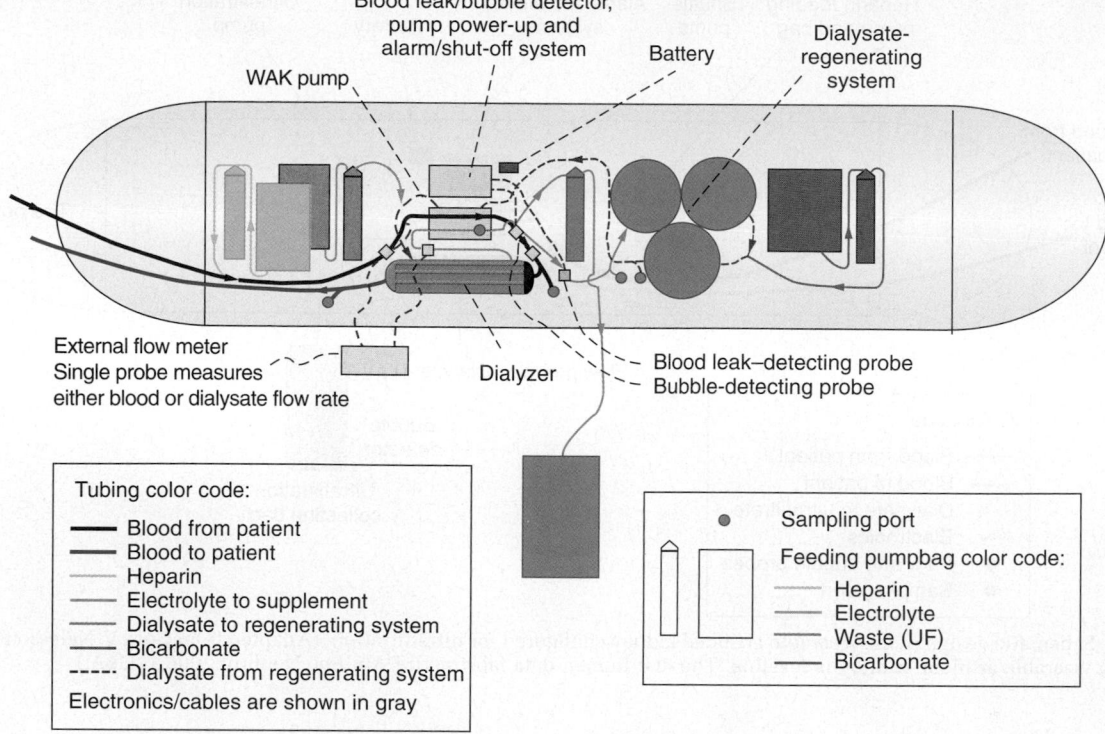

FIGURE 260-4. Schematics of the V1.2 wearable artificial kidney. U.S. patent 6,960,179.

TABLE 260-2

Summary of Findings in Animal Studies of Wearable Artificial Kidney V1.1*

BIOCHEMICAL INDEX	FINDING
Effective urea clearance (mL/min)	39.8 ± 2.7
Effective creatinine clearance (mL/min)	40.9 ± 2.3
Total urea removal (g)	15.3 ± 4.4
Total creatinine removal (g)	1.7 ± 0.2
Total phosphate removal (g)	1.83 ± 0.70
Total potassium removal (mmol)	150.5 ± 16.7
Extrapolated standard Kt/V	7.7 ± 0.5

*In anesthetized uremic pigs subjected to 8 hours of dialysis. Values are means ± SD.
Data from Gura V, Beizai M, Ezon C, Polaschegg HD: Pulsatile blood and dialysate counter phase flows, increased sorbent capacity and a high flux membrane explain the high efficiency of the wearable artificial kidney (WAK). J Am Soc Nephrol 2005;16:38A-39A.

tion of a continuous sodium bicarbonate infusion. The WAK Version 1.1 (V1.1) delivered even higher clearances of urea and creatinine,[17] as shown in Table 260-2.

The optimization of the pH leads to an improvement in the amount of urea removed from the dialysate per gram of sorbent. The pH of the dialysate after the initial conversion of urea to ammonia and CO_2 is very low, effectively preventing bacterial growth and lending further support to the continued sterility of the dialysate. On the other hand, it is important to optimize the pH of the dialysate entering the dialyzer. This will not only avoid aggravating the acidosis of ESRD patients but actually provide a source of badly needed buffer for these patients. The amounts of phosphorus and potassium removed in the initial animal

studies suggest that if similar rates of removal are achieved in humans with continuous use, use of phosphate binders and dietary potassium intake limitations may become obsolete.

The development of the WAK pump brought into perspective the unique opposed-phase pulsating mechanism of both blood and dialysate. In this pump, both fluids circulate in separate parallel channels.[17] The pump has two compressible elastic chambers with valve mechanisms at both ends. The valve motor moves through a gear box with two arms that alternately compress both chambers so that when one chamber is being compressed and the fluid is propelled out of the chamber (as in the heart in systole), the other chamber is recovering its original form and filling up (as in diastole). This mechanism provides for a very high convective force across the dialyzer membrane, because a tide of blood entering a hollow fiber creates an excess volume in its lumen. Also, because blood is a liquid and as such is not compressible, the hollow fiber is rigid, and the valves in the pump prevent retrograde flow, the excess volume has nowhere to go but through the membrane pores, creating a higher-magnitude convective drag. The increased convection, in turn, is conducive to an increase in β_2-microglobulins. Accumulation of these middle-molecular-weight molecules constitutes an important marker of developing uremia, and their removal is a desirable goal of treatment for patients with ESRD. Bench studies showed effective β_2-microglobulin clearance from human blood to dialysate and removal of these molecules from the dialysate by the activated charcoal component of the sorbent system.[18] The effective performance of hemodiafiltration and removal of middle-molecular-weight molecules with this platform suggests that this extracorporeal circulation modality may become a useful tool in critically ill patients requiring CRRT in the ICU as well. Ongoing

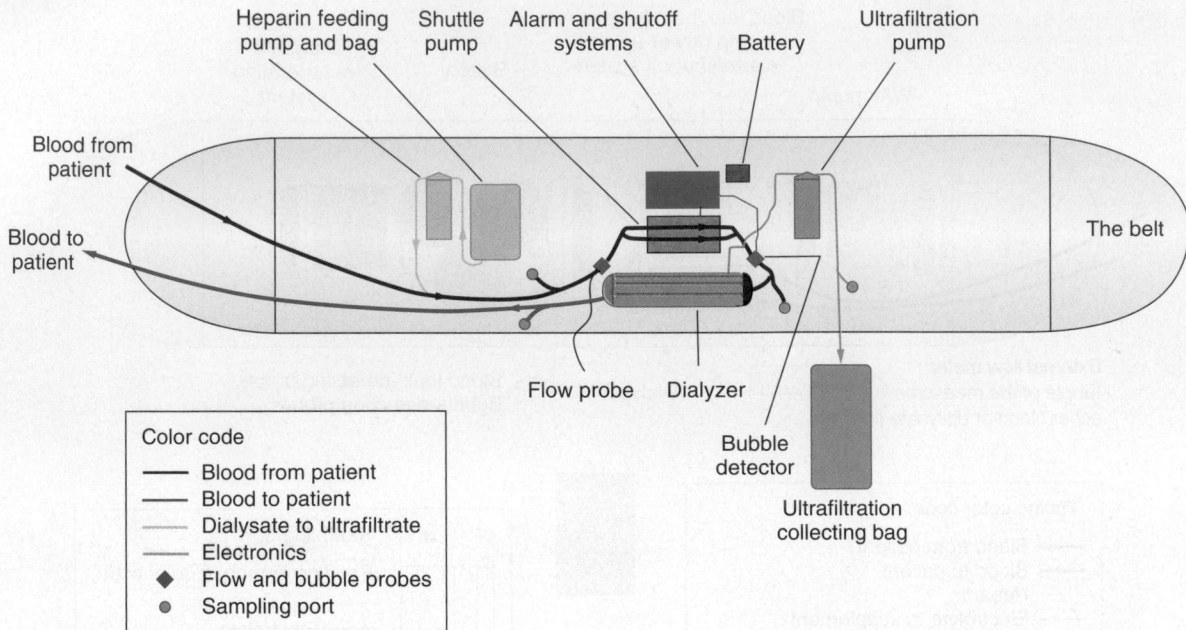

FIGURE 260-5. Schematic design of the wearable artificial kidney configured for ultrafiltration. (Adapted from Gura V, Nalesso F, Brendolan A, et al: The wearable artificial kidney is feasible. The first human data [abstract]. J Am Soc Nephrol 2006;17:59A.)

clinical studies in humans are being conducted with the intention to develop this technology into a useful tool for the practicing nephrologist.

The WAK, like any other CRRT device, can be used for continuous hemofiltration (Fig. 260-5). Mounting evidence in the literature points to this modality as an effective means of alleviating fluid overload, mostly in patients with decompensated congestive heart failure (CHF).[19-21] All data accumulated to date derive from single sessions in acutely ill patients. Ultrafiltrate from patients with CHF has been shown in vitro to have a myocardial depressant effect.[22] Lung functional capacity and urine output improved, and hyponatremia decreased, with hemofiltration in patients with CHF, and of greatest importance, renal function was preserved.[23,24] In the Acute Decompensated Heart Failure National Registry (ADHERE), which tracked data for more than 100,000 patients with CHF,[25] patients with a serum creatinine level below 2 mg had less than half the mortality of those with a serum creatinine above 2 mg. Further data have confirmed that mortality in patients with CHF increases with decline in glomerular filtration rate.[26] Diuretics are by far the most frequently used agents for treatment of decompensated CHF, but their use has been documented to cause a decrease in renal function. This deficit may well push a patient from the lower-mortality-risk group, with a serum creatinine below 2 mg, beyond the threshold into a higher-mortality-risk group. Although the greater mortality associated with higher creatinine is well documented, data are lacking on whether the use of diuretics in CHF actually increases the mortality associated with this condition. Although the evidence suggests that urine output improves, it is unclear whether kidney function may get better with hemofiltration.

Hemofiltration can be performed with currently available dialysis and CRRT machines, and a hemofiltration machine is now available specifically for hemofiltration in CHF, but no device is available for continuous ambulatory hemofiltration outside a hospital or clinic setting. The WAK was configured for hemofiltration intended for continuous ambulatory hemofiltration without impeding the performance of activities of daily living in fluid-overloaded patients, with the hope of maintaining them euvolemic, free of the stigmata of CHF, and avoiding as many hospitalizations as possible. In initial animal studies,[27] the WAK removed up to 700 mL of ultrafiltrate per hour. Attempts to remove fluid at a higher hourly rate were limited by the increased hematocrit inside the hollow fibers, resulting in their temporary occlusion. The average removal rate was 100 mL/hour.

A phase I feasibility study was conducted in 6 patients with fluid overload treated for 6 hours with no untoward effects.[28] In this study, the WAK removed an average of 170 mL/hour with a blood flow of 120 mL/minute, and the patients were able to ambulate with no impediment while undergoing slow continuous hemofiltration (Table 260-3). Plasma ultrafiltrate is considered iso-osmotic and as such contains 0.9 gr% of salt. Thus, the amount of salt removed was estimated to be 9.8 g. This considerable amount is of particular importance because patients will replace ultrafiltrate removed in the process by drinking water and not normal saline solution. The resulting sodium deficit would have to be made up by allowing the addition of generous amounts of salt to the diet of patients with fluid overload due to CHF. The impact on their quality of life would be quite obvious. Undoubtedly, many more studies are in order to adequately evaluate the true impact of continuous ambulatory hemofiltration on actual outcomes in patients with CHF, specifically in terms of reducing morbidity and mortality.

The same issues remain open for the continued ambulatory use of the WAK in patients with ESRD and the application of double-pulsation hemodiafiltration technology in critically ill patients. Nevertheless, a pressing need remains for the nephrology community to develop more creative therapies to answer the needs of the growing population of patients with ESRD. A WAK may well be the technological solution to this challenge.

TABLE 260-3

Summary of Clinical Results with Ultrafiltration Using the Wearable Artificial Kidney*

PATIENT NO.	Q$_B$ (mL/min)	Q$_F$ (mL/hr)	HEPARIN (U/hr)	TREATMENT TIME (hr)	TOTAL VOLUME (mL)	SALT REMOVED (g)
1	134.2	120	758.3	6	770	6.9
2	118.9	288	300	4	984	8.8
3	121.9	120	1000	6	708	6.4
4	106.1	250	500	6	1610	14.5
5	106.8	175	533.3	6	1233	11.1
6	108.6	200	1000	6	1201	10.8
Average	116.1	192.1	682.0	5.7	1084.3	9.7
SD	±11.1	±68.3	±286.1	±0.8	±335.4	±3.0

*In 6 patients who underwent continuous ultrafiltration for 6 hours.
Q$_B$, blood flow rate; Q$_F$, filtrate (dialysate) flow rate.
Data from Gura V, Nalesso F, Brendolan A, et al: The wearable artificial kidney is feasible. The first human data [abstract]. J Am Soc Nephrol 2006;17:59A.

Key Points

1. Prolonged and frequent or daily dialysis treatments are a much-desired goal in the treatment of end-stage renal disease, yet logistically are very difficult to accomplish.
2. The wearable artificial kidney provides a practical and feasible solution to satisfy this need.
3. The wearable artificial kidney double-pulsation pump in opposite phases provides for hemodiafiltration and adds a significant convective force across the dialyzer membrane that makes the device more efficient.
4. Mounting evidence indicates that ultrafiltration is useful in treating the fluid overload of patients with congestive heart failure.
5. The wearable artificial kidney can be configured to treat the fluid overload of congestive heart failure on an ambulatory setting.

Key References

5. Mohr PE, Neumann PJ, Franco SJ, et al: The case for daily dialysis: Its impact on costs and quality of life. Am J Kidney Dis 2001;37:777-789.
13. Gura V, Beizai M, Ezon C, Polaschegg HD: Continuous renal replacement therapy for end-stage renal disease: The wearable artificial kidney (WAK). In Ronco C, Brendolan A, Levin NW (eds): Cardiovascular Disorders in Hemodialysis. Basel, Karger, Contrib Nephrol 2005;149:325-333.
17. Gura V, Beizai M, Ezon C, Polaschegg HD: Pulsatile blood and dialysate counter phase flows, increased sorbent capacity and a high flux membrane explain the high efficiency of the wearable artificial kidney (WAK). J Am Soc Nephrol 2005; 16:38A-39A.
27. Gura V, Beizai M, Ezon C, Rambod E: Continuous renal replacement therapy for congestive heart failure: The wearable continuous ultrafiltration system. ASAIO J 2006;52:59-61.
28. Gura V, Nalesso F, Brendolan A, et al: The wearable artificial kidney is feasible. The first human data [abstract]. J Am Soc Nephrol 2006;17:59A.

See the companion Expert Consult website for the complete reference list.

CHAPTER 261

The Bioartificial Kidney

H. David Humes

OBJECTIVES

This chapter will:
1. Present the scientific rationale for renal stem cell and progenitor cell therapy.
2. Describe an extracorporeal approach to renal cell replacement therapy.
3. Summarize preclinical and clinical data on the effects of the bioartificial kidney.

CELL THERAPY IN ACUTE RENAL FAILURE

Cell therapy is a new and exciting approach to the management of acute and chronic diseases.[1-3] The potential success of this treatment approach is indicated by the growing appreciation that most disease processes are not due to the lack of a single protein but result from alterations in the complex interactions of a variety of cell products.

H. David Humes is founder and shareholder of Nephrion, Inc, and Innovative BioTherapies, Inc, biotechnology spinoff companies of the University of Michigan.

Growing evidence suggests that acute renal failure (ARF) is not merely a surrogate marker for severity of disease but also an independent predictor of death and a separate pathogenic entity, even when nearly physiological levels of small-molecule clearance are administered. This possibility gives rise to the hypothesis that the native kidney has clinically important functions that are not replaced by dialysis or hemofiltration. These functions may include synthesis of cytokines,[4-7] antigen presentation, reclamation of glutathione, synthesis of glutathione reductase, oxidative deamination and gluconeogenesis, 1,25-dihydroxyvitamin D_3 hydroxylation, trace mineral and element reclamation, and other, as-yet-undiscovered entities.[8]

Human renal cells have been isolated from cadaveric kidneys and cultured for the purpose of integrating them within a filtration device to provide more complete renal replacement.[9,10] These tubule cells, obtained from adult tissue and having stem cell–like characteristics, are grown in confluent monolayers along the inner surface of the hollow fibers in a conventional hemofiltration cartridge. The resulting construct containing these living cells is called a *bioartificial renal tubule assist device* (RAD).[11]

RENAL TUBULE ASSIST DEVICE

The RAD is clearly feasible when conceived of as a combination of living cells supported on polymeric substrata acting as scaffolds for the cells. The renal tubule progenitor cells were cultured on the biomatrix-coated, hollow-fiber membrane of a standard high-flux hemofiltration cartridge. The membrane is both water- and solute-permeable, allowing for differentiated vectorial transport and metabolic and endocrine activity. Immunoprotection of cultured progenitor cells is achieved concurrently with long-term functional performance so long as conditions support tubule cell viability.[12] Studies of RADs populated with porcine renal proximal tubule progenitor cells have demonstrated that the cells retain vectorial fluid transport properties as a result of Na^+,K^+-ATPase; other differentiated active transport properties, including active glucose and bicarbonate transport; differentiated metabolic activities, including intraluminal glutathione breakdown, constituent amino acid uptake, and ammonia production; and the important capacity for endocrinological conversion of 25-hydroxy-vitamin D_3 (25-OH-D_3) to 1,25-dihydroxy-vitamin D_3 (1,25-(OH)$_2$-D_3).[13]

BIOARTIFICIAL KIDNEY

The bioartificial kidney consists of a filtration device (a conventional high-flux hemofilter) connected in series to the RAD (Fig. 261-1). Blood pumped out of the patient enters the fibers of the hemofilter, where ultrafiltrate is formed and delivered into the fibers of the tubule lumens within the RAD, downstream of the hemofilter. Processed ultrafiltrate exiting the RAD is collected and discarded as "urine." The filtered blood exiting the hemofilter enters the RAD through the extracapillary space port and disperses among the fibers of the device. Upon exiting the RAD, the processed blood is returned to the patient's body by means of a third pump. The RAD is oriented horizontally and kept in a 37° C temperature-controlled environment to ensure optimal functionality of the cells.

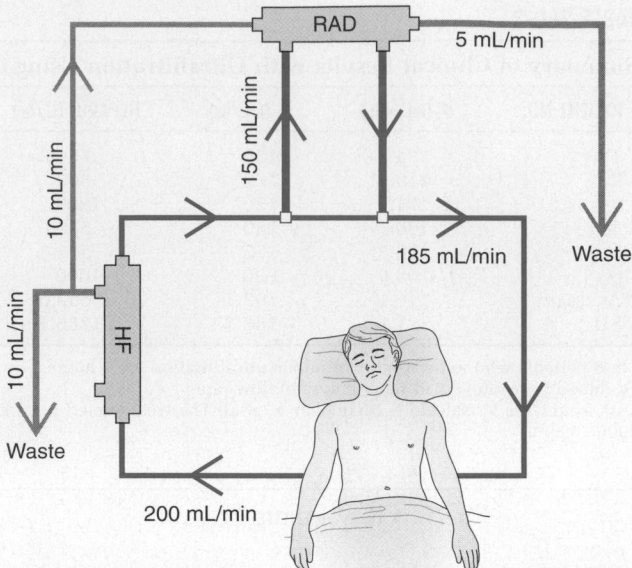

FIGURE 261-1. Schematic of the extracorporeal circuit for perfusion of the bioartificial kidney that was used in the phase I/II clinical trial described in the text. HF, hemofilter; RAD, renal tubule assist device. (Redrawn from Humes HD, Weitzel WF, Bartlett RH, et al: Initial clinical results of the bioartificial kidney containing human cells in ICU patients with acute renal failure. Kidney Int 2004;66:1578-1588 [Nature Publishing Group].)

Studies have shown that the bioartificial kidney using a RAD consisting of either porcine or human cells replaces filtration, transport, metabolic, and endocrine functions of the kidney in acutely uremic dogs after bilateral nephrectomies.[14,15] The dogs were treated with hemofiltration using either a RAD cartridge containing tubule cells or a sham control cartridge containing no cells. Fluid and small solutes, including urea, creatinine, and electrolytes, were adequately controlled in both groups. Potassium and blood urea nitrogen (BUN) levels were more easily controlled during RAD treatment than during sham treatment. Furthermore, active reabsorption of K^+, HCO_3^-, and glucose and excretion of ammonia were accomplished only in RAD treatments. Glutathione reclamation from the ultrafiltrate was greater than 50% in the RAD. Finally, uremic animals receiving cell therapy attained normal 1,25-(OH)$_2$-D_3 levels, whereas sham treatment resulted in a further decline from the already low plasma levels.[14]

In a series of animal experiments investigating whether the bioartificial kidney can protect against the high mortality risk associated with sepsis complicated by ARF, surgically nephrectomized dogs were intravenously administered endotoxin and treated with continuous venovenous hemofiltration (CVVH) incorporating either a RAD or an identically prepared sham cartridge containing no cells. Mean arterial pressures were found to be significantly higher in animals in the RAD treatment group. Mean peak levels of an anti-inflammatory cytokine, interleukin (IL)-10, also were significantly higher in these animals. Levels of a pro-inflammatory cytokine, tumor necrosis factor-α (TNF-α), were on average lower among animals in the RAD treatment group than among those in the sham treatment group, but the difference was not statistically significant.[16]

To further assess the effect of the bioartificial kidney in ARF with bacterial sepsis, dogs were nephrectomized and 48 hours later were given an intraperitoneal injection of 3×10^{11} *Escherichia coli* cells per kilogram of body weight.[17] Immediately after bacteria administration, animals were placed in a CVVH circuit with either a RAD with cells or a sham cartridge without cells. Compared with sham therapy, RAD treatment maintained better cardiovascular performance, as determined by mean arterial blood pressure and cardiac output, for longer periods. All animals that received sham therapy expired within 2 to 10 hours after bacteria administration, whereas all those that received RAD treatment survived longer than 10 hours. Plasma cytokine levels of IL-10 were significantly higher in the RAD group than in the control group.[17]

In another study, pigs with normal kidney function were administered an intraperitoneal injection of 3.0×10^{11} E. coli cells/kg. One hour later, animals were placed in a CVVH circuit containing either a RAD with cells or a sham cartridge without cells. ARF with anuria developed within 2 to 4 hours after bacteria administration in all animals. Compared with sham therapy, RAD treatment maintained better cardiovascular performance, as determined by cardiac output and renal blood flow, for longer periods. Animals in the RAD treatment group consistently had significantly longer survival times than control animals. RAD treatment was associated with significantly lower plasma circulating pro-inflammatory cytokine levels of IL-6 and interferon-γ. Taken together, these data and those from the studies in dogs demonstrate that septic shock results in early ARF and that RAD treatment in a bioartificial kidney circuit improves cardiovascular performance associated with changes in cytokine profiles and confers a significant survival advantage.[18]

CLINICAL ASSESSMENT OF THE BIOARTIFICIAL KIDNEY

These encouraging preclinical animal data led to a U.S. Food and Drug Administration (FDA)-approved phase I-II clinical trial to evaluate the safety and efficacy of this new system in 10 critically ill patients with ARF and multiple organ failure receiving CVVH.[19] The predicted hospital mortality rates for these patients averaged greater than 85%. The devices used in this study were seeded with human renal proximal tubule cells isolated from kidneys donated for cadaveric transplantation but found to be unsuitable because of anatomical or fibrotic defects. The RAD perfusion pump system was connected in series to a CVVH extracorporeal pump system, following the principles tested in the preclinical animal studies, but with a minor adaptation of the circuit to maintain the original CVVH prescription in terms of blood flow rate from the patient and ultrafiltration rate from the hemofilter. The postfiltered blood from the CVVH circuit was pumped with a peristaltic pump system at a rate of 150 mL/minute to the extracapillary space of the RAD and dispersed among the fibers of the device. Upon exiting the RAD, the processed blood traveled through an additional pump and was delivered back to the patient. The ultrafiltrate formed from the synthetic hemofilter was delivered into the fibers of the tubule lumen within the RAD downstream to the hemofilter at a rate of 10 mL/minute. The hydraulic pressures within the RAD were adjusted to reabsorb and return ultrafiltrate to the patient at a rate of 5 mL/minute. Processed ultrafiltrate exiting the luminal space of the RAD was collected and discarded as "urine."

The results of this clinical trial demonstrated that the experimental treatment could be delivered safely under study protocol guidelines for up to 24 hours when used in conjunction with CVVH.[19] The clinical data also indicate that the RAD maintains and exhibits viability, durability, and functionality in this clinical setting. Cardiovascular stability of the patients was maintained, and increased native kidney function, as determined by elevated urine output, was temporally correlated with RAD treatment. The device also demonstrated differentiated metabolic and endocrinologic activity, with glutathione reclamation and endocrinological conversion of 25-OH-D_3 to 1,25-(OH)$_2$-D_3. All but one treated patient with more than a 3-day follow-up period showed improvement, as assessed by acute physiological scores. Six of the 10 treated patients survived past 28 days with kidney function recovery. One patient expired within 12 hours after RAD treatment owing to his family's request to withdraw ventilatory life support. Three other patients died of fatal complications unrelated to RAD therapy and ARF: toxic megacolon in one patient, fungal pericarditis and vancomycin-resistant enterococcal septicemia in a second patient, and ischemic colitis with bowel perforations in the third patient. Plasma cytokine levels suggest that RAD therapy produces dynamic and individualized responses in patients depending on their unique pathophysiological condition. For the subset of patients who had excessive pro-inflammatory cytokine levels, RAD treatment resulted in significant declines in granulocyte colony-stimulating factor, IL-6, IL-10, and especially IL-6/IL-10 ratios, suggesting a greater decline in IL-6 relative to IL-10 levels and a less active pro-inflammatory state.

These favorable phase I-II trial results led to an FDA-approved, randomized, controlled, open-label phase II investigation at 12 clinical sites to determine whether this cell therapy approach alters patient mortality. This phase II study involved 58 patients, of whom 40 were randomized to receive RAD therapy and 18 made up a control group with comparable demographics and severity of illness. The early results have been as compelling as the phase I-II results. Renal cell therapy improved the 28-day mortality rate from 61% in the conventional hemofiltration treatment control group to 34% in the RAD treatment group.[20,21] This survival impact continued through the 90- and 180-day follow-up periods ($P < .04$), with the Cox proportional hazard ratio indicating that the risk of death was 50% of that observed in the conventional continuous renal replacement therapy (CRRT) group. This survival advantage with renal cell therapy was observed for ARF of various causes and regardless of organ failure number (1 to 5+) or the presence of sepsis.

The results of these clinical trials have shown a safety profile comparable to that for CVVH alone. Hypoglycemia and hypotension, both treatable in the intensive care unit, have been observed and were due to insulin release from cell culture media during maintenance of the RAD in manufacturing and the increase in extracorporeal blood volume required by the second cell-containing cartridge, respectively. The addition of a second cell-containing cartridge necessitates an additional extracorporeal pump system to maintain adequate filtrate and blood flow to the cells. This pump system requires additional expertise to maintain safe functionality and interface with the standard CVVH circuit.

CONCLUSION

ARF is a common complication in the ICU setting. The loss of kidney function, including fluid and electrolyte homeostasis and control of metabolic, endocrine, and immunological activities, leads to further deterioration and increased mortality in septic patients. Despite advances in current CRRT, which improves only the fluid and electrolyte homeostasis function of the kidney, mortality rates have remained stable over the last 2 decades. These therapies fail to address the complicated pathophysiology of ARF. Cell therapy has the potential to overcome many of the limitations of existing treatments. The bioartificial kidney, a cell therapy approach to renal replacement therapy, has been tested in large animal studies and phase I-II and phase II clinical trials. The results to date have demonstrated the RAD's ability to replace multiple kidney functions and show a survival advantage in ARF associated with multiple organ dysfunction, apparently due to modulation of inflammatory mediators. Further studies are required to confirm these results and elucidate detailed mechanisms underlying the effects of the RAD.

Key Points

1. Cell therapy has the potential to provide critically important functions of the native kidney that are not replaced by dialysis or hemofiltration.
2. A renal tubule assist device has been developed using either adult human or porcine renal tissue.
3. A bioartificial kidney consisting of the renal tubule assist device (containing either human or porcine cells) and a conventional filtration device has been found to replace filtration, transport, metabolic, and endocrine functions in acutely

uremic large animals and to improve survival of septic animals.
4. In a phase I-II clinical trial, the renal tubule assist device in conjunction with continuous venovenous hemofiltration was used safely and maintained viability, durability, and functionality for up to 24 hours in patients with acute renal failure.
5. An open-label phase II trial demonstrated decreased mortality in patients with acute renal failure receiving renal tubule assist device therapy compared with those receiving sham renal tubule assist device therapy.

Key References

8. Humes HD: Bioartificial kidney for full renal replacement therapy. Semin Nephrol 2000;20:71-82.
13. Humes HD, MacKay SM, Funke AJ, Buffington DA: Tissue engineering of a bioartificial renal tubule assist device: In vitro transport and metabolic characteristics. Kidney Int 1999;55:2502-2514.
14. Humes HD, Buffington DA, MacKay SM, et al: Replacement of renal function in uremic animals with a tissue-engineered kidney. Nat Biotechnol 1999;17:451-455.
18. Humes HD, Buffington DA, Lou L, et al: Cell therapy with a tissue-engineered kidney reduces the multiple-organ consequences of septic shock. Crit Care Med 2003;31:2421-2428.
19. Humes HD, Weitzel WF, Bartlett RH, et al: Initial clinical results of the bioartificial kidney containing human cells in ICU patients with acute renal failure. Kidney Int 2004;66:1578-1588.

See the companion Expert Consult website for the complete reference list.

CHAPTER 262

Information Technology and Therapy Delivery in Continuous Renal Replacement Therapies

Francesco Paolini, Pier Paolo Manzini, Francesco Garzotto, Fabio Grandi, and Claudio Ronco

OBJECTIVES

This chapter will:
1. Outline the main tasks of the intensive care unit.
2. Relate these tasks to the usefulness of and need for information technology in the intensive care unit.
3. Review trends in information technology and general technical infrastructure.
4. Present sample clinical applications packages for therapy order entries and therapy monitoring.

INTENSIVE CARE UNIT TASKS: OVERVIEW

Today, intensive care units (ICUs) are complex, high-technology domains in which clinicians routinely integrate huge numbers of discrete data points with life support systems providing a coherent picture of their patients' status, as well as sophisticated therapies.[1] Critical care patients often are affected by impairment or failure of

TABLE 262-1

Some Devices Used at the Bedside in the Intensive Care Unit

Monitoring
Cardiovascular
Respiratory
Central venous system monitors
Gastrointestinal tract
Musculoskeletal system monitoring
Metabolic
Portable x-ray units
Life Support Systems
Mechanical ventilation
Infusion pumps
Intra-aortic balloon pump
Left ventricular assist device
Renal support systems
Liver support systems
Hemodepuration

TABLE 262-2

Clinical and Biochemical Parameters and Sources of Information Monitored at the Bedside in the Intensive Care Unit*

Cardiovascular	Central Nervous System
Heart rate and blood pressure (systolic, diastolic)	EEG
	Evoked potentials
Pulmonary artery pressure	Intracranial pressure
Central venous pressure	Epidural pressure
Ejection fraction; cardiac output and cardiac index	Cerebral perfusion pressure
	Cortical oxygen saturation
Aortic flow	Jugular bulb saturation
Ventricular pressure-volume loops	**Gastrointestinal**
	Esophageal pH and sphincter tone
ECG	
Ankle-brachial index	**Musculoskeletal**
SvO_2	Intra-abdominal pressure
Blood volume change	Muscular compartment pressure
Respiratory	External skin pressure
Respiratory rate	Skin shear stress
Tidal volume	**Metabolic**
Respiratory flow	Temperature
Mean airway pressure	Oxygen consumption
Mean intrathoracic pressure	CO_2 production
Minute volume	Blood chemistries
End-tidal CO_2	Fluid balance
Oxygen saturation	
Breathing work	

*All parameters are potentially available for automatic recording.
ECG, electrocardiography; EEG, electroencephalography; SvO_2, venous oxygen saturation.
Adapted from Booth FV: Computerized physiological monitoring. Crit Care Clin 1999;15:3548-3562.

several organs at once (multiorgan dysfunction syndrome [MODS]), requiring concurrent use of multiple monitoring devices and life support systems. Table 262-1 lists various monitoring and life support systems available today for different organs, which may mean dealing with dozens of medical devices in a single patient. Indeed, a look at Table 262-2 will show the numerous parameters that can now be monitored, often giving the bedside the appearance of a well-lighted Christmas tree.[2]

In current practice, these instruments typically are self-contained devices capable of stand-alone operation under manual control of an operator. Each instrument will have a prominently displayed "operations panel." It is essential, however, to assess the patient's status from a global perspective, whereas the readout for each instrument provides only a small portion of the big picture.[3] Overall patient status, then, must be reconstructed, rather like a jigsaw puzzle, by the clinician. The task here involves not only recovery of the different data and entry into the patient's medical record but also analysis of the results.

Two further dimensions characterizing the ICU environment are *time* and *number of caregivers*. Near-instantaneous detection of any critical alterations in patient status must be followed by an appropriate and immediate response, such as initiating or terminating a therapeutic modality or changing the choice or dose of medication. In this setting, it is of paramount importance to discriminate a key change from mere artifact, assessment of which can steal precious seconds. Clinicians are faced with the need to differentiate between data points that are relevant and those that are irrelevant in a particular situation; this has been called the *significance of data* problem.[4]

Time also is of the essence with respect to number of caregivers. In fact, implementation of continuous therapies lasting up to several hours or days is necessarily based on the assumption that different caregivers will manage the same patient during a single treatment session. This point also bears out the issue of potential incoherence and misinterpretation of orders and reports from different physicians.[5]

Health care will certainly be affected by the pervasive influence of computing technologies. A look at the most important trends in information technology (IT) will readily suggest which technologies can be applied to the

ICU environment, and how such implementation can be accomplished.[6]

This chapter explores why and how IT can help caregivers in their routine tasks in a number of ways, with particular applications in continuous renal replacement therapies (CRRTs): from IT infrastructures, to data acquisition and storage, to understanding and recoding the units of single information into chunks of status information, to translating the monitored data into prescription, coherent order entry, and surveillance of therapy delivery.

INFORMATION TECHNOLOGY IN THE INTENSIVE CARE UNIT

The amount of single information units that can be received and transferred in one transaction is strongly limited. In 1956, George Miller[7] published a review showing that the upper limit at which someone can match the responses to the stimuli provided (*channel capacity*) magically approaches the number 7. Let's say, then, that a subject is able to discriminate no more than 7 alternatives in sounds or loudness or the position of a point in a line. But Miller also pointed out that this limit is overcome by purposeful exploitation of further capabilities, such as dimensionality (e.g., the channel capacity of a point in a square is higher than in a line), correlation between information sources, recoding of single information into chunks, and time to exposure (or length of memory), which can shift the limit several times over.

This limitation stands in stark contrast with the hundreds of variables encountered by clinicians in the ICU environment. The mismatch between human limitation and excess information almost certainly contributes to unnecessary variation in clinical practice, clinical error, and poor compliance with guidelines.

IT in the ICU environment can overcome many of these limitations:

1. It allows for increasing the dimensionality of information by providing access to several parameters at the same time.
2. It allows for recoding the several single sources of information into more powerful, physiologically related information (e.g., weight loss and blood volume change during CRRT can be recoded to discriminate poor plasma refillers from good plasma refillers, or to discriminate between a dehydrated patient and an overhydrated one), or into diagnostic tools (e.g., severity scores).
3. It allows for lengthening the exposure time to a source of a single information unit.

INFORMATION TECHNOLOGY TRENDS IN INTENSIVE CARE UNITS

The first reported use of a computer in an ICU was in 1964 at the University of Southern California in Los Angeles.[8] Jensen and coworkers connected an IBM 1620 digital computer through an analog-to-digital converter to bedside devices that measured and collected values for arterial and venous pressure, body and air temperatures, and urinary output, as well as an electrocardiogram. The computer calculated derived values for cardiac output and other variables related to dye dilution techniques. Of interest, in the discussion portion of their paper, these investigators envisioned most of the potential benefits linked to the use of digital computers and what would be called, many years later, *information technology*.

The research experience with computing in academic ICUs inspired manufacturers of physiological monitoring systems to offer commercial ICU computer systems. Based on a central minicomputer connected to bedside terminals, the system automatically acquired and displayed data from the patients' physiological monitors. However, the minicomputer architecture and crude user interface, which relied on keypads and complex menus, could not meet the demands of clinicians for a fast, easy-to-use system that was seamlessly integrated with the flow of clinical work.

Second-generation systems comprise a majority of the ICU computing systems currently in use. The core clinical functionality is the emulation of the bedside flowsheet.[6] One of the most important issues preventing acceptance of second-generation systems is the difficulty in querying the patient database to support unit management, clinical cost accounting, and clinical research. Performing meaningful database searches requires advanced database skills, forcing the clinician either to learn arcane database languages, such as Structured Query Language (SQL), or to hire a database programmer.

Third-generation information systems offer much of the same clinical functionality of second-generation systems, with well-developed flowsheet presentations of vital signs, medications, fluids, and laboratory results.

Graphic displays and user interface are arguably better with these systems. Software interface libraries substantially diminish the need to pay for expensive customized programming to acquire data automatically from bedside devices.

Third-generation systems are better than second-generation ones in supporting queries against cumulative patient data, but much work still needs to be done before the typical clinician can do this easily.[6]

CURRENT INFORMATION TECHNOLOGY INFRASTRUCTURE

The schematic for single-patient care management presented in Figure 262-1 highlights that caregivers interface with information sources on three different levels[3]: The first level is intradepartmental and includes all of the medical devices directly connected to the bedside, patient data storage, and resident medical applications; the second level is the hospital level, which includes laboratories, the pharmacy, dietary sources, the billing department, and so on; the third level includes Internet databases (registries) and Web-based applications.

A typical network configuration is shown in Figure 262-2. Each bed in the critical care room is equipped with several diagnostic interfaces and therapeutic devices that allow caregivers access to appropriate records and information sources and permit the delivery of therapies. All of the devices can either be directly connected to the local area network (LAN), which is the "bone marrow" of the ICU IT system, or to a local ICU server by way of Ethernet or RS232 connections. The ICU LAN can be facilitated by the introduction of wireless technology that enables mobile computing devices and peripherals to be connected to each other and to network access points to a wider area. Key local wireless technologies include the Infrared Data Associations protocol (iRDA), for the shortest data transmission distance, and Bluetooth and Institute for Electrical and Electronic Engineers (IEEE) 802.11 protocols, for longer distances and broader bandwidths.

The LAN is served with a records server that provides centralized storage of the data generated within the ICU area or as resident applications server to calculate or analyze ICU-specific parameters (medical calculators or decision support systems).

The ICU LAN is separated from the traffic on the hospital intranet and acts as a firewall restricting access to the LAN, or translates the message formats used both inside and outside the LAN. Typically, the LAN is based on Ethernet technologies, to which all of the instruments and medical devices transfer data by wired connection to local servers using proprietary protocols.

At the LAN level, the transmission proprietary protocols have unfortunately been the impediment to even faster growth of IT systems in ICUs. Recently, this issue has been addressed by the IEEE by setting a new standard, IEEE 1073, aimed at providing plug-and-play interoperability among point-of-care medical devices, and devices and systems that manage their operations.[9]

The second network level is the hospital intranet, which is the way of exchanging data among and between several departments (e.g., laboratories, the pharmacy). The intranet is again separated by the next network level by a gateway that acts as firewall to the Internet level, restricting the

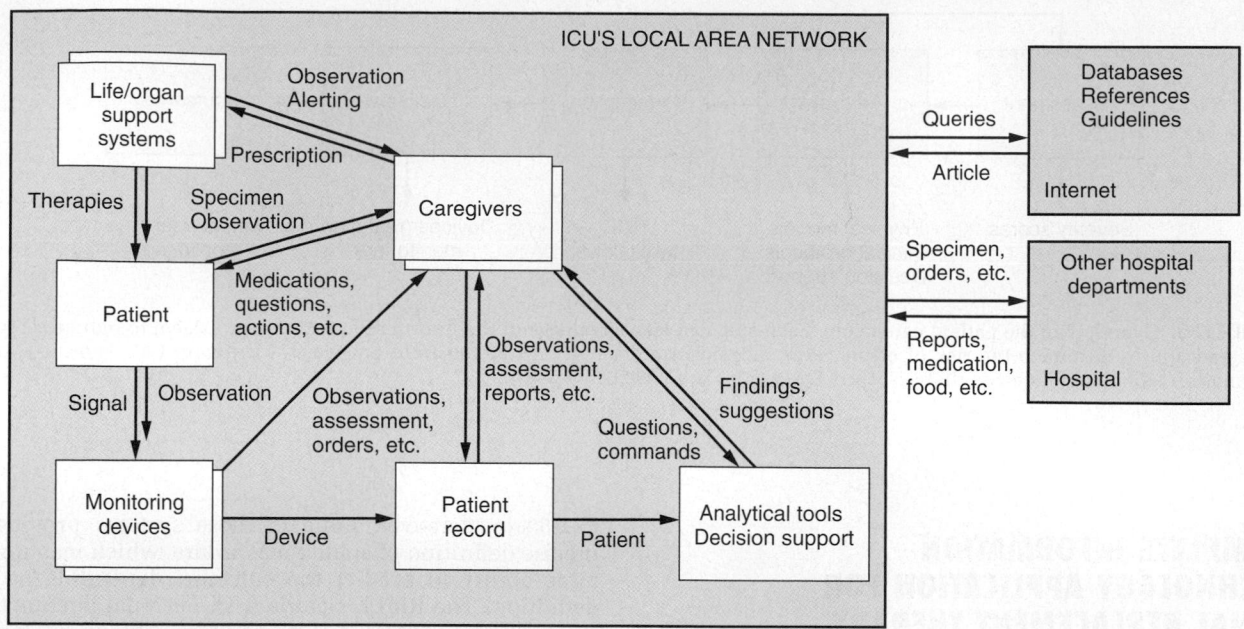

FIGURE 262-1. Schematic diagram of the ICU environment and gateways to information from the caregivers divided by network area. ICU, intensive care unit. (Adapted from Craft RL: Trends in technology and the future intensive care unit. Crit Care Med 2001;29: N151-N158.)

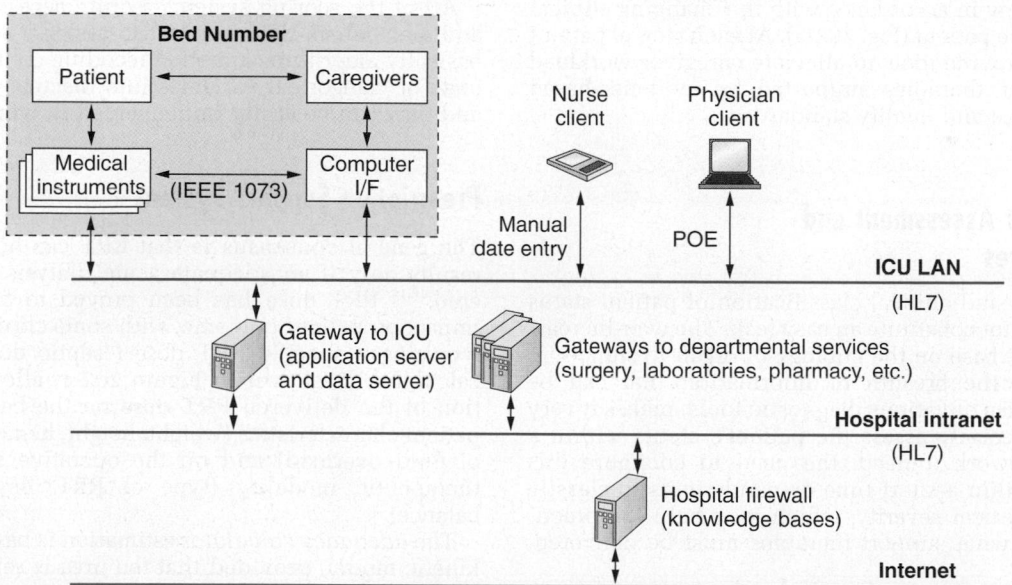

FIGURE 262-2. Typical information technology system infrastructure with three network levels. HL7, Health Standard 7; ICU, intensive care unit; IEEE 1073, Institute for Electrical and Electronic Engineers standard 1073; I/F, interface; LAN; local area network.

access to the intranet network. Software applications of the intranet usually exchange data using the Health Level 7 (HL7) standard, a structured, message-oriented protocol framework for computer communication between health care application systems.

Finally, the third network level is Internet-based. At this level, data are exchanged to wide databases (registries) or to knowledge-based databases (forums) for use in clinical

trials or for rapid exchange of clinical experiences. The data export process should be based on an encrypted data system to guarantee that all patient-related information remains anonymous and blinded to external processing and analysis. This third level also allows for the acquisition of information from Web-based clinical practice guidelines such as the Acute Dialysis Quality Initiative (ADQI).[10]

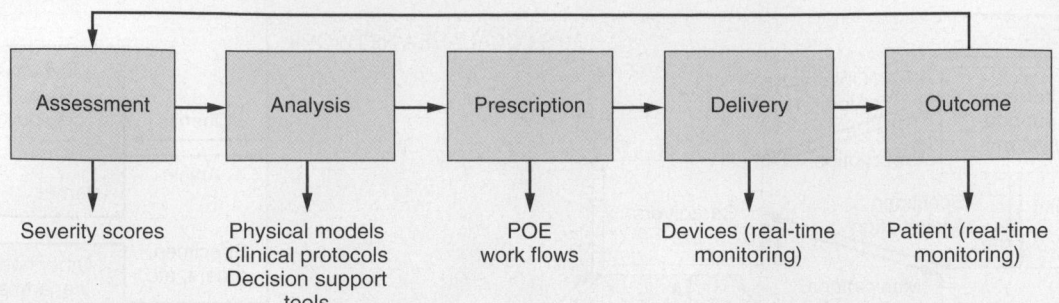

FIGURE 262-3. Overview of the patient care cycle. Each step can take advantage of the information technology system to reduce caregiver workload and to minimize the risk of errors. POE, physician order entry. (Adapted from Savage B, Marquardt GW, Paolini F, et al: Information technology in acute dialysis. Curr Opin Crit Care 2002;8:544-548.)

COMPLETE INFORMATION TECHNOLOGY APPLICATION FOR RENAL REPLACEMENT THERAPY

The patient care cycle is a precise sequence of actions in which information flow begins with the patient's clinical assessment, moves forward to the start of therapy, and proceeds to patient outcome and back to the assessment level, where appropriate feedback directs delivery of time-adjusted therapy in accordance with the changing clinical condition of the patient (Fig. 262-3). At each step of patient care, IT can provide tools to alleviate caregiver workload and to deliver therapies supported by evidence-based clinical practice and quality standards.[11]

Initial Patient Assessment and Severity Scores

The definition and clinical classification of patient status in the ICU do not constitute an easy task. The ever-increasing knowledge base on the etiology of organ dysfunction, coupled with the breadth of information that can be derived with use of various diagnostic tools, makes it very difficult to precisely assess the patient's status within a clinical framework. Indeed, the need to configure this framework within a short time demands tools to classify patients by clinical severity, which may help the practitioner decide what support therapies must be delivered, and when.

The Applied Physiology and Chronic Health Evaluation (APACHE) scales represent the best-known and most widely applied scoring system.[12] The aim of this scoring system is to permit classification of patients into groups for which the survival potential can be established a priori and for which more aggressive care may be beneficial. When used in large populations across several ICUs, the power to correctly predict the outcome was demonstrated to be very high. Like the APACHE scale, additional models, such as the Simplified Acute Physiology Score (SAPS) and Sepsis-Related Organ Failure Assessment (SOFA), were developed to increase predictability of patient survival or to describe the sequence of complications in critically ill patients.[13,14] As applied in CRRT, APACHE, SAPS, and SOFA take renal function into account, but the weight on the overall scores is relatively low (at approximately 12%

to 15%). Moreover, none of these systems provides a precise definition of acute renal failure, which may undermine ability to predict the outcome, depending on the definition. The RIFLE criteria (*r*isk for renal dysfunction, *i*njury to the kidney, *f*ailure of kidney function, *l*oss of kidney function, and *e*nd-stage kidney disease) for classification of acute kidney injury constitute a scoring system developed to overcome this limitation.[15] Despite the lack of clinical data regarding initiation of therapy and outcome, this scoring system has been used for time of initiation and follow-up purposes.[16,17]

All of the scoring systems require access to anamnesis and metabolism data in order to assign a score. They are basically algorithms aimed at recoding continuous or discrete or categorical variables into discrete numeral ones, and they can be easily implemented in worksheets.

Prescription Support System

The general consensus is that RRT can achieve optimal results only if an adequate acute dialysis dose is delivered.[18,19] RRT dose has been proved to have a clinical impact on patient outcome, with some clinical conditions requiring a specific RRT dose ("septic dose").[20] A dose calculator, as shown in Figure 262-4, allows for estimation of the delivered RRT dose on the basis of primary patient characteristics (weight, height, hematocrit, amount of fluid overload) and on the operative settings of the therapeutic modality (type of RRT, flow rates, fluid balance).[21]

The *adequacy calculator* estimation is based on the urea kinetic model, provided that the urea is representative of low-molecular-weight uremic toxins. The calculator prescribes the dialysis dose after the calculated urea clearance, expected treatment time, and body weight are entered.

The main concern with such a calculator is its accuracy in predicting the effective delivered dialysis dose. The adequacy calculator has been found to be fairly accurate, to the extent that the Pearson correlation coefficient was 0.97, even though it showed a tendency to underestimate the effective dose when the urea clearance is higher than 60 mL/minute, but always below the 15% variation coefficient.[21]

A further example of a dialysis calculator has been recently described by Vitale and associates.[22] These investigators used a modified continuous venovenous hemodiafiltration (CVVHDF) (i.e., continuous venovenous

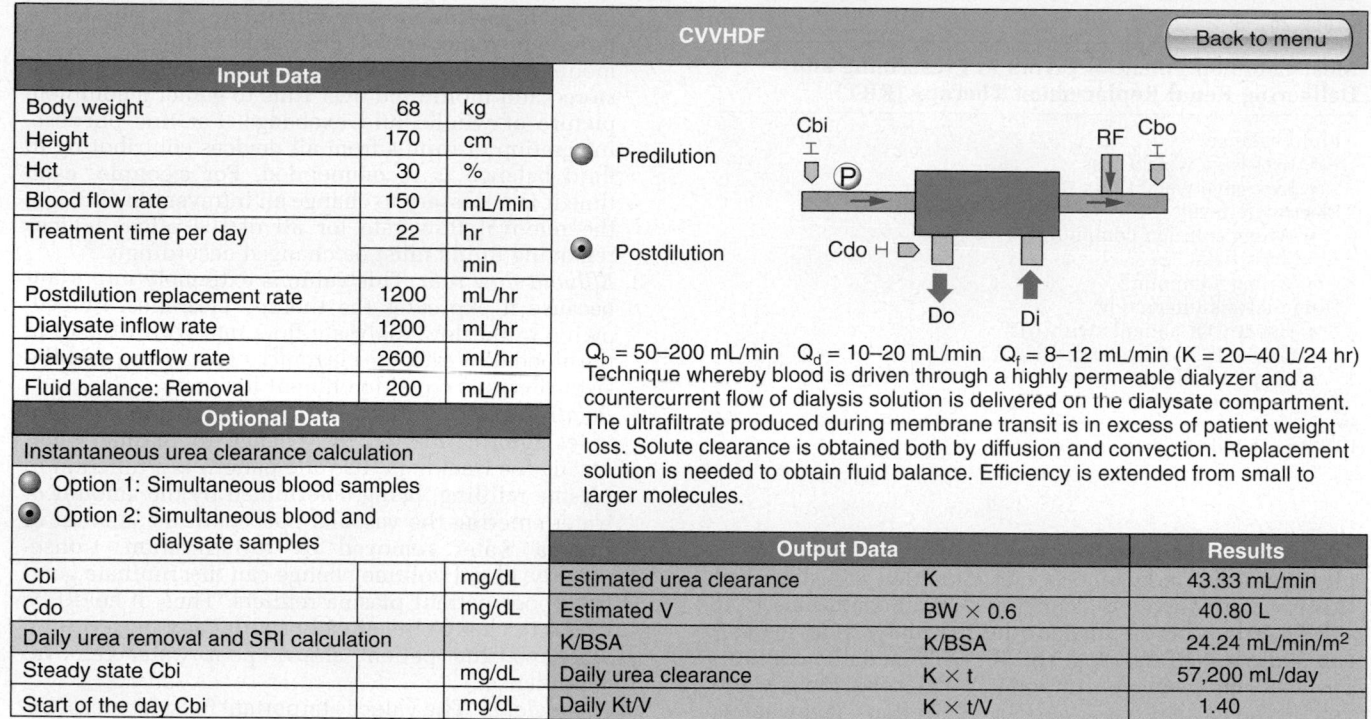

CVVHDF

Back to menu

Input Data		
Body weight	68	kg
Height	170	cm
Hct	30	%
Blood flow rate	150	mL/min
Treatment time per day	22	hr
		min
Postdilution replacement rate	1200	mL/hr
Dialysate inflow rate	1200	mL/hr
Dialysate outflow rate	2600	mL/hr
Fluid balance: Removal	200	mL/hr
Optional Data		
Instantaneous urea clearance calculation		

○ Option 1: Simultaneous blood samples

◉ Option 2: Simultaneous blood and
dialysate samples

Cbi		mg/dL
Cdo		mg/dL
Daily urea removal and SRI calculation		
Steady state Cbi		mg/dL
Start of the day Cbi		mg/dL

○ Predilution

◉ Postdilution

Q_b = 50–200 mL/min Q_d = 10–20 mL/min Q_f = 8–12 mL/min (K = 20–40 L/24 hr)
Technique whereby blood is driven through a highly permeable dialyzer and a countercurrent flow of dialysis solution is delivered on the dialysate compartment. The ultrafiltrate produced during membrane transit is in excess of patient weight loss. Solute clearance is obtained both by diffusion and convection. Replacement solution is needed to obtain fluid balance. Efficiency is extended from small to larger molecules.

Output Data		Results
Estimated urea clearance	K	43.33 mL/min
Estimated V	BW × 0.6	40.80 L
K/BSA	K/BSA	24.24 mL/min/m²
Daily urea clearance	K × t	57,200 mL/day
Daily Kt/V	K × t/V	1.40

FIGURE 262-4. Adequacy dose calculator. This tool can be used to prescribe continuous renal replacement therapy and to estimate the delivered dose according to the patient's clinical condition (body weight [BW], hematocrit [Hct], fluid excess) and procedure-specific requirements. BSA, body surface area; Cbi, concentration at blood inlet; Cdo, concentration at blood outlet; Do, dialysate outlet; Di, dialysate inlet; K, clearance; Q_b, blood flow rate; Q_d, dialysate flow rate; Q_f, flow rate; SRI, solute removal index. (Adapted from Ricci Z, Salvatori G, Bonello M, et al: In vivo validation of the adequacy calculator for continuous renal replacement therapy. Crit Care 2005;9: R266-R273.)

acetate-free biofiltration [CVVAFB]) protocol in which the acid-base correction was obtained by infusing, in predilution mode, a sterile solution of sodium bicarbonate at a concentration of 167 mEq/L. The composition of the dialysate was completely buffer-free. This compelling hemodiafiltration technique needs to be tailored to the patient's acid-base status; the infusate and dialysate flow rates must be adjusted to achieve a steady-state bicarbonatemia at an HCO_3^- concentration of approximately 28 to 30 mEq/L. The computer program then calculates these two parameters by mathematical modeling of plasma sodium and bicarbonate. The input data are patient weight, height, hematocrit, and endogenous fixed acid generation and additional metabolic parameters, as well as therapy-specific parameters such as blood, dialysate, infusate, and ultrafiltration flow rates; the output data are the estimated final values of plasma sodium and bicarbonate. The accuracy of the model in predicting the actual plasma values of Na^+ and HCO_3^- was high ($y = x - 0.55$; $r = 0.61$; $P = .021$ for Na^+; $y = x - 1.61$; $r = 0.87$; $P < .001$ for HCO_3^-).

Even more complex is modeling the flow rates in the regional anticoagulation technique based on sodium citrate. This is a very attractive technique suited for use in patients at high risk for bleeding (such as postsurgical patients) or at potential risk for heparin-induced thrombocytopenia. The technique's main drawback lies in the fact that unadjusted blood, substitution, and dialysate flow rates can easily result in hypernatremia, alkalosis, and hypocalcemia. Hence, a computer program capable of accurately defining the level of all flow rates used in CVVHDF with sodium citrate would be ideal. Unfortunately, models of this task are lacking.

Renal Replacement Therapy Physician Order Entry

Based on the assumption that human decision making is inherently limited, the likelihood of medication errors increases at a rate at least proportional to the amount of excess information clinicians need to process. Medication errors are reported to result in nearly 1% of adverse reactions and in nearly 7% of potential adverse reactions. The correlated cost has been estimated at approximately $2000 per event and $2 billion per year at a national level.[23] Computer-based decision-making support systems and computerized physician order entry (POE) can maximize efficient and accurate integration of data, potentially resulting in better prescription compliance, error rate reduction, and improved health care quality.[24]

POE systems are IT tools by which clinicians can enter medical orders on line in a database integrating clinical practice with patient data. As an example, POE can avoid prescription of drugs for which the patient is known to be at risk for an adverse reaction, or of multidrug regimens that carry increased potential for drug-drug interactions.

The most common errors in RRT are listed in Table 262-3. These RRT errors may be associated with various adverse effects such as signs and symptoms (e.g., nausea, vomiting, cramps, hypotension, severe arrhythmias, severe acidosis or alkalosis, filter clotting) occurring during the dialysis session but also may potentially result in ineffective treatment or, worse, in organ impairment or injury. Moreover, ready access to computerized prescription orders may be especially relevant in RRT because the treat-

TABLE 262-3

Most Common Potential Errors in Prescribing and Delivering Renal Replacement Therapy (RRT)

Fluid balance
- Excessive weight loss
- Excessive weight loss rate

Electrolyte levels
- Wrong solution compound

Acid-base balance
- Wrong compound

Drug-dialysis interaction
- Heparin in patients with HIT
- Citrate in patients with liver failure
- Drug pharmacokinetics

RRT underdosage

HIT, heparin-induced thrombocytopenia.

ment may extend over multiple caregiver shifts. Unambiguous orders and reports may facilitate adjustment of therapy components to changing clinical conditions.[26]

RRT orders can be loaded into the dialysis device and can address the following: specific RRT modality continuous venovenous hemofiltration (CVVH), continuous venovenous hemodialysis (CVVHD), continuous venovenous hemodiafiltration (CVVHDF), slow continuous ultrafiltration (SCRUF), plasma exchange, or hemoperfusion), the eventual pre- or post-infusion mode, anticoagulation regimen (type and mode of delivery), disposable set, weight loss, and weight loss rate. For each parameter, a preset monitor configuration can be used; in some instances, certain operating limits (e.g., flow rates) can be selected, or preset alarms are included, making the therapy even safer. POE also allows for the designation of unambiguous and appropriate RRT protocols in terms of filter types, compounds, and anticoagulants.

POE must be traceable both during the prescription phase and whenever a change in the prescription is submitted in a treatment session.

ONLINE THERAPY MONITORING

CRRT monitoring is essential because such therapy is a long and complex process that includes several parameters and alarms, often with data acquired from different devices. The main parameters available for data transfer from CRRT monitors to ICU data storage are the following:

1. *Weight loss rate.* The desired rate of weight loss specifies the amount of fluid to be removed hourly from the patient's body. This value must be set at the beginning of the CRRT session according to the estimated fluid overload associated with overhydration of the patient or medication-induced overload. It is advisable to set an upper limit alarm because the risk of hypovolemia-induced hypotension increases as the weight loss rate increases.

2. *Fluid balance.* The fluid balance accounts for the total fluid delivered to the patient and the total fluid removed. The fluid balance must account also for body weight loss. This value must be accurately monitored to avoid excess fluid removal from the patient or to prevent fluid overload.[25] CRRT monitors usually can automatically calculate the fluid balance, so each time the clinical status dictates, for example, the need to increase the amount of fluid replaced to the patient

(as in high-volume hemofiltration), the amount of fluid to be removed will change accordingly. Of paramount importance, however, these data must be stored and monitored over time to gather a complete picture of whole fluid exchange. For this purpose, integration of inputs from all devices contributing to fluid balance is recommended. For example, each time it is necessary to change an intravenous therapy, the removal flow rate for all of the other devices removing fluids must be changed accordingly.[25]

3. *Effluent flow rate.* This value is extremely important because it expresses the therapy clearance. Indeed, owing to the low dialysate flow rate with respect to the blood flow rate, the clearance of small and middle-size solutes is equal to effluent flow rate.

4. *Relative blood volume change.* This parameter provides information on the change in plasma water during the treatment. Its time pattern is a function of plasma refilling, being determined by the amount of water entering the vascular space and the amount of plasma water removed by ultrafiltration. Consequently, blood volume change can discriminate good from poor patient plasma refillers. Thus, it could be useful to change the already set therapy prescription whenever the patient shows poor water removal compliance.

5. *Hemoglobin.* The value is important for safety reasons, particularly when the patient begins CRRT therapy with low hemoglobin values. It also is used for monitoring the oxyhemoglobin concentration.

6. *Transmembrane pressure.* This parameter is closely related to the treatment setting, particularly for convection at the filter and amount of anticoagulant used. The transmembrane pressure becomes extremely important when low heparin dosage or heparin-free treatments are delivered to a patient at high risk for bleeding. Close monitoring of the transmembrane pressure may prevent clotting of the extracorporeal circuit, which otherwise could result in termination of the treatment session with loss of the blood inside the circuit.

7. *Access (or arterial) and return (or venous) pressures.* These parameters are useful for monitoring access function. The access pressure should not be excessively negative; otherwise, recirculation within the access site itself would be favored, reducing overall treatment efficiency. Negative pressure also can highlight incorrect positioning of the vascular access. On the other hand, return pressure should not be excessively positive. Such values can be an indication of high return-flow resistance, incorrect access positioning, or thrombus formation.

8. *Alarms.* Many of the foregoing parameters must be supervised with use of specific alarms to alert caregivers to the occurrence of wide deviations from preset values. Many of these alarms must be individualized, being patient-dependent, such as for weight loss rate, relative blood volume changes, and access and return pressures.

CONCLUSION

The ICU environment is complex, requiring an IT infrastructure capable of integrating multiple sources of information and making the data readily accessible and applicable. IT can help caregivers to efficiently and accurately assess the clinical status of critically ill patients in order to deliver an appropriate therapeutic protocol or to change components of therapy in an easier and more functional way.

Key References

3. Craft RL: Trends in technology and the future intensive care unit. Crit Care Med 2001;29:N151-N158.
5. Bates DW, Teich JM, Lee J, et al: The impact of computerized physician order entry on medication errors prevention. J Am Med Inform Assoc 1999;6:313-321.
6. Seiver A: Critical care computing: Past, present, future. Crit Care Clin 2000;16:601-621.
11. Savage B, Marquardt GW, Paolini F, et al: Information technology in acute dialysis. Curr Opin Crit Care 2002;8:544-548.
21. Ricci Z, Salvatori G, Bonello M, et al: In vivo validation of the adequacy calculator for continuous renal replacement therapy. Critical Care 2005;9:R266-R273.

See the companion Expert Consult website for the complete reference list.

CHAPTER 263

Adjustment of Antimicrobial Regimen in Septic Patients Undergoing Continuous Renal Replacement Therapy in the Intensive Care Unit

Dingwei Kuang, Chang Yin Chionh, and Claudio Ronco

OBJECTIVES

This chapter will:
1. Review the current status of sepsis and antimicrobial therapy strategy in the intensive care unit.
2. Discuss the effects of sepsis, acute renal failure, and continuous renal replacement therapy on the pharmacological properties of antimicrobials.
3. Present the rationale for and principles of adjustment of antimicrobial regimens in critically ill patients undergoing continuous renal replacement therapy.

Critically ill patients are at increased risk for the development of bacteremia as a result of alterations in their host defense mechanisms caused by the precipitating disease, the extensive use of invasive procedures, and coexisting endogenous or exogenous immunosuppression. Accordingly, infection is a common problem in the intensive care unit (ICU). Furthermore, a study by de Lalla demonstrated that the infection rate among patients in the ICU was 5 to 10 times higher than among general ward patients, and that infections acquired in these units account for more than 20% of all nosocomial infections.

Acute renal failure (ARF) represents a frequent, severe complication in critically ill patients, and it is increasingly seen as part of the multiple organ dysfunction syndrome (MODS), which is the most frequent cause of death in patients admitted to ICUs. From the available data, severe sepsis and septic shock are the primary causes of MODS. In the past several decades, a dramatic evolution in extracorporeal blood purification (ECBP) technology has led to new machines and new techniques for the therapy of critically ill patients in the ICU.[1] Now, continuous renal replacement therapy (CRRT) is widely used in the management of septic patients with or without ARF in ICU because it offers several advantages over conventional intermittent hemodialysis and peritoneal dialysis.[2]

At present, delivery of effective and safe antimicrobial therapy poses one of the greatest challenges to the intensivist in the management of septic patients in the ICU, with persistently high mortality and morbidity rates observed in clinical practice.[3] Of increasing relevance in this setting, sepsis, ARF, and CRRT may have profound effects on the pharmacological properties of various antimicrobials. This chapter reviews the current status of sepsis, ARF, and ECBP therapies in the ICU, considers the impact of these factors on the pharmacological properties of antimicrobials, and explores adjustment of the antimicrobial regimen in critically ill patients.

INFECTION AND SEPSIS IN THE INTENSIVE CARE UNIT: CURRENT STATUS

Definition

The presence of infection is recognized to be an important determinant of outcome for patients requiring ICU admission. *Infection* is the invasion of a tissue or organ by a pathogenic microorganism and generally is characterized by the organism responsible and the organ concerned. *Sepsis* is the complex, systemic inflammatory response to this infection. *Severe sepsis* and *septic shock* are defined according to the degree of organ involvement.[4] Although a number of published systems have suggested working definitions for such terms and concepts, universally agreed-upon definitions of infection are lacking. Therefore, the International Sepsis Forum recently convened an international consensus conference to formulate a set of definitions of infections that occur commonly in the ICU, to improve the quality and comparability of clinical trials of sepsis therapies.[5]

Epidemiology

According to the European Prevalence of Infection in Intensive Care (EPIC) report, 44.8% of patients in ICUs had a microbiologically confirmed infection on the day of their evaluation, and an ICU-acquired infection was found in 20.6% of the patients. The most common type of infection acquired in an ICU was pneumonia (46.9%); other infections included lower respiratory tract infections (17.8%), urinary tract infections (17.8%), and bloodstream infections (12%). Members of Enterobacteriaceae (34.4%), *Staphylococcus aureus* (30.1%), and *Pseudomonas aeruginosa* (28.7%) were the most common pathogens associated with infection.

In the United States, a survey by Rechards and colleagues of data for a total of 498,998 patients admitted to 205 ICUs showed that pneumonia was the most frequent nosocomial infection (31%), followed by urinary tract infection (23%) and primary bloodstream infection (14%). The most common pathogens recovered from these three sites were *S. aureus* (17%), *Escherichia coli* (19%), and coagulase-negative staphylococci (39%).

A multicenter study by Alberti and coworkers involving 28 ICUs was conducted in six European countries, Israel, and Canada. Of the total of 14,364 patients, 21.1% were infected on admission. Respiratory, digestive, urinary tract, and primary bloodstream infections represented approximately 80% of all cases. Approximately 28% of infections were associated with sepsis, 24% with severe sepsis, and 30% with septic shock. The crude in-hospital mortality rates ranged from 16.9% for noninfected patients to 53.6% for patients with hospital-acquired infections.

More recently, Harrison and associates presented the results of the secondary analysis of a high-quality clinical database, the ICNARC Case Mix Programme Database, containing data for 343,860 patients admitted to 172 ICUs in England, Wales, and Northern Ireland from 1996 to 2004. The percentage of patients with severe sepsis during the first 24 hours rose from 23.5% in 1996 to 28.7% in 2004, reflecting an increase from an estimated 18,500 to 31,000 admissions to all ICUs. The in-hospital mortality rate for patients with severe sepsis decreased from 48.3% in 1996 to 44.7% in 2004.

Studies by Angus and colleagues in 192,980 patients with severe sepsis in the 847 nonfederal hospitals in seven U.S. states indicated that the average costs per case were $22,100, with annual total costs of $16.7 billion nationally. Recently, Padkin and Martin and coworkers found that the sepsis syndromes and their sequelae are associated with mortality rates of 30% to 45% and consumption of 45% of ICU and 33% of hospital bed-days.

Antimicrobial Therapy Strategy

Appropriate antibacterial therapy to achieve effective active drug concentrations that result in clinical cure while avoiding drug-associated toxicity is still the most fundamental and important aspect of management of septic patients.[4] It is important not only in ensuring an optimal clinical outcome but also in controlling the emergence of resistance among pathogenic microorganisms and in containing costs. Selection of such an appropriate antimicrobial regimen in this setting involves many considerations, including the site of infection, the patient's clinical status, the presumptive pathogen(s), the kind of antimicrobial agent (single or combination), the dosage and dosing interval of the antimicrobial agent, and so on. Inadequate empirical antimicrobial therapy has been recognized as an independent risk factor for in-hospital mortality. Recent studies by MacArthur and associates showed that adequate antimicrobial therapy influences outcome for patients in ICUs, because mortality was significantly higher for those receiving inadequate than for those receiving adequate therapy.

ACUTE RENAL FAILURE IN THE INTENSIVE CARE UNIT

Definition

ARF occurs frequently as a part of MODS in the ICU. The most controversial aspect of ARF is the definition. Indeed, more than 30 definitions appear in the recent literature. The variability of definitions used in clinical studies is an important determinant of the wide range in reported occurrence rates and associated mortality rates for ARF. In fact, the lack of a uniform definition for ARF is believed to be a major impediment to research in this field. In order to establish a uniform definition for ARF, the Acute Dialysis Quality Initiative (ADQI) group proposed the RIFLE classification of acute kidney injury (risk, injury, failure, loss of function, end-stage disease) and recently updated the modified RIFLE criteria. This classification defines three grades of increasing severity of ARF (risk, injury, and failure), and two outcome variables (loss and end-stage kidney disease).[6] A unique feature of the RIFLE classification is that it provides for three grades of severity of renal dysfunction on the basis of a change in serum creatinine or urine output from the baseline condition. RIFLE is a newer classification system; nevertheless, several studies by Bell and Herget and coworkers have suggested that RIFLE is a valid predictor of clinical outcomes and correlates with existing biomarkers of ARF.

Epidemiology

The Beginning and Ending Supporting Therapy for the Kidney (BEST Kidney) Study, which was conducted in 54 centers (23 countries) around the world, found that among 29,269 critically ill patients, the period prevalence of ARF during their ICU stay is 5.7% all over the world. Of the patients with ARF, 72.5% patients were treated with renal replacement therapy (RRT), and CRRT is the most common initial modality used (80.0%). The most common contributing factor for ARF was septic shock (47.5%). Overall in-hospital mortality rate was 60.3%. Rate of dialysis dependence at hospital discharge was 13.8% for survivors. Independent risk factors for hospital mortality included use of vasopressors, mechanical ventilation, septic shock, cardiogenic shock, and hepatorenal syndrome.

The incidence of ARF depends on the definition used and the population studied. Combining other recently published results for ARF in the ICU, sepsis is demonstrated to be the leading cause of ARF in the ICU, occurring in approximately 19% of patients with moderate sepsis, 23% of those with severe sepsis, and 51% of those with septic shock when blood cultures are positive. The incidence of ARF is 10% to 25%. Overall mortality rate in patients who are admitted with ARF or in whom ARF develops in the ICU is 23% to 80%. Patients with ARF not requiring RRT have a mortality rate of 10% to 53%. However, patients in whom ARF requiring RRT develops have a higher mortality rate of 57% to 80%.[7] Of those patients with ARF who receive RRT and survive, only 5% to 30% require longer-term dialysis. This wide variation in published results is due in part to various problems not specifically addressed in a majority of studies: variable definition of ARF and inclusion criteria, significant heterogeneity of the population in terms of severity of illness and demographics, different incidence rates for renal injury and mortality with different disease processes, variable duration of outcome analysis, and so on.

EXTRACORPOREAL BLOOD PURIFICATION THERAPY IN THE INTENSIVE CARE UNIT: BEYOND RENAL REPLACEMENT THERAPY

Different Choices of Dialytic Modality in Critically Ill Patients

Traditional cornerstones of RRT for critically ill patients with ARF have included intermittent hemodialysis and peritoneal dialysis. However, studies by Schiffl and coworkers indicated that daily intermittent hemodialysis was better than alternate-day intermittent hemodialysis in critically ill patients who require RRT, improving the time to resolution and survival at 14 days. Several advances have been made in this area, particularly with respect to volumetrically controlled machines with precise ultrafiltration control, variable sodium concentration, bicarbonate-buffered dialysate, and online production of ultrapure or sterile dialysis or substitution fluids. Peritoneal dialysis techniques continue to occupy a small niche for RRT, particularly in pediatric patients. In our opinion, peritoneal dialysis is not suited to the care of critically ill adult patients in a modern ICU. Not only does it require surgical placement of a catheter into the peritoneum, but it also is associated with a high rate of peritoneal infection, achieves inadequate solute clearances, and cannot maintain optimal uremic control. Moreover, peritoneal dialysis also impedes diaphragmatic movement, is associated with abdominal wall leaks, and induces rapid glucose absorption with unpredictable and highly variable levels of glycemia.[8]

In the early 1980s, when ARF changed its epidemiological pattern and involvement of other organs became more and more common, contemporary methods for provision of CRRT have emerged as a new form of artificial renal support in the ICU.[9] Use of CRRT is much more common in Europe, although its use is highly variable between centers, and CRRT is the predominant choice in Australia. In the United States, CRRT is now being used at ever-increasing rates, up from more than 25% of all patients with ARF before 1999 to 60% recently. Because current evidence is insufficient to permit strong conclusions regarding the choice of mode for RRT in critically ill patients, it is noteworthy that currently the choice of intermittent or continuous therapy is largely based on the availability of CRRT and not on evidence-based indications. Nevertheless, CRRT has several theoretical advantages compared with intermittent hemodialysis, including enhanced hemodynamic stability, increased solute removal, greater ultrafiltration capacity, and the possibility of a favorable effect on the inflammatory response.[8,9]

Timing and Criteria for Starting Continuous Renal Replacement Therapy in the Intensive Care Unit

No absolute rules have emerged regarding when CRRT should begin, but too early is better than too late, and the treatment should be started before complications occur.[8] Indications for immediate treatment in critically ill patients with ARF include hyperkalemia (causing significant electrocardiographic changes), severe pulmonary edema, uremic acidosis (causing cardiac compromise), and gross uremia (Table 263-1).

Recent Advances in Continuous Renal Replacement Therapy Technology in the Intensive Care Unit

Two interesting aspects of the evolution of RRT in the ICU over the past decade are represented by the definition of an "adequate" dose of dialysis in ARF and the potential application of high-dose therapies for the treatment of sepsis.[1] In a landmark clinical trial by Ronco and

TABLE 263-1

Criteria for Starting Continuous Renal Replacement Therapy (CRRT) in the Intensive Care Unit

- Oliguria (urine output <200 mL/12 hours)
- Anuria (urine output <50 mL/12 hours)
- Severe acidemia (pH <7.1) due to metabolic acidosis
- Azotemia ([urea] >30 mmol/L)
- Hyperkalemia ([K^+] >6.5 mmol/L or rapidly rising [K^+])
- Suspected uremic organ involvement (pericarditis, encephalopathy, neuropathy, myopathy)
- Severe dysnatremia ([Na^+] >160 or <115 mmol/L)
- Hyperthermia (core temperature >39.5° C)
- Clinically significant organ edema (especially lung)
- Drug overdose with dialyzable toxin
- Coagulopathy requiring large amounts of blood products in patient at risk for development of pulmonary edema or ARDS

Meeting one of the criteria constitutes sufficient grounds for initiating CRRT. Meeting two of the criteria makes CRRT essentially mandatory. Combined derangements suggest the initiation of CRRT even before some of the above-mentioned "limits" have been reached.
ARDS, acute respiratory distress syndrome.

coworkers, the first of a dialysis dose of 35 mL/kg per hour improves survival, whereas higher doses do not seem to give additional benefits in the general population. The second concept introduces the rationale for high-volume hemofiltration (HVHF) in critically ill patients with ARF and sepsis. HVHF is a variant of CVVH that requires greater-surface-area hemofilters and uses ultrafiltration volumes of 35 to 80 mL/kg per hour. The high dose that characterizes HVHF can be delivered either using a constantly high exchange rate or by delivering a "pulse" (for 6 to 8 hours) of very HVHF (85 to 100 mL/kg per hour), followed by standard doses.[10]

One of the most important advances of the past decade is the combined use of adsorbent techniques in systems. Coupled plasma filtration and adsorption (CPFA), which has been shown to have beneficial effects in septic patients, is a combined therapy in which plasma is separated from blood and circulated through a sorbent bed. After this purification phase, blood is reconstituted and dialyzed with standard techniques. The final effect is an increased removal of protein-bound solutes and large-molecular-weight toxins. Nonspecific removal of a broad range of inflammatory mediators by HVHF and CPFA may be beneficial, as recently suggested on the basis of the *peak concentration hypothesis*. Given the available data, it is possible to speculate that immunomodulation using HVHF will be most useful in the early stages of severe sepsis and septic shock, when high levels of inflammatory mediators appear in the circulation. Nonetheless, research is needed to evaluate the effect of HVHF and CPFA on clinical outcome, or the effect of different modalities of CRRT on length of hospital or ICU stay and recovery of renal function in critically ill patients with sepsis.[1]

ARF is not the only clinical disorder observed in ICU patients, nor is it any longer regarded as an isolated syndrome. ECBP management of such patients cannot focus solely on RRT. In these cases, conventional RRT no longer represents an adequate form of therapy. In accordance with current knowledge of the molecular biology of sepsis, a "humoral" theory of MODS makes pathophysiological sense, with a corollary that specifies the need to consider ECBP techniques as multiple organ support therapy (MOST), rather than merely single organ support.[9]

BASIC PHARMACOLOGICAL PARAMETERS OF ANTIMICROBIAL AGENTS: PHARMACOKINETICS AND PHARMACODYNAMICS

A constellation of pathophysiological changes can occur in patients with sepsis, along with related organ failure and the need for organ-supportive therapy, the effects of which complicate antimicrobial dosing. Knowledge of the pharmacokinetic and pharmacodynamic properties of the antimicrobials used for the management of sepsis is essential for selecting the optimal antimicrobial dosage regimen. Rational and optimal dosing of anti-infective therapy must consider the related pharmacokinetic and pharmacodynamic principles.

Pharmacokinetic Parameters

Pharmacokinetics refers to the study of concentration changes of a drug over a given period. The primary pharmacokinetic parameters of importance to antimicrobials include the following[3]:
- Plasma protein binding (PPB)
- Volume of distribution (V_d)
- Clearance (Cl)
- Half-life ($T_{1/2}$)
- Peak serum drug concentration achieved by a single dose (C_{max})
- Minimum serum drug concentration during a dosing period (C_{min})
- Area under the serum concentration-time curve (AUC)

These factors can be used to determine whether appropriate concentrations of the antimicrobial agents are being delivered to the target area.[11]

Pharmacodynamic Parameters

Pharmacodynamics is the study of the biochemical and physiological effects of drugs and their mechanisms of action. Pharmacodynamic parameters relate the pharmacokinetic factors to the ability of an antimicrobial to kill or inhibit the growth of the infecting organism. Pharmacodynamic parameters include the following[3]:
- Time for which the serum concentration of a drug remains above the minimum inhibitory concentration (MIC) for a dosing period (T > MIC)
- Ratio of the maximum (peak) antimicrobial concentration, C_{max}, to MIC (C_{max}/MIC)
- Ratio of the AUC during a 24-hour period to MIC (AUC_{24}/MIC)
- Postantibiotic effect (PAE)

Pharmacodynamically, the rate and extent of the bactericidal activity of an antimicrobial agent are dependent on the interaction between and among drug concentration at the site of infection, bacterial load, phase of bacterial growth, and the MIC for the pathogen.[11] It follows that a change in any of these factors will alter the activity of the antimicrobial agent against a particolar pathogen and may affect the outcome of therapy.

Kill Characteristics of Antimicrobial Agents

Different antimicrobial classes appear to have different types of "kill characteristics," or lethal effects on bacteria.[3] The β-lactam group of antimicrobials have a time-dependent (or concentration-independent) kill characteristic, with T > MIC being the best predictor of efficacy. These agents appear to have improved antimicrobial efficacy when the exposure time, rather than concentration, is maximized. Other representative agents in this group include aztreonam, carbapenems, macrolides, clindamycin, and vancomycin. By contrast, aminoglycosides, metronidazole, and daptomycin have a concentration-dependent (or time-independent) kill characteristic. More effective killing is observed with higher concentrations. C_{max}/MIC and AUC/MIC ratios are the parameters correlating with clinical efficacy for this group of agents. Fluoroquinolones are more complex and initially were reported to be C_{max}/MIC–dependent, although subsequent studies also have found that AUC_{24}/MIC is important. In determining dosing frequency, consideration also should be made for those antimicrobials that exhibit a PAE, or prolonged activity observed even when concentrations fall below the MIC.

IMPACT OF SEPSIS ON PHARMACOLOGICAL CHARACTERISTICS OF ANTIMICROBIAL AGENTS: BASED ON PATHOPHYSIOLOGICAL CHANGES

The appropriate prescription of antimicrobials requires a detailed knowledge of the pathophysiological and subsequent pharmacokinetic changes that occur throughout the course of sepsis. Concomitant patient factors to be considered that may influence the pharmacological characteristics include changes in total body water, albumin and acute-phase protein levels, muscle mass, blood pH, bilirubin concentration, as well as renal, hepatic, and cardiac function. Changes in V_d and clearance of the antimicrobials have been noted in sepsis, which will affect the antimicrobial concentration at the target site. It follows that the pharmacodynamic parameters that determine antimicrobial efficacy, which can vary between antimicrobial classes, also may be affected.[3]

Various endogenous inflammatory mediators are produced during the development of sepsis. These mediators may affect the vascular endothelium directly or indirectly, resulting in maldistribution of blood flow, endothelial damage, and increased capillary permeability, which will cause fluid shifts from the intravascular compartment to the interstitial space. This will increase V_d of water-soluble antimicrobials, which decreases their serum drug concentration. In addition, an interesting possibility is that the serum concentration of albumin may change in these critically ill patients, because acute-phase reactant proteins (e.g., α_1-acid glycoproteins) are synthesized preferentially. The binding affinity of drugs to albumin also may decrease as a result of uremia.

Hypotension is very common as a result of the inflammatory response associated with sepsis. Inotropic agents often are prescribed in septic patients who fail to respond to administration of intravenous fluids, resulting in an increased cardiac index and renal preload. Consequently, serum creatinine and drug clearance are increased in patients without kidney or liver dysfunction. This increase in clearance is the major reason for the different dosing requirements between patients requiring ICU management and those managed on general hospital wards.[12]

As a serious complication, MODS often occurs in patients with sepsis and results in a consequent decrease in antimicrobial clearance, which prolongs elimination $T_{1/2}$ and may increase antimicrobial concentrations or lead to the accumulation of metabolites. The effects of renal dysfunction and RRT on the pharmacological parameters are discussed later on. Of note, these pathophysiological changes will reverse with recovery from sepsis. Furthermore, because the physiology of these patients may change over a relatively short period of time, ongoing evaluation of severity is indicated to allow timely adjustment of antimicrobial dosing.[3]

IMPACT OF ACUTE KIDNEY INJURY ON PHARMACOLOGICAL CHARACTERISTICS AND DOSAGE ADJUSTMENT OF ANTIMICROBIAL AGENTS: DIFFERENCE FROM CHRONIC KIDNEY DISEASE

Many drugs pass through the glomeruli from the circulation, especially if they are water-soluble; therefore, impaired renal function may have profound effects on the pharmacokinetics and pharmacodynamics of renal-excreted antimicrobials, necessitating modification of the dosage regimen in order to avoid toxicity through accumulation of the parent or its metabolites. The most universal pharmacokinetic equation is[13]

$$T_{1/2} = 0.693 \times V_d/Cl \qquad [1]$$

Because $T_{1/2}$ is reciprocal to the clearance, an interpolation for any degree of renal impairment can be made from the extreme values for normal kidney function and anuria. $T_{1/2}$ is the pharmacokinetic characteristic most profoundly changed with renal dysfunction. For example, the normal $T_{1/2}$ is 2 hours for ceftazidime but 24 hours with anuria. If renal function is reduced to 50%, a $T_{1/2}$ of 12 hours can be interpolated.[13]

Although the V_d for most drugs rises slightly because of water retention, these discrepancies are considerably smaller than the total volume of body fluid; as a result, the influence on pharmacokinetics is limited. Large inter- and intraindividual variations in actual V_d, however, have been described in critically ill patients with ARF. A difference in PPB also has been found as a result of reduction in net protein content and accumulation of various kinds of uremic toxins.

Neither renal failure nor ECBP therapy requires adjustment of the loading dose, which depends solely on V_d. Maintenance doses for drugs that undergo considerable renal excretion should be adapted to the reduced renal clearance, however.[14] Two different approaches are used in adjusting drug dosage in accordance with degree of impairment of renal function in nondialyzed patients: the Dettli rule and the Kunin rule. *Dettli's proportional dose reduction rule* adjusts the maintenance dosage in proportion to the reduced clearance. Alternatively, *Kunin's half-dosage rule* is derived from the elimination $T_{1/2}$. The normal starting dose is given, and one half of the starting dose is repeated at an interval corresponding to one $T_{1/2}$. The Dettli rule results in an AUC that is the same as in normal subjects. With the Kunin rule, the peak levels are identical (C_{max}), but the AUC and the C_{min} are higher than in normal subjects.[13]

Because the adjustment of antimicrobial regimen depends mainly on the glomerular filtration rate (GFR) of the patient, a precise estimate of GFR is rather important. In clinical practice, it is customary to estimate the GFR based on serum creatinine concentration if the patient's renal function is stable, using the Cockcroft-Gault equation. A newer equation derived from the Modification of Diet in Renal Disease (MDRD) study has been found to provide a significantly more accurate estimate of the GFR than estimates obtained with other commonly used equations. Of note, however, a comparative analysis demonstrated statistically significant differences between the Cockcroft-Gault and the MDRD equations, resulting in different antimicrobial dosing recommendations in 21% to 37% of patients. Therefore, the MDRD equation should not be advocated as the preferred method to estimate renal function to make critical decisions about medication dosing.[15]

If the patient is anuric or in ARF, the MDRD equation will not give a true reflection of GFR. It is still difficult to obtain an accurate measurement of GFR in patients with ARF in non–steady-state conditions. Convenient biochemical markers such as serum creatinine or blood urea nitrogen are not accurate reflections of renal function, owing to the lag time in rapidly fluctuating renal function. Each of these variables, however, has limitations for use as a marker of GFR in patients with ARF. Urine output also may be misleading in view of the different phases (oliguric, diuretic, and recovery) in the natural progression of ARF. Among newer markers, although some studies have found serum cystatin C to be an early and reliable marker of ARF in patients in ICUs, it has not yet been well validated as a GFR indicator in ARF.

Several pharmacotherapeutic recommendations regarding adjustment of antimicrobial regimens according to renal impairment are available.[16-18] These recommendations often are considered reliable and are in common use. Of note, however, studies by Vidal and colleagues demonstrated remarkable variation between these sources, with no adjustment recommended for a specific drug in one source versus a designation as contraindicated in renal failure in another source, for example. In the clinical setting, it is important to identify specific categories of renal impairment for dose or interval adjustment and then carefully choose a regimen suitable for the clinical condition.

Nevertheless, a point worthy of emphasis is that all of these recommendations are based on chronic renal dysfunction and pharmacokinetic data derived from studies conducted in healthy volunteers, or even in patients in the stable phase of a disease process. Thus, the findings cannot be extrapolated readily to application in critically ill patients with ARF due to sepsis. Consequently, drug handling in such patients remains largely unpredictable, and calculations based on data in the literature yield only rough estimates of drug dosage adaptation.

IMPACT OF CONTINUOUS RENAL REPLACEMENT THERAPY ON PHARMACOLOGICAL CHARACTERISTICS AND DOSAGE ADJUSTMENT OF ANTIMICROBIAL AGENTS: HOW TO ACHIEVE AN ACCURATE REGIMEN

The past 3 decades have seen a dramatic evolution of CRRT from the initial arteriovenous hemofiltration (CAVH) driven by the patient's arteriovenous pressure difference to more sophisticated modalities using pump-driven devices: continuous venovenous hemofiltration (CVVH), continuous venovenous hemodialysis (CVVHD), continuous venovenous hemodiafiltration (CVVHDF), and continuous venovenous high-flux hemodialysis (CVVHFHD). CRRT can be expected to have a profound effect on the pharmacokinetics of antimicrobials, with multiple variables affecting drug clearance. Those factors governing the extent of drug removal from the extracorporeal system can be broadly classified into two major categories: (1) factors specific to the antimicrobial agent and (2) technical factors specific to the extracorporeal modality.

Pharmacological Factors Specific to the Antimicrobial Agent

Molecular Weight

Most antimicrobial agents have molecular weights up to 500 daltons (D). Generally, it is easier for drugs of smaller molecular size (less than 500 D) to pass through a membrane and be removed more readily. But large-molecule drugs such as vancomycin, at 1448 D, can easily pass through typical high-flux membranes. Only cuprophane and some other cellulose-based membranes with small pores make a significant filtration barrier to unbound drugs.[19]

Volume of Distribution

Removal of agents with a large V_d by CRRT is minimal despite efficient clearance, because of the small proportion of total body drug present in the systemic circulation. Because total body water constitutes approximately 67% of the body weight, a drug that distributes well to all fluid compartments (intracellular, interstitial, and intravascular fluid) would have a V_d of close to 0.7 L/kg. Accordingly, a V_d greater than 0.8 L/kg probably signifies tissue binding, so the drug is not likely to be efficiently removed by CRRT.

Plasma Protein Binding

Only the unbound drug present in plasma water is pharmacologically active and can be removed by ECBP. Therefore, antimicrobials with a high degree of PPB (greater than 80%) will be poorly cleared by CRRT.[14] Many factors may alter the fraction of unbound drug, such as systemic pH, heparin therapy, hyperbilirubinemia, concentration of free fatty acids, relative concentration of drug and protein, and other drugs that may act as competetive displacers. Thus, the reported unbound fraction in healthy volunteers and in patients with chronic renal insufficiency may differ substantially from that in critically ill patients receiving CRRT.[20]

Fractional Extracorporeal Clearance

Total body clearance of an antimicrobial agent is the sum of clearances from different sites in the body, which may include hepatic, renal, and other metabolic pathways and ECBP therapy. But ECBP elimination, measured as fractional extracorporeal clearance (Fr_{EC}), is considered clinically significant only if its contribution to total body clearance exceeds 25% to 30%.[21]

$$Fr_{EC} = Cl_{EC}/(Cl_{EC} + Cl_{NR} + Cl_R) \qquad [2]$$

where Cl_{EC} is extracorporeal drug clearance, Cl_{NR} is nonrenal drug clearance, and Cl_R is renal drug clearance. This also explains why ECBP elimination will not be clinically relevant for drugs with predominantly nonrenal clearance. Although it often is difficult to estimate residual renal function (RRF) in ARF, such remaining function also needs to be taken into account in determining total body clearance. Moreover, significant RRF reduces the fraction that is removed by ECBP procedures, which may render ECBP elimination negligible.

Of note, ECBP elimination replaces only glomerular filtration. By contrast, Cl_R includes glomerular filtration, tubular secretion, and reabsorption. Therefore, any attempt to determine the extracorporeal creatinine clearance using the same dosage guidelines as in patients with reduced renal function cannot be recommended, especially with drugs largely eliminated by tubular secretion.[14]

Drug Charge

The Gibbs-Donnan effect may have a significant effect on polycationic drugs. Because large anionic molecules such as albumin do not pass through membrane readily, and retained proteins on the blood side of the membrane make the membrane negatively charged, they may partially retard the transmembrane movement of polycationic drugs (e.g., aminoglycosides). This drug charge and membrane interaction may explain in part the discrepancy between PPB and observed sieving coefficient (S_c).

Technical Factors Specific to Extracorporeal Blood Purification Therapies

Membrane

Drug clearance is directly proportional to the surface area of the dialytic membrane or hemofilter, which usually is in the range of 0.5 to 2.0 m². The pore size of the filter is the other crucial factor determining the extent of drug removal. In general, the pore size of conventional dialytic membranes made up of natural substances (cellulose or cuprophane) is relatively small, permitting passage of fluid and small solutes (molecular size less than 500 D) only. High-flux dialytic membranes usually are made up of biosynthetic material (polysulfone, polyacrylonitrile, polyamide) with relatively larger pore sizes (5000 to 20,000 D). Even-larger pore sizes are used in hemofilters (20,000 to 50,000 D).

Diffusion (Hemodialysis)

The efficiency of solute removal based on diffusion in hemodialysis is determined by the concentration gradient, in addition to the porosity and surface area of the dialytic membrane. Compared with convective clearance, diffusive clearance will decrease as molecular weight increases.[21] Owing to the lower diffusive permeability, greater influence of molecular weight on diffusive clearance is found with conventional dialysis membranes than with the synthetic membranes used in CRRT.[14]

In CVVHD, the countercurrent flow of dialysate is always considerably smaller than blood flow, resulting in complete equilibration between blood serum and dialysate. Therefore, the dialysate leaving the filter will be 100% saturated with at least the small, easily diffusible, solutes. Diffusive clearance of small unbound solutes will equal the dialysate flow rate (Q_d). Dialysate saturation (S_d) represents the capacity of a drug to diffuse through a dialysis membrane and saturate the dialysate and is calculated by dividing drug concentration in the dialysate (C_d) by its plasma concentration (C_p):

$$S_d = C_d/C_p \qquad [3]$$

Consequently, diffusive drug clearance (Cl_{HD}) is calculated by multiplying Q_d by S_d:

$$Cl_{HD} = Q_d \times S_d \qquad [4]$$

Because either a higher molecular weight decreases the speed of diffusion or a higher Q_d decreases the time available for diffusion, an increase in each of them will give rise to a decrease in S_d.[21] S_d can theoretically be influenced by drug-membrane interactions and by protein adsorption to the membrane. When extracorporeal drug clearance is calculated, S_d can be approximately replaced by the unbound fraction. Of note, however, S_d does not remain constant, and a serious error would result if the same S_d were used in different Q_d flows.

Convection (Hemofiltration)

Convective solute removal used in hemofiltration is not affected by molecular weight up to the cutoff value for sieving of the membrane. Continuous hemofiltration usually uses highly permeable membranes, with high cutoff values (20,000 to 50,000 D). Because most drugs fall in the lower- to middle-molecular-size category, molecular weight will have little impact on drug sieving with hemofiltration. The capacity of a drug to pass through the membrane of a hemofilter is expressed mathematically in the S_c term, which is the relation between drug concentration in the ultrafiltrate (C_{uf}) and in plasma (C_p).

$$S_c = C_{uf}/C_p \qquad [5]$$

For most antimicrobials, S_c can be estimated by the extent of the unbound fraction ($S_c \approx 1 - PPB$). Moreover, an excellent correlation was found between S_c and the unbound fraction. S_c is a dynamic parameter, however, and is dependent on the age of the membrane and the filtration fraction (Q_{uf}/Q_b). A loss of S_c will be approximately 20% for drugs such as vancomycin after use of the membrane over 12 hours. Given a Q_b of 100 mL/minute, an increase in Q_{uf} from 14 mL/minute to 28 mL/minute will decrease the S_c for drugs like vancomycin by approximately 30%.[12]

There are two basic dilutional modes (pre- and postdilution) for the substitution fluid, which may influence the solute removal efficiency. In the postdilution mode, the convective clearance of an antimicrobial agent ($Cl_{post-HF}$) can thus be easily obtained by multiplying the ultrafiltration rate (Q_{uf}) by its S_c:

$$Cl_{post-HF} = Q_{uf} \times S_c \quad [6]$$

If hemofiltration is used in predilution mode, however, the drug concentration in the plasma entering the dialyzer is lower than the plasma drug concentration in the patient's circulation. The drug concentration in the ultrafiltrate is the same as that in the plasma water of the blood inside the dialyzer.[19] So the correction of predilutional effect must be integrated in the clearance equation:

$$Cl_{pre-HF} = Q_{uf} \times S_c \times [Q_b/Q_b + Q_{uf})] \quad [7]$$

As a newer technical innovation in CRRT, HVHF or pulse HVHF (pHVHF) is increasingly used in critically ill patients in the ICU. In order to achieve the balance between greater solute clearance and fewer associated complications such as circuit clotting, predilution and postdilution often are used simultaneously or, in a certain percentage of cases, sequentially.[10] This makes it more complicated to calculate the drug clearance.

Combination with Diffusion and Convection (Hemodiafiltration)

In hemodiafiltration, solutes are removed by both diffusion and convection. The calculation of drug clearance during this combination therapy is extremely difficult, especially at different Q_{uf} and Q_d rates. Drug clearance with CVVHDF (Cl_{HDF}) in postdilution phase may be estimated by calculating the convective clearance and diffusive clearance from the following equation:

$$Cl_{HDF} = Q_{uf} \times S_c + Q_d \times S_d \quad [8]$$

Greater overestimation will result if S_d is replaced by the unbound fraction. Davies and coworkers measured the extracorporeal clearance of several antimicrobials during continuous hemodiafiltration with a Q_{uf} of 400 mL/hour and a Q_d of 1 and 2 L/hour. Compared with the calculated clearances based on the unbound fraction reported in healthy volunteers, the results show that the difference between calculated and measured clearance rates is not clinically significant with a low Q_d, but with a high Q_d, the calculated clearance may be overestimated by up to 100%.

Because an interaction between diffusive and convective solute transfer has been demonstrated in intermittent high-flux hemodiafiltration by protein layer formation on the blood side of the capillary, it also gives the possibility for the two processes to interact in such a manner in CVVHDF that solute removal is significantly less than what would be expected if the individual components were simply added together. In CVVHDF, as the presence of convection-derived solute in the dialysate decreases the concentration gradient, the driving force for diffusion, the S_d, can be lowered even further. The diffusive clearance of a drug during CVVHDF is difficult to predict and will depend on its MW, Q_b, Q_d, and Q_{uf} and the membrane used.

In CAVHDF, Vos and Vincent found a close exponential correlation of a drug's diffusive mass transfer coefficient (K_{rel}) through membranes:

$$K_{rel} \times K_d/K_{cr} = (MW/113)^{-0.42} \quad [9]$$

where K_d and K_{cr} are the diffusive mass transfer coefficients for the drug and creatinine, respectively, and 113 is the molecular weight of creatinine.

The drug clearance of CAVHDF may be estimated as follows:

$$Cl_{CAVHDF} = Q_{uf} \times S_c + Q_d \times S_d \times K_{rel} \quad [10]$$

Using this equation to estimate CVVHDF clearance, Kroh and associates found very good correlation between observed and estimated clearances ($y = 0.004 + 0.96x$). However, whether CAVHDF also is suitable for all antimicrobial agents has not been investigated thus far.

Adsorption to Membrane

Adsorption to filter membranes leads to increased drug removal from plasma and the various filters have different adsorptive capacity. Some dialysis membranes such as polyacrylonitrile (PAN) may adsorb a substantial amount of drugs to their surface. For example, Kronfol and Tian and coworkers found that PAN membranes have a high adsorbent capacity to bind aminoglycosides and levofloxacin. Adsorption is a saturant process, however, so the influence on drug removal will depend on the frequency of filter changes.[20] Adsorption of drugs onto the membrane may lead to a reduction in membrane permeability and filtration rate over time. Although dosing adjustment will not account for adsorption effects, using drug-adsorbing membranes for CRRT usually is not recommended.[19]

HIGH-VOLUME CONTINUOUS RENAL REPLACEMENT THERAPY

High-volume CRRT (HV-CRRT), such as HVHF, is increasingly used in septic patients with ARF in the ICU. Nevertheless, the different effects on pharmacological characteristics of antimicrobial removal between HV-RRT and low-volume CRRT (LV-CRRT) have been understated.

Pharmacokinetic experiments have found that many antimicrobials exhibit two- and three-compartment characteristics. The central compartment often is referred to as the plasma space, whereas the other compartments are peripheral compartments representative of various tissues in the body. In standard LV-CRRT, the rate-limiting step of drug clearance has been Q_d or Q_{uf}, because Q_b greatly exceeds Q_d or Q_{uf}. Consequently, no appreciable rebound occurs after LV-CRRT stops because drug transfers to the central compartment at least as fast as it is being removed by CRRT. At HV-CRRT initiation, the central compartment becomes rapidly stripped of unbound drug. The rate-limiting step for any further drug removal becomes the rate at which drug can transfer from the peripheral compartments into the center compartment for removal by HV-RRT.[22]

As mentioned earlier, an increase in Q_{uf} from 14 mL/minute to 28 mL/minute will decrease the S_c for drugs like vancomycin by approximately 30%. However, as Q_d increased from 8.3 mL/minute up to 33.3 mL/minute, a 30% decline in vancomycin S_d and an 8% decline in urea S_d were seen with use of AN69 hemodiafilters. Available data indicate that doubling Q_d from standard low-volume flows to higher dialysate flows may result in substantially less than a doubling of solute dialytic clearance, particularly for larger solutes. Increasing Q_d (to greater than 2000 mL/hour) should result in decreasing S_d, but the rate of S_d decline is filter-dependent.[22] Therefore, the drug clearance calculation during HV-CRRT is rather complex, and the changed S_c and S_d should be further considered.

Adjustment of Antimicrobial Regimen

In patients with concomitant renal failure on CRRT, underdosing may lead to inadequate anti-infective therapy, with increased mortality risk, whereas overdosing may lead to drug accumulation and unnecessary toxicities. Drug dosing adjustments during CRRT can be guided by using available drug-dosing recommendations, by measuring or estimating CRRT drug clearance, or by monitoring drug serum concentrations.

Available Drug-Dosing Recommendations

Drug-dosing recommendations for patients with ARF receiving CRRT have not kept pace with the advances in CRRT technology and the speedy development of newer antimicrobial agents. Nonetheless, published drug-dosing recommendations for ARF patients on CRRT are becoming available but still limited.[17,18,21,23,24] After searching the literature and reviewing recent clinical investigations, we adopted some of these recommendations. Then we summarized the pharmacokinetic characteristics and dosing recommendations of 60 antimicrobials most commonly used in critically ill patients undergoing CRRT into a complete dosing guide (Table 263-2).

All of these recommendations, however, have unavoidable inherent shortcomings that influence their clinical practicability to some extent. First, all of these dosing recommendations are based on low Q_{uf} and Q_d with old dialysis membranes or hemofilters. Second, pharmacokinetic data on which calculations are based are obtained mainly from databanks obtained from healthy persons or patients with stable chronic kidney disease. Third, some recommendations were derived from CRRT conducted in arteriovenous mode. Fourth, the filters, Q_{uf} and Q_d, and treatment time are considerably different among these recommendations. Finally, most of these recommendations are based on very limited clinical data, and in many cases, dosing recommendations are extrapolations from clinical experience. Additional clinical data are urgently needed to support such extrapolations, and these recommendations should not supersede sound clinical judgment.[24]

It is widely recognized that the extent of drug removal during CRRT in critically ill patients with ARF is dependent on numerous factors of patient, illness, drug, and the operational modality of CRRT. These parameters vary widely among different patients, or even at different moments in time in the same patient. CRRT does not always yield stable conditions, because Q_b and Q_{uf} are quite variable during the therapeutic process. Moreover, the renal function and sepsis may reverse under effective treatment during the disease course. Therefore, it is extremely difficult and almost impossible to devise a comprehensive dosing guide for various antimicrobials that encompasses all of the potentially changing variables involved in CRRT for all patients, as well as for the various combinations of prescriptions, machines, filters, and other variables. Therapy must be individualized to the needs of each patient.

Estimation by Mathematical Equation

Making these estimates is time-consuming, requiring a careful search for basic pharmacokinetic data. Based on the understanding of the principles of drug removal by CRRT and the pharmacokinetics of various antimicrobial agents, the drug dosage and dosing interval may be estimated using mathematical equations for application in individualized therapy. Drug clearance must be calculated to determine a maintenance dose. The serum concentration at steady state (C_{pss}) multiplied by the Cl_{EC} provides the clinician with the amount of drug specifically removed by ultrafiltration per hour under steady-state conditions. Therefore, the amount of drug removed by CRRT (D_{EC}) can be calculated using the following equation:

$$D_{EC} = C_{pss} \times Cl_{EC} \times T_{dur} \qquad [11]$$

where T_{dur} is the duration of CRRT.

Cl_{EC} can be calculated using Equations 4, 6 to 8, and 10, as shown previously, according to treatment modality. The total amount of drug required during CRRT (D) may be calculated using the following equation, including the typical anuric dose (D_{anur}) in addition to D_{EC}[25]:

$$D = D_{anur} + D_{EC} = D_{anur} + C_{pss} \times Cl_{EC} \times T_{dur} \qquad [12]$$

Besides Equation 12, the drug dose during CRRT in an anuric patient also may be estimated using the following equation[19]:

$$D = D_{anur} \times [1 + Cl_{EC}/Cl_{NR}/2(\text{interval/half-life})] \qquad [13]$$

where *half-life* is the $T_{1/2}$ of the drug in an anuric nondialyzed patient and *interval* is the dose interval in an anuric nondialyzed patient.

At present, there is an increasing tendency to start CRRT earlier in the course of illness, and RRT may contribute to drug clearance. According to Dettli's equation and the related investigation by Keller and associates, the estimated dose during CRRT in a patient with RRT may be calculated as follows[20]:

$$D_{EC} = D_n \times [P_x + (1 - P_x) \times Cl_{CRtot}/Cl_{CRn}] \qquad [14]$$

where D_n is the normal dose, $P_x = Cl_{NR}/Cl_N$ (in which Cl_N = normal drug clearance), Cl_{CRtot} is the sum of renal and extracorporeal creatinine clearance, and Cl_{CRn} is the normal creatinine clearance. This equation uses the patient's actual creatinine clearance to estimate drug clearance and drug dosing, and dose estimates will automatically be adjusted as changes occur in renal function.

Although complex mathematical models have been proposed, an accurate and usable equation remains unavailable. Because the data on drug dose in ARF are rare and the calculation of drug clearance in various modes of CRRT also is complicated, the approach to estimate the dose with the dosing regimen used in chronic kidney disease and to apply a dosing multiplication factor to account for extracorporeal clearance was found to result in serious dosing errors.[22] Most mathematical models are demonstrated to be suitable for use only with certain drugs on a conditional basis; their application in clinical practice is still limited.

Whether it may be more appropriate to increase the drug dose or to shorten the dosing interval in critically ill patients during CRRT is dependent on anti-infective mechanisms of action and the kill characteristics of the various classes of antimicrobial agents. For concentration-dependent kill characteristic antimicrobial agents, it is better to increase the drug dose, because their

TABLE 263-2

Adjustment of Antimicrobial Regimen for Different Drugs in Patients with Acute Renal Failure Undergoing Continuous Renal Replacement Therapy (CRRT)

DRUG	MW (D)	PPB	V_D (L/kg)	$T_{1/2normal}$ (h)	$T_{1/2anuria}$ (h)	NORMAL DOSAGE	DOSAGE ADJUSTMENT ON CRRT
Aminoglycoside Antibiotics							
Amikacin	585.6	0-11%	0.25-0.4	2.0-3.0	30-90	7.5 mg/kg q12h	7.5 mg/kg q24h (CVVHD/ CVVH/CVVHDF: Q_d 1 L/h, Q_{uf} 1 L/h)
Gentamicin	477.6	<5%	0.26-0.4	2.0-3.0	20-60	1.7 mg/kg q8h	2.0 mg/kg q24h (CVVHD/ CVVH/CVVHDF: Q_d 1 L/h, Q_{uf} 1 L/h)
Netilmicin	475.6	<5%	0.25-0.4	2.0-3.0	35-70	2.0 mg/kg q8h	2.0 mg/kg q12h (CVVHF: Q_d 0.5-1.8 L/h, Q_{uf} 100-400 mL/h, predilution, 0.6 m² AN69)
Tobramycin	467.5	<5%	0.26-0.4	2.0-3.0	30-60	1.7 mg/kg q8h	2.0 mg/kg q24h (CVVHD/ CVVH/CVVHDF: Q_d 1 L/h, Q_{uf} 1 L/h)
Carbapenem Antibiotics							
Imipenem	299.3	13-21%	0.23	1	4	0.25-1.0 g q6h	0.5 q6-12h (CVVHD/CVVH/ CVVHDF: Q_d 1 L/h, Q_{uf} 1 L/h, 0.9 m² AN69)
Meropenem	383.5	2%	0.35	1	7	0.5-1.0 g q6h	1.0 g q12h (CVVHD: Q_d 1 L/h) 1.0 g q12h (CVVH: Q_{uf} 1-2 L/h, postdilution, 0.9 m² AN69) 1.0 g q8h (CVVH: Q_{uf} 2.6 L/h, postdilution, 0.43 m² high-flux PS) 1.0 g q12h (CVVHDF: Q_d 1-1.5 L/h, Q_{uf} 1-1.5 L/h, pre/ postdilution, 0.9 m² AN69)
Cephalosporin Antibiotics							
Cefaclor	367.8	23.50%	0.24-0.35	1	3	250-500 mg q8h	500 mg q8-12h (CVVHD/CVVH: Q_d 1.5 L/h, Q_{uf} 1.5 L/h)
Cefamandole	475.6	75%	0.16-0.25	0.5	6.0-11	0.5-1.0 g q4-8h	1.0 g q18h (CVVHD/CVVH: Q_d 1.5 L/h, Q_{uf} 1.5 L/h)
Cefazolin	454.5	84%	0.13-0.22	2	40-70	0.5-1.5 g q6h	2.0 g q12h (CVVHD/CVVHDF: Q_d 1 L/h, Q_{uf} 1 L/h) 1.0-2.0 g q12h (CVVH: Q_{uf} 1-2 L/h) 1.0 g q8h (CVVH: Q_{uf} 3 L/h)
Cefepime	480.6	<20%	0.71	4.6	8.1	0.25-2.0 g q8h	1.0-2.0 g q12h (CVVHD/CVVH/ CVVHDF: Q_d 1 L/h, Q_{uf} 1 L/h, postdilution, 0.6 m² AN69)
Cefmenoxime	511.6	45-75%	0.27-0.37	1	6.0-12	1.0 g q6h	1.0 g q24h (CVVH: Q_{uf} 1 L/h)
Cefoperazone	645.7	90%	0.14	2	3	1.0-2.0 g q12h	1.0-2.0 g q24h (CVVHD/CVVH: Q_d 1.5 L/h, Q_{uf} 1.5 L/h)
Cefotaxime	455.5	37%	0.35	2	15-35	1.0 g q6h	2.0 g q12h (CVVHD/CVVHDF: Q_d 1 L/h, Q_{uf} 1 L/h) 1.0 g q6-8h (CVVH: Q_{uf} 1-2 L/h) 2.0 g q8h (CVVH: Q_{uf} 3 L/h)
Cefoxitin	427.4	40.75%	0.31	1	13-23	1.0-2.0 g q6-8h	1.0 g q18h (CVVHD/CVVH: Q_d 1.5 L/h, Q_{uf} 1.5 L/h)
Cefpirome	512	<10%	0.32	2	14.5	2.0 g q12h	2.0 g q8h (CVVH: Q_{uf} 3 L/h, postdilution, 0.7 m² high-flux PS)
Cefradine	349.4	8-17%	0.25-0.46	0.7-1.3	6.0-15	1.0-2.0 g q6h	1.0 g q12h (CVVHD/CVVH: Q_d 1.5 L/h, Q_{uf} 1.5 L/h)
Ceftazidime	546.6	17%	0.28	2	13-25	1.0-2.0 g q8h	2.0 g q12h (CVVHD/CVVHDF: Q_d 1 L/h, Q_{uf} 1 L/h) 1.0-2.0 g q12h (CVVH: Q_{uf} 1 L/h) 2.0 g q8h (CVVH: Q_{uf} 3 L/h, postdilution, 0.7 m² high-flux PS)
Ceftriaxone	554.6	95%	0.12-0.18	6.0-9.0	12.0-24.0	0.5-1.0 g q12h	2.0 g q12-24h (CVVHD/CVVH/ CVVHDF: Q_d 1 L/h, Q_{uf} 1 L/h)
Cefuroxime	424.4	50%	0.19	1.5	17	0.75-1.5 g q8h	0.5 g q8h (CVVHD/CVVH: Q_d 1.5 L/h, Q_{uf} 1.5 L/h)
Cephalexin	347.4	14%	0.35	1	16	250-500 mg q6h	0.5 g q12h (CVVHD/CVVH: Q_d 1.5 L/h, Q_{uf} 1.5 L/h)

TABLE 263-2

Adjustment of Antimicrobial Regimen for Different Drugs in Patients with Acute Renal Failure Undergoing Continuous Renal Replacement Therapy (CRRT)—cont'd

DRUG	MW (D)	PPB	V_D (L/kg)	$T_{1/2normal}$ (h)	$T_{1/2anuria}$ (h)	NORMAL DOSAGE	DOSAGE ADJUSTMENT ON CRRT
Fluoroquinolone Antibiotics							
Ciprofloxacin	331.3	20-40%	1.9-2.8	4.4	8.7	400 mg q12h	200 mg q8-12h (CVVHD: Q_d 1-2 L/h, 0.43 m² AN69) 200 mg q12h (CVVH: Q_{uf} 1 L/h, postdilution, 0.6 m² AN69) 200 mg q12h (CVVHDF: Q_d 1 L/h, Q_{uf} 1 L/h, postdilution, 0.6 m² AN69) 200 mg q8h (CVVHDF: Q_d 1 L/h, Q_{uf} 2 L/h, predilution, 0.6 m² AN69)
Enoxacin	320.3	40%	1.6	3.0-6.0	15-25	400 mg q12h	400 mg q24h (CVVHD/CVVH: Q_d 1.5 L/h, Q_{uf} 1.5 L/h)
Levofloxacin	361	24-38%	1.09-1.26	6.3	76	500-750 mg q24h	250 mg q24h (CVVHD/CVVH/ CVVHDF: Q_d 1 L/h, Q_{uf} 1 L/h, postdilution, 0.6 m² AN69)
Moxifloxacin	401.4	47%	3.3	12	12	400 mg q24h	400 mg q 24h (CVVHD/CVVH/ CVVHDF: Q_d 1 L/h, Q_{uf} 1 L/h, pre/postdilution, 0.6 m² AN69)
Ofloxacin	361.4	20-25%	1.5-2.5	4.0-7.0	40-50	200-400 mg q12h	400 mg q24h (CVVH: Q_{uf} 3 L/h, postdilution, 0.7 m² high-flux PS)
Pefloxacin	333.4	20-30%	1.8	8.6	12.0-15.0	400-800 mg q24h	400-800 mg q24h (CVVHD/ CVVH: Q_d 1.5 L/h, Q_{uf} 1.5 L/h)
Macrolide Antibiotic							
Erythromycin	734	84%	0.9	1.5	6	150-300 mg q6h	250-500 mg q12-24h (CVVHD/ CVVH: Q_d 1.5 L/h, Q_{uf} 1.5 L/h)
Miscellaneous Antibiotic							
Aztreonam	435.4	55%	0.25	2	6.0-8.0	1.0-2.0 g q8-12h	2.0 g q12h (CVVHD/CVVHDF: Q_d 1 L/h, Q_{uf} 1 L/h) 1.0 g q8h (CVVH: Q_{uf} 1 L/h) 2.0 g q12h (CVVH: Q_{uf} 2 L/h) 2.0 g q8h (CVVH: Q_{uf} 3 L/h)
Chloramphenicol	323.1	53%	0.9	4	3.0-7.0	12.5 mg/kg q6h	12.5 mg/kg q6h (CVVHD/ CVVH: Q_d 1.5 L/h, Q_{uf} 1.5 L/h)
Clindamycin	425	60-95%	0.7	2.5	4	150-300 mg q6h	600-900 mg q8h (CVVHD/ CVVH/CVVHDF: Q_d 1 L/h, Q_{uf} 1 L/h)
Colistin	1750	55%	0.34	2	7.5	2.5 mg/kg q24hr	2.5 mg/kg q48h (CVVHD/ CVVH/CVVHDF: Q_d 1 L/h, Q_{uf} 1 L/h)
Daptomycin	1619.7	92%	0.13	8	29.3	4-6 mg q24h	4-6 mg q48h (CVVHD/CVVH/ CVVHDF: Q_d 1 L/h, Q_{uf} 1 L/h)
Linezolid	337.3	31%	0.6-0.8	4.4-5.5	7.0-8.0	600 mg q12h	600 mg q12h (CVVHD/CVVH/ CVVHDF: Q_d 1-2 L/h, Q_{uf} 1-2 L/h, pre/postdilution)
Metronidazole	171.2	20%	0.8	6.0-14	7.0-21	7.5 mg/kg q6h	7.5 mg/kg q24h (CVVHD/ CVVH: Q_d 1.5 L/h, Q_{uf} 1.5 L/h)
Teicoplanin	1879.7	>90%	0.34-0.89	30-140	157-567	400 mg q24h	200 mg q48h (CVVHD/CVVH/ CVVHDF: Q_d 1 L/h, Q_{uf} 1 L/h)
Trimethoprim	290.3	30-50%	1-2.2	11	20-50	100-200 mg q12h	100-200 mg q12h (CVVHD/ CVVH: Q_d 1.5 L/h, Q_{uf} 1.5 L/h)
Vancomycin	1449.3	10-55%	0.64	6	200-250	500 mg q6h/1.0 g q12h	1.0 g q24h (CVVHD/CVVHDF: Q_d 1 L/h, Q_{uf} 1-2 L/h) 1.0 g q48h (CVVH: Q_{uf} 1-1.5 L/h)
Penicillins							
Amoxicillin	365.4	15-25%	0.37	1	5.0-20	250-500 mg q8h	1.0 g q12h (CVVHD/CVVH: Q_d 1.5 L/h, Q_{uf} 1.5 L/h)
Ampicillin/ (sulbactam 2:1)	349.4	20%	0.22	1	7.0-20	1.5-3.0 g q6h	3.0 g q8h (CVVHD/CVVHDF: Q_d 1 L/h, Q_{uf} 1 L/h) 3.0 g q12h (CVVH: Q_{uf} 1 L/h)
Azlocillin	461.5	20-46%	0.29	1.3-1.5	6	2.0-3.0 g q4h	3.0 g q24h (CVVHD/CVVH: Q_d 1.5 L/h, Q_{uf} 1.5 L/h)
Flucloxacillin	453.9	95%	0.54	1	3	1.0-2.0 g q6-8h	2.0 g q24h (CVVHD/CVVH: Q_d 1.5 L/h, Q_{uf} 1.5 L/h)

TABLE 263-2

Adjustment of Antimicrobial Regimen for Different Drugs in Patients with Acute Renal Failure Undergoing Continuous Renal Replacement Therapy (CRRT)—cont'd

DRUG	MW (D)	PPB	V_D (L/kg)	$T_{1/2normal}$ (h)	$T_{1/2anuria}$ (h)	NORMAL DOSAGE	DOSAGE ADJUSTMENT ON CRRT
Mezlocillin	539.6	20-46	0.26	1.3	3.0-5.0	1.5-4.0 g q4-6 h	2.0 g q24h (CVVHD/CVVH: Q_d 1.5 L/h, Q_{uf} 1.5 L/h)
Nafcillin	414.5	85%	0.35	1	2	1.0-2.0 g q4-6h	2.0 g q4-6h (CVVH/CVVHD/ CVVHDF: Q_d 1 L/h, Q_{uf} 1 L/h)
Oxacillin	435.9	92-96%	0.19-0.33	0.5	?	0.25-1.0 g q4-6h	1.0 g q8h (CVVHD/CVVH: Q_d 1.5 L/h, Q_{uf} 1.5 L/h)
Penicillin G	334.4	6-20%	0.3	0.5	6.0-20	0.8-4.0 million U q4-6h	2.0 million U q12h (CVVHD/ CVVH: Q_d 1.5 L/h, Q_{uf} 1.5 L/h)
Piperacillin/ (tazobactam 8:1)	516.5	30%	0.3	1	3.0-5.1	3.375 g q6h	2.25 g q6-8h (CVVHD, Q_d 1-1.5 L/h, AN69)

2.25 g q4-6h (CVVH/CVVHDF, Q_d 1 L/h, Q_{uf} 1-2 L/h, postdilution, 0.7 m² PS) |
| Ticarcillin/ (clavulanate 30:1) | 384.4 | 45-60% | 0.14-0.22 | 2.2 | 11.0-17.0 | 3.1 g q4-6h | 3.1 g q6h (CVVHD/CVVHDF: Q_d 1 L/h, Q_{uf} 1 L/h)

2.0 g q6-8h (CVVH: Q_{uf} 1 L/h) |
Tetracycline Antibiotic							
Doxycycline	444.4	>90%	0.75	15-20	18-25	100 mg q24h	100 mg q24h (CVVHD/CVVH: Q_d 1.5 L/h, Q_{uf} 1.5 L/h)
Antifungal Antibiotics							
Amphotericin B lipid complex	924.1	>90%	1.7-3.9	173	173	5 mg/kg q24h	3.0-5.0 mg/kg q24h (CVVHD/ CVVH/CVVHDF: Q_d 1 L/h, Q_{uf} 1-2 L/h)
Fluconazole	306.3	12%	0.7	37	100	200-400 mg q24h	400-800 mg q24h (CVVHD/ CVVHDF: Q_d 1 L/h, Q_{uf} 1 L/h)

200-400 mg q24h (CVVH: Q_{uf} 1 L/h) |
Flucytosine	129.1	<10%	0.6	3.0-6.0	75-200	37.5 mg/kg q6h	37.5 mg/kg q12h (CVVHD/ CVVH: Q_d 1.5 L/h, Q_{uf} 1.5 L/h)
Itraconazole, IV	705.6	99.80%	10	21	25	100-200 mg q12h	100-200 mg q12h (CVVHD/ CVVH: Q_d 1.5 L/h, Q_{uf} 1.5 L/h)
Voriconazole, IV	349.3	58%	4.6	12	13.7	6 mg/kg q12h twice, then 4 mg/kg q12h	6 mg/kg q12h twice then 4 mg/ kg q12h (CVVHDF: Q_d 1 L/h, Q_{uf} 0.5 L/h, predilution, 0.9 m² AN69)
Antituberculous Antibiotics							
Ethambutol	204.3	20-30%	1.6	4	20	15-25 mg/kg q24h	10-15 mg/kg q24-48h (CVVHD/ CVVH: Q_d 1.5 L/h, Q_{uf} 1.5 L/h)
Isoniazid	137.1	4-30%	0.75	1.0-4.0	1.0-17	300 mg q24h	300 mg q24h (CVVHD/CVVH: Q_d 1.5 L/h, Q_{uf} 1.5 L/h)
Rifampin	823	89%	0.9	3.5	9	600 mg q24h	600 mg q24h (CVVHD/CVVH: Q_d 1.5 L/h, Q_{uf} 1.5 L/h)
Antiviral Agents							
Acyclovir, IV	225.2	9-33%	0.7	2.5	20	5.0 mg/kg q8h	5.0-7.5 mg/kg q24h (CVVHD/ CVVH/CVVHDF: Q_d 1 L/h, Q_{uf} 1 L/h)
Amantadine	151.2	67%	4.0-5.0	10.0-14.0	7-10 days	100 mg q12h	100-200 mg q60h (CVVHD/ CVVH: Q_d 1.5 L/h, Q_{uf} 1.5 L/h)
Ganciclovir	256.2	1-2%	0.47	3	30	5.0 mg/kg q12h	5.0 mg/kg q48h (CVVHD/ CVVHDF: Q_d 1 L/h, Q_{uf} 0.3 L/ h, postdilution)

CRRT, continuous renal replacement therapy; CVVH, continuous venovenous hemofiltration; CVVHD, continuous venovenous hemodialysis; CVVHDF, continuous venovenous hemodiafiltration; MW, molecular weight; PPB, plasma protein binding; Q_d, dialysate flow rate; Q_{uf}, ultrafiltrate rate; V_d, apparent volume of distribution; $T_{1/2anuria}$ = plasma half-life in anuric nondialyzed patients; $T_{1/2normal}$ = normal plasma half-life; ?, data not available.

antimicrobial effects correlate with the C_{max}. For example, low doses of aminoglycosides used in anuric nondialyzed patients result in low C_{max} with low bacterial killing efficiency, although the risk of toxic adverse effects also is low. A preferable approach, however, is to increase the single daily dose to achieve the higher C_{max} in CRRT, although the minimum (trough) drug concentration (C_{min}) is decreased by CRRT and the risk of side effects is con-

siderably reduced. By contrast, for time-dependent kill characteristic antimicrobial agents such as β-lactam antibiotics, it is better to shorten the drug dosing interval, because their antibiotic effects correlate with T > MIC. The shorter dosing interval during CRRT may be estimated from the following equation, and the individual dose remains unchanged from that used in anuric nondialyzed patients:[19]

$$Iv_{EC} = Iv_{anu} \times [Cl_{NR}/Cl_{EC} + Cl_{NR})] \qquad [15]$$

where Iv_{EC} is the interval during CRRT and Iv_{anu} is the interval in an anuric patient.

Drug Serum Concentration Monitoring

Not only are pharmacokinetics and pharmacodynamics often less predictable in critically ill patients, but it also has not been consistently shown that convincing results may be obtained from current drug dosing recommendations or be estimated accurately using available mathematical equations. Therefore, serum drug concentration monitoring is highly recommended whenever possible, especially for those drugs with a narrow therapeutic range. Although the monitoring of total drug concentrations is considered a reasonable strategy to enhance optimal dosing and minimize toxic side effects, it is not readily available for all medications. The following equation often is used to estimate the required dose (D_{requir}) to achieve the desired peak concentration (C_{max}) from the actual trough (or any) concentration (C_{actual}):

$$D_{requir} = (C_{max} - C_{actual}) \times V_d \times \text{Body weight} \qquad [16]$$

CONCLUSION

Appropriate anti-infective therapy remains an essential approach in decreasing persistently high morbidity and mortality rates in the ICU. In septic patients with ARF, often also at high risk of MODS, CRRT is increasingly accepted as an effective ECBP therapy to be used in these critically ill patients. Considerable data are available to demonstrate that sepsis, ARF, and CRRT each may have profound effects on the pharmacokinetic and pharmacodynamic characteristics of various antimicrobial agents commonly used in the ICU. The extent of alteration is dependent on multiple mechanical and drug factors during the treatment of sepsis. An understanding of these interactions, fundamental pharmacological principles, and drug clearance during CRRT is important to adjust the antimicrobial regimen in critically ill patients. Awareness of the kill characteristics of the antimicrobials in question helps determine the optimal mode of administration; meanwhile, monitoring drug serum concentrations is still mandatory whenever clinically feasible. Drug dosing guidelines are available but are unlikely to fit all patients as well as all methods of treatment. More pharmacokinetic simulation modeling and clinical studies are needed to provide accurate guidance on appropriate dosage adjustment under different circumstances.

<hr>

Key Points

1. Delivery of effective and safe antimicrobial therapy poses one of the greatest challenges to the intensivist in the management of septic patients in the intensive care unit.
2. Sepsis, acute renal failure, and different modalities of continuous renal replacement therapy each have profound effects on the pharmacological characteristics of various antimicrobial agents commonly used in the intensive care unit.
3. Drug dosing recommendations are available, but it is still difficult to find a dosing guideline to fit different patients with individualized therapy.
4. Based on an understanding of the principles of drug removal by continuous renal replacement therapy, individual antimicrobial dosage and dosing interval may be estimated by mathematical equation.
5. Monitoring drug serum concentrations remains mandatory, especially with use of antimicrobials that possess a narrow therapeutic range.

<hr>

Acknowledgment

This work was made possible in part through the International Society of Nephrology–funded fellowship of Dr. Dingwei Kuang.

Key References

17. Aronoff GR, Berns JS, Brier ME, et al (eds): Drug Prescribing in Renal Failure: Dosing Guidelines for Adults. Philadelphia, American College of Physicians, 1999.
18. Ashley C, Currie A (eds): The Renal Drug Handbook, 2nd ed. Oxford, Radcliffe Medical Press, 2004.
19. Boiler J, Donauer J, Keller F: Pharmacokinetic principles during continuous renal replacement therapy: Drugs and dosage. Kidney Int 1999;56(Suppl 72):S24-S28.

See the companion Expert Consult website for the complete reference list.

SECTION 19

Peritoneal Dialysis in the Intensive Care Unit

CHAPTER 264

The Peritoneal Dialysis System

Claudio Ronco

OBJECTIVES

This chapter will:
1. Describe the anatomical characteristics of the peritoneal dialysis system.
2. Discuss peritoneal microcirculation.
3. Explain the mesothelial membrane.
4. Discuss the dialysate compartment and the influence of different dialysate flow/dwell times on efficacy of treatment.

Several factors affect the delivery of therapy in peritoneal dialysis. They are the amount of fluid utilized, the frequency of exchanges, the dwell time, and the type of solution employed. However, the final efficacy of the therapy depends on the anatomical and functional components of the dialytic system, such as the peritoneal circulation (blood compartment), the mesothelium (peritoneal membrane), and the dialysate compartment. Once these components are clearly described, different parameters of each technique become the foundations for an adequate therapy prescription and a crucial factor in treatment delivery.

THE PERITONEAL DIALYSIS SYSTEM

Since the beginning of dialytic therapy, diffusion and convection have been combined in an attempt to replace renal function.[1] The knowledge about diffusion came from industrial chemistry, and dialyzers were designed to be ideal countercurrent exchangers.[2] Only later was convection used in clinical practice, showing potential advantages.[3,4] Although ultrafiltration was employed first to treat overhydrated patients,[5] convective was subsequently used to enhance solute removal.[6-9] In peritoneal dialysis, such mechanisms of solute removal are employed with the same objectives as hemodialysis.

The peritoneal dialysis system has three major components, the peritoneal microcirculation, the peritoneal membrane, and the dialysate compartment, which includes the composition of the solution and the modalities of delivery. All of these components may have an important effect on the final performance of the technique (Fig. 264-1).[10]

THE DIALYSATE COMPARTMENT

The dialysate compartment is represented by the peritoneal cavity and the amount of fluid infused in one exchange. Basically, the compartment can be divided into a bulk region and a boundary layer of fluid, close to the peritoneal membrane. Furthermore, several variables should be taken into account, such as the time of infusion and drainage, the dwell time, the flow of dialysate, its temperature and composition, and the possible use of tidal techniques.

In Figure 264-2, urea clearance is plotted against dialysate flow rate. The curve identifies three specific regions. The first region consists of the dialysate flow rates typical for continuous ambulatory peritoneal dialysis (CAPD) (3-5 exchanges/day). In this region, the correlation is very steep, and clearance displays significant changes even in the presence of minimal changes in the dialysate flow. However, minimal variations in dialysate flow rate may require changing from four to five exchanges per day. This region is therefore dialysate flow–dependent or flow-limited, because the volume of dialysate per day is the factor that chiefly limits the clearance value. In this region, it would be theoretically simple to increase the dialysate flow by a few milliliters per day to achieve much higher clearances and, consequently, significant increases in Kt/V. However, although theoretically possible, this process would not be feasible in practice because it would mean carrying out 6 to 10 exchanges per day. The only possible way to increase the dialysate flow without raising the number of exchanges is to increase the volume of solution per exchange. To achieve the same fractional clearance in patients weighing 60 and 90 kg, one must schedule four exchanges per day, with 2-L and 3-L bags, respectively. The impact of possible intraperitoneal pressure rise must be carefully checked to avoid middle- to long-term complications such as hernias, respiratory problems, and decreased ultrafiltration. In conclusion, a typical CAPD technique is basically dialysate flow–limited.

The second part of the curve is the typical region of automated or intermittent peritoneal dialysis. The dialysate flows may vary significantly owing to a variation of the dwell time from 30 min to 0 and in the number of exchanges per day. Based on a 30-minute dwell time with 20 minutes for influx and outflow, 12 two-for-one exchanges can be performed overnight for an overall duration of 10 hours. The clearance will be 19 mL/min or 11.4 L/day. When the dwell time is reduced to 0 and the dialysate flow is therefore increased, the clearance rises to 22 to 30 mL/min with a total clearance per day of 18 L/day. This would result in a rise in the weekly Kt/V in a 60-kg patient from 2.21 to 3.50. However, this treatment, which could be defined as high-flux automated peritoneal dialysis (HFAPD), would require 60 L of dialysis solution, and the cost would become excessive. A good compromise could be the use of a tidal volume of solution, which may increase the dialysate volume artificially and enable better utilization of the surface area available for the exchanges.

The third part of the curve is the region where the plateau is reached, and further increases in dialysate flow rates do not result in parallel increases in clearance. This region has been explored experimentally, especially utilizing continuous flow peritoneal dialysis (CFPD) performed with double lumen peritoneal catheters[11] and theoretical mathematical models based on mass transfer-area coefficient (MTC) calculation.[12] The value of the mass transfer coefficient is a function of the product of the overall permeability of the peritoneum and the available surface area of the membrane. This parameter is based on the calculation made for each single subject of the maximal clearance theoretically achievable at infinite blood and dialysate flow rates, i.e., at a constantly maximal gradient for diffusion.

The regions of the curve just discussed describe the relationship between dialysate flow and solute transport. Other factors, such as dialysate temperature, intraperitoneal volume, and dialysate osmolality, are further factors affecting solute transport, either by increasing the diffusion process or by adding some convective transport because of increased ultrafiltration rates.

The Peritoneal Dialysis Membrane

The peritoneal dialysis membrane is a living structure that can be considered more a functional barrier than a precisely defined anatomical structure. On the basis of the flow/clearance curve described previously, the following question may arise: Why is the value of the mass transfer coefficient (MTC) so low in peritoneal dialysis compared with other dialysis treatments, and is the membrane involved in such limitations?

The three-pore model of peritoneal transport has been proposed by Rippe and associates[13] to explain the peculiar behavior of the peritoneal membrane in relation to macromolecules, micromolecules, and water transport. According to this model, human peritoneum appears to behave as a membrane with a series of differently sized pores as follows: large pores (25 nm; macromolecule transport), small pores (5 nm; micromolecule transport), and ultra-small pores (water transport). The anatomical structure of these ultra-small pores corresponds to the "water channels" created by a specific protein "aquaporin" acting as a carrier for water molecules. This model locates the main resistance to transport at the level of the capillary wall,

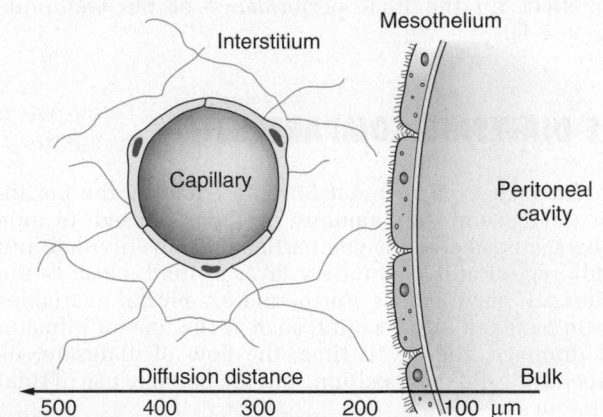

FIGURE 264-1. The peritoneal dialysis system: capillary, interstitium, mesothelium, and peritoneal cavity with the dialysate compartment.

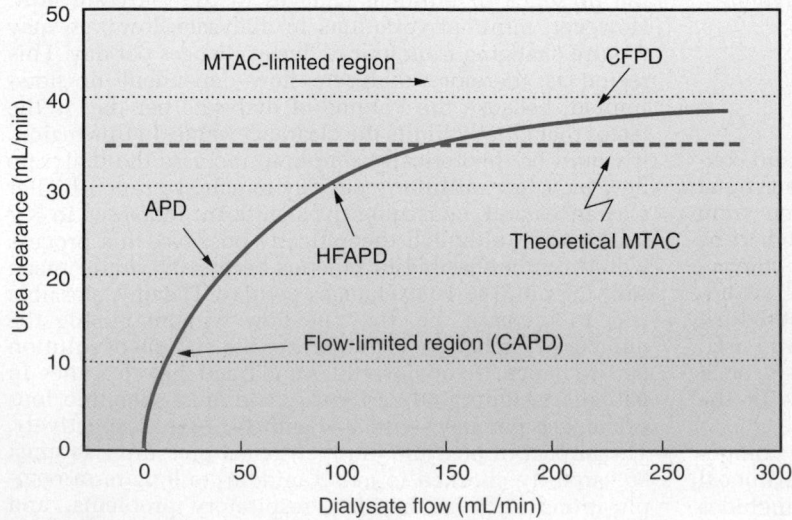

FIGURE 264-2. Dialysate flow rate/urea clearance domain map in peritoneal dialysis. A progressive increase in clearance is displayed with a parallel increase in dialysate flow. The phenomenon reaches a plateau at which no further clearance increases can be observed. APD, automated peritoneal dialysis; CAPD, continuous ambulatory peritoneal dialysis; CFPD, continuous-flow peritoneal dialysis; HFAPD, high-flow automated peritoneal dialysis; MTAC, mass transfer-area coefficient.

regarding all other anatomical structures as a negligible site of resistance. Later the interstitium was added as an additional site of resistance.

A controversial opinion is offered by the so-called "distributed model" offered by Dedrick and colleagues.[14] In this model, the main resistance to transport is apparently located in the interstitial tissue. This anatomical entity consists of a double-density material containing water and glycosaminoglycans in different proportions. The interstitial matrix seems to act as the main site of resistance to solute and water transport from the bloodstream to the peritoneal cavity. The solute diffusivity in free water is greater than that in the tissue by more than one order of magnitude. Accordingly, not only the structure of the interstitium but also the thickness of the glycosaminoglycan layer may play an important role in restricting the diffusive transport of solutes. There is a certain discrepancy between the two models, and overall transport

process is probably governed by a more complex and integrated series of events, each with a remarkable but not absolute importance. The pressures applied to the system that contribute to the generation of the transmembrane pressure are shown in detail in Figure 264-3. It is evident that the osmotic pressure generated by the glucose contained in the dialysate is by far the most important. Nevertheless, as shown in Figure 264-4, because the peritoneal membrane is not a perfect barrier for the employed osmotic agent (glucose), the transmembrane pressure gradient is continuously varying in relation to the velocity of reabsorption of glucose from dialysate into the blood compartment. Furthermore, capillaries, which are located at different distance from the mesothelial barrier, may be exposed to different concentrations of readsorbed glucose with different levels of cell damage (Fig. 264-5).

The Peritoneal Microcirculation

Despite several lines of evidence suggesting that peritoneal blood flow should be high enough to avoid any limitation in solute clearances and ultrafiltration, the real impact of effective blood flow on the efficiency of the peritoneal dialysis system is still controversial.[15] Experimental work has in fact suggested that peritoneal ultrafiltration and solute clearances might be blood flow–limited at least in some condition.[16]

Mesenteric blood flow averages 10% of cardiac output, but the peritoneal capillary blood flow seems to vary between 50 and 100 mL/min. The "effective" amount of flow involved in peritoneal exchanges is unknown, however, and could be much lower. Gas clearance studies have suggested that peritoneal blood flow may be as high as 68 to 82 mL/min,[17] whereas other studies have suggested a much lower value for "effective" blood flow.[18] Gas

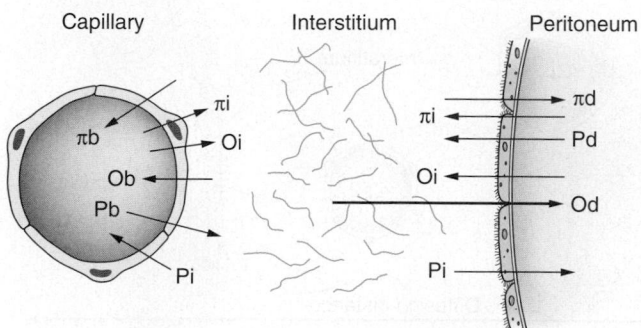

FIGURE 264-3. Depiction of the different pressures contributing to the generation of the transmembrane pressure: b, blood; d, dialysate; i, interstitium; O, osmotic; P, hydrostatic; π, oncotic.

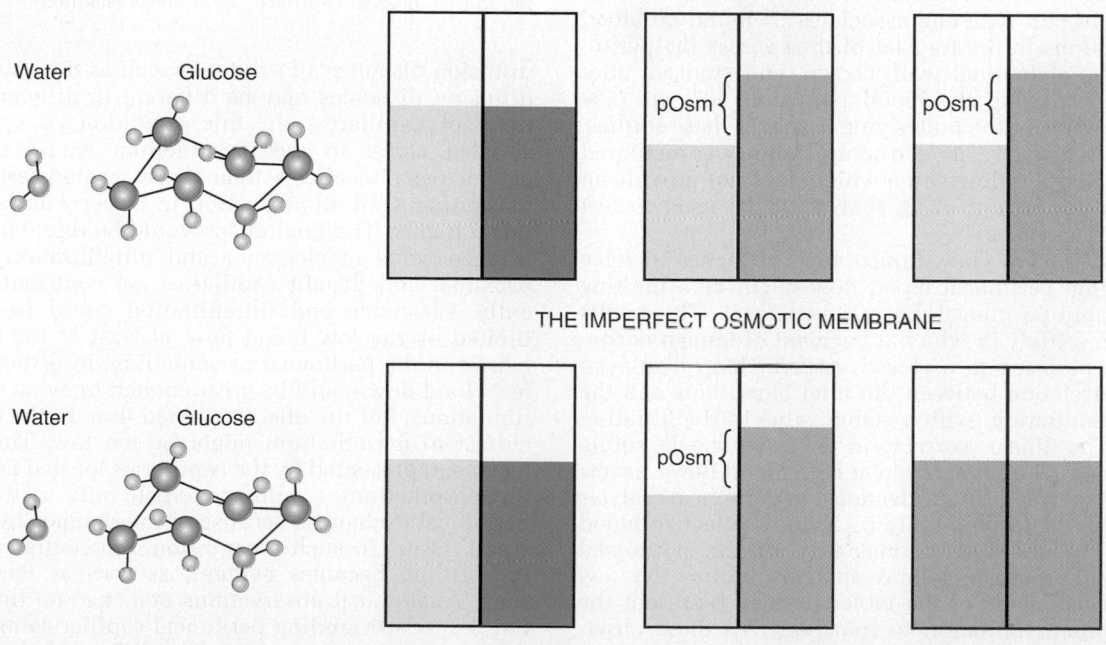

FIGURE 264-4. Graphic representation of perfect and imperfect osmotic membranes. After a time, the imperfect membrane allows a back-diffusion of the osmotic agent, and equilibrium is reached. The initial osmotic effect is achieved only because of the different diffusion velocities between glucose molecules and water molecules.

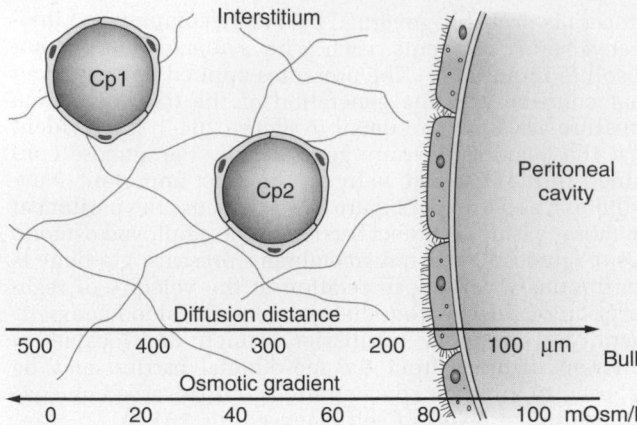

FIGURE 264-5. Graphic representation of a three-dimensional distribution of peritoneal microcirculation. Capillaries may have various distances from the mesothelial barrier, and this is the difference between the two.

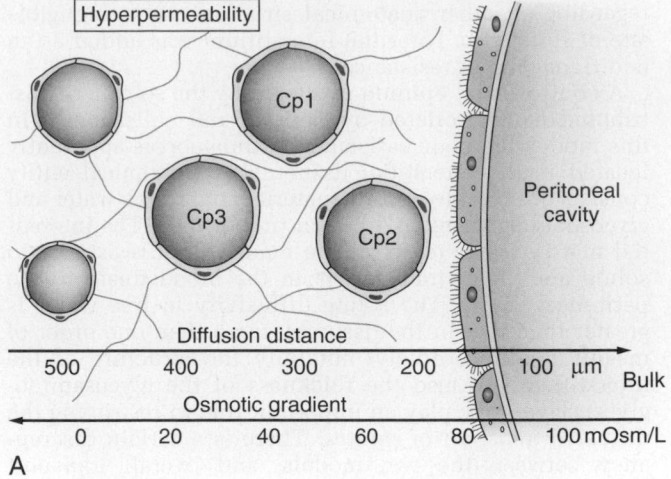

A

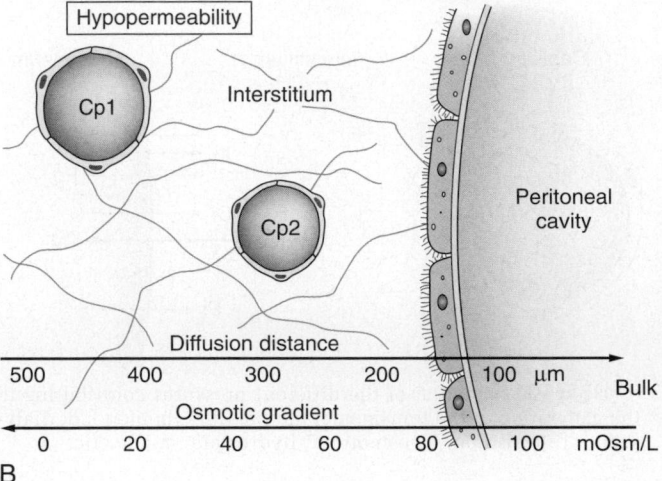

B

FIGURE 264-6. Graphic representations of the possible anatomical bases of hyperpermeability (**A**) and hypopermeability (**B**) according to the "nearest capillary" hypothesis (see text).

clearance studies were based on the assumption that peritoneal gas clearance is equivalent to effective blood flow, and this assumption may not necessarily represent the actual condition. Ronco and colleagues[19] have obtained an indirect measure of "effective" blood flow of between 25 and 45 mL/min.

In conclusion, controversy exists about whether the blood supply to the peritoneum and subperitoneal tissues limits the transport of solutes between the peritoneal cavity and the blood. Using a distributed model approach, Waniewski and coworkers[20] predicted the following marked changes in the mass transfer-area coefficient (MTAC, mL/min) for small solutes when the tissue blood perfusion rate (Q_b) was changed from 0.5 mL/min/g tissue to 0.1: $MTAC_{urea}$ decreases from 23 to 14, $MTAC_{creatinine}$ decreases from 17 to 11, and $MTAC_{glucose}$ decreases from 13 to 8. Unfortunately, there are no direct measurements of Q_b during peritoneal dialysis to test these calculations. In a study in rats, Kim and associates[21,22] found no blood flow limitations in the transfer of urea across the peritoneum of the abdominal wall, cecum, and stomach after suddenly decreasing the blood perfusion 60% to 72% from its baseline in the underlying tissue. In these studies, the blood perfusion relative to control value was measured with laser Doppler flowmetry, which does not provide an absolute measurement of Q_b that could be used to test Waniewski's assertion.

As an alternative view, Ronco and colleagues[18,19] have proposed that peritoneal blood flow might be a limiting factor in rapid peritoneal dialysis exchanges. The results obtained in a study in which a fragment of human peritoneum was perfused in a closed vascular loop displayed a linear correlation between the inlet blood flow and the rate of ultrafiltration, with a stable value of the filtration fraction. The linear correlation between small solute clearance and blood flow, even at high blood flows, seems to suggest that small solute clearance in peritoneal dialysis can probably be limited more by the low effective blood flow than by the low permeability of the peritoneal membrane. For larger solutes such as inulin, the low diffusion coefficients of the molecule may represent the most important limitation to transport. All these observations led to the formulation of the *nearest capillary hypothesis*.[23]

Because the peritoneal microvasculature is a network of capillaries with a three-dimensional distribution and different distances from the mesothelium (Fig. 264-5), the

diffusion distances of solutes as well as the glucose back-diffusion distances may be different in different populations of capillaries. In this condition, the capillaries situated closer to the mesothelium would experience greater osmotic effects than those located farther away, presenting a filtration fraction in closer capillaries to be much higher. The final effect would be represented by an average value of clearance and ultrafiltration to which proximal and distant capillaries are contributing differently. Clearance and ultrafiltration could be definitely limited by the low blood flow, at least in the capillaries closest to the peritoneal mesothelium. In distant capillaries, blood flow could be great enough to avoid significant limitations, but the effective blood flow in the capillaries closest to mesothelium might be too low. The vascular reserve, represented by the capillaries located farther from the mesothelium, would participate only partially in the peritoneal exchanges because of interference by the interstitial tissue. In such a condition, the central role of the interstitium becomes evident, as well as its hydration state. Anatomical observations demonstrate that interstitial tissue surrounding peritoneal capillaries may vary in thickness from 15 to 300 µm. The different locations of the capillary network in this tissue and the varying distances from the mesothelium may therefore help explain the different transport rates observed in different portions of the human peritoneum.[23]

The nearest capillary hypothesis may also help explain the pathological conditions of hyperpermeability and hypopermeability of the peritoneal membrane. Hyperpermeability could occur from reduction in the interstitial spaces and a consequent crowding of the capillaries in a position close to the mesothelium (Fig. 264-6A). Hypopermeability could occur in the case of interstitial hyperhydration or in pathological processes that affect the capillaries proximal to the mesothelium (Fig. 264-6B).

CONCLUSION

This chapter discussed the major factors influencing the efficiency of peritoneal dialysis, focusing on the anatomical and functional components of the peritoneal dialysis system. Other factors, such as patient and staff compliance, significantly influence treatment efficacy. Nevertheless, understanding the dialytic process in peritoneal dialysis starts with an understanding of the different components of the system and their specific function.

Key Points

1. Peritoneal dialysis relies on a semipermeable membrane (the peritoneum), which is a living structure and so presents significant variations in performance.
2. The peritoneal dialysis system comprises the microcirculation of the peritoneal area, the meso-

thelium, and the peritoneal cavity with the infused solution.
3. The microcirculation can become a crucial factor when rapid exchanges are utilized, and blood flow may become a limiting factor under certain circumstances.
4. The mesothelium has different levels of permeability in different subjects. Furthermore, it is not a perfect osmotic barrier.
5. The dialysate compartment is the component with a broader spectrum of possibilities in terms of variations of volume, flows, and other manipulations.

Key References

10. Ronco C, Brendolan A, La Greca G: The peritoneal dialysis system. Nephrol Dial Transplant 1998;13(Suppl 6):94-99.
12. Ronco C: Limitations of peritoneal dialysis. Kidney Int 1996;50(Suppl 56):69-74.
13. Rippe B, Simonsen O, Stelin G: Clinical implications of a three pore model of peritoneal transport. Perit Dial Int 1991;7:3-9.
14. Dedrick RL, Flessner MF, Collins JM, Schultz JS: Is the peritoneum a membrane? ASAIO J 1982;5:1-8.
23. Ronco C: The nearest capillary hypothesis: A novel approach to peritoneal transport physiology. Perit Dial Int 1996;16:121-125.

See the companion Expert Consult website for the complete reference list.

CHAPTER 265

Indications, Contraindications, and Complications of Peritoneal Dialysis in Acute Renal Failure

Stephen R. Ash

OBJECTIVES

This chapter will:
1. Present data on the clinical effectiveness of peritoneal dialysis in acute renal failure.
2. Compare clinical benefits of acute peritoneal dialysis with those of other modalities of dialysis for support of patients with acute renal failure.
3. Explain some particular benefits of peritoneal dialysis, especially in removal of middle-molecular-weight toxins, protein-bound toxins, and fluid.
4. Detail the clearance benefits of continuous-flow peritoneal dialysis and methods by which it can be performed currently in patients with acute renal failure.
5. Discuss the particular disadvantages of peritoneal dialysis in the treatment of acute renal failure, including peritonitis, and compare its risks with those of other therapies.

OVERALL SUCCESS OF ACUTE PERITONEAL DIALYSIS IN ADULTS

When choosing treatment for an adult with acute renal failure (ARF), nephrologists generally think of continuous venovenous hemodialysis (CVVHD) or intermittent hemodialysis (IHD), but not peritoneal dialysis (PD). This tendency makes acute PD a considerably underused therapy,[1] in spite of numerous problems encountered with the extracorporeal therapies that can be eliminated by the use of the peritoneal membrane. In fact, PD could be considered the perfect and natural version of continuous arteriovenous hemofiltration (CAVH) and dialysis.

As with all dialysis procedures, PD was first used in therapy of ARF.[2] Now continuous ambulatory peritoneal dialysis (CAPD) or PD cycler therapy supports about 10% of patients with end-stage renal disease (ESRD) in the United States[3] and a higher percentage of patients than are

TABLE 265-1

Comparison of Mortality in Acute Renal Failure: Peritoneal Dialysis (PD) versus Hemodialysis (HD)

			Mortality (%)	
STUDY*	YEAR	NO. PATIENTS	PD	HD or CVVH
Orofino et al[8]	1976	82	52	62
Firmat[9]	1979	1,101	50	50
Ash[2]	1983	97	38	48
Swartz[10]	1980	77	44	60
Struijk[11]	1980	45	45	(same)
Struijk[†]	1986-1999	50	78	(same)
Phu[12]	2002	70	47	15
Chitalia et al[13]	2002	82[‡]	7[§]	—

*Superscript numbers indicate chapter references.
[†]Personal communication, 2000.
[‡]Tidal peritoneal dialysis and continuous equilibrium PD.
[§]All hypercatabolic patients.

supported by hemodialysis in some countries. PD was once a more common choice for treatment of ARF in adults.[4] In ARF, PD is appropriate for the same types of patients for which CAVH is chosen: those with heart failure and low cardiac index who cannot tolerate the rapid fluid removal rate of standard hemodialysis. PD has a risk of complications in the range of or lower than that for CVVHD (as discussed later). PD is still the mainstay in treatment of ARF in infants and children.[5,6] For PD in pediatric patients with the use of a surgically placed Tenckhoff catheter, incidence of all types of complications during the course of renal failure was only 9%, compared with 49% for patients in whom catheters were placed percutaneously at the bedside.[7] With chronic peritoneal dialysis, complications are measured in number per year rather than number per week. Regarding patient outcomes, a number of prospective and retrospective studies and some randomized studies have compared PD and hemodialysis in the treatment of ARF. With the acknowledging that the patient populations in the various studies are not exactly the same, most studies have shown outcomes to be at least as good for PD as for hemodialysis, as shown in Table 265-1.[8-13]

Except for the study by Phu and colleagues,[12] all studies summarized in Table 265-1 have shown that in patients with ARF treated with PD, mortality and incidence of renal recovery are roughly equivalent to those in similar patients treated with hemodialysis. Firmat and Zucchini,[9] reviewing literature reports involving more than 1100 patients, concluded that the mortality rate was identical for patients with ARF receiving PD and those receiving hemodialysis. Most of these studies were performed in the 1970s and 1980s. However, Struijk continued analyzing patients treated with each modality at the Academic Free Hospital in Amsterdam from 1986 through 1999 (DG Struijk, personal communication, 2000). In these studies, mortality in patients treated with PD was identical to that of patients treated with hemodialysis. In the study by Chitalia and associates,[13] both tidal PD (TPD) and manual-exchange PD were adequate for treatment of patients with ARF and mild to moderate hypercatabolism. Death occurred in hypercatabolic patients, but overall mortality rate was still very low (7%).

In the study by Phu and colleagues,[12] 70 adult patients with ARF, due to severe falciparum malaria in 48 and to sepsis in 22, were randomly assigned to treatment by PD or by CVVH. The mortality was significantly higher in the group treated with PD (47%), as well as a lower rate of renal recovery than in the group treated with hemofiltration (mortality 15%). The PD schedule was very aggressive (70 L of fluid per day). Urea clearance of urea with PD was about equal to that with CVVH, but creatinine clearance with PD was about half that with CVVH.[12] What is most unusual about the Phu study is the exceedingly low mortality of the group treated with CVVH, rather than an unusually high mortality in the group treated with PD. As Daugirdas[14] pointed out, it is possible that the heparin anticoagulation of CVVH was of benefit to the many patients with malaria in this study. Also, hyperglycemia may have stimulated malarial growth in the liver or red cells, or high osmolality may have diminished white cell function. Failure to correct acidosis may have been due to use of acetate rather than lactate or bicarbonate as buffer in the PD solution.

None of the studies summarized in Table 265-1, except for the study by Phu and colleagues,[12] was randomized or prospectively controlled, and there was bias in patient selection. However, this bias worked both for and against patients treated by PD. Patients with ARF who have abdominal trauma, are awaiting abdominal surgery, or have abdominal drains or severe ileus cannot be treated by PD. In general, however, patients with ARF after surgery have a higher rate of recovery from ARF than patients with other causes of ARF, such as sepsis and shock. In these studies, PD was often chosen for patients with hypotension or cardiovascular instability that would make hemodialysis dangerous, a practice that also selected a group with a potentially worse outcome. The techniques used for PD in most of the studies were antiquated by today's standards. In many studies, semirigid acute PD catheters were used. Such catheters have irregular outflow characteristics, and many must be removed and re-inserted every 3 days. Each insertion increases the risk of bowel puncture and outflow failure. PD fluid was infused from bottles in many of the studies, and there were no Y-sets to allow drainage and infusion of PD fluid though a single catheter connection. In spite of all of these disadvantages, PD patients in these studies recovered renal function and survived at least as frequently as patients treated with hemodialysis, with the notable exception of the study by Phu and colleagues.[12]

In many of the studies comparing PD with hemodialysis for ARF, the improved survival in the PD group correlated with a higher rate of renal recovery. Very few patients with ARF recover general health but fail to recover renal function, leaving the hospital with ESRD to be supported by dialysis. In patients with ESRD, treatment by CAPD results in better preservation of intrinsic renal function than treatment with IHD.[15-18] This preservation of renal function is important in ESRD because it maintains the endocrine function of the kidneys, diminishes the clearance requirements for dialysis, minimizes required ultrafiltration during dialysis, and thus diminishes physiological stress during dialysis. IHD is known to have the following nephrotoxic effects: (1) generation of inflammatory mediators by the extracorporeal circuit, (2) concomitant and rapid decrease in osmolality and vascular volume, which diminish renal perfusion, and (3) hypotensive episodes, which result in fresh ischemic lesions in the kidneys.[19]

By contrast, the effects of CAPD therapy help maintain renal perfusion, as follows: (1) smaller daily variation in body weight, (2) more constant blood pressure, (3) continued mild overhydration, with higher mean pulmonary arterial pressure,[20] (4) persistent high blood osmolality, due partly to glucose,[20] and (5) continued removal of proteins from the blood, including β_2-microglobulin, albumin, plasminogen activator inhibitor type 1, and immunoglobulins.[14,21,22]

Given the beneficial effects of PD, it is not surprising that some patients started on PD for what appears to be ESRD recover intrinsic renal function and no longer need dialysis (3.3%). Given the negative physiological effects of hemodialysis, it is also not surprising that very few patients with ESRD who are treated with IHD recover renal function (0.8%).[20] Recovery of renal function is most common in patients whose renal failure was caused by uncontrolled hypertension, cardiac failure, nephrotic syndrome, rapidly progressive renal failure, analgesic nephropathy, urinary obstruction, or cholesterol emboli.[20] Many of these underlying conditions are better corrected by CAPD than by hemodialysis, because of the former's continuous chemical removal, better preservation of renal perfusion and glomerular filtration rate,[20] and slow removal of immunoglobulins. These same physiological and chemical benefits may account for the higher recovery of renal function, in most studies, in patients with ARF treated with PD than with hemodialysis.[14-19,23]

There is general consensus that continuous dialysis therapies such as CVVH and CVVHD are the most chemically effective therapies for ARF, with the fewest adverse physiological effects. These "gentle" forms of therapy remove fluid at a slow rate and cause less decrease in cardiac output than hemodialysis. They do not adversely affect pulmonary function or significantly activate the complement cascade.[6] CAVH was first described in 1967.[24] Pump-assisted CVVH and CVVHD were developed to make the rate of blood flow through the hemofilter more consistent, improve clearances, and render the therapy more nearly continuous. Continuous blood therapies also have a number of disadvantages in comparison with IHD and PD. CVVH requires considerable attention from nurses to ensure adequate blood flow, monitor anticoagulation status, adjust ultrafiltration rate, and calculate patient fluid balance. The patient is immobilized during the treatment. Continuous heparin administration increases risk of bleeding. Central venous or femoral catheters often provide insufficient blood flow and carry risks for infection and sepsis.[4-6] In spite of the name and intent, the average duration of individual treatments with "continuous" blood therapies is 20 hours before clotting of the system or need for discontinuation to transport the patient for diagnostic

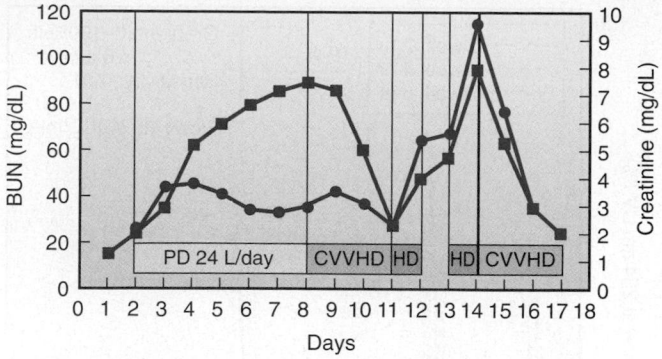

FIGURE 265-1. Blood urea nitrogen (BUN; *circles*) and serum creatinine (*squares*) concentrations in a single patient with acute renal failure treated successively with high-volume peritoneal dialysis, continuous venovenous hemodialysis (CVVHD), hemodialysis (HD), hemodialysis, and CVVHD. (From Amerling R: Peritoneal dialysis in treatment of acute renal failure. Presented at CRRT Conference, San Diego, 2005.)

or therapeutic procedures. Some centers previously performing CVVH or CVVHD for acute dialysis have begun using sustained low-efficiency dialysis with extended duration (6-8 hours/day) to avoid many of the problems of CVVH or CVVHD, limiting heparin use and immobility of the patient while keeping the advantages of vascular stability and improved clearances.[25] By contrast, PD is a truly continuous dialysis therapy, requiring less risk and less nursing effort than CVVH or CVVHD and allowing more patient mobility during therapy.

The major criticism of PD, of course, is a low clearance of uremic toxins, and clearance of low-molecular-weight toxins is in fact lower than that with other therapies. For continuous therapies, the time-averaged clearance is the same as the immediate clearance. For intermittent therapies, the time-averaged clearance is diminished in proportion to the time between dialysis sessions. Although blood urea nitrogen clearance is lower with PD than with either CVVH or hemodialysis, creatinine clearance with PD can be close to that with CVVH if the peritoneal fluid flow is high enough. Figure 265-1 compares blood urea nitrogen and creatinine levels in a patient treated with high-volume PD, then CVVH, then hemodialysis.[26] Although the blood urea nitrogen level rose to approximately 80 mg/dL during days of PD, the creatinine values with PD and CVVHD were comparable and were lower than the creatinine value with IHD.

The clearance of PD appears more effective with observation of large molecule removal. Clearance rate for phosphorus is close to that for creatinine. PD is quite effective in removing various anionic organic compounds that function as middle molecules (Fig. 265-2).[21] In ARF, clinical experience confirms that PD results in equal or higher rates of resolution of uremic symptoms and patient survival in comparison with the other therapies (described previously). This fact may be due to removal of numerous middle-size organic molecules.

In addition to removal of uremic toxins, of course, dialysis for ARF must remove fluid and salt from the patient. With a properly functioning PD catheter, exchanges of 2 L of dialysate with 2.5% or 4.25% glucose concentration provides daily fluid removal at a rate the same as or greater than that of other regimens, without causing hypotension

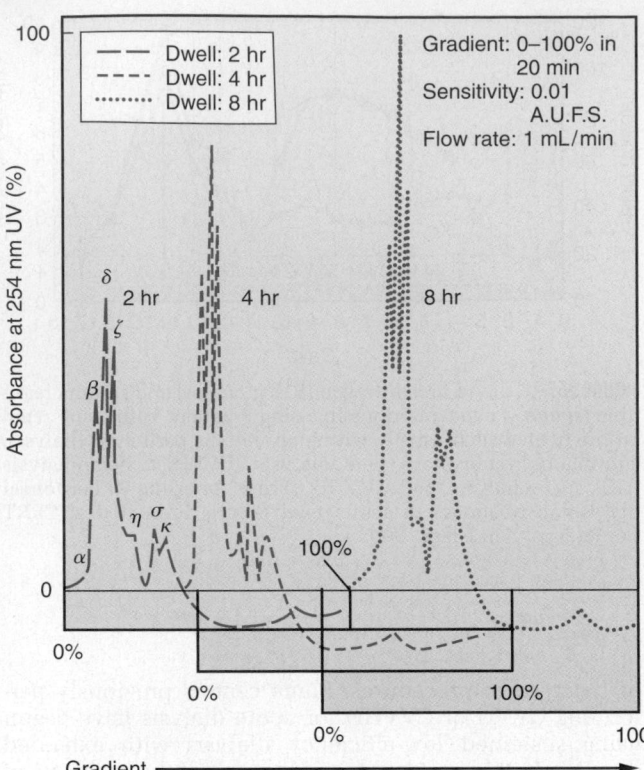

Anion exchange chromatograms of 2 L of peritoneal fluid removed from one patient after dwells of 2, 4, and 8 hours

FIGURE 265-2. Increase in anionic organic compounds within peritoneal dialysis fluid, over periods of 2 hours, 4 hours, and 8 hours, in a patient with end-stage renal disease. Chromatograms generated by direct anion exchange chromatography, without protein removal. (From Ash SR, Bungu ATJ, Regnier FE: Dependence of middle molecular clearance on protein concentration of peritoneal fluid. In Maher JF, Winchester JF (eds): Frontiers in Peritoneal Dialysis. New York, Field, Rich and Associates, 1986, pp 56-63.)

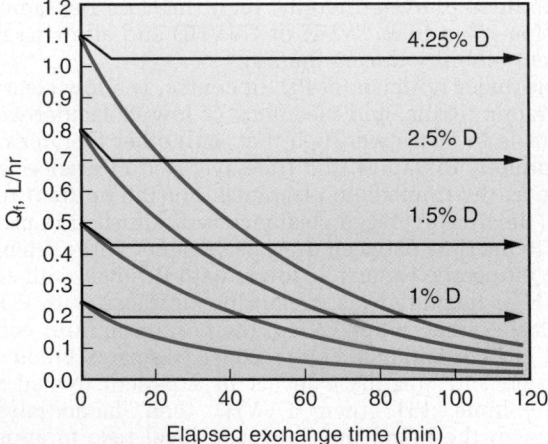

FIGURE 265-3. Fluid removal rate (Q_f) with batch exchanges of peritoneal dialysis fluid (*blue lines*) and continuous-flow peritoneal dialysis (*black arrows*). (From Gotch FA: Kinetic modeling of continuous flow peritoneal dialysis. Semin Dial 2001;14:378-383.)

in most patients. In patients with refractory congestive heart failure, fluid removal is the main goal, and with PD therapy and hypertonic dialysate, improvement in clinical symptomatology and left ventricular function is routine. In one study of 20 patients with resistant congestive heart failure, all improved after PD with only 12 inflow/outflow cycles.[27] As demonstrated by Gotch,[28] fluid removal rates with batch exchanges are initially 0.2 to 1.0 L/hour (Fig. 265-3). With continuous-flow peritoneal dialysis (CFPD; discussed later), fluid removal can be maintained at the initial rate of batch exchanges.

Just as with CVVHD, the small molecule clearance of PD can be greatly increased by raising the flow rate of dialysate to 1.5 to 2 L/hr or more. Tidal PD (TPD) can easily deliver 2 L/hr into and out of the peritoneum, and with use of a cycler, automated TPD is only a little more complicated than manual in/out exchanges. In one study of patients with ARF, a peritoneal dialysate flow rate of 2 L/hr produced an average normalized creatinine clearance of 68.5 L per week per 1.73 m² of body surface area (BSA) and a urea clearance value (Kt/V) of 2.43, versus average values for "equilibrium" PD, 58.9 L/wk/1.73m² BSA and a Kt/V of 1.80. Both TPD and manual-exchange PD were adequate for treatment of patients with ARF and mild to moderate catabolism, but insufficient in some patients with hypercatabolism.[21]

Future implementation of PD for ARF will have much higher urea and creatinine clearances, through the use of an "old but good" idea, CFPD. This modality utilizes two access points to the peritoneum, one for inflow of dialysate and the other for outflow. Because there is no interruption of inflow to allow outflow, flow rates are determined only by the rate at which the draining catheter can reproducibly drain the abdomen. With CFPD, dialysate flow rates of up to 300 mL/min can be maintained through the peritoneum.[29] With use of an external dialyzer to "regenerate" the dialysate, clearances for urea, creatinine, and urate average 57, 35, and 39 mL/min, respectively in adult patients.[30] At 170 mL/min of dialysate flow, urea and creatinine clearances have averaged 31 and 23 mL/min, respectively.[23] Studies using dialyzer-regenerated PD fluid and dual Tenckhoff catheters have confirmed urea clearances of 50 mL/min or more in several patients with ARF.[31]

CFPD has also been used effectively for treating massive fluid overload, much like isolate ultrafiltration. In six pediatric patients with ARDS due to sepsis or systemic inflam-

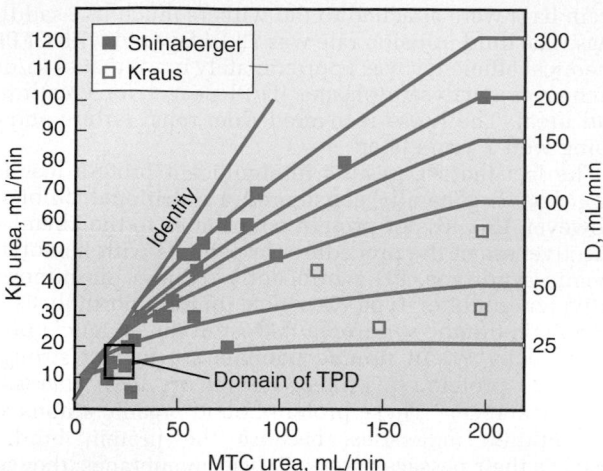

FIGURE 265-4. Analysis of published urea clearances (K_p) and peritoneal mass transfer coefficient (MTC) at varying peritoneal dialysate flow rates (D) during continuous-flow peritoneal dialysis. (Data from Kraus; and Shinaberger et al.[30]) (From Gotch FA: Kinetic modeling of continuous flow peritoneal dialysis. Semin Dial 2001;14:378-383.)

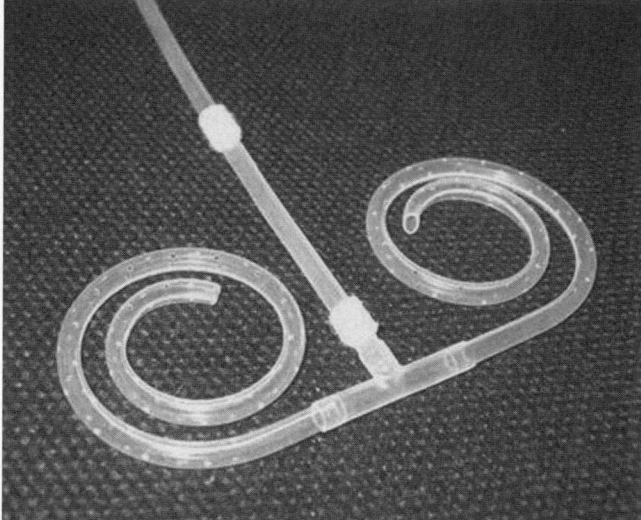

FIGURE 265-5. The MaxFlow peritoneal dialysis catheter (Ash Access Technology, Inc., Lafayette, IN). The limbs are straightened before placement; after placement of the catheter through a single hole in the peritoneum via either dissection or peritoneoscopy and the Quill guide, the limbs uncoil against the parietal peritoneum.

matory response syndrome, CFPD at 10 to 30 mL/kg/hr with two Tenckhoff catheters resulted in an average 33% decrease in body weight and an improvement in alveolar-arterial oxygen gradient.[32] With CFPD, the time-averaged clearance of urea with PD can theoretically exceed that with daily 4-hour hemodialysis and come close to those with CVVH or CVVHD—approaching the K_oA or maximal clearance theoretically obtainable from the peritoneum, as shown in Figure 265-4.[33] Dialysate flow rates of 200 to 300 mL/min seem unrealistic today only because nephrologists are accustomed to using expensive, prepackaged dialysate and gravity flow. However, if PD machines reappear that proportion fluid on site, or if sorbent-based regenerative systems are commercialized,[34-36] peritoneal dialysate will be available at just about any flow rate desired. Clearances of urea by CFPD may approach the theoretical limit of the peritoneal membrane and far exceed those of TPD (as in Fig. 265-4). However, there is a considerable variation in clearance, especially at lower flow rates. This variance probably relates to day-to-day variations in intraperitoneal volume or to channeling between catheters, problems that must still be solved for CFPD to be a reliable therapy.[37]

For CFPD to be successful, there must be effective drainage of the peritoneum at relatively high flow rates. Theoretically this goal is not difficult, because the standard Tenckhoff catheter can drain the abdomen at 300 mL/min or more under gravity flow in CAPD during the early part of outflow. However, flow from Tenckhoff catheters is somewhat variable and much slower toward the end of outflow. A diminution in flow during CAPD exchanges represents merely a slower outflow and some inconvenience. In CFPD at 300 mL/min, it is possible to build up an extra liter of fluid in the peritoneum in only a few minutes. The Advantage T-fluted peritoneal catheter (Ash Access Technology, Lafayette, IN) is a newer catheter for chronic PD that has grooves rather than holes on two limbs that lie against the parietal peritoneum. The catheter provides higher flow rate and more complete drainage of peritoneal fluid than the standard Tenckhoff catheter. The use of this catheter may make performance of PD easier in patients with ARF, even if they have mild ileus.[38,39] The

catheter may also provide faster and more reliable drainage for CFPD, using a second site for infusion of fluid into the peritoneum or one limb of the T-shaped catheter for infusion and one for drainage.[40] A potential improvement on this catheter is the MaxFlow catheter, being developed by Ash Access Technology, which consists of two limbs that are shaped like the ends of curled Tenckhoff catheters (Fig. 265-5). These limbs open and lie against the peritoneal surface as the catheter is placed (with a Quill Guide or through dissection). Flow with the MaxFlow catheter appears to be as high as or higher than flow with the Advantage catheter. Resistance to omental attachment and outflow failure with the MaxFlow appears to be very low, from initial clinical experience. If flow of the catheter is as expected, it may serve effectively as the drainage limb of a CFPD system.

For CFPD to be successful, the intraperitoneal volume or pressure must also be controlled. In an animal study, Ash[41] demonstrated that there is an optimal peritoneal volume for highest efficiency of the peritoneum in CFPD, about 1.5 L in the dog. With in-and-out manual PD, the abdomen is drained fairly well at the end of each outflow cycle. With CFPD, as with TPD, the amount of fluid going into and out of the abdomen may be known, but the intraperitoneal volume is unknown because of the variability of ultrafiltration rate. In TPD, the abdomen is drained in the middle of an 8-hour treatment, so as to restart the treatment with a near-zero intraperitoneal volume.

With CFPD, a simpler approach is to control the intraperitoneal pressure, which is related to intraperitoneal volume. Because the compliance of the peritoneum is relatively constant and symptoms relate to pressure rather than volume, controlling the pressure in the peritoneum provides a relatively constant volume and a modest decrease in cardiac output and vital capacity (Fig. 265-6).[42,51] To provide a constant peritoneal pressure using an Advantage catheter or other well-functioning catheter in a supine patient with ARF is fairly easy. Infusion of peritoneal fluid through a second site is performed at up to 1.5 to 3 L/hr, and the Advantage catheter is attached to a drain bag that lies flat upon a bedside stand, 6 cm above the umbilicus (Fig. 265-7). With a well-functioning drainage catheter, this arrangement provides an intraperitoneal pressure of 6 to 8 cm. One can measure ultrafiltration rate by intermittently weighing the PD drain bag and subtracting the inflow bag weight. This method is relatively simple to perform manually but would be even simpler with automated, regenerating PD equipment.

Pressure-controlled CFPD has been performed in a patient using an Advantage catheter for drainage in the left mid-quadrant and a straight Tenckhoff catheter for infusion into the right lower quadrant.[29] Fluid removal was consistent, and clearances equaled those of in/out exchanges of similar volume. CFPD has also been used in a full-grown horse with nonoliguric ARF and a creatinine level of 16 mg/dL.[43] The draining catheter was a large chest tube in the lower abdomen, and for pressure control, the

drain bags were attached to the withers much like saddlebags. The fluid infusion rate was 72 L/day, and with CFPD, chemical efficiency was approximately twice that of in/out exchanges (Dialysate/plasma [D/P] near 1 for creatinine and urea). The horse recovered from renal failure and is doing well 2 years later.

The fact that PD results in significant protein loss (5-20 g/day) is generally considered a nutritional problem. However, this loss of protein contributes to the chemical effectiveness of the procedure. In patients with hemolytic uremic syndrome, PD significantly reduces plasminogen activator inhibitor type 1, which inhibits fibrinolysis in hemolytic uremic syndrome.[44] Most of the organic anions removed by PD in uremic patients are in fact strongly bound to protein, so protein output or "loss" increases their clearance.[29] These protein-bound organic anions act like middle molecules, because the protein binding restricts their passage across dialysis membranes; they are still accumulating in peritoneal dialysate at 8 hours of dwell time (see Fig. 265-2). The presence of protein within the dialysate facilitates the transfer of these compounds into the peritoneum. The peritoneal transfer of protein can be increased by application of hypertonicity and pharmacotherapy; the globulin removal by PD on a daily basis could equal or exceed that of daily therapeutic plasmapheresis.[30]

Every therapy for ARF has some risks. In ARF the success and risks of various dialysis modalities relate in part to the access devices needed to provide them. If acute catheters are used in PD, each catheter can be used for only 3 days without high risk of peritonitis or bowel perforation, and each successive catheter carries a higher risk of these complications. For acute PD to be performed effectively and safely, a chronic tunneled PD catheter must be the access device. Chronic PD catheters were used in the studies by Ash and colleagues[21] and Struijk and colleagues[11] but rigid acute catheters were used in the study by Phu.[12]

Chronic PD catheters can be placed at the bedside in the ICU, in procedure rooms, or via surgery using local anesthesia. With use of the peritoneoscopic technique and local anesthesia, it takes only 15 to 30 minutes to place a chronic two-cuff Tenckhoff catheter, just as is done for patients with ESRD.[45] Peritoneoscopically placed catheters are usually placed at the lateral border of the rectus muscle and can be directed to lie against the parietal peritoneum in a direction that avoids adhesions and bowel loops. The parietal peritoneal surface provides a more consistent flow

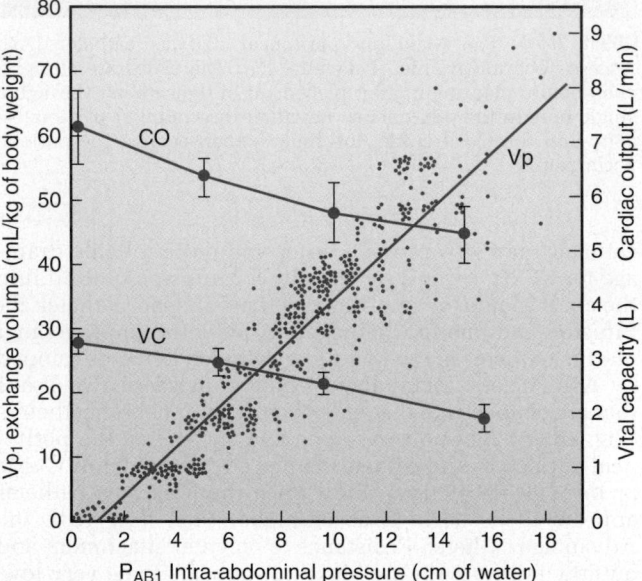

FIGURE 265-6. Relationship among intraperitoneal pressure (P_{AB1}; measured versus umbilicus, with patient reclining), intraperitoneal volume (Vp) vital capacity, and cardiac output. (From Ash SR, Carr DJ, Diaz-Buxo JA, Crabtree JH: Peritoneal access devices: Design, function, and placement techniques. In Nissenson AR, Fine RN [eds]: Clinical Dialysis, 4th ed. New York, McGraw-Hill, 2005.)

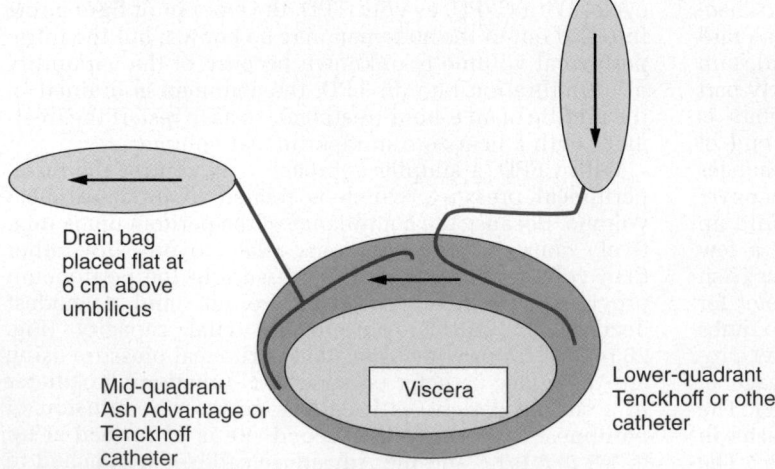

FIGURE 265-7. Simplified method for controlling intraperitoneal pressure and volume during continuous-flow peritoneal dialysis by placing the drain bag above the umbilicus.

of fluid from the abdomen during outflow. Peritoneoscopically placed catheters have the highest rate of successful hydraulic function in the first few weeks of use as well as over years of use.[46] With a properly functioning chronic peritoneal access, the effectiveness of PD is increased and risks are considerably diminished, because one catheter is used for the duration of ARF therapy. Tenckhoff catheters allow peritoneal access for years, rather than the days of safe use for acute PD catheters. Advantage catheters can also be placed peritoneoscopically by expansion of the initial 2-mm puncture site to a 9-mm diameter.[41,47] During the same procedure, a second small infusion catheter can also be placed with an entry to the peritoneum several inches or more from the Advantage catheter and directed toward the opposite quadrant.

Among therapies for ARF, PD has the unique risk of causing peritonitis. However, in patients in whom infection is suspected as a cause of ARF, performing PD can be helpful in ensuring that peritonitis is not present. In other patients, if peritonitis is detected, diagnostic tests can be implemented to determine the source, and antibiotic therapy begun to treat the infection. Nurses who are properly trained for PD soak the connectors with polyvinylpyrrolidone-iodine, put on a mask and nonsterile gloves, and use care in performing connections. The risk of contamination of PD fluid is minimal during each exchange. The incidence of peritonitis in PD therapy of ARF is much different from that in CAPD therapy. If peritonitis is detected during therapy of ARF with PD, it usually occurs within 2 or 3 days of the start of therapy.[16,48] Therefore, PD may reveal contamination of the peritoneum that predated the implementation of PD. The organisms causing peritonitis in patients with ARF are much different from those causing peritonitis in patients undergoing CAPD. There is predominance of *Staphylococcus epidermidis* and *Candida* species in PD, which are not usually seen in peritonitis in patients undergoing CAPD (Table 265-2), and mixed infection is common.[49] If peritonitis occurs during PD therapy, it causes cloudy dialysate and sometimes local symptoms but does not usually result in septicemia in the patient with ARF. This is a much different outcome from that of catheter infection during hemodialysis or CVVH, which always results in septicemia.

The complications of PD and hemodialysis for ARF have been compared in one center providing both types of therapy.[42] In this study reported by Swartz and colleagues,[10] the patients treated by hemodialysis had a high incidence of severe hypotension and severe hemorrhage, acidosis, and shunt clotting. Patients undergoing PD had a high incidence of hyperglycemia, poor catheter drainage, and asymptomatic peritonitis (Table 265-3). The major causes of death in patients with ARF were also different for patients treated by hemodialysis and with PD. Death from sepsis unrelated to dialysis was higher for the hemodialysis group, but cardiac deaths were higher in the PD group owing to the more frequent implementation of this therapy in patients with underlying heart disease (Table 265-4).

When one compares the overall risks of each type of therapy for ARF, there are marked differences among CVVH, CVVHD, hemodialysis, and PD (Table 265-5). The blood treatment therapies have a significant risk of septicemia, low flow from the blood access, hypotension, membrane clotting, and bleeding. PD therapy involves risks of PD catheter outflow failure, hyperglycemia, and asymptomatic peritonitis. Peritonitis is the only one with potential to adversely affect the patient; however, if the initiation of PD reveals a preexisting peritonitis, antibiotic or surgical therapy may resolve the infection that caused the ARF. In patients treated with PD during ARF, recognition and therapy of preexisting peritonitis contribute to the improved outcome of these patients.

There are no studies comparing the costs of performing these four uremic therapies, or the cost of treatment of various complications (other than the study by Phu,[12] in which all therapies were relatively inexpensive). Nurses who perform acute PD will confirm that this therapy is simple; every 2 to 4 hours, a clamp is opened to drain the peritoneum, a new bag is attached to the inflow line, and the inflow clamp is opened. The costs of the therapy are only the cost of 6 to 12 bags of peritoneal dialysate each day, plus that of the labor of an ICU nurse to open a clamp to drain the peritoneum, then attach and infuse the volume of a new bag. Data collection is simple; the outflow volume is measured and recorded, and the fluid is inspected to determine whether it is clear or cloudy. Much more nursing time is required for procedures and measurements related to CVVH, CVVHD, and hemodialysis treatments.

PD for ARF has a number of other advantages, summarized by Golper[50] as follows:

- Procedure is widely available and technically easy to perform.
- Large amounts of fluid can be removed in hemodynamically unstable patients; this fluid removal may also permit the administration of parenteral nutrition.
- Dysequilibrium syndrome is not precipitated because of slow solute removal.
- Acid-base and electrolyte imbalances are corrected easily and gradually.
- PD access placement is relatively easy, particularly in children.
- Arterial or venous puncture and anticoagulation are not required.
- PD is a highly biocompatible technique requiring no systemic anticoagulation.

TABLE 265-2

Bacteriology of Peritonitis in Peritoneal Dialysis of Acute Renal Failure

ORGANISM	NUMBER OF PATIENTS	PERCENTAGE OF PATIENTS
Staphylococcus aureus	2	7
Staphylococcus epidermidis	7	26
Multiple gram-negative organisms	4	15
Escherichia coli	1	4
Other gram-negative organisms	2	7
Multiple (gram-positive and -negative) organisms	2	7
Candida sp.	7	26
Culture-negative specimens	2	7
Total	27	100

From Sharma RK, Kuma J, Gupta A, Gulati S: Peritoneal infection in acute intermittent peritoneal dialysis. Ren Fail 2003;25:975-980.

TABLE 265-3

Complications of Dialysis in Acute Renal Failure*

	HEMODIALYSIS	PERITONEAL DIALYSIS
Number of dialyses	240	65
Number of patients	34	43
Severe hypotension[†]	85/240 (35%)	8/65 (12%)
Severe hemorrhage[‡]	15/34 (44%)	2/43 (5%)
Metabolic complications:		
Hyperglycemia (250 mg/dL)		37/65 (57%)
Hypernatremia (150 mEq/L)		2/65 (3%)
Acidosis	9/34 (26%)	
Neurologic complications:		
Seizures	1/34 (3%)	3/43 (7%)
Deterioration in state of consciousness		9/65 (14%)
Mechanical complications:		
Mild bleeding		17/65 (26%)
Poor drainage, leaking		34/65 (52%)
Shunt clotting	11/34 (32%)	
Infections:		
Shunt infection	2/34 (6%)	
Peritonitis		4/34 (12%)
Asymptomatic positive peritoneal culture results		19/65 (29%)

*Expressed as a fraction of total dialysis or total patients.
[†]Blood pressure <90 mm Hg systolic, requiring blood products or vasopressor administration.
[‡]Requiring transfusion.
From Swartz RD, Valk TW, Brain AJW, Hsu CH: Complications of HD in ARF. ASAIO J 1980;3:98.

TABLE 265-4

Causes of Death from Acute Renal Failure*

	HEMODIALYSIS (N = 34)	PERITONEAL DIALYSIS (N = 43)
Causes not related to dialysis:	16 (48%)	14 (33%)
Sepsis	11	2
Cardiac	2	7[†]
Hemorrhage	3	3
Hepatorenal	4	2
Other	1	0
Dialysis-related causes:	4 (12%)	5 (12%)
Sepsis[‡]	3	3
Cardiac	3	22
Hemorrhage	2	0

*Several patients died from more than one cause.
[†]Of the 9 cardiac deaths in the PD group, 7 occurred in patients with underlying heart disease (p < 0.05).
[‡]Shunt sepsis in HD; peritoneal sepsis in PD.
From Swartz RD, Valk TW, Brain AJW, Hsu CH: Complications of HD in ARF. ASAIO J 1980;3:98.

TABLE 265-5

Risks of Various Dialysis Therapies for Acute Renal Failure*

RISK	CONTINUOUS ARTERIOVENOUS HEMOFILTRATION	CONTINUOUS VENOVENOUS HEMODIALYSIS	HEMODIALYSIS	PERITONEAL DIALYSIS
Septicemia	+	+	+	−
Vascular occlusion	+	+	+	−
Hypotension	−	−	+	−
Membrane clotting	+	+	+	−
Bleeding due to anticoagulant	+	+	+	−
Peritoneal dialysis catheter outflow failure				+
Hyperglycemia				+
Asymptomatic peritonitis, often preexisting				+

*Plus sign indicates that risk applies to modality; minus sign indicates that risk does not apply to modality.

Some of the indications for the use of PD as summarized by Golper[50] are as follows:

- Hemodynamically unstable patients
- The presence of a bleeding diathesis or hemorrhagic conditions
- Difficulty in obtaining blood access
- Removal of high-molecular-weight toxins (>10 kDa)
- Clinically significant hypothermia hyperthermia
- Heart failure refractory to medical or management

There are also a number of contraindications to PD for ARF that are relative rather than absolute[50]:

- Recent abdominal and/or cardiothoracic surgery
- Diaphragmatic peritoneum-pleura connections
- Severe respiratory failure
- Life-threatening hyperkalemia
- Extremely high catabolism
- Severe volume overload in a patient not on a ventilator
- Severe gastroesophageal reflux disease
- Low peritoneal clearance rates
- Fecal or fungal peritonitis
- Abdominal wall cellulitis
- ARF in pregnancy

CONCLUSION

When a properly functioning chronic peritoneal access device is placed, PD is a safe, effective, and inexpensive modality for the treatment of ARF. This modality is greatly under-utilized for treatment of ARF in the United States. When improvements in chemical efficiency, such as with CFPD, have been implemented, PD will become a much more widely used therapy for ARF.

Key Points

1. Clinical outcomes of acute renal failure, such as recovery of renal function and patient sur-vival, are similar for peritoneal dialysis and hemodialysis.
2. The chemical function of peritoneal dialysis is equivalent to or better than that of intermittent acute hemodialysis, though less effective than that with continuous venovenous hemodialysis or continuous hemodialysis.
3. Fluid removal by peritoneal dialysis is continuous, offering clinical advantage over intermittent therapies.
4. Continuous-flow peritoneal dialysis, which offers the potential to greatly improve the chemical effectiveness of acute peritoneal dialysis, can be performed with the use of currently available catheters and bagged solutions.
5. The unique adverse effects of peritoneal dialysis include peritonitis and increased intraperitoneal pressure; to minimize risk of these complications, certain patients with acute renal failure should not be treated with this modality.

Key References

13. Chitalia VC, Almeida AF, Rai H, et al: Is peritoneal dialysis adequate for hypercatabolic acute renal failure in developing countries? Kidney Int 2002;6:747-757.
29. Roberts M, Ash SR, Lee DBN: Innovative peritoneal dialysis: Flow-through and dialysate regeneration. ASAIO J 1999;45: 372-378.
31. Amerling R, Glezerman I, Savransky E, et al: Continuous flow peritoneal dialysis: Principles and applications. Semin Dial 2003;16:335-340.
47. Ash SR: Chronic peritoneal dialysis catheters: Procedures for placement, maintenance, and removal. Semin Nephrol 2002;22:221-236.
50. Golper TA: Use of peritoneal dialysis for the treatment of acute renal failure. UpToDate, 2006. Available at www.uptodate.com/

See the companion Expert Consult website for the complete reference list.

CHAPTER 266

Peritoneal Access for Acute Peritoneal Dialysis

Claudio Ronco and Roberto Dell'Aquila

OBJECTIVES

This chapter will:
1. Review the history of peritoneal catheters.
2. Explore peritoneal catheter designs and materials.
3. Explain the differences between the most popular peritoneal catheters.
4. Discuss the choice of peritoneal catheter for acute renal failure.

Over the last decade, significant advances have been made in the availability of different dialysis methods for replacement of renal function. Although the majority have been developed for patients with end-stage renal disease, there has been an increase in their application for the treatment of acute renal failure (ARF). Renal replacement therapy for ARF must be able to (1) maintain fluid, electrolyte, acid-base and solute homeostasis, (2) prevent worsening of renal function, (3) promote renal recovery, and (4) allow other support measures, such as nutrition, without limiting fluid volume.

A growing number of patients affected with ARF need to be treated in an intensive care unit because ARF occurs as a complication of a medical or surgical misfortune, or as part of the multiple-organ failure syndrome. The presence of more than one organ failure adversely affects the overall prognosis and creates additional management problems, such as respiratory failure, cardiovascular instability, inadequate cerebral perfusion, coagulation disturbances, specific nutritional needs, and the continuous threat of infections. Among various dialysis therapies for ARF in the adult, today's nephrologists favor continuous extracorporeal treatment over peritoneal dialysis (PD), making acute PD a considerably underused therapy.[1]

REASONS FOR UNDERUSE OF PERITONEAL DIALYSIS

There are several reasons for a less frequent use of peritoneal dialysis in ARF today. First, there has been a change in the spectrum of patients in whom ARF develops. The underlying diseases are much more serious than in the past, sepsis and hypercatabolism are often present, the patients are older, and ARF often develops quite late in the development of the multiple-organ failure syndrome. The lower efficiency of peritoneal dialysis, compared with extracorporeal dialysis, in removing solute and fluid limits its use in patients with ARF who require significant volume and solute removal (i.e., catabolic patients).

Second, ARF often occurs in patients who have had intra-abdominal surgery, in whom the insertion of an intraperitoneal catheter may cause problems of leakage and can be considered a source of infection. Third, by increasing the intra-abdominal pressure, peritoneal dialysis may compromise lung function and may therefore not be feasible in patients with acute respiratory distress syndrome.

And last, continuous extracorporeal renal replacement modalities have become more common therapeutic options for treatment of ARF in the intensive care unit. Reasons for its greater popularity include greater ease and convenience of use, a slow and continuous mode of volume control and blood purification, applicability in patients with low or unstable blood pressure, and lack of induction of hemodynamic instability.

WHY PERITONEAL DIALYSIS?

PD is a safe, effective, low-cost intracorporeal renal replacement modality with some inherent advantages. The peritoneal membrane is a biocompatible, internally located dialyzer. In fact, the peritoneum can be considered the "perfect" membrane, because it provides the following:
- Natural membranes located within the body
- Permeability to uremic toxins and limited passage of albumin and tightly bound toxins
- Limited passage of antibodies that cause kidney failure in some patients
- Infallible blood access with blood flow rate of about 200 mL/min
- Controllable ultrafiltration rate
- Biocompatibility of blood pathways, obviating need for anticoagulants

- Impermeability to bacteria in dialysate, preventing septicemia after dialysate contamination
- Permeability to white cells into dialysate if there is bacterial contamination, to limit proliferation and provide a visible sign of contamination
- Passage of the components of the PD fluid, such as glucose and/or various nutrients, through the peritoneal membrane directly to the liver (where metabolic conversion of lactate to bicarbonate takes place when lactate-based solutions are used)
- Ease of use, allowing continuous 24-hour dialysis through mere intermittent infusion and draining of modest volumes of sterile dialysate through a permanent access

Like other dialysis procedures, PD was first used in the therapy of ARF.[2] PD is appropriate for the same types of patients with ARF for whom continuous extracorporeal treatment is chosen—namely, patients affected with heart failure and low cardiac index who cannot tolerate the rapid fluid removal rate of standard hemodialysis.[3] PD is still the mainstay of treatment of ARF in infants and children.[4,5] In one study in which PD was performed in pediatric patients through a surgically placed Tenckhoff catheter, incidence of all types of complications during the course of renal failure were only 9%, versus 49% in adult patients in whom transcutaneous catheter placement was performed at the bedside immediately before dialysis.[6]

Patients with ARF who have abdominal trauma or who have undergone abdominal surgery and in whom drains are still in place, and patients with severe ileus cannot be treated by PD and they may have a higher mortality rate.

PD therapy has effects that help to maintain renal perfusion: they are smaller daily variation in body weight, more constant blood pressure, continued mild overhydration with higher mean pulmonary arterial pressure,[7] persistent high blood osmolality partly due to glucose,[7] and continued removal of proteins from the blood, including β_2-microglobulin, albumin, plasminogen activator inhibitor type 1, and immunoglobulins.[8-10]

There is general consensus that continuous dialysis therapies are the most chemically effective therapies for ARF with the fewest adverse physiological effects. These "gentle" forms of therapy remove fluid at a slow rate and therefore do not decrease cardiac output. They also do not adversely affect pulmonary function or activate the complement cascade.[5] Continuous blood therapies, however, require considerable attention from nurses to guarantee adequate blood flow, monitor anticoagulation status, adjust the ultrafiltration rate, and calculate the patient's fluid balance. The patient is generally immobilized during the treatment. Continuous heparin administration increases risk of bleeding. Vascular access catheters often provide insufficient blood flow and impose a risk of infection leading to sepsis.[3-5]

The success of peritoneal dialysis in end-stage renal disease and sustained low-efficiency dialysis (SLED) in acute dialysis would indicate that higher-molecular-weight toxins are more likely to be the real causes of uremic illness. Peritoneal dialysis is quite effective in removing various anionic organic compounds that function as middle-molecular-weight molecules. In ARF, clinical experience confirms that PD, like other therapies, achieves equal or higher rates of resolution of uremic symptoms and patient survival.

Besides removal of uremic toxins, of course, dialysis must also remove fluid and salt from the patient. With a properly functioning PD catheter, exchanges of 2 L of dialysate with 2.5% or 4.25% glucose concentration provide daily fluid removal at the same or a higher rate as other regimens, without causing hypotension in most patients. In patients with refractory congestive heart failure, fluid removal is the main goal; PD therapy in such patients, with hypertonic dialysate, routinely results in improvement in clinical symptomatology and left ventricular function. In one study involving 20 patients with resistant congestive heart failure, all improved with only 12 in/out PD cycles.[11]

Probably, continuous-flow peritoneal dialysis (CFPD) represents the future of peritoneal dialysis for ARF.[12-16] This technique (see later) allows the contemporaneous inflow and outflow of dialysate through the use of a double peritoneal access. High urea and creatinine clearances may be obtained with this technique, balancing fill volumes and flow rates; small abdominal fill volumes less the impact of dialysis on respiratory status.

PERITONEAL ACCESS

Brief History of the Peritoneal Catheter

In the 1960s it was discovered that silicone rubber is less irritating to the peritoneal membrane than other plastics, and in 1968, Tenckhoff and Schechter used a Dacron felt cuff to safely seal the catheter to the tissues, reducing the occurrence of leakage. This was the most important innovation in the history of peritoneal devices.

The Tenckhoff catheter has become the gold standard for peritoneal access. Some of these investigators' original recommendations for catheter insertion, such as an arcuate subcutaneous tunnel with downward directions of both intraperitoneal and external exits, are still considered very important elements of catheter implantation.

Peritoneal Catheters
Catheter Design and Materials

The four designs of the intraperitoneal portion of a peritoneal catheter are as follows (Table 266-1)[17]:

TABLE 266-1

Designs for Intraperitoneal Portion of Catheter for Peritoneal Dialysis

Straight and coiled Tenckhoff catheters	Straight
	Straight with discs (Toronto Western Hospital)
	Straight with weight (Di Paolo)
	Straight short (Vicenza)
	Coiled
	Balloon (Valli)
	T-fluted (Ash Advantage, Ash Access Technology, Lafayette, IN)
Swan-neck catheters	Swan-neck abdominal catheter
	Swan-neck Tenckhoff straight and coiled
	Swan-neck Missouri straight and coiled
	Moncrief-Popovich catheter
	Swan-neck presternal catheter
	Swan-neck Missouri catheter

- Straight Tenckhoff, with an 8- or 16-cm portion containing sideholes; the 16-cm catheter is available with or without a 12-g tungsten weight in the tip
- Curled Tenckhoff, with a coiled 16-cm portion containing sideholes
- Straight Tenckhoff, with perpendicular silicone discs (Toronto-Western Hospital [TWH] or Oreopoulos-Zellerman catheter)
- T-fluted catheter (Ash Advantage, Ash Access Technology, Lafayette, IN): a T-shaped catheter with grooved limbs positioned against the parietal peritoneum

The three basic shapes of the subcutaneous portion between the muscle wall and the skin exit site are (1) straight or a gently curved straight catheter, (2) a permanent 150-degree bend or arc (swan-neck), and (3) a permanent 90-degree bend, with another 90-degree bend at the peritoneal surface (pail handle or Cruz catheter).

The three positions and designs for Dacron (polyester) cuffs are as follows:

- Single cuff around the catheter, usually placed in the rectus muscle but sometimes on the anterior surface of the rectus (depending on the procedure used to implant the catheter)
- Dual cuffs around the catheter, one in the rectus muscle and the other in subcutaneous tissue
- Disc-ball deep cuff, with parietal peritoneum and posterior rectus sheath sewn between a Dacron disc and a silicone ball and a second subcutaneous cuff (TWH and Missouri catheters)

The adult PD catheter has an outer diameter of approximately 5 mm; various types of catheters have one of three internal diameters, as follows:

- 2.6 mm, the standard Tenckhoff catheter size: also swan-neck catheter, Missouri swan-neck catheter, and TWH catheter
- 3.1 mm: Cruz catheter
- 3.5 mm: Flex-Neck catheter (Medigroup, Inc., Oswego, IL), Ash Advantage catheter

Two materials are used to construct PD catheters; most are made of silicone rubber, and some are made of polyurethane (e.g., Cruz catheter).

A study by Nielsen and colleagues[18] demonstrated a longer 3-year survival rate for coiled than for straight Tenckhoff catheters. If properly placed, dual-cuff Tenckhoff catheters have a lower incidence of exit site infection and longer life span than single-cuff catheters.[19] Curled Tenckhoff catheters have a lower incidence of outflow failure than straight catheters. Swan-neck catheters appear to have a lower incidence of exit site infection than catheters with straight subcutaneous segments.[20]

The Ash Advantage Catheter

The design of the Ash Advantage catheter (Fig. 266-1) ensures a stable catheter position without extrusion of the deep cuff or erosion of the exit site.[21,22] Advantage catheters demonstrate a 1-year survival of 90%. During follow-up of 42 patients with Advantage catheters in place for up to 4 years, only 1 patient had a pericatheter leak, and no patient has experienced a pericatheter hernia or late exit infection. Outflow rate of PD fluid is on average equal to that of the best-functioning Tenckhoff catheters, including Flex-Neck catheters, which have a large internal diameter. The negative features of the Advantage catheter include the fact that it is somewhat more complicated to insert. Also, if the peritoneal fluid contains a considerable amount of blood or fibrin, the small openings between the fluted

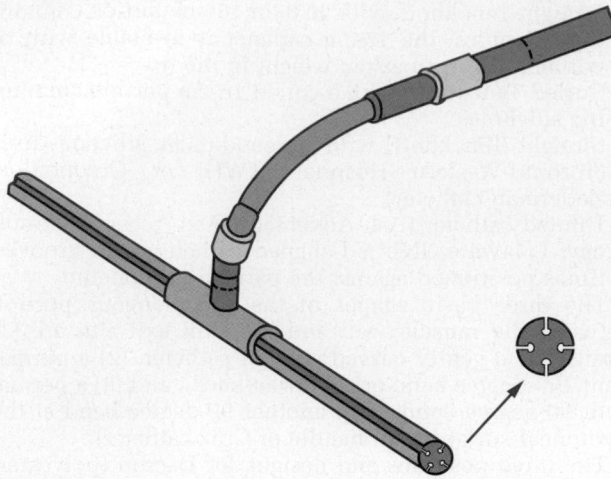

FIGURE 266-1. The Ash Advantage catheter. (From Stephen R. Ash, with permission.)

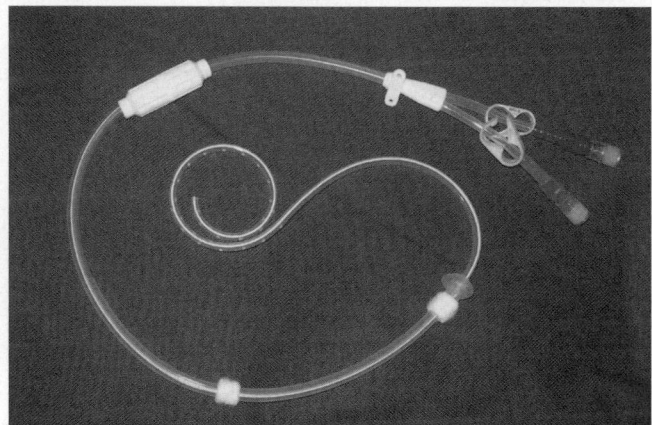

FIGURE 266-2. The Ronco catheter for continuous-flow dialysis.

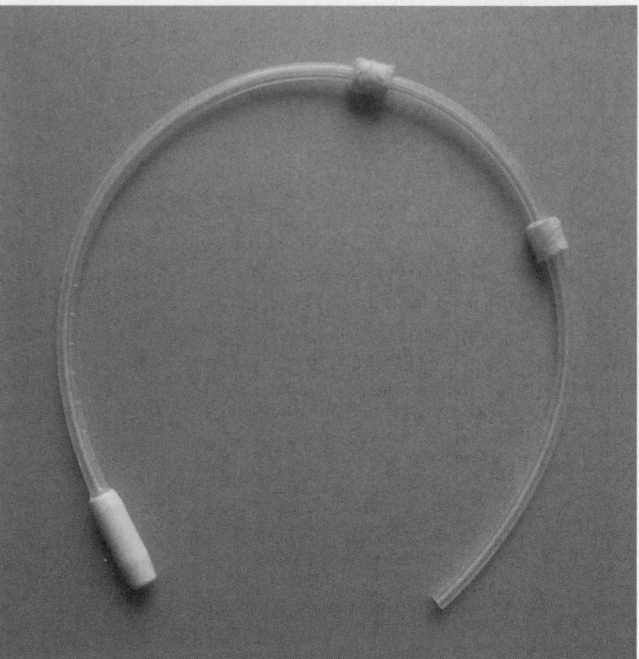

FIGURE 266-3. Di Paolo self-locating peritoneal dialysis catheter.

limbs and the central T portion of the Ash Advantage catheter can become blocked.

The Ronco Catheter for Continuous-Flow Peritoneal Dialysis

Probably the future of peritoneal dialysis for ARF may be CFPD.[13-17] This technique may utilize either two different access points or one double-lumen access, in which one lumen is for inflow of dialysate and the other for outflow (Fig. 266-2). Double-lumen catheters were originally designed with one branch short and another long of straight and of spiral shape. Ash and coworkers designed a catheter with a T configuration in order to maximize distance between the tips of the two lumens. Ronco and colleagues[23,24] have designed a novel catheter for CFPD. The catheter has a double cuff and a thin-walled silicone diffuser to gently diffuse the inflow dialysate into the peritoneum. To eliminate the problem of recirculation, the diffuser design and hole locations (Fig. 266-3) disperse the high-flow dialysate fluid at 360 degrees, reducing trauma to the peritoneal walls and allowing the dialysate to mix into the peritoneum; the dispersed fluid infused into the

peritoneal cavity is then drained through the second lumen, the tip of which is placed into the lower Douglas cavity. The results so far achieved seem to offer advantages in terms of high flows, minimal pressure regimens, and negligible recirculation. Further design features include a removable hub with two spikes to be adapted to the double-lumen cannula and to be applied after the catheter has been extracted from the skin through a small but adequate hole, and a new tunnelizer.

High urea and creatinine clearances may be obtained through a combination of flow rate and abdominal resident fill volume. Low abdominal fill volumes favorably reduce the impact of PD on respiratory status. Because there is no interruption of inflow to allow outflow with the Ronco catheter, flow rates are determined only by the rate at which the draining catheter can reproducibly drain the abdomen. With CFPD, dialysate flow rates of up to 300 mL/min can be maintained through the peritoneum.[25] With use of an external dialyzer to "regenerate" the dialysate, urea, creatinine, and urate clearances average 57, 35, and 39 mL/min, respectively, in adult patients.[26] These high dialysate flow rates seem unrealistic today only because current clinicians are accustomed to using expensive, prepackaged dialysate and gravity flow. However, if PD machines allowing fluid production on site are manufactured, or if sorbent-based regenerative systems are commercialized,[27-29] peritoneal dialysate will be available at just about any flow rate desired, allowing the low abdominal fill volumes that reduce PD's effect on respiratory status.

The cost of the therapy is only the cost of 6 to 12 bags of peritoneal dialysate each day, plus the labor of an ICU nurse to open a clamp to drain the peritoneum, remove the old bag, and attach and infuse the volume of a new bag. Afterwards, data collection is simple; the outflow volume is measured and recorded, and the fluid is inspected to determine whether it is clear or cloudy. Much more nursing time is required for extracorporeal treatments.

The Toronto Western Hospital Catheter

Sikaneta and associates[30] retrospectively studied charts for 192 patients receiving PD therapy with TWH catheters. Depending on whether catheter removal because of peritonitis was considered a catheter failure or a censored event, 1- and 3-year actuarial survival rates were 0.8536, 0.7406, and 0.9182 respectively. There was no difference in survival rates between diabetic and nondiabetic patients, males and females, and patients older and younger than 65 years. The 349 catheter complications occurred during 4845.3 catheter months of follow-up:

- 38 catheters were associated with more than one episode of peritonitis
- 27 catheters required removal because of recurrent, refractory, fungal, or tuberculous peritonitis
- 26 catheters were associated with two or more exit site infections
- Obstructions developed more than once in 7 catheters
- 9 catheters required replacement after intervention failed to relieve the obstruction, but intervention was successful in the other 57 catheter obstructions
- Malfunction was diagnosed and led to catheter replacement in 8 cases
- The leaks that occurred in 5 catheters developed at an average of 30.9 months after catheter insertion

These investigators concluded that most studies "have generally shown results similar to those of TWH catheters.[31,32] It seems likely, therefore, that factors other than choice of catheter are what affect survival and complication rates. Indeed, the absence of any convincing prospective data showing superiority of any peritoneal catheter has led some authors to suggest that practical considerations such as cost or availability be the factors that govern catheter choice.[33]"

Di Paolo Self-locating Catheter

The self-locating catheter, designed by Di Paolo, has been increasingly used in Italy and elsewhere since 1994; currently, this catheter is implanted in about a thousand patients every year. Twelve grams of tungsten inserted in the tip of the conventional Tenckhoff catheter keep the tip firmly in the Douglas cavity (see Fig. 266-3).[34-37]

In 2004, Di Paolo and associates[38] published results of a multicenter controlled study that lasted 24 months and was conducted in 16 Italian nephrology departments with 962 uremic patients undergoing peritoneal dialysis, 216 (2678 patient-months) of whom had Tenckhoff catheters and 746 (10,444 patient/months) self-locating catheters.[38] These investigators assessed the following parameters: number of displacements per year, catheter life in months, number of cuff extrusions per year, number of leakages per year, number of exit site infections per year, number of peritonitis episodes per year, number of peritoneal sclerosis events per year. The results of the study showed statistically significantly lower rates of displacements, peritonitis, tunnel infection, cuff extrusion, obstruction, and early and late leakage with the self-locating catheter.

The Vicenza "Short" Peritoneal Catheter

The Vicenza catheter is a modified straight double-cuff Tenckhoff with a inner shaft of 8 cm instead of the normal 15 cm (Fig. 266-4).[39,40] In a 2005 study, Dell'Aquila and coworkers[41] evaluated 701 of the 726 Vicenza catheters

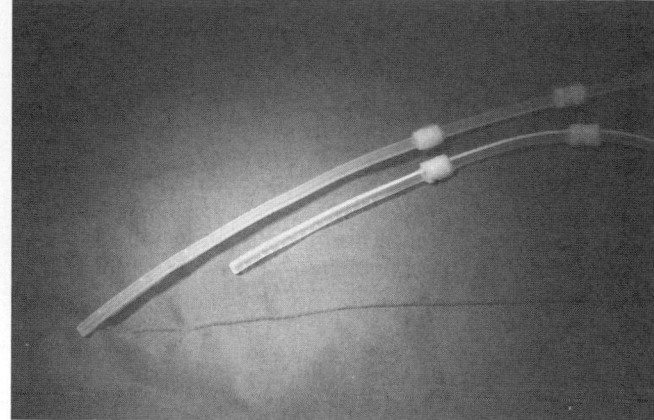

FIGURE 266-4. The Vicenza "short" catheter shown in comparison with the classic Tenckhoff catheter.

implanted at their institution since 1985, in terms of rate of removal due to infection, rate of removal due to infection in obese patients, and catheter dislocation. Of the 701 catheters with available data, a prospective analysis on 233 catheters implanted from 1995 to 2000 was carried out with particular regard to catheter survival; 2-year survival was 94.3%, and 5-year survival 91.5 %. These investigators opined that their high survival figures were probably due to meticulous attention to the care of the exit site and early antibiotic treatment of infections. From 1985 to 2005, the rate of infections per patient-year decreased from 0.7 to 0.2, and the number of removed catheters per patient-year decreased from 0.63 to 0.03. All of these data demonstrate that the development of a good experience in exit site care is one of the most important factors in reducing the incidence of infectious complications and catheter removal.[42]

In 1986 these investigators had 26 prevalent patients with a catheter dislocation rate of 22%; in 2005, data on 102 prevalent patients showed a removal rate of only 4%. In 2005, the authors of this chapter evaluated a total of 27 abdominal radiographic examinations of malfunctioning devices and observed that catheters with exit sites on the left side of the abdomen (18/27) had a higher rate of migration than those with the exit on the right side (9/27). Also, the catheters with exit site on the right side could be relocated more easily after enhancement of peristalsis; in this situation, the clockwise direction of the peristalsis allows the tip of the catheter to relocate.

CONCLUSION

Even if some shapes of catheters have demonstrated better performances in terms of survival, reduction of rates of displacements, peritonitis, tunnel infection, cuff extrusion, obstruction, and early and late leakage, none of the most commonly used catheters discussed in this chapter is completely free of these complications. Some researchers believe that catheter design is important in the risk of complications, but probably there are other conditions leading to these complications. Medical and nursing staff must pay special attention to implantation technique, tunnel and exit site construction, and early care of complications.

Key Points

1. Peritoneal dialysis is a safe, effective, low-cost intracorporeal renal replacement modality with some inherent advantages.
2. There are many different peritoneal catheter designs and materials.
3. All devices present some complications, such as dislocation, infection, and infusion or drainage failure.
4. It is particularly important to choose the best catheter for the patient. Nevertheless, medical and nursing staff must pay special attention to implantation technique, tunnel and exit site construction, and early care of complications.

Key References

13. Ronco C, Gloukhoff A, Dell'Aquila R, Levin NW: Catheter design for continuous flow peritoneal dialysis. Blood Purif 2002;20:40-44.
20. Eklund BH, Honkanen EO, Kala A-R, Kyllonen LE: Peritoneal dialysis access: Prospective randomized comparison of the swan neck and Tenckhoff catheters. Perit Dial Int 1995;15: 353-356.
31. Ortiz AM, Fernandez MA, Troncoso PA, et al: Outcome of peritoneal dialysis: Tenckhoff catheter survival in a prospective study. Adv Perit Dial 2004;20:145-149.
38. Di Paolo N, Capotondo L, Sansoni E, et al: The self-locating catheter: Clinical experience and follow-up. Perit Dial Int 2004;24:359-364.
41. Dell'Aquila R, Chiaramonte S, Rodighiero MP, et al: The Vicenza "short" peritoneal catheter: A twenty year experience. Int J Artif Organs 2006;29:123-127.

See the companion Expert Consult website for the complete reference list.

CHAPTER 267

Solute and Water Transport across the Peritoneal Membrane

Michael F. Flessner

OBJECTIVES

This chapter will:
1. Describe the structure of the peritoneal barrier.
2. Review the physiology of solute and water transport under normal conditions.
3. Discuss the effects of the special conditions in the intensive care unit on transperitoneal solute and water transport.

Acute renal failure commonly develops in patients in either surgical or medical intensive care units because of these patients' underlying problems. The presence of acute renal failure in the intensive care unit (ICU) in the setting of multiple-organ dysfunction increases the risk of mortality to 50% to 100%, depending on the number of organs in failure.[1] There are several ways to manage this type of renal failure. One is intermittent hemodialysis, which is performed with a standard hemodialysis machine. Another technique is continuous renal replacement therapy, performed with smaller dialysis machines that constantly process the blood. Typically, hemodialysis requires one-to-one nursing to monitor the blood pump and ensure the security of all blood lines.

Although used infrequently in the United States, peritoneal dialysis (PD) is a distinct alternative to provide renal support in the ICU. The major advantage of PD is that there is no need for anticoagulation, which is contraindicated in patients with bleeding diathesis or hemorrhagic conditions. The process can be carried out manually or with a programmable cycler, which does not require one-to-one nursing. If the catheter becomes obstructed or the machine malfunctions, the ICU nurse can merely turn off the machine until dialysis personnel are called to correct the situation. PD tends to be gentler on the cardiovascular system and is useful in hemodynamically unstable patients, such as those with heart failure.[2] A more thorough discussion of the indications for, contraindications to, and complications of PD in acute renal failure can be found in Chapter 293.

PD can be used to deliver drugs or remove toxins owing to the peritoneum's permeability to both small solutes and higher-molecular-weight proteins. Dobutamine, insulin, antibiotics, and other chemotherapeutic agents may be given intraperitoneally[3,4]; indeed there is a significant pharmacokinetic advantage to local delivery of a drug when the target is located in the abdominal cavity.[5] In addition, the PD fluid can be simultaneously utilized as a nutritional delivery system, by means of glucose, amino acids, and any other nutrients placed in the solution.[6] These substances are absorbed chiefly into the gut, the circulation of which drains via the portal system directly into the liver.

Besides the clinical considerations, the physician must weigh carefully whether the technique will accomplish the desired outcome. Because PD uses parts of the patient's body to carry out the dialysis, assessments of the fundamental physiology and the impact of pathologic conditions on the dialysis process are important to the successful outcome. Patients with abdominal trauma or intraperitoneal bleeding diathesis obviously cannot undergo this mode of dialysis. Occasionally, cardiothoracic surgery or recent abdominal surgery may be a contraindication because of multiple drains in the chest and peritoneal

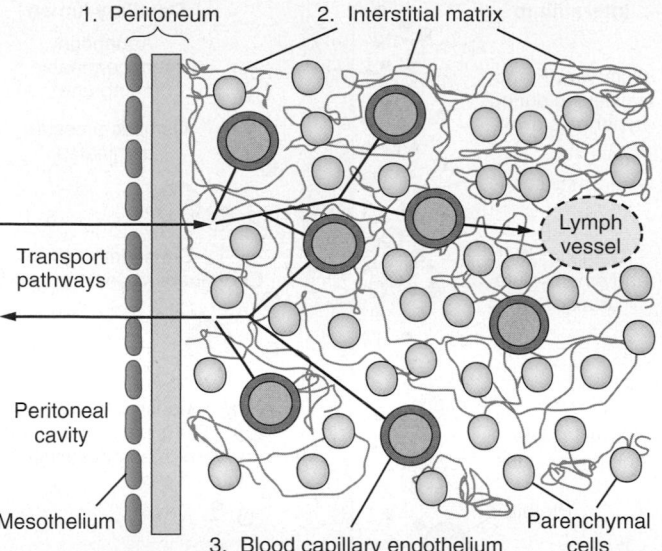

FIGURE 267-1. Potential barriers separating the dialysis solution in the peritoneal cavity and plasma flowing within the microvasculature distributed within the subperitoneal tissue.

cavity, which may increase the risk of infection and also result in leaks from the cavity. Diaphragmatic peritoneal pleural connections may be present and may result in pleural effusions when dialysis fluid is placed in the cavity.[7] PD increases intra-abdominal pressure,[8] potentially impeding the descent of the diaphragm and compromising ventilation or respiration.

This chapter describes the basic structure and function of the peritoneum and the special considerations needed for utilization of the peritoneal cavity as a dialyzer in the ICU.

STRUCTURE OF THE PERITONEAL BARRIER AND TRANSPORT PRINCIPLES

Distributed Nature of the Barrier

Figure 267-1 displays the elements of the peritoneal barrier, which is much more complex than the concept of a single "peritoneal membrane." As illustrated, the barrier actually has the following three components: (1) the anatomical peritoneum, (2) interstitial matrix, and (3) blood capillary endothelium, which is distributed within the tissue. The anatomical peritoneum consists of a single layer of mesothelial cells overlying several layers of connective tissue. The visceral peritoneum has been dissected and measured to be 90 μm thick in the normal state.[9] Although many nephrologists consider the anatomical peritoneum the barrier to transport, experiments in both humans and rodents have demonstrated that the peritoneum is not a barrier to solute and water transport.[10] Complete destruction of the peritoneum in rodents has had no effect on the transfer of small solutes or the osmotic filtration of fluid from the peritoneal cavity into a transport chamber.[10] There have been parallel findings in patients who undergo extensive peritonectomy for treatment of peritoneal carcinomatosis; in one report, clearance of

mitomycin C from the peritoneal cavity was not significantly affected by an extensive peritoneal resection.[11]

The two other major components of the peritoneum, therefore, make up the barrier. The cell-interstitial matrix restricts movement of solutes and water between the blood capillary walls and the peritoneal cavity,[12] slowing transport and making it less efficient than if the blood vessels were in direct contact with the dialysis solution. Because the muscle of the abdominal wall and the gut constitute the vast majority of the peritoneal surface in contact with the dialysis solution,[13] the vessels of these tissues dominate transport. The endothelium of most smooth muscles, capillaries, and venules is known to be size selective.[14] As illustrated in Figure 267-1, these vessels through which the blood flows are distributed within these tissues, which are surrounded by cells and the interstitial matrix.[15]

Effects of the Interstitial Matrix on Transport

The interstitial matrix, once considered to be inert, "sticky" mucopolysaccharides and termed "ground substance," is now known to be an orderly structure of the tissue.[16] Collagen fibers, which provide the skeleton of the interstitial network, are linked to interstitial cells and possibly pericytes through adhesion molecules such as β_1-integrins.[17] These collagen fibers can stretch and contract as the cells to which they are attached are stimulated in different ways.[18] Wrapped around the collagen fibers and, in some cases, attached to them are large (1-40 megadaltons) molecules of hyaluronan, with proteoglycan molecules bound to the hyaluronan molecules. The hyaluronan molecules within the collagen matrix are highly negatively charged, imbibe large amounts of water, and restrict the passage of negatively charged proteins.[19] Proteins are typically restricted to about 50% of the interstitial space,[20] which translates into a protein space of 6% to 10% of the entire tissue space available to proteins for transport if the typical interstitial space is only 12% to 20%.[21]

The rates of transport through the tissue depend on the interstitial matrix. Transport includes diffusion, which can be described by the effective diffusivity as follows:

$$D_{eff} = \frac{D_{isf}\theta_{isf}}{\tau} \qquad [1]$$

where D_{eff} is effective tissue diffusivity; D_{isf} is diffusion coefficient in the interstitium; θ_{isf} is the interstitial fraction (fraction of the total tissue space available to the solute); and τ is tortuosity (factor to account for the convoluted path of the solute around cells and through the interstitial matrix).[22] For water transport and substances that are transported chiefly through convection or solvent drag, the hydraulic connectivity of the tissue space (K_{tiss}) has been shown to depend on the interstitial fraction and the concentrations of collagen, proteoglycan, and hyaluronan.[21]

Dialysis solutions infused into the peritoneal cavity typically cause intraperitoneal hydrostatic pressures (IPP) above 3 or 4 mm Hg, which alter the surrounding tissue space.[23] Intraperitoneal pressures depend on the size and position of the patient, and on the infusion volume used (Fig. 267-2A).[8,24] IPPs of 4 mm Hg would seem to be a very small increase, but the tissue responds by absorbing significant amounts of fluid.[25] This absorption occurs particularly in the abdominal wall, where there is a positive-pressure gradient from the serosa to the subcutaneous space (Fig.

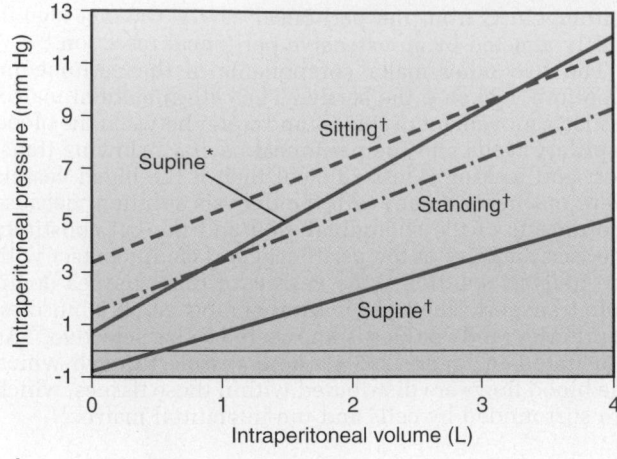

A

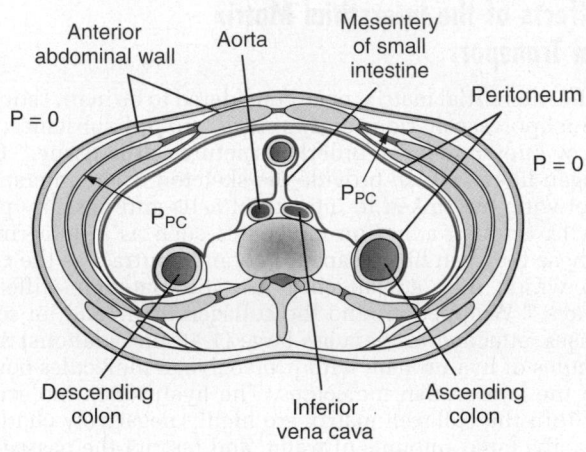

B

FIGURE 267-2. A, Intraperitoneal hydrostatic pressure versus volume instilled. *Data from Gotloib L, Mines M, Garmizo L, Varka I: Hemodynamic effects of increasing intra-abdominal pressure in peritoneal dialysis. Peritoneal Dial Bull 1981;1:41-43. [†]Data from Twardowski ZJ, Prowant BF, Nolph KD: High volume, low frequency continuous ambulatory peritoneal dialysis. Kidney Int 1983;23:64-70. **B,** Abdominal cross section demonstrating pressure gradient from the cavity into local tissue and, in particular, the abdominal wall. P, pressure at skin surface; P_{PC}, peritoneal hydrostatic pressure.

267-2B).[26] Studies in rats have demonstrated that the extracellular space doubles with a rise in IPP from zero to 3 mm Hg,[27] and the hydraulic conductivity increases four to five times.[28] In experiments in the rat, sampling of the interstitial fluid after 4 hours of dialysis showed a 50% decrease in colloid osmotic pressure.[29] Expansion of the interstitial space and decreases in collagen and hyaluronan concentrations raise the rates of diffusion and convection within the tissue.

Nature of the Endothelial Barrier

The endothelial barrier is depicted in Figure 267-3 as a transcellular pore, called an *aquaporin*, and different intercellular gaps lined with matrix material, called the *glycocalyx*[30]; this concept represents a necessary modification of the three-pore model of peritoneal transport[31] to account for alterations in pathological states. The aquaporin permits only water through its channel and is respon-

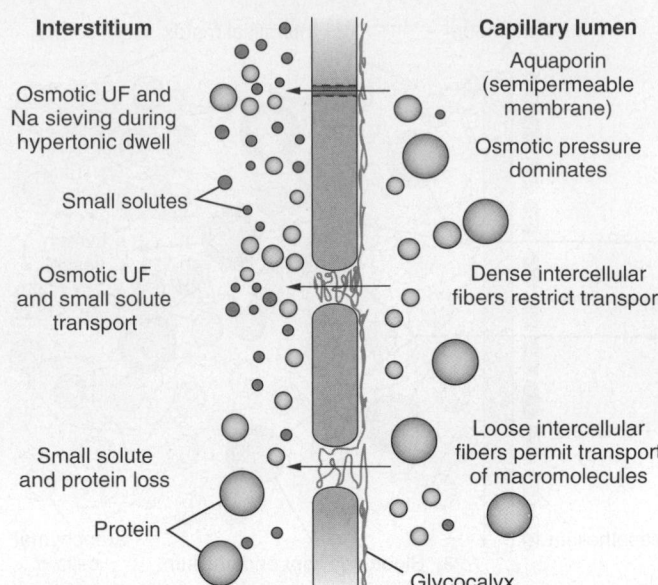

FIGURE 267-3. Pore-fiber-matrix concept of the blood capillary endothelial barrier. UF, ultrafiltration.

sible for much of the osmotically induced filtration from the plasma.[32] Intercellular gaps lined by the glycocalyx are the second portion of the barrier, which permit the transfer of solutes and water, depending on the density of the glycocalyx.

The discovery of aquaporins by Agre and colleagues[33] has brought new understanding to the transfer of water across blood capillaries into the tissue and subsequently into the peritoneal cavity. Because the aquaporin does not permit any solute to transfer, it represents the perfect semipermeable membrane across which any solute concentration difference exerts osmotic pressures that result in filtration. The functional significance of the aquaporins has been demonstrated in numerous experiments. Carlsson and associates[34] showed that in vivo inhibition of aquaporins with mercuric chloride resulted in a significant decrease in volume of osmotically filtered fluid from the tissue. Sixty-six percent inhibition of water flow through the aquaporins was verified subsequently by Yang and coworkers[32] in aquaporin 1–knockout mice. When mice were dialyzed with a hypertonic solution, the filtration in the knockout mice was 40% of that in normal mice. Another study in rodents has demonstrated both the structural appearance and the functionality of the endothelial aquaporins.[35]

Solute transport depends on the density of the glycocalyx in the intercellular gap.[36] A denser glycocalyx restricts the passage of larger solutes (functionally equivalent to the "small pore" of the three-pore model), with a less dense glycocalyx allowing protein leakage (the equivalent of the "large pore" of the three-pore model). In the normal situation, the vast majority of the intercellular spaces are densely packed with glycocalyx and restrict the passage of macromolecules, making up 95% of the total capillary permeable area[37]; these spaces are responsible for 40% to 50% of the osmotic filtration. The remainder of the capillary is made up of intercellular junctions, which permit proteins to leak out.

The rate of transfer from the plasma to the interstitial space of the surrounding tissue can be represented in a simplified fashion as follows[38]:

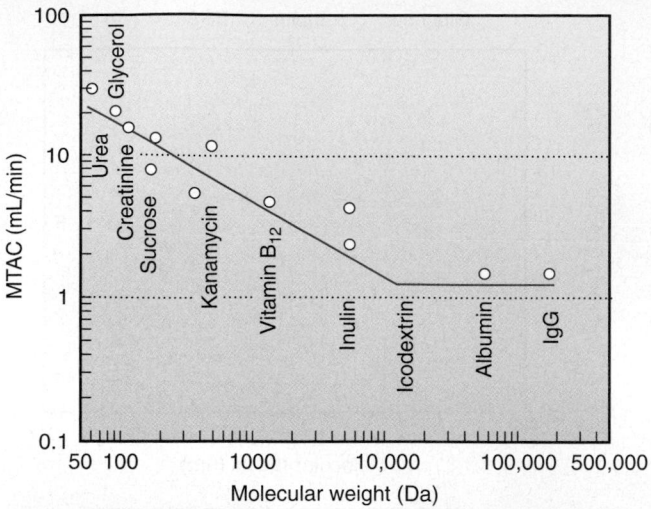

FIGURE 267-4. Mass transfer-area coefficient (MTAC) versus molecular weight. (Adapted from Flessner MF: Intraperitoneal drug therapy: Physical and biological principles. In Beelen RH [ed]: Multidisciplinary Management of Peritoneal Carcinomatosis. New York, Springer, 2006.)

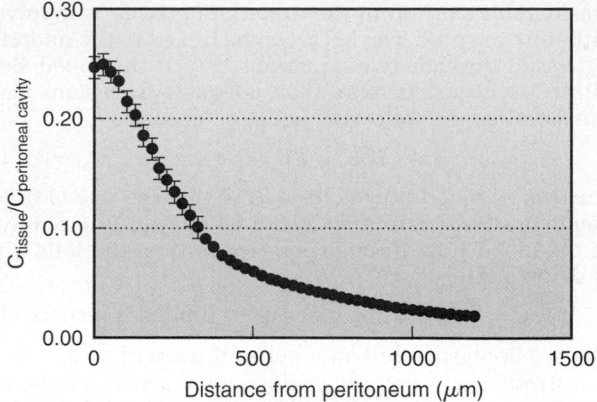

FIGURE 267-5. Concentration (C) profile of mannitol (equivalent to that of dextrose) in the abdominal wall of the rat. (Adapted from Flessner MF, Deverkadra R, Smitherman J, et al: In vivo determination of diffusive transport parameters in a superfused tissue. Am J Physiol Renal Physiol 2006;291:F1096-F1103.)

$$J_{endo} = pa(C_{plasma} - C_{isf}) \qquad [2]$$

where J_{endo} is solute transfer rate across the endothelium (mass/time/tissue mass); p is overall endothelial permeability, including the effect of all intercellular passages; a is capillary surface area/mass of tissue; C_{plasma} is solute concentration in plasma; and C_{isf} is solute concentration in interstitial fluid. More complicated mathematical approaches can be employed to include the three elements of the endothelial barrier.[22,39]

PHYSIOLOGY OF TRANSPORT: NORMAL CONDITIONS

The overall rate of mass transfer can be described by the following equation[38]:

$$\frac{dM_{cavity}}{dt} = MTC \times A_{contact}(C_{plasma} - C_{cavity}) \qquad [3]$$

where M_{cavity} is solute mass in the peritoneal cavity (equal to the product of the solute concentration in cavity—C_{cavity}—and the volume in the cavity); t = time; MTC is the overall mass transfer coefficient across the peritoneal barrier; $A_{contact}$ is the area of the peritoneum in contact with the dialysis solution; and C_{plasma} is solute concentration in the plasma. In experiments in rodents, four major surfaces within the peritoneal cavity have been shown to have very similar MTCs,[40] thus justifying the use of one value for the overall MTC. MTC has been shown to be very similar in different rodent species as well and likely is similar in other mammals.[41] $A_{contact}$ is typically not measured in humans, and its product with the MTC is termed the *mass transfer-area coefficient* (MTAC).[42] The overall clearance or MTAC is plotted in Figure 267-4.

Importance of the Surface Contact Area

As can be observed in equation 3, the contact area ($A_{contact}$) is a major determinant of the rate of solute transfer. As can be seen in Figure 267-1, if the solution does not make contact with the tissue, transfer from the blood capillaries to the peritoneal cavity cannot occur. That the rate of transfer is directly proportional to this surface contact area is apparent from equation 3. This relationship has also been shown both in animals[43] and in patients undergoing PD.[44,45]

Keshevian and associates[46] carried out one of the first studies in humans, in which they determined the MTAC (MTC × $A_{contact}$) in 10 patients who were dialyzed with different solution volumes varying from 0.5 to 3.5 L. Upon increasing the fill volume from 0.5 to about 3 L, these investigators observed a linear rise in the MTAC, which was attributed to an increase in surface area. Chagnac and associates[45] dialyzed patients with a radiographic contrast agent injected intraperitoneally and employed computed tomography with special stereographic techniques to calculate the area; they found that with 2 L in a typical patient, the area covered was about 0.55 m² or about one third of the total anatomic area.[47] When the fill volume was raised to 3 L, the investigators also observed an increase in the measured contact area of 18% and obtained a 25% increase in MTAC.[44] When the peritoneal volume is maximized to about 3.0 L of standard solution, $A_{contact}$ approaches a maximum, ensuring maximal rates of transfer. Unfortunately, larger volumes also increase the IPP (see Fig. 267-2A)[8] and may compromise respiration or net ultrafiltration.[23]

Solute Transfer across the Peritoneal Barrier

The functional proof for the concept of the peritoneal barrier as a distributed microvasculature within a tissue space is derived from the solute profile data shown in Figure 267-5. Concentration profiles for mannitol (equivalent to glucose) are plotted in Figure 267-5, demonstrating solute transporting from the cavity into the tissue over hundreds of microns. Because the normal human peritoneum is less than 100 μm thick, the extension of the concentration profile over 500 to 1000 μm implies that a considerable portion of the underlying tissue is involved with the transport. The MTC can be linked to the underlying tissue through two equations.[3,38,42] If the blood flow within the tissue is more than adequate to sustain mass transfer, then the following equation applies:

$$MTC = \sqrt{D_{eff}(pa)} \qquad [4]$$

However, if blood flow is limited so that the rate of diffusion in the tissue is limited by the solute supply or removal by the blood flow through the tissue, then the following equation applies:

$$MTC = \sqrt{D_{eff} \times q} \text{ for blood-flow limited transport} \quad [5]$$

where q is plasma flow rate per unit mass of tissue.

In theory, very low blood flows may actually limit the transfer of small solutes such as urea (molecular weight 60 Da). Experiments in rats, however, demonstrated that lowering the perfusion in local tissues in individual organs to 20% or 30% of the original level did not change mass transfer rates of urea across the peritoneum of the cecum, stomach, or abdominal wall; however, solute transfer across the liver was significantly altered with the decrease in blood flow.[48] In analogous experiments, a decrease in blood flow across these organs did result in reductions in the transfer of water through osmotic filtration, but the results were not statistically significant except in the liver.[49] One can therefore conclude that under normal circumstances, the transfer of solutes and water should not be restricted by the blood flow but are probably limited by the rate of diffusion through the tissue and the perfused capillary area (a) and permeability (p). From this theory, offered by Dedrick and colleagues[38] in 1982, for the diffusion-limited solute with a molecular weight of less than 6000 daltons, the steady-state concentration profile can be defined as follows:

$$\frac{C_{isf} - C_{plasma}}{C_{cavity} - C_{plasma}} = \exp^{-\sqrt{\frac{(pa)}{D_{eff}}}x} \qquad [6]$$

where x is the distance from the peritoneum into the tissue. The fitting of equation 6 to measured profiles during the dialysis in rodents has permitted the estimation of both D_{eff} and (pa).[42] The perfused capillary surface area per unit volume of tissue was measured, and the actual p was calculated from the (pa) factor. Figure 267-6A is a plot of the derived diffusivities, and Figure 267-6B shows values for capillary permeability (p) from data described by Dedrick and colleagues.[38] The capillary area-density "a" of muscle capillary is about 70 cm² per gram of tissue,[50] and that of the abdominal wall is 600 cm² per mL of abdominal wall tissue.[42]

Water Flow and Calculation of Net Ultrafiltration

There are many theories as to how water is extracted from the body during PD, but none of them fully explains the phenomena of net ultrafiltration (net UF).

Net UF is defined as follows[23]:

$$\text{Net UF} = \frac{\text{Drain volume} - \text{Fill volume}}{\text{Dwell time}} \qquad [7]$$

This equation does not identify what forces govern the transfer of fluid. Ultrafiltration across a blood capillary follows the classic Starling equation:

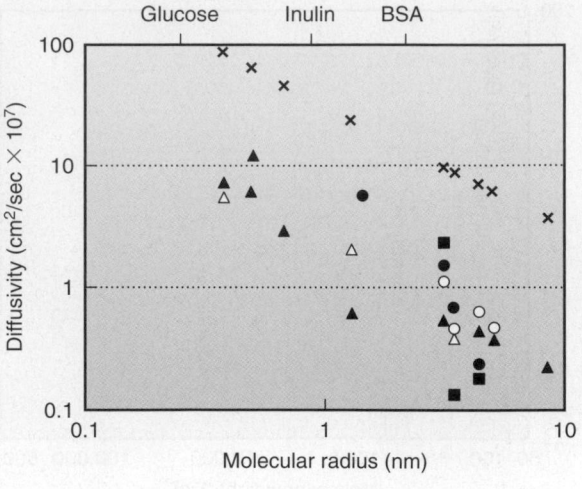

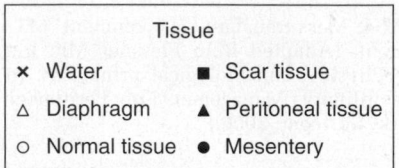

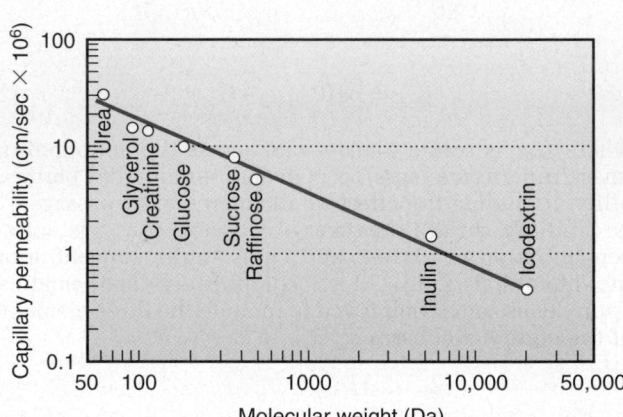

FIGURE 267-6. **A,** Solute diffusivities in water and various tissues versus solute molecular radius. The plot demonstrates the order of magnitude differences between the diffusion coefficients in water and those in tissues. BSA, bovine serum albumin. (Data from Dedrick RL, Flessner MF, Collins JM, Schultz JS: Is the peritoneum a membrane? ASAIO J 1982;5:1-5; Dedrick RL: Interspecies scaling of regional drug delivery. J Pharm Sci 1986;75:1047-1052; and Flessner MF: Peritoneal transport physiology: Insights from basic research. J Am Soc Nephrol 1991;2:122-135.) **B,** Capillary permeability versus molecular weight of solutes. (Data from Dedrick RL, Flessner MF, Collins JM, Schultz JS: Is the peritoneum a membrane? ASAIO J 1982;5:1-5.)

$$\text{Fluid transport rate} = K_f a \times [P_{plasma} - P_{isf} - (\pi_{plasma} - \pi_{isf})] \quad [8]$$

where: K_f is membrane filtration coefficient; P is hydrostatic pressure; and π is effective osmotic pressure. However, the integration of this equation into the distributed model concept cannot easily be accomplished because of the uncertainty of the true osmotic forces in the interstitium and the variable concentration of the osmotic solute (see Fig. 267-5). At this time, most models are semi-empirical in nature and often resort to fitting the model to patient data.

The net UF is made up of two components as follows:

$$\text{Net UF} = \text{Osmotically driven filtration} - \text{Fluid loss} \quad [9]$$

Fluid loss is fluid transfer from the cavity, which is equal to direct lymph flow plus the hydrostatic pressure–driven convection to the surrounding tissues. From the tissue, transfer into the blood capillaries or intra-tissue lymphatics carries the fluid back to the plasma compartment.[3,23] The lymphatic flow is a minor part of the fluid loss term.

Lymphatic Drainage from the Peritoneal Cavity

The lymphatic system draining the peritoneal cavity is divided into two parts. The subdiaphragmatic lymphatic system drains 70% to 80% of the lymphatic flow from the peritoneal cavity.[51] The diaphragm acts as a pumping mechanism that pulls fluid from the lower parts of the peritoneal cavity toward the diaphragm. As the diaphragm moves upward in expiration, the lymphatic plexus expands, and a negative pressure is established in the lymphatic vessels. Lacunae, or penetrations in the basement membranes, open via stomata to take in fluids, solutes, and particles up to 25 µm in diameter. For this reason, bacteria are rapidly taken up from the cavity and transported toward the venous system in the neck. When the diaphragm contracts, the tension in the lymphatic wall is released, the stomata are closed, and pressure is exerted on the lacunae.[52] The fluid is propelled upward toward the right lymphatic duct or into the thoracic duct.

The remaining 20% to 30% of lymph flow from the peritoneal cavity is absorbed into the visceral lymphatics. These drain to the mesenteric lymphatics and to the cisterna chyli at the base of the thoracic duct. This duct subsequently drains into the left venous system.[53] Under normal conditions in stable patients undergoing PD, the rate of lymphatic flow varies between 7 and 20 mL/hr,[23] with the total peritoneal fluid loss between 60 and 91 mL/hr.[54-56]

Clinical Effects of Intraperitoneal Pressure

Durand and colleagues[57] demonstrated the importance of intraperitoneal hydrostatic pressure (IPP) in determining the fluid loss from the cavity. They carried out a careful study of the effect of IPP on the net UF in 34 patients. All patients were placed in supine position to minimize changes of IPP during dialysis with 3.86% dextrose solution. After 2 hours, the net UF was measured; it was shown to vary indirectly with the intraperitoneal hydrostatic pressure and to have a net fluid absorption rate from the peritoneal cavity between 31 and 36 mL/hr per cm H_2O of IPP.[57] Rusthoven and associates[58] have verified the measurements published by Durand and associates[57] in children and have demonstrated an inverse correlation between change in IPP and the body's surface area.

Both animal data and human data have shown that fluid loss during PD—that is, flow back to the patient—can amount to 1.5 to 2 L per day. Increases in intraperitoneal dwell volume increase the IPP and may lead to a decrease in net UF. This decrease can greatly affect the child with

a small body surface area and has been shown to have a negative correlation with body surface area.

Alteration of the Transport Barrier: Normal Physiology

As discussed previously, enhancement of solute transport can be accomplished by increasing the contact surface area through larger peritoneal volumes.[44,46] This approach may be impossible for some patients in the ICU because of respiratory or ventilatory difficulties. If the concentration of the surfactant diacetyl sodium sulfosuccinate in the PD solution is relatively high,[13,59] 100% of the anatomic peritoneum is in contact with the solution; however, such a high concentration is toxic and should not be used in humans. If surfactant materials are to be used, they must have been very carefully tested and proven to be nontoxic to patients.

A second way to raise the rate of transfer is to increase the perfused capillary surface area. Nitroprusside, when placed in the dialysis solution, has been shown to significantly enhance transport.[60-62] Unfortunately, intraperitoneal nitroprusside appears to be limited by a loss of effect after approximately five exchanges. In addition, there may be some decrease in blood pressure with the use of this drug. Vasoconstrictors have been demonstrated to reduce the perfused endothelial area and significantly decrease mass transfer.[42]

ACUTE PERITONEAL DIALYSIS IN THE INTENSIVE CARE UNIT: SPECIAL CONDITIONS

Hypotension and Peritoneal Blood Supply

Severe trauma or sepsis often results in hypotension, which leads to generalized vasoconstriction that might compromise the circulation supplying the tissues adjacent to the peritoneum. Blood flow limitation is observed when delivery of solute in the plasma to the exchange vessels is less than the rate of solute transfer across the capillaries into the interstitium. In a previous study in normotensive rodents, reducing the blood flow locally to 20% to 30% of baseline did not limit solute transfer but did decrease fluid transfer.[48,49] Additional studies have demonstrated that use of high doses of vasoconstrictors (1 mg/mL of norepinephrine) locally reduces the perfused vascular area, resulting in a marked decrease in the rate of mass transfer and osmotic ultrafiltration.[42] Other researchers have shown, however, that if an animal is put into shock by bleeding,[63] the mass transfer coefficient is reduced by 25% after the mean arterial blood pressure decreases from 133 to 61 mm Hg.[63] The perfused vascular area was not measured in this study, but the perfusion, as measured by laser Doppler flowmetry, was reduced by 50%, in turn resulting in a 25% reduction in the mass transfer of labeled ethylenediaminetetra-acetic acid (EDTA). From this information, one may conclude that the condition of circulatory shock with severe hypotension may have a modest effect on PD solute transfer, which may be further compromised by the presence of endogenous or exogenously administered high levels of vasoconstrictors.

Dehydration and Hypotension

Occasionally patients in the ICU may be extremely dehydrated, because of heat exhaustion, severe diarrheal illness, or profound diuresis. Such was the case in one patient with severe heart failure who had been given massive amounts of diuretics, which resulted in renal failure, hyperosmolality, and hypotension (blood pressure approximately 90 mm Hg systolic, 50 mm Hg diastolic). After placement of a peritoneal catheter, the patient was started on a 90-minute 2 L dwell of 1.5% dextrose solutions; the 2L volume returned 1000 mL. The solution was changed to 2 L of 2.5% dextrose solution, with the same result. Subsequently, the solution was changed to a 4.25% dextrose dialysis solution with a positive output. It is well known that dehydration lowers the interstitial pressure from about 0 mm Hg to a *negative* value (−5 to −10 mm Hg[64]); this event in the patient likely set up a very large positive-pressure difference between the cavity and abdominal wall tissue (see Fig. 267-2). The 2 L of fluid absorbed in the first two exchanges not only increased the mean arterial pressure but also hydrated the tissue surrounding the peritoneal cavity and raised the tissue pressure, in turn decreasing the fluid loss rate. Although solute transfer was not compromised in this case, the osmotic ultrafiltration failed until the peritoneal tissue was hydrated and the patient's blood pressure rose to a normal range.

Practical Limits of Solute Transfer

Maximal rates of mass transfer in any ICU renal replacement therapy ensure adequate therapy. As discussed previously, vasodilators such as nitroprusside enhance the rate of mass transfer for several exchanges but then lose their effectiveness and may further compromise systemic blood pressure.[61] The dwell volume can be increased to improve the contact area, but this approach increases the IPP, potentially causing either leakage around the recently placed catheter or compromise of ventilation. Under conditions prevalent in the ICU, it would appear that the nephrologist would have little control over the perfused vascular area. However, use of innovations such as continuous-flow PD[65] in postoperative chemotherapy[66] has achieved marked increases in mass transfer with the use of dual catheters and continuous circulation of a heated solution (40° C). The mass transfer rates for small substances, such as glucose and creatinine, increased to approximately twice that of the normal clearance and approached the region of the "MTAC-limited area" outlined in Figure 267-7.[67] This marked elevation was likely due to a combination of increased peritoneal contact area and the recruitment of blood vessels by the heated fluid.

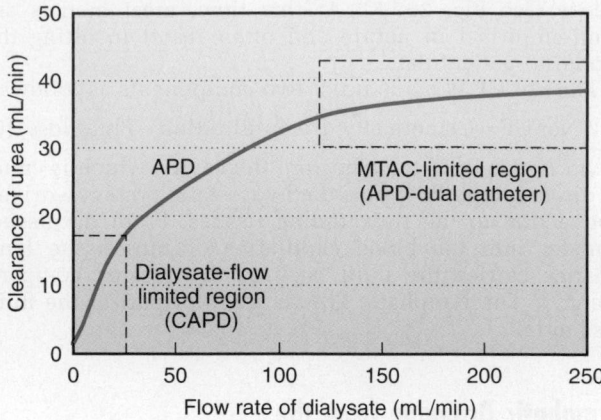

FIGURE 267-7. Urea clearance versus dialysate flow rate. (Adapted from Ronco C: Limitations of peritoneal dialysis. Kidney Int 1996;50[Suppl 56]:S69-S74.)

3. Although the rate of water and mass transfer is directly proportional to the peritoneal area in direct contact with the dialysis solution, only one third of the anatomical peritoneum is typically exposed to 2 to 3 L at any moment during dialysis.
4. Increasing the volume in the cavity generally enlarges the contact area and raises the rate of mass transfer but may also increase intraperitoneal pressure and lead to a reduction in net ultrafiltration.
5. Raising the osmotic pressure in the cavity generally raises the rate of fluid removal from the body.
6. Peritoneal dialysis can be used in the intensive care unit as a mode of renal replacement therapy, with the advantages of improved hemodynamic stability and no requirement for anticoagulation.

Acknowledgment

This work was supported by U.S. Public Health Service Grant RO1-DK-048479.

Key References

3. Flessner MF: The transport barrier in intraperitoneal therapy. Am J Physiol 2005;288:F433-F442.
30. Vink H, Duling BR: Identification of distinct luminal domains for macromolecules, erythrocytes, and leucocytes within mammalian capillaries. Circ Res 1996;79:581-589.
32. Yang B, Folkesson HG, Yang J, et al: Reduced osmotic water permeability of the peritoneal barrier in aquaporin-1 knock-out mice. Am J Physiol 1999;276:C76-C81.
44. Chagnac A, Herskovitz P, Ori Y, et al: Effect of increased dialysate volume on peritoneal surface area among peritoneal dialysis patients. J Am Soc Nephrol 2002;13:2554-2559.
57. Durand P-Y, Chanliau J, Gamberoni J, et al: Hydrostatic intraperitoneal pressure and volume of ultrafiltration in CAPD. Adv Perit Dial 1993;9:46-48.

See the companion Expert Consult website for the complete reference list.

Key Points

1. The normal anatomical peritoneum is not a significant barrier to solute and water transport during dialysis.
2. The functional transport barrier in peritoneal dialysis is made up of size-selective capillary endothelia that are distributed within the cell-interstitial matrix of subperitoneal tissue.

CHAPTER 268

Choice of Peritoneal Dialysis Technique: Intermittent or Continuous

Raymond T. Krediet

OBJECTIVES

This chapter will:
1. Describe continuous and intermittent techniques of peritoneal dialysis with their advantages and disadvantages.
2. Discuss the advantages and disadvantages deriving from short dwells.
3. Describe a typical continuous ambulatory peritoneal dialysis schedule.
4. Analyze the potential of continuous-flow peritoneal dialysis.

CONTINUOUS VERSUS INTERMITTENT TECHNIQUES

A *continuous dialysis* therapy represents a period of treatment spanning a full 24-hour period, and is usually applied for several days in a row. Intermittent dialysis has a distinct beginning and end of therapy and is usually performed within a period measured in hours.[1] Using these definitions for peritoneal dialysis (PD) in acute renal failure, however, makes it almost impossible to distinguish between the two modalities. In the early days of PD in patients presenting with severe uremia, the treatment often consisted of hourly exchanges during a period of 72 hours as maximum, because a longer duration was associated with a higher risk of peritonitis.[2,3] It should be noted, however, that these results were obtained with stylet catheters placed percutaneously at the bedside.[4] These restrictions do not apply to the polymeric silicone (Silastic) Tenckhoff catheters currently used, especially when they are inserted via mini-laparotomy or laparoscopy. It follows from these considerations that PD in the intensive care unit (ICU) should be continuous whenever possible. This chapter focuses on the duration of the dialysis dwells.

ADVANTAGES OF SHORT DWELLS

The growing use of automated PD has stimulated the development of cyclers, which allow PD to be performed on a continuous basis in patients in the ICU without investment of much additional nursing time and with precise adjustments of inflow, dialysis, and drainage times. The peritoneal clearance of solutes depends on their molecular weights. Boen has shown, in patients with acute renal failure, that the maximum urea clearance, 28.5 mL/min, was obtained with a dialyzed volume of 3.5 L/hr.[5] However, using a markedly lower volume, 2.5 L/hr, resulted in an almost similar urea clearance, 26 mL/min. The clearances of other solutes and clearance rates are given in Table 268-1. It follows from the clearance ratio that the potassium clearance is 80% of that of urea, and the clearances of solutes with molecular weights between 100 and 200 Da average 60% of that of urea. In comparison, hemodialysis for 4 hours per day results in an equivalent urea clearance of 33 mL/min when expressed per 24 hours, and a creatinine clearance of 24 mL/min. Although these small solute clearances are still higher than achieved by PD, beneficial effects on outcome have not been found, probably because of the need for anticoagulation during hemodialysis and a greater tendency for cardiovascular instability. A comparison of PD with continuous filtration techniques is beyond the scope of this chapter.

DISADVANTAGES OF SHORT DWELLS

Short dwells during PD are advantageous regarding the removal of low-molecular-weight solutes. However, they also have disadvantages. The strengths and weaknesses of short dwells are summarized in Table 268-2. It is well established that the loss of plasma proteins in effluent is greater with PD using hourly exchanges than with a standard continuous ambulatory peritoneal dialysis (CAPD) regimen.[6,8] The reason is that peritoneal transport of all solutes, including macromolecules, is higher during the first hour of a dialysis dwell than in the subsequent hours,[9] probably owing to instillation of the dialysis fluid.

The dialysate sodium concentration decreases during the first 1 to 2 hours of a dialysis dwell with hypertonic dialysis solutions, especially those with an osmolarity above 400 mOsmol/L.[10] This so-called sodium sieving is caused by glucose-induced transport of free water through the water channel aquaporin-1.[11] Therefore, more water than sodium is removed during short exchanges,[12] possibly leading to hypernatremia.[13] The contribution of free water transport to total fluid removal during 3.86% glucose exchanges averages 40% during the first hour and decreases to 20% after 4 hours.[14]

TABLE 268-1

Peritoneal Solute Clearances (mL/min) during Hourly Exchanges and 4-Hour Exchanges

SOLUTE	MOLECULAR WEIGHT (kDa)	Hourly Exchanges*		4-Hour Exchanges†	
		2.5 L/hr (= 60 L/24 hr)	CLEARANCE RATIO	2 L/4 hr (= 12 L/24 hr)	CLEARANCE RATIO
Urea	60	26	1.0	9	1.0
Potassium	39	21	0.81	8	0.89
Creatinine	113	15	0.58	6	0.67
Phosphorus	98	16	0.62	5	0.56
Uric acid	168	14	0.55	6	0.67

*Data from Boen ST: Kinetics of peritoneal dialysis. Medicine 1961;40:243-287.
†Data from Kagan A, Bar-Khayim Y, Schafer Z, Fainara M: Kinetics of peritoneal protein loss during CAPD. 1: Different characteristics for low and high molecular weight proteins. Kidney Int 1990;37:971-979.
The clearance ratio is the clearance relative to that of urea.

TABLE 268-2

Comparison between a Peritoneal Dialysis Schedule Using Short Exchanges Only and a Continuous Ambulatory Peritoneal Dialysis (CAPD)–Like Schedule

	ADVANTAGE OF SHORT DWELLS ONLY	ADVANTAGE OF CAPD SCHEDULE ONLY
Small solute removal	+	–
Middle-size molecule removal	+	+
Sodium removal	–	+
Water removal	+	+
Use of icodextrin	–	+
Protein losses in effluent	–	+
Local host defense	–	+

The glucose molecules are mainly connected at the α1-4 binding sites. A 7.5% icodextrin solution is slightly hypotonic to plasma and induces ultrafiltration by colloid osmosis.[15] This process takes place through the small pore system. Therefore, the transport of water and sodium is proportional, leading to the absence of sodium sieving,[16] so icodextrin does not induce hypernatremia. However, owing to its composition, its effects on ultrafiltration are especially marked with long dwell (>8 hours) exchanges.[16,17]

Cells exposed to fresh dialysis solutions develop severe functional deficiencies (reviewed by Topley and colleagues[18]). Peritoneal cells are removed during each drainage procedure. They consist mainly of macrophages. The *ex vivo* function of these macrophages depends on the dwell time.[19] The lowest phagocytosis capacity is present after a dwell of 1.5 hours. Macrophages obtained after an overnight dwell have essentially normal immunoeffector functions.[20] It is not known whether a continuous treatment with short dialysis cycles influences the risk of the development of peritonitis in patients with acute renal failure in the ICU, but one cannot exclude the possibility that the high peritonitis incidence reported earlier with

use of a stylet catheter for more than 72 hours is a consequence of impaired host defense due to drainage of macrophages.

A CONTINUOUS AMBULATORY PERITONEAL DIALYSIS SCHEDULE

The original schedule for CAPD consists of four 4-hour exchanges and one 8-hour exchange. Average clearance values are given in Table 268-1. Compared with high-volume, short-dwell dialysis, the dialysate volume during a CAPD-like schedule is reduced to 20% and the urea clearance to 40%. Yet such a schedule allows equilibrium among urea generation, urea removal, and plasma urea in noncatabolic patients.[21] Assuming a protein equivalent of nitrogen appearance (nPNA) of 1.1 g per kg body weight per 24 hrs, the urea removal (UR) in the dialysate (mmoL/day) is calculated as follows[22]:

$$UR = 4 \times body\ weight\ (kg) - 70$$

The drained volume (DV) necessary to achieve this is calculated as follows:

$$DV = \frac{(4.5 \times BW - 70)}{Plasma\ urea}$$

It can be calculated from the preceding equations that for a patient of 70 kg treated with a classic CAPD schedule, drainage of 9.4 L dialysate per day is required to maintain a stable plasma concentration of 25 mmol/L.[21] It is evident that such a schedule does not apply in hypercatabolic patients.

CONTINUOUS-FLOW PERITONEAL DIALYSIS

Continuous-flow PD (CFPD) can be considered the opposite of CAPD. Owing to the continuous dialysate flow of

100 of 300 mL/min, this modality mimics hemodialysis. CFPD was described already 40 years ago[23] but has never been applied on a large scale because of the need for two catheters and for large amounts of a sterile dialysis solution. The development of on-line preparation of dialysis solutions and of double-lumen PD catheters has led to a renewed interest in CFPD.[24,25] Owing to the absence of saturation of the dialysate, a doubling of peritoneal creatinine clearance has been described.[26] Also, ultrafiltration rates are higher because the initial glucose concentration gradient remains. A review of CFPD has been published.[27]

Up to now, CFPD has been a technique still in development. Once the logistics are well established, it could be considered in hypercatabolic patients. Effects of CFPD on local host defenses and mortality are not known.

CONCLUSION

With the current technology, continuous treatment is the preferred form of PD in patients in the ICU with acute renal failure. Short exchanges are more effective than long exchanges for the removal of low-molecular-weight solutes like urea. However, when possible, an 8- to 12-hour icodextrin exchange performed every 24 to 48 hours should be considered to enhance sodium removal and preserve local peritoneal host defense. A CAPD schedule can be effective in noncatabolic patients. In this situation, the required drained volume can be calculated. CFPD should still be considered an experimental treatment.

Key Points

1. Continuous peritoneal dialysis techniques are preferred whenever possible.
2. Short exchanges are especially effective for the removal of urea.
3. A long dwell time with the use of icodextrin improves sodium removal and may be advantageous for local host defenses.
4. A continuous ambulatory peritoneal dialysis–like schedule is effective in noncatabolic patients.
5. Continuous-flow peritoneal dialysis should still be considered an experimental treatment.

Key References

9. Imholtz ALT, Koomen GCM, Struijk DG, et al: Fluid and solute transport in CAPD patients using ultralow sodium dialysate. Kidney Int 1994;46:333-340.
10. Nolph KD, Twardowski ZJ, Popovich RP, Rubin J: Equilibration of peritoneal dialysis solutions during long-dwell exchanges. J Lab Clin Med 1979;93:246-256.
14. Parikova A, Smit W, Struijk DG, et al: The contribution of free water transport and small pore transport to the total fluid removal in peritoneal dialysis. Kidney Int 2005;68:1849-1856.
16. Ho-dac-Pannekeet MM, Schouten N, Langedijk MJ, et al: Peritoneal transport characteristics with glucose polymer based dialysate. Kidney Int 1996;50:979-986.
27. Ronco C, Amerling R: Continuous flow peritoneal dialysis: Current state-of-the-art and obstacles to further development. Contrib Nephrol 2006;150:310-320.

See the companion Expert Consult website for the complete reference list.

CHAPTER 269

Technology of Peritoneal Dialysis in the Intensive Care Unit

José A. Diaz-Buxo

OBJECTIVES

This chapter will:
1. Show that peritoneal dialysis is a viable option for the treatment of acute renal failure in the intensive care unit.
2. Describe the technological advances in this modality that may be of benefit in the environment of the intensive care unit and the treatment of acute renal failure.
3. Correlate specific technological advances in equipment and solutions with potential benefits of peritoneal dialysis to patient care.

Peritoneal dialysis (PD) is a viable and well-tested option for the treatment of acute renal failure (ARF). It was used extensively in the acute intensive hospital setting before hemodialysis, hemofiltration, and other modalities of continuous renal replacement therapy (CRRT) became available. The first patient ever treated with PD was a woman with ureteral obstruction due to uterine carcinoma reported by Ganter[1] in 1923. Boen[2] summarized the interesting evolution of PD for the treatment of acute, reversible renal failure throughout the first three decades of clinical use.[2] By 1950, more than 100 patients had been treated with PD, of whom approximately two thirds had had ARF.[3] It is interesting to note that their survival was around 50%, a

TABLE 269-1

Use of Various Forms of Dialysis in Intensive Care Units in Two Periods: 1994-1995 and 1999-2000

THERAPY	Patients Receiving Therapy (%)	
	1994-1995	*1999-2000*
Peritoneal dialysis	8	3
Intermittent hemodialysis	83	71
Continuous renal replacement therapy	9	26

Adapted from Hyman A, Mendelssohn DC: Current Canadian approaches to dialysis for acute renal failure in the ICU. Am J Nephrol 2002;22:29-34.

figure quite similar to current results with modern therapy. Many clinicians favor PD for the treatment of infants and small children with ARF, mostly owing to difficulties in securing adequate vascular access for hemodialysis and in matching the extracorporeal circuit volume to a child's body surface area.

The current utilization of PD for the treatment of ARF in the intensive care unit (ICU) has diminished since the advent of extracorporeal CRRT and a partial shift in delivery of therapy from the nephrologist to the intensivist. A survey conducted by mail questionnaires sent to all adult academic and community registered Canadian nephrology centers that offer treatment for ARF was performed to evaluate modality utilization during two periods, 1994-1995 and 1999-2000.[4] The largest increase between the two periods was in use of CRRT (9% vs. 26%, respectively). Utilization of both intermittent hemodialysis and PD decreased (Table 269-1). In the second period, the predominant CRRT methods utilized venovenous access (continuous venovenous hemofiltration) (80%); during the first period, continuous arteriovenous hemofiltration had been most common (52%). Notwithstanding a lack of definitive evidence of superior outcomes with CRRT over older methods, the utilization of CRRT has been dramatically growing for the treatment of ARF in many developed countries.

TECHNOLOGICAL ADVANCES IN PERITONEAL DIALYSIS AND THEIR APPLICATION IN THE INTENSIVE CARE UNIT

The technological advances made in PD have been a response to the needs of the patient undergoing long-term home treatment. However, the advancements readily apply to the ICU environment and the patient with ARF as well—the cyclers, biocompatible solutions, and bicarbonate-based solutions. Another important area is the development of equipment and supplies specifically designed for pediatric patients, because neonates constitute a significant proportion of the patients treated with acute PD in the ICU.

Cyclers

When PD is used for the treatment of renal failure in the ICU, the utilization of cyclers, rather than manual exchanges, is almost universal. Peritoneal cyclers make possible the automated delivery of multiple exchanges/cycles of a prescribed volume of commercial PD solution. Modern software has made it simple to select the modality of PD desired, whether continuous cyclic PD or one of its variants or tidal peritoneal dialysis with variable tidal volumes. Progress in computer science and hydraulic systems has improved the precision, reliability, and safety of cyclers. The shift from an empirical approach to an analytical one in cycler design has improved data collection, data analysis, and the incorporation of quality assessment programs. The extensive list of features of a modern cycler and their application to the ICU setting are summarized in Table 269-2.

The evolution of the cycler and its adaptability to the ICU reflect the progress and availability of miniaturized, reliable, and inexpensive hydraulic devices. The essential components of a cycler are as follows: pumps, occluders to control fluid transit, manifolds, a heater cabinet or plate, hardware to process electronic data, software to collect and analyze data, and the display screen or control board. The vast majority of cyclers used to rely on gravity for both infusion and drainage. Many modern cyclers have incorporated active pumping of fluid and pump-assisted drainage in order to improve fluid dynamics and to make hydraulic control more precise and efficient (Fig. 269-1). The traditional rotary pumps, valves, and occluders have been replaced by complex disposable flow circuits built into disposable cassettes and devices that create changes in pressure in the cassette chambers and conduits. An example of this concept is a cassette containing two fluid chambers and a series of channels for solution flow (Fig. 269-2). Air pressure is applied to one chamber to generate positive pressure, thus pressing fluid out of the chamber and into the patient or the drain line, depending on the function (inflow or prime) selected (Fig. 269-3). Negative pressure draws fluid in from the patient (during drain) or from the heater bag. For the safety and comfort of the patient, the amount of negative pressure applied should approximate the natural gravity pressure observed in continuous ambulatory peritoneal dialysis. Air is also used to open and close the valves that control the flow of solution. The measurement of fluid volume flowing through the cassette can also be used for volumetric control.

Connectors

Several developments in the field of connection design may prove beneficial in ICU use of PD. Barcode labels can be used to identify specific PD solutions. The label is read by a laser beam incorporated in the cycler above the manifold tray of certain cyclers (Fig. 269-4). Automated connections, using a stationary manifold and a moving tray (connection rail) to attach the bag lines to the cassette, are now possible.

The combined use of barcodes, programs to profile glucose use and predict ultrafiltration, and automated mechanical connections may result in safer connections with less peritonitis, reduction in prescription and procedural errors, and better recordkeeping. Upon termination of the cycling session, the patient line can be disconnected and capped using sterile technique, using external occlusion, or with connectors that automatically occlude the

TABLE 269-2

Characteristics of Modern Cyclers and Their Importance in the Intensive Care Unit

CHARACTERISTIC	COMMENTS
Functionality	
Performs all prescriptions (continuous cyclic, tidal, and intermittent peritoneal dialysis)	
Delivers high total volume of dialysate (>50 L)	Less procedural time, fewer interruptions
Delivers large number of cycles	Less procedural time, fewer interruptions
Delivers minimum fill volume of 50 mL	For infants and prematures
Delivers fluid in small increments (10-20 mL)	For infants and prematures
Delivers large fill volumes (≥4 L)	Improves efficiency
Allows fast drainage (≥200 mL/min)	Improves efficiency
Pumps effluent to either bags or drain	
Records ultrafiltration by cycle and for entire treatment	
Variable alarm volume according to severity of malfunction	Reduces nuisance alarms
Programmable option for total treatment time with broad limits for fill, dwell, and drain	Individualized prescriptions
Automatic flush-before-fill as part of setup	Reduces contamination
Automatic priming of the patient line	Reduces errors
Fast and efficient warming of solutions	Important with rapid cycling
Appropriate fields for entry of pertinent laboratory parameters in treatment history	
Easy to follow step-by-step tutorial	Facilitates nurse training
Mechanical and Physical Characteristics	
Small footprint	Space saver
Low weight (≤25 lb)	Easy portability
Capability to hold a broad range of bag sizes (up to 6 L)	Time and cost saver
Noise level ≤30 dBA at maximum pumping	
120 V and 240 V AC power choices	Flexibility
User Interface	
Control panel that is easy to read and easy to use, with variable brightness and color display	
User-friendly, user-driven menu and graphics	
Safety Features	
Lockout option to prevent unauthorized changes in settings	
Stability (no tipping while holding up to 30 L)	
Locking wheels and non-slip feet	To prevent rolling and sliding
Underwriters Laboratories, Inc., Canadian Standards Association, and Conformité Européene approvals	For worldwide use
Easily disinfected with common agents	
Sealed outer case	Prevents penetration of liquids
Reliability	
Built to withstand stresses of daily use	
Can withstand extreme temperatures (−25 to +130° F)	
Information Technology	
Onboard modem	To allow wireless connection
Two or more USB ports	For memory stick, blood pressure monitors, scales, etc.
Instructions and screens in multiple languages	
Sufficient memory	For information downloads
Patient data management programs	
Full therapy data management	
Administrative module	
Prescription modeling module	
Continuous quality improvement program	
"Help" feature with online access to service	
Secured data communication	
Disposables	
Single-use, sterile components	
One-step loading (cassette)	
Advanced connection technology	Elimination of clamps
Good visualization of effluent and sample port	
Adequate organizer for operator's use	

lumen of the tubing with a pin to prevent leakage of dialysate or contamination.

Solutions

Perhaps more important than any other technological improvement is the development of more biocompatible solutions, especially those based on bicarbonate. Biocompatible solutions are manufactured using double-chambered bags to separate an acid solution containing glucose from an alkaline solution containing the buffer base. With this innovative packaging, a neutral pH solution results from mixing of the contents of the two compartments, along with low or minimal generation of glucose degradation products (GDPs) during heat sterilization. Both of

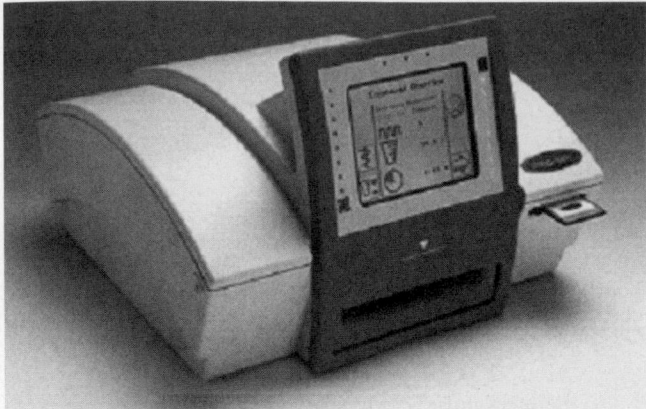

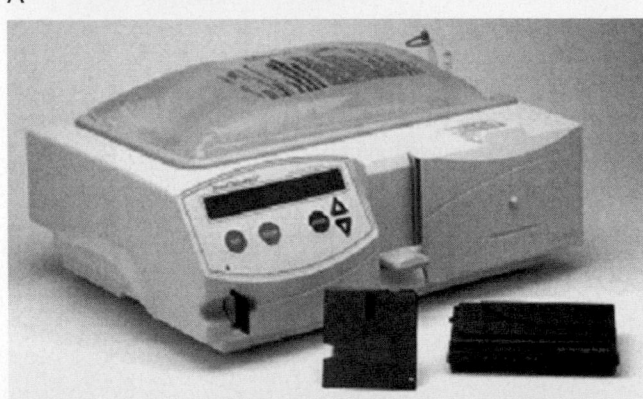

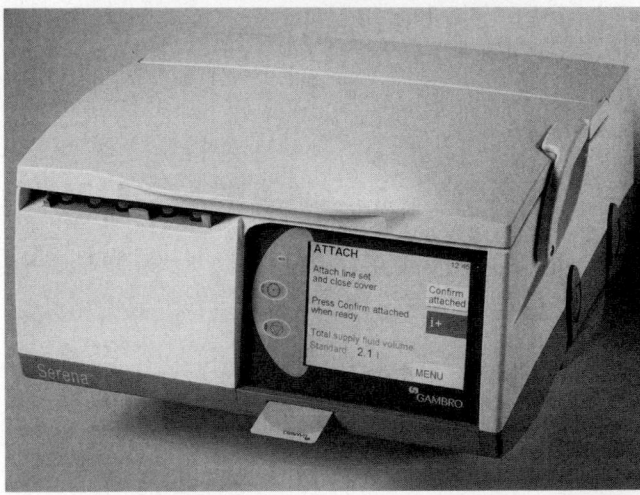

FIGURE 269-1. Modern cyclers using active infusion and drainage of peritoneal dialysis fluid. **A,** Sleepsafe cycler (Fresenius Medical Care AG, Bad Homburg, Germany). **B,** HomeChoice PRO with PD Link cycler (Baxter Healthcare Corporation, McGaw Park, IL). **C,** Serena cycler (Gambro Renal Care, Lund, Sweden).

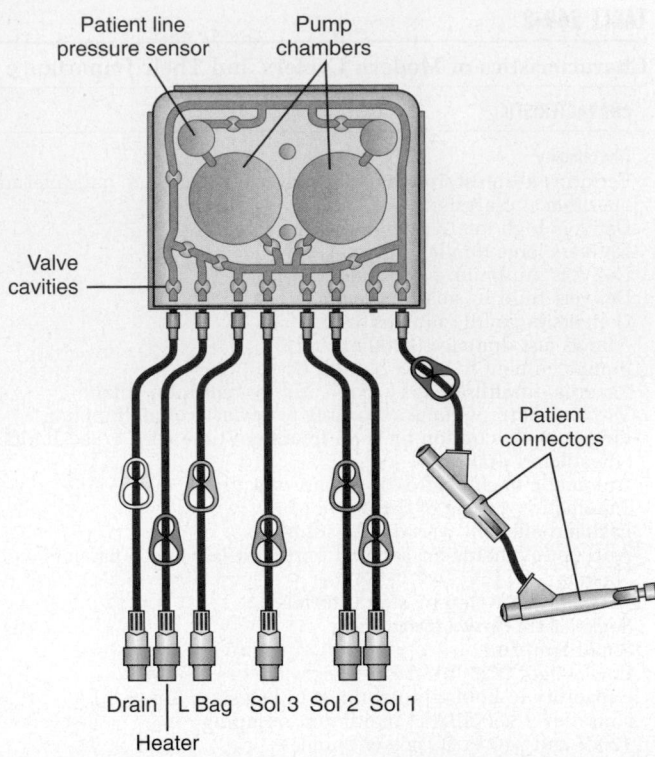

FIGURE 269-2. Cassette with heating circuit, dual fluid chambers, ports for automated bag connectors, and drainage lines. L bag, last bag; Sol, peritoneal dialysis solution.

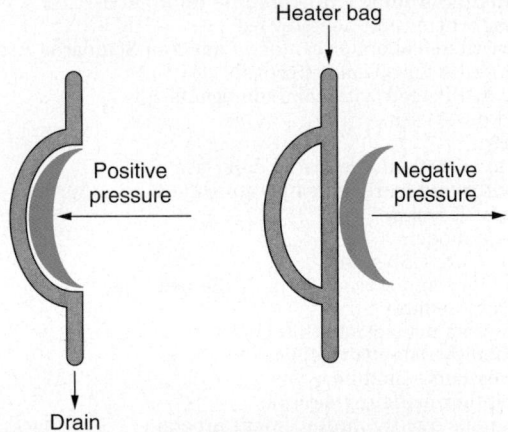

FIGURE 269-3. Diagram of cassette fluid chambers. *Left,* Positive pressure caused by air results in infusion of solution into the patient or into the drain. *Right,* The effect of negative pressure inside the chamber, which causes influx of solution from the patient and into the heating circuit.

these features have been shown to improve biocompatibility.[5] An abundance of experimental data and a few clinical experiences show better biocompatibility, improved hemodynamics, and excellent correction of metabolic acidosis with use of these novel solutions.[6-12] There are also laboratory and preliminary clinical data to suggest improved host defenses with the use of neutral pH, low-GDP, bicarbonate-based solutions.

The use of low-GDP solutions has been shown to improve monocyte, polymorphonuclear cell, and macrophage function in vitro.[13-15] Low pH has also been shown to exert an independent negative effect on phagocytosis and cytokine production by peritoneal cells.[15] Exposure of polymorphonuclear cells to fluids at pH 5.2 resulted in a lactate concentration–dependent reduction in phagocytosis.[16] Preliminary clinical reports also suggest a reduction in the risk of peritonitis with the use of neutral pH, low-

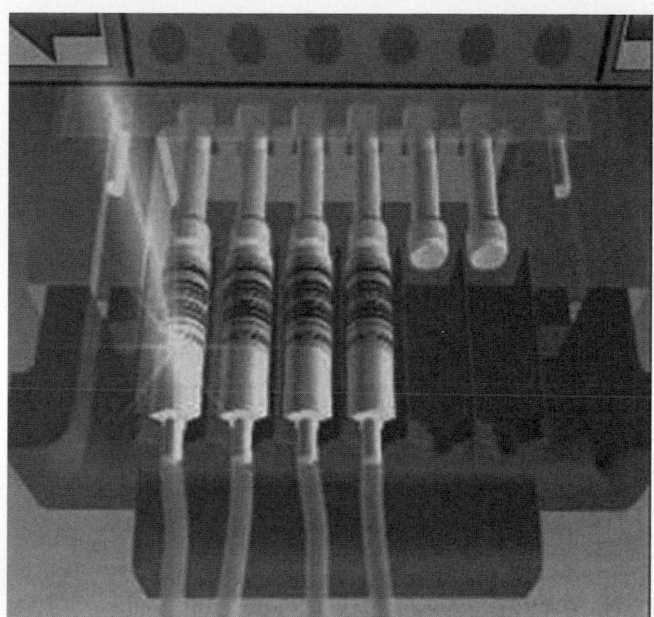

FIGURE 269-4. Automated connection device showing open tray with four bag lines connected to the cycler and barcode reader.

GDP, bicarbonate-based solutions.[17] All these features are quite relevant in the treatment of patients with unstable cardiovascular systems, multiple-organ failure (particularly liver insufficiency), severe metabolic acidosis, and impaired metabolism of lactate, such as neonates, patients with diabetic acidosis, and patients with liver cirrhosis.

CONCLUSION

The rate of use of PD for the treatment of the acutely ill patient with renal failure is low, but technological advances in this modality have made it an efficient mode of renal replacement therapy that can provide adequate treatment for a much larger number of patients. The most significant technological developments are sophisticated delivery systems with features that enhance the quality of therapy, improved recordkeeping in a simple and highly automated manner, safer and simpler connection design, and highly biocompatible solutions. There is limited literature describing clinical experiences with PD therapy in the ICU using modern equipment and solutions, but on the basis of the optimistic reports of clinical outcomes with the use of these devices and solutions for chronic therapy, prospective studies comparing PD with CRRT in the ICU setting are encouraged.

Key Points

1. Peritoneal dialysis is a viable and well-tested option for the treatment of acute renal failure.
2. The utilization of both intermittent hemodialysis and peritoneal dialysis for the treatment of acute renal failure has diminished, whereas that of continuous renal replacement therapies has dramatically increased in most developed countries. This trend is not evidence-based.
3. The technological advances in peritoneal dialysis can be readily applied in the intensive care unit and the patient with acute renal failure as well.
4. Progress in computer science and hydraulic systems has improved the precision, reliability, and safety of cyclers.
5. The development of more biocompatible solutions, especially those based on bicarbonate, may turn out to be the most important technological improvement in this area.

Key References

4. Hyman A, Mendelssohn DC: Current Canadian approaches to dialysis for acute renal failure in the ICU. Am J Nephrol 2002;22:29-34.
8. Mortier S, De Vriese A, Passlick-Deetjen J, Lameire N: Hemodynamic effects of conventional and new peritoneal dialysis (PD) solutions on the microcirculation of the rat peritoneal membrane (PM). Perit Dial Int 2001;21(Suppl 2):S18-S29.
9. Feriani M, Kirchgessner J, La Greca G, Passlick-Deetjen J: Randomized long-term evaluation of bicarbonate-buffered CAPD solution. Kidney Int 1998;54:1731-1738.
12. Montenegro J, Saracho RM, Martinez IM, et al: Long-term clinical experience with pure bicarbonate peritoneal dialysis solutions. Perit Dial Int 2006;26:89-94.
17. Montenegro J, Munoz RI, Martinez I, et al: Important decrease of peritonitis incidence using new double-chamber bicarbonate solution in CAPD. J Am Soc Nephrol 2003;14;480A.

See the companion Expert Consult website for the complete reference list.

CHAPTER 270

Correction of Fluid, Electrolyte, and Acid-Base Derangements by Peritoneal Dialysis in Acute Renal Failure

Laura A. Kooienga and Isaac Teitelbaum

OBJECTIVES

This chapter will:
1. Describe the key components of an acute peritoneal dialysis prescription in the intensive care unit.
2. Explore the role of acute peritoneal dialysis in the management of patients with volume overload in the intensive care unit.
3. Discuss the correction of electrolyte abnormalities with the use of acute peritoneal dialysis.
4. Summarize the role of this modality in the correction of acid-base derangements.
5. Detail potential metabolic complications of acute peritoneal dialysis in the intensive care unit.

Acute renal failure (ARF) is a common problem in the intensive care unit (ICU) and represents a clinically diverse entity. It is associated with significant morbidity, mortality, and financial expenditure.[1-4] Management involves the appropriate control of fluid balance, electrolyte status, and acid-base balance and the initiation of renal replacement therapy when appropriate. Numerous treatment options are available, although there is no consensus in the literature on the best method or ideal dialysis dose in the setting of ARF in the ICU. Unlike in many developing countries, where peritoneal dialysis (PD) constitutes the mainstay of therapy for ARF, in the United States this modality is typically reserved for those patients with end-stage renal disease. This often-overlooked modality for dialytic support should be considered a viable option for the treatment of selected patients with ARF in the ICU. This chapter details the role of PD in correction of fluid, electrolyte, and acid-base derangements in the patient with ARF.

PRESCRIPTION FOR ACUTE PERITONEAL DIALYSIS

Once the decision is made to initiate PD, a prescription must be formulated on the basis of the particular clinical situation and therapeutic goals (Table 270-1). The details of the therapy instituted, in addition to fluid balance, should be recorded meticulously on flow sheets to facilitate future decisions about the patient's PD regimen. The PD prescription should be reviewed frequently and appropriate adjustments made on the basis of the patient's laboratory and clinical parameters.

The length and the technique of PD must be determined. Session lengths can vary greatly depending on the etiology and duration of ARF as well as the presence or absence of underlying chronic kidney disease. The length of the dialysis sessions also depends on the goals of fluid and solute removal. PD can be performed intermittently or continuously, either manually or with an automated cycling device. Techniques available for the treatment of ARF include acute intermittent PD, continuous equilibrating peritoneal dialysis, continuous-flow PD, and tidal PD.

Once the technique of PD is decided upon, consideration must be given to the composition of the dialysate to be used for treatment. Standardized peritoneal dialysate solutions are commercially available. They are typically composed of dextrose as the osmotic agent and lactate as the buffer. In addition, they also contain sodium, chloride, magnesium, and calcium. Standard dextrose concentrations available in the United States are 1.5%, 2.5%, and 4.25%. It is the concentration of dextrose that determines the osmotic strength of the dialysate and, hence, the level of ultrafiltration obtained. Therefore, the initial choice of dextrose concentration is determined in part by the patient's volume status. In patients with more severe volume overload, a reasonable choice of dextrose solution would be 4.25%; for patients who are hemodynamically unstable with only slight volume overload, an initial dialysis dextrose solution of 1.5% or 2.5% might be more appropriate. Dextrose-containing solutions can provide a substantial source of caloric intake in the critically ill patient and may require an intensive insulin regimen to prevent the development of hyperglycemia. On the other hand, the use of dextrose-containing PD solutions should be used with caution in the patient with severe respiratory failure, in whom administration of such solutions might worsen respiratory failure through the greater production of carbon dioxide.[5]

Standard dialysate solutions use lactate (35-40 mmol/L) as the bicarbonate-generating base because of its high stability in the presence of calcium and magnesium. However, in patients with reduced lactate metabolism, such as those with hepatic failure, lactic acidosis, or severe septic shock, lactate-buffered solutions should be avoided, and bicarbonate-buffered solutions used. Such preparations are available through use of a two-compartment bag system to keep the bicarbonate separate from the calcium and magnesium until just before administration.

TABLE 270-1

Components of an Acute Peritoneal Dialysis Prescription

Length of dialysis session
Dialysate composition
Dialysate additives
Exchange volume
Number of exchanges
Inflow period
Dwell time
Outflow period

Another approach to PD is through the simultaneous use of both glucose-based and amino acid–based dialysates that are mixed immediately prior to administration with an automated device. This approach has the theoretical advantage of reducing amino acid loss and improving nitrogen balance. The amino acid–based dialysate is used only for one or two exchanges per day, because these solutions have been found to cause mild acidosis and to contribute to elevations in urea concentrations,[6] which may not be well tolerated in a critically ill patient with ARF. Amino acid–based solutions have not been studied in adults with ARF; however, they have been evaluated in children with ARF. In a retrospective analysis of the use of PD solutions with amino acids, Vande Walle and associates[7] found that glucose reabsorption and protein loss were significantly lower than glucose-based solutions alone when mixed amino acid solutions were used, although they observed no significant difference in serum albumin levels.

Icodextrin is yet another solution available for use in PD. It is a mixture of high-molecular-weight glucose polymers that exerts a stable colloid osmotic pressure. In patients with end-stage renal disease, icodextrin has been found to produce greater ultrafiltration rates with improved urea and creatinine clearances than dialysate with 2.5% dextrose.[8] This mixture has also been shown, in a multicenter, randomized, double-blind trial of its use in patients with end-stage renal disease, to produce superior ultrafiltration in high-average and high-transporters compared to that obtained with 4.25% dextrose.[9] Icodextrin may play a role in the treatment of ARF with PD but has not been studied in this setting so its efficacy is not known.

The standard dialysate contains calcium in concentrations ranging from 1.25 to 1.75 mmol/L (2.5-3.5 mEq/L). Such concentrations of calcium typically result in the movement of calcium from the PD solution to the extracellular fluid, potentially helping to support blood pressure in the critically ill patient. Standard dialysate does not contain potassium but does contain sodium (132 mEq/L) and magnesium (0.5-1.5 mEq/L). Other agents, such as heparin, insulin, antibiotics, epoetin alpha, and potassium, may be added to the dialysate as the clinical situation dictates.

Another key component of the dialysis prescription is determining the appropriate *exchange volume*—the amount of dialysate solution instilled into the peritoneal cavity during an exchange. This volume is influenced by several factors, including technique of PD being used, concomitant medical problems such as the presence of hernias or respiratory disease, the estimated size of the patient's peritoneal cavity, and any noted leakage of dialysate around the PD catheter. For example, in acute intermittent PD, an exchange volume for an average-size person without respiratory failure might be 2 L, whereas in a larger patient,

it might be as much as 3.5 L. On the other hand, an exchange volume for a small person with acute respiratory distress syndrome might be only 0.5 to 1.5 L to prevent compromise of the diaphragmatic excursions and respirations. Dialysate solutions should be warmed to body temperature prior to infusion to avoid discomfort and enhance solute transport. The temperature of the PD dialysate can be especially advantageous in the management of both hyperthermia and hypothermia.[10]

The number of exchanges is determined by the overall goals of fluid and solute removal. Increasing the number of exchanges serves to augment both fluid and solute removal. A usual number of exchanges for acute PD is 24 per day; 4 to 6 exchanges per day are common with the use of continuous equilibrating PD. The *inflow period* is the time required to instill the dialysate into the peritoneal cavity. For manual exchanges, gravity is the primary determinant of this period, although the exchange volume, elevation of the dialysate bag, and presence of inflow resistance also play roles. In order to maximize the efficiency of PD, the inflow period must be kept to a minimum. A typical inflow period is 10 to 15 minutes. The *outflow period* is defined as the time needed to drain the peritoneal cavity of the effluent dialysate, which averages 20 to 30 minutes. This period consists of an initial fast segment lasting a few minutes, in which time approximately 80% of dialysate is drained; this segment is followed by a slower segment in which the remainder is emptied. Like the inflow period, the outflow period must also be kept to a minimum and is determined primarily by gravity. The time between the inflow and outflow period is referred to as the *dwell time*—the period in which the exchange volume remains in the peritoneal cavity. The standard dwell time for acute PD is approximately 30 minutes, the time in which the gradients for fluid and urea are most favorable. For continuous equilibrating PD, the usual dwell time ranges from 3 to 6 hours; for continuous-flow PD, a large volume of dialysate is instilled and drained in a continuous manner.

FLUID REMOVAL

Fluid balance is a critical component of the care of patients in the ICU who have ARF. In fact, in a study by Ronco and coworkers[11] collecting data from 345 nephrology centers on five continents, continuous renal replacement therapy (CRRT) was used in 52% of centers for indications other than ARF. Of these, the two most commonly reported conditions, which accounted for approximately half of the uses, were congestive heart failure and fluid overload.[11] Overall fluid balance depends on the amount of fluid intake, which is countered by the amount removed by both any remaining urine output and ultrafiltration. The titration of fluid removal with PD is not as easily achieved as that with hemodialysis or CRRT, because fluid removal occurs with PD through an osmotic gradient for water from the patient's blood to the peritoneum. Ultrafiltration is generally well tolerated with less hemodynamic instability than seen in other forms of renal replacement therapy because of the continuous nature of the therapy. This improved hemodynamic stability may at least theoretically lessen the insult to the acutely damaged kidneys. Fluid removal with PD may also permit the administration of parenteral nutrition to help counter protein losses through the peritoneum, even in patients who otherwise may not have been able to tolerate the fluid load.

Large amounts of fluid can be removed in patients treated with acute PD, through a combination of larger fill volumes, higher number of exchanges, and greater tonicity of the dialysate. When this technique is employed, close attention must be paid to the serum sodium because hypernatremia may result from a phenomenon known as *sodium sieving*. Sodium sieving occurs as a consequence of transcellular water transport through aquaporins during the first phase of the dwell time, which removes relatively more water than sodium and hence can lead to significant hypernatremia in the setting of repeated rapid exchanges with hypertonic dextrose solutions. After this initial phase of water transport through the aquaporin channels, sodium transport increases continuously through diffusive and convective transport into the peritoneal cavity. Therefore, sodium sieving is more marked during short dwell times. Furthermore, those treatment regimens with high dialysate flow and relatively short dwell times may be associated with impaired sodium removal even if they achieve better small solute clearances.

Although acute PD has the capacity to remove large amounts of fluid, its use should probably be avoided in cases of severe volume overload with impending respiratory failure in patients who are not supported by mechanical ventilation. On the other hand, patients with congestive heart failure (CHF) refractory to medical management may benefit from the use of acute PD. The acute treatment prescription of patients with CHF consists of initial small volumes, such as 0.5 to 1 L of hypertonic dextrose solution, with short dwell times, 1 to 2 hours.[12,13] PD as treatment of CHF improves fluid status and reduces pulmonary capillary wedge pressure, increases cardiac output, and improves hyponatremia, and quality of life; however, it is not known whether this therapy affects survival.[14,15] It is important to remember that, in the setting of CHF as well as other diseases associated with ascites, intraperitoneal third space extravasation may dilute the dialysate, altering its concentration and effectiveness.

Although the use of icodextrin has not been studied specifically in the setting of CHF with ARF, its use has been reported in two patients with CHF. Bertoli and colleagues[16] used a single nocturnal dwell of icodextrin in two elderly subjects with moderate to severe chronic renal failure; in both patients, the treatment significantly increased creatinine clearance, reduced morbidity and the need for hospitalization, along with improvement in or stability of ejection fraction and quality of life.[16] These cases suggest a possible benefit for patients with CHF and renal impairment, but that has yet to be proven.

ELECTROLYTE ABNORMALITIES

PD can be used to correct electrolyte abnormalities in blood urea, creatinine, potassium, and sodium serum concentrations. This modality enables the continuous correction of electrolyte imbalances with the gradual removal of nitrogenous waste products without the risk of dysequilibrium syndrome. In a prospective randomized study, Arogundade and coworkers[17] managed 40 patients with ARF, who were matched for age and clinical diagnosis, with either intermittent PD or hemodialysis. These investigators found that patients treated with PD had significant reductions in concentrations of urea (from 29.2 ± 7.2 mmol/L to 13.2 ± 4.6 mmol/L), creatinine (from 1693.7 ± 580.5 µmol/L to 796.0 ± 458.0 µmol/L), and potassium (from 4.8 ± 1.2 mmol/L to 3.3 ± 0.6 mmol/L). There were no signifi-

cant differences in the reduction of these parameters between the two treatment groups. However, the hemodialysis group required more blood transfusions ($P < .05$), and their treatments involved overall greater cost of dialysis and total cost of hospitalization, compared with the PD group.[17]

Acute PD may not be preferred, although it may be the only option in some developing countries, for cases of severe hypercatabolism or life-threatening hyperkalemia. Nonetheless, it is of benefit in managing cases of hyperkalemia other than those that are life-threatening. PD not only allows for the gradual removal of potassium but also enhances the intracellular movement of potassium through the correction of metabolic acidosis and the stimulation of insulin production by the administration of intraperitoneal glucose. It is equally important to remember that with longer durations of dialysis, hypokalemia may ensue because standard PD solutions do not contain potassium. Hypokalemia can be corrected through the addition of potassium to the dialysate fluid or with oral or peripheral administration of potassium supplement.

PD can also be used for the correction of sodium abnormalities associated with problems with urinary dilution and urinary concentration that are frequently encountered in ARF. In a study by Inagaki and associates,[18] correction of severe abnormalities of serum sodium was obtained through the use of individualized PD solutions. These researchers were able to successfully lower the serum sodium concentration to 138 mEq/L in a severely hypernatremic patient with an initial value of 170 mEq/L through the administration of hypotonic (Na, 70 mEq/L) peritoneal solution. Likewise, in two patients with hyponatremia (serum sodium concentrations of 113 mEq/L and 121 mEq/L), Inagaki and associates[18] raised serum sodium concentrations to the normal range through the administration of PD solutions with a sodium concentration of 190 mEq/L. Similarly, hypercalcemia can be ameliorated through the use of PD dialysate either without calcium or with a lower calcium concentration than that of a standard solution.

ACID-BASE DERANGEMENTS

Correction of metabolic acidosis with PD in the setting of ARF occurs through the gain of alkali from the absorption of either lactate or bicarbonate from the PD dialysate. In the case of lactate-buffered solutions, lactate absorbed into the bloodstream can be converted to bicarbonate via the enzyme pyruvate dehydrogenase, which is found principally in the liver and muscles. A randomized study has examined the efficacy of both lactate and bicarbonate-buffered solutions in the correction of metabolic acidosis in patients both with and without shock. Thongboonkerd and colleagues[19] studied a group of 20 subjects requiring acute PD who were further classified by the presence or absence of shock. They were then randomly assigned to treatment with either bicarbonate- or lactate-buffered PD solutions with an average exchange volume of 1.4 ± 0.01 L with a dwell time of 30 minutes. By cycle 12, subjects in the shock group treated with bicarbonate-buffered solutions had a more rapid improvement and significantly higher blood pH (7.30 ± 0.03 vs. 7.05 ± 0.04; $P < .05$) and serum bicarbonate (21.2 ± 1.8 mmol/L vs. 14.3 ± 1.3 mmol/L; $P < .05$) values. These improvements remained statistically significant between the two groups through cycle 36. Overall lactate levels were significantly lower in the group receiving the bicarbonate-buffered solution in both the patients with shock (3.6 ± 0.4 mmol/L vs. 5.2 ± 0.3 mmol/L) and without shock (2.9 ± 0.2 mmol/L vs. 3.4 ± 0.2 mmol/L). However, the patients without shock had comparable improvements in both blood pH and serum bicarbonate with either solution, and peritoneal urea and creatinine clearances were similar in all of the subgroups.[19] Results of this study suggest that ARF associated with poor perfusion states, such as shock, lactic acidosis, and multiple-organ failure, should be managed with the use of bicarbonate-buffered solutions rather than lactate solutions. In line with findings in this study, Inagaki and associates[18] reported successful treatment of two cases of lactic acidosis with a fluid mixed with distilled water, 10% sodium chloride, and 7% sodium bicarbonate. This therapy allowed for the diffusion of lactic acid from the extracellular fluid into the PD fluid and diffusion of bicarbonate from the PD fluid into the extracellular space.

PD can also be used to correct metabolic alkalosis. A study by Inagaki and associates[18] also examined nine patients who had either ARF or CRF and in whom hemodialysis was unable to correct metabolic alkalosis. These researchers found that by administering normal saline as the primary component of the dialysate, they were able to correct the metabolic alkalosis through shift of bicarbonate from the extracellular space into the PD solution and of chloride from the PD solution into the bloodstream.[18]

UPDATE

As this chapter went to press another important study was published. Gabriel and colleagues[20] reported the results of a randomized prospective trial comparing outcomes in 120 patients with acute kidney injury (77% in ICU) treated with either daily hemodialysis (DHD) or high volume peritoneal dialysis (HVPD). The DHD patients underwent treatment for at least 3 hours 6 times per week achieving a mean weekly Kt/V of 4.7; the HVPD patients underwent 18-22 two-liter exchanges every day (dwell times ranged from 35 to 50 minutes), achieving a mean weekly Kt/V of 3.6. The rates of hospital survival and recovery of renal function were comparable in the two groups, as were control of acidosis, potassium, and azotemia. This study clearly supports a role for peritoneal dialysis in the treatment of patients with acute kidney injury.

CONCLUSIONS

Acute PD is an often-overlooked therapy for dialytic support in patients with ARF in the ICU. When used in the appropriate clinical setting, this modality has the capacity to correct fluid balance disturbances, electrolyte abnormalities, and acid-base derangements. One of the keys to successful implementation of this form of renal replacement comes from the careful attention to all components of the PD prescription along with meticulous monitoring of the therapy. Furthermore, it has the distinctive advantage of better hemodynamic stability secondary to its continuous nature without the need for anticoagulation.

Key Points

1. The peritoneal dialysis prescription for acute renal failure must be individualized to fulfill the specific and often changing needs of the critically ill patient, particular attention being paid to volume status, respiratory status, and the presence of any metabolic abnormalities.
2. Bicarbonate-buffered dialysate solutions are preferred over lactate-buffered solutions in the setting of impaired lactate metabolism such as that seen in shock, lactic acidosis, and hepatic failure.
3. Short dwell times, which are often used in the clinical setting of volume overload, may place the patient at risk for significant hypernatremia as a result of sodium sieving.
4. Peritoneal dialysis may be efficacious in settings other than acute renal failure in the intensive care unit, such as for treatment of hypothermia, hyperthermia, and congestive heart failure.
5. Through individualized prescription, peritoneal dialysis is a viable and safe option for the correction of severe abnormalities of serum sodium and calcium concentrations, metabolic acidosis, and metabolic alkalosis.

Key References

8. Wolfson M, Piraino B, Hamburger RJ, Morton AR: A randomized controlled trial to evaluate the efficacy and safety of icodextrin in peritoneal dialysis. Am J Kidney Dis 2002; 40:1055-1065.
11. Ronco C, Zanella M, Brendolan A, Milan M: Management of severe acute renal failure in critically ill patients: An international survey in 345 centers. Nephrol Dial Transplant 2001;16:230-237.
12. Mehrotra R, Khanna R: Peritoneal ultrafiltration for chronic congestive heart failure: Rationale, evidence and future. Cardiology 2001;98:177-182.
15. Bargman JM: Nonuremic indications for peritoneal dialysis. Perit Dial Int 1993;S159-S164.
18. Inagaki Y, Miyazaki T, Amano I: Peritoneal dialysis as therapy for electrolyte and acid base disorders. Int J Artif Organs 1998;12:632-637.
20. Gabriel DP, Caramori JT, Martim LC, et al: High volume peritoneal dialysis vs daily hemodialysis: A randomized, controlled trial in patients with acute kidney injury. Kid Int 2008;73:S87-S93.

See the companion Expert Consult website for the complete reference list.

CHAPTER 271

Efficiency and Adequacy of Peritoneal Dialysis in Acute Renal Failure

Ashutosh Shukla and Joanne M. Bargman

OBJECTIVES

This chapter will:
1. Review the role of peritoneal dialysis in the management of acute renal failure.
2. Discuss the mechanical complications resulting from insertion of a peritoneal dialysis catheter in the acutely ill patient.
3. Explain the prescription of acute peritoneal dialysis to optimize ultrafiltration and solute removal.
4. Discuss the measurement and assessment of the adequacy of acute peritoneal dialysis in the acutely ill patient.

Although the initial descriptions of peritoneal dialysis (PD) in renal failure were of its performance in patients with acute renal failure (ARF), PD has become an important modality of renal replacement therapy (RRT) in patients with stable chronic renal failure. The decline in the use of PD for ARF has resulted from the development of other continuous extracorporeal therapies described elsewhere in this book, and perhaps also from the overall loss of expertise and faith in peritoneal dialysis in general by the medical community in many countries. However, the very characteristics of PD—gentle clearance that avoids metabolic fluxes and dysequilibrium, minor or no interference with hemodynamics, lack of requirement for anticoagulation, the notion that it does more than merely clear the small solutes (clearance of middle-molecular-weight molecules and cytokines), and its simplicity and efficacy—make it an attractive contender for RRT in ARF in general and in the intensive care unit (ICU) specifically. This chapter discusses the role of peritoneal dialysis in the treatment of ARF in critically ill patients.

ROLE OF PERITONEAL DIALYSIS IN THE INTENSIVE CARE UNIT

Before considering the application of PD in ARF in the intensive care unit (ICU), one must understand the issues involved in managing any RRT in the ICU. More than three quarters of patients with advanced renal insufficiency have multiple-organ dysfunction, and many have evidence of dysfunction in four or five organ systems.[1] In such a severely sick population, a cause-and-effect relationship between various disease manifestations and particular organ system failure is difficult to determine; in many cases, different insults affect outcome synergistically. These factors also affect determination of the treatment options, with the possibility of both undertreatment and overzealous therapy, which lead to even more complications. Therefore, indications for dialysis in the setting of critical illness can be difficult to define, and unproven markers are sometimes used for the determination of dialysis need as well as its efficacy and safety.

The first decision in the patient with ARF is the need for dialysis. This issue has been discussed in previous sections of the book so it is merely summarized here. Data from published studies are inadequate to support definitive recommendations regarding the optimal timing of initiation of RRT in ARF. There is little controversy about its use in presence of imminent metabolic threat—for example, for the treatment of refractory hyperkalemia, fluid overload refractory to diuretic therapy, severe metabolic acidosis, or overt uremic symptoms. The precise extent or duration of renal dysfunction warranting initiation of RRT in the absence of absolute indications has been difficult to define, however.

A large part of the evidence comes from the small retrospective case series from the previous decades. Few prospective data are available, and even those are from studies that involved small patient numbers and were usually uncontrolled or nonrandomized. Most of these studies have examined the level of uremia as reflected by the blood urea nitrogen (BUN) concentration. However, BUN concentration alone may be inadequate to gauge the severity of renal failure. With these limitations in mind, some investigators have suggested that in the absence of symptoms, advanced uremia, reflected by a BUN of 80 to 100 mg/dL, substantiates the need for dialysis[2]; this range is not an absolute value, however, and the decision must be made according to the individual patient's clinical condition. Prophylactic dialysis has lately been studied in the context of continuous renal replacement therapy (CRRT), with equivocal results.[3] Although it is reasonable to assume that early initiation of dialysis may avoid complications of renal failure, many patients with ARF recover without dialytic therapy. The institution of dialysis when the kidneys are recovering could have its own complications. Further evaluation of this issue with appropriately powered, multicenter, randomized studies is needed. Once the decision to initiate RRT has been made, however, the precise modality of dialysis performed is affected by various medical and administrative factors.

Peritoneal dialysis for the treatment of uremia was first realized by Georg Ganter in the early 20th century; he performed it in a patient with obstructive renal failure with the help of a rigid catheter and saline solution as the PD fluid.[4] Use of PD grew in the late 1950s, when a rigid trocar–based PD cannula replaced the surgical tubes for access to the peritoneal cavity. In later decades, the development of the Tenckhoff flexible catheters[5] and the use of PD as a continuous modality increased the acceptance of this modality.

In the 1970s, intermittent PD (IPD) by means of a rigid catheter was widely used in patients with ARF. In this process, rapid exchanges were carried out over 10 to 24 hours. At the end of this time, the patient was left without any dialysate dwell until the next session of peritoneal dialysis. With the advent over the last two decades of technical advances in hemodialysis involving proportioning machines, controlled ultrafiltration, and better anticoagulation strategies, there has been a reduction in PD utilization for ARF. With the availability of better tolerated hemodialysis, the concept of higher dialysis dose for better patient survival was introduced, and PD was considered "inadequate" for this challenge. It was reserved mainly for children and patients with coagulation abnormalities and hemodynamic instability.[6] Developments in CRRTs (principally venovenous therapy) during the 1990s, along with availability of bicarbonate-based dialysis solutions, have resulted in further erosion into the classic "PD pool" of patients. In fact, only 10% of 831 U.S. nephrologists surveyed in 2002 thought that PD was as efficient as IHD in management of ARF.[6] Although similar opinions have resonated from other parts of the developed world, and only about 20% of facilities offer the option of peritoneal dialysis in patients of ARF, its utilization is far less than that figure indicates.[7,8] PD is a more prominent treatment modality for ARF in the developing world, although a similar trend of decline is evident in many urban areas.[9]

Given these developments, the questions remain whether peritoneal dialysis is truly inferior to the other modalities of dialysis and whether its use in developing countries is justified only by financial incentives. On the other hand, is an overzealous embrace of the expensive, glamorous new technologies determining the choice of modality? Certainly, similar assumptions regarding PD in patients with chronic kidney disease (CKD) have now been proven wrong. Outcomes of PD in patients with end-stage renal disease (ESRD) are equal if not superior to those of hemodialysis, and PD provides a better quality of life. In addition, PD is technically simple, economically sounder, and medically less interfering with other comorbidities. It also avoids anticoagulation, a significant hazard in many critically ill patients. In many parts of the underdeveloped world and a large part of the developed world, economic factors by themselves have driven the therapy of ARF, with PD being a primary mode of RRT in ARF, especially in patients with hemodynamic compromise.[9-11]

DEFINING THE EFFICACY OF PERITONEAL DIALYSIS IN ACUTE RENAL FAILURE

There is no consensus in the literature regarding the universal marker for estimating either the extent of renal dysfunction or the efficacy of dialysis in ARF. BUN and serum creatinine concentrations most commonly are used to estimate renal dysfunction. However, their values vary with nonrenal factors, limiting their ability to accurately reflect the extent of renal dysfunction. In ARF and in the absence of steady-state metabolism, the value of the BUN value to determine the extent of renal dysfunction is further compromised by an inadequate supply of nutritional substrates, loss of nutritional substrates during dialysis, increased circulating concentrations of catabolic hormones, gastrointestinal bleeding, systemic inflammatory response syndrome, administration of corticosteroids, and exposure to bioincompatible dialysis apparatus.[12] The serum creatinine concentration is commonly used in routine clinical practice for estimating the extent of renal dysfunction in patients with ARF. However, its value as such a marker is significantly compromised as well because of changes in gastrointestinal and renal handling of creatinine that occur with ARF. Thus, decisions are based not on absolute values of these markers but on their trend over time, along with the clinical state of the patient. In addition, no definitive data exist regarding the target levels for these markers, even though both BUN and creatinine concentrations have been loosely used in clinical studies of ARF.[13,14]

The concept of hemodialysis adequacy based on urea kinetic modeling (UKM) was put forth in the 1980s. UKM utilizes certain steady-state assumptions, and Kt/V is the volume-averaged clearance achieved during a particular dialysis session. Kt/V_{urea} in HD is calculated with the help of predialysis and post-dialysis blood sampling. Many studies have applied UKM and Kt/V in ARF. However, UKM has significant limitations. Variations in urea generation, sometimes from hour to hour in ARF, require a dynamic model of urea kinetics, and the steady-state assumptions as used in the stable population with CKD do not apply in these situations. In addition, computation of the urea distribution volume (V) from the standard formulas may not be applicable owing to retention of excess water and the tendency of V to change frequently in critically ill patients.[15] In the end, urea kinetics during hemodialysis may in fact have multicompartment rather than single- or dual-compartment characteristics in patients with critical illness.[16] Thus, Kt/V cannot be validated for ARF. Evanson and colleagues[17] have elegantly shown the large discrepancy between prescribed and delivered doses of dialysis when UKM and Kt/V_{urea} are used. Urea clearance (mL/min) has been used in studies involving continuous venovenous hemodialysis/filtration.[18]

Fortunately, these limitations are not major for peritoneal dialysis. PD is a continuous therapy (even in automated dialysis) with good equilibration between various body compartments, reducing the effects of multicompartment complications. In addition, the Kt/V measurement in patients undergoing PD (although perhaps not the best way to measure adequacy in PD; see later) is achieved through measurement of urea in the dialysate and, hence, has much less tendency to differ from the true delivered dose.[9]

However, the strength of PD lies in other areas than simply the removal of small solutes. Indices of small solute clearance, such as Kt/V_{urea}, bear little correlation with the adequacy of peritoneal dialysis[19] and survival in patients with CKD.[20] These changes in understanding have been duly recognized in updates of adequacy guidelines for PD, in which greater emphasis has been placed on evaluation of multiple clinical and biochemical parameters.[21] Among the other studied markers, solute reduction indices (SRIs) and urea nitrogen appearance (UNA) have drawn significant attention. SRI_{urea} is the ratio between the amount of urea removed and the total body urea content.

SRI is especially advantageous in patients undergoing hemodialysis, because the calculation is made from the dialysate compartment and avoids the computation from blood values, negating the effect of compartmentalization.[22] Collection of the dialysate effluent makes its routine calculation difficult, though newer hemodialysis machines with on-line measurement of effluent concentration may be useful in such situations. In addition, this approach still does not address the variable urea generation and fallacies in calculation of V in ARF. UNA more closely reflects the protein catabolism in patients with ARF and better defines the need for small solute clearance. However, the cumbersome nature of the routine calculations of these markers, especially in patients undergoing hemodialysis, makes them less desirable. Owing to these limitations, few units measure the dose of dialysis in ARF.[23] Other, non-nitrogenous biochemical parameters (e.g., potassium, phosphate, uric acid, acidosis) and the patient's clinical condition are frequently used to define the level of impairment and judge the need for change in dialysis dose. These parameters may be especially suitable for patients undergoing PD, because no single index of adequacy accurately reflects its efficacy.

ADEQUACY AND OUTCOMES OF PERITONEAL DIALYSIS IN ACUTE RENAL FAILURE

The primary goal of any therapy is to neutralize the insult caused by the disease process and, if possible, promote the eventual recovery of the body to its predisease state. *Acute renal failure* is defined as abrupt cessation or decline of renal function leading to retention of nitrogenous waste products. Along with the decline of renal function, most patients with ARF also have a catabolic state resulting in degradation of body proteins. Accumulation of these waste products has various metabolic and systemic effects. Thus, in simplistic terms, adequate dialytic therapy for ARF would clear the body of these excess waste products so as to nullify their harmful effects and limit further insult pending eventual renal recovery.

Several studies have demonstrated the efficacy of PD and its equivalence to hemodialysis in terms of morbidity and mortality.[24-34] Most of these studies were small, retrospective case series. Also, patients receiving PD in the studies were usually sicker than their counterparts undergoing hemodialysis. In one of the earliest reports, Cameron and associates[13] studied the efficacy of PD performed with exchanges of 1 to 3 L/hour in patients with hypercatabolic ARF secondary to burns or to cardiac or aortic surgery. These investigators concluded that satisfactory clinical control of uremia was achieved in the majority of the patients (defined as blood urea concentration less than 200 mg/dL, which is equivalent to a BUN 100 mg/dL) and that hypercatabolism by itself not be a contraindication to PD.

The benefit of peritoneal dialysis was subsequently shown in a variety of diseases causing ARF as PD was increasingly utilized and studied in both relative eubolic and hypercatabolic states. Indraprasit and colleagues,[35] in their 1988 report on 10 patients with hypercatabolic ARF treated with PD, demonstrated that the treatment achieved adequate waste product control and fluid and electrolyte balance for 2 to 30 days. They suggested an equivalence between urea clearance of approximately 12 mL/min with peritoneal dialysis and a clearance of 120 mL/min with alternate-day hemodialysis for 5-hour sessions. It is now understood that PD with even lower mathematical urea clearance has equivalent outcome compared to thrice weekly hemodialysis in patients with ESRD.

Not all researchers have agreed with this assertion of PD being equivalent to hemodialysis, however.[6,23] In certain diseases that cause ARF—sepsis with multiple-organ dysfunction syndrome, snake bite, tumor lysis, intoxications, poisoning—there is a much higher level of catabolism, which may lead to a higher solute load. PD may not be suitable in such conditions.

However, since the older concept of the quantification of dialysis dose and adequacy has been challenged, the adequacy of peritoneal dialysis has been regarded differently. As indicated earlier, much of the confusion arises from the fact that currently, there is no universally accepted standard of dialysis dose and adequacy in ARF. With improvement in hemodialysis and CRRT technology, the concept that a higher dialysis dose leads to better survival has been put forth. Many authorities believe that there is a close relationship between morbidity, mortality, and dialysis dose in ARF,[36-38] despite the absence of satisfactory markers of adequacy. Concerns have been raised about the ability of PD to adequately control the level of uremia, especially considering its lower small solute clearance in comparison with hemodialysis. However, the concerns about small solute clearance do not correctly reflect the clearance of PD and also may not apply in ARF.

Since the advent of CRRT, studies involving PD in ARF have decreased in the developing world. Most of the latest literature about the use of PD in ARF comes from developing countries, where the use of PD in ARF is still prevalent. Most studies have evaluated intermittent peritoneal dialysis with manual cycling. The investigators have used an open drainage system, and many have used rigid catheters.

In the only available randomized trial comparing PD with continuous venovenous hemofiltration, Phu and colleagues[10] enrolled 70 adults (48 with severe falciparum malaria and 22 with sepsis), randomly assigning them to undergo hemofiltration (34 patients) or PD (36 patients). The primary outcome (mortality) was higher in the PD group (47%) than in the hemofiltration group (15%; $P = .05$). The secondary outcomes, such as correction of acidosis and solute clearance (serum creatinine value and rate of its decrease), were better ($P < .05$) in the hemofiltration group. However, this study had several methodological problems. PD was performed with a rigid peritoneal catheter, which has been found inferior as to outcomes (flow rates, clearance, complications, etc.).[39-41] Also, the manual exchange method with open drainage system was used for PD cycling—both of which are associated with higher risks of infections.[42] In fact, these researchers reported only one case of peritonitis during the study period, but cloudy dialysate was observed in 42% of the patients at some time during dialysis. This finding can be explained by the very short cycle, which obscures true peritonitis and could also have affected outcomes. In addition, a 30-minute dwell time was used. With administration of 70 L/day of peritoneal dialysate, most of the time was consumed by manual exchanges with inflow and outflow times rather than actual contact of dialysis fluid with the peritoneal membrane.

Another problem with this study is that the investigators used locally prepared dialysate with a sodium concentration of 141 mmol/L. This feature could lead to poorly controlled fluid status and ongoing hypervolemia, both of which could have affected both clearance and outcomes. Use of low-sodium dialysate would have countered the sieving effect occurring during the frequent cycling (especially with the ultra-short cycles used). In addition, they used acetate-buffered PD solutions, which have largely been replaced in most of the developed world by lactate-based or, in some cases bicarbonate/lactate-based solutions, which have been shown to be more biocompatible.[43] In summary, the comparison of state-of-the-art technology and knowledge for CRRT with an improperly designed PD procedure may have contributed to the observed outcomes. In fact, in an earlier study, the same group of researchers had shown substantial reduction of mortality and improved outcomes with the use of PD in patients of ARF due to falciparum malaria.[44]

In addition, many other studies have demonstrated successful application of PD in similar situations. Chitalia and associates[9] conducted a randomized crossover trial in 87 patients with mildly to moderately hypercatabolic ARF in which they compared continuous equilibrating PD with tidal PD in 236 sessions (118 in each treatment). These investigators concluded that both modalities provide reasonable options for treatment of mildly to moderately hypercatabolic ARF, although mortality data were not provided. Furthermore, in the absence of adequacy markers for ARF, they compared the dialysis dose with adequacy guidelines used for patients in stage V CKD and suggested that it fell just short of adequacy. With the improved understanding of peritoneal dialysis, adequacy guidelines have been revised[45]; according to the new guidelines even the urea clearance achieved with continuous equilibrating PD is adequate. In their review of the topic, Gabriel and coworkers[46] have highlighted their prospective experience with 30 patients with ARF who received 236 sessions of CPD. They reported encouraging results for metabolic, electrolytic, and acid-base control with a sufficient dialysis dose, showing higher values than described in other studies.

Better data are available in the pediatric literature comparing PD with other dialysis modalities. PD has been shown to be beneficial in all age groups of pediatric patients with a variety of causes of ARF.[47-56] Ease of administration, avoidance of anticoagulation, excellent hemodynamic tolerance, and equivalent outcomes are the principal reasons for its popularity. In fact, PD has been suggested to be a preferred modality of RRT in neonatal and infantile ARF even when the availability of hemodialysis and hemofiltration are not an issue.[57,58] For ARF in older children, PD is still used more than in adult populations, although the rate has been affected by the emergence of alternative therapy[59] without convincing data that it offers particular survival advantage over PD.

Despite many reviews arguing against the role of PD in patients with ARF, studies substantiating such arguments are isolated and uncontrolled. It is well established that conventional PD provides a slower solute clearance and is probably unsuitable for conditions requiring more immediate control of metabolic or volume disturbances—for example, hyperkalemia with cardiac manifestations, poisonings or intoxications, severe pulmonary edema, and tumor lysis syndrome. These conditions require some form of acute hemodialysis for control. Wiwanitkit[60] reported on outcome of ARF secondary to snakebite in ten patients needing dialysis; eight patients underwent hemodialysis, and two PD. The only patients who died were the two who had received peritoneal dialysis, so this author recommended that PD be contraindicated in ARF secondary to snakebite. However, PD is commonly offered in much sicker populations in developing countries, and it is quite likely that the severity of disease in these two patients before dialysis led to the adverse outcomes, rather than the dialytic modality itself. There have been few dis-

senting notes from the pediatric literature as well with some data suggesting evidence of better fluid control or solute clearance indices with PD. Nevertheless, none was able to show significant difference in any of the survival endpoints.[61,62]

Most of the arguments against the PD in ARF are borne out of concern about small solute clearance. Clearance in PD is limited by individual peritoneal transport characteristics, amount of the dialysate, and dwell time. Although the first factor cannot be changed, the other two are amenable to modification. Dialysis can be augmented with frequent cycling in an attempt to improve the clearance. Most studies using PD in ARF have utilized frequent cycling. However, with more frequent cycles, the amount of time spent in exchange procedures lengthens, and the dwell time of dialysis (contact of PD fluid with peritoneum) decreases. This approach can limit the benefits of increasing the frequency and, eventually, dialysate volume. Few modifications of the existing PD procedures have been tried in an attempt to reduce this "dead time." They include tidal PD (TPD) and continuous-flow PD (CFPD). TPD was originally developed to counter the "dead time," allowing a continual contact between the peritoneal membrane and residual peritoneal fluid during the time of exchange. In the only available report of TPD in ARF, Chitalia and colleagues[9] compared the effects of TPD and continuous equilibration PD in a randomized crossover fashion and concluded that, for a similar volume of PD fluid, TPD effected higher small solute clearance and lower glucose absorption in a much shorter time but was associated with greater protein loss.

With the new interest among nephrologists in increasing dialysis dose to improve the outcomes in both ESRD and ARF, the interest in CFPD has also been regenerated. It has many differences from conventional PD and has some similarities to hemodialysis. Access to peritoneal cavity is achieved via either two separate catheters or a double-lumen peritoneal catheter with tips placed far apart providing separate portals for inflow and outflow of PD fluid. Modifications in catheter designs have been tried,[64] and preliminary data have suggested significantly higher small solute clearance, comparable to that in daily hemodialysis and significantly higher than that with conventional PD IHD.[65,66] However, in view of the poor correlation between small solute clearance in PD and survival, its role may be limited to patients with CKD.[67] In ARF, however, PD may add significant flexibility in times of need for higher small solute clearance.[68] The principal drawbacks of CFPD are significant streaming and recirculation of the PD solutions.[69] Despite these theoretical advantages, no outcome data comparing CFPD with other modalities of dialysis are available.

Most studies comparing PD with HD in ARF have not accounted for the contribution of residual renal function (RRF). However, RRF has been proven to play a major role in survival of ESRD patients undergoing PD, and PD may be beneficial in preserving this function.[70] PD may also be associated with better chances of recovery in ARF, because its use avoids sudden hemodynamic changes, especially in patients with marginal renal blood flow. Several reports have suggested a better chance of recovery with PD than with hemodialysis in patients with ARF secondary to atheroembolic renal disease.[71,72] Avoidance of anticoagulation (decreasing the chances of further atheroembolism) in addition to the hemodynamic benefits may have contributed to this advantage. Katz and associates[73] reported a beneficial role for PD in terms of recovery of renal function in patients with ARF due to malignant hypertension. Although attractive as a hypothesis, this assertion awaits formal testing in a clinical trial.

To summarize, there are no satisfactory head-to-head trials comparing PD with any modality of hemodialysis in the adult population. However, the majority of trials of PD in ARF have shown outcomes comparable to those of then-prevalent hemodialysis and CRRT. Thus, the question arises as to why PD is a "nonpreferred" therapy for ARF in developed countries. Three factors influence this assertion. First, in absence of an adequacy index correctly reflecting the contribution of PD, indices of small solute clearance principally developed to reflect the role of HD are used in clinical practice and judgments. Second, the physician bias toward hemodialysis has been suggested to be a principal factor affecting declining rates of PD for the treatment of ESRD. This bias also leads to a decline in local expertise in PD, further reducing its use in more acute situations. Many experts in the field of PD have repeatedly argued about the adequacy of PD in ARF and its greater role in the treatment of this disorder.[74,75]

In the end, it is well recognized that ARF requiring dialysis support has significantly poor outcome in patients with critical illness. In most studies, these outcomes have been found to be related to the patients' burden of disease. The higher number of failed organs, need for vasopressors, preexisting illness, and need for RRT are the major outcome determinants. The modality of RRT has not been found to be a major determinant in these critically ill patients. In a retrospective analysis of the outcomes in 454 elderly patients (>60 years) with ARF, Mahajan and colleagues[11] compared different RRTs. They concluded that underlying chronic illness, presence of cardiac failure, sepsis, oliguria, need for RRT, and increasing number of failed organs were associated with poor outcome; choice of dialytic modality did not affect survival. Bunchman and coworkers[76] retrospectively examined 226 children who underwent RRT from 1992 to 1998 to compare the outcomes of different dialytic modalities in pediatric ICUs. Factors influencing patient survival were low blood pressure (BP) at onset of RRT, use of pressors anytime during RRT, and diagnosis of renal failure. Although they did find better survival in patients undergoing hemodialysis than in those undergoing continuous therapies (40% survival with HF, 49% survival with PD, 81% survival with hemodialysis; $P < .01$ for hemodialysis vs. PD or HF), these investigators found this improvement to be correlated with the use of vasopressors rather than with RRT modality. They suggested that the use of pressors, rather than RRT modality, was the strongest predictor of survival. Since their study, many trials have compared CRRT with IHD in randomized fashion.

SPECIAL CONSIDERATIONS FOR PERITONEAL DIALYSIS IN ACUTE RENAL FAILURE

Other important parameters may affect feasibility and outcomes of peritoneal dialysis in patients with ARF. As previously explained, most newer data about the efficacy of PD in ARF emanate from the developing world. In many cases, there are problems with the optimal use of PD related to financial constraints. Advancements in PD could be used for the better application of this modality in ARF.

Peritoneal Dialysis Catheter

Early in the development of PD, various surgical instruments and tubes were used to obtain access to the peritoneal cavity. Subsequently, a rigid PD catheter was inserted by a trocar. With the advancement of medicine and development of the flexible silicone catheter pioneered by Tenckhoff and Schechter in the late 1960s,[5] the use of a rigid PD catheter declined. Flexible PD catheters are associated with better catheter survival as well as lower rates of infection and occlusion. Currently, the use of rigid catheters for PD is obsolete in the developed world. However, in the developing world, economic considerations moderate the decision-making.

Peritoneal Dialysis Catheter Insertion

Improvements in catheter placement techniques have increased the options for performing PD in patients with renal failure. The majority of catheters placed for long-term treatment are placed by surgeons in operating rooms. Placement of PD catheters by surgeons at the bedside is common practice in some ICUs. Surgical catheter placements have the advantage of direct visualization of the peritoneum and optimum guidance of the catheter in the pelvic space. Insertion via laparoscopy also allows for insertion of the catheter in difficult situations, including patients with previous history of abdominal procedures, insertion in an atypical site, and the need for limited lysis of peritoneal adhesions.

Timing of Peritoneal Dialysis Catheter Insertion

PD catheters are inserted well in advance in patients with ESRD who are starting peritoneal dialysis, in order to promote wound healing and avoid development of leak. However, in patients with ARF, this practice is not possible. Use of low-volume exchanges in the early period after insertion of a PD catheter may be helpful in these patients. Percutaneous techniques for catheter insertion are especially useful. Abdominal aortic and certain cardiovascular procedures are associated with high risk for development of ARF and the need for dialysis. Prophylactic insertion of a PD catheter may be advised if the peritoneal cavity is likely to be intact in such instances.[77]

Solutions for Peritoneal Dialysis
Sodium Concentration

Sodium sieving occurs during the early part of the PD cycle owing to the removal of water from the vascular compartment via aquaporin channels. This effect is negated later in the dwell by means of transport of the sodium along its own concentration gradient. Frequent PD exchanges result in excessive removal of water in the ultrafiltrate compared with sodium. The resultant hypernatremia leads to higher water intake and ineffective ultrafiltration or fluid overload. Newer PD solutions with lower sodium concentration (126-128 mEq/L) have been designed to partially negate this effect via generation of higher sodium efflux and better "true" ultrafiltration.[78]

Low-sodium dialysate should be considered in the treatment of a patient who is likely to undergo frequent cycling for a prolonged duration or when there is suboptimal control of the hypervolemia.

Nutritional Aspects

Conventional PD solutions contain glucose (dextrose) as the osmotic agent. Typical solutions are available in three strengths of dextrose monohydrate, 1.5%, 2.5%, and 4.25% (in North American nomenclature, corresponding to 1.36%, 2.26%, or 3.86% of dextrose anhydrous in European nomenclature). Absorption of glucose leads to obligatory caloric intake in patients undergoing PD. Although the exact amount of the glucose absorbed varies with individual transport characteristics, strength and volume of PD fluid used, and dwell time, extensive clinical data show that patients on average can acquire 20% to 30% of their daily caloric intake through this route.[79] Limited data are available on the glucose load in ARF. In one of the studies using 10 to 40 L of (4.25% or 2.5%) PD fluid daily, estimated dextrose absorption ranged between 331 and 754 g/day (1125 to 2563 kcal/day).[80] This glucose load can provide much needed calories in some ARF patients with depleted glycogen stores (e.g., those with falciparum malaria or liver failure) or with negative energy balance, but it has the potential to cause hyperglycemia and may generate the need for insulin therapy. Plasma glucose concentration must be checked regularly in patients with critical illness and ARF who are started on PD, given the association of hyperglycemia with death.[81]

In addition to glucose dynamics, patients undergoing PD lose on average 10-12 gm of protein in the dialysate, which may lead to negative protein balance. A single 6 hr exchange with 1.1% amino acid solution corrects this negative nitrogen balance in chronic dialysis patients, although the effect on patient outcomes is unknown. The efficacy of the amino acid solution in the ARF dynamics has not been studied but carries the risk of generating higher nitrogenous waste products and exacerbating metabolic acidosis and is not currently advised.

Alternative Osmotic Agents

In addition to the amino acid solutions previously discussed, icodextrin is the most commonly used non-dextrose PD solution. It is used principally for the longer cycle of the continuous PD prescription (night cycle of CAPD or day cycle of CCPD), because the use of dextrose in such situations leads to negative ultrafiltration (reabsorption of peritoneal content back into the body with loss of glucose gradient). The use of Icodextrin is normally restricted to one exchange a day for fear of causing accumulation of mannose. Ultrafiltration is slower with icodextrin, so this agent is not useful in conditions with fluid overload requiring urgent fluid removal, although it could be used for the control of uremia in stable patients with ARF.

Types of Peritoneal Dialysis

Peritoneal dialysis can be carried out with various dosing schedules. Many studies have performed as a standard PD

procedure, principally because of the lifetime of the rigid peritoneal dialysis catheter. However, with the flexible PD catheter, a continuous PD schedule can be used because it allows better control over uremia with higher clearance. The need for frequent cycling can be determined from the metabolic and volemic status of the patient. In such patients, CCPD or some modification of it can be utilized, on the basis of local administrative constraints. Continuous equilibration PD is ideal for the patient with stable metabolism because it is associated with attractive economics, minimal nursing burden, and better clearance of middle-molecular-weight molecule clearance. TPD is usually reserved for patients with infusion pain but may be utilized in patients on rapid cycling in ARF. No clinical data are currently available for CFPD in patients with severe hypercatabolic renal failure, and it may be safer to use IHD for such patients with a very high need for small solute clearance.

PROPOSED GUIDELINES FOR PERITONEAL DIALYSIS IN ACUTE RENAL FAILURE

In the absence of good clinical data on peritoneal dialysis in ARF and its comparison with other modalities of dialysis, recommendations for utilization of peritoneal dialysis in ARF can only be opinion-based level C recommendations. The following list contains proposed guidelines for the use of PD in ARF.

- Choice of RRT should be made in the individual patient on the basis of clinical condition and associated comorbidities.
- Conventional peritoneal dialysis seems efficacious and adequate in most instances of ARF, as long as the peritoneal cavity is intact, but should be considered especially in patients with coagulopathies, poor cardiovascular status, advanced noncorrectable heart failure, pancreatitis, post–cardiovascular surgery ARF, poor vascular access, or potentially recoverable ARF (e.g., secondary to atheroembolic renal disease, thrombotic microangiopathies), in children, and in elderly patients with multiple comorbidities. PD should not be used in a patient with intrusion into the peritoneal cavity or intra-abdominal sepsis.
- Percutaneous placement of the PD catheter should be considered in patients with critical illness who need immediate dialysis, if the local expertise is available.
- PD prescription varies according to patient size and clinical situation. Automated peritoneal dialysis can be used in all patients, especially in ICUs, because it can deliver individualized prescription with accurate measurements and minimize the need for additional dialysis nursing staff. However, a manual exchange should be undertaken at the outset to exclude leak of dialysate.
- Peritoneal fill volume varies according to patient size and comfort. The patient undergoing PD should be in a supine/reclining position, and low fill volumes should be used immediately after catheter insertion to prevent leak.
- Clearance needs must be determined individually. In the absence of any measure linking the dose of PD to outcomes, clearance goals should at least be those

desired for patients with ESRD, although no single index can be taken as absolute.

• On the basis of current data, PD provides adequate options for management of most patients with ARF except those with severe hypercatabolism. PD is currently not recommended for certain patients with ARF, such as those with severe hypercatabolism, poisoning/intoxication, severe left ventricular failure with frank pulmonary edema, or tumor lysis syndrome. These conditions require either IHD or large-volume hemofiltration. The role of CFPD in such situations has not been studied adequately to allow definitive recommendations to be made. Clinical, biochemical, and nutritional monitoring of the patient should be performed regularly to assess the adequacy of therapy and the need for change.

CONCLUSION

With the advent of CRRTs, the utilization of older therapies such as IHD and PD has decreased. However, proving the advantage of one modality over the other has been difficult. Despite multiple arguments produced against it, no convincing data have been reported that support either the superiority or the inferiority of PD for the management of ARF. Given these facts, consideration should be given to PD because of its simplicity, economy, and efficiency.

Key Points

1. PD offers unique advantages as the dialysis modality in the ICU, including obviating the need for anticoagulation.
2. Measurement of clearance adequacy is fraught with pitfalls and target clearances are unknown.
3. A functioning catheter is crucial for the successful implementation of PD in the ICU.
4. The role of PD in ARF associated with a hypercatabolic state is less well-defined but should be avoided if possible.

Key References

10. Phu NH, Hien TT, Mai NT, et al: Hemofiltration and peritoneal dialysis in infection-associated acute renal failure in Vietnam. N Engl J Med 2002;347:895-902.
35. Indraprasit S, Charoenpan P, Suvachittanont O, et al: Continuous peritoneal dialysis in acute renal failure from severe falciparum malaria. Clin Nephrol 1988;29:137-143.
50. Flynn JT, Kershaw DB, Smoyer WE, et al: Peritoneal dialysis for management of pediatric acute renal failure. Perit Dial Int 2001;21:390-394.
75. Rao P, Passadakis P, Oreopoulos DG: Peritoneal dialysis in acute renal failure. Perit Dial Int 2003;23:320-322.

See the companion Expert Consult website for the complete reference list.

CHAPTER 272

Clinical Results and Complications of Peritoneal Dialysis in Acute Renal Failure

Ravindran Visvanathan and Vijay Kher

OBJECTIVES

This chapter will:
1. Explore the role that peritoneal dialysis may play in the management of acute renal failure in the current era.
2. Discuss some of the clinical trials of peritoneal dialysis in acute renal failure vis-à-vis the other modalities of treatment, namely, intermittent hemodialysis and continuous renal replacement therapy.
3. Describe the complications of acute peritoneal dialysis.

The incidence of acute renal failure (ARF) has risen in the past two decades,[1] with a shift in the spectrum from isolated cases of ARF to a picture that is complex, involving multiple systems and seen mainly in intensive care units.[1,2]

Correspondingly, renal replacement therapy for ARF has also evolved, with rapid advances in medical technology leading to the development of the various continuous extracorporeal therapies that are now able to provide dialysis for more complicated and unstable patients. This development has led to a change in renal replacement modality patterns over the last decade. On the basis of surveys from 1999 and 2000, more traditional renal replacement therapy techniques, especially peritoneal dialysis, have been replaced by newer continuous therapies.[3-5] Even in the pediatric community, in which peritoneal dialysis was originally the treatment of choice,[6] the preferential use of continuous therapy appears to be increasing with a diminishing role for PD.

Some of the major concerns about peritoneal dialysis include unpredictable solute and fluid removal, risk of peritonitis, diaphragmatic splinting with possible compromise of ventilation, and fluctuations in glycemic control.[7]

With this apparent underutilization of peritoneal dialysis in ARF, at least in developed countries, there has been a scarcity of data in recent literature, and most studies of this modality date back to the 1970s and 1980s.[8] However, this impression may be misleading because of under-reporting of current practices in other parts of the world. In developing countries, the epidemiology of ARF, although beginning to follow the spectrum of the more developed nations, still demonstrates a significant number of cases of ARF secondary to medical causes such as dehydration, to infections like leptospirosis, malaria, and dengue fever, and to drugs such as herbal medication.[1,9]

Peritoneal dialysis, which uses a simple technology that is easily accessible and relatively less costly, is being utilized for the management of ARF in many developing countries that lack resources for more technologically advanced equipment and highly trained personnel. Thus, peritoneal dialysis still constitutes the mainstay of therapy in many of the developing countries.[9-13]

Chow and associates compared cases of ARF in a single center in Malaysia during two time periods (1994 and 2004); they found that the etiology of ARF and the dialysis modality remained unchanged over that 10 years (YW Chow, personal communication, 2007). Prerenal ARF accounted for 43.6% of cases in 1994 and 53.5% of cases in 2004, and peritoneal dialysis was the main dialysis modality in both time periods (being used in 69.2% and 74.3% of cases, respectively.[13]

HISTORICAL PERSPECTIVE

The initial description of peritoneal dialysis for the management of ARF is credited to Professor G. Ganter, a German clinical investigator who in 1923 used this technique to treat a woman with uremia and suffering from obstructive uropathy. His recommendations then formed the basis for what later became known as intermittent peritoneal dialysis (IPD).[14]

In March 1946, Fine and colleagues[15] reported the successful application of peritoneal dialysis in a case of antibiotic-induced ARF. This report also established the closed dialysis system as well as the constituents of the dialysis solution, use of which became the standard for peritoneal dialysis. A number of reports followed that reviewed the literature during that period and confirmed the usefulness of peritoneal dialysis in uremia.[16,17]

By the 1970s, IPD was established as an effective form of renal replacement therapy. Subsequently, as interest in peritoneal dialysis grew, the treatment underwent further improvement, with the development of better peritoneal access and the use of automated peritoneal dialysis machines.[18]

EFFECT ON MORTALITY

There is a paucity of data concerning the effects on mortality of peritoneal dialysis and intermittent hemodialysis or continuous therapies. However, a number of studies published in the 1960s and 1970s compared intermittent hemodialysis with peritoneal dialysis. The results suggested that mortality and the incidence of renal recovery with acute peritoneal dialysis were at least comparable to those with hemodialysis,[19-23] even though peritoneal dialysis was often chosen to treat unstable patients for whom hemodialysis was not suitable.[19] Unfortunately, most of these reports typically involved only patients from single institutions and were retrospective in design. None of

these studies was randomized or prospectively controlled. In one 1990 study reviewing the records of 246 elderly patients, survival rates between those treated with peritoneal dialysis and those treated with hemodialysis were also not different.[24]

However, more recently, Phu and associates[25] conducted an open randomized trial comparing continuous venovenous hemofiltration with peritoneal dialysis in patients with infection-associated ARF; 48 of the patients had falciparum malaria, and 22 were septic. The mortality was significantly higher in patients treated with peritoneal dialysis (47%) than in those patients treated with continuous venovenous hemofiltration (15%; $P < .005$). These results contrast with those of a previous study by the same investigative team showing a significant reduction in mortality in patients with malaria-related ARF who were treated with acute peritoneal dialysis.[12] Improved survival in the hemofiltration group in the later study may be explained on the basis of the modality's superior solute clearance, but it is also possible that some adverse factors in the peritoneal dialysis group—the use of acetate as buffer, the use of rigid catheters, presence of a cloudy dialysate suggesting infection in 42% of patients, and other technical and specific factors—could have attributed to the poorer outcome.[26] These factors must be considered before one can conclude that peritoneal dialysis is inappropriate for infection-associated ARF.[26,27]

DIALYSIS ADEQUACY

Traditionally, IPD has been held to be potentially inadequate to control azotemia, especially in hypercatabolic patients.[28] This perception was reflected in a survey among nephrologists to determine modalities in the treatment of ARF; 90% of those surveyed believed that solute clearance with peritoneal dialysis was inadequate.[3]

In contrast to these expectations, however, a number of early studies evaluating peritoneal dialysis in patients with ARF who were deemed hypercatabolic reported satisfactory control of fluid and metabolic derangements.[29-33] These studies had major limitations. The majority of the study populations were small in numbers, were not randomized, and did not use appropriate measurements of dialysis adequacy and catabolic rate.[27]

Chitalia and colleagues[9] conducted a randomized, prospective, crossover trial comparing adequacies of both tidal peritoneal dialysis (TPD) and continuous equilibration peritoneal dialysis (CEPD) in 87 patients with mild to moderate hypercatabolic ARF (Table 272-1). Compared with CEPD, TPD produced higher solute clearance in a smaller dialysis volume. Comparing adequacy indices (Kt/V, normalized creatinine clearances, solute reduction indices), these investigators concluded that both TPD and CEPD are reasonable options for mild to moderate catabolic ARF even though CPD fell short of the adequacy standard. With TPD offering better clearances at lower cost and time, developing countries that have access to PD cyclers should consider TPD for the treatment of hypercatabolic ARF. One of the limitations of the study, however, was that the patient base was different from most of the studies dealing with hypercatabolic ARF; therefore, the results may not be applicable to critically ill patients, especially in developed countries. The major limitation of the use of TDP is the high protein loss.

The study by Phu and colleagues mentioned earlier demonstrated that the rate of resolution of acidosis as well as the decline in serum creatinine was more than twice as high in the hemofiltration group as in the peritoneal dialysis group ($P < .005$). However, solute clearance and dialysis adequacy were not reported in the two study groups.[25] Table 272-2 shows dialysis prescriptions and adequacy parameters in various studies utilizing PD in acute renal failure.

RENAL RECOVERY

Recovery of renal function after an episode of ARF is an important determinant of morbidity. In many of the older studies comparing peritoneal dialysis with hemodialysis for ARF, the reason for improved survival in the peritoneal dialysis group was related to a higher rate of renal recovery.[19] There are no randomized trials to date, but several published reports suggest that patients with ARF secondary to atheroembolic disease may have a better chance of renal recovery with peritoneal dialysis than with hemodialysis.[34] The reasons for the apparent benefit were attributed to less hemodynamic fluctuation and the absence of anticoagulation during peritoneal dialysis.

TABLE 272-1

Adequacies of Both Tidal Peritoneal Dialysis (TPD) and Continuous Equilibration Peritoneal Dialysis (CEPD) in 87 Patients with Mild to Moderate Hypercatabolic Acute Renal Failure

PARAMETER	TPD (MEAN)	CEPD (MEAN)
Urea clearance (mL/min)	19.85 + 1.95	10.63 + 2.62
Creatinine clearance (mL/min)	9.94 + 2.93	6.74 + 1.63*
Kt/V	2.43 + 0.87	1.8 + 0.32

*$P < .001$.
From Chitalia AC, Almeida AF, Rai H, et al: Is peritoneal dialysis adequate for hypercatabolic acute renal failure in developing countries? Kidney Int 2002;61:747-757.

Katz and associates,[35] who conducted a retrospective study in patients with renal failure secondary to malignant hypertension, reported that 55% of patients undergoing peritoneal dialysis recovered renal function, compared with none undergoing hemodialysis. This finding suggests that peritoneal dialysis may be beneficial in patients whose renal failure is due to malignant hypertension.

FUTURE TRENDS

There is now renewed interest in continuous-flow peritoneal dialysis, which can provide higher solute clearances.[36] Several small clinical studies using this modality reported better peritoneal clearances for urea and creatinine than with conventional peritoneal dialysis.[37,38] With continuous-flow peritoneal dialysis, dialysate flow rates up to 300 mL/min can be maintained through the peritoneum; this modality may become an attractive alternative in the intensive care unit for the treatment of ARF.[39]

COMPLICATIONS OF ACUTE PERITONEAL DIALYSIS

Although acute peritoneal dialysis has been described as a safe and effective form of renal replacement therapy,[19] only a few reports have been published that discuss complications of this procedure. Peritoneal dialysis is associated with a set of unique complications not dissimilar to those with CAPD, which can be broadly classified into infectious and noninfectious.

Infectious Complications

Peritonitis is a serious complication, with a reported incidence between 1% and 12% of procedures performed.[40]

TABLE 272-2

Dialysis Protocol Prescription and Adequacy Parameters in Different Studies on Peritoneal Dialysis in Acute Renal Failure

	Studies				
PARAMETER	KATIRZOGLOU ET AL[30]	CAMERON ET AL[31]	INDRAPARASIT ET AL[32]	CHITALIA ET AL[9]	PHU ET AL[25]
N	12	90	10	87	36
Method	CPD	IPD	CPD	CPD vs tidal PD	CPD
Catheter	Rigid	Rigid	Flexible	Flexible Flexible	Rigid
Dialysate fluid (per cycle; mL)	2000	1000-3000	1000-3000	2000 2000	2000
Dwell time (min)	180-240	30	30	210 10	15-30
Total volume dialysate (per session; L)	10-14	24-36	24-72	26 26	70
Duration of session (hr)	24	24	24	48 12	24
Duration per cycle (min)	240-300	60	60-120	240 20	30-60
Total exchanges (per session)	5-7	24	24	12 36	24-35
Tonicity (glucose; %)	1.5-2.5	1.5-2.5	1.5-2.5	2.5 2.5	1.5-4.25
Flow rate (mL/min)	7.0-9.8	16.7-25	16.7-50	9 36	48
Post-dialysis BUN level (mean; mg/dL)	75	<100	60-80	64 50	NC
Urea clearance (mean; mL/min)	NC	13-35	12	11 20	NC
Creatinine clearance (mean; mL/min)	NC	NC	NC	6.8 10	NC
Weekly Kt/V	NC	NC	NC	1.8 2.4	NC
Ultrafiltration (L/session)	NC	NC	NC	2.9 2	NC

BUN, blood urea nitrogen (concentration); CPD, continuous peritoneal dialysis; IPD, intermittent peritoneal dialysis; N, total sample size; NC, not calculated; TPD, tidal peritoneal dialysis.
From Gabriel DP, Nascimento GVR, Caramori JT, et al: Peritoneal dialysis in acute renal failure. Ren Fail 2006;28:451-456.

The risk of peritonitis frequently occurs within 48 to 72 hours of treatment,[41] and the leading cause of peritonitis continues to be contamination at the time of peritoneal dialysis exchange.[42]

In a prospective study, Valeri and associates[43] examined the epidemiology of peritonitis in acute IPD. They reported a higher incidence of peritonitis in the study subset than in patients from the National CAPD registry.[44] There was also a higher rate of early peritonitis (<48 hours after dialysis). The use of a closed system reduced the incidence of both early and system-related peritonitis. Gram-positive infections accounted for a substantial percentage of the cases of peritonitis, but in addition, there was a shift toward more gram-negative and fungal organisms, probably owing to the wide use of broad-spectrum antibiotics.[43]

Occasionally, if symptoms persist, ultrasonography or computed tomography may be of value in localizing and draining infected collections in patients with peritonitis.

Peritoneal Catheter–Related Infections

Catheter infections include both exit site and tunnel infections. The use of silicon-cuffed catheters is reported to be associated with fewer complications. Exit site infections can manifest as erythema and tenderness with or without purulent discharge. On the basis of studies of CAPD, *Staphylococcus aureus* accounts for more than 50% of exit site infections, followed by *Staphylococcus epiderdermidis* (20%), *Pseudomonas aeruginosa* (8%), and *Escherichia coli* (4%).[45]

Catheter tunnel and cuff infections are generally an extension of exit site infections, and the distribution of pathogens is usually similar. Tunnel infections are associated with edema, erythema, or tenderness over the subcutaneous track with or without discharge around the exit site. Occult tunnel infections can be detected by ultrasonography of the subcutaneous pathway.

Revised guidelines for the treatment of CAPD peritonitis have been published; these guidelines can also be applied to peritonitis due to acute peritoneal dialysis and catheter-related infections.[46]

Noninfectious Complications

The noninfectious complications of peritoneal dialysis can be classified as follows: surgical, mechanical, related to increased intra-abdominal pressure, and metabolic complications, and noninfectious cause of cloudy peritoneal dialysate.

Surgical Complications

Postoperative bleeding around the catheter placement site is usually mild. However, more severe bleeding into the peritoneum has been reported. This complication was particularly common if the insertion was performed via a blind technique using rigid catheters. Mital and coworkers[47] reported a rate of 2% for major bleeding complications associated with peritoneal dialysis catheter insertion.[47] Visceral perforations of the bladder and bowel have also been reported.[40]

Mechanical Complications

Inflow pain has been attributed to the position of the catheter, solution's acidity or low temperature, introduction of air, and additives such as antibiotics.[48] Mactier and associates[49] conducted a randomized, double-blind, crossover study to compare the effects of novel bicarbonate and a bicarbonate/lactate solution in patients who had experienced infusional pain with the current lactate solution. Both of the new solutions caused less infusion pain than the control (original solution), but the bicarbonate/lactate solution appeared to be more effective.[49]

INFLOW/OUTFLOW DIFFICULTY. Malposition of the catheter is suspected if there is inflow but no outflow. Other causes are omental wrap and constipation. Total obstruction to both inflow and outflow suggests obstruction within the catheter lumen by fibrin, cellular debris, or blood clots.

Complications Related to Increased Intra-abdominal Pressure

Dialysate leaks can occur around the exit site and from the peritoneal cavity.[50] They can manifest as edema of the abdominal or genital wall, with a higher incidence in men owing to a patent processus vaginalis.[51] Diagnosis can be made with computed tomography of the peritoneum using iodinated contrast agent mixed with the dialysate and instilled into the abdominal cavity.[51] Using lower volumes of exchange may help.

HYDROTHORAX. Associated with a defect in the tendinous part of the diaphragm or occurring via the lymphatics, hydrothorax tends to occur more in women and on the right side of the chest. Large effusions may compromise respiration. Chest radiography is usually diagnostic. In uncertain cases, thoracocentesis and fluid analysis help in demonstrating a transudate and a very high glucose concentration.[50,51]

ALTERED MECHANICS OF BREATHING. Respiratory function may be compromised in peritoneal dialysis, especially with high-volume exchanges. Studies in stable patients undergoing CAPD have demonstrated reduction in lung volumes, including functional residual capacity and reduced forced vital capacity (FVC), of up to 42% when patients were supine.[51] In contrast, Epstein and colleagues[52] found that although dialysate reduced pulmonary volume, vital capacity and expiratory volume in their subjects remained unaltered.[52]

Metabolic Complications

Dextrose content in dialysis solutions provides the osmotic gradient for fluid removal. A significant proportion of the dextrose is absorbed into the circulation. Frequent exchanges with high-dextrose fluids can give rise to significant overfeeding. This in turn contributes to fatty liver and increases in carbon dioxide consumption and minute ventilation that lead to respiratory decompensation, especially in patients with limited ventilatory reserve.[53] Hyperglycemia can also predispose to further complications.[54]

FLUID AND ELECTROLYTE DISORDERS. Hypernatremia due to aggressive ultrafiltration may occur with frequent use of hypertonic exchanges. Significant hypokalemia can also develop, as there is no potassium in the peritoneal dialysis fluid.

ACID-BASE BALANCE. Standard peritoneal dialysis solutions contain lactate as the buffer, posing problems for patients with hepatic failure and those with severe lactic acidosis, in whom peritoneal dialysis may worsen the acidosis. Thongboonkerd and associates[55] reported a randomized controlled study comparing bicarbonate and a lactate solution in terms of correction of metabolic acidosis, hemodynamics, and systemic host defense in patients with or without septic shock who were undergoing acute peritoneal dialysis. In the septic group, significant improvement was seen in blood pH, serum bicarbonate level, and mean arterial pressure ($P < .05$) in the bicarbonate arm compared with the lactate arm of the study. However, the serum bicarbonate and blood pH levels in the nonseptic groups were comparable. Also, lactic acidosis was more rapidly corrected with bicarbonate solution in both groups ($P < .05$).[55]

PROTEIN LOSSES. Protein losses via the dialysate can be as high as 10 to 20 g daily and even higher during peritonitis. Blumenkrantz and colleagues[56] reported that up to 48 g of total protein and 26 g of albumin can be lost in 24-hour IPD during peritonitis.[56] This loss should be accounted for to prevent undernutrition in critically ill patients.

Culture-Negative Cloudy Peritoneal Dialysate

In the patient with culture-negative peritonitis, other etiologies should be considered in the differential diagnosis.[57] These include chemical peritonitis, eosinophilia of the effluent, hemoperitoneum, malignancy (rare), and chylous effluent.

CONCLUSION

Peritoneal dialysis, although marginalized as a form of renal replacement therapy in the developed world, still plays a major role in the management of acute renal failure in developing countries. Peritoneal dialysis has been shown to be safe, effective, and inexpensive. Technological advances in peritoneal dialysis have led to better outcomes in patients undergoing continuous ambulatory peritoneal dialysis. Applying these new developments to the management of acute renal failure requires further research.

Future clinical trials should focus on ways to optimize the potential of peritoneal dialysis through (1) appropriate patient selection, (2) utilizing the capabilities of the latest automated cyclers, (3) use of biocompatible solutions, and (4) determination of appropriate methods of measuring peritoneal dialysis adequacy. As knowledge evolves, peritoneal dialysis may play a bigger role in the management of acute renal failure in the future.

Key Points

1. Peritoneal dialysis is currently underutilized in the management of acute renal failure in the developed world but still plays a major role in treating this disorder in the developing world.
2. Peritoneal dialysis has been shown to be comparable to intermittent hemodialysis in certain populations, although the evidence is not strong.
3. There is evidence to suggest that tidal peritoneal dialysis is a reasonable option for patients with mildly to moderately hypercatabolic acute renal failure.
4. Future research should be directed at optimizing the potential of peritoneal dialysis in acute renal failure.

Acknowledgment

We thank Dr. Ghazali Ahmad and Dr. Wong Hin Seng for reviewing the manuscript and offering valuable guidance.

Key References

8. Lameire N: Principles of peritoneal dialysis and its application in acute renal failure. In Ronco C, Bellomo R (eds): Critical Care Nephrology. Norwall, MA, Kluwer Academic Publishers, 1998, pp 1357-1371.
18. Gabriel DP, Nascimento GVR, Caramori JT, et al: Peritoneal dialysis in acute renal failure. Ren Fail 2006;28:451-456.
19. Ash SR: Peritoneal dialysis in acute renal failure of adults: The under-utilized modality. Contrib Nephrol 2004;144:239-254.
46. Pirano B: Peritoneal dialysis related infections recommendations: 2005 Update. Perit Dial Int 2005;25:107-131.
48. Passadakis P, Oreopoulos D: Peritoneal dialysis in acute renal failure. Int J Artif Organs 2003;26:265-277.

See the companion Expert Consult website for the complete reference list.

CHAPTER 273

Treatment of Peritonitis and Other Clinical Complications of Peritoneal Dialysis in the Critically Ill Patient

Wai-Kei Lo, Man-Fai Lam, Terence Pok-Siu Yip, and Sing-Leung Lui

OBJECTIVES

This chapter will:
1. Discuss the common complications of peritoneal dialysis in the critically ill patient.
2. Describe the preventive measurements and management of such complications.

Peritoneal dialysis (PD) is an effective supportive therapy for patients with acute renal failure and for critically ill patients with renal failure. However, the occurrence of complications related to PD would make the supportive treatment fail and raise patient's risk of death. Proper technique and preventive measures are important in the performance of PD.

Complications arising from PD are as follows:
- Peritonitis and catheter-related infections
- Complications related to catheter insertion: bleeding from insertion wound, intraperitoneal or visceral bleeding, external leakage
- Complications related to obstructed or poor flow of peritoneal dialysate
- Complications related to increased intraperitoneal pressure: diaphragmatic tenting, hydrothorax
- Metabolic complications: hyperglycemia, electrolyte disturbances, lactate accumulation, metabolic acidosis
- Fluid balance complications: inadequate ultrafiltration, hypotension

PERITONITIS AND CATHETER-RELATED COMPLICATIONS

Compared with the early days in the development of PD, the risk of peritonitis has been much reduced. However, peritonitis is probably the most important and most common serious complication of PD.

Diagnosis of Peritonitis

The cardinal features of peritonitis are cloudy effluent, fever, and abdominal pain. The diagnosis is confirmed with a dialysate white cell count greater than 100 cells/mm³ with more than 50% neutrophils.[1] Although the efflu-ent is almost always cloudy during peritonitis, fever and abdominal pain may not be present, particularly if the peritonitis is mild or in critically ill, sedated, or ventilated patients. Therefore, patients with cloudy effluent should be presumed to have peritonitis, and a specimen of the effluent should be collected for differential cell count, gram staining, and microbiological culture. Antibiotic therapy should be given promptly. Very occasionally, abdominal pain may precede the onset of cloudy effluent[2]; in this situation, a high index of suspicion with appropriate investigations is required.

Cloudy effluent may sometimes be due to peritoneal eosinophilia, which usually occurs shortly after insertion of a PD catheter and commencement of intermittent PD.[3] It is characterized by increases in numbers of polymorphs in effluent dialysate, with more than 10% being eosinophils. The pathogenesis of peritoneal eosinophilia is obscure, possibly related to the introduction of air into the peritoneal cavity in rapid cycles or to plasticizers from the dialysate bags. The condition is benign and self-limiting. It usually subsides rapidly with a change to continuous PD using longer cycles. Specific treatment is not required. Occasionally, however, the eosinophilia is associated with fungal peritonitis; therefore, regular peritoneal effluent culture for microorganisms and monitoring of changes in white cell differential counts in the effluent are required.

Causative Organisms in and Risk Factors for Peritonitis

Conventionally, gram-positive organisms like *Staphylococcus aureus* and *Staphylococcus epidermidis* (coagulase-negative *Staphylococcus*) are the most common causative organisms in PD-related peritonitis. The portal of entry of the organisms is mainly through the connection during exchange procedures, particularly if the PD procedures are performed manually with the single bag and spike system. However, if the exchange procedure is performed with proper aseptic technique by nurses, the risk of peritonitis should be very low. The employment of the flush-before-fill technique or the use of an automated PD cycler in acute PD significantly reduces the chance of acquiring gram-positive peritonitis through the exchange procedure in chronic PD[4,5]; this is probably also the case for acute PD. The risk of peritonitis is much higher if an uncuffed rigid PD catheter is used, particularly if the catheter is used for more than 48 hours. If the requirement for PD is expected to last for more than 48 hours, a cuffed

TABLE 273-1

Antibiotic Dosing Recommendations for Acute Peritoneal Dialysis Using Rapid Cycles*

ANTIBIOTIC	INTRAVENOUS LOADING DOSE IN SEPTIC PATIENTS	INTRAPERITONEAL LOADING IF A 6-hr DWELL TIME ALLOWS (mg/L)	INTRAPERITONEAL CONTINUOUS DOSE (mg/L), ALL EXCHANGES
Aminoglycosides			
Amikacin	5 mg/kg	2 mg/kg	12
Netilmicin	1.5 mg/kg	0.6 mg/kg	4
Tobramycin	1.5 mg/kg	0.6 mg/kg	4
Cephalosporins			
Cefazolin	1000 mg	15 mg/kg	125
Cefepime	1000 mg	1 g	125
Cephalothin	1000 mg	15 mg/kg	125
Ceftazidime	1000 mg	15 mg/kg	125
Penicillins			
Ampicillin	500 mg	500 mg	125
Vancomycin	1 g	1 g	25
Imipenem/cilastatin	500 mg	500 mg	200

*Modified from Piraino B, Bailie GR, Bernardini J, et al; ISPD Ad Hoc Advisory Committee: Peritoneal dialysis-related infections recommendations: 2005 update. Perit Dial Int 2005;25:107-131.

catheter such as a Tenckhoff catheter, whether single- or double-cuffed, should be used.

Apart from gram-positive organisms, the critically ill patient is susceptible to peritonitis from endogenous sources, such as gram-negative organisms from the gut flora and fungal peritonitis (in particular *Candida* peritonitis), as a result of the severe impairment of the immune system and disturbance of gut flora after broad-spectrum antibiotic therapy.[6,7] Gram-negative peritonitis may also follow acute pancreatitis, intestinal obstruction, perforation, or ischemia, none of which is uncommon in critically ill patients. Such patients being treated in intensive care units are also highly susceptible to hospital-acquired infection by organisms like *Pseudomonas* and *Acinetobacter* species.[8,9]

Route of Administration of Antibiotics

In chronic PD, the administration of antibiotics—continuous intraperitoneal, intermittent once daily, or intraperitoneal intravenous (mainly for vancomycin)—is well established. The optimal dwell time for intraperitoneal antibiotics should be at least 4 to 6 hours to allow them to be absorbed systemically.[10] In acute PD for the critically ill, however, short rapid cycles are often employed, allowing insufficient time for systemic antibiotics to diffuse back into peritoneal fluid and achieve an antibiotic level above minimal inhibitory concentration (MIC). In such cases, a continuous intraperitoneal antibiotics regimen should be used instead of intermittent once-daily or intravenous regimens, and an intraperitoneal loading dose for a continuous regimen may not be possible. Instead, additional intravenous loading is preferred to achieve an adequate serum level promptly, particularly in patients who have severe peritonitis with septicemia. Such an approach is also suitable for tidal PD and continuous-flow PD.

Choice of Antibiotics

Before the Gram staining result is available, an antibiotic should be given that can cover the common gram-positive and gram-negative organisms. A common regimen is a combination of a first-generation cephalosporin and an

aminoglycoside. The use of vancomycin should be restricted to minimize the risk for development of vancomycin-resistant *Enterococcus* and vancomycin-resistant *S. aureus*.[11] However, in centers where methicillin-resistant staphylococcal infection is prevalent, a policy on choosing vancomycin as first-line peritonitis treatment should be developed, with the benefits and risks seriously considered.

In the very ill or septic patient, broad-spectrum and potent antibiotics should be considered for first-line antibiotic treatment. This approach would involve the early use of vancomycin, third-generation cephalosporins, or the carbapenem group of antibiotics. In cases in which there is deterioration of the patient's condition or absence of signs of resolution of peritonitis within 1 or 2 days, a change of antibiotics to a more potent and more broad-spectrum regimen is desirable. When the causative bacteria and its antibiotic sensitivity are known, the antibiotic regimen may be modified accordingly. Table 273-1 shows the dosage of antibiotics as adopted from the 2005 update of the International Society for PD's recommendations for PD–related infections.[10] Antibiotic therapy should last 14 days or for at least 5 days after complete resolution of signs and symptoms of peritonitis; for more severe peritonitis or *Pseudomonas* peritonitis, a 3-week antibiotic course is often recommended. If peritonitis is becoming more severe or does not respond to the antibiotic regimen, the dialysis catheter should be removed and the patient should be switched to another mode of dialysis with continuation of the appropriate antibiotics given intravenously.

Fibrin formation may be severe during an episode of peritonitis, causing catheter blocking. Intraperitoneal heparin is often added, at a dose of 500 to 1000 units/L, to prevent catheter blocking during severe peritonitis.

In the patient with fungal peritonitis, immediate removal of the catheter should be considered, because of the extremely low rate of success for antifungal therapy without catheter removal. This condition should be treated with appropriate antifungal agents, most commonly intravenous amphotericin B with or without intravenous or oral flucytosine. Amphotericin B is nephrotoxic and may reduce the chance of renal recovery of patients with acute renal failure. Fluconazole, given intravenously or orally, may be used if the causative organism is *Candida albicans*, which is generally sensitive to fluconazole, although resistance has been noted. The use of this agent in infections with other *Candida* species is less reliable because of a higher incidence of fluconazole resistance with such organisms.[12] Other antifungal agents, like caspofungin and voriconazole, may be considered for filamentous fungi and fluconazole-resistant *Candida* species. Voriconazole should be given only orally because the intravenous solubilizing agent (sulfobutylether-β-cyclodextrin), not voriconazole itself, can accumulate in the patient with renal failure.

Catheter-Related Infection

Infection can occur around the exit site of the PD catheter. The signs are acute erythema and purulent discharge. The risk of catheter exit site infection is increased with the use of uncuffed catheters, with insertion without proper aseptic technique, or in an inappropriate insertion setting. One randomized controlled study showed that prophylactic antibiotics given prior to catheter insertion may help reduce exit site infection in chronic PD, vancomycin being more effective than cefazolin.[13] On the basis of this experience, routine prophylactic pre-insertion antibiotic therapy should be used in critically ill patients. The choice between vancomycin and cephazolin prophylaxis should be decided locally, with consideration of the risk of emergence of vancomycin-resistant *Enterococcus*. However, many critically ill patients may have been undergoing some sort of antibiotic therapy already and therefore may not need an additional antibiotic prophylaxis if the preceding therapy has covered gram-positive organisms. Postoperatively, routine application of mupirocin ointment or gentamicin ointment prophylaxis to the exit site may be considered, as both agents have been shown to be effective in reducing exit site infection and peritonitis in patients undergoing chronic PD.[14,15]

The signs of acute exit site infections include erythema, swelling, and purulent discharge. Formation of granulation tissue takes longer to develop. Such infections should be treated with vigorous systemic antibiotic therapy, either oral or parenteral. Because most acute infections of the exit site are caused by *S. aureus*, they should be treated with first-generation cephalosporins or cloxacillin unless there is a high local prevalence of methicillin-resistant *Staphylococcus*. However, in the intensive care unit setting, *Pseudomonas* and *Acinetobacter* infections are also very common. When the exit site swab culture result is available, antibiotic therapy should be adjusted accordingly. The clinician must also remember to adjust the dosage of antibiotics according to the patient's renal function.

In the more severe exit site infection, tunnel track infection may develop. The catheter should be removed to prevent development of peritonitis. The possibility of underlying bowel disease must also be considered, particularly with gram-negative polymicrobial peritonitis. Further investigations and surgical exploration may be required.

COMPLICATIONS RELATED TO CATHETER INSERTION

Complications may arise during catheter insertion. Perforation of the bowel or bladder may occur. The risk of the latter is increased particularly if the bladder is not emptied during insertion. Intraperitoneal bleeding may arise from abdominal wall vessel puncture, omental tear, or even, very rarely, aorta perforation when a rigid sharp stylet is used for insertion of a PD catheter. If bleeding is minor, intraperitoneal heparin may be added to prevent clot formation from blocking the catheter. Intravenous desmopressin (DDAVP) may be used to help hemostasis by promoting of von Willebrand factor release and shorten bleeding time.[16] In the worst cases, surgical exploration is needed to identify the bleeding site and achieve hemostasis.

Leaking not uncommonly follows insertion of a PD catheter. The chance of leakage with immediate initiation of PD is high after insertion of a straight rigid uncuffed catheter or the use of a trocar and cannula for insertion of a cuffed Tenckhoff catheter via the midline. Paramedian surgical mini-laparotomy insertion with tight pursestring sutures around the peritoneal opening or percutaneous insertion with Seldinger technique with or without peritoneoscopy are both associated with very low risk of leakage, even with immediate commencement of PD.[17] In case of leakage, the dwell volume must be reduced or PD be temporarily suspended. However, such interventions may prevent the patient from receiving adequate dialysis, so another means of dialysis may be needed. The catheter must be removed and a new catheter inserted to allow PD to carry on. Fibrin glue, which has been reported to be useful for both treatment and prevention of early pericatheter leakage, can be considered.[18,19]

COMPLICATIONS RELATED TO OBSTRUCTION OF FLOW

Intraperitoneal bleeding may cause formation of clot, which then blocks the catheter. When intraperitoneal heparin fails to prevent clot formation and catheter blocking, intracatheter instillation of urokinase may help dissolve the clot and restore flow. Catheter blocking may also be caused by fibrin clots. Intraperitoneal heparin may help prevent or reduce the blockage. Intracatheter instillation of urokinase may also help dissolve the fibrin clot and restore flow. A dose of 75,000 units of diluted urokinase infused into the catheter followed by flushing of the catheter with peritoneal dialysate has been reported to be effective in dissolving fibrin clot and restoring dialysate flow without systemic side effects.[20]

Outflow obstruction with minimal inflow obstruction is a classic feature of omental wrapping of the catheter tip. This development often requires laparoscopic omentectomy, which in the critically ill may not be possible. Inserting a new catheter at another site with or without removing the original catheter may allow PD to proceed. Retaining the original omentum-wrapped catheter in situ may have the theoretical advantage of keeping the omentum "busy," thus minimizing further omental wrapping of the new catheter.

COMPLICATIONS RELATED TO INCREASED INTRAPERITONEAL PRESSURE

Although most adult patients can tolerate a 2-L peritoneal dwell in the supine position, some may experience complications related to the increased intraperitoneal pressure. The susceptible patients are those with pulmonary disease. Peritoneal fluid may hamper the movement of the diaphragm, reducing expansion or compliance of the lung and resulting in inadequate ventilation. This possibility is particularly likely when a higher dwell volume is used or in tidal PD. Reducing the dwell volume may be useful, with caution used to avoid inadequate dialysis.

Hydrothorax not uncommonly occurs in patients undergoing chronic PD, as a result of a pleural peritoneal communication developed through a congenitally weak point in the diaphragm, usually on the right side.[21] This complication usually develops quickly and is marked by sudden reduction in ultrafiltration and acute onset of shortness of breath. However, its occurrence during acute PD in the critically ill patient is extremely rare, owing to the lower intraperitoneal pressure in a supine position compared with ambulatory PD. If hydrothorax occurs, PD must be stopped, and therapeutic drainage of pleural fluid may be needed if the fluid is compromising ventilation function.

Hernia formation not uncommonly complicates chronic PD. This complication is rare in acute PD because patients are in a supine position and do not ambulate, although it may occur in patients with preexisting hernias.

METABOLIC COMPLICATIONS

Hyperglycemia

Because of the absorption of glucose through the peritoneal cavity, diabetic patients may demonstrate hyperglycemia, especially when peritoneal dialysate with higher glucose concentration (e.g., 4.25%) is used to increase fluid removal. The amount of glucose absorbed through the peritoneal cavity is often overlooked. Given that critically ill patients are in a stressed condition, hyperglycemia is even more likely to develop. The blood glucose level must be closely monitored, and the insulin dosage adjusted accordingly. In patients who have been taking oral hypoglycemic agents, change to insulin is often needed. Intravenous insulin drip or subcutaneous short-acting insulin in multiple doses is preferred over intraperitoneal administration, because the majority of intraperitoneally administered insulin is adsorbed into the plastic tubing of the PD system,[22] and the rapid cycle of acute PD does not allow time for insulin to be absorbed, making its absorption very unpredictable.

On the other hand, hypoglycemia may occur when peritoneal dialysate is changed from a high to a lower glucose content (e.g., when fluid overload is corrected) or when PD is stopped or the cycle frequency is reduced but the insulin dosage is not adjusted in a timely manner.

Hypernatremia

In PD with aggressive ultrafiltration using dialysate with very high glucose concentration (e.g., 4.25%), water is removed in excess of sodium in the first hour of a cycle. This is called the *sodium sieving effect*.[23] In rapid-cycle PD using dialysate with high glucose content, this effect would lead to water loss in excess of sodium loss, resulting in a rapid rise in serum sodium concentration or even hypernatremia. This possibility should be watched for by means of frequent monitoring of plasma sodium level. If the sodium level is rising rapidly, part of the ultrafiltration

should be replaced by water, given either orally or intravenously in a dextrose solution.

Hypokalemia and Hyperkalemia

Compared with hemodialysis, PD is much less effective in removing potassium. Therefore, hyperkalemia may not be easily corrected, particularly in a hypercatabolic patient. Other means of correction or prevention of hyperkalemia may be needed in addition to PD. Hypokalemia, however, may still occur, particularly in patients who already have low serum potassium level to start with and in patients with poor oral intake. Potassium, 3.5 to 4 mmol/L, may be added to PD fluid to prevent or correct hypokalemia.

Metabolic Acidosis

The conventional peritoneal dialysate fluid uses lactate as the base buffer. Lactate absorbed during PD is then converted into bicarbonate to correct metabolic acidosis. However, in patients with liver insufficiency or lactic acidosis, this process may lead to or may perpetuate lactic acidosis. In this condition, the multi-chambered PDF containing bicarbonate at physiologic pH would help.

FLUID BALANCE COMPLICATIONS

Inadequate Ultrafiltration

Unlike hemodialysis, in which the amount of ultrafiltration can be easily adjusted by a change in transmembrane pressure, PD allows much less precise ultrafiltration control. The ultrafiltration amount can be controlled through the use of different dialysate glucose concentrations, but it still varies substantially among individuals. Factors contributing to variation in ultrafiltration include peritoneal transport characteristics, effective peritoneal membrane area, and position of the dialysis catheter. Attention must be paid to fluid removal and balance, particularly in patients who were given large amounts of intravenous fluid, such as those who need parenteral alimentation and those who are receiving high-dose inotropic therapy, colloid, or large amounts of saline infusion.

Hypotension and Dehydration

Because of the slower ultrafiltration rate in PD, hypotension is less likely than in hemodialysis, but prolonged, excessive ultrafiltration may still lead to this complication. Accurate assessment of the target amount of fluid removal and adjustments in concentration of PD fluid are needed to prevent hypotension and over-dehydration.

CONCLUSION

Complications of acute PD in the critically ill patient, and their management, differ somewhat from those in chronic PD. Complications include the potential causative organisms of peritonitis, antibiotic choice, dosing and route of administration, risk of leakage, blood sugar fluctuations, and electrolyte and hemodynamic disturbances. Prevention of complications is very important to the success of PD therapy in critically ill patients.

Key Points

1. Peritonitis complicating peritoneal dialysis in the critically ill patients should be treated promptly with intraperitoneal antibiotics. Intravenous antibiotic loading should be considered in patients with severe sepsis.
2. The pattern of organisms causing peritonitis in the critical ill may be quite different from that in regular chronic peritoneal dialysis patients.
3. Exit site infection may be prevented with local mupirocin or gentamicin ointment prophylaxis.
4. Many mechanical complications of peritoneal dialysis are related to the method of insertion and types of peritoneal dialysis catheter.
5. Metabolic complications are more subtle and require attention in prevention.

Key References

8. Vincent JL, Bihari DJ, Suter PM, et al: The prevalence of nosocomial infection in intensive care units in Europe: Results of the European Prevalence of Infection in Intensive Care (EPIC) Study. EPIC International Advisory Committee. J Am Med Assoc 1995;274:639-644.
9. National Nosocomial Infections Surveillance (NNIS) report, data summary from October 1986-April 1996, issued May 1996: A report from the National Nosocomial Infections Surveillance (NNIS) System. Am J Infect Control 1996;24:380-388.
10. Piraino B, Bailie GR, Bernardini J, et al; ISPD Ad Hoc Advisory Committee: Peritoneal dialysis-related infections recommendations: 2005 update. Perit Dial Int 2005;25:107-131.
14. Tacconelli E, Carmeli Y, Aizer A, et al: Mupirocin prophylaxis to prevent *Staphylococcus aureus* infection in patients undergoing dialysis: A meta-analysis. Clin Infect Dis 2003;37:1629-1638.
22. Quellhorst E: Insulin therapy during peritoneal dialysis: Pros and cons of various forms of administration. J Am Soc Nephrol 2002;13(Suppl 1):S92-S96.

See the companion Expert Consult website for the complete reference list.

CHAPTER 274

Comparison of Peritoneal Dialysis with Other Treatments for Acute Renal Failure

Georges Saab, Ramesh Khanna, and Karl Nolph

OBJECTIVES

This chapter will:
1. Compare solute clearances of peritoneal dialysis and other dialysis modalities in acute renal failure.
2. Discuss the relative costs of the use of peritoneal dialysis and other dialysis modalities in acute renal failure.
3. Consider the technical aspects of the use of peritoneal dialysis and those of other dialysis modalities in acute renal failure.
4. Describe the additional benefits of peritoneal dialysis, independent of solute clearance, fluid removal, and metabolic control.
5. Discuss the potential complications of the use of peritoneal dialysis in acute renal failure.

Acute renal failure (ARF) in the intensive care unit is common and is associated with higher mortality. Indeed, in a 2005 multinational, multicenter, prospective observational study, the mean prevalence of oliguric ARF was approximately 6% and was associated with an overall mortality of about 60% in critically ill patients.[1] Although the severity of illness certainly plays a role in the higher risk of death, the development of oliguric ARF appears to be an independent risk factor for death.[2,3]

The poor outcomes with oliguric ARF may be related to several metabolic derangements, such as hyperkalemia and metabolic acidosis, that ultimately may require the initiation of renal replacement therapy. Other factors are also likely playing a role. Fortunately, a number of different modalities for renal replacement therapy have been developed to help manage some of these complications, including intermittent hemodialysis (IHD), continuous renal replacement therapy (CRRT), sustained low-efficiency dialysis (SLED), and acute peritoneal dialysis (PD). Despite the inherent differences among these modalities, the superiority of one over the other has not been clearly demonstrated.

No clear benefit has been shown, but the preferential use of CRRT in oliguric ARF has been rising and that of acute PD and IHD have been falling.[4,5] Although an excellent modality for metabolic control, CRRT is not universally available and requires significant time and resources. Furthermore, vascular access for CRRT may be limited, particularly among critically ill infants and small children, or may be difficult to obtain, such as in patients with coagulation disorders or significant vascular disease. The need for continuous anticoagulation is also a concern because it may raise bleeding risk and is associated with

TABLE 274-1

Comparison of Peritoneal Dialysis, Continuous Renal Replacement Therapy, and Intermittent Hemodialysis

FEATURE	PERITONEAL DIALYSIS	CONTINUOUS RENAL REPLACEMENT THERAPY	INTERMITTENT HEMODIALYSIS
Solute clearance	Adequate, but less than with other modalities	Adequate	Adequate
Cost	Low	High	Moderate
Technical expertise required	Low	High	Moderate
Availability	Wide	Less	Moderate
Hypotensive patients	Yes	Yes	Maybe
Need for systemic anticoagulation	No	Yes	Yes
Need for central venous access	No	Yes	Yes
Delivers nutrition	Yes	No	No
Administers medications	Yes	No	No
Treatment of severe acute hyperkalemia	No	Maybe	Yes
Treatment of severe volume overload	Yes	Yes	Yes
Infections	Yes—peritonitis	Yes—line sepsis	Yes—line sepsis

greater utilization of resources for monitoring adequacy of anticoagulation. Despite these concerns, many nephrologists are turning to CRRT to manage critically ill patients with ARF.

In centers that lack the resources and expertise in CRRT, acute PD may be a viable option for the management of ARF in critically ill patients. It may be better tolerated than IHD among patients who are hemodynamically unstable or have severe congestive heart failure. Furthermore, the use of continuous PD therapy in ARF appears to provide both adequate control of metabolic derangements in catabolic patients and significant solute removal.[6] This chapter reviews the use of PD in ARF and how it compares with other renal replacement modalities (Table 274-1).

SOLUTE/VOLUME CONTROL AND OVERALL OUTCOMES

There is significant controversy as to the definition of adequate dialysis in ARF and what parameters best represent this adequacy. Currently, most data suggest that use of a higher dialysis dose in CRRT or IHD for the patient with ARF is associated with better survival.[7-9] Although not all studies have consistently found this result,[10] it is likely that, at the very least, inadequate dialysis is associated with poorer outcomes. Consequently, because of the lower daily solute clearance with PD, many investigators have argued that PD may not be a viable option for critically ill patients with ARF, particularly those who are highly catabolic.

Several studies have documented adequate solute control with PD in ARF[11-14] but have been criticized for their small sample sizes and lack of assessment of catabolic rate. Perhaps the best study addressing this issue was conducted by Chitalia and associates,[6] who compared continuous equilibrating peritoneal dialysis (CEPD) with tidal peritoneal dialysis (TPD) in patients with hypercatabolic ARF. In this study, patients were classified as having mild, moderate, or severe hypercatabolic ARF according to severity of catabolism, which was based on estimation of excess urea nitrogen appearance (UNA). Patients with mildly to moderately hypercatabolic ARF were subsequently randomly assigned to undergo TPD or CEPD with a total volume of approximately 26 L per session in both arms. TPD was associated with lower post-dialysis BUN

and creatinine concentrations and higher creatinine and urea clearances than CEPD. The per-session and weekly Kt/V urea achieved with TPD were 0.34 ± 0.14 and 2.43 ± 0.87, respectively—significantly higher than those with CEPD. Although blood kinetic measurement of Kt/V may overestimate urea removal in the setting of ARF,[15] it does not appear to do so in PD. The major limiting factor Chitalia and associates[6] found was significant protein loss with TPD.

The Kt/V achieved with TPD is significantly less than that reported in IHD or CRRT,[7,10] but there is no consensus on what adequate Kt/V is in ARF. Most experts would recommend achieving a dose at least equal to that in patients with end-stage renal disease undergoing PD. The National Kidney Foundation's Kidney Disease Outcomes Quality Initiative (K/DOQI) guidelines for 2006 recommend a weekly peritoneal dialysis Kt/V of 1.7 for anuric patients,[16] a goal easily achieved with TPD in this study. Unfortunately, no direct comparison of TPD with CRRT or IHD in ARF has been performed.

Continuous venovenous hemofiltration (CVVH) has been compared with intermittent PD in a randomized controlled trial. In a study from Vietnam, Phu and colleagues[17] examined 70 patients with ARF from malaria or sepsis randomly assigned to renal replacement therapy with CVVH or PD. PD consisted of 2-L exchanges using an acetate-based dialysis fluid with a 30-minute dwell time (approximately 70 L/day). PD access was accomplished with a rigid PD catheter. CVVH consisted of a lactate-based replacement fluid given pre-filter for approximately 25 L/day. Patients randomly assigned to CVVH had a more significant decline in serum creatinine, better correction of acidosis, and improved survival than those who underwent PD. Other noncontrolled studies have documented similar results. In a retrospective study of children with ARF after cardiac surgery, Fleming and coworkers[18] found better urea and creatinine reduction as well as greater propensity toward negative fluid balance in patients treated with CVVH or continuous arteriovenous hemofiltration than in those who underwent PD. This latter study was limited in that there was not a standard treatment protocol for each modality. Although neither study accurately documented solute removal, solute clearance in these two studies appears to have been significantly lower in patients treated with PD. These findings may demonstrate superiority of CRRT over PD, but they may also simply reflect the fact that inadequate dialysis is associated with poorer outcomes.

In addition to decreased solute removal, other factors related to PD itself may have contributed to the worse outcomes in the study by Phu and colleagues.[17] First, peritoneal access was achieved with a rigid catheter, which is associated with more complications than polymeric silicone (Silastic) catheters, including outflow obstruction, peritonitis, and bowel perforation.[20] Risk of dialysis solution leak with subsequent higher infection risk is further enhanced by the multiple manual exchanges that were performed during PD. Although the reported incidence of peritonitis was low, the fluid was said to be cloudy in approximately 40% of patients. Second, the better control of the acid/base abnormalities with CVVH may be partially attributed to the use of acetate in the PD arm. Use of acetate in PD has been discontinued since the mid-1980s. Use of lactate- or bicarbonate-based replacement solutions has been shown to be superior to acetate-based solutions in correcting metabolic acidosis in patients treated with CVVH.[21,22] Acetate has also been associated with the development of sclerosing peritonitis, which may have also contributed to the adverse outcomes. Although the better solute clearance in CVVH may have accounted for some of the improved outcomes with this technique, suboptimal PD may also have contributed. A direct comparison of TPD with CRRT or IHD would be of great interest.

Clearances with continuous-flow peritoneal dialysis (CFPD) may be superior to those in TPD, and CFPD may be particularly useful in ARF.[23] In this modality, large volumes of intraperitoneal fluid are continuously replenished with dialysis solution in constant contact with the membrane. There are two modes of CFPD, continuous infusion and removal of sterile dialysate solution (called single-pass CFPD) and recirculation of the dialysate (in which the peritoneal effluent, and not blood, is "dialyzed" through a hemodialysis or CRRT circuit against an external dialysate and then returned to the patient). Obviously, this technique requires either two catheters or a catheter with dual lumens. Physical separation of catheter lumens is important to minimize recirculation. Urea clearances of 30 to 50 mL/min are usually achieved with this technique, with the potential for even greater clearances.[24] Such clearances are equal or superior to those achieved with CRRT. Unfortunately, no studies have directly compared CFPD with other modalities in patients with ARF. The overall cost of CFPD may also be limiting and may preclude its routine use in ARF, particularly at centers with limited resources. Further studies of the use of CFPD in ARF are required for this promising PD modality.

Volume overload is commonly encountered in critically ill patients with ARF. Hypotension oftentimes limits the rate at which fluid can be removed, making IHD less desirable for many nephrologists. Although most nephrologists would prefer CRRT in these cases, PD offers an alternative. Exchanges using 4.25% dextrose can yield approximately 1 L per 4-hour exchange and even more with hourly exchanges, so rates of sodium and water removal can be quite high with PD. Hypernatremia is a risk with rapid PD ultrafiltration, because of sodium sieving, but not with IHD or CRRT. However, low-sodium PD solutions can be prepared to yield very high rates of ultrafiltration with balanced Na and water removal.

COST

Chitalia and associates[6] found TPD and CEPD to be relatively inexpensive. They reported that (at the time of publication in 2002) a 12-hour treatment with TPD cost approximately $160 and 48 hours of CEPD cost $175; these figures would yield weekly rates of approximately $1100 for TPD and $600 for CEPD. In comparison, the weekly cost of SLED is about $1200 to $1400, that of CRRT with heparin anticoagulation about $2000 to $2500, and that of CRRT with citrate anticoagulation about $2500 to $3500.[25,26] The significantly higher costs of CRRT are secondary to greater nursing time, higher equipment costs, and larger need for anticoagulation.

VASCULAR ACCESS

Obtaining venous access may be difficult in some patients, and thus, PD may be the only modality that is acceptable in such situations. Such is the case with small children and infants, in whom the central venous system may not be suitable for IHD or CRRT access. Indeed, our personal clinical experience with acute PD in infants and small children has found it an excellent mode of RRT in such patients. Furthermore, although both venous access and peritoneal access can result in infection, central venous access is also associated with the development of venous thrombosis, particularly in the femoral and subclavian veins, putting patients at risk for embolic events. In addition, the placement of central venous access can lead to central venous stenosis, which can have significant long-term sequelae, particularly for children.

Peritoneal access, however, may not be uniformly achievable, particularly in patients who have recently undergone bowel surgery. In such patients, PD is probably contraindicated. In addition, critically ill patients with ARF may have bacteremia, raising their risk for development of peritonitis with the placement of PD access. Having a PD catheter in place is in itself a risk factor for peritonitis, but concomitant bacteremia will probably raise this risk. Given the high rates of hospital-acquired bacteremia, particularly in the intensive care unit, the issue of peritoneal seeding and peritonitis should be considered when PD is being considered for renal replacement therapy.

POTENTIAL BENEFITS FAVORING PERITONEAL DIALYSIS

The use of continuous or extended dialysis usually requires some level of anticoagulation. The use of heparin anticoagulation can lead to bleeding and may be contraindicated in patients with a bleeding diathesis or recent surgery. Monitoring of partial thromboplastin time adds to nursing and laboratory costs. Furthermore, patients treated with heparin sometimes develop heparin antibodies, precluding its use. The use of citrate can ameliorate some of these problems with heparin but adds further to complexity and cost. In PD, anticoagulation is not necessary.

When high volumes of replacement fluid are used in CRRT, hypothermia can develop because the fluid temperature is much lower than the body core temperature. This effect can often be treated with the use of a blood warmer or warming of the dialysate (when dialysis is added in addition to hemofiltration), but hypothermia is much less likely with acute PD. In fact, acute PD using a warmed dialysate has been reported to be a successful treatment for acute hypothermia.[27]

Adequate nutrition is important in critically ill patients, particularly those who are hypercatabolic. Enteral and parenteral feedings can be used for nutritional support. The latter requires additional central access, raising the risk of infection, particularly fungemia. Peritoneal dialysis using dialysate containing amino acids can potentially provide nutritional support and has been shown to enhance nitrogen balance in patients undergoing chronic or acute PD.[28,29] Furthermore, the addition of amino acids may reduce the glucose exposure, and subsequently insulin requirements, in acutely ill hypercatabolic patients with ARF. The high glucose exposure is certainly one of the potential disadvantages of acute PD in ARF.

Dosing of medications is difficult in critically ill patients. Factors such as intestinal edema, liver dysfunction, and renal dysfunction significantly affect the absorption and metabolism of such medications. Clearances for a number of medications via both CRRT and IHD have been described and have led to recommendations for dosage and frequency of administration adjustments when these modalities are administered. However, fluctuations in drug levels still probably occur, which may lead to periodic subtherapeutic levels. In PD, a number of medications can be given intraperitoneally, and they have much more steady absorption via this route. This feature may lead to more constant steady-state levels of drugs and possibly greater efficacy.

POTENTIAL LIMITATIONS FAVORING OTHER MODALITIES

Although PD may be able to achieve adequate solute removal and may have additional potential benefits that cannot be provided with CRRT or IHD, it is associated with certain unique complications that are not seen with CRRT or IHD. These complications should not preclude the use of PD in ARF, but their consideration and management are crucial in the planning for acute PD.

Pulmonary function may be compromised in patients undergoing PD owing to an elevation in intra-abdominal pressure, particularly in small children and infants. Indeed, Bunchman and colleagues[30] described the PD treatment of four infants with ARF who were undergoing mechanical ventilation. These investigators found that increased midcycle intra-abdominal pressure correlated with reduced pulmonary compliance and increased airway resistance. The increased abdominal pressure may be partially avoided by using more frequent cycling of lower dialysate volumes. Other pulmonary complications are the development of pleural effusions from migration of peritoneal fluid into the thorax, which can be managed with lower dialysate volumes and supine dialysis.

Complications from PD catheter insertion include bowel perforation, intraperitoneal hemorrhage, and peritonitis. Although there is usually some bleeding with catheter insertion, large-volume bleeding can also occur. These complications are most often seen with rigid PD catheters but can also be seen with nonrigid catheters. Peritonitis is a known complication of both chronic and acute renal

failure. Given the high rate of hospital-acquired infections, particularly in the intensive care unit, proper sterile technique should be adhered to and intensive care nurses should receive focused instruction in its performance, particularly if a cycler is unavailable.

CONCLUSION

Acute renal failure requiring renal replacement therapy is associated with significant morbidity and mortality. Although solute clearances and metabolic control are easy to achieve with CRRT and IHD, these modalities are not universally available and require a certain technical expertise. Furthermore, the risks of anticoagulation and the need for central access may preclude their use. PD may be an option in these situations. PD can achieve adequate solute clearances in mildly to moderately hypercatabolic ARF and at a lower cost than CRRT and IHD. Direct comparisons between these modalities and PD are few and have significant technical limitations. Further studies are required to address these issues. PD is a viable option in the management of ARF.

Key Points

1. Although solute clearances are generally less than with other modalities, acute peritoneal dialysis can achieve adequate solute clearances in most patients.
2. Acute peritoneal dialysis is significantly less expensive than other modalities and requires less technical expertise.
3. Acute peritoneal dialysis is more readily available than other modalities, particularly in smaller centers and developing countries.
4. Infectious complications of this modality are common and great care must be taken to adhere to sterile technique.

Key References

6. Chitalia VC, Almeida AF, Rai H, et al: Is peritoneal dialysis adequate for hypercatabolic acute renal failure in developing countries? Kidney Int 2002;61:747-57.
11. Cameron JS, Ogg C, Trounce JR: Peritoneal dialysis in hypercatabolic acute renal failure. Lancet 1967;1(7501):1188-1191.
17. Phu NH, Hien TT, Mai NT, et al: Hemofiltration and peritoneal dialysis in infection-associated acute renal failure in Vietnam. N Engl J Med 2002;347:895-902.
27. Vella J, Farrell J, Leavey S, et al: The rapid reversal of profound hypothermia using peritoneal dialysis. Ir J Med Sci 1996;165:113-114.
29. Tjiong HL, van den Berg JW, Wattimena JL, et al: Dialysate as food: Combined amino acid and glucose dialysate improves protein anabolism in renal failure patients on automated peritoneal dialysis. J Am Soc Nephrol 2005;16:1486-1493.

See the companion Expert Consult website for the complete reference list.

CHAPTER 275

Continuous-Flow Peritoneal Dialysis as Acute Therapy

Richard Amerling and Aicha Merouani

OBJECTIVES

This chapter will:
1. Elucidate the rationale for continuous-flow peritoneal dialysis and its underlying physiology.
2. Review the historical perspective of continuous-flow peritoneal dialysis.
3. Discuss the techniques of this modality: single-pass versus recirculation, dual-lumen catheter versus two catheters, ultrafiltration control, and dose of dialysis
4. Review the special considerations in and clinical experience of continuous-flow peritoneal dialysis in pediatric acute renal failure.
5. Describe the clinical experience with this modality in acute renal failure.
6. Discuss the advantages of and indications for continuous-flow peritoneal dialysis.
7. Consider the future directions of this modality.

RATIONALE AND PHYSIOLOGY

Peritoneal dialysis (PD) has been used in the treatment of acute renal failure (ARF) for a generation, and its details described elsewhere. Use of PD in ARF has declined largely because the slow solute clearance it renders it inadequate to deal with the modern hypercatabolic patient with ARF who has multiple–organ system failure (MOSF). Urea clearance in acute PD is limited, even under optimal circumstances, to 10 to 15 mL/min.[1] This limitation is not due to membrane surface area, permeability, or blood flow, which should be more than capable of delivering clearances of 40 to 80 mL/min.[2] Solute clearance is limited by the fill-dwell-drain cycle of standard PD.

Figure 275-1 depicts an idealized PD exchange. Dialysis, or solute flux across the membrane, requires dialysate contact with the membrane, which makes the fill and drain segments extremely inefficient. Flux (J) is defined mathematically as the permeability coefficient of the membrane or mass-transfer area coefficient (MTAC) multiplied by the difference between the solute concentration in the blood (C_B) and that in the dialysate (C_D), or concentration gradient, as shown in the following equation:

$$J = MTAC (C_B - C_D)$$

In standard PD, the concentration gradient decreases continuously as solute transport occurs during a dwell, steadily reducing the flux, or rate of transport (see Fig. 275-1).

CFPD works by constantly replenishing the dialysate, either with fresh, sterile dialysate in single-pass mode, or by externally purifying the dialysate with a hemodialysis (or sorbent) system in recirculation mode. In either case the net effect is to lower C_D and to keep it low throughout the treatment. This greatly enhances clearance and allows the system to perform up to the level of its inherent permeability/blood flow limitations (Fig. 275-2). CFPD has been mathematically modeled in vitro and in vivo.[3] Clearance approaches the MTAC as intraperitoneal solute concentration approaches zero. Clearance varies with intraperitoneal volume, rate of dialysate flow through the peritoneum (Q_P), and efficiency of the external regenerating circuit, which in turn depends on external dialysate flow rate or Q_D (Fig. 275-3).

HISTORICAL PERSPECTIVE

Our work in CFPD is based largely on the pioneering observations of James A. Shinaberger and colleagues,[4] who in 1965 reported on the first successful series of patients treated with this technique. They compared intermittent PD (IPD), then the standard of care, with CFPD in five patients. They used two catheters, one placed deep within the pelvis and the other near the diaphragm. A 2-L to 3-L intraperitoneal reservoir was drained via the pelvic catheter, recirculated through a primitive extracorporeal circuit consisting of a twin-coil dialyzer sitting in a 50-L vat of dialysate, and returned to the patient through the subdiaphragmatic catheter (Fig. 275-4). Dialysate flow was varied between 20 and 300 mL/min. At flows of 200 to 300 mL/min, urea clearances ranging from 46 to 125 mL/min were obtained.

Other researchers reported experiences over the next 15 years using different setups and homebuilt dual catheters.[5-10] Most of these investigators reported urea clearances of around 30 mL/min. The 1980s were dominated by continuous ambulatory PD (CAPD) and continuing cycling PD (CCPD), and little work was done on CFPD until the mid-1990s, which coincided with the end of the honeymoon with CAPD. At that time, CFPD was rediscovered.[11-15]

THE TECHNIQUE

CFPD can be performed in single-pass mode using sterile dialysate or in recirculating mode with external purification. A peritoneal flow rate (Q_P) of at least 100 mL/min requires 6 liters of dialysate per hour, or 60 L per 10-hour treatment. This is a prohibitively large volume, both from the practical perspective of cost and because of the potential for clinically significant protein losses. An exception

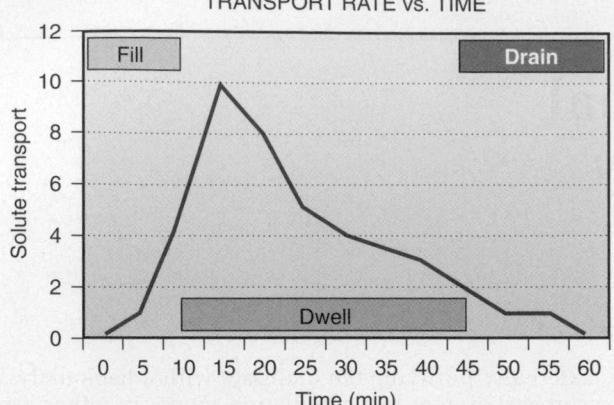

FIGURE 275-1. An idealized PD exchange: Solute flux is poor during inflow/outflow, and falls off rapidly during dwell as concentration gradient dissipates.

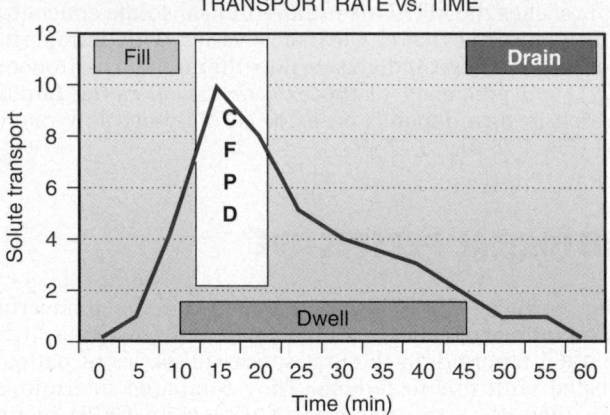

FIGURE 275-2. Continuous-flow peritoneal dialysis (CFPD) operates at maximal concentration gradient, greatly improving solute flux.

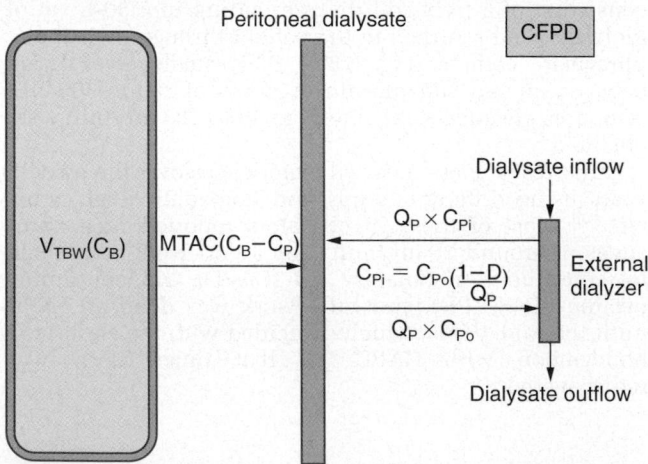

FIGURE 275-3. The continuous-flow peritoneal dialysis (CFPD) two-compartment model with solute transport across the peritoneal membrane governed by peritoneal mass-transfer area coefficient (MTAC) and the concentration gradient across the membrane. External clearance depends on rate of dialysate flow through the peritoneum (Q_P) and the dialysance (D) of the external circuit. C_B, solute concentration in the blood; C_D, solute concentrate in the dialysate; C_{Pi}, solute concentration in peritoneal inflow; C_{Po}, solute concentration in peritoneal outflow; Q_D, external dialysate flow rate; V_{TBW}, volume of total body water. (Courtesy of Frank Gotch.)

is in pediatric ARF, in which delivered volumes are much lower (see later). Recirculation of sterile dialysate with external regeneration is the only practical approach to CFPD in the acute (or chronic) setting. Although sorbent-based systems can and have been used,[16] we and most others have preferred hemodialysis technology to regenerate dialysate. Any hemodialysis machine can be adapted for CFPD.

As with all forms of renal replacement therapy, access is crucial. This is particularly true in CFPD, in which there is great potential for streaming of fresh dialysate directly to the draining catheter across a channel within the peritoneal fluid reservoir, generating internal recirculation and losing efficiency (Fig. 275-5).[17] A dual-lumen catheter would have to ensure minimal streaming and maximal mixing of fresh dialysate with dwelling volume. Drainage from a pelvic catheter (à la Shinaberger) with return through a diffuser positioned near the diaphragm should provide this situation (Fig. 275-6). We are currently testing a catheter designed for chronic CFPD that could eventually serve in the ICU setting (Fig. 275-7).[18] In the interim, acute CFPD can be successfully performed through the use of two catheters placed percutaneously or surgically. Care should be taken to position the intraperitoneal ports as far away from each other as possible. A short, straight Tenckhoff catheter oriented toward the diaphragm and a swan-neck coiled catheter in the pelvis can be placed through the same incision.[19]

Once access is obtained, 1.5 to 3.0 L of sterile dialysate is infused, depending on patient size, body habitus, and ventilator parameters. If tolerated, larger volumes are preferred because they are associated with less chance of streaming and more membrane surface area is in contact with dialysate. If cells or fibrin are present (e.g., if the patient has ascites), heparin, 2000 U/L, should be added to prevent clotting in the dialyzer. The catheters are connected via standard saline-primed hemodialysis tubing to the machine, and purification of the dialysate is initiated through an artificial kidney at 200 to 300 mL/min. External clearance is optimal with a 1.5- to 2.0-m² kidney and Q_D of 500 mL/min.[20]

Ultrafiltration remains a challenge in recirculating CFPD. With single-pass CFPD, Cruz and associates[14] and Freida and coworkers[21] achieved ultrafiltration rates of 16 mL/min and 2 to 8 mL/min with 1.5% and 1.36% dextrose, respectively. In recirculating mode, the external dialysis rapidly removes dextrose and its osmotic gradient. A true CFPD machine would deliver a constant glucose concentration, controlled by the external dialysate composition. Ideally this could be varied to produce different rates of internal (transperitoneal) ultrafiltration. External ultrafiltration rate can then be roughly matched by assessing intraperitoneal pressure. Because standard dialysis machines are not equipped for this requirement, alternative approaches are required. One approach is simply to interrupt CFPD with a 2- to 6-hour exchange using 4.25% dextrose solution, or icodextrin. Another would be to combine CFPD with peripheral venovenous hemofiltration. Our experience with CFPD in ARF (see later) has been limited to patients with ascites.[22] In this setting, ultrafiltration of ascites via the external circuit is straightforward. The subsequent concentration of protein within the residual ascites effectively "pulls" peripheral edema, and net fluid removal is accomplished.

Monitoring a CFPD treatment requires some attention. It is a low-resistance circuit, so "arterial" and "venous" pressures on the dialysis machine should be near zero. On a true CFPD machine, these sensors would be recalibrated

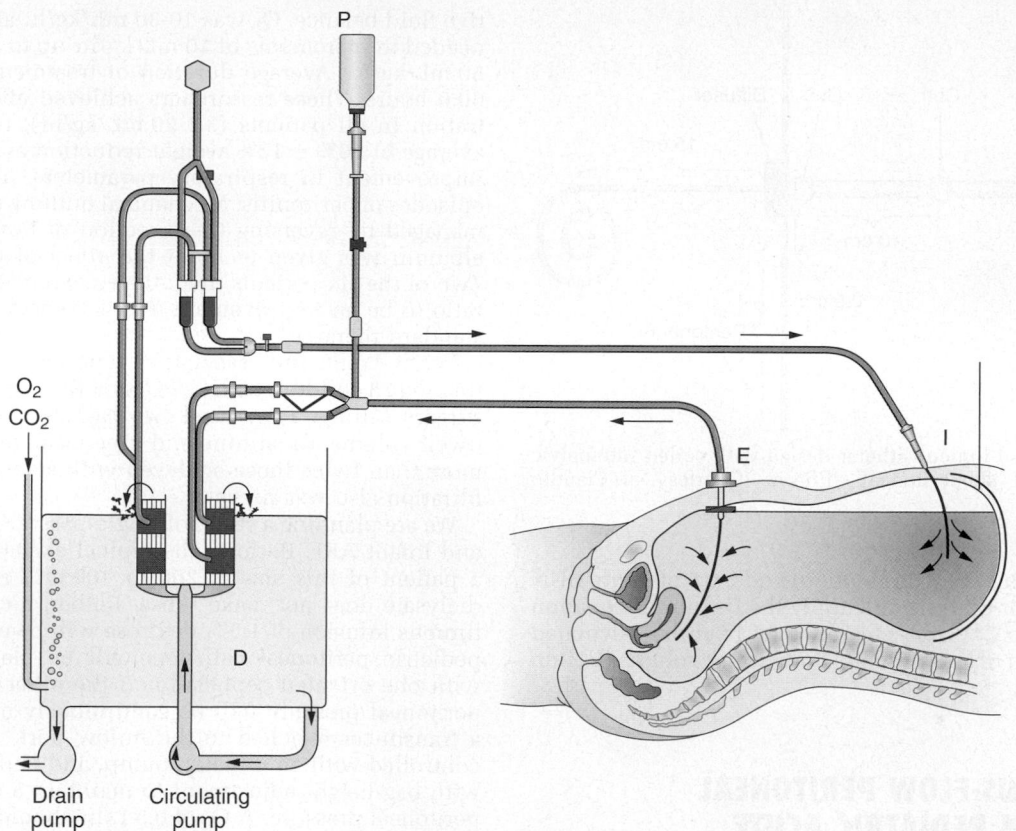

FIGURE 275-4. Original setup for continuous-flow peritoneal dialysis, with two catheters and an external circuit consisting of a twin-coil dialyzer in a vat of dialysate. D, external dialysate; E, outflow catheter; I, inflow catheter; P, peritoneal dialysate. (Adapted from Shinaberger JH, Shear L, Barry KG: Peritoneal-extracorporeal recirculation dialysis: A technique for improving efficiency of peritoneal dialysis. Invest Urol 1965;2:555-565.)

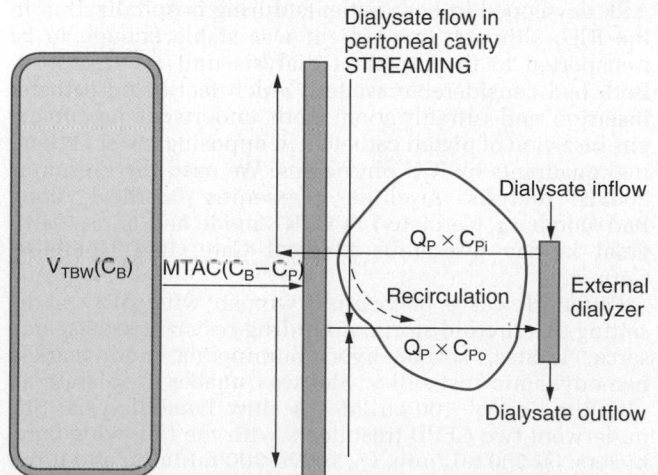

FIGURE 275-5. Intraperitoneal recirculation, or "streaming," detracts from the efficiency of continuous-flow peritoneal dialysis. C_B, solute concentration in the blood; C_D, solute concentrate in the dialysate; C_{Pi}, solute concentration in peritoneal inflow; C_{Po}, solute concentration in peritoneal outflow; Q_D, external dialysate flow rate; MTAC, mass-transfer area coefficient; Q_P, rate of dialysate flow through the peritoneum; V_{TBW}, volume of total body water. (Courtesy of Frank Gotch.)

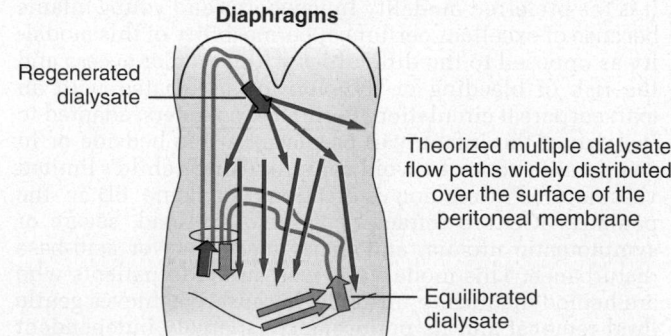

FIGURE 275-6. Ideal port position to limit intraperitoneal streaming. (Courtesy of Frank Gotch.)

to optimally detect pressures in the range of 0 to 20 cm H_2O. Ultrafiltration is assessed from changes in patient weight. Clearance can be measured directly in single-pass CFPD by collecting the dialysate, measuring the urea nitrogen and/or creatinine concentration, dividing this number by the average BUN or creatinine concentration during the treatment, and multiplying the result by the total drained

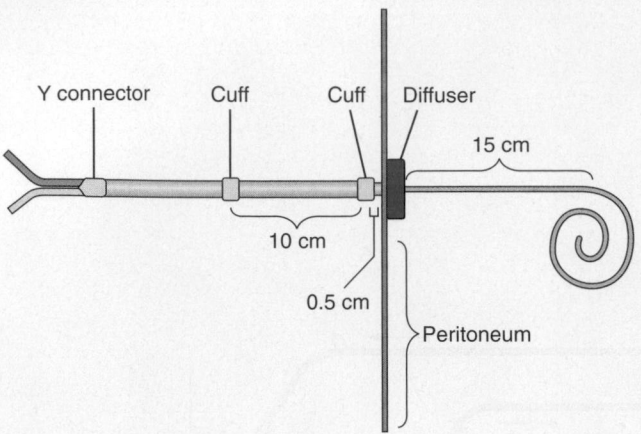

FIGURE 275-7. Dual-lumen catheter design with coiled intrapelvic drain port and subperitoneal diffuser. (Courtesy of Claudio Ronco.)

dialysate volume. In recirculation mode, we measure BUN before and after dialysis and apply the Daugirdas equation to estimate Kt/V.[23] Urea clearance (K_u) can be calculated by substitution of an estimated body water volume (V) into the equation.

CONTINUOUS-FLOW PERITONEAL DIALYSIS IN PEDIATRIC ACUTE RENAL FAILURE

Renal replacement therapy in children differs from that in adults because of the variation in size and weight of the patients as well as child-specific indications such as inborn errors of metabolism. It requires special expertise because of the lower incidence of pediatric ARF and the size-specific modes of treatment.[24]

Acute PD is frequently used in pediatric ARF and is regarded by many authorities as the preferred modality.[25] It is the preferred modality in newborns and young infants because of excellent peritoneal permeability of this modality as opposed to the difficulties with vascular access and the risk of bleeding or hypotension associated with an extracorporeal circulation. Peritoneal catheters, adapted to the size of the infant, can be placed at the bedside or in an operating room, to avoid compromising a child's limited vasculature.[26] Common indications for acute PD in the pediatric ICU are refractory volume overload, severe or symptomatic uremia, and major electrolyte or acid-base disturbance. This modality is well suited to patients who are hemodynamically unstable, because it achieves gentle fluid removal and its performance is largely independent of blood pressure.[27]

Two major disadvantages of PD in the child are (1) relatively poor solute clearance and (2) marked variation in intra-abdominal volume and pressure with possible impairment of ventilation. The latter problem often forces a reduction in dwell volume with further loss of clearance.[28] Both problems are addressed by CFPD.

Sagy and Silver[29] treated six patients aged 18 ± 37 months who had acute respiratory distress syndrome by means of single-pass CFPD using two tunneled Tenckhoff catheters placed surgically and 2.5% dextrose solution. The patients had been ventilated for an average of 8 days before treatment was initiated and were in strongly posi-

tive fluid balance. Q_P was 10-30 mL/kg/hr and adjusted as needed in increments of 10 mL/kg/hr up to a maximum of 50 mL/kg/hr. Average duration of treatment was 126.7 ± 60.0 hours. These researchers achieved effective ultrafiltration in all patients (3.1-20 mL/kg/hr), resulting in an average of 30% ± 12% weight reduction and a significant improvement in respiratory parameters. There were no episodes of peritonitis. Mechanical outflow problems were managed by reversing the direction of flow. Intravenous albumin was given to blunt the effect of protein losses. Two of the six patients died; the researchers believed this ratio to be an improvement over expected outcome with standard therapy.

Vande Walle and associates[30] reported their experience treating 28 children with CFPD for ARF in the post–cardiac surgery setting. They used two catheters and a minimal dwell volume. Creatinine and urea clearance values were more than twice those achieved with standard PD. Ultrafiltration also was higher.

We are planning a study of single-pass CFPD in neonatal and infant ARF. Because the typical exchange volume in a patient of this size is 200 to 400 mL, regeneration of dialysate does not make sense. Rather, a controlled continuous infusion of 1.5% dextrose will be employed. Two pediatric peritoneal catheters will be placed surgically with one oriented cephalad and the other caudad. Intraperitoneal pressure will be continuously monitored with a transducer attached to the inflow port. Inflow will be controlled with an infusion pump, and outflow by gravity with bag height adjustment to maintain a constant intraperitoneal pressure. A Q_P of 0.5 L/hr should deliver excellent dialysis at the cost of a single 10-L bag of dialysate per day.

CLINICAL EXPERIENCE WITH CONTINUOUS-FLOW PERITONEAL DIALYSIS IN ACUTE RENAL FAILURE

We have had two experiences treating ARF with CFPD. ARF developed in both patients during hospitalization in the ICU, although one patient was stable enough to be transported to the inpatient dialysis unit for treatment. Both had considerable ascites, which facilitated catheter insertion and ultrafiltration. Both underwent percutaneous insertion of pigtail catheters in opposing lower abdominal quadrants by ICU physicians. We used the Fresenius 2008H dialysis machine (Fresenius Medical Care, Bad Homburg, Germany) in CRRT mode and an F80 artificial kidney (Fresenius Medical Care, Bad Homburg, Germany).

Patient 1 was a 66-year-old woman with ARF in the setting of a thyroid storm, multidrug-resistant sepsis, anasarca, ascites, severe hypoalbuminemia, and marked hemodynamic instability. She was unable to tolerate an ultrafiltration of 100 mL/hr via slow hemodialysis. She underwent two CFPD treatments with the following parameters: Q_P 200 mL/min, Q_D 100 to 300 mL/min, and ultrafiltration rate 50 to 200 mL/hr. In the first treatment, 3.6 L were removed in 24 hours. The BUN value decreased from 54 to 22 mg/dL, for a urea reduction ratio of 59%. Applying the Daugirdas equation yielded a Kt/V of 1.11 and a urea clearance (V = 40 L) of 31 mL/min. The procedures were well-tolerated, but peritonitis developed and the catheters were removed. The patient died about a month later, with no further attempts at renal replacement.[22]

Patient 2, a 65-year-old man with cirrhosis, had acute renal failure, likely from drug-induced allergic interstitial nephritis. He presented with oliguria, severe ascites, and peripheral edema, all of which were refractory to diuretics. He underwent 3 consecutive days of CFPD, for 5 to 8 hours a day via percutaneous pigtail catheters placed in the ICU (Figs. 275-8 and 275-9). Q_P was 250 to 300 mL/min, Q_D 500 mL/min, and ultrafiltration flow rate 400 to 500 mL/

hr. More than 10 kg of fluid was removed by ultrafiltration of the ascites during the treatment. The patient was hemodynamically stable throughout. Urea clearance averaged 50 mL/min (Table 275-1), and BUN and creatinine concentrations declined with each treatment (Fig. 275-10). The catheters were removed after 3 days. The patient's renal function recovered, and he was transferred to another institution for liver transplantation.

In the dialysis of ascitic fluid, as in these two cases, clearance of the blood compartment is delayed by 30 to 60 minutes, the time it takes to remove enough solute from the ascitic fluid to create a diffusion gradient across the peritoneal membrane (Figs. 275-11 and 275-12).

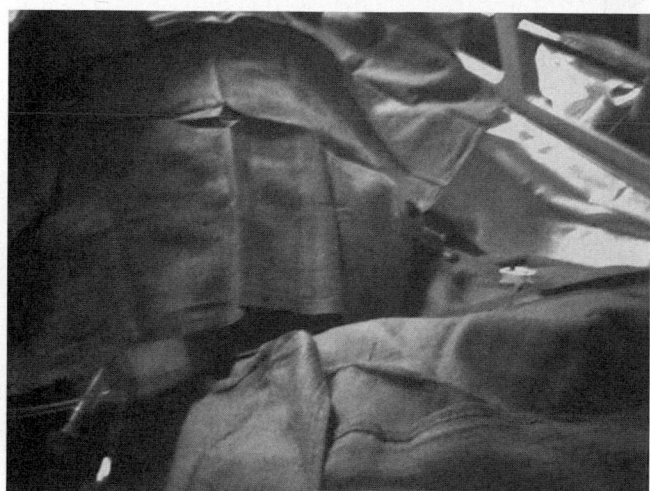

FIGURE 275-8. Patient 2 with dual pigtail catheters attached to dialysis machine for continuous-flow peritoneal dialysis in the Inpatient Dialysis Unit.

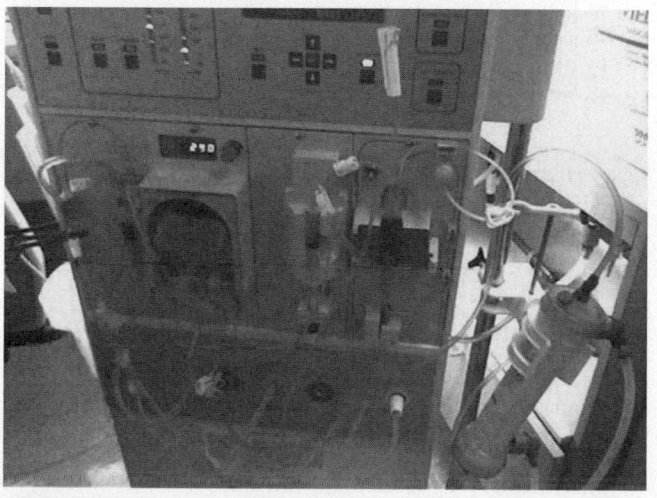

FIGURE 275-9. Continuous-flow peritoneal dialysis in progress in Patient 2 with a Fresenius 2008H dialysis machine (Fresenius Medical Care, Bad Homburg, Germany).

ADVANTAGES AND INDICATIONS FOR CONTINUOUS-FLOW PERITONEAL DIALYSIS IN ACUTE RENAL FAILURE

CFPD combines the safety, simplicity, and hemodynamic stability of PD with the clearance of continuous venovenous hemofiltration or hemodialysis. CFPD should be the preferred renal replacement therapy in the unstable patient, particularly if blood access is problematic. Pediatric ARF is, we believe, an ideal indication. Other likely indications are ARF associated with ascites, acute pancreatitis, congestive heart failure with hemodynamic instability, and bleeding diathesis. In the patient with pancreatitis, single-pass CFPD should initiate treatment in order to effectively lavage the peritoneum.

Once ultrafiltration control is perfected, CFPD would be appropriate for any form of ARF in which peritoneal access is possible. Disadvantages are the requirement for two catheters or a double-lumen catheter, and the previously mentioned issues surrounding ultrafiltration. Other risks are exactly those of standard PD: peritonitis, mechanical drainage issues, transdiaphragmatic leakage, viscus perforation, and hyperglycemia.

CONCLUSION AND FUTURE DIRECTIONS

CFPD has great promise for treatment of ARF, especially in children with ARF, in whom the peritoneal route has significant advantages, and relatively low fluid requirements permit the single-pass mode to be used. The ability to offer clearances comparable to that for other forms of continuous renal replacement therapy, with the safety of peritoneal rather than blood access, makes a compelling argument to pursue this therapy. Ultrafiltration and access

TABLE 275-1

Summary of Three Continuous-Flow Peritoneal Dialysis Treatments in Patient 2*

DATE	ULTRAFILTRATE VOLUME (L)	URR (%)	Kt/V	VOLUME (mL)**	TREATMENT TIME (min)	TOTAL UREA CLEARANCE (mL/min)
9 Nov	2	18	0.26	72,000	354	52.88
10 Nov	3.7	23	0.35	70,000	485	50.52
11 Nov	4.4	18	0.29	68,000	400	49.30

*Kt/V was calculated from predialysis and postdialysis blood urea nitrogen concentrations using the Daugirdas[23] equation. Average urea clearance was 50 mL/min.
**Volume = TBW volume estimated as weight in ks × 0.6.

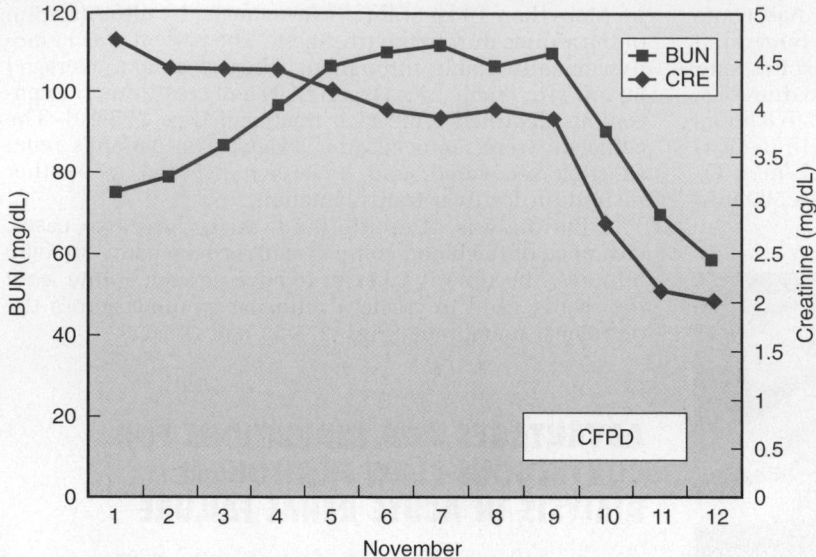

FIGURE 275-10. Evolution of blood urea nitrogen (BUN) and creatinine (CRE) concentrations in Patient 2, who has acute renal failure, with 3 consecutive days of treatment with continuous-flow peritoneal dialysis (CFPD).

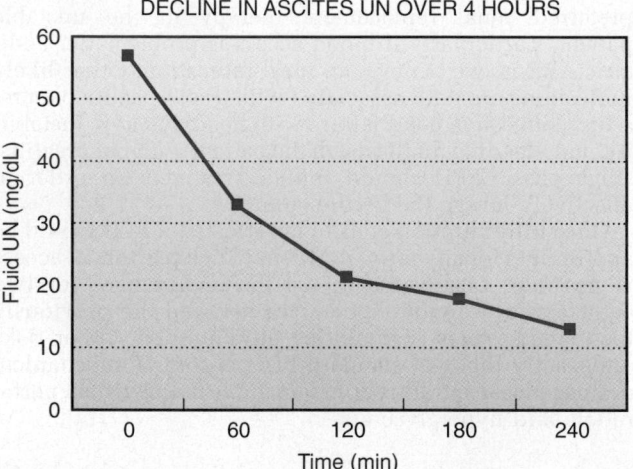

FIGURE 275-11. Decline in ascitic urea nitrogen concentration (UN) takes up to 60 minutes, delaying the onset of significant transperitoneal solute clearance.

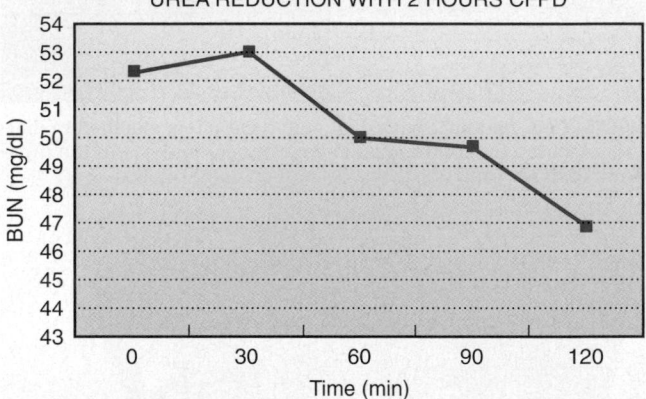

FIGURE 275-12. Decline in blood urea nitrogen (BUN) concentration with CFPD of ascites delayed due to need to lower ascitic UN.

issues will be worked out "in the field," and it is hoped that machine manufacturers will add modifications to permit CFPD. Sorbent-based dialysis systems could also easily be adapted, as could hemodiafiltration machines that manufacture sterile dialysate.[31] Use of CFPD in the outpatient setting is also being investigated but is beyond the scope of this text.

Key Points

1. The technique of traditional peritoneal dialysis underutilizes the transport characteristics of the peritoneal membrane. Continuous-flow peritoneal dialysis overcomes these limitations by maximizing transperitoneal solute gradients throughout the treatment cycle.
2. Continuous-flow peritoneal dialysis has been used clinically since 1965 but was replaced by the much simpler continuous ambulatory peritoneal dialysis approach.
3. Continuous-flow peritoneal dialysis offers considerable advantages over standard peritoneal dialysis in the treatment of acute renal failure, particularly in pediatric patients.
4. This modality requires a dual-lumen catheter (or two catheters) capable of delivering the high flow rates of peritoneal dialysate. Treatment mode can be either single-pass or recirculating, with external regeneration of dialysate.
5. Continuous-flow peritoneal dialysis has been used successfully for treatment of acute renal failure in both children and adults.

Key References

2. Korthuis RJ, Granger DN: Role of the peritoneal microcirculation in peritoneal dialysis. In Nolph KD (ed): Peritoneal Dialysis, 3rd ed. New York, Kluwer Academic, 1989, pp 28-47.

4. Shinaberger JH, Shear L, Barry KG: Peritoneal-extracorporeal recirculation dialysis: A technique for improving efficiency of peritoneal dialysis. Invest Urol 1965;2:555-565.
20. Amerling R, Glezerman I, Savransky E, et al: Continuous flow peritoneal dialysis: Principles and applications. Semin Dial 2003;16:335-340.
29. Sagy M, Silver P: Continuous flow peritoneal dialysis as a method to treat severe anasarca in children with acute respiratory distress syndrome. Crit Care Med 1999;27:2532-2536.

31. Ronco C, Amerling R: Continuous flow peritoneal dialysis: Current state-of-the-art and obstacles to further development. Contrib Nephrol 2006;150:310-320.

See the companion Expert Consult website for the complete reference list.

CHAPTER 276

Nursing Issues and Procedures in Acute Peritoneal Dialysis

André Luís Balbi, Estela Regina Pereira, Daniela Ponce Gabriel, and José Carolino Divino-Filho

---

OBJECTIVES

This chapter will:
1. Describe peritoneal dialysis routine procedures in the treatment of acute renal failure.
2. Support the indication for peritoneal dialysis as an option in the treatment of acute renal failure.
3. Reinforce the importance of the dialysis nursing team in the care of patients with acute renal failure treated with peritoneal dialysis.

Peritoneal dialysis (PD) is a continuous and simple renal replacement therapy; therefore, it should not be discarded as a therapeutic option for a selected group of patients with acute renal failure (ARF).[1-3]

There have not been many studies in the later medical literature evaluating the utilization of PD in ARF, and their results have been conflicting.[1,4-9] Chitalia and colleagues[8] have evaluated the use of two PD modalities, tidal and continuous, in patients with ARF who have mild to moderate catabolism. These researchers concluded that both modalities are reasonable options in relation to dialysis dose measured by the solute removal index (SRI) and to weekly urea clearance (Kt/V urea).

Phu and associates[7] reported, in a prospective study, that PD was not adequate in treating patients with ARF because it kept blood urea nitrogen (BUN) levels above 75 mg/dL and because the mortality rate was significantly higher in patients undergoing PD than in patients treated with continuous venovenous hemofiltration (CVVH). However, it is extremely important to note that in this study, the PD modality utilized was intermittent with the use of rigid PD catheters, manual exchanges, and very short dwell times, whereas the continuous venovenous hemofiltration used modern technology. This PD technique is not used anymore in the developed world or many of the developing countries, because automated PD (APD) with the use of permanent flexible PD catheters, closed and flexible PD systems, and automated cyclers are

now available. The technique and prescription mode used by Phu and associates[7] are naturally prone to significantly increase the rates of mechanical and infectious complications as well as to significantly reduce the efficiency of the therapy; therefore, this model should not be pursued in any country where flexible catheters and automated cyclers are available.

Peritonitis is the most common PD-related complication, with an incidence of 12% to 25% in the literature and a predominance of gram-positive microorganisms and fungi.[10,11] Among the mechanical complications, dialysate leakage occurs in less than 10% of cases and is usually due to the use of the catheter immediately after implantation.[8,9,12-14] Protein losses, even though significant, do not reduce serum albumin levels.[9,15]

Gabriel and coworkers[9] have demonstrated, in a prospective study with 236 PD sessions in 30 patients with ARF, that high-volume continuous PD (CPD) performed with a cycler and using Tenckhoff catheters is an effective therapy leading to adequate metabolic and volemic control. The prescription details and adequacy parameters are shown in Tables 276-1 and 276-2.

Because CPD is a continuous dialytic method, it must be performed by a multiprofessional team, with the practical aspects coordinated by the nursing staff.

PRACTICAL ASPECTS OF THE UTILIZATION OF PERITONEAL DIALYSIS IN ACUTE RENAL FAILURE

CPD can be initiated right after catheter implantation with exchanges being performed automatically by the cycler, or even manually, with an initial infusion volume of 1500 mL, with the patient in the supine position and the glucose concentration in the PD solutions varying (from 1.5% thru 4.25%) according to the patient's volume status and needs. With the use of these procedures, the occurrence of leakages is reduced. As Gabriel and coworkers[9] have shown, the flexible PD catheter can be implanted percutaneously

TABLE 276-1

Characteristics of 476 Continuous Peritoneal Dialysis Sessions in 30 Patients

Dialysate fluid/cycle (mL)	2000 mL
Inflow time	10 min
Dwell time	35-50 min
Outflow time	20 min
Duration/cycle	65-80 min
Total exchanges per session	18-22
Total duration of session	24 hrs
Total volume of dialysate per session	36-44 L
Flow rate	25-30 mL/min
Glucose (%):	1.5-4.25
With 14 bags	1.5
With 6 bags	2.0*
With 7 bags	2.5
With 3 bags	3.4[†]

*Mix of 1.5% and 2.5% glucose bags.
[†]Mix of 2.5% and 4.25% glucose bags.
Data from Gabriel DP, Nascimento GV, Caramori JT, et al: High volume peritoneal dialysis for acute renal failure. Perit Dial Int 2007;27:277-282.

TABLE 276-2

Parameters of 476 Continuous Peritoneal Dialysis Sessions in 30 Patients

PARAMETER	MEDIAN ± SD
Creatinine clearance per session	15.8 ± 4.16 mL/min
Urea nitrogen clearance per session	17.3 ± 5.01 mL/min
Prescribed Kt/V:	
Per session	0.65
Weekly	4.5
Delivered Kt/V:	
Per session	0.55 ± 0.12*
Weekly	3.85 ± 0.62*
Normalized creatinine clearance	110.6 ± 22.5 L/week/ 1.73 m² body surface area
Solute reduction index	41 ± 9.9

*Not significantly different from prescribed.
Data from Gabriel DP, Nascimento GV, Caramori JT, et al: High volume peritoneal dialysis for acute renal failure. Perit Dial Int 2007;27:277-282.

at the bedside, under aseptic conditions, with local anesthesia and light sedation, by a nephrologist. Besides providing dialysis parameter information, the cycler may also lower the incidence of peritonitis by reducing the number of connections and because it is a closed system.

The nursing staff provides continuous patient and catheter care support from the moment of catheter implantation throughout PD dialysis treatment time. The PD catheter must be monitored in regard to eventual bleedings, leakages, and signs of infection in the catheter exit site. The nursing staff also checks the dialysis prescription at initiation of the cycler or manual exchange session and monitors the infusion and drainage volumes, visual aspects of the drained effluent (clear, bloody, cloudy), and also any medication additions (for example, heparin, insulin, potassium) to the PD solutions.[16,17] Heparin is used whenever fibrin appears in the effluent and/or there is a problem with the infusion and/or drainage. Insulin and potassium may be added according to individual patients' needs.

According to the experience reported by Gabriel and coworkers,[9] with the utilization of automated high-volume CPD, the nursing staff is responsible, after a medical pre-

scription is made, for the daily setup of the cycler as well as for blood and drained dialysate sampling used for diagnostic and adequacy evaluations. A daily medical and nursing staff meeting for a global evaluation of each PD-treated patient is important, especially for planning the next hours of the PD session.

The systematic collection of blood and dialysate samples during and after the sessions enables evaluation of the prescription and quantification of the dialysis doses prescribed and delivered. The dialysate sampling may also help in the diagnosis of peritonitis. In the presence of peritonitis, the nursing team collects a specific drained dialysate sample for culture and white blood cell (WBC) count as well as performs daily monitoring of the evolution of peritonitis through observation of the patient's clinical condition (fever, abdominal pain), visual inspection of the drained PD fluid (looking for clearing), and PD effluent WBC count.

Some studies have extensively described the blood and dialysate sampling routine for laboratory analysis necessary for evaluation of the PD adequacy in ARF.[8,9] It is possible, through the use of CPD, to obtain a high weekly dialysis dose in the patient with ARF, as quantified by Kt/V urea and solute removal index. Gabriel and coworkers[9] have proposed (1) daily blood sampling for urea, creatinine, potassium concentrations as well as venous blood gas levels (pH and bicarbonate) and (2) sampling every 3 days for evaluation of total protein and albumin levels. Three daily dialysate samplings—performed every 8 hours, corresponding to the start, middle, and end of every PD session—of 3 mL each should be made in order to measure creatinine and urea levels. Furthermore, measurements of dialysate cell count, total proteins, and albumin as well as dialysate cultures may also be performed after sampling of the PD effluent every 3 days.

CONCLUSION

This chapter describes the feasibility and capacity of CPD as a dialysis option and the importance of nursing care in the accomplishment and success of this dialytic therapy for patients with ARF. In a selected group of patients with ARF, PD is capable of promoting adequate metabolic and volemic control, with low incidence of mechanical and infectious complications, when a flexible PD catheter, a cycler, and continuously high-volume PD solutions are used. The success of this procedure is fundamentally based on active participation of the nurses in coordination with the medical team.

Key Points

1. There are very few published studies on the treatment of acute renal failure with peritoneal dialysis and its modern technical developments.
2. Peritoneal dialysis is a therapeutic option for a selected group of patients with acute renal failure.
3. Peritoneal dialysis should preferably be performed with a flexible catheter (for example, Tenckhoff type) and an automated cycler.
4. High-volume continuous peritoneal dialysis should be the preferable dialysis option in the treatment of acute renal failure.

5. Nursing care throughout the dialytic treatment of acute renal failure is of utmost importance to the success of the therapy.

Key References

1. Gabriel DP, Nascimento GV, Caramori JT, et al: Peritoneal dialysis in acute renal failure. Ren Fail 2006;28:451-456.
3. Ash SR, Bever LS: Peritoneal dialysis for acute renal failure: The safe, effective and low cost modality. Adv Ren Replace Ther 1995;2:160-163.
7. Phu NH, Hien TT, Mai NT, et al: Hemofiltration and peritoneal dialysis in infection-associated acute renal failure in Vietnam. N Engl J Med 2002;347:895-902.
8. Chitalia V, Almeida AF, Rai H, et al: Is peritoneal dialysis adequate for hypercatabolic acute renal failure in developing countries? Kidney Int 2002;61:747-757.
9. Gabriel DP, Nascimento GV, Caramori JT, et al: High volume peritoneal dialysis for acute renal failure. Perit Dial Int 2007;27:277-282.

See the companion Expert Consult website for the complete reference list.

Extracorporeal Blood Purification Techniques beyond Dialysis

CHAPTER 277

Plasmapheresis in Critical Illness

John H. Reeves

OBJECTIVES

This chapter will:
1. Review the development of plasmapheresis as a therapeutic tool.
2. Explain the theory and rationale of plasmapheresis.
3. Examine the current role of plasmapheresis in critical illness.

Plasmapheresis is "the removal of blood plasma from the body by the withdrawal of blood, its separation into plasma and cells in a centrifuge, and the reintroduction of the cells suspended in a harmless medium."[1] Experts put forward alternative definitions for terms such as plasmapheresis and plasma exchange.[2,3] *Plasma exchange* is plasmapheresis in which the volume of plasma exchanged approaches or exceeds the estimated plasma volume. The general term *therapeutic apheresis* has now become favored. For simplicity, the term *plasmapheresis* is used generically in this chapter.

The aim of this chapter is to review plasmapheresis in critical illness, with an emphasis on those conditions for which proven benefit has been demonstrated in randomized controlled trials (RCTs). Novel techniques in which plasma is purified after separation from red cells and reintroduced to the patient are dealt with in other chapters.

HISTORY

The term plasmapheresis was first used in 1920 by G. H. Whipple and associates[4] in a landmark series of animal experiments investigating the pathophysiology of shock: "Bleeding a dog from a large artery and . . . simultaneous replacement of a red blood cell in Locke solution mixture may be called plasma depletion or plasmapheresis."

In 1952, plasmapheresis was introduced as a means of repeatedly harvesting plasma from human donors.[5] In the same year, plasmapheresis was attempted as treatment in a patient with multiple myeloma.[6] Five hundred milliliters of whole blood was removed and refrigerated for 24 hours. Plasma was decanted, and the erythrocytes were re-infused into the patient. The procedure had only minimal effects on the level of abnormal proteins. Successful treatment of Waldenström's macroglobulinemia with plasmapheresis was reported in 1960.[7]

Plasmapheresis was first reported as a treatment for hepatic coma in 1968,[8] for Goodpasture's syndrome in 1975,[9] for thrombotic thrombocytopenic purpura in 1977,[10] and for meningococcal sepsis in 1979.[11] By 1983, plasmapheresis had been evaluated for use in immune-mediated neurological diseases such as myasthenia gravis, multiple sclerosis, acute and chronic-relapsing Guillain-Barré syndromes, polymyositis, and dermatomyositis.[12] RCTs began to appear in the 1980s.[13-18] Important landmark studies are discussed here along with specific indications.

THEORY AND RATIONALE

The goal of plasmapheresis is the removal of pathogenic substances present in plasma. Putative pathogenic factors include autoreactive antibodies, immune complexes, paraproteins, lipoproteins, and inflammatory mediators such as cytokines.

Clearance

Clearance is defined as the volume of plasma from which a substance has been completely removed in a given time. Using a single-compartment exponential washout model, one can predict that a one plasma volume exchange should reduce the level of the substance by 63%. But the kinetics of plasmapheresis is more complex. In reality, there are at

TABLE 277-1

Relative Density of Blood Components

COMPONENT	DENSITY RELATIVE TO H_2O
Plasma	1.025-1.029
Platelets	1.040-1.045
Lymphocytes	1.050-1.061
Granulocytes	1.087-1.092
Erythrocytes	1.078-1.114

From El-Ghariani K, Unsworth DJ: Therapeutic apheresis—plasmapheresis. Clin Med 2006;6:343-347.

TABLE 277-2

Molecular Weight of Selected Plasma Components Removed by Plasmapheresis

SUBSTANCE	MOLECULAR MASS (Da)
Immunoglobulins	
IgM	900,000
IgG	150,000
IgA monomer	162,000
IgD	172,000
IgE	196,000
Coagulation Factors	
Factor VIII	$0.83-20 \times 10^6$
Von Willebrand factor:	
Monomer	280×10^3
Multimer	Up to 12×10^6
Fibrinogen	340,000
Factor V	330,000
Factors II, III, VII, IX, X, XII	$50-80 \times 10^3$
Antithrombin III	58,000
Protein C and protein S	$62-69 \times 10^3$
Inflammatory Mediators	
Tumor necrosis factor trimer	$(17 \times 3) = 51 \times 10^3$
Interleukin-1	23×10^3
Interleukin-6	23×10^3
C-reactive protein	110,000
C1 complement	900,000
C3 complement	185,000
Endotoxin (lipopolysaccharide)	10,000
Lipopolysaccharide-binding protein	$58-60 \times 10^3$
Shiga toxin	70×10^3
Other	
Cold agglutinins	450,000
Albumin	66,500

least two "compartments," intravascular and extravascular. Plasma levels may be maintained by ongoing synthesis and/or redistribution between compartments. For example, 80% of immunoglobulin (Ig) M is intravascular, compared with 45% of IgG.[19] One plasma volume (50 mL/kg) plasma exchange causes a 50% reduction in IgM levels, and three treatments reduce the IgM level by 80% to 90%.[20] In contrast, a significant proportion of IgG is extravascular, so its clearance by plasmapheresis is less efficient.

If the synthesis of pathogenic substances is supported by feedback mechanisms, extracorporeal elimination by plasmapheresis may simply drive ongoing production. In fact, when plasmapheresis is stopped, the accelerated production may result in rebound of plasma levels and increase in disease severity. There are examples of this phenomenon when plasmapheresis is employed in autoimmune disease such as systemic lupus erythematosus. Therefore, plasmapheresis must be combined with other treatments aimed at modulating underlying disease processes.

Separation of Plasma from Cells

Plasma is separated from cells by centrifugation, which is based on density (Table 277-1), or ultrafiltration, which is based on molecular size (Table 277-2). Continuous centrifugal plasma separators are usually employed by the hematology or nephrology service. Citrate is commonly used for anticoagulation. Large-pore hemofilters, called *plasmafilters*, are now being employed to separate plasma from the formed elements of the blood. Plasmafiltration uses technology (vascular access, pumps, and lines) developed for renal replacement therapy in the intensive care unit, and it is often initiated and conducted by staff in that unit. Anticoagulation is usually performed with heparin or low-molecular-weight heparin.[21,22] Plasmafilters have a pore size of around 0.3 to 0.5 μm (around 10 times as large as conventional hemofilter pores), which allow the ultrafiltration of molecules up to a maximum molecular weight of approximately 3×10^6 Da. The extent to which molecules are filtered is described by the sieving coefficient—the ratio of concentration of substance in the filtrate to that in plasma. Sieving coefficients for a number of substances during plasmafiltration have been published.[21]

Substances removed by plasmafiltration include all of the nonformed elements of the blood up to the specified cutoff molecular weight. In contrast, centrifugal separators have the capacity to remove larger molecules (e.g., unusually large multimers of von Willebrand factor in thrombotic thrombocytopenic purpura (TTP) and cellular components such as activated platelets and white blood cells. Discussion of cytapheresis techniques is beyond the scope of this chapter.

Replacement Solutions

There is no consensus regarding replacement solutions for plasmapheresis. Only one RCT has specifically investigated replacement solutions in plasmapheresis.[23] The ideal replacement solution regimen should (1) maintain normovolemia, (2) avoid significant reductions in plasma oncotic pressure, (3) avoid serious depletion of clotting factors, and (4) maintain normal plasma electrolyte concentrations. The choice of solutions includes crystalloids, semisynthetic colloids (hetastarch, gelatin, dextrans), human albumin solutions, liquid stored plasma, fresh-frozen plasma, and cryoprecipitate. The replacement solutions most commonly used are liquid stored plasma and human albumin solution. Reduction in circulating immunoglobulins caused by plasmapheresis may be a therapeutic goal or an unwanted side effect of plasmapheresis necessitating administration of intravenous immune globulin. In some diseases, the replacement solution may be as therapeutic as the plasmapheresis itself.[24]

Complications

The complications of plasmapheresis include those due to large-bore vascular access to the circulation, such as bleeding, infection, air embolus, and damage to local structures; those due to removal of important substances from the

TABLE 277-3

Indications for Plasmapheresis

EVIDENCE BASE	DISEASE	FACTOR(S) REMOVED
Accepted benefit	Cryoglobulinemia	Cryoglobulin
	Hyperviscosity	Paraprotein
	Thrombotic thrombocytopenic purpura (TTP)	Antimetalloproteinase
		Von Willebrand factor multimers
	Goodpasture's disease	Anti–basement membrane
	Pauci-immune glomerular nephritis	?Antineutrophil cytoplasmic antibody
		?Other factors
	Focal segmental glomerulosclerosis	Permeability factor
	Guillain-Barré syndrome	?Antiganglioside
	Chronic inflammatory demyelinating polyneuropathy	?
	Myasthenia gravis	Anti-acetylcholine receptor
Possible benefit	Renal allograft rejection	Anti-ABO, anti-HLA
	Paraprotein-associated neuropathy	Paraprotein
	Multiple sclerosis	Cytokines
	Hyperlipidemia	Low-density lipoprotein
Doubtful value	Systemic lupus erythematosus	Immune complexes
	Myeloma protein–induced renal damage	Paraprotein
Unknown	Sepsis	?Cytokines

From El-Ghariani K, Unsworth DJ: Therapeutic apheresis—plasmapheresis. Clin Med 2006;6:343-347.

plasma, such as coagulopathy from factor depletion and immunosuppression from reduced immunoglobulin levels; and those associated with replacement solutions, such as fluid balance errors, electrolyte and acid-base disturbances, and transmission of infection from blood products. During prolonged extracorporeal therapy, heat loss from the circuit can cause hypothermia. Finally, the extracorporeal circuit, plasmafilter, or centrifuge may damage platelets and/or activate complement, kinin/bradykinin, and other inflammatory pathways, causing hypotension and/or thrombocytopenia. Centrifugal separators may be more biocompatible than plasmafilters in this respect.[25]

OVERVIEW OF INDICATIONS AND EVIDENCE

Indications for plasmapheresis have evolved significantly over the past 25 years. The Canadian Apheresis registry published its experience of more than 100,000 plasma exchanges between 1981 and 1997.[26] In 1981, 55% of procedures were performed for five core indications—myasthenia gravis (MG), systemic lupus erythematosus, TTP, Guillain-Barré syndrome (GBS), and Waldenström's macroglobulinemia—and 45% were performed for other, miscellaneous diseases. By 1997, systemic lupus erythematosus had been dropped as an indication, and chronic inflammatory demyelinating neuropathy had been added. In 1997, the five core indications—MG, TTP, GBS, chronic inflammatory demyelinating neuropathy, and Waldenström's macroglobulinemia—accounted for 81.1% of procedures. An international registry for apheresis, begun in 2002, will provide more up-to-date information on treatment patterns and facilitate multicenter international RCTs.[27] Indications for plasmapheresis have been categorized according to efficacy by the American Society for Apheresis,[28] and this information has been summarized by El-Ghariani and Unsworth (Table 277-3).[20]

The evidence for therapeutic apheresis has been reviewed in extensive detail.[29] Shehata and colleagues[29] used a validated scale to score 88 controlled trials of therapeutic apheresis from 1 to 5. The average score was 2.64 ± SD 0.96. Studies scoring 2 points or less were more likely to report larger (perhaps exaggerated) treatment effects than studies scoring 3 points or more.[29] It was clear that there is still insufficient high-quality evidence for some of the common indications for plasmapheresis.

SPECIFIC DISEASES

Neurological Disorders

The use of plasmapheresis in neuroimmunological diseases has been reviewed comprehensively.[31,32] Only those diseases that may require management in the intensive care unit are discussed here.

Guillain-Barré Syndrome

GBS is an acute demyelinating inflammatory polyneuropathy preceded in many cases by an infective illness. *Campylobacter jejuni* is detectable in approximately one fourth of cases.[33] Lipopolysaccharides of *C. jejuni* isolated from patients with GBS have a ganglioside-like epitope, possibly provoking cross-reacting antibodies by molecular mimicry. Cytomegalovirus is the most common viral antecedent infection.[34]

GBS, possibly the best-studied indication for plasmapheresis, was shown to be superior to simple supportive care in two large French controlled trials.[23,35] The treatment groups became independent of mechanical ventilation more quickly, were able to walk unassisted sooner, and had a higher rate of full muscle strength at 1 year than controls. One of these studies also showed that replacement of discarded plasma with albumin was equivalent to replacement with fresh-frozen plasma.[23] In 1997, a dose-response study established that 2 plasma exchanges were superior to none in mild GBS, 4 plasma exchanges were superior to 2 exchanges in moderately severe GBS, but that

6 plasma exchanges were not superior to 4 in severe GBS.[36] Meanwhile, two large Dutch controlled trials showed that therapy with intravenous immune globulin was at least as effective as plasmapheresis in GBS.[24,37] Finally, it was shown that the combination of plasmapheresis and intravenous immune globulin was not superior to either treatment alone.[38] Currently, intravenous immune globulin is favored as initial therapy for GBS because of its lower risk of side effects.

Myasthenia Gravis

MG is an autoimmune disease associated with antibodies to the postsynaptic acetylcholine receptor (AChR).[39] It is characterized by muscle weakness and fatigability. Treatment includes thymectomy, acetylcholine esterase inhibitors, corticosteroids, immunosuppressants, and plasmapheresis. Plasmapheresis may be employed for acute myasthenic crises and in the perioperative care of patients undergoing thymectomy, but the evidence for these indications is limited. A systematic review[40] identified only one controlled trial of plasmapheresis in MG. In this review, there was no significant benefit when plasmapheresis was added to prednisolone for the therapy of MG.

Multiple Sclerosis and Acute Demyelinating Diseases of the Central Nervous System

MS is a relapsing inflammatory disease of the central nervous system. The pathogenesis consists of activation of self-reactive T cells that target the central nervous system and activate B cells and macrophages, causing the release of cytokines and antibodies and the activation of complement. Autoantibodies to myelin basic protein and myelin oligodendrocyte glycoprotein have been detected in some patients with MS. Immunoglobulins are synthesized predominantly intrathecally. An early trial of plasmapheresis in 54 patients with chronic progressive MS suggested a clinical benefit.[41] A subsequent larger trial (168 patients) compared three treatments—daily cyclophosphamide and prednisone, alternate-day cyclophosphamide/prednisone with weekly plasma exchange, and placebo medications combined with sham plasmapheresis.[42] There was no difference in outcome at 6 months among the three groups. In contrast, plasmapheresis may be beneficial in disorders involving acute demyelination of the central nervous system, such as acute disseminated encephalomyelitis (ADEM), that fail to respond to high-dose corticosteroids.[43]

HEMATOLOGICAL DISORDERS

Thrombotic Microangiopathies
Pathogenesis

TTP and hemolytic uremic syndrome (HUS) are microvascular occlusive disorders characterized by thrombocytopenia, microangiopathic hemolytic anemia, and systemic or intrarenal aggregation of platelets.[44] Patients with TTP present with fever, neurological symptoms, acute renal failure, thrombocytopenia, and hemolytic anemia. Patients with HUS often present with more marked acute renal failure and less severe neurological manifestations. Platelet aggregation in TTP is caused by the presence of unusually large multimers of von Willebrand factor in the circulation, due to a deficiency or blocking of the enzyme ADAMTS-13, which normally cleaves the multimers during synthesis and secretion of von Willebrand factor by endothelium. The abnormality in ADAMTS-13 is probably due to autoimmune antibodies triggered by infection. The pathogenesis of HUS is more complex. It usually follows infection with enteropathogenic *Escherichia coli* that produce Shiga toxins. Shiga toxins are absorbed across damaged gut epithelium into the circulation. They then bind avidly to receptors on gut, cerebral, and glomerular endothelia, where they provoke a complex inflammatory response that culminates in thrombocytopenia, hemolytic anemia, and acute renal failure. HUS is not usually associated with a decrease in levels or activity of ADAMTS-13.

Treatment

Mortality of TTP without treatment approaches 100%. Encouraging case reports of improved outcome with exchange transfusion and plasma infusion led to the performance of a large RCT by the Canadian Apheresis Study Group.[45] They compared treatment with aspirin/dipyridamole/plasma infusion to treatment with aspirin/dipyridamole/plasmapheresis. Outcome was better in the group that received plasmapheresis. However, patients in the plasmapheresis group received more than three times as much plasma (21.5 L vs 6.7 L), a difference that may have been important in replacing depleted ADAMTS-13. A smaller trial compared fresh-frozen plasma replacement with cryosupernatant plasma in TTP.[46] There was no significant difference in outcome between the treatment groups.

In contrast to treatment of TTP, that of HUS is generally supportive. Although Shiga toxins should be removed by plasmapheresis, HUS usually responds poorly to plasmapheresis.[47] Renal replacement therapy is used only as needed for patients who also have acute renal failure. Antibiotics are relatively contraindicated in HUS because they may release more Shiga toxins, increasing disease severity.

Thrombotic syndromes can develop secondary to other diseases, such as sepsis, transplantation, HELLP (hemolysis, elevated liver enzymes, and low platelets) syndrome, drug exposure, and pancreatitis, but the evidence for plasmapheresis in these settings is scant.[48] In the setting of severe sepsis, an acquired deficiency of ADAMTS-13 may be associated with the thrombocytopenia.[49]

Hyperviscosity Syndromes

Hyperviscosity syndromes are potentially life-threatening conditions. Patients may present with bleeding, visual disorders, neurological disturbances and congestive cardiac failure. The three categories of hyperviscosity syndromes are as follows:

- Pleocytosis, in which there is an excess number of formed elements of the blood, such as polycythemia rubra vera and leukemia.
- Sclerocitic, in which there is an abnormality in the deformability of red cells, such as sickle cell anemia.

- Sieric, in which there is an abnormality of plasma proteins such as myeloma, Waldenström's macroglobulinemia, and cryoglobulinemia. Symptoms occur when plasma viscosity is at least four times that of normal serum, corresponding to serum IgM level greater than 3 g/L, an IgG level greater than 4 g/L, or an IgA level greater than 6 g/L.[50] The intrinsic viscosity of IgM is great because of its high molecular weight and unique structure (five arms extending out from a central core).

The treatment of pleocytotic and sclerotic hyperviscosity syndromes may involve acute cytapheresis as well as specific therapy of the underlying disorder; further discussion of this issue is outside the scope of this chapter. Plasmapheresis has a central role in the acute treatment of dysproteinemias, but it must be followed by specific treatment of the underlying disorder. Waldenström's macroglobulinemia, characterized by elevations of serum IgM, accounts for 85% to 90% of sieric hyperviscosity syndromes. A 3-L plasma exchange with albumin replacement solution causes a 50% to 60% reduction in circulating IgM. Three to four treatments are usually given in the first 2 weeks, then one treatment per week until chemotherapy suppresses paraprotein production.[19]

Rheumatological and Nephrological Disorders

Both rheumatoid arthritis and systemic lupus erythematosus are autoimmune diseases that are modified by immune suppression, but RCTs of plasmapheresis have shown no benefit in either condition.[29] Renal allograft rejection is a significant complication of kidney transplantation. Plasmapheresis has been used in an attempt to remove anti-donor antibodies. Four RCTs have compared conventional anti-rejection therapy to standard anti-rejection therapy plus plasmapheresis; no overall treatment benefit was demonstrated.[29]

Rapidly progressive glomerulonephritis may be caused by Goodpasture's syndrome, Wegener's granulomatosis, microscopic polyarteritis, and other vasculitides. Pathogenic factors include anti–glomerular basement membrane (anti-GBM) antibodies, anti–neutrophil cytoplasmic antibodies (ANCAs) and immune complexes. Plasmapheresis has been combined with immunosuppressive drugs (cyclophosphamide and prednisolone) to accelerate the reduction of anti-GBM antibodies. In the only RCT of plasmapheresis for Goodpasture's syndrome, plasmapheresis with albumin and fresh-frozen plasma replacement was performed every third day until anti-GBM antibody levels were lower than 5% or patients were stable on hemodialysis.[51] A benefit for plasmapheresis was shown serologically and pathologically, the mean serum creatinine in the exchange group being less than half that in the controls. The evidence for plasmapheresis in rapidly progressive glomerulonephritis *not* associated with anti-GBM antibodies is less compelling. Only two of six RCTs showed a statistically significant improvement in renal function in patients randomly assigned to plasmapheresis.[29]

Sepsis and Multiple-Organ Failure

Severe sepsis is a generalized inflammatory response caused by infection. It has both cellular and humoral immune components. The deleterious effects of severe infection may be due to both the direct effects of bacterial toxins and the self-injurious effects of excessive generalized inflammation. Extracorporeal depurative techniques such as plasmapheresis are intuitively attractive for treatment of sepsis, because they potentially remove harmful endogenous (inflammatory) and exogenous (infective) factors. They may also constitute a form of immune modulation, smoothing out the peak concentration of inflammatory mediators in plasma.[21,52] Numerous case reports have been published describing the apparently salutary effect of plasmapheresis in sepsis. These early experiences were summarized in 2002 by Reeves[53]; more than 40 patients with severe sepsis (including meningococcemia) were given rescue therapy with plasmapheresis. The survival rate was more than 70%, although it had been expected to be less than 50%. A large case series of plasma exchange as rescue therapy in multiple-organ failure was published the next year. Stegmayr and colleagues[54] described 76 patients with multiple-organ failure, due in 66 to severe sepsis, who underwent plasma exchange by continuous centrifugation. Fluid replacement was performed with liquid stored plasma and anticoagulation therapy consisted of heparin. The observed survival rate was 82%, but these investigators did not estimate expected survival. Both of these studies were nonrandomized and therefore lacked contemporaneous controls.

Other researchers have proposed plasmapheresis as therapy for multiple-organ failure, especially when it is associated with sepsis and/or "secondary thrombotic syndrome."[48,55] One difficulty with such a proposal is obtaining a uniform group of patients to study in controlled trials. Multiple-organ failure is usually due to sepsis but may have a number of other causes as well. In the large series reported by Stegmayr and colleagues,[54] 10 of 76 cases of multiple-organ failure had nonseptic causes. Nevertheless, at least one controlled trial of intensive plasmapheresis in thrombocytopenia-associated multiple-organ failure in children has been published.[56] Ten patients with platelet counts lower than 100,000 cells/mm[3] and three or more organs failing were randomly assigned to conventional therapy with or without daily plasmapheresis until resolution of organ failure. Survival was higher in the treated group (5/5) than the control group (1/5; $P < .05$).

Two RCTs of plasmapheresis in sepsis have been performed. The first was a small study of continuous plasmafiltration in sepsis.[21] Thirty patients with sepsis syndrome were randomly assigned to receive protocol-driven intensive care support with or without 34 hours of continuous plasmafiltration, during which five plasma volumes were replaced with a mixture of fresh-frozen plasma and albumin electrolyte solution. The anticoagulant was heparin. There was no significant difference in mortality between the treatment group and controls, but there was a trend toward fewer organs failing in the treatment group. Several inflammatory mediators were assayed. All passed freely into the plasmafiltrate, but the plasma kinetics of most was not modified by plasmafiltration. Only the acute-phase response was significantly attenuated.

A larger RCT of plasmapheresis in sepsis randomly assigned 106 patients with severe sepsis and septic shock to conventional intensive care with or without plasmapheresis. Those receiving plasmapheresis underwent one or two plasma exchanges of approximately 30 to 40 mL/kg (just less than one plasma volume) in the 24 hours after presentation. Replacement solutions were fresh-frozen plasma and 5% human albumin solution. The anticoagulant was heparin. Eighteen of the 54 patients (33%) in the treatment group died, as did 28 of the 52 patients (54%)

in the control group ($P = 0.05$). Multiple logistic regression analysis showed there was a nonsignificant trend toward better outcome in the treatment group (odds ratio 0.41; 95% confidence interval 0.15-1.09; $P = .07$).

Results of both studies suggested a trend toward better outcome in the groups treated with plasmapheresis. There is a strong argument for a large trial of plasmapheresis in sepsis, but obtaining adequate albumin solution and fresh-frozen plasma for replacement solutions remains a significant barrier. Perhaps the future lies in reprocessing of plasma using techniques such as coupled plasmafiltration adsorption.[57]

CONCLUSION

Plasmapheresis is a major undertaking that should be reserved for severe illness. After encouraging results in individual cases, the only way forward is the performance of high-quality randomized controlled trials.[58] This step is difficult (but not impossible) with rare conditions and often requires international cooperation.[27] The questions that ideally should be addressed in relation to plasmapheresis in any specific illness are as follows:

- Is plasmapheresis efficacious?
- What is the correct dose?
- What is the correct replacement solution?
- Is membrane separation or centrifugal separation better?
- What form of anticoagulation should be used?
- Is there a simpler and safer therapy that works just as well?

These questions have been answered in only a small proportion of conditions currently treated with plasmapheresis, but they form a basis for ongoing research in this fascinating area.

Key Points

1. Plasmapheresis removes plasma containing pathogenic substances.
2. Blood components are separated by centrifugation or ultrafiltration.
3. Discarded plasma must be replaced, usually with a protein-electrolyte solution or donor plasma.
4. 80% of plasmaphereses are performed for the following five core indications: thrombotic thrombocytopenic purpura, Guillain-Barré syndrome, chronic inflammatory demyelinating polyneuropathy, myasthenia gravis, and Waldenström's macroglobulinemia.
5. New indications for plasmapheresis, such as sepsis and multiple-organ failure, merit investigation with large randomized controlled trials.

Key References

26. Clark WF, Rock GA, Buskard N, et al: Therapeutic plasma exchange: An update from the Canadian Apheresis Group. Ann Intern Med 1999;131:453-462.
29. Shehata N, Kouroukis C, Kelton JG: A review of randomized controlled trials using therapeutic apheresis. Transfus Med Rev 2002;16:200-229.
31. Lehmann HC, Hartung HP, Hetzel GR, et al: Plasma exchange in neuroimmunological disorders. Part 1: Rationale and treatment of inflammatory central nervous system disorders. Arch Neurol 2006;63:930-935.
32. Lehmann HC, Hartung HP, Hetzel GR, et al: Plasma exchange in neuroimmunological disorders. Part 2: Treatment of neuromuscular disorders. Arch Neurol 2006;63:1066-1071.

See the companion Expert Consult website for the complete reference list.

CHAPTER 278

Sorbents: From Basic Structure to Clinical Application

Dingwei Kuang, Chang Yin Chionh, Dinna N. Cruz, and Claudio Ronco

OBJECTIVES

This chapter will:
1. Describe the nature, structure, and composition of sorbent materials.
2. Characterize the mechanisms of the adsorption process.
3. Discuss the potential for the application of sorbents in extracorporeal blood purification techniques.
4. Summarize some of the advances achieved by the use of sorbents in specific clinical syndromes.

The possibility of removing solutes from blood to obtain blood purification has mainly focused over the years on classic hemodialysis. However, both the characteristics of some solutes that make their removal difficult and the limited efficiency of some dialysis membranes have spurred a significant interest in the use of further mechanisms of solute removal, such as adsorption.[1,2] Materials with high capacity for adsorption (sorbents) have been used for about 50 years in extracorporeal blood treatments. The evolution in knowledge and clinical use of sorbents can be summarized as shown in Table 278-1.

TABLE 278-1

Development of Sorbents in Extracorporeal Blood Therapies

1850	First inorganic aluminosilicates (zeolites) used to exchange NH_4 and Ca
1910	Water softeners using zeolites display instability in presence of mineral acids
1935	Adams and Holmes synthesize the first organic polymer ion exchange resin
1950	Application of synthetic porous polymers (styrene or acrylic acid–based) (Spherical beads: trade names Amberlyte, Duolite, Dowex, Ionac, and Purolite)
1960	Manipulation of physiochemical characteristics (commercial use)
1970	Application in blood purification techniques such as hemoperfusion
1980-2000	Improved design and coating for better hemocompatibility of adsorbent materials
2000 and beyond	Search for new sorbent materials and new possibilities of application

The analysis of the molecular structure of a sorbent as well as the study of the chemical and physical mechanisms involved in the process of adsorption are fascinating and may contribute to understanding of the potential for its clinical application.[3,4]

BASIC PRINCIPLES

The mixing of chemicals to form a mixture is a spontaneous, natural process accompanied by an increase in entropy or randomness. The inverse process—separation of that mixture into its constituent species—is not a spontaneous process and requires an expenditure of energy. If the mixture occurs in two or more immiscible phases, gravity, pressure or electrical fields may be used, but if it exists in a single homogeneous phase, different processes must be applied to achieve separation, such as:
- Phase addition or creation (distillation, crystallization, desublimation)
- A barrier (reverse osmosis, dialysis, microfiltration, ultrafiltration)
- A solid agent (adsorption, chromatography, ion exchange)
- An external field or gradient (electrodialysis, electrophoresis)

In clinical settings, blood purification techniques mostly rely on the second and third groups of processes.[4,5] Although diffusion and convection are used mostly for membrane filtration processes, adsorption is generally employed in blood detoxification techniques such as hemoperfusion. Diffusion may be limited by the diffusion coefficients of the molecules or by other factors such as temperature, surface area, and distance. Convection, on the other hand, is limited mostly by the sieving properties of the membrane and the flux of solvent obtained in response to a positive pressure gradient. When these processes are inadequate to remove the target molecules from patient's blood, the use of adsorbents may become the alternative pathway for blood purification. *Hemoperfusion* is in fact a technique in which patient's blood is circulated through a unit containing a sorbent material. Blood purification is obtained through adsorption of molecules onto the sorbent particles. Sorbents can be synthetic or natural.

In the past, problems related to hemoperfusion were due mostly to the incompatibility of the biomaterial used as a sorbent. The first sessions of hemoperfusion were accompanied by chills, fever, cutaneous rush, thrombocytopenia, leukopenia, and aluminum load. Today, these reactions are prevented in two ways: (1) separating plasma from red cells and circulating only the separated plasma through the sorbent bed, and (2) making the sorbent biocompatible or hemocompatible by coating the particles with specific biomaterials.[6]

While the use of sorbents is quite justified in poisoning or acute intoxications, there may exist a rationale for the use of sorbents in chronic or acute blood purification techniques.[7] The efficiency of membrane separation processes in hemodialysis is limited by membrane permeability. To overcome this problem, high-flux membranes have been introduced. However, the efficiency of such membranes for solutes of middle to high molecular weight is limited by the low diffusion coefficients of those solutes. A further improvement has come with hemodiafiltration and even better with on-line hemodiafiltration, in which the high rate of ultrafiltration significantly increases clearance of middle- to high-molecular-weight solutes. Nevertheless, the possible selectivity of adsorptive processes, and the possibility of placing the sorbent in direct contact with blood may be seen as further steps toward improving the efficiency of the blood purification process.[8] However, the sorbent must be hemocompatible and adequately coated. Also, size-dependent, nonselective adsorption may cause unwanted losses, and kinetics for middle to large molecules could be expected to be completely different from that commonly observed in hemodialysis.

To make an adequate adsorbent therapy, one needs an effective and safe sorbent material, an adequately designed sorbent cartridge, and, finally, optimal utilization of the available surface of the sorbent.[1]

MATERIALS AND STRUCTURE OF SORBENTS

Sorbents can be found in nature as raw materials or can be synthetically produced in the laboratory. Natural sorbents such as zeolites (aluminosilicates) are inorganic porous polymers with porosity deriving from their crystal structure (today they can be synthetically modified to control the structure of the internal pore system). Other typical sorbents, such as porous carbons, are cellulose-derived organic polymers prepared by controlled thermal oxidation (Fig. 278-1).

Synthetic sorbents are constituted by different polymers of synthetic origin. Almost all polymerizable monomers can be built up into large molecules via a multitude of reactions. Difunctional monomers tend to aggregate in linear polymeric structures, while highly functional monomers tend to polymerize in cross-linked structures. Divinylbenzene is generally used as a potent cross-linker (Fig. 278-2). Synthetic sorbents can also exist in forms of granules or fibers that are functionalized with specific substances (Fig. 278-3).

Sorbents exist in granules, spheres, cylindrical pellets, flakes and powder. They are solid particles with single-particle diameter between 50 µm and 1.2 cm. The ratio of surface area to volume is extremely high in sorbent particles,

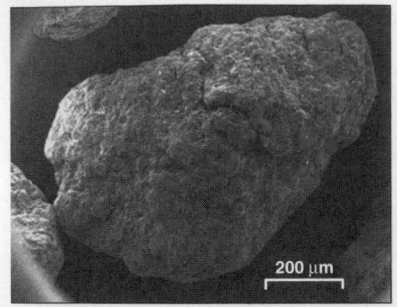
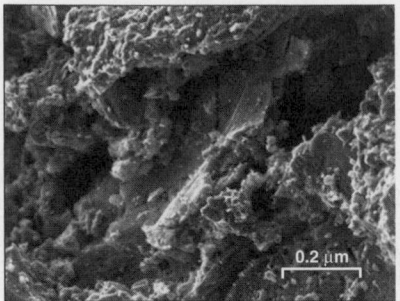
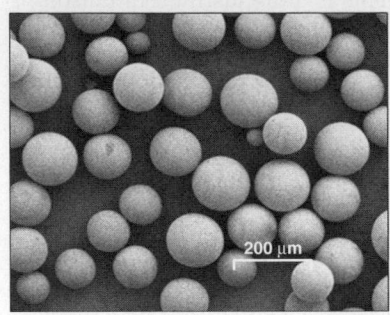
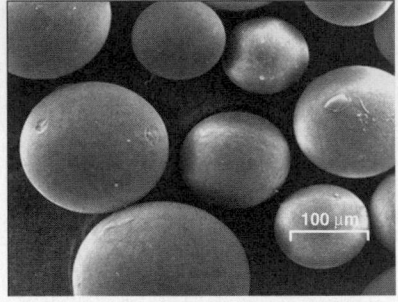

FIGURE 278-1. Scanning electron microscopic view of a natural sorbent (uncoated charcoal) at different magnifications (*top panels*) and of a synthetic polymer in granules (*bottom panels*).

SORBENTS

NATURAL	SYNTHETIC

Zeolites (alumino silicates)

Inorganic porous polymers with porosity deriving from their crystal structure (today synthetically made to control the structure of the internal pore system)

Porous Carbons

Cellulose-derived organic polymers prepared by controlled thermal oxidation

Almost all polymerizable monomers can be built up into large molecules via a multitude of reactions.

Difunctional Monomers

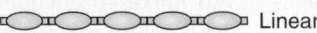 Linear

High Functional Monomers

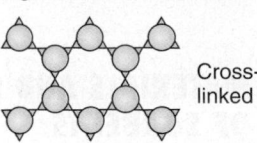

Cross-linked

Divinylbenzene (potent cross-linker)

FIGURE 278-2. Description of sorbent characteristics and distinction between natural and synthetic sorbents.

with a surface area varying from 300 to 1200 m²/g. They can also be defined according to pore size, as follows:

Macroporous: pore size >500 Å (50 nm)
Mesoporous: pore size 20-500 Å
Microporous: pore size <20 Å.

The ratio of surface area (S) to volume (V) is enormous and is generally described by the following equation:

$$\frac{S}{V} = \pi d_p L \left(\frac{\pi d_p^2 L}{4} \right) = 4 d_p \qquad [1]$$

where d_p is pore diameter and L is pore length. If ε_p is fractional particle porosity and ρ_p is particle density, the specific surface area per unit of mass (S_g) is expressed as follows:

$$S_g = \frac{4\varepsilon_p}{\rho_p d_p} \qquad [2]$$

For example, if:

$$\varepsilon_p = 0.5,$$

$$\rho_p = 1 \text{ g/cm}^3 = 1 \times 10^6 \text{ g/m}^3,$$

and

$$d_p = 20 \text{ Å } (20 \times 10^{-10} \text{ m}),$$

then

$$S_g = 1000 \text{ m}^2/\text{g}$$

In other words, one gram of sorbent material provides a potential surface for adsorption that measures 1000 m². Not all the surface is utilized, however, and many factors contribute to the fraction of surface used for adsorption in different conditions.

REQUIREMENTS FOR A SORBENT

A suitable sorbent material must have high selectivity or affinity to enable sharp separation and high capacity to minimize the amount of sorbent employed to make a commercial product. The sorbent should have a favorable

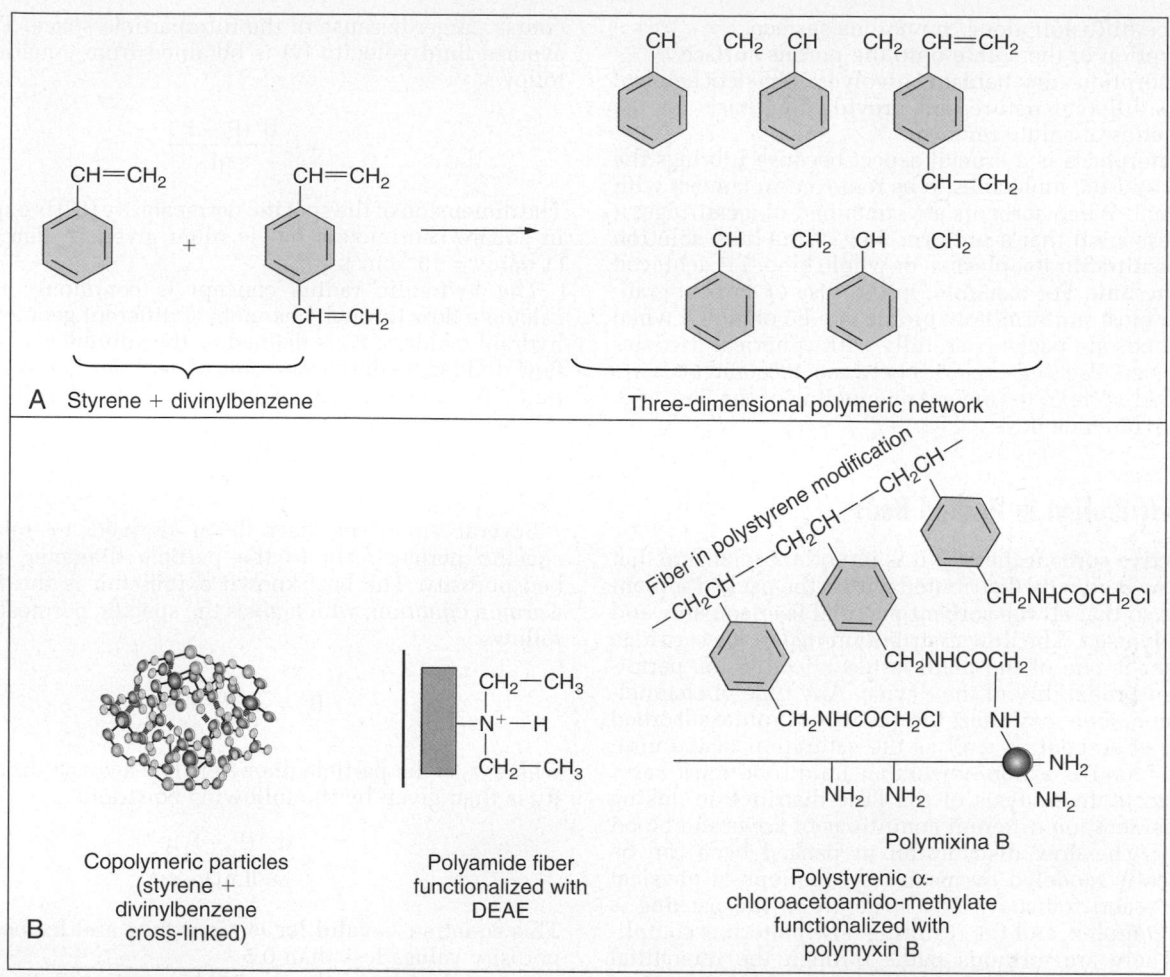

FIGURE 278-3. A, In most synthetic sorbents, styrene is cross-linked by divinylbenzene, forming solid gels in spherical or granular form (40 mm-1.2 cm). The characteristics are peculiar: ionic functional groups attached; typical moisture content (water saturated), 40-65 wt%; particle density, 1-1.5 g/cm³ (water swollen); bulk density, 0.5-1 g/cm³ when packed in beds; fractional bed porosity, 0.3-0.4. **B,** Other forms of synthetic sorbents can be generated beyond the mixture styrene-divinylbenzene (*left*); adsorbent materials can also be represented by polymeric substrates possibly functionalized with specific chemical substances, such as polyamide fibers functionalized with DEAE (diethylaminoethyl-) (*center*) and polystyrenic α-chloroacetoamide-methylate functionalized with polymyxin B (*right*).

kinetics and transport properties for rapid adsorption of the target solutes, chemical and thermal stability, low solubility in the contacting fluid, and mechanical strength to prevent crushing or erosion. In a sorbent cartridge made for clinical purposes, the material must have a free-flowing tendency for ease of filling and emptying of the packed bed, high resistance to fouling for long adsorption life, and maximal biocompatibility with no tendency to promote undesirable chemical reactions or side effects. Finally the sorbent must be cost effective, and the possibility of regeneration should be explored for possible multiple uses. Unwanted losses of hormones, proteins, and drugs when the sorbent is used must be identified and addressed as potential side effects. Adequate anticoagulation should also be scheduled to prevent clotting or platelet losses.

MECHANISM OF ADSORPTION OF SOLUTES IN POROUS MEDIA

For the adsorption of a solute onto the porous surface of an adsorbent, the following steps are required (Fig. 278-4):

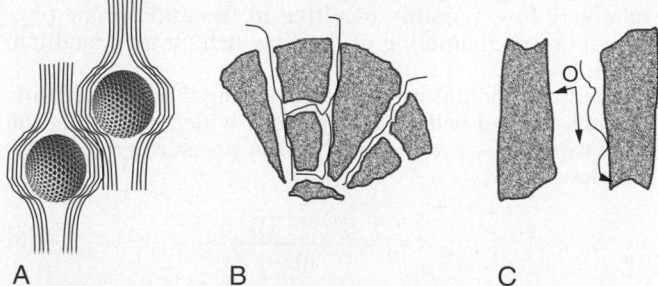

FIGURE 278-4. Mechanisms of mass transport from the bulk solution to the sorbent surface. **A,** External (interphase) mass transfer of the solute from the bulk fluid by convection through a thin film or boundary layer to the outer surface of the sorbent. **B,** Internal (intraphase) mass transfer of the solute by pore diffusion from the outer surface of the adsorbent to the inner surface of the internal porous structure. **C,** Surface diffusion along the porous surface and adsorption of the solute onto the porous surface.

1. External (*interphase*) mass transfer of the solute from the bulk fluid by convection through a thin film or boundary layer, to the outer surface of the sorbent.
2. Internal (*intraphase*) mass transfer of the solute by pore diffusion from the outer surface of the adsorbent to the inner surface of the internal porous structure.

3. Surface diffusion along the porous surface.

4. Adsorption of the solute onto the porous surface.

The adsorption mechanism involves physicochemical forces of different nature and provides the basis for the final kinetics of solute removal.[6,8]

The interphase is a crucial aspect because it brings the solution and the molecules to be removed in contact with the sorbent. When sorbents are contained in a cartridge, it is quintessential that a uniform flow of the bulk solution (it can be ultrafiltrate, plasma, or whole blood) is achieved inside the unit. For example, in the case of sorbent granules, the most uniform flow profile can be obtained when sorbent beds are packed carefully with spherical particles of equal size. Packing densities between 40% and 60% are considered optimal to prevent channeling of the flow and, thus, loss of efficiency.

Flow Distribution in Packed Beds

For effective sorbent therapy it is important to ensure that blood flow is equally distributed within the packed sorbent particles so that all the sorbent material is adequately and effectively used. The flow distribution inside the cartridge of sorbent is one of the main issues affecting the performance and reliability of the device. Any type of channeling phenomenon may affect the quantity of solute adsorbed per unit of sorbent as well as the saturation of the unit. Because blood is a non-newtonian fluid, one must carry out an accurate analysis of the flow distribution, taking into consideration different conditions of flows and blood viscosity. The flow distribution in packed beds can be theoretically modeled by means of equations of physical chemistry and transport. The structure of the packing is usually complex, and the resulting flow pattern is complicated. There are tortuous paths through the interstitial space of the bed, which consists of channels (pores) of various diameters. In well-packed beds, the diversity of channel diameters and velocities in the individual channels is small. In such cases, the packed bed can be approximated as a bundle of tortuous capillary tubes. In practice, some wide-diameter channels and gaps in the packing structure may be present, and the local flow velocity is relatively low, possibly resulting in the undesirable phenomenon of channeling of the flow, which may facilitate clotting.[9]

The fundamental principle governing the flow of fluids through packed beds is *Darcy's law*, which states that the flow velocity is proportional to the pressure gradient, as follows:

$$v_o = \frac{B^o(P_o - P_i)}{\eta L} \qquad [3]$$

Where P_o and P_i are the pressures at the outlet and at the inlet of the cartridge, respectively, η is the viscosity, L is the length of the conduit, B^o is the *specific permeability coefficient*, and v_o is the so-called *superficial velocity*, or the average linear velocity the fluid would have in the cartridge if no packing were present. Superficial velocity is calculated by dividing the volume flow rate by the cross-sectional area of the empty cartridge (specific permeability coefficient for open tubes is equal to $r^2/8$, where r is the radius).

The free cross section of the bed is expressed by the *interparticle porosity* (ε). Random packing of equal-size particles usually results in an ε value of 0.4 ± 0.03. The *total porosity* of beds packed with porous particles is, of course, larger because of the intraparticle space. The true average fluid velocity (v) is obtained from equation 1 as follows:

$$v = \frac{B^o(P_o - P_i)}{\varepsilon \eta L} \qquad [4]$$

The dimension of the specific permeability (B^o) is expressed in square centimeters but is often given in darcy units ($1\ \text{darcy} = 10^{-8}\ \text{cm}^2$).

The hydraulic radius concept is commonly used to calculate flow through channels of different geometry. The hydraulic radius, r_n, is defined as the volume available for flow divided by the surface area of particles in contact with fluid. The average flow velocity is expressed as follows:

$$v = \frac{(P_o - P_i)r_n^2}{2\eta L} \qquad [5]$$

Several equations have been derived to relate the specific permeability to the particle diameter and the bed porosity. The best known expression is the *Kozeny-Carman equation*, which gives the specific permeability as follows:

$$B^o = \frac{d_p^2 \varepsilon^3}{180(1-\varepsilon)^2} \qquad [6]$$

where d_p is the particle diameter. The average fluid velocity is then given by the following equation:

$$v = \frac{d_p^2(P_o - P_i)\varepsilon^2}{180 L \eta (1-\varepsilon)^2} \qquad [7]$$

This equation is valid for laminar flow and for beds with porosity values less than 0.5.

For packed beds, the Reynolds number (Re), which is dimensionless, is calculated with particle diameter substituted for tube diameter, as follows:

$$Re = \frac{\rho v d_p}{\eta} \qquad [8]$$

where v is the fluid velocity (cm/sec), ρ is the fluid density (g/cm^3), d_p is the particle diameter (cm), and η is the fluid viscosity (poise).

Turbulence and the transition from laminar to turbulent flow are not nearly as well defined in packed beds as in open tubes. It is assumed that turbulence in packed beds develops gradually as Re increases from 1 to 100. Actually, even at low Reynolds numbers, in packed tubes there is a lateral movement of the fluid elements as a result of stream splitting. At high flow velocities, this movement amounts to a substantial "convective diffusivity," which is analogous to the eddy diffusivity in turbulent flow. The flow profile can then be approximated as plug flow.

The most uniform flow profile can be obtained when beds are packed carefully with spherical particles of equal size. A ratio of the tube diameter to the particle diameter less than 100 may have a significant effect on the flow profile.

In commercial cartridges, the ratio of tube diameter to particle diameter is far from the above-mentioned ranges; the diameter of the cartridge is about 5 cm, and the diameter of the particle is around 1,000 μm. In some experimental analyses, the flow observed is quite close to optimal, and it can easily be compared to a plug flow with absence of channeling phenomena (Fig. 278-5). This results in an easy calculation of the saturation time and the maximal solute removal per unit of sorbent. From these data, the optimal amount of sorbent utilized in one unit can be calculated according to the treatment duration, the average concentration of the solute at the beginning of the session, and the volume of distribution of the solute in the body.

The internal mass transfer, or intraphase, can be seen as a convective transport of the solute through the structure of the sorbent. This once again depends on the packing density, the differential pressure, and the permeability coefficient of the particle. Very seldom this phase is fully optimized, and the sorbent is generally used only minimally, in part because of insufficient permeation of the bulk solution in the structure of the particle (Fig. 278-6).[9]

Finally, the physicochemical mechanisms regulating molecular surface adsorption are multiple. Once the molecule is brought to the surface of the sorbent, different chemical and physical forces are involved, such as van der Waals forces generated by the interaction between electrons of one molecule and the nucleus of another molecule; these are weak and generally reversible. Ionic bonds are generated by electrostatic attraction between positively charged and negatively charged ions; these are typical of exchange ion resins. Hydrophobic bonds are also present and generated by the hydrophobic affinity of the sorbent and the solute molecules (Fig. 278-7).

EFFICIENCY OF ADSORPTION

Porous polymers can be designed and constructed with varying internal surface selectivity and varying pore sizes so that molecules can be separated from one another on the basis of size, geometry, and individual binding properties.

To make a selective or partially selective process of adsorption, one must know the properties of the molecules to be separated or removed. If the information is lacking, the properties of the molecules under analysis can be ascertained by combining a number of available analytical measurements to develop an understanding of the molecular structures or by trial and error through adsorption iso-

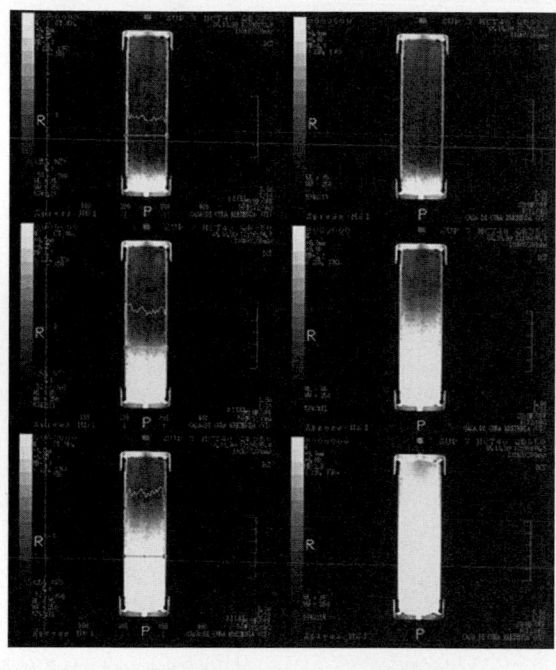

Q_b 250   Q_b 350

FIGURE 278-5. Computed tomography scans of a sorbent cartridge during injection of blood with contrast medium to study the flow distribution within the packed sorbent bed. Q_b, blood flow rate.

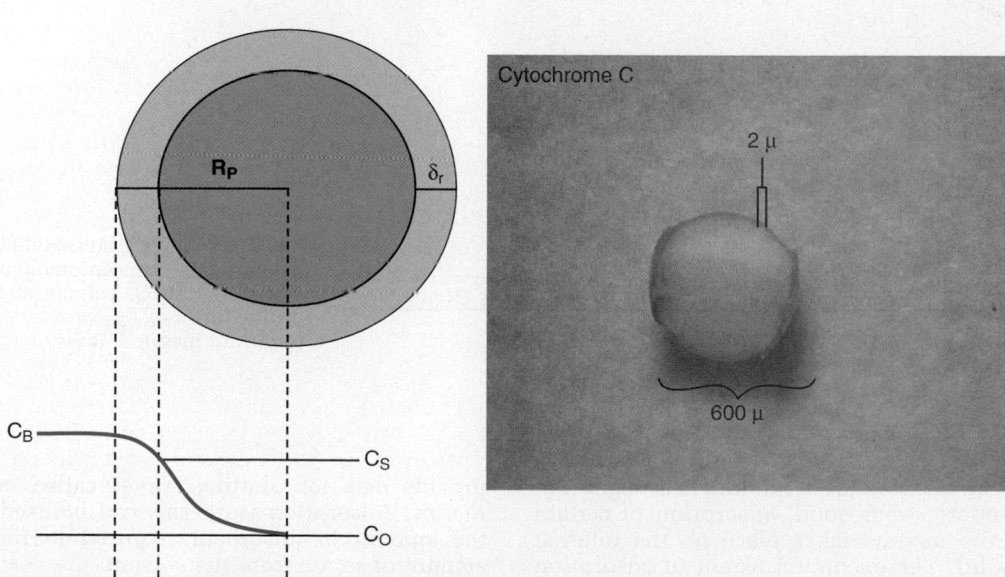

FIGURE 278-6. *Left,* The intraphase or internal mass transfer is described by the difference between the concentration of a solute in the blood (C_B) and the concentration in different internal zones of the sorbent particle (from C_S at the surface to C_O in the innermost zone); δr, surface penetration; R_P, radius of particle. *Right,* A practical example with cytochrome C in a sorbent particle. Surface penetration depends on surface shear rate, coating, hydration, and molecular diffusion coefficient. (Image on right courtesy of Dr. James Winchester, Beth Israel Medical Center, New York.)

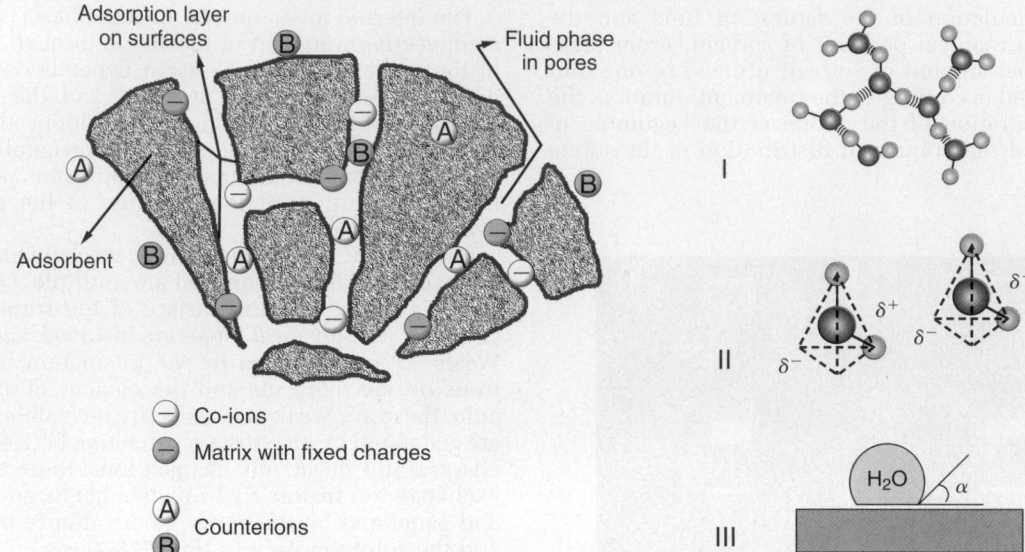

FIGURE 278-7. *Left,* Physicochemical mechanisms regulating molecular surface adsorption. *Right,* Once the molecule is brought to the surface of the sorbent, different chemical and physical forces play the final role: **I,** Van der Waals forces generated by the interaction between electrons of one molecule and the nucleus of another molecule (weak and generally reversible); **II,** ionic bonds generated by electrostatic attraction between positively charged and negatively charged ions (typical of exchange ion resins); **III,** hydrophobic bonds generated by the hydrophobic affinity of the sorbent and the solute molecules.

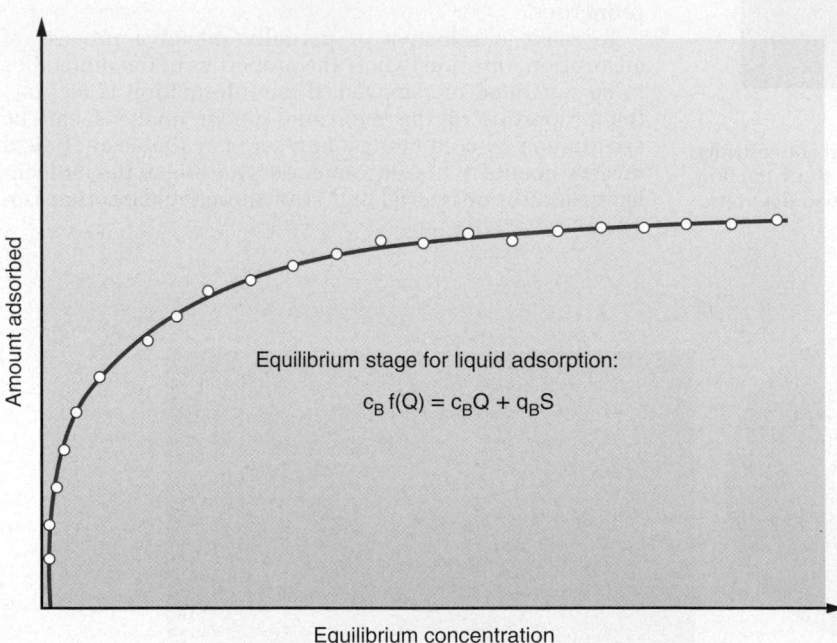

Equilibrium stage for liquid adsorption:

$$c_B f(Q) = c_B Q + q_B S$$

FIGURE 278-8. Typical example of an adsorption isotherm. c_B, concentration of solute in the carrier liquid; Q, volume of liquid (constant during process); q_B, concentration of adsorbate (mol/unit mass); S, mass of adsorbent.

therms (Fig. 278-8). When a liquid mixture is brought into contact with a microporous solid, adsorption of certain components in the mixture takes place on the internal surface of the solid. The maximum extent of adsorption occurs when equilibrium is reached. No theory for predicting adsorption curves is universally embraced. Instead, laboratory experiments must be performed at fixed temperature (separation processes are energy intensive and affect entropy) for each liquid mixture and adsorbent to

provide data for plotting curves called *adsorption isotherms.* Adsorption isotherms can be used to determine the amount of adsorbent required to remove a given amount of solute from the solvent.

Another measure of the efficiency of the unit is obtained through the use of marker molecules to determine the so-called mass transfer zone. The mass transfer zone is the portion of the cartridge length that goes from a fully saturated sorbent to a completely unsaturated condition. In

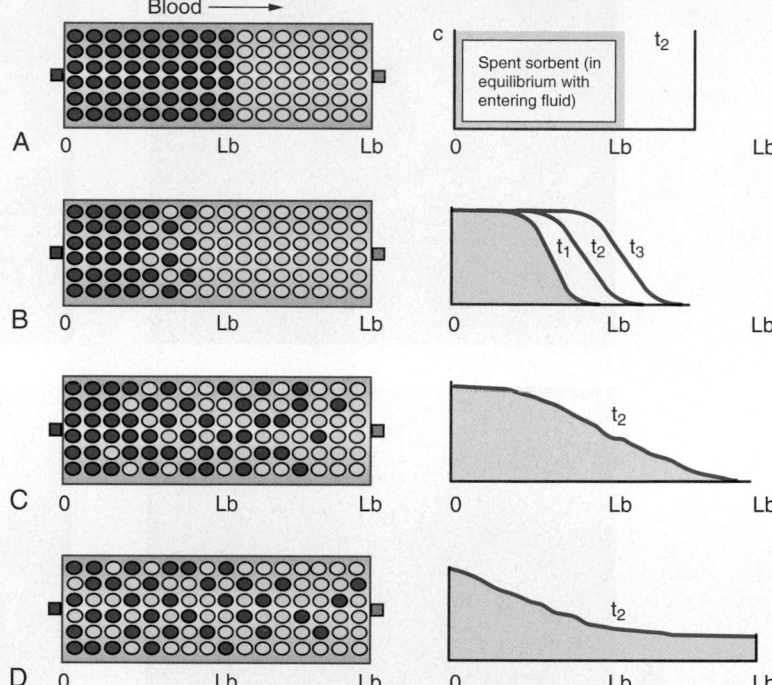

FIGURE 278-9. Evaluation of unit efficiency by determination of mass transfer zones. For this test, concentration of a colored marker molecule (c) is generally used. **A,** The mass transfer zone is near 0; and this is the ideal stoichiometric front for a fixed bed adsorption. **B,** Uneven concentration front builds mass transfer zones, but the dimension of each mass transfer zone at each time is less than 1/3 of the length of the unit (Lb). **C,** The mass transfer zone occupies the entire length of the unit; in this situation, the flow-through condition is obtained immediately after the beginning of the treatment. **D,** The mass transfer zone is larger than the length of the unit; this condition describes a poor design, the presence of channeling phenomena, or a sorbent material with poor efficiency and leads to typical breakthrough conditions.

Figure 278-9, different possibilities are described to define the characteristics of the unit. Determining the mass transfer zone also helps define the design of the unit and the expected duration of efficacy before saturation.

BIOCOMPATIBILITY OF SORBENTS

The biocompatibility of a system utilizing sorbents for extracorporeal therapies should be studied from different aspects. First, the sorbent must be resilient and must have a structure that prevents delivery of microparticles or fragments of the material. To further prevent dissemination of small particles in the body, cartridges contain a screen that allows free passage of blood but retains particles and their fragments (Fig. 278-10). A derivate measure of biocompatibility in this sense is given by the behavior of the end-to-end pressure drop in the unit throughout the treatment. Fouling of the screens due to cell or albumin trapping may result in greater resistance to flow and, thus, in an increased pressure drop inside the cartridge. Second, the intrinsic structure of the sorbent material must be determined; if the material comes into direct contact with blood, then it must be hemocompatible—that is, it must not cause unwanted reactions (from complement activation to cytokine release), leukopenia, thrombocytopenia, or adsorption of albumin beyond a certain limit. All of these effects can be partially prevented by coating the surface of the granules or the fibers with a biocompatible material such as polysulfone. The coating may render the sorbent less efficient, however, because it may negatively affect the intraphase component of the transport. To avoid this inconvenience, some techniques include a plasma separation process so that cells do not come into contact with the sorbent, the plasma is circulated through the sorbent bed, and, finally, blood is reconstituted after an extracorporeal single-pass treatment.[10]

RATIONALE FOR THE USE OF ADSORPTION IN CLINICAL SETTINGS

Is there a rationale for the use of sorbents in acute critical illness and kidney injury? The question has already been posed for patients with chronic kidney disease, and the answers are multiple: Assuming that the patient has a humoral disorder that depends on circulating molecules and that the final target of a therapy is to remove them, the process of adsorption seems to offer some specific benefits. The membrane separation processes (hemodialysis and hemofiltration) have limited efficiency owing to both molecule-dependent and membrane-dependent factors. In this case, an extra mechanism of solute removal in addition to diffusion and convection may provide extra efficiency. With an adsorptive process, selectivity or size exclusion can be included so that specific substances can be removed from the circulation. Also, in some cases the sorbent can be placed in direct contact with blood, facilitating the adsorption process. On the other hand, one must consider the limitations imposed by the use of sorbents, including the fact that sorbent must be hemocompatible or adequately coated to prevent reactions. Size-dependent, nonselective adsorption may cause unwanted losses; also, sorbents might alter the requirement for heparin in the extracorporeal circuit. Nevertheless, the use of sorbents in clinical practice offers some interesting advantages, some of which have already become evident.[2]

TYPICAL MODALITIES OF THE UTILIZATION OF SORBENTS

Typical modalities for the utilization of sorbents in extracorporeal therapies are represented in Figure 278-11.

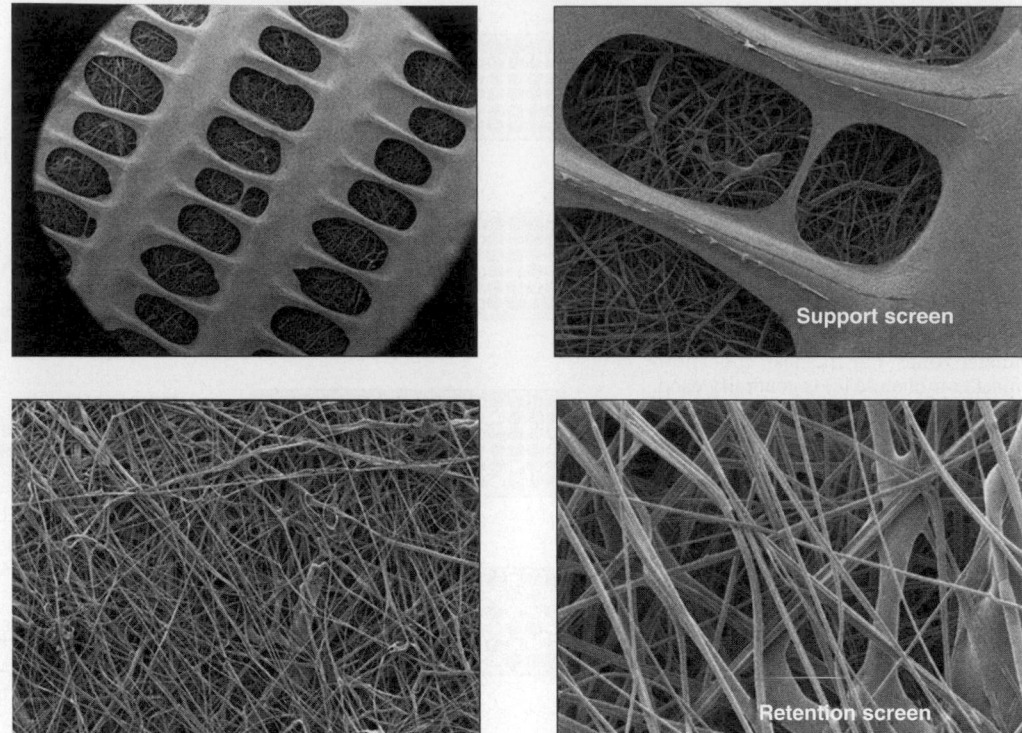

FIGURE 278-10. Screens are used in cartridges to prevent dissemination of sorbent particles and fragments into the circulation. *Top panels* depict support screens, and *bottom panels* depict retention screens. (Images courtesy of Professor P. M. Ghezzi.)

These techniques have been applied to the management of both acute and chronic renal failure.[11-16]

Hemoperfusion

Classically, hemoperfusion has been described as a technique in which the sorbent is placed in direct contact with blood in an extracorporeal circulation.[17] Hemoperfusion has the advantage of a much simpler circuit, but it requires a very biocompatible sorbent because of the direct contact with blood, particularly blood cells. Charcoal has a high adsorbing capacity, especially for low-molecular-weight waste products that accumulate during kidney or liver failure. Its use in hemoperfusion, however, requires a coating of the sorbent surface to make it biocompatible. Coated charcoal, although biocompatible, has a remarkably reduced adsorptive capacity owing to the cutoff of the coating material. Synthetic polymers have been introduced that have remarkable capacity for adsorption. The size selectivity is determined only by the size of the pores on the surface of the granular elements, not by the material itself. Nevertheless, specific advantages of such polymers have been experimentally demonstrated in the removal of poisons, cytokines, and even endotoxins. For specific types of hemoperfusion, consult the relevant chapters in this book.

Hemoperfusion Coupled with Hemodialysis

Sorbents have also been used in conjunction with hemodialysis (hemoperfusion-hemodialysis [HPHD]). In this modality, the sorbent unit is placed in series with the dialyzer, just ahead of it.[18] The reason for this placement is that the dialyzer adjusts for temperature or other abnormalities induced by the sorbent (e.g., acidosis). In this setting, the sorbents are hemocompatible and they are mostly utilized in the attempt to remove molecules such as β_2-microglobulin, which are poorly removed by dialysis.

Another approach consists of the use of sorbents in "uncoated" form. These, however, cannot be placed in direct contact with whole blood, so they are used for the on-line treatment of the ultrafiltrate or the plasmafiltrate.

Double-Chamber Hemodiafiltration

With double-chamber hemodiafiltration, plasma water is separated from whole blood, and after passing through the sorbent, the plasma water is re-infused into the blood circuit to reconstitute the- whole blood structure.[19] This technique has mostly been used in chronic dialysis as a particular form of hemodiafiltration.

Coupled Plasmafiltration-Adsorption

Coupled plasmafiltration-adsorption (CPFA) is a modality of blood purification in which plasma is separated from whole blood and circulated in a sorbent cartridge. After the sorbent unit, plasma is returned to the blood circuit, and the whole blood undergoes hemofiltration or hemodialysis.[12] The rationale of this modality is to attempt adequate removal of molecules that are not removed by other

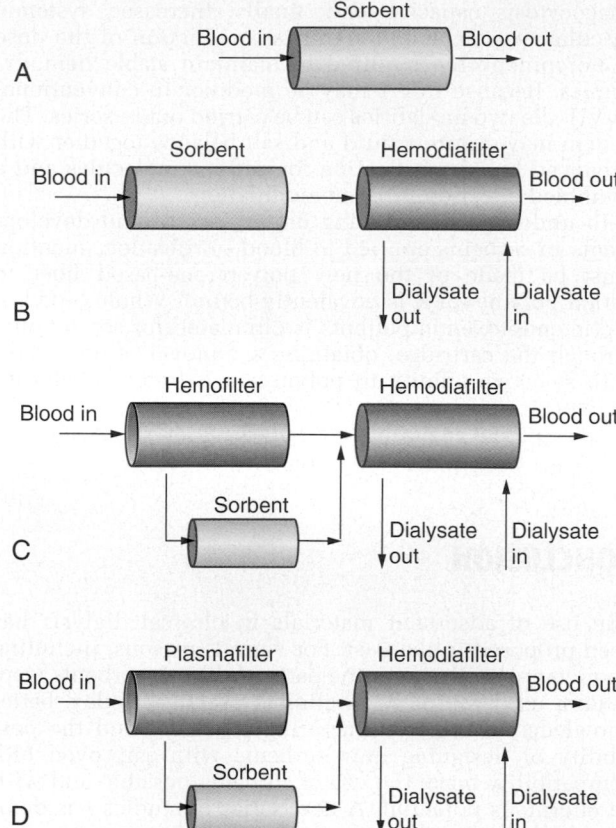

FIGURE 278-11. Possible modes of sorbent application. **A,** Hemoperfusion (HP). **B,** In hemoperfusion-hemodialysis (HPHD), the sorbent unit is placed in series before the hemodialyzer. **C,** The sorbent unit is placed on-line in the ultrafiltrate produced from a hemofilter. The hemofilter is placed in series with the hemodialyzer. The system, used for on-line hemodiafiltration in patients undergoing long-term treatment, is called paired filtration dialysis with sorbent (HFR). **D,** The sorbent unit is placed on-line in the plasmafiltrate produced from a plasmafilter. The plasmafilter is placed in series with the hemodiafilter. The system, which is used for critically ill patients with septic shock, is called coupled plasmafiltration-adsorption (CPFA).

hemofiltration or hemodialysis techniques. The advantages are that the blood cells do not come into contact with the sorbent and that endogenous plasma can be re-infused after undergoing nonselective simultaneous removal of different sepsis-associated mediators, so there is no need for donor plasma. One must balance the sparing effect of this modality on endogenous plasma compared with the potential unwanted losses of autologous plasma compounds.

This technique has mostly been used in septic patients,[11,12] in whom it has shown specific advantages of blood purification, restoration of hemodynamics, and immunomodulation (refer to relevant chapter in this book).

In another technique using uncoated sorbents (detoxification-plasmafiltration [DTPF], HemoCleanse, Inc., West Lafayette, IN), a hemodiabsorption mechanism is associated with a push-pull plasmafiltration system (a suspension of powdered sorbents surrounding 0.5-μm plasma

filter membranes). Bidirectional plasma flow (at 80-100 mL/min) across the plasmafiltration membrane provides direct contact between plasma proteins and powdered sorbents as well as clearance of cytokines (tumor necrosis factor-α [TNF-α], interleukin-1β [IL-1β], and IL-6.[20-22]

A major criticism may be raised concerning the removal of beneficial substances or drugs through the mechanism of adsorption. Reiter and colleagues[23] assessed different adsorptive properties of a hydrophobic resin for the most commonly used antibiotics. Except for vancomycin, for which a modest removal was observed, the levels of antibiotics such as tobramycin or amikacin tended to remain stable over time.

SORBENTS IN SEPSIS

Efficiency and adequacy of treatment, known milestones in the extracorporeal treatment for chronic renal failure, are now being reconsidered in critical care nephrology. The complex scenario of sepsis must not be underestimated. Nevertheless, 20 years or so after the first descriptions, we all face a disease with an ever-rising incidence and unacceptably high mortality. Innovative techniques address the importance of dedicated extracorporeal systems for sepsis, in which acute renal failure is just one of the pathologic complications. This wider approach to the concept of blood purification opens new perspectives in a revisited strategy for the application of extracorporeal treatments.

The cellular and humoral responses of the host to bacterial invasion result in a series of symptoms and organ derangements that are affected by the presence of chemical mediators. Continuous renal replacement therapies have gained greater popularity for their ability to ensure the removal of excess fluid and waste products in septic patients with acute kidney injury. However, removal rates and clearances of the different pro-inflammatory cytokines (IL-1, TNF) and lipid mediators (platelet-activating factor) are hindered by poor membrane passage.

Innovative approaches include high-volume hemofiltration and the use of superpermeable membranes. The latter are still under investigation for possible excess leakage of albumin. Plasmafiltration techniques have shown an increase in TNF clearance by two orders of magnitude and have demonstrated some improved survival in septic animals. However, plasmapheresis can hardly be regarded as a continuous renal replacement therapy.

The combined requirements of a continuous renal replacement therapy with high sieving capacity and possible selective removal of sepsis-associated mediators seem to find an answer in the application of sorbents. The most interesting experience with sorbents in sepsis has been with CPFA. This modality has been utilized with the rationale of re-infusing endogenous plasma after nonselective simultaneous removal of different sepsis-associated mediators without the need for donor plasma. In vitro studies demonstrated that removal rates of cytokines differed according to the sorbent tested. More importantly, when sorbents were tested at different linear velocities, their efficiencies in removing cytokines greatly exceeded the mass of individual cytokines calculated on the basis of the highest levels detected in the plasma of septic patients.

In rabbits injected with lipopolysaccharide, CPFA resulted in a significantly higher survival (85%) ($P = .0041$)

at 72 hours than was seen in rabbits not treated with coupled plasmafiltration-adsorption.[24] It must be emphasized that the overall net effect on survival could be due to the removal not only of the TNF or platelet-activating factor but also of many other mediators not monitored in the study.

In a prospective randomized crossover trial aimed at comparing clinical and biological effects of CPFA and continuous venovenous hemofiltration (CVVH) in critically ill septic patients, significant improvements were observed after 10 hours of CPFA. Despite the fact that all patients had relatively low plasma concentrations of cytokines (TNF-α, IL-1β), the sorbent adsorbed almost 100% of the cytokines in the plasmafiltrate. In all patients at the start of the treatment, the in vitro TNF production of circulating monocytes to exogenous lipopolysaccharide was remarkably impaired in relation to monocytes from healthy subjects. When the same patient was studied after 5 and 10 hours treatment with CPFA, the ability of monocytes to produce TNF-α was restored in the range seen for normal monocytes. Co-incubation experiments with a monoclonal antibody directed against IL-10 could abrogate (60%) monocyte unresponsiveness. In CVVH, abrogation of monocyte unresponsiveness was only partial compared with CPFA and occurred significantly later (after 10 hours of treatment). At the hemodynamic level, all patients (Acute Physiology and Chronic Health Evaluation [APACHE] score >20) showed greater peripheral vascular resistances that allowed a significant reduction in the dose of vasopressor drugs after 5 hours of CPFA and remained steadily low after 10 hours. The reduction of vasopressor drugs was not observed in patients undergoing CVVH. These data suggest that CPFA may ensure better hemodynamics in highly unstable patients than CVVH. Because CPFA may be modular to conventional CVVH, the former system may ensure a fluid and salt balance together with enhanced blood purification.

In the concept of using extracorporeal therapies for sepsis, there has been a widespread tendency to remove "bad factors" rather than to attempt to bring about a restoration of balance of physiological factors. Often, too much emphasis has been put on individual markers. The results obtained with CPFA suggest that treatments should focus more carefully on a "balancing hypothesis" in an attempt to restore a correct equilibrium between immunological suppression and activation.

The results obtained in clinical practice were in fact the basis for the formulation of the "peak concentration hypothesis" and to offer a possible explanation of the beneficial effects of sorbents in septic patients. The unselective but continuous removal of the peak concentrations of both pro-inflammatory and anti-inflammatory mediators may in fact lead to a kind of immunomodulation with partial restoration of the immunohomeostasis.

The rationale for exposing the plasma to the sorbent in a plasmafiltration system is to exclude the blood cells from contact with the sorbent and to re-infuse endogenous plasma after it has undergone nonselective simultaneous removal of different sepsis-associated mediators without the need for donor plasma. The main issue concerns balancing the sparing effect of CPFA on endogenous plasma as compared with potential unwanted losses of autologous plasma compounds.

The major advantages of CPFA can be summarized as a restoration of cell responsiveness to exogenous lipopolysaccharides, improvement of the pathological apoptosis detected in sepsis, improved HLA-DR expression as a measure of the immunoresponse of the patient, improved

phagocytosis capacity, and, finally, increased systemic vascular resistance and significant reduction of the dose of norepinephrine required to maintain stable hemodynamics. Because CPFA may be modular to conventional CVVH, the two modalities can be carried out in series. The system may ensure a fluid and salt balance together with enhanced blood purification for various molecules and a combined effect on immunomodulation.

To underline the growing importance of and developments in sorbents applied to blood purification, mention must be made of the new polystyrene-based fiber to which polymyxin B is covalently bound. Whole blood of septic endotoxemic patients is circulated for some hours through the cartridge, obtaining a removal of endotoxin with selective affinity to polymyxin B (refer to relevant chapter).

New sorbent materials are appearing on the scene and will soon be available for clinical trials.[25]

CONCLUSION

The use of adsorbent materials in clinical dialysis has been proposed in the past. For various reasons, including poor compatibility with the patient's blood, sorbents were seldom used routinely in clinical practice. Today, better knowledge of the manufacturing processes and the possibility of designing new sorbents with improved biocompatibility make the use of sorbents possible and with an enormous potential. A new series of studies has demonstrated the feasibility, safety, and advantages of using sorbent alone or in combination with other techniques. The future should see further developments in this area.

Key Points

1. Conventional extracorporeal treatments have some limitations in capacity to remove protein-bound compounds or solutes in the molecular range beyond the membrane cutoff. For this reason, in addition to diffusion and convection, the classic mechanisms used in membrane separation processes, adsorption is used to remove solutes from the circulating blood.

2. Natural and synthetic sorbents are used in clinical practice. They must have high selectivity/affinity to enable sharp separation, high and rapid capacity of adsorption, chemical and thermal stability, low solubility in the contacting fluid, mechanical strength to prevent crushing and erosion, resistance to fouling, and good biocompatibility.

3. Different chemical and physical forces are involved in adsorption, including van der Waals forces generated by atomic and molecular interactions, ionic bonds generated by electrostatic forces, and hydrophobic bonds.

4. Sorbents can be applied in different modes depending on the technique: A) Hemoperfusion (HP), where there is direct contact of the sorbent with blood. B) Hemoperfusion-hemodialysis

(HPHD), in which the sorbent unit is placed in series before the hemodialyzer. C) Paired filtration dialysis with sorbent, in which the sorbent unit is placed on-line in the ultrafiltrate obtained from a hemofilter. D) Coupled plasmafiltration adsorption (CPFA), in which the sorbent unit is placed on-line in the plasmafiltrate produced from a plasmafilter.

Key References

21. Tetta C, Cavaillon JM, Schulze M, et al: Removal of cytokines and activated complement components in an experimental model of continuous plasmafiltration coupled with sorbent adsorption. Nephrol Dial Transplant 1998;13:1458-1464.

22. Menegatti E, Ronco C, Winchester JF, et al: Absence of NF-kB activation by a new polystyrene-type adsorbent designed for hemoperfusion. Blood Purif 2005;23:91-98.
23. Reiter K, Bordoni V, Dall'Olio G, et al: In vitro removal of therapeutic drugs with a novel adsorbent system. Blood Purif 2002;20:380-388.
24. Tetta C, Gianotti L, Cavaillon JM, et al: Coupled plasma filtration adsorption in a rabbit model of endotoxic shock. Crit Care Med 2000;28:1526-1533.
25. Winchester JF, Ronco C, Brady JA, et al: The next step from high-flux dialysis: Application of adsorbent technology. Blood Purif 2002;20:81-86.

See the companion Expert Consult website for the complete reference list.

CHAPTER 279

Hemoperfusion

Rafael Ponikvar

OBJECTIVES

This chapter will:
1. Define hemoperfusion.
2. Discuss the use of sorbents in hemoperfusion.
3. Describe the indications for hemoperfusion.

Since 1960, sorbents (activated charcoal and ion exchange resin) have been used for the removal of uremic toxins, hepatic toxins, drugs, and chemical poisons.[1,2]

Hemoperfusion is the extracorporeal procedure in which the anticoagulated patient's blood passes through a column that contains adsorbent material. A hemodialysis monitor with blood lines is commonly used to bring blood to the hemoperfusion column and back to the patient. The anticoagulant used is usually heparin (to achieve whole blood clotting time between 20 and 30 minutes). Citrate can offer advantages over heparin—no systemic anticoagulation, less platelet activation, and better biocompatibility. Vascular access is achieved by either a double-lumen catheter or two single-lumen hemodialysis catheters; in patients in the intensive care unit, use of the femoral vein could be preferable. Blood flow is usually set at 250 to 300 mL/min, and hemoperfusion is performed for about 4 hours, when saturation of the column occurs. Transient leukopenia (complement activation), thrombocytopenia, hypocalcemia, and hypoglycemia are common side effects of hemoperfusion. In order to avoid hypocalcemia, metabolic acidosis, hypoglycemia, and hypothermia, simultaneous performance of hemoperfusion and hemodialysis is a better choice than hemoperfusion alone (Fig. 279-1).

SORBENTS

Formerly, hemoperfusion devices consisted of activated charcoal, ion-exchange resins, or non-ionic macroporous resins. Early hemoperfusion systems contained uncoated activated charcoal; because of incompatibility, they are no longer in clinical use. Most of the currently used hemoperfusion devices use coated activated charcoal. Granular charcoal is coated with cellulose nitrate (collodion), albumin, or heparin; extruded charcoal is coated with cellulose acetate (e.g., Adsorba, Gambro AB, Stockholm) (Fig. 279-2) or with methacrylic hydrogel (e.g., Hemacol, Smith, and Nephew, London); spherical charcoal is derived from petroleum and is coated with polyhema solution (e.g., Hemosorba, Asahi Medical, Tokyo). Clinically used charcoal devices contain up to 500 g of sorbent with large surface areas, about 1000 m²/g. The solute enters the coating membrane and then proceeds through the macropores (radius ≥500 Å) and is trapped in the mesopores (radius 20-500 Å) and micropores (radius <20 Å). Binding of the solute to the charcoal is irreversible.

Ion-exchange resins may be used as adsorbents because they exchange one ion for another. Their drawback is that they also remove calcium, magnesium, and potassium from plasma. The non-ionic resins consist of macroporous cross-linked polystyrene Amberlite material (e.g., XAD-2, XAD-4), which is formed into beads by agglomeration of microspheres. Surface area of these resins is about 300 to 500 m^2/g. Adsorption is more reversible with resins than with activated charcoal.[3] Some currently available hemoadsorption columns are listed in Table 279-1.

INDICATIONS FOR HEMOPERFUSION

Poisoning

One of the most important indications for hemoperfusion, the treatment of poisoning with drugs and chemicals, is described in detail elsewhere in this book.

Uremia

In 1964, when dialysis technology and technique were rather undeveloped, Yatzidis[1] introduced charcoal hemoperfusion for removal of uremic compounds from the blood of uremic patients. Unfavorable side effects of hemoperfusion and the efficient elimination of uremic toxins by modern dialysis eliminated hemoperfusion from clinical use in patients with uremia.

Hepatic Encephalopathy

The first use of charcoal hemoperfusion to treat fulminant hepatic failure with encephalopathy had promising results,[4] although in a small group of patients.[5] However, O'Grady and colleagues[6] conducted two randomized controlled trials that did not find any difference in the survival rate between patients with 5 hours and 10 hours of daily charcoal hemoperfusion (survival rate was 51.3% vs. 50.0%, respectively) as well as no difference in survival rate between patients receiving no hemoperfusion and those receiving 10 hours of daily charcoal hemoperfusion (survival rate was 39.3% vs. 34.5% respectively).[6] Accord-

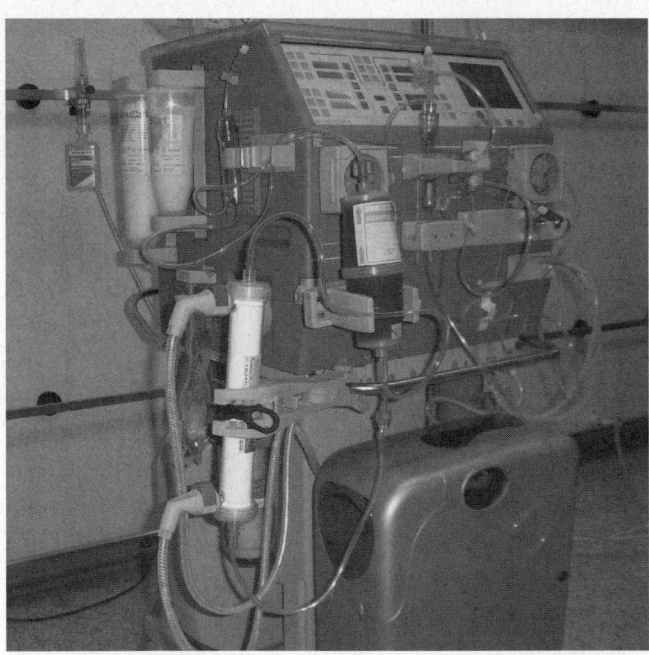

FIGURE 279-1. Charcoal column and dialyzer connected in series, using a hemodialysis monitor together with a portable water softener and reverse osmosis, prepared for use in the intensive care unit.

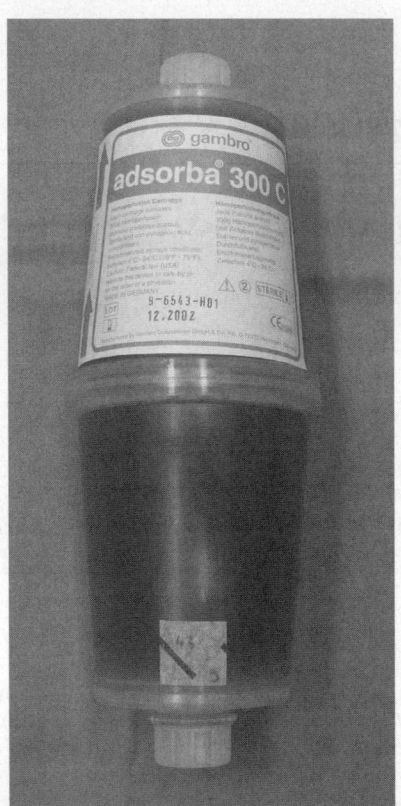

FIGURE 279-2. Hemoperfusion column containing activated charcoal coated with cellulose acetate (Adsorba, Gambro AB, Stockholm).

TABLE 279-1

Some Hemoperfusion Cartridges Used in Poisoning, Dialysis-Related Amyloidosis, and Gram-Negative Sepsis

CARTRIDGE	SORBENT/AMOUNT	MANUFACTURER	INDICATION	DURATION OF HP
Adsorba	Charcoal/300 g	Gambro AB, Stockholm	Poisoning	4 hours
Hemosorba	Charcoal/170 g	Asahi Medical, Tokyo	Poisoning	4 hours
Lixelle	Cellulose beads/150-350 mL	Kaneka Corporation, Tokyo	Hemodialysis-related amyloidosis	During hemodialysis
Toraymyxin	Polymyxin B/370 mg	Toray Medical, Tokyo	Gram-negative sepsis	2 hours; 1-2 procedures/day

ing to these results, hemoperfusion no longer has a place in the treatment of hepatic encephalopathy.

Dialysis-Related Amyloidosis

Dialysis-related amyloidosis is a special form of amyloidosis that occurs as a late complication of dialysis treatment. It appears in 70% of patients after 10 years of dialysis, in 90% of the patients after 15 years, and in all patients after 20 years. The most common clinical manifestations are carpal tunnel syndrome and shoulder pain. Symptoms and signs are due to accumulation of β_2-microglobulin (β_2M) and the modification of β_2-microglobulin by advanced glycation end products in tissues around the joints, tendons, and fasciae of the muscles, and accumulation of β_2M in the bones and also in the heart, gastrointestinal tract, lung, and liver. Bone cysts, which can be signs of amyloidosis, can cause pathological fractures of long bones. Paraplegia, quadriplegia, and even death can be observed when compressive fractures of the spine occur.[7]

β_2M, a globular protein with a molecular weight of about 11,800 Daltons, is negatively charged in the serum and is derived from the surfaces of the nucleated cells. The normal serum concentration of β_2M in healthy humans is 1 to 2.7 mg/L, and the generation rate is 0.13 mg per kg of body weight per hour, about 220 mg/day in a 70-kg human. Elimination of β_2M (about 220 mg/day) is carried out by the kidneys via its destruction in tubular cells. In anuric patients undergoing dialysis, elimination of β_2M is severely impaired, and the protein is therefore deposited in the targeted tissue. Accumulation of 400 to 600 g of β_2M in the tissue is associated with the onset of dialysis-related amyloidosis.[7]

Small, uncontrolled studies have reported a subjective improvement of the symptoms of dialysis-related amyloidosis after treatment with high-flux hemodialysis. In one study, however, autopsy did not detect a significant difference in appearance of dialysis-related amyloidosis between patients treated with hemodialysis, hemofiltration, and continuous ambulatory peritoneal dialysis.[8]

Much more promising is the elimination of β_2M along with improvement of clinical symptoms and signs after the treatment with selective β_2M sorbent. An adsorbent column (Lixelle, Kaneka Corporation, Tokyo) for direct hemoperfusion has been available in Japan since 1996. The Lixelle S-15 cartridge contains 150 mL, and the Lixelle S-35 cartridge 350 mL, of porous cellulose adsorbent beads with a diameter of about 460 μm, in which a hexadecyl group with high hydrophobicity is used as a ligand. The column adsorbs hydrophobic proteins (such as β_2M) with a molecular weight of 4000 to 20,000 Da. The beads in the column have the capacity to adsorb 1 mg of β_2M per 1 mL of beads. The Lixelle S-35 can therefore remove 200 to 350 mg of β_2M per session.

Abe and colleagues[9] treated 17 patients with the Lixelle S-35 during each dialysis session, for 1 year, with the column and the dialyzer connected in line. Patients had been undergoing hemodialysis for 13 to 29 years (mean 20.2 ± 4.5 years) prior to the study and had been treated, prior to Lixelle therapy, with high-flux hemodialysis for 1 year. At the start of hemodialysis, the β_2M mean concentration was 34.6 ± 9.3 mg/mL; this value did not change during hemodialysis treatment and remained the same at the end of the year (34.5 ± 8.4 mg/mL). That was the starting concentration when Lixelle therapy was instituted for the next year. At the end of the second year, the β_2M concentration was significantly lower, at 28.8 ± 7.3 mg/mL. During one combined Lixelle/hemodialysis procedure, β_2M was reduced on average by 22 mg/L (from 29.9 ± 7.7 mg/L to 7.9 ± 1.7 mg/L), a reduction of 74% ± 6%. Along with reduction of serum β_2M concentration, clinical improvement was also observed after 1 year. The patients demonstrated significant increase in pinch strength and significant reductions in median motor terminal latency, joint pain, and nocturnal awakenings.

The Lixelle column has also been reported to remove other biologically active substances, such as interleukin-1 (IL-1), interleukin-6, tumor necrosis factor-α, endotoxins, and peptidoglycans. Removal of these inflammatory mediators may also modify (decrease) generation of β_2M.[10,11] Lixelle hemoperfusion could be an additional therapeutic tool for hemodialysis in patients with dialysis-related amyloidosis.

Sepsis

The mortality rate of septic patients with multiple-organ dysfunction syndrome (MODS) and multiple-organ failure (MOF) has been reported to be between 30% and 80%.[12,13] A major contributor to lethality from gram-negative sepsis is endotoxin itself, through systemic activation of host-derived inflammatory mediators, the most important of which are proinflammatory cytokines, activated neutrophils, monocytes, endothelial cells, the complement system, the extrinsic coagulation cascade and the fibrinolytic system, platelet-activating factor, the kinins, prostaglandins, and leukotrienes, reactive oxygen radicals, and nitric oxide. The endotoxin molecule itself is not intrinsically toxic; septic shock is in fact an exaggerated host response to systemic release of endotoxin by gram-negative bacteria. Bactericidal antimicrobial agents paradoxically exacerbate the harmful effects of endotoxin, which is released by the outer membrane of gram-negative bacteria during bacteriolysis. Therefore, treatment strategies that destroy bacteria on the one hand and diminish quantity of immunological active endotoxin on the other hand could be useful in the management of patients with systemic gram-negative bacterial infection. Unfortunately, the same defense system that protects the patient in localized bacterial infection may react in the form of a generalized, potentially fatal systemic inflammatory response to the presence of gram-negative bacteria in the bloodstream. Therefore, removal of endotoxin, rather than cytokines, which are part of the patient's defense system, is one of the main goals of the prevention and treatment of septic shock.[14-16]

Attempts to prevent and treat septic shock have been based on the therapies that interrupt the synthesis of endotoxin, prevent endotoxin interaction with host effector cells, interfere with endotoxin-mediated signal transduction pathways, and bind endotoxin and neutralize its activity.[16] Blood purification extracorporeal procedures have been used to remove endotoxin from the blood of septic patients, with varying efficacy.

Adsorption on the hemofilter's membrane was the mode of action in continuous renal replacement therapies, however, the results were not clinically important.[17,18] Highly permeable super-flux hemofilters, used later, have high convective clearance also for cytokines and presumably endotoxin, but with an expense of additional substantial loss of albumin.[19,20] Membrane plasma exchange has been used successfully, although not widely, to treat septic patients and to improve their survival rate.[21,22]

Direct hemoperfusion using polymyxin B–immobilized polystyrene-derived fibers (PMX-F) is among the most effective extracorporeal therapies that remove endotoxin from blood of septic patients. It is more potent than anion sorbent columns and cellulose sorbents. Polymyxin B is a cyclic basic polypeptide that acts as a cationic, surface-active detergent to disrupt the permeability of both the outer and cytoplasmic membranes of gram-negative bacteria. This agent has an affinity for the lipid A, the biologically active moiety of lipopolysaccharide that actually mediates the direct toxic effect of endotoxin. Chemical decomposition of endotoxin with an acid, alkali, or oxidizing agent, which is performed in vitro, cannot be used in vivo. Besides, polymyxin B is nephrotoxic and neurotoxic, so cannot be applied to the systemic circulation. The only approach to eliminate endotoxin from blood is therefore adsorption using an extracorporeal device.

Polymyxin B is covalently bound via its amino group to an α-chloracetamide-methylated polystyrene insoluble fiber. The amount of polymyxin B released from the fiber is very small (1 ppb) and is not toxic. Reversible thrombocytopenia and transient leukopenia are the common side effects of PMX-F hemoadsorption. In vitro studies demonstrated very efficient removal of endotoxin from human plasma. However, cytokine production was not completely inhibited, thus indicating that bacterial products other than endotoxin contribute to sepsis and therefore, to some extent, limit the efficacy of polymyxin B hemoperfusion in the therapy of sepsis.[23]

Since 1994, PMX-F direct hemoperfusion (Toraymyxin, Toray Industries, Inc., Tokyo) (Fig. 279-3) has been commercially available and approved for use in Japan as a blood purification device for endotoxin removal. The adsorbent column is a 170-mL polypropylene tube containing 53 g of PMX-F covalently bound to 370 mg polymyxin B (7 mg polymyxin B/1 g fiber). PMX-F hemoperfusion is usually carried out for 2 hours, once or twice a day, with blood flow at about 100 mL/minute.[24,25] Anticoagulant could be heparin or, in patients with bleeding tendency or in heparin-induced thrombocytopenia (HIT), nafamostat mesylate (available in Japan) or citrate.

In a prospective uncontrolled clinical trial reported by Kodama and associates,[26] 42 septic patients were treated by PMX-F hemoperfusion. Endotoxin concentration dropped significantly immediately after the procedure (from 85 pg/mL to 57 pg/mL) and even 24 hours after the procedure (to 28 pg/ml), suggesting prolonged effect of the hemoperfusion. The 14-day all-cause mortality rate was 48% for patients undergoing PMX-F hemoperfusion therapy.[26] In another study, PMX-F hemoperfusion substantially and significantly reduced endotoxin concentration in 16 septic patients, from 76 pg/mL to 21 pg/mL. Patients' hemodynamics improved, and the 14-day survival rate was 56%; 43% of the patients were discharged from the hospital.[27] Nakamura and coworkers reported that 10 out of 14 septic patients (71%) treated with PMX-F hemoperfusion survived, compared with 5 out of 12 septic patients (42%) who survived with conventional therapy without PMX-F hemoperfusion. The PMX-F group had significantly lower concentrations of endotoxin after two consecutive procedures than the conventionally treated group.[28] Although mortality and survival rates of PMX-F treated patients was similar to those of comparable septic patients treated the conventional way, results of PMX-F therapy were impressive in terms of reducing concentrations of endotoxin and cytokines. The impact on improvement of survival might have been greater in this study if the procedure had been instituted earlier in the course of the patients' disease.

CONCLUSION

Although the main indication for hemoperfusion is still poisoning with drugs and chemicals, it has also been used to treat some other diseases. Early in the use of hemodialysis treatment, hemoperfusion was used to eliminate uremic toxins. However, modern hemodialysis technique made hemoperfusion obsolete and unnecessary. Hemoperfusion no longer has a place in the treatment of hepatic encephalopathy. Other efficient procedures are currently available and are discussed elsewhere in this book.

Dialysis-related amyloidosis is a serious problem in the patients who have been treated with dialysis for more than 10 years. Elimination of β_2-microglobulin with high-flux dialysis is not sufficient to prevent symptoms and signs of this disease. Results of clinical studies of the use of specific β_2-microglobulin sorbent in Lixelle cartridges have been encouraging and convincing enough to recommend use of the device as complementary to hemodialysis, at least in patients with overt clinical symptoms of dialysis-related amyloidosis.

Gram-negative sepsis and septic shock with multiple-organ dysfunction syndrome are still serious clinical problems with high mortality rates that have not declined in recent years. Several attempts have been made to eliminate endotoxin and cytokines from the circulation of the patient, mostly without affecting the course of the disease or survival rate. The clinical use of PMX-F cartridges in septic patients achieved efficient removal of endotoxin from the blood and significant improvement of hemodynamics. Although survival rate did not improve in spite of the use of the PMX-F hemoperfusion device, it is a promising procedure in septic patients and might be more helpful if applied earlier in the course of sepsis.

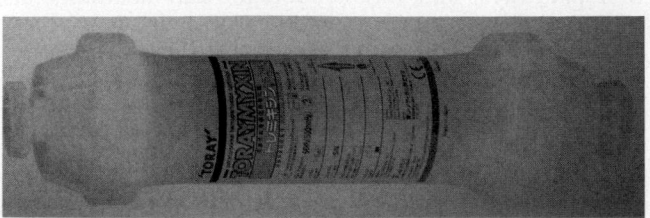

FIGURE 279-3. PMX-F (polymyxin B–immobilized polystyrene-derived fibers) cartridge for the treatment of patients with gram-negative sepsis and septic shock (Toraymyxin, Toray Medical, Tokyo).

Key Points

1. The main indication for hemoperfusion is poisoning with some drugs and chemicals.
2. Hemoperfusion is obsolete in the treatment of uremia and hepatic encephalopathy.
3. Hemoperfusion with a specific column for β_2-microglobulin adsorption efficiently removes this substance from uremic plasma and may have a role in patients with dialysis-related amyloidosis.

4. Hemoperfusion with polymyxin B cartridges efficiently removes endotoxin from blood, but so far has demonstrated no survival benefit in patients with gram-negative sepsis.
5. Hemoperfusion is usually performed with a hemodialysis monitor, with a hemoperfusion cartridge and dialyzer connected serially.

Key References

3. Winchester JF: Dialysis techniques: Hemoperfusion. In Horl WH, Koch KM, Lindsay RM, et al (eds): Replacement of Renal Function by Dialysis, 5th ed. New York, Kluwer Academic, 2004, pp 725-738.
9. Abe T, Uchita K, Orita H, et al: Effect of β2-microglobulin adsorption column on dialysis-related amyloidosis. Kidney Int 2003;64:1522-1528.
11. Tsuchida K, Takemoto Y, Nakamura T, et al: Lixelle adsorbent to remove inflammatory cytokines. Artif Organs 1998;22:1064-1069.
26. Kodama M, Aoki H, Tani T, Hanasawa K: Hemoperfusion using a polymyxin B immobilized fiber column for the removal of endotoxin. In Levin J, Alvin CR, Munford RS, Stutz PL (eds): Bacterial Endotoxin: Recognition and Effector Mechanisms. Amsterdam, Elsevier Science, 1993, pp 389-398.
28. Nakamura T, Kowagoe Y, Suzuki T, et al: Changes in plasma interleukin-18 by direct hemoperfusion with polymyxin B-immobilized fiber in patients with septic shock. Blood Purif 2005;23:417-420.

See the companion Expert Consult website for the complete reference list.

CHAPTER 280

Albumin Dialysis with Molecular Adsorbent Recirculating System in the Treatment of Liver Failure

Steffen R. Mitzner and Jan Stange

OBJECTIVES

This chapter will:
1. Explain the rationale for albumin dialysis as a liver support method.
2. Describe the structure and function of albumin dialysis with the Molecular Adsorbent Recirculating System.
3. Discuss the major indications for this treatment.
4. Describe clinical effects and safety aspects of the modality.

Artificial liver support techniques carry the prospect of removing liver-bound toxins and thus permitting autoregeneration of the liver. The fact that most of the potential liver toxins, such as hydrophobic bile acids, bilirubin, and plasmatic nitric oxide, use albumin as their transport protein has led to the development of albumin dialysis.

The concept of albumin dialysis aims at specific clearance of albumin-bound toxins (ABTs) from the blood of patients with liver failure without losing valuable plasma compounds. It is based on the assumption that secondary organ failures can be avoided or reversed if plasma concentrations of ABTs can be kept sufficiently low during a given critical time frame of several days, thus allowing for liver regeneration or liver transplantation. The most important albumin dialysis technique is the Molecular Adsorbent Recirculating System (MARS; developed by Teraklin and now manufactured by Gambro AG, Lund, Sweden). The system was developed at Rostock University, Germany,

in the early 1990s and has now become the most commonly used liver support system.

TECHNOLOGY

The MARS is a liver support method consisting of elements from extracorporeal renal replacement techniques like hemodialysis and ultrafiltration as well as adsorption. It contains no biological components (e.g., hepatocytes). The method uses an albumin-enriched dialysate to facilitate the removal of ABTs. The three different fluid compartments ("circuits") are the blood circuit, an albumin circuit, and an open-loop, single-pass dialysate circuit (Fig. 280-1). The MARS requires a standard dialysis machine or a continuous venovenous hemofiltration monitor to run the blood and dialysate circuits and an extra device (MARS Monitor) to run and monitor the closed-loop albumin circuit.

The blood circuit uses a venovenous access (double-lumen catheter) and is driven by the blood roller pump of the dialysis machine continuous venovenous hemofiltration monitor. The blood flow rate is 150 to 250 mL/min, depending on the patient's hemodynamic status. Blood is passed through a non–albumin-permeable, high-flux dialysis membrane (MARS Flux) (Fig. 280-2). The albumin circuit, containing 600 mL of 20% human serum albumin, is driven by a roller pump of the MARS monitor at 150 mL/min. The dialysate human serum albumin is passed through the dialysate compartment of the blood

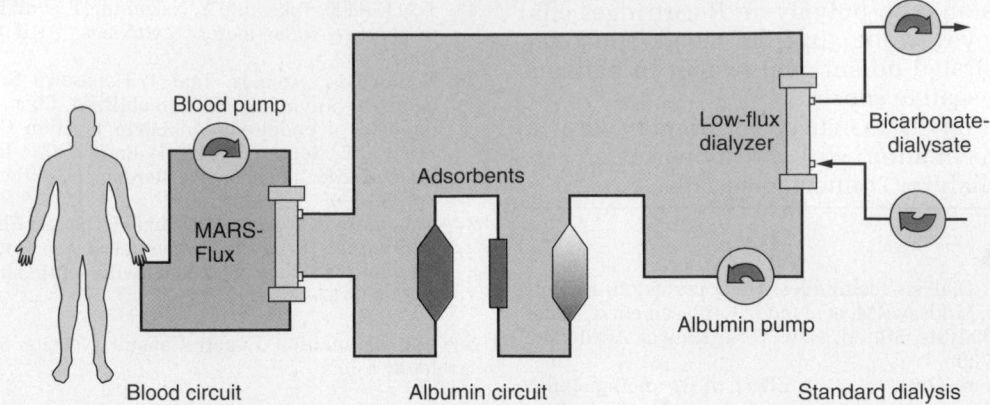

FIGURE 280-1. Schematic drawing of the Molecular Adsorbent Recirculating System (MARS) method.

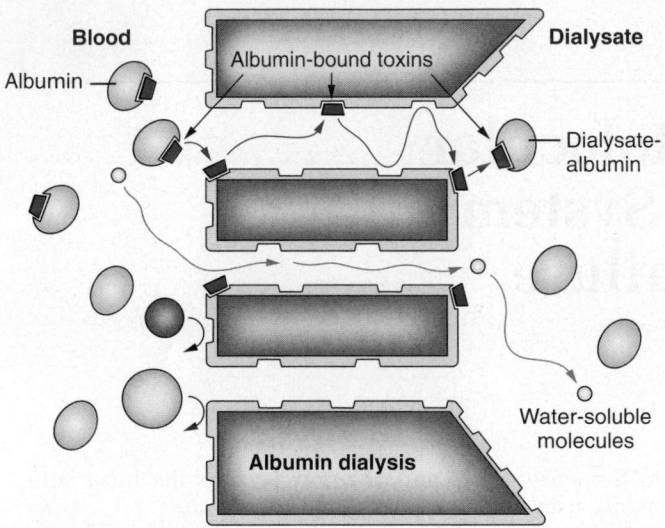

FIGURE 280-2. Structure of Molecular Adsorbent Recirculating System membrane and transmembrane transport.

dialyzer (MARS Flux) and subsequently regenerated by dialysis in the diaFLUX Dialyzer (i.e., a low-flux dialyzer) against a bicarbonate-buffered dialysate (dialysate circuit) followed by passage through a column with uncoated charcoal and a second column with an anion exchange resin. Flow directions in the MARS Flux—as well as in the diaFLUX Dialyzer—are countercurrent to maintain a maximum transmembrane toxin gradient. Typically, heparin is used as an anticoagulant. Activated clotting time is kept between 160 and 190 seconds throughout the treatment. Treatment time ranges between 6 and 24 hours.

INDICATIONS FOR ALBUMIN DIALYSIS

During more than 10 years of clinical experience with MARS, a stable spectrum of indications has evolved. Acute decompensation of chronic liver disease (acute-on-chronic liver failure [ACLF]) and acute liver failure (ALF) account

for more than three quarters of the treatments. Decompensation is typically caused by bleeding, infection, adverse drug reactions, or acute excessive alcohol intake (alcoholic hepatitis). Progressive jaundice, hepatorenal syndrome, and hepatic encephalopathy are typical complications in ACLF.

In ALF, precipitating events typically are acute infection (hepatitis B/C or other), drug overdose and intoxication (chemicals, poisonous mushrooms), idiosyncratic drug reaction, Wilson's disease, or unknown causes.[1]

The use of MARS in primary nonfunction or poor hepatic function in patients who have received liver transplants,[2] liver failure after liver resection,[3] and ischemic liver failure secondary to heart failure is under investigation.[4] Liver failure secondary to multiple-organ failure and sepsis represents another indication,[5] as does the improvement of quality of life in chronic cholestatic syndromes. Especially the treatment of intractable hepatic pruritus is an emerging indication for liver support (see details later). A down-scaled version of MARS with a smaller extracorporeal blood volume was successfully used in pediatric liver failure.[1,6]

A BRIDGE TO LIVER TRANSPLANTATION

The primary aim in patients with ALF and other patients on the transplantation waiting list was to create a safe bridge to support the patients until liver transplantation (LTx). Not only was the treatment reported to be safe but the patients' condition improved markedly in a substantial number to such an extent that sustained liver regeneration was achieved. In rare cases, anhepatic patients were supported by MARS until transplantation.[1] Koivusalo and associates[7] reported on use of MARS in 56 patients with ALF (29 toxic, 22 unknown, 5 other). All fulfilled LTx criteria or had ingested a lethal dose of a known toxic agent (e.g., paracetamol, *Amanita phalloides*). A mean number of three MARS treatments was performed per patient, and target treatment duration was 22 hours per session. The 1-year survival was 84%. Recovery of native liver function occurred in 30 patients (1-year survival, 79%). In the patients who underwent transplantation, 1-year survival was 94%. The recovery rate was 76% in the subgroup of patients with toxic ALF, and 23% in the sub-

TABLE 280-1

Substances Cleared by the Molecular Adsorbent Recirculating System

SUBSTANCE	CHAPTER REFERENCE(S)
Ammonia	1, 5, 9, 11-13, 20, 24, 25
Aromatic amino acids (increase in Fischer ratio)	1, 24, 25
Benzodiazepam-like substances	24
Bile acids	1, 5, 9, 12, 14, 16, 20, 25, 28, 34
Bilirubin	1, 2, 5, 8-10, 12-15, 18, 20, 25, 27, 34
Copper	1
Creatinine	1, 2, 5, 9, 13, 14, 25, 27, 34
Diazepam	1
Interleukin-1β	20
Interleukin-6	1, 5, 20
Interleukin-8	5
Interleukin-10	5, 9, 19, 21
Lactate	13
Medium- and short-chain fatty acids	1
Nitric oxide	5, 17, 18
Tumor necrosis factor-α	1, 5, 9, 20
Tryptophan	24
Urea/blood urea nitrogen	1, 12, 20, 34

group with ALF of unknown origin.[7] Camus and coworkers[8] found similar results in their LTx candidates. They treated patients twice with 8-hour sessions and found a LTx-free survival of 29%.[8] A number of other groups reported safe and successful "bridging" to LTx or even recovery of native liver function in their patients treated with MARS,[9-12] among others in children.[6] However, not all groups observed native liver recovery.[12] MARS as a bridge to LTx in ALF is currently being studied in a multicenter randomized clinical trial in France.

SUBSTANCE REMOVAL

ABTs are significantly removed by MARS.[6,9,12-15] Beyond the removal of total bile acids, MARS induces a shift toward more hydrophilic bile acids in patients' blood.[16] Aromatic amino acids are removed, leading to a rise in Fischer's index.[1] Plasmatic nitric oxide (NO), transported as a nitrosothiol by albumin, is of central importance for the typical hemodynamic changes of liver failure (hyperdynamic hypotension). Removal of nitric oxide is a consistent finding in the clinical use of MARS.[17,18] Beyond the group of ABTs, much attention has been paid to the clearance of circulating cytokines. Significant removal of a number of pro-inflammatory and anti-inflammatory cytokines was observed.[5,9,18-20] However, this removal did not always lower blood cytokine levels.[17,21]

Removal of both water-soluble and albumin-bound drugs—for example, antibiotics—must be considered in the planning of medical treatment. Basic handling recommendations include dosage application after treatment and therapeutic drug monitoring for blood level surveillance.[1] Table 280-1 lists the substances that are cleared by the MARS method.

CLINICAL EFFECTS OF MARS

Typical complications of liver failure are hemodynamic insufficiency, hepatic encephalopathy, renal failure, and synthetic dysfunction leading to disorders of plasmatic coagulation. Patients with chronic cholestatic syndromes suffer from impaired quality of life, especially fatigue or pruritus. The impact of MARS on the different complications was studied in detail. Findings are summarized here.

Hemodynamic Insufficiency and Hyperdynamic Hypotension

One of the key features of MARS is the improvement of the hemodynamic state of patients, both those with ALF as well as those with ACLF. Initial finding of a rise in the systemic vascular resistance index during MARS treatments[1] have been confirmed.[9,18] Several groups of investigators have described an increase in mean arterial pressure, too.[1,2,14,18] In patients with ALF, Schmidt and colleagues[22] found a significant increase in both the systemic vascular resistance index and mean arterial pressure, leading to a significant decrease in the cardiac index and heart rate.

The blood perfusion of single organs improved during MARS treatments. A central phenomenon is the decrease in portal pressure in ACLF[23] and the improvement in renal blood flow.[1] Increased cerebral perfusion pressure has also been described in patients with ACLF undergoing MARS theapy.[24]

Hepatic Encephalopathy and Intracranial Hypertension

A significant improvement in hepatic encephalopathy for patients with both chronic and with acute liver failure has been reported since the first applications of albumin dialysis. The Glasgow Coma Scale score also improved significantly (for review, see Mitzner and associates[24]). A multicenter randomized clinical trial studying MARS in 70 patients with ACLF and hepatic encephalopathy grade III or IV showed significant differences in the cumulative number of two-grade improvements in hepatic encephalopathy favoring MARS.[25] This finding was confirmed in another randomized control trial[17] and in several case series.[2,8,9,12,14,15]

A drop in intracranial pressure during the clinical use of MARS has been reported by different groups.[1,24] Sen and coworkers[26] investigated this phenomenon in a randomized study using an ALF model based on devascularized pigs. MARS, initiated 2 hours after hepatic devascularization, significantly attenuated the ICP increase. The MARS treatment group had a significantly lower brain water content and brain ammonia concentration.[26]

Liver Synthesis

A number of trials found a significant improvement in liver synthesis function during treatment with MARS.[8,9,14] However, this was not a uniform finding in all reports.

There are no trials reporting further decrease in synthesis parameters.[1] One study reported that the plasma clearance of indocyanine green increased significantly after MARS treatment.[2]

Kidney Function and Hepatorenal Syndrome

Several groups reported improvement of kidney function during MARS treatments. This improvement included decrease in serum creatinine and urea concentrations, a rise in urine output, and resolution of hepatorenal syndrome.[1,2,14,15] Results were confirmed in a small randomized controlled trial in patients with hepatorenal syndrome type I.[27] The reason for the improved function is currently unknown. However, a significant drop in plasma renin was found in patients with ACHF and renal failure who were treated with MARS.[28] This is not an effect of the substance being cleared by the system but might reflect improved renal blood perfusion.

Therapy-Resistant Hepatic Pruritus

Patients with unbearable pruritus resistant to medical therapy have been reported to have good response to MARS treatments. Underlying liver diseases in such patients were cholestatic forms of liver disease, such as primary biliary cirrhosis and primary sclerosing cholangitis, as well as chronic viral hepatitis. Typically, two single treatments lowered pruritus impressively, as documented by the Visual Analog Scale. The relief lasted from several weeks up to 3 months.[12,29] The phenomenon cannot be explained fully. However, selective removal of hydrophobic bile acids, leading to a longer-lasting shift in the bile acid pattern of the patients, may be a potential mechanism.[16]

SAFETY PROFILE

There are numerous reports that the MARS procedures run smoothly and safely even in critically ill patients.[2,8,11,15] The risk profile of albumin dialysis seems to be comparable to that of kidney dialysis and constitutes a slight but significant drop in platelet count during the procedure.[1] Bleeding is a rare complication. Apparently, patients with ALF can tolerate a worse coagulation state before the commencement of MARS than patients with ACLF. Moreover, the presence of infection and sepsis has a negative impact on the coagulation status and might lead to more complications associated with extracorporeal treatments. The number of treatments seems to correlate with the rate of bleeding episodes observed. A fixed protocol with, for instance, seven treatments per week is not appropriate today. In patients with ACLF who have active bleeding or platelet counts below 50,000 cells/mL should not undergo immediate commencement or progression of treatment.

Last, but not least, the mode of anticoagulation obviously affects the severity of bleeding complications.[21,30] The use of citrate in adapted dosage and with close monitoring of ionized calcium levels seems feasible and advantageous (compared with heparin) even in advanced cirrhosis.[31]

SURVIVAL DATA

Influence of MARS on survival has been evaluated in a number of small randomized controlled trials. In one trial, 13 patients with hepatorenal syndrome type I showed improvement in survival after treatment. Seven-day survival was 67% in the MARS group compared with 0% in the control group; 30-day survival was 25% in the MARS group.[27] In another randomized trial, MARS was used in patients who had postoperative liver failure after heart surgery in a cardiac intensive care setting. In a preliminary report, a clear tendency toward better survival in the MARS group was observed (7 survivors of 8 patients in the MARS group compared with 1 survivor of 4 patients in the control group).[4]

Finally, in 24 patients with ACLF and severe cholestasis (mean bilirubin level >30 mg/dL), a significant improvement in 30-day survival was found (92% in the MARS group vs. 50% in the control group; $P < .05$).[14]

In clinical cohort trials in ACLF, the MARS group showed significantly better 3-month outcomes[15] and 3-year survival in comparison with patients given standard medical care, with a favorable cost-to-benefit ratio.[32]

A Cochrane Biliary Group analysis of liver support systems published in 2003 found a significant 33% reduction in mortality in patients with ACLF who were treated with MARS.[33]

MOLECULAR ADSORBENT RECIRCULATING SYSTEM AND OTHER LIVER SUPPORT SYSTEMS

Other liver support systems have been developed that have albumin regeneration as a central therapeutic goal. These are single-pass albumin dialysis (SPAD), the modular extracorporeal liver support system (MELS), selective plasma exchange therapy (SEPET), and the Prometheus System (Fresenius Medical Care, Bad Homburg, Germany).[34] Among these, the Prometheus System is the one studied best. Clinical trials comparing it with MARS revealed differences in removal of substances and clinical effects. The two systems showed similar results with regard to general clearance of ABT and cytokines.[16,21] The Prometheus System had superior clearance rates for ammonia, urea, and creatinine.[35] MARS removed more hydrophobic bile acids.[16] Patient hemodynamics improved with MARS but not with the Prometheus System.[18] Because of its albumin-permeable membrane, the Prometheus System is less selective in substance removal than MARS. Accordingly, significant loss of procoagulant and anticoagulant factors was observed with the Prometheus System.[36]

TREATMENT RECOMMENDATIONS

From today's perspective, the correct timing of liver support treatment is of utmost importance for clinical success. Clearly not every patient with ACLF is a good candidate for albumin dialysis. In general, liver support should be considered in patients with ACLF that does not respond to standard medical care. For ALF with a high expected mortality rate, commencement of MARS treatment is recommended as soon as the diagnosis is made. Beyond the indications discussed in detail here, it is important to consider the following points:

- ALF and ACLF represent rather different indications for liver support, so different inclusion and exclusion criteria must be applied.
- The absence or presence of sepsis and severe disseminated intravascular coagulation seem to divide patients with ACLF into good and bad candidates for MARS. We recommend early and sufficiently aggressive antibiotic treatment of infections as well as antibiotic prophylaxis in patients without infections.
- Patients with ACLF, very low platelet count, high International Normalized Ratio (INR) value (>2.3), and advanced kidney failure requiring dialysis or hemofiltration represent a subgroup that might not benefit from treatment.
- In the patient with ACLF, the total dosage of treatment should be prescribed flexibly, with days of no treatment interspersed between treatments, especially if the platelet count is decreasing to low values or the INR exceeds 2.3. The mode should be intermittent rather than continuous, with treatment lengths of 6 to 8 hours per day.
- In the patient with ALF, the need for treatment is much greater, and continuous treatment with few breaks is probably most efficient.
- Patients with ALF can tolerate much worse INR values than patients with ACLF, probably because of the difference in pathogenesis of the INR increase (synthesis defect and hypercoagulation, respectively). Cautious anticoagulation with either low-dose heparin or citrate is recommended.

CONCLUSION

The MARS approach seems to allow for safe "bridging" to liver transplantation and better outcome in primary hepatic nonfunction after transplantation. An encouraging number of patients recover native hepatic function before transplantation. Moreover, there is convincing evidence that severe decompensation of chronic liver disease represents a good indication for the treatment.

The use of a non–albumin-permeable synthetic membrane seems to be a key feature for clinical success. Such a membrane facilitates good hemocompatibility and selectivity of the detoxification procedure.

Currently, MARS represents the most frequently used liver support method. It allows the safe and effective removal of albumin-bound as well as water-soluble substances. Clinically, this removal is often accompanied by

stable or improved single-organ function and better overall clinical status. Several small randomized controlled trials and case-control studies have reported statistically significant increases in survival for patients treated with MARS in comparison with those receiving standard medical care. The performance of larger randomized trials will add greatly to our knowledge of this method of liver support.

Key Points

1. Albumin is the key transporter of liver failure toxins and, therefore, of paramount interest for modern liver support methods.
2. Albumin dialysis with the Molecular Adsorbent Recirculating System is the most frequently used liver support method at present.
3. This modality efficiently removes both water-soluble and albumin-bound toxic compounds.
4. The Molecular Adsorbent Recirculating System has a profound impact on clinical course and outcome of patients with different forms of liver failure.
5. The method is easy to use, technically safe, and well tolerated.

Key References

1. Mitzner SR, Stange J, Klammt S, et al: Extracorporeal detoxification using the Molecular Adsorbent Recirculating System for critically ill patients with liver failure. J Am Soc Nephrol 2001;12(Suppl 17):S75-S82.
14. Heemann U, Treichel U, Loock J, et al: Albumin dialysis in cirrhosis with superimposed acute liver injury: A prospective, controlled study. Hepatology 2002;36:949-958.
18. Laleman W, Wilmer A, Evenepoel P, et al: Effect of the Molecular Adsorbent Recirculating System and Prometheus devices on systemic haemodynamics and vasoactive agents in patients with acute-on-chronic alcoholic liver failure. Crit Care 2006; 10:R108.
25. Hassanein T, Tofteng F, Brown RS, et al: A prospective, controlled study of the clinical efficacy of albumin dialysis using the Molecular Adsorbent Recirculating System (MARS) for the treatment of patients with hepatic encephalopathy. Hepatology 2007;46:1853-1862.
27. Mitzner SR, Stange J, Klammt S, et al: Improvement of hepatorenal syndrome with extracorporeal albumin dialysis MARS: Results of a prospective, randomized, controlled clinical trial. Liver Transpl 2000;6:277-286.

See the companion Expert Consult website for the complete reference list.

CHAPTER 281

Clinical Outcomes with the Molecular Adsorbent Recirculating System

Alexander Chiu and Sheung Tat Fan

OBJECTIVES

This chapter will:
1. Discuss the clinical outcome of the Molecular Adsorbent Recirculating System in specific complications of liver failure.
2. Review the clinical outcomes of treatment using this system in different subtypes of liver failure.
3. Describe the factors affecting outcome of treatment with Molecular Adsorbent Recirculating System: timing and initiation, bilirubin as a surrogate marker.
4. Discuss the potential complications of this system.

The Molecular Adsorbent Recirculating System (MARS; developed by Teraklin and now manufactured by Gambro AG, Lund, Sweden) is an extracorporeal detoxification system that can remove both albumin-bound and water-soluble toxins present in the patient with liver failure. The system was first launched at the University of Rostock, Germany, in 1993, according to the prototype designed by Mitzner and Stange.[1] Clinical application of MARS started in 2000, and within a few years, the system became one of the most commonly used artificial liver support devices around the world. The desired effect of MARS is to reduce the hepatotoxin load in the body in order to prevent or reverse complications of liver failure and to "bridge" patients to spontaneous recovery or liver transplantation.

TOXINS REMOVED BY MOLECULAR ADSORBENT RECIRCULATING SYSTEM

The special design of the MARS membrane allows albumin-bound toxins to be adsorbed onto it and transported into the albumin dialysate through a non–energy-dependent process of ligandification and deligandification. Toxins of large molecular size are removed through the charcoal adsorption column, whereas those that carry a negative charge are removed through the cholestyramine column. Water-soluble toxins, excessive fluid, electrolytes, and hydrogen ions can traverse across the MARS membrane freely and can be regulated through the renal replacement circuit. A list of toxins documented in the literature to be removed by MARS is shown in Table 281-1.

TREATING SPECIFIC COMPLICATIONS OF LIVER FAILURE

Hepatorenal Syndrome

Type 1 hepatorenal syndrome is a complication with a high mortality rate. Many patients succumb before they can undergo liver transplantation. The use of MARS to treat hepatorenal syndrome has been shown in a randomized controlled trial to have a survival benefit.[2] The prolongation of survival was significant albeit not remarkable (25.2 ± 34.65 days with MARS vs. 4.6 ± 1.8 days without it). Nevertheless, if prolonging survival increases the patient's chance for liver transplantation, the potential benefit of MARS is much amplified. The limitations of this study are that the sample size is small (13 patients) and that there is no difference in mortality rates between the treatment and control groups after 3 months. Another important point is that hemofiltration was included as part of standard medical therapy, implying that the improvement observed was not due to the renal replacement component of MARS alone. Other investigators have suggested that the mechanism by which MARS improves hepatorenal syndrome may be related to modulation of nitric oxide metabolism in the circulation.[3]

Hepatic Encephalopathy

MARS has been the only treatment other than lactulose that has shown a consistent benefit in the management of hepatic encephalopathy. The effect of MARS on this disorder has been described indirectly in previous reports, which demonstrated its ability to remove albumin-bound neurotoxins.[4,5] Other studies have demonstrated that MARS improves neuronal activity, cerebral hemodynamics, and cerebral oxygen consumption in patients with hepatic encephalopathy.[6,7] Clinical improvement in grade of hepatic encephalopathy has been described in many reports, despite the fact that most of them are case series with small numbers of patients. A multicenter randomized controlled trial investigating the effect of MARS on high-grade hepatic encephalopathy with objective neuropsychiatric tests in end-stage liver failure suggested that MARS significantly improves hepatic encephalopathy faster and more frequently than standard medical therapies.[8] In most published series, the etiology of liver failure in which hepatic encephalopathy showed a favorable response to MARS had been mostly alcoholic liver disease.[9-11] At Queen Mary Hospital, Hong Kong, where the majority of patients suffered from cirrhosis secondary to viral hepatitis, the response to the treatment was less satisfactory.

Portal Hypertension

MARS has been shown to have a portal hypotensive effect in patients with severe alcoholic hepatitis and chronic liver failure.[12,13] The hepatic venous pressure gradient decreased rapidly by more than 20% and reached 12 mm Hg in a significant proportion of patients who had undergone MARS treatment, a threshold known to have a protective effect in preventing variceal rebleeding.[14] The reduction in the hepatic venous pressure gradient was also found to have lasted for up to 18 hours after treatment.

CLINICAL OUTCOME IN DIFFERENT SUBTYPES OF LIVER FAILURE

The clinical outcome of MARS dialysis depends on the following three factors: potential of spontaneous recovery, underlying hepatic reserve, and timing of initiation. The

TABLE 281-1

Toxins Removed by the Molecular Adsorbent Recirculating System

Water-soluble toxins	Urea
	Ammonia
Albumin-bound toxins	Bilirubin
	Bile acids
	Tryptophan
	Short- and medium-chain fatty acids
	Gamma-aminobutyric acid–like substances
	Aromatic acids
	Copper
	Manganese
	Mercaptans

availability of liver transplantation is a confounding factor that affects overall survival. Table 281-2 shows the outcomes of patients treated with MARS in major clinical studies published since 2000.

Acute liver failure (ALF) has the greatest potential for spontaneous recovery among all causes of liver failure, and the use of MARS in the treatment of patients with ALF has shown promising results. Lahdenpera and associates[15] reported that the transplantation-free survival of patients with ALF who were treated with MARS approached 51%. The prognosis appeared even better in a subgroup of patients in whom cause of ALF was intoxication. Given the results of these previous reports, the fact that transplant patients have to face lifelong immunosuppression and its associated hazards and that avoidable transplantation could reserve the precious organs for other patients in need, it is worthwhile to use MARS dialysis in patients with ALF as an auxiliary treatment in hopes of achieving spontaneous recovery during the wait for liver transplantation. The treatment course of a patient with ALF who has undergone MARS is illustrated in Figure 281-1.

In acute-on-chronic liver failure (ACLF), the underlying hepatic reserve and availability of liver transplantation determine the patients' outcome. The primary role of MARS is to gain time for (act as a bridge for) these patients during the wait for liver transplantation. Most reports on this topic demonstrated improved short-term survival but none provided in-depth investigations of long-term survival.[16,17] Our experience indicates that patients with ACLF commonly revert to continued deterioration rather than remain in a steady state once MARS dialysis has been stopped. Long-term support does not appear to be a feasible option, because MARS achieves only detoxification and does not provide other important hepatic functions. Patients with ACLF undergoing MARS therapy should therefore be constantly evaluated to determine whether continuation of treatment is worthwhile. The treatment course of a patient with ACLF who has undergone multiple MARS treatments is shown in Figure 281-2.

Post-hepatectomy liver failure occurs when the post-resection liver reserve is not able to support the patient's metabolic demand. MARS, in theory, can support the body until adequate hepatic regeneration occurs. In practice, such a target is difficult to achieve, because the regeneration process could be protracted, especially if renal failure

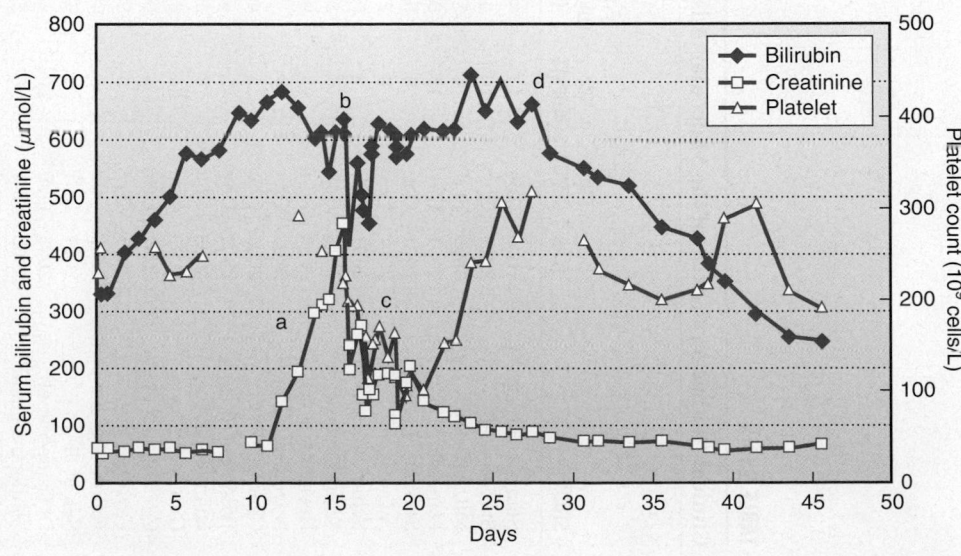

FIGURE 281-1. Graph showing serum bilirubin (*diamonds*) and creatinine (*squares*) concentrations and platelet count (*triangles*) in a 30-year-old woman with drug-induced acute liver failure who was transferred to our center for consideration of liver transplantation. She developed type one hepatorenal syndrome (a) while waiting for a cadaveric graft. She was subjected to 3 courses of MARS treatment (b) and her renal function improved shortly afterward (c). The bilirubin level fell but rebounded after each MARS session. Then, it decreased gradually after a lag phase, during which she developed a nosocomial sepsis (d) with a transient rise in the bilirubin level.

TABLE 281-2

Clinical Studies on the Use of the Molecular Adsorbent Recirculating System in Liver Failure

STUDY	YEAR	STUDY DESIGN	NO. PATIENTS	OVERALL SURVIVAL (%)	Patients with Acute Liver Failure			Patients with Acute-on-Chronic Liver Failure			Patients with GD			Patients with PH		
					NO.	SURVIVORS AFTER OLT	SURVIVORS AFTER MARS	NO.	SURVIVORS AFTER OLT	SURVIVORS AFTER MARS	NO.	SURVIVORS AFTER OLT	SURVIVORS AFTER MARS	NO.	SURVIVORS AFTER OLT	SURVIVORS AFTER MARS
Stange et al[29]	1999	Obv	13	69.0				13	0	9						
Stange et al[19]	2000	Obv	26	65.4				26	0	17						
Mitzner et al[2]	2000	RCT	8	75.0				8	0	6						
Lamesch et al[30]	2001	Obv	17	52.9	4	0	3	9	3	5	2	1	0	2	0	1
Sorkine et al[31]	2001	Obv	8	62.5				8	1	4						
Awad et al[32]	2001	Obv	9	22.2	4	0	1	3	0	0	2	1	0			
Schmidt et al[33]	2001	Obv	8	50.0				8	0	4						
Kellersmann et al[34]	2002	Obv	5	20.0							3	0	1	2	0	0
Heemann et al[11]	2002	RCT	12	91.6				12	0	11						
Novelli et al[35]	2002	Obv	34	79.4	9	3	3	10	1	6	15	4	9			
Chen et al[36]	2002	Obv	25	48.0				25	0	12						
Wilmer et al[37]	2002	Obv	13	38.0	5	0	3	6	0	1	2	0	1			
Jalan et al[38]	2003	Obv	8	50.0				8	1	3						
Guo et al[39]	2003	Obv	24	37.5	11	1	4	13	3	1						
Covic et al[40]	2003	Obv	6	66.7	6	0	4									
Faybik et al[41]	2003	Obv	6	83.3	5	2	2	1	0	1						
van de Kerkhove et al[18]	2003	Obv	5	20.0										5	0	1
Sen et al[5]	2004	RCT	9	44.4				9	0	4						
Di Campli et al[42]	2005	Obv	20	50.0	3	2	0	13	2	2	4	0	2			
Lahdenpera et al[15]	2005	Obv	88	58.0	45	13	23	31	5	2	8	3	3			
Lai et al[43]	2005	Obv	10	30.0	10	2	3									
Koivusalo et al[44]	2005	Obv	101	61.4	56	16	30	35	5	3	10	3	5			
Inderbitzin et al[45]	2005	Obv	7	71.4				1	0	1	2	1	1	4	0	2
Tsai et al[46]	2005	Obv	10	30.0	10	1	2									
Chiu et al[47]	2006	Obv	22	27.3	2	1	1	12	2	0	4	0	0	4	0	0

GD, graft dysfunction; MARS, Molecular Adsorbent Recirculating System; Obv, observation; OLT, orthotopic liver transplantation; PH, post-hepatectomy; RCT, randomized controlled trial.

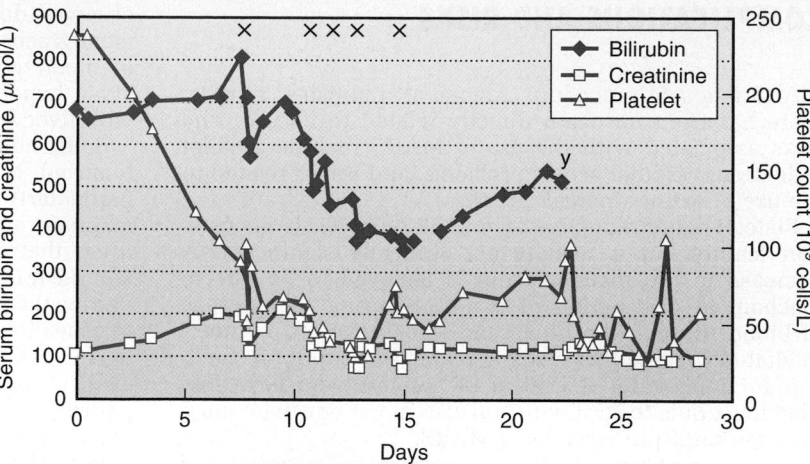

FIGURE 281-2. Graph showing serum bilirubin (*diamonds*) and creatinine (*squares*) concentrations and platelet count (*triangles*) in a 50-year-old man with a history of Child C hepatitis B-related cirrhosis in whom acute-on-chronic liver failure developed due to hepatitis virus reactivation. The patient received 5 courses of MARS treatment (X) and the bilirubin level fell from 800 to 350 μmol/L. During this period, the patient did not lapse into hepatic encephalopathy or hepatorenal syndrome and did not need mechanical ventilation or inotropic support. He was finally bridged to liver transplantation (y) 2 weeks after initiation of MARS and made a full recovery afterward.

or sepsis has occurred. Patients frequently succumb to these complications before their livers have recovered. There have been only isolated reports on the use of MARS in post-hepatectomy liver failure, and the outcomes were mostly dismal.[18] Our center has also attempted to treat a few patients with post-hepatectomy liver failure using MARS. Although their serum biochemistry parameters improved with treatment, worsening coagulopathy and superimposed sepsis eventually led to the patients' death.

Post-transplantation liver failure represents a wide range of conditions, from primary nonfunction to chronic rejection. MARS is considered a salvage therapy when retransplantation is not possible. Hetz and coworkers[19] evaluated the effect of MARS on early allograft dysfunction after orthotopic liver transplantation and reported a 66% survival with no patient requiring retransplantation. In Hong Kong, where there is a significant organ shortage, MARS is often the only choice and offers an invaluable opportunity to evaluate the effect of this modality on allograft recovery. With the exception of patients with primary hepatic nonfunction, recovery of graft function has been observed in some patients, and retransplantation avoided.

A few case reports have demonstrated that in liver failure associated with multiple-organ failure and conditions such as sepsis[20] and cardiogenic shock,[21] the use of MARS reverses liver failure and improves survival. MARS is used in these conditions principally to modulate inflammatory mediators; this concept of blood purification has been called *multi-organ support therapy*. On the basis of current evidence, MARS can be regarded only as an experimental treatment in multi-organ failure, but it is an interesting topic that is worth further research.

INITIATION, TIMING, AND EVALUATION OF EFFICACY

Timing of initiation is a pertinent factor that determines the outcome of patients undergoing MARS. To date, there have been no clear-cut criteria for initiation of MARS therapy. Circumstances in which MARS is started include onset of complications of liver failure, such as hepatorenal syndrome and hepatic encephalopathy, and a high serum bilirubin level associated with raised parenchymal liver enzyme levels or coagulopathy. The serum bilirubin level indicating the initiation of MARS varies between 250 and 500 μmol/L in the literature. There have been questions, however, about whether starting MARS at such a bilirubin level is early enough. In fact, when MARS is commenced late in the course of liver failure, the cascade of complications induced by liver failure often leads to disappointing results.

In our opinion, the rapidity of deterioration in liver function rather than an arbitrarily determined biochemical value is more important in governing the initiation of MARS. A serum bilirubin level of 200 μmol/L in a patient with ALF would warrant MARS dialysis if the deterioration occurred within a short time. From our experience, early application of MARS lessens the need for mechanical ventilation and inotropic support, and, hence, indirectly improves outcome. MARS should be considered a treatment to arrest deterioration rather than to salvage devastation. In practice, the opportunity of early intervention is commonly jeopardized by delayed referral. Education of the general medical community to increase the awareness of this treatment is therefore important.

As shown in various studies, removal of bilirubin by MARS ranges from 10% to 90%. The amount of bilirubin removed is often regarded as a surrogate marker of the efficacy of the system, because other albumin-bound toxins are rarely measured in routine clinical practice. Bilirubin is not a good marker, however, because its removal is affected by the presence of delta-bilirubin—bilirubin molecules bound to albumin with tight covalent bonds. They account for a significant proportion of total bilirubin in patients with severe cholestatsis.[22] Although MARS can effectively eliminate free bilirubin molecules and albumin-bound bilirubin by noncovalent bonds, it fails to remove delta-bilirubin.[23] A second factor that affects bilirubin removal is the slow equilibration of bilirubin between the intravascular and extravascular pools.[24] MARS can remove bilirubin only within the intravascular compartment, whereas tissue bilirubin is constantly released into the intravascular pool to attain a new equilibrium. Along with the concurrent production of bilirubin by the body, a rebound phenomenon is observed after each MARS session. With successive MARS treatments, the amount of bilirubin stored within the extravascular pool diminishes and the serum bilirubin level gradually falls as well.

COMPLICATIONS AND RISKS

MARS is a safe procedure. Among all published reports, there has been no death directly related to its use. The risks associated with the use of MARS include platelet reduction, vascular access problems, and issues related to the use of extracorporeal circuits.

Platelet count reduction after MARS dialysis is a consistent feature but is usually not clinically significant. A decrease in the platelet count is believed to be due to mechanical destruction of platelets during the passage of blood through the filters and lines or to an immune-mediated process that leads to platelet disruption.[25] Such a reduction could be critical in patients who have low platelet counts to start with and also in patients who must undergo multiple sessions of MARS.

The femoral vein is the preferred vascular access for MARS in our center because of the ease of puncture, adequate blood flow, and ready compressibility after catheter removal. Vascular access could be a problem in patients with coagulopathies and who require multiple sessions of MARS, and meticulous nursing care is necessary to keep the dialysis catheter clean and to avoid infection. The puncture site must be observed closely for oozing and bruises, both during dialysis and after removal of the catheter, because extensive hematoma may form and may be unnoticed for a long time unless checked for.

Complications associated with the use of an extracorporeal circuit include embolism, infection, loss of thermoregulation, and clogging of blood in the system.

In patients with liver failure, the use of anticoagulation for the extracorporeal circuit must be balanced carefully against the risk of bleeding. Systemic heparin infusion has been shown in many centers to be a safe and effective anticoagulation method, but it may pose problems in patients with coagulopathies. The alternative approach is the use of heparin only for priming the blood side of the system but not during dialysis. Heparin coating appears to reduce the incidence of platelet activation and thrombosis over the artificial surface. Heparin priming has been adopted by our center as the means of anticoagulation, and the result is satisfactory. Other centers have used regional citrate and prostacyclin with variable success. For patients in whom anticoagulation is absolutely contraindicated, regular bolus saline flushing alone may be used.

Monitoring of the patient's coagulation status during MARS with commonly used laboratory tests, such as prothrombin time, partial thromboplastin time, and platelet count, are of limited use because of the long "turnaround time" for results. Our center uses activated clotting time, which is a rapid measurement that can be conveniently performed at the bedside, although the result may be affected by conditions such as hemodilution, platelet dysfunction, and hypothermia. Thromboelastography is a global assessment of whole blood homeostasis. It is a dynamic test that yields information relating to the cumulative effect of the many components of coagulation, including platelet function. Its use in MARS has been evaluated, and in patients with complicated hemostatic issues, the coagulopathy may be corrected according to the results of thromboelastography before MARS treatment.[26]

Glucose, being water soluble and having a low molecular weight, traverses the MARS membrane with ease and is constantly removed from the dialysate fluid by the adsorption chambers. Asymptomatic hypoglycemia with a serum glucose level of less than 4 mmol/L has been observed during the course of MARS dialysis if replacement glucose is not given.[27] Hourly monitoring by means of blood glucose fingersticks is therefore necessary to avoid hypoglycemia that may be detrimental in patients with liver failure.

Both albumin-bound and water-soluble drugs are removed by MARS dialysis. Administration of drugs, particularly antibiotics, must be carefully planned to maintain an adequate level in the blood.[28] In principle, drugs that are highly albumin bound would require re-administration after MARS dialysis. For drugs with a narrow therapeutic window, drug assays may be necessary to gauge the dosage needed.

The patients' physical and psychological needs must also be addressed, because the treatment requires the patients to lie flat on the bed for a significant time. Careful explanation before the treatment as well as constant attention to the patients' discomfort, such as back pain and muscle cramps, are of utmost importance to obtain cooperation and achieve the best results. The ambient temperature should be kept high, because the patients frequently feel cold owing to heat loss from the extracorporeal circuit.

CONCLUSION

The main criticism of MARS dialysis is that most of the studies that have been conducted to assess it are retrospective and observational in nature; only a handful of randomized controlled trials have been performed, and none of these provides adequate data to show survival benefit. There are also no standardized indications or criteria determining in whom and when MARS should be applied or for how long the treatment should be continued. Because liver failure is a disease with a high mortality rate and heterogeneous etiology, only large-scale multiple-center collaborations would unveil the mechanisms. At present, without such answers, the use of MARS must be evaluated according to the possible risks and benefits of the treatment in individual patients with liver failure.

Key Points

1. On the basis of observational evidence, the Molecular Adsorbent Recirculating System has been shown to have a beneficial effect in the management of hepatic encephalopathy and hepatorenal syndrome.
2. When applied to patients with acute liver failure, this modality can bring about spontaneous recovery in certain cases.
3. When applied to patients with acute-on-chronic liver failure, treatment with the Molecular Adsorbent Recirculating System is likely to function as a means to support the patients until they can undergo liver transplantation.
4. In post-hepatectomy and post-transplantation liver failure, the Molecular Adsorbent Recirculating System is best regarded as a salvage therapy.
5. The key to successful treatment with this modality lies in the timing of initiation.

6. The initiation of such treatment should be based on the rapidity of deterioration rather than any arbitrarily set biochemical value.

7. Early initiation of Molecular Adsorbent Recirculating System therapy reduces the body's hepatotoxin load, lessens the chance of complications of liver failure, and hence indirectly improves patient outcome.

8. If this modality is initiated late in the course of liver failure, the result is frequently not satisfactory.

9. Use of the Molecular Adsorbent Recirculating System is a safe procedure but carries potential complications such as platelet reduction, hypoglycemia, and other risks of extracorporeal circuitry exist.

10. Albumin-bound drugs given before treatment with this modality would have to be re-administered after dialysis.

11. Given the limited available data, use of the Molecular Adsorbent Recirculating System can be regarded only as an experimental procedure

to be used in highly specialized liver treatment units.

Key References

1. Stange J, Mitzner S, Ramlow W, et al: A new procedure for the removal of protein bound drugs and toxins. ASAIO J 1993;39:M621-M625.
2. Mitzner S, Stange J, Klammt S, et al: Improvement of hepatorenal syndrome with extracorporeal albumin dialysis MARS: Results of a prospective, randomized, controlled clinical trial. Liver Transpl 2000;6:277-286.
5. Sen S, Davies NA, Mookerjee RP, et al: Pathophysiological effects of albumin dialysis in acute-on-chronic liver failure: A randomized controlled study. Liver Transpl 2004;10:1109-1119.
23. Evenepoel P, Maes B, Wilmer A, et al: Detoxifying capacity and kinetics of the molecular adsorbent recycling system: Contribution of the different inbuilt filters. Blood Purif 2003;21:244-252.
47. Chiu A, Fan ST: MARS in the treatment of liver failure: Controversies and evidence. Int J Artif Organs 2006;29:660-667.

See the companion Expert Consult website for the complete reference list.

CHAPTER 282

Extracorporeal Blood Purification Techniques beyond Dialysis: Coupled Plasmafiltration-Adsorption

Marco Formica, Sergio Livigni, and Claudio Ronco

OBJECTIVES

This chapter will:
1. Discuss the use of extracorporeal blood purification techniques within the clinical picture of sepsis.
2. Provide a rationale based on in vitro and animal studies for the use of coupled plasmafiltration-adsorption in human sepsis.
3. Analyze early clinical results of this approach in terms of hemodynamics, respiratory function, immune status, and survival.

Sepsis is one of the main causes of morbidity and mortality in intensive care units worldwide and the tenth leading cause of death in the United States.[1] Mortality of sepsis has been estimated to range from 20% to 80%—depending to a large extent on the severity of the clinical picture, the involvement of one or more organs (the so-called multiple-organ dysfunction syndrome [MODS]), the study design (and reporting methods), and the timing of treatment initiation. Multiple-organ dysfunction syndrome and renal

failure often result from the exaggerated host response to infection.[2,3] Although several attempts have targeted specific components of the inflammatory cascade, no improvements in outcome have been reported in clinical trials.[4]

Sepsis is the leading cause of acute kidney injury (AKI), the prevalence of which ranges from 19% in sepsis, to 23% in severe sepsis, to 51% in septic shock.[5]

Sepsis involves two important pathways, the pro-inflammatory response and an immunosuppressive (or immunodysfunctional) response. The first is aimed at the delivery of mediators with a pro-inflammatory action, such as tumor necrosis factor-α, interleukin-1, interleukin-6, and the other releases cytokines with a predominant anti-inflammatory activity, such as interleukin-10 and interleukin-4. Both responses may take place at the same time, and not in sequence as previously considered.[6]

It is hypothesized that inflammatory molecules are responsible for diffuse endothelial injury, inducing vasoparalysis and driving selective permeability with important ramifications on systemic hemodynamics and multiple-organ dysfunction syndrome. On the other hand, monocytes lose their ability to synthesize and deliver cytokines as a consequence of inflammatory stimuli, leading to an "immunoparalytic" state characterized by monocyte deactivation.[7,8] The substantial failure of the first interventional trials targeting specific components of the pro-inflammatory cascade, such as tumor necrosis factor-α, moved attention to different targets, for example, to blood purification techniques, which may remove several mediators simultaneously, positively affecting the outcome in septic shock.[9]

Of the extracorporeal treatments as a whole, "classic" continuous renal replacement therapies show intrinsic limitations tied to constrained exchange volumes and a low sieving coefficient of the molecules affected (with an approximate molecular weight ranging from 5 to 50 kDa), which leads to low removal rates and clearances.[10] In vitro studies have shown that employing a large-pore membrane may enhance the convective transfer of soluble pro-inflammatory and anti-inflammatory mediators, leading to increased clearance of nonselective cytokines.[11-13]

In order to overcome some of these problems, a new extracorporeal blood purification system was developed, coupled plasmafiltration-adsorption (CPFA), which uses a resin cartridge along with a second hemofiltration system that allows convective exchange. The system exploits the nonselective removal of inflammatory mediators by means of a hydrophobic styrenic resin. The resin has high affinity and a large capacity for many cytokines and mediators.[14] The rationale for sorbent adsorption is to re-infuse the endogenous plasma after nonselective, simultaneous removal of different sepsis-associated mediators by means of processing it through a specific cartridge.[15]

CPFA is performed with the use of a four-pump modular treatment (Lynda, Bellco, Mirandola, Italy) consisting of a plasmafilter—0.45 m² polyethersulfone with approximate cutoff of 800 kDa and absorption on a unselective hydrophobic resin cartridge (140 mL)—with a surface of about 700 m²/g, and a final passage of the reconstituted blood through a synthetic, high-permeability, 1.4-m² polyethersulfone hemofilter in which convective exchanges may be applied in a post-dilutional mode (Fig. 282-1).

The advantage in processing the plasma and not the blood through the sorbent cartridge is related to the fact that the plasma flow is lower than blood flow, allowing for a longer contact time with the sorbent.[16] Other advantages of using plasma are that there are no bioincompatibility issues and the problem of having to "coat" the resin with a biocompatible matrix, which often decreases efficacy, is avoided.

The post-dilution reinfusion rate can be set for up to 4 L/hr. The blood flow is usually 150 to 180 mL/min, and the plasmafiltration rate is maintained at a fractional filtration of the blood flow (approximately 15%-20%). The treatment is usually run for approximately 10 hours, after which the cartridge begins to show saturation by the mediators.

Early studies of CPFA used a prototype machine and cartridge with less resin that needed to be changed more often. Ronco and colleagues,[17] who tested the first clinical treatments of CPFA using the prototype machine, reported that a single CPFA treatment lasting 10 hours showed better hemodynamic improvement than continuous venovenous hemodiafiltration (referring to an improvement in mean arterial pressure and a decrease in norepinephrine requirement). Furthermore, this study provided very interesting biological data: Monocytes in plasma drawn after passage through the sorbent cartridge were again able to respond to the lipopolysaccharide challenge with tumor

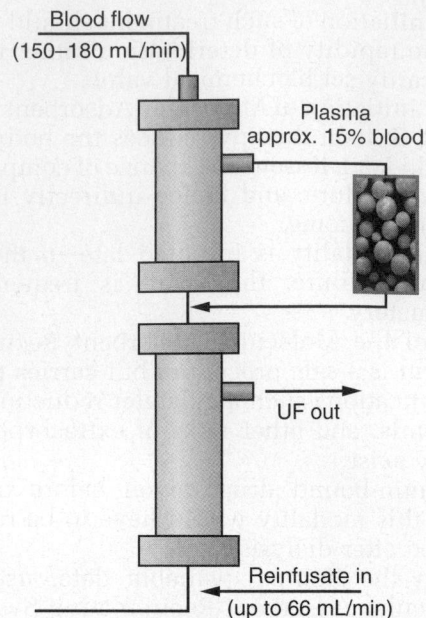

FIGURE 282-1. Schematic diagram of coupled plasmafiltration-adsorption.

necrosis factor-α production at a magnitude significantly greater than with continuous venovenous hemodiafiltration (Fig. 282-2). According to these preliminary data, CPFA was suggested to have a potential role for blood purification in septic shock treatment, modulating the immune response and resetting the balance between pro-inflammatory and anti-inflammatory mediators. This concept was novel in that it suggested a role for extracorporeal therapies in actual purification of blood to remove inflammatory mediators, reaching beyond the traditional role of support for patients with renal failure.

Still employing the prototype machine, Formica and associates[18] evaluated the hemodynamic performance of CPFA. Their study had two unique features: (1) repeated application of the technique during the course of the septic shock (a mean of ten 10-hour sessions were applied) and (2) use in patients without concomitant AKI. Improvements have been reported in the main hemodynamic and respiratory parameters, such as mean arterial pressure, cardiac index, peripheral vascular resistance, and ratio of oxygen arterial pressure to inspired oxygen fraction ratio, as well as in levels of some mediators and severity of illness scores (Fig. 282-3). Norepinephrine was progressively tapered and stopped with different timings in the patient's population. Hence, it may have been stopped in one patient after three sessions and in another after eight sessions. The mean among the patients was five sessions.

No untoward clinical effects were recorded during the procedures, thus underlying the safety of the technique, which may be applied irrespective of the presence of AKI. The sessions had been originally planned for a duration of 10 hours, but the mean delivery time was about 8 hours 45 minutes. Reasons for shorter sessions related to clinical requirements (radiological procedures, emergency surgery) and to technical problems (circuit coagulation, plasmafilter malfunction). The issue of coagulation with CPFA has been further addressed in a study performed in a particular AKI population.[19]

These technical problems have greatly delayed the introduction of a new machine that contained seven pressure transducers to monitor the transmembrane pressure and

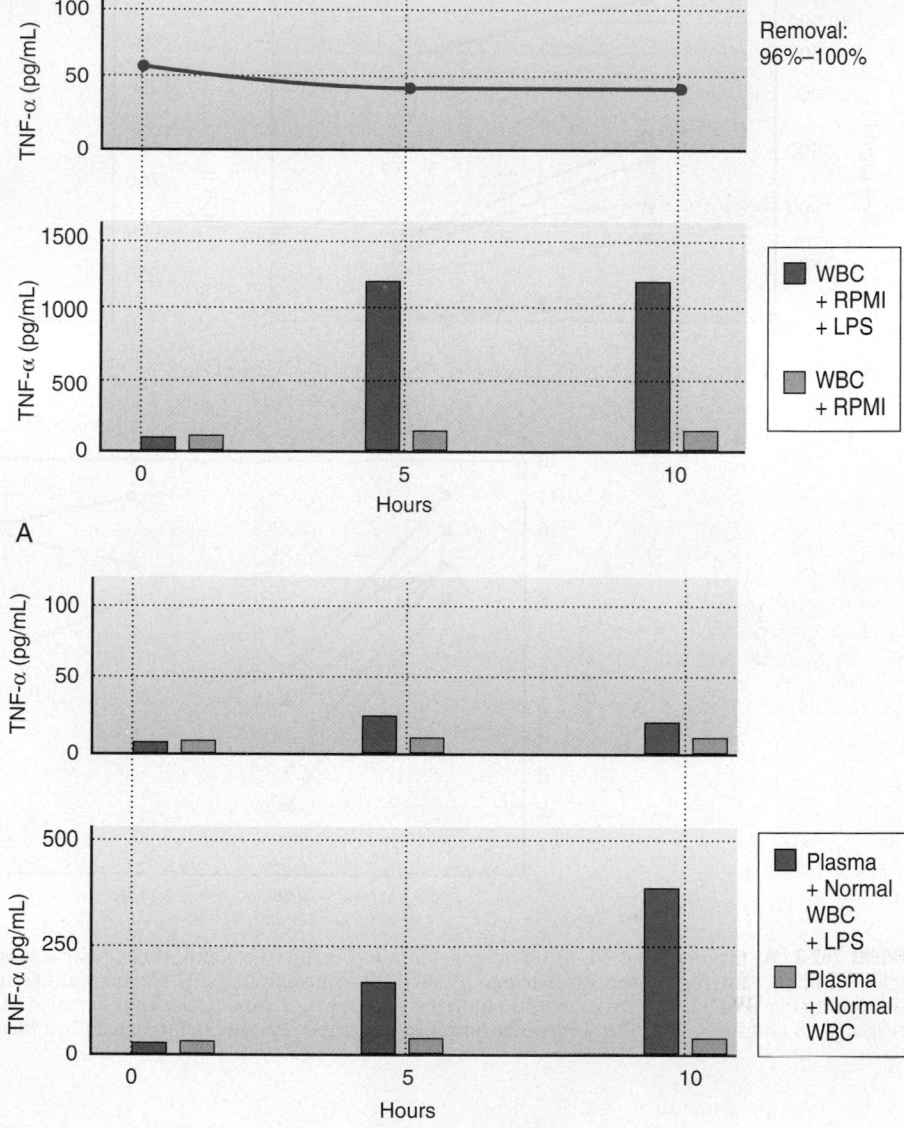

FIGURE 282-2. *A,* In vitro production of tumor necrosis factor-α (TNF-α) after lipopolysaccharide challenge at different times during coupled plasmafiltration-adsorption (CPFA). *Top,* plasma TNF-α level; *bottom,* in vitro production. *Dark blue bar* indicates white blood cells plus lipopolysaccharide; *light blue bar* indicates white blood cells plus RPMI medium only. *B,* Effect of septic plasma on normal white blood cell production of TNF-α during CPFA treatment. *Top,* pre-cartridge plasma; *bottom,* post-cartridge plasma. *Dark blue bar* indicates plasma plus normal white blood cells plus lipopolysaccharides; *light blue bar* indicates plasma plus normal white blood cells. (Data from Ronco C, Brendolan A, Lonnemann G, et al: A pilot study of coupled plasma filtration with adsorption in septic shock. Crit Care Med 2002;30:1250-1255.).

pressure drops of the plasmafilter, hemofilter, and adsorptive cartridge in real time. Several pilot studies are currently under way to evaluate the role of mediator removal during barotraumas induced by mechanical ventilation and the role of CPFA versus pulsed high-volume hemofiltration in sepsis-induced apoptosis (C. Ronco, personal communication, 2006).

CONCLUSION

The prognosis of patients admitted to intensive care units with septic shock and multiple-organ dysfunction syndrome has still today a burden of high mortality, and all attempts to find a "magic bullet" to restore the immune derangements have failed owing to the complex interactions between pro-inflammatory and anti-inflammatory responses during sepsis, along with the clinical course of the disease.

Interest in the use of extracorporeal blood purification techniques in sepsis has been growing.[20] Of all techniques, CPFA has been demonstrated to be a feasible and safe treatment, with positive results in terms of improved systemic hemodynamics and respiratory functions paralleled by a quick tapering of the need for vasoactive drugs. Also of interest is the improvement in splanchnic perfusion, evaluated by means of tonometry of gastric-mucosal PCO_2 diffusion, which could further emphasize the resolution of the hyperdynamic-vasoparalytic state displayed in septic shock.[21]

Thus, CPFA is a treatment targeted to the nonselective removal of soluble mediators involved in the septic shock scenario. One can further speculate that the association of different removal mechanisms (diffusion/convection/adsorption) in this modality may play a role in reestablishing a new immune balance (*immunomodulation*) with a significant reduction in acute-phase reactants achieved by hampering their peak levels.[22,23] The results may be related to the ability to restore leukocyte responsiveness to immu-

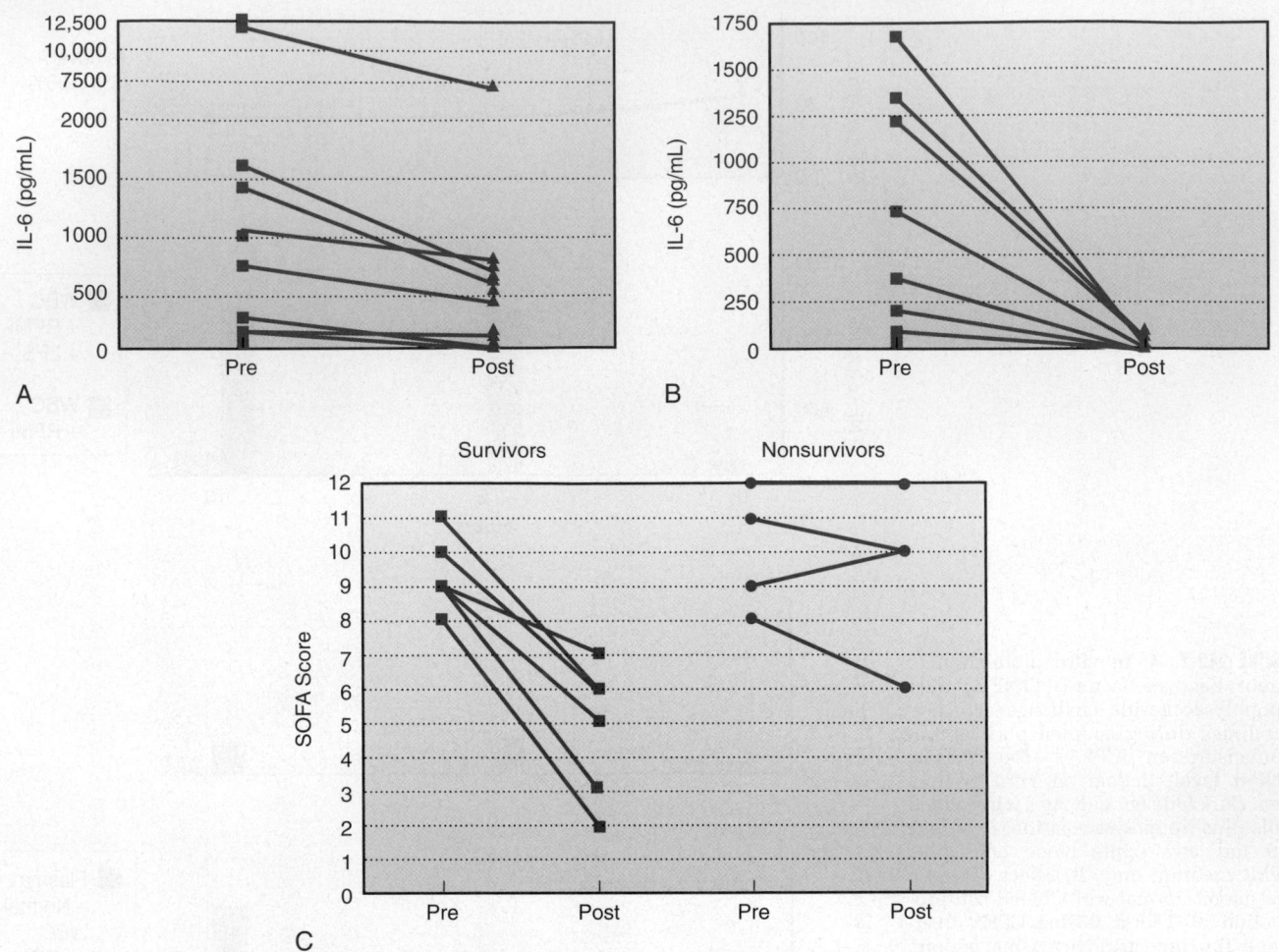

FIGURE 282-3. A, Interleukin-6 (IL-6) blood concentration before (Pre) and after (Post) a session of coupled plasmafiltration-adsorption (CPFA). **B,** Pre-cartridge and post-cartridge plasma IL-6 concentrations. **C,** Sequential Organ Failure Assessment (SOFA) scores before (Pre) and after (Post) CPFA treatment in survivors and nonsurvivors. (Data from Formica M, Olivieri C, Livigni S, et al: Hemodynamic response to coupled plasmafiltration-adsorption in human septic shock. Intensive Care Med 2003;29:703-708.).

noactive stimuli, which may be clinically beneficial because of the link to hemodynamic improvement.[17,24] Considering the still high morbidity and mortality rates in patients admitted to intensive care units with septic shock, this new blood purification technique seems to exert its benefits best when applied early in the course of sepsis and also when used in patients without concomitant AKI, suggesting that it can be performed to prevent rather than treat AKI.[18] With these premises, if confirmed, it is reasonable to propose to extend this technique also to early stages of septic shock (such as severe sepsis or systemic inflammatory response syndrome—along with pancreatitis).

Despite the fact that some clinical results of CPFA treatment appear quite good, they must be regarded with caution because of the small sample sizes in the studies. One must emphasize, however, that these good outcome results, where achieved, fueled the relationship between the nephrologists and the intensivists in managing these very complex, critically ill patients.

Further studies may provide evidence that clarifies issues regarding the potential utility of blood purification systems such as CPFA in patients with sepsis. Among these, one study is investigating clinical outcome in septic patients with AKI who are randomly assigned either to

CPFA and pulsed high-volume hemofiltration (C. Ronco, personal communication, 2006).

Furthermore, a large Italian multicenter study, identified by the acronym COMPACT (COMbined Plasmafiltration and Adsorption Clinical Trial)—registered on Clinical Trial.gov with the identifier NCT00332371 and on www. ISRCTN.org with the code ISRCTN24534559—has been initiated. It is evaluating the treatment of patients with septic shock by means of early initiation (within 6 hours of diagnosis) of CPFA (Fig. 282-4). The objectives of the study are to compare hospital and intensive care unit mortality and morbidity rates in a group given CPFA in addition to standard medical care and a control group receiving standard medical care alone. The sample size needed to show a mortality difference of 25% between the two arms is 330 patients. The study was started in December 2006.

Key Points

1. Continuous plasmafiltration-adsorption is a feasible, safe, and well-tolerated treatment for critically ill patients with sepsis.

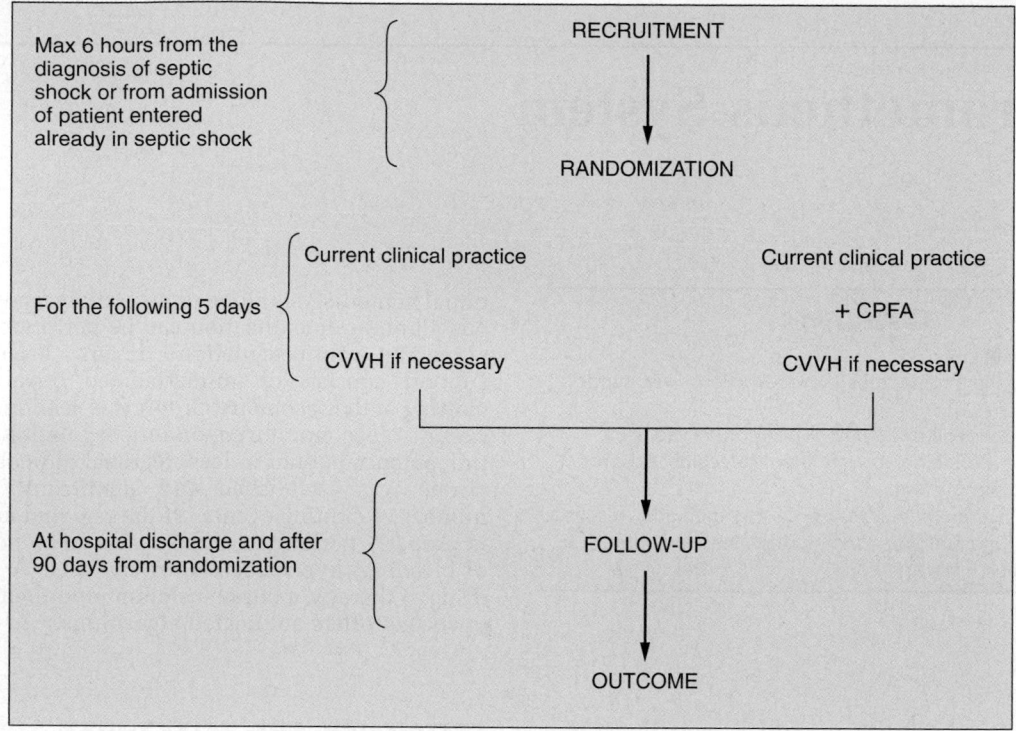

FIGURE 282-4. Flow chart of the COMbined Plasmafiltration and Adsorption Clinical Trial (COMPACT). CPFA, coupled plasmafiltration-adsorption; CVVH, continuous venovenous hemofiltration.

2. This procedure has been shown to improve hemo-dynamics (mean arterial pressure, cardiac index, vascular peripheral resistance) and pulmonary function (ratio of oxygen arterial pressure to inspired oxygen fraction), to reduce norepineph-rine requirement, and to restore immune balance (improvement of monocyte deactivation).

3. Continuous plasmafiltration-adsorption allows a nonselective binding of a wide array of pro-inflammatory and anti-inflammatory mediators, cutting down their peak concentrations and showing an effective body clearance beyond a reduced inflammatory state.

4. This technique can be used in combination with other therapies, such as continuous venovenous hemofiltration, but it may also be of use in patients without acute kidney injury in order to *prevent* the renal involvement.

5. Despite some anecdotal data on improved survival, more large-scale trials are needed to support the potential benefits of continuous plasmafiltra-tion-adsorption in treating septic patients. A large multicenter trial is currently under way to evalu-ate the survival effects of this modality in patients with septic shock.

Acknowledgments

We are grateful to Mary Lou Wratten, PhD, for her labora-tory work and for her invaluable assistance in interpreting data and revising the manuscript.

Key References

12. Tetta C, Gianotti L, Cavaillon JM, et al: Continuous plasma-filtration coupled with sorbent adsorption in a rabbit model of endotoxic shock. Crit Care Med 2000;28:1526-1533.

17. Ronco C, Brendolan A, Lonnemann G, et al: A pilot study of coupled plasma filtration with adsorption in septic shock. Crit Care Med 2002;30:1250-1255.

18. Formica M, Olivieri C, Livigni S, et al: Hemodynamic response to coupled plasmafiltration-adsorption in human septic shock. Intensive Care Med 2003;29:703-708.

21. Cesano G, Livigni S, Vallero A, et al: Trattamento dello shock settico con l'impiego della CPFA (plasmafiltrazione ed assor-bimento associate): Impatto sull'emodinamica valutata con il sistema Picco. G Ital Nefrol 2003;20:258-263.

23. Ronco C, Tetta C, Mariano F, et al: Interpreting the mecha-nisms of continuous renal replacement therapy in sepsis: The peak concentration hypothesis. Artif Organs 2003;27:792-801.

See the companion Expert Consult website for the complete reference list.

CHAPTER 283

The Prometheus System

Kinan Rifai

OBJECTIVES

This chapter will:
1. Describe the Prometheus extracorporeal liver support system.
2. Summarize available clinical data on Prometheus.
3. Compare Prometheus with the Molecular Adsorbent Recirculating System.
4. Provide a critical discussion of the methods, results, possible indications, and further needed data for Prometheus.

Patients with liver failure have a high mortality if liver transplantation is not available in time.[1] Therefore, the development of extracorporeal liver support devices has been attempted for a long time. Of these, bioartificial systems ("biolivers") contain hepatocytes in a bioreactor that seeks to replace full liver function. In contrast, artificial systems ("liver dialysis") aim at only supporting liver detoxification by using different filtration techniques that remove toxic substances.[2] However, a substantial improvement in patient outcome could not be demonstrated by any system or method. The field of artificial liver support systems has now regained attention as new devices such as the Molecular Adsorbent Recirculating System (MARS; Gambro AG, Lund, Sweden) were developed.[3] These systems combine the removal of albumin-bound and water-soluble substances and are therefore often referred to as "albumin dialysis."

THE PROMETHEUS SYSTEM

The Prometheus system (Fresenius Medical Care, Bad Homburg, Germany) is a novel artificial liver support device. The purification method of fractionated plasma separation and adsorption (FPSA) that it uses was developed by Falkenhagen and colleagues.[4] The combined removal of albumin-bound substances and water-soluble substances is achieved by a different method from that in MARS, which uses an *albumin-impermeable* membrane, so that toxins are removed by diffusion.[5] In Prometheus, an *albumin-permeable* polysulfone membrane (AlbuFlow) separates the albumin fraction with all bound substances of the patient's blood and passes it into the secondary circuit (Fig. 283-1). There, special adsorbers (Prometh01, Prometh02) directly purify the plasma from albumin-bound toxins. Thereafter, water-soluble substances are removed by conventional high-flux dialysis (FX50) inside the primary circuit. A modified hemodialysis unit (4008H) integrates the two circuits of the Prometheus system, which are run separately by the unit. Thus, either conven-tional hemodialysis alone or hemodialysis with simultaneous albumin detoxification can be performed.

Usually, anticoagulation during Prometheus liver support consists of unfractionated heparin.[6] However, clotting of the secondary circuit was seen in some patients despite close monitoring of anticoagulation. To overcome this potential albumin loss, regional anticoagulation with citrate was established and significantly reduced the number of clotting events.[7] If the regional anticoagulation is properly performed, there seems to be no elevated risk of bleeding, hypocalcemia, or acidosis. To ease the handling of therapy, a citrate-calcium module has been developed that offers automated algorithms.

EFFICIENCY AND SELECTIVITY OF REMOVAL

Toxin clearance by Prometheus was studied in detail by Evenepoel and coworkers.[8] In nine patients with acute-on-chronic liver failure, these investigators measured concentrations of different substances at different times in the arterial line and inside the secondary circuit during 6 hours of treatment with Prometheus. Blood clearances declined during treatment as the capacity of the adsorption columns became saturated. Overall, removal rates for total bilirubin, conjugated bilirubin, bile acids, creatinine, and urea were between 41% and 68%. Only the removal rate for serum ammonia was lower (17%), which can possibly be explained by a high generation or redistribution rate of ammonia.

Rifai and colleagues[9] evaluated the removal selectivity of the Prometheus device. In nine patients with liver failure, no significant effect of Prometheus therapy on closely monitored blood levels of cytokines (e.g., tumor necrosis factor-α), coagulation factors (e.g., factors II and V) or other plasma proteins (e.g., fibrinogen) was observed. One can therefore assume that the filters and adsorbers used have a high selectivity for albumin-bound toxins and water-soluble substances.

A prospective comparison of the in vivo extraction capacities of the Prometheus system and MARS was performed by Krisper and associates[10] in eight patients with acute-on-chronic liver failure. The trial was a crossover study; that is, each patient was treated two times with each system. Clearance rates and reduction ratios for both protein-bound and water-soluble substances were higher with Prometheus treatment than with MARS therapy. Furthermore, unconjugated bilirubin as a marker of strong protein binding was removed only by the Prometheus system. The investigators concluded that the Prometheus system delivers a higher treatment dose than the MARS.

Another study retrospectively compared the blood clearances and reduction ratios for various substances with the Prometheus system and MARS in 18 patients

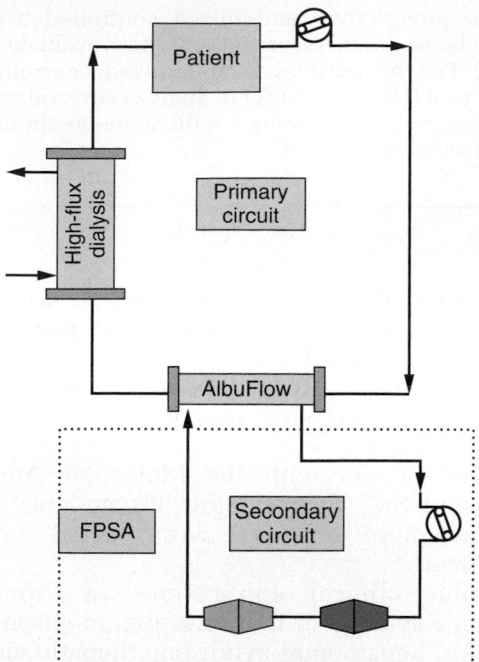

FIGURE 283-1. Schematic of Prometheus system. The system consists of a primary circuit and a secondary circuit that are separated by an albumin-permeable polysulfone membrane (AlbuFlow). From the membrane, the patient's albumin fraction is filtered into the secondary circuit, where direct purification from albumin-bound toxins by different adsorbers (Prometh01, Prometh02) takes place. Afterwards, conventional high-flux dialysis (FX50) is performed inside the primary circuit. FPSA, fractionated plasma separation and adsorption.

with acute-on-chronic liver failure.[11] As Krisper and associates[10] found, blood clearances and reductions ratios for all substances except bile acids were higher with Prometheus than with MARS therapy. Furthermore, the decline in blood clearances of protein-bound substances over time was significantly higher with MARS than with Prometheus, suggesting a more rapid saturation of the MARS adsorber.

SAFETY

The pilot trial of the Prometheus system was especially conducted to evaluate the safety of the device.[6] Eleven patients with various types of acute-on-chronic liver failure and concomitant renal failure were treated with Prometheus for 4 to 6 hours on two consecutive days instead of their regular dialysis sessions. In general, Prometheus treatment was safe. However, a reversible decrease in mean arterial pressure during Prometheus treatment was observed, especially in two patients with systemic inflammatory response syndrome. Because the separated plasma inside the secondary circuit adds to the extracorporeal volume in Prometheus, the decrease in blood pressure could be more pronounced with this system than with conventional dialysis.

A randomized study in 18 patients with acute-on-chronic liver failure compared the effect of Prometheus, MARS, and standard medical therapy on systemic hemodynamics.[12] Mean arterial pressure and peripheral resis-

tance improved only in patients treated with MARS. This finding may be related to a removal of vasoactive agents such as renin and nitric oxide only by MARS and not by the Prometheus system.

Another side effect of Prometheus therapy during the pilot trial was a reversible increase in white blood cell count.[6] No other signs of systemic inflammation were observed, so a transient leukocyte activation by the Prometheus membrane is probable. On the other hand, the rate of treatment-related thrombopenia seems to be significantly lower with Prometheus therapy than with MARS therapy. Furthermore, no treatment-related bleeding episodes have been reported to date.

Regarding a possible loss of the patient's albumin during Prometheus therapy, findings are inconsistent.[6,8,9]

CLINICAL DATA

The first published reports of clinical application of Prometheus by Kramer and associates[13] described the case of a 27-year-old man with acute liver failure. Because the liver failure was due to ecstasy and cocaine intoxication, he was regarded as not eligible for liver transplantation. When multiple-organ failure and advanced cerebral edema with transtentorial herniation developed, continuous Prometheus treatment was initiated. The therapy rapidly normalized ammonia levels, and subsequently, the cerebral edema disappeared and hepatic function recovered. The patient was discharged with only minor neurological deficits.

In a study by Skwarek and colleagues,[14] Prometheus was used in 16 patients with acute liver failure. The major causes of liver failure were paracetamol ($n = 5$), *Amanita* intoxication ($n = 4$), and unknown ($n = 5$). All patients fulfilled the King's College Hospital Criteria for urgent liver transplantation. Five patients died before transplantation because of a lack of grafts ($n = 4$) or consent ($n = 1$). Seven patients were supported with Prometheus therapy ("bridged") until transplantation, and 4 survived without transplantation.

Regarding patients with acute-on-chronic liver failure, the pilot trial demonstrated the efficacy of the Prometheus system by showing a significant improvement in serum concentrations of various protein-bound and water-soluble substances.[6] Liver detoxification was demonstrated by the removal of bilirubin, bile acids, and ammonia. Parameters of renal function, such as serum creatinine, urea, and blood pH, improved as well. However, for clinical parameters such as hepatic encephalopathy and Child-Pugh Score, the improvement did not reach statistical significance. In-hospital patient mortality was high without any evidence of treatment-related complications. In interpretation of the clinical results, the small number of treatments given during the pilot trial must be considered.

For patients with severe hepatorenal syndrome, the Prometheus system offers a new therapeutic option for the combination of liver support and renal replacement therapy. The removal of important protein-bound and water-soluble substances was confirmed in 10 patients with combined liver and renal failure.[15]

Further clinical experience with Prometheus therapy has been gained in the successful support ("bridging") of adult and pediatric patients awaiting liver transplantation.[16] The longest bridging period so far was 51 days with 23 Prometheus sessions in a 38-year-old patient with liver failure and hepatorenal syndrome.[17]

TABLE 283-1

Possible Indications for and Contraindications to Prometheus Therapy

Possible indications	Acute liver failure
	Acute-on-chronic liver failure
	Acute alcoholic hepatitis
	Hepatorenal syndrome
	Hepatic encephalopathy
	"Bridging" to liver transplantation
	Refractory cholestatic pruritus
	Intoxication with protein-bound drugs
Contraindications	Uncontrolled bleeding
	Severe hemodynamic instability
	Uncontrolled septicemia
	Disseminated intravascular coagulation
	Severe thrombocytopenia

Severe refractory cholestatic pruritus is another emerging indication for Prometheus therapy. Rifai and colleagues[18] treated seven patients with various types of severe cholestatic pruritus that was refractory to all medical treatments. All patients with elevated serum bile acid levels (6 of 7) reported a marked improvement of pruritus after three to five Prometheus sessions. In four of the six patients, the benefit lasted more than 4 weeks. Overall, a visual analogue scale score as a subjective measure of pruritus intensity and serum bile acid levels significantly improved. Interestingly, all patients without sustained response presented without significant elevation of serum bilirubin values. Possible indications for and contraindications to Prometheus therapy are summarized in Table 283-1.

CONCLUSIONS

Fractionated plasma separation and adsorption is used in Prometheus as a new concept for extracorporeal liver support in patients with liver failure. The system is safe and useful and has a high potential to remove both protein-bound and water-soluble substances. Thus, if needed, liver support and renal replacement therapy can be combined in one treatment. The dose delivered by the Prometheus system seems to be higher than that delivered by the MARS. So far, there are no signs of unselective removal except for a possible small albumin loss.

A meta-analysis has demonstrated a survival benefit for patients with acute-on-chronic liver failure after treatment with artificial liver support devices.[19] However, there is a need for prospective randomized controlled trials that involve large numbers of patients and evaluate patient survival. For this purpose, a randomized, controlled multicenter trial (HELIOS study) to analyze survival with Prometheus treatment in patients with acute-on-chronic liver failure has been initiated.

Key Points

1. The Prometheus system is a novel extracorporeal liver support system based on fractionated plasma separation and adsorption.
2. Initial studies proved its safety, feasibility, and efficacy in removing protein-bound and water-soluble toxins.
3. In comparison with the Molecular Adsorbent Recirculating System, the Prometheus system seems more effective with regard to toxin removal.
4. Possible clinical applications of Prometheus include acute liver failure, acute-on-chronic liver failure, hepatorenal syndrome, hepatic encephalopathy, "bridging" to liver transplantation, refractory pruritus, and intoxication with protein-bound substances.
5. The ongoing HELIOS trial will provide further information regarding a potential benefit for patient survival.

Key References

6. Rifai K, Ernst T, Kretschmer U, et al: Prometheus—a new extracorporeal system for the treatment of liver failure. J Hepatol 2003;39:984-990.
10. Krisper P, Haditsch B, Stauber R, et al: In vivo quantification of liver dialysis: Comparison of albumin dialysis and fractionated plasma separation. J Hepatol 2005;43:451-457.
12. Laleman W, Wilmer A, Evenepoel P, et al: Effect of the Molecular Adsorbent Recirculating System and Prometheus devices on systemic hemodynamics and vasoactive agents in patients with acute-on-chronic alcoholic liver failure. Crit Care 2006;10:R108.
18. Rifai K, Hafer C, Rosenau J, et al: Treatment of severe refractory pruritus with fractionated plasma separation and adsorption (Prometheus). Scand J Gastroenterol 2006;41:1212-1217.
19. Kjaergard LL, Liu J, Als-Nielsen B, Gluud C: Artificial and bioartificial support systems for acute and acute-on-chronic liver failure: A systematic review. JAMA 2003;289:217-222.

See the companion Expert Consult website for the complete reference list.

CHAPTER 284

Toraymyxin and Other Endotoxin Adsorption Systems

Gualtiero Guadagni, Dinna N. Cruz, Hisataka Shoji, and Claudio Ronco

---

OBJECTIVES

This chapter will:
1. Describe the role of endotoxin in septic patients.
2. Define the possibility of measuring endotoxins.
3. Describe the evolution of endotoxin-targeted therapy of sepsis, from drugs to medical devices.
4. Discuss the characteristics of Toraymyxin endotoxin adsorption.
5. Evaluate the importance and accuracy of measurement and removal of endotoxins as a feasible theranostic approach for septic shock.

ROLE AND MEASUREMENT OF ENDOTOXIN IN SEPTIC PATIENTS

Endotoxin, also known as lipopolysaccharide, is a major cell wall constituent of gram-negative bacteria and the primary gram-negative bacterial product responsible for septic shock (Fig. 284-1). Endotoxin in the blood comes from one of two sources, a bacterial infection or bacteria that reside normally in the gastrointestinal tract from which endotoxin has translocated into the bloodstream.[1-3] Endotoxin causes the release of cytokines such as interleukin-1 and tumor necrosis factor-α and activates complements and coagulation factors. Endotoxin is considered one of the principal biological substances that cause gram-negative septic shock.[3]

High levels of endotoxin in the blood are responsible for many of the symptoms seen during a serious infection or inflammation, such as fever and elevated white blood cell count. Severe sepsis occurs when the body is overwhelmed by the inflammatory response and body organs begin to fail. Sepsis may develop as a result of infections acquired in the community, such as pneumonia, or may be a complication that develops during the treatment of trauma or cancer or after major surgery. Increased levels of endotoxin can be associated with other conditions in critically ill patients, such as shock and hypoxemia. Endotoxemia has pathogenic properties in patients who have liver disease, who have undergone surgery, or who are undergoing cardiopulmonary bypass.

The historical assay for the detection of lipopolysaccharide in non–blood-based or non–plasma-based fluids has been the *limulus* amebocyte lysate proteolytic coagulation cascade. This assay performs well in matrices such as crystalloids, in which endotoxin is not bound by specific substances. In plasma and in whole blood, however, lipopolysaccharide binds to lipopolysaccharide-binding protein and some substances, such as protein and lipopro-

tein, so various extraction and pre-treatment strategies have been developed to attempt to release lipopolysaccharide from its binding sites in whole blood or plasma and to neutralize poorly defined inhibitors that confound *limulus* amebocyte lysate–based technologies. These changes have not been successful in overcoming all issues, however. In fact the *limulus* amebocyte lysate test has never been approved by regulatory agencies in North America for clinical use in humans.

The EAA Endotoxin Activity Assay (Spectral Diagnostics Inc, Toronto) is a new diagnostic test approved by the U.S. Food and Drug Administration for the measurement of endotoxin in whole blood. The test relies on the following factors:
- The endotoxin reacts with antibody specific to its lipid A portion.
- The antibody-antigen complex is amplified by the patient's neutrophils in whole blood.

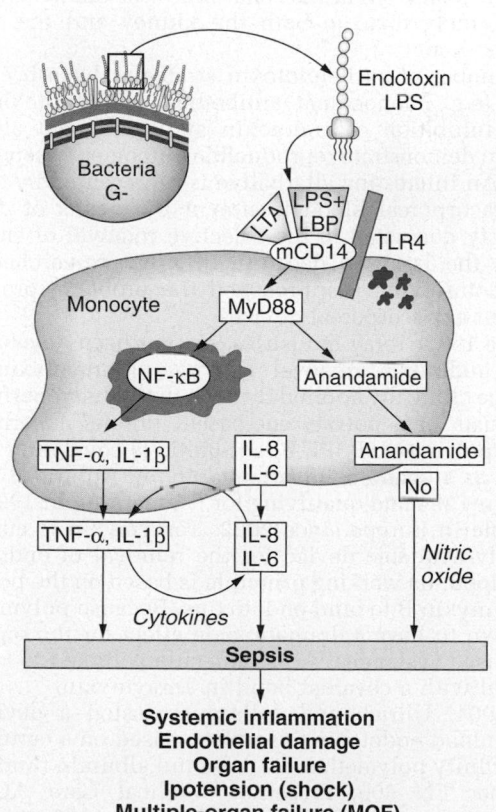

FIGURE 284-1. Role of endotoxin in sepsis. Endotoxin triggers the release of inflammatory mediators and nitric oxide, a major endogenous vasodilator.

- The amplification results in an enhanced respiratory burst in the presence of zymosan; the burst is detected by luminal chemiluminescence.
- The magnitude of the priming influence is proportional to the concentration of antigen-antibody complex.

The test is feasible, accurate, and reliable, providing in less than 40 minutes a quick measurement of blood endotoxin concentration. In a multicenter clinical trial involving more than 1000 patients, the test was shown to have excellent test characteristics in critically ill patients with suspected sepsis and its results correlated strongly with adverse outcomes, including death and organ dysfunction.[4] Elevations of endotoxin are significantly associated with the development of a clinical diagnosis of severe sepsis. When endotoxin levels are moderately high, the odds ratio for development of severe sepsis is 2.0; when endotoxin levels are high, the odds ratio rises to 3.0. These values are equivalent to 100% and 200% increased risks, respectively. Results of this trial suggest that EAA could be used as a marker of the risk for development of sepsis as well as a trigger for endotoxemia-directed therapies.

THERAPIES AGAINST ENDOTOXINS: FROM DRUGS TO MEDICAL DEVICES

Many efforts have been made in the last three decades to assess therapies against endotoxin, the primary trigger of the inflammatory process, as a drug target.[5] The idea started in the middle 1970s, when polymyxin B was discovered to be protective against endotoxin-induced hemodynamic shock but at the same time was demonstrated to be extremely toxic to both the kidney and the central nervous system.[6]

A number of anti-endotoxin strategies have been proposed (e.g., monoclonal antibodies, antiendotoxin vaccines, inhibition of endotoxin synthesis), but all have failed to demonstrate reproducible outcomes in septic subjects.[5] An interesting alternative is represented by the use of extracorporeal blood treatment by means of devices expressly dedicated to the selective removal of endotoxins; in the last two decades, different researchers and manufacturers have approached the problem, proposing different extracorporeal devices.

Since 1983, Toray Industries Inc. has been developing a blood endotoxin removal cartridge (Toraymyxin) that could be clinically applied through direct hemoperfusion.[4] It consists of a polystyrene-based, fibrous adsorbent in which polymyxin B (PL-B) antibiotic is covalently immobilized as a ligand to adsorb endotoxin. Approved first in Japan in 1994 and qualifying for CE marking in 1998, and available in Europe since 2002, Toraymyxin is currently the only available device for the removal of endotoxins from blood. Its working principle is based on the potential of polymyxin B to bind endotoxins. Because polymyxin B is known to have a dramatic side effect for the organism when used systemically, its molecule is linked to an inert material with a covalent bond in Toraymyxin.

In 2001, Ullrich and colleagues tested a device for whole-blood endotoxin adsorption based on a cartridge of high-affinity polymethacrylate-bound albumin (Endotoxin Adsorber EN 500, Fresenius Medical Care AG, Bad Homburg, Germany).[7] Results of the pilot study were interesting, but a large multicenter randomized trial reported by Reinhart in 2004 did not demonstrate a benefit of this absorber, probably because of non-optimal timing and definition of inclusion criteria.[8]

Bengsch and colleagues in 2005 proposed that the use of an apheresis system derived from H.E.L.P. and based on a diethylaminoethyl-cellulose absorber is capable of reducing the plasma concentration of endotoxin in patients with severe sepsis.[9] The treatment is based on 5 to 10 consecutive apheresis treatments of 1.6 L of plasma. The researchers described the experience of a pilot observational trial, reporting encouraging results in terms of reduction in endotoxins as well as consequent reduction in inflammatory mediators.

THE TORAYMYXIN SYSTEM: CONCEPT AND MANUFACTURING PROCESS

Toraymyxin is a device principally made of covalently immobilized polymyxin B fiber (PMX-F) used as an adsorbent bed.[4] PL-B, a polycationic antibiotic, is well known to bind endotoxin and neutralize its toxicity. The binding site of PL-B to endotoxin is reported to be a lipid A portion, with binding via ionic and hydrophobic interactions. Lipid A is the toxic moiety of endotoxin, and its structure is much more conserved among gram-negative bacterial species and strains. The intravenous use of PL-B is contraindicated, owing to its nephrotoxicity and neurotoxicity. Therefore, for the new device, the PL-B was immobilized on the surface of an insoluble carrier material, so that it maintained its affinity for endotoxin, to obtain a selective adsorbent.

Polystyrene and polypropylene conjugated fibers were produced by a melt spinning process, with island-sea–type conjugated fibers and polypropylene (island component) to provide reinforcement of the fibers (Fig. 284-2). A bundle of the insoluble fibers was knitted into a fabric, and the polystyrene component of the fibers was chemically modified to obtain α-chloroacetoamide methyl groups; these act as functional groups to fix PL-B. The developers of this device found that the higher the number of active primary amino groups in the fixed PL-B, the more the endotoxin removal capacity of PMX-F was increased. PL-B was fixed so that there were three to four active primary amino groups after the immobilization reaction. Because primary amino groups are positively charged, they appear to play a major role in the ionic binding to the lipid A portion of endotoxin (see Fig. 284-2).

The endotoxin adsorption capacity of PMX-F was evaluated in an in vitro setting and was compared with the carrier fiber without immobilized PL-B.[10] One gram of PMX-F or carrier fibers without PL-B was added to a test tube containing 30 mL of calf serum solution with 10 ng/mL purified lipopolysaccharide (E. coli 0111:B4). After 2 hours of incubation, the serum endotoxin level of each test tube was measured with the limulus amebocyte lysate assay.[11] PMX-F sharply reduced the endotoxin level, but the carrier fiber was not effective. The endotoxin adsorption capacity of Toraymyxin was also evaluated. A calf serum solution of purified Escherichia coli lipopolysaccharide was circulated through a Toraymyxin cartridge and also a carrier fiber cartridge (with no PL-B) at a flow rate of 100 mL/min. After 2 hours of circulation, the endotoxin level was compared; only Toraymyxin could reduce the level of endotoxin.

Jaber and coworkers[12,13] evaluated the in vitro efficacy of Toraymyxin in a model of 10% human plasma after in vitro characterization of the cytokine-inducing potency of gram-negative bacterial or endotoxic challenges. Heparinized blood was obtained from healthy volunteers. The blood was used to harvest peripheral blood mononuclear cells and a 10% plasma solution was prepared from the residue. Cytokine production by peripheral blood mononuclear cells incubated with 10% plasma before and after in vitro hemoperfusion was used as the index of endotoxin removal. After 2 hours of hemoperfusion, tumor necrosis factor-α production by peripheral blood mononuclear cells was decreased in both samples. These investigators suggested an impressive in vitro removal of endotoxin by Toraymyxin. They also found, using the same experimental method, that *Staphylococcus aureus* lipoteichoic acid–induced production of TNF-α was significantly suppressed by Toraymyxin. These investigators suggested that this suppression might be due to stoichiometric binding of lipoteichoic acids to PL-B.

Various animal studies were used to assess the biocompatibility of the device[14] as well as to determine the optimal polymyxin concentration, which is 3.0 mg per 1-g of fibers.[3] Biocompatibility was excellent, although a slight reduction in platelet count was noted during the treatment, as has been observed in other canine models of hemodialysis.[14]

CLINICAL EXPERIENCE WITH ENDOTOXIN ADSORPTION

Toraymyxin has been applied clinically since 1994 in Japan by means of the health insurance system. Patients must fulfill the following three conditions simultaneously

in order for the use of Toraymyxin to be paid by health insurance:

- Endotoxemia or suspected gram-negative infection.
- Two or more of the following conditions[15]: fever (oral temperature >38° or <36° C), tachycardia (heart rate >90 beats/min), tachypnea (respirations >24 breaths/min), and leukocytosis/leukopenia (>12,000 leukocytes/mm³, <4000 leukocytes/mm³, or 10% band count).
- Septic shock necessitating vasopressor therapy.

Toraymyxin treatment is usually performed for 2 hours at a blood flow rate of 80 to 100 mL/min by direct hemoperfusion. Nafamostat mesylate is often used as the anticoagulant, owing to its short half-life in the blood, although heparin can also be used safely. Since 1994, more than 60,000 patients have been treated with Toraymyxin. A number of incidents during Toraymyxin treatment, such as decreased platelet count and decreased blood pressure, have been reported as adverse effects. However, the frequency of these incidents is small, and no serious side effects have been reported since 1994.

Despite the well-documented capacity to lower blood endotoxin levels, the impact of PMX-F therapy on clinical endpoints has not been well-defined. Because PMX-F does not directly address the source of sepsis, physiological endpoints such as reduction in vasopressor or ventilatory support, improvement in hemodynamics or oxygenation, and reduction in severity scores, rather than mortality, may be more appropriate outcome measures. We recently performed a systematic review to describe the published experience with DHP-PMX.[6] The primary endpoints of interest were the effects of DHP-PMX on blood pressure, use of vasoactive drugs, and oxygenation; the secondary endpoints were the effects on endotoxin levels and mortality. Of 118 abstracts identified on literature search over the past 10 years, we identified 28 published studies reporting relevant endpoints.[16-20]

This systematic review of the published literature, which involved almost 1400 patients treated in seven countries, demonstrated multiple beneficial benefits of direct hemoperfusion with PMX-F in comparison with conventional medical therapy for patients who had sepsis or septic shock (Table 284-1). Briefly, the mean arterial pressure increased by 19 mm Hg (95% confidence interval [CI], 16-22 mm Hg; $P < .001$) after PMX-F, and the dopamine/dobutamine dose decreased by 1.8 µg/kg/min (95% CI, 0.4-3.3 µg/kg/min; $P = .01$). Although we did not find sufficient data for analyzing more specific hemodynamic parameters, such as systemic vascular resistance, cardiac output, or cardiac index, pooled data seem to indicate that PMX-F therapy increases blood pressure while simultaneously reducing the dose of vasoactive agents,[16,21] strongly suggesting a clinically significant improvement in hemodynamic status. The positive effects are thought to be due to reductions in endotoxin levels after DHP-PMX (weighted mean difference −22 pg/mL; 95% CI, −18.1 to −25.8 pg/mL). The pooled estimate also suggests that PMX-F

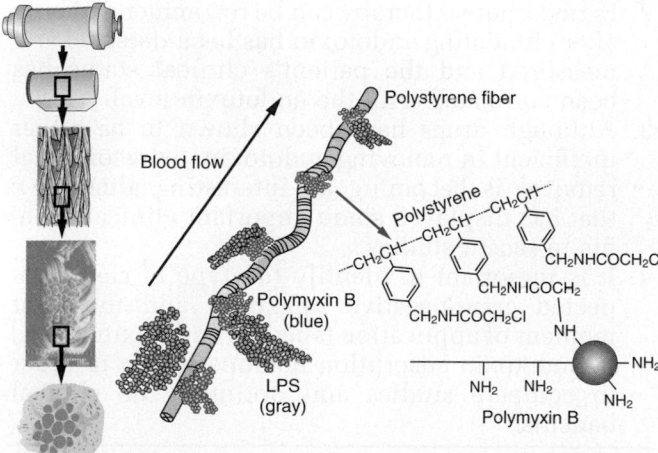

FIGURE 284-2. An adsorbent compartment of a Toraymyxin cartridge; Figure 2 illustrates the schema of the cross section of island-sea type conjugated fiber filament shows an electron micrograph of the cross section of a fiber filament. The schematic diagram of the immobilization of polymyxin B on the surface of polystyrene-based carrier fiber through a covalent bond.

TABLE 284-1

Summary of Systematic Reviews of the Clinical Effects of Polymyxin B–Immobilized Fiber Column in Sepsis

PARAMETER	NO. OF STUDIES	NO. OF PATIENTS	EFFECT SIZE	95% CONFIDENCE INTERVAL	OVERALL EFFECT (*P* VALUE)
Change in mean arterial pressure (mm Hg)	12	275	+19	15, 22	<.001
Change in dopamine/dobutamine dose (µg/kg/min)	4	96	−1.8	−3.3, −0.4	.01
Change in PaO₂/FiO₂ ratio (units)	7	151	+32	23, 41	<.001
Change in endotoxin level (pg/mL)	17	435	−22	−25.8, −18.1	<.001
Mortality (risk ratio)	15	885	0.54	0.44, 0.67	<.001

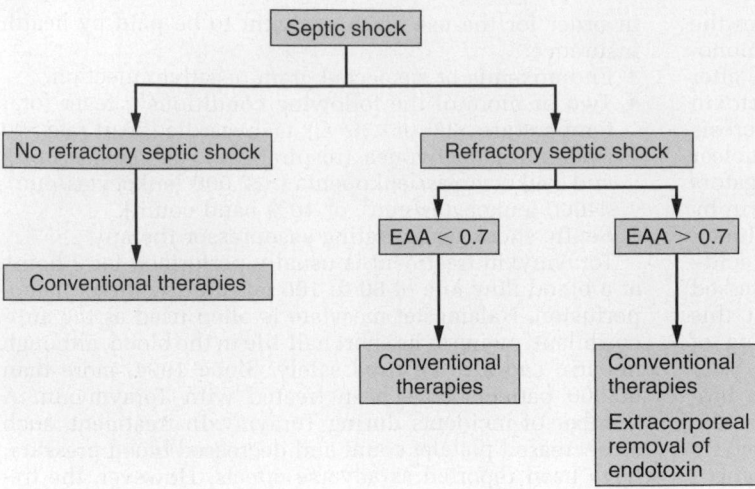

FIGURE 284-3. Possible algorithm for recommendation for the clinical use of extracorporeal endotoxin removal on the basis of available evidence.

improves gas exchange, as represented by the PaO_2/FiO_2 ratio (weighted mean difference 32 units; 95% CI, 23-41 units), although the single RCT that reported this outcome showed only a nonsignificant positive trend.[17] In addition, there appeared to be a beneficial effect on mortality (relative risk [RR], 0.54 relative to standard medical therapy; 95% CI, 0.44-0.67). However, this finding must be interpreted with caution because very few of the studies reviewed were planned or powered to specifically assess mortality. Overall, these putative benefits remain to be determined definitively in a prospective trial with appropriate clinical endpoints.

MEASUREMENT AND REMOVAL OF ENDOTOXINS: A FEASIBLE THERANOSTIC APPROACH FOR SEPTIC SHOCK

Despite the wide (Japanese) experience, PMX was never considered for inclusion in international guidelines for sepsis treatment, neither as rescue therapies in refractory septic shock (for which surviving sepsis guidelines suggest to start considering experimental therapies) nor as a preventive therapy. Because we are convinced that a definitive randomized trial to assess the clinical benefit of PMX is needed, we suggest that one should begin to consider the use of extracorporeal endotoxin adsorption as an experimental therapy in *endotoxin sustained refractory septic shock*.

The a.m. "MEDIC study" showed that the EAA is useful for identifying endotoxemia-related risk in patients in Japanese intensive care units. An elevated EAA value positively predicted the occurrence of hemodynamic abnormalities such as septic shock and correlated well with the patient's clinical condition. The efficacy of endotoxin removal in patients receiving extracorporeal Toraymyxin column treatment was reflected by a lowering of EAA levels after treatment. On the basis of the available studies and experience, the next step should be to evaluate the possibility of using PMX hemoperfusion under the conditions shown in Figure 284-3. Results of ongoing clinical

trials may eventually expand recommendations for the use of PMX hemoperfusion at an earlier stage of sepsis and for a broader range of indications.

Key Points

1. The sepsis syndrome is generally caused by circulating endotoxin and its subsequent biological cascade.
2. Extracorporeal therapy can be recommended only after circulating endotoxin has been detected and measured and the patient's clinical status has been correlated with the endotoxin level.
3. Although drugs have been shown to be rather inefficient in removing endotoxin, extracorporeal removal is becoming an interesting alternative that has displayed some important clinical benefits in recent studies.
4. It is important to identify the type of case (suspected gram-negative infection) and the right moment of application (specific endotoxin levels) of endotoxin adsorption hemoperfusion in order to compare studies and optimize the clinical benefits.

Key References

3. Shoji H, Tani T, Hanasawa K, Koidama M: Extracorporeal endotoxin removal by polymyxin B immobilized fiber cartridge: Designing and antiendotoxin efficacy in the clinical application. Ther Apher 1998;2:3-12.
4. Marshall JC, Foster D, Vincent JL, et al: Diagnostic and prognostic implications of endotoxemia in critical illness: results of the MEDIC study. J Infect Dis 2004;190:527-534. Epub 2004 Jul 2.
5. Opal SM, Glück T: Endotoxin as a drug target. Crit Care Med 2003;31(1 Suppl):S57-S64. Review.
6. Cruz DN, Perazella MA, Bellomo R, et al: Effectiveness of polymyxin B-immobilized fiber column in sepsis: A systematic review. Crit Care 2007;11:R47.

See the companion Expert Consult website for the complete reference list.

CHAPTER 285

The Plasmafiltration-Adsorption-Dialysis System

Federico Nalesso and Claudio Ronco

OBJECTIVES

This chapter will:
1. Describe the possibility of combining convection, diffusion, and adsorption to improve the efficiency of extracorporeal depurative techniques.
2. Discuss plasma as a substrate and a medium of blood purification.
3. Describe utilization of the patient's plasma as "dialysate" to perform a new type of high-permeability-cutoff plasma dialysis.

Molecules are present in the plasma or in plasma water or are bound to specific or unspecific carriers. The most important carrier in plasma is albumin. According to their characteristics of solubility, plasma molecules are present as solution in the plasma water, if water soluble, or bound to carriers, if hydrophobic.

Techniques such as hemodialysis, hemofiltration, and their combination (hemodiafiltration and high-flux dialysis) are able to remove small molecules (urea and creatinine) and medium-sized molecules (β_2-microglobulin) acting on plasma water and its solutes. Depending on the membrane cutoff value and the volume of infusion, they can remove more high-molecular-weight molecules than small molecules such as urea and creatinine. In order to improve the efficiency of molecule removal, convective and/or diffusive processes may be combined with adsorption on specific materials.

Adsorption allows removal of a wide range of hydrophobic and higher-molecular-weight substances, such as bilirubin, salt acids, cytokines, and myoglobin. The possibility of using specific physical interactions in some molecule adsorbers (ion exchange, chemical affinity, van der Waals forces) allows the removal of specific molecule targets, such as cytokines in the patient with sepsis and bile acids and bilirubin in the patient with liver failure. The adsorption process acts on protein-bound substances (bilirubin and drugs) and high-molecular-weight toxins present in the plasma. Convection and diffusion cannot achieve good clinical clearances of high-molecular-weight or hydrophobic molecules owing to their theoretical and practical limitations (volume of infusion and permeability limits of the membrane).

Summarizing all these concepts allows one to appreciate the central role of plasma as a transporter of toxic molecules and its potential function in the purification of blood. Through its intrinsic capacity to bind and transport molecules, plasma is the best fluid to perform a purification process. In physiological and pathological conditions, all molecules are present and are transported by the plasma (in plasma water or bound to selective/unselective carriers). It seems useful to combine the physical and chemical principles of purification (diffusion, convection, and adsorption) to improve and obtain the best removal of substances.

According to this view, coupled plasmafiltration-adsorption combines plasma adsorption with hemofiltration. The adsorption is specific to removal of cytokines, and the convective process is able to reestablish fluid balance, acid-base status, and electrolytes balance. Clinical applications of coupled plasmafiltration-adsorption are sepsis, septic shock, and systemic inflammatory response syndrome (SIRS). Further evolution of a combined system is the Molecular Adsorbent Recycling System (MARS; Gambro AG, Lund, Sweden). This technique bases its mechanism on the transporter role of albumin. The closed loop of albumin is used as a medium to transport albumin-bound toxins from whole blood to the sites of purification (cartridges and a dialyzer with a low-permeability-cutoff membrane, where hemofiltration or hemodialysis of albumin is performed). Albumin from donors in the closed loop is regenerated and used continuously. The clinical application of the MARS is liver failure and hepatorenal syndrome.

In these latter two techniques, plasma is viewed as a substrate of purification and the albumin, one of its components, is used as a medium of purification (MARS). The combination of more principles allows coupled plasmafiltration-adsorption and MARS to improve the clearance and total removal of the substances implicated in the pathophysiology of diseases for which they are designed. According to this evolution of purification, it is possible to use plasma in a new blood purification process.

The plasmafiltration-adsorption-dialysis (PFAD) system combines high-volume hemofiltration directly on plasma with plasma adsorption on a specific adsorber. The regenerated patient's plasma is used in two ways. It can be returned to the patient through the venous line or used as a dialysate in a new process of "plasma dialysis" through a membrane with a very high-permeability-cutoff.

THE PROCESS OF PLASMAFILTRATION-ADSORPTION-DIALYSIS

PFAD technology is based on a new principle of purification that utilizes a tricompartmental dialyzer (TD) to purify the patient's blood through a combination of three sequential techniques: convection and adsorption, both on plasma, followed by a process of "whole blood dialysis" provided by the patient's regenerated plasma (Figs. 285-1 and 285-2).[1]

The tricompartmental dialyzer is the core of this new technology (Fig. 285-3). It is composed of hollow fibers

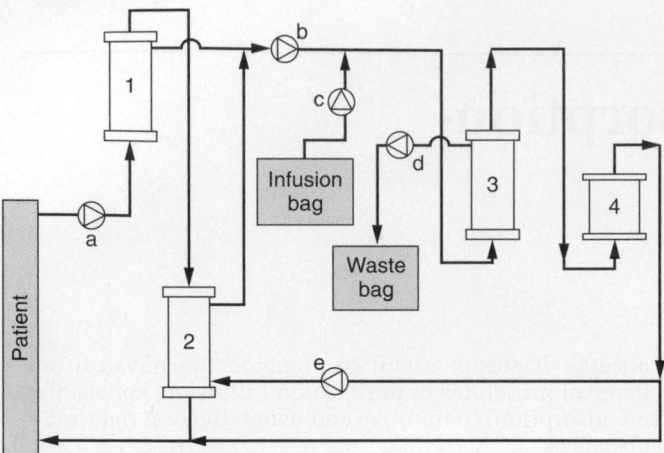

FIGURE 285-1. Schematic representation of the plasmafiltration-adsorption-dialysis system: a, blood pump (blood flow = Q_B); b, plasma (plasma flow = Q_P); c, infusion pump (re-infusion flow = Q_R); d, ultrafiltration pump; e, plasma dialysate pump (dialysate flow = Q_D); 1, plasma separator (second compartment); 2, dialyzer (third compartment); 3, filter to perform convection on plasma; 4, adsorber. The second and third compartments are described as separate devices to simplify the explanation of a single process.

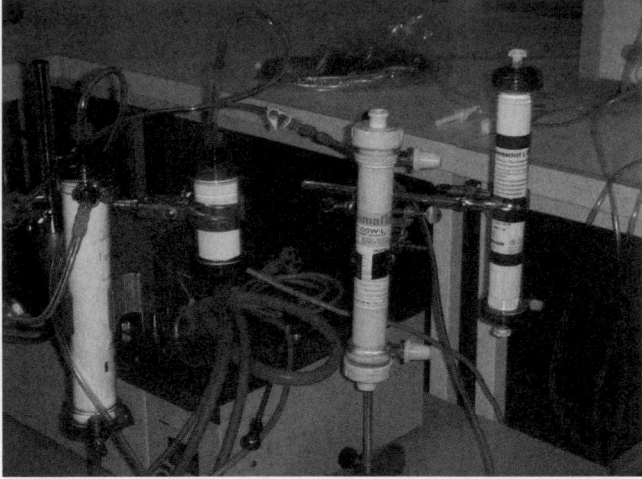

A

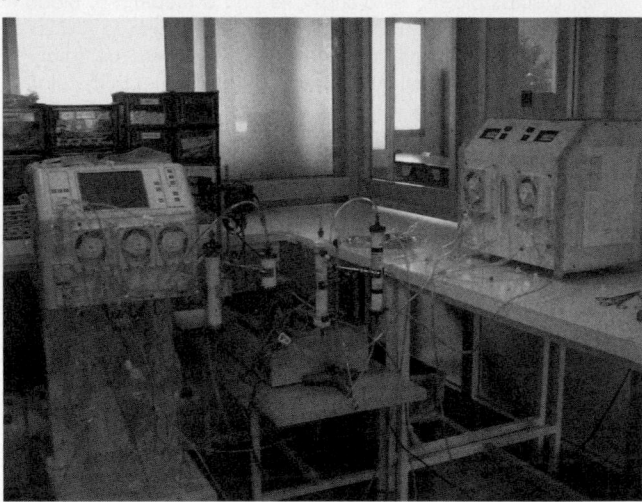

B

FIGURE 285-2. A, The three compartments of the tricompartmental dialyzer, the filter for the convective process, and the adsorber. **B,** The prototype plasmafiltration-adsorption-dialysis system.

like those in a regular hemodialyzer. The compartments are located in different areas, each with its own particular function. The hollow fibers form three compartments along the extension of the dialyzer (see Fig. 285-3). The first compartment is formed by the inner space of hollow fibers in which the blood goes through the whole fibers' length thanks to a roller pump (blood pump). The internal compartment of the dialyzer is divided into two more compartments separated by a wall along the extension of the hollow fibers; the second compartment forms a stage for filtering plasma, and the third compartment forms a stage for dialysis. The second compartment is the delineated space where the patient's plasma can be filtered from the whole blood across the hollow-fiber membrane (see Fig. 285-1, 1). The third compartment is the space where the patient's regenerated plasma performs a process of purification based on a "diffusive and binding process"; in this way, the regenerated patient's plasma is used as a dialysate in a countercurrent to purify the blood flowing in the first compartment (see Fig. 285-1, 2). The second and third compartments have a specific permeability cutoff value of hollow-fiber membranes according to their specific function, and their area is able to ensure the processes that occur (filtration and dialysis). The second and the third compartments communicate through a particular opening in the arterial end of dialyzer (see Fig. 285-3; not shown in Fig. 285-1 or 285-4). In the first human prototype of this system, the second and the third compartments are separated and formed by two different devices, as shown in the figures.

The first step of the process aims to separate the plasma from whole blood (see Fig. 285-1; Table 285-1). This process determines the plasmafiltration from the inner space of hollow fibers to the space of the second compartment. The plasma obtained from the patient goes from the second compartment to the plasma purification circuit, where it is purified by two different and separated methods, convection (see Fig. 285-1, 3) and adsorption (see Fig. 285-1, 4). The plasma flow is performed by a roller pump (see Fig. 285-1, b).

The plasma purification circuit is composed of two separate processes in order to remove first the water-soluble and dialyzable toxic molecules by convection and then the hydrophobic and nondialyzable molecules by adsorption on a specific adsorber (see Fig. 285-1, 3 and 4). Convection is obtained through high-volume hemofiltration directly on plasma. It is known that high-volume ultrafiltration using a super-high-flux filter has achieved better cytokine clearances than those currently achieved by urea during standard continuous renal replacement therapy.[2] The convective process is able to reestablish electrolyte balance, acid-base equilibrium, and fluid balance by acting directly on plasma water.

After convective purification, the plasma is adsorbed by a specific adsorber to remove hydrophobic or nondialyzable molecules (see Fig. 285-1, 4). The adsorber is specific for the molecules implicated in the patient's disease (sepsis, hepatorenal syndrome, acute and chronic liver failure, etc.). The cartridge for adsorption has good pressure-flow performance and excellent mechanical and chemical stability in order to perform the best adsorption of the plasma.

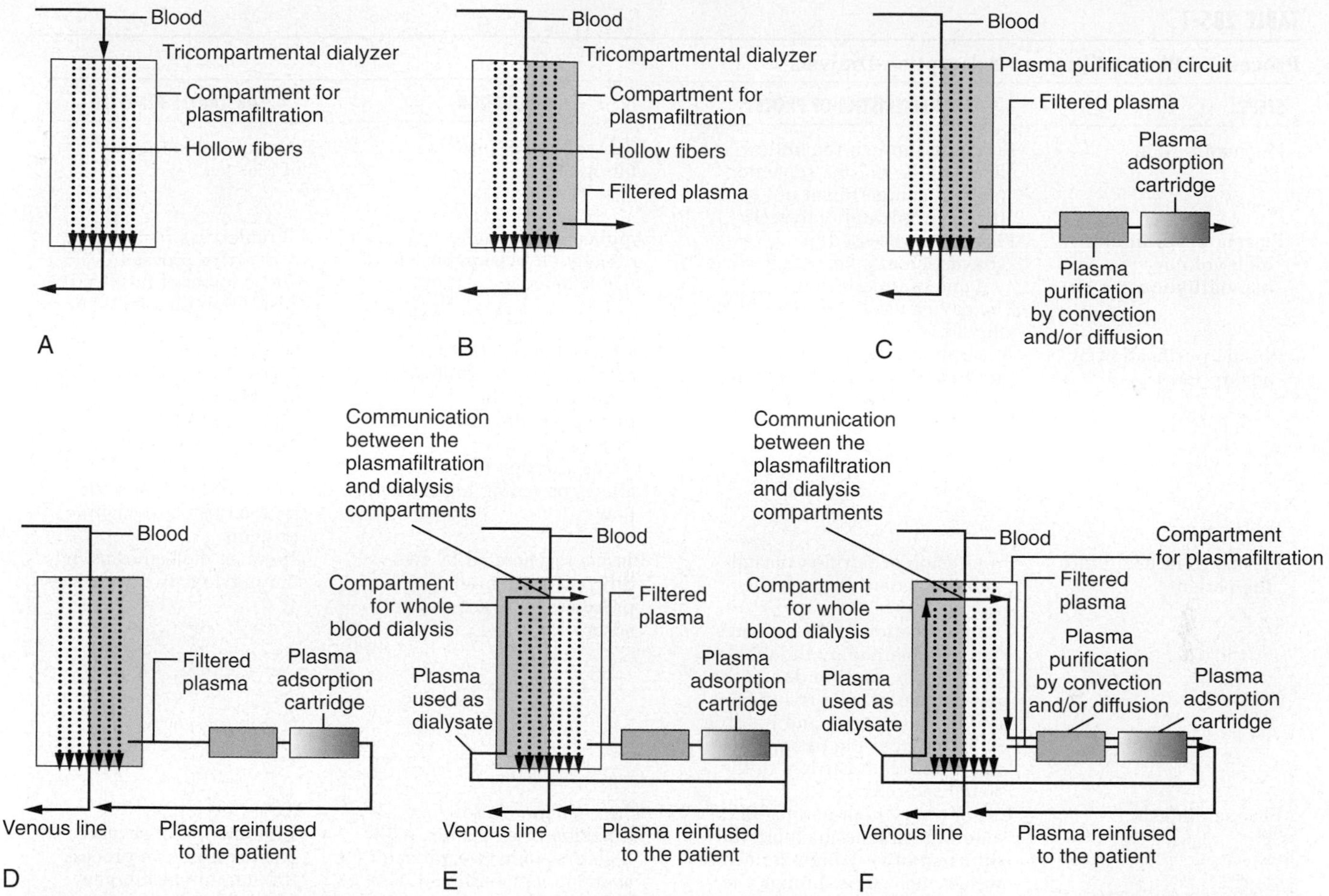

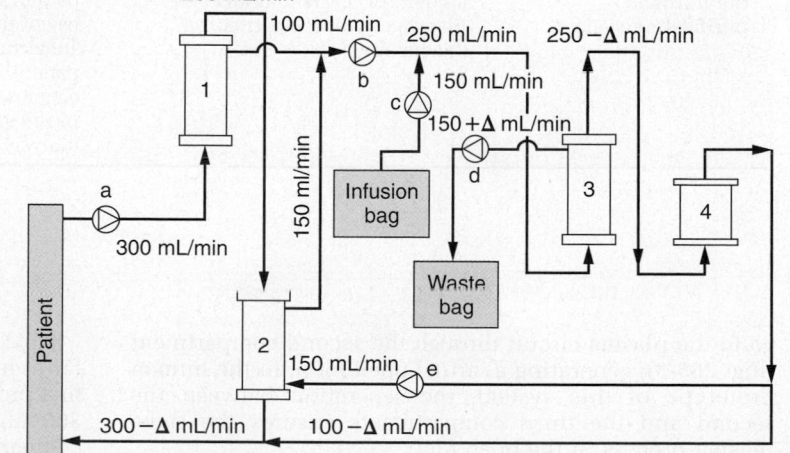

FIGURE 285-3. The tricompartmental dialyzer and the purification processes. **A,** First compartment; **B,** second compartment; **C,** plasma purification; **D,** plasma re-infusion; **E,** plasma dialysis; **F,** recycling virtual system. The second and third compartments are described as separate devices to simplify the explanation of a single process.

FIGURE 285-4. Standard flows during a plasmafiltration-adsorption-dialysis treatment. a, blood pump (blood flow = Q_B); b, plasma (plasma flow = Q_P); c, infusion pump (re-infusion flow = Q_R); d, ultrafiltration pump; e, plasma dialysate pump (dialysate flow = Q_D); 1, plasma separator (second compartment); 2, dialyzer (third compartment); 3, filter to perform convection on plasma; 4, adsorber. The second and third compartments are described as separate devices to simplify the explanation of a single process. Δ, weight loss during treatment.

After these two different processes, the purified plasma can go either of two ways (see Fig. 285-1). In the first, the purified plasma returns to the patient through the venous line. In the second, the patient's regenerated plasma is used as dialysate in the compartment of the TD, in order to perform the dialysis procedure based on diffusion and binding. In this step, the filtrated patient's plasma from the whole blood and the exhausted dialysate from the third compartment can be purified again in the plasma circuit (see Fig. 285-1). In fact, there is a connection between the second and the third compartments at the arterial end of the TD; thus, the exhausted dialysate can

TABLE 285-1

Process of Plasmafiltration-Adsorption-Dialysis

STEPS	CHARACTERISTICS OF PROCESS	INNOVATION	SUBSTANCES REMOVED
Plasmafiltration	Filtration through the hollow fibers of the plasma separator (second compartment of tricompartmental dialyzer)	High volume of plasma filtration	Not applicable (production of plasma)
Plasma purification by high-volume hemofiltration	Plasma is processed by convection of a very high volume in predilution The device used is a super-high-flux filter	Application of convection directly on plasma instead of whole blood	All molecules removed by convective process A little quota of unselective adsorption on membrane surface
Plasma purification by adsorption	Adsorption as a specific adsorber The adsorber is specific to remove the target molecules	The absorber is chosan according to the molecules implicated in the pathophysiology of patient's disease The new design of cartridge allows obtaining high plasma flow	Depending on the specific adsorber: cytokines, myoglobin, lipopolysaccharide, bilirubin, salt acids, immune complex, autoantibodies, specific high-molecular-weight proteins
Plasma re-infusion into the patient	Re-infusion of purified plasma into the patient through the venous line The purification of the patient's body is obtained by the whole blood toxin dilution due to the regenerated plasma re-infusion and by the shifting and binding of toxins from the tissues due to the regenerated carriers in the re-infused plasma	Plasma regenerated by two different sequential processes, convection and adsorption	The same molecules as in the previous two processes
Plasma dialysis	Use of a very high-permeability-cutoff membrane to obtain the diffusion of very high-molecular-weight molecules through the membrane Driving force of regenerated plasma in order to shift and bind toxins from whole blood	The membrane allows diffusion of molecules with high molecular weight such as immunoglobulins M, G, and more Plasma used as dialysate in a diffusive process Driving force of plasma carrier used as a medium of purification	According to the combination of several factors: diffusive process through the membrane, plasma driving force and previous plasma purification by specific adsorption
Recycling of plasma in the plasma purification system	The system is recycling a virtual amount of plasma because the plasma circuit is open at the venous line	The possibility of obtaining patient's plasma avoids the use of donor albumin The virtual amount of patient's plasma recycling enables high dialysate flows in the system for the plasma dialysis	It allows the plasma dialysis process described previously to be obtained

go to the plasma circuit through the second compartment (Fig. 285-3), generating a virtual open loop. In the human prototype of this system, the separation between the second and the third compartments ensures the same plasma process in the open loop.

Because the plasma circuit is an open circuit, the dialysis system is not working in closed recycling modality but receiving fresh regenerated plasma from the plasma circuit every time (see Fig. 285-1). The peculiarity of the plasma circuit is that to obtain the dialysate in the third compartment, the plasma flow is a virtual flow inside the open plasma loop and can exceed the plasma filtration flow from the first compartment, being a recycling flow, as shown in the figures.

PFAD is a technique that can be performed continuously for at least 8 hours or longer each day. The results of the first prototype show that the standard blood flow (Q_B) was 300 mL/min and the plasma flow (Q_P) from the second compartment was 100 mL/min (6 L/hr); the dialysate flow (Q_D) was 150 mL/min (9 L/hr) and the flow of re-infusion fluid (Q_R) for convection was 150 mL/min (Fig. 285-4). Plasma purification by convection was achieved through predilution of a standard solution for hemodiafiltration at the same flow as the Q_D. The circuit heparinization was mandatory and required at least 300 to 800 U/hr, depending on the patient's clinical condition. Thermal balance was maintained or modified through changes in the temperature of fluids used in the plasma purification circuit.

TABLE 285-2

Clearance and Removal Rates Achieved by the Plasmafiltration-Adsorption-Dialysis System

SUBSTANCES	REMOVAL RATE
Substances Cleared	
Urea	89 mL/min
Creatinine	96 mL/min
Inulin	118 mL/min
Myoglobin	84 mL/min
Substances Removed	
Lipopolysaccharide	84%
Potassium	34%

PRELIMINARY DATA FROM IN VITRO STUDIES

The special geometry of the sorbent used in the first prototype allowed very high plasma flows (up to 250 mL/min). We measured single-pass clearances of urea, creatinine, inulin, and myoglobin (Table 285-2). The specific solution was as follows: urea 100 mg/dL, creatinine 10 mg/dL, inulin 20 mg/dL, potassium 6 mEq/L, and myoglobin 10.000 ng/mL; lipopolysaccharide removal (2.5 UI/mL solution). The treatment settings were Q_B 300 mL/min, Q_P 100 mL/min, Q_R 150 mL/min, and Q_D 150 mL/min. According to our preliminary data, the adsorber was able to adsorb a very high amount of lipopolysaccharide (84%). This mechanism of purification is improved by the whole blood dialysis performed by the regenerated plasma from the patient, which, when used as a dialysate, is able to shift and bind lipopolysaccharide and cytokines from the whole blood. The same mechanism acts within the tissues in the human body, when the regenerated plasma is re-infused into the patient. The plasma hemofiltration in predilution and the plasma dialysis are also able to substitute for renal function. Therefore the plasma is both a substrate for and a medium of purification, and it can improve total purification by the plasma dialysis process. The results highlight the importance of this device as continuous renal replacement therapy for the critically ill patient in the intensive care unit who has sepsis, SIRS, or multiple-organ failure syndrome.

DISCUSSION

PFAD combines three different processes in order to purify the patient's whole blood using the patient's plasma. In this technology, the plasma is both a medium and a substrate of purification. Thanks to its intrinsic characteristic as a molecule carrier, the purified plasma can be used as a new ideal fluid to purify pathological whole blood or plasma.

This technology allows for the removal of molecules from plasma water and protein-bound plasma through the sequential combination of convective treatment and adsorption. PFAD can remove both diffusible and nondiffusible molecules, such as tumor necrosis factor-α and other cytokines according to their water solubility and molecular weight, through the combination of specific techniques. In the first step, water-soluble and diffusive

molecules can be removed by convection. This purification process can improve the selection of successive adsorption, which is able to remove hydrophobic and high-molecular-weight molecules. In the plasma circuit, the patient's plasma is the substrate of purification, but when it is re-infused or used as dialysate, it becomes the medium of purification. The purified plasma is able to re-establish electrolyte balance, acid-base status, and fluid balance through its actions on whole blood flowing in the third compartment (dialysis). After the purified plasma is re-infused into the patient, it acts along with the dialyzed blood to reestablish electrolyte balance, acid-base status, and fluid balance by the reequilibration of ions, solutes (urea, creatine, etc.) and water among tissues and in the bloodstream. It is important to highlight the double role of plasma as both vector and substrate of purification. The regenerated albumin and carriers are able to bind toxic ligands according to the law of mass action—an important physical process that allows ligands to be shifted from the whole blood and tissues and bound to the regenerated carriers across the TD or capillary membrane in the PFAD system and patient's body, respectively.

In the specific case of sepsis and septic shock, PFAD can support or substitute for renal function and remove the high levels of pro-inflammatory and anti-inflammatory cytokines responsible for the pathophysiology of organ injury and failure.[3] This is possible by means of the association of convective purification and specific adsorption for cytokines and lipopolysaccharide, improved by the plasma dialysis.

Another extremely important clinical problem relates to patients affected by liver failure, in whom, as the pathology progresses, kidney failure (hepatorenal syndrome) inevitably develops along with all the complications caused by retention of liver toxins. The accumulation of albumin-bound toxins has been demonstrated during liver failure; these toxins are responsible, to variable extents, for multiple-organ dysfunction (kidney, cardiovascular instability, etc.).[4] The functions of albumin as a transporter and as a possible purification vector have been described in albumin dialysis; the removal of these molecules through the process improves the clinical condition of the patient. The best-known and most widely used extracorporeal device for liver function support is the MARS,[5] which uses albumin only to perform purification by adsorption and by classic dialysis. The current literature demonstrates that this approach is capable of improving patient survival.[6,7] Moreover, this type of approach is useful for intoxications caused by exogenous pathogens that are scarcely water-soluble but are plasma protein–bound.

In all of these disorders (sepsis, hepatorenal syndrome, SIRS), there is an involvement of cytokines, and much of the damage that affects the various organs and systems that are not primarily involved in the basic pathological process are determined by molecular factors that circulate in the blood or are either dissolved in the plasma water or bound by albumin. The PFAD system is able to reestablish electrolyte balance and acid-base equilibrium acting directly on plasma water in the plasma circuit. The specificity of the adsorber used for the plasma adsorption is important to remove the toxic molecules retained or produced during sepsis, SIRS, acute-on-chronic liver failure, chronic liver failure, primary liver dysfunction, and hepatorenal syndrome. In these cases, one or more adsorbers with high selectivity for cytokines, unconjugated and conjugated bilirubin, phenols, and other retained molecules can be used.

PFAD is the latest technology that can combine the best processes of blood/plasma purification in order to determine a selective and effective purification of molecules implicated in disease, such as sepsis, SIRS, and liver failure.

5. The combination of one or more principles of purification (convection, adsorption, diffusion) with use of regenerated plasma as purification fluid (plasma dialysis) can achieve the best results in the purification process.

Key Points

1. The combination of convection with adsorption improves the total removal of toxic molecules implicated in the pathophysiology of diseases that are treated by extracorporeal therapy.
2. All toxic molecules that are present are transported by the plasma, in the plasma water, or bound to some carriers.
3. Plasma is the medium of transportation of toxins, and acting directly on it can improve total purification.
4. Purified plasma is the best fluid to perform purification of the whole blood or pathological plasma.

Key References

1. Nalesso F: Machine for plasma purification combined with plasma adsorption-perfusion by using a tricompartmental dialyzer. Patent WO/2004/091694, 2004.
2. Uchino S, Bellomo R, Goldsmith D, et al: Super high flux hemofiltration: A new technique for cytokine removal. Intensive Care Med 2002;28:651-655.
3. Ronco C, Bonello M, Bordoni V, et al: Extracorporeal therapies in non-renal disease: Treatment of sepsis and the peak concentration hypothesis. Blood Purif 2004;22:164-174.
4. Sen S, Jalan R, Williams R: Liver failure: Basis of benefit of therapy with the molecular adsorbents recirculating system. Int J Biochem Cell Biol 2003;35:1306-1311.
5. Sen S, Williams R, Jalan R: Emerging indications for albumin dialysis. Am J Gastroenterol 2005;100:468-475.

See the companion Expert Consult website for the complete reference list.

CHAPTER 286

Slow Plasma Exchange plus CHDF for Liver Failure and CHDF Alone for Severe Acute Pancreatitis

Hiroyuki Hirasawa, Shigeto Oda, Hidetoshi Shiga, Kenichi Matsuda, Tomohito Sadahiro, and Masataka Nakamura

OBJECTIVES

This chapter will:
1. Explore the mechanism of the beneficial effect of continuous hemodiafiltration using a polymethyl methacrylate membrane hemofilter in the treatment of acute hepatic failure.
2. Explain why use of a high-dialysate-flow version of this modality plus slow plasma exchange is necessary for patients with acute hepatic failure.
3. Discuss recent concepts of the pathophysiology of severe acute pancreatitis.
4. Describe the efficacy of continuous hemodiafiltration using a polymethyl methacrylate membrane hemofilter in the treatment of severe acute pancreatitis.

Acute hepatic failure (AHF) remains one of the critical conditions causing death in the intensive care unit despite advances in critical care and modern technology of artificial support and monitoring systems. The mortality rate of AHF in the United States remains as high as 30%.[1] The application of orthotopic liver transplantation, especially from living donors, has improved the survival rate of patients with AHF dramatically.[2] However, this treatment option is costly, and the limited supply of suitable liver grafts seriously reduces the availability of this option to all the patients who would benefit from it[3]—especially in Japan, where cadaveric liver grafting is seldom available for many reasons, such as religious opposition. Therefore, medical critical care including artificial liver support (ALS) with various types of blood purification remains one of the mainstays of the treatment of patients with AHF.[4] Such patients often experience acute failure of other organs as well, such as acute renal failure and acute respiratory failure; therefore, these patients are treated with many kinds of artificial supports, such as artificial kidneys and mechanical ventilators, much like patients with multiple organ failure. Furthermore, the general condition of patients undergoing orthotopic liver transplantation should be kept stable, and ALS with blood purification plays an important role as a bridge to transplantation.

Many kinds of ALS are applied clinically to patients with ALS, such as plasma exchange (PE), the Molecular Adsorbent Recirculating System (Gambro AG, Lund, Sweden), and newly developed plasmafiltration systems.[5-7] ALS for AHF should fulfill the following purposes: (1) removal of causative substances of hepatic coma and accumulated waste products for the recovery from hepatic coma,[8] (2) supply of the coagulation factors and opsonic proteins to prevent hemorrhagic complication and immunodeficiency, (3) removal of harmful humoral mediators to accelerate liver regeneration and to prevent remote organ failure, and (4) maintenance of homeostasis.

To fulfill such purposes, PE alone or the Molecular Adsorbents Recirculating System alone is not effective enough. Furthermore, one study has reported that hypercytokinemia plays an important role in the pathophysiology of AHF.[9] Also, Nakada and colleagues[10] reported that continuous hemodiafiltration (CHDF) using a polymethyl methacrylate (PMMA) membrane hemofilter (PMMA-CHDF) can remove a variety of cytokines from the bloodstream of patients continuously and effectively. Taking these considerations into account, we developed a new ALS system consisting of slow plasma exchange (SPE) plus high-dialysate-flow PMMA-CHDF.

Since the introduction of the pathophysiological concept of systemic inflammatory response syndrome,[11] many changes have been proposed for the pathophysiology of severe acute pancreatitis (SAP). It is now well known that hypercytokinemia plays a central role in the pathophysiology of SAP.[12,13] Therefore, we applied PMMA-CHDF to patients with SAP regardless of renal function as an effective countermeasure against hypercytokinemia. Thus, in this chapter, we report on the efficacy of (1) SPE plus CHDF for AHF and (2) CHDF for SAP.

SLOW PLASMA EXCHANGE PLUS HIGH-DIALYSATE-FLOW CHDF

In Japan, PE is still most commonly applied as ALS. Usually, fresh-frozen plasma (FFP) equal to one plasma volume of the patient is used as replacement fluid, and one session of PE is commonly finished within 2 to 3 hours. However, we have noticed that if a PE session is finished within 2 to 3 hours in a patient with AHF, more severe PE-induced complications, such as hypernatremia, metabolic alkalosis, and abrupt drop in colloid osmotic pressure, easily develop.[14] We also found that the amount of bilirubin removed by one session of PE is larger when PE is performed more slowly, over 6 to 8 hours, than by a PE session performed conventionally for 2 to 3 hours. Therefore, now we perform every session of PE slowly for 6 to 8 hours to exchange one plasma volume of FFP. This modality is called slow PE (SPE).

As for the CHDF, we noticed that the PMMA hemofilter is superior to the hemofilters made from other membrane materials, such as polyacrylonitrile and polysulfone, in terms of cytokine-removing ability.[10,15] The major mechanism of cytokine removal with PMMA-CHDF is the adsorption of cytokine to the hemofilter membrane, and among hemofilters made from various membrane materials, the PMMA hemofilter has the greatest ability to adsorb cytokines. Therefore, we use only PMMA hemofilters when we perform CHDF for removal of cytokines.

When we apply CHDF as a part of our ALS, we use a dialysate flow of 500 mL/min. The dialysate flow is usually 1000 to 2000 mL/hr when PMMA-CHDF is used for cytokine removal in patients who do not have AHF. Because the major mechanism of cytokine removal with PMMA-CHDF is the adsorption of cytokine to the hemofilter mem-

brane, we do not need to use a high-filtration volume in CHDF to remove the cytokines, as proposed by others who use hemofilters of materials other than PMMA.[16] However, we noticed that when we use PMMA-CHDF with a dialysate flow of 1000 to 2000 mL/hr, sometimes intracranial pressure cannot be controlled in patients with AHF. The intracranial pressure can be controlled when dialysate flow in PMMA-CHDF is increased from 500 mL/min to 1000 to 2000 mL/hr. The reason may be that intracranial pressure is raised by an increase in small- to medium-molecular-weight substances, which can be removed effectively by more vigorous PMMA-CHDF.[17]

To remove small- to medium-molecular-weight substances, high-volume-filtration CHDF may be effective. However, application of high-volume-filtration CHDF causes some problems. Large amounts of sterile replacement fluid would be needed, and the life of the hemofilter might be shortened. Therefore, we typically choose to increase dialysate flow instead of the filtration rate to enhance the ability of removal of small- to medium-molecular-weight substances even though there are some differences between the substances removed with high-dialysate-flow CHDF and substances removed with high-filtration-volume CHDF.

Figure 286-1 shows the changes in the ALS system used in our intensive care unit. Originally we applied conventional PE with FFP equal to one plasma volume. Then we switched to SPE plus PMMA-CHDF. Now we routinely apply high-dialysate-flow PMMA-CHDF (HFCHDF) using a bedside console for maintenance hemodialysis whenever we apply PMMA-CHDF as a part of ALS. Figure 286-2 shows a photo and flow diagram of the use of SPE plus high-dialysate-flow PMMA-CHDF. In this ALS, we use a relatively low filtration rate, such as 200 to 500 mL/hr.

EFFICACY IN ACUTE HEPATIC FAILURE

The efficacy of slow PE plus HFCHDF is very impressive. Figure 286-3 compares rates of recovery from hepatic coma and 28-day survival among patients treated by three different types of ALS: conventional PE alone, SPE plus PMMA-CHDF, and SPE plus HFCHDF. Especially among patients with fulminant hepatic failure of the subacute type—in which hepatic coma develops between 10 days and 8 weeks after the onset of initial hepatitis-related symptoms, such as nausea, fatigue, elevated liver enzyme values, and hyperbilirubinemia—rates of recovery from hepatic coma and 28-day survival were higher than those in AHF patients who were treated with the other two approaches.[14] Furthermore, the incidence of adverse effects of PE, such as hypernatremia, metabolic alkalosis, and sudden drop of colloid osmotic pressure, which developed with rapid transfusion of FFP as replacement fluid during conventional PE, decreased dramatically in patients treated with SPE plus PMMA-CHDF and completely disappeared in patients treated with SPE plus HFCHDF, as shown in Figure 286-4. These effects of slow SPE plus high-dialysate-flow PMMA-CHDF are clinically relevant, since they can cause deterioration in patient consciousness, and such deterioration is very harmful even in patients undergoing liver transplantation.[18]

We did not systematically check the changes in various blood cytokine levels in patients undergoing the various

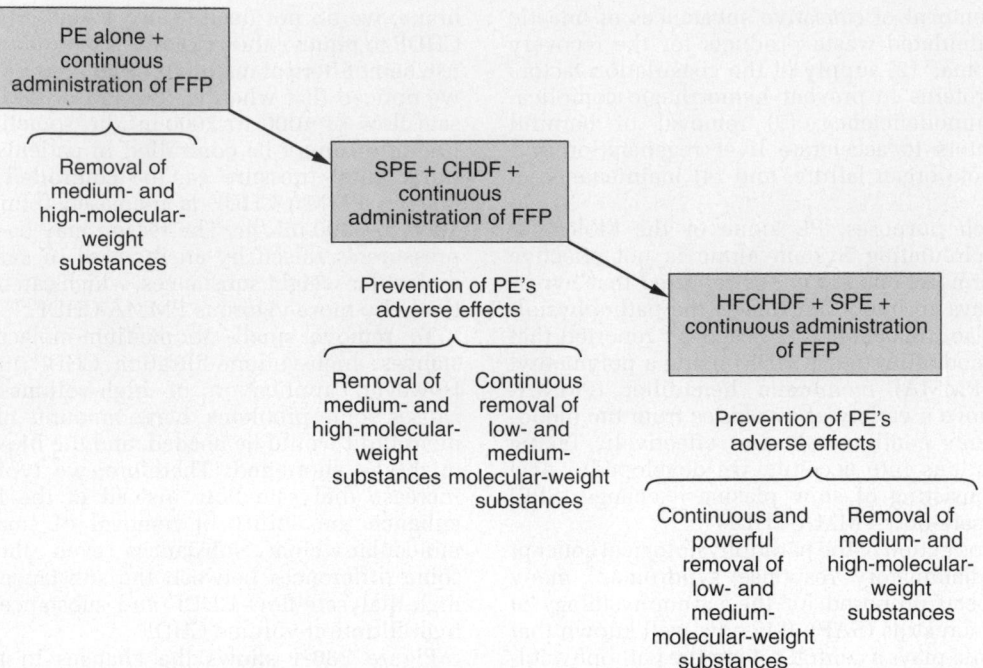

FIGURE 286-1. Changes in artificial liver support system for acute hepatic failure in the Intensive Care Unit of Chiba University Hospital. CHDF, continuous hemodiafiltration; FFP, fresh-frozen plasma; HFCHDF, high-dialysate-flow continuous hemodiafiltration; PE, plasma exchange; SPE, slow plasma exchange.

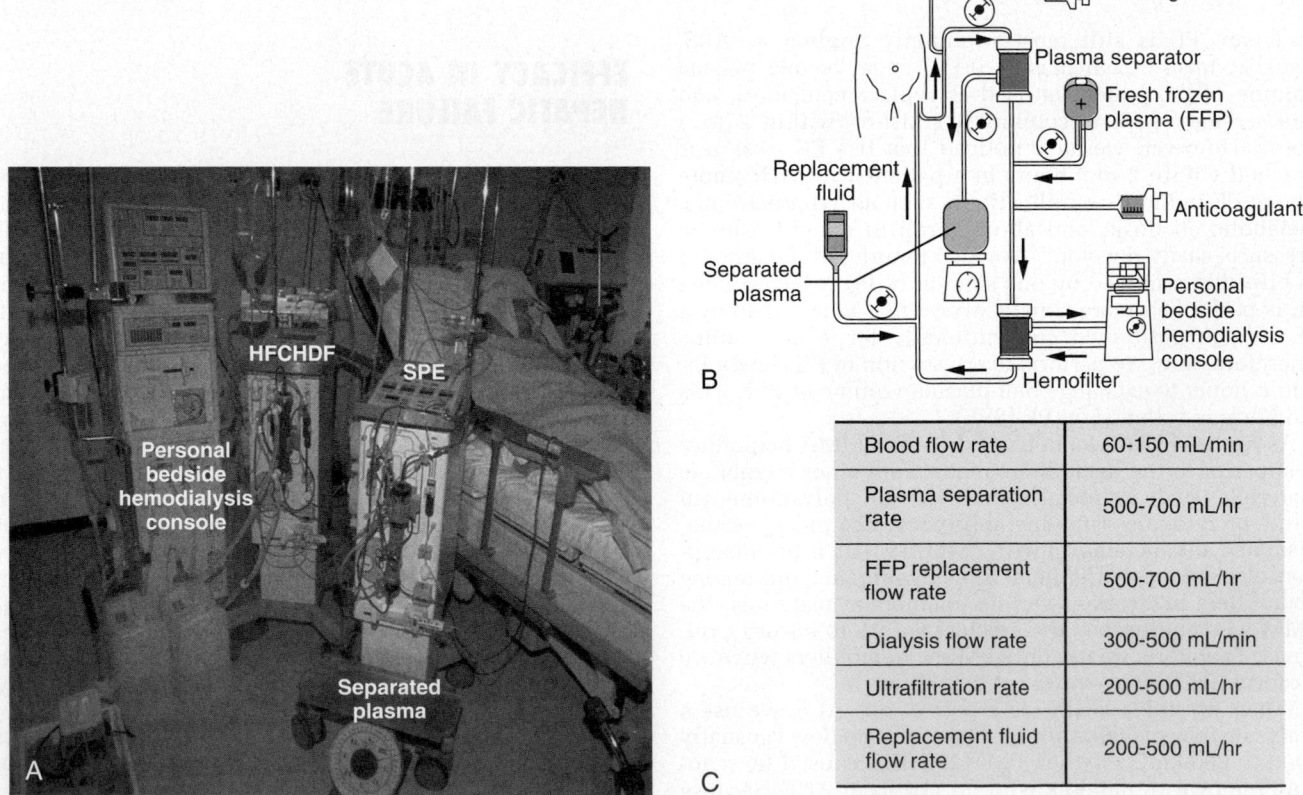

Blood flow rate	60-150 mL/min
Plasma separation rate	500-700 mL/hr
FFP replacement flow rate	500-700 mL/hr
Dialysis flow rate	300-500 mL/min
Ultrafiltration rate	200-500 mL/hr
Replacement fluid flow rate	200-500 mL/hr

FIGURE 286-2. Photograph (**A**) and flow diagram (**B**) of slow plasma exchange (SPE) plus high-dialysate-flow continuous hemodiafiltration (HFCHDF). **C,** Table of operative conditions.

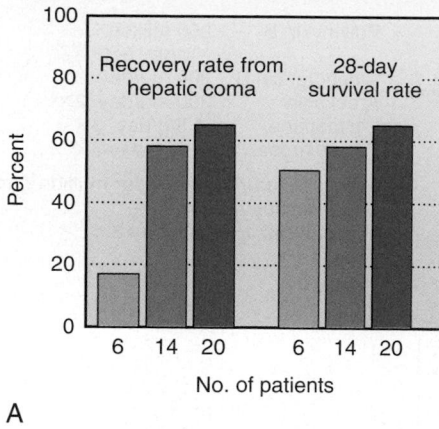
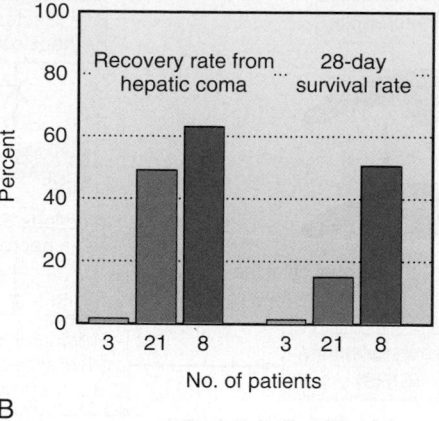

FIGURE 286-3. Comparison of recovery rates from hepatic coma and 28-day survival in acute (**A**) and subacute (**B**) hepatic failure among patients treated with three different artificial liver support systems. *Ligh blue* bars indicate plasma exchange (PE) alone; *medium blue* bars indicate slow PE (SPE) plus continuous hemodiafiltration (CHDF); *dark blue* bars indicate SPE plus high-dialysate-flow continuous hemodiafiltration.

FIGURE 286-4. Comparison of the incidence (%) of adverse effects during artificial liver support with three different support systems. *Light blue* bars indicate plasma exchange (PE) alone; *medium blue* bars indicate slow PE (SPE) plus continuous hemodiafiltration (CHDF); *dark blue* bars indicate SPE plus high-dialysate-flow continuous hemodiafiltration.

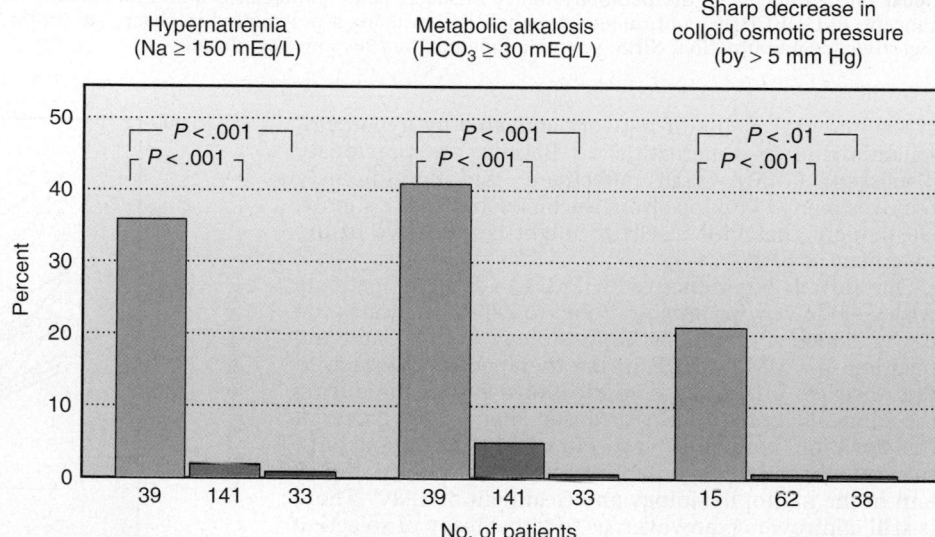

forms of ALS. However, we have previously reported that PMMA-CHDF could remove a variety of cytokines from the bloodstream of critically ill patient, such as patients with severe sepsis, septic shock, septic multiple organ failure, and acute respiratory failure, and that PMMA-CHDF could reduce the blood levels of a variety of cytokines in those patients.[10,15,19] From these data, we can safely assume that PMMA-CHDF removes cytokines from the bloodstream of patients with AHF and that such cytokine removal is one of the mechanisms of the beneficial effect of ALS using SPE plus HFCHDF in patients with AHF. These data clearly indicate that SPE plus HFCHDF is a very effective ALS, fulfilling many of the purposes for which ALS is performed. Such a powerful ALS is useful as a bridge to transplantation in the era of living orthotopic liver transplantation for AHF.

PATHOPHYSIOLOGY OF SEVERE ACUTE PANCREATITIS AND USE OF PMMA-CHDF AS A COUNTERMEASURE

Conventionally, it is widely accepted that digestive enzymes released from an injured or inflamed pancreas and entering the systemic circulation play a central role in the pathophysiology of SAP, causing remote organ failure such as acute respiratory failure. However, since the pathophysiological concept of the systemic inflammatory response syndrome in 1992,[11] much has changed concerning the pathophysiology of SAP. Now SAP is thought to be caused by severe systemic inflammatory response syndrome initially caused by acute pancreatitis or SAP is thought to be caused by the overwhelming activation

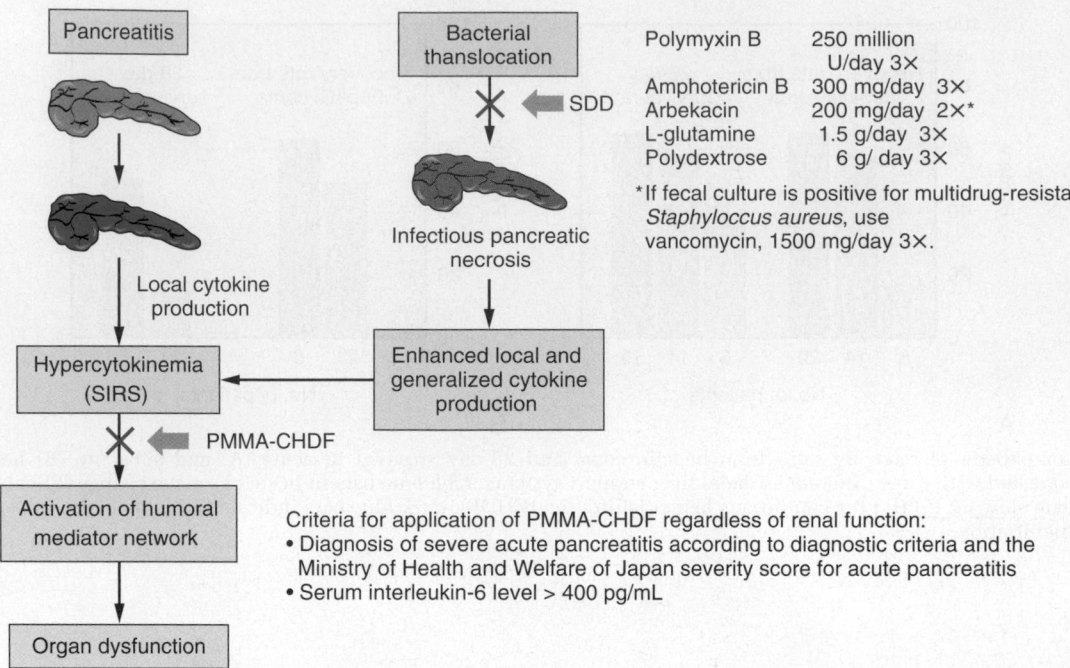

FIGURE 286-5. Concept of the pathophysiology of severe acute pancreatitis and a therapeutic approach to the disorder according to the concept. PMMA-CHDF, continuous hemodiafiltration using a polymethyl methacrylate (PMMA) membrane hemofilter; SDD, selective digestive decontamination; SIRS, systemic inflammatory response syndrome.

of the humoral mediator network activated by hypercytokinemia due to pancreatitis.[12,13] Because, as previously discussed, PMMA-CHDF effectively and continuously removes many cytokines from the bloodstream of patients, we thought that PMMA-CHDF might be effective in the treatment of SAP.

Our initial experience with PMMA-CHDF in patients with SAP is very promising.[20] Figure 286-5 illustrates the newer concept of the pathophysiology of SAP and the position of PMMA-CHDF in the therapeutic approach to this disease. Infectious complications that occur during the clinical course of SAP, caused mainly via bacterial translocation, which is very effectively prevented with selective digestive decontamination, are also very important in the pathophysiology and treatment of SAP.[21] There is still controversy, however, as to the efficacy of selective digestive decontamination in patients with SAP.[22]

Abdominal compartment syndrome (ACS) is also important in the pathophysiology of SAP. Because PMMA-CHDF is very effective in controlling body water balance, this modality could be also very effective in the treatment and/or prevention of ACS in patients with SAP. Furthermore, CHDF is also very useful as renal replacement therapy in the treatment of SAP, because acute renal failure often develops in patients with SAP. Taking these factors into consideration, we now routinely apply PMMA-CHDF in patients with SAP, even those without renal failure.[23]

The efficacy of PMMA-CHDF in patients with SAP is striking. Sixty-one of 65 patients (94%) with SAP who were treated with PMMA-CHDF during a 10-year period survived. Figure 286-6 shows the change in blood interleukin-6 (IL-6) levels in patients with SAP treated with PMMA-CHDF; the IL-6 level significantly decreased with PMMA-CHDF.[23]

In Japan, PMMA-CHDF has become a standard therapeutic approach to SAP even though its efficacy has not been confirmed in randomized controlled trials.

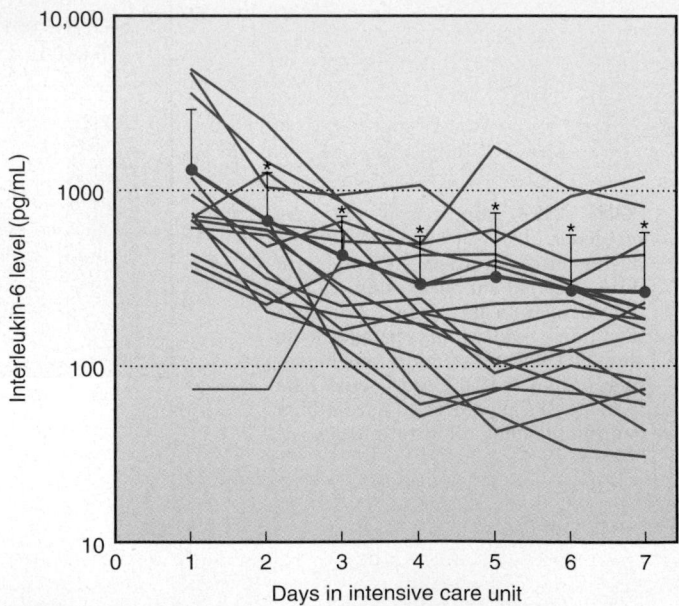

FIGURE 286-6. Change in blood interleukin-6 levels in patients with severe acute pancreatitis who were treated with continuous hemodiafiltration using a polymethyl methacrylate membrane hemofilter. Repeated one-way analysis of variance; $P < .0001$. $*P < .001$ compared with day 1 (Fischer's projected least significant difference).

Key Points

1. Simultaneous application of continuous hemodiafiltration when plasma exchange is used as an artificial liver support system is essential to overcome the complications of plasma exchange, such

as hypernatremia, metabolic alkalosis, and abrupt drops in colloid osmotic pressure.

2. The combination of slow plasma exchange and high-dialysate-flow continuous hemodiafiltration using a polymethyl methacrylate membrane hemofilter is preferable to enhance the efficacy of the artificial liver support system.

3. Artificial liver support using this combination approach achieves higher rates of recovery from hepatic coma and survival than use of plasma exchange alone.

4. Hypercytokinemia plays an important role in the pathophysiology of severe acute pancreatitis and,

therefore, continuous hemodiafiltration using a polymethyl methacrylate membrane hemofilter, as cytokine modulator, is very effective in the treatment of severe acute pancreatitis.

5. Continuous hemodiafiltration using a polymethyl methacrylate membrane hemofilter could be applied in a variety of disorders in which hypercytokinemia plays a central role.

See the companion Expert Consult website for the complete reference list.

CHAPTER 287

Multiple-Organ Support Therapy for the Critically Ill Patient

Alessandra Brendolan, Rinaldo Bellomo, and Claudio Ronco

OBJECTIVES

This chapter will:
1. Describe the complexity of derangements occurring in multiple-organ dysfunction syndrome.
2. Present the potential benefits of different forms of extracorporeal therapies in this syndrome.
3. Characterize the different modalities of extracorporeal support therapy and their specific functions.

The incidence of the multiple organ dysfunction syndrome (MODS) in intensive care units (ICUs) is rapidly rising.[1,2] MODS is usually combined with sepsis[3,4] and is the most common cause of death in the patients treated in the ICU.[5] The nature of ICU cases has changed over the last years. It includes a variety of severe cases due to major surgical interventions, trauma, hemodynamic instability, sepsis and so on, but also an older population than previously. All of these factors can easily lead to MODS. In previous years, the only available and efficient therapy was renal replacement therapy (RRT) for acute renal failure (ARF), but the development of technology has provided devices to support the other systems as well. The adequacy of any artificial organ support system is evaluated by how closely it mimics the flexibility and efficacy of the organ system it seeks to replace or support.

In a cataract of events, such as that created by sepsis and MODS, all of these criteria should be applied at the same time but for different organs and different tasks. RRT, and especially continuous renal replacement therapies (CRRTs), provided extracorporeal treatment in critically ill patients with hypercatabolism and fluid overload[5] and achieved excellent hemodynamic stability. New techniques in CRRT, such as high-volume hemofiltration, have

been applied in septic patients, with very promising results.[6,7] These observations give rise to a question: Can extracorporeal blood purification have a positive affect on different organ systems? A possible answer might come from the simple observation that all organs have one thing in common—contact with blood. All extracorporeal therapies also have one thing in common—treatment of blood. On the basis of these observations and knowledge of the molecular biology of sepsis, a "humoral" theory of MODS makes pathophysiological sense, and its consequence becomes the need to regard extracorporeal therapy as multiple-organ support therapy (MOST), not just as single-organ support.

MULTIPLE-ORGAN SUPPORT THERAPY

A hemofilter can perform RRT supporting one organ, whereas a more complex extracorporeal support system with a multitasking machine platform and additional devices could perform MOST. The common ground for this approach is modulation of the composition of blood. Thus, the final effect would be a reduction in the physiological disorders derived from multiple-organ failure, and at the same time, a return to the "internal milieu" facilitating the recovery of organ function. Can MOST be practically applied? Theoretically, we need an integrated approach to serve as a platform for different therapeutic options (Fig. 287-1).The tasks of this approach, based on the needs of the critically ill patients, are as follows:

1. Blood purification and renal support
2. Temperature control
3. Acid-base control
4. Fluid balance control

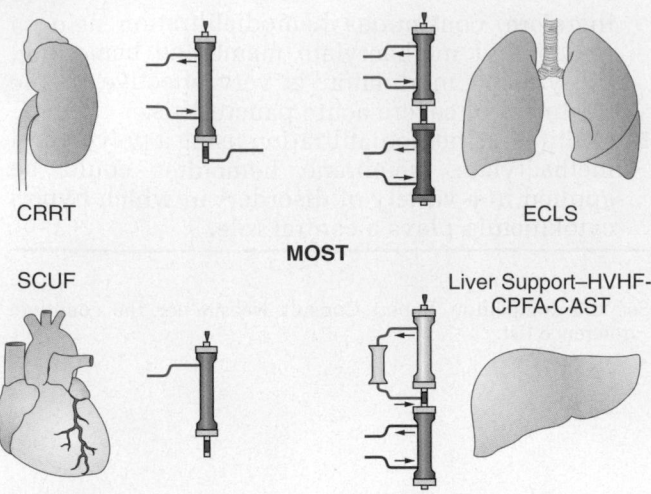

FIGURE 287-1. The platform for multiple-organ support therapy (MOST) should have enough flexibility to make possible the application of different extracorporeal techniques such as continuous renal replacement therapy (CRRT), slow continuous ultrafiltration (SCUF), extracorporeal lung support (ECLS), and liver support with all other therapies for immunomodulation. The new machine for MOST should be a multifunctional platform with the possibility of using different circuit layouts and different devices with specific functions. CAST, continuous attenuating sepsis therapy; CPFA, coupled plasmafiltration-adsorption; HVHF, high-volume hemofiltration.

5. Cardiac support
6. Protective lung support
7. Brain protection
8. Bone marrow protection
9. Blood detoxification and liver support
10. Therapy of sepsis, immunomodulation, and endothelial support

Blood Purification and Renal Support

Extracorporeal therapies have traditionally been employed to replace lost renal function in ARF, definitely the most common use of CRRT in the ICU. In the last 20 years, evidence has accumulated to support the concept that CRRT is efficient, safe, and well tolerated.[5] Progress from the arteriovenous circulation to venovenous pumped systems has improved efficiency and increased clearance to 2 or even 3 L/hr. Such a clearance results in values of daily Kt/V ranging from 1 to 1.5. If one disregards for a moment the concept that dose and outcome are correlated, the end result of an efficient therapy such as CRRT is blood purification similar to that obtained by the native kidney. Therefore, task #1 can reasonably be considered accomplished.

Thermal Energy Balance

The extracorporeal circulation can be a potent modulator of body temperature and overall thermal balance. With the extracorporeal fluxes used for continuous venovenous hemofiltration (CVVH) and continuous venovenous hemodialysis (CVVHD), a negative thermal balance of up to −100 kJ/hr can be obtained, depending on the length of the

blood lines, the room temperature, and the dialysate or replacement fluid temperature. Such a negative balance might contribute to modulating the inflammatory response as well as oxygen demand in several organs, with the possibility of using such a mechanism for specific clinical targets. Thus, task #2 can reasonably be considered accomplished.

Homeostatic Equilibration

Most imbalances of sodium and other electrolyte imbalances can be corrected by increasing or restricting free water intake. Other electrolyte imbalances can be medically corrected. When disorders are life-threatening or refractory to medical corrections, extracorporeal therapy is the treatment of choice. The use of convection applied to the extracorporeal circulation is the same as that used by the human glomerulus. The ultrafiltrate contains crystalloids in the same concentration as in plasma water, but not cells or colloids. This mechanism is guaranteed by the use of a highly permeable membrane mounted on the hemofilter with permeability characteristics similar to those of the human glomerulus. The function of the renal tubules and the interstitium is accomplished, during hemofiltration, by the re-infusion of a tailored replacement solution. With this mechanism, a final solute and electrolyte balance can be achieved meeting the desired goals.

The advantage of such a system, in comparison with the use of diuretics, is the possibility of dissociating the removal of water from that of sodium or other electrolytes. Because of the slow and gentle rate of fluid exchange, the treated blood operates in continuous equilibrium with peripheral tissues and organs, and the entire organism may benefit from a rapid and effective restoration of water, sodium, and electrolyte homeostasis. This restoration of homeostasis is particularly true for acid-base control (because administration of bicarbonate can be easily titrated to the necessary acid-base goals), intracellular/extracellular potassium and phosphate equilibrium, and water fluxes between interstitium and the intracellular space. For these tasks, hemofiltration is physiologically superior to hemodialysis because accurate balances can be planned and obtained. Thus, tasks #3 and #4 on the list can reasonably be considered accomplished.

Fluid Balance and Cardiac Support

Myocardial dysfunction is common in the critically ill. It may be a consequence of a myocardial dilatation with reduced contractility, ventricular stiffness with diastolic dysfunction, or myocardial injury or circulating myocardial depressant factors, as seen in sepsis. In all cases, cardiac support can be achieved by the optimization of fluid balance, the reduction of organ edema, and the restoration of desirable levels of preload and afterload.[8] Several reports have shown that myocardial elastance can improve after hemofiltration with restoration of adequate fluid balance. In such conditions, the continuity of the extracorporeal therapy allows remarkable cardiovascular stability with maintenance of hemodynamic parameters, including mean arterial pressure, heart rate, and systemic vascular resistance. Such stability, which is achieved through slow continuous ultrafiltration and continuous refilling of the intravascular volume from the interstitium, allows stability of circulating blood volume and the preservation of organ perfusion, which are crucial in facilitating renal recovery during ARF. Thus, task #5 can, to an extent, reasonably be considered accomplished.

Protective Lung Support

The fundamental concept in patients with acute lung injury is to provide adequate gas exchange without causing further barotrauma or volutrauma to the lungs and also decrease extravascular lung water. Mechanical ventilation is typically needed in the treatment of acute lung injury but is injurious to the lungs. The possibility of removing carbon dioxide from the circulating blood in such conditions by means of extracorporeal methods has been previously explored.[9] Today, the idea of using a special carbon dioxide–removing cartridge in series with the hemofilter might represent, in selected patients, a new chance to reduce the requirement for invasive mechanical ventilation, allowing instead for a noninvasive approach. Special membranes are under evaluation that use a dry/wet gas exchange process leading to significant values of carbon dioxide clearance in the extracorporeal circuit. Such systems might reduce the morbidity and mortality of acute lung injury in the future. Furthermore, by optimizing the patient's volume status and offering the ability to remove interstitial fluid, extracorporeal therapy may give additional support to the failing lung. Thus, although it is still far from being an ideal system, we are already offering an important level of lung support. Thus, task #6 can reasonably be considered accomplished.

Brain Protection

Cerebral edema is a consequence of rapid solute movement during intermittent hemodialysis.[10] The arrival of CRRT has eliminated this risk.[10] The accumulation of uremic toxins from inadequate blood purification is a known cause of encephalopathy. The use of CRRT in the ICU has eliminated this risk. The development of hypotension can induce brain injury. The use of CRRT with its associated hemodynamic stability has decreased the risk. The accumulation of amino acid derivatives might be responsible for the encephalopathy of sepsis. By removing such excessive soluble derivatives and decreasing imbalances between amino acids, CRRT may also have an effect on the encephalopathy of sepsis. Acidemia induces changes in the function of cerebral enzymes involved in glucose utilization and may be responsible for changes in conscious state. The correction of acidemia by CRRT might also be another way of protecting the brain from injury. Thus, although a long way from the ideal, a significant degree of brain protection is already available. Thus, task #7 can reasonably be considered accomplished.

Bone Marrow Support

Bone marrow function is depressed by sepsis and uremia. Red blood cell production and platelet function are affected by the accumulation of uremic toxins. Although other important events affect bone marrow function, the removal of uremic toxins is an important way in which extracorporeal therapies already offer bone marrow support. Of course, this support can be improved with the use of recombinant human erythropoietin. Thus task #8 can reasonably be considered accomplished.

Extracorporeal Liver Support

Liver dysfunction may be superimposed on ARF and may require management of associated metabolic intoxication. The healthy liver is a detoxifying organ with secretory function for coagulation factors, proteins, and hormones. The liver hydrolyzes several toxins, making their excretion through the kidneys possible. When this function is impaired, protein-bound hydrophobic substances tend to accumulate in blood, and specific blood purification systems are required.

The ideal blood purification system for liver support should have a blood flow of at least 600 to 800 mL/min, should be capable of removing lipid-soluble, water-soluble, and protein-bound toxins, and should achieve clearances of these toxins at a minimum rate of 600 to 700 mL/min. A complete liver support system should have a detoxification component and a secretory component, possibly capable of metabolic activity. Although detoxification can be accomplished by an inert mechanical system, secretion can be performed only by a hybrid artificial organ containing a mixture of synthetic materials and living hepatocytes. Nevertheless, the detoxifying component can be sufficient to perform liver support and to support patients during recovery of the native organ or liver transplantation.

Different systems are now available for liver support to perform such a task.[11] Some of them utilize the hemoperfusion technique, applying the direct contact of blood with adsorbent materials. This approach can be utilized in series with standard hemofiltration procedures, but it has the limitations imposed by the partial adsorptive capacity of the sorbents. In fact, in order for the sorbent to be placed in contact with blood, its material must be coated to improve biocompatibility, and this process of coating often reduces the efficiency of the adsorptive process. On the other hand, more effective sorbent materials can be utilized and placed in contact with plasma, if the blood cells are previously separated through a plasma filter or an albumin-permeable filter. In such condition, protein- and albumin-bound toxins can be removed by the adsorbent, and blood can be reconstituted downstream after the plasma has been purified.[12] In these circumstances, uncoated resins and carbons can be utilized without any problem of bioincompatibility, because the sorbent never directly contacts the blood cells. This technique has been performed in series with high-flux hemodialysis in the Prometheus System (Fresenius Medical Care, Bad Homburg, Germany) using a standard hemodialysis machine.[13]

Other modern technologies include cascade plasmapheresis and the Molecular Adsorbent Recirculating System (MARS; Gambro AG, Lund, Sweden).[14] MARS is an extracorporeal liver support system designed to remove albumin-bound toxic molecules. Based on albumin dialysis principle, dialysis membranes used are impermeable to albumin but able to clear toxic substances bound to albumin when an albumin-rich dialysate is used. The dialysate also contains electrolytes and bicarbonate and is regenerated by passage through an anionic exchange resin, charcoal adsorption, and sequential hemodialysis.

The final expected physiological effects can be an improved neurological state, clearance of unconjugated bilirubin at 20 to 40 mL/min or higher, clearance of some aromatic amino acids, a decrease in serum ammonia, and removal of some cytokines. Thus, although large, properly designed clinical trials of this modality are needed, we are already making the first important steps toward clinically relevant liver support. Thus task #9 can reasonably be considered accomplished.

Therapy of Sepsis and Immunomodulation

Most patients treated with RRT for ARF have an underlying septic syndrome. Thus, many patients with sepsis receive extracorporeal therapies. Various observations have reported beneficial, clinically visible effects in patients with sepsis treated with CRRT.[15-17] These effects may reflect the possible changes in mediator activity induced by this therapy. According to this "humoral theory of sepsis" in physiological conditions, the biological activity of sepsis-associated mediators is under the control of specific inhibitors that may act at different levels. In sepsis, the homeostatic balance is altered, and a profound disturbance of relative production and release of different mediators occurs. The spillover of mediators into the circulation generates systemic effects, including endothelial damage, hemodynamic shock, and vasomotor paralysis. Furthermore, monocytes from septic humans display a profound inability to produce cytokines when they are challenged with different stimuli ex vivo. Thus, although the pathophysiology of sepsis was initially described as an overproduction of pro-inflammatory factors, the concept of sepsis as a simply pro-inflammatory event has been challenged.[18,19]

To describe the excessive anti-inflammatory counterpart of systemic inflammatory response syndrome (SIRS), Bone and colleagues[20] coined the acronym CARS, for compensated anti-inflammatory response syndrome. Terms such as monocyte deactivation, immunoparalysis, and more simply, cell hyporesponsiveness have all been used to indicate the inability of cells to respond ex vivo to lipopolysaccharide stimuli. These researchers also proposed that at a given time, SIRS or CARS predominates in patients, inducing either shock or immune depression. However, much evidence now suggests that, in many patients, SIRS and CARS may coexist but in different compartments (Fig. 287-2).

Other investigators had proposed that the events associated with sepsis/SIRS may occur in sequence (the sequential or serial sepsis theory),[21,22] whereby pro-inflammatory and anti-inflammatory mediators are alternatively produced in high or low generation periods, thus leading to SIRS and/or CARS simultaneously (the parallel sepsis theory), and SIRS and CARS may coexist in different districts or systems (Fig. 287-3).

In intensive care medicine, blocking one mediator has not led to measurable outcome improvement in patients with sepsis. Possibly more clearly defined subgroups would gain from treatments that block tumor necrosis factor (TNF). On the other hand, antagonizing a cytokine may lead to deleterious consequences resulting in substantially higher mortality. A low-level TNF response seems to be necessary for the host defense against infection, whereas high levels of TNF must be modulated by anti-inflammatory feedback. Because sepsis does not fit a one-insult model but shows the complex behavior of mediator levels that change over time, neither single mediator–directed nor one-time interventions seem appropriate. Therefore, one of the major criticisms attributed to continuous blood purification treatments in sepsis—its lack of specificity—could turn out to be a major strength. Nonspecific removal of soluble mediators, be they pro-inflammatory or anti-inflammatory, without complete elimination of their effects may be the most logical and adequate approach to a complex and long-running process like sepsis (Fig. 287-4).

The issue whether hemofiltration can remove inflammatory mediators has been controversial for some time. Numerous ex vivo as well as animal and human studies have shown that synthetic filters can extract nearly every substance involved in sepsis to a certain extent. Prominent examples are complement factors, TNF, interleukins 1, 6, and 8, and platelet-activating factor (PAF). The decrease in plasma cytokine levels with hemofiltration appears to be only minor. Some studies showed no influence of CRRT on cytokine plasma levels. On the other hand, significant clinical benefits, in terms of hemodynamic improvement, have been achieved even without measurable decreases in cytokine plasma levels.

The removal of substances other than the measured cytokines might have been responsible for the achieved effect. In this context a further step in clarifying the immu-

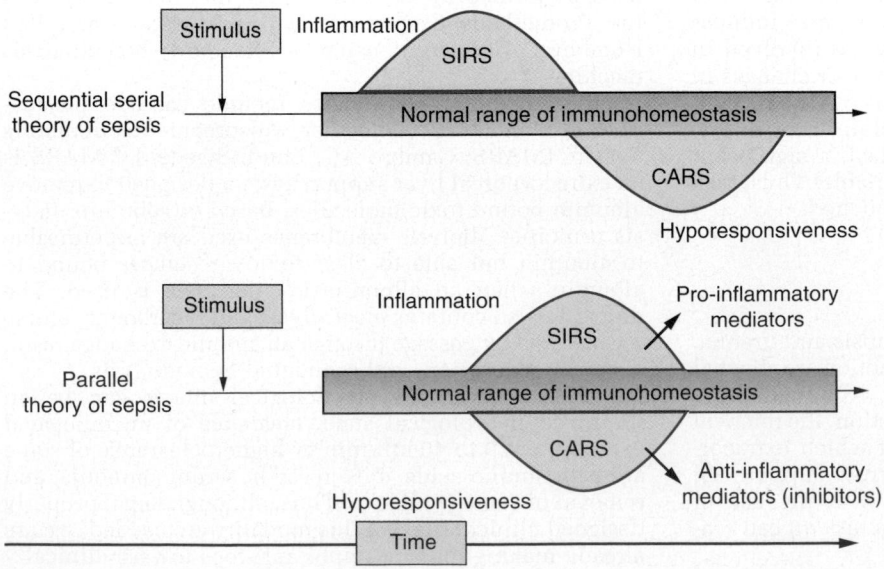

FIGURE 287-2. The humoral theory of sepsis implies either sequential inflammation and counter-inflammation (serial or sequential theory of sepsis) or the simultaneous presence of the two processes in the body (parallel theory of sepsis). In the first possibility, the sequence of events starts temporally with a stimulus, such as endotoxin dissemination, and a systemic inflammatory response syndrome follows with a spillover into the circulation of several pro-inflammatory mediators. Subsequently, a potent inhibition of the inflammatory process and a consequent cell hyporesponsiveness occur. In the parallel theory, both processes occur simultaneously and a parallel synthesis of pro-inflammatory and anti-inflammatory mediators exists in different locations in the body. CARS, compensated anti-inflammatory response syndrome; SIRS, systemic inflammatory response syndrome.

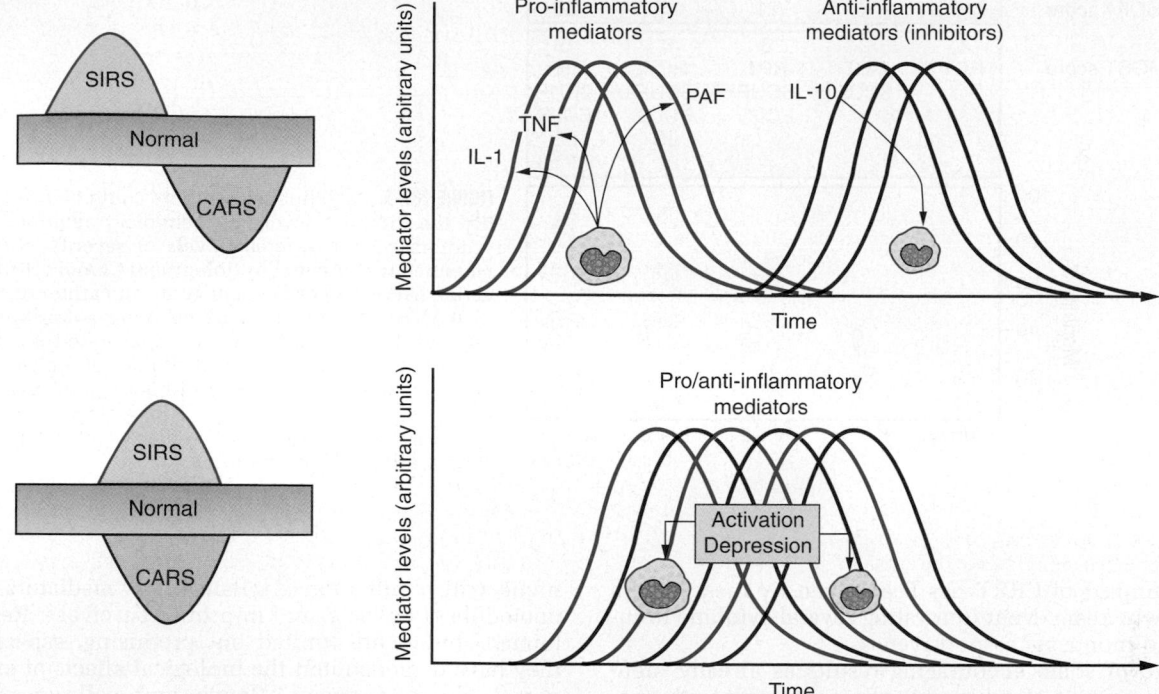

FIGURE 287-3. In the sequential theory of sepsis, provided that the immunological condition of the patient allows a rapid response, specific remedies can be prescribed. In the parallel theory of sepsis, simultaneous activation and depression of the immunological system are present, and therefore a specific therapy is impossible. In the sequential theory, peaks of proinflammatory mediators are followed by peaks of anti-inflammatory mediators. In the parallel theory, there is a mixture of pro-inflammatory and anti-inflammatory mediators. CARS, compensated anti-inflammatory response syndrome; SIRS, systemic inflammatory response syndrome; IL-, interleukin-; PAF, platelet-activating factor; TNF, tumor necrosis factor.

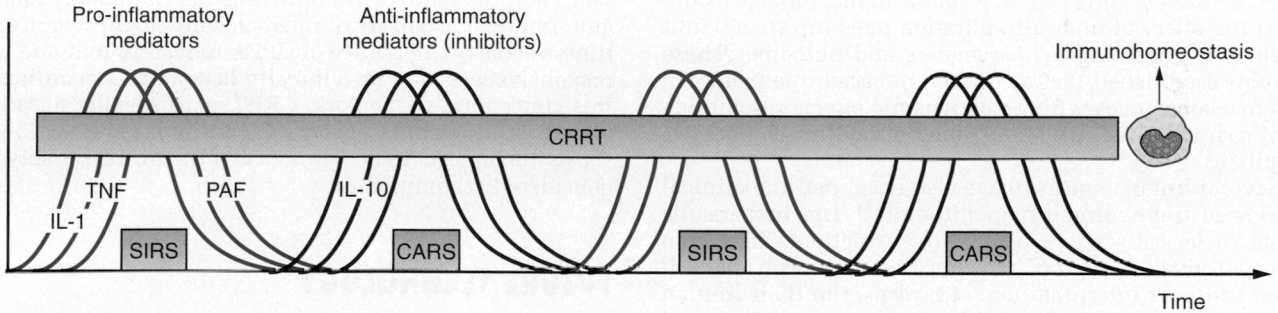

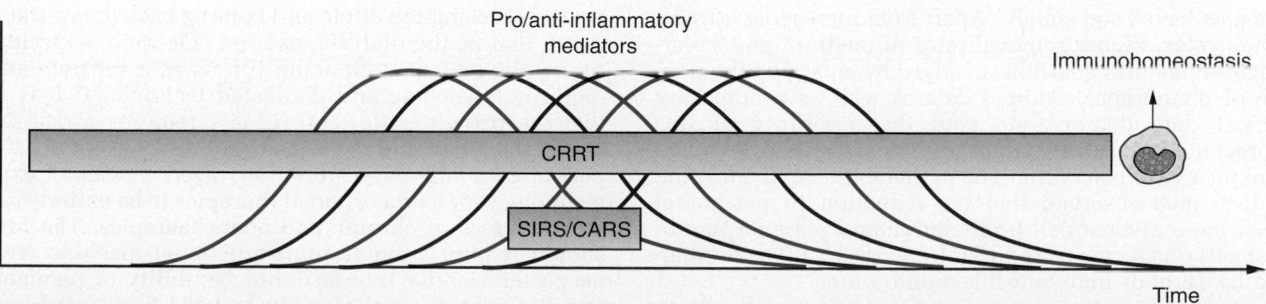

FIGURE 287-4. Continuous attenuation sepsis therapy (CAST) can be successful in both conditions of sepsis (sequential and parallel; see Fig. 287-2) because of the specific removal of pro-inflammatory and anti-inflammatory mediators. The sequential theory leads to the conclusion that, if pro-inflammatory and anti-inflammatory activities could be monitored, specific therapies could be targeted for selected actions at different points during the course of the syndrome. In the parallel theory, any therapy could be effective on one side but deleterious on another. In both theories (sequential and parallel), the concept introduced by the peak concentration hypothesis suggests that a nonselective control of the inflammation peaks and immunoparalysis may contribute to diminishing the patient's disease and increase the host defenses induced by a nearly normal immunohomeostasis.

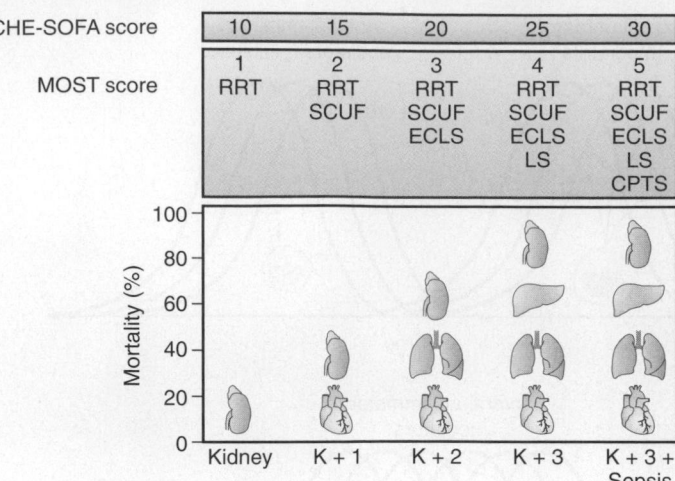

FIGURE 287-5. A technological score could be used to identify the different levels of technology required to treat syndromes with different levels of severity. Severity as measured with Acute Physiology and Chronic Health Evaluation (APACHE) or Sequential Organ Failure Assessment (SOFA) score must be paralleled by a Multiple-Organ Support Therapy (MOST) score that describes the complexity of technology to be instituted for a given level of organ involvement. CPTS, continuous protective therapy of sepsis; ECLS, extracorporeal lung support; K, kidney; LS, liver support; RRT, renal replacement therapy; SCUF, slow continuous ultrafiltration.

nologic impact of CRRT has been taken by measuring a more downstream event integrating several cytokine influences and monocyte responsiveness.

In spite of some encouraging results as already mentioned, the extent of achievable clinical benefit with conventional CRRT (using conventional filters and flow rates) in sepsis has generally been disappointing. Consequently, attempts have been made to improve the efficiency of soluble mediator removal in sepsis by increasing the amount of plasma water exchange—in other words, increasing ultrafiltration rates. Animal studies provide great support of this concept. Starting in the early 1990s, several studies using different septic animal models examined the effect of high ultrafiltration rates (up to 200 mL/kg/hr) on physiological parameters and outcome. These studies established that a convection-based treatment can remove substances with hemodynamic effects resembling septic shock when sufficiently high ultrafiltration rates are applied.

Several human studies have also examined the clinical effects of high-volume hemofiltration.[12] The first results seem to be satisfactory, especially in patients in whom poor survival was predicted. Results of these trials still need cautious interpretation with respect to their limited design, but they do offer evidence of the feasibility and efficacy needed to set the stage for a large-scale trial of high-volume hemofiltration in sepsis.

Other approaches to achieve higher mediator clearance in sepsis have been sought. Apart from increasing ultrafiltration rates, higher removal rates of medium-molecular-weight molecules could be achieved by enlarging the pore size of membranes. Animal data as well as preliminary clinical data demonstrate both the feasibility of this approach and probable superior removal rates of selected cytokines with use of more open membranes. In addition, studies have observed that the reduction in peripheral blood mononuclear cell proliferation and polymorphonuclear cell phagocytosis induced by sepsis could be normalized by 12-hour high-cutoff hemofiltration.

A further step to improve mediator removal has been achieved by modifying the circuit to favor adsorption. Coupled plasmafiltration-adsorption (CPFA) uses a plasma filter that isolates plasma and redirects it through a synthetic resin cartridge before returning it to the blood. A further filter can be coupled to provide standard RRT. Animal studies have confirmed the efficacy of this technique, with elimination of inflammatory mediators, immunomodulatory effects, and improved survival.[23] Results of human studies are limited but promising, especially as they have demonstrated the biological effects of extracorporeal blood treatment. Ronco and colleagues[24] have shown that CPFA achieves better unselective cytokine removal, hemodynamics, and leukocyte responsiveness than hemodiafiltration. After 10 hours of CPFA, not only was the capacity of monocytes to produce TNF-α in response to lipopolysaccharide restored but phagocytosis was also returned to near-normal levels. In a second study,[25] CPFA used in septic patients with and without renal failure resulted in improvements in hemodynamics and impressive survival rates despite high severity of illness scores. The ability of CPFA to restore immune cell responsiveness may be clinically beneficial. According to this conceptual framework, CRRT with specific filtration and adsorption could become a continuous attenuation of sepsis therapy (CAST). Thus task #10 can reasonably be considered accomplished.

FUTURE TECHNOLOGY

Many years ago, Ronco and Bellomo suggested the design of a new machine for patients with ARF.[26] As machines became more complex, the question arose as to whether we were closing the circle and coming back to our starting point, that is, the dialysis machine. Or were we trying to regard the patient with acute illness as a separate entity requiring a specific and dedicated technology? It is true that the patient with acute illness requires a dedicated series of devices and machines, and the concept of MOST perfectly fits this description; however, we cannot expect technology for extracorporeal therapies to be entirely separate for cases of chronic and acute therapies. The future should require a single multifunctional machine with a very user-friendly interface and flexibility of parameters and prescription so that it can be used to respond to different medical needs with the use of different disposable layouts. The question who should be using such machines will be answered by the simplicity of the interface and the operating characteristics. As personal computers today do not require computer experts to perform complex tasks, so the new generation of machines should be usable by different operators in various hospitals and settings. In the meantime, an intermediate series of machines already exist: They are not hemodialysis machines, but they still require an experienced operator. They can perform different treatments and tasks, but they still require specific programming and dedicated disposables. Given this view of MOST, the machine will be a platform with different options and an easy-to-use interface so that severity scores can be paralleled by a "technology score" required to restore homeostasis (Fig. 287-5).

Key Points

1. The multiple-organ dysfunction syndrome is the leading cause of death in critically ill patients and is responsible for much health care expenditure.
2. Because the probability of death is directly correlated to the number of failing organs beyond the kidney and the extent of physiological derangement, a clinically sensible approach is to broaden the spectrum of physiological endpoints targeted by extracorporeal therapy.
3. Blood is the vital element that regulates all body systems from cellular to organ level. Continuous

renal replacement therapy has direct access to blood and thus to all organ systems.
4. The evolution of continuous renal replacement therapy from simple renal re-placement to a multiple-organ support therapy is logical and should be the gold standard of extracorporeal blood purification in the intensive care unit.

Key References

3. Bone RC, Balk RA, Cerra FB, et al: Definitions for sepsis and organ failure and guidelines for the use of innovative therapies in sepsis. The ACCP/SCCM Consensus Conference Committee. American College of Chest Physicians/Society of Critical Care Medicine. Chest 1992;101:1644-1655.
4. Camussi G, Montrucchio G, Dominioni L, Dionigi R: Septic shock—the unravelling of molecular mechanisms. Nephrol Dial Transplant 1995;10:1808-1813.
5. Bellomo R, Ronco C: Indications and criteria for initiating renal replacement therapy in the intensive care unit. Kidney Int 1998;53(Suppl 66):S106-S109.
18. Cavaillon JM, Munoz C, Fitting C, et al: Circulating cytokines: The tip of the iceberg? Circ Shock 1992;38:145-152.

See the companion Expert Consult website for the complete reference list.

Part IV

Special Topics in Critical Care Nephrology

Critical Care Nephrology in Pediatrics

CHAPTER 288

Pathophysiology of Pediatric Acute Kidney Injury

Prasad Devarajan

OBJECTIVES

This chapter will:
1. Present an overview of the morphological, hemodynamic, and tubulodynamic alterations in acute kidney injury.
2. Describe the alterations in tubule cell structure and metabolism in acute kidney injury.
3. Review the evidence for a role for apoptosis in human acute kidney injury, and outline the pathomechanisms involved.
4. Discuss the role of the microvasculature and the inflammatory response in acute kidney injury.
5. Identify novel therapeutic approaches to acute kidney injury based on pathophysiological mechanisms.

Acute renal failure (ARF) is a common clinical problem, with increasing incidence, serious consequences, and unsatisfactory therapeutic options in both children and adults.[1,2] ARF may be classified as *prerenal* (the functional response of structurally normal kidneys to hypoperfusion), *intrinsic* or intrarenal (involving structural damage to the renal parenchyma), and *postrenal* (urinary tract obstruction). The focus of this chapter is on intrinsic ARF, which is the most common and clinically significant subtype in hospitalized patients and can be associated with acute tubular necrosis. The prognosis for patients with intrinsic ARF remains poor, with a mortality rate of 40% to 80% in the intensive care unit (ICU) setting. Two major problems have plagued the field. First, well over 20 definitions for ARF have been used in published studies, ranging from "dialysis requirement" to "subtle increases in serum creatinine." In an attempt to standardize the definition, the term *acute kidney injury* (AKI) has been proposed.[3] This clinical entity is a complex disorder with multiple causative factors that occurs in a variety of settings, with diverse clinical manifestations ranging from a minimal elevation in serum creatinine to anuric renal failure. In this chapter, use of the term *acute tubular necro-*

sis is avoided, and the designations AKI and intrinsic ARF are used preferentially and interchangeably.

The second problem is an incomplete understanding of the cellular and molecular mechanisms underlying AKI. Current advances in basic and translational research that hold promise for elucidation of the pathogenesis of human AKI are reviewed later in the chapter. Although the emphasis is on ischemic AKI, additional mechanisms pertinent to nephrotoxins and sepsis also are briefly explored. Of note, however, AKI in the ICU setting frequently is multifactorial, with concomitant ischemic, nephrotoxic, and septic components, and with overlapping pathophysiological mechanisms.

MORPHOLOGICAL ALTERATIONS

The term *acute tubular necrosis* is a misnomer, because frank tubule cell necrosis is rarely encountered in human ARF. Prominent morphological features of AKI in humans include effacement and loss of proximal tubule brush border, patchy loss of tubule cells, focal areas of proximal tubular dilatation and presence of distal tubular casts, and areas of cellular regeneration.[4] Necrosis is inconspicuous and restricted to the highly susceptible outer medullary regions. By contrast, apoptosis is a consistent finding in both distal and proximal tubules in both ischemic and nephrotoxic forms of human AKI.[5] In addition, peritubular capillaries display a striking vascular congestion, endothelial damage, and leukocyte accumulation.[6] The mechanisms underlying these morphological findings, and their implications for the ensuing profound renal dysfunction, are detailed next.

HEMODYNAMIC ALTERATIONS

An intense and persistent renal vasoconstriction that reduces overall renal blood flow to approximately 50% of

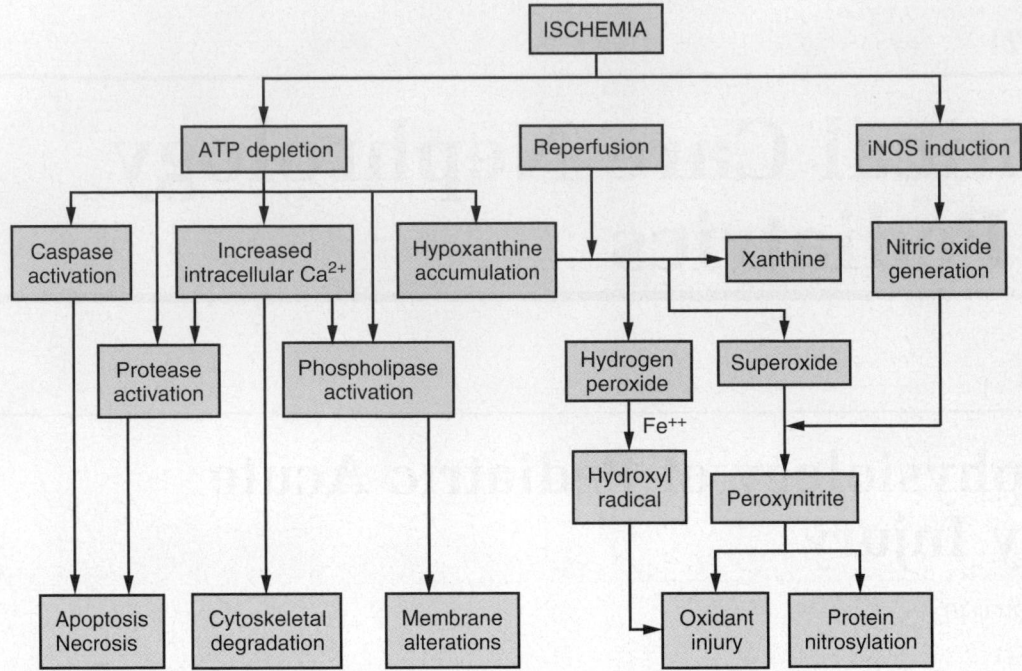

FIGURE 288-1. Alterations in tubule cell metabolism. The initiation phase of acute kidney injury is characterized by ATP depletion, which activates a number of oxidative and cell death mechanisms. During the extension phase, reperfusion propels these pathways to completion. iNOS, inducible nitric oxide synthase.

normal has long been considered a hallmark of intrinsic ARF.[1] In addition, the postischemic kidney displays regional alterations in blood flow patterns.[6] Marked congestion and hypoperfusion of the outer medulla are seen that persist even though cortical blood flow improves during reperfusion after an ischemic insult, leading to prolonged cellular injury and cell death in these predisposed tubule segments. Mechanisms underlying these hemodynamic alterations relate primarily to endothelial cell injury.[6] The result is a local imbalance of vasoactive substances, with enhanced release of vasoconstrictors such as endothelin and decreased abundance of vasodilators such as endothelium-derived nitric oxide. Endothelin receptor antagonists ameliorate ischemic AKI in animals, but human data are lacking. Similarly, carbon monoxide and carbon monoxide–releasing compounds are protective in animal models of ischemic AKI, probably through vasodilatation and preservation of medullary blood flow, but this approach has not been tested in humans. These hemodynamic abnormalities, however, cannot fully account for the profound loss of renal function, and several human trials of vasodilators such as dopamine have failed to demonstrate improvement in glomerular filtration rate in established ARF despite augmentation of overall renal blood flow.

ALTERATIONS IN TUBULE DYNAMICS

Known derangements in tubule dynamics include obstruction, backleak, and activation of tubuloglomerular feedback. The consistent histological findings of proximal tubular dilatation and distal tubular casts in human biopsy specimens indicate that obstruction to tubular fluid flow certainly occurs in ischemic AKI. The intraluminal casts contain Tamm-Horsfall protein, which normally is secreted by the thick ascending limb as a monomer. Conversion

into a gel-like polymer is promoted by the increased luminal sodium concentration typically encountered within the distal tubule in AKI. This provides an ideal environment for cast formation, with desquamated tubule cells and brush border membranes contributing to obstruction. It is unlikely, however, that obstruction alone can account for the intense renal dysfunction, because human studies using forced diuresis did not demonstrate an impact on survival and renal recovery rates in patients with ARF.

A role for activation of tubuloglomerular feedback has been proposed. The increased delivery of sodium chloride to the macula densa due to cellular abnormalities in the proximal tubule would be expected to induce afferent arteriolar constriction by means of A_1 adenosine receptor (A1AR) activation, thereby decreasing glomerular filtration rate. In recent studies, however, a knockout of the A1AR resulted in a paradoxical worsening of ischemic AKI, and exogenous activation of A1AR was protective.[7] Thus, tubuloglomerular feedback activation secondary to ischemic injury may represent a beneficial phenomenon that limits delivery of ions and solutes to the damaged proximal tubules, thereby reducing the demand for adenosine triphosphate (ATP)-dependent reabsorptive processes. Any salutary effect of exogenous A1AR activation in human AKI remains to be determined.

ALTERATIONS IN TUBULE CELL METABOLISM

A profound reduction in intracellular ATP content invariably occurs early after ischemic renal injury, which sets in motion a number of critical metabolic consequences in tubule cells[4,8] (Fig. 288-1). Oxygen deprivation leads to a rapid degradation of ATP to adenosine diphosphate (ADP) and adenosine monophosphate (AMP). With prolonged ischemia, AMP is further metabolized to adenine nucleotides and to hypoxanthine. Adenine nucleotides freely diffuse out of cells, and their depletion precludes resynthesis of intracellular ATP during reperfusion. Nevertheless, although provision of exogenous adenine nucleotides or thyroxine (which stimulates mitochondrial ATP regeneration) can mitigate AKI in animal models, this approach has yielded disappointing results in human ARF.

ATP depletion leads to impaired calcium sequestration within the endoplasmic reticulum, as well as diminished extrusion of cytosolic calcium into the extracellular space, resulting in increased free intracellular calcium after AKI. Potential downstream complications include activation of proteases and phospholipases and cytoskeletal degradation. Calcium channel blockers may provide some protection from renal injury in the transplantation setting, but evidence for their efficacy in other forms of human AKI is lacking.

The role of reactive oxygen species in the pathogenesis of AKI is supported by substantial evidence. During reperfusion, the conversion of accumulated hypoxanthine to xanthine generates hydrogen peroxide and superoxide. In the presence of iron, hydrogen peroxide forms the highly reactive hydroxyl radical. Concomitantly, ischemia induces nitric oxide synthase in tubule cells. The nitric oxide generated interacts with superoxide to form peroxynitrite, which results in cell damage via oxidant injury as well as protein nitrosylation.[4,8] Collectively, reactive oxygen species cause renal tubule cell injury by oxidation of proteins, peroxidation of lipids, damage to DNA, and induction of apoptosis. A recent study has documented a dramatic increase in oxidative stress in humans with ARF, as evidenced by depletion of plasma protein thiols and increased carbonyl formation.[9] Scavengers of reactive oxygen molecules (such as superoxide dismutase, catalase, and N-acetylcysteine) protect against ischemic AKI in animals, but human studies have been inconclusive. A promising new advance in the field is the protective effect of edaravone, a potent scavenger of free radicals and inhibitor of lipid peroxidation, observed with administration at the time of reperfusion in a rat model of ischemic AKI.[10] Edaravone has been approved for human use in the treatment of cerebral ischemia, and results with its use in human AKI are awaited.

Free iron derived from red cells or other injured cells is one of the most potent factors in the generation of reactive oxygen species, and the iron scavenger deferoxamine alleviates ischemia-reperfusion injury in animal models. The systemic toxicity (primarily hypotension) of this agent, however, precludes its routine clinical use in human AKI. Two major advances have come to light in the area of iron chelation. The first is the availability of human apotransferrin, an iron-binding protein, which protects against AKI in animals by abrogating renal superoxide formation.[11] Apotransferrin has been successfully used for the reduction of redox-active iron in patients undergoing hematologic stem cell transplantation without any adverse effects. The second is the discovery of neutrophil gelatinase-associated lipocalin (NGAL), a major iron-transporting protein complementary to transferrin, as one of the most highly induced genes and proteins in the kidney after AKI.[12] Administration of NGAL provides remarkable structural and functional protection in animal models.[13] The potential use of these endogenous agents (apotransferrin and NGAL) in human AKI is under investigation.

ALTERATIONS IN TUBULE CELL STRUCTURE

The structural response of the tubule cell to injury is multifaceted and includes loss of cell polarity and brush borders, cell death, de-differentiation of viable cells, proliferation of tubule cells, and restitution of a normal epithelium (Fig. 288-2). Cellular ATP depletion leads to a rapid disruption of the apical actin cytoskeleton and redistribution of actin from microvilli into the cytoplasm.[14] The ensuing alterations in microvillar structure lead to formation of membrane-bound, free-floating extracellular vesicles, or "blebs," that are either internalized or lost into the tubular lumen. Brush border membrane components released into the lumen contribute to cast formation and obstruction. These casts and vesicles containing actin and actin-depolymerizing factor (ADF), also known as cofilin, have been detected in urine in animal as well as human AKI.[14] ADF (cofilin) is a cytosolic protein that normally is maintained in the inactive phosphorylated form by Rho GTPases. In cultured tubule cells, ATP depletion leads to Rho GTPase inactivation, with resultant activation and relocalization of ADF to the surface membrane and membrane-bound vesicles. Concomitantly, ATP depletion dissociates the actin-stabilizing proteins tropomyosin and ezrin, allowing the activated ADF to now bind and consequently sever actin, which in turn leads to microvillar breakdown. Thus, inactivation of ADF may represent a promising but unexplored direction in AKI.

Disruption of the apical cytoskeleton by ATP depletion also results in loss of tight (zonula occludens) junctions and zonula adherens junctions. Reduced expression, redistribution, and abnormal aggregation of a number of key proteins that constitute the tight and adherens junctions have been documented after ischemic injury in cell culture, animal models, and human studies.[4] The consequent loss of tight junction barrier function can potentially magnify the transtubular backleak of glomerular filtrate induced by obstruction.

Ischemia results in the early disruption of at least two basolaterally polarized proteins—namely, Na$^+$,K$^+$-ATPase and integrins. The Na$^+$,K$^+$-ATPase normally is tethered to the spectrin-based cytoskeleton at the basolateral domain by the adapter protein ankyrin. In cell culture, animal models, and human studies, ischemia leads to a reversible cytoplasmic accumulation of Na$^+$,K$^+$-ATPase, ankyrin, and spectrin in viable cells.[15] The mislocated Na$^+$,K$^+$-ATPase remains bound to ankyrin but is devoid of spectrin. Postulated mechanisms for loss of Na$^+$,K$^+$-ATPase polarity include hyperphosphorylation of ankyrin, with consequent loss of spectrin binding, and cleavage of spectrin by ischemia-induced activation of proteases such as calpain. A physiological consequence of the loss of basolateral Na$^+$,K$^+$-ATPase is an impairment in proximal tubular sodium reabsorption and a consequent increase in fractional excretion of sodium, which are diagnostic signatures of intrinsic ARF.

The β_1 integrins are normally polarized to the basal domain, where they mediate cell-substratum adhesions. Ischemic injury leads to a redistribution of integrins to the apical membrane, with consequential detachment of viable cells from the basement membrane. The exfoliated cells display abnormal adhesion within the tubular lumen, mediated by an interaction between apical integrin and the Arg-Gly-Asp (i.e., RGD) motif of integrin receptors. Administration of synthetic RGD compounds attenuates tubular obstruction and renal impairment in animal models, and

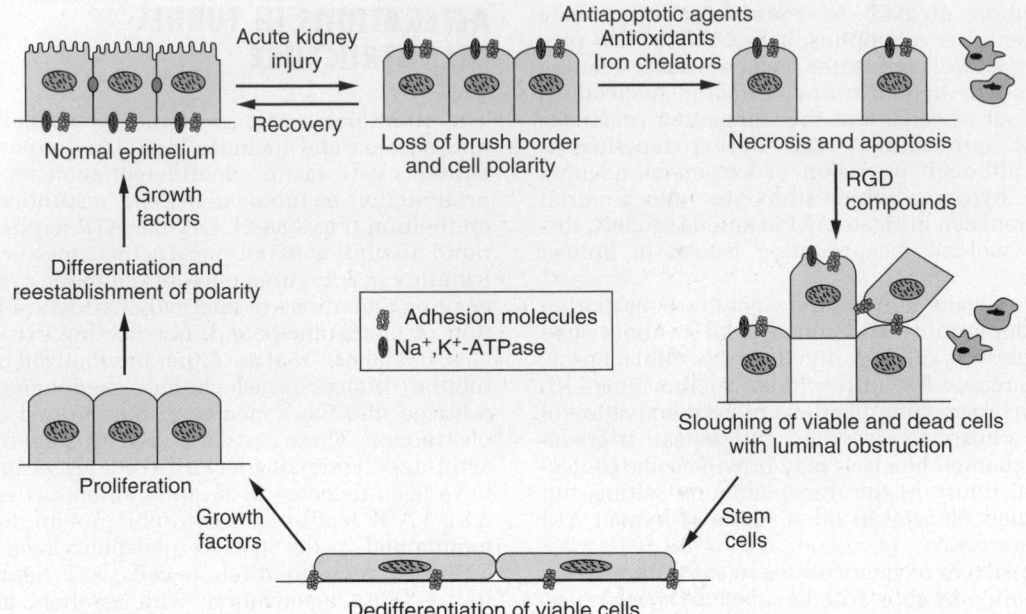

FIGURE 288-2. Alterations in tubule cell structure. The initiation phase of acute kidney injury (AKI) leads to sublethal injury, with loss of cell polarity and brush borders. If the injury is alleviated at this stage, complete recovery is usual. If not checked, the injury progresses to the extension phase, with onset of apoptosis and necrosis. Anti-apoptotic, antioxidant, and iron chelator therapies hold promise for treatment of AKI at this stage. Subsequent desquamation of cells leads to obstruction, which may be prevented by RGD (i.e., Arg-Gly-Asp) peptides. The maintenance phase is characterized by a balance between tubule cell death and regeneration. Acceleration of the repair process using stem cells or growth factors may hasten recovery.

the recent development of orally active integrin antagonists holds promise for clinical application in human AKI.[16]

ALTERATIONS IN CELL VIABILITY

Injured tubular epithelial cells can suffer one of three distinct fates after AKI. A majority of cells remain viable, suggesting that they either escape injury entirely or are only sublethally injured and undergo recovery. A subset of tubule cells display patchy cell death resulting from at least two pathophysiological mechanisms: *Necrosis* is an explosive, chaotic process characterized by loss of membrane integrity, cytoplasmic swelling, and cellular fragmentation. *Apoptosis* is a quiet, orderly demise typified by cytoplasmic and nuclear shrinkage, DNA fragmentation, and breakdown of the cell into membrane-bound apoptotic bodies that are rapidly cleared by phagocytosis. These two forms of cell death can coexist and are considered to present the two ends of a spectrum. In AKI, the mode of cell death depends primarily on the severity of the insult and the resistance of the cell type. Necrosis occurs after more severe injury and in the more susceptible nephron segments, whereas apoptosis predominates after less severe injury and especially in the ischemia-resistant distal nephron segments. Apoptosis can be followed by "secondary necrosis," especially if the apoptotic cells are not rapidly removed.

Apoptosis is the major mechanism of early tubule cell death in contemporary clinical ARF, and considerable attention has been directed toward dissecting out the molecular mechanisms involved.[5,17] Several pathways, including the intrinsic (Bcl-2 family, cytochrome *c*, caspase

9), extrinsic (Fas, FADD, caspase 8), and regulatory (p53, NF-κB) factors, appear to be activated by ischemic AKI. The role of the Fas-FADD pathway in animal models was suggested by demonstration of upregulation of these proteins in apoptotic tubule cells after ischemia,[18] and the functional protection afforded by small interfering RNA duplexes targeting the Fas gene. Convincing human data are lacking, however, because the induction of the Fas gene shown in one study of human cadaveric kidney transplants was not reproduced in two subsequent publications.[5,17] On the other hand, growing evidence implicates an imbalance between the pro-apoptotic (Bax, Bid) and anti-apoptotic (Bcl-2, Bcl-xL) members of the Bcl-2 family in both animals and humans so affected.[5,17] The proapoptotic transcription factor p53, among the regulatory factors, is induced at the mRNA and protein levels, and inhibition of p53 by pifithrin-α suppresses ischemia-induced apoptosis by inhibiting transcriptional activation of Bax and mitochondrial translocation of p53.[19] Pifithrin-α is an unlikely candidate for therapeutic consideration in humans, however, because generalized inhibition of p53-dependent apoptosis is likely to promote survival of damaged or mutation-bearing cells in other organ systems.

Inhibition of apoptosis holds significant promise for clinical application in human AKI.[20] Caspase activation is by and large the final common "execution" step in apoptosis, and cell-permeant caspase inhibitors have provided particularly attractive targets for study. Currently available inhibitors have largely been investigated only in animals, provide only partial protection, and are most effective when administered before the insult. Erythropoietin, $α_1$-acid glycoprotein, minocycline, tumor necrosis factor-α (TNF-α) antagonists, A_1 adenosine receptor agonists, peroxisome proliferator–activated receptor-β ligands, geranylgeranylacetone, and poly(ADP-ribose) polymerase inhibitors all have provided encouraging functional protection from AKI, with inhibition of apoptosis and inflammation.[4] Some of these agents are already widely available and have been safely used in other human conditions, and results with their use in AKI should be forthcoming. Challenges for the future clinical use of apoptosis inhibition in AKI include determining the best timing of therapy, optimizing the specificity of inhibitor, minimizing the extrarenal side effects, and tubule-specific targeting of the apoptosis-modulatory maneuvers.

The mechanisms whereby a majority of tubule cells escape cell death and either emerge unscathed or recover completely after AKI remain under active investigation. Heat shock proteins (HSPs) have surfaced as prime mediators of this cytoprotection. Induction of HSPs is part of a highly conserved innate cellular response that is swiftly and robustly activated subsequent to ischemic AKI. The heat shock response is particularly robust in immature kidneys and may form the basis for the common observation that subsequent ARF is less likely to develop in premature infants than in adults. HSPs promote cell survival by inhibiting apoptosis, and liposomal delivery of HSP72 into cultured renal tubule cells blocks ischemia-induced apoptosis. HSPs also facilitate the restoration of normal cellular function by acting as molecular chaperones that assist in the refolding of denatured proteins, as well as proper folding of nascent polypeptides. In cultured tubule cells, inhibition of the heat shock response by gene silencing techniques has been shown to produce profound impairment of cellular integrity and Na^+,K^+-ATPase polarity, and overexpression of HSP70 was noted to mitigate the loss of Na^+,K^+-ATPase polarity after ATP depletion.[21] Collectively, these findings suggest that maneuvers that enhance the innate HSP response have potential benefit in human AKI.

Surviving renal tubule cells possess a remarkable ability to regenerate and proliferate after AKI. Morphologically, repair is heralded by the appearance of de-differentiated epithelial cells that express vimentin, a marker for multipotent mesenchymal cells. These cells most likely represent surviving tubule cells that have de-differentiated. In the next phase, the cells upregulate genes encoding a variety of growth factors, such as insulin-like growth factor-1 (IGF-1), hepatocyte growth factor (HGF), and fibroblast growth factor (FGF), and undergo marked proliferation. In the final phase, cells express differentiation factors such as NCAM and osteopontin and undergo redifferentiation until the normal fully polarized epithelium is restored. Thus, during recovery, renal tubule cells recapitulate phases and processes very similar to those during normal kidney development.[22] Understanding the molecular mechanisms of repair may provide clues toward accelerating recovery from ARF. For example, HGF is renoprotective and renotrophic in animal models of AKI, as a consequence of its proliferative, antiapoptotic, and anti-inflammatory actions. The use of HGF in humans, however, has been hampered at least in part by the widespread expression of its receptor, raising the possibility of serious extrarenal side effects.[23] In the case of IGF-1, enthusiasm for its renoprotective effects has been dampened by its exacerbation of inflammation and neutrophilic infiltration in the kidney after ischemia in animals. Human trials with recombinant IGF-1 have not demonstrated a beneficial effect.

Identification of the source of multipotent mesenchymal cells involved in the regeneration and repair processes has been a matter of intense contemporary research. Evidence for an extrarenal progenitor—namely, bone marrow–derived mesenchymal stem cells (MSCs)—comes from detection of tagged MSCs in the recipient kidney after cross-gender transplantation or systemic infusion. Administered MSCs clearly enhance recovery from ischemic AKI in animals, but the mode of protection may be related not to transdifferentiation processes but rather to powerful anti-inflammatory and anti-apoptotic mechanisms that are being uncovered.[24] Because bone marrow–derived MSCs are easily accessible, this therapeutic approach holds promise in human AKI. The overall balance of evidence, however, is now in favor of the notion that restoration of the tubule epithelium after AKI occurs predominantly by means of proliferation of endogenous renal cells.[25]

ALTERATIONS IN THE MICROVASCULATURE

In recent years, the role of endothelial alterations in the initiation and extension of AKI has received increasing attention.[6] Morphologically, disruption of the actin cytoskeleton and junctional complexes, similar to those previously described in tubule epithelial cells, have now been documented in endothelial cells in experimental AKI. Consequent endothelial cell swelling, blebbing, and death, with detachment of viable cells, have been observed, and circulating endothelial cells have been demonstrated in humans with septic shock. Sites of endothelial denudation are prone to prolonged vasoconstriction, and in one study, systemic or intrarenal administration of fully differentiated endothelial cells into postischemic rat kidneys resulted in functional protection.[4] Furthermore, ischemic injury leads to a marked upregulation of angiostatin, a well-known antiangiogenic factor that induces apoptosis of endothelial cells. Collectively, these findings provide a rationale for the use of proangiogenic agents that can increase the pool or mobilization of endothelial progenitor cells, such as erythropoietin, bone morphogenic protein, vascular endothelial growth factor (VEGF), and statins.

AKI also leads to increased endothelial expression of a variety of adhesion molecules that promote endothelium-leukocyte interactions. These include intercellular adhesion molecule-1 (ICAM-1), P-selectin, and E-selectin. Although ablation of the ICAM-1 gene and pretreatment with ICAM-1 antibody was shown to render mice resistant to ischemic AKI, human trials with anti-ICAM-1 monoclonal antibody administered after ischemic insult did not prevent AKI in cadaveric transplant recipients. Similarly, gene knockouts, monoclonal antibodies, and pharmacological inhibitor studies have suggested a role for E- and P-selectins.[4] However, subsequent studies have shown that it is platelet P-selectin, and not endothelial P-selectin, that is the key component leading to AKI. Possible mechanisms include (1) adhesion of platelets to the endothelium, with subsequent leukocyte adhesion, and (2) adhesion of platelets to neutrophils, with consequent aggregate formation and trapping in narrow peritubular capillaries.[4] These abnormalities, combined with other derangements in the coagulation cascade such as alterations in tissue-type plasminogen activator and plasminogen activator inhibitor-1 in the kidney, may account for the fibrin deposits characteristically found in the renal microvasculature after ischemic injury.

ALTERATIONS IN THE INFLAMMATORY RESPONSE

A growing body of evidence indicates that the inflammatory response plays a major role in ischemic AKI. Inflammatory cascades initiated by endothelial dysfunction can be augmented by the generation of a number of potent mediators by the ischemic proximal tubule, which is thought to represent a "maladaptive response."[26] These include pro-inflammatory cytokines (such as TNF-α, interleukin [IL]-6, IL-1β, and transforming growth factor-β [TGF-β], and chemotactic cytokines (such as monocyte chemoattractant protein-1 [MCP-1], IL-8, and RANTES). Elegant human studies have recently demonstrated that the levels of the pro-inflammatory cytokines IL-6 and IL-8 in the plasma predict mortality in patients with AKI, and the levels of CXCR3-binding chemokines in the urine predict AKI after kidney transplantation, attesting to the clinical significance of these mechanisms.[4] Toll-like receptor 2 (TLR2) may represent a major component of this pro-inflammatory response.[27] Renal tubular expression of TLR2 is enhanced after ischemic AKI, and *TLR2* gene silencing by knockout and antisense treatment prevents ischemia-induced renal dysfunction, neutrophil influx, tubule apoptosis, and induction of MCP-1, TNF-α, IL-6, and IL-1β.

Morphologically, several leukocyte subtypes have been shown to aggregate in peritubular capillaries and interstitial space and even within tubules after ischemic AKI, and their relative roles remain under investigation. Neutrophils are the earliest to accumulate in the postischemic kidney. Neutrophil depletion or blockade of neutrophil function provides partial functional protection in some but not all animal models. Furthermore, neutrophils are not a prominent feature of ischemic AKI in humans, casting doubt on the clinical significance of neutrophil infiltration.

Macrophages are the next to accumulate in animal models, in response to upregulation of MCP-1 in tubule cells and induction of its cognate receptor CCR2 on macrophages. Selective macrophage depletion ameliorates ischemic AKI, but the induction of tissue injury by macrophages appears to additionally require the coordinated action of T cells and neutrophils. T cells have been identified in animal as well as human models of ischemic AKI, and T cell depletion is protective in experimental AKI.[28] Double–CD4$^+$/CD8$^+$ knockout mice are protected from ischemic AKI, and adoptive transfer of wild-type T cells into the null mice abrogates this protective effect. Inconsistencies exist, however, and recent data suggest that the role of T cells in ischemic AKI may be complex, with the identification of both protective (T$_H$2 phenotype) and deleterious (T$_H$1 phenotype) subtypes of T cells. Moreover, animals deficient in both T and B cells are not protected from ischemic AKI, and depletion of peripheral CD4$^+$ T cells fails to bestow protection from ischemic AKI.

The potential role of B cells in ischemic AKI is intriguing. Compared with wild-type animals, B cell–deficient mice are partially protected from structural and functional ischemic renal injury, despite comparable neutrophil and T cell infiltrations. Wild-type serum transfer, but not B cell transfer, into B cell–deficient mice was shown to restore susceptibility to ischemic AKI, implicating a soluble serum factor as a mechanism by which B cell deficiency confers renal protection.[4]

Activation of the complement system in AKI, with resultant amplification of the inflammatory response in the kidney, has received widespread attention in recent years. Whereas ischemia-reperfusion injury in most organs activates the complement cascade along classic pathways, studies in animals and humans have implicated the alternative pathway in AKI.[4] This evidence remains debatable, however, because other reports have identified a role for the mannose-binding lectin pathway after animal and human ischemic AKI. Also controversial is the identification of the final active complement component. Although earlier studies pointed to the C5b-directed formation of a membrane attack complex, recent observations have identified a predominant role for C5a in ischemic AKI.[29] C5a is a powerful chemoattractant that recruits inflammatory cells such as neutrophils, monocytes, and T cells. The kidney is one of the few organs in which the C5a receptor normally is expressed, in proximal tubule epithelial cells as well as in interstitial macrophages. C5a receptor expression in tubule epithelial cells is markedly upregulated after ischemia-reperfusion injury and sepsis. Inhibition of C5a generation using monoclonal antibodies was found to protect against renal dysfunction induced by ischemia, and in turn to inhibit neutrophil and macrophage influx in experimental models. Of importance, pretreatment with orally active small molecule C5a receptor antagonists substantially reduced the histological and functional impairment induced by ischemic AKI in animal models.[30] Small-molecule antagonists for C5a receptor currently are undergoing a phase II clinical trial in rheumatoid arthritis and represent promising agents for the treatment or prevention of ischemic AKI.

Other strategies that modulate the inflammatory response also may provide significant beneficial effects in human AKI, and several have already been tried in experimental situations. For example, IL-10 is a potent anti-inflammatory cytokine that has been shown to provide functional protection against ischemic AKI by inhibiting maladaptive cytokine production by Th1 cells. Administration of a monoclonal antibody against the pro-inflammatory cytokine IL-6 ameliorated structural and functional consequences of ischemic AKI, decreased neutrophil infiltration, and reduced pro-inflammatory cytokine production. Bimosiamose, a novel pan-selectin inhibitor, was shown to provide protection from ischemic AKI in a kidney transplant model by reducing infiltration of macrophages and T cells and inhibiting intragraft expression of chemokines and cytokines. In addition to cholesterol lowering in humans, widely used statins possess several properties that may be beneficial in ischemic AKI, including profound anti-inflammatory effects, inhibition of reactive oxygen species, and stimulation of endothelial nitric oxide production. In fact, several investigators have reported impressive structural and functional protection from ischemic AKI by short-term pretreatment with statins.[31] Similarly, erythropoietin, extensively used in people for stimulating erythropoiesis, also has prominent antiapoptotic and anti-inflammatory actions and has been used successfully for functional amelioration of ischemic AKI in animals.[32] Finally, α-melanocyte-stimulating hormone (α-MSH), an anti-inflammatory cytokine, protects against ischemic AKI by inhibiting the maladaptive activation of genes that cause inflammatory and cytotoxic renal injury. Of interest, α-MSH potentiates the beneficial effect of erythropoietin, remains effective even when administered after the renal ischemia, and also protects against the distant lung injury that occurs after ischemic AKI.[33] The overall safety records with some of these interventions render them promising candidates for the prevention and treatment of ischemic AKI.

ALTERATIONS IN GENE EXPRESSION

Attempts at unraveling the molecular basis of the myriad pathways activated by AKI have been facilitated by recent advances in functional genomics and complementary DNA (cDNA) microarray-based technologies.[22] Several investigators have used these techniques in human and animal models of AKI to obtain expression profiles of thousands of genes. When combined with bioinformatics tools, these studies have identified novel genes with altered expression, new signal transduction pathways that are activated, and even new drug targets and biomarkers in AKI. One of the first induced molecules to be identified in the postischemic kidney using genomic approaches was kidney injury molecule 1 (KIM-1). KIM-1 protein was subsequently demonstrated to be upregulated in postischemic animal and human kidney tubules, predominantly on the apical membranes of proximal tubule epithelial cells, where it may play a role in renal regeneration. An ectodomain is shed into the urine, making KIM-1 a promising noninvasive urinary biomarker of ischemic human AKI.[34]

Another recent example is NGAL, one of the most highly induced genes in the early postischemic kidney.[35] NGAL protein is markedly upregulated in kidney tubules very early after ischemic AKI in animals and humans and is rapidly excreted in the urine, where it represents a novel, sensitive, early biomarker of ischemic AKI.[36] In the postischemic kidney tubule, NGAL protein is highly expressed in tubule cells that are undergoing proliferation, suggesting a protective or regenerative role subsequent to AKI. Exogenous administration of NGAL in experimental models before, during, or even shortly after ischemic or nephrotoxic injury provides remarkable protection at the functional and structural levels, with induction of proliferation and striking inhibition of apoptosis of tubule epithelial cells.[13] In this context, NGAL mitigates iron-mediated toxicity by providing a reservoir for excess iron and may provide a regulated source of intracellular iron to promote regeneration and repair. Exogenously administered NGAL also markedly upregulates heme oxygenase-1 (HO-1), a proven multifunctional protective agent in experimental AKI that works by limiting iron uptake, promoting intracellular iron release, enhancing production of antioxidants such as biliverdin and carbon monoxide, and inducing the cell cycle–regulatory protein p21. Because of its multifaceted protective action, NGAL has emerged as a potential therapeutic target in AKI.

Another maximally induced gene identified very early after ischemic injury is Zf9, a Kruppel-like transcription factor involved in the regulation of a number of downstream targets. Zf9 protein is markedly upregulated in the postischemic tubule cells, along with its major transactivating factor, TGF-β1. Gene silencing of Zf9 was shown to abrogate TGF-β1 overexpression and mitigate the apoptotic response to ATP depletion in vitro.[37] Relevant studies have thus identified a hitherto unrecognized pathway that may play a critical role in the early tubule cell death that accompanies ischemic renal injury.

NEPHROTOXIC ACUTE KIDNEY INJURY

Drugs contribute to approximately 15% of all cases of ARF in the adult critical care setting, but children in general are less prone to experience nephrotoxicity.[38] The nephrotoxic potential of pharmacological agents is significantly increased in patients in the ICU setting, in whom renal blood flow may already be compromised by sepsis, cardiac dysfunction, AKI, or dehydration. Thus, nonsteroidal anti-inflammatory drugs commonly induce a hemodynamically mediated ARF by inhibiting cyclooxygenase (COX), the enzyme required for the synthesis of intrarenal vasodilatory prostaglandins. Vasopressors commonly used to support blood pressure and organ perfusion also can lead to a hemodynamically mediated ARF as a result of their direct renal vasoconstricting actions. On the other hand, antibiotics such as aminoglycosides and antineoplastic agents such as cisplatin are primarily proximal tubular toxins. Radiocontrast agents represent one of the most common causes of nephrotoxic AKI. Radiocontrast agent–induced nephrotoxicity is thought to result from at least four pathophysiological mechanisms: (1) direct toxic effects on tubule epithelial cells, (2) intrarenal vasoconstriction, (3) increased viscosity of the intrarenal blood flow, and (4) microshowers of atheroemboli.

ACUTE KIDNEY INJURY IN SEPSIS

Sepsis is one of the most common causes of AKI in the critical care setting. ARF occurs in more than 50% of patients with septic shock, in whom the mortality rate exceeds 70%. Sepsis-related ARF is primarily hemodynamically mediated, resulting from a potent combination of systemic vasodilation and renal vasoconstriction.[39] The generalized arterial vasodilatation characteristic of sepsis is mediated at least in part by cytokines that enhance the expression of inducible nitric oxide synthase (iNOS) in the vasculature. The arterial underfilling leads to activation of the renin-angiotensin-aldosterone axis and to the nonosmotic release of vasopressin, all of which result in compromised renal perfusion. In addition, direct renal vasoconstriction results from cytokines such as TNF-α, which induces endothelin release. Of note, however, a trial of a monoclonal antibody against TNF-α in sepsis did not improve patient survival, suggesting that other pathways contribute to sepsis-induced ARF. These include glomerular and vascular microthrombosis due to disseminated intravascular coagulation, generation of reactive oxygen species, activation of complement pathways, and hyperglycemia-induced alterations in the inflammatory response. Recent clinical trials of activated protein C to combat the procoagulant state, insulin for improved glycemic control, and antagonists of the C5a receptor have provided encouraging results in terms of improved survival in sepsis.[39]

CLINICOPATHOLOGICAL CORRELATIONS

The clinical course of AKI has classically been divided into three phases: initiation, maintenance, and recovery. To this paradigm, the addition of an "extension" phase following the initiation phase has been proposed, primarily to reflect previously underestimated amplification processes.[4,6] Recent advances in the pathogenesis of AKI allow postulation of temporal relationships between the clinical phases and the cellular alterations detailed in this chpater.

The *initiation* phase is the period during which initial exposure to the ischemic insult occurs, kidney function begins to fail, and parenchymal injury is evolving but not fully entrenched. Intracellular ATP depletion is profound, sublethal injury to the tubule epithelial and endothelial cells predominates, generation of reactive oxygen molecules is initiated, and activation of inflammatory mechanisms commences. Intrarenal protective mechanisms such as induction of heat shock proteins in tubule cells also are brought to play during the initiation phase. If the injury is alleviated at this stage, complete restitution and recovery are the rule.

Prolongation of ischemia followed by reperfusion ushers in the *extension* phase. Blood flow returns to the cortex, and tubules undergo reperfusion-dependent cell death but also commence the regeneration process. By contrast, medullary blood flow remains severely reduced, resulting in more widespread tubule cell death, desquamation, and luminal obstruction. Injured endothelial and epithelial cells amplify the raging inflammatory cascades, and the endothelial denudation potentiates the intense vasoconstriction. The glomerular filtration rate continues to decline. This phase probably represents the optimal window of opportunity for early diagnosis and active therapeutic intervention.

During the *maintenance* phase, parenchymal injury is established, and the glomerular filtration rate is maintained at its nadir even though renal blood flow begins to normalize. Both cell injury and regeneration occur simultaneously, and the duration and severity of this phase may be determined by the balance between cell survival and death. Repair of both epithelial and endothelial cells appears to be critical to overall recovery. Measures to accelerate the endogenous regeneration processes may be effective during this phase.

The *recovery* phase is characterized functionally by improvement in glomerular filtration rate and structurally by reestablishment of tubule integrity, with fully differentiated and polarized epithelial cells. The repair process may be incomplete, however, and both microvascular and tubular dropout have been demonstrated in animal studies.

Key Points

1. Acute kidney injury is a potentially lethal condition in the intensive care unit setting with multiple pathophysiological mechanisms that interplay with and amplify one another.
2. Acute kidney injury in the intensive care unit setting frequently is multifactorial, with concomitant septic, ischemic, and nephrotoxic components, and with overlapping mechanisms.
3. Recent advances have brought new insights into the roles of apoptosis, oxidant- and iron-mediated injury, endothelial changes, and the inflammatory response in the pathogenesis of acute kidney injury.
4. Conquering acute kidney injury will require a comprehensive approach, including making an early diagnosis and executing a multifaceted therapeutic approach based on a better understanding of the pathophysiology.
5. Novel strategies that have emerged from recent findings hold tremendous promise for the proactive treatment of human acute kidney injury.

Key References

1. Lameire N, Van Biesen W, Vanholder R: Acute renal failure. Lancet 2005;365:417-430.
2. Uchino S, Kellum JA, Bellomo R, et al for the Beginning and Ending Supportive Therapy for the Kidney (BEST Kidney) Investigators: Acute renal failure in critically ill patients: A multinational, multicenter study. JAMA 2005;294:813-818.
4. Devarajan P: Update on mechanisms of ischemic acute kidney injury. J Am Soc Nephrol 2006;17:1503-1520.
6. Molitoris BA, Sutton TA: Endothelial injury and dysfunction: Role in the extension phase of acute renal failure. Kidney Int 2004;66:496-499.

See the companion Expert Consult website for the complete reference list.

CHAPTER 289

Epidemiology of Pediatric Acute Kidney Injury

Stuart L. Goldstein

> ## OBJECTIVES
>
> This chapter will:
> 1. Review the major causes of acute kidney injury in critically ill pediatric patients.
> 2. Describe pediatric acute kidney injury seen in different subpopulations, including infants in the postoperative period after corrective congenital heart surgery, stem cell transplant recipients, and patients with multiple organ dysfunction syndrome.
> 3. Preview new diagnostic measures for pediatric acute kidney injury, including classification systems and biomarkers.

Interpretation and extrapolation of findings reported in the epidemiology literature on pediatric acute kidney injury (AKI) have been hampered by numerous factors, including lack of a consistent definition of AKI, increased survival of critically ill children with multiorgan dysfunction and AKI due to advances in care, the wide range of patient size distribution in pediatrics, and limited access to renal replacement therapies and tertiary care in developing countries. Although multicenter epidemiological pediatric AKI data are lacking, single-center studies from the 1980s and early 1990s report hemolytic uremic syndrome,[1,2] other primary renal causes, sepsis, and burns as the most prevalent causes of pediatric AKI. Many pediatric AKI studies from the 1990s and early 2000s, with the exception of those in infants who received peritoneal dialysis after corrective congenital heart surgery, are composed solely of literature reviews.[3,4] In fact, little published literature exists currently to describe the baseline incidence of pediatric AKI in most populations. Recent epidemiology of pediatric AKI has been studied mainly in acutely ill hospitalized patients, because nonoliguric forms of AKI may be self-limited and go undetected in the outpatient setting. In developing countries with limited or no access to intensive care resources, published reports detail experiences with trauma-associated AKI induced by rhabdomyolysis[5] or with AKI secondary to epidemic disease such as hemolytic uremic syndrome or poisonings.[6]

This chapter is concerned with AKI in the critically ill child, with data derived for the most part from studies in patients who received renal replacement therapy. Also presented are emerging AKI definition concepts and biomarkers expected to change pediatric AKI epidemiological assessment in the near future. Because AKI of a severity necessitating renal replacement therapy provision often is viewed as an outcome measure, changes in the incidence

of need for and in the modalities of renal replacement therapy used in pediatric patients with AKI are discussed in a subsequent chapter (Chapter 336).

PEDIATRIC ACUTE KIDNEY INJURY EPIDEMIOLOGY: CURRENT STATE OF KNOWLEDGE

Recent single-center data detail the underlying causes of pediatric AKI in large cohorts of children and demonstrate an epidemiological shift wherein AKI more often is now a concomitant of another underlying disease or systemic process, or its treatment, instead of a primary renal disease. This shift was concurrent with technological improvements in pediatric, neonatal, and cardiovascular intensive care. Accordingly, critically ill children who require renal replacement therapy have been the most-studied pediatric AKI cohort in the past decade.[7] Bunchman reported data for 226 children with AKI treated with renal replacement therapy, the most common causes of AKI being congenital heart disease, acute tubular necrosis (ATN), and sepsis.[8] Hui-Stickle and colleagues performed a retrospective review of 248 patients aged birth to 21 years with a diagnosis of AKI on discharge or death summary.[9] AKI was then verified by an estimated creatinine clearance of 75 mL/minute/1.73 m², determined using the Schwartz formula.[10] This study found ATN and nephrotoxic medicines to be the most common cause of acute renal failure (ARF) for all age groups and patient sizes, whereas primary kidney disease was cited in only 7% of the cases. Table 289-1 combines data from these two large studies to describe the underlying causes of pediatric AKI that necessitate subsequent renal replacement therapy.

Many single-center studies report data on the experience with pediatric AKI for 10 years or longer and compare different periods at the same institution or geographical region. Of interest, all studies demonstrate a slight male predominance in pediatric AKI. Vachvanichsanong and colleagues assessed pediatric AKI epidemiology in 311 children (318 episodes) from 1983 through 2004 at a Thailand tertiary referral center.[11] These investigators reported an incidence of AKI of 0.5 to 0.9 case per 1000 pediatric patients younger than 18 years of age who were admitted to their institution. This report also divided AKI epidemiology into three different eras: 1983 to 1995, 1995 to 2000, and 2000 to 2004. In each era, sepsis was the most common underlying cause of AKI, whereas hypovolemic ATN decreased from 16.1% of cases in the early era to 8.3% in the latter era. Of interest, this study reports a high incidence of other infections, including leptospirosis and

TABLE 289-1

Causes of Pediatric Acute Renal Failure Leading to Renal Replacement Therapy*

DIAGNOSIS	N	%
Bone marrow transplantation/malignancy	48	15.7
Heart transplantation	16	5.3
Acute tubular necrosis	56	18.4
Sepsis	39	12.8
Congenital heart disease	61	20.0
Hemolytic uremic syndrome/ glomerulonephritis	19	6.2
Liver transplantation	22	7.2
Nephrotoxins	40	13.1

*Aggregate data combined (N = 304) from two separate studies: Bunchman TE, McBryde KD, Mottes TE, et al: Pediatric acute renal failure: Outcome by modality and disease. Pediatr Nephrol 2001;16: 1067-1071; and Hui-Stickle S, Brewer ED, Goldstein SL: Pediatric ARF epidemiology at a tertiary care center from 1999 to 2001. Am J Kidney Dis 2005;45:96-101.

TABLE 289-2

Pediatric Modified RIFLE Criteria

RIFLE SCALE COMPONENT	eCCL*	URINE OUTPUT
Risk	Decrease by 25%	<0.5 mL/kg/hour for 8 hours
Injury	Decrease by 50%	<0.5 mL/kg/hour for 16 hours
Failure	Decrease by 75%, or <35 mL/min/1.73 m^2	<0.3 mL/kg/hour for 24 hours or anuric for 12 hours
Loss	Persistent failure >4 weeks	
End-stage disease	End-stage renal disease (persistent failure >3 months)	

*Estimated by the Schwartz formula (as discussed by Schwartz and coworkers[10]).
eCCl, estimated creatinine clearance.
Data from Arikan AA, Washburn K, Loftis L, et al: Evaluation of the RIFLE criteria in critically ill children with acute kidney injury [abstract]. J Am Soc Nephrol 2005;16:534A.

dengue hemorrhagic shock syndrome. Poststreptococcal glomerulonephritis and systemic lupus erythematosus accounted for a majority of primary renal AKI causes, with combined incidence increasing from 19.3% of cases in the early era to 24.8% of cases in the latter era.

Williams and colleagues evaluated 228 consecutive pediatric AKI cases in critically ill children from Richmond, Virginia, between 1979 and 1998.[12] These investigators divided their epidemiological assessment into the earlier and latter decades studied and compared underlying causes leading to AKI in survivors and in nonsurvivors. In the earlier era, hemolytic uremic syndrome, sepsis, and burns were cited as the most common causes leading to AKI, whereas hematological-oncological and pulmonary causes replaced burns as a common cause of AKI in the second era. Higher mortality rates were observed in the latter era in patients after cardiac surgery or with pulmonary or hematological-oncological comorbid conditions.

The Prospective Pediatric Continuous Renal Replacement Therapy (ppCRRT) Registry Group[13] reported epidemiology and outcome for 116 patients with multiple organ dysfunction syndrome (MODS) who received continuous renal replacement therapy (CRRT) at seven U.S. pediatric centers.[14] Sepsis (49.2%) and cardiogenic shock (20%) were the most common causes of AKI. The most common comorbid conditions were stem cell transplantation (15.5%) and solid nonrenal organ transplantation (6.9%).

ACUTE KIDNEY INJURY EPIDEMIOLOGY: FUTURE DIRECTIONS

Toward a Useful Definition of Pediatric Acute Kidney Injury

Lack of a uniform and multidimensional classification system of ARF has been a very real barrier to generalization of single-study findings. Furthermore, because most definitions of AKI are based on a relatively large, readily measurable rise in serum creatinine, significant renal injury may escape recognition, with resultant delay in

treatment. Chertow and colleagues recently demonstrated that "small" increases in serum creatinine of 0.3 mg/dL could be associated with increased patient mortality, even when outcome is controlled for significant patient comorbidity.[15] Preliminary data showed a rise in serum creatinine of 0.3 mg/dL or greater in 60 pediatric patients with acute decompensated heart failure; such patients demonstrated a seven-fold increased mortality risk.[16] Collaborative multicenter efforts to study the potential association between a small serum creatinine rise and patient outcome should be a priority for the pediatric nephrology community.

These data argue for a graded AKI classification system that can identify patients at risk for the development of significant renal insult and metabolic disturbance. The Acute Dialysis Quality Initiative (ADQI) (www.adqi.net) recently proposed a multidimensional system termed the RIFLE criteria (risk, injury, failure, loss of function, and end-stage disease) that classify the degree of renal insult by changes in serum creatinine or duration of oliguria, or both.[17]

RIFLE is an empirical classification system that has only recently undergone clinical validation. Two preliminary pediatric prospective studies have assessed application of the RIFLE criteria. Arikan and colleagues evaluated RIFLE criteria modified for children (pRIFLE) (Table 289-2) in critically ill pediatric patients receiving mechanical ventilation to describe the pattern of pediatric AKI and to determine if pRIFLE provides sufficient sensitivity and specificity in this clinical setting.[18] In a majority of patients in whom AKI was diagnosed by pRIFLE criteria, AKI developed within the first 7 days of ICU admission. Patients in whom AKI was diagnosed by pRIFLE criteria within the first 14 days had increased Pediatric Risk of Mortality (PRISM II)[19] scores on ICU admission. Failure to reach RIFLE-defined levels in the first 7 days after ICU admission resulted in a 98% negative predictive value of developing AKI after 7 days. The pRIFLE criteria also were helpful in classifying patients who had reversible AKI (prerenal) versus persistent AKI (i.e., ATN), because one third recovered renal function as measured by pRIFLE criteria within 48 hours.

Phan and colleagues applied the RIFLE criteria to 1047 patients admitted to pediatric ICUs, irrespective of severity of illness.[20] AKI was diagnosed by RIFLE criteria in 3.14% of admissions, and the most common causes of AKI were hemolytic uremic syndrome (18.2%), hematological-oncological diseases (18.2%), cardiac surgery (11.4%), and sepsis (9.1%).

Urinary Biomarkers of Acute Kidney Injury: The Search for "Renal Troponin I"

As noted in the previous section, small increases in serum creatinine may reflect significant renal insult and be associated with significant morbidity in patients with AKI. Intensive investigation has led to the identification of several potential urinary biomarkers that may herald AKI before a rise in serum creatinine occurs. Pediatric patients constitute an important population for study, because they usually do not have significant comorbid illnesses, such as hypertension, atherosclerosis, and diabetes, that affect kidneys in adults.

Infants with congenital heart disease undergoing corrective surgery provide an important population for study of putative urinary AKI biomarkers, because the duration of renal ischemia (i.e., cardiopulmonary bypass) is known, and these children can be studied prospectively for development of AKI. Mishra and colleagues[21] assessed the incidence of AKI in this population and assayed urine for appearance of neutrophil gelatinase-associated lipocalin (NGAL), to determine if increased urinary NGAL concentration after cardiopulmonary bypass preceded and predicted increases in serum creatinine. In a total of 71 patients, AKI (defined as a doubling of serum creatinine) was found to develop in 20 of the infants. Urinary NGAL increased at least 50-fold, and the NGAL increase preceded serum creatinine rise by at least 24 hours in all patients in whom AKI developed.

Parikh and colleagues compared urinary interleukin (IL)-18 concentrations between healthy control subjects and adult patients with ATN. Median urinary IL-18 concentrations were significantly greater in patients with ATN than in healthy control subjects—644 pg/mg creatinine (mean, 814 ± 151 pg/mg creatinine) versus 16 pg/mg creatinine (mean, 23 ± 9 pg/mg creatinine) ($P < .0001$).[22] IL-18 may not be present early in the AKI course. Both kidney injury molecule-1 (KIM-1) and IL-18 need to be studied in children, with larger patient numbers and across all disease classes.

Preliminary studies of NGAL and IL-18 have been performed in critically ill children to evaluate for potential associations between these biomarkers and ultimate AKI development and severity by day 14 of ICU stay. Pilot data are available for 103 children admitted to the pediatric ICU who received mechanical ventilation and vasoactive medications and in whom urine was obtained for NGAL assessment.[23] Urinary samples for this purpose were obtained in 61 patients before AKI development as assessed by pRIFLE. Urinary NGAL was significantly higher in patients in pRIFLE category I or F than in RIFLE category R or control patients, and significantly more patients in RIFLE category I or F had urinary NGAL levels greater than 1 ng/mg creatinine. Pilot data from a cohort of 22 patients in the same study population (consisting of 7 control patients and 5 each of patients in RIFLE categories R, I, and F) showed that patients in RIFLE category F had higher peak urinary IL-18 levels compared with control patients.[24] Thus,

urinary biomarkers may be helpful in predicting both the development and severity of pediatric AKI. Other biomarkers currently under study in children include serum cystatin C[25] and urinary KIM-1.[26]

CONCLUSION

Over the past decade, pediatric AKI epidemiology in the critically ill has undergone a transition in most centers from primary renal diseases to kidney disease resulting from other systemic illnesses and their treatment. The epidemiological shift has occurred as a result of advances in intensive care for all pediatric patients and in capability to provide renal replacement therapy to children of all sizes. Almost all data are derived from single-center reports, however, so further multicenter study is required to validate these recent observations. Another epidemiological shift in pediatric AKI can be expected over the next decade as pRIFLE or other multidimensional classification systems and urinary biomarkers change the ways in which pediatric nephrologists and critical care physicians define and detect pediatric AKI, respectively.

Key Points

1. The epidemiology of acute kidney injury in the critically ill child has changed from primary renal disease to kidney involvement secondary to another organ system illness or its treatment.
2. Hypoxic-ischemic injury and nephrotoxic medications are the most common causes of pediatric acute kidney injury in the current era.
3. Few data exist to classify all-cause pediatric acute kidney injury, and most data derive from studies of children who receive acute renal replacement therapy.
4. Most critically ill children with acute kidney injury who require renal replacement therapy receive continuous renal replacement therapy.
5. Multidimensional acute kidney injury classification systems and new potential biomarkers can be expected to lead to more sensitive and specific detection of pediatric acute kidney injury.

Key References

1. Moghal NE, Brocklebank JT, Meadow SR: A review of acute renal failure in children: Incidence, etiology and outcome. Clin Nephrol 1998;49:91-95.
2. Wong W, McCall E, Anderson B, et al: Acute renal failure in the paediatric intensive care unit. N Z Med J 1996;109:459-461.
8. Bunchman TE, McBryde KD, Mottes TE, et al: Pediatric acute renal failure: Outcome by modality and disease. Pediatr Nephrol 2001;16:1067-1071.
9. Hui-Stickle S, Brewer ED, Goldstein SL: Pediatric ARF epidemiology at a tertiary care center from 1999 to 2001. Am J Kidney Dis 2005;45:96-101.
12. Williams DM, Sreedhar SS, Mickell JJ, et al: Acute kidney failure: A pediatric experience over 20 years. Arch Pediatr Adolesc Med 2002;156:893-900.

See the companion Expert Consult website for the complete reference list.

CHAPTER 290

Treatment of Acute Kidney Injury in Children: Conservative Management to Renal Replacement Therapy

Timothy E. Bunchman

OBJECTIVES

This chapter will:
1. Review the etiology of pediatric acute kidney injury, correlated with reversibility and outcome.
2. Outline the components of conservative management of pediatric acute kidney injury.
3. Present an approach to dialytic management of pediatric acute kidney injury.

Management of acute kidney injury (AKI) in a child should begin with a thorough etiological evaluation to pinpoint the underlying cause or causes and an assessment of the potential for reversibility of the renal impairment, as well as its likely duration. This information is crucial in predicting severity and outcome of AKI.

This chapter describes both nondialytic (conservative) and dialytic management of children with AKI.

ETIOLOGY

As in adults, the etiology of AKI in children can be divided into prerenal, intrarenal, and postrenal causes. The initial evaluation is straightforward, with assessment of volume status and cardiac output and careful examination for evidence of volume depletion, to detect a prerenal component of AKI. Evaluation by hemodynamic monitoring as well as determination of the fractional excretion of sodium (FeNa) may be helpful to diagnose renal dysfunction in this etiological category.[1]

The postrenal causes of AKI can readily be evaluated by renal ultrasound imaging. An ultrasound examination can easily be completed at the bedside to look for an obstructive pattern, at the level of either the bladder or the ureters. Identifying whether the patient has solitary or bilateral kidneys also is helpful.

The remaining causes of AKI are intrarenal (intrinsic) processes. With advances in technology and medical care in Western medical centers, intrinsic kidney disease often is related to drug toxicity, acute tubular necrosis (ATN), or an acute process with underlying chronic kidney disease (CKD).[2] In other areas of the world, the primary cause of intrarenal AKI continues to be hemolytic uremic syndrome.[3] The diagnosis of hemolytic uremic syndrome can easily be made by evaluation of a peripheral smear, looking for subnormal cell counts and presence of schistocytes, with worsening anemia and uremia. This clinical picture should be distinguished from that in sepsis or disseminated intravascular coagulation (DIC), which can include the same findings. In the absence of hemolytic uremic syndrome, drug-induced AKI, or ATN, renal biopsy is indicated to identify the cause and perhaps to direct therapy.

GENERAL APPROACH TO CONSERVATIVE MANAGEMENT

Removal or Correction of the Offending Cause

With intrarenal or intrinsic disease, it is important to look for all possible offending causes. Many of the newer agents that are useful for pain management (e.g., nonsteroidal anti-inflammatory drugs [NSAIDs]), in transplantation (e.g., calcineurin inhibitors), or for general medical care may be beneficial in relief or prevention of symptoms but detrimental to renal function. A review of the patient's current medications, therefore, can potentially identify an etiological factor that can be adjusted or removed in order to minimize the AKI.

Enhancement of cardiac output also is in order. Evidence to date from studies in adult patients has shown that renal-dose dopamine is not beneficial for preservation of urine output or recovery of renal function.[4] This aspect of management of AKI has never been adequately looked at in the pediatric population, however. Data from both adult critical care and animal models now support the concept of "renal-dose norepinephrine." In both human studies and septic animal models, low-dose norepinephrine has been shown to improve splanchnic blood flow, improve renal perfusion, and enhance urine output by maximizing cardiac output and vascular tone.[5,6] The result of this beneficial effect may be avoidance of the need for renal replacement therapy (RRT). Nesiritide and fenoldopam were introduced in the past decade and have been touted as drugs that have renal-protective mechanisms while enhancing urine output.[7] These agents have yet to be found to be beneficial in the pediatric population.[8]

The use of albumin versus saline to preserve intravascular volume integrity is the subject of ongoing debate.

The sentinel study by Finfer and colleagues, involving a hypovolemic comparison of 4% albumin versus saline, showed no difference in AKI or in need for RRT between the two treatment groups.[9] In the subset of patients with sepsis or burns, a preferential benefit was observed in the albumin treatment group. In a recent study, Dubois and associates noted that in patients with a low plasma albumin, replacement of albumin as compared with saline will improve splanchnic blood flow, as evidenced by the patient's ability to tolerate enteral feedings.[10] Therefore, enhancement of cardiac output by volume replacement or use of norepinephrine and enhancement of vascular tone by means of norepinephrine have now become common practice in the management of AKI in adults. None of this has been adequately studied in the pediatric population, however, so many physicians continue to rely on data derived from clinical experience in adults for decisions about the care of pediatric patients.

Attention to Solute and Fluid Status

To avoid the need for RRT in a patient with AKI, consideration of both solute and fluid status is essential. Specific attention to drug dosing and nutrition delivery based on renal clearance is in order. Antibiotics such as aminoglycosides or vancomycin can be used safely in patients with AKI with careful attention to serum drug levels. Toxicity of these drugs can be avoided by careful monitoring and adjusting the dose in accordance with the patient's changing renal function status.

Nutrition is important in patients with AKI as part of ongoing care. Either the parenteral or the enteral route can be used for delivery of nutritional formulas. The evidence to date in both adult and pediatric patients has clearly shown an advantage of enteral nutrition over parenteral nutrition. As supported by clinical experience in many programs, specialized formulas can be delivered to patients with AKI to maximize nutrition and minimize both solute and fluid excess. To this end, the use of "adult-based formulas" such as Renalcal (Nestle, Glendale, CA), Suplena (Ross, Columbus, OH), Nepro (Ross, Columbus, OH), or Magnacal (Novartis, East Hanover, NJ) can provide high-calorie nutrition, with either low or high protein and low or no electrolytes. All of these formulas deliver 2 cal/mL, with either no electrolytes (Renalcal) or low electrolytes (specifically, potassium and phosphorus) for nutritional supplementation. These formulas can be given either orally or by feeding tube to provide adequate caloric intake. Because these formulas are hyperosmolar (600 mOsm), they may induce a hyperosmolar diarrhea that may be detrimental to nutrition absorption. If the patient can tolerate these feedings, then adequate dietary supplementation can be easily provided with a minimal risk for need for RRT (Fig. 290-1).

Volume Status

Attention to the patient's volume status is essential throughout the hospital stay. Many programs focus exclusively on intake and output measurements as a way to monitor volume status. This approach, however, does not take into account insensible losses. Therefore, obtaining daily weight measurements on the same scale is paramount and, in combination with vital signs, heart rate, and blood pressure, will give the clinician a better sense of the patient's volume status.

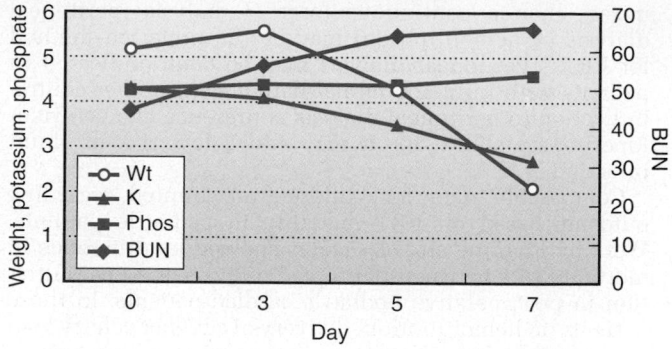

Calories/kg/day = 107; Protein/kg/day = 2.1 g

FIGURE 290-1. "Insensible loss" nutrition with an "adult-based formula" (Renalcal) in an anuric infant. BUN, blood urea nitrogen (mg/dL); K, potassium (mmol/L); Phos, phosphate (mg/dL); Wt, weight.

Diuretics

Diuretics can be used to augment urine output but will not enhance solute clearance. Comparison of loop diuretics given as an intermittent bolus or by continuous infusion shows that the use of continuous infusion involves less exposure to these potentially toxic agents with the same amount of urine output.[11,12] Thiazide-like diuretics (e.g., oral metolazone or intravenous chlorothiazide) can be given to enhance the effectiveness of loop diuretics.[13] Of note, urinary flow does not reflect effective solute clearance. Accordingly, increased urine output does not correlate with improvement of renal function or with improvement of solute clearance.

In summary, for successful nondialytic treatment of AKI in children, it is essential to pinpoint the cause of the renal impairment, to estimate its probable duration, and to identify interventions that may be necessary for reversal of the renal injury (e.g., high-dose Solu-Medrol for crescentic glomerulonephritis, which would increase catabolism), as well as methods to enhance recovery of function. Other important considerations include mechanisms to enhance cardiac output and renal blood flow (renal-dose norepinephrine) and attention to volume status by monitoring daily weights. Finally, attention to nutrition supplementation is in order to maximize nutrition and minimize solute excess and volume excess.

DIALYTIC THERAPIES

If the blood urea nitrogen (BUN) level rises above 70 mg/dL, or if volume excess is greater than 10%, or if a classic indication for RRT, such as metabolic acidosis, hyperkalemia, or pulmonary edema, is present, intervention with dialytic therapy should be considered.[14-18]

RRT in a critical care setting can be carried out using intermittent hemodialysis, continuous peritoneal dialysis, or a continuous hemofiltration protocol.[19,20] Hemodialysis can be done in either a convective or a diffusive mode, or a combination of both. The evidence to date does not suggest that one modality is superior to another in terms of outcome. In patients who are less hemodynamically compromised and are receiving primarily enteral feedings, intermittent hemodialysis may be the most appropriate form of RRT. If patients are hemodynamically compromised, then a continuous form of dialysis (peritoneal dialysis or hemofiltration) may be the preferred method for RRT.[21] Peritoneal dialysis may be contraindicated in patients with intra-abdominal pathology. Another contraindication to peritoneal dialysis is presence of a ventriculoperitoneal shunt, for it may add a low risk of shunt infection.

Comparable data for children are limited regarding outcome based on RRT modality in pediatric patients. Work by Fleming and associates showed no difference in mortality rate between peritoneal dialysis and hemofiltration in postoperative pediatric cardiac patients. In those patients on hemofiltration, delivery of a higher calorie load was possible, but this had no impact on mortality rate.[22]

In later work, Maxvold and coworkers used a retrospective database to compare hemodialysis and hemofiltration. These investigators found that mortality rate was not related to the modality of RRT but was influenced by the severity of illness as measured by pressor use.[23] A more recent study looked at a large series of children on intermittent hemodialysis, peritoneal dialysis, or hemofiltration, extending the work of Maxvold's group. Again, this report demonstrated that the modality had minimal impact on outcome, but the severity of illness predicted survival versus nonsurvival in this population.[21]

Thus, with use of RRT in patients with AKI, work as early as 1994 by Lane and colleagues demonstrated that volume excess may be a predictor of nonsurvival.[15] These investigators demonstrated that in bone marrow transplant recipients with a volume excess greater than 10%, those with a higher volume excess at the initiation of RRT had a worse survival. In hemofiltration-specific studies, Goldstein and colleagues in 2001,[16] Foland and associates in 2004,[17] Gillespie and coworkers in 2004,[24] and the Prospective Pediatric Continuous Renal Replacement Therapies (pPCRRT) study group in 2005[18] all demonstrated the same effect of higher volume excess in patients at the initiation of RRT: a negative impact on survival.

In summary, no controlled studies in pediatric patients to date have compared modality differences in outcome, or have assessed the relative benefits of convection versus diffusion in hemofiltration modalities. Ongoing research by the pPCRRT study group is in progress to begin evaluating outcome in certain patient subgroups, such as bone marrow transplant recipients, in whom use of a convective modality may be beneficial.

Finally, long-term follow-up evaluation of patients who had recovered from AKI demonstrated evidence of ongoing risk of progressive loss of kidney function over time in a small subset of patients. In a group of children who had survived acute renal failure and RRT with clinical recovery, Askenzai and colleagues found evidence of microalbuminuria, increased glomerular filtration rate such as hyperfiltration syndrome, and hypertension. Resolution of AKI after RRT is no longer needed does not mean that these patients are left with no long-term risk factors.[25]

CONCLUSION

The care of the child with AKI need not begin with RRT, but initiation of specific interventions is indicated at the earliest identification of the renal impairment. Attention to volume status, nutrition, and drug delivery, as well as avoidance of nephrotoxins, is important in this setting. Some form of RRT should be instituted in patients with a rising BUN or a BUN in excess of 70 mg/dL, a volume status greater than 10% excess, or one of the more classic indications, which include malignant hypertension, pulmonary edema, hyperkalemia, and metabolic acidosis.

Key Points

1. The etiology of acute kidney injury in children can be divided into prerenal, intrarenal, and postrenal causes.
2. For management of children with acute kidney injury, enhancement of cardiac output is essential, as is specific attention to drug dosing and nutrition delivery based on renal clearance.
3. Diuretics can be used to augment urine output in these patients but will not enhance solute clearance.
4. Intervention with dialytic therapy may be indicated for patients with blood urea nitrogen in excess of 70 mg/dL or greater than 10% of volume excess, or if metabolic acidosis, hyperkalemia, or pulmonary edema is present.

Key References

12. Luciani GB, Nichani S, Chang AC, et al: Continuous versus intermittent furosemide infusion in critically ill infants after open heart operations. Ann Thorac Surg 1997;64:1133-1139.
17. Foland JA, Fortenberry JD, Warshaw BL, et al: Fluid overload before continuous hemofiltration and survival in critically ill children: A retrospective analysis. Crit Care Med 2004;32:1771-1776.
18. Goldstein SL, Somers MJ, Baum MA, et al: Pediatric patients with multi-organ dysfunction syndrome receiving continuous renal replacement therapy. Kidney Int 2005;67:653-658.
21. Bunchman TE, McBryde KD, Mottes TE, et al: Pediatric acute renal failure: Outcome by modality and disease. Pediatr Nephrol 2001;16:1067.
25. Askenazi DJ, Feig DI, Graham HM, et al: 3-5 year longitudinal follow-up of pediatric patients after acute renal failure. Kidney Int 2006;69:184-189.

See the companion Expert Consult website for the complete reference list.

CHAPTER 291

Technical Aspects of Pediatric Continuous Renal Replacement Therapy

Carl H. Cramer II, Richard Hackbarth, and Patrick D. Brophy

OBJECTIVES

This chapter will:
1. Outline the basic principles of continuous renal replacement therapy as they apply in pediatric patients.
2. Delineate the particular aspects of pediatric continuous renal replacement therapy that differ from adult continuous renal replacement therapy in terms of prescription, thermic control, access, and anticoagulation.
3. Review the concept of the blood priming–bradykinin release phenomenon and its importance in infant continuous renal replacement therapy using polyacrylonitrile membranes.
4. Describe the methods and techniques available to avoid the bradykinin release phenomenon.

Critically ill children with acute oliguric renal failure are a challenging group of patients to manage. These patients often are poorly suited to hemodialysis and peritoneal dialysis because of the tenuous nature of their hemodynamic and pulmonary status. Hemodialysis may remove fluid too quickly for the child to tolerate, and peritoneal dialysis may interfere with ventilation or venous return and is relatively inefficient for fluid and solute removal. Continuous renal replacement therapy (CRRT), by virtue of its continuous nature and the fine control of fluid balance it permits, often is ideally suited to management of the critically ill child who requires fluid or solute removal.

The basic principles of CRRT are similar for adults and for children. Applying these modalities in children, however, requires recognition of the unique technical aspects of pediatric CRRT, including weight-based fluid calculations for solutions, anticoagulation, blood flow, extracorporeal blood volume, blood priming, temperature control, access options, filter size and properties.

Historically, arteriovenous modalities of CRRT were the standard methods used in practice.[1] Although this technique offers the advantage of simplicity, it poses considerable challenges for use in the pediatric population. The lower mean arterial blood pressure and higher hematocrit in children, as well as the higher resistance and flow limitations of smaller-diameter catheters, have limited the practical application of this technique in children. Another disadvantage of arteriovenous techniques is the requirement for both venous and arterial access and the potential risk of limb ischemia from the arterial line.[2]

The development of precision-volumetric fluid pumps with air leak detectors and pressure monitors, as well as pediatric-specific dialysis catheters, has made venovenous techniques preferable to arteriovenous methods. As a result, CRRT has become not only feasible but practicable in infants and children.

PRESCRIPTION

The CRRT prescription in the pediatric patient follows the same principles as those in an adult patient, but with dosing based on weight or body surface area. The flow rate of dialysate (Q_d) or filter replacement fluid (Q_f) can be referred to as the *dialysis dose*. The optimal dialysis dose is not known, but the trend has been toward increased dialysis dose in adults on CRRT. Ronco and colleagues demonstrated that in adult patients with acute renal failure, a Q_f of at least 35 mL/kg per hour was associated with improved patient survival.[3] A subset of these patients was reevaluated and in the setting of sepsis, a Q_f of 45 mL/kg per hour was associated with improved patient survival. The maximum dialysis dose may be limited by the total ultrafiltration rate allowed by the filter. In most children, a comparable dialysis dose rate of 2 to 4 L/1.73 m² per hour is readily achievable.

Even though continuous venovenous hemodialysis (CVVHD) is primarily a diffusion-based therapy, some degree of convection will be present because of the prescribed net fluid balance and ongoing removal of intravenous fluids from the patient. Goldstein and colleagues described a mean contribution by convective clearance of 17% to the total dose of dialysis in patients on CVVHD.[4] Net patient fluid removal usually is between 0.5 and 2.0 mL/kg per hour, depending on patient volume status and hemodynamics. This rate is a direct extrapolation from work on hemodialysis by Donckerwolcke and Bunchman, who demonstrated this to be a safe and effective ultrafiltration rate in pediatric hemodialysis.[5] In the severely edematous and hemodynamically marginal patient, increasing pressor support to optimize mean arterial blood pressure may allow for more aggressive ultrafiltration in the initial 24 to 48 hours of CRRT, resulting in improved cardiac and pulmonary function as volume overload is reduced.

BLOOD PRIMING

As in infant hemodialysis, the relationship of the patient's blood volume to the extracorporeal volume of the CRRT circuit needs to be taken into consideration. Patients weighing less than 10 kg have blood volumes of approximately 80 mL/kg, whereas larger children have blood volumes closer to 70 mL/kg. If the circuit volume is in excess of 10% of the patient's total blood volume, blood priming often becomes necessary.

Blood priming has its own set of potential problems. Banked blood has an inherently low pH and low ionized calcium concentration related to the presence of anticoagulant. In addition, high potassium content develops during prolonged storage. Another concern is that this low pH potentiates the bradykinin release when an AN-69 membrane is used. This unphysiological blood prime may potentially cause further hemodynamic instability in the child during initiation of CRRT. A couple of different approaches can be used to prevent a serious decrease in the patient's hematocrit while avoiding hemodynamic instability.

One approach involves *direct transfusion of blood* into the patient at the time of dialysis initiation. The packed red cells obtained from most blood banks possess a high hematocrit of approximately 50% to 60% and should be reconstituted to a hematocrit of 30% to 35% with 0.9% saline or 5% albumin, to minimize risk of clotting the circuit. The blood can be directly infused through the venous port of the dialysis catheter. This infusion should occur simultaneously with initiation of CRRT, the circuitry for which has been primed with 0.9% normal saline. As the patient's blood infuses into the circuit from the arterial port, the primed saline is drained into a collection bag that has been temporarily connected to the venous end of the filter system. Once blood has reached the venous collection bag, then the CRRT machine is temporarily paused. The collection bag is then removed, and the venous end of the filter system is connected to the venous port of the dialysis catheter. Sodium bicarbonate boluses can be used to help minimize cardiac instability secondary to a "membrane reaction" during the initiation of CRRT.[6]

Another approach involves the *zero balance ultrafiltration* ("Z-BUF") technique.[7] The CRRT machine is primed according to the manufacturer's recommendations. Banked blood, diluted to an approximate hematocrit of 30% to 35% with 5% albumin, is then used to prime the circuit. Before the circuit is connected to the patient, the arterial and venous ends of the circuit are connected to each other, and the circuit is hemofiltered or dialyzed on itself using a physiological solution of electrolytes such as Normocarb. Calcium chloride is added to the solution to improve the ionized calcium of the prime. The blood flow rate is set to 100 mL/minute, and the circuit is then ultrafiltered at a rate of 2 L/hour for 15 to 20 minutes while a neutral circuit volume (zero balance) is maintained. Hemofiltration or hemodialysis of the circuit seems to be equally effective at normalizing pH and electrolyte content of the prime. This technique also may help blunt the initial bradykinin-type reaction seen with initiation of CRRT. Careful monitoring of the pressures in the circuit is essential. Once the blood has circulated for the allotted time, the machine is placed in pause, and the arterial and venous lines are connected to the patient. The circuit flow is then resumed.

TEMPERATURE CONTROL

Infants and small children have large body surface area–to–weight ratios. This feature, coupled with the significant amount of blood volume that resides in the extracorporeal circuit at any given time, places these small patients at substantial risk for the development of hypothermia. Simple techniques such as use of radiant warmers may help but often are not enough to maintain body temperature. With the new dialysis machines, line warmers may be available for purchase, such as the Prismatherm II (Gambro Renal Products, Lakewood, CO). In-line fluid warmers, such as the Hotline warmer (Smiths-Level 1 Inc., Rockland, MA), also are very effective but add additional priming volume to the circuit. Other warmers have been adapted, such as heating pads or nondialysis blood line warmers. Some of these options require extension of the tubing from the dialysate or replacement fluid bag to the appropriate access point through the warmer. This "excess" tubing is at risk for partial kinking, which will result in triggering of the machine's alarm. If the problem is not appropriately addressed, then excessive fluid may be removed from the patient as the dialysis machine attempts to maintain the programmed total fluid removal goal.

BLOOD FLOW

Blood flow rates for CRRT in children are related to patient size, which will dictate the size of the catheter used, but also are influenced by the vascular access pressures. Poiseuille's law,

$$Q = \frac{\pi r^4 P}{8 \eta L}$$

describes the determinants of flow for newtonian fluids and provides the basis for understanding the potential limitations to blood flow in the pediatric CRRT circuit. The hematocrit in infants and particularly newborns is higher than in older children, which increases the viscosity (η), which will in turn resist flow. The ideal access for optimal flow is a short, large-bore catheter.[8] The catheter diameter size that can be used in young children is by far the greatest limitation to blood flow. A typical blood flow prescription for CVVHD is a rate of 3 to 5 mL/kg per minute,[9] with higher blood flow rates (6 to 10 mL/kg per minute) preferred in patients for whom anticoagulation is contraindicated or to optimize access pressures in the machine. Blood flow rates range from 10 to 50 mL/minute in the infant weighing less than 5 kg, 30 to 85 mL/minute in the child weighing 5 to 15 kg, 50 to 125 mL/minute in the child weighing 16 to 25 kg, and often 100 to 250 mL/minute in the larger child.

ACCESS

The primary goal of vascular access for CRRT is to have adequate flow to provide optimal therapy with minimal interruption. A free-flowing catheter allows for more efficient hemofiltration and less tendency for circuit loss due to clotting. In general, maintenance of a venous access pressure less than 200 mm Hg is desirable. Although recirculation is a common consideration with hemodialysis, it is less of an issue with continuous modalities. Classically, dual-lumen catheters were sufficient for CRRT, but with the trend toward citrate anticoagulation, an additional separate central line port for calcium infusion has become necessary. This has spawned interest in triple-lumen pediatric dialysis catheters to accommodate the extra port. Obviously, such catheters will be limited to larger French

TABLE 291-1

Suggested Vascular Access Devices for Use in Continuous Renal Replacement Therapy in Pediatric Patients

PATIENT SIZE	CATHETER SIZE/SOURCE(S)*	SITE OF INSERTION
Neonate	Single-lumen 5 Fr/Cook	Femoral artery or vein
	Dual-lumen 7.0 Fr/Cook, Medcomp	Internal/external jugular, subclavian, or femoral vein
3-6 kg	Dual-lumen 7.0 Fr/Cook, Medcomp	Internal/external jugular, subclavian, or femoral vein
	Triple-lumen 7.0 Fr/Medcomp, Arrow	Internal/external jugular, subclavian, or femoral vein
6-30 kg	Dual-lumen 8.0 Fr/Kendall, Arrow	Internal/external jugular, subclavian, or femoral vein
>15 kg	Dual-lumen 9.0 Fr/Medcomp	Internal/external jugular, subclavian, or femoral vein
>30 kg	Dual-lumen 10.0 Fr/Arrow, Kendall	Internal/external jugular, subclavian, or femoral vein
>30 kg	Triple-lumen 12 Fr/Arrow, Kendall	Internal/external jugular, subclavian, or femoral vein

*Arrow International, Reading, PA; Cook Vascular Inc., Vandergrift, PA; Kendall International, Inc., Mansfield, MA; Medcomp/Medical Components, Inc., Harleysville, PA.

sizes so as not to compromise blood flow by decreasing lumen size. The alternative is to establish a second central access, or calcium can be "Y-ed" into the return line of a double-lumen dialysis catheter. The latter is a less desirable solution because of the increased risk of clotting in the return port.

Access can be placed in the internal jugular, subclavian, or femoral vessels, with the choice based on patient size, local anatomy, hemostasis considerations, and operator comfort. Many nephrologists avoid use of subclavian catheters with the corresponding risk of subclavian artery stenosis, because subsequent development of end-stage renal disease, as occurs in some patients, may necessitate creation of a fistula later on. Any subtle kinking of the catheter between the first rib and the clavicle may affect access pressure and blood flow. The advantage of the internal jugular catheter is that it is independent of the patient's motion and appears to give adequate blood flow with minimal resistance. The disadvantages of the internal jugular catheter are the potential for pneumothorax or hemothorax and the risk of inadvertent carotid artery puncture at the time of placement. These risks may be minimized by the use of ultrasound imaging during venipuncture. The femoral line may carry a lower risk of complications at the time of placement and afford easier hemostasis compared with a "high line." The disadvantages, however, are greater risk of infection; the potential for catheter kinking with flow problems in an awake, uncooperative patient; and the risk of thrombosis of the vein, complicating future renal transplantation.

Table 291-1 lists appropriate catheters for pediatric patients based on size.

SOLUTIONS

The type of modality to be used, diffusive or convective, needs to be considered in choosing the type of dialysis solution for CRRT. At present, the use of countercurrent dialysis solution versus filter replacement fluid or both is based on the local standard of care.

The U.S. Food and Drug Administration (FDA) considers anything that is placed into the vascular space to be a drug. Normocarb (Dialysis Solutions Inc. [DSI], Richmond Hills, Ontario) currently is the only commercially available solution approved for use as a sterile filter replacement fluid. In the late 1990s, an FDA ruling allowed for local standard of practice in using drugs for which no safe alternative exists. Some programs use normal saline (NS),

lactated Ringer's (LR), or custom (prepared by the local pharmacy) solutions as the standard replacement fluid. Both NS (pH of 5.4) and LR (lactate load) may give rise to metabolic acidosis. Local pharmacy–made solutions lack industry standards of quality assurance, and fatal or near-fatal complications due to errors in compounding the solutions have been reported.[10]

Dialysis solutions are considered devices rather than drugs because they are not infused intravascularly. The FDA has therefore approved them for use in CVVHD (Table 291-2). In the United States, several FDA-approved solutions for dialysis are currently available. These include the bicarbonate-based solutions Normocarb, PrismaSate (Gambro Renal Products, Lakewood, CO), Accusol (Baxter Health Care, McGaw, IL), and Duosol (Braun, Bethlehem, PA). Options outside the United States include Hemosol L0 and B0 (Gambro Hospal, Huntingdon, UK), which are available as lactate- and bicarbonate-based dialysis solutions, respectively. PrismaSate also comes in a lactate-based formula. Alternatively, pharmacy-prepared bicarbonate-based customized solutions may be used. The use of bicarbonate concentrations of 25 mEq/L in customized solutions will help maintain acid-base balance in most clinical situations. If acidosis needs to be aggressively treated, then a separate sodium bicarbonate drip (150 mEq/L) can be infused into the patient at 40 to 80 mL/m^2 per hour. These custom solutions may be phosphorus-based or calcium-based. If calcium-depleted solutions are used, calcium must be infused into the patient. When phosphorus-depleted solutions are used, phosphorus must be given as a continuous infusion, starting at 0.5 to 2 mmol/kg per 24 hours. As an alternative, Troyanov and colleagues have shown that 6 mmol of potassium phosphate can be added to 5-L bags of Hemosol LG2 or Hemosol B0 (both have calcium concentrations of 1.75 mmol/L) without evidence of precipitation or patient complications.[11]

ANTICOAGULATION

Activation of the clotting cascade occurs in CRRT circuits as a result of contact of the circulating blood with artificial surfaces. A low blood flow rate, turbulent blood flow, and high hematocrit will exacerbate this effect. Various methods of anticoagulation have been suggested for CRRT. Adult studies support a longer filter life span with use of citrate rather than heparin; however, one prospective pediatric study did not demonstrate any difference in filter life

TABLE 291-2

Comparison of Common Dialysis Solutions*

COMPONENT OR FEATURE	NORMOCARB (DSI)	PrismaSate (Gambro)			ACCUSOL (BAXTER)	DUOSOL (BRAUN)	CUSTOM (PHARMACY-PREPARED)
		BK0/3.5	BKK2/0	B25GK4/0			
Na (mEq/L)	140	140	140	140	140	140	135
Ca (mEq/L)	0	3.5	0	0	3.5	3	0
K (mEq/L)	0	0	2	4	0-4	0-4	0-4
Mg (mEq/L)	1.5	1	1	120.5	1.0-1.5		1.5
Cl (mEq/L)	107	109.5	108	120.53	109.5-116.3	109-113	110
Phosphate (mmol/L)	0	0	0	0	0	0	0.75-1.50
Lactate (mEq/L)	0	3	3	3	0	0	0
Bicarbonate (mEq/L)	25/35	23/32	23/32	22	30-35	35	25
Glucose (mg/dL)	0	0	110	110	0-100		0
FDA approval	Yes (D, FRF)	Yes (D)			Yes (D)	Yes (D)	No (D, FRF)

*Not all-inclusive of the various formulas available; visiting each individual company's Web site or directly contacting the company for complete information is recommended.

D, dialysate (Q_d); FDA, U.S. Food and Drug Administration; FRF, filter replacement fluid (Q_f).

span between heparin and citrate.[12] Historically, either anticoagulation for CRRT was heparin-based, or no anticoagulation was given, with use of intermittent NS flushes to maintain patency of the filter. More recently, citrate anticoagulation has gained acceptance owing to its ease of administration and favorable patient side effect profile compared with heparin.[12-15] The individual circumstances of the patient dictate the anticoagulation regimen to be used.

The use of no anticoagulation has been shown repeatedly to be associated with a shorter circuit life.[12] This approach typically is used in a patient with fulminant disseminated intravascular coagulation (DIC). Of note, however, DIC may deplete anticoagulant factors as well, leading to a hypercoagulable state, which would benefit from regional anticoagulation to prevent the CRRT system from clotting.

Heparin is one option for anticoagulation. Heparin is infused in the CRRT system at a prefilter point and is used to anticoagulate the system. Anticoagulation is optimized by measuring a postfilter partial thromboplastin time (PTT) or an activated clotting time (ACT). Heparin monitoring targets an ACT between 180 and 220 seconds or the PTT between 1.5 and 2 times normal. This usually is accomplished by initially giving a 20- to 30-unit/kg bolus followed by a continuous intravenous infusion of 10 to 20 units/kg per hour of heparin. The advantage of heparin is its familiarity to medical personnel. The disadvantage of heparin is systemic anticoagulation with increased risk for bleeding. An additional risk is that of heparin-induced thrombocytopenia (HIT), which can increase the potential for bleeding and thrombosis. In many patients with multiorgan system failure (MOSF) necessitating renal replacement therapy, systemic heparinization may be a detriment and should be avoided.

Citrate anticoagulation has been used by adult programs since the 1990s and has subsequently been adopted by pediatric programs. Infusing citrate prefilter starting at 1.5 times the blood flow rate allows for regional anticoagulation of the CRRT system. Coagulation is a calcium-dependent process; therefore, binding calcium minimizes clot formation in the circuit. Hypocalcemia is avoided by infusing calcium back into the patient through a central venous access separate from the CRRT system access. Citrate anticoagulation can be conceptualized as two processes. The first process is management of the citrate anticoagulant infusion in the circuit to target a postfilter ionized calcium between 0.25 and 0.40 mmol/L. The second process is the infusion of calcium chloride back into the patient, titrated to achieve a serum ionized calcium level between 1.10 and 1.30 mmol/L. Although many protocols exist, either a 4% trisodium citrate (TSC) solution or an ACD-A (Baxter Healthcare, Deerfield, IL) solution is available. An equimolar amount of ACD-A has a lower amount of citrate (67% TSC and 33% citric acid) compared with 4% TSC, resulting in a lower risk of metabolic acidosis and a lesser sodium load.

Side effects are more frequent in pediatric patients, necessitating close monitoring for development of increased anion gap metabolic acidosis, metabolic alkalosis, citrate toxicity, hypocalcemia, hyperglycemia, and hypernatremia.[13] The metabolic acidosis and alkalosis often are related to citrate metabolism by the liver: Under normal circumstances, 1 mmol of citrate is metabolized into 3 mmol of bicarbonate, potentially resulting in a metabolic alkalosis. This complication used to be more common with use of higher-concentration bicarbonate-based replacement and dialysis solutions. Recently, the concentration of bicarbonate in these solutions has been decreased. Metabolic alkalosis can be readily corrected by decreasing the citrate infusion rate, increasing the dialysate rate to increase the clearance of citrate, or infusing saline as a filter replacement fluid (e.g., 0.9% NS, pH 5.4 to 5.8, infusing at 25% citrate rate in mL/hr) back to the patient. If the patient is on total parenteral nutrition, the chloride-to-acetate ratio also can be adjusted to help avoid alkalosis. Anion gap metabolic acidosis from citrate is rare and generally occurs only in the setting of extreme liver failure, in which citrate cannot be metabolized. The clearance rate of citrate (sieving coefficient of 0.88 to 1.00) is related to both the clearance properties of the hemofilter (either convective or diffusive) and hepatic metabolism.[16] This phenomenon, termed *citrate lock*, becomes apparent when the patient's total calcium (albumin-calcium complex + citrate-calcium complex + ionized calcium = total calcium) rises while the patient's ionized calcium is stable or dropping. Citrate levels can be measured, but results of these tests are not immediately available. A ratio of total calcium to ionized calcium greater than 2.5 supports a diagnosis of citrate lock. If this phenomenon occurs, the citrate infusion is discontinued for 30 minutes and reinitiated at 70% of the previous rate. Citrate can be used in hepatic insuf-

TABLE 291-3

Filters* for Use in Continuous Renal Replacement Therapy in Pediatric Patients

PATIENT SIZE (kg)	HEMOFILTER†	MEMBRANE MATERIAL	BODY SURFACE AREA (m²)	FILTER PRIMING VOLUME (mL)‡
<10	Minifilter Plus	Polysulfone	0.07	15
>10	HF 400		0.30	28
>20	HF 700		0.71	53
>30	HF 1200		1.25	83
>35	HF 2000		1.98	132
>10	PAN 0.3	Polyacrylonitrile	0.3	33
>20	PAN 0.6		0.6	63
>30	PAN 1.0		1.0	87

*Filter only—no connection to tubing.
†A sample of various filters available in the United States is presented here. See manufacturer's specification sheet for complete details.
‡The arterial and venous line volumes vary depending on manufacturer. For example, adult lines (110 mL) and pediatric lines (64 mL) are available to use with the HF series.

TABLE 291-4

Filter Systems* for Use in Continuous Renal Replacement Therapy in Pediatric Patients

PATIENT SIZE (kg)	HEMOFILTER†	MEMBRANE MATERIAL	BODY SURFACE AREA (m²)	FILTER PRIMING VOLUME (mL)	SET VOLUME (mL)
<5	M 10	Acrylonitrile and sodium	0.042	3.5	50
>5	M 60	methallyl sulfonate	0.6	42	84
>15	M 100	copolymer‡	0.9	65	107
>20	HF 1000	Poly-arylethersulfone	1.15		165
>30	HF 1400		1.40		186

*Filter attached to venous and arterial tubing.
†A sample of various filter systems available in the United States is presented here. See manufacturer's specification sheet for complete details.
‡AN-69 membranes.

ficiency, but the initial rate of citrate infusion should be 50% to 70% of the usual starting rate and monitored in the same fashion as in patients with normal hepatic function. Blood flow also can be decreased, allowing for a proportional decrease in overall citrate infusion.

Hypocalcemia can be a life-threatening event, and judicious monitoring of the patient's ionized calcium concentration is imperative. Hyperglycemia is more frequent in smaller infants because of the glucose in the ACD-A solution (2.45 g/dL), and these patients may require adjustment in the dextrose concentration in the TPN and possibly a concomitant insulin infusion. Hypernatremia can occur but is less common with the use of ACD-A (220 mEq/L) solution compared with the 4% TSC solution (440 mEq/L). Vigilant monitoring of electrolytes can minimize the occurrence of metabolic derangements and allow for timely correction of any developing anomalies.

hypotension develops on initiation of CRRT, especially in the smaller child. The phenomenon is pH-dependent and can be ameliorated by normalizing the pH of the patient's blood prime, and of the patient, before initiation of CRRT. Hemodynamic instability also may develop with use of other biocompatible membranes for which the bradykinin response is not chemically evident.[7,17]

The use of banked blood at the initiation of CRRT increases the risk of cardiac instability, related to a low pH (approximately 6.3), hyperkalemia, hypocalcemia, and bioactive components in the banked blood. The cardiac instability can be minimized by using one of the techniques described earlier under "Blood Priming." Prefilter alkalinization with sodium bicarbonate and use of bicarbonate-based dialysate or replacement fluid also will help to minimize hemodynamic alterations during the initiation of CRRT.[6,18]

MEMBRANES

The hemofilters used in pediatric CRRT have chemical properties identical with those used in adults, and size and material options often are limited to those compatible with the CRRT machine being used. The patient's body surface area needs to be considered in selecting a filter size (Tables 291-3 and 291-4). The biocompatibility of both hemofilters and hemodialysis membranes has improved in recent decades. The AN-69 membrane (polyacrylonitrile membrane) has resulted in decreased complement activation and improved overall patient outcome but has the potential to cause the *bradykinin release phenomenon*, wherein

CONCLUSION

CRRT affords the critically ill pediatric patient an efficient, reliable, and safe form of renal replacement therapy in the setting of appropriate monitoring. CRRT use is expanding within the pediatric critical care community as the technology has become better adapted to the pediatric patient. The proper timing of initiation of therapy, the most appropriate dialysate dose and modality for particular disease processes, and effect on outcome continue to be studied. Once the determinants of survival for critically ill infants and children with acute renal failure and metabolic disorders are better established, it is likely that CRRT will assume a greater role in the overall approach to treatment. The continued cooperation of manufacturers and nephrologists, intensivists, and other members of the health care team is mandatory to maximize the usefulness of CRRT in the pediatric patient.

Key References

4. Goldstein SL, Somers MJG, Baum MA, et al: Pediatric patients with multi-organ dysfunction syndrome receiving continuous renal replacement therapy. Kidney Int 2005;67: 653-658.
6. Brophy PD, Mottes TA, Kudelka TL, et al: AN-69 membrane reactions are pH-dependent and preventable. Am J Kidney Dis 2001;38:173-178.
7. Hackbarth RM, Eding D, Gianoli SC, et al: Zero balance ultra-filtration (Z-BUF) in blood primed CRRT circuits achieves electrolyte and acid-base homeostasis prior to patient connection. Pediatr Nephrol 2005;20:1328-1333.
12. Brophy PD, Somers MJG, Baum MA, et al: Multi-centre evaluation of anticoagulation in patients receiving continuous renal replacement therapy. Nephrol Dial Transplant 2005; 20:1416-1421.
13. Bunchman TE, Maxvold NJ, Barnett J, et al: Pediatric hemo-filtration: Normocarb® dialysate solution with citrate anticoagulation. Pediatr Nephrol 2002;17:150-154.

See the companion Expert Consult website for the complete reference list.

CHAPTER 292

Multiple Organ Dysfunction in the Pediatric Intensive Care Unit

Stefano Picca and Isabella Guzzo

OBJECTIVES

This chapter will:
1. Define multiple organ dysfunction, with a focus on peculiarities and problems encountered in the pediatric patient.
2. Present an overview of the epidemiology of multiple organ dysfunction in the pediatric intensive care unit.
3. Discuss the etiology of pediatric multiple organ dysfunction, including systemic inflammatory response syndrome, sepsis, and related pathogenic mechanisms.
4. Summarize various scoring systems in use for predicting prognosis and outcome in critically ill children.
5. Review the recent evidence on outcome, treatment, and prevention of multiple organ dysfunction, including survival related to systemic inflammatory response syndrome and sepsis, immunomodulation, and renal replacement therapy in children.

DEFINITION OF MULTIPLE ORGAN DYSFUNCTION

As in adult patients, pediatric *multiple organ dysfunction* (MOD) usually is described as the simultaneous occurrence of dysfunction in at least two organs or systems.[1] Adult organ dysfunction criteria often have been applied to pediatric populations, although these criteria lack validity in children because of the physiological changes occurring in the pediatric age group. Consequently, age-related criteria for the definition of MOD have been created.

In 2005, at an International Pediatric Consensus Conference, adult definitions of the sepsis continuum and MOD were modified for children.[2] Age-related variations of physiological and laboratory variables were adopted in order to reach this definition (Table 292-1). Seven organs or systems were considered in defining this clinical entity: cardiovascular and respiratory (dysfunction of at least one

TABLE 292-1

Pediatric Organ Dysfunction Criteria

Cardiovascular
Despite administration of intravenous fluid bolus ≥40 mL/kg in 1 hour:
- Decrease in BP to values under the 5th percentile for age, or systolic BP <2 SD, or
- Need for vasoactive drug (dopamine >5 µg/kg/minute) or
- Two of the following:
  Unexplained metabolic acidosis (base deficit >5.0 mEq/L)
  Increased arterial lactate to more than twice the upper limit of normal
  Urine output <0.5 mL/kg/hour
  Prolonged capillary refill: >5 seconds
  Core to peripheral temperature gap >3° C

Respiratory
- PaO$_2$/FIO$_2$ ratio <300 or
- PaCO$_2$ >65 mm Hg, or 20 mm Hg over baseline, or
- >50% FIO$_2$ to maintain saturation ≥92% or
- Need for mechanical ventilation

Neurological
- GCS score ≤11 or
- Acute change in mental status with decrease in GCS score by 3 or more

Hematological
- Platelet count <80,000/mm^3, or a decline of 50% in platelet count, or
- INR >2

Renal
- Serum creatinine ≥2 times upper limit of normal for age or twofold increase from baseline

Hepatic
- Total bilirubin ≥4 mg/dL (not applicable to newborn) or
- ALT twice the upper limit of normal for age

ALT, alanine transaminase; BP, blood pressure; GCS, Glasgow Coma Scale; INR, international normalized ratio; SD, standard deviation.
Modified from Goldstein B, Giroir B, Randolph A: International Pediatric Sepsis Consensus Conference: Definitions for sepsis and organ dysfunction in pediatrics. Pediatr Crit Care Med 2005;6:2-8.

of these two systems was a criterion), neurological, hematological, renal, hepatic, and gastrointestinal systems. A distinction between primary and secondary MOD also is accepted in children.[3] Primary MOD is regarded as a consequence of a specific insult and is defined as the simultaneous occurrence of two-organ dysfunction within the first week after admission to a pediatric intensive care unit (PICU). Secondary MOD is considered to represent an effect of the host response, in which organ dysfunction appears more than 7 days after admission to the PICU. Most cases of MOD are primary, and only 12% of children diagnosed with MOD were reported to have secondary MOD. Compared with children with primary MOD, those with secondary MOD had a longer duration of organ dysfunction, a more extended PICU stay, and a higher mortality rate.[3]

EPIDEMIOLOGY

The incidence of and mortality rate for MOD depend mainly on association with the systemic inflammatory response syndrome (SIRS) or sepsis, PICU population characteristics, and the country of the study population. In fact, the reported incidence of MOD ranges from 18% to 56.5% of the PICU population.[3-7] The impact of sepsis due to locally predominant infections plays a determinant role in MOD epidemiology. As an example, in a study performed in Montreal, Canada, MOD was identified in 18% of the PICU population, and the mortality rate among children with MOD was 36% (sepsis was present in 21% of the patients). Mortality rates differed between patients with and those without SIRS (12% versus 40%).[3] Conversely, different percentages and etiological factors may be reported in studies performed in developing countries. In a study from Peru, 56.5% of children admitted to the PICU during a period of 6 months had MOD, and sepsis was present in 31% of them.[5] In this study, patients with associated sepsis had 53% mortality rate, as opposed to 28.9% in those without sepsis. In another study concerning the etiology of MOD, Khilnani and coworkers reported that in 184 children from India, 83.6% had sepsis; 38.6% of the septic children had dengue shock or malaria.[6]

From these data, it appears that MOD epidemiology is heavily affected by local and selection characteristics.

ETIOLOGY

In the 2005 International Pediatric Consensus Conference, the definitions of *systemic inflammatory response syndrome* (SIRS), *sepsis*, *severe sepsis*, *septic shock*, and *MOD* as a continuum (see Table 292-1) were delineated.[1] A direct benefit of this improvement was etiological clarification. In fact, multiple organ dysfunction syndrome (MODS) may correspond to the final and possibly most severe stage of an uncontrolled SIRS or sepsis. SIRS represents an inflammatory response mediated by cytokines to various insults: infections, trauma, burns, pancreatitis, shock, and so on. Sepsis defined a systemic inflammatory response similar to SIRS but specifically related to an infection induced by bacterial, mycotic, or viral toxins. Although SIRS, sepsis, and septic shock usually are connected to bacterial infection, bacteremia cannot be detected in half of the episodes thought to be septic. Therefore, an infection is the inciting stimulus in only half of the cases of MOD.[4]

The pathophysiology of sepsis and MOD is quite complex and involves many inflammatory cells and mediators. The initial process is the linkage of the circulating toxins from the bacterial wall to a protein called lipopolysaccharide-binding protein (LBP). The complex lipopolysaccharide (LPS)-LBP binds to the mCD14 receptor present on monocyte-macrophages, inducing synthesis of inflammatory mediators—cytokines and chemokines. In particular, cytokines induce further activation of the cellular immunity. T lymphocytes are stimulated and play a different role according to the specific population activated. T-helper 1 (T$_H$1) cells are involved in the synthesis of pro-inflammatory cytokines: tumor necrosis factor-α (TNF-α), interleukin (IL)-2, interferon (INF)-γ; T-helper 2 (T$_H$2) cells produce anti-inflammatory cytokines: IL-4 and IL-10. The target of the pro-inflammatory cytokines is the endothelial cells, which in turn produce vasoactive mediators such as arachidonic acid metabolites, nitric oxide, endothelin, and platelet-activating factor, with local and systemic effects. The anti-inflammatory cytokines, usually synthesized in a second moment, limit inflammation and prevent organ dysfunction and septic shock. Thus, inflammation is controlled by a balance between pro- and anti-inflammatory mediators. An excessive production of pro-inflammatory substances is implicated in organ dysfunction, whereas a disproportionate anti-inflammatory response leads to anergy and death.[8] Apoptotic or necrotic cell death modulates the immunity response. Necrotic lymphocytes induce T_H1, producing pro-inflammatory mediators, whereas apoptotic lymphocytes stimulate T_H2, producing anti-inflammatory cytokines. Widespread apoptosis of the lymphoid cell population in the spleen and colon has been reported in patients who died from sepsis and MOD.[9]

SCORING SYSTEMS

Using survival as a single endpoint, severity composite scores have been created in order to predict (prognostic scores) or to describe (outcome scores) the outcome in patients in intensive care units (ICUs). Basically, different clinical, laboratory, and other variables recorded at different times in the ICU course are used to measure how far indices of function for selected altered organs or systems are from the normal range. A *prognostic score* is used both for the evaluation of effectiveness and efficiency of intensive care and for investigation purposes. An *outcome score* describes the severity of illness during the ICU stay. Consequently, it also can be used as a surrogate for death as an outcome (much less frequent in PICUs than in adult ICUs). In both cases, a baseline evaluation is made (on ICU admission or at randomization). Subsequent reevaluations

are used in outcome scores to increase sensitivity in assessment of changes in the patient's condition.

Since 1986, severity scores also have been applied to children.

Predictive Scores

The Pediatric Risk of Mortality (PRISM) system is the de facto standard scoring system used in a majority of studies on pediatric intensive care. It derives from the Physiologic Stability Index (PSI) published in 1986[10] and was therefore named PRISM II in its first version. As shown in Table 292-2, it contains 14 variables, which are documented as the most abnormal values recorded in the first 24 hours of intensive care. Although widely used and relatively accurate, PRISM II presents some problems. First, its discrimination capacity is falsely high: Because 40% of deaths occur in the first 24 hours,[11] the worst variables recorded in the same period may reflect the condition closest to death, rather than representing a prediction score. Second, it tends to blunt qualitative differences between PICUs. This tendency may significantly affect scores of both mildly and severely ill patients, with consequent underevaluation of mortality rate in low-level PICUs or overevaluation of mortality rate in high-level

TABLE 292-2

Variables and Validity* of Major Pediatric Severity Scores

FEATURE	Scoring System[†]					
	PRISM II	**PRISM III**	**PIM**	**PIM2**	**PELOD**	**P-MODS**
Variables considered	Systolic blood pressure	Systolic blood pressure	Systolic blood pressure	Systolic blood pressure	Systolic blood pressure	pLactic acid
	Diastolic blood pressure	Heart rate	Pupillary reaction	Pupillary reaction	Heart rate	PaO_2/FIO_2
	Heart rate	GCS score	PaO_2/FIO_2	PaO_2/FIO_2	GCS score	pBililirubin
	Respiratory rate	Pupillary reaction	BE	BE	Pupillary reaction	Fibrinogen
	PaO_2/FIO_2	Temperature	Mechanical ventilation	Mechanical ventilation	Mechanical ventilation	BUN
	PCO_2	pH	Elective admission	Elective admission	PCO_2	
	GCS score	CO_2	High-risk diagnosis	High-risk diagnosis	PaO_2	
	Pupillary reaction	PCO_2		Recovery postsurgery	pCreatinine	
	PT/PTT	PaO_2		Bypass	ALT	
	pBililirubin	pGlucose			PT	
	pPotassium	pPotassium			WBC	
	pCalcium	pCreatinine			PLTs	
	pGlucose	BUN				
	pBicarbonate	WBC				
		PLTs				
		PT				
		PTT				
Discrimination capacity (area under the ROC curve)	0.92	0.94	0.90	0.90	0.91	0.81
Calibration (Hosmer-Lemeshow goodness-of-fit test)	>0.95	0.55	0.37	0.17	<0.0001	0.64

*The validity of a score is evaluated by *discrimination* and *calibration*. Discrimination is the capacity of the score to differentiate patients who meet the outcome from those who do not. It is evaluated by the area under the receiver operating characteristic (ROC) curve (AUC = 1 means perfect discrimination, AUC = 0.5 means discrimination no better than that resulting from chance). Calibration measures the goodness of fit at different levels of probability between the predicted and the verified outcomes. Its analysis is done with the Hosmer-Lemeshow test. A *P* value greater than 0.10 indicates a good calibration.

[†]PELOD, Paediatric Logistic Organ Dysfunction; PIM, Pediatric Index of Mortality; PIM2, Pediatric Index of Mortality 2003 revision; P-MODS, Pediatric Multiple Organ Dysfunction Score; PRISM-II, Pediatric Risk of Mortality (derived from Physiologic Stability Index [PSI]); PRISM-III, Pediatric Risk of Mortality, 1996 revision. See text for details.

ALT, alanine transaminase; BE, base excess; BUN, blood urea nitrogen; FIO_2, fraction of inspired oxygen; GCS, Glasgow Coma Scale; PLTs, platelets; PT, prothrombin time; PTT, partial thromboplastin time; WBC, white blood cell count.

PICUs. In an attempt to overcome such problems, PRISM III was created in 1996.[12] PRISM III is calculated from 17 variables, and it can be evaluated during the first 12 hours (PRISM III-12) or during the first 24 hours (PRISM III-24). Both methods have yielded good results.[1] Two important problems are recognized, however: The increase in number of variables to be recorded generally has been poorly accepted by potential users. Moreover, the equation used to predict the mortality rate is not in the public domain, and a fee is charged for use of the algorithms. This requirement has made PRISM III unpopular outside the United States.

In 1997, the Pediatric Index of Mortality (PIM) was proposed.[13] Its main difference from PRISM was that only seven variables were required at entry, thereby avoiding the risks related to variations that may occur in the first 12 or 24 hours of the PICU stay. An update of PIM was published in 2003 as PIM2,[14] in which three new variables were introduced. This refinement improved the established standard of care, compared with PIM1 and PRISM III. PIM2 discriminated between death and survival better than PRISM III (area under the ROC curve, 0.90 versus 0.87). Moreover, the PIM score calculations are available on the Internet.

Outcome Scores

Both in adults and in children, it has been shown that mortality rate increases with the number of organs failing. The lack of consensus on MOD definition in children complicated matters, however (see earlier). In fact, the "binary" approach (i.e., organ failure versus function) induced lack of sensitivity. A new approach is found in the Paediatric Logistic Organ Dysfunction (PELOD) score.[15] PELOD takes into account both the number of failing organs and the degree of organ dysfunction by a scoring system, assigning increasing scores to four levels of severity for each of the 18 considered variables. A daily PELOD (dPELOD) also was proposed in 2003.[16] dPELOD measurement provides an additional index of the course of illness and a surrogate measure for death as an outcome in clinical trials. Moreover, dPELOD can be integrated by the "delta-PELOD" (difference between the worst dPELOD after randomization and dPELOD at day of randomization). Finally, PELOD is the only outcome score validated in a multicenter study. Unfortunately, the researchers recently reported a mistake published in the original paper of 2003, and a poor calibration of PELOD ($P < .0001$) was discovered.[17] More evidence is needed in the validation of the PELOD score.

Recently, Graciano and colleagues[18] proposed an outcome score named Pediatric Multiple Organ Dysfunction Score (P-MODS). In this model, no neurological dysfunction was taken into consideration, on the assumption that reliability of this evaluation in heavily sedated patients is low. Although tested in a large pediatric population ($N = 6456$), the area under the ROC curve was lower than that of PELOD (0.81 versus 0.91). Moreover, its reproducibility is unknown, because data were collected in a single center.

In conclusion, predictive and outcome scores in children with MOD are in their early days. Their potential application is of paramount importance to pediatric intensivists, for both clinical and investigation purposes. The main limitations at present seem to be the lack of validation in a significant number of countries and in children with SIRS or sepsis or in the long term. The main limita-

tion in the future probably will be the need for continuous updating owing to changes in PICU populations over time.

OUTCOME

Mortality rates in critically ill children with MOD are variably reported between 30% and 80%. Among children with secondary MOD, the mortality rate is 6.5 times greater than in those with primary MOD.[3] As previously reported, MOD frequently is the end stage of sepsis, but the relationship among SIRS, sepsis, severe sepsis, and septic shock with respect to mortality rate is less well defined than in the adult population. Proulx and coworkers reported a 36% mortality rate among 191 of 916 children who presented with MOD. In this series, the association of SIRS or septic shock with MOD did not induce significant changes in mortality rate (40% versus 52%).[3] Similarly, Wilkinson and associates observed comparable mortality rates in children with MOD with sepsis and in those with MOD without sepsis (46% versus 47%).[19] Therefore, in contrast with adult patients, sepsis did not seem to significantly increase the risk of death among children with MOD. Subsequent studies, however, reported opposite conclusions. In 84 children with MOD, Goh and Lum reported a higher mortality in the presence of sepsis (22%), severe sepsis (65%), and septic shock (80%).[20] In a more recent study, 87 of 156 children with MOD had sepsis, and the mortality rate (51.7%) was greater than in those patients who did not present with sepsis (28.9%).[5] Conversely, a link between MOD and death in septic children has been demonstrated, and 90% to 100% of septic children who die in PICUs have MOD.[21] From these data, it seems that the association of MOD and sepsis affects mortality in a non-univocal way: A septic child in whom MOD develops has a higher risk of death than a child with MOD who becomes septic.

An important contribution to the definition of the outcome of MOD has come from severity scores and serological markers. Proulx and coworkers reported that three markers had been identified as independent predictors of death in 85 children with MOD: higher number of organs or systems with simultaneous failure during the PICU stay, age of 12 months or younger, and a worse PRISM score on the day of admission.[7] Also, Leclerc and associates demonstrated in 269 children with MOD an increased risk of death with increasing severity of MOD, as evaluated by the PELOD score or the number of dysfunctional organs.[22] Finally, Khilnani and colleagues observed mortality rates of 9%, 29%, 58%, and 100% in patients with OFI (Organ Failure Index) scores of 2, 3, 4 to 5, and greater than 5, respectively.[6]

Recently, the importance of fluid accumulation during ICU stay has been demonstrated in outcomes for children with MOD receiving continuous renal replacement therapy (CRRT). In 116 children with MOD treated with CRRT (data from the Prospective Pediatric CRRT Registry Group), Goldstein and coworkers demonstrated a strong association between the degree of fluid accumulation from PICU admission to CRRT initiation and mortality rate. This association was more significant than with traditional variables as influential as patient age and weight or pressor dosage.[23] Moreover, risk of death was proportional to the percentage of fluid overload category.[24] Future evaluation of children with MOD will have to take into account the fluid overload variable.

The prognostic value of some biomarkers measured at ICU admission has been recently reported. Procalcitonin (PCT), IL-10, and TNF levels at PICU admission were higher in children with worse multiorgan system failure (MOSF) scores and elevated mortality. PCT measurements after 24 hours decreased significantly in patients with a better prognosis.[25] Similarly, blood levels of C-reactive protein (CRP) have been investigated as an indicator of organ failure and mortality risk in the PICU setting.[26]

In conclusion, MOD in children usually occurs early, and sepsis increases mortality. Secondary MOD negatively affects outcomes. Negative prognostic factors are number of organs involved, younger age, worse prognostic scores, and fluid overload in children who received CRRT. Serial measurements of some serological markers may have prognostic significance and also may alter the therapeutic approach.

TREATMENT AND PREVENTION

MOD may be considered to represent the terminal stage of the imbalance between pro- and anti-inflammatory mediators regulating host humoral defense mechanisms. After this uncontrolled activation of the immune system, MOD may result. Immunomodulation aims to ameliorate the early hyperinflammatory phase to avoid the development of MOD. Experience with immunomodulation in children includes renal replacement therapy (RRT), plasma filtration, immunonutrition, and the use of some recent specific immunomodulators.

CRRT provides both metabolic control and *removal of inflammatory mediators* in critically ill patients. Proinflammatory mediators (TNF-α, thromboxane B$_2$, IL-1, and platelet-activating factor) have been detected in the outflow dialysate and on membrane surfaces during CRRT.[27] Convective clearance and membrane adsorption both are involved in removing pro-inflammatory mediators. Mediator removal by hemofiltration in children also has been reported,[28,29] although no study demonstrating an association between mediator removal by CRRT and survival in children has been published. In 1996, Journois and coworkers reported that in children who had undergone cardiac surgery and were managed with zero-fluid balance hemofiltration, amelioration of secondary endpoints, such as need for pressors, time to extubation, or postoperative blood loss, was observed, while C3a, IL-1, IL-6, IL-8, IL-10 and TNF-α levels decreased.[30] In this series, improvement did not seem to be a consequence of fluid removal but evidently was due to cytokine clearance. No definite evidence for a beneficial effect of CRRT in patients without renal failure is available, however.

Plasma filtration has been proposed as an alternative to cytokine removal. In a recent trial, 30 patients with sepsis, of whom 13 were children, were randomized to receive plasma filtration for 34 hours or supportive therapy alone. No statistically significant difference in the all-cause 14-day mortality rate emerged between the two groups. Nevertheless, a trend toward failure of fewer organs was observed in the plasma filtration treatment group. Plasma filtration effected a reduction in the acute-phase response without any effect on the cytokine response.[31]

The rationale for use of *immunonutrition* is based on the double assumption that both an increased energy requirement and the use of specific nutrients (glutamine, *n*3-polyunsaturated fatty acids, nucleotides) may enhance a positive immune response. Results with use of immuno-nutrition showed an improvement with respect to secondary endpoints such as nosocomial infections[32] and duration of mechanical ventilation and of hospital stay,[33] rather than changes in mortality rate. In children managed with immunonutrition, a reduction in IL-6 levels was demonstrated without any significant change in mortality.[34]

The use of *steroids* in pediatric MOD is controversial. In the 2003 Surviving Sepsis Campaign Guidelines for Management of Severe Sepsis and Septic Shock,[35] the administration of 1 to 2 mg/kg hydrocortisone is recommended for stress coverage after diagnosis of adrenal insufficiency. Studies in children with post–cardiopulmonary bypass SIRS failed to demonstrate the efficacy of higher steroid dosages.[36,37]

Granulocyte-macrophage colony-stimulating factor is recommended for children with demonstrated neutropenic sepsis or white blood cell primary immune deficit.[38]

Activated protein C administration has been shown to be effective and safe in reducing the 28-day mortality rate in adult patients.[39] The results of a large multicenter study including 187 children have been recently published.[40] Although no definite conclusion regarding the efficacy of this treatment was possible, owing to the lack of a control group, lowest post-treatment protein C levels were associated with highest 28-day mortality rates. A high incidence (27.7%) of bleeding complications was reported, however, and two patients died of postinfusion brain hemorrhage.

Besides the treatment of sepsis, MOD therapy is supportive. Although all therapeutic strategies to treat pediatric MOD per se should be considered, clear-cut evidence of efficacy of specific and nonspecific treatments for MOD in children is lacking, and further randomized controlled trials are needed.

Key Points

1. Multiple organ dysfunction is the simultaneous occurrence of dysfunction of at least two organs or systems. In children, age-related criteria are needed to define organ dysfunction.
2. Reported incidence of multiple organ dysfunction in pediatric intensive care units is between 18% and 56.5%. This wide range is due to local and selection characteristics.
3. PRISM II is the most utilized prognostic severity score in children. In children, outcome scores are useful for clinical course measuring and may be used as surrogate outcome of death.
4. In children, the mortality rate for multiple organ dysfunction is between 30% and 80%. Secondary multiple organ dysfunction carries a higher risk of death than primary multiple organ dysfunction, and sepsis developing after primary multiple organ dysfunction significantly worsens the outcome.
5. Evidence of efficacy of several forms of treatment and prevention of pediatric multiple organ dysfunction is still lacking.

Key References

1. Lacroix J, Cotting J, for the Pediatric Acute Lung Injury and Sepsis Investigators (PALISI) Network: Severity of illness and organ dysfunction scoring in children. Pediatr Crit Care Med 2005;6(3 Suppl):S126-S134.

2. Goldstein B, Giroir B, Randolph A: International Pediatric Sepsis Consensus Conference: Definitions for sepsis and organ dysfunction in pediatrics. Pediatr Crit Care Med 2005; 6:2-8.
11. Pollack MM, Ruttimann UE, Getson PR: Pediatric Risk of Mortality (PRISM) score. Crit Care Med 1988;16:1110-1116.
16. Leteurtre S, Martinot A, Duhamel A, et al: Validation of the Paediatric Logistic Organ Dysfunction (PELOD) score: Pro-

spective, observational, multicentre study. Lancet 2003;362: 192-197.
23. Goldstein SL, Somers MJ, Baum MA, et al: Pediatric patients with multi-organ dysfunction syndrome receiving continuous renal replacement therapy. Kidney Int 2005;67:653-658.

See the companion Expert Consult website for the complete reference list.

CHAPTER 293

Drug Dosing in Pediatric Acute Kidney Insufficiency and Renal Replacement Therapy

Jeffrey F. Barletta and Gina-Marie Barletta

OBJECTIVES

This chapter will:
1. Describe the pharmacokinetic alterations that occur in critically ill children with acute kidney insufficiency that may affect drug dosing.
2. Review the limitations of the various methods used to calculate drug doses in children receiving continuous renal replacement therapy.
3. Identify the factors that influence drug removal through continuous renal replacement therapy modalities that use convection.
4. Identify the factors that influence drug removal through continuous renal replacement therapy modalities that use diffusion.
5. Present an appropriate dosing regimen for critically ill children on continuous renal replacement therapy.

Drug dosing in the pediatric population can be a challenging task and is particularly problematic in the child with acute kidney insufficiency (AKI). Data regarding optimal dosing in pediatrics are limited; therefore, many dosing regimens are extrapolated from either clinical experience or the adult literature. Published drug information references are useful guides, albeit with limitations, and variability in their recommendations has been noted.[1]

The discipline that describes how medications are absorbed, distributed throughout various organs or tissues, metabolized, and eliminated from the body is termed *pharmacokinetics*. Several physiological changes that occur during maturation can affect drug pharmacokinetics, making dosing extrapolations from the adult literature inaccurate.[2] For example, bioavailability is variable owing to changes in gastric acidity, motility, and enzymatic activity. Volume of distribution (V_d), which is the mathematical concept representing the nonphysiological compartment in which a drug disperses, is higher in children, particu-

larly for drugs that are highly water soluble (e.g., aminoglycosides). Protein binding is reduced, thereby increasing the free fraction or pharmacologically active portion of the drug at the site of action. Drug metabolism (both phase I and phase II reactions) and elimination (through glomerular filtration and tubular secretion) are immature at birth but generally reach adult levels within 1 year.[2,3] For a complete discussion of these alterations, the reader is referred to other excellent reviews.[2,3]

ESTIMATION OF CREATININE CLEARANCE

Quantification of kidney function is important in critically ill children in order to properly adjust the dosage of medications that are eliminated by the kidneys. The glomerular filtration rate (GFR) represents a direct overall measure of kidney function and may be significantly diminished before the onset of overt signs or symptoms of kidney insufficiency or failure.[4,5] GFR is a measure of the renal clearance of a substance from plasma and is expressed as the volume of plasma that is cleared of that substance over 1 minute—in absolute values (mL/minute) or in relative values (mL/minute/1.73 m^2), after correction for body surface area.[4-6] Glomerular filtration must be monitored closely in the setting of acute kidney insufficiency, especially in those children receiving potentially nephrotoxic agents, which typically are eliminated by the kidneys. GFR is most accurately measured by evaluating the urinary or plasma clearance of exogenous filtration markers such as inulin, iohexol (^{99m}Tc-diethylenetriaminepenta-acetic acid), ^{51}Cr-ethylenediaminetetra-acetic acid (EDTA), or iothalamate.[4,5,7,8] These infusion techniques, however, are impractical in clinical situations, in which merely a reliable approximation of GFR is required in order to adjust medication dosages or to evaluate a trend in variable kidney function. As an alternative, equations that use

TABLE 293-1

Common Equations to Assess Renal Function in Pediatric Patients

Timed Urine Specimen Creatinine Clearance

CrCl = [Ucr × (Vur/SCr)] × [1.73/BSA]

CrCl, creatinine clearance(mL/min/1.73 m²); Ucr, urine creatinine (mg/dL); Vur, total urine volume (mL) divided by the duration of the collection (min); SCr, serum creatinine (mg/dL), (when midpoint values are not available, use average serum creatinine values from start and end of collection period); BSA, body surface area (m²).

Schwartz

Estimated GFR = kL/SCr

GFR, glomerular filtration rate (mL/min/1.73 m²); k, proportionality constant (0.33 for low birth weight during first year of life, 0.45 for term-appropriate gestational age during first year of life, 0.55 for children and adolescent girls, 0.7 for adolescent boys); L, length (cm); SCr, serum creatinine (mg/dL).

Counahan-Barratt

Estimated GFR = (0.43 × L)/SCr

GFR, glomerular filtration rate (mL/min/1.73 m²); L, length (cm); SCr, serum creatinine (mg/dL).

Cystatin C Formula

log(GFR) = 1.962 + [1.123 × log(1/cystatin c)]

GFR, glomerular filtration rate (mL/min/1.73 m²).

Data from Schwartz GJ, Brion LP, Spitzer A: The use of plasma creatinine concentration for estimating glomerular filtration rate in infants, children, and adolescents. Pediatr Clin North Am 1987;34:571-590; Counahan R, Chantler C, Ghazali S, et al: Estimation of glomerular filtration rate from plasma creatinine concentration in children. Arch Dis Child 1976;51:875-878; and Filler G, Lepage N: Should the Schwartz formula for estimation of GFR be replaced by cystatin C formula? Pediatr Nephrol 2003;18:981-985.

serum creatinine levels are routinely implemented by clinicians to estimate GFR.[4,6-9]

Creatinine is an endogenous metabolic product derived primarily from the metabolism of creatine and phosphocreatine in muscle. Creatinine typically is present at relatively stable serum levels and reflects overall muscle mass.[5,8,10] Creatinine is freely filtered by glomeruli; however, it also is secreted into urine by renal proximal tubular cells.[5,8] Because creatinine is filtered primarily through the glomerular capillary wall, a common approach to estimating GFR in pediatric and adult patients is to measure the 24-hour urinary creatinine clearance (CrCl).[10,11] CrCl is calculated by analyzing creatinine levels obtained from serum and from a 24-hour urine sample (Table 293-1).[8,10,12] Overall, CrCl consistently overestimates GFR by roughly 10% to 40% in healthy persons, owing to the renal tubular secretion of creatinine.[5,8,13] Although consistent discrepancies in CrCl as an estimate of GFR are recognized, measured 24-hour CrCl is classically used as a method to approximate GFR in order to adjust drug dosages.[14,15] In the critical care setting, however, medical decision making and institution of therapy typically occur before completion of such prolonged evaluations. Timed urine collections, therefore, can be impractical and cumbersome and frequently are incomplete, leading to inaccurate data.

Because medication dosing decisions typically are made before the completion of a prolonged 24-hour urine collection, some clinicians have investigated the accuracy of shorter collection periods.[10,16,17] For example, one study of critically ill pediatric patients demonstrated that a 12-hour CrCl was as accurate as the standard 24-hour CrCl. A study of critically ill adult patients, however, demonstrated a poor correlation with 24-hour CrCl with use of urine collections obtained over a period less than 8 hours.[16]

To overcome the need to perform timed urine collections, several equations have been developed to provide a rapid estimation of GFR or CrCl (see Table 293-1). Such equations typically incorporate patient weight, length, age, and gender. In addition, they assume that renal function is stable, with steady-state serum creatinine kinetics. In the pediatric population, the *Schwartz equation* has been broadly evaluated and used as an estimate of GFR.[4,6,9,10] The Schwartz equation originally was derived in 1976 from data obtained in 186 non–critically ill pediatric patients using factors such as patient length, plasma creatinine, and urine creatinine.[6] Subsequently, the Schwartz equation underwent several revisions for estimating GFR using patient length, serum creatinine level, and a constant that varies with the age and gender of the patient.[4] This formula has demonstrated adequate correlation with measured CrCl, along with sufficient accuracy for clinical use in pediatric patients without acute critical illness. A second equation that is commonly used is the *Counahan-Barratt equation*.[18] The Counahan-Barratt equation uses the plasma creatinine and patient length to estimate body surface area-adjusted GFR (mL/minute/ 1.73 m²).[18] Both the Schwartz and the Counahan-Barratt equations are simple techniques to estimate GFR and remain the standard for rapid assessment of GFR in non–critically ill pediatric patients. However, several studies have demonstrated that the Schwartz equation is not an accurate indicator of kidney function in critically ill pediatric patients.[10,15,19]

Some studies have suggested that serum or plasma cystatin C may represent a marker of GFR that is superior to serum creatinine in pediatric and adult patients.[20-22] In fact, one study using a cystatin C–based GFR equation provided an improved estimate of GFR in non–critically ill children compared with that obtained with the Schwartz equation.[21] This equation, however, has not been evaluated in critically ill children with AKT.

The evaluation of kidney function in critically ill pediatric patients represents an exceptional challenge owing to the significant variability in kidney function, altered body composition or muscle mass, inconsistent or poor nutritional status, irregular volume status, and hemodynamic instability seen in this population. As a result of such wide inconsistency, steady-state serum creatinine kinetics cannot be readily achieved, limiting the accuracy particularly of creatinine-based equations for evaluation of kidney function. In addition, such formulas do not account for obligate renal tubular secretion of creatinine, which may represent a greater overall proportion of total observed clearance at lower GFR.[11] Furthermore, an increase in serum creatinine typically is delayed behind the actual decrease in overall kidney function, so equations that estimate CrCl may not detect declining kidney function until a significant proportion of that function is lost. An accurate equation for estimating GFR has yet to be validated for use in critically ill pediatric patients. Therefore, in view of the numerous limitations of many of the equations that are available to estimate kidney function in critically ill pediatric patients, the completion of a timed urinary creatinine clearance collection (12 or 24 hours) has been advocated as a more acceptable measure to estimate GFR and may be especially useful in adjusting dosage for agents that have a narrow therapeutic index.[10,16]

PHARMACOKINETIC ALTERATIONS WITH ACUTE KIDNEY INSUFFICIENCY

The typical pharmacokinetic parameters that are evaluated in making drug dosing decisions are bioavailability, volume of distribution (V_d), elimination half-life, and clearance. Renal failure can have a profound effect on many of these parameters, and failure to recognize these changes can lead to inappropriate dosing regimens and possibly treatment failure.

The V_d can be significantly altered in critically ill children with renal failure.[23] Such alterations most commonly are due to increased extracellular volume, intravascular fluid shifts, and decreased protein binding. An increase in fluid volume from either fluid resuscitation or oliguria can increase the V_d, particularly for hydrophilic drugs such as the aminoglycosides. Accordingly, larger loading doses would be necessary to achieve similar peak serum concentrations. Conversely, the V_d of digoxin is known to be lower in patients with renal disease as a result of competitive inhibition of tissue binding.[23] Loading doses, therefore, should be reduced.

Plasma protein concentrations can change in children with renal failure, influencing V_d by altering the free or unbound portion of drug available at the site of action.[24] The three major plasma proteins that influence protein binding are albumin, α_1-acid glycoprotein (AAG), and lipoproteins. Acidic drugs such as furosemide, theophylline, and phenytoin are bound primarily to albumin, whereas basic drugs such as lidocaine are bound to AAG.[23] Albumin concentrations typically are reduced in children with AKI, so the unbound fraction of drug is increased. AAG, on the other hand, often is increased in AKI, so unbound drug may be lower and the clinical effects are reduced.

Although renal failure naturally will affect the clearance of drugs that are eliminated primarily by the kidney, it also can affect the clearance of drugs that are not. Hepatic metabolism can be significantly reduced in patients with end-stage or chronic kidney disease, but in patients with AKI, it can be highly variable.[25] In fact, some studies have demonstrated higher nonrenal clearance values for drugs in patients with AKI than in those with chronic kidney disease who have similar CrCl values.[26,27] For example, the nonrenal clearance of imipenem was 95 ± 13.8 mL/minute for adult patients with AKI, compared with 51.1 ± 10.5 mL/minute for those with chronic kidney disease ($P < .02$).[27] In a second study, vancomycin nonrenal clearance was strongly correlated with total clearance ($r = 0.94$, $P < .0005$) and decreased significantly with each day of renal replacement therapy.[26] The extrapolation of drug doses recommended for patients with chronic kidney disease to those used in AKI should be done with caution because of the associated risk for underdosing; additional studies that are specific to pediatric patients are needed to address this concern.

With medications that are renally eliminated, it is important to recognize that AKI will increase the half-life of not only the parent compound but also its active metabolites. This consideration is of particular concern with drugs that have a narrow therapeutic window. For example, the active metabolite of midazolam, 1-OH-midazolam-glucuronide, has been shown to accumulate in patients with renal failure, leading to prolonged sedation.[28] In fact, one study noted levels of 1-OH-midazolam-glucuronide in a child with renal failure that were twice that of the population mean.[29] Of interest, 1-OH-midazolam-glucuronide is

TABLE 293-2

Relationship between Creatinine Clearance (CrCl) and Total Body Clearance for Selected Drugs

DRUG	TOTAL BODY CLEARANCE (mL/min)
Acyclovir	3.37 (CrCl) + 0.41
Amikacin	0.6 (CrCl) + 9.6
Aztreonam	0.8 (CrCl) + 26.6
Cefepime	0.96 (CrCl) + 10.9
Ceftazidime	1.15 (CrCl) + 10.6
Ciprofloxacin	2.83 (CrCl) + 363
Digoxin	0.88 (CrCl) + 23
Gentamicin	0.983 (CrCl)
Lithium	0.235 (CrCl)
Ofloxacin	1.04 (CrCl) + 38.7
Penicillin G	3.35 (CrCl) + 35.5
Piperacillin	1.36 (CrCl) + 1.5
Teicoplanin	7.09 (CrCl) − 16.2
Tobramycin	0.801 (CrCl)
Vancomycin	0.69 (CrCl) + 3.7

Data from Matzke GR, Comstock TJ: Influence of renal function and dialysis on drug disposition. In Burton ME, Shaw LM, Schentag JJ, Evans WE (eds): Applied Pharmacokinetics and Pharmacodynamics: Principles of Therapeutic Drug Monitoring, 4th ed. Philadelphia, Lippincott Williams & Wilkins, 2006, pp 187-212; and Frye RF, Matzke GR: Drug therapy individualization for patients with renal insufficiency. In DiPiro JT, Talbert RL, Yee GC, et al (eds): Pharmacotherapy: A Pathophysiologic Approach, 6th ed. New York, McGraw-Hill, 2005, pp 919-935.

effectively removed with both continuous venovenous hemofiltration (CVVH) and continuous venovenous hemodialysis (CVVHD), whereas midazolam (the parent drug) is not.[30,31]

DOSING CONSIDERATIONS WITH RENAL FAILURE

Several key principles must be considered in establishing a dosing regimen for a critically ill child with renal failure. The first such consideration is the proportion of renal clearance for a given medication in relation to total body clearance (Table 293-2). Generally, when renal clearance accounts for less than 30% of total body clearance, AKI will have minimal impact on drug removal.[32] Dosing adjustments, therefore, are not required. A second consideration addresses the balance between a need for aggressive therapy with the adverse effect profile of the individual agent. Depending on the severity of disease, it may not always be appropriate to choose drug doses that are at the lower end of the dosing range, particularly for medications that generally are considered safe (e.g., beta-lactam antibiotics). In fact, some investigators have recommended increasing the renally adjusted dose by 30% for drugs with a low degree of toxicity.[33] It is important to individualize each regimen in accordance with the safety profile of the medication and the severity of disease. Finally, the pharmacodynamic properties of the medication should be considered. Pharmacodynamics is the study of the relationship between the concentration of a drug and the response that is obtained in the patient. Although pharmacodynamic principles apply for all medications used in the intensive care unit (ICU), they have been most thoroughly studied with antibiotics.

Antibiotics typically are categorized as having either concentration-dependent or time-dependent activity (Table 293-3). The activity of *concentration-dependent*

TABLE 293-3

Pharmacokinetic/Pharmacodynamic Parameters of Renally Eliminated Anti-Infective Drugs

Concentration-Dependent	Time-Dependent	Hepatically Eliminated
Amikacin	Acyclovir	Caspofungin
Ciprofloxacin	Ampicillin	Ceftriaxone
Daptomycin	Aztreonam	Clindamycin
Gentamicin	Cefazolin	Linezolid
Levofloxacin	Cefepime	Metronidazole
Tobramycin	Cefotaxime	Micafungin
	Ertapenem	Moxifloxacin
	Fluconazole	Nafcillin
	Imipenem	Oxacillin
	Meropenem	
	Piperacillin	
	Ticarcillin	
	Vancomycin	
	Voriconazole	

antibiotics (e.g., aminoglycosides, fluoroquinolones) increases as the peak serum concentrations of drug increase. Dosing adjustments for renal failure, therefore, most often consist of prolonging the dosing interval with use of the same dose. By contrast, *time-dependent* antibiotics (e.g., beta-lactams) kill at the same rate regardless of the peak concentration that is achieved. The primary concern with these agents is to maintain a serum concentration that is above the minimum inhibitory concentration (MIC) for the infecting organism throughout most or all of the dosing interval. Thus, dosing adjustments for these agents should entail using a lower dose but maintaining a frequent dosing interval.

DOSING CONSIDERATIONS WITH RENAL REPLACEMENT THERAPY

Continuous Renal Replacement Therapy

Continuous renal replacement therapy (CRRT) is becoming the most popular modality for dialysis in the critically ill patient with AKI.[34] Optimizing drug dosing for CRRT can be extremely challenging because pharmacokinetic studies in children are limited. Dosing guidelines are available for the adult population, but it is essential to recognize their limitations, especially in extrapolating these recommendations for the pediatric population. First, many of these recommendations are based on pharmacokinetic studies conducted in otherwise healthy adults with chronic kidney disease on intermittent hemodialysis.[25] They fail to account for the differences in nonrenal clearance that are observed in patients with AKI. Even guidelines that are specific to pharmacokinetics with CRRT may be of limited relevance owing to the use of higher ultrafiltration rates and advanced dialysis filter technology. Furthermore, differences in drug removal may exist based on the method of clearance utilized as the efficiency of each mode can vary with each medication and its physical or chemical properties (i.e., molecular weight, water versus lipid solubility, and so on). Finally, the dialysis prescription used in pediatric patients can provide greater clearance than that achievable with the same prescription used in adults. Because the dialysis prescription typically is measured by urea kinetic modeling (i.e., Kt/V where k =

dialyzer clearance of urea, t = time of dialysis and, v = total body water) and V naturally is smaller in pediatric patients, greater clearance (and increased drug removal) can be obtained, because K and t do not vary.

Several factors that affect drug removal by CRRT include the characteristics of the drug, the mode of dialysis used (i.e., CVVH, CVVHD, or continuous venovenous hemodiafiltration [CVVHDF]) and the dialysis prescription within each mode.[25,32,35] One factor that affects drug removal, independent of the mode of dialysis, is V_d. Drugs that have a smaller V_d (i.e., less than 0.6 L/kg) are removed more effectively than drugs with a larger V_d. Drugs with a smaller V_d generally are confined to the plasma, which in pharmacokinetic terms is known as the central compartment. Only solutes present in the plasma are removed by CRRT (Fig. 293-1). Drugs with a larger V_d, on the other hand, distribute within deeper tissues. With rapid clearance from the central compartment during CRRT, equilibration will ultimately occur as the drug is transferred back into the central compartment from the deeper tissues. The rate-limiting step in this case is not the rate at which the drug can be eliminated by means of CRRT, but the rate at which the drug can transfer from the auxiliary compartment into the central compartment. An important point is that many patients with AKI will be fluid-overloaded secondary to oliguria, which will increase the V_d, particularly for water-soluble drugs (e.g., aminoglycosides). Removal of this fluid using CRRT will therefore lower the V_d and increase drug removal.

Drug removal through CVVH occurs by convection. One drug-specific factor that markedly affects clearance by means of CVVH is the sieving coefficient. The *sieving coefficient* is a measure of a solute's ability to cross the dialysis membrane and is calculated as the ultrafiltrate solute concentration divided by the simultaneous arterial solute concentration. The sieving coefficient is highly influenced by the degree of protein binding, which tends to be more readily available (e.g., from the package insert) and therefore can be used as an alternative for most medications (i.e., the sieving coefficient is equal to 1 minus the percent protein bound)[36] (Table 293-4). Drugs that are highly protein bound (i.e., greater than 80%) typically are not removed by CRRT.

During CVVH, drug removal is directly proportional to the ultrafiltration rate (Fig. 293-2). Furthermore, the method by which replacement fluids are administered can influence drug removal. Administration of replacement fluids proximal to the filter can dilute the concentration of solutes in the blood and reduce clearance by up to 15%.[37] This limitation usually can be overcome, however, by the use of additional ultrafiltration volume.

With CVVHD, drug removal occurs by diffusion. In this CRRT modality, clearance is affected by dialysate flow rate but also is strongly influenced by the drug's molecular weight (see Fig. 293-2).[37] Drugs that have a lower molecular weight are more effectively removed with CVVHD, and increases in dialysate flow rate have a more profound effect on their clearance. By contrast, clearance is not as efficient for drugs that have a higher molecular weight (e.g., vancomycin), and increasing the dialysate flow rate has less of an effect. Therefore, CVVH may be more efficient for larger-molecular-weight medications, because clearance is not significantly altered until molecular weight reaches 10,000 Daltons. Vancomycin, which is considered to be a drug with one of the largest molecular weights, is approximately 1450 Daltons.

Whereas sieving coefficients are used to calculate drug removal during CVVH, *saturation coefficients* are used for

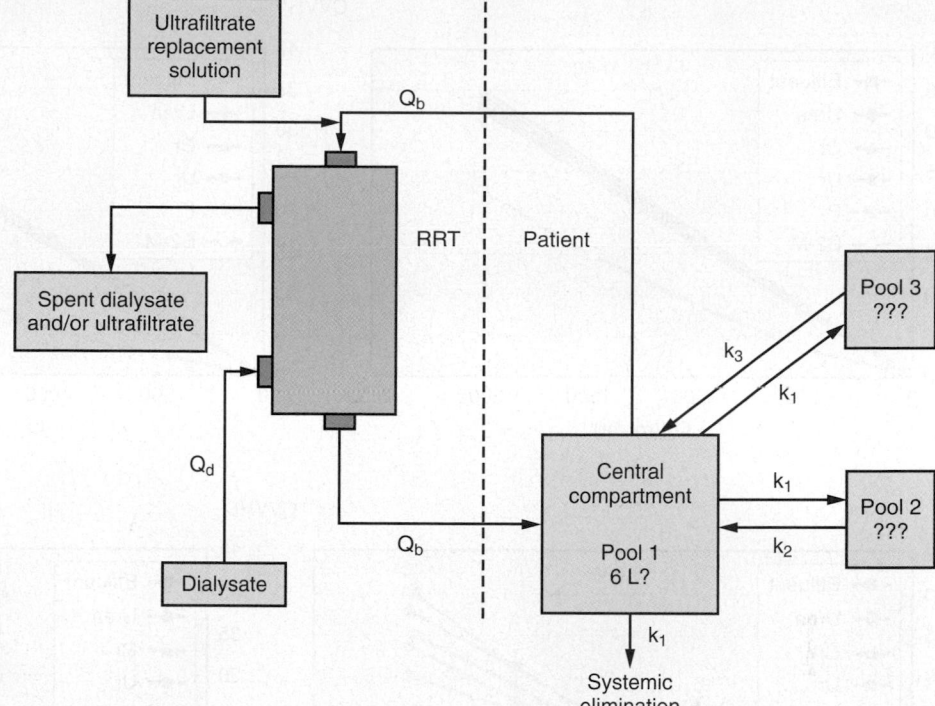

FIGURE 293-1. Pharmacokinetics of drug removal through continuous renal replacement therapy (RRT). Q_b, blood flow rate; Q_d, dialysate flow rate; K, rate of transfer. (Adapted from Mueller BA, Pasko DA, Sowinski KM: Higher renal replacement therapy dose delivery influences on drug therapy. Artif Organs 2003;27:808-814.)

TABLE 293-4

Sieving Coefficients of Commonly Used Medications in Continuous Renal Replacement Therapy

	Sieving Coefficient	
DRUG	**PREDICTED**	**MEASURED**
Amikacin	0.95	0.88-0.95
Amphotericin B	0.1	0.3-0.4
Amphotericin (Liposomal)	0.1	0.1
Ampicillin	0.8	0.69
Cefepime	0.82	0.72
Cefotaxime	0.62	0.51-1.06
Cefoxitin	0.3	0.3
Ceftazidime	0.9	0.9
Ceftriaxone	0.1	0.2-0.82
Cefuroxime	0.66	0.57-0.87
Ciprofloxacin	0.6	0.5-1.02
Clindamycin	0.4	0.49-0.98
Digoxin	0.75	0.96
Erythromycin	0.3	0.37
Fluconazole	0.88	1
Gentamicin	0.95	0.81
Imipenem	0.8	0.78
Meropenem	0.98	0.6-1
Metronidazole	0.8	0.86
Nafcillin	0.2	0.54
Phenobarbital	0.6	0.86
Phenytoin	0.1	0.45
Procainamide	0.86	0.86
Theophylline	0.47	0.85
Tobramycin	0.95	0.78-0.9
Vancomycin	0.9	0.5-0.8

Data from Golper TA: Update on drug sieving coefficients and dosing adjustments during continuous renal replacement therapies. Contrib Nephrol 2001;(132):349-353; and Joy MS, Matzke GR, Armstrong DK, et al: A primer on continuous renal replacement therapy for critically ill patients. Ann Pharmacother 1998;32:362-375.

CVVHD. The saturation coefficient is equal to the dialysate solute concentration divided by the simultaneous arterial solute concentration. With low-volume CRRT, the saturation coefficient closely approximates the sieving coefficient.[25] With high-volume CRRT, on the other hand, the difference between the saturation coefficient and the sieving coefficient may be more substantial, specifically for larger-sized molecules.

Drug clearance also will vary in accordance with the type of dialysis filter used. For example, vancomycin clearance was significantly greater with use of a polymethylmethacrylate filter, compared with an acrylonitrile and sodium methallyl sulfonate copolymer 0.6 m^2 (AN69) or polysulfone filters when dialysate flow rates exceeded 25 mL/minute[38] (Fig. 293-3). Drug clearance with CVVH, however, was not affected by filter type.

Many institutions use a combination of diffusive and convective mechanisms (e.g., CVVHDF). A combination protocol presents the most challenging scenario for optimizing drug dosing because of the lack of pharmacokinetic literature specific to pediatric patients and the variability in pharmacokinetics (as previously noted) related to drug clearance. Specifically, although both convection and diffusion are efficient in removing small particles, convection is more effective in removing middle- to larger-sized molecules. Unfortunately, combining the two methods does not always yield solute removal equivalent to the sum of the clearances for both methods used alone. In one study, clearance of smaller particles by CVVHDF using an M-60 filter was moderately reduced compared with the sum of the individual clearances.[37] Clearance values using an M-100 filter, on the other hand, were similar to the sum of both convective and diffusive clearance measured separately. By contrast, clearance of larger particles was markedly lower with both filters. In fact, the addition of diffusion did not increase clearance beyond that

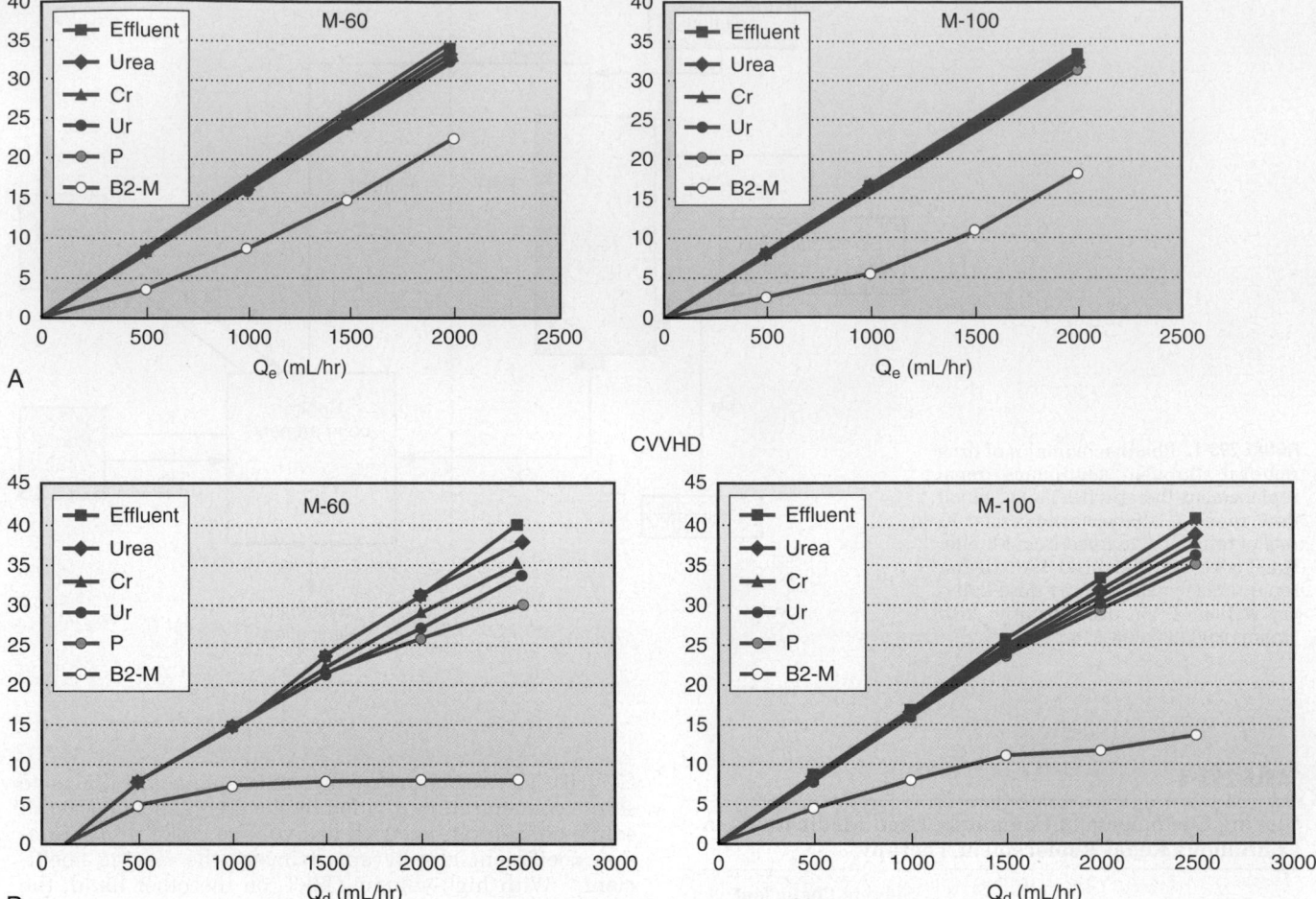

FIGURE 293-2. **A,** Convective clearances by means of CVVH for various solutes. **B,** Diffusive clearances by means of CVVHD for various solutes. B2-M, β_2-microglobulin; Cr, creatinine; CVVH, continuous venovenous hemofiltration; CVVHD, continuous venovenous hemodialysis; M-60, Multiflow 60; M-100, Multiflow 100; P, phosphate; Q_d, dialysate flow rate; Q_e, effluent flow rate; Ur, urate. (Adapted from Brunet S, Leblanc M, Geadah D, et al: Diffusive and convective solute clearances during continuous renal replacement therapy at various dialysate and ultrafiltration flow rates. Am J Kidney Dis 1999;34:486-492.)

achieved with convection alone. This limitation can have considerable impact in use of medications with a larger molecular weight, such as vancomycin.

The preferred method for developing dosing regimens in critically ill children on CRRT is to use data from published pharmacokinetic studies specific to the pediatric population. It is important that the dialysis filter type and fluid rates (i.e., dialysis fluid and ultrafiltrate fluid) used in the study be similar to that used in the clinician's individual practice. Unfortunately, this literature is limited, and extrapolations from adult-based guidelines or studies often must be made. In such instances, the pharmacokinetic alterations specific to children and the shortcomings of these studies themselves (regarding filter type, dialysis fluid rates, residual clearance, and so on) must be considered.

In many cases, an individualized approach should be sought. Two basic strategies for drug dosing during CRRT can be used.[33,39] The first begins with the dose recommended for normal renal function and adjusts downward. The second begins with the dose recommended for chronic kidney disease and adjusts upward. Both methods have their limitations, but the former may be preferable to the latter, especially for medications with a higher sieving coefficient.[25] One such approach is described in Figure 293-4.

Intermittent Hemodialysis

The predominant mechanism for drug removal by hemodialysis is diffusion. Three main factors influence a particular drug's removal: drug characteristics, the dialysis filter, and the dialysis prescription.[23] Drug characteristics that favor elimination through hemodialysis are a small V_d, a low degree of protein binding, high water solubility, and a low molecular weight.[23,32,35] The impact of molecular weight, however, has changed substantially with the availability of newer, high-flux dialysis filters. These filters have larger pore sizes, allowing for passage of molecules up to 20,000 daltons. Conventional filters typically are impermeable to molecules larger than 1000 daltons. Thus, vancomycin (approximately 1450 daltons in size) is not adequately removed with conventional hemodialysis but is extensively removed by high-flux techniques.

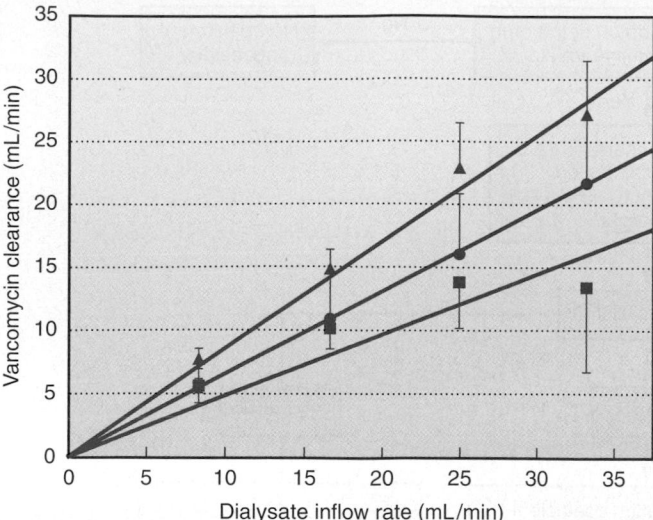

FIGURE 293-3. Vancomycin clearance by means of continuous venovenous hemodialysis (CVVHD) for the AN69 (■), PS (●), and PMMA (▲) filters at constant blood flow (Q_b) of 100 mL/minute. (Adapted from Joy MS, Matzke GR, Frye RF, Palevsky PM: Determinants of vancomycin clearance by continuous venovenous hemofiltration and continuous venovenous hemodialysis. Am J Kidney Dis 1998;31:1019-1027.)

After a hemodialysis session, occurrence of a "rebound" effect is not uncommon when the transfer rate of drug from blood to dialysate exceeds the transfer rate from the tissues to blood. For example, one study in adult patients demonstrated an increase in gentamicin serum concentration of approximately 27% within 1.5 hours after dialysis.[40] Caution is in order regarding interpretation of single post-dialysis drug concentrations in blood drawn immediately after dialysis, because the effectiveness of clearance can be overestimated. This error can lead to supratherapeutic doses and potentially increased toxicity.

In establishing drug regimens in the critically ill patient on hemodialysis, doses typically begin with the appropriate dose based on the estimated degree of residual renal function. Supplemental doses are therefore administered for medications that are adequately eliminated through hemodialysis. If doses are extrapolated from adult guidelines, a greater degree of drug removal for the pediatric patient should be considered.[41] Careful coordination of drug administration and the dialysis schedule is necessary to ensure that optimal drug concentrations are maintained. For example, administration of medications for which a high degree of clearance occurs through hemodialysis should be scheduled after the dialysis session has been completed. Greater clearance has been noted even for drugs that have a large V_d (and therefore minimal expected clearance) if they are administered immediately before or during dialysis, before distribution to the deeper tissues has been completed.

THERAPEUTIC DRUG MONITORING

Therapeutic drug monitoring can be particularly useful in optimizing dosing regimens for drugs that have a narrow therapeutic index. Some important considerations arise, however, in evaluating serum concentrations in patients with AKI. First is whether or not the serum concentration represents a steady-state level. Typically, it takes approximately 4 to 5 half-lives to reach steady state, but in the patient with AKI, half-life is significantly prolonged. Second is the timing of the level in relation to the dose. The most appropriate time for assessment (e.g., peak versus trough) will vary for each individual drug. It is essential to confirm that the blood sample was actually drawn at the time intended. For peak levels, adequate time for distribution must be allowed; otherwise, artificially high levels will be recorded. Samples for trough levels should be drawn within 1 hour before the next dose. A third factor is the timing of sampling in relation to dialysis and the potential for drug rebound. Finally, the severity of disease and specific pharmacodynamic principles (e.g., peak to MIC ratio for antibiotics) must be considered in determining the necessary therapeutic range.

CONCLUSION

A multitude of factors may affect drug dosing in critically ill children with renal failure who are undergoing renal replacement therapy. These factors can be drug-specific, practitioner-specific, or patient-specific. Failure to appreciate this variability can lead to suboptimal drug dosing, potentially increasing the risk for treatment failure or drug toxicity. Unfortunately, the literature evaluating drug dosing in renal failure that is specific to pediatric patients is limited. Extrapolations from the adult literature, clinical guidelines, and published references (electronic and print) must be made with caution, in view of the shortcomings of these recommendations and the advances in dialysis therapy since their publication. An individualized approach should be sought, with consideration of the clinician's personal preferences and practices. Therapeutic drug monitoring should be used when applicable.

Key Points

1. Pharmacokinetic alterations that occur in critically ill children with renal failure can be the source of significant error in dosing extrapolations from pharmacokinetic studies in healthy volunteers (and the adult literature), leading to inappropriate drug dosages in these patients.
2. Key considerations in establishing a dosing regimen in critically ill children with renal failure include the proportion of renal clearance in relation to total body clearance, balance between a need for aggressive therapy and the adverse effect profile for the medication, and the pharmacodynamic properties of the drug.
3. Factors that affect drug removal during continuous renal replacement therapy are the characteristics of the drug (e.g., volume of distribution, degree of protein binding, molecular weight), the mode of dialysis used (i.e., continuous venovenous hemofiltration, continuous venovenous hemodialysis, or continuous venovenous hemodiafiltration), and the dialysis prescription within each mode.
4. Dialysis prescriptions that use both convective and diffusive mechanisms represent the most dif-

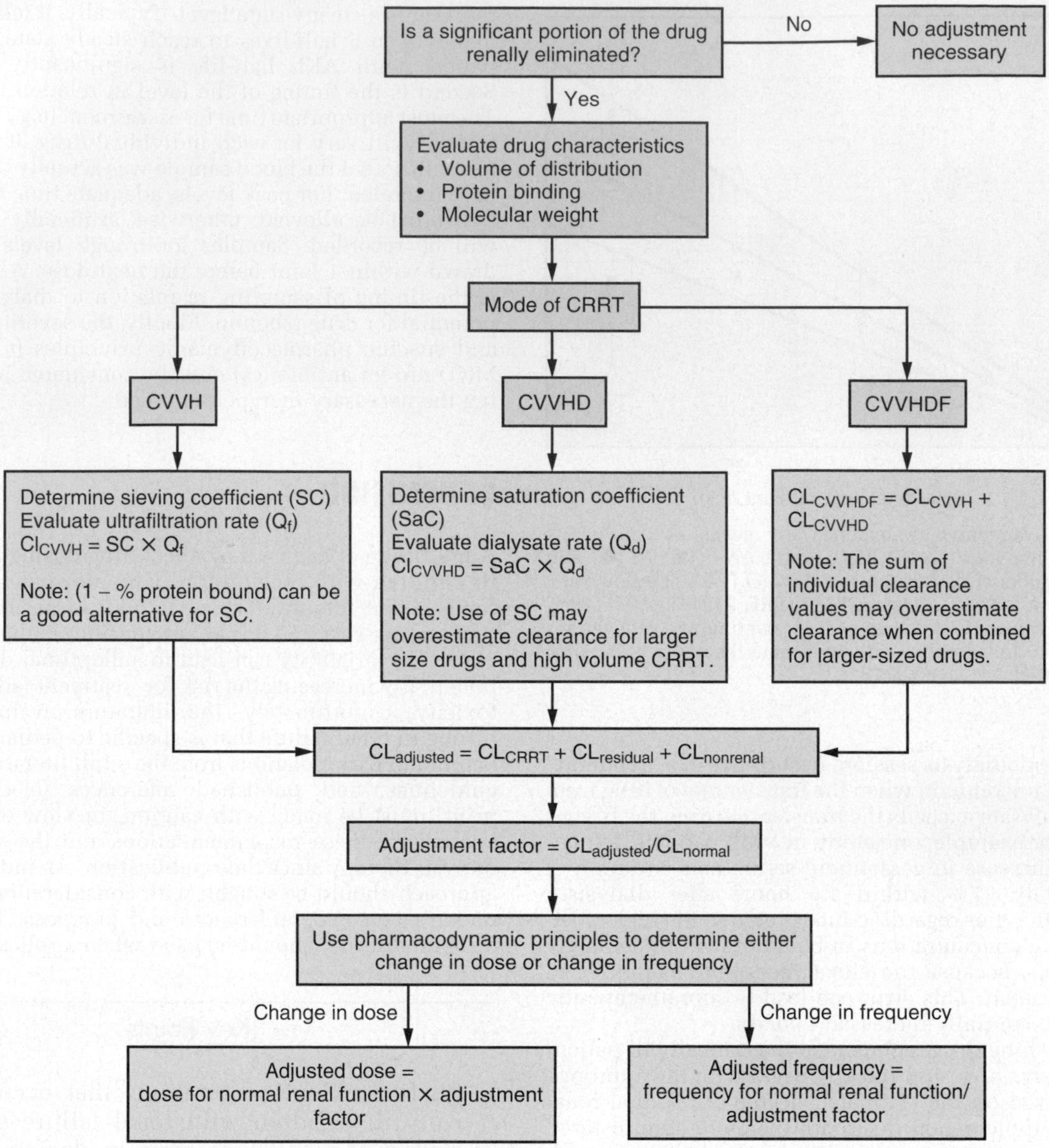

FIGURE 293-4. Algorithm for individualized drug dosing and continuous renal replacement therapy (CRRT). CVVH, continuous venovenous hemofiltration; CVVHD, continuous venovenous hemodialysis; CVVHDF, continuous venovenous hemodiafiltration.

ficult scenarios for drug dosing, because combining the two methods may not always yield solute removal equivalent to the sum of removal with both methods alone.

5. The availability of newer, high-flux dialysis filters has allowed for removal of drugs with much larger molecular weights, such as vancomycin.

6. Therapeutic drug monitoring should be used to optimize dosing regimens for drugs that have a narrow therapeutic index.

Key References

5. Thomas L, Huber AR: Renal function—estimation of glomerular filtration rate. Clin Chem Lab Med 2006;44:1295-1302.

25. Mueller BA, Pasko DA, Sowinski KM: Higher renal replacement therapy dose delivery influences on drug therapy. Artif Organs 2003;27:808-814.

32. Bugge JF: Influence of renal replacement therapy on pharmacokinetics in critically ill patients. Best Pract Res Clin Anaesthesiol 2004;18:175-187.

35. Golper TA, Marx MA: Drug dosing adjustments during continuous renal replacement therapies. Kidney Int Suppl 1998;66:S165-S168.

43. Joy MS, Matzke GR, Armstrong DK, et al: A primer on continuous renal replacement therapy for critically ill patients. Ann Pharmacother 1998;32:362-375.

See the companion Expert Consult website for the complete reference list.

CHAPTER 294

Nutrition of Critically Ill Children with Acute Renal Failure

Michael Zappitelli, Norma J. Maxvold, and Leticia Castillo

OBJECTIVES

This chapter will:
1. Summarize important background information on managing nutrition in pediatric acute renal failure and during renal replacement therapy.
2. Review important relevant pediatric studies on nutrition in children with acute renal failure.
3. Present suggested nutritional guidelines for use in critically ill children with acute renal failure.

Malnutrition is prevalent among critically ill patients with a prolonged or protracted clinical course.[1,2] Supplying adequate and optimal nutrition for the critically ill child with acute renal failure (ARF) is an important and elusive goal. Malnutrition in ARF generally is a result of starvation due to poor nutritional support but may also be a component of the hypermetabolic state often present in critically ill patients with ARF.[3-6] Nutritional intake in ARF must meet the complex demands imposed by this condition and the consequent stress response in these patients.

Adequate nutrition in critically ill children with ARF is a crucial component of their treatment. Critically ill children, particularly infants, are at especially high risk for the development of protein-energy malnutrition, or of specific nutritional deficiencies, because of their proportionately higher nutritional needs for growth and maintenance.[3,7] The percent body mass accounted for by protein, decreases with age, placing very young children at high risk for protein malnutrition. In addition, the inverse relationship between energy expenditure and body weight leads to higher energy needs per kilogram of body weight in younger children.[3,7]

ARF poses special challenges in providing adequate nutrition in the pediatric intensive care unit (PICU). Critically ill children with uremia demonstrate substantial declines in anthropometric measures at PICU discharge.[8] ARF in children often is associated with increased severity of illness,[9] which contributes to the high risk for serious nutritional deficits. Moreover, children with ARF often have chronic conditions predisposing them to poor baseline nutritional status.[9,10] The additional need for continued growth in the setting of prolonged illness marks adequate nutrition as particularly important for these children.[11-15] Furthermore, renal replacement therapy (RRT) contributes to additional nutritional losses.

Data on specific nutritional needs of critically ill children, including patients with ARF, are limited. To date, no evidence-based guidelines for nutrition of pediatric ARF have been reported. Thus, the nutritional management of these children is based on knowledge acquired from adult literature, concepts of alterations in nutrient utilization known to be present in ARF, and the limited available data on critically ill children without ARF. The general goal of nutritional management is to avoid catabolism, with consequent growth retardation and underfeeding, while avoiding overfeeding in the context of the metabolic abnormalities present in ARF. For a detailed description of basic concepts of energy and protein metabolism in ARF of critical illness and of nutrition of the critically ill child, the reader is referred to appropriate chapters in Part I, Section 8, of this book. This chapter presents an approach to nutritional assessment and management of pediatric patients with acute renal failure.

EVALUATING BASELINE NUTRITIONAL STATUS

Assessment of nutritional status in the child with ARF is an important component of evaluation but is very difficult to achieve. Clinicians use a combination of anthropometric and laboratory data to diagnose malnutrition.[8] Carefully elicited past history with details of weight gain, dietary history, recent illness, and medications allows identification of risk factors for preadmission malnutrition. Height-for-age or weight-for-height values less than the 90th percentile for age and gender suggest poor baseline nutritional status.[1] Weight on hospital admission is important and may be the only estimate of the actual dry weight before the capillary leak syndrome and fluid retention lead to edema and weight gain. When admission weight cannot be established with certainty, ideal body weight can be used for nutritional calculations. Triceps skinfold thickness and midarm muscle circumference are difficult to interpret. Furthermore, biochemical parameters such as albumin, prealbumin, and visceral proteins also will be altered by fluid shifts. Weight changes during the ICU stay should be interpreted in the context of fluid therapy, diuresis, or other causes of altered fluid status. Physical examination can be directed to look for specific signs of nutritional and metabolic deficiencies. Hair, skin, eyes, mouth, and extremities may reveal stigmata of protein-energy malnutrition or vitamin and mineral deficiencies.[1]

NUTRITIONAL APPROACH

Estimating nutritional requirements in critically ill children is a challenging endeavor. Fluid overload is an important factor in the early phase of critical illness, and it limits nutritional intake. Intolerance to lipid and glucose administration and increased protein breakdown add to the challenge of providing adequate nutritional support. Yet recovery from critical illness will require adequate protein synthesis and metabolic support.

Recommendations for pediatric nutritional requirements traditionally have focused on the supply of nutrients for growth. Current recommendations for nutritional requirements of the critically ill child with ARF are derived from limited data, based on studies in healthy children and on limited methodological approaches.[16] Although the Food and Agricultural Organization (FAO) and the World Health Organization (WHO) have recommended that energy requirements and dietary recommendations be based on measurements of energy expenditure, adherence to this recommendation is difficult in the critically ill child with ARF. Ideally, determination of initial nutrient requirements and its prescription requires careful assessment of (1) initial nutritional status and (2) extent of injury or insult during current ICU admission.

Early institution of enteral nutrition should always be attempted for all critically ill children, unless contraindicated.[17-19] Enterally administered feedings meet nutritional requirements in critically ill children with a functional gastrointestinal system and have the advantages of low cost, manageability, safety, and preservation of gastrointestinal function. Early introduction of enteral feeding in critically ill patients helps to achieve positive protein and energy balance and restores nitrogen balance during the acute hypermetabolic state of illness. In addition, enteral nutrition maintains gut integrity and elicits release of growth factors and hormones that also maintain gut integrity and function.[20]

Children with ARF are at high risk for the development of hyperphosphatemia and hyperkalemia; therefore, enteral formulas designed for patients with renal disease (e.g., Suplena, Nepro) should be used. These formulas are concentrated to minimize fluid intake without sacrificing protein and caloric intake. If continuous renal replacement therapy (CRRT) is initiated, regular pediatric formulas generally can be instituted, with close monitoring of serum potassium and phosphate, and full awareness of the added electrolyte burden during nondialysis periods (e.g., for CRRT circuit change). Because children with ARF requiring dialysis often are affected by contraindications to use of enteral feeding alone, the use of parenteral nutrition often will be required. An attempt should be made to maintain enteral feedings, even if they are only for trophic purposes. Once contraindications are resolved, enteral feedings should be instituted, even during RRT.

ENERGY PROVISION

The measurement of resting energy expenditure (REE) in critically ill children has been broadly investigated. By using indirect calorimetry (with a bedside metabolic cart), REE in ventilated children is readily obtainable,[13,21] with the same limitations as in adults.[12,21] When large endotracheal tube leaks are present, alternative isotope methods may be used, which are not affected by air leaks or the fraction of inspired oxygen (FIO_2).[22,23] Concerns have emerged regarding the validity of measuring REE in patients receiving RRT, particularly CRRT. These problems are related to bicarbonate fluxes that occur at the level of the hemodialysis membrane: Use of bicarbonate-based dialysis solutions may lead to "bicarbonate enrich-

ment" in the patient, which converts to CO_2, potentially leading to false elevation of expired CO_2, with consequent overestimation of REE. The converse may be true when bicarbonate-free solutions are used.[24-26] The extent to which this phenomenon actually affects REE measurements has not been defined. Further study on the use of stable isotope methods for measuring REE in patients receiving RRT may clarify this uncertainty.

The literature on predictive equations for REE in critically ill children is extensive.[21,27-31] Comparisons with measured energy expenditures have led to unanimous consensus on the inaccuracy of these predictive equations.[28,31-33] Nevertheless, they frequently are used in the PICU setting as a reference point for determination of basal energy needs.

Controversy also exists regarding whether critically ill children have elevated REE, with some authors reporting REE as high as 25% above expected basal metabolic needs[14,33,34] and others reporting that REE is not affected by critical illness or diagnostic categories (such as sepsis).[5,21,22,31,35,36] The range of mean REE values reported in critically ill pediatric patients has been between 35 and 65 kcal/kg per day (0.15 and 0.27 MJ/kg per day), probably owing to differences in severity of illness and patient populations. No studies have examined the relationship between REE and pediatric ARF, so the contribution of ARF to the hypermetabolic state is unknown.

It has been suggested that caloric intake 20% to 30% above the estimated requirement will provide adequate calories in most children with ARF,[4] without significant risk of overfeeding and associated complications.[7] This intake will often differ from that recommended for adults of 35 kcal/kg per day.[37,38] Under physiological conditions, a close interrelationship exists between protein and energy (glucose and fat) metabolism. Excess carbohydrate loads may induce lipogenesis.[39,40] An increase in the energy supply will not promote nitrogen retention unless the amino acid supply is adequate, and conversely, an increased amino acid supply will not be useful if energy is limited—hence the importance of providing adequate energy and protein intake. Thus, the energy provision should consist of approximately 20% to 25% carbohydrates (with insulin as needed to maintain normal serum glucose levels), in order to avoid excess CO_2 with subsequent ventilatory burden and hyperglycemia.[7] Lipid supplementation, in the form of 20% lipid emulsions, consisting of 30% to 40% of total energy needs, should be provided, as in other critically ill children. The remainder of energy needs should be provided by protein.

PROTEIN INTAKE

Abnormal amino acid metabolism in ARF resuts from a number of factors to by factors related to severe critical illness (including increased hepatic gluconeogenesis, relative insulin resistance, metabolic acidosis, and elevated stress hormones),[11,41] altered protein metabolism associated with ARF, and losses incurred with RRT. Protein turnover is highest in younger children and is associated with increased REE.[24] In ARF, the kidney's role in synthesis and metabolism of amino acids is reduced, also contributing to amino acid imbalances.[41-43] This hypercatabolism can manifest as protein malnutrition, muscle wasting, weight loss, a high rate of urea nitrogen appearance (180 to 250 mg/kg per day),[4,15] and a net negative nitrogen balance.

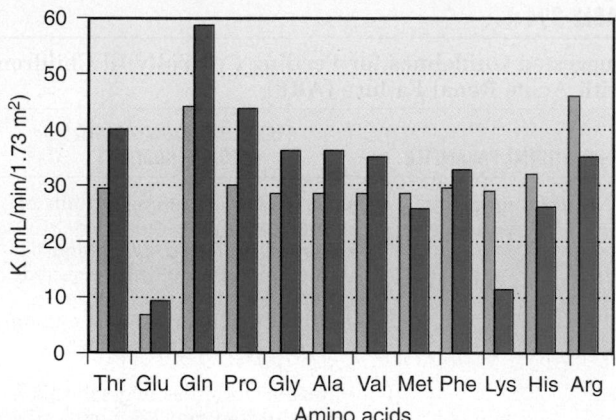

FIGURE 294-1. Clearance (K) of essential amino acids by continuous renal replacement therapy in critically ill children with acute renal failure. *Light blue bars* represent amino acid clearance achieved by continuous venovenous hemofiltration,[4] and *dark blue bars,* clearance by continuous venovenous hemodialysis.[44] Thr, threonine; Glu, glutamic acid; Gln, glutamine; Pro, proline; Gly, glycine; Ala, alanine; Val, valine; Met, methionine; Phe, phenylalanine; Lys, lysine; His, histidine; Arg, arginine. (Data from Maxvold NJ, Smoyer WE, Custer JR, Bunchman TE: Amino acid loss and nitrogen balance in critically ill children with acute renal failure: A prospective comparison between classic hemofiltration and hemofiltration with dialysis. Crit Care Med 2000;28:1161-1165; and Zappitelli M, Castillo L, Coss-Bu J, et al: Continuous veno-venous hemodialysis leads to amino acid, trace element, and folate clearance in critically ill children. J Am Soc Nephrol 2006;17:767A.)

During acute illness, it is difficult to decrease protein breakdown, but protein synthesis can be increased by supplying amino acids.[13,14,20] Of note, however, critically ill children without ARF had a negative nitrogen balance despite the provision of 2.5 g/kg per day in one study.[13] The task of achieving positive nitrogen balance becomes even more difficult in the presence of RRT, as a result of the additional losses of amino acids through the hemofilter. As in adults, amino acid losses by continuous venovenous hemofiltration (CVVH),[4,15] continuous venovenous hemodiafiltration (CVVHDF),[4] and continuous venovenous hemodialysis (CVVHD)[44] can be anywhere from 10% to 20% of the amount provided in the parenteral nutrition (PN) solution, which is associated with the development of negative nitrogen balance.[4]

The clearance of amino acids by CRRT generally is in the range of 20 to 40 mL/minute/1.73 m², similar to urea clearance (Fig. 294-1); however, a higher clearance of glutamine,[4,44] which is not included in most pediatric PN solutions, has been observed. In one pediatric study, glutamine losses during CRRT accounted for approximately 25% of all amino acid losses.[4] Multiple adult clinical trials of glutamine supplementation in critical illness suggest some benefit of modulating the catabolic state, including reduction in infectious morbidity and decrease in length of stay. Interstudy findings have been controversial, however.[45-49] Thus, glutamine supplementation may be beneficial in the setting of prolonged CRRT, but further study is required. Only one pediatric study describes serum amino acid levels just before initiation of CRRT[44]: Although some amino acid levels were on average decreased (arginine and serine, as expected, owing to the kidney's role in their synthesis),[50,51] it is unlikely that serum levels adequately reflect body stores or amino acid

utilization. Future studies evaluating the actual utilization of amino acids provided to children in ARF must be performed, using stable isotope–labeled amino acid studies,[42,43] in order to elucidate the regulatory mechanisms of protein homeostasis under conditions of pediatric ARF, and to what extent additional protein supply is beneficial for protein turnover.

In view of the age-associated baseline elevated protein needs of children and the presence of abnormal amino acid synthesis and increased protein catabolism in critical illness and ARF, daily protein intake in these children should be on the order of at least 2 to 3 g/kg per day. During RRT, commensurate adjustment of protein intake must be made to account for losses in the dialysate (10% to 20% of amino acid intake). It has been recommended to aim for serum urea nitrogen levels in the range of 40 to 80 mg/dL as a guide to determining whether protein intake is sufficient during RRT. No specific pediatric amino acid solutions for ARF currently are available; however, future research is likely to reveal that such parenteral solutions may be beneficial.

ELECTROLYTES

Electrolyte disturbances caused by ARF in children are similar to those due to ARF in adults: hyperkalemia, hyponatremia of variable degree, hypocalcemia, hyperphosphatemia, hypermagnesemia, and metabolic acidosis[52] and are covered extensively elsewhere in this book. Of note, however, children with ARF often are nonoliguric, particularly if the primary etiological factor is exposure to nephrotoxic medication.[9,52] Moreover, pediatric-specific diagnoses, such as cystic dysplasia or nephrogenic diabetes insipidus, may be associated with frank polyuria, which can lead to significant losses of sodium and other electrolytes, free water, or both. Thus, serum electrolytes must be extremely closely monitored and replaced, if needed, in these settings.

VITAMINS AND TRACE ELEMENTS

Very little literature exists on vitamin and trace element metabolism in pediatric critical illness, and none in pediatric ARF. In adults with severe ARF, profound deficiencies in water-soluble and fat-soluble vitamins have been found, vitamin K being the exception.[53] Levels of water-soluble vitamins often are low in the setting of RRT losses,[53,54] and changes in several trace elements have been found in association with ARF in adults.[53,54]

For children with ARF managed by CRRT, losses of water-soluble vitamins are likely. Thus, for children receiving CRRT for prolonged periods, serum levels should be monitored, and additional supplementation may be required. An exception is vitamin C; because of a concern for the development of oxalosis, no more than 200 g/day should be provided.

In one pediatric study evaluating the clearance of five trace elements—manganese, copper, selenium, chromium, and zinc—in 14 critically ill children receiving CRRT, approximately 50% of the patients had low serum zinc levels and approximately 25% had low serum copper levels, whereas other serum levels were in the normal range, before CRRT initiation.[44] Serum zinc and copper levels, however, are difficult to interpret owing to their

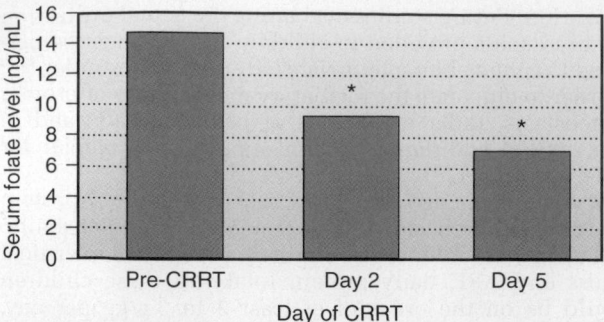

FIGURE 294-2. Clearance of folate by continuous venovenous hemodialysis in critically ill children with acute renal failure. CRRT, continuous renal replacement therapy; *, serum levels significantly reduced from pre-CRRT levels. (Data from Zappitelli M, Castillo L, Coss-Bu J, et al: Continuous veno-venous hemodialysis leads to amino acid, trace element, and folate clearance in critically ill children. J Am Soc Nephrol 2006;17:767A.)

association with other factors such as serum albumin (zinc) and the presence of inflammation (copper and zinc).[53] Most of these patients had been receiving PN solutions with standard additional trace element pediatric preparations at the time of CRRT initiation; thus, the presence of normal serum selenium and chromium concentrations suggests that the supplementation was adequate. The clearance achieved by CVVHD for each of the trace elements generally was below 10 mL/minute/1.73 m², except for chromium, which had a clearance of approximately 25 mL/minute/1.73 m². Moreover, clearance rates were stable on days 2 and 5 of the CRRT regimen, but serum levels were unchanged. The extent to which additional trace element supplementation should be provided in children with ARF is still unclear.

In the aforementioned pediatric study, folate clearance also was measured and found to be approximately 16 mL/minute/1.73 m² (in keeping with properties of a moderate volume of distribution and protein binding but relatively small size of the folate molecule) and was stable on days 2 and 5 of CRRT initiation. Although serum folate levels decreased by approximately 50% from CRRT initiation to 5 days after initiation, serum levels were still in the normal range on day 5 (Fig. 294-2). Therefore, it is possible that additional folate supplementation is needed in children who are receiving CRRT for prolonged periods. Until more research is performed in the area of vitamin and trace element metabolism in ARF and on the effect of losses due to RRT, we recommend providing the recommended daily allowances in standard pediatric formulations, as well as monitoring water-soluble vitamin, trace element, and folate levels in children receiving prolonged RRT.

CONCLUSION

The principles of nutritional care of critically ill children with ARF are based mostly on those of nutrition in critically ill children and from adult studies of ARF. Of note, however, children with ARF often have prolonged illness, chronic conditions, or increased severity of illness, so they are at high risk for the development of specific nutritional deficiencies or protein-energy malnutrition. The need for support for continued growth constitutes an additional

---

TABLE 294-1

Suggested Guidelines for Feeding Critically Ill Children with Acute Renal Failure (ARF)

NUTRITIONAL PARAMETER	LEVEL 3 EVIDENCE–BASED RECOMMENDATIONS
Nutrition modality	• Early enteral feeding (within 24 hours of admission) • Enteral preferred; parenteral nutrition often will be required • Renal formulas are used in children who are uremic and not receiving renal replacement therapy • Regular formulas may be used for children on CRRT, but monitor electrolytes and change to renal formulas if CRRT is stopped
Total energy	• Approximately 20% to 30% above basal metabolic needs as measured on metabolic cart or estimated with equations
Energy composition	• 20% to 25% as carbohydrates (insulin as needed); 30% to 40% lipid formulations (20% lipid emulsions); 40% to 50% protein
Protein	• 2 to 3 g/kg/day with ARF • Increase intake if on CRRT (by 20%)
Vitamins	• Daily recommended intake • Monitor serum folate, water-soluble vitamin levels ± replacement with prolonged CRRT (more than 1 week) • Activated vitamin D may be needed in prolonged ARF
Trace elements	• Daily recommended intake
Monitoring	• Resting energy expenditure, nitrogen balance, electrolytes, vitamins, trace elements

CRRT, continuous renal replacement therapy.

challenge in management of the critically ill pediatric patient. Nutrition is an integral component of care for these children. Indeed, nutritional needs are an indication for initiation of dialysis.[55,56] A summary of the suggested recommendations for feeding children with ARF is presented in Table 294-1. Future research on the effects of RRT on specific nutritional losses and on the abnormalities in substrate utilization in ARF may reveal more specific nutritional requirements in this select population.

Key Points

1. Critically ill children with acute renal failure are at very high risk for the development of protein-energy malnutrition because of a frequent association with poor baseline nutritional status, increased severity of illness, abnormal amino acid metabolism, elevated protein and energy needs, and the requirement for continued growth.

2. The preferred mode of feeding children with acute renal failure is use of the enteral route.
3. Ten percent to 20% of amino acids (relative to intake) are lost through the dialysis membrane during pediatric continuous renal replacement therapy, which must be accounted for in prescribing the nutritional regimen.
4. Total energy provision should be approximately 20% to 30% above resting energy expenditure, and protein intake should be at least 2 to 3 g/kg per day.
5. The nutritional management of children with acute renal failure must be performed in a multidisciplinary fashion (involving the physician, a nutritionist, and a pharmacist) and must be reassessed frequently.

Key References

1. Bettler J, Roberts KE: Nutrition assessment of the critically ill child. AACN Clin Issues 2000;11:498-506.
4. Maxvold NJ, Smoyer WE, Custer JR, Bunchman TE: Amino acid loss and nitrogen balance in critically ill children with acute renal failure: A prospective comparison between classic hemofiltration and hemofiltration with dialysis. Crit Care Med 2000;28:1161-1165.
5. Oosterveld MJ, Van Der Kuip M, De Meer K, et al: Energy expenditure and balance following pediatric intensive care unit admission: A longitudinal study of critically ill children. Pediatr Crit Care Med 2006;7:147-153.
6. Rogers EJ, Gilbertson HR, Heine RG, Henning R: Barriers to adequate nutrition in critically ill children. Nutrition 2003; 19:865-868.
7. Agus MS, Jaksic T: Nutritional support of the critically ill child. Curr Opin Pediatr 2002;14:470-481.

See the companion Expert Consult website for the complete reference list.

CHAPTER 295

Continuous Renal Replacement Therapies in Combination with Other Extracorporeal Therapies

Matthew L. Paden and James D. Fortenberry

OBJECTIVES

This chapter will:
1. Describe the use of continuous renal replacement therapy in neonatal and pediatric patients on extracorporeal membrane oxygenation support.
2. Discuss practical aspects and concerns in using continuous renal replacement therapy with extracorporeal membrane oxygenation in neonatal and pediatric age groups.
3. Review considerations in the use of continuous renal replacement therapy in combination with other extracorporeal therapies for severe septic shock.

RATIONALE FOR USE OF CONTINUOUS RENAL REPLACEMENT THERAPY WITH EXTRACORPOREAL SUPPORT

Failure of the cardiac or respiratory system is a common problem in critically ill patients in pediatric and neonatal intensive care units (PICUs and NICUs). When conventional management fails to improve the child's condition, extracorporeal life support techniques such as extracorporeal membrane oxygenation (ECMO) can provide lifesaving temporary heart and lung support.[1] Illnesses leading to respiratory failure can require large-volume fluid resuscitation, and once on ECMO, patients can receive large amounts of blood products. Renal failure often compli-

cates care of these critically ill children on ECMO, leading to accumulation of fluid and volume overload that can worsen their heart and lung disease.[2,3] Reported rates of acute renal failure (ARF) requiring renal replacement therapy in patients on ECMO range from 40% to 69%, depending on the population studied and the definition of renal insufficiency used.[2,4-6] Weber and Kountzman[2] described development of renal failure in 10 (18%) of 55 children on ECMO. However, 38 (69%) of these patients received ultrafiltration or hemodialysis for control of renal failure or fluid overload that could not be adequately managed with diuretics alone. In a recent large cohort of children with congenital heart disease whose management included ECMO, transient renal insufficiency developed in 41 (49%) of 94 patients.[4] Elevated creatinine was seen in 53 of 100 adult patients on ECMO in a University of Michigan review.[6] Consensus is lacking regarding the optimal method of treatment of ARF during ECMO; center-specific trends range from fluid restriction and diuretic therapy to aggressive early institution of continuous renal replacement therapy (CRRT) concomitant with institution of ECMO. The development of ARF during ECMO support is an independent risk factor associated with increased mortality.[6-8] Presence of ARF before cannulation, however, is not considered an absolute contraindication to ECMO.

The presence of fluid overload is associated with pulmonary edema, worsening lung injury, and increased incidence of multiple organ failure in critically ill patients.[9,10] Recent studies have suggested that improved fluid balance may be associated with improved outcomes in critically ill patients.[11,12] Restrictive fluid management has been demonstrated to improve patient outcomes in acute lung injury.[10] In patients receiving other extracorporeal therapies, CRRT can be used either in its usual role as a treatment for renal failure or as a tool for meticulous fluid management and correction of massive volume overload. The institution of CRRT in patients on ECMO can potentially allow minute-to-minute control of fluid balance by providing continuous fluid, electrolyte, and toxin clearance even in the absence of adequate native renal function. CRRT allows restoration of positive fluid balance in patients who are in a resuscitative phase requiring additional intravascular volume, as well as providing a means for slow removal of fluid without resultant hypotension once the patient stabilizes.

spective nature) suggests that fluid overload is a risk factor for death in pediatric critically ill patients. Of note, however, children on ECMO were excluded from these studies. Data on fluid overload and mortality in patients on ECMO are lacking. Decreasing fluid overload has been associated with improved outcomes in retrospective studies of neonates[15] and children on ECMO.[15,16] In addition, it has been suggested that degree of fluid overload may correlate with duration of ECMO support for neonates.[17] The cumulative experience of these studies supports a judicious approach to fluid management in an attempt to avoid fluid overload.

FLUID OVERLOAD IN PEDIATRIC CRITICAL ILLNESS

Goldstein and associates[12] noted a correlation between fluid overload and mortality in a small study of 21 pediatric patients with ARF requiring CRRT. Percent fluid overload at the time of CRRT initiation was defined as ([fluid in − fluid out]/PICU admission weight) × 100. Survivors had significantly less fluid overload compared with nonsurvivors (median, 16% versus 34%); the association was independent of risk-adjusted mortality. A larger study of 77 children with ARF[13] confirmed this association, finding that greater than 10% fluid overload at initiation of CRRT was associated with a threefold increase in death over that associated with low or no fluid overload (Fig. 295-1). A retrospective analysis by Foland and coworkers[11] of outcomes in 113 pediatric patients who received CRRT supported previous findings and also demonstrated that percent fluid overload was independently associated with survival from three-organ or greater multiple organ dysfunction syndrome (MODS). In the first-reported multicenter experience from the seven-center Prospective Pediatric CRRT Registry[14] members, 116 patients demonstrated significantly less fluid overload in CRRT survivors compared with nonsurvivors (median, 14% versus 25%). The weight of the evidence (although limited by its retro-

MANAGEMENT OF FLUID BALANCE IN EXTRACORPOREAL LIFE SUPPORT

During resuscitation, patients often require intravenous volume replacement, blood products, and medications, all of which can rapidly lead to fluid overload. In these critically ill patients, renal insufficiency with oliguria or anuria also can develop before or during the ECMO course. Management often uses fluid restriction, which decreases optimal caloric intake, which in turn is potentially detrimental to overall outcomes.[18] Treating or preventing fluid overload in this setting can require aggressive use of diuretics. Use of diuretics has been associated with worsened outcomes in critically ill adults with renal failure,[19] although the significance of this association is controversial.[20] Continuous venovenous hemofiltration (CVVH) allows meticulous, minute-to-minute control of fluid balance by providing continuous fluid, electrolyte, and toxin clearance, even in the absence of adequate native renal function. Thus, the addition of CVVH to the ECMO circuit offers a potential solution for improved fluid homeostasis.

Several series have directly described a benefit for use of CVVH in neonatal[15] and pediatric[16] ECMO. In a single-center experience, Hoover and colleagues[21] compared 26 pediatric patients with respiratory failure receiving CVVH

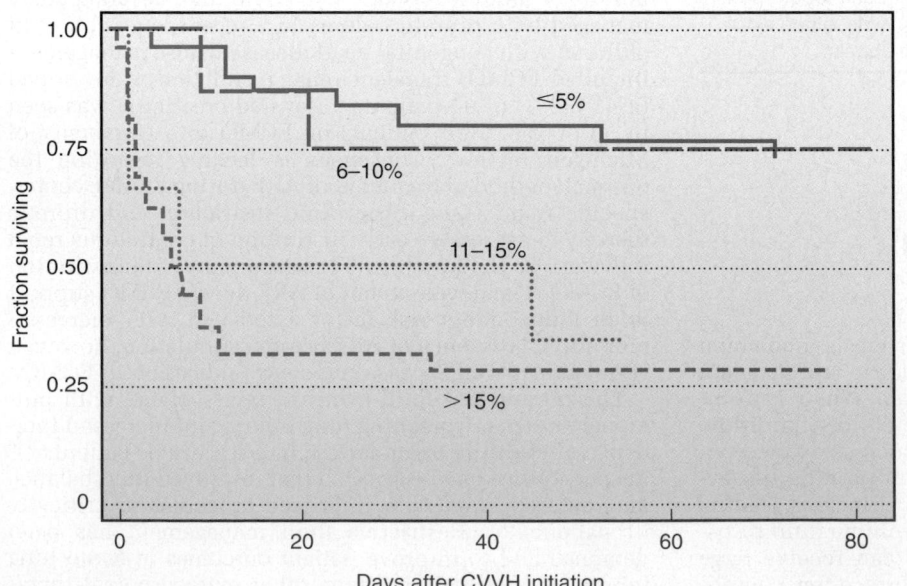

FIGURE 295-1. Kaplan-Meier survival estimates for pediatric patients receiving continuous renal replacement therapy, by degree of fluid overload. *Individual lines* represent fraction of patients surviving after CVVH initiation for each level of percent fluid overload, as described in text. (From Gillespie RS, Seidel K, Symons JM: Effect of fluid overload and dose of replacement fluid on survival in hemofiltration. Pediatr Nephrol 2004;19:1394-1399, with permission.)

during their ECMO run (in 15 with CVVH, for greater than 40% of total ECMO run) with case-matched controls not receiving CVVH. All patients receiving CVVH while on ECMO had significantly less fluid overload on ECMO when calculated for CVVH days alone (median fluid balance, +25 mL/kg per day versus +40 mL/kg per day; $P = .022$). Among the survivors, patients on ECMO plus CVVH had less fluid overload for the overall ECMO course compared with patients on ECMO without CVVH (median, +25 mL/kg per day; range −40 to +71, versus +40 mL/kg per day, range +1.1 to +135; $P = .028$). Overall ECMO duration and ventilator days were not different with CVVH. Of note, however, patients on ECMO plus CVVH had shorter time to desired caloric intake (median, 1 day versus 5 days; $P < .001$) and less daily furosemide use (median, 0.67 mg/kg versus 2.11 mg/kg; $P < .009$).[21]

PRACTICAL ASPECTS OF CONTINUOUS RENAL REPLACEMENT THERAPY WITH EXTRACORPOREAL MEMBRANE OXYGENATION

Many centers using CVVH in patients on ECMO add a traditional hemofiltration machine to the ECMO circuit. Although both the arterial and the venous sides of the oxygenator have been used, the current standard is to place the hemofilter before the oxygenator to reduce the likelihood of embolism to the patient. Although the specific configuration of ECMO circuits varies across centers, the method used at our institution (Children's Healthcare of Atlanta) uses the pre-membrane technique. Blood is removed from a catheter attached to the circuit bladder, circulated through a hemofilter using a CRRT delivery system (Diapact, Braun, Bethlehem, PA), and reinfused into the circuit by way of a pre-bladder pigtail catheter. This creates an element of recirculation of previously hemofiltered blood back to the hemofilter but the amount is clinically insignificant owing to the overall high circuit flows achieved in ECMO. This arrangement creates no difference between set pump flow and pump flow delivered to the patient. Anticoagulation is maintained by the heparin regimen used for ECMO. No adjustment in activated clotting time is necessary with the addition of hemofiltration. No adjustment to routine blood flow calculation is necessary so long as venous return is adequate. Precipitation of calcium salts occurs as the fluid passes the heater on the hemofiltration device when used with ECMO. The etiology of this phenomenon is unclear, but the problem can be prevented by removing calcium from the replacement fluid and running it as a separate infusion. At our institution, management of hemofiltration using a traditional hemofiltration machine is the responsibility of the patient's nurse, who must be specially trained in its use.

Alternatively, continuous hemofiltration can be provided to patients on ECMO by means of a simplified in-line hemofilter device. This technique decreases cost, complexity, and nursing requirements compared with additional hemofiltration machinery. Hemofiltration is driven by ECMO pump flow, rather than by an additional CRRT delivery system pump (Fig. 295-2). In this standardized procedure, previously described by Weber and Kountzman,[2] a primed hemofiltration circuit is inserted in line with the existing ECMO circuit. The hemofiltration circuit is constructed using a hemofilter with CRRT tubing.

Blood is removed before the oxygenator, or through a pigtail on the bottom of the oxygenator, and then is driven through the hemofilter and returned into the bladder. Blood flow leaving the ECMO circuit for hemofiltration exits after the roller head pump and is returned proximal to the roller head pump, creating a difference in the set pump flow and the flow delivered to the patient. Postoxygenator ultrasound flow monitoring allows measurement of delivered flow to the patient, as well as allowing determination of the amount of blood flow in the hemofiltration circuit. As with a separate hemofiltration device inline, no change in anticoagulation is needed. Ultrafiltrate from the hemofilter is removed using intravenous fluid infusion tubing and an intravenous pump, which is intended to control the hourly fluid removal rate. Ultrafiltrate is measured by a urine drainage system (urometer). Hourly management of this method of hemofiltration is the responsibility of the ECMO specialist.

ISSUES IN CONCOMITANT USE OF CONTINUOUS RENAL REPLACEMENT THERAPY AND EXTRACORPOREAL MEMBRANE OXYGENATION

Several potential issues arise with use of an in-line hemofiltration approach in patients on ECMO support. Close attention is required to assess the patient's level of hydration, because some inaccuracy in intravenous pump delivery of replacement fluid volume is possible, creating the potential for excessive fluid removal. Clinical experience has suggested that significant differences between prescribed and observed fluid removal rates can occur, leading to inadvertent patient dehydration out of proportion to intended fluid removal. In preliminary observations of replacement fluid pumps using an in-line system, inaccuracy in replacement fluid volume of up to 12.5% has been reported.[22,23] This inaccuracy has discouraged some ECMO centers from using this technique. One approach to combat this problem is to weigh both ultrafiltrate and replacement fluid bags each hour to determine actual fluid volume removal by weight.[24] Careful clinical observation of the patient's vital signs and physical examination, evaluating particularly for signs of dehydration, can diminish potential safety issues associated with this technique.

Concern also has been raised that aggressive use of CRRT in patients on ECMO, instead of conventional treatment with fluid restriction and diuretics, increases the likelihood of subsequent development of chronic renal failure or need for prolonged artificial kidney support in ECMO survivors. This possibility has not been demonstrated in case series experience, however. In the largest published pediatric review to date, Meyer and coworkers[16] found complete renal recovery in 14 of 15 (93%) ECMO survivors who received CRRT for renal insufficiency. The only patient in this series requiring chronic support had underlying vasculitis producing both pulmonary and renal disease. In a significantly larger case experience[25] from 1997 to 2005 at Children's Healthcare of Atlanta at Egleston, 56 survivors received CRRT and ECMO for either renal insufficiency, volume overload, or electrolyte abnormalities. Fifty-four (96%) of those patients had normal creatinine without need for renal replacement therapy at time of discharge. Two patients had abnormal creatinine

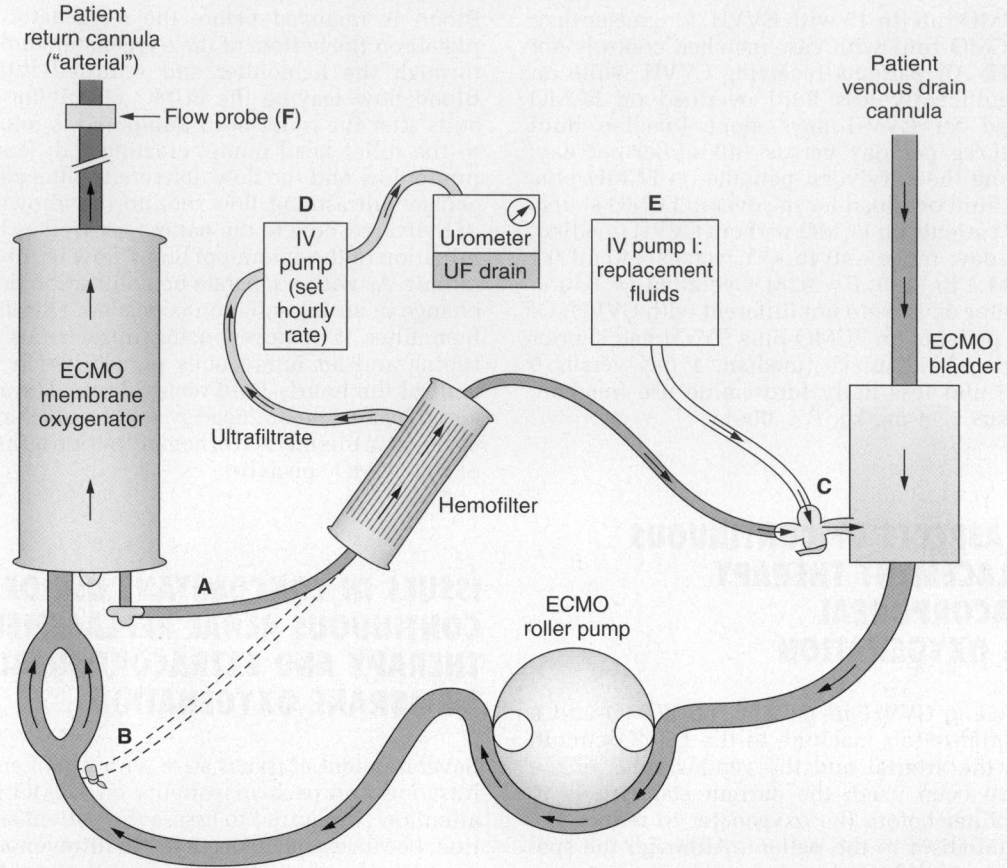

FIGURE 295-2. Schematic diagram illustrating arrangement for in-line hemofiltration on ECMO utilizing intrinsic ECMO roller pump flow, as used at Children's Healthcare of Atlanta. ECMO, extracorporeal membrane oxygenation; UF, ultrafiltrate.

levels associated with primary renal disease caused by small-vessel vasculitis. Multiple studies[26-28] have included patients who received concomitant ECMO and CRRT; however, many reports do not detail outcome data for renal recovery. In studies that do provide such data,[6,29,30] significant chronic renal failure is not described in survivors. On the basis of these findings, concern about causing chronic renal failure by concomitant use of CRRT and ECMO appears to be unwarranted.

USE OF EXTRACORPOREAL THERAPIES IN CONJUNCTION WITH CONTINUOUS RENAL REPLACEMENT THERAPY FOR SEPTIC SHOCK

As intensive care support in critical illness associated with severe septic shock has improved, so have efforts to offer other therapies to patients in whom conventional support was inadequate to treat more severe multiple organ failure. In particular, patients with septic shock and multiple organ failure have been increasingly offered extracorporeal support, with variable outcomes.[2,31,32] Several advanced extracorporeal approaches have been developed, all of which can use CRRT in combination.

Extracorporeal Life Support

Current expert consensus clinical recommendations include consideration of ECMO in the treatment of neonatal and pediatric septic shock. The American College of Critical Care Medicine (ACCM) Consensus Conference has presented practice parameters for septic shock support.[33] For neonates, the committee concluded that level II evidence (i.e., reasonably justifiable by scientific evidence and strongly supported by expert critical care opinion) existed to recommend ECMO for refractory shock unresponsive to catecholamines. For pediatric septic shock, consensus opinion on use was less definitive, recommending only to "consider ECMO" in patients with persistent catecholamine-resistant shock failing directed therapies to attain adequate cardiac output. The use of ECMO in septic patients serves two potential benefits. The obvious immediate benefit would be to provide direct hemodynamic support to the failing cardiorespiratory system. ECMO also could indirectly provide benefit by allowing patient stabilization to provide a "platform" allowing access for addition of CRRT, plasma exchange, coupled plasma filtration-adsorption (CPFA), and other novel extracorporeal therapies.

Of any extracorporeal therapy, CRRT enjoys the greatest amount of clinical support for use in septic patients. In addition to the benefits of preventing fluid overload and treating renal failure as described earlier, CRRT may potentially provide other theoretical immunomodulatory benefits in septic patients on ECMO. Use of CRRT could enhance removal and adsorption of undesirable inflammatory mediators in patients on ECMO. The membrane oxygenator and the extracorporeal circuit activate cytokine, chemokine, complement, and thrombotic pathways.[34-36] Use of hemofiltration in ECMO has been suggested to diminish cytokine concentrations, possibly by increased mediator clearance or by adsorption on the hemofilter itself. Skogby and associates,[37] using an experimental ECMO model, found that addition of a hemofilter to the circuit markedly diminished any increase in interleukin-8 and interleukin-6 concentrations compared with control circuit elevations. Although quantitative mediator reductions can be documented, the potential effects of reducing inflammatory mediators in ECMO on patient outcome are difficult to determine.

Further research trials of other emerging technologies are needed, however, before they can be routinely advocated for therapy for sepsis. Several techniques that can be used in combination with CRRT are described next.

Plasma-Based Therapies

Plasmapheresis is a term often used broadly to describe therapeutic techniques involving separation of plasma from whole blood. Plasma most commonly is separated by either a centrifugal or a filter-based technique. Once the plasma has been separated, any of numerous variations of these techniques can be used. A complete review of these therapies is beyond the scope of this discussion. Combination therapies such as CPFA or plasma exchange plus CRRT may have potential uses in sepsis.

Replacement of the separated plasma with donor plasma, often referred to as *plasma exchange*, is a nonspecific therapy aimed at overall reduction in levels of mediators of sepsis and restoration of plasma coagulation factors depleted by consumption. Plasma exchange has been most successfully used as a treatment for thrombotic thrombocytopenic purpura (TTP), a microangiopathy with multiorgan involvement and a high mortality rate.[38-40] Sepsis-associated coagulopathy—in particular, thrombocytopenia-associated multiple organ failure (TAMOF)[41]—also results in significant thrombotic end-organ damage. TTP and sepsis-associated DIC both feature excessive concentrations or activation of procoagulant mediators and decreased levels and activity of antithrombotic mediators. Increasing work has been undertaken to evaluate the role of plasma exchange in sepsis, with conflicting results. Various animal models, case reports, case series, and retrospective reviews either have suggested benefit from plasma exchange[42,43] or have found no benefit for or potential harm[44,45] from this modality. Few prospective randomized controlled trials have been conducted.

Stegmayr and coworkers[46] retrospectively described there experience using plasma exchange as rescue therapy in a series of 76 adults with profound organ failure. Predicted survival was very poor, based either on historical controls (less than 20%) or on APACHE (Acute Physiology and Chronic Health Evaluation) II score (33%). Actual survival with plasma exchange in this series, however, was 82% ($P < .0001$). A combined effect of CVVH with plasma exchange also has been described. In a prospective cohort of 19 septic adult surgical patients, no overall difference in mortality was seen with use of CVVH and

plasma exchange, in comparison with 24 matched historical control subjects who did not receive extracorporeal therapy.[43] A significant decrease in mortality rate, however, was seen in patients in the treatment group who had initial APACHE II scores of 21 to 25 (17% versus 40%; $P < .05$), single-organ failure (0 versus 25%, $P < .0001$), or two-organ failure (17% versus 42%; $P < .0001$), suggesting that early institution of plasma exchange may offer greater benefit. Of note, both studies used plasma exchange as a filtration method rather than centrifugation. As suggested in a review of several other published case series, patients who received centrifugation evidently had better outcomes than those receiving filtration.[47]

Busund and associates[48] performed the largest prospective randomized trial comparing plasma exchange with conventional therapy for septic shock. In a Russian study of 106 adults, the 28-day mortality rate was significantly decreased from that observed in the control (conventional treatment) group (33.3% versus 53.8%; $P = .05$). Controlling for age and infection site differences negated statistical significance, but in patients with abdominal infections, plasma exchange was associated with a significant decrease in mortality rate (33% versus 69%; $P < .05$).

A preliminary trial by Nguyen and colleagues[49] randomized 10 pediatric patients with TAMOF to receive either plasma exchange or conventional therapy. The study was terminated after interim analysis demonstrated a significant benefit from plasma exchange. Paediatric Logistic Organ Dysfunction (PELOD) scores[50] markedly decreased (approximately 30-fold) at 28 days for patients receiving plasma exchange, whereas PELOD scores rose threefold in children receiving conventional therapy alone. No patients in the plasma exchange group died by 28 days, whereas 4 of 5 patients receiving conventional therapy died. Since preliminary study completion, patients meeting TAMOF criteria at Children's Hospital of Pittsburgh have been offered plasma exchange. Sixty patients have undergone plasma exchange, with a 10% 28-day mortality rate and a 20% mortality rate at 1 year. Among 16 patients who chose not to receive plasma exchange, the 28-day mortality rate was 80% (J. Carcillo, personal communication). A prospective multicenter registry (Directed from Children's Healthcare of Atanta) is accruing data to evaluate outcomes with pediatric TAMOF, including use of plasma exchange.

Coupled Plasma Filtration-Adsorption

CPFA is a nonselective extracorporeal method combining the benefits of adsorption with renal replacement therapy. In CPFA, blood is removed and passed through a filter for plasma separation, followed by passage through a cartridge that removes mediators by means of adsorption. Plasma returns to combine with the blood, which can subsequently be passed through a renal replacement hemofilter if needed. The specific adsorbent material used in the CPFA cartridge is biocompatible and effective at typical blood flow rates and binds multiple mediators of sepsis. A review of its development and chemistry is beyond the scope of this discussion but has been described elsewhere.[51]

CPFA has been shown in vitro and in animal models of sepsis to be effective in reducing cytokine levels. In addition, CPFA was shown to reduce mortality in a rabbit model of endotoxin-mediated shock.[52] In an early-phase human clinical study, Formica and associates[53] examined the hemodynamic response to 10 CPFA treatments, each of 10 hours' duration, in a consecutive series of 10 mechanically ventilated patients in septic shock with multiorgan failure, vasopressor dependence, and various degrees of ARF. Statistically significant improvement in mean arterial pressures, systemic vascular resistance, and PaO_2/FIO_2 ratio was seen for both individual treatments and over the entire treatment course. The 28-day survival rate was 90%, compared with 60% APACHE II–predicted. A larger phase II controlled, randomized study of CPFA is ongoing and should provide useful information regarding this promising therapy.

In accordance with Ronco and Bellomo's "peak concentration hypothesis,"[54] CPFA has traditionally been described using a nonselective adsorption cartridge with additional high-volume hemofiltration or hemodiafiltration if needed to reduce mediators to the normal physiological range. Similar nonspecific mediator reduction methods[55,56] have been designed by combining plasma exchange, rather than adsorption, with renal replacement therapy, originally as a treatment for liver failure, but with a possible role in the management of septic shock.

CONCLUSION

The use of CRRT in combination with other extracorporeal therapies is increasing in pediatric patients. Concomitant use of ECMO and CRRT has been demonstrated to be safe and effective for the treatment of renal failure. The development of renal failure in patients on ECMO is a poor prognostic sign, often heralding the onset of multiple organ system failure; however, survivors who have received ECMO and CRRT do not appear to be at increased risk for the development of chronic renal failure. An expanded indication for CRRT is as a fluid management tool in critically ill patients without renal failure who are on ECMO. In the child with refractory septic shock, use of ECMO as a platform for multiple extracorporeal therapies may be lifesaving. Finally, published evidence supporting the use of many of these therapies is lacking. Research is needed not only to determine the efficacy of these novel therapies but also to identify those patients most likely to benefit from such treatment.

Key Points

1. Continuous renal replacement therapy can be safely used with extracorporeal membrane oxygenation in neonatal and pediatric populations.
2. Continuous renal replacement therapy provides a novel technique for fluid management in critically ill children on extracorporeal membrane oxygenation.
3. Concomitant use of continuous renal replacement therapy and extracorporeal membrane oxygenation does not increase rates of chronic renal failure in survivors.
4. Clinical assessment of fluid balance is essential to avoid complications of continuous renal replacement therapy in patients on extracorporeal membrane oxygenation.
5. Continuous renal replacement therapy, alone or in combination with other extracorposeal therapies, may have a therapeutic role in severe septic shock.

Key References

14. Goldstein SL, Somers M, Baum M, et al: Pediatric patients with multi-organ dysfunction syndrome receiving continuous renal replacement therapy. Kidney Int 2005;67:1-6.
16. Meyer RJ, Brophy PD, Bunchman TE, et al: Survival and renal function in pediatric patients following extracorporeal life support with hemofiltration. Pediatr Crit Care Med 2001;2: 238-242.
47. Carcillo JA, Kellum JA: Is there a role for plasmapheresis/ plasma exchange therapy in septic shock, MODS, and thrombocytopenia-associated multiple organ failure? We still do not know, but perhaps we are closer. Intensive Care Med 2002;28:1373-1375.
48. Busund R, Koukline V, Utrobin U, Nedashkovsky E: Plasmapheresis in severe sepsis and septic shock: A prospective, randomized, controlled trial. Intensive Care Med 2002;28: 1434-1439.
49. Nguyen TC, Han YY, Kiss JE, et al: Intensive plasma exchange increases ADAMTS-13 activity and reverses organ dysfunction in children with thrombocytopenia-associated multiple organ failure. Critical Care Medicine, 2008, in press.

See the companion Expert Consult website for the complete reference list.

Outcome of Pediatric Acute Kidney Injury

Stuart L. Goldstein

OBJECTIVES

This chapter will:

1. Compare mortality rates observed in various critically ill pediatric populations in which acute kidney injury develops.
2. Analyze outcomes for children who acquire acute kidney injury in terms of need for renal replacement therapy.
3. Identify clinical variables associated with increased mortality in critically ill children with acute kidney injury who receive renal replacement therapy.
4. Review long-term sequelae in children who survive an episode of acute kidney injury.

The study of pediatric acute kidney injury (AKI) outcomes has undergone an increased focus in the past decade, with significant attention paid to children who receive renal replacement therapy (RRT). Most data come from retrospective single-center studies, however, so very little evidence is available regarding therapeutic measures that may prevent or ameliorate pediatric AKI. Three different pediatric outcome measures are addressed in this chapter: (1) mortality, (2) the need for RRT, and (3) long-term sequelae in patients who survive an AKI episode.

THE CRITICALLY ILL PEDIATRIC PATIENT

As noted in Chapter 329, the epidemiology of pediatric AKI has changed from predominantly primary renal diseases to AKI caused by other underlying systemic illness or their treatment. Hui-Stickle and colleagues noted that 185 of 246 patients (75%) diagnosed with AKI from 1999 to 2001 on hospital discharge or death summary documents had been admitted to an intensive care unit (ICU).[1]

Overall survival rates for critically ill pediatric patients are remarkably similar across different countries and studies. Hui-Stickle and colleagues noted a 70% survival rate in their study in the United States of 246 patients but also found significantly lower survival among patients younger than 1 year of age than among older children (60% versus 77%; $P < .0001$).[1] Vachvanichsanong and colleagues reported a 64% survival rate in 311 patients, but they did not note a similar association between younger patient age and mortality.[2] This Thailand study spanned 21 years of hospitalizations, and the investigators did note a trend toward improved survival over 3 eras (1982 to

1995: 53%; 1995 to 2000, 57%; and 2000 to 2004: 65%; $P = .12$). Williams and coworkers noted a stable survival rate of 71% to 73% over their 20-year study of 228 cases of pediatric AKI in Richmond, Virginia.[3] Of interest, large pediatric AKI studies before 1990 show similar survival rates of 58% to 75%.[4,5] Although this finding could be interpreted to reflect lack of improvement in the care of children with AKI, it is more likely to reflect the provision of care for a greater number of critically ill children who acquire AKI than was the case in earlier decades.

As might be expected, patients with multiorgan system dysfunction or other nonrenal system involvement demonstrated worse survival in all studies than that observed for children with primary renal causes of AKI. Williams and coworkers noted that the survival rate decreased from 87% to 12% as the number of affected organs increased from 2 to 4.[3] Hui-Stickle and colleagues noted that survival was worse in patients with sepsis (41%) or cardiac disease (65%) than in those with renal disease alone (95%).[1]

THE CRITICALLY ILL PATIENT REQUIRING RENAL REPLACEMENT THERAPY

An understanding of the pattern of pediatric multiple organ dysfunction syndrome (MODS) will lend insight into some of the shortcomings and strengths of pediatric ARF outcome data presented later in the chapter. Proulx and associates demonstrated that severe and life-threatening MODS developed very early in the ICU course in children, in contrast with adult patients. In 87% of the children, the maximum number of organ failures occurred within 72 hours of ICU admission, and the children who died with MODS did so very early in the ICU course, with 88.4% of deaths occurring within 7 days of MODS diagnosis.[6,7] Thus, methods to quickly identify children at risk for the development of MODS would allow early and aggressive initiation of supportive measures, including renal replacement therapy to treat or prevent ARF sequelae, presumably with improved outcomes in pediatric patients.

Unfortunately, many issues plague the pediatric ARF outcome literature: a relative lack of prospective study, the mixture of RRT modalities used, with a lack of modality stratification in subject populations studied, and the inconsistent use of methods to control for patient illness severity in outcome analysis. A few studies have considered the effect of a clinical variable on outcome. Smoyer and associates reviewed outcomes for 98 infants and children with ARF who received either arteriovenous or venovenous modalities of continuous renal replacement therapy (CRRT) and found higher mortality in patients on pressors.[8] Subsequent work by Bunchman and colleagues upheld this finding, showing a survival rate of only 35% for patients requiring pressors versus 89% for those without a pressor requirement in the course of AKI treatment.[9] As a result, pressor use has been construed as a surrogate for worse patient illness severity in the pediatric population requiring CRRT.

Few pediatric outcome studies use a standardized scoring system to control for patient illness severity, which may result from the fact that published data provide contradictory conclusions with respect to the utility of various illness severity scoring systems in predicting death in pediatric patients with ARF. Faragson demonstrated significant overlap in Pediatric Risk of Mortality (PRISM) scores between surviving and nonsurviving children who received intermittent hemodialysis and therefore concluded that PRISM scores should not be used to differentiate patients who would benefit from those who would not be likely to benefit from dialysis initiation.[10] Zobel and coworkers demonstrated that children who received CRRT with worse illness severity by PRISM score had increased mortality, but this study included patients who received both arteriovenous and venovenous CRRT therapies and did not stratify by modality.[11]

A recent study[12] examined outcomes in 22 critically ill children who received only venovenous CRRT modalities and used the PRISM II score to control for illness severity at ICU admission and CRRT initiation. Neither mean PRISM scores at the time of PICU admission nor time of CRRT initiation differed between survivors and nonsurvivors. Of the clinical variables studied, only the degree of fluid overload at the time of CRRT initiation differed between survivors (16.4% ± 13.8%) and nonsurvivors (34.0% ± 21.0%; P = .03), even with use of a multiple regression model to control for severity of illness by PRISM score. In addition, 75% of nonsurvivors died within 21 days of ICU admission.

Numerous single-center studies have since demonstrated a similar association between fluid overload and mortality. Lowrie and colleagues demonstrated that CRRT performed better to prevent fluid overload and improve survival in children with AKI.[13] Foland and associates studied 77 children with AKI who received CRRT in their ICU and found that survivors with involvement of three or more organs had significantly lower fluid overload before CRRT initiation compared with nonsurvivors (9.2% versus 15.5% [8.3, 28.6]; P = .01), and lesser degree of fluid overload was independently associated with survival even with initiation of control for patient illness severity.[14] Gillespie and colleagues found that children with greater than 10% fluid overload before CRRT initiation had a 3.02 greater risk of death than that in children who had less than 10% fluid overload at CRRT initiation.[15] Williams and coworkers noted that nonsurvivors had significantly lower serum albumin concentrations compared with survivors immediately before RRT initiation (2.6 ± 0.7 g/dL versus 3.3 ± 0.9 g/dL; P < .05).[3] Serum albumin is affected by many factors, including inflammation status and nutrition, but also can be a marker of fluid status.

One multicenter study, performed by the Prospective Pediatric CRRT Registry Group, examined 116 patients with MODS at seven U.S. centers and demonstrated a similar association between fluid overload and mortality at CRRT initiation.[16] This study also noted that nonsurvivors had significantly higher central venous pressures and mean airway pressures. One interpretation of these data is that nonsurvivors may have received excess fluid before CRRT initiation.

The findings from the foregoing studies, coupled with the predilection for early multiorgan system failure and death in critically ill children with AKI, argue for early and aggressive initiation of CRRT. Further prospective study, including use of goal-directed fluid resuscitation strategies, is clearly warranted to substantiate the findings of these retrospective efforts.

INFANTS

CRRT has been prescribed since the mid-1980s for treatment of ARF in critically ill infants.[17,18] The first CRRT modalities were arteriovenous in configuration, because the extracorporeal volumes were small in these circuits, and ultrafiltration was driven by patient perfusion pressure, thereby reducing the risk of hypotension from too much ultrafiltration. Introduction of more accurate machines with volumetric control has increased the use of venovenous-modality CRRT in pediatric patients, including neonates and infants. Zobel and coworkers noted[18] that technical problems occurred with continuous venovenous hemofiltration (CVVH) only in a 1991 study of early neonatal outcome in which patients received either continuous arteriovenous hemofiltration (CAVH) or CVVH. Symons and associates reported data[19] from a more recent retrospective multicenter study evaluating the CVVH course for 90 infants weighing less than 10 kg from 1993 through 2001, which demonstrate very few technical complications using newer CVVH machinery. Infant survival among patients receiving CRRT has also been consistent over the past decade at 35% to 38%, which is similar to survival rates as noted previously for older pediatric patients,[18,20] although patients weighing less than 3 kg exhibited a trend toward worse survival (24%) when compared with infants larger than 3 kg (41%).[20]

CONGENITAL HEART DISEASE

Infants in whom ARF develops after corrective surgery for congenital heart problems constitute a well-studied cohort,[20-26] for good reason: In these patients, the timing of the event leading to ARF—namely, cardiopulmonary bypass (CPB)—is precisely known. In this sense, children undergoing CPB are akin to adults receiving nephrotoxic radiocontrast agents or undergoing emergency surgery for aortic aneurysms: In all of these patient groups, the clinical scenario provides an opportunity to follow the time course of ARF from beginning to end in patients without significant underlying renal disease.

The incidence of infant AKI after CPB ranges from 2.7% to 5.3%, with survival rates ranging from 21% to 70%.[20,21,24] Risk factors for death include increasing underlying complexity of the congenital heart disease and poor cardiac function.[20,24] A recent trend toward providing peritoneal dialysis therapy earlier in the post-CPB course has been reported, with one study of 20 patients demonstrating 80% patient survival.[25] Although improved survival with early initiation of peritoneal dialysis may result from prevention of fluid overload, some investigators posit[26] improved survival with early peritoneal dialysis results from increased clearance of CPB-induced pro-inflammatory cytokines, although further study is required to support this hypothesis. In our center, patients with an underlying diagnosis of hypoplastic left heart syndrome, transposition of the great arteries, or anomalous pulmonary venous return receive peritoneal dialysis immediately postoperatively in order to prevent fluid accumulation.

LONG-TERM OUTCOME WITH PEDIATRIC ACUTE KIDNEY INJURY

Most critically ill patients who survive an AKI episode regain renal function. Hui-Stickle and colleagues found that 66% of patients recovered renal function completely, 29% had improved but not normal renal function, and 5% required renal replacement therapy at the time of hospital discharge.[1] Vachvanichsanong and coworkers found that 174 of 196 (88%) survivors recovered renal function completely, and chronic renal failure developed in the remainder.[2]

The long-term sequelae of pediatric AKI have recently been studied. Askenazi and colleagues[27] found 3- to 5-year patient survival rate after an AKI episode to be 56.8%; 59% of these patients demonstrated evidence of chronic kidney injury. The investigators recommend routine evaluation of all survivors of pediatric AKI for evidence of chronic kidney disease, hypertension, or microalbuminuria. Garg and associates performed a meta-analysis of studies with 10 or more patients who suffered from diarrhea-associated HUS.[28] This analysis demonstrated that nearly 25% of patients have some renal sequelae after HUS, and that long-term prognosis was worse in patients with increased severity of illness, central nervous system involvement, or need for dialysis. Finally, Abitbol and coworkers studied long-term renal function (mean follow-up period, 7 years) in 20 low-birth-weight infants who survived an AKI episode.[29] In this study, 45% of infants demonstrated chronic renal failure and proteinuria, with serum creatinine greater than 0.6 mg/dL at 1 year of age; larger patients in this cohort were found to have chronic kidney disease.

Key References

1. Hui-Stickle S, Brewer ED, Goldstein SL: Pediatric ARF epidemiology at a tertiary care center from 1999 to 2001. Am J Kidney Dis 2005;45:96-101.
9. Bunchman TE, McBryde KD, Mottes TE, et al: Pediatric acute renal failure: Outcome by modality and disease. Pediatr Nephrol 2001;16:1067-1071.
12. Goldstein SL, Currier H, Graf C, et al: Outcome in children receiving continuous venovenous hemofiltration. Pediatrics 2001;107:1309-1312.
14. Foland JA, Fortenberry JD, Warshaw BL, et al: Fluid overload before continuous hemofiltration and survival in critically ill children: A retrospective analysis. Crit Care Med 2004;32:1771-1776.
16. Goldstein SL, Somers MJ, Baum MA. et al: Pediatric patients with multi-organ dysfunction syndrome receiving continuous renal replacement therapy. Kidney Int 2005;67:653-658.

See the companion Expert Consult website for the complete reference list.

CHAPTER 297

Renal Replacement Therapy for the Critically Ill Infant

Jordan M. Symons

The expanding role of renal replacement therapy in the care of critically ill children extends to the smallest pediatric patients. Infants with oliguria, volume overload, multiorgan dysfunction, and metabolic disorders can be managed successfully with techniques that have been established in larger children and adults. Renal replacement therapy for infants presents special challenges. Data regarding dialysis support for infants in the intensive care unit (ICU) are limited, and recommendations often are based on clinical experience. Overall, the need is relatively uncommon, but dialysis is potentially lifesaving

TABLE 297-1

Potential Indications for Renal Replacement Therapy in Infants

Volume Overload or Metabolic/Electrolyte Abnormalities Related to Decreased Kidney Function

Diminished effective circulating volume: "prerenal" states
- Volume depletion
- Hemorrhage/blood loss
- Fluid redistribution ("third spacing")
- Diminished cardiac output (e.g., congenital heart disease)
- Hypotension/shock (e.g., sepsis syndrome)

Urinary obstruction: "postrenal" states
- Bladder outlet obstruction (e.g., posterior urethral valves)
- Bladder dysfunction (e.g., neurogenic bladder)
- Obstructing tumor or mass
- Congenital obstruction of ureters
- Solitary functioning kidney with obstruction

Intrinsic renal disease or injury: "intrarenal" states
- Ischemic injury
- Tubular toxicity (e.g., drugs, myoglobin)
- Vascular thrombosis
- Hemolytic uremic syndrome
- Congenital renal diseases (e.g., renal dysplasia)

Multiorgan dysfunction

Intoxication

Endogenous intoxication (e.g., hyperammonemia of the newborn)

Exogenous intoxication (e.g., drug intoxication)

Renal Support

Suboptimal kidney function limiting delivery of nutrition and medical therapy

RENAL FAILURE AND OTHER INDICATIONS FOR RENAL REPLACEMENT THERAPY

Indications for renal replacement therapy in the critically ill infant parallel those seen in older children and adults (Table 297-1). Acute renal failure is a common complication seen in the neonatal period and has been recently reviewed.[1-3] Causes for renal failure in the newborn period can include urinary obstruction, so-called prerenal conditions with diminished perfusion, and intrinsic renal disease including congenital abnormalities. A majority of infants with acute kidney injury will experience recovery of renal function without the need for therapy beyond supportive care. When conservative measures fail, renal replacement therapy can be considered for the newborn with renal dysfunction. Renal replacement in this setting provides the parallel needs of metabolic control and fluid balance, identical to those required by an older child or adult with acute kidney injury. Rarely, a patient will present in infancy who requires renal replacement therapy for chronic kidney disease. Indications are similar to those in older children or adults, with the additional need to

begin treatment in the setting of suboptimal growth or inability to provide sufficient nutrition to the infant due to fluid limitations.

Acute intoxications, either with endogenous toxins as seen with inborn errors of metabolism or exogenous toxins due to iatrogenic events, represent another clinical scenario that may necessitate treatment by dialysis. Hemodialysis can rapidly remove toxins and often is the therapy of choice for severe intoxication in older children and adults. For infants, hemodialysis is similarly more efficient than peritoneal dialysis in this setting and should be considered for the treatment of intoxication.[4]

The concept of "renal support" has been applied in a study including older patients[5] to describe the use of renal replacement therapies before the development of absolute indications such as fluid overload or uremia. Fluid restriction as part of conservative management for a patient with mild renal dysfunction may potentially lead to reduced nutrition. Renal replacement therapy can reduce the total fluid burden related to daily fluid input and also permits maximal medical support. The infant with renal dysfunction can benefit from this approach as well, and the use of renal replacement therapy should be considered early in the course of acute kidney injury.

PERITONEAL DIALYSIS

Despite technological improvements that have opened the possibility of use of all modalities of renal replacement therapy in the critically ill infant, peritoneal dialysis remains an effective renal replacement modality and may represent a superior alternative for infants who require renal replacement therapy.[6] Even the most experienced centers may have difficulty achieving vascular access in infants, limiting options for the use of hemodialysis and continuous renal replacement therapy (CRRT). Children with vascular abnormalities, certain types of cardiac disease, or hemodynamic issues may be suboptimal candidates for extracorporeal perfusion. In such circumstances, peritoneal dialysis can be the best choice for renal replacement therapy.

Indications

Peritoneal dialysis is an effective method for achieving metabolic control and fluid balance in the infant with renal failure. The technique is relatively straightforward, and protocols for therapy in the newborn are well established. Peritoneal dialysis often is considered the preferred method of management for infants who have undergone cardiac surgery and can be a useful adjunct to maintaining fluid balance in those patients who have low cardiac output.[7]

Technique

To perform peritoneal dialysis, a dialysis catheter must be placed in the infant's abdomen. These catheters come in various sizes, and smaller catheters are available for use in the newborn or small infant. Either a surgically placed catheter or a percutaneously inserted temporary catheter may be used. Some evidence suggests fewer complications with surgically placed catheters.[8-10] Local practice often determines who will insert the catheters when they are

when circumstances warrant. Careful preparation, communication, and coordination between various hospital specialists, including nephrologist, neonatologist, surgeon, nurse, nutritionist, and pharmacist, can maximize the likelihood of a good outcome for these critically ill infants.

needed; the procedure requires expertise to ensure proper function of the catheter.

Peritoneal dialysate comes in standardized concentrations that are available commercially. These formulations usually are acceptable for use in the critically ill infant. In the United States, peritoneal dialysate is available in standard dextrose concentrations of 1.5%, 2.5%, and 4.25%, with lactate used as the base. Lactate absorption can lead to complications in critically ill infants and the hospital pharmacy may need to specially prepare dialysate with bicarbonate,[11] although in our experience, standard lactate-based dialysate usually is acceptable. Outside of the United States, bicarbonate-based peritoneal dialysate is available commercially. Peritoneal dialysate should be warmed to body temperature before use in infants, to prevent hypotension associated with cold dialysate infusion.

Initial exchanges with a newly placed peritoneal dialysis catheter should use relatively lower volumes of 10 to 20 mL/kg (200 to 500 mL/m²) of dialysate, to limit the chance of leak from the catheter insertion site. Low-volume peritoneal dialysis can be an effective method in the infant, successfully achieving ultrafiltration goals.[12] Exchanges of dialysate can be performed throughout the day in the ICU, thereby increasing time on dialysis compared with that typical with peritoneal dialysis performed in the ambulatory setting. This more frequent exchange helps achieve metabolic balance even with use of lower dialysate volumes. For those patients who require greater mass transfer after successful initiation, fill volumes may increase gradually to 1000 to 1100 mL/m².

Shorter dwell times often are used for infants in the critical care setting. Although longer dwell periods provide more time for equilibration of dialysate and for ultrafiltration, shorter dwell periods may permit more dialysis and ultrafiltration in a 24-hour period by allowing more exchanges per day. Initial dwell periods of 15 to 30 minutes in the newborn can be adjusted later in accordance with clinical status.

Programming limitations may prevent the use of a cycler for infants who require very small fill volumes or very short dwell times. In such circumstances, peritoneal dialysis must be performed manually. Premade tubing systems for hand dialysis in the neonate are available commercially, or caregivers familiar with the modality may extemporaneously assemble a system using intravenous tubing. In either case, bedside care providers must take care to maintain sterility through a closed system.

Disadvantages and Complications in the Infant

This modality requires placement of a peritoneal catheter and a sufficiently maintained intra-abdominal status for success. Infants who have undergone abdominal surgery or have had abdominal complications or abnormalities, such as diaphragmatic hernia, omphalocele, or necrotizing enterocolitis, may be poor candidates for peritoneal dialysis.

Dialysate can fail to fill or drain through the dialysis catheter as a result of kinking, fibrin plugs, omental obstruction, or catheter malposition. The catheter can perforate abdominal or pelvic structures, either during placement or later on.[9] Although perforation is a relatively uncommon event, significant morbidity can result.

Fluid leak most often is seen with dwell volumes that are too large, especially in the period immediately after catheter placement.[13] This complication is of particular concern in the critically ill patient and in the newborn. Fluid leak into the thorax can compromise respiration. External fluid leak around the catheter increases infection risk. Peritonitis is a significant complication and can prove fatal in the critically ill infant receiving peritoneal dialysis. Careful attention to sterile technique reduces the likelihood of infection.

Infants on peritoneal dialysis can lose protein into the dialysate and may require increased nutritional support over that needed in older children and adults. The high dextrose concentrations in the dialysate can cause hyperglycemia, necessitating administration of insulin. Indwelling dialysate causes increased intra-abdominal pressure that can complicate care of the critically ill patient by limiting diaphragmatic excursion, reducing venous return, or causing gastroesophageal reflux.

Vande Walle and colleagues[14] have proposed that low-volume peritoneal dialysis with frequent exchanges, as often performed in the infant, can lead to diminished sodium transport despite apparently adequate ultrafiltration. This problem may potentially result in volume overload and hypernatremia. These investigators performed peritoneal dialysis in infants using lower sodium concentrations in their dialysate (127 mmol/L) and noted improved sodium extraction with maintained ultrafiltration.

INTERMITTENT HEMODIALYSIS

The technique for intermittent hemodialysis for pediatric patients is well established.[15,16] Intermittent hemodialysis offers the advantages of high efficiency for rapid metabolic correction and fluid removal. Hemodialysis in infants is particularly challenging; a majority of the devices and materials are designed for larger patients, and special techniques are required. Successful treatment can be achieved but requires experienced personnel and careful attention to detail.[17,18]

Indications

Hemodialysis usually is considered the best modality for rapid particle removal because of its high efficiency, making it a good choice for the treatment of toxic ingestions, many serious drug overdoses, and metabolic derangements that lead to the overproduction of endogenous toxins such as ammonia.[19-23] Consequently, intermittent hemodialysis is an important modality to consider in the treatment of hyperammonemia of the newborn, in whom rapid reduction of ammonia levels is essential to preserving neurological outcome.[4,24]

The hemodialysis system can perform ultrafiltration more rapidly than any other renal replacement modality, making it the best choice for the treatment of critical volume overload. Profound metabolic imbalance, such as seen with critical hyperkalemia, can be corrected most quickly with intermittent hemodialysis.

Technique

Successful hemodialysis requires a functional vascular access. This requirement remains a significant obstacle to use of this modality in small patients. Physical limitations

TABLE 297-2

Catheter Options for Hemodialysis and Continuous Renal Replacement Therapy in Infants

- Single-lumen 5 Fr (in small neonates)
- Double-lumen 7 Fr (in infants weighing 3 to 6 kg)
- Triple-lumen 7 Fr (provides option for infusion)
- Umbilical catheters (single-lumen)
  - 5 Fr umbilical artery for source
  - 5 Fr or larger umbilical vein for return

of small blood lines greatly limit the rate of blood flow for dialysis.[25] Umbilical catheters do not have favorable flow qualities for hemodialysis, although larger sizes (e.g., at least 5 Fr for each lumen) sometimes can be used successfully. Catheter options for hemodialysis in infants are summarized in Table 297-2. Small double-lumen hemodialysis catheters (7 Fr) can provide acceptable blood flow between 25 and 50 mL/minute, sufficient for adequate hemodialysis in a newborn. Placement of even these small catheters can be challenging in the tiniest babies, and use of two separate single-lumen access tubes (e.g., 5 Fr) may be preferable. If the available dialysis machine offers a single-needle option, this approach also can be successful in a small neonate and can limit the need for additional or more complex vascular access. In view of the difficulties in achieving vascular access in a small infant, this should be attempted by the most skilled practitioner available to reduce the likelihood of complications and increase chances for success.

Most patients receiving intermittent hemodialysis will require heparin for anticoagulation. In the neonate, heparin requirements for dialysis must be balanced with the risks of systemic anticoagulation. Neonatology and nephrology personnel should discuss the anticoagulation plan and consider the best option for the individual patient. Some patients may successfully tolerate dialysis with little or no heparin, as a result of poor clotting status related to their systemic disease. The risk of circuit clotting is increased with heparin-free dialysis, however.

In the smallest patients, smaller dialyzers are used to limit extracorporeal blood volume and to reduce the risk of dialyzer clotting with slower blood flow rates. These small dialyzers have a lower theoretical clearance than is possible with use of which the circuit has a larger surface area. However, because of the low blood flow used for infant dialysis, mass transfer through small and through large dialyzers becomes roughly equivalent.

Neonatal-specific tubing sets are available for hemodialysis machines. Even using low-volume tubing and a small dialyzer, the extracorporeal circuit can still represent 30% or more of the infant's intravascular volume. In view of the relatively large extracorporeal volume in a hemodialysis circuit, infants usually require priming of the hemodialysis circuit with reconstituted whole blood. This can be accomplished with a blend of packed red blood cells and 5% albumin. As a result of the nonphysiological properties of banked blood used for blood priming (low pH, high potassium content, low calcium content, citrate load), infants can be at risk for metabolic instability at dialysis initiation. These factors must be considered when a blood prime is to be used.

The development of dialysis machines with volumetric ultrafiltration control allows for accurate and safe hemodialysis in neonates and infants, in whom small inaccuracies in ultrafiltration volumes may potentially lead to severe fluid imbalances.

Disadvantages and Complications

The principal disadvantage of intermittent hemodialysis is the requirement for vascular access. As noted previously, difficulties with vascular access are magnified in the smallest patients. Complications related to the access can include infection, bleeding, and thrombosis. Relatively large catheters placed in vessels of small infants can occlude venous flow.

Infants undergoing hemodialysis are at increased risk for hemodynamic instability. This can occur at the time of hemodialysis initiation as a result of exposure to the blood prime as noted earlier, or may be due to rapid expansion of the blood volume and dilution of vasoactive medications, or to rapid ultrafiltration related to the shorter hemodialysis sessions. The care provider must give careful consideration to these potential problems and be prepared to intervene with blood pressure support or discontinuation of the hemodialysis session.

Infants undergoing intermittent hemodialysis for ongoing renal replacement therapy in the ICU require special attention to fluid and electrolyte balance. Potassium and phosphorus delivery should be limited because the intermittent nature of the treatment makes it difficult to determine amounts administered. Similarly, total daily fluids also may need to be limited, because ultrafiltration occurs only intermittently. Fluid and electrolyte balance is of particular concern in the critically ill infant, who will receive high volumes of fluid to deliver daily medications and nutrition and to simply maintain patent vascular access. Medication doses and schedule may require adjustment owing to poor excretion with renal failure and subsequent rapid removal on dialysis.

CONTINUOUS RENAL REPLACEMENT THERAPY

First applied to infants as described in an early series by Ronco and colleagues[26] using the nonpumped arteriovenous technique, CRRT use in critically ill children continues to expand. Technological improvements in catheters, blood pumps, ultrafiltration control mechanisms, and venovenous technique permit the application of CRRT to even the smallest infants.[27]

Indications

As a result of the slow, continuous removal of fluid, CRRT is particularly well suited to the treatment of volume overload in neonates and infants, for whom rapid removal of fluid may be poorly tolerated. CRRT is useful to maintain metabolic balance through ongoing removal of unwanted particles. CRRT can be used as a secondary method to maintain metabolic balance after rapid correction with hemodialysis, as may be necessary in hyperammonemia in the newborn with ammonia rebound.[24]

CRRT can serve as a method for renal support for infants with diminished renal function, permitting administration of the daily load of fluids required to deliver medication and nutrition. This can be useful in the infant for whom peritoneal dialysis is unsuitable.

Technique

As with intermittent hemodialysis, successful CRRT requires adequate vascular access (see Table 297-2). The same difficulties apply in the CRRT setting, with the added issue of continuous use of the vascular access and associated risk for inadequate function, infection, and hemorrhage. In infants, priming of the CRRT circuit with blood-albumin mix may be required.[28] Blood flow rates for an infant on CRRT would be similar to those seen for intermittent hemodialysis, that is, 25 to 50 mL/minute, limited by the flow through the vascular access, the CRRT device, and the clinical status of the patient.

Systemic heparinization has been the traditional form of anticoagulation used in CRRT. Infants may be at increased risk for hemorrhage with continuous systemic anticoagulation. Neonates may suffer intracranial hemorrhage as part of their overall critical illness, and the likelihood rises with systemic heparinization. Careful coordination between neonatology and nephrology services is warranted. As an alternative, regional citrate anticoagulation is becoming increasingly popular for CRRT in both adult and pediatric patients. Several protocols have been developed for regional citrate anticoagulation in CRRT,[29,30] to include use in pediatric patients.[31] Citrate anticoagulation can be used successfully in the infant on CRRT, but careful attention must be paid to electrolyte and acid-base balance.

Many brands of hemofilter are available for CRRT. Some CRRT devices require the use of a proprietary hemofilter, whereas others are open systems that permit the use of a hemofilter from any manufacturer. Hemofilter size and material must be considered in performing CRRT in infants. In particular, hypotensive events related to the use of the AN69 membrane have been reported.[32,33] This reaction is thought to be related to the release of bradykinin in response to the low pH of blood used to prime the CRRT circuit. Infants may be at highest risk for this reaction, termed the *bradykinin release syndrome*, because blood priming frequently is used in these patients. Maneuvers to adjust pH within the circuit, with the aim of limiting this reaction, have been described.[33,34] Some institutions avoid the use of the AN69 membrane in infants, choosing to use a larger hemofilter, if necessary, made from a different material. Alternatively, a prototype of a low-volume device for hemodialysis and CRRT in small infants has been described[35] that can provide therapy to an infant weighing less than 1000 g without the need for circuit priming. Such an approach may prove useful in the future if the technique can be developed for more widespread use.

Disadvantages and Complications

As with intermittent hemodialysis, a significant obstacle to successful CRRT in infants is the requirement for vascular access, and similar caveats apply. Continuous extracorporeal perfusion and anticoagulation carry increased risks of bleeding and infection. Hemodynamic instability can develop despite the slow, continuous method of ultrafiltration. Continuous exposure to heparin runs the risk of hemorrhage or heparin-induced thrombocytopenia. Citrate anticoagulation may cause acid-base disturbance or hypocalcemia. Citrate overload can cause low patient ionized calcium with normal or high total calcium levels—the so-called *calcium gap* or *citrate lock*.[31,36,37] In our experience, infants are particularly susceptible to electrolyte compli-

cations during CRRT, related to both citrate anticoagulation and excess loss of electrolytes through the hemofilter. This susceptibility may be due to smaller body mass relative to citrate delivery and clearance capabilities. Careful monitoring and adjustment to CRRT prescription, intravenous fluids, and nutritional support are warranted. Attention must be paid to appropriate replacement of electrolytes lost through CRRT. Similarly, nitrogen losses on CRRT can be high,[38] and infants will require thorough nutritional evaluation with increased delivery of protein and calories. Coordination between ICU and nephrology staff is essential to establish appropriate goals for fluid removal and metabolic control.

CONCLUSION

The requirement for renal replacement therapy in infants represents a special challenge in clinical management. Any modality available for older children and adults may be used for the infant; choice of modality may depend on clinical status of the patient and local expertise. Careful attention to fluid and electrolyte balance, appropriate nutritional support, and close interaction between critical care and nephrology personnel will yield the best outcomes.

Key Points

1. Peritoneal dialysis remains an excellent form of acute renal replacement therapy for infants and often is the preferred method.
2. Hemodialysis is the modality of choice for rapid correction of metabolic imbalance, such as seen in hyperammonemia of the newborn.
3. Continuous modalities can provide effective treatment for infants requiring renal replacement therapy.
4. Infants receiving renal replacement therapy require careful monitoring of fluid and electrolyte balance and nutritional needs.
5. Coordination between critical care and nephrology staff is essential to successful management of infants requiring renal replacement therapy.

Key References

6. Flynn JT, Kershaw DB, Smoyer WE, et al: Peritoneal dialysis for management of pediatric acute renal failure. Perit Dial Int 2001;21:390-394.
24. McBryde KD, Kershaw DB, Bunchman TE, et al: Renal replacement therapy in the treatment of confirmed or suspected inborn errors of metabolism. J Pediatr 2006;148:770-778.
26. Ronco C, Brendolan A, Bragantini L, et al: Treatment of acute renal failure in newborns by continuous arterio-venous hemofiltration. Kidney Int 1986;29:908-915.
27. Symons JM, Brophy PD, Gregory MJ, et al: Continuous renal replacement therapy in children up to 10 kg. Am J Kidney Dis 2003;41:984-989.
31. Bunchman TE, Maxvold NJ, Barnett J, et al: Pediatric hemofiltration: Normocarb dialysate solution with citrate anticoagulation. Pediatr Nephrol 2002;17:150-154.

See the companion Expert Consult website for the complete reference list.

CHAPTER 298

Inborn Errors of Metabolism and Continuous Renal Replacement Therapy

Scott Walters and Patrick D. Brophy

> **OBJECTIVES**
>
> This chapter will:
> 1. Review the rationale for use of continuous renal replacement therapy in the management of inborn errors of metabolism.
> 2. Outline the differences from acute renal failure management in terms of blood and dialysate flows, prescription, and thermic control.

Individual inborn errors of metabolism are rare, but with emerging diagnostic capabilities, many specific disorders can now be identified. The neonatal period is a critical time for detection as well as treatment of a significant proportion of disorders due to inborn errors of metabolism. The initial diagnosis of such disorders often is delayed as a result of the nonspecificity of presenting signs and symptoms, which may include poor feeding, vomiting, hypotonia, irritability, and somnolence. Inborn errors of metabolism are strongly suggested, however, by findings of hyperglycemia or hypoglycemia and hyperammonemia or ketoacidosis on common blood chemistry studies, including comprehensive metabolic panels. The clinical presentation of urea cycle disorders may be that of a severely ill child with hyperammonemia and a low blood urea nitrogen (BUN) concentration with respiratory alkalosis, whereas patients with organic acidemias or congenital lactic acidosis commonly demonstrate laboratory results consistent with metabolic acidosis or ketoacidosis with hyperammonemia. For many disorders, screening tests have little impact on management or prognosis, because results are unavailable at the time of presentation.[1] Many abnormalities are acutely treatable, particularly hyperammonemia; therefore, any delay in initiating treatment can lead to permanent neurological damage.

The main goals of therapeutic interventions for the treatable inborn errors of metabolism are early recognition and prompt treatment, with the aim of preventing progressive neurological damage and limiting morbidity and mortality.[2] Along with appropriate clinical examination and correction of dehydration (which almost always is present in these patients) or any electrolyte abnormalities, the use of continuous renal replacement therapy (CRRT) for treatment of inborn errors of metabolism (such as urea cycle defects) (Fig. 298-1) has become standard practice when dietary and medical interventions fail to produce improvement.

Hyperammonemia results from the inability of the body to excrete nitrogenous waste, as seen during inborn errors of metabolism involving the urea cycle or organic acidemias (Fig. 298-2). Both ammonia, levels of which are elevated in urea cycle defects and some organic acidemias, and branched-chain amino acids, levels of which are elevated in maple syrup urine disease, have been shown to be effectively cleared by CRRT, demonstrating this to be an efficient adjuvant therapy for acute management of inborn errors of metabolism.[3-6]

Eight identified inborn errors of ureagenesis (seven autosomal recessive and one X-linked) have a combined estimated prevalence of 1 in 30,000 live births and together constitute the most common cause of neonatal hyperammonemia.[7] These disorders typically manifest within 12 to 72 hours of birth. To prevent permanent brain damage and death secondary to the extensive neurotoxicity of increased levels of ammonia, the current recommended guidelines for initial treatment include (1) restriction of nitrogen supply; (2) inhibition of endogenous catabolism by providing adequate calories; (3) substitution of missing metabolites; (4) increased clearance of toxic compounds; and (5) in patients not responsive to medical therapy alone, extracorporeal removal of metabolites through dialysis.[2]

Treatment of severe hyperammonemia (serum ammonia levels greater than 1000 µmol/L) should begin with hemodialysis when medically appropriate and tolerated, because CRRT has an efficacy of only 5% to 15% of that achieved with hemodialysis. Once serum ammonia levels are less than 200 µmol/L, transition to CRRT is appropriate.[8] This combined use of initial hemodialysis followed by CRRT has been shown to result in improved control of hyperammonemia and prevents the rebound of serum ammonia levels seen with intermittent therapy alone.[9] CRRT alone may be used as an initial therapy in patients with less severe hyperammonemia (serum ammonia levels less than 500 µmol/L), but in the event that levels increase during CRRT, use of hemodialysis must be considered. Peritoneal dialysis has little role in the treatment of these disorders.

Because the goal of any treatment in patients with inborn errors of metabolism is rapid removal of toxic metabolites (such as ammonia or branched-chain amino acids), appropriate pharmacological therapy needs to be initiated as soon as possible to control the primary disease, in addition to the initiation of hemodialysis or CRRT, or both. CRRT prescriptions should be altered to maximize clearance of the toxic molecules. Recommendations are for blood flow rates to increase by 100% from 4 to 5 mL/kg per minute to 8 to 10 mL/kg per minute and for dialysate flow rates to increase by 50% to 100% from 2000 mL/1.73 m^2 to 3000 to 4000 mL/1.73 m^2, when possible. With increased flow

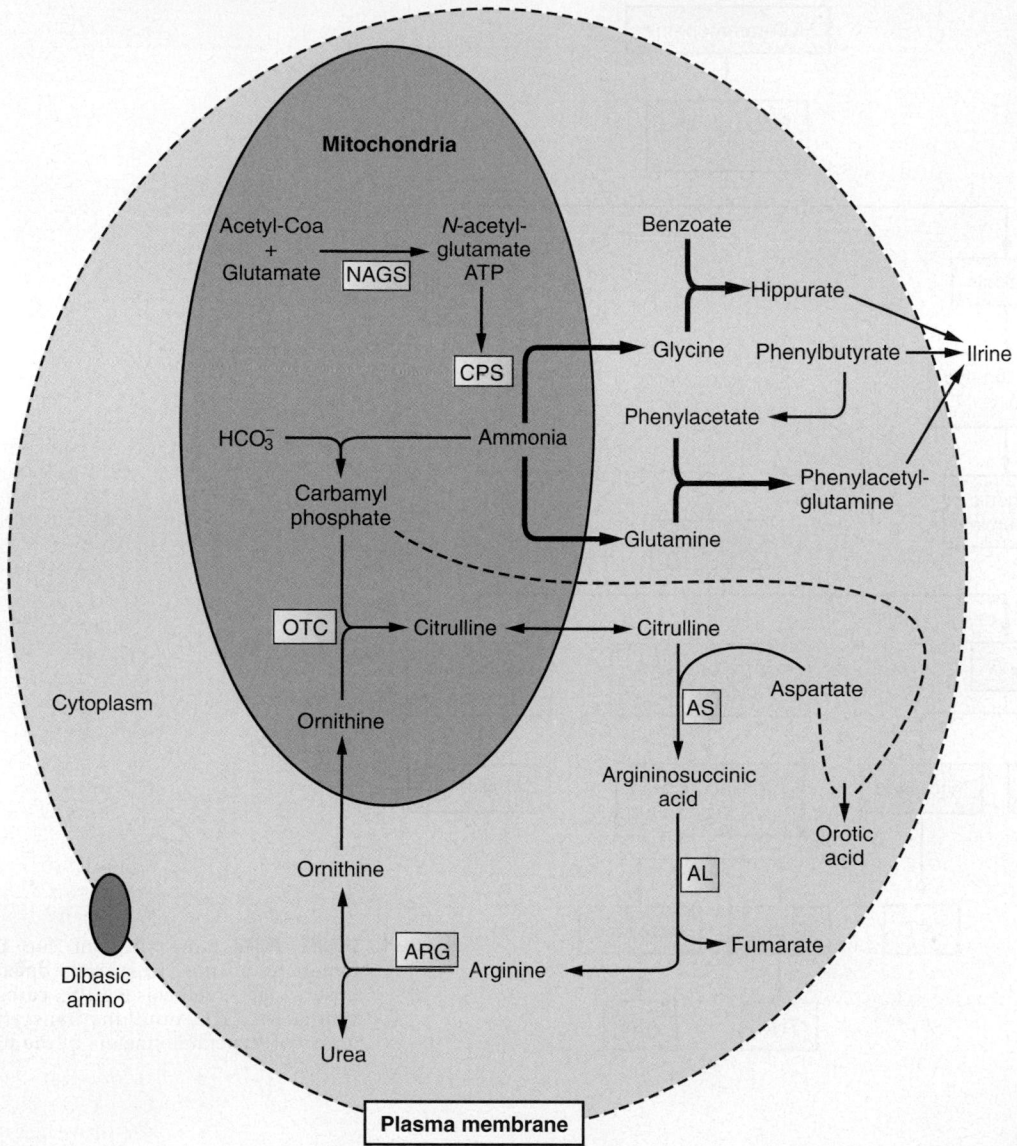

FIGURE 298-1. Urea cycle pathway. *Thin arrows* indicate primary pathway. *Thick arrows* show alternative pathways used to eliminate nitrogen in patients with urea cycle defects. Enzymes are in *boxes*. Acetyl-CoA, acetyl-coenzyme A; AL, argininosuccinate lyase; ARG, arginase; AS, argininosuccinate synthetase; CPS, carbamoylphosphate synthetase; NAGS, *N*-acetylglutamate synthase; OTC, ornithine transcarbamoylase.

rates effectively increasing clearance, electrolytes should be monitored frequently (every 6 hours), and care must be taken to prevent the development of any abnormalities, particularly hypophosphatemia.[10] Patients with inborn errors of metabolism who do not have acute oliguric or anuric renal failure will routinely require potassium- and phosphate-containing dialysate during renal replacement therapy (hemodialysis or CRRT).

Studies continue to demonstrate that a lower presenting serum ammonia concentration (less than 200 μmol/L) is associated with improved survival and fewer or milder neurological sequelae, and a high presenting plasma ammonia concentration (greater than 200 μmol/L) demonstrates a trend toward decreased survival and more severe neurological deficits.[11] Deodato and colleagues, with limited data, showed short-term prognosis to be related to the duration of hyperammonemic coma.[2] With the very

young age at presentation for most inborn errors of metabolism involving hyperammonemia, the outcome is highly dependent on the speed with which the diagnosis is made (or suggestive abnormalities are detected) and treatment initiated.[1]

Complications related to CRRT in the treatment of inborn errors of metabolism can be associated with cardiovascular compromise (hypotension or arrhythmias) or hypothermia. McBryde and associates observed that the most common complication was hypotension.[11] The high risk of hypothermia in patients with inborn errors of metabolism and severe hyperammonemia is a result of the combination of small patient size (generally these patients are infants), low blood volumes, and increased blood flow rates required for adequate toxic metabolite clearance. Implementation of preventive measures such as use of heat lamps or warming blankets, warming of the circuit tubing,

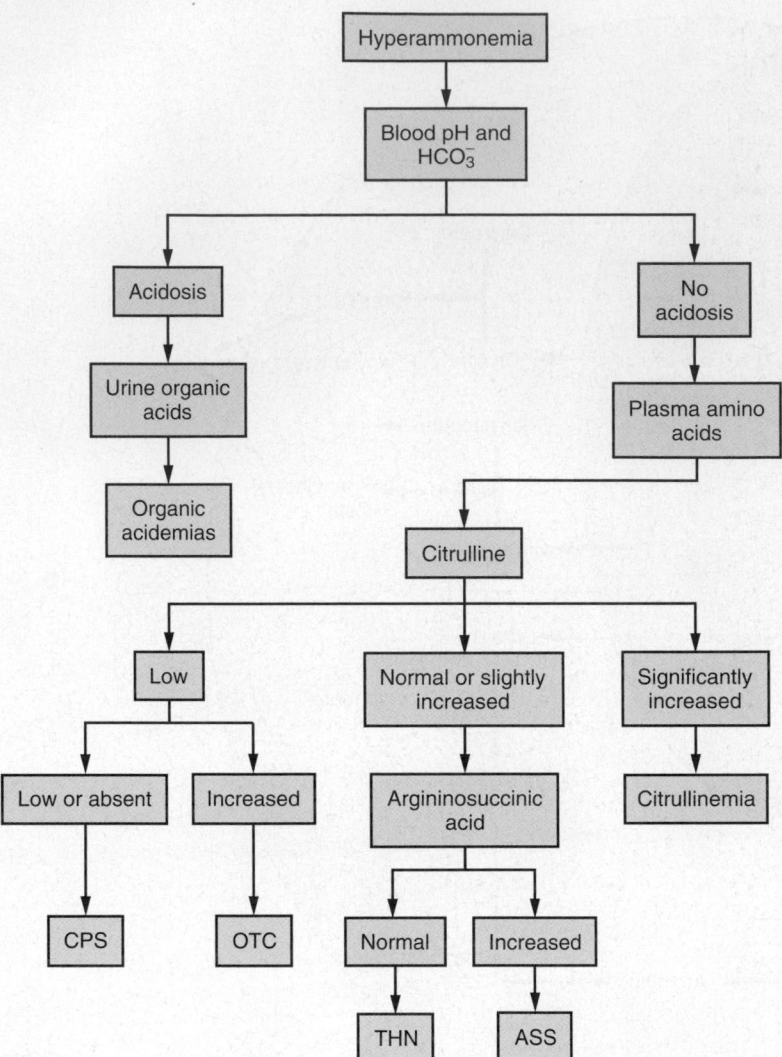

FIGURE 298-2. Flow diagram for the etiology of hyperammonemia. Urea cycle defects: ASS, argininosuccinate synthetase; CPS, carbamoylphosphate synthetase; OTC, ornithine transcarbamylase; THN, transient hyperammonemia of the newborn.

or use of an in-line blood warmer should be considered with the initiation of CRRT.[12]

CRRT has been shown to clear pharmacologically created substrates that provide alternative pathways of nitrogen removal, such as glutamine and glycine.[13-14] It also has been demonstrated that pharmacological agents (e.g., sodium benzoate, sodium phenylacetate or phenylbutyrate, arginine hydrochloride) used to treat metabolic disorders are substantially cleared with these therapies, and the administration of increased doses of these agents should be considered when they are used with CRRT or hemodialysis.[15]

Unlike the management of acute renal failure, in which nutritional supplementation is required, the treatment of inborn errors of metabolism often requires that protein be significantly restricted at presentation. Depending on the duration of CRRT, long-term protein intake may range anywhere from 0.5 to 2 g/kg per day, to prevent development of a catabolic state. Increased clearance of glucose and amino acids in supplemented intravenous fluids, total parenteral nutrition solutions, or enteral feedings that occurs with CRRT needs to be taken into account. This consideration, along with the fact that many of these infants and children have otherwise appropriate renal function, necessitates careful attention to composition of the dialysate or filter replacement fluid composition in order to provide homeostatic electrolytes.

Key Points

1. The main goal of therapy of inborn errors of metabolism is early recognition with prompt treatment to prevent progressive neurological damage and limit morbidity and mortality.
2. Continuous renal replacement therapy is an efficient adjuvant therapy for the acute treatment of inborn errors of metabolism.
3. Continuous renal replacement therapy prescriptions should be individualized to maximize clearance of toxic molecules created during inborn errors of metabolism.

Key References

1. Leonard JV, Morris AAM: Diagnosis and early management of inborn errors of metabolism presenting around the time of birth. Acta Paediatr 2006;95:6-14.

3. Ponikvar R, Kandus A, Urbancic A, et al: Continuous renal replacement therapy and plasma exchange in newborns and infants. Artif Organs 2002;26:163-168.

11. McBryde KD, Kershaw DB, Bunchman TE, et al: Renal replacement therapy in the treatment of confirmed or suspected inborn errors of metabolism. J Pediatr 2006;148:770-778.

13. McBryde KD, Gregory M, Brophy PD, et al: Renal replacement therapy in metabolic disease. Pediatr Nephrol 2000.

See the companion Expert Consult website for the complete reference list.

CHAPTER 299

Modified Ultrafiltration in Pediatric Heart Surgery

Massimo A. Padalino and Giovanni Stellin

OBJECTIVES

This chapter will:
1. Present a rationale for use of modified ultrafiltration in pediatric cardiac surgery.
2. Review the pathophysiological changes leading to the systemic inflammatory response syndrome with use of cardiopulmonary bypass.
3. Summarize the benefits of modified ultrafiltration for pediatric cardiac surgery.
4. Provide guidelines for the modified ultrafiltration procedure based on clinical experience.

Pediatric heart surgery is an area of new frontiers. Many infants and children born with congenital heart defects are now discovering an encouraging future. The invention of the heart-lung machine, with development of techniques for cardiopulmonary bypass (CPB), along with new strides in technology and surgical procedures, has provided new hope for the possibility of repairing complex defects in pediatric patients. Such procedures entail open-heart surgical repair, requiring CPB, which is not without risks. Despite technical improvements that have significantly reduced postoperative morbidity, use of CPB may expose infants to extremes of hemodilution and hypothermia, often associated with tissue ischemia, as well as initiating a systemic inflammatory response, with significant accumulation of excess body water.

One of the most challenging problems related to use of CPB is hemodilution. In fact, the bypass pump must be primed with solutions to provide an air-free circuit. Despite use of blood-derived products during bypass, these solutions are introduced into the patient's vascular space, causing hemodilution and a consequent decrease in the patient's hematocrit level, platelets, and clotting factors. These changes in turn cause increased bleeding, need for transfusions, prolonged intubation time, and increased length of stay in the intensive care unit (ICU). Hemodilution also decreases the patient's colloid osmotic pressure, which causes fluid to move into the extravascular tissues, producing edema.

In addition, a cardiac surgical procedure, much like a traumatic injury, triggers an acute inflammatory response, but the continuous exposure of heparinized blood to non-endothelial cell surfaces, followed by reinfusion and circulation within the body, greatly magnifies this response in procedures in which CPB is used. This inflammatory response is extremely pronounced in neonates and infants, in whom it is expressed as the *systemic inflammatory response syndrome* (SIRS) and *capillary leak syndrome*. The resulting edema affects many organs, including the brain, kidneys, liver, and lungs.

Therefore, it is necessary to use all possible means to limit these extra fluids, to decrease hemodilution. Continuous hemofiltration, delivered in either arteriovenous or venovenous mode, is nowadays a safe and effective extracorporeal treatment modality not only to limit azotemia but also to control electrolytes and fluid balance in critically ill adults as well as pediatric patients with acute renal failure and hemodynamic instability who cannot tolerate conventional methods of dialytic treatment.[1-5] Both conventional and modified ultrafiltration are techniques derived from hemofiltration that are currently used during and after CPB to combat the aforementioned inevitable adverse effects, which are more pronounced in neonates and infants.

HISTORICAL BACKGROUND

Ultrafiltration is a direct derivation of dialytic filtration. In 1974 Silverstein and colleagues[6] modified the extracorporeal dialytic circuit by introducing an additional filter that could eliminate water and proteins with a molecular weight lower than 50,000 Daltons. With this modification, ultrafiltration could now be used to treat conditions of chronic water retention or pulmonary edema; the filtration circuit was designed to be separate from and independent of the dialysis circuit. In 1979, Darup and coworkers[7] applied hemofiltration to CPB in 10 patients with reduced or borderline kidney function undergoing cardiac surgery. During the 1980s, ultrafiltration was used as an adjunct to CBP only in patients with preoperative renal failure or edema. The concept of ultrafiltration arose as a response to the observation of an accumulation of total body water associated with open heart surgery. In the later 1980s and early 1990s, the hypothesis that tissue edema was causing organ dysfunction postoperatively stimulated the idea that removal of water from the body toward the end of CPB would result in improved organ function and perhaps better outcomes. Introduction of ultrafiltration during and after CPB came right after this recognition. Naik and coworkers in 1991[8] were the first to report results with the use of *modified ultrafiltration* (MUF) in pediatric patients (Table 299-1). Their randomized study, which included 50 children, showed that this technique decreased need for blood products and colloids, reduced the amount of body fluid, and improved postoperative cardiac function. Several later studies have confirmed these results.

INFLAMMATORY RESPONSE TO CARDIOPULMONARY BYPASS

CPB in cardiac surgery unleashes a broad and intense acute inflammatory response of variable degree. This acute inflammatory response, together with microembolization, is responsible for most of the morbidity of CPB. The inflammatory response to CPB is initiated by contact between heparinized blood and nonendothelial cell surfaces, with continuous recirculation of blood that is sequentially in contact with the wound, the perfusion circuit, and the intravascular compartment, to which is added the washout from reperfused ischemic organs and tissues.[9] Blood contact with nonendothelial cell surfaces in the wound and in the perfusion circuit activates plasma zymogens and cellular blood elements that constitute part of the body's defense reaction to all noxious substances, (including infectious agents, toxins, foreign antigens, allergens) and also injuries. All surgery, like traumatic injury, triggers an acute inflammatory response, but the continuous exposure of heparinized blood to nonendothelial cell surfaces followed by reinfusion and circulation within the body greatly magnifies this response in procedures in which CPB is used.

Although far from fully elucidated, this predominantly "blood" injury is known to produce a unique response that differs from that caused by other threats to homeostasis. The principal blood elements involved in this acute defense reaction are contact and complement plasma protein systems, neutrophils, monocytes, endothelial cells, and, to a lesser extent, platelets. When activated during CPB, the principal blood elements release vasoactive and cytotoxic substances; produce cell signaling inflammatory and inhibitory cytokines; express complementary cellular receptors that interact with specific cell signaling substances and other cells; and generate a host of vasoactive and cytotoxic substances for release into the circulation.[10] Blood circulating during clinical cardiac surgery with cardiopulmonary bypass is a stew of vasoactive and cytotoxic substances, activated blood cells, and microemboli. Shear stress, turbulence, cavitation, and other rheologic forces and complement components cause hemolysis of some red cells. Complement anaphylatoxins, bradykinin formed by activation of the contact proteins, and pro-inflammatory cytokines stimulate endothelial cells to contract, allowing extravasation of intravascular fluid into the extravascular space.[11] As neutrophils and monocytes migrate across the endothelial cell barrier, stromal and parenchymal cells are exposed to a cytotoxic environment mediated by neutral proteases, collagenases, and gelatinases, reactive oxidants, lipid peroxides, complement components, and other cytotoxins.[12]

The clinical manifestations of the inflammatory response include systemic signs and symptoms such as malaise, fever, increased heart rate, mild hypotension, interstitial fluid accumulation,[13] and temporary organ dysfunction, particularly of the brain, heart, lungs, and kidneys. The magnitude of this defense reaction during and after CPB is influenced by many exogenous factors, including the surface area of the perfusion circuit, the duration of blood contact with extravascular surfaces, general health and preoperative organ function of the patient, extent of blood loss and replacement, organ ischemia and reperfusion injury, sepsis, different degrees of hypothermia, periods of circulatory arrest, the patient's genetic profile, and use of corticosteroids or other pharmacological agents. Several methods have been proposed to control the acute inflammatory response to CBP, and MUF is one of them; other methods include the following:

- *Off-pump cardiac surgery:* This appears to reduce the acute inflammatory response but does not prevent it.[14]
- *Perfusion temperature:* Release of mediators of inflammation is temperature sensitive. Normothermic CPB increases the release of cytokines and other cellular and soluble mediators of inflammation, whereas hypothermia reduces production and release of these mediators until rewarming begins.[15] Perfusion at tepid temperatures between 32° C and 34° C is a reasonable compromise for many operations requiring 1 to 2 hours of CPB.
- *Perfusion circuit coatings:* Ionic- or covalent-bonded heparin perfusion circuits are the most widely used surface coatings; however, differences in efficacy remain to be demonstrated.
- *Leukocyte filtration:* The role of neutrophils in the acute inflammatory response has led to development of leukocyte-depleting filters for the CPB circuit. Evidence of consistent efficacy in reducing markers of neutrophil activation and of improvement in respiratory or renal function is lacking. Most clinical studies fail to document significant leukocyte depletion or clinical benefits.
- *Complement inhibitors:* The central role of complement in the acute inflammatory response with CPB provides ample rationale for inhibition. C1 inhibitor (a natural inhibitor of complement components C1s and C1r), factor XIIa, kallikrein, and factor XIa, factor H, and C4BP, C3 and C5 convertase subunit inhibitors are not effective as inhibitors of induced activation of the complement system. The sequential activation cascade with convergence of the classic and alternative pathways at C3 offers many opportunities for inhibition by recombinant proteins. Although any effective and safe inhibitor is welcome, C3 may be a better target for inhibition because both activation pathways are blocked at the point of convergence and because C3 concentrations in plasma are 15 times greater than those of C5.[16]
- *Glucocorticoids:* Many investigators have used glucocorticoids to suppress the acute inflammatory response to CPB and clinical cardiac surgery, but beneficial effects have been inconsistent.[17] Steroids reduce release of rapid-response cytokines, tumor necrosis factor-α (TNF-α), and interleukin (IL)-1β from macrophages; enhance release of IL-10; and suppress expression of endothelial cell selectins and neutrophil integrins.[18]
- *Protease inhibitors:* Aprotinin is a natural serine protease inhibitor in the kinine superfamily that strongly inhibits plasmin and weakly inhibits kallikrein.[18] The anti-inflammatory effects of aprotinin are more difficult to quantitate and may reflect multiple mechanisms,

TABLE 299-1

Guidelines for Performance of Modified Ultrafiltration (MUF)

- MUF after CPB must be performed by a certified clinical perfusionist.
- To use MUF, the perfusionist who operates the heart-lung machine first modifies the pediatric bypass circuit to incorporate the MUF system.
- MUF for patients who weigh less than 15 kg is implemented immediately after CPB ceases.
- MUF typically is performed for 20 minutes, to remove an approximate volume of filtrate determined using the following equation: $F = (P + Ca + Cr) - (Cuf + D)$, where F is filtrate volume, P is priming crystalloid volume, Ca is cardioplegia volume, Cr is crystalloid volume added during CPB, Cuf is ultrafiltrate volume removed during CUF, and D is diuresis volume.
- Approximately 10 to 20 mL/kg per minute of fluid is removed from the patient, which averages between 400 and 600 mL, depending on the patient's weight, amount of time the MUF system is deployed, and the surgeon's preference.

Goals
1. Reduce "third space" edema, thereby increasing end-organ perfusion.
2. Improve hemodynamic stability.
3. Optimize the patient's post-bypass hematocrit.
4. Remove inflammatory mediators.

Procedure
Set-up
1. Before priming the CPB circuit, the perfusionist adds a roller head, hemoconcentrator, extra tubing, and connectors to the circuit to incorporate the MUF line. The pump and these extra supplies then are primed to ensure a bubble-free circuit.
2. The MUF line is a PVC tube with dimensions of 2.8 mm × 4.2 mm × 150 cm; both ends are connected to a "male" Luer-Lok connector.
3. Insert a three-way stopcock on the primed arterial filter.
4. Connect the MUF line to the CPB circuit.
5. Pass the MUF line to the sterile field.
6. At the sterile field, the nurse clamps and cuts the venous line to add a Luer-Lok connector.
7. Discuss with the nursing staff the types of connectors required (usually ¼-inch connector–Luer-Lok–¼-inch connector–venous cannula) before starting CPB.
8. It is essential to account for all pieces of ¼-inch tubing required to complete the connections.
9. Flush the MUF line with blood prime from the CPB circuit while on pump to "debubble" it.
10. The MUF line coming from the pump will be attached to the Luer-Lok connector by the surgeon. Take care in avoiding air bubbles in lines.

Initiation of MUF
1. After termination of CPB, the patient remains fully heparinized. It is best to refrain from giving blood products until MUF is completed.
2. Clamp out the venous line just distally to the Luer-Lok at which the MUF line is connected.
3. Drain the venous line blood. For safety, the venous line can be siphoned. The venous return then can be used for the patient.
4. When the venous (superior vena cava or right atrial) line is in place, bubble-free and secure, hemofiltration can begin.
5. Set the timer; the estimated time for the procedure is 20 minutes.
6. Plan to remove an approximate volume of filtrate determined using the following formula: $F = (P + Ca + Cr) - (Cuf + D)$, where F is filtrate volume, P is priming crystalloid volume, Ca is cardioplegia volume, Cr is crystalloid volume added during CPB, Cuf is ultrafiltrate volume removed during CUF, and D is diuresis volume.
7. Observe patient hemodynamics closely. Specifically look at maintaining a designated CVP, constant MAP, and, more important, a consistently stable positive pressure in the arterial line. To do so will require a continual "shuffle" between the pump monitor and the patient monitor.
8. If necessary, turn on suction on the hemoconcentrator once flow has started.
9. As systemic pressure falls, turn on the arterial pump head slowly to stabilize. **Remember:** *Never* increase the arterial pump head more than the MUF roller pump head.
10. As the venous reservoir is depleted, up to 500 mL of crystalloid can be added to flush the circuit of blood.
11. The procedure should take 20 minutes. The limiting factor is volume in the venous reservoir.
12. If volume remains in the venous reservoir after MUF is discontinued, continue to flush the circuit and hemoconcentrate; then bag the blood. Once the arterial line is clamped, the recirculating line will need to be opened.
13. The optimal flow through the hemoconcentrator is 8 to 10 mL/kg per minute, but the patient may or may not tolerate this rate of volume removal.
14. Follow pressures closely—ensure a positive pressure in the arterial line at all times. Note the pressures (i.e., arterial line pressure as well as the MAP). **Remember:** If the arterial line pressure becomes negative or a quick drop in positive pressure occurs, air may be drawn across the membrane and into the circuit.

Termination of MUF
1. Ask for the arterial line to be removed, and perform hemoconcentration as the blood is returned.
2. Maintain a primed filter and circuit, as usual.
3. Once the superior vena cava or right atrial line is removed, bag the hemoconcentrated blood from the MUF line as completely as possible.

Supplies Required
- Hemoconcentrator
- Hemoconcentration tubing pack
- Two perfusion adapters: ¼-inch Luer-Lok, ¼-inch connectors (2 inches of ¼-inch tubing)
- Sterile blade and alcohol
- Effluent container with measuring capability (i.e., urometer)

Note:
- When arterial pump flow is used to supplement MUF, *never* increase arterial pump flow to a rate greater than that of MUF pump flow.

CPB, cardiopulmonary bypass; CUF, continuous ultrafiltration; CVP, central venous pressure; MAP, mean arterial pressure; PVC, polvinylchloride.

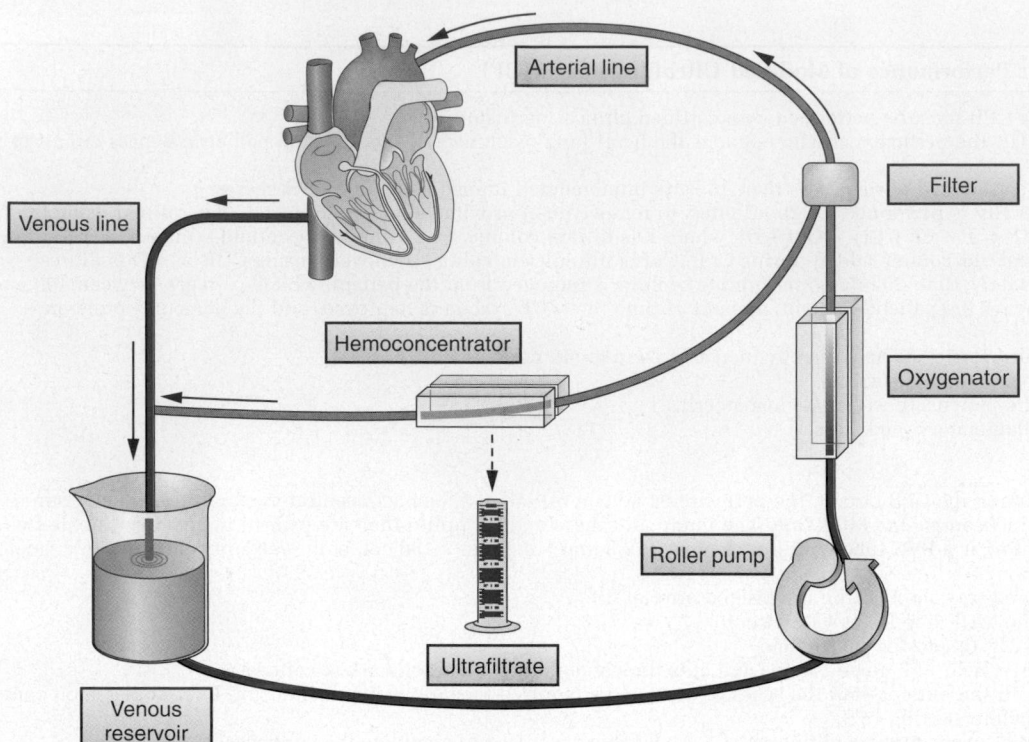

FIGURE 299-1. Diagram showing continuous ultrafiltration (CUF) circuit (arteriovenous). The hemoconcentrator is connected by means of a Luer-Lok connector to the arterial filter. During cardiopulmonary bypass, part of the oxygenated blood is bypassed to the ultrafilter, from which filtered blood reaches the venous line and is stored in the venous reservoir. Filtrate fluid is stored in a separate waste container, to be discarded later.

including partial kallikrein inhibition, direct effects, and inhibition of nuclear factor (NF)-κB. Clinically, aprotinin reduces circulating TNF-α, IL-6, IL-8, and neutrophil CD11b expression and synergistically increases IL-10 synthesis.[19] Nevertheless, low- or high-dose aprotinin used in large, randomized controlled clinical trials fails to show a reduction in pro-inflammatory cytokines, activated complement, neutrophil elastase, and myeloperoxidase.[20] Thus, the efficacy of aprotinin as an anti-inflammatory agent remains unresolved.

MODIFIED ULTRAFILTRATION

Recently, MUF has been used in pediatric cardiac surgery to limit deleterious effects of CPB. The recognized benefits of MUF are reduction in total body water accumulation seen after CPB, improved left ventricular function, increase in hematocrit with concomitant reduction of transfused blood products, improved hemostasis, dynamic pulmonary compliance, and modification of complement activation. Ultrafiltration is a technique that removes plasma water and low-molecular-weight solutes by a convective process involving hydrostatic forces acting across a semipermeable membrane; substances with a molecular mass less than the membrane pore size are filtered because of the transmembrane gradient. The composition of filtrate is dependent on the pore size of the hemofilter. Continuous ultrafiltration (CUF) usually is performed during the rewarming phase of CPB to decrease the excess of total body water and limit postoperative edema (Fig. 299-1).

The increase in total body water is caused by the relatively large volume of pump prime compared with the circulating blood volume, especially in small children. SIRS triggered by CPB increases capillary permeability and further aggravates the increase in total body water. CUF has failed to produce a consistent reduction in postoperative total body water or in transfusion requirements because of frequent addition of crystalloid or blood to the circuit to maintain an adequate reservoir level and CPB while on support. These unsatisfactory results with CUF in consistently preventing an increase in total body water and reversing hemodilution after CPB in children were the stimulus for the development of MUF by Naik and associates,[8] as mentioned earlier. In a preliminary study, these investigators compared the efficacy of no ultrafiltration, CUF, and MUF in preventing accumulation of excess total body water.[21] For MUF, the CPB circuit is altered so that blood is pumped retrograde from the aortic cannula, through the hemoconcentrator, and returned to the right atrium. This design results in return of warmed hemoconcentrated oxygenated blood to the heart and pulmonary vasculature (Fig. 299-2). The absolute volume of ultrafiltrate that should be removed to obtain maximal hemodynamic and end-organ functional improvement is not well defined. Endpoints differ among institutions: Some remove a specific volume (mL/kg) of ultrafiltrate; others perform MUF for a predetermined period of time (usually 15 to 20 minutes) or to achieve a specific hematocrit (usually greater than 40%).

Effectiveness of MUF has been quantified by Maehara and colleagues,[22] who validated the use of bioelectrical impedance as a noninvasive means of determining changes

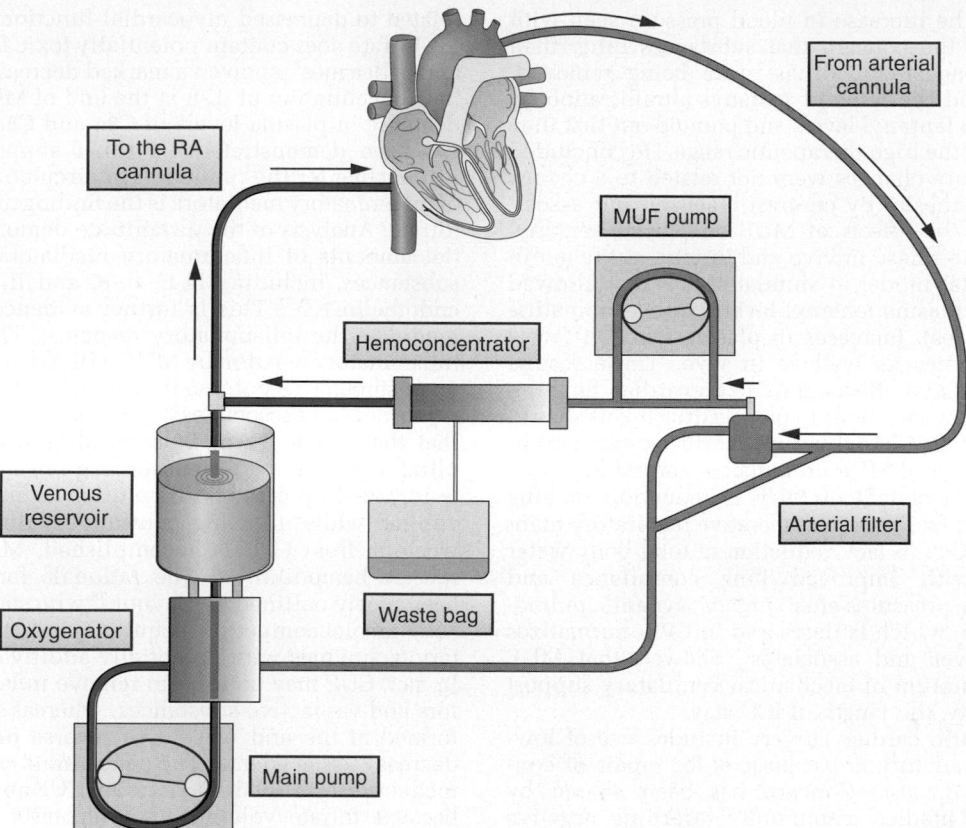

FIGURE 299-2. Diagram showing modified ultrafiltration (MUF) circuit. Ultrafilter/hemoconcentrator is connected by means of a Luer-Lok connector to the arterial filter. When cardiopulmonary bypass is off, a roller pump drives blood from aorta to the ultrafilter-hemoconcentrator, from which filtered blood reaches the venous line and returns to the right atrium (RA). In this case, the venous reservoir line is clamped. Filtrate fluid is stored in a separate waste container, to be discarded later.

in total body water associated with CPB. The same group of investigators have demonstrated an increase in total body water of 11% to 18% higher than pre-CPB levels. Thus, the optimal filtrate volume could be assessed by impedance evaluation before and after CPB. In fact, the benefits of MUF versus standard ultrafiltration (CUF) were first shown by the GOS group[8,21] as measured by bioelectrical impedance. The volume of ultrafiltrate that could be removed during MUF was significantly greater than that during CUF; MUF significantly reduced the postoperative increase in total body water, whereas the response to CUF was neither uniform nor reproducible.

The beneficial effects of MUF are multiple and have been demonstrated by several groups of investigators. Naik and associates[8] demonstrated a decrease in postoperative blood loss and consequently a reduction in blood products usage after MUF when compared with no ultrafiltration during CPB. A significant decrease in blood loss and blood transfusion requirements has been demonstrated by others.[23] In addition, MUF resulted in an unexpected increase in arterial blood pressure, increase in cardiac index, and decrease in pulmonary vascular resistance, without changes in systemic vascular resistance. These hemodynamic benefits correlated directly with the increasing hematocrit and thus the degree of hemoconcentration.[24]

Gaynor and coworkers[25] showed that increase in myocardial cross-sectional area seen after CPB can be reversed after MUF. Davies and colleagues[26] confirmed that MUF

improves intrinsic left ventricular systolic function, improves diastolic compliance, increases blood pressure, and decreases inotropic drug use in the early postoperative period. In a randomized study in 21 infants undergoing CPB, an ultrasound dimension transducer was used to measure the anteroposterior minor axis diameter, and a left ventricular micromanometer was applied as well. Left ventricular systolic function was assessed by means of the slope of the preload-recruitable stroke work index. Myocardial cross-sectional area was measured by echocardiography. In the MUF group, the filtrate volume was 363 ± 262 mL. The hematocrit value increased from 26.0% ± 2.7% to 36.7% ± 9.5% (P = .018), myocardial cross-sectional area decreased from 3.72 ± 0.35 cm^2 to 3.63 ± 0.36 cm^2 (P = .04), end-diastolic length increased from 25.6 ± 9.0 mm to 28.8 ± 9.9 mm (P = .01), and end-diastolic pressure fell from 5.6 ± 0.8 mm Hg to 4.2 ± 0.8 mm Hg (P = .005), suggesting an improved diastolic compliance. In the control group, these parameters were unchanged. The demonstration of increased left ventricular end-diastolic length and decreased end-diastolic pressure is consistent with improved left ventricular compliance secondary to decreased myocardial edema.

Daggett and colleagues[27] confirmed the superiority of MUF to conventional ultrafiltration and no filtration in reducing total body weight gain, lessening myocardial edema, raising mean arterial pressure, and improving left ventricular contractility in neonatal piglets undergoing cardiopulmonary bypass and cardioplegic arrest.

The cause of the increase in blood pressure seen with MUF has raised the concern that substances other than water, such as anesthetic drugs, were being removed. Elliott[28] addressed the issue of fentanyl ultrafiltration by measuring serum fentanyl levels and pointed out that they remained within the high therapeutic range. He concluded that blood pressure changes were not related to a change in depth of anesthesia. By contrast, Taenzer and associates[29] examined the effects of MUF on plasma fentanyl levels using a two-phase in vivo and in vitro study (an in vitro experimental model to simulate MUF that allowed measurement of plasma fentanyl levels while eliminating biological variables). Increases in plasma fentanyl levels were found in vitro as well as in vivo. These results confirm the beneficial effects of MUF on cardiac function and emphasize that variations in plasma drug levels should be taken into account in delivering anesthetic care and in analyzing the effect of MUF on outcome variables.

Another proven benefit of MUF is reduction in lung water, which will facilitate postoperative respiratory management in the ICU. In fact, reduction in total body water is associated with improved lung compliance and decreased airway pressures after surgery. Dynamic pulmonary compliance, which is decreased in CPB, normalizes after MUF.[30] Sever and associates[31] showed that MUF decreases the duration of mechanical ventilatory support and, subsequently, the length of ICU stay.

Current pediatric cardiac surgery includes use of low-flow CPB or circulatory arrest periods for repair of congenital cardiac disease. Concern has been shared by members of the medical community regarding negative effects of these often necessary techniques. Skaryak and coworkers[32] investigated the effect of MUF on cerebral metabolic recovery after deep hypothermic circulatory arrest on 1-week-old piglets that were supported by CPB and after 90 minutes of circulatory arrest followed by rewarming to 37° C. After being weaned from CPB, animals were divided into three groups: a control group, an MUF group, and a group in which transfusion with hemoconcentrated blood was given. Global cerebral blood flow was measured by xenon-133 clearance methods. Cerebral metabolic rate of oxygen consumption, cerebral oxygen delivery, and hematocrit were calculated before CPB, after CPB discontinuation, and after completion of MUF. These investigators showed an increase in cerebral oxygen consumption from baseline, suggesting that the decrease in cerebral metabolism seen immediately after CPB is reversible. High levels of cerebral metabolic rate of oxygen consumption may be necessary to repay the oxygen debt incurred during circulatory arrest. After MUF, cerebral oxygen delivery and metabolic rate of oxygen consumption both increase, showing that brain recovery from metabolic dysfunction after deep hypothermic circulatory arrest can be improved with MUF. Proposed mechanisms for this improvement include decrease in cerebral edema as a reflection of the decrease in total body water, removal of vasoactive substances, and alteration of leukocyte-mediated injury.

As mentioned, the inflammatory response stimulated by exposure of blood to the nonendothelialized surfaces of the CPB pump, especially if coupled with hypothermia or circulatory arrest, contributes to capillary leakage. Several studies have explored the role of MUF in mediating activation of the inflammatory response seen with CPB. Dagget and associates[27] demonstrated in their neonatal swine model that MUF was effective in preventing accumulation of total body water and myocardial edema and resulted in improved cardiac function. Reinfusion of the filtrate was

related to depressed myocardial function, suggesting that the filtrate does contain potentially toxic factors. El Habbal and colleagues[33] showed a marked decrease in the circulating concentration of IL-8 at the end of MUF. A significant decrease in plasma levels of C3a and C5a after MUF also has been demonstrated.[34] Further support that MUF is responsible for the reduction in circulating plasma levels of inflammatory mediators is the finding of C5a in the ultrafiltrate. Analysis of the ultrafiltrate demonstrated substantial amounts of inflammatory mediators and vasoactive substances, including IL-6, IL-8, and IL-10, TNF-α, and endothelin-1.[35-37] This is further evidence that MUF may modulate the inflammatory response. Thus, limiting the inflammatory reaction by MUF will have significant effects on postoperative pulmonary and myocardial function.

Journois and associates[36] reported a modification of CUF that they called "zero balance ultrafiltration," in which ultrafiltration is performed during rewarming and filtrate is replaced by crystalloid solution to maintain reservoir volume while allowing continuous ultrafiltration. After weaning from CPB is accomplished, MUF is started to reverse hemodilution. The rationale for doing this has been nicely outlined by Gaynor,[38] who states that CUF and MUF are not competing techniques but rather complementary techniques with potentially additive positive effects. In fact, CUF may be used to remove inflammatory mediators and vasoactive substances, whereas MUF can be performed at the end of CPB to reverse hemodilution and decrease tissue edema. The concentration of inflammatory mediators does not differ between CUF and MUF; however, because filtrate volume is significantly greater in MUF, removal of mediators is correspondingly greater. Thus, the optimal use of ultrafiltration in children undergoing open heart surgery will likely result from a combination of these two techniques.

Finally, concerns have been raised about potential risks and complications of MUF due to technical errors or mishaps leading to changes in the delicate balance of the CPB circuit: improper assembly of the modified ultrafiltration pump, introduction of air into the patient's vascular system, line rupture, and hypotension due to exceedingly quick volume depletion caused by MUF itself, if appropriate volume replacement (i.e., fresh frozen plasma) is not effected. Neurological deficits also may be potentially associated with modified ultrafiltration if the blood flow through the system is too high, causing a decrease in blood flow to the brain. An early concern was that MUF would lead to hemodynamic instability secondary to withdrawal of blood from the arterial cannula immediately after CPB. Actually, the converse has proved true: MUF results in an increase in arterial blood pressure, with decreased filling pressure and improved cardiac function. Multiple studies have demonstrated, however, that all concerns over possible complications are primarily theoretical. In a review of 22 centers, Darling and associates[39] found no reports of MUF-related morbidity or mortality.

In conclusion, modified ultrafiltration has proved to be a safe and effective technique to improve the postoperative course in children undergoing open heart surgery. As reported by Groom and coworkers[40] in a recent survey of data for 76 hospitals in North America, modified ultrafiltration was used in 75% of the centers surveyed. Thus, the beneficial effects of MUF are currently recognized and MUF is used by most pediatric cardiac surgeons. No study has yet established a definite relationship between removal of inflammatory mediators and improved outcome, however, and the mechanisms by which ultrafiltration results in improved organ function require additional elucidation. Further studies are needed to identify which patients are most likely to benefit from MUF and to define the best protocols for rational use of this technique.

Key Points

1. Modified ultrafiltration currently is used in pediatric cardiac surgery to limit deleterious effects of cardiopulmonary bypass.
2. The recognized benefits of modified ultrafiltration are reduction in total body water accumulation seen after cardiopulmonary bypass, improved left ventricular function, increase in hematocrit with concomitant reduction in need for transfused blood products, improved hemostasis and dynamic pulmonary compliance, and modification of complement activation.
3. Modified ultrafiltration is a safe and effective technique that does not add either additional risk or excessive cost to the procedure of cardiopulmonary bypass.
4. Modified ultrafiltration after cardiopulmonary bypass must be performed by a certified clinical perfusionist.
5. Modified ultrafiltration after cardiopulmonary bypass may be used with hemofiltration during cardiopulmonary bypass to maximize beneficial effects for the patient.

Acknowledgments

We thank our perfusion team at the University of Padua, especially Enrico Ceccherini, CP, and Fabio Zanella, CP, for their invaluable help, either in the preparation of the manuscript for this chapter or in our everyday work in the operating room.

Key References

8. Naik SK, Knight A, Elliott MJ: A prospective randomized study of a modified technique of ultrafiltration during pediatric open-heart surgery. Circulation 1991;84(Suppl): III422-III431.
25. Gaynor JW, Tulloh RMR, Owen CH, et al: Modified ultrafiltration reduces myocardial edema and reverses hemodilution following cardiopulmonary bypass in children. J Am Coll Cardiol 1995;200A.
26. Davies MJ, Nguyen K, Gaynor JW, Elliott MJ: Modified ultrafiltration improves left ventricular systolic function in infants after cardiopulmonary bypass. J Thorac Cardiovasc Surg 1998;115:361-369.
35. Bando K, Turrentine MW, Vijay P, et al: Effect of modified ultrafiltration in high risk patients undergoing operations for congenital heart disease. Ann Thorac Surg 1998;66:821-828.
38. Gaynor JW: Use of ultrafiltration during and after cardiopulmonary bypass in children. J Thorac Cardiovasc Surg 2001;122:209-211.

See the companion Expert Consult website for the complete reference list.

Kidney Transplantation and Critical Care

CHAPTER 300

Patient Selection and Pretransplantation Care for Kidney Transplant Recipients

Jerry McCauley, Nirav Shah, Mark Unruh, and Christine Wu

OBJECTIVES

This chapter will:
1. Outline an overall approach to evaluating renal transplant recipients.
2. Identify risk factors for graft loss and death after transplantation.
3. Identify renal diseases known to recur after transplantation.
4. Identify the basic cardiac evaluation for transplant recipients.
5. Identify appropriate waiting periods for patients with malignancies before transplantation.

Innovations in transplantation have led to progressive improvement in patient and graft survival after renal transplantation. In most transplant centers, the criteria for the referral and acceptance of patients with end-stage renal disease (ESRD) have broadened. Guidelines have now been advanced by the American Society of Transplantation (AST), the Canadian Society of Transplantation (CST), and the European Association of Urology (EAU).[1-3] Both the AST and the CST used a system developed by the Canadian Task Force on Preventive Health Care to grade their recommendations as follows[4]:

A—There is good evidence to support the recommendation that the condition be considered in the evaluation process.

B—There is fair evidence to support the recommendation that the condition be considered in the evaluation process.

C—There is poor evidence regarding the inclusion of the condition in the evaluation process, but recommendations may be made on other grounds.

D—There is fair evidence to support the recommendation that the condition be excluded from consideration in the evaluation process.

E—There is good evidence to support the recommendation that the condition be excluded from consideration in the evaluation process.

Although this is a qualitative scheme that may leave room for clinical judgment, it does set common ground for patient evaluation. We will, therefore, use the AST grading in discussing the evaluation of renal transplant recipients in this chapter.

REFERRING PATIENTS FOR KIDNEY TRANSPLANTATION

Preparation for renal transplantation should begin once progression to ESRD can be predicted (C). The process of evaluation for transplantation begins when patients are referred to the transplant center. Preemptive transplantation may generate superior graft and patient survival in renal transplant recipients.[5] Both the CST and the AST recommend preemptive transplantation (C), but the CST recommends waiting until the glomerular filtration rate (GFR) is 20 mL/min or less.

The importance of early transplantation was illustrated in a study comparing patients undergoing early (<6 months on dialysis) versus late (>24 months on dialysis) kidney transplantation; at 60 months, graft survival was 78% versus 58% in the two groups, respectively.[6] A further study by Ojo and colleagues demonstrated that the long-term risk of death can be reduced by renal transplantation compared with remaining on dialysis.[7] Given these studies and others, there is little justification for delaying referral of patients for transplantation.

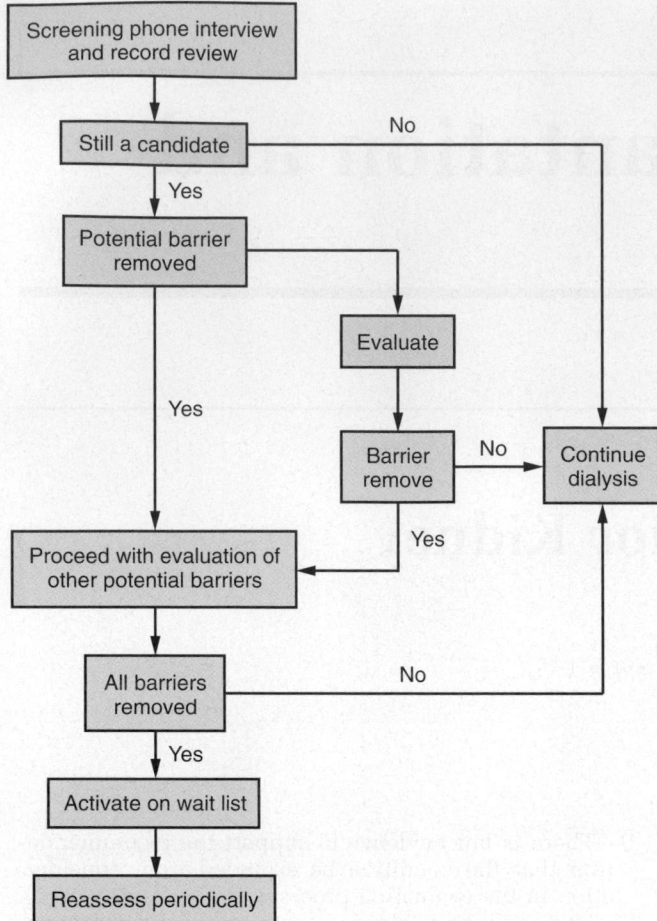

FIGURE 300-1. Transplant recipient evaluation process. (Adapted from Kasiske BL, Cangro CB, Hariharan S, et al: The evaluation of renal transplant candidates: Clinical practice guidelines. Am J Transplant 2001;1[Suppl 2]:1-95.)

TABLE 300-1

Contraindications to Transplantation

Noncompliance (nonadherence to therapy)
Active infection
Active or incurable malignancy
Psychiatric illness preventing decision making or compliance
Illicit drug abuse
Primary oxalosis (without prior liver transplantation)
Severe uncorrectable impairment of other organs (e.g., liver failure, cardiovascular disease, pulmonary disease)
Severe obesity (body mass index >40)

TABLE 300-2

Evaluation Protocol for Renal Transplantation

Professional evaluations	Social Worker, Nurse Coordinator, Financial Coordinator, Dentist, Surgeon, Nephrologist
General laboratory studies	BUN, creatinine, electrolytes, calcium, phosphorus, AST, ALT, GGTP, alkaline phosphatase, cholesterol, triglyceride, LDH, amylase, albumin, total protein, CBC, platelet count, PT, PTT, RPR
Viral infection screen	Cytomegalovirus (IgG and IgM), hepatitis B (HBsAb/Ag), hepatitis C, HIV, Epstein-Barr virus, herpes zoster, herpes simplex, varicella
Other routine studies	Chest radiograph, ECG, PPD + controls, urine culture and sensitivity
Urologic studies	Ultrasound of both kidneys and right upper quadrant; PSA (men ≥40 years)
Screening studies for women	Mammogram (≥40 years); gynecology examination, PAP
Immunology studies	ABO type and screen, HLA and DR typing, PRA, circulating antibodies, crossmatch
Gastrointestinal evaluation	Colonoscopy (≥50 years)

ALT, alanine transaminase; AST, aspartate transaminase; BUN, blood urea nitrogen; CBC, complete blood count; ECG, electrocardiogram; GGTP, gamma-glutamyl transpeptidase; HBsAb/Ag, hepatitis B surface antibody/antigen; HIV, human immunodeficiency virus; HLA, human leukocyte antigen; Ig, immunoglobulin; LDH, lactate dehydrogenase; PAP, Papanicolaou smear; PPD, purified protein derivative; PRA, panel-reactive antibody; PSA, prostate-specific antigen; PT, prothrombin time; PTT, partial thromboplastin time; RPR, rapid plasma reagin test.

THE RECIPIENT EVALUATION PROCESS

Evaluation of patients is costly, is time-consuming for patients, and expends limited healthcare resources. For these reasons, the process should attempt to eliminate contraindications to transplantation early in the process. Figure 300-1 illustrates the flow of events in evaluating potential candidates. An initial screening history is taken before the patient is scheduled for a visit to the center. Special attention is given to problems that would contraindicate transplantation (Table 300-1). Patients with known contraindications should be eliminated at that point, and appropriate patients should be scheduled for a visit to the center. During the evaluation process, potential barriers to transplantation are reviewed and measures to remove them are performed if possible. If a prohibitive barrier cannot be removed, the patient should continue dialysis. The protocol for recipient evaluation is outlined in Table 300-2. In many centers, the patients and their referring physicians are given a list of routine studies that could be performed before the visit. This may expedite transplantation, but expensive or potentially risky studies should be withheld until after the visit to the transplant center. Once the patients have been seen at the transplant center, a multidisciplinary professional approach is begun.

Detailed examinations are performed by the professional staff, looking for medical, surgical, or psychosocial problems. Patients who are unable to consistently take medications or appear for clinic visits are more likely to develop acute rejection and graft failure. Typically, compliance with therapy for 6 to 12 months is required before placement on the waiting list. Drug or alcohol abuse has been reported in 25% of patients being evaluated for renal transplantation and may indirectly jeopardize long-term graft survival.[8] Common practice and the ATC guidelines (C) require that all patients with chemical dependence be evaluated and treated for this problem in addition to having a documented drug- or alcohol-free period of 6 months before being listed for transplantation.

Most centers obtain screening studies for viral infections and immunology studies during the clinic visit, but the general laboratory studies, other routine studies, urological and cancer screening studies (prostate-specific antigen, mammogram, gynecology examination, Papanicolaou smear, and colonoscopy) can be performed at the patient's referring center and are most efficiently performed before the visit at the transplant center.

EVALUATING RISKS TO SUCCESSFUL TRANSPLANTATION

The goal of the preliminary pretransplantation evaluation is to identify risks to successful transplantation and to long-term patient and graft survival. Improvements in transplantation continue to ameliorate conditions previously considered to be absolute contraindications (see Table 300-1). Generally accepted contraindications include continued noncompliance, active infection, some untreated malignancies, uncontrolled psychiatric illness, and continued illicit drug abuse. Primary oxalosis without prior liver transplantation remains a contraindication in most centers. Severe uncorrectable liver failure, cardiac disease, or pulmonary disease is also a contraindication at most centers, although many centers attempt transplantation in patients with advanced but end-stage nonrenal disease. Patients with near–end-stage nonrenal organ failure may be candidates for transplantation of these organs before kidney transplantation is undertaken.

If there are no contraindications to transplantation, the remainder of the evaluations center on measures to reduce perioperative risk and to improve long-term survival of the patient and allograft.

Elderly Recipients

During the past decade, the number of elderly patients accepted for ESRD care has steadily grown. In 2004, 49% of patients starting renal replacement therapy were 65 years of age or older. However, only 1% of these older patients were transplanted.[9] Advances in transplantation have resulted in excellent graft and patient survival for elderly recipients. These improvements in elderly patients can largely be attributed to more careful patient selection and more rigorous pretransplantation medical evaluation. Principal among these measures is a detailed cardiovascular and peripheral vascular examination. The minimum cardiovascular evaluation should include a pharmacological cardiac stress test and angiography in high-risk patients. Symptoms and signs of peripheral vascular disease should be sought. Symptoms of claudication and diminished peripheral pulses should prompt an evaluation consisting of arterial Doppler studies and angiography of the lower extremities if necessary. Uncorrected peripheral vascular disease may prevent an adequate vascular anastomosis during the surgery, jeopardize perfusion of the extremity, and increase the risk of thrombosis of the allograft after transplantation. Many centers require carotid artery Doppler studies routinely or angiography for selected elderly patients. Vascular disease of all types should be corrected, if possible, before transplantation.

Many centers have arbitrarily instituted an age limitation for transplantation at approximately 70 years. As with all patients, the number of comorbid illnesses has a major impact on outcomes. Some centers have successfully transplanted patients in the ninth decade of life without major complications.

Race and Ethnicity

Race and ethnicity are factors in patient survival on dialysis and after transplantation. Disparities in access to transplantation and clinical outcomes have been documented in many countries. In the United States, African-American patients survive longer on dialysis than whites but have inferior graft survival after transplantation.[10,11] African Americans in the United States and other ethnic minorities worldwide also wait longer for deceased donor organs. Although well-documented biological factors contribute to poor survival after transplantation in African Americans, there is a growing recognition that socioeconomic factors may explain the majority of the differences in outcomes.[12] These problems may pose formidable barriers to transplantation, and solutions should be intensively sought before transplantation.

Obesity

Many studies have demonstrated that obesity is an important risk factor after transplantation.[13] Obese patients experienced more infections, wound complications, admissions to the intensive care unit, new-onset diabetes, and mortality than nonobese patients. Delayed graft function and long-term graft failure are more common in obese patients.[14] For these reasons, weight reduction is usually advised before transplantation. Morbidly obese patients may benefit from gastric bypass or other weight-reduction surgery. The CST recommend supervised weight reduction with a target body mass index of less than 30 (B), but, due to limited data, they were unable to recommend which patients should be denied transplantation. Underweight patients also have increased risk of graft loss and other complications.[15] Figure 300-2 illustrates the risk imposed by variation from ideal weight. Underweight patients should be evaluated for underlying medical and psychiatric illnesses.

RECURRENCE OF PRIMARY RENAL DISEASE AFTER TRANSPLANTATION

Recurrence of the primary renal disease after transplantation is an important consideration in the recipient evaluation. Glomerular diseases are the most common lesions to recur. Table 300-3 illustrates the risks of recurrence and graft loss in glomerular and nonglomerular diseases. In most cases, recurrence of disease does not preclude further transplantation, because the patients may obtain many dialysis-free years with subsequent grafts.

Focal segmental glomerulosclerosis (FSGS) recurs in approximately 20% to 30% of patients. Graft loss is approximately 50% in primary grafts, but the rate increases once recurrence has occurred and may approximate 100% in patients with prior recurrence. No measures reduce the risk of recurrence. Prophylactic plasma exchange has been used, but the data are insufficient to recommend it (C). Despite this gloomy picture, patients with FSGS benefit from renal transplantation, and it is

TABLE 300-3

Recurrence of Renal Disease after Transplantation

RENAL DISEASE	RECURRENCE RATE (%)	GRAFT LOSS (%)
Idiopathic Glomerular Diseases		
FSGS	20-30	40-50
Membranous glomerulonephritis	10-20	50
Type I MPGN	20-30	30-40
Type II MPGN	80-100	10-20
IgA nephropathy	40-50	6-33
Anti-GBM nephritis	10	Rare
Secondary Glomerular Diseases		
Henoch-Schönlein purpura	15-35	10-20
Lupus nephritis	<10	Rare
HUS/TTP	28	40-50
Diabetic nephropathy	100	<5
Amyloidosis	30-40	Unknown
Wegener's granulomatosis	17	<10
Essential mixed cryoglobulinemia	50	"Frequent"
Nonglomerular Diseases		
Oxalosis	90-100	Majority
Cystinosis	~0	Rare
Fabry's disease	100	Rare
Sickle cell nephropathy	Rare	Unknown
Scleroderma	20	"Often"
Alport's syndrome	~0 (anti-GBM)	~0

FSGS, focal segmental glomerulosclerosis; GBM, glomerular basement membrane; HUS, hemolytic uremic syndrome; IgA, immunoglobulin A; MPGN, membranoproliferative glomerulonephritis; TTP, thrombotic thrombocytopenic purpura.
From Kasiske BL, Cangro CB, Hariharan S, et al. The evaluation of renal transplantation candidates: Clinical practice guidelines. Am J Transplant 2001;1 Suppl 2:3-95.

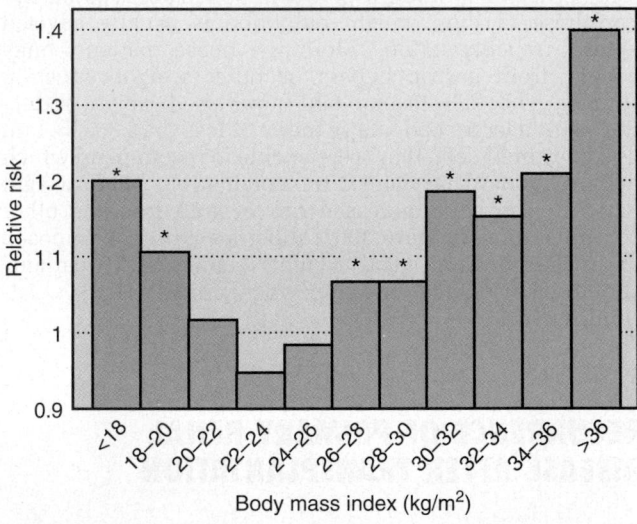

Events = 15,676   Overall *P* < .0001
n = 51,927   **P* < .005

FIGURE 300-2. Relative risk for graft loss by body mass index. (Adapted from Meier-Kriesche HU, Arndorfer JA, Kaplan B: The impact of body mass index on renal transplant outcomes: A significant independent risk factor for graft failure and patient death. Transplantation 2002;73:70-74.)

recommended after patients are warned about the risk of recurrence (C).

The recurrence rate of membranous glomerulonephritis is 10% to 20%. Graft loss due to recurrence develops in 50%. No treatment reverses the recurrent membranous disease. Patients should be informed of the risk of recurrence but should be offered transplants (C).

Patients with membranoproliferative glomerulonephritis (MPGN) type I have been found to have recurrence rates of 20% to 30%,[16] but others have reported rates as high as 70% in primary grafts.[17] The histological picture of transplant glomerulopathy is similar to MPGN type I, and this may have led to overestimation of recurrence in earlier studies. Serum complement levels are usually normal in recurrent disease compared with primary MPGN type I.[18] Graft loss develops in 30% to 40% of patients with recurrence.

In type II MPGN, recurrence is almost universal after transplantation. Reported rates are 80% to 100%.[19] Loss of grafts due to recurrence has been reported in 10% to 20% of cases, although graft loss rates approximating 50% have also been reported. Risk factors for graft loss included younger age and the presence of crescents at presentation.[20]

IgA nephropathy recurs in 40% to 50% of patients.[21] Patients with living related transplants and those with B35 and DR4 human leukocyte antigens (HLA) may also be at greater risk for recurrence.[22] However, graft loss due to recurrence develops in less than 6% to 33% of patients. The type of immunosuppression does not affect recurrence.[23]

Anti–glomerular basement membrane (GBM) disease recurs in approximately 10% of renal transplants, but graft loss appears to be rare. Renal transplantation should be delayed until circulating anti-GBM antibodies are undetectable (C).

Clinically evident Henoch-Schönlein purpura recurs in less than 15% to 35% of recipients by 5 years, and the graft failure rate is 11%. Recurrence may be higher in children (75% to 88%) and in recipients of living related transplants.

Recurrent lupus nephritis should be uncommon (10%) if patients are not transplanted until the disease is inactive

(C). Serological evidence for inactivity and clinical quiescence characterizes what has been turned "burned out" lupus. Graft loss is rare in appropriately selected cases.

Hemolytic uremic syndrome (HUS) and thrombotic thrombocytopenia purpura (TTP) recurs in 28% of recipients, with graft failure developing in 50%. Recurrence may be reduced by use of antiplatelet agents such as low-dose aspirin, dipyridamole, or ticlopidine (C). Development of HUS/TTP in a prior transplant should not preclude retransplantation (B).

Diabetic nephropathy is the most commonly recurring glomerular disease after transplantation. Histological recurrence can be seen in as many as 100% of cases.[24] However, few patients develop clinically evident diabetic nephropathy. Loss of graft function to recurrence of diabetic nephropathy is less than 5%.

Other forms of glomerular disease are less common, and evidence often consists of relatively small case series. Amyloidosis recurs in 30% to 40% of recipients, and the graft loss rate is unknown due to small sample sizes. Wegener's granulomatosis recurs in 17% with less than 10% graft loss. Essential mixed cryoglobulinemia recurs in 50% with "frequent" loss of grafts.

The nonglomerular causes of renal failure have also been reported to recur. Oxalosis recurs in 100% of renal recipients if not preceded by liver transplantation. Isolated kidney transplantation can be attempted in patients without severe systemic disease (B). Preemptive liver transplantation alone before ESRD or simultaneous liver/kidney transplantation should be considered for some patients (B).

Cystinosis is primarily a pediatric disease and is caused by an inborn error of metabolism that leads to deposition of cystine crystals in the renal interstitium. Because the transplanted kidney corrects the deficiency, recurrence or graft loss does not develop. Fabry's disease is caused by a hereditary deficiency of α-galactosidase that leads to accumulation of glycophospholipids in the kidney and other organs. It was initially hoped that a transplanted kidney could provide sufficient enzyme to correct the disturbance, but this is not the case. Histological recurrence develops in 100% of cases, but graft loss is rare.

Sickle cell disease is associated with ESRD due to chronic interstitial fibrosis or FSGS. Recurrence of these diseases and graft loss are rare after transplantation, but the risk of long-term graft failure is greater in African American patients without sickle cell disease. Transplantation is the treatment of choice for these patients (C), and there are few data supporting the practice of delaying surgery in patients with frequent sickle cell crisis (C).

Scleroderma is an uncommon cause of renal failure. The recurrence rate is therefore based on relatively small case series. Recurrence develops in 20%, and graft loss occurs "often." Renal transplantation is believed to be the treatment of choice for patients without severe disease precluding surgery (B).

THE GASTROINTESTINAL EVALUATION

Evaluation of the gastrointestinal tract gains great importance because postoperative complications can be life-threatening. Patients with a previous history of peptic ulcer disease should undergo upper gastrointestinal endoscopy before transplantation (C). The prevalence may be as high as 25% of potential recipients, and 10% of patients develop peptic ulcer disease de novo after transplantation. Routine endoscopy is not warranted in asymptomatic patients without a prior history.

Colonic perforation is most commonly caused by diverticulitis and occurs in 0.5% to 2.0% patients after transplant, with a mortality rate of 17% to 43%.[25] Routine screening is not warranted (D), but patients 50 years of age or older should have a colonoscopy for cancer screening. Patients with a prior history of diverticulitis should have a colonoscopy and should be considered for elective partial colectomy before transplantation (C).

The evaluation and management of cholelithiasis remains controversial. Some centers screen all patients and perform elective pretransplantation cholecystectomy if cholelithiasis is found. Others do not screen and only remove the gallbladder if symptoms are present. The incidence is 5% to 10% for nondiabetics but 25% in diabetics. The ATC guidelines suggest that (1) patients with a history of cholecystitis should have an ultrasound examination with consideration given to cholecystectomy (C) and (2) diabetics should have an ultrasound examination and should be offered cholecystectomy if gallstones are found (C).

Preexisting liver disease requires close attention during the evaluation. Liver disease develops in 7% to 24% of kidney recipients in the early postoperative period and is the cause of late death in 8% to 28% of patients.[26,27] Hepatitis B (HBV) and hepatitis C (HCV) are the leading causes of viral hepatitis, and all patients should be screened for these infections (C). Patients with HBV and active viral replication and patients who are carriers of the HBV surface antigen (HBsAg) should be offered lamivudine before transplantation (C). A positive anti-HCV serology result should prompt testing for viral replication; if that result is positive, patients should be offered interferon-α therapy (C). Advanced liver disease is usually a contraindication to renal transplantation, but appropriate patients should be referred for combined liver/kidney transplantation (C).

THE CARDIAC EVALUATION

Cardiovascular disease is the leading cause of death after transplantation, with a relative risk between 3 and 10 times that in the general population.[28] The cardiac evaluation can be expensive, and angiography carries significant risk. Most programs have instituted attempts to apply risk stratification models. The ATC guidelines suggest the following: (1) patients at high risk (e.g., diabetic nephropathy, prior intermittent hemodialysis) should have cardiac stress testing (B); (2) patients with positive stress tests should have angiography (B); and (3) revascularization should be performed in those with critical coronary lesions before transplantation (B).

MALIGNANCIES

Malignancies are more prevalent in patients with ESRD than in the general population. Age-appropriate screening should be performed for all patients before they are placed on the waiting list.[29] Most centers perform abdominal ultrasound examinations that include the kidneys to detect renal carcinoma, given the increased prevalence in ESRD patients.

TABLE 300-4

Minimum Recommended Cancer-Free Waiting Period Based on American Society of Transplantation (AST) Guidelines

TUMOR	RECOMMENDED WAIT (yr)	AST CATEGORY*
Renal cell cancers		
Incidental renal cancer (<5 cm)	None	B
Symptomatic	2	B
Lesions >5 cm	5	B
Testicular	2	B
Cervix or uterus	2	B
Thyroid	2	B
Lymphoma	2	B
Leukemias	2	B
Wilms'	2	B
Colon	5	B
Prostate	2	B
Breast	5	B
Bladder	2	B
In situ	None	B
Melanoma	5	B
Basal cell skin	None	C
Other nonmelanoma skin	Unknown	C
Myeloma	Unknown	C

AST category B—There is fair evidence to support the recommendation that the condition be considered in the evaluation process; AST category C—There is poor evidence regarding the inclusion of the condition in the evaluation process, but recommendations may be made on other grounds.
From Kasiske BL, Cangro CB, Hariharan S, et al: The evaluation of renal transplantation candidates: Clinical practice guidelines. Am J Transplant 2001;1(Suppl 2):3-95.

An appropriate waiting period should be observed in patients with prior malignancy (Table 300-4) before listing. Most cancers require 2 years of waiting ("2-year rule"), but others, such as large renal cell, breast, colon, and melanoma cancers, may demand at least 5 years before attempting transplantation. Insufficient information is available to determine an appropriate waiting period for nonmelanotic skin cancers and myeloma. Patients with in situ lesions of all cancers probably can be listed earlier than the standard period, but patients should be informed that the risk of recurrence after transplantation is uncertain. Patients with incidentally found renal cell cancers and basal cell skin cancers can usually be listed without waiting.

ORGAN ALLOCATION SYSTEMS

Once patients have been placed on the waiting list for kidney transplantation, the organs are allocated based on models developed by national organizations which are usually monitored by their governments. The models are constantly evolving, and any attempt at delineating them will be quickly outdated. In Eurotransplant International

Foundation,[30] UK Transplant,[31] and France Transplant,[32] among others, oversee the process. In the United States, the United Network of Organ Sharing[33] assumes this responsibility. Current policy can be found on the Web sites of these and other organizations.

CONCLUSION

Evaluation of potential renal transplant recipients is increasingly challenging, but careful attention to elimination of potential barriers has resulted in continued improvements in patient and allograft survival.

Key Points

1. Given evidence that earlier transplantation can result in improved long-term survival, prominent guidelines for renal transplant support preemptive transplantation, but many also recommend waiting until the glomerular filtration rate is less than 20 mL/min.
2. Chemical dependency is an indicator of adverse outcomes in renal transplantation. In general and as specified in specific guidelines, patients with chemical dependence are required to be drug and alcohol free for at least 6 months before receiving a renal allograft.
3. Many centers limit transplant candidacy to persons younger than 70 years and those who have a body mass index lower than 30.
4. Cardiac evaluation is an important part of the workup for patients being evaluated for renal transplant because cardiovascular disease is an important co-morbidity in patients with end-stage renal disease. When indicated, coronary revascularization should be performed before renal transplant.

Key References

1. Kasiske BL, Cangro CB, Hariharan S, et al: The evaluation of renal transplantation candidates: Clinical practice guidelines. Am J Transplant 2001;1(Suppl 2):3-95.
2. Knoll G, Cockfield S, Blydt-Hansen T, et al: Canadian Society of Transplantation: Consensus guidelines on eligibility for kidney transplantation. CMAJ 2005;173:S1-S25.
13. Srinivas TR, Meier-Kriesche HU: Obesity and kidney transplantation. Contrib Nephrol 2006;151:19-41.
19. Choy BY, Chan TM, Lai KN: Recurrent glomerulonephritis after kidney transplantation. Am J Transplant 2006;6:2535-2542.
28. Ojo AO: Cardiovascular complications after renal transplantation and their prevention. Transplantation 2006;82:603-611.

See the companion Expert Consult website for the complete reference list.

CHAPTER 301

Kidney Support and Perioperative Care in Kidney Transplantation

Jerry McCauley, Nirav Shah, Christine Wu, and Mark Unruh

OBJECTIVES

This chapter will:
1. Describe the evaluation of patients immediately before transplantation.
2. Describe the evaluation and management of patients immediately after surgery.
3. Describe the management of hypertension and of mineral and electrolyte problems after surgery.
4. Describe the identification and management of surgical complications in the perioperative period.
5. Describe specific issues related to dialysis and the care of the allograft.

PRETRANSPLANTATION EVALUATION

Perioperative management of kidney transplant recipients begins when they are initially admitted for transplantation. At that time, a complete review of the patient's prior history, current medical conditions, and any recent events that could increase the risks associated with transplantation should be assessed. A complete physical examination should be performed, searching for active illnesses that could preclude surgery.

If no active problems are present, attention centers on laboratory studies drawn preoperatively. In particular, the serum potassium concentration should be normal; if it is high, the patient should be considered for hemodialysis before surgery if time allows. Patients with elevated serum potassium before surgery frequently develop worsening values intraoperatively and postoperatively. Patients undergoing peritoneal dialysis tend to be hypokalemic and seldom require preoperative dialysis. The decision to perform dialysis preoperatively is usually based on physician preference unless absolute indications are present. Some surgeons and nephrologists prefer to have all patients dialyzed before surgery so that dialysis after transplantation can be delayed if the allograft does not function immediately. Others, perhaps most, prefer to avoid adding cold ischemia time by doing dialysis and want to take the patient directly to surgery if possible. Many also fear that hemodialysis immediately before transplantation may adversely affect graft function postoperatively. There are very few studies to support an evidence-based decision. Theoretically, preoperative hemodialysis with a bioincompatible filter with volume removal may delay recovery of graft function. Bioincompatible dialysis filters (cellulose and others) induce a host inflammatory response, which leads to activation of the alternative complement pathway and activation of cytokines (interleukin-1, tumor necrosis factor, and others). More biocompatible synthetic filters (polyacrylonitrile and others) have gained favor because these problems are less extensive. Van Loo and colleagues[1] compared graft recovery in patients treated with dialysis 24 hours before transplantation with biocompatible or incompatible filters and with or without ultrafiltration. They found that graft recovery was best in patients treated with biocompatible filters without fluid removal by ultrafiltration. Fontana and colleagues[2] found no difference in graft recovery with hemodialysis versus peritoneal dialysis before transplantation. If dialysis is required, it should be heparin free and brief (2 hours) if possible, and volume removal should be avoided ideally.

Hypertension can usually be managed easily intraoperatively. Intraoperative intravenous labetalol is popular but can pose a risk of severe hyperkalemia in hemodialysis patients with long cold ischemia times and low intraoperative and postoperative urine outputs.[3] Labetalol should be avoided in any patient who is expected to have delayed graft function (e.g., donor after cardiac death, elderly donor) and in those with long cold ischemia times. Most would favor the use of perioperative beta blockers and continuation of statins, because both have been associated with reduced perioperative mortality in a variety of settings.[4] All medications should be closely reviewed before surgery, and agents that are likely to cause complications after transplantation should be stopped. In particular, angiotensin inhibitors are withheld by many programs, because they may predispose to hyperkalemia, anemia, and elevated creatinine. Given the long-term advantages of these drugs, many would restart them once the patient is stable weeks to months later.

IMMEDIATE POSTOPERATIVE ASSESSMENT

Patients should be evaluated immediately after returning to the recovery room. In addition to the usual postoperative care, patients should be evaluated for early allograft function (urine output), hemodynamic status (both hypotension and hypertension are common), and status of serum potassium. Table 301-1 illustrates a checklist of items to be evaluated in the first 24 hours after transplantation, and Figure 301-1 is a copy of the postoperative orders used in the University of Pittsburgh kidney and pancreas transplant programs.

Many patients are transferred from the recovery room to the intensive care unit (or step-down unit) for close monitoring if they have been unstable during the operation or if they have known cardiovascular disease or other conditions that could pose risk during the first 24 hours. Most patients can be transferred directly from the recovery room to a routine hospital bed.

TABLE 301-1

Checklist of Items to Be Evaluated during the First 24 Hours after Transplantation

Hemodynamic State
Blood pressure (both hypotension and hypertension are common)
Respiratory Status
Extubation
Underlying pulmonary disease?
Pulmonary embolus?
Volume Status
Volume given during operation
Cardiac Status
Kidney Status
Urine output
Vascular anastomoses (Doppler ultrasound examination within 24 hr)
Electrolytes and Minerals
Potassium (in recovery room and daily)
Creatinine and blood urea nitrogen
Phosphorus
Calcium
Magnesium
Dialysis Access
Arteriovenous fistula functioning
Peritoneal membrane disrupted during surgery?

Hemodynamic Status

Close monitoring of the hemodynamic status of patients after surgery is vital, because aberrations may represent threats to the patient or the allograft. Volume overload can cause pulmonary edema, and hypotension can lead to graft thrombosis or predispose to a cardiac event or stroke. Hypertension is very common in dialysis patients and is often exacerbated by increased intravascular volume or by withholding of the patient's routine antihypertensive medications before surgery. The best strategy to control hypertension in most patients is to restart most or all of their pretransplantation medications and to use agents such as clonidine or, rarely, intravenous infusions for short-term management. Few patients should chronically require clonidine, given its predictable complications of somnolence and impotence. Patients with volume expansion should have their intravenous replacement fluids decreased. Renal artery stenosis is a relatively late complication which develops after weeks to months, but compression of the renal artery by a fluid collection rarely may lead to worsening hypertension and delayed graft recovery in the early postoperative period.

Respiratory Status

The respiratory status is closely monitored after surgery, and patients can usually be extubated in the recovery room. Overzealous attempts to extubate patients early by giving insufficient anesthesia may lead to great pressure on the wound when the patient coughs, which can cause wound dehiscence or even partial extrusion of the allograft. Adequate oxygenation is usually ensured by pulse oximetry in the recovery room, and this may be continued on the floor in patients with known pulmonary disease.

Volume Status

A brisk urine output after surgery is the goal after renal transplantation, and most programs administer large amounts of intravenous fluids to patients with good function after surgery. This can cause significant volume overload in many patients if they are not monitored closely and timely adjustments are not made. For patients with a urine output that is less than 300 mL/hr, fluids are usually replaced at a rate of 1 mL saline for each 1 mL urine output during the first 24 hours (see Figure 301-1). Those producing greater than 300 mL/hr of urine are given 4 to 5 mL per milliliter of urine output. The reduction in replacement is made to avoid "chasing your tail" by giving large volumes of fluid in patients with large urine outputs. This could be a serious problem in patients with significant azotemia (e.g., blood urea nitrogen [BUN] 200 mg/dL) and a living donor or excellent deceased donor leading to urine volumes of 10 to 15 L/day. Such patients experience an early osmotic diuresis from the azotemia, which would resolve if the fluid replacement were adjusted appropriately. If they continue to receive equal-volume replacement, their urine output could be maintained at 10 to 15 L/day indefinitely.

Many programs no longer routinely insert central venous pressure catheters to assist in volume management. When such catheters are used, they are usually removed during the first 24 to 48 hours postoperatively. In most cases, estimation of the patient's volume status can be effectively made based on physical examination. The central venous pressure catheter may be invaluable, however, in patients with poor cardiac function before surgery, who may be prone to develop congestive heart failure when relatively large volumes of fluid are administered during and after the operation.

Cardiac Assessment

Renal transplant recipients have a high prevalence of cardiovascular disease, and close attention must be given to this area after surgery. Patients without a known history of cardiac disease and those without risk factors for cardiac disease (other than renal disease) usually are given routine monitoring after surgery. For those with known cardiovascular disease and at least two additional risk factors, very close attention is required. This is particularly important for diabetics with preexisting cardiac disease and for those with at least 25 years of diabetes. Such patients are often declared to be at high cardiac risk and are placed directly into the intensive care unit or a monitored unit after surgery. In such patients, unexplained hypotension may be the only sign of a myocardial infarction. Serial troponin levels are often monitored in addition.

Electrolytes and Minerals

Routine measurement of electrolytes and minerals is important, because abnormalities in this area can be expected in patients with renal failure. As discussed earlier, hyperkalemia is common before and during surgery. It is perhaps even more prevalent after transplantation, particularly in patients with poor allograft function. A serum potassium concentration of 5.5 mg/dL or greater should be considered to be a medical emergency, because the potassium may be rising rapidly and poses a threat to the patient's survival.

Kidney / Pancreas Transplant Postop - Physician Order Set

Nursing Unit: _____ Attending Physician: _____

Status Post: ☐ Deceased Donor Kidney Transplant Recipient   ☐ Deceased Donor Pancreas Transplant Recipient
☐ Living Donor Kidney Recipient

Allergies: _____   Condition: _____

Check All Orders that Apply with a ☒ *& All Handwritten Orders Should be* __BLOCK PRINTED__ *for Clarity*

Communication Orders

☐ Notify physician for the following:

- T > 38.5° C.
- HR < 60 or > 120 beats/minute
- SBP > 160 or DBP > 100 mm Hg
- Urine Output < _____ ml/hour or > _____ ml/hour
- Unrelieved pain
- Other: _____
- O$_2$ Saturation < 92%

☐ For living renal recipient, the __postop__ nursing RN is to document the start __and__ finish time of Alemtuzumab (**Campath**) (administered preop)

Vital Signs

☐ Vital signs every 1 hour × 24 hours, then every 2 hours × 24 hours, then routine

Activity

☐ Bedrest   ☐ OOB ad lib   ☐ OOB to chair and ambulate   ☐ Encourage mobilization as tolerated
☐ Ambulate qid when alert.

Patient Care

☒ Intake and Output: every 1 hour × 24 hours, then every 4 hours × 24 hours, then routine.
☐ If Pancreas Recipient: Capillary blood sugar every 1 hour × 24 hours, then every 6 hours
☐ Strict intake and output   ☐ Patient may **NOT** Shower
☐ Weigh patient daily   ☐ SCD's while in bed
☐ Elevate head of bed - 30 degrees   ☐ Wound Care: Keep dry and clean and exposed
☐ Turn, cough and deep breathe every 2 hours until ambulatory   ☐ Foley catheter to gravity drainage
☐ Discontinue nasogastric tube in PACU unless nauseated.   ☐ Irrigate Foley with 50 ml Sodium Chloride prn
☒ Ask MD about plans for removing __any__ current indwelling parenteral catheters/lines prior to discharge (dialysis catheter, etc.)

Nutritional Services

☐ NPO   ☐ Clear Fluids po

Continuous Infusions

☐ For Deceased Donor Kidney Tx: Replace Urine output that is < 300 ml/hour with 1 ml:1 ml of the following: _____
☐ For Deceased Donor Kidney Tx: Replace Urine output that is > 300 ml/hour with 4/5 ml/ml with the following: _____
☐ For Living Related Kidney Tx: Dextrose 1% in 0.45% normal saline with 10 mEq of Sodium Bicarbonate - 1 ml:1 ml
☐ For Pancreas Transplant/Pancreas After Kidney Tx Only: 0.45% Sodium Chloride at _____ ml/hour

_____   _____
(Print Name)   (Signature)

Date / Time: _____   Pager # _____

FIGURE 301-1. Postoperative orders sheet used at the University of Pittsburgh Medical Center.

Figure 301-2 illustrates the order sheet used at the University of Pittsburgh Medical Center for standardized management of hyperkalemia. Once the potassium has reached 5.5 mg/dL, this protocol in instituted; it consists initially of close patient electrocardiographic and laboratory monitoring with appropriate treatment. All medications and dietary sources of hyperkalemia are sought and discontinued. Treatment is based on severity of hyperkalemia and graft function. Patients with excellent early graft function may be managed with increased diuresis, with insulin and glucose in addition to sodium bicarbonate treatment (particularly if the patient has a metabolic acidosis). Polystyrene sulfonate (Kayexalate) should never be used during the first month after renal transplantation, because its use has been associated with intestinal perforation and death.[5,6]

Instead, hemodialysis should be performed in patients with life-threatening hyperkalemia.

Renal Function

Renal function is initially assessed by urine output. After some hours, the serum creatinine and BUN will begin to fall in patients with good graft function. There is little value in monitoring these parameters more frequently than once or twice per day. In patients with slow graft recovery, a decrease in the rate of rise in creatinine may herald impending recovery. In such patients, dialysis should be deferred unless there is a life-threatening reason such as hyperkalemia or pulmonary edema.

Hyperkalemia Management for Renal Transplant Patients with Serum Potassium ≥ 5.5

Check All Orders that Apply with a   ☒   *& All Handwritten Orders Should be <u>BLOCK PRINTED</u> for Clarity*

STAT Orders
☒ **STAT** repeat serum potassium, if not already done   ☒ **STAT** ECG, if not already done
☒ **STAT** fingerstick glucose, if not already done   ☐ **STAT** ABG (consider when potassium > 6.5 mEq/L)
☐ Transfer patient to monitored bed *(consider when potassium > 6.5 mEq/L or ECG changes consistent with hyperkalemia [see following form])*

Patient Care
☒ Vital Signs q 4 hours   ☒ I & O q 2 hours   ☐ Low potassium diet
☐ Blood sugar (fingerstick glucoses) q 30 minutes × 2, then q 1 hour × 2 after insulin has been given

Labs
☒ Repeat Serum Potassium q 2 hours until < 5.5 mEq/L

Communication Orders
☒ Call MD if the Repeat potassium is > 6.0 mEq/L; pulse < 50 or > 120 bpm; BP < 90/50 or > 160/90 mmHg; BS < 100 or BS > 400

Discontinue potassium sources:
☒ Discontinue Potassium from all IV fluids
☒ Discontinue the following medications which may contribute to elevated Potassium *(see following form for example)*
☐ _____   ☐ _____

Select one of the following treatments for Potassium ≥ 5.5 mEq/L:
☐ No treatment *(Note: for potassium between 5.5–6.0 mEq/L, merely removing potassium-increasing medications may be sufficient)*
☐ Patient is dialysis dependent.   Contact renal fellow for emergent dialysis.
☐ Furosemide (**Lasix**)____mg PO / IV *(circle one)* × 1 *(consider when CrCl > 30 mL/min; usual start dose 20–40 mg)*
☐ Sodium Bicarbonate_____ mEq IV push over 2–5 minutes × 1 *(criteria for use: pH < 7.3)*
   ▪ If pH is < 7.3, give 100 mEq   ▪ If pH is < 7.2, give 150 mEq

Do not use sodium polystyrene sulfonate in renal transplant patients less than 30 days post transplant or patients at risk for colonic perforation, fluid overload or those requiring sodium restriction.

For severe hyperkalemia, and ONLY for patients MORE THAN THIRTY DAYS post transplant:
☐ Sodium polystyrene sulfonate* (Kayexalate) PO q 4 hrs prn bowel movement and Potassium < 5.5 mEq/L *(max duration = 12 hrs)*
   Select dose: ☐ 30 gm   ☐ 60 gm   ☐ Other:_____
☐ Sodium polystyrene sulfonate* (Kayexalate)_____ grams **retention enema** PR × 1. *(Use rectal balloon catheter, patient to retain enema ≥ 30–60 min)*

IN ADDITION, if <u>potassium > 6.9</u>, patient is <u>symptomatic</u>, or has <u>ECG changes</u>, select one or more of the following: *
☐ Calcium chloride 1 gram IV push over 5–10 minutes × 1 *(criteria for use: digoxin toxicity is <u>NOT</u> suspected)*
☐ Albuterol 10 mg via nebulizer over 10 minutes q 2 hours prn Potassium > 5.5 mEq/L *(use only if pt is NOT hypertensive and does NOT have CAD)*
☐ Fludrocortisone acetate (**Florinef**) 0.1 mg po every 12 hours
☐ Insulin **plus** Glucose as follows (**see CAUTION on following form**):
   ▪ Regular insulin 6 units IV × 1 (**hold** if last dose of subcutaneous regular or rapidly-acting insulin was < 2 hours ago)
   ▪ If BS is 130–200, start Dextrose 10% IV infusion at 100 ml/hour
   ▪ If BS < 130, give 1 amp Dextrose 50% IV push **and** start Dextrose 10% IV infusion at 100 ml/hour
   ▪ <u>After</u> insulin has been given, check BS q 30 minutes × 2, then q 1 hour × 2
   ▪ If any <u>repeat</u> BS is < 100, give 1 amp Dextrose 50% IV push **and** start Dextrose 10% IV infusion at 100 ml/hour
   ▪ Discontinue Dextrose 10% IV infusion after 3 hours <u>OR</u> if any repeat BS > 300

**** Not necessarily applicable for patients who are dialysis dependent. Please contact renal fellow for advice.**

_____   _____
(Print Name)   (Signature)

                 Date / Time: _____ Pager # _____

FIGURE 301-2. Hyperkalemia management order sheet used at the University of Pittsburgh Medical Center.

Calcium Phosphorus and Magnesium

Dialysis patients frequently have hyperparathyroidism resulting in potentially rapid changes in calcium-phosphorus metabolism after surgery. Hypophosphatemia and hypercalcemia (or hypocalcemia) are common in patients with good graft function and hyperparathyroidism. Many patients are admitted taking cinacalcet (Sensipar). Most centers elect to continue this agent after surgery. Limited information is available on the role of this agent after renal transplantation, but it has been demonstrated to control the hypercalcemia of hyperparathyroidism is some patients.[7] Some studies have observed an increased serum creatinine level in patients treated with cinacalcet, but this effect has been small and reversible.[8,9]

Hypomagnesemia is also common in patients treated with calcineurin inhibitors.[10,11] The mechanism appears to be increased urinary excretion of magnesium and calcium

TABLE 301-2

Causes of Early Renal Dysfunction

Acute tubular necrosis
Arterial or venous thrombosis
Obstruction
Nephrotoxicity
Calcineurin inhibitors
Angiotensin-converting enzyme inhibitors
Angiotensin receptor blockers
Volume depletion
Hyperacute or subacute rejection
Acute cellular rejection (usually after 1 wk)

TABLE 301-3

Risk Factors for Delayed Graft Function

Increased cold ischemia time
Increased donor age
Increased panel reactive antibody
African-American ethnicity
Diabetes
Human leukocyte antigen mismatch
Duration of long-term dialysis
Expanded criteria donor

due to these agents and is independent of parathyroid function.[12] Diuretics and resolution of the acute renal failure also contribute to hypomagnesemia. Magnesium should be replaced intravenously, because many patients have an ileus or slow intestinal function in the early period after surgery.

Dialysis Access

The status of dialysis access should be assessed in the early post-transplantation period, because patients with arteriovenous fistulas or synthetic grafts often experience thrombosis of the grafts after surgery. These grafts may have been inadvertently occluded during surgery or during transport to or from the operating room. Thrombosed grafts often have anatomical defects such as stenoses or aneurysms that predispose them to this problem. Even if the renal allograft is functioning well, the access should be evaluated by vascular surgery, because many of them can be salvaged.

In patients with peritoneal catheters, the surgeon should be queried to determine if the peritoneal membrane was disrupted during surgery. If the patient requires dialysis after transplantation, peritoneal dialysis may be the preferred option. However, if the peritoneal membrane was punctured, a leak of peritoneal fluid can be expected once fluid is instilled. Some surgeons attempt to oversew the peritoneal opening if it is discovered during surgery. If this has been the case, low-volume exchanges (1 to 1.5 L) can be attempted, with close attention to signs of a leak. If the peritoneum was disrupted and not oversewn, it is probably prudent to wait approximately 2 weeks before attempting peritoneal dialysis.

EARLY GRAFT DYSFUNCTION AND DELAYED GRAFT FUNCTION

The pathophysiology of acute allograft dysfunction and that of acute renal failure in kidney transplant recipients are discussed in other chapters. Here, we concentrate on the practical management of delayed recovery of renal function immediately after transplantation. Table 301-2 illustrates the causes of early renal dysfunction. Some degree of renal dysfunction develops in most renal allografts. Clinically, it may improve rapidly after renal transplantation, but a range of renal dysfunction may be observed, from anuria to a slowly falling serum creatinine concentration (slow graft function, SGF).[13]

Delayed graft function (DGF) is a term commonly used to describe initial poor allograft function. DFG is important because it has been associated with inferior long-term graft and patient survival and increased risk of acute rejection.[14] In large transplant registries, DGF is often operationally defined as the requirement for dialysis during the first postoperative week. Most publications use this definition. The decision to institute dialysis is subjective and varies widely by transplant center. The lack of uniform criteria for DGF has led to a wide variation in reported incidences, which range from 5% to 40%.[15] Alternative definitions have not enjoyed wide acceptance. Table 301-3 illustrates risk factors for DGF.[16,17] The most common cause is acute tubular necrosis. This is a direct effect of ischemia of the allograft after donor nephrectomy. Warm ischemia time (WIT) is defined as the time (in minutes) from the moment when the renal vessels are ligated until the allograft is warmed to 4° C. Cold ischemia time (CIT) is the period from when the allograft is paced at 4° C until the vascular anastomosis is completed. Increased WIT and increased CIT both increase the risk of DGF. Since the introduction of donation after cardiac death (DCD), centers have been faced with relatively long WIT and higher rates of DGF. These grafts sustain increased WIT because the acquisition of organs does not begin until cardiac function ceases. Although DGF is more common in deceased donor allografts (23%), it may also be seen uncommonly after living donation (6%). The histological findings in acute tubular necrosis–related DGF are similar to those found in native kidneys. Solez and associates found that DGF biopsies had less tubular casts, some necrosis of complete tubular cross-sections, less tubular dedifferentiation and regeneration, and more isometric vacuolization.[18]

Other donor-related factors associated with DGF are older donor (>50 years),[19] high panel reactive antibody (PRA), African-American ethnicity, and the presence of diabetes. Donor-recipient human leukocyte antigen (HLA) mismatch is associated with DGF and inferior long-term graft survival. The duration of long-term dialysis before transplantation has been associated with DGF, poor long-term graft survival, and increased long-term mortality. The best short- and long-term outcomes are in patients receiving preemptive transplantation.[20,21] The type of dialysis has variably been reported to affect the rate of DGF. Some studies found lower rates of DGF with peritoneal dialysis and an increased risk of graft thrombosis and early graft loss compared to hemodialysis, but others found no difference in outcomes.[22-25]

The shortage of renal allografts has led to acceptance of previously unacceptable donors. The United Network of Organ Sharing (UNOS) in the United States now defines a population of donors termed expanded criteria donors

MORTALITY RISK

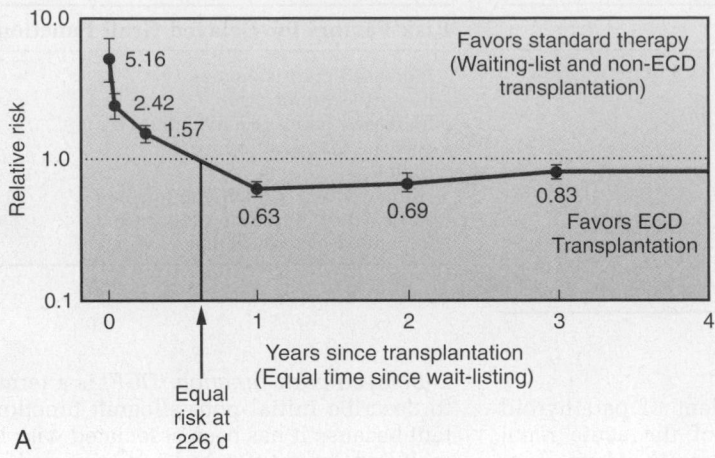

A

Equal
risk at
226 d

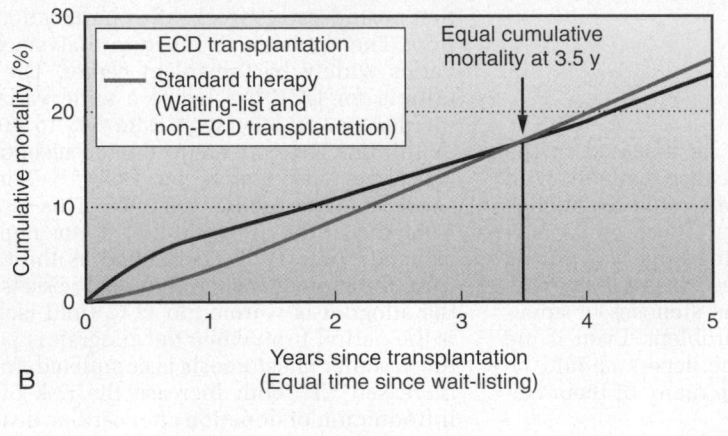

B

No. at risk						
ECD transplantation	7790	6250	5014	3403	2900	2053
Standard therapy	109127	90046	73392	55407	41092	29711

FIGURE 301-3. Time to equal risk of mortality (**A**) and time to equal cumulative mortality (**B**) for expanded criteria donor (ECD) kidney recipients versus patients receiving standard therapy. (Adapted from Merion RM, Ashby VB, Wolfe RA, et al: Deceased-donor characteristics and the survival benefit of kidney transplantation. JAMA 2005;294:2726-2733.)

(ECD). The definition of ECD includes age 60 years or older or 50 to 59 years of age and at least two of the following medical conditions: a history of hypertension, serum creatinine level greater than 1.5 mg/dL, and cerebrovascular event as the cause of death.[26] Merion and coworkers found that recipients of organs from ECDs experienced higher postoperative mortality and DGF (Figure 301-3).[27] The risk of perioperative mortality was 5.2 times higher during the first 2 weeks compared to standard criteria donors. The mortality risk decreased slowly thereafter and became equal to that observed with standard donors at 33 weeks. Thereafter, the risk of death was lower than for recipients of standard criteria donor kidneys. Overall, mortality did not become equal until 3.5 years due to the high early mortality in ECD recipients. These patients require careful management of cardiovascular risk, volume management, and attention to other comorbid illnesses. Few ECD organs are offered to younger, otherwise healthy patients and Merion and colleagues recommended that they be offered only to non-Hispanic patients 40 years of age or older who have diabetes and have been on the waiting list for longer than 1350 days.

When to Do Dialysis in Patients with Delayed Graft Function

Patients with DGF by definition require dialysis. Determining when to perform dialysis remains a controversial subject. All would agree that life-threatening hyperkalemia (unresponsive to medical management) and volume overload leading to pulmonary edema (without an adequate response to diuretics) are absolute indications for dialysis. In other settings, there is great variability in the timing of dialysis. For most, the problem centers on the observation that urine output typically falls after hemodialysis treatments. Many have developed the impression that hemodialysis delays recovery of DGF, particularly in patients with some urine output and in those who develop early recovery of renal function. As mentioned earlier, hemodialysis membranes stimulate cytokines and activate complement, which may have a direct effect on an injured renal allograft. Little direct evidence exists to confirm that hemodialysis itself is harmful to the recovering graft. Dialysis is usually performed for indications, so that randomization of patients to hemodialysis or no hemodialysis

TABLE 301-4

Prevalence of Thrombophilic Disorders Causing Vascular Thrombosis after Renal Transplantation

DISORDER	GENERAL POPULATION (%)	PATIENTS WITH FIRST VTE (%)	RENAL TRANSPLANT RECIPIENTS (%)
Antithrombin deficiency	0.04	1	NA
Protein C deficiency	0.3	3	NA
Protein S deficiency	0.1	3	NA
Hyperhomocysteinemia	5	10	50-90
Factor V Leiden	5	20	4-6
Prothrombin gene mutation	3	6	3.7
High factor VIII levels	10	25	NA
Antiphospholipid antibodies	2	15	19-28

NA, not available; VTE, venous thromboembolism.
From Kujovich JL: Thrombophilia and thrombotic problems in renal transplant patients. Transplantation 2004;77:959-964.

is not a feasible study design given the risk to the untreated groups. Dialysis should be performed before patients have uremic symptoms, but there is currently no consensus on the optimal level of azotemia before uremia at which dialysis would be advantageous in patients with DGF. Unfortunately, oversight agencies using the current definition of DGF may encourage transplant centers to delay dialysis until after 1 week, because the rate of DGF is now considered to be a quality measure for transplant programs in the United States.

Early Surgical Complications

Most surgical complications develop early in the post-transplantation period.[28] Problems such as renal artery stenosis are usually detected weeks to months later. Vascular complications can be some of the most dramatic early problems. Prompt recognition of vascular complications may provide an opportunity to salvage the allografts in these patients with high graft loss rates.

Renal Artery Thrombosis

Arterial thrombosis may develop shortly after the renal vascular anastomosis or days later. The reported incidence ranges from 0.5% to 6.2%, and it usually results in graft loss.[29] Life-threatening complications include allograft rupture, hemorrhage, and pulmonary embolus. This problem usually manifests with sudden oliguria and a rapidly rising serum creatinine concentration. The rate of graft loss is determined by the location and degree of thrombosis. Thrombosis of the main renal artery usually leads to graft loss, but thrombosis limited to segmental vessels may provide an opportunity for salvage if detected and treated quickly. The most useful diagnostic study is Doppler ultrasound examination, which is noninvasive and universally available in transplant centers. Most centers routinely perform a screening Doppler ultrasound study on all patients within the first 24 hours precisely to detect arterial and venous thrombosis. Emergent re-exploration is required if arterial thrombosis is suspected.

Renal artery thrombosis is usually caused by technical or mechanical problems during recovery or during the transplant operation, including kinking or torsion of the vessels, trauma to vessels during recovery causing an intimal flap, vessel size disparities, and atherosclerosis of the donor or recipient vessels. Hyperacute or subacute rejection may also manifest as an arterial thrombus. Hypotension, inducing slow arterial flow, is one of the most

common causes of graft thrombosis, and this can be avoided by close hemodynamic monitoring and timely corrective measures.

Thrombophilic disorders are also common causes of vascular thrombosis after transplantation.[30] Table 301-4 lists the major thrombophilic disorders causing thrombosis after renal transplantation. These disorders may cause arterial or venous thrombosis after transplantation. The incidence of several of these are unknown after renal transplantation but others (e.g., hyperhomocysteinemia, antiphospholipid antibodies) are much more common in transplant recipients. Patients with recurrent deep vein thrombosis with or without embolism, recurrent thrombosed vascular access, or prior venous or arterial thrombosis should be screened for thrombophilic disorders before transplantation. Such patients usually require anticoagulation in the perioperative period.

Renal Vein Thrombosis

Renal vein thrombosis also usually develops during the early post-transplantation period and typically leads to graft loss. The clinical presentation includes a tender, swollen allograft and hematuria. As with arterial thrombosis, technical causes are common and include kinking or angulation of the vessels, but renal vein thrombosis also may result from compression of hematomas or lymphoceles or extension of a deep vein thrombus from a lower extremity. Thrombophilic disorders should be considered in patients who are without an obvious technical cause for thrombosis. The diagnosis can be confirmed by Doppler ultrasound, and urgent re-exploration is required if salvage is to be successful; as with arterial thrombosis, graft rupture may threaten the patient's life.

Other Surgical Complications

Other early surgical complications include obstruction, urine leaks and urinomas, hematomas, and, rarely, wound dehiscence.[31] Early obstruction may be caused by blood clots blocking the Foley catheter, kinking of the ureter, or hematomas occluding the ureter. Obstruction usually manifests as a rising serum creatinine concentration. Patients who have been anuric for many years may have a very small bladder that does not expand with filling by urine. In these patients, the tiny bladder fills rapidly once the Foley catheter is removed, leading to reflux into the new ureter and functional obstruction. Management centers on prolonged (weeks) placement of the Foley catheter and "training" of the bladder by allowing progressive increases in bladder pressure and volume using intermittent clamping. Urine leaks usually develop at the bladder anastomosis and may be caused by ischemia that occurs when the donor surgeon unnecessarily devascularizes the ureter. Other causes include increased tension due to a short donor ureter and trauma to the ureter during procurement.

Hemorrhage is an uncommon complication that is usually caused by unligated vessels in the hilum of the graft or leaks from small retroperitoneal vessels. Rapid bleeding typically manifests as a falling hematocrit, tachycardia, and hypotension. Slower bleeding usually causes perinephric hematomas, which may become large enough to occlude arteries, veins, or the ureter. Patients with rapid bleeding should undergo urgent re-exploration. Hematomas not causing obstruction of major structures or a progressive fall in hematocrit can be monitored.

Wound complications are possible in all patients, so the wound should be examined closely until complete healing has occurred. Obese patients have the greatest incidence of these complications.[32] Infection and superficial wound breakdown are the most common causes. Wound dehiscence is a rare complication that is more common in obese patients and those patients treated with sirolimus. Most transplant programs withhold sirolimus in the early postoperative period to avoid this dramatic complication.[33]

Key Points

1. Perioperative management of the kidney transplant recipient begins with a pretransplant evaluation.

2. In recent years postoperative management of renal allograft recipients has been outside the intensive care unit except for patients with severe preoperative disease or with intraoperative instability.

3. Key areas of concern following renal transplantation include cardiovascular (both hypo- and hypertension are common), volume status, cardiac and respiratory function, fluid and electrolyte balance, and renal allograft function.

4. The lack of uniform criteria for delayed graft function (DGF) has led to wide variation in reported prevalence. The most common cause of DGF is acute tubular necrosis, but other causes, including technical problems (e.g., vascular anastomotic problems) and acute rejection, are important to rule out.

Key References

4. Feringa HH, Bax JJ, Poldermans D: Perioperative medical management of ischemic heart disease in patients undergoing noncardiac surgery. Curr Opin Anaesthesiol 2007;20:254-260.
16. Halloran PF, Hunsicker LG: Delayed Graft Function: State of the Art, November 10-11, 2000. Summit Meeting, Scottsdale, Arizona. Am J Transplant 2001;1:115-120.
28. Akbar SA, Jafri SZ, Amendola MA, et al: Complications of renal transplantation. Radiographics 2005;25:1335-1356.
30. Kujovich JL: Thrombophilia and thrombotic problems in renal transplant patients. Transplantation 2004;77:959-964.
31. Humar A, Matas AJ: Surgical complications after kidney transplantation. Semin Dial 2005;18:505-510.

See the companion Expert Consult website for the complete reference list.

CHAPTER 302

Short- and Long-Term Management after Kidney Transplantation

Jerry McCauley, Nirav Shah, Christine Wu, Mark Unruh, and Jose Bernardo

---

OBJECTIVES

This chapter will:
1. Identify clinical issues and management strategies in the short term following renal transplantation.
2. Determine the appropriate schedules for short-term and long-term follow-up of renal transplant recipients.
3. Identify clinical issues and management strategies in the long term following renal transplantation.
4. Identify the level of chronic kidney disease in renal transplant recipients, and devise appropriate management strategies.
5. Identify the major causes of graft loss and patient death after renal transplantation, and devise strategies to improve survival of the organs and patients.

Renal transplantation is the most successful and frequently performed form of organ replacement. The short- and long-term graft and patient survival rates are superior to those for liver, heart, and lung transplantation. The management of these patients has evolved from intense inpatient care to what is primarily outpatient support. During the late 20th century, the length of hospital stay for renal transplant recipients was approximately 1 month. Improvements in surgical technique, immunosuppression, and medical management led to progressive reductions in morbidity and mortality, which allowed a steady decline in the time required in hospital. Most uncomplicated renal transplantation patients now are discharged from the hospital within 1 week after surgery, and many programs routinely discharge them 3 to 4 days after surgery.[1] Many

TABLE 302-1

Short- and Long-Term Surgical and Urological Complications after Renal Transplantation

Hematomas
Arteriovenous fistulas and pseudoaneurysms
Urinary obstruction
Ureteral stricture
Lymphocele
Infection and abscess
Renal artery stenosis
Infarction
Renal calculi
Renal cancer

TABLE 302-2

Causes of Short- and Long-Term Graft Dysfunction

Acute or subacute rejection
Urological or surgical complications
Calcineurin inhibitor toxicity
Volume depletion
Donor preexisting renal dysfunction
Other nephrotoxic agents
Cardiac failure

TABLE 302-3

Causes of Death after Transplantation

CAUSE	≤1 YR (%)	>1 YR (%)
Infection	33-37	17.6
Cardiovascular	35-37	36
Cerebrovascular	7-7.4	6.2
Hemorrhage	2.4-4.3	—
Malignancy	2.7-4.9	9.2
Other	16.1	30.9

transplant programs have developed "day hospital settings" in which patient are treated after discharge. They routinely arrive between 6 and 7 AM, when blood samples and vitals are obtained. The patients are seen by a physician once the laboratory studies are available. Adjustments to medications, wound care, and other procedures are performed. Patients are typically free to leave by noon. This streamlined approach to patient management assumes that the team has a detailed understanding of potential medical or surgical problems encountered during this period.

SHORT-TERM (0 TO 12 MONTHS AFTER TRANSPLANTATION)

During the immediate postdischarge period, continued management of potential perioperative complications is important. Potential surgical complications developing in the short and long term are listed in Table 302-1.[2,3] Most surgical complications may be encountered after discharge from hospital but seldom are seen past 1 month after transplantation. Arterial and venous thromboses typically develop in the early posttransplant period and seldom are encountered after approximately 2 weeks. Hematomas due to localized hemorrhage are common and may arise within days after surgery or may develop at any time due to allograft biopsy or trauma. Most are small and subclinical, requiring no therapy. Large hematomas that are rapidly expanding or causing obstruction of vessels or the ureter should be evacuated. Old hematomas found during an evaluation of fever may require aspiration to rule out infection. The diagnosis is typically made with ultrasound or, less often, with computed tomography.

Arteriovenous fistulas or pseudoaneurysms are usually complications of allograft biopsy performed to identify rejection, or they may be caused by partial disruption of an arterial anastomosis.[4] These problems may develop at any time after the first postoperative week. Most centers delay renal biopsies until after the first week, because the risk of complications is greater and rejection is seldom seen before the first week. These lesions are usually asymptomatic but may cause mild to severe hematuria and hypotension. The diagnosis can be made with Doppler ultrasound, but magnetic resonance imaging may be needed in technically difficult cases. Most arteriovenous fistulas and pseudoaneurysms can be managed conservatively, but progressively expanding pseudoaneurysms may require embolic therapy such as absorbable gelatin sponges (Gelfoam) or steel coils.

Graft Dysfunction

Graft dysfunction occurring during the first 12 months may be caused by ischemic ATN during the first weeks after transplantation. Rejection typically does not develop before 7 to 10 days after surgery unless there are preformed antibodies against donor antigens that have been missed. Preoperative serologic screening usually detects antibodies to these antigens, which are classified as "unacceptable antigens," and the organ is not offered to such recipients. Rarely, these unacceptable antigens are not defined preoperatively, placing the patient at risk for early rejection. Other causes of early renal dysfunction include volume depletion due to overzealous use of diuretics. In addition, with increasing use of older donors, renal dysfunction may be present, particularly with donors older than 60 years of age. In addition, calcineurin toxicity or nephrotoxic agents should be sought when renal dysfunction cannot be explained. Angiotensin-converting enzyme (ACE) inhibitors may be used in the early post-transplantation period, but they can be a common reason for persistent renal dysfunction, particularly in volume-depleted patients. Unsuspected cardiac failure is common in older patients. The expected 20:1 BUN-to-creatinine ratio may be attributed to early steroid use (Table 302-2).

Early and Late Patient Mortality

The causes of death during the first year and late mortality after transplantation are listed on Table 302-3.[5,6] During the first year, the risk of death due to infection or hemorrhage is greater; the late mortality risk is greater for malignancy and other causes. Cardiovascular and cerebrovascular disease is more common in patients older than 60 years of age and is rare in those 25 years of age or younger. During the early or late periods, mortality is strongly associated with the number and type of comorbid illnesses. The greatest mortality occurs in older patients with significant comorbidity who receive ECD allografts. These patterns of mortality can assist in long-term management, and a new organ allocation system may incorporate increasing risks of death in older patients in determining who will receive grafts.

Hypertension

Hypertension is common in dialysis patients and in renal transplant recipients. Table 302-4 lists potential causes of hypertension after transplantation. Prednisone causes hypertension particularly with doses greater than 10 mg/day. The mechanisms of calcineurin-related hypertension include direct vasoconstriction and increased intravascular volume, and it can be dose dependent.

Hypertension developing from disease in the allograft is usually related to chronic allograft nephropathy, calcineurin toxicity, and recurrence of primary renal diseases including diabetic nephropathy. Renal artery stenosis is also a common cause of hypertension, and a sudden onset of severe hypertension or worsening of stable hypertension should suggest this diagnosis. Renal artery stenosis in the native kidneys is an uncommon cause of hypertension after transplantation, and when present, may be cured with nephrectomy. Perhaps the most common cause of post-transplantation hypertension is persistence of preexisting hypertension from the recipient; use of deceased donors with preexisting hypertension may increase the risk of worsening hypertension after transplant.

The treatment of post-transplantation hypertension must take into consideration both the pathophysiology of hypertension and potential drug interactions with calcineurin inhibitors. The preferred first-line agents are probably beta blockers, given their proven efficacy, lack of

interactions with calcineurin inhibitors, and potential of reducing cardiac risk. Second-line drugs include calcium channel blockers. The dihydropyridines do not affect calcineurin inhibitor blood levels and are very effective in lowering blood pressure. Diltiazem and verapamil may increase calcineurin inhibitor blood levels. They have been used to lower the dosage of these agents by approximately 50%. Centrally acting agents (clonidine) may be effective with no drug interactions, but they may be poor long-term agents for older patients due to somnolence. The role of ACE inhibitors remains controversial, but most believe that they should be used frequently, given their potential advantage of delaying progression of renal disease and reducing proteinuria. The routine side effects of hyperkalemia, anemia, and increased creatinine should be expected, and these drugs should not be used in patients with poorly controlled hyperkalemia, severe anemia, or unstable renal function. They also should not be used in patients with renal artery stenosis, because acute renal failure may develop.

LATE (MORE THAN 1 YEAR AFTER TRANSPLANTATION)

Renal transplantation increases life expectancy by as much as 20 years, but the burden of comorbid illnesses and problems associated with transplantation require close attention by those monitoring the patients in the long term. It is now clear that transplant centers are not capable of managing these patients without the assistance of nontransplant nephrologists and primary care physicians. Recently, several attempts have focused on setting guidelines for long-term care.[7,8] The Lisbon Conference was an international meeting convened to develop recommendations aimed at improving long-term outcomes in renal transplant recipients. Table 302-5 illustrates the timing and frequency of clinical and laboratory evaluations. The frequencies of laboratory studies were divided into basic, desired, and potentially advantageous categories. Basic routine studies should be performed at least every 3 months in the second year, every 6 months in years 3 through 5, and every 12 months after 5 years. This very low frequency of laboratory studies is inadequate for most patients. We perform clinical evaluations every 6 to 12 months and laboratory studies every month in stable patients. In our experience, most patients do not need to be seen more frequently if they are also under the care of a nontransplant nephrologist and/or primary care physician. Unstable patients should be seen as frequently as their clinical condition dictates.

All renal recipients should benefit from age-appropriate routine screening studies to detect malignancy and prevent cardiovascular disease. Most of these studies should be

TABLE 302-4

Causes of Hypertension in Renal Transplant Recipients

CAUSE	EXAMPLES
Immunosuppressive therapy	Steroids
	Calcineurin inhibitors (acute vascular effect)
Diseases in the renal allograft	Chronic allograft nephropathy
	Chronic calcineurin toxicity
	Recurrent or de novo glomerulonephritis
	Recurrent diabetic nephropathy
High renin output of native kidneys	Renal artery stenosis of native kidneys
	Allograft
Recurrent essential hypertension	Recurrent/persistent systemic disease
	Transplantation of a predisposed graft

TABLE 302-5

Timing and Frequency of Post-transplantation Laboratory and Clinical Evaluations after 1 Year

YEAR AFTER TRANSPLANTATION	Basic (mo)		Desired (mo)		Potentially Advantageous (mo)	
	CLINICAL	LABORATORY	CLINICAL	LABORATORY	CLINICAL	LABORATORY
Year 2	Every 3	Every 3	Every 2	Every 2	Every 1	Every 1
Years 3-5	Every 6	Every 3	Every 4	Every 2	Every 2	Every 1
Years 6+	Every 12	Every 6	Every 6	Every 3	Every 4	Every 2

performed by the primary care physician, but transplant physicians must monitor to ensure they are being performed and must be informed of the results. For example, a patient with a newly diagnosed malignancy may benefit from reduction of immunosuppression therapy. Close cooperation between the nontransplant physician and the transplant center is vital.

Reproduction and Pregnancy

Renal transplantation improves sexual function and the ability of women to successfully reproduce. Pregnancy should be delayed until at least 1 year after successful transplantation. Contraception should be started before transplantation and continued without interruption for the first year. After the first year, a woman who wants to become pregnant should address the topic in advance with the transplant center and her obstetrician. She should be monitored closely by a high-risk obstetrician and a transplant physician. The Lisbon Conference reviewed the recommendations by the AST and other groups including the World Health Organization; the important features are summarized in Table 302-6.

Infection

Infection is one of the most common serious complications after transplantation.[9,10] Figure 302-1 illustrates the timing of common infections. Infections are more common in transplant recipients during the early post-transplantation period, when the immune system is most at risk. During the first month, bacterial infections such as wound infections and pneumonia are common. Fungal infections are frequent in programs using high-dose steroids but uncommon in steroid-free programs. Patients with preexisting

TABLE 302-6

Recommended Conditions before Conception and Appropriate Care for Pregnant Women after Renal Transplantation

PARAMETER	RECOMMENDATION
Interval after transplantation before pregnancy	1-2 yr
Kidney function	Creatinine <133 µmol/L
Proteinuria	<500 mg/day
Blood pressure	Normal
Allograft ultrasound study	Normal
Rejection history	None recent
Immunosuppression dosing	Stable
Care providers	High-risk obstetrician and transplant physician
Initial visit frequency	Every 2-4 mo
Third-trimester visit frequency	Every 1-2 wk
Postpartum follow-up	To 3 mo after delivery
Laboratory frequency	Every 2-4 wk
Blood pressure checks	Daily (self)
Fetal monitoring	Every 2 wk during third trimester

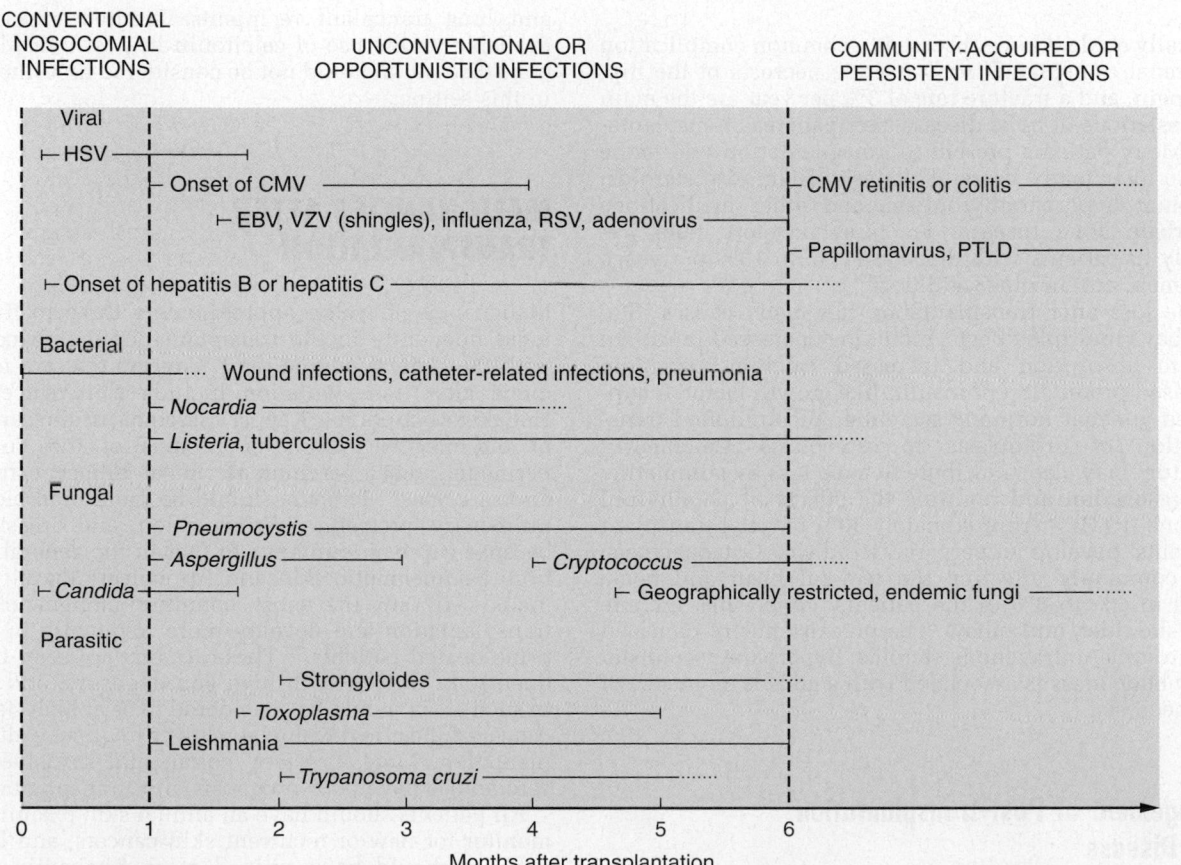

FIGURE 302-1. Infections after transplantation. CMV, cytomegalovirus; EBV, Epstein-Barr virus; HSV, herpes simplex virus; PTLD, posttransplantation lymphoproliferative disorder; RSV, respiratory syncytial virus; VZV, varicella-zoster virus. (Adapted from Fishman JA, Rubin RH: Infection in organ transplant recipients. New Engl J Med 1998;338:1741-1751.)

viral hepatitis may develop increased viral replication and clinical liver disease. After the first month, opportunistic infections such as *Pneumocystis, Listeria,* and *Aspergillus* begin. Most programs use Bactrim prophylaxis against *Pneumocystis* for the first year, and many continue it indefinitely. Epstein-Barr virus may predate transplantation, or patients may acquire it as a primary infection from the donor. It is associated with post-transplantation lymphoproliferative disease (PTLD). This usually develops in the setting of aggressive immunosuppression in patients at risk (new or preexisting exposure). Reduction or cessation in immunosuppression may be sufficient to cure many patients, although others may require chemotherapy. Patients with prior papillomavirus infection may develop rapid growth in venereal warts or malignant cervical lesions. Treatment of venereal warts should include surgery or other local treatment. Use of imiquimod has been effective in other settings but should probably be avoided until post-transplantation studies have been performed, because its mode of action is to stimulate cytokine production and other immune mediators to control the lesions. Not only is the efficacy questionable in a patient receiving immunosuppressive therapy, but there is added fear that the drug may induce rejection.

The risk of serious post-transplantation infections can be reduced by avoiding excessive immunosuppression. Appropriate long-term tapering of immunosuppression and avoidance of repeated rejection treatment in poorly functioning grafts are the hallmarks.

BONE DISEASE

Clinically evident bone disease is a common complication after renal transplantation.[11] Aseptic necrosis of the hip, bone pain, and a fracture rate of 3% per year are the main manifestations of bone disease after pancreas transplantation. Many patients present to transplantation with bone disease after many years of dialysis. High-dose steroids, persistent hyperparathyroidism, and other medications exacerbate bone disease. Fractures develop more frequently in patients with diabetes (11% to 13% per year), in women, and in older adults.[12,13]

Bone loss after transplantation has many causes. Steroids have multiple effects, including decreased intestinal calcium absorption and increased calcium excretion, decreased production of insulin-like growth factor 1, suppressed gonadal hormone secretion, and inhibited transformation of protoblasts to osteoblasts. Calcineurin inhibitors may also contribute to bone loss by stimulating bone resorption and blunting the effects of parathyroid hormone (PTH).[14] Approximately 30% of renal transplant recipients develop hyperparathyroidism. Osteonecrosis, most commonly affecting the femoral head and neck, occurs in 6% to 8% of the patients. Other sites include knee, shoulder, and elbow. The preexistence of damaged bone, trauma, intravenous steroids, hyperparathyroidism, or low bone mass is associated with a greater incidence of osteonecrosis.

Management of Post-transplantation Bone Disease

Management should begin with early ambulation and encouragement of physical exercise. All patients (with and without bone disease) should have a routine weight-bearing exercise program which can directly increase bone density.[15] Bone density should be evaluated before transplantation and annually thereafter with dual energy x-ray absorptiometry. Hyperphosphatemia usually resolves with a functioning graft but may persist in patients with DGF or chronic allograft nephropathy and should be aggressively controlled to avoid worsening hyperparathyroidism.[16] Oral calcium and vitamin D supplements are also suggested to prevent steroid-induced osteoporosis.

Parathyroidectomy may be required in patients with severe persistent hypercalcemia unresponsive to conservative measures. Most patients with moderate hypercalcemia due to secondary hyperparathyroidism do not require parathyroidectomy. The classic approach has been to delay surgery for approximately 1 year to allow involution of the glands. However, if the hypercalcemia is severe (>12.5 mg/day) or is causing severe bone disease, surgery should be performed earlier. The calcimimetic agent (cinacalcet) may offer a new approach to control of hypercalcemia and reduction of PTH levels after transplantation. In a recent study by Kruse and colleagues, this agent normalized serum creatinine in most renal transplant recipients with persistent hyperparathyroidism, but some continued to have persistent hypercalcemia.[17] A subsequent report demonstrated that the drug can be used to treat symptomatic hypercalcemia in renal transplant recipients, with improvement in symptoms and PTH levels.[18] This promising agent may become very useful in managing persistent hypercalcemia after kidney and pancreas transplantation, but confirmation of its efficacy should await larger, well-designed studies in patients with transplants. Bisphosphonates may be effective in reducing steroid-induced bone disease and bone fractures in kidney, liver, and lung transplant recipients. Limited experience is available on the use of calcitonin in post-transplantation bone disease. It should not be considered first-line therapy in this setting.

MALIGNANCIES AFTER TRANSPLANTATION

Malignancies develop approximately three to five times more frequently in the transplant population compared with the general population.[19] Cancers that are more frequent after transplantation include skin cancers, non-Hodgkin's lymphoma, Kaposi's sarcoma, in situ carcinomas of the uterine cervix, carcinomas of the vulva and perineum, renal carcinomas, hepatobiliary carcinomas, and sarcomas.[20] Patients should be monitored closely for pulmonary, prostatic, uterine, colon, and breast cancer, because survival is inferior to that in the general population. Nonmelanotic skin and lip cancers (basal or squamous cell) are the most common malignancies after transplantation and develop more frequently in azathioprine-treated patients.[21] These lesions are seen most frequently in regions with high sun exposure, and patients in such areas should be considered to be at high risk. Some cancers appear to develop at a lower frequency after transplantation. Lung, prostate, colon, and invasive uterine carcinomas have poor prognosis after transplantation.[22]

All patients should have an annual skin examination to monitor for new or recurrent skin cancers, and high-risk patients should be examined more frequently. Routine digital rectal examinations should be performed annually after 40 years of age. Sigmoidoscopy should be encouraged at 50 years of age and every 3 to 5 years thereafter. Pelvic

TABLE 302-7

Stages of Chronic Kidney Disease (CKD) and Action Plan in Renal Transplant Recipients

STAGE	DEFINITION (GFR IN mL/min)	CLINICAL PLAN
1	≥90	Slow progression, treat comorbid illnesses
2	60-89	Above, and monitor progression
3	30-59	Above, and treat complications of CKD
4	15-29	Above, and prepare for dialysis or retransplantation
5	<15	Dialysis if uremic, retransplantation

GFR, glomerular filtration rate.
From Abbud-Filho M, Adams PL, Alberu J, et al: A report of the Lisbon Conference on the care of the kidney transplant recipient. Transplantation 2007;83:S1-S22.

examinations and Papanicolaou (Pap) smears should be performed annually in women age 20 to 65 years and earlier in sexually active teens. Routine mammograms should be performed every 2 years in women beginning at approximately 35 years of age.

CHRONIC KIDNEY TRANSPLANT DYSFUNCTION

Although renal transplantation is a highly effective treatment for ESRD, a few patients have normal renal function and should be classified as having chronic kidney disease (CKD), similar to patients before dialysis. Causes of CKD in transplant recipients include, among others, chronic allograft nephropathy, calcineurin nephrotoxicity, recurrent or de novo glomerular disease, polyoma (BK) nephropathy, and, with aging donors, preexisting donor renal insufficiency.

All renal transplant recipients should have measures instituted aimed at delaying progression of renal disease regardless of the stage (Table 302-7). These include excellent blood pressure control, minimization of nephrotoxic agents (including calcineurin inhibitors), and the use of ACE inhibitors. Control of comorbid illnesses such as hyperlipidemia is particularly important in all stages. Avoiding nonadherence to medications is vital in young patients and in those with low socioeconomic status who may not be able to afford expensive immunosuppression. Despite these measures, many patients progress to stage 4 or 5. Such patients should be prepared for dialysis or, preferably, retransplantation.

The Failing Allograft

Once a patient has developed stage 4 CKD and returned to dialysis, immunosuppression should be reduced or discontinued. If the transplantation was performed within the previous year, most centers proceed to an allograft nephrectomy, because 50% of these patients will require nephrectomy due to rejection if weaning of immunosuppression is attempted. Patients with longer-surviving grafts can undergo slow weaning. The general approach to weaning once patients have started dialysis includes the following:

TABLE 302-8

Indications for Allograft Nephrectomy

INDICATION	COMMENTS
Acute late rejection after withdrawal of immunosuppression	Graft pain, fever, abdominal pain
Recurrent or de novo glomerulonephritis with severe nephrotic syndrome symptoms	Refractory to conservative management
Persistent urinary tract infection associated with calculi, pyelonephritis, hydronephrosis	Inability to produce sterile urine due to urological abnormalities
To allow rapid withdrawal of immunosuppression	Patients with nonrenal infection, cancer, or other reasons to avoid immunosuppression
Allograft renal artery stenosis	Persistent moderate to severe hypertension in dialysis patient with nonfunctioning graft

prednisone doses are slowly tapered (by approximately 2.5 to 5 mg/mo depending on the starting dose); mycophenolic acid, rapamycin, and azathioprine can be stopped immediately; and calcineurin inhibitors are reduced by 50%. All agents should be progressively reduced so that most patients are off all immunosuppressants by 6 to 8 months. Patients losing their grafts to severe refractory rejection may benefit from nephrectomy regardless of the time after transplantation. Some clinicians would instead plan a delayed weaning schedule.

Nephrectomy

The indications for allograft nephrectomy are listed in Table 302-8. Some patients develop graft pain, fever, hematuria, and abdominal pain during weaning of immunosuppression. This usually indicates acute rejection and requires nephrectomy, because there is usually little value in treating it with more immunosuppression. Patients with recurrent severe nephrotic syndrome due to recurrence of glomerulonephritis may obtain rapid relief from the symptoms of nephrotic syndrome after nephrectomy. Patients with persistent urinary tract infections involving the allograft should undergo nephrectomy, as should any other patient for whom rapid withdrawal of immunosuppression would be beneficial.

Key Points

1. The number and type of co-morbid illnesses complicate the early and late management of renal transplant recipients and are major determinants of morbidity, mortality, and graft survival.
2. The length of hospital stay after transplantation is short, leading to the majority of care being conducted in the outpatient settings.
3. Rejection seldom develops before 1 week after transplantation unless there are preformed antibodies to the donor.
4. The vast majority of successful renal transplant recipients have chronic kidney disease and should

be managed similar to patients who had renal disease before developing end-stage renal disease.

5. Infectious complications can be minimized by avoiding excessive immunosuppression in both the short and the long term.

Key References

3. Humar A, Matas AJ: Surgical complications after kidney transplantation. Semin Dial 2005;18:505-510.
7. Saifu MO, Tedla F, Markell MS: Management of the well renal transplant recipient: Outpatient surveillance and treatment recommendations. Semin Dial 2005;18:520-528.

8. Abbud-Filho M, Adams PL, Alberu J, et al: A report of the Lisbon Conference on the care of the kidney transplant recipient. Transplantation 2007;83:S1-S22.
10. Fishman JA, Rubin RH: Infection in organ transplant recipients. N Engl J Med 1998;338:1741-1751.
11. Heaf JG: Bone disease after renal transplantation. Transplantation 2003;75:315.
19. Dantal J, Pohanka E: Malignancies in renal transplantation: an unmet medical need. Nephrol Dial Transplant 2007; 22(Suppl 1):4-10.

See the companion Expert Consult website for the complete reference list.

CHAPTER 303

Acute Renal Failure in Kidney Transplant Recipients

Paolo Cravedi, Norberto Perico, and Giuseppe Remuzzi

OBJECTIVES

This chapter will:

1. Discuss the causes and risk factors of delayed graft function (DGF).
2. Describe the pathophysiology of ischemia/reperfusion damage.
3. Address the question of whether DGF is associated with an increased risk of acute rejection and long-term graft dysfunction.
4. Discuss strategies to prevent ischemia/reperfusion injury and DGF.
5. Discuss future therapeutic perspectives.

Delayed graft function (DGF) is a form of acute renal failure after kidney transplantation that results in post-transplantation oliguria, increased allograft immunogenicity, and risk of acute rejection. Rarely, a graft never functions (primary nonfunction). Experimental studies have shown that both ischemia and reinstitution of blood flow in ischemically damaged kidneys after hypothermic preservation activate a complex sequence of events that sustain renal injury and play a pivotal role in the development of DGF.[1]

The incidence of DGF has been variously reported to occur in 8% to 50% of primary cadaveric renal transplants in the United States[2] and in 35% of cadaveric transplants in a European multicenter study report.[3] According to the United Network for Organ Sharing (UNOS) Renal Transplant Registry, the frequency of DGF in cadaver transplants declined only slightly, from about 29% to 23% during the 1990s,[4] despite improvements in donor and recipient management and in diagnostic and therapeutic tools. This can be partly explained by the expansion of criteria for acceptable donors, including use of marginal and older donors,[5] as well as recipients that may be more predisposed to develop DGF.

CAUSES AND RISK FACTORS OF DELAYED GRAFT FUNCTION

Prerenal, renal, or postrenal factors may cause DGF (Table 303-1). Recipient hypovolemia is the most common prerenal cause of DGF, and it is generally reversible with proper fluid management. One rare form of prerenal DGF, which is yet a major cause of early graft failure, is vascular thrombosis.[6,7] Risks associated with graft loss from thrombosis are increased with a pediatric recipient or donor, with prolonged cold ischemia time, and with acute tubular necrosis (ATN). OKT3 monoclonal antibody treatment may also increase the risk of thrombosis by inducing the expression of tissue factor on endothelial cells and monocytes.[8] The primary causes of DGF in renal transplantation are hyperacute rejection, ATN, and calcineurin inhibitor nephrotoxicity. Postrenal causes of DGF, found in up to 4% of kidney recipients, are usually related to ureteral leakage rather than obstruction.[9]

Risk Factors Related to the Donor

The source of donors is particularly important (see Table 303-1). ATN, for example, is remarkably higher in recipients of cadaveric kidney transplants than in those receiving a living kidney. The difference is mainly accounted for by the massive release of cytokines and growth factors associated with brain death that contributes to ischemia and inflammation[10] of the kidney and, together with the hemodynamic instability, leads to ATN. The modality of organ procurement represents another important risk factor for donor-related DGF. The growing shortage of organs for transplantation has increased interest in using non–heart-beating and expanded criteria donors. Renal grafts from non–heart-beating donors[11] have twice the risk for DGF as those from heart-beating donors, despite similar outcomes at 1 year. There are now considerable data and experience to support the policy that no marginal or sub-

TABLE 303-1

Risk Factors for Delayed Graft Function

Procurement Factors
Kidney from non–heart-beating donor
Inotropic support of the donor
Cold storage preservation
Cold ischemia time
Donor Factors
Age (>55 yr)
Marginal kidney from diabetic or hypertensive donor
Recipient Factors
Prerenal
Recipient hypovolemia
Intraoperative albumin administration
Nocturnal hemodialysis
Hemodialysis with ultrafiltration within 24 hr before
   transplantation
Recipient or donor body weight
Number of previous transplants
Renal
Inherited thrombophilia
Factor V Leiden mutation
OKT3 monoclonal antibody therapy
Antiphospholipid antibodies
Preformed antidonor antibodies
Acute tubular necrosis
Cyclosporin nephrotoxicity
Postrenal
Ureteral leakage
Ureteral obstruction

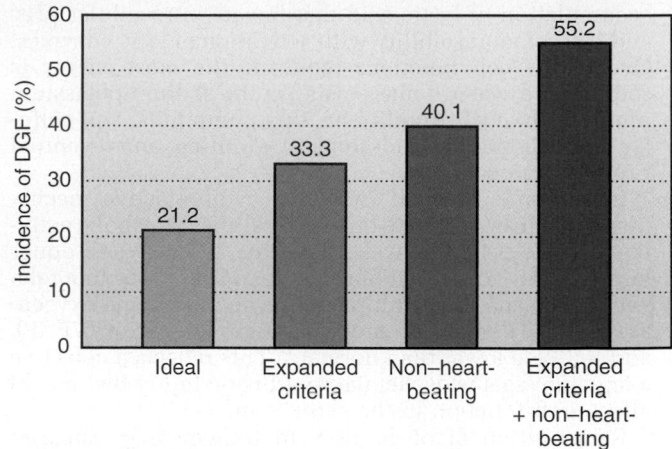

FIGURE 303-1. Incidence of delayed graft function (DGF) in kidney transplant recipients from ideal, expanded criteria, non–heart-beating and non–heart-beating with expanded criteria donors between 2000 and 2004 in the United States. Expanded criteria donors were all donors aged 60 years or older and those between 50 and 59 years of age with at least two of the following criteria: serum creatinine concentration greater than 1.5 mg/dL, history of hypertension, or cerebrovascular accident as cause of death. (From U.S. Department of Health and Human Services. 2005 Annual Report of the U.S. Organ Procurement and Transplantation Network and the Scientific Registry of Transplant Recipients: Transplant Data 1995-2004. Rockville, MD: Health Resources and Services Administration, Healthcare Systems Bureau, Division of Transplantation, 2005.)

optimal graft should be discarded due to donor age, diabetes, or hypertension, providing that the pretransplantation kidney biopsy is acceptable.[12] Over the short term, the use of marginal kidney donors has resulted in successful increased utilization of organs that normally would not be considered for transplantation, particularly kidneys from older donors. Nevertheless, the successful use of marginal donors has been associated with a significant increased risk of DGF (Fig. 303-1), an event that is expected to become more important in the future.[13,14]

Organ preservation also plays a role (see Table 303-1). Pulsatile perfusion has been reported to be superior to simple cold storage preservation.[9] Moreover, prolonged cold ischemia time, now more common in organ transplantation, appears to be an additional independent risk factor for DGF.[15] This is supported by data from the U.S. Renal Data System Registry that demonstrated a 23% increase in risk of DGF for every 6 hours of cold ischemia.[2] Improved allocation policies that reduce ischemia times therefore represent a central instrument to reduce the incidence of DGF in the near future.[16] Donor age is a further important risk factor for DGF. Analysis of the U.S. Scientific Renal Transplant Registry from 1990 to 1998 showed a doubling of DGF risk for recipients of kidneys from donors 55 years of age or older.[17] Of note, kidneys from older donors are also more susceptible to damage from cold ischemia.

Risk Factors Related to the Recipient

Allosensitization of the recipient represents one of the key factors influencing early graft function. Almost all patients (90%) with pretransplantation panel reactive antibodies (PRA) greater than 50% required post-transplantation dial-

ysis, compared with 45% of those with PRA 10% to 50% and 27% of those with PRA less than 10%.[18] Based on capillary deposition of complement component C4d, it has been suggested that humoral reactivity may contribute to DGF in as many as 50% of cases.[19]

Nonimmunological factors may additionally contribute to enhance the risk of DGF. In 158 consecutive living-related kidney transplant recipients, the mean recipient/donor weight was significantly higher in patients with DGF compared to those without DGF.[20] Dialysis modality at the time of transplantation and race have also been recognized as risk factors for DGF.[21] In one study, after adjustment for confounding factors, the relative risk of oliguria in the first week after surgery was 60% higher in hemodialyzed African-American patients than in those on peritoneal dialysis. This finding was not confirmed by others.[22] Additional recipient risk factors include the number of previous transplants, poor quality of reperfusion, absence of intraoperative diuresis, pretransplantation anuria or oliguria,[3] and lower mean perioperative diastolic blood pressure,[23] possibly reflecting the exacerbation of ischemia in hypotensive patients (see Table 303-1).

PATHOPHYSIOLOGY OF RENAL ISCHEMIA-REPERFUSION INJURY

Ischemia starves the tissue of oxygen and nutrients and causes accumulation of metabolic waste products. At the cellular level, the biochemical changes occurring during ischemia induce rapid anaerobic glycolysis, resulting in accumulation of lactic acid that lowers intracellular pH[24] and lysosomal instability with activation of lytic enzymes. One of the cell functions requiring the most energy is sodium and water homeostasis via the sodium-potassium pump. In hypoxic conditions, this pump fails, and cellular, mitochondrial, and nuclear swelling and eventual rupture can occur.[25]

In response to renal ischemia, cytoprotective mechanisms, such as a rapid decrease of cellular metabolic activity,[26] are activated as well. However, in cadaveric donor kidneys, the expression of genes encoding for factors relevant to the adaptive graft response, such as heme-oxygenase-1 (HO-1), vascular endothelial growth factor (VEGF), and Bcl-2, is lower than normal.[27] This reflects a defective adaptation against ischemia/reperfusion injury that would affect graft function in the short term.

Reinstitution of blood flow in ischemically damaged kidneys after hypothermic preservation activates a sequence of events that sustain renal injury and play a pivotal role in the development of DGF. This reperfusion injury is mediated by an array of inflammatory mechanisms that cause direct tissue damage by initiating a cascade of deleterious cellular responses. In the reperfusion phase, the adherent leukocytes plug capillaries, generate proteolytic enzymes, and release cytokines. The vasa recta become congested, peritubular capillary perfusion is impaired, and endothelial permeability is increased.[28] Activated leukocytes, particularly the polymorphonuclear cells, generate oxygen free radicals and ultimately infiltrate renal tissue. The complex interplay among reactive oxygen radicals, chemokines/cytokines, complement factors, adhesion receptors, and leukocytes leads to an inflammatory process that eventually damages renal epithelial cells, particularly those of the proximal tubule. These mechanisms may impair graft function beyond the injury associated with ischemia itself.

ISCHEMIA-REPERFUSION INJURY ENHANCES ALLOGRAFT IMMUNOGENICITY

Risk of Acute Rejection

Ischemic renal injury increases the risk of acute rejection because of the effects of innate immunity in response to injury on the foreign tissue of the graft.[29] Ischemia upregulates the expression of major histocompatibility complex (MHC) class I and II molecules on the kidney,[9] predominantly in tubular cells for class I and in interstitial cells for class II. MHC antigens are responsible for alloreactivity, either via direct recognition of MHC alloantigen molecules on the surface of the graft or via indirect recognition of processed peptides derived from those molecules and presented to the recipient immune system by recipient antigen-presenting cells.[30] Consequently, acute rejection occurs more frequently in patients who experience DGF than in those with immediate function,[31] although this is not a uniform finding.[32] In 308 recipients of cadaveric renal transplants, the incidence of acute rejection was 53% in those with DGF and 46% in those without DGF.[33] However, detection of acute rejection in the kidney with DGF is difficult because the rising serum creatinine concentration and oliguria cannot be used to make the diagnosis, and only protocol biopsy every 7 to 10 days, as is done in some centers, can be of help.

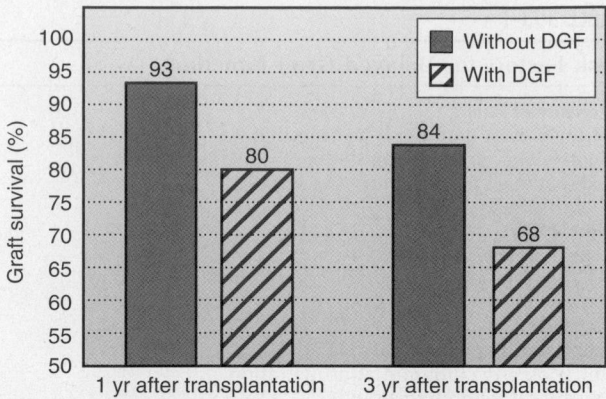

FIGURE 303-2. Kidney graft survival at 1 and 3 years for recipients with or without delayed graft function (DGF). (From U.S. Department of Health and Human Services. 2005 Annual Report of the U.S. Organ Procurement and Transplantation Network and the Scientific Registry of Transplant Recipients: Transplant Data 1995-2004. Rockville, MD: Health Resources and Services Administration, Healthcare Systems Bureau, Division of Transplantation, 2005.)

Risk of Long-Term Graft Dysfunction

Recovery from ischemic damage may initiate a cascade of events leading to chronic graft injury. Experimental studies of kidney transplantation in rats documented that ischemia/reperfusion injury and uni-nephrectomy may interact to produce progressive fibrotic changes in the graft.[34] In the clinical setting, data show an association between the occurrence of DGF and impaired long-term graft function (Fig. 303-2). In the precyclosporine era, a multicenter analysis to address this issue reported a significant correlation between early post-transplantation renal function (at day 1 and week 1) and long-term graft survival.[35] Despite an overall improvement of kidney graft survival with cyclosporine use, the effect of DGF was still evident, with lowering of 1-year graft survival by 20% to 30% in most single center studies.[36] A multivariate analysis confirmed DGF as an independent predictor of graft loss and showed a relative risk of graft loss 2.9 times greater for DGF compared with immediate kidney function.[37] The importance of DGF in long-term graft outcome is further supported by findings that, in cadaver transplants from 1994 to 1998 in the United States, the half-life of kidneys with no DGF was 11.5 years, compared to 7.2 years with DGF.[17] Multivariate analysis of factors affecting graft survival confirmed that DGF was significantly associated with graft loss, independent of other factors, including donor age and human leukocyte antigen (HLA) mismatches.[17] Other studies confirmed that the presence as well as the duration of DGF negatively affects long-term graft function. In addition, the analysis from the U.S. Renal Data System, involving more than 37,000 primary cadaveric renal transplants, revealed that DGF was independently predictive of 5-year graft loss (relative risk, 1.53), and the presence of both DGF and early acute rejection further reduced the rate of 5-year graft survival.[2]

This observation opens one of the most controversial issues, namely whether DGF is harmful in the absence of rejection. It can be a difficult interaction to dissect, because kidneys with DGF have a higher incidence of acute rejection, and biopsy is not always performed during the DGF period, so rejection may be underdiagnosed. Nevertheless, in a multicenter study of 57,000 first cadaveric transplants reported to the UNOS registry, DGF showed a strong effect independent of rejection.[38] In the presence of rejection, the effect of DGF was even stronger, with graft half-life decreasing from 9.4 to 6.2 years.[38] The impact of DGF alone or in combination with acute rejection on kidney graft survival in the long term was recently analyzed.[39] At 10 years after transplantation, the actuarial graft survival rate was 64% in patients with no history of DGF or rejection episodes, 44% in those with DGF, 36% in those with history of rejection, and 15% if both risk factors were present, further suggesting an additive negative effect on graft outcome.

Not all studies, however, concur with the conclusion that DGF is a strong predictor of long-term outcome of the graft. Indeed, some investigators reported that DGF was an independent risk factor for graft loss in the first 6 months but not later on.[40] Similarly, others found DGF to be associated with increased graft loss during the first year but not in the later post-transplantation period.[41] In a cohort of 3800 cadaveric renal transplant recipients, patients with well-recovered graft function by 1 month after DGF had a significantly reduced 4-year graft survival rate, compared with patients with no prior history of DGF.[42] However, patients with a history of DGF but good graft function at 6 months showed long-term graft survival similar to that of patients with no history of DGF.

The discrepancies among these studies can be at least partly explained by the presence of different policies on performing biopsies during the anuria period in different centers. Therefore, to evaluate the relative impact of DGF and acute rejection on long-term graft outcomes, future studies should include per protocol biopsies within 7 to 10 days after transplantation, to exclude the occurrence of acute rejection in those patients who develop DGF.

STRAGEGIES TO PREVENT ISCHEMIA-REPERFUSION INJURY AND DELAYED GRAFT FUNCTION

The improvement in understanding of the pathophysiology of renal ischemia and reperfusion injury has contributed to the evolution of strategies to decrease the rate of DGF which have focused on donor management, organ procurement and preservation techniques, recipient fluid management, and pharmacological agents (Table 303-2).

Preservation Solutions

Regardless of the method of kidney storage, preservation solutions have been designed to minimize ischemic damage (see Table 303-2). Particular components are added to these solutions to decrease cell swelling, maintain calcium homeostasis, decrease free radical generation, and provide high-energy substrates. The University of Wisconsin solution of Belzer and Southard[43] has emerged as the standard, effective preservation solution; it has proved superior to the EuroCollins solution in reducing DGF rates at all but the shortest cold ischemia times.[44] Modified solutions that omit the hydroxyethyl starch seem equally effective but are potentially less expensive.[45] A new solution, Celsior, is already used for heart, lungs, and liver transplants and has recently been proposed for kidney preservation. In a multicenter trial on 187 renal

TABLE 303-2

Proposed Strategies to Prevent Ischemia-Reperfusion Injury and Delayed Graft Function

Preservation Solutions
University of Wisconsin solution
Histidine-tryptophan-ketoglutarate solution
Celsior solution
Pulsatile perfusion machine
Recipient Fluid Management
Fluid expansion with colloid or crystalloids
Mannitol or furosemide
Vasodilatory Agents
Calcium-channel blockers
Prostacyclin
Atrial natriuretic peptide
Selective and nonselective endothelin receptor antagonists
Antioxidants
Heme-oxygenase-1 induction or overexpression in the graft
N-Acetylcysteine
Propionyl-L-carnitine
Inhibitors of inducible nitric oxide synthase
Anti-inflammatory Agents
Antagonists of platelet-activating factor receptor
Monoclonal antibodies to TNF-α
Inhibitors or antagonists of cytokines: interleukins 1, 10, and 13; CXCL-8; MCP-1
Monoclonal antibodies to ICAM-1 and leukocyte function-associated antigen 1
Soluble P-selectin glycoprotein ligand
Immunosuppressants (CTLA4-Ig fusion protein, mycophenolate mofetil)
Complement inhibitors
Statins
Growth Factors
Insulin-like growth factor
Cell Therapy

CTLA4, cytotoxic T-lymphocyte antigen 4; CXCL-8, interleukin-8; ICAM-1, intercellular adhesion molecule 1; Ig, immunoglobulin; MCP-1, monocyte chemotactic protein 1; TNF, tumor necrosis factor.

transplants in a clinical setting, the preservation of kidneys in Celsior solution resulted in a DGF rate similar to that observed with the use of University of Wisconsin solution (31.3% versus 33.9%).[46] Similar results were obtained using the Solution de Conservation des Organes et des Tissus (SCOT), a solution that combines an extracellular-like composition with 20-kDa polyethylene glycol, which is known for its cell-protection properties.[47] Research on preservation is now focused on additives that could supplement the standard solutions, such as trimetazidine,[48] dextrans,[49] and bioflavonoids.[50]

The method of preservation may also have a role in decreasing DGF, but whether a pulsatile perfusion machine is superior to simple cold storage is still controversial. When two kidneys from each donor were split between pulsatile perfusion and cold storage, no significant improvement in early graft function was found in the perfusion group, even with cold ischemia times greater than 24 hours.[51] However, more recent studies have shown that the use of pulsatile perfusion may decrease the rate of DGF, particularly in the setting of expanded criteria donor kidneys.[52]

Recipient Fluid Management

Patients are often volume contracted before surgery because of recent dialysis. Fluid expansion with colloid or crystalloids[53] under central venous monitoring can reduce the incidence of DGF. The role of adequate hydration of the recipient is supported by the finding of lower DGF rates in patients previously receiving peritoneal rather than hemodialysis treatment. In the normal setting, mannitol, because of its diuretic and antioxidant properties, has been shown to improve early graft function when given to the recipient just before reperfusion.[54] Furosemide is often given during the vascular anastomosis to promote diuresis, although whether it actually improves early function or simply increases urine output from a functioning kidney is unclear.[55]

Immunosuppressive Management of Delayed Graft Function

Many centers change their immunosuppression regimen when faced with DGF or a high risk of DGF. A common change is to reduce or delay the introduction of calcineurin inhibitors and to switch to a depleting antibody, because cyclosporine may negatively affect recovery from ATN and may increase the risk of dysfunction or even failure of the graft. Furthermore, the fact that poorly functioning kidneys complicate the differential diagnosis of rejection[56] makes treatment with antibody induction therapy attractive. Studies have evaluated the effects of Thymoglobulin (rabbit antithymocyte globulin, or RATG) and monoclonal antibodies such as anti-CD3 antibodies (OKT3), which are devoid of appreciable nephrotoxicity but are powerful immunosuppressants.[57] A clinical trial documented that intraoperative administration of RATG in adult cadaveric renal transplant recipients was associated with a significant decrease in DGF, better early allograft function in the first month after transplantation, and a decreased post-transplantation hospital length of stay, compared with postoperative treatment.[58] Previous studies suggested that the intraoperative administration of RATG may help to prevent DGF by blocking adhesion molecules, because this polyclonal agent contains antibodies to a variety of adhesion molecules.[59] The clear short-term advantage of RATG may, however, be offset to some extent by an increased risk of opportunistic infections and post-transplantation lymphoproliferative disease (PTLD).[60] As an alternative, the novel monoclonal antibodies to block interleukin-2 receptor (IL-2R) on T cells (basiliximab, daclizumab) have been shown to be extremely safe in transplantation, with encouraging although not always consistent results in DGF.[61] In addition, recent findings indicate that, under induction therapy with basiliximab, early or delayed introduction of cyclosporine results in similar function in renal transplant patients regardless of DGF risk level.[62] Add-on therapy with anti-IL-2R antibody in an induction protocol based on the use of low-dose RATG has been also proposed as a rational strategy to fully inhibit T-cell function even without achieving a complete T-cell depletion. Very promising are the results of a pilot, explorative study performed to test the possibility that basiliximab, given to kidney transplant recipients who are at increased immunological risk or who have DGF, in combination with low-dose RATG, is at least as effective as RATG at standard dose but has a more favorable safety profile.[63]

As an alternative to cyclosporine, mammalian target of rapamycin (mTOR) inhibitors such as sirolimus and everolimus have been proposed, because they lack known nephrotoxicity.[64] However, in a retrospective analysis of 132 consecutive cases of DGF at the University of California, San Francisco, sirolimus appeared to prolong recovery from DGF.[65] Similarly, a randomized prospective study in kidney transplant recipients showed that the addition of sirolimus to low-dose cyclosporine, corticosteroids, and basiliximab delayed the recovery from DGF but did not affect graft function at 1 year, compared to triple therapy with conventional cyclosporine dose, mycophenolate mofetil, and corticosteroids.[66] These observations indicate that sirolimus may not be the optimal immunosuppressive agent in the DGF setting.

FUTURE THERAPEUTIC PERSPECTIVES

While these approaches are finalized to accelerate recovery from DGF, effective treatments for preventing its occurrence are still lacking. Several new drugs show promise in animal studies in preventing or ameliorating ischemia/reperfusion injury and possibly preventing DGF, but definite clinical trials are lacking (see Table 303-2). In various experimental models, pharmacological manipulation of cytokine and chemokine activities through specific antibodies or receptor antagonists has been reported to attenuate postischemic injury.[67] The goal of monotherapy for the prevention or treatment of DGF may, however, be unattainable, and multidrug approaches or single drugs targeting multiple signals may be the next step to reduce post-transplantation injury and DGF.

An increasing body of evidence has also revealed that injury to a target organ may be sensed by bone marrow stem cells which migrate to the site of damage, undergo differentiation, and promote structural and functional repair. This remarkable stem cell plasticity has been shown to be effective in repairing injured kidney in mouse models of ischemia/reperfusion or toxic injury, in which bone marrow–derived hematopoietic or mesenchymal stem cells differentiated into tubular epithelial cells, eventually restoring renal structure and function.[68,69] The evidence that mesenchymal stem cells, by virtue of their renoprotective property, can restore renal tubular structure and also ameliorate renal function during experimental acute renal failure provides opportunities for novel therapeutic interventions for DGF.

Key Points

1. Delayed graft function is a form of acute renal failure that results in post-transplantation oliguria and has been associated with an increased risk of acute rejection episodes and decreased long-term survival.
2. Prerenal, renal, and postrenal factors related to the transplant donor or the recipient can cause delayed graft function.
3. Experimental studies have shown that both ischemia and reinstitution of blood flow in ischemically damaged kidneys after hypothermic preservation activate complex sequences of events that sustain renal injury and play a pivotal role in the development of delayed graft function.
4. Strategies to decrease the rate of delayed graft function are focused on donor management, organ procurement and preservation techniques, recipi-

ent fluid management, and pharmacological agents (vasodilators, antioxidants, and anti-inflammatory agents).

5. Multidrug approaches and cell therapy will be the next steps to reduce post-transplantation injury and delayed graft function.

Key References

1. Perico N, Cattaneo D, Sayegh MH, Remuzzi G: Delayed graft function in kidney transplantation. Lancet 2004;364:1814-1827.
52. Matsuoka L, Shah T, Asward S, et al: Pulsatile perfusion reduces the incidence of delayed graft function in expanded

criteria donor kidney transplantation. Am J Transplant 2006;6:1473-1478.
58. Goggins WC, Pascual MA, Powelson JA, et al: A prospective, randomized, clinical trial of intraoperative versus postoperative Thymoglobulin in adult cadaveric renal transplant recipients. Transplantation 2003;76:798-802.
62. Kamar N, Garrigue V, Karras A, et al: Impact of early or delayed cyclosporine function in renal transplant recipients: A randomized, multicenter study. Am J Transplant 2006;6:1042-1048.
65. McTaggart RA, Gottlieb D, Brooks J, et al: Sirolimus prolongs recovery from delayed graft function after cadaveric renal transplantation. Am J Transplant 2003;3:416-423.

See the companion Expert Consult website for the complete reference list.

CHAPTER 304

Infectious Complications of Renal Transplantation

Ali Al-Khafaji and Peter K. Linden

OBJECTIVES

This chapter will:
1. Describe the typical timeline of opportunistic infections after kidney transplantation.
2. Describe the epidemiology, risk factors, and usual presentations of infections due to common opportunistic pathogens.
3. Describe the common surveillance, preemptive, and prophylactic strategies used to monitor for and prevent infection.

Current 1-year patient and renal allograft survival rates have risen to 98% and 92%, respectively, in the United States. The success of renal transplantation largely depends on technically competent surgery and preventing or treating allograft rejection and post-transplantation infectious complications. Although advances in the quality and monitoring of immunosuppression play a large part in improved patient and renal allograft survival, a fine balance exists between the quantity of immunosuppression needed to prevent rejection and the superimposed risk of opportunistic infection. Infection in such immunocompromised hosts may also be characterized by a broad spectrum of opportunistic pathogens, fulminant or atypical presentations, and a poor outcome if there are delays in the appropriateness of anti-infective or surgical treatments.

This chapter summarizes the risk factors, differential diagnosis, possible prevention measures, and treatment for infectious complications after kidney transplantation.

TIME LINE OF INFECTION AFTER KIDNEY TRANSPLANTATION

Infectious complications after transplantation can be roughly categorized based on their temporal relation to the time of the transplantation procedure (Fig. 304-1). However, significant variance may occur due to epidemiologic exposures, necessity for greater immunosuppression, and the effects of anti-infective chemoprophylaxis.

Early Period (During the First Month)

Infections occurring during the first month after transplantation are usually related to the surgery itself; they include technical complications such as perinephric hematomas, leakage of the ureteral anastomosis, vascular anastomotic complications, superficial wound infection, nosocomial infection (e.g., central venous catheter infection), urinary tract infection, pneumonia, and *Clostridium difficile* colitis. The dominant pathogens during this time are either endogenous flora or antimicrobial-resistant modified endogenous flora: methicillin-resistant *Staphylococcus aureus* (MRSA), vancomycin-resistant enterococcus (VRE), multiresistant gram-negative bacilli, and *Candida* spp. Reactivation of herpes simplex virus (HSV) may also manifest during this early period due to the effects of iatrogenic immunosuppression. Patients with poorly controlled diabetes and other significant comorbidities are also at enhanced risk of infection during this time.

Middle Period (Between 1 and 6 Months)

Infections relating to cumulative immunosuppression occur commonly between months 1 and 6 after transplan-

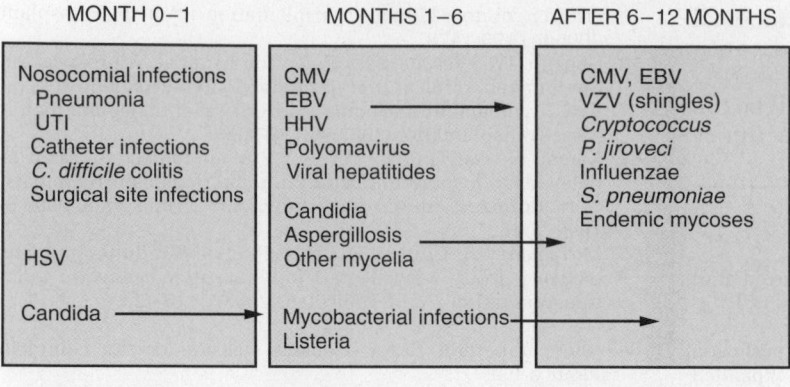

MONTH 0–1

MONTHS 1–6

AFTER 6–12 MONTHS

Nosocomial infections
  Pneumonia
  UTI
  Catheter infections
  C. difficile colitis
  Surgical site infections

HSV

Candida

CMV
EBV
HHV
Polyomavirus
  Viral hepatitides

Candidia
Aspergillosis
Other mycelia

Mycobacterial infections
Listeria

CMV, EBV
VZV (shingles)
Cryptococcus
P. jiroveci
Influenzae
S. pneumoniae
Endemic mycoses

——————▶ May occur with higher immunosuppression or high risk exposure

FIGURE 304-1. Time line of opportunistic infections in the renal transplant recipient. CMV, cytomegalovirus; EBV, Epstein-Barr virus; HHV, human herpesviruses; HSV, herpes simplex virus; UTI, urinary tract infections; VZV, varicella-zoster virus.

tation. They are caused by dormant organisms that were previously held in check by intact cellular immunity (e.g., cytomegalovirus [CMV], other herpesviruses), mycobacteria, endemic fungi (*Histoplasma capsulatum, Coccidioides immitis, Pneumocystis jiroveci, Toxoplasma gondii, Strongyloides stercoralis*), or exposure to exogenous pathogens (*Cryptococcus neoformans, Aspergillus* and other mycelial fungi, *Nocardia, Listeria monocytogenes, Legionella*).

Late (After 6 Months)

After the first 6 months, many of the observed infections in kidney transplant recipients are similar to those seen in the general community, such as pyogenic bacterial infections, influenza and other respiratory viral diseases, and varicella zoster virus (VZV) reactivation (shingles). However, patients with a prior or ongoing high immunosuppressive requirement may continue to have infections observed during the earlier time periods.

General Risk Factors for Infection

Advanced age, malnutrition, and chronic illnesses such as diabetes, cirrhosis, or cardiac failure pose higher risks for infection after transplantation than in recipients without such comorbidities. The invasive nature of surgical procedure itself and the frequent use of instruments such as urinary catheters and central venous catheters provide potential sources of infection. The renal graft function is a main predictor of infection, which is likely related to the intensity of the immunosuppressant agents used. Patients with poor graft function have the highest risk of development of opportunistic infections, whereas patients with normal graft function have almost the same risk of developing infections as in the general population.[1,2]

SPECIFIC INFECTIONS: PRESENTATION AND TREATMENT

Bacterial Infections

Bacterial infection can cause urinary tract infection (UTI), pneumonia, meningitis, and deep and superficial wound infections. UTI is the most common bacterial infection in renal transplant recipients, with an incidence of more than 30%.[3-6] Female gender, retransplantation, urinary catheters and stents, trauma to the kidney or ureter during surgery, neurogenic bladder, diabetes, and graft rejection are major risk factors for UTI.[7-9] Common bacterial urinary pathogens in renal transplant recipients include *Escherichia coli, Enterococcus, Pseudomonas aeruginosa, Serratia marcescens, Proteus* spp., *S. aureus, Staphylococcus epidermidis, Enterococcus* spp. and *Enterobacter cloacae.* Recurrent episodes of UTI should increase suspicion of anatomical abnormalities.[10] UTI can be prevented by the routine use of oral trimethoprim-sulfamethoxazole (TMP-SMX) daily for 6 to 12 months after transplantation. Alternatively, oral ciprofloxacin, 250 mg twice a day, can be used in patients who do not tolerate TMP-SMX or have sulfa allergy.

Bacterial pneumonia may arise from a diverse spectrum of pathogens. Mechanistically, the most common pathogens cause pneumonia similarly in these patients and in immunocompetent hosts, via colonization of the upper airways followed by microaspiration and overwhelming of the lower airway defenses. *S. aureus, Pseudomonas,* and the enteric gram-negative bacilli comprise the majority of cases in the nosocomial setting, whereas *S. pneumoniae* is the most common community-acquired bacterial respiratory pathogen. Both sporadic and, rarely, epidemic *Legionella* infections have been described after renal transplantation. High-dose corticosteroid therapy for the treatment of acute rejection may predispose patients to legionellosis with a high mortality rate. Nocardiosis is relatively uncommon and may manifest as multiple cavitary or noncavitary pulmonary lesions with or without associated hematogenous spread to skin, central nervous system, or other viscera. Therapy requires a prolonged course (6 to 12 months) of two to three agents with in vitro activity against the infecting *Nocardia* strain. The incidence of nocardiasis has fallen, possibly secondary to improved immunosuppression practices or the standard use of TMP-SMX prophylaxis for UTI and pneumocystosis.

Mycobacterium tuberculosis affects approximately 1% of kidney transplant recipients and is associated with high mortality. Patients may present with fever, malaise, night sweats, and weight loss. The diagnosis needs to be made clinically, because only 25% of recipients have a positive tuberculin skin test. A diverse spectrum of clinical and radiological findings including both cavitary and noncavitary lesions can be seen. However, a sputum culture, bronchoalveolar lavage (BAL), or other lung tissue specimen with demonstrable acid-fast bacilli and/or a positive culture for *M. tuberculosis* must be obtained for a confirmed diagnosis. Combination treatment with isoniazid, rifampin, and pyrazinamide for 9 to 12 months is the most common treatment regimen employed, but all definitive treatment should be guided by the results of susceptibility testing and the toxicity risks of the individual patient. Consideration of active *M. tuberculosis* should automatically prompt respiratory isolation in a negatively pressured, externally vented single room to avoid patient-to-patient spread. Renal recipients exposed to an active case of *M. tuberculosis* should be offered isoniazid prophylaxis.

Atypical mycobacteria (*Mycobacterium kansasii, Mycobacterium-avian* complex, *Mycobacterium fortuitum,* and *Mycobacterium xenopi*) may produce similar presentations and also require prolonged treatment tailored to susceptibility testing but do not require continued isolation once *M. tuberculosis* is excluded.

Viral Infections

Viral infections in renal transplant patients have both short-term and potential long-term sequelae, such as allograft dysfunction, rejection, and malignancy. Exposure to viruses may constitute a "primary" infection if the recipient has no prior viral-specific immunity or may represent a "secondary" infection, whereby a dormant strain from a distant prior exposure reactivates as a result of iatrogenic immunosuppression.

Primary infections due to CMV transmitted via the renal allograft or blood transfusions are more likely to produce symptomatic disease and other sequelae including graft dysfunction and rejection. Most herpesvirus infections in adult transplant recipients are caused by reactivation because of the high seroprevalence of prior infection.

The herpesvirus family includes HSV-1, HSV-2, CMV, VZV, Epstein-Barr virus (EBV), human herpesvirus 6 (HHV-6), HHV-7, and HHV-8. Other important viral pathogens are the polyoma JC/BK viruses, parvovirus B-19, adenovirus, and the viral hepatitides.

Cytomegalovirus

CMV is the single most important viral infection in renal transplant recipients, although aggressive antiviral preemptive and prophylaxis strategies have partially reduced its impact in recent years. After transplantation, a CMV-seronegative recipient (R–) who develops a primary infection from a CMV-seropositive donor (D+) is at the highest risk for symptomatic CMV disease (Table 304-1). However

approximately 70% to 80% of the adult population is CMV seropositive, and CMV disease may develop either from reactivation of a prior infection or from superinfection with the CMV donor strain.

CMV-seropositive recipients (R+) who receive OKT3, antithymocyte globulin, or other antilymphocyte therapy are at enhanced risk for CMV superinfection. Most significant CMV disease does not occur during the first month after transplantation, but evidence of asymptomatic CMV viral shedding may be present as early as 2 to 3 weeks when measured by the detection of circulating CMV early antigens or DNA.

Symptoms of CMV disease are protean and vary widely in severity. The mildest presentation is termed "syndrome" and may include nonlocalizing constitutional symptoms such as fever, malaise, headache, myalgia, and arthralgia. Leukopenia and a rightward shift in the differential may also be observed. The most serious and common tissue-invasive disease is CMV pneumonitis, which is usually heralded by a diffuse interstitial radiographic pattern and associated dyspnea and increased alveolar-arterial oxygen difference. Both upper (gastroduodenitis) and lower (colitis) gastrointestinal disease can produce significant hemorrhage. Other disease manifestations include hepatitis, retinitis, pancreatitis, cerebritis, nephritis, and disseminated disease involving two or more noncontiguous sites. Definitive diagnosis is usually made by tissue biopsy, which may demonstrate CMV-typical intranuclear inclusions, or by the demonstration of CMV antigens/genome.

CMV is an immunomodulatory virus that can increase susceptibility to opportunistic infections such as *Pneumocystis* and *Aspergillus*. In addition, CMV infection can lead to acute and/or chronic allograft dysfunction modulated both by an increase in human leukocyte antigen (HLA) class II antigen expression and the tapering or withdrawal of iatrogenic immunosuppression. A direct immune fluorescent stain of CMV pp65 antigen in circulating leukocytes, shell vial culture, and polymerase chain reaction (PCR) are all techniques currently used for the diagnosis of CMV infection.

Prevention of CMV disease can be achieved by either prophylactic or preemptive therapy coupled to regular surveillance monitoring with a molecular technique.[11,12] The wide variety of approaches are summarized in Table 304-2. Whether prophylaxis or preemption is superior in preventing CMV disease is still not established.[13] The preemptive approach requires a regular (one to two times weekly) blood monitoring technique (usually DNA detection with PCR or early viral antigen detection with an immunofluorescent staining technique such as CMV pp65). Patients found to have a threshold load of viral DNA or antigen are treated preemptively, usually with a course of parenteral ganciclovir or oral valganciclovir to prevent

TABLE 304-1

Risk Stratification for Cytomegalovirus (CMV) Infection in Renal Transplant Recipients

RISK CATEGORY	CMV DONOR/RECIPIENT STATUS	IMMUNOSUPPRESSION	OTHER VARIABLES
High	D+/R–	Antilymphocyte therapy (ALG, OKT3, ATG)	Coinfection with other immunomodulatory viruses (HIV-1, HCV, EBV)
Moderate	D+/R+ D–/R+	Antilymphocyte therapy (ALG, OKT3, ATG)	Coinfection with other immunomodulatory viruses (HIV-1, HCV, EBV)
Lowest	D–/R–		High transfusion burden with CMV + products

ALG, antilymphocyte globulin; ATG, antithymocyte globulin; EBV, Epstein-Barr virus; HCV, hepatitis C virus; HIV, human immunodeficiency virus.

TABLE 304-2

Chemoprophylaxis for Common Pathogens in the Renal Transplant Recipient

TYPE OF INFECTION	TARGET PATHOGENS	THERAPEUTIC AGENTS
Wound infection	*Staphylococcus aureus*, gram-negative bacilli	Ampicillin-sulbactam, piperacillin-tazobactam
Urinary tract infection	Enteric gram-negative bacilli, enterococci	TMP-SMX, quinolone
Viral infection	Herpes simplex virus	Acyclovir
	Cytomegalovirus	Valganciclovir, ganciclovir
Fungal infection	*Candida* spp.	Fluconazole
	Pneumocystis jiroveci	TMP-SMX, atovaquone. aerosolized pentamidine

TMP-SMX, trimethoprim-sulfamethoxazole.

progression to invasive disease. Repeat episodes of CMV shedding are not uncommon during the first 6 months after transplantation.

A second approach is prophylaxis administered to all patients, which may be stratified to their risk status. High-risk patients (CMV D+/R–) should receive CMV prophylactic therapy with oral valganciclovir, 900 mg daily for 3 months, or with intravenous ganciclovir adjusted for renal function for 3 weeks, followed by oral ganciclovir 3 g/day for 3 months. Higher doses of valganciclovir or ganciclovir should be used in high-risk patients who received antilymphocyte agents during immunosuppression induction or acute rejection. Intermediate-risk recipients (CMV D–/R+ or CMV D+/R+) should receive either prophylactic or preemptive therapy with valganciclovir or ganciclovir.

Intermediate-risk recipients (CMV D–/R+ or CMV D+/R+) who receive induction therapy or treatment of acute rejection with antilymphocyte agents should receive prophylactic therapy with intravenous ganciclovir while hospitalized, followed by oral ganciclovir; alternatively, they can receive oral valganciclovir. Low-risk recipients (D–/R–) do not require prophylaxis[11,14]; however, monitoring by PCR or pp65 should be done for 3 months, with preemptive treatment instituted for a positive test.

If the diagnosis of CMV disease is confirmed, treatment is initiated with intravenous ganciclovir for 14 to 21 days, followed by oral treatment for 3 to 6 months. Dose reduction or temporary cessation of ganciclovir may be needed if leukopenia or thrombocytopenia develops. CMV hyperimmune globulin may be a helpful addition to ganciclovir therapy in patients with organ involvement.[15]

To prevent relapse, treatment with intravenous ganciclovir should continue for at least 1 week after the CMV viral load becomes undetectable.

The routine use of prophylactic and preemptive CMV therapy has decreased the incidence and severity of CMV infections, but at the expense of the emergence of ganciclovir-resistant CMV. The overall incidence of ganciclovir-resistant CMV infection ranges between 1% and 13% among kidney and kidney/pancreas transplant recipients, respectively. High viral load, high level of immunosuppression, CMV D+/R– serologic status, universal prophylaxis, and suboptimal serum drug concentrations are all associated with increased risk for ganciclovir resistance. Ganciclovir-resistant CMV is treated with foscarnet or cidofovir.

Epstein-Barr Virus

EBV infections in renal transplant recipients can cause mononucleosis-like symptoms such as malaise, fever, headache, and sore throat. Post-transplantation lympho-proliferative disease (PTLD) is the life-threatening complication of EBV infection and occurs with an incidence of 1% to 3%.[16-18] EBV primary infection (D+/R–), a high EBV viral load, CMV sero-mismatch (D+/R–), and use of OKT3 increase the risk of PTLD.[19] Patients at greater risk are whites, younger than 25 years of age, during the first years after transplantation.[20] PTLD can occur months to years after transplantation, particularly in heavily immunosuppressed recipients. Immunosuppression impairs the ability of virus-specific cytotoxic T lymphocytes to control the expression of EBV-infected transformed B cells, leading to polyclonal and monoclonal proliferation of B-lymphocytes. PTLD may manifest in nodal tissue, extranodal viscera, or both.

Before treatment is started, the diagnosis should be confirmed by tissue biopsy. Treatment includes a decrease or discontinuation of immunosuppression, together with administration of antiviral agents, anti-CMV immune globulin, anti-CD20 antibody (rituximab), or conventional lymphoma chemotherapy.[21,22] Complete withdrawal of immunosuppression may precipitate allograft failure and the need for hemodialysis.

Herpes Simplex Virus

Primary HSV infections are rare, but reactivation is common, especially in patients who receive antilymphocyte or corticosteroid inductions. Reactivation may occur as early as the first month after transplantation. HSV is highly prevalent, with approximately 90% of the population having a positive serologic test, but only a fraction exhibit clinical symptoms of infection. The most common manifestation of HSV infection in the immunosuppressed patient is mucocutaneous lesions of the oropharynx or genital regions. Lesions may persist for weeks, and dissemination to the esophagus, colon, bladder, cornea, and retina may rarely occur. HSV hepatitis can occur as early as 4 to 20 days after transplantation. Diagnosis of HSV infection is clinical, with direct observation of the characteristic lesions, but definitive diagnosis of active infection requires isolation of the virus in cell cultures of vesicular fluid, mucosal swabs, cerebrospinal fluid, or urine. PCR testing is the preferred technique for cerebrospinal fluid. A Tzanck smear of scrapings from the base of the vesicle provides simple and quick diagnosis of a herpesvirus infection, but it is not specific for HSV. Immunofluorescence staining with specific antisera is preferred.

Treatment for mucocutaneous HSV infections is with oral acyclovir 400 mg four times per day. The dose should be reduced based on renal function. In disseminated HSV hepatitis or meningoencephalitis, immunosuppression should be reduced and intravenous acyclovir

(10 mg/kg every 8 hours for 7 to 14 days) should be administered.

Varicella-Zoster Virus

Most renal transplant recipients are VZV seropositive as a result of childhood chickenpox infection. Approximately 5% to 10% of recipients develop reactivated VZV infection. These patients may develop unidermatomal shingles or disseminated cutaneous zoster involving both sides or multiple dermatomes. Up to 33% of untreated cases disseminate, causing hemorrhagic pneumonia, encephalitis, pancreatitis, hepatitis, and disseminated intravascular coagulation.

The diagnosis is frequently made clinically, but VZV can be cultured, and direct immunofluorescent antibody staining or Tzanck preparation can be used. VZV requires systemic therapy with acyclovir 10 mg/kg every 8 hours for 7 to 14 days. Varicella-zoster immune globulin might play a role in treating seronegative recipients and for passive prophylaxis of exposed VZV-seronegative recipients; however, recent supply shortages of this preparation have reduced its availability.

Polyomavirus

The polyomaviruses belong to the Papovavirus family. Three species are known to infect humans: BK virus, JC virus, and Simian virus (SV40). Serological studies have shown that up to 90% of humans have been exposed to polyomavirus by adulthood, but clinical disease occurs only in the immunocompromised. Initial infection is usually asymptomatic and probably occurs via the respiratory route or as a bloodborne infection.

Multiple rejection episodes treated with potent immunosuppressive agents in the setting of a seropositive donor and/or recipient are the main risk factors leading to polyomavirus nephropathy (PVN). Because PVN can be confused with acute cellular rejection, it is essential to perform a graft biopsy to confirm the diagnosis.[23] Urine or plasma polyomavirus viral load may help in diagnosis and treatment follow-up. The treatment of PVN is achieved by reducing immunosuppression.[24] Intravenous immunoglobulin, cidofovir, leflunomide, and quinolone antibiotics have been used in treatment, especially for PVN that is progressive and refractory to immunosuppression dose reduction.

Human Herpesviruses

HHV-6 and HHV-7 are recently discovered immunomodulatory viruses that can lead to opportunistic infections, graft dysfunction, and a variety of clinical presentations such as bone marrow suppression, encephalitis, pneumonitis, and hepatitis.[25] The diagnosis is usually established by qualitative and quantitative molecular assays of tissue or blood.

HHV viremia is often asymptomatic and has been shown to be present in 38% to 55% of renal recipients, usually between the second and fourth weeks after transplantation. Treatment is achieved by reduction of immunosuppression and use of ganciclovir or foscarnet. HHV-8 is the viral etiological agent associated with Kaposi's sarcoma, a vascular endothelial tumor that can cause a cutaneous mucosal or visceral disease and is particularly common in transplant recipients of Mediterranean or Middle Eastern origin. Transmission of HHV-8 has been shown to occur via the renal allograft itself.[26]

Community-Acquired Respiratory Viruses

Important community-acquired respiratory virus infections in immunocompromised hosts include influenza virus types A and B, respiratory syncytial virus, parainfluenza viruses, adenoviruses, and rhinoviruses. Transmission is via contact for all viruses except influenza, which is transmitted by respiratory droplets. Common cold, upper respiratory tract infection, pharyngitis, laryngitis, tracheobronchitis, influenza-like syndromes, bronchiolitis, and pneumonia are common syndromes. In the immunocompromised host, viral shedding may persist for months. Oseltamivir (Tamiflu) may shorten the duration of viral shedding and symptoms in influenza. Seasonal influenza vaccination is recommended.

Fungal Infections

Among all solid organ transplant recipients, renal recipients have the lowest rates of fungal infection, although the case-fatality rate is the highest for fungal infection than for any other pathogen categories.[27,28] Most fungal infections occur within the first 6 months after transplantation, although a longer period of risk may occur in more heavily immunosuppressed recipients. The incidence can be as high as 14%, and more than 90% of cases are caused by *Candida* spp. *Candida albicans* and *Candida tropicalis* are the two most common species responsible for serious infection, although *Candida glabrata* is becoming more prevalent, particularly in patients with prior azole exposure and long length of hospital stay. Central venous catheters, surgical drains, urinary catheters, diabetes mellitus, use of corticosteroids or broad-spectrum antibiotics, and length of hospital stay are important risk factors for the development of *Candida* infection in the immunosuppressed recipient.[27,28]

Candidiasis can be categorized as either superficial or deep. Commonly involved superficial sites are the oral cavity, esophagus, and bladder. Oral candidiasis manifests as single or multiple, white, raised, plaque-like lesions over the tongue and oropharyngeal mucous membranes. Oral candidiasis can progress distally and can lead to esophageal involvement that may manifest as odynophagia or dysphagia or may be asymptomatic. Esophageal candidiasis, if untreated, can lead to esophageal bleeding, perforation, and disseminated candidiasis. Candiduria may represent asymptomatic colonization in renal recipients with indwelling bladder catheters or lower or upper tract infection. Candiduria in a renal transplant recipient can theoretically lead to ascending infection with involvement of the ureteral anastomosis, so a clinical bias to treat even asymptomatic candiduria in the recent renal recipient is rational. Therapeutic options include fluconazole, caspofungin, or amphotericin B bladder irrigation.

Deep-seated candidiasis can manifest with persistent fever or cryptogenic sepsis in patients who are receiving antibacterial therapy or have other risk factors for candidiasis. Isolation of *Candida* from one or more blood cultures should always be considered to represent a true pathogen. Candidemia may represent a catheter-related infection or a manifestation of deep tissue-invasive candidiasis. The absence of candidemia does not exclude the latter, however, because no more than 30% of patients with tissue-invasive candidiasis have documented candidemia. In the renal transplant recipient, candidemia can lead to metastatic infection at the renal vascular anastomosis or in the renal parenchyma itself. Other signs of dissemination include eye pain, red eye, photophobia, and visual loss, which might signify *Candida* endophthalmitis; skin lesions; and spread to the bones or joints. Such signs are indicative of hematogenous dissemination and the requirement for a longer, more aggressive course of antifungal treatment.

Involvement of the renal vascular anastomosis or renal allograft parenchyma usually requires allograft nephrectomy, cessation of immunosuppression, and a prolonged course of treatment with either a polyene (amphotericin B or a lipid formulation of amphotericin B) or a chitin-synthetase inhibitor (caspofungin, micafungin, anidulafungin). *Candida*-directed antifungal prophylaxis (usually fluconazole) is often prescribed for high-risk patients (i.e., those with prolonged broad-spectrum antibiotics, high levels of immunosuppression, or technical allograft complications requiring surgery) during the first several months after transplantation.

Aspergillus infections are acquired by airborne transmission of spores to the sinuses or respiratory tract, and outbreaks have been reported among patients in proximity to hospital construction sites. The most common species are *Aspergillus fumigatus*, *Aspergillus flavus*, and *Aspergillus terreus*. The lungs are the most common initial site of infection, which may manifest as solitary or multiple nodules or cavitary lesions, pulmonary infarction due to vascular invasion, and intrapulmonary hemorrhage. Hematogenous dissemination to organs with high blood flow, particularly the middle cerebral artery territory of the brain, vertebral bodies, and other viscera, can result in dissemination, which carries a very high mortality rate.

Voriconazole, with or without a second active agent (caspofungin, lipid amphotericin B), has emerged as the first-line treatment for aspergillosis, coupled with withdrawal of immunosuppression and occasionally with surgical resection of isolated lung or brain lesions.

Other, less common mycelial fungi of clinical importance include those causing zygomycosis (*Mucor, Rhizomucor*), *Pseudallescheria boydii*, dematiaceous (pigmented molds), *Fusarium*, and others.

Cryptococcus neoformans is a ubiquitous encapsulated yeast found in the soil, in pigeon feces, and in the skin of some fresh fruits and vegetables. Although the main portal of entry is the respiratory tract, *Cryptococcus* pneumonia is rare. More commonly, hematogenous spread to the central nervous system with seeding of the leptomeninges can lead to subacute or chronic meningitis. Diagnosis requires the detection of *Cryptococcus* in the cerebrospinal fluid by India ink staining, identification of cryptococcal antigen by latex agglutination, or culture. Treatment requires combination therapy with amphotericin B or lipid formulation amphotericin B and 5-flucytosine.

Based on taxonomic evidence, *P. jiroveci* (formerly called *Pneumocystis carinii*) has been reclassified as a fungus rather than a protozoan. This pathogen can cause interstitial pneumonia occurring relatively late after transplantation, although its incidence has been drastically reduced due to the uniform use of TMP-SMX or other chemoprophylactic agents. Symptoms include fever, dyspnea, and nonproductive cough. A chest radiograph reveals the presence of interstitial infiltrates. Silver or Giemsa staining of BAL fluid can establish the diagnosis

in more than 90% of cases, and lung biopsy is rarely needed. Therapy consists of intravenous TMP-SMX (dosage adjusted according to kidney function) or, in case of sulfa hypersensitivity, pentamidine or dapsone. *P. jiroveci* pneumonia, like most other severe infections, requires reduction or temporary cessation of immunosuppression. *P. jiroveci* infection can be prevented with the use of TMP-SMX (80 mg and 400 mg, respectively) daily for 6 to 12 months. Alternatively, oral dapsone (100 mg/day), oral atovaquone, or aerosolized pentamidine (300 mg monthly) can be used in TMP-SMX–intolerant individuals, although breakthrough cases of *Pneumocystis* have been observed more frequently with these alternative regimens.

The endemic mycoses should be considered in enigmatic pulmonary, cutaneous, or complex disseminated presentations in patients who were (or are) native to one of the geographic areas where the prevalence of such fungi is more common: Ohio and Mississippi River valleys (histoplasmosis), southwestern United States (coccidioidomycosis), and southeastern United States (blastomycosis).

PREVENTION OF INFECTION

The major chemoprophylaxis strategies to reduce the incidence of infection in the renal transplant recipient are summarized in Table 304-2. It should be emphasized that there may be significant variance pertaining to the specific agent, duration of therapy, and patient selection criteria across transplant centers. The most common vaccination strategies include the polyvalent pneumococcal vaccine (Pneumovax), seasonal influenza immunization, and hepatitis B vaccination programs. Passive immunoprophylaxis has been employed with hyperimmune CMV globulin (Cytogam) for seronegative recipients at high risk for CMV and EBV infection and disease.

Key Points

1. A typical temporal pattern exists for some infections during the post-transplantation period.
2. The risk for specific opportunistic pathogens is the product of the patient's epidemiological exposure and net immunosuppressive state.
3. Urinary tract infection is the most common bacterial infection; however, its incidence can be reduced substantially with antibiotic prophylaxis.
4. Cytomegalovirus is the most frequent post-transplantation pathogen and can cause tissue-invasive infection, graft rejection and dysfunction, and opportunistic infection.
5. Preemptive and prophylactic antiviral strategies are both efficacious approaches to reduce the clinical impact of cytomegalovirus infection and disease in high- and moderate-risk patients.
6. Candidiasis is the most common fungal pathogen; it arises as a result of technical complications, heavy immunosuppression, and the presence of invasive catheters.

Key References

2. Fishman JA, Rubin RH: Infection in organ-transplant recipients. N Engl J Med 1998;338:1741-1751.

11. Kalil AC, Levitsky J, Lyden E, et al: Meta-analysis: The efficacy of strategies to prevent organ disease by cytomegalovirus in solid organ transplant recipients. Ann Intern Med 2005;143:870-880.

14. Hodson EM, Jones CA, Webster AC, et al: Antiviral medications to prevent cytomegalovirus disease and early death in recipients of solid-organ transplants: A systematic review of randomised controlled trials. Lancet 2005;365:2105-2115.

20. Smith JM, Rudser K, Gillen D, et al: Risk of lymphoma after renal transplantation varies with time: An analysis of the United States Renal Data System. Transplantation 2006; 81:175.

23. Hirsch HH, Brennan DC, Drachenberg CB, et al: Polyomavirus-associated nephropathy in renal transplantation: Interdisciplinary analyses and recommendations. Transplantation 2005;79:1277-1286.

See the companion Expert Consult website for the complete reference list.

Special Kidney Problems in the Intensive Care Unit

CHAPTER 305

Management of Patients with Diabetes in the Intensive Care Unit

Monica Beaulieu and Adeera Levin

OBJECTIVES

This chapter will:
1. Describe the epidemiology of diabetic kidney disease and the burden of illness in the intensive care unit (ICU) setting.
2. Illustrate the spectrum of renal disease observed in patients with diabetes in the ICU.
3. Describe the metabolic abnormalities observed in patients with diabetes in the ICU.
4. Review the risks and benefits of intensive glycemic control in the ICU.
5. Recommend treatment strategies for patients with diabetes in the ICU.

WHAT IS KNOWN AND WHAT IS NOT KNOWN

Despite recognition of diabetes mellitus (DM) as a risk factor for acute kidney injury (AKI), the inclusion of DM in stratifying patients within large databases is not consistent. In reviewing several recent papers describing the *R*isk of renal failure, *I*njury to the kidney, *F*ailure of kidney function, *L*oss of kidney function, and *E*nd-stage renal failure (RIFLE) and Acute Physiology And Chronic Health Evaluation (APACHE) scores and the use of new biomarkers for AKI, we were surprised to find that DM was not overtly identified in the demographics of any of the published studies.[1-4] Nonetheless, in other studies, DM is a well-recognized risk factor for AKI, and the coexistence of DM in the critical care population raises unique management challenges for clinicians. This chapter reviews key issues related to the incidence, prevalence, and care of patients with diabetes in critical care settings.

EPIDEMIOLOGY AND BURDEN OF ILLNESS

The worldwide prevalence of diabetes for all age groups was estimated to be 2.8% in 2000, comprising 171 million people. There is an international epidemic of diabetes, with a predicted doubling to 4.4% of the population by 2030.[5] The United States will have more than 30 million affected persons, but the most significant increases are expected to occur in the Middle East, sub-Saharan Africa, and India. This high prevalence and increasing incidence is important in that these patients are at high risk for AKI in a multitude of settings.

Patients with diabetes frequently require hospital admission for both diabetic and nondiabetic complications. Despite focus on optimal diabetic management, there is ongoing evidence that complications including myocardial infarction, congestive heart failure, stroke, peripheral vascular disease, AKI, and infections will continue to increase.[5] Diabetics with evidence of kidney disease (proteinuria, abnormal kidney function) are at greater risk of AKI than those without renal involvement. Retinopathy, neuropathy, coronary disease, and peripheral vascular disease are more prevalent in patients with nephropathy.[6] Patients with diabetes may require intensive care, most commonly for treatment of conditions other than diabetes. Once hospitalized, diabetic patients have a longer duration of stay than nondiabetics.[7,8] Therefore, efficient and effective treatment for these patients is increasingly important from both a patient outcome and a cost perspective.

DIABETIC KIDNEY DISEASE: KIDNEYS AT RISK

Diabetic nephropathy is common in both type 1 and type 2 DM. In type 1 diabetes, earlier literature reported a 16% chance of developing end-stage renal disease within 30 years after the initial diagnosis.[9,10] Historically, type 2 diabetics were believed to have a better renal prognosis, but recent epidemiological studies have suggested that the renal risk of a patient with type 2 DM is similar to that of a type 1 diabetic.[11] Type 2 diabetes, which is 10 to 15 times more common than type 1, is the leading cause of end stage renal disease in the Western world.[12,13]

Hyperfiltration: Missing Those at Risk

The initial stages of diabetic nephropathy are characterized by hyperfiltration and renal hypertrophy. Glomerular filtration rates (GFRs) during these stages may be 25% to 50% greater than normal. This hyperfiltration may be more pronounced in type 1 diabetics, with GFRs often exceeding 150 mL/min; the appearance of supranormal GFR (or very low creatinine values) should raise suspicion of hyperfiltration. Patients who develop glomerular hyperfiltration appear to be at increased risk for progressive diabetic renal disease.[14] Because many patients present to the intensive care unit (ICU) in these stages of diabetic renal disease, clinicians must be vigilant, recognizing that, for many diabetics, a normal creatinine or GFR may represent hyperfiltration or early kidney disease. Corroboration with urinalysis (presence of proteinuria) and previous laboratory tests is recommended.

Given the impaired kidney autoregulation, the often overwhelming burden of illness, and the susceptibility to damage, the current literature suggests that strict glycemic and blood pressure control, as well as minimizing nephrotoxin exposure, are key strategies to reduce AKI in acute settings.

Acute Kidney Injury

The prevention of AKI in critically ill patients is crucial, because renal failure in the ICU setting has repeatedly been identified as an independent predictor of mortality.[15,16] Patients with diabetes are at increased risk of AKI in the ICU due to several factors, including extracellular fluid volume contraction, diabetic ketoacidosis, nonketotic hyperosmolar coma, other kidney diseases, papillary necrosis, and obstruction. In addition, many of these patients are taking angiotensin-converting enzyme (ACE) inhibitors or angiotensin II receptor blockers before their ICU admission, which may be a factor in their AKI.

Patients with diabetes who are nephrotic, and therefore extracellular fluid volume contracted, are at increased risk of prerenal insults and acute tubular necrosis. Acute diabetic complications such as diabetic ketoacidosis and nonketotic hyperosmolar coma, which are characterized by profound extracellular fluid volume contraction and absolute or relative insulin lack, can lead to AKI. Patients with diabetic nephropathy are also at increased risk of contrast-induced nephropathy because of a number of factors, most of which were listed earlier. Cholesterol embolization should also be considered in a patient with AKI, because many patients with diabetes also have a significant atherosclerotic burden.

In the case of acute changes in kidney function in a patient with diabetes, nondiabetic glomerular diseases must also be considered. Clinical findings of hematuria, changes in proteinuria, and blood pressure control have been described in patients with a nondiabetic primary glomerular disease and have been well documented in diabetic patients. Membranous nephropathy has generally been considered the most commonly associated nephropathy.[17] If there is an acute deterioration in renal function, a rapidly progressing glomerulonephritis should be considered. Nondiabetic glomerular disease should be considered in the diabetic patient with AKI if the patient has a short duration of diabetes, no previous documented proteinuria, no retinopathy, red blood cells on urinalysis, and rapidly deteriorating renal function.

Urinary Tract Infections

Urinary tract infections are more common in patients with diabetes, especially those infections caused by gram-negative organisms; many of these infections are documented in the absence of symptoms.[18] Complications such as acute pyelonephritis with associated perinephric abscesses and emphysematous pyelonephritis are also more common in diabetics. Renal papillary necrosis, caused by low flow states and ischemia-induced sloughing of the papilla, is also common in long-standing diabetes and is described in the setting of urinary tract infection or infection more commonly.[19] Although early treatment of urinary tract infections has decreased this complication, it should still be considered in the diabetic patient with rapidly progressing acute renal failure.

Progressive Diabetic Renal Disease

Patients with diabetes may have progression of their underlying kidney disease during their hospitalization. Alternatively, an episode of AKI superimposed on preexisting chronic kidney disease can leave patients with further reduced kidney function when they leave the ICU or hospital. It is increasingly recognized that minimizing AKI in these patients is important to reduce the long-term morbidity related to the accelerated progression of chronic kidney disease, which can be exacerbated by episodic AKI.

Metabolic Acidosis

Patients with diabetes in the ICU often present with or develop metabolic acidosis, which may be related to the acute illness requiring ICU admission (e.g., lactic acidosis secondary to decreased perfusion) or, on occasion, may be more readily attributable to diabetes itself. Causes related directly to the diabetic state include preexisting renal tubular acidosis (RTA), an acute deterioration of diabetic control, and a drug-induced disorder such as metformin ingestion.

Drug-Induced Acidosis (Biguanides)

Oral hypoglycemic treatment with metformin (and previously phenformin) has been associated with the development of type B lactic acidosis in a subgroup of patients.[20,21] Risk factors including impaired kidney function (serum creatinine >132 μmol/L), liver disease, congestive heart failure, and excessive alcohol consumption have been reported. Importantly, most cases occur in the context of rapid change in kidney function, without concomitant adjustment of this renally excreted medication. Patients taking metformin who develop a severe illness requiring

ICU admission (e.g., shock), in combination with abrupt reductions of kidney function, are at even greater risk of developing severe lactic acidosis.

Metformin is associated with lactic acidosis because of interference with pyruvate dehydrogenase function and subsequent decrease in lactate consumption. In patients with rapid reduction of kidney function, reduced excretion and subsequent increase in serum lactate levels cause the acidosis, which can be profound. A recent Cochrane database systematic review evaluated all prospective and observational cohort studies from 1966 to August 2005 that evaluated type 2 diabetics treated with metformin compared with another hypoglycemic agent or placebo.[22] This review of 206 trials, representing 47,846 patient-years of metformin use, documented no cases of fatal or nonfatal lactic acidosis. In addition, no difference in lactate levels was found in groups treated with metformin versus non-metformin. The authors concluded that, under study conditions, metformin is not associated with an increased risk of lactic acidosis compared with other antihyperglycemic treatments. Nonetheless, it is the risk of AKI that more likely predicts the risk of metformin-induced metabolic acidosis, not the use of the drug per se.

Although not causative, the permissive impact of metformin use on diabetic outcomes raises a number of questions. The number of diabetics treated with metformin continues to rise, and many patients may still be prescribed metformin despite reduced kidney function.[23] Cases of patients with profound lactic acidosis related to metformin use continue to be reported.[24]

Treatment of metformin-associated lactic acidosis includes supportive therapy and hemodialysis, if necessary. Both conventional intermittent hemodialysis and continuous venovenous hemodiafiltration (CVVHDF) have been used with success.[24,25]

Unique Problems: Type 4 Renal Tubular Acidosis

A subset of patients with diabetes have an underlying type 4 RTA (hyporeninemic hypoaldosteronism) characterized by hyperkalemia and baseline low bicarbonate (average, approximately 18 mEq/L). The causes of this RTA are multifactorial but include interstitial fibrosis associated with progressive decline in kidney function. A few diabetics with normal kidney function also have this RTA.[26] Diabetics with this underlying disorder may present with a mixed disorder of a more profound acidosis that could be explained on clinical circumstances alone. However, an intercurrent illness requiring ICU admission may unmask or even exacerbate the disorder. It is important to recognize this preexisting disorder (chronic metabolic acidosis, compensated), because it may affect a patient's response to therapy for these electrolyte abnormalities, and it may change treatment strategies.

Mixed Disorders

In addition to preexisting RTA and metformin-induced lactic acidosis, diabetic patients may be acidotic for a number of other reasons. Diabetic ketoacidosis is a common cause of severe anion-gap acidosis, often requiring ICU admission for correction of the severe volume depletion and metabolic abnormalities that accompany the lack of insulin. It should be remembered that a moderate degree of lactic acidosis, in addition to the recognized ketoacidosis, is also observed in some patients,[27,28] potentially due to the severe hypovolemia.

TREATMENT

General Principles

The general principles of managing diabetes in the ICU include maintenance of normoglycemia and correction of other metabolic abnormalities. In addition, to minimize the risk of AKI, prompt recognition of diabetics who have or are at risk of having diabetic kidney disease is also important. Over-reliance on the serum creatinine concentration is problematic because of the issues mentioned earlier regarding hyperfiltration, and the utility of a urinalysis should be emphasized in the evaluation of these patients.

Avoidance of nephrotoxins (e.g., aminoglycosides), nonsteroidal anti-inflammatory drugs, and other drugs in the ICU and use of intravenous contrast only if no alternatives are available and with appropriate renal protection are important measures to reduce the incidence and subsequent morbidity of diabetic AKI.

Glycemic Control in Acute Care Settings

Patients with acute illness often present with hyperglycemia and insulin resistance. This is observed even in patients without preexisting diabetes.[29] Factors responsible for this hyperglycemia include increased levels of stress hormones and pro-inflammatory cytokines.[30] Adverse effects of hyperglycemia include but are not limited to fluid and electrolyte shifts, decreased wound healing, immune dysfunction, and endothelial dysfunction.[31] Recent evidence has highlighted the benefits of strict glycemic control in critically ill patients[32,33] and after acute myocardial infarction.[34] In a randomized trial of 1548 patients in a surgical ICU, tight glucose control with an insulin infusion (target glucose concentration, 4.4 to 6.1 mmol/L) resulted in a 42% lower mortality rate (4.6% versus 8%; $P < .04$) than standard care (intravenous insulin only if glucose levels exceed 11.8 mmol/L).[32] Notably, the intensive treatment arm also required significantly less dialysis. This study protocol was recently repeated in a medical ICU.[33] In-hospital mortality in this study was not different between the groups as a whole, but for the prespecified group of patients who remained in the ICU for longer than 3 days, a decrease in mortality was observed in the intensive treatment group (43% versus 52.5%). Morbidity was also decreased in the intensive treatment group, including improved renal status and a reduced duration of mechanical ventilation.

A major challenge of intensive management is the risk of hypoglycemia, the symptoms and signs of which may be masked in the critically ill. In both of the trials just mentioned, hypoglycemia (<2.2 mmol/L) was increased in the intensive treatment group. The short- and long-term consequences of hypoglycemia in the ICU have not been described. Although tight glycemic control is important, attempts must be made to minimize hypoglycemic events and to correct hypoglycemia promptly if it occurs.

Although most studies of strict glycemic control in critically ill patients have suggested improved outcomes, including better kidney outcomes, several questions remain unanswered. Specifically, the exact glycemic target and the patient population most likely to benefit remain unknown. Ongoing trials are expected to help answer these questions.[35]

As general recommendations, hyperglycemia in the critical care setting should be treated, although the exact target blood glucose level remains unknown. Intravenous insulin infusions are preferred to subcutaneous injections in the critical care setting. If a patient required insulin before admission, then a basal level of insulin must be maintained, especially if the patient is prone to ketosis. Every attempt must be made to avoid hypoglycemia. Once a patient leaves the ICU, follow-up of glycemic control is important, especially if the patient was not previously known to be diabetic.

CONCLUSION

The incidence and prevalence of DM continues to increase worldwide, and the number of patients who have diabetic kidney disease, or who are at risk for severe illness that may precipitate AKI, will also continue to rise. Patients with diabetes often require hospital admission, and a subset require critical care for both diabetic complications (diabetic ketoacidosis and hyperosmolar coma) and, more commonly, nondiabetic cardiac, vascular, and infectious conditions. Many diabetic patients are at increased risk of AKI, for a number of reasons—including under-recognition of the problem due to an over-reliance on the serum creatinine measurement and no review of urinalyses, hypovolemia due to osmotic diuresis, and diarrhea.

Early identification of at-risk individuals, avoidance of nephrotoxins, and prompt treatment are crucial to attenuate the increase in both short- and long-term morbidity and mortality associated with AKI in the ICU. Future studies of AKI should always include diabetes in their stratification systems, given the importance and uniqueness of this group of patients.

Key Points

1. The incidence and prevalence of diabetes mellitus is rising.
2. Diabetic nephropathy remains a leading cause of end-stage renal disease. Diabetic patients often require critical care admission for both diabetic and nondiabetic complications.
3. Diabetic patients are at substantial risk of acute kidney injury in the intensive care unit, and avoidance of nephrotoxins should be stressed in this population.
4. Metabolic acidosis is common in diabetics. Specific causes include preexisting renal tubular acidosis, drug-induced disorders, and decompensated diabetes.
5. Intensive insulin therapy to treat hyperglycemia has resulted in decreased mortality and morbidity in some groups of patients in the intensive care setting.

Key References

2. Hoste EAJ, Clermont G, Kersten A, et al: RIFLE criteria for AKI are associated with hospital mortality in critically ill patients: A cohort analysis. Critical Care 2006;10:R73.
30. Schetz M, Van den Berghe G: Glucose control in the critically ill. In Ronco C, Bellomo R, Brendolan A (eds): Sepsis, Kidney and Multiple Organ Dysfunction. Contrib Nephrol 2004;144:119-131.
32. Van den Berghe G, Wouters P, Weekers F, et al: Intensive insulin therapy in critically ill patients. N Engl J Med 2001;345:1359-1367.
33. Van den Berghe G, Wilmer A, Hermans G, et al: Intensive insulin therapy in the medical ICU. N Engl J Med 2006;354:449-461.

See the companion Expert Consult website for the complete reference list.

CHAPTER 306

Acute Renal Failure in the Elderly Critically Ill Patient

Monica Bonello, Dimitris Petras, Zaccaria Ricci, Nereo Zamperetti, and Claudio Ronco

OBJECTIVES

This chapter will:
1. Define the epidemiology and pathogenesis of acute renal failure and multiple-organ failure in the elderly critically ill patient.
2. Describe renal replacement therapy and multiple-organ support therapy in the elderly critically ill patient.
3. Analyze bioethical problems regarding the elderly in intensive care.

Acute renal failure (ARF) affects 5% to 7% of all hospitalized patients[1-3] and continues to be associated with poor outcome.[4-10] This syndrome is common in the intensive care unit (ICU), with a reported incidence of 1% to 25%,[11,12] depending on the population being studied and the criteria used to define its presence. Uncomplicated ARF can usually be managed outside the ICU setting and carries a good prognosis, with mortality rates ranging from 5% to 10%.[13] In contrast, ARF complicating nonrenal organ system failure in the ICU setting is associated with a mortality rate of 50% to 70%, which has remained relatively constant over the last decades.[14-19] Furthermore, evidence exists that ARF is a specific, independent risk factor for poor prognosis in the critically ill patient.[20]

It is well known that a substantial proportion of patients admitted to the ICU are older than 65 years of age, and a particular discipline has arisen within critical care medicine for critical care of the elderly patient. This new discipline now deals with the unprecedented spectrum of clinical problems associated with the profound physiological derangements of critical illness and advanced age. Patients who would previously have died before they could develop ARF are now surviving longer, and older patients, who are more susceptible to ARF, are making up an increasing percentage of the ICU population. Older people are also more likely to develop dysfunction of individual organ systems and therefore are more at risk for multiple-organ dysfunction syndrome (MODS).

The same pathophysiological factors involved in the development of ARF are also incriminated in the failure of other organs, so that ARF is generally part of the MODS.[19] It is evident that patients with ARF as part of MODS have the highest mortality rate. Additionally, critically ill patients, and especially elderly critically ill patients, are affected by variously combined causes and risk factors for ARF, including all conditions that reduce the effective circulating volume.

This chapter discusses the epidemiology, pathogenesis, treatment, and bioethical problems of the management of ARF and MODS in the elderly critically ill patient.

EPIDEMIOLOGY OF ACUTE RENAL FAILURE AND MULTIPLE-ORGAN DYSFUNCTION SYNDROME IN THE ELDERLY

Elderly patients are frequently admitted to ICUs, and an increasing proportion of patients in ICUs are older than 65 years of age. Of the 17,440 patients in medical and surgical ICUs from 40 institutions in the United States, the proportion of patients older than 65 years of age was 48%; 25% were between 65 and 74 years, 17.2% were 75 to 84 years, and 5.3% were older than 85 years of age.[21]

Hospital survival for elderly patients ranges from 60% to 85%, depending on the type of ICU and enrollment criteria.[22-24] Most studies reviewed indicated that survival for patients older than 65 years was significantly lower than for younger patients, and some suggested that age is a risk factor for death due to critical illness.

The incidence of acute respiratory failure, a diagnosis that almost uniformly requires ICU admission, increases almost exponentially with age. According to a cohort drawn from 904 hospitals in the United States, the incidence of acute respiratory failure in the 65- to 84-year age group was almost twice that of the 55- to 64-year age group and more than three times that of younger age groups.[25]

Acute lung injury and acute respiratory distress syndrome (ARDS) are more severe forms of respiratory failure that carry a higher overall burden of illness for patients. Two studies suggested that age is an important factor in survival from these conditions.[26,27]

In a large study to determine whether provision of less aggressive care is a factor in the higher short-term mortality for seriously ill elderly patients, the investigators in the Study to Understand Prognoses and Preferences for Outcomes and Risks of Treatments (SUPPORT) examined sur-

vival over a period of 180 days for 9105 patients who were enrolled in the study.[28] Patients in the five participating institutions were enrolled based on having one of nine serious diagnoses and an expected 6-month mortality risk of 50% or less. Adjusting for sex, ethnicity, income, baseline functional status, severity of illness, and aggressiveness of care, each additional year of age increased the hazard of death by 1.0% for patients 18 to 70 years of age and by 2.0% for patients older than 70 years of age. For SUPPORT patients with average severity of illness and treatment intensity, estimates of age-specific 6-month mortality rates were 44%, 48%, 53%, and 60% for patients aged 55, 65, 75, and 85 years, respectively. It should be noted, however, that the severity of acute physiological abnormalities and diagnoses were much stronger contributors to prognosis than age.

Age is a well-known risk factor in trauma patients, as well. Preexisting medical conditions in older age and impaired age-dependent physiological reserve contributing to a worse outcome in elderly patients with multiple injuries are hypothesized as reasons for increased mortality. A recent retrospective clinical study[29] of a statewide trauma dataset from 1993 through 2000 included 5375 patients with an Injury Severity Score (ISS) greater than 16 who were stratified by age. Mortality in this series increased beginning from age 56 years, and that increase was independent of the ISS. The mortality rate among patients with an ISS between 16 and 24 increased from 7.3% for those 46 to 55 years of age to 13.0% for those aged 56 to 65 years; in these same age groups, mortality increased from 23.8% to 32.1% among those with an ISS between 25 and 50, and from 62.2% to 82.1% in those with an ISS between 51 and 75 ($P < .05$). Severe traumatic brain injury was the most frequent cause of death, with a significant peak in patients older than 75 years.

ARF usually appears as a consequence in patients with ARDS, sepsis, or trauma and is associated with a high mortality rate, especially in elderly patients. Furthermore, ARF is a specific independent risk factor for prognosis in critically ill patients.[20]

PATHOGENESIS OF ACUTE RENAL FAILURE AND MULTIPLE-ORGAN DYSFUNCTION SYNDROME IN THE ELDERLY

Although the pathogenesis of ARF and MODS is the same in elderly and in younger patients, it seems that the elderly are more susceptible to develop these conditions. There are no controlled, randomized trials to support this hypothesis but only indirect data. One fact is that, despite improvements in dialytic technology, there has been no effective change in the high mortality rates associated with ARF. The change in the population of patients seems to be the main possible explanation. Additionally, critically ill patients, and especially elderly critically ill patients, are affected by variously combined causes and risk factors for ARF, including all conditions that reduce effective circulating volume and lead to decreased mean arterial pressure and renal perfusion pressure. These conditions include hypovolemia, hypotension, hypoxia, sepsis,[30] rhabdomyolysis,[31] diabetes mellitus, positive-pressure ventilation, and exposure to nephrotoxins, in addition to preexisting renal, hepatic, or cardiac dysfunction. In the perioperative setting, ARF risk factors include prolonged aortic clamping,[32] emergency rather than elective surgery, use of higher volumes (>100 mL) of intravenous contrast media, and raised intra-abdominal pressure.

Over the last 3 decades, several experimental models have identified pathophysiological mechanisms associated with ARF and enhanced understanding of the disease.[33-35] It is evident that ARF can result from alterations in renal perfusion, glomerular filtration, and tubular function and that correction of these factors can ameliorate the effects of ARF.[36,37] It is well known that these three systems are impaired in elderly patients and that ischemic injury can occur more easily. Elderly patients usually have reduced renal blood flow, and autoregulation of the glomerular filtration rate may be lost, leading to hypoxia in the cortex and the medulla in the early onset of MODS. Furthermore, the same pathophysiological factors involved in the development of ARF are also incriminated in the failure of other organs, so that ARF is generally part of the MODS.[19]

Elderly patients are more susceptible to inflammation because their immune system is inadequate, atherosclerotic lesions are present, and glucose metabolism is impaired. Therefore, they are more susceptible to oxidative stress-mediated apoptosis. There are also existing data indicating that cells in elderly people are more vulnerable to apoptosis.

Despite great improvements in the field of the pathophysiology, the mechanisms that are involved in the development of ARF and MODS are still not known, but it is clear that elderly, critically ill patients are more susceptible than younger patients to development of ARF and MODS.

RENAL REPLACEMENT THERAPY IN ACUTE RENAL FAILURE AND MULTIPLE-ORGAN DYSFUNCTION SYNDROME

Renal replacement therapy (RRT) has evolved from the concept of treating the dysfunction of a single organ (the kidney). As ICUs have become more and more complex, it has become clear that the majority of patients, especially the older ones, who have ARF also have dysfunction of several other organs. To facilitate single-organ support in this setting, continuous renal replacement therapy (CRRT) techniques have been developed. The proper goal of extracorporeal blood purification in the ICU should be multiple-organ support therapy (MOST). MOST represents the most logical future conceptual and practical evolution of CRRT: Its biological rationale is provided by animal and clinical evidence that confirms the need to move rapidly in this direction theoretically, practically, and technologically. CRRT techniques and MOST are described in detail in other chapters of this book.

The number of failing organs other than the kidney is significant in elderly, critically ill patients because of preexisting injuries due to atherosclerotic lesions, impaired glucose metabolism, and other conditions associated with increased age. A clinically sensitive approach should try to broaden the spectrum of physiological end points targeted by extracorporeal therapy and should attempt to reduce the number of dysfunctional organs, degree of severity, loss of homeostasis, and, ultimately, effect on outcome. Because the severity of the physiological disorder (score) in the first 24 hours after admission to the ICU "drives" prognosis at hospital discharge, early and adequate correction of disorders is critical for outcome. The adequacy of any artificial organ support is, therefore, measured by how closely it mimics the flexibility, versatility, and efficacy of the organ system it seeks to replace or support.

POTENTIAL USES OF MULTIPLE-ORGAN SUPPORT THERAPY

Kidneys

Extracorporeal therapies have traditionally been employed to replace lost renal function in ARF, and this is the most common use of CRRT in the ICU. In the last 20 years, evidence has accumulated to support the concept that CRRT is efficient, safe, and well tolerated even in older patients.[38]

Temperature

With the extracorporeal fluxes used for continuous venovenous hemofiltration and hemodialysis (CVVH and CVVHD, respectively), a negative thermal balance of up to –100 kJ/hr can be obtained, depending on the length of the blood lines, the room temperature, and the dialysate or replacement fluid temperature. This cooling effect might contribute to modulation of the inflammatory response as well as oxygen demand in several organs, with the possibility of using such a mechanism for specific clinical targets.

Acid-Base and Electrolyte Balance

Most imbalances of sodium and other electrolytes can be corrected by increasing or restricting free water intake; other electrolyte imbalances can be medically corrected. When disorders are life-threatening or refractory to medical corrections, extracorporeal therapy is the treatment of choice. The advantage of such therapy in comparison to the use of diuretics is the possibility of dissociating the removal of water from that of sodium or other electrolytes. Because of the slow and gentle rate of fluid exchange, the treated blood operates in continuous equilibrium with peripheral tissues and organs, and the entire organism may benefit from a rapid and effective restoration of water, sodium, and electrolyte homeostasis. This benefit of restoration of homeostasis is particularly true for acid-base control (because the administration of bicarbonate can be easily titrated to the necessary acid-base goals), for intracellular/extracellular potassium and phosphate equilibrium, and for water fluxes between the interstitium and the intracellular space. It is especially important in elderly, critically ill patients in whom blood flow is impaired due to atheromatosis.

Heart

Cardiac support can be achieved by optimization of fluid balance, reduction of organ edema, and restoration of desirable levels of preload and afterload. Furthermore, the continuity of the extracorporeal therapy allows re-markable cardiovascular stability, with maintenance of hemodynamic parameters including mean arterial pressure, heart rate, and systemic vascular resistance. Such stability, which is achieved through slow, continuous ultrafiltration and continuous refilling of the intravascular volume from the interstitium, allows stability of circulating blood volume and preservation of organ perfusion. Such stability is essential in elderly patients, who usually have preexisting cardiac dysfunction and in whom even small reductions of mean arterial pressure can be fatal.

Brain

Cerebral edema is a consequence of rapid solute movement during intermittent hemodialysis.[39] The advent of CRRT has eliminated this risk. The accumulation of uremic toxins from inadequate blood purification is a known cause of encephalopathy. This is not the case during the use of CRRT in the ICU. It is well known that a degree of encephalopathy often preexists in elderly patients, so that worsening of this condition can produce serious damage in the brain. The development of hypotension can induce brain injury. As pointed out earlier, the use of CRRT, with its associated hemodynamic stability, has decreased this risk. The accumulation of amino acid derivatives may be responsible for the encephalopathy of sepsis. By removing such excessive soluble derivatives and decreasing imbalances between amino acids, CRRT may also have an effect on the encephalopathy of sepsis. Acidemia induces changes in the function of cerebral enzymes involved in glucose utilization and may be responsible for changes in conscious state.[40] The correction of acidemia by CRRT might be another way of protecting the brain from injury. Therefore, a significant degree of brain protection is provided by CRRT.

Liver

The general principles for use of a blood purification system for liver support are the same as for other organs, but it must be kept in mind that liver function in the elderly has a greater chance of becoming impaired due to preexisting factors, mainly drugs that elderly patients usually receive.

Sepsis and Septic Shock

High-volume hemofiltration and plasmafiltration coupled with adsorption and followed by dialysis or filtration (coupled plasmafiltration-adsorption, or CPFA)[41] is beneficial in elderly critically ill patients, who are more susceptible to infection and sepsis due to impaired reaction of their immune system.

MULTIPLE-ORGAN DYSFUNCTION SYNDROME IN THE ELDERLY: BIOETHICAL PROBLEMS

Caring for elderly patients with MODS can pose important bioethical questions, which must be carefully addressed and correctly managed. The most important features of the situation can be summarized as follows:

1. The pathological insult is very severe by definition, and the prognosis is usually worsened by coexisting chronic pathologies (e.g., diabetes, hypertension, chronic obstructive pulmonary disease) and multiple-organ subclinical derangements.
2. Very elderly patients can already be beyond the physiological limits of life expectancy and near the natural end of their life.

3. Finally, the overall standard of care needed by these patients can be extremely burdensome, long, and painful, as well as very expensive.

The consequent core question is, How intensive and prolonged should the care be for an elderly patient with MODS? Do existing published data help clinicians make a correct decision?

Published data are too heterogeneous to draw easy conclusions. This happens because of the great variability among patients. Actually, biology and biography very seldom coincide, and a chronological age of 75 years can have totally different meanings in two patients with different biological status. Coexisting diseases can make differences even more relevant.

A good policy would be to plan a timely course of treatment for every patient, involving the patient and his or her relatives as soon as possible in the decision-making process. Ideally, every patient should be admitted to the ICU with a clear plan of action in which the patient's wishes, attitudes, and moral/religious beliefs are clarified and the intended therapeutic goal is specified. In this way, it is possible give the right sense to every intended intervention and to make sound decisions even in case of unexpected or unplanned situations. Of course, as clinical conditions change, the therapeutic goal can be updated, but it should always be clear, well-known, and shared by everyone involved in the patient's care. Unfortunately, all of this happens very rarely in the real world, even though decisions have to be made daily.

For a correct decision, at least three key factors are relevant:

1. *The clinical data:* The diagnosis and the prognosis should be ascertained as reasonably as possible. A decision based on wrong or incomplete data is both clinically and morally questionable.
2. *The patient:* The person's wishes concerning the intensity of care should be clarified, hopefully before starting intensive care. If competence is questionable, advance directives (when available) can help. In case of refusal of possibly meaningful nonfutile care, the patient's position should be carefully evaluated and weighed against the patient's view of life and moral and religious beliefs (as witnessed by the patient's relatives and friends), in order to assess its acceptability and to do what the patient really wishes to be done.
3. *The environment:* The presence and the position of a caring and loving family is usually a key factor in making a correct decision. Indeed, the patient's relatives can play a fundamental role in the decision-making process, supporting the conscious patient or helping clinicians to assess the wishes of an unconscious one. After the at least partial failure of large and expensive trials as the SUPPORT study, the La Crosse experience deserves great attention.[42] Two of the most important features of this prehospital, community-based study were that the focus of end-of-life decision making was on facilitating discussion about values and preferences, not completion of documents, and that such a discussion was refocused away from autonomy toward family relationships.[43]

In practice, the best decision is the one that best promotes the patient's dignity, keeping in mind that excellence in ICU care is measured by the quality of ICU survivals and of ICU deaths as well. Obviously, the patient's position, as to the definition of an acceptable level of care and of (residual) life, is mandatory.[44]

Whatever the final decision, every patient has the right to be protected against pain and any form of physical and psychological suffering.

Key Points

1. The number of older people admitted to intensive care units is increasing.
2. Survival of older patients is significantly lower than for younger patients.
3. Older patients are more susceptible to acute renal failure.
4. Acute renal failure is a specific independent risk factor for prognosis in critically ill patients.
5. The pathogenesis of acute renal failure and multiple-organ dysfunction syndrome is the same in elderly as in younger patients.
6. Renal replacement therapy has evolved from the concept of treating the dysfunction of a single organ—the kidney.
7. The proper goal of extracorporeal blood purification in the intensive care unit should be multiple-organ support.
8. Elderly critically ill patients are affected by variously combined causes and risk factors for acute renal failure.
9. Very elderly patients may already be beyond the physiological limits of life expectancy.
10. The patient's dignity must be considered.
11. Every patient has the right to be protected against pain and any form of physical and psychological suffering.

See the companion Expert Consult website for the complete reference list.

CHAPTER 307

Anticancer Drugs and the Kidney

Ilya G. Glezerman and Richard Amerling

OBJECTIVES

This chapter will:
1. Characterize major nephrotoxic chemotherapy agents and their effects on kidney function and electrolyte homeostasis.
2. Describe strategies aimed at preventing and alleviating chemotherapy-induced acute renal failure.
3. Provide guidelines for administration of chemotherapeutic agents to patients undergoing renal replacement therapy.

The kidneys are the major elimination pathway for many chemotherapeutic agents and are vulnerable to the toxic effects of chemotherapy. Antineoplastic agents are known to cause acute and chronic renal failure as well as a variety of electrolyte abnormalities. Dose, patient characteristics, and coadministration of other nephrotoxins determine the degree of renal impairment. In addition to direct nephrotoxicity, cancer therapy may cause tumor lysis syndrome and neutropenia, leading to sepsis and acute renal failure; these topics are covered elsewhere in this text (see Chapters 80, 183).

CISPLATIN

Cisplatin, a platinum-based compound, is widely used as first-line chemotherapy for a variety of solid tumors. After intravenous administration, more than 90% of cisplatin is protein-bound, and only 10% to 40% is eliminated by the kidneys in the first 24 hours via glomerular filtration and tubular secretion.[1] Cisplatin antineoplastic effects are mediated by intrastrand DNA cross-linking and inhibition of DNA replication. Its active metabolites can cause mitochondrial damage, cell cycle arrest, inhibition of adenosine triphosphatase activity, alterations of cellular transport, and, ultimately, apoptosis or necrosis and cell death. These mechanisms are responsible for the nephrotoxic effects of cisplatin. The S3 segment of the proximal tubule in the corticomedullary region is the most common site of cisplatin nephrotoxicity in rats. More distal sites may also be affected in humans while glomeruli remain un-affected. Cisplatin can cause ototoxicity, neurotoxicity, and bone marrow suppression, but nephrotoxicity is the major dose-limiting side effect of this drug.[2,3]

Cisplatin causes decreases in renal function in a dose-dependent fashion. Single doses smaller than 50 mg/m^2 rarely cause clinically significant ARF. Acute nonoliguric renal failure occurs with higher doses, usually 3 to 5 days after exposure, and is associated with minimal proteinuria (<0.5 g/day). Function usually returns to baseline within 2 to 4 weeks, although recovery may be delayed for several months.[4] Chronic renal failure may also develop after prolonged exposure, particularly with total doses exceeding 850 mg, but few patients progress to end-stage renal disease.[5] Cisplatin has been linked to hemolytic uremic syndrome (HUS) when administered as a single agent or in combination with bleomycin and vinblastine. Signs of HUS, such as azotemia, elevated lactate dehydrogenase (LDH), anemia, schistocytosis, and thrombocytopenia usually occur 1 to 4 months after exposure.[6]

Several electrolyte abnormalities have been described with cisplatin. Renal salt wasting may result in significant morbidity, including severe hyponatremia, orthostatic hypotension, mental status changes, and prerenal azotemia. This syndrome usually develops 2 to 4 months after cisplatin is started. Salt wasting nephropathy is treated with vigorous hydration with normal saline and oral sodium supplementation where feasible.[7,8] Several authors also report hyponatremia as a consequence of the syndrome of inappropriate secretion of antidiuretic hormone (SIADH), which usually occurs after a few days of therapy. Postchemotherapy nausea may also contribute to high levels of antidiuretic hormone. Hypertonic saline, restriction of free water, and loop diuretics have been used to treat patients with cisplatin-induced hyponatremia.[9,10] Selective vasopressin receptor inhibitors have been used successfully to treat hyponatremia due to SIADH[11]; however, no data exist for treatment of the cisplatin-induced disorder.

Magnesium wasting is present in almost all patients treated with multiple courses of cisplatin. Cisplatin impairs magnesium reabsorption in the ascending limb of the loop of Henle and in distal tubules, resulting in hypermagnesuria despite low serum magnesium concentrations. Hypomagnesemia may also be exacerbated by coadministration of aminoglycosides, amphotericin, loop diuretics, foscarnet, and other drugs. Cisplatin-induced hypomagnesemia may persist for up to 6 years. Both hypokalemia and hypocalcemia have been described in patients with cisplatin-induced hypomagnesemia. The former is believed to be caused by proximal tubular injury leading to increased distal delivery of sodium, potassium, and water, which results in enhanced potassium secretion. The latter is caused by direct inhibition of parathyroid hormone (PTH) secretion as well as end-organ PTH resistance. Vigorous oral magnesium supplementation is needed to overcome cisplatin-induced magnesium wasting.[12]

Various strategies have been employed for prophylaxis of cisplatin-induced ARF. The most effective to date is solute diuresis induced by normal saline and mannitol infusion, which is initiated 12 to 24 hours before drug administration and titrated to achieve at least 125 mL/hr of urine output. Cisplatin is then infused in isotonic saline over 3 hours, followed by another 24 hours of normal saline infusion. Cisplatin is given in divided doses over 5 days, with a cumulative dose of less than 120 mg/m^2. Higher doses cause an unacceptable incidence and degree of nephrotoxicity.[3,6]

Amifostine, an inorganic thiophosphate, is renoprotective, most likely via a free radical scavenging mechanism and intracellular binding of the drug. Amifostine is selectively taken up by normal tissue and does not diminish the anticancer effect of cisplatin.[2] Recent reports suggest that inhibition of intracellular pro-apoptotic pathways in tubular cells protects against cisplatin-induced injury.[3] In mice, granulocyte colony-stimulating factor administered before cisplatin exposure blunted renal injury and accelerated renal recovery.[13]

Carboplatin is another platinum-containing antineoplastic agent. Its dose-limiting toxicity is myelosuppression, with the maximum tolerated dose being 1200 mg/m^2. Higher doses (up to 2.1 g/m^2) require stem cell transplant rescue and may lead to nephrotoxicity. High-dose carboplatin–induced renal toxicity is a transient but frequent complication that occasionally requires renal replacement therapy, although irreversible renal failure is infrequent.[6]

METHOTREXATE

Methotrexate (MTX) is a folic acid antagonist antimetabolite that is used for treatment of many malignancies, including acute lymphocytic leukemia, lymphoma, osteosarcoma, breast, and head and neck carcinomas. When given at doses that exceed 1 g/m^2, MTX has a tendency to precipitate in the renal tubules, especially in the setting of an acidic pH. This may lead to crystal-induced nonoliguric, nonproteinuric renal failure 1 to 2 days after initial exposure. Because MTX is excreted by the kidney, renal failure leads to toxic MTX blood levels. The accumulation of MTX places patients at risk for prolonged myelosuppression, severe mucositis, and hepatitis. Vigorous intravenous saline and, if necessary, loop diuretics are administered to maintain high urine flow during infusion and afterward, until nontoxic levels of MTX (<0.1 µmol/L) are achieved. Sodium bicarbonate is infused concomitantly to alkalinize the urine and inhibit crystal formation.[14] When appropriate preventive measures are employed, MTX-induced ARF is relatively rare. Only 1.8% of patients treated with high-dose MTX for osteosarcoma develop grade 2 or greater nephrotoxicity. However, once ARF develops, the mortality rate is 4.4%.[15]

Because ARF is usually self-limited and resolves in a mean of 12 days (standard deviation, ±7 days),[16] the goal of therapy is to prevent extrarenal MTX toxicity. Diuresis and urinary alkalinization are maintained to facilitate MTX renal excretion. Intravenous leucovorin is given at doses ranging from 100 to 1000 mg/m^2 every 3 to 6 hours, depending on the MTX level, and until such level is below the toxic threshold.[14] Leucovorin is converted in vivo into folinic acid, which bypasses the enzymatic step inhibited by MTX, thereby minimizing extrarenal toxicity. Recently, the cloned enzyme carboxipeptidase-G$_2$ was shown to selectively hydrolyze MTX to inactive metabolites and to lower MTX levels by a median of 97% (range, 73% to 99%) within 15 minutes after administration.[17] Hemodialysis, high-flux hemodialysis, charcoal-based hemoperfusion, and hemofiltration have also been used to remove MTX in patients with ARF. High-flux hemodialysis appears to be most effective, with a median MTX reduction ratio of 75.5% (range, 42% to 94%). All modalities exhibited significant postprocedure rebound.[15] Patients who develop MTX renal toxicity can be successfully rechallenged once renal failure resolves.[18]

GEMCITABINE

Gemcitabine is a nucleoside analogue with antineoplastic activity against a variety of solid tumors, including pancreatic, non–small cell lung, bladder, ovarian, and breast carcinomas. The primary toxicity of gemcitabine is myelosuppression and liver function abnormalities. HUS is a well-described complication with an incidence of 0.31%. The presentation is subacute, with insidious onset of renal dysfunction, hemolytic anemia, hypertension, and thrombocytopenia. Left unrecognized, progression to fulminant acute renal failure and hypertensive crisis can occur.[19,20] A report of 29 patients with gemcitabine-induced HUS treated at a single institution is instructive. Gemcitabine was discontinued in all patients as soon as HUS was recognized. Patients were treated with supportive therapy and hemodialysis when indicated. Nineteen patients achieved full or partial renal recovery, seven progressed to end-stage renal disease, and three developed chronic renal failure but did not require dialysis.[21]

MITOMYCIN C

Mitomycin C is used as salvage therapy for many solid malignancies. It is an alkylating agent isolated from *Streptomyces caespitosus*. In addition to pulmonary and bone marrow toxicity, mitomycin C is associated with HUS at total cumulative doses greater than 40 to 60 mg/m². HUS usually occurs within 4 to 8 weeks after the last dose and carries a poor prognosis; most patients die within 4 months due to renal or pulmonary failure or from progression of cancer.[22]

IFOSFAMIDE

Ifosfamide is an alkylating agent that is a nitrogen mustard analogue. Its active metabolite, acrolein, is toxic to urinary epithelium and causes hemorrhagic cystitis. Ifosfamide also has significant renal toxicity, with proximal tubular damage resulting in Fanconi's syndrome with urinary phosphorus and potassium wasting, non–anion gap metabolic acidosis (proximal renal tubular acidosis), glycosuria at normal serum glucose levels, and aminoaciduria. Distal tubular defects may also be present, causing nephrogenic diabetes insipidus and distal tubular acidosis.[23,24] Acute as well as chronic renal failure has been reported.[25]

Moderate to severe nephrotoxicity occurs in 18% to 28% of patients treated with ifosfamide. Risk factors for the development of renal dysfunction include prior or concurrent cisplatin administration, unilateral nephrectomy, and cumulative dose of the drug greater than 60 to 72 g/m².[24] A safe dose limit has not been established, and doses as low as 6 g/m² given over 2 days have been reported to be toxic.[26] Age younger than 5 years has also been reported as a risk factor, but recent reports indicate that adults may be equally susceptible to ifosfamide renal toxicity.[24,27]

Saline infusion has been used for prevention of ifosfamide nephrotoxicity and hemorrhagic cystitis. Mesna compound (2-mercaptoethane sulfonic acid) given orally or intravenously is converted into active metabolites that bind acrolein and prevent the development of hemorrhagic cystitis; they are ineffective against renal toxicity.[28]

CYCLOPHOSPHAMIDE

Cyclophosphamide is another nitrogen mustard analogue known to cause hemorrhagic cystitis, but, unlike ifosfamide, has not been reported to cause nephrotoxicity. Cyclophosphamide can cause SIADH which develops within hours after administration of the drug and resolves in 24 to 48 hours. Conservative management with fluid restriction is usually adequate in patients without neurological signs or symptoms. A fatal outcome has been reported.[29-31]

BISPHOSPHONATES

Pamidronate and zoledronic acid are intravenous bisphosphonates used in oncology for treatment of hypercalcemia of malignancy and lytic metastatic bone lesions. Both drugs are renally excreted unchanged and have been associated with significant nephrotoxicity. Acute tubular necrosis has been reported with both agents.[32,33] Pamidronate also has been linked to focal segmental glomerulosclerosis with nephrotic syndrome and renal failure.[34] In clinical trials, between 9% and 15% of the patients who received zoledronic acid developed renal dysfunction manifested by elevated serum creatinine levels. Of patients who developed ARF, 25% had received only a single dose of the drug.

Risk factors for nephrotoxicity include advanced cancer, previous exposure to bisphosphonates, use of nonsteroidal anti-inflammatory drugs, and duration and dose of the infusion.[35,36] Careful monitoring of renal function in patients treated with intravenous bisphosphonates is mandatory. According to the manufacturers, pamidronate should not be given to patients with a serum creatinine concentration of 3 mg/dL or greater, and zoledronic acid should be avoided in patients with a creatinine clearance of 30 mL/min or less. Treatment should be discontinued if renal function deteriorates. Patients may be rechallenged with the drug once renal function returns to within 10% of baseline.[37]

BEVACIZUMAB

Targeted and biological therapies are increasingly being used in the treatment of cancer. They offer potential for low systemic toxicity and improved patient outcome. Bevacizumab is a humanized monoclonal antibody directed against vascular growth factor. In clinical trials, it has been associated with increased incidence of hypertension and proteinuria. Careful monitoring of blood pressure and proteinuria is necessary. Hypertension generally can be managed with standard oral antihypertensive therapy, although the drug should be discontinued in patients who develop a hypertensive crisis. Similarly, proteinuria is usually mild, but nephrotic syndrome has been reported and should prompt discontinuation of therapy.[38]

CANCER CHEMOTHERAPY AND DIALYSIS

Well over 300,000 patients are undergoing chronic hemodialysis in the United States, and this number is expected to increase. Currently, 6% of patients initiating hemodialysis carry a concurrent diagnosis of cancer. Furthermore, patients with chronic kidney disease have an increased incidence of cancer.[39] Table 307-1, adapted from Tomita and colleagues,[40] provides recommendations for administration of chemotherapy to a growing population of dialysis patients with cancer. As noted earlier, bisphosphonates are commonly used in cancer patients. Pamidronate, at a dose of 30 mg daily on 3 consecutive days, was used safely in a patient undergoing hemodialysis for treatment of hypercalcemia of malignancy.[41] Table 307-2 summarizes recommendations for chemotherapy dose adjustments in

TABLE 307-1

Recommendations for Dosage Adjustment of Antineoplastic Drugs in Patients Receiving Hemodialysis

DRUG	RECOMMENDATION AND COMMENTS
Paclitaxel	Pharmacokinetics are not altered by HD in anephric patients; use the same dose schedule as in patients with normal renal function.
Cisplatin	Reduce dose by 50% and carry out HD immediately after administration.
Carboplatin	A delay of 16 hr is recommended between drug administration and initiation of HD. Dosage should be determined based on the AUC-directed method.*
Etoposide	Poorly dialyzable; 40% of the dose is renally excreted. Reduce dose by 60% in HD patients.
Fluorouracil	Metabolized by liver and other tissues; no dose adjustment is required.
Methotrexate	Rate of elimination is increased during dialysis, but high drug levels persist for several days; prolonged rescue with folinic acid is recommended.
Cyclophosphamide	HD should not be initiated earlier than 12 hr after infusion, preventing drug removal in the early distribution phase but still correcting for the prolonged terminal elimination phase.
Ifosfamide	HD may be helpful if intoxication causes encephalopathy, but ifosfamide should not be used in this patient group.
Antibiotics (mitomycin, dactinomycin)	Because of strong tissue binding and very long plasma half-life (slow excretion in feces and urine), HD is unlikely to be successful.
Anthracyclines (doxorubicin, epirubicin, daunorubicin)	Nondialyzable due to large volume of distribution and long half-life.
Vinca alkaloids (vincristine, vinblastine, vindesine)	Nondialyzable due to large volume of distribution, high metabolic rate, and long half-life.

AUC, area under concentration-time curve; GFR, glomerular filtration rate; HD, hemodialysis.
*Dose determined by Calvert Formula: Dose (mg) = [AUC (mg/mL × min)] × [GFR (mL/min) + 25]. The target AUC is 5-7 mg/mL × min. Assume that GFR = 0 mL/min in HD patients. (See ref. 43.)
Adapted from Tomita M, Aoki Y, Tanaka K: Effect of hemodialysis on pharmacokinetics of antineoplastic drugs. Clin Pharmacokinet 2004;43:515-527.

TABLE 307-2

Adjustment of Dose Based on Glomerular Filtration Rate

DRUG	Glomerular Filtration Rate (mL/min)		
	30-60	10-30	<10
Bleomycin	50	Omit	Omit
Carboplatin	*	*	*
Cisplatin	50	Omit	Omit
Cyclophosphamide	NC	NC	50
Cytosine arabinose	50	Omit	Omit
Dacarbazine	75	50	Omit
Etoposide	NC	NC	50
Fludarabine	75	50	Omit
Hydroxyurea	75	75	50
Ifosfamide	75	50	Omit
Melphalan (IV)	75	75	50
Methotrexate	50	Omit	Omit
Mithramycin	75	50	Omit
Mitomycin	75	50	Omit
Nitrosoureas	Omit	Omit	Omit
Pentostatin	50	Omit	Omit
Topotecan	75	50	Omit

NC, no change.
*Dose determined by Calvert Formula: Dose (mg) = [AUC (mg/mL × min)] × [GFR (mL/min) + 25]. The target AUC is 5-7 mg/mL × min. (See ref. 43.)

patients with stage III to stage V chronic kidney disease who do not yet require renal replacement therapy. These recommendations are based on direct toxicity or percentage of renal clearance.[42]

Despite the progress made in recent decades, nephrotoxicity of antineoplastic agents continues to be a signifi-

cant clinical challenge in the treatment of cancer. Appropriate prophylactic measures, dose adjustments, and early recognition of toxicity can significantly reduce renal morbidity and permit more effective treatment of the underlying neoplasm.

Key Points

1. The kidneys are the major pathway for elimination of chemotherapy agents and are vulnerable to direct toxicity.
2. Acute renal failure and electrolyte abnormalities are major side effects of many chemotherapeutic agents.
3. Hemolytic uremic syndrome is an unusual complication of certain anticancer agents.
4. Novel targeted cancer therapies present new challenges in management of renal complications of anticancer drugs.
5. Careful dose adjustment and avoidance of certain chemotherapies is necessary when treating patients with advanced stages of chronic kidney disease.

Key References

1. Lugones F, Leblanc M: Acute renal failure in cancer patients. In Cohen E (ed): Cancer and the Kidney. Oxford, Oxford University Press, 2005, pp 55-91.
4. Flombaum C: Nephrotoxicity of chemotherapy agents and chemotherapy administration in patients with renal isease. In Cohen E (ed): Cancer and the Kidney. Oxford, Oxford University Press, 2005, pp 127-167.

6. Kintzel P: Anticancer drug-induced kidney disorders. Drug Safety 2001;24:19-38.
40. Tomita M, Aoki Y, Tanaka K: Effect of hemodialysis on pharmacokinetics of antineoplastic drugs. Clin Pharmacokinet 2004;43:515-527.

42. Patterson W, Reams G: Renal and electrolyte abnormalities due to chemotherapy. In Perry M (ed): Chemotherapy Source Book. Philadelphia, Lippincott Williams & Wilkins, 2001.

See the companion Expert Consult website for the complete reference list.

CHAPTER 308

Anti-inflammatory Drugs and the Kidney

Andrew A. House and Claudio Ronco

OBJECTIVES

This chapter will:
1. Identify the mechanisms of renal damage induced by nonsteroidal anti-inflammatory drugs (NSAIDs) and coxibs.
2. Describe the incidence and epidemiology of NSAID-induced acute kidney injury.
3. Describe the risk factors for NSAID-induced acute vasomotor renal injury and NSAID-induced nephrotoxicity.

Nonsteroidal anti-inflammatory drugs (NSAIDs) are widely prescribed in clinical practice. NSAIDs, including the more selective inhibitors of cyclooxygenase 2 (coxibs), are potentially nephrotoxic and can have significant side effects, including salt and water retention, acute tubular necrosis, acute interstitial nephritis, proteinuria, hyperkalemia, and various degrees of renal damage evolving into chronic kidney disease (CKD).[1] Although the potential for these side effects is relatively low, the widespread use of these drugs and the availability of some without prescription make the incidence of complications frequent.[2] Among the various clinical complications, the effects on the kidney are probably the most common and severe. It has been reported that 37% of drug-associated acute renal failure (ARF) is associated with the use of NSAIDs, and NSAID-induced ARF accounts for 7% of overall cases of ARF.[3]

There is an increased risk of developing renal damage in patients who regularly consume NSAIDs. This risk increases with advanced age and other comorbidities. Age-related changes in renal function predispose to nephrotoxicity, especially when there is a decreased glomerular filtration rate (GFR), decreased renal blood flow, and increased renal vascular resistance, dehydration, or impaired liver function. In addition, with age and comorbidity the pharmacokinetics of NSAIDs may be affected. In all these conditions, the risk for renal dysfunction is further enhanced by the presence of sepsis, multiple organ dysfunction, and critical illness in general. In a recent analysis of a large general practice database in the United Kingdom, current users of NSAIDs faced a relative risk of ARF of 3.2 (95% confidence interval [CI], 1.8 to 5.8). This risk increased with comorbid illness, and in particular it rose dramatically, to 11.6 (95% CI, 4.2 to 32.2), when concomitant diuretics were being taken.[4] At the moment of admission to the hospital or intensive care unit, careful attention must be paid to completely understand the medical history of the patient and his or her pharmacological history, especially in relation to the consumption of prescription or nonprescription NSAIDs.[5]

MECHANISMS OF RENAL DAMAGE INDUCED BY NONSTEROIDAL ANTI-INFLAMMATORY DRUGS

Acute kidney injury (AKI) is a well-described complication of NSAID use. There are two main mechanisms of renal damage induced by NSAIDs: One is hemodynamically mediated, and the other is derived from a direct toxicity of the drugs on the renal parenchyma.

Hemodynamically Mediated Acute Kidney Injury

AKI can result from an alteration of intrarenal microcirculation (and, consequently, of glomerular filtration) caused by inhibition or blockage of endogenous prostanoids, particularly in those conditions in which kidney microperfusion and function are highly dependent on their augmented serum concentration.[4] NSAID-induced AKI is not common, but it may occur with increased incidence in patients at risk. Risk factors for this disorder include volume and salt depletion, advanced age, renal insufficiency, liver dysfunction, diabetes, and congestive heart failure.[6,7] In these patients, side effects involving the kidney can occur both with classic nonselective NSAIDs, and also with coxibs.[8] The explanation for the increased incidence of AKI in volume-depleted patients is based on the fact that under euvolemic conditions there is typically very little synthesis of prostaglandins, so intrarenal circulation is not dependent on these substances for maintenance of GFR.

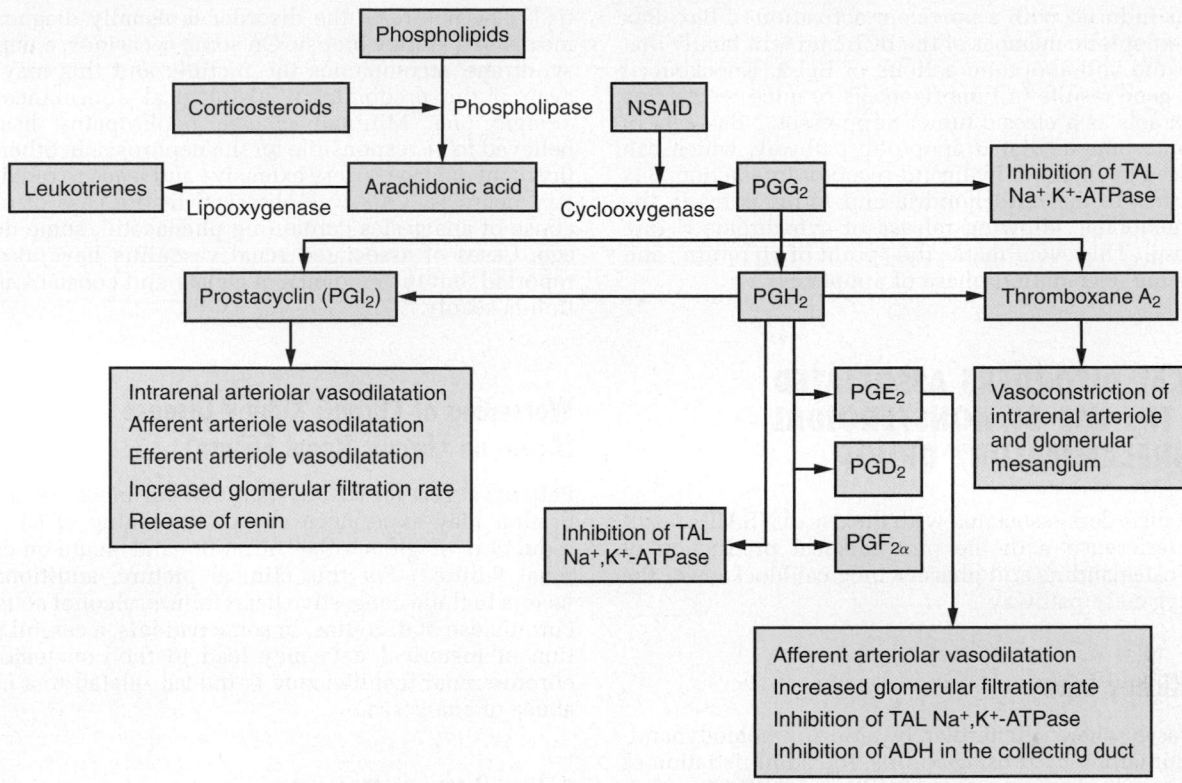

FIGURE 308-1. Arachidonic acid pathway and site of action of nonsteroidal anti-inflammatory drugs (NSAID). ADH, antidiuretic hormone; Na+,K+-ATPase, sodium-potassium adenosine triphosphatase; PG, prostaglandin; TAL, thick ascending limb of Henle.

In turn, the inhibition of prostaglandin synthesis by NSAIDs very seldom affects renal circulation and function. On the contrary, in volume-depleted and hemodynamically unstable patients, prostaglandin synthesis is enhanced, significantly mitigating the vasoconstriction induced by angiotensin II and the effects of vasopressin on the collecting tubular epithelium.[9] The consequence of inhibiting endogenous prostaglandin synthesis with NSAIDs is removal of this counterbalancing force, which leads to increased vascular tone with significant antidiuresis and antinatriuresis. A complete overview of the arachidonic acid metabolic pathways and the roles of the various metabolites in renal function is presented in Figure 308-1.

Kidneys produce a mixture of autacoids with vasodilating action (prostaglandin E2 [PGE2], PGI2) and vasoconstricting action (PGF2α, thromboxane A2). Such substances contribute to the regulation of intrarenal blood flow, tubular sodium handling, tubular water transport, and renin release. In Figure 308-1, the actions of these metabolites of arachidonic acid are described. A delicate feedback system leads to hemodynamically mediated activation of prostaglandin secretion in response to the vasoconstriction induced by angiotensin II, endothelin, catecholamines, leukotrienes, and vasopressin. Furthermore, in patients with underlying ischemic or inflammatory renal injury (e.g., sepsis), the consumption of NSAIDs may produce a catastrophic event mediated not only by a blockage of vasodilatory prostaglandin production but also by a nonenzymatic stimulation of vasoconstrictor metabolites in a setting in which free oxygen radical production is enhanced.[10]

Nephrotoxic Acute Kidney Injury

Interstitial nephritis can occur in association with NSAIDs due to allergic reaction, direct cellular toxicity, alteration of metabolic pathways, and possibly obstruction. These complex and multifactorial mechanisms may also combine with hemodynamic perturbations. In some cases, the damage becomes extensive, leading to papillary necrosis. The use of NSAIDs is often associated with worsening of mild to moderate CKD, with significant reduction of GFR and evolution of CKD toward more advanced stages.[11] Direct toxicity to the tubules is manifested by loss of polarity, loss of tight junctions, loss of cell substrate adhesion, exfoliation of viable cells from the tubular basement membrane, and aberrant renal cell-cell adhesion. Further damage may lead to altered gene expression, cellular dedifferentiation, and lethal injury such as necrosis or apoptosis.[12] Tubular necrosis is characterized by severe depletion of cellular stores of adenosine triphosphate, reduced activity of membrane transport pumps, cell swelling, increase in intracellular free calcium, activation of phospholipases and proteases, glycine depletion, and plasma and subcellular membrane injury.[13]

Renal parenchymal cells may be triggered to undergo programmed cell death, or apoptosis. Apoptosis is generally characterized by a significant depletion of guanosine triphosphate in the cells and may be activated via the death receptor pathway, in which a combination of physiological activators such as cytokines and the deficiency of renal growth factors may jointly activate the pre-caspase 8 or the activation caspase pathway.[14] In the cell injury pathway, an altered equilibrium in the BCL2 protein family is induced with a prevalent activation of Bax. Bax is a pro-apoptotic member of the BCL2 protein family that inhibits the anti-apoptotic actions of Bcl-2. Knockout of the Bax gene results in tumorigenesis in mice, suggesting that Bax acts as a classic tumor suppressor.[15] Bax acts in the apoptosome-mediated apoptotic pathway, which can be induced by injury or by ligand-receptor interaction. Bax translocates to the mitochondria and forms pores in the outer membrane, allowing release of cytochrome C into the cytosol. This event marks the "point of no return" and leads to the degradation phase of apoptosis.[16]

CLINICAL DISORDERS ASSOCIATED WITH THE USE OF NONSTEROIDAL ANTI-INFLAMMATORY DRUGS

Clinical disorders associated with the use of NSAIDs result from interference with the physiological production of renal prostaglandins and pharmacological blockade of the cyclooxygenase pathway.

Acute Kidney Injury

In all cases where glomerular filtration is hemodynamically maintained by prostaglandins, the administration of NSAIDs can lead to reduction of GFR and ARF. The clinical picture begins typically with a functional and reversible disorder characterized by avid sodium and water retention, and renal function often improves simply on stopping the drug. In some cases, however, the disorder evolves into frank parenchymal damage with overt renal failure. Elderly patients and those with comorbid conditions seem to be at increased risk for renal side effects of NSAIDs due to predisposing concomitant factors (Table 308-1).[6,7]

Acute Interstitial Nephritis

In several cases, ARF caused by NSAID administration has been found to be associated with acute interstitial nephri-

TABLE 308-1

Risk Factors for NSAID-Induced Renal Side Effects in the Elderly Population

Age-related Changes in Renal Function
Decreased renal functional reserve
Decreased glomerular filtration rate
Decreased total renal blood flow
Increased renal vascular resistance
Diabetes Mellitus
Altered Pharmacokinetics
Increased free drug concentration
Dehydration
Reduced drug distribution volume
Hypoalbuminemia
Decreased elimination of the drug via alternative pathways
Interaction with Other Drugs
Diuretics
ACE inhibitors
Beta Blockers

ACE, angiotensin-converting enzyme; NSAID, nonsteroidal anti-inflammatory drug.

tis.[17] The nature of the disorder is usually diagnosed by means of a kidney biopsy. On some occasions, a nephrotic syndrome accompanies the picture, and this may occur even if the predominant histological appearance is an allergic one. Minimal change nephropathy has been believed to be responsible for the nephrosis. In other cases, the renal damage is very extensive and leads to renal papillary necrosis. This was observed in the case of chronic abuse of analgesics containing phenacetin, some decades ago. Cases of associated renal vasculitis have also been reported, but the evidence of a clear and constant association is scanty.[18]

Worsening of Chronic Kidney Disease (Acute on Chronic Renal Failure)

Patients at risk for AKI by virtue of advanced age or dehydration may experience abrupt worsening of CKD with reduction of glomerular filtration and acute-on-chronic renal failure.[19] For this clinical picture, additional risk factors include congestive heart failure, alcohol abuse, and chronic use of diuretics. In some patients, a careful collection of historical data may lead to the conclusion that chronic renal insufficiency is indeed related to a chronic abuse of analgesics.

Salt and Water Retention

Sodium retention is the most common renal side effect associated with NSAID therapy. The syndrome is clearly related to inhibition of the potent natriuretic and diuretic effects induced by prostaglandins, especially in those conditions in which high renin activity is present.[20]

Hypertension

New onset or worsening hypertension is a frequent complication of NSAID use, and it occurs in patients in whom sodium and water retention has upset the delicate hemodynamic equilibrium. Furthermore, inhibition of the counterbalancing mechanisms involved in systemic vascular relaxation may be invoked as a triggering mechanism.[21]

Hyperkalemia

In patients with diabetes mellitus or CKD or both, hyperkalemia may develop after administration of NSAIDs. A further aggravating factor may be simultaneous consumption of potassium-sparing diuretics, angiotensin-converting enzyme inhibitors or angiotensin receptor blockers, and beta blockers. In these circumstances, hyperkalemia may be accompanied by a mild metabolic acidosis and a deterioration in renal function.[22]

CONCLUSION

Selective and nonselective NSAIDs (including coxibs) are an important class of drugs that can have significant renal side effects. These unwanted and potentially hazardous clinical effects may be exaggerated by advanced age, preexisting renal conditions, comorbid illnesses, and concomitant use of other drugs such as diuretics or anti-hypertensives. The ubiquitous use of these agents makes it essential to carefully monitor renal function when they are administered to patients at increased risk or for a prolonged period of time.

Key Points

1. Nonsteroidal anti-inflammatory drugs (NSAIDs) and selective cyclooxygenase 2 inhibitors (coxibs) enjoy widespread use in clinical practice, leading to a remarkable frequency of unwanted renal side effects.
2. Most cases of NSAID-induced acute renal failure or acute kidney injury are hemodynamically mediated.
3. Clinical syndromes associated with NSAID use include acute renal failure, acute interstitial nephritis, worsening of chronic kidney disease, salt and water retention, and hypertension.

4. Careful monitoring of renal function is advisable in patients at increased risk, such as elderly individuals, cardiac-compromised patients, and diabetics.

Key References

2. Bennett WM, Henrich WL, Stoff JS: The renal effects of non-steroidal anti-inflammatory drugs: Summary and recommendations. Am J Kidney Dis 1996;28(1 Suppl 1):S56-S62.
6. Gambaro G, Perazella MA: Adverse renal effects of anti-inflammatory agents: Evaluation of selective and nonselective cyclooxygenase inhibitors. J Intern Med 2003;253:643-652.
8. Schneider V, Levesque LE, Zhang B, et al: Association of selective and conventional nonsteroidal antiinflammatory drugs with acute renal failure: A population-based, nested case-control analysis. Am J Epidemiol 2006;164:881-889.
11. Gooch K, Culleton BF, Manns BJ, et al: NSAID use and progression of chronic kidney disease. Am J Med 2007;120: 280.e1-280.e7.
20. Harris RC Jr: Cyclooxygenase-2 inhibition and renal physiology. Am J Cardiol 2002;89(6A):10D-17D.

See the companion Expert Consult website for the complete reference list.

CHAPTER 309

Antibiotics and Antiviral Drugs in the Intensive Care Unit

Rosanna Coppo, Licia Peruzzi, and Alessandro Amore

OBJECTIVES

This chapter will:
1. Point out the clinical conditions in patients in the intensive care unit (ICU) that deserve particular attention in regard to potential antibiotic related kidney toxicity and the choices that can be made to minimize the risk.
2. Report the interactions between antibiotics and other drugs given to critically ill patients in the ICU.
3. Discuss the choice and dosage of antimicrobial drugs in patients in the ICU undergoing continuous replacement therapy.

The patients in the intensive care unit (ICU) often need antibiotic or antifungal drugs, because infectious complications increase the risk of unfavorable outcomes, particularly if renal function is decreased. Such treatments in this setting require careful choices as far as both drug and dosage are concerned.

WHY ATTENTION MUST BE PAID WHEN A PATIENT IN AN ICU NEEDS ANTIBIOTIC OR ANTIFUNGAL THERAPY

The patient in an ICU is always a critically ill subject, often suffering from chain complications superimposed on pre-existing chronic organ dysfunctions. High attention should be paid to detect early renal function impairment and to avoid worsening to overt acute renal failure (ARF).[1] Even a moderate degree of ARF not requiring dialysis increases by fivefold the risk of death, and the need for dialysis dramatically increases the death rate up to 90%.[2,3] Preexisting reduced renal functional reserve,[4] comorbidities (mainly cardiovascular, hepatic, or hematological), diabetes mellitus, and the extremes of age (either advanced or neonatal) provide increased risk.[5] Surgical patients are particularly at risk to develop ARF because of the tissue insult of surgery in association with preexisting comorbidities and sepsis.[6] Other risk factors include hypothermia, hypoxia, unstable hemodynamics, and cardiopulmonary bypass. In these clinical settings so exposed to the risk of ARF, infectious complications are common and dangerous; not infrequently, they are severe and life-threatening. The need for antimicrobial drugs represents an additional risk, because it may favor worsening of an instable borderline renal function into fully expressed ARF, thus limiting the possibilities of successful outcome even if there is successful healing of the primary illness.

Prevention of antibiotic-induced ARF requires knowledge of the clinical setting, as summarized in Table 309-1.

Patient Conditions That Increase the Risk for Acute Renal Failure

When a potentially nephrotoxic drug has to be prescribed, the patient's risk of increased susceptibility to renal damage due to preexisting conditions favoring ARF should be considered. Anesthesia by itself, hypotension, hematological volume loss or overload and heart failure, and peripheral shunting of blood due to vasodilatation from sepsis are the most common situations that may determine a reduction in renal function. The possibility of ARF due to obstructive nephropathy should be considered in gynecological or abdominal oncological surgery. Intrinsic causes (mainly acute tubular necrosis of ischemic or toxic origin) account for approximately 30% of inpatient ARF. Sodium-depleted subjects have increased risk due to impaired renal hemodynamics and activation of the renin-angiotensin system.

Other aspects to be taken into account in choosing an antibiotic for an ICU patient are the blood gas analysis, because acidosis may exacerbate intrarenal crystal deposition, and hypoalbuminemia, which may limit protein binding of the drug, thus increasing the active free drug concentration.[7] Preexisting renal injury and chronic renal damage represent diffuse risk factors for faster and more severe decrements in renal function.

Correct Evaluation of Renal Function

Evaluation of renal function is needed both to indicate developing ARF and because several antimicrobial and antifungal drugs are eliminated through the kidney, and dosage adjustment is needed in case of decreased renal function (Table 309-2). This task is not easy: The creatinine clearance in patients with highly reduced renal function overestimates the glomerular filtration rate (GFR) because of the increased contribution of tubular excretion. Moreover, in the critically ill patient, a wasted muscular mass may determine a lower serum creatinine level, leading to overestimation of GFR.[8] To overcome these problems, several formulas have been produced.

The Cockcroft-Gault formula is used to calculate GFR in adult men[9]:

$$GFR = (140 - Age) \times Body\ weight \div (72 \times sCr)$$

where the unit of GFR is mL/min, Age is given in years, Body weight is in kilograms, and sCr is the serum creatinine concentration (mg/dL). For women, the result is

TABLE 309-1

Effective Measures for Preventing Antibiotic-Induced Acute Renal Failure in a Patient in the Intensive Care Unit Needing Potentially Nephrotoxic Antibiotic or Antifungal Drugs

1. Knowledge of patient's risk factors for acute renal failure
2. Correct evaluation of renal function and early recognition of renal injury
3. Knowledge of risk factors related to antibiotics/antifungals
4. Consideration of alternative therapies for antibiotics with potential nephrotoxicity
5. Appropriate antibiotic dosing adapted to altered kinetics
6. General and specific preventive measures for nephrotoxicity

TABLE 309-2

Pharmacokinetics and Pharmacodynamic Parameters of Antibiotics Used in the Intensive Care Unit

DRUG	PROTEIN BINDING CAPACITY (%)	PRIMARY ROUTE OF ELIMINATION	VOLUME OF DISTRIBUTION (L/kg)	HALF-LIFE WITH NORMAL RENAL FUNCTION (hr)	TIME- OR CONCENTRATION-DEPENDENT KILLING	TARGET TROUGH LEVEL (mg/L)
Acyclovir	15	Renal	0.6	2-4	Time	NA
Aztreonam	56	Renal	0.2	1.7-2.9	Time	8
Ceftazidime	21	Renal	0.23	1.6	Time	8
Ceftriaxone	90	Hepatic	0.15	8	Time	8
Ciprofloxacin	40	Renal	1.8	4.1	Concentration	1
Clavulanic acid	30	Hepatic	0.3	1	Not assessed	NA
Fluconazole	12	Renal	0.65	30	Time	8-16
Imipenem	20	Renal	0.23	1	Time	4
Levofloxacin	24-38	Renal	1.09	7-8	Concentration	2
Linezolid	31	Hepatic	0.6	4.8-5.4	Time	4
Meropenem	2	Renal	0.25	1	Time	4
Piperacillin	16	Renal	0.18	1	Time	16
Tazobactam	20-23	Renal	0.8-0.33	1	Not assessed	4
Vancomycin	55	Renal	0.7	6	Time	10
Voriconazole	58	Hepatic	4.6	12	Time	0.5

NA, not available.

multiplied by 0.85. A second widely used formula is that of Schwarz, which calculates GFR in children[10]:

$$GFR = 0.55 \times Body\ length \div sCr$$

where body length is given in centimeters.

However, in particular settings, the GFR values obtained through these calculations may be overestimated. In patients older than 65 years of age who have a reduced body mass, who are obese, or who are diabetic, both creatinine clearance and the Cockcroft-Gault formula may overestimate GFR. In these cases, the Modification of Diet in Renal Disease (MDRD) formula may better represent GFR[11]:

$$GFR = 186 \times sCr^{-1.154} \times Age^{-0.203}$$

for an adult man; this value is multiplied by 0.742 for a female patient and by 1.210 for a male or female African-American patient.

In obese patients, none of the available formulas is completely satisfactory. Estimation based on the cystatin C value, if available, may overcome this problem.[12]

Risk Factors Related to Use of Antibiotics

Antibacterial, antifungal, and antiviral drugs possess an intrinsic nephrotoxic potential, which is mostly dose dependent for drugs inducing crystal deposition and for drugs that act directly on tubular cells or on intrarenal hemodynamics. Prolonged duration of treatment increases the nephrotoxicity of aminoglycosides and amphotericin. Once-daily dosing is effective and actually less toxic than multiple daily doses, because several drugs have a proximal tubule saturable uptake.[13,14]

The rate of administration is important for drugs that cause crystal-induced nephropathy. Amphotericin infusion over 45 minutes did not induce more nephrotoxicity than an infusion over 4 hours, and a continuous infusion appeared to be safer than a 4-hour infusion. The nephrotoxicity of amphotericin B is related to renal vasoconstriction and direct tubular damage by deoxycholate, which is used as a solubilizing agent. Several randomized clinical studies have shown decreased nephrotoxicity with lipid formulations of amphotericin. There is level I evidence that the risk of nephrotoxicity is lower with liposomal amphotericin than with amphotericin lipid complex.[15-18]

Specific drug combinations may result in synergistic nephrotoxicity, such as certain cephalosporins and aminoglycosides, the combination of vancomycin and aminoglycosides, or the combination of cephalosporin and acyclovir (see later discussion).

Alternative Therapies for Drugs with Potential Nephrotoxicity

The simplest way to prevent drug-induced ARF is not to administer potentially nephrotoxic drugs. When aminoglycosides are appropriate, empirical therapy in patients with sepsis is increasingly being questioned. Other antifungal drugs belonging to the classes of azoles (voriconazole) or echinocandins (caspofungin, micafungin) have been shown to be equally effective or even superior to amphotericin in certain indications and potentially less toxic.[19-21] Concerning the potential nephrotoxicity of vancomycin, at this time there is not any strong evidence to avoid it based only on this reason.

Appropriate Drug Dosing Adapted to Altered Kinetics

The key pharmacokinetic principles include clearance, volume of distribution, half-life, and protein binding. The alterations of pharmacokinetics induced by organ failure and critical illness must be considered and are particularly important for drugs with a small volume of distribution or high protein binding or both. For example, the extracellular fluid space is the volume of distribution of aminoglycosides and includes edema, ascites, and effusion fluids.[22-24] A standard per-kilogram loading dose would be inadequate in patients with these conditions, so the amount of excess extracellular fluid should be estimated and the dose increased accordingly. Alternatively, extracellular volume depletion reduces the aminoglycoside volume of distribution, and a standard per-kilogram loading dose would be excessive. This may explain the increased incidence of aminoglycoside nephrotoxicity in obese patients, who have a reduced fraction of total body weight that is extracellular water. In addition to the nature of the infection (location, medical versus surgical therapy, life-threatening versus less serious), the suspected organism and its minimum inhibitory concentration (MIC) should be considered. For example, *Pseudomonas* has an MIC for gentamicin or tobramycin that is usually less than 2 mg/L. If a ratio of 10 times the MIC is desired for efficient pseudomonal killing, a peak concentration of 10 to 20 mg/L will be required.

The ideal body weight (IBW) in kilograms can be calculated from the height (H) in inches or centimeters, as follows:

$$IBW\ male = 50 + 2.3(H_{inches} - 60) = 0.9(H_{cm}) - 88$$

$$IBW\ female = 45.5 + 2.3(H_{inches} - 60) = 0.9(H_{cm}) - 97$$

For each kilogram of edema, ascites, or effusion fluid, an additional 20 mg aminoglycoside may be added to the usual dose of 5 to 7 mg/kg.

For aminoglycoside dosing in the morbidly obese, a similar strategy applies: The dosing weight is the IBW plus $0.4 \times$ (Total body weight − IBW). The next dose should occur when the serum concentration is 1 mg/L or less.

The extended dose interval should probably not exceed 48 hours, because of the increased risk of bacterial regrowth. In patients with a low GFR, this interval will be too long; in this setting, one should reassess whether alternative antibiotics would be equally efficacious, because they probably would be less nephrotoxic. Whether therapeutic drug monitoring can reduce the nephrotoxicity of aminoglycosides or vancomycin remains a matter of debate and probably depends on the patient population, with high-risk patients benefiting more.[25] Individualized pharmacokinetic monitoring of aminoglycosides has been shown to be associated with less nephrotoxicity.

Preventive Measures for Nephrotoxicity

In many clinical settings, the need for a nephrotoxic treatment outweighs the risk of causing kidney dysfunction. In these situations, measures are required to prevent or at least minimize drug-induced renal damage. General preventive measures for nephrotoxicity include addressing all the previously mentioned risk factors that can be corrected or modified. Besides correct dosing and reassessment of concomitant medications, ensuring adequate hydration is of utmost importance before the administration of nephrotoxic drugs. The evidence for preventive hydration is mostly from observational studies, but it is questionable whether more rigorous studies will ever be conducted. The importance of hydration has been shown for amphotericin, for foscarnet, and for drugs that cause crystal-induced nephropathy.[26-28] Sodium administration is useful to prevent amphotericin B nephrotoxicity. Intervention on urinary pH with urinary alkalinization may reduce crystal precipitation of some drugs such as sulfadiazine, whereas acidification reduces indinavir precipitation.[29]

INTERACTIONS OF ANTIBIOTIC AND ANTIFUNGAL DRUGS

Patients in intensive care, particularly those who have an underlying chronic kidney disease or carry a grafted kidney, are frequently prescribed a large number of medications, increasing the risk for interactions with antibiotic or antifungal drugs and enhancing their potential nephrotoxicity.[30-32]

Pharmacodynamic interactions include those that result in additive or antagonistic pharmacological effects. They include induction or inhibition of metabolizing enzymes in the liver or other organs involved in drug metabolism, modification of drug-plasma protein binding and gastrointestinal absorption, and competition in active renal secretion. The pharmacodynamic interactions are relatively predictable, because the pharmacology of any given drug is known. The liver plays a major role in performing oxidative reactions, which are the initial step (phase I) in drug biotransformation, mediated by the cytochrome P-450 (CYP) system. These enzymes may be induced or inhibited by other agents, leading to important modifications in the metabolism of the primary drug. In the subsequent phase II reactions, drug metabolites are converted into more water-soluble compounds to be eliminated by the kidneys. CYP may be induced (e.g., by barbiturates) or inhibited (e.g., by cimetidine, fluconazole, erythromycin). The risk of nephrotoxicity of macrolides, cephalosporins, and amphotericin is highly modulated by the contemporary use of other drugs enhancing CYP activity. A noncompetitive enzyme inhibition induced by a second agent can reduce the metabolism of the first drug, favoring higher plasma drug concentrations and a risk for toxicity. In the case of competitive inhibition, the metabolism of both drugs can be reduced, resulting in higher than expected concentrations of each drug.

Drugs may exist in plasma either reversibly bound to plasma proteins or in the free (unbound) state. The primary drug-binding plasma proteins are albumin and α_1-acid glycoprotein. The pharmacological effect is exerted by the free drug component. A competition for plasma protein binding sites may occur, and one drug may displace another that was previously bound to a protein. The result is an increase in the free form of the drug in the blood, often resulting in toxicity. Some drugs normally exist in a state of high protein binding, often exceeding 90%. With these, even a small decrease in protein binding could significantly increase the free drug concentration. As an example, nonsteroidal anti-inflammatory drugs are provided with a very high binding to plasma protein, and their use may increase the effect of nephrotoxic antibiotics (e.g., vancomycin, amphotericin) by increasing the level of free and active drug up to a nephrotoxic level. The

reduction in albumin concentration, frequently observed in ICU patients, favors a decreased binding of drugs to albumin, thus increasing their potential nephrotoxicity (see Table 309-2).

Most drugs eliminated by the kidney are excreted via passive glomerular filtration. Only some drugs are eliminated via active tubular secretion, including penicillins, cephalosporins, and most diuretics. The reduction of renal function alters the drug elimination, resulting often in toxicity and necessity of dose reduction. The potential interaction between diuretics and aminoglycosides could result in worsening of renal function.

Elderly patients are more disposed to experience drug interactions because of reduced hepatic and renal function.

Drugs that require careful dose titration to maintain efficacy and avoid toxicity must be monitored particularly carefully for drug interactions. Most drug interactions can be avoided or managed by substitution of one or more agents or by more intense monitoring for the potential result. Important strategies for clinicians to limit drug interactions include separation of doses of interacting agents (e.g., ciprofloxacin and calcium) and adjustment of doses. The clinical significance of drug interaction is variable. A moderate interaction may be responsible for a deterioration in the patient's clinical status. A significant interaction may potentially be life-threatening or may lead to definitive renal damage. The most relevant interactions are listed in Table 309-3.

ANTIMICROBIAL DRUGS IN PATIENTS RECEIVING CONTINUOUS RENAL REPLACEMENT THERAPY

Continuous renal replacement therapy (CRRT) is frequently used to treat critically ill patients with ARF or chronic renal failure. CRRT is better tolerated by hemodynamically unstable patients and is as effective at removing solutes during a 24- to 48-hour period, compared with a single session of conventional hemodialysis. Solute removal is particularly relevant to antimicrobial therapy, because many critically ill patients with ARF have serious infections and require treatment with more than one antimicrobial agent.[33] The rate of drug clearance during CRRT can be highly variable in critically ill patients.

The most common modalities of CRRT currently used in the ICU are continuous venovenous hemofiltration, hemodialysis, and hemodiafiltration (CVVH, CVVHD, and CVVHDF, respectively). Before calculating an adjusted antimicrobial dose for a patient undergoing CRRT, the antibiotic must be one that is at least 25% renally eliminated, because drugs cleared from the blood through nonrenal mechanisms are not significantly affected by CRRT. The pharmacokinetics of drug removal in critically ill patients receiving CRRT is complex, with multiple variables affecting clearance. These variables make generalized dosing recommendations difficult. Drug-protein complexes have a larger molecular weight; therefore, antibiotics with low protein binding capacity in serum are removed by CRRT more readily. Similarly, antibiotics that penetrate and bind to tissues have a larger volume of distribution, reducing the quantity removed during CRRT. Sepsis itself increases the volume of distribution, extends drug half-life, and alters the protein binding capacity of many antimicrobials. CRRT mechanical factors may also

TABLE 309-3

Most Relevant Drug Interactions That May Occur in a Patient in the Intensive Care Unit Needing Antibiotic or Antifungal Therapy

DRUG	INTERACTING DRUG	POTENTIAL EFFECT	MANAGEMENT
Aminoglycosides	Cephalosporins	Increased risk of nephrotoxicity	Monitor aminoglycoside concentrations and kidney function.
	Loop diuretics	Increased risk of ototoxicity	Avoid excessive doses. Monitor aminoglycosides. Use alternative antibiotic if possible.
	Penicillins	Inactivation of aminoglycosides	Do not mix drugs in same solution. Separate administration times.
Macrolides	Digoxin	Increased concentrations of digoxin	Monitor signs/symptoms of digoxin toxicity. Decrease digoxin dose if necessary.
	Rifamycin	Decreased effects of clarithromycin; increased adverse effects of rifamycin	Monitor for increased adverse effects and decreased response. Use alternatives.
	CyA/Tac	Increased concentration of CyA/Tac	Monitor CyA concentration. Adjust CyA/Tac dose during therapy.
	Warfarin	Increased effects of warfarin	Monitor INR. Decrease warfarin dose if necessary.
Quinolones	Iron salts	Decreased GI absorption	Avoid combination.
	Phosphate binders	Decreased GI absorption	Separate administration by at least 2 hr.
	CyA	Increased risk of nephrotoxicity	Monitor CyA concentration. Use alternative quinolones (levofloxacin).
Imipenem	CyA	Increased CNS adverse effects of both drugs	Use alternative antibiotics if interaction is suspected.
Metronidazole	Barbiturates	Therapeutic failure of metronidazole	Increase metronidazole dose. Use higher initial metronidazole dose.
TMP-SMX	CyA	Decreased effects of CyA; increased risk of nephrotoxicity	Avoid combination if possible. Monitor CyA concentration and adjust dose.
	Warfarin	Increased effects of warfarin	Monitor INR. Decrease warfarin dose if necessary.
Vancomycin	Muscle relaxants	Increased effects of nondepolarizing muscle relaxant (prolonged respiratory depression)	Avoid combination if possible. Monitor respiratory function. Adjust muscle relaxant dose.
Azole antifungal	CyA/Tac	Increased concentration of CyA	Monitor CyA concentration and signs/symptoms of toxicity. Adjust dosage according to azoles therapy.
	Indinavir, ritonavir, saquinavir	Increased concentration of protease inhibitor	Decrease protease inhibitor dose if necessary.
	Prednisolone	Increased effects of methylprednisolone	Decrease steroid dose if necessary.
	Warfarin	Increased effects of warfarin	Monitor INR. Decrease warfarin dose if necessary.
Voriconazole	Barbiturates	Decreased concentration of voriconazole	Avoid combination.
	Carbamazepine	Decreased concentration of voriconazole	Avoid combination.
	CyA/Tac/sirolimus	Increased concentration of CyA/Tac/sirolimus	Strictly monitor CyA/Tac/sirolimus blood levels
Caspofungin	Tac	Decreased concentration of Tac	Monitor Tac concentration. Adjust Tac dose.
Foscarnet	CyA	Increased risk of renal failure	Avoid combination if possible. Strictly monitor renal function.
Ganciclovir	Zidovudine	Increased risk of life-threatening hematological toxicity	Avoid combination. Use foscarnet instead.
Indinavir, ritonavir	Azole antifungals	Increased concentration of protease inhibitor	Decrease protease inhibitor dose.
	Rifamycins	Decreased concentration of indinavir; increased concentration of rifamycin	Avoid combination if possible. Increase indinavir if necessary.

CNS, central nervous system; CyA, cyclosporine; GI, gastrointestinal; INR, International Normalized Ratio; Tac, tacrolimus; TMP-SMX, trimethoprim/sulfamethoxazole.

TABLE 309-4

Antibiotic Dosing in Patients Receiving Continuous Renal Replacement Therapy

DRUG	CVVH		CVVHD or CVVHDF	
	DOSE	FREQUENCY	DOSE	FREQUENCY
Amphotericin B				
Deoxycholate	0.4-1.0 mg/kg	q24h	0.4-1.0 mg/kg	q24h
Lipid complex	3-5 mg/kg	q24h	3-5 mg/kg	q24h
Liposomal	3-5 mg/kg	q24h	3-5 mg/kg	q24h
Acyclovir	5-7.5 mg/kg	q24h	5-7.5 mg/kg	q24h
Aztreonam	1-2 g	q12h	2 g	q12h
Ceftazidime	1-2 g	q12h	2 g	q12h
Ceftriaxone	2 g	q12-24h	2 g	q12-24h
Ciprofloxacin	200 mg	q12h	200-400 mg	q12h
Clavulanic acid				
Fluconazole	200-400 mg	q24h	400-800 mg	q24h
Imipenem	250 mg	q6h	250 mg	q6h
	OR 500 mg	q8h	OR 500 mg	q8h
			OR 500 mg	q6h
Levofloxacin	250 mg	q24h	250 mg	q24h
Linezolid	600 mg	q12h	600 mg	q12h
Meropenem	1 g	q12h	1 g	q12h
Piperacillin-tazobactam	2.25 g	q6h	2.25-3.375 g	q6h
Ticarcillin-clavulanate	2 g	q6-8h	3.1 g	q6h
Vancomycin	1 g	q48h	1 g	q24h
Voriconazole	4 mg/kg PO	q12h	4 mg/kg PO	q12h

CVVH, continuous venovenous hemofiltration; CVVHD, continuous venovenous hemodialysis; CVVHDF, continuous venovenous hemodiafiltration. From Trotman RL, Williamson JC, Shoemaker DM, Salzer WL: Antibiotic dosing in critically ill adult patients receiving continuous renal replacement therapy. Clin Infect Dis 2005;41:1159-1166.

affect drug clearance. Increasing the blood or dialysate flow rate can change the transmembrane pressure and increase drug clearance. The dialysate concentration may also affect drug removal in hemofiltration. Lastly, the membrane pore size is directly proportional to the degree of drug removal by CRRT, often expressed as a sieving coefficient. In general, biosynthetic membranes have larger pores than conventional filters, allowing removal of drugs with a larger molecular weight. These patient, drug, and mechanical variables significantly diminish the utility of routine pharmacokinetic calculations for determining antimicrobial dosing during CRRT.[34]

The Medline-referenced literature was recently reviewed[35] to formulate dosing recommendations for antibiotics frequently used to treat critically ill adult patients undergoing CRRT (Table 309-4). The pharmacokinetic and pharmacodynamic properties of each antimicrobial agent and the typical susceptibilities of relevant pathogens were considered (see Table 309-2). In most cases, the recommended "target" drug concentration corresponds to the upper limit of the MIC range for susceptibility. The goal of the dosing recommendation is to keep the concentration above the target MIC for an optimal proportion of the dosing interval, reflecting known pharmacodynamic properties (time-dependent versus concentration-dependent killing), while minimizing toxicity due to unnecessarily high concentrations. These recommendations should serve only as a guide until more data are available, and they should not replace clinical judgment.

Key Points

1. Infectious complications of patients in the intensive care unit increase the risk of unfavorable outcome.

2. Attention should be paid to the antibiotic drugs, to potential kidney toxicity, and to the clinical settings that amplify the risk, including correct evaluation of the renal function, drug volume distribution, and increased free drug concentration due to hypoalbuminemia.

3. Choices of individual drugs and medication associations should be made to minimize the risk.

4. In patients in the intensive care unit who are receiving continuous replacement therapy, large volumes of solute removal may modify the rate of drug clearance and the actual concentrations in the body fluids.

Key References

1. Liano F, Junco E, Pascual J, et al: The spectrum of acute renal failure in the intensive care unit compared with that seen in other settings. The Madrid Acute Renal Failure Study Group. Kidney Int Suppl 1998;66:S16-S24.
3. Silvester W, Bellomo R, Cole L: Epidemiology, management, and outcome of severe acute renal failure of critical illness in Australia. Crit Care Med 2001;29:1910-1915.
23. Pinder M, Bellomo R, Lipman J: Pharmacological principles of antibiotic prescription in the critically ill. Anaesth Intensive Care 2002;30:134-144.
34. Bellomo R, Ronco C, Kellum J, et al; and the ADQI Workgroup: Acute renal failure definition, outcome measures, animal models, fluid therapy and information technology needs: The Second International Consensus Conference of the Acute Dialysis Quality Initiative (ADQI) group. Crit Care 2004;8:R204-R212.
35. Trotman RL, Williamson JC, Shoemaker DM, Salzer WL: Antibiotic dosing in critically ill adult patients receiving continuous renal replacement therapy. Clin Infect Dis 2005;41:1159-1166.

See the companion Expert Consult website for the complete reference list.

CHAPTER 310

Calcineurin Inhibitors and Other Immunosuppressive Drugs and the Kidney

Francesco Paolo Schena, Silvia Porreca, and Giovanni Pertosa

OBJECTIVES

This chapter will:
1. Define potential mechanisms underlying nephrotoxicity of immunosuppressive drugs in the intensive care unit (ICU).
2. Analyze the pharmacological interactions among immunosuppressive agents and other drugs used in ICU patients.
3. Evaluate clinical outcomes after adjustment or reduction of the immunosuppressive regimen.

Drug-induced nephrotoxicity is a common cause of acute renal failure (ARF) in patients in the intensive care unit (ICU). Several renal disorders are caused by drug toxicity, including direct tubular damage (tubular cell apoptosis and necrosis), interstitial inflammation (interstitial nephritis), vascular injury (thrombotic microangiopathy), and alteration of tubular cell functions (i.e., decreased membrane transport, defective mitochondrial function, and increased level of oxidative stress species).[1] However, the progression from functional impairment to renal failure usually requires additional factors, such as metabolic disorders associated with diabetes, sepsis, hypovolemia, or use of contrast media.[2] Several drugs have been reported as responsible for renal damage in ICU patients, including antibiotics (aminoglycosides) and antimycotic agents. In addition, recent evidence suggests the importance of the action of immunosuppressive drugs in the development of renal injury in ICU patients. The most used immunosuppressive drugs are glucocorticoids, calcineurin inhibitors (cyclosporine, tacrolimus), inhibitors of nucleotide synthesis (mycophenolate mofetil, mycophenolic acid), antimetabolites (azathioprine), mammalian target of rapamycin (mTOR) inhibitors (rapamycin), and monoclonal and polyclonal antibodies (Table 310-1). The pathogenesis of immunosuppressive-induced nephrotoxicity is multifactorial and is linked to the various mechanisms of action of these drugs.

NEPHROTOXICITY INDUCED BY CALCINEURIN INHIBITORS

Patients treated with calcineurin inhibitors (CIs) have a higher risk of developing both acute and chronic renal injury.[3] In particular, it has been demonstrated that acute nephrotoxicity secondary to CI treatment is dose dependent and reversible after adjusting or reducing the dosage.

On the other hand, the development of chronic renal damage is usually irreversible.[4-6]

Mechanisms involved in acute CI nephrotoxicity include endothelial damage with reduced release of L-arginine nitric oxide (NO) and prostaglandin E (PGE), increased production of transforming growth factor beta-1 (TGF-β1), and increased production of vasoconstrictory substances such as thromboxane and endothelin 1. Increased sympathetic tone may also be present,[7] although renal vasoconstriction occurs even in denervated kidneys. The reduced glomerular filtration rate (GFR) and renal plasma flow secondary to vasoconstriction seems to correlate with the dosage and time of administration.[8,9] In addition, activation of the intrarenal renin-angiotensin system plays an essential role in the pathogenesis of chronic cyclosporine (CsA) nephrotoxicity because of the increasing release of renin from the afferent and efferent arterioles and the glomerular capillaries.[10] Several reports indicate that the decrease in renal plasma flow and GFR can be antagonized by calcium channel blockers through an inhibition of endothelin-mediated calcium entry into vascular smooth muscle cells. This suggests an important role for calcium channel blockers in the antihypertensive strategy used in ICU patients treated with CsA.

It has been reported that chronic administration of CIs is responsible for several serum electrolyte impairments, such as hypercalcemia, hypomagnesemia, and hyperkalemia. These conditions need to be controlled to avoid important clinical complications in critically ill patients. The concomitant administration of drugs commonly used in ICU patients may increase these secondary effects. In particular, hyperkalemia secondary to CsA administration may be potentiated after concomitant administration of angiotensin-converting enzyme (ACE) inhibitors, angiotensin receptor blockers (ARBs), or beta blockers and may become life-threatening.[11] Moreover, hypercalcemia and, especially, hypomagnesemia may predispose to seizures with secondary effects on the clinical outcome of ICU patients.

Another uncommon clinical complication associated with CI treatment is represented by acute vascular damage. This condition may easily be misclassified, and it needs a careful diagnosis to discriminate it from hemolytic uremic syndrome and thrombotic thrombocytopenic purpura, which are often observed in the ICU.

The nephrotoxicity that occurs with CI treatment may be responsible for the development of chronic renal damage. The interstitial fibrosis, exacerbating preexisting renal alterations, may determine a rapid decline of the renal function leading to end-stage renal disease (ESRD). Several studies have been designed to define a common mechanism responsible for the chronic CI nephrotoxicity,

TABLE 310-1

Classification of Immunosuppressive Drugs

Glucocorticoids
Calcineurin Inhibitors
Cyclophilin-binding drugs (e.g., cyclosporine)
FKBP12-binding drugs (e.g., tacrolimus)
Inhibitors of Nucleotide Synthesis
Mycophenolate mofetil
Mycophenolic acid
TOR Inhibitors
Sirolimus
Everolimus
Antimetabolites
Azathioprine
Depleting Antibodies (against T cells, B cells, or both)
Polyclonal antibody (e.g., horse or rabbit antithymocyte
    globulin)
Mouse monoclonal anti-CD3 antibody (e.g., muromonab-CD3
    or OKT3)
Intravenous Immune Globulin
Nondepleting Antibodies and Fusion Proteins
Humanized or chimeric monoclonal anti-CD25 antibody
    (e.g., daclizumab, basiliximab)
New Immunosuppressive Drugs
Sphingosine-1-phosphate–receptor antagonists (e.g., FTY720)
Pyrimidine synthesis (DHODH) inhibitors (e.g., leflunomide)
Humanized monoclonal anti-CD52 antibody (e.g.,
    alemtuzumab)
B-cell–depleting monoclonal anti-CD20 antibody (e.g.,
    rituximab)
T-cell costimulatory blockers
Chemokine blockers

DHODH, dihydro-orotate dehydrogenase; FKBP12, FK506 (tacrolimus)
binding protein 12; TOR, target of rapamycin.

TABLE 310-2

Drugs That Interfere with Cyclosporine (CsA)

DRUGS THAT INCREASE CsA BLOOD CONCENTRATIONS	DRUGS THAT LOWER CsA BLOOD CONCENTRATIONS
Allopurinol	Carbamazepine
Amiodarone	Nafcillin
Bromocriptine	Octreotide
Cimetidine	Orlistat
Clarithromycin	Phenobarbital
Colchicine	Phenytoin
Danazol	Rifabutin
Diltiazem	Rifampin
Erythromycin	Ticlopidine
Fluconazole	
Itraconazole	
Ketoconazole	
Lansoprazole	
Methylprednisolone	
Metoclopramide	
Nicardipine	
Rabeprazole	
Verapamil	

but several issues still need to be addressed. Evidence has been reported associating the development of interstitial fibrosis with increased expression of osteopontin (a potent macrophage chemoattractant secreted by tubular epithelial cells),[12] chemokines (a class of cytokines that are strong chemoattractants for a variety of hematopoietic cells),[13] and TGF-β (a powerful stimulator of extracellular matrix production).[14,15] The increased TGF-β gene and protein expression appears to result from decreased secretion of NO as well as increased local concentrations of angiotensin II. This may explain the beneficial effect of ACE inhibitors and ARB antagonists to attenuate the evolution of chronic renal injury in this setting. Indeed, several studies clearly demonstrated that concomitant administration of ACE inhibitor and ARB significantly reduces arteriolopathy, interstitial fibrosis, and tubular atrophy and improves blood pressure levels.[16,17]

CIs are metabolized by the hepatic cytochrome P-450 enzyme CYP3A, and several drugs used in the ICU may interfere with their metabolism, thereby influencing CI blood concentrations, efficacy, and toxicity. Any of the drugs listed in Table 310-2 should be used with caution in patients receiving CsA. An increased CsA plasma concentration after introduction of some antibiotics (i.e., azithromycin, clarithromycin, erythromycin, norfloxacin, imipenem, and quinupristin/dalfopristin) has been observed. This event may be responsible for important clinical complications such as progression of renal dysfunction (in concomitant administration with ciprofloxacin, gentamicin, tobramycin, vancomycin, and trimethoprim-sulfamethoxazole), reduction of immunosuppressive effects (in the presence of ciprofloxacin) and secondary toxic effects such as central nervous system disturbances and seizures (in the presence of imipenem).

Even if these secondary effects are well recognized in clinical practice, the question whether there is a "safe" chronic dose of CsA that is effective immunologically but does not cause progressive renal dysfunction is difficult to answer, because there is still a lack of controlled clinical trials. Short-term (1-year) studies in patients receiving CsA for nonrenal autoimmune diseases (e.g., early insulin-dependent diabetes mellitus, uveitis) suggest that a maintenance dose of less than 5 mg/kg/day may not lead to progressive chronic nephrotoxicity.[18] However, a longer (2-year) trial in which 5 mg/kg/day was given for uveitis reported a mean elevation in plasma creatinine concentration of 0.4 mg/dL (35 μmol/L) and a fall in mean GFR from 116 to 75 mL/min. Tacrolimus (FK506) is also metabolized by the CYP3A enzyme and should therefore be susceptible to many of the drug interactions noted for CsA.[19] Early detection of renal dysfunction is recommended to stop the progression of critical renal damage. Even in patients with normal renal function, initial signs of nephrotoxicity should be carefully investigated through laboratory testing, and it is highly recommended that frequent measurement of plasma concentrations of these drugs be included in the monitoring of CI therapy.

OTHER IMMUNOSUPPRESSIVE DRUGS INDUCING NEPHROTOXICITY

Glucocorticoids

Glucocorticoids are frequently used to treat ICU patients for their potent anti-inflammatory effect.[20] Despite its efficacy, steroid therapy is characterized by a broad range of toxic effects such as hypertension, glucose intolerance, and cardiovascular disease, which contribute to the increased risk of premature death from atherosclerotic heart disease, particularly in renal transplant recipients.

Other reported toxic effects include lymphoproliferative disorders, dyslipidemia, weight gain with central obesity, peptic ulcer formation, pancreatitis, cataract formation, diabetes, osteoporosis with avascular necrosis of bone,[21] growth retardation,[22] and personality disorders. In addition, it has been well established that corticosteroid therapy increases the patient's risk of life-threatening infections and metabolic abnormalities.

To avoid the development of these complications, it is necessary to taper the drug as soon as the disease being treated appears to be under control. Tapering must be done carefully to avoid both recurrent activity of the underlying disease and possible cortisol deficiency resulting from suppression of the hypothalamic-pituitary-adrenal axis during the period of steroid therapy.

Combinations of the new immunosuppressants make it feasible for most patients to avoid corticosteroids or to withdraw early from these drugs.[23]

Inhibitors of Nucleotide Synthesis and TOR Inhibitors

The introduction of drugs such as mycophenolate mofetil (MMF), mycophenolic acid (MPA), and the mTOR inhibitors sirolimus and everolimus has increased the use of CI-free and/or steroid-free immunosuppressive therapy. MMF is a prodrug that requires an active intracellular metabolism to become effective. The immunosuppressive mechanism is principally based on the inhibition of inosine monophosphate dehydrogenase, a key enzyme in de novo synthesis of purine nucleotides. Based on its pharmacokinetics and pharmacodynamics, this drug may be safely used in patients with renal disorders, because it is associated with a decreased relative risk of renal failure[24] and significant protection against long-term deterioration of renal function.[25]

The most common adverse events are related to the gastrointestinal tract. Neurotoxicity and hepatotoxicity have not been observed with MMF. MPA is not metabolized through the CYP3A enzyme system, and it can be administered in combination with other drugs metabolized by this enzymatic complex. MMF is primarily absorbed by intestinal cells and should not be administered simultaneously with antacids, cholestyramine, or oral ferrous sulfate. In addition, MMF may modify the tubular secretion of several drugs used in the ICU (acyclovir, valacyclovir, ganciclovir, and valganciclovir) and thus increase their blood levels.

Regarding adverse effects of MMF, there are no large studies examining the incidence of infections that could be important for patients treated with this drug who are admitted to an ICU. The existing studies[26] are too small to allow generalizations. However, a large number of patients with solid organ transplants have been treated with MMF. Regarding viral infections, in one study of heart transplant recipients, a higher incidence of herpes zoster was associated with MMF.[27] Of greater concern, however, is the risk of cytomegalovirus infection.

The mTOR is a key regulator kinase in the process of cell division. The term *TOR inhibitor* refers to two similar immunosuppressant drugs whose mechanism of action is closely linked to inhibition of this kinase. Sirolimus, also known as rapamycin, is a macrolide antibiotic compound that is structurally related to tacrolimus. Everolimus is a similar compound with a shorter half-life. Sirolimus was originally developed as an antifungal agent; it was later found to have immunosuppressive and antiproliferative properties that may be useful to treat or prevent proliferative diseases such as tuberous sclerosis, psoriasis, and malignancy.

The mTOR inhibitors can be tubulotoxic and can produce hypokalemia and hypomagnesemia as a result of kaliuresis and magnesuria. However, dosage adjustment of sirolimus is not required in the presence of renal impair-

ment, considering the low level of nephrotoxicity of this drug. On the contrary, dosage reductions of approximately one-third the normal maintenance dose should be used for patients with hepatic impairment. The use of these drugs in critically ill patients requires monitoring of hemoglobin and other blood cell counts, because anemia, thrombocytopenia, and leukopenia can be caused by sirolimus. In addition, the frequent measurement of drug concentration in the blood is welcome.

Azathioprine

Azathioprine is an antimetabolite, an imidazole derivate of 6-mercaptopurine. It has been used in clinical transplantation for more than 30 years. The most important side effects of this drug that could have an importance for critically ill patients and require careful monitoring are thrombocytopenia and leukopenia. Azathioprine is converted to inactive 6-thiouric acid by xanthine oxidase. This enzyme is inhibited by allopurinol, so this drug combination must be avoided. In the presence of renal impairment, the azathioprine dose must be reduced by 75% when the creatinine clearance rate is between 10 and 50 mL/min and by 50% when it is less than 10 mL/min.

Intravenous Immune Globulin

Another immunosuppressive drug–induced nephrotoxicity is ARF associated with intravenous immune globulin (IVIG), which has been reported in approximately 100 ICU patients.[28,29] Most of the reported cases occurred with IVIG preparations that contained sucrose as a stabilizing agent. Older patients and patients with preexisting renal impairment or diabetes mellitus are predisposed to nephrotoxicity from IVIG.[30] The clinical picture consists of oliguric renal failure requiring renal replacement therapy in up to 33% of the patients. In more than 80% of these cases, ARF appears to be reversible. Renal damage in these patients was suggested to be the result of sucrose tubular uptake, as a consequence of the infusion of sucrose-containing IVIG, leading to osmotic cellular swelling and damage. Prevention consists in avoiding sucrose-containing IVIG preparations in older patients and in those with renal impairment or diabetes. Additional protection can be achieved by limiting the dose applied or lengthening the dosing interval.

Monoclonal Antibodies

The monoclonal antibody muromonab-CD3 (OKT3) is an immunoglobulin G, a monoclonal antibody produced by the hybridization of murine antibody-secreting B lymphocytes. This drug is usually employed in the treatment of steroid-resistant acute allograft rejection. Renal function may deteriorate during the early days of OKT3 administration; a previously nonoliguric patient may even require dialysis. This deterioration is typically transient and is followed by an adequate diuresis. Infection, most commonly with cytomegalovirus, may be a late adverse sequela of OKT3 use.

Rituximab is a monoclonal antibody directed against CD20 that is active especially in the treatment of lymphoid malignancies. Use of rituximab may be associated with severe renal toxicity, including ARF, in patients with high levels of circulating tumor cells (>25,000/mm³) or a high tumor burden, who experience tumor lysis syndrome.[31,32]

Although there are no formal published guidelines, rituximab should probably be discontinued in patients who develop a rising serum creatinine value or oliguria during treatment.

CONCLUSION

Drug-induced nephrotoxicity is a relatively common cause of ICU-acquired ARF and can be induced by a variety of drugs with different mechanisms. Prevention leads to decreased morbidity and a reduction in length and cost of hospital stay. Keys to prevention include minimization of use of potential nephrotoxins, especially in high-risk patients, and early detection of ARF with subsequent rapid cessation of the offending agent.

CIs are associated with efficacy-limiting adverse events, particularly nephrotoxicity, which may modify their benefits for long-term renal survival. To obtain significant improvement in renal outcomes, it may be necessary to adopt new immunosuppressive regimens that rely less on CIs. The use of MMF in CsA- and tacrolimus-sparing regimens is associated with improved renal function while maintaining adequate immunosuppression. Finally, it is important to adjust the dosage of immunosuppressant agents according to their plasma concentration, which should be monitored constantly.

Key Points

1. It is increasingly common for intensive care physicians to be involved in the care of patients treated with immunosuppressive therapy for various pathologies, such as allograft recipients.

2. It is important that intensive care physicians be familiar with immunosuppressive drugs that have been introduced in recent years and know their potential nephrotoxicity.

3. Common immunosuppressants include calcineurin inhibitors (cyclosporine and tacrolimus), antimetabolites (mycophenolate mofetil, mycophenolate sodium, and azathioprine), and inhibitors of the mammalian target of rapamycin (sirolimus and everolimus).

4. Protocols for avoidance, minimization, and/or withdrawal of immunosuppressive drugs should be used in the intensive care unit, taking into consideration the frequent measurement of plasma concentrations of these drugs.

Key References

6. Olyaei AJ, de Mattos AM, Bennett WM: Nephrotoxicity of immunosuppressive drugs: Long-term consequences and challenges for the future. Am J Kidney Dis 2000;35:333-339.
20. Kirwan JR, Hickey SH, Hallgren R, et al: The effect of therapeutic glucocorticoids on the adrenal response in a randomized controlled trial in patients with rheumatoid arthritis. Arthritis Rheum 2006;54:1415-1421.
25. Meier-Kriesche HU, Steffen BJ, Hochberg AM, et al: Mycophenolate mofetil versus azathioprine therapy is associated with a significant protection against long-term renal allograft function deterioration. Transplantation 2003;75:1341-1346.

See the companion Expert Consult website for the complete reference list.

CHAPTER 311

Alternative Medicine and Chinese Herbs and the Kidney

Kian Bun Tai and Alex W. Yu

OBJECTIVES
This chapter will:
1. Define complementary and alternative medicine.
2. Present general treatment principles of Chinese herbal medicine.
3. Provide an overview of mechanisms of nephrotoxicity with exposure to alternative medicine, with specific examples of herb-related nephrotoxicity.
4. Discuss possible therapeutic roles of alternative medicines in renal disease.

DEFINITIONS

Complementary and alternative medicine (CAM) involves therapies that are not usually taught in Western medical schools. It includes a broad range of therapies and beliefs such as acupuncture, chiropractic care, relaxation techniques, massage therapy, and herbal remedies. According to the National Center for Complementary and Alternative Medicine (NCCAM) of the U.S. National Institutes of Health, *complementary and alternative medicine* is defined as a group of diverse medical and health care systems, practices, and products that are not presently considered to be part of conventional medicine. Although complementary medicine is usually used together with conventional medicine, whereas alternative medicine is used to replace conventional medicine, studies indicate that many patients who use alternative medicines also seek conventional treatment and vice versa. Therefore, the terms "complementary and alternative" are used either together (CAM) or interchangeably. Sometimes, the term *integrative medicine* is used to indicate the combination of mainstream medical therapies with CAM

TABLE 311-1

Classification of Complementary and Alternative Medicine

CATEGORY	DESCRIPTION	EXAMPLES
Alternative medical systems	Built on complete systems of theory and practice	Traditional Chinese medicine Ayurveda Homeopathic medicine Naturopathic medicine
Mind-body interventions	Designed to enhance the mind's capacity to affect bodily function and symptoms	Meditation Prayer Mental healing Art therapy Music therapy
Biologically based therapies	Use substances found in nature	Vitamin or dietary supplements Natural products (e.g., shark cartilage and *Ling Zhi* to treat cancer)
Manipulative and body-based methods	Involve body manipulation and/or movement of one or more parts of the body	Chiropractic/osteopathic manipulation Body massage
Energy therapies	Involve use of energy fields	Qi-gong Reiki Therapeutic touch

therapies that have some scientific evidence of safety and effectiveness.

Edzard Ernst commented in the *Medical Journal of Australia* that "about half the general population in developed countries use complementary and alternative medicine."[1] In the United Kingdom, the annual expenditure on alternative medicine is as high as 230 million U.S. dollars.[2] CAM therapies are classified by NCCAM into five categories (Table 311-1). Traditional Chinese medicine includes acupuncture, acupressure, herbal medicine, tai chi, and qi-gong. The common characteristic of these diverse therapies is an emphasis on maximizing the body's inherent healing ability and on treating of the "whole" person by addressing their physical, mental, and spiritual attributes rather than focusing on a specific pathogenic process, as is emphasized in conventional medicine.

Herbs have been used for medicinal purposes for thousands of years in the developing world. The use of botanical medicine by far accounts for the majority of traditional remedies. Traditional medicine accounts for a substantial proportion of primary health care in Africa, Asia, and Latin America. In China, as much as 30% to 50% of the total medicinal consumption consists of traditional herbal preparations. Just as with the conventional drugs, all herbal products are associated with adverse reactions. Indeed, the association of alternative therapies and kidney injury is well recognized. It is beyond the scope of this chapter to present an exhaustive list of possible side effects after intake of all the different types of herbs and plants. Instead, we will highlight certain important examples and discuss the possible therapeutic roles of traditional drugs in renal disease.

GENERAL TREATMENT PRINCIPLES OF CHINESE HERBAL MEDICINE

The concept of disease in Chinese medicine is different from that of conventional Western medicine. Disease is regarded as an imbalance between the health *qi* and pathogenic factors. This *qi* runs within the vessels and has a nutritive action. Sickness is also a result of *yin-yang* dis-

harmony between different parts of the body (*zang-fu*, internal organs) and in the whole body. Therefore, the primary therapeutic principle of Chinese medicine is to strengthen the health *qi*, eliminate the pathogenic factors, and restore the *yin-yang* harmony of the body parts as well as with the environment. On the whole, Chinese medicine takes on a more holistic approach besides the use of herbs. Treatment targeting at the kidney may not consist of treating illness arising from kidney dysfunction. Diarrhea can be stopped by herbs that "warm" the kidney with *yang* deficiency. Sexual impotence can also be treated by "warming" the kidney to revitalize *yang*. On the other hand, diuresis can be induced by warming the kidney with some other herbs in relieving edema caused by kidney *yang* deficiency.

MECHANISMS OF NEPHROTOXICITIES OF HERBAL MEDICINE

The kidney is responsible for the excretion of chemicals and drugs. The high blood flow rate, large endothelial surface area, active uptake by tubular cells, and medullary concentration of toxins make the kidney vulnerable to the toxicity of drugs. A toxin may achieve a very high concentration in the renal tubules because of their concentrating capabilities. Herbal and plant products are among the most frequent causes of acute renal failure in Africa.[3]

Herbal pharmacopoeias usually include active and useful compounds as well as toxic substances. The relative paucity of professional surveillance, the lack of industrial standardization, and the often undisclosed secret formulas pose significant hazards to consumers.[4-7] Furthermore, commercial plant products may lack purity or potency due to variability in the amount of ingredients.[8] Herbal medicine may be the source of kidney injury via a number of mechanisms:

1. Known herb with unknown or underestimated toxicity
2. Toxic effect related to wrong preparation or use of substitute
3. Contaminants or adulteration
4. Indirect toxicity related to drug-drug interaction

TABLE 311-2

Kidney Syndromes Associated with the Use of Alternative Medicines

Acute tubular necrosis	Traditional African medicine: toxic plants (*Securidaca longepedunculata, Euphorbia matabalensis, Crotalaria laburnifolia, Heliotropium, Symphytum, Senecio* plants, *Callilepsis laureola, Atractylis gummifera,* Cape Aloes) or adulteration by dichromates
	Sri Lankan traditional Ayurvedic pharmacopoeia: toxic plants (*Crotalaria* spp., *Cassia auriculata, Hollarrhena antidysenterica*)
	Asian rural areas: raw carp bile
	Saudi Arabia: raw sheep bile
	China: *Taxus celebrica*
	Hydrazine sulfate
	Mentha spicata
	Chinese herbs contaminated with arsenic (*Niu Huang Chieh tu Pien*)
	Morocco: *Takaout roumia* (PPD)
	Sudan: henna adulterated with PPD
	Cantharidin
	Chelation therapy with EDTA
Proximal tubulopathy (Fanconi's syndrome)	*Glycyrrhiza* spp. (herbal cough mixtures, Chinese herbal teas, gancao, Boui-ougi-tou)
	Chinese herbs contaminated with cadmium
Distal tubular toxicity	Germanium
Acute interstitial nephritis	Traditional African medicine: toxic plants (Cape Aloes)
	Peruvian medicine (*Uno degatta*)
	China: *Taxus celebrica*
	Chinese herbs adulterated with NSAIDs (*Tung Shueh* pills)
	Hypericum, Iedum
Analgesic nephropathy, papillary necrosis	Willow bark (*Salix* spp.)
	Chinese herbs adulterated with NSAIDs (indomethacin, diclofenac, mefenamic acid, phenylbutazone): *Chuifong Tuokuwan, Tung Shueh* pills, others
Hypertension	*Glycyrrhiza* spp. (herbal cough mixtures, Chinese herbal teas, gancao, Boui-ougi-tou)
	Ephedra-containing herbal preparations (*Ma Huang,* dietary supplements containing ephedra alkaloids)
Kidney stones	Ephedra-containing herbal preparations (*Ma Huang,* dietary supplements containing ephedra alkaloids)
	Cranberry juice (oxalate)
	Chinese herbs contaminated with cadmium
Urinary retention	Niger: *Datura* spp. (Sobi-lobi)
	Chinese herbs: *Rhododendron molle, Rehmannia glutinosa, Carthamus tinctorius, Atropa belladonna, Hyoscyamus niger, Datura* spp.
Chronic tubulointerstitial nephritis with fibrosis	Chinese herbs containing *Aristolochia* sp.: Belgian slimming regimen, Mokutsu, Boui
	China: *Jia Wey Guo Sao* pills (herbal mixtures without Aristolochia)
Urinary tract carcinoma	Chinese herbs containing *Aristolochia* sp.: Belgian slimming regimen
Acute rejection of kidney transplant	Drug interaction with alternative medicine: St. John's wort
	Immunostimulating drugs: alfalfa (*Medicago sativa*)

EDTA, ethylenediamine tetra-acetic acid; NSAIDs, nonsteroidal anti-inflammatory drugs; PPD, paraphenylenediamine.
From Colson CR, De Broe ME: Kidney injury from alternative medicines. Adv Chronic Kidney Dis 2005;12:261-275.

They may result in a variety of clinical manifestations and/or pathological changes in the kidney (Table 311-2).

HERBS WITH KNOWN TOXICITY

Licorice (*Glycyrrhiza glabra*)

Licorice roots contain 5% to 9% glycyrrhizic acid, a glycoside that is much sweeter than sugar. Derivatives from licorice can be used to treat peptic ulcer disease.

Aqueous extracts of licorice contain 10% to 20% glycyrrhizic acid. Glycyrrhizic acid is hydrolyzed by intestinal flora to glycyrrhetic acid, which inhibits 11β-hydroxysteroid dehydrogenase in the kidney. This enzyme catalyzes inactivation of cortisol; hence, the use of licorice may result in a state of pseudohyperaldosteronism.[5,6] Tox-

icity may manifest as headache, sodium and water retention, hypokalemia, heart failure, and even cardiac arrest.

Glycyrrhizic acid is mainly used as a flavoring and sweetening agent for bitter drugs, beverages, candies, and chewing gum. It may also be present in some cough and cold mixtures. Many health products and Chinese herbal teas contain considerable amounts of glycyrrhizic acid. Excessive intake of these products may result in Fanconi's syndrome.[9-11]

Ma Huang

Ma Huang is a Chinese herbal preparation that contains ephedra. The vasoconstrictive effects of ephedra (primarily from ephedrine and pseudoephedrine) render it useful in conditions characterized by edematous tissues and congested membranes. Although it is used to treat patients with respiratory symptoms and common cold, it also is in widespread use as a weight loss aid (appetite suppressant) and euphoria agent (for its central nervous system stimulant properties). The most common toxic effects are usually those resulting from its sympathomimetic activitis, such as hypertension, palpitation, tachycardia, and stroke.[5] It may cause damage to the kidney secondary to ephedrine nephrolithiasis.[5,12]

Flavonoid Drugs

Flavonoids are plant constituents that are used to treat disorders of the peripheral circulation, liver diseases, phalloides intoxication, and intolerance to radiation therapy in Europe. They have been widely used around the world for many years. In China, extracts of *Taxus celebica,* which contains sciadopitysin, a flavonoid compound, is used in traditional medicine to treat diabetes mellitus.[6]

Intoxication manifests with fever and gastrointestinal upset several hours after taking a large dose of a flavonoid compound. This is followed by oliguric renal failure, cola-colored urine, and jaundice. Patients may develope hemolysis, cholestatic hepatitis, and disseminated intravascular coagulopathy. Biopsy shows acute interstitial nephritis with acute tubular necrosis.[13] The exact mechanism of flavonoid-induced renal failure is unknown. Acute tubulointerstitial nephritis and tubular necrosis could be the result of tubular toxicity of hemoglobulin from intravascular hemolysis. Direct nephrotoxicity through accumulation and uptake into tubular cells may be responsible and may explain why some patients develop renal failure after taking flavonoids for a prolonged period.

USE OF WRONG PREPARATION OR SUBSTITUTE

Plants may look alike and may even be considered to be interchangeable in certain traditional remedies. Furthermore, plants may get mixed up because they have similar names. A well-known example occurred in Brussels, Belgium, and involved the use of incorrectly identified herbs in slimming pills. In 1992, there was an outbreak of severe nephritis among young women in Brussels. Epidemiological survey identified a total of nine cases of renal failure among women who had undergone a slimming regimen in the same medical clinic.[14] Biopsy of the kidneys revealed extensive interstitial fibrosis, while the glomeruli were relatively spared. Patients progressed rapidly to end-stage renal failure (ESRF). Retrospectively, it was found that the clinic had changed the weight reduction regimen and introduced powdered extracts of Chinese herbs in the slimming pills. Subsequently, the syndrome was named Chinese herb nephropathy (CHN). Further investigation suggested that one of the herbs in the formula, *Stephania tetrandra,* was replaced by *Aristolochia* species due to misidentification.[14,15]

After publication of the index cases, similar cases were reported all around the world.[16-18] As a result of this episode, aristolochic acid (*Aristolochia* spp.) is probably the most notorious and best studied nephrotoxic herb-related agent. The major histological finding of the renal biopsy from affected kidneys is interstitial fibrosis with relative sparing of glomeruli.[19] Aristolochic acid nephrop-

athy is characterized by a lower proteinuria, more severe anemia, and faster progression to renal failure than other interstitial nephropathies.[16] Many patients developed ESRF and required maintenance dialysis or renal grafting. In Japan, aristolochic acid was reported to be associated with Fanconi's syndrome.[6] Proximal tubular cells were probably the primary target in this nephropathy.[5]

Exposure to aristolochic acid is also associated with a high incidence of uroepithelial tumorigenesis.[5,20] Attention was drawn to carcinogenicity after the discovery of cellular atypia throughout the urothelium of native kidneys removed at the time of transplantation in three patients with aristolochic acid nephropathy. Subsequently, in another 39 patients with aristolochic acid nephropathy who were being treated with dialysis or underwent transplantation, prophylactic surgical removal of native kidneys and ureters was performed. Among them, 18 cases of urothelial carcinoma were found, and mild-to-moderate dysplasia was found in 19 of the 21 remaining patients.[20] Regular cystoscopy was therefore recommended for patients with aristolochic acid nephropathy.

CONTAMINANTS AND ADULTERANTS

Impurities or the unexpected presence of chemicals or medication in alternative formulas is no rare finding.

Heavy Metals

Heavy metals may be introduced during manufacturing or by natural means due to the ubiquitous problem of soil and water pollution in certain regions. High levels of lead and cadmium have been found in some herbal medicines.[21] Furthermore, minerals or other adulterants may be added to traditional medicines for therapeutic purposes. Cadmium, lead, mercury, and arsenic have been identified in this context.[6,15] Details of nephrotoxicity due to heavy metal ingestion can be found in textbooks related to poisoning and drug overdose.[22]

Other nephrotoxic contaminants that have been identified in various reports include mefanamic acid, ephedrine, phenylbutazone, and paraphenylenediamine (PPD).[5,6,23] They have been found in the Chinese herbal mixtures (*Chuifong Tuokuwan),* Chinese herbal pills (*Tung Shueh),* and some other herbal preparations for arthralgia. Their presence has resulted in various types of renal injury, including interstitial nephritis, bilateral papillary necrosis, and kidney failure.

DRUG INTERACTIONS

One of the problems of the use of alternative medicine is multipharmacy. Many patients take herbs as supplementary medicine in addition to whatever they have been prescribed. This is especially alarming in patients with underlying renal disease and in those who have undergone transplantation, who are usually taking multiple conventional medications.

St. John's wort (*Hypericum perforatum*) is promoted as an antidepressant and anxiolytic agent. The active constituents are believed to be hypericins or hyperforins.[7,24] The proposed mechanism of action lies in the inhibition of serotonin, dopamine, and norepinephrine reuptake in the central nervous system. A number of systemic reviews and randomized trials have supported the efficacy of St. John's wort in patients with depression.[7,25] Although St. John's wort has a good safety profile as monotherapy,[25] concerns have been raised with regard to the possibility of important drug interactions.[26,27] Coadministration of St. John's wort reduces the plasma levels or efficacy of various conventional medicines. Induction of the cytochrome P-450 isoenzyme CYP3A4 and P-glycoprotein has been proposed as the underlying mechanism.[7] There are reports of acute graft rejection after renal transplantation, presumably due to decreased cyclosporine or tacrolimus activities after taking St. John's wort.[28,29]

OTHER ALTERNATIVE THERAPIES

Other alternative therapies may also be associated with renal injury.

Body Massage

Body massage is a type of CAM used to relieve pain or improve quality of life. It is considered relatively safe. However, recently there was a report of acute renal failure secondary to body massage. Rhabdomyolysis was induced by too vigorous body massage in an elderly man with diabetes mellitus.[30] Inadequate water intake potentiating the effect of rhabdomyolysis was postulated.

Mesotherapy

Mesotherapy is a form of CAM that involves multiple microinjections of homeopathic medication into mesoderm. It is used as a form of treatment for osteoarticular disease and has recently been used also as part of slimming regimens and cosmetic procedures. A case of ESRF due to rapidly progressive interstitial fibrosis after mesotherapy has been reported. An advanced degree of tubular loss and atrophy with tubulointerstitial fibrosis and progression to ESRF was observed. Inadvertent use of nephrotoxin for injection was suspected.[31]

Chelation Therapy

Chelation therapy is a process involving use of chelating agents to remove heavy metals from the body. It is a form of therapy with application in conventional as well as alternative medicine. Ethylenediamine tetra-acetic acid (EDTA) chelation therapy is used as a form of alternative therapy for atherosclerotic heart disease. Its effect is achieved by improving metabolic function and blood flow through blocked arteries throughout the body. This form of therapy has been reported to be associated with acute renal failure due to acute tubular necrosis.[31] The mechanism of nephrotoxicity is unknown but release of heavy metals with subsequent deposition in the tubulointerstitium may be the cause. Patients with pre-existing renal disease are more prone to the risk of nephrotoxicity.

Easy access to multiple chemicals or alternative medical agents via the Internet contributes to the diversity of kidney injury. For example, cases of renal failure after use of an alternative cancer remedy[32] and ingestion of an aromatic therapy mixture[33] purchased via the Internet were reported. A thorough history of chemicals or drugs taken is imperative in any patients suffering from renal injury.

THERAPEUTIC ROLES OF ALTERNATIVE THERAPIES IN RENAL FAILURE

Herbal medicine does not necessarily lead to nephrotoxicity. More than 50% of drugs used in the Western pharmacopoeia owe their origin to herbs and chemicals derived from plants.[5,34] Herbs may be of benefit to kidney health. Many herbs have been employed for their diuretic and renal protective actions for centuries. Studies are ongoing with regard to the use of herbs as treatment for renal failure.

Cs

Cs is a blade-shaped fungus that derives its nutrients from the larvae of *Lepidoptera* spp. found at high altitudes. In Chinese medicine, Cs is used as a kidney tonic. In vitro studies demonstrated antioxidant activity and inhibition of mesangial cell proliferation.[34] Human trials are limited, and more clinical studies are needed to fully evaluate the role and toxicity of this traditional and valued medication from ancient China.[35]

Rhubarb

Rhubarb root is used in Chinese medicine. It is a strong cathartic agent and is thought to increase excretion of waste products through the intestines. Many patients develop diarrhea after taking rhubarb root. In animal studies, it decreases proteinuria and glomerulosclerosis.[36]

Others

Salvia miltiorrhiza root contains many phenolic compounds with strong antioxidant actions. It is used in Chinese traditional formulas for renal failure. *Astragalus* species are also used in numerous Chinese recipes for renal disorders, and diuretic actions have been observed.[34] Ginsenoside-Rd demonstrated a renal protective effect in animal models.[37,38]

On the whole, the risk-benefit profile and the efficacy of herbal remedies are matters of concern. Further experiments are necessary to determine the roles of these medicines in the treatment of renal disease.

Key Points

1. Complementary and alternative medicine (CAM) is widely used all over the world.
2. Herbs are the most common example of CAM.
3. CAM-induced renal injury may be due to known drugs with nephrotoxicity, wrong con-

stituents, contaminants and adulterants, or drug interactions.

4. Aristolochic acid is believed to be the agent responsible for Chinese herb nephropathy. Licorice, *Ma Huang,* St. John's wort, heavy metals, and flavonoids can cause renal damage.
5. Therapeutic values of many herbs for renal disease are still under study.
6. Today's easy access to various chemicals and remedies with acclaimed therapeutic values results in increasing numbers and varieties of renal intoxication.
7. Enquiry regarding the use of CAM should be included in the patient history and assessment of renal failure.

Key References

5. Isnard Bagnis C, Deray G, Baumelou A, et al: Herbs and the kidney. Am J Kidney Dis 2004;44:1-11.
6. Colson CR, De Broe ME: Kidney injury from alternative medicines. Adv Chronic Kidney Dis 2005;12:261-275.
15. Wojcikowski K, Johnson DW, Gobe G: Medicinal herbal extracts: Renal friend or foe? Part 1: The toxicities of medicinal herbs. Nephrology (Carlton) 2004;9:313-318.
17. Yang CS, Lin CH, Chang SH, Hsu HC: Rapidly progressive fibrosing interstitial nephritis associated with Chinese herbal drugs. Am J Kidney Dis 2000;35:313-318.
34. Wojcikowski K, Johnson DW, Gobe G: Herbs or natural substances as complementary therapies for chronic kidney disease: Ideas for future studies. J Lab Clin Med 2006; 147:160-166.

See the companion Expert Consult website for the complete reference list.

CHAPTER 312

Environment, Smoking, Obesity, and the Kidney

Filippo Aucella, Mauro Cignarelli, Olga Lamacchia, and Loreto Gesualdo

OBJECTIVES

This chapter will:
1. Review the effects of environmental injury, smoking, and obesity in the critically ill.
2. Unravel the main pathophysiological mechanisms of these effects.
3. Suggest preventive and therapeutic measures.

ENVIRONMENT

The kidney is especially vulnerable to toxic injury because it receives about one quarter of the cardiac output and it transports and concentrates potentially toxic compounds within its parenchyma. The main mechanisms of nephrotoxicity are vasoconstriction, altered intraglomerular hemodynamics, tubular cell toxicity, interstitial nephritis, crystal deposition, thrombotic microangiopathy, and osmotic nephrosis. In the intensive care unit (ICU), many drugs are potential nephrotoxins. Here, we briefly review the roles of some environmental nephrotoxins (for heavy metals, see Chapter 313).

Environmental Nephrotoxins

Exposure to organic solvents has been suggested to cause or exacerbate renal disease.[1] Cellular toxicity appears to derive largely from metabolic activation within cells of free radical toxic metabolites, with initiation of lipid peroxidation reactions causing deleterious effects on cellular membrane structure and function. Moreover, nephrotoxins may themselves become covalently bound in damaging fashion to cellular macromolecules. However, methodological concerns regarding previous studies preclude firm conclusions. The results from a recent nationwide, population-based study do not support the hypothesis of an adverse effect of organic solvents on development of chronic renal failure in general, although detrimental effects from subclasses of solvents on specific renal diseases cannot be ruled out.[2]

Mycotoxins such as ochratoxin A, aflatoxin B, and the immunosuppressive agent cyclosporine may be nephrotoxic, and clinical syndromes have been documented.[3] Ochratoxin A is a ubiquitous nephrotoxic and carcinogenic mycotoxin considered to be involved in the etiology of Balkan endemic nephropathy.[4] The occurrence of this human fatal disease that appears in regions of Bosnia, Herzegovina, Bulgaria, Croatia, Romania, Serbia, and Montenegro correlates with a very high incidence of otherwise rare urothelial tumors of the renal pelvis and ureters. Although ochratoxin A was found more frequently or in higher concentration in the food and blood of inhabitants in regions with Balkan endemic nephropathy than in other regions, the involvement of ochratoxin A in the development of Balkan endemic nephropathy is still an open question.

Acute ethylene glycol intoxication is a medical emergency that, if not diagnosed correctly and treated aggressively, leads to serious neurological, cardiopulmonary, and renal dysfunction and may result in death.[5] Ethylene glycol toxicity is characterized by severe metabolic acidosis, with high anion and osmolal gaps, and calcium oxalate crystals in the urine. Early recognition of ethylene glycol intoxication and rapid, aggressive use of large amounts of sodium bicarbonate, ethanol infusion, and hemodialysis may improve the chance of survival.

Summary

Acute renal damage by environmental nephrotoxins should require admittance to the ICU. Clinicians need to be aware of this possibility, because correct diagnosis and management are critical to allow time for renal function to improve.

SMOKING

Smoke and the Patient in Intensive Care

Cigarette smoking is associated with excessive morbidity and mortality in various diseases, most prominently cardiovascular and lung diseases. It induces a variety of effects on the vascular and hormonal systems and is involved in the development of atherosclerosis, thrombogenesis, and vascular occlusion, all conditions that greatly influence the outcome of the critically ill patient admitted to the ICU. In fact, smokers experience an increased incidence of respiratory complications during anesthesia, increased risk of intraoperative and postoperative complications, and increased risk of postoperative ICU admittance.[6] Even passive smoking is associated with increased risk at operation. There is increasing evidence that it is also a risk factor for infection and wound-related complications. Long-term tobacco smoking (>50 pack-years) carries a higher risk of postoperative admission to the ICU, and there seems to be a dose relationship between the amount of tobacco consumed and the risk of postoperative ICU admission. Preoperative smoking cessation 6 to 8 weeks before surgery can reduce the risk of complications significantly. Four weeks of abstinence from smoking seems to improve wound healing. An intensive, individualized approach to smoking intervention results in a significantly better postoperative outcome. Future research should focus on the effect of a shorter period of preoperative smoking cessation. All smokers admitted for surgery should be informed of the increased risk, be advised of the benefits of preoperative smoking cessation, and be offered a smoking intervention program whenever possible.[7]

Smoking as a Renal Risk Factor

Despite increasing evidence, cigarette smoking has not been sufficiently acknowledged as a major renal risk factor, either in the general population or in ICU patients.[8] Smoking is reported to be associated with renal damage in the general population; particularly in men and in the elderly, it increases the albumin excretion rate, even in a range below the level of microalbuminuria.[9] Moreover, it is now clear that smoking increases not only the risk of albuminuria/proteinuria but also that of renal functional deterioration.[9]

Diabetologists were the first to recognize the adverse effects of smoking on the kidney. In both type 1 and in type 2 diabetes, smoking increases the risk of nephropathy development and almost doubles the rate of progression to end-stage renal failure (ESRF). In fact, in diabetic patients, smoking not only increases the risk of developing

TABLE 312-1

Smoking-Related Renal Damage: Main Potential Pathophysiological Mechanisms

Increased sympathetic activity: ↑ BP, ↑ HR
Alterations in intrarenal hemodynamics: ↓ GFR, ↓ FF, ↓ RPF, ↑ RVR
Cellular: ↑ oxidative stress, ↓ NO, ↑ ET-1
Hormonal imbalance: ↑ insulin resistance, ↑ vasopressin

↑, increase; ↓, decrease; BP, blood pressure; HR, heart rate; GFR, glomerular filtration rate; FF, filtration fraction; RPF, renal plasma flow; RVR, renal vascular resistance; NO, nitric oxide; ET-1, endothelin 1.

microalbuminuria[10] but also accelerates the rate of progression from microalbuminuria to manifest proteinuria,[11] and eventually to renal failure.[12]

Smoking has also been shown to increase the risk of progression to ESRF in patients with primary renal disease, whether inflammatory or noninflammatory (e.g., immunoglobulin A glomerulonephritis, polycystic kidney disease).[13,14]

Potential Mechanisms of Smoking-Related Nephrotoxicity

Several potential mechanisms of smoking-induced renal dysfunction and damage have been discussed,[8,14] but the precise nature of the nephrotoxic effect of smoking is not well understood (Table 312-1).

Smoking may induce albuminuria and abnormal renal function through advanced glycation end products (AGE). It is known that AGE are responsible for enhanced vascular permeability and that they accelerate the vasculopathy of diabetic ESRF. Moreover, aqueous extracts of tobacco and cigarette smoke contain glycotoxins, highly reactive glycation products that can rapidly induce in vitro and in vivo formation of AGE on proteins.[15] It is reasonable to expect that the AGE formed by the reaction of glycotoxins from cigarette smoke with serum and tissue proteins affect the systemic and renal vasculature.

Insulin resistance may be another possible mechanism underlying the pathophysiological effects of smoking-induced renal damage.[14] Several investigators have found smoking to be causally related to insulin resistance in nondiabetic persons. Insulin resistance has been known to be related to both albuminuria and abnormal renal function. Both of these mechanisms (AGE and insulin resistance) might act through endothelial dysfunction; that is, by inducing an imbalance between the contracting and relaxing substances produced by the endothelium. The plasma concentration of endothelin has been shown to be increased in smokers compared with nonsmokers, and further indirect evidence supports a disturbance of endothelin, prostacyclin, or nitric oxide release on stimulation in smokers. Smoking, by the induction of hypoxic stress, may interfere with vascular endothelial growth factor (VEGF) synthesis and activity; VEGF is a potent mitogen for endothelial cells, plays a central role in the regulation of vasculogenesis and vascular permeability, and seems to be involved in diabetic complications.

Moreover, smoke has also been shown to induce structural damage to the renal tissue. Smokers had a smoking dose-dependent increase in glomerular basement membrane width, which, along with mesangial expansion and arteriolar hyalinosis, is the structural hallmark of diabetic nephropathy.[16] Recently, Jaimes and colleagues demonstrated that human mesangial cells are endowed with the nicotinic acetylcholine receptors (nAChRs) α_4, α_5, α_7, β_2, β_3, β_4, and β_5.[17] In this manner, nicotine may accelerate and promote the progression of kidney disease. Moreover, smoking may be associated with podocyte injuries in patients with early diabetic nephropathy. More podocytes are excreted in the urine of smokers with microalbuminuria, compared to nonsmokers with microalbuminuria. Urinary podocytes disappeared after 3 years in 10 of 13 patients who stopped smoking, whereas urinary podocyte excretion increased in all patients who continued to smoke.[18]

The nicotine-induced increase in blood pressure and heart rate via sympathetic activation and vasopressin release appears to be a major mechanism contributing to the adverse renal effects of smoking.[8] Nicotine, apart from the cellular effects already cited, directly stimulates catecholamine release from peripheral sympathetic nerve endings and the adrenal medulla. On the basis of these vasoactive effects of smoking, it has been hypothesized that repeated episodes of acute renal hypoperfusion induced by smoking may favor structural alterations of preglomerular vessels and glomerular obsolescence, thus leading to hypertrophy and hyperfiltration of remnant glomeruli.[19] This would explain the elevated glomerular flow rate (GFR) that is observed in current smokers, compared with nonsmokers and former smokers. GFR is a predictor of glomerular basement membrane thickening, which is an early marker of kidney disease in diabetes.

Cigarette smoke exerts an inhibitory effect on components of the L-arginine–nitric oxide pathway. Therefore, potential effects of cigarette smoking on the availability of intracellular L-arginine may be one mechanism adversely influencing the survival of endothelial cells in the setting of oxidative stress and progressive atherosclerosis. Therefore, excessive or prolonged signaling induced by cigarette smoking may contribute to pathological fibrosis, scarring, and matrix deposition (i.e., remodeling) in a surprising variety of diseases—including, above all, diabetic nephropathy.[20]

Whether a genetic susceptibility determines an increased renal risk in smokers is an issue that deserves further investigation. In this context, a result of the Bergamo NEphrologic DIabetes Complications Trial (BENEDICT) is noteworthy: A genetic predisposition of smokers to develop albuminuria was found in carriers of the DD-genotype of the angiotensin-converting enzyme gene.[21]

Summary

In conclusion, smoking is clearly a risk factor for kidney involvement in critically ill patients. Smoking cessation is an opportunity after critical illness. Smokers make up a high percentage of patients admitted to the ICU, and the directive to stop smoking is one message that should be clearly given to recovering patients. The recovery period provides an important opportunity for patients to quit smoking, because the period of sedation and ventilation allows patients to start nicotine withdrawal.

OBESITY

Obesity and the Patient in Intensive Care

Critically ill obese patients are at increased risk of morbidity and mortality compared with nonobese patients.[22,23]

Obstructive airway disease, pneumonia, and sepsis are the main reasons for admission to the ICU in the morbidly obese group. Morbidly obese patients admitted to ICUs have higher rates of mortality, nursing home admission, and ICU complications, including sepsis, nosocomial pneumonia, acute respiratory distress syndrome, catheter infection, tracheostomy, and acute renal failure. Moreover, they have longer stays in the ICU and longer time on mechanical ventilation.[22,23] The care of critically ill obese patients is often complicated by the derangements in cardiovascular, respiratory, metabolic, and kidney function, all features of chronic obesity. In this regard, drug administration may be affected, depending on the lipophilicity of the molecule administered. The ability to gain vascular access is often impaired because of large body habitus and should be aided with ultrasound guidance. The fidelity of blood pressure monitoring can also be adversely affected, necessitating the use of direct intra-arterial monitoring.[24] However, in recent years the outcome of obese ICU patient seems to be improved.[24]

Obesity Is an Independent Risk Factor for Renal Damage

Obesity is a well-recognized risk factor for diabetes and hypertension, so the global obesity epidemic translates into substantially heightened risk factors for chronic kidney disease (CKD) worldwide. Obesity, especially abdominal obesity, not only increases the risk of hypertension but also makes hypertension more resistant to treatment. The higher blood pressures associated with overweight and obesity are probably due to multiple factors and include activation of the sympathetic nervous and renin-angiotensin systems, increased serum leptin levels, volume expansion, and sleep apnea. Uncontrolled hypertension in obese adults may certainly accelerate loss of kidney function over time, especially when compounded by the additional risks for CKD that accompany obesity.[25]

Aside from its link with traditional CKD risk factors, obesity itself may increase susceptibility to CKD via several potential mechanisms. Over the past several years, several cross-sectional and longitudinal studies from diverse populations have secured the importance of higher body weight for height as a risk factor in the prevalence and progression of CKD.[26,27] This causal association has mechanisms quite different from that of the so-called inverse epidemiology of ESRF, a condition in which a paradoxical association between higher body weight for height and survival has been found[28]; the latter finding is almost certainly explained by residual confounding due to malnutrition and competing mortality risks in the years preceding ESRF. The relation between excess weight and risk of CKD and ESRF appeared to persist even after accounting for the presence or absence of baseline diabetes and hypertension. Obesity, while having the strongest association with diabetic nephropathy, also carried a twofold to threefold increased risk for all major subtypes of chronic renal failure. Analyses that were confined to strata without hypertension or diabetes revealed a threefold increased risk among patients who were overweight at age 20 years, whereas the twofold observed risk elevation among those who had a highest lifetime BMI of greater than 35 was statistically nonsignificant.[27] So, obesity seems to be an important, potentially preventable, risk factor for chronic renal failure, with additional pathways different from those of hypertension and type 2 diabetes.

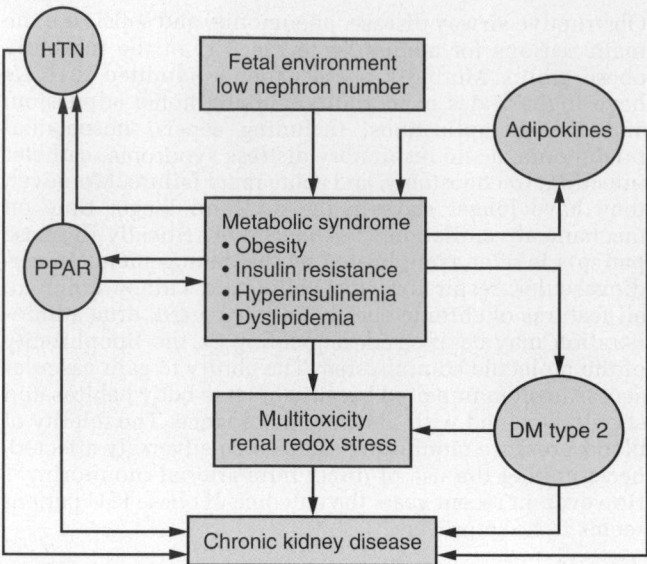

FIGURE 312-1. Obesity-related renal damage. DM, diabetes mellitus; HTN, hypertension; PPAR, peroxisome proliferator activated receptor. (Modified from Abrass CK. Overview: Obesity: What does it have to do with kidney disease? J Am Soc Nephrol 2004;15:2768-2772.)

Pathophysiological Mechanisms of Obesity-Related Renal Damage

Several molecular mechanisms have been proposed for obesity-related renal damage[29] (Fig. 312-1). First, adipose tissue is now recognized as an active endocrine organ that can affect the function of other organs and an important source of proinflammatory cytokines, chemokines, growth factors, and complement proteins called adipokines. Almost all of these influence the cardiovascular system, and many influence kidney function; they should be related to the outcome of the obese patient, especially among the critically ill. In this regard, leptin is the hallmark of these substances. In fact, it stimulates activity of the sympathetic nervous system, endocapillary cell proliferation, and mesangial collagen deposition; its renal effects are a natriuretic property and the ability to stimulate reactive oxygen species. So, leptin exerts a deteriorative impact on the cardiovascular system and kidneys by significant contributions to the pathogenesis of obesity-related hypertension and nephropathy.[29] On the other hand, in the ICU patient, leptin secretion is closely linked to the functions of the hypothalamic-pituitary-adrenal (HPA) axis and the immune system, both of which are crucial in influencing the course and outcome of critical illness. Both leptin and interleukin 6 (IL-6) are hypersecreted in acute critical illness (e.g., sepsis). Leptin inhibits, and IL-6 stimulates, the HPA axis. The negative relation between IL-6 and leptin is of paramount clinical importance, because high IL-6 levels are associated with poor outcome in critically ill patients, whereas plasma leptin levels are increased in survivors of acute sepsis; relatively low leptin levels may impair sympathetic system and immune functions.[30]

Another potential pathophysiological link between obesity and renal damage may be the metabolic syndrome. The fact that central adiposity modifies the association between overweight and obesity and measures of CKD points to the potential role of the metabolic syndrome. Central adiposity is frequently accompanied not only by hypertension but also by hypertriglyceridemia, low high-density lipoprotein (HDL) cholesterol, inflammation, and a prothrombotic state. These metabolic changes reflect a state of insulin resistance and its interaction with obesity.[29] Evidence linking metabolic syndrome and renal disease has only recently emerged. We can speculate on mechanisms of early renal damage in obesity-initiated metabolic syndrome.[31] Several possibilities, acting singly or in combination, deserve consideration: (1) adverse effects of adaptations to increased body mass/excretory load, (2) adverse effects of adaptations to obesity-induced sodium retention, (3) direct or indirect effects of hyperinsulinemia/insulin resistance, and (4) renal lipotoxicity.

Metabolic syndrome represents hyperinsulinemia, which may lead to structural renal changes.[25,32] Increased metabolic demands on the kidney may also mediate increased CKD risk in overweight and obesity. Weight gain increases the work of each individual nephron. Body size is positively correlated with glomerular size, GFR, and effective renal plasma flow. Increased filtration fraction in overweight and obese individuals, in the presence of increased blood flow, suggests the potential existence of increased glomerular capillary pressure. As an individual gains weight, single-nephron GFR must increase, and this occurs at the expense of increased capillary pressures.[33] These changes predispose the glomerular capillary wall to hemodynamic injury and glomerular hypertrophy. In the setting of obesity, there are multiple stimulants of transforming growth factor 1 (TGF-1), including increased levels of insulin and angiotensin II, heightened glomerular volume, and increased capillary pressures. These factors all interact and promote structural changes and glomerular damage. Individuals with reduced nephron mass possess a high risk for CKD in the setting of overweight and obesity. The compensatory glomerular hypertrophy among individuals with reduced nephron mass is compounded by the increased metabolic load imposed on the kidney by overweight and obesity. These individuals are also at high risk for subsequent development of other CKD risk factors, including hypertension and diabetes. However, this cascade of CKD risk factors can be avoided if these individuals with reduced nephron mass maintain an ideal body weight.

Obesity, especially morbid obesity, has been linked with focal segmental glomerulosclerosis (FSGS).[34] Obesity itself is unlikely to be the sole mediator of secondary FSGS, given the rarity of this disease in the general population, in contrast to the high prevalence of obesity. However, within a background of genetic susceptibility and perhaps other clinical risk factors including sleep apnea and reduced nephron number, obesity could potentiate development of secondary FSGS.

Summary

Obesity has clear pathophysiological effects on the kidneys. A thorough knowledge of the unique pathophysiological changes that occur in this population will allow prevention and more effective treatments.

Key Points

1. Environment is a possible source of acute nephrotoxic damage.
2. Smoking may induce albuminuria and abnormal renal function.

3. Obesity is an independent risk factor for chronic kidney disease.
4. Smoking habit and obesity influence the outcome of patients in the intensive care unit.

Key References

2. Fored CM, Nise G, Ejerblad E, et al: Absence of association between organic solvent exposure and risk of chronic renal failure. J Am Soc Nephrol 2004;15:180-186.
17. Jaimes E, Tian RX, Raij L: Nicotine: The link between cigarette smoking and the progression of renal injury? Am J Physiol Heart Circ Physiol 2007;292:H76-H82.
25. Kramer H: Obesity and chronic kidney disease. Contrib Nephrol 2006;151:1-18.

See the companion Expert Consult website for the complete reference list.

CHAPTER 313

Lead and Heavy Metals and the Kidney

Paolo Lentini, Lusine Poghosyan, and Claudio Ronco

OBJECTIVES

This chapter will:
1. Discuss the mechanisms of the renal toxicity related to heavy metals exposure.
2. Describe the clinical features of poisoning by heavy metals.
3. Analyze the therapeutic approaches to heavy metal intoxication.

There are more than 30 metals that can cause renal damage through occupational, therapeutic, or accidental exposure. The more common substances involved in renal damage are arsenic, barium, cadmium, cobalt, copper, lead, lithium, mercury, and platinum. Small amounts of these elements are necessary for good health, because they are important factors and cofactors in many biochemical reactions.

Heavy metals are used in industrial applications such as production of pesticides, batteries, alloys, and textile dyes. Excessive exposure may lead to specific disorders. The use of cisplatinum for cancer therapy and that of barium during radiological examinations, also can produce unexpected forms of toxicity due to heavy metals.

Heavy metals may enter into the human body through food, water, or air; acute poisoning can occur as the result of accidental contamination, suicide attempt, or an inappropriate use of some therapeutic measures.

MECHANISM OF HEAVY METALS TOXICITY

The kidney is a target organ in heavy metal toxicity because of its ability to reabsorb and concentrate divalent metals. The extent of renal damage depends on the nature, the dose, and the time of exposure. In general, acute damage differs from chronic damage in its mechanism of toxicity. As a consequence, the clinical features and therapeutic approach are also different.[1]

Heavy metals in plasma exist in both nondiffusible (protein-bound) and diffusible (complexed and ionized) forms. The luminal fluid in the early proximal tubule can contain both the bound form and the free form. The ionized form is toxic and produces direct cellular toxicity; the mechanism consists of membrane rupture and uncoupling of mitochondrial respiration, with the release of numerous death signals such as reactive oxygen species and cytokines.[2]

Metals are quickly cleared from the blood and are sequestered in many tissues; in acute intoxication, the main site of reabsorption is the apical membrane of the first zone of the proximal tubule, but also the loop of Henle and the terminal segments can participate in reabsorption of heavy metals. During chronic intoxication, on the other hand, the bound, inert form is conjugated with metallothionein and glutathione, which are then released into the blood by the liver and the kidney. These compounds are subsequently reabsorbed through an endocytotic process in segment S1 of the proximal tubule.[1,2]

THERAPEUTIC APPROACH

Treatment regimens include chelation therapy, decontamination procedures (e.g., charcoal, cathartics, emesis, gastric lavage), supportive care (e.g., intravenous fluids, cardiac stabilization, mechanical ventilation, exchange transfusion), and extracorporeal therapy. The choice of treatment depends on clinical parameters such as age; preexisting pathologies of the liver and kidney (affecting endogenous clearance); cardiovascular disease; toxicological parameters such as total body, liver, and renal clearances; elimination half-life; molecular weight; toxic dose; protein binding; and the apparent distribution volume.[3]

The remainder of this chapter presents specific considerations for some of the most common metals (Table 313-1).

TABLE 313-1

Therapy in Acute Heavy Metal Toxicity

METAL	HD	PD	CVVH	CVVHDF	TPE	HP	CHELATORS
Aluminum	No	No	?	?	No	Yes	DFO
Arsenic	HD + DMSA or HD + BAL	PD + DMSA or PD + BAL	?	?	?	?	BAL, DMSA, D-penicillamine
Barium	Yes	Yes	?	Yes	?	?	—
Bismuth	Yes	Yes	?	?	?	?	BAL, DMSA, DMPS
Cadmium	No	No	No	No	No	No	Calcium-EDTA
Chrome	No	No	No	No	No	No	—
Copper	HD + D-penicillamine	?	?	CVVHDF + D-penicillamine	No	Yes	D-penicillamine, BAL
Lead	No	No	No	No	?	No	Calcium-sodium-EDTA, BAL, DMSA
Lithium	Yes	Yes	Yes	Yes	No	No	No
Mercury	No	No	No	CVVHDF + DMPS	?	No	BAL, DMSA, DMPS (inorganic only)
Platin	Yes	Yes	?	?	Yes	No	No
Thallium	HD + Prussian blue	?	?	?	No	No	Prussian blue

BAL, dimercaprol; CVVH, continuous venovenous hemofiltration; CVVHDF, continuous venovenous hemodiafiltration; DFO, desferrioxamine; DMPS, dimercapo-1-propane sulfonate; DMSA, dimercaptosuccinic acid; EDTA, ethylenediamine tetra-acetic acid; HD, hemodialysis; HP, hemoperfusion; PD, peritoneal dialysis; TPE, therapeutic plasma exchange.

LEAD

Lead (Pb) is one of the oldest occupational toxins, and evidence of lead poisoning can be found dating back to Roman times. Lead is the most ubiquitous of the nephrotoxic metals, and humans are exposed to this agent in air, food, and water.

Source of Exposure

Lead exists in three different forms: metallic lead, inorganic lead (water-soluble lead salts), and organic lead such as tetramethyl lead, which is more toxic than the inorganic form.

Acute Exposure

Acute intoxication is extremely rare and occurs after accidental or intentional ingestion of water-soluble inorganic lead salts or inhalation of tetramethyl lead.

Chronic Exposure

Lead paint, drinking water, lead-glazed ceramics, and herbal remedies from Asia are potential sources of lead exposure. Workers in certain occupations are exposed to high levels of lead, including manufacture of ammunition, batteries, sheet lead, bronze plumbing, radiation shields, and intravenous pumps. Lead also contaminates emissions from motor cars with antiknock additives (tetramethyl lead).[4]

Mechanism of Kidney Damage
Acute Exposure

Acute lead poisoning disrupts the proximal tubular architecture, with histological changes featuring eosino-philic intranuclear inclusions in tubular cells consisting of lead-protein complexes as well as mitochondrial swelling.[5]

Chronic Exposure

The damage extends both to the proximal tubule and to the distal tubule with increased urate secretion, vasoconstriction, and glomerulosclerosis with hypertension and interstitial fibrosis.[6]

Clinical and Laboratory Features
Acute Exposure

Lead poisoning produces a metallic taste in the mouth, nausea, vomiting, diffuse abdominal pain, paresthesias, muscle weakness, and severe anemia with acute hemolytic crisis. Renal impairment may manifest as acute tubular necrosis with hematuria, casts, and aminoaciduria and may be so severe as to progress to frank acute renal failure. This damage occurs in 1 or 2 days. Severe toxicity, with a blood lead level of 50 μg/dL or more, also affects the central and peripheral nervous systems, with frank paralysis, tremors, decreased nerve conduction velocity, and papilledema.[6]

Chronic Exposure

Patients present with myalgias, fatigue, dyspnea, nonspecific abdominal pain, and anorexia. Renal damage includes glycosuria, aminoaciduria, and phosphaturia (Fanconi-like syndrome).

Laboratory Tests

Normochromic or hypochromic anemia with basophilic stippling; elevated reticulocyte count; elevation of blood urea nitrogen (BUN), creatinine, and serum uric acid; with amino acids, glucose, and ALA in the urine (proximal tubule damage) are common laboratory features.

The lead level in the whole blood is an indicator of recent exposure; the selected diagnosis to evaluate the lead level is the ethylenediamine tetra-acetic acid (EDTA) lead mobilization test.[5]

Treatment of Acute Lead Intoxication
Supportive Measures

Gastric lavage and decontamination with activated charcoal are indicated if lead salts have been ingested. Fluid-electrolyte balance must be maintained. Diuretic therapy is indicated, not to eliminate lead but to remove the chelators.[7]

Chelating Agents

In an inorganic lead intoxication, there is an indication to use EDTA, dimercaprol (BAL), dimercaptosuccinic acid (DMSA), and D-penicillamine.

Extracorporeal Therapies

Extracorporeal detoxification measures are ineffective because 95% of lead is stored in the erythrocytes; however, chelators, which are nephrotoxic, can be effectively removed by hemodialysis.[7] The half-life of lead in blood is 9 hours during combined hemodialysis and EDTA and 96 hours when EDTA is given alone.[8] Peritoneal dialysis, hemoperfusion, continuous renal replacement therapies (CRRT), and therapeutic plasma exchange are generally ineffective.

MERCURY

Mercury (Hg) is a silvery white liquid that is volatile at room temperature because of its high vapor pressure. Mercury exists in three forms: elemental, inorganic, and organic.

Source of Exposure

The general population is primarily exposed to this metal from dental amalgam and the diet; amalgam fillings are the most important source of inorganic mercury, and fish are the most important source of the organic one. Occupational exposure occurs in dentistry, in thermometer factories, and in the alloys and chloralkali industries.[9]

Mechanism of Kidney Damage

Mercury accumulates in the kidney and induces epithelial injury and necrosis in the pars recta of the proximal tubule.[10] After acute exposure to mercury, acute tubular necrosis appears, usually accompanied by oligoanuria.

Clinical and Laboratory Features
Acute Exposure

Elemental mercury in vapors produces symptoms after a few hours such as chills, vomiting, diarrhea, acute dyspnea with the occasional fatal form of interstitial pneumonitis, and neurological symptoms with hypotension and profuse salivation.

Chronic Exposure

Organic mercury gives skin manifestations and neurological disturbances such as ataxia, paresthesias, deafness. Mercury is now recognized as causing different types of kidney damage, such as nephrotic syndrome with membranous nephropathy pattern and tubular dysfunction with elevated urinary excretion of albumin, transferrin, retinol binding protein, and β-galactosidase.[10]

Laboratory Tests

A mercury concentration greater than 45 mg/dL in blood suggests acute poisoning.

Treatment of Acute Mercury Exposure
Supportive Measures

Immediate elimination of the metal by gastrointestinal decontamination and rapid administration of chelators, followed by intensive monitoring of hemodynamics and breathing, is necessary.

Chelating Agents

Treatment with chelators should be considered in patients with acute symptoms arising from the central nervous system. The antidotes currently available are BAL, dimercapo-1-propane sulfonate (DMPS), and DMSA.

Extracorporeal Therapies

Plasma protein binding of mercury is 95%, and the toxin is distributed in a large apparent volume of distribution; for these reasons, hemodialysis, peritoneal dialysis, and hemoperfusion with charcoal are poorly efficient.[7] On the other hand, hemodialysis is useful to eliminate chelators that are highly water-soluble. Continuous venovenous hemofiltration (CVVH) is more effective in removing the complex mercury-DMPS than is hemodialysis.[11] Among the extracorporeal elimination methods, plasma exchange appears to be the most efficient treatment to remove inorganic mercury and could be useful in association with chelation therapy.[12]

CADMIUM

Cadmium (Cd) can cause severe toxicity in humans. There are many cases of chronic intoxication due to exposure to cadmium but only a few cases of acute poisoning from oral ingestion or accidental inhalation of cadmium-containing fumes.

Sources of Exposure

Exposure to cadmium mainly results from eating contaminated food, smoking cigarettes, and working in cadmium-contaminated work places. Major industrial applications for cadmium are in the production of alloys and batteries.

Mechanism of Kidney Damage

Acute Exposure

The ionized, free form is primarily responsible for acute intoxication. It induces cellular toxicity by reduction of phosphate and glucose transport and by inhibition of mitochondrial respiration with membrane rupture of the proximal tubular cells of the nephron.[5]

Chronic Exposure

After ingestion or inhalation, cadmium is transported to the liver and to the kidney by metallothionein, which binds cadmium. A chronic tubular-interstitial nephropathy is produced by the accumulation of this metal in the S1 segment of the proximal tubule and in the medulla. Signs of cell apoptosis and cytokine pathway activation are common in this syndrome.

Clinical and Laboratory Features

Acute Exposure

The toxic symptoms include dyspnea, nausea, vertigo and vomiting, hypotension, shock, and acute renal and liver failure.

Chronic Exposure

Emphysema, cough, chronic kidney damage, and gastrointestinal ulcerations occur during chronic exposure. Renal damage by cadmium may result in tubular proteinuria with renal glycosuria, aminoaciduria, hyperphosphaturia, hypercalciuria, and polyuria with loss of concentration capacity.

Laboratory Tests

Exposure to cadmium is commonly determined by measuring 24-hour urinary cadmium excretion; an elevated urinary excretion of β_2-microglobulin has proved to be useful in detecting the more subtle signs of cadmium nephrotoxicity.[13]

Treatment of Acute Cadmium Exposure

Supportive Measures

Within 3 hours from the ingestion, it is recommended that gastrointestinal decontamination be performed, with support for cardiac and pulmonary function. Forced diuresis is not indicated, because cadmium is highly nephrotoxic.

Chelating Agents

Very soon after absorption, cadmium is stored in the erythrocytes and bound with metallothionein. There are no antidotes for cadmium intoxication. In contrast to the other heavy metals, chelators may actually increase cadmium nephrotoxicity.

Extracorporeal Therapies

The extracorporeal measures of detoxification are ineffective, because cadmium is fixed to cells; peritoneal dialysis, hemodialysis, and CRRT are used to remove chelators in acute renal failure caused by cadmium.[7]

CISPLATIN

Cisplatin is an antineoplastic agent that is used against various types of solid and hematological tumors; however, cisplatin is a drug with potential side effects, including nephrotoxicity, neurotoxicity, myelotoxicity, and ototoxicity.

Sources of Exposure

The typical source of exposure is chemotherapy.

Mechanism of Kidney Damage

The toxicity is dose-related. Cisplatin is a strong renal tubular toxin that can damage the S3 segment cells of the proximal tubule; the distal nephron may also be involved. The earliest change in tubule function is decreased protein synthesis due to the formation, via cytochrome P-450 enzymes, of highly reactive hydroxyl radicals that produce injury by DNA binding.[14]

Clinical and Laboratory Features

Accidental overdose of cisplatin may manifest as severe nausea, vomiting, loss of hearing, and oligoanuria with hematuria and casts in the urine. The urine osmolality is similar to that of plasma; this concentrating defect reflects platinum-induced damage to the loop of Henle.

Laboratory Tests

Liver damage, as indicated by elevated aspartate transferase (AST), alanine transferase (ALT), gamma-glutamyl transferase (GGT), and bilirubin values, and elevated renal dysfunction markers are common findings during acute cisplatin intoxication. Cisplatin is frequently associated with anemia due to erythropoietin deficiency induced by kidney injury.

Treatment of Acute Cisplatin Intoxication
Supportive Measures

The most common measures used to prevent cisplatin-induced nephrotoxicity are hydration with electrolyte replacement, forced diuresis, and antiemetic therapy; severe myelosuppression often requires the administration of granulocyte colony-stimulating factors.[15]

Chelating Agents

There is no specific chelation therapy for cisplatin intoxication. Amifostine, an organic thiophosphate, may diminish cisplatin-induced toxicity by donating a protective thiol group.

Extracorporeal Therapies

Hemodialysis is able to reduce free cisplatin in plasma, but the metal binds to plasma proteins after administration very quickly and cannot be further eliminated by this procedure. There is also a large rebound of cisplatin into plasma from an exchangeable pool after hemodialysis.

Plasmapheresis appears capable of removing both the protein-bound fraction and the cisplatin free form; Practical experiments have been conducted using a plasma filter and the substitution of 3 L of plasma for three to four sessions.[15]

ARSENIC

Arsenic (As) exists in inorganic forms (arsine gas, arsenite, and arsenate) and in organic forms (the trivalent and pentavalent forms). Acute high-dose exposure to arsenic can cause severe systemic toxicity and death.

Source of Exposure

Trivalent arsenic or arsenite compounds are considered the most toxic forms; common sources of exposure are pesticides, herbicides, homeopathic remedies, and contaminated water and food supplies.

Mechanism of Kidney Damage

Arsenic compounds are well absorbed after ingestion or inhalation. On entering the circulation, arsenic strictly binds hemoglobin. After 24 hours, it is accumulated in soft tissue; after 2 weeks, arsenic is incorporated in hair and nails.

Trivalent (+3) arsenic, the most toxic form, avidly binds to sulfhydryl groups and interferes with numerous enzyme systems, such as those of cellular respiration, with uncoupling oxidative phosphorylation.[7]

Clinical and Laboratory Features
Acute Exposure

Acute exposure can occur after ingestion or acute inhalation of high levels of arsenic dusts or fumes and in suicide or poisoning attempts. Acute toxicity symptoms include nausea, vomiting, abdominal pain, and diarrhea. These symptoms are soon followed by a diffuse pruritic macular rash, dehydration, hemodynamic instability, and acute respiratory distress syndrome. Renal injury can lead to oligoanuria, proteinuria, hematuria, and acute tubular necrosis; renal damage is intensified by hemoglobinuria due to hemolysis and hypotension.[16]

Chronic Exposure

In chronic poisoning, peripheral neuropathy and encephalopathy with cognitive impairment are the predominant manifestations.

Laboratory Tests

ACUTE EXPOSURE. Measurements of arsenic levels in the urine are more significant than those in the blood, because arsenic is rapidly cleared from the blood. Excretion of more than 200 µg in a 24-hour urine collection is suggestive of arsenic overload.

CHRONIC EXPOSURE. Chronic arsenic exposure can be confirmed by a 24-hour urine collection and arsenic concentration determination.

Treatment of Acute Arsenic Intoxication
Supportive Measures

The first step is the elimination of further exposure. Gastrointestinal decontamination with charcoal and forced emesis is recommended, with careful assessment of the intravascular volume and administration of fluids and electrolytes. Moreover, because arsenic is well eliminated by urine, it is useful to force diuresis.

Chelating Agents

In a severely ill patient with acute arsenic poisoning, chelation may be required; BAL and DMSA are the most frequently used agents.

Extracorporeal Therapies

Hemodialysis has very limited capacity in arsenic removal, but it can be used to remove chelators that are nephrotoxic. Furthermore, hemodialysis and other extracorporeal blood purification techniques should be used if acute renal failure develops. CVVH-CVVHDF with a large-pore membrane is preferred to help maintain greater hemodynamic stability. In association, exchange transfusion has been used in severe arsenic intoxication, providing some benefit.[7]

Peritoneal dialysis and hemoperfusion are inefficient and are not indicated.

LITHIUM

Lithium (Li) carbonate is commonly prescribed for the treatment of bipolar manic-depressive disorder. Either during chronic maintenance therapy or in acute treatment/overdose, lithium may lead to severe toxicity

Sources of Exposure

Lithium ingestion can occur accidentally or in suicide attempts. Antidepressive therapy may also lead to excessive exposure.

Mechanism of Kidney Damage

Lithium carbonate is almost completely absorbed by the tissues within the 8 hours after distribution into the intravascular space; therefore, there is a rapid disappearance from the plasma and a slow excretory phase. In fact, 95% of a dose is excreted in urine—30% to 60% during the first 12 hours and 70% to 40% during the next 10 to 14 days. Lithium is a small ion that does not bind to proteins; however, lithium diffusion between intracellular and extracellular compartments is slow.[7]

Clinical and Laboratory Features

The patient with acute lithium intoxication has stupor, tremor, confusion, hemodynamic instability, vomiting, diarrhea, hyperreflexia, and acute renal failure, sometimes with polyuria and casts in the sediment. Chronic lithium ingestion is a common cause of nephrogenic diabetes insipidus, renal tubular acidosis, nephrotic syndrome (minimal change or focal-segmental glomerulosclerosis), and chronic interstitial nephropathy.[17]

Laboratory Tests

The serum lithium therapeutic range is 0.4 to 1.2 mmol/L. Values exceeding this range are significant for intoxication; however, values in the normal range do not exclude excessive exposure.

Treatment of Acute Lithium Intoxication
Supportive Measures

Gastric lavage and administration of emetics should be carried out within 8 hours after acute overdose. Patients with normal renal function should initially be treated with a rapid infusion of saline with sodium bicarbonate to increase the urinary lithium output. If the patient has a severe intoxication with coma, convulsions, and acute renal failure, the only treatment should be the application of renal replacement therapy. Cardiac monitoring and mechanical ventilation are recommended during acute intoxication.

Chelating Agents

There are no chelating agents specific for acute lithium intoxication.

Extracorporeal Therapies

To accelerate lithium clearance when levels are higher than 3.5 mmol/L, as in the case of acute intoxication,

various modalities of extracorporeal blood purification may provide adequate results.

HEMODIALYSIS. Being a small, non–protein-bound molecule, lithium is rapidly removed by hemodialysis with simultaneous correction of acid-base and electrolyte disorders. High-efficiency bicarbonate dialysis is recommended. Mixed diffusive-convective therapies such as hemodiafiltration and dialysis with high-flux membranes (e.g., polysulfone, polyamide, polymethylmethacrylate [PMMA]), seem to be even more efficient, and they represent the first-choice therapy for severe acute lithium intoxication.[18] The efficiency of extracorporeal removal is limited by a high postdialysis rebound of lithium levels due to compartmentalization of the molecule.

PERITONEAL DIALYSIS. Lithium can be removed by peritoneal dialysis, although its clearance is much lower than in hemodialysis. Peritoneal dialysis can be considered an alternative when hemodialysis is not available.[18]

HEMOPERFUSION. Because the adsorption of lithium with activated charcoal or resins is very limited, the technique of hemoperfusion is poorly efficient.

CONTINUOUS RENAL REPLACEMENT THERAPIES. CRRT can result in a remarkable blood purification, removing also intracellular lithium by preventing postdialysis rebound. However, CRRT in cases of acute intoxication does not reduce the lithium level as rapidly as hemodialysis does. The best treatment for acute lithium intoxication appears to be the combination of hemodialysis for rapid lithium removal, followed by continuous hemodiafiltration to prevent postdialysis rebound.[18]

OTHER HEAVY METALS

Few papers in the literature report about acute renal failure caused by other heavy metals such as uranium, bismuth salts, hexavalent chromium, aluminum, vanadium, and copper. Treatment for poisoning by these agents is not well codified, and evidence for various therapies is scanty.

CONCLUSION

Thanks to improvements in industrial safety, cases of acute heavy metal poisoning are less frequent, but they remain a cause of acute renal failure that should always be considered in suicide attempts, cases of accidental contamination, and environmental or industrial disasters.

Key Points

1. Acute toxicity differs completely from chronic toxicity in its clinical, diagnostic, and therapeutic aspects.
2. The extracorporeal treatments, even if not always as decisive as chelation, are nevertheless the key strategy in accelerating detoxification and improving the outcome of patients with acute poisoning; these treatments also play an important role in renal detoxification related to nephrotoxicity of chelating agents.
3. The use of continuous renal replacement therapy, particularly continuous venovenous hemofiltration and hemodiafiltration, as yet not well codi-

fied, appears to offer particular advantages under the conditions of hemodynamic instability that characterize the poisoning state, without reducing the purifying effect.

Key References

1. Sabolic I: Common mechanisms in nephropathy induced by toxic metals. Nephron Physiol 2006;104:107-114.
2. Barbier O, Jacquillet G, Tauc M, Cougnon M: Effects of heavy metals on and handling by the kidney. Nephron Physiol 2005;99:105-110.

7. Seyfart G: Poison Index: Heavy Metals Intoxication, 4th ed. Berlin, Pabst Science Publishers, 1997, pp 90-97, 390-410.
9. Clarkson TW, Magos L, Myers GJ: The toxicology of mercury—current exposures and clinical manifestations. N Engl J Med 2003;349:1731-1737.
15. Hofman G, Bauernhofer T, Krippl P, et al: Plasmapheresis reverses all side-effects of a cisplatin overdose: A case report and treatment recommendation. BMC Cancer 2006;6:1-7.

See the companion Expert Consult website for the complete reference list.

CHAPTER 314

Statins and the Kidney

A. D. Booth and Adeera Levin

OBJECTIVES

This chapter will:
1. Discuss the role of statins in inflammatory atherosclerotic disease.
2. Explore the potential benefits of statins on vascular disease in patients with kidney disease.
3. Explain the potential beneficial effect of statins on kidney function.
4. Discuss whether the benefits of statins extend beyond their cholesterol-lowering effects.

Cardiovascular events and renal failure are common conditions, the management of which frequently requires admission to intensive care units with associated patient and economic costs.[1] There is a clear need to reduce cardiovascular risk and preserve renal function. The 3-hydoxy-3-methylglutaryl coenzyme A (HMG-CoA) reductase inhibitors (statins) are a group of lipid-lowering agents that reduce mortality in patients who are at risk for or have cardiovascular disease.[2] Patients with chronic kidney disease (CKD) are at particular risk for cardiovascular events and progression to renal failure.[3] It has been suggested that the clinical benefit of statins extends beyond that attributable to the reduction in low-density lipoprotein (LDL) and LDL cholesterol levels, the so-called pleiotropic effects.[4] This review discusses the potential benefits of statins on both cardiac and renal outcomes in patients with CKD.

ATHEROSCLEROSIS: AN INFLAMMATORY DISEASE

Atherosclerosis is considered to be a systemic inflammatory disease in which endothelial dysfunction is a key early finding. In vitro studies have shown that reduced bioavailability of endothelial-derived nitric oxide (NO) is associated with increased expression of endothelial-derived adhesion molecules, such as selectins, intracellular adhesion molecules (ICAM-1), and vascular cell adhesion molecule 1 (VCAM-1). Leukocyte margination, adhesion, and migration into the subendothelial space occurs under the influence of chemotactic stimulants such as monocyte chemoattractant factor 1 (MCP-1) and is influenced by vascular smooth muscle cells.[5] There is increased expression of cytokines, such as tumor necrosis factor α (TNF-α), interleukin 6 (IL-6), and interferon-γ. Plaque formation is augmented by uptake of lipid by the infiltrating macrophages and formation of oxidized LDL.[6] Matrix metalloproteases (MMPs) and leukocyte-derived myeloperoxidases may also influence plaque stability.[7]

In vivo, circulating C-reactive protein (CRP), an acute-phase reactant, independently predicts risk in patients with cardiovascular disease and in healthy individuals. TNF-α and IL-1 are also associated with increased cardiovascular risk.[8] Endothelial dysfunction independently predicts cardiovascular events.[9] Vasomotor endothelial dysfunction, reflecting reduced bioavailability of NO, has been reported in patients with cardiovascular risk factors such as diabetes, hypertension, hypercholesterolemia, and smoking.[10-13] Inflammation and endothelial dysfunction have been linked in in vivo experimental models of induced acute inflammation and in clinical conditions such as rheumatoid arthritis and systemic vasculitis.[14]

Potential therapeutic targets in the management of atheromatous disease include LDL levels, inflammation, and endothelial dysfunction—all processes exacerbated by traditional risk factors such as hypertension, smoking, diabetes, and hyperlipidemia.

STATINS, ATHEROSCLEROSIS, AND INFLAMMATION

Statins reduce cholesterol levels by inhibiting HMG-CoA reductase, the rate-limiting step in cholesterol synthesis. Statins reduce mortality in patients who are at risk or who have cardiovascular disease. A 30% to 50% reduction in LDL levels has been reported in large trials, depending on the dose and nature of the drug used.[2] It remains unclear whether the absolute reduction in the level of LDL or the alteration in lipid composition (high-density lipoprotein, triglycerides, or LDL microparticles) is important. In addition to the lipid-lowering effects, statins have also been shown to influence inflammatory activity.[4] They reduce circulating CRP and plaque levels of TNF-α, IL-1 and IL-6, MCP-1, and expression of nuclear factor κB (NF-κB), the factor controlling cytokine expression. Furthermore, statins may also reduce expression of endothelial adhesion molecules, leukocyte chemotaxis/proliferation, and monocyte differentiation into macrophages. These drugs also stabilize and increase endothelial nitric oxide synthase (eNOS) expression in humans. This has been supported by improvement in endothelial-dependent vasodilatory responses (NO-mediated vasomotor function). The anti-inflammatory effects of statins are thought to occur through interference with the synthesis of isoprenoid compounds. The resulting inhibition of isoprenylation leads to influences on the guanosine triphosphatases Ras, Rac, and Rho, factors known to influence cell activation and proliferation.[15]

STATINS AND CARDIOVASCULAR RISK IN PATIENTS WITH CHRONIC KIDNEY DISEASE

The major cause of morbidity and mortality in patients with CKD is cardiovascular disease. This risk is particularly high in these patients compared with an age-matched population.[3] Furthermore, the cardiac event rate rises as the estimated glomerular filtration rate (eGFR) falls, and in patients undergoing dialysis, 40% of deaths are attributed to cardiovascular causes.[3,16] Both traditional and nontraditional risk factors, such as anemia, proteinuria, dyslipidemia, hyperphosphatemia, and CRP, are more prevalent in patients with CKD. The influence of traditional and nontraditional risk factors on cardiovascular risk and the interactions among these factors remain unclear. Most of the large cardiovascular outcome studies (randomized, controlled trials) using statins have excluded patients with significant renal disease, and, although it is tempting, there is a danger in extrapolating the benefits of statin therapy from the general population to those patients with eGFR less than 60 mL/min/1.73 m². Indeed, loss of GFR is associated not only with intimal-mediated atherogenesis but also with medial calcification. Vascular smooth muscle cells are transformed into osteoblast-like cells that are capable of producing a matrix of bone collagen and noncollagenous proteins. Calcification may then result. In more severe renal disease, the degree of calcification correlates with the cardiovascular mortality rate.[17] The resulting "inflammatory vasculopathy" suggests an alteration in the pathophysiology as GFR declines.

Statins significantly improve lipid profiles of patients with CKD, lowering levels of total cholesterol by 18%, LDL by 24%, and triglycerides by 13%. It remains unclear whether the absolute level of LDL or the alteration in lipid composition is important in patients with renal disease and atherosclerosis. Retrospective studies in patients undergoing hemodialysis have suggested that statin use is associated with a reduction in cardiac death by 36%.[18] However, the only reported randomized, controlled trial in diabetic patients with end-stage renal failure, the so-called 4D study, assessed the effect of 20 mg atorvastatin in diabetics undergoing hemodilalysis.[19] A 4-year follow-up of this patient group demonstrated a 42% reduction in LDL but no change in the composite endpoint of nonfatal myocardial infarction and cardiovascular mortality. There is an ongoing trial of rosuvastatin (10 mg daily) in 2000 patients with end-stage renal failure (the Aurora Study).[20] The Study of Heart and Renal Protection (SHARP) is an international, multicenter, randomized, controlled trial that aims to determine the effects of lowering blood cholesterol with a combination of simvastatin (20 mg daily) and the cholesterol-absorption inhibitor ezetimibe (10 mg daily) on the risk of major vascular events among 9000 patients with CKD who do not have established coronary heart disease.[21] The presence of the control limb containing a cholesterol-lowering arm may allow the pleiotropic effects of the statin to be determined.

STATINS AND CHRONIC KIDNEY DISEASE

Hyperlipidemia is associated with initiation and progression of kidney disease through the process of atherogenesis or the direct toxic effects of lipids on renal cells, or both. Studies in vitro and in animals have shown an association between hyperlipidemia and mesangial, glomerular, and tubular cell injury. Mesangial matrix expansion is stimulated by LDL and accompanied by leukocyte recruitment, expression of endothelial adhesion molecules (VCAM-1 and ICAM-1), and increased IL-6, TNF-α, and MCP-1. Statins reduce the levels of both LDL and inflammatory mediators.[22] Furthermore, reduction in the cytotoxicity of oxidized LDL on mesangial cells and increased NO bioavailability have been shown.

Statins may also reduce proteinuria, a major determinant of progression in both experimental and human nephropathies. Reduction in proteinuria is associated with improvement in renal and cardiovascular outcomes.[23] High levels of urinary proteins, which reflect excess protein trafficking through the glomerulus, are associated with a faster course of disease.[24] Experimental observations suggested mechanisms whereby enhanced tubular reabsorption of proteins contributes substantially to promote interstitial inflammatory and fibrogenic reactions that evolve to renal scarring. Statins have been shown, first, to reduce protein filtration at the glomerulus through improvement in podocyte function. Second, they block receptor-mediated endocytosis of filtered protein through inhibition of prenylation. Third, they may also act to reduce inflammation. The resulting degree of proteinuria is therefore a balance between the expected short-term increase in tubular protein loss and the longer-term reduction in proteinuria. A number of randomized, controlled trials have attempted to determine whether the in vitro benefit of statins translates into the clinical situation. Only one of the four trials in diabetic nephropathy suggested a reduction in microalbuminuria, and in that study the placebo arm was associated with an increase in proteinuria. Of the nine trials in patients with nondiabetic nephropathy reviewed by Agarwal, six showed that statins have beneficial effects on proteinuria.[25] It is unclear whether this is a class effect, a dose effect, or both. Furthermore, rosuvastatin has been associated with increased tubular protein loss in 12% of patients at higher doses.

Statins may also have beneficial effects on eGFR. A meta-analysis of 13 small, prospective trials demonstrated a slowing in the decline of GFR (–0.16 mL/min/mo; 95% confidence interval, 0.03 to 0.29 mL/min/mo; P = .008). Post hoc analysis of three randomized, placebo-controlled trials in patients with high cardiovascular risk suggested that statins are associated with improved renal outcome in such patients.[26] The Cholesterol and Recurrent Events (CARE) study (N = 690), using pravastatin (40 mg daily), demonstrated a reduced rate of decline in eGFR, which was most beneficial for the lower eGFR group (baseline, <50 mL/min/1.73 m²) over a period of 4.9 years. The Heart Protection Study (N = 20,000) showed a slower rise in serum creatinine over 4.6 years in the simvastatin group. The Greek Atorvastatin and Coronary Heart Disease Evaluation Study (N = 1600) suggested a 12% increase in creatinine clearance associated with atorvastatin.[26] Although there are large inherent problems in extrapolating results from post hoc analyses, these findings suggest that statins may be associated with potential renoprotection.

STATINS AND ACUTE KIDNEY INJURY

Animal models have shown potential benefits of statins in reducing ischemia/reperfusion injury independent of cholesterol levels. The partial inhibition of Rho, activation of eNOS, and higher availability of NO after statin treatment are thought to play a major role in this protection. Whether this potential benefit translates into clinical improvement in renal endpoints remains unknown.

Statin use is rarely associated with rhabdomyolysis (see Chapter 75). A systematic review of 20 randomized, controlled trials showed that the incidence of rhabdomyolysis was 3.4 (range, 1.6 to 6.5) per 100,000 person-years.[27] The case-fatality rate was 10%. Incidence was higher among patients treated with statins metabolized by the cytochrome P-450 isoenzyme CYP3A4, such as lovastatin, simvastatin, or atorvastatin. Sixty percent of cases involved drugs known to inhibit CYP3A4, such as erythromycin and azole antifungals, and 19% involved fibrates.

ARE THE "PLEIOTROPIC EFFECTS" OF STATINS INDEPENDENT OF CHOLESTEROL LOWERING?

Although there are increasing reports of anti-inflammatory, immunomodulatory, and vascular effects of statins, it is not clear that these observations are independent of the lipid-lowering effects or that they contribute additional cardiovascular risk reduction beyond that expected from the degree of LDL lowering. Few studies have had a control arm containing a cholesterol-lowering treatment such as ezetimibe or fibrates. Indeed, in humans, a single LDL apheresis has been shown to improve endothelial function in hypercholesterolemic patients.[28] Fibrates have been shown to improve endothelial function and to reduce oxidative stress. Cholesterol reduction per se may reduce inflammation through alteration in the membrane composition of lipid rafts (cell signaling domains). This in turn, may alter endothelial function and leukocyte signaling.[29] Furthermore, large-scale studies in hypercholesterolemic patients have shown that coadministration of ezetimibe with a statin results in greater CRP reduction than does statin therapy alone. The SHARP study should address this concern in renal progression.[21]

CONCLUSION

The impact of the cholesterol-lowering effects of statins in patients with CKD remains undetermined. Once this effect is controlled for in large trials, then the pleiotropic effects of statins can be explored and the impact of these on patients with CKD and end-stage renal failure determined. Although benefit is unproven, it is logical to offer statin therapy as part of an aggressive cardiovascular risk-reduction strategy in patients with CKD. Statins are rarely associated with acute renal injury, and initiating therapy in patients with acute renal failure from other causes needs careful consideration.

Key Points

1. Statins improve morbidity and mortality in patients who are at risk for or have cardiovascular disease.
2. Post hoc analysis of randomized, controlled trials suggests that these benefits should also accrue to patients with chronic kidney disease, but one such trial failed to show benefit in dialysis; results of the SHARP study are awaited.
3. Statins may influence the progression of kidney disease through effects on proteinuria and glomerular filtration rate.
4. Beneficial effects of statins beyond cholesterol lowering are suggested but not proven.
5. Animal studies suggesting potential protective effects of statins in acute kidney injury have not yet been shown to have clinical benefit.

Key References

2. Gotto AM Jr, LaRosa JC: The benefits of statin therapy: What questions remain? Clin Cardiol 2005;28:499-503.
10. Makimattila S, Liu ML, Vakkilainen J, et al: Impaired endothelium-dependent vasodilation in type 2 diabetes: Relation to LDL size, oxidized LDL, and antioxidants. Diabetes Care 1999;22:973-981.
15. Wolfrum S, Jensen KS, Liao JK: Endothelium-dependent effects of statins. Arterioscler Thromb Vasc Biol 2003;23:729-736.
19. Wanner C, Krane V, Marz W, et al; German Diabetes and Dialysis Study Investigators: Atorvastatin in patients with type 2 diabetes mellitus undergoing hemodialysis. N Engl J Med 2005;353:238-248.
21. Baigent C, Landry M: Study of Heart and Renal Protection (SHARP). Kidney Int Suppl 2003;(84):S207-S210.
29. Mason RP, Walter MF, Jacob RF: Effects of HMG-CoA reductase inhibitors on endothelial function: Role of microdomains and oxidative stress. Circulation 2004;109(21 Suppl 1):II34-II41.

See the companion Expert Consult website for the complete reference list.

CHAPTER 315

Erythropoietin Therapy in Critically Ill Patients

Anton Verbine and Claudio Ronco

OBJECTIVES

This chapter will:
1. Review available evidence on the use of erythropoietin (EPO) in the intensive care unit population.
2. Discuss practical benefits and drawbacks of correction of "anemia of critical illness" with EPO.
3. Explore nonhematological actions of EPO and the potential use of recombinant human EPO in acute renal failure as a renoprotective hormone.

Human erythropoietin (EPO) is a 30.4-kDa glycoprotein hormone that was originally isolated as a hematopoietic growth factor. It is widely accepted that EPO promotes the survival, proliferation, and differentiation of erythroid precursor cells. Binding of EPO to its receptor on burst-forming and colony-forming units of early erythroid precursors changes the balance of proapoptotic and antiapoptotic factors via the BCL2 family of genes. As a result, large numbers of erythrocyte precursors survive and progress to mature erythrocytes.

EPO is primarily produced by interstitial cells (fibroblasts) of the renal cortex. Normally, low baseline levels of EPO in plasma are sufficient to maintain erythropoiesis. Anemia and tissue hypoxia cause release of hypoxia-inducible factor 1 (HIF-1), with resulting increase in both expression of the EPO gene and EPO production by a thousand times. There is an inverse relationship between serum EPO and hemoglobin concentrations in chronic anemia, and levels of EPO remain elevated until anemia is corrected.

The EPO gene was successfully cloned in 1985, and nowadays recombinant human EPO (rHuEPO), with its longer-acting hyperglycosylated analogue, is widely available commercially. Meanwhile, in contrast to the extensive clinical experience with rHuEPO for correction of various chronic anemias, its use in acute settings continues to be controversial, and no large trials have been completed.

RECOMBINANT HUMAN ERYTHROPOIETIN AND ANEMIA OF CRITICAL ILLNESS

Anemia is extremely common in the intensive care unit (ICU) patient population. Large cohort studies across the United States and Western Europe indicate that 20% to 53% of critically ill patients require blood transfusions, with a mean of about 5 units of red blood cells (RBCs) transfused during the ICU stay.[1-3]

Although anemia is usually multifactorial, with contributing blood loss from frequent blood sampling, various procedures, occult gastrointestinal bleeding, and other causes, the iron deficiency component cannot explain the severity of anemia in most cases. Patients with sepsis are known to have a greater decline in hemoglobin and continuous progression of anemia during their hospital stay, compared with other nonbleeding ICU patients.[4]

An important contributor to decreasing hemoglobin levels, known as *anemia of critical illness*, is usually linked to sepsis or major tissue injury and presumably results from an acute inflammatory response. Elevated levels of C-reactive protein, interferon-γ, tumor necrosis factor-α, interleukin 10, interleukin 13, and other inflammatory mediators are also known to be associated with increased resistance to exogenous EPO in patients with chronic kidney disease.[5,6] Anemia of critical illness shares many laboratory and clinical features with anemia of chronic disease, including low serum iron, low serum transferrin, high serum ferritin, blunted erythropoietic response to EPO, and relative decrease of EPO production,[7,8] and may represent an acute variant of that condition.

Acute renal failure (ARF) is closely linked to necrosis, apoptosis, and dysfunction of both endothelial and parenchymal cells in renal cortex. It appears, however, that damage to renal fibroblasts and subsequent decreased EPO production is not the major mechanism of anemia in ARF and cannot by itself explain the extent of hemoglobin decrease during the course of critical illness.

Some studies have provided insight about the pattern of EPO concentration change during the progression of acute illness. During the first 1 or 2 days of critical illness, the concentration of EPO was found to be increased to supranormal serum levels in critically ill patients with ARF.[9] High EPO concentration in patients with multiple organ failure seemed to correlate with higher Acute Physiology and Chronic Health Evaluation (APACHE) score, an acute inflammatory response, and the presence of ARF. By day 3 and until the recovery from ARF, blood EPO levels were in the low-normal range.[9,10] When compared to the response to iron deficiency, this EPO secretion is inappropriately low for the degree of anemia—a so-called blunted EPO response. This phenomenon occurs in sepsis as well as in ARF, and a number of authors have suggested that inflammatory mediators have a role in its development.[11]

Exogenous rHuEPO was able to overcome some effects of inflammatory mediators on erythropoietic marrow, and it was known to improve hemoglobin levels in anemia of chronic disease resulting from AIDS, chronic autoimmune diseases, and nonmyeloid cancers. It was also capable of modulating iron metabolism in critically ill patients, at

TABLE 315-1

Summary of the Effects of Recombinant Human Erythropoietin (rHuEPO) in Patients in the Intensive Care Unit

Increased reticulocyte count (on average by week 2)

Higher rise in hemoglobin and hematocrit from baseline (on average by weeks 3-6)

Higher level of hemoglobin and hematocrit compared with controls (usually iron only) by the end of the study

Significant reduction in the number of RBC transfusions (on average 1-3 RBC units per patient)

No increase in complications that could be attributed to EPO (e.g., thrombosis, pure RBC aplasia) so far

No benefit in mortality or ICU length of stay reported.

EPO, erythropoietin; ICU, intensive care unit; RBC, red blood cell.

least by increasing the level of serum transferring receptors.[12] So, there were logical reasons to try exogenous EPO in anemia of critical illness, particularly in cases with coexisting ARF.

The half-life after subcutaneous administration of rHuEPO in ICU patients (mean, 15.0 ± 6.12 hours) is comparable to that in healthy subjects[13] and seems to depend mostly on adsorption, rather than elimination, because the terminal half-life of rHuEPO is longer after subcutaneous administration.

At least six prospective randomized studies, involving from 21 to more than 1000 patients, have evaluated the effects of rHuEPO in the ICU patient population.[11-17] Trials utilized various doses and dosing schedules (from one to three times weekly) for either subcutaneously or intravenously administered rHuEPO (average, 40,000 to 120,000 U/wk), but the results were remarkably similar in many ways (Table 315-1).[11] Administration of rHuEPO was able to overcome the blunted response to EPO in all studies of anemia of critical illness. Significantly higher reticulocyte counts and a significantly higher rise in hemoglobin and hematocrit were noted in rHuEPO-treated subjects. Significantly higher hemoglobin and hematocrit levels were reached in the treated groups at the end of the studies, despite administration of fewer RBC transfusions. However, none of these studies was able to show a decrease in mortality, hospital length of stay, or ICU length of stay in rHuEPO-treated subjects. Neither did rHuEPO affect the rate of renal recovery in a retrospective cohort study of patients with ARF who required renal replacement therapy.[17]

Blood transfusion is given in an attempt to increase oxygen delivery and, as a result, to decrease tissue hypoxia and damage from necrosis and apoptosis. Meanwhile, improving oxygen delivery does not guarantee increase in tissue oxygenation or oxygen utilization. Neither can higher hemoglobin levels ensure decreased morbidity and mortality. At least two observational studies[1,2] reported independent positive associations between the number of transfusions and higher morbidity and mortality. The randomized, controlled study of Hebert and colleagues showed a decrease in mortality for critically ill patients with a restrictive transfusion strategy (hemoglobin transfusion threshold, approximately 7 g/dL), particularly for younger and less sick patients.[18] Currently, only surrogate measures of tissue oxygenation are available, and there is limited understanding of the complex relationship between oxygen delivery and survival. The harm from extremely low hemoglobin levels is well studied in cardiopathic and

transfusion-refusing patient populations. However, the exact balance of the benefits and risks of a rising hemoglobin level (either by transfusion or by EPO administration) in the average ICU patient remains unclear, and no guidelines endorsing a "critical" hemoglobin level as a transfusion trigger or as a goal for rHuEPO therapy are available so far.

Perhaps avoiding some RBC transfusions will reduce the risk of pathogen transmission and various noninfectious complications. Meanwhile, with respect to viral, bacterial, parasitic, and prion diseases in Western countries, RBC transfusions are quite safe.[19] Various immunological phenomena such as immunosuppression, acute and delayed hemolytic transfusion reactions, alloimmunization, and transfusion-related acute lung injury (TRALI) might be more common than infectious complications,[19] but their incidence, extent, and significance vary in different clinical settings. Certainly, not transfusing on average 1 unit of RBC during the ICU stay in prospective studies would avoid the possible complications and errors of transfusion, but the cost-effectiveness of administering 2 to 3 doses of rHuEPO instead is questionable (i.e., \$800 to \$1200 for rHuEPO versus \$300 to \$400 for RBC pack).[17]

Furthermore, the lag between the start of rHuEPO therapy and reticulocytosis was approximately 3 weeks, and another 3 to 4 weeks was needed for "normalization" of the hematocrit in studies.[11] Therefore, even if the decision to use rHuEPO to alleviate anemia of critical illness is judged cost-effective in certain patient groups, it might be useful to have some prediction rules for selecting appropriate patients for preemptive intervention.[20]

NONHEMATOLOGICAL EFFECTS OF RECOMBINANT HUMAN ERYTHROPOIETIN

The discovery of EPO receptors as well as evidence of local EPO secretion in various cells and tissues and the need for EPO in the normal development of heart, blood vessels, and brain have stimulated research on the nonhematopoietic actions of EPO, such as activation of intracellular "survival" pathways.

At least part of these EPO effects are hypoxia induced and serve to protect tissues by inhibition of apoptosis, stimulation of cellular regeneration, angiogenesis, and vascular repair.[21] For example, in a well-studied area of EPO neuroprotection, the neutralization of endogenous EPO augmented brain damage, and systemic EPO administration significantly reduced ischemic brain injury in animal models.

The identification of EPO receptors in different cell types in kidney (proximal tubular epithelial cells, mesangial cells, endothelial cells) led to numerous studies of EPO effects in animal models of ARF.[22-25] Many of these investigated ischemic ARF in a rat ischemia/reperfusion model that is associated with renal tubular expression of both proapoptotic (Bad, p53, FADD, Bak) and antiapoptotic (BCL2 family) proteins. The balance between proapoptotic and antiapoptotic factors early during renal injury has been shown to affect the severity of damage and dysfunction, so the antiapoptotic action of EPO could explain the beneficial results seen (Tables 315-2 and 315-3). Proposed pathways of interaction between EPO and expression of apoptotic genes are represented in Figure 315-1.

TABLE 315-2

Summary of Renal Tissue Responses to Recombinant Human Erythropoietin (rHuEPO) in Various Animal Models of Acute Renal Failure

Reduced oxidative stress
Reduced lipid peroxidation
Reduced caspase activation and apoptosis in renal tubular cells
Decreased necrosis of renal tubular cells
Increased regeneration of renal tubular cells
Increased expression of renal aquaporins, sodium-hydrogen exchanger, and thiazide-sensitive cotransporter
Decreased kidney myeloperoxidase and malondialdehyde
Decreased histological renal injury

TABLE 315-3

Summary of Physiological Kidney Responses to Recombinant Human Erythropoietin (rHuEPO) in Various Animal Models of Acute Renal Failure

Increased functional recovery
Increased glomerular filtration rate
Increased renal blood flow
Decreased plasma blood urea nitrogen and creatinine
Decreased fractional excretion of sodium (Fe_{Na})
Decreased polyuria
Decreased tubular cast formation

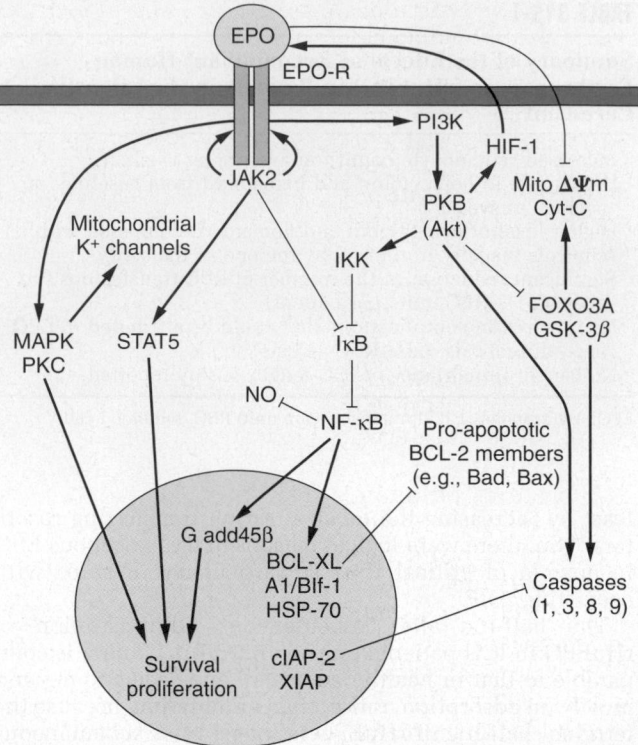

FIGURE 315-1. Proposed pathways of renoprotection provided by erythropoietin (EPO). A1/Bif-1, endophilin A1/endophilin B1; Bad, BCL2-antagonist of cell death; Bax, BCL2-associated X protein; BCL2, B-cell CLL/lymphoma/leukemia 2; BCL-XL, BCL2-like 1; cIAP-2, cellular inhibitor of apoptosis protein 2; Cyt-C, cytochrome C; EPO-R, erythropoietin receptor; FOXO3A, forkhead box O3A; Gadd45β, growth arrest and DNA damage–inducible 45β; GSK3β, glycogen synthase kinase 3β; HIF-1, hypoxia-inducible factor 1; HSP-70, heat shock protein 70; IKK, IκB kinase; IκB, inhibitor of κB; JAK2, Janus tyrosine kinase 2; K^+, potassium ion; MAPK, mitogen-activated protein kinase; Mito. Δψm, mitochondrial membrane potential; NF-κB, nuclear factor κB; NO, nitric oxide; PI3K, phosphotidylinositol-3′-kinase; PKB (Akt), protein kinase B; PKC, protein kinase C; STAT5, signal transducer and activator of transcription 5; XIAP, X-linked inhibitor of apoptosis protein. (Adapted from Johnon DW, Forman C, Vesey DA: Novel renoprotective actions of erythropoietin: New uses for an old hormone. Nephrology 2006;11:306-312.)

The detailed mechanism of EPO-related renoprotection is complex and unclear (see reviews in references 22 through 26). For example, activation of the classic EPO receptor (EPO-R) yields more than 40 binding sites, some targets for which are known and are involved in protecting the kidney from injury. One of the main molecules that bind to it and induce intracellular signaling is Janus tyrosine kinase 2 (JAK2). The signal transducer and activator of transcription 5 (JAK2-STAT5) transcription factor pathway exerts hematopoietic EPO actions and protects erythroid precursors from apoptosis; it is a likely candidate for a "survival" pathway in nonhematopoietic cell lines.

Another important result of EPO-R stimulation is the induction of protein kinase B (Akt) phosphorylation, with increased expression of BCL2 and BCL-xL (BCL2L1), important antiapoptotic proteins that prevents mitochondrial depolarization.[27] Influences of the Akt pathway on programmed cell death seem to be pivotal for cytoprotective EPO actions, because prevention of Akt phosphorylation abolished the beneficial effects of rHuEPO in settings of experimental cardiovascular or neuronal injury.[28] The role in cytoprotection of other EPO-related pathways that are not linked to hematopoiesis (e.g., protein kinase C, heat shock proteins, mitogen-activated protein kinase [MAPK]) is studied less and remains to be clarified. There might be additional receptor complexes that mediate EPO tissue protection, different from the hematopoietic receptor, because carbamylated modification of EPO that does not affect erythropoiesis still can protect neurons from apoptosis.[29] Investigation of possible cytoprotective EPO actions via actions on mitochondria and inhibition of cytochrome C release, also independent of the EPO-R, remains to be done.[22]

Some experimental animal studies involved much higher EPO doses than those used in clinical practice (3000 to 9000 U/kg in single or multiple doses versus 75 to 300 U/kg/wk).[22-25,28-30] Theoretically, such doses in humans could increase the risk of thrombosis and other unwanted effects of EPO. However, in some experimental ARF studies done on rats, either pretreatment or treatment with rHuEPO in doses comparable to those routinely used in humans resulted in decreased apoptosis in renal tubular cells.[30,31] Hematologically noneffective doses of darbepoetin (equivalent to 20 to 50 U/kg of rHuEPO) in a 5/6 nephrectomy chronic kidney disease model in rat were able not just to reduce kidney dysfunction but also to increase animal survival.[27] The presumed mechanism for this beneficial effect, reduced apoptosis in endothelial and epithelial glomerular cells with resulting improvement in kidney microcirculation, lessening ischemia, and glomerular and tubulointerstitial sclerosis,[28] might also be relevant for modulating the pathogenesis of ARF.

Therefore, if a planned intervention or diagnostic procedure is linked to a high risk of causing ARF, for example in diabetic and vasculopathic patients prepared for major surgery, cardiopulmonary bypass, or intravenous contrast studies, preemptive administration of EPO is feasible and needs to be studied. Even if the insulting injury already occurred some time ago, there still might be the opportunity for an EPO trial in established ARF.[22,23] The results of animal studies have prepared the ground for human trials of rHuEPO to evaluate possible preservation and improved regeneration of kidney tissue in ARF resulting from various causes.

Key Points

1. There is evidence that recombinant human erythropoietin (rHuEPO) can overcome the blunted response to erythropoietin in critically ill patients.
2. In studies on anemia of critical illness, rHuEPO therapy significantly raised the hemoglobin and hematocrit and resulted in fewer red blood cell transfusions.
3. No study has been able to demonstrate benefit for intensive care or hospital length of stay or for mortality, and the cost-effectiveness of correcting hemoglobin level in intensive care patients by rHuEPO administration remains questionable.
4. Erythropoietin is able to reduce apoptosis in non hematopoietic tissues via activation of several salvage pathways.

5. Animal studies of experimental acute renal failure demonstrated decreased renal injury and increased regeneration of renal tubular cells after either pretreatment or treatment with rHuEPO.
6. No evidence of rHuEPO-induced renoprotection from human studies is available yet.

Key References

11. Stubbs JR: Alternatives to blood product transfusion in the critically ill: Erythropoietin. Crit Care Med 2006;34:S160-S169.
13. Vincent J-L, Spapen HDMH, Creteur J, et al: Pharmacokinetics and pharmacodynamics of once-weekly subcutaneous epoetin alfa in critically ill patients: Results of a randomized, double blind, placebo controlled trial. Crit Care Med 2006;34:1661-1667.
15. Corwin HL, Gettinger A, Rodriguez RM, et al: Efficacy of recombinant human erythropoietin in the critically ill patient: A randomized, double-blind, placebo-controlled trial. Crit Care Med 1999;27:2346-2350.
22. Johnson DW, Forman C, Vesey DA: Novel renprotective actions of erythropoetin: New uses for an old hormone. Nephrology 2006;11:306-312.
24. Sharples EJ, Yaqoob MM: Erythropoetin in experimental acute renal failure. Nephron Exp Nephrol 2006;104:e83-e88.

See the companion Expert Consult website for the complete reference list.

CHAPTER 316

Activated Protein C Therapy and Sepsis-Associated Acute Kidney Injury

William L. Macias, Akanksha Gupta, G. Matthew Vail, and Brian W. Grinnell

OBJECTIVES

This chapter will:
1. Discuss the association of acute kidney injury with severe sepsis.
2. Describe the potential role of protein C deficiency in the pathophysiology of sepsis-associated acute kidney injury (AKI).
3. Review preclinical studies of sepsis-associated AKI and treatment effects associated with activated protein C therapy.
4. Discuss the potential role of activated protein C in patients with sepsis-associated AKI.

The constellation of infection and resulting organ dysfunctions, inclusive of acute kidney injury (AKI), comprises the diagnosis of severe sepsis.[1,2] In patients with severe sepsis who are without AKI at diagnosis, those who develop AKI have an increased risk of death compared to those who do not develop AKI over the course of their illness.[3-6] The etiology of sepsis-associated AKI is unclear but may involve alterations in renal blood flow, soluble mediator–induced injury (e.g., from circulating cytokines, endothelins, reactive oxygen species), and endothelial dysfunction.[7,8]

Recently, Chawla and colleagues demonstrated that a markedly elevated level of interleukin 6 (IL-6) and an elevated Acute Physiology and Chronic Health Evaluation

(APACHE II) score at diagnosis were associated with an increased risk for developing AKI in patients with severe sepsis.[9] These investigators also demonstrated that measures of cardiovascular dysfunction were not predictors of sepsis-associated AKI. Additionally, Vail and coworkers demonstrated that severe protein C deficiency (<40% of normal control values) predicted the development of AKI in patients with severe sepsis.[10] Taken together, these data suggest that sepsis-associated AKI results directly from the pro-inflammatory and procoagulant host response to infection and not solely as a consequence of sepsis-induced hypotension and renal hypoperfusion.[9]

Protein C levels are rapidly depleted in patients with severe sepsis, and protein C deficiency (<80% of normal control values) is common at the time of diagnosis. Patients with severe protein C deficiency are at very high risk of death.[11] Protein C is a member of the vitamin K–dependent family of blood hemostasis proteins and circulates as an inactive zymogen. Thrombin, complexed to thrombomodulin on the endothelial surface, converts the inactive zymogen to activated protein C (aPC).[12] aPC provides feedback inhibition of thrombin generation by inactivating activated factors V and VIII.[12] Additionally, aPC has direct anti-inflammatory and cytoprotective effects mediated by binding to the endothelial protein C receptor (EPCR), which is present not only on the endothelium but on circulating neutrophils, eosinophils, monocytes, and some epithelial cells.[13]

By these means, aPC plays a fundamental role in a coordinated system for controlling thrombosis, limiting inflammatory responses, and potentially decreasing endothelial cell apoptosis in response to inflammatory cytokines and ischemia.[14] In severe sepsis, the beneficial effects of endogenous aPC may be compromised because of decreased levels of the protein C zymogen and a potential inability to convert it to the active moiety related to decreased endothelial expression of EPCR and thrombomodulin.[15] These observations raise the possibility of a potential role for protein C deficiency in the etiology of sepsis-associated AKI and the potential utility of aPC replacement as therapy.

PRECLINICAL STUDIES OF ACTIVATED PROTEIN C IN ACUTE KIDNEY INJURY

The potential of aPC as therapy for AKI has been investigated in a number of preclinical models. Krishnamurti and colleagues first investigated the potential role of aPC in endotoxin-treated rabbits, a model characterized by high levels of plasminogen activator inhibitor 1 (PAI-1) and fibrin deposition in the kidney.[16] They demonstrated that bovine-derived aPC, coadministered with human tissue-type plasminogen activator (tPA), markedly inhibited fibrin deposition in the kidney. Endogenous PAI-1 activity was completely inhibited by aPC. The potential role of aPC was also investigated in a model of ischemia/reperfusion injury.[17] Multiple renal parameters were assessed, including renal microvascular permeability, renal blood flow, histopathology, myeloperoxidase activity, and serum levels of fibrin degradation products. The intravenous administration of human plasma-derived aPC markedly reduced changes induced by ischemia/reperfusion in all parameters, whereas administration of dansyl glutamyl-glycylarginyl chloromethyl ketone-treated factor Xa

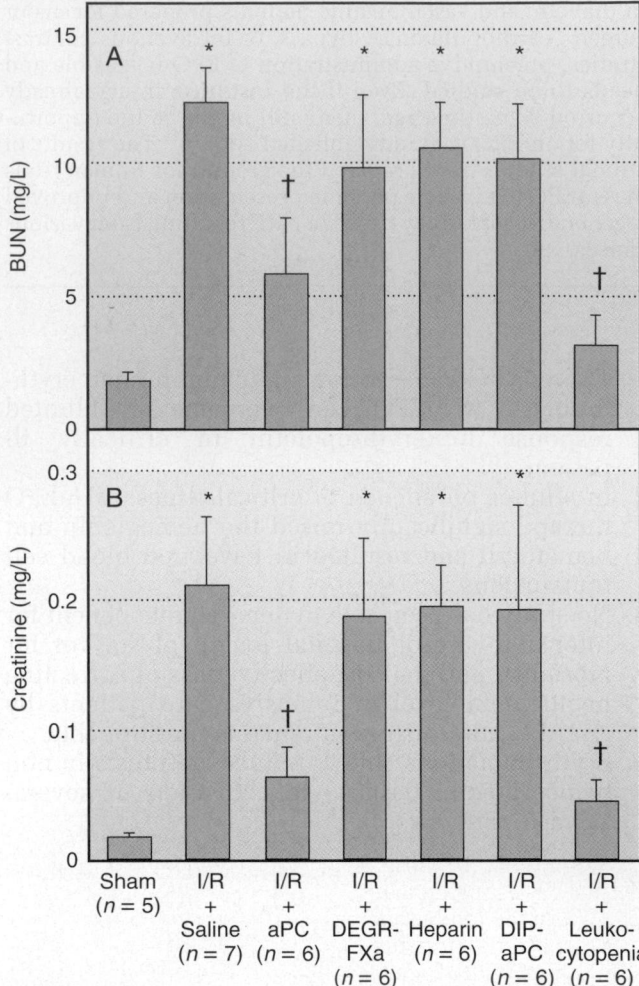

FIGURE 316-1. Effects of saline, activated protein C (aPC), active-site–blocked factor Xa (DEGR-FXa), heparin, inactivated aPC (DIP-aPC), and leukocytopenia on measures of renal function after ischemia and reperfusion (I/R). Serum levels of blood urea nitrogen (BUN) and creatinine were measured 24 hours after reperfusion in rats subjected to 60 minutes of renal ischemia. Data are expressed as mean ± standard deviation of the mean. *$P < .01$ compared to sham-operated animals; †$P < .01$ compared to saline-treated group. (From Mizutani A, Okajima K, Uchiba M, Noguchi T: Activated protein C reduces ischemia/reperfusion-induced renal injury in rats by inhibiting leukocyte activation. Blood 2000;95:3781-3787.)

(DEGR-FXa; active-site–blocked factor Xa), heparin, or diisopropyl fluorophosphates (DIP)–treated aPC (inactivated aPC) had no effect (Fig. 316-1). Induction of leukopenia prior to the ischemia/reperfusion injury also markedly reduced the extent of injury, suggesting that the mechanism of aPC-induced improvement in renal function resulted in part from inhibition of neutrophil-mediated injury.

In similar experiments, these investigators assessed the effects of human plasma–derived aPC on endotoxin-induced hypotension and nitric oxide (NO) production in the rat.[18] Intravenous administration of aPC prevented the endotoxin-induced hypotension and diminished the increase in plasma levels of NO^{2-}/NO^{3-}, an indicator of NO production in vivo. These effects were accompanied by decreases in lung levels of inducible nitric oxide synthase (iNOS) and tumor necrosis factor-α (TNF-α) activity,

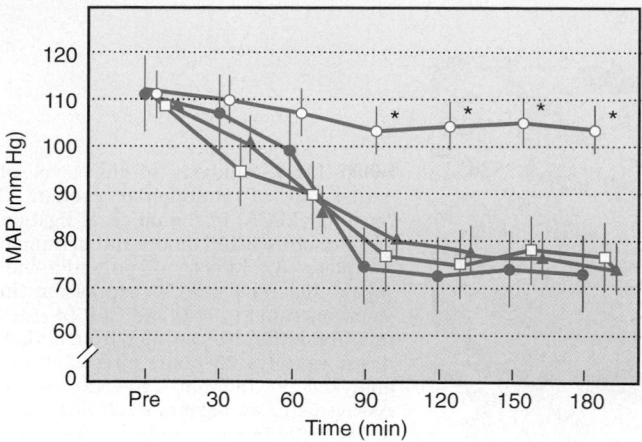

FIGURE 316-2. Effects of saline, activated protein C (aPC), active-site–blocked factor Xa (DEGR-FXa), and inactivated aPC (DIP-aPC) on mean arterial pressure (MAP) after intravenous administration of endotoxin. Treatment with aPC *(open circles)* resulted in prevention of endotoxin-induced hypotension ($P < .01$) compared to treatment with saline *(solid circles).* Administration of DEGR-FXa *(open squares)* or DIP-aPC *(solid triangles)* did not prevent the decrease in MAP. (From Isobe H, Okajima K, Uchiba M, et al: Activated protein C prevents endotoxin-induced hypotension in rats by inhibiting excessive production of nitric oxide. Circulation 2001;104:1171-1175.)

apparently related to decreased production of messenger RNAs (mRNA) for these molecules. The administration of DEGR-FXa or inactivated aPC did not affect any endotoxin-induced alterations, including the endotoxic effects on mean arterial pressure (Fig. 316-2). However, induction of leukopenia produced effects similar to those observed with aPC administration. Although these findings were not specific to the kidney, they do suggest that administration of aPC can reduce leukocyte-mediated upregulation of NO and TNF-α, both of which may play a role in AKI in critically ill patients.[19,20]

More recently, Grinnell and colleagues[21,22] have completed a number of investigations of the potential role of acquired protein C deficiency and aPC therapy in a rat cecal ligation and puncture (CLP) model of polymicrobial sepsis. In this model, rats undergo early death or late death or are considered permanent survivors. Severe protein C deficiency, defined as a level less than 60% of baseline, demonstrated 100% sensitivity and 100% specificity for early death by receiver operating characteristics (ROC) analysis.[21,22] The decline in protein C levels was in part due to a decreased expression of protein C mRNA, indicating decreased production of protein C by the liver.[22] In rats with severe protein C deficiency, there was a highly significant increase in blood urea nitrogen (BUN), whereas CLP rats without protein C deficiency demonstrated no change in BUN.[23] Additionally, protein C–deficient rats had significantly higher levels of neutrophil gelatinase–associated lipocalin (Ngal), an early biomarker of AKI,[24] compared to sham-treated and CLP rats without protein C deficiency. These laboratory markers correlated with pathological evidence of AKI in protein C–deficient rats.

These data suggest that the development of protein C deficiency is associated with AKI in the rat with polymicrobial sepsis. Interestingly, the development of severe protein C deficiency and AKI in this model was also associated with an increase in EPCR mRNA expression and a corresponding increase in protein expression in the microvasculature (Fig. 316-3). Levels of EPCR mRNA and protein in CLP rats that were not protein C deficient did not differ from those of sham-operated controls. Supporting the rat sepsis model, an analysis of kidney sections in human AKI revealed a similar increase in the expression of EPCR in the glomerular and tubular microvessels after injury (see Fig. 316-3B). Because the anti-inflammatory and cytoprotective effects of aPC are mediated by binding of aPC to EPCR, the finding of increased EPCR expression may represent a compensatory response to severe protein C deficiency.

In this model, the effect of administration of rat aPC (12-hour intravenous infusion beginning 10 hours after CLP) was investigated. At 10 hours after CLP, BUN was significantly increased in aPC-treated versus sham controls. From 10 to 22 hours, BUN decreased in aPC-treated rats compared with saline-treated rats, in which BUN remained unchanged.[23] The effect of aPC appeared to be most pronounced in rats with marked elevations in BUN at 10 hours. An improvement in renal pathology scores was also observed in aPC-treated rats. Similar to the findings of Isobe and colleagues,[18] administration of rat aPC was also associated with a reduction in iNOS mRNA expression in the kidney. Levels of iNOS correlated highly with levels of renal Ngal.

The potential beneficial effects of aPC administration were also investigated in a rat model of endotoxemia.[25] Endotoxemia was induced by administration of intravenous *Escherichia coli* lipopolysaccharide (LPS) and was assessed for the development of systemic hypotension and AKI. AKI was characterized by obstruction of peritubular capillary flow, increased leukocyte rolling and adhesion, increased endothelial permeability injury, tubular damage, and tubular obstruction. The administration of rat aPC, compared to administration of a pyrogen-free saline control, significantly improved peritubular capillary flow, downregulated iNOS mRNA levels, decreased production of NO byproducts, and decreased leukocyte rolling and adhesion in the kidney. BUN levels in aPC-treated rats were similar to those in sham controls at 24 hours after LPS treatment. The finding that aPC reduced leukocyte-endothelial interactions (i.e., rolling and adhesion) was also reported in other vascular beds in endotoxin-challenged animals.[26,27]

The importance of the protein C system in preserving renal function in sepsis and endotoxemia has been demonstrated by a number of studies using wild-type and heterozygous protein C–deficient mice.[28-31] Levi and colleagues studied heterozygous protein C–deficient mice rendered endotoxic by the intraperitoneal administration of *E. coli* endotoxin.[28] Compared to wild-type controls, heterozygous mice developed more severe disseminated intravascular coagulation (DIC), more severe liver and kidney injury, and higher mortality. Histological evaluation of the kidneys of heterozygous mice showed more extensive fibrin deposition compared to wild-type controls. Ganopolsky and Castellino exposed protein C–deficient mice to CLP.[29] In wild-type mice, CLP was associated with the development of hypotension and liver injury, as assessed by aspartate aminotransferase (AST). Twenty-four hours after CLP, BUN and creatinine levels did not differ from baseline. Heterozygote protein C–deficient mice developed significantly more systemic hypotension, a similar degree of liver injury, and significantly increased levels of serum BUN and creatinine at 24 hours after CLP. These investigators also utilized genetic engineering to produce protein C–deficient mice of varying

HUMAN KIDNEY

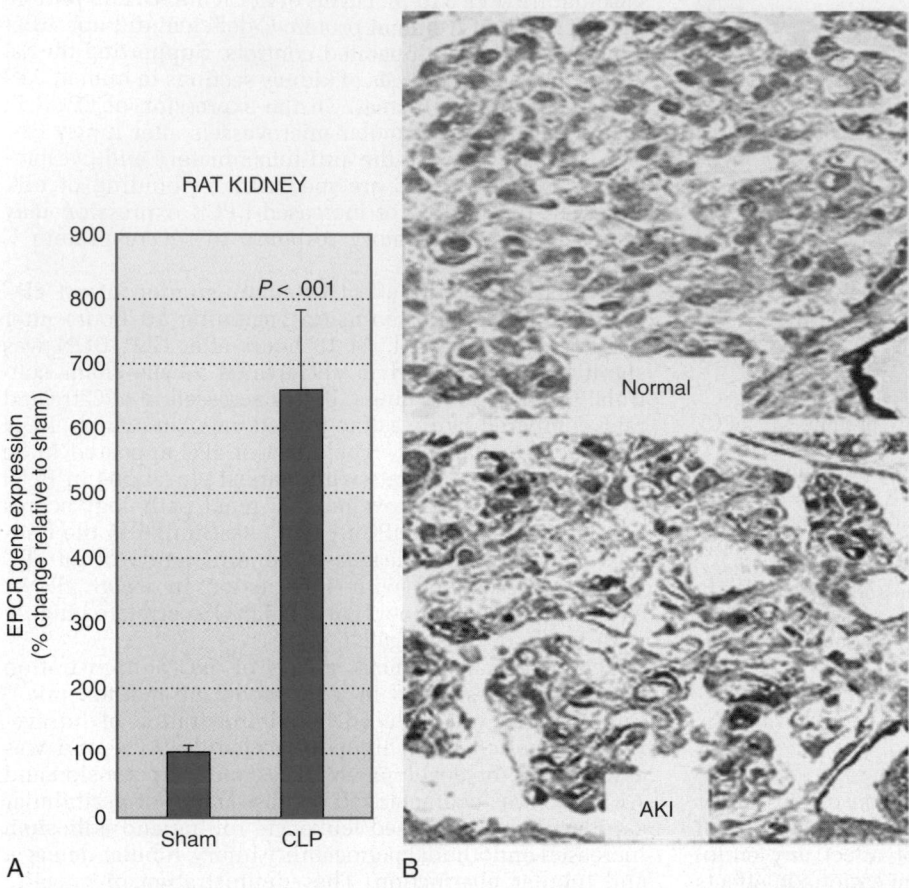

FIGURE 316-3. Analysis of the level of expression of endothelial protein C receptor (EPCR) in the rat cecal ligation and puncture (CLP) model and in human samples. **A,** Effect of polymicrobial sepsis on renal EPCR expression in sham-operated ($n = 8$) and CLP ($n = 10$) rats. Total RNA was purified from kidney tissue samples 22 hours after CLP and analyzed by TaqMan Gene Expression Assays using endogenous 18S ribosomal RNA (rRNA) as control. Data are expressed as mean ± standard error of the mean. **B,** Examination of EPCR expression by immunohistochemistry in samples from patients with normal kidney and acute kidney injury (AKI). Human tissue specimens were retrieved from the tissue bank of the Cooperative Human Tissue Network using an institutional review board–approved protocol and stained for EPCR expression. The AKI samples had documented increases in blood urea nitrogen (BUN) or creatinine, or both, before harvest. Increased expression of EPCR in the microvessels of AKI samples is indicated by the brown staining. (From Gupta A, Berg DT, Gerlitz B, et al: Role of protein C in renal dysfunction following polymicrobial sepsis. J Am Soc Nephrol 2007;18:860-867.)

degrees (1%, 3%, 5%, 18%, and 50% of wild-type protein C levels).[31] Administration of intraperitoneal *E. coli* endotoxin was associated with higher mortality in the more severely protein C–deficient mice. Additionally, genetically protein C–deficient mice were more prone to the development of hypotension, DIC, and organ injury, including increased apoptosis of the kidney. The administration of recombinant human aPC, known as drotrecogin alfa (activated) or DrotAA, improved the endotoxin-induced hypotension and reduced mortality.

In models of polymicrobial sepsis or endotoxemia, protein C deficiency is associated with increased hypotension, organ dysfunction (including AKI), and mortality compared to animals that either do not have protein C deficiency at baseline or fail to develop protein C deficiency. Administration of aPC consistently improves hypotension and the function of renal and other organs and reduces mortality in these models. The potential mechanism involved is unclear but almost certainly involves aPC binding to its receptor (EPCR), a consequent decrease in leukocyte-endothelial interactions and a downregulation of iNOS mRNA production. How binding of aPC to its receptor signals intracellularly is unclear but may involve interactions with protease-activated receptor 1 (PAR-1).[13] Furthermore, it appears that the cytoprotective effects of aPC can be separated from its antithrombotic effects, because genetically engineered aPC variants without antithrombotic properties have been shown to improve survival in endotoxemic mice.[32]

CLINICAL STUDIES OF ACTIVATED PROTEIN C

As discussed earlier, preclinical data strongly support a role for protein C deficiency in the pathophysiology of sepsis-associated AKI. Whether protein C deficiency is associated with AKI of nonsepsis origin is unclear. Clinical data from healthy subjects administered an endotoxin challenge (either intravenous or endobronchial) and DrotAA or from patients with severe sepsis administered DrotAA demonstrate many of the effects of aPC observed in animal models of sepsis-associated AKI. However, human studies specifically investigating the efficacy of DrotAA as therapy for AKI are lacking.

Kalil and colleagues studied the effect of DrotAA on the systemic response of healthy subjects administered an intravenous endotoxin challenge.[33] In this study, the administration of DrotAA prevented the development of endotoxin-induced hypotension. This observation was similar to the findings in the Recombinant Human Activated Protein C Worldwide Evaluation in Severe Sepsis (PROWESS) study, in which the administration of DrotAA to patients with severe sepsis, compared with placebo, was associated with a statistically significant improvement in cardiovascular function and resolution of hypotension.[34] Nick and coworkers investigated the effect of DrotAA in healthy subjects administered endotoxin endobronchially.[35] Compared with placebo, the administration of

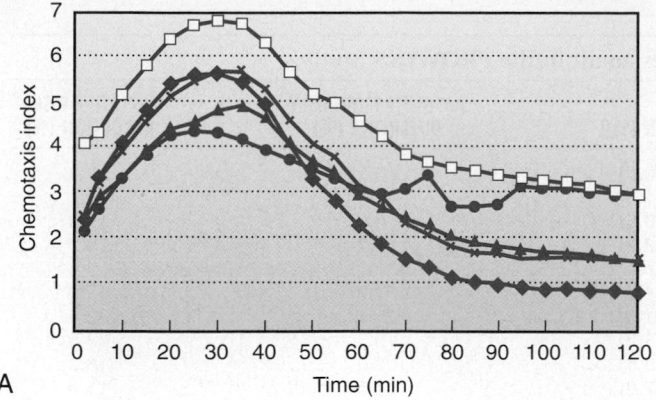

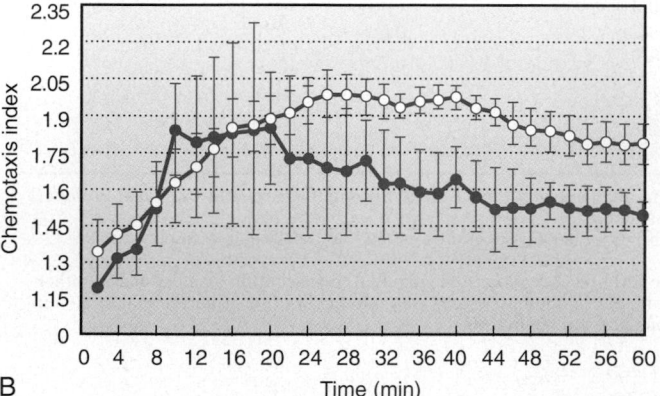

FIGURE 316-4. Blockade of interleukin 8 (IL-8)–induced migration after exposure to drotrecogin alfa (activated) (DrotAA). **A,** Effect of no treatment *(open squares)*, and treatment with 10^{-4} g/mL *(solid diamonds)*, 10^{-6} g/mL *(asterisks)*, 10^{-8} g/mL *(solid triangles)*, and 10^{-10} g/mL *(solid circles)* DrotAA on neutrophil migration. Treatment with DrotAA resulted in a statistically significant reduction of migration at all concentrations tested ($P = .01$ for 10^{-10} g/mL and $P < .0001$ for the three higher concentrations), compared with no treatment. Plot depicts the mean chemotaxis index for five experiments. For reference, plasma concentrations of DrotAA in patients with severe sepsis are approximately 10^{-7} g/mL (reported by Macias et al.[40]). **B,** Effect of intravenous administration of DrotAA on neutrophil migration assessed ex vivo. Neutrophils obtained from DrotAA-treated subjects *(solid circles)*, n = 3, demonstrated a significant reduction in migration compared with neutrophils obtained from placebo-treated subjects *(open circles)*, n = 4 ($P = .012$). Neutrophils were isolated from bronchoalveolar lavage fluid obtained from subjects 16 hours after endobronchial endotoxin administration. (From Nick JA, Coldren CD, Geraci MW, et al: Recombinant human activated protein C reduces human endotoxin-induced pulmonary inflammation via inhibition of neutrophil chemotaxis. Blood 2004;104:3878-3885.)

DrotAA significantly reduced leukocyte accumulation in the air spaces. Neutrophils recovered from the bronchoalveolar lavage fluid of DrotAA-treated subjects demonstrated decreased chemotaxis ex vivo, which was confirmed in in vitro experiments (Fig. 316-4). These data indicate that the same effects of aPC observed in animals exposed to endotoxin or polymicrobial sepsis are observed in humans administered a therapeutic dose of DrotAA.

Post hoc analyses from the PROWESS study investigating the efficacy of DrotAA in patients with severe sepsis suggested that severe protein C deficiency is associated with an increased risk of developing sepsis-associated AKI.[10,36] Additionally, for those patients who are severely protein C deficient, the administration of DrotAA was associated with decreased incidences of AKI, need for dialysis, and mortality. Exploratory analyses of the PROWESS dataset confirmed that renal dysfunction is associated with a marked increase in mortality for placebo-treated patients, regardless of whether dysfunction was classified by oliguria alone, by renal Sequential Organ Failure Assessment (SOFA) score, calculated creatinine clearance, or APACHE II score classification for acute renal failure (Table 316-1). A larger treatment effect, by both absolute and relative benefit, was observed with DrotAA therapy in patients with moderate renal insufficiency. Less effect was observed in the population of patients with a renal SOFA score of zero or with a calculated creatinine clearance of 50 mL/min or greater. However, a conclusion that the treatment effect associated with DrotAA might vary by baseline renal function assessment, other than that related to severity of illness, awaits prospective validation.

FUTURE STUDIES OF ACTIVATED PROTEIN C IN ACUTE KIDNEY INJURY

Prospective studies of DrotAA for AKI are somewhat problematic to design. DrotAA has antithrombotic and profibrinolytic properties which increase the risk of bleeding complications. Furthermore, DrotAA has a relatively high acquisition cost, and cost-effectiveness would need to be established. Therefore, inclusion criteria must identify a population of patients at very high risk of developing AKI and must do so early in the clinical course, so that intervention might be both beneficial and cost-effective. These requirements are probably applicable to all new therapies, because most therapeutic agents will be at least relatively expensive compared to other medications used in the intensive care unit. Currently, many measures of early renal injury and decreased renal function are available. However, none offers the sensitivity and specificity to predict those patients who will develop severe renal dysfunction sufficient to prompt initiation of a potentially expensive therapy or a therapy with clinically important side effects.

Additionally, it is not clear what the primary endpoint should be for studies designed to investigate the benefit of therapies to prevent or treat AKI in critically ill patients.[37] All-cause mortality is the most comprehensive endpoint and probably the one most readily accepted by regulatory authorities. This endpoint is appropriate for studies designed to treat established AKI.[37] The appropriate endpoint for studies of therapies designed to prevent AKI or to diminish the extent of early kidney injury is less clear. In this setting, use of a mortality endpoint would assume that development of AKI is the major contributor to mortality in critically ill patients, an assumption that has not yet been prospectively validated.

The potential to study AKI within specific settings, such as sepsis-associated AKI or contrast-induced nephropathy, may offer the best opportunity for success. Although multiple risk factors for the development of AKI have been identified, the presence of infection appears to raise the risk for kidney injury across a spectrum of patient-specific characteristics,[38,39] and this may make sepsis-associated AKI a more preferable target. Because severe protein C

TABLE 316-1

28-Day All-Cause Mortality by Baseline Renal Function Assessment in the PROWESS Study

POPULATION	DrotAA (N [%])	PLACEBO (N [%])	ABSOLUTE MORTALITY DIFFERENCE (%)	RELATIVE RISK REDUCTION (%)
All patients*	850 (24.7)	840 (30.8)	6.1	19.8
Renal dysfunction†				
Yes	357 (32.5)	353 (40.5)	8.0	19.8
No	493 (19.1)	487 (23.8)	4.7	19.7
Renal SOFA score				
0	323 (19.8)	323 (21.4)	1.6	7.5
1	235 (21.3)	241 (31.5)	10.2	32.4
2	188 (33.0)	176 (43.2)	10.2	23.6
3	73 (31.5)	52 (38.5)	7.0	18.2
4	30 (33.3)	45 (37.8)	4.5	11.9
Baseline creatinine clearance (mL/min)‡				
≥50	478 (18.4)	484 (19.4)	1.0	5.2
≥20 to <50	278 (31.7)	278 (46.8)	15.1	32.3
<20	67 (41.8)	63 (46.0)	4.2	9.1
APACHE II classification for acute renal failure				
Yes	180 (38.3)	192 (50.5)	12.2	24.2
No	668 (21.0)	644 (25.0)	4.0	16.0

APACHE, Acute Physiology and Chronic Health Evaluation; DrotAA, drotrecogin alfa (activated); PROWESS, Recombinant Human Activated Protein C Worldwide Evaluation in Severe Sepsis; SOFA, Sequential Organ Failure Assessment.
*Statistical comparison is provided only for the primary analysis ($P = .005$). Mortality rates for subgroups defined by baseline assessment of renal dysfunction are provided for descriptive purposes only.
†Renal dysfunction was defined as urine output <0.5 mL/kg/hr despite adequate fluid resuscitation. Adequate fluid resuscitation was defined as either (1) the administration of an intravenous fluid bolus (≥500 mL crystalloid solution, ≥20 g albumin, or ≥200 mL other colloid) over an interval of 30 min or less; or (2) pulmonary artery wedge pressure ≥12 mm Hg; or (3) central venous pressure ≥8 mm Hg.
‡Creatinine clearance was calculated by the Cockcroft-Gault equation.
Data on file, Eli Lilly and Company; clinical report for study F1K-MC-EVAD.

deficiency has been associated with increased risk of developing AKI in the septic population, the possibility that the administration of aPC might ameliorate the extent of renal injury warrants prospective investigation.

CONCLUSION

The development of AKI in patients with severe sepsis is associated with a substantial increase in mortality. Studies in both humans and animals demonstrate that sepsis-associated AKI results from the host response to infection and not solely from decreased renal perfusion with ischemia. Acquired protein C deficiency is common in severe sepsis and is associated with a higher incidence of AKI and mortality, potentially as a result of decreased generation of endogenous aPC. Endogenous aPC plays a fundamental role in a coordinated system for controlling thrombosis, limiting inflammatory responses and potentially decreasing endothelial cell apoptosis in response to inflammatory cytokines and ischemia. The administration of aPC appears to improve renal perfusion, decrease leukocyte-endothelial interactions, downregulate iNOS mRNA production, and improve renal function in a variety of animal models of AKI, including endotoxin and polymicrobial sepsis. Studies evaluating the administration of DrotAA in critically ill patients with early AKI are warranted.

Key Points

1. Acute kidney injury is common in severe sepsis. Sepsis-associated acute kidney injury may result directly from the pro-inflammatory and procoagulant host response to infection and not solely as a consequence of sepsis-induced hypotension and renal hypoperfusion.

2. In patients with severe sepsis, protein C deficiency is common, and severe protein C deficiency is associated with a higher risk of developing acute kidney injury, as well as a higher risk of death.

3. Animal models of acute endotoxemia or polymicrobial sepsis demonstrate that protein C deficiency is associated with mortality and organ dysfunction, including acute kidney injury.

4. The administration of activated protein C to animals with renal injury induced by ischemia/reperfusion, endotoxemia, or polymicrobial sepsis is associated with an improvement in renal perfusion, a decrease in leukocyte-endothelial interactions, a downregulation of inducible nitric oxide synthase (iNOS) messenger RNA production, and improved function.

5. Studies of drotrecogin alfa (activated) as therapy for critically ill patients with early acute kidney injury warrants investigation.

See the companion Expert Consult website for the complete reference list.

CHAPTER 317

Vasoactive Drugs and Renal Function

Giorgio Della Rocca and Manuela Lugano

OBJECTIVES

This chapter will:

1. Discuss acute renal failure in critically ill patients as a frequent complication of gram-negative sepsis with a high risk of mortality.
2. Evaluate the most used drugs in the intensive care unit, the vasoconstrictor and vasodilator drugs with various inotropic functions, such as norepinephrine, epinephrine, dobutamine, levosimendan, and dopamine.
3. Discuss whether nonpharmacological strategies are more effective than drug infusion to prevent acute renal failure or progression of renal damage.

In critically ill patients, acute renal failure (ARF) is a frequent complication of gram-negative sepsis with a high risk of mortality. Endotoxemia causes a systemic elaboration of inflammatory cytokines, which play a critical role in lipopolysaccharide (LPS)–mediated reduction in systemic vascular resistance, potentially producing hypotension and shock.[1] This reduction in systemic vascular resistance culminates in renal vasoconstriction and reduction in renal perfusion pressure. If this condition is sufficiently prolonged or severe, ischemic tubular necrosis and apoptosis can supervene.[2] Specific components of the sepsis-related inflammatory cascade can amplify acute tubular injury and intrarenal inflammation, exacerbating ischemic ARF.[3]

In patients with shock, either cardiogenic or vasodilatory, maintenance of adequate mean arterial pressure and cardiac output is fundamental to achieve adequate perfusion and function of vital organs.[2] The treatment of hypotension or shock with administration of fluid and vasoconstrictor drugs may induce amplification of renal ischemia and tubular injury.[2]

Beyond fluid resuscitation, vasoactive drugs such as dopamine, norepinephrine, and epinephrine are often administered in patients with shock to improve either cardiac output or mean arterial pressure and to achieve optimization of organ perfusion and therefore renal perfusion.[4,5] With the exception of dopamine, there have been no randomized controlled trials of sufficient statistical power to detect differences in clinical outcome and renal protection.[4] It is still unclear what hemodynamic manipulation is appropriate to obtain renal protection and ameliorate renal perfusion.[4] Most intensive care unit (ICU) patients received continuous infusion of two or more vasoactive drugs at the same time. In ICU patients, the goal is to maintain organ perfusion, first with fluid challenge, and

secondly with infusion of drugs. The most used drugs in the ICU are vasoconstrictors and vasodilators with various inotropic functions, such as norepinephrine, epinephrine, dobutamine, levosimendan, and dopamine.

The more important discussion is whether nonpharmacological strategies are more effective than drug infusion to prevent ARF or progression of renal damage.[6]

VASOCONSTRICTOR DRUGS

Dopamine

Dopamine has been the first drug used in ICUs since the first clinical description of its use in patients with congestive heart failure.[7] Dopamine acts on two populations of dopamine receptors, D_1 and D_2, which are located on cells of the vascular smooth muscle of the kidney, the mesentery, and the coronary, cerebral, gastric, and hepatic arteries. The binding of dopamine to these receptors results in localized arterial vasodilatation, an increased glomerular filtration rate, increased renal blood flow (RBF), and increased sodium excretion.[8] At low doses (1-3 µg/kg/min), there is evidence of β_1-adrenoreceptor recruitment, manifested as increased cardiac output and heart rate.[8] At higher doses, dopamine stimulates dopaminergic and adrenergic receptors such as beta receptors (at 3-5 µg/kg/min) and alpha receptors (>5 µg/kg/min), with inotropic and vasoconstrictive actions.[9]

Use of low-dose dopamine has been widely accepted in common clinical practice in attempts to prevent or treat renal dysfunction. Nevertheless, a systematic review of 58 studies concluded that there is no evidence, despite its widespread use, to support the prescription of low-dose dopamine to prevent or treat ARF.[9]

The improvement in urine output, in patients without shock, is an expression only of the diuretic effect of dopamine, rather than a protective effect on renal function.[10] Furthermore, this diuretic effect wanes by 48 hours after the start of continuous infusion.[11] In oliguric patients, however, dopamine failed to reverse oliguria or hypotension and did not significantly modify the clearance of creatinine, incidence of ARF, need for dialysis, or patient survival.[12] Particularly in critically ill patients, dopamine has some potential disadvantages, such as earlier onset of gut ischemia, tissue necrosis, and digital gangrene. A meta-analysis by Kellum and colleagues excluded any effect of dopamine on the risk of ARF, although dopamine was totally inefficacious in preventing or treating renal dysfunction.[9]

The only dopamine effect that has been confirmed is the temporary increase in glomerular filtration rate in patients with septic shock, caused by reversal of the vaso-constrictive action of vasopressor drugs used in these patients.[13] The natriuretic effect of dopamine increases solute delivery to the distal tubular cells, which may increase medullar oxygen consumption and exacerbate the ischemia during hypotension. This effect could explain why increases in RBF are not protective.[4] The Australian and New Zealand Intensive Care Study (ANZICS) analyzed the use of dopamine in 324 critically ill patients with systemic inflammatory response syndrome and oliguria and confirmed that there were no differences in mortality, ARF, renal replacement therapy requirement, length of hospital stay, or peak serum creatinine.[13]

Renal-dose dopamine may increase the risk of post-operative atrial fibrillation, especially in critically ill patients, in whom impaired renal clearance of dopamine results in high plasma levels that stimulate postsynaptic D_2 receptors.[14] Because of the increase in atrioventricular conduction rate, dopamine infusion results in a rapid ventricular response and hemodynamic instability.[15] Even low-dose dopamine can worsen renal perfusion in patients with ARF, which adds to the rationale for abandoning the routine use of low-dose dopamine in critically ill patients.[16]

Norepinephrine

Norepinephrine is a very common drug used in patients with septic shock. It has only a moderate β_1- and β_2-adrenergic effect but a strong α-adrenergic effect that causes vasoconstriction in all vascular beds. The postsynaptic α_1-receptor activity sustains arterial blood pressure and peripheral vascular resistance but induces vasoconstriction that can compromise renal, splanchnic, and mesenteric blood flows. Dopamine may counteract the norepinephrine-induced decrease in RBF in healthy volunteers.[8] However, there are insufficient data to define the effect on the kidney, either in normal subjects or under septic conditions.[4]

The restoration of adequate blood pressure by norepinephrine is associated with increased urine output, but this is achieved with any drug that improves blood pressure, and probably also RBF and glomerular filtration rate.[4]

There is no reason to avoid norepinephrine administration because of concern that it could have a specific adverse effect on renal function. When compared to high-dose dopamine, norepinephrine is more effective in restoring mean arterial pressure. For this reason, it is a vasopressor of choice in vasodilated hypotensive states with preserved or increased cardiac output.[4] Norepinephrine was more effective in restoring normotension in 32 patients with hyperkinetic and hypotensive septic shock, compared with high-dose dopamine.[17]

There are no controlled data to define the effects of norepinephrine on the kidney in the clinical context. However, many patient series have not been published. The clinical experience in septic patients and in cardiac patients with inflammatory or pharmacological vasodilatation is also positive. At this time, there is no reason to fear the effects of norepinephrine. If it is used to support a patient with vasodilation after adequate intravascular filling has occurred and after a normal or increased cardiac output has been established, it is likely to be a friend and not a foe.[18]

Phenylephrine

Phenylephrine, a predominant α_1-adrenergic receptor–mediated agonist, increases blood pressure mainly by increasing the systemic vascular resistance. In septic patients, it appears not to have adverse effects on the kidney and produces a stable serum creatinine concentration and increased urine output.[4] The same effects have been noted in postoperative patients undergoing cardiopulmonary bypass.[4]

Vasopressin

Vasopressin has been proposed as an alternative to catecholamine for persistent hypotension in septic shock, because, in patients with catecholamine hyporesponsiveness, peripheral vessels respond surprisingly, even supranormally, to intravenous injection of vasopressin.[19]

Vasopressin in healthy patients has only a little effect on vascular tone, but it successfully restores blood pressure in vasodilating conditions such as septic shock or hepatorenal syndrome.[19] Vasopressin acts via three types of receptors: The V_{1a} receptor, located on vascular smooth muscle cells, mediates vasoconstriction; the V_2 receptor, mainly located on the distal convoluted tubules and medullary collecting ducts of the kidney, mediates water movements; and the V_3 receptor, mainly located in the anterior hypophysis, is involved in the control of corticotrophin release. In addition, vasopressin is capable of closing activated adenosine triphosphate (ATP)–sensitive potassium channels.[19] In a septic model, organ blood flow in the left ventricle, right ventricle, ventricular septum, kidney, liver, spleen, and skeletal muscle was measured with the use of radioisotope-tagged microspheres in two groups of patients treated with vasopressin or norepinephrine. Vasopressin increased RBF and decreased hepatic arterial blood flow, whereas norepinephrine did not.[20]

A multicentric, open-label, randomized trial in early hyperdynamic septic shock found that high-dose vasopressin used as a single vasopressor agent initially failed to maintain the mean arterial pressure higher than 70 mm Hg.[21]

Terlipressin

Terlipressin (triglycyl lysine-vasopressin) is the synthetic analogue of vasopressin.[22] In a randomized study, terlipressin was compared to norepinephrine in regard to effects on creatinine clearance and urine flow in septic patients; the authors concluded that renal function was improved with both drugs.[22] Earlier, Morelli and colleagues demonstrated that terlipressin decreases oxygen consumption, although the measurement was not performed independently from cardiac output.[23] Because it has been speculated that terlipressin might exhibit anti-inflammatory effects that decrease oxygen demand of the tissues, this reduction of oxygen consumption may be interpreted as a positive consequence of terlipressin action.[24] Terlipressin is the drug of choice in hepatorenal syndrome: It reverses hepatorenal syndrome in half of the treated patients and appears to be safe and well tolerated.[25]

Epinephrine

Epinephrine acts simultaneously on alpha and beta receptors. At low doses, it has β-adrenergic effects and increases cardiac output. At higher doses, its α-adrenergic effect causes vasoconstriction, particularly in the splanchnic and renal vascular beds, and results in elevated systemic vascular resistance and elevated blood pressure.[26] One of the most important uses of epinephrine in the ICU is in septic shock, and it is also used in cardiopulmonary resuscitation.[27]

Epinephrine infusion was associated with a significant increase in renal vascular resistance and decrease in RBF. The absolute RBF index, renal oxygen consumption, creatinine clearance, and urine output remained constant.[4]

Epinephrine, despite an increase in mean arterial pressure, may cause undesirable splanchnic effects on ICU patients such as lower splanchnic flow and oxygen uptake, lower mucosal pH, and higher hepatic vein lactates.[5]

The data are very limited concerning renal effects of epinephrine compared with placebo or other vasoactive drugs. The data available on renal effects of epinephrine are level III or IV evidence or data from animal studies, and knowledge about renal effects of epinephrine is still limited.[4]

INOTROPIC DRUGS

Dobutamine

Dobutamine is the drug of choice in case of acute heart failure or shock with low cardiac output.[28] In ICU patients, the concurrent use of norepinephrine and dobutamine is most frequent in cases of septic shock to maintain mean arterial pressure and tissue perfusion.

Dobutamine is a partial agonist on $β_1$- and $β_2$-adrenoceptors with little effect on α-adrenoceptors; it increases heart rate, cardiac index, and oxygen delivery within a therapeutic range of 2 to 15 µg/kg/min. The inotropic and chronotropic actions of dobutamine are associated with therapy-derived tachycardia, which would bear the potential for increasing myocardial oxygen consumption and ischemic injury.[29] In normovolemic patients, dobutamine increases the cardiac index with no change or increase in systemic blood pressure. In hypovolemic patients, the use of dobutamine may induce reduction in mean arterial pressure ($β_2$ effect) and an increase in oxygen consumption[30] because of potent vasodilation through activation of β-adrenergic receptors.[28]

The specific renal effect is probably dependent on the ability to increase cardiac output. The additive effect of the cardiac $α_1$ and $β_1$ agonist activities gives dobutamine a strong cardiac inotropic action. Because of the vasodilatory $β_2$ effect, dobutamine is rarely used as a single agent in critically ill patients, and it is difficult to assess the effect of this drug alone on the kidney.[4]

The increase in cardiac output and consequent increase in RBF have a beneficial effect on renal function, but there are insufficient data to recommend the use of dobutamine to provide renal protection.[4]

Dopexamine

Dopexamine increases splanchnic and renal perfusion via a dopaminergic effect.[4] Dopexamine has a marked intrinsic agonist activity on $β_2$-adrenergic receptors and weak agonist activity on D_1 and D_2 dopaminergic and $β_1$-adrenergic receptors.[31] A total of 351 articles were analyzed in a systematic review: 3 articles investigated the effect of dopexamine on renal function in elective high-risk surgery, and 1 of these investigated renal perfusion in critically ill patients.[31] Despite some authors' suggestions that dopexamine may protect renal function in patients undergoing cardiac surgery, there is no evidence to suggest a protective role in critically ill patients.[31] Some protective effects may be attributable to a vasodilating action that unmasks a covert hypovolemia, necessitating the use of additional volume expansion. This fluid excess administered to the patient may explain some of the beneficial effects attributed to dopexamine.[31]

On the other hand, flaws in study methodology further compound interpretation of results, and the review authors concluded that there was insufficient evidence to recommend the use of dopexamine for protection of either hepatosplanchnic or renal perfusion in critically ill patients or in high-risk surgical patients.[31]

In a randomized, controlled trial, 102 critically ill patients showed no benefit for creatinine clearance in ARF requiring renal replacement therapy.[32]

Levosimendan

Levosimendan, a new cardiac inotrope, may also have a role in endotoxemic ARF. It is a myocardial calcium sensitizer and may offset sepsis-induced reduction in myocardial function; it may also improve systemic hemodynamics, augment renal perfusion via blockade of ATP-sensitive potassium channels, and mitigate LPS-induced inflammatory states.[2]

Levosimendan was able to protect against endotoxemic ARF in a rodent model, because of 70% reductions in blood urea nitrogen (BUN) and plasma creatinine concentrations in levosimendan-treated compared with placebo-matched endotoxemic mice.[2] Levosimendan protection arose from the downstream consequences of an LPS-mediated inflammatory response and a blunting of its secondary renal hemodynamic alterations. In fact, endotoxemic mice develop ARF in the absence of overt tubular injury or glomerular thromboses. It is reasonable to postulate that levosimendan-mediated protection results from reduction in renal vascular resistances, because of abrogation of the major cause of sepsis-mediated ARF (i.e., the vasoconstrictor state). This mechanism is mediated by reduction of mesangial cell contraction and theoretically should increase the renal glomerular filtrate.[2]

On the other hand, despite recent data about the effects of levosimendan on kidney, Oldner and associates showed that pretreatment with levosimendan in pigs with septic shock did not affect the RBF.[33]

VASODILATOR DRUGS

Nitroglycerin

Nitroglycerin is a potent dilator on vascular smooth muscle, because it inhibits vascular smooth muscle contraction by increasing cyclic guanosine monophosphate (cGMP).[34] Nitroglycerin produces venodilation at very low dosages, with little additional vasodilation of the venous circulation with increasing dosage. Nitrates increase arterial diameter and improve arterial conductance; at higher doses, they produce dilation of the arteriolar or resistance vessels of the body.[34] Despite this, RBF remains essentially unchanged or only slightly decreased after nitroglycerin infusion, although reflex sympathetic activity may cause secondary vasoconstriction.[34] This failure of systemic administration of nitroglycerin to increase RBF has been demonstrated in both animals and humans with heart failure. The findings indicate a selective vasodilatory effect of nitroglycerin on renal conductance but not on resistance blood vessels.[35] During infusion of nitroglycerin in patients with chronic heart failure, renal sympathetic activity decreased despite reductions in arterial pressure and cardiac filling pressure. This phenomenon is not observed in healthy volunteers.[36] The attenuation of the renal sympathetic response contributes to the beneficial effect of nitroglycerin in patients with chronic heart failure.[36]

Sodium Nitroprusside

Sodium nitroprusside is a peripheral vasodilator that acts directly as an arterial and venous smooth muscle relaxant, like nitroglycerin.[37] Its metabolism leads to cyanmethemoglobin formation and free cyanide ions. In relation to the kidney, it increases renin release and contributes to overactivity of the sympathetic nervous system, which causes vasoconstriction and reduction in RBF.[37]

Fenoldopam

Fenoldopam is a selective D_1 agonist that at low doses (0.03 to 0.1 μg/kg/min) causes D_1 receptor–mediated vasodilatation, preferentially at afferent arterioles, and then reduces renal vascular resistances and improves RBF, fractional excretion of sodium, and free water clearance.[4,38] Fenoldopam is six times more effective as a renal vasodilator than dopamine and causes no activation of other adrenergic receptors. At a dose of 0.1 μg/kg/min, no significant decrease in systolic blood pressure was observed, but at higher doses fenoldopam is a potent vasodilator.[38]

In a study in renal transplant recipients, there seemed to be no differences in the effects of dopamine versus fenoldopam, probably because these two drugs do not work on denervated kidney or because the sample sizes were too small to explain statistical differences. There was a superior trend in urine output, serum creatinine, and renal vascular resistance in the fenoldopam group.[19]

In critically ill patients, a continuous infusion of fenoldopam did not cause any clinically significant hemodynamic impairment and improved renal function, compared with renal-dose dopamine.[38] In early acute renal dysfunction, before severe renal failure has occurred, the attempt to reverse renal hypoperfusion with fenoldopam is more effective than with low-dose dopamine.[38] Fenoldopam may help to prevent the progression to established ARF or accelerate the recovery of renal function in critically ill patients.[38]

Fenoldopam seemed to be effective in preventing renal damage when administered prophylactically in patients undergoing elective aortic surgery or cardiopulmonary bypass.[39] Moreover, fenoldopam seemed to preserve renal function, counterbalancing the renal vasoconstrictive effects of cyclosporine in kidney[40] and liver[41,42] transplant recipients. It is not clear whether this promising effect would lead to a reduction in morbidity and mortality and a consequent reduction in the cost of medical care.[38]

CONCLUSION

The prophylactic and therapeutic uses of dopamine, the most studied vasoactive drug, actually have not been supported. For all other vasoactive drugs, the data at this moment are contradictory, and few conclusions can be made. To protect renal function, despite the wide use of vasoactive drugs, only the maintenance of adequate volume replacement and perfusion pressure may be recommended with certainty. Because the use of vasoactive drugs is a pervasive practice in the ICU, suitably powered, multicenter, randomized, placebo-controlled, double-blind studies are needed to provide more rational indications for clinical practice.

Key Points

1. Low-dose dopamine is not useful in prevention or treatment of acute renal failure.
2. Fenoldopam presents a promising trend in preventing acute renal failure.
3. Vasoconstrictor drugs may be used also in early acute renal failure in critically ill patients.
4. Attention to hemodynamics and optimization of fluids are the only appropriate strategies to prevent acute renal failure or progression of renal damage.
5. More studies are necessary to provide more rational indications for clinical practice.

Key References

4. Lee RWC, Di Giantomasso, May C, Bellomo R: Vasoactive drugs and the kidney. Best Pract Res Clin Anaesth 2004;18:53-74.
5. Girbes AR: Prevention of acute renal failure: Role of vasoactive drugs, mannitol and diuretics. Int J Artif Organs 2004;27:1049-1053.
6. Kellum JA, Leblanc M, Gibney RT, et al: Primary prevention of acute renal failure in the critically ill. Curr Opin Crit Care 2005;11:537-541.
16. Lauschker A, Teichgräber M, Frei U, Eckardt K-U: Low-dose dopamine worsens renal perfusion in patients with acute renal failure. Kidney Int 2006;69:1669-1674.
18. Bellomo R: Nordrenalin: Friend or foe? Heart Lung Circ 2003;12(Suppl 2):S42-S48.

See the companion Expert Consult website for the complete reference list.

CHAPTER 318

Drug Dosing in Patients with Acute Kidney Injury and in Patients Undergoing Renal Replacement Therapy

Kevin M. Sowinski and Bruce A. Mueller

OBJECTIVES

This chapter will:
1. Detail how critically ill patients with acute kidney injury (AKI) may have abnormalities in drug absorption, distribution, metabolism, and elimination.
2. Explain why published dosing recommendations derived in studies of patients with chronic kidney disease may not be applicable to patients with AKI.
3. Explain why drugs with larger volumes of distribution may not be removed effectively by high-volume continuous renal replacement therapy.
4. Explain why phenytoin serum concentrations should be monitored using unbound phenytoin assay methods in patients with AKI.

The provision of renal replacement therapy for patients with chronic kidney disease (CKD) has been reasonably standardized for decades. Debates regarding dialysis membrane type[1] and the fractional clearance (Kt/V) achieved[2] have occurred, but thrice-weekly hemodialysis has been used as the standard for as long as most nephrologists have been in practice. Consequently, drug dosing in dialysis-dependent CKD is relatively well understood. In contrast, consensus has not yet been reached on the optimal type and amount of renal replacement therapy (RRT) for patients with acute kidney injury (AKI), as can be seen by the many chapters in this text that describe different RRT modalities. As a result of this variability in practice, drug dosing in AKI also remains a moving target, particularly because these patients are much more dynamic than the typically stable, dialysis-dependent patient with CKD.

DOSING CONSIDERATIONS IN ACUTE KIDNEY INJURY

Mehta described RRT in AKI patients as providing needed "renal support" until the kidneys could recover on their own.[3] The pharmacotherapy in AKI patients should be similarly supportive. Effective drug therapy is often compromised when many of the RRTs are applied to patients with AKI. For example, sepsis is a leading cause of AKI in the intensive care unit (ICU). Pharmacological treatment of sepsis is difficult in the best of circumstances,[4] and

these difficulties may be compounded by the many aggressive extracorporeal therapies that have been suggested as adjunctive therapies in sepsis.[5,6] What is usually lacking in these descriptions of high-volume convective therapies in septic patients is how to properly dose antimicrobial agents (possibly the most important aspect of treatment). Similar pharmacotherapeutic challenges are faced in treating patients who are undergoing plasma exchange therapies, high-flux hemodialysis, slow daily dialysis regimens, and so on.

The patient with AKI provides other drug dosing challenges. Not only do we want to correctly dose medications for their RRT and residual renal function, but the choices of drug therapy may be limited compared to what can be used in patients with CKD. Because the patient with AKI is being supported until endogenous renal function recovers, the tendency for most clinicians is to avoid using nephrotoxic agents as much as possible. Radiocontrast dye usage is typically limited in these patients, with some clinicians going so far as to remove the dye by hemofiltrative therapies.[7] Whenever possible, nephrotoxic agents such as aminoglycosides and amphotericin B are avoided in favor of β-lactam antibiotics and echinocandins, respectively. These are not aspects of drug therapy that are much considered in the treatment of CKD stage V patients. The effects of nephrotoxic agents in AKI patients receiving RRT have not been well studied. Their use in these patients is presumed to adversely affect patient outcome, but supporting data are surprisingly sparse. However, nephrotoxic agents are used extensively in the ICU. Our group reported that 21.6% of all drug orders in the adult ICUs at a large tertiary care hospital were for potentially nephrotoxic agents.[8] This percentage rose to 39.9% for all orders in the pediatric ICUs. With all of these constraints on choices of drug therapy, clinicians need solid dosing information to ensure that the pharmacotherapeutic decisions that are made for these critically ill patients are appropriate.

ADAPTATION OF PUBLISHED DOSING GUIDELINES

Numerous drug information resources are available to clinicians to aid drug dosing in patients with renal disease. In general, these sources are inconsistent in their dosing recommendations; their definitions of kidney disease vary; and often they are not evidence based.[9] A recent study compared the renal drug dosing recommendations of four commonly used published tertiary references.[9] The authors reported a surprisingly high level of disagreement among the four references, both for dosing recommendations and in their definitions of renal impairment. There were several instances in which one resource stated that use of a drug in patients with renal impairment required no dosage adjustment but another resource indicated that the drug was contraindicated in that situation. Finally, most of the current recommendations are based on dosing information in patients with CKD, not AKI. In texts, most of the recommendations for dosing were based on patients receiving intermittent, thrice-weekly hemodialysis, not the almost daily hemodialysis sessions required by critically ill patients with AKI.[10] In general, drug dosing recommendations for daily hemodialysis or other RRTs are not well described and are likely to be quite different from those for intermittent hemodialysis.

When drug dosing guidelines are available for continuous renal replacement therapy (CRRT), they are usually based on older, lower-volume (1000 mL/hr) CRRT techniques. In lower-dose CRRT, the blood flow rate (Q_B) greatly exceeds the dialysate flow rate (Q_D) and/or the ultrafiltrate production rate (Q_{UF}). Consequently, the rate-limiting step for drug clearance in these therapies is Q_D and/or Q_{UF}. With higher-volume CRRT, a situation similar to intermittent hemodialysis occurs, in which Q_{UF} and Q_D are usually much higher than the transfer of drug from the peripheral or deeper compartments into the plasma compartment. When higher-volume CRRT is initiated, unbound drug in the plasma compartment is rapidly removed, due to high dialytic clearance. The rate-limiting step for any further drug removal becomes the rate at which drug can be transferred from the deeper or peripheral compartments into the plasma compartment.

Similarly, the size of the apparent volume of distribution (deep or peripheral compartments) of each drug also influences actual drug removal. Because it is difficult or impossible to sample from these compartments, the transfer rates between compartments and the peripheral or deep compartment volumes of distribution are very difficult to determine (Fig. 318-1). However, clinicians should recognize that drug removal may change during the course of higher-volume CRRT, so serum concentration monitoring is essential whenever possible.

DOSING CONSIDERATIONS IN RENAL REPLACEMENT THERAPY

Drug clearances via low-volume ($\leq$1000 mL/hr) continuous hemodialysis and hemofiltration are thought to be so similar that most clinicians consider them to be equivalent. Continuous dialysis therapies operating at these low Q_D are slow enough that solute concentrations between blood and dialysate are able to reach equilibrium. Whereas large-molecular-weight substances may be more readily cleared with convection than diffusion, these differences are thought to be negligible at slow Q_D or Q_{UF}. Indeed, at low flows, drug-dosing recommendations for low-volume CRRT have not differentiated between diffusive and convective clearance.

In continuous venovenous hemofiltration (CVVH), the appropriate measure of a solute's ability to cross the membrane is the sieving coefficient (SC), which is the ratio of ultrafiltrate concentration to the simultaneous arterial solute concentration. The SC is generally thought to be unchanged despite changes in Q_{UF}, and this seems to be the case in published assessments of SC.[11] In contrast, in the calculation of dialytic clearance, the saturation coefficient (SA), at a given set of blood and dialysate flow rates, is equal to the ratio of drug concentration in the spent dialysate and the average of simultaneously obtained arterial and venous solute concentrations. Early dosing guidelines, based on low-volume continuous venovenous hemodialysis (CVVHD), suggested that SA is equal to

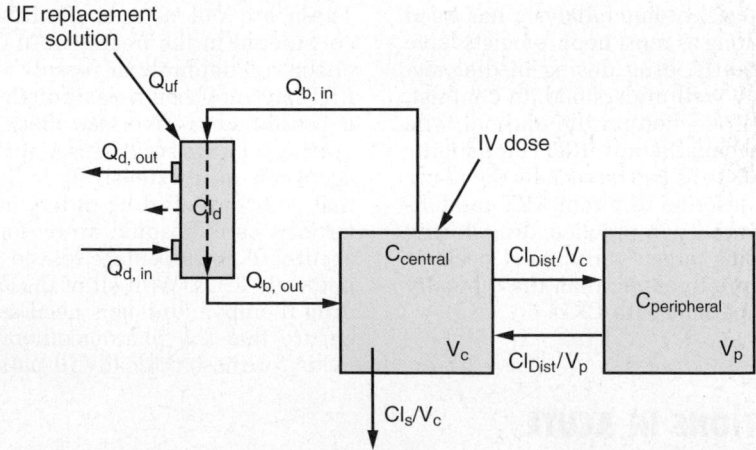

FIGURE 318-1. Schematic representation of a two-compartment open pharmacokinetic model in concert with drug removal by renal replacement therapy (RRT). Most drugs exhibit multicompartmental characteristics, consisting of a central compartment and one or more peripheral compartments. In this figure, only one peripheral compartment is depicted. Solutes are assumed to be removed from the central compartment either by RRT or through endogenous means. In high-volume RRT, drugs are rapidly cleared from the first compartment, possibly even faster than they can equilibrate from other, deeper compartments. In this scenario, the rate-limiting step for drug removal becomes the rate at which the drug can transfer to the central compartment from these deeper compartments. $C_{central}$, concentration of drug in the central compartment; $C_{peripheral}$, concentration of drug in the peripheral compartment; Cl_s, systemic clearance (sum of all endogenous clearances, renal and nonrenal); Cl_{Dist}, distribution clearance or intercompartmental clearance; Cl_d, dialytic clearance; IV, intravenous; $Q_{b,in}$, blood flow rate into the dialyzer; $Q_{b,out}$, blood flow rate out of the dialyzer; $Q_{d,in}$, dialysate flow rate into the dialyzer; $Q_d$out, dialysate flow rate out of the dialyzer; Q_{uf}, ultrafiltrate flow rate; V_c, volume of distribution of drug in the central compartment; V_p, volume of distribution of drug in the peripheral compartment.

SC.[12,13] This assumption is appropriate with low-volume CVVHD because Q_D is slow enough to allow almost complete equilibrium of solute concentration between the dialysate and blood sides of the dialysis membrane. However, this assumption is almost certainly incorrect with high-volume CVVHD. Few studies have been conducted on the issue of SA and SC differences in high-volume CRRT, but one report suggested a marked difference between the two.[11] The difference probably is more pronounced with larger-molecular-weight substances, because diffusivity is inversely related to molecular size. As molecular size increases, the difference between SA and SC should grow, although this difference is also dependent on hemofilter characteristics. Clinically, this separation of SA and SC is likely to be seen with solutes of larger molecular weight.

The SAs of urea and vancomycin were determined in an in vivo study conducted in CKD patients receiving experimental CVVHD at varying dialysate flow rates.[14] At relatively low Q_D (8.3 mL/min), the SA for urea was between 0.71 and 0.88, and that for vancomycin was between 0.63 and 0.9. The variation of SA was found to be hemodiafilter dependent. However, as Q_D increased from 8.3 to 33.3 mL/min, the SA of each solute changed from a 9% increase to a 30% decline. The largest decline in SA (vancomycin 30%, urea 8%) was seen with AN69 hemodiafilters. Using the same filter, Brunet found that increasing the Q_D to greater than 1000 mL/hr did not enhance clearance of β_2-microglobulin.[15] In contrast, smaller volume drugs such as ceftazidime tend to have increased dialytic clearance when Q_D is increased.[16] These data indicate that doubling of the Q_D, from a standard low-volume flow (1000 mL/hr) to a higher flow (2000 mL/hr), may result in substantially less than a doubling of clearance, particularly for larger solutes. Increasing Q_D ($\geq$2000 mL/hr) should result in decreasing clearance, but the rate of SA decline is hemodiafilter dependent.[14] Finally, therapies that combine convection and diffusion, such as continuous venovenous hemodiafiltration (CVVHDF), are likely to have different clearances than either modality alone. Data regarding other techniques, such as sustained low-efficiency dialysis (SLED), are even more limited.[17-20]

PHARMACOKINETICS IN PATIENTS WITH ACUTE KIDNEY INJURY

In addition to the previous description of issues related to the effect of CRRT on drug pharmacokinetics and the obvious, although unpredictable, effect that reduced and unstable renal function have on renally cleared drugs, critically ill AKI patients also exhibit pharmacokinetic alterations related to their illness. For this reason, the extensive body of pharmacokinetic data obtained in patients with CKD may not apply to AKI patients. Many reviews are available describing changes in pharmacokinetics that exist in patients with CKD[21,22] and, to a much lesser extent, changes that occur in AKI. Pharmacokinetic investigations in patients with AKI are difficult to conduct, and there are few studies in the literature. This is partially due to the extreme difficulty of enrolling and maintaining these patients in clinical trials. In studies that have been completed, the unstable nature of the enrolled patients makes interpretation of the results challenging.

Drug pharmacokinetics are dependent on multiple processes, including absorption, distribution, metabolism,

and excretion, and alterations in any of these processes may affect drug concentrations in biological fluids and subsequent dosing requirements. In patients with underlying CKD, acute changes may compound alterations that are already present. Acute critical illness is known to alter the intestinal absorption of drugs and nutrients via alterations in gastrointestinal perfusion, intestinal atrophy, and gastrointestinal motility.[23] In addition, absorption of drugs in patients with critical illness may be caused by drug-drug or drug-nutrient interactions. For example, we showed that the absorption of fluoroquinolone antibiotics is reduced when they are concomitantly administered with enteral nutrition.[24,25] Historically, there are also data to suggest that phenytoin oral absorption may be affected by enteral nutrition, although this is controversial.[26] Little else is known regarding drug absorption in critical illness specifically affecting patients with AKI.

Drug distribution describes the process by which drugs leave the systemic circulation and are transported to the extravascular spaces of the body. *Volume of distribution* is a term that relates the amount of drug in the body to the concentration of drug in the plasma or blood. Volume of distribution is apparent and not a true physical volume. The rate and extent of drug distribution throughout the body is determined by several factors: blood flow and tissue permeability, plasma protein binding, and tissue binding. These factors determine the steady-state volume of distribution of a drug, and all of them can, in theory, be altered in critically ill patients with AKI receiving CRRT.

For hydrophilic drugs, such as aminoglycoside antibiotics, which have relatively small volumes of distribution and are not highly protein or tissue bound, the volume of distribution is highly dependent on blood or plasma volume, and dose adjustment may be necessary in the hypervolemic patient. This is the most common issue in AKI patients receiving RRT, particularly CRRT. These patients may require larger loading doses to achieve adequate peak concentrations. However, initiation of CRRT in the hypervolemic patient with AKI may result in a loss of 20 kg in the first week. Clearly, the maintenance doses of hydrophilic drugs with small volumes of distribution (e.g., aminoglycosides) will need to be reduced to achieve the same desired peak and trough plasma concentration in these patients with changing volume status.

Protein binding alterations caused by drug interactions or physiological conditions usually have little importance clinically, because drug exposure is not affected by changes in protein binding.[27] The most commonly cited drug in which protein binding is thought to have a clinical effect in patients with renal disease is phenytoin. Phenytoin is highly protein-bound (90%), primarily to albumin. Renal failure is associated with a decrease in protein binding of phenytoin, because uremia causes hypoalbuminemia and/or reduced affinity of albumin for phenytoin. Both situations result in reduced free fraction of phenytoin, but, because of the nature of phenytoin metabolism, there is no change in the concentration of unbound phenytoin, which is the form responsible for the drug's effect. However, the total phenytoin concentration will be reduced, and, unless clinicians either apply a "correction" to the measured phenytoin concentration or use the free concentration for therapeutic drug monitoring, errors in drug dosing may result.[28]

Drug elimination refers to the irreversible removal of drug from the body by all routes of elimination. This concept is typically divided into two major physiological components; metabolism and excretion. *Metabolism,* or biotransformation, is the process by which drugs are changed or transformed into their metabolites. Clearance processes are both nonrenal and renal. Nonrenal clearance mechanisms may include metabolic processes, among others. The act of hemodialysis itself has been shown to affect drug metabolic pathways in patients with CKD. Hemodialysis acutely improves metabolic processes that involve the cytochrome P-450 (CYP) CYP3A isoenzyme.[29] Considerable research has been conducted to evaluate the impact of CKD on renal clearance, but changes in nonrenal clearance have also been studied.[21] There are limited data in AKI, but it seems clear that nonrenal drug clearances are not necessarily the same in CKD as in AKI. There are examples for vancomycin[30] and imipenem[31] that indicate nonrenal clearances substantially higher in AKI than in CKD for these two drugs. The assumption that nonrenal clearance will be the same as in CKD can result in severe underdosing of these antibiotics in patients with AKI.

Finally, in addition to the obvious but difficult-to-predict changes that CRRT may have on drug removal, clinicians must consider also the contributions of any residual renal function. Some patients are initiated on RRT even though they have residual renal function. Patients with AKI may have improving or declining renal function, occasionally on the same day! This dynamic effect on clearance can certainly make drug dosing very difficult in these patients.

CONCLUSION

Drug dosing tables for patients with reduced renal function undergoing the most common forms of RRT have been published.[32] Reviews of the considerations for dosing in pediatric patients have also been published,[33] so yet another listing of these recommendations will not be made here. However, knowledge of the patient and RRT-specific factors affecting drug distribution, as outlined earlier, will help the clinician proactively adjust doses as the situation changes. The Key Points listed at the end of this chapter provide important practical considerations when determining a pharmacotherapeutic regimen for a patient with AKI.

Drug dosing in patients with AKI is complicated. Successful pharmacotherapy requires real-time knowledge about the drug, the patient, and any RRT being employed. In most cases, the initial dose and dosing regimen is likely to change during the course of therapy as volume status and renal function change. Drug dosing requires continuous monitoring by a multidisciplinary team to maximize therapeutic outcomes.

Key Points

1. Patients with acute kidney injury (AKI) are in a dynamic situation: the drug volume of distribution must be assessed and reassessed as volume status changes, and urine output and laboratory markers of renal function must be monitored closely as endogenous renal function fluctuates.

2. Nonrenal clearance in the critically ill AKI patient may differ substantially from published values derived in patients with chronic kidney disease (CKD) and from what is observed in other AKI patients; it may also change as AKI persists.

3. Drug clearance by renal replacement therapy is likely to be lower in the critically ill AKI patient compared with stable CKD patients due to differences in tolerated blood flow rate (Q_B), so literature estimates of clearance should be viewed with caution.

4. When possible, serum concentrations of drugs should be monitored, and measurement of the free drug concentrations should be ordered when available (especially for phenytoin).

5. If published dosing guidelines for a drug in patients undergoing continuous renal replacement therapy (CRRT) are available, ensure that the guideline addresses the CRRT parameters that your patient is receiving—same dialysate flow rate (Q_D) and/or ultrafiltrate production rate (Q_{UF}) and same hemodiafilter type.

6. If CRRT dosing guidelines are not available, a reasonable dosage in an AKI patient with no residual renal function may be estimated by assuming that $Q_{UF} + Q_D$ = estimated creatinine clearance, using the manufacturer's recommended dose for that creatinine clearance estimate, and following up with serum concentration monitoring.

Key References

4. Roberts JA, Lipman J: Antibacterial dosing in intensive care: Pharmacokinetics, degree of disease and pharmacodynamics of sepsis. Clin Pharmacokinet 2006;45:755-773.
9. Vidal L, Shavit M, Fraser A, et al: Systematic comparison of four sources of drug information regarding adjustment of dose for renal function. BMJ 2005;331:263.
22. Churchwell MD, Mueller BA: Selected pharmacokinetic issues in patients with chronic kidney disease. Blood Purif 2007;25:133-138.
23. Boucher BB, Wood GC, Swanson JM: Pharmacokinetic changes in critical illness. Crit Care Clin 2006;22:255-271.
33. Veltri MA, Neu AM, Fivush BA, et al: Drug dosing during intermittent hemodialysis and continuous renal replacement therapy: Special considerations in pediatric patients. Paediatr Drugs 2004;6:45-65.

See the companion Expert Consult website for the complete reference list.

CHAPTER 319

Dialysis for Acute Renal Failure in Developing Countries

Mani John Panat

OBJECTIVES

This chapter will:
1. Spell out the essentials of safe and adequate, inexpensive dialysis using nonproprietary technology.
2. Describe simpler ways to accomplish high manual reuse, heparin modeling, water plant design, ultrafiltration control, peritoneal dialysis, and continuous therapies.

The topic of dialysis in developing countries has to be approached with trepidation, because many of the opinions expressed do not have precedent in the literature, and much of the experience developed by workers in the field have not been published in standard sources.

Dialytic care of renal failure was, from the beginning, a major technical exercise wherein the nephrologist also had to be a skilled technician. Current medical techniques with hierarchies of specialization have made such skills redundant in developed countries, but they are still relevant in underdeveloped countries. There are 64 countries, with a total population of about 2 billion, in which the per capita income is less than $800 per year (Table 319-1).[1] It is important to find methods that can bring dialysis therapies to such places without either following unrealistically high standards or compromising on dialysis safety.

Developing countries may have prescribed standards for health care, generally imported wholesale from the developed world, that make the application of cost-effective, improvised methods impossible. Reuse is forbidden in many countries, but the United States has permitted reuse and has a standard protocol for it, and this protocol can be adopted as the standard in many Third World countries.[2] If the United States were to ban reuse, then pressure would bear upon authorities for a similar ban in the Third World, with major cost burdens for the patients to follow.

The use of nonproprietary technology is to be encouraged, especially in the underdeveloped countries, because the marketing and service network required for many patented technologies simply does not exist. Patented technologies are hard to obtain and expensive to maintain; they discourage understanding of the technology that goes into the development of the product and also prevent free discussion and improvement in its use. An example is an automated reuse machine, the working of which is unknown to the operator, that uses expensive chemicals such as Renalin sterilant (Renal Systems, Minntech Corp., Minneapolis, MN). The situation is akin to the movement in the computer industry for open source and free software, wherein knowledge is freely shared among users, compared with closed proprietary computer software.

The nephrologist in a developing country is under pressure to find ways of delivering dialysis modalities to a needy population that does not have money to pay for the usual therapies and yet without falling afoul of the laws of the country. Such methods can be developed for both hemodialysis and peritoneal dialysis. This chapter describes methods which can be freely adapted for use everywhere, in both developed and less developed countries.

HEMODIALYSIS

Overall Planning of Hemodialysis Unit

It is better to plan for a larger number of dialysis machines in a hospital setting. Labor costs are not as significant in developing countries as they are in developed countries. Larger units can have training programs to provide more desperately needed staff. Cheap refurbished machines can be obtained and will provide benefit to more patients than small numbers of highly sophisticated machines, the majority of the functions of which will lie unused (e.g., high-flux dialysis, single-needle dialysis). A mixture of older machines, for the usual stable patient with chronic disease, and a few modern machines, intended for the acutely ill and also for providing specialized therapies, can provide the right blend.

General or industrial-purpose water treatment equipment often provides for much larger capacity at lower cost than do plants made for dialysis specifically (Fig. 319-1). The parts tend to be more generic and more widely available as well. These scaled-up plants enable more economies of operation, so that cheap and plentiful amounts of water are available for both dialysis and reuse.

Planning for chronic patients ensures good utilization of the resources of staff, water plant, and equipment on a continuous basis, compared with dependence on sporadic numbers of patients with acute renal failure.

Dialysis Machines

Current dialysis machines are very sophisticated with various subsystems and online monitoring of hematocrit and efficacy of treatment (Kt/V). They require highly trained staff for their maintenance. In contrast, older dialysis machines such as the Centry 3 series (Cobe Laboratories, Lakewood, CO) can be maintained by the dialysis technicians and hospital-based staff, and parts for these machines often can be improvised from equipment available in local markets. Such machines can be obtained at minimal cost from sources of refurbished machines internationally. There do not seem to be legal barriers to the

TABLE 319-1

Economic Classification of Countries

GROUP	NO. OF COUNTRIES	TOTAL POPULATION (BILLIONS)	ANNUAL PER CAPITA GROSS NATIONAL PRODUCT (US$)
High	50	0.93	>9265
Upper middle	38	0.57	2996-9265
Low middle	55	2.28	755-2995
Low	64	2.05	<755

Report in the World Bank: 2000. New York, Oxford University Press, 2000, pp 270-335.

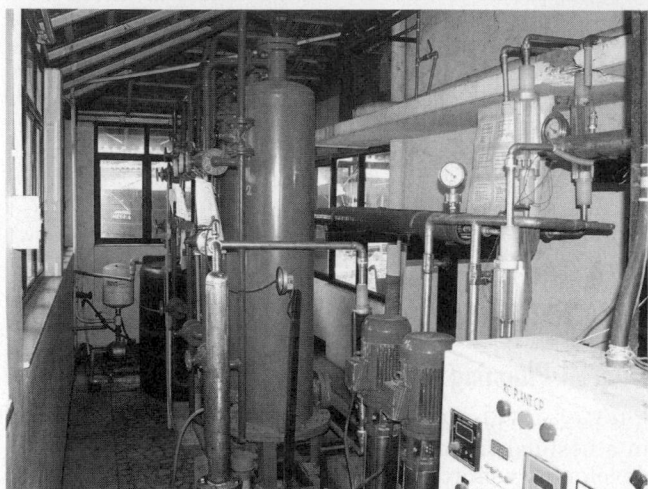

FIGURE 319-1. An industrial reverse osmosis (RO) water plant with 1000 L water output per hour has been adapted for use in a dialysis unit using stainless steel supply lines.

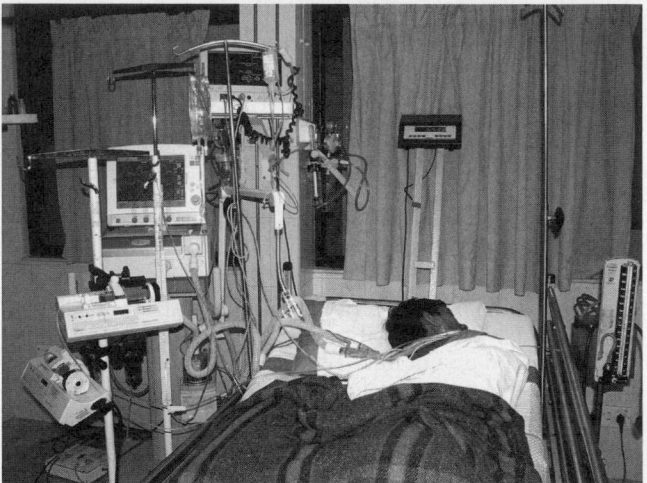

FIGURE 319-2. A bed-weighing scale made from local components is used to monitor the weight of a patient during continuous venovenous hemodiafiltration (CVVHDF).

use of such machines, although the import of used dialysis machines may require special sanctions in various countries. If such cheap machines are used, it is possible to have a quality-care dialysis unit with many more machines, with major implications for patient care. It may be better to have more machines running in fewer shifts than to have a small number of machines running around the clock. An analysis of the data from the United States Renal Data System (USRDS) has shown higher mortality for elderly patients being dialyzed in the afternoon compared with morning or evening treatments, which may be relevant in this case.[3]

Access Methods

The Scribner shunt may still have advantages over the current venous catheters, because it is cheap and can be produced locally. Moreover, it can be used to initiate dialysis in a patient with chronic renal failure, and the shunt subsequently can be converted to a fistula after arterialization of the vein with a higher success rate than creation of a primary fistula. The Teflon vessel tips are no longer in production, however.

Ultrafiltration Control

The biggest advantage with the newer dialysis machines is the availability of ultrafiltration control, which makes

for safer dialysis. The accuracy demanded for ultrafiltration control is 0.1%, which far exceeds the limits of flow meters and requires other mechanisms.[4] Machines that give complicated ultrafiltration profiles are expensive compared with those that have only negative pressure control. If the patient's weight is directly monitored using a bed fitted with a load cell device, changes of weight of 25 g can be detected. Such a bed, in conjunction with a simple negative pressure control machine (e.g., Centry 2) can lead to accuracy equal to that of ultrafiltration control devices. Because the patient's weight is directly monitored, this system also takes into account any fluids ingested or lost by the patient, which the machine with ultrafiltration control cannot detect. Such a system has been shown to be robust, very economical, and reliable[5] and can be constructed using readily available local technology with off-the-shelf components.

The combination of older, reconditioned dialysis machines without ultrafiltration control and a bed-weighing system constructed from local resources (Fig. 319-2) can prove to be very cost-efficient and acceptable for quality care as well. High-flux dialysis cannot be performed by this system.

Water Treatment Systems

The availability of large quantities of dialysis-quality water, both for dialysis and for reuse, is essential. The cost of running such a plant is lower if industrial-type plants are used. Dialysis units often have specially dedicated medical-grade water plants which are prohibitively expensive. Often, local industries such as electronics plants and pharmaceutical industries have water plants that are of equivalent quality and may be cheaper to run and maintain. Such manufacturers may not be aware of the role of such plants in dialysis units; they may have a wrong idea about the standards required for such plants and therefore do not design for dialysis units. The nephrologist should get in contact with local suppliers and discuss the standards required; the aim should be to obtain a plant that will be considerably more robust than an equivalent medical-grade plant. The importance of obtaining a dialysis water plant using locally available equipment cannot be overemphasized. It is often possible to attain very high standard distribution lines, such as stainless steel (medical grade 316), with Venturi systems for minimizing dead ends, and permanent hot recirculation systems in the reverse osmosis (RO) plants obtained from local suppliers, rather than the very expensive dialysis dedicated plants made by multinational companies.[6] For legal purposes, the water output standards can be used as justification.

Reuse

A lot has been published about reuse of dialyzers. A study in 2005 suggested no change in mortality with reuse.[7] Reuse can be done effectively using simple chemicals and pressurized water to obtain good standard reuse. In acute renal failure, reuse is not of paramount importance, but a system that enables good reuse will also maintain the quality of the dialysis reuse even in the first few times, enabling good clearances and also safer reuse. Most centers achieve low reuse, often in single figures, and the key to improvement is to install a constant-pressure tank (Table 319-2, Fig. 319-3).

Heparin Modeling

Every unit should have its own setup for measuring activated clotting time (ACT). This could be done using machines that check ACT using proprietary technology. These devices add appreciably to the cost of dialysis and hence are not appropriate for low-cost techniques. A generic method has been devised based on these principles.[8] It requires a warm water bath, pipette, and stopwatch, along with tissue thromboplastin reagent, and can ensure multiple measurements of clotting time cheaply (Fig. 319-4). The use of methods such as those published by Ouseph and Ward[9] to calculate heparin dosing based on these measurements can ensure minimal use of heparin based on the heparin sensitivity of the individual. This also increases the life of dialyzers and hemofilters. The method is detailed in Table 319-3.

In summary, the combination of larger dialysis centers, reconditioned older-generation machines, low-flux dialysis, bed-weighing systems rather than ultrafiltration control machines, industrial-scale water treatment RO plants, and good reuse using robust manual techniques can ensure the lowest operational costs for dialysis in both acute and chronic settings. Such a unit can operate various smaller satellite dialysis units with one or two machines using scaled-down technologies on a similar basis.

TABLE 319-2

Low-Cost Reuse System (Manual Method)*

Requirements: High-capacity low–running cost RO plant (suggested 1000 L capacity per hour for every 15 dialysis machines), diaphragm-type constant-pressure tank (see Fig. 319-3), hydrogen peroxide 3%, formalin 4%.

Step 1. Flush dialyzer with water pressure at 1.6 kPa (20 psi), with RO water with the constant-pressure water tank in the water treatment line. This will ensure adequate pressure even if all dialyzers are connected together (see Fig. 319-3).

Step 2. Perform reverse-pressure cleaning with one dialyzer port closed, from the dialyzer side to the blood compartment side, for 5 minutes.

Step 3. Fill with hydrogen peroxide 3% in the dialyzer compartment and close all ports for 5 minutes.

Step 4. Repeat flushing with water in both ports simultaneously.

Step 5. Fill and seal with formalin 4%.

Step 6. Before next use, perform the pressure test and check for fiber-bundle leaks manually.

RO, reverse osmosis.
*With this method, reuse in excess of 45 times for high-flux dialyzers and 28 times for ordinary dialyzers has been achieved with 80% of initial fiber-bundle volumes and absence of blood leaks. Because the chemicals used are cheap and manual methods are used, the cost is very low in comparison to that of the dialyzer.
From Mani PJ, Parameswaran H: How we do it: Multiple dialyser reuse using manual methods [abstract]. Indian J Nephrol 2003;12:175); method modified from Association for the Advancement of Medical Instrumentation: Recommended Practice for Reuse of Hemodialyzers. Arlington, VA, AAMI, 1993.

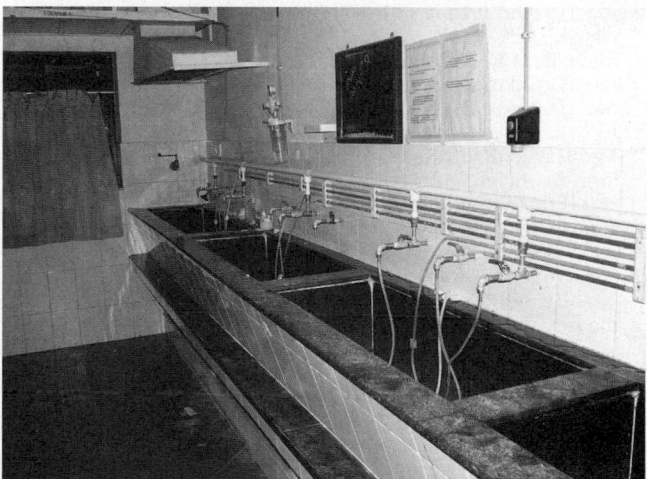

FIGURE 319-3. Manual reuse unit is designed for high reuse.

CONTINUOUS THERAPIES

Continuous renal replacement therapies (CRRTs) can be administered in various ways. The oldest method of direct arterial cannulation for the arterial line and filtration without a pump can be tried in places where the patient in renal failure cannot be shifted to a major dialysis center. In dialysis centers, techniques with pumps are preferred. The dedicated CRRT machines are the best, but they cannot be used for other purposes and may be difficult to justify when cost constraints are present. Possible alternatives include the following.

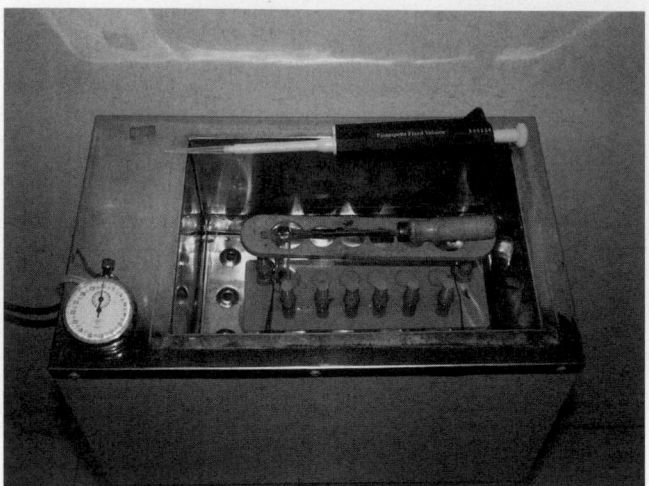

FIGURE 319-4. Water bath, pipette, and stopwatch are used to measure activated clotting time.

TABLE 319-3

Heparin Modeling Method

Equipment needed: Water bath, pipette, stopwatch, tissue thromboplastin reagent (used for measuring activated partial prothrombin time).

Step 1. Measure whole blood activated clotting time (ACT)—method of Mani & Parameswaran[6] (see Fig. 319-4).

Step 1A. Take 0.4 mL blood in the pipette and keep in test tube in the water bath at 37° C for 2 min.

Step 1B. Add 0.2 mL of tissue thromboplastin reagent; visually inspect for signs of clotting after 30 sec and thereafter for clotting.

Step 1C. Take basal ACT sample.

Step 1D. Measure ACT after 15 min of dialysis.

Step 1E. Measure 30 min before closing dialysis.

Step 2. Calculate bolus dose and infusion dose from the formula, Loading dose = 1600 + 10 × (Wt − 76), subtracting 300 if the patient has diabetes and 100 if the patient is a smoker. The infusion rate is 1750 IÚ/hr.

Step 3. Modify the calculated dose according to the measured ACT to bring it to 1.6 times the basal level. Usually, the dose is achieved after three measurements so the infusion rate will be corrected on the second dialysis session.

From Ouseph R, Ward J: Anticoagulation for intermittent hemodialysis. Semin Dial 2000;13:181-187.

1. A standard machine may be used in bypass mode, so that hemodialysis concentrate is not needed. Peritoneal dialysis fluid is allowed to gravitate at 1 L/hr. The peritoneal dialysis fluid is more expensive. The blood pump module of the dialysis machine may be used in isolation for such purposes.

2. Pharmacy-based bicarbonate-based fluids have been used.[10] This involves considerable setup and machinery that may be absent in the Third World. One working method can be to use a hemodialysis machine to generate about 50 L of fluid in a separate run. This fluid can be passed through a low-flux dialyzer so as to filter out pyrogens and then used immediately during CVVHD. This will keep the cost of replacement fluids at the lowest (method developed along with G. K. Ninan).

3. Some centers in the Third World have manufactured isolated blood pumps with air detectors alone, and these can be used for continuous arteriovenous hemodiafiltration (CAVHDF).

4. The bed-weighing system mentioned earlier must be used with all of these systems to keep track of the fluids infused and removed.

In summary, a low-cost CAVHDF system consists of a standard dialysis machine used in bypass mode so that concentrate is not needed, with separately generated hemodialysis fluid and a bed-weighing system. Isolated blood pumps can be used if air detection systems are present. Bedside monitoring of clotting time, by the method described later, ensures longer life of hemofilters.

PERITONEAL DIALYSIS

Peritoneal dialysis is an attractive option by virtue of its simplicity. It is not necessarily the most effective or cheaper than hemofiltration, however. A study from Vietnam showed that peritoneal dialysis, even using hospital pharmacy-based fluid, was more expensive than hemofiltration.[11] The Weston Roberts catheter is popular because it is simple to insert: The abdominal wall is punctured using a metal stylet in the catheter.[12] Because the catheter leads to peritoneal infection within 3 days, current recommendations in the developed world are to use chronically placed catheters for acute dialysis.[13] This increases the cost several-fold, because the cost of the Tenckhoff catheter is about 35 times that of the Roberts catheter in India, rivaling the cost of the entire dialysis itself. The other major costs are for fluids and for nursing care in the intensive care unit. Hence, the lowest-cost strategy is to use the Roberts catheter with glass or plastic bottled peritoneal dialysis fluid for acute dialysis lasting less than 3 days. If the patient needs longer dialysis, placement of a Tenckhoff catheter is a better option. The Tenckhoff catheter can be inserted using percutaneous or peritoneoscopic techniques by skilled nephrologists without additional surgical help. The dialysis can be done in the same fashion as with the Roberts catheter.

It is estimated that each patient will need about 140 L of fluid (2 L/hr for 72 hours). If this is done with standard continuous ambulatory peritoneal dialysis (CAPD) bags, it represents a formidable cost. Two liters of peritoneal dialysis fluid in a glass or plastic bottle costs only about one third as much as a CAPD bag in India. Hence, the choice for low-cost continuous equilibrated peritoneal dialysis (CEPD) for less than 3 days would be to use such fluids rather than CAPD bags.

Hospitals could use their own peritoneal dialysis fluids, because their guidelines are available in standard pharmacopeias, and existing manufacturers of intravenous fluids could easily convert some of their production to such fluids, as shown by a published Nigerian experience.[14]

Concerns with adequacy of dialysis, safety, and reduced nursing requirements have prompted the use of cyclers. However, peritoneal dialysis in acute renal failure has been considered inadequate therapy in view of the low clearances achieved.

Tidal peritoneal dialysis (with 750 mL) fluid removed every 20 minutes after a 2-L fill using a cycler was shown to produce adequate clearances in mild to moderate hypercatabolic conditions, as did standard CEPD.[15] However, tidal peritoneal dialysis achieved greater solute clearance at lower fluid quantity. The cost for tidal peritoneal dialysis can be reduced considerably by using lower-cost bags and fluids with locally produced cyclers.

Peritoneal dialysis fluids can be sourced in two ways. The older and considerably cheaper option is to use fluid available from manufacturers of intravenous fluids in plastic bags or bottles with spike connecting systems and a rigid peritoneal dialysis catheter. The fluid costs about $1 for a 2-L bag; acetate or, less commonly, lactate is used as the base. The more expensive option is to use fluid from dedicated CAPD manufacturing companies; this will be $3 to $4 per bag. There are still hospitals that have their own dedicated manufacturing units for intravenous fluids, and peritoneal dialysis fluids made by such units can be cheaper than outside manufacture. Pharmacopeia guidelines are available for the standards required by peritoneal dialysis fluids and should be followed rather than guidelines set by CAPD companies, which are often in excess of the pharmacopeia and outside the reach of the poorer countries. This would be a nice approach to cut costs and yet not to compromise safety.

5. Bedside monitoring of clotting time with simple generic equipment, using heparin sensitivity measurements, ensures longer life of dialyzers and safer dialysis.
6. A low-cost continuous arteriovenous hemodiafiltration (CAVHDF) system consists of use of a standard dialysis machine in bypass mode so that concentrate is not used, with separately generated hemodialysis fluid and a bed-weighing system; isolated blood pumps can be used if air detection systems are present.
7. Peritoneal dialysis is an attractive option for low-cost dialysis. It can be used in more peripheral centers and also for some patients with hypercatabolic renal failure. Costs can be kept low by using peritoneal dialysis fluids sourced from intravenous fluid manufacturers rather than from dedicated continuous ambulatory peritoneal dialysis units. Pharmacopeia guidelines should be followed.

Key Points

1. Large dialysis units using a mixture of ultrafiltration control machines for high-flux dialysis and older, reconditioned machines may achieve both variety and economies of operation.
2. Industrial-grade water plants with high-capacity and high-quality delivery systems are the basis for efficient reuse and economical operation of dialysis units.
3. Manual reuse methods[16] using cheap chemicals can achieve safe and efficient multiple reuse.
4. Cheap ultrafiltration control can be achieved with older, negative-pressure dialysis machines, with bed-weighing systems constructed using local resources.

Key References

5. Mani PJ, Parameswaran H: New method of ultrafiltration control in dialysis [abstract]. Indian J Nephrol 2003;12:184.
7. Fan Q, Liu J, Ebben JP, Collins AJ: Reuse-asssociated mortality in indigent hemodialysis patients in the United States, 2000-2001. Am J Kidney Dis 2005;46:661-668.
9. Ouseph R, Ward J: Anticoagulation for intermittent hemodialysis. Semin Dial 2000;13:181-187.
15. Almeida AF, Rai H, Bapat M, et al: Is peritoneal dialysis adequate for hypercatabolic acute renal failure in developing countries. Kidney Int 2002;61:747-757.
17. Association for the Advancement of Medical Instrumentation: Recommended Practice for Reuse of Hemodialyzers. Arlington, VA, AAMI, 1993.

See the companion Expert Consult website for the complete reference list.

CHAPTER 320

Medical Informatics in Disaster Response

Maury N. Pinsk and Kim Solez

OBJECTIVES

This chapter will:
1. Explain the role of information technology in developing an appropriate disaster response.
2. Discuss the limitations and fallibilities of communication systems that may be employed in a disaster response.
3. Explain the obstacles that currently limit effective information transfer during a medical response to disaster.

The provision of acute nephrology care in disaster zones involves mobilization of resources to provide acute dialysis care for victims of disasters and for chronically ill patients displaced by the disaster chaos. The delivery of nephrology care has improved with experience from catastrophes of the past, and plans for international aid have been discussed in the literature.[1-3] However, recent events in Southeast Asia, and more recently in the Gulf Coast of the United States, show that, even when many people are eager to help and many resources are available to provide relief, there may be a fundamental lack of efficient, accurate information gathering to facilitate decision-making, deployment, and administration of relief. Medical informatics is the discipline devoted to improving the methods and technologies used to gather, process, and analyze medical information. The role of medical informatics in disaster response planning is seminal, because the choice of technology and communications systems determines the success of the disaster response effort.

INFORMATION TECHNOLOGY DEFINED

Information technology should be robust and reliable so that it functions in difficult conditions, often in sites dangerous to personnel. The technology should provide accurate information about the nature of the disaster and the needs of those requiring medical intervention, so that appropriate relief services can be deployed. Any technology used in emergency sites must be easy to use, because it is likely to be used by semiskilled relief and aid workers. The transmission of medical information must maintain aspects of security, privacy, and confidentiality for the patients involved. Each of these points represents ideals of what medical technology should bring to the disaster relief effort. In practical terms, choosing the correct technology to meet these aims has proved difficult because of the unpredictable nature of disasters. To a large extent, the technology used in disaster zones for information transfer and retrieval has been whatever remained usable or could be mobilized to the area. However, common themes develop in what constitutes useful technology.

Miyamoto and associates[4] described the use of information technology after a 7.4 Richter scale earthquake occurred in the Hanshin-Awaji region of Japan in 1995. The authors described the functionality, deployment, and shortcomings of information technology in 52 medium- to large-sized hospitals. They found that most information systems were not damaged but were nonfunctional because of damage to power grids within the area. Power restoration occurred anywhere from within 30 minutes to 11 days after the onset of the earthquake. As a result, 36 of the responding hospitals could no longer use their computers, and 16 ultimately sought to transfer patients out of the area because of their inability to continue providing patient care. The primary modes of communication in the Hanshin-Awaji earthquake defaulted to battery-powered radios and direct person-to-person communication. The integrity and usability of this information soon became suspect, because inaccurate information was often broadcast on public radio systems concerning where to find daily necessities and which hospitals were receiving patients. For example, misinformation resulted in many hemodialysis patients' appearing at closed hospitals seeking hemodialysis treatment. Individuals used available functional technology to provide and collect information, including portable battery-powered telephones, cell phones, e-mail, wireless computer networks, and fax machines. This posed a substantial obstacle, because each of these communication systems, with the exception of e-mail, quickly became overwhelmed with the number of users on communication networks and ceased to work reliably. Even available satellite telephone systems were unusable due to damage to power grids and unavailability of backup generators. Interestingly, e-mail became the best means of disseminating information out of the disaster zone 3 days after the disaster struck in hospitals where the computer networks remained intact. The technology of routing e-mail messages through alternative server nodes resulted in successful delivery of e-mails by avoiding damaged areas of the network. The system did not become overwhelmed, because e-mails were batched and routed, rather than being sent in real time.

Indeed, e-mail can be a robust means of communicating information out of disaster zones. In the experience with Hurricane Katrina in the Gulf Coast of 2005, existing e-mail networks (listserves) operated by CyberNephrology/National Kidney Foundation assumed many roles that facilitated information transfer. These listserves developed to facilitate information exchange among nephrology professionals. During Hurricane Katrina relief efforts, they allowed institutions to be identified that would accept patient transfers out of the disaster zone.[5] Health care providers could also identify required resources in the disaster zone and facilitate mobilization of these resources using existing aid distribution networks. The most unexpected development was the use of the NephKids listserve, a system that was set up to provide information about kidney disease to families, which evolved into a network of tracking families within the disaster zone and ensuring that the NephKids family remained intact.[6] The utility of the listserve technology was recognized by the Kidney Community Emergency Response Coalition, which published recommendations in 2006 including the establishment of a Kidney Community Emergency Listserve[7] for use in future disaster situations affecting the renal community. The listserves are operated by CyberNephrology,[8] and the National Kidney Foundation via offices in New York and Edmonton, Alberta, to provide reliable functionality for all users and prevent vulnerability resulting from provision of services by a single center alone.

PROACTIVE DESIGN OF RELIABLE INFORMATION TECHNOLOGIES

Aid workers within a disaster zone develop creative applications of existing usable technologies to help disseminate information. However, there is an essential need to proactively develop communication systems to ensure disaster preparedness. Components of such a system may draw on multiple technologies and may challenge users to integrate systems to provide redundancy, ultimately resulting in seamless information transfer should one part of the network collapse.

Simmons and colleagues[9] studied communication networks based at the East Carolina University during a mock disaster in 2002. The purpose was to demonstrate that existing information infrastructure, coupled with additional technologies linked into this network, could provide a useful basis for further system design. The study reported that significant obstacles existed in using technologies such as land-based telephones and cell phones. These communication systems quickly became overwhelmed during the disaster, impairing communication to and between hospitals. Satellite teleconference systems, however, were not utilized, despite the ability to mobilize these technologies quickly and the fact that the technologies already existed in the hospital systems. The authors noted that portable satellite communication networks, similar to those used to broadcast television feeds from remote locations, were employed in the field to both survey the environment and communicate with emergency response personnel triaging patients. Although the authors endorsed the use of telehealth technologies for communication among hospitals and with personnel in the field, they were also quick to point out that none of the existing telehealth networks had power generation backup, and all would be likely to fail if the power grids were disrupted.

Other technologies that have a role in the creation of a viable disaster information system include wireless networks to capture data, speech/sound, and video from remote sites. Using this technology, information could be relayed from central wireless nodes over public Internet links or dedicated local area networks. This would enable teleconferencing, even if data transmission occurred over Internet protocol networks. Although this technology could, in theory, be overwhelmed with the transfer of large data files associated with real-time communications, it would be extremely useful for transmitting asynchronous data, such as pictures or datasets. Many commercially available recorders can provide this functionality, providing video, sound, global positioning system (GPS) location, and even chemical and environmental data from the disaster scene.[10]

ENSURING DATA ACCURACY

Extracting information from a disaster scene is a difficult job and is influenced by adverse environmental factors and inexperienced personnel. Information technology, if inadequate, can impair the ability to retrieve and interpret information from the field and significantly hamper decision-making abilities, particularly in providing care to patients. As an example, Strode and colleagues[11] performed a trial of technology to test transmissibility via satellite and through wireless networks. The authors trialed a portable ultrasound unit used to assess patients in the field and reviewed the interpretability of the images, either static or cine-loop movies at three locations: at the site of imaging, after transmission through a wireless network 1500 m in radius, and after the image was further transmitted through a satellite transmission Internet protocol network. They reported that image quality was comparable at the site of image acquisition and after transmission through the wireless network. However, further transmission through satellite feeds and Internet routing resulted in a significant drop in image quality, with resulting increase in noninterpretability of images. With respect to renal anatomy, this translated in a drop of interpretability rate, from 67% at the site of imaging to 17% after satellite and Internet transmission. Although this does illustrate the limitations of high-resolution data transmission over similarly structured networks, it does not eliminate the important role that this information technology could have in the transmission of low-resolution data from the field.[12] Similarly, the study demonstrated that high-resolution information can be transmitted successfully over broadband wireless networks like those commercially available today. Formal evaluation of these technologies in information transmission from disaster zones is still under investigation.

ENSURING SECURITY AND CONFIDENTIALITY

In the setting of disaster response with delivery of renal services, access to medical information, either from the hospital or from the field, can be life-saving. Current regulations in the United States, under the jurisdiction of Health Insurability and Portability and Accountability Act (HIPAA),[13] protect patient confidentiality by limiting access to patient information to only those involved in direct care. However, for disaster planning and management to be effective, often mass epidemiological data must be sent outside of the current jurisdiction of public health to effectively locate and provide services. O'Connor and colleagues[14] argued that new relationships must continue to be developed between emergency service providers and public health workers so that information transfer is not hindered for the benefit of the greater good.

On a different level, bedside management of patients in hemodialysis units also requires sharing of information among facilities and aid workers. Health care monitoring and patient tracking in disaster zones face the obstacles of transmitting patient information in a timely fashion, with accuracy, and following the patient throughout care. In a system reminiscent of tracking a person's location by his or her credit card utilization, technologies for patient identification are available that allow rapid triage, transport, and delivery of medical care using a wristband encoded with personal health care information.[12] As patients move through the triage system and receive care, the identification number is scanned and information is updated. Similarly, patients can be tracked with radiofrequency emitters that similarly create a mobile information system for tracking patients. As well, mobile patient monitoring systems that allow wireless transmission of patient information, such as vital signs, can occur in real time. These technologies can be linked with electronic health records to ensure that health information is available immediately to multiple users, either on site or remotely from the point of care. However, this requires significant investment in electronic health record charting, which is currently being used by only about 10% to 25% of United States physicians.[15] Even within those institutions using electronic charting, there is just now an evolving appreciation for standards of data handling, including aspects of diagnostic coding, information transfer protocols, and standards for information storage. Still, the ability to separate the ability to track a patient in the health care system from access to the detailed medical record creates opportunity for aid workers to remain integrally involved in the provision of care without compromising patient confidentiality.

CONCLUSION

The Health Metrics Network defined the use of information technology in emergency zones as "a set of data collection platforms implemented by a coordinated group of humanitarian actors generating information to support strategic decisions, monitor changes, prioritize action, allocate resources, manage programs, scale up or scale down operations, advocate, and formulate concerns in relation to an emergency context."[16] Clearly, no technology is perfect for every situation, but a clear understanding of the limitations of technologies and the ability to develop parallel networks of communication help ensure that communication networks remain robust in disaster zones. Technologies will continue to be developed that enable more sophisticated and accurate data gathering. However, the utility of this information is only as good as the infrastructure that is in place to analyze and manage it. It is in this area that much work needs to be done to facilitate information sharing with the right people at the right time.

Key Points

1. Medical response to disasters requires the ability to gather accurate information and analyze it in a timely fashion to facilitate aid response.
2. Communication systems that are used on a routine basis often fail during emergency response exercises because of technical failure or overwhelming of networks due to overuse.
3. Technologies exist to facilitate patient tracking throughout the emergency aid system, and they would be greatly augmented by being allowed to link with electronic health records. Exceptions

to the usual privacy rules may need to be considered.
4. Relationships among public health and emergency response teams are being developed and will greatly improve the ability to gather and access information for response planning.

Key References

1. Solez K, Bihari D, Collins AJ, et al: International dialysis aid in earthquakes and other disasters. Kidney Int 1993;44: 479-483.
3. Solez K: Disaster management and communications as viewed from 2003: Taking the long view. Adv Ren Replace Ther 2003;10:85-86.
4. Miyamoto M, Sako M, Kimura M, et al: Great earthquakes and medical information systems, with special reference to telecommunications. JAMA 1999;6:252-258.
7. Kidney Community Emergency Emergency Preparedness and Response. Final Report of the Eight Response Groups Created at the January Disaster Summit, July 1, 2006. Available at www.nraa.org (accessed May 14, 2008).

See the companion Expert Consult website for the complete reference list.

Index

Note: Page numbers followed by the letter f refer to figures, and those followed by t refer to tables.